Fleisher & Ludwig's

Textbook of Pediatric Emergency Medicine

Seventh Edition

Senior Editors

Kathy N. Shaw, MD, MSCE
Professor and Associate Chair
Department of Pediatrics
Perelman School of Medicine at the University of Pennsylvania
The Nicholas Crognale Endowed Chair in Emergency Medicine
The Children's Hospital of Philadelphia
Philadelphia, Pennsylvania

Richard G. Bachur, MD
Professor of Pediatrics
Associate Professor of Emergency Medicine
Harvard Medical School
Chief
Division of Emergency Medicine
Boston Children's Hospital
Boston, Massachusetts

Associate Editors

James M. Chamberlain, MD
Division Chief
Department of Emergency Medicine
Children's National Health System
Professor of Pediatrics and Emergency Medicine
George Washington University School of Medicine and Health Sciences
Washington, DC

Jane Lavelle, MD
Associate Professor of Pediatrics
Department of Pediatrics
Perelman School of Medicine at the University of Pennsylvania
Medical Director, Associate Division Chief Emergency Medicine
Medical Director, Pathway Program
Office of Continuous Quality Improvement
The Children's Hospital of Philadelphia
Philadelphia, Pennsylvania

Joshua Nagler, MD, MHPEd
Assistant Professor of Pediatrics and Emergency Medicine
Harvard Medical School
Fellowship Director and Director of Medical Education
Division of Emergency Medicine
Boston Children's Hospital
Boston, Massachusetts

Joan E. Shook, MD
Professor
Department of Pediatrics
Baylor College of Medicine
Chief Safety Officer and Chief Clinical Information Officer
Texas Children's Hospital
Houston, Texas

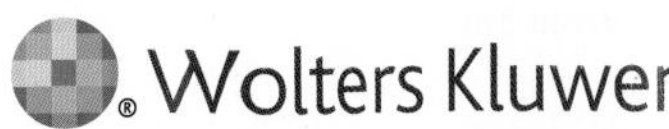

Philadelphia • Baltimore • New York • London
Buenos Aires • Hong Kong • Sydney • Tokyo

Acquisitions Editor: Jamie M. Elfrank
Product Development Editor: Ashley Fischer
Editorial Assistant: Brian Convery
Marketing Manager: Stephanie Kindlick
Production Project Manager: Bridgett Dougherty
Design Coordinator: Holly McLaughlin
Manufacturing Coordinator: Beth Welsh
Prepress Vendor: Aptara, Inc.

7th Edition

9 8 7 6 5 4 3 2

Printed in China

Library of Congress Cataloging-in-Publication Data
Textbook of pediatric emergency medicine
Fleisher & Ludwig's textbook of pediatric emergency medicine / senior editors, Kathy N. Shaw, Richard G. Bachur; associate editors, James Chamberlain, Jane Lavelle, Joshua Nagler, Joan E. Shook. – 7th edition.
p. ; cm.
Fleisher and Ludwig's textbook of pediatric emergency medicine
Preceded by: Textbook of pediatric emergency medicine / editors, Gary R. Fleisher, Stephen Ludwig. 6th ed. c2010.
Includes bibliographical references and index.
ISBN 978-1-4511-9395-4 (alk. paper)
I. Shaw, Kathy N., editor. II. Bachur, Richard G., editor. III. Title. IV. Title: Fleisher and Ludwig's textbook of pediatric emergency medicine.
[DNLM: 1. Child. 2. Emergencies. 3. Critical Care. 4. Emergency Treatment. 5. Infant. WS 205]
RJ370
618.92′0025—dc23

2015028445

LWW.com

CCS0217

DEDICATION

I'd like to dedicate this book to all my colleagues, nationally and internationally, in Emergency Medicine and Pediatrics that care for ill and injured children. I hope this new edition will help in our mission to provide high-quality care. To the many students, residents, fellows, and junior colleagues whom I have taught and have taught me, thank you for your dedication. Finally, and most importantly, my love and gratitude to my family for their support: my husband Ben Green and our children Andrew, Becca, and Eric.

Kathy N. Shaw

Upon reflecting on this endeavor, I first need to thank my extraordinary mentor, Gary Fleisher, who bestowed this editorial position on me and provided strong guidance and support throughout my career. Taking the reins from Steve and Gary on this symbolic tool of our field is one of the highest honors of my career. To Bernadette, Ryan, and Abby, thank you for your love and encouragement. As we release this 7th edition, I am extremely hopeful that this textbook continues to be a tremendous resource for all those dedicated to emergency care for children.

Richard G. Bachur

I would like to dedicate this work to my lovely wife, Pamela Berry, and my three amazing children, Daniel, Michael, and Meghan. You give me the "strength to do what needs to be done." I'd like to thank my colleagues, fellows, and patients, from whom I relearn daily the joys of practicing medicine.

James M. Chamberlain

To my Mom and Dad, thanks for inspiring me to follow my passion and for instilling in me a strong work ethic and the importance of contributing to the world in some small way. To my incredible family, Drew, Adam, and Jamie, thanks for the adventures.

Jane Lavelle

What a remarkable opportunity to take part in creating this next edition of Gary's book (Steve's book for those with ties closer to Philly), under Rich and Kathy's incredibly thoughtful oversight. Thank you to the impressive group of contributors—from junior faculty who will soon influence this field to the most senior clinicians who already have. Finally, a special thanks to Jan, Maddie, and Jack who graciously integrated "TPEM" into the craziness of our regularly scheduled programming.

Joshua Nagler

I would like to recognize my family—Jeff, Nathan, Matthew, and Hannah Starke—without you my life would lose its meaning. I also would like to recognize the residents, fellows, and colleagues I have had the opportunity to teach and work with—your dedication to children is the bedrock of our specialty and an inspiration. And above all, thank you to the children and families whom we have the privilege to serve.

Joan E. Shook

CONTRIBUTING AUTHORS

Alyssa M. Abo, MD
Director of Emergency Ultrasound Fellowship
Associate Director of Emergency Ultrasound
Assistant Professor of Pediatrics and Emergency Medicine
Division of Emergency Medicine
Children's National Medical Center
The George Washington University School of Medicine and Health Sciences
Washington, DC

Cynthia M. Adams, MD
Instructor in Pediatrics
Harvard Medical School
Division of Emergency Medicine
Boston Children's Hospital
Boston, Massachusetts

Michael S.D. Agus, MD
Associate Professor
Department of Pediatrics
Harvard Medical School
Chief, Division of Medicine Critical Care
Department of Medicine
Boston Children's Hospital
Boston, Massachusetts

Kiyetta H. Alade, MD, RDMS, FAAP
Assistant Professor
Department of Pediatrics
Baylor College of Medicine
Director, Pediatric Point-of-Care Ultrasound
Department of Pediatrics
Texas Children's Hospital
Houston, Texas

Dolores H. Albert, BSN, RN, CPEN
Clinical Nurse Expert
Emergency Department
The Children's Hospital of Philadelphia
Philadelphia, Pennsylvania

Elizabeth R. Alpern, MD, MSCE
Professor
Department of Pediatrics
Northwestern University
Attending Physician
Department of Pediatrics
Ann and Robert H. Lurie Children's Hospital of Chicago
Chicago, Illinois

Angela C. Anderson, MD, FAAP
Director, Pediatric Pain and Palliative Care
Hasbro Children's Hospital
Associate Professor of Pediatrics and Emergency Medicine
Alpert School of Medicine at Brown University
Providence, Rhode Island

Nickie Niforatos Andescavage, MD
Assistant Professor
Division of Neonatology
Children's National Health System
Washington, DC

Paul L. Aronson, MD
Assistant Professor of Pediatrics
Associate Director, Pediatric Residency Program
Section of Emergency Medicine, Department of Pediatrics
Yale School of Medicine
New Haven, Connecticut

Magdy W. Attia, MD, FAAP, FACEP
Professor of Pediatrics,
The Sidney Kimmel College of Medicine at Thomas Jefferson University
Philadelphia, Pennsylvania
Associate Director Emergency Medicine
Nemours/Alfred I. duPont Hospital for Children
Wilmington, Delaware

Jeffrey R. Avner, MD, FAAP
Professor
Department of Pediatrics
Albert Einstein College of Medicine
Chief
Pediatric Emergency Medicine
Children's Hospital at Montefiore
Bronx, New York

Richard G. Bachur, MD
Professor of Pediatrics
Associate Professor of Emergency Medicine
Harvard Medical School
Chief
Division of Emergency Medicine
Boston Children's Hospital
Boston, Massachusetts

Pamela J. Bailey, MD
Assistant Professor of Pediatrics
Baylor College of Medicine
Attending Physician
Department of Pediatrics
Texas Children's Hospital
Houston, Texas

Fran Balamuth, MD, PhD, MSCE
Assistant Professor of Pediatrics
Perelman School of Medicine at the University of Pennsylvania
Department of Pediatrics, Division of Emergency Medicine and Center for Pediatric Clinical Effectiveness
The Children's Hospital of Philadelphia
Philadelphia, Pennsylvania

Mark N. Baskin, MD
Assistant Professor of Pediatrics
Harvard Medical School
Division of Emergency Medicine
Service Chief, Short Stay Unit
Boston Children's Hospital
Boston, Massachusetts

Theresa M. Becker, DO
Assistant Professor of Pediatrics
Harvard Medical School
Executive Network Director
Division of Emergency Medicine
Boston Children's Hospital
Boston, Massachusetts

Robert A. Belfer, MD
Professor
Department of Pediatrics
Perelman School of Medicine at the University of Pennsylvania
The Children's Hospital of Philadelphia
Philadelphia, Pennsylvania

Frances Turcotte Benedict, MD, MPH
Assistant Professor
Department of Emergency Medicine and Pediatrics
Alpert Medical School of Brown University
Hasbro Children's Hospital
Providence, Rhode Island

Deena Berkowitz, MD, MPH
Assistant Professor of Pediatrics and Emergency Medicine
Children's National Health System and
George Washington University School of Medicine and Health Sciences
Washington, DC

Steven S. Bin, MD
Associate Clinical Professor
Departments of Emergency Medicine and Pediatrics
Director
Pediatric Emergency Department
UCSF Benioff Children's Hospital – San Francisco
San Francisco, California

Mercedes M. Blackstone, MD
Attending Physician, Emergency Medicine
Associate Professor of Clinical Pediatrics
Department of Pediatrics
Perelman School of Medicine at the University of Pennsylvania
The Children's Hospital of Philadelphia
Philadelphia, Pennsylvania

Robert G. Bolte, MD
Professor of Pediatrics
Division of Pediatric Emergency Medicine
University of Utah
Department of Pediatrics
Primary Children's Hospital
Salt Lake City, Utah

Alison St. Germaine Brent, MD
Associate Professor
Department of Pediatrics
University of Colorado School of Medicine
Aurora, Colorado
Section of Emergency Medicine
Children's Hospital Colorado
Aurora, Colorado

Marisa B. Brett-Fleegler, MD
Assistant Professor of Pediatrics
Harvard Medical School
Division of Emergency Medicine
Boston Children's Hospital
Boston, Massachusetts

Kathleen M. Brown, MD
Associate Professor of Pediatrics and Emergency Medicine
The George Washington University School of Medicine
Children's National Medical Center
Washington, DC

Linda L. Brown, MD, MSCE
Assistant Professor
Departments of Pediatrics and Emergency Medicine
Alpert Medical School of Brown University
Attending Physician
Pediatrics Emergency Department
Departments of Pediatrics and Emergency Medicine
Hasbro Children's Hospital
Providence, Rhode Island

Beth Bubolz, MD
Assistant Professor
Department of Pediatrics
Baylor College of Medicine
Texas Children's Hospital
Houston, Texas

Michele M. Burns, MD, MPH
Assistant Professor of Pediatrics and Emergency Medicine
Harvard Medical School
Director, Massachusetts and Rhode Island Poison Control Center
Division of Emergency Medicine
Boston Children's Hospital
Boston, Massachusetts

Rebekah A. Burns, MD
Assistant Professor
Department of Pediatrics, Division of Emergency Medicine
University of Washington School of Medicine
Seattle Children's Hospital
Seattle, Washington

Robyn L. Byer, MD
Assistant Professor of Pediatrics
Harvard Medical School
Division of Emergency Medicine
Boston Children's Hospital
Boston, Massachusetts

Diane P. Calello, MD
Director of Medical Toxicology
Division of Pediatric Emergency Medicine, Department of Emergency Medicine
Morristown Medical Center
Morristown, New Jersey

James M. Callahan, MD
Professor of Clinical Pediatrics
Department of Pediatrics
Perelman School of Medicine at the University of Pennsylvania
Vice Director, Pediatric Residency Program
Department of Pediatrics, Division of Emergency Medicine
The Children's Hospital of Philadelphia
Philadelphia, Pennsylvania

Kerry Caperell, MD, MS
Assistant Professor of Pediatrics
Department of Pediatrics
University of Louisville
Kosair Children's Hospital
Louisville, Kentucky

Leslie Castelo-Soccio, MD, PhD
Assistant Professor of Pediatrics and Dermatology
Perelman School of Medicine at the University of Pennsylvania
The Children's Hospital of Philadelphia
The University of Pennsylvania
Philadelphia, Pennsylvania

Theodore J. Cieslak, MD
Defense Department Liaison Officer
Centers for Disease Control and Prevention
Atlanta, Georgia

James M. Chamberlain, MD
Division Chief
Department of Emergency Medicine
Children's National Health System
Professor of Pediatrics and Emergency Medicine
George Washington University School of Medicine and Health Sciences
Washington, DC

Laura L. Chapman, MD
Assistant Professor
Department of Pediatric Emergency Medicine
Alpert Medical School of Brown University
Providence, Rhode Island

Aaron Chen, MD
Associate Professor of Clinical Pediatrics
Department of Pediatrics and Pediatric Emergency Medicine
Perelman School of Medicine at the University of Pennsylvania
The Children's Hospital of Philadelphia
Philadelphia, Pennsylvania

Vincent W. Chiang, MD
Associate Professor of Pediatrics
Harvard Medical School
Chief, Inpatient Services and Vice Chair for Finance
Department of Medicine
Boston Children's Hospital
Boston, Massachusetts

Maryanne R.K. Chrisant, MD
Associate Clinical Professor of Pediatrics
Medical Director, Pediatric Cardiac Transplant, Heart Failure and Cardiomyopathy
The Heart Institute
Joe DiMaggio Children's Hospital
Hollywood, Florida

Cindy W. Christian, MD
Professor
Department of Pediatrics
Perelman School of Medicine at the University of Pennsylvania
Chair
Child Abuse and Neglect Prevention
The Children's Hospital of Philadelphia
Philadelphia, Pennsylvania

Jennifer H. Chuang, MD, MS
Assistant Professor of Clinical Pediatrics
Craig-Dalsimer Division of Adolescent Medicine
Perelman School of Medicine at the University of Pennsylvania
The Children's Hospital of Philadelphia
Philadelphia, Pennsylvania

Bruno P. Chumpitazi, MD, MPH
Associate Professor
Deparment of Pediatrics
Baylor College of Medicine
Director of Neurogastroenterology
Director of Motility
Pediatric Gastroenterology
Texas Children's Hospital
Houston, Texas

Corrie E. Chumpitazi, MD
Assistant Professor of Pediatrics
Department of Pediatric Emergency Medicine
Baylor College of Medicine
Texas Children's Hospital
Houston, Texas

Thomas H. Chun, MD, MPH
Associate Professor
Department of Emergency Medicine and Pediatrics
Alpert Medical School of Brown University
Providence, Rhode Island

Sarita Chung, MD
Assistant Professor of Pediatrics
Harvard Medical School
Division of Emergency Medicine
Boston Children's Hospital
Boston, Massachusetts

Joanna S. Cohen, MD
Assistant Professor of Pediatrics and Emergency Medicine
Department of Pediatrics, Division of Emergency Medicine
The George Washington University School of Medicine and Children's National Medical Center
Washington, DC

Keri A. Cohn, MD, MPH, DTM&H
Assistant Professor of Clinical Pediatrics
Perelman School of Medicine at the University of Pennsylvania
Attending Physician
Division of Emergency Medicine
The Children's Hospital of Philadelphia
Philadelphia, Pennsylvania

Joy L. Collins, MD, FAAP
Assistant Professor of Clinical Surgery
Department of Surgery
Perelman School of Medicine at the University of Pennsylvania
Attending Surgeon
Department of General and Thoracic Surgery
The Children's Hospital of Philadelphia
Philadelphia, Pennsylvania

Erika Constantine, MD
Assistant Professor
Department of Pediatrics and Emergency Medicine
Alpert Medical School of Brown University
Attending Physician
Division of Pediatric Emergency Medicine
Rhode Island Hospital/Hasbro Children's Hospital
Providence, Rhode Island

Jacqueline B. Corboy, MD
Assistant Professor of Pediatrics
Feinberg School of Medicine
Department of Emergency Medicine
Ann and Robert H. Lurie Children's Hospital of Chicago
Chicago, Illinois

Kathleen M. Cronan, MD
Associate Professor
Department of Pediatrics
Jefferson Medical College
Philadelphia, Pennsylvania
Attending Physician, Emergency Department
Director of Health Content Integration
Nemours Center for Children's Health Media
Nemours A. I duPont Hospital for Children
Wilmington, Delaware

Stacy E. Croteau, MD, MMS
Instructor of Pediatrics
Harvard Medical School
Division of Hematology/Oncology
Boston Children's Hospital
Boston, Massachusetts

Andrea T. Cruz, MD, MPH
Assistant Professor
Department of Pediatrics
Baylor College of Medicine
Chief of Research
Pediatric Emergency Medicine
Department of Pediatrics
Texas Children's Hospital
Houston, Texas

Beth M. D'Amico, MD
Instructor, Department of Pediatrics
Section of Emergency Medicine
Texas Children's Hospital/Baylor College of Medicine
Houston, Texas

Valerie Davis, MD, PhD
Assistant Professor
Department of Pediatrics, Division of Emergency Medicine
University of Alabama at Birmingham
Birmingham, Alabama

J. Kate Deanehan, MD, RDMS
Assistant Professor of Pediatric Emergency Medicine
Division of Pediatric Emergency Medicine
Johns Hopkins Children's Center
Baltimore, Maryland

Atima C. Delaney, MD
Instructor of Pediatrics
Harvard Medical School
Division of Emergency Medicine
Boston Children's Hospital
Boston, Massachusetts

Eva M. Delgado, MD
Assistant Professor of Clinical Pediatrics
Perelman School of Medicine at the University of Pennsylvania
Division of Emergency Medicine
The Children's Hospital of Philadelphia
Philadelphia, Pennsylvania

Karen J. DiPasquale, DO, MPH
Clinical Associate Professor of Pediatrics
Department of Emergency Medicine
The Children's Hospital of Philadelphia
Philadelphia, Pennsylvania

Aaron Donoghue, MD, MSCE
Associate Professor of Critical Care Medicine and Pediatrics
Perelman School of Medicine at the University of Pennsylvania
Attending Physician
Divisions of Critical Care Medicine and Emergency Medicine
The Children's Hospital of Philadelphia
Philadelphia, Pennsylvania

Shanna R. Dooley, BSN, RN, CPEN
Clinical Nurse, Level III
Emergency Department
The Children's Hospital of Philadelphia
Philadelphia, Pennsylvania

Kate Dorney, MD
Instructor of Pediatrics and Emergency Medicine
Harvard Medical School
Division of Emergency Medicine
Boston Children's Hospital
Boston, Massachusetts

Cara B. Doughty, MD, Med
Assistant Professor
Department of Pediatrics
Baylor College of Medicine
Attending Physician
Section of Pediatric Emergency Medicine
Texas Children's Hospital
Houston, Texas

Nanette C. Dudley, MD
Clinical Professor
Department of Pediatrics
Division of Pediatric Emergency Medicine
University of Utah School of Medicine
Salt Lake City, Utah

Karen E. Dull, MD
Assistant Professor of Pediatrics
Harvard Medical School
Division of Emergency Medicine
Boston Children's Hospital
Boston, Massachusetts

Yamini Durani, MD
Assistant Professor of Pediatrics
The Sidney Kimmel Medical College at Thomas Jefferson University
Division of Emergency Medicine
Alfred I. duPont Hospital for Children
Wilmington, Delaware

Matthew Eisenberg, MD
Instructor of Pediatrics and Emergency Medicine
Harvard Medical School
Division of Emergency Medicine
Boston Children's Hospital
Boston, Massachusetts

Edward M. Eitzen Jr., MD, MPH
Senior Partner
Biodefense and Public Health Programs
Martin-Blanck and Associates
Alexandria, Virginia

Angela M. Ellison, MD, MSc
Assistant Professor of Pediatrics
Perelman School of Medicine at the University of Pennsylvania
Division of Emergency Medicine
The Children's Hospital of Philadelphia
Philadelphia, Pennsylvania

Karan McBride Emerick, MD, MSCI
Associate Professor of Pediatrics
Division of Pediatric Gastroenterology, Hepatology and Nutrition
Connecticut Children's Medical Center
Hartford, Connecticut

Mirna M. Farah, MD
Attending Physician and Professor of Pediatrics
Department of Pediatrics, Division of Emergency Medicine
Perelman School of Medicine of the University of Pennsylvania
The Children's Hospital of Philadelphia
Philadelphia, Pennsylvania

Karen S. Farbman, MD, MPH
Instructor of Pediatrics
Harvard Medical School
Division of Emergency Medicine
Boston Children's Hospital
Boston, Massachusetts

Joel A. Fein, MD, MPH
Professor
Departments of Pediatrics and Emergency Medicine
Perelman School of Medicine at the University of Pennsylvania
Attending Physician
Emergency Department
The Children's Hospital of Pennsylvania
Philadelphia, Pennsylvania

Zameera Fida, DMD
Director of Predoctoral Pediatric Dentistry
Department of Development Biology
Harvard School of Dental Medicine
Boston, Massachusetts

Andrew M. Fine, MD, MPH
Assistant Professor of Pediatrics and Emergency Medicine
Harvard Medical School
Division of Emergency Medicine
Boston Children's Hospital
Boston, Massachusetts

Julie C. Fitzgerald, MD, PhD
Assistant Professor of Anesthesia and Critical Care Medicine
Department of Anesthesia and Critical Care Medicine
Perelman School of Medicine at the University of Pennsylvania
The Children's Hospital of Philadelphia
Philadelphia, Pennsylvania

Eric W. Fleegler, MD, MPH
Assistant Professor of Pediatrics
Harvard Medical School
Division of Emergency Medicine
Boston Children's Hospital
Boston, Massachusetts

Gary R. Fleisher, MD
Egan Family Foundation Professor
Department of Pediatrics
Harvard Medical School
Physician-in-Chief, Pediatrician-in-Chief, and Chairman
Department of Medicine
Boston Children's Hospital
Boston, Massachusetts

Todd A. Florin, MD, MSCE
Assistant Professor of Pediatrics
Attending Physician
Department of Pediatrics
Division of Pediatric Emergency Medicine
Cincinnati Children's Hospital Medical Center
University of Cincinnati College of Medicine
Cincinnati, Ohio

Warren D. Frankenberger, PhD, RN, CCNS
Clinical Nurse Specialist
Department of Emergency
The Children's Hospital of Philadelphia
Philadelphia, Pennsylvania

Janet H. Friday, MD
Clinical Professor
Department of Pediatrics
University of California, San Diego
La Jolla, California
Attending Physician
Pediatric Emergency Department
Rady Children's Hospital
San Diego, California

Eron Y. Friedlaender, MD, MPH
Associate Professor of Clinical Pediatrics
Department of Pediatrics
Perelman School of Medicine at the University of Pennsylvania
Attending Physician
Department of Pediatrics
The Children's Hospital of Philadelphia
Philadelphia, Pennsylvania

Mary Kate Funari, MSN, RN, CPEN
Education Nurse Specialist
Department of Emergency Nursing
The Children's Hospital of Philadelphia
Philadelphia, Pennsylvania

Ronald A. Furnival, MD
Professor of Pediatrics and Emergency Medicine
University of Minnesota Medical School
Medical Director, Emergency Services
University of Minnesota Masonic Children's Hospital
Minneapolis, Minnesota

Payal K. Gala, MD
Assistant Professor of Clinical Pediatrics
Department of Pediatrics
Perelman School of Medicine at the University of Pennsylvania
Attending Physician
Division of Pediatric Emergency Medicine
The Children's Hospital of Philadelphia
Philadelphia, Pennsylvania

Eric W. Glissmeyer, MD
Assistant Professor
Department of Pediatrics
University of Utah School of Medicine
Division of Pediatric Emergency Medicine
Primary Children's Hospital
Salt Lake City, Utah

Nicolaus W.S. Glomb, MD, MPH
Post-doctoral Fellow
Department of Pediatrics
Baylor College of Medicine
Post-doctoral Fellow, Pediatric Emergency Medicine
Department of Pediatrics
Texas Children's Hospital
Houston, Texas

Marc H. Gorelick, MD, MSCE
Professor of Pediatrics
Medical College of Wisconsin
Chief Operating Officer and Executive Vice President
Children's Hospital of Wisconsin
Milwaukee, Wisconsin

Monika K. Goyal, MD, MSCE
Assistant Professor of Pediatrics and Emergency Medicine
Department of Pediatrics
Children's National Health System
The George Washington University
Washington, DC

Rose C. Graham, MD, MSCE
Pediatric Gastroenterology
Durham, North Carolina

Matthew P. Gray, MD, MS
Assistant Professor
Department of Pediatrics, Division of Emergency Medicine
Medical College of Wisconsin
Children's Hospital of Wisconsin
Milwaukee, Wisconsin

Toni K. Gross, MD, MPH
Clinical Associate Professor
Department of Child Health
University of Arizona College of Medicine-Phoenix, Phoenix Children's Hospital
Phoenix, Arizona

Megan Hannon, MD
Instructor of Pediatrics
Harvard Medical School
Division of Emergency Medicine
Boston Children's Hospital
Boston, Massachusetts

Sanjiv Harpavat, MD, PhD
Assistant Professor
Department of Pediatrics
Baylor College of Medicine
Assistant Professor
Department of Pediatrics
Texas Children's Hospital
Houston, Texas

Melissa M. Hazen, MD
Instructor
Boston Children's Hospital
Department of Medicine
Divisions of General Pediatrics and Rheumatology
Harvard Medical School
Boston, Massachusetts

Marissa A. Hendrickson, MD
Assistant Professor of Pediatrics
Department of Pediatrics, Division of Pediatric Emergency Medicine
University of Minnesota Masonic Children's Hospital
Minneapolis, Minnesota

Erin B. Henkel, MD
Pediatric Emergency Medicine Fellow, Instructor of Pediatrics
Department of Pediatric Emergency Medicine
Texas Children's Hospital/Baylor College of Medicine
Houston, Texas

Fred M. Henretig, MD
Professor Emeritus of Pediatrics
Perelman School of Medicine at the University of Pennsylvania
Director, Section of Clinical Toxicology
The Children's Hospital of Philadelphia
Philadelphia, Pennsylvania

Hilary A. Hewes, MD
Assistant Professor
Department of Pediatrics, Division of Pediatric Emergency Medicine
University of Utah
Primary Children's Medical Center
Salt Lake City, Utah

Eric C. Hoppa, MD
Assistant Professor of Pediatrics
University of Connecticut School of Medicine
Attending Physician
Pediatric Emergency Department
Connecticut Children's Medical Center
Hartford, Connecticut

Deborah Hsu, MD, MEd
Associate Professor
Department of Pediatrics, Section of Emergency Medicine
Baylor College of Medicine
Attending Physician
Department of Pediatrics, Section of Emergency Medicine
Texas Children's Hospital
Houston, Texas

Joel D. Hudgins, MD
Instructor of Pediatrics and Emergency Medicine
Harvard Medical School
Division of Emergency Medicine
Boston Children's Hospital
Boston, Massachusetts

Elizabeth S. Jacobs, MD
Assistant Professor
Departments of Pediatrics and Emergency Medicine
Alpert Medical School of Brown University
Hasbro Children's Hospital/Rhode Island Hospital
Providence, Rhode Island

Cynthia R. Jacobstein, MD, MSCE
Associate Professor of Clinical Pediatrics
Department of Pediatrics, Division of Emergency Medicine
Perelman School of Medicine at the University of Pennsylvania
The Children's Hospital of Philadelphia
Philadelphia, Pennsylvania

Lenore R. Jarvis, MD, MEd
Adjunct Instructor of Pediatrics
Department of Pediatrics
The George Washington University School of Medicine and Health Sciences
Fellow
Division of Emergency Medicine
Children's National Health System
Washington, DC

Andrew Jea, MD
Associate Professor
Department of Neurosurgery
Baylor College of Medicine
Director, Neuro-spine Program
Director, Educational Programs
Division of Pediatric Neurosurgery
Texas Children's Hospital
Houston, Texas

Melinda Jen, MD
Assistant Professor of Pediatrics and Dermatology
Perelman School of Medicine at the University of Pennsylvania
The Children's Hospital of Philadelphia
Philadelphia, Pennsylvania

Mark D. Joffe, MD
Associate Professor of Pediatrics
Division of Emergency Medicine
Perelman School of Medicine at the University of Pennsylvania
Director, Community Pediatric Medicine
The Children's Hospital of Philadelphia
Philadelphia, Pennsylvania

Rahul Kaila, MD
Assistant Professor of Pediatric Emergency Medicine
Division of Pediatric Emergency Medicine
University of Minnesota Masonic Children's Hospital
Minneapolis, Minnesota

Ron L. Kaplan, MD
Associate Professor
Department of Pediatrics
University of Washington School of Medicine
Attending Physician
Emergency Department
Seattle Children's Hospital
Seattle, Washington

Emily R. Katz, MD
Assistant Professor (Clinical)
Departments of Psychiatry and Human Behavior
Alpert Medical School of Brown University
Director, Child and Adolescent Psychiatry Consultation-Liaison Service
Department of Psychiatry
Rhode Island Hospital/Hasbro Children's Hospital
Providence, Rhode Island

Young-Jo Kim, MD, PhD
Associate Professor of Orthopedic Surgery
Department of Orthopedic Surgery
Boston Children's Hospital
Boston, Massachusetts

Amir A. Kimia, MD
Assistant Professor of Pediatrics
Harvard Medical School
Division of Emergency Medicine
Boston Children's Hospital
Boston, Massachusetts

Christopher King, MD, FACEP
Professor
Department of Emergency Medicine and Pediatrics
Albany Medical College
Chair
Department of Emergency Medicine
Albany Medical Center
Albany, New York

Susanne Kost, MD, FAAP, FACEP
Clinical Professor of Pediatrics
The Sidney Kimmel Medical College at Thomas
Jefferson University
Philadelphia, Pennsylvania
Medical Director, Day Medicine Unit and Sedation Service
Attending Physician
Department of Anesthesia and Pediatrics
Division of Pediatric Emergency Medicine
Nemours/Alfred I. duPont Hospital for Children
Wilmington, Delaware

Nathan Kuppermann, MD, MPH
Professor and Bo Tomas Brofeldt Endowed Chair
Department of Emergency Medicine
UC Davis School of Medicine
Sacramento, California

Jane Lavelle, MD
Associate Professor of Pediatrics
Department of Pediatrics
Perelman School of Medicine at the University of Pennsylvania
Medical Director, Associate Division Chief Emergency Medicine
Medical Director, Pathway Program
Office of Continuous Quality Improvement
The Children's Hospital of Philadelphia
Philadelphia, Pennsylvania

Megan Lavoie, MD
Assistant Professor of Clinical Pediatrics
Department of Pediatrics
Division of Emergency Medicine
Perelman School of Medicine at the University of Pennsylvania
The Children's Hospital of Philadelphia
Philadelphia, Pennsylvania

Gi-Soo Lee, MD, EdM
Instructor
Department of Otology and Laryngology
Harvard Medical School
Associate in Otolaryngology and Communication Enhancement
Boston Children's Hospital
Boston, Massachusetts

Lois K. Lee, MD, MPH
Assistant Professor of Pediatrics and Emergency Medicine
Harvard Medical School
Division of Emergency Medicine
Boston Children's Hospital
Boston, Massachusetts

Alex V. Levin, MD, MHSc, FRCSC
Chief, Pediatric Ophthalmology and Ocular Genetics
Robison D. Harley, MD Endowed Chair in Pediatric Ophthalmology and Ocular Genetics
Wills Eye Hospital
Professor, Departments of Ophthalmology and Pediatrics
The Sidney Kimmel Medical College at Thomas
Jefferson University
Philadelphia, Pennsylvania

Jason A. Levy, MD, RDMS
Assistant Professor of Pediatrics and Emergency Medicine
Harvard Medical School
Associate Clinical Director
Division of Emergency Medicine
Boston Children's Hospital
Boston, Massachusetts

Danica B. Liberman, MD, MPH
Assistant Professor of Clinical Pediatrics
Department of Pediatrics
Division of Emergency and Transport Medicine
Children's Hospital Los Angeles/Keck School of Medicine of the University of Southern California
Los Angeles, California

Erica L. Liebelt, MD, FACMT
Professor of Pediatrics and Emergency Medicine
Department of Pediatrics, Division of Pediatric Emergency Medicine
University of Alabama Birmingham School of Medicine
Children's of Alabama
Birmingham, Alabama

Henry C. Lin, MD
Assistant Professor
Department of Pediatrics
Perelman School of Medicine at the University of Pennsylvania
Attending Physician
Department of Pediatrics
The Children's Hospital of Philadelphia
Philadelphia, Pennsylvania

Galina Lipton, MD
Instructor of Pediatrics
Harvard Medical School
Division of Emergency Medicine
Boston Children's Hospital
Boston, Massachusetts

John M. Loiselle, MD
Associate Professor
Department of Pediatrics
The Sidney Kimmel Medical College at Thomas Jefferson University
Philadelphia, Pennsylvania
Chief, Emergency Medicine
Alfred I. duPont Hospital for Children
Wilmington, Delaware

Patricia Lopez, MSN, CRNP
Nurse Practitioner
Division of Emergency Medicine
The Children's Hospital of Philadelphia
Philadelphia, Pennsylvania

Naomi Love, BSN, RN, CPEN
Registered Nurse
Emergency Department
The Children's Hospital of Philadelphia
Philadelphia, Pennsylvania

David A. Lowe, MD
Clinical Assistant Professor
Herbert Wertheim College of Medicine
Florida International University
Attending Physician
Department of Emergency Medicine
Nicklaus Children's Hospital
Miami, Florida

Dennis P. Lund, MD
Professor of Surgery and Chief Medical Officer, Lucile Packard Children's Hospital
Associate Dean of the Faculty for Pediatrics and Obstetrics, Stanford University School of Medicine
Department of Surgery
Lucile Packard Children's Hospital/Stanford University School of Medicine
Palo Alto, California

James M. Madsen, MD, MPH, FCAP, FACOEM COL, MC-FS
Adjunct Associate Professor of Preventive Medicine and Biometrics
Assistant Professor of Pathology
Uniformed Service, University of the Health Sciences
Bethesda, Maryland
Deputy Director of Academics and Training
Chemical Casualty Care Division
US Army Medical Research Institute of Chemical Defense (USAMRICD)
APG-South, MB

Vincenzo Maniaci, MD
Clinical Assistant Professor
Herbert Wertheim College of Medicine
Florida International University
Fellowship Director
Department of Emergency Medicine
Nicklaus Children's Hospital
Miami, Florida

Rebekah Mannix, MD, MPH
Assistant Professor of Pediatrics and Emergency Medicine
Harvard Medical School
Division of Emergency Medicine
Boston Children's Hospital
Boston, Massachusetts

Ronald F. Marchese, MD, PhD
Assistant Professor of Clinical Pediatrics
Department of Pediatrics, Division of Emergency Medicine
Perelman School of Medicine at the University of Pennsylvania
The Children's Hospital of Philadelphia
Philadelphia, Pennsylvania

Constance M. McAneney, MD, MS
Professor
Department of Pediatrics
University of Cincinnati College of Medicine
Associate Director
Division of Emergency Medicine
Cincinnati Children's Hospital Medical Center
Cincinnati, Ohio

Patrick J. McMahon, MD
Assistant Professor of Pediatrics and Dermatology
Department of Pediatric Dermatology
The Children's Hospital of Philadelphia
Philadelphia, Pennsylvania

Julie K. McManemy, MD, MPH
Assistant Professor of Pediatrics
Department of Pediatric Emergency Medicine
Baylor College of Medicine
Texas Children's Hospital
Houston, Texas

Alisa McQueen, MD
Associate Professor of Pediatrics
Department of Pediatrics, Section of Pediatric Emergency Medicine
University of Chicago Comer Children's Hospital
Chicago, Illinois

Chris Merritt, MD, MPH
Assistant Professor
Department of Emergency Medicine and Pediatrics
Alpert Medical School of Brown University
Attending Physician
Department of Pediatric Emergency Medicine
Hasbro Children's Hospital/Rhode Island Hospital
Providence, Rhode Island

Rakesh D. Mistry, MD, MS
Attending Physician
Section of Emergency Medicine
Children's Hospital Colorado
Associate Professor of Pediatrics
University of Colorado School of Medicine
Denver, Colorado

Manoj K. Mittal, MD, MRCP(UK)
Associate Professor of Clinical Pediatrics
Department of Pediatrics
Division of Emergency Medicine
Perelman School of Medicine at the University of Pennsylvania
The Children's Hospital of Philadelphia
Philadelphia, Pennsylvania

Matthew R. Mittiga, MD
Assistant Professor of Clinical Pediatrics
Department of Pediatrics
University of Cincinnati College of Medicine
Attending Physician
Division of Emergency Medicine
Cincinnati Children's Hospital Medical Center
Cincinnati, Ohio

Cynthia J. Mollen, MD, MSCE
Associate Professor and Attending Physician
Department of Pediatrics
Division of Emergency Medicine
Perelman School of Medicine at the University of Pennsylvania
The Children's Hospital of Philadelphia
Philadelphia, Pennsylvania

Jennifer Molnar, MSN, RN, PNP-BC, CPNP-AC, SANE-P
Pediatric Nurse Practitioner
Department of Emergency Department
The Children's Hospital of Philadelphia
Philadelphia, Pennsylvania

David P. Mooney, MD, MPH
Associate Professor of Surgery
Harvard Medical School
Department of Surgery
Children's Hospital Boston
Boston, Massachusetts

Sage R. Myers, MD, MSCE
Assistant Professor of Pediatrics
Perelman School of Medicine at the University of Pennsylvania
Attending Physician
Department of Pediatrics
Division of Emergency Medicine
The Children's Hospital of Philadelphia
Philadelphia, Pennsylvania

Frances M. Nadel, MD, MSCE
Professor of Clinical Pediatrics
Department of Pediatrics
Perelman School of Pennsylvania at the University of Pennsylvania
Attending Physician
The Children's Hospital of Philadelphia
Philadelphia, Pennsylvania

Joshua Nagler, MD, MHPEd
Assistant Professor of Pediatrics and Emergency Medicine
Harvard Medical School
Fellowship Director
Division of Emergency Medicine
Boston Children's Hospital
Boston, Massachusetts

Michael L. Nance, MD
Templeton Professor of Surgery
Department of Surgery
The Children's Hospital of Philadelphia and Perelman School of Medicine at the University of Pennsylvania
Philadelphia, Pennsylvania

Howard L. Needleman, DMD
Senior Associate/Clinical Professor
Department of Dentistry, Developmental Biology (Pediatric Dentistry)
Harvard School of Dental Medicine
Boston Children's Hospital
Boston, Massachusetts

Douglas S. Nelson, MD, FACEP, FAAP
Professor
Department of Pediatrics
University of Utah School of Medicine
Medical Director
Emergency Department
Primary Children's Hospital
Salt Lake City, Utah

Kyle Nelson, MD, MPH
Assistant Professor of Pediatrics and Emergency Medicine
Harvard Medical School
Division of Emergency Medicine
Boston Children's Hospital
Boston, Massachusetts

Linda P. Nelson, DMD, MScD
Assistant Clinical Professor
Department of Dentistry, Developmental Biology (Pediatric Dentistry)
Harvard School of Dental Medicine
Senior Attending
Department of Pediatric Dentistry
Boston Children's Hospital
Boston, Massachusetts

Mark I. Neuman, MD, MPH
Associate Professor of Pediatrics and Emergency Medicine
Harvard Medical School
Research Director
Division of Emergency Medicine
Boston Children's Hospital
Boston, Massachusetts

Thuy L. Ngo, DO, MEd
Assistant Professor
Department of Pediatrics
Division of Pediatric Emergency Medicine
Johns Hopkins University
Baltimore, Maryland

Michelle L. Niescierenko, MD
Instructor of Pediatrics and Emergency Medicine
Harvard Medical School
Division of Emergency Medicine
Boston Children's Hospital
Boston, Massachusetts

Katherine A. O'Donnell, MD
Instructor of Pediatrics
Harvard Medical School
Hospital Medicine and Toxicology
Boston Children's Hospital
Boston, Massachusetts

Lila O'Mahony, MD, FAAP
Assistant Professor
Department of Pediatrics
Division of Emergency Medicine
University of Washington School of Medicine
Seattle Children's Hospital
Seattle, Washington

Kevin C. Osterhoudt, MD, MSCE
Medical Director
The Poison Control Center
Division of Emergency Medicine
The Children's Hospital of Philadelphia
Philadelphia, Pennsylvania

Bonnie L. Padwa, DMD, MD
Associate Professor of Oral and Maxillofacial Surgery
Harvard School of Dental Medicine
Oral Surgeon-in-Chief
Department of Plastic and Oral Surgery
Boston Children's Hospital
Boston, Massachusetts

Jan Paradise, MD
Pediatrician
Easton, Massachusetts

Shilpa Patel, MD, MPH
Assistant Professor of Pediatrics and Emergency Medicine
Division of Emergency Medicine
Children's National Health System
The George Washington University School of Medicine
Washington, DC

Ronald I. Paul, MD
Professor of Pediatrics
Division of Pediatric Emergency of Medicine
University of Louisville
Kosair Children's Hospital
Louisville, Kentucky

Denis R. Pauzé, MD, FACEP
Vice Chairman, Operations
Associate Professor of Emergency Medicine and Pediatrics
Department of Emergency Medicine
Albany Medical College
Albany, New York

Faria Pereira, MD
Assistant Professor
Department of Pediatrics
Baylor College of Medicine
Faculty
Department of Pediatrics
Texas Children's Hospital
Houston, Texas

Marissa J. Perman, MD
Assistant Professor
Department of Pediatrics, Section of Dermatology
The Children's Hospital Of Philadelphia and The University of Pennsylvania
Philadelphia, Pennsylvania

Catherine E. Perron, MD
Assistant Professor of Pediatrics
Harvard Medical School
Director of Quality Assurance and Patient Safety
Division of Emergency Medicine
Boston Children's Hospital
Boston, Massachusetts

Holly E. Perry, MD
Assistant Professor
Department of Emergency Medicine
Tufts University School of Medicine
Boston, Massachusetts
Attending Physician
Emergency Medicine
Baystate Medical Center
Springfield, Massachusetts

Andrew E. Place, MD, PhD
Instructor
Department of Pediatrics
Harvard Medical School
Attending Physician
Pediatric Hematologic Malignancy Program
Dana-Faber Cancer Institute &
Boston Children's Hospital
Boston, Massachusetts

Jeannine Del Pizzo, MD
Assistant Professor of Clinical Pediatrics
Department of Pediatrics
Perelman School of Medicine at the University of Pennsylvania
Attending Physician
Division of Emergency Medicine
The Children's Hospital of Philadelphia
Philadelphia, Pennsylvania

Jill C. Posner, MD, MSCE, MSEd
Professor of Clinical Pediatrics
Perelman School of Medicine at the University of Pennsylvania
Division of Emergency Medicine
The Children's Hospital of Philadelphia
Philadelphia, Pennsylvania

Debra A. Potts, MSN, RN, CPEN, CEN
Nurse Manager
Emergency Department
The Children's Hospital of Philadelphia
Philadelphia, Pennsylvania

Carla M. Pruden, MD, MPH
Attending Physician
Associate Professor of Pediatrics
Simulation Program Co-Director
Division of Pediatric Emergency Medicine
Connecticut Children's Medical Center
Hartford, Connecticut

Casandra Quiñones, MD
Assistant Professor
Department of Pediatric Emergency Medicine
Baylor College of Medicine
Texas Children's Hospital
Houston, Texas

Ann Marie Reardon, MSN, CRNP
Nurse Practitioner
Department of Emergency Medicine
The Children's Hospital of Philadelphia
Philadelphia, Pennsylvania

Rachel G. Rempell, MD, RDMS
Instructor of Pediatrics and Emergency Medicine
Harvard Medical School
Director of Emergency Ultrasound
Division of Emergency Medicine
Boston Children's Hospital
Boston, Massachusetts

Mark G. Roback, MD
Director, Division of Pediatric Emergency Medicine
Professor of Pediatrics and Emergency Medicine
University of Minnesota Masonic Children's Hospital
Minneapolis, Minnesota

Bonnie Rodio, RN, BSN, CEN, CPHQ
Unit Based Safety & Quality Coordinator
Emergency Department
The Children's Hospital of Philadelphia
Philadelphia, Pennsylvania

Brent D. Rogers, MD
Fellow
Department of Pediatrics, Division of Emergency Medicine
Nemours/Alfred I. duPont Hospital for Children
Wilmington, Delaware

Steven C. Rogers, MD
Attending Physician
Associate Professor of Pediatrics and Emergency Medicine
Division of Pediatric Emergency Medicine
Connecticut Children's Medical Center
University of Connecticut School of Medicine
Hartford, Connecticut

Christine Roper, BSN, RN
Staff Nurse
Emergency Department
The Children's Hospital of Philadelphia
Philadelphia, Pennsylvania

Cindy G. Roskind, MD
Assistant Professor of Pediatrics
Department of Pediatrics, Division of Emergency Medicine
Columbia University College of Physicians and Surgeons
New York, New York

Richard M. Ruddy, MD
Professor of Pediatrics
University of Cincinnati College of Medicine
Medical Director
Cincinnati Children's Hospital—Liberty Campus
Cincinnati Children's Hospital Medical Center
Cincinnati, Ohio

Marideth C. Rus, MD
Clinical Instructor of Pediatric Emergency Medicine
Baylor College of Medicine
Texas Children's Hospital
Houston, Texas

Eric A. Russell, MD
Clinical Instructor
Department of Pediatric Emergency Medicine
Baylor College of Medicine
Texas Children's Hospital
Houston, Texas

Richard A. Saladino, MD
Professor of Pediatrics
University of Pittsburgh School of Medicine
Chief, Pediatric Emergency Medicine
Department of Pediatrics
Children's Hospital of Pittsburgh
Pittsburgh, Pennsylvania

Margaret Samuels-Kalow, MD, MPhil, MSHP
Instructor
Department of Pediatrics
Perelman School of Medicine at the University of Pennsylvania
The Children's Hospital of Philadelphia
Philadelphia, Pennsylvania

Richard J. Scarfone, MD
Associate Professor
Department of Pediatrics
Perelman School of Medicine at the University of Pennsylvania
Medical Director
Emergency Preparedness
The Children's Hospital of Pennsylvania
Philadelphia, Pennsylvania

Aileen Schast, PhD
Clinical Psychologist
Perelman School of Medicine at the University of Pennsylvania
The Children's Hospital of Philadelphia
Philadelphia, Pennsylvania

Dana A. Schinasi, MD
Assistant Professor of Pediatrics
Division of Pediatric Emergency Medicine
Ann and Robert H. Lurie Children's Hospital of Chicago
Northwestern University Feinberg School of Medicine
Chicago, Illinois

Suzanne Schmidt, MD
Assistant Professor in Pediatrics
Division of Pediatric Emergency Medicine
Ann and Robert H. Lurie Children's Hospital of Chicago
Northwestern University Feinberg School of Medicine
Chicago, Illinois

Deborah Schonfeld, MD, FRCPC
Assistant Professor
Department of Pediatrics
University of Toronto
Associate Staff Physician
Division of Emergency Medicine
The Hospital for Sick Children
Toronto, Ontario

Mary Schucker, RN, MSN, CRNP
Course Director
School of Nursing at the University of Pennsylvania
Pediatric Nurse Practitioner
Department of Emergency Medicine
The Children's Hospital of Philadelphia
Philadelphia, Pennsylvania

Sara A. Schutzman, MD
Assistant Professor of Pediatrics and Emergency Medicine
Harvard Medical School
Division of Emergency Medicine
Boston Children's Hospital
Boston, Massachusetts

Philip V. Scribano, DO, MSCE
Professor, Clinical Pediatrics
Department of Pediatrics
Perelman School of Medicine at the University of Pennsylvania
Director, Safe Place: Center for Child Protection and Health
Division of General Pediatrics
The Children's Hospital of Philadelphia
Philadelphia, Pennsylvania

Desiree M. Seeyave, MBBS
Assistant Professor
Division of Emergency Medicine
The George Washington University School of Medicine
Children's National Medical Center
Washington, DC

Jeffrey A. Seiden, MD
Assistant Professor of Clinical Pediatrics
Department of Pediatrics, Division of Emergency Medicine
Perelman School of Medicine at the University of Pennsylvania
The Children's Hospital of Philadelphia
Philadelphia, Pennsylvania

Steven M. Selbst, MD
Professor of Pediatrics
Vice Chair for Education
Director, Pediatric Residency Program
The Sidney Kimmel Medical College at Thomas Jefferson University
Philadelphia, Pennsylvania
Attending Physician, Division of Emergency Medicine
Nemours/Alfred I. duPont Hospital for Children
Wilmington, Delaware

Sonal N. Shah, MD, MPH
Instructor of Pediatrics
Harvard Medical School
Division of Emergency Medicine
Boston Children's Hospital
Boston, Massachusetts

Kathy N. Shaw, MD, MSCE
Professor and Associate Chair
Department of Pediatrics
Perelman School of Medicine at the University of Pennsylvania
The Nicholas Crognale Endowed Chair in Emergency Medicine
The Children's Hospital of Philadelphia
Philadelphia, Pennsylvania

Rohit P. Shenoi, MD
Associate Professor
Department of Pediatrics
Baylor College of Medicine
Attending Physician, Emergency Center
Department of Pediatrics
Texas Children's Hospital
Houston, Texas

Stephen Shusterman, DMD
Dentist-in-Chief Emeritus
Clinical Associate Professor
Harvard School of Dental Medicine
Department of Dentistry
Boston Children's Hospital
Boston, Massachusetts

Lamia Soghier, MD, FAAP
Assistant Professor of Pediatrics
Department of Neonatology
Children's National Health System
The George Washington University School of Medicine and Health Sciences
Washington, DC

Aun Woon Soon, MD
Fellow
Deparmtent of Pediatric Emergency Medicine
Northwestern University
Ann and Robert H. Lurie Children's Hospital of Chicago
Chicago, Illinois

Philip Spandorfer, MD, MSCE
Attending Physician
Department of Pediatric Emergency Medicine
Children's Healthcare of Atlanta at Scottish Rite, Pediatric Emergency Medicine Associates
Atlanta, Georgia

Anne M. Stack, MD
Associate Professor of Pediatrics and Emergency Medicine
Harvard Medical School
Clinical Chief
Division of Emergency Medicine
Boston Children's Hospital
Boston, Massachusetts

Michelle D. Stevenson, MD, MS, FAAP
Associate Professor of Pediatrics
University of Louisville
Louisville, Kentucky

Gregory E. Tasian, MD, MSc, MSCE
Assistant Professor
Department of Surgery, Division of Urology
Perelman School of Medicine at the University of Pennsylvania
Attending Physician
Department of Surgery, Division of Urology
The Children's Hospital of Pennsylvania
Philadelphia, Pennsylvania

Khoon-Yen Tay, MD
Assistant Professor of Pediatrics
Department of Pediatrics
Perelman School of Medicine at the University of Pennsylvania
Philadelphia, Pennsylvania
Attending Physician
Division of Emergency Medicine
The Children's Hospital of Philadelphia
Philadelphia, Pennsylvania

Stephen J. Teach, MD, MPH
Professor and Chair
Department of Pediatrics
The George Washington University School of Medicine
Children's National Health System
Washington, DC

Amy D. Thompson, MD, FAAP, FACEP
Attending Physician
Emergency Medicine
Alfred I. duPont Hospital for Children
Wilmington, Delaware
Assistant Professor
Department of Pediatrics
The Sidney Kimmel Medical College at Thomas Jefferson University
Philadelphia, Pennsylvania

Rachel Thompson, MD
Assistant Professor of Pediatrics
Department of Pediatrics, Division of Pediatric Emergency Medicine
Boston University School of Medicine
Boston Medical Center
Boston, Massachusetts

Sharon Topf, RN, BSN, CPEN
Clinical Supervisor
Emergency Department
The Children's Hospital of Philadelphia
Philadelphia, Pennsylvania

Susan B. Torrey, MD
Associate Professor of Emergency Medicine and Pediatrics
Department of Emergency Medicine
New York University School of Medicine
New York, New York

James R. Treat, MD
Associate Professor of Pediatrics and Dermatology
Perelman School of Medicine at the University of Pennsylvania
The Children's hospital of Philadelphia
Philadelphia, Pennsylvania

Nicholas Tsarouhas, MD
Professor of Clinical Pediatrics
Department of Pediatrics
Perelman School of Medicine at the University of Pennsylvania
Medical Director, Transport Team
Attending Physician of Emergency Medicine
Department of Pediatrics
Division of Emergency Medicine
The Children's Hospital of Philadelphia
Philadelphia, Pnnsylvania

Lisa Tyler, MS, RRT-NPS, CPFT
Manager
Respirating Care
The Children's Hospital of Philadelphia
Philadelphia, Pennsylvania

Leah Tzimenatos, MD
Associate Clinical Professor
Department of Emergency Medicine
UC Davis School of Medicine
Sacramento, California

Christopher F. Valente, MD
Fellow, Pediatric Emergency Medicine
Department of Pediatrics
Perelman School of Medicine at the University of Pennsylvania
Fellow, Pediatric Emergency Medicine
Department of Pediatrics
Division of Emergency Medicine
The Children's Hospital of Philadelphia
Philadelphia, Pennsylvania

Cheryl Vance, MD
Professor, Emergency Medicine and Pediatrics
Department of Emergency Medicine
UC Davis School of Medicine
Sacramento, California

Robert J. Vinci, MD
Chief of Pediatrics
Department of Pediatrics
Boston University School of Medicine
Boston Medical Center
Boston, Massachusetts

Theresa A. Walls, MD, MPH
Assistant Professor of Pediatrics
Department of Pediatrics, Division of Emergency Medicine
The George Washington University School of Medicine
Children's National Health System
Washington, DC

Jinsong Wang, MD, PhD
Orthopaedic Surgeon
New Hampshire Orthopaedic Center
Badford, New Hampshire

Vincent J. Wang, MD, MHA
Associate Division Head
Division of Emergency Medicine
Children's Hospital Los Angeles
Associate Professor of Pediatrics
Keck School of Medicine of the University of Southern California
Los Angeles, California

Sarah N. Weihmiller, MD, FAAP, FACEP
Clinical Assistant Professor of Pediatrics
Division of Pediatric Emergency Medicine
The Sidney Kimmel Medical College at Thomas
Jefferson University
Nemours/Afred I. duPont Hospital for Children
Wilmington, Delaware

Debra L. Weiner, MD, PhD
Assistant Professor of Pediatrics
Harvard Medical School
Division of Emergency Medicine
Boston Children's Hospital
Boston, Massachusetts

Dana A. Weiss, MD
Assistant Professor of Surgery in Urology
Division of Urology
The Children's Hospital of Philadelphia
University of Pennsylvania
Philadelphia, Pennsylvania

Scott L. Weiss, MD, MSCE
Assistant Professor
Department of Anesthesiology and Critcial Care Medicine
Perelman School of Medicine at the University of Pennsylvania
Attending Physician
Department of Anesthesiology and Critcial Care Medicine
The Children's Hospital of Philadelphia
Philadelphia, Pennsylvania

T. Bram Welch-Horan, MD
Assistant Professor of Clinical Pediatrics
Department of Pediatrics
Perelman School of Medicine at the University of Pennsylvania
Division of Emergency Medicine
The Children's Hospital of Philadelphia
Philadelphia, Pennsylvania

Heidi C. Werner, MD, MSHPEd
Assistant Professor
Department of Pediatrics
Boston University School of Medicine
Attending Physician
Division of Pediatric Emergency Medicine
Boston Medical Center
Boston, Massachusetts

James F. Wiley II, MD, MPH
Clinical Professor of Pediatrics and Emergency Medicine/Traumatology
Departments of Pediatrics and Emergency Medicine/Traumatology
University of Connecticut School of Medicine
Farmington, Connecticut

Emily L. Willner, MD
Assistant Professor of Pediatrics and Emergency Medicine
Division of Emergency Medicine
The George Washington University School of Medicine
Children's National Medical Center
Washington, DC

Michael Witt, MD, MPH
Clinical Assistant Professor of Medicine
Geisel School of Medicine at Dartmouth
Hanover, New Hampshire
Attending Physician
Pediatric Emergency Medicine
New Hampshire's Hospital for Children
Elliot Health System
Manchester, New Hampshire

Margaret Wolff, MD
Assistant Professor
Department of Emergency Medicine and Pediatrics
University of Michigan
Ann Arbor, Michigan

Joanne N. Wood, MD, MSHP
Assistant Professor of Pediatrics
Division of General Pediatrics
Perelman School of Medicine at the University of Pennsylvania
The Children's Hospital of Philadelphia
Philadelphia, Pennsylvania

George A. Woodward, MD, MBA
Division Chief of Emergency Medicine
Medical Director, Transport Services
Professor of Pediatrics
Department of Pediatrics
University of Washington School of Medicine
Seattle Children's Hospital
Seattle, Washington

Loren G. Yamamoto, MD, MPH, MBA
Professor
Department of Pediatrics
University of Hawaii John A. Burns School of Medicine
Chief of Staff and Pediatric Emergency Medicine
Attending Physician
Kapi'olani Medical Center for Women & Children
Honolulu, Hawaii

Albert C. Yan, MD, FAAP, FAAD
Chief, Section of Pediatric Dermatology
The Children's Hospital of Philadelphia
Professor, Pediatrics and Dermatology
Perelman School of Medicine at the University of Pennsylvania
Philadelphia, Pennsylvania

Katelyn N. Young, RN, MSN, CPEN
Registered Nurse
Emergency Department
The Children's Hospital of Philadelphia
Philadelphia, Pennsylvania

Shabana Yusuf, MD
Assistant Professor of Pediatrics
Section of Emergency Medicine, Department of Pediatrics
Baylor College of Medicine
Texas Children's Hospital
Houston, Texas

Lauren E. Zinns, MD, FAAP
Assistant Professor of Clinical Pediatrics
Perelman School of Medicine at the University of Pennsylvania
Division of Emergency Medicine
The Children's Hospital of Philadelphia
Philadelphia, Pennsylvania

Mark R. Zonfrillo, MD, MSCE
Assistant Professor
Department of Emergency Medicine
Alpert Medical School of Brown University
Hasbro Children's Hospital
Providence, Rhode Island

Joseph Zorc, MD, MSCE
David Lawrence Atlschuler Professor
Department of Pediatrics
Perelman School of Medicine at the University of Pennsylvania
Director
Emergency Information Systems
Emergency Department
The Children's Hospital of Philadelphia
Philadelphia, Pennsylvania

ACKNOWLEDGMENTS

In taking over the responsibility for producing the 7th edition of the Textbook of Pediatric Emergency Medicine, we would like to acknowledge the dedication and extraordinary efforts of the former editors, Drs. Stephen Ludwig and Gary Fleisher. In developing this textbook in the 1980s, they recognized the importance of defining and disseminating the rapidly evolving knowledge of pediatric emergency medicine. Through six prior editions over three decades, this reference has guided thousands of physicians in the care of children across the globe. For each edition, they identified expert clinicians to provide the most current evidence and practical clinical guidelines, and, in so doing, they have contributed to the evolution of pediatric emergency medicine. The newest edition with its format changes, online availability, and focus on quality is a direct extension of Steve and Gary's high standards and original goals for the textbook—namely, the promotion of optimal emergency care for children.

We also want to recognize the current associate editors, James M. Chamberlain, Jane Lavelle, Joshua Nagler, and Joan E. Shook, for their tremendous effort to produce the 7th edition. All of these editors are true leaders in pediatric emergency medicine, and each volunteered their precious time for the common goal of producing the best reference for pediatric emergency care.

Kathy N. Shaw, MD, MSCE and Richard G. Bachur, MD
Senior Editors

CONTENTS

e To view this chapter please access the eBook bundled with this text. Please see the inside front cover for eBook access instructions.

(e) To view this chapter please access the eBook bundled with this text. Please see the inside front cover for eBook access instructions.

(e) **To view this chapter please access the eBook bundled with this text. Please see the inside front cover for eBook access instructions.**

INTRODUCTION
High Quality Emergency Care for Children

Kathy N. Shaw, MD, MSCE and Richard G. Bachur, MD

GOALS OF EMERGENCY CARE

Our primary goal as practitioners is to provide high-quality, safe care for each child who arrives in our emergency department. The ability to stay current with pediatric medical literature across all possible conditions and injuries is impossible for any clinician. Furthermore, the evidence may be poor, inconsistent, or changing for the management of many diseases or injuries. This leads to a wide variation in practice, high rates of inappropriate care, patient harm, and wasted resources. With this new edition of the Textbook of Pediatric Emergency Medicine, we provide easy web-based access for use in practice, clinical pathways based on the latest evidence and expert consensus, and a new, streamlined format that emphasizes the goals of quality care and links to the corresponding "Signs and Symptoms" algorithms and Clinical Pathways.

KEY POINTS

- Standardization of care by using evidence-based clinical pathways or guidelines reduces variation in practice and decreases the rates of inappropriate care for children
- Easily accessed web-based resources aid clinicians in reducing medical errors due to cognition
- Teamwork, communication, and a nonpunitive reporting environment are key to providing safe care for children in EDs.
- Both the systems at the "blunt end" and the practices of the clinicians at the "sharp" end must be consistently monitored and improved to provide highly reliable care

QUALITY AND ITS MEASUREMENT IN PEDIATRIC EMERGENCY MEDICINE

KEY POINTS

- Pediatric Quality Improvement Coordinators and Committees are essential to providing safe care for children in EDs
- Monitoring pediatric indicators across the six domains of quality and instituting improvement when needed are essential to providing the highest value and safest care for children in our EDs

Current Evidence and Practice

The quality and safety of pediatric emergency medicine vary widely. In addition to unexplained variations in care related to individual providers and hospitals, there is likely a bimodal relationship between volume and quality. In other words, providers in EDs where pediatric volumes are low lack familiarity with pediatric diseases and may also lack basic equipment and supplies to care for children. In contrast, overcrowding in EDs with very high pediatric volumes may result in delays in care and failure to identify the one truly sick child among many who are not critically ill. In an effort to improve the quality of care for children in our nation's EDs, the American Academy of Pediatric, American College of Emergency Physicians, and the Emergency Nursing Association issued a joint policy statement "Guidelines for Care of Children in Emergency Departments" Table INT.1. This statement provides guidelines for the following: policies, procedures, and protocols; clinical and professional competency of staff; and the necessary pediatric equipment, supplies, medications, and services. Table INT.1 is a reproduction of a checklist developed as part of the policy statement (http://www2.aap.org/visit/Checklist_ED_Prep-022210.pdf). Additionally, the policy statement stresses the need for a physician and nurse pediatric coordinator to assure that there is continuous monitoring of quality indicators and process improvement in place for pediatric patients. EDs with a pediatric quality coordinator are more likely to have the equipment, policies, and protocols than those without pediatric champions.

The Institute of Medicine defines six domains of quality: care that is safe, timely, efficient, effective, equitable, and patient centered. Essentially, high-quality care increases the potential for the best health outcome in the shortest amount of time, at the lowest possible cost, with the lowest risk, while being respectful of the wishes of the patients, and not varying care based on personal characteristics. Ultimately, this provides the best value to patients as value in healthcare can be defined as quality/cost.

Most pediatric ED quality metrics and initiatives have concentrated on timeliness or patient flow. This focus on ED flow stems from the national issue of ED overcrowding that threatens many aspects of high-quality care as overcrowding is associated with medical errors, prolonged length of stay, and decreased patient satisfaction. Although metrics such as arrival to triage, door to doctor, admission decision to inpatient bed, and overall length of stay are important, the other domains of quality need to also be monitored and addressed. Consensus and review of the literature by a diverse panel of experts and consumers prioritized pediatric

TABLE INT.1

GUIDELINES FOR CARE OF CHILDREN IN THE EMERGENCY DEPARTMENT

Guidelines for Care of Children in the Emergency Department

This checklist is based on the American Academy of Pediatrics, the American College of Emergency Physicians, and the Emergency Nurses Association 2009 joint policy statement "Guidelines for Care of Children in the Emergency Department," which can be found online at ttp://aappolicy.aappublications.org/cgi/reprint/pediatrics;124/4/1233.pdf. Use the checklist to determine if your emergency department (ED) is prepared to care for children.

Appointed Pediatric Physician and Nurse Coordinator

- ❍ Pediatric physician coordinator is a specialist in pediatrics, emergency medicine, or family medicine, appointed by the ED medical director, who through training, clinical experience, or focused continuing medical education demonstrates competence in the care of children in emergency settings including resuscitation. See policy statement for details.
- ❍ Pediatric Nurse coordinator is a registered nurse (RN), appointed by the ED nursing director, who possesses special interest, knowledge, and skill in the emergency medical care of children. See policy statement for details.

Physicians, Nurses and Other Healthcare Providers Who Staff the ED

- ❍ Physicians who staff the ED have the necessary skill, knowledge, and training in the emergency evaluation and treatment of children of all ages who may be brought to the ED, consistent with the services provided by the hospital.
- ❍ Nurses and other ED health care providers have the necessary skill, knowledge, and training in providing emergency care to children of all ages who may be brought to the ED, consistent with the services offered by the hospital.
- ❍ Baseline and periodic competency evaluations completed for all ED clinical staff, including physicians, are age specific and include evaluation of skills related to neonates, infants, children, adolescents, and children with special health care needs. Competencies are determined by each institution's medical staff privileges policy.

Guidelines for QI/PI in the ED

The pediatric patient care-review process is integrated into the ED QI/PI plan.

- ❍ Components of the process interface with out-of-hospital, ED, trauma, inpatient pediatric, pediatric critical care, and hospital-wide QI or PI activities.

Guidelines for QI/PI in the ED, Continued

Clinical and Professional Competency

Below are the potential areas for the development of pediatric competency and professional evaluations.

- ❍ Triage
- ❍ Illness and injury assessment and management
- ❍ Pain assessment and treatment, including sedation and analgesia
- ❍ Airway management
- ❍ Vascular access
- ❍ Critical care monitoring
- ❍ Neonatal and pediatric resuscitation
- ❍ Trauma care
- ❍ Burn care
- ❍ Mass-casualty events
- ❍ Patient- and family-centered care
- ❍ Medication delivery and equipment safety
- ❍ Training and communication
- ❍ Mechanisms are in place to monitor professional performance, credentials, continuing education, and clinical competencies.

Guidelines for Improving Pediatric Patient Safety

The delivery of pediatric care should reflect an awareness of unique pediatric patient safety concerns and are included in the following policies or practices:

- ❍ Children are weighed in kilograms.
- ❍ Weights are recorded in a prominent place on the medical record.
- ❍ For children who are not weighed, a standard method for estimating weight in kilograms is used (e.g., a length-based system).
- ❍ Infants and children have a full set vital signs recorded (temperature, heart rate, respiratory rate) in the medical record.
- ❍ Blood pressure and pulse oximetry monitoring are available for children of all ages on the basis of illness and injury severity.

Produced by the AAP, the EMSC National Resource Center, and Children's National Medical Center

- ❍ A process for identifying age-specific abnormal vital signs and notifying the physician of these is present.
- ❍ Processes in place for safe medication storage, prescribing, and delivery that includes precalculated dosing guidelines for children of all ages.
- ❍ Infection-control practices, including hand hygiene and use of personal protective equipment, are implemented and monitored.
- ❍ Pediatric emergency services are culturally and linguistically appropriate.
- ❍ ED environment is safe for children and supports patient- and family-centered care.
- ❍ Patient-identification policies meet Joint Commission standards
- ❍ Policies for the timely reporting and evaluation of patient safety events, medical errors, and unanticipated outcomes are implemented and monitored.

Guidelines for ED Policies, Procedures, and Protocol

Policies, procedures, and protocols for the emergency care of children should be developed and implemented in the areas listed below. These policies may be integrated into overall ED policies as long as pediatric specific issues are addressed.

- ❍ Illness and injury triage
- ❍ Pediatric patient assessment and reassessment
- ❍ Documentation of pediatric vital signs and actions to be taken for abnormal vital signs
- ❍ Immunization assessment and management of the under-immunized patient
- ❍ Sedation and analgesia for procedures, including medical imaging
- ❍ Consent including when parent or legal guardian is not immediately available
- ❍ Social and mental health issues
- ❍ Physical or chemical restraint of patients
- ❍ Child maltreatment and domestic violence reporting criteria, requirements, and processes.
- ❍ Death of the child in the ED
- ❍ Do not resuscitate (DNR) orders
- ❍ Families are involved in patient decision-making and medication safety processes
- ❍ Family presence during all aspects of emergency care
- ❍ Patient, family, and caregiver education
- ❍ Discharge planning and instruction
- ❍ Bereavement counseling
- ❍ Communication with the patient's medical home or primary care provider
- ❍ Medical imaging policies that address pediatric age- or weight-based appropriate dosing for studies that impart radiation consistent with ALARA (as low as reasonably achievable) principles.
- ❍ All-hazard disaster-preparedness plan that addresses the following pediatric issues:
- ❍ Availability of medications, vaccines, equipment, and trained providers for children
- ❍ Pediatric surge capacity for injured and non-injured children
- ❍ Decontamination, isolation, and quarantine of families and children
- ❍ Minimization of parent–child separation (includes pediatric patient tracking, and timely reunification of separated children with their family)
- ❍ Access to specific medical and mental health therapies, and social services for children
- ❍ Disaster drills which includes a pediatric mass casualty incident at least every 2 years
- ❍ Care of children with special health care needs
- ❍ Evacuation of pediatric units and pediatric subspecialty units.
- ❍ Interfacility transfer policy defining the roles and responsibilities of the referring facility and referral center.
- ❍ Transport plan for delivering children safely and in a timely manner to the appropriate facility that is capable of providing definitive care.
- ❍ Process for selecting the appropriate care facility for pediatric specialty services not available at the hospital (may include critical care, reimplantation or digits or limbs, trauma and burn care, psychiatric emergencies, obstetric and perinatal emergencies, child maltreatment, rehability for recovery from critical conditions).
- ❍ Process for selecting an appropriately staffed transport service to match the patient's needs
- ❍ Process for patient transfer (including obtaining informed consent)
- ❍ Plan for transfer of patient information (medical record, copy of signed transport consent), personal belongings, directions and referral institution information to family'
- ❍ Process for return transfer of the pediatric patient to the referring facility as appropriate.

Guidelines for ED Support Services

- ❍ Radiology capability must meet the needs of the children in the community served
- ❍ A process for referring children to appropriate facilities for radiological procedures that exceed the capability of the hospital is established.
- ❍ A process for timely review, interpretation, and reporting of medical imaging by a qualified radiologist is established.
- ❍ Laboratory capability must meet the needs of the children in the community served, including techniques for small sample sizes.
- ❍ A process for referring children or their specimens to appropriate facilities for laboratory studies that exceed the capability of the hospital is established.

Produced by the AAP, the EMSC National Resource Center, and Children's National Medical Center

TABLE INT.2

TOP 10 EMSC NATIONAL RESOURCE CENTER PEDIATRIC QUALITY INDICATORS

Rank	Name	Donabedian framework	IOM domain(s)	Diagnostic category
1	Timely administration of fluids in patients with septic shock	Process	Timely, effective	Critical illness
2	All pediatric equipment present in the ED (per ACEP, AAP, ENA policy statement)	Structure	Effective, safe	General
3	Confirming endotracheal tube placement by the end-tidal CO_2 method	Process	Effective, safe	Critical illness
4	Timely treatment with antiepileptic drugs for patients in status epilepticus	Process	Timely, effective	Seizures
5	Medication error rates	Outcome	Safe	Crosscutting
6	Early definitive airway management in children with head trauma and a GCS <8	Process	Effective, safe	Head trauma
7	Protocol for suspected child abuse in place	Structure	Effective, safe	Child abuse
8	Systemic corticosteroids in asthma patients with acute exacerbation	Process	Effective	Asthma
9	Measuring weight in kilograms for ED patients <18 yrs of age	Process	Effective, safe	General
10	Handwashing rates	Process	Safe	General

Data from www.childrensnational.org/EMSC/PubRes/OldToolboxPages/Hospital-based_Performance_Measures.aspx.

ED quality indicators (Table INT.2) with more emphasis on processes that lead to more effective care (services based on scientific knowledge) such as time to intravenous fluids for patients in shock, time to anticonvulsants for those in status epilepticus, confirming end-tidal CO_2 for intubations, and steroids for status asthmaticus. Most EDs have patient satisfaction surveys, while few are adding patient or parents to their quality and safety committees. Safe practices include weighing children in kilograms to avoid medication errors and having all necessary pediatric equipment. Efficiency of care metrics such as reducing unnecessary antibiotic use for viral illness and CTs for children with minor head trauma are important metrics that some EDs are beginning to track, and will become more common practice with the emergence of Accountable Care. Many of these quality metrics should be subanalyzed by patient characteristics such as insurance status or ethnicity to assure equitability of care. In this new edition, goals of emergency care will stress many of these quality domains for each medical and surgical emergency chapter and are prominently listed for each clinical pathway.

In order to provide high-quality care for children, EDs must adopt the principles of high-reliability organizations and acknowledge that providers are human beings who fail to communicate well and make cognitive errors, especially in a stressful environment. A brief discussion of these issues and how this textbook can be used to aid the clinician follows.

High Reliability and Patient Safety

KEY POINTS

- Clinicians are human beings who will make mistakes; everyone must be aware of this and accept oversight and suggestions from colleagues and defer to the person with the most expertise
- Report and take action on near miss events—this will prevent future errors

High-reliability organizations are ones that operate under trying conditions yet manage to have relatively low frequency of safety events. The ED environment, by nature, is perpetually operating under challenging conditions with no regulation of patient arrival or acuity and frequent workflow interruptions. Furthermore, children add unique challenges such as the lack of standardization of dosing and need to calculate dosing and choose equipment based on weight and size, the inability of young or disabled children to communicate their complaints, and unique developmental and physical characteristics that may affect treatment strategies.

To provide highly quality care for children in EDs, the principles of high-reliability organizations must be embraced (Table INT.3). Such organizations understand that human beings have limitations and systems have to be proactively designed to help them avoid error. Examples of a systems-based approach include the standardization of processes or procedures as guided by evidence or consensus rather than by individual preference. Use of clinical pathways accessible from the electronic medical record with linked computerized order sets and the use of checklists before starting a procedure are examples of standardization of practice. Another high-reliability principle is the concept that each caregiver is fallible and thus is preoccupied with preventing harm to patients. Frontline clinicians should be willing to have others cross-check their work, defer to the person with the most expertise in a situation, and use structured and open communication. HROs have procedures for detecting, reporting, and taking corrective action for pediatric safety events. Best practices for detection and reporting include having unit-based patient safety walk-rounds or huddles and a safety event reporting system in place. Resultant information is reported to and subsequent actions taken by the ED Quality and Safety Committee and ED leadership. The effectiveness of any reporting system depends on active campaigns to develop a culture of safety, nonpunitive responses to errors, and both open and anonymous assessments of the environment and leadership.

TABLE INT.3

CHARACTERISTICS OF HIGH-RELIABILITY ORGANIZATIONS

5 principles of high-reliability organizations	
A safety culture	
Preoccupation with failure	Operating with a chronic wariness of the possibility of unexpected events
Deference to expertise	Decision-making authority migrates to the person with the most expertise with the problem at hand, regardless of rank
Sensitivity to operations	Paying attention to what is happening on the frontline
Structure for prevention, reporting, and action	
Commitment to resilience	Developing capabilities to detect, contain, and bounce back after errors
Reluctance to simplify interpretations	Taking deliberate steps to question assumptions

Adapted from Weick KE, Sutcliffe KM. Managing the unexpected: resilient performance in an age of uncertainty. 2nd ed. San Francisco, CA: Jossey-Bass, 2007.

Teamwork and Communication

KEY POINTS

- The physician, as team leader, sets the tone by introducing themselves by name and openly inviting input from others on the team
- Simulations and team training require all disciplines to participate (e.g., nurses, respiratory therapists, pharmacists, clinical assistants) in addition to physicians
- Use a structured handoff, preferably interdisciplinary and at the bedside, provides the highest standard of care

As in other high-risk workplaces, team training is imperative in providing high-quality care. The aviation industry adopted the behavioral principles of Crew Resource Management (CRM) that team communication and coordination behaviors are identifiable and teachable and the Institute of Medicine in its 1999 report recommended that healthcare organizations "establish interdisciplinary team training programs that incorporate proven methods for team management, such as CRM." Team training and simulation exercises that include all disciplines and practice pediatric resuscitation and stabilization scenarios for different ages are critical to keeping children safe in our EDs. Structured communication, especially during the multiple handoffs of care, is a key tool in reducing error. Examples of such tools in EDs include SBAR (Situation, Background, Assessment, and Recommendation) and SHOUT (Sick or not sick; History and Hospital Course; Objective data; Upcoming plan or disposition; and To do) (Table INT.4). Situational awareness improves if the team is introduced including first names and roles. Use of checklists before procedures and medication double checks for high-risk medications are also examples of methods to ensure good communication and teamwork.

TABLE INT.4

EXAMPLES OF STRUCTURED HAND-OFF MNEMONICS FOR EMERGENCY MEDICINE

ISBARQ	SHOUT
I: Introduction	S: Sick or not sick
S: Situation	H: History, ED course
B: Background	O: Objective data
A: Assessment	U: Upcoming plan, disposition
R: Recommendations	T: To do
Q: Questions	

Cognitive Error

KEY POINTS

- Stop and make yourself think "what else could this be" and "what would prove me wrong" to help avoid diagnostic error
- Reliance on intuition and experience are often effective but more likely to lead to diagnostic error

Cognitive error is considered the next frontier of patient safety. Although systems errors contribute to diagnostic errors and delays, the use of electronic medical records and better access to technology are reducing this source of error. Cognitive error, or how clinicians think, is more difficult to control. In a busy ED, many clinicians rely on their memory instead of quickly checking online resources. This new edition is available online and can be downloaded to your personal device. In trying to make a diagnosis, one may not know what disease or injury to look up—needing instead to find the possible diagnoses through the signs and symptoms that are presented and the age and sex of the child. Often one should start with the "Signs and Symptoms" algorithms provided in this text. With this new edition, we are aiming to provide easy access to an evidence-based resource for pediatric emergency care.

In making clinical decisions, the human mind works in one of two modes, intuitive or analytical. We prefer to use the faster, intuitive mode that is often effective, but prone to causing unconscious mistakes or cognitive biases. When in this mode, we take short cuts and often quickly "pattern match" to past experience. The analytic mode requires more time and resources, and is thus less preferred, but is more reliable and less prone to error. In order to reduce diagnostic or decision-making error, we must try and train ourselves to slow down and verify our intuitive thoughts by adding some analytical ones. This is particularly important in high-risk situations. Our ability to make decisions or diagnoses is influenced by

TABLE INT.5

EXAMPLES OF COMMON COGNITIVE BIASES IN EMERGENCY MEDICINE

Type of bias	Definition/example
Anchoring bias	Premature closure; failure to consider reasonable alternatives once diagnosis has been made: *Examination and labs consistent with acute abdomen; pneumonia not considered despite new data of tachypnea and cough*
Availability bias	Judge things as being more likely if they readily come to mind: *Fever, vomiting, and benign abdominal examination must be viral enteritis*
Blind obedience	Authority effect inhibits trainees: *Medical student worried about high heart rate—told its "OK" and patient has myocarditis*
Diagnostic momentum	Once labels are attached, they become "sticky": *Colleague signed out patient with "gastroenteritis" and you miss appendicitis despite concerning labs and evolving examination*
Framing	Clinician accepts framing provided by others: *Patient is triaged as low acuity so must not be sick*
Judgmental	Stereotyping: *This young mother does not have insurance and keeps seeking ED care—the child does not have a "real" problem*
Listening omission	Hearing only the opening statement and conclusion and accepts it as full story: *20th case presented by trainee of child with vomiting*
Wait and see	Not actively seeking an answer: *wait and see if the child can drink and what happens when the fever resolves*

both environmental and individual factors. If the ED is particularly chaotic or understaffed or if we are tired, stressed, or cognitively overloaded, we are more likely to make errors. Our gender, past experiences, personality, and background may also impact our decision making. Some common types of cognitive biases are listed in Table INT.5.

Strategies to reduce cognitive bias and improve decision making include thinking out loud and encouraging others to add their impressions or thoughts. Identification of one's assumptions, avoiding "premature" closure when making complex or critical decisions, and challenging oneself about what would prove one wrong are critical steps to avoid cognitive errors. What else could it be? Is something else going on? Is there anything that does not fit? Seeking feedback on your decisions by following up on patients after admission or discharge and attending morbidity and mortality conferences improve diagnostic ability. Continuing to look up information as you practice or after a shift is part of deliberate practice and reinforces the importance of not relying on experience alone.

CONCLUSION

Reflecting on all these elements of quality emergency care for children, we hope this edition of the textbook will serve as a valuable resource for all emergency medicine practitioners with its improved accessibility to key information and attention to quality measures for each clinical condition.

Suggested Readings and Key References

Alessandrini E, Varadarajan K, Alpern ER, et al; Pediatric Emergency Care Applied Research Network. Emergency department quality: an analysis of existing pediatric measures. *Acad Emerg Med* 2011; 18(5):519–526.

American Academy of Pediatrics, Committee on Pediatric Emergency Medicine, American College of Emergency Physicians, et al. Joint policy statement—guidelines for care of children in the emergency department. *Pediatrics* 2009;124(4):1233–1243.

American Academy of Pediatrics, Committee on Pediatric Emergency Medicine. Overcrowding crisis in our nation's emergency departments: is our safety net unraveling? *Pediatrics* 2004;114(3):878–888.

Chamberlain JM, Krug S, Shaw KN. Emergency care for children in the United States. *Health Affairs (Millwood)* 2013;32(12):2109–2115.

Committee on Pediatric Emergency Medicine, American Academy of Pediatrics, Krug SE, et al. Patient safety in the pediatric emergency care setting. *Pediatrics* 2007;120(6):1367–1375.

Croskerry P, Singhal G, Mamede S. Cognitive debiasing 1: origins of bias and theory of debiasing. *BMJ Qual Saf* 2013;0:1–7.

Institute of Medicine. *Emergency care for children: growing pains.* Washington, DC: National Academies Press, 2006.

Institute of Medicine, Committee on the Quality of Health Care in America. *Crossing the quality chasm: A new health system for the 21st century.* Washington, DC: National Academies Press, 2001:39–60.

KaiserPermanenteofColorado.n.d.SBARTechniqueforCommunication: A situational briefing model. Institute for Healthcare Improvement. Available at: www.ihi.org/IHI/topics/patientsafety/safetygeneral/toolsSBARTechniqueforCommunicationASituationalBriefingMode. Accessed September 8, 2015.

Neale G, Hogan H, Sevdalis N. Misdiagnosis: analysis based on case record review with proposals aimed to improve diagnostic processes. *Clin Med* 2011;114:317–321.

Pediatric Emergency Department Performance Indicators. Available at: http://emscnrc.org/EMSC_Resources/ED_Pediatric_Performance_Measures_Toolbox.aspx. Accessed September 7, 2015.

Weick KE, Sutcliffe KM. Managing the unexpected: resilient performance in an age of uncertainty. 2nd ed. San Francisco, CA: Jossey-Bass, 2007.

SECTION I
Resuscitation and Stabilization

CHAPTER 1 ■ A GENERAL APPROACH TO ILL AND INJURED CHILDREN

MIRNA M. FARAH, MD, KHOON-YEN TAY, MD, AND JANE LAVELLE, MD

BACKGROUND

Children account for approximately 20% to 25% of all emergency department (ED) visits in the United States. In 2010, 25 million children <18 years of age were evaluated in EDs, comprising 20% of the 128 million total ED visits. The vast majority of children (96%) were treated and discharged from the ED. Younger children have the highest utilization rate; although infants <1 year old represent just 5% of the pediatric population, they comprised 12% of treat-and-release ED visits and almost 23% of inpatient admission. Children 1 to 4 years of age comprise 22% of this population, but account for 32.8% of all pediatric treat-and-release ED visits and 26.3% inpatient admissions. Approximately 5% of children will have severe illness. Over the past decades, as the application of new medical knowledge has eradicated many diseases and rendered others curable, trauma has emerged as the leading cause of morbidity and mortality. Children of all ages remain susceptible to infection. There are also more children with complicated health issues that depend on readily available sophisticated medical care. It is vital that emergency medicine clinicians can promptly recognize ill child and execute life-saving interventions.

PEDIATRIC DIFFERENCES

The medical evaluation of an infant or child can be challenging for all providers, but especially so for those who do not routinely care for children. Knowledge of development assists the clinician in determining the overall severity of illness. Fear or anxiety in acute situations is common and may be contributed to changes in mental status (MS) and vital signs (VSs). Preverbal infants and toddlers are less able to localize pain or discomfort. Children have remarkable resilience; initial signs of severe illness may be subtle; thus it is important to recognize warning signs of deterioration and intervene in a timely way. Clinicians must rely on parental and/or other caretaker accounts and perceptions of the history. Parental concerns must be considered carefully during care of the child. The approach to the care of the sick child, by nature must be family-centered. Ultimately, the task is the same for all emergency clinicians; rapid, accurate identification of serious, life-threatening illnesses, with swift intervention to reduce morbidity and mortality. This chapter outlines a standard approach to assist in achieving this goal.

RECOGNITION OF ILLNESS

Identifying the critically ill child is challenging. The defining principle of critical illness is the presence of an existing or potential threat to delivery of oxygen to meet the demands of the tissues. This is almost always the final common pathway that various childhood diseases lead to morbidity and mortality. The body's oxygen delivery system is separated into the respiratory system (brings oxygen to the arterial blood) and the circulatory system (controls flow of oxygenated blood to the tissues). Critical illness leads to a global threat to oxygen delivery to all tissues of the body. The exceptions to this rule are diseases that compromise oxygen delivery to the central nervous system (CNS). By keeping the concept of life-threatening illnesses compromising oxygen delivery through respiratory, circulatory, or neurologic failure, clinicians can better evaluate and treat ill children. You will encounter this theme in the other chapters in this section, including the Chapter 2 Approach to the Injured Child, Chapter 3 Airway, Chapter 4 Cardiopulmonary Resuscitation, and Chapter 5 Shock.

Children with decreased or failured oxygen delivery to the skin, brain, kidneys, and cardiovascular system exhibit clinical findings in each of these organ systems. Manifestations of CNS hypoxia include irritability, confusion, delirium, seizures, and unresponsiveness. Cardiovascular manifestations include tachycardia, diaphoresis, bradycardia, and hypotension. Cutaneous manifestations include pallor, cyanosis, mottling, and poor capillary refill. In Chapter 4 Cardiopulmonary Resuscitation, Figure 4.2 shows the progression of physical examination findings associated with inadequate tissue oxygenation for each of these organ systems.

More than half of children with critical illness have disease affecting the respiratory system. Approximately 25% of children have diseases affecting the circulatory system presenting with hypovolemic, distributive, obstructive, or cardiogenic shock (see Chapter 5 Shock). CNS failure accounts for the final 25%. Table 1.1 lists examples of diseases that may cause severe illness in children, along with common medications and interventions needed to restore oxygen delivery and support vital function. Although there is overlap among organ system

TABLE 1.1

RECOGNITION OF CRITICAL ILLNESS BY ORGAN SYSTEM

	Respiratory 30–50%	Circulatory 10–30%	Neurologic 10–30%
Disease	Croup/epiglottis Foreign body Artificial airway Asthma/bronchiolitis Pneumonia Poisoning/overdose Postseizure apnea Chronic lung disease Chronic ventilation	Dehydration/hypovolemic Shock Septic shock Hemorrhagic shock Distributive shock/anaphylaxis Congenital heart disease Structural Arrhythmia Acquired heart disease Myocarditis Pericarditis Cardiomyopathy	Head trauma Meningitis/encephalitis Stroke, venous thrombosis Intracranial hypertension Mass Spinal cord injury Status epilepticus Hypoxic ischemic Encephalopathy
Treatment and specific procedures	Oxygen Positioning Suctioning Accessory airways Bag-valve-mask ventilation High flow nasal cannula Nasal CPAP Bi-PAP Endotracheal intubation Bronchodilators Antibiotics Sedation, paralytic medications Decontamination	Normal saline/lactated ringers Dopamine Epinephrine Norepinephrine Milrinone Atropine Amiodarone Adenosine Magnesium Antibiotics	C-spine immobilization Head elevation 30 degrees Hypertonic saline 3% Hyperventilation Glucose Sedation medications Seizure medications Antibiotics Surgical decompression LP, EEG
Common procedures	Continuous cardiorespiratory, oxygen saturation, and $ETCO_2$ monitoring Frequent BP (q15min), assessment of capillary refill, I/O Access: IV, US-guided IV, IO, central line Foley, nasogastric tube, C-spine immobilization Temperature maintenance Cardioversion, defibrillation		
Associated chapters	Airway (Chapter 3) Pulmonary Emergencies (Chapter 107) Toxicologic Emergencies (Chapter 110) Infectious Disease Emergencies (Chapter 102)	Dehydration (Chapter 17) Shock (Chapter 5) Cardiac Emergencies (Chapter 94) Cardiopulmonary Resuscitation (Chapter 4)	Neurologic Emergencies (Chapter 105) Infectious Disease Emergencies (Chapter 102)

failures, in this table, the diseases are categorized by the primary organ system failure.

Triage

An organized triage system is a key component for early identification of children at risk for significant illness. The majority of pediatric EDs use the 5-level Emergency Severity Index (ESI) Triage system. Children are triaged to ESI 1, 2 by an experienced nurse by quick evaluation of MS, VSs, concerning chief complaints, and presence of high-risk conditions. Children triaged as ESI 1 require immediate evaluation, often by an organized rapid response team; those triaged as ESI 2 should ideally be assessed by clinicians within 30 minutes (see Chapter 73 Triage). Table 1.2 lists chief complaints, conditions, or characteristics of patients who may be at increased risk for respiratory, circulatory, or neurologic failure when they present to triage.

VITAL SIGNS

Measured VSs (heart rate [HR], respiratory rate, temperature, and pulse oximetry) significantly outside of the age-specific norms often signify potential for severe illness. Ready access to age-specific VS parameters is ideal as VS parameters vary significantly with age of the child. Temperature >38°C (100.4°F) in a neonate (<56 days) is considered a fever. VS

TABLE 1.2

HIGH-RISK PATIENTS WITH INCREASED RISK FOR RESPIRATORY, CIRCULATORY, OR NEUROLOGIC FAILURE

Respiratory	Apparent life-threatening event with history of cyanosis, change in mental status (MS), tone
	Tracheostomy, ventilator dependence, difficult/critical airway
	Suspected button battery ingestion
	Ingestion/foreign body with distress
	Asthma/bronchiolitis with hypoxemia, altered MS
	Respiratory distress with hypoxemia/change in MS
Circulatory	Hematology/oncology patient with fever
	BMT or solid organ transplants
	Sickle cell patient with fever or pain, other patients with asplenia
	Immune compromised, suppression
	Petechial, purpuric rash
	Erythroderma
	Posttonsillectomy and adenoidectomy with bleeding
	Infants less than 56 days (8 weeks) with fever/hypothermia
	Bleeding disorder with significant trauma
	Peritonitis/bilious emesis
	Cardiac patient with change in baseline pulse oximetry level, change in behavior/MS or perfusion
	Extremity trauma with neurovascular changes, compartment syndrome
Neurologic	Not acting right, irritability, stiff neck
	VP shunt with headache, fever, change in MS, vomiting
	Diabetic with altered mental status
	Hypoxic ischemic encephalopathy
	Frequent or prolonged seizure
	Focal neurologic symptoms, signs
	Acute onset of severe HA
	Suicidal, homicidal ideation, delirium, psychosis

reassessment is important to monitor evolving disease and response to interventions. VS abnormalities are sensitive warning signs of deterioration alerting the clinician team to intervene (Table 1.3).

SYSTEMS FOR A STANDARDIZED STRUCTURED RESPONSE

Patients triaged to ESI 1 (critical) are often best cared for in well-designed, fully stocked resuscitation room. These spaces allow immediate access to necessary equipment, medications, and ancillary services such as radiology. There is more room for staff to perform necessary interventions. It is optimal to care for children triaged as ESI 2 (emergent) in an ED examination room with monitors, oxygen and suction, and basic bedside equipment.

TABLE 1.3

HIGH-RISK VITAL SIGNS BY AGE

Age	Tachycardia[a]	RR[a]	Systolic BP hypotension	Systolic BP 50th percentile
1 month to 1 yr	>180	>34	<75	85–95
>1–5 yrs	>140	>22	<74	88–95
>5–12 yrs	>130	>18	<83	96–106
>12 to 18 yrs	>120	>14	<90	108–118

Remember, heart rate is affected by pain, anxiety, medications and hydration status.
[a]>95th percentile.

TEAM COMPOSITION

Ideally, children with critical illnesses are evaluated and treated by an organized, practiced team of providers. The physician team leader directs the overall assessment, interventions, and treatment. They receive input from the resuscitation team members, physiologic monitoring, and laboratory/radiographic data. Members of the resuscitation team include right and left bedside RN/Technician, a respiratory therapist, an RN documenter, and an RN or pharmacist to prepare medications. The roles of these providers should be explicitly defined in the ED Resuscitation Team Policy to assure an organized approach. Other physicians/CRNPs assist with physical examination, reassessments, and performance of necessary procedures. Child Life Specialists are helpful in distraction and calming techniques for fully conscious, not sedated patients. Social Workers or Charge RNs can accompany the family during the resuscitation and offer emotional support as well as an explanation of resuscitation events.

An automated communication alert to notify members of the resuscitation team allows for rapid response. A communication system to alert specialists, such as trauma, neurosurgery, critical care, anesthesiology, or otolaryngology physicians, should their assistance be needed emergently is also helpful. A clinical pharmacist is a valuable addition to the resuscitation team to assist with pediatric weight-based dosing. Special aids are available to provide pediatric weight-based doses and recommended equipment size based on the patient's height/length or weight (see Figure 4.13, in Chapter 4 Cardiopulmonary Resuscitation). Skilled personnel (parent or provider) cannot accurately estimate a child's weight on the basis of appearance. However, length is easily measured and tapes with precalculated medication doses and resuscitation equipment for various patient lengths have been clinically validated. Preparation of equipment ahead of time using precalculated weight-based doses of resuscitation medications and equipment sizes reduces error.

RAPID ASSESSMENT

A structured approach enables the team to assess the severity of illness and prioritize interventions. Although this rapid assessment is divided into the primary and secondary survey, it is a continuous and dynamic process with frequent reassessment.

Tertiary diagnostic testing, subspecialty consultation, and timely transfer to the definitive care setting follow.

PRIMARY SURVEY

The goal of the primary survey is to identify and treat impending or existing respiratory, circulatory, and/or neurologic failure. This is initiated as soon as the patient arrives to the ED and is ideally completed in less than 5 minutes. Importantly, early recognition and treatment of a patient with deficiencies in ventilation, perfusion, or neurologic function frequently prevents deterioration to respiratory or cardiac arrest. It is important to monitor and reassess patients following interventions in order to quickly recognize deterioration. The physician performing the survey should be loud, clear, organized, and confident while verbalizing the ABCDE assessment of the patient; other team members perform life-saving procedures based on the findings of the surveyor (see Chapter 3 Airway, Chapter 4 Cardiopulmonary Resuscitation, Chapter 5 Shock, and Chapter 94 Cardiac Emergencies; Tables 1.4 and 1.5).

TABLE 1.4

PRIMARY SURVEY COMPONENTS

A	Airway Cervical spine	Determine if the airway is patent Note obstruction, complete or partial Reposition, suction, consider artificial airways, continuous positive pressure Assess need for C-spine immobilization
B	Breathing	Check for increased or poor respiratory effort Place on continuous CR monitor, pulse oximetry, $ETCO_2$ Administer oxygen, assist ventilation with BVM Consider need for ETT, have LMA ready Decrease gastric distension Needle thoracostomy and chest tube as indicated
C	Circulation	Assess HR, BP, rhythm Peripheral pulses and capillary refill, pallor, cyanosis
D	Disability Dextrose Decontamination	Assess mental status, pupils, motor activity, and symmetry Cardioversion, defibrillation, pericardiocentesis AVPU Score, note lateralizing signs Treat hypoglycemia, seizures, increased ICP Drug overdoses, or electrolyte abnormalities
E	Exposure Environment	Undress patient, log roll Check temperature, skin, and evidence of trauma Prevent hypothermia

TABLE 1.5

AVPU MNEMONIC FOR LEVEL OF CONSCIOUSNESS

	Level of arousal	GCS
A	Alert	15
V	Voice	13
P	Pain	8
U	Unresponsive	3

See Table 2.2, in Chapter 2 Approach to the Injured Child for GCS and Infant Coma Scales.

Airway/Breathing

The respiratory system is divided into the extrathoracic airway (nostrils to trachea), the respiratory pump (muscles, pleura, respiratory control center), and the lung and intrathoracic airways. Respiratory failure due to extrathoracic obstruction presents with inspiratory stridorous or sonorous sounds along with decreased air entry and suprasternal retractions. Diseases that narrow the lumen of the intrathoracic airway cause expiratory wheezing. Diseases that increase airway resistance or decrease lung, or chest wall, compliance require greater effort on the child's part to maintain alveolar ventilation. Children most often respond by reducing their tidal volume and increasing their respiratory rate. Even at the lower tidal volumes, negative pleural pressures must be greater than normal to suck open the intrathoracic airways or diseased lung to overcome the obstruction. Thus, intercostal and supraclavicular retractions are noted. Small infants depend more on diaphragmatic motion and may manifest seesaw motion. During inspiration the diaphragm descends/abdomen bulges and the chest collapses from lower pleural pressures. During expiration, the glottis closes, in infants and young children, grunting occurs when air escapes through an actively closed glottis in an attempt to maintain FRC. Respiratory center disease manifests as an irregular respiratory pattern with pauses or apnea. The most common cause of hypoxemia in children are hypoventilation and ventilation/perfusion mismatch. $ETCO_2$ measurement may help to distinguish between them. With VQ mismatch the end tidal is normal or low in contrast to hypoventilation where the end tidal will be high. Diseases of the extrathoracic airway or the respiratory pump usually lead to hypoventilation with hypercarbia out of proportion to hypoxemia. Diseases of the lung and pump result in VQ mismatch with much greater hypoxemia than hypercarbia.

Treatment of extrathoracic airway includes airway positioning, suctioning, and NP/OP airways (Figure 4.4, in Chapter 4 Cardiopulmonary Resuscitation). Positive pressure and ETI may be required to overcome the obstruction. When disease primarily involves the lung and the intrathoracic airways, supplemental oxygen and positive end expiratory pressure are the main treatments. In addition, specific therapies such as bronchodilators, vasoconstrictors, anti-inflammatories or antibiotics target the underlying cause.

Circulation

The circulatory system includes the heart, the blood, the blood vessels, and the autonomic controls in the central and the peripheral nervous system. There is no single physical or laboratory finding that will identify shock, however, the physical signs exhibited by the patient in shock are ultimately due to insufficient oxygen and substrate delivery to the tissues. Recall that cardiac output (CO) is equal to mean arterial pressure divided by the systemic vascular resistance (MAP/SVR). Additionally, CO is also the product of the stroke volume (SV) and HR, (SV × HR), thus, MAP = HR × SV × SVR (see discussion in Chapter 5 Shock). HR and BP are easily measured, and the SVR can be assessed by physical examination of pulses, extremity temperature, color, and capillary refill. The physical manifestations vary with type of shock but include tachycardia, decreased skin perfusion, and hypotension; or tachycardia, bounding pulses and flushed skin with hypotension. If cardiogenic shock is present, HR may be normal or only modestly elevated. Remember that hypotension is a late finding requiring 50% decrease in the circulating volume. Treatment includes crystalloid infusion; increasing preload to increase SV. Contractility agents are considered if volume resuscitation 60 mL per kg is not effective. Afterload reduction may also be needed to treat cardiac dysfunction. It is important to correct hypoxemia acidosis and electrolyte abnormalities and provide other specific therapies to treat the underlying cause.

Disability

CNS failure is manifest by altered MS or focal neurologic deficit. Recall that the CNS is composed of the brain, the blood vessels, and the cerebrospinal fluid. Many diseases that cause CNS failure cause compartment physiology. Examples of primary CNS disease include intracranial hypertension/hemorrhage and status epilepticus. The CNS may also be secondarily affected by respiratory or circulatory disease. The AVPU scale (Table 1.5) and GCS (Table 2.2, in Chapter 2 Approach to the Injured Child) are used to measure level of consciousness in a standardized way. Interventions to treat CNS failure include modest hyperventilation, maintenance of MAP and oxygenation, hypertonic therapy, avoidance of hyperthermia, and potentially induce hypothermia. Other therapies aimed at the underlying cause include anticonvulsants, antibiotics, and surgical decompression.

Exposure/Environment

A complete physical examination requires removal of all clothing, log rolling, and checking axillary areas of the patient. Monitor and maintain body temperature using increased ambient temperature, warm blankets, and warmed fluids and oxygen. The use of therapeutic hypothermia in arrested pediatric patients remains controversial, however, hyperthermia should be treated aggressively. Lowering of core body temperature to 32 to 34 degrees during the first few hours after cardiac arrest is associated with improved neurologic outcomes and decreased mortality in adults with an out-of-hospital cardiac arrest. In children, evidence is very limited. The use of therapeutic hypothermia may be considered for children with out-of-hospital arrest and persistent coma or those with ventricular fibrillation or pulseless ventricular tachycardia.

IV Access

Vascular access in peripheral veins of the upper extremity with a large bore short catheter is preferred. For patients in pulseless arrest, with severe hypotension, or difficult access in which immediate access is ideal, intraossesous access provides a quick, reliable route to provide fluid resuscitation and medications. The ED clinicians should have an IV escalation plan in place with resources to assure timely IV access. This has become more important aspect of care due to the increasing numbers of children with difficult IV access due to success in treating chronic illnesses (Table 1.6).

TABLE 1.6

IV ESCALATION PLAN

- Establish 2 large bore IVs and begin NS fluid resuscitation within the first 15 min
- Implement IV escalation pathway considering individual patient
- Use any existing Broviac, port, PICC line
- Give antibiotics and pressors through central access, when available
- Ill patients require a second access at a peripheral site

Minutes	Access procedure
0–5	First peripheral IV with largest gauge possible Consider IO immediately in severely ill patients
5–10	Second peripheral attempt Consider US-guided peripheral IV Consider EJ (US guided) Notify vascular access specialist (IV team)
10–15	If still no access EZ-IO EJ (consider US guided) Central line (consider US guided) or Call PICU to assist at bedside Consider Chief Surgical Fellow as additional resource

Fluid Resuscitation

Deliver isotonic fluids (normal saline or lactated ringers) rapidly in 20 mL per kg aliquots up to 1,000 mL and reassess VS, MS, and skin perfusion. The push–pull technique using a 30-mL syringe with a macrodrip setup with a three-way stopcock and a T-connector is useful for rapid fluid resuscitation in children <50 kg. For children >50 kg, fluids can be infused using a pressure bag or a rapid infuser. To date, evidence has not shown benefit for the use of albumin or synthetic colloids in pediatric septic shock, cardiopulmonary arrest, or trauma. Dextrose-containing solutions should not be used for initial resuscitation due to risk for hyperglycemia and secondary osmotic diuresis and neurologic injury. Bedside glucose testing is important, treat hypoglycemia with D10 or D25 and follow with an infusion of fluids including dextrose. Other critical electrolyte abnormalities should be treated.

The choice of laboratory and imaging studies is guided by the patient's differential diagnosis (Table 1.7). Medications commonly used in pediatric resuscitation are listed in Table 4.6 of Chapter 4 Cardiopulmonary Resuscitation.

When time is limited in obtaining a pediatric history, providers can remember the acronym "SAMPLE," to briefly obtain key elements (Table 1.8). Other important information may include medications available in the home, travel history, immunizations, social history and stressors, suicide risk, substance abuse, and sexual assault.

TABLE 1.7

PRIMARY SURVEY: DIAGNOSTIC STUDIES AND PROCEDURES

Laboratory tests	Point-of-care glucose	Blood, urine culture
	iSTAT	Drug screen
	CBC, CMP, ESR, CRP	Beta-HCG
	Type and screen, PT/PTT	
	CPK, troponin, BNP	
Imaging	Bedside US	CXR
	Head US/CT	Abdominal US/CT
Procedures	ECG	
	NG Tube	
	Foley	

SECONDARY SURVEY

The goal of the secondary survey is to identify the definitive cause of the respiratory, circulatory, and/or neurologic abnormalities treated during the primary survey.

A systematic head-to-toe examination is performed with special attention to specific organ systems associated with the patient's chief complaint. Elements of the secondary survey may be skipped or deferred, depending on the clinical situation, patient acuity, and patient stability (Table 1.9).

FAMILY PRESENCE

Family presence (FP) during resuscitation and procedures has become an increasingly common practice; and is endorsed by the AAP, ACEP, and ENA. Family members who were at the side of a loved one during the final moments of life believe that their presence was beneficial to the patient and to themselves, and was helpful in their adjustment and grieving process. FP also promotes good communication with the clinician team. It allows parents to comfort and support their child, allowing children to be more cooperative so the evaluation and treatments go more smoothly. Studies have also shown that in the overwhelming majority, FP is not disruptive, and does not create stress among staff or negatively affect their performance. In general, the more experience healthcare providers have with FP and dealing with distressed families, the higher their acceptance and success of FP. Parents often fail to ask, but healthcare providers are obligated to offer the opportunity whenever possible. Written institution-specific guidelines, and resources including dedicated family support person (FSP) during resuscitation, are among the crucial initial steps toward a successful FP experience. The FSP assesses and prepares family members prior to treatment and remains with the family to provide comfort and answer questions. The family is initially escorted to a designated area within the treatment room away from the bedside; they can then be brought to the head of the bed at the completion of the secondary survey and all urgent procedures. The designated FSP can be a social worker, nurse, or chaplain who has no direct patient care responsibility, has a good knowledge of grief reactions, and is assigned exclusively to assist the family. If family members become overwhelmed or interfere with patient care, the FSP should respectfully escort them out of the treatment room. Families can also choose to leave the room at any time, and may stay or leave during invasive procedures or resuscitations. Patients who choose not to have family members present, or family members who desire not to participate must be supported in their decision without judgment. The AAP recommends that all EDs have a policy and procedure in place to support this.

TABLE 1.8

SAMPLE HISTORY

Sign and symptoms	What were the signs/symptoms that were exhibited by the patient prior to presentation?
Allergies	Any drug or food allergies?
Medications	What medications does the patient take on a regular basis? Was the patient given any medications prior to arrival?
Past medical history	What medical problems does the patient have?
Last meal	What time did the patient last take anything by mouth?
Events leading to presentation	What were the events immediately preceding the decision to present to the emergency room/call emergency services?

QUALITY AND COMPETENCY

The vast majority (>80%) of children are seen in community (nonpediatric) EDs; 50% of US EDs see fewer than 10 children per day. Critically ill children may only be encountered a few times per year. The Emergency Medical Services for Children (EMSC), a federal program designed to ensure that all children have access/receive appropriate care in an emergency, completed a national assessment with the Pediatric Readiness Survey in March 2013. Over 80% of EDs responded to the survey. EDs with low-volume pediatric visits (<1,800 per year) were the least pediatric ready (average score of 62/100), and EDs with higher-volume pediatric visit (>10,000 per year) were the most pediatric ready (average score of 84/100). The average score across over 4,000 hospitals was 69.

There are several strategies that can be implemented in general EDs in order to increase readiness for child patients and help to standardize key components of pediatric care for common medical diseases. Evidence- and concensus-based guidelines from the American Academy of Pediatrics as well as individual institutional pathways facilitate translation of evidence into bedside care. Some examples include AAP guidelines for bronchiolitis, acute otitis media and febrile UTI, IDSA guidelines for skin and soft tissue infection and community-acquired pneumonia, and NHBLI guidelines for asthma. Additionally, several pediatric institutions developed pathways; Seattle Children's Hospital and The Children's Hospital of Philadelphia have made these available to all clinicians on the Internet.

It is also important to provide opportunities for the ED clinicians to maintain resuscitation skills. Workshops with simulation for hands-on practice of key resuscitation skills should

TABLE 1.9

SECONDARY SURVEY: FINDINGS AND IMPLICATIONS

Secondary survey	Exam finding (examples)	Potential disease implications (examples)
Head	Hematomas, lacerations	Occult traumatic brain injury
	Ventriculoperitoneal shunt	Shunt malfunction/increased intracranial pressure (ICP)
	Bulging fontanel	Increased ICP
	Sunken fontanel	Dehydration
Eyes	Pupil examination: size, reactivity, symmetry	Toxidromes, increased ICP, ruptured globe
	Extraocular movement palsies	Increased ICP, Lyme disease, orbital cellulitis
	Proptosis or exophthalmos	Orbital cellulitis; thyroid dysfunction, intraorbital or retrobulbar bleed
	Scleral icterus	Biliary dysfunction, hemolysis
	Papilledema	Increased ICP
Ears	Mastoid tenderness or ear proptosis	Mastoiditis
	Tympanic membrane abnormalities: bulging, perforation, hemotympanum	Acute otitis media; tympanic membrane perforation; basilar skull fractures
Nose	Nasal flaring	Respiratory distress
Throat	Dry mucous membranes	Dehydration
	Exudative pharyngitis	Streptococcal pharyngitis; infectious mononucleosis
	Tonsillar and uvular deviation; trismus	Peritonsillar abscess (PTA)
	Lesions: vesicles, papules, Koplik spots, ulcerations	Viral processes: HSV, coxsackie, measles
	Drooling	Peritonsillar or retropharyngeal abscess, epiglottitis, bacterial tracheitis
Neck	Meningismus	Meningitis
	Neck pain with movement, especially rotational	Retropharyngeal abscess, neck injury
Chest	Intercostal, subcostal, suprasternal retractions	Respiratory distress
Lungs	Decreased air entry	Obstructive process (e.g., asthma)
	Wheezing	Obstructive process (e.g., asthma)
	Rales	Lower respiratory tract illness (e.g., pneumonia), congestive heart failure (CHF)
	Inspiratory stridor	Croup, airway foreign body
Heart	Murmurs	Congenital heart disease, valvular dysfunction, anemia
	Rubs	Pericarditis, pericardial effusion
	Gallops	CHF, cardiomyopathy
	Tachycardia	Supraventricular tachycardia, sinus tachycardia
Abdomen	Distension	Ileus, obstruction, volvulus
	Hepatomegaly	CHF; oncologic processes
	Splenomegaly	Splenic sequestration, CHF, oncologic processes
	Tenderness to palpation (location dependent)	Appendicitis (RLQ), pancreatitis (epigastric), cholecystitis (RUQ), ovarian torsion (RLQ or LLQ)
	Peritoneal signs	Peritonitis
Genitourinary	External vaginal examination	Imperforate hymen
	Testicular examination	Testicular torsion
	Pelvic examination	Pelvic inflammatory disease; ectopic pregnancy, ovarian torsion
Extremities	Joint swelling	Septic arthritis
	Edema	CHF, liver failure, renal disease
	Poor perfusion	Sepsis, dehydration, shock
Skin	Petechiae/purpura	Idiopathic thrombocytopenic purpura (ITP), oncologic process, Henoch–Schoenlein purpura (HSP), meningococcemia
	Urticaria	Anaphylaxis
	Characteristic rashes	Viral exanthems, Lyme disease, erythema multiforme, Stevens–Johnson syndrome
	Erythema, induration, fluctuance, pain	Abscess, cellulitis, necrotizing fasciitis

(*continued*)

TABLE 1.9

SECONDARY SURVEY: FINDINGS AND IMPLICATIONS (*CONTINUED*)

Secondary survey	Exam finding (examples)	Potential disease implications (examples)
Neurologic	CN palsies	Increased ICP, intracranial masses, meningitis, cerebrovascular accident (CVA)
	Altered mental status	Encephalopathy, meningitis, encephalitis, drug effects, seizure, demyelinating diseases, vasculitides, dehydration, intussusception
	Weakness	CVA, increased ICP, intracranial mass, Guillain–Barré syndrome
	Sensory deficits	CVA, transverse myelitis, intracranial mass
	Uncoordinated/unbalanced	Intracranial mass, postinfectious cerebellitis, drug effects
Psychiatric	Flat affect	Depression
	Suicidal ideation	Drug ingestion, suicidal attempt
	Hallucinations	Schizophrenia, psychosis, drug effects

be offered throughout the year. It is also valuable for the ED team members to practice using resuscitation simulation scenarios in their own resuscitation room, ideally with members of the multidisciplinary team. In addition to cognitive and skill practice, these simulation sessions provide a venue to improve team collaboration and communication. Clinicians may also benefit from maintaining PALS, ACLS, and ATLS certification.

Quality improvement initiatives for pediatric resuscitations can take multiple forms. Videotaped resuscitations can be reviewed by a multidisciplinary team to identify areas for system improvements, opportunities for targeted clinician education, and improved teamwork and communication. Resuscitation cases can be reviewed in advanced case conferences for in-depth discussion around medical including the most recent evidence. Data can be extracted from the EMR for process and outcome quality measures to further improve/inform care.

SUMMARY

The critically ill child manifests signs related to potential or existing threat to the delivery of oxygen to meet the demands of tissues. This is the final common pathway that leads to morbidity and mortality in the majority of childhood diseases.

KEY POINTS

- Clinicians should rapidly assess the ABCDE (airway, breathing, circulation, disability, exposure) components of the primary survey while performing lifesaving procedures
- An efficient, targeted history and secondary survey can offer clues to the assessment and diagnosis of an acutely ill child.
- Healthcare providers should offer the family the opportunity to be present during resuscitations and procedures whenever a family support person is available.
- Institutions should invest time and resources into periodic multidisciplinary training sessions for their providers to refresh and practice pediatric resuscitation skills in their own environment with their own equipment and resources.
- Many modalities exist for monitoring the quality and competency of pediatric care delivered to acutely ill children and can serve to improve that care on an ongoing basis.

Suggested Readings and Key References

American Academy of Pediatrics, American College of Emergency Physicians. In: Fuchs S, Yamamoto L, eds. *APLS: The pediatric emergency medicine resource.* 5th ed. Sudbury, MA: Jones and Bartlett Learning, 2012.

Gauche-Hill M, Schmitz C, Lewis RJ. Pediatric preparedness of US emergency departments: a 2003 survey. *Pediatrics* 2007;120(6):1229–1237.

Hazinski MF, Samson RA, Schexnayder SM, eds. *Pediatric advanced life support provider manual.* Dallas, TX: American Heart Association, 2012.

Lavelle JM, Costarino AT, Ludwig S. Recognition and Management of the Ill Child. *Compr Ther* 1995;21(12):711–718.

Sinha M, Lezine MW, Frechette A, et al. Weighing the pediatric patient during trauma resuscitation and its concordance with estimated weight using Broselow Luten Emergency Tape. *Pediatr Emerg Care* 2012;28:544–547.

So TY, Farrington E, Absher RK. Evaluation of the accuracy of different methods used to estimate weights in the pediatric population. *Pediatrics* 2009;123:e1045–e1051.

2010 American Heart Association Guidelines for Cardiopulmonary Resuscitation and Emergency Cardiovascular Care Science. Circulation 2010.

CHAPTER 2 ■ APPROACH TO THE INJURED CHILD

MEGAN LAVOIE, MD AND MICHAEL L. NANCE, MD

RELATED CHAPTERS

Injuries are commonly seen in the emergency department (ED), thus clinicians caring for children and adolescents in this setting should be prepared to manage a range of injuries. Although pediatric trauma victims have needs distinguishing them from adults, it is only since the mid-1990s that investigators have begun to systematically look at the care of the injured child. The goal of this chapter is to help prepare ED clinicians for the triage, assessment, and initial management of pediatric trauma patients along the spectrum of minor to life-threatening injuries.

EPIDEMIOLOGY

Injury remains the leading cause of death in children 1 to 19 years old in the United States accounting for more than 50% of all childhood deaths. In 2012, more than 11,000 children and adolescents <19 years died from unintentional and nonaccidental injury. Nearly 22 million children are injured annually; and there are approximately 10 million primary care office visits, 9 million ED visits, and 500,000 hospitalizations yearly. Injuries are the leading cause of ED visits and account for approximately one-third of all visits for children younger than 15 years. It has been estimated that the cost of unintentional pediatric injuries is $347 billion every year: $17 billion in medical costs, $72 billion in future work lost, and $257 billion in lost quality of life.

Motor vehicle crashes continue to be the most common cause of injury-related death and resulted in >4,000 deaths in 2012. Rates for childhood homicide tripled and rates for childhood suicide quadrupled between 1950 and 1993; and are the second and third leading cause for death in ages 0 to 19 years respectively. In 2012, firearms were reported to be involved in 2,683 deaths. Homicide rates in children have two peaks: from age 0 to 3 years and from 14 to 18 years. In black teenagers, homicide from firearms is the leading cause of death. Although less fatal, falls, drowning, poisoning, and fire/burn injuries are significant causes of morbidity.

The societal impact of years of life lost from childhood unintentional injury is staggering. In a 10-year period, more than 50,000 unintentional injury deaths are reported in children <5 years. Annually, there are >70,000 injuries as a result of automobile crashes in the same population. Crash mortality statistics show that the youngest occupant in an automobile is the most vulnerable to injury. Children from 5 to 9 years of age are most likely to be pedestrian injury victims. Overall, pediatric pedestrian injury accounts for 46% of motor vehicle fatalities. Boys in densely populated urban areas represent the largest group at risk. Injury from bicycle crashes is particularly common in children 6 to 16 years. Societal violence as a cause of death in children is increasing at an alarming rate. An estimated 8,625 child maltreatment fatalities occurred in the 50 states and the District of Columbia from 1999 to 2002.

Blunt trauma is the predominant mechanism of major injury in children; only 10% to 20% experience penetrating injury. Although the mortality rate for children requiring hospitalization is less than 1% in many pediatric trauma centers, 80% of all childhood trauma deaths occur at the scene or in the ED. As many as 18% of hospital trauma deaths are avoidable with correct diagnosis and treatment. Brain injury is responsible for 80% of trauma mortality. Failure to secure the airway is the most common cause of preventable death. Multisystem injury occurs in more than 50% of victims and requires a coordinated approach by a team of specialists with immediate access to varied diagnostic and treatment modalities including the OR, ICU, or rapid skilled transport.

Attention to pediatric differences in anatomy and physiology of children is key: multisystem trauma is more likely as impact is distributed more widely throughout the body; compensatory mechanisms to volume loss make hypotension a late finding; greater surface area relative to body size causes increased heat and insensible fluid loss. Children have higher energy requirements, and fluid and nutrition requirements vary by age and stage of growth. Finally, varying developmental stages can present challenges in assessment.

This chapter provides a framework for the emergency management of pediatric injuries, isolated and multiple, mild to life-threatening, with emphasis on the rapid, systematic evaluation by the ED and trauma team specialists.

SPECTRUM OF TRAUMA AND INITIAL TRIAGE

Trauma causes injuries that range from mild to life- or limb-threatening. During initial triage several categorizations of

TABLE 2.1

CLASSIFICATION AND DISPOSITION OF TRAUMA BY SEVERITY

		Physical examination			
Category	History	Vital signs	Local findings	Laboratory radiographic studies	Probable disposition
Mild	Minimal force	Normal	Superficial only	Few	Discharge
Moderate	Significant force	Normal	Suspicious for internal injury	Intermediate	Evaluate
Severe	Critical force	Abnormal	Indicative of internal injury	Many	Immediate therapy; admit

injury are useful: (1) extent—multiple or isolated; (2) nature—blunt or penetrating; and (3) severity—mild, moderate, or severe.

Surgeons have standardized the definition of multiple trauma as documented significant injury to two or more body areas in order to meaningfully compare patient outcomes. For the ED clinician, multiple trauma is defined as apparent injury to two or more body areas of any severity (forehead laceration and forearm fracture). Isolated trauma involves one anatomic region of the body regardless of severity. The distinction between isolated and multiple trauma may be challenging as (1) serious injuries often evolve over time; (2) children may be difficult to examine because of development stage; (3) injury may have been intentional so true mechanism is unclear; (4) drugs or alcohol exposure may coexist. Differentiation between isolated and multiple trauma is thus a dynamic process, and the emergency physician's first impression may change as new evidence accumulates. The nature of the injury, blunt or penetrating also guides the evaluation based on the specific force and the expected internal injuries. Table 2.1 provides classification of injury severity based on history and physical examination, as well as a general schema for disposition, based on extent of laboratory and imaging required to evaluate the patient. Initial severity categorization depends on the history and the physical examination. Assessment of severity is essential in the ED as it determines the need for immediate intervention, the extent of diagnostic evaluation, and patient disposition.

ORGANIZATION OF THE TRAUMA SERVICE

The regionalization of trauma care in the United States continues to evolve. In many areas, hospitals are stratified on the basis of their capability and desire to care for the multiply injured child; in other areas, no such stratification exists. The goal of trauma center designation, under the guidance of the American College of Surgeons Committee on Trauma, is the triage of injured children to appropriate, qualified facilities. Because of the relative scarcity of pediatric trauma centers, approximately 70% of injured children still receive care in general facilities. Another 77% of all children are within 60 minutes of a pediatric trauma center by air or ground transportation. The availability of rapid pediatric transport services and pre-existing transfer agreements may accelerate the needed regionalization of pediatric trauma care.

The effective management of pediatric trauma requires the integration of a multidisciplinary team, including surgeons, emergency physicians, critical care physicians, emergency and intensive care nurses, respiratory therapists, radiologists, and various subspecialty services (neurosurgery, orthopedic surgery, anesthesia etc.), as well as the ready availability of diagnostic and operating room resources. Each institution must develop its own organizational response for pediatric trauma with a well-established chain of command and a designated leader, a responsibility that may change hands as additional personnel arrive for resuscitation in the ED. The leader accepts responsibility for patient care and organizes the multiple specialists needed to care for the patient with multisystem injury. Such organization begins at the scene of an injury and EMS transport, continues throughout patient triage after initial evaluation, and care once the patient arrives in the ED. After ED resuscitation and stabilization, the decision to transfer the child to a hospital with a higher level of capability, admit to the ward or to the intensive care unit, or proceed to the operating room is made by the team leader after consultation with the specialists involved. If it becomes clear that the predominant injury is to a single-body system, it may be appropriate for the team leader to transfer patient care responsibility to the designated leader of a given subspecialty (e.g., orthopedics, neurosurgery). Figure 2.1 demonstrates a flow diagram of a response to the seriously injured child, an example of organizational schema put into action when or before a victim of serious trauma arrives in the ED. Mock resuscitations with members of the multidisciplinary trauma team allows a venue to practice resuscitation interventions and utilize special

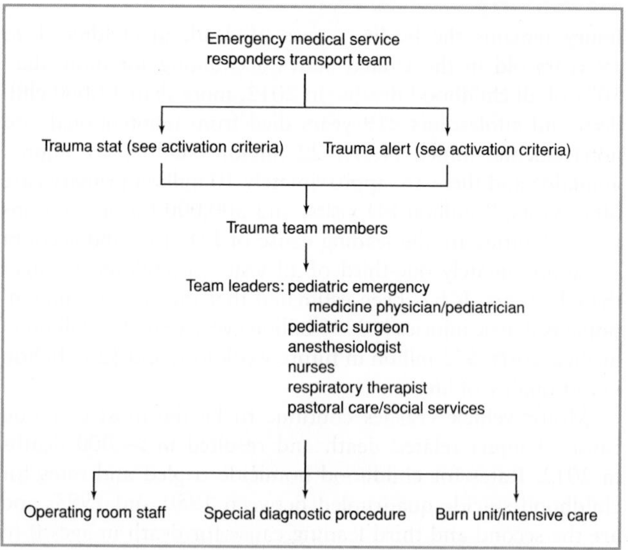

FIGURE 2.1 Sample flow diagram of a response from the emergency medical services team that is placed into action when or before a victim of serious trauma arrives in the emergency department.

CH The Children's Hospital of Philadelphia®

Trauma Activation and Consult Criteria and Response

	Level I Activation	Level II Activation	Trauma Consult
Criteria	• Respiratory Distress • Severe maxillo-facial trauma • Unstable airway • Cardiac arrest • Current Glasgow Coma scale ≤8 • Unstable vital signs (age appropriate) • Lateralizing neurologic signs or worsening neurologic exam • Evidence of shock (age appropriate) • Severe uncontrolled hemorrhage • SBP <80 that does not respond to fluid resuscitation • Patients with airway compromise • Major vascular injuries, including signigicant crush or amputation above the elbow or knee with a high probability of operative intervention • Penetrating injury to the head, neck and torso. (may downgrade to a level II if trajectory obviously tangential) • Burns ≥25% TBSA with/without inhalation innjury • Spinal Cord Injury with persistent neurologic signs or symptoms and/or unstable vertebral factures	• GCS ≥9 and ≤13 • Hypotension prior to transport, resolved during transport • Blunt abdominal trauma with abnormal exam • Blunt chest trauma with >2 rib fractures • Significant penetrating trauma to upper extremities or distal to the groin • Significant crush or amputation distal to the elbow or knee with a high probability of operative intervention • Patients with transient neurologic changes (i.e. "stingers") • **High Index of Suspicion** The Emergency Department Attending, Trauma Attending or Trauma Chest may initiate a Level II activation based on a high index of suspicion. This can be upgraded or downgraded as more information is obtained.	No obvious life threatening injuries and vital signs are stable.

FIGURE 2.2 Trauma Activation and Consult Criteria at The Children's Hospital of Philadelphia.

bedside equipment, assures that necessary personnel and processes are in place, and importantly allows team discussion around leadership, roles, and communication.

Upon notification of a patient's impending arrival, the ED physician determines the risk for severe injury, and whether activation of the trauma team is necessary. Early activation is optimal to prepare for the patient arrival. The three levels of trauma team activation (variably named) include trauma stat (major trauma), trauma alert (moderate trauma), and trauma consult (minor trauma). Notification necessitates an in-the-field determination of likelihood of severe injury. Historically, trauma activation criteria have been based on mechanism of injury. In a mechanism of injury trauma activation system, patients who meet certain criteria are automatically triaged as major traumas. However, triaging systems based on mechanism have led to "overtriaging" of pediatric trauma patients, leading to unnecessary use of personnel and resources and costs, as well as disruption of other hospital care and procedures. For injured pediatric patients, activation based on anatomic and physiologic has been shown to be a more accurate method of triaging patients (see Fig. 2.2).

GENERAL PRINCIPLES OF MANAGEMENT

Triage

Definitive care may occur in the prehospital setting (e.g., endotracheal intubation), in the ED (e.g., chest tube placement), in the intensive care unit, or operating room. Triage is a process of patient assessment, prioritization of treatment, and selection of appropriate treatment location. In the early stages of patient assessment, the precise diagnosis of anatomic injury is often impossible. To identify patients with a potential for major morbidity or death, various physiologic scoring systems have been developed. The most useful are the Glasgow Coma Scale (GCS) (see Table 2.2), the Trauma Score (TS, which includes GCS) and the Pediatric Trauma Score (PTS) (see Table 2.3). Prehospital triage to a designated pediatric

TABLE 2.2

PEDIATRIC COMA

	Glasgow Coma Scale	Infant Coma Scale	Score
Eye opening	Spontaneous	Spontaneous	4
	To voice	To voice	3
	To pain	To pain	2
	None	None	1
Verbal response	Oriented	Coos, babbles	5
	Confused	Irritable cry, consolable	4
	Inappropriate	Cries to pain	3
	Garbled	Moans to pain	2
	None	None	1
Motor response	Obeys commands	Normal movements	6
	Localizes pain	Withdraws to touch	5
	Withdraws to pain	Withdraws to pain	4
	Flexion	Flexion	3
	Extension	Extension	2
	Flaccid	Flaccid	1

TABLE 2.3

PEDIATRIC TRAUMA SCORE[a]

	Category		
Component	**+2**	**+1**	**–1**
Size	>20 kg (40 lb)	10–20 kg	<10 kg
Airway	Normal	Maintainable	Unmaintainable
Systolic blood pressure	>90 mm Hg	50–90 mm Hg	<50 mm Hg
Central nervous system	Awake	Obtunded/loss of consciousness	Coma/decerebrate
Skeletal	None	Closed fracture	Open/multiple fractures
Cutaneous	None	Minor	Major/penetrating sum (pediatric trauma score)

[a]Pediatric trauma score for prehospital and in-hospital use.
From Tepas JJ III, Ramenofsky ML, Mollitt DL, et al. The pediatric trauma score as a predictor of injury severity: an objective assessment. *J Trauma* 1988; 28:425–429. Copyright Lippincott Williams & Wilkins. Reprinted with permission.

trauma center is indicated in any patient with a GCS <12, a TS <12, or a PTS <8. Field studies of the TS showed that at night, it is difficult to assess capillary refill and respiratory effort. Therefore, the most common tool used in prehospital triage is the revised trauma score (RTS), which deletes these two variables. Triage to a pediatric trauma center is then indicated for any of the following criteria: GCS <12, low systolic blood pressure, or abnormal respiratory rate for age. In the ED setting, a complete TS or PTS is usually obtained. The RTS is the most commonly used tool when evaluating outcomes. The PTS emphasizes the importance of patient size and ability to maintain the airway. Studies confirm the validity of the PTS as a predictor of outcome: 9% mortality for PTS >8 and 100% mortality for PTS <0. From 0 to 8, there is a linear relationship between lower PTS and an increased potential for mortality. Nevertheless, studies comparing TS, RTS, and PTS do not show any statistical advantage of PTS for the purposes of triage. In fact, many children with significant solid organ injuries have a normal PTS. Therefore, whichever physiologic scoring system is selected, it should be used consistently and sequentially to measure how the patient is responding to interventions.

Initial Evaluation

Advanced Trauma Life Support (ATLS) established by the American College of Surgeons outlines a standard approach to evaluation and treatment of the trauma victim. After prehospital evaluation and care, the injured child is transported to the hospital. Trauma level notification based on physiologic criteria from the scene determines the need for trauma team activation. The indication for team activation varies depending on local personnel but should include all children with anatomic or physiologic signs of significant injury (Fig. 2.2). In the ED assessment includes a primary survey, resuscitation, secondary survey, and subsequent transfer to definitive care (Table 2.4). A rapid, reproducible schema of immediate, simultaneous, and subsequent evaluation and treatment principles are applied to every child who may potentially have major or multiple trauma (Table 2.5). The principles of crisis resource management are utilized to guide the flow of the evaluation and resuscitation. Two key principles are followed in the initial assessment of the trauma patient. First, if any physiologic threat to the patient is identified, this threat is treated immediately. The order of priority is airway, breathing, circulation, disability, exposure and environment (ABCDE) (Table 2.6). In reality, with a highly organized trauma team, activities continue in parallel, rather than in series. Second, if at any point in the patient's secondary survey or subsequent care there is unexpected physiologic deterioration; the primary survey is rapidly repeated in order of priority (ABCDE).

Primary Survey

The goal of the primary survey is to assess the ABCDEs, identify life-threatening injuries, and initiate interventions to preserve cardiovascular function. The potential for cervical spine injury is assumed present in all patients with major trauma. The chin-lift or jaw-thrust maneuver is the preferred method to open the airway while clearing secretions or preparing for intubation to minimize cervical spine movement. All patients with major trauma should receive supplemental oxygen therapy; endotracheal intubation is established as

TABLE 2.4

INITIAL ASSESSMENT AND MANAGEMENT GUIDELINES FOR INJURED CHILDREN

Primary survey	Secondary survey
Airway maintenance	Head
Cervical spine control	Neck
Breathing	Chest
Circulation	Abdomen
Disability	Extremities
Exposure	Neurologic
Resuscitation	Urinary catheter, nasogastric tube placement
Oxygenation, airway management, and ventilation	Triage
Shock management	Imaging, laboratory studies
Venous access	

TABLE 2.5

MANAGEMENT OF SEVERE MULTIPLE TRAUMA

Time (min)	Phase	Action	Phase description
0	1	A	Airway, respiration, pulse, active hemorrhage, capillary refill, level of consciousness (AVPU or GCS score)
		T	Airway management with stabilization of cervical spine (bag-valve-mask, endotracheal intubation) (Surgical airway PRN)
			Ventilation with F_{IO_2} = 1.00, mild hyperventilation
			Cardiac compression (cardiopulmonary resuscitation) as needed
			Intravenous access/volume infusion
			Decompress pneumothorax/thoracostomy, tube placement as needed
			Relieve tamponade, control major hemorrhage
			Elevated head of bed to 30 degrees if no signs of shock
			Exposure—remove all clothing
			Wrap/bind pelvis
		M	Respiratory rate, pulse oximetry
			Heart rate (electrocardiogram)
			Blood pressure (mercury or Doppler)
		D	Complete blood cell count, type and cross-match, chemistries (glucose, amylase, alanine transaminase, aspartate transaminase)
5	2	A	Adequacy of airway, breathing, and circulation
			Level of consciousness (AVPU or GCS score)
			Temperature
			Penetrating wounds
		T	Nasogastric tube (orogastric if suspected midface fracture)
			Intravenous access, intraosseous, central catheter, or cut down as needed
			Thoracotomy or thoracostomy tube as needed
			Pericardiocentesis as needed
			Drug therapy (e.g., epinephrine)
			Blood transfusion/volume
			Prevent or treat increased ICP
		M	Heart rate, respiratory rate, pulse oximetry, blood pressure
			ET_{CO_2} if intubated
			Temperature (especially infants)
		D	ABGs PRN
10	3	A	Adequacy of airway, breathing, and circulation
		T	Additional venous access PRN/volume
			Urinary catheter (except in suspected urethral disruption)
			Arterial access as needed
			Thoracotomy as needed
			Drug therapy, including for pain management
			Avoid hypothermia
			Operating suite as needed
		M	Heart rate, respiratory rate, pulse oximetry, blood pressure
			ET_{CO_2} if intubated
			Temperature (especially infants)
		D	ABGs PRN
20	4	A	Adequacy of airway, breathing, and circulation
			GCS score, neurologic assessment
			Repeat full examination
		T	Cervical traction as needed
			Splint fractures
			Drug therapy (e.g., tetanus toxoid or tetanus immune globulin, antibiotics)
		M	Heart rate, respiratory rate, pulse oximetry, blood pressure
			Consider ICP bolt if severe head injury
		D	Repeat laboratory studies PRN

A, assessment; T, treatment; M, monitoring; D, diagnostics; AVPU, *a*lert, *v*erbal stimuli response, *p*ainful stimuli response, *u*nresponsive; GCS, Glasgow Coma Scale; ICP, intracranial pressure; ET_{CO_2}, end-tidal carbon dioxide; ABG, arterial blood gas; PRN, as needed.

TABLE 2.6

EMERGENCY DEPARTMENT ASSESSMENT AND MANAGEMENT PLAN FOR INJURED CHILD

Assessment	Diagnosis	Management	Evaluation study
Airway/breathing		Clear airway	
		Ventilate	
		Intubate	
Cardiac function		External cardiac massage	Cardiorespiratory monitor
Shock	External hemorrhage	Direct pressure	CBC count
	Internal hemorrhage	Trendelenburg position	CBC count
		Establish intravenous/intraosseous access	
Head/neck injury	Closed head injury	Normal perfusion, ventilation	CT scan, head
	Possible cervical spine fracture	Cervical spine immobilization	Lateral neck radiograph
Chest injury	Cardiac contusion	Pericardiocentesis	Chest radiograph
	Hemopneumothorax	Tube thoracostomy	Electrocardiogram
	Flail chest	Intubation/ventilation	Oxygen saturation monitor
	Sucking wound	Sterile dressing	Arterial blood gas
Abdominal injury	Penetrating injury	Wound exploration	Triple-contrast CT scan
		Operating room	Laparoscopy
	Blunt injury	Serial examination	Abdominal CT scan
		Paracentesis with lavage	FAST examination
			Amylase/liver function tests
			Serial CBC count
Renal/urinary injury	Renal contusion/laceration	Bladder catheterization	Urinalysis
			Abdominal CT scan
	Bladder/urethral injury	Delayed catheterization	Retrograde urethrogram
			Voiding cystourethrogram
Musculoskeletal injury	Dismembered part	Salvage, irrigate, and cool	Extremity radiographs
			Operating room
Soft tissue injury	Compound fracture	Sterile dressing; splint	Distal neurologic assessment
		Splint, traction	Distal perfusion assessment
	Bony injury	Irrigate, debride	Radiograph to exclude foreign body
		Primary versus delayed repair	

CBC count, complete blood cell count; CT, computed tomography.

clinically necessary. It is imperative to anticipate a "difficult airway" prior to intubation. If this is anticipated, the most experienced clinician in airway management should secure the airway. Difficult airway equipment (video laryngoscopes) should be available. Findings suggesting a difficult airway include a small mouth, inability to open the mouth, temporomandibular joint abnormalities, narrow receding mandible, protuberant maxilla (overbite), large tongue, distance <6 cm between the mandible and thyroid prominence, inability to place in the "sniffing position" (such as with suspected cervical spine injury), patients with a short, full, or bull neck, patients with a neck mass such as a large hematoma or significant penetrating trauma to the face or neck. If a difficult airway is suspected, management with bag-valve-mask ventilation or placement of a laryngeal mask may be preferred until a definitive airway can be established in a controlled environment. In children younger than 8 years, the choice of surgical airway is most often a needle cricothyroidotomy. An emergent airway should be converted into a more stable airway in the operating room as soon as is clinically practical (see Chapter 3 Airway).

After the airway has been secured, breathing is assessed to assure adequate air exchange. Continuous oxygen saturation measurement and end-tidal CO_2 monitoring in both the intubated and nonintubated patients allows for continued assessment of oxygenation and ventilation. Compromise of ventilatory function most often occurs secondary to a depressed sensorium. Other causes include airway occlusion, restriction of lung expansion, and direct pulmonary injury (see Chapter 123 Thoracic Trauma). Compromise of diaphragmatic excursion is a special hazard in children because of the increased importance of their diaphragms in ventilation. Gastric distention, a common event in an injured child, may significantly limit diaphragmatic excursion and impair ventilation; early use of a nasogastric or orogastric tube to decompress the stomach may assist ventilation. Prompt recognition of and attention to a hemothorax or pneumothorax, especially with mediastinal shift is essential. Thoracic subcutaneous emphysema is a sign of pneumothorax until determined otherwise.

Circulation is assessed by examining the character of the pulse, skin color, and capillary refill time. Presence of a palpable peripheral pulse typically correlates with a pressure

TABLE 2.7

AVPU METHOD FOR ASSESSING LEVEL OF CONSCIOUSNESS

A—*A*lert	P—*P*ainful stimuli, responds to
V—*V*oice, responds to	U—*U*nresponsive

greater than 80 mm Hg; an absent peripheral pulse with a palpable central pulse correlates with a pressure greater than 50 to 60 mm Hg. In a normovolemic patient, the capillary refill time is less than 2 seconds. External hemorrhage should be controlled by direct pressure or pneumatic splints. Application of an extremity tourniquet to stop bleeding, while becoming more common in adult trauma patients, remains to be evaluated in children.

Disability is assessed by completing a rapid neurologic examination to establish level of consciousness and pupillary response (Table 2.7). The GCS (Table 2.2) provides a quantitative measure of the level of consciousness and is useful for following the evolution of the injury.

The patient is then fully exposed to complete the initial assessment; attention to the maintenance of body temperature is especially important in children. Radiant warmers, warm blankets, air shields, and IV fluid warmers are useful tools for accomplishing this goal.

Resuscitation

Vascular access is an early but often challenging necessity in resuscitation. Percutaneous cannulation of bilateral upper extremity veins with two large-bore cannulas is ideal. However, the size of the available veins guides the choice of cannulas. Successful placement of a 22- or 20-gauge cannula is preferable to failed attempts to place larger cannulas. Relatively large volumes of fluids and blood can be given through a small, short cannula. Improvement in vascular volume may then permit the placement of a larger cannula at an alternative site. Intraosseous access provides a quick, easy alternative during early resuscitation especially in children with cardiovascular compromise (see Chapter 141 Procedures). In a hypotensive child in whom initial attempts at peripheral access or IO access are unsuccessful, the femoral vein provides a safe site for the insertion of a central catheter using the standard Seldinger guidewire technique. However, a long, narrow, standard central catheter may be less effective than a large peripheral IV catheter for rapid fluid resuscitation. Rapid cutdown access is best done on a basilic vein at the elbow or the saphenous vein either at the ankle or in the groin just below the saphenofemoral junction. Central vein cannulation above the diaphragm, although necessary at times, is not a preferred emergency access route in children due to the risk of significant complications; this should be done by experienced personnel. The use of ultrasound guidance may also increase success in obtaining vascular access at peripheral and central sites. Blood should be sent immediately for a type and cross-match, a complete blood count, and coagulation and chemical parameters.

Shock after major trauma is most often due to acute loss of ≥40% of the blood volume. Cardiogenic, neurogenic (spinal cord injury), and obstructive (tension pneumothorax, cardiac tamponade) can also be present. Shock secondary to isolated brain injury is more common than previously believed, but other etiologies must be excluded first. Assume shock is present in any injured patient with cold skin and tachycardia until proven otherwise. Reliance on the hematocrit alone is unreliable as initial near-normal hematocrit level does not exclude the possibility of significant blood loss.

Classification of hemorrhagic shock is used to determine severity using physiologic parameters to estimate volume loss (see Table 2.8). Class I hemorrhage, estimated blood loss of 15% (up to a 250 mL in a 20 kg child), causes minimal physiologic changes. A single 20 mL per kg IV fluid bolus should stabilize the circulation. Class II hemorrhage, estimated blood loss of 15% to 30% (250 to 500 mL in a 20 kg child), causes tachycardia, tachypnea, a fall in pulse pressure, and increase in peripheral vascular resistance due to circulating catecholamines. Patients have impaired capillary refilling and early signs of poor mentation. A 20 to 40 mL per kg of IV crystalloid is needed to stabilize these patients. Class III hemorrhage, estimated blood loss of 30% to 40% (500 to 650 mL of blood in a 20 kg child) causes obvious signs of shock including altered mental status, tachycardia, tachypnea, and measurable fall in systolic pressure. Crystalloid resuscitation should begin immediately; most patients will require blood products. Class IV hemorrhagic shock, estimated blood loss 40%, is immediately life-threatening. Patients are mentally depressed, cold, pale, and have profound tachycardia and tachypnea, with narrow pulse pressure. Immediate transfusion is required; these patients often require prompt operative intervention to stop ongoing blood losses.

Cardiogenic shock from myocardial contusion is rare. Obstructive shock from cardiac tamponade or tension pneumothorax is also rare. Dilated neck veins in a patient with a decelerating injury, sternal contusion, or penetrating thoracic trauma should arouse suspicion. Neurogenic shock classically causes hypotension without tachycardia or vasoconstriction. Isolated head injuries may be associated with shock, though other causes be considered first. Septic shock rarely occurs immediately after injury, even in the face of abdominal contamination.

Crystalloid isotonic solution and Ringer's lactate or normal saline are the initial resuscitative fluids of choice for treatment of hypovolemic shock. The initial crystalloid infusion is given as rapidly as possible in a dose of 20 mL per kg with careful monitoring of the physiologic response. Table 2.8 emphasizes the anticipated fluid needs, depending on the degree of shock; formulation is based on the premise that the patient requires 300 mL of crystalloid for each 100 mL of blood loss. To simplify the approach, treat shock with an immediate, rapid 20 mL per kg of crystalloid; if no response, proceed with a second 20 mL per kg of crystalloid; and if there is no response, give a third 20 mL per kg of crystalloid or 10 mL per kg of packed red blood cells (PRBCs). In adults with hemorrhagic shock, this resuscitation strategy is inferior to blood plus fresh-frozen plasma (FFP) resuscitation; this therapy has not yet been evaluated in children. No response to 60 mL per kg in children suggests the need for operative intervention. Failure to respond to crystalloid resuscitation with a suspected source of hemorrhage is an indication for early transfusion. The restoration of vital signs and perfusion may be clinically assessed, although in unusual situations, invasive monitoring with elective placement of a central venous catheter may be helpful after patient

TABLE 2.8

THERAPEUTIC CLASSIFICATION OF HEMORRHAGIC SHOCK IN PEDIATRIC PATIENT

	Class I	Class II	Class III	Class IV
Blood volume loss[a]	Up to 15%	15–30%	30–40%	≥40%
Pulse rate	Normal	Mild tachycardia	Moderate tachycardia	Severe tachycardia
Blood pressure	Normal/increased	Normal/decreased	Decreased	Decreased
Capillary blanch test	Normal	Positive	Positive	Positive
Respiratory rate	Normal	Mild tachypnea	Moderate tachypnea	Severe tachypnea
Urine output	1–2 mL/kg/hr	0.5–1.0 mL/kg/hr	0.25–0.5 mL/kg/hr	Negligible
Mental status	Slightly anxious	Mildly anxious	Anxious/confused	Confused/lethargic
Fluid replacement (3:1 rule)	Crystalloid	Crystalloid	Crystalloid% blood	Crystalloid% blood

[a]Assume blood volume to be 8–9% of body weight (80–90 mL/kg).

transition. The urinary output is also a measure of circulating volume; physiologic target is 1 mL/kg/hr in children >1 year, 2 mL/kg/hr in children <1 year.

Blood transfusion is done preferably with fully cross-matched, warmed blood. In the face of a transient or absent response to a rapid crystalloid infusion, type-specific, or type O-negative blood can be given as a whole-blood transfusion. Fluid and blood are given rapidly enough to maintain stable vital signs and adequate urine output. Vasopressors, steroids, and sodium bicarbonate do not play a role in the initial treatment of hypovolemic shock. In massive transfusion situations in adults, resuscitation with a ratio of FFP to packed RBCs of 1:1 leads to the best survival.

A urinary catheter should be placed in patients who need ongoing close monitoring of organ perfusion. Although urethral injuries are rare in children, urinary catheterization should not be attempted if urethral integrity is questionable based on blood at the urethral meatus or in the scrotum, or if there is abnormal prostate placement on rectal examination. Urine is immediately analyzed for the presence of gross or microscopic blood. Patients with significant abdominal injury and those with inadequate airway protection should have a nasogastric or orogastric tube placed. In the presence of a basilar skull fracture, care must be taken in inserting a nasogastric tube to avoid passage into the brain through a cribriform plate fracture. An orogastric tube is preferred in such patients.

Secondary Survey

A rapid, systematic head to toe examination with assessment of organ systems is performed after completing the ABCs. An AMPLE history should be performed indicating allergies, medications, past illnesses, time of last meal, and events preceding the injury.

Head examination includes evaluation of pupillary size and response, examination of the eye for hemorrhage or penetrating injury, and a quick assessment of visual acuity. Visualization of blood in the external auditory canal or behind the tympanic membrane raises suspicion for a basilar skull fracture. Thorough palpation of skull and mandible may detect fractures and dislocations, but if the airway is secure, further evaluation of maxillofacial bony trauma is of lesser priority.

Injury to the cervical spine is comparatively uncommon in children, but risk of injury is always considered, especially with trauma above the clavicles. For young children, other higher risk mechanisms include fall from ≥1 floor, pedestrian versus motor vehicle at 30 mph or more, and unrestrained or poorly restrained occupants of a motor vehicle involved in a significant crash. In older children, sports injuries are the second most common cause of cervical spine injury. In alert, cooperative children with no neurologic abnormalities and low risk for cervical spine injury, the neck can be cleared with a normal clinical examination similar to the adult NEXUS criteria. Patients with a normal neurologic examination without tenderness over the cervical vertebrae, are asked to rotate the neck as able 45 degrees to each side, this is followed by flexion and then extension. If there are no symptoms or signs of spasm, guarding, pain, or tenderness, a decision can be made with a high degree of certainty that there is no fracture, ligamentous instability, or cord injury. Otherwise, adequate cervical spine radiographs are required to evaluate for a bony injury. Ligamentous disruption and dislocations of the cervical spine without radiographic evidence of bony (SCIWORA) injury occur in children due to ligamentous laxity and incomplete development of the bony spine. In patients with a high-risk mechanism of trauma or pain, obtain three-view C-spine series (AP, lateral, and odontoid). If the patient has an altered sensorium, a semirigid cervical collar is left in place even if the three survey radiographs show negative findings, until the patient recovers sufficiently to permit a full evaluation of the neck. For patients with prolonged coma: Normal plain radiographs with the addition of either a cervical spine magnetic resonance imaging within 48 hours or normal flexion and extension views with simultaneous brain stem evoked potentials are performed to clear the cervical spine (see Chapter 120 Neck Trauma).

Two situations require further discussion. First, if a seriously injured child has had an endotracheal tube placed, computed tomographic (CT) scan of C1 and C2 during head CT imaging, replaces the need for the odontoid view. Second, if a patient is brought to the hospital with a helmet in place and no condition requiring immediate intubation, an initial cervical spine radiographic series can be performed before helmet removal. If it is necessary to remove the helmet before the neck is cleared, a two-person technique ensuring neck immobilization is recommended.

Visual inspection of the chest identifies the rare sucking chest wound, best treated by immediate application of a sterile occlusive dressing; even more rarely, a major flail component, treated by splinting or endotracheal intubation; or a penetrating wound. Auscultation may not reveal a pneumothorax or hemothorax secondary to the broad transmission of breath sounds in a child. A prompt chest radiograph is helpful in demonstrating these conditions in stable patients. The diagnosis of tension pneumothorax is supported by contralateral tracheal shift and distended neck veins, in addition to diminished breath sounds. Anterior needle thoracostomy provides temporary relief, but tube thoracostomy with the placement of the tube to suction should follow. Cardiac tamponade is suggested by muffled heart sounds, distended neck veins, and a narrow pulse pressure and should be relieved by prompt pericardiocentesis. Bedside ultrasound is useful in detecting tamponade as well as pneumothorax or hemothorax (see Chapter 141 Procedures). Impaled object anywhere on the body are best left in place until definitive operation. If the history suggests a severe deceleration injury and the chest radiograph demonstrates a widened mediastinum with or without a fractured first rib, a thoracic aortic injury is suggested. In the stable patient, a thoracic CT angiogram is promptly indicated (see Chapter 123 Thoracic Trauma).

The secondary abdominal examination establishes whether visceral injury exists. Visceral injury is suspected in the presence of abdominal wall contusion, distention, abdominal or shoulder pain, signs of peritoneal irritation, gross hematuria, and/or shock. Hemodynamically stable patients are evaluated with abdominal CT scan as soon as possible. Gastric distention may lead to left upper quadrant tenderness, even in patients with injuries remote to their abdomen. The passage of a nasogastric or orogastric tube may relieve this condition and prevent the need for imaging. Diagnostic peritoneal lavage (DPL), previously a mainstay of emergency trauma evaluation, is rarely performed in the pediatric patient with blunt trauma. The performance of a DPL prior to abdominal CT scan may introduce air, decreasing the ability of CT to diagnose this life-threatening condition. DPL has been supplanted by the focused abdominal sonography for trauma (FAST) examination, which may demonstrate intraperitoneal free fluid suggesting injury. Most importantly, large majority of children with documented intra-abdominal or retroperitoneal injury do not require surgery, thus avoiding unnecessary DPL is optimal (see Chapter 111 Abdominal Trauma).

A rectal examination provides valuable information in the setting of real or potential spinal cord injury or perineal trauma. However, in the majority of trauma patients, the utility of this examination is limited and is stressful for the child.

A thorough extremity examination assesses for deformity, contusions, abrasions, penetration, and perfusion, including pulse palpation. Although the presence of a distal extremity pulse does not exclude a concomitant proximal arterial injury, the presence of equal Doppler blood pressures makes it much less likely. Inspect soft tissue injuries for foreign bodies and devitalized tissue. Apply pressure to the pubis and anterior iliac spines for pelvic stability. Palpate long bones for point tenderness and crepitance, sensation, strength, pulses and capillary refill and evidence of compartment syndrome. Severe extremity angulations should be straightened and immobilized, and traction splints should be applied followed by repeat examination of distal neurologic function and perfusion. Open fracture sites should be covered with sterile dressings. Generous irrigation and debridement of open wounds not associated with fractures or joint injuries are beneficial in early wound care to minimize contamination before considering primary or delayed wound closure (see Chapter 119 Musculoskeletal Trauma).

Hypothermia is a special risk in injured children, due to their larger surface area. Hypothermia can develop in the prehospital setting and worsen in the ED, as proper assessment and treatment requires exposure of the patient. The dangers of hypothermia include impaired hemodynamics and coagulation, increased peripheral vascular resistance, and increased metabolic demand. Use of overhead radiant warmers, warm blankets, and warmed IV solutions assist in maintaining adequate body temperature.

Neurologic assessment includes a reevaluation of the level of consciousness, a repeat pupillary examination, and a thorough sensorimotor examination. Serial reassessment with GCS is critical to detect changes (Table 2.3). It is important to carefully reassess and document the neurologic deficits in patients with suspected spinal cord injury as these findings change over time; maintain the patient in a semirigid cervical collar (see Chapter 120 Neck Trauma).

Supplemental studies are performed after the secondary survey, as indicated by a history and physical examination. Tetanus prophylaxis and antibiotics should be administered as clinically indicated.

Imaging the Pediatric Trauma Patient

Traditionally, the radiologic survey for major trauma patients included cervical spine, chest, and pelvic radiographs. More recent studies have demonstrated that patients with a GCS score of 15, no distracting injury, no pain in the pelvic region, and a normal examination of their pelvis have a low incidence of fractures obviating the routine use of pelvic plain films. The need for cervical spine imaging is described above. Additional radiographs of the thoracolumbar spine and extremities are indicated by clinical findings and mechanism of trauma.

The findings from the primary and secondary survey guide the need for more definitive imaging studies. Cranial CT is recommended in the presence of an abnormal GCS or focal neurologic findings; it should be considered in patients with bleeding disorders, posttraumatic seizure, or prolonged lethargy. Abdominal CT is indicated in stable patients with blunt trauma if there is physical signs of intra-abdominal injury or gross hematuria; or if there is a significant mechanism of injury in a child with depressed mental status. Abdominal CT for trauma is usually performed with IV contrast alone; oral contrast delays the test and increases the risk for aspiration. If a Foley catheter is in place, it should be clamped during the abdominal CT scan to provide information about the bladder. The likelihood of positive findings on abdominal CT scans is significantly increased if three or more of the following indicators are present: (i) Gross hematuria, (ii) lap belt injury, (iii) assault or abuse as a mechanism of trauma, (iv) abdominal tenderness, and (v) TS ≤12. Certain indicators alone, such as positive abdominal findings, worrisome mechanism of trauma (e.g., ejected from a motor vehicle), and neurologic compromise (e.g., GCS score of less than 10) may warrant abdominopelvic CT scan to exclude clinically occult intra-abdominal or retroperitoneal injury. In general, the accuracy of CT scans in diagnosing intraperitoneal or retroperitoneal injuries is 95% or better. The use of ultrafast and multiplanar CT scans increases the diagnostic accuracy by limiting motion artifact and improving contrast enhancement. Ultrasound has been used successfully in the evaluation of the adult trauma patient using the FAST examination. In the hands of an experienced examiner, it can be performed in the ED and will document approximately 70% of the injuries to the liver, spleen, and/or kidneys through the demonstration of free intraperitoneal fluid. This may be an alternative when emergency CT scans of the abdomen are not available; however, its utility in the pediatric trauma patient is still evolving. Free intraperitoneal fluid alone in a child does not necessitate operative exploration.

The major limitation of abdominal CT is its inability to reliably detect hollow viscus injuries such as perforation of the bowel and bladder. Free intraperitoneal air is seen in only 25% of patients with a bowel perforation. Free fluid in the abdomen without solid organ injury, bowel wall thickening, and a mesenteric hematoma are seen on CT scan in a minority of patients with documented bowel injury. Serial abdominal examinations may indicate need for repeat CT imaging.

Selective urologic contrast studies are indicated in two situations. A retrograde urethrogram is indicated if there is gross blood at the meatus, especially if clinical and radiographic studies suggest a pelvic fracture. If the urethra is damaged, a surgical or urologic consultation is essential. If the urethra is not damaged, a cystogram may be performed after carefully advancing the catheter into the bladder. Second, a one-shot IV pyelogram may be performed in the operating room if a patient with blunt or penetrating abdominal trauma is too unstable for CT. An abdominal film is obtained 5 minutes after IV administration of a bolus of 2 to 4 mL per kg of 50% diatrizoate sodium (Hypaque; Winthrop Laboratories). This study will usually confirm the function or malfunction of both kidneys and occasionally the upper ureters (see Table 2.6).

Massive Transfusion Protocol

Children who experience severe, multiple trauma are at high risk for trauma-induced coagulopathy; those with traumatic brain injury are especially at risk. Tissue injury, hemorrhagic shock, dilution, acidosis, and hypothermia trigger the coagulation cascade. Trauma-induced coagulopathy has been associated with increased morbidity and mortality in children and adults alike. A process for monitoring alterations in coagulation and a process to provide massive transfusion is necessary in every trauma center. Coagulation monitoring includes early testing of prothrombin time (PT), activated partial thromboplastin time (aPTT), INR, fibrinogen, and D-dimer. A massive transfusion protocol is initiated when an injured child requires ongoing transfusions to maintain stable hemodynamics. This typically requires the administration of multiple blood products, including PRBCs, platelets, and FFP. Based on extensive military experience, transfusion ratios have evolved to deliver products in a ratio of 1 unit PRBC:1 unit platelets:1 unit FFP. However, as yet, similar data are not available in the pediatric population to make a similar recommendation. Early use of platelets and FFP in addition to PRBCs is likely beneficial. Administration of procoagulant concentrates may also be helpful, including fibrinogen, recombinant factor VIIa, and factor IX complex, though there are no clearly defined pediatric indications for these.

APPLYING THE ATLS FRAMEWORK TO CHILDREN WITH MULTIPLE TRAUMA BY SEVERITY OF INJURY

Mild Multiple Trauma

The ATLS framework is applied to the evaluation and management of the child with apparent mild multiple trauma in order to confirm the absence of severe injuries. The ABCDEs are assessed rapidly, and if there is concern for more severe injury, IV access, laboratory and radiographic screening studies and consultation are implemented. However, in cases that obviously seem to involve mild trauma, the physician can proceed directly to the examination. This includes a full set of vital signs with capillary refill, attention to the child's mental status and neurologic examination, and complete head to toe examination with full body exposure to assure that no injuries have been missed. A child with a history of mild multiple trauma and a normal examination usually requires no laboratory or radiographic studies.

Moderate Multiple Trauma

The child with moderate multiple trauma requires immediate evaluation using the ATLS framework which determines the need for further diagnostic evaluation and interventions. During the primary survey, assess the need for oxygen vascular access, consider the need for C-spine immobilization, and assess for life-threatening injury. If the vital signs and primary survey are normal for age, the physician should then proceed with a thorough examination, as outlined in mild multiple trauma.

Most patients with moderate multiple trauma require ancillary studies as part of their evaluation. These include a CBC count, urinalysis, amylase/lipase, and/or liver function tests and radiographs of the chest, cervical spine, and/or pelvis. A type and cross for red blood cells is indicated if ongoing hemorrhage is suspected or the need for operative intervention is anticipated. Depending on the history and physical examination, CT scans of the head, abdomen, pelvis, and/or spine may be indicated. In fully awake patients, a completely normal examination may be sufficient to exclude the need for screening studies. Many patients in this category will require admission to the hospital. However, an older child with a history of a moderately severe impact, who has an unremarkable examination and normal studies, may be discharged from the ED after observation for several hours.

Severe Multiple Trauma

The management of the child with severe multiple trauma demands immediate action in hospitals with a trauma center, with the highest level alert. The initial approach identifies either obvious life-threatening injury or a reasonable likelihood that such an injury exists. An alteration of vital signs (hypotension, tachycardia), diaphoresis, or depressed consciousness automatically categorizes the injury as severe. Although helpful as an initial guide, mechanism alone (e.g., a fall from a two-storey building) is not a highly accurate predictor of the risk of sustaining significant injuries. To adequately manage the child with severe multiple trauma, the physician must understand the need to institute treatment frequently before a full examination has been completed and to continually intersperse detailed reassessments after intervention. Table 2.5 provides an outline for organizing the initial approach to severe multiple trauma in the ED. It uses a four-pronged strategy: Assessment, treatment, monitoring, and diagnostic testing. The protocol is laid out over time in an idealized fashion; obviously, limitations in the number of personnel or unusually difficult technical procedures may slow the progression of the evaluation and management.

Monitoring, Measuring, and Maintaining Quality and Competency

Injured children must be stabilized in the ED where they present. Hospitals that are not trauma centers must ensure that their physicians, nurses, and ancillary staff are able to initiate interventions necessary to stabilize the patient. After stabilization, the child with multiple injuries should be transferred to a trauma center. Periodic multidisciplinary training sessions and simulation assist clinicians in pediatric and general EDs to review the primary and secondary survey, resuscitation interventions, and identification of potential life- or limb-threatening injuries allowing for hands-on practice. Skills-based training sessions reinforce competency in skills that are performed rarely such as intraosseous access, performing endotracheal intubation, tube thoracostomy, and splinting extremities. Periodic review of the process of coordinated communication and transfer of patients needing care in a trauma center is ideal. Providers who regularly care for injured patients should be certified in ATLS and participate in trauma-continuing medical education.

Finally, quality improvement initiatives for pediatric trauma resuscitations can take several forms. Cases can be reviewed at morbidity and mortality conferences to evaluate systems to expedite care, recognize the severely injured child sooner and discuss ways to improve management. Trauma resuscitations can be video recorded and reviewed to evaluate teamwork, communication, and time to key interventions. The trauma flow sheet or electronic medical record can be reviewed if video recording is not available to ensure that care of the injured patient is timely, appropriate, and occurring in parallel.

SUMMARY

Injuries ranging from mild to severe frequently present to the ED; the challenge lies in executing a thorough evaluation so that injuries are not missed while obtaining the appropriate radiologic and/or laboratory studies in a timely fashion. This chapter describes a standard approach that can be applied systematically to all the children with trauma providing a common mental model that can be shared by all team members which serves as a platform for assessment, evaluation, and communication.

CLINICAL PEARLS AND PITFALLS

- Ideal assessment of the injured child requires strong collaboration between many clinicians. Explicit processes should be in place for triage, trauma notification, availability of blood, pediatric radiographic dosing, and availability for OR interventions, and safe transfer to definitive care.
- Children can present with mild to severe, single to multiple, trauma. In any injured child, an immediate assessment must be made to identify risk for serious injury.
- Children with multiple or severe trauma require systematic evaluation and resuscitation, beginning with rapid assessment of injuries, determination of management priorities, and performance of critical interventions. Immediate establishment of airway, breathing, and circulation must occur.
- Imaging should occur based on findings in the primary and secondary survey. CT is recommended for any child with an altered mental status, signs of closed head injury or a severe mechanism of injury. Cervical spine imaging is necessary if the C-spine cannot be clinically cleared.

Suggested Readings and Key References

American College of Surgeons Committee on Trauma. *Advanced trauma life support for doctors*. Chicago, IL: American College of Surgeons, 2012.

Avarello JT, Cantor RM. Pediatric major trauma: An approach to evaluation and management. *Emerg Med Clin North Am* 2007;25(3):803–836.

Capraro AJ, Mooney D, Waltzman ML. The use of routine laboratory studies as screening tools in pediatric abdominal trauma. *Pediatr Emerg Care* 2006;22(7):480–484.

Cotton BA, Nance ML. Penetrating trauma in children. *Semin Pediatr Surg* 2004;13(2):87–97.

Eppich WJ, Zonfrillo MR. Emergency department evaluation and management of blunt abdominal trauma in children. *Curr Opin Pediatr* 2007;19(3):265–269.

Holmes JF, Gladman A, Chang CH. Performance of abdominal ultrasonography in pediatric blunt trauma patients: A meta-analysis. *J Pediatr Surg* 2007;42(9):1588–1594.

National Center for Injury Prevention and Control. Web-based Injury Statistics Query and Reporting System (WISQARS). cdc.gov/injury/wisqars. Accessed October 15, 2008.

Rees MJ, Aickin R, Aolbe A, et al. The screening pelvic radiograph in pediatric trauma. *Ann Emerg Med* 2003;41(2):497–500.

Slack SE, Clancy MJ. Clearing the cervical spine of paediatric trauma patients. *Emerg Med J* 2004;21(2):189–193.

Viccellio P, Simon H, Presmann BD, et al. NEXUS Group. A prospective multicenter study of cervical spine injury in children. *Pediatrics* 2001;108(2):E20.

CHAPTER 3 ▪ AIRWAY

AARON DONOGHUE, MD, MSCE, JOSHUA NAGLER, MD, MHPEd, AND LOREN G. YAMAMOTO, MD, MPH, MBA

GOALS OF EMERGENCY THERAPY

Tracheal intubation (TI) is a fundamental procedure during resuscitation of a critically ill child. The goals of therapy are the placement of an artificial airway in the trachea in a safe, expedient fashion, while simultaneously avoiding physiologic deterioration (hypoxia, hypercapnia, bradycardia, hypotension).

TI is indicated for any clinical state where existing or impending failure exists of oxygenation, ventilation, neuromuscular respiratory drive, or airway protective reflexes. Reports in pediatrics have shown that the most frequent indications for TI in children involve neurologic failure (traumatic brain injury, cardiac arrest, status epilepticus) as opposed to primary respiratory failure, with trauma accounting for more than half of all cases of pediatric TI in the ED. TI should be considered the definitive method of managing existing or impending respiratory failure from any cause in the ED (see Chapter 4 Cardiopulmonary Resuscitation).

Pediatric anatomy and physiology has direct influence on intubation technique, equipment selection, and prevalence of adverse physiologic events during TI. Table 3.1 summarizes the anatomic and physiologic features in children that are important to consider when approaching TI in a child. The summary effects of the various respiratory physiologic phenomena described above are a greater tendency for hypoxemia and arterial desaturation, which must be kept in mind during the preintubation and intubation phases of the procedure.

Quality and Safety

Despite the fact that TI is a fundamental, essential skill for emergency providers, pediatric TI is an uncommon occurrence when measured at the level of an individual provider. A recent survey of pediatric ED directors found that the annual incidence of TI in the PED ranged from 12 to 64 cases per year. Sixty-two percent of surveyed PED directors believed that their faculty did not encounter sufficient exposure to TI in their clinical duties to maintain competence at this essential procedure. Additionally, the same survey found that there was a negligible difference in the median number of TI cases per faculty at the PEDs where their directors thought exposure was insufficient (five cases per faculty per year) and those where their directors thought exposure was sufficient (seven cases per faculty per year). Data from tertiary PEDs published in the past few years has shown low-frequency exposure to TI for PED faculty, with fewer than half of PED faculty performing TI during a year of typical clinical experience, and supervising TI performance a median of four times per year.

Published data on exposure to pediatric TI among trainees in pediatrics and pediatric EM also shows scant—and possibly diminishing—experience. Multiple studies have shown that pediatric residents are exposed to opportunities for attempting TI less often. A study of video recorded TI attempts from a tertiary PED demonstrated success rates of 33% for residents and 50% for PEM fellows. Multihospital registry data on pediatric TI in the ICU has shown a significant positive association between residents attempting TI and the occurrence of adverse events. In 2013, the Accreditation Council for Graduate Medical Education removed nonneonatal TI from the core competencies for housestaff training in pediatrics.

Finally, while historically reported as uncommon, physiologic deterioration during intubation may be more common than previously appreciated in children. In the previously mentioned study of video recorded cases of pediatric emergency intubation, oxyhemoglobin desaturation (defined as pulse oximetry of <90%) has been shown to occur in up to one-third of cases of emergency TI in the PED. Cardiovascular instability (bradycardia, hypotension) have been noted to occur in up to 8% of patients, with cardiac arrest from asphyxia occurring in 2%. This combination of high clinical risk, infrequent occurrence, and dwindling exposure among trainees has led to widespread reconsideration of what operators are appropriate to perform TI in the PED. Careful attention should be paid to training exposure and cumulative clinical experience among personnel in the PED who may be required to perform TI on children.

Bridging the gap between the infrequent nature of TI and the need for ongoing skill maintenance is a challenge to be met as PEM moves forward. Multiple novel approaches to this challenge have been reported in published literature. The use of retrospective review of TI data from individual centers and multicenter databases, both from medical records and from video-recorded patient encounters, has been reported as a technique to identify areas for improvement. Simulation education is well suited to this uncommon, high-stakes procedure; data on the effectiveness of simulation in educational and affective outcomes (e.g., learner satisfaction) have been promising, but additional research is necessary to determine the optimal means of using simulation to improve clinical outcomes in the PED during TI.

EQUIPMENT

Anticipating the need for increasing airway support and having necessary advanced airway equipment available is critical. An oxygen supply source, devices for passive oxygen delivery, and a bag-valve-mask device are needed for preparation as well as during advanced airway management procedures. Adjunctive devices such as oral and nasal airways should be available. Equipment in a range of sizes suitable for children from birth to adolescence should be available. Monitoring equipment including capnography should be available. For advanced airway management, additional equipment should include

TABLE 3.1

ANATOMIC AND PHYSIOLOGIC FEATURES IN CHILDREN PERTINENT TO LARYNGOSCOPY AND INTUBATION

Anatomy

- **Size**—airway structures are smaller and field of vision is more narrow.
- **Adenoidal hypertrophy** is common in young children.
- **Developing teeth**—while young infants are edentulous, the underlying alveolar ridge contains developing tooth buds that are susceptible to disruption.
- **Primary teeth** in young children can be easily avulsed and/or aspirated.
- **Tongue is large** relative to size of oropharynx.
- **Superior larynx**—often referred to as "anterior," the laryngeal opening in infants and young children is actually located in a *superior* position (in infants, the larynx is opposite C3–C4 as opposed to C4–C5 in adults). This makes the angle of the laryngeal opening with respect to the base of the tongue more acute and visualization more difficult.
- The **hyoepiglottic ligament** (connects base of tongue to epiglottis) has less strength in young children—thus, a laryngoscope blade in the vallecula will not elevate the epiglottis as efficiently as in an adult.
- The **epiglottis** of children is narrow and angled acutely with respect to the tracheal axis; thus the epiglottis covers the tracheal opening to a greater extent and can be more difficult to mobilize.
- The **narrowest point** occurs at the level of the **cricoid cartilage.**

Physiology

- **Lung**—smaller and fewer alveoli, decreased gas exchange surface area, absent collateral channels of ventilation.
- **Respiratory mechanics**—the cartilaginous chest wall in children has poor elastic recoil and leads to increased compliance. The closing volume (CV), the volume at which terminal bronchioles collapse as a result of extrinsic pressure exceeding intrabronchial pressure + elastic recoil forces is frequently higher than functional residual capacity (FRC), leading to a greater tendency for atelectasis and collapse.
- **Cellular physiology**—increased oxygen consumption in infants; prone to significant increase with physiologic perturbation (e.g., fever, hypothermia).
- **Cardiovascular**—high vagal tone, greater tendency for bradycardia with hypoxia, laryngeal stimulation.

endotracheal (ET) tubes, stylets, and traditional laryngoscope blades and handles and/or an indirect or videolaryngoscope.

Endotracheal Tubes

Both cuffed and uncuffed ET tubes are available for use in pediatrics. Historically, uncuffed tubes were preferentially used in young children to allow use of the maximal tube size that would be accommodated by the anatomic narrowing at the level of the subglottis. More recent bronchoscopic and radiologic data suggest that the pediatric airway may be more elliptically shaped at this level rather than circumferentially narrowed. In addition, newly designed cuffed pediatric ET tubes are manufactured with balloons that are low profile and moved distally on the tube to avoid laryngeal structures when appropriately positioned. Use of these new cuffed tubes has been shown to decrease the need for tube exchange secondary to inappropriate sizing, with no increase in postextubation stridor, need for racemic epinephrine, or long-term complications. Pediatric Advanced Life Support Guidelines as well as anesthesia literature now supports that, beyond the newborn period, cuffed ET tubes are equally as safe as uncuffed tubes. In addition, cuffed tubes are favored in clinical circumstances where airway diameter may change over the course of treatment (e.g., inhalational injury, angioedema), as a protective measure for children at risk for aspiration, and in any child in whom underlying lung disease may necessitate high ventilator pressures (e.g., bronchiolitis, status asthmaticus, chronic lung disease). The risk associated with the use of cuffed ET tubes is inadvertent excessive cuff pressures, which could lead to ischemia of the tracheal mucosa. Various recommendations suggest that pressures higher than 20 to 30 cm H_2O should be avoided. This can be achieved either through listening for an air leak while applying positive pressure through the ET tube, or by using an ET tube cuff manometer.

ET tube sizes are reported based on the internal diameter, measured in millimeters (mm). Available sizes range from 2.5 mm (suitable for a preterm infant) to adult sizes of 7.0 mm or more. Resistance to airflow as well as risk of tube obstruction are both increased in smaller tubes. Tube selection in pediatrics therefore aims to balance these risks associated with smaller tubes, with the need to select a tube that will pass easily through the vocal cords and not create excessive pressure on the tracheal wall. Methods of selecting the appropriate tube size include use of a length-based resuscitation tape, pediatric sizing programs available online or on mobile devices, and use of an age-based formula. Each has been shown to be effective, though inclusion of options for cuffed tube sizing is not offered in each. For *uncuffed* ET tube sizing, the age-based formula: **4 + (age in years/4)** has been shown to be accurate in children. For newer, low profile cuffed ET tubes, selecting a tube one-half size smaller is recommended. Thus, for cuffed tubes, the formula is **3.5 + (age in years/4)**. Regardless of the method chosen in selecting the initial tube size, it is important to have additional tubes available, one size smaller in the event that tube passage is difficult and one size larger if a large air leak results in inadequate ventilation, despite inflation of the cuff where appropriate.

ET tube stylets provide rigidity and shape to the ET tube, offering facility in guiding the tube through the glottic opening. Various sizes exist to accommodate both pediatric- and adult-sized ET tubes. Most stylets are manufactured with a friction reducing surface coating, however water-soluble lubricant can be utilized to facilitate passage as needed. The stylet should not project past the tip of the tube or through the Murphy eye.

Bending the stylet over the adapter at the proximal end of the tube prevents inadvertent movement during intubation.

Direct Laryngoscopes

There are two components to traditional direct laryngoscopes, the handle and the blade. Pediatric- and adult-sized handles are available that differ in diameter and length. Smaller diameter handles tend to be favored with smaller blades, though selection is ultimately based on operator's preference. Laryngoscope blades are either curved or straight. The choice of curved or straight blade is best made based on the experience and preference of the operator. Curved blades are designed to follow the base of the tongue into the vallecula. They often have a beaded tip to allow pressure against the hyoepiglottic ligament which helps elevate the epiglottis. They also have a large flange which facilitates displacement of the tongue. Straight blades allow direct lifting of the epiglottis to expose the glottic opening. This type of blade may be preferred in infants and younger children in whom the epiglottis is often larger and more likely to fall into the line of sight.

Selecting the appropriate laryngoscope blades size allows the operator to control the tongue and reach the glottic structures. A number of approaches can be used to select the appropriate sized equipment for airway management. Resources include age-based guidelines, length-based resuscitation tapes, anatomic landmarks, and electronic applications. Although size 00 and 0 blades are used in neonatology, blades smaller than size 1 are rarely required in emergency medicine. Size 1 blades can be used in patients less than 2 years of age. Size 2 blades are commonly used in children starting at 2 years of age. Size 3 blades are commonly used beginning around 10 to 12 years of age. Selecting a laryngoscope blade that approximates the distance between the upper incisors and the angle of the mandible can be used as a guide in patients whose age is not known or when the anatomy appears incongruous with proposed blade size based on other available references.

Videolaryngoscopy

Videolaryngoscopy (VL) involves the incorporation of video and optical technology to laryngoscopy for the purpose of assisting in TI. Traditional direct laryngoscopy requires the creation of a direct line of sight through the mouth to the glottic opening. This is achieved by positioning the patient in the sniffing position to align the oral, pharyngeal, and tracheal axes and then lifting the tongue and soft tissue into the mandibular block using a laryngoscope. Videolaryngoscopy provides a vantage point from behind the base of the tongue, through a camera or lens built into the device. As such, operators can indirectly visualize the glottis around the natural curvature of the upper airway, obviating the need to align the axes or displace the tongue. Data support that videolaryngoscopes commonly offer improved laryngeal views over direct laryngoscopy, and may be particularly valuable in cases where creating a direct line of sight may be challenging. Some studies suggest that intubation success rates are higher with videolaryngoscopy compared to direct laryngoscopy, though benefits may not be noted in routine cases performed by experienced providers, in whom direct laryngoscopy success rates are high. Currently, no relevant studies on pediatric patients exist regarding use outside the operating room. Data regarding time to successful intubation using videolaryngoscopes is varied in pediatric populations. Benefits in terms of timing seem to be most notable: (1) When devices are used by novice operators who may not have developed skill with direct laryngoscopy as a comparison, and (2) in patients with difficult airways where the ability to gain an adequate view is favored by a video-enhanced approach.

An additional advantage of videolaryngoscopy is the ability for multiple practitioners to view the procedure simultaneously. This allows for real-time guidance and supervision during TI. Finally, it is worth recognizing that the role for videolaryngoscopy is emerging and dependent on clinical setting. Oftentimes in emergency medicine, patients require rapid airway management without the benefit of prescreening or comprehensive airway assessments, and by providers who have less frequent occasions to perform invasive airway procedures. Therefore, the recognized advantages of videolaryngoscopy may be more likely to be actualized in all ER pediatric airway cases and not only when used with potential difficult cases or as a rescue approach following failed direct laryngoscopy.

A number of videolaryngoscopic devices are available for use in pediatrics, varying in their cost, design, reusability, and technique for use. Currently, only a few offer sizing that allows for use across the entire spectrum of ages, from neonates through to adolescents (e-Table 3.1). Each design offers unique advantages but also have nuances in technique. The decision regarding which device to use is ultimately based on availability, operator preference and experience, and patient-specific attributes that may favor a given approach. It is important to note that although each is designed to facilitate laryngoscopy and intubation, the technique varies amongst the devices. Therefore, skill acquisition with multiple devices is challenging given the infrequency with which most emergency medicine providers perform pediatric advanced airway management.

MEDICATIONS

Sedatives

Sedatives used for intubation should render the patient rapidly unconscious (Table 3.2). They should ideally have minimal side effects on hemodynamics or intracranial pressure (ICP); however, all sedatives have adverse effects and efficacy limitations. The optimal sedative depends on the clinical situation with regard to benefits, limitations, and adverse effect risk. A thorough understanding of the side effects of various drugs is essential so that the best option for a given patient's situation can be determined.

Etomidate is the most commonly used sedative for intubation in the ED. Its advantages are rapid and effective sedation, reliable pharmacokinetics, and minimal cardiovascular side

TABLE 3.2

SEDATIVES

Medication	Dose
Benzodiazepines (midazolam, lorazepam)	0.2–0.3 mg/kg
Narcotics (fentanyl)	1–2 mcg/kg
Ketamine	1–3 mg/kg
Etomidate	0.3 mg/kg
Propofol	1–4 mg/kg

effects. Despite its common use and its advantages, some studies have demonstrated poorer outcomes in patients receiving etomidate. Etomidate is an inhibitor of 11-beta hydroxylase and is known to suppress adrenal corticosteroid synthesis. While the clinical significance of this side effect from a single intubating dose is unclear, multiple authors and provider groups have raised caution in its use. The current recommendations of the American Heart Association Pediatric Advanced Life Support guidelines state that etomidate should be avoided in children being intubated as a result of septic shock.

Propofol is the most commonly used sedative in general, yet its role in ED RSI is unclear. Propofol is a potent vasodilator and myocardial depressant; even a single dose of propofol frequently results in hypotension which makes it unsuitable for hypovolemic patients, children in shock, or patients in whom maintenance of cerebral perfusion is essential. While some sources have described propofol as having cerebroprotective properties, the primary source proof of this and substantiation in human studies is difficult to find.

Ketamine is a dissociative anesthetic with reliable and rapid onset. It has the potentially beneficial effects of increasing heart rate, right atrial pressure, and systemic vascular resistance, making it the theoretical drug of choice for patients who are hypotensive and/or in shock. Ketamine also preserves airway reflexes and respiratory drive. Ketamine is used very frequently as a procedural sedative/analgesic in children, and significant adverse events that have been reported during ketamine administration include vomiting in 5% to 10% of patients, apnea and/or laryngospasm (both very rare), and emergence delirium. In the context of airway management (with the co-administration of a paralytic agent) these side effects are of negligible significance. Ketamine increases oral secretions (a sialogogue); the co-administration of atropine is sometimes recommended to counter this side effect (see below). Early clinical data suggested that ketamine causes an increase in ICP. This has led to the widespread belief that ketamine is relatively contraindicated in head trauma which, as mentioned earlier, remains the most frequent indication for TI in a child in the ED. Newer studies in adults and children have shown that the effect of ketamine on ICP is variable, and its role in head trauma may be underappreciated. Ketamine is reported to have bronchodilator properties which favors its selection in status asthmaticus; however, this evidence is weak.

Benzodiazepines are generally considered safer with anticonvulsant and amnestic effects, reversibility (flumazenil), and less cardiovascular depression. However, dosing is variable in that a standard dose of a benzodiazepine (e.g., 0.1 mg/kg) does not reliably result in inducing unconsciousness in a child. Higher doses are often required which have a slower onset and place the patient at higher cardiovascular risk.

It should be noted that all sedatives can result in cardiovascular collapse in patients with marginal cardiovascular function such as in hypotension, hypovolemia, myocardial dysfunction, and sepsis. In severe hemodynamic compromise (e.g., hemorrhagic shock, septic shock), consider that no sedative might be preferable, especially if the patient is already unconscious to prevent cardiovascular collapse.

Neuromuscular Blocking Agent (Paralyzing Agent)

The neuromuscular blocking agent (NMBA) used to facilitate intubation should render the patient completely flaccid, negating the effects of laryngeal reflexes on passage of an ET tube (Table 3.3). Ideally, its onset should be rapid and its duration should be short in case the patient cannot be intubated so that spontaneous ventilation can resume. However, spontaneous ventilation is not always a sufficient "rescue" for the inability to intubate since the patient is generally being intubated for a reason.

TABLE 3.3

NEUROMUSCULAR BLOCKING AGENTS (PARALYTICS)

Medication	Dose
Succinylcholine	1–2 mg/kg
Rocuronium	0.6–1.2 mg/kg
Vecuronium	0.1–0.2 mg/kg
Cisatracurium	0.1–0.2 mg/kg

Succinylcholine is considered the standard since it is the oldest and most rapid onset paralyzing agent. It has an onset time of 30 to 60 seconds and a duration of 3 to 8 minutes. It is a "depolarizing" paralyzing drug, causing muscle fasciculation prior to the onset of paralysis. This can cause muscle pain, myoglobin release, potassium release (hyperkalemia), histamine release, and a higher risk of malignant hyperthermia. It also frequently results in transient bradycardia; atropine premedication is often recommended to minimize this effect (see below). Succinylcholine carries a "black-box" warning pertaining to the risk of hyperkalemic cardiac arrest in children; this was the result of a series of cases of children with undiagnosed skeletal muscle myopathies receiving succinylcholine. The incidence of this severe side effect in routine use in the pediatric ED is exceedingly rare, and succinylcholine remains in widespread use in pediatrics.

Nondepolarizing NMBAs do not cause fasciculations and their attendant side effects. While several different medications in this class are available, rocuronium and vecuronium are the most frequently used in emergency airway management. Rocuronium has an onset time of 1 to 3 minutes and a duration of 30 to 45 minutes. Larger doses have faster onset times, but longer durations. Vecuronium has been observed to have a slightly longer onset time, but with a similar dose dependency (i.e., higher doses shorten the onset time and lengthen the duration of effect).

The longer duration of action of nondepolarizing NMBAs may be perceived to be a disadvantage. However, in most instances, maintenance of the paralysis is preferable for imaging, ventilator management, vascular access, etc. Succinylcholine requires repeated doses or conversion to a longer-acting agent (generally a nondepolarizing NMBA) to maintain paralysis when needed. Paralyzing drugs with longer durations require maintenance of sedation as well to avoid conscious paralysis.

Adjunctive Agents

Atropine

Atropine is a vagolytic medication which reduces the risk of bradycardia resulting from laryngoscopy or succinylcholine use, a physiologic phenomenon more commonly observed in infants and younger children. Atropine reduces oral secretions

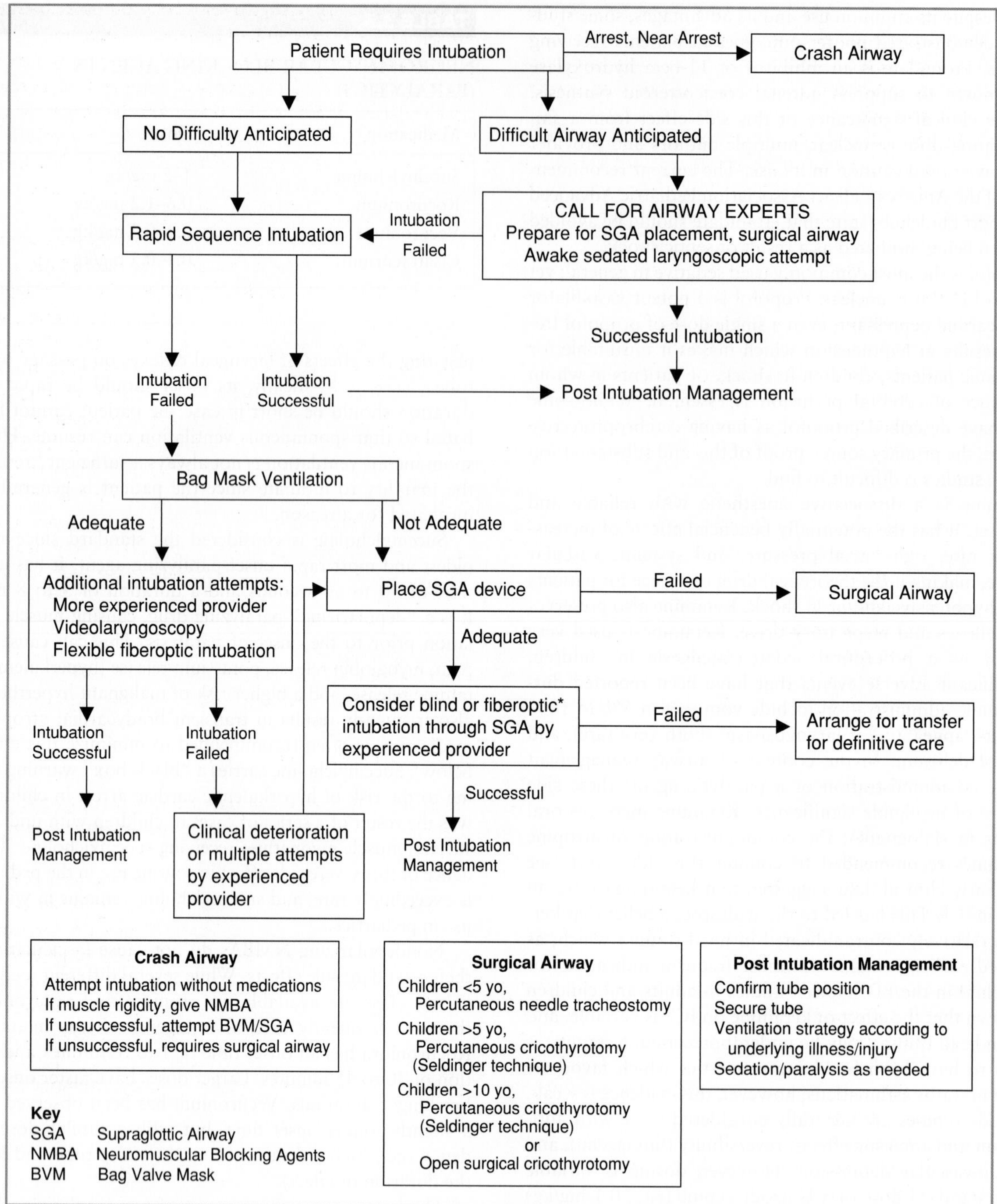

FIGURE 3.1 Approach to the difficult airway. SGA, supraglottic airway; NMBA, neuromuscular blocking agents; BVM, bag-valve mask.

if ketamine is going to be given. Data on atropine premedication during pediatric intubation in the ED has not clearly demonstrated a benefit in terms of reducing the incidence of bradycardia during laryngoscopy. Nonetheless, the American College of Emergency Physicians (ACEP) recommends premedication with atropine for children less than 1 year old, children being intubated with succinylcholine as their NMBA, or patients with preprocedure bradycardia.

Lidocaine

Lidocaine is administered to blunt the autonomic effects of laryngoscopy on hemodynamics and ICP during laryngoscopy. Historically, it has been recommended for patients undergoing intubation as a result of traumatic brain injury. Meta-analyses in adults have failed to demonstrate a benefit of lidocaine premedication during intubation, although data in pediatric patients is lacking (see Fig. 3.1).

POSTPROCEDURE MANAGEMENT

Immediately following intubation, correct placement of the ET tube in the trachea must be confirmed. Studies have shown that 5% to 10% of intubation attempts in emergent settings result in esophageal tube placement, with even higher rates reported when performed on children or in the prehospital setting. Therefore, a systematic approach to confirming tube placement is warranted.

End-tidal carbon dioxide detection, either colorimetric or capnographic, is a rapid and reliable method for confirming tracheobronchial positioning of the ET tube (e-Fig. 3.1). This means of confirmation has been endorsed by position statements and recommendations from professional societies within emergency medicine, anesthesiology, and critical care; it is the current gold standard method according to American Heart Association Pediatric Advanced Life Support guidelines. Single use, colorimetric devices qualitatively detect CO_2 in the ET tube. Following tube placement, the end-tidal detector is attached and six positive pressure breaths are delivered. The device will change color in the presence of CO_2 during exhalation. Capnography involves the generation of a continuous quantitative measurement of exhaled CO_2 levels. The presence of a regular waveform has nearly 100% sensitivity in confirming tracheobronchial tube position in patients with a perfusing cardiac rhythm. As a quantitative measurement of end-tidal CO_2, capnography also offers a means to adjust ventilatory parameters as indicated in recently intubated patients. Rarely, initial breaths may show evidence of CO_2 in an esophageal patient who has been previously bagged with resultant gastric insufflation, or in a patient who has consumed large volumes of carbonated beverages. However, in these rare circumstances, the concentration of CO_2 would be expected to fall quickly. Conversely, a tube in the hypopharynx may lead to CO_2 detection with each breath, but without an appropriately secured airway.

Direct or video-assisted visualization of the ET tube passing through the vocal cords, or above the posterior cartilages in cases of suboptimal view is fundamental to success, and is included in national emergency medicine guidelines. However, laryngoscopic view may be compromised by blood, vomitus or secretions, or when swelling, habitus, or anatomic anomalies prevent visualization of the glottic apertures. In addition, even when the view is adequate, less-experienced providers may misidentify anatomic structures. Finally, even after successful placement the ET tube may become dislodged. Therefore, it is recommended that tube position be verified by secondary means, even in circumstances where it has been witnessed to pass successfully through the cords.

Expected clinical findings when the position of the tube is within the tracheobronchial tree include visible rise of the chest wall, auscultation of breath sounds in both hemithoraces, absence of air movement over the stomach, and condensation within the ET tube. However, clinical evaluation is not always accurate. Auscultation can be challenging amidst the extraneous noises that are common in critical resuscitations. In addition, practical experience and case reports suggest that localizing sounds can be difficult, with providers interpreting breath sounds in cases of esophageal intubation. Therefore confirmatory devices should also be used.

Continuous pulse oximetry should be used to detect adequate oxygenation. Developing or sustained hypoxia after intubation may suggest incorrect tube placement, if equipment issues or underlying disease do not provide an alternative explanation. In most cases, desaturation in children will develop quickly, however studies have shown that in some cases there is a significant lag time before hypoxia develops. This potential delay precludes relying on pulse oximetry as a means for early detection of a missed intubation.

Postintubation imaging with a chest radiograph is considered standard of care; this is necessary to confirm midtracheal placement of the tip of the ET tube. Newer data suggest that bedside ultrasound may play a role in rapidly detecting tracheal tube position. Small studies in children and adults have shown that ultrasound imaging can allow direct visualization of the tube in the trachea, or can be used to evaluate for lung sliding and/or diaphragmatic excursion bilaterally as an indirect measure of lung inflation. In addition, the ability to evaluate each hemithorax independently allows for the detection of asymmetry, suggesting endobronchial intubation which would not be recognized by end-tidal detection alone. Until more data exists regarding the accuracy of ultrasound for this indication, a postprocedure anterior–posterior chest radiograph should be obtained. Radiographs are used to confirm the location of the tip of the ET tube, as well to assess for any complications secondary to the procedure. The goal for tube positioning is for the tip to be midtrachea, ideally a minimum of 1 to 3 cm above the carina and below the thoracic inlet. The decision to adjust the tube position based on the radiograph should be made in the clinical context.

RESCUE DEVICES IN PEDIATRIC AIRWAY MANAGEMENT

When to Use

Protocols for airway management set forth by the American Society of Anesthesia include rescue devices as an option for sustaining effective assisted ventilation in the 'can't intubate, can't ventilate' scenario, when a facemask is ineffective (e-Fig. 3.2). All rescue devices have in common that they are not definitive airways, that is, they do not isolate the trachea from the esophagus, thus the risk of gastric contents being regurgitated and aspirated remains significant when these devices are used. In most emergent situations, a rescue device is used to avert life-threatening desaturation while at the same time as mobilizing appropriate support (personnel and/or equipment) for subsequent attempts at securing a definitive airway.

Laryngeal Mask Airways

Laryngeal mask airways (LMAs) are the mainstay of rescue devices for adults and children. They consist of a teardrop-shaped inflatable cuff around an aperture at the end of a tube; when properly inserted the cuff sits in the hypopharynx above and behind the glottis opening; air flow through the device is directed anteriorly through the glottis into the lungs. LMAs are manufactured in a range of sizes that are suitable for patients throughout the pediatric age spectrum, including newborns and infants. Multiple models of LMAs are available and, while the numerical sizing conventions are nonuniform among manufacturers, all LMAs have information on both their packaging and the device itself displaying the correct patient size and volume of air for cuff inflation a given device requires. Studies in anesthesia, emergency medicine, and pediatrics have shown that LMAs are easy to place, require very little training to use effectively, and have a very low complication rate.

Clinical data on LMA use on adults with cardiac arrest in the prehospital arena and depressed newborns in the delivery suite have demonstrated comparable effectiveness and equivalent or improved clinical outcomes when compared with prehospital TI and bag-valve-mask ventilation, respectively.

Other Supraglottic Devices

The following list describes several additional available options for rescue devices during emergency airway management. All of these devices have in common that they are lacking in clinical data outside the operating room demonstrating ease of use or relative efficacy in pediatric patients.

Esophageal Combination Tube (CombiTube)

The CombiTube is a dual lumen tube with two inflatable cuffs, a larger proximal one and a smaller distal one. When blindly inserted, the device usually enters the esophagus (>95% of attempts), but is designed in such a way that ventilation can be accomplished with either esophageal or tracheal placement, depending on which port is attached to the bag-valve device. CombiTubes only exist in sizes small enough to accommodate a patient 1.2 m in height; thus the pediatric application of CombiTubes is limited to older children.

Laryngeal Tube

The laryngeal tube is designed for blind placement in the esophagus, with a single port that inflates a dual cuff (one above and one below the opening for airflow) which secures the device in the hypopharynx and directs airflow anteriorly into the glottis. Laryngeal tubes are made in sizes small enough to be suitable for patients weighing as little as 12 kg.

Perilaryngeal Airway

The perilaryngeal airway is a device with an inflatable cuff proximal to a widened distal end, designed to sit posterior to the larynx. Randomized trials in anesthetized patients (including children) have demonstrated comparable speed and ease of placement when compared with LMAs. Perilaryngeal airways are also suitable for bronchoscopy and intubation through the distal end when correctly placed.

Suggested Readings and Key References

American College of Emergency Physicians. Verification of endotracheal intubation: Policy statement. Revised 2009. Available online at: http://www.acep.org/practres.aspx?id=29846 (Accessed August 15, 2014).

Chan CM, Mitchell AL, Shorr AF. Etomidate is associated with mortality and adrenal insufficiency in sepsis: A meta-analysis. *Crit Care Med* 2012;40(11):2945–2953.

Filanovsky Y, Miller P, Kao J. Myth: Ketamine should not be used as an induction agent for intubation in patients with head injury. *CJEM* 2010;12(2):154–157.

Kerrey BT, Rinderknecht AS, Geis GL, et al. Rapid sequence intubation for pediatric emergency patients: Higher frequency of failed attempts and adverse effects found by video review. *Ann Emerg Med* 2012;60(3):251–259.

Kim JT, Na HS, Bae JY, et al. GlideScope video laryngoscope: A randomized clinical trial in 203 paediatric patients. *Br J Anaesth* 2008; 101(4):531–534.

Kleinman ME, Chameides L, Schexnayder SM, et al. Part 14: Pediatric advanced life support: 2010 American Heart Association Guidelines for Cardiopulmonary Resuscitation and Emergency Cardiovascular Care. *Circulation* 2010;122:S876.

Lee-Jayaram JJ, Yamamoto LG. Alternative airways for the pediatric emergency department. *Pediatr Emerg Care* 2014;30(3):191–199.

Losek JD, Olson LR, Dobson JV, et al. Tracheal intubation practice and maintaining skill competency: Survey of pediatric emergency department medical directors. *Pediatr Emerg Care* 2008;24(5):294–299.

Mittiga MR, Geis GL, Kerrey BT, et al. The spectrum and frequency of critical procedures performed in a pediatric emergency department: Implications of a provider-level view. *Ann Emerg Med* 2013;61(3): 263–270.

Sagarin MJ, Chiang V, Sakles JC, et al. National Emergency Airway Registry (NEAR) investigators. Rapid sequence intubation for pediatric emergency airway management. *Pediatr Emerg Care* 2002;18(6): 417–423.

Weiss M, Dullenkopf A, Fischer JE, et al. Prospective randomized controlled multi-centre trial of cuffed or uncuffed endotracheal tubes in small children. *Br J Anaesth* 2009;103(6):867–873.

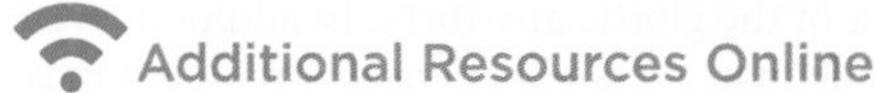

CHAPTER 4 ■ CARDIOPULMONARY RESUSCITATION

SAGE R. MYERS, MD, MSCE, DANA A. SCHINASI, MD, AND FRANCES M. NADEL, MD, MSCE

GOALS OF EMERGENCY THERAPY

CPR is a series of interventions aimed at restoring and supporting vital function after apparent death. The immediate goal of resuscitation is to reestablish substrate delivery to meet the metabolic needs of the myocardium, brain, and other vital organs. The overall goal is to return the child to society without morbidity related to the underlying disease or the resuscitation process. Given the poor prognosis of children who have arrested, primary prevention efforts are crucial in improving childhood mortality. This chapter will focus on the management of the critically ill child and neonate based on the 2010 American Heart Association (AHA) CPR Resuscitation Guidelines, Pediatric Advanced Life Support (PALS) principles, the literature, and our experience. Of note, the next edition of the AHA Guidelines are expected in the fall of 2015.

INCIDENCE

It is estimated that of the 10,000 children who suffer an out-of-hospital cardiac arrest (OHCA) annually, only 5% to 12% will survive, most with significant neurologic injury. U.S. mortality rates related to age in years for 2010 and 2011 are shown in Table 4.1. Of note, mortality rates of children less than 1 year old approach the rates of people over 54 years old. Table 4.2 describes the leading causes of death for children and young adults. After the first year of life, unintentional injury is the most common cause of death and therefore, preventable.

RELATED CHAPTERS

Resuscitation and Stabilization
- A General Approach to Ill and Injured Children: Chapter 1
- Approach to the Injured Child: Chapter 2
- Airway: Chapter 3
- Shock: Chapter 5
- Interfacility Transport and Stabilization: Chapter 6

Medical Emergencies
- Cardiac Emergencies: Chapter 94

Procedures and Appendices
- Prehospital Care: Chapter 139

PATIENT CHARACTERISTICS

Age

Children less than 1 year of age have a much higher incidence and worse rate of survival from OHCA than older children or teens. In large population-based studies of children who were resuscitated by the Emergency Medical Services (EMS) after an OHCA, 39% to 44% are infants. Pediatric CPR education should focus on anatomic and physiologic characteristics of the young child; but the emergency department (ED) staff must be prepared to cope with the full spectrum of age and size. In fact, in the Children's Hospital of Philadelphia Emergency Department, 4% of the patients requiring resuscitative services were adults.

Etiology

OHCA encountered in the ED results from trauma (20% to 30% of cases), sudden infant death syndrome (SIDS), or other causes. Though the literature varies in defining the cause of arrest, a primary cardiac etiology occurs in about 13% of children, as compared to 72% of adults. Approximately 10% of OHCA patients have ventricular tachycardia (VT) or ventricular fibrillation (VF). Children with congenital anomalies, chronic sequelae of prematurity or birth trauma, and those with chronic relapsing disease are also seen in the ED, as increasing numbers of children have survived the neonatal period, transplantation, complex surgery, and cancer therapy and have been discharged from the hospital.

Pediatric cardiopulmonary arrest follows one of two pathways: (1) Respiratory distress followed by respiratory failure and secondary cardiac arrest; or (2) primary cardiac arrest due to cardiac disease. In our experience, the majority of children suffer an asphyxial arrest (Fig. 4.1).

Demographics

There are few demographic studies to identify socioeconomic, ethnic/racial, familial, or community characteristics of children who require life support interventions. A recent multi-city study of children older than a year showed a predominance of males and children of black race. In addition, the majority of pediatric arrests occurred in private residences; less than half were witnessed arrests. It is difficult to generalize this information as the sample was limited to an urban population. National demographic studies are important however for developing profiles of high-risk patient populations for subsequent development of surveillance or prevention programs, as well as targeted community-based education initiatives. Some states have begun child death review efforts that shed light on prevention strategies. On a national level, the Cardiac Arrest Registry to Enhance Survival (CARES) is an EMS-based registry for OHCA in 29 participating US cities. Data on both pediatric and adult OHCA events and outcomes are collected with the goal to improve resuscitative care. On a local level, hospital-based quality improvement programs can help to track the population of patients drawn from one hospital's catchment area.

TABLE 4.1

DEATHS AND DEATH RATES, BY AGE, UNITED STATES[a]

	2011		2010	
Age	Number	Rate	Number	Rate
All ages	2,513,171	806.6	2,468,435	799.5
Under 1 yr	23,910	598.3	24,586	623.4
1–4 yrs	4,236	26.2	4,316	26.5
5–14 yrs	5,377	13.1	5,279	12.9
15–24 yrs	29,624	67.6	29,551	67.7
25–34 yrs	43,631	104.4	42,259	102.9
35–44 yrs	69,746	171.7	70,033	170.5
45–54 yrs	182,994	409.2	183,207	407.1
55–64 yrs	323,015	848.7	310,802	851.9
65–74 yrs	414,792	1,845.0	407,151	1,875.1
75–84 yrs	625,860	4,750.3	625,651	4,790.2
85 yrs and over	789,854	13,767.3	765,474	13,934.3

[a]Age—specific rates are per 100,000 population in specified group. Age-adjusted rates are per 100,000 U.S. standard population.
Adapted from Hoyert DL and Xu J. *Deaths: Preliminary data for 2011*. National vital statistics reports. Vol 61. No. 6. Hyattsville, MD: National Center for Health Statistics, 2012.

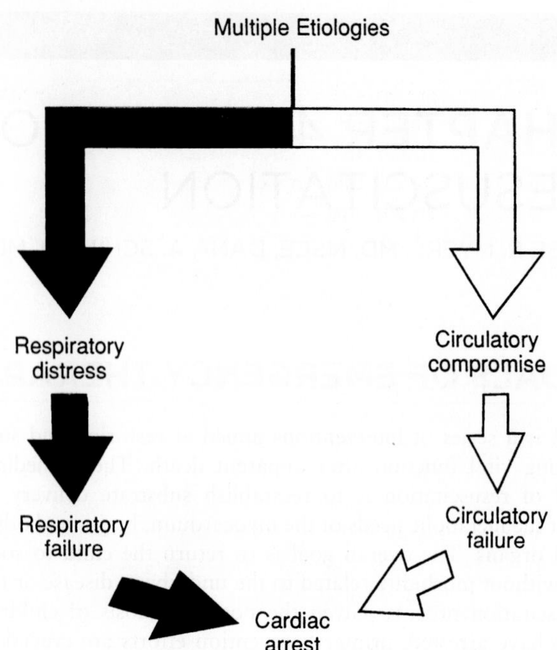

FIGURE 4.1 Pathophysiologic pathways from etiologies to cardiac arrest. (Adapted from PALS, American Heart Association.)

TABLE 4.2

10 LEADING CAUSES OF DEATH BY AGE GROUP, UNITED STATES, 2012

	Age groups in years				
Rank	<1	1–4	5–9	10–14	15–24
1	Congenital anomalies 30.0%	Unintentional injury 44.3%	Unintentional injury 42%	Unintentional injury 36.4%	Unintentional injury 47.6%
2	Short gestation 25.5%	Congenital anomalies 16.4%	Malignant neoplasms 24.9%	Malignant neoplasms 21.3%	Suicide 19.5%
3	SIDS 10.1%	Malignant neoplasms 12.8%	Congenital anomalies 9.4%	Suicide 13.8%	Homicide 18.4%
4	Maternal pregnancy comp. 9.1%	Homicide 11.1%	Homicide 7.8%	Homicide 7.8%	Malignant neoplasms 6.3%
5	Unintentional injury 7.1%	Heart disease 5.0%	Heart disease 3.8%	Congenital anomalies 7.2%	Heart disease 3.8%
6	Placenta cord membranes 6.2%	Influenza and pneumonia 3.0%	Chronic low respiratory disease 3.6%	Heart disease 4.9%	Congenital anomalies 1.7%
7	Bacterial sepsis 3.4%	Septicemia 2.0%	Benign neoplasms 2.7%	Chronic low respiratory disease 2.5%	Diabetes mellitus 0.78%
8	Respiratory distress 3.1%	Cerebrovascular 1.8%	Influenza and pneumonia 2.5%	Cerebrovascular 2.3%	Cerebrovascular 0.73%
9	Circulatory system disease 3.0%	Benign neoplasms 1.8%	Cerebrovascular 1.9%	Influenza and pneumonia 1.8%	Complicated pregnancy 0.67%
10	Neonatal hemorrhage 2.6%	Chronic low respiratory disease 1.7%	Septicemia 1.5%	Benign neoplasms 1.8%	Influenza and pneumonia 0.59%
Total	16,498	3,056	1,769	2,214	25,042

From National Vital Statistics System, National Center for Health Statistics, CDC.

TREATMENT OVERVIEW

Pediatric CPR presents the emergency physician with many challenges. The child may arrive from EMS without the same level of field treatment that adult patients receive routinely.

The overwhelming majority of cardiac/respiratory arrests occur in adults so paramedics have limited exposure, a lower comfort level and less success in advanced life skills for children. The wide spectrum of age, weight, and diagnoses adds additional complexity and equipment needs (see Chapter 139 Prehospital Care).

The chain of survival after an OHCA arrest includes rapid access to EMS, rapid CPR, rapid defibrillation when indicated, and rapid advanced care. Once in the ED, resuscitation is best accomplished with an effective leader who organizes and directs a skilled team. The American College of Surgeons divides trauma resuscitation into the primary and secondary surveys (see Chapter 2 Approach to the Injured Child), and the application of this technique to medical resuscitation can allow for rapid, thorough assessment of the patient in an orderly manner. The primary survey is the assessment of airway, breathing, circulation, and disability (ABCDs). The secondary survey is a head-to-toe examination to determine the etiology of the arrest, while concurrently, diagnostic studies are done, consultants are called, and arrangements for definitive care are completed (see Chapter 1 A General Approach to Ill and Injured Children). The ABCDs are reassessed frequently throughout the resuscitation.

Our experience shows that careful management of airway and breathing is extremely important in children. Because the cause of the arrest is most often related to respiratory failure and the child's myocardium is relatively resilient to hypoxemia, the rapid correction of hypoxemia may be all that is necessary to restore circulation. Bag-valve-mask (BVM) ventilation is an effective way to rapidly address hypoxemia and, in the prehospital setting, BMV alone (without subsequent intubation) has been shown to improve outcomes for patients with respiratory arrest in urban settings.

For those patients who do not respond to airway and breathing management alone, life support interventions are more complex. In the ED, the lack of an immediate patient response usually predicts a need for multiple drug interventions.

Vascular access is a major challenge in severely ill pediatric patients. Peripheral intravenous access may be difficult to establish quickly. The intraosseous (IO) route is a safe, effective method to obtain access rapidly. In fact, PALS recommends immediate IO access for a patient in cardiac arrest. Central lines are useful for longer-term access but require advanced skills and often take more time to place.

Arrhythmia management is a relatively infrequent problem in pediatric life support. The absence of atherosclerotic vascular disease makes the child's myocardium less susceptible to arrhythmias; and a minority of arrested children present with a shockable rhythm. As a result, antiarrhythmic medications and defibrillation are infrequently used. The most common cardiac rhythms to be recognized and managed in pediatric arrest are sinus bradycardia, pulseless electrical activity (PEA), and asystole. The exceptions to this are those children with congenital heart disease and those who have sustained direct myocardial trauma (see Chapter 94 Cardiac Emergencies). These children may have unusual and difficult arrhythmias that require subspecialist expertise to achieve a successful outcome.

Finally, there remains much to be learned on how to care for children requiring resuscitation. Researchers in CPR face many challenges. In the past, much of the work was done at single sites retrospectively. The creation of research networks and CPR registries has greatly expanded the possibility for prospective, large, multicentered trials. CPR research has unique ethical and legal considerations. Exception from informed consent is an evolving concept in studies of children with a life-threatening condition that has furthered recent work. Patient populations, characteristics, terminology, and methodology vary among studies, making it difficult to compare results. To address these concerns, experts developed and issued the Utstein Criteria that has brought some uniformity to CPR research terminology.

PROGNOSIS

Survival after CPR in children is variable. Despite advances in medical care of the critically ill child and improved EMS systems, OHCA survival remains poor. Less than 10% of children who suffer an OHCA survive, usually with significant neurologic injury (Table 4.3). Unfortunately, about 60% to 88% of OHCA are unwitnessed events and only about ⅓ of children receive bystander CPR, which may contribute to their poor prognosis. However, if a hospitalized child has respiratory arrest that is recognized rapidly and managed skillfully, immediate survival may be as high as 90%. Overall, children resuscitated after an in-hospital arrest (IHA) have a more

TABLE 4.3

OUTCOME FOR OUT-OF-HOSPITAL PEDIATRIC CARDIOPULMONARY ARREST

	% of Patients (% Survival)			
	Donoghue (2005)	Young (2004)	Sirbaugh (1999)	Young (1999)
Witnessed	31 (13)	34 (16)		31 (19)
Bystander CPR	31 (9)	31	26	30 (26)
ROSC	23	29	11	
Survival to hospital admission	24	25		
Survival to hospital discharge	6.7	8	2	8
Good neurologic outcome	2	31	17	

CPR, cardiopulmonary resuscitation; ROSC, return of spontaneous circulation.

TABLE 4.4

OUTCOME FOR IN-HOSPITAL PEDIATRIC CARDIOPULMONARY ARREST

	% Patients		
	Meaney (2006) $n = 464$	Nadkarni (2006) $n = 880$	Reis (2002) $n = 129$
ROSC	50	52	64
Survival to hospital discharge	23	27	16
Good neurologic outcome	64[a]	65[a]	90[a]

ROSC, return of spontaneous circulation.
[a]Percent of those patients who survived to hospital discharge with good neurologic outcome.

favorable outcome with about 30% or more of children surviving to hospital discharge (see Table 4.4). Earlier recognition of prearrest phases, advances in medical care and education, and rapid response teams have likely contributed to the improved survival over time seen in IHA.

CLINICAL MANIFESTATIONS

The clinical manifestations of persons requiring immediate life support are most often related to failure of oxygen delivery to the skin, brain, kidneys, and cardiovascular system. One can identify most potential or existing life-threatening conditions by assessing a child's general appearance and abnormalities in their airway, breathing, and circulation (ABCs) as outlined in Chapter 1 A General Approach to Ill and Injured Children (Fig. 4.2). It is essential to identify patients who are *at risk* for failure of substrate delivery as early intervention prevents respiratory failure and subsequent cardiovascular collapse.

MANAGEMENT

Management Sequence

Figure 4.3 outlines an efficient tool to rapidly assess and manage critically ill or injured patients.

C-A-B Versus ABC. For basic life support, the 2010 AHA guidelines recommend that the rescuer begin chest compressions first in an effort to remove obstacles associated with airway interventions and decrease delays in resuscitation. Healthcare providers should tailor all resuscitation recommendations to meet the needs of the individual patient; thus interventions occur simultaneously using ABC approach.

AIRWAY

Evaluation

The overwhelming majority of pediatric arrests are due to asphyxia; the recognition and treatment of airway obstruction and respiratory failure is crucial.

Despite good evidence that prehospital intubation in children does not improve outcomes over BVM ventilation in areas without prolonged transit time, many children are still intubated in the field. When a child arrives in the ED with an ETT in place, verify position immediately. For stable patients, measured end-tidal CO_2 ($ETCO_2$) (continuous is optimal) and chest radiograph confirms placement. In arrested patients, interpretation of $ETCO_2$ and breath sounds may be unreliable; in addition to these strategies, tube placement is confirmed by direct laryngoscopy. All patients should have continuous pulse oximetry, $ETCO_2$, and cardiorespiratory monitors placed immediately.

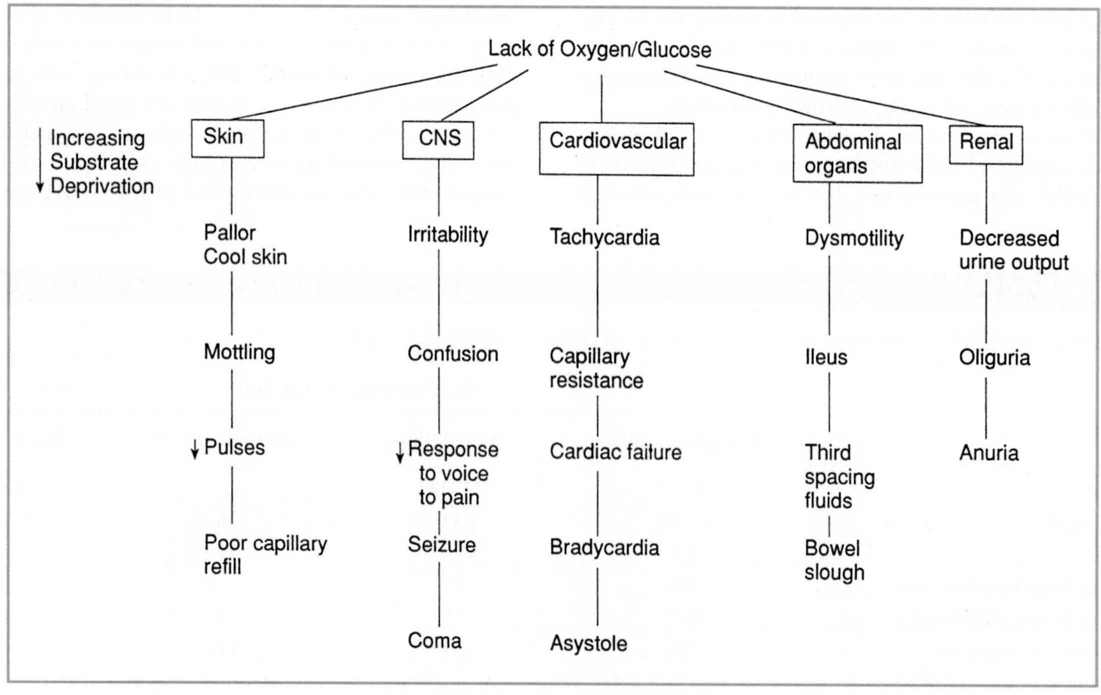

FIGURE 4.2 Signs and symptoms of lack of substrate delivery to vital organ systems. CNS, central nervous system.

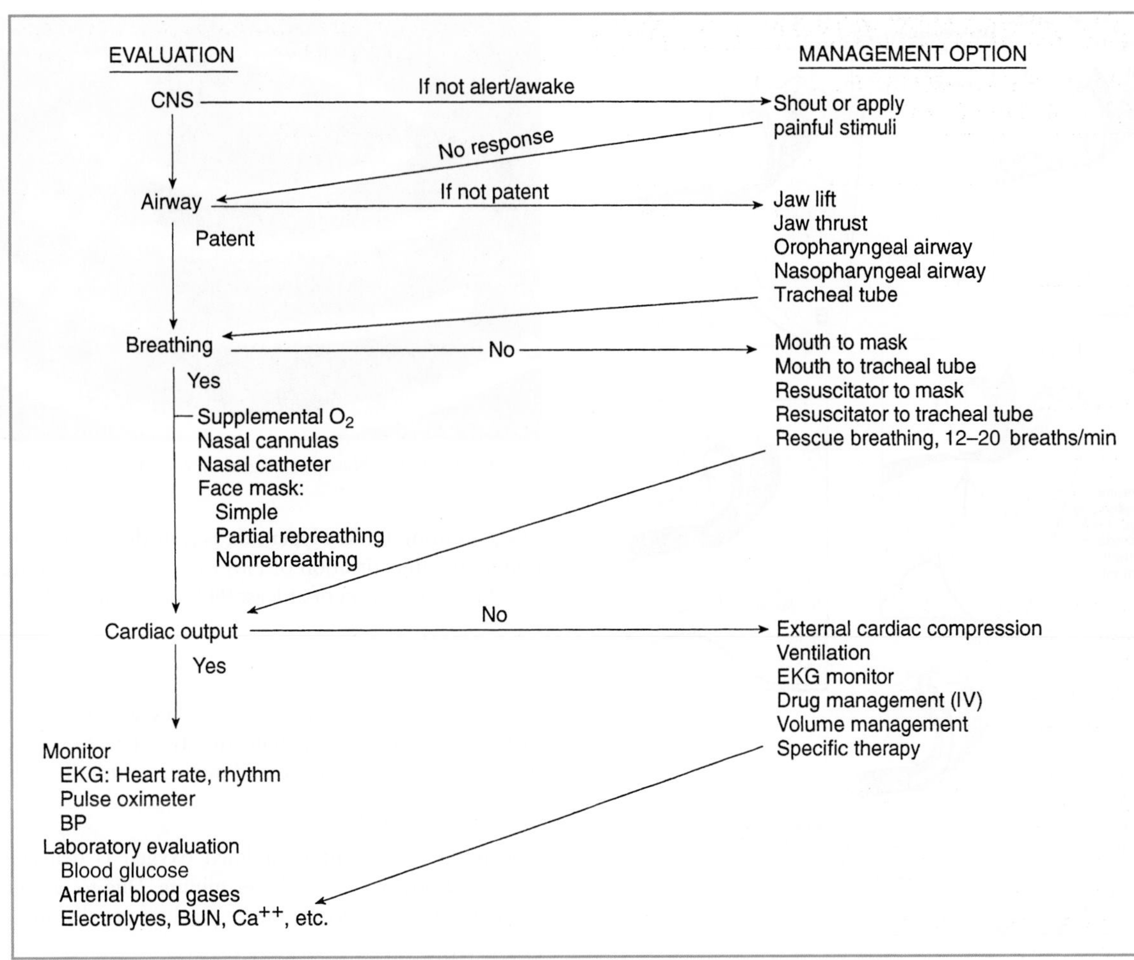

FIGURE 4.3 Management sequence for pediatric life support. CNS, central nervous system; EKG, electrocardiogram; BP, blood pressure; BUN, blood urea nitrogen; Ca^{++}, calcium.

MANAGEMENT

Airway Positioning

If cervical trauma is suspected, the head and cervical spine must be stabilized (during all airway maneuvers). Airway obstruction is most often related to relaxation of the jaw and neck muscles causing the tongue and mandibular tissues to fall posteriorly against the posterior wall of the hypopharynx. Airway positioning maneuvers, such as the head tilt–chin lift and the jaw thrust, are used first to relieve obstruction (Fig. 4.4). Jaw thrust alone is used if cervical stabilization is needed.

Artificial Airways

If airway positioning fails to relieve obstruction, oropharyngeal (OPA) or nasopharyngeal artificial airways (NPA) may be used.

Oropharyngeal Airways

Estimate OPA size by placing it against the side of the child's face; with the flange at the corner of the mouth assuring that the tip ends just proximal to the angle of the mandible; place it using a tongue depressor (Fig. 4.5). OPAs are used in unconscious patients only. If not inserted properly or too short, the OPA may push the tongue backward into the posterior pharynx, aggravating airway obstruction. If the OPA is too long, it may touch the larynx and stimulate vomiting or laryngospasm.

Nasopharyngeal Airways

The correct NPA size covers the distance from the nares to the tragus of the ear (Fig. 4.6). The NPA can be used in conscious patients. The NPA may lacerate the vascular adenoidal tissue, thus adenoidal hypertrophy and bleeding diatheses are relative contraindications to the use of these airways.

Endotracheal Tubes

ET tubes are used to overcome upper airway obstruction, isolate the larynx from the pharynx, allow mechanical aspiration of secretions from the tracheal bronchial tree, and facilitate mechanical ventilation or end-expiratory pressure delivery (see Chapter 3 Airway).

BREATHING

Evaluation

Breathing is assessed through observation of chest wall movement and auscultation. Gas exchange is confirmed by auscultation and monitoring of $ETCO_2$ and pulse oximetry.

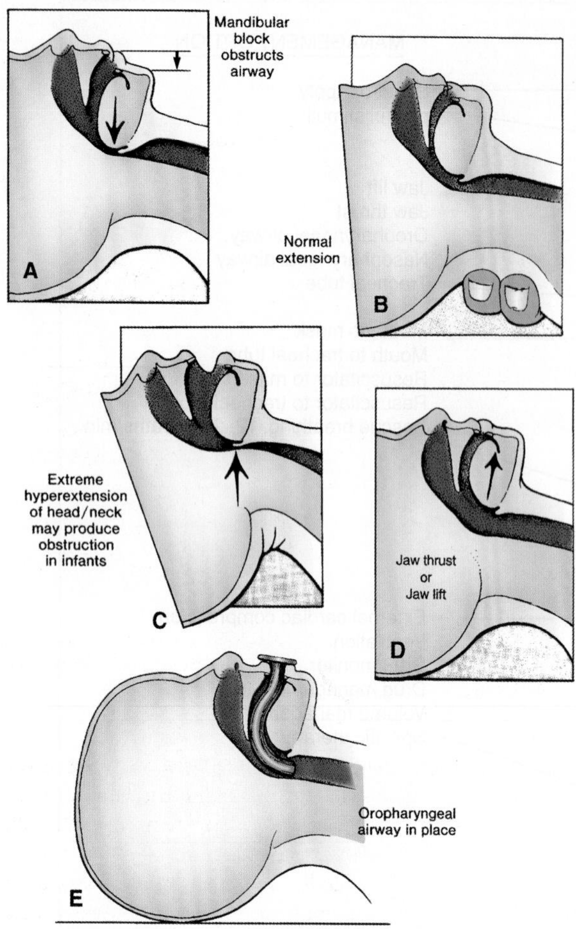

FIGURE 4.4 **A:** Upper airway obstruction related to hypotonia. **B:** Partial relief of airway obstruction by means of head extension (danger of cervical spine injury in cases of trauma). **C:** Extreme hyperextension causing upper airway obstruction. **D:** Fully open airway through use of jaw thrust or jaw lift. **E:** Oropharyngeal airway stenting mandibular block off of posterior pharyngeal wall.

MANAGEMENT

Spontaneous Ventilation

Supplemental oxygen is administered to the spontaneously breathing ill patient. If the patient is not breathing spontaneously, positive pressure ventilation is required. Though the optimal concentration is not known, it is reasonable to provide 100% oxygen during CPR. Hyperoxia is a mediator of postresuscitation injury, thus titration of Fio_2 to the minimum concentration to achieve saturation of at least 94% is recommended.

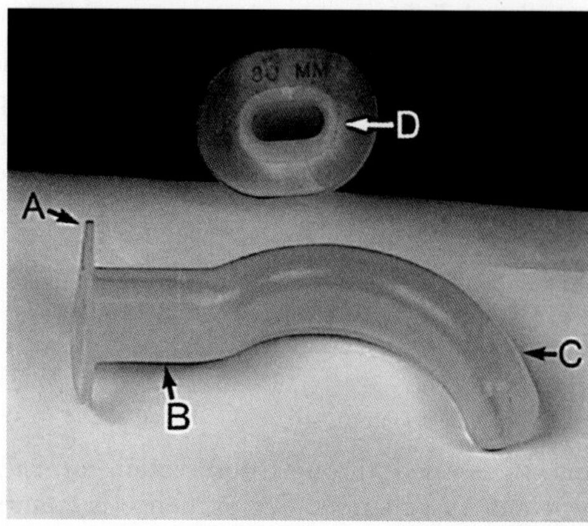

FIGURE 4.5 Oropharyngeal airway: flange (A), bite block (B), stent (C), and gas exchange or suction conduit (D).

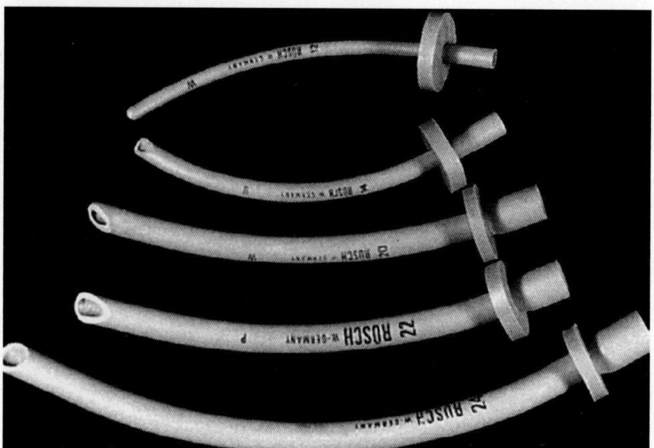

FIGURE 4.6 Nasopharyngeal airways in a variety of sizes.

Oxygen Delivery Devices

A variety of oxygen delivery devices are available for use in patients who have patent airways. The oxygen delivered depends on the child's size and minute ventilation.

Nasal Cannulas

One hundred percent humidified oxygen is delivered to the nares at a flow of 4 to 6 L per minute. Due to entrainment of room air, the final oxygen delivery is low, usually 30% to 40%.

High Flow Nasal Cannulas

High flow nasal cannula (HFNC) allows the delivery of humidified and warmed oxygen/gas at flow rates up to 12 L per minute in infants and 30 L per minute in children. This increased flow allows for noninvasive continuous positive airway pressure (CPAP) and has been used as an alternative to CPAP devices, especially for infants with bronchiolitis.

Oxygen Masks

There are several types of oxygen masks that offer a wide range of inspired oxygen concentrations.

Simple Masks. The simple face mask delivers a moderate Fio_2 that varies from 35% to 60%.

Partial Rebreathing Masks. Partial rebreathing masks allow reliable delivery of an Fio_2 of 50% to 60%. When the flow in the reservoir bag is greater than the patient's minute ventilation and the oxygen is adjusted so the bag does not collapse during inhalation, there is negligible CO_2 rebreathing allowing for more reliable oxygen delivery.

Nonrebreathing Masks. These masks have nonrebreathing valves incorporated into the face mask and the reservoir bag and reliably provide oxygen concentrations up to 95% with high flow rates 10 to 15 L per minute.

Continuous Positive Airway Pressure Devices

CPAP provides positive pressure to stent open the child's airways leading to improved ventilation and oxygenation. CPAP can be applied with large nasal prongs, a nasal mask which covers just the nose of the patient, or a full face mask which covers the mouth and nose.

Assisted Ventilation

BLS rescue breathing rates in infants and children with respiratory arrest is 12 to 20 breaths per minute, with higher rates for infants and younger children. Newly born infants may need a rate of 40 to 60 breaths per minute. For children and infants who require CPR, the recommended respiratory rate is 8 to 10 breaths per minute. Ventilations are asynchronous with chest compressions when an advanced airway is in place. Ventilations are coordinated with chest compressions with a rate of 15 compressions to 2 ventilations (100 to 120 compressions per minute) when an advanced airway is not in place. With all ventilation techniques, the force and volume needed to just see the chest rise is recommended. Overventilation is a common error in resuscitation; in the AHA 2013 Consensus Statement, a ventilation rate of less than 12 and a ventilation volume that causes no more than minimal chest wall rise during CPR is emphasized.

Because of risk of infection transmission, mouth-to-mouth resuscitation is no longer recommended. Instead, rescue breathing should be done with a pocket mask. Placement of the mask over the mouth alone, over the mouth and nose, or over a tracheostomy site depends on the patient and the equipment available.

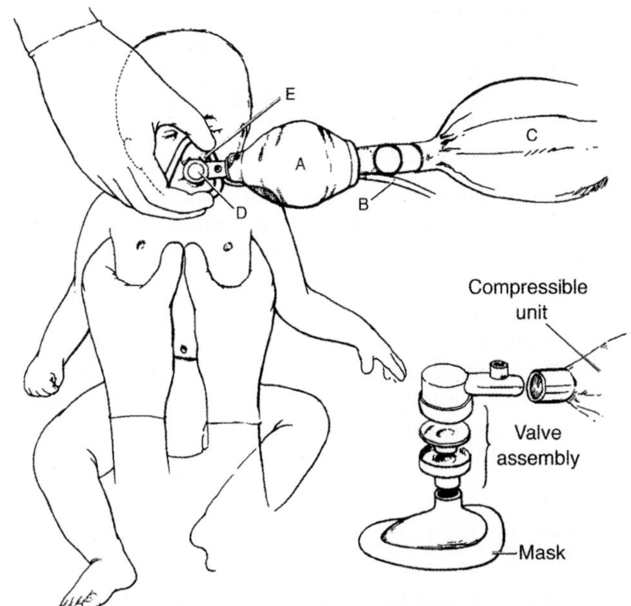

FIGURE 4.7 Self-inflating hand-powered resuscitator: compressible unit (**A**), oxygen source (**B**), oxygen reservoir (**C**), one-way valve assembly (**D**), and mask with transparent body (**E**).

Expired Air Techniques

Bag-valve-mask ventilation is an essential skill for all emergency medicine clinicians and provides a rapid means to provide oxygenation and ventilation for children with respiratory and/or circulatory failure.

Masks

The properly fit mask covers the tip of the chin, the mouth, and the nose allowing for a tight seal against the skin. Masks with a pneumatic cuff design allow for the easiest and most efficient fit that avoids air leaks. When enough personnel are available, a two-person technique may improve oxygen delivery and ventilation. One person uses both hands to correctly position the mask on the face creating a good seal, while the other squeezes the bag paying attention to ensure appropriate chest rise and ventilation.

Hand-squeezed, Self-inflating Resuscitators

Hand-squeezed, self-inflating resuscitators are easy to use and do not require a gas source. The elasticity of a self-inflating bag allows it to refill with oxygen or room air as the gas intake valve opens. During compression the gas intake valve closes, and a second valve opens to allow flow into the patient. A valve between the mask and the bag allows for patient exhalation into the atmosphere. Most self-inflating bags are equipped with a pressure-limiting pop-off valve that is preset at 35 cm H_2O to prevent barotrauma; if not, an inline manometer should be used (Fig. 4.7). To deliver oxygen concentrations 60% to 90%, use a flow rate of 10 to 15 L per minute. Use a minimum of a 500-mL bag for infants and children.

Anesthesia Bags

Anesthesia breathing circuits (sometimes called a Mapleson circuit) consist of a source of fresh gas flow attached to a reservoir bag with an adjustable pressure-limiting (APL) valve (Fig. 4.8). These devices are favored by many for several reasons. When there is no significant leak at the mask-to-patient interface, CPAP can be provided to the patient airway and the pressure adjusted with the APL valve. Positive pressure ventilation can also be provided by squeezing the bag. The respiratory effort can be observed through changes in the filling and emptying of the reservoir bag. Additionally, if the fresh gas flow is provided through an oxygen blender, any desired concentration of oxygen may be provided. However, there are several disadvantages with this type of bag. First, a high-pressure source of fresh gas flow is necessary for the system to function at all. Second, significant experience in maintaining a complete seal at the mask-to-patient interface is needed in order to maintain positive airway pressure and positive pressure ventilation can occur. The operator must adjust the fresh gas flow rate and the APL opening with the patient ventilation to balance rate of gas escape from circuit to prevent over or under filling. If the bag is removed from a leak-tight patient application, it promptly deflates and one must wait for the reservoir to refill. Alternatively, overfilling the bag may result in dangerously high-pressure transmission to the lung and stomach. Third, exhaled gases return to the circuit and bag which can lead to hypercarbia unless the fresh gas flow is

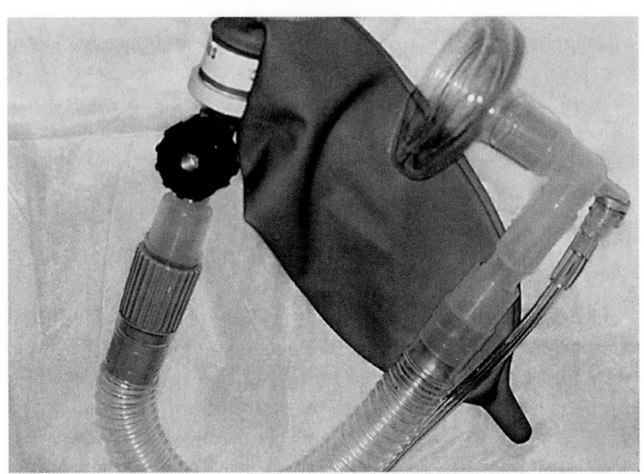

FIGURE 4.8 Anesthesia bag.

great enough (generally twice the patient's minute ventilation) to "washout" the circuit. These disadvantages have prompted many to recommend the primary use of the self-inflating resuscitator bag as the primary mode of ventilation.

Mechanical Ventilators

In children who require prolonged or relatively high minute ventilation, inspiratory pressures, or positive end-expiratory pressures (PEEPs), the use of a mechanical ventilator may provide better management compared to manual ventilation. Care must be taken to assure that the appropriate tidal volumes and pressures are set for patient size and treatment goals. We recommend the use of mechanical ventilator only if the providers are skilled in the use of the device or in consultation with a pediatric expert and appropriate support from Respiratory Therapy.

CIRCULATION

The 2010 AHA guidelines emphasize immediate, high-quality chest compressions. Adult cardiac arrest survival has improved with immediate chest compressions and rapid defibrillation. Pediatric primary asphyxial arrest requires a different strategy including rapid recognition of prearrest signs and well-executed airway management and immediate chest compressions at the onset of circulatory arrest.

Evaluation

The 2010 AHA guidelines minimize the importance of the pulse check by healthcare providers as it is neither quickly nor reliably assessed. A clinician should take no more than 10 seconds to determine the presence of a brachial, femoral, or carotid pulse. Evaluate the effectiveness of circulation by observing skin and mucous membrane color, and checking capillary refill (Fig. 4.9). Continuous electrocardiogram (EKG) monitoring and frequent blood pressure measurements are required. Most modern defibrillators have "quick-look" paddles to allow for rapid evaluation of cardiac rhythm. Defibrillator adhesive pads provide both continuous EKG monitoring and defibrillation and can remain in place while external cardiac compression (ECC) is being performed.

Management

Management may be divided into five phases: (i) Cardiac compression, (ii) establishment of an intravascular access, (iii) use of primary drugs, (iv) use of secondary drugs, and (v) defibrillation.

EXTERNAL CARDIAC COMPRESSION

Well-executed ECC is the primary treatment for cardiopulmonary arrest. The AHA 2010 Guidelines and 2013 Consensus Statement recommend the following: push hard (⅓ chest diameter), push fast (at least 100 per minute), allow full chest recoil, minimize interruptions (<10 seconds) in chest compressions, avoid hyperventilation (8 to 10 beats per minute

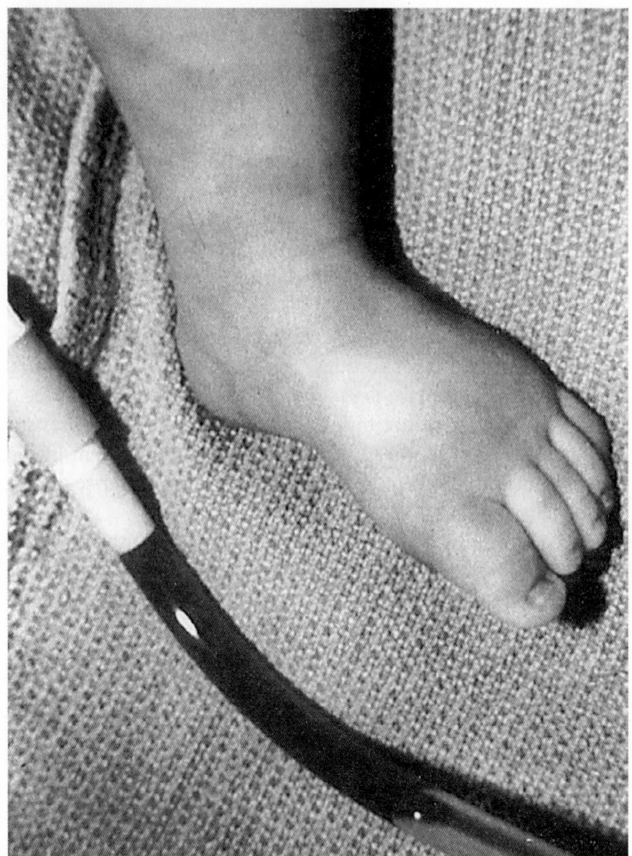

FIGURE 4.9 Delayed capillary refill.

[bpm]), and change rescuers at least every 2 minutes. With the patient on a firm surface, compress the lower half of the sternum, avoiding the xiphoid process. The compression depth is about one-third to one-half the AP diameter of the chest or 2 in in children and 1½ in in infants. For infants (<1 year), the Thaler or two thumb-encircling hands technique is the preferred method for healthcare providers (Fig. 4.10). The recommended rate of compressions for all ages except neonates is at 100 to 120 compressions per minute. The duration of the compression and the relaxation phases should be equal. Blood flow and cardiac output are impaired by incomplete chest wall release that occurs when the rescuer leans over the patient or does not pause at the end of the compression phase. Prior to intubation, compressions and ventilations should be coordinated in a 15:2 ratio (Table 4.5). Once the airway has been secured, coordination of compressions and rescue breathing is no longer necessary. Interruptions in chest compressions result in diminished cardiac output and are associated with poorer outcomes.

Previously, ED rescuers had little more than the presence of the femoral artery pulse with compressions as a means of quickly assessing the adequacy of ECC. Newer techniques such as $ETCO_2$ monitors and accelerometer sensors allow for the rapid and continuous monitoring of ECC quality. Exhaled CO_2 rises as pulmonary blood flow and cardiac output increases; an $ETCO_2$ of less than 10 mm Hg may indicate inadequate chest compression technique. Patients who have return of spontaneous circulation (ROSC) often first demonstrate an abrupt increase in $ETCO_2$ to 35 mm Hg or greater. An accelerometer/force sensor monitor provides real-time

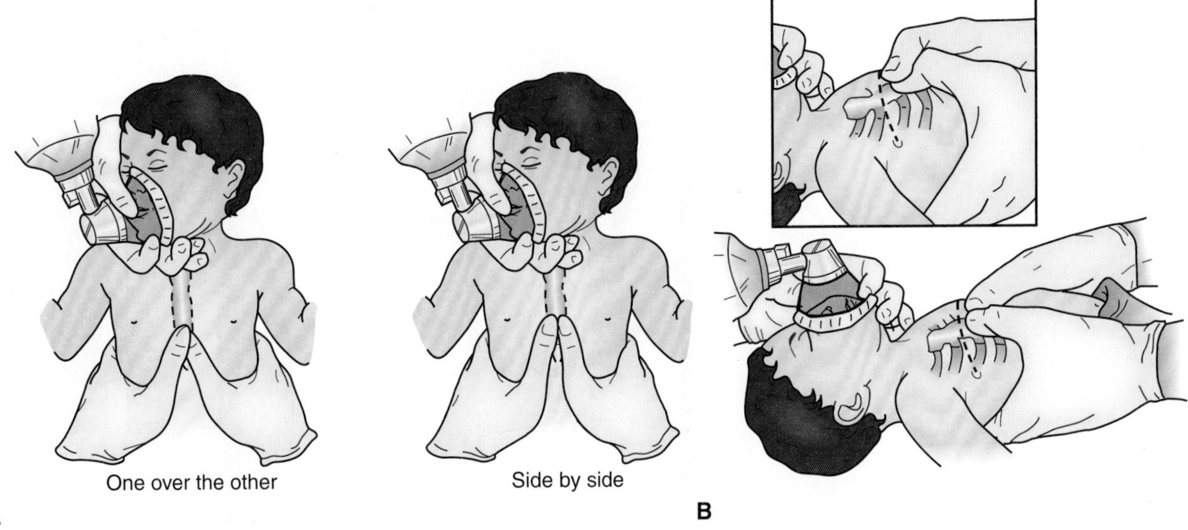

FIGURE 4.10 External cardiac compression using the Thaler method of thumbs encircling the chest. **A:** Infant receiving chest compressions with thumb 1 fingerbreadth below the nipple line and hands encircling chest. **B:** Hand position for chest encirclement technique for external chest compressions in neonates. Thumbs are side by side over the lower third of the sternum. In the small newborn, thumbs may need to be superimposed (*inset*).

feedback of CPR quality. A sensor puck is placed on the child's chest and provides visual and verbal feedback about ECC quality. Though previously only available for children >8 years old, new pediatric electrodes with CPR rate and depth sensor capabilities are now available for infants and children less than 8 years old.

In the newly arrested child, vigorous, high-quality chest compressions generate approximately one-third of the normal cardiac output. This generates a coronary artery perfusion pressure (CPP) of approximately 10 to 20 mm Hg. CPP determines the blood flow to the myocardium and is equivalent to the difference between the aortic pressure and the right atrial pressure. A minimum CPP of 5 to 10 mm Hg is needed to produce any myocardial blood flow. Increased CPP to levels that allow for myocardial perfusion during CPR is associated with ROSC. Pauses in CPR result in lower CPPs, supporting recent AHA efforts to minimize interruptions in compressions during resuscitation.

The mechanism by which blood moves during CPR continues to be the subject of investigation. Techniques that augment this forward flow could potentially improve the rates of successful ROSC and neurologic survival. "Direct compression" and "thoracic pump" describe the current mechanisms that explain blood flow during CPR (see Fig. 4.11). In the "direct compression" model, the heart is squeezed between the sternum and the posterior vertebrae. During compression (systole), blood moves through the AV valves and the aorta. During relaxation (diastole), blood fills the myocardium in preparation for the next systole. In the "thoracic pump" model, the heart is viewed as a conduit. During compression, venous valves at the thoracic inlet close preventing retrograde flow, the venous side of the circulation is compressed, and blood moves forward through the AV valves and the aorta. During relaxation, negative intrathoracic pressures suck blood into the pulmonary bed and heart in preparation for the next systole. In practice, both methods likely contribute to blood

TABLE 4.5

CHEST COMPRESSION PARAMETERS

Age	Rate	Depth	Technique	Location	CC:Ventilation
Newly born[a]	90	⅓ AP chest diameter	Thaler method	Lower ⅓ sternum	3:1
Infant	≥100	1.5 in (4 cm) ⅓ AP chest diameter	Thaler or 2 fingers	Just below nipple line	30:2[b] 15:2[c]
1 yr to puberty	≥100	2 in (5 cm) ⅓ AP chest diameter	1 or 2 hands	Lower ½ sternum	30:2[b] 15:2[c]
Adult	≥100	2 in (5 cm)	2 hands	Lower ½ sternum	30:2[b] 15:2[c]

[a]Outside the delivery room, providers may choose to use infant guidelines for chest compressions for the newly born.
[b]Single rescuer, no advanced airway.
[c]Two rescuers, no advanced airway.
CC, chest compression.
Adapted from the American Heart Association 2010 Guidelines for Cardiopulmonary Resuscitation and Emergency Cardiovascular Care.

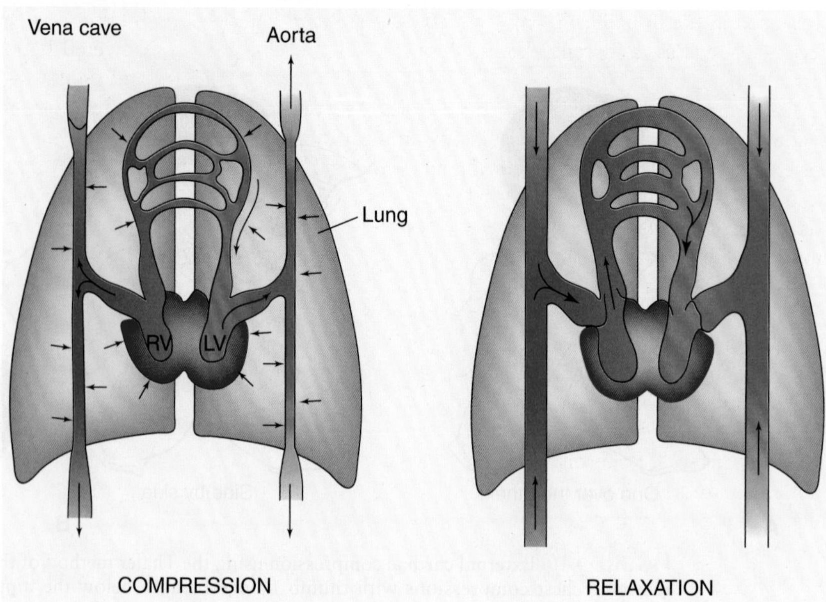

FIGURE 4.11 Blood flow during external cardiac compression. RV, right ventricle; LV, left ventricle.

flow. Because of the compliance and elasticity of the chest wall and the intrathoracic structures, direct compression may play a larger role in the pediatric patient.

Based on the previous data, investigators have explored different techniques to increase blood flow through the aorta and the coronary arteries. These have included high-frequency compression rates (more than 100 compressions per minute), interposed abdominal compression CPR (IAC-CPR), active compression–decompression CPR (ACD-CPR) using a suction device applied to the chest, vest CPR, open chest massage, simultaneous ventilation–compression CPR, and use of automated feedback devices that monitor the quality of CPR. To date, compression rates and automated performance feedback have been the most promising. The other techniques are not supported by pediatric data and their use is not indicated.

Compression rates affect the cardiac output. During CPR, CPP rises during consecutive chest compressions and falls during pauses. Compression rates of more than 100 have been shown to improve cardiac output, CPP, and 24-hour survival when compared with rates less than 80. Although the optimal compression rate remains unknown, compression rate of at least 100 per minute is now recommended for all ages beyond the neonatal period. There is some evidence in adults that compression-only CPR (no ventilation) produces similar survival rates. Because of the etiology of pediatric arrest, in addition to a higher metabolic rate and lower functional residual capacity, this practice is not recommended for children with an asphyxial arrest.

The optimal duty cycle (compression:relaxation) also remains unknown. To date, a duty cycle of 50% is believed to provide the highest flow rates. Leaning or incomplete decompression of the chest during the relaxation phase occurs commonly and may affect the cardiac output generated by CPR by decreasing venous return.

Open cardiac massage provides better blood flow to vital organs in animals and in adults when compared with CPR. However, because of the compliance of the thoracic structures in children, this technique may not offer any benefit. There is inadequate data to recommend its use in the resuscitation of children who have suffered a medical cause of their arrest.

In the newly arrested patients, CPR should be provided immediately to establish a minimum of circulation to the brain and heart, as this is associated with improvements in both survival and outcome. Though healthcare providers may assume mastery of this seemingly basic skill, many studies have demonstrated that the quality of CPR administered in both OHCA and IHA meets the AHA standards <50% of the time. Providers fail to adhere to recommended chest compression rate and depth; interruptions, overventilation, and leaning are common. In a case series of out-of-hospital arrests, paramedics provided chest compressions only half of the available time. In adults, ROSC is associated with a higher chest compression rate and an increased depth of compression and decreased pre- and postcompression pauses related to defibrillation. Survivors are more likely to have received rates between 85 and 100 and the average depth of compression 2.4 mm deeper than nonsurvivors.

Though a rescuer may not feel fatigued, chest compression quality deteriorates within the first 2 minutes of chest compressions, leading to the current recommendation of switching providers every 2 minutes. However, frequent changes in providers cause an interruption in compressions and new compressors may be more likely to lean during the first compressions. Some providers may maintain high-quality compressions beyond the recommended 2-minute limit. Using a real-time CPR feedback system may provide objective information regarding when to change compressors. In Bobrow's study of adults with an OHCA, chest compression rate, depth, ventilation rate, and preshock pause were all improved when audiovisual feedback was used in combination with rescuer retraining. Most importantly, feedback and training improved survival by 30%.

INTRAVENOUS ACCESS

The site used for vascular access depends on the patient's condition and the provider's experience. The most common sites used in the ill pediatric patient include peripheral venous access, IO access, and central venous access via the femoral vein.

In the arrested patient, IO access is indicated and can be accomplished quickly (30 to 60 seconds) and provides a route for all drugs and fluids needed during resuscitation. The onset of action of drugs administered via this route is comparable to that of drugs administered into the central circulation. Adenosine, which is rapidly metabolized once administered, may not work when given via the IO. Manual pressure, a push–pull fluid delivery system or use of a pressure bag is necessary when giving fluids to restore the vascular volume in order to overcome the resistance of the marrow venous plexus. The preferred site in children is the medial surface of the tibia 1 to 3 cm below the tibial tuberosity Alternative sites include the anterior surface of the distal femur, proximal to the medial malleolus, and the anterior iliac spine (Fig. 4.12). There are several types of rigid, styletted needles commercially available for this procedure in infants and children. There are also semi-automated IO devices available for use in children. The bone injection gun (BIG) is a spring-loaded device that can be used in adolescents/adults and can effectively penetrate the thicker bony cortex. The EZ-IO (Vidacare, San Antonio, TX) a battery-powered handheld drill, is available for use in both children and adults. Further research is needed to evaluate efficacy of the semiautomated IO placement devices as compared to manual IO needles. Contraindications to IO placement include recently fractured bone, osteogenesis imperfecta, and osteopetrosis. Complications are rare and have been reported in less than 1% of patients. These have included extravasation, epiphyseal injury, fracture, compartment syndrome, fat embolism, and thrombosis (see Chapter 141 Procedures).

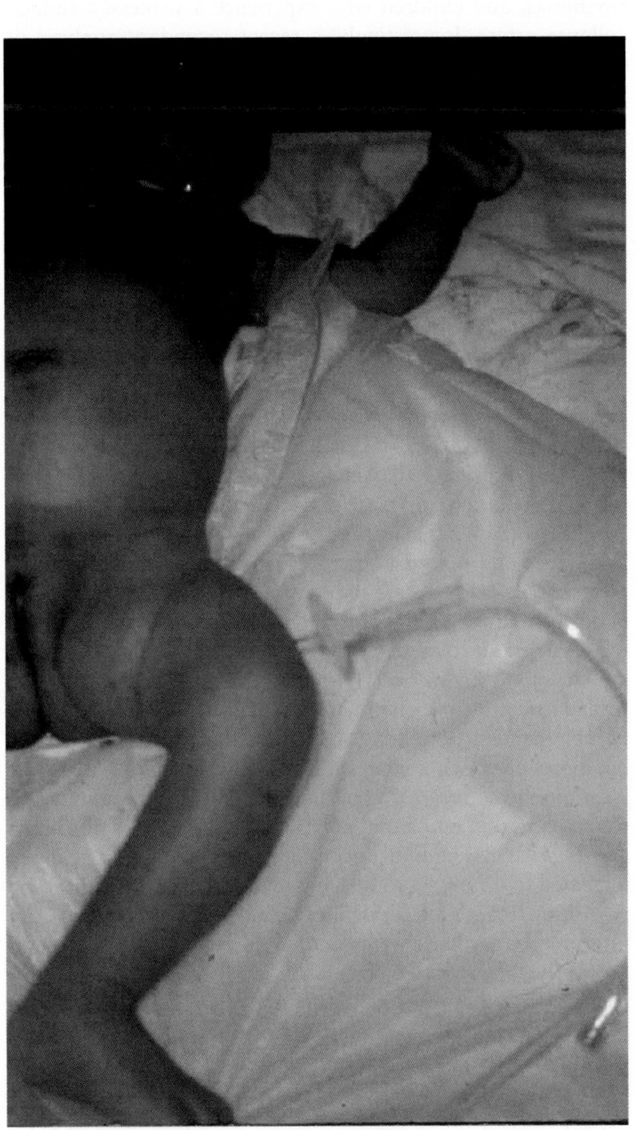

FIGURE 4.12 Intraosseous needle placed in distal femur.

Peripheral venous access provides an adequate route for prearrest resuscitations. Veins of the hands, forearm, and ankle are most commonly used. Prolonged unsuccessful attempts at IV access in critically ill or injured children delay fluid or medication administration as well as interfere with other life-saving procedures; use of the IO should not be delayed. Recent advances in the use of bedside ultrasound by the emergency clinician have increased the placement of ultrasound-guided peripheral IVs, especially in patients with difficult IV access. An IV escalation plan should be developed and in place (see Chapter 142 Ultrasound).

The femoral vein is the easiest central vein to access in the critically ill child and has less complications. Central venous access provides a more secure route, allows the capability of monitoring central venous pressure, and allows for blood sampling. In adults, this route has been shown to provide more rapid onset of action and higher peak drug levels that theoretically could affect outcome. This has not been shown to be the case in the pediatric patient. In a child with uncompensated shock or arrest, IO access is obtained first for rapid initial resuscitation and central venous access may follow (see Chapter 141 Procedures).

DRUGS OF RESUSCITATION

Estimating Body Weight

Drug doses, fluid therapy, and equipment size is weight and size based. The 50th percentile weight from a standardized growth curve can be used to estimate weight based by known/estimated age. The Broselow tape allows a simple, accurate method of estimating the weight and drug doses based on the measured height (Fig. 4.13). In the absence of compelling research, AHA currently recommends using the actual or tape-based weight for obese children rather than an ideal weight. Drug doses should never exceed the adult maximum dose. Many handheld computer programs are available to calculate pediatric resuscitation drug doses (see Table 4.6 for doses and comments on common resuscitation medications).

Alternative Routes of Medication Administration

Intravenous administration, including IO, is the preferred route for medications. However, the pulmonary bed provides a surface for absorption of lipid-soluble drugs and can be used if vascular access is unavailable. Currently, lidocaine, epinephrine, atropine, and naloxone (LEAN) can be used via this route. The optimal drug dosage remains unknown as absorption likely varies widely due to its dependence on pulmonary blood flow. Animal studies have shown that standard doses

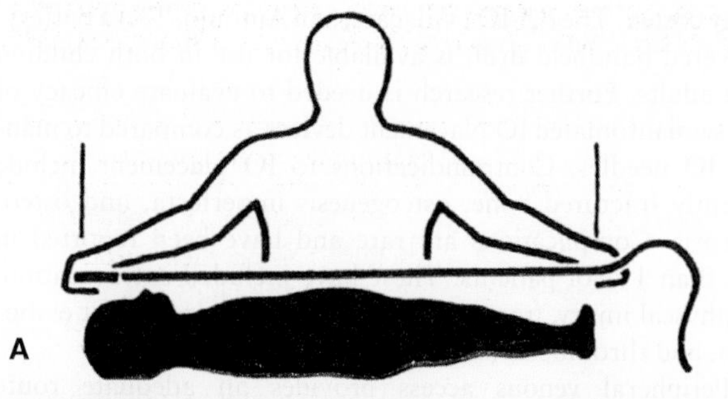

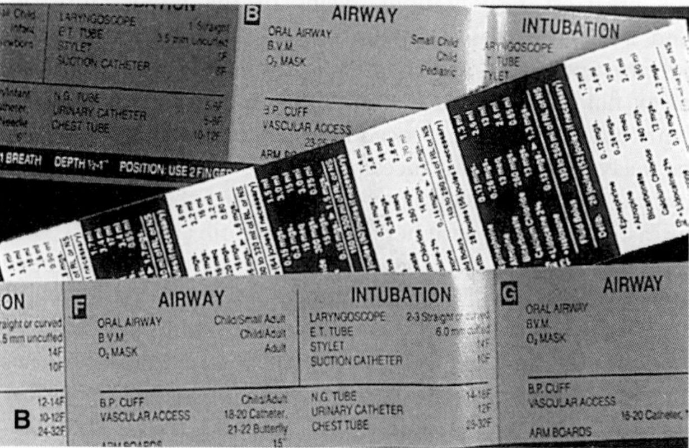

FIGURE 4.13 Broselow tape for determining drug dosage schedule based on patient length. **A:** Placement of tape. **B:** Equipment size and drug dosage schedule printed on tape.

of epinephrine (0.01 mg per kg) achieve serum levels that are approximately 10% of those achieved by the intravascular route. Thus, the recommended dose of epinephrine to be given via the ET tube is 0.1 mg per kg, 10 times the recommended IV dose. Larger doses of the LEAN drugs are also recommended ranging from 2 to 10 times the IV dose. All drugs are diluted in 5 mL of saline and given with five manual ventilations to distribute it across the alveolar surface. Other routes of medication administration for patients for which vascular access has not yet been obtained include intramuscular (epinephrine for anaphylaxis), subcutaneous (terbutaline for status asthmaticus), and transmucosal, including rectal mucosa, buccal mucosa, and nasal mucosa (benzodiazepines for status epilepticus).

FLUID RESUSCITATION

Isotonic crystalloids (normal saline or lactated Ringer solution) in 20 mL per kg aliquots remain the mainstay of acute volume resuscitation. Dextrose solutions should not be used in the initial phases of fluid resuscitation. For children, it is important to recognize signs of shock (poor end organ perfusion) and treat with isotonic crystalloid boluses even if the blood pressure is normal.

Hypertonic saline causes an osmotic shift of fluid from the intracellular and interstitial spaces to the extracellular compartment, providing rapid volume expansion with less interstitial edema. In addition, less volume is required, which can be given over a shorter period of time. Hypertonic solutions are also believed to reduce ICP by establishing an osmotic gradient across the blood–brain barrier that draws water from the brain into the vascular space. Conversely, potential ill effects include continued hemorrhage from injured blood vessels, and increased ICP due to leakage of sodium through a disrupted blood–brain barrier. Currently, data does not support the use of hypertonic saline over isotonic crystalloid for the resuscitation of patients.

Serum albumin concentration has been shown to be inversely related to mortality risk. Thus, its use in the resuscitation of ill patients has been explored. It is 30 times more expensive than crystalloid solutions and has limited availability. Systematic reviews have failed to show benefit from its administration. Albumin is believed to have some anticoagulant properties and may leak across the capillary wall promoting edema.

DEFIBRILLATION AND CARDIOVERSION

The true prevalence of VT and VF in children with cardiopulmonary arrest in published reports is approximately 10% in both IHA and OHCA pediatric arrest (Table 4.7). An additional 10% to 15% will develop VT/VF as a subsequent rhythm. Although the need for defibrillation is relatively uncommon, it must always be considered in older children, children with a history of congenital heart disease or dysrhythmias, and children who experience a witnessed sudden collapse arrest. Interestingly, a recent secondary analysis of the CARES registry found that though younger children (1 to 8 years) with OHCA had a relatively low incidence of an initial shockable rhythm (11%) as expected, older children (9 to 18 years old) had an incidence of an initial shockable rhythm similar to that of adults (32%).

Defibrillation is the asynchronous delivery of a shock to the myocardium in an attempt to produce simultaneous depolarization of a critical mass of myocardial cells to allow spontaneous repolarization and the resumption of a perfusing cardiac rhythm. Most defibrillators deliver biphasic wave forms allowing for successful defibrillation at a lower energy of 150 J. Standard adult paddles, 8 to 13 cm in diameter and pediatric paddles 4.5 cm in diameter, are available with most defibrillators. The correct paddle size is that which makes complete uniform contact with the chest wall. The large paddle can usually be used for infants older than 1 year of age and/or weighing more than 10 kg. Larger paddle surfaces result in decreased intrathoracic impedance and optimize the energy reaching the myocardium. Electrode paste decreases impedance and prevents skin injury. Paddles are applied anteriorly at the right, upper chest below the clavicle and to the left of the nipple in the anterior axillary line directly over the heart; they are applied with pressure and should never touch each other. Most defibrillators also have disposable hands-free adhesive pads that allow both rhythm recognition and shock delivery. These can be applied in the same location on the arrested child immediately at the beginning of the resuscitation and aid in preventing delays in rhythm checks and treatment. The initial dose for defibrillation is 2 J per kg, increased to 4 J per kg if the first attempt is unsuccessful.

Automated external defibrillators (AEDs) automatically interpret the cardiac rhythm and, if pulseless VT/VF is present, advise the operator to deliver a charge. They are small, easy to use, and have batteries that last for 5 years. For patients with pulseless VT/VF, early rapid defibrillation is the treatment of choice. AEDs have been proven to be highly sensitive and specific when used on adults, and there is good evidence that its use in the out-of-hospital setting has resulted in a dramatic improvement in survival of adults with VF.

TABLE 4.6

DRUGS OF RESUSCITATION

Drug	Dose	Route	Action	Indications/comments/side effects
Epinephrine 1:10,000 STANDARD	0.01 mg/kg/dose 0.01 mL/kg/dose Max dose: 1 mg	IV, IO	α-β agonist, α most prominent at higher doses Intense vasoconstriction increasing CPP, CBF Augments myocardial contractility Increases intensity of fine VF for increased defibrillation success	PEA, asystole, severe hypotension SE: hypertension, tachycardia, widened pulse pressure, malignant dysrhythmias, and excessive vasoconstriction Consider infusion for postarrest hypotension or calcium blocker overdose
Epinephrine 1:1,000 HIGH DOSE	0.1 mg/kg/dose 0.1 mL/kg/dose Max dose: 10 mg	ETT		PEA, Asystole no venous access NOT recommended for IV/IO, associated with worse outcomes
Vasopressin	40 IU/kg	IV, IO	Acts at V_1 receptors, causes intense vasoconstriction in skeletal muscle, intestine, and skin and slightly less vasoconstriction in coronary and renal vessels with vasodilatation in cerebral vessels	Not enough pediatric data to support its use
Sodium bicarbonate	0.5–1 mEq/kg	IV, IO	Treats metabolic acidosis via increased CO_2 excretion Requires adequate ventilation to work	NOT recommended in arrest resuscitations May cause harm Indicated treatment of hyperkalemia, hypermagnesemia, tricyclic antidepressant overdose, calcium channel blocker overdose SE: hyperosmolarity, hypernatremia, left shift of oxyhemoglobin dissociation curve, increased lactate production, catecholamine inactivation, decrease CPP
Atropine	0.02 mg/kg/dose Min 0.1 mg/dose Child 0.5 mg/dose Teen 1 mg/dose ETT 0.3 mg/kg/dose	IV, IO ETT	Parasympatholytic with peripheral and central effects Peripheral—vagolytic, increased sinus, atrial pacemakers, and increased conduction through the AV node Centrally—stimulates medullary vagal nucleus causing bradycardia (low dose)	Vagally mediated bradycardia Primary heart block Consider preparation for pacing
Glucose 10% Glucose 25%	0.5–1 g/kg Infant/child $D_{25}W$ 2–4 mL/kg Teen $D_{50}W$ 1–2 mL/kg	IV, IO	Needed substrate for myocardium, brain Higher needs due to high metabolic rate and decreased glycogen stores	Treat documented hypoglycemia Follow with IVF containing glucose Avoid hyperglycemia, implicated in postarrest CNS injury
Adenosine		IV, IO	Short-acting purine nucleoside, blocks AV node adenosine receptors, slows conduction and blocks reentry circuits, depresses the automaticity of primary pacemaker cells	Stable and unstable SVT, metabolized by adenosine deaminase on RBCs, has an extremely short half-life Rapid IV bolus, proximal vein if possible SE: facial flushing, chest pain, anxiety, and dyspnea bronchospasm or apnea, accelerated ventricular rhythm, wide complex tachycardia, and brief asystole

(continued)

TABLE 4.6

DRUGS OF RESUSCITATION (*CONTINUED*)

Drug	Dose	Route	Action	Indications/comments/side effects
Amiodarone	5 mg/kg/dose push May repeat ×2 Max 300 mg Perfusing VT 5 mg/kg over 20–60 min	IV, IO	Class III antiarrhythmic, blocks K^+ channels which prolongs phase 3 of the cardiac action potential and prolongs the refractory period. Some sodium channel and beta-adrenoreceptor blockade	Pulseless VT, VF Liver metabolism, protein bound, rapid distribution SE: Prolongs QT interval, bradycardia, tachydysrhythmias, and hypotension
Lidocaine	1 mg/kg/dose Max 3 mg/kg/dose	IV, IO, ETT	Class I antiarrhythmic blocks sodium channel reducing slope of phase 4, decreases automaticity, and suppresses ventricular dysrhythmias	Has been replaced by amiodarone in pediatric algorithms SE: myocardial depression, CNS depression, seizures, and muscle twitching
Calcium chloride 100 mg/mL 27.2 mg/mL of elemental calcium	10–20 mg/kg Max 1 g 0.14–0.28 mEq/kg Max 14 mEq	IV, IO Centrally preferred	Vascular smooth muscle excitation–contraction coupling Enhances systolic function and systemic vascular resistance via vascular smooth muscle contraction	Routine administration is NOT recommended, may cause harm, associated with poorer outcomes Used for treatment of hypocalcemia, hypermagnesemia, hyperkalemia, and calcium channel overdose
Calcium gluconate	30–100 mg/kg Max 3 g 0.28–0.45 mEq/kg Max 13.5 mEq	IV, IO Can give peripherally		
Magnesium sulfate	25–50 mg/kg Max 2 g	IV, IO	Inhibits calcium channels, decreasing intracellular calcium resulting in smooth muscle relaxation	Indicated for hypomagnesemia, torsades de pointe and severe asthma SE: Hypotension Infuse over 20 min

CNS, central nervous system; ET, endotracheal; IO, intraosseous; IV, intravenous; IVF, intravenous fluid; PEA, pulseless electrical activity; RBCs, red blood cells; SVT, supraventricular tachycardia; VF, ventricular fibrillation; VT, ventricular tachycardia.

TABLE 4.7

PRESENTING RHYTHM IN PEDIATRIC PATIENTS WITH OUT-OF-HOSPITAL CARDIOPULMONARY ARREST AND IN-HOSPITAL CARDIOPULMONARY ARREST (%)

PATIENTS WITH OUT-OF-HOSPITAL CARDIOPULMONARY ARREST (%)				
	n	Asystole	VT/VF	PEA
Young (1999)	548	67	9	24
Sirbaugh (1999)	300	83	4	12
Diechmann (1995)	65	83	9	8
Young (2004)	3,097	75	10	
Donoghue (2005)	2,734	78	8	13
Gerein (2006)	503	77	4	16
Atkins (2009)	503	82	7	
PATIENTS WITH IN-HOSPITAL CARDIOPULMONARY ARREST (%)				
Reis[a] (2002)		55	1	11
Nadkarni (2006)		40	14	24

[a]Children with heart disease not in the study population.

Pediatric-based EKG rhythm analysis algorithms for AEDs are 99% sensitive and specific for determining shockable and nonshockable pediatric rhythms.

Available AEDs deliver a standard adult charge between 150 and 200 J, they can be used for children >1 year of age. An attenuating pediatric electrode system is available which decreases the charge delivered to 50 J and is preferred if available for children 1 to 8 year olds. For infants <1 year, a manual defibrillator is preferred, but an AED equipped to deliver pediatric charge doses may be used. If neither of these is available, an AED may be used.

Synchronous cardioversion is delivered with the patient's R wave, reducing the risk of VF by avoiding delivery of the charge during the T wave. This is indicated for treatment of perfusing rhythms, when a pulse is present, such as stable VT or SVT. The initial charge for synchronized cardioversion is 0.5 to 1 J per kg. This dose can be doubled to 2 J per kg if the tachydysrhythmia persists. Sedation and analgesia should be considered during this procedure.

SPECIFIC RESUSCITATION SCENARIOS

In the 2010 AHA resuscitation guidelines, an international expert panel updated guidelines for pediatric prearrest/arrest

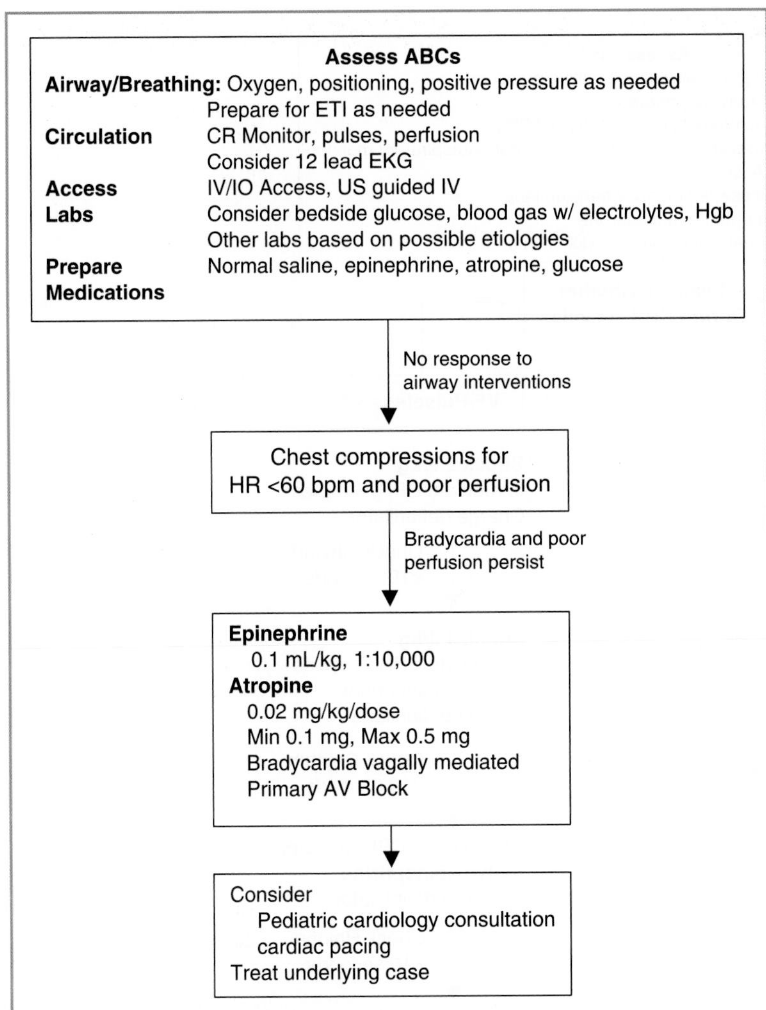

FIGURE 4.14 PALS Bradycardia Algorithm. ABCs, A, airway, B, breathing, C, circulation; AV, atrioventricular; CR, cardiorespiratory; EKG, electrocardiogram; ETI, endotracheal intubation; Hgb, hemoglobin; HR, heart rate; IV/IO, intravenous/intraosseous. (*Source:* American Heart Association, Inc.)

scenarios. Figures 4.14–4.16 summarize these guidelines along with the following commentary. It is important to remember that no algorithm can cover every clinical situation; the treating team of healthcare professionals must consider the many etiologies of arrest and modify therapies accordingly for the individual patient. Early recognition and immediate treatment of respiratory and circulatory failure and frequent reassessment are the foundation of successful resuscitation efforts for all scenarios encountered in the ED.

Bradycardia with a Pulse and Poor Perfusion

Bradycardia most commonly results from impending or existing respiratory failure (Fig. 4.14). As always, early recognition and intervention to support the respiratory system and other vital functions reduces morbidity and may be life-saving. Other etiologies of bradycardia include heart block, heart transplant, increased ICP, hypoglycemia, hypercalcemia, drug effect, increased parasympathetic tone, and hypothermia. The first step in the treatment of children with bradycardia is airway management. Remember that because increase in heart rate is the primary mechanism by which children increase their stroke volume, bradycardia readily leads to hypotension. Chest compressions should begin when perfusion is inadequate. Assess the rhythm on the cardiac monitor. If the bradycardia is believed to be due to increased vagal tone or heart block, atropine is an appropriate intervention. For most situations, epinephrine is the drug of choice. In children with heart block, cardiac pacing may be necessary.

Pulseless Arrest

Asystole and PEA are the most common arrest scenarios encountered in children (Fig. 4.15). In the pulseless child, the rhythm must be identified so the correct intervention can be instituted. In a witnessed, sudden collapse arrest, primary cardiac etiologies should be considered. For asystole and PEA, standard dose epinephrine is the drug of choice. Always consider treatment of reversible causes such as hypovolemia, hypothermia, electrolyte abnormalities, poisonings, tension pneumothorax, and cardiac tamponade.

Treatment for pulseless VT/VF is immediate CPR and defibrillation. In the 2005 guidelines, the recommendation for single defibrillation replaced the recommendation for three successive shocks. Biphasic defibrillators have a higher first shock success rate and the administration of three successive shocks leads to delays in CPR that is associated with decreased survival. Cardiac compressions are interrupted only for rhythm checks and shock delivery. If defibrillation is unsuccessful, standard

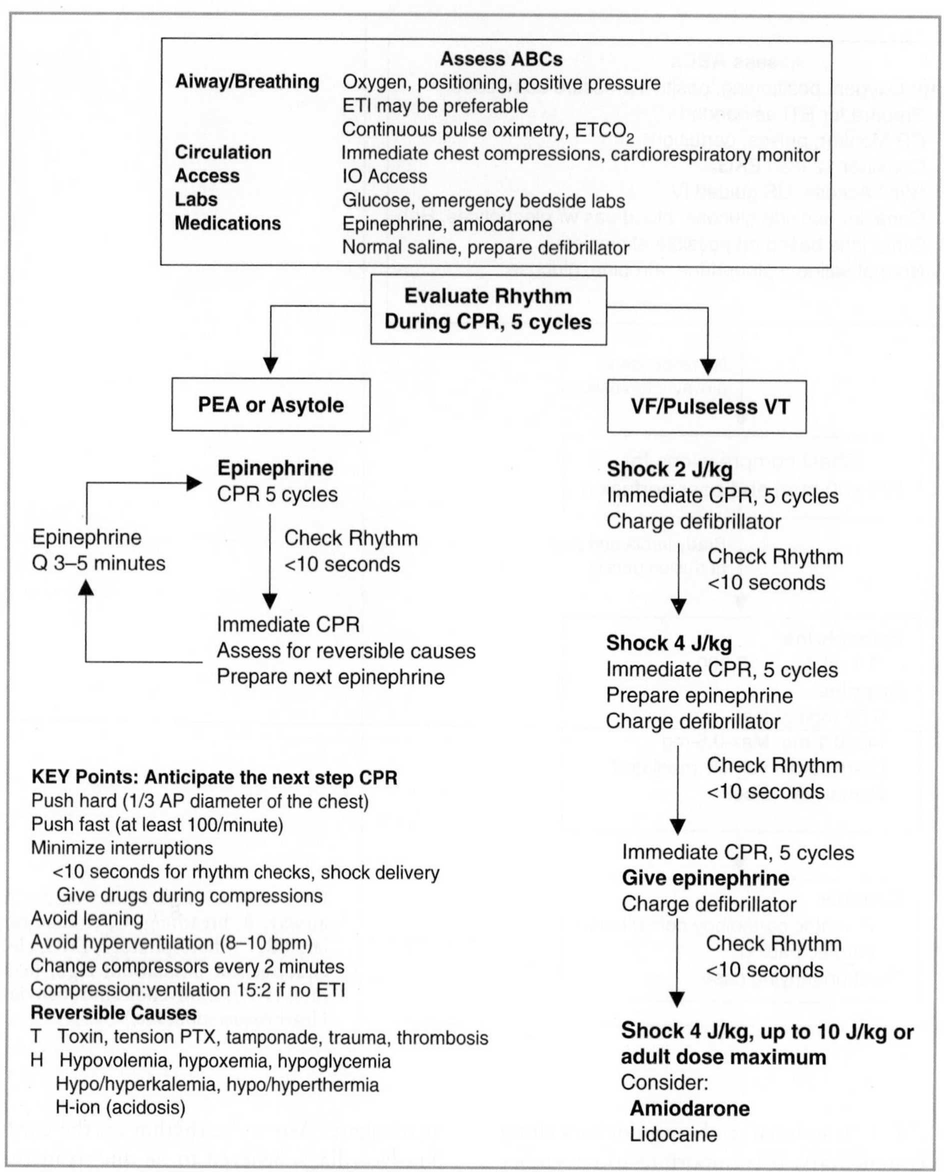

FIGURE 4.15 PALS Pulseless Arrest Algorithm. ABCs, A, airway, B, breathing, C, circulation; CPR, cardiopulmonary resuscitation; $ETCO_2$, end tidal CO_2; ETI, endotracheal intubation; IO, intraosseous; IV, intravenous; PEA, pulseless electrical activity; PTX, pneumothorax; ROSC, return of spontaneous circulation; VF, ventricular fibrillation; VT, ventricular tachycardia. (*Source:* American Heart Association, Inc.)

dose epinephrine is the drug of choice. The use of vasopressin may be considered. Amiodarone is the preferred drug for refractory pulseless VT/VF Magnesium is indicated if the rhythm is torsades de pointes VT. The pattern of interventions is CPR→ rhythm check→ resume CPR while charging defibrillator → deliver single shock→ resume CPR→ brief rhythm check → resume CPR as drug is prepared and administered. Interruptions in CPR should be held to very brief periods to check the rhythm and to administer shocks. The resuscitation team should anticipate the need for the next interventions.

Tachydysrhythmias with a Pulse and Poor Perfusion

The differential diagnosis of tachycardias includes sinus tachycardia (ST), SVT, and VT. Narrow complex morphology and beat-to-beat variability are usually present in children with ST (Fig. 14.16). Rates rarely exceed 220 bpm in infants and 180 bpm in children. Common causes of ST include hypoxemia, hypovolemia, hyperthermia, metabolic abnormalities, and pain/anxiety. Therapy is directed at treating the underlying cause.

SVT can be distinguished from ST by its lack of beat-to-beat variability and rate (most often >220 bpm in infants, and >180 bpm in children). In children, aberrant conduction yielding a wide complex rhythm SVT occurs less than 10% of the time. SVT is most commonly caused by accessory reentry pathways. Patients with stable SVT have adequate oxygenation and perfusion; those with unstable SVT have inadequate perfusion and thus require rapid intervention. Chemical or electrical conversion can be used for the treatment of unstable SVT. Because of the efficacy and safety of adenosine in the treatment of SVTs, it is the drug of choice when vascular or IO access is available. In infants, verapamil can cause myocardial depression or arrest and should be used only in

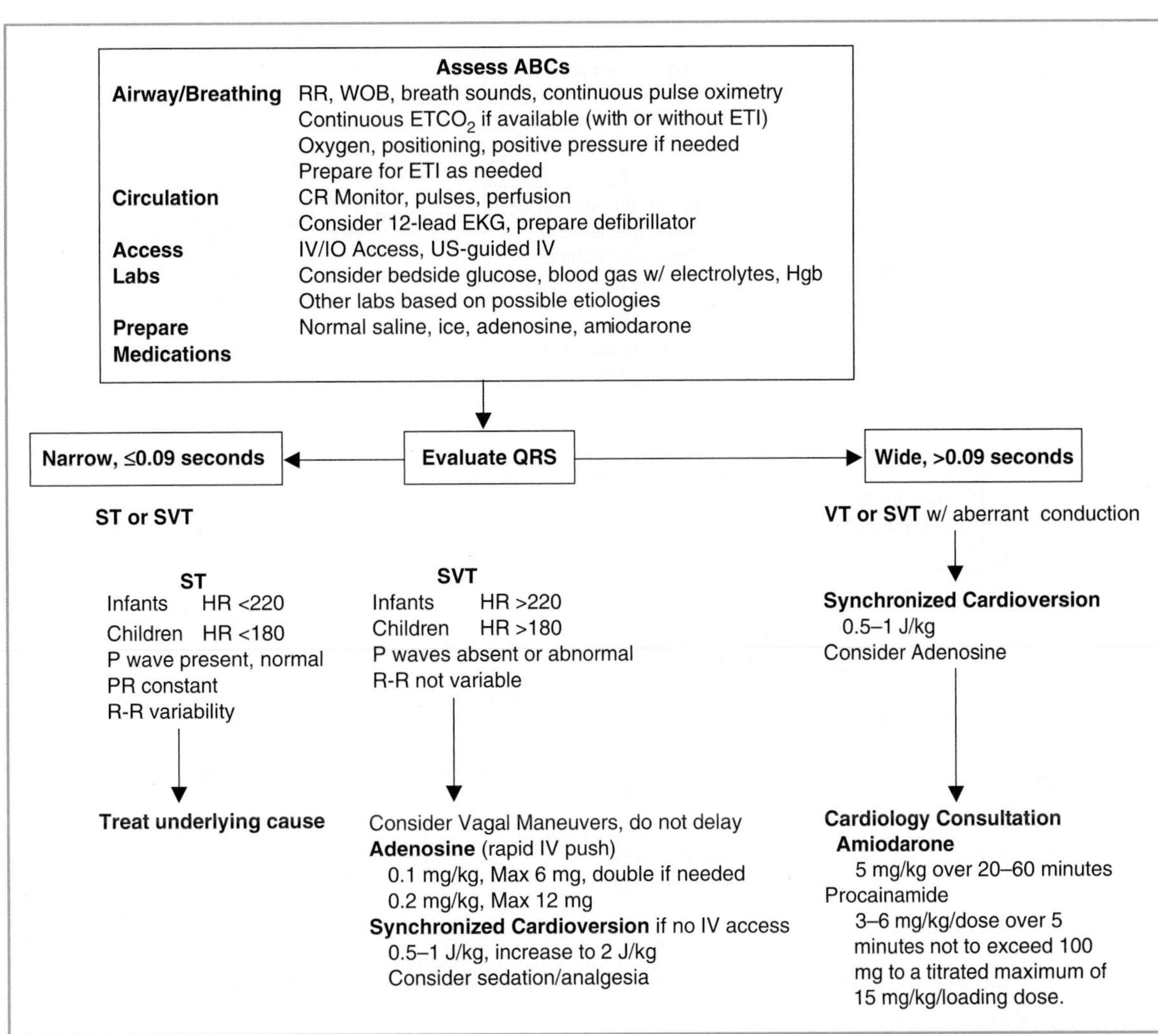

FIGURE 4.16 PALS Tachycardia with Pulses and Poor Perfusion Algorithm. ABCs, A, airway, B, breathing, C, circulation; CBC, complete blood count; CR, cardiorespiratory; EKG, electrocardiogram; $ETCO_2$, end tidal CO_2; ETI, endotracheal intubation; Hgb, hemoglobin; HR, heart rate; IV/IO, intravenous/intraosseous; RR, respiratory rate; SVT, supraventricular tachycardia; VT, ventricular tachycardia; WOB, work of breathing. (*Source:* American Heart Association, Inc.)

consultation with a cardiologist. It is optimal to obtain a 12-lead EKG prior to and during treatment to aid in the diagnosis. If the patient fails to convert to sinus rhythm after two doses of adenosine, synchronized cardioversion (0.5 J per kg) is recommended. Use of sedation/analgesia should be considered. Vagal maneuvers were reintroduced in the 2000 AHA guidelines for stable SVT. In infants and young children, ice may be applied to the face; in older children, carotid massage and Valsalva maneuvers, such as knee to chest or forceful blowing on an obstructed straw, may be attempted. Ocular pressure should be avoided. Use of other therapies such as procainamide, digoxin, and beta-blockers may be considered after pediatric cardiology consultation.

VT is characterized by wide complex (QRS >0.08 second) and typically has a rate ranging from 120 to 200 bpm. Etiologies of VT include prolonged QT syndrome, structural heart disease, myocarditis, cardiomyopathy, and poisonings. In children presenting with stable VT, close monitoring and immediate consultation with a pediatric cardiologist to determine etiology and definitive treatment is the best management. For children with unstable VT, begin with synchronized cardioversion. For hemodynamically stable patients, consider chemical conversion using amiodarone or procainamide in conjunction with consultation with an expert.

EXTRACORPOREAL CARDIOPULMONARY RESUSCITATION

There is now some information regarding the use of extracorporeal CPR (E-CPR) through the use of extracorporeal membrane oxygenation (ECMO) or cardiopulmonary bypass following CPR to treat refractory cardiac arrest in children presenting to an ED setting. Currently, it is an option available in large, tertiary care Children's Hospitals. The majority of the literature to date comes from the treatment of inpatients with primary cardiac disease. Use of E-CPR for these patients following a witnessed arrest seems to increase the chance for favorable outcome. The 2010 Guidelines state "There is insufficient evidence to recommend the routine use of ECPR for patients in cardiac arrest. However in settings where ECPR is readily available, it may be considered when the time without blood flow is brief and the condition leading to the cardiac

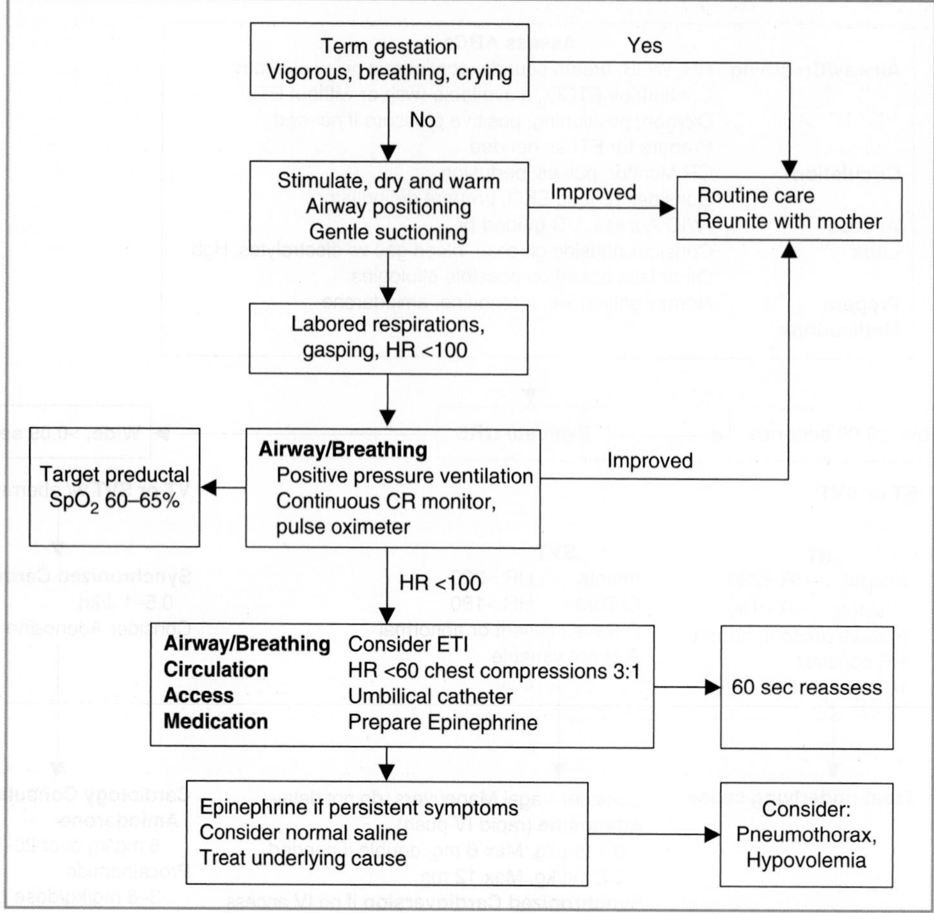

FIGURE 4.17 Newborn Resuscitation Algorithm. CR, cardiorespiratory; CPAP, continuous positive airway pressure; ETI, endotracheal intubation; HR, heart rate. (*Source:* American Heart Association, Inc.)

arrest is reversible or amenable to heart transplantation or revascularization." Use of E-CPR may be considered for children who have had a short downtime and have received high-quality CPR and a cardiac etiology is suspected when the resources and personnel are available.

NEWLY BORN INFANT RESUSCITATION

Guidelines for CPR in the newly born child and for newborns in the neonatal intensive care unit (NICU) differ from guidelines for CPR of the young infant presenting to the ED (Fig. 4.17). To avoid confusion, the AHA recommends that the PALS CPR algorithm be used for all nonnewly born pediatric patients presenting in arrest to the ED, PICU, and other non-NICU settings given that there is no scientific evidence to support the use of either algorithm over the other in these patients.

Though rare, the ED team must be prepared for the resuscitation of the newly born. Fortunately, 90% of neonates transition from intrauterine to extrauterine life without resuscitative needs beyond simple warming and stimulation. However, the remaining 10% require some assistance, and 1% will require extensive resuscitative efforts. Resuscitative needs vary greatly by birth weight. Approximately 6% of term newborns will require resuscitation at birth, compared with nearly 80% of infants weighing less than 1,500 g. The key to a successful newborn resuscitation for the ED team includes preparedness of staff and equipment and anticipation of high-risk births.

Emergency Department Preparedness

Early notification allows time to assemble important team members. Education of staff, necessary equipment, and specific policies and procedures are critical for preparedness. Multiple trained personnel must be available for high-risk deliveries. In addition to a standard obstetric tray, every ED should have a newborn resuscitation kit that is readily accessible, maintained, and rapidly restocked after use. Necessary equipment and medications are listed in Table 4.8. A medication dosing chart by weight and a radiant warmer are invaluable. Because neonatal resuscitations in the ED are uncommon, simulations and mock codes allow staff to remain familiar with neonatal resuscitation skills and supplies. Most births that occur outside the delivery room have high-risk components such as trauma-induced labor and unexpected or teenage pregnancy. Important history includes prematurity, multiple gestation, meconium-stained amniotic fluid, and maternal drug use. The team can then anticipate the need for assisted ventilation, simultaneous resuscitations, tracheal suctioning, or pharmacologic interventions. Table 4.9 lists other risk factors associated with the need for neonatal resuscitation.

TABLE 4.8

NEONATAL RESUSCITATION EQUIPMENT AND DRUGS

Equipment

Gowns, gloves, and masks for universal precautions
Radiant warmer with temperature probe
Warm towels and blankets
Bulb syringe
Suction equipment with manometer
Suction catheters (5F, 8F, and 10F)
Meconium aspirator
Oxygen with flow meter and tubing
Oxygen/air blender
Self-inflating resuscitation bag (500 mL) with oxygen reservoir or anesthesia (flow-inflating) bag with manometer (must be capable of delivering 90–100% oxygen and be no larger than 750 mL)
Face masks (premature, newborn, and infant sizes)
Oral airways (sizes 000, 00, and 0)
Endotracheal tubes (2.5, 3.0, 3.5, and 4.0) and small stylets
Laryngoscope handles and straight blades (nos. 0 and 1)
Extra batteries and laryngoscope bulbs
Laryngeal mask airways (size 1 and 1.5)
Stethoscope
Tape
Scissors
Sterile umbilical catheterization tray
Umbilical catheters (3.5F and 5F)
Three-way stopcocks
Needles and syringes
Nasogastric feeding tubes (8F and 10F)
Small electrocardiographic leads
Pulse oximeter with newborn probe
End-tidal CO_2 detector
Chest tubes (8F and 10F)
Magill forceps, small

Drugs

Weight-based resuscitation chart
Epinephrine 1:10,000 (0.1 mg/mL)
Dextrose in water, 10%
Isotonic crystalloid: normal saline, Ringer lactate

TABLE 4.9

NEONATAL HIGH-RISK PROFILE

Prenatal	Natal	Postnatal
Maternal	**Maternal**	**Fetal**
Older than 35 yrs of age	Hypotension	Respiratory distress
Younger than 16 yrs of age	Prolonged labor (>24 hrs)	Asphyxia
	Precipitous labor	
Diabetes	Placenta previa	Hypotension
Hypertension (chronic or pregnancy-induced)	Abruptio placenta	Meconium staining
	Prolonged rupture of membranes (>18 hrs)	
Second- or third-trimester bleeding	Drugs	Prematurity
Infection	Cesarean section	Small for dates
	Chorioamnionitis	
	General anesthesia	
Premature rupture of membranes	**Fetal**	
Drug ingestion or therapy	Abnormal presentation	
Drug abuse	Prolapsed cord	
Anemia	Abnormal heart rate	
Rh sensitization	Meconium-stained fluid	
Cardiac, liver, or renal disease	Polyhydramnios or oligohydramnios	
Previous fetal/neonatal death		
No prenatal care	Forceps/vacuum delivery	
Preeclampsia, eclampsia		
	Nonreassuring heart rate tracing	
Fetal		
Fetal distress on monitor		
Multiple gestation		
Meconium-stained amniotic fluid		
Premature labor		
Postmature labor		
Intrauterine growth retardation		
Fetal malformation		
Diminished fetal activity		

Pathophysiology

Physiology of Intrauterine Development

Full alveolar development and sufficient surfactant production is not complete until 34 weeks' gestation. Prior to 23 to 24 weeks' gestation, there is a lack of surfactant and terminal airways have not developed, therefore resuscitation prior to 23 to 24 weeks is generally futile.

Changes at Birth

The fetus has two large right-to-left shunts: One from the right atrium to the left atrium through the foramen ovale, and the second from the pulmonary artery to the aorta across the ductus arteriosus. At birth, two major changes occur that eliminate these shunts: the umbilical cord is clamped, and then respirations are initiated. Expansion of the lungs increases the neonate's Pao_2 and pH, which causes pulmonary vasodilation and a fall in pulmonary vascular resistance. The initial breaths taken by the infant must inflate the lungs and effect a change in vascular pressures so that the lung water is absorbed into the pulmonary arterial system and cleared from the lung. This inflation pressure is a powerful mechanism for the release of pulmonary surfactant, which increases compliance of the lung and establishes functional residual capacity.

Asphyxia

Neonatal asphyxia can result from multiple factors. The initial response to asphyxia is hyperpnea and sinus tachycardia. If there is no significant increase in Pao_2, after 2 to 3 minutes, respirations will stop (primary apnea). During primary apnea, stimulation such as drying or slapping of the feet will restart breathing. If the apnea is prolonged (more than 1.5 minutes), the infant becomes bradycardic and may attempt gasping, nonrhythmic respiratory efforts while the heart rate continues to fall. Soon thereafter, the child ceases to gasp (secondary apnea) and stimulation will not cause the infant to resume breathing. Ventilatory support must be initiated for the newborn to survive. Brain and other organ damage progresses rapidly beyond this point.

Management

Initiation and Termination of Resuscitation

Noninitiation of resuscitation is appropriate in conditions associated with high mortality or poor outcome such as a gestational age less than 23 weeks or birth weight of less than 400 g or anencephaly. For conditions associated with a high rate of survival and acceptable morbidity such as gestational age ≥25 weeks and most congenital anomalies, resuscitation should be initiated. Though the often-precipitous nature of ED births may make it difficult, it is important to include parents in the discussion regarding the initiation and continuation of resuscitative efforts. Resuscitative efforts should be performed on any term infant; if there is any question of viability of premature infants, it is probably best to initiate resuscitative efforts.

After 10 minutes of a well-executed resuscitation, if the heart rate remains undetectable, it is reasonable to stop resuscitative efforts. Consultation with a neonatal expert may be helpful in making such a decision.

Initial Management Priorities

The initial assessment and management occur quickly and often simultaneously. For the term, vigorous baby, routine care and reunification with the mother are all that is usually necessary. The initial steps of neonatal resuscitation include positioning and clearing the airway, drying and warming with prevention of heat loss, stimulating, and repositioning. These steps occur within 30 seconds and are followed immediately by an evaluation of respirations, heart rate, and color. When possible, all resuscitation equipment should be ready for use, the radiant warmer on, and a team with preassigned roles assembled. Figure 4.17 is a flow diagram of neonatal resuscitation.

Thermoregulation

Ambient temperature in the ED is lower than ideal for a newborn. All infants, especially very low–birth-weight (VLBW) and premature babies, are at great risk of hypothermia because of their greater body-surface-area-to-weight ratio, minimal fat stores, and thinner epidermis and dermis. Hypothermia increases metabolic needs and produces hypoxia, hypercarbia, metabolic acidosis, and hypoglycemia and delays normal transition.

As the patient is dried and placed under a radiant warmer, the temperature should be monitored via the axillary route using electronic thermometers with a disposable tip. Normal axillary temperatures fall between 36.5°C and 37.4°C. Rectal temperatures are reserved for infants whose core temperature may be in question. Alternative methods of warming infants, particularly while awaiting a radiant warmer in the case of an unexpected delivery, include warm blankets and towels. Placing the dried infant naked against the mother's body and covering both mother and infant with blankets may also warm the stable infant. For VLBW infants, additional methods of warming include wrapping the baby in food grade plastic wrap, using exothermic mattresses or a radiant heater and increasing the room's ambient temperature. Monitor the temperature carefully as these methods may lead to hyperthermia. Although preventing heat loss is vital, hyperthermia should be avoided because it is associated with perinatal respiratory depression and hypoxic-ischemic injury may be worsened.

Suctioning

Many newborns have excessive secretions, including amniotic fluid, cervical mucus, and meconium that can generally be removed by placing the infant on his or her side and gently suctioning the mouth and then the nose with a bulb syringe. Mechanical suction with an 8F or 10F suction catheter may also be used. To avoid soft tissue injury, negative pressure from mechanical suctioning should not exceed 100 mm Hg. Suctioning of the oropharynx in a newborn is likely to cause vagally mediated bradycardia and/or apnea. Excessive suctioning may also contribute to atelectasis. Therefore, suctioning is reserved for the newly born with obvious obstruction to breathing or those requiring positive pressure ventilation (PPV).

Stimulation

Most newborns will begin effective breathing during stimulation from routine drying and suctioning. Other methods of safe stimulation include flicking the heels and rubbing the back of the newborn infant. More vigorous methods of stimulation are unnecessary and may be associated with harmful consequences. If, after a brief period of stimulation, suctioning, and drying (no more than 30 seconds) effective respirations have not been established, PPV is initiated (Fig. 4.17).

Airway Positioning

If airway obstruction persists after routine suctioning, reposition the airway. Correct positioning, with the neck slightly extended in the "sniffing position," aligns the posterior pharynx, larynx, and trachea and facilitates air entry. This maneuver may also be accomplished by placing a towel or blanket beneath the upper back of the supine infant. Avoid flexion or hyperextension of the newborn's neck, which is likely to exacerbate airway obstruction.

Administration of Oxygen. Recent studies have shown better survival for newborns resuscitated with air compared to 100% oxygen. Sustained high levels of oxygen may be toxic. The AHA recommends newborns SpO_2 should correlate with a range of normal values as described in Table 4.10. To achieve the targeted SpO_2, clinicians should use air or blended oxygen when available, titrating the amount of oxygen based on the pulse oximetry. If the baby remains bradycardic after 90 seconds of air or blended oxygen, 100% oxygen should be started. Deliver warm, humidified oxygen when possible to maintain temperature.

Airway and Breathing

One large observational study noted that initial management steps and ventilation were effective in establishing normal vital signs in more than 99% of newly born infants. Therefore, particular attention must be paid to providing skilled ventilation interventions for compromised newborns in the ED.

Bag-valve-mask Ventilation

If initial management interventions are unsuccessful and the newborn is still not breathing or is gasping, or the heart rate is less than 100 bpm, PPV must be initiated. For the infant's first breath, a relatively higher inflation pressure, between 25 and 40 cm H_2O, delivered slowly over several seconds is commonly used. Subsequent ventilations typically require less pressure (15 to 20 cm H_2O for normal lungs and 20 to 40 cm H_2O for diseased or immature lungs), and are best judged by good chest wall rise and breath sounds and heart rate response. An assisted ventilatory rate of 40 to 60 breaths per minute will provide effective ventilation and oxygenation.

TABLE 4.10

TARGETED PREDUCTAL SPO_2 AFTER BIRTH

1 min	60–65%
2 min	65–70%
3 min	70–75%
4 min	75–80%
5 min	80–85%
10 min	85–90%

PPV is similar to infants and children with a few caveats. First, relatively small volumes of air (approximately 4 to 6 mL per kg) are delivered to the newly born. A 450-mL self-inflating bag rather than the larger bags should be used to avoid complications from barotrauma. Many self-inflating bags have a pressure-limiting pop-off valve set at 30 to 45 cm H_2O, occlusion of this valve may be necessary if initial high inflation pressures are needed for the first breath.

If bag-valve-mask ventilation is required for longer than several minutes, an orogastric tube should be placed to decompress the stomach. If respirations are restored and the heart rate is >100 bpm, PPV may be slowly discontinued. If respirations remain inadequate or the HR <100 bpm, assisted ventilation must be continued and endotracheal (ET) intubation must be considered.

Endotracheal Intubation

In the event that there is a prolonged need for PPV or mask ventilation has not been effective in restoring vital functions, ET intubation is indicated. Chapter 3 Airway reviews advanced airway management in depth and this generally applies to the newly born with a few differences. Sizes of airway equipment can be determined by birth weight (Table 4.11). ET tube size can be estimated by gestational age: ETT size in mm = Gestational age in weeks divided by 10. Thus, a 35-week premature infant would require a 3.5-mm ET tube. Proper ET tube insertion depth is estimated as follows: Total cm at gum line = 6 + Weight of the infant in kg.

End Expiratory Pressure

For centers skilled in the respiratory management of neonates, CPAP may be an alternative to ET intubation in a spontaneously breathing preterm newborn with respiratory distress.

Laryngeal Mask Airways

LMAs can be successfully used for ventilating full-term or near-term newborns, particularly in cases of ineffective

TABLE 4.11

SELECTION OF AIRWAY EQUIPMENT BY WEIGHT

Weight (g) or gestational age (wk)	Endotracheal tube size (mm)	Suction catheter (F)	Oral airway	Laryngoscope straight blade
<1,000 or <28	2.5	5, 6	000	0
1,000–2,000 or 28–34	3.0	6, 8	000 or 00	0
2,000–3,000 or 34–38	3.5	8	00 or 0	0, 1
>3,000 or >38	3.5, 4.0	8 or 10	0	1

TABLE 4.12

MEDICATIONS FOR NEONATAL RESUSCITATION

Medication	Concentration	Dosage	Route	Comment
Epinephrine	1:10,000	0.1–0.3 mL/kg	IV, ET, IO	Rapid push, dilute with 2 mL saline via ET tube
Dextrose	10%	2–5 mL/kg	IV, IO	Correction of hypoglycemia
Crystalloid/pRBCs		10 cc/kg	IV, IO	Volume expansion

ET, endotracheal; IV, intravenous; IO, intraosseous; pRBCs, packed red blood cells.

bag-valve-mask ventilation or failed ET intubation. Although LMAs may be used as a secondary device to ventilate newborns by healthcare practitioners skilled in their use, data supporting use of LMAs in preterm infants are insufficient to routinely recommend their use in this scenario.

Circulation

Chest Compressions. Chest compressions are needed in less than 0.1% of all births. Bradycardia and asystole are virtually always a result of respiratory failure, hypoxemia, and tissue acidosis and are successfully treated with airway management. Chest compressions are indicated if the heart rate remains less than 60 bpm despite 30 seconds of PPV.

The chest compression:ventilation ratio in the newly born is 3:1 aiming for 90 chest compressions and 30 ventilations in 1 minute (rate of 120 events per minute) (Table 4.5). The Thayer technique is the preferred means of ECC (Fig. 4.10).

Vascular Access. The umbilical vein is considered the preferred site for vascular access during neonatal resuscitation; it is easily located and cannulated, and medication delivery requires insertion only to the point at which blood can be aspirated (usually 2 to 4 cm) (see Chapter 141 Procedures). Vascular access may also be obtained by placing peripheral catheters in the extremities or scalp. IO lines may also be used. A 20- or 22-gauge spinal needle may replace the 16- or 18-gauge larger IO needles; however, the procedure for line placement in the proximal tibia is the same as for older children. Recall that premature infants have a small IO space. Finally, the ET tube may be used for administration of epinephrine when vascular access has not yet been established.

Medications and Volume Expanders for Acute Resuscitation

Epinephrine

Standard dose epinephrine is indicated when the newborn's heart rate remains less than 60 bpm, despite 30 seconds of effective ventilation with 100% oxygen and another 30 seconds of coordinated chest compressions and ventilation (see Table 4.12 for dosing). It may be administered via an umbilical venous catheter, a peripheral IV, an IO line, or the ET tube and repeated every 3 to 5 minutes. Intravenous epinephrine should be administered as rapidly as possible and followed by a 1-mL normal saline flush. High-dose epinephrine is not recommended and may cause harm.

Volume Expanders

Crystalloid (lactated Ringer or normal saline) is administered intravenously over 5 to 10 minutes in 10 mL per kg aliquots to avoid an increased risk of intracranial hemorrhage. Administration of O-negative red blood cells (cross-matched with mother's blood if time allows) may be needed for large volume blood loss or poor response to crystalloid infusion. Albumin-containing solutions are not recommended because of cost, limited availability, risk of infection, and potential increased mortality.

Other Medications

ED stabilization should focus on basic resuscitation interventions outlined above. Other medications such as buffers, narcotic antagonist, vasopressors, or surfactant therapy are rarely given in ED phase of care.

Sodium Bicarbonate

Bicarbonate therapy may contribute to respiratory acidosis and a worsening intracellular acidosis, which may actually impair myocardial and cerebral function. In prolonged resuscitations, after establishment of adequate ventilation, bicarbonate may be given to treat documented metabolic acidosis or hyperkalemia using arterial blood gases and serum chemistries to guide administration. Use 0.5 mEq per mL (4.2%, half-strength) solution to decrease effects of hypertonicity. Little research data exist to support the choice of other buffers, such as tris(hydroxymethyl)aminomethane (THAM), for documented metabolic acidosis; practitioners may use this to reduce the occurrence of hypernatremia.

Naloxone Hydrochloride

Naloxone is a narcotic antagonist that reverses narcotic-induced respiratory depression. Naloxone is not recommended for the initial resuscitation attempts in the newly born. The focus of the resuscitation remains the same, providing adequate respiratory support to correct abnormalities in ventilation and circulation. Naloxone given to the newborn of a mother suspected of narcotic addiction may precipitate acute narcotic withdrawal and seizures.

Atropine

Atropine is not recommended for acute neonatal resuscitation as vagal stimulation does not cause bradycardia in neonates. Furthermore, many investigators believe that the vagally mediated bradycardia response to hypoxia is a valuable reflex to guide resuscitative efforts and should not be pharmacologically abolished by atropine.

Glucose

Hypoglycemia in the neonate is associated with increased risk for brain injury and adverse outcomes with hypoxic-ischemic events. Therefore, the administration of IV glucose infusion should be considered as early as is practical after initial resuscitative measures. The goal of glucose infusion should be to maintain euglycemia.

Artificial Pulmonary Surfactant

Newborns who require intubation due to the respiratory distress associated with insufficient surfactant production may benefit from replacement therapy with an artificial surfactant product. Prematurity of less than 35 weeks is the most common indication for surfactant use. Replacement surfactant is delivered to the pulmonary bed via an ET tube. Use of surfactant in the ED should be done in consultation with a neonatologist.

Antibiotics

Chorioamnionitis is usually due to Group B streptococcal or *Escheria coli* infections. Ampicillin and gentamycin are reasonable empiric antibiotics in a newly born infant with suspected chorioamnionitis (see Chapters 87 Fever in Infants and 102 Infectious Disease Emergencies).

Special Situations

Induced Hypothermia and Hypoxic-ischemic Encephalopathy in Newly Born Infants

Data from large, multicenter, randomized controlled trials have demonstrated that systemic or selective head cooling hypothermia initiated within 6 hours of life, in infants ≥36 weeks reduced death or neurologic disability in infants with moderate or severe hypoxic-ischemic encephalopathy. In a 2012 meta-analysis of 7 studies, induced hypothermia resulted in a 24% decrease in the relative risk of death or major neurodevelopmental disability. The American Academy of Pediatrics Committee on Fetus and Newborn and the AHA guidelines recommend that infants ≥36 weeks' gestation who have moderate to severe hypoxic encephalopathy be offered therapeutic hypothermia. Currently, hypothermia therapy is not recommended for infants less than 36 weeks' gestation but clinical trials are ongoing for this age group.

Induced hypothermia should be done at a facility able to provide comprehensive neonatal care, following studied protocols, initiated within 6 hours of birth and continued for 72 hours. For infants born at centers unable to provide such care, early identification of potential candidates and consultation with experts is critical. Table 4.13 defines criteria for moderate to severe encephalopathy. Ideally, medical centers skilled in hypothermia management and community hospitals should develop educational programs and procedures for transfer.

Meconium

Management of meconium-stained amniotic fluid has changed substantially over the last 2 decades. Meconium staining of the amniotic fluid complicates 12% of all pregnancies; the risk of meconium-related complications increases to nearly 30% in infants born after 42 weeks' gestation. Approximately 2% to 5% of infants born with meconium in the amniotic fluid will experience some degree of aspiration syndrome, ranging from mild tachypnea to very severe pneumonitis with persistent pulmonary hypertension (Fig. 4.18).

When meconium staining is detected during an ED delivery, the infant should be immediately transferred to the resuscitation team without intrapartum suctioning of the infant's mouth and nose (Fig. 4.19). This recommendation is a change from previous guidelines after a multicenter randomized trial showed no decrease in the risk of meconium aspiration syndrome when suctioning was performed after delivery of the infant's head but before delivery of the body.

Current guidelines for further management of newborns with meconium in the amniotic fluid are based on the status of the newborn rather than the consistency of the meconium. If meconium is present and the infant has depressed respirations, muscle tone, or a heart rate <100 bpm—direct suctioning of the trachea soon after delivery is indicated before many respirations have occurred. After delivery, place the infant in a warm environment, and before other resuscitative efforts, intubate the trachea to facilitate suctioning of the lower airway. Because the ET tube itself is the largest diameter item placed in the trachea, it is the most

TABLE 4.13

INDUCED HYPOTHERMIA FOR NEWBORNS

Criteria for moderate to severe encephalopathy[a]
For newly born infant of gestational age ≥36 wks, ≤6 hrs of life
And
1. pH ≤7.0 or base deficit ≥16 mmol/L within 60 min of birth
2. APGAR ≤5 at 10 min after birth or continued need for resuscitation at 10 min after birth
3. Moderate to severe encephalopathy on clinical examination
4. Abnormal EEG

[a]Specific criteria may vary based on individual center's policies.
Adapted from Committee of Fetus and Newborn of American Academy of Pediatrics.

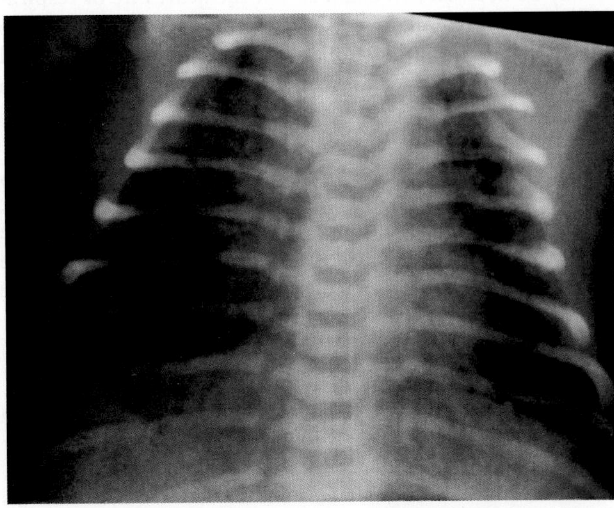

FIGURE 4.18 Meconium aspiration radiograph.

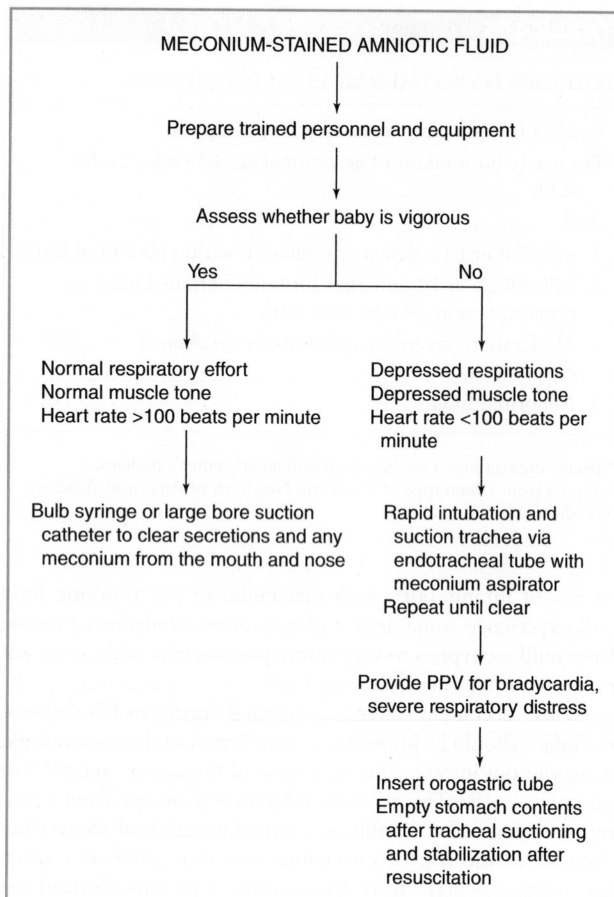
MECONIUM-STAINED AMNIOTIC FLUID
Prepare trained personnel and equipment
Assess whether baby is vigorous
Yes
No
Normal respiratory effort
Normal muscle tone
Heart rate >100 beats per minute
Depressed respirations
Depressed muscle tone
Heart rate <100 beats per minute
Bulb syringe or large bore suction catheter to clear secretions and any meconium from the mouth and nose
Rapid intubation and suction trachea via endotracheal tube with meconium aspirator
Repeat until clear
Provide PPV for bradycardia, severe respiratory distress
Insert orogastric tube
Empty stomach contents after tracheal suctioning and stabilization after resuscitation

FIGURE 4.19 Management of infant born with meconium-stained amniotic fluid. PPV, positive-pressure ventilation.

effective means of suctioning meconium. A meconium aspirator (Fig. 4.20) directly attached between the ET tube and mechanical suction provides a means of meconium removal. Negative pressure is applied by occluding the opening on the side of the aspirator with a finger. Mechanical suctioning should not exceed 100 mm Hg. Repeat intubation and suctioning with another ET tube may be required until the aspirated material is clear. After initial tracheal suctioning, it may be necessary to begin PPV if the heart rate or respirations are severely depressed, despite persistent meconium in the airway. Wait until completion of tracheal suctioning and resuscitation to place an orogastric tube to empty meconium from the newborn's stomach.

When meconium is present and the baby is vigorous (normal respiratory effort and muscle tone, and HR >100 bpm), a bulb syringe or large-bore (12F or 14F) suction catheter is used to clear secretions and any meconium from the mouth and nose. Tracheal suctioning should not be done in vigorous infants, regardless of the consistency of the meconium.

Prematurity

Early involvement of neonatologists and neonatal centers adept in the management of low–birth-weight infants is crucial to improve outcome. Hospitals without neonatal units need easily available guidelines and established relationships

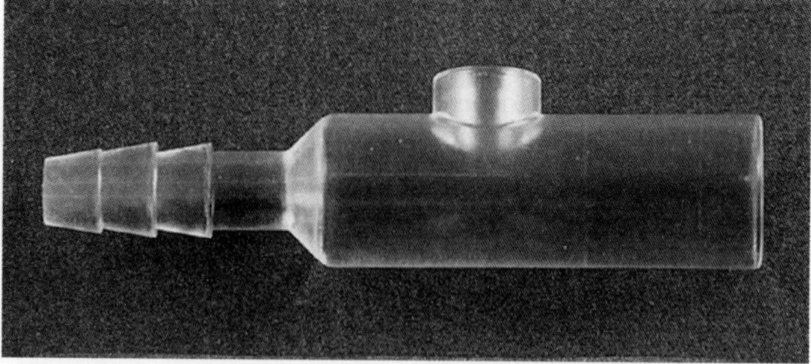

FIGURE 4.20 Meconium aspirator.

for accessing neonatal consultation and transport. Premature infants are at greater risk for bacterial infections, heat loss, inadequate ventilation, and intraventricular hemorrhage. They are more likely to develop respiratory distress and require assisted ventilation. Hyperoxia may lead to complications such as retinopathy of prematurity so beginning the resuscitation with less than 100% inspired oxygen is a reasonable option. If no improvement in heart rate or color occurs by 90 seconds, the fraction of inspired oxygen should be increased. Once the infant is stabilized after initial resuscitative care, the fraction of inspired oxygen can be decreased while monitoring pulse oximetry.

The germinal matrix of the preterm infant's brain is vulnerable to bleeding. Factors contributing to subsequent intracranial hemorrhage include excessive pressure or osmolality delivered to an already maximally dilated vascular bed. Subsequently, in premature infants, hyperosmolar solutions such as 25% dextrose or 8.4% sodium bicarbonate should be avoided. Volume expanders, dextrose, and half-strength sodium bicarbonate solutions, when indicated, should be administered slowly to minimize injury to these vascular beds.

Pneumothorax

Pneumothorax is a potentially lethal problem in the neonate because it can rapidly progress to a tension pneumothorax. It is often the result of PPV, PEEP, or resuscitation. Pneumothorax is also more common in premature infants with surfactant deficiency or meconium aspiration. If significant respiratory distress is present and a pneumothorax is suspected, rapid decompression may be achieved with a large syringe, 20-gauge needle or catheter over needle using a three-way stopcock. The needle is advanced at the fourth intercostal space in the anterior axillary line or the second interspace in the midclavicular line. Subsequently, a chest tube (8F) may be placed using a standard technique (see Chapter 141 Procedures).

Diaphragmatic Hernia

Diaphragmatic hernia is a true neonatal emergency; the diagnosis is confirmed by a chest radiograph showing bowel gas within the thorax (Fig. 4.21). Infants with diaphragmatic hernias require ET intubation to avoid excessive amounts of air accumulation in the bowel. A nasogastric tube should be rapidly placed to decompress the stomach. The infant must be rapidly evaluated by a pediatric surgeon after ventilation is stabilized and venous access is achieved.

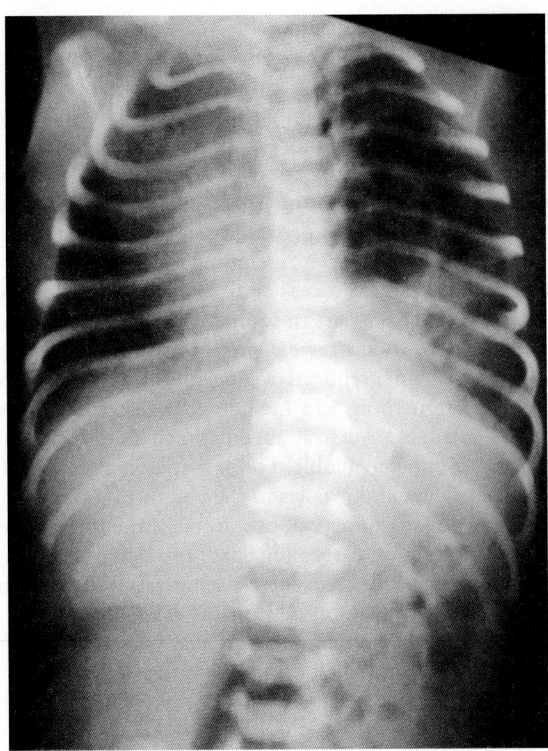

FIGURE 4.21 Left diaphragmatic hernia radiograph.

Stabilization and Transport

After appropriate resuscitative efforts, continuous monitoring and anticipation of complications must occur until the patient is safely transported to a neonatal unit or a facility with a neonatal unit. Priority must be given to thermoregulation. If mechanical ventilation is required, a pressure ventilator should be used. Peak pressures are determined by clinical evaluation of adequate chest wall rise and blood gas analyses. A good starting point for peak pressure is that needed for good chest wall rise and breath sounds during hand ventilation as shown on the manometer, usually between 15 and 30 cm H_2O. Use the lowest pressure necessary for good clinical response and continue to monitor closely. Excessive positive pressure decreases venous return to the heart and thus cardiac output, and causes injury to lung tissue. The patient should be transported by personnel with appropriate expertise along with appropriate equipment and medications.

TEAMWORK IN RESUSCITATION FOR ALL PEDIATRIC PATIENTS

The new PALS and ACLS curricula have incorporated learning modules on leadership, role clarity, and communication. Effective leaders and team members must have cognitive skills (fund of knowledge), technical and procedural skills, and behavioral skills. Postresuscitation team debriefing is increasingly recognized as a critical component in maintaining effective teamwork and communication skills in pediatric resuscitations. Recent information reveals lack of effective teamwork skills and their negative impact on outcomes. Effective education includes challenging active exercises, such as high-fidelity simulation. Video-recording of resuscitation provides another venue for identifying opportunities for improving care processes and for providing constructive feedback on team management skills. Maintenance of competency for physicians working in ED settings includes procedural competency and leadership competency. Developing and maintaining the ability to effectively lead a multidisciplinary team in a high-stakes, high-risk, error-prone environment is necessary and must be thoughtfully considered in this era of decreasing frequency of individual exposure to these patients.

Finally, parental presence in the resuscitation room is recommended by the AAP and should be routine practice. All EDs should have a written policy and a process in place; and all families should be offered this opportunity (see Chapter 1 A General Approach to Ill and Injured Children).

DISCONTINUATION OF LIFE SUPPORT IN CHILDREN

If well-executed resuscitative measures fail to achieve ROSC, resuscitative efforts should be discontinued. There is now good evidence to support that there is no chance for meaningful survival in patients who remain unresponsive to aggressive airway intervention, chest compressions, and two doses of epinephrine after unwitnessed cardiac arrest. Thus, a brief, well-executed resuscitation is indicated for the child who arrives to the ED with cardiopulmonary arrest. This includes definitive airway management; vigorous, monitored chest compressions; IO access; and one to two doses of epinephrine. During this time, the leader of the resuscitation can review the history and complete the primary and secondary survey. Prolonged resuscitation efforts past 20 minutes, without ROSC, are usually futile unless other treatable problems exist such as hypothermia, drug overdose, or VT/VF. Prolonged resuscitation may be indicated for witnessed collapsed arrest, with short onset of effective BLS/ACLS, especially if a cardiac etiology is suspected. Ultimately, the diagnosis of death and subsequent discontinuation of resuscitative efforts is a judgment that is made by the team leader in conjunction with the team. A decision not to begin resuscitation is generally not made in the ED unless there is a written do-not-resuscitate (DNR) document provided by the child's parent or guardian.

A well-prepared ED should consider and have a plan in place for issues such as advanced directives, palliative care, bereavement measures and postmortem care, survivor follow-up, and request for autopsy and organ donations as outlined in the recent AAP guidelines. Proper documentation of a death is essential, as is notification of medical legal authorities, donor programs, and referring physicians and consultants.

CEREBRAL RESUSCITATION

Permanent brain damage following arrest is determined by many factors and includes arrest time (no-flow state), CPR time (low-flow state), and temperature. Cardiopulmonary–cerebral resuscitation is needed to prevent brain injury. Oxygen stores are depleted within 20 seconds following arrest, and glucose and adenosine are depleted within 5 minutes. During no-flow states, multiple complex chemical derangements occur that contribute to the death of neurons. With ROSC, there is impaired cerebral blood flow. Circulatory and pharmacologic interventions to prevent postanoxic brain injury have yielded disappointing results to date.

Hypothermia

The use of mild hypothermia after OHCA due to VF in adults has been associated with improved neurologic outcome and is generally tolerated without significant complication. Current AHA recommendations are to begin therapeutic hypothermia for all adult patients after VT/VF arrest with ROSC to a goal temperature of 32 to 34°C for 12 to 24 hours. The AHA also recommends the use of therapeutic hypothermia in adult patients with ROSC after arrest from other nonshockable rhythms. Data from large, multicenter, randomized controlled trials have demonstrated that therapeutic hyphothermia for asphyxiated newly born infants ≥36 weeks' gestation can reduce death and neurologic disability when initiated within 6 hours of birth. AHA guidelines recommend that all such infants with moderate to severe hypoxic-ischemic encephalopathy be offered therapeutic hypothermia.

However, the data for pediatric patients is less clear. Current AHA guidelines state that therapeutic hypothermia may be considered for children who remain comatose after return of spontaneous circulation following cardiac arrest to a level of 32° to 34°C. It is most reasonable to consider for adolescent patients who are resuscitated from a sudden witnessed VT/VF arrest. Fever adversely affects recovery from ischemic brain injury, and should be treated aggressively; avoiding T >38°C is recommended. A large, multicenter, randomized controlled trial of therapeutic hypothermia after out-of-hospital arrest (published after the most recent AHA guidelines) comparing therapeutic hypothermia to therapeutic normothermia found no difference on survival with good functional outcome.

QUALITY IMPROVEMENT

EDs represent a high-risk environment for the medical care of patients due to factors such as clinical uncertainty, frequent interruptions, and the need for haste. Children are at particular risk in emergency care because of their physical and developmental vulnerabilities, their inability to accurately describe symptoms or past medical history, the complexity of weight-based treatment, and the relative discomfort of some providers in treating pediatric patients. This risk is particularly heightened during emergency resuscitation, which is a team-dependent and information-intensive process of rapidly treating acute life-threatening and organ-threatening diseases. The medical resuscitation environment is especially prone to medical errors due to its fast-paced, complex and information-technology poor environment. Therefore, ongoing surveillance of resuscitation events, with an eye to process and system changes which could support the resuscitation team, minimize distraction from patient care and maximize protocol adherence is vital. A video review process in which all resuscitation events are video recorded, and a subset are reviewed in detail by an open, multidisciplinary committee provides an opportunity to improve. The review process focuses on time to critical events (completion of primary/secondary survey, vascular access, fluid/med administration, etc.), adherence to expected protocols, teamwork measures (including closed loop communication, ambient noise, anticipation of medications and equipment, etc.), specific role performance, and identification of barriers and facilitators to care. Specific resuscitation events are chosen for review through a combination of provider request and identification of the highest-risk scenarios, including the most complex and least common events. Process and system issues, educational deficits, and other barriers to protocol-compliant care identified through the video review process are addressed on an ongoing basis. Interventions to improve quality of care in the resuscitation room can include changes in the physical resources available, such as medications, fluids and equipment, or personnel available. For example, movement of the EZ-IO introducer and needles to the bed during room preparation prior to patient arrival can decrease the time to vascular access. Assigning a second senior physician to supervise CPR and other procedures in resuscitation events requiring CPR, can decrease the burden on the leader physician and increase protocol compliance with CPR. Other interventions to improve care may include simulated resuscitative events to allow for practice of uncommon events. Multidisciplinary simulations that occur in the actual resuscitation environment are most likely to maximize learning and may identify latent barriers to care. In addition, participation in video review, itself, allows for participants to experience patient resuscitations that simulate cognitive decision making for the viewer. Finally, intermittent group review of important findings from the quality improvement efforts, targeted group education modules and personal feedback on given resuscitation events can support improvements in provider behavior to maximize protocol adherence and decrease variability in resuscitation care. It is important that EDs identify a feasible means to monitor resuscitation care and provide ongoing local quality improvement to insure that optimal care is provided in this high-stakes, error-prone environment.

ETHICAL ISSUES IN PEDIATRIC CARDIOPULMONARY RESUSCITATION

There are many ethical issues surrounding pediatric resuscitation: When are resuscitation attempts futile? Is the ED physician obligated to provide care at the families' insistence? How do family religious beliefs play a role in decision making? What is the role of parental presence? Should procedures be performed on the recently dead? Can resuscitation research be performed without informed consent? Some of these issues have been addressed in policy statements made by professional organizations, but each question needs to be considered in discussions that occur at the local ED level.

In response to these varied, complex, and often highly charged issues, postresuscitation debriefing has become a vital component of the pediatric resuscitation. Consider taking a few minutes for critical reflection following the completion of the resuscitation event; this has the potential to enhance teamwork and communication, and provides an opportunity to improve future performance through group reflection on the shared experience.

KEY POINTS

- The vast majority of pediatric cardiac arrests are asphyxia and both survival and neurologic outcome is poor.
- Recognition of impending respiratory and circulatory failure and immediate intervention can be truly life-saving.
- VT/VF is estimated to occur in approximately 10% of OHCA.
- IO is the preferred access for arrested patients, and patients with severe hypotension or other severely ill patients where attempt at IV access is prolonged.
- Airway management and high-quality chest compressions are the key resuscitation interventions.
- All EDs should have program for continuous quality improvements around the care of critically ill children.
- Strong leadership and teamwork with closed loop communication is essential.
- EDs should have practice simulations and skills sessions to assure competency in knowledge and critical resuscitation skills.

Suggested Readings and Key References

Abella BS, Alvarado JP, Myklebust H, et al. Quality of cardiopulmonary resuscitation during in-hospital cardiac arrest. *JAMA* 2005; 293(3):305–310.

Abella BS, Aufderheide TP, Eigel B, et al. Reducing barriers for implementation of bystander-initiated cardiopulmonary resuscitation: a scientific statement from the American Heart Association for healthcare providers, policymakers, and community leaders regarding the effectiveness of cardiopulmonary resuscitation. *Circulation* 2008;117:704–709.

American Academy of Pediatrics, American Heart Association. *PALS provider manual*. Dallas, TX: AHA publication, 2011.

American Heart Association Guidelines 2010 for Cardiopulmonary Resuscitation and Emergency Cardiovascular Care [Supplement]. *Circulation* 2010;122.

Atkins DL, Everson-Stewart S, Sears GK, et al. Epidemiology and outcomes from OHCA in children: The Resuscitation Outcomes Consortium Epistry–Cardiac Arrest. *Circulation* 2009:119(11): 1484–1491.

Atkins DL, Scott WA, Blaufox AD, et al. Sensitivity and specificity of an automated external defibrillator algorithm designed for pediatric patients. *Resuscitation* 2008;76(2):168–174.

Aufderheide TP, Lurie KG. Death by hyperventilation: a common and life-threatening problem during cardiopulmonary resuscitation. *Crit Care Med* 2004;32(9):S345–S351.

Badaki-Makun O, Nadel F, Donoghue A, et al. Chest compression quality over time in pediatric resuscitations. *Pediatrics* 2013;131(3): e797–e804.

Baren JM, Mahon M. End-of-life issues in the pediatric emergency department. *Clin Pediatr Emerg Med* 2003;4:265–272.

Berger TM. Neonatal resuscitation: foetal physiology and pathophysiological aspects. *Eur J Anaesthesiol* 2012;29(8):362–370.

Blumberg SM, Gorn M, Crain EF. Intraosseous infusion: a review of methods and novel devices. *Pediatr Emerg Care* 2008;24(1):50–56.

Bobrow BJ, Vadeboncoeur TF, Stolz U, et al. The influence of scenario-based training and real-time audiovisual feedback on out-of-hospital cardiopulmonary resuscitation quality and survival from out-of-hospital cardiac arrest. *Ann Emerg Med* 2013;62(1): 47–56.e1.

Chalkias A, Xanthos T, Syggelou A, et al. Controversies in neonatal resuscitation. *J Matern Fetal Neonatal Med* 2013;26(suppl 2): 50–54.

Chamberlain JM, Slonim A, Joseph J. Reducing errors and promoting safety in pediatric emergency care. *Ambul Pediatr* 2004;4(1): 55–63.

Chisholm CD, Dornfeld AM, Nelson DR, et al. Work interrupted: a comparison of workplace interruptions in emergency departments and primary care offices. *Ann Emerg Med* 2001;38(2):146–151.

Chitty H, Wyllie J. Importance of maintaining the newly born temperature in the normal range from delivery to admission. *Semin Fetal Neonatal Med* 2013;18(6):362–368.

Committee on Fetus and Newborn, Papile LA, Baley JE, Benitz W, et al. Hypothermia and neonatal encephalopathy. *Pediatrics* 2014; 133(6):1146–1150.

Dawson JA, Kamlin CO, Vento M, et al. Defining the reference range for oxygen saturation for infants after birth. *Pediatrics* 2010; 125(6):e1340–e1347.

Dingeman RS, Mitchell EA, Meyer EC, et al. Parent presence during complex invasive procedures and cardiopulmonary resuscitation: a systematic review of the literature. *Pediatrics* 2007;120:842–854.

Donoghue AJ, Nadkarni V, Berg RA, et al. Out-of-hospital pediatric cardiac arrest: an epidemiologic review and assessment of current knowledge. *Ann Emerg Med* 2005;46:512–522.

Donoghue AJ, Nadkarni VM, Elliott M, et al. Effect of hospital characteristics on outcomes from pediatric cardiopulmonary resuscitation: a report from the national registry of cardiopulmonary resuscitation. *Pediatrics* 2006;118:995–1001.

Duncan JM, Meaney P, Simpson P, et al. Vasopressin for in-hospital pediatric cardiac arrest: Results from the AHA National Registry of CPR. *Pediatr Crit Care Med* 2009;10(2):191–195.

Edelson DP, Abella BS, Kramer-Johansen J, et al. Effects of compression depth and preshock pauses predict defibrillation failure during cardiac arrest. *Resuscitation* 2006;71:137–145.

Ewy GA. Cardiac resuscitation—when is enough enough? *N Engl J Med* 2006;355:510–512.

Fearon DM. Ethical issues in pediatric resuscitation. In: Cahill JD, ed. *Updates in emergency medicine*. New York, NY: Kluwer Academic/Plenum Publishers, 2003:56–63.

Gerein RB, Osmond MH, Stiell IG, et al. What are the etiology and epidemiology of out-of-hospital pediatric cardiopulmonary arrest in Ontario, Canada? *Acad Emerg Med* 2006;13:653–658.

Hallstrom A, Ornato JP, Weisfeldt M, et al. Public-access defibrillation and survival after out-of-hospital cardiac arrest. *N Engl J Med* 2004; 351:637–646.

Hutchings FA, Hillard TN, Davis PJ. Heated humidified high-flow nasal cannula therapy in children. *Arch Dis Child* 2014;0:1–5.

Idris AH, Guffey D, Aufderheide TP, et al. Relationship between chest compression rates and outcomes from cardiac arrest. *Circulation* 2012;125(24):3004–3012.

Johnson MA, Grahan BJ, Haukoos JS, et al. Demographics, bystander CPR, and AED use in out-of-hospital pediatric arrests. *Resuscitation* 2014;85(7):920–926.

Kapadia VS, Wyckoff MH. Drugs during delivery room resuscitation–what, when and why? *Semin Fetal Neonatal Med* 2013;18(6):357–361.

Kattwinkel J, Perlman JM, Aziz K, et al. Part 15: neonatal resuscitation: 2010 American Heart Association Guidelines for Cardiopulmonary Resuscitation and Emergency Cardiovascular Care. *Circulation* 2010; 122(suppl 3):S909–S919.

Kessler DO, Cheng A, Mullan PC. Debriefing in the emergency department after clinical events: a practical guide. *Ann Emerg Med* 2014;65(6):690–698.

Lerner EB, Dayan PS, Brown K, et al. Characteristics of the pediatric patients treated by the Pediatric Emergency Care Applied Research Network's affiliated EMS agencies. *Prehosp Emerg Care* 2014;18(1):52–59.

Martin JA, Hamilton BE, Osterman MJ, et al. Births: final data for 2012. *Nat Vital Stat Rep* 2013;62:9.

McDonald CH, Heggie J, Jones CM, et al. Rescuer fatigue under the 2010 ERC guidelines, and its effect on cardiopulmonary resuscitation (CPR) performance. *Emerg Med J* 2013;30(8):623–627.

McInnes AD, Sutton RM, Orioles A, et al. The first quantitative report of ventilation rate during in-hospital resuscitation of older children and adolescents. *Resuscitation* 2011;82(8):1025–1029.

Mildenhall LF, Huynh TK. Factors modulating effective chest compressions in the neonatal period. *Semin Fetal Neonatal Med* 2013;18(6): 352–356.

Meaney PA, Bobrow BJ, Mancini ME, et al. Cardiopulmonary resuscitation quality: improving cardiac resuscitation outcomes both inside and outside the hospital: a consensus statement from the American Heart Association. *Circulation* 2013;128(4):417–435.

Meaney PA, Nadkarni VM, Cook EF, et al. Higher survival rates among younger patients after pediatric intensive care unit cardiac arrests. *Pediatrics* 2006;118:2424–2433.

Mentzelopoulos SD, Malachias S, Chamos C, et al. Vasopressin, steroids, and epinephrine and neurologically favorable survival after in-hospital cardiac arrest: a randomized clinical trial. *JAMA* 2013;310(3):270–279.

Moler FW, Silverstein FS, Holubkov R, et al. Therapeutic hypothermia after out-of-hospital cardiac arrest in children. *N Engl J Med* 2015;372:1898–1908.

Niles D, Nysaether J, Sutton R, et al. Leaning is common during in-hospital pediatric CPR, and decreased with automated corrective feedback. *Resuscitation* 2009;80(5):553–557.

Ong ME, Pellis T, Link MS. The use of antiarrhythmic drugs for adult cardiac arrest: a systematic review. *Resuscitation* 2011;82(6):665–670.

Raymond TT, Cunnyngham CB, Thompson MT, et al. Outcomes among neonates, infants, and children after extracorporeal cardiopulmonary resuscitation for refractory inhospital pediatric cardiac arrest: a report from the National Registry of Cardiopulmonary Resuscitation. *Pediatr Crit Care Med* 2010;11(3):362–371.

Raymond TT, Stromberg D, Stigal W, et al. Sodium bicarbonate use during in-hospital pulseless cardiac arrest – A report from the American Heart Association Get with the Guidelines-Resuscitation. *Resuscitation* 2015;89:106–115.

Reis AG, Nadkarni V, Perondi MB, et al. A prospective investigation into the epidemiology of in-hospital pediatric cardiopulmonary resuscitation using the international Utstein reporting style. *Pediatrics* 2002;109:200–209.

Samson RA, Nadkarni VM, Meaney PA, et al. Outcomes of in-hospital ventricular fibrillation in children. *N Engl J Med* 2006; 354(22):2328–2339.

Sayre MR, Berg RA, Cave DM, et al. Hands-only (compression-only) cardiopulmonary resuscitation: a call to action for bystander response to adults who experience out-of-hospital sudden cardiac arrest: a science advisory for the public from the American Heart Association Emergency Cardiovascular Care Committee. *Circulation* 2008;117:2162–2167.

Srinivasan V, Morris MC, Helfaer MA, et al. Calcium use during in-hospital pediatric cardiopulmonary resuscitation: a report from the National Registry of Cardiopulmonary Resuscitation. *Pediatrics* 2008;121:e1144–e1151.

Stiell IG, Brown SP, Christenson J, et al. What is the role of chest compression depth during out-of-hospital cardiac arrest resuscitation? *Crit Care Med* 2012:40(4):1192–1198.

Sutton RM, French B, Nishisaki A, et al. AHA CPR quality targets are associated with improved arterial blood pressure during pediatric cardiac arrest. *Resuscitation* 2013;84(2):168–172.

Sutton RM, Maltese MR, Niles D, et al. Quantitative analysis of chest compression interruptions during in-hospital resuscitation of older children and adolescents. *Resuscitation* 2009;80(11): 1259–1263.

Sutton RM, Wolfe H, Nishisaki A, et al. Pushing harder, pushing faster, minimizing interruptions but falling short of 2010 CPR targets during in-hospital pediatric and adolescent resuscitation. *Resuscitation* 2013;84(12):1680–1684.

Tagin MA, Woolcott CG, Vincer MJ, et al. Hypothermia for neonatal hypoxic ischemic encephalopathy: an updated systematic review and meta-analysis. *Arch Pediatr Adolesc Med* 2012;166(6):558–566.

Valdes SO, Donoghue AJ, Hoyme DB, et al. Outcomes associated with amiodarone and lidocaine in the treatment of in-hospital pediatric cardiac arrest with pulseless ventricular tachycardia or ventricular fibrillation. *Resuscitation* 2014;85(3):381–386.

Wallace SK, Abella BS, Becker LB. Quantifying the effect of cardiopulmonary resuscitation quality on cardiac arrest outcome: a systematic review and meta-analysis. *Circ Cardiovasc Qual Outcomes* 2013; 6(2):148–156.

Wik L, Kramer-Johansen J, Myklebust HB, et al. Quality of cardiopulmonary resuscitation during out-of-hospital cardiac arrest. *JAMA* 2005;293(3):299–304.

Yilidzdas D, Horoz OO, Erdem S. Beneficial effects of terlipressin in pediatric cardiac arrest. *Pediatr Emerg Care* 2011;27(9):865–868.

Young KD, Gausche-Hill M, McClung CD, et al. A prospective, population-based study of the epidemiology and outcome of out-of-hospital pediatric cardiopulmonary arrest. *Pediatrics* 2004;114: 157–164.

Young KD, Seidel J. Pediatric cardiopulmonary resuscitation: a collective review. *Ann Emerg Med* 1999;33:195–205.

CHAPTER 5 ■ SHOCK

FRAN BALAMUTH, MD, PhD, MSCE, JULIE FITZGERALD, MD, PhD, AND SCOTT L. WEISS, MD, MSCE

DEFINITION OF SHOCK

Normal circulatory function is maintained by a complex interplay between the central pump (heart) and blood flow at the regional level (microcirculation) for the purpose of delivering oxygen and nutrients to tissues and removing metabolic by-products (e.g., carbon dioxide). *Shock* can be defined as an acute syndrome of cardiovascular dysfunction in which the circulatory system fails to provide adequate oxygen and nutrients to meet the metabolic demands of vital organs. This definition recognizes that shock can and does exist without hypotension, especially in children. Furthermore, as knowledge of the pathophysiology of the shock state has evolved, it is now clear that inadequate cellular metabolism of oxygen and nutrients also contributes to the clinical manifestations and outcomes observed in patients with shock.

GOALS OF EMERGENCY THERAPY

All physicians who care for ill children will be faced with managing the clinical syndrome of shock. Many common childhood illnesses, such as trauma, gastroenteritis, infection, and accidental drug ingestions, can lead to shock. Ultimately, without timely medical intervention, the child in shock will follow a common pathway to multiorgan system failure and death. Early recognition and appropriate therapy are vital if we hope to reduce the morbidity and mortality associated with this serious syndrome.

The goals of emergency therapy in pediatric shock are threefold:

- Prompt recognition
- Shock reversal
- Transfer to definitive care

This chapter is devoted to addressing each of these goals in turn. We begin with a discussion of clinical and pathophysiologic considerations in pediatric shock, followed by a description of different etiologic types of shock including hypovolemic, cardiogenic, obstructive, distributive (septic), and dissociative shock (Fig. 5.1). The remainder of the chapter is focused on pediatric shock recognition and clinical management including diagnostic testing, fluid resuscitation, vasoactive agent choice, source control, treatment of refractory shock, and transfer to definitive care. Because increasing evidence has accumulated indicating that care for patients with septic shock can be improved through the utilization of protocolized or bundled goal-directed therapy, we include a discussion on quality improvement initiatives utilizing a bundled approach for septic shock.

RELATED CHAPTERS

Resuscitation and Stabilization
- A General Approach to Ill and Injured Children: Chapter 1

Signs and Symptoms
- Dehydration: Chapter 17
- Fever: Chapter 26
- Septic Appearing Infant: Chapter 68
- Tachycardia: Chapter 72
- Triage: Chapter 73

Clinical Pathways
- Fever in Infants: Chapter 87
- Shock: Chapter 91

Medical/Surgical/Trauma Emergencies
- Allergic Emergencies: Chapter 93
- Cardiac Emergencies: Chapter 94
- Infectious Disease Emergencies: Chapter 102
- Metabolic Emergencies: Chapter 103
- Toxicologic Emergencies: Chapter 110
- Neck Trauma: Chapter 120

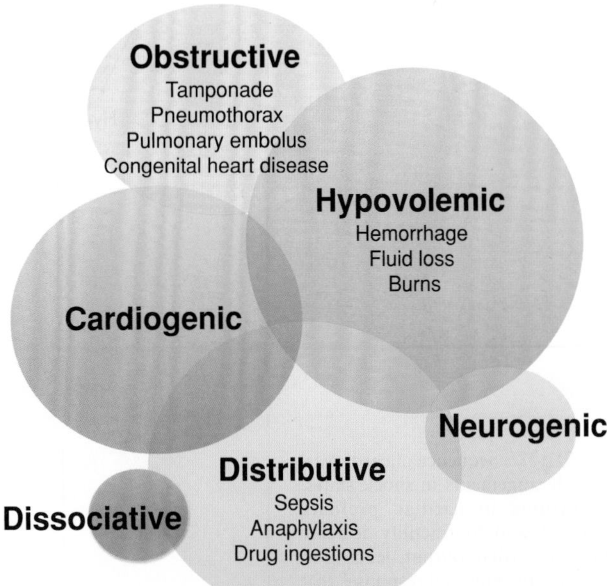

FIGURE 5.1 Etiologic types of shock. The size of each circle is proportional to the incidence of each shock type. Although distinct etiologies are evident, there is considerable overlap in the clinical presentation and underlying pathophysiology between categories.

CLINICAL AND PATHOPHYSIOLOGIC CONSIDERATIONS

Delivery of oxygen and nutrients is predominantly regulated by cardiac output and microvascular blood flow. Cardiac output is calculated by multiplying the stroke volume (volume of blood ejected by the left ventricle) by the heart rate (ejection cycles per minute). The stroke volume depends on the filling volume of the ventricle (preload), myocardial contractility and rhythm, and the systemic vascular resistance (SVR) against which the ventricle is pumping blood to the body (afterload). Heart rate, preload, contractility, rhythm, and afterload are regulated through a variety of neurohumoral and metabolic factors, including the sympathetic nervous system, endogenous catecholamine release, tissue pH and oxygen tension, nitric oxide, reactive oxygen species, and calcium homeostasis, that themselves respond to changes in blood volume, circulating inflammatory cytokines, and endothelial cell activation (Fig. 5.2). Infants require special consideration, as they have relatively little reserve myocardial contractility to increase stroke volume and thus depend almost exclusively on heart rate to increase cardiac output.

Blood pressure is determined by both cardiac output and SVR and is generally used as a clinical surrogate for tissue perfusion. While low blood pressure will reduce oxygen and nutrient delivery to tissues, the absence of hypotension in children should not be taken to mean that organ perfusion is adequate since efforts to compensate for changes in cardiac output and SVR may initially preserve blood pressure. Early signs of shock with a normal blood pressure, referred to as *compensated shock,* include tachycardia, mild tachypnea, slightly delayed capillary refill (more than 2 to 3 seconds), cool extremities, orthostatic changes in blood pressure or pulse, decreased urine output, and subtle changes in mental status (e.g., mild irritability or sleepiness). In some cases of distributive shock, such as sepsis or anaphylaxis, a fall in SVR due to peripheral vasodilation may lead to the findings of "bounding" pulses, flash capillary refill, and widened pulse pressure. In addition to these clinical signs, biochemical changes such as an increased base deficit or blood lactate level, may also signal diminished organ perfusion early in shock.

As shock continues, early compensatory mechanisms fail to maintain cardiac output and SVR and blood pressure falls. Shock with hypotension is referred to as *uncompensated shock*. In addition to hypotension, clinical signs include worsening tachycardia (or bradycardia in infants) and tachypnea, mottled skin, cold extremities, and markedly delayed capillary refill (>4 seconds). Tachypnea and respiratory distress may herald underlying pulmonary disease, but may also reflect an increase in minute ventilation (to decrease $PaCO_2$) to compensate for an increasing metabolic acidosis. Signs of organ dysfunction are typically evident, including further alterations in mental status (agitation, confusion, lethargy, stupor), gastrointestinal ileus, azotemia, coagulopathy, thrombocytopenia, and hyperbilirubinemia.

All types of shock encompass some degree of absolute or functional hypovolemia. Absolute hypovolemia exists in cases of dehydration from fluid losses (e.g., diarrhea, severe emesis, hyperthermia), hemorrhage, and "third spacing" of fluid due to increased vascular permeability, as in sepsis. Functional hypovolemia exists when vascular capacity increases, as in septic shock, spinal cord injury, anaphylaxis, or certain

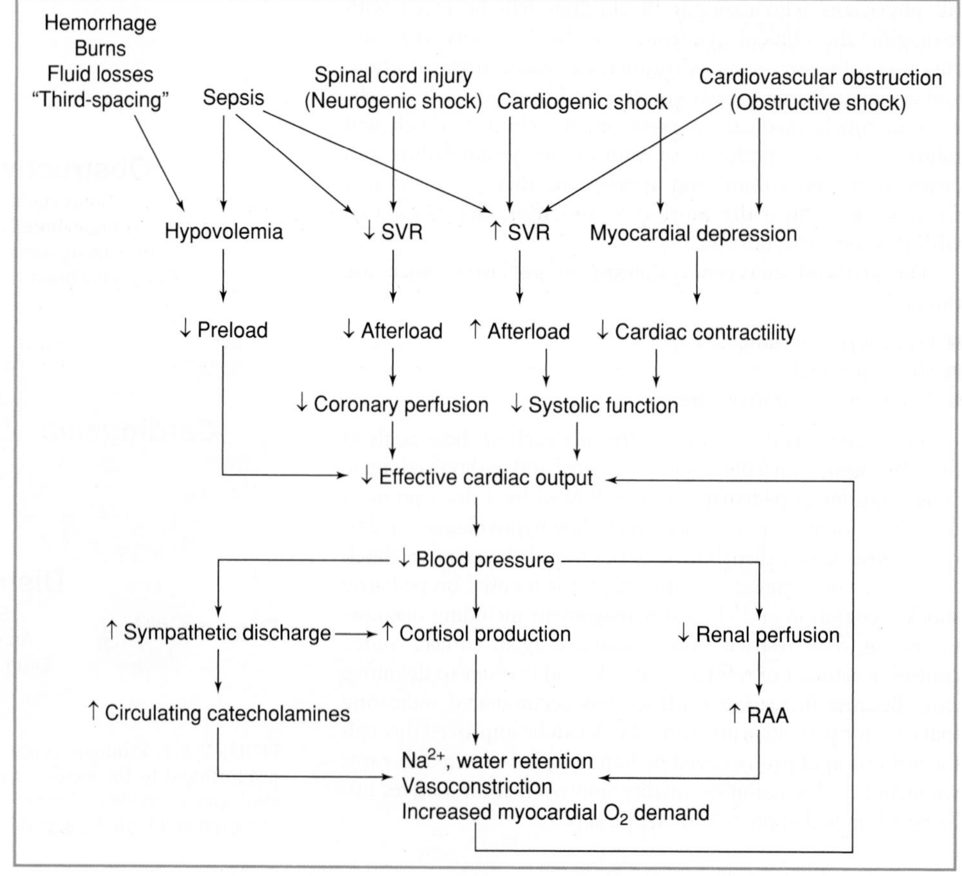

FIGURE 5.2 Sequence of cardiovascular derangements in shock states. Alterations in cardiac preload, afterload, and contractility decrease effective cardiac output, leading to several neurohumoral responses that attempt to restore organ perfusion. As the shock state progresses, these compensatory mechanisms fail to maintain effective cardiac output and clinical deterioration from *compensated* to *uncompensated* shock becomes evident.

medication effects. In addition to volume loss, microcirculatory dysfunction is characterized by a maldistribution of capillary blood flow and is common to all types of shock. Even with reestablishment of global circulation, the activation of inflammatory cytokines in response to pathogen-associated molecular patterns (PAMPs) from invading microorganisms in sepsis and danger-associated molecular patterns (DAMPs) from cell injury in trauma, as well as endothelial cell activation and microthrombi formation, leads to regional changes in blood flow within and across organ systems. This contributes to local tissue ischemia that fuels a vicious cycle of tissue injury and inflammation that can result in the multiorgan dysfunction syndrome (MODS). Furthermore, a second wave of *reperfusion injury* may occur due to an increase in oxidant and nitrogenous stress even after the primary insult of decreased tissue perfusion in shock is corrected.

The inability of cells to efficiently utilize oxygen to produce energy in the form of ATP has been termed "cytopathic hypoxia" and is largely attributable to mitochondrial bioenergetic dysfunction. The inability of mitochondria to use oxygen to sustain ATP production results in an energy deficit that can impair cellular metabolism and, ultimately, organ function. Mitochondrial dysfunction has been postulated to explain the increasingly recognized paradox of progressive organ injury following shock (particularly in sepsis and after trauma) despite minimal cell death even after restoration of tissue oxygen delivery.

TYPES OF SHOCK

Table 5.1 compares clinical findings by type of shock including some common examples.

Hypovolemic Shock. Hypovolemia (decreased circulating blood volume) is the most common cause of shock in children. Volume losses from vomiting and diarrhea secondary to gastrointestinal infections are most prevalent etiology of *hypovolemic shock* worldwide. Other causes of hypovolemic shock include hemorrhage (trauma, postsurgical, gastrointestinal), plasma losses (burns, hypoproteinemia, pancreatitis), and extragastrointestinal water losses (glycosuric diuresis, heat stroke). Acute hypovolemia results in decreased cardiac output due to a fall in preload with a compensatory increase in heart rate and SVR. A fall in blood pressure detected within the baroreceptors of the carotid sinus leads to an increase in the sympathetic nervous system activity, stimulating cardiac chronotropy and vascular smooth muscle constriction as well as epinephrine release from the adrenal medulla. Upregulation of the renin–angiotensin–aldosterone (RAA) system and release of antidiuretic hormone (ADH) from the posterior pituitary gland promote sodium and water retention by the kidneys. Angiotensin II is also a direct vasoconstrictor, contributing to the observed increase in SVR.

Cardiogenic Shock. The term *cardiogenic shock* is generally reserved for a decrease in cardiac output resulting from a decrease in myocardial contractility. Shock due to obstruction of blood flow from certain types of congenital heart lesions is better classified as *obstructive shock* (see below). Although myocardial depression can occur in all forms of shock, primary deficits in myocardial contractility leading to cardiogenic shock are caused by viral myocarditis, anomalous left coronary artery arising from the pulmonary artery (ALCAPA), incessant arrhythmias, drug ingestions (e.g., cocaine), metabolic derangements (e.g., hypoglycemia), and postoperative complications of cardiac surgery. Characteristic signs of cardiogenic shock are congestive heart failure, including pulmonary rales, a gallop cardiac rhythm, hepatomegaly, jugular venous distention, pitting peripheral edema, and cardiomegaly on chest radiograph. Laboratory findings of elevated creatine kinase, troponin, or brain natriuretic protein (BNP) levels may herald myocardial dysfunction, but are not universally present. As in hypovolemic shock, upregulation of the sympathetic nervous system, RAA system, and ADH, as well as the natriuretic peptides (BNP and atrial natriuretic peptide) raise SVR to compensate for a low cardiac output. Unlike hypervolemia, however, the volume deficit

TABLE 5.1

CLINICAL CHARACTERISTICS BY TYPE OF SHOCK

Shock type	Examples	HR	BP	CO	Capillary refill	Extremity temperature	SVR	Treatment
Hypovolemic	Hemorrhage Dehydration	↑	↓	↓	Delayed	Cool	High	Stop bleeding Fluid resuscitation
Cardiogenic	Myocarditis Dysrhythmia	↑	↓	↓	Delayed	Cool	High	Inotropes Caution with fluids ECMO
Distributive	Sepsis Anaphylaxis	↑	↓	↓ or ↑	Flash or delayed	Warm or cool	Low or high	Antibiotics, fluids Epinephrine
Neurogenic	Spinal cord injury Traumatic brain injury	↓	↓	↓	Flash or normal	Warm	Low	Fluid resuscitation Vasopressors
Obstructive	Tamponade Tension pneumothorax	↑	↓	↓	Delayed	Cool	High	Pericardiocentesis Chest tube
Dissociative	Carbon monoxide Cyanide	↑	Normal or ↑	↑	Normal	Normal	Low to normal	Antidotes Hyperbaric therapy

HR, heart rate; BP, blood pressure; CO, cardiac output; SVR, systemic vascular resistance.

is functional (decreased effective circulating blood volume) rather than absolute (see Chapter 94 Cardiac Emergencies).

Obstructive Shock. An acute mechanical obstruction to ventricular outflow can result in *obstructive shock*. Causes include proximal pulmonary embolus, cardiac tamponade, tension pneumothorax, and obstructive lesions of the left side of heart (hypertrophic left heart syndrome, aortic coarctation, interrupted aortic arch, and critical aortic valve stenosis). An acute increase in SVR results from a sudden decrease in cardiac output and functional hypovolemia. Rapid recognition of the cause of obstructive shock is critical in order to implement the correct therapy. Congenital heart lesions typically present at 1 to 3 weeks postnatal age, following closure of the ductus arteriosus.

Distributive Shock. *Distributive shock* results from inappropriate vasodilation and pooling of blood in the peripheral vasculature. Common causes in children are sepsis, anaphylaxis, and drug ingestions (e.g., atypical antipsychotics). Rarely is distributive shock present without other types of shock, most notably hypovolemic shock.

Pediatric sepsis is defined as the *systemic inflammatory response syndrome (SIRS),* which includes either an abnormal temperature or leukocyte count along with tachycardia/bradycardia and/or tachypnea, in the presence of a confirmed or suspected invasive infection. Severe sepsis is defined as sepsis plus (1) cardiovascular dysfunction, (2) acute respiratory distress syndrome, or (3) ≥2 organ system dysfunctions. Septic shock refers to the subset of patients with cardiovascular dysfunction. In 2005, approximately 75,000 children were hospitalized with severe sepsis in the United States at $4.8 billion in healthcare costs and an estimated mortality of 8.9%. Although many patients who appear to have sepsis, severe sepsis, or septic shock have negative cultures, exposure to microbial components (e.g., endotoxin, lipoteichoic acid, viral proteins) is believed to trigger a cascade of inflammatory, coagulation, and vascular mediators that result in severe capillary leak (causing hypovolemia), myocardial depression, and vasomotor instability. Although classic septic shock results in hyperdynamic cardiac function and low SVR that manifest as "warm" shock, more than half of children with septic shock exhibit low cardiac output and elevated SVR, or "cold" shock.

In anaphylaxis, the sudden release of preformed histamine, proteases (tryptase, chymase), and proteoglycans (heparin) in mast cells followed by prostaglandins and leukotrienes leads to the classic symptoms of the skin and respiratory tract, as well as a profound vasodilatory response resulting in a low SVR state along with capillary leak causing hypovolemia. The resulting neurohumoral response leads to an increase in heart rate and contractility that raise cardiac output (see Chapter 93 Allergic Emergencies).

Neurogenic Shock. *Neurogenic shock* is a special cause of distributive shock resulting from the sudden disruption of sympathetic nerve stimulation to the vascular smooth vessel leading to a profound decrease in SVR. Unlike other types of shock, the unopposed vagal activity classically results in bradycardia or, at least, absence of the usual tachycardic response to hypotension. Neurogenic shock can be seen following severe traumatic brain or cervical spine injury (see Chapter 120 Neck Trauma).

Dissociative Shock. Dissociative shock is a special category of shock that occurs as a consequence to a toxic metabolite or drug that severely impairs cellular oxygen delivery or utilization despite sustained or supranormal tissue perfusion. Examples include severe anemia, methemoglobinemia, and carbon monoxide poisoning (see Chapter 110 Toxicologic Emergencies).

CLINICAL CONSIDERATIONS IN SHOCK RECOGNITION

An ongoing clinical challenge is the early recognition of children with compensated shock. We include here a detailed discussion about early septic shock recognition, but the principles discussed can be applied to multiple shock types. Because hypotension is a late finding in pediatric shock, children often present with tachycardia alone. Although adults have often used vital sign criteria based on the SIRS to identify patients with compensated shock, the high prevalence of SIRS in the pediatric emergency setting in patients without sepsis, as well as the overall rarity of sepsis in children with infectious illness, precludes using these vital sign–based criteria alone to recognize sepsis.

Vital Signs

Despite the challenges of identifying the pediatric patient with compensated septic shock, which is often described as "finding a needle in a haystack," there is increasing interest from hospitals, professional medical societies, and legislative bodies to put systems in place to improve sepsis recognition. Vital sign–based sepsis alert systems that are embedded in the electronic medical record are one such mechanism. Although there is evidence that such alerts can improve the sensitivity of sepsis recognition, the use of such alerts must be accompanied by a detailed physician evaluation at the bedside. In addition, the impact of vital sign–based electronic alerts on sepsis overidentification, antibiotic overuse, and other balancing measures in the emergency department, remains to be fully evaluated.

History and Physical Examination Findings

In addition to vital signs, there are elements of history and physical examination that should be assessed to recognize compensated and decompensated shock.

Hypovolemic Shock

Hemorrhagic Shock. Determine by history whether there was possible trauma, and if so whether it was blunt or penetrating. The provider should also determine whether any source of bleeding was recognized prior to arrival (e.g., hematemesis, hemoptysis, vaginal bleeding, hematochezia). The emergency provider also needs to have a high index of suspicion for nonaccidental trauma in a child presenting in shock with no other preceding symptoms.

- Trauma or suspected trauma patients should undergo a full trauma evaluation including the primary and secondary surveys as detailed in Chapter 2 Approach to the Injured Child.
- Careful evaluation for evidence of bleeding including assessment of open fontanelles, all orifices, and thorough abdominal examination.

Dehydration. Determine if volume loss may be due to decreased intake or increased output (vomiting, diarrhea). On physical examination, one should assess the following:

- Mental status/level of activity
- Sunken fontanelle and/or eyes
- Skin turgor
- Capillary refill
- Urine output

Cardiogenic Shock. Cardiogenic shock is often difficult to distinguish from other shock states, as a prolonged history of worsening symptoms is less common in children as compared to adult heart failure. Historical information should be obtained regarding chest pain, syncope, known cardiac abnormalities, and cardiac medications. On physical examination, one should assess the following:

- Neck: Jugular venous distention
- Cardiac: Murmur, gallop, perfusion abnormalities including delayed capillary refill, diminished or bounding pulses
- Respiratory: Respiratory distress, rales to suggest pulmonary edema
- Abdomen: Hepatomegaly
- Extremities: Peripheral edema, delayed capillary refill

Obstructive Shock. On physical examination, one should assess the following:

- Neck: Jugular venous distention
- Cardiac: Murmur, gallop
- Respiratory: Unilateral decreased breath sounds suspicious for tension pneumothorax
- Abdomen: Hepatomegaly
- Extremities/skin: Poor perfusion, cyanosis in unrepaired congenital heart disease including differential perfusion, and cyanosis between the upper and lower extremities to indicate interrupted aortic arch or critical aortic coarctation
- Beck triad in cardiac tamponade: Distended neck veins, hypotension, diminished heart sounds

Distributive Shock

Septic Shock. The provider should determine by history whether the patient has any underlying conditions which may predispose them to septic shock including neonatal age, innate or acquired immunodeficiency or immunosuppression (including malignancy, sickle cell disease and other causes of asplenia, bone marrow or solid organ transplant), or the presence of an indwelling central venous catheter or other invasive hardware. In addition, they should evaluate carefully for evidence of end-organ dysfunction on physical examination as described by organ system below (and summarized in Table 5.2):

- Cardiac: Poor perfusion (including diminished or bounding pulses, flash capillary refill or delayed >3 seconds, and abnormally cool or warm extremities)

TABLE 5.2

ORGAN DYSFUNCTION DEFINITIONS (ADAPTED FROM INTERNATIONAL CONSENSUS CONFERENCE STATEMENT)

Organ system	Definition of dysfunction
Cardiovascular	Despite administration of isotonic IV fluid bolus of at least 40 mL/kg in 1 hr, presence of ANY of the following: • Hypotension <5th percentile for age • Need for vasoactive medication to maintain normal blood pressure • Two of the following: ▪ Unexplained metabolic acidosis (base deficit >5 mEq/L) ▪ Increased arterial lactate >2× upper limit of normal ▪ Oliguria: Urine output <0.5 mg/kg/hr ▪ Prolonged capillary refill >5 s ▪ Core to peripheral temperature gap >3°C
Respiratory	Presence of ANY of the following: • PaO_2/FiO_2 <300 in absence of cyanotic heart disease or pre-existing lung disease • $PaCO_2$ >65 Torr or 20 mm Hg over baseline $PaCO_2$ • Proven need for >50% FiO_2 to maintain saturation >92% • Need for nonelective invasive or noninvasive mechanical ventilation
Neurologic	Presence of EITHER: • Glasgow coma score ≤11 • Acute change in mental status with a decrease in Glasgow Coma Score ≥3 points from abnormal baseline
Hematologic	Presence of EITHER: • Platelet count <80,000/mm^3 • Decline of 50% platelet count from highest value recorded over past 3 days (for chronic hematology/oncology patients) • International normalized ratio >2
Renal	Presence of EITHER: • Serum creatinine ≥2× upper limit of normal for age • Twofold increase in baseline creatinine
Hepatic	Presence of EITHER: • Total bilirubin ≥4 mg/dL (not applicable for newborn) • ALT 2× upper limit of normal for age

- Respiratory: Tachypnea, signs of respiratory distress or failure
- Hematologic: Rashes suspicious for disseminated intravascular coagulation such as petechiae or purpura; or a toxin-mediated process manifested as erythroderma
- Neurologic: Altered mental status
- Renal: Decreased urine output

Anaphylaxis. The provider should determine by history whether the patient has any known or suspected allergies to food, medications, or environmental allergens, as well as evaluate for the following physical findings:

- HEENT: Facial or mouth/tongue swelling
- Cardiac: Poor perfusion, hypotension as above
- Respiratory: Respiratory distress, wheezing, stridor
- Skin: Urticarial rash

Diagnostic Testing in Septic Shock. Laboratory testing in suspected septic shock is focused on determining evidence of end-organ dysfunction and recommended testing is listed by organ system below (and is summarized in Table 5.3):

- Cardiac: Lactate, base deficit, central venous oxygen saturation ($ScvO_2$) (if central line present) measured by cooximetry
- Respiratory: Blood gas if clinically indicated
- Hematologic: Complete blood count to assess for leukopenia, anemia, thrombocytopenia, coagulation studies
- Renal: Serum creatinine
- Hepatic: Transaminases, bilirubin

TABLE 5.3

RECOMMENDED LABORATORY TESTING IN SUSPECTED SEPSIS

Recommended laboratory testing in suspected sepsis	
Source testing	• Blood culture • Urinalysis, urine culture • Consider other cultures based on suspected source (e.g., lumbar puncture, drainage of abscess, or fluid collection) • CXR and other focused radiologic studies • Influenza and other viral testing • Consider procalcitonin, C-reactive protein as biomarkers for presence of infection
Perfusion	• Lactate • Base deficit • Central venous oxygen saturation ($ScvO_2$)
Respiratory	• Blood gas if clinically indicated
Hematologic	• Complete blood count • Coagulation studies (PTT, PT/INR, fibrinogen, D-dimer)
Renal	• Serum creatinine
Hepatic	• Transaminases (ALT, AST) • Bilirubin • Albumin

- Microbiologic: Blood culture, other bacterial testing based on suspected source (e.g., urinalysis, urine culture, chest x-ray, lumbar puncture, etc.)

There have been efforts to determine whether additional laboratory testing including white blood cell count, immature neutrophils, C-reactive protein (CRP), and procalcitonin may have predictive value in children with compensated shock. Increased procalcitonin and CRP have both been associated with an increased likelihood of bacterial infection. Serum lactate levels in the emergency department have also been used to stratify risk of organ dysfunction in pediatric sepsis and risk of death at the time of pediatric intensive care unit (PICU) admission. While these biomarkers may suggest a patient is more likely to require treatment for bacterial sepsis, optimal thresholds and their clinical utility have yet to be demonstrated rigorously.

Attempts have also been made to risk stratify critically ill pediatric patients with sepsis using RNA-based gene expression profiling to identify clinically useful protein biomarkers. Using genome-wide association studies, a pediatric sepsis biomarker risk model has been developed and validated to predict mortality in a cohort of critically ill children with septic shock and includes the following panel of serum biomarkers: Chemokine ligand 3, interleukin 8, heat shock protein 70 KDa 1B, granzyme B, and metallopeptidase 8.

Neurogenic Shock. Assess for evidence of spinal cord injury or severe traumatic brain injury.

Neonates with Shock. Very young infants (<28 days) can present with shock from a variety of causes, and are mentioned separately here due to challenges in shock recognition and differences in treatment in this vulnerable population. Neonates with shock can decompensate very rapidly. They certainly can present in a similar fashion to older children with the signs and symptoms described above, but also can present in a decompensated state with hypothermia, apnea, and bradycardia. A broad differential diagnosis should be maintained including sepsis, undiagnosed congenital heart disease (Chapter 68 Septic Appearing Infant), metabolic disease, and trauma (accidental or nonaccidental).

PRINCIPLES OF SHOCK MANAGEMENT

The mainstays of shock treatment are rapid recognition of the compensated or uncompensated shock state, rapid reversal of shock, and identification and treatment of the underlying etiology of shock. Important aspects of shock reversal include assessment of airway patency and adequacy of breathing, provision of supplemental oxygen, establishment of vascular access, restoration of the circulating blood volume, support of the cardiac and vascular system with appropriate vasoactive agents when necessary, and frequent reassessment of the patient's response. The management strategies discussed in the following sections apply to all shock types, with additional discussion at the end of the section for type-specific management recommendations.

Vascular Access

Intravenous (IV) access should be established immediately, preferably with two large bore peripheral IVs. If peripheral IV access cannot be obtained within the first 5 minutes of shock recognition, intraosseous access should be established until more definitive vascular access can be obtained. Central venous access should be strongly considered if the patient has fluid refractory shock (e.g., remains in shock despite rapid administration of at least 60 mL per kg of fluid resuscitation) or if vasoactive agents are initiated. For those in refractory shock, central venous access also allows for monitoring of important goal-directed therapy targets, such as central venous pressure (CVP) and $ScvO_2$. Arterial blood pressure monitoring with an intra-arterial line is also recommended for children in fluid refractory shock. An arterial catheter provides continuous monitoring of the arterial blood pressure to aid in titration of fluid resuscitation and vasoactive infusions and enables access to serially monitor arterial blood gases to follow acidosis and lactate that can help to guide adequacy of resuscitation. Although central venous access and arterial access are more commonly established following transfer to definitive care in the PICU, advanced vascular access could be obtained in the ED setting if immediate transfer to definitive care is not feasible and there is a provider available experienced in the placement of these devices in children in shock.

Volume Resuscitation

Several studies of pediatric shock have shown decreased mortality with early and aggressive fluid resuscitation, and the current recommendation is to administer fluid in 20 mL per kg boluses pushed over 5 minutes, with reassessment of perfusion and vital signs during and after each fluid bolus. Fluid boluses totaling up to and over 60 mL per kg should be administered if the child remains in shock, with a goal of delivering at least 60 mL per kg in the first 20 to 60 minutes if shock persists. Additional fluid resuscitation should be reconsidered if hepatomegaly or signs of pulmonary edema develop. In addition, caution should be taken with rapid fluid resuscitation in neonates <30 days of age, and in patients with known or suspected cardiac or renal disease or suspected cardiogenic shock. For these patients, smaller boluses of 5 to 10 mL per kg are prudent with frequent reassessment to determine clinical response. The recent FEAST trial in sub-Saharan Africa, which is discussed in more detail below, has called into question the paradigm of aggressive fluid resuscitation in pediatric septic shock, and more study is warranted to fully answer this question.

Fluid should be administered via IV push or a rapid infuser system to achieve the time goals set by the Surviving Sepsis Campaign. IV push delivery may be facilitated by attaching a large syringe with a three-way stopcock to the IV tubing from the IV fluid bag, creating a so-called "push–pull system" that allows the user to rapidly draw up fluid into the syringe and then administer via IV push without repeatedly disconnecting and reconnecting the syringe to the patient's IV. In larger patients >50 kg, a pressure bag or rapid infuser may be used to rapidly administer large volumes of fluid through a large gauge peripheral IV over the goal of 5 minutes.

The optimal fluid choice for resuscitation remains a matter of debate. While Maitland et al. showed reduction in mortality in shock related to malaria with albumin versus crystalloid resuscitation and the adult SAFE study showed a trend toward improved survival in subgroup analysis of patients with septic shock receiving albumin versus crystalloid, many other studies have shown no differences in outcome with a colloid versus crystalloid resuscitation strategy. Furthermore, the SAFE study showed worse outcomes in the subgroup analysis of patients with traumatic brain injury who received colloid resuscitation. Until further data become available, use of crystalloids (0.9% saline or lactated Ringer solution) is generally more common for initial fluid resuscitation due to their availability, ease of administration, and low cost. There is increasing evidence supporting a risk of renal injury with the use of synthetic colloids, such as hydroxyethyl starch, and its use is currently not recommended by the Surviving Sepsis Campaign.

The use of blood products for volume expansion is another important consideration, especially in hemorrhagic shock. The *Advanced Trauma Life Support* guidelines recommend resuscitation with crystalloid and blood products for Class III and IV hemorrhagic shock (see Chapter 2 Approach to the Injured Child for more details on trauma). Based on the Rivers et al. study of adult septic shock, and a follow-up pediatric study by Oliveira et al., packed red blood cells should also be administered to maintain a goal hemoglobin >10 g per dL and an $ScvO_2$ >70% for children with *fluid-refractory* septic shock during the early stages of resuscitation.

As mentioned above, there are several instances in which the provider should be very cautious about using aggressive fluid resuscitation, as it may worsen the shock state. If signs of hepatomegaly or pulmonary edema develop, ongoing fluid resuscitation should be reevaluated. It is also important to perform ongoing clinical assessment of the patient response to fluid administration. If there is underlying congenital heart disease, fluid administration could precipitate or worsen congestive heart failure. Similarly, if myocarditis is suspected, fluid administration should proceed cautiously, with initial volumes of 5 to 10 mL per kg rather than 20 mL per kg. Finally, in patients with pre-existing oliguric or anuric renal failure judicious fluid administration is important as the child may not be able to mobilize the administered fluid after shock reversal.

Vasoactive Agents

Dopamine, norepinephrine, and epinephrine are all considered first-line therapies for fluid-refractory shock. Table 5.4 describes the mechanism of action and considerations for use of vasoactive agents. They may be run initially via peripheral IV or an IO in dilute concentrations, but should be quickly transitioned to a larger vein once central venous access is obtained.

The decision to add a second vasoactive agent in the ED setting should be considered for patients in whom hypotension persists despite titration of the initial vasoactive therapy. For patients with "warm" shock, if initially receiving dopamine, addition of norepinephrine is warranted. Patients who do not respond to norepinephrine infusion may receive epinephrine or vasopressin. Case reports, case series, and one trial indicate that administration of vasopressin is associated with an increase in mean arterial blood pressure and urine output in children with fluid-refractory, catecholamine-resistant septic shock. However, in a multicenter trial of 65 children with vasodilatory shock, low-dose vasopressin did not decrease the time to hemodynamic stability off of vasoactive agents versus placebo (49.7 vs. 47.1 hours) and there was a concerning trend toward increased mortality in the vasopressin group (30% vs. 16%, $p = 0.24$).

For patients with "cold" shock, priority should be given to improving cardiac contractility with inotropes. First-line therapy with dopamine or low-dose epinephrine (≤0.1 μg/kg/min)

TABLE 5.4

VASOACTIVE AGENTS

Agent	Dose range	Mechanism	Use	Considerations
Dopamine	5–10 µg/kg/min	α_1, β_1, β_2, D_1 stimulation	Fluid-refractory shock	Variable stimulation of receptors based on dose Inotrope and chronotrope, vasoconstrictor at higher doses
Epinephrine	0.05–1 µg/kg/min	α_1, β_1, β_2 stimulation	Fluid-refractory shock Cold shock	β effects predominate at lower doses (vasodilation), α effects predominate at higher doses (vasoconstriction) Inotrope and chronotrope Inhibits insulin and effects lactate metabolism
Norepinephrine	0.05–1 µg/kg/min	α_1, β_1 stimulation	Warm shock with low blood pressure	Inotrope and vasopressor
Vasopressin	0.0002–0.004 units/kg/min, maximum 0.04 units/min	Stimulates vasoconstriction via V1a receptor, independent of adrenergic receptors	Catecholamine-resistant shock	Third line, not well studied in pediatrics Increases intracellular calcium
Dobutamine	2.5–20 µg/kg/min	β_1 stimulation, mixed α agonist/antagonist	Cold shock with normal blood pressure or in addition to norepinephrine for cold shock with low blood pressure and $ScvO_2$ <70%	Inotrope and chronotrope Increases myocardial oxygen demand
Milrinone	0.25–1 µg/kg/min	Type III phosphodiesterase inhibitor	Cold shock with normal blood pressure	Long half-life Use caution with impaired renal function

is recommended. Once the patient is transferred to the ICU, $ScvO_2$ is often monitored. If $ScvO_2$ remains <70% in septic shock, addition of agents with additional inotropic properties along with afterload reduction (dobutamine, milrinone) may also be helpful.

In the setting of myocardial dysfunction, such as cardiogenic shock from myocarditis, early initiation of inotropic therapy with dopamine and/or epinephrine should be considered. These agents should be carefully titrated, as they may contribute to arrhythmias and increase myocardial oxygen demand.

Electrolyte Abnormalities

Electrolyte abnormalities such as hypoglycemia or hypocalcemia may precipitate or worsen existing shock. Blood glucose and ionized calcium can both be measured rapidly via bedside point of care testing and should be measured during the initial resuscitation. If present, hypoglycemia and hypocalcemia should be corrected during the initial resuscitation.

If an inborn error of metabolism is known or suspected, diagnostic evaluation should also include measurement of serum ammonia levels. This includes neonates with shock of unknown etiology, as their initial presentation may be due to metabolic crisis. With the exception of children with glucose-6-phosphate dehydrogenase deficiency, all children with inborn errors of metabolism in shock should receive dextrose-containing fluids (at least D_{10}) to aid in the conversion from catabolic to anabolic state. Any center treating a patient with known or suspected inborn error of metabolism should consult immediately with a specialty center while resuscitating with volume and dextrose as above.

Airway Management

Supplemental oxygen should be provided to increase oxygen delivery while rapidly obtaining IV access, administering fluid, and initiating vasoactive infusions. Use of a 100% nonrebreather mask provides the highest amount of noninvasive supplemental oxygen delivery. Indications for intubation and mechanical ventilation are discussed below in the section on refractory shock. If the patient has respiratory failure in addition to shock, extra caution needs to be taken during intubation and the transition from negative pressure to positive pressure ventilation. Positive pressure ventilation will decrease venous return in a patient who is already hypovolemic, which could precipitate cardiovascular collapse. It is therefore prudent to have fluid boluses readily available and vasoactive agents started or immediately ready to administer during this transition.

Source Control

While IV access is obtained and fluid resuscitation to reverse shock is undertaken, early consideration of source control to treat the etiology of shock is necessary.

Hypovolemic Shock. Hemorrhagic shock should be treated with a combination of crystalloid and blood product administration, as discussed above. For definitive treatment, the source of bleeding must be found and controlled. Ultrasound and computed tomography are important modalities for diagnosis of hemorrhagic shock. Interventional radiology procedures to find and control sources of bleeding are also becoming increasingly available in children, though early surgical consultation is recommended as part of the primary and secondary surveys.

Shock related to hypovolemia from etiologies such as gastroenteritis and dehydration should primarily be treated with fluid resuscitation. Patients with gastroenteritis are at risk for ongoing fluid losses and may need prolonged replacement of fluid losses until symptoms improve. It is important to check electrolytes in this setting as electrolyte abnormalities, especially abnormalities in sodium handling, are common.

Cardiogenic Shock. Children with congenital heart disease, cardiomyopathies, or myocarditis may present with cardiogenic shock. Presence of ductal-dependent congenital heart disease should be suspected in the neonate or young infant (typically <2 to 3 weeks of age) presenting in shock. Prostaglandin infusion should be considered if a ductal-dependent cardiac lesion is suspected. Imaging with chest radiography and echocardiography may aid in diagnosis and a pediatric cardiologist should be consulted early in the treatment course. Rapid transfer to a tertiary care center with a pediatric cardiovascular intensive care unit should be arranged.

Distributive Shock. The Surviving Sepsis Campaign recommends the administration of broad-spectrum antibiotics within 1 hour of sepsis recognition, and this is a key quality metric for septic shock treatment. Several adult studies have shown increased mortality with delays in rapid antibiotic administration in patients with septic shock, and there is emerging pediatric evidence supporting this association as well. Initial antibiotic choice should be broad and tailored to the local antibiogram and patient age (Table 5.5). Seasonal patterns in virus activity should also be considered and antiviral agents for influenza should be included in the initial antimicrobial regimen during influenza season. Intramuscular administration of antibiotics should be considered if access to the IV or intraosseous route is delayed.

In addition to the common community-acquired pathogens, infants under 2 to 3 months are at risk for infections with Group B *Streptococcus,* coagulase-negative *Staphylococcus, Listeria monocytogenes*, gram-negative organisms such as *Escherichia coli* and *Haemophilus influenza,* and herpes simplex virus. They are also at increased risk for central nervous system infections, so initial antibiotic choice should include coverage for these organisms and adequate doses to penetrate the central nervous system.

For anaphylactic shock, epinephrine is the definitive treatment, and epinephrine infusion may be needed for those with shock refractory to intermittent dosing of epinephrine.

PROTOCOL-BASED CARE FOR SEPTIC SHOCK (SEE CHAPTER 91 SHOCK)

Although the goal of rapid shock recognition and reversal applies to all types of shock, there has been a recent national focus on improving recognition and care of pediatric patients with septic shock. The following discussion is thus focused on sepsis, although the general principles likely apply to other shock types as well.

Timely Antimicrobial and Fluid Resuscitation Therapy

Timely antimicrobial therapy and fluid resuscitation are essential in the treatment of severe sepsis and septic shock. In critically ill adults with sepsis, evidence suggests that delays in appropriate antimicrobial therapy increase mortality. Recent data also demonstrate that delays in antibiotic administration are associated with increased mortality and prolonged organ dysfunction in pediatric sepsis. In addition, these studies demonstrate the importance of appropriate antibiotic selection in improving sepsis outcomes. Institutional antibiograms can help to facilitate antibiotic

TABLE 5.5

EXAMPLE OF INITIAL ANTIMICROBIAL CHOICES IN SEPTIC SHOCK

Patient history	Antibiotic choices	Additional considerations
Previously healthy child with community acquired infection	Ceftriaxone and vancomycin	Oseltamivir during influenza season Add clindamycin if toxin-mediated syndrome suspected
Suspected intra-abdominal source of infection	Piperacillin/tazobactam and vancomycin OR Ceftriaxone, metronidazole, and vancomycin	
Immunocompromised patient, history of cancer, chronic medical conditions, recent hospitalization or resides in a long-term care facility, indwelling central line present	Cefepime and vancomycin Include gentamicin for patients with history of cancer	Consider antifungal coverage for those patients already on broad-spectrum antibiotics
Neonate	Ampicillin and gentamicin	Consider acyclovir

selection in sepsis, and are typically based on host factors, suspected source, and local microbial susceptibility patterns.

In addition to antimicrobial therapy, rapid shock reversal via fluid resuscitation and appropriate vasoactive medications is essential to improve outcomes in septic shock. Multiple studies have demonstrated improved survival after septic shock in adults with early goal-directed therapy aimed at reversing shock, though the optimal method by which to measure successful resuscitation is not clear. The recently completed ProCESS trial found no difference in outcomes whether shock reversal was measured by CVP/$ScvO_2$ or hypotension/shock index reversal. Pediatric studies have also demonstrated improved survival with timely fluid resuscitation, and continuous monitoring of $ScvO_2$, though large-scale prospective studies of fluid resuscitation and bundled sepsis care in pediatrics have not yet been performed in the United States.

Global Considerations

The efficacy of fluid resuscitation in pediatric sepsis has been questioned in the FEAST trial which demonstrated increased mortality in children with septic shock who received rapid and large volume fluid resuscitation. Several concerns have been raised that these findings were specific to the local host population with a high prevalence of malaria, severe anemia, and low availability of critical care interventions, and also that the definition of shock may differ between this study and others. However, this study was a robust trial, and certainly raises the possibility that caution should be taken with fluid resuscitation in certain populations of children with sepsis, especially those with severe anemia and malnutrition.

Surviving Sepsis Campaign Recommendations

Based on available data, the Surviving Sepsis Campaign currently recommends antibiotic administration within 1 hour of recognition of septic shock, as well as prompt fluid resuscitation in adults and children. In addition, timely sepsis care has been identified as a quality metric at many pediatric institutions in the United States. Several pediatric institutions have successfully implemented protocol-based sepsis care and have demonstrated associated improvements in the delivery of timely sepsis care. These improvements have been associated with improved ICU and hospital length of stay.

Quality Metrics in Pediatric Sepsis

Quality improvement initiatives in pediatric sepsis have focused largely on process metrics such as time to initial antimicrobial administration and fluid resuscitation for which clear improvement has occurred after the institution of sepsis protocols. There are now multiple organizations focused on quality improvement in sepsis care including the American Academy of Pediatrics, Surviving Sepsis Campaign, the World Federation of Pediatric Intensive and Critical Care Societies, and the World Health Organization. Outcome metrics include mortality, severity and progression of organ dysfunction, and ICU/hospital length of stay. To date, significant reductions in both ICU and hospital length of stay have been demonstrated in the presence of bundled sepsis care in pediatric septic shock. Ongoing multi-institutional efforts through the American Academy of Pediatrics Septic Shock Collaborative are helping to implement bundled sepsis care at 25 pediatric hospitals and track associated improvements in both process and outcome metrics.

CLINICAL PARAMETERS OF SHOCK REVERSAL

Several clinical and laboratory parameters should be frequently reassessed to determine response to initial resuscitative efforts for shock (Tables 5.6 and 5.7). Clinical signs of successful resuscitation include a decrease in heart rate and respiratory rate, increase in blood pressure, improved urine output to >0.5 mL/kg/hr, normalization of mental status, decreased capillary refill time, and warmth of distal extremities. If a central venous catheter has been inserted, an increase in CVP to 8 to 12 mm Hg in nonventilated and 12 to 15 mm Hg in ventilated patients in the absence of pulmonary hypertension or right ventricular heart dysfunction suggests satisfactory initial fluid therapy, though perfusion may be adequate in the setting of a lower CVP in many patients. Despite limitations of static ventricular filling pressure as a surrogate for adequacy of fluid resuscitation, measurement of CVP is currently the most readily obtainable target of fluid responsiveness and a low CVP generally supports that additional volume loading is indicated if perfusion remains inadequate by other indices. Although CVP monitoring at the SVC–right atrial (RA) junction is preferred, the trend in pressure changes measured from a catheter in the femoral vein may also be useful if concurrent intra-abdominal hypertension is not present.

Serial measurements of venous oxygen saturation and lactate can also be useful. $ScvO_2$ measured from the SVC–RA junction <70% is evidence for increased tissue oxygen extraction and inadequate oxygen delivery to meet demand. In shock, $ScvO_2$ <70% should prompt consideration to further improve oxygen delivery either through additional fluid administration, vasoactive therapy, or an increase in arterial blood oxygen content (i.e., increase inspired oxygen or red blood cell transfusion if hemoglobin is <10 g per dL). Although $ScvO_2$ may also be low if metabolic demand is high (e.g., fever in sepsis), an $ScvO_2$ <70% is evidence that oxygen delivery is lower than oxygen demand, and thus the shock state remains. An elevated blood lactate concentration may also indicate that tissue perfusion is inadequate, even if hypotension is not present (so-called *cryptic shock*). Two randomized trials in adult sepsis have shown that a 10% to 20% decrease in lactate over 1 to 2 hours is associated with reduced mortality. Blood pH and base deficit may also be used as laboratory surrogates for improved tissue perfusion, but these may be affected by hyperchloremia that commonly develops following fluid resuscitation or changes in ventilation.

Several non- or minimally invasive monitoring devices are available to further assess volume status, cardiac output, and tissue perfusion. Bedside echocardiography (commonly referred to as cardiac ultrasound in the hands of a noncardiologist) to serially measure inferior vena cava diameter and collapsibility and right ventricular diameter has been associated with overall volume status and can predict clinical responsiveness to subsequent volume loading. Although cardiac ultrasound is increasingly available, results are prone to individual provider variability. More objective devices are available that use pulse contour analysis to calculate cardiac output based on the relationship among blood pressure, stroke volume, arterial compliance, and SVR. However, these devices require

TABLE 5.6

CLINICAL AND LABORATORY PARAMETERS OF IMPROVEMENT IN SHOCK

Parameter	Comment	Target
Heart rate	Tachycardia can be a sign of hypovolemia or ongoing shock; bradycardia can be a sign of shock in infants or neurogenic shock in older children	Age-related (Table 5.7)
Respiratory rate	Tachypnea indicates pulmonary disease or reflects an increasing metabolic acidosis	Age-related (Table 5.7)
Systolic blood pressure	Hypotension may not be evident early in compensated shock, especially in infants/young children. A wide pulse pressure (>30–50 mm Hg) indicates low SVR (distributive or neurogenic shock)	Age-related (Table 5.7)
Mean arterial blood pressure		Age-related (Table 5.7)
Diastolic blood pressure		Age-related (Table 5.7)
Capillary refill	Flash capillary refill can be seen in warm shock, delayed capillary refill can be seen in cold shock	1–2 s
Extremity temperature	Warm extremities can be seen in warm shock, cool extremities can be seen in cold shock	Normal extremity temperature
Mental status	Lethargy, confusion, agitation, or stupor can be a sign of poor end-organ perfusion	Alert and appropriate for age
Urine output	Inadequate urine output is one sign of poor end-organ perfusion	<30 kg: >1 mL/kg/hr ≥30 kg: ≥30 mL/hr
Central venous pressure	Most accurately measured from percutaneous central venous catheter with tip at the SVC-RA junction. Femoral catheter or PICC measurements are less reliable, but trends may be useful	8–12 cm H_2O (natural airway) 12–15 cm H_2O (mechanical ventilation)
Lactate	Elevated lactate >4 mmol/L may be sign of shock with inadequate oxygen delivery	<4 mmol/L *or* ≥10% decrease every 1–2 hrs

placement of an arterial catheter, which limits their use for initial resuscitation. Other devices that measure bioimpedance, which is the change in voltage of a current applied across the thorax, are available to estimate cardiac output without an arterial catheter, though pediatric experience is limited. Cutaneous near-infrared spectroscopy (NIRS) measures venous-weighted oxyhemoglobin saturation in an underlying tissue bed (e.g., renal, splanchnic, brain) and displays a number (rSO_2) that varies with local oxygen delivery and extraction. A decrease in NIRS rSO_2 has been correlated with a fall in local tissue perfusion in animal models of shock, decreased cardiac output in infants following cardiac surgery, and predicted fluid responsiveness in dehydrated children.

TABLE 5.7

AGE-SPECIFIC VITAL SIGN TARGETS

Age	HR	RR[a]	SBP[b]	MAP	DBP[b]
0–7 days	100–160	<60	>60	>40	>30
8–30 days	100–160	<60	>65	>45	>30
31 days–<2 yrs	90–160	<50	>70	>50	>35
2–<6 yrs	<140	<30	>75	>50	>40
6–<13 yrs	<130	<24	>85	>60	>45
>13 yrs	<110	<20	>90	>65	>50

[a]Nakagaw S, Shime N. Respiratory rate criteria for pediatric systemic inflammatory response syndrome. *Pediatr Crit Care Med* 2014;15:182.
[b]Five percentile SBP and DBP based on National High Blood Pressure Education Program Working Group on High Blood Pressure in Children and Adolescents. The fourth report on the diagnosis, evaluation, and treatment of high blood pressure in children and adolescents. *Pediatrics* 2004;114(2 suppl 4th Report):555–576.
HR, heart rate (beats per minute); RR, respiratory rate (breaths per minute); SBP, systolic blood pressure (mm Hg); MAP, mean arterial pressure (mm Hg); DBP, diastolic blood pressure (mm Hg).

FLUID-REFRACTORY AND CATECHOLAMINE-RESISTANT SHOCK

Fluid-refractory, catecholamine-resistant shock is defined as insufficient tissue perfusion despite at least 60 mL per kg of fluid resuscitation and dopamine ≥10 μg/kg/min and/or direct-acting catecholamines (epinephrine, norepinephrine). Principles of management for children with refractory shock include treatment of reversible etiologies, combination vasoactive drug therapy, reducing metabolic demand through mechanical ventilation, stress-dose corticosteroid therapy for patients with absolute adrenal insufficiency, and extracorporeal membrane oxygenation (ECMO) support.

Reversible Etiologies. Treatment of reversible etiologies includes relieving causes of obstructive shock (tamponade, pneumothorax), prostaglandins for a closing ductus arteriosus, controlling hemorrhage (often requires surgical intervention), relieving intra-abdominal hypertension through drainage of ascites or surgery, and specific therapy for anaphylaxis.

Identification and removal of an infectious source (e.g., infected catheter, empyema, abdominal abscess) may also enhance resuscitative efforts in septic shock.

Mechanical Ventilation. Sedation and endotracheal intubation reduce the work of breathing which can divert cardiac output away from the muscles of respiration and improve perfusion to other organs. Of the sedative agents available for intubation, ketamine is generally preferred in patients without contraindications (e.g., increased intracranial pressure). As several studies have reported adverse outcomes following intubation with etomidate, pediatric septic shock guidelines now recommend against using etomidate in these patients.

Stress-dose Corticosteroids. For patients with septic shock, absolute or relative adrenal insufficiency is a common condition that is frequently associated with refractory shock. Stress doses of hydrocortisone (50 to 100 mg per m^2) are recommended for patients with risk factors for adrenal insufficiency (e.g., septic shock with purpura, prior steroid therapy for chronic illness, known pituitary or adrenal abnormalities). If possible, a serum cortisol level should be obtained prior to hydrocortisone administration. Even patients without risk factors may develop *critical illness–related corticosteroid insufficiency* with an inadequate adrenal response and, although evidence for a clinical benefit is not clear, stress-dose hydrocortisone is recommended for children with fluid-refractory, catecholamine-resistant shock without a reversible etiology.

ECMO. ECMO has been used to support neonates and children with refractory septic shock with reported survival rates of ~70% for newborns and ~50% for older children. Recent studies suggest that central cannulation via sternotomy may achieve survival rates of 74%. In cardiogenic shock due to myocarditis, survival rates of 70% have been reported following ECMO. Although counterintuitive due to the need for systemic anticoagulation, ECMO has also been used successfully in hemorrhagic shock in small series. In most cases of refractory shock, venoarterial ECMO is preferred over venovenous due to the presence of hemodynamic instability. Given the risk of ECMO-related complications, the optimal timing for ECMO cannulation remains unclear.

CONSIDERATIONS FOR INTENSIVE CARE AND TRANSPORT

After initial resuscitation in the emergency department, children with shock should be managed by clinicians with the appropriate critical care and trauma expertise in a setting that has the necessary resources to provide pediatric intensive care. Individuals requiring significant fluid resuscitation, vasoactive infusions, noninvasive/invasive mechanical ventilation, or high risk for recurrent hemorrhage should be considered for admission to a PICU. Children with shock who present to facilities without the necessary resources to treat shock-associated organ dysfunction (e.g., acute kidney injury requiring dialysis) following the initial resuscitation period should undergo timely transfer to an appropriate facility once cardiopulmonary stability has been achieved. Use of a pediatric specialized team is associated with improved patient survival and fewer adverse effects during transport. Thus, the use of pediatric specialized teams for transport of children with shock is recommended whenever it is available.

OUTCOMES

Overall, mortality following pediatric shock has declined dramatically over the past several decades with improved recognition and implementation of goal-directed resuscitation protocols. Recent estimates suggest ~5% mortality for pediatric patients presenting to an emergency department with shock from all etiologies. The World Health Organization reports that hypovolemic shock due to diarrhea accounts for 760,000 deaths in children less than 5 years each year. In the United States, estimates of inhospital mortality following pediatric septic shock range from 4.2% to ~20% depending on the patient population and how the diagnosis of sepsis is determined (e.g., billing codes vs. chart review). Infants <1 year and bone marrow transplant recipients have the highest risk of death following sepsis. Mortality following hemorrhagic shock due to trauma is estimated at 16%, but these data are largely from injuries in combat areas.

There is increasing emphasis on long-term outcomes, including quality of life (QOL), following shock. Most studies evaluating pediatric patients following admission to an intensive care unit report good QOL scores but lower than their community peers. The ongoing Life After Pediatric Sepsis Evaluation (LAPSE) study will determine long-term health-related QOL changes following sepsis, but data following nonseptic causes of shock are lacking.

CLINICAL PEARLS AND PITFALLS

The keys to treating the child with shock are (1) early recognition of shock, (2) aggressive treatment to rapidly reverse shock, and (3) rapid diagnosis and correction of the underlying cause of shock. The principles described in this chapter are broadly applicable to children with various causes of shock, and comprise the basic management strategies for emergency stabilization. The most common pitfalls in emergency stabilization of the child with shock are the following:

- Delayed recognition of shock. Shock is a state of decreased tissue perfusion, but hypotension does not need to be present and is a late finding in children.
- Incomplete reversal of shock etiology. The underlying cause of shock must be treated to ultimately reverse shock. Important considerations are hemorrhagic shock in which the source of bleeding must be controlled, the use of epinephrine for anaphylactic shock, and caution with fluid administration in cardiogenic shock.
- Delayed establishment of access for fluid and medication administration. If peripheral IV access cannot be obtained rapidly, intraosseous access should be obtained and used until definitive access is obtained.

Suggested Readings and Key References

Arlt M, Philipp A, Voelkel S, et al. Extracorporeal membrane oxygenation in severe trauma patients with bleeding shock. *Resuscitation* 2010;81(7):804–809.

Balamuth F, Weiss SL, Neuman MI, et al. Pediatric severe sepsis in US children's hospitals. *Pediatr Crit Care Med* 2014;15(9):798–805.

Brierly J, Carcillo JA, Choong K, et al. Clinical practice parameters for hemodynamic support of pediatric and neonatal septic shock:

2007 update from the American College of Critical Care Medicine. *Crit Care Med* 2009;37(2):666–688.

Carcillo JA, Davis AL, Zaritsky A. Role of early fluid resuscitation in pediatric septic shock. *JAMA* 1991;266(9):1242–1245.

Ceneviva G, Paschall JA, Maffei F, et al. Hemodynamic support in fluid-refractory pediatric septic shock. *Pediatrics* 1998;102(2):e19.

Chakravarti SB, Mittnacht AJ, Katz JC, et al. Multisite near-infrared spectroscopy predicts elevated blood lactate level in children after cardiac surgery. *J Cardiothorac Vasc Anesth* 2009;23(5):663–667.

Choong K, Bohn D, Fraser DD, et al. Canadian Critical Care Trials Group. Vasopressin in pediatric vasodilatory shock: a multicenter randomized controlled trial. *Am J Respir Crit Care Med* 2009;180(7): 632–639.

Cruz AT, Perry AM, Williams EA, et al. Implementation of goal-directed therapy for children with suspected sepsis in the emergency department. *Pediatrics* 2011;127(3):e758–e766.

Cruz AT, Williams EA, Graf JM, et al. Test characteristics of an automated age- and temperature-adjusted tachycardia alert in pediatric septic shock. *Pediatr Emerg Care* 2012;28(9):889–894.

Dellinger RP, Levy MM, Rhodes A, et al. Surviving sepsis campaign: international guidelines for management of severe sepsis and septic shock: 2012. *Crit Care Med* 2013;41(2):580–637.

Dugas MA, Proulx F, de Jaeger A, et al. Markers of tissue hypoperfusion in pediatric septic shock. *Intensive Care Med* 2000;26(1):75–83.

Ferrer R, Artigas A, Suarez D, et al. Effectiveness of treatments for severe sepsis: a prospective, multicenter, observational study. *Am J Respir Crit Care Med* 2009;180(9):861–866.

Ferrer R, Martin-Loeches I, Phillips G, et al. Empiric antibiotic treatment reduces mortality in severe sepsis and septic shock from the first hour: results from a guideline-based performance improvement program. *Crit Care Med* 2014;42(8):1749–1755.

Finfer S, Belloma R, Boyce N, et al. The SAFE Investigators. A comparison of albumin and saline for fluid resuscitation in the intensive care unit. *N Engl J Med* 2004;350(22):2247–2256.

Fisher JD, Nelson DG, Beyersdorf H, et al. Clinical spectrum of shock in the pediatric emergency department. *Pediatr Emerg Care* 2010;26(9): 622–625.

Gaieski DF, Mikkelsen ME, Band RA, et al. Impact of time to antibiotics on survival in patients with severe sepsis or septic shock in whom early goal-directed therapy was initiated in the emergency department. *Crit Care Med* 2010;38(4):1045–1053.

Gatti G, Forti G, Bologna A, et al. Rescue extracorporeal membrane oxygenation in a young man with a stab wound in the chest. *Injury* 2014; 45(9):1509–1511.

Gebara BM. Values for systolic blood pressure. *Pediatr Crit Care Med* 2005;6(4):500–501.

Goldstein B, Giroir B, Randolph A, et al. International pediatric sepsis consensus conference: definitions for sepsis and organ dysfunction in pediatrics. *Pediatr Crit Care Med* 2005;6(1):2–8.

Hanson SJ, Berens RJ, Havens PL, et al. Effect of volume resuscitation on regional perfusion in dehydrated pediatric patients as measured by two-site near-infrared spectroscopy. *Pediatr Emerg Care* 2009;25(3):150–153.

Hartman M, Lin JC. Functional outcomes for children with severe sepsis: is a "good save" good enough? *Pediatr Crit Care Med* 2013;14(9): 893–894.

Hartman ME, Linde-Zwirble WT, Angus DC, et al. Trends in the epidemiology of pediatric severe sepsis. *Pediatr Crit Care Med* 2013;14(7): 686–693.

Hotchkiss RS, Karl IE. The pathophysiology and treatment of sepsis. *N Engl J Med* 2003;348:138–150.

Jones AE, Shapiro NI, Trzeciak S, et al. Lactate clearance vs central venous oxygen saturation as goals of early sepsis therapy: a randomized clinical trial. *JAMA* 2010;303(8):739–746.

Kissoon N, Carcillo JA, Espinosa V, et al. World Federation of Pediatric Intensive Care and Critical Care Societies: global sepsis initiative. *Pediatr Crit Care Med* 2011;12(5):494–503.

Kumar A, Roberts D, Wood KE, et al. Duration of hypotension before initiation of effective antimicrobial therapy is the critical determinant of survival in human septic shock. *Crit Care Med* 2006;34(6):1589–1596.

Larsen GY, Mecham N, Greenberg R. An emergency department septic shock protocol and care guideline for children initiated at triage. *Pediatrics* 2011;127(6):e1585–e1592.

MacLaren G, Butt W, Best D, et al. Central extracorporeal membrane oxygenation for refractory pediatric septic shock. *Pediatr Crit Care Med* 2011;12(2):133–136.

Maitland K, Kiguli S, Opoka RO, et al. Mortality after fluid bolus in African children with severe infection. *N Engl J Med* 2011;364(26): 2483–2495.

Marik PE. Noninvasive cardiac output monitors: a state-of-the-art review. *J Cardiothorac Vasc Anesth* 2013;27(1):121–134.

Nahum E, Skippen PW, Gagnon RE, et al. Correlation of near-infrared spectroscopy with perfusion parameters at the hepatic and systemic levels in an endotoxemic shock model. *Med Sci Monit* 2006;12(10): BR313–BR317.

Odetola FO, Gebremariam A, Freed GL. Patient and hospital correlates of clinical outcomes and resource utilization in severe pediatric sepsis. *Pediatrics* 2007;119(3):487–494.

Ogawa Y, Grant JA. Mediators of anaphylaxis. *Immunol Allergy Clin North Am* 2007;27(2):249–260, vii.

Oliveira CF, Nogueira de Sá FR, Oliveira DS, et al. Time- and fluid-sensitive resuscitation for hemodynamic support of children in septic shock: barriers to the implementation of the American College of Critical Care Medicine/Pediatric advanced life support guidelines in a pediatric intensive care unit in a developing world. *Pediatr Emerg Care* 2008;24(12):810–815.

Patregnani JT, Borgman MA, Maegele M, et al. Coagulopathy and shock on admission is associated with mortality for children with traumatic injuries at combat support hospitals. *Pediatr Crit Care Med* 2012;13(3):273–277.

Paul R, Melendez E, Stack A, et al. Improving adherence to PALS septic shock guidelines. *Pediatrics* 2014;133(5):e1358–e1366.

Paul R, Neuman MI, Monuteaux MC, et al. Adherence to PALS Sepsis Guidelines and hospital length of stay. *Pediatrics* 2012;130(2): e23–e280.

Puskarich MA, Kline JA, Summers RL, et al. Prognostic value of incremental lactate elevations in emergency department patients with suspected infection. *Acad Emerg Med* 2012;19(8):983–985.

Puskarich MA, Trzeciak S, Shapiro NI, et al. Association between timing of antibiotic administration and mortality from septic shock in patients treated with a quantitative resuscitation protocol. *Crit Care Med* 2011;39(9):2066–2071.

Puskarich MA, Trzeciak S, Shapiro NI, et al. Prognostic value and agreement of achieving lactate clearance or central venous oxygen saturation goals during early sepsis resuscitation. *Acad Emerg Med* 2012;19(3):252–258.

Rhee C, Gohil S, Klompas M. Regulatory mandates for sepsis care–reasons for caution. *N Engl J Med* 2014;370(18):1673–1676.

Rivers E, Nguyen B, Havstad S, et al. Early goal-directed therapy in the treatment of severe sepsis and septic shock. *N Engl J Med* 2001; 345(19):1368–1377.

Romero-Bermejo FJ, Ruiz-Bailen M, Gil-Cebrian J, et al. Sepsis-induced cardiomyopathy. *Curr Cardiol Rev* 2011;7(3):163–183.

Scott HF, Donoghue AJ, Gaieski DF, et al. The utility of early lactate testing in undifferentiated pediatric systemic inflammatory response syndrome. *Acad Emerg Med* 2012;19(11):1276–1280.

Teele SA, Allan CK, Laussen PC, et al. Management and outcomes in pediatric patients presenting with acute fulminant myocarditis. *J Pediatr* 2011;158(4):638–643e1.

van den Bosch CM, Hulscher ME, Natsch S, et al. Development of quality indicators for antimicrobial treatment in adults with sepsis. *BMC Infect Dis* 2014;14:345.

Weiss SL, Fitzgerald JC, Balamuth F, et al. Delayed antimicrobial therapy increases mortality and organ dysfunction duration in pediatric sepsis. *Crit Care Med* 2014;42(11):2409–2417.

Weiss SL, Parker B, Bullock ME, et al. Defining pediatric sepsis by different criteria: discrepancies in populations and implications for clinical practice. *Pediatr Crit Care Med* 2012;13(4):e219–e226.

Wong HR. Genetics and genomics in pediatric septic shock. *Crit Care Med* 2012;40(5):1618–1626.

Wong HR. Clinical review: sepsis and septic shock—the potential of gene arrays. *Crit Care* 2012;16(1):204.

Wong HR, Cvijanovich N, Allen GL, et al. Genomic expression profiling across the pediatric systemic inflammatory response syndrome, sepsis, and septic shock spectrum. *Crit Care Med* 2009;37(5): 1558–1566.

Wong HR, Cvijanovich NZ, Hall M, et al. Interleukin-27 is a novel candidate diagnostic biomarker for bacterial infection in critically ill children. *Crit Care* 2012;16(5):R213.

Wong HR, Cvijanovich N, Lin R, et al. Identification of pediatric septic shock subclasses based on genome-wide expression profiling. *BMC Med* 2009;7:34.

Wong HR, Dalton HJ. The PICU perspective on monitoring hemodynamics and oxygen transport. *Pediatr Crit Care Med* 2011; 12(4 suppl):S66–S68.

Wong HR, Salisbury S, Xiao Q, et al. The pediatric sepsis biomarker risk model. *Crit Care* 2012;16(5):R174.

Wong HR, Weiss SL, Giuliano JS Jr, et al. Testing the prognostic accuracy of the updated pediatric sepsis biomarker risk model. *PLoS One* 2014;9(1):e86242.

Wong HR, Weiss SL, Giuliano JS Jr, et al. The temporal version of the pediatric sepsis biomarker risk model. *PLoS One* 2014;9(3): e92121.

Yealy DM, Kellum JA, Huang DT, et al. A randomized trial of protocol-based care for early septic shock. *N Engl J Med* 2014;370(18): 1683–1693.

Zhang Z, Xu X. Lactate clearance is a useful biomarker for the prediction of all-cause mortality in critically ill patients: a systematic review and meta-analysis. *Crit Care Med* 2014;42:2118–2125.

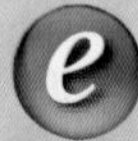

To view this chapter please access the eBook bundled with this text. Please see the inside front cover for eBook access instructions.

CHAPTER 6 ■ INTERFACILITY TRANSPORT AND STABILIZATION

GEORGE A. WOODWARD, MD, MBA AND NICHOLAS TSAROUHAS, MD

SECTION II
Signs and Symptoms

CHAPTER 7 ■ ABDOMINAL DISTENSION

JEFFREY R. AVNER, MD, FAAP

Distension may occur in any structure that has an encircling and restricting wall; abdominal distension is generally defined as an increase in the breadth of the abdominal cavity. Often, the distension is large and thus easily noticeable to the child or parent. However, subtle increases in abdominal girth may be first appreciated by the child's sensation of abdominal pressure, fullness, or bloating. In general, abdominal distension is often due to an increase in intra-abdominal volume by air, fluid, stool, mass, or organomegaly. Nevertheless, care should be taken not to confuse true abdominal distension with certain conditions that cause an *apparent* increase in abdominal girth such as poor posture, the natural exaggerated lordosis of childhood, abdominal wall weakness, obesity, and pulmonary hyperinflation. Examination of the patient in both the supine and upright positions assists the clinician in recognizing these factors before considering diagnoses that truly increase the volume of the abdominal cavity.

Abdominal distension is a nonspecific sign. That is, the causes of abdominal distension are numerous (Table 7.1). Even when the discussion is limited to the more common causes (Table 7.2) or emergent and urgent causes of abdominal distension (Table 7.3), the list is long. When confronted with a patient with abdominal distension, one approach is to divide the causes into the following generic categories: *distended bowel, extraluminal gas* (e.g., free air), *extraluminal fluid, massive hepatomegaly, massive splenomegaly,* and *other causes* (e.g., mass, cyst, pregnancy). This categorization is more easily described on paper than discerned at the bedside. A large cystic mass can be easily mistaken for ascitic fluid. A Wilms tumor may feel much like splenomegaly. Another difficulty in the clinical application of this categorization is that many pathologic processes that lead to abdominal distension do so through several of the previously mentioned categories. For example, kwashiorkor causes abdominal distension secondary to hepatosplenomegaly and ascites. For these reasons, the reader is urged to regard this initial categorization, when used at the bedside, as tentative, pending confirmation from plain radiograph, ultrasound, computed tomography (CT), or other imaging studies.

DIFFERENTIAL DIAGNOSIS

Bowel distension occurs secondary to mechanical or functional intestinal obstruction, aerophagia, malabsorption, or obstipation. Mechanical obstruction most commonly occurs in infants secondary to congenital malformations (atresia, volvulus, Hirschsprung disease), incarcerated hernia, duplication cysts, or intussusception. At any age, a history of previous abdominal surgery usually suggests intra-abdominal adhesions as the cause of intestinal obstruction. The amount of bowel distension is often related to the level of obstruction. After several hours, most of the gas distal to the obstruction is passed, leaving an airless segment distally. Therefore, the lack of air in the rectum and sigmoid colon on a prone cross-table lateral radiograph of the abdomen supports the diagnosis of mechanical obstruction. Functional obstruction, or paralytic ileus, is suggested by tympanitic abdominal distension with the absence of bowel sounds. In general, all parts of the gastrointestinal (GI) tract are dilated, but the colon is usually more distended than the small intestine. Paralytic ileus may occur secondary to numerous causes. Signs such as involuntary guarding and pain with movement suggest peritoneal irritation secondary to infection, pancreatic enzymes, bile, or blood. Fever without peritoneal signs suggests intestinal inflammation, gastroenteritis, systemic infection, or anticholinergic poisoning (see Chapters 102 Infectious Disease Emergencies and 110 Toxicologic Emergencies). Various poisonings (atropinics), toxins (botulism), antimotility drugs (loperamide), and metabolic abnormalities (hypokalemia, hypercalcemia, uremia, acidosis) may also result in an ileus. These will most likely occur in the patient who has no abdominal findings other than tympanitic abdominal distension. In these cases, the abdomen is usually distended but nontender. Toxic megacolon, an extensive dilatation of the colon, is a potentially fatal complication of severe colitis. Children with toxic megacolon appear ill and have abdominal distension along with diarrhea, pain, fever, dehydration, and possibly sepsis. Similar clinical symptoms are seen with enterocolitis, which may present as a life-threatening complication of Hirschsprung disease. Infants with acute food protein–induced enterocolitis syndrome (FPIES), a non–IgE-mediated food hypersensitivity, present with profuse emesis soon after ingestion of the trigger food, followed by lethargy, diarrhea, abdominal distension, and, in severe cases, hypotension. It is important to note that some conditions such as sepsis and peritonitis may cause a combination of functional and mechanical obstruction. Finally, gastric dilatation may result from several causes, including localized paralytic ileus (due to gastroenteritis or a pulmonic process), aerophagia, and iatrogenic reasons (bag-valve-mask ventilation or esophageal intubation). The resulting gastric distension is an extremely important entity that may result in significant respiratory embarrassment secondary to upward pressure on the diaphragm unless decompressed through a nasogastric tube or other means.

Bulky, foul-smelling, or diarrheal stools suggest malabsorption secondary to many causes, which may include formula

TABLE 7.1

DIFFERENTIAL DIAGNOSIS OF ABDOMINAL DISTENSION

Spurious
- Poor posture
- Obesity
- Pulmonary hyperinflation
- Lordotic posture of childhood
- Abdominal muscle weakness/hypotonia

Bowel distension
- Aerophagia
  - Postprandial
  - Post–positive-pressure ventilation with bag-valve-mask device
  - Tracheoesophageal fistula
- Intestinal obstruction (mechanical)
  - Volvulus
  - Incarcerated hernia
  - Intussusception
  - Adhesive bands
  - Duplications and other masses
  - Meconium ileus
- Ileus
  - Toxic megacolon
  - Food protein–induced enterocolitis syndrome (FPIES)
  - Infection
    - Abscess
    - Appendicitis
    - Peritonitis
    - Botulism
    - Gastroenteritis
    - Pneumonia
    - Sepsis
    - Necrotizing enterocolitis
- Intraperitoneal blood (trauma, ruptured ectopic pregnancy, aneurysm)
- Electrolyte abnormalities
  - Hypokalemia
  - Hypercalcemia
- Poisoning/medications (e.g., anticholinergic, opiate, loperamide, botulism)
- Trauma
- Shock
- Severe pain secondary to
  - Biliary colic
  - Renal colic
- Malabsorption
  - Congenital causes
  - Bacterial overgrowth
  - Parasites
  - Formula enteropathy
  - Lactose intolerance
  - Celiac disease
- Obstipation
  - Functional
  - Hirschsprung disease
  - Hypothyroidism

Free peritoneal air
- Intestinal perforation
- Pneumomediastinum

Extraluminal fluid
- Hypoproteinemia
  - Malnutrition
  - Nephrotic syndrome
  - Renal failure
  - Cirrhosis
  - Protein-losing enteropathy
  - Congenital syphilis and TORCH infections
- Blood
  - Hepatic laceration
  - Splenic laceration
- Peritoneal inflammation
  - Bile peritonitis
  - Peritonitis
  - Leukemia
  - Tuberculosis
  - Pancreatitis
- Cirrhosis
  - Biliary atresia
  - Chronic active hepatitis
  - Wilson disease
  - α_1-Antitrypsin disease
  - Tyrosinemia
  - Galactosemia (late)
- Portal hypertension
- Chylous ascites
- Congestive heart failure/pericarditis
- Budd–Chiari syndrome

Hepatomegaly
- Congestive heart failure/constrictive pericarditis (chronic)
- Budd–Chiari syndrome
- Biliary atresia
- Inflammation
  - Abscess
  - AIDS
  - Hepatitis
  - Tyrosinemia
  - Galactosemia
  - Wilson disease
  - Congenital syphilis and TORCH infections
- Neoplastic disease
  - Hodgkin disease
  - Neuroblastoma
  - Leukemia
  - Lymphoma (non-Hodgkin's)
  - Hepatoblastoma
- Storage disease
- Hemolytic anemia
  - Sickle cell
  - β-Thalassemia
  - Malaria
- Hepatic laceration (subcapsular hematoma)

Splenomegaly
- Portal hypertension
- Neoplastic disease
  - Hodgkin disease
  - Leukemia
  - Lymphoma (non-Hodgkin's)
- Hemolytic anemia
  - Sickle cell
  - Spherocytosis
  - β-Thalassemia
  - Malaria
- Inflammation
- AIDS
- Storage diseases
- Hemorrhage
  - Trauma (subcapsular hematoma)
- Sequestration (sickle cell)

Mass
- Cysts
  - Choledochal cyst
  - Ovarian cyst
  - Mesenteric cyst
  - Peritoneal cyst
  - Omental cyst
  - Polycystic kidneys
- Obstructive uropathy
- Uterine enlargement
  - Pregnancy
  - Hematocolpos
- Neoplastic disease
  - Wilms tumor
  - Ovarian tumor
  - Teratoma
- Inflammatory masses
  - Regional enteritis

TABLE 7.2

COMMON CAUSES OF ABDOMINAL DISTENSION[a]

Aerophagia (crying, feeding)
Gastroenteritis
Obstipation
Pregnancy
Traumatic ileus
Intestinal obstruction (mechanical)
Obstructive uropathy (infants)
Pneumonia/sepsis
Peritonitis
Intra-abdominal bleeding
Hemolytic disease
Congestive heart failure
Hepatitis

[a]Listed in approximate order of frequency.

TABLE 7.3

LIFE-THREATENING CAUSES OF ABDOMINAL DISTENSION

Infectious
Peritonitis
Sepsis/pneumonia
Botulism
Pancreatitis
Congenital syphilis
Hepatitis
Tuberculosis
Congenital
Tyrosinemia
Galactosemia
Hemolytic disease
Traumatic
Intra-abdominal bleeding
Neoplastic
Leukemia and other malignancies
Other
Intestinal obstruction (mechanical)
Electrolyte abnormality
Renal failure
Poisoning
Necrotizing enterocolitis
Intestinal perforation
Shock
Budd–Chiari syndrome
Congestive heart failure
Pericarditis
Portal hypertension
AIDS
Toxic megacolon
Food protein–induced enterocolitis syndrome (FPIES)

enteropathies, bacterial overgrowth, parasites, and cystic fibrosis (see Chapters 99 Gastrointestinal Emergencies and 102 Infectious Disease Emergencies). In lactose intolerance, bacterial metabolism of unabsorbed lactose produces intestinal gas causing abdominal distension, cramping, flatulence, and diarrhea. The severity of the symptoms is related primarily to the quantity of lactose ingested. Celiac disease may present with prominent abdominal distension, especially in children younger than 2 years, along with nonspecific GI symptoms and poor weight gain. Obstipation is a common cause of abdominal distension. The patient usually has a history of irregular stooling or chronic constipation. This is often due to a severe functional disturbance, but pathologic processes, including Hirschsprung disease and other defects in bowel enervation, and hypothyroidism should be excluded (see Chapter 13 Constipation).

Extraluminal gas usually causes abdominal distension only when present as free peritoneal air. This may result from intestinal perforation (due to trauma, inflammation, ulcer, foreign body ingestion, or other causes) or secondary to a pneumomediastinum. It is demonstrated with an upright or cross-table lateral radiograph of the abdomen or on an upright chest radiograph to detect free air under the diaphragm. An ileus generally contributes to the abdominal distension.

Extraluminal fluid in the abdomen may be an effusion, blood, chyle, bile, urine, or pus. The most common reason in pediatrics for the accumulation of fluid in the abdominal cavity is secondary to a low serum albumin. This may be the result of protein loss due to nephrotic syndrome or protein-losing enteropathy, or due to decreased protein synthesis such as that which occurs in cirrhosis and malnutrition. There is usually associated peripheral edema and pleural effusion. Increased venous and lymphatic resistance through the portal and hepatic veins may also cause accumulation of abdominal fluid. Obstruction of blood flow through the liver is suggested by distended abdominal wall veins, a history of hemoptysis, and an enlarged spleen. Although cirrhosis evolves gradually, its clinical presentation may be abrupt. It results from Wilson disease, α_1-antitrypsin disease, biliary atresia, and other congenital problems, or occasionally, from chronic active hepatitis. Decreased clotting factors would be among the many laboratory findings of cirrhosis. Obstruction of flow at the hepatic veins or above occurs as a result of Budd–Chiari syndrome, CHF, or constrictive pericarditis. The liver is engorged, resulting in hepatomegaly and right upper quadrant tenderness in each of these entities. Finally, a diseased peritoneum from infectious, inflammatory, or malignant causes can also cause an intra-abdominal effusion.

A history of recent trauma and signs of shock point to intraperitoneal bleeding, usually due to a splenic or hepatic laceration. An ileus secondary to both peritoneal inflammation and shock likely contributes to the abdominal distension. Trauma in the recent past suggests chylous ascites. Finally, a diffusely tender abdomen suggests infectious peritonitis, pancreatitis, or bile peritonitis.

Extreme hepatomegaly that develops acutely occurs secondary to inflammation, congestion due to increased central venous pressure or vascular obstruction, or trauma (see Chapter 99 Gastrointestinal Emergencies). There will be marked right upper quadrant tenderness and general systemic toxicity. Causes include hepatitis, CHF, constrictive pericarditis, and congenital enzyme deficiencies. Neoplastic disease, especially the proliferative blood cell disorders (leukemia, lymphoma), commonly causes significant hepatomegaly and splenomegaly.

Extreme splenomegaly without marked hepatomegaly in the toxic-appearing child suggests intraparenchymal bleeding with an intact capsule, sickle cell sequestration crisis, or malaria (see Chapters 101 Hematologic Emergencies and 102 Infectious Disease Emergencies). In the nontoxic child, portal hypertension, neoplastic disease, and chronic hemolysis should be suspected. Neoplastic disease often results in a spleen with an irregular surface. Chronic hemolysis secondary to sickle cell disease, β-thalassemia, and hereditary spherocytosis may also result in a very large spleen. In the case of hemoglobin "SS" disease, but not hemoglobin "SC" disease or sickle-thalassemia, splenic enlargement is followed by splenic atrophy beyond 5 years of age. A peripheral blood smear generally identifies this group of causes of massive splenomegaly (see Chapter 101 Hematologic Emergencies).

Other causes of abdominal distension include cysts, masses, tumors, uterine enlargement, obstructive uropathy, bowel duplication, and inflammation. Cystic lesions include ovarian cysts; mesenteric, omental, or peritoneal cysts; choledochal cysts; and polycystic kidneys. These conditions generally present with a subacute history and physical examination. The exception is torsion of the large ovarian cyst, which produces vomiting and marked abdominal pain. Abdominal ultrasound generally identifies intra-abdominal cysts readily. Renal abnormalities are probably the most common cause of abdominal masses in early infancy. Renal cystic disease is the most common cause of flank mass in the neonate. Hydronephrosis due to ureteral–pelvic junction obstruction or posterior urethral valves may also cause abdominal distension in the neonate. Confirmation of renal anomalies is made by ultrasound. Tumors such as neuroblastoma, Wilms tumor, an ovarian tumor, and a teratoma generally can be palpated easily as firm, discrete abdominal masses by the time they are causing frank abdominal distension (see Chapter 106 Oncologic Emergencies). Bowel duplication can be a subtle diagnosis until a complication such as mechanical bowel obstruction or hematochezia develops. Finally, a midline pelvic mass should suggest pregnancy or hematocolpos.

EVALUATION AND DECISION

History

The history should attempt first to differentiate acute from chronic symptomatology by focusing on the rate of progression, recent trauma, weight loss, or weight gain. Progressive distension suggests accumulating ascites, intra-abdominal tumor, or increasing hepatosplenomegaly. Parents may note early, subtle changes in these symptoms before they become apparent to the clinician. Next, systemic signs such as fever, anorexia, edema, and lethargy further define the acuteness of the problem and, to some degree, narrow the diagnostic possibilities. One must always be on alert, however, for an acute complication superimposed on a more subtle chronic condition. Next, symptoms relative to specific organs, including the GI, renal, cardiac, and gynecologic systems, should be pursued. These include questions about nausea, vomiting (bilious or nonbilious), abdominal pain, change in bowel habits, stool history (color, consistency), shortness of breath, cough, hemoptysis, urine output (including strength of stream and any abnormality of urinary color or foamy urine), menstrual history, and sexual activity. Other important historical information includes stress or anxiety (associated with aerophagia), previous abdominal surgery, and recent medication use (including laxatives and antidiarrheal agents). Finally, a family history of anemia, early infant death among relatives or metabolic disease, a travel history, and a careful newborn history may be revealing.

Physical Examination

After ruling out life-threatening respiratory embarrassment and shock, the physical examination should focus on determining whether the cause of the abdominal distension is related to bowel (air or stool) (Fig. 7.1), free fluid (Fig. 7.2), massive hepatomegaly (Fig. 7.3), massive splenomegaly (Fig. 7.4), inspissated stool, or a discrete mass (Fig. 7.5). A tympanitic abdomen suggests bowel distension (either by a mechanical obstruction or an ileus) or, especially in a toxic-appearing child, free air. A fluid wave or shifting dullness (more reliable in younger children) suggests ascites. Palpable loops of bowel or a palpable descending colon suggests stool. Massive hepatomegaly and splenomegaly generally are defined easily by palpation. However, care should be taken to begin palpation in the pelvic area and advance superiorly so as not to overlook the liver edge. Furthermore, the examiner must be cautious since other masses may mimic hepatomegaly and, in particular, splenomegaly. Thus, it is important to note not only the location of the mass, but also whether it is firm, fixed (suggesting retroperitoneal origin), cystic, smooth, or nodular. Other key physical findings include signs of CHF, abdominal tenderness, peripheral edema, signs of trauma or easy bruising, lymphadenopathy, pallor, and jaundice. A rectal examination for a mass, tenderness, gross (frank blood, currant jelly stool) or occult blood, and the presence or absence of stool is also helpful. More specific findings may be pursued once an initial hypothesis is made based on the algorithms in this chapter.

Laboratory

The initial laboratory evaluation of abdominal distension is determined by the clinical findings and may include complete blood count with smear, reticulocyte count, erythrocyte sedimentation rate, and C-reactive protein; liver function tests, including serum albumin and clotting studies; electrolytes with BUN, creatinine, lipase, and amylase; a urinalysis with reducing substances; and an upright chest radiograph and a two-view abdomen plain radiograph. The radiographs are helpful in determining the intestinal gas pattern, presence of free intra-abdominal air, and presence of intra-abdominal calcifications. If intestinal obstruction is suspected, one of the plain radiographs should be a prone cross-table lateral view to determine the presence or absence of air in the rectum and sigmoid colon. The addition of a left lateral decubitus view to the supine radiograph of the abdomen adds to the diagnostic utility if an intussusception is suspected, although ultrasonography has a higher overall sensitivity.

Often, after the initial history, physical examination, and laboratory evaluation, further imaging studies will be necessary. Ultrasound is an excellent first step since it is portable, has no ionizing radiation, is inexpensive, and can usually determine the presence and characteristics of a mass, organomegaly, and ascites (see Chapter 142 Ultrasound). It is also fairly accurate in the diagnosis of GI obstruction, malrotation, and intussusception. Furthermore, physical examination findings (site of maximal tenderness and/or distension) can be correlated with ultrasound findings. An abdominal CT scan is the preferred study in the

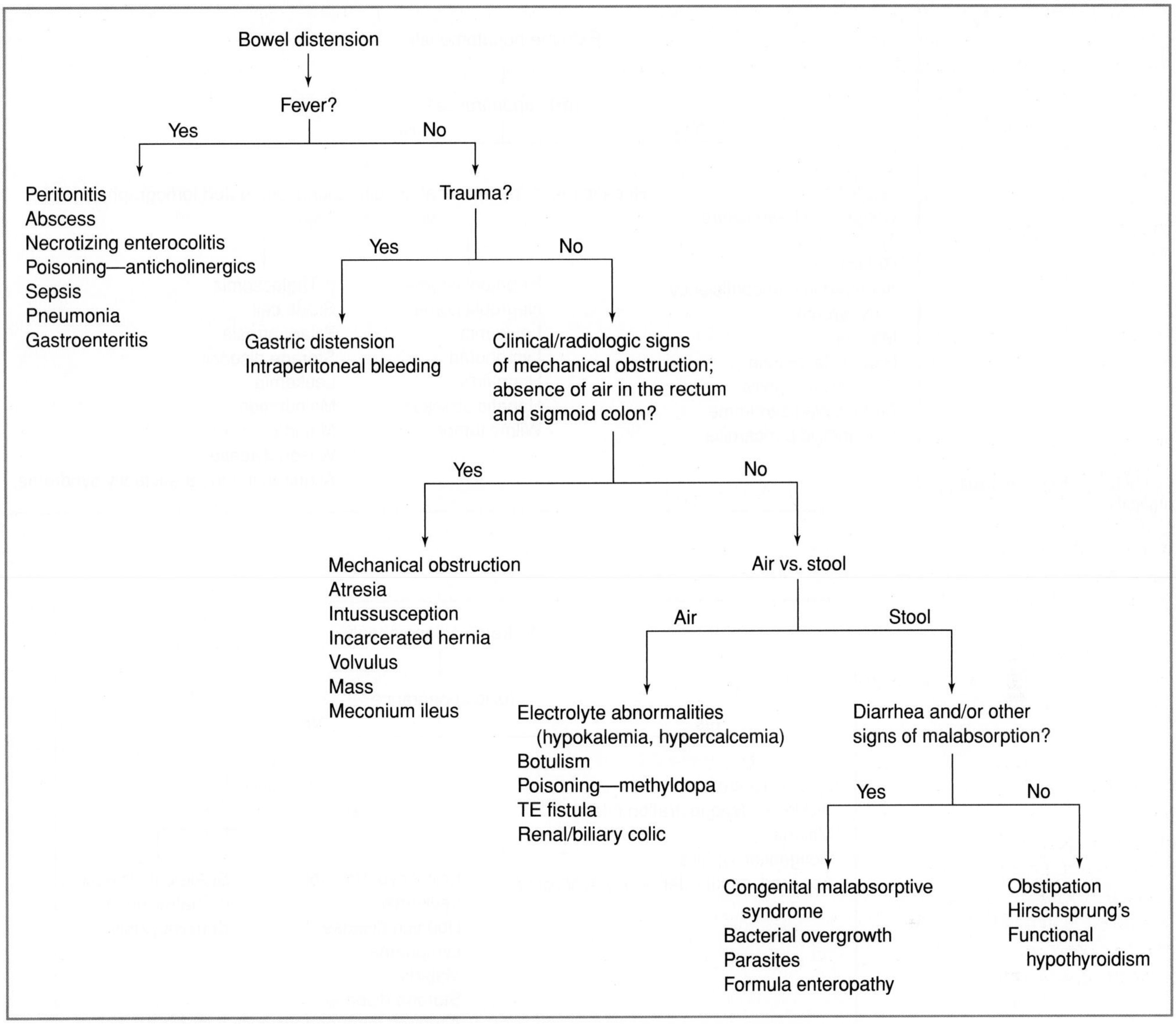

Bowel distension
Fever?
Yes
No
Peritonitis
Abscess
Necrotizing enterocolitis
Poisoning—anticholinergics
Sepsis
Pneumonia
Gastroenteritis
Trauma?
Yes
No
Gastric distension
Intraperitoneal bleeding
Clinical/radiologic signs of mechanical obstruction; absence of air in the rectum and sigmoid colon?
Yes
No
Mechanical obstruction
Atresia
Intussusception
Incarcerated hernia
Volvulus
Mass
Meconium ileus
Air vs. stool
Air
Stool
Electrolyte abnormalities (hypokalemia, hypercalcemia)
Botulism
Poisoning—methyldopa
TE fistula
Renal/biliary colic
Diarrhea and/or other signs of malabsorption?
Yes
No
Congenital malabsorptive syndrome
Bacterial overgrowth
Parasites
Formula enteropathy
Obstipation
Hirschsprung's
Functional hypothyroidism

FIGURE 7.1 Bowel distension. TE, tracheoesophageal.

Fluid (ascitic, blood)
Tender?
No
Yes
Low serum albumin?
Yes
No
PLE
Nephrotic syndrome
Malnutrition
Portal hypertension
Tyrosinemia
Congenital syphilis
Cirrhosis
Portal hypertension
TB peritonitis
Chylous ascites
Renal failure
Leukemia
Hodgkin's
Obstructive uropathy[b]
Wilson disease
Hematocolpos[b]
Peritonitis
Pancreatitis
CHF[a]
Constructive pericarditis[a]
Bile peritonitis
Hepatitis[a]
Budd–Chiari syndrome[a]
Intraperitoneal bleeding (trauma, ectopic pregnancy)
Hepatic abscess

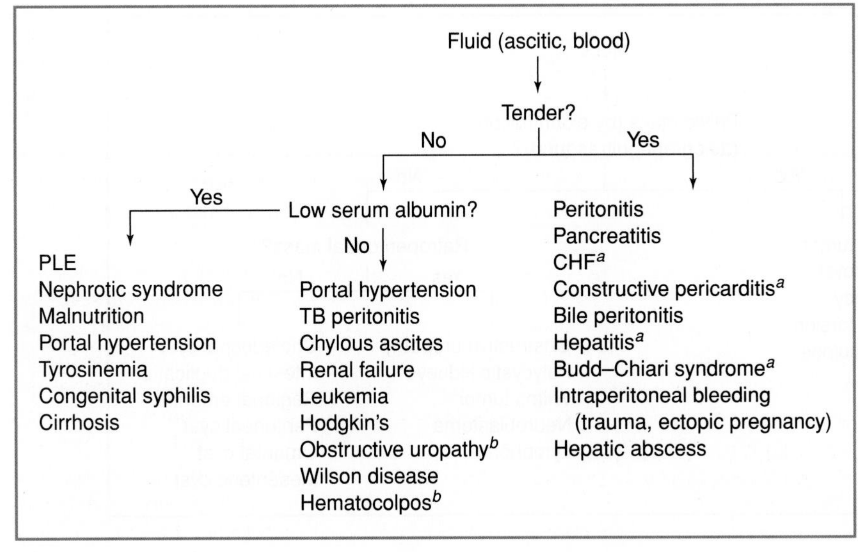

FIGURE 7.2 Fluid (ascitic, blood). PLE, protein-losing enteropathy; TB, tuberculosis; CHF, congestive heart failure. [a]Right upper quadrant tenderness; [b]newborn period only or primarily.

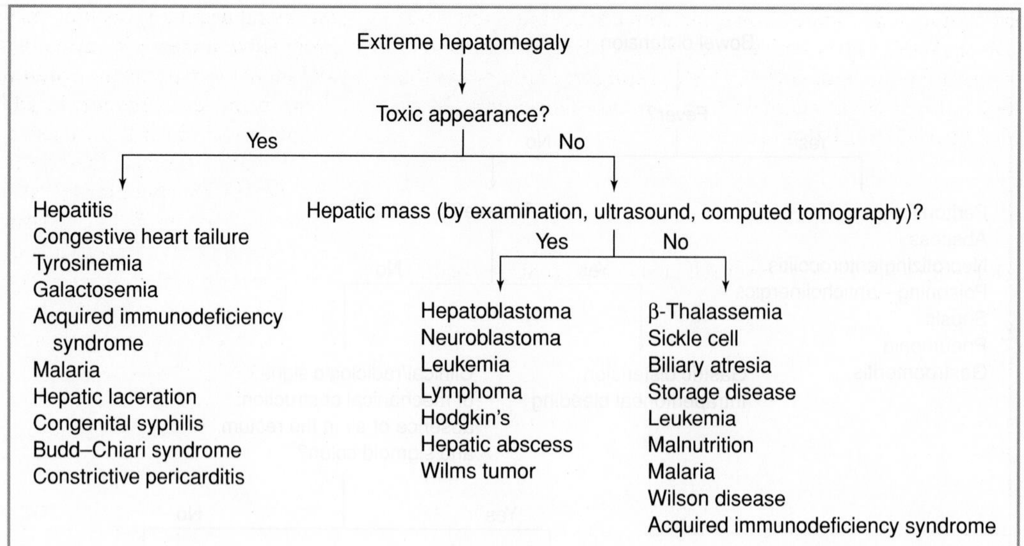

FIGURE 7.3 Extreme hepatomegaly.

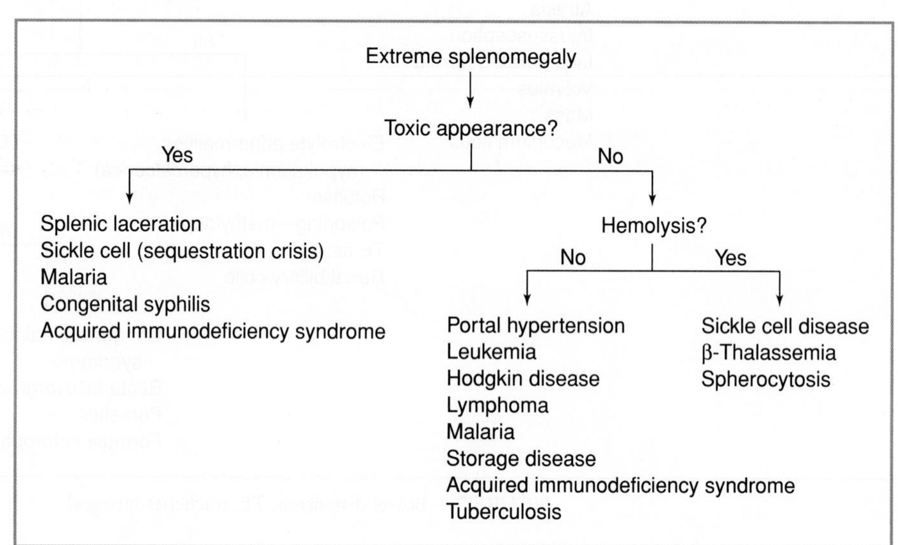

FIGURE 7.4 Extreme splenomegaly.

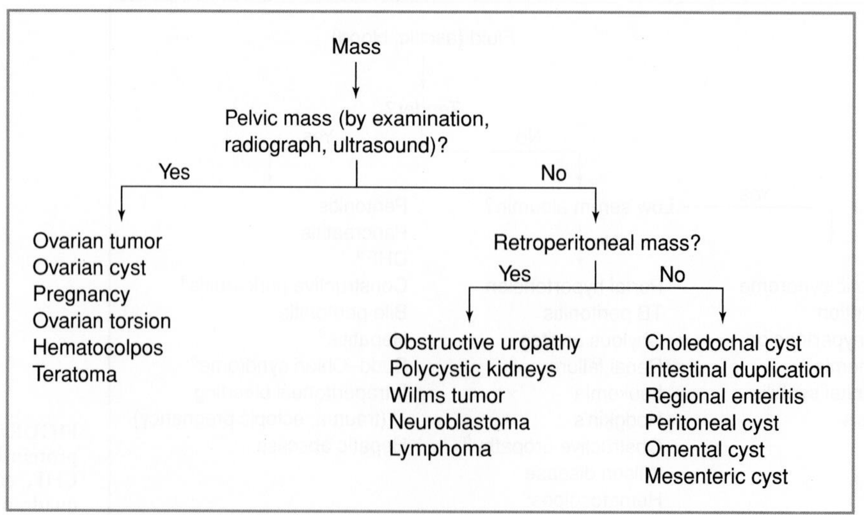

FIGURE 7.5 Mass.

evaluation of abdominal distension if an ultrasound is inconclusive or unable to be obtained (i.e., obesity). Focused abdominal sonography for trauma (FAST) is a useful screening tool in the initial evaluation of abdominal trauma in pediatrics (see Chapter 111 Abdominal Trauma).

Management

Abdominal distension by itself may represent a medical emergency. First, this occurs when the distension is so severe that diaphragmatic excursion is compromised. For example, gastric and bowel distension secondary to aerophagia and ileus posttrauma may significantly impair a child's respiratory status. Massive ascites and free peritoneal air may also compromise respiration. Therefore, the first step in management is to assess and stabilize the child's respiratory status, including the use of positive-pressure ventilation and/or emergent relief of distension, if needed. Passage of a nasogastric or orogastric tube may also result in dramatic improvement in the child's respiratory status.

The second, far less common situation in which abdominal distension may represent an emergent situation in itself is compression of the inferior vena cava (IVC), resulting in a compromised cardiovascular status. For example, occasionally, a child with severe obstipation may present with weak pulses and cool extremities. In this situation, rapid infusion of intravenous fluids, as well as disimpaction, will improve the patient's perfusion status rapidly. Managing the child in the lateral decubitus position may relieve pressure on the IVC. Progressive increase in intra-abdominal pressure may lead to abdominal compartment syndrome (ACS) that resultant end-organ damage of the gut, in addition to affecting the renal, pulmonary, and cardiovascular systems. ACS may be seen in the setting of trauma (massive hemorrhage or volume resuscitation) or in conditions that result in massive ascites or bowel wall edema. If ACS is suspected, immediate abdominal decompression with nasogastric and rectal tubes should be performed as well as surgical consultation. When the airway, breathing, and circulation have been stabilized, the diagnostic evaluation can proceed with laboratory and imaging studies as discussed previously.

Suggested Readings and Key References

Fonio P, Coppolino F, Russo A, et al. Ultrasonography (US) in the assessment of pediatric nontraumatic gastrointestinal emergencies. *Crit Ultrasound J* 2013;5(1):1–10.

Holmes JF, Gladman A, Chang CH. Performance of abdominal ultrasonography in pediatric blunt trauma patients: a meta-analysis. *J Pediatr Surg* 2007;42(9):1588–1594.

Mandeville K, Chien M, Willyerd FA, et al. Intussusception: clinical presentations and imaging characteristics. *Pediatr Emerg Care* 2012; 28(9):842–844.

Nowak-Węgrzyn A, Konstantinou G. Non-IgE-mediated food allergy: FPIES. *Curr Pediatr Rep* 2014;2:135–143.

Rasquin A, Di Lorenzo C, Forbes D, et al. Childhood functional gastrointestinal disorders: child/adolescent. *Gastroenterology* 2006; 130(5):1527–1537.

CHAPTER 8 ■ AGITATED CHILD

LAURA L. CHAPMAN, MD, EMILY R. KATZ, MD, AND THOMAS H. CHUN, MD, MPH

This chapter presents an approach for the diagnosis of the acutely agitated or aggressive child. Additional details of management of the conditions discussed here are found in Chapter 134 Behavioral and Psychiatric Emergencies.

DIFFERENTIAL DIAGNOSIS

A wide variety of medical and psychiatric conditions can lead to a child's development of significant agitation and aggression. These disorders are listed in Table 8.1 and include severe psychiatric disturbances, life-threatening medical conditions, and minor aberrations in the child's ability to respond to stressful events.

Medical Conditions

Agitation, especially in the presence of disorientation, abnormal vital signs, or decreased level of consciousness, should be attributed to an emergent medical cause until proven otherwise. Clinicians should resist the temptation to immediately ascribe agitation or aggression to psychiatric causes, even in children with a pre-existing psychiatric diagnosis. These children remain susceptible to medical illness and are at even higher risk than their peers for engaging in substance use and high-risk behaviors. The first step in evaluating a child with a chief complaint of sudden personality change or confusion is to rule out any potentially life-threatening medical causes.

TABLE 8.1

DIFFERENTIAL DIAGNOSIS OF AGITATION AND AGGRESSION IN CHILDHOOD

- Anxiety
- Adjustment reaction of childhood or adolescence
- Disruptive behavioral disorders (ADHD, oppositional defiant disorder, conduct disorder)
- Depression
- Mania/mixed manic–depressive states
- Medical illness (including delirium)
- Pervasive developmental disorders (e.g., autism)
- Personality disorders
- Psychosis caused by:
  - Medical illness
  - Ingestion of toxic substance
  - Primary psychotic disorder
  - Other psychiatric disorders (e.g., depression, anxiety, trauma)
- Trauma

The history and physical examination can provide multiple diagnostic clues to help the emergency physician differentiate medical from psychiatric causes (Table 8.2). In general, medical causes of agitation have an acute onset and the patient is likely to be disoriented, particularly with regard to time and place. Recent memory can be impaired. In addition, hallucinations may be visual, tactile, or gustatory, rather than auditory in nature (auditory hallucinations are less common). In contrast, psychiatric causes of agitation and confusion typically have a gradual onset, often following a prolonged period of progressive social and emotional withdrawal. Hallucinations with psychiatric conditions are most frequently auditory.

Table 8.3 lists medical conditions that can induce agitation in a child. Most of these diagnoses present acutely. For example, a patient with closed head trauma or a cerebral hemorrhage will present with an acute change in mental status and agitation that worsens over a period of minutes to hours. These patients may also be acutely intoxicated, making the evaluation challenging. Careful assessment of vital signs, and, in this case, head imaging and toxicologic screening will lead to the correct diagnosis. Other medical conditions, such as thyroid disease, diabetes mellitus, and electrolyte imbalances, will present subacutely. These disorders are usually preceded by medication changes or by a period of weeks to months of symptoms such as weight change, hair loss, diarrhea or vomiting, or fatigue. A patient with a chronic condition such as heart or renal disease can present with agitation during a period of acute worsening of their chronic illness. It is therefore critically important to obtain an accurate history of current and previous medical problems.

TABLE 8.2

DIFFERENTIATING FEATURES OF ORGANIC AND PSYCHIATRIC PSYCHOSIS[a]

Evaluation feature	Organic psychosis	Psychiatric psychosis
Onset	Acute	Gradual
Pathologic autonomic signs[b]	May be present	Absent
Vital signs	May be abnormal	Normal
Orientation	Impaired	Intact
Recent memory	Impaired	Intact
Intellectual ability	May be impaired	Intact
Hallucinations	Visual	Auditory

[a]Children with both functional and organic psychoses may have impaired reality testing, inappropriate affect, thought disorder, poor behavior control, and disturbed relating ability.
[b]Increase or decrease in heart rate, respiratory rate, blood pressure, and temperature; miosis or mydriasis; and skin color changes.

TABLE 8.3

MEDICAL CONDITIONS THAT MAY LEAD TO AGITATION AND DELIRIUM

Central nervous system lesions
Tumor
Brain abscess
Cerebral hemorrhage
Meningitis or encephalitis
Temporal lobe epilepsy
Closed head trauma
Cerebral hypoxia
Pulmonary insufficiency
Severe anemia
Cardiac failure
Carbon monoxide poisoning
Metabolic and endocrine disorders
Electrolyte imbalance
Hypoglycemia
Hypocalcemia
Thyroid disease (hyper and hypo)
Adrenal disease (hyper and hypo)
Uremia
Hepatic failure
Diabetes mellitus
Porphyria
Reye syndrome
Wilson disease
Collagen-vascular diseases
Systemic lupus erythematosus
Polyarteritis nodosa
Infections
Malaria
Typhoid fever
Subacute bacterial endocarditis
HIV and complicating infections
Pain

A special consideration in pediatrics, especially in the preverbal, autistic, or mentally delayed child, is pain. These children may appear agitated, when in fact they have an acute medical condition or an acute injury. A careful physical examination and a broad diagnostic workup are necessary to fully evaluate these children. Child abuse should always be considered, especially in the autistic or mentally delayed child, as these children have been shown to be at higher risk.

Toxicologic Ingestion or Withdrawal

Acute ingestion of a toxicologic substance, or in the case of a chronic user, withdrawal from a substance, commonly leads to agitation and may lead to psychosis (Table 8.4). In obtaining a history, a frequent important clue in drug intoxication is the acute onset of disordered thinking in the presence of visual hallucinations. A history of drug abuse and the availability of toxic substances are other important historical clues. Intoxication with alcohol, sedatives, antidepressants, anticholinergic agents, and heavy metals can be life-threatening if enough of the agent has been ingested. Withdrawal syndrome in patients habituated to alcohol or sedative-hypnotic agents may likewise result in severe agitation, psychosis, seizure, and death (see Chapter 110 Toxicologic Emergencies).

TABLE 8.4

EXOGENOUS SUBSTANCES CAUSING AGITATION AFTER INGESTION OF SIGNIFICANT QUANTITY OR OVERDOSE, OR DURING WITHDRAWAL WHEN HABITUATED

Intoxication/overdose
Alcohol
Marijuana and synthetic cannabinoids
Cocaine
Opioids (e.g., heroin, methadone)
Amphetamines
Methamphetamines/MDMA (ADHD medications, ecstasy)
Hallucinogens—LSD, peyote, mescaline
Corticosteroids (adverse therapeutic effect)
Phencyclidine (PCP)
Barbiturates
Methaqualone (Quaalude)
Anticholinergic compounds
Antipsychotics (e.g., phenothiazines)
Withdrawal
Alcohol
Barbiturates
Benzodiazepines
Other sedative-hypnotic agents

Delirium

Delirium can be broadly defined as acute, fluctuating global cerebral dysfunction due to a medical condition. The presentation can be quite variable, but the core feature is a disturbance in consciousness with a decreased ability to focus, sustain, or shift attention (Table 8.5). While many delirious patients may be agitated or suffering from hallucinations, others can

TABLE 8.5

CLINICAL DISTURBANCES OF DELIRIUM

Consciousness	Decreased awareness of the environment
Attention	Impaired ability to focus, sustain, or shift attention
Cognition	Disorientation, disorganization, thought disturbance (e.g., paranoia, confusion, language, or memory deficit)
Perception	Hallucinations (especially tactile and visual), illusions, misperceptions
Sleep	Sleep–wake cycle disturbances, fluctuating symptoms (i.e., "sundowning"—waxing and waning symptoms)
Behavior	Agitation, hyper- or hypoactivity, restlessness
Mood/affect	Anxious, depressed, irritable, labile
Neurologic	Diffuse EEG slowing, myoclonus, asterixis, abnormal tone

TABLE 8.6

"I WATCH DEATH" MNEMONIC FOR DELIRIUM

Infection	Meningoencephalitis, HIV, sepsis, abscess
Withdrawal	Alcohol, barbiturates, benzodiazepines, other sedative hypnotics
Acute metabolic disturbance	Acidosis, alkalosis, electrolyte abnormality, hepatic or renal failure
Trauma	Head injuries, heatstroke, postoperative complications, severe burns
CNS pathology	Increased intracranial pressure (e.g., hydrocephalus), seizures, neoplasms, vasculitis
Hypoxia	Anemia, carbon monoxide poisoning, cardiopulmonary failure, impaired cerebral circulation
Deficiencies	Vitamins B_{12}, B_1 (thiamine), B_3 (niacin), folate
Endocrine disturbances	Hyper- and hypocortisol states, hyper- and hypoglycemia, myxedema, hyperparathyroidism
Acute vascular events	Stroke, arrhythmia, shock, hypertensive encephalopathy
Toxins/drugs	Illicit drug use, prescription drugs, pesticides, solvents
Heavy metals	Lead, mercury, manganese

Adapted from Wise MG, Terrell CD. Delirium in the intensive care unit. In: Hall JB, Schmidt GA, Wood LD, eds. Principles of critical care. 2nd ed. New York, NY: McGraw-Hill; 1998:969–972.

appear hypoactive, quiet, and withdrawn. Irritability, mood fluctuation, and anxiety are common findings in pediatric patients suffering from delirium. If delirium is present, priorities should be maintaining the patient's safety while evaluating and treating the underlying cause (Table 8.6).

Psychiatric Conditions

A number of psychiatric conditions can present with agitation or aggression. Agitation or aggressive behavior may be the final common pathway for a number of psychiatric conditions. These conditions are discussed below and in greater detail in Chapter 134 Behavioral and Psychiatric Emergencies.

Psychotic Disorders

Psychosis refers to a mental state in which major disturbances in thinking, relating, and reality testing occur. They may have hallucinations, delusions (fixed, false beliefs), and/or grossly disorganized behavior and speech. Psychotic patients do not express themselves clearly and have difficulty answering direct questions. They also may be extremely suspicious and hostile. Primary psychotic disorders include brief psychotic disorder, schizophreniform disorder, schizophrenia, delusional disorder, and schizoaffective disorder. These illnesses share core diagnostic criteria but differ primarily based on duration of symptoms. It is important to note that in children, psychosis is less likely to be due to a primary psychotic disorder such as schizophrenia and more likely due to a medical illness or another psychiatric disorder that can present with psychotic symptoms (e.g., severe anxiety, posttraumatic stress disorder [PTSD], depression, or mania).

TABLE 8.7

"SIGECAPS" MNEMONIC FOR DEPRESSION

Sleep (decreased, increased, or disturbed sleep)
Interests (loss of interests, morbid preoccupations)
Guilt (excessive guilt)
Energy (decreased energy)
Concentration (decreased or problems with concentration)
Appetite (decrease or increase in appetite)
Psychomotor functioning (decreased or problems with functioning)
Suicidal ideation

Adapted from Caplan JP, Stern TA. Mnemonics in a nutshell: 32 aids to psychiatric diagnosis. *Curr Psychiatr* 2008;7:27.

It is useful to assess the child presenting with psychotic symptoms for their level of premorbid functioning as well as any recent stressors. Primary psychotic disorders can present in children who have been previously well adjusted or may have had mild to moderate emotional problems but have been exposed to acute or chronic unmanageable stressor(s) such as trauma or abuse. For children who present with a prolonged prodromal period of progressive social and emotional withdrawal, an eventual diagnosis of a chronic disorder such as schizophrenia is more likely.

Depression

The depressed child who presents to the ED may appear sad, hopeless, anxious, anhedonic, or withdrawn. However, some depressed children present with irritability as their main symptom and deny feeling sad. This irritability can, in turn, lead to agitated and aggressive behavior. Thus, the emergency physician should ask about other common symptoms of depression including depressed mood and a disturbance in "SIGECAPS" (Table 8.7), a family history of mood disorders, and any major recent changes in the child's life. While depression and resulting irritability can occur in the absence of any major apparent stressors, common precipitants of depression and a sense of hopelessness may include parental divorce or separation, loss of a parent through death, a recent devaluation of personal abilities through poor academic performance, peer rejection, or the onset of significant physical illness. Once depression is identified, it is extremely important to inquire about the presence and nature of any suicidal ideation.

Manic/Mixed Episodes

While mania is primarily associated with elation or elevated mood, the main symptom, especially in children, can be irritability. In fact, signs of elation may be completely absent. As with depression, the irritability can be severe and judgment can be so impaired that children can become aggressive and violent. A manic episode is defined as a 7-day period (or shorter if hospitalization is required) of a persistently elevated or irritable mood along with symptoms of distractibility, indiscretions/hypersexuality, grandiosity, flight of ideas, increased goal-directed activity, rapid or pressured speech, and decreased need for sleep (Table 8.8). Some children will have a mixed episode, simultaneously meeting criteria for mania and depression. Irritability, agitation, violent acts, and suicidality are more likely to occur when mixed symptoms are present. Children

TABLE 8.8

"DIG FAST" MNEMONIC FOR MANIA

Distractibility (attention too easily drawn to unimportant or irrelevant external stimuli)
Indiscretion (excessive involvement in pleasurable activities that have a high potential for painful consequences such as buying sprees/shoplifting, sexual indiscretions, or driving recklessly)
Grandiosity (excessively inflated self-esteem, feeling invincible, reporting they have or are planning to achieve wildly unrealistic goals)
Flight of ideas (rapidly leaping from one idea to the next or subjective experience that thoughts are racing)
Activity increase (socially, at school, or at home) or psychomotor agitation
Sleep deficit (decreased need for sleep while still feeling rested or energized)
Talkativeness/pressured speech (difficult or impossible to interrupt)

Adapted from Caplan JP, Stern TA. Mnemonics in a nutshell: 32 aids to psychiatric diagnosis. *Curr Psychiatr* 2008;7:27.

and adolescents experiencing mixed or manic symptoms may be difficult to engage in an interview. They tend to speak rapidly and have pressured speech, have difficulty staying still, and find it difficult or impossible to concentrate long enough to answer questions. As with all presentations of psychiatric symptoms, a high suspicion for an organic etiology should be maintained, especially if abnormal vital signs, confusion, and/or disorientation exist.

Anxiety

Children with anxiety disorders can become quite agitated and even aggressive in an effort to avoid something they are afraid of. For example, children with separation anxiety may become violent—kicking and punching caregivers, destroying property—in their increasingly desperate attempts to prevent their parents from dropping them off at day care. Children with obsessive-compulsive disorder (OCD) can become agitated and/or aggressive when they are kept from carrying out a compulsion. Agitation and aggression tend to escalate as the fear of the event or activity draws near and may resolve rather precipitously when the event has passed. For example, the child with a school phobia may become increasingly irritable as the weekend draws to a close. It may worsen to the point of trying to jump out of a moving school bus. However, that same child may then appear perfectly safe and happy within 15 minutes of starting the school day. Typically, children whose anxiety leads to severe irritability or aggression will have a long-standing history of anxiety symptoms, and the patient or their parents are usually able to give a clear history of precipitating events. In the absence of such a history and/or a clear precipitating event, suspicion for an organic contribution should be raised.

Trauma

Children and adolescents who have been victims of past or ongoing physical or sexual abuse or other severe trauma may develop acute agitation brought on by PTSD. The symptoms of this disorder include fluctuating behavior with episodes of excitement, fearfulness, or irritability; recurrent nightmares or flashbacks; and lack of involvement in usual friendships or activities. Children who experience posttraumatic reactions often avoid or refuse to talk about the trauma, and thus, parents may be confused about the reasons for the child's disturbed behavior. If parents are aware of the traumatic event, they may be upset or feel guilty about its occurrence.

Alternatively, one or more of the child's parents may be the perpetrators of the trauma. Parents and children should thus be asked about trauma separately, as part of the diagnostic assessment. Children who are upset about a previous trauma may be particularly difficult to evaluate. They will appear frightened, may behave erratically, and may be uncomfortable with discussing previous traumatic events. A quiet environment and gentle support from the physician may help these children express their thoughts and fears.

Disruptive Behavior Disorders

Disruptive behavior disorders include attention-deficit/hyperactivity disorder, oppositional defiant disorder, and conduct disorder; these disorders are discussed in greater length in Chapter 134 Behavioral and Psychiatric Emergencies. Children with each of these disorders commonly present with out-of-control, agitated, and/or violent behavior. Acute agitation or aggression that requires an ED visit is likely to result from some consequences of the child's difficulties at school or at home. Usually their presenting symptoms fit into a long-standing pattern of similar behaviors. Children with disruptive behavior disorders are at increased risk for substance abuse and suffering trauma-related injuries. Therefore, any acute change in behaviors, especially if accompanied by any physical symptoms or abnormal vital signs, should raise suspicion of a medical contribution to the patient's presentation.

Adjustment Disorders

Adjustment disorder is characterized by a deterioration of functioning from a previously higher level. The decline in function occurs in the presence of some precipitating event or situation that leads to significant emotional or behavioral distress or a symptomatic response in excess of what would be expected given the specific stressor. At times, the precipitant may be a developmental event, such as enrollment in a new school, increased peer pressure, or the emergence of secondary sexual characteristics during puberty. The precipitant also may be an acute event such as the loss of a parent through death or divorce. Children with adjustment reactions can present with anxiety, depressed mood, and/or behavioral disturbances.

The child with an adjustment reaction is oriented and usually can explain his or her problems well, although those who present with behavioral disturbances may be quite angry and difficult to engage. In order for a diagnosis of adjustment disorder to be made, the patient's symptoms must not meet criteria for any other major psychiatric disorder. The agitation and aggression of an adjustment reaction can be as dangerous and require intensive intervention as other psychiatric disorders. As such, patients with adjustment reactions need to be screened for suicidality, homicidality, and safety to return home.

Pervasive Developmental Disorders Including Autism

These disorders are discussed in greater length in Chapter 134 Behavioral and Psychiatric Emergencies. Children with pervasive developmental disorders (PDD) who present with agitation or aggression can pose a significant diagnostic and treatment challenge. The range of causes of such behavior is extremely broad, and the patient's ability to report his or her current symptoms can be severely impaired. Clinicians should pay special attention to questioning caregivers about any recent changes in the patient's life or behaviors, no matter how insignificant they may initially appear. Small changes in the patient's routine or apparently minor medical ailments such as constipation can lead to severe behavioral disturbances including self-injurious behavior. Suspicion for medical causes/contributions to the patient's presentation must be extremely high and consultation with the patient's primary clinicians should be sought whenever available. While interventions for agitated and aggressive behavior will be discussed in detail later in this chapter and in Chapter 134 Behavioral and Psychiatric Emergencies, it should be noted that special care should be taken with PDD spectrum patients. Caregivers should be consulted in order to ascertain what calming/distracting techniques have been useful for the patient in the past, and clinicians should use caution when dosing sedative medications, as patients with PDD spectrum often require smaller doses than other children and are especially sensitive to medication side effects.

EVALUATION AND DECISION

The emergency assessment of the agitated or withdrawn child or adolescent involves three complementary areas. The first is determination of whether the problematic behavior is caused by some medical condition or organic state. Potential life-threatening effects of the medical condition must be recognized and treated. Second, the psychiatric manifestations of the presenting condition, whether organic or psychiatric, are assessed. Third, the family system and social support for the child are assessed. Once these three areas have been evaluated, the physician can make an appropriate decision regarding disposition and further treatment.

General Approach/Initial Stabilization

The first priority when approaching an agitated and/or aggressive patient is to ensure the safety of both the patient and the ED staff. Pharmacologic and nonpharmacologic interventions that can be employed are discussed in Chapter 134 Behavioral and Psychiatric Emergencies.

Medical Conditions

First, to determine whether the child's agitation or withdrawal is organically based, the physician should bear in mind the differential diagnosis of these behaviors, which include psychiatric as well as organic origins (Table 8.1). A complete history of the acute events that led up to the ED visit, including any changes in behavior or functioning of the child, should be obtained. The possibility of drug use or ingestions should be explored with the parents and with the child. The child's medical history should be documented carefully, and any previous episodes of the current behavior should be reviewed. In general, organically based problems are acute in onset and result from an ingestion, an injury, or the worsening of a medical condition. The differentiating features of organic psychoses and psychiatric psychoses have already been discussed and are listed in Table 8.2.

TABLE 8.9

MEDICAL EVALUATION OF THE AGITATED CHILD

Baseline evaluation
Physical examination including neurologic examination
If intoxication suspected
Toxicologic screening
Specific drug testing
Anion/osmolar gap
Blood gas
If suggested by history or physical examination
CBC
ESR
Urinalysis
Electrolytes
Blood glucose
BUN
Ammonia
LFTs
Pregnancy test
Thyroid function tests
EKG
If trauma or mass lesion suspected
Head CT or MRI

CBC, complete blood cell count; ESR, erythrocyte sedimentation rate; BUN, blood urea nitrogen; LFTs, liver function tests; EKG, electrocardiogram; CT, computed tomography; MRI, magnetic resonance imaging.

The medical evaluation of agitation and withdrawal requires that each child who presents to the ED with these behaviors receive a complete physical examination, including full neurologic evaluation. This makes it possible to detect most significant ongoing organic illnesses and neurologic disease of traumatic, infectious, or structural origin. Mild incoordination, abnormalities of rapid alternating movements, and impaired tandem gait may be present in children with an attention-deficit disorder. In situations in which an acute intoxication is being considered, blood and urine should be obtained and sent for specific drug determination or toxic screening, as appropriate. Additional laboratory studies should be pursued in accordance with the findings of the physical examination (Table 8.9).

Psychiatric Evaluation

The second major area in the ED approach to an agitated or withdrawn child involves assessment of psychiatric manifestations of the presenting condition. This is achieved through a thorough history of present illness (HPI), mental status examination (MSE), in conjunction with an evaluation of the child's previous level of adjustment, past psychiatric history, and family psychiatric history. In older children and adolescents, the Folstein "Mini-Mental Status Examination" (MMSE) can be a useful screening tool. In younger children who cannot complete the tasks of the MMSE, bedside observation and questioning of parents (or nursing staff) will be the mainstay of assessment. All patients should be asked whether their thinking is confused, whether they are seeing or hearing any strange things, and about any homicidal or suicidal ideation. The ED physician can obtain much of the MSE during the history and physical examination. Other areas will require direct questioning of the child by the physician.

The categories of the MSE, as described in Chapter 134 Behavioral and Psychiatric Emergencies, are also summarized here. The child's appearance will have already been noted. Orientation to person, place, time, and situation should be determined. Short- and long-term memory should be tested, as should cognitive functions, which include intelligence, fund of knowledge, and the ability to reason and think clearly. The child's behavior should be assessed for activity level and age appropriateness. Particularly important in the emergency assessment of the child are affect and thinking. Affect refers to the predominant feelings displayed by the child. The examiner should observe the nature of the affect (e.g., happy, sad, angry, flat), its degree of appropriateness to the situation, and how it changes as various subjects are discussed. Thinking includes thought processes and thought content. The coherence and goal directedness of verbal communication are assessed, and loose associations and speech that lack internal consistency are noted.

Evaluation of thought content involves identifying the child's major themes and concerns. Preoccupations, such as hallucinations, delusions, and ideas of reference (present in psychosis), or sadness, hopelessness, and feelings of depression (present in depression) should also be sought. The child's strengths can be assessed from spontaneous statements and from forthrightness in answering specific questions. The child's insight into the current problem should be noted, and their capacity to suggest a plan for the present crisis should be evaluated.

Determining the presence or absence of suicidal or homicidal ideation and intent is an essential part of the MSE and provides an opportunity to ask about past attempts. The circumstances and intent of any previous suicidal or homicidal attempts should be explored thoroughly and should include questioning about how the patient feels about the fact that prior attempts have failed. If the patient reports suicidal or homicidal ideation, they should be asked whether they have a plan, if they have the means to carry out that plan, what they think will happen if they carry it out, and what, if anything, has kept them from acting on their plan already. The most effective way of determining such intent is by asking the child directly. Such an approach opens the subject in a way that is often reassuring, thereby enabling the discussion to proceed.

While interviewing the patient, physicians should pay attention to the feelings they experience when interacting with the child, as this can be a rich source of useful information. Recognition of the feelings engendered by a patient can be useful in helping physicians summon empathy and prevent themselves from acting in a counter-therapeutic or unnecessary manner (i.e., being overly aggressive with physical restraints).

Evaluation of Support Systems

Finally, emergency evaluation includes assessment of the family and social support system. Information about who lives at home with the child, the nature of their relationships with each other, and any recent changes in family composition or in the child's living situation help in understanding the current problem and in determining treatment.

The physician can gain information about the family through observation and direct questioning. Information about family relationships, including the parents' level of concern and their ability to appreciate the child's current situation, is obtained. The parents' description of the child during the history taking offers insight into how the child is perceived in the family. The extent to which the parents try to engage a withdrawn child or to calm and set limits with an agitated child should be noted, as well as the child's response to these efforts.

As the child is questioned by the physician, the parents' responses are also informative. Do the parents answer for the child and interrupt when he or she tries to speak? The parental response suggests the degree to which the child's independent thinking and behavior are encouraged. If the child is not cooperative during the psychiatric or physical examinations, how effective are the parents in telling the child that he or she must cooperate? The parents' success in gaining the child's cooperation during the ED visit may offer a valuable clue about their ability to manage their child effectively at home.

The physician can assess the degree of coping by the family, in part, by the way in which the family members describe problems. Responses that suggest that the parents are overwhelmed and disorganized should lead the physician to consider psychiatric consultation and possible hospitalization. The openness of the family in discussing recent difficulties also is important. Some families are extremely guarded and deny problems, despite the presence of a major crisis that they are unable to manage. Other families offer a more balanced view of family functioning, instilling greater confidence in the physician. If the child's parents are divorced, assessing the relationship between the parents is important. Arguments and disagreements, as well as the possibility of violence, lead to a lack of safety and security for the child in crisis. The degree of support that a single parent receives from extended family and neighbors is also an important factor in evaluating family support and capacity.

Before discharge, the physician should be confident that the child is safe; otherwise, social work or psychiatric consultation should be obtained.

Disposition

In determining the disposition of a child with a psychiatric problem in the ED (Fig. 8.1), the physician should be guided by the severity of the problem and by the ability of the family to manage the child on an outpatient basis. The physician should inquire about what social supports are available to the parents. If extended family or close friends are available and the parents believe that their participation would be helpful, the physician should encourage the parents to enlist such help. If other agencies are working with the family, their efforts should be coordinated with those of the hospital or mental health facility at which the child receives treatment. Many families express a clear preference about whether their child should be hospitalized. The physician should keep this preference in mind, but should make the decision based on the data about the child's physical and emotional well-being and the assessment of the family support system.

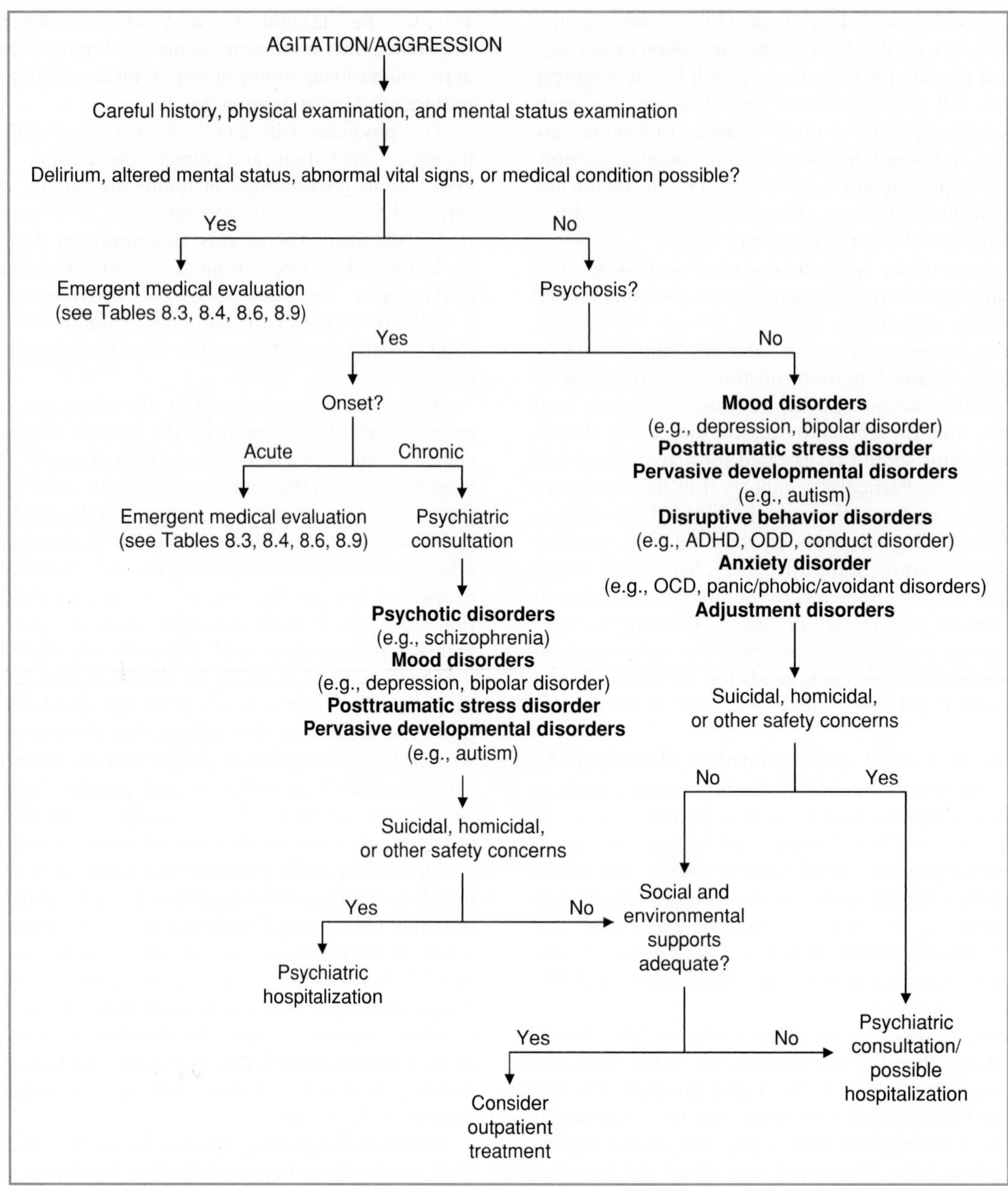

FIGURE 8.1 Approach to the diagnosis and initial disposition of the acutely agitated child.

When organic etiologies are suspected or delirium is present, full medical evaluation, observation, and treatment of the underlying condition is required. This is best accomplished through medical hospitalization. Psychiatric consultation is indicated in all cases of psychiatric psychosis, mania, and/or suicidal or homicidal intent. Social work or child protection team consultation is indicated whenever abuse or neglect is suspected.

Psychotic patients who are not suicidal, homicidal, or aggressive and who are able to engage in normal activities of daily living may be referred for ongoing outpatient treatment after a positive response to antipsychotic medication (see Chapter 134 Behavioral and Psychiatric Emergencies).

Patients who have suicidal or homicidal intent are usually hospitalized, as are patients who are unable to maintain their own safety. Patients with disruptive behavior disorders sometimes require brief inpatient hospitalization when current outpatient and community supports are inadequate to prevent further violence. In the absence of suicidal ideation, homicidal ideation, impaired decision making leading to unsafe behaviors, inability to carry out basic daily functions, or extreme acts of aggression, the ability of the family and social support system to control the child's behavior and prevent further emotional and physical harm should be assessed. If the support system is adequate and timely and appropriate treatment is available, referral to outpatient treatment may be appropriate. When the support system is not adequate and/or appropriate outpatient treatment options are not available, psychiatric hospitalization may be necessary, especially with such behaviors as fire setting, persistent aggressiveness, or failure of prior or current outpatient treatment. The Joint Commission 2014 National Patient Safety Goals for Behavioral Health recommends that as part of assessment and disposition planning, providers conduct a risk assessment of the individual or the environment that may increase or decrease the risk of suicide; address the patient's immediate safety needs; and provide suicide prevention information (such as a crisis hotline) at the time of discharge.

If a child is already in treatment, every effort should be made to contact the child's providers in order to obtain their assessment as to the appropriate disposition and to attempt to arrange for follow-up as close to ED discharge as possible. The physician who discharges a child for outpatient psychiatric treatment should help the family develop short-term measures to manage the child and relieve his or her distress until outpatient psychiatric treatment begins.

Suggested Readings and Key References

Autism/Pervasive Developmental Disorders

McGonigle JJ, Vekat A, Beresford C, et al. Management of agitation in individuals with autism spectrum disorders in the emergency department. *Child Adolesc Psychiatr Clin N Am* 2014;23(1):83–95.

Delirium

Turkel SB, Tavaré CJ. Delirium in children and adolescents. *J Neuropsychiatry Clin Neurosci* 2003;15(4):431–435.

General

Chun TH, Katz ER, Duffy SJ. Pediatric mental health emergencies and special health care needs. *Pediatr Clin North Am* 2013;60(5): 1185–1201.

Dolan MA, Fein JA; Committee on Pediatric Emergency Medicine. Pediatric and adolescent mental health emergencies in the emergency medical services system. *Pediatrics* 2011;127(5):e1356–e1366.

Interview/Mental Status Examination

Folestein MF, Folstein SE, McHugh PR. A practical method for grading the cognitive state of patients for clinicians. *J Psychiatr Res* 1975; 12(3):189–198.

Lempp T, de Lange D, Radeloff D, et al. The clinical examination of children, adolescents and their families. In: Rey JM, ed. *IACAPAP e-Textbook of child and adolescent mental health.* Geneva: International Association for Child and Adolescent Psychiatry and Allied Professions, 2012.

Psychosis

American Academy of Child and Adolescent Psychiatry. Practice parameters for the assessment and treatment of children and adolescents with schizophrenia. *J Am Acad Child Adolesc Psychiatry* 2013;52(9):976–990.

Sikich L. Diagnosis and evaluation of hallucinations and other psychotic symptoms in children and adolescents. *Child Adolesc Psychiatr Clin N Am* 2013;22(4):655–673.

Quality/Safety Measures

Rhodes AE, Bethell J, Newton AS, et al. Developing measures of quality for the emergency department management of pediatric suicide-related behaviors. *Pediatr Emerg Care* 2012;28(11): 1124–1128.

CHAPTER 9 ▪ APNEA

THUY L. NGO, DO, MEd AND SUSAN B. TORREY, MD

Neonates and infants can experience apneic episodes in response to a variety of physiologic and pathophysiologic processes not seen later in life. Differences in maturity of the central nervous system (CNS), respiratory drive and reserve, and susceptibility to infectious agents are among the factors that interact to make the very young patient susceptible. The causes of apnea in older children are similar to those in adults, although, those in infants and younger children, are different. In this chapter, the neonate and the young infant are emphasized, but for completeness, the older child also is considered.

Apnea is defined as a respiratory pause of greater than 20 seconds, or of any duration if there is associated pallor or cyanosis and/or bradycardia. Apnea must be distinguished from periodic breathing, which is a common respiratory pattern in young infants and is characterized by cycles of short respiratory pauses followed by an increase in respiratory rate. Normal newborn infants display respiratory patterns that vary by gender and by conceptual age, as well as by sleep state. Studies have demonstrated that premature infants typically have more apneic episodes than do term infants. Normal-term infants experience significantly more episodes of nonperiodic apnea during rapid eye movement (REM) sleep than during non-REM sleep, although respiratory failure occurs more often during non-REM sleep. Apnea can occur in the setting of an acute life-threatening event (ALTE), in which the apneic episode is accompanied by change in color, muscle tone, or mental status, or by choking.

PATHOPHYSIOLOGY

Respiratory centers in the pons and medulla control respiration through output to the upper airway and bellows apparatus. Peripheral modulators of respiration include hypoxia, hypercarbia, and laryngochemical stimulation. The immature response of the neonate and infant to these influences, in comparison to that of the older child, accounts for some of the vulnerability of these young patients. The adult response to hypoxemia is to increase respiratory rate in proportion to the decrease in oxygen partial pressure (PO_2). Tachypnea is maintained for the duration of the hypoxic stimulus. In contrast, the neonate demonstrates a brief increase in respiratory rate followed by depression of respiratory drive and, often, apnea. As an example, hypoxemia during sleep may not cause arousal in infants. Hypoxemia also results in less of a response to rising arterial carbon dioxide tension ($PaCO_2$) with further depression of respiratory drive. Therefore, mildly hypoxic infants tend to breathe periodically or develop apneic spells.

Feeding affects ventilation in young infants. Poor coordination of sucking and breathing can result in apnea. Furthermore, infants can develop apnea with hypoxia and bradycardia as the result of exaggerated laryngeal chemical reflexes and laryngospasm in response to regurgitation. Mild hypoxia, as can occur in association with feeding or sleep, exacerbates this response.

A number of exogenous factors, including toxins and metabolic derangements, affect respiratory control by causing medullary depression. Clinical experience demonstrates that newborns and very young infants are particularly sensitive to these factors; for example, hypoglycemia can be manifested as apnea in young infants, and apnea can be related to anemia in premature babies. The young infant is susceptible to bellows failure on a purely mechanical basis. The infant's thoracic cage is extremely pliable, which can cause the chest wall to collapse during inspiration. More muscular effort is then required to produce an adequate tidal volume, resulting in increased work of breathing. In addition, the diaphragmatic muscles have limited glycogen stores and tire easily, resulting in greater vulnerability to respiratory failure as a result of respiratory distress.

DIFFERENTIAL DIAGNOSIS

The differential diagnosis of apnea is extensive (Table 9.1). Gastroesophageal reflux is frequently diagnosed in infants with an apparent life-threatening event (ALTE), with or without a history of vomiting. Several infectious processes can cause apnea. Meningitis, even in the absence of fever, must be included in the differential diagnosis. Respiratory syncytial virus, the predominant cause of bronchiolitis, may cause apnea in infants who were premature or have preexisting lung disease or congenital heart disease. Pertussis can cause apnea in small infants. Infant botulism is a diagnosis that will hopefully be made before apnea occurs. It must be suspected on the basis of age, symptoms, and clinical findings. Apnea may be the only clinical manifestation of seizure activity. This may be particularly difficult for emergency physicians to identify if they did not witness the episode and neurologic examination may be normal in the postictal period. Apnea may be a symptom of several systemic disease processes, including metabolic abnormalities that result in hypoglycemia, and sepsis. Congenital abnormalities must always be considered in newborns and in young infants. Prolongation of the QT interval can cause a dysrhythmia that is manifested as an ALTE. Finally, there have been well-substantiated reports of ALTE as the result of life-threatening child abuse such as Munchhausen's by proxy or inflicted head injury. Frequently, no cause for the ALTE is identified.

The risk of sudden infant death syndrome (SIDS) for an infant who has an unexplained ALTE is of great concern to both parents and physicians. Multiple studies have identified no causal relationship between ALTE and SIDS. Furthermore, although the rate of SIDS in the United States has dropped dramatically since 1992 when the American Academy of Pediatrics recommended that infants be placed supine or on the

TABLE 9.1

DIFFERENTIAL DIAGNOSIS OF APNEA

	Neonate, infant	Older child
Central nervous system	Infection (meningitis, encephalitis)	Infection
	Seizure	Toxin
	Prematurity	Tumor
	Inflicted head injury	Seizure
	Increased intracranial pressure (ICP)	Increased ICP (trauma, hydrocephalus)
	Congenital anomaly (e.g., Arnold–Chiari)	Idiopathic hypoventilation ("Ondine's curse")
	Breath-holding spell	
Upper airway	Laryngospasm (e.g., gastroesophageal reflux)	Obstructive sleep apnea
	Infection (e.g., croup, pertussis)	Infection (epiglottitis, croup)
	Congenital anomaly (e.g., Down syndrome)	Foreign body
Lower airway	Infection (pneumonia, bronchiolitis)	Infection
	Congenital anomaly	Asthma
Other	Infant botulism	Guillain–Barré syndrome
	Hypocalcemia, hypoglycemia	Spinal cord injury
	Anemia	Flail chest
	Sepsis	Dysrhythmia
	Dysrhythmia	Ingestion

side during sleep, there has been no change in the incidence of ALTEs. In addition, the vast majority of SIDS events occur at night, whereas infants typically experience ALTEs during the day. The peak incidence of ALTEs is during the first 2 months of life while SIDS occurs most frequently in older infants between 2 and 4 months of life.

EVALUATION AND DECISION

Initial Stabilization

The first priority of the emergency physician, after immediate resuscitation of the patient, is to identify life-threatening conditions (Fig. 9.1) such as persistent or recurrent apnea, hypoxia, septic shock, or hypoglycemia. In addition to assessment of the vital signs, including a rectal temperature and blood pressure, the general appearance and mental status should be noted. Regardless of the cause, apnea is life threatening; therefore, a diagnostic investigation, guided by history and physical findings, should be performed to evaluate the child for several common etiologies (Table 9.2). The next phase of evaluation addresses two key questions: (i) Is this episode of clinical significance? (ii) What is the risk of recurrence? Factors to consider include signs of another acute illness, the age of the child, other possible risk factors for clinically significant or recurrent apnea, and family history of congenital, metabolic, respiratory, or cardiac diseases (Table 9.3).

Has a Significant Apneic Episode Occurred?

The key to answering the two questions is invariably in the history (Table 9.3). A clear initial history from a first-hand observer without the predictable influence of repeated questions is vital. This may not be a simple task, considering the observer's recent stressful experience. The following details should be included: (i) where the event took place; (ii) how long the event lasted; (iii) whether the infant was awake or asleep; (iv) whether there was an associated color change and, if so, to what colors and in what order; (v) description of associated movements, posture, or changes in tone; (vi) what resuscitative efforts were made and the infant's response to them; (vii) when the infant was last fed; (viii) how quickly the infant returned to baseline behavior. The response to these questions may provide the physician with clues to the diagnosis. As an example, an 8-month-old infant who was interrupted in a favorite activity, began to cry, turned red and blue, and finally had several seconds of tonic–clonic motor activity likely had a breath-holding spell. In contrast, a history of 40 minutes of cyanosis and apnea in a now well-appearing child may be unreliable. Other recent events that should be documented are symptoms of other illnesses, including changes in behavior, activity, and appetite, as well as recent trauma and immunizations.

In many cases, the description of the event may be concerning, although the child appears well. In this situation, hospitalization for further workup, as outlined next, is warranted. A typical case might be the previously well 5-week-old child who was noted by the parents to be apneic during a nap. The infant was described as limp and blue and "looked like he was dead." There was no response to tactile or verbal stimulation for 5 to 10 seconds, but after 15 to 20 seconds of mouth-to-mouth breathing, the child coughed, gagged, and began to breathe. His color improved over the next 30 seconds, and the parents rushed him to the emergency department (ED). Although the baby now looks entirely normal, he may be at grave risk for experiencing another ALTE.

The medical history also may provide important information regarding infants at risk for significant or recurrent

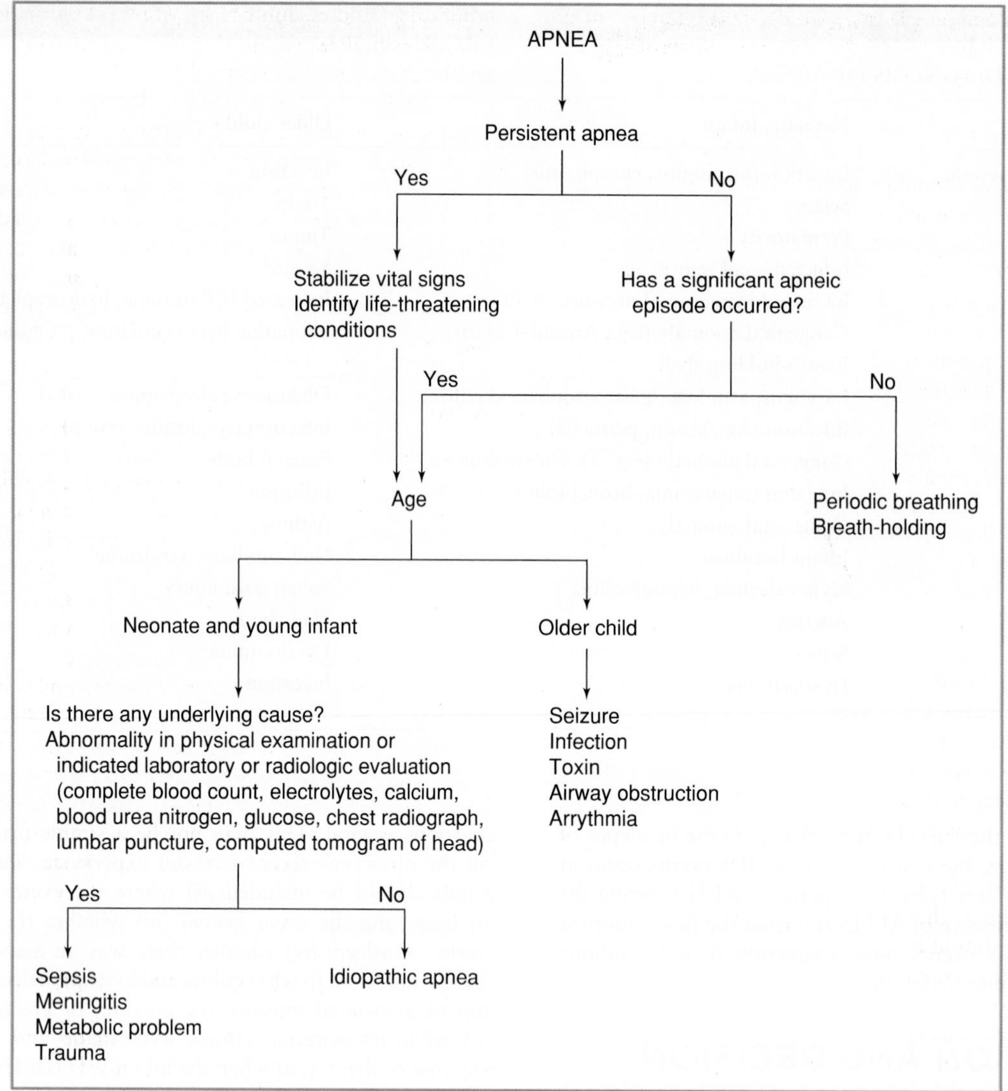

FIGURE 9.1 Approach to the diagnosis and management of apnea.

apnea. The physician should ask specifically about previous similar episodes. Information about prenatal and perinatal events, including gestational age (birth weight), labor and delivery, maternal health and medication exposures, and nursery course, is helpful. A family history with specific reference to seizures, infant deaths, and serious illnesses in young family members also should be included. Finally, information regarding medications, including those available over the counter,

TABLE 9.2

COMMON LIFE-THREATENING CONDITIONS THAT CAUSE APNEA

Pneumonia
Sepsis/meningitis
Hypoglycemia
Seizures
Intracranial hypertension
Shock
Ingestion (e.g., analgesics, sedatives, muscle relaxants)

TABLE 9.3

HISTORICAL FEATURES OF APNEA

History	Significant apnea
Duration of event	Greater than 20 s or of any duration associated with pallor, cyanosis, and/or bradycardia
Was child asleep or awake?	Either, but apnea during sleep is more worrisome
Color change	Pallor or cyanosis
Associated movements, posture, or change in tone	Seizure activity Hypotonia "He/she looked dead"
Resuscitative efforts and response	Color change or hypotonia requiring cardiopulmonary resuscitation to improve
Interval since last feeding	If shortly after feeding, consider gastroesophageal reflux
Where event occurred	Association with sleep, trauma

and poisons available in the household may be important in treating an older child.

Is There an Underlying Cause?

A careful physical examination identifies many treatable acute illnesses that can cause apnea. One clue to serious systemic disease is fever or hypothermia. Tachypnea suggests either a respiratory problem or a metabolic problem. Shock may be secondary to sepsis or hypovolemia from occult trauma. Evaluation of the nervous system should include notation of mental status, palpation of the fontanelles, and funduscopic examination. Dysmorphic features might suggest an underlying congenital abnormality. Bruising may be indicative of non-accidental trauma or abusive head injury. However, an entirely normal physical examination provides no reassurance that the described event was clinically insignificant and will not recur.

Laboratory evaluation should be guided by the history and physical examination. Tests to consider in the ED include a measurement of blood glucose and serum electrolytes. Any indication that the infant could have a serious infection should be pursued with cultures of blood, urine, and cerebrospinal fluid. Urine and blood for toxicologic analysis should be obtained from patients who may have been exposed to toxic substances or medications. Noninvasive pulse oximetry is adequate to identify hypoxemia, and significant metabolic acidosis will be identified through analysis of serum electrolytes. The arterial or venous blood gas examination does not serve as a screening test for a serious event and should be obtained on the basis of specific indications. Radiologic studies (such as of the lateral neck, chest, abdomen, or computed tomography of the head) should be performed as indicated by the history and physical examination. An electrocardiogram (EKG) may also be performed to evaluate for dysrhythmias.

The tasks of the emergency physician faced with a young patient who has had an apneic episode are to identify whether he/she should be hospitalized and to treat underlying conditions. If a careful history and physical examination suggest that a significant apneic episode has not occurred, the diagnosis of periodic breathing or breath-holding can be made, and the patient can be discharged after appropriate counseling of the parents and arrangements for close follow-up. The evaluation of a young child with apnea, however, rarely will be so straightforward. If historical information indicates that significant apnea has occurred, the infant is at risk for a recurrence of this potentially life-threatening event. An aggressive search for an underlying cause is necessary and may include laboratory studies, lumbar puncture, chest radiograph, and EKG. Hospital admission should be arranged for observation and further diagnostic evaluation.

A significant apneic episode in the absence of systemic disease leaves the emergency physician in a quandary. There may not be an explanation for the event that satisfies the physician or the anxious parents. Thus, it is judicious to refer the family to an available specialist or center. There is considerable practice variation in the inpatient evaluation and management of an ALTE. The approach that is usually pursued is designed to identify known causes of primary apnea. It generally includes in-hospital observation with monitoring, a chest radiograph, and/or an EKG. More significant events warrant further evaluation. This may include an evaluation of the CNS with an electroencephalogram (EEG), and some type of sleep study. Respiratory function is evaluated with a pneumogram. Gastroesophageal reflux is often recognized clinically, though a barium swallow and esophageal pH study can be utilized if the diagnosis is unclear. An ultrasound can identify hydrocephalus or intraventricular hemorrhage, though a CT or MRI would be indicated if inflicted head injury is suspected. Home cardiorespiratory monitoring is beyond the scope of emergency practice, but is not routinely recommended.

In many instances, a thorough history and careful physical examination with appropriate laboratory studies will suggest that a significant apneic event has not occurred and that there is no serious underlying illness. In this situation, the emergency physician should reassure and educate the family before discharging the patient. Good medical practice dictates that the parents also should be given specific instructions regarding indications for another emergent ED visit and a close follow-up visit to a primary care provider.

Suggested Readings and Key References

Jawdeh E, Martin R. Neonatal apnea and gastroesophageal reflux (GER): is there a problem? *Early Human Develop* 2013;89S1: S14–S16.

Kaji A, Claudius I, Santillanes G, et al. Apparent life-threatening event: Multicenter prospective study to develop a clinical decision rule for admission to the hospital. *Ann Emerg Med* 2013;61:379–387.

Kant S, Fisher JD, Nelson D, et al. Mortality after discharge in clinically stable infants admitted with a first-time apparent life-threatening event. *Am J Emerg Med* 2013;31:730–733.

Schroeder A, Mansbach J, Stevenson M, et al. Apnea in children hospitalized with bronchiolitis. *Pediatrics* 2013;132:e1194–1201.

Tieder J, Altman R, Bonkowsky J, et al. Management of apparent life-threatening events in infants: A systematic review. *J Pediatr* 2013; 163:94–99.

CHAPTER 10 ■ ATAXIA

JANET H. FRIDAY, MD

Acute childhood ataxia is an uncommon presenting complaint in the emergency department. *Ataxia* is defined as a disturbance in coordination of movements and may be manifested as an unsteady gait. When it occurs, it is a distressing problem to both parent and clinician. It is important to establish the sign because true ataxia may be difficult to differentiate from clumsiness in toddlers. Parents are generally more sensitive to gait abnormalities in this age group. In older children, ataxia may be confused with weakness or vertigo. Life-threatening causes of pure ataxia are rare in children. After consideration of these, the problem may be approached in an orderly, stepwise fashion.

PATHOPHYSIOLOGY

The cerebellum coordinates complex activities such as walking, talking, and eye movements. Ataxia may be caused by either a focal or global pathologic condition within the cerebellum or by disruptions in the afferent or efferent pathways. Anatomically, the cerebellum is located in the posterior cranial fossa, separated from the cerebrum by the tentorium. The ventral borders of the cerebellum form the roof of the fourth ventricle. Space-occupying lesions such as posterior fossa tumors and cerebellar hemorrhage may impede cerebrospinal fluid (CSF) flow, leading to hydrocephalus and increased intracranial pressure (ICP). Conversely, direct pressure on the cerebellar peduncles may cause ataxia.

The cerebellum links with other portions of the central nervous system through the superior, middle, and inferior peduncles via the midbrain, pons, and medulla. Proprioceptive and sensory afferent impulses from muscles, joints, and tendons are carried via inferior peduncles to the cerebellar cortex. Labyrinthine afferent input is also conducted through the inferior peduncles. Connections from frontal motor cortex travel through the middle cerebellar peduncles. The superior peduncles carry efferent output to musculoskeletal tracts from the nuclei of the cerebellum.

The cerebellum is composed of two hemispheres. Because of the decussation patterns, a lesion that affects only one side of the cerebellum will result in movement abnormalities of the ipsilateral side, with distal movements more affected than proximal ones. Midline lesions lead to truncal ataxia, with swaying during standing, sitting, and walking, and/or with titubations (small rhythmic movements) of the head and neck. Finally, the intrinsic function of the cerebellum may be disrupted by toxins and autoimmune and metabolic disorders.

DIFFERENTIAL DIAGNOSIS

Ataxia as a presenting sign invokes a broad differential diagnosis (Table 10.1). Distinguishing among acute, intermittent, and chronic progressive and nonprogressive ataxia may be helpful, although some diagnoses have overlap in their time course at presentation. Fortunately, common causes of pure ataxia (Table 10.2) are not rapidly progressive. Acute cerebellar ataxia or postinfectious cerebellitis is truncal in nature and occurs 8 days to 3 weeks after an infectious illness (see Chapters 102 Infectious Disease Emergencies and 105 Neurologic Emergencies). Children of ages 1 to 3 years are most commonly affected. Varicella is the classically identified culprit. Other prodromal infections include mumps, Epstein–Barr virus, and mycoplasma. Nystagmus, while not seen commonly, may be a feature. The ataxia is most severe at its onset. Complete recovery usually is noted after several weeks, but rarely symptoms may last several months. CSF may show mild lymphocytosis and increased protein. Imaging studies are normal. In contrast, acute cerebellitis has abnormal neuroimaging. In the most severe cases, hydrocephalus and cerebellar edema occur, and outcomes are less favorable. Acute disseminated encephalomyelitis (ADEM) may have cerebellar components, but the CNS lesions are widespread.

Ingestions of anticonvulsants, alcohol, or sedative-hypnotics generally cause depressed mental status (see Chapter 110 Toxicologic Emergencies) and may have associated ataxia. However, for certain substances (phenytoin, carbamazepine, primidone), ataxia may be the most remarkable feature of intoxication.

When a seemingly ataxic patient presents with weakness and areflexia, Guillain–Barré syndrome may be present. If ophthalmoplegia and areflexia are prominent, the Miller Fisher variant can be suspected. Neuroimaging is normal, and the CSF may show a mild leukocytosis and elevated protein. Tick paralysis may present similarly, with the discovery of an engorged tick (which may be hidden by long hair), as the diagnostic finding.

Ataxia may be an early prominent sign of posterior fossa tumors (especially medulloblastoma) and other conditions associated with increased ICP, including hydrocephalus and supratentorial tumors (see Chapter 106 Oncologic Emergencies). Labyrinthitis and benign paroxysmal vertigo are rarely seen in young children but are occasionally encountered in adolescents. The sensation of loss of balance classically produces a wide-based gait. Usually, vertigo can be differentiated from ataxia in that vertigo causes a sensation that the room is spinning. Conversion disorder should be suspected in a patient who walks with a narrow gait and has elaborate "near falls."

Life-threatening causes of ataxia (Table 10.3) rarely present as ataxia alone. In a few cases, bacterial meningitis has been reported with ataxia as the first symptom. Acute cerebellitis can be distinguished from acute cerebellar ataxia by abnormal neuroimaging. Neuroblastoma may present with titubations, myoclonic ataxia, and chaotic eye movements (opsoclonus). The syndrome is immune mediated. It should be suspected in patients with acute ataxia that waxes and wanes over several days. One should consider vertebrobasilar occlusion in a patient with neck trauma and ataxia, cerebellar hemorrhage

TABLE 10.1

DIFFERENTIAL DIAGNOSIS

Acute or recurrent ataxia
Acute cerebellar ataxia (postinfectious)
Guillain–Barré syndrome[a]
Tick paralysis[a]
Drug intoxication
Labyrinthitis[a]
Vasculitis or Kawasaki disease
Vertebrobasilar occlusion
Meningitis
Acute cerebellitis
Intracranial hemorrhage
Postconcussion syndrome
Benign paroxysmal vertigo[a]
Conversion reaction
Multiple sclerosis
Acute disseminated encephalomyelitis
Migraine
Epilepsy (pseudoataxia)
Transient ischemic attacks
Metabolic diseases
Hartnup disease
Wilson disease
Maple syrup urine disease
Pyruvate decarboxylase deficiency
Episodic ataxia type 1 (paroxysmal ataxia and myokymia)
Episodic ataxia type 2 (acetazolamide-responsive ataxia)
Chronic or progressive
Hydrocephalus
Posterior fossa tumors
Cerebellar hemangioblastoma (von Hippel–Lindau disease)
Chiari I malformation
Vermal aplasia (Dandy–Walker malformation and Joubert syndrome)
Spinocerebellar degenerations
Basilar impression
Cerebellar hemisphere hypoplasia or agenesis
Abetalipoproteinemia (vitamin E deficiency)
Friedreich ataxia
Metabolic diseases
Juvenile sulfatide lipodosis
Juvenile GM_2 gangliosidosis
Refsum disease
Hartnup disease
Ataxia telangiectasia
Ataxia with oculomotor apraxia
Familial periodic ataxia
Marinesco–Sjögren syndrome

[a]Indicates weakness or vertigo that may mimic ataxia.

with ataxia and headache, and vasculitis in a child with features of Kawasaki disease.

Migraine, seizure, transient ischemic attack, and metabolic disease are the most common causes for intermittent ataxia.

TABLE 10.2

COMMON CAUSES OF ACUTE ATAXIA

Acute cerebellar ataxia
Drug ingestion
Guillain–Barré syndrome[a]

[a]Indicates weakness or vertigo that may mimic ataxia.

Chronic progressive ataxias may have a basis in metabolic defects, some of which are treatable. When a progressive ataxia acutely worsens, this may signify severe hydrocephalus or hemorrhage into a posterior fossa tumor. A variety of familial, metabolic, and congenital causes exist for chronic nonprogressive ataxias.

EVALUATION AND DECISION

The approach to the problem should begin with a thorough history and physical examination. Once the duration and progression of illness is established, the ataxia is defined as acute, intermittent, or chronic. Chronic ataxia should be further divided into progressive or nonprogressive. Key historical points include recent illnesses such as varicella or other infectious diseases and access to medications or alcohol (Table 10.4). Family history may be helpful in recurrent or genetic causes.

Physical examination should focus on signs of increased ICP (papilledema, bradycardia, hypertension, abnormal respirations), meningeal irritation (nuchal rigidity, Kernig or Brudzinski sign), fever, rash, attached tick, and evidence of middle ear disease. A detailed neurologic examination should document level of consciousness, cranial nerve function, strength, tone, reflexes, sensation, proprioception, and presence or absence of nystagmus. Romberg test will be positive. Observation of the actual movements will help sharpen the diagnosis because particular syndromes have more truncal versus distal involvement or unilateral versus bilateral involvement. Specific testing of cerebellar function is impossible in young children. However, a cooperative older child can be asked to perform a finger–nose–finger test, heel–shin test, and rapid alternating movements to further delineate neurologic dysfunction.

The decision to pursue specific laboratory testing is outlined in the algorithm shown in Figure 10.1. Patients with

TABLE 10.3

LIFE-THREATENING CAUSES OF ATAXIA

Meningitis
Drug intoxication
Brain tumor
Neuroblastoma
Cerebral vascular accident (stroke)
Intracranial hemorrhage
Hydrocephalus
Labyrinthitis[a]
Middle ear trauma[a]

[a]Indicates weakness or vertigo that may mimic ataxia.

TABLE 10.4

DRUGS AND TOXINS THAT MAY CAUSE ATAXIA

Phenytoin
Alcohol
Carbamazepine
Benzodiazepines
Tricyclic antidepressants
Antihistamines
Dextromethorphan
Lead
5-Fluorouracil
Ethylene glycol
Primidone
Phenothiazines
Topiramate
Risperidone
Gabapentin

an acute presentation, focal neurologic deficits, recent head trauma, or signs of increased ICP warrant urgent evaluation with neuroimaging, which may reveal intracranial hemorrhage, hydrocephalus, or posterior fossa tumor. Neurosurgical involvement should be sought. If the imaging study is normal, the diagnosis may be postconcussion syndrome for patients with head trauma. Consultation with a neurologist may be indicated if physical examination findings other than ataxia persist.

If the patient has fever or nuchal rigidity, emergent imaging of the head is indicated because cerebellar tonsil herniation may cause neck stiffness. If imaging results are negative, a lumbar puncture can be performed safely. When bacterial meningitis is strongly suspected, appropriate antibiotics may be administered before the testing is done. MRI is the imaging of choice to detect acute cerebellitis.

When other causes have been eliminated, it is prudent to consider drug or alcohol ingestion (Table 10.4). With the exception of benzodiazepines, the routine toxicologic screen of urine will not detect many of these drugs. Thus, specific blood levels are indicated when intoxication is suspected.

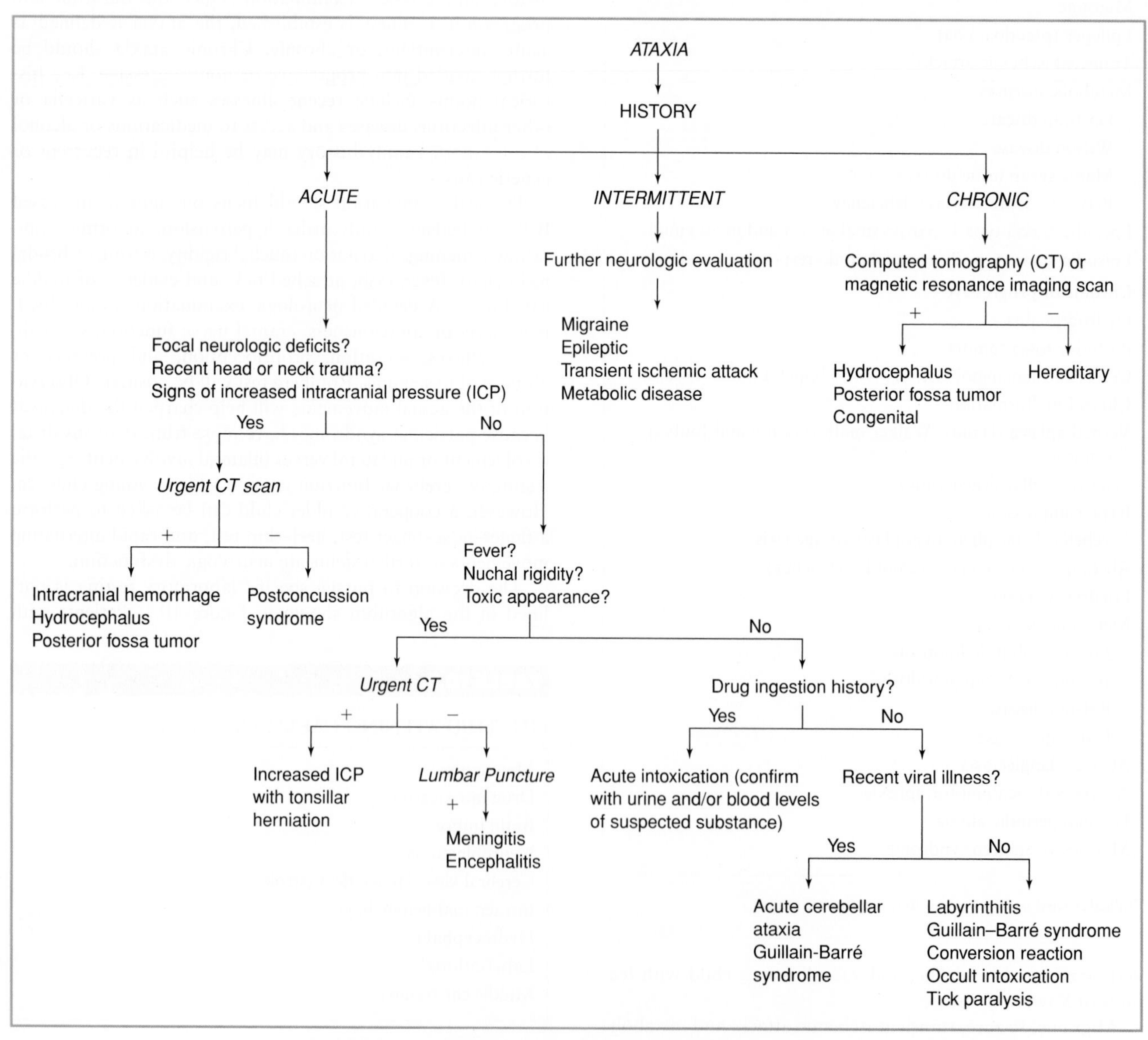

FIGURE 10.1 The diagnostic approach to the child with ataxia.

Management of ataxia in children is directed at the underlying cause. Fortunately, the most common cause, acute cerebellar ataxia, is a self-limiting illness that resolves completely in most cases. During periods of significant ataxia, head protection may be warranted because of the risk of falling. Also, special caution with sedatives is necessary because their effect may be greatly heightened.

Suggested Readings and Key References

Desai J, Mitchell WG. Acute cerebellar ataxia, acute cerebellitis, and opsoclonus-myclonus syndrome. *J Child Neurol* 2012;27:1482–1488.

Pina Garza E, Fenichel GM, eds. Ataxia. In: *Clinical pediatric neurology: a signs and symptoms approach,* 7th ed. St. Louis, MO: Saunders, 2012:215–235.

CHAPTER 11 ▪ BREAST LESIONS

RAKESH D. MISTRY, MD, MS

Complaints related to the breast usually involve pain, discharge, and either discrete or diffuse enlargement. Presentation of a breast lesion in a pediatric patient in the emergency setting is uncommon; however, pediatric emergency physicians must be able to distinguish etiologies that require immediate intervention from those that are more appropriately handled by referral to a specialist or close follow-up with a general pediatrician. Fortunately, most breast lesions in children and adolescents are benign and self-limited. However, many patients and their families will benefit from reassurance that neoplastic diseases of the breast are extremely rare in all pediatric age groups. This chapter covers the spectrum of disorders that pediatric emergency physicians are likely to encounter, focuses on the diagnostic approach to breast lesions, and discusses the management of common etiologies.

DIFFERENTIAL DIAGNOSIS

Breast lesions in children are typically divided into the following categories: infections, benign cysts or masses, malignant masses, abnormal nipple secretions, lesions associated with pregnancy and lactation, and miscellaneous causes, including both anatomic and physiologic entities (Table 11.1). A complete history and physical examination are essential to narrow the differential diagnosis and usually provides sufficient information to guide management. With few exceptions, most breast lesions require little diagnostic testing in the emergency department (ED) and typically can be evaluated using outpatient referral to an appropriate specialist. The commonly encountered disorders (Table 11.2) are almost always benign, but consideration must be given to potentially life-threatening processes (Table 11.3).

Breast Infections

Infection in the breast may take the form of a mastitis, cellulitis, or abscess. The incidence of breast infection occurs bimodally, with the early peak in the neonatal age group and the later, more common, peak in postpubertal females. Neonatal breast infection (mastitis neonatorum) most frequently presents in the first few weeks of life, commonly resulting from infection of the already enlarged breast bud produced by intrauterine maternal estrogen stimulation. As a result, mastitis neonatorum is more likely to occur in full-term, as opposed to premature infants. In some cases, excessive handling of the hypertrophied tissue by concerned caregivers may facilitate introduction of bacteria. The most common infecting organism is *Staphylococcus aureus* in >75% of cases; however, gram-negative enterics, as well as group A or group B streptococci may be isolated. More recent studies have demonstrated an increased incidence of community-associated methicillin-resistant *S. aureus* (CA-MRSA), and the presence of anaerobic bacteria in neonatal, adolescent, and adult breast infections.

The clinical presentation of neonatal breast infection is characterized by local signs of inflammation, such as edema, erythema, and warmth. Fever may be present in just 22% to 38% of cases and, although systemic symptoms are uncommon, the potential exists for seeding and associated invasive infections, including bacteremia, osteomyelitis, and pneumonia. For this reason, a complete evaluation for sepsis should be strongly considered in the presence of neonatal breast mastitis or abscess under the age of 2 months, especially in the setting of ill or toxic appearance. For older, well-appearing neonates, the emergency physician may elect to perform only a blood culture, and culture of purulent discharge, if present. Initial ED therapy consists of empiric broad-spectrum intravenous antibiotic for *S. aureus,* including CA-MRSA if indicated by local resistance rates, streptococcal organisms, and gram-negative enterics. Appropriate initial choices may include coverage for gram-positive organisms (vancomycin or clindamycin), with or without additional third-generation cephalosporins for gram-negative coverage. Subsequent antibiotic therapy can be guided by the results of a Gram stain and lesion culture. For cases where a breast abscess has developed, removal of purulent material is indicated. However, great care must be taken to avoid damaging the breast bud; therefore, surgical consultation is recommended, and needle aspiration is preferred to incision and drainage of the abscess cavity.

Breast infection in postpubertal females can be further classified as lactational or nonlactational. Lactational mastitis is discussed later in this chapter. Nonlactational mastitis and, less commonly, breast abscess, can develop in the central or peripheral regions of the breast usually resulting from introduction of skin bacteria into the ductal system. Infections in the central region of breast, proximal to the nipple, are more likely in the setting of obesity, nipple piercings, or poor hygiene, while peripheral mastitis is more likely to be associated with trauma or systemic illness. Other predisposing factors for mastitis include previous radiation therapy, foreign body, sebaceous cysts, hidradenitis suppurativa, and trauma to the periareolar area. Signs and symptoms of infection include local erythema, warmth, pain, and tenderness; dimpling of the overlying skin; and purulent nipple discharge. Systemic signs, including fever, are less commonly present. Organisms commonly implicated in this age group include both methicillin-sensitive and resistant *S. aureus,* streptococcal species, *Enterococcus, Pseudomonas* species, and anaerobic organisms such as *Bacteroides* species.

Recommended treatment for mastitis in the postpubertal female includes initiation of antistaphylococcal oral antibiotic therapy and warm compresses. Patients should be instructed to keep the area as clean and dry as possible, to wear a clean cotton bra to help prevent excessive sweating, and to avoid skin creams or talcum powders. The majority of patients may be managed as outpatients, but require a follow-up appointment in 24 to 48 hours to ensure the infection is improving.

TABLE 11.1

BREAST ENLARGEMENT/MASSES

I. Inflammatory conditions
  A. Cellulitis and mastitis
  B. Breast abscess
II. Noninflammatory conditions
  A. Infancy
    1. Physiologic hypertrophy
    2. Tumor (rare)
  B. Childhood
    1. Premature thelarche
    2. Precocious puberty
    3. Prepubertal gynecomastia (male)
    4. Malignancy (rare)
  C. Adolescence
    1. Male
      a. Postpubertal (physiologic) gynecomastia
      b. Exogenous hormonal stimulation
      c. Drug exposure
        i. Phenothiazines
        ii. Opiates
        iii. Cannabis (tetrahydrocannabinol)
        iv. Anabolic steroids
        v. Antiretroviral therapy
        vi. Tricyclic antidepressants
        vii. Calcium channel blockers or digoxin
      d. Endocrinopathy
      e. Nipple cyst
      f. Malignancy (rare)
    2. Female
      a. Isolated, benign cyst
      b. Fibroadenoma
      c. Fibrocystic disease
      d. Juvenile hypertrophy
      e. Hematoma/fat necrosis (posttraumatic)
      f. Papillomatosis
      g. Cystosarcoma phylloides and other cancers (rare)

TABLE 11.2

COMMON BREAST LESIONS

Newborn
Physiologic hypertrophy
Mastitis (mastitis neonatorum)

Prepubertal Child
Premature thelarche (female)

Pubertal/Postpubertal Male
Pubertal gynecomastia

Pubertal/Postpubertal Female
Enlargement/galactorrhea secondary to pregnancy
Mastitis and breast abscess
Fibroadenoma
Fibrocystic disease
Benign, isolated cysts

TABLE 11.3

LIFE-THREATENING BREAST LESIONS

Newborn
Mastitis (mastitis neonatorum)

Prepubertal Child
Breast enlargement with precocious puberty (secondary to hormonal secretion by a tumor)

Postpubertal Male
Breast enlargement with abnormal sexual development (secondary to hormonal secretion by a tumor)

Postpubertal Female
Neoplastic mass
Galactorrhea secondary to prolactin-secreting tumor

For patients with systemic symptoms, those who appear toxic, or demonstrate a lack of response to outpatient antibiotics, hospital admission for intravenous antibiotics is indicated. If a breast abscess is suspected, confirmation via ultrasonography is preferred. Breast abscesses should be drained via needed aspiration by a surgical specialist; incision and drainage are only occasionally necessary.

Benign Cysts and Masses

Enlargement of breast tissue may occur at any age, even in the neonatal period. As previously discussed, the male and female neonatal breast bud is hypertrophied in the first few weeks of life secondary to in utero maternal estrogen stimulation. This is a normal physiologic response that abates over time; treatment is not required and caregivers should be instructed to avoid manual stimulation. In preschool age girls, a temporary unilateral or bilateral enlargement of the breast bud may occur. This is typically consistent with isolated premature thelarche in the absence of other manifestations or development of secondary sexual characteristics: Reassurance should be provided as the enlargement will most likely spontaneously resolve, though close follow-up with a primary care physician is prudent. The presence of breast enlargement in the setting of secondary sexual characteristics, such as pubic hair (precocious puberty) in girls, or any breast enlargement in young boys (prepubertal gynecomastia), is atypical, and a specific cause should be aggressively pursued. Careful history and examination focused on the presence of adrenal, ovarian, or hypothalamic pathology, including hormone-secreting tumors and intracranial tumors, are indicated in these cases. Recent medication usage should be reviewed as several medications can cause gynecomastia (Table 11.1). Unless an intracranial mass is suspected, most children can be referred for outpatient workup with an experienced physician or endocrinologist.

Fibroadenomas are the most common benign breast lesion (>75%) in the adolescent age group. When present in adolescent girls, these lesions are sometimes called juvenile fibroadenomas. Fibroadenomas are usually discovered by self-examination and present as well-circumscribed, solitary, mobile, rubbery, mildly tender masses of the upper outer quadrants of the breast that are typically <2 to 3 cm in size. These lesions are benign and do not require extensive evaluation; ultrasonography is most helpful and is recommended in the ED to secure the diagnosis, and exclude more severe pathologies. Fibroadenomas can be observed over time, and reassurance that the exceedingly low malignant potential should be provided. Treatment is required for giant fibroadenomas (>5 cm), referral to a pediatric or breast surgeon for excisional biopsy is preferred to prevent destruction of healthy breast tissue.

Fibrocystic disease is a benign, progressive process generally seen in women during the reproductive years, but may also present in adolescence. Fibrocystic masses may be solitary or multiple, unilateral or bilateral, feel nodular within the breast tissue, and are most prominent in the upper outer quadrants of the breast. Frequently, presentation is that of cyclically painful masses, that change in size or nodularity during the course of the menstrual cycle, with the maximal symptoms during the premenstrual phase. Nipple discharge is rarely present and is typically nonbloody, green, or brown. Importantly, in the adolescent population, these lesions are not precancerous. Breast ultrasonography can be used to confirm the diagnosis; neither needle aspiration nor breast biopsy is required. Treatment is largely symptomatic with breast support, nonsteroidal analgesics, and avoidance of caffeine. Oral contraceptive agents can reduce symptoms in severe cases for adults, but are not typically prescribed for fibrocystic disease in adolescence. Follow-up and subsequent evaluation by a primary care physician is recommended; referral to a surgeon for needle aspiration or excisional biopsy is indicated for painful, large, solitary lesions.

Nipple masses represent another group of generally benign breast masses. Benign intraductal papillomatosis is the most common etiology and can be seen in prepubertal or pubertal boys and girls, often coming to attention because of bleeding from the nipple. Occasionally, the lesion may obstruct the nipple and causing pain and possibly infection. In extremely rare instances, a nipple mass can represent an intraductal carcinoma. In these cases, cytologic examination of the bloody nipple discharge can be of diagnostic value. Therefore, expedient referral to a breast surgeon or pediatric surgeon is indicated after detection. In cases of benign nipple masses, careful observation for several weeks by an experienced primary care physician or surgical specialist is indicated. If the nipple mass or bleeding persists, excision is the treatment of choice.

Trauma to the breast can lead to hematomas and fat necrosis, both of which are palpated as firm, well-circumscribed breast masses. Initially, these lesions may be tender. If left untreated, they may develop into areas of scar tissue that are affixed to the skin. Fat necrosis is relatively common, but the differentiation from other more serious lesions may be difficult, requiring consultation with a surgeon in cases of uncertainty.

Malignant Masses

Primary cancers of the breast have been reported in children, but are exceedingly rare, with an incidence of 1 in 1,000,000 females less than age 20 years. In children, breast tumors accounting for less than 1% of all malignancies and less than 0.1% of all breast cancers occur in the pediatric age group. Metastatic disease is far more common than primary breast tumors, and may be secondary to Hodgkin and non-Hodgkin lymphoma, neuroblastoma, and leukemia, and rhabdomyosarcoma. Adolescent or childhood breast tumors are often classified as secretory carcinomas that behave more benignly than breast cancers in adults. Other histologic classifications of breast malignancies reported in children and adolescents include carcinomas, sarcomas, and cystosarcoma phylloides, which can have both benign and malignant features. Physical examination characteristics suggestive of malignancy include a hard, nontender, solitary mass with ambiguous margins. The mass may be fixed to surrounding tissues, and overlying skin changes such as edema, warmth, skin dimpling, and/or nipple retraction may be present. Other signs include bleeding from the nipple and local lymphadenopathy. The appropriate treatment for suspected malignant lesions is the same as that for a benign mass—prompt referral to a pediatric or breast surgeon for definitive workup, usually consisting of excisional biopsy. Among the strongest risk factors for malignant breast masses in the pediatric population include chest irradiation, particularly when incurred during high-dose treatment for Hodgkin disease or with radioiodine treatment for thyroid cancer. Radiation exposure between ages 10 to 16 years is most harmful. In girls treated for Hodgkin lymphoma, there is a higher incidence of breast cancer within 20 years of treatment. Children with a strong familial history of breast malignances, such as those who are offspring of women with inherited cancer syndromes, are also more susceptible to developing breast malignancy. Important for detection of potential malignant breast masses is self-examination of the breast; adolescents should be encouraged to routinely perform self-examinations, especially if they are at increased risk of developing breast cancer. For children at particularly high risk, routine screening with magnetic resonance imaging should be considered.

Abnormal Secretions (Nipple Discharge)

There are multiple etiologies of abnormal nipple secretions in children and adolescents. These can be divided according to their potential for surgical management. Nonsurgical causes typically present as nonspontaneous discharges. The most common example is discharge fluid expressed during breast self-examination. The fluid may be milky, multicolored, and sticky and is a normal, physiologic discharge of little concern. When breast infection (mastitis or abscess) is present, a purulent discharge may be expressed or occur spontaneously.

Galactorrhea is the most common spontaneous nipple discharge and usually occurs bilaterally. Pregnancy and lactation are typical causes of galactorrhea; however, in the absence of these conditions, increased prolactin states should be suspected. Structural lesions of the hypothalamus and pituitary (e.g., adenomas) and exogenous medications can cause increased prolactin levels. Drugs implicated include oral contraceptives, tricyclic antidepressants, phenothiazines, metoclopramide, α-methyldopa, anabolic steroids, and cannabis. As mentioned earlier, in utero estrogen exposure can lead to breast bud hypertrophy in neonates; in addition, this hypertrophy can be accompanied by a colostrum-like material that has been referred to as "witch's milk." This discharge occurs temporarily, until maternal estrogen levels decline, and is not considered pathologic.

Other nonsurgical spontaneous nipple discharges have been described as multicolored, grossly bloody, serous, or clear and watery. Nonbloody discharges are rarely indicative of malignancy. Mammary duct ectasia, traumatic nipple erosions (e.g., "jogger's nipple"), and eczema are among the more common causes of nonbloody discharges. These disorders can be treated with nipple hygiene, warm compresses, and topical antibiotics, if necessary. When nipple discharge is described as serosanguinous or frankly bloody, or when it tests positive for occult blood, the potential for surgical pathology increases, particularly when a mass is palpable below the nipple. However, surgical etiologies are rare, with malignancy only present in 6% of bloody nipple discharges. Any pediatric patient with spontaneous nipple discharge not explained by an obvious cause (e.g., jogger's nipples) should be referred to a breast or surgical specialist for close follow-up and further diagnostic and therapeutic evaluation.

Lesions Associated with Pregnancy and Lactation

Significant changes occur in the female breast as a result of pregnancy, most prominently an increase in breast size and weight. Although pregnant patients may have any of the breast lesions seen in nonpregnant patients, they are prone to develop some unique conditions. The most frequent of these is puerperal (lactational) mastitis, which develops in up to one-third of lactating women, usually within the first few weeks postpartum. Lactational mastitis is likely to result from infection with *S. aureus*, with an increasing incidence of CA-MRSA. *Streptococcus* species, gram-negative organisms, mycobacteria, *Candida*, and *Cryptococcus* have all been implicated as causative organisms of lactational mastitis. Breast abscess may also arise, and frequently requires drainage of purulent material. Treatment of lactational mastitis consists of warm compresses, antistaphylococcal antibiotic therapy, and frequent evacuation of breast milk. Breast engorgement may exacerbate the symptoms of breast infection; therefore, continued feeding or pumping is recommended. The risk of mother-to-infant transmission of infection is rare and breast-feeding can typically continue. In cases where there is substantial pain, or the infant does not like the taste of infected milk, feeding can proceed in the opposite breast. Mastitis within the first 2 weeks postpartum is often a result of cracked nipples, infant attachment difficulties and anatomic abnormalities (e.g., cleft lip or palate); later onset is usually a result of poor hygiene or inadequate emptying of the breast with subsequent milk stasis, engorgement, and colonization of bacteria within the milk.

Pregnant patients may also have simple milk-filled cysts called galactoceles, which are often tender and located on the periphery of the breast. Ice packs, breast support, and aspiration may be needed to relieve the obstruction of the milk-filled ducts.

Nonlactating pregnant patients may develop bloody discharge from the nipple during the second or third trimester, representing a benign condition from epithelial cell proliferation. If the discharge persists after delivery, a more thorough investigation for alternate etiologies is recommended. Fibroadenomas often increase in size during pregnancy and may result in significant pain. Excision is often advised for any solitary mass and the patient should be expediently referred to a breast surgeon. The number of cases of breast malignancy diagnosed during pregnancy is very low.

Miscellaneous Breast Lesions

Congenital Lesions

Supernumerary breasts (polymastia) and supernumerary nipples (polythelia) are congenital conditions that are unlikely to present as chief complaints in the ED, but that may be discovered incidentally on examination. Polymastia results from failure of the embryonic mammary ridges to regress and is present at birth, often resembling skin tags or nevi, and may not be noticed until the tissue is hormonally influenced. Supernumerary breasts are most commonly found in the axillae but have been reported to occur in several locations. This ectopic tissue may become tender with menses and has been reported to develop the same range of pathology as normal breast tissue, necessitating excision under certain circumstances.

Polythelia occurs both sporadic and familial, and is most commonly found on the left, inferior to the normal nipple. In newborns, polythelia may appear as small, wrinkled lesions with or without pigmentation. Polythelia is typically of little significance, though there is a possible association with unsuspected urologic anomalies. For this reason, patients with polythelia should be referred for at least a primary screening of underlying urologic disease. Otherwise, this disorder requires no treatment unless the diagnosis is uncertain (e.g., the lesion looks like a possible melanoma) or is perceived as a cosmetic problem.

Premature Thelarche

Premature thelarche refers to isolated breast development without other signs of puberty. Minimum acceptable age for thelarche is 8 years; appearance of breast tissue prior to this age should prompt consultation with an endocrinologist. Typically appearing within the first 2 years of life in its most common form, premature thelarche is a benign, transient condition of unknown etiology. Cases of premature thelarche usually present to the ED secondary to concern raised by parents of prepubertal girls, and reassurance is usually all that is required. However, premature thelarche may be the first sign of true precocious puberty or pseudopuberty, or exposure to exogenous estrogens, and careful follow-up with the primary physician is required.

Juvenile Breast Hypertrophy

Juvenile breast hypertrophy is a rare disorder characterized by sudden, rapid, massive breast enlargement at a time of intense endocrine stimulation, usually between 8 and 16 years of age, after onset of menarche. It is believed to result from end-organ hypersensitivity to estrogen. The hypertrophy is usually bilateral and asymmetric and may progress at an alarming rate over 36 months. The differential diagnosis of this lesion includes cystosarcoma phylloides, juvenile fibroadenoma, and precocious puberty; however, true endocrine or neoplastic lesions are uncommon. In some cases, the hypertrophy regresses in 1 to 3 years, but referral to a breast surgeon is always indicated; breast reduction or even total ablation may become necessary. This disorder is often associated with extreme emotional and psychosocial distress for patients and families.

Gynecomastia

Gynecomastia is a term commonly used to describe a broad spectrum of clinical breast lesions in boys, including excess breast tissue, breast enlargement, and masses of tissue below the nipple that are discrete and nonadherent to the chest wall, and may occur unilaterally or bilaterally. Gynecomastia has been described as the male equivalent of fibrocystic changes in the female breast, based on histologic evidence. Typically, local breast tissue demonstrates evidence of mild estrogen–testosterone hormone imbalance, resulting from physiologic changes (neonatal, puberty, aging); exogenous medications;

tumors of the testes, adrenal glands, and lungs; metabolic conditions (cirrhosis, hyperthyroidism, renal disease); or hypogonadism.

From a clinical perspective, gynecomastia occurs in about 50% of all boys between the ages of 11 and 18 years and typically lasts about 2 years. It can be associated with growth spurts and can also cause a significant degree of pain. The glandular enlargement is about 4 cm and resembles the early stages of female breast budding. More commonly, gynecomastia presents to the emergency physician because of associated anxiety in adolescent boys. If the patient has normal-sized genitalia and none of the predisposing conditions listed earlier, reassurance is all that is required, though inquiry about both prescription and illicit use of drugs should be sought. There is often particular concern about gynecomastia in obese boys, since they may appear to have an overabundance of fatty tissue in the breast region. Of note, the incidence of true gynecomastia is not increased in boys who are obese, compared with those who are not obese. Rarely, a few conditions can be mistaken for physiologic gynecomastia, such as lipomastia, a round adipose tissue mass, or neoplasm. If there is any concern for these entities or systemic diseases, then the patient should be urgently referred to an endocrinologist. Overall, gynecomastia is best managed by referral to the primary care physician for continued follow-up.

Physiologic Mastalgia

During the first trimester of pregnancy, some teenage girls may complain of breast fullness, though nongravid patients may experience breast pain as well, likely related to the hormonal milieu of the breast throughout the menstrual cycle. Mastalgia is often described as a bilateral, poorly localized, dull, achy pain that radiates to the axillae. The pain is often worse with activity and relieved with the onset of menses. In general, there are no abnormal physical findings, except tender, nodular breasts. Most patients will improve with reassurance, analgesics such as nonsteroidal anti-inflammatory medications, warm compresses, and breast support. If the pain is refractory to these measures, other suggested therapies include caffeine avoidance, salt restriction, and diuretics. Danazol, a synthetic androgen, is reserved for severe, debilitating pain.

EVALUATION AND DECISION

History and Physical Examination

Initial evaluation of a breast lesion begins with a careful history and physical examination (Table 11.4). The two most common categories of breast lesions presenting in children are infections and structural or mass lesions. In the absence of infection, evaluation of mass lesions requires a detailed menstrual history and a chronology of the development of secondary sexual characteristics. Features of intracranial masses, including headaches or visual changes, should be assessed. Pregnant or lactating patients may also present to a pediatric ED. These patients should be queried regarding breast-feeding or breast-feeding attempts, as well as about general symptoms related to changes in the breast tissue. Medications may have an effect on the growth of certain breast lesions and may also affect hormonal pathways, leading to abnormal breast secretions (Table 11.1). Few breast disorders may have a familial pattern; however, a careful family history can be helpful.

TABLE 11.4

IMPORTANT HISTORICAL AND PHYSICAL EXAMINATION COMPONENTS IN THE EVALUATION OF A BREAST LESION

History
Onset and duration of lesion
Pain
Nipple discharge
Relationship of lesion with menses
Complete menstrual and sexual development history, including sexual activity and previous pregnancies
Family history of breast disease
Diet
Medications and illicit drugs
Concomitant medical disorders
Systemic symptoms: fever, weight loss, sweating, headaches, visual changes
Physical Examination
Breasts: symmetry, skin appearance, temperature, areola, nipples, secretions, masses, chest wall, axillae
Lymph nodes
Hair distribution
Genitalia

A comprehensive physical examination should be performed on any pediatric patient who complains of a breast mass or lesion. Premature appearance of secondary sexual characteristics, hirsutism, or abnormal skin coloring may indicate the presence of an endocrinopathy. A detailed evaluation of the breasts and adjacent structures is essential. The chest wall should be inspected for any gross deformities, asymmetry, or skin changes. The physician should have the patient lean forward with hands on hips and again observe for any asymmetry or skin retraction. With the patient supine with arms above the head, the physician should palpate each breast in a series of concentric circles radiating outward from the nipple, looking and feeling for nodules, cysts, masses, or inconsistencies in the breast tissue. Each areola should be gently compressed to assess for masses or nipple discharge. If present, the color, character, and odor of any discharge should be noted. The physician should feel for the presence of any masses or lymphadenopathy in both axillae.

Diagnostic Testing

The majority of patients presenting to the ED will not require intensive laboratory or radiologic testing. All postmenarchal girls should have a pregnancy test performed; breast tenderness and swelling are among the earliest signs of pregnancy. The most helpful test in the emergency setting is breast ultrasonography, which is useful in distinguishing between masses and cystic lesions as well as the presence of abscess with mastitis. Other imaging studies are rarely helpful. Mammography is of little value in children and adolescents, owing to the high proportion of fibroglandular tissue within the breast. Chest radiography is rarely helpful, except when the examiner elicits signs and symptoms from the lungs or chest wall that may be referred to the breast. If nipple discharge is present, Gram

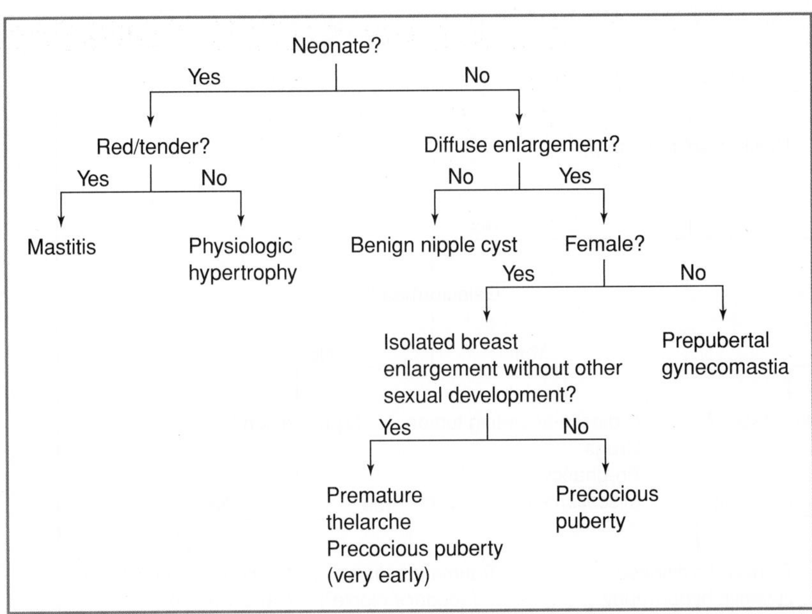

FIGURE 11.1 Approach to breast complaints in the prepubertal child.

stain, culture, and rarely cytology can be of value. Fine-needle aspiration is used in a limited fashion in children and adults, since the majority of lesions are typically benign. Serum endocrinology testing may be indicated for some breast lesions, although these generally take place outside the ED.

APPROACH

The approach to the patient with complaints related to the breast primarily depends first on whether the patient is prepubertal or pubertal/postpubertal. Among patients who are pubertal/postpubertal, the considerations vary greatly between boys and girls. Finally, unique considerations pertain to the pregnant or lactating girl, as discussed earlier in this chapter.

Prepubertal Child

Among prepubertal children (Fig. 11.1), the most common breast disorders are physiologic hypertrophy in the newborn period and premature thelarche in young girls. When physiologic hypertrophy is noted in newborns, erythema or tenderness should be assessed, and mastitis and potential serious bacterial infection should be considered. Breast development in prepubertal girls, without other signs of puberty, particularly in those younger than 2 years of age, is likely due to the common and benign condition of premature thelarche. Since this may be the first sign of precocious puberty, urgent follow-up with the primary care physician and/or an endocrinologist for additional testing is recommended. Also among prepubertal children, isolated lesions underneath the nipple may be noted and are usually benign cysts.

Pubertal/Postpubertal Male

The adolescent male (Fig. 11.2) may complain of breast pain, yet have no clearly palpable breast enlargement. This sensation may be caused by minor chest trauma in a boy with early pubertal gynecomastia or may represent underlying chest pain (see Chapter 50 Pain: Chest). Most often, adolescent males will present for bilateral (sometimes asymmetric) enlargement diffusely throughout the breast tissue, which usually represents (physiologic) pubertal gynecomastia, in the setting of normal sexual development. Unilateral, discrete masses or bilateral, diffuse enlargement with abnormal sexual development require subspecialty referral and additional diagnostic evaluation.

Pubertal/Postpubertal Female

The initial step in evaluating the adolescent girl (Fig. 11.3) is to obtain a pregnancy test, which, when positive, points to a number of conditions that are specific to the gravid state (see earlier discussion). Both pregnant and nonpregnant girls may experience a myriad of disorders related to the breast. The emergency physician's primary goal is to distinguish underlying disorders that are causing chest rather than breast pain (see Chapter 50 Pain: Chest) and to assess for a few relatively

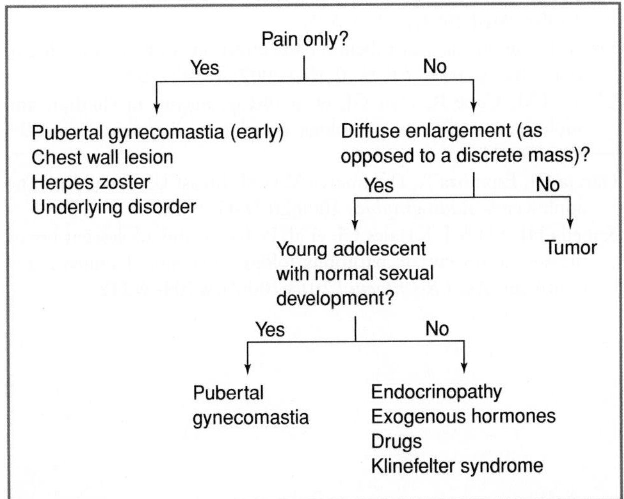

FIGURE 11.2 Approach to breast complaints in the pubertal/postpubertal boy.

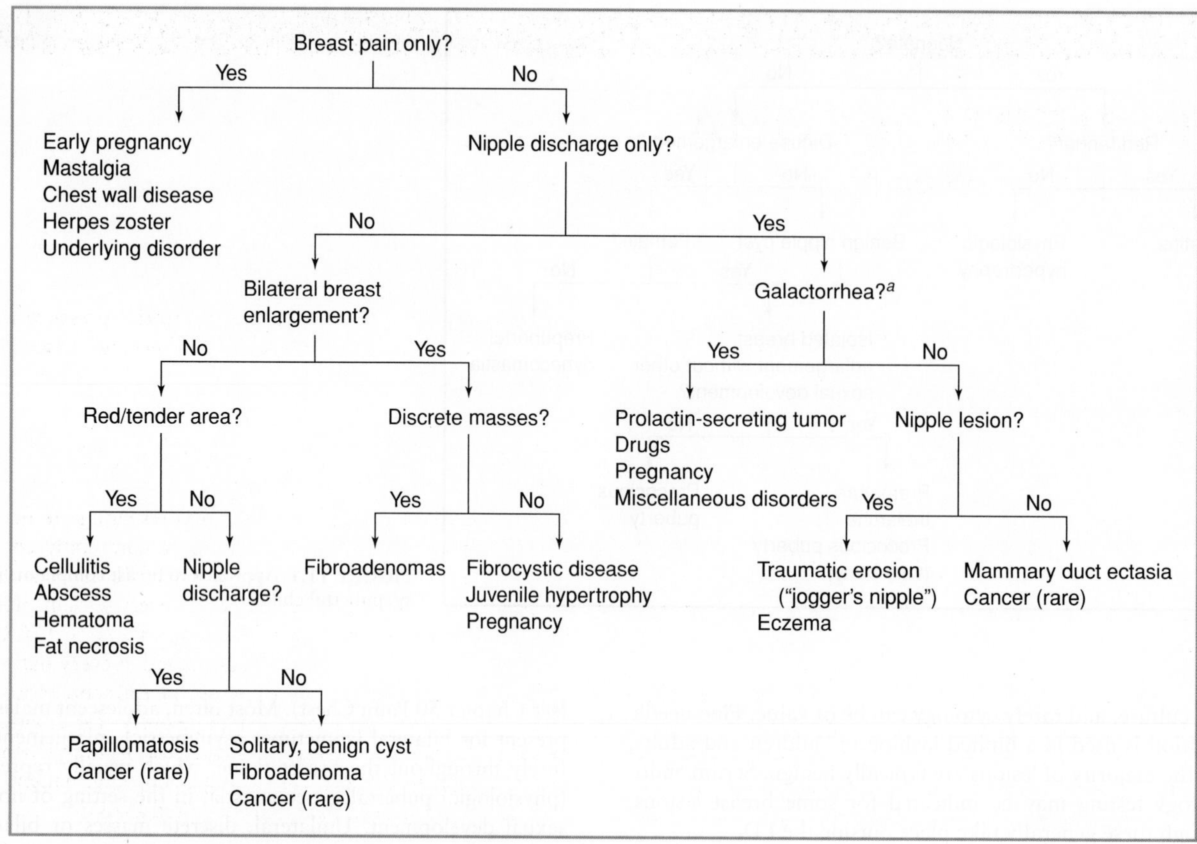

FIGURE 11.3 Approach to breast complaints in the pubertal/postpubertal girl. [a]Galactorrhea refers to milky, as opposed to bloody, serous, or purulent discharge.

minor problems, including cellulitis, abscess, hematoma, and traumatic erosions. In cases where there is concern for deeper infection or an irregular or large breast mass, breast ultrasonography can be used to rule out severe, life-threatening etiologies. Less severe causes of breast enlargement, masses, and discharge require outpatient follow-up and evaluation by an appropriate specialist.

Suggested Readings and Key References

Arca MJ, Caniano DA. Breast disorders in the adolescent patient. *Adolesc Med* 2004;15:473–485.

Brook I. Cutaneous and subcutaneous infections in newborns due to anaerobic bacteria. *J Perinat Med* 2002;30:197–208.

Chung EM, Cube R, Hall GJ, et al. Breast masses in children and adolescents: radiologic-pathologic correlation. *Radiographics* 2009; 29:907–931.

Garcia CJ, Espinoza A, Dinamarca V, et al. Breast US in children and adolescents. *Radiographics* 2000;20:1605–1612.

Kaneda HJ, Mack J, Kasales CJ, et al. Pediatric and adolescent breast masses: a review of pathophysiology, imaging, diagnosis, and treatment. *Am J Roentgenol* 2013;200(2):W204–W212.

Kennedy RD, Boughey JC. Management of pediatric and adolescent breast masses. *Semin Plas Surg* 2013;27:19–22.

Lazala C, Saenger P. Pubertal gynecomastia. *J Pediatr Endocr Metab* 2002;15:553–560.

Merlob P. Congenital malformations and developmental changes of the breast: a neonatological view. *J Pediatr Endocr Metab* 2003; 16:471–485.

Michie C, Lockie F, Lynn W. The challenge of mastitis. *Arch Dis Child* 2003;88(9):818–821.

Neinstein LS. Breast disease in adolescent and young women. *Pediatr Clin North Am* 1999;46(3):607–629.

Scott-Conner CE, Schorr SJ. The diagnosis and management of breast problems during pregnancy and lactation. *Am J Surg* 1995;170: 401–405.

Spencer JP. Management of mastitis in breastfeeding women. *Am Fam Physician* 2008;78:727–732.

Stafford I, Hernandez J, Laibl V, et al. Community-acquired methicillin-resistant staphylococcus aureus among patients with puerperal mastitis requiring hospitalization. *Obstet Gynecol* 2008;112:533–537.

Stricker T, Navrath F, Sennhauser FH. Mastitis in early infancy. *Acta Paediatr* 2005;94:166–169.

Templeman C, Hertweck SP. Breast disorders in the pediatric and adolescent patient. *Obstet Gynecol Clin North Am* 2000;27(1):19–34.

CHAPTER 12 ■ COMA

ERIC W. GLISSMEYER, MD AND DOUGLAS S. NELSON, MD, FACEP, FAAP

Consciousness refers to the state of being awake and aware of oneself and one's surroundings. It is a basic cerebral function that is not easily compromised; impairment of this faculty may therefore signal the presence of a life-threatening condition. An altered level of consciousness (ALOC) is not in itself a disease but a state caused by an underlying disease process. *Coma* refers to a state lacking wakefulness and awareness from which a patient cannot be roused; this represents the most extreme form of ALOC. The term *coma* is often modified with descriptors such as light or deep. Lesser levels of impairment are described using other terms whose meanings may overlap. *Lethargy* refers to depressed consciousness resembling a deep sleep from which a patient can be aroused but into which he or she immediately returns. A patient is said to be stuporous or obtunded when he or she is not totally asleep but demonstrates greatly depressed responses to external stimuli. Not all ALOC states produce a diminished mental state, but may include abnormal activation of consciousness such as in delirium (see Chapter 8 Agitated Child). Because neurologic status may vary dramatically over time, it may be difficult to summarize such symptoms using a single descriptor and, as noted above, meanings of terms may overlap. Therefore, recording the comatose patient's specific response (e.g., body movement, type of vocalization) to a defined stimulus (e.g., a sternal rub) is usually preferable (Table 12.1).

PATHOPHYSIOLOGY

The state of wakefulness is mediated by neurons of the ascending reticular activating system (ARAS) located in the brainstem and pons. Neural pathways from these locations project throughout the cortex, which is responsible for awareness. If the function of these neurons is compromised or if both cerebral hemispheres are sufficiently affected by disease, an ALOC will result.

Proper function of the ARAS and cerebral hemispheres depends on many factors, including the presence of substrates needed for energy production, adequate blood flow to deliver these substrates, absence of abnormal serum concentrations of metabolic waste products or extraneous toxins, maintenance of body temperature within normal ranges, and the absence of abnormal neuronal excitation or irritation from seizure activity or central nervous system (CNS) infection.

Disorders that produce coma by raising intracranial pressure (ICP) increase the volume of an existing intracerebral component such as brain or cerebrospinal fluid (CSF) within the confined space of the cranial cavity. Alternatively, a new component such as a tumor or extravasated blood may be introduced. The brain can initially compensate for this altered volume relationship by regulating blood flow and CSF production. When the limits of these compensatory mechanisms are reached, ICP will rise abruptly, decreasing cerebral perfusion pressure (defined as mean arterial pressure minus ICP) and placing the patient at risk for herniation (see Chapter 121 Neurotrauma).

DIFFERENTIAL DIAGNOSIS

A differential diagnosis for children presenting in or near coma is shown in Table 12.2. The more commonly encountered causes of coma are listed in Table 12.3. These most likely causes of coma should be considered in every patient presenting with this condition. Life-threatening causes of ALOC are listed in Table 12.4 and must be considered in every patient. If present, these disorders require emergent treatment. More than one problem may be present simultaneously; for example, a victim of submersion injury may incur head trauma when falling into a swimming pool, or a deeply postictal patient with known seizure disorder may have ingested a toxin.

Primary Central Nervous System Disorders

Trauma

Coma-producing brain lesions that result from trauma include subdural and epidural hematomas, intraparenchymal and subarachnoid hemorrhage, penetrating injuries, cerebral contusion, diffuse cerebral edema, and concussion (see Chapter 121 Neurotrauma). Though most pediatric head injuries are blunt in nature and are accompanied by a history of trauma, abusive head trauma is also common and may present with nonspecific complaints. Patients suffering head trauma may present in a comatose state or may be alert for variable periods after impact.

ALOC resulting from diffuse cerebral edema and diffuse axonal injury is common in children and is less amenable to neurosurgical intervention than epidural and subdural hematomas. Characteristic CT findings of loss of gray–white interface may not be visible for 12 to 24 hours after the trauma was sustained. When radiographic abnormalities appear, they may be similar to those produced by hypoxia.

Concussion is an inexact term for a transient alteration in normal neurologic function after experiencing head trauma. A postconcussion syndrome may last for hours to days and is characterized by nausea, vomiting, dizziness, headache, and lethargy, with some symptoms lasting for weeks in some patients. Neuroimaging studies are normal, yet patients may be symptomatic enough to require admission for observation and intravenous (IV) hydration.

Seizures

Consciousness is greatly diminished both during and after periods of seizure activity. Although generalized seizure activity is readily recognizable by the rhythmic motor activity accompanying

TABLE 12.1

GLASGOW COMA SCALE AND MODIFICATIONS FOR INFANTS AND CHILDREN

	Score	Infant	Child	Adult
Eye opening	4	Spontaneous	Spontaneous	Spontaneous
	3	To speech	To speech	To speech
	2	To pain	To pain	To pain
	1	None	None	None
Best verbal response	5	Coos and babbles	Oriented, appropriate	Oriented
	4	Irritable, cries	Confused	Confused
	3	Cries in response to pain	Inappropriate words	Inappropriate words
	2	Moans in response to pain	Incomprehensible sounds	Incomprehensible sounds
	1	None	None	None
Best motor response	6	Moves spontaneously and purposefully	Obeys commands	Obeys verbal command
	5	Withdraws in response to touch	Localizes painful stimulus	Localizes
	4	Withdraws in response to pain	Withdraws in response to pain	Withdraws
	3	Abnormal flexion posture to pain	Flexion in response to pain	Abnormal flexion
	2	Abnormal extension posture to pain	Extension in response to pain	Extensor response
	1	None	None	None

Adapted from the American Heart Association. 2010 Handbook of Emergency Cardiovascular Care.

TABLE 12.2

ETIOLOGY OF ACUTE-ONSET COMA/ALTERED LEVEL OF CONSCIOUSNESS

I. Conditions arising from head trauma or primary central nervous system disease
  A. Trauma
    1. Intracranial hematoma (subdural, epidural, subarachnoid)
    2. Cerebral contusion
    3. Diffuse cerebral edema
    4. Concussion
  B. Seizures
    1. Status epilepticus (convulsive, nonconvulsive)
    2. Postictal state
  C. Infection
    1. Meningitis
    2. Encephalitis
    3. Focal infections (brain abscess, subdural empyema, epidural abscess)
  D. Neoplasms
    1. Tumor (edema, hemorrhage, blockage of CSF flow)
  E. Vascular disease
    1. Cerebral infarct (thrombotic, hemorrhagic, embolic)
    2. Cerebral sinovenous thrombosis
    3. Subarachnoid hemorrhage
    4. Vascular malformation/aneurysm
  F. Hydrocephalus
    1. Obstructive (from tumor or other cause)
    2. Cerebrospinal fluid shunt malfunction

II. Conditions affecting the brain diffusely
  A. Vital sign abnormalities
    1. Hypotension, hypertension
    2. Hypothermia, hyperthermia
  B. Hypoxia
    1. Pulmonary disease
    2. Severe anemia
    3. Methemoglobinemia
    4. Carbon monoxide
    5. Posthypoxic encephalopathy
  C. Intoxications
    1. Sedative drugs: antihistamines, barbiturates, benzodiazepines, ethanol, gamma-hydroxybutyrate (GHB), and analogs, narcotics, phenothiazines
    2. Tricyclic and other antidepressants
    3. Antipsychotics (i.e., risperidone, quetiapine, olanzapine)
    4. Antiepileptics
    5. Salicylates
  D. Metabolic abnormalities
    1. Hypoglycemia (sepsis, insulin overdose, ethanol intoxication)
    2. Hyperglycemia (diabetic ketoacidosis, hyperglycemic hyperosmolar syndrome)
    3. Metabolic acidosis
    4. Metabolic alkalosis
    5. Hyponatremia, hypernatremia
    6. Hypocalcemia, hypercalcemia
    7. Hypomagnesemia, hypermagnesemia
    8. Hypophosphatemia
    9. Uremia (kidney failure)
    10. Liver failure
    11. Acute toxic encephalopathy (Reye syndrome)
    12. Inherited metabolic disorders
  E. Other
    1. Intussusception
    2. Hemolytic uremic syndrome
    3. Dehydration
    4. Sepsis
    5. Rheumatologic conditions (SLE, Behçet's)
    6. Psychiatric conditions

TABLE 12.3

COMMON CAUSES OF COMA/ALTERED LEVEL OF CONSCIOUSNESS

Subdural hematoma
Epidural hematoma
Cerebral edema
Postictal state
Hypotension
Posthypoxic/ischemic insult
Hypoglycemia
Toxic ingestions
Meningitis

TABLE 12.4

LIFE-THREATENING CAUSES OF COMA/ALTERED LEVEL OF CONSCIOUSNESS

Intracranial hemorrhage
Cerebral edema
Brain neoplasms
Cerebral infarctions
Cerebrospinal fluid shunt
Malfunction
Meningitis, encephalitis
Toxic ingestions
Hypotension
Hypoxia
Sepsis

an ALOC, partial or absence seizure activity may present in a more subtle fashion with staring, tremors, eye blinking, rhythmic nodding, or other inappropriate repetitive motor activity. Seizures of all types, except absence and simple partial seizures, are usually followed by a postictal period, during which obtunded patients gradually regain consciousness. Patients in nonconvulsive status epilepticus may present in coma, and if other causes have been ruled out, comatose patients should have an electroencephalogram (EEG) performed.

The diagnostic approach toward a patient with ALOC from seizure activity varies based on whether seizures have occurred in the past and the progression or resolution of his or her neurologic abnormalities (see Chapter 67 Seizures). Posttraumatic or new focal seizures are assumed to reflect an intracranial lesion until proven otherwise. Children taking antiepileptic medications benefit from drug-level measurement (if available for the medication) during an observation period. Subtherapeutic antiepileptic drug levels are one of the most common causes of seizures in this population. Subtherapeutic levels result in convulsions with postictal ALOC, whereas supratherapeutic levels less commonly result in seizure, but often produce ALOC of a different appearance based on the medication involved. The presence of fever may indicate that a febrile seizure has occurred or, if normal consciousness is not regained, that the patient has contracted a CNS infection such as meningitis or encephalitis (see Chapters 102 Infectious Disease Emergencies and 105 Neurologic Emergencies). The new onset of afebrile generalized seizures requires a more elaborate evaluation, as detailed in Chapter 67 Seizures.

Infection

Coma-inducing infections of the CNS may involve large areas of the brain and surrounding structures, as in meningitis or encephalitis, or they may be confined to a smaller region, as in the case of cerebral abscess or empyema (see Chapter 102 Infectious Disease Emergencies). Bacterial meningitis remains the most common infection severe enough to produce severe ALOC. Despite the overall decrease in cases since the introduction of vaccines effective against *Haemophilus influenzae* and *Streptococcus pneumoniae,* infections with the latter organism and *Neisseria meningitidis* still occur and are now the most common etiologic agents after the neonatal period. In some regions, *Borrelia burgdorferi* is a common cause of meningitis as part of Lyme disease. Meningitis may also be caused by viral (enteroviruses, herpes), fungal (*Candida, Cryptococcus*), mycobacterial (tuberculosis), and parasitic (cysticercosis) organisms. These nonbacterial infections usually have a slower onset of symptoms. The incidence of viral meningitis peaks in late summer, when enterovirus infections are most common.

Encephalitis, or inflammation of brain parenchyma, may also involve the meninges (see Chapter 102 Infectious Disease Emergencies). It occurs most commonly as a result of viral infection or immunologic mechanisms. Mumps and measles viruses were common etiologic agents before immunizations against these diseases, and they still occur in unimmunized individuals. Varicella encephalitis occurs 2 to 9 days after the onset of rash. The incidence of arthropod-borne encephalitides varies by geographic location but usually peaks in late summer and early fall. The herpes simplex virus remains the most common devastating cause of encephalitis, causing death or permanent neurologic sequelae in more than 70% of patients. It affects the temporal lobes most severely (outside the neonatal period), leading to seizures and parenchymal swelling, which can cause uncal herniation.

Focal CNS infections include brain abscesses, subdural empyemas, and epidural abscesses (see Chapter 102 Infectious Disease Emergencies). Brain abscesses occur most often in patients with chronic sinusitis, chronic ear infection, dental infection, endocarditis, or uncorrected cyanotic congenital heart disease. One-fourth of the cases of brain abscess occur in children younger than 15 years of age, with a peak incidence between 4 and 7 years of age. Subdural empyema also occurs secondary to chronic ear or sinus infection, but it is most commonly seen as a sequela of bacterial meningitis. Cranial epidural abscess is rare, but most cases occur from extension of sinusitis, otitis, orbital cellulitis, or calvarial osteomyelitis.

Neoplasms

Alterations in consciousness as a result of intracranial neoplasms (see Chapter 106 Oncologic Emergencies) may be caused by seizure, hemorrhage, increases in ICP caused by interruption of CSF flow, or direct invasion of the brainstem by the malignancy. The location of the tumor determines additional symptoms: Ataxia and vomiting for infratentorial lesions versus seizures, hemiparesis, and speech or intellectual difficulties resulting from supratentorial neoplasms. Hydrocephalus caused by tumor growth most commonly presents with headache (especially morning headache), lethargy, and vomiting.

Vascular

Coma of cerebrovascular origin is caused by interruption of cerebral blood flow (stroke) as a result of hemorrhage, thrombosis, or embolism (see Chapter 105 Neurologic Emergencies). Hemorrhage is often nontraumatic, stemming from an abnormal vascular structure such as an arteriovenous malformation (AVM), aneurysm, or cavernous hemangioma. Rupture of an AVM is the most common cause of spontaneous intracranial bleeding among pediatric patients. The hemorrhage is arterial in origin and located within the parenchyma, but it can rupture into a ventricle or the subarachnoid space. Aneurysm rupture is less common and is unusual in that repetitive episodes of bleeding may occur ("sentinel bleeds"), with rising morbidity and mortality from each subsequent episode of bleeding. Subarachnoid blood may be present in either case, although more commonly with aneurysm rupture. Cavernous and venous hemangiomas are lower-flow lesions that produce a less acute onset of symptoms.

Stroke may also occur from thrombosis or embolism of a normal vessel. Cerebral infarction caused by occlusion of the anterior, middle, or posterior cerebral artery usually produces focal neurologic deficit rather than coma. Acute occlusion of the carotid artery, however, may produce sufficient unilateral hemispheric swelling to cause herniation and coma. Cerebral sinovenous thrombosis is most commonly seen with hypercoagulable states or as a sequela of infections of the ear or sinus.

Swelling or hemorrhage from infarcted brain can cause increased ICP, leading to decreased parenchymal blood flow and resultant coma. Focal symptoms vary based on the size and location of brain with inadequate blood supply. Vascular accidents in the cerebellum present with combinations of ataxia, vertigo, nausea, occipital headache, and resistance to neck flexion. Coma is an unusual early sign of infarction of cerebral structures but becomes more common as lower anatomic centers are affected. Occlusion of the basilar artery may result in upper brainstem infarction, resulting in rapid onset of coma, as does hemorrhage or infarction of the pons. Posterior reversible encephalopathy syndrome (PRES, a.k.a. reversible posterior leukoencephalopathy syndrome [RPLS]) causing ALOC is associated with autoimmune disease, sepsis, nephrotic syndrome, or immunosuppressive agents.

Cerebrospinal Fluid Shunt Problems

Children with congenital or acquired hydrocephalus as a result of prematurity, neoplasm, or trauma depend on the continued function of a neurosurgically placed shunt to drain CSF and to prevent rises in ICP (see Chapter 130 Neurosurgical Emergencies). The most common shunt type is ventriculoperitoneal (VP), draining CSF from a lateral cerebral ventricle, through a small hole in the skull, through a valve with an attached reservoir beneath the scalp and into the peritoneum via tubing placed under the skin of the neck, chest, and abdomen. CSF shunts may malfunction for many reasons, including tubing rupture, valve malfunction, tubing blockage, tubing disconnection, and shunt infection. The risk of failure is greatest during the first 6 months after shunt placement or revision.

Systemic Abnormalities

The second major category of disorders causing coma listed in Table 12.2 arises in organs other than the CNS and affects the brain diffusely. These abnormalities alter neuronal activity by a variety of mechanisms, including decreasing metabolic substrates required for normal function (e.g., hypoxia, hypotension, hypoglycemia, other electrolyte abnormalities), altering the rate of intracellular chemical reactions (e.g., hypothermia, hyperthermia), and introducing extraneous toxins into the CNS. Children with autoimmune disease such as systemic lupus erythematosus, Behçet disease, multiple sclerosis, and acute disseminated encephalomyelitis (ADEM, a.k.a. postinfectious encephalitis) may present with ALOC due to inflammation of brain parenchyma.

Hypoxia

Oxygen delivery to the brain may be adversely affected by disorders that compromise a patient's airway, breathing, or circulation. Neurons are the cells most sensitive to oxygen deprivation, and they will cease to function within seconds after being deprived of adequate levels of oxygen. Hypoxic coma may result from airway obstruction, pulmonary disease, severe acute anemia, severe methemoglobinemia, carbon monoxide poisoning, or asphyxia (e.g., drowning). Permanent CNS dysfunction results from total anoxia lasting more than 4 to 5 minutes at normal body temperatures; lesser degrees of hypoxia may be tolerated for longer periods. Submersion in near-freezing water may cool the brain sufficiently to exert a neuroprotective effect, but the information available in the emergency department is insufficient to make reliable prognoses about the extent of neurologic damage. Hypercarbia may accompany hypoxia and also be responsible for neurologic depression and coma.

Cardiovascular Abnormalities

ALOC may be produced by poor cerebral perfusion resulting from insufficient cardiac output or hypotension, as in hemorrhage, dehydration, septic shock, arrhythmia, and intoxication. Hypertensive encephalopathy is distinguished by headache, nausea, vomiting, visual disturbance, ALOC, or coma in the presence of a blood pressure greater than the 95th percentile for age and gender (see Chapter 33 Hypertension). The acute onset of severe hypertension may reflect ongoing renal (e.g., unilateral renal artery stenosis, acute glomerulonephritis), endocrine (e.g., pheochromocytoma), or cardiac (e.g., aortic coarctation) pathology, or it may be the result of a toxic ingestion (e.g., cocaine). Hypertension accompanied by bradycardia may be caused by increased ICP.

Disorders of Thermoregulation

Hypothermia or hyperthermia in the pediatric patient is usually caused by prolonged environmental exposure to temperature extremes, such as those found in cold water or in a closed car in sunlight (see Chapter 98 Environmental Emergencies, Radiological Emergencies, Bites and Stings). The child who becomes comatose as a result of abnormal core temperature will have multiple organ system abnormalities in addition to CNS dysfunction. Mental impairment is progressive as body temperature is lowered because each fall of 1°C produces a 6% decline in cerebral blood flow. At 29° to 31°C, confusion or delirium is present, as is muscular rigidity. Patients with core temperatures of 25° to 29°C are comatose with absent deep tendon reflexes and fixed, dilated pupils. CNS findings in hyperthermia include headache, vomiting, and obtundation, leading to coma and/or seizures, especially above 41°C. Nonenvironmental causes of hyperthermia include neuroleptic malignant syndrome, serotonin syndrome, and malignant hyperthermia.

Toxic Ingestions

Pediatric toxic ingestions are often unwitnessed and are usually complicated by the young patient's inability to provide information on the quantity or identity of the substance ingested (see Chapter 110 Toxicologic Emergencies). Table 12.2 lists many drug classes that cause coma with overdose. Exogenous toxins may impair neuronal function directly or by causing hypoxia, acidosis, enzyme inhibition, hypoglycemia, or seizures. Overdoses of street drugs, resulting in coma, have been reported in young children coerced into "body packing" drugs in their intestines. Severe ALOC can occur after direct intrathecal injection of medication such as baclofen resulting from intrathecal pump malfunction, or in the immediate postoperative setting after receipt of an inadvertent intraoperative bolus of baclofen.

Metabolic Alterations

Abnormal serum concentrations of any substrate or product involved in neuronal metabolism can produce ALOC leading to coma. Hypoglycemia is the most common disorder in this category, especially in infants and young children, whose capacity for hepatic gluconeogenesis is limited. Disorders known to produce hypoglycemia include serious bacterial infections, sepsis, dehydration, and toxic ingestions (especially ethanol, beta blockers, and oral hypoglycemics). Diabetes mellitus, especially of new onset, may present with profoundly depressed consciousness from the combination of hyperosmolarity, dehydration, hypotension, and metabolic acidosis. Patients under treatment for diabetic ketoacidosis may also develop cerebral edema and ALOC. Patients with type 2 diabetes may have coma as part of hyperglycemic hyperosmolar nonketotic syndrome, which can be complicated by malignant hyperthermia.

Metabolic acidosis or alkalosis of sufficient degree produces ALOC. The most common disorder of this type in children is severe dehydration leading to metabolic acidosis. Abnormal concentrations of any serum electrolyte, including sodium, calcium, magnesium, and phosphorus, can also produce altered mental status. The degree of resulting neurologic compromise will be affected by the duration and severity of the electrolyte disturbance and concurrent disorders. Severe dehydration alone may also produce profound lethargy in infants and children, even in the absence of significant electrolyte abnormalities.

Other causes of metabolic coma in the pediatric age group include kidney or hepatic failure, both of which may result in progressive apathy, confusion, and lethargy. Urea cycle defects may present with ALOC and hyperammonemia in young infants (see Chapter 103 Metabolic Emergencies). Acute toxic encephalopathy (Reye syndrome) is a rare but devastating illness caused by mitochondrial injury of unknown origin that affects all organs of the body, particularly the brain and liver (see Chapter 105 Neurologic Emergencies). An epidemiologic association exists between the disorder and an antecedent viral illness (including varicella) from which a patient is recovering. Patients with Reye syndrome typically develop severe vomiting, followed by combative delirium that progresses to coma. Cerebral edema, increased ICP, and central herniation may occur.

Miscellaneous Conditions

Other causes of coma or ALOC in children are less easily categorized. Children with intussusception, the most common cause of bowel obstruction in childhood, may have significant apathy and lethargy in addition to vomiting, intermittent abdominal pain, and bloody stools. As a result, they are often treated for dehydration, sepsis, or meningitis before the appropriate diagnosis is discovered. CNS involvement in hemolytic uremic syndrome may produce a comatose state because of cerebral infarction, most commonly occurring in the basal ganglia. Breastfed infants of vegan mothers have presented in coma, suffering from severe vitamin B_{12} deficiency. Children with adrenoleukodystrophy may present acutely with coma.

Psychiatric disorders may produce a true stuporous state. More commonly, neurologically intact patients attempt to feign unresponsiveness, and they may be remarkably successful at remaining immobile despite painful stimuli. The nature of their illness may be discovered by a detailed neurologic examination. Conscious patients will usually avoid hitting their face with a dropped arm, may resist eyelid opening, will raise their heart rate to auditory or painful stimuli, and will have intact deep tendon, oculovestibular, and oculocephalic reflexes.

EVALUATION AND DECISION

An approach for the evaluation of pediatric patients presenting with coma is summarized in Figure 12.1. All patients need rapid assessment of their airway, breathing, and circulation, followed by a focused history, physical examination, and consideration of laboratory and imaging studies. This approach is based on the selective use of the following critical clinical and laboratory findings: (i) Vital signs; (ii) a history of recent head trauma, seizure activity, or ingestion; (iii) signs of increased ICP or focal neurologic abnormality; (iv) fever; (v) laboratory results; (vi) brain CT scan results; and (vii) CSF analysis. The evaluation of the comatose patient should follow an orderly series of steps, addressing the more life-threatening problems of hypoxia, hypotension, or increased ICP before investigating less urgent disorders. If one or more of the former are present, immediate resuscitative efforts are begun.

History and Physical Examination

Focused, goal-directed questioning pertaining to suspected diagnoses is required to treat coma quickly. Specific queries regarding current medications, medications and substances available to ingest, seizures, fever, headache, irritability, vomiting, changes in gait, and behavioral abnormalities should be made. The most important historical finding in a comatose patient is a history of recent head trauma. If no history of head trauma is present, it should continue to be considered as a potential cause of ALOC, since many cases are unwitnessed.

A patient's vital signs will reveal the presence of fever, hypotension, or hypertension. The consciousness of a neurologically impaired patient may initially be evaluated using a simple AVPU scale, representing four major levels of alertness: Alert, responsive to Verbal stimuli, responsive to Painful stimuli, and Unresponsive. Elements of a more detailed neurologic evaluation are discussed in the following section.

The patient should be carefully examined for physical findings consistent with head trauma, including retinal hemorrhage, hemotympanum, CSF otorrhea or rhinorrhea, postauricular hematoma (Battle sign), palpable or visual damage to scalp or skull, and periorbital hematoma ("raccoon eyes"). Child abuse should be suspected if unexplained bruising is

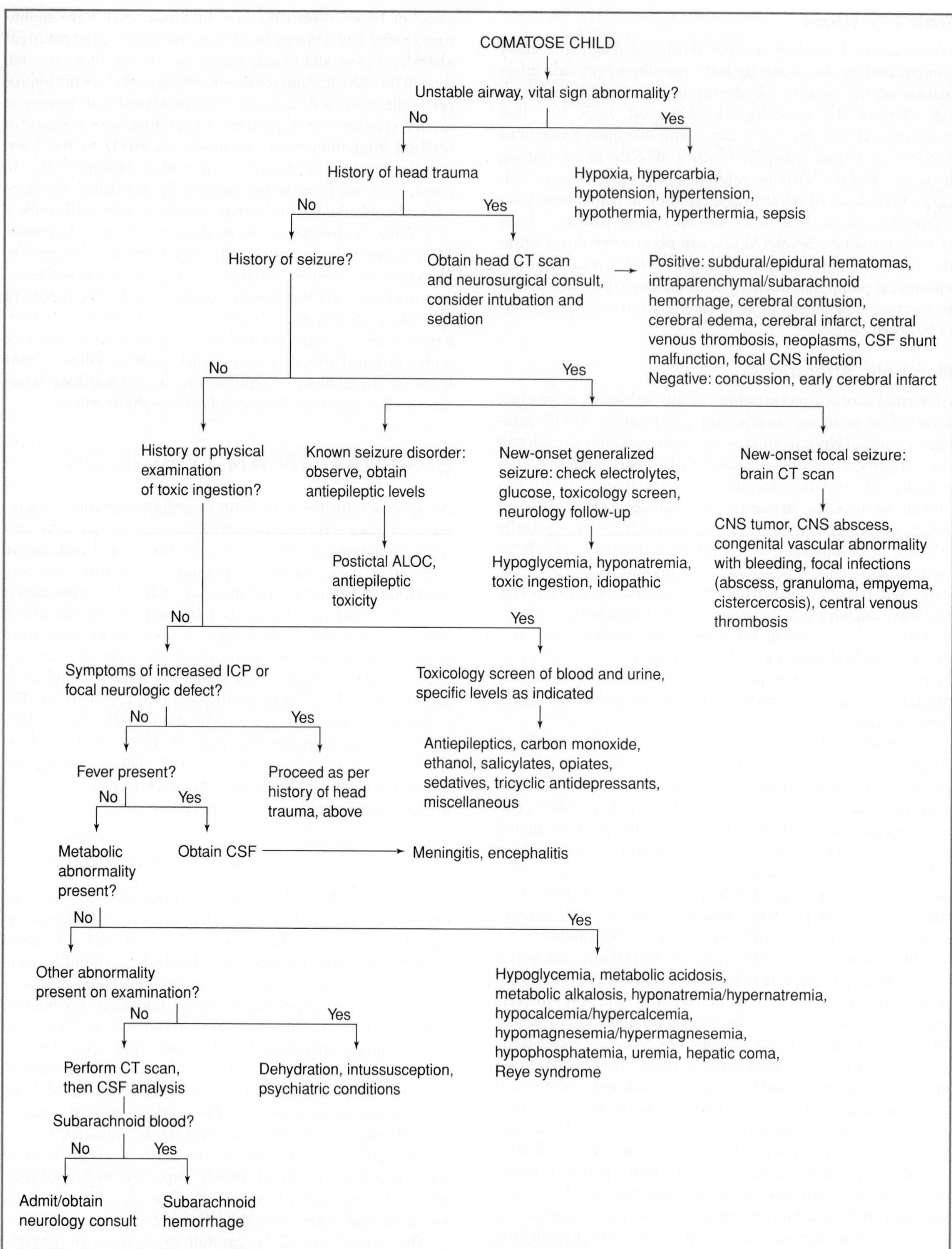

FIGURE 12.1 Evaluation of the comatose child. CT, computed tomography; CSF, cerebrospinal fluid; CNS, central nervous system; ALOC, altered level of consciousness; ICP, intracranial pressure.

present or the stated mechanism of injury is disproportionate to the degree of physical damage present or to the developmental level of the child (e.g., 1-month-old "rolled off bed"). Bruising on the face, head, and ears in nonambulatory children is of great concern for abusive head trauma ("those who don't cruise, rarely bruise"). Other significant physical findings include anisocoria, absent or reduced pupil reactivity, papilledema, and nuchal rigidity. Purpuric or varicelliform rashes may signify the presence of systemic infections with CNS involvement. Incontinence of urine or stool may indicate that an unwitnessed seizure has occurred.

Neurologic Examination and Scoring

The neurologic examination of the comatose patient should include standard tests of eye opening, responsiveness to verbal and tactile stimuli, and deep tendon reflexes as well as the more specialized examinations described in this section. Any focal (unilateral) abnormal finding is always significant because it may indicate a structural CNS lesion. Abnormal findings on neurologic examination reflect the underlying pathologic condition causing coma and may allow localization of a lesion within the brain.

Patients with ALOC benefit from quantification of their impairment using standard measurements. This allows evaluation of patients' changing neurologic status over time and the recording of this information in the medical record. The effect of medical interventions may then be more easily assessed. The use of accepted scoring systems also facilitates communication with consultants such as neurologists and neurosurgeons. In addition, many outcome measures of neurologically injured patients rely on scales used to assess neurologic function. Although originally developed for trauma, a widely used measurement of consciousness is the Glasgow Coma Scale (GCS) shown in Table 12.1. Patients are graded on three areas of neurologic function: Eye opening, motor response, and verbal responsiveness. A GCS score of 3 is the minimum score possible and represents complete unresponsiveness; a GCS score of 15 is assigned to fully alert patients. Modifications of the GCS are available for preverbal children and infants.

Pupillary responses provide the most direct window to the brain of a comatose patient. A unilaterally enlarging pupil (greater than 5 mm) that becomes progressively less reactive to light indicates either progressive displacement of the midbrain or medial temporal lobe, or downward displacement of the upper brainstem. Bilateral enlarged and unreactive ("blown") pupils indicate profound CNS dysfunction and are most commonly seen with posttraumatic increases in ICP. Nontraumatic conditions affecting the brain diffusely usually spare pupillary responses. Exceptions include maximal constriction of pinpoint pupils caused by opiate intoxication and minimal constriction of widely dilated pupils caused by intoxication with anticholinergic agents.

Other ocular signs noted in patients with depressed consciousness are the roving side-to-side conjugate eye movements seen in lighter stages of metabolic coma. Persistent conjugate deviation of the eyes to one side may be caused by focal seizure activity, its resultant postictal state, or focal lesions within the brain. Ongoing seizure activity is usually apparent because of the jerking ocular movements present. Most structural brainstem lesions abolish conjugate eye movements, but it is rare for a metabolic disorder to do so. Deepening ALOC may also be measured by the reduction and loss of spontaneous blinking, then loss of blinking caused by touching the eyelashes, and finally loss of blink with corneal touch. Both eyes should be tested to detect asymmetry.

Limb movement and postural changes seen in comatose patients include the bilateral restless movements of the limbs of patients in light coma. Unilateral jerking muscular movements may indicate focal seizure activity or generalized convulsions in a patient with hemiparesis. Decerebrate rigidity refers to stiff extension of limbs with internal rotation of the arms and plantar flexion of the feet. It is not a posture that is held constantly; it usually occurs intermittently in patients with midbrain compression, cerebellar lesions, or metabolic disorders. Decorticate rigidity, when arms are held in flexion and adduction and legs are extended, indicates CNS dysfunction at a higher anatomic level, usually in cerebral white matter or internal capsule and thalamus. Signs of meningeal irritation include Kernig sign, resistance to bent knee extension with the hip in 90 degrees flexion, and Brudzinski sign, involuntary knee and hip flexion with passive neck flexion.

The abnormal breathing pattern most commonly seen in comatose patients is Cheyne–Stokes respirations, where intervals of waxing and waning hyperpnea alternate with short periods of apnea. Other abnormal breathing patterns that occur with brainstem lesions include central neurogenic hyperventilation, which can produce respiratory alkalosis, and apneustic breathing, in which a 2- to 3-second pause occurs during each full inspiration.

Laboratory and Radiologic Studies

Immediate bedside glucose determination should be performed on every patient with nontraumatic ALOC. Other laboratory tests indicated for evaluation of coma in the absence of trauma include electrolytes, blood urea nitrogen, creatinine, blood gas, hemoglobin, hematocrit, osmolality, ammonia, and antiepileptic levels. Toxicologic screening of both blood and urine should be obtained in patients with ALOC of unknown origin. A noncontrast CT scan of the brain can reveal many causes of coma, such as cerebral edema, hydrocephalus, malignancy, hematomas, and abscesses. Infarction, thrombosis, and inflammatory conditions may require the addition of contrast or the use of magnetic resonance imaging.

Vital Sign Abnormalities

Evaluation and treatment of airway, breathing, and circulatory compromise always take precedence in the child with ALOC. Both airway patency and respiratory effort may be compromised by decreased mental status and may result in hypoxia and/or hypercarbia. The former may be readily measured using pulse oximetry, although values will be inaccurate if a toxic hemoglobinopathy, such as methemoglobinemia or carboxyhemoglobinemia, is present. The adequacy of ventilation can be assessed clinically with a stethoscope and can be quantified by continuously monitoring end-tidal CO_2 (see Chapter 16 Cyanosis). Arterial blood gas analysis with co-oximetry is useful to quantify respiratory status and to identify altered hemoglobin states.

The numerical definition of hypotension varies with age, but pallor and evidence of poor peripheral perfusion, with prolonged capillary refill time, is recognizable even before placement of a sphygmomanometer cuff. Immediate administration of IV crystalloid therapy starting with 20 mL per kg of normal saline or lactated Ringer solution is indicated, followed by additional boluses and vasopressors if needed (see Chapter 3 Airway). Of the empiric antidotal therapies often used in adults, only glucose (0.25 to 0.5 g per kg) is routinely administered to children. An empiric trial of naloxone (0.1 mg per kg, max 2 mg per dose) is sometimes justified, whereas flumazenil and thiamine are given only for specific indications (see Chapter 110 Toxicologic Emergencies).

Severe hypertension is less easily discerned on physical examination. If confirmed in more than one extremity, antihypertensives should be administered via the IV route (see Chapters 33 Hypertension and 108 Renal and Electrolyte Emergencies). Mental status should improve after blood pressure is lowered to high normal levels. Patients in hypertensive crises are at risk for hemorrhagic stroke and should be evaluated with a head CT scan if they are neurologically abnormal after blood pressure lowering. Hypertension in the comatose patient after traumatic injury may represent a physiologic response to increased ICP to allow maintenance of cerebral perfusion pressure by raising mean arterial pressure. In this context, elevated blood pressure should not be lowered with antihypertensives, instead treatment should be aimed at decreasing ICP.

Hypothermia and hyperthermia are readily recognized once a core (rectal) temperature less than 35°C or greater than 41°C is obtained. The mental status of these patients should begin to improve as body temperature approaches the normal range. A significant percentage of patients with abnormal core temperatures have drowned, fallen through ice, or were engaged in sporting activities in extreme environments. Adolescents with hypothermia may have associated ethanol toxicity. Head trauma, hypoxia, and/or cervical spine injury may be present in these patients.

History of Head Trauma

The patient with deeply depressed consciousness (GCS score less than 9) after head trauma is presumed to have increased ICP until proven otherwise. Rapid sequence intubation is indicated to protect the airway and to maintain effective ventilation. Cervical spine injury should be assumed and cervical immobilization maintained at all times. An emergent noncontrast brain CT scan should be obtained and neurosurgery consulted. In cases when immediate but necessary neurosurgical intervention is not possible for intracranial hemorrhage (e.g., extended transport time) or in cases of diffuse cerebral edema, 3% saline or mannitol may be helpful to treat elevated ICP. Elevation of the head of the bed to 30 degrees and maintenance of the midline position of the head are simple nonpharmacologic maneuvers to try to reduce ICP. At this time there is insufficient evidence to recommend therapeutic hypothermia in children.

History of Seizures

The patient with ALOC in the absence of trauma should be evaluated for recent seizure activity with current postictal state (see Chapters 67 Seizures and 105 Neurologic Emergencies). A history of previous seizures, witnessed convulsive activity, and ALOC consistent with previous postictal periods are valuable clues to this etiology of coma. Ongoing seizure activity may be revealed by the presence of muscular twitching, increased tonicity, nystagmus, or eyelid fluttering. Patients with subtle or completely nonconvulsive forms of status epilepticus may exhibit tachycardia but may require an EEG to diagnose. The mental status examination of the postictal patient should gradually improve over several hours. Although temporary focal neurologic deficits may follow seizures, they must be presumed to indicate the presence of focal CNS lesions until proven otherwise.

The evaluation of neurologically depressed patients with seizures varies based on the patient's history, type of seizure, and presence or absence of fever. Patients with a history of seizures should have serum antiepileptic concentrations measured and be observed until they approach their neurologic baseline. Children who have had a simple febrile seizure (see Chapter 67 Seizures) should return to their baseline state soon, usually within 1 hour. Those who remain lethargic or irritable past this point (especially after antipyretics have been administered) should be suspected of having meningitis and are candidates for lumbar puncture.

Patients with new-onset generalized seizures who are afebrile warrant additional evaluation. Depending on recent history (e.g., vomiting or diarrhea), it may be advisable to check serum electrolytes or a toxicologic screen, for example. Depending on local resources and practice, patients with newly diagnosed afebrile seizures will generally receive EEG testing and CT or MR imaging of the brain. Consultation with a neurologist who treats children is important to coordinate this workup (see Chapters 67 Seizures and 105 Neurologic Emergencies).

The new onset of focal seizures, with or without the presence of fever, should be evaluated with a head CT scan to determine the presence of a focal lesion such as a tumor, abscess, or hemorrhage. Only after the results of this study are known should a lumbar puncture be performed. If neuroimaging is unavailable and meningitis or encephalitis is a concern, empiric treatment for bacterial meningitis or herpetic encephalitis may be administered and lumbar puncture deferred (see Chapter 102 Infectious Disease Emergencies).

History of Toxic Ingestions

If no history or physical examination findings suggestive of head trauma or seizures are present, a toxic ingestion should be considered, especially in toddlers and adolescents. The availability of any substances capable of depressing CNS function should be thoroughly explored. In general, coma from toxic ingestions is of slower onset than that from trauma and may be preceded by delirium or other abnormal behaviors.

Chapter 110 Toxicologic Emergencies lists major toxidromes that result from ingestions that produce CNS depression. The pupils of a poisoned comatose patient are a particularly valuable source of information. Miosis occurs with ingestions of narcotics, clonidine, organophosphates, gamma-hydroxybutyrate (GHB), phencyclidine, phenothiazines, and occasionally, barbiturates and ethanol. Mydriasis is produced by ingestions of anticholinergic agents (e.g., atropine, antihistamines, and tricyclic antidepressants) and sympathomimetic compounds (e.g., amphetamines, caffeine, cocaine, LSD, and nicotine). Nystagmus may indicate the ingestion of barbiturates, ketamine, phencyclidine, or phenytoin. Pupillary responses are likely to be preserved in toxic or metabolic comas. Systemic toxins do not cause unequal pupils; anisocoria in the setting of ALOC should be pursued with neuroimaging.

A toxicologic screen of blood and urine should be considered in all children with coma of unknown origin. Table 12.5

TABLE 12.5

POISONS UNDETECTED BY TYPICAL DRUG SCREENING THAT CAUSE COMA/ALTERED LEVEL OF CONCIOUSNESS

Miosis present
Bromide
Chloral hydrate
Clonidine
Gamma-hydroxybutyrate (GHB)
Methadone, buprenorphine
Organophosphates
Phenobarbital
Pilocarpine and tetrahydrozoline eye drops
Phenothiazines
Valproic acid
Mydriasis present
Anoxia caused by cyanide, carbon monoxide, or methemoglobinemia
LSD

lists compounds capable of causing coma that are not typically detected by routine drug screening; the compounds are grouped by pupillary effects.

The poisoned patient with depressed consciousness should be intubated with a cuffed endotracheal tube for airway protection before gastrointestinal decontamination. Naloxone may be administered as empiric antidotal therapy for coma-producing toxic ingestions involving unknown medications. Flumazenil should not be given routinely to these patients because seizures may result. Its use is limited to pure benzodiazepine overdoses in patients with no history of seizures or drug habituation.

Increased Intracranial Pressure or Focal Neurologic Defect

Nontraumatic causes of increased ICP or focal neurologic deficits include neoplasms, CSF shunt malfunction, cerebral abscess, and hemorrhage (see Chapters 105 Neurologic Emergencies and 130 Neurosurgical Emergencies). These patients may present with a history of headache, vomiting, confusion, lethargy, meningismus, focal neurologic dysfunction, or seizure activity, or may present with sudden onset of deep coma. Initial physical signs of increased ICP include a bulging fontanelle in infants and sluggishly reactive pupils. More severe and prolonged increases in ICP produce a unilaterally enlarged pupil, other cranial nerve palsies (III, IV, VI), papilledema, and Cushing triad of hypertension, bradycardia, and periodic breathing. All may signal impending or progressive herniation. From the standpoint of the emergency physician, which type of herniation is present is unimportant; all are life-threatening, and the initial treatment is identical for all. Endotracheal intubation using rapid sequence induction is performed to gain airway and breathing control. Evaluation should parallel that for traumatic head injury, bearing in mind the increased desirability of using IV contrast for CT imaging. Comatose patients with a CSF shunt may need their shunt reservoir or ventricle tapped emergently to treat increased ICP.

Fever

Coma accompanied by fever may indicate CNS infection (see Chapters 26 Fever and 102 Infectious Disease Emergencies). Resistance to neck flexion is the most important physical finding in meningitis, the most common infection of this type, although children younger than 2 years of age may lack this finding. Historical data may also include a steadily increasing headache, irritability, vomiting, and worsening oral intake. Kernig and Brudzinski signs may be present. Other useful physical clues to CNS infection are the rashes that accompany meningococcemia, varicella, and Rocky Mountain spotted fever. The historical and physical findings in encephalitis are similar to those in meningitis; meningismus may be absent, however. Seizures are particularly common if herpes simplex is the causative agent.

A history of localized CNS dysfunction or seizures before the onset of febrile coma or the presence of concomitant focal neurologic signs may indicate the presence of a focal cerebral infection such as an abscess or subdural empyema. In addition, either diffuse or focal infections may present with signs of increased ICP secondary to cerebral edema or blockage of CSF flow. If this is the case, a head CT scan should be obtained before lumbar puncture is performed. A contrast-enhanced study is desirable if concern about focal infection is present. The ill-appearing patient should receive antibiotics before neuroimaging is performed.

CSF analysis remains the key to establishing the diagnosis of CNS infection. Abnormalities of CSF white blood cell count (pleocytosis), glucose, and protein occur in roughly predictable patterns with bacterial or viral meningitis, and pathogens may be visible using Gram and other stains (see Chapter 102 Infectious Disease Emergencies). Rapid testing with agglutination studies or polymerase chain reaction tests might also be used to identify pathogens. CSF pleocytosis in encephalitis is variable and, if present, is usually mild (less than 500 cells per mm^3), with normal levels of glucose and protein being common. Bloody or xanthochromic CSF under increased pressure in the absence of signs of infection indicates subarachnoid hemorrhage.

Metabolic Abnormalities

The presence of a metabolic disorder leading to coma is usually apparent once the results of routine laboratory tests are available. These values for glucose, sodium, potassium, bicarbonate, calcium, magnesium, and phosphorus make any deficiency or excess of these serum components readily apparent and treatable. Blood gas analysis for evaluation of acidosis or alkalosis from metabolic or respiratory causes may also be indicated. Decreased consciousness caused by diabetic ketoacidosis may initially worsen because of a paradoxical temporary decrease in CSF pH and/or cerebral edema complicating the disease.

Renal and hepatic functions should be quantified with analysis of blood urea nitrogen, creatinine, and ammonia. Markedly elevated serum blood urea nitrogen and creatinine, oliguria, hypertension, anemia, acidosis, and hypocalcemia indicate the presence of uremic coma as a result of renal failure. Hyperammonemia with decreased mental status may be caused by hepatic failure, acetaminophen ingestion with resultant hepatotoxicity, valproic acid toxicity, Reye syndrome, or

TABLE 12.6

COMMON ERRORS IN THE EVALUATION AND MANAGEMENT OF CHILDREN WITH COMA

Assuming no head trauma has taken place if no such history is given
Neglecting to secure the airway before imaging studies are performed
Hyperventilating intubated patients to a Pco_2 well below 35 mm Hg
Not sedating patients once they are paralyzed and intubated
Believing that a toxic ingestion has not occurred because the "tox screen" is negative

inborn metabolic errors. The hyperammonemia of Reye syndrome is accompanied by a history of antecedent viral illness resolving within the past week and likely treated with aspirin (see Chapter 105 Neurologic Emergencies). Unremitting vomiting is soon accompanied by encephalopathy, in the absence of jaundice, scleral icterus, focal neurologic signs, or meningeal irritation. Hyperammonemia without accompanying liver failure in the young infant may indicate the presence of a congenital urea cycle defect.

Coma of Unknown Origin

Patients with coma of unknown origin not falling into any of the diagnostic categories discussed previously usually benefit from a noncontrast brain CT scan, CSF analysis, and neurologic consultation, in that order. The emergence of new infectious diseases such as West Nile virus and eastern equine encephalitis virus means that diagnosis may require consultation with infectious disease experts and the Centers for Disease Control. The CDC now lists six mosquito-borne viral encephalitides. If meningeal irritation is present without fever or other signs of infection, a subarachnoid hemorrhage may be the cause. Common avoidable errors in the evaluation and management of children with coma are listed in Table 12.6.

Suggested Readings and Key References

Cohen BH, Andrefsky JC. In: Maria BL, ed. *Current management in child neurology,* 4th ed. Hamilton, Ont. Shelton, Conn. People's Medical Pub. House: BC Decker; 2009:669–680.

Herman BE, Makoroff KL, Corneli HM. Abusive head trauma. *Pediatr Emerg Care* 2011;27(1):65–69.

Kirkham FJ, Ashwal S. Coma and brain death. *Handb Clin Neurol* 2013;111:43–61.

Taylor DA, Ashwal S. In: Swaiman KF, ed. *Pediatric neurology: principles & practice,* 5th ed. Philadelphia, PA: Elsevier/Saunders, 2012: 1062–1086.

CHAPTER 13 ■ CONSTIPATION

ROSE C. GRAHAM, MD, MSCE

Constipation is an important problem in the pediatric emergency department for many reasons. It is one of the most common pediatric complaints, accounting for 3% of primary care visits. There are many causes for constipation (Table 13.1), some rare and some very common (Table 13.2). Most constipation in children is functional, meaning that no underlying medical disease is responsible. Occasionally, the presentation of constipation is atypical, with chief complaints that superficially seem unrelated to the gastrointestinal tract (Table 13.3). Although relatively rare, some causes of constipation are potentially life-threatening and need to be recognized promptly by the emergency physician (Table 13.4). In addition, constipation may produce symptoms that mimic other serious illnesses such as appendicitis.

DEFINITION

Although constipation most commonly is defined as decreased stool frequency, there is not one simple definition. The stooling pattern of children changes based on age, diet, and other factors. Average stooling frequency in healthy infants is approximately four stools per day during the first week of life, decreasing to 1.7 stools per day by 2 years of age, and approaching the adult frequency of 1.2 stools per day by 4 years of age. Nevertheless, normal infants can range from seven stools per day to one stool per week. Older children can defecate every 2 to 3 days and be normal.

It is easier to define constipation as a problem with defecation. This may encompass infrequent stooling, passage of large and/or hard stools associated with pain, incomplete evacuation of rectal contents, involuntary soiling (encopresis), or inability to pass stool at all.

PHYSIOLOGY

The passage of food from mouth to anus is a complex process that relies on input from intrinsic nerves, extrinsic nerves, and hormones. The colon is specialized to transport fecal material and balance water and electrolytes contained in the feces. When all is functioning well, the fecal bolus arrives in the rectum formed but soft enough for easy passage through the anus. Normal defecation requires the coordination of the autonomic and somatic nervous systems and normal anatomy of the anorectal region. The internal anal sphincter is a smooth muscle, innervated by the autonomic nervous system and tonically contracted at baseline. It relaxes involuntarily in response to the arrival of a fecal bolus in the rectum, allowing stool to descend to the portion of the anus innervated by somatic nerves. At this point, the external anal sphincter, striated muscle under voluntary control, tightens until the appropriate time for fecal passage. Before defecation, squatting or sitting straightens the angle between the rectum and anal canal, allowing easier passage. Voluntary relaxation of the external anal sphincter and increasing intra-abdominal pressure via Valsalva allow passage of the feces.

EVALUATION AND DECISION

The evaluation of the child presumed to have constipation should begin with a thorough history and physical examination. Special attention should be paid to the age of the patient, duration of symptoms, timing of first meconium passage after birth, changes in frequency and consistency of stool, stool incontinence, pain with defecation, rectal bleeding, presence of abdominal distention and/or palpable feces, and a rectal examination to assess anal position, sphincter tone, widening of the rectal vault, and presence of hard stool. Signs and symptoms that raise concern for more serious underlying diagnoses include onset of constipation in the first month of life, delayed meconium passage >48 hours, ribbon-like stools, blood in stool without anal fissure, failure to thrive, bilious emesis, fever, severe abdominal distention, abnormally positioned/appearing anus, or abnormal neurologic examination.

A complaint of constipation is not sufficient for diagnosis. A decrease in stool frequency or the appearance of straining is often interpreted as constipation. The physician should be aware of the grunting baby syndrome, or infant dyschezia, in which an infant grunts, turns red, strains, and may cry while passing a soft stool. This is the result of poor coordination between Valsalva and relaxation of the voluntary sphincter muscles. Examination reveals the absence of palpable stool in the rectum or abdomen. Complaints of constipation not supported by history or physical examination are called pseudoconstipation (Fig. 13.1).

Acute Constipation

Constipation is not a disease; it is a symptom of a problem. Constipation is acute when it has occurred for less than 1 month's duration. The patient's age and the duration of the constipation are important when determining the cause and significance of the problem.

The infant younger than 6 months of age with acute constipation is particularly concerning. Potential causes include dehydration, malnutrition, infant botulism, and anorectal malformations. A recent viral illness accompanied by dehydration from vomiting, diarrhea, fever, and increased respiratory rate can precipitate acute constipation in an infant. Adynamic ileus or decreased intake after gastroenteritis may slow transit through the colon, leading to hard stools. Dietary protein allergy (i.e., cow's milk protein allergy) may present with constipation. Anal fissures and/or diaper rash after a bout of diarrhea may precipitate painful defecation, resulting in stool retention.

TABLE 13.1

ETIOLOGY OF CONSTIPATION

- **I. Functional**
  - A. Fecal retention
  - B. Depression
  - C. Harsh toilet training
  - D. Toilet phobia
  - E. Avoidance of school bathrooms
  - F. Fecal soiling
  - G. Anorexia nervosa
- **II. Pain on defecation**
  - A. Anal fissure
  - B. Foreign body
  - C. Sexual abuse
  - D. Laxative overuse
  - E. Proctitis
  - F. Rectal prolapse
  - G. Rectal polyps
  - H. Perianal streptococcal infection
- **III. Mechanical obstruction**
  - A. Hirschsprung disease
  - B. Imperforate anus
  - C. Abdominal/pelvic mass
  - D. Upper bowel obstruction
  - E. Anal/rectal stenosis
  - F. Anal atresia (newborn)
  - G. Meconium ileus (newborn)
  - H. Pregnancy
- **IV. Decreased sensation/motility**
  - A. Drug induced
  - B. Viral "ileus"
  - C. Neuromuscular disease
    - 1. Hypotonia
    - 2. Werdnig–Hoffmann disease
    - 3. Cerebral palsy
    - 4. Down syndrome
    - 5. Chronic intestinal pseudoobstruction
  - D. Metabolic abnormalities
    - 1. Hypothyroidism
    - 2. Hyperparathyroidism
    - 3. Hypercalcemia
    - 4. Hypokalemia
    - 5. Diabetes mellitus
    - 6. Diabetes insipidus
    - 7. Renal tubular acidosis
    - 8. Heavy metal poisoning
  - E. Infant botulism
  - F. Spinal cord abnormality (tumor, tethered cord)
  - G. "Prune belly" syndrome
- **V. Stool abnormalities**
  - A. Dietary
  - B. Dehydration
  - C. Malnutrition
  - D. Celiac disease
  - E. Cystic fibrosis
- **VI. Pseudoconstipation**
  - A. Breast-fed infant
  - B. Normal variation in stool frequency

TABLE 13.2

COMMON CAUSES OF CONSTIPATION

Functional
Anal fissure
Viral illness with ileus
Dietary

Inadequate fluid intake and malnutrition should be uncovered by dietary history. Recent medications may cause constipation (Table 13.5). Ingestion of lead is also a potential and serious reason for constipation. Infant botulism presents with acute constipation, weak cry, poor feeding, and decreasing muscle tone (see Chapter 105 Neurologic Emergencies). Acute constipation can also be a symptom of a bowel obstruction, but usually a less prominent feature than other symptoms (see Chapter 124 Abdominal Emergencies).

Acute constipation in the child ≥6 months of age occurs for many of the same reasons as in the young infant. History may reveal dietary factors such as introduction of solid foods or excessive intake of cow's milk, recent viral illness or use of medication, as well as the presence of underlying illness, such as neuromuscular disease. Physical examination will rule out anal malformations and other physical problems that could result in trouble defecating.

Chronic Constipation

Constipation of more than 1 month's duration in a young infant <6 months of age, although likely to be a functional problem, is especially concerning and should prompt consideration of an underlying illness. Spinal muscular atrophy, amyotonia, congenital absence of abdominal muscles, dystonic states, and spinal dysraphism, cause problems with defecation and can be readily diagnosed with history and physical examination.

Anorectal anomalies occur in approximately 1 in 2,500 live births. Imperforate anus presents at birth with absence of any anal opening. Anal stenosis causes the passage of ribbon-like stools with intense effort and is diagnosed by rectal examination demonstrating a tight, constricted canal. In "covered anus," the anus can be covered by a flap of skin, leaving only a small opening for passage of stool. Anterior displacement of the anus may cause constipation by creating a pouch at the posterior portion of the distal rectum that catches the stool and allows only overflow to be expelled after great straining. The treatment may be medical or surgical.

TABLE 13.3

SOME ATYPICAL PRESENTATIONS OF CONSTIPATION

Anorexia
Headaches
Lethargy
Limp
Refusal to walk
Seizure-like activity (shaking, staring spells)
Urinary retention
Urinary tract infection

TABLE 13.4

LIFE-THREATENING CAUSES OF CONSTIPATION

Acute constipation
Mechanical obstruction
Dehydration
Infantile botulism
Chronic constipation
Hirschsprung disease
Abdominal/pelvic mass
Anorexia nervosa

Hirschsprung disease, or congenital intestinal aganglionosis, is rare (1 in 5,000 live births) but must be considered in the constipated infant because it has the potential to cause life-threatening complications. The distal aganglionic segment remains tonically contracted while the segment proximal to the blockage dilates with stool buildup. This can lead to megacolon which, in turn, can cause life-threatening enterocolitis that may present with abdominal distention, explosive sometimes bloody stools, and fever progressing to sepsis and hypovolemic shock.

Of infants with Hirschsprung disease, 80% are diagnosed within the first year of life. A history of late passage of meconium >48 hours after birth is often but not always noted (Table 13.6). However, if the involved segment is relatively short, the diagnosis may be delayed. Abdominal examination in Hirschsprung's often yields a suprapubic mass of stool that may extend throughout the abdomen. Rectal examination reveals a constricted anal canal with the absence of stool in the rectal vault, commonly followed by expulsion of stool when the finger is removed. The combination of palpable abdominal feces and an empty rectal vault is abnormal and must be further investigated. Diagnosis is supported by unprepped barium enema showing a transition zone where the narrow distal bowel transitions to a dilated proximal bowel. When only a short segment of bowel is involved, barium enema may miss the transition zone and anal manometry aids in diagnosis. Confirmation is made by rectal biopsy (see also Chapter 99 Gastrointestinal Emergencies).

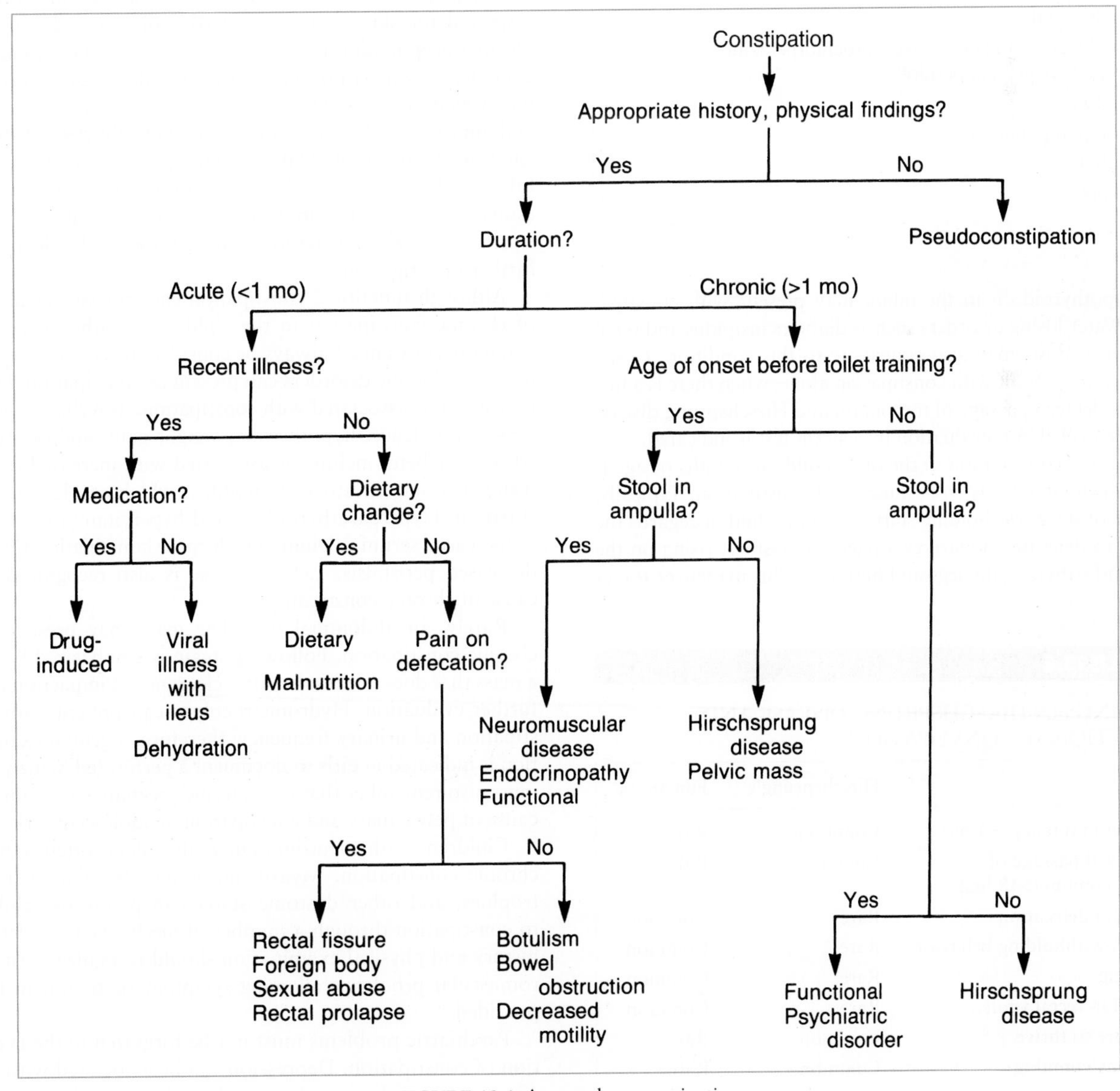

FIGURE 13.1 Approach to constipation.

TABLE 13.5

SOME MEDICATIONS ASSOCIATED WITH CONSTIPATION

Aluminum
Amiodarone
Amitriptyline
Anticholinergic agents (benztropine, glycopyrrolate, promethazine)
Antineoplastic agents (procarbazine, vincristine)
Benzodiazepines
β-Blockers
Calcium salts
Calcium channel blockers
Cholestyramine
Diazoxide
H2 receptor antagonists (ranitidine)
Iron
Mesalamine
Ondansetron
Opioids
Phenobarbital
Phenothiazines and derivatives (prochlorperazine, promethazine, haloperidol)
Phenytoin
Proton pump inhibitors
Sucralfate
Ursodiol

Hypothyroidism in the infant may present with constipation. Water-losing disorders such as diabetes insipidus and renal tubular acidosis may also contribute to this condition. Cystic fibrosis can present with constipation alone; when there is a history of delayed passage of meconium and Hirschsprung disease has been ruled out, evaluation by a sweat test is indicated.

Chronic constipation in the older child ≥6 months of age is overwhelmingly likely to be functional constipation. Typically, a cycle of stool withholding starts when the child disregards the signal to defecate and strikes a retentive posture, rising on the toes and stiffening the legs and buttocks. This maneuver forces the stool back into the rectum, which subjects the fecal bolus to further water absorption and enlargement leading to painful and traumatic defecation. This reinforces stool-withholding behavior. Over time, the rectum dilates and sensation diminishes. Eventually, the child loses the urge to defecate altogether. Proximal watery stool can leak around the large fecal mass, causing involuntary soiling or encopresis. This may be misconstrued as diarrhea or as regression in the toilet-trained child. Many parents consult a physician at this point. Other reasons parents seek medical attention for their children are abdominal pain, anorexia, vomiting, and irritability.

TABLE 13.6

FINDINGS IN HIRSCHSPRUNG DISEASE AND FUNCTIONAL CONSTIPATION

	Hirschsprung's	Functional
Onset in infancy (<1 mo)	Common	Rare
Delayed passage of meconium (>48 hrs)	Common	Rare
Painful defecation	Rare	Common
Stool-withholding behavior	Rare	Common
Soiling	Rare	Common
Stool in rectal vault	Rare	Common
Failure to thrive	Common	Rare
Bilious vomiting	Common	Rare

Peak times for functional constipation to develop are when routines change such as occurs during toilet training and starting school. Play time may distract a child from the signal to defecate. Painful defecation from streptococcal perianal disease or sexual abuse must be remembered as potential precipitants of stool withholding. Functional constipation can also be associated with dysfunctional urinary voiding and recurrent urinary tract infections.

A history supportive of functional constipation includes retentive posturing, infrequent passage of very large stools, and involuntary soiling. Physical examination typically reveals palpable stool in the abdomen. The sacrum should be inspected for skin changes suggestive of spinal dysraphism. Normal deep tendon reflexes and lower extremity strength in conjunction with a normal anal-wink reflex make neurologic impairment unlikely. The anus should be normal in placement and appearance. Rectal examination typically yields a dilated vault filled with stool. Abdominal flat-plate x-ray can be helpful if the diagnosis of fecal impaction is unclear but is not necessary (Fig. 13.2). Failure to thrive is not typically associated with functional constipation and, if present, should prompt further investigation.

Although functional constipation encompasses most cases of chronic constipation in the child ≥6 months of age, less common causes must always be considered. As in the younger infant, endocrine disorders can present as constipation. Hypothyroidism is associated with constipation, as well as sluggishness, somnolence, hypothermia, weight gain, and peripheral edema. Diabetes mellitus is associated with increased urinary water loss and intestinal dysmotility, which can lead to constipation. Hyperparathyroidism and hypervitaminosis D lead to increased serum calcium, which cause constipation through decreased peristalsis. Celiac disease is also recognized as a cause of chronic constipation.

Rarely, an abdominal or pelvic mass may present with chronic constipation. Follow-up again is emphasized because a mass that does not resolve after clearance of impaction needs further evaluation. Hydrometrocolpos can present with constipation and urinary frequency; therefore, a genital examination is indicated in girls to document a perforated hymen. One must also remember that intrauterine pregnancy is a common cause of pelvic mass and constipation in adolescent girls.

Children with neuromuscular disorders often develop chronic constipation. Myasthenia gravis, the muscular dystrophies, and other dystonic states can predispose children to constipation through a number of mechanisms. A detailed history and physical examination should recognize most neuromuscular problems, allowing symptomatic treatment to be provided.

Psychiatric problems must not be forgotten in the evaluation of constipation. Depression can be associated with constipation secondary to decreased intake, irregular diet, and

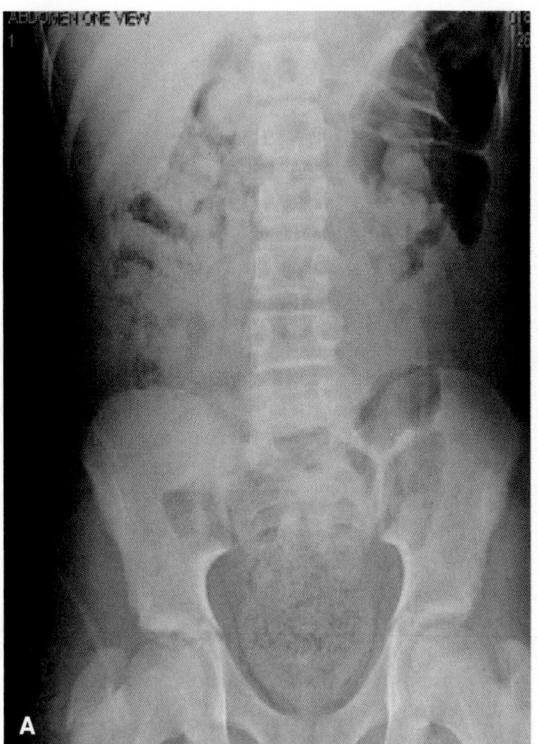

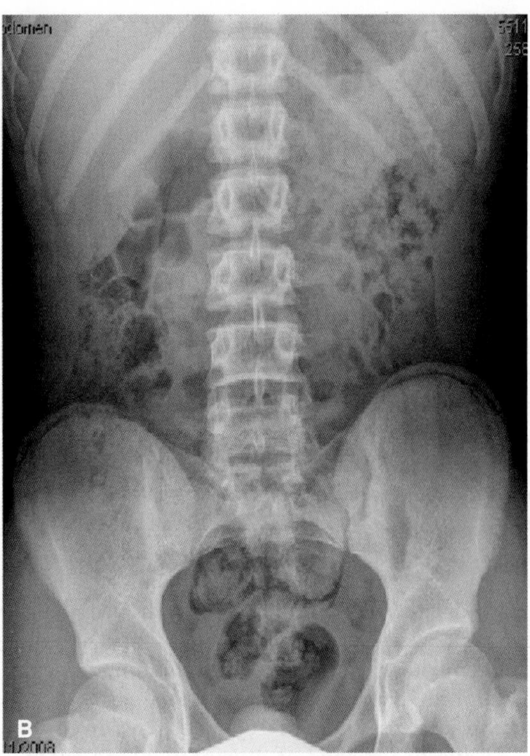

FIGURE 13.2 Both abdominal radiographs demonstrate evidence of constipation with extensive retained fecal material throughout the colon and rectum. The rectum in figure (**A**) is widened and contains a large fecal impaction while that in figure (**B**) is less widened and the stool is less compacted.

decreased activity. Many psychotropic drugs can cause constipation. Anorexia nervosa may present with constipation because of decreased intake or metabolic abnormalities, and laxative abuse can cause paradoxical constipation.

TREATMENT

Simple acute constipation in an infant <1 year of age should be treated initially with dietary changes (Table 13.7). Decreasing consumption of cow's milk, possible formula change to a protein hydrolysate, and increasing fluid intake when appropriate may be enough to alleviate the symptoms. In addition, supplementing with sorbitol-containing juice such as prune, pear, white grape, or apple juice can be helpful to soften the stool and improve stool passage. If dietary measures are insufficient, lactulose or polyethylene glycol (PEG) 3350 (MiraLax, GlycoLax) may be useful as osmotic agents. Historically, Karo corn syrup was used, but its use fell out of favor due to concerns that the syrup may contain spores of *Clostridium botulinum*. Stool lubricants such as mineral oil should not be used in children <3 years of age and should also be avoided in children at risk for aspiration. PEG solutions have gained increased use in the outpatient setting (see discussion below). When perianal irritation or anal fissures are present, local perianal care may decrease painful defecation, which, in turn, may decrease stool-retentive behavior. Follow-up is the most important aspect of treating simple constipation.

Therapy for acute functional constipation in the child ≥1 year of age is similar to that for the infant, with dietary changes and stool softeners as mainstays; however, attention

TABLE 13.7

TREATMENT STEPS FOR FUNCTIONAL CONSTIPATION: "DEFECATE"

D—Disimpact
Oral route: PEG 3350 (MiraLax), PEG electrolyte solution, magnesium hydroxide, magnesium citrate, lactulose, sorbitol, senna, or bisacodyl
Rectal route: saline enema (Fleet), mineral oil enema, glycerin suppository (infants), bisacodyl suppository (children)
E—Evacuate/empty bowel
PEG 3350 (MiraLax), PEG electrolyte solution (GoLYTELY), lactulose, senna, bisacodyl
F—Fluids
Increase fluid intake, decrease caffeine intake
E—Eat fiber
Foods high in fiber or fiber supplements, increase nonabsorbable carbohydrates (i.e., sorbitol)
C—Cathartics, softeners, and lubricants (maintenance)
PEG 3350 (MiraLax), lactulose, lubricants (mineral oil, Kondremul, and Milkinol [>3 yrs])
A—Album (diary/journal)
Daily record of bowel movements with details
T—Toileting
Set bathroom time after meals, proper height of toilet with foot support, reward systems/positive reinforcement, local perineal care, ointment, sitz baths
E—Education and early follow-up critical for success of therapy

should also be paid to psychological factors such as recent stress that may be complicating the situation.

Treatment for chronic constipation in the infant <1 year of age should include dietary measures such as use of pureed fruits and vegetables, sorbitol-containing juices, and possible formula change. If dietary measures alone are insufficient, a daily stool softener such as lactulose can be used to help maintain soft stool passage and a glycerin suppository can be used on occasion to disimpact the rectum, although this should not be used routinely. Although safety data are still emerging, PEG may also be a safe and effective treatment for chronic constipation in infants. Loening-Baucke et al. studied 20 children and Michail et al. studied 12 children younger than 1 year of age, who were safely and successfully treated with PEG used for several months or more. Although more safety data is needed to make specific recommendations, PEG will likely become one of the therapeutic options for use in infants.

Treatment (Table 13.7) for chronic functional constipation in the child older than 1 year of age begins with disimpaction and evacuation of the stool remaining in the colon. This is accomplished with either oral or rectal therapy or a combination of the two. Youssef et al. demonstrated that in fecally impacted children whose palpable stool mass did not extend above the level of the umbilicus, PEG 3350 at a dose of 1 to 1.5 g/kg/day (up to a maximum of 100 g per day) given for 3 days was an effective method of disimpaction and evacuation. Other oral options include lactulose, sorbitol, senna, bisacodyl, PEG electrolyte solution, magnesium hydroxide, and magnesium citrate. A combination of oral osmotic and stimulant agents may be effective for disimpaction. Oral phosphosoda was removed from the US market due to serious adverse events. Rectal disimpaction can be accomplished with saline (Fleet or Pedialax) enemas or bisacodyl suppositories. A mineral oil enema administered the night before the first saline enema may soften existing stool, allowing less painful passage. Saline enemas are typically dosed at one adult-sized enema (118 mL) for patients ≥3 years, and one pediatric-sized enema (59 mL) for those 1 to 3 years of age. The enema may be repeated, spaced 24 hours apart, with a maximum of three total doses. Subsequent doses should only be given if evacuation of the previous dose has occurred. Phosphate enemas are no longer available due to life-threatening adverse events. Tap water and soapsuds enemas should be avoided because of the possibility of water intoxication. Milk and molasses enemas have also fallen out of favor due to cases of serious adverse events. If there is no response after 3 days, more aggressive disimpaction under physician supervision is indicated.

The long-term maintenance phase of therapy, which is equally as important as the disimpaction and evacuation phase, involves nonstimulant osmotic laxatives, lubricants, fluids, fiber, and behavioral therapy. Laxatives include hyperosmolar agents such as PEG 3350 and lactulose. Lubricants such as mineral oil and Kondremul are helpful to lubricate the intestine for easier passage of stool. These should only be used in children ≥3 years of age and those without a high risk for aspiration. Increasing fluid and fiber intake is also critical to long-term success in treating constipation. Table 13.8 outlines the recommended daily fiber intake by age. Fiber should be increased gradually toward goal to minimize flatulence. Regular toileting should be encouraged with positive reinforcement in the school-aged child. Toilet training should be discontinued in the training toddler until retentive behaviors improve. Education of patients and parents about the pathophysiology of constipation, the etiology of encopresis when present, and the expectations of therapy is vital. Close follow-up is a mainstay of treatment. Successful therapy may take several months to years to complete.

TABLE 13.8

RECOMMENDED FIBER DOSE IN GRAMS PER DAY

Toddler	8–10
Preschool	12–14
School age	14–16
Adult	20–35

Approach to the Patient with Severe Chronic Constipation

Disimpaction and evacuation of stool in the patient with severe chronic constipation or one who has failed simple therapy presents a challenge, particularly in the emergency department setting. A series of saline enemas in conjunction with an oral disimpaction regimen may not be sufficient to disimpact a larger stool mass. Use of PEG with electrolytes solution (GoLYTELY) as a lavage either orally or via nasogastric tube at a dose of 10 to 25 mL/kg/hr up to 1,000 mL per hour until stool is clear may be helpful to treat more severe impactions. This method should be done in the hospital under supervision of a physician with close monitoring of the patient's volume and cardiovascular status and electrolytes. Risks may be higher in patients with complex medical conditions such as cardiac disease. Gastrografin or *N*-acetylcysteine enemas may be an additional method of disimpaction, especially in the case of distal intestinal obstructive syndrome as occurs in patients with cystic fibrosis. In cases of very severe fecal impaction, surgical disimpaction may be necessary. Milk and molasses enemas have fallen out of favor as a result of safety concerns following several case reports of serious adverse events, including one death. The other components of constipation therapy apply as outlined previously and in Table 13.7.

Suggested Readings and Key References

Gordon M, Naidoo K, Akobeng AK, et al. Osmotic and stimulant laxatives for the management of childhood constipation (Review). *Evid Based Child Health* 2013;8(1):57–109.

Loening-Baucke V, Krishna R, Pashankar DS. Polyethylene glycol 3350 without electrolytes for the treatment of functional constipation in infants and toddlers. *J Pediatr Gastroenterol Nutr* 2004;39: 536–539.

Michail S, Gendy E, Preud'Homme D, et al. Polyethylene glycol for constipation in children younger than eighteen months old. *J Pediatr Gastroenterol Nutr* 2004;39:197–199.

Tabbers MM, DiLorenzo C, Berger MY, et al. Evaluation and treatment of functional constipation in infants and children: evidence-based recommendations from ESPGHAN and NASPGHAN. *J Pediatr Gastroenterol Nutr* 2014;58:258–274.

Youssef N, Peters JM, Henderson W, et al. Dose response of PEG 3350 for the treatment of childhood fecal impaction. *J Pediatr* 2002; 141(3):410–414.

CHAPTER 14 ■ COUGH

TODD A. FLORIN, MD, MSCE

Cough is a common pediatric complaint with a variety of causes. Although cough is usually a self-limited symptom associated with upper respiratory illnesses, it occasionally indicates a more serious process. Under most circumstances, history and physical examination can accurately determine the cause.

PATHOPHYSIOLOGY

Cough is a reflex designed to clear the airway. Although a cough can be initiated voluntarily, it is usually elicited by stimulation of receptors located throughout the respiratory tract, from the pharynx to the bronchioles, in addition to the paranasal sinuses, stomach, and external auditory canal. Receptors may be triggered by inflammatory, chemical, mechanical, and thermal stimuli. Direct (central) stimulation of a cough center in the brain occurs more rarely. The reflex consists of a forced expiration and sudden opening of the glottis, which rapidly forces air through the airway to expel any mucus or foreign material.

DIFFERENTIAL DIAGNOSIS

The causes of cough differ in the type of stimulus and the site of involvement in the respiratory tract (Table 14.1). The common causes of cough are listed in Table 14.2. Potentially life-threatening causes are listed in Table 14.3.

In distinguishing the etiologies of cough, the clinician must consider features that are atypical for simple upper respiratory infections (URIs) or routine asthma. Although pertussis exists as a URI in the catarrhal phase, infants with paroxysms of coughing, color change, significant posttussive emesis, or apneic episodes should be tested and managed as possible pertussis. Similarly, toddlers and young children with new-onset wheezing following a choking episode, those infants with wheezing unresponsive to usual therapy, and those with persistent lobar pneumonia should be evaluated for a foreign body. Cough associated with expectoration of blood (hemoptysis) should prompt evaluation for infection, vasculitis, pulmonary vascular disorders, trauma, congenital heart defects, neoplasm, or coagulopathy. Finally, children who present with cough and associated stridor may have croup, but those with recurrent stridor, associated dysphagia, or chronic hoarseness must be evaluated for a foreign body, extrinsic compression of the trachea (vascular ring, tumor), or laryngeal pathology (papilloma, hemangioma).

EVALUATION AND DECISION

The history and physical examination are the keys to establishing a diagnosis in a patient with cough. The first priority is to recognize and treat any life-threatening conditions. Patients with significant respiratory distress should receive supplemental oxygen and rapid assessment of their airway and breathing (Fig. 14.1).

History

Cough can occur as an acute or chronic symptom, depending on the underlying process. Most common and serious causes of cough have an acute onset (Fig. 14.1). Certain conditions, such as asthma, may present with an acute or a chronic history of cough.

The relationship of the cough to other factors is helpful. Cough in the neonate must raise the possibility of congenital anomalies, gastroesophageal reflux, congestive heart failure, and atypical pneumonia (e.g., *Chlamydia*). If the cough began with other upper respiratory tract symptoms or fever, an infectious cause is likely. A cough that started with a choking or gagging episode, especially in an older infant or toddler, suggests a foreign-body aspiration (see Chapter 27 Foreign Body: Ingestion and Aspiration). Concern for button battery and peanut aspirations require emergent evaluation and removal when present. Cough associated with exercise or cold exposure, even in the absence of wheezing, may be a sign of reactive airway disease. A primarily nocturnal cough often stems from allergy, sinusitis, or reactive airway disease. Systemic complaints should also be considered in patients with a cough: Headache, fever, facial pain or pressure (sinusitis), acute dyspnea (asthma, pneumonia, cardiac disease), chest pain (asthma, pleuritis, pneumonia), dysphagia (esophageal or pharyngeal foreign body), dysphonia (laryngeal edema or tracheal mass), or weight loss (malignancy or tuberculosis).

The quality of the cough may also be helpful in determining etiology. A barking, seal-like cough, with or without stridor, supports the diagnosis of laryngotracheitis (croup). A paroxysmal cough associated with an inspiratory "whoop," cyanosis, or apnea is characteristic of pertussis. Infants younger than 6 months of age with pertussis may present with severe cough, poor feeding, apnea, or bradycardia without the classic whooping paroxysms of cough. Tracheitis gives a deep "brassy" cough, whereas conditions accompanied by wheezing (asthma or bronchiolitis) typically produce a high-pitched "tight" (often termed *bronchospastic*) cough. Vocal cord dysfunction can result in cough and audible wheeze that may mimic asthma, and should be considered in older children and adolescents with multiple cough and wheezing episodes that do not respond to repeated courses of standard asthma therapy. Determining whether a cough is productive can be difficult in young children who often swallow, rather than expectorate, their sputum. Although a productive-sounding cough may be seen with uncomplicated URIs, sinusitis and lower respiratory tract infections are more commonly accompanied by a productive cough. Contrary to popular belief, the color of expectorated sputum does not necessarily indicate infectious or bacterial etiology.

TABLE 14.1

CAUSES OF COUGH IN CHILDREN

Infection
Upper respiratory infection
Sinusitis
Tonsillitis
Laryngitis
Laryngotracheitis (croup)
Tracheitis/tracheobronchitis
Bronchiolitis
Acute bronchitis
Pneumonia/empyema
Pleuritis/pleural effusion
Bronchiectasis/pulmonary abscess
Inflammation/allergy
Allergic rhinitis
Laryngeal edema
Reactive airway disease
Chronic bronchitis
Cystic fibrosis
Vocal cord dysfunction
Mechanical or chemical irritation
Foreign-body aspiration
Neck/chest trauma
Chemical fumes
Inhaled particulates
Smoking
Neoplasm
Pharyngeal or nasal polyp
Hemangioma of the larynx or trachea
Papilloma of the laryrnx or trachea
Lymphoma compressing airway
Mediastinal tumors
Congenital anomalies
Cleft palate
Laryngotracheomalacia
Laryngeal or tracheal webs
Tracheoesophageal fistula
Vascular ring
Pulmonary sequestration
Miscellaneous
Gastroesophageal reflux
Congestive heart failure
Swallowing dysfunction
Granulomatous diseases (e.g., pulmonary tuberculosis)
Vasculitis (e.g., Wegener granulomatosis)
Psychogenic cough
Foreign body in otic canal
Medications (e.g., angiotensin-converting enzyme inhibitors)

Typically, the onset of cough with rhinorrhea suggests a viral URI or bronchiolitis. However, if a child with an apparent URI becomes more ill or has persistent symptoms, secondary bacterial infections in the lungs or sinuses, pertussis, as well as noninfectious etiologies should be considered.

TABLE 14.2

COMMON CAUSES OF COUGH

Upper respiratory infection
Sinusitis
Laryngotracheitis (croup)
Bronchiolitis
Acute bronchitis
Pneumonia
Allergic rhinitis
Reactive airway disease

Expectoration of bloody sputum, or hemoptysis, poses a particular diagnostic challenge. Blood-streaked sputum, particularly with fever, may suggest tracheobronchitis or pneumonia. Tracheal foreign bodies may cause hemoptysis, usually associated with a choking episode. Hematuria associated with hemoptysis suggests a pulmonary-renal vasculitis, such as Wegener granulomatosis. Other easy bleeding or bruising may accompany the hemoptysis if due to a coagulopathy, such as von Willebrand disease or platelet disorders.

Physical Examination

Patients with a cough require evaluation of the entire respiratory system. Usually, the cause of the cough can be localized to the upper or lower respiratory tract based on the physical examination. Physical examination should include inspection of the nares, otic canal, and oropharynx and auscultation of the chest. Young infants may have respiratory distress with localized upper airway congestion, but distress in older infants and children usually signifies lower respiratory tract disease (except in the obvious case of stridor). Rhinorrhea, congestion, swollen turbinates, sinus tenderness, and pharyngitis are all signs of upper respiratory tract involvement. Allergic features include boggy nasal mucosa, an allergic nasal crease, and allergic "shiners." An otoscopic examination may reveal a small foreign body (e.g., hair) in the otic canal, which may cause chronic cough. Visualizing the posterior pharynx with a tongue blade will often elicit an episode of coughing, allowing the practitioner to gauge the quality of the cough. Laryngitis

TABLE 14.3

LIFE-THREATENING CAUSES OF COUGH

Reactive airway disease
Laryngotracheitis (croup)
Bronchiolitis
Foreign body
Pneumonia
Laryngeal edema
Pertussis
Toxic inhalation
Congestive heart failure
Bacterial tracheitis
Significant pulmonary bleeding (e.g., arteriovenous malformation)

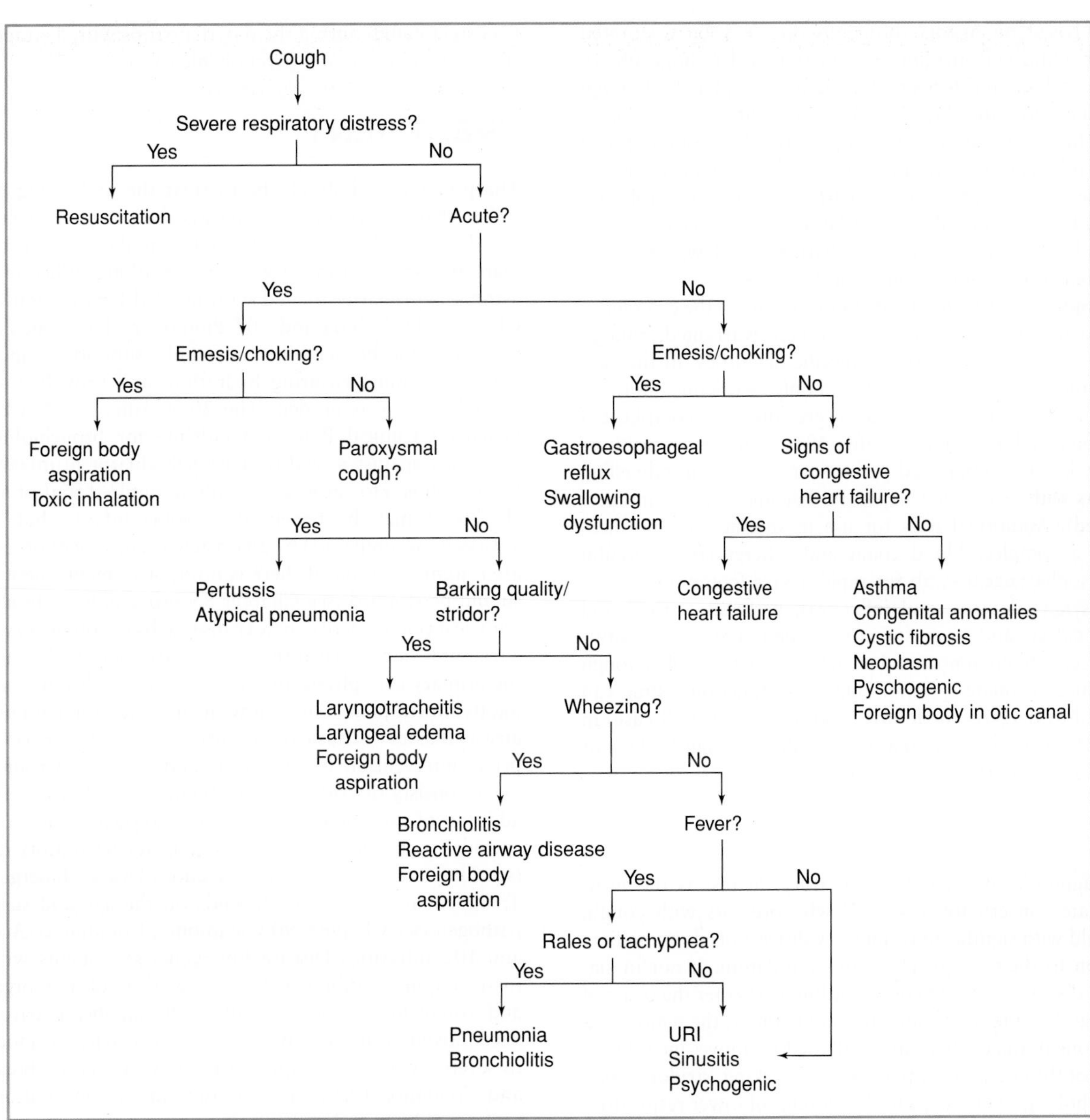

FIGURE 14.1 Approach to the child with cough.

and/or stridor generally imply inflammation or obstruction at the level of the trachea or larynx. Unequal breath sounds, wheezes, rhonchi, and rales are signs of lower respiratory tract disease. Wheezing may indicate bronchiolitis, asthma, or, rarely, foreign-body aspiration. Patients with asthma may complain only of cough and deny any wheezing. Careful auscultation during forced exhalation may detect wheezing or a prolonged expiratory phase. In an older child, significant lower airway obstruction can be measured with a handheld peak flow meter. Asymmetric, or focal, wheezing is seen with lower airway masses and foreign bodies. A careful cardiac evaluation should be performed to detect evidence of congestive heart failure, and any clubbing should be noted, as this finding is suggestive of a chronic, cyanotic condition such as cystic fibrosis.

Ancillary Studies

For most children with a cough, the history and physical examination should be sufficient to make a diagnosis. The 2011 Infectious Diseases Society of America/Pediatric Infectious Diseases Society pediatric pneumonia guidelines recommend that routine chest radiographs are not necessary to confirm suspected pneumonia in children well enough to be treated in the outpatient setting (see Chapter 90 Pneumonia, Community-Acquired). These guidelines recommend anteroposterior and lateral chest radiographs in patients with hypoxia, significant respiratory distress, in those who failed initial antibiotic therapy for pneumonia, in all patients hospitalized for pneumonia, those with concern for complications of pneumonia, such as empyema or abscess, and in those in whom the diagnosis is in question. Furthermore, in patients with unexplained cough or significant or persistent pulmonary signs, a chest radiograph is warranted. In children with an uncomplicated exacerbation of their asthma, a radiograph is unnecessary. Inspiratory and expiratory or decubitus films have traditionally been recommended if a radiolucent foreign body is suspected; however, these studies have been found to have only fair-to-moderate sensitivity and specificity and thus their clinical utility is unknown. If the suspicion for aspiration is high based on history, bronchoscopy may be warranted without additional imaging beyond standard radiographs to identify radiopaque foreign bodies (see Chapter 27 Foreign Body: Ingestion and Aspiration). All patients with hemoptysis should have chest radiographs performed. Chest computed tomography is indicated in patients with persistent or moderate-to-severe hemoptysis, particularly if chest radiographs are normal. Other studies that could be useful in selected patients include lateral neck radiographs, barium swallow, and computed tomography of the sinuses, neck, or chest.

Laboratory testing for a patient presenting to the emergency department with cough is not routinely warranted, though may be useful or necessary for specific diagnoses. In the case of pneumonia, blood cultures should only be obtained in those hospitalized with moderate-to-severe disease, complicated pneumonia, failure to improve after 48 to 72 hours of antibiotic therapy, immunosuppressed patients or those with indwelling catheters with fever (see Chapter 90 Pneumonia, Community-Acquired). Additional tests for use in specific circumstances include a complete blood count and differential, tuberculin test, nasopharyngeal swab for rapid assays (commonly respiratory syncytial virus, and influenza), pertussis testing, and sputum culture and Gram stain (neutrophils and gram-positive diplococci with pneumococcal pneumonia) in those old enough to produce adequate sputum. Pulmonary function testing can be useful to diagnose or follow obstructive airway disease. In cases of airway masses, airway anomalies, foreign bodies, or atypical pneumonias, bronchoscopy may be necessary.

Approach

The magnitude of a child's respiratory distress is the most immediate concern for any child who presents with cough. Any child with significant respiratory distress needs immediate attention to their oxygenation and ventilation. If not in significant distress, the next consideration is whether the onset of the cough is acute or chronic. If acute in onset, the major considerations in the evaluation, as alluded to above, include the quality of the cough (e.g., paroxysmal, barking, stridor), associated choking or emesis, and the findings of lower respiratory tract signs or fever (Fig. 14.1). Most patients with cough of acute onset will have a simple URI, asthma, bronchiolitis, or pneumonia. Although rales, decreased breath sounds, or focal wheezing are signs associated with pneumonia, a small proportion of patients with pneumonia may not have any findings by auscultation. Therefore, in cases of significant cough, especially in very young children and those with high fever or elevated white blood cell counts, a chest radiograph may be useful to exclude the diagnosis of pneumonia.

Children with chronic cough are likely to have reactive airway disease, allergic rhinitis, or sinusitis. In young children with failure to thrive or recurrent pulmonary infections, cystic fibrosis (see Chapter 107 Pulmonary Emergencies) should be considered. Chronic cough with a history of recurrent pneumonias or chronic bronchitis can also be suggestive of immunodeficiency or anatomic lesions (see Chapters 107 Pulmonary Emergencies, 132 Thoracic Emergencies). Choking with feeding or emesis followed by cough or wheezing in young infants is typical of gastroesophageal reflux. Newborns who exhibit a cough deserve special consideration for airway anomalies, atypical pneumonias, and congestive heart failure (see Chapters 102 Infectious Disease Emergencies, 107 Pulmonary Emergencies, and 126 ENT Emergencies). Persistent cough during the day that stops with distraction or sleep is supportive of a psychogenic cause.

TREATMENT

The primary goal should be to treat the underlying process rather than to attempt to suppress the cough. Patients with any distress or hypoxia need supplemental oxygen and immediate assessment of the airway and breathing. Wheezing from asthma is primarily treated with inhaled beta-2 agonists (see Chapters 84 Asthma and 107 Pulmonary Emergencies). The treatment for bronchiolitis is mainly supportive, including nasal suctioning, ensuring hydration, and providing supplemental oxygen as needed. The 2014 American Academy of Pediatrics Clinical Practice Guideline for bronchiolitis recommends against a trial of a bronchodilator in infants with bronchiolitis. However, a carefully monitored trial of a bronchodilator may be beneficial in some infants, but should always be accompanied by an objective assessment of response after administration. If there is no improvement, these agents should be stopped (see Chapter 85 Bronchiolitis). In children with suspected reactive airway disease based on history alone, a trial of bronchodilator therapy is warranted. Follow-up with the primary care physician is crucial for establishing an ongoing treatment plan. Children with suspected foreign bodies or airway masses (intrinsic or extrinsic to the airway) need appropriate intervention for diagnosis and removal. Croup treatment consists of corticosteroid therapy in all cases, and the addition of racemic epinephrine and oxygen for more severe episodes with stridor at rest or significant respiratory distress (see Chapters 70 Stridor, 102 Infectious Disease Emergencies). Treatment of pneumonia depends on the age and suspected pathogen (see Chapters 90 Pneumonia, Community-Acquired and 102 Infectious Disease Emergencies). Patients with pertussis require antibiotics for eradication of the organism, and young infants or any child with significant paroxysms need hospitalization. Patients with recurrent or moderate-to-severe hemoptysis require attention to airway, breathing, and circulation first and foremost. Timely consultation with otolaryngology and pulmonology is warranted to assist in medical and procedural treatment of persistent bleeding.

Antitussive medications have limited value and should not be used routinely in young infants. It is better to give specific therapy (e.g., bronchodilators in asthma, antibiotics in sinusitis) and avoid suppressing a cough in conditions with increased sputum production (e.g., asthma, pneumonia). In children older than 1 year of age, honey may be a useful treatment for symptomatic relief of acute cough. In older children with a nonproductive cough that interrupts sleep, antitussives can be prescribed. Using cool mist humidifiers and elevating the head during sleep can be beneficial for coughs associated with viral URIs.

Suggested Readings and Key References

Asilsoy S, Bayram E, Agin H, et al. Evaluation of chronic cough in children. *Chest* 2008;134(6):1122–1128.

Bradley JS, Byington CL, Shah SS, et al. The management of community-acquired pneumonia in infants and children older than 3 months of age: clinical practice guidelines by the Pediatric Infectious Diseases Society and the Infectious Diseases Society of America. *Clin Infect Dis* 2011;53(7):617–630.

Brown JC, Chapman T, Klein EJ, et al. The utility of adding expiratory or decubitus chest radiographs to the radiographic evaluation of suspected pediatric airway foreign bodies. *Ann Emerg Med* 2013;62(6):604–608.

Chang AB. Cough. *Pediatr Clin North Am* 2009;56(1):19–31.

Chang AB, Glomb WB. Guidelines for evaluating chronic cough in pediatrics: ACCP evidence-based clinical practice guidelines. *Chest* 2006;129(1 suppl):260S–283S.

Klig JE. Current challenges in lower respiratory infections in children. *Curr Opin Pediatr* 2004;16(1):107–112.

Litowitz T, Whitaker N, Clark L, et al. Emerging battery-ingestion hazard: clinical implications. *Pediatrics* 2010;125(6):1168–1177.

Mackey JE, Wojcik S, Long R, et al. Predicting pertussis in a pediatric emergency department population. *Clin Pediatr (Phila)* 2007;46(5): 437–440.

Mikita JA, Mikita CP. Vocal cord dysfunction. *Asthma Allergy Proc* 2006;27(4):411–414.

Oduwole O, Meremikwu MM, Oyo-Ita A, et al. Honey for acute cough in children. *Cochrane Database Syst Rev* 2012;3:CD007094.

Quinonez RA, Garber MD, Schroeder AR, et al. Choosing wisely in pediatric hospital medicine: five opportunities for improved healthcare value. *J Hosp Med* 2013;8(9):479–485.

Ralston SL, Lieberthal AS, Meissner C, et al. Clinical practice guideline: the diagnosis, management, and prevention of bronchiolitis. *Pediatrics* 2014;134(5):e1474–e1502.

Vernacchio L, Kelly JP, Kaufman DW, et al. Cough and cold medication use by US children, 1999–2006: results from the slone survey. *Pediatrics* 2008;122(2):e323–e329.

CHAPTER 15 ■ CRYING

EMILY L. WILLNER, MD AND SHILPA PATEL, MD, MPH

For the purposes of this chapter, we limit our discussion to crying in early infancy, that is, the first 3 months of life.

Infant crying is a nonspecific response to discomfort, with causes ranging from normal hunger and desire for company to life-threatening illness. Many common minor irritations and illnesses can be elucidated by careful history and physical examination. Often, however, a normal, thriving baby will develop a pattern of unprovoked daily paroxysms of irritability and crying known as colic. Colic usually begins in the second to third week of life, with complete resolution by 3 months of age. Crying may last for several hours each day and is more common in the late afternoon or evening. A typical episode is described as sudden fussiness that develops into a piercing scream, as if the baby were in pain. The infant may draw up the legs, the abdomen may appear distended, bowel sounds are increased, and flatus may be passed, leading parents to be concerned that their baby has abdominal distress. Only when crying episodes are repeated and stereotypical, and other causes of crying are excluded, can a diagnosis of colic be made with certainty. When colic is suspected, the emergency physician must have an orderly approach in order to rule out severe, life-threatening illnesses, detect common medical etiologies, and provide preliminary guidance to the family.

PATHOPHYSIOLOGY

Any unpleasant sensation can cause an infant to cry. Pain or an altered threshold for discomfort (irritability) may be caused by many physical illnesses. Those most likely to present abruptly in a young infant are listed in Table 15.1. Numerous unproven theories abound about the etiology of colic, including cow's milk allergy, immaturity of the gastrointestinal tract or central nervous system, parental anxiety, maternal smoking during pregnancy, poor feeding technique, and individual temperament characteristics. Gastroesophageal reflux has been suggested as a possible etiology of infant colic; however, studies have shown antireflux medications are not superior to placebo in reducing colicky crying. Moreover, there is poor correlation between crying and reflux episodes documented by pH probe. The search for a specific cause of colic continues.

No single theory (or therapy) has gained uniform acceptance. Colic may be a syndrome that represents the manifestations of some or all these factors in varying degrees in a population of babies whose tendency to cry varies along a normal distribution. Multiple studies have documented crying in early infancy. They show that crying tends to cluster in the evening, and daily crying times increase from birth to a peak of approximately 3 hours per day at 6 to 8 weeks, followed by a rapid decline. Although there are variations in the literature, most agree that a reasonable definition for colic embraces Wessel criteria: An infant younger than 3 months of age with more than 3 hours of crying per day occurring more than 3 times per week for more than 3 weeks.

EVALUATION AND DECISION

A careful history, physical examination, and rarely, additional studies, should enable the physician to diagnose identifiable illnesses or injuries causing severe paroxysms of crying (Table 15.1).

The history should elicit the onset of crying and any associated events—particularly trauma, fever, use of medications, or recent immunization (extreme irritability lasting up to 24 hours has been described after pertussis vaccination). Because feeding is vigorous exercise for the young infant, irritability with feeds may indicate ischemic heart disease. Alternatively, yeast infections of the mouth, or severe reflux, may cause infants to cry with feeding. Parents may recall a pattern of crying after maternal ingestion of specific foods in infants who are breast-feeding. Irritability on being picked up ("paradoxic irritability") may indicate a fractured bone or meningeal inflammation. Crying with manipulation of an arm may indicate a clavicle fracture sustained during birth.

Physical examination must be thorough, with the infant completely undressed. Vital signs may reveal either low or high temperature, suggesting infection, or hyperpnea (see Chapter 87 Fever in Infants), suggesting metabolic acidosis (see Chapter 103 Metabolic Emergencies) or increased intracranial pressure. The head should be explored for evidence of trauma and the fontanel should be palpated. Eyes must be examined with fluorescein to look for corneal abrasion, even in infants with no symptoms referable to the eyes. In addition, eversion of the upper eyelids can exclude a foreign body. Fundoscopy should be attempted (retinal hemorrhages are common signs of abuse, especially in shaken baby syndrome). Careful otoscopy is required to visualize the tympanic membranes. The heart should be evaluated for signs of congestive failure or arrhythmia (Table 15.1, I.C). Abdominal examination must be performed to detect signs of peritonitis (see Chapter 124 Abdominal Emergencies) or incarcerated umbilical hernia. The diaper must be removed and the area examined for incarcerated inguinal hernia, testicular torsion, hair tourniquet of the genitalia, or anal fissure. Careful palpation of all long bones may reveal subtle signs of fracture, even in the absence of external signs of trauma. Each finger and toe should be inspected to look for strangulation by hair or thread.

Consideration of laboratory or radiographic evaluation is made in light of the clinical findings. Crying may be the primary symptom of an occult urinary tract infection (see Chapter 92 UTI, Febrile), therefore urinalysis and culture of a sterile specimen of urine should be considered. A low threshold for urine toxicology screening is warranted in the persistently irritable baby, given that intoxication (see Chapter 110 Toxicologic Emergencies) with, or withdrawal from, illicit drugs may cause

TABLE 15.1

CONDITIONS ASSOCIATED WITH ABRUPT ONSET OF INCONSOLABLE CRYING IN YOUNG INFANTS

I. Discomfort caused by identifiable illness
- A. Head and neck
  1. Meningitis[a]
  2. Skull fracture/subdural hematoma[a]
  3. Glaucoma
  4. Foreign body (especially eyelash) in eye[b]
  5. Corneal abrasion[b]
  6. Otitis media[b]
  7. Caffey disease (infantile cortical hyperostosis)
  8. Child abuse[a]
- B. Gastrointestinal
  1. Aerophagia (improper feeding/burping technique)
  2. Gastroenteritis[b]
  3. Gastrointestinal surgical emergency (e.g., volvulus)[a]
  4. Anal fissure[b]
  5. Constipation[b]
  6. Cow's milk protein intolerance
  7. Gastroesophageal reflux/esophagitis
- C. Cardiovascular
  1. Congestive heart failure[a]
  2. Supraventricular tachycardia[a]
  3. Coarctation of the aorta[a]
  4. Anomalous origin of left coronary artery from pulmonary artery[a]
- D. Genitourinary
  1. Torsion of the testis
  2. Incarcerated hernia[a]
  3. Urinary tract infection
- E. Integumentary
  1. Burn
  2. Strangulated finger, toe, penis (hair tourniquet)
- F. Musculoskeletal
  1. Child abuse[a]
  2. Extremity fracture
  3. Musculoskeletal infection (septic joint or osteomyelitis)[a]
- G. Toxic/metabolic
  1. Drugs: antihistamines, atropinics, adrenergics, cocaine (including passive inhalation), aspirin[a]
  2. Metabolic acidosis, hypernatremia, hypocalcemia, hypoglycemia[a]
  3. Pertussis vaccine reactions
  4. Prenatal/perinatal drug exposure/withdrawal

II. Colic—recurrent paroxysmal attacks of crying[b]

[a]Life-threatening causes.
[b]Common causes.

irritability. Examination of the stool for blood and eosinophils may help to diagnose milk allergy. Infants with unexplained, incessant crying, even after an observation period in the ED, may require an extensive evaluation and hospitalization.

Many infants will have a completely normal emergency department evaluation, and the history (or subsequent follow-up) will be suggestive of colic. Over the time in which the crying attacks recur, the infant must demonstrate adequate weight gain (average 5 to 7 oz per week in the first months of life) and absence of physical disorders on several examinations before underlying illnesses can be excluded and colic can be diagnosed confidently (Fig. 15.1). When it becomes clear that an infant is experiencing colic, the practitioner faces the challenge of advising the family. No dramatic cure is currently available, however the symptoms almost invariably resolve by 3 months of age. Furthermore, many studies on the etiology and treatment of colic have methodologic weaknesses, making it difficult for clinicians to interpret results.

There is no safe and effective pharmacologic treatment for colic. The efficacy of simethicone is not supported by good-quality trials, but there have been no reported side effects and it is widely used. Methylscopolamine is neither effective nor safe. Dicyclomine, once believed to be effective, is no longer recommended in infants younger than 6 months because it can cause apnea, seizures, and coma. Studies of maternal hypoallergenic diets while breast-feeding have yielded mixed results whereas a systematic review of hypoallergenic formulas did show a reduction in crying time. Since only approximately 4% of infants have true cow's milk protein allergy, further studies are needed. Herbal tea mixtures appear to reduce crying times, though there are multiple drawbacks, including compromised nutrition due to the large volume required for symptomatic relief and lack of standardized dosing and strength. In addition, there is a potential for parental misidentification of recommended ingredients, causing GI or neurotoxicity. Several small studies have shown that adding a probiotic dietary supplement to breast-fed infants' diets decreases crying time. In contrast, a recent double blind placebo-controlled randomized clinical trial (RCT) evaluating *Lactobacillus reuteri* found that the probiotic did not benefit a mixed sample of breast-fed and formula-fed infants with colic. A subsequent meta-analysis of all published RCT data demonstrated that *L. reuteri* does reduce crying in predominantly breast-fed infants. *L. reuteri* is safe in immunocompetent infants and may have a role in reducing crying time in breast-fed infants, however further trials are needed since most studies have been conducted outside of the United States, and the evidence for formula-fed infants is inconclusive. Chiropractic manipulation has been shown to decrease parent-reported crying time, but all studies are small and methodologically prone to bias. The safest and most effective course of treatment at this time seems to be empathy, and counseling to respond quickly to the crying infant. The physician can reassure the parents that their baby is thriving and will outgrow the colic and develop normally, and that the crying is not due to their parenting.

Colic is not dangerous and does not last forever, but it will be a nuisance for several weeks. Exhaustion of the parents may be dangerous for the infant, both psychologically and physically. The National Center for Shaken Baby Syndrome (http://www.DONTSHAKE.org) acknowledges that excessive crying is a risk factor for abuse. The physician should assess the parents' emotional state, investigate the status of available support systems, and recommend a respite for the primary caregivers if possible. For amelioration of crying at the time of the ED visit, no drug therapy or feeding change is recommended. Rather, most colicky babies derive some temporary relief from rhythmic motion, such as rocking, being carried, or riding in a car; from continual monotonous sounds, such as those from a washing machine or electric fan; and from

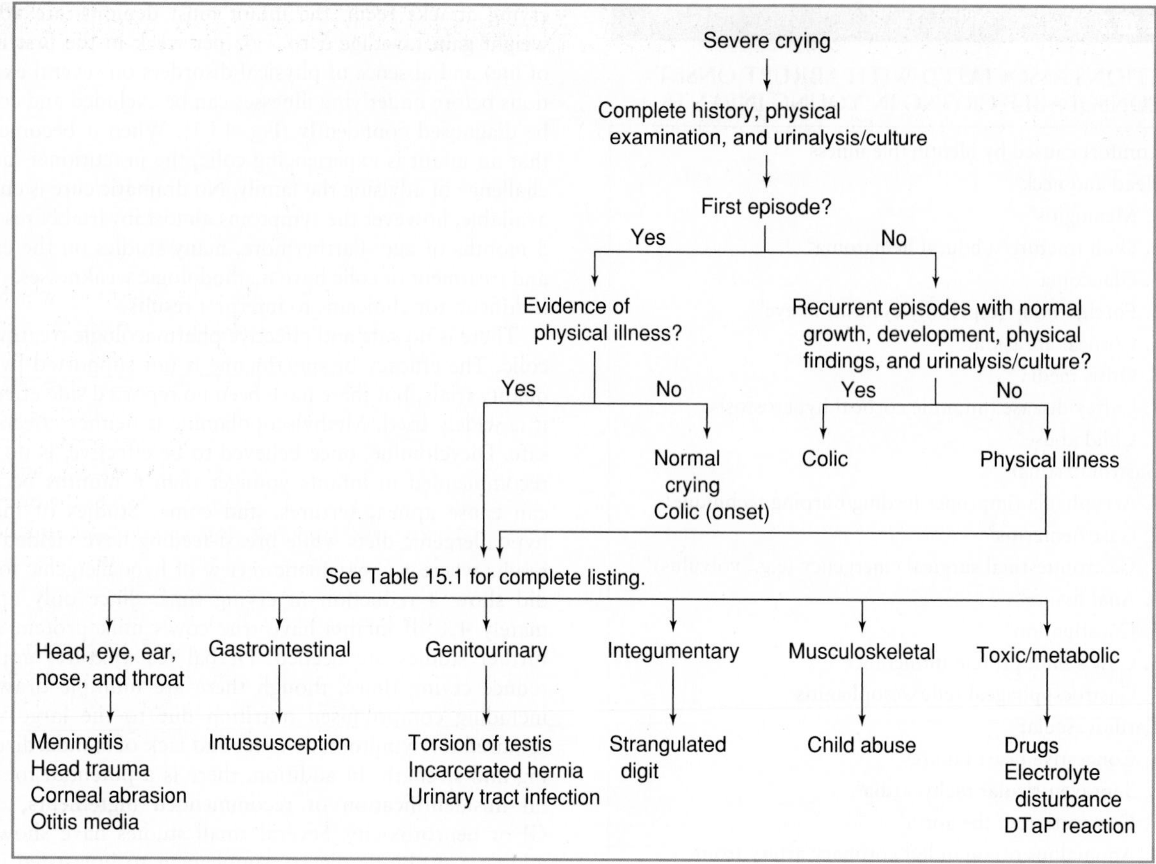

FIGURE 15.1 Approach to abrupt onset of severe crying in infancy. DTaP, diphtheria–pertussis–tetanus (vaccine).

nonnutritive sucking. Because the differential diagnosis of infant crying is broad, referral to a pediatrician for follow-up is extremely important.

ACKNOWLEDGMENTS

The authors gratefully acknowledge the contributions of Barbara B. Pawel, MD and Fred M. Henretic, MD to the content of this chapter.

Suggested Readings and Key References

Barr RG. Changing our understanding of infant colic. *Arch Pediatr Adolesc Med* 2002;156:1172–1174.

Brazelton TB. Crying in infancy. *Pediatrics* 1962;29:579–588.

Brotherton H, Philip RK. Anomalous left coronary artery from pulmonary artery (ALCAPA) in infants: a 5-year review in a defined birth cohort. *Eur J Pediatr* 2008;167:43–46.

Dobson D, Lucassen PL, Miller JJ, et al. Manipulative therapies for infantile colic. *Cochrane Database Syst Rev* 2012;12:CD004796.

Evanoo G. Infant crying: a clinical conundrum. *J Pediatr Health Care* 2007;21:333–338.

Fireman L, Serwint J. Colic. *Pediatr Rev* 2006;27:357–358.

Garrison MM, Christakis DA. A systematic review of treatments for infant colic. *Pediatrics* 2000;106:184–190.

Hardoin RA, Henslee JA, Christenson CP, et al. Colic medication and apparent life-threatening events. *Clin Pediatr* 1991;30:281–285.

Herman M, Le A. The crying infant. *Emerg Med Clin North Am* 2007; 25:1137–1159.

Reijneveld SA, Brugman E, Hirasing RA. Excessive infant crying: the impact of varying definitions. *Pediatrics* 2001;108:893–897.

Savino F. Focus on infantile colic. *Acta Paediatr* 2007;96:1259–1264.

Savino F, Pelle E, Palumeri E, et al. Lactobacillus reuteri (American type culture collection strain 55730) versus simethicone in the treatment of infantile colic: a prospective randomized study. *Pediatrics* 2007;119(1):e124–e130.

Sondergaard C, Henriksen TB, Obel C, et al. Smoking during pregnancy and infantile colic. *Pediatrics* 2001;108:342–346.

St James-Roberts I. Persistent infant crying. *Arch Dis Child* 1991;31(3): 653–655.

Wessel MA. Paroxysmal fussing in infancy, sometimes called "colic." *Pediatrics* 1975;14:421–435.

CHAPTER 16 ■ CYANOSIS

DAVID A. LOWE, MD AND ANNE M. STACK, MD

Cyanosis, a bluish-purple discoloration of the tissues, is a disturbing condition commonly confronted by the pediatric emergency physician. It is most easily appreciated in the lips, nail beds, earlobes, mucous membranes, and locations where the skin is thin and may be enhanced or obscured by lighting conditions and skin pigmentation.

PATHOPHYSIOLOGY

The three factors that ultimately determine the occurrence of cyanosis are the total amount of hemoglobin (Hb) in the blood, the degree of Hb oxygen saturation or qualitative changes in the Hb, and the state of the circulation.

Oxygenated Hb is bright red, and deoxygenated Hb is purple. Cyanosis is evident when the total reduced or deoxygenated Hb in the blood exceeds 5 g per dL or when oxygen saturation approaches 85%. When the total amount of Hb is decreased, as in anemia, the patient may not appear cyanotic even in the presence of unsaturated Hb. Conversely, polycythemic patients may appear ruddy because of the increased red cell mass, and the relative increase in unsaturated Hb will add a blue hue to the skin.

The degree of Hb saturation is determined by several factors, including the partial pressure of oxygen (Po_2) in the alveoli, the ability of oxygen (O_2) to diffuse across the alveolar wall into the red cell and the Hb molecule itself. First, if the level of alveolar ventilation falls, so does the alveolar Po_2, resulting in a fall in arterial Po_2, resulting in desaturation and subsequent cyanosis. Second, the ability of O_2 to diffuse across the alveolar wall into the red cell, or blood–gas barrier, is greatly affected by the circumstances of the barrier itself. According to *Fick's law,* any condition that diminishes alveolar surface area and/or increases the thickness will decrease gas diffusion and hence arterial Po_2. Third, the Hb molecule itself has unique properties that affect the amount of oxygen it can carry. The color of whole blood is determined in part by the state of the Hb molecule. Under normal circumstances, oxygen binds reversibly to the iron molecule of the Hb subunit, changing its conformation from a purple deoxygenated form to a bright red oxygenated Hb. Consequently, factors that affect O_2 binding to Hb will affect the color of the blood. For example, carbon monoxide competitively binds to hemoglobin at an affinity 200 times more than that of oxygen to form carboxyhemoglobin. This abnormal form of Hb has a cherry red color, despite the fact that little oxygen is bound to the Hb molecule. Another important conformational change in Hb occurs when heme iron is oxidized from its normal ferrous to a ferric state, to form methemoglobin. Hemoglobin in this state is brownish-purple in color, is incapable of binding O_2, and results in cyanosis if the level exceeds 10% to 15% of total Hb.

The state of the circulation plays an important role in the presence and degree of cyanosis. Cyanosis can result from shunting. A *shunt* is defined as a mechanism by which deoxygenated blood that has not traveled through the ventilated alveolar capillary bed mixes with oxygenated arterial blood, hence reducing the arterial Po_2. If the shunt is large, the reduction in arterial Po_2 can be severe, leading to marked cyanosis. Oxygen is unloaded to the tissues as blood travels through a capillary, with the relative concentration of unsaturated Hb increasing from one end of the capillary bed to the other. Poor perfusion states and cold temperature favor the unloading of oxygen and thus increase the amount of unsaturated Hb in the tissue capillaries. In an upright lung, the apex is ventilated more than the base, and the base is perfused more than the apex resulting in ventilation/perfusion (V/Q) mismatch. In healthy subjects, this is not clinically relevant; however, in patients with diseased lungs, the contribution of V/Q inequality to lowering of blood Po_2 can be significant.

DIFFERENTIAL DIAGNOSIS

The most common causes of cyanosis are cardiac and respiratory diseases but many other conditions can also cause a patient to appear blue (Tables 16.1 and 16.2). Consideration of the pathophysiologic framework outlined previously allows an orderly approach to the differential diagnosis of cyanosis. Life-threatening causes of cyanosis are summarized in Table 16.3.

Polycythemia, as in newborns with twin–twin transfusion, infants of diabetic mothers or children with high erythropoietin states, may give the appearance of cyanosis. This can occur even with a normal saturation because absolute the amount of unsaturated Hb is above 5 g per dL, however that makes up only a small percentage of the total Hb.

The degree of Hb saturation is affected by many factors, which can be grouped conveniently by systems. First is the significant contribution from respiratory conditions. Any circumstance leading to a decrease in the concentration of inspired oxygen, such as a house fire, confinement to a small unventilated space, or high altitude, can lead to diminished arterial Po_2 and cyanosis. Upper airway obstruction, as with a foreign body, croup, epiglottitis, bacterial tracheitis, tracheal/bronchial disruption, or congenital airway abnormalities, must be severe to cause hypoxemia and consequent cyanosis. Age, events leading to presentation, and examination features, such as barking cough, can help distinguish amongst these diagnoses. Cyanosis ensues rapidly when chest wall movement or lung inflation is impeded. This condition is often a result of trauma and includes external chest compression, flail chest, or hemothorax. Tension pneumothorax, whether traumatic or as a result of preexisting lung disease such as asthma or cystic fibrosis, is diagnosed by dyspnea, deviated trachea, and possibly distended neck veins with diminished breath sounds on the affected side. Empyema or pleural effusion caused by infection, malignancy,

TABLE 16.1

CAUSES OF CYANOSIS

- I. Respiratory
  - A. Decrease in inspired O_2 concentration
  - B. Severe upper airway obstruction
    1. Foreign body
    2. Croup
    3. Epiglottitis
    4. Bacterial tracheitis
    5. Traumatic disruption
    6. Congenital anomalies (e.g., vascular malformation, hypoplastic mandible, laryngotracheomalacia)
  - C. Chest wall
    1. External compression
    2. Flail chest
  - D. Pleura
    1. Pneumothorax
    2. Hemothorax
    3. Empyema/effusion
    4. Diaphragmatic hernia
  - E. Lower airway
    1. Asthma
    2. Bronchiolitis
    3. Cystic fibrosis
    4. Pneumonia
    5. Acute respiratory distress syndrome
    6. Foreign body/aspiration
    7. Congenital hypoplasia
- II. Vascular
  - A. Cardiac
    1. Cyanotic congenital defects
       - a. Tetralogy of Fallot
       - b. Transposition of the great vessels
       - c. Truncus arteriosus
       - d. Pulmonary atresia
       - e. Severe pulmonary stenosis with patent foramen
       - f. Tricuspid atresia
       - g. Ebstein's anomaly
       - h. Total anomalous pulmonary venous drainage
       - i. Atrioventricular canal defect
    2. Congestive cardiac failure
    3. Cardiogenic shock
  - B. Pulmonary
    1. Pulmonary edema
    2. Primary pulmonary hypertension of the newborn
    3. Pulmonary hypertension
    4. Pulmonary embolism
    5. Pulmonary hemorrhage
  - C. Peripheral
    1. Moderate cold exposure
    2. Shock: septic/cardiogenic
    3. Acrocyanosis of the newborn
    4. Complex regional pain syndrome
- III. Neurologic
  - A. Drug or toxin-induced respiratory depression (e.g., morphine, barbiturates)
  - B. Central nervous system lesions (e.g., intracranial hemorrhage, contusion)
  - C. Seizure
  - D. Breath holding
  - E. Neuromuscular disease (e.g., Guillain–Barré, spinal muscular atrophy)
- IV. Hematologic
  - A. Polycythemia
  - B. Methemoglobinemia
- V. Dermatologic
  - A. Blue dye
  - B. Pigmentary lesions
  - C. Tattoos
  - D. Amiodarone therapy

or large chylothorax may be associated with fever, respiratory distress, dullness to percussion, and asymmetric breath sounds on auscultation. Importantly, any lung dysfunction that directly affects pulmonary gas exchange can lead to cyanosis. The most common conditions in children are asthma, bronchiolitis, pneumonia, cystic fibrosis, foreign body aspiration, and pulmonary edema.

TABLE 16.2

COMMON CAUSES OF CYANOSIS

- I. Local cyanosis
  - A. Acrocyanosis of the newborn
  - B. Moderate cold exposure
- II. Generalized cyanosis
  - A. Respiratory dysfunction
  - B. Congenital heart disease

Circulatory or vascular conditions leading to diminished arterial P_{O_2} are also associated with cyanosis. One of the most common causes of cyanosis in children is congenital heart disease. Although most newborns with cyanotic congenital heart disease are discovered in utero or while in the newborn nursery, on occasion, such a newborn will initially present to the emergency department (ED) in the first few days or weeks of life with cyanosis. One condition particularly prone to such late presentation is tetralogy of Fallot with pulmonary atresia. When the ductus closes, profound cyanosis ensues. Rarely, an infant with mild tetralogy of Fallot (or "pink tet") may present with intermittent cyanosis during a "tet" or "hypercyanotic" spell. These self-limited episodes are caused by increased right-to-left shunting and decrease in pulmonary blood flow. The causes of cyanotic congenital heart disease are listed in Table 16.1 (II, A).

Cyanosis may also be caused by pulmonary congestion from cardiac failure or left-to-right cardiac lesions leading to increased pulmonary blood flow and diminished diffusion of O_2 across the blood–gas barrier (see Chapter 94 Cardiac

TABLE 16.3

LIFE-THREATENING CAUSES OF CYANOSIS

I. Respiratory
  A. Decreased inspired O_2 concentration
  B. Upper airway obstruction/disruption
  C. Chest wall immobility
  D. Tension pneumothorax
  E. Massive hemothorax
  F. Lung disease leading to hypoxemia
II. Vascular
  A. Cardiac
    1. Cyanotic congenital defects
    2. Congestive heart failure
    3. Cardiogenic shock
  B. Pulmonary
    1. Pulmonary edema
    2. Primary pulmonary hypertension of the newborn
    3. Pulmonary embolism
    4. Pulmonary hemorrhage
  C. Peripheral
    1. Septic shock
III. Other
  A. Neurologic conditions leading to hypoxemia
  B. Severe methemoglobinemia

Emergencies). Several pulmonary vascular abnormalities can also lead to cyanosis. These include primary pulmonary hypertension of the newborn or pulmonary hypertension from other causes. When pulmonary pressures are high, blood is shunted away from the lungs and the child becomes hypoxemic. Pulmonary embolism and pulmonary hemorrhage, although rare in children, also impair lung perfusion and must be considered.

Low perfusion states may lead to local cyanosis, particularly of the hands, feet, and lips. Moderate cold exposure, for example, can result in local blueness. Patients in septic or cardiogenic shock may have perfusion-related cyanosis as a result of pump failure. Poor perfusion can also result from hyperviscous states such as polycythemia or leukemia. Acrocyanosis, or blueness of the hands and feet with preserved pinkness centrally, is seen commonly in newborns and is related to variable perfusion in the extremities. It is seen in well-appearing babies and resolves within the first few days of life.

Neurologic conditions can also lead to Hb desaturation and cyanosis. Patients who hypoventilate because of central nervous system (CNS) depression, whether from primary CNS lesions or drugs/toxins that depress the respiratory center, are often centrally cyanotic at presentation to the ED. Episodic blue spells in infants and young children who are otherwise well may be caused by breath holding, especially when associated with a sudden insult such as fright, pain, frustration, or anger (see Chapter 134 Behavioral and Psychiatric Emergencies). Seizures are often associated with cyanosis from inadequate respiration during the convulsion. A variety of neuromuscular diseases that affect chest wall or diaphragmatic function may ultimately lead to hypoventilation.

With respect to the Hb molecule itself, methemoglobinemia is an unusual but not rare reason for presentation to the pediatric ED. Methemoglobinemia can be either congenital or acquired. Congenital methemoglobinemia is caused by either Hb variants designated M hemoglobins or deficiency of NADH-dependent methemoglobin reductase. The more common acquired form occurs when red blood cells are exposed to oxidant chemicals or drugs. Methemoglobinemia has also been associated with diarrheal illnesses in children. Young infants are particularly susceptible to the development of methemoglobinemia as a result of immature enzyme systems required to reduce Hb. Even at low levels, skin discoloration is prominent, often with intense or "slate gray" cyanosis from the presence of methemoglobin beneath the skin (see Chapter 101 Hematologic Emergencies).

Other conditions leading to a blue appearance of the skin may be confused with cyanosis. A rare but perplexing presentation is that of the well-appearing child with unusually localized cyanosis, which can be related to blue dye of clothing. Slate blue discoloration of the face, neck, and arms has been noted in patients on chronic amiodarone therapy. Certain pigmentary lesions such as Mongolian spots can be confused with cyanosis, especially when uncharacteristically large or in unusual locations. Adolescents will occasionally "tattoo" areas of the body that may appear as local cyanosis.

EVALUATION AND DECISION

A careful yet rapid history and physical examination are critical to the approach to the cyanotic patient because timely correction may be lifesaving. Many historical features can help narrow the differential diagnosis and lead to prompt evaluation and treatment. The onset and pattern, location, quality, temporal nature, and presence of palliative or provocative features must be explored. Age of the patient with respect to onset of cyanosis, whether at birth, shortly after birth, or acquired later, is critical. In newborns, congenital cardiac and respiratory diseases are the most common causes of cyanosis. Special attention must also be paid to known preexisting heart or lung disease that may predispose to the acute onset of cyanosis. History of exposure to environmental conditions or toxins, such as cold, trauma, smoke inhalation, confinement to an airtight space, drugs, or chemicals, is crucial. Known patient or family history of methemoglobinemia may lead directly to the cause of cyanosis. A history of sudden pain or fright with crying or seizure occurrence should be sought.

The physical examination must include a complete general examination, with special attention paid to the vital signs, oxygen saturation, and cardiovascular and pulmonary systems. An immediate and key physical examination feature is the presence or absence of respiratory distress. In general, children with respiratory distress are likely to have respiratory dysfunction, and careful examination of the airway, breathing, and circulation should be rapidly initiated. A temperature should be obtained. Presence of cough, "sniffing position," stridor, retractions, or fever should be determined. Lung examination may reveal adventitious (e.g., wheezing or rales) or diminished breath sounds. Presence of a cardiac murmur often suggests cardiac disease. Careful attention to the peripheral circulation, including pulses and capillary refill is also helpful. A rapid neurologic examination should be performed.

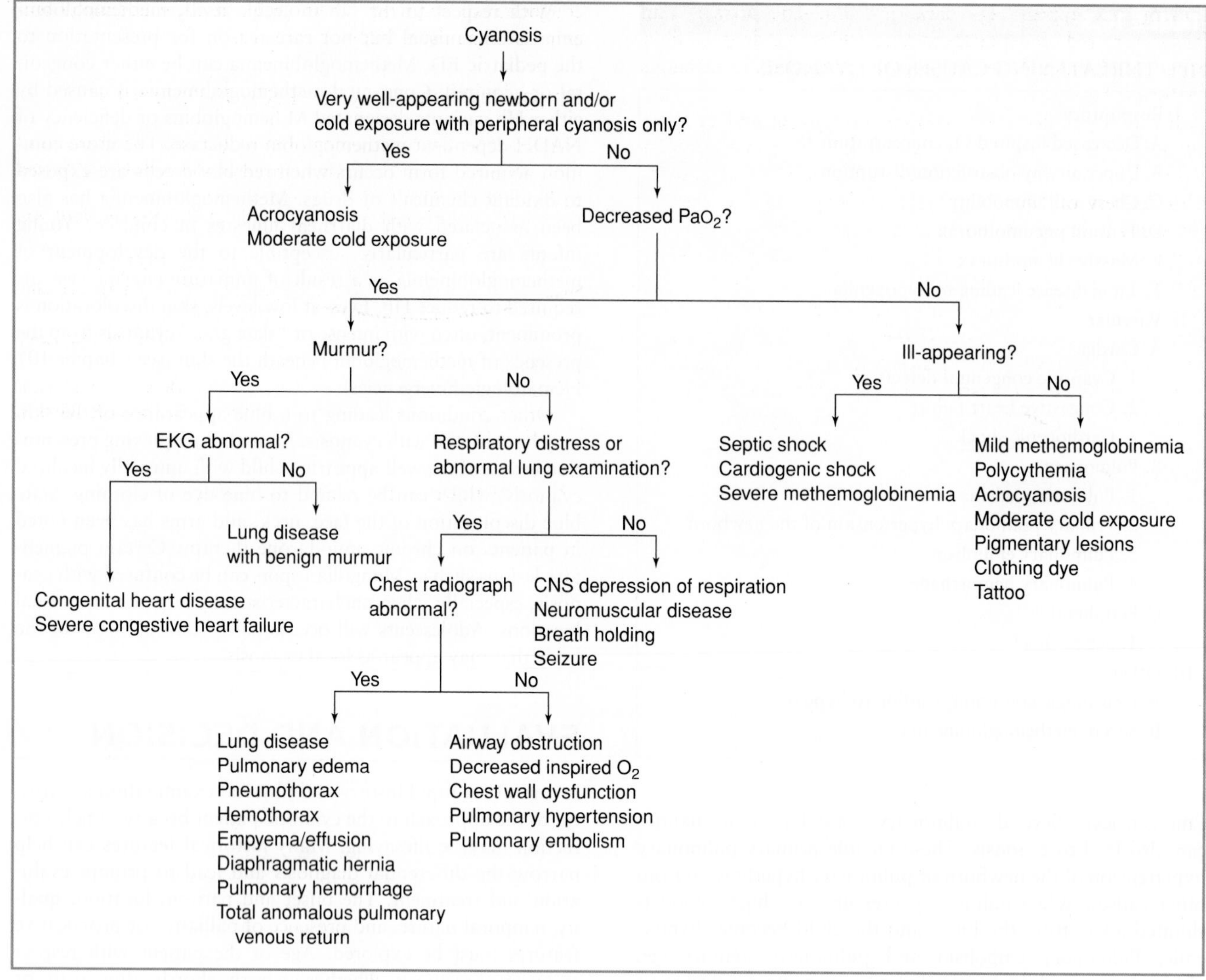

FIGURE 16.1 Laboratory evaluation of cyanosis. EKG, electrocardiogram; CNS, central nervous system.

Location of cyanosis helps determine its cause. Central cyanosis is noted in the mucous membranes, tongue, trunk, and upper extremities. It is most often the result of decreased arterial Po_2 but can also result from severe methemoglobinemia or polycythemia. If the cyanosis is peripheral only (hands, feet, lips), moderate cold exposure, newborn acrocyanosis (e-Figs. 16.1 and 16.2), shock states, or mild methemoglobinemia may be the cause. Local blue discoloration of a single extremity corresponds to compromise of distal circulation or autonomic tone as seen in traumatic vascular lesions or complex regional pain syndrome. Cyanosis and swelling of just the head may be seen with superior vena cava syndrome. In addition, a local blue hue to the skin may also be a result of simple phenomena such as pigmentary lesions or blue clothing dye. If blue coloring appears on an alcohol swab wiped across the discolored area of skin, dye is responsible. Differential cyanosis of the lower body versus the upper body may indicate high pulmonary vascular resistance with right-to-left shunting via the ductus arteriosis. Transposition of the great arteries with pulmonary-to-aortic shunt of oxygenated blood through the ductus arteriosis is represented in the rare instance that the upper body is blue and the lower body pink.

Laboratory evaluation is determined based on the historical features and physical findings established on initial encounter (Fig. 16.1). All patients, except very well-appearing newborns and well-appearing cold-exposed patients with peripheral cyanosis only, require measurement of arterial Po_2. (Oxygen saturation by pulse oximetry may be helpful in determining if hypoxemia is the cause of cyanosis, but it may also be misleading when abnormal forms of Hb such as methemoglobin or carboxyhemoglobin are present.)

If the Po_2 is normal, the laboratory evaluation is determined by the degree of ill appearance. Well-appearing oxygenated children with cyanosis usually have less urgent conditions, such as polycythemia, mild methemoglobinemia, cold exposure, newborn acrocyanosis, or dermatologic findings. In this case, laboratory evaluation might include a methemoglobin level and complete blood count (CBC), or no further investigation may be warranted. Despite a normal Po_2, an ill-appearing cyanotic patient may have a more emergent condition such as severe methemoglobinemia or septic or cardiogenic shock and may require aggressive laboratory investigation. This might include CBC, methemoglobin level, co-oximetry, blood cultures, and blood chemistry. Blood with high methemoglobin content may appear very dark or "chocolate brown" and fails to turn red on exposure to air, such as in a drop on filter paper. Methemoglobinemia may improve with intravenous methylene blue.

If the Po_2 is decreased, oxygen therapy should be instituted. In general, cyanosis caused by decreased alveolar ventilation or diffusional abnormalities often improves with delivery of 100% O_2. However, hypoxemia caused by decreased pulmonary perfusion or shunt will have minimal response to oxygen therapy. Next, a chest radiograph should be obtained. Abnormalities of the lungs may confirm pulmonary disease, and changes in the cardiac size or silhouette may suggest cardiac causes. If the chest radiograph is normal, other reasons for diminished arterial Po_2, such as CNS- or chest wall–related respiratory depression, upper airway obstruction, or pulmonary perfusion abnormalities, must be entertained. If a concomitant murmur or other concern for cardiac disease exists, an electrocardiogram (EKG) is essential. Abnormal EKGs may suggest cardiac etiologies, either congenital or acquired (Table 16.1). Echocardiography will help establish the definitive diagnosis.

Suggested Readings and Key References

Bradberry SM. Occupational methaemoglobinaemia. Mechanisms of production, features, diagnosis and management including the use of methylene blue. *Toxicol Rev* 2003;22(1):13–27.

Driscoll DJ. Evaluation of the cyanotic newborn. *Pediatr Clin North Am* 1990;37:1–23.

Lundsgaard C, Van Slyke DD. Cyanosis. *Medicine* 1923;2:15.

Steinhorn RH. Evaluation and management of the cyanotic neonate. *Clin Pediatr Emerg Med* 2008;9(3):169–175.

Umbreit J. Methemoglobin—it's not just blue: a concise review. *Am J Hematol* 2007;82(2):134–144.

West JB. Gas transport to the periphery. In: West JB, ed. *Physiological basis of medical practice,* 12th ed. Baltimore: Williams & Wilkins, 1990:538–559.

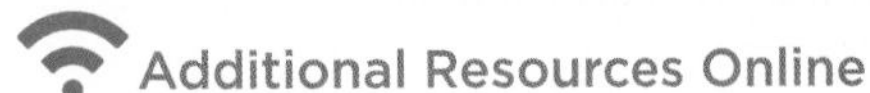

CHAPTER 17 ▪ DEHYDRATION

PHILIP R. SPANDORFER, MD, MSCE

Dehydration is not a disease itself, rather a symptom of another process. Infants have higher morbidity and mortality from dehydration and are more susceptible to it because of their larger water content, three times higher metabolic turnover rate of water than adults, renal immaturity, and inability to meet their own needs independently. Children with various illnesses and circumstances will present to the emergency department (ED) with signs of dehydration (Table 17.1).

PATHOPHYSIOLOGY

Dehydration is a reduction in the water content of the body. Over two-thirds of the total body water is intracellular and one-third is in the extracellular space. Of the extracellular fluid, three-fourths is interstitial and only 25% is in the intravascular space as plasma. Early in the process of dehydration, the majority of the water loss is from the extracellular compartment, which contains 135 mEq per L of sodium and negligible potassium. However, with time, there is an equilibration from the extracellular compartment to the intracellular compartment, which has 150 mEq per L of potassium and negligible sodium. As the electrolyte composition of extracellular fluid and intracellular fluid varies greatly, an understanding of this process helps the clinician gauge the optimal composition and rate of fluid deficit correction (see Chapter 108 Renal and Electrolyte Emergencies).

Dehydration is often categorized by the serum osmolarity and severity (degree of fluid deficit), which is helpful in determining fluid therapy. Based on the initial serum sodium, most children have isonatremic dehydration (also referred to as isotonic dehydration, serum sodium 130 to 150 mEq per L), whereas others have hypernatremic dehydration (hypertonic dehydration, serum sodium greater than 150 mEq per L) or hyponatremic dehydration (hypotonic dehydration, serum sodium less than 130 mEq per L). Severity is judged by the amount of body fluid lost or the percentage of weight loss, and is typically characterized as mild (less than 50 mL per kg, or less than 5% of total body weight), moderate (50 to 100 mL per kg, or 5% to 10% of total body weight), and severe (greater than 100 mL per kg, or greater than 10% of total body weight).

DIFFERENTIAL DIAGNOSIS

Fluid imbalance in dehydration results from (i) decreased intake; (ii) increased output secondary to insensible, renal, or gastrointestinal (GI) losses; or (iii) translocation of fluid such as occurs with major burns or ascites (Table 17.1). Gastroenteritis is the most common cause of dehydration in infants and children, and is the leading cause of death worldwide in children younger than 4 years of age. In the United States, an average of 300 children younger than 5 years of age die each year, and an additional 200,000 are hospitalized, secondary to diarrheal illnesses with dehydration. Prior to widespread use of the rotavirus vaccine, rotavirus gastroenteritis was responsible for about half of the gastroenteritis cases and is generally more severe than nonrotavirus cases. Other common causes of dehydration in children include vomiting, stomatitis, or pharyngitis with poor intake secondary to pain, febrile illnesses with increased insensible losses and decreased intake, and diabetic ketoacidosis (Table 17.2). More severe or life-threatening causes are listed in Table 17.3.

EVALUATION AND DECISION

The first step in evaluating a child with dehydration is to assess the severity or degree of dehydration, regardless of the cause (Table 17.4). Most children with clinically significant dehydration will have two of the following four clinical findings: (i) capillary refill greater than 2 seconds, (ii) dry mucous membranes, (iii) no tears, and (iv) ill appearance. The more dehydrated a patient is, the more hypovolemic they are and the more likely they are progressing toward shock. Mild, moderate, and severe dehydration correspond to impending, compensated, and uncompensated states of shock, respectively (see Chapter 3 Airway). If there is severe dehydration or uncompensated shock, the child must be treated immediately with isotonic fluids to restore intravascular volume, as detailed later in this chapter.

History

A thorough history is needed to assess the child with dehydration to determine the cause and degree of dehydration (Fig. 17.1). Attention should be paid to the child's output and intake of fluids and electrolytes. Overt GI losses from diarrhea and vomiting are the most common causes of dehydration in children (see Chapters 18 Diarrhea and 77 Vomiting). The child may not be drinking because of physical restriction (e.g., dependence on a caregiver, pain, altered consciousness, anorexia). Fever, high ambient temperatures or bundling a baby, sweating, and hyperventilation may cause increased insensible losses. It is important to note whether there is any underlying disease that would contribute to dehydration (e.g., cystic fibrosis, diabetes, hyperthyroidism, renal disease).

Asking the parents about documented weight loss, amount of urine output, and the presence or absence of tears is helpful in determining the severity of the dehydration. Although decreased urine output is an early sign of dehydration, only 20% of patients with the complaint of decreased urine output will be dehydrated. All ingested fluids should be noted because diluted juices or water can be associated with hyponatremic

TABLE 17.1

CAUSES OF DEHYDRATION

- Decreased intake
  - Physical restriction
    - Infant
    - Central nervous system depression
  - Anorexia
  - Voluntary or imposed cessation of drinking
    - Pharyngitis, stomatitis
    - Respiratory distress
    - Child abuse
  - Hypothalamic hypodipsia
- Increased output
  - Insensible losses
    - Fever
    - Sweating
    - Heat prostration
    - High ambient temperature/low humidity
    - Hyperventilation
    - Cystic fibrosis
    - Thyrotoxicosis
  - Renal losses
    - Osmotic
    - Diabetic ketoacidosis
    - Acute tubular necrosis
    - High protein feeds
    - Mannitol usage
  - Nonosmotic
    - Diabetes insipidus
    - Sustained hypokalemia–hypercalcemia
    - Sickle cell disease
    - Chronic renal disease
    - Bartter syndrome
  - Sodium-losing
    - Congenital adrenal hypoplasia
    - Diuretics
    - Sodium-losing nephropathy
    - Pseudohypoaldosteronism
  - Gastrointestinal losses
    - Diarrhea (see Chapter 18 Diarrhea)
      - Secretory vs. nonsecretory
    - Vomiting (see Chapter 77 Vomiting)
      - Obstructive vs. nonobstructive
- Translocation of fluids
  - Burns
  - Ascites (e.g., nephrotic syndrome)
  - Intraintestinal
    - Paralytic ileus
    - Postabdominal surgery

dehydration, whereas excess salt intake or low liquid intake may indicate hypernatremic dehydration. Further, inquiring how the infant formula is prepared may lead to the discovery of electrolyte abnormalities with dehydration if too little or too much water is added.

TABLE 17.2

COMMON CAUSES OF DEHYDRATION

Gastroenteritis	Febrile illness
Stomatitis/pharyngitis	Diabetic ketoacidosis

Physical Examination

Vital signs are an important and objective assessment of dehydration (Table 17.4). There are several scoring systems that have been designed to aid in determining the degree of dehydration. A simple 4-point dehydration score that has been shown to be valid and reliable is presented in Table 17.5. The 4-point score is very useful clinically whereas other scoring systems are more useful in research. The first sign of mild dehydration is tachycardia, whereas hypotension is a very late sign of severe dehydration. In mild to moderate dehydration, the respiratory rate is usually normal. As a child becomes more acidotic and fluid is depleted, the respiratory rate increases and the breathing pattern becomes hyperpneic. Unfortunately, vital signs alone are not always reliable. Tachycardia also may be caused by fever, agitation, or pain; respiratory illness affects respiratory rates; and orthostatic signs are difficult to obtain in babies and young children.

Age of the child, nutritional status, and type of dehydration may also affect clinical assessment, which is critical to effective management of the acutely dehydrated child. In general, older children show signs of dehydration sooner than babies do because of their lower levels of extracellular water. Babies with excess subcutaneous fat may look less dehydrated than they really are, whereas severely malnourished babies may appear to be more dehydrated secondary to wasted supporting tissues. Signs of dehydration may be less evident or appear later in hypernatremic dehydration. Excessive irritability with increased muscle tone, and doughy or smooth and velvety skin, often are noted with this type of dehydration. Conversely, signs of dehydration may be more pronounced or appear sooner in hyponatremic dehydration. Keeping these observations in mind, particular attention should be paid to the overall appearance, mental status, eyes, and skin on physical examination. The mildly dehydrated child usually appears well or may be tired, have decreased tearing and a slightly dry mouth. Dry mucous membranes are an early sign of dehydration, but this finding is affected by rapid breathing and ingestion of fluids. Conversely, the severely dehydrated baby classically appears quite ill with lethargy or irritability, a dry

TABLE 17.3

LIFE-THREATENING CAUSES OF DEHYDRATION

Gastroenteritis (especially infants)	Heat prostration
Diabetic ketoacidosis	Gastrointestinal obstruction
Burns over 25% of body surface area	Cystic fibrosis
Thyrotoxicosis	Diabetes insipidus
Congenital adrenal hyperplasia	Child abuse

TABLE 17.4

CLINICAL ESTIMATION OF DEGREE OF DEHYDRATION[a,b]

Clinical finding	PPV	NPV	Sensitivity (95% CI)	Specificity (95% CI)
Decreased skin elasticity	0.57	0.93	0.35 (0.23–0.49)	0.97 (0.92–0.99)
Capillary refill >2 s	0.57	0.94	0.48 (0.35–0.61)	0.96 (0.90–0.99)
Ill appearance (tired, listless)	0.42	0.95	0.59 (0.46–0.71)	0.91 (0.84–0.95)
Absent tears	0.40	0.96	0.67 (0.53–0.78)	0.89 (0.82–0.94)
Abnormal respirations	0.37	0.94	0.43 (0.30–0.56)	0.86 (0.78–0.91)
Dry mucous membranes	0.29	0.99	0.80 (0.67–0.89)	0.78 (0.70–0.85)
Sunken eyes	0.29	0.95	0.60 (0.47–0.72)	0.84 (0.76–0.90)
Abnormal radial pulse	0.25	0.93	0.43 (0.30–0.56)	0.86 (0.78–0.91)
Tachycardia (>150)	0.20	0.93	0.46 (0.32–0.61)	0.79 (0.72–0.87)
Decreased urine output (parental report)	0.17	0.97	0.85 (0.73–0.93)	0.53 (0.44–0.62)

[a]The 10-point dehydration score listed in descending PPV.
[b]One to two findings indicate mild dehydration <5% total body weight, three to six findings indicate moderate dehydration (5–10% total body weight), and seven to ten findings indicate severe dehydration (>10% total body weight).
PPV, positive predictive value; NPV, negative predictive value; CI, confidence interval.
Reproduced by permission of *Pediatrics* 1997;99(5):e6.

mouth, sunken fontanel, and absent tears. Moderate states of dehydration, however, require careful evaluation. One of the more objective measures of dehydration is assessment of skin perfusion by measuring capillary refill time (Fig. 17.2). Although the child's body temperature does not predictably affect capillary refill time, it may be falsely prolonged when measured on the foot or in a cool room.

Laboratory

In general, laboratory values are not helpful in diagnosing dehydration, rather the history and physical examination should be used. However, in children who are judged to have moderate to severe dehydration that requires intravenous (IV) rehydration, laboratory tests of electrolytes, glucose, blood urea nitrogen, and creatinine are usually obtained to determine osmolarity and renal function. Approximately one-third of moderately to severely dehydrated children will have hypoglycemia less than 60 mg per dL. The acid–base status may be assessed further with an arterial or venous blood gas. The quantity and quality of urine produced are also important indicators of the cause or degree of dehydration. If the physical examination indicates significant dehydration and there is dilute or copious urine, a renal or adrenal origin is most likely. In addition, polyuria and the presence of glucose and ketones may indicate diabetic ketoacidosis, whereas a history of disorders of the central nervous system (CNS) suggests diabetes insipidus.

Diagnostic Approach

In approaching the patient with presumed dehydration, the initial assessment serves to determine whether compensated or uncompensated shock is present. If the child appears to be in shock, resuscitation should begin and a number of life-threatening disorders need to be considered, as listed in Table 17.3 and discussed in Chapter 3 Airway. Patients with obvious burns or diseases that disrupt the integument in the same way (e.g., scalded skin syndrome) are presumed to have become dehydrated through transudation of fluid through the skin.

A history of vomiting (see Chapter 77 Vomiting) or diarrhea (see Chapter 18 Diarrhea) should be sought. Most children with vomiting or diarrhea have viral gastroenteritis, but many diseases (Table 17.1) produce these symptoms. Oral intake should be assessed as several common minor infections, such as pharyngitis and stomatitis, as well as more serious disorders of the CNS, cause dehydration as a result of voluntary or involuntary limitation of fluids taken orally.

Next, the history should address the nature and quantity of the urine output. With dehydration, one expects to find oliguria or anuria if normal renal concentrating function remains intact. Severe oliguria or anuria may also, however, be manifested if severe dehydration and shock has led to acute renal failure (see Chapter 108 Renal and Electrolyte Emergencies). The unexpected discovery of polyuria points to diabetes mellitus or insipidus, adrenal insufficiency, diuretic use, or renal injury or disease with resultant loss of concentrating ability (Fig. 17.1).

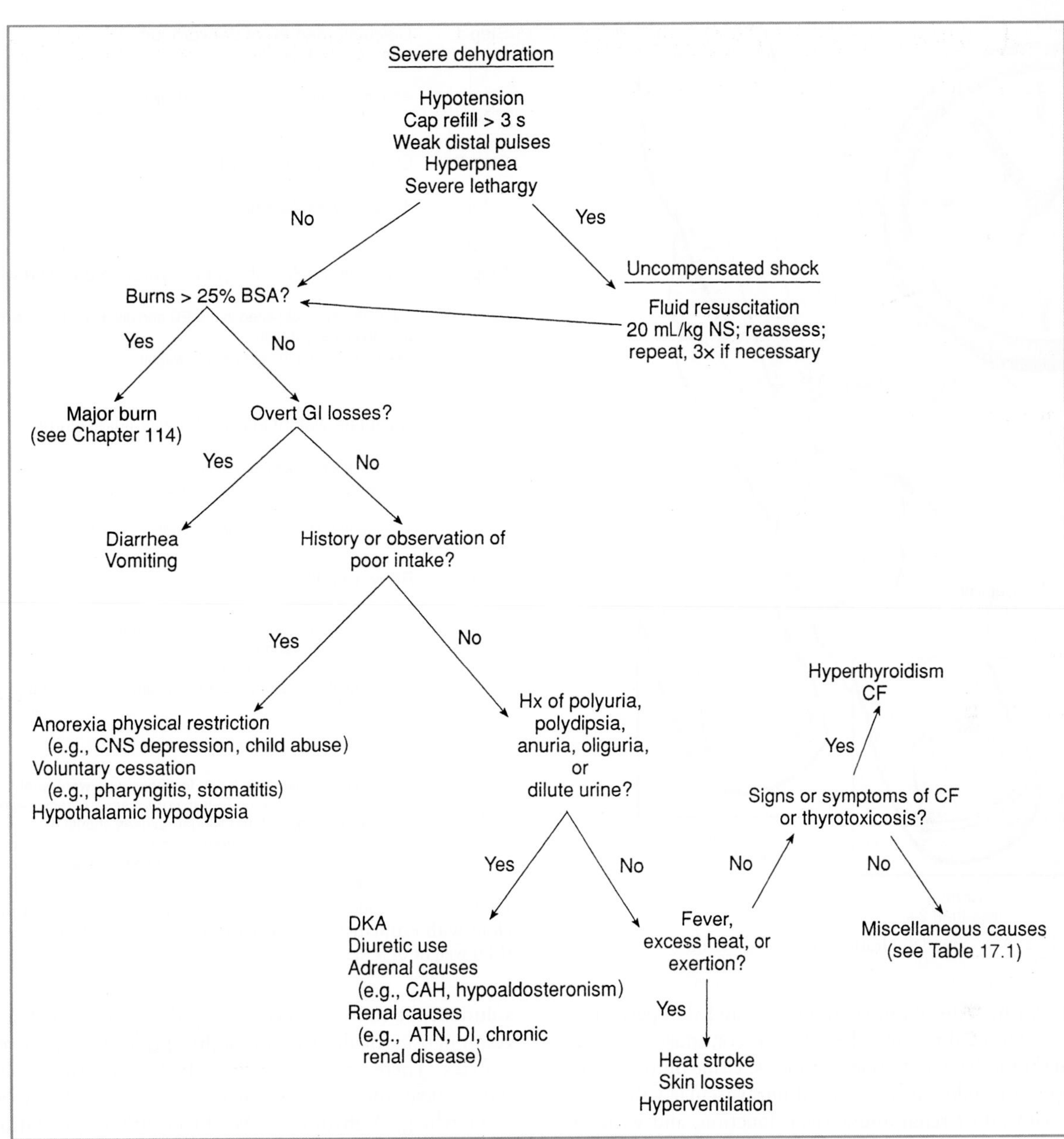

FIGURE 17.1 Suspected dehydration. BSA, body surface area; NS, normal saline; GI, gastrointestinal; CNS, central nervous system; Hx, history; DKA, diabetic ketoacidosis; CAH, congenital adrenal hyperplasia; ATN, acute tubular necrosis; DI, diabetes insipidus; CF, cystic fibrosis.

By this point, the physician will have established a diagnosis in most patients. Hot weather or when there is prolonged fever, skin losses must be considered. Patients with cystic fibrosis (see Chapter 107 Pulmonary Emergencies) are prone to dehydration because of a high concentration of sodium in the sweat (the finding of hyponatremic dehydration seemingly unexplained by the estimated fluid loss should suggest this diagnosis). Additional considerations are listed in Table 17.1.

TABLE 17.5

4-POINT DEHYDRATION SCALE

Clinical finding	Interpretation
Ill appearance	0 feature = not dehydrated
Dry mucous membranes	1 feature = mild dehydration
Decreased tears	2–3 features = mild to moderate dehydration
Capillary refill >2 s	4 features = severe dehydration

Reproduced by permission of *Pediatrics* 1997;99(5):e6.

Initial Management

The dehydrated child must be examined immediately for the degree of dehydration or state of hypovolemic shock. If there is severe dehydration or uncompensated shock, the patient is treated acutely with isotonic fluids to restore intravascular volume regardless of serum osmolarity or cause of the dehydration (Fig. 17.3). Normal saline or Ringer lactate is given via an IV or intraosseous line in 20 mL per kg aliquots over approximately 15 to 30 minutes, or as quickly as possible if there is uncompensated shock. Reassessment is paramount after each fluid bolus. When blood pressure is restored, heart rate

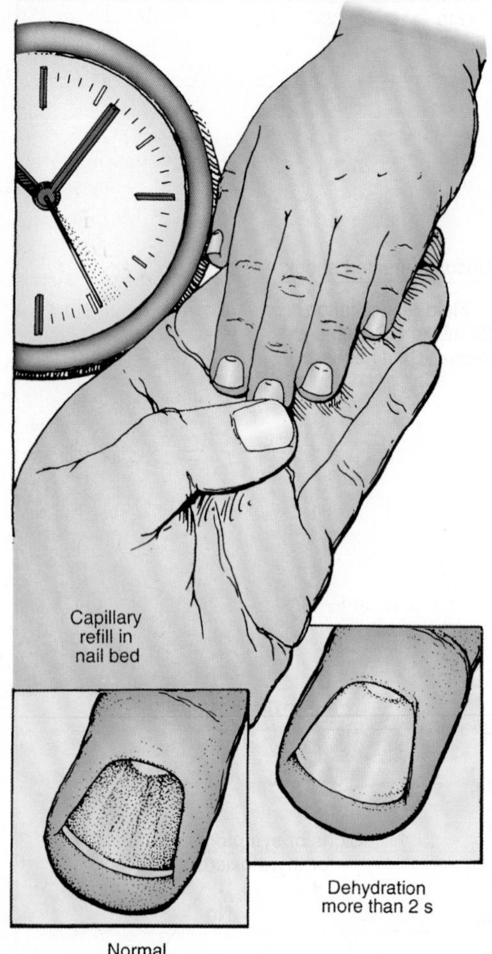

FIGURE 17.2 Assessing dehydration by capillary refill.

Step 1: Calculate degree of dehydration.
(see Table 17.4 and text)

Assume a patient is moderately dehydrated (10% dehydration).

⇩

Step 2: Obtain weight in the ED.

The patient weighs 9 kg.

⇩

Step 3: Calculate back to the predehydration baseline weight.

Take the weight obtained in the ED and divide by 1 minus the proportion dehydration.
(9 kg)/(1 – 0.1) = 10 kg baseline weight

⇩

Step 4: Calculate weight loss and deficit fluid volume.

10 kg – 9 kg = 1 kg weight loss
1 kg is equivalent to 1,000 mL deficit

This patient has a 1,000 mL fluid deficit (100 cc/kg).

⇩

Step 5: Rehydrate the child.

Oral rehydration therapy is first-line therapy for mild and moderate dehydration and should be administered as 2 cc/kg of baseline weight for the moderately dehydrated patient (1 cc/kg of baseline weight for the mildly dehydrated patient) every 5 min over a 4-h period.

2 cc/kg × 10 kg = 20 cc every 5 min orally

Administer intravenous fluids for those who were unable to tolerate oral rehydration therapy or for severe dehydration. Normal saline or lactated Ringer boluses should be administered for the emergency phase (20 cc/kg). Half of the remaining fluid deficit is given in the first 8 hrs and the remainder over the next 16 hrs.

FIGURE 17.3 Calculation of deficit therapy using the example of a child with estimated 10% dehydration and emergency department (ED) weight of 9 kg.

returns to normal, distal pulses strengthen, and skin perfusion improves, isotonic fluids may be safely discontinued. Careful attention should be paid to ongoing losses. Urine output is the most important indicator of restored intravascular volume in patients with intact renal and adrenal function, and without diabetes mellitus or insipidus, and should be a minimum of 1 mL/kg/hr. If dextrose is needed initially for low serum glucose, 0.5 to 1 g per kg is given in a single bolus of 10% or 25% dextrose and the serum level is rechecked.

Oral Rehydration Therapy

If the child is determined to be mildly or moderately dehydrated, then oral rehydration therapy (ORT) is the therapeutic option of choice. ORT is the frequent administration of small volumes of an appropriate rehydration solution, typically with an oral syringe. The use of ondansetron, a serotonin $5HT_3$ selective receptor antagonist, has clearly been shown to improve the success of rehydration with ORT (Table 17.6). An appropriate rehydration solution has the correct balance of glucose and sodium, which enables the body to absorb the water passively via the sodium glucose cotransport mechanism in the small intestine. The glucose-to-sodium ratio is an important determinant in the acceptability of these solutions. Optimal solutions have a 1:1 or a 2:1 glucose:sodium ratio. When additional sweetener is added to the rehydration solution, the ratio of glucose to sodium is distorted and may result in osmotic diarrhea or inappropriate absorption of electrolytes. There are two categories of rehydration solutions: initial rehydration solutions that contain 60 to 90 mEq per L of sodium (e.g., Rehydralyte, World Health Organization oral rehydration solutions) and maintenance solutions that contain 40 to 60 mEq per L of sodium (e.g., Pedialyte). If the etiology of the dehydration is presumed to be due to cholera, then the higher sodium concentration is appropriate because there is a large sodium loss in the diarrhea stools of cholera patients. However, if the etiology of the dehydration is presumed to be viral gastroenteritis, then the lower sodium concentration solutions would be appropriate and are more readily available. Both rehydration and maintenance solutions have approximately 20 mEq per L of potassium and a low glucose concentration of 2% to 2.5%. Soda, juice, popsicles, sports drinks, and soups are inappropriate rehydration

TABLE 17.6

ONDANSETRON DOSING FOR GASTROENTERITIS

Patient weight (kg)	Dose
<10	2 mg orally disintegrating tablet (½ tablet)
≥10	4 mg orally disintegrating tablet

solutions in dehydrated infants and children and should be strongly discouraged. These fluids do not have the appropriate glucose-to-sodium ratio and are not absorbed as easily as electrolyte solutions.

The amount of fluid to be administered is dependent on the degree of dehydration. Mild dehydration reflects up to 5% weight loss, so 5% of the child's body weight (50 mL per kg) should be administered as small-volume frequent feeds. Moderate dehydration represents up to 10% weight loss, so 10% of the child's weight (100 mL per kg) should be administered. An easy rule of thumb to remember is that a mildly dehydrated patient can receive 1 mL per kg every 5 minutes and a moderately dehydrated patient can receive 2 mL per kg every 5 minutes. As the child tolerates the feeds, the volume can be increased as well as the frequency. The rehydration should be completed over a 4-hour time frame (Fig. 17.3). ORT has been shown to be equivalent to IV fluid therapy in terms of rehydration efficacy and it has been shown that it takes less time to institute therapy with ORT (i.e., teach the parents how to administer the fluids) than to start an IV line in a child, and there is less staff time involved in administering care to these patients as well as shorter ED stays. There are a significant number of patients with gastroenteritis who will be unable to perform ORT and will subsequently require alternative methods for rehydration. Nasogastric (NG) tube use is an acceptable alternative as it has been shown to be as effective as IV hydration. They are relatively easy to place and the patient does not need to remain awake while receiving the rehydration solution. A small feeding tube is better tolerated for fluid administration than a larger NG tube. Since NG tubes are considered a very noxious intervention, practitioners and parents may choose parenteral rehydration over NG.

Parenteral Rehydration

Approximately 20% of patients will be unable to tolerate oral syringe administration of ORT because of persistent vomiting, high stool outputs, or inability to cooperate. If the patient is unable to tolerate ORT or is severely dehydrated, then administration of 20 mL per kg boluses of isotonic saline or lactated Ringer solution intravenously would be appropriate. The number of boluses required depends on the patient's physiologic response to the fluid that has been administered. Once the initial resuscitation phase is completed, an IV fluid is determined for the maintenance phase (see Chapter 108 Renal and Electrolyte Emergencies). The initial fluid often is D5–1/2NS with 20 mEq per L of potassium chloride. Notable exceptions include major burn patients who continue to require isotonic fluids (see Chapter 112 Burns), children with diabetic ketoacidosis who do not require dextrose initially (see Chapter 97 Endocrine Emergencies), and children with severe electrolyte disturbances, such as may occur with pyloric stenosis or severe hypernatremic dehydration (see Chapter 108 Renal and Electrolyte Emergencies). There are recent studies advocating for the use of isotonic fluids for all patients who require maintenance of hydration. The benefit of isotonic solutions (such as normal saline) is to avoid fatal hyponatremia.

The fluid rate is determined by the estimated fluid deficit and ongoing losses (Fig. 17.3). Usually, 50% of the child's fluid deficit is given over the first 8 hours in addition to one-third of the daily maintenance fluid requirements. In hypertonic states, after initial stabilization with isotonic fluids, the replacement solution is given more slowly to allow equilibration across the blood–brain barrier (see Chapter 108 Renal and Electrolyte Emergencies).

Parenteral rehydration via an IV catheter has been used extensively. The advantages of IV rehydration are numerous including familiarity with the procedure, widespread acceptance, and direct vascular access to rehydrate a patient. There are disadvantages associated with IV catheter use, primarily difficulty in obtaining access in dehydrated children, particularly those younger than 3 years, pain associated with placement, and the time and resources required for placement. Subcutaneous rehydration is a method to deliver fluids parenterally that was common prior to the widespread use of IV catheters. There is evidence that using human recombinate hyaluronidase (Hylenex) with a subcutaneous catheter may be an alternative for mild and moderately dehydrated children who have failed ORT. It is a method that can also be used as a bridge to getting IV access in severely dehydrated patients. Hyaluronidase temporarily dissolves hyaluronic acid and allows fluid to be administered subcutaneously, which is subsequently absorbed into the vascular system. Advantages of subcutaneous fluid administration include ease of placement and decreased pain with insertion. More research in this new modality is required.

In all types of dehydration and their methods of treatment, the patient must be monitored closely. Physical examination and vital signs should be reassessed continually, urine output monitored closely, ongoing losses quantified and replaced, and therapy individualized. Patients should be considered for admission if they are severely dehydrated, unable to adequately keep up with the ongoing losses, if they are persistently hypoglycemic, appropriate care cannot be provided as an outpatient, or if the etiology of the dehydration is unclear and further workup is required.

Suggested Readings and Key References

Allen CH, Etzwiller LS, Miller MK, et al. Subcutaneous hydration in children using recombinant human hyaluronidase: safety and ease of use. *Ann Emerg Med* 2008;52(4 suppl):S75–S76.

American Academy of Pediatrics, Provisional Committee on Quality Improvement, Subcommittee on Acute Gastroenteritis. Practice parameter. The management of acute gastroenteritis in young children. *Pediatrics* 1996;97:424.

Atherly-John YC, Cunningham SJ, Crain EF. A randomized trial of oral vs intravenous rehydration in a pediatric emergency department. *Arch Pediatr Adolesc Med* 2002;156:1240.

Finberg L, Kravath RE, Hellerstein S, eds. *Water and electrolytes in pediatrics: physiology, pathophysiology, and treatment.* 2nd ed. Philadelphia, PA: WB Saunders, 1993.

Fonseca BK, Holdgate A, Craig JC. Enteral vs. intravenous rehydration therapy for children with gastroenteritis. *Arch Pediatr Adolesc Med* 2004;158:483–490.

Freedman SB, Adler M, Seshadri R, et al. Oral ondansetron for gastroenteritis in a pediatric emergency department. *N Engl J Med* 2006; 354(16):1698–1705.

Freedman SB, Parkin PC, Willan AR, et al. Rapid versus standard intravenous rehydration in paediatric gastroenteritis: pragmatic blinded randomized clinical trial. *BMJ* 2011;343:d6976.

Gorelick MH, Shaw KN, Murphy KO. Validity and reliability of clinical signs in the diagnosis of dehydration in children. *Pediatrics* 1997;99:1. Available online at: http://www.pediatrics.org/cgi/content/full/99/5/e6.

Hartling L, Bellemare S, Wiebe N, et al. Oral versus intravenous rehydration for treating dehydration due to gastroenteritis in children. *Cochrane Database Syst Rev* 2006;3:CD004390.

King CK, Glass R, Bresee JS, et al. Managing acute gastroenteritis among children: oral rehydration, maintenance, and nutritional therapy. *MMWR* 2003;52(RR-16):1–16.

Moritz ML, Ayus JC. Prevention of hospital-acquired hyponatremia: a case for using isotonic saline. *Pediatrics* 2003;111:227–230.

Spandorfer PR, Alessandrini EA, Joffe M, et al. Oral vs. intravenous rehydration of moderately dehydrated children: a randomized controlled trial. *Pediatrics* 2005;115:295–301.

Spandorfer PR, Mace SE, Okada PJ, et al. A randomized clinical trial of recombinant human hyaluronidase facilitated subcutaneous versus intravenous rehydration in mild to moderately dehydrated children in the emergency department.*Clin Therapeut* 2012;34(11):2232–2245.

World Health Organization. *The treatment of diarrhoea. A manual for physicians and other senior health workers.* WHO/CDD/SER/80.2. 4th ed. Geneva: Division of Diarrhoeal and Acute Respiratory Disease Control, World Health Organization, 2005.

CHAPTER 18 ▪ DIARRHEA

FARIA PEREIRA, MD AND DEBORAH HSU, MD, MEd

Diarrhea, defined as a decrease in the consistency of the stool (loose/watery) and/or greater than three stools in a 24-hour period, is a common presenting complaint to the emergency department (ED). Infants and children have variability in frequency and type of stools; therefore, any deviation from the usual stooling pattern should arouse at least a mild concern, regardless of the actual number of stools or their water content. An acute diarrheal illness typically lasts less than 5 days. In the United States, diarrhea accounts for approximately 1.5 million annual outpatient visits. Although most bouts of illness are self-limited, approximately 200,000 patients are hospitalized and 300 die each year. Since the introduction of the rotavirus vaccine in 2006, the number of hospitalizations due to diarrheal disease has been reduced.

DIFFERENTIAL DIAGNOSIS

Diarrhea may be the initial manifestation of a wide spectrum of disorders as outlined in Table 18.1. The most common etiology for diarrhea in pediatric patients presenting to the ED is viral gastroenteritis, with rotavirus and norovirus being the most common agents. Other causes include bacterial and parasitic infections, parenteral diarrhea (nongastrointestinal infection such as otitis media), and antibiotic induced. The emergency physician must be vigilant in recognizing the few children who have diseases that are likely to be life-threatening from among the majority of children who have self-limiting infections. Particularly urgent are intussusception, hemolytic uremic syndrome (HUS), pseudomembranous colitis, and appendicitis (Table 18.2). In addition, children may develop severe dehydration with diarrhea secondary to any etiology.

Intussusception is a potentially life-threatening condition that can present with bloody diarrhea, although this is not the typical presenting complaint. Intussusception peaks in frequency between 5 and 10 months of age and tapers off rapidly after 2 years of age unless there is a predisposing pathologic condition. This topic is covered in more detail in Chapter 48 Pain: Abdomen.

HUS should also be considered in a child presenting with bloody diarrhea. HUS is an uncommon but potentially life-threatening disease that typically presents with the classic triad of microangiopathic hemolytic anemia, thrombocytopenia, and acute kidney injury. Children are affected most often in the first 3 years of life. They often present with abdominal pain, vomiting, and diarrhea that become bloody. Five to 10 days after onset of diarrhea, children with HUS develop pallor, petechiae, and decreased urine output. The most common cause of HUS is Shiga-like toxin-producing *Escherichia coli* (*E. coli* 0157:H7).

Pseudomembranous colitis is another serious disorder that may cause bloody diarrhea. Clinically, the child with pseudomembranous colitis appears ill with prostration, abdominal distention, and blood in the stool. This disease results from an overgrowth of toxin-producing *Clostridium difficile,* usually as a result of destruction of the normal intestinal microflora. It may occur at any age but is uncommon in early childhood. Although the incidence of pseudomembranous colitis is highest after treatment with clindamycin, studies have shown that exposure to any antibiotic increases susceptibility to *C. difficile* infection. In fact, because of its common use, amoxicillin is responsible for most cases of pseudomembranous colitis in childhood, even though overall incidence of *C. difficile* infection after therapy with this agent is low. Occasional cases occur in children with no recent usage of antibiotics.

Appendicitis manifests primarily with abdominal pain. Common presentation is periumbilical abdominal pain that migrates to the right lower quadrant, followed by anorexia, vomiting, and/or fever. Less commonly, appendicitis may cause diarrhea. The presumed mechanism for the diarrhea is irritation of the colon by the inflamed appendix. Particularly in very young children or among patients of any age who have a perforated appendix and a long duration of illness, the diagnosis of appendicitis as the cause of diarrhea may be delayed because the classic constellation of signs and symptoms is often absent. However, the examiner will usually be able to elicit abdominal tenderness greater than would be expected with gastroenteritis.

Toxic megacolon is a life-threatening condition that can occur as a complication of a number of conditions including inflammatory bowel disease (IBD), shigella infection, pseudomembranous colitis, and Hirschsprung disease. It is characterized by a dilated colon and abdominal distention with abdominal pain and fever that may progress to shock.

EVALUATION AND DECISION

The history and physical examination are paramount in determining if the child with diarrhea has a mild self-limiting illness or a condition that is potentially life-threatening. Further, the physician must also identify if the diarrheal illness is acute or chronic as the etiologies can be different.

In evaluating a child with diarrhea, a rapid assessment is necessary to determine the need for urgent or emergent fluid resuscitation. Historical information that should be elicited include detailed questions about the onset of illness, frequency (number of diarrheal stools per day), quantity (smear in the diaper or stool fills and overflows the diaper in infants), and characteristics (e.g., bloody, mucoid, black) of stools, presence of concurrent vomiting, the amount of liquid taken orally, and the frequency or volume of urination (number of wet diaper changes in the infant).

A diagnostic approach to the pediatric patient with diarrhea is outlined in Figure 18.1. Inquiry about associated symptoms may be helpful in determining possible causes and need for other acute interventions. The presence of vomiting and fever

TABLE 18.1

CAUSES OF DIARRHEA

Infections
Enteral
Viruses: rotavirus, caliciviruses (norwalk and sapporo viruses), enteroviruses, adenoviruses, astroviruses
Bacteria: *Salmonella, Shigella, Yersinia, Campylobacter,* pathogenic *Escherichia coli, Aeromonas hydrophila, Vibrio* spp., *Clostridium difficile,* tuberculosis
Parasites: *Giardia lamblia, Entamoeba histolytica, Cryptosporidia*
Nongastrointestinal (parenteral diarrhea): otitis media, pneumonia, urinary tract infection
Dietary disturbances
Overfeeding, food allergy, starvation stools
Anatomic abnormalities
Intussusception, Hirschsprung disease, partial obstruction, appendicitis, blind loop syndrome, intestinal lymphangiectasia, short bowel syndrome
Inflammatory bowel disease
Ulcerative colitis, Crohn disease
Malabsorption or increased secretion
Cystic fibrosis, celiac disease, disaccharidase deficiency, acrodermatitis enteropathica, secretory neoplasms
Systemic illnesses
Immunodeficiency
Endocrinopathy: hyperthyroidism, hypoparathyroidism, congenital adrenal hyperplasia
Psychogenic disturbances (irritable bowel syndrome)
Miscellaneous
Antibiotic-induced diarrhea, secondary lactase deficiency, neonatal drug withdrawal, toxins (e.g., organophosphate ingestion), hemolytic uremic syndrome

may help determine infectious versus noninfectious causes. Vomiting in association with diarrhea is very suggestive of viral gastroenteritis, whereas bilious vomiting in isolation is more concerning for intestinal obstruction. Bloody diarrhea points particularly to bacterial enteritis but occasionally occurs with viral infections and may also herald the onset of HUS or pseudomembranous colitis. The combination of episodic abdominal pain and blood in the stool characterizes intussusception. The presence of abdominal pain should raise the index of suspicion for appendicitis and intussusception. A history of ear pain, cough, or dysuria should alert to the possibility of nonintestinal infections as the etiology of the diarrhea.

TABLE 18.2

LIFE-THREATENING CAUSES OF DIARRHEA

Intussusception
Hemolytic uremic syndrome
Pseudomembranous colitis
Appendicitis
Salmonella gastroenteritis (with bacteremia in the neonate or immunocompromised host)
Hirschsprung disease (with toxic megacolon)
Inflammatory bowel disease (with toxic megacolon)

Pre-existing conditions in the child may account for the diarrhea or predispose him or her to unusual causes; in particular, the emergency physician should search for a history of gastrointestinal surgery or chronic illnesses, such as ulcerative colitis or regional enteritis. Immunodeficiency syndromes, neoplasms, and immunosuppressive therapy all lead to an increased susceptibility to infection. Institutionalized children and those recently returning from underdeveloped countries are more likely to harbor bacterial or parasitic pathogens. A history of daycare exposure suggests a viral infection whereas recent antibiotic use may suggest antibiotic-associated diarrhea or pseudomembranous colitis. A child who presents with chronic diarrhea (more than 5 days) may suggest other etiologies such as IBD, irritable bowel disease, bacterial infections, Hirschsprung disease, human immunodeficiency infection (HIV), and assorted malabsorptive and secretory disorders. With the possible exception of bacterial enteritis in a febrile or toxic-appearing patient, such conditions, if uncomplicated, do not require a definitive diagnosis emergently, but rather an evaluation over time.

A complete physical examination is essential for determining the severity of the dehydration in the child with diarrheal illness as well as for determination of potential etiologies for the diarrhea (see Chapters 17 Dehydration and 108 Renal and Electrolyte Emergencies). Various clinical scales have been developed and validated to determine the degree of dehydration. Scales that are commonly used in the acute care setting include the Gorelick scale, the Clinical Dehydration Scale (CDS), and the World Health Organization (WHO) scale. See Figure 18.2 for these scales.

Altered mental status may be seen in children with severe dehydration, hypovolemic shock, and intussusception. Pallor and petechiae may denote HUS or malignancy. On abdominal examination, the findings of a mass (IBD, intussusception, malignancy) or evidence of obstruction (abdominal distention, pain, and paucity of bowel sounds) is important. A rectal examination should be performed in the child who has chronic diarrhea. With overflow stools secondary to prolonged constipation, the rectal ampulla often contains a large amount of hard stool, but it is usually empty in the patient with Hirschsprung disease.

Routine diagnostic testing is not necessary in pediatric patients with suspected self-limiting diarrheal disease. If a history of significant stool output accompanied by poor oral intake is obtained, bedside point of care glucose check should be performed to evaluate for possible hypoglycemia, especially in infants and toddlers. Electrolytes, BUN, and creatinine should be obtained only if the history and/or physical examination are concerning for potential electrolyte abnormalities or impaired renal function. Plain abdominal films should be performed in patients with suspected gastrointestinal obstruction, but are frequently normal in children with intussusception and gastroenteritis. Because of its high diagnostic sensitivity and lack of ionizing radiation, ultrasound (US) has replaced contrast enema as the diagnostic test of choice in children with suspected intussusception. US may also be helpful in the diagnosis of the patient with appendicitis. When HUS is suspected, a complete blood count, renal function studies including serum creatinine, urinalysis, coagulation studies, and peripheral smear should be performed. The peripheral blood smear, in addition to reduced numbers of platelets, may show evidence

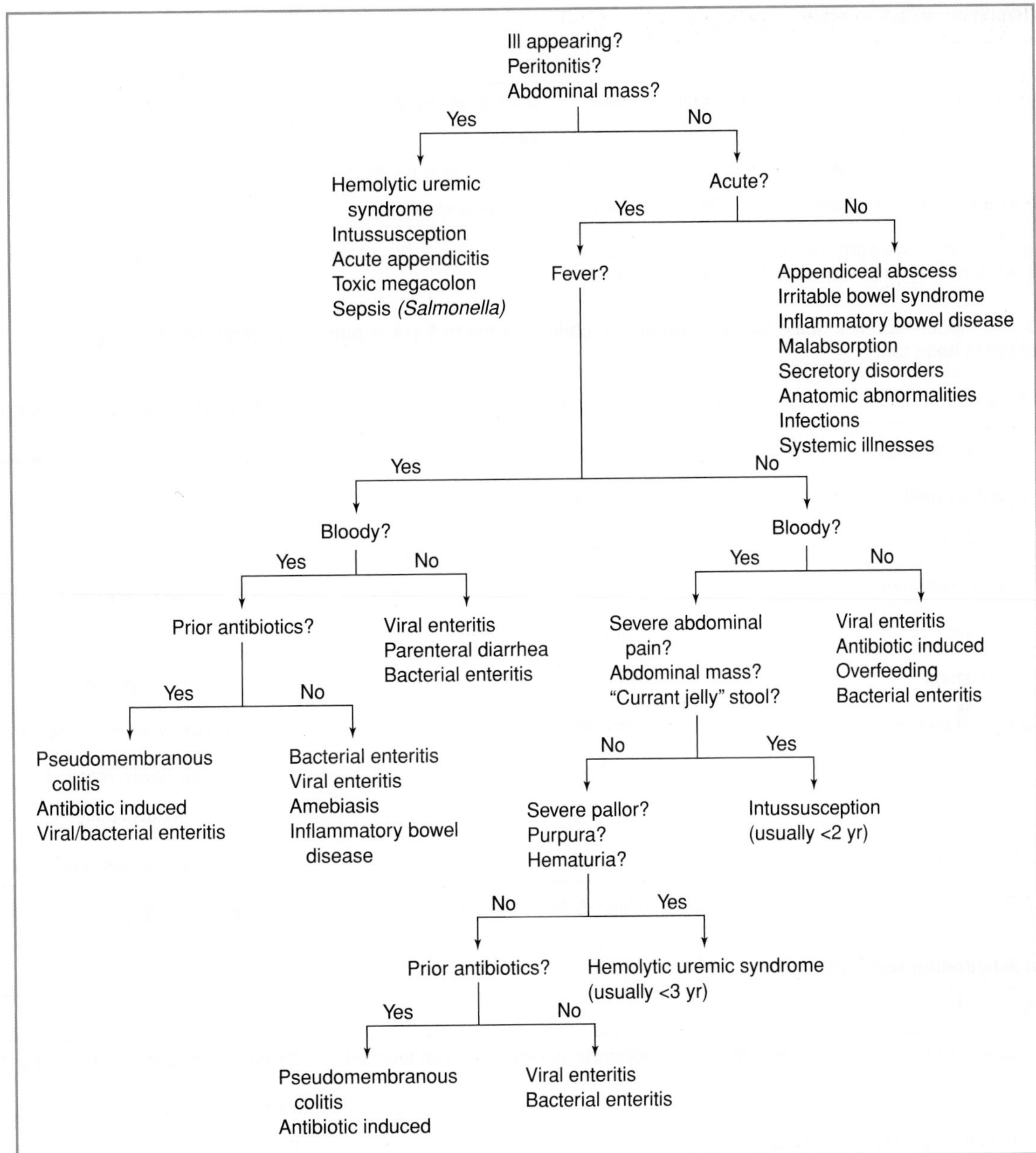

FIGURE 18.1 Diagnostic approach to the immunocompetent child with diarrhea.

of intravascular hemolysis, including helmet cells and schistocytes. The urinalysis shows hematuria (dipstick detection of free hemoglobin) and proteinuria. In patients with suspected pseudomembranous colitis, stool toxin analysis provides the mainstay of diagnosis. Polymerase chain reaction (PCR) has been shown to have higher sensitivities for toxin A and B than enzyme immunoassay (EIA). Testing for fecal leukocytes is neither sensitive nor specific for inflammatory diarrhea; fecal lactoferrin is a more sensitive marker but not specific for detection of particular pathogens. When selected bacterial or parasitic pathogens are strongly suspected, appropriate microbiologic studies should be collected.

TREATMENT

The treatments for the different causes of diarrhea are covered in the medical and surgical sections of this book; however, the therapy for viral gastroenteritis or parenteral diarrhea merits a summary. All children with circulatory compromise and many children with moderate to severe dehydration need intravenous rehydration with isotonic (normal saline or lactated Ringer's) fluids, given rapidly in increments of 20 mL per kg boluses. Infants and children who are symptomatically hypoglycemic should receive IV glucose. However, most pediatric patients with acute gastroenteritis can be managed with oral solutions. Most children will tolerate small feedings given frequently. Fluids may also be delivered via a nasogastric tube if needed.

Optimal oral rehydration therapy emphasizes the use of appropriate glucose and electrolyte solutions, as well as the early reintroduction of feeding. Ideal oral rehydration solutions, based on formulas carefully tested by the WHO, have a carbohydrate:sodium ratio that approaches 1:1. Although some recommend, particularly for young infants, initial oral rehydration with a solution that contains 75 to 90 mEq per L

World health organization scale.

	A	B	C
Look at condition	Well, alert	Restless, irritable	Lethargic or unconscious
Eyes	Normal	Sunken	Sunken
Thirst	Drinks normally, not thirsty	Thirsty, drinks eagerly	Drinks poorly or not able to drink
Feel: Skin pinch	Goes back quickly	Goes back slowly	Goes back very slowly

A Scoring: Fewer than two signs from column B and C: no signs of dehydration, <5%; ≥2 signs in column B: moderate dehydration, 5–10%; ≥2 signs in column C; severe dehydration, >10%.

The 10- and 4-point Gorelick Scale for dehydration: for children 1 mo to 5 yrs; 4-point scale physical exam signs highlighted in italic font

Characteristic	No or minimal dehydration	Moderate to severe dehydration
General appearance	*Alert*	*Restless, lethargic, unconscious*
Capillary refill	*Normal*	*Prolonged or minimal*
Tears	*Present*	*Absent*
Mucous membranes	*Moist*	*Dry, very dry*
Eyes	Normal	Sunken; deeply sunken
Breathing	Present	Deep; deep and rapid
Quality of pulses	Normal	Thready; weak or impalpable
Skin elasticity	Instant recoil	Recoil slowly; recoil >2 s
Heart rate	Normal	Tachycardia
Urine output	Normal	Reduced; not passed in many hours

B Scoring: Presence of <3 signs: <5% dehydration; 3–5 signs: 5–9% dehydration; ≥6 signs: 10% or more dehydration.

Clinical dehydration scale (CDS).

Characteristic	0	1	2
General appearance	Normal	Thirsty, restless, or lethargic, but irritable when touched	Drowsy, limp, cold, sweaty, and/or comatose
Eyes	Normal	Slightly sunken	Very Sunken
Mucous membranes	Moist	"Sticky"	Dry
Tears	Tears	Decreased tears	Absent tears

C Scoring: 0: no dehydration <3%, 1–4: some dehydration ≥3–6%, 5–8: moderate dehydration ≥6%.

FIGURE 18.2 Dehydration scales. **A:** WHO Dehydration scale. (From Jauregui J, Nelson D, Choo E, et al. External validation and comparison of three pediatric clinical dehydration scales. *PloS One.* 2014;9(5):e95739.) **B:** Gorelick scale. (From Pringle K, Shah SP, Umulisa I, et al. Comparing the accuracy of the three popular clinical dehydration scales in children with diarrhea. *Int J Emerg Med.* 2011;4:58.) **C:** CDS dehydration scale. (From Jauregui J, Nelson D, Choo E, et al. External validation and comparison of three pediatric clinical dehydration scales. *PloS One.* 2014;9(5):e95739.)

of sodium (i.e., WHO 2003 oral rehydration salts solution) and subsequent maintenance with a more hypotonic formulation (i.e., Pedialyte), most clinicians use a single preparation during the course of routine, brief illnesses. Older children with mild gastroenteritis tolerate juices and other commercial products, even though the carbohydrate:sodium ratio deviates from the WHO standard. Feeding with age-appropriate diet, including breast-feeding for infants, is recommended as soon as rehydration is complete. Doing so appears to reduce stool output and duration of the diarrheal disease. Foods with complex carbohydrates, lean meats, fruits, and vegetables are better tolerated than those that contain fat and simple sugars. The commonly recommended restriction to clear liquid and BRAT (bananas, rice, applesauce, toast) diets provide suboptimal nutrition and are no longer recommended.

Use of probiotics (Lactobacillus GG strain most commonly used) in children with presumed infectious diarrhea may reduce the duration and frequency of diarrheal stools. Lactobacillus should not be given to immunocompromised children due to potential for lactobacillus sepsis. Antibiotics are not routinely recommended, even for bloody diarrhea, because acute diarrheal illnesses are usually self-limited. Antibiotics should only be used when diagnostic tests reveal a treatable bacterial or parasitic etiology. In general, antidiarrheal agents are ineffective, have potentially serious side effects, and therefore have no role in the treatment of infectious gastroenteritis. Antimotility drugs, opiate receptor agonists (e.g., loperamide), reduce intestinal mobility and delay transit time, thereby prolonging course of illness. Toxic side effects of these medications include lethargy and paralytic ileus. Antisecretory drugs like bismuth subsalicylate have limited efficacy and have potential for salicylate toxicity. Adsorbents (e.g., hydrated aluminomagnesium silicates and kaolinpectin), while having potential to bind digestive mucus and reduce water loss, have not been shown to reduce diarrheal duration, frequency, or volume.

Suggested Readings and Key References

Bryant K, McDonald LC. *Clostridium difficile* infection in children. *Pediatr Infect Dis J* 2009;28:145.

Centers for Disease Control and Prevention. Delayed onset and diminished magnitude of rotavirus activity – United States, November 2007–May 2008. *MMWR Morb Mortal Wkly Rep* 2008;57(25): 697–700.

Denno DM, Shaikh N, Stapp JR, et al. Diarrhea etiology in a pediatric emergency department: a case control study. *Clin Infect Dis* 2012; 55:897–904.

Gerber A, Karch H, Allerberger F, et al. Clinical course and the role of Shiga toxin-producing *Escherichia coli* infection in hemolytic-uremic syndrome in pediatric patients, 1997–2000 in Germany and Austria: a prospective study. *J Infect Dis* 2002;186:493–500.

Goldman RD, Friedman JN, Parkin PC. Validation of the clinical dehydration scale for children with acute gastroenteritis. *Pediatrics* 2008;122:545–549.

Gorelick MH, Shaw KN, Murphy KO. Validity and reliability of clinical signs in the diagnosis of dehydration in children. *Pediatrics* 1997;99:E6.

Horwitz JR, Gursoy M, Jaksic T, et al. Importance of diarrhea as a presenting symptom of appendicitis in very young children. *Am J Surg* 1997;173:80–82.

King CK, Glass R, Bresse JS, et al. Managing acute gastroenteritis among children: oral rehydration, maintenance and nutritional therapy. *MMWR Recomm Rep* 2003;52:1–20.

Lochhead A, Jamjoom R, Ratnapalan S. Intussusception in children presenting to the emergency department. *Clin Pediatr (Phila)* 2013; 52(11):1028–1033.

Van Niel CW, Reudtner C, Garrison MM, et al. Lactobacillus therapy for acute infectious diarrhea in children: a meta-analysis. *Pediatrics* 2002;109:678.

CHAPTER 19 ▪ DIZZINESS AND VERTIGO

THERESA A. WALLS, MD, MPH AND STEPHEN J. TEACH, MD, MPH

Dizziness can be a vague term that patients use to describe nonvertiginous disturbances (pseudovertigo) such as lightheadedness, presyncope, intoxication, ataxia, visual disturbances, unsteadiness, weakness, stress, anxiety, hyperventilation, depression, and fear. True vertigo is the perception that the environment is rotating relative to the patient or that the patient is rotating relative to the environment. It can be immensely disturbing, even frightening, to patients and their families. Preverbal children, unable to articulate the sensation, may be irritable, may vomit, or may prefer to lie still. Even older children and adults may have difficulty describing the sensation.

Patients may present with dizziness as an isolated complaint or as part of a constellation of symptoms related to an underlying illness. When evaluating a child complaining of dizziness, the practitioner should listen carefully to the details of the history as these may allow him or her to distinguish true vertigo from pseudovertigo. The key element in the history that strongly suggests true vertigo is the subjective sense of rotation. Often, the best response to a chief complaint of being dizzy is to say, "Tell me what you mean by 'dizzy'." Initially vague complaints often become increasingly concrete, and the underlying diagnosis may become increasingly clear.

PATHOPHYSIOLOGY

True vertigo arises from a disturbance in either the peripheral or central components of the vestibular system. The two peripheral sensory organs of the system (together known as the labyrinth) are the semicircular canals (stimulated by rotary motion of the head) and the vestibule (stimulated by gravity). Both organs lie near the cochlea within the petrous portion of the temporal bone. The proximity of the vestibular and cochlear apparatus explains the frequent association of vertigo with hearing impairment.

Afferent impulses from these organs travel via the vestibular portion of the eighth cranial nerve to the vestibular nuclei in the brainstem and in the cerebellum. Efferent impulses travel through the vestibulospinal tract to the peripheral muscles (helping to maintain balance and position sense) and also within the medial longitudinal fasciculus to cranial nerves III, IV, and VI (accounting for the oculovestibular reflexes). Almost all patients complaining of true vertigo should have nystagmus, at least when the vertiginous symptoms are peaking. The fast component of the nystagmus is almost always in the same direction as the perceived rotation.

DIFFERENTIAL DIAGNOSIS

As discussed earlier, dizziness is best divided into vertiginous conditions (true vertigo) and nonvertiginous conditions (pseudovertigo). Table 19.1 lists the differential diagnosis of true vertigo and highlights the life-threatening causes. Table 19.2 lists the most common causes of vertigo. Table 19.3 lists numerous nonvertiginous conditions that may initially be described as dizziness. Because the spectrum of nonvertiginous conditions is so broad, the following discussion will concentrate on true vertigo.

Vertigo follows a dysfunction of the vestibular system within the semicircular canals, vestibule, or vestibular nerve (peripheral vertigo), or within the brainstem, cerebellum, or cortex (central vertigo). It can also be divided into conditions in which hearing is impaired (usually peripheral causes) and into conditions in which hearing is spared (usually central causes). Finally, vertigo can be divided into acute (usually infectious, postinfectious, traumatic, or toxic) and chronic-recurrent groups (usually caused by seizures, migraine, or benign paroxysmal vertigo of childhood).

Infections

Both acute and chronic bacterial and viral infections of the middle ear, with or without associated mastoiditis, may cause vestibular and auditory impairment (see Chapters 30 Hearing Loss and 53 Pain: Earache). Severe, untreated, acute suppurative otitis media with effusion may extend directly into the labyrinth. Even without direct invasion of the pathogens, inflammation can cause labyrinthitis.

Chronic and recurrent otitis media can produce a cholesteatoma of the tympanic membrane, an abnormal growth of keratinizing squamous epithelium caused by repeated cycles of perforation and healing. Cholesteatomas can erode the temporal bone and the labyrinth, producing a draining fistula from the labyrinth that presents as vertigo, nausea, and hearing impairment. Computed tomography (CT) scan or magnetic resonance imaging (MRI) shows destruction of the temporal bone.

Viral infections can directly affect the labyrinth or the vestibular nerve, together these conditions are known as *vestibular neuronitis*. Known pathogens include mumps, measles, and the Epstein–Barr virus. Herpes zoster infection of the ear canal and facial palsy (Ramsay Hunt syndrome) may also involve the eighth nerve. More commonly, a nonspecific upper respiratory tract infection may precede the illness. Onset is usually acute and can be severe. Nystagmus is usually present. Patients prefer to lie motionless with their eyes closed. Recovery is from 1 to 3 weeks. Early use of prednisone may shorten the course.

Migraine

Vertigo may be a prominent feature of classic migraine, or of a migraine equivalent, in which there is no associated headache (see Chapters 54 Pain: Headache and 105 Neurologic Emergencies). Nearly 20% of children with migraine may have vertiginous symptoms during their aura. Basilar migraine presents as a throbbing occipital headache following signs and symptoms of brainstem dysfunction

TABLE 19.1

CAUSES OF VERTIGO IN CHILDREN

Peripheral causes	Central causes
Ingestions[a]	Tumor[a]
Temporal bone fracture[a]	Meningitis[a]
Suppurative or serous labyrinthitis	Encephalitis[a]
External ear impaction (especially cerumen)	Trauma[a]
Ramsay Hunt syndrome (Varicella zoster infection)	Stroke[a]
Cholesteatoma	Increased intracranial pressure[a]
Perilymphatic fistula	Multiple sclerosis
Vestibular neuronitis	Seizure (usually complex partial)
Benign paroxysmal vertigo	Migraine
Posttraumatic vestibular concussion	Motion sickness
Ménière disease	Paroxysmal torticollis of infancy

[a]Life-threatening causes of vertigo.

(including vertigo, ataxia, tinnitus, and dysarthria). Vertigo from migraine equivalent (without pain) is typically seen in patients with a family history of migraine headache and is associated with other transient neurologic complaints (e.g., weakness, dysarthria).

The differential diagnosis of headache and vertigo also includes a brainstem or cerebellar mass, hemorrhage, and infarction. These uncommon disorders are best assessed by MRI.

Benign Paroxysmal Vertigo of Childhood

Considered by many to be a form of migraine, benign paroxysmal vertigo of childhood is most common in children between the ages of 1 and 5 years. Patients have recurrent attacks, usually one to four per month, and occasionally in clusters. Onset is sudden—the child often cries out at the start of each episode—and is associated with emesis, pallor, sweating, and nystagmus. Episodes are brief, lasting up to a few minutes, and may be mistaken for seizures. Consciousness and hearing are preserved, and the neurologic examination is otherwise normal. The electroencephalogram (EEG) is normal. The disorder spontaneously remits after 2 to 3 years.

TABLE 19.2

COMMON CAUSES OF VERTIGO

Suppurative or serous labyrinthitis
Benign paroxysmal vertigo
Migraine
Vestibular neuronitis
Ingestions
Seizure
Motion sickness

TABLE 19.3

COMMON CAUSES OF PSEUDOVERTIGO

Depression
Anxiety
Hyperventilation
Orthostatic hypotension
Hypertension
Heat stroke
Arrhythmia
Cardiac disease
Anemia
Hypoglycemia
Pregnancy
Ataxia
Visual disturbances
Psychogenic disturbance

Ototoxic Drugs

Most agents that disturb vestibular function will also disturb auditory function. Specific agents include aminoglycoside antibiotics, furosemide, ethacrynic acid, streptomycin, minocycline, salicylates, and ethanol. Toxic doses of certain anticonvulsants and neuroleptics can produce measurable disturbances of vestibular function, although associated complaints of vertigo are rare.

Trauma

Several mechanisms account for posttraumatic vertigo. The most obvious is fracture through the temporal bone with damage to the labyrinth (see Chapters 114 ENT Trauma and 121 Neurotrauma). Presentation includes vertigo, hearing loss, and hemotympanum. CT scanning or MRI of the temporal bone should be obtained when there is hemotympanum or posttraumatic evidence of vestibular dysfunction.

More subtle causes of posttraumatic vertigo include trauma-induced seizures, migraine, or a postconcussive syndrome. Vestibular concussion typically follows blows to parietooccipital or temporoparietal regions and presents with headache, nausea, vertigo, and nystagmus. Although it generally remits with time, intermittent and recurrent episodes can occur. Hyperextension and flexion ("whiplash") injuries can be associated with vestibular dysfunction, probably caused by basilar artery spasm with subsequent impairment of their labyrinth and cochlear connections. Symptoms may mimic basilar artery migraine or cerebellar stroke.

Seizures

Two types of seizures are associated with vertigo: vestibular seizures (seizures causing vertigo) and vestibulogenic seizures ("reflex" seizures brought on by stimulating the semicircular canals or vestibules by sudden rotation or caloric testing). Vestibular seizures, the more common type, consist of sudden onset of vertigo with or without nausea, emesis, and headache, and are followed by loss or alteration of consciousness. The EEG is abnormal and anticonvulsants may be of benefit.

Motion Sickness

Motion sickness is precipitated by a mismatch in information provided to the brain by the visual and vestibular systems during unfamiliar rotations and accelerations. The most common situation occurs when a child travels in a car or airplane and is deprived of a visual stimulus that confirms movement. Symptoms include vertigo, nausea, and nystagmus. Attacks can be prevented by allowing patients to watch the environment move in a direction opposite to the direction of body movement (such as encouraging a child to look out the window while riding in a car).

Ménière Disease

Uncommon in children younger than 10 years, Ménière disease is characterized by episodic attacks of vertigo, hearing loss, tinnitus, nystagmus, and autonomic symptoms of pallor, nausea, and emesis. The underlying cause is believed to be an overaccumulation of endolymph within the labyrinth, which causes a rupture (endolymphatic hydrops). Typical attacks last from 1 to 3 hours and usually begin with tinnitus, a sense of fullness within the ear, and increasing hearing impairment. The patient may have intermittent attacks for years, and there may be permanent hearing loss.

Miscellaneous Causes

Vertigo may occur at any point in the clinical course of multiple sclerosis when the central demyelination interferes with the vestibular nuclei in the brainstem or its efferents or afferents. Diagnosis is confirmed by MRI and lumbar puncture. Paroxysmal torticollis of infancy consists of spells of head tilt associated with nausea, emesis, pallor, agitation, and ataxia. Episodes are brief and self-limited and may recur for months or years. The cause is unclear, although some authors see it as a prelude to benign paroxysmal vertigo. Perilymphatic fistula is an abnormal communication between the labyrinth and the middle ear, with leakage of perilymphatic fluid through the defect. It may be congenital or acquired by trauma, infection, or surgery. The diagnosis may be suspected when vertigo is provoked by sneezing or coughing, actions that can increase perilymphatic drainage. Diagnosis is confirmed by middle ear exploration. Benign paroxysmal positional vertigo (BPPV) is rare in children, but has been reported in the literature in a patient as young as 3 years old. Patients typically complain of vertigo with changes in head position, especially upon waking in the morning and sitting up in bed. Episodes usually last less than 1 minute. Finally, vertigo may be associated with diabetes mellitus and chronic renal failure.

EVALUATION AND DECISION

Differentiation of True Vertigo and Pseudovertigo

Evaluation of children with dizziness begins by distinguishing between those with true vertigo and those with pseudovertigo (Tables 19.1 and 19.3). True vertigo is always associated with a subjective sense of rotation of the environment relative to the patient or of the patient relative to the environment. All vertigo is made worse by moving the head, and acute attacks are usually accompanied by nystagmus.

True Vertigo

History and Physical Examination. Once true vertigo (Fig. 19.1) is identified, its severity, time course, and pattern must be established. In general, the most severe attacks of vertigo have peripheral causes, whereas central causes tend to be more recurrent, chronic, and progressive. Sudden onset of sustained vertigo suggests central or peripheral trauma, infection, stroke, or ingestion. Recurrent episodic attacks suggest seizures, migraine, or benign paroxysmal vertigo. More persistent episodes suggest brainstem or cerebellar mass lesions.

Recurrent, transient, altered mental status suggests seizure or basilar migraine. Episodes of prior head injury suggest concussion syndromes. Recent upper respiratory tract infections may suggest vestibular neuronitis. History of ototoxic drug or intoxicant use is important, as is a family history of migraine. Age of the patient is especially useful—benign paroxysmal vertigo is unusual after age 5 years, whereas Ménière disease is unusual before age 10 years. The physical examination focuses on the middle ear and on neurologic and vestibular testing. Visualization of the external ear canal may reveal cerumen impaction, foreign body, or zoster lesions (Ramsay Hunt syndrome). Perforation or distortion of the tympanic membrane should be noted. A pneumatic bulb will enable the examiner to see whether abrupt changes in the middle ear pressure trigger an episode of vertigo, a suggestion that a perilymphatic fistula may be present (Hennebert sign).

The neurologic examination must be complete, focusing closely on the auditory, vestibular, and cerebellar systems. Both vestibular and cerebellar disorders may present with an unsteady gait. If there is a unilateral lesion, the child will fall toward the side of the lesion. The two may at times be distinguishable by the nature of the nystagmus (described below). If cerebellar dysfunction is present, the patient may have dysmetria and ataxia. All cases of suspected vestibular or cerebellar dysfunction require close follow-up evaluation because of the risk of a posterior fossa mass.

Nystagmus is a highly specific sign for both central and peripheral vertiginous disorders. A patient complaining of dizziness with vertigo may not have nystagmus at the time that he or she is examined. Tests to elicit positional vertigo and nystagmus can therefore be helpful in identifying and even distinguishing central and peripheral vestibular dysfunction, particularly if the tests elicit or increase the patient's complaint.

Nystagmus should be sought in all positions of gaze and with changes in head position. The Nylen–Hallpike test can be used to elicit nystagmus if not apparent on initial examination. It is performed by moving a child rapidly from a sitting to a supine position with the head 45 degrees below the edge of the examining table and turned 45 degrees to one side. Nystagmus and a vertiginous sensation may result as the vestibular system is stressed. Certain features of nystagmus may be helpful in distinguishing central from peripheral vestibular dysfunction. In central dysfunction, for example, onset of nystagmus is immediate; in peripheral vestibular disorders, it is delayed. Central lesions are characterized by nystagmus with the fast component toward the affected side and reversal of the

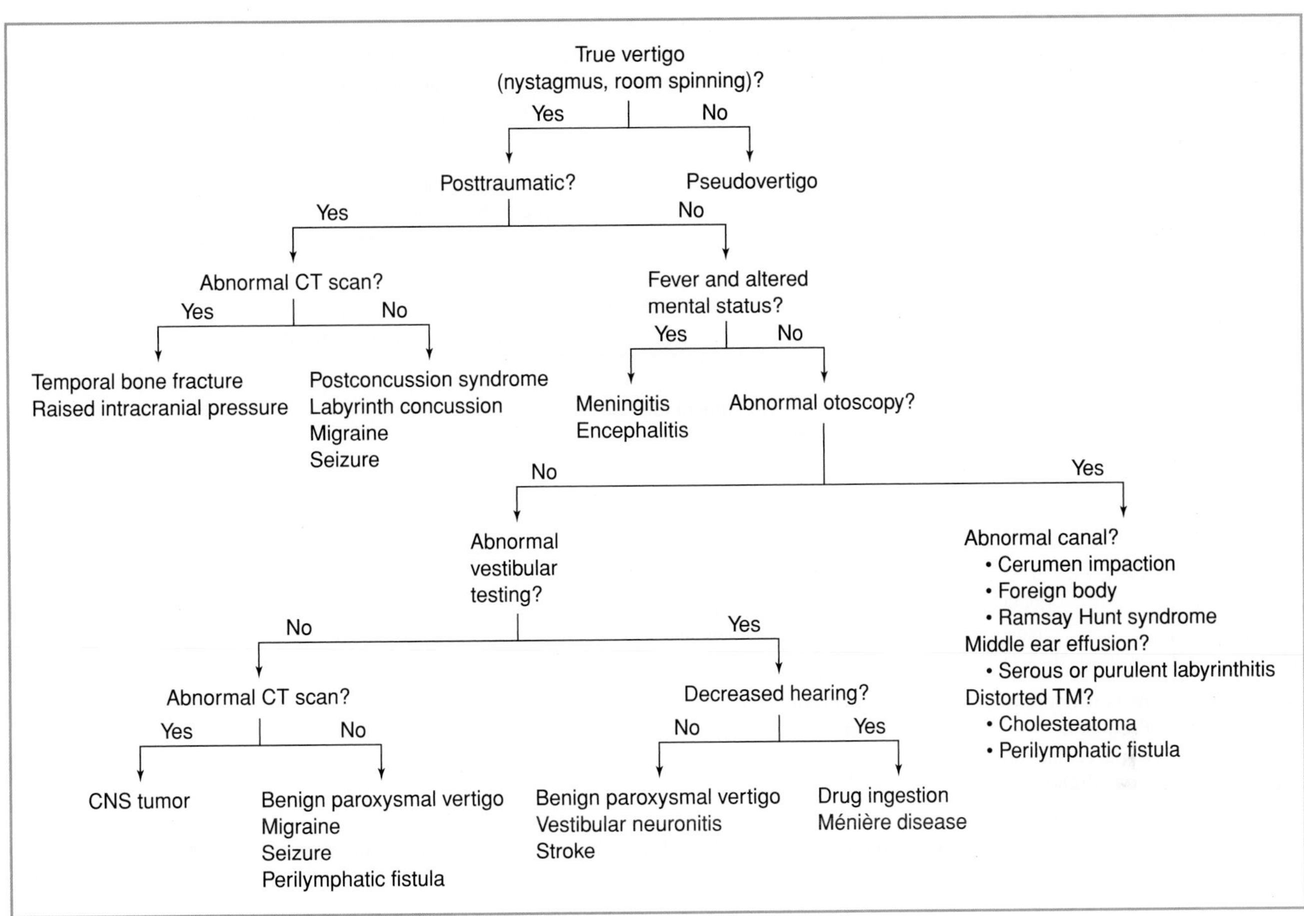

FIGURE 19.1 Approach to the child with true vertigo. CT, computed tomography; TM, tympanic membrane; CNS, central nervous system.

fast component when changing from right to left lateral gaze. Peripheral vestibular disorders are characterized by a "jerk" nystagmus with the slow component toward the affected side. Finally, visual fixation does not affect nystagmus from central causes, but tends to dampen peripheral nystagmus.

The cold caloric response tests for integrity of the peripheral vestibular system. Slow and careful irrigation of either 100 mL of tap water 7°C below body temperature or 10 mL of ice water into the external ear canal through a soft plastic tube, with the child lying about 60 degrees recumbent, should induce a slow movement of the eyes toward the stimulus and a fast movement away. Instillation of warm water (44°C) will cause an inverse reaction. Vestibular damage will suppress the response on the affected side. Absence of nystagmus indicates absence of peripheral vestibular function. The test is contraindicated if the tympanic membrane is perforated.

Ancillary Tests. Laboratory investigations have a limited role in the evaluation of vertigo. Useful initial tests include complete blood count, serum glucose, and an electrocardiogram. Together, these may help identify patients with pseudovertiginous conditions caused by anemia, hypoglycemia, and rhythm abnormalities. Further laboratory testing may reveal diabetes or renal failure, both of which have been associated with vertigo. Toxicologic testing including specific anticonvulsant levels and an ethanol level, if indicated, may be helpful. A lumbar puncture is indicated in cases of suspected meningitis or encephalitis.

Radiologic imaging of the central nervous system, preferably by MRI for adequate visualization of the posterior fossa and brainstem, is indicated in cases of chronic and recurrent vertigo to exclude mass lesions. Children with vertigo and an underlying bleeding diathesis or a predisposition toward ischemic stroke (i.e., sickle cell disease) may also need an emergent cranial CT or MRI. Posttraumatic vertigo, especially when accompanied by hearing loss or facial nerve paralysis, is best assessed by CT that includes adequate images of the temporal bone.

Some children with true vertigo will require referral for more extensive testing. An EEG is indicated when vertigo accompanies loss of consciousness or other manifestations of a seizure. Audiometry is indicated when vertigo accompanies otalgia, hearing loss, or tinnitus. Specialized testing for nystagmus, including electronystagmography, which measures eye movements at rest and at extremes of gaze, can separate central from peripheral vestibular disorders. It may be combined with caloric and positional testing.

Management. Most causes of vertigo remit spontaneously without therapy, but specific disorders require treatment. Suppurative labyrinthitis, for example, is treated with antibiotics if a bacterial etiology is suspected. An erosive cholesteatoma requires surgical removal. Anticonvulsants may diminish vestibular and vestibulogenic seizures. Motion sickness may respond to simple behavioral changes (e.g., encouraging children to look out the window).

Subspecialist consultation is indicated in certain situations. Neurosurgical evaluation after trauma may be indicated in cases of suspected basilar skull fracture. Suspected perilymphatic fistula, cholesteatoma, traumatic rupture of tympanic membrane, or complicated otitis media may merit

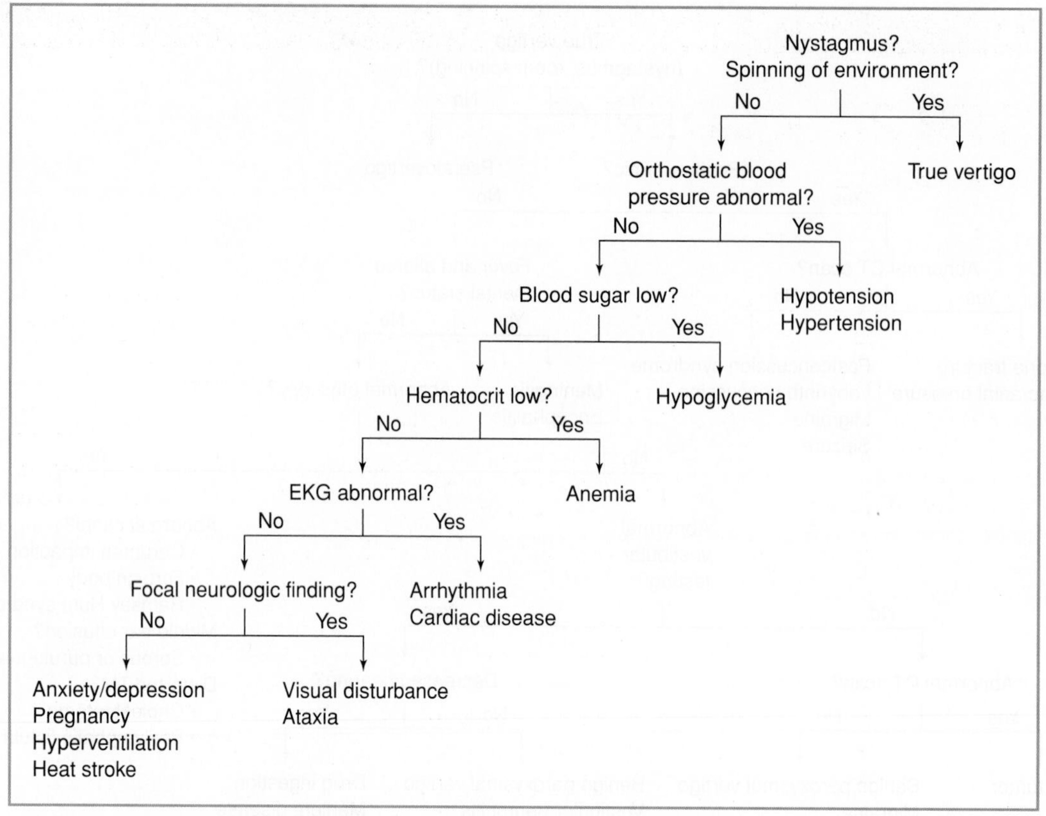

FIGURE 19.2 Approach to the child with pseudovertigo. EKG, electrocardiogram.

otorhinolaryngologic evaluation. Neurologists may be helpful in cases of suspected seizure or migraine.

Children with severe or recurrent attacks of vertigo may require treatment with specific medications. The antihistamines dimenhydrinate (12.5 to 25 mg orally every 6 to 8 hours, maximum dose 75 mg per day for ages 2 to 6 years and 25 to 50 mg every 6 to 8 hours for ages 6 to 12 years, maximum dose 150 mg per day) and meclizine (12.5 to 25 mg orally every 12 hours in children older than 12 years of age) may be helpful. Concomitant use of a benzodiazepine such as diazepam (0.1 to 0.3 mg/kg/day orally divided every 6 to 8 hours, maximum 10 mg per dose) as a sedative may be necessary in severe cases.

Pseudovertigo

Pseudovertigo (Fig. 19.2) refers to a broad array of symptoms such as lightheadedness, presyncope, intoxication, ataxia, visual disturbances, unsteadiness, stress, anxiety, and fear. Uniformly absent are a sense of rotation and ocular nystagmus. Underlying causes are numerous; several of the most common causes are listed in Table 19.3 (see also discussions of syncope in Chapter 71 Syncope). Careful consideration of the patient's age, gender, detailed history, and physical examination, together with a limited number of ancillary tests, may help establish the specific diagnosis.

Suggested Readings and Key References

Bower CM, Cotton RT. The spectrum of vertigo in children. *Arch Otolaryngol Head Neck Surg* 1995;121:911–915.

Lewis DW. Pediatric migraine. *Pediatr Rev* 2007;28:43–53.

MacGregor DL. Vertigo. *Pediatr Rev* 2002;23:10–16.

Phillips JO, Backous DD. Evaluation of vestibular function in young children. *Otolaryngol Clin North Am* 2002;4:765–790.

Tusa RJ, Saada AA, Niparko JK. Dizziness in childhood. *J Child Neurol* 1994;9:261–274.

CHAPTER 20 ■ EDEMA

LINDA L. BROWN, MD, MSCE

Edema is defined as the abnormal swelling of tissues from the accumulation of fluid in the extravascular space. This fluid may appear as generalized or localized swelling. Frequently in pediatrics, edema occurs as a localized response to injury or inflammation and, in this setting, is often benign and self-limited. However, it is important to recognize that edema may be the result of a variety of causes and the initial presentation of generalized edema may be quite subtle. When significant edema is present, collections of fluid may be visualized as pericardial or pleural effusions, or as ascites. When edema is profound and generalized, the patient is described as having anasarca. The completion of a careful history and a thorough physical examination will not only help to identify these patients early, but may also lead to a definitive diagnosis in some cases.

PATHOPHYSIOLOGY

The occurrence of edema in healthy individuals is usually prevented by the balance of oncotic and hydrostatic pressures between the intravascular and interstitial spaces, as well as the normal function of the lymphatic system. Any imbalance in this system may lead to increased interstitial fluid and eventual tissue swelling. Edema may occur as a result of decreased intravascular oncotic pressure, increased vascular permeability, increased hydrostatic pressure, lymphatic dysfunction, or a combination of these factors.

Tightly controlled levels of circulating proteins, especially albumin, maintain normal intravascular oncotic pressure. Hypoalbuminemia may arise from the decreased production of proteins caused by hepatic disease, as a result of protein malnutrition or, more commonly, from losses of protein through gastrointestinal, renal, or dermal conditions. When the albumin level is less than 2.5 g per dL, the oncotic pressure in the vascular space is reduced enough for fluid to move freely into the soft tissues and, if not corrected, generalized edema may result.

Edema can also result from changes in vascular (capillary) permeability, mediated by intrinsic cytokines and other inflammatory factors. This is seen most commonly in patients with burns, sepsis, or hypersensitivity reactions. In certain cases, the swelling may be rapid, localized, and potentially life-threatening. In patients with a severe allergic reaction, such as that associated with anaphylaxis, this edema may involve the tissues adjacent to the airway leading to potential airway compromise.

When intravascular albumin levels are within the normal range and vascular permeability is preserved, edema can result from increased hydrostatic pressures that overcome the oncotic pressure, forcing fluid out of the vascular space. This can occur as a result of changes in sodium and water retention from cardiac failure, renal failure or estrogen–progesterone excess, or from venous obstruction. Lymphatic dysfunction, either congenital or acquired, can also result in edema.

DIFFERENTIAL DIAGNOSIS

A myriad of disease processes can result in either localized or generalized edema (Table 20.1). Localized edema in children is often caused by an allergic reaction, with the most severe reactions resulting from exposure to nuts, shellfish, or hymenoptera venom. Idiopathic nephrotic syndrome, although rare (occurring in just 2 to 3 of every 100,000 children annually), is the most common cause of generalized edema (Table 20.2). Overall, most children who develop edema will have a benign diagnosis and a self-limited course. However, potentially life-threatening conditions (Table 20.3) causing edema can also occur, including severe allergic reactions, sepsis (see Chapter 102 Infectious Disease Emergencies), venous thrombosis, and kidney, liver, or cardiac disease.

EVALUATION

When evaluating the child with edema it is necessary to obtain a thorough history and perform a complete physical examination, including the assessment of vital signs. It is important to remember that the onset of symptoms is often gradual and subtle for causes of generalized edema. In fact, a 10% to 15% weight gain may be accumulated, with symptoms existing for weeks to months, before a patient presents for medical care. It is, therefore, essential to inspect for edema around the eyes, scrotum or labia, as well as the distal extremities, as these areas may be the only locations with perceptible swelling.

It is also helpful to classify the swelling as localized or generalized (Fig. 20.1) and to determine the location of the edema (facial vs. extremities), as well as any associated symptoms including fever, shortness of breath, pain, or recent illness. The duration of the symptoms and the patient's age may help to narrow down the potential diagnoses, as certain disorders will present in the newborn period (congenital lymphedema, Turner syndrome) while others occur more frequently in school-age children or adolescents (nephrotic syndrome, vasculitis). A thorough medical history, including a dietary history and a family history, is helpful to identify patients with chronic conditions, such as protein malnutrition, or inherited disorders, such as hereditary angioedema. Current and recent medications and allergies may also assist in clarifying the diagnosis.

LOCALIZED EDEMA

Localized edema is a more common presenting complaint in pediatrics than generalized edema. Usually, areas of localized

TABLE 20.1

CAUSES OF EDEMA

Decreased oncotic pressure
Protein loss
Protein-losing enteropathy
Nephrotic syndrome
Reduced albumin synthesis
Liver disease
Malnutrition
Increased hydrostatic pressure
Increased blood volume from water and sodium retention
Congestive heart failure
Primary renal sodium retention
Acute glomerulonephritis
Henoch–Schönlein purpura
Nephrotic syndrome
Renal failure
Premenstrual edema or edema of pregnancy
Venous obstruction
Constrictive pericarditis
Acute pulmonary edema
Portal hypertension
Budd–Chiari syndrome
Local venous obstruction
Thrombophlebitis/deep venous thrombosis
Increased capillary permeability
Allergic reaction
Hereditary angioedema
Inflammatory reactions
Burns
Cellulitis
Sepsis
Pit viper envenomation
Vasculitis
Lymphatic dysfunction/other
Hypothyroidism (myxedema)
Lymphedema
Milroy disease
Meige disease (lymphedema praecox)
Turner syndrome
Noonan syndrome
Epstein–Barr virus infectious mononucleosis (upper eyelid edema)

TABLE 20.2

COMMON CAUSES OF EDEMA

Localized
Allergic reaction
Cellulitis
Trauma
Generalized
Nephrotic syndrome
Allergic reaction

TABLE 20.3

LIFE-THREATENING CAUSES OF EDEMA

Localized
Allergic reaction with airway involvement
Hereditary angioedema
Cellulitis (with bacteremia)
Pit viper envenomation
Superior vena cava syndrome
Venous thrombosis
Generalized
Cardiac disease
Congestive heart failure
Pericardial effusion
Hepatic failure
Renal disease
Nephrosis
Nephritis
Sepsis

swelling are caused by minor trauma, infection, or secondary to an allergic reaction. Historical factors and physical examination findings will often lead to a particular diagnosis without the need for further testing. Tenderness to palpation and associated bruising points to trauma, while fever, erythema, and overlying warmth more commonly occur with an infectious cause (Table 20.4). On the face and distal extremities, insect bites may produce swelling and warmth, which can be difficult to distinguish from cellulitis. A therapeutic response to an oral antihistamine or to an intramuscular dose of epinephrine can help to differentiate an allergic reaction from other causes of localized swelling.

Localized bilateral upper eyelid edema (Hoagland sign) may be found in up to 50% of patients with Epstein–Barr virus (EBV) infectious mononucleosis. It is not associated with any significant discomfort, is seen only for the first few days of the illness, and is very specific for EBV so that it may be used to trigger further laboratory evaluation to confirm the diagnosis.

When a child presents with severe or recurrent facial edema, especially if there is a family history of similar symptoms, the diagnosis of hereditary angioedema (see Chapter 93 Allergic Emergencies) should be considered. When a patient with localized edema of the head or neck presents for care, it is crucial that the physician evaluate the child carefully for concurrent airway involvement. Facial edema may also be caused by oral, dental, or sinus infections, including acute sinusitis, orbital cellulitis, or dental abscess. Often these patients will present with a history of dental or facial pain, sinus congestion, erythema, or fever. A history of environmental exposure should lead to the diagnosis of other common causes of localized swelling including sunburn, frostbite, and plant-induced dermatitis (poison ivy). Although rarely seen, pit viper envenomation may cause rapid onset of painful swelling at the site of injury (see Chapter 98 Environmental Emergencies, Radiological Emergencies, Bites and Stings). Occasionally, an infant will present with unexplained, localized swelling of an extremity that has been present since birth. In this situation, the possibility of an injury secondary to birth trauma should

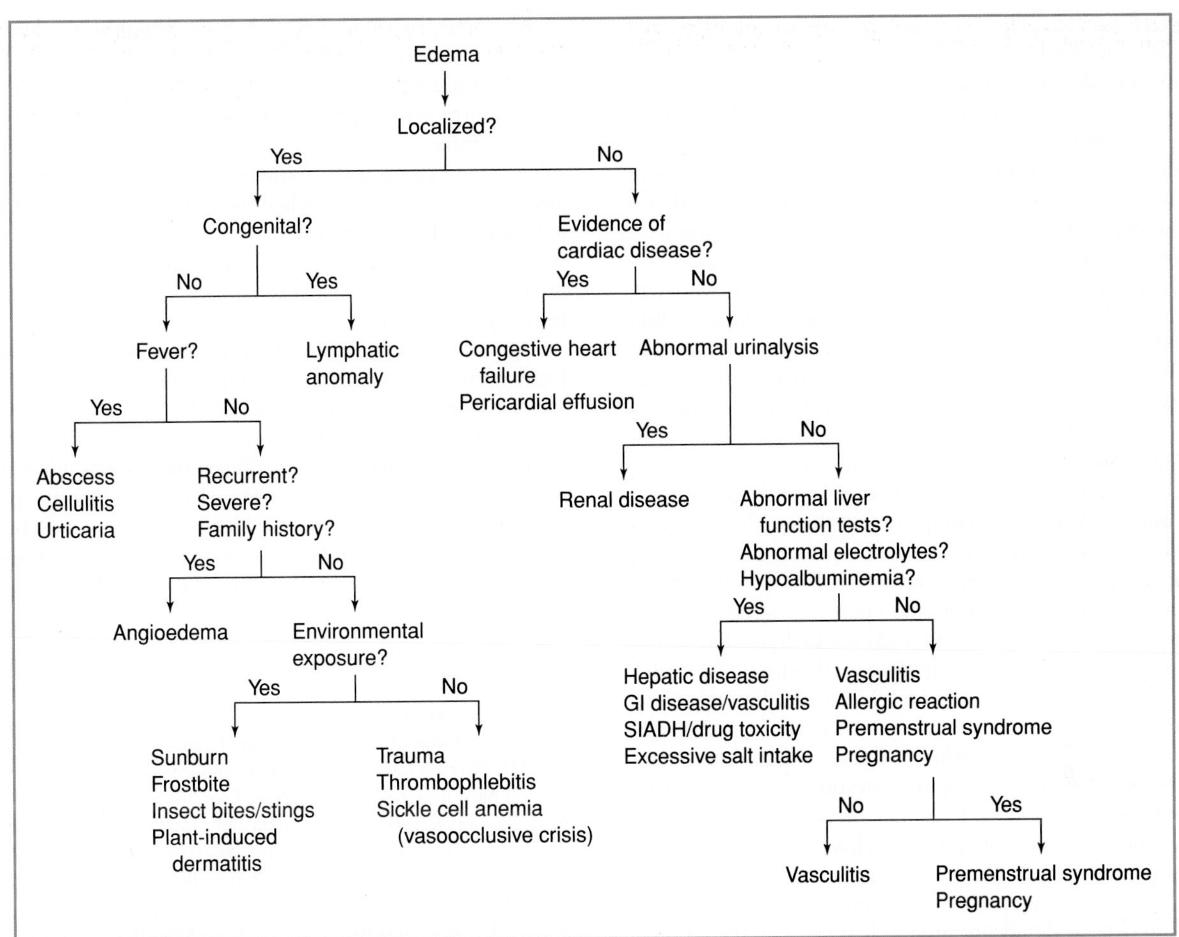

FIGURE 20.1 Edema in children. GI, gastrointestinal; SIADH, syndrome of inappropriate secretion of antidiuretic hormone.

be explored. Less commonly, congenital lymphedema (Milroy disease), Turner syndrome (bilateral leg edema), and Noonan syndrome (pedal edema) should be considered. Meige disease (lymphedema praecox) is a hereditary disorder that also results in lymphedema, but patients will present later in childhood or around puberty, usually with swelling of the feet or lower legs.

Sickle cell anemia may cause swollen and painful digits in young children, referred to as dactylitis (see Chapter 101 Hematologic Emergencies). Thrombophlebitis or deep venous thrombosis rarely occurs in the prepubertal child but may affect adolescents; inherited hypercoagulable states, weight-lifting, indwelling catheters, and the use of oral contraceptive pills predispose patients to this condition. Evaluation of these patients should include an ultrasound of the venous system of the affected limb and a thorough laboratory evaluation. Superior vena cava syndrome is a medical emergency caused by obstruction of blood flow through the vessel, resulting from compression from a tumor, thrombosis, or neoplastic invasion. This usually presents with shortness of breath and swelling to the head, neck, or upper extremities, often with some degree of cyanosis or plethora.

GENERALIZED EDEMA

Generalized edema, with an otherwise normal examination, occurs most commonly in patients with renal disease, particularly nephrotic syndrome (see Chapter 108 Renal and Electrolyte Emergencies). The initial diagnosis is based on significant proteinuria (3+ or 4+ or >300 mg/dL on a urinalysis). A urinalysis should therefore be included early in the evaluation of any pediatric patient presenting with

TABLE 20.4

DIFFERENTIATION AMONG THE COMMON CAUSES OF LOCALIZED EDEMA

	Fever	Local tenderness	Local warmth	Lesion/color
Allergic reaction	No	No	Yes	Erythematous
Trauma	No	Yes	No	Violaceous
Infection	Usually	Yes	Yes	Erythematous or violaceous

SIGNS AND SYMPTOMS

generalized edema. The presence or absence of urine red blood cells, white blood cells, or casts in the urine, along with further laboratory testing including chemistries, albumin, total protein, complement and triglyceride levels may help to confirm the diagnosis. Various factors, including the presence of hypertension or significant fluid collections in the pleural or peritoneal spaces, must be considered to determine the appropriate initial management of these patients.

Other forms of renal disease or vasculitis, including glomerulonephritis, hemolytic uremic syndrome, or Henoch–Schönlein purpura (HSP) may cause generalized edema. In the child with HSP, the swelling primarily affects the lower extremities, where the purpuric rash predominates, or is isolated to specific joints when arthritis is present. The purpuric rash, despite normal platelet count and coagulation studies (consistent with a vasculitis), is usually, but not universally, present.

The evaluation of the child presenting with generalized edema must also include a complete and thorough cardiovascular examination. Patients with CHF, pericarditis, myocarditis, or cardiomyopathy may present with edema, but these children will often have additional signs and symptoms. An edematous child presenting with a gallop, tachycardia, tachypnea, inspiratory crackles, or hepatomegaly should be evaluated for cardiac disease (see Chapter 94 Cardiac Emergencies).

In an edematous patient with a normal cardiac examination and no proteinuria, further evaluation should include a search for hepatic and other gastrointestinal diseases, as well as other forms of vasculitis. Patients with protein-losing enteropathy, from milk protein allergy, celiac disease, giardiasis, or inflammatory bowel disease, can present with generalized edema with few other physical examination findings. These patients may have significant protein loss through the GI tract and will often present with hypoalbuminemia. An initial laboratory evaluation, including liver function tests, electrolytes, erythrocyte sedimentation rate, and measurement of total protein and albumin, may reveal abnormalities. However, further evaluation, including more specific blood, urine, and stool testing, is often required to definitively diagnose the etiology of edema in this subset of patients.

As noted throughout this chapter, generalized edema may be a sign of a serious underlying disease. However, less serious conditions may be causative as well. Certain medications (oral contraceptive pills, corticosteroids, lithium, nonsteroidal anti-inflammatory agents, calcium channel blockers, and others) may cause some patients to become edematous. This swelling usually resolves when the drug is discontinued. Cyclical edema related to menstruation occurs frequently in young women. The etiology of this edema is likely hormonally mediated, although the exact mechanisms are unclear. Pregnancy may result in edema as well.

In conclusion, it is important to remember that a complete history and physical examination of the patient with either localized or generalized edema may be enough to arrive at a likely diagnosis. It is of particular importance to focus on the renal, cardiovascular, and gastrointestinal systems when searching for an etiology for generalized edema. Commonly, patients presenting with symptoms of localized edema will have an allergic, traumatic, or infectious etiology and, with appropriate management, will have resolution of their symptoms without serious sequelae.

Suggested Readings and Key References

Braamskamp MJ, Dolman KM, Tabbers MM. Clinical practice. Protein-losing enteropathy in children. *Eur J Pediatr* 2010;169:1179–1185.

Hsu DT, Pearson GD. Heart failure in children: Part I: history, etiology, and pathophysiology. *Circ Heart Fail* 2009;2:63–70.

Katz BZ. Epstein-Barr virus infections. In: Long SS, Pickering LK, Prober CG, eds. *Principles and practice of pediatric infectious disease,* 3rd ed. New York, NY: Churchill Livingstone, 2008: 1036–1044.

Kidney Disease: Improving Global Outcomes (KDIGO) Glomerulonephritis Work Group. KDIGO Clinical Practice Guideline for Glomerulonephritis. *Kidney Inter* 2012;2:139–274.

Rockson SG. Lymphedema. *Am J Med* 2001;110:288–295.

Sardana N, Craig TJ. Recent advances in management and treatment of hereditary angioedema. *Pediatrics* 2011;128:1173–1180.

WHO. *Guideline: Updates on the management of severe acute malnutrition in infants and children.* Geneva: World Health Organization, 2013.

CHAPTER 21 ■ EPISTAXIS

EVA M. DELGADO, MD AND FRANCES M. NADEL, MD, MSCE

Epistaxis (nose bleeding) is a common symptom in young children and may be alarming to parents who often overestimate the amount of blood loss. It is usually noted first at about age 3 years and increases in frequency until peaking before or in adolescence. An orderly approach to the history and physical examination is necessary to identify the small minority of patients who require emergent hemorrhage control, laboratory investigation, or consultation with an otorhinolaryngologist (ORL) for further management.

PATHOPHYSIOLOGY

Minor trauma, nasal inflammation, desiccation, and congestion, as well as the rich vascular supply of the nose, contribute to the frequency of nosebleeds in otherwise normal children. The nose is a favored site for recurrent minor trauma, especially habitual, often absent-minded picking. The nasal mucosa is closely applied to the perichondrium and periosteum of the nasal septum and lateral nasal walls giving little structural support to its supply of small blood vessels. These vessels join to form plexiform networks like Kiesselbach plexus in Little's Area of the anterior nasal septum, about 0.5 cm from the tip of the nose and a frequent source of epistaxis blood (see Fig. 126.9).

DIFFERENTIAL DIAGNOSIS

Local Causes

Epistaxis is most often the result of local inflammation, irritation, infection, or trauma (Table 21.1). The most common causes of epistaxis are found in Table 21.2. Acute upper respiratory infections, whether localized as in colds or secondary to more generalized infections such as measles, infectious mononucleosis, or influenza-like illnesses, contribute to the onset of epistaxis. Nasal colonization with *Staphylococcus aureus* may predispose to a more friable mucosa and to furuncles, both of which can cause epistaxis. Allergic rhinitis may also be a factor. *Rhinitis sicca* refers to desiccation of the nasal mucosa, often occurs in cold winter climates with low ambient humidity prompting the use of dry hot-air heating systems, and increases the risk of epistaxis. Rhinitis sicca is also important to consider in the differential of a child with dependence on any respiratory device that instills dry air into the nares such as nasal cannula, nasal BiPAP, or other similar systems.

Inspection may reveal a nasal foreign body, which is sometimes suspected by history of insertion or by reports of chronic or recurrent unilateral epistaxis accompanied by a mucopurulent drainage or foul breath. Also discoverable by examination are telangiectasias (Osler–Weber–Rendu disease), hemangiomas, or evidence of other uncommon tumors that cause nosebleeds. Juvenile nasopharyngeal angiofibromas may be seen in adolescent boys with nasal obstruction, mucopurulent discharge, and severe epistaxis. These benign tumors may bulge into the nasal cavity, sometimes causing problems by invading adjacent structures. A rare childhood malignant tumor, nasopharyngeal lymphoepithelioma, may cause a syndrome of epistaxis, torticollis, trismus, and unilateral cervical lymphadenopathy. Other rare local causes of epistaxis include nasal diphtheria and Wegener granulomatosis.

Systemic Causes

Children rarely present with a nosebleed as their only manifestation of a more systemic disease, though there are several conditions that can increase the risk for epistaxis (Table 21.1). In children with severe or recurrent nosebleeds, a concerning family history, or constitutional signs and symptoms, the physician should consider a systemic process. Von Willebrand disease and platelet dysfunction are two of the more common systemic diseases that cause recurrent or severe nosebleeds. Less common systemic factors include hematologic diseases such as leukemia, hemophilia, and clotting disorders associated with severe hepatic dysfunction or uremia. Arterial hypertension rarely is a cause of epistaxis in children. Increased nasal venous pressure secondary to paroxysmal coughing, which can occur in pertussis or cystic fibrosis, occasionally may cause nosebleeds. *Vicarious menstruation* refers to a condition occasionally found in adolescent girls in whom monthly epistaxis related to vascular congestion of the nasal mucosa occurs concordant with menses and is presumably related to cyclic changes in hormone levels. Nosebleeds in infants, especially preambulatory children, are rare, and one should consider the possibility of child abuse or some systemic disorder.

EVALUATION AND DECISION

Rarely are nosebleeds in children life-threatening or require more than simple measures to gain control of hemorrhage. However, one's evaluation should begin with hemorrhage control and identification of children who are unstable by noting alterations in the patient's general appearance, vital signs, airway, color, and mental status. Steady pressure and efforts to calm the family often provide sufficient treatment. The child can sit on a parent's lap with the head tilted slightly forward and using some distraction such as a toy or video while the adult provides pressure to the anterior nose for 5 to 10 minutes to achieve hemostasis. This is usually effective since most bleeding in children is from the anterior nasal septum, but may be helped by the use of a cotton (dental) roll under the upper lip to compress the labial artery. The addition

TABLE 21.1

DIFFERENTIAL DIAGNOSIS OF EPISTAXIS

Local predisposing factors
Trauma, direct and picking
Local inflammation
Acute viral upper respiratory tract infection (common cold)
Bacterial rhinitis/sinusitis
Congenital syphilis
β-Hemolytic streptococcus
Foreign body
Acute systemic illnesses accompanied by nasal congestion, measles, infectious mononucleosis, acute rheumatic fever
Allergic rhinitis
Nasal polyps (cystic fibrosis, allergic, generalized)
Staphylococcal furuncle
Vascular malformations (telangiectasias as in Osler–Weber–Rendu disease, hemangiomas)
Juvenile angiofibroma[a]
Other tumors, granulomatosis, ectopic nasal tooth (rare)[a]
Rhinitis sicca
Systemic predisposing factors
Hematologic diseases[a]
Platelet disorders
Quantitative: idiopathic thrombocytopenic purpura, leukemia, aplastic anemia
Qualitative: von Willebrand disease, Glanzmann disease, uremia
Hemophilias
Clotting disorders associated with severe hepatic disease, disseminated intravascular coagulation (DIC), vitamin K deficiency
Drugs: aspirin, nonsteroidal anti-inflammatory drugs (NSAIDs), warfarin, valproic acid rodenticide
Vicarious menstruation
Hypertension[a]
Arterial (unusual cause of epistaxis in children)
Venous: superior vena cava syndrome or with paroxysmal coughing seen in pertussis and cystic fibrosis

[a]Life-threatening condition.

of cotton pledgets moistened with a few drops of epinephrine (1:1,000) or application of topical thrombin will occasionally be required to help achieve hemostasis. Nasal packing or the use of expandable nasal tampons can help in severe epistaxis, as can cautery of an anterior bleeding site with a silver nitrate stick (see Chapter 141 Procedures sections on Nasal Cauterization and Nasal Packing—Anterior and Posterior). Patients who require nasal tampons face the risk of toxic shock syndrome and so need ORL follow-up. More severe epistaxis may require surgical or angiographic intervention.

TABLE 21.2

COMMON CAUSES OF EPISTAXIS

Trauma
Foreign body
Allergic rhinitis
Rhinitis sicca
Viral rhinitis

While working to control bleeding, one should also seek its origin. A posterior bleed is important to identify since these bleeds are often harder to control and warrant more intensive therapy. Blood seen in the oropharynx, blood in both nares, difficulty controlling bleeding despite adequate anterior pressure, and a normal anterior examination are more characteristic of a posterior nasal bleed but can be found with an anterior causative site. Bleeding seen at any site in a child who has undergone tonsillectomy and/or adenoidectomy in the preceding 1 to 2 weeks is concerning and should prompt immediate evaluation by ORL (see Chapter 126 ENT Emergencies). Patients with hemorrhagic diathesis will require correction of their underlying disorder in addition to procedural approaches described above to achieve hemostasis.

After treating any emergent problems, the evaluation should then proceed with a thorough history. One should elicit frequency of nosebleeds, degree of difficulty in achieving hemostasis, frequency of upper respiratory infections and/or allergic discharge, symptoms of obstruction, and contributing factors such as recurrent trauma from nose picking or other cause. Often asking children which finger they pick their nose with will elicit a more honest answer. Other symptoms sometimes reported are sequelae of swallowed blood such as hematemesis or melena. Since the differential diagnosis for these conditions includes systemic hemorrhagic disorders, one should elicit further history including family history of bleeding. Menstrual history and any relation to epistaxis in adolescent girls is worth noting.

Physical examination must include a complete general examination with special attention paid to vital signs, including heart rate and blood pressure, evidence of hematologic disease (enlarged nodes, organomegaly, petechiae, or pallor), and inspection of the nasal cavity after reasonable efforts to stop the bleeding. To facilitate the nasal examination, ask the child to blow his nose or use suction to clear the nares. Using one's thumb, the tip of the nose is pushed upward to allow examination of the vestibule, the anterior portion of the septum, and anterior portion of the inferior turbinate in search of the site of bleeding, mucosal color, excoriations, discharge, foreign body or other mass, or septal hematoma. A good light source, body fluid precautions, and in some cases, a topical vasoconstrictor or decongestant can help. A more thorough examination requires the use of a nasal speculum, which when passed vertically into the nares and opened, allows examination of the septum, turbinates, and middle meatus. A topical anesthetic, involvement of a child life specialist, anxiolytic medications, or restraints may be necessary for such an examination in young children.

No laboratory workup is indicated in children without clinical evidence of severe blood loss, in whom systemic factors are not suspected, and for whom an anterior site of bleeding is identified and stopped readily with local pressure. Reassurance and education about appropriate at-home management needs to be provided. Home therapies may include use of a cool mist vaporizer to lessen rhinitis sicca. An emollient, such as petroleum jelly or a topical antibiotic cream, placed in the nostrils twice daily, and saline nasal spray also are useful for maintaining normal moistness of the nasal mucosa. Instructing parents

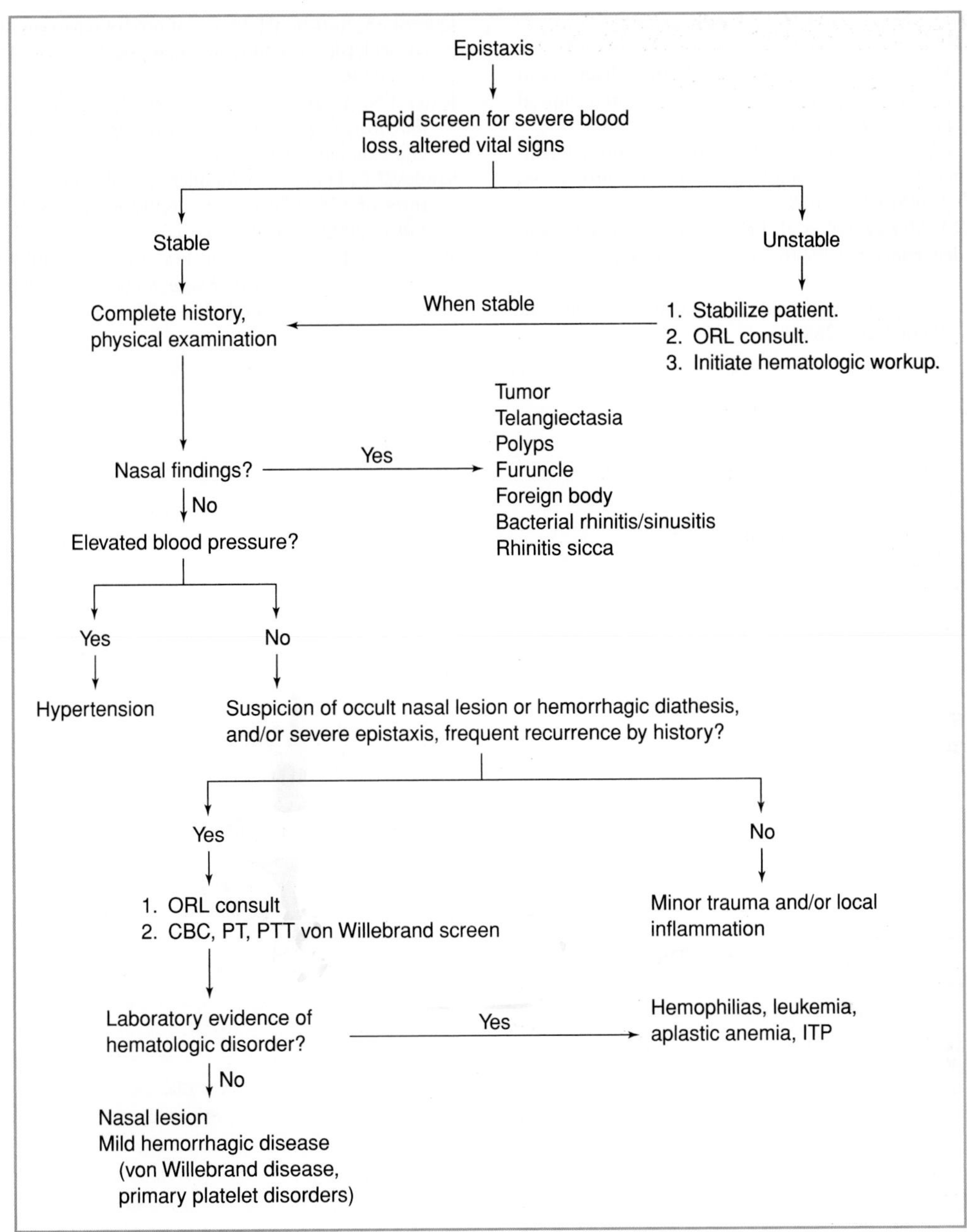

FIGURE 21.1 Approach to diagnosis of epistaxis. ORL, otorhinolaryngologist; CBC, complete blood count; PT, prothrombin time; PTT, partial thromboplastin time; ITP, idiopathic thrombocytopenic purpura.

to keep the child's fingernails short is also helpful. Occasionally, recurrent epistaxis during an acute upper respiratory infection or flare-up of allergic rhinitis may be lessened with use of an antihistamine–decongestant preparation, although care must be taken not to dry the nose excessively. Potential side effects of these combination products argue against their use in children younger than 6 years.

Evaluation for hemorrhagic diathesis should be performed in any child with pertinent positive findings on history, family history, or physical examination. This usually would include prothrombin time, partial thromboplastin time, complete blood cell count, and screening study for von Willebrand disease. Although the yield would be low in the absence of corroborative clinical features, some children with isolated epistaxis that is severe or frequently recurrent might also deserve such screening. They may have mild bleeding abnormalities and a referral to a pediatric hematologist may be helpful. Certain medications, such as valproate, have been associated with epistaxis. These considerations are outlined in the epistaxis algorithm (Fig. 21.1).

All patients discharged from the emergency department (ED) after evaluation for significant epistaxis should be given specific instructions on nares compression and indications for repeat evaluation. For patients with specific local abnormalities, such as tumors, polyps, or telangiectasias, referral to an ORL is necessary. Such referral might also be considered, even with questionable findings on the ED nasal examination, if bleeding was severe, recurrent, or suspected to be posterior in origin. When epistaxis is noted in patients with a recent tonsillectomy/adenoidectomy, the otolaryngologist should be involved in the child's care before determining if it is safe to discharge them home.

Suggested Readings and Key References

Elden L, Reinders M, Witmer C. Predictors of bleeding disorders in children with epistaxis: value of preoperative tests and clinical screening. *Int J Pediatr Otorhinolaryngol* 2012;76(6):767–771.

McIntosh N, Mok JY, Margerison A. Epidemiology of oronasal hemorrhage in the first 2 years of life: implications for child protection. *Pediatrics* 2007;120(5):1074–1078.

Pallin DJ, Chng YM, McKay MP, et al. Epidemiology of epistaxis in US emergency departments, 1992 to 2001. *Ann Emerg Med* 2005; 46(1):77–81.

Pimpinella RJ. The nasopharyngeal angiofibroma in the adolescent male. *J Pediatr* 1964;64:260–267.

Qureishi A, Burton MJ. Interventions for recurrent idiopathic epistaxis (nosebleeds) in children. *Cochrane Database Syst Rev* 2012;(9): CD004461.

Ritter FN. Vicarious menstruation. In: Strome M, ed. *Differential diagnosis in pediatric otolaryngology.* Boston, MA: Little, Brown and Company, 1975:216.

Sandoval C, Dong S, Visintainer P, et al. Clinical and laboratory features of 178 children with recurrent epistaxis. *J Pediatr Hematol Oncol* 2002;24(1):47–49.

Whymark AD, Crampsey DP, Fraser L, et al. Childhood epistaxis and nasal colonization with *Staphylococcus aureus. Otolaryngol Head Neck Surg* 2008;138(3):307–310.

CHAPTER 22 ▪ EYE: RED EYE

ATIMA C. DELANEY, MD AND ALEX V. LEVIN, MD, MHSc, FRCSC

"Red eye" is a generic term that refers to any condition in which the "white of the eye" appears red or pink. A red eye may be caused by local factors, intraocular disease, or systemic problems. Tables 22.1, 22.2, and 22.3 list common and life-threatening causes of red eye. The cause of a red eye can often be identified by the history alone. The history should include the presence or absence of pain, foreign-body sensation, itching, discharge, tearing, photophobia, onset, visual disturbances, recent illnesses, and trauma. The examination should include visual acuity, pupil shape and reactivity, the gross appearance of the sclera and conjunctiva, extraocular muscle function, and palpation of preauricular nodes. The evaluation often requires fluorescein staining and slit lamp examination by an experienced provider.

Discussion here, of chemical conjunctivitis or irritation caused by agents such as smoke or trauma, is limited because the history often makes the diagnosis clear. The management of these disorders is discussed in Chapters 122 Ocular Trauma and 131 Ophthalmic Emergencies.

PATHOPHYSIOLOGY

The term *conjunctivitis* should be reserved for disorders in which the conjunctiva is inflamed. Inflammation may be caused by direct irritation, infection, abnormalities of underlying or contiguous structures (e.g., cornea), immune phenomena, or processes secondary to abnormalities of the lid and lashes. Inflammation within the anterior chamber affecting the iris (iritis) may also result in secondary inflammation of the conjunctiva.

The sclera may become inflamed (scleritis). An intermediate layer, the episclera, lies beneath the conjunctiva's substantia propria and another largely avascular fascial layer (Tenon's fascia), where it is firmly attached to the sclera. The episclera is more vascularized than the sclera and may become inflamed either in a diffuse or localized fashion (diffuse, sectorial, or nodular episcleritis).

A tear film, which prevents desiccation, is constantly present over the surface of the eye. A disruption in the function of the anatomic structures of the tear film may cause desiccation of the ocular surface, resulting in irritation and inflammation (dry eye syndrome).

Innervation of the conjunctiva and cornea comes from the first division of the trigeminal nerve (V1). Abnormalities on the ocular surface may give rise to pain or a foreign-body sensation. The reflex arc that involves the afferent trigeminal nerve and the efferent facial nerve results in a rapid blink, with contraction of the orbicularis oculi muscle, to protect the surface of the eye in response to noxious stimuli. Two other reactions to noxious stimuli may occur: tearing and discharge. Tearing (epiphora) may accompany virtually any conjunctival inflammation or irritation. Tearing may even be a part of some forms of dry eye syndrome, as the lacrimal gland attempts to compensate for ocular surface. Discharge from the eye results either from conjunctival exudation or precipitation of mucus out of the tear film. The latter occurs when the tear film is not flowing smoothly (e.g., nasolacrimal duct obstruction), causing misinterpretation as infection when the problem is actually mechanical. Although discharge may be a nonspecific finding, the nature of the discharge may be helpful in the cause of an inflammation or infection. The presence of membranes or pseudomembranes (Fig. 22.1) is more common with adenovirus infection or Stevens–Johnson syndrome. These white or white–yellow plaques are caused by loosely or firmly adherent collections of inflammatory cells, cellular debris, and exudate.

EVALUATION AND DECISION

The approach to the child who presents in the emergency department with a red eye is outlined in the flowchart shown in Figure 22.2.

Any child who wears contact lenses regularly, even if the lens is not in the eye at the time of the examination, should be referred to an ophthalmologist within 12 hours if he or she has red eye. Red, and often painful, eyes of a person who wears contact lenses may represent potentially blinding corneal infection (corneal ulcer) or the breakdown of the corneal epithelium, which would predispose the person to subsequent corneal infection. Other than removing the contact lens when possible (topical anesthesia may be helpful), further diagnostic or therapeutic interventions by the pediatric emergency physician are not indicated in these patients without direct consultation with an ophthalmologist. Decisions regarding starting empiric antibiotics should be made with an ophthalmologist, as there may be benefit to waiting until corneal cultures can be obtained. The presence of a white spot on the cornea of a contact lens wearer with inflamed conjunctiva is an ominous sign that may represent an ulcer. The absence of such a spot does not rule out corneal ulcer. Other causes of red eye in a contact lens wearer include contact lens solution allergy (which may develop even after years of using the same regimen), overwearing of contact lenses, overly tight fit, foreign body, or a damaged contact lens. Examination by an ophthalmologist is perhaps the only way to ensure that a corneal ulcer is not missed by ascribing the red eye to one of these other etiologies. It is therefore recommended that all contact lens wearers with a red eye be seen by an ophthalmologist.

Numerous systemic diseases may be associated with ocular inflammation. A representative sample can be found in Table 22.3. In some systemic diseases, the associated ocular abnormality involves intraocular inflammation (iritis, vitritis), which can then cause secondary conjunctival infection or inflammation. Patients with these diseases may also have coincidental ocular inflammation unrelated to their underlying conditions. Ophthalmology consultation may be helpful

TABLE 22.1

COMMON CAUSES OF RED EYE[a]

Conjunctivitis
Infectious: Viral (including herpes), bacterial, chlamydial
Allergic or seasonal
Chemical (or other physical agents such as smoke)
Systemic disease (Table 22.3)
Trauma
Corneal or conjunctival abrasion
Iritis
Foreign body
Subconjuctival hemorrhage
Dry eye syndromes
Abnormalities of the lids and/or lashes
Blepharitis
Trichiasis due to epiblepharon
Stye or chalazion (external or internal hordeolum)
Molluscum of lid margin
Periorbital or orbital cellulitis
Contact lens–related problems
Infectious keratitis (corneal ulcer)
Allergic conjunctivitis
Corneal abrasion
Poor fit
Overwear

[a]Not listed in order of frequency. List not complete.

in making this distinction. For example, in Kawasaki disease, the inflammation of the conjunctiva may be associated with mild iritis. More often, the conjunctiva is inflamed in isolation as part of the systemic mucous membrane involvement. The conjunctivitis of Kawasaki disease is usually confined to the bulbar conjunctiva, often with limbal sparing (Fig. 22.3), with little or no discharge. In contrast, the bulbar and palpebral conjunctiva are inflamed in infectious conjunctivitis (Fig. 131.7).

Direct ocular trauma may result in a red eye due to corneal or conjunctival abrasion, hyphema, iritis, or rarely, traumatic glaucoma (see Chapter 122 Ocular Trauma). If there is no fluorescein staining of the conjunctiva or cornea and there is no obvious evidence of severe intraocular injury (e.g., hyphema, ruptured globe), the examiner may need to consider the possibility of noxious material coming in contact with the eyeball at the

TABLE 22.2

LIFE-THREATENING CAUSES OF RED EYE[a]

Systemic disease (Table 22.3)
Child abuse
Blunt trauma
Covert instillation of noxious substances (medical child abuse [Munchausen syndrome by proxy])
Traumatic intracranial arteriovenous fistula (very rare)

[a]List not meant to be complete.

TABLE 22.3

SYSTEMIC CONDITIONS THAT MAY BE ASSOCIATED WITH RED EYE[a]

Collagen vascular disorders
Juvenile rheumatoid arthritis
Infectious diseases
Varicella, rubeola, otitis media
Kawasaki disease
Inflammatory bowel disease
Cystic fibrosis
Vitamin A deficiency
Cystinosis
Leukemia
Ectodermal dysplasia
Trisomy 21
Cornelia de Lange syndrome
Status postradiation therapy, including ocular field
Bone marrow transplantation
Stevens–Johnson syndrome

[a]Not a complete list: Intended to demonstrate multiorgan representation.

time of trauma. Both acidic and alkaline substances may cause a red eye (see Chapter 131 Ophthalmic Emergencies). Likewise, a foreign body may cause ocular pain and inflammation. Foreign bodies often can be difficult to see on brief, superficial examination, especially if the foreign body is smaller than what the naked eye can see. To enhance visualization, spin the focusing wheel of a direct ophthalmoscope to the black or green number 10 or more. This will turn the instrument into a self-illuminated handheld magnifier. All the recesses and redundant folds of the conjunctiva must be inspected. The upper eyelid should be everted (see Chapter 122 Ocular Trauma). The lower eyelid should be pulled down from the globe as the patient looks upward so the inferior fornix can be inspected. The patient should be asked to adduct the affected eye when the lateral canthus (junction of the upper and lower eyelid laterally) is stretched laterally to allow inspection of the lateral fornix. There is no analogous medial fornix. In addition to direct trauma, head injury can rarely cause the development

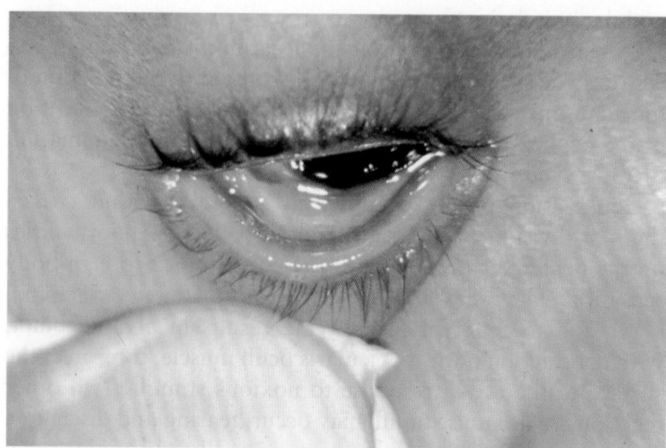

FIGURE 22.1 Pseudomembrane on lower lid palpebral conjunctiva and extending into the inferior fornix in patient with epidemic keratoconjunctivitis (adenovirus).

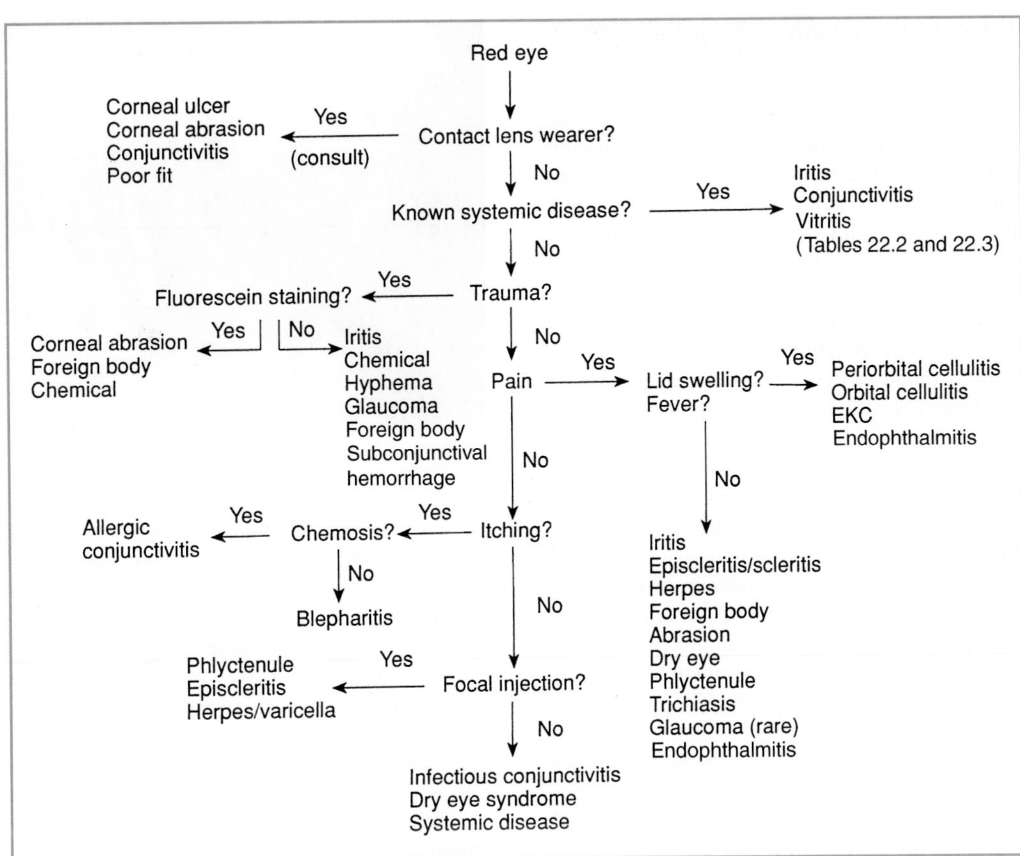

FIGURE 22.2 Diagnostic evaluation of red eye. EKC, epidemic keratoconjunctivitis.

of an intracranial arteriovenous fistula that may present with proptosis, chemosis, red eye, corkscrew conjunctival blood vessels, and decreased vision.

It is wise to inspect the position of the eyelashes before performing lid eversion and examining the conjunctival fornices. Eyelashes that turn against the ocular surface (trichiasis) may cause a red eye that is accompanied by pain or foreign-body sensation in the absence of lid swelling. Although corneal fluorescein staining may reveal the effect on the corneal epithelium, the condition may be so mild that it would only be detected by slit lamp biomicroscopy despite significant symptoms. Trichiasis is particularly common in patients who have had prior injury or surgery to the eyelid and in patients of Asian background. In the latter case, a prominent fold of skin (epiblepharon) may be found medially just below the eyelid margin, causing the lower lid medial eyelashes, and less commonly the upper lid lashes, to rotate toward the eyeball.

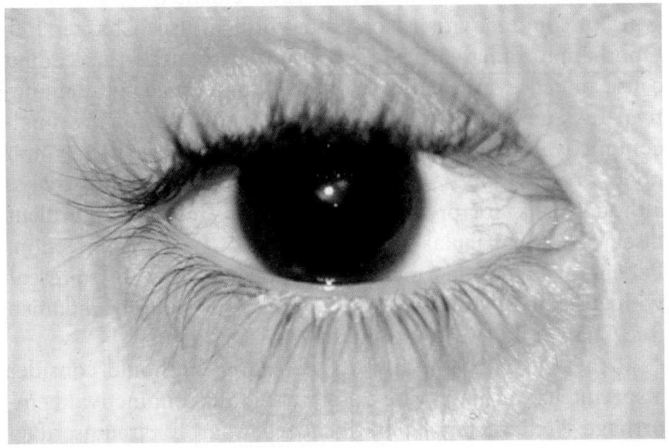

FIGURE 22.3 Bulbar conjunctival injection in patient with Kawasaki disease.

In the absence of cornea/conjunctiva abrasion, foreign body, and trichiasis, the painful red eye caused by trauma may have iritis. This may not present for up to 72 hours after the trauma. Photophobia and vision blurring may also occur. The ipsilateral pupil may be smaller. Occasionally, one will see a cloudy inferior cornea caused by the deposition of inflammatory cells and debris on the inner surface (keratoprecipitates). This finding may be easier to recognize with the direct ophthalmoscope focused as a magnifier (see above). Hypopyon, layered pus or white cells in anterior chamber, may be seen in extremely severe iritis. Iritis may also occur in association with systemic disease or as an isolated idiopathic ocular finding. Iritis associated with juvenile idiopathic arthritis (formerly known as juvenile rheumatoid arthritis) is characterized by the distinct absence of signs or symptoms until the disease has progressed significantly, thus underscoring the need for routine screening of these patients. Other systemic causes of iritis include sarcoidosis, tuberculosis, inflammatory bowel disease, collagen vascular disorders, systemic lupus erythematosis, Wegener's, tubular interstitial nephritis uveitis (TINU) syndrome, and leukemia. Traumatic iritis and nontraumatic iritis often are indistinguishable except by history. All causes of iritis, regardless of the etiology, require ophthalmologic consultation and follow-up. The diagnosis of iritis requires slit lamp examination by a skilled provider. Prescription of topical steroids should be reserved for ophthalmologists.

Episcleritis and scleritis may also cause a painful red eye. Episcleritis is more commonly seen in young adults while scleritis occurs more commonly in adult females. Although episcleritis is usually an isolated, self-limited ocular abnormality, scleritis is often associated with an underlying systemic disease, particularly the collagen vascular disorders. Both entities may present with focal or diffuse inflammation. A focal nodular or diffuse elevation may be seen. The eye is often tender, especially with scleritis, where the inflamed area may have a bluish hue. There may also be pain on attempted movement of the eye. Scleritis is much less common than conjunctivitis and episcleritis. Diagnosis and treatment require slit lamp examination and ophthalmologic consultation.

Herpetic corneal infection is another cause of painful red eye. This may be caused by either the simplex or varicella-zoster viruses. Usually, there are no concomitant lesions except in association with chickenpox, when a unilateral or bilateral lesion may be seen on the conjunctiva (usually near or just on the edge of the cornea) with focal injection. Most often, no treatment is required for a conjunctival pox lesion, but herpetic corneal ulcers require urgent treatment to prevent corneal scarring and vision loss (see Chapter 131 Ophthalmic Emergencies). Patients with herpetic corneal ulcers may have a history of prior recurrent painful red eye, although herpes occasionally can be painless because of induced corneal hypoesthesia. Herpes simplex is virtually always unilateral and sometimes associated with vesicles in the distribution of the ophthalmic branch of the trigeminal nerve, involving the forehead, periorbital area, and tip of the nose. Fluorescein staining of the cornea may reveal a linear branching pattern referred to as dendrites (Fig. 131.9).

If the infected area is located eccentrically on the corneal surface, the injection may be localized to the quadrant of conjunctiva adjacent to the lesion. If eye pain is relieved by a drop of topical anesthetic (see Chapter 122 Ocular Trauma), the patient most likely has a surface problem (e.g., foreign body, abrasion). If the pain is not relieved and periorbital swelling and fever are present, the red eye may be caused by periorbital or orbital cellulitis which are emergent conditions (see Chapter 131 Ophthalmic Emergencies). Eye pain and marked lid swelling also may be associated with epidemic keratoconjunctivitis (EKC) secondary to adenovirus (Fig. 131.7). When questioned further, patients may reveal that they actually have a sandy foreign-body sensation rather than true ocular pain. Pseudomembranes are a fairly diagnostic sign when present (Fig. 22.1). Low-grade fever and tender preauricular adenopathy may also occur, making it difficult to distinguish EKC from periorbital cellulitis. EKC usually affects the eyes consecutively and bilaterally as opposed to the unilateral nature of periorbital cellulitis. There also may be associated prominent photophobia and tearing in adenoviral conjunctivitis, which is not usually seen in cellulitis.

Itching is another important diagnostic symptom. When it is associated with swelling of the conjunctiva, giving it the appearance of a blister-like elevation (chemosis, Fig. 131.8), one should suspect acute allergic conjunctivitis. Unlike chronic, recurrent, seasonal, allergic conjunctivitis in which patients often have coexisting nonocular signs of seasonal allergy, there are usually no associated systemic symptoms. Acute chemosis is usually due to an exposure and occurs without systemic signs of allergy. Often, there is no known causative agent, and there may be associated periocular swelling. The condition may be unilateral or bilateral and usually has an acute or hyperacute onset. Photophobia, tearing, and lid swelling may also occur.

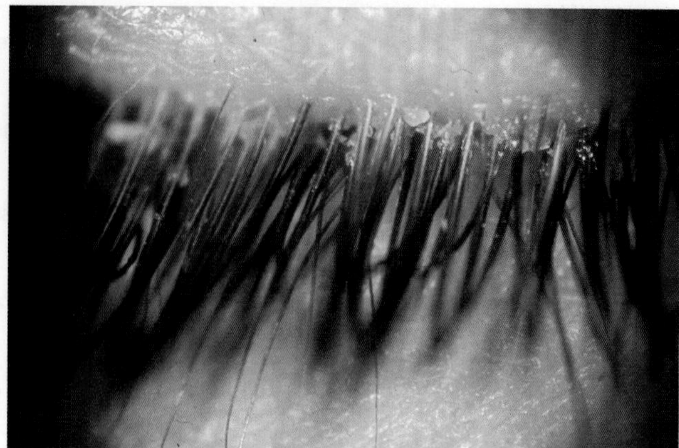

FIGURE 22.4 Blepharitis. Note crusts and flakes at base of eyelashes.

Itching may also accompany blepharitis, an idiopathic disorder in which there is suboptimal flow of secretions from the meibomian glands normally present in the eyelids resulting in an abnormal tear film and rapid corneal desiccation. Symptoms are aggravated by activities associated with prolonged staring and a decreased blink rate (reading, television or computer viewing, and video games) or going outside on windy days. Patients may have photophobia and a sandy foreign-body sensation. To compensate for the tear film deficiency, reflex excess tearing may occur from the lacrimal gland. The most characteristic sign is erythema of the eyelid margins and flaking and crusting at the base of the eyelashes (Fig. 22.4). This can be well visualized with the direct ophthalmoscope as a magnifier (see above). Left untreated, the reduced flow of the meibomian glands may allow for proliferation of the coagulase-negative staphylococci, which are normally present. This overgrowth may lead to an immune response causing an inflamed elevated white spot(s) on the conjunctiva (phlyctenule) or peripheral corneal infiltrates associated with a red eye. Slit lamp examination is helpful in making these diagnoses and is most helpful to rule out the presence of corneal involvement.

The absence of itching and pain should lead one to suspect an infectious cause of conjunctivitis. Conjunctivitis usually causes diffuse unilateral or bilateral inflammation of the conjunctiva, with rare exception (e.g., sectoral herpes keratitis). The differentiation of bacterial, viral, chlamydial, and other types of conjunctivitis is sometimes difficult (see Chapter 131 Ophthalmic Emergencies). Viral conjunctivitis is the leading cause of red eye in children. It is characterized by conjunctival hyperemia, a watery discharge, and occasionally small conjunctival hemorrhages. A palpable preauricular lymph node strongly supports the diagnosis of viral conjunctivitis, although it is not present in the majority of cases. Purulent discharge is particularly characteristic of bacterial infection. Patients with nasolacrimal duct obstruction can also present with discharge; however, the conjunctiva is rarely inflamed (see Chapter 131 Ophthalmic Emergencies).

If the injection is localized, the examiner should consider a specific list of diagnostic possibilities. Subconjunctival hemorrhage is characterized by localized, sharply circumscribed acute redness (Fig. 22.5). There is no pain, visual disturbance, or discharge. It is uncommon in children who do not have

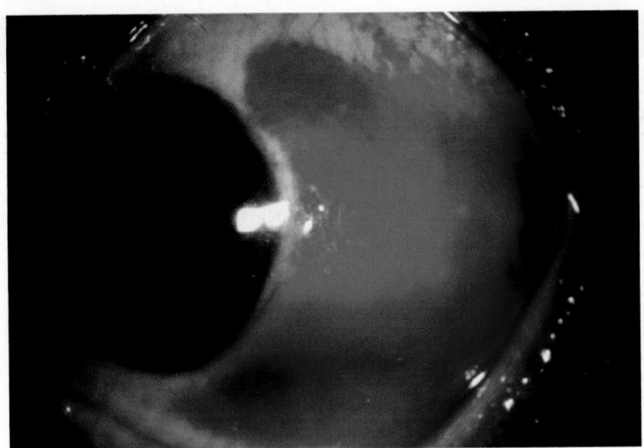

FIGURE 22.5 Subconjunctival hemorrhage. (From Rapuano CJ. Wills Eye Institute – Cornea. 2nd ed. Philadelphia, PA: Lippincott Williams & Wilkins, 2011.)

a history of a direct blow to the eye. Subconjunctival hemorrhage in a young child should evoke a workup coagulopathy, or the possibility of nonaccidental trauma or suffocation. Pertussis infection can result in 360-degree unilateral or even bilateral prominent subconjunctival hemorrhage, which is not expected to occur with other causes of cough. Conjunctival petechia can rarely be seen after strong Valsalva but usually with additional petechia elsewhere on the face. Herpes keratitis phlyctenule, episcleritis, and scleritis may present with focal involvement, as previously discussed. Localized injection of the conjunctiva may be an indicator of an embedded foreign body, varicella, or other focal processes that require the attention of an ophthalmologic consultant.

Acute acquired glaucoma causes a painful red eye, sometimes associated with corneal clouding and decreased visual acuity. Acquired glaucoma, is most often associated with trauma, other anatomic abnormalities, or iritis that would be apparent on examination. Because it is difficult to determine intraocular pressure in children, ophthalmologic consultation may be required if emergency medicine providers do not have experience with this procedure.

Suggested Readings and Key References

Greenberg MF, Pollard ZF. The red eye in childhood. *Pediatr Clin North Am* 2003;50:105–124.

Klig JE. Ophthalmic complications of systemic disease. *Emerg Med Clin North Am* 2008;26:217–231.

Leibowitz HM. The red eye. *N Engl J Med* 2000;343:345–351.

Mahmood AR, Narang AT. Diagnosis and management of the acute red eye. *Emerg Med Clin North Am* 2008;26:35–55.

Prentiss KA, Dorfman DH. Pediatric ophthalmology in the emergency department. *Emerg Med Clin North Am* 2008;26:181–198.

CHAPTER 23 ■ EYE: STRABISMUS

ATIMA C. DELANEY, MD AND ALEX V. LEVIN, MD, MHSc, FRCSC

Strabismus refers to any misalignment of the eyes such that they are not viewing in the same direction. *Esotropia* refers to eyes that are turned in (cross-eyed). *Exotropia* refers to eyes that are turned out (wall eyed). The terms *hypertropia* and *hypotropia* refer to a higher or lower eye, respectively. By convention, vertical misalignment of the eyes is always categorized by the higher eye (e.g., right hypertropia), unless it is known that a specific abnormal process is causing one eye to be held in a lower position (e.g., left hypotropia). Many children with strabismus require a formal evaluation by an ophthalmologist for definitive diagnosis and management, but the emergency physician should attempt to answer two questions: (1) "Is the strabismus an emergency?" and, if so, (2) "What is the most likely cause?"

PATHOPHYSIOLOGY

Six muscles surround each eyeball (Fig. 23.1). Although several of these muscles may individually move the eye in more than one direction, knowledge of the primary action of these muscles allows for the definition of diagnostic positions of gaze (Table 23.1). This can be helpful in pinpointing specific muscle dysfunction. For example, if a muscle that primarily governs abduction (e.g., lateral rectus) is impaired, the eye is unable to abduct and will usually lie in a position of adduction (esotropia). Likewise, if a muscle that is involved with downward gaze (e.g., inferior rectus) is impaired, the eye will have a tendency to remain in relative upward gaze (ipsilateral hypertropia).

Strabismus is categorized into misalignment as a result of impaired muscle function or misalignment in the presence of full-normal muscle function. In general, there are only two emergent reasons why the function of a particular muscle might be impaired: Neurogenic palsy or muscle restriction.

Three cranial nerves are responsible for the innervation of the six extraocular muscles (Table 23.1). The sixth cranial nerve innervates the ipsilateral lateral rectus muscle. This nerve exits the ventral pons and then travels on the wall of the middle cranial fossa (clivus), reaching the sphenoid ridge, along which it travels until entering the cavernous sinus. The course of this nerve allows it to be injured by vascular or neoplastic changes in the midbrain, increased intracranial pressure (ICP), large anterior midline craniofacial tumors (e.g., nasopharyngeal carcinoma), otitis media (OM) with involvement of the petrous portion of the sphenoid (Gradenigo syndrome), and any abnormality that involves the cavernous sinus. An abnormality of the sixth cranial nerve will cause a reduction in ipsilateral abduction (Fig. 23.2) resulting in a possible ipsilateral esotropia.

The fourth cranial nerve innervates the superior oblique muscle. It is the only cranial nerve that completely decussates and has a dorsal projection over the midbrain. This position renders the fourth cranial nerve particularly vulnerable to blunt head trauma, one of the most common causes of fourth nerve palsy. The fourth cranial nerve also has a relatively long intracranial course, which makes it particularly susceptible to increased ICP and parenchymal shifts caused by cerebral edema. It also runs through the cavernous sinus. Fourth cranial nerve palsy may be congenital but asymptomatic for several years during childhood until the brain is no longer able to compensate. Acquired or congenital palsy of this cranial nerve causes the eyes to become misaligned vertically (ipsilateral hypertropia). Patients with congenital fourth cranial nerve paresis compensate by tilting their head to the ipsilateral side, which allows for a rebalancing of the eye muscles such that alignment may be achieved. Old photographs may demonstrate this tilt. Facial asymmetry can also be seen after years of this compensatory tilting. Ophthalmic consultation is usually needed to differentiate between congenital and acquired palsy.

The third cranial nerve supplies the remaining four extraocular muscles. It is involved with downgaze, upgaze, and adduction. Parasympathetic innervation to the pupil (see Chapter 24 Eye: Unequal Pupils) and innervation to the eyelid muscle (levator palpebrae) are also carried in the third cranial nerve. A complete third cranial nerve palsy results in an eye that is positioned down (from the remaining action of the unaffected superior oblique muscle) and out (from the remaining action of the unaffected lateral rectus muscle) with ipsilateral ptosis and ipsilateral pupillary dilation (Fig. 23.3). Because the third cranial nerve divides into a superior and an inferior division just as it enters the orbit from the cavernous sinus and because the fibers to individual muscles are segregated within the nerve throughout its course, partial third cranial nerve palsies may occur with or without ptosis and/or pupillary dilation. This may leave the patient with complex strabismus, which is best left to the ophthalmology consultant. The differential diagnosis of third cranial nerve palsies is summarized in Chapter 24 Eye: Unequal Pupils.

The action of a muscle may also be impaired by restriction. The muscle can become infiltrated with substances that might restrict its action or cause fibrosis. Children with hyperthyroid eye disease (e.g., Graves) can have large, tight eye muscles. An eyeball may also be restricted in its movements by tumors or infection in and around the globe. Orbital tumors, cellulitis, or abscesses that cause restriction may be associated with proptosis or a displacement of the entire eyeball, either vertically or horizontally. After blunt trauma to the eyeball, the globe may be translocated posteriorly, causing an increased intraorbital pressure that may result in a "blowout" fracture of the bony orbital wall. When an orbital wall fracture occurs, the muscle or surrounding tissues that run along that wall may become entrapped within that fracture, tethering the eyeball so the eye cannot look in the direction opposite the fracture. Children with orbital floor or medial orbital wall fracture are

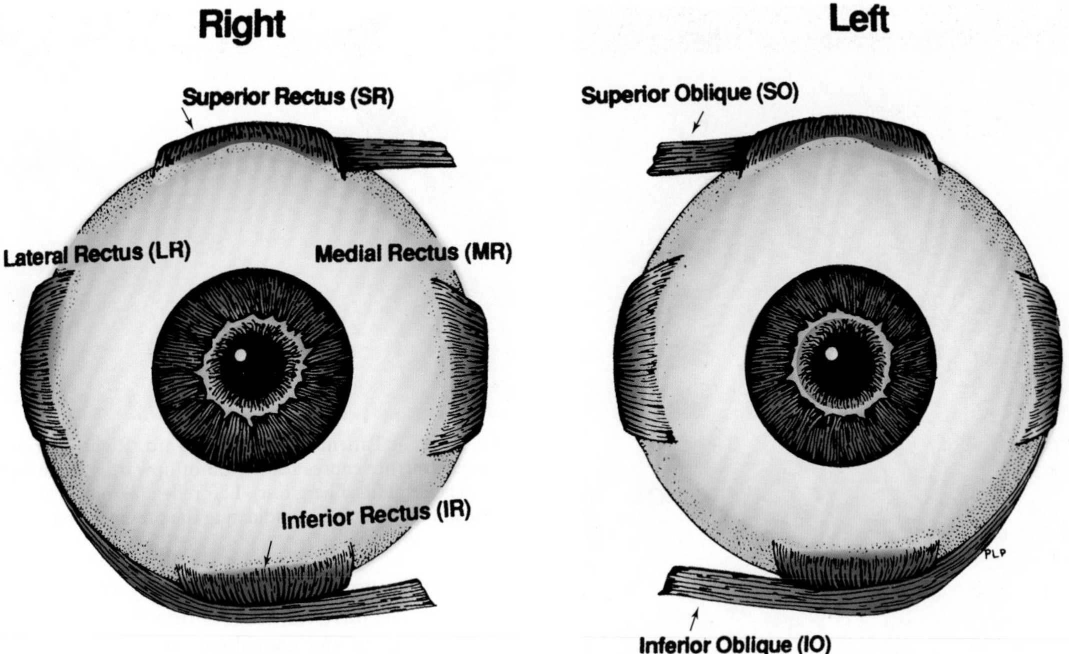

FIGURE 23.1 Normal extraocular muscle anatomy.

prone to entrapment of the inferior or medial rectus muscles, respectively. This may not be noticeable until eye movements are attempted. For example, fractures of the orbital floor may entrap the inferior rectus muscle, tethering the eye downward so upgaze is restricted (Fig. 23.4). Less commonly, the eye may have a limitation of movement in the direction of the fracture. Orbital wall fractures may also be associated with enophthalmos, in which the eye appears to be sunken in the orbit, or proptosis caused by orbital hemorrhage. All patients with orbital fractures must receive a complete ophthalmic examination to rule out accompanying ocular injury. The most common fracture involves the inferior and/or medial walls of the orbit. The lateral wall is rarely fractured. Fracture of the superior wall (orbital roof) is particularly worrisome because it may allow communication between the orbit and the subfrontal intracranial space.

The remaining types of strabismus fall into the category where eye muscle function is unimpaired (nonrestrictive and nonparalytic). These problems are not emergent. The eyes may be misaligned as a result of failure of the brain to use both eyes simultaneously in a coordinated fashion (idiopathic), a need for glasses, or the presence of poor vision in one eye. Uncorrected farsightedness (hyperopia) can result in accommodative esotropia, which may have an acute onset, usually between the ages of 2 and 6 years, with the misalignment often worse at near viewing. Uncorrected nearsightedness (myopia) can result in exotropia, especially when the patient views in the far distance. Both types of misalignment may be treated with glasses.

Checking the vision in both eyes (see Chapter 131 Ophthalmic Emergencies) is essential in all cases of strabismus with full eye movements to rule out the presence of uncorrected refractive error or a poorly seeing eye. The latter may be due to serious eye problems such as retinoblastoma or cataract. Strabismus is the second most common presenting sign of retinoblastoma after leukocoria.

TABLE 23.1

EXTRAOCULAR MUSCLES

Muscle[a]	Cranial nerve	Action[b]	Eye position in palsy
Medial rectus	III (inferior division)	Adduction	Exotropia
Inferior rectus	III (inferior division)	Downward gaze	Hypertropia
Lateral rectus	VI	Abduction	Esotropia
Superior rectus	III (superior division)	Upward gaze	Hypotropia
Superior oblique	IV	Downward gaze	Hypertropia
Levator palpebrae[c]	III (superior division)	Eyelid	Ptosis (lid)

[a]Inferior oblique not included for simplicity. Isolated palsy of the inferior oblique is extremely rare.
[b]Action in the horizontal or vertical field only. Cyclorotatory movements not included.
[c]By definition, not truly an extraocular muscle.

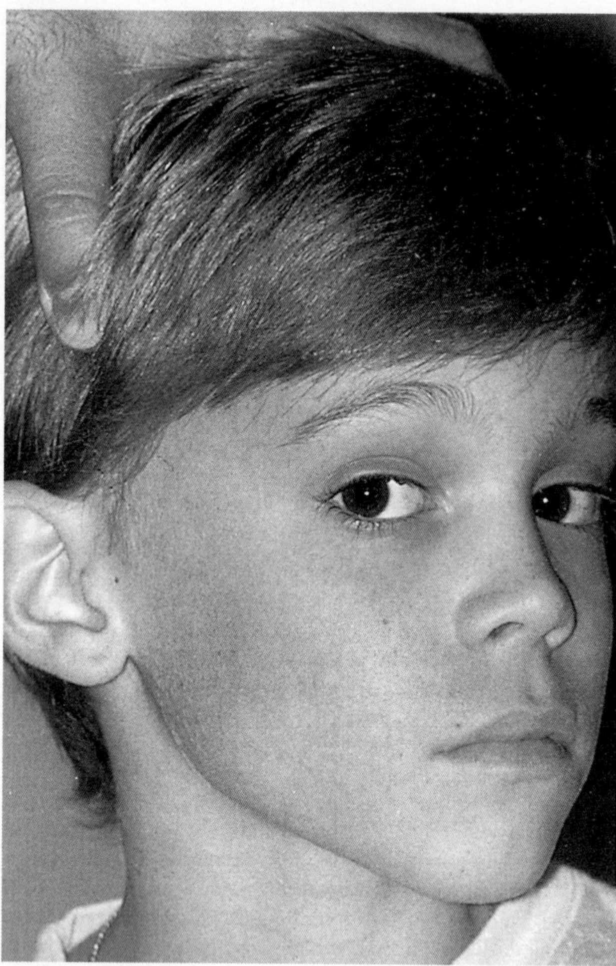

FIGURE 23.2 Patient's head is being rotated passively to patient's left as he looks straight ahead. This causes displacement of eyes into right gaze. Left eye adducts fully, showing no visible sclera medially. Subtle right sixth nerve palsy demonstrated by failure of right eye to abduct fully: Sclera is still visible laterally on right eye.

EVALUATION AND DECISION

The history should include period of onset, progression, duration and severity, family history of strabismus and amblyopia,

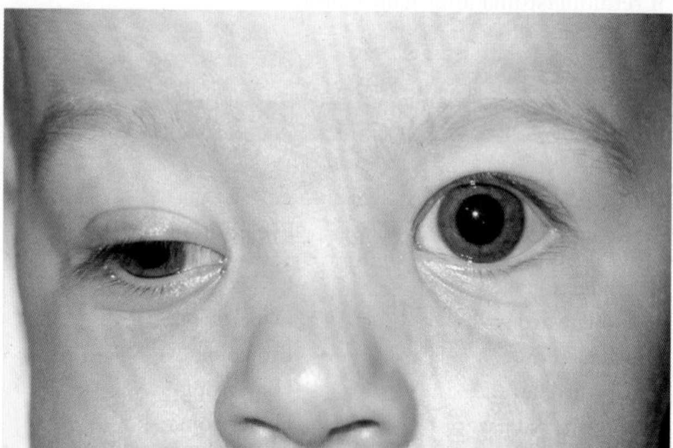

FIGURE 23.3 Right third cranial nerve palsy. When looking straight ahead with left eye, right eye rests in a hypotropic and exotropic position. Note right ptosis. Right pupil is involved (mydriatic), but both pupils were dilated pharmacologically by examiner just before this photograph was taken.

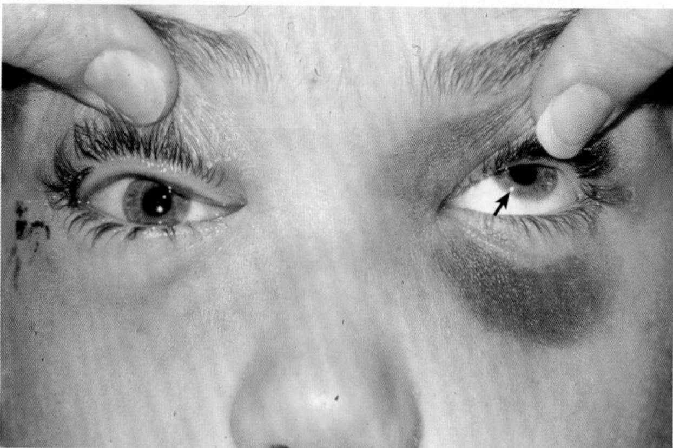

FIGURE 23.4 Patient is looking upward. Right inferior orbital wall blowout fracture causes restriction of upward gaze in right eye. Note light reflexes (Hirschberg test). Left reflex (*arrow*) is lower in reference to pupil than right reflex, indicating the presence of a right hypotropia.

history of trauma, as well as history of any other medical problems. The physical examination should be complete, with specific focus on the neurologic and ophthalmologic evaluation. The ophthalmologic examination should include visual function, pupillary activity, and extraocular movement. The presence or absence of ptosis, lid retraction, proptosis, or enophthalmos should be noted. The Hirschberg light reflex test can be helpful in determining whether strabismus is present. The physician should shine a penlight or direct ophthalmoscope light at the patient's eyes from 2 to 3 ft while the patient is told to look at the other end of the room. In younger children, the patient may choose to look at the light itself, but all efforts should be made to distract the child with a more distant target. The examiner should observe the white dot light reflex that appears to be located on the cornea, overlying the iris or pupil of each eye. In the normal state, the light reflex should be located in a nearly symmetric position and falls slightly off-center in the nasal direction in both eyes (Fig. 23.5). If the eyes are misaligned, symmetry would not be preserved (Figs. 23.4 and 23.6).

Two findings are helpful in assessing whether strabismus is emergent: (1) The presence or absence of double vision and (2) the status of the eye movements. Although young children may not complain of diplopia, this symptom often indicates an

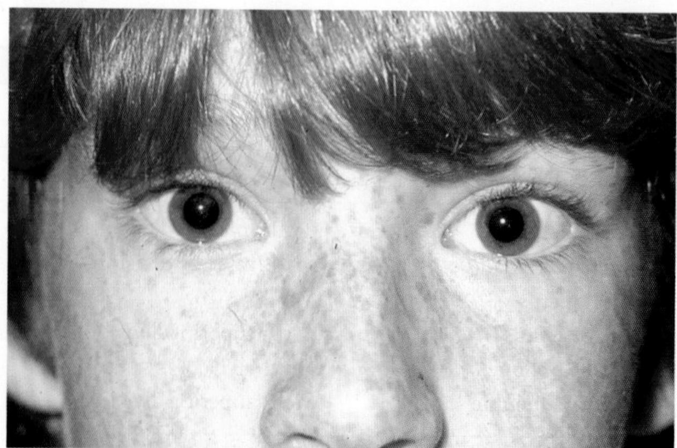

FIGURE 23.5 Normal Hirschberg light reflex test. Light reflexes fall symmetrically in each eye. The reflex in the patient's left eye is a bit nasal to the center, but still within normal limits.

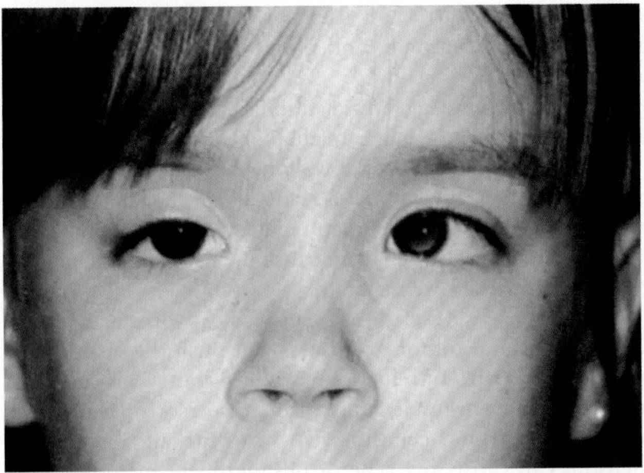

FIGURE 23.6 Left esotropia. Note lateral displacement of Hirschberg light reflex in the left eye. Photograph demonstrates right ptosis. Pupils are pharmacologically dilated. Asymmetry of red reflex is caused by misalignment of the eyes.

acute or subacute onset of ocular misalignment. Nonemergent childhood strabismus is usually not associated with double vision because the brain becomes adept at suppressing the misaligned nonfixing eye. If a child complains of diplopia, ophthalmology consultation is appropriate, even if no strabismus appears on examination by the emergency physician.

If the eye movements are completely full and symmetric, a neurogenic palsy or restrictive phenomenon can be ruled out, and one can be virtually certain that the strabismus is not emergent. Problems that cause emergent strabismus do so by impairing the action of one or more muscles. If there are any questions about subtle reductions in extraocular movement or if there is prominent nystagmus elicited in one particular field of gaze (more than the few beats of normal end point nystagmus known as gaze paretic nystagmus), ophthalmology consultation is most likely appropriate.

Depending on age and clinical circumstance, some children may not cooperate fully with portions of the examination. If a child will not follow an examiner's target but will fix on the examiner, the examiner can ask the parent to gently move the patient's head to each side and then up and down. The examiner can also guide the child by putting one hand on the child's head (Fig. 23.2), although care must be used to avoid heightening the anxiety for some patients. As the patient continues to look straight ahead when the head is being turned, the eyes are moving passively in reference to the head and orbit. When the head is turned to the left, the eyes move into right gaze to maintain fixation straight ahead (Fig. 23.2). If the head is tilted up, the eyes are moved into relative downgaze. Essentially, this is the "doll's eye" maneuver used in the assessment of comatose patients. If the eyes move symmetrically and fully on passive movement of the head, this rules out the presence of a neurogenic or restrictive problem with the same accuracy as if the patient had voluntarily followed a target.

Computed tomography (CT) scan of the orbit with both coronal and axial views is the imaging modality of choice when there is limited extraocular motility in patients in whom orbital fracture is suspected (see Chapters 115 Facial Trauma and 122 Ocular Trauma).

The causes of pediatric strabismus are summarized in Tables 23.2 to 23.4. The first considerations (Figs. 23.4 and 23.6) are restrictive strabismus and neurogenic palsies. Myasthenia gravis and thyroid eye disease can mimic virtually any strabismus with deficiency of extraocular movement and must always be considered in the differential diagnosis in any pattern of ocular misalignment. Myasthenia may cause intermittent strabismus and variable ptosis, whereas thyroid disease

TABLE 23.2

DIFFERENTIAL DIAGNOSIS OF STRABISMUS[a]

Neurogenic palsies
III Cranial nerve palsy (partial or complete)
IV Cranial nerve palsy
VI Cranial nerve palsy
Traumatic extraocular muscle palsy
Myasthenia gravis
Internuclear ophthalmoplegia
Skew deviation
Restrictive strabismus
Orbital wall fracture
Orbital hemorrhage, tumor, infection, or abscess
Thyroid eye disease
Nonthyroid extraocular muscle infiltration (e.g., metastasis)
Orbital cellulites
Nonneurogenic nonrestrictive strabismus
Idiopathic childhood strabismus
Strabismus caused by refractive errors (e.g., accommodative esotropia)
Sensory strabismus (unilateral visual loss)

[a]Not listed in order of frequency.

TABLE 23.3

COMMON CAUSES OF STRABISMUS[a]

Esotropia
Congenital infantile or acquired (with or without farsightedness), nonparalytic, nonrestrictive
Long-standing unilateral visual loss
Medial orbital wall fracture
VI Cranial nerve palsy
Exotropia
Nonparalytic nonrestrictive idiopathic childhood exotropia
Long-standing unilateral visual loss
III Cranial nerve palsy
Hypertropia
Dissociated vertical deviation (a nonparalytic nonrestrictive childhood deviation)
Idiopathic over action or the inferior oblique muscle (affected eye rises in adduction)
Inferior or superior orbital wall fracture
IV Cranial nerve palsy: congenital or acquired
Hypotropia
Brown syndrome (tight superior oblique tendon)
Inferior or superior orbital wall fracture

[a]Not listed in order of frequency.

TABLE 23.4

LIFE-THREATENING CAUSES OF STRABISMUS[a]

Intracranial mass	Head trauma
Elevated intracranial pressure	Meningitis
Myasthenia gravis	Neoplastic infiltration of extraocular muscles
Orbital tumor	Superior orbital wall fracture
Orbital cellulitis	Retinoblastoma causing visual loss

[a]Not listed in order of frequency.

causes retraction of the upper lid. The pupils are not involved in either condition.

ESOTROPIA EMERGENCIES

Figure 23.7 summarizes the approach to a patient with esotropia and exotropia. Patients with a restrictive or neurogenic esotropia (deficiency of abduction) may adopt an abnormal head position to place the eyes in the position of best alignment to avoid double vision. By turning the face in the direction of the deficiency (e.g., right face turn for right sixth nerve palsy) when looking straight ahead, the eyes are aligned and appear straight. The patient's head must be held in the straight ahead position to notice that the affected eye is actually crossed.

Esotropia following orbital trauma may be due to lateral rectus injury, hemorrhage, medial or lateral wall fracture. Fracture of the medial orbital wall may cause entrapment and restriction of the medial rectus. Fracture of the lateral wall—usually part of a tripod fracture that involves the zygoma and inferior lateral wall—may cause orbital hemorrhage that would displace the eye medially.

The presence of proptosis suggests an orbital process. A lateral orbital tumor or abscess can push the eye toward the nose or restrict abduction. Any infiltrative process that involves the eye muscles may also cause esotropia through restriction. Orbital cellulitis, with or without abscess formation, can cause any type of misalignment including esotropia. A contrast CT scan of the orbit with coronal and axial views is the diagnostic procedure of choice in these situations.

Lateral rectus palsy (sixth cranial nerve palsy) occurs most commonly secondary to head trauma (see Chapter 121 Neurotrauma) or increased ICP. Other CNS signs, such as papilledema, may be present. A CT of the brain may be the first imaging choice to evaluate for intracranial hemorrhage given its rapid availability, however magnetic resonance imaging (MRI) of the brain is the imaging study of choice to further investigate the ophthalmologic findings. Sixth cranial nerve palsy can also occur rather precipitously after the placement

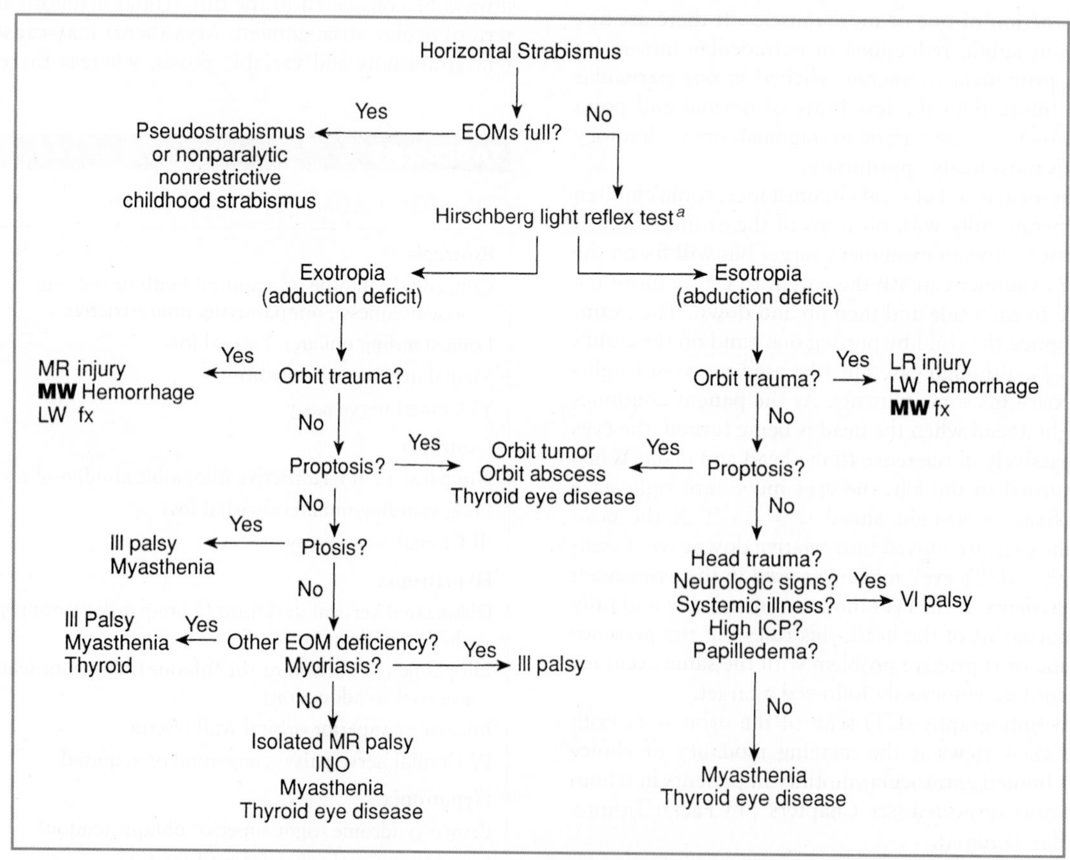

FIGURE 23.7 Evaluation of horizontal strabismus. [a]With head held in straight ahead position. EOM, extraocular muscle movement; MR, medial rectus; LW, lateral orbital wall; MW, medial orbital wall; fx, fracture; LR, lateral rectus; ICP, intracranial pressure; INO, internuclear ophthalmoplegia.

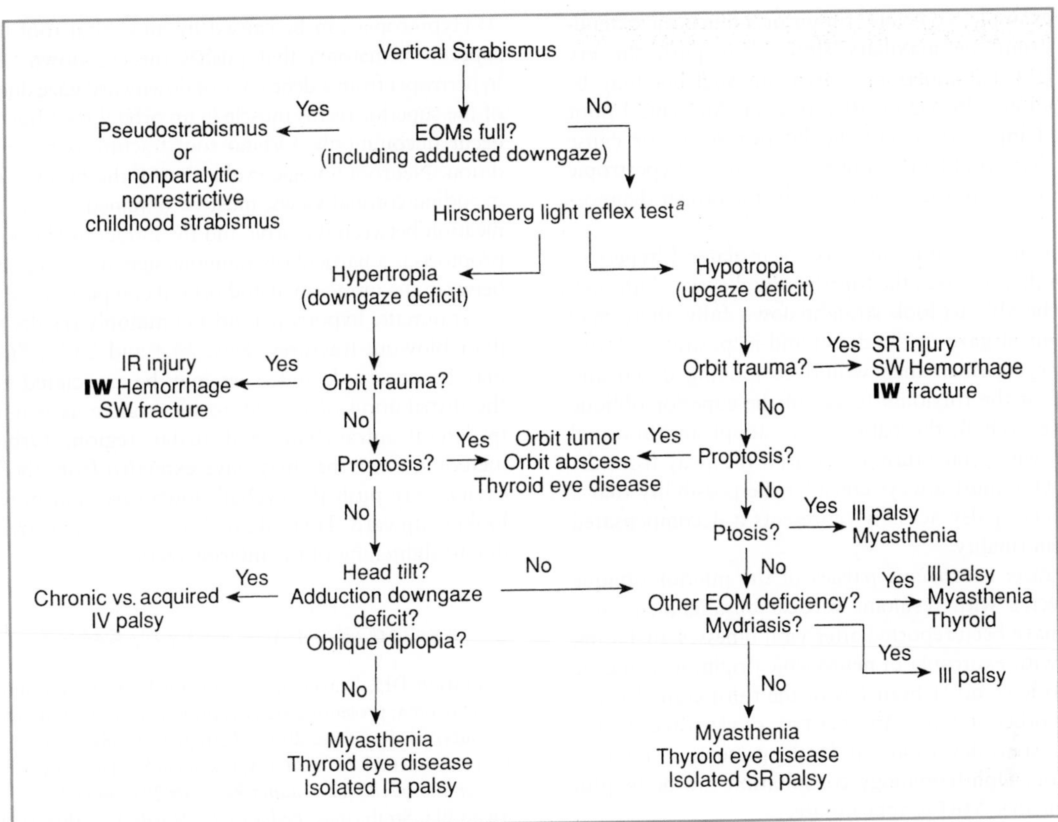

FIGURE 23.8 Evaluation of vertical strabismus. [a]With head held in straight ahead position. EOM, extraocular muscle movement; IR, inferior rectus; SW, superior orbital wall; IW, inferior orbital wall; SR, superior rectus.

of ventricular shunts designed to relieve increased ICP even if the palsy was not obvious preoperatively. Sixth cranial nerve palsy may be bilateral, resulting in bilateral esotropia with reduced ability to abduct bilaterally which required careful examination to detect. Asymmetric presentations are more likely to be readily identified.

EXOTROPIA EMERGENCIES

Orbital cellulitis, thyroid eye disease, and orbital tumors may also cause exotropia. Trauma very rarely results in exotropia because lateral wall fractures rarely cause entrapment. Orbital hemorrhage (with or without medial wall fracture) can have a mass effect, causing the eye to be turned out.

Isolated paresis of the medial rectus muscle, resulting in a deficiency of adduction and exotropia, is quite unusual because other muscles are also innervated by the same branch of the third cranial nerve. One should look for accompanying ptosis, pupillary dilation, or deficiencies of upgaze or downgaze to confirm third cranial nerve involvement, even if these findings are subtle.

Unilateral isolated deficiency of adduction may be the result of an intranuclear ophthalmoplegia secondary to a brainstem injury that involves the interconnecting pathways between the third and sixth cranial nerves. Bilateral isolated deficiency of adduction is virtually diagnostic of this condition. MRI of the brainstem should be ordered emergently. The provider should also look for prominent nystagmus on attempted abduction of the contralateral eye.

HYPERTROPIA/HYPOTROPIA EMERGENCIES

Paretic or restrictive vertical eye muscle imbalance must be referred to an ophthalmologist. Figure 23.8 summarizes the approach to the patient with vertical ocular misalignment. To determine whether it is the higher or lower eye that is abnormal, the examiner must have the patient look upward and then downward. If one eye is unable to look downward fully, the patient has a hypertropia of that eye. If one eye is unable to look upward fully, that eye is hypotropic (Fig. 23.4). Patients may adopt abnormal head positions to compensate for this misalignment. By lifting the chin to look straight ahead, the eyes are placed in relative downward gaze, thus indicating that the strabismus is worse when the patient looks up. Likewise, the patient may adopt a chin down position to look straight ahead, indicating that the strabismus is worse in downward gaze. A chin up or chin down position does not prove strabismus as there may be other causes (e.g., chin up position as compensation for ptosis, or to lessen nystagmus). When a patient has an anomalous head position, it can be useful to examine the patient with the head in the opposite position to better highlight the abnormality for which the spontaneous head position is trying to compensate. For example, if the patient presents with a chin up position, the eyes may appear to be aligned in that position. If the head is moved by the examiner into a chin down position, the vertical misalignment of the eyes will be more apparent. An eye may become hypertropic for several reasons. Any mass underneath the eyeball—for example, an orbital tumor or a mucocele extending upward from the maxillary sinus—may push the eye upward. A tightened superior rectus is unusual but may be seen in thyroid eye disease or after trauma. An orbital floor fracture could injure (weaken) the inferior rectus or cause hemorrhage that would push the eye up into a hypertropic position. A CT scan of the orbit would be the proper diagnostic modality.

Perhaps the most important cause of ipsilateral hypertropia is a lesion that involves the fourth cranial nerve. Although the eye may be able to look straight down fully, there may be a restriction of gaze in the down-and-in position relative to the other eye (which then would be looking down and out). Because of the torsional forces of the superior oblique muscle on the eyeball, the patient may adopt an abnormal head position with a face turn and a head tilt away from the affected eye. One must always consider the possibility that a new fourth nerve palsy actually represents a decompensated congenital abnormality.

Although rare, neurogenic palsies of the inferior oblique or inferior rectus with resultant vertical misalignment may occur. These have been reported after viral illnesses, including varicella. As with exotropia of neurogenic origin, it would be more likely to have other branches of the third cranial nerve involved with other findings. Another type of vertical eye muscle imbalance, skew deviation, can be the presenting sign of a midbrain lesion. Ophthalmology consultation can be helpful in deciding whether MRI is appropriate.

Hypotropia can be caused by an orbital roof fracture with superior hematoma that pushes the eye down. Alternatively, hypertropia from a deficiency of downward gaze due to tethering of the superior rectus muscle in an orbital roof fracture can also occur uncommonly. Orbital roof fracture is an emergent condition. Neuroradiologic evaluation of the brain and the orbits, including coronal views, must be obtained to rule out communication between the orbit and the intracranial cavity. Pulsating proptosis is a particularly ominous sign indicating direct contact between the intracranial and orbital compartments.

Traumatic hypotropia most commonly results from orbital floor blowout fractures (Figs. 23.4 and 23.8). Enophthalmos may be observed, and there may be associated numbness in the distribution of the infraorbital nerve as it innervates the ipsilateral infraorbital and malar region. Orbital lesions, including those that may have extended from the intracranial cavity, may push the eyeball downward and prevent it from looking upward. Thyroid eye disease also can cause hypotropia due to tightening of the inferior rectus.

Suggested Readings and Key References

Abramson DH, Beaverson K, Sangani P, et al. Screening for retinoblastoma: presenting signs as prognosticators of patient and ocular survival. *Pediatrics* 2003;112(6 pt 1):1248–1255.

Oppenheimer AJ, Monson LA, Buchman SR. Pediatric orbital fractures. *Craniomaxillofac Trauma Reconstr* 2013;6(1):9–20.

Ticho BH. Strabismus. *Pediatr Clin North Am* 2003;50(1):173–188.

CHAPTER 24 ■ EYE: UNEQUAL PUPILS

ELIZABETH S. JACOBS, MD AND ALEX V. LEVIN, MD, MHSc, FRCSC

Abnormalities of the pupils can be helpful diagnostically when assessing central nervous system, autonomic nervous system, orbital, and ocular problems. Pupillary disorders can be divided into two categories: Disorders in which the size of one or both pupils is abnormal and disorders in which the shape of one or both pupils are abnormal. The pupil can also be malpositioned (*corectopia*). Congenital or acquired (e.g., after trauma) corectopia generally requires ophthalmology consultation. When the pupils are different in size, the term applied is *anisocoria*. An abnormally dilated pupil is called *mydriasis*. *Miosis* refers to an abnormally constricted pupil. Figure 24.1 represents a flowchart for an approach to anisocoria.

PATHOPHYSIOLOGY

The pupillary dilator muscle receives sympathetic innervation. The pupillary sphincter receives parasympathetic innervation that also supplies the ciliary muscle of the eye that governs focusing (accommodation) of the lens.

The first-order sympathetic neurons extend from the hypothalamus through the midbrain, pons, and medulla into the spinal cord, where they synapse with the second-order neurons just before exiting the cord at roots C8–T2. The cervicothoracic sympathetic trunk then travels over the apex of the lungs to the superior cervical ganglion in the neck, where synapses are made with the third-order neurons. Sympathetic innervation to the face departs from the superior cervical ganglion or at the bifurcation of the common carotid artery. Therefore, complete unilateral anhidrosis in association with unilateral miosis suggests damage to the second-order neurons or superior cervical ganglion. The third-order neurons travel with the internal carotid artery into the cranial vault, where the fibers gain access to the orbit via the nasociliary branch of the first division of the trigeminal nerve. They then travel through the ciliary ganglion in the orbit without synapse. Fibers extend to the iris dilator via the ciliary nerves. Disruption of sympathetic innervation anywhere along its course results in ipsilateral miosis (Horner syndrome) and is often accompanied by mild ptosis, enophthalmos, with or without ipsilateral anhidrosis. The lower lid may be higher than the contralateral side ("upside down ptosis").

Parasympathetic neurons originate in the Edinger–Westphal nuclei, located on the dorsal aspect of the third cranial nerve nucleus. These neurons travel with the third cranial nerve, exiting the midbrain on its ventral aspect and passing between the posterior cerebral artery and the superior cerebellar arteries at the circle of Willis. The nerve then runs anteriorly and enters the cavernous sinus superiorly and laterally. Just before entering the posterior orbit through the superior orbital fissure, the third cranial nerve splits into a superior and an inferior division. The latter contains the parasympathetic fibers that then pass into the ciliary ganglion, where they synapse. Short ciliary nerves then carry the postsynaptic fibers to the pupillary sphincter muscle and the ciliary muscle (behind the iris). Unilateral mydriasis can be caused by damage to the parasympathetic fibers anywhere along their course. With the exceptions noted next, it is distinctly unusual for the parasympathetic fibers to be damaged without other evidence of third cranial nerve palsy (a deficit in the ability of the eye to adduct, look upward, and/or look downward, and/or ptosis; see Chapter 23 Eye: Strabismus).

Local factors can also cause physical changes in the iris or in the surrounding structures that may result in miosis or mydriasis.

EVALUATION AND DECISION

When testing pupillary size, it is essential that the patient be instructed to look at a *distant* target that does not involve reading letters or numbers. This prevents the eyes from needing to accommodate. Because the innervation for accommodation is the same as that for the pupillary sphincter, the accommodating patient also has reflex contraction of the pupils, particularly when focusing at near. Focusing on a near object also stimulates convergence of the eyes toward each other. Crying or forced eyelid closure may also induce miosis.

ANISOCORIA

When evaluating the patient with anisocoria, the emergency physician must answer two critical questions: (1) Which pupil is abnormal, the smaller or the larger? and (2) Is this abnormality acute or chronic?

To establish which pupil is abnormal, the relative difference in pupillary size should be noted under conditions of bright and dim illumination. Using the largest diameter circle of the direct ophthalmoscope or a bright penlight, both pupils should be illuminated simultaneously in a room with the lights on. The room lights should then be turned off and the handheld light source held tangentially from below or from above so the eyes are illuminated only enough that the examiner can note the pupillary size.

Normally, the pupils constrict equally in response to bright illumination and dilate equally in dim illumination. If the relative difference in pupillary size increases under bright illumination, the larger pupil is the abnormal pupil: The larger pupil is not constricting normally (Fig. 24.2). If the relative difference in pupillary size increases under dim illumination, the smaller pupil is the abnormal pupil: The smaller pupil is not dilating normally. If the relative difference in pupillary size is the same in both dim and bright illumination, the patient does *not* have an abnormal pupil (Fig. 24.3). Rather, the patient has physiologic anisocoria. Approximately 20% of people with normal pupils have a difference in the size of their pupils in excess of 0.4 mm.

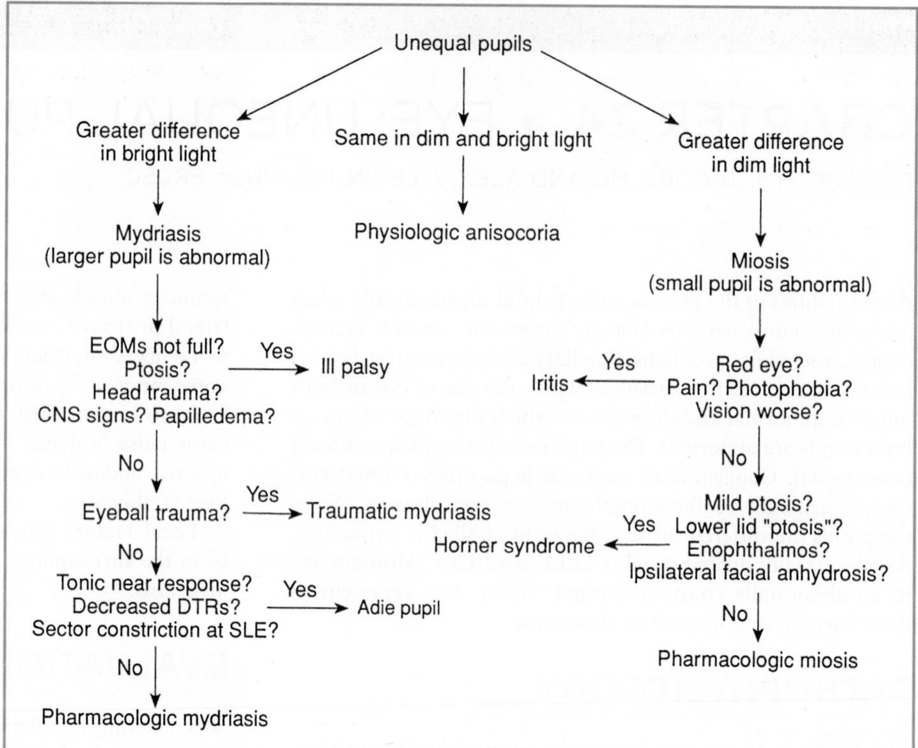

FIGURE 24.1 Unequal pupils. EOM, extraocular muscle movement; CNS, central nervous system; III, third cranial nerve; DTR, deep tendon reflex; SLE, slit lamp examination.

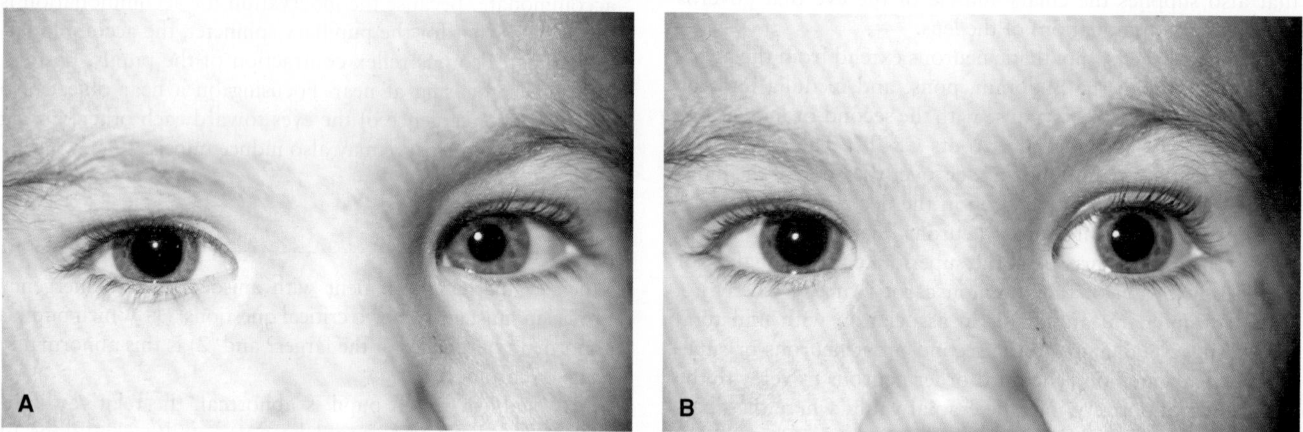

FIGURE 24.2 Patient with right mydriasis. Relative difference between the pupil size is greater in bright illumination (A) than in dim illumination (B).

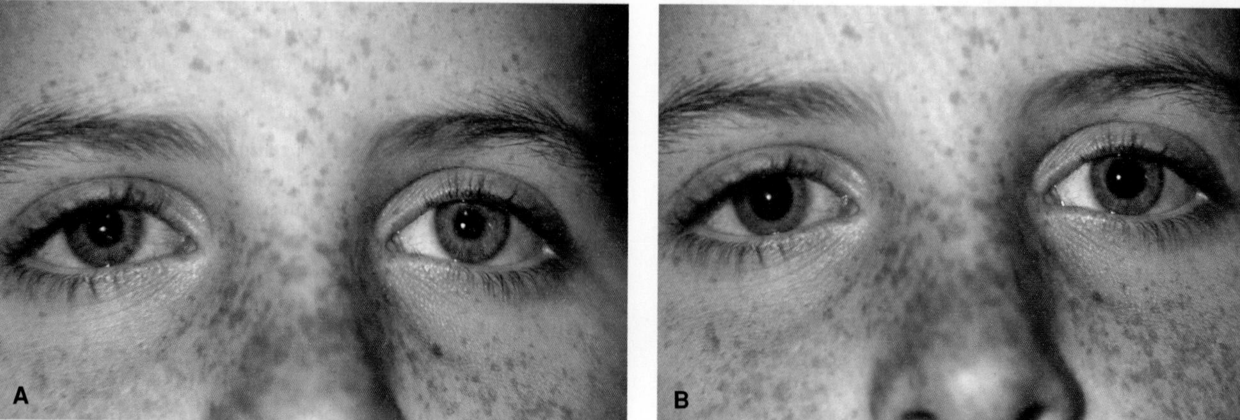

FIGURE 24.3 Physiologic anisocoria. Relative difference in pupil size is the same in bright illumination (A) and dim illumination (B).

TABLE 24.1

DIFFERENTIAL DIAGNOSIS OF UNEQUAL PUPILS[a]

Physiologic anisocoria
Pharmacologic (miotics or mydriatics)
Local factors
Miosis: iritis, surgical trauma
Mydriasis: trauma
Abnormal pupil shape from scar formation following prior iritis or trauma
Neurologic causes
Miosis: Horner syndrome
Mydriasis: third cranial nerve palsy, Adie pupil
Congenital abnormalities
Iris coloboma
Anterior chamber dysgenesis syndromes (e.g., Axenfeld–Rieger)

[a]Not listed in order of frequency.

When trying to establish whether the anisocoria is of relatively recent or acute onset, as opposed to long-standing anisocoria, it is helpful to view old photographs. Sometimes, chronic physiologic anisocoria will not have been noticed previously. The direct ophthalmoscope can be used to provide magnification and illumination of the photograph so the pupils can be viewed. Set the focusing dial on progressively higher black (or green) numbers until adequate magnification has been achieved while viewing through the direct ophthalmoscope. It is also important to note any other symptoms that accompanied the onset of anisocoria (headaches, pain, double vision, or blurred vision). The causes of anisocoria are summarized in Tables 24.1 to 24.3.

MIOSIS

Local Factors

An irritated or inflamed iris sphincter muscle will result in miosis. Iritis, secondary to trauma or other factors, is a common cause (see Chapter 22 Eye: Red Eye). The eye is usually injected, and there are symptoms of eye pain, photophobia, tearing, with or without decreased vision. Injection may surround the cornea for 360 degrees, creating a ring of erythema ("ciliary blush"). More diffuse injection may also occur. Traumatic iritis is often not apparent for 12 to 72 hours after eye trauma. Children with juvenile idiopathic arthritis may not have these classic symptoms associated with their iritis; in fact, they may have no symptoms at all and may have delayed diagnoses. Iritis from any cause, especially when longstanding (as is often seen in juvenile idiopathic arthritis) can result in scar tissues between the pupil edge and the lens just behind the pupil (posterior synechia), which prevent pupillary dilation or cause asymmetric irregular dilation of one or both pupils. The diagnosis of iritis is confirmed by slit lamp biomicroscopy. This technique is described in Chapter 122 Ocular Trauma. Ophthalmology consultation is important for evaluation and treatment.

Other local factors include surgical irritation of the iris and pharmacologically induced unilateral miosis. Mechanical contact with the iris during any intraocular surgical procedure may result in transient postoperative unilateral miosis. Parasympathomimetic or sympatholytic systemic medications and topical drops can also result in transient miosis. It is helpful to remember that most topical ophthalmic miotics are supplied in bottles that have green caps.

TABLE 24.2

COMMON CAUSES OF UNEQUAL PUPILS[a]

Physiologic anisocoria
Miosis
Iritis secondary to trauma, juvenile rheumatoid arthritis, or idiopathic
Abnormal pupil shape from scar formation following prior iritis or trauma
Horner syndrome (Table 24.4)
Mydriasis
Trauma
Third cranial nerve palsy
Adie pupil
Congenital abnormalities
Iris coloboma

[a]Not listed in order of frequency.

TABLE 24.3

LIFE-THREATENING CAUSES OF UNEQUAL PUPILS[a]

Miosis
Intracranial mass lesion or vascular insult
Spinal cord tumor or compression
Intrathoracic tumor
Aneurysm
Cavernous sinus inflammation, thrombosis, or tumor
Mydriasis
Increased intracranial pressure
Intracranial mass lesion
Aneurysm
Cavernous sinus inflammation, thrombosis, or tumor
Orbital tumor

[a]Not listed in order of frequency.

Neurologic Factors

Congenital Horner syndrome may result from brachial plexus injury and is often associated with ipsilateral iris hypopigmentation. This sign is not as helpful in the first few months of life when both eyes are normally relatively hypopigmented. More than 50% of children with congenital Horner syndrome have a history of difficult extraction at delivery. Congenital varicella infection may also be a cause.

If the presence of Horner syndrome is questioned, one drop of topical 4% cocaine can be instilled into both eyes. This testing is best performed by ophthalmology or neurology consultants. Because cocaine prevents reuptake of norepinephrine at the terminal myoneural junction of the sphincter muscle, pupillary dilation will occur normally. Failure of the miotic pupil to dilate is diagnostic of Horner syndrome. Knowledge

TABLE 24.4

CAUSES OF ACQUIRED HORNER SYNDROME IN CHILDREN[a]

First-order neuron
Brainstem glioma or other tumor
Brainstem vascular insult (aneurysm, infarct)
Spinal cord tumor
Syringomyelia
Poliomyelitis
Head or spinal trauma
Postsurgical
Second-order neuron
Intrathoracic tumor (neuroblastoma, ganglioneuroma, metastatic)
Intrathoracic aneurysm
Cervical tumor or adenitis
Trauma (especially brachial plexus trauma)
Postsurgical
Third-order neuron
Internal carotid thrombosis or aneurysm
Internal carotid or head trauma
Otitis media
Nasopharyngeal malignancy
Cavernous sinus thrombosis, tumor, or inflammation
Postsurgical

[a]Not listed in order of frequency.

of the sympathetic system anatomy can be exploited through the use of other topically applied diagnostic agents to localize the site of the lesion. Table 24.4 summarizes the causes of acquired Horner syndrome in children. All children who have Horner syndrome should receive a complete evaluation unless congenital Horner syndrome is known to be present, based on history, old photographs, and examination.

MYDRIASIS

Local Factors

Both trauma and topical agents can cause unilateral mydriasis. Blunt trauma (and, less commonly, intraocular surgery) can result in a fixed dilated pupil. Traumatic mydriasis usually occurs in a setting in which a clear history of trauma and other intraocular injuries, such as hyphema, are noted. The pupil may be somewhat irregular in shape if the sphincter has irregular tears that appear as V-shaped notches in the pupil margin best seen using the direct ophthalmoscope as a magnifier. Sometimes, pigment deposition can be seen on the anterior surface of the lens.

Topical parasympatholytics and sympathomimetics can also cause mydriasis. Most of these drops are supplied in bottles that have red caps. Systemic medications from the same classes (e.g., phenylephrine, atropine, scopolamine) can cause bilateral pupillary dilation. Inhaled medications (e.g., ipratropium) can also cause transient mydriasis, often presenting unilaterally. Also certain plants with anticholinergic properties (e.g., jimson weed) have been reported to cause isolated mydriasis.

Neurologic Factors

When a child with unilateral mydriasis arrives in the emergency department, the initial concern is often cerebral herniation leading to compression and stretching of the third cranial nerve. A rapid neurologic assessment usually is sufficient to diagnose herniation because most patients will have a decreased level of consciousness, abnormal vital signs, or focal findings in addition to a dilated pupil, and usually deficiencies of eye movements and/or ptosis (see Chapter 23 Eye: Strabismus). Once the physician is certain that increased intracranial pressure (ICP) is not present, a more careful evaluation is appropriate.

Examination by an ophthalmologist is often indicated to help define patterns of extraocular muscle deficit and strabismus, as well as to assess for the possible presence of papilledema. This can help determine alternative etiologies for mydriasis. In children, head trauma is the most common cause of acquired third cranial nerve palsy. Meningitis and increased ICP have been associated with mydriasis from third cranial nerve involvement without abnormalities of the extraocular muscles. Other causes are listed in Table 24.5. Neuroradiologic investigation is almost always indicated.

Other problems may mimic the eye muscle imbalance of third nerve palsy. For example, an inferior orbital wall blowout fracture (see Chapter 23 Eye: Strabismus) may cause a deficiency in the eye's ability to look up. Trauma may also result in unilateral mydriasis. Together, these findings may mimic a third cranial nerve palsy. Complex etiologies such as this underscore the importance of ophthalmology consultation when pathologic unilateral mydriasis and/or eye muscle deficits are present. Diagnostic clues to the presence of a long-standing third cranial nerve palsy include phenomena associated with aberrant regeneration of the oculomotor nerve. Examples include eyelid elevation when the patient looks down and pupillary constriction when the patient looks upward, downward, or into adduction.

Adie pupil is most often unilateral. It is caused by parasympathetic denervation at the myoneural junction of the pupillary sphincter muscle. It may be associated with deep tendon hyporeflexia. Also known as tonic pupil, an Adie pupil constricts

TABLE 24.5

CAUSES OF THIRD CRANIAL NERVE PALSY IN CHILDREN[a]

Head trauma
Congenital (isolated or with other cranial nerves involved)
Brain/meningeal tumor
Meningitis/encephalitis
Postviral syndromes
Hydrocephalus
Migraine
Cavernous sinus thrombosis
Aneurysm
Benign idiopathic ("cryptogenic")

[a]Not listed in order of frequency.

slowly to near convergence and then redilates deliberately. Slit lamp examination may reveal serpentine microundulations or asymmetries on constriction to light. Adie pupil usually has an acute or subacute onset. It has been reported after trauma and viral illnesses, including varicella. In conjunction with ophthalmology consultation, weak pilocarpine (0.125% or 0.1%) drops can be instilled into both eyes. This concentration is too weak to cause constriction of the normal pupil, though the denervated Adie pupil will become miotic. Acutely, this test may be falsely negative.

A common misconception is that poorly seeing eyes have large pupils. Even an eye with very poor vision (light perception) or total blindness may have normal pupil size.

CORECTOPIA AND IRREGULAR PUPILS

Pupils that are located eccentrically rather than centrally are often bilaterally abnormal and represent congenital anomalies. A corectopic pupil can also be due to a progressive change in iris anatomy. Congenital corectopia may be associated with other holes in the iris (polycoria), abnormal iris strands that may be adherent to the cornea, or alterations in iris color. These abnormalities may also be associated with glaucoma and systemic malformations such as dental and umbilical abnormalities (Axenfeld–Rieger spectrum). Progressive changes in pupil location may be secondary to adherence to surrounding tissue, either progressive formation of scar tissue after eye surgery or posterior synechia. After trauma, the presence of corectopia, or a teardrop-shaped pupil, is particularly ominous because this may indicate an underlying associated rupture of the eyeball (see Chapter 122 Ocular Trauma).

The direct ophthalmoscope can be helpful in identifying iris anomalies. The focusing dial should be turned so the iris is in focus (less than 6 in away from the patient). The dial will be turning in the direction of increasingly higher black (or green) numbers to provide increasing magnification at shorter distances from the eye. The red reflex test (see Chapter 122 Ocular Trauma) can also be helpful when the pupil does not appear as a perfect circle.

Perhaps the most familiar disorder of pupillary shape and/or location is the congenital iris coloboma. This "keyhole" pupil (Fig. 24.4) represents a failure of proper embryologic development of the iris tissue. By itself, iris coloboma is usually asymptomatic and not associated with a functional deficit. Associated colobomatous defects of the retina or optic nerve may exist, and these can result in serious visual compromise. An eye with coloboma may be smaller (microphthalmia).

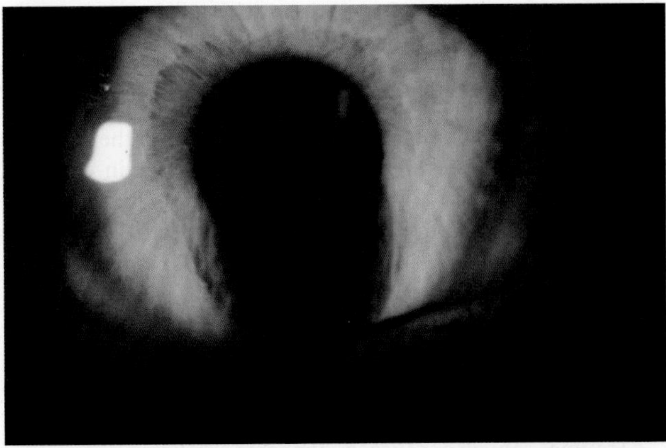

FIGURE 24.4 Iris coloboma creating a "keyhole" pupil. The iris defect is always inferior or inferior-nasal.

Occasionally, when dilating drops are instilled initially, the pupil may begin to dilate irregularly and asymmetrically. This is of no concern provided the ultimate shape of the dilated pupil is round. Otherwise, it is wise to seek ophthalmology consultation in all situations of corectopia or irregular pupillary shape.

UNEQUAL PUPILLARY REACTIVITY

Both pupils should be equally brisk in their constricting reaction to a penlight (or direct ophthalmoscope light). When asymmetry in pupillary reactivity is found, it is always the more sluggish pupil that is abnormal. Often, the more sluggish pupil will be a unilaterally dilated pupil. If both pupils are symmetric in their baseline positions, an abnormally sluggish pupil may indicate the presence of a serious retinal or optic nerve problem that is impairing the ability of the affected eye to perceive the light source equally. Testing visual acuity is essential under these circumstances. A Marcus Gunn pupil (also known as afferent pupillary defect [APD]) occurs when there is unequal perception of light between the two eyes, usually due to a unilateral or asymmetric optic neuropathy, which could be due to trauma, tumor (e.g., glioma in neurofibromatosis type 1), genetic optic neuropathies (e.g., Leber hereditary optic neuropathy), demyelinating disease, or inflammation of the optic nerve (papillitis). The reader is referred elsewhere for details of the "swinging flashlight test" used to evaluate for a Marcus Gunn pupil.

The pupil should not be pharmacologically manipulated in the ED if there is a concern about a pupil abnormality. Rather, direct referral to an ophthalmologist is appropriate so the pupils may be observed unaltered.

Suggested Readings and Key References

American Academy of Pediatrics, Section on Ophthalmology, American Association for Pediatric Ophthalmology And Strabismus, et al. Red reflex examination in neonates, infants, and children. *Pediatrics* 2008; 122:1401–1404.

Biousse V, Newman NJ. *Neuro-ophthalmology illustrated.* Stuttgart, Germany: Thieme Verlag, 2009.

Brazis PW. Localization of lesions of the oculomotor nerve: recent concepts. *Mayo Clin Proc* 1991;66:1029–1035.

Brodsky MC, Baker RS, Hamed LM. *Pediatric Neuro-Ophthalmology.* New York, NY: Springer, 1996.

Hamed LM. Associated neurologic and ophthalmologic findings in congenital oculomotor nerve palsy. *Ophthalmology* 1991;98: 708–714.

Jeffery AR, Ellis FJ, Repka MX, et al. Pediatric Horner syndrome. *J AAPOS* 1998;2:159–167.

Miller NR. Solitary oculomotor nerve palsy in childhood. *Am J Ophthalmol* 1977;83:106–111.

Thompson HS, Pilley SF. Unequal pupils. A flow chart for sorting out the anisocorias. *Surv Ophthalmol* 1976;21:45–48.

Young TA, Levin AV. The afferent pupillary defect. *Pediatr Emerg Care* 1997;13:61–65.

CHAPTER 25 ▪ EYE: VISUAL DISTURBANCES

KAREN E. DULL, MD

Sudden loss or deterioration of vision (or diplopia) can be caused by numerous diseases and injuries (Tables 25.1–25.3). A systematic approach is necessary to reach a correct diagnosis and to minimize the risk of permanent visual impairment. The patient's age, underlying disease conditions, visual history, and history of possible injury must be determined. The extent of the visual impairment, the rapidity of its onset, and the association with other systemic findings are vital pieces of information. It is important to remember that visual acuity improves with age in children. The normal visual acuity for a toddler is 20/40 and gradually improves to the normal adult acuity of 20/20 by age 5 or 6 years. A careful eye examination, including gross and ophthalmoscopic examination, determination of extraocular movement, and visual acuity, together with the history, leads to correct diagnosis and management of the patient.

Few ocular conditions in the pediatric population are truly emergent (Table 25.4), but many are urgent; most can be treated by the emergency physician or can be referred for appropriate follow-up with an ophthalmologist. Many conditions seen by a pediatric ophthalmologist are not discussed here because they rarely are seen in the emergency department (ED). Conditions that are more likely to be seen in the ED are emphasized in this chapter.

PATHOPHYSIOLOGY

Vision may be impaired through interference at any point in the visual pathway. Light must reach the eye, pass through the cornea and the anterior chamber, be focused by the lens, pass through the posterior chamber, and reach the retina. The retina must react to the visual stimuli, generate electrical impulses, and transmit these impulses along the optic nerve and eventually to the visual cortex for interpretation. In addition, for binocular vision, the movement of both eyes must be coordinated and smooth. Loss of clarity of the visual media or damage to the conductive tissues anywhere along the visual pathway can lead to decreased vision.

DIFFERENTIAL DIAGNOSIS

Trauma and infections are the two most common causes of acute visual impairment that can interfere with any part of the visual pathway (Tables 25.1 and 25.2). The total spectrum of diseases that cause visual impairment can be understood best if the visual pathway is divided into its parts, and each part is considered sequentially (Table 25.1).

Vision may be limited by periorbital diseases such as periorbital cellulitis, tumor, infection, or allergic swelling of the eyelids. Orbital cellulitis should be considered if decreased visual acuity, proptosis, ophthalmoplegia, or pain with eye movements is present.

Blunt trauma to the eye may cause a blowout fracture of the orbit. The weakest portion of the orbit, the floor, most commonly breaks, and this may entrap the extraocular muscles. Visual impairment may be limited to double vision when looking in a certain direction, particularly upward. Testing the extraocular movements reveals the limitation. Careful inspection of the globe is also necessary.

Diseases of the cornea that cause visual impairment are predominantly infectious or traumatic. Infections of the cornea and conjunctiva can be caused by bacteria, viruses, and fungi (see Chapters 22 Eye: Red Eye and 131 Ophthalmic Emergencies). All these diseases may present as a unilateral or bilateral process, usually affecting only the conjunctiva and cornea. Onset is variable but usually occurs over 1 or 2 days, and vision is not greatly impaired. In the newborn period, gonococcal, chlamydial, and herpetic infections must be considered. *Staphylococcus* species are the leading cause of bacterial keratitis. *Pseudomonas* species is the most commonly isolated bacteria in patients who wear contact lenses. In the United States, the most common corneal infection that causes permanent visual impairment is herpes simplex keratoconjunctivitis, whereas trachoma infection is the most common cause worldwide. A careful ophthalmoscopic or slit lamp examination will reveal the characteristic dendritic ulcers of herpes simplex infection after the eye has been stained with fluorescein. Unless this disease is excluded, steroid-containing medications should not be used. With a recent eye injury or foreign-body intrusion, fungal infections are possible.

There are various types of traumatic injuries to the cornea. Injury secondary to alkali burns constitute one of the true ophthalmologic emergencies. Alkali burns in general carry a worse prognosis than acid burns. Immediate copious irrigation of the eye with normal saline is imperative to prevent permanent visual impairment and to preserve visual acuity. Both ultraviolet and infrared light can cause damage to the cornea, resulting in severe pain and photophobia within 24 hours of exposure. Lacerations with perforation of the cornea usually affect other parts of the eye as well and can lead to significant visual impairment. Careful inspection of the globe with associated lid trauma is mandatory.

The anterior chamber of the eye consists of the aqueous humor, the iris, and the lens. Acute iritis is rare in children, and the cause is often uncertain. There is a sudden onset of pain, redness, and photophobia that usually affects one eye only. The degree of visual impairment varies with the severity of inflammation. Certain diseases, such as juvenile idiopathic arthritis, have associated iritis. Blunt trauma can also cause iritis, but vision is only slightly impaired unless other structures are involved. Traumatic iritis often presents 24 to 72 hours after the trauma.

Trauma can also cause a hyphema or hemorrhage into the anterior chamber. This can result in little to severe visual impairment in the affected eye, depending on the extent of

TABLE 25.1

CAUSES OF ACUTE VISUAL DISTURBANCES

	Traumatic	Nontraumatic
Periorbital	Eyelid hematoma, edema from trauma	Orbital or periorbital cellulitis, tumor, allergic edema
Cornea and conjunctiva	Chemical burns, thermal burns, ultraviolet or infrared burns, laceration of cornea	Conjunctivitis (bacterial, viral, fungal)
Anterior chamber	Traumatic iritis, hyphema, posttraumatic cataract, dislocation of lens, glaucoma	Acute iritis, glaucoma, uveitis
Posterior chamber	Vitreous hemorrhage	Endophthalmitis
Retina	Severed retinal artery, retinal tears or detachment, commotio retinae	Retinal vein or artery obstruction, spontaneous
Cortex	Head trauma	Optic neuritis, toxins, hysteria, hypoglycemia, leukemia, cerebrovascular accidents, migraine, multiple sclerosis, acute disseminated encephalomyelitis, meningitis, encephalitis, seizure, cerebral venous sinus thrombosis, idiopathic intracranial hypertension, posterior reversible encephalopathy syndrome
Other	Carotid artery trauma	Poisoning Shunt malfunction Vitamin A deficiencies Measles Neoplasm

bleeding and associated trauma. Complications of hyphema include rebleeding, which typically occurs within the first 5 days after injury, and increased intraocular pressure potentially leading to glaucoma. Previously, all patients with hyphema were hospitalized on strict bed rest. However, this was not shown to improve outcome, but close follow-up with an ophthalmologist is recommended. Despite lack of definitive evidence, most ophthalmologists recommend cycloplegic and corticosteroid drops to reduce pain and possibly reduce inflammatory complications. Nonsteroidal anti-inflammatory drugs (NSAIDs) should be avoided. The risk of vision loss is highest in patients with sickle cell disease or trait, when greater than 20% of the visual field is affected, with rebleeding, and when residual blood lasts beyond 3 to 4 days duration.

Traumatic injuries can lead to cataract formation, usually within a few days of injury, but onset may be delayed for years. Dislocation of the lens after trauma causes significant visual impairment but can be recognized easily with a careful examination. Glaucoma and retinal detachment may be late complications of blunt trauma. Pain around the eye, blurred vision, and occasionally, nausea and vomiting in a patient with glaucoma or with a recent eye injury may represent an acute attack of glaucoma. If any one of these is noted as a primary complaint or an incidental finding, immediate referral is required.

The uvea consists of the iris, ciliary body, and choroid. One or all portions of the uvea may become inflamed, causing uveitis. Iritis and iridocyclitis may be called anterior uveitis, whereas inflammation of the choroid is often called posterior uveitis. The etiologies may be divided into infectious and noninfectious. Infectious uveitis may be caused by viruses, bacteria, fungi, or helminths. The most common cause of posterior uveitis in children is toxoplasmosis. Noninfectious causes include juvenile idiopathic arthritis, trauma, ankylosing spondylitis, Behçet disease, idiopathic intracranial hypertension (IIH, pseudotumor cerebri), peripheral uveitis, sarcoidosis, and sympathetic ophthalmia. Vogt–Koyanagi–Harada syndrome is a panuveitis with meningeal and cutaneous findings. Prompt treatment of this syndrome is necessary for optimal visual outcome.

TABLE 25.2

COMMON CONDITIONS THAT CAUSE ACUTE VISUAL DISTURBANCES

Trauma
Migraine
Chemical burns
Hyphema
Ruptured globe
Periorbital infection
Conjunctivitis

TABLE 25.3

CAUSES OF ACUTE DIPLOPIA

Blowout fractures
Poisoning
Central nervous system pathology (tumor, bleed, idiopathic intracranial hypertension)
Shunt malfunction
Arnold–Chiari malformation
Myasthenia gravis
Head trauma

TABLE 25.4

EMERGENT CONDITIONS THAT CAUSE VISUAL DISTURBANCES

Alkali or acid burns
Central retinal artery occlusion
Ruptured globe

In addition to blurred vision in one or both eyes, anterior uveitis is also associated with pain in the affected eye, headache, photophobia, and conjunctival injection. On gross examination, the pupil may be constricted and have a ring of redness surrounding the cornea. A slit lamp examination is used to confirm the diagnosis. Anterior uveitis may be confused with conjunctivitis or an acute attack of glaucoma. In posterior uveitis, the pain and photophobia may be less pronounced, but there may be a more pronounced visual impairment.

The posterior chamber is composed of the vitreous humor. The vitreous gel is usually clear, and any diseases that affect the clarity will impair vision. Certain chronic conditions such as uveitis can cause deposits in the vitreous humor, but the visual impairment is very gradual. Infections inside the eye (endophthalmitis) usually result from a penetrating injury, surgery, or extension of a more superficial infection. Bacterial infections develop more rapidly than do fungal infections. The child will have severe pain in or around the eye and, with bacterial infections especially, may have fever and leukocytosis. The process is usually unilateral, and vision is severely compromised. Purulent exudate is formed in the vitreous humor, and ophthalmoscopic examination may reveal a greenish color with the details of the retina lost. A hypopyon—accumulation of pus in the anterior chamber—is usually present.

Either penetrating or blunt trauma (see Chapter 122 Ocular Trauma) to the eye can lead to vitreous hemorrhage, but this is uncommon in children. Diabetes mellitus, hypertension, sickle cell disease, and leukemia may cause vitreous hemorrhage as well as retinal tears, and central retinal vein occlusion. There is a sudden loss or deterioration of vision in the affected eye. This may present as strabismus and nystagmus in younger preverbal patients. Findings on examination depend on the degree of hemorrhage. Blood clots may be visible with the ophthalmoscope, or the fundus reflex may be black, obscuring the retina in more severe cases.

Retinal vein and artery obstruction are also uncommon in pediatric patients. With central retinal artery occlusion, there is a sudden, painless, total loss of vision in one eye. If only a branch is occluded, a field loss will result. Ophthalmoscopic examination reveals the cherry-red spot of the fovea, the optic nerve appears pale white, and the arteries are narrowed significantly. A Marcus Gunn pupil (relative afferent defect) may be present and may be diagnosed by shining a light in one eye, then in the other. When the light is shone in the normal eye, both pupils will constrict. When light is shone in the damaged eye, the pupil will dilate. The retinal artery may be severed by trauma or obstructed by emboli, as in a patient with endocardial thrombi or arterial obstructions in systemic lupus erythematosus (SLE) and in diseases with hypercoagulability, such as sickle cell disease. The arterial spasm associated with migraine may also lead to retinal artery obstruction.

As with retinal artery occlusion, retinal vein occlusion causes a painless loss of vision. Visual loss may be severe, with total occlusion of the central retinal vein, or less pronounced, with branch obstruction. Examination of the retina reveals multiple hemorrhages with a blurred, reddened optic disc. The arteries are narrowed, the veins engorged, and patchy white exudates may be evident. These findings will be limited to one area in branch occlusion. Retinal vein obstruction, although rare, may occur with trauma or diseases such as leukemia, cystic fibrosis, or retinal phlebitis.

As mentioned, a tear in the retina may lead to vitreous hemorrhage, causing decreased vision in the affected eye. If the tear is in the macula, the visual loss will be severe. A tear in the retina may not cause immediate visual impairment. Retinal detachment from a retinal tear may be delayed for years. The visual impairment may go unnoticed if the detachment is peripheral. As the detachment progresses or when it involves more central areas, the patient will complain of cloudy vision with lightning flashes (photopsia). This may be followed by a shadow or curtain in the visual field. Visual acuity may remain normal if the macula is not involved. Examination of the eye will reveal a lighter-appearing retina in the area of detachment, and it may have folds. Flashing lights or visual field defects, after trauma, should raise the suspicion of retinal detachment. Retinoschisis, splitting of the layers of the retina, may be seen in shaken baby syndrome.

Commotio retinae, or Berlin edema, is edema of the retina that may follow blunt ocular trauma by 24 hours. The visual loss is variable, and the retina will appear pale gray because of the edema, but the macula is usually spared.

The optic nerve transmits visual signals to the cortex. Optic neuritis is involvement of the optic nerve by inflammation or demyelination. The process is usually acute and may be unilateral or bilateral. Loss of vision may take from hours to days, and visual impairment ranges from mild loss to complete blindness. Patients often complain of disturbance of color vision. Pain may be absent or present on movement of the eye or palpation of the globe. It is rarely an isolated event in children. Causes include meningitis, viral infections, immunizations, encephalomyelitis, Lyme disease, and demyelinating diseases. Multiple sclerosis uncommonly occurs in childhood, but may present with sudden onset of intermittent episodes of optic neuritis associated with gait disturbances, paresthesias, and dysesthesias. Exogenous toxins and drugs (e.g., lead poisoning, long-term chloramphenicol treatment) may also cause optic neuritis.

IIH or pseudotumor cerebri, which is characterized by increased intracranial pressure with normal cerebrospinal fluid content, normal neuroimaging, absence of neurologic signs except cranial nerve VI palsy, and often without discernable cause, can also present with visual loss. Visual acuity loss and/or visual field defects can be reversed with appropriate therapy.

Pressure on the optic nerve from a neoplastic lesion, such as an optic glioma or craniopharyngioma, may cause visual field loss as an early finding. Optic nerve gliomas can occur anywhere along the optic nerves, chiasm, and optic tract. Optic nerve gliomas are slow growing, and patients present with proptosis, unilateral or bilateral visual loss, strabismus, optic atrophy, or nystagmus. Children with craniopharyngiomas often present with nonspecific complaints of headaches or progressive visual loss of unknown cause. They may also present with endocrine abnormalities related to pituitary dysfunction.

Various toxins are capable of causing impaired vision. The loss may be gradual or sudden, depending on the particular toxin. Toxins usually act on ganglion cells of the retina or on optic nerve fibers, causing contraction of the peripheral field, central visual defect, or a combination. Methyl alcohol, when ingested, may cause bilateral sudden blindness, which may be complete and permanent or may have a more gradual onset. With methyl alcohol ingestion, associated symptoms include nausea, vomiting, abdominal pain, headache, dizziness, delirium, and convulsions. Other toxins include halogenated hydrocarbons, sulfanilamide, quinine, mercury, and quinidine. Large doses of salicylates may cause amblyopia. Digitalis may cause transient amblyopia, visual blurring, or the perception of yellow halos around light (xanthopsia).

Visual impairment may also result from interference with the visual cortex of the brain. Cortical blindness has many causes (Table 25.5). Head trauma (see Chapters 36 Injury: Head and 121 Neurotrauma) may cause total loss of vision soon after the event. This has been called "footballer's migraine" because of its association with head trauma in soccer. Even trivial head trauma has been known to cause blindness. The physical examination may be completely normal. There may be a delay of onset, but the entire course is usually brief, lasting minutes to hours. This form of blindness is often confused with hysterical blindness, the latter being a diagnosis of exclusion. Monocular blindness may be caused by trauma to the carotid artery on the affected side.

Cerebral venous sinus thrombosis may present with headache, diplopia, nausea, vomiting, blurred vision, and photophobia. It may be associated with hypercoagulable states.

Migraine headaches are a common cause of visual loss in children. Ophthalmoplegic migraine, which occurs primarily in children, affects the third cranial nerve causing ptosis, pupillary dilation, exotropia and diplopia, and blurred vision

TABLE 25.5

CAUSES OF CORTICAL BLINDNESS

Cardiac arrest
Status epilepticus
Hypoxia
Perinatal asphyxia
Cerebral infarction
Meningitis
Encephalitis
Subacute sclerosing leukoencephalitis
Hypoglycemia
Uremia
Hydrocephalus
Shunt malfunction
Head trauma
Cardiac surgery
Posterior reversible encephalopathy syndrome
Cerebral or vertebral angiography
Drugs (steroids)
Carbon monoxide poisoning
Occipital epilepsy
Postictal states
Hypertensive crisis

as the headache ends and takes days to weeks to resolve. Basilar migraine are typically occipital, associated with visual disturbances and accompanied by blurred or tunnel vision, dizziness, ataxia, diplopia, and vomiting. Retinal migraine is characterized by sudden loss of vision associated with a headache. Headache and nausea after such an episode are very common.

Seizures may also present with visual changes, which sometimes manifest as a migraine-like episode. Visual disturbances may also be the only clinical manifestation of childhood occipital epilepsy, but are more commonly associated with more typical seizure activity. Posterior reversible encephalopathy syndrome should be considered if a child presents with hypertension, altered mental status, seizures, and visual changes. It is typically seen with patients with renal, oncologic, and autoimmune diseases and characteristic edema of the posterior cerebral region is seen on radiographic imaging. Prompt neurologic consultation should be obtained if a child presents with this constellation of symptoms as rapid recognition and treatment is essential to help prevent complications.

EVALUATION AND DECISION

The absolute ophthalmologic emergencies are alkali burns, a ruptured globe, and retinal artery occlusion. The diagnosis of the first is by history, and therapy must be initiated promptly to minimize the damage to the eye. If there is any doubt about the actual substance to which the eyes have been exposed, treatment for an alkali burn is always prudent. The eye should be anesthetized with topical therapy and then irrigated with copious amounts of normal saline until the pH of the tears is less than 7.5. The pH should be repeated to ensure it remains normal. A ruptured globe must be suspected with any possible penetrating injury to the eye. The injury may be subtle, and the vision may be normal. If a possibility of a ruptured globe exists, the patient should have immediate evaluation by an ophthalmologist. The eye should be protected with an eye shield and the head of bed should be elevated to 30 degrees. Avoid ocular medication drops, such as fluorescein, and aggressive examination of the eye. Intravenous antiemetics such as ondansetron, antibiotics, pain medications, and sedation should be considered. Retinal artery thrombosis is rare in children, but it should be suspected when there is sudden, unilateral painless loss of vision, and a predisposing condition. Predisposing conditions include those associated with emboli, such as endocardial thrombi or amniotic fluid; conditions with arteritis leading to obstruction, as in SLE; disease states associated with hypercoagulability, such as sickling hemoglobinopathies; and conditions with arterial spasm, such as severe hypertension.

If alkali burns, a ruptured globe, and retinal artery occlusion can be excluded, the patient may be evaluated more carefully before instituting therapy. Significant historical information includes episodes of recent trauma, unilateral or bilateral nature of the loss, and association of pain in or around the eye (Fig. 25.1). Child abuse may present with any of a variety of traumatic injuries. Retinal hemorrhages in a child are almost always caused by nonaccidental trauma. Most children seen in the ED will have a traumatic or infectious process.

If hysterical blindness is suspected, the mirror test may be used. A mirror that is large enough to prevent the patient from looking around it is placed in front of the patient's face

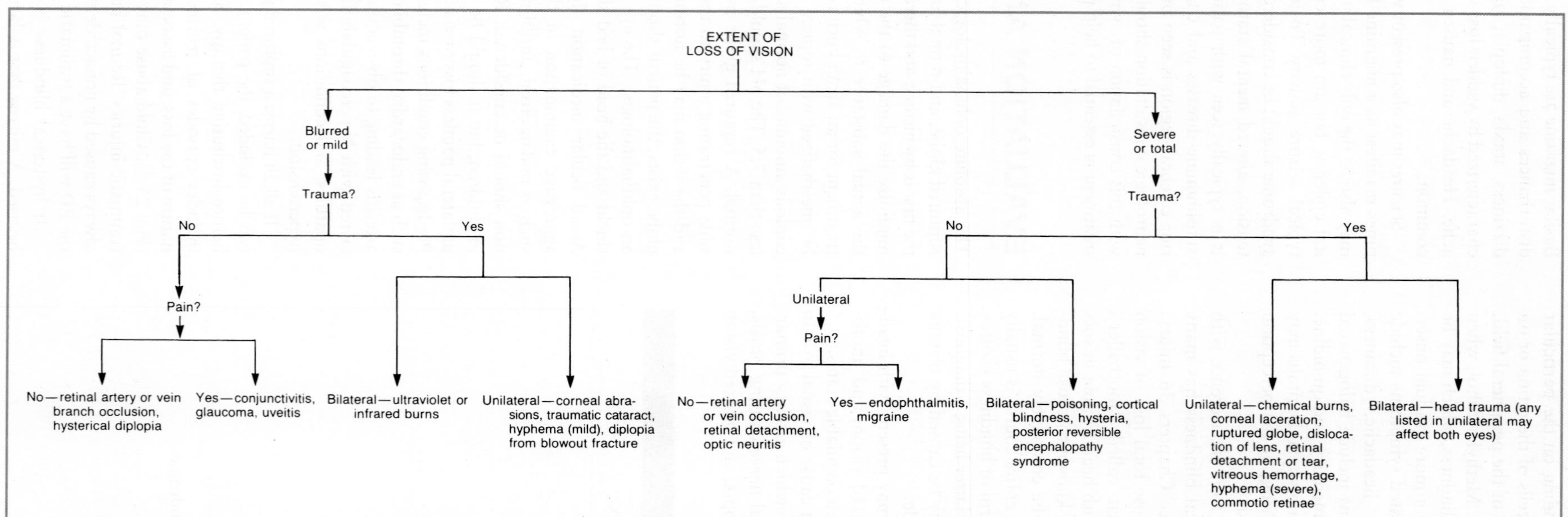
EXTENT OF LOSS OF VISION
Blurred or mild
Trauma?
No
Yes
Pain?
No—retinal artery or vein branch occlusion, hysterical diplopia
Yes—conjunctivitis, glaucoma, uveitis
Bilateral—ultraviolet or infrared burns
Unilateral—corneal abrasions, traumatic cataract, hyphema (mild), diplopia from blowout fracture
Severe or total
Trauma?
No
Yes
Unilateral
Pain?
No—retinal artery or vein occlusion, retinal detachment, optic neuritis
Yes—endophthalmitis, migraine
Bilateral—poisoning, cortical blindness, hysteria, posterior reversible encephalopathy syndrome
Unilateral—chemical burns, corneal laceration, ruptured globe, dislocation of lens, retinal detachment or tear, vitreous hemorrhage, hyphema (severe), commotio retinae
Bilateral—head trauma (any listed in unilateral may affect both eyes)

FIGURE 25.1 Diagnostic approach to visual disturbances.

and is slowly rocked back and forth. The examiner should observe the patient from above to see if the patient is able to suppress the tendency to follow the mirror or hide a response to another visual stimulus, such as a funny face made by the examiner.

Severe Visual Loss Associated with Trauma

Severe bilateral visual loss associated with head trauma is likely cortical blindness. This condition usually is totally reversible in less than a few hours. Any of the traumatic injuries that cause severe unilateral loss of vision may cause bilateral loss if both eyes are involved. If there is any possibility of a penetrating injury or rupture of the globe, the involved eye should be protected from further damage by covering the eye with a hard shield after a brief physical examination, and arranging emergent ophthalmologic evaluation. The head of the bed should be elevated 30 degrees. Administration of intravenous antiemetics, such as ondansetron, antibiotics, pain control, and sedation should be considered. Instillation of topical medications such as fluorescein should be avoided. If the globe is intact and no penetration by a foreign body occurred, an ophthalmoscopic or slit lamp examination usually leads to the correct diagnosis. These conditions include chemical burns of the cornea, hyphema, dislocation of the lens, vitreous hemorrhage, detachment or tear of the retina, and commotio retinae.

Severe Visual Loss Not Associated with Trauma

With severe bilateral visual loss not associated with trauma, the possibility of toxins must be explored. Also, cortical blindness may cause a similar picture, but this is rare and generally associated with another problem, such as hypoglycemia, leukemia, and cerebrovascular or anesthetic accidents. If severe visual loss is unilateral and painful, endophthalmitis must be suspected, but once again, such loss is usually the result of a previous penetrating injury or an extension of a local infectious process. If a headache is associated with the visual loss, migraine may be implicated. If the severe loss is unilateral and painless, retinal artery or vein occlusion, or retinal detachment, may be diagnosed by ophthalmoscopic examination. Optic neuritis will also present this way.

Mild Visual Loss with Trauma

If the visual loss is unilateral, not severe, and if trauma recently occurred, corneal abrasions, traumatic cataracts, and small hyphemas should be sought. A blowout fracture may cause diplopia, but if each eye is examined individually, the visual acuity should be normal. If the process is bilateral, exposure to ultraviolet or infrared light should be considered.

Mild Visual Loss without Trauma

When the visual loss is mild and nontraumatic, and if the process is unilateral and painful, conjunctivitis, uveitis, and acute attacks of glaucoma are possible. If the process is painless, retinal vein or artery branch occlusion may be suspected. Any of these processes may also be bilateral.

Suggested Readings and Key References

Albert DM, Miller JW. *Albert and Jakobiec's principles and practice of ophthalmology.* 3rd ed. Philadelphia, PA: Saunders Elsevier; 2008.

Beauchamp GR. Causes of visual impairment in children. *Pediatr Ann* 1980;9(11):414–418.

Caraballo RH, Cersosimo RO, Fejerman N. Childhood occipital epilepsy of Gastaut: a study of 33 patients. *Epilepsia* 2008;49(2): 288–297.

Chabas D, Strober J, Waubant E. Pediatric multiple sclerosis. *Curr Neurol Neurosci Rep* 2008;8(5):434–441.

Chen TH, Lin WC, Tseng YH, et al. Posterior reversible encephalopathy syndrome in children: case series and systematic review. *J Child Neurol* 2013;28(11):1378–1386.

Chew E, Morin JD. Glaucoma in children. *Pediatr Clin North Am* 1983; 30(6):1043–1060.

Cinciripini GS, Donahue S, Borchert MS. Idiopathic intracranial hypertension in prepubertal pediatric patients: characteristics, treatment, and outcome. *Am J Ophthalmol* 1999;127(2):178–182.

Cologno D, Torelli P, Manzoni GC. Transient visual disturbances during migraine without aura attacks. *Headache* 2002;42(9):930–933.

Datner EM, Jolly BT. Pediatric ophthalmology. *Emerg Clin North Am* 1995;13(3):669–679.

Ganesh A, Al-Zuhaibi S, Pathare A, et al. Orbital infarction in sickle cell disease. *Am J Ophthalmol* 2008;146(4):595–601.

Harrison DW, Walls RM. Blindness following minor head trauma in children: a report of two cases with a review of the literature. *J Emerg Med* 1990;8(1):21–24.

King MA, Barkovich AJ, Halbach VA, et al. Traumatic monocular blindness and associated carotid injuries. *Pediatrics* 1989;84(1): 128–132.

Kump LI, Cervantes-Castaneda RA, Androudi SN, et al. Analysis of pediatric uveitis cases at a tertiary referral center. *Ophthalmology* 2005;112(7):1287–1292.

Kwartz J, Leatherbarrow B, Davis H. Diplopia following head injury. *Injury* 1990;21(6):351–352.

Levin AV. Retinal hemorrhage in abusive head trauma. *Pediatrics* 2010;126(5):961–970.

Lotze TE, Northrop JL, Hutton GJ, et al. Spectrum of pediatric neuromyelitis optica. *Pediatrics* 2008;122(5):e1039–e1047.

Mackay MT, Chua ZK, Lee M, et al. Stroke and nonstroke brain attacks in children. *Neurology* 2014;82(16):1434–1440.

Recchia FM, Saluja RK, Hammel K, et al. Outpatient management of traumatic microhyphema. *Ophthalmology* 2002;109(8):1465–1470; discussion 1470–1471.

Salvin JH. Systematic approach to pediatric ocular trauma. *Curr Opin Ophthalmol* 2007;18(5):366–372.

Spector J, Fernandez WG. Chemical, thermal, and biological ocular exposures. *Emerg Med Clin North Am* 2008;26(1):125–136.

Spirn MJ, Lynn MJ, Hubbard GB 3rd. Vitreous hemorrhage in children. *Ophthalmology* 2006;113(5):848–852.

Wagner RS, Aquino M. Pediatric ocular inflammation. *Immunol Allergy Clin North Am* 2008;28(1):169–188.

Wall M. Idiopathic intracranial hypertension: mechanisms of visual loss and disease management. *Semin Neurol* 2000;20(1):89–95.

Williams JR. Optic neuritis in a child. *Pediatr Emerg Care* 1996;12(3): 210–212.

Wong VC. Cortical blindness in children: a study of etiology and prognosis. *Pediatr Neurol* 1990;7(3):178–185.

Woodward GA. Posttraumatic cortical blindness: are we missing the diagnosis in children? *Pediatr Emerg Care* 1990;6(4):289–292.

CHAPTER 26 ▪ FEVER

FRAN BALAMUTH, MD, PhD, MSCE, FRED M. HENRETIG, MD, AND ELIZABETH R. ALPERN, MD, MSCE

Fever, the abnormal elevation of body temperature, has been recognized for centuries by physicians as a sign of disease. The problem of the febrile child is one of the most commonly encountered in clinical pediatrics, accounting for as many as 20% of pediatric emergency department (ED) visits. The problem of appropriate clinical and laboratory evaluation of febrile children, however, remains a major challenge. The approach outlined in this chapter helps the physician evaluate and treat a febrile child in the ED, proceeding systematically with the appropriate diagnostic steps and management. The principal causes of fever in children are listed in Table 26.1.

PATHOPHYSIOLOGY

Fever is a complex process, involving the highly coordinated interplay of autonomic, neuroendocrine, and behavioral responses to a variety of infectious and noninfectious inflammatory challenges. Fever is believed to be an adaptive response that is ubiquitous in animals. Exogenous pyrogens (e.g., toxins, infectious agents, etc.) from many sources produce fever by inducing the production of endogenous pyrogens (e.g., interleukin-B1, interleukin-6, etc.). These pyrogens interact with specialized receptor neurons of the hypothalamus. This leads to the production of prostaglandins as the critical mediators of the febrile response, resetting the hypothalamic thermostat to elevate body temperature. There is some evidence that increased body temperature impairs replication of microbes and may aid phagocytic bactericidal activity. Additionally, the febrile response includes adaptive neuroendocrine and metabolic effects that further enhance the host's response to microbial invasion. Rarely, fever results from central nervous system (CNS) dysfunction (e.g., hypothalamic tumor, infarction) that alters the thermostatic set point directly, rather than via pyrogen induction. Finally, sometimes hyperpyrexia is not due to altered hypothalamic regulation, but rather to increased heat production (e.g., stimulant drug overdose; see Chapter 110 Toxicologic Emergencies) or exposure to excess environmental heat (heat stroke; see Chapter 98 Environmental Emergencies, Radiological Emergencies, Bites and Stings).

It is difficult to pinpoint the lowest temperature elevation considered to be definitely abnormal for all children under all circumstances. Some children normally have rectal temperatures as low as 36.2°C (97.2°F) or as high as 38°C (100.4°F). Children, like adults, also have diurnal variations in temperature, with the peak usually occurring between 5 pm and 7 pm. Factors such as excessive clothing, physical activity, hot weather, and ovulation can raise temperature in the absence of disease. For the appropriately dressed child who has been at rest for 30 minutes, a rectal temperature of 38°C (100.4°F) is defined as fever for this discussion.

Using the proper technique to record temperature is important for maximum accuracy. Rectal thermometry combines attributes of being the least invasive way to most approximate core temperature compared to other invasive methods, such as esophageal or bladder thermometry. Optimal technique for rectal thermometry includes appropriate positioning and restraint in infants (prone, supine, or on the side with hips slightly flexed), depth of insertion (about 2 to 3 cm), and time for equilibration (2 to 3 minutes with glass thermometers or several seconds with electronic digital probes). The thermometer should not be placed directly into a fecal mass because the fecal temperature may not have equilibrated with rapid fluctuations in core temperature and thus may be falsely low as temperature rises rapidly. Other noninvasive methods have varying accuracy and precision with most being shown to overestimate at lower body temperatures and underestimate at higher temperatures. Oral and axillary temperatures are usually about 0.6°C (1°F) and 1.1°C (2°F) lower than rectal temperatures, respectively. More recent attempts to measure temperature with less invasive techniques include temperature-sensitive pacifiers and forehead strips, both of which have been found to be unreliable. Infrared tympanic membrane (aural) thermometry, based on the premise that the tympanic membrane shares vascular supply with the hypothalamus, has also shown inadequate accuracy and precision in both afebrile and febrile children and is not useful in healthcare settings. Temporal artery thermometry, which uses similar infrared technology to measure heat produced by the temporal artery, has more recently been studied. The temporal artery technique has been shown to more closely approximate rectal temperatures; however, it has still been found to underestimate high temperatures and overestimate low ones. As even a low-grade fever may be clinically significant in young infants <60 days of age, and as there is at least some doubt about the reliability of axillary, tympanic, or temporal artery measurements in this age group, rectal temperatures should be obtained in this population.

EVALUATION AND DECISION

The importance of fever lies in its role as a sign of disease. The physicians caring for a febrile child should concentrate on discovering the cause of the fever and treating the underlying illness. Although any degree of fever may indicate an important infectious etiology, the risk of serious bacterial infection is slightly higher with hyperpyrexia (defined as a temperature of 41.1°C) in children and a thorough assessment for possible bacterial etiology (e.g., pneumonia, bacteremia, or meningitis) should be seriously considered. However, the magnitude of reduction of fever in response to antipyretics does not distinguish children with serious bacterial illnesses from those with viral diseases. If no specific treatment for the determined diagnosis is necessary, the physician's goal is then to provide appropriate supportive care and follow-up. Because many parents

TABLE 26.1

PRINCIPAL CONDITIONS IN CHILDREN ASSOCIATED WITH FEVER

- Infections
  - Central nervous system
    - Meningitis
    - Encephalitis
    - Brain abscess
  - Ocular
    - Periorbital (preseptal) cellulitis
    - Orbital cellulitis/abscess
  - Airways and upper respiratory tract
    - Common cold (upper respiratory infection)
    - Pharyngitis/tonsillitis
    - Otitis media
    - Acute cervical adenitis
    - Acute sinusitis
    - Peritonsillar, retropharyngeal, lateral pharyngeal wall abscess
    - Croup
    - Epiglottitis
  - Oral cavity and salivary glands
    - Alveolar abscess
    - Viral stomatitis (herpangina, herpetic gingivostomatitis)
    - Parotitis (mumps, acute suppurative parotitis)
  - Pulmonary
    - Bronchiolitis
    - Pneumonia
    - Bronchitis
    - Pulmonary tuberculosis
    - Lung abscess
  - Cardiac
    - Myocarditis
    - Endocarditis
    - Pericarditis
  - Gastrointestinal
    - Acute gastroenteritis (viral, salmonella, shigella)
    - Appendicitis
    - Peritonitis
    - Pancreatitis
    - Acute mesenteric adenitis
    - Hepatitis
    - Cholangitis
    - Intra-abdominal abscesses
  - Genitourinary
    - Urinary tract infection/pyelonephritis
    - Perinephric abscess
    - Acute salpingitis, tuboovarian abscess
    - Acute prostatitis
    - Epididymitis, orchitis
  - Musculoskeletal
    - Septic arthritis
    - Osteomyelitis
    - Myositis
  - Skin and soft tissue/lymphoid
    - Abscess (methicillin-resistant *Staphylococcus aureus*, methicillin-sensitive *S. aureus*, group A *Streptococcus*)
    - Cellulitis
    - Necrotizing fasciitis
    - Exanthems (systemic infections usually associated with prominent rashes)
      - Viral: roseola, rubeola, rubella, varicella, hand–foot–mouth disease (Coxsackievirus)
      - Bacterial toxin: scarlet fever
      - Syphilis (secondary)
      - Meningococcemia (occasionally other primary septicemia)
      - Rocky Mountain spotted fever
      - Lymphadenitis
  - Systemic infections
    - Bacterial sepsis (primary—especially meningococcemia)
    - "Occult bacteremia" (especially pneumococcal)
    - Viruses (Epstein–Barr, adenovirus)
    - Lyme disease
    - Rickettsial (Rocky Mountain spotted fever, ehrlichiosis), chlamydial, fungal, parasitic, and unusual bacterial infections
    - Toxic shock syndrome
    - Miliary tuberculosis
- Vasculitis syndromes and hypersensitivity phenomena
  - Acute rheumatic fever
  - Juvenile rheumatoid arthritis
  - Systemic lupus erythematosus
  - Polyarteritis nodosa
  - Kawasaki syndrome
  - Dermatomyositis/polymyositis
  - Mixed connective tissue disease
  - Henoch–Schönlein purpura
  - Serum sickness
  - Stevens–Johnson syndrome
  - Drug and immunization reactions
- Neoplasms
  - Leukemia
  - Neuroblastoma
  - Lymphoma
  - Ewing sarcoma
- Poisonings and drug reactions
  - Sympathomimetics (e.g., amphetamines, cocaine)
  - Anticholinergics (e.g., antihistamines, tricyclic antidepressants, atropinic alkaloids)
  - Salicylates
  - Malignant hyperthermia
  - Serotonin syndrome
  - Neuroleptic malignant syndrome
  - Alcohol/sedative–hypnotic withdrawal
- Central nervous system (CNS) disorders
  - CNS lesions in hypothalamus/brainstem
  - Prolonged seizures
  - Riley–Day syndrome
- Metabolic diseases
  - Thyrotoxic crisis
  - Etiocholanolone fever
  - Acute intermittent porphyria
- Miscellaneous conditions
  - Dehydration
  - Intravascular hemolysis
  - Hemorrhage into an enclosed space
  - Anhidrotic ectodermal dysplasia
  - Extreme environmental heat excess
  - Hereditary periodic fever syndromes
  - PFAPA (periodic fever, aphthous stomatitis, pharyngitis, adenitis)
  - Cyclic neutropenia
  - Sarcoidosis
  - Inflammatory bowel disease
  - Factitious
  - Major trauma (crush injuries)
  - Other rare causes

have "fever phobia," instructions that explain the importance of fever as an indicator of disease, not as an inherently harmful entity, should be given.

A complete *history and physical examination* will provide the most important clues in determining the diagnosis of children with febrile illnesses. The age of the infant or child should be carefully considered as it significantly impacts the risk of fever source and etiology. Very young infants' rate of serious bacterial illnesses is higher than other age groups and children under 24 months have distinct risks of certain infectious causes of fever (see Chapter 102 Infectious Disease Emergencies). The *general impression* obtained in the first few moments of an evaluation is extremely important in the recognition of potentially life-threatening causes of fever (Table 26.2). A great deal of information can be attained by visual assessment of the child while in the arms or lap of the parent. The severity of the illness may become apparent if the child is agitated or uninterested in the surroundings while in this comfortable, safe position. If the child appears nontoxic, observation of the child while the *history* of the present illness and medical history is being discussed may provide further insight into the diagnosis. Specifics of fever have different management implications for distinct subsets of children. Therefore, a clear understanding of the degree, mode of measurement, and duration of fever is especially important in the initial evaluation. The physician should ask questions concerning associated signs and symptoms, medications being given (including antipyretics and antibiotics), presence of ill contacts, travel history, and pet or insect exposures. The medical history should focus on recurrent febrile illnesses and the presence of any diseases or drug regimens that would compromise normal host defenses, such as sickle cell anemia, asplenia (functional, congenital, or surgical), malignancy (noting particularly chemotherapeutic or radiation treatments), human immunodeficiency virus (HIV), renal disease, prolonged steroid use, or indwelling catheters or ventriculoperitoneal shunts. Personal immunization status as well as known exposure to unimmunized individuals should also be determined. An understanding of prior evaluation and treatments during this illness may be helpful.

As stated above, the *physical examination* of the young febrile patient begins during the interview with the caregiver. The physician should note the child's alertness, responsiveness to persons and objects, work of breathing, color, feeding activity, and age-related appropriateness of social interaction and gross motor functions. The *febrile infant who appears irritable and/or lethargic* while being held by a parent before the examination has the possibility of having a serious infection such as meningitis or sepsis. The complaint or observation that a child's crying increases with parental attempts to comfort is critical because "paradoxical irritability" is an important sign of meningitis in infancy.

Other signs of severe or life-threatening infections heralded by fever should be sought early in the examination. CNS infections may be marked by fever with altered sensorium, convulsion, meningismus, or focal neurologic deficits. However, infants younger than 2 months of age with meningitis may not have meningismus. They may instead have irritability, somnolence, a bulging fontanel, or nonspecific symptoms such as anorexia, lethargy, or vomiting. Severe upper airway infections may present with stridor, excessive drooling, and tripod positioning. A child with pneumonia, pericarditis, endocarditis, or sepsis syndrome may display tachycardia, dyspnea or tachypnea, cyanosis or pallor, poor perfusion or hypotension, as well as altered mental status. Hemorrhagic rashes may signal bacterial or rickettsial infections such as meningococcemia or Rocky Mountain spotted fever.

Careful assessment of the vital signs can provide early important clues to more severe illnesses. Severe sepsis and septic shock are defined as infection with organ dysfunction (see Chapter 5 Shock). It is important to note, however, that hypotension is a late finding in children, and that prompt recognition of the child with compensated septic shock is critical in the ED. That said, recognition of compensated shock can be quite challenging in children, as the prevalence of systemic inflammatory response syndrome (SIRS) defined by fever, tachycardia, and tachypnea is high in pediatric patients, the

TABLE 26.2

LIFE-THREATENING ACUTE FEBRILE ILLNESSES

- Infection
  - Central nervous system
    - Acute bacterial meningitis
    - Encephalitis
  - Upper airway
    - Acute epiglottitis
    - Retropharyngeal abscess
    - Laryngeal diphtheria (rare)
    - Croup (severe)
  - Pulmonary
    - Pneumonia (severe)
    - Tuberculosis, miliary
  - Cardiac
    - Myocarditis
    - Bacterial endocarditis
    - Suppurative pericarditis
  - Gastrointestinal
    - Acute gastroenteritis (fluid/electrolyte losses)
    - Appendicitis
    - Peritonitis (other causes)
  - Musculoskeletal
    - Necrotizing myositis (gas gangrene)/fasciitis
  - Systemic
    - Meningococcemia
    - Other bacterial sepsis
    - Rocky Mountain spotted fever
    - Toxic shock syndrome
- Collagen-vascular
  - Acute rheumatic fever
  - Kawasaki syndrome
  - Stevens–Johnson syndrome
- Miscellaneous
  - Thyrotoxicosis
  - Heat stroke
  - Acute poisonings and drug reactions: sympathomimetics, anticholinergics, salicylate, serotonin syndrome, neuroleptic malignant syndrome, malignant hyperthermia, alcohol/sedative–hypnotic withdrawal
  - DRESS: Drug Rash with Eosinophilia and Systemic Symptoms
  - Malignancy

majority of whom are not critically ill. However, close observation of children with fever and tachycardia is warranted. If the tachycardia resolves with antipyretics and/or oral hydration, and the child is well appearing with normal perfusion and mental status, the child should undergo an evaluation based on the algorithms presented in Clinical Pathway Chapters 87 Fever in Infants and 88 Fever in Children. If tachycardia persists, the child is ill appearing, has a high-risk condition, poor perfusion, or altered mental status, more aggressive treatment for sepsis may be indicated including rapid fluid resuscitation and antimicrobial therapy.

Although the index of suspicion for serious febrile illness must be high throughout the evaluation of each child, most childhood illnesses with fever are minor and self-limiting. Once the physician has ascertained that the child is not in immediate danger, the examination should focus on sites of common pediatric infections, including the ears, nose, and throat; cervical lymph nodes; respiratory, gastrointestinal, and genitourinary tracts; and skin, joints, and skeletal system (Table 26.3). Evaluation of each child is developed with an understanding of the common infectious entities that affect that child's age group and the presenting signs and symptoms or lack thereof in each infectious entity (see Chapter 102 Infectious Disease Emergencies).

Some febrile exanthems are characteristic enough to be diagnostic (see Chapter 65 Rash: Papulosquamous Eruptions). Varicella, rubeola, scarlet fever, and coxsackievirus can all be identified by their pathognomonic rashes. However, if a child with chickenpox presents several days into the illness with a new fever, the possibility of group A β-hemolytic streptococcal or *Staphylococcus aureus* superinfection should be considered. Children with *fever and petechiae* may have invasive meningococcal disease, disseminated streptococcal infection, or Rocky Mountain spotted fever; however, they may simply have a less serious viral infection or streptococcal pharyngitis. Differentiation of these entities is crucial and is based on clinical appearance of the patient and laboratory evaluation. A child with only a few petechiae (especially if only above the nipple line), normal white blood cell (WBC) count, normal platelet count, and well appearance is less likely to have invasive disease. However, any child who appears ill, has distinctly abnormal laboratory results, or has a rapidly progressive petechial rash needs a more complete evaluation for sepsis or meningitis and should receive empiric antibiotics. A patient with fever and diffuse erythroderma should be evaluated carefully for hemodynamic instability or other signs and symptoms of toxic shock syndrome. Fever associated in a young child with severe skin blistering and exfoliation may be toxin-mediated staphylococcal scalded skin syndrome.

On physical examination, acute otitis media is identified by the acute onset of otalgia or fever with changes in the tympanic membranes, such as redness, bulging, decreased mobility, loss of landmarks and light reflex, air–fluid level behind the tympanic membrane, or purulent drainage from a perforation. Careful examination of the head and neck may reveal rhinorrhea and signs of inflammation, suggesting a viral upper respiratory infection (URI). The oropharynx may reveal pharyngitis or stomatitis (see Chapters 47 Oral Lesions and 69 Sore Throat). Children with a history of a recent respiratory infection may have reactive, tender, swollen cervical lymph nodes; asymmetric enlargement of nodes especially with tenderness and overlying erythema might indicate bacterial

TABLE 26.3

COMMON CAUSES OF FEVER

- Infections
  - Central nervous system
    - Acute bacterial meningitis
    - Viral meningoencephalitis
  - Ocular
    - Periorbital cellulitis
    - Orbital cellulitis
  - Upper respiratory tract
    - Common cold
    - Pharyngitis/tonsillitis
    - Cervical adenitis
    - Croup
    - Acute sinusitis
    - Otitis media
  - Oral cavity and salivary glands
    - Alveolar abscess
    - Herpangina
    - Herpetic gingivostomatitis
    - Mumps (unimmunized child)
  - Pulmonary
    - Acute tracheobronchitis
    - Bronchiolitis
    - Pneumonia
  - Gastrointestinal
    - Acute gastroenteritis
    - Appendicitis
  - Genitourinary
    - Urinary tract infection
    - Acute salpingitis
    - Tuboovarian abscess
  - Musculoskeletal
    - Septic arthritis
    - Osteomyelitis
  - Skin and soft tissue/lymphoid
    - Abscess
    - Cellulitis
    - Lymphadenitis
    - Miscellaneous systemic infections associated with prominent rash (e.g., meningococcemia and Rocky Mountain spotted fever)
    - Scarlet fever
    - Viral exanthems (especially varicella, measles if unimmunized)
  - Systemic
    - Primary septicemia—especially meningococcemia
    - "Occult" bacteremia
    - Viral syndromes
    - Vector-borne disease—especially Lyme disease
    - Toxic shock syndrome
- Miscellaneous
- Drug and vaccine reactions, including serum sickness
- Kawasaki syndrome
- Amphetamine, cocaine, salicylate poisoning

lymphadenitis. Croup is readily identified by a barky cough with or without stridor in young children, whereas a distinctive "hot potato voice" with unilateral tonsillar swelling in adolescents indicates a peritonsillar abscess. Wheezing, tachypnea, and fever in infants younger than 2 years of age usually mark bronchiolitis. Pneumonia often presents with cough, fever, tachypnea, auscultatory findings, and hypoxemia. Mild abdominal pain or tenderness, vomiting, and/or diarrhea most often suggests viral gastroenteritis but early hepatitis, appendicitis, or pancreatitis should also be considered. More severe findings, particularly the occurrence of peritoneal signs, may indicate appendicitis, intra-abdominal abscess, or peritonitis from other causes (see Chapters 48 Pain: Abdomen, clinical pathway, 82 Abdominal Pain in Postpubertal Girls, 83 Appendicitis (Suspected), and 124 Abdominal Emergencies). However, in children, fever with abdominal pain may also represent lower lobe pneumonia, streptococcal pharyngitis, urinary tract infection (UTI), gastroenteritis, or mesenteric adenitis. Additional findings in UTI may include suprapubic or costovertebral angle tenderness (see clinical pathway Chapter 92 UTI, Febrile). Adolescent girls with pelvic or abdominal pain and fever should be evaluated for pyelonephritis and pelvic inflammatory disease (see clinical pathway Chapter 82 Abdominal Pain in Postpubertal Girls). A close skin examination may reveal an abscess or cellulitis associated with community-acquired methicillin-resistant *S. aureus* or *Streptococcus pyogenes*. Differentiation of these diverse diagnoses depends on a thorough history, physical examination, and at times, well-directed laboratory evaluation.

Continued advancements in *immunizations* have changed the frequency and risk of certain febrile illness in children. The Centers for Disease Control and Prevention reported that the *Haemophilus influenzae* type B (Hib) vaccine has drastically changed the risk and causative agents for meningitis in children with a 94% reduction in the incidence of *H. influenzae* meningitis and a shift in the median age of those affected from 15 months to 25 years of age. The current rarity of epiglottitis in children is also due to this decline in *H. influenzae* infections. In addition, the conjugate pneumococcal vaccine (PCV) has significantly decreased the overall risk of invasive pneumococcal diseases in children. However, after the initial heptavalent PCV vaccine introduction, there was noted a small, but not inconsequential increase in invasive bacterial infections in children due to nonvaccine pneumococcal serotypes. The current 13-valent vaccine, with expanded serotype coverage, has continued to decrease invasive pneumococcal disease in children, especially those less than 2 years of age. Recognition of these epidemiologic changes is crucial in evaluating and treating the febrile child. These findings obviously influence the evaluation and treatment of febrile children with signs of meningitis, as well as those young children without an identified source of infection after thorough historical and physical examination.

Although vaccines have significantly changed the risk and epidemiology of infectious diseases in children, the clinician must be aware of increasing and important outbreaks of vaccine-preventable illnesses in children. Although measles was declared eliminated (without year-round endemic transmission) in the United States in 2000, there have been recent significant outbreaks due to worldwide travel from endemic areas and infection in unvaccinated (due to personal choice, missed vaccine opportunities, or in children too young to receive the primary vaccine series) individuals in the United States. For example, clinicians must continue to consider measles in suspicious cases with the constellation of fever, rash, cough, coryza, and conjunctivitis, especially in un- or underimmunized patients.

Given these general considerations, an algorithmic *approach to the child with an acute* (less than 5 days) *febrile illness* can be formulated, using the following *key features:* overall degree of *toxicity* and presence of signs or symptoms of life-threatening disease, immunocompromised *host status,* patient's *age,* unusual *risk factors* (immunization status, travel, animal exposures), and presence of *localizing features* on history and physical examination (see clinical pathway Chapters 87 Fever in Infants and 88 Fever in Children). Laboratory studies are indicated only for selected situations as defined by clinical features. Most older febrile children do not need routine laboratory testing.

Infants younger than 2 months of age are at increased risk of serious bacterial infections and bacteremia and are more difficult to assess clinically than older children. The management of febrile young infants is particularly challenging because of the relatively high prevalence of serious bacterial infections (up to 15%) and the inability to easily distinguish those with serious bacterial disease or herpes simplex virus from those with uncomplicated, common viral illnesses such as respiratory syncytial virus (RSV), parainfluenza, influenza, adenovirus, human metapneumovirus, or enteroviruses.

Thus, for children with fevers of 38°C (100.4°F) or higher who are younger than 2 months of age, many authorities recommend a laboratory investigation for serious infection ("sepsis workup"), including complete blood count (CBC), blood culture, urine analysis, urine culture, and lumbar puncture with cerebrospinal fluid (CSF) for cell count, glucose, protein, Gram stain, and culture. Some of these authorities support the same evaluation for infants up to 3 months of age; regardless of the exact age parameter, most clinicians base their approach on one of the several published guidelines for managing febrile infants. Clinical examination alone, without further laboratory evaluation, is generally not considered sensitive enough to identify serious illness in these very young infants. In addition, the peripheral blood WBC count has been shown to be inadequate as an indicator of young febrile infants at risk for meningitis. Herpes simplex virus polymerase chain reaction (PCR) or culture from blood and CSF with presumptive antiviral treatment should be considered in acutely ill neonates less than 3 weeks of age and in those with historical concerns or physical findings of skin, eye, or mouth lesions; respiratory distress; seizures; signs of sepsis; or CSF pleocytosis. Stool for leukocytes and culture should be obtained if diarrhea is present. Respiratory findings are good predictors of clinically significant positive chest radiographs in children younger than 3 months; therefore, chest radiographs may be obtained only when there are clinically evident respiratory signs. During local enteroviral season, CSF enterovirus PCR testing has been shown to decrease length of hospitalization and unnecessary antibiotic use in neonates and young febrile infants. Other respiratory viral testing may also be informative as febrile infants younger than 60 days with influenza have lower risk of serious bacterial infections but still have substantial risk of UTI. Biomarkers, including procalcitonin and C-reactive protein, have been recently evaluated as predictors of serious bacterial infection in febrile young infants and may help to identify populations at low risk for serious bacterial infection.

Further evaluations of these markers alone and in combination with existing algorithms are needed to determine if they will provide improved prediction of serious bacterial infection in newborns and young infants.

Special consideration has been given to the evaluation of the febrile young infant with signs and symptoms suggestive of bronchiolitis. Several studies showed that bacteremia is unlikely in the face of a clinical diagnosis of bronchiolitis. In the well-appearing child with bronchiolitis who is to be treated as an outpatient, the risk of meningitis or occult bacteremia is exceedingly low. However, the rate of occult UTI is still significant in children with concurrent bronchiolitis. Therefore, evaluation for UTI should still be considered in the very young infant with fever and clinical signs of bronchiolitis.

An additional dilemma involves the very young infant who presents to the ED with a description of either tactile fever alone or fever confirmed by rectal temperature at home but who is afebrile on arrival. This situation was studied by Bonadio et al., who found that the history of tactile fever in such infants did not correlate with subsequent fever, whereas an elevated rectal temperature at home correlated with subsequent fever in 20% of such patients. However, all infants who were found to have serious bacterial infections (including five who were afebrile on presentation) were observed to have had an abnormal initial clinical profile and/or laboratory workup. Although there is no consensus on the approach to this situation, it seems prudent to consider a careful clinical evaluation in all young infants with a history of fever, including one or more repeat temperatures over 1 to 2 hours in the ED after the baby is unbundled. If there is a reliable history of elevated rectal temperature, a sepsis workup should be seriously considered, as described above, along with a subsequent disposition based on the clinical findings and laboratory results. The infant with only a history of tactile fever whose repeated temperatures are normal and who has an entirely normal clinical evaluation may be assessed as not requiring laboratory studies. All such infants discharged home warrant close follow-up and appropriate short-term monitoring of rectal temperature. An additional conundrum is the young infant with fever who recently received vaccinations. One study addressed this question and recommends that children with recent vaccinations and fever be treated similarly to those who have not recently received vaccinations, mainly due to risk of UTI.

Infants younger than 1 month are usually admitted to the hospital for observation with presumptive antibiotic therapy after full evaluation as noted above in the ED. Acyclovir should be considered for febrile infants younger than 21 days of age or in those with risk factors or findings concerning for HSV (including ill appearance, vesicular rash, hepatitis, or seizures). Studies have found that children between 1 and 2 months of age, who are not pretreated with any antibiotics and who have a completely normal physical examination and completely benign laboratory evaluation, may be safely discharged home with careful observation and close follow-up. For such a disposition, parents should be able to watch the infant closely for changes in symptoms, should have ready access to health care, and should be willing to return for evaluation. These studies found that either close observation without antibiotics or after empiric ceftriaxone are safe and effective management strategies in this age group.

The *febrile child between 2 and 24 months of age* with signs suggesting a serious focal infection (e.g., irritability, meningismus, tachypnea, flank tenderness) should be evaluated with the appropriate diagnostic tests and treated for any identified source. Of course, any child with signs or symptoms of lower pulmonary disease should be evaluated with a chest x-ray. An association between pneumonia and fever greater than 39°C with a WBC greater than 20,000 per mm^3 in the absence of signs of pulmonary disease has also been suggested. Therefore, if a CBC has been obtained and there is marked increase in WBC count, in a child without otherwise identified source of fever, a chest x-ray should be considered. If the child has neither clinical findings of pulmonary disease nor the constellation of high fever associated with leukocytosis, there is no need to perform a chest x-ray.

Young children with fever but no identifiable source on examination are at risk for occult infections including occult bacteremia or UTI. Although in older children, UTIs are accompanied by signs and symptoms such as dysuria, frequency, urgency, incontinence, vomiting, or abdominal, suprapubic, and/or flank pain, in young children fever may be the only sign of a UTI. Studies have established the overall prevalence of occult UTI in young children without an identified source of infection to be between 3% and 9%, with a pooled prevalence estimate of 5%. The risk is highest in febrile non–African-American girls younger than 2 years of age and in uncircumcised boys who are not toilet trained. Renal scarring is associated with a febrile UTI in young children and may lead to further sequelae such as hypertension and renal insufficiency. Therefore, laboratory testing to evaluate for occult UTI is indicated for at-risk young febrile children without an identifiable focus of infection. Certainly any febrile child with a history of UTI should be considered to be at risk for a recurrence. For children without a prior history or overt signs of UTI, one approach is to obtain a urinalysis and urine culture in febrile boys younger than 6 months of age and in any age febrile boy who is uncircumcised and not yet toilet trained. Febrile girls younger than 2 years of age should be considered for urine studies if any three of the following characteristics are present: fever of 39°C (102.2°F) or higher, 1 year of age or younger, non–African-American race, fever lasting 2 days or longer, or no identifiable source of infection. Urine dipstick and culture should be performed for all children at significant risk for occult UTI. Screening urinalysis may be obtained via catheterization, or bag specimen as opposed to catheterized specimen in children older than 6 months of age. If the bag specimen UA is positive, a catheterized urine specimen must be obtained for culture. In children who are not toilet trained, aseptic urethral catheterization or suprapubic aspiration is the appropriate method to obtain urine for the diagnostic urine cultures.

If the child between 2 and 24 months of age with a temperature of 39°C (102°F) or higher does not have localizing symptoms or laboratory/radiograph results (when performed) indicative of definitive focal infection, the child should be assessed for the risk of occult bacteremia especially if younger than 6 months of age or not fully immunized for Hib and *Streptococcus pneumoniae*. A "well" clinical appearance does not decrease the risk for occult bacteremia (otherwise the bacteremia would not be "occult"). Children with occult bacteremia are at risk to develop serious bacterial infections such as septic arthritis, osteomyelitis, meningitis, or sepsis. Historically, some febrile children, 2 to 24 months of age, with temperatures greater than 39°C (102°F) and no clear source of infection were evaluated with a CBC and blood culture for risk of occult bacteremia. The WBC count was used by some to determine the risk of occult bacteremia and guide empiric antibiotic use. However, as the risk of occult bacteremia has decreased, the previous strategy of screening has become less valuable. As mentioned previously, with the licensure of the PCV, rates of invasive pneumococcal infections including occult bacteremia have decreased. Studies from the post-Hib vaccine and post-PCV era indicate the risk of occult bacteremia in immunized children to be less than 1%. Currently, in an immunized population, a detailed history and physical examination and close follow-up is advocated over screening laboratory evaluations. Additional laboratory testing in children 2 to 24 months of age who are well appearing without focal source of fever is not recommended.

Rapid viral testing may be helpful in evaluating patients with specific symptoms or signs of a viral illness and complex medical situations, but in general are not indicated in most children without significant comorbidities. Several recent investigations have shown a decreased risk of bacterial infections with positive rapid tests for specific viruses. Despite positive viral tests, children should be evaluated for secondary bacterial infection through careful examination, especially those patients who have an atypical course based on their duration or severity of their symptoms. Caution should be taken when interpreting results of rapid tests for influenza, which have been shown to have poor sensitivity and positive predictive value, particularly when clinical suspicion of disease is high.

Children *older than 24 months of age* can usually be managed on the basis of degree of irritability, evidence of meningeal signs, and/or other foci of infection found on history and physical examination. These children need not be screened routinely for occult bacteremia or other occult infections. After excluding meningitis, there are several important infections that may be present in ill-appearing, febrile children in this age group, without obvious initial focus. These include meningococcemia, Rocky Mountain spotted fever, and pyelonephritis. Early institution of presumptive therapy may be lifesaving in some of these situations, so their possibility must be borne in mind with toxic, febrile children at any age. Additionally, one should consider history of travel and animal/insect exposure in the evaluation of the febrile child and broaden the differential diagnosis accordingly (clinical pathway Chapter 88 Fever in Children). Several emerging infections deserve mention in this category including mosquito born West Nile virus, Ebola virus, and novel coronaviruses such as those implicated in severe acute respiratory syndrome (SARS), or Middle Eastern Respiratory Syndrome (MERS).

Simple febrile seizures occur in 3% to 5% of all children (see Chapter 67 Seizures). They are defined as generalized tonic–clonic seizures without focal neurologic findings, occurring only once per febrile illness (usually in the first 12 hours of onset of fever) in children 6 months to 5 years of age and lasting less than 15 to 20 minutes in duration. By definition, they are seizures accompanied by fever that occur in children without CNS infection or other underlying cause. The dilemma that faces the emergency physician is to decide whether a febrile seizure is truly such, or if a child presenting with a fever and seizure requires a lumbar puncture to rule out meningitis. The American Academy of Pediatrics published guidelines in 2011, which address this critical issue. The decision to perform a lumbar puncture should be determined by the presence of signs or symptoms of meningitis or other CNS infection. As such, any child with irritability, lethargy, abnormal mental status findings after a usual postictal period, or signs of meningitis such as bulging fontanel, should have a lumbar puncture performed. Because of the difficulty in recognizing signs and symptoms of meningitis in very young infants, particular care should be taken in the assessment of children younger than 12 months of age (especially in infants who have not received their scheduled immunizations or in whom immunization status cannot be determined), and in children pretreated with antibiotics (because symptoms of partially treated meningitis may be minimal or absent). Children with atypical or complex febrile seizures should be closely evaluated for CNS infection. Neuroimaging, electroencephalogram (EEG), and routine laboratory testing should not be performed in the evaluation of a neurologically healthy child with simple febrile seizure.

Other causes of acute febrile episodes should be kept in mind, including intoxications, environmental exposure, immunization reactions, and autoimmune/inflammatory disease processes. *Toxic exposures,* particularly aspirin, anticholinergics, and sympathomimetics (e.g., amphetamines, cocaine, and methylenedioxymethamphetamine or "ecstasy"), may present with severe hyperpyrexia (see Chapter 110 Toxicologic Emergencies). Additional uncommon febrile drug reactions include the *serotonin syndrome* occurring with the combined use of monoamine oxidase inhibitors and analgesic, antitussive, or psychotropic serotonergic medications (e.g., meperidine, dextromethorphan, fluoxetine), and the *neuroleptic malignant syndrome.* History of environmental heat exposure preceding severe hyperpyrexia may represent *heat stroke* rather than an infectious cause for the increased temperature (see Chapter 98 Environmental Emergencies, Radiological Emergencies, Bites and Stings). Therapeutic exposure to the antiepileptic drug zonisamide can result in oligohydrosis and severe resultant heat stroke. *Immunizations* (such as the conjugate pneumococcal or diphtheria, tetanus, acellular pertussis vaccine) are associated with fever that usually occurs within 48 hours. Fever, at times accompanied by a faint rash, may occur 7 to 10 days after immunization with the live-attenuated measles vaccine or the measles–mumps–rubella vaccine. In addition, autoimmune and inflammatory processes should be considered including but not limited to juvenile idiopathic arthritis (JIA), familial recurrent fever syndromes, and Kawasaki disease, a vasculitis of childhood of unknown origin which can result in cardiac complications if untreated (see Chapter 94 Cardiac Emergencies).

Fevers of unknown origin (FUOs) are defined as daily temperatures of 38.5°C (101.3°F) or higher for at least 2 weeks without discernible cause. Many children evaluated for FUOs actually have consecutive unrelated viral illnesses or unusually prolonged courses of common viral illnesses. Infections commonly causing prolonged fever in children include Epstein–Barr virus infections, osteomyelitis, *Bartonella henselae* infections (cat-scratch disease), UTIs, and Lyme disease. Although consecutive viral illnesses are the most common etiology for recurrent fevers in a child, occasional cases are due to *periodic fever syndromes* that are marked by recurrence of fever at regular intervals, affecting the child over a period of years. PFAPA (periodic fever, aphthous stomatitis, pharyngitis, and cervical adenitis), familial Mediterranean fever, or cyclic neutropenia is in the differential for the diagnosis of the child with recurrent, intermittent fevers.

Additional noninfectious causes of prolonged fever include neoplasms, collagen vascular diseases, and inflammatory disorders (ulcerative colitis or Crohn disease).

SYMPTOMATIC TREATMENT

In general, antipyretic therapy should parallel the pathophysiologic basis of the fever. When the fever is caused by altered hypothalamic set point, as in infection, antigen–antibody reactions, and malignancy, attempts to reset the "thermostat" with antipyretic medications are most likely to enhance patient comfort. Antipyretics work via the inhibition of hypothalamic prostaglandin synthesis. If fever is caused by imbalance of heat production and heat loss mechanisms, such as in heat stroke, urgent cooling by physical removal of heat is necessary and antipyretics will not help (see Chapter 98 Environmental Emergencies, Radiological Emergencies, Bites and Stings). However, children at risk for recurrent febrile seizures do not, unfortunately, tend to be protected by rapid use of "prophylactic" antipyretics at first sign of fever.

Acetaminophen and ibuprofen are currently the most commonly used pediatric antipyretic medications in the United States (aspirin is no longer recommended for routine antipyretic use in children because of its potential to cause severe gastrointestinal bleeding and its implication as an etiologic risk factor for Reye syndrome). The current dosage recommendation for acetaminophen is 10 to 15 mg per kg given every 4 to 6 hours, with a maximum of four doses per day, resulting in 40 to 60 mg/kg/day. Several reports and reviews have stressed that, although very rare, repetitive dosing of acetaminophen at the upper limit of, or just slightly above, recommended dosages may result in severe or fatal fulminant hepatic failure. This is particularly the case for children who were fasting (e.g., because of vomiting or diarrhea with febrile illness), younger than age 2 years, treated for several days, or treated with adult-intended preparations.

Ibuprofen is typically dosed at 5 to 10 mg/kg/dose, given every 6 to 8 hours, with a maximum of four doses per day (e.g., 30 to 40 mg/kg/day). Several studies have found that ibuprofen is more effective in reducing fever, especially in single-dose comparisons at 4 and 6 hours after administration, than acetaminophen at commonly used doses of each agent. However, the difference narrows and is of little clinical significance for most patients when antipyretic therapy is used repetitively over 12 to 24 hours or more, as typically prescribed for most childhood febrile illnesses. Acetaminophen is available in both rectal and intravenous formulations, and thus can be an option in children who cannot tolerate oral medication. The intravenous formulation of acetaminophen has been shown to have similar pharmacokinetics to the oral form in phase I trials, though there is minimal published experience in the ED setting. Theoretical concern that widespread use of ibuprofen in children might manifest a significantly increased incidence of serious gastrointestinal bleeding, renal failure, or allergic reactions relative to acetaminophen has not been borne out in large, prospective studies. Nevertheless, ibuprofen has been rarely associated with acute renal dysfunction when it was used in children with dehydration. An additional concern with ibuprofen is that its anti-inflammatory activity in the treatment of routine febrile illnesses, particularly varicella, might predispose to invasive bacterial, particularly streptococcal, disease. Although not proven to be causally related, it might still be prudent to avoid ibuprofen in such cases of suspected or at-risk streptococcal disease, as well as for children at risk of dehydration. Several epidemiologic studies have noted an association between acetaminophen use in young children and increased risk of asthma. This association has been confirmed in one large meta-analysis, but no randomized controlled trials have been performed to confirm this finding. Several studies in the past decade have evaluated the practice of combining or alternating ibuprofen and acetaminophen. In general, these have found modest increments in antipyretic effect without an increase in observed short-term drug toxicity. However, many commentators have noted that "real-world" safeguards are not equivalent to those enforced in prospective studies, that such complicated regimens pose considerable potential for parental confusion and overdosing, and that they may well add to unreasonable "fever phobia." Thus, our practice is to avoid prescribing such regimens for routine antipyresis, but rather to consider dual therapy in exceptional cases. If instituted, it may be prudent to use submaximal doses of each agent and to provide very detailed instructions and precautions.

It is important to remember that many parents greatly fear even moderately high fever in their children and require reassurance that the fever itself, in its usual range of severity does not cause damage. They need education about appropriate indications for antipyretic treatment, particularly seeking to reduce fever-associated discomfort, rather than a modestly elevated temperature itself. They need further education about appropriate, safe antipyretic dosing regimens, the lack of urgency in treating fever (unless temperature goes above 41.1°C [106°F] or there are febrile seizures), and most important, the concept that the overall well-being of the child, in context with age, is usually far more important than the temperature per se.

Suggested Readings and Key References

Pathophysiology and Thermometry

Allegaert K, Casteels K, Van Gorp I, et al. Tympanic, infrared skin, and temporal artery scan thermometers compared with rectal measurement in children: a real-life assessment. *Curr Ther Res Clin Exp* 2014;76:34–38.

Barnason S, Williams J, Proehl J, et al. Emergency nursing resource: noninvasive temperature measurement in the emergency department. *J Emerg Nurs* 2012;38(6):523–530.

Hasday JD, Fairchild KD, Shanholtz C. The role of fever in the infected host. *Microbes Infect* 2000;2(15):1891–1904.

Jean-Mary MB, Dicanzio J, Shaw J, et al. Limited accuracy and reliability of infrared axillary and aural thermometers in a pediatric outpatient population. *J Pediatr* 2002;141(5):671–676.

Evaluation/Decision

Black S, France EK, Isaacman D, et al. Surveillance for invasive pneumococcal disease during 2000–2005 in a population of children who received 7-valent pneumococcal conjugate vaccine. *Pediatr Infect Dis J* 2007;26(9):771–777.

Byer RL, Bachur RG. Clinical deterioration among patients with fever and erythroderma. *Pediatrics* 2006;118(6):2450–2460.

Gastañaduy PA, Redd SB, Fiebelkorn AP, et al. Measles – United States, January 1- May 23, 2014. *MMWR Morb Mortal Wkly Rep* 2014;63(22):496–499.

Kaplan SL, Barson WJ, Lin PL, et al. Serotype 19A is the most common serotype causing invasive pneumococcal infections in children. *Pediatrics* 2010;125(3):429–436.

Kaplan SL, Barson WJ, Lin PL, et al. Early trends for invasive pneumococcal infections in children after the introduction of the 13-valent pneumococcal conjugate vaccine. *Pediatr Infect Dis J* 2013;32(3): 203–207.

Kaplan SL, Schutze GE, Leake JA, et al. Multicenter surveillance of invasive meningococcal infections in children. *Pediatrics* 2006; 118(4):e979–e984.

Larru B, Gerber J. Cutaneous bacterial infections caused by Staphylococcus aureus and Streptococcus pyogenes in infants and children. *Pediatr Clin North Am* 2014;61:457–478.

Mahajan P, Ramilo O, Kuppermann N. The future possibilities of diagnostic testing for the evaluation of febrile infants. *JAMA Pediatr* 2013;167(10):888–898.

Maniaci V, Dauber A, Weiss S, et al. Procalcitonin in young febrile infants for the detection of serious bacterial infections. *Pediatrics* 2008;122(4):701–710.

Moran GJ, Krishnadasan A, Gorwitz RJ, et al. Methicillin-resistant S. aureus infections among patients in the emergency department. *N Engl J Med* 2006;355(7):666–674.

Singleton RJ, Hennessy TW, Bulkow LR, et al. Invasive pneumococcal disease caused by nonvaccine serotypes among Alaska native children with high levels of 7-valent pneumococcal conjugate vaccine coverage. *JAMA* 2007;297:1784–1792.

Tan TQ. Pediatric invasive pneumococcal disease in the United States in the era of pneumococcal conjugate vaccines. *Clin Microbiol Rev* 2012;25(3):409–419.

Trautner BW, Caviness AC, Gerlacher GR, et al. Prospective evaluation of the risk of serious bacterial infection in children who present to the emergency department with hyperpyrexia (temperature of 106 degrees F or higher). *Pediatrics* 2006;118(1): 34–40.

Whitney CG, Farley MM, Hadler J, et al. Decline in invasive pneumococcal disease after the introduction of protein-polysaccharide conjugate vaccine. *N Engl J Med* 2003;348:1737–1746.

Young Infant

Bachur RG, Harper MB. Predictive model for serious bacterial infections among infants younger than 3 months of age. *Pediatrics* 2001; 108(2):311–316.

Baker MD, Bell LM, Avner JR. Outpatient management without antibiotics of fever in selected infants. *N Engl J Med* 1993;329(20): 1437–1441.

Bonsu BK, Harper MB. Utility of the peripheral blood white blood cell count for identifying sick young infants who need lumbar puncture. *Ann Emerg Med* 2003;41(2):206–214.

Bramson RT, Meyer TL, Silbiger ML, et al. The futility of the chest radiograph in the febrile infant without respiratory symptoms. *Pediatrics* 1993;92(4):524–526.

Byington CL, Enriquez FR, Hoff C, et al. Serious bacterial infections in febrile infants 1 to 90 days old with and without viral infections. *Pediatrics* 2004;113(6):1662–1666.

Byington CL, Reynolds CC, Korgenski K, et al. Costs and infant outcomes after implementation of a care process model for febrile infants. *Pediatrics* 2012;130(1):e16–e24.

Corey L, Wald A. Maternal and neonatal herpes simplex virus infections. *N Engl J Med* 2009;361:1376–1385.

Dewan M, Zorc JJ, Hodinka RL, et al. Cerebrospinal fluid enterovirus testing in infants 56 days or younger. *Arch Pediatr Adolesc Med* 2010;164(9):824–830.

Ferrera PC, Bartfield JM, Snyder HS. Neonatal fever: utility of the Rochester Criteria in determining low risk for serious bacterial infections. *Am J Emerg Med* 1997;15(3):299–302.

Garra G, Cunningham SJ, Crain EF. Reappraisal of criteria used to predict serious bacterial illness in febrile infants less than 8 weeks of age. *Acad Emerg Med* 2005;12(10):921–925.

King RL, Lorch SA, Cohen DM, et al. Routine cerebrospinal fluid enterovirus polymerase chain reaction testing reduces hospitalization and antibiotic use for infants 90 days of age or younger. *Pediatrics* 2007;120(3):489–496.

Levine DA, Platt SL, Dayan PS, et al. Risk of serious bacterial infection in young febrile infants with respiratory syncytial virus infections. *Pediatrics* 2004;113(6):1728–1734.

Long SS, Pool TE, Vodzak J, et al. Herpes simplex virus infection in young infants during 2 decades of empiric acyclovir therapy. *Pediatr Infect Dis J* 2011;30(7):556–561.

Pantell RH, Newman TB, Bernzweig J, et al. Management and outcomes of care of fever in early infancy. *JAMA* 2004;291(10):1203–1212.

Zorc JJ, Levine DA, Platt SL, et al. Clinical and demographic factors associated with urinary tract infection in young febrile infants. *Pediatrics* 2005;116(3):644–648.

Young Child

Alpern ER, Alessandrini EA, Bell LM, et al. Occult bacteremia from a pediatric emergency department: current prevalence, time to detection, and outcome. *Pediatrics* 2000;106(3):505–511.

American Academy of Pediatrics, Subcommittee on Febrile Seizures. Clinical practice guideline: febrile seizures: guideline for the neurodiagnostic evaluation of the child with a simple febrile seizure. *Pediatrics* 2011;127:389–394.

Carstairs K, Tasnen D, Johnson AS, et al. Pneumococcal bacteremia in febrile infants presenting to the emergency department before and after the introduction of the heptavalent pneumococcal vaccine. *Ann Emerg Med* 2007;49:772–777.

Finnell SM, Carroll AE, Downs SM; Subcommittee on Urinary Tract Infection. Technical report—Diagnosis and management of an initial UTI in febrile infants and young children. *Pediatrics* 2011;128(3):e749–e770.

Gomez B, Bressan S, Mintegi S, et al. Diagnostic value of procalcitonin in well-appearing young febrile infants. *Pediatrics* 2012;130(5): 815–822.

Gorelick MH, Shaw KN. Clinical decision rule to identify febrile young girls at risk for urinary tract infection. *Arch Pediatr Adolesc Med* 2000;154(4):386–390.

Herz AM, Greenhow TL, Alcantara J, et al. Changing epidemiology of outpatient bacteremia in 3- to 36-month-old children after the introduction of the heptavalent-conjugated pneumococcal vaccine. *Pediatr Infect Dis J* 2006;25:293–300.

Kimia AA, Capraro AJ, Hummel D, et al. Utility of lumbar puncture for first simple febrile seizure among children 6 to 18 months of age. *Pediatrics* 2009;123(1):6–12.

Murphy CG, van de Pol AC, Harper MB, et al. Clinical predictors of occult pneumonia in the febrile child. *Acad Emerg Med* 2007; 14(3):243–249.

Nigrovic LE, Kuppermann N, Malley R. Children with bacterial meningitis presenting to the emergency department during the pneumococcal conjugate vaccine era. *Acad Emerg Med* 2008;15(6): 522–528.

Shaikh N, Morone NE, Bost JE, et al. Prevalence of urinary tract infection in childhood: a meta-analysis. *Pediatr Infect Dis J* 2008;27(4): 302–308.

Shaikh N, Morone NE, Lopez J, et al. Does this child have a urinary tract infection? *JAMA* 2007;298(24):2895–2904.

Wilkinson M, Bulloch B, Smith M. Prevalence of occult bacteremia in children aged 3 to 36 months presenting to the emergency department with fever in the postpneumococcal conjugate vaccine era. *Acad Emerg Med* 2009;16:220–225.

Wolff M, Bachur R. Serious bacterial infection in recently immunized young febrile infants. *Acad Emerg Med* 2009;16:1284–1289.

Yo CH, Hsieh PS, Lee SH, et al. Comparison of the test characteristics of procalcitonin to C-reactive protein and leukocytosis for the detection of serious bacterial infections in children presenting with fever without source: a systematic review and meta-analysis. *Ann Emerg Med* 2012;60(5):591–600.

Treatment

Curtis N. Non-steroidal anti-inflammatory drugs may predispose to invasive group A streptococcal infections. *Arch Dis Child* 1996;75:547.

Etminan M, Sadatsafavi M, Jafari S, et al. Acetaminophen use and the risk of asthma in children and adults: a systematic review and metaanalysis. *Chest* 2009;136(5):1316–1323.

Evered LM. Does acetaminophen treat fever in children? *Ann Emerg Med* 2003;41:741–743.

Hay AD, Costelloe C, Redmond NM, et al. Paracetamol plus ibuprofen for the treatment of fever in children (PITCH): randomised controlled trial. *BMJ* 2008;337:a1302.

Kramer LC, Richards PA, Thompson AM. Alternating antipyretics: antipyretic efficacy of acetaminophen versus acetaminophen alternated with ibuprofen in children. *Clin Pediatr* 2008;47:907–911.

Lesko SM, O'Brien KL, Schwartz B, et al. Invasive group A streptococcal infection and nonsteroidal antiinflammatory drug use among children with primary varicella. *Pediatrics* 2001;107:1108–1115.

McBride JT. The association of acetaminophen and asthma prevalence and severity. *Pediatrics* 2011;128(6):1181–1185.

Sarrell EM, Wielunsky E, Cohen HA. Antipyretic treatment in young children with fever: acetaminophen, ibuprofen, or both alternating in a randomized, double-blind study. *Arch Pediatr Adolesc Med* 2006;160(2):197–202.

CHAPTER 27 ■ FOREIGN BODY: INGESTION AND ASPIRATION

AUN WOON SOON, MD AND SUZANNE SCHMIDT, MD

Through play, experimentation, and daily activities, children are likely to place foreign bodies just about anywhere. Once an object or foodstuff is in a child's mouth, it can lodge in the nasopharynx, respiratory tract, or be ingested. According to the American Association of Poison Control Centers' National Poison Data System, more than 110,000 foreign-body exposures were reported in the United States in 2012, and of these, 88% occurred in the pediatric population. Young children, age 6 months to 4 years, are at an increased risk for foreign-body aspiration or ingestion due to their inquisitive nature and tendency to explore objects with their mouths. Often, a "choking episode" will clear the foreign body; however, serious sequelae of an aspirated object can range from an acute life-threatening event to a slowly evolving pneumonia. The severity of an ingested foreign body is determined by the nature of the object (e.g., blunt, long, sharp, battery, magnetic) and its location in the gastrointestinal (GI) tract. Generally, most ingested foreign material is well tolerated, and may pass unnoticed by the family and child.

PATHOPHYSIOLOGY

There are three main pathophysiologic considerations for aspirated and ingested foreign bodies: the anatomic determinants of lodgment site, the physical properties of the foreign body (size, shape, and composition), and the local tissue reaction to the foreign body.

The respiratory tract gradually narrows distal to the larynx, whereas the GI tract has several sites of anatomic or functional narrowing. An ingested foreign body may lodge in three distinct esophageal sites, may be unable to pass through the pylorus, or may become impacted in the duodenum, appendix, ileocecal valve, rectum, or any other location of congenital or acquired narrowing.

The nature of the foreign body (size, shape, and composition) and the ability of the tissue to distend influence the site of lodgment within the respiratory or GI tract. Depending on the location in the airway, an aspirated object may minimally, intermittently, or completely impede airflow. The composition of the foreign body also determines the local tissue reaction and the evolution of complications. A button battery can erode through the esophageal wall rapidly compared with the slow tissue reaction to a coin. In the bronchial tree, the fatty oils in some aspirated foods (e.g., peanuts) create a more severe inflammatory reaction than a similarly sized nonorganic object. While the ingestion of a single blunt magnet may cause little problem, the ingestion of more than one can lead to magnetic attraction across bowel walls, resulting in bowel necrosis, perforation, or volvulus.

DIFFERENTIAL DIAGNOSIS

Gastrointestinal Foreign Body

Esophagus

The esophagus is the most common site of lodgment for an ingested foreign body and may have serious complications. Most childhood esophageal foreign bodies are round or spherical objects, with coins accounting for 50% to 75% of these (Fig. 27.1). This contrasts with adults, whose impacted esophageal foreign bodies tend to be foodstuffs (meat) and bones (e.g., fish or chicken), and are often associated with underlying conditions of the esophagus (e.g., strictures, dysmotility, extrinsic compression). Most children with esophageal impactions have a structurally and functionally normal esophagus. Children with acquired esophageal strictures (e.g., secondary to caustic ingestions) or repaired congenital conditions (e.g., esophageal atresia, tracheoesophageal fistula) are at increased risk for recurrent esophageal impactions, including foodstuffs (e.g., hot dogs, chicken).

Foreign bodies of the esophagus tend to lodge at three sites. The thoracic inlet (Fig. 27.1) is the most common location, accounting for 60% to 80% of esophageal foreign bodies. The next most common sites are the gastroesophageal junction (10% to 20%) and the level of the aortic arch (5% to 20%). The level of lodgment in children with underlying esophageal conditions depends on the location of the constricting lesion.

Foreign bodies that remain lodged in the esophagus may lead to potentially serious complications including respiratory distress, upper airway compromise, esophageal perforation, mediastinitis, and aortic or tracheal fistula formation. Therefore, it is imperative that the physician consider the possibility of esophageal foreign bodies, especially in young children 6 months to 4 years of age.

Stomach and Lower Gastrointestinal Tract

Objects that pass safely into the stomach generally traverse the remainder of the GI tract without complication. Safe passage has been documented in hundreds of cases involving various foreign objects, including sharp objects such as screws, tacks, and staples. This may not be true in the younger child when long (greater than 5 cm) objects are unable to negotiate the turns and may become impacted in the duodenum and ileocecal region. However, no definitive age or length guidelines exist. This also may not be true of some very sharp objects (e.g., bones, needles, pins) that may perforate the hollow viscera, resulting in peritonitis, abscess formation, or hemorrhage.

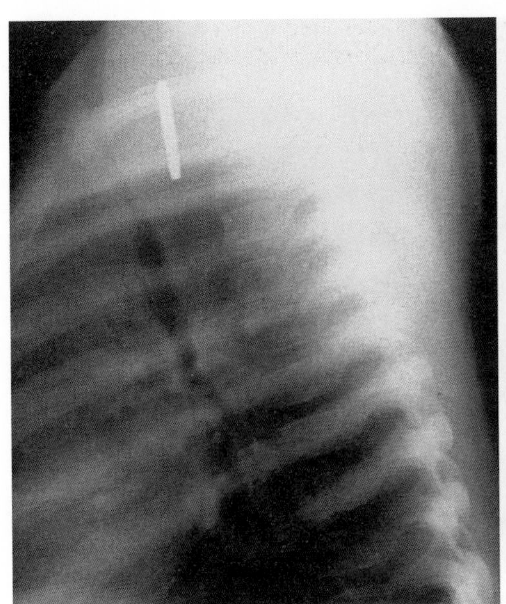

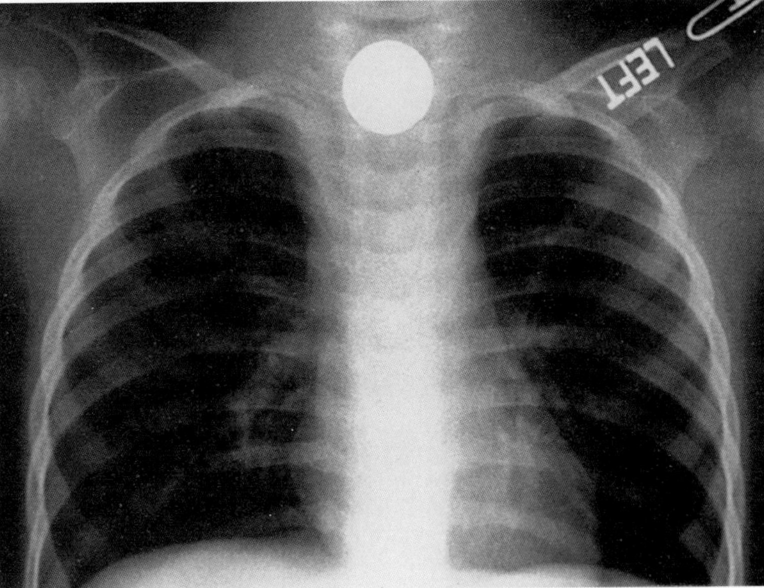

FIGURE 27.1 Two-view chest radiograph demonstrating impacted esophageal coin located at the thoracic inlet.

Respiratory Foreign Body

Upper Airway

Foreign bodies that lodge in the upper airway can be immediately life-threatening. According to the National Safety Council, choking was the fourth leading cause of unintentional injury death in the United States in 2007. In 2009, 4,600 deaths were reported from unintentional ingestion or inhalation of food or objects that resulted in airway obstruction. Most children with aspirated foreign bodies are younger than 3 years of age. The most common foods responsible for fatalities include hot dogs, candy, meat, and grapes. Childhood fatality from aspiration of manmade objects is less common. These objects tend to be conforming objects, with balloons, small balls, and beads accounting for most cases. Children with foreign bodies in their upper airways may present with acute respiratory distress, stridor, or complete obstruction of their upper airway. In patients with complete airway obstruction, emergency treatment depends on proper application of basic life-support skills. Back blows and chest compressions are used in infants, and the Heimlich maneuver is used in toddlers, children, and adolescents while the patient remains conscious. Cardiopulmonary resuscitation should be initiated if the patient becomes unresponsive. If these methods fail to dislodge the foreign body, rapid progression to direct visualization and manual extraction or an emergency airway is necessary (see Chapters 3 Airway and 4 Cardiopulmonary Resuscitation).

Lower Respiratory Tract

Childhood foreign bodies of the lower tracheobronchial tree represent a diagnostic challenge due to the ubiquitous nature of the presenting symptoms (e.g., cough, wheezing, respiratory distress), the frequency of the asymptomatic presentation, and the potential for false-negative and false-positive screening radiographs.

Foreign bodies of the lower respiratory tract occur more commonly in young children, with a slight propensity to lodge in the right lung (52%). Organic matter accounts for 81% of aspirations, with nuts and seeds (sunflower and watermelon) being the most common, followed by other food products (apples, carrots, and popcorn), plants, and grasses. Plastics and metals make up a minority of aspirated objects (Fig. 27.2), and coin aspiration has rarely been reported.

The diagnosis of lower airway foreign-body aspiration is often delayed due to nonspecific symptoms, and these patients may be incorrectly diagnosed with an asthma exacerbation, pneumonia, or bronchiolitis. One study found the classic clinical triad for an aspirated foreign body (cough, focal wheeze, and decreased breath sounds) was present in only 14% of patients. The most common symptoms were persistent cough (81%), difficulty breathing (60%), and wheezing (52%). A history of a witnessed choking event is highly suggestive of acute aspiration with a sensitivity of up to 93%. It is therefore important to inquire about a choking history because this is a crucial clue to diagnosis.

EVALUATION AND DECISION

Unknown Location

Generally, the symptom complex and history that surround the event provide the clues necessary to decide whether to evaluate the respiratory or GI tract. Foreign bodies in both locations may present with airway symptoms, gagging, or vomiting. Symptoms of cough and respiratory distress with tachypnea, retractions, stridor, wheezing, or asymmetric aeration suggest a foreign body in the airway. Symptoms of gagging, vomiting, drooling, dysphagia, or pain suggest esophageal impaction. Diagnosis is further complicated in that foreign bodies in either location may be asymptomatic. If the history and physical examination do not provide the necessary clues, initial evaluation should include a chest radiograph (including the neck and upper abdomen) to screen for a radiopaque foreign body. Coupling this with an expiratory chest radiograph or lateral decubitus films (as outlined later) screens for an aspirated foreign body (Fig. 27.3).

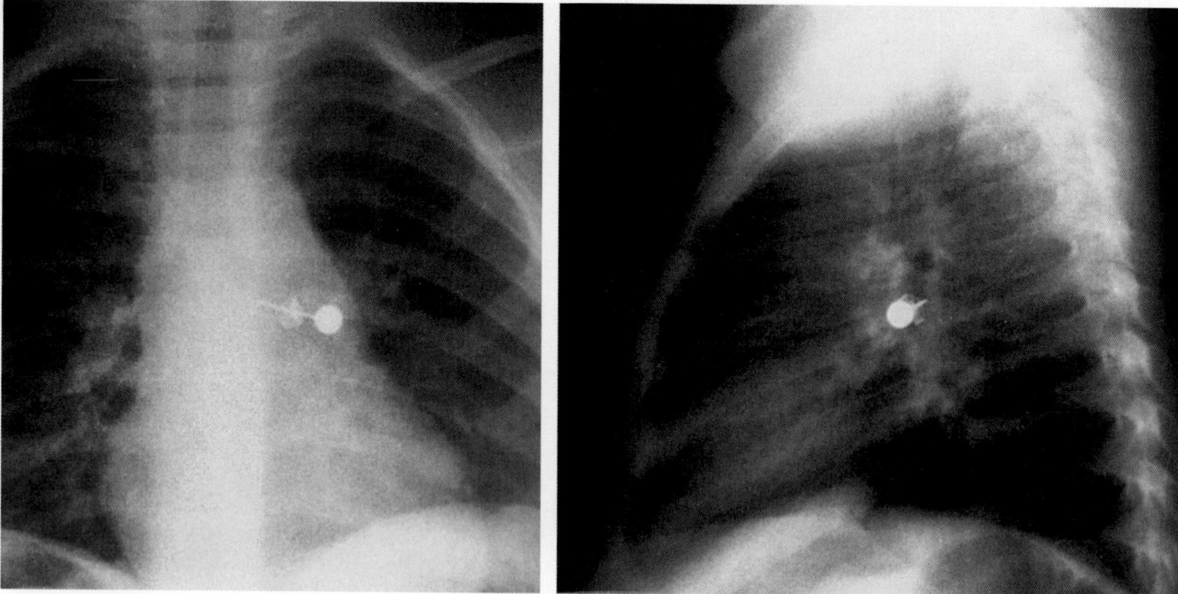

FIGURE 27.2 Two-view chest radiograph demonstrating aspirated radiopaque foreign body—an earring—located in the left bronchus.

Gastrointestinal Foreign Body

Esophageal Foreign Body: Diagnosis

Children with esophageal foreign bodies often have a history of having swallowed the foreign body. Symptoms associated with esophageal impaction include dysphagia, refusal to eat, foreign-body sensation or localization, drooling, and vomiting. When these symptoms are associated with a history of foreign-body ingestion, the diagnosis is straightforward. In the absence of an ingestion history, the diagnosis may be challenging because these same symptoms occur with common childhood ailments such as acute gastroenteritis, pharyngitis, or gingivostomatitis. Any patient with swallowing difficulty requires a thorough examination of the mouth, oropharynx, neck, chest, and abdomen. Radiographic evaluation may be needed in some cases (see Chapter 51 Pain: Dysphagia).

The approach to a child with foreign-body ingestion is outlined in Figure 27.4. Children may be asymptomatic with an esophageal foreign body. Since 40% of children with coins impacted in the esophagus are asymptomatic in the emergency department, it is suggested that most children with a history of ingested foreign bodies undergo radiographic evaluation. In the asymptomatic patient, this evaluation is urgent but not emergent; however, button battery ingestions and multiple magnet ingestions are exceptions as discussed in the "Button Battery Ingestion" and "Magnet Ingestions" sections below. If the patient's symptoms suggest esophageal impaction, endoscopy is recommended for visualization and removal of the object. Oral contrast studies should be avoided due to the risk of aspiration and contrast material obscuring visualization on endoscopy. CT scan may be considered in special circumstances. Children with a predisposing condition (tracheoesophageal

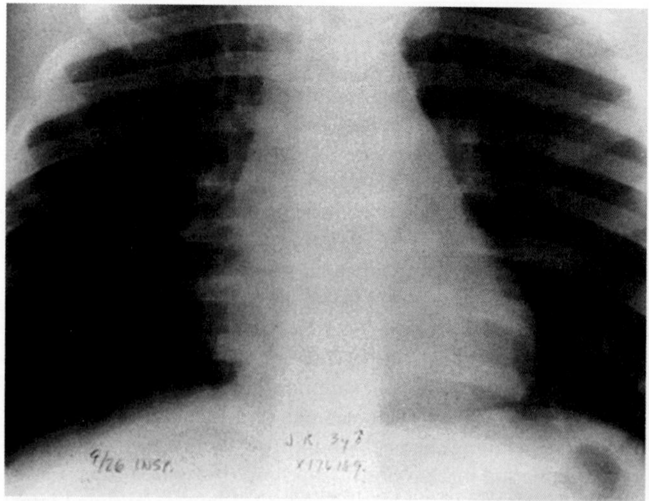

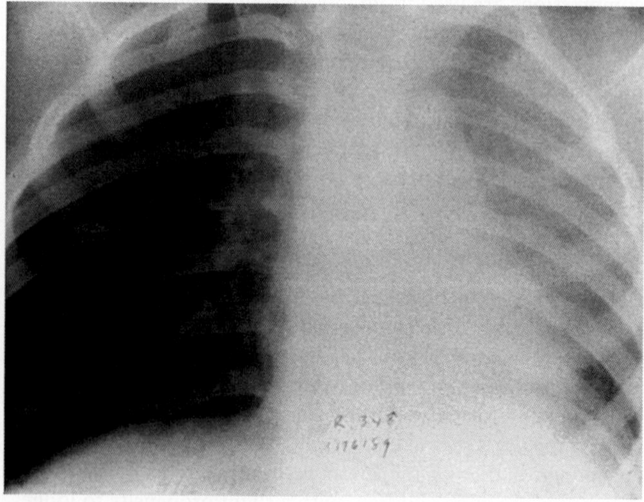

FIGURE 27.3 Inspiratory and expiratory chest radiographs demonstrating air trapping in the right lung during expiration, indicating likely right-sided foreign body. A peanut was removed at bronchoscopy.

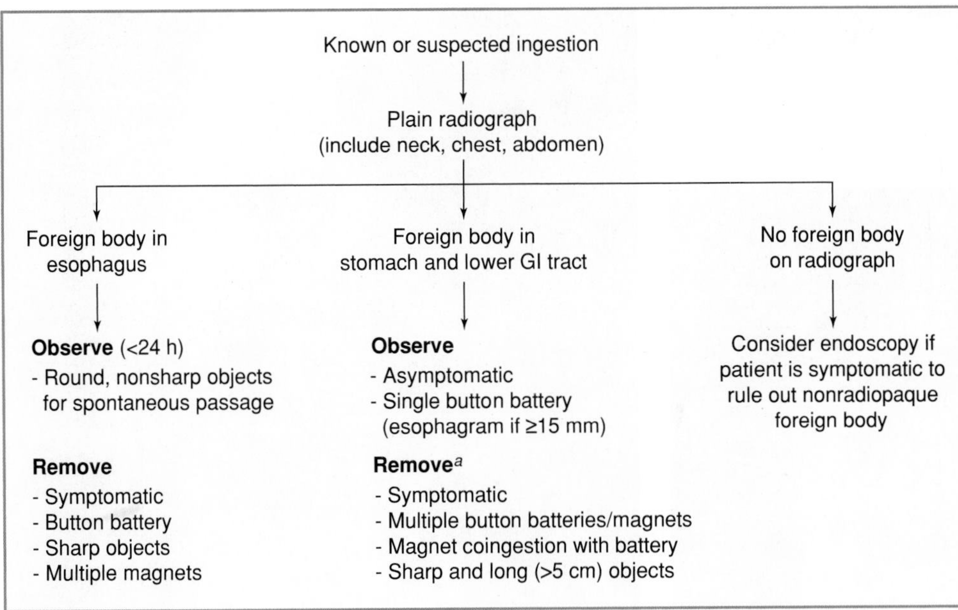

FIGURE 27.4 Management of ingested foreign body. GI, gastrointestinal.
[a]Remove with endoscopy, consult general surgery if object is not within reach and patient is symptomatic.

fistula repair, esophageal stricture, eosinophilic esophagitis) are more likely to have food or foreign-body impaction.

Handheld metal detectors have been used as an initial screen when coin ingestion is suspected, as an alternative to radiographs. Though these devices compare favorably with radiography in determining presence or absence of a coin and its location, they are less reliable in detecting foreign bodies in obese patients and noncoin metallic objects. Users would need to gain experience with the device using x-ray confirmation before abandoning radiography, and ensure patient follow-up as some objects may be missed with this method.

Esophageal Foreign Body: Removal

In general, once an esophageal foreign body is detected, it should be removed promptly. This is especially true of sharp esophageal foreign bodies and button batteries. A button battery should be removed emergently as it may cause esophageal injury within a few hours of ingestion, leading to permanent sequelae. Location of the foreign body within the esophagus influences the likelihood of spontaneous passage. Asymptomatic esophageal coins in the distal third of the esophagus are most likely to pass into the stomach spontaneously with a 47% rate of passage. Those in the proximal or middle third of the esophagus had a 26% and 10% rate of spontaneous passage. Of those patients who had spontaneous passage of a coin, approximately half occurred within 6 hours and the rest within 19 hours. When evaluating an acute esophageal impaction (within a few hours of ingestion), it is reasonable to allow an observation period of 8 to 16 hours for spontaneous passage of round, noncorrosive foreign bodies (e.g., coins) in the asymptomatic patient, with no history of esophageal disease.

Removal techniques for impacted esophageal foreign bodies vary regionally and depend on the duration of impaction, associated symptoms, and the nature of the foreign body. Traditional removal methods include rigid esophagoscopy and flexible endoscopy under anesthesia. Endoscopy has been proven to be safe and efficacious and is applicable to all types of foreign bodies, allows for direct examination of the esophageal lumen, and can be used in patients with respiratory distress. Other methods have been employed for the retrieval of coins and similar objects, including a balloon-tipped catheter under fluoroscopic guidance to extract the coin, bougienage to advance the coin into the stomach, Magill forceps with direct laryngoscopy for coins located in the proximal esophagus, or fluoroscopic-guided grasping endoscopic forceps covered by a soft rubber catheter. These methods have reported high success rates with removal options being determined by local opinion and referral pattern. The balloon-tipped catheter technique has been criticized because of poor control of the foreign body during extraction, inadequate visualization of the esophagus, and potential for esophageal perforation. These alternative removal or advancement methods, though less costly than endoscopy, should be attempted only by clinicians familiar with the techniques. They are generally recommended only for noncorrosive, blunt esophageal foreign bodies that have been impacted for less than 2 days.

Use of medications (e.g., glucagon) to reduce muscular tone, to enhance esophageal motility, or to relax the lower esophageal sphincter has been suggested to facilitate foreign-body passage from the esophagus. Success with these methods is mostly anecdotal, and there is little data comparing the use of medications with spontaneous, nonmedicated, passage rates. One study of impacted esophageal coins demonstrated similar passage rates when 1-mg intravenous glucagon was compared with placebo.

Stomach and Lower Gastrointestinal Tract

Watchful waiting is appropriate for most foreign bodies of the stomach and lower GI tract if the patient is asymptomatic. Though most sharp objects will pass through the GI tract without complications, endoscopic removal should be considered if the object is located in the stomach due to risk of perforation. Long objects (greater than 5 cm) should also be removed from the stomach. In addition to perforation, they can cause pressure necrosis and obstruction. If the long or sharp object has passed out of the stomach of an asymptomatic patient at the time of evaluation and is not within the

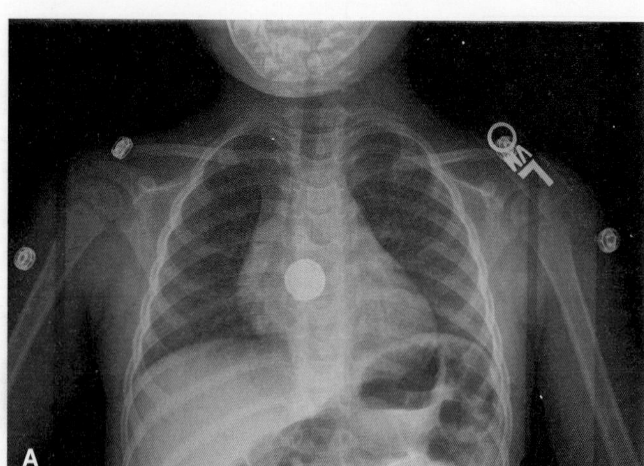

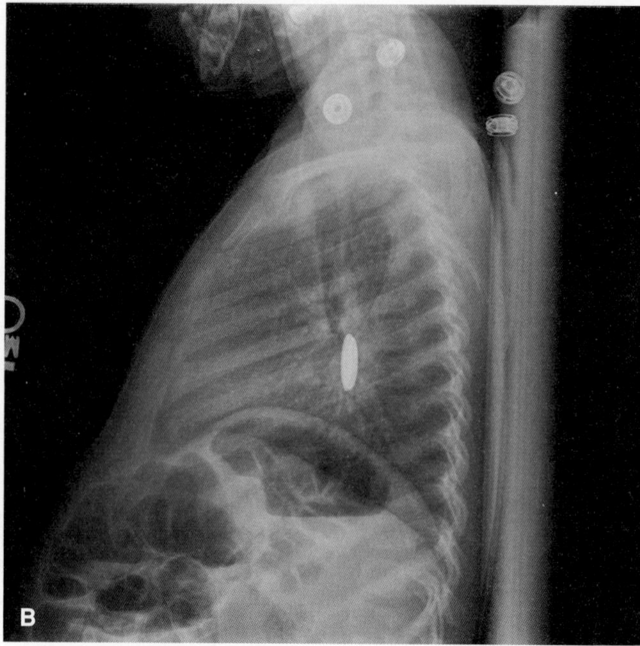

FIGURE 27.5 Two-view chest radiograph demonstrating a button battery in the esophagus. Note the "double rim" or "halo" effect on the AP radiograph (**A**) and step-off pattern on the lateral view (**B**).

reach of the endoscope, serial abdominal radiographs every 2 to 3 days and serial examinations should be considered to ensure uneventful passage. Most round objects (e.g., coins) will traverse the GI tract in 3 to 8 days without any complications. Some providers advocate parental examination of the stool for the foreign body with a follow-up radiograph in 2 weeks if the foreign body has not passed. Occasionally, some innocuous objects (e.g., quarter) remain in the stomach for a long duration. A prolonged time, up to a few weeks, can be allowed for passage of inert objects out of the stomach before surgical or endoscopic removal is necessary. If the patient with an ingested foreign body becomes symptomatic, endoscopic or surgical intervention may be necessary.

Button Battery Ingestion

Button batteries are the power source for many household items, including watches, cameras, calculators, and hearing aids, leaving them within reach of children. From 1985 to 2009, there was a 6.7-fold increase in the percentage of button battery ingestions with major or fatal outcomes, according to the National Poison Data System. This is due to the emergence of the 20-mm lithium cell as a popular household battery, which is responsible for 92.1% of serious or fatal ingestions. All fatalities and most major morbidities occurred in children younger than 4 years of age. Button batteries with other cell chemistries (manganese dioxide, zinc-air, silver oxide, and mercuric oxide) were not associated with significant injuries or death. The mechanisms of injury include direct pressure necrosis, generation of an external electrolytic current resulting in liquefaction necrosis, and leakage of material causing direct caustic injury. Button batteries in the esophagus should be identified and removed emergently, ideally within 2 hours of ingestion. Care should be taken when evaluating a disc-shaped foreign object on radiograph, as ingested button batteries may be mistaken for being a coin ingestion. Findings that suggest a button battery are a "double rim" or "halo" effect on an AP radiograph, or a step-off pattern on a lateral chest radiograph (Fig. 27.5). Button batteries in the stomach or beyond should be left to pass spontaneously if the patient is asymptomatic. For large (≥15 mm) batteries that have passed into the stomach, an esophagram should be performed to evaluate the esophagus for injury, especially when the time of ingestion is unknown. Parents should be advised to inspect the stool and a radiograph should be repeated in 4 days (for ≥15-mm batteries) or 10 to 14 days (for <15-mm batteries) if the battery has not yet passed. A coingested magnet mandates prompt removal, even in the asymptomatic patient. Complications after removal of the battery include tracheoesophageal fistula, esophageal stricture or perforation, mediastinitis, and vocal cord paralysis. The most common cause of death is secondary to an aortoesophageal fistula. Only sporadic cases of systemic absorption of battery contents have been suggested in the literature, and no serious toxicities have been reported.

Magnet Ingestions

Though most magnets that are ingested tend to be small and blunt, they pose a unique hazard to children. Single magnet ingestions can be treated like other GI ingestions but multiple magnet ingestions can be potentially dangerous. If they connect in the stomach and travel as a single foreign body, there is generally little need for concern. If they traverse the GI tract separately, they may magnetically attract each other across the bowel wall, trapping bowel in between the magnets. Continued magnetic adherence can result in bowel obstruction, pressure necrosis, and bowel perforation. Removal of a single magnet should be considered if the patient is at risk for further ingestions. Parents should be advised to remove small metallic and magnetic objects from the child's environment. All ingestions involving multiple magnets require surgical consultation. Multiple magnets located in the esophagus or stomach should be removed by endoscopy. For the asymptomatic patient with multiple magnets located beyond the stomach, serial radiographs and abdominal examinations can be performed to monitor progression. If the patient is symptomatic and the magnets are beyond the stomach, surgical intervention is indicated.

Respiratory Foreign Body

Lower Respiratory Tract: Diagnosis

A high clinical index of suspicion is necessary to diagnose foreign-body aspiration accurately and promptly. Symptoms seen in pediatric foreign-body ingestions are also present in other common diseases such as upper respiratory tract infection, bronchiolitis, pneumonia, and asthma. Radiographs serve as important diagnostic aids, but when the clinical suspicion of foreign-body aspiration is high (good history for aspiration, acute onset of symptoms and signs), the lack of confirmatory radiographic studies should not dissuade the clinician from pursuing bronchoscopy for diagnosis and treatment. Findings on a chest radiograph suggestive of a foreign body include air trapping, atelectasis, mediastinal shift, and consolidation. The more time that has elapsed since the aspiration event, the more likely the chest radiograph will be abnormal and the greater the percentage of patients who exhibit consolidation and atelectasis.

Inspiratory and expiratory films comparing the relative deflation of the two lungs may demonstrate unilateral air trapping indicative of a foreign body (Fig. 27.3). In the young or uncooperative child in whom obtaining an adequate expiratory film may be difficult, bilateral lateral decubitus chest radiographs (both obtained during inspiration) comparing the relative deflation of the dependent lung may be a useful adjunct. In one study of 1,024 children with foreign-body aspiration, inspiratory and expiratory chest radiographs were found to be normal in 15% of cases. If available, chest fluoroscopy may also be useful for diagnosis, demonstrating evidence of focal air trapping on the side of the foreign body or a mediastinal shift away from the affected side on expiration. More recently, chest CT scan has been used to diagnose aspirated foreign bodies. This appears to be more reliable than either plain radiography or fluoroscopy with sensitivity of 91% or higher, though it is associated with increased radiation exposure.

The approach to diagnosing foreign-body aspiration is outlined in Figure 27.6. In instances in which a respiratory foreign body is being considered, the patient should be given nothing by mouth until the disposition is determined due to the possible need for bronchoscopy. The patient should first be evaluated with inspiratory and expiratory or lateral decubitus chest radiographs. If these studies are normal, the aspiration history is poor, the material uncommonly aspirated, and the patient has mild or no symptoms without focal findings on physical examination, then discharge with follow-up in a few days is appropriate. If diagnosis is still unclear after plain films and there is a historical or clinical suspicion of aspiration, fluoroscopy or chest CT may be considered. In some instances, despite normal radiographic or fluoroscopic evaluation, bronchoscopy is indicated to confirm the presence or absence of a foreign body when there is a high clinical index of suspicion (choking history with typically aspirated foods—nuts, seeds,

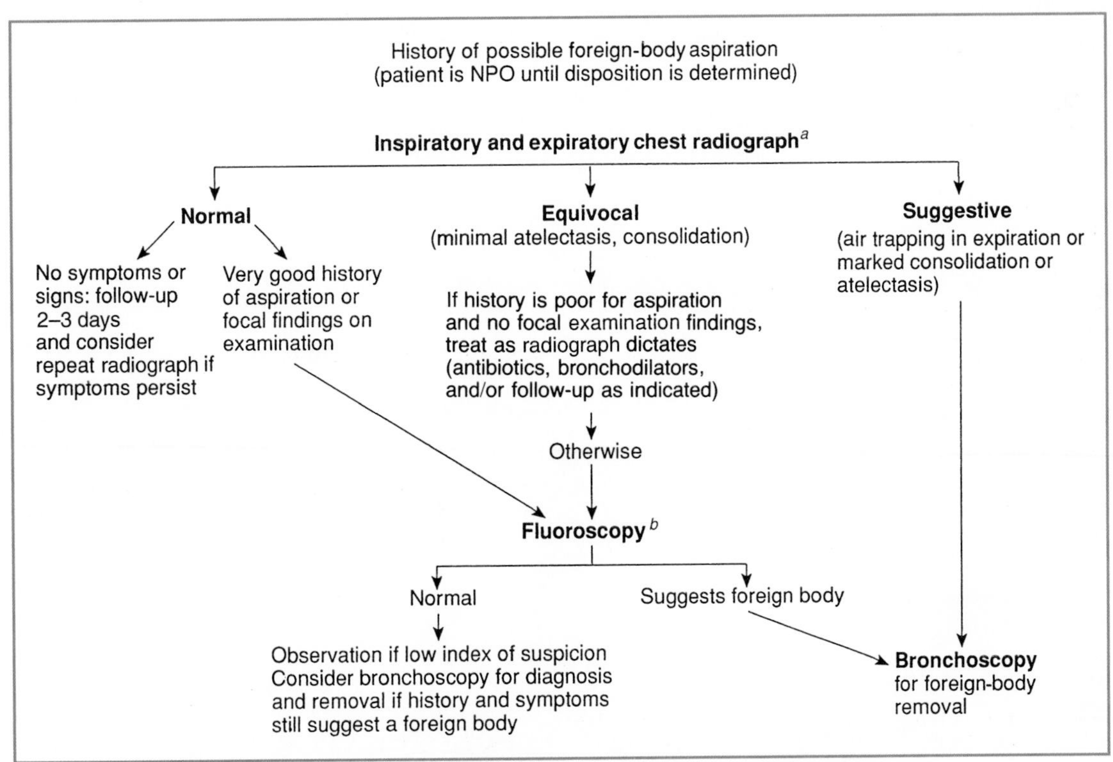

FIGURE 27.6 Guidelines for management of the child with suspected foreign-body aspiration.
[a]Lateral decubitus chest radiographs or fluoroscopy may substitute in younger or uncooperative patients.
[b]Fluoroscopy is not necessary if there is an acute onset of focal physical findings (unilateral wheeze, decreased aeration) or a convincing aspiration history. The patient may proceed directly to bronchoscopy.

apples, etc.). It is reasonable to proceed directly to bronchoscopy if there is an acute onset of focal physical findings (unilateral wheeze, decreased aeration) or a convincing aspiration history.

A history of aspirated foreign bodies should be sought in all cases of new-onset respiratory distress, stridor, wheezing, or cough, especially in young children aged 6 months to 4 years. History taking should include questions about recent choking episodes, especially when eating nuts, seeds, apples, and carrots. The differential diagnosis of foreign-body aspiration includes many common childhood diseases, including viral upper respiratory tract infections, bronchiolitis, pneumonitis, and reactive airway disease.

Lower Respiratory Tract: Removal

Rigid bronchoscopy performed under general anesthesia is still the most common technique used to remove an airway foreign body with a success rate of more than 98%. It is rare to require a tracheostomy or thoracotomy. Bronchoscopy can often be performed on an outpatient surgery basis, although any preoperative or postoperative concerns about the patient's respiratory status mandate inhospital observation after the procedure. Potential postoperative complications after removal of an aspirated foreign body include atelectasis, pneumonia, stridor, bronchospasm or laryngospasm, and retained foreign body.

ACKNOWLEDGMENTS

The authors thank Dr. Mariam Kappil and Dr. Marina Doliner for their radiographic contributions to this chapter.

Suggested Readings and Key References

Ingested Foreign Bodies

Arana A, Hauser B, Hachimi-Idrissi S, et al. Management of ingested foreign bodies in childhood and review of the literature. *Eur J Pediatr* 2001;160(8):468–472.

Mehta D, Attia M, Quintana E, et al. Glucagon use for esophageal coin dislodgment in children: a prospective, double-blind, placebo-controlled trial. *Acad Emerg Med* 2001;8:200–203.

Sharpe SJ, Rochette LM, Smith GA. Pediatric battery-related emergency department visits in the United States, 1990–2009. *Pediatrics* 2012;129(6):1111–1117.

Waltzman ML, Baskin M, Wypij D, et al. A randomized clinical trial of the management of esophageal coins in children. *Pediatrics* 2005;116:614–619.

Wright CC, Closson FT. Updates in pediatric gastrointestinal foreign bodies. *Pediatr Clin North Am* 2013;60(5):1221–1239.

Aspirated Foreign Bodies

Altkorn R, Chen X, Milkovich S, et al. Fatal and non-fatal food injuries among children (aged 0–14 years). *Int J Pediatr Otorhinolaryngol* 2008;72:1041–1046.

Fidkowski CW, Zheng H, Firth PG. The anesthetic considerations of tracheobronchial foreign bodies in children: a literature review of 12,979 cases. *Anesth Analg* 2010;111(4):1016–1025.

Gang W, Zhengxia P, Hongbo L, et al. Diagnosis and treatment of tracheobronchial foreign bodies in 1024 children. *J Pediatr Surg* 2012;47(11):2004–2010.

Heyer CM, Bollmeier ME, Rossler L, et al. Evaluation of clinical, radiologic, and laboratory prebronchoscopy findings in children with suspected foreign body aspiration. *J Pediatr Surg* 2006;41:1882–1888.

Paksu S, Paksu MS, Kilic M, et al. Foreign body aspiration in childhood: evaluation of diagnostic parameters. *Pediatr Emerg Care* 2012; 28(3):259–264.

CHAPTER 28 ■ GASTROINTESTINAL BLEEDING

LENORE R. JARVIS, MD, MEd AND STEPHEN J. TEACH, MD, MPH

Gastrointestinal (GI) bleeding is a relatively common problem in pediatrics. Over one 12-month study period at a large urban pediatric emergency department, complaints of rectal bleeding accounted for 0.3% of all visits. Upon the patient's arrival, the emergency physician must first assess the need for cardiovascular resuscitation and stabilization. However, most children who arrive in the ED with an apparent GI bleed have an acute, self-limited GI hemorrhage and are hemodynamically stable.

In most cases of upper and lower GI bleeding, the source of the bleeding is inflamed mucosa (infection, allergy, drug induced, stress related, or idiopathic). The emergency physician must be vigilant in differentiating inflammatory conditions that are often self-limited from causes that may require emergent surgical or endoscopic intervention, such as ischemic bowel (intussusception, volvulus), structural abnormalities (Meckel diverticulum, angiodysplasia), and portal hypertension (esophageal varices). Acute GI bleeding rarely represents a surgical emergency. In the previously noted study, only 4.2% of 95 patients required a blood transfusion or an operative intervention.

INITIAL ASSESSMENT

The clinician should sequentially assess the patient through the following questions:

1. Is the patient in hemorrhagic shock (see Chapter 5 Shock for signs of hemorrhagic shock)?
2. Is the patient really bleeding? Is the bleeding coming from the GI tract? If so, how severe is the bleeding?
3. Is it upper or lower GI bleeding?
4. What is the age-related differential diagnosis based on pertinent history, physical examination, and diagnostic tests?

GI Bleed Imitators

Many substances ingested by children may simulate fresh or chemically altered blood. Red food coloring (found in cereals, antibiotics and cough syrups, Jell-O, and Kool-Aid), as well as fruit juices and beets, may resemble blood if vomited or passed in the stool. Medications such as antibiotics (cefdinir—which can cause "brick red" stools), iron supplementation, and bismuth (in Pepto-Bismol) may cause the stool to look melanotic or bloody. Foods such as dark chocolate, spinach, cranberries, blueberries, grapes, or licorice may also produce dark-colored stools. In these cases, confirmation of the absence of blood with Gastroccult (vomitus) or Hemoccult (stool) tests will allay parental anxiety, as well as prevent unnecessary concern and testing.

A careful search for other causes of presumed GI bleeding (recent epistaxis, dental work, menses, and hematuria) should be sought. *Hematemesis* (vomiting of blood) also needs to be differentiated from *hemoptysis* (bleeding from the airways).

Severity of Bleeding

Estimation of blood loss (a few drops, a spoonful, a cupful, or more) should be ascertained on initially although this can be difficult and inaccurate. Hemoglobin and hematocrit are also unreliable estimates of acute blood loss because of the time required for hemodilution to occur after an acute hemorrhage. The estimated volume of blood loss should be correlated with the patient's clinical status. In pediatrics, a patient may lose 15% of their circulating blood volume prior to changes in the vital signs. The presence of resting tachycardia, pallor, prolonged capillary refill time, and metabolic acidosis point to significant enteral blood loss. Hypotension is a late finding in young children, typically after greater than 30% of blood volume has been lost, and should be treated as hemorrhagic shock demanding immediate resuscitative measures (intravenous fluids and blood transfusion).

Children with only a few drops or flecks of blood in the vomit or stool should not be considered "GI bleeders" if their history and physical examinations are otherwise unremarkable. Caution must be taken, however, as small amounts of blood (whether in emesis or passed per rectum) may be the harbinger of more extensive enteral bleeding.

Establishing the Level of Bleeding

There are two general categories of GI bleeding: upper and lower. *Upper GI bleeding* refers to bleeding proximal to the ligament of Treitz. Twenty percent of GI bleeds in pediatrics are from the upper GI tract. *Lower GI bleeding* is distal to the ligament of Treitz. In most cases, the clinical findings along with nasogastric lavage will delineate the cause of bleeding within the GI tract. *Hematemesis,* defined as the vomiting of blood, can range from fresh and bright red to old and dark with the appearance of "coffee grounds" (due to the effect of gastric acidity). *Hematochezia,* the passage of bright red blood per rectum, suggests lower GI bleeding or upper GI bleeding with a very rapid enteral transit time (such as in infants). *Melena,* the passage of stool that is shiny, black, and sticky, reflects bleeding from either the upper GI tract or the proximal large bowel. In general, the darker the blood in the stool, the higher it originates in the GI tract (or, alternatively, the longer it has resided in the GI tract). "Currant jelly" stools indicate vascular congestion and hyperemia of the colon with passage of blood mixed with mucus, as seen with intussusception. Maroon-colored stools generally occur with a voluminous bleed anywhere proximal to the rectosigmoid area, such as seen with a Meckel diverticulum.

Patients with a significant bleeding episode should have a nasogastric tube placed for a diagnostic saline lavage (Fig. 28.1). In patients with hematemesis or melena, a nasogastric aspirate yielding blood confirms an upper source of GI bleeding, whereas

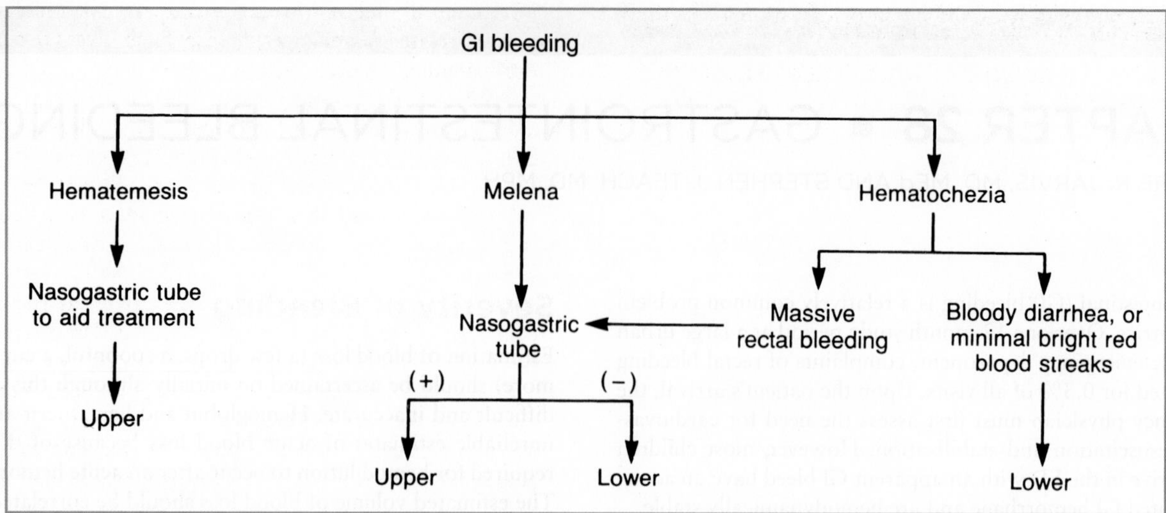

FIGURE 28.1 Establishing level of gastrointestinal (GI) bleeding.

a negative result almost always excludes an active upper GI bleed. Occasionally, a postpyloric upper GI lesion, such as a duodenal ulcer, bleeds massively without reflux into the stomach, resulting in a negative aspirate. In such a case, an upper GI endoscopy will detect such a lesion. Patients with significant hematochezia or melena should likewise have a nasogastric tube placed. As noted above, because blood can exert a cathartic action, brisk bleeding from an upper GI lesion may induce rapid transit through the gut, thus preventing blood from becoming melanotic. In patients with hematochezia manifested as bloody diarrhea or minimally blood-streaked stools, a lower GI source should be investigated.

UPPER GASTROINTESTINAL BLEEDING

Differential Diagnosis

As seen in Table 28.1, there is considerable overlap between age groups and causes of upper GI bleeding. Mucosal lesions, including esophagitis, gastritis, gastric and duodenal ulcers, and Mallory–Weiss tears, are the most common sources of GI bleeding in all age groups (Table 28.2; see Chapter 99 Gastrointestinal Emergencies). Of all cases of upper GI bleeding in children, 95% are related to mucosal lesions and esophageal varices. Coagulation disorders (e.g., disseminated intravascular coagulation, Von Willebrand disease, hemophilia, thrombocytopenia, liver failure, uremia, and factor deficiencies) should also be considered for all age groups as a cause of bleeding, but will not be discussed in detail in this chapter (see Chapter 101 Hematologic Emergencies for further details on coagulation disorders). Life-threatening causes of upper GI bleeding are listed in Table 28.3.

Neonatal Period (0 to 1 Month)

Hematemesis in a healthy newborn most likely results from swallowed maternal blood either at delivery or during breast-feeding. In the breast-fed neonate with new onset of hematemesis and maternal history of cracked nipples, who is well appearing and with normal examination, one approach is to allow the mother to nurse (or use a breast pump) in the

TABLE 28.1

ETIOLOGY OF UPPER GASTROINTESTINAL BLEEDING BASED ON AGE[a]

Neonatal period (<4 wks)	Infancy (<2 yrs)	Preschool age (2–5 yrs)	School age (>5 yrs)
Swallowed maternal blood	Gastritis	Epistaxis	Gastritis
Gastritis	Esophagitis	Gastritis	Mallory–Weiss tear
Peptic ulcer	Mallory–Weiss tear	Esophagitis	Peptic ulcer
Idiopathic	Peptic ulcer	Mallory–Weiss tear	Stress ulcer
Vitamin K–deficient bleeding	Foreign body	Toxic ingestion	Toxic ingestion
Esophagitis	Pyloric stenosis (<2 mo of age)	Peptic ulcer	Esophagitis
Intestinal duplication	Vascular malformation	Foreign body	Esophageal varices
Vascular malformations	Toxic ingestion	Vascular malformation	Vascular malformation
Pyloric stenosis	Intestinal duplication	Esophageal varices	Hemobilia
		Hemobilia	

[a]In approximate order of frequency of occurrence.

TABLE 28.2

COMMON CAUSES OF UPPER GASTROINTESTINAL BLEEDING BASED ON AGE

Neonatal period
Swallowed maternal blood
Infancy
Gastritis
Esophagitis
Mallory–Weiss tear
Preschool age
Epistaxis
Gastritis
Esophagitis
Mallory–Weiss tear
School age
Gastritis
Mallory–Weiss tear
Peptic ulcer

ED. Often, when the infant has been at the breast for a few moments and then is pulled away, obvious bleeding from the mother's nipple is apparent, providing reassurance to both physicians and parents.

Although less common, gastritis (from stress, sepsis, cow's milk intolerance, and trauma from nasogastric tube insertion), necrotizing enterocolitis (NEC), and coagulation disorders should be considered. If vitamin K was not administered in the immediate postpartum period, vitamin K–deficient bleeding (previously known as hemorrhagic disease of the newborn) should be considered. Maternal drugs that cross the placenta, including aspirin, phenytoin, and phenobarbital, may also interfere with clotting factors and cause hemorrhage.

Infancy (1 Month to 2 Years)

Common, and often less severe, causes of bleeding in this age group are gastritis and reflux esophagitis. Significant and sometimes massive upper GI hemorrhage in a newborn may occur with no demonstrative anatomic lesion or only "hemorrhagic gastritis" at endoscopy. This is usually a single, self-limited event that is benign if treated with appropriate blood replacement and supportive measures. Other causes of significant hemorrhage may include pyloric stenosis (often at less than 2 months of age, preceded by significant nonbloody emesis), peptic ulceration, a duplication cyst, foreign body, or caustic ingestion.

TABLE 28.3

LIFE-THREATENING CAUSES OF UPPER GASTROINTESTINAL BLEEDING

Ulcer
Esophageal varices
Vascular malformation
Intestinal duplication

Critically ill children of any age are at risk for developing stress-related peptic ulcer disease. Such ulcers occur with life-threatening illnesses, including shock, respiratory failure, hypoglycemia, dehydration, burns (Curling ulcer), intracranial lesions or trauma (Cushing ulcer), renal failure, and vasculitis. These ulcers may develop within minutes to hours after the initial insult and primarily result from ischemia. Hematemesis, hematochezia, melena, and/or perforation of the stomach or duodenum may accompany stress-associated ulcers.

Hematemesis secondary to gastroesophageal reflux and esophagitis is uncommon but should be considered in patients who are severely symptomatic with vomiting or aspiration. Hematemesis following the acute onset of vigorous vomiting or retching at any age suggests a Mallory–Weiss tear. These tears occur at the gastroesophageal junction due to a combination of mechanical factors (e.g., retching) and gastric acidity.

Preschool Period (2 to 5 Years)

Idiopathic peptic ulcer disease is a common cause of GI bleeding in preschool and older children. Most preschool children with idiopathic ulcers develop GI bleeding (hematemesis or melena). Complications, including obstruction and perforation, may occur. Younger children have less characteristic symptoms, often localize abdominal pain poorly, and may have vomiting as a predominant symptom. Older children and adolescents describe epigastric pain in a pattern typical of adults. *Helicobacter pylori* infection has emerged as a leading cause of secondary gastritis, particularly in older children. Nonsteroidal anti-inflammatory drugs (NSAIDs) and acetylsalicylic acid can also be a cause of gastritis in this age group.

School Age through Adolescence Period

In older children, the possibility of bleeding esophageal varices must be considered in the differential diagnosis of upper GI bleeding. Esophageal and gastric varices associated with portal hypertension due to hepatic and vascular disorders are the most common causes of severe upper GI hemorrhage in older children. One-half to two-thirds of these children have an extrahepatic presinusoidal obstruction, often resulting from portal vein thrombosis, as the cause of portal hypertension. Omphalitis with or without a history of umbilical vein cannulation, dehydration, and a number of other factors may contribute. Other children with portal hypertension have hepatic parenchymal disorders such as neonatal hepatitis, congenital hepatic fibrosis, cystic fibrosis, or biliary cirrhosis associated with biliary atresia. Two-thirds of patients with portal hypertension develop bleeding before 5 years of age, and 85% do so by 10 years of age.

Evaluation and Decision: Upper Gastrointestinal Bleeding

History and Physical Examination

Pertinent historical elements to be sought include a history of umbilical catheterization or sepsis in the neonatal period, previous episodes of bleeding from the GI tract or other sites, and past hematologic disorders and liver disease. A family history of peptic ulcer disease can be found in up to 30% of patients with idiopathic ulcers. The presence of prior epigastric pain may suggest more long-standing esophagogastritis or ulcer disease. Ingestions including theophylline, aspirin, iron, NSAIDs, alcohol, and steroids should be sought as a possible cause. Massive hemorrhage associated with right upper quadrant pain and jaundice in the posttrauma patient indicates bleeding into the biliary tract (hemobilia).

The physical examination should include visualization of the anterior nose and pharynx to eliminate epistaxis as a source of bleeding. Epigastric pain suggests peptic ulcer disease. Signs of liver disease and/or portal hypertension with esophageal varices may include icterus, abdominal distention, prominent abdominal venous pattern, hepatosplenomegaly, cutaneous spider nevi, and ascites. As previously mentioned, gastric lavage examination can help to diagnose an upper GI bleeding source. A rectal examination for the detection of melena, hematochezia, and occult blood is crucial in all cases of GI bleeding.

Laboratory Evaluation

If concerned about significant bleeding, a clinician should obtain a type and cross, complete blood count, blood urea nitrogen, serum creatinine, transaminases, and coagulation profile. Laboratory tests are not useful for identifying a precise cause of upper GI bleeding, but can aid in narrowing the differential diagnosis.

Gastroccult tests can confirm the presence of blood in the vomitus. Gastroccult is a specific and sensitive assay, and can detect as little as 300 mcg per dL of hemoglobin. The Apt–Downey test can differentiate neonatal from maternal hemoglobin, but obtaining sufficient vomited blood to perform this test may be difficult. Vitamin K–deficient bleeding in neonates should be considered with prolongation of the prothrombin time. A low mean corpuscular volume and hypochromic, microcytic anemia suggests chronic mucosal bleeding. Initial low white blood cell and platelet counts may be seen in either hypersplenism from portal hypertension or sepsis with associated mucosal ulceration due to stress. Abnormal hepatic studies, including an elevation of serum bilirubin, transaminases, and prothrombin time, and a low serum albumin, are suggestive of esophageal varices. A blood urea nitrogen to creatinine ratio greater than 30 may indicate blood resorption and an upper GI source of bleeding.

Diagnostic Approach

If a significant upper GI bleed has occurred, and once hemodynamic stability is restored, identification of the specific age-related disorder is the next step (Table 28.1 and Fig. 28.2). If the bleeding is mild and self-limited or the gastric aspirate is negative, a minor mucosal lesion is likely. Although mucosal lesions such as esophagitis, gastritis, or peptic ulcer disease can present with severe bleeding, most often bleeding from mucosal lesions is self-limiting and will respond to conservative medical management.

In patients with persistent or recurrent hemorrhage, emergent endoscopy for diagnosis (location of bleeding and biopsies as needed) and treatment may be necessary if the bleeding is life-threatening (continued transfusion requirement, hemodynamic instability). In this setting, endoscopy should be considered prior to the use of contrast radiography in which contrast material obscures the bleeding source. Endoscopy can now diagnose the cause of upper GI bleeding in more than 90% of patients. In the small percentage of patients in whom bleeding is massive, making endoscopic visualization impossible, angiography or radionuclide studies (Technetium-sulfur colloid/Tc-labeled red blood cells) may be indicated. In rare emergencies, a surgeon may also be needed for diagnosis and treatment of severe bleeding.

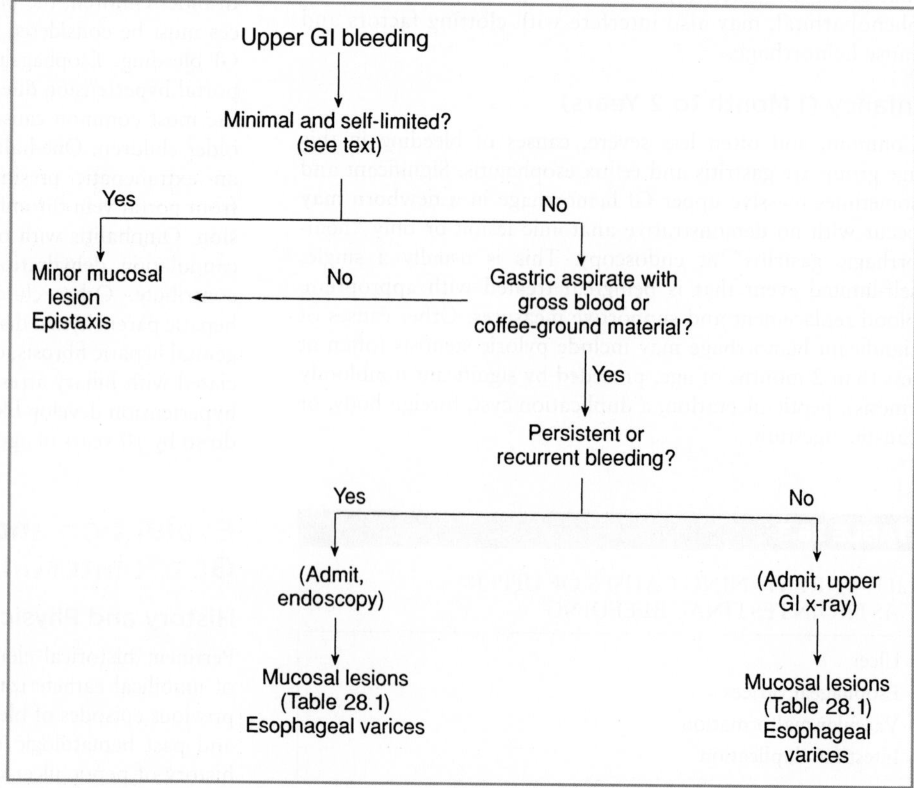

FIGURE 28.2 Diagnostic approach to upper gastrointestinal (GI) bleeding.

TABLE 28.4

ETIOLOGY OF LOWER GASTROINTESTINAL BLEEDING BASED ON AGE[a]

Neonatal period	Infancy (1 mo–2 yrs)	Preschool age (2–5 yrs)	School age (>5 yrs)
Typically well-appearing			
Swallowed maternal blood	Anal fissure	Anal fissure	Infectious colitis
Infectious colitis	Infectious colitis	Infectious colitis	Polyps
Allergic colitis	Allergic colitis	Juvenile polyps	Inflammatory bowel disease
Hemorrhagic disease	Nonspecific colitis	Intussusception	Hemorrhoids
Duplication of bowel	Juvenile polyps	Henoch–Schönlein purpura	Meckel diverticulum
Meckel diverticulum	Intussusception	Meckel diverticulum	Hemolytic uremic syndrome (HUS)
Typically ill-appearing			
Infectious colitis	Meckel diverticulum	HUS	Pseudomembranous colitis
Midgut volvulus	Duplication	Inflammatory bowel disease	Ischemic colitis
Hirschsprung disease	HUS	Peptic ulcer	Peptic ulcer
Disseminated coagulopathy	Inflammatory bowel disease	Pseudomembranous enterocolitis	Angiodysplasia
Necrotizing enterocolitis	Pseudomembranous enterocolitis		
Intussusception	Ischemic colitis	Ischemic colitis	
Congestive heart failure	Lymphonodular hyperplasia	Angiodysplasia	
	FPIES		

[a]In approximate order of frequency of occurrence.

Treatment of specific mucosal conditions and esophageal varices is discussed in Chapter 99 Gastrointestinal Emergencies.

Eighty percent to 85% of upper GI bleeding stops spontaneously, regardless of the source, before or early in the hospital course. In stable patients who have stopped bleeding, an upper GI contrast study and endoscopy provide valuable and often complementary information. In this group of patients, endoscopy need not be performed on an emergent basis and may be done electively in the first 12 to 24 hours after admission. Elective endoscopy should be performed in patients who stop bleeding spontaneously but who have required transfusion and/or have a history of previously unexplained upper GI bleeding episodes.

LOWER GASTROINTESTINAL BLEEDING

Differential Diagnosis

As previously mentioned, rectal bleeding is common in children. Similar to upper GI bleeding, there is significant overlap among age groups in the etiology of lower GI bleeding (Table 28.4). The most common disorders by age group are listed in Table 28.5, and the life-threatening causes are listed in Table 28.6. Of note, many cases of lower GI bleeding resolve spontaneously without a specific diagnosis being established.

Neonatal Period (0 to 1 Month)

As is true for upper GI bleeding, a common cause of blood in the stool in well-appearing neonates is the passage of maternal blood swallowed either at delivery or during breastfeeding from a fissured maternal nipple. Infectious diarrhea can occur in very young infants, and stools may contain blood or mucus. Common bacterial pathogens in this age group include *Campylobacter jejuni* and *Salmonella.*

In ill-appearing neonates with lower GI bleeding, midgut volvulus, NEC, and Hirschsprung disease should be considered (Table 28.4). Malrotation with midgut volvulus is most common during this period presenting initially with bilious vomiting, abdominal distention, and pain. Melena is seen in 10% to 20% of patients with midgut volvulus and signifies vascular compromise. NEC, most common in preterm infants (although 10% occur in term infants), signifies sections of bowel tissue necrosis. The diagnosis of Hirschsprung disease should be considered in any newborn who does not pass meconium in the first 24 to 48 hours of life. Twenty-five percent of neonates with Hirschsprung disease have enterocolitis that may present with GI bleeding.

TABLE 28.5

COMMON CAUSES OF LOWER GASTROINTESTINAL BLEEDING BASED ON AGE

Neonatal period
Swallowed maternal blood
Infectious colitis
Allergic colitis
Infancy
Anal fissure
Infectious colitis
Allergic colitis
Preschool age
Anal fissure
Infectious colitis
School age
Infectious colitis
Intestinal polyp

TABLE 28.6

LIFE-THREATENING CAUSES OF LOWER GASTROINTESTINAL BLEEDING

Necrotizing enterocolitis
Midgut volvulus
Intussusception
Meckel diverticulum
Hemolytic uremic syndrome
Pseudomembranous colitis
Ischemic colitis
Peptic ulcer
Angiodysplasia
FPIES
Toxic megacolon

The risk of enterocolitis remains high until about 6 months of age.

Infancy (1 Month to 2 Years)

In the first 2 years of life, anal fissures and colitis (including infectious and allergic) are among the most common causes of rectal bleeding. Anal fissures are usually associated with constipation or trauma (rarely, this trauma can be nonaccidental). Infectious enterocolitis as a cause of bloody diarrhea is common in all age groups. Pseudomembranous colitis should be considered in any infant or child with bloody stools and a history of recent antibiotic therapy. "Nonspecific colitis" is a common cause of hematochezia in infants younger than 6 months of age and may represent a variation in the colonic response to viral invasion.

Milk- or soy-allergic enterocolitis causes bloody diarrhea and usually occurs during the first month of life, but can occur in older children depending on food exposure. Trialing a change in formula from cow's milk or soy protein to an elemental formula (Nutramigen, Alimentum, Pregestimil) can also help to assess for milk protein allergy. Breast-fed infants whose mothers drink cow's milk may develop an allergic colitis that responds to removal of cow's milk from the mother's diet.

Food protein–induced enterocolitis syndrome (FPIES) represents a rare (affects up to 0.34% of infants) but severe, non–IgE-mediated food hypersensitivity that occurs within hours of offending food ingestion. Symptoms, including hypovolemic shock, typically begin in the first month of life, with a mean age at initial presentation of 5.5 months. Infants typically react to one or two specific foods with the most common being soy and cow's milk, and, less commonly, rice, vegetables, fruits, meats, oats, egg, and fish. Most children develop tolerance to the offending food trigger by 3 years of age.

Meckel diverticulum should be suspected in infants or young children who present with intermittent painless rectal bleeding (dark or red blood) that may cause massive GI hemorrhage. Sixty percent of complications from Meckel diverticulum (hemorrhage and intestinal obstruction) occur in patients younger than 2 years of age. Idiopathic intussusception may occur in infancy, with 80% occurring before 2 years of age. Lymphonodular hyperplasia is an uncommon cause of rectal bleeding in this age group and may cause mild, painless hematochezia that is self-limited. Intestinal duplications are also an uncommon cause of lower GI bleeding and, when diagnosed, are usually found in children younger than 2 years of age. Duplications can be found anywhere in the GI tract but are most common in the distal ileum and usually present with obstruction and lower GI bleeding.

Preschool Period (2 to 5 Years)

The most common conditions to cause bleeding in children 2 to 5 years of age are anal fissures, juvenile polyps, and infectious enterocolitis. Most polyps in childhood are often multiple and inflammatory in nature without significant malignant potential. Polyps typically present with painless rectal bleeding in this age group, and significant bleeding is unusual. In children older than 3 years with intussusception, a lead point (polyp, Meckel diverticulum, or hypertrophied lymphoid patch) is more often found than in younger children. Infectious causes of colitis are similar to those discussed in younger age groups.

Hematochezia may be a manifestation of systemic diseases such as hemolytic uremic syndrome (HUS) and Henoch–Schönlein purpura (HSP). HUS is the most prevalent of these conditions reported in infants and children up to 3 years of age. Bloody diarrhea due to *Escherichia coli* O157:H7 may precede the development of renal and hematologic abnormalities in HUS. GI manifestations of HSP occur in 50% of patients and include colicky abdominal pain, melena, and bloody diarrhea. These symptoms precede the characteristic rash in 20% of patients. GI complications among patients with HSP include hemorrhage (5%), intussusception (3%), and rarely, intestinal perforation.

Angiodysplasia is a rare cause of GI bleeding but can be associated with massive hemorrhage. Vascular lesions of the GI tract may have a congenital basis. Several recognized syndromes, including Rendu–Osler–Weber syndrome and Turner syndrome, may be associated with intestinal telangiectasia.

School Age through Adolescence Period

For the most part, the diagnostic considerations relevant to the preschool child apply to school-age and adolescent children. In this age group, colorectal polyps become more frequent, with a prevalence of 12% in children with lower GI bleeding undergoing colonoscopy. Solitary juvenile polyps are the most common type, but up to 26% of patients may have multiple juvenile or adenomatous polyps. Inflammatory bowel disease is also unique to the age group, and is rare before the age of 10 years. Rectal bleeding is a common presentation of both ulcerative colitis and Crohn disease. Massive lower GI bleeding occurs in 2% to 5% of children with Crohn disease. Fulminant colitis and toxic megacolon are life-threatening presentations of both ulcerative colitis and Crohn disease.

Evaluation and Decision: Lower Gastrointestinal Bleeding

History and Physical Examination

Symptoms of an acute abdominal process with bowel obstruction, including abdominal pain, distention, and vomiting, should be elicited. Cases of NEC present with nonspecific signs of sepsis (temperature instability, apnea, and/or bradycardia) and with specific GI tract findings, such as vomiting, abdominal distention, tenderness, and abdominal wall erythema.

It is also important to elicit a history of blood-streaked firm stools compared to bloody diarrhea and whether pain is present. A history of constipation in a young infant with acute onset of bloody diarrhea suggests enterocolitis associated with Hirschsprung disease. Bloody diarrhea with pain may indicate infectious or allergic colitis, intussusception, IBD, or HUS. Paroxysmal pain of intussusception may be associated with occult blood, hematochezia, or "currant jelly stools." Lethargy alone (without pain) has been recognized as a presenting symptom of intussusception in young children. Firm stool streaked with bright red blood or blood seen on the toilet paper characterizes anal fissures associated with constipation. Colonic polyps often present with painless rectal bleeding. Extraintestinal manifestations of inflammatory bowel disease, including weight loss, anorexia, and arthralgias, may be predominant symptoms in school-age children.

Eliciting a dietary history in the setting of bloody diarrhea may suggest features of milk or soy protein intolerance and/or FPIES. These infants can present with chronic diarrhea and failure to thrive, with stools containing blood or mucus, or less commonly, with fulminant colitis and shock. FPIES presents with profuse vomiting, lethargy, pallor, and bloody diarrhea that develops within a few hours of food ingestion. Up to 20% of these infants present in hypovolemic shock with need for fluid resuscitation and 26% have hypothermia.

A detailed family history (bleeding diathesis, familial polyposis) and drug history (NSAIDs, salicylates, iron) or antibiotics (pseudomembranous colitis) are important in patients with lower GI bleeding. A past medical history of abnormal bleeding may signify a coagulopathy.

Physical examination to detect abdominal obstruction (abdominal tenderness, distention, palpable mass, peritoneal signs, hyperactive [early] or hypoactive [late] bowel sounds) is the most urgent task of the evaluating physician. Careful separation of the buttocks with eversion of the anal mucosa may reveal a fissure. Prominent or multiple perianal skin tags may raise suspicion of Crohn disease. Between 30% and 40% of rectal polyps are palpable on rectal examination. Cutaneous lesions may provide important diagnostic clues in patients with GI bleeding. Eczema may be associated with milk allergy, whereas erythema nodosum is the most common skin manifestation of IBD. Mucocutaneous pigmentation (Peutz–Jeghers syndrome) and cutaneous or subcutaneous tumors (Gardner syndrome) indicate intestinal polyposis. Petechiae or bruising is seen in HUS and palpable purpura in HSP.

Laboratory Evaluation

Many causes of lower GI tract bleeding are easily identifiable and do not require laboratory testing. If needed, Hemoccult tests can help to confirm the presence of blood in the stool. Fecal alpha-1 antitrypsin can also be elevated in patients with GI blood loss and is more sensitive and specific than a guaiac test. Bacterial causes (*Salmonella, Shigella, Campylobacter,* pathogenic *E. coli,* and *Yersinia enterocolitica*) should be identified with stool cultures. Stool testing may also be performed if there is concern for *Clostridium difficile.* In symptomatic infants and children, the presence of leukocytes in a stool smear (or fecal lactoferrin) may aid in preliminary diagnosis. Anemia, leukocytosis, thrombocytosis, elevated ESR/CRP, decreased albumin, and elevated fecal leukocytes support the diagnosis of IBD. Infants with FPIES can present with a metabolic acidosis, leukocytosis, thrombocytosis, hypoalbuminemia, and methemoglobinemia. HUS can be identified by microangiopathic hemolytic anemia, thrombocytopenia, and renal injury.

Diagnostic Approach

Rectal bleeding presents in all pediatric age groups (Table 28.4 and Fig. 28.3). The causes of lower GI bleeding vary significantly with age, and are often transient and benign. Occasionally, lower GI bleeding reflects a life-threatening

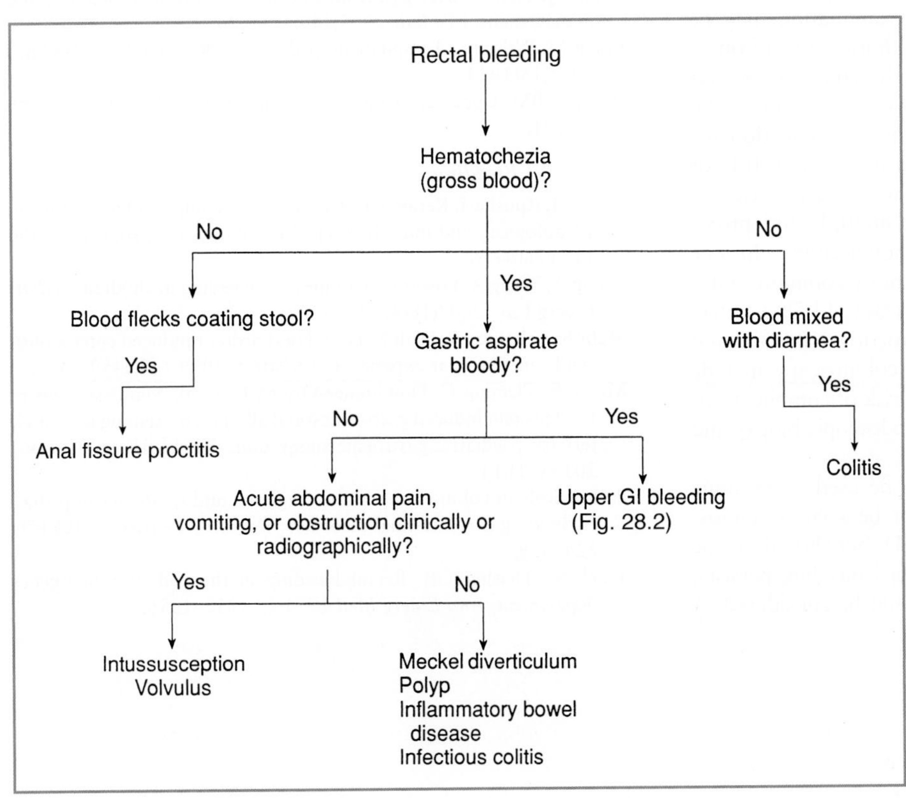

FIGURE 28.3 Diagnostic approach to lower gastrointestinal (GI) bleeding.

pathologic condition, and establishment of a specific diagnosis becomes urgent.

The priority in evaluating the patient with lower GI bleeding is to identify lower tract bleeding associated with intestinal obstruction and with other causes of large volume bleeding such as a Meckel diverticulum. Intussusception and a late presentation of midgut volvulus secondary to malrotation are the major types of intestinal obstruction associated with lower GI hemorrhage. All causes of abdominal obstruction (e.g., adhesions, incarcerated hernia, and appendicitis) eventually result in bleeding if diagnosis is delayed and vascular compromise occurs.

Severe lower GI bleeding leading to hemodynamic instability or requiring transfusion is rare in pediatrics, and gastric lavage is essential in these cases to rule out a possible upper GI tract source. Meckel diverticulum is the most common cause of severe lower GI bleeding in all age groups. Following Meckel diverticulum, Crohn disease and arteriovenous malformation are prominent causes of massive lower GI bleeding in adolescents.

The urgency and extent of evaluation of patients with lower GI bleeding will depend on the amount of bleeding, the patient's age, and associated physical findings. In a healthy infant with a few streaks of blood in the stool and a normal examination, a limited evaluation and observation are reasonable. If more significant hematochezia is found and if a nasogastric aspirate is negative, then significant pathology must be sought. Flat and upright abdominal radiographs should be performed if an obstructive process (e.g., intussusception, volvulus) is suspected by history or physical examination. The absence of radiographic findings should not, however, deter the physician from pursuing further diagnostic evaluation. Upper GI contrast radiography with small bowel series can often define the level of small bowel obstruction. Ultrasound and computed tomography (with intravenous and enteral contrast) has been increasingly used to identify etiologies of obstruction. An air or barium enema examination may be diagnostic and therapeutic in children with intussusception.

If obstruction is not considered likely, colonoscopy has become a standard procedure in the diagnosis of lower GI bleeding. Hematochezia is the most common indication for pediatric colonoscopy, and is often used to diagnose IBD or suspected colonic polyps. Colonoscopy is frequently used to locate polyps (especially those that are multiple and proximally located) and for colonoscopic polypectomy. In one study, juvenile polyp (20.5%) was the most common endoscopic diagnosis, followed by Crohn disease (13.5%), infectious or nonspecific colitis (10.0%), proctitis (10.0%), and angiodysplasia (0.6%). The benefits of colonoscopy include identification of the site of bleeding, low risk of complications of the procedure, and the possibility of endoscopic biopsy and intervention.

Wireless capsule endoscopy can also be used to examine areas of the small intestine that cannot be seen by endoscopy/colonoscopy for ulcerations and IBD, but should not be used in a bleeding emergency. If undefined bleeding persists, radionuclide studies or angiography should be considered. A technetium scan may detect ectopic gastric mucosa as seen in Meckel diverticulum, whereas angiography will help identify bleeding vascular malformations in the GI tract. Ongoing, undiagnosed GI hemorrhage accounts for fewer than 10% of cases in infants and children. Exploratory laparotomy may be necessary and lifesaving in these circumstances.

SUMMARY

Management of acute GI bleeding often requires a team approach, including the emergency physician, surgeon, gastroenterologist, and radiologist. The primary goals of ED evaluation of patients with GI bleeding are establishment of hemodynamic stability and determination of level of bleeding. Patients with nontrivial upper GI bleeding should generally be admitted for observation and further evaluation. If an acute abdominal process is suspected, surgical consultation and diagnostic workup should be instituted. If rectal bleeding is mild and self-limited and the history and physical examination is unremarkable, further investigation with the primary care provider or a gastroenterologist is recommended.

Suggested Readings and Key References

Overview

Boyle JT. Gastrointestinal bleeding in infants and children. *Pediatr Rev* 2008;29:39–52.

Fox VL. Gastrointestinal bleeding in infancy and childhood. *Gastroenterol Clin North Am* 2000;29:37–66.

Saliakellis E, Borrelli O, Thapar N. Paediatric GI emergencies. *Best Pract Res Clin Gastroenterol* 2013;27(5):799–817.

Upper GI Bleeding

Chelimsky G, Czinn S. Peptic ulcer disease in children. *Pediatr Rev* 2001;22:349–355.

Czinn SJ. Helicobacter pylori infection: detection, investigation, and management. *J Pediatr* 2005;146:S21–S26.

Friedt M, Welsch S. An update on pediatric endoscopy. *Eur J Med Res* 2013;18(1):24.

Rodgers BM. Upper gastrointestinal hemorrhage. *Pediatr Rev* 1999; 20:171.

Lower GI Bleeding

Arvola T, Ruuska T, Keränen J, et al. Rectal bleeding in infancy: clinical, allegological, and microbiological examinations. *Pediatrics* 2006; 117:e760–e768.

Leung A, Wong A. Lower gastrointestinal bleeding in children. *Pediatr Emerg Care* 2002;18(4):319–323.

Mehr S, Kakakios A, Frith K, et al. Food protein-induced enterocolitis syndrome: 16-year experience. *Pediatrics* 2009;123:e459–e464.

Meyer R, Fleming C, Dominguez-Ortega G, et al. Manifestations of food protein induced gastrointestinal allergies presenting to a single tertiary paediatric gastroenterology unit. *World Allergy Organ J* 2013;6(1):13.

Park J. Role of colonoscopy in the diagnosis and treatment of pediatric lower gastrointestinal disorders. *Korean J Pediatr* 2010;53(9): 824–829.

Teach SJ, Fleisher GR. Rectal bleeding in the pediatric emergency department. *Ann Emerg Med* 1994;23:1252–1258.

CHAPTER 29 ■ GROIN MASSES

EVA M. DELGADO, MD AND RONALD F. MARCHESE, MD, PhD

There are many different causes of inguinal swelling in children, ranging from inconsequential to serious (Table 29.1). Although hernia is the most common etiology, other important causes include local lymphadenitis, benign or malignant tumors, and pathology related to conditions in which the testicle is found outside the scrotum (retractile, undescended, ectopic, and dislocated); these conditions are discussed in this section. Testicular torsion, scrotal masses, and infections such as epididymitis and orchitis are addressed in Chapter 57 Pallor on scrotal pain, and approach to the incarcerated inguinal hernia is more completely addressed in Chapter 124 Abdominal Emergencies.

GENERAL APPROACH

In evaluating an inguinal mass, consider duration of symptoms, presence/absence of pain, symptoms of obstruction, signs of systemic disease and/or local infection, change in mass with changes in intra-abdominal pressure, trauma and past medical history such as prematurity, abdominal or urogenital malformation, and connective tissue disorder. Careful history and physical examination and judicial use of laboratory tests and ultrasound confirm the diagnosis. The next section includes more detail about common pediatric inguinal mass diagnoses and characteristics specific to each of their presentations. Figure 29.1 reviews the approach to the differential diagnosis.

DIFFERENTIAL DIAGNOSIS

Lymphadenopathy and Lymphadenitis

There are two groups of inguinal nodes: Superficial and deep. The superficial nodes are subdivided into a horizontal chain that runs parallel to the inguinal ligament and a vertical chain located laterally. The horizontal group drains the skin of the lower abdominal wall, perineum, gluteal region, penis and scrotum or the mucosa of the vagina, and the lower anal canal. The vertical group drains lymph from the gluteal region, the penis and deep structures of the scrotum, the anterior and lateral areas of the thigh and leg, and the medial portions of the foot. The deep inguinal nodes, which lie beneath the fascia lata medial to the femoral vein, drain all the superficial nodes, the clitoris or glans of the penis, the medial thigh and leg, and the lateral portion of the foot.

Normal inguinal nodes are less than 1.5 to 2 cm long, and are oval, firm, slightly moveable, and nontender. Lymphadenopathy describes enlarged, nontender nodes, and can be regional or generalized (see Chapter 42 Lymphadenopathy). Isolated inguinal lymphadenopathy may be unilateral or bilateral, and typically develops in response to a local irritation or infection. Inguinal lymphadenopathy associated with generalized lymphadenopathy is associated with systemic diseases including infectious (e.g., human immunodeficiency virus, Epstein–Barr virus), malignant, rheumatologic, or inflammatory processes. Local tumors, such as testicular tumors, can metastasize to the inguinal nodes causing a localized lymphadenopathy.

Isolated inguinal adenopathy most often results from inflammation or infection of the gluteal region, perineum, genitalia, or lower extremities, and therefore, these areas should be examined carefully. Chronic eczema, tinea cruris, or an innocuous inflammation (e.g., an insect bite, diaper rash) may produce lymphadenopathy. In such cases, treatment of the underlying condition suffices.

Lymphadenitis presents as an enlarged, tender node with or without overlying erythema, suppuration, or ulceration. Skin flora, such as Group A β-hemolytic streptococcus and *Staphylococcus aureus,* are often the source of infection. Children without significant systemic symptoms, pain, or other comorbidities can be treated as outpatients with oral antibiotics effective against these organisms and follow-up. If there is a concern for suppuration, ultrasound is helpful in identifying the presence of phlegmon or abscess (Fig. 29.2). Incision and drainage is the treatment of choice for abscess. If drainage is inadequate, or there is overlying cellulitis an antibiotic effective against MRSA is indicated (see Chapter 102 Infectious Disease Emergencies). Children with severe symptoms from lymphadenitis/cellulitis should be admitted and treated with intravenous antibiotics.

Lymphadenitis can also be associated with zoonotic or sexually transmitted infections. Animal and insect bites occurring on the lower extremity can cause inguinal adenopathy or adenitis. Catscratch disease (*Bartonella henselae*) results in regional lymphadenopathy that is often red, indurated, and warm. Lymphadenopathy resolves spontaneously within 2 to 4 months. Antibiotic treatment for immune-competent children with mild disease is of uncertain value (see Chapter 102 Infectious Disease Emergencies). *Yersinia pestis* transmitted via flea bites carries a high mortality and is rare in the United States. Bubonic plague, the most common form, causes regional exquisitely tender lymphadenitis (bubo) with overlying erythema in the area of the bite; the inguinal nodes are the most common site. Ulceroglandular tularemia is transmitted by tick bites and can cause inguinal adenopathy and adenitis that often precedes the appearance of a small papule that later ulcerates at the portal of entry on the lower extremity. Both plague and tularemia exist in pneumonic forms that have become agents of bioterrorism (see Chapter 136 Biological and Chemical Terrorism). Filariasis, a parasitic disease transmitted by fly or mosquito bites and found in the tropics, can produce adenopathy or adenitis associated with lower extremity lymphedema and scrotal pathology. Treatment is dependent on the extent of disease. (See treatment options in Table 29.2.)

Sexually transmitted infections can result in inguinal adenopathy or adenitis (see Chapter 100 Gynecology Emergencies).

TABLE 29.1

CAUSES OF INGUINAL MASSES

Painful
[a]Torsion of an undescended testicle
[a]Trauma (e.g., dislocated testicle)
[a]Incarceration or strangulation of an indirect or direct inguinal hernia
Herniation of the ovary and/or fallopian tube
Herniation of appendicitis
Lymphadenitis
Usually or comparatively painless
Hernia
Hydrocele
Lymphadenopathy
Tumor, benign or malignant
Retractile or undescended testicle

[a]Urgent or emergent condition.

Herpes simplex is a common cause of genital ulcerations and bilateral lymphadenitis. Occasionally, enlarged lymph glands precede the appearance of vesicles. The chancre of primary syphilis is painless and has a raised, indurated border and a clean surface. Bilateral (70%) or unilateral, nontender inguinal adenopathy is common. Chancroid, more common in developing countries than in the United States, is caused by *Haemophilus ducreyi*, which is hard to isolate and requires selective media. Unlike syphilis, the chancroid ulcer is painful and nonindurated, and has serpiginous borders and a friable base covered with a gray or dirty yellow exudate. About one-half of patients develop painful adenitis, usually unilaterally. The node or nodes often suppurate and drain spontaneously, but may require needle aspiration or surgical incision.

Lymphogranuloma venereum, which occurs mostly in tropical and subtropical countries, is caused by *Chlamydia trachomatis*. The genital papule, vesicle, or ulcer is often missed because it is painless, inconspicuous, and transitory. One or more unilaterally enlarged, moderately tender, fluctuant nodes are characteristic. If left untreated, these nodes can drain and form fistulae.

Granuloma inguinale is usually sexually transmitted, and while rare in the United States, it is important to consider when evaluating inguinal adenopathy since an untreated infestation can generate multiple subcutaneous granulomas (pseudobuboes) in the inguinal area that mimic adenopathy. (See Table 29.2 for recommended treatment.)

Inguinal Hernias

Hernias may be direct or indirect; they may be intermittent, reducible, or incarcerated. Indirect hernias are far more common in children and present as a smooth, firm mass that emerges through the external inguinal ring, lateral to the pubic tubercle, and results in swelling in the scrotum or labia. Parents or older children may first notice an inguinal hernia when an increase in

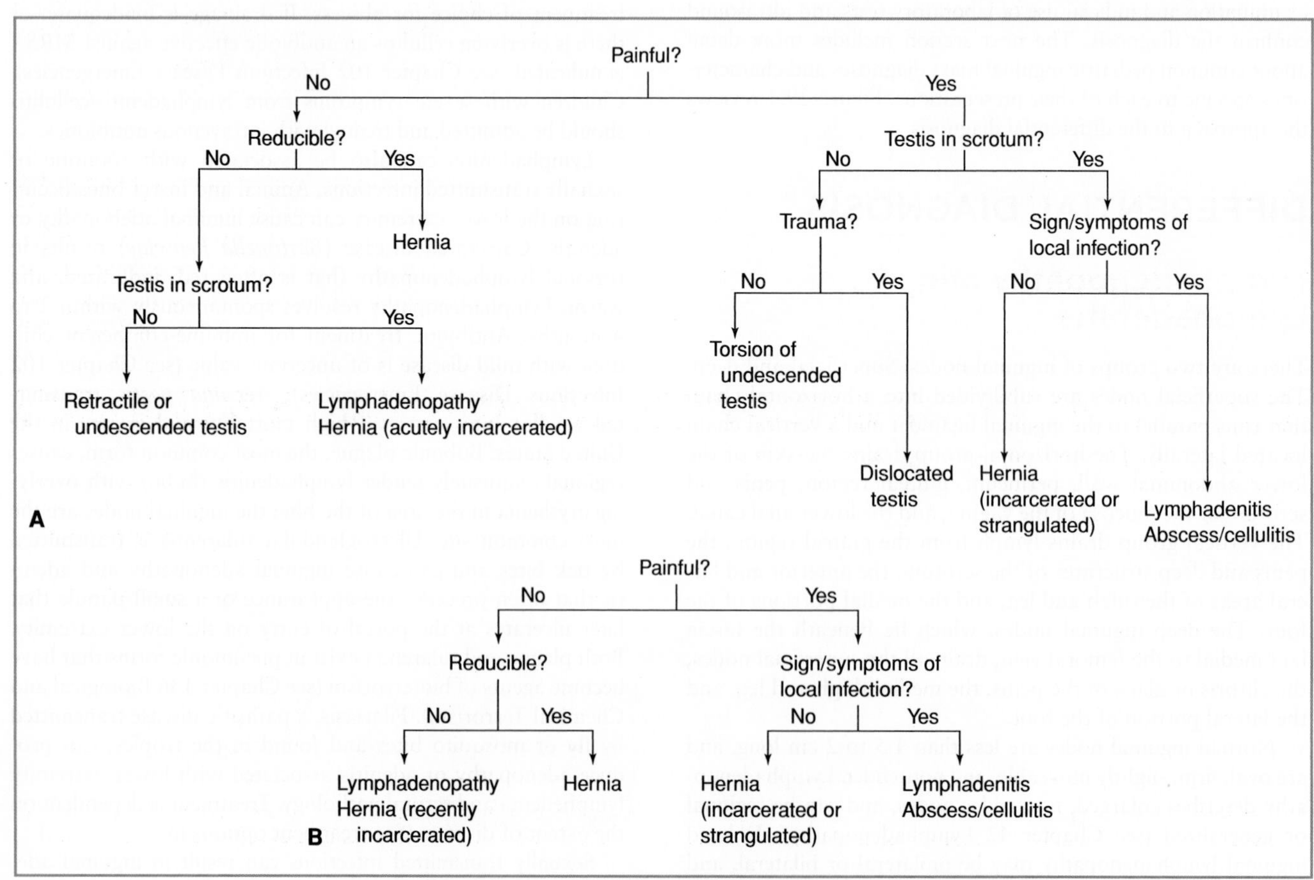

FIGURE 29.1 **A: Inguinal masses in males. B: Inguinal masses in females.**

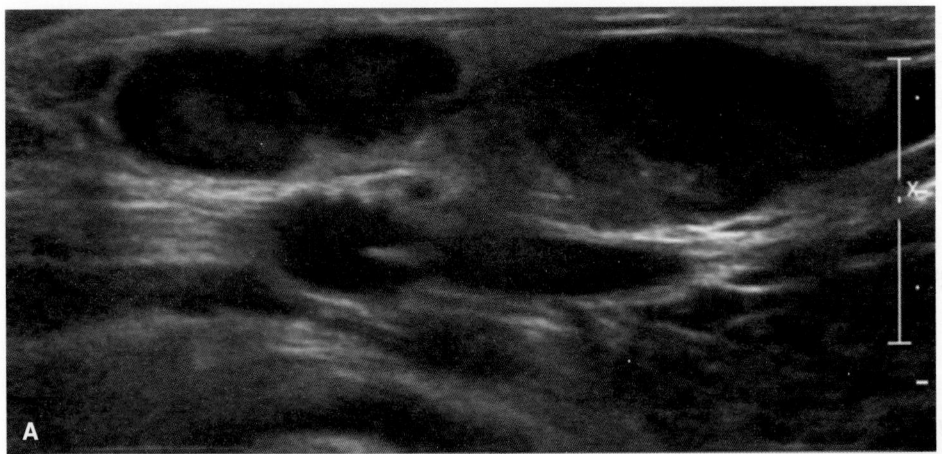

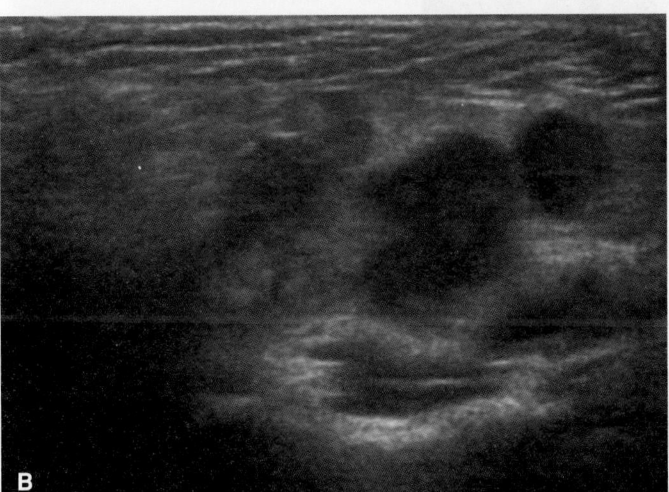

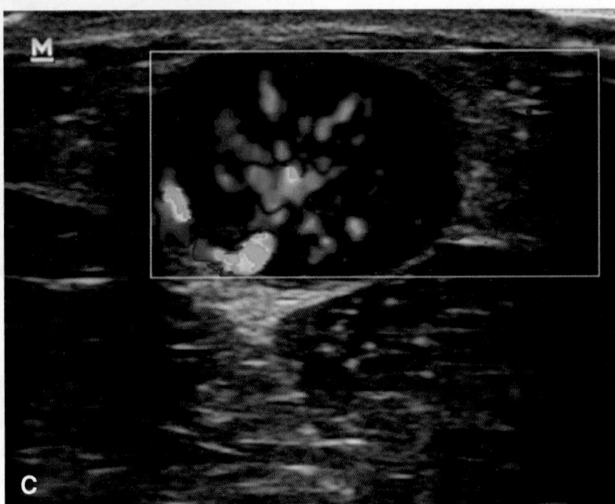

FIGURE 29.2 Sonographic findings of inguinal masses. **A:** Multiple enlarged inguinal lymph nodes in catscratch disease. **B:** Cellulitis and phlegmon formation, multiple reactive lymph nodes. **C:** Vascular stalk on Doppler identifying inguinal lymph node.

intra-abdominal pressure during crying or passing gas provokes the inguinal swelling that resolves when the abdomen relaxes. Hernias result from a persistent patent processus vaginalis. This peritoneal outpouching extends through the internal inguinal ring and accompanies the testis into the scrotum in males as shown in Figure 29.3, and extends through the inguinal canal into the labia majora in females. Indirect inguinal hernias occur in up to 5% of full-term newborns, with a male to female ratio of 6:1; the incidence is much higher, up to 30%, in very low birth weight and very preterm infants. Ultrasound imaging can be helpful in distinguishing hernia from other causes of scrotal swelling (see Chapters 56 Pain: Scrotal, and 127 Genitourinary Emergencies).

TABLE 29.2

RECOMMENDED THERAPEUTIC AGENTS FOR INGUINAL INFECTIONS

Infection	Antibiotic/Antiviral agent
Skin and soft tissue infections	Clindamycin or trimethoprim/sulfamethoxazole
Yersinia pestis (plague)	Trimethoprim/sulfamethoxazole, aminoglycosides, cefotaxime, or fluoroquinolones
Ulceroglandular tularemia	Streptomycin or gentamicin
HSV	Acyclovir[a]
Syphilis	Benzathine Penicillin G: 2.4 million units IM
Haemophilus ducreyi (chancroid)	Azithromycin 1 gm PO or ceftriaxone 250 mg IM
Lymphogranuloma venereum (*Chlamydia trachomatis*)	Doxycycline or erythromycin[b]
Granuloma inguinale (*Klebsiella granulomatis*)	Doxycycline, trimethoprim/sulfamethoxazole, or erythromycin[b]

[a]To shorten symptoms of primary disease; therapy cannot affect frequency/severity of recurrence.
[b]Three-week treatment course.

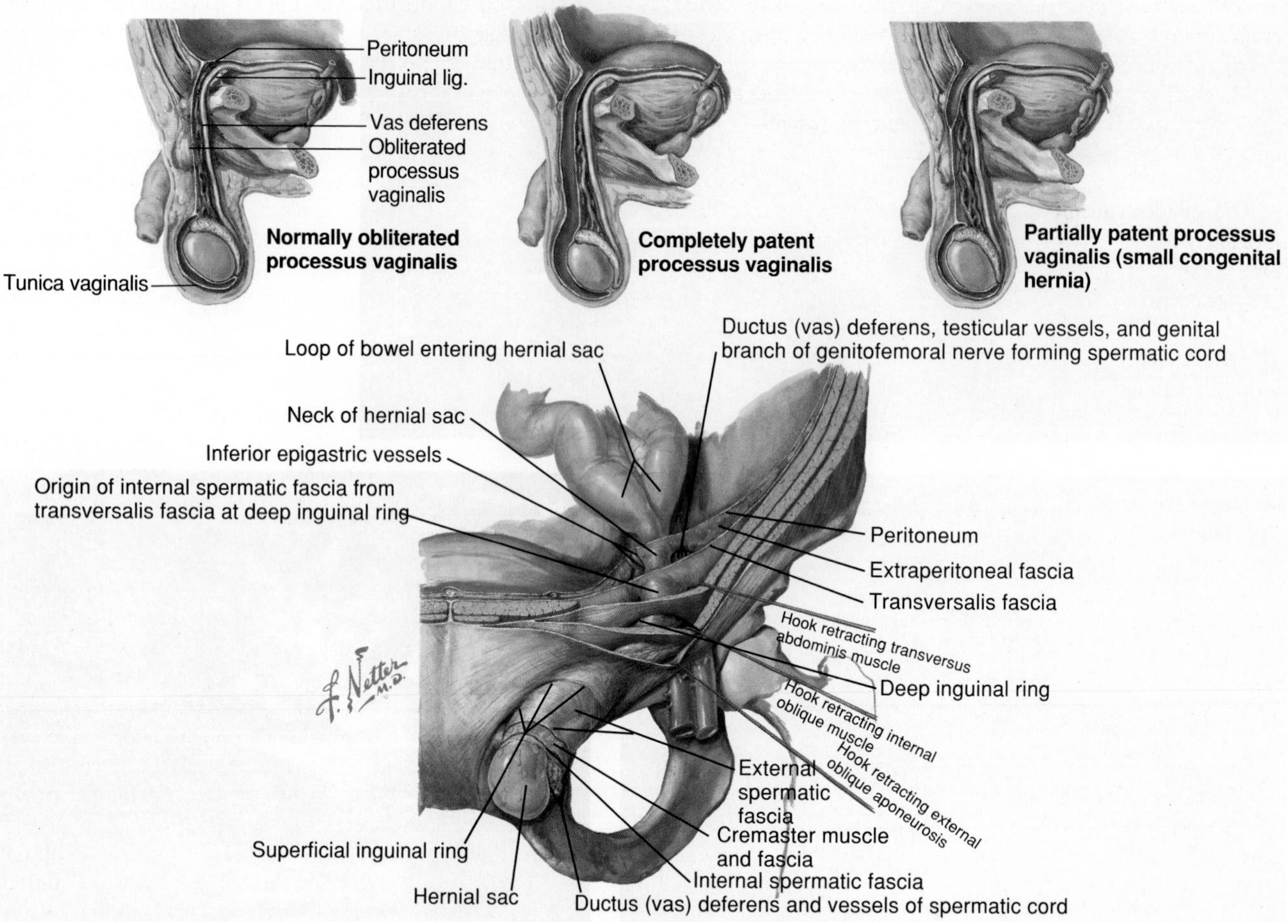

FIGURE 29.3 Indirect inguinal hernia.

Incarcerated inguinal hernias are associated with a persistent inguinal mass, significant discomfort, and/or vomiting. Gentle, steady pressure on the mass will fail to reduce the contents of the hernia back into the abdominal cavity placing its contents at risk for ischemia.

Incarceration is more common in infants; 25% of inguinal hernias occur in children <6 months. The contents of the hernia sac include small bowel, omentum, and rarely the appendix. In females, the hernia sac can include the ovary and/or the fallopian tube which increases risk for torsion and ischemia. The ischemia of hernia contents is known as strangulation, and a manual reduction can be attempted to prevent this outcome when an incarcerated hernia is identified. The approach to reduction may be dependent on the preferences of surgical consultants, and some would like to be involved for this step (see Chapters 124 Abdominal Emergencies, 127 Genitourinary Emergencies, and 141 Procedures). Emergency surgery is indicated for incarcerated hernias; patients with reducible hernias should be referred for scheduled surgery to avoid future complications.

Retractile, Undescended, Ectopic, and Traumatically Dislocated Testes

When an inguinal mass is associated with an empty scrotum, it is likely a retractile or undescended testis. A retractile testis is pulled into an abnormally high position by a hyperactive cremasteric reflex and can be maneuvered back into the scrotum by the examiner. When the testicle is retractile, the scrotum appears fully developed. Although it may retract again, it will ultimately assume a normal position; therefore, no treatment is needed (see Chapter 127 Genitourinary Emergencies). Failure of at least one testicle to descend, cryptorchidism, occurs in 2% to 4% of full-term males. Cryptorchidism incidence correlates inversely with gestational age: it is 10 times more common in premature males, and occurs in almost all newborns weighing less than 900 g at birth. The incidence falls to 0.8% by 1 year of age with spontaneous descent unlikely to occur thereafter since the frequency in adult men is similar. The testis can lodge anywhere along its natural line of descent: In the abdomen, inguinal canal, or just outside the external inguinal ring. Of note, an intra-abdominal testicle is not palpable, and the scrotum appears underdeveloped. Cryptorchidism is right-sided in 50% of patients, left-sided in 20%, and bilateral in 30%. There is a right-sided predominance as the right testicle descends later than the left during embryologic development. Bilateral cryptorchidism occurs more often in premature males and in conjunction with some anatomic, enzymatic, and chromosomal disorder. There is an increased incidence of cryptorchidism among family members. The testis can also be located ectopically—for example, in a superficial pouch near the external ring, or less commonly, in the suprapubic, perineal, or femoral areas.

Cryptorchidism left untreated results in various complications, including testicular underdevelopment, infertility, malignancy, hernia, torsion, and traumatic injury. Regarding infertility, germ cell depletion increases after 15 months of age, and further degenerative changes, such as Leydig cell atrophy, hypotrophy of the seminiferous tubules, and peritubular fibrosis develop over time. These histologic abnormalities are worse in testicles located more proximally. The incidence of malignancy (usually a seminoma or a nonseminomatous germ cell tumor) is increased four- to sevenfold compared with men who have normally descended testes. An undescended testicle located in the inguinal region is more likely to be injured from trauma. Testicular torsion occurs more often in cryptorchid testes. Finally, approximately 90% of undescended testicles are associated with a patent processus vaginalis, increasing the possibility that a hernia will develop.

Early referral to a urologist is warranted for all patients with undescended testes. Laparoscopy is the preferred way to locate a nonpalpable testis or to identify a missing or malformed testis. Although specific clinical scenarios may require the use of ultrasound prior to laparoscopy, ultrasound identification of the "missing" testis is not highly sensitive. Orchiopexy (laparoscopic and/or surgical) is the translocation of the testis, spermatic cord, and vascular structures into the scrotum with ligation of a patent processus vaginalis, and is generally performed around 1 year of age, although some urologists recommend earlier treatment. Although it was hoped that earlier orchiopexy would decrease the incidence of malignancy and/or facilitate earlier diagnosis, this remains unclear. In certain cases, early orchiopexy may improve the chances for fertility. Hormonal therapy (e.g., human chorionic gonadotropin, luteinizing hormone-releasing hormone) to promote testicular descent may benefit a few select cases, however, cannot overcome anatomic alterations of the inguinal canal which prevent descent.

Finally, a traumatically dislocated testicle may be discovered in the inguinal. Testicular dislocation occurs primarily in the older adolescent and young adult but is rare even then. It usually follows major trauma—for example, a deceleration straddle injury in a motorcyclist. Often an associated injury, such as a pelvis or femur fracture, is found. Despite swelling, ecchymosis, and tenderness, the scrotum feels empty. As mentioned, sometimes the testis is palpated in an abnormal location, most often in the inguinal in the superficial pouch anterior to the external oblique aponeurosis. Occasionally, the testis can be manually reduced, but if this is unsuccessful, surgery is necessary (see Chapter 127 Genitourinary Emergencies).

EVALUATION AND DECISION

In evaluating an inguinal mass, one needs to consider age and gender of the child, presence or absence of pain, location of the testis (in males), response to attempted reduction, history of trauma, and findings of local infection.

In males, testicular pain often heralds a potentially emergent condition. Begin the evaluation by carefully palpating the scrotum. An empty scrotum may point to a dislocated testis after trauma or spontaneous torsion of an undescended testis, diagnoses that can be ruled out with palpable, bilateral descended testes. An isolated, painful inguinal mass may also be an incarcerated or strangulated inguinal hernia, an emergent condition which must be evaluated in both male and female patients. This is particularly important to consider in females with a painful inguinal mass since the presence of an ovary within a hernia sac places it at risk for torsion. The ability to reduce the mass with gentle pressure confirms this diagnosis, but failure to reduce the mass cannot rule it out and may even suggest an incarcerated or strangulated hernia warranting surgical consultation. When a painless mass is irreducible, an acutely incarcerated hernia that has not yet become painful (particularly involving an ovary) is a possible cause, but a painless, irreducible mass may also be an enlarged lymph node. Reduction can be attempted for painless masses to help both diagnose and treat the underlying pathology. In general, painless inguinal masses are usually not urgent. The finding of penile or vaginal lesions, such as those of herpes or syphilis, evidence of soft tissue infection localized to the perineum, or insect bites, eczema, or infected wounds on the legs or lower abdomen, may identify the source of inguinal adenopathy or adenitis.

With equivocal physical findings, ancillary tests may be helpful to establish the diagnosis. Laboratory tests should be used judiciously and on a case-by-case basis; for example, complete blood count and CRP can help differentiate between infectious and oncologic processes and reflect severity of illness. Various microbiologic assays may be used to make definitive diagnoses and direct treatment. Ultrasonography can also be useful when the physical examination is indeterminate and is considered the imaging modality of choice for suspected inguinal abnormalities. Sonographic images can identify evidence of soft tissue infectious changes (i.e., cellulitis) as distinct from drainable fluid collections (i.e., abscess). Ultrasound can differentiate between such fluid collections and lymph nodes, which is important in planning procedures or consultation with surgical specialists. This modality can also characterize tumors and identify hernias. Bedside ultrasound may be useful for directing procedures and to locate important neighboring structures (i.e., blood vessels) (Fig. 29.2).

Suggested Readings and Key References

Lymphadenopathy and Lymphadenitis

Hammerschlag MR, Rawstron SA. Sexually transmitted infections. In: Jenson H, Baltimore RS, eds. *Pediatric infectious diseases: principles and practice.* Philadelphia, PA: WB Saunders, 2002:1009.

Pickering L, ed. *Red book: 2006 report of the Committee on Infectious Diseases.* 27th ed. Elk Grove Village, IL: American Academy of Pediatrics, 2006.

Tunnessen WW Jr. Lymphadenopathy. In: Roberts KR, ed. *Signs and symptoms in pediatrics.* Philadelphia, PA: JB Lippincott, 1999:63.

Twist CJ, Link MP. Assessment of lymphadenopathy in children. *Pediatr Clin North Am* 2002;49:1009.

Hernias

Aiken JJ, Oldham KT. Inguinal hernias. In: Kliegman RM, Behrman R, Jenson HB, et al., eds. *Nelson's textbook of pediatrics.* Philadelphia, PA: Saunders Elsevier, 2007:1644.

Fitch MT, Manthey DE. Abdominal hernia reduction. In: Custalow C, Chanmugam A, Chudnofsky CR, et al., eds. *Roberts and Hedges clinical procedures in emergency medicine,* 5th ed. Philadelphia, PA: Saunders Elsevier, 2010:790.

Retractile, Undescended, and Ectopic Testicle

Esposito C, Caldamone AC, Settimi A, et al. Management of boys with nonpalpable undescended testis. *Nat Clin Pract Urol* 2008;5:252–260. Available at http://www.nature.com/clinicalpractice/uro

Husmann DA. Cryptorchidism. In: Belman B, King L, Kramer S, eds. *Clinical pediatric urology.* London: Martin Dunitz, 2002:1125.

Hutson JM, Clarke MC. Current management of the undescended testicle. *Semin Pediatr Surg* 2007;16:64.

Petterson A, Richiardi L, Nordenskjold A, et al. Age at surgery for undescended testis and risk of testicular cancer. *N Engl J Med* 2008; 356:18.

Tasian GE, Copp HL, Baskin LS. Diagnostic imaging in cryptorchidism: utility, indications, and effectiveness. *J Ped Surg* 2011;46: 2406–2413.

Yang DM, Kim HC, Lim JW, et al. Sonographic finding of groin masses. *J Ultrasound Med* 2007;26:605–614.

Scrotal Trauma

Chang KJ, Sheu JW, Chang TH, et al. Traumatic dislocation of the testes. *Am J Emerg Med* 2003;21:247.

CHAPTER 30 ■ HEARING LOSS

ROBERT J. VINCI, MD

Hearing loss during early childhood may compromise the ability to attain normal language. Therefore, early recognition of hearing loss, with appropriate evaluation and treatment, is crucial to avoid cognitive impairment, which may negatively impact school performance, socialization, and emotional development.

Acute hearing loss is of two main types: conductive and sensorineural. Conductive hearing loss is caused by abnormal transmission of sound waves to the inner ear, whereas sensorineural hearing loss is caused by defective processing of sound waves (Table 30.1). Etiologies may be congenital or acquired. Hearing loss can occur as an isolated symptom or in association with auditory or central nervous system (CNS) dysfunction. The emergency physician must identify the etiology of hearing loss, especially those disorders that are associated with serious systemic disease.

PATHOPHYSIOLOGY

Normal hearing is dependent on an intricate series of properly aligned anatomic and physiologic connections. The auricle or outer ear is designed to receive sensory transmission, or "sound waves," from the child's environment. When patent, the external ear canal transmits sound waves to the tympanic membrane and vibrations of the membrane produce movement of the middle ear ossicles, which result in the transmission of fluid waves to the inner ear fluid within the cochlea. Here the specialized receptors, hair cells in the spiral organ of Corti, convert this mechanical energy to nerve impulses that are transmitted by the cochlear (acoustic) nerve, the auditory portion of the eighth cranial nerve, to the brain. These nerve impulses are integrated by the brain and transformed into what is perceived as sound. It is important to note that anatomically the acoustic apparatus is closely related to the vestibular system, which is concerned with the proprioceptive senses of posture and equilibrium. Therefore, abnormalities in the inner ear may cause both auditory and vestibular symptoms.

DIFFERENTIAL DIAGNOSIS

Conductive Hearing Loss

In children, conductive hearing loss occurs when there is a decrease in the transmission of sound waves from the external environment to the cochlea or inner ear. Commonly, middle ear effusion (either acute or chronic), impacted cerumen, foreign body of the external ear canal, and infections of the external ear canal (otitis externa) may produce conductive hearing loss. Less commonly, fixation or disruption of the middle ear ossicles may cause conductive hearing loss (Table 30.1). In children with chronic recurrent/otitis media (OM), a cholesteatoma—an epidermal inclusion cyst of the middle ear—may develop and cause a slowly progressive conductive hearing loss. Acute head injury, especially in association with a basilar skull fracture, may produce a conductive hearing loss caused by hemotympanum, rupture of the tympanic membrane, or disruption of the inner ear ossicle. Perforation of the tympanic membrane can occur from a self-inflicted injury from a cleaning device such as a cotton swab. Rarely, the conductive hearing loss may be secondary to congenital malformations of the external or middle ear.

Congenital Sensorineural Hearing Loss

Approximately 1.4 in 1,000 infants are born with congenital hearing loss. Diagnostic possibilities include genetic disorders, chromosomal abnormalities, metabolic and storage diseases, and abnormal development of the auditory apparatus (Table 30.1). Sensorineural hearing loss has been described in more than 70 syndromes, including Waardenburg syndrome (facial dysmorphism, white forelock), Jervell and Lange-Nielsen syndrome (prolonged Q-T syndrome), Usher syndrome (retinitis pigmentosa and sensorineural hearing loss) as well as the chromosomal disorders caused by trisomies (especially trisomies 13 to 15, 18, and 21). Many of these patients are diagnosed because of anatomic features associated with each of these disorders, although the hearing loss that occurs may be present at birth or may develop over time. Overall, one-third of patients with congenital hearing loss have associated clinical symptoms of a known syndrome. Recent advances in genetic testing have begun to elucidate gene abnormalities in patients with nonsyndromic hearing loss.

Acquired Sensorineural Hearing Loss

Although acquired sensorineural hearing loss occurs less commonly than congenital sensorineural hearing loss, the absence of associated symptoms may make it a more difficult diagnosis. An array of clinical problems can produce sensorineural hearing loss during childhood.

Acute Infection

Bacterial meningitis is the most common cause of acquired sensorineural hearing loss. Reported in 10% to 20% of patients with meningitis, the hearing loss is usually profound and often bilateral. The hearing loss associated with meningitis is organism specific and most commonly associated with *Streptococcus pneumoniae* but was also associated with infections caused by *Haemophilus influenzae* and *Neisseria meningitidis*. Vaccine programs that have led to a decrease in the

TABLE 30.1

DIFFERENTIAL DIAGNOSIS OF HEARING LOSS

I. Conductive hearing loss
- A. Congenital or neonatal
  1. Malformation of the auricle or external ear canal
  2. Atresia of the ossicle chain
- B. Acquired
  1. Middle ear effusion (acute or chronic)
  2. Impacted cerumen
  3. Foreign body of external ear canal
  4. Otitis externa
  5. Ossicle dysfunction (fixation)
  6. Cholesteatoma
  7. Acute trauma
     - a. Hemotympanum
     - b. Rupture of the tympanic membrane
     - c. Disruption of the ossicles

II. Sensorineural hearing loss
- A. Congenital or neonatal
  1. Anatomic abnormalities
     - a. Aplasia of the inner ear (Michel aplasia)
     - b. Abnormal cochlear development
  2. Syndromes (more than 70 described with hearing loss)
     - a. Waardenburg syndrome
     - b. Jervell and Lange-Nielsen syndrome (prolonged Q-T syndrome)
     - c. Usher syndrome
     - d. Alport syndrome
  3. Chromosomal abnormalities
     - a. Trisomy 13–15
     - b. Trisomy 18
     - c. Trisomy 21
  4. Infections
     - a. TORCH
     - b. Congenital syphilis
  5. Metabolic
     - a. Hypothyroidism
     - b. Storage disorders
  6. Neonatal
     - a. Birth asphyxia
     - b. Kernicterus
     - c. Use of ototoxic drugs
     - d. Extreme prematurity
- B. Acquired
  1. Infection
     - a. Bacterial meningitis
     - b. Viral labyrinthitis
     - c. Acute otitis media
  2. Vascular insufficiency
     - a. Sickle cell disease
     - b. Diabetes mellitus
     - c. Polycythemia
  3. Trauma
     - a. Temporal bone fracture
     - b. Noise-induced injury
     - c. Barotrauma, perilymphatic fistula
     - d. Lightning
  4. Tumor
     - a. Acoustic neuroma
     - b. CNS tumors
     - c. Leukemic infiltrates
     - d. Neurofibromatosis
  5. Autoimmune disease
  6. Functional hearing loss
  7. Miscellaneous
     - a. Kawasaki disease
     - b. Hypothyroidism
     - c. Hypoparathyroidism
     - d. Ototoxic drugs (e.g., gentamicin)
  8. Idiopathic

TORCH, toxoplasmosis, other (infections), rubella, cytomegalovirus (infection), and herpes (simplex); CNS, central nervous system.

incidence of these bacterial pathogens have been instrumental in decreasing the occurrence of this complication. For patients with acute bacterial meningitis, adjunctive therapy with dexamethasone may decrease the incidence of neurologic sequelae, including hearing loss.

Congenital infection caused by cytomegalovirus (CMV) is the most common intrauterine infection that produces sensorineural hearing loss. Congenital infection from rubella, syphilis, toxoplasmosis and perinatally acquired herpes simplex infections are also associated with acquired sensorineural hearing loss. The hearing loss associated with these infections may occur in infants without other manifestations of congenital infection, and may not develop until early childhood. Thus, many experts advocate for universal newborn hearing screening and regular monitoring of children with known congenital infections or high-risk infants such as neonatal intensive care unit patients.

Viral infections of the labyrinth caused by mumps, parainfluenza, adenovirus, herpes simplex, CMV, and rubeola have been described and confirmed by serologic studies. Labyrinthitis usually has symptoms related to inflammation of the inner ear and involvement of the vestibular apparatus, and patients may complain of vomiting, tinnitus, and vertigo.

Vascular Insufficiency

Sudden hearing loss caused by vascular insufficiency has been described in the pediatric patient. Vascular insufficiency may compromise blood flow to the cochlea, producing a hypoxic insult to the sensitive nerve cells in the organ of Corti. Once injured, these nerve cells may not regenerate and profound sensorineural hearing loss can develop. In children, sickle cell disease, long-standing diabetes mellitus, and hyperviscosity states associated with polycythemia can compromise cochlear blood flow and produce sudden hearing loss.

Perilymphatic Fistula

Anatomic defects in the bony or membranous enclosure of the perilymphatic space may produce a perilymphatic fistula and result in an anomalous communication between the middle and inner ear compartment and lead to acute sensorineural hearing loss. A perilymphatic fistula can occur at any age and symptoms may include tinnitus, vertigo, dizziness, and nystagmus. Antecedent trauma usually underlies the development of a fistula, and may include vigorous exercise or changes in barometric pressure associated with airplane travel or scuba diving. Although unilateral hearing loss is most common, bilateral hearing deficits have been described. Occasionally, a perilymphatic fistula will develop in a child with previously abnormal hearing. Therefore, this diagnosis needs to be considered in any patient who has sudden onset of hearing loss, fluctuation in hearing, or complaints of progressive hearing loss, regardless of baseline hearing function. Patients with a perilymphatic fistula generally have a normal otoscopic examination. If a tympanogram is performed, middle ear effusion is usually absent. Emergent referral to an otolaryngologist is warranted because surgery may be required for closure of the anatomic defect.

Head Trauma

Both the vestibular and cochlear nerves can be injured with fractures of the temporal bone. Assessment of audiologic function should be considered in any child with major head trauma; computed tomography (CT) or magnetic resonance imaging (MRI) scan may be required to diagnose these injuries.

Acoustic Trauma

Immediate, severe, and permanent hearing loss can follow even a short period of exposure to sound greater than 120 dB. Exposure to sounds in the 80- to 100-dB range can produce hearing loss with chronic exposure and is most commonly diagnosed in adolescents. Rock concerts, stereo headphones, machinery, and explosive devices are capable of producing sound at the intensity required to produce this condition.

Chronic/Recurrent Otitis Media

A history of chronic/recurrent OM may predispose patients to the development of sensorineural hearing loss as a result of inflammatory changes in the inner ear. Because middle ear effusions produce a conductive hearing loss, the clinician must be aware of the possibility of OM producing a mixed picture.

Functional Hearing Loss

Functional hearing loss may occur in patients who have a psychological component to their presentation. Most commonly occurring during adolescence, functional hearing loss should be considered in patients who present with other manifestations of psychiatric illness. Often, these patients will have a normal physical examination and inconsistent findings with bedside hearing tests.

Miscellaneous

Acoustic neuroma, CNS tumors, and leukemic infiltrates are also associated with sensorineural hearing loss. Other considerations in pediatric patients include Kawasaki disease, hypothyroidism, lightning injury, hyperlipidemia, and hyperbilirubinemia, or the use of ototoxic drugs in the neonatal period. Finally, some children will have no demonstrable cause for their hearing loss.

TABLE 30.2

COMMON CAUSES OF ACUTE HEARING LOSS

Conductive hearing loss	Sensorineural hearing loss
Middle ear effusion	TORCH infections
Impacted cerumen	Birth asphyxia
Foreign body of external ear canal	Viral labyrinthitis
	Bacterial meningitis
	Perilymphatic fistula
	Trauma
	Acoustic neuroma

TORCH, toxoplasmosis, other (infections), rubella, cytomegalovirus (infection), and herpes (simplex).

EVALUATION AND DECISION

Any complaint of hearing loss requires prompt evaluation. Common causes of acute hearing loss are listed in Table 30.2. Life-threatening causes of acute hearing loss are rare in pediatric patients (Table 30.3). The initial step is to confirm the presence of acute hearing loss (Fig. 30.1). Although sophisticated hearing tests are best performed by an audiologist, the emergency physician should attempt bedside testing of gross hearing function. In young children, behavioral responses to loud stimuli can be assessed by delivering an auditory stimulus (e.g., vigorous hand clapping or ringing a bell) to the child. Eye blinking or turning toward the stimulus represents a positive response and suggests some degree of intact hearing. In older children or adolescents, hearing can be assessed by asking the patient if they hear a low-intensity sound such as a soft whisper or fingers rubbing together. Because hearing dysfunction can be subtle and can occur over the entire range of auditory frequencies, these bedside tests may underestimate the degree of hearing impairment. Therefore, an abnormal test should be considered a confirmation of hearing impairment; a negative test needs to be interpreted in the context of the chief complaint of the patient. If the history remains strongly suggestive of hearing loss, the physician should assume some degree of hearing loss despite the results of bedside testing, and formal audiology follow-up is required.

Critical elements of the medical history should include the onset of the hearing loss and the duration of symptoms. Family history of hearing loss may suggest the diagnosis of a genetic disorder with delayed presentation. A history of birth

TABLE 30.3

LIFE-THREATENING CAUSES OF ACUTE HEARING LOSS

Acute head injury
Brain tumor
Leukemic infiltrate
Vascular insufficiency

SIGNS AND SYMPTOMS

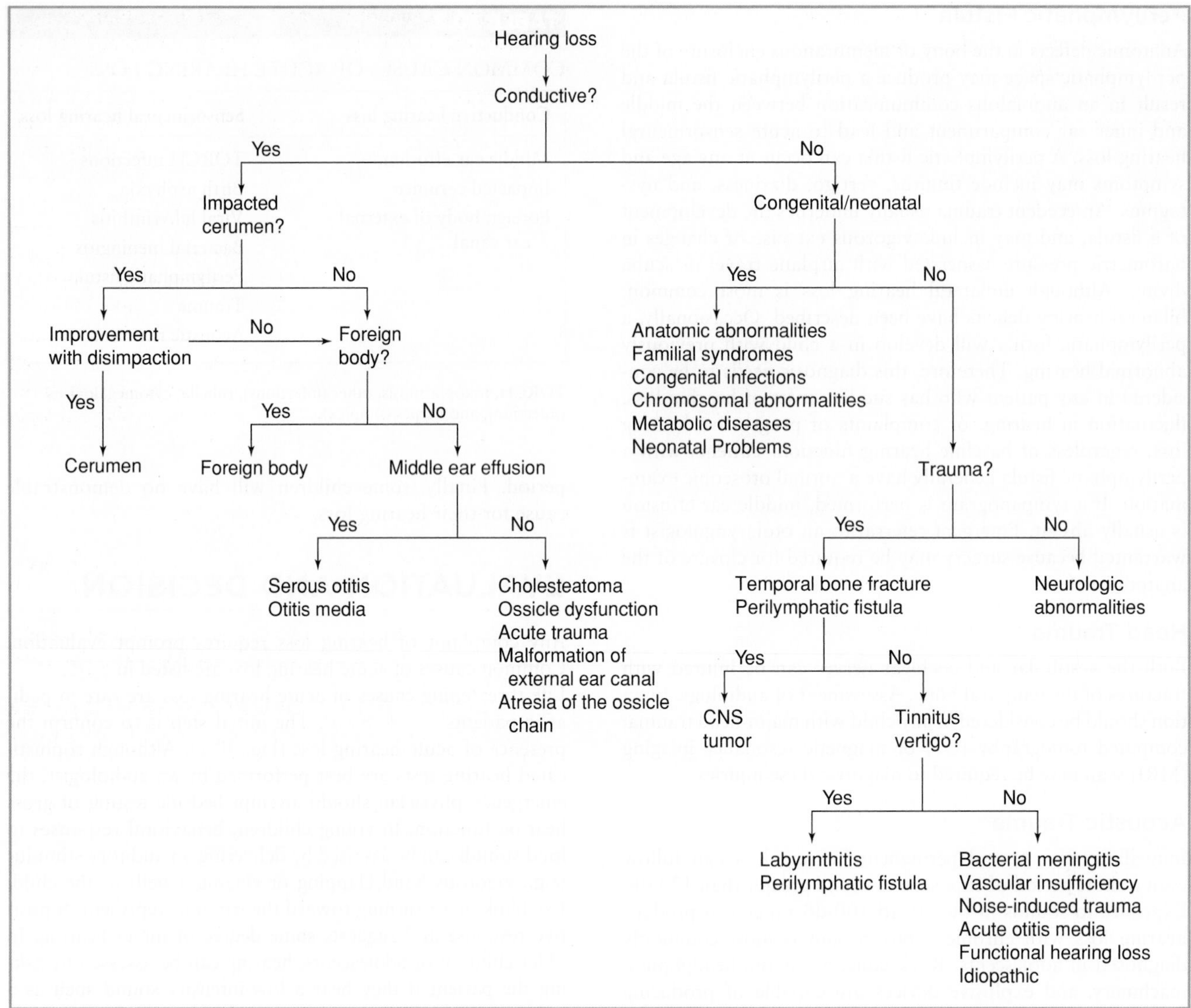

FIGURE 30.1 Evaluation of hearing loss.

asphyxia, prematurity, hyperbilirubinemia, or maternal infection points to a neonatal cause. A more recent history of head trauma or barotrauma (e.g., scuba diving) may suggest the diagnosis of perilymphatic fistula. Fever and otalgia suggest a diagnosis of acute OM. Associated neurologic symptoms such as tinnitus, vertigo, and dizziness suggest inner ear disease or CNS involvement. Headache can be a marker for tumor of the CNS or extension of middle ear infection (Fig. 30.1).

On physical examination, the presence of fever may suggest an infection such as OM or viral labyrinthitis. A detailed otoscopic examination to detect the presence of a middle ear effusion, impacted cerumen or evidence of an external ear infection, perforated tympanic membrane, foreign body, or other abnormality of the tympanic membrane is a priority. Tympanometry can be used to supplement the physical examination, especially if the otoscopic examination suggests the presence of middle ear disease. A careful neurologic examination is required and must include evaluation of vestibular function and the presence of nystagmus.

Once hearing loss is established, the next step is to differentiate conductive from sensorineural hearing loss with the use of tuning fork tests (Fig. 30.1). Conductive hearing loss can be confirmed by the Weber test. In the Weber test, a vibrating, 512-Hz tuning fork is placed in the midline of the patient's forehead. Patients with hearing loss will report that the vibrations of the tuning fork lateralize to the side with the conductive hearing loss (vibrations are felt better in the bad ear) or away from the side with the sensorineural hearing loss (vibrations are felt better in the good ear). For the Rinne test, the vibrating tuning fork is placed against the mastoid process. When the patient signals that the vibration has ceased, the tuning fork is placed adjacent to that ear to determine whether the patient can hear the sound of the still-vibrating tuning fork. Patients with conductive hearing loss will not be able to hear the tuning fork. This is a negative Rinne test (bone conduction greater than air conduction). Sensorineural hearing loss shows up as a positive Rinne test (air conduction greater than bone conduction). Finally, a test by confrontation is performed by placing a tuning fork at a point equidistant from both ears. Regardless of the type of hearing loss, the patient will report the sound to be higher on the side with normal hearing.

Laboratory evaluation is seldom necessary in the ED; when needed, it should focus on a diagnosis that may be contemplated after obtaining a detailed history and physical examination. Complete blood cell (CBC) count and peripheral blood smear, renal function tests, serologic tests for syphilis, TORCH titers, and bacteriologic cultures should be performed only if the history and physical examination suggest an associated diagnosis. Thyroid function tests, lipid profile, and serum calcium levels should be individualized in the context of clinical findings. Referral for genetic testing may be indicated for children with congenital sensorineural hearing loss.

In children with the clinical suspicion of intracranial pathology, a radiologic evaluation assists in the diagnosis. Patients with known or suspected congenital malformation of the middle and inner ears should be evaluated with a CT scan because bony detail is essential for diagnosis. Inner ear abnormalities have been demonstrated in 8% to 20% of patients with sensorineural hearing loss. A CT scan should also be performed in patients with suspected fracture of the temporal bone. MRI is indicated for the accurate diagnosis of an acoustic neuroma or for any patient with suspected retrocochlear pathology.

Most children with decreased hearing in the ED have a conductive hearing loss. If impacted cerumen is seen on examination, it must be removed because it may be the cause of the decreased hearing and prevents further otoscopic evaluation. Children whose hearing improves after disimpaction and who have a normal otoscopic examination need no further treatment. Patients without impacted cerumen and those who fail to improve after removal of cerumen may have a foreign body in the ear canal. Only large objects that completely obstruct the external auditory canal should impair hearing; thus, this diagnosis is easily established during otoscopic examination.

The next step in the evaluation is a careful examination of the tympanic membrane, including pneumatic otoscopy. Many patients will show evidence of a middle ear effusion, the most common cause of hearing loss seen in the ED. Rarely, a cholesteatoma may be seen through the translucent tympanic membrane. Sensorineural hearing loss is seen less often in the ED. In patients with acquired sensorineural hearing loss, a history of significant trauma may suggest the diagnosis of temporal bone fracture or a perilymphatic fistula. If there is no preceding trauma, a careful neurologic examination should be performed, looking for evidence of CNS tumors. The most common cause of acquired sensorineural hearing loss seen in children in the ED without a history of trauma is viral labyrinthitis. These patients usually have associated tinnitus, vertigo, and vomiting but no focal neurologic abnormalities. Most of the remaining causes of hearing loss are idiopathic. Vascular insufficiency merits consideration in children with sickle cell anemia, diabetes mellitus, and collagen vascular disease. If the cause of the hearing loss remains uncertain, otolaryngologic consult and evaluation should be considered.

Suggested Readings and Key References

Brouwer MC, McIntyre P, Prasad K, et al. Corticosteroids for acute bacterial meningitis. *Cochrane Database Syst Rev* 2013;(Issue 6): CD004405.

Kutz JW, Simon LM, Chennupati SK, et al. Clinical predictors for hearing loss in children with bacterial meningitis. *Arch Otolaryngol Head Neck Surg* 2006;132(9):941–945.

Mafong DD, Shin EJ, Lalwani AK. Use of laboratory evaluation and radiologic imaging in the diagnostic evaluation of children with sensorineural hearing loss. *Laryngoscope* 2002;112(1):1–7.

Simons JP, Mandell DL, Arjmand EM. Computed tomography and magnetic resonance imaging in pediatric unilateral and asymmetric sensorineural hearing loss. *Arch Otolaryngol Head Neck Surg* 2006;132(2):186–192.

Tarshish Y, Leschinski A, Kenna M. Pediatric sudden sensorineural hearing loss: diagnosed causes and response to intervention. *Int J Pediatr Otorhinolaryngol* 2013;77(4):53–59.

CHAPTER 31 ■ HEART MURMURS

LILA O'MAHONY, MD, FAAP

A heart murmur is the audible vibration of turbulent blood flow through the cardiovascular system. It can be normal or abnormal, congenital or acquired and upward of 90% of children will have an audible murmur at some point in their life. Fortunately, the vast majority of murmurs have no clinical significance and less than 1% is due to congenital heart defects (CHDs). Murmurs without clinical significance are referred to as "normal," "flow," "functional," or "innocent"; whereas, abnormal murmurs, commonly referred to as "pathologic," are clinically significant, often associated with structural heart defects and/or dysfunction and can lead to acute cardiopulmonary compromise (Table 31.1). A wide variety of cardiac and extracardiac conditions can be associated with heart murmurs (Table 31.2).

When evaluating a newly identified murmur in the emergency department (ED), the primary objective is not to diagnose a cardiac lesion, but to determine whether the murmur is clinically significant and if so, whether the murmur indicates that the child has significant heart disease that requires intervention or consultation by a pediatric cardiologist.

DIFFERENTIAL DIAGNOSIS

History

Unless the patient is in extremis, a focused history is always the starting place and the examiner should include questions related to cardiac disease or dysfunction.

- Infant specific
  - History of abnormal in utero ultrasound findings?
  - Significant prenatal and maternal history? (Advanced maternal age, maternal diabetes, intrauterine alcohol and drug/medication exposure as well as intrauterine infections are all associated with increased risk of CHD)
  - Easily fatigues, sweats, difficulty breathing, or skin color changes with feeding?
  - History of poor growth?
- Child >1 year
  - Tires easily when playing? Daily activities limited by fatigue or breathing difficulties? Does the child squat after walking? Climb stairs? Have cyanotic "spells"?
- All patients
  - Has the murmur been identified previously? What were the findings?
  - Is there a history of cardiac surgery?
  - Recent illness, sore throat, upper respiratory infection, or fevers?
  - Weight gain or loss? Edema? Hypertension? Chest pain? Syncope? Joint symptoms?
  - Family history of sudden death in children, congenital malformations, or heart disease/defects in children?

Examination

The evaluation should consist of a complete physical examination with special attention to the cardiovascular system and associated signs of cardiac dysfunction or compromise.

General Assessment

First, determine the cardiopulmonary stability of the patient following Pediatric Advanced Life Support guidelines (see Chapter 4 Cardiopulmonary Resuscitation). Specific attention should be paid to the child's skin color, presence or absence of cyanosis, mental status, work of breathing, and perfusion. Vital signs should be obtained including heart rate, blood pressure, respiratory rate, temperature, and oxygen saturation by pulse oximetry. Vital sign abnormalities may be the first indication for further and/or emergent cardiopulmonary evaluation. For example, lower extremity blood pressures are normally measured 10 to 40 mm Hg higher than upper pressures and an elevated systolic blood pressure in the upper compared to the lower extremities may indicate a coarctation or obstruction of the aorta; hyperthermia may be associated with infectious etiologies or contribute to high blood flow state contributing to nonpathologic flow murmur whereas hypothermia may be associated with cardiogenic shock. Finally, oxygen desaturation that does not improve with supplemental oxygen may indicate cardiac pathology, and it has been shown that in the neonatal period pulse oximetry screening increases the detection of life-threatening CHD. Finally, infants and children with pre-existing or congenital heart disease may have abnormal oxygen saturations. Always ask their caregiver or parent what is normal for their child.

Precordial Examination

Inspect for left- or right-sided chest bulge which could indicate cardiac hypertrophy or dilation, palpate for thrills and clicks and points of maximal impulse, listen carefully for the heart sounds and adventitial sounds. If present, the third and fourth sounds, opening snaps, valve-associated clicks, pericardial rub, and unusual rhythms can be confused for murmurs and therefore are possible confounding factors in the precordial evaluation.

Murmur Characteristics

The range of characteristics will be briefly defined here:

- *Timing and duration:* Is the murmur systolic, diastolic, or continuous? Early, mid, late, or throughout (holosystolic) the specific cardiac cycle?
- *Intensity (loudness):* Graded from barely audible (grade I) to accompanied by a palpable thrill (grade IV) to audible with stethoscope off the chest (grade VI).
- *Shape:* Describes the murmur's change in intensity over the cardiac cycle. Common terms used to characterize these volume flow patterns are plateau (constant intensity),

TABLE 31.1

CHARACTERISTICS USUALLY ASSOCIATED WITH A MURMUR

	Normal	Pathologic
Timing	Midsystole	Diastole, continuous
Intensity	Grades I through III, varies with position	Grades III and above
Location of maximal intensity	Left sternal border	Variable
Radiation	Possibly faint to the precordium and neck, but rarely the back	Variable to carotids, axilla, or back
Quality	"Twangy" or "vibratory"	Harsh
Heart sounds	Readily definable, including splitting of S_2	Variable, may be obscured

crescendo, decrescendo, and crescendo–decrescendo (diamond shaped).

- *Quality:* Common terms used are musical, blowing, rumbling, harsh, vibratory, twang, soft, rough, grating, and click.
- *Pitch:* Described qualitatively as low (associated with low pressure gradient), medium, or high (associated with high pressure gradient).
- *Location and radiation:* Location is the point of maximum intensity (upper, lower, middle left, or right sternal margin; apex; midclavicular or axillary line). Radiation refers to the area of maximal sound transmission (back, neck, axilla, or throughout entire precordium).

Variation with maneuvers: An innocent murmur's intensity often changes significantly with change in position, such as from supine to sitting or vice versa. Two important exceptions are hypertrophic cardiomyopathy (HCM) and mitral valve prolapse (MVP), both of which have intensity changes based on position and are both pathologic.

Associated Signs and Symptoms

Skin Color. Central cyanosis (see Chapters 16 Cyanosis and 107 Pulmonary Emergencies) is diffuse and is best differentiated from peripheral cyanosis by involvement of the

TABLE 31.2

CONDITIONS THAT MAY BE ASSOCIATED WITH PRESENCE OF A CARDIAC MURMUR[a]

I. Infancy
- A. Cardiac
  - 1. Noncyanotic
    - a. Normal/innocent murmur
    - b. Congenital defects
      - (1) Patent ductus arteriosus
      - (2) Atrial septal defect
      - (3) Ventricular septal defect
      - (4) Aortic stenosis
      - (5) Coarctation of aorta
      - (6) Pulmonary stenosis
      - (7) Partial anomalous pulmonary venous drainage
    - c. Myocarditis
    - d. Primary myocardial disease
  - 2. Cyanotic
    - a. Congenital defects
      - (1) Tetralogy of Fallot
      - (2) Transposition of the great vessels
      - (3) Truncus arteriosus
      - (4) Pulmonary atresia
      - (5) Severe pulmonary stenosis with patent foramen
      - (6) Tricuspid atresia
      - (7) Ebstein anomaly
      - (8) Total anomalous pulmonary venous drainage
      - (9) Atrioventricular canal defect
      - (10) Hypoplastic left heart
      - (11) Primary pulmonary hypertension
  - 3. Congestive cardiac failure
    - a. Secondary to any of the previous as well as noncardiac causes listed as follows
- B. Extracardiac
  - 1. Severe anemia
  - 2. Arteriovenous malformation
  - 3. Pulmonary insufficiency (including infection, hypoperfusion, pulmonary arterial hypertension)
  - 4. Hyperpyrexia

II. Older child
- A. Cardiac
  - 1. Normal murmur
  - 2. Congenital defect (same list as for infancy—both cyanotic and noncyanotic)
  - 3. Mitral valve prolapse
  - 4. Myocarditis (viral, collagen, toxic, endocrine, genetic)
  - 5. Acute rheumatic fever
  - 6. Healed rheumatic carditis
  - 7. Subacute bacterial endocarditis
  - 8. Congestive cardiac failure (associated with any of previous or following noncardiac diseases)
- B. Extracardiac
  - 1. Severe anemia
  - 2. Arteriovenous malformation
  - 3. Pulmonary insufficiency (with incidental murmur)
  - 4. Thyrotoxicosis
  - 5. Hyperpyrexia

[a]It should be kept in mind that *any* pediatric problem may be coincidentally associated with the presence of a normal cardiac murmur or with one of the other conditions in this table.

tongue. Central cyanosis due to a cardiac lesion may be differentiated from cyanosis due to pulmonary disease by administering 100% oxygen to the child while monitoring pulse oximetry. Those with pulmonary disease may improve their oximetry reading while those with cardiac lesions often will not. In older children, if clubbing of the distal fingers is present; cyanosis is probably chronic and persistent.

Other Skin Findings. Note midline surgical scars, look for petechiae, including in the conjunctivae and under the fingernails. Check for erythema marginatum and subcutaneous nodules. Severe pallor related to marked anemia may be associated with high output cardiac failure.

Potential Signs of Cardiac Failure. (See Chapter 94 Cardiac Emergencies)

- *Edema:* More likely to be dependent and pitting in cardiac disease. In the preambulant child, dependent edema may be best appreciated along the posterior trunk and periorbital areas, rather than the lower extremities.
- *Neck veins:* Notable distention infrequent. Evaluate with the patient lying flat or propped at a 45-degree angle.
- *Respiratory effort:* Tachypnea, grunting, subcostal retractions, tracheal tug, and orthopnea. Listen for crackles and wheeze, usually symmetric compared to primary lung disease which is often asymmetric.
- *Organ enlargement:* Palpate for a soft, engorged liver, particularly the left lobe, which becomes palpable early in right-sided congestive heart failure (CHF). Check for splenomegaly.

Remaining Examination

- *Joints:* Check for tenderness, redness, warmth, and swelling (see Chapter 55 Pain: Joints).
- *Neurologic:* Check cranial nerve function.
- *Nutritional evaluation:* Are the child's height and weight reasonable compared with the parents'? Is the weight percentile significantly different than that for height?

Ancillary Diagnostic Aids

Chest radiographs and electrocardiograms, specifically, are not routinely indicated in the evaluation of a murmur in asymptomatic patients, as they have not been found to add significant diagnostic or clinical information in these patients and may even be misleading. Therefore, they should be ordered selectively if clinical assessment of the child does not allow a satisfactory conclusion regarding the significance of the murmur or in patients who are symptomatic.

Electrocardiography (EKG or ECG). A 12-lead electrocardiogram, using age- and size-appropriate electrodes, should be readily available for screening and evaluation purposes. The emergency physician should be able to assess significant rhythm disturbances, ischemic changes, and gross hypertrophy understanding that normal EKG parameters vary with the age group of the child (see Chapter 94 Cardiac Emergencies).

Chest Radiograph (CXR). Films should be taken in both posteroanterior (PA) and lateral views. The physician should look for gross cardiac enlargement in the PA views, which may be determined in older children by a transverse diameter greater than 50% of the width of the thoracic cage. In infants, the diameter normally may be considerably wider than that ratio. Thymic shadows, scoliosis, rib abnormalities, and less than full inspiration may be confounding factors. The lung fields should be evaluated for infiltrates and for increased or diminished pulmonary vascular flow. Rib notching may be present secondary to long-standing coarctation of the aorta. Familiarity with specific CXR patterns associated with CHD may be helpful.

Echocardiography. Echocardiography is recommended for symptomatic patients with clinical evidence of heart failure or disease and asymptomatic patients with presumed pathologic murmurs and/or abnormal CXR or EKG findings. The echocardiogram allows definitive diagnosis for many congenital cardiac lesions, determination of the severity of cardiac failure, differentiation of myocarditis from pericardial effusion, evaluation of intrathoracic pressure phenomena (tamponade, effusion, tumors), and discovery of coronary artery malpositions or coronary dilatation, as in Kawasaki disease. Pediatric echocardiograms require special expertise to interpret and usually should be obtained in conjunction with pediatric cardiology consultation.

Blood Studies. Screening tests should be obtained based on what is found on the history and physical examination. Studies that might be of value under specific circumstances include a complete blood cell count with differential, erythrocyte sedimentation rate and/or C-reactive protein, arterial blood gas measurements, co-oximetry, blood culture, antistreptolysin titer, sickle cell screening, troponin, brain natriuretic protein (bnp), and antinuclear antibody.

EVALUATION AND DECISION

Neonates and infants (defined herein as <1-year-old) with heart disease present differently than older children. It makes sense to divide murmur evaluations into two patient age groups: from birth to 1 year of age (Fig. 31.1A,B) and older than 1 year of age (Fig. 31.2A,B). Table 31.2 lists conditions that may be associated with cardiac murmurs.

Infants with Cardiac Murmur

Neonates and infants younger than 1 year of age who present with a murmur require extremely careful assessment. This is particularly true in the first weeks of life when the ductus arteriosus closes and ductal-dependent cardiac defects (see Chapter 94 Cardiac Emergencies), often associated with cyanosis, become clinically significant.

Cyanotic Infants

Any infant who has a murmur and appears cyanotic (Fig. 31.1A) should have a thorough physical examination, pulse oximetry, EKG, CXR, and echocardiography following assessment and support of their ABCs.

If the *physical examination is normal,* except for the perceived cyanosis and the murmur, and the *EKG, CXR, and pulse oximetry are normal,* the infant probably has a clinically insignificant murmur and a noncardiac cause of his cyanosis (peripheral acrocyanosis, polycythemia, methemoglobinemia). These patients do not require emergent cardiology consultation.

If an otherwise *well-appearing cyanotic infant has an abnormal EKG, CXR, and diminished oxygen saturation,* the baby probably has cyanotic heart disease. The differential diagnosis for such a patient includes tetralogy of Fallot, transposition of

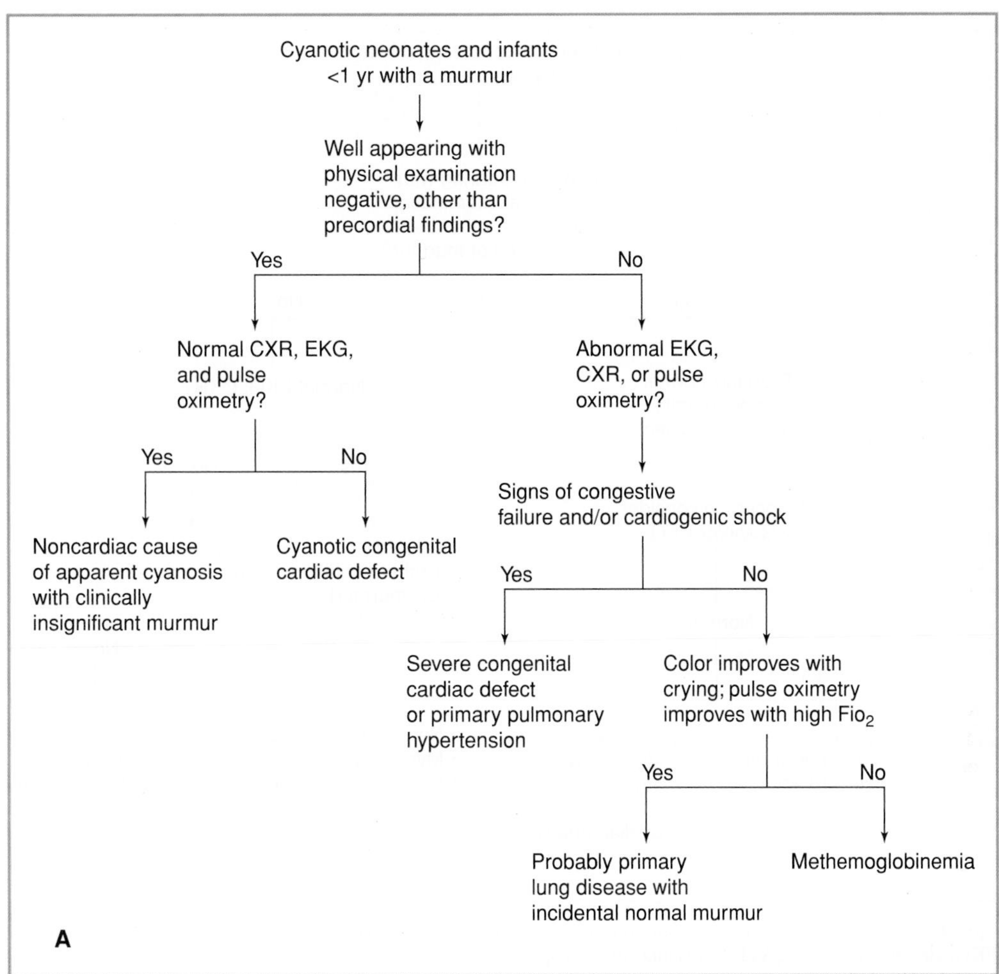

FIGURE 31.1 **A:** Assessment of a cyanotic infant younger than 1 year of age in whom a murmur is heard.

the great vessels with single ventricle, truncus arteriosus, Ebstein anomaly, tricuspid atresia with patent foramen ovale, anomalous pulmonary venous drainage, or moderately severe pulmonary stenosis with right-to-left shunting through an atrial or ventricular septal defect or a patent ductus. Pediatric cardiology consultation should be obtained for all of these patients and neonates admitted to the hospital for evaluation and treatment.

If the *cyanotic infant is ill appearing,* pulse oximetry, CXR, and/or EKG will likely be abnormal. If the findings on examination suggest CHF and/or cardiogenic shock, the infant likely has severe cyanotic congenital heart disease or an extremely severe acyanotic defect with the cyanosis related to poor perfusion and failure. Primary pulmonary hypertension should also be considered and steps initiated toward treatment with either inhaled NO or extracorporeal membrane oxygenation. See Table 31.3 for differential diagnosis of potential cardiac defects. Survival of patients with these severe lesions is dependent on maintaining patency of the ductus arteriosus. Early infusion therapy with prostaglandin E1 (Alprostadil) under carefully controlled monitoring and emergent cardiology consultation is recommended (see Chapter 94 Cardiac Emergencies).

In the older cyanotic infant, additional considerations include large arteriovenous malformation, atrioventricular canal defect, and large ventricular septal defect. These infants should be admitted to the hospital or transferred to a pediatric cardiac center for further evaluation and treatment.

If the evaluation of the *ill-appearing cyanotic infant* does not suggest CHF or shock, and the saturation improves with crying and oxygen, the infant likely has primary lung disease due to infection, hypoperfusion, or pulmonary arteriolar hypertension. These infants should be admitted for further evaluation and treatment with concurrent close monitoring of the murmur. If an infant without cardiac disease presents with persistent low oxygen saturation despite supplemental oxygen, methemoglobinemia should be considered and co-oximetry blood gas studies performed (see Chapter 98 Environmental Emergencies, Radiological Emergencies, Bites and Stings).

Infants Who Are Not Cyanotic

Acyanotic, well-appearing neonates and infants (Fig. 31.1B) with a nonspecific physical examination, except for their murmur, likely have a clinically insignificant murmur that represents a small cardiac defect (small patent ductus, atrial or ventricular septal defect, mild aortic or pulmonary stenosis, partial anomalous pulmonary venous drainage) or a normal flow murmur. These children can be followed by their primary care provider. If uncertainty exists about the clinical significance of the murmur, an EKG and CXR can be obtained. If these studies are normal, then the murmur is likely innocent. Peripheral pulmonary stenosis, related to angulation of the distal pulmonary arteries, is a common cause of normal murmurs in neonates, transmits well to the back and may be loud, but will disappear in time. Consultation with a pediatric cardiologist can be helpful in guiding subsequent evaluation of these babies.

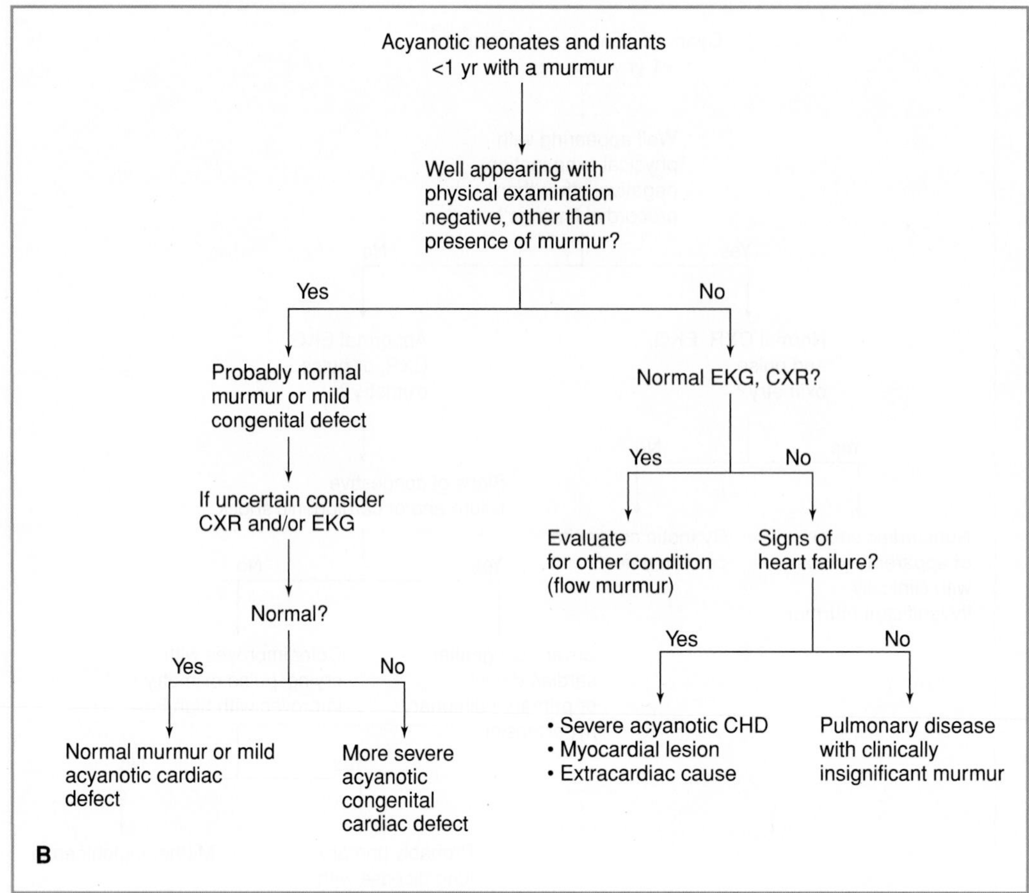

FIGURE 31.1 **B:** Assessment of a noncyanotic infant younger than 1 year of age in whom a murmur is heard. EKG, electrocardiogram; VH, ventricular hypertrophy.

If the *EKG and CXR are abnormal in the acyanotic, well-appearing infant,* a more clinically significant manifestation of the same acyanotic defects, or possibly an acyanotic (or "silent") tetralogy of Fallot, is possible. Consultation with a pediatric cardiologist should ensue.

If the *acyanotic infant with a murmur appears ill,* an EKG and CXR should be obtained. If these are normal, the murmur is likely to be inconsequential, and the infant should be evaluated for an underlying medical or surgical illness. If these studies are *abnormal and/or there are signs of cardiac failure,* emergent cardiac consultation should be obtained with concern for severe acyanotic congenital cardiac defect such as a large ventricular septal defect, large patent ductus, or severe aortic or pulmonary stenosis. In the neonate, and in consultation with a pediatric cardiologist, consider indomethacin or an accepted alternative therapy to close the ductus arteriosus and lessen the left-to-right shunting. Additional considerations include myocarditis, primary myocardial disease, anomalous origin of the left coronary artery, or an extracardiac problem causing high cardiac output (severe anemia, large arteriovenous malformation). All of these infants need hospital admission or transfer to a tertiary pediatric center.

If the *infant appears ill but does not have signs suggestive of cardiac failure,* primary pulmonary disease should be considered. In this case, the murmur is either normal or represents a milder acyanotic defect. Hospital admission for further evaluation and therapy is recommended.

TABLE 31.3

LIFE-THREATENING CARDIAC LESIONS IN THE ILL AND/OR DEEPLY CYANOTIC NEONATE[a]

Hypoplastic left heart
Severe coarctation of the aorta
Critical aortic stenosis
Critical pulmonary stenosis
Pulmonary atresia with intact ventricular septum
Tricuspid atresia with closed foramen

[a]Emergency cardiac consultation should be requested and consideration given to immediate infusion therapy with prostaglandin E1 to ensure patency of the ductus arteriosus.

Children Greater than 1 Year of Age with Murmur

By the time children who live in areas with easy access to medical care reach 1 year of age, most severe congenital lesions have been identified and many have been surgically repaired. Therefore, acquired cardiac and noncardiac etiologies constitute a larger proportion of new murmurs in this age group.

Normal murmurs are by far the most commonly discovered murmurs in an older child.

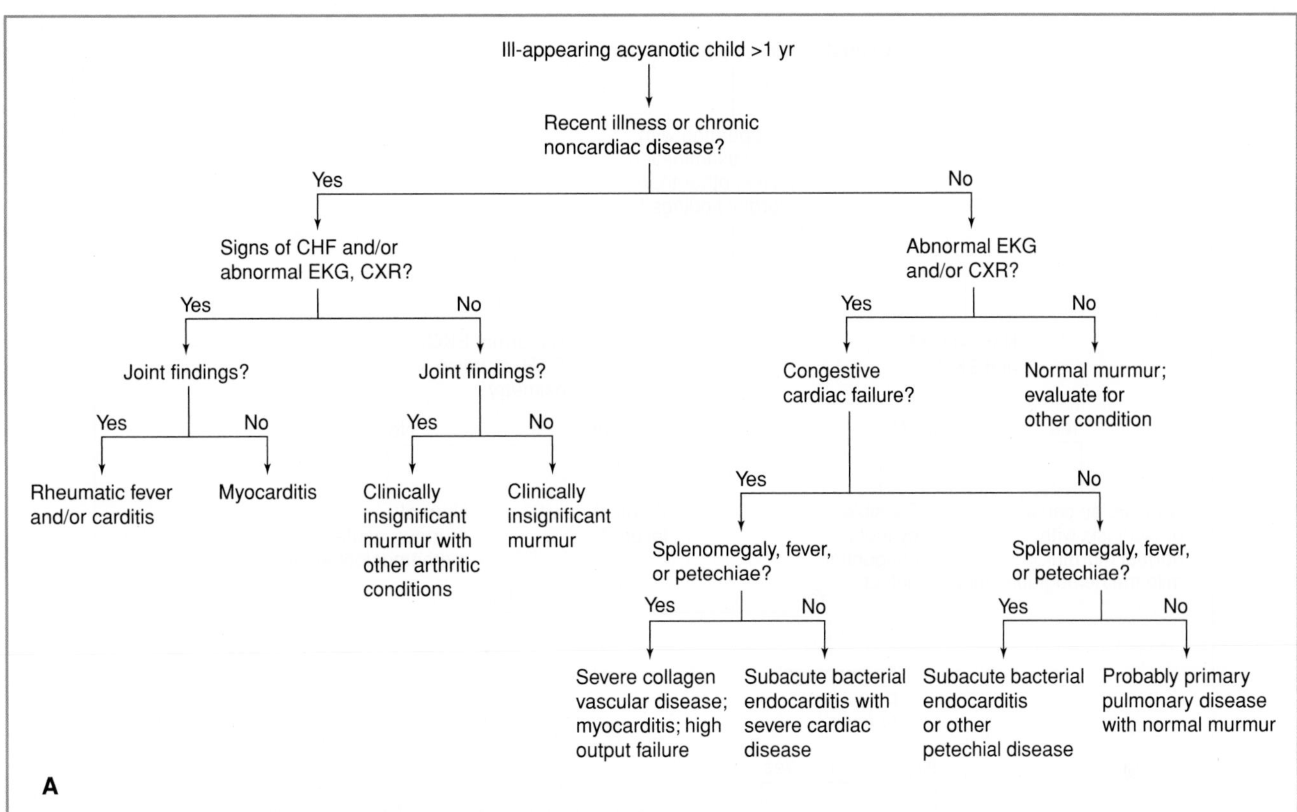

FIGURE 31.2 **A:** Assessment of a noncyanotic, sick child 1 year or older in whom a murmur is heard.

Acyanotic Children Greater than 1 Year of Age

The *acyanotic child with a murmur who appears well* and has an otherwise normal physical examination, most likely has a clinically insignificant murmur, including mild acyanotic cardiac lesions such as small atrial or ventricular septal defects. If the examining provider is satisfied that the murmur is normal or benign, further workup and specialty consultation is not indicated while the child is in the ED. Additional evaluation can be determined by the child's outpatient primary care provider. If uncertainty exists, an EKG and CXR can be ordered. If these are normal, one has further assurance that primary care follow-up is all that is necessary. If these are abnormal, a more severe acyanotic defect is possible and echocardiography should be obtained. Referral should be made to a pediatric cardiologist on a nonemergency basis for further characterization.

If the *acyanotic child appears acutely ill* (Fig. 31.2A), has a history of recent illness, swollen, red, or tender joints, and signs or symptoms of heart failure, acute rheumatic fever should be strongly considered. The child should be hospitalized for evaluation of acute rheumatic fever (see Chapter 94 Cardiac Emergencies) including cardiology consultation and echocardiography. In contrast, the *acyanotic ill-appearing child* with joint findings but without signs of cardiac failure or EKG changes, is more likely to have a normal murmur with a concurrent illness such as septic, reactive or rheumatologic arthritis. These children need diagnostic evaluation of their acute illness but only primary care follow-up for their murmur.

The *ill-appearing acyanotic child* with a murmur and a history of chronic or recent illness, but no joint findings, may have myocarditis or pericarditis. EKG and CXR should be obtained and if abnormal, echocardiography, in consultation with a pediatric cardiologist. These children should be admitted for ongoing monitoring and therapy.

The *ill-appearing acyanotic child* who has a murmur but no chronic or recent illness but who shows signs of CHF, may have severe acyanotic congenital heart disease, myocarditis, or high output failure secondary to severe anemia, large arteriovenous malformation, or thyrotoxicosis (Fig. 31.2A). This child requires further evaluation and admission.

If the *ill-appearing acyanotic child with a murmur has a fever,* he should be examined carefully for splenomegaly and petechiae. If present, infectious endocarditis is of immediate concern and the child should be admitted for antibiotics, pediatric cardiology consultation, and echocardiography (see Chapter 94 Cardiac Emergencies). In addition to infectious endocarditis, consideration must also be given to other conditions characterized by petechiae, such as meningococcemia, idiopathic thrombocytopenic purpura (ITP), rickettsial infection, hemolytic uremic syndrome (HUS), or Henoch–Schönlein Purpura (HSP). Blood cultures and other appropriate labs should be drawn, treatment initiated, and the child admitted for further evaluation and monitoring.

If the *acyanotic ill-appearing child with a murmur is not in failure, has no splenomegaly or petechiae,* and has a normal EKG, the murmur is most likely normal or associated with the high cardiac output of hyperpyrexia or anemia. These children should be evaluated for underlying noncardiac conditions.

Cyanotic Children Greater than 1 Year of Age

As with infants, cyanotic older children (Fig. 31.2B) with heart murmurs should have an EKG, CXR, pulse oximetry, and blood gas after a careful history and complete physical examination. If these are normal, except for the cyanosis and

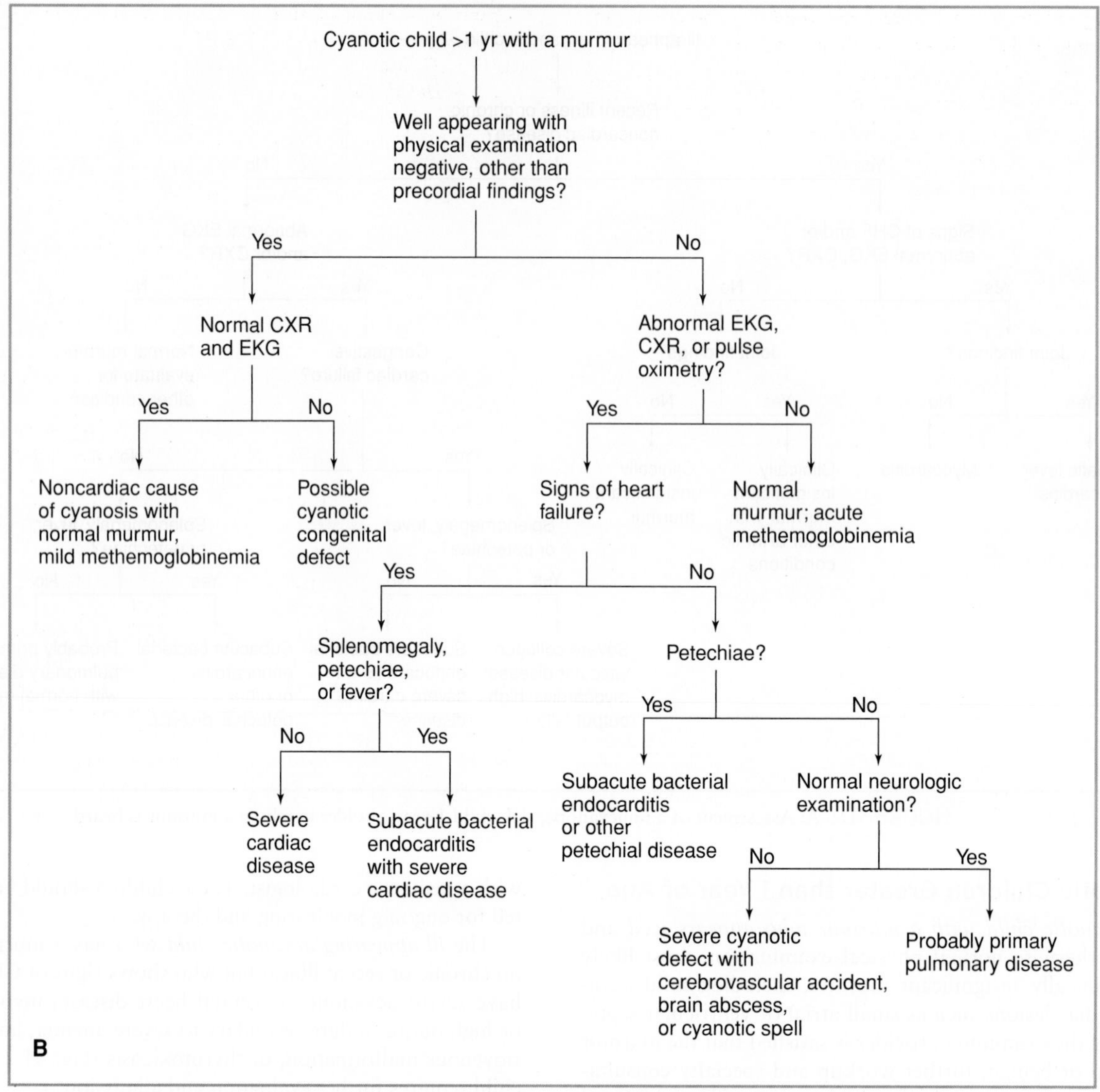

FIGURE 31.2 **B:** Assessment of a cyanotic child 1 year of age or older. EKG, electrocardiogram.

murmur, the child probably does not have cardiac-associated cyanosis. The murmur may be normal or associated with a small acyanotic congenital defect. Entities such as polycythemia and methemoglobinemia should be considered and the primary condition further investigated. If uncertainty exists about a noncardiac etiology once the studies are obtained, an echocardiogram should be performed in consultation with a pediatric cardiologist.

The *cyanotic child who is well appearing* but has an abnormal EKG, CXR, and pulse oximetry likely has cyanotic heart disease that may ultimately require surgical intervention. The child should be referred to a pediatric cardiologist for further evaluation, including echocardiography.

If the *cyanotic child appears acutely ill and has signs of CHF,* severe cardiac disease is present. The etiologies include a congenital cardiac defect with associated progressive cardiac compromise, in which case the cyanosis is intense (Table 31.2), or cardiac failure secondary to acquired disease, in which the cyanosis is related to hypoperfusion and is usually less intense. These children need to be admitted for therapy and further cardiac evaluation.

A careful neurologic examination should be part of the evaluation of every ill child with cyanotic heart disease. If findings are abnormal, complications of hypoxemic "spells," cerebrovascular accident ("stroke"), or, if febrile, brain abscess must be considered.

Regardless of whether there are signs of CHF, in the *cyanotic child with a murmur, if there is fever, splenomegaly, and/or petechiae,* blood cultures should be drawn given the concern for infective endocarditis. If the child is not in failure and petechiae are found, infective endocarditis is still a possibility, but other noncardiac causes of petechial presentations must be considered (meningococcemia, Valsalva maneuvers, HUS, ITP, HSP). Appropriate laboratory studies should be obtained and the child hospitalized.

If the *ill-appearing cyanotic child* has an abnormal CXR but shows significantly improved oxygen saturations with supplemental oxygen, the child most likely has primary pulmonary disease. The murmur may be related to tricuspid regurgitation secondary to the high right ventricular pressure. These children need admission for evaluation and treatment.

In the *cyanotic child* who has a normal EKG and chest film, but abnormal pulse oximetry with normal arterial Po_2, the possibility of acute toxin-induced methemoglobinemia must be considered, with the murmur being clinically insignificant. Co-oximetry blood gas studies should be obtained.

SUMMARY

This chapter provides recommendations for the initial assessment and disposition of infants and children in whom a murmur is discovered in the ED. Although diagnostic pathways have been suggested herein, it has also been shown that definitive diagnosis of the underlying cardiac defect is not the primary aim of ED evaluation, careful assessment of the patient and safe disposition are. The emphasis, in other words, is on the patient and less so on the murmur.

Suggested Readings and Key References

Barrett MJ, Lacey CS, Sekara AE, et al. Mastering cardiac murmurs: the power of repetition. *Chest* 2004;126:470–475.

Biancaniello T. Innocent murmurs. *Circulation* 2005;111:e20–e22.

Bonow RO, Carabello BA, Chatterjee K, et al. 2008 Focused update incorporated into the ACC/AHA 2006 guidelines for the management of patients with valvular heart disease: a report of the American College of Cardiology/American Heart Association Task Force on Practice Guidelines (Writing Committee to Develop Guidelines for the Management of Patients with Valvular Heart Disease). *Circulation* 2008;118:e523–e661.

Etoom Y, Ratnapalan S. Evaluation of children with heart murmurs. *Clin Pediatr* 2014;52(2):111–117.

Fuerst RS. Use of pulse oximetry. In: King C, Henretig FM, eds. *Textbook of pediatric emergency procedures*. 2nd ed. Philadelphia, PA: Wolters Kluwer, 2008:749–754.

Gardiner S. Are routine chest x-ray and ECG examinations helpful in the evaluation of symptomatic heart murmurs? *Arch Dis Child* 2003; 88:638–642.

Gersony WM. Major advances in pediatric cardiology in the 20th century. *J Pediatr* 2001;139(2):328–333.

Gladman G. Management of asymptomatic heart murmurs. *Pediatr Child Health* 2012;23(2):64–68.

Goldmuntz E. The epidemiology and genetics of congenital heart disease. *Clin Perinatol* 2001;28:1–10.

Hoffmann JIE. Cardiology. In: Rudolph CD, Hoffmann JIE, Rudolph AM, eds. *Pediatrics*. 21st ed. New York, NY: McGraw-Hill, 2003: 1780–1842.

Iyer SB. The electrocardiogram in infants and children. In: King C, Henretig FM, eds. *Textbook of pediatric emergency procedures*. 2nd ed. Philadelphia, PA: Wolters Kluwer, 2008:693–703.

Johnson R, Holzer R. Evaluation of asymptomatic heart murmurs. *Curr Paediatr* 2005;15:532–538.

Keane JE, Fyler DK, Lock JF, eds. *Nadas' pediatric cardiology*. 2nd ed. Philadelphia, PA: Elsevier, 2006.

Kwiatkowski D, Wang Y, Cnota J. The utility of outpatient echocardiography for evaluation of asymptomatic murmurs in children. *Congenit Heart Dis* 2012;7:283–288.

Maher K, Reed H, Cuadrado A, et al. B-Type natriuretic peptide in the emergency diagnosis of critical heart disease in children. *Pediatrics* 2008;121:e1484.

Mahle WT, Newburger JW, Matherne GP, et al. Role of pulse oximetry in examining newborns for congenital heart disease: a scientific statement from the AHA and AAP. *Pediatrics* 2009;124:823–836.

Menashe V. Heart murmurs. *Pediatr Rev* 2007;28:e19–e22.

Noponen A, Lukkarinen S, Angerla A, et al. Phono-spectographic analysis of heart murmur in children. *BMC Pediatr* 2007;7:23.

Section on Cardiology and Cardiovascular Surgery; American Academy of Pediatrics. Guidelines for pediatric cardiovascular centers. *Pediatrics* 2002;109(3):544–549.

Shaddy RE, Wernovsky G, eds. *Pediatric heart failure*. London: Taylor & Francis, 2005.

Tanel RE. ECGs in the ED. *Pediatr Emerg Care* 2008;24:586–587.

Thomas RL, Parker GC, Van Overmeire B, et al. A meta-analysis of ibuprofen versus indomethacin for closure of patent ductus arteriosus. *Eur J Pediatr* 2005;164:135–140.

Yi MS, Kimball TR, Tsevat J, et al. Evaluation of heart murmurs in children: cost-effectiveness and practical implications. *J Pediatr* 2002; 141:504–511.

CHAPTER 32 ■ HEMATURIA

ERICA L. LIEBELT, MD, FACMT AND VALERIE DAVIS, MD, PhD

Hematuria, the presence of red blood cells (RBCs) in the urine, is a presenting complaint in the emergency department (ED). The required evaluation for hematuria (either gross or microscopic) in the ED and its urgency is dictated by the patient's history and clinical presentation. Recent literature has demonstrated that isolated gross hematuria in children and adolescents most often has a benign cause (hypercalciuria without nephrolithiasis or no apparent etiology) and long-term prognosis is good. Disease processes manifested by gross hematuria accompanied by other symptoms (e.g., acute onset of edema, headache, and hypertension), or with a history of trauma, are the context in which hematuria requires urgent/emergent evaluation in the ED. Microscopic hematuria (more than five RBCs per high-power field [HPF]) may be accompanied by other signs and symptoms or may be completely asymptomatic; it can usually be evaluated in the outpatient setting. In addition, asymptomatic microscopic hematuria in children is rarely indicative of serious illness and may warrant only a limited or even no diagnostic evaluation.

Red or brown urine does not always indicate hematuria. Several foods, substances, and drugs may color the urine; therefore, it is important to document the presence of blood in the urine. Reagent strips can be used as the initial screening test for hematuria. Heme-positive reagent strips must be confirmed by microscopic examination for the presence of RBCs because both hemoglobinuria and myoglobinuria can cause a positive reaction in the absence of RBCs. The evaluation of a child with hematuria must take into consideration the clinical presentation, patient and family histories, physical examination, and complete urinalysis so that a logical, orderly, and cost-effective approach can be undertaken.

PATHOPHYSIOLOGY

The pathophysiology of hematuria can be explained by categorizing it as either glomerular or nonglomerular. Immune-mediated inflammatory damage to the glomerular filtration surface, as seen in postinfectious nephritis, causes disruption of the glomerular basement membrane with subsequent leakage of RBCs and protein. Glomerular bleeding that results in gross hematuria may be brown, smoky, or cola or tea colored. RBCs may become enmeshed in the protein matrix to form RBC casts, a sensitive indicator of glomerular hematuria. The renal papillae are sites of nonglomerular bleeding that are susceptible to microthrombi and anoxia in patients with sickle cell disease or trait. Inflammation of the tubules and interstitium caused by antibiotics can result in hematuria, proteinuria, and eosinophiluria. Nonsteroidal agents can produce hematuria from both tubulointerstitial nephritis and inhibition of prostaglandin synthesis. Grossly bloody urine that is bright red or pink with or without clots is more likely to be originating from the lower urinary tract, usually the bladder or urethra. Hematuria from trauma to the kidney or bladder is caused by contusions, hematomas, or lacerations anywhere along the tract. Increased vascularity from infection or chemical irritation can lead to leakage of RBCs into the urine. Exercise-related hematuria results from ischemic injury as well as direct trauma. Benign familial hematuria, a principal cause of asymptomatic hematuria, is caused by leakage of RBCs through a thin glomerular basement membrane and rarely comes to the attention of the emergency physician except as an incidental finding.

DIFFERENTIAL DIAGNOSIS

The differential diagnosis of hematuria is vast and can be categorized on the basis of whether the cause of bleeding is disease restricted to the urinary system or secondary to a systemic process (Table 32.1). The most common causes of hematuria (Table 32.2) are urinary tract infection (UTI), hypercalciuria without nephrolithiasis, acute poststreptococcal glomerulonephritis, and trauma; the latter two also being the most common of the potentially life-threatening causes. Other potentially serious causes of hematuria include hematologic disorders, renal stones with obstruction, tumors, and hemolytic uremic syndrome (HUS). Other glomerular causes of hematuria that are primary renal diseases include nonstreptococcal postinfectious glomerulonephritides, membranous glomerulonephritis, immunoglobulin A (IgA) nephropathy, and Alport syndrome (hereditary nephritis). Hematuria as a manifestation of a systemic condition is most commonly seen in children with a vasculitis such as Henoch–Schönlein purpura, or systemic lupus erythematosus (SLE) (Table 32.3).

Extraglomerular causes of hematuria include congenital anomalies such as diverticula of the urethra and bladder; hemangiomas in the bladder; cysts of the kidneys, as in polycystic or multicystic kidney; and obstruction of the ureteropelvic junction. In addition to congenital anomalies, renal vein thrombosis secondary to a coagulation disorder or to the placement of an umbilical catheter is a cause of hematuria in the neonate. Wilms tumor is a common childhood solid tumor associated with hematuria. Nephrolithiasis should be considered if there is a family history or a predisposing condition such as recurrent infection, bladder dysfunction (seen in myelomeningocele), or chronic diuretic therapy. Hypercalciuria and cystinuria are metabolic diseases that also predispose patients to renal stones and hematuria. Finally, urethral prolapse may present with vaginal bleeding that can contaminate a collected urine specimen and be misinterpreted as hematuria.

EVALUATION AND DECISION

The initial evaluation of hematuria must begin with the confirmation of blood in the urine. Further investigation of the

TABLE 32.1

PRINCIPAL CAUSES OF HEMATURIA IN CHILDREN

Urinary tract
Extraglomerular
- Trauma
- Urinary tract infection (cystitis, pyelonephritis)
- Hemorrhagic cystitis (bacterial, viral, drugs)
- Stones
- Hypercalciuria
- Interstitial nephritis
- Polycystic kidney disease
- Renal vein thrombosis
- Papillary necrosis
- Wilms tumor
- Posterior urethral valves
- Hydronephrosis
- Ureteropelvic junction obstruction
- Urethritis
- Urethral diverticula
- Urethral prolapse
- Foreign body
- Hemangiomas

Glomerular
- Acute poststreptococcal glomerulonephritis
- Other postinfectious glomerulonephritis
- IgA nephropathy
- Alport syndrome (hereditary nephritis)
- Exercise
- Familial benign hematuria
- Other chronic nephritides (membranoproliferative, membranous)
- Nutcracker syndrome (compression of the left renal vein)

Systemic
Coagulation disorders—hemophilia, platelet disorders
Sickle cell disease or trait
Anticoagulant therapy
Drugs—aspirin, nonsteroidal anti-inflammatory drugs, phenacetin, penicillins, cephalosporins, cyclophosphamide
Leukemia
Serum sickness
Henoch–Schönlein purpura
Hemolytic uremic syndrome
Systemic lupus erythematosus
Polyarteritis nodosa
Subacute bacterial endocarditis
Shunt nephritis
Tuberculosis
Hepatitis

cause and treatment includes detailed patient and family histories, careful physical examination, and microscopic urinalysis. A specific diagnosis may or may not be made in the ED, and the patient may require further diagnostic testing. The most important role for the emergency physician in evaluating a child with hematuria is to identify serious, treatable, and progressive conditions such as trauma, nephritis associated with hypertension, bleeding disorders, and infection.

TABLE 32.2

COMMON CAUSES OF HEMATURIA

Urinary tract infection—cystitis, pyelonephritis	Hypercalciuria without nephrolithiasis
Trauma (kidney, bladder, urethra)	Benign hematuria
Acute poststreptococcal glomerulonephritis	Urethritis
Sickle cell disease or trait	No defined etiology

Blood in the urine may come from sources outside the urinary tract. Vaginal hemorrhage in the female secondary to infection, foreign body, urethral prolapse, or trauma (sometimes secondary to abuse) may contaminate the urine. In addition, parents may report finding blood in the urine when, in fact, a rectal fissure has caused a small hemorrhage, producing a mixture of blood and urine in the diaper or underwear.

Urine dipsticks yielding positive result for blood require microscopic examination of the urine. Hemoglobinuria from hemolysis and myoglobinuria from rhabdomyolysis will cause a positive dipstick reaction for blood and an absence of RBCs on urine microscopic examination. Many dyes, drugs, and pigments will change the urine color to pink, red, brown, or black but will not yield a positive dipstick test result for blood. A partial list includes beets, blackberries, urates, aniline dyes, bile pigments, porphyrin, diphenylhydantoin, phenazopyridine (Pyridium), rifampin, deferoxamine, phenolphthalein, ibuprofen, methyldopa, chloroquine, homogentisic acid, and *Serratia marcescens* infection. False-positive dip reactions may be seen from certain cleaners, such as those containing hypochlorite and iodine, or other strong oxidizers.

The history taking for infants and neonates with hematuria should include questions about umbilical vessel catheters (renal venous or arterial thrombosis), passage of clots on voiding (hemorrhagic disorders), abdominal swelling or palpable mass (tumor, polycystic disease, ureteropelvic junction obstruction, posterior urethral valves), and significant birth asphyxia (corticomedullary necrosis). Urate crystals are commonly seen in the newborn/neonatal period as pink/salmon-colored spotting on the diaper. In the absence of other symptoms, no further evaluation is needed when the history and observation are suggestive of this etiology. Dysuria or urinary frequency in children and adolescents suggests cystitis, whereas flank, abdominal, or back pain suggests trauma, genitourinary infection, or stones as the cause. Sore throat, upper respiratory tract infection, or pyoderma (preceding or appearing concurrently with the onset of hematuria) points

TABLE 32.3

LIFE-THREATENING CAUSES OF HEMATURIA

Trauma (kidney, bladder, spleen)	Tumor
Acute glomerulonephritis	Hematologic disorders
Hemolytic uremic syndrome	Toxin/xenobiotic
Renal stones with obstruction	

to acute postinfectious glomerulonephritis. A history of gross hematuria with a concomitant viral upper respiratory tract or gastrointestinal tract infection may also suggest IgA nephropathy. Hematuria associated with systemic disorders may be uncovered by eliciting a history of skin rashes and arthralgia or arthritis as seen in Henoch–Schönlein purpura and SLE. Both sickle cell anemia and sickle cell trait are associated with chronic, asymptomatic gross hematuria. Finally, a history of drug use, especially the use of nonsteroidal anti-inflammatory drugs, penicillins, and cephalosporins, may point to interstitial nephritis as the cause. Antibiotic-associated tubulointerstitial nephritis is associated with high-dose, long-term antibiotic therapy and is characterized clinically by fever, rash, eosinophilia with pyuria, eosinophiluria, hematuria, proteinuria, and nonoliguric renal failure. Family history of renal stones, deafness, nephritis, renal anomalies, or hematologic disease may suggest a diagnosis in the child such as Alport syndrome, sickle cell anemia, or hemophilia.

Physical examination of a child with hematuria should always include a blood pressure measurement. Hypertension may accompany glomerulonephritis, obstructive uropathy, Wilms tumor, polycystic kidney, or vascular disease. Periorbital edema and facial swelling may be the first physical sign of nephritis. Urethral prolapse presents as a doughnut-shaped mass at the site of the urethral meatus, which is usually hyperemic and friable with scant bloody drainage.

Bruising of the abdomen, flank, or back should raise suspicion of trauma, including child abuse, as a cause of hematuria. Tenderness of the flank or lower abdomen may signal pyelonephritis, obstructed kidney, or lower UTI. Flank or abdominal masses suggest Wilms tumor or hydronephrosis, hydroureter, or polycystic kidney. Petechial or purpuric lesions on the skin and arthritis may accompany hematuria seen in vasculitic syndromes such as Henoch–Schönlein purpura. The "nutcracker syndrome," or compression of the left renal vein, may present with hematuria, left flank pain, and abdominal or groin pain. Pallor may be a sign of anemia from chronic renal insufficiency, HUS, hemoglobinopathy, leukemia, or tumors.

A careful, detailed urinalysis plays an essential role in the evaluation of the child with hematuria. Several clues in the urinalysis can help localize the site of hematuria. RBC casts, cellular casts, tubular cells, tea-colored or smoky-brown urine, and proteinuria 2+ or more by a dipstick test all point to glomerular bleeding. The presence of dysmorphic RBCs has been used as markers of glomerular bleeding In contrast, nonglomerular bleeding is suggested by red or pink urine, blood clots, no proteinuria (or less than 2+ in the absence of gross hematuria), and normal morphology of erythrocytes. Calcium oxalate crystals may be seen in the urine of patients with renal stones. Suspicion for disease processes that may cause eosinophiluria requires examination of the urine with Hansel's stain to specifically delineate eosinophils. Interpretation of catheterized urinary specimens must take into account that the catheterization itself might produce a small amount of trauma and cause a small number of RBCs (<10 RBCs/HPF).

Other blood studies may be useful in selected cases and include a complete blood cell (CBC) count, prothrombin time (PT), partial thromboplastin time (PTT), erythrocyte sedimentation rate (ESR), blood urea nitrogen (BUN), serum creatinine, complement levels (C3 and C4), and streptococcal serologies (antistreptolysin O, anti-DNase B, and antihyaluronidase titers). The history and physical examination should direct the emergency physician to those additional tests that are needed, if any.

A clinical algorithm for evaluating hematuria in the ED is shown in Figure 32.1. The first step is to confirm the presence of true hematuria. If a traumatic cause for the hematuria is suspected on the basis of history or physical findings, emergent evaluation for serious anatomic lesions must be initiated. Parenchymal contusions, lacerations, renal transections, and pedicle disruptions are possible injuries. Hematuria is the cardinal marker of renal injury, with the magnitude of hematuria paralleling the severity of injury (except for renal pedicle injuries, which may have no associated hematuria). Hematuria may also signal traumatic injury to adjacent organs such as the spleen. Patients presenting with blunt trauma associated with microscopic hematuria and no other associated injuries who are hemodynamically stable do not require radiologic evaluation because significant renal injuries are unlikely. The presence of gross hematuria or significant microscopic hematuria (more than 50 RBCs/HPF) in the context of significant mechanisms of injury necessitates emergent imaging (see Chapter 111 Abdominal Trauma). Hematuria disproportionate to the injury may indicate a congenital renal anomaly or tumor.

If there is no history of trauma, then coagulopathies should be considered as the cause. However, the medical history alone usually will point to this cause because the sudden occurrence of isolated hematuria in a previously healthy child is unlikely with either a congenital or an acquired bleeding disorder. Hematuria in a child known to have hemophilia or a related disorder often requires minimal investigation and is managed in accordance with standard protocols. If an acquired coagulopathy is suspected, a CBC count, PT, and PTT is warranted.

If trauma and coagulopathies are considered unlikely, identifying the site of bleeding as either glomerular or nonglomerular (based on urinalysis and other signs or symptoms) can direct further evaluation and diagnosis. Acute glomerulonephritis characterized by hypertension, edema, RBC casts, proteinuria, and tea-colored urine most often follows a streptococcal infection and merits serious consideration in the ED because it may cause significant hypertension and pulmonary edema requiring immediate intervention. HUS is a serious disorder that may present with glomerular-induced hematuria and proteinuria as well as a characteristic microangiopathic hemolytic anemia, thrombocytopenia, and renal failure. Laboratory studies useful in children suspected of having nephritis include a CBC, ESR, BUN, serum creatinine, complement levels, and antistreptococcal antibodies. Other nephritides associated with vasculitis may require further diagnostic evaluation before a specific diagnosis is made (see Chapter 109 Rheumatologic Emergencies).

Most children without a history of trauma who are evaluated for gross and/or microscopic hematuria in the ED have a UTI. The infection may be either in the upper tract (e.g., pyelonephritis, characterized by fever, chills, flank pain, vomiting, and dysuria) or in the lower tract (e.g., cystitis, characterized by dysuria, frequency, and occasionally, abdominal pain and fever). The cause of a UTI is either bacterial or viral. Acute hemorrhagic cystitis is often associated with adenovirus. The findings of pyuria and bacteriuria on urinalysis suggest an infectious cause, although their absence does not exclude either pyelonephritis or cystitis; thus, a urine culture is essential if no other cause has been uncovered. If the clinical suspicion is high for a bacterial UTI,

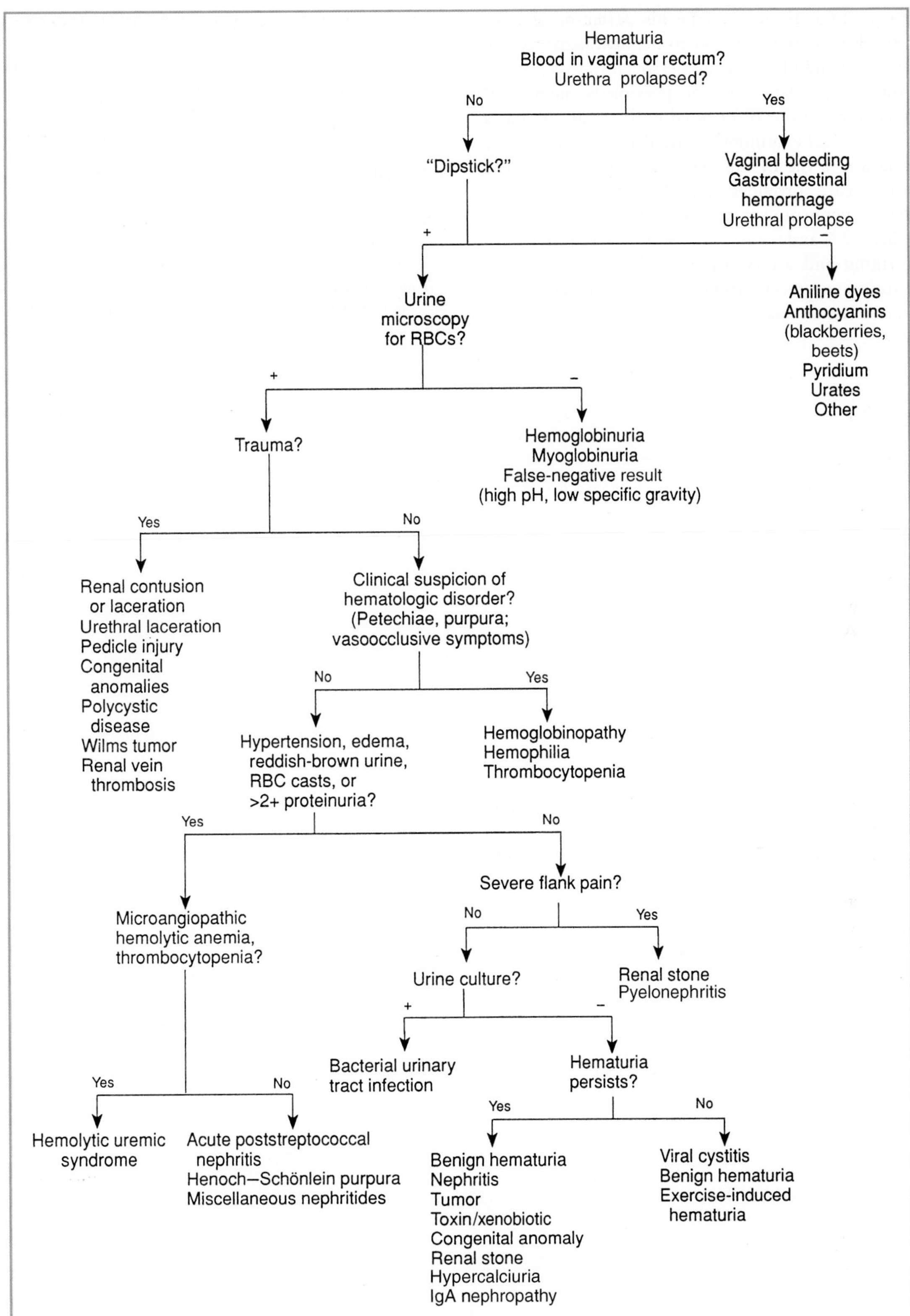

FIGURE 32.1 Approach to hematuria in the emergency department.

presumptive antimicrobial treatment should be initiated (see Chapter 102 Infectious Disease Emergencies).

Severe flank pain radiating to the groin is characteristic of renal colic from calculi, which may present with either gross or microscopic hematuria. Stones may occur in children with metabolic abnormalities or stasis secondary to obstruction and in premature infants taking furosemide. Topiramate is also associated with an increased risk of nephrolithiasis. Crystals may be seen on urinalysis; further investigation with renal ultrasound or computed tomography usually confirms stones if a plain abdominal radiograph does not reveal the presence of radiopaque material. Hypercalciuria is an important cause of hematuria in children and may be idiopathic or secondary to another disease and can lead to nephrocalcinosis (see Chapter 108 Renal and Electrolyte Emergencies).

Hematuria that persists after the previously mentioned causes have been ruled out or deemed unlikely on the basis of history and physical examination usually does not require further evaluation in the ED and should be pursued by the primary health care provider, possibly in collaboration with a pediatric nephrologist. These additional causes are listed in Figure 32.1 and Table 32.1 and may require more extensive imaging and interventions such as renal biopsy, metabolic studies, or serial urinalyses (benign hematuria, exercise-induced hematuria).

Suggested Readings and Key References

Bergstein J, Leiser J, Andreoli S. The clinical significance of asymptomatic gross and microscopic hematuria in children. *Arch Pediatr Adolesc Med* 2005;159:353–355.

Greenfield SP, Williot P, Kaplan D. Gross hematuria in children: a ten-year review. *Urology* 2007;69:166–169.

Patel HP, Bissler JJ. Hematuria in children. *Pediatr Clin North Am* 2001; 48:1519–1537.

Saunders F. Best evidence topic report: investigating microscopic haematuria in blunt abdominal trauma. *Emerg Med J* 2002;19: 322–323.

Youn T, Trachtman H, Gauthier B. Clinical spectrum of gross hematuria in pediatric patients. *Clin Pediatr* 2006;45:135–141.

CHAPTER 33 ■ HYPERTENSION

ERIKA CONSTANTINE, MD AND CHRIS MERRITT, MD, MPH

Until recently, the prevalence of hypertension in the pediatric population had been relatively low. Recent trends in childhood obesity, however, appear to be linked to the observation of an overall increase in blood pressure values seen in children. The Fourth Report on High Blood Pressure in Children and Adolescents, a national consensus statement published in 2004, suggests that a child with three or more blood pressure measurements above the 95th percentile for age, height, and gender should be considered hypertensive. *Stage 1 hypertension* is defined as blood pressure values that range from the 95th percentile to 5 mm Hg above the 99th percentile. Those with blood pressure measurements of 5 mm Hg or more above the 99th percentile are considered to have *stage 2 hypertension* (Table 33.1). *Hypertensive urgency* is a significantly elevated blood pressure level that may be potentially harmful but is without evidence of end-organ damage or dysfunction. *Hypertensive emergency* describes an elevated blood pressure level associated with evidence of secondary organ damage such as hypertensive encephalopathy or acute left ventricular failure. Hypertensive urgencies ordinarily develop over days to weeks, whereas hypertensive emergencies generally develop over hours.

Standard blood pressure nomograms in children are based on auscultatory measurements of blood pressure levels using the right arm supported at the level of the heart. Appropriate blood pressure cuff size is essential for accurate measurement. The inflatable rubber bladder should be long enough to completely encircle the circumference of the arm (overlap is acceptable). Bladder width should be approximately 40% of the arm circumference at a point halfway between the acromion and the olecranon. A narrow cuff can produce falsely elevated readings, while an overly broad cuff may produce readings that are falsely low.

Auscultation remains the recommended method for blood pressure determination in children. Current guidelines recommend that the disappearance of the fifth Korotkoff sound should be used to define diastolic blood pressure. In the emergency department (ED) setting, however, sphygmomanometer readings are sometimes difficult to perform, particularly in neonates and very young children. In such cases, an oscillometric device, which measures the mean arterial pressure and calculates systolic and diastolic blood pressure values, may be used. Because blood pressure calculations by this method may vary widely from device to device, any abnormal reading should be repeated by auscultation.

In the ED, where children are often stressed or agitated by an unfamiliar environment or underlying illness, abnormally high blood pressure readings are not uncommon. These measurements should be repeated after a brief period of quiet rest.

PATHOPHYSIOLOGY/ DIFFERENTIAL DIAGNOSIS

Hypertension may be either primary or secondary in nature. Primary, or essential, hypertension is a condition in which no underlying disease can be identified. The increasing frequency of primary hypertension in the pediatric population is believed to be largely attributable to the increases in body mass index, sedentary lifestyle, and high-salt and high-calorie diets of today's children. Nonetheless, essential hypertension is a diagnosis of exclusion and is rarely the cause of hypertensive urgencies or emergencies.

Secondary hypertension can be the result of an underlying pathologic process, such as a cardiovascular, renal, endocrine, toxic, or central nervous system disturbance. Disruptions in the renin–angiotensin system, volume overload or sympathetic stimulation by tumors, drugs, or other processes, may all contribute to the development of hypertension.

The differential diagnosis of hypertension changes with the age of a child (Table 33.2), with younger children being more likely to have a discernable cause for their hypertension (Table 33.3). In adolescent girls, oral contraceptive pills may be a cause of hypertension, and in all age groups, drug- or toxin-induced hypertension should be considered.

EVALUATION AND DECISION

Children with a persistently elevated blood pressure level in the ED require a brief but thorough history and physical examination, with emphasis on detecting an underlying cause for hypertension and eliciting signs and symptoms of end-organ damage resulting from the hypertensive process. In the absence of concerning findings in the history or physical examination, the child with mild or moderate hypertension should be referred for follow-up with the primary care physician. Although it is appropriate to initiate the process of patient education in the ED regarding weight loss, dietary salt reduction, and exercise, a definitive diagnosis of hypertension should not be offered until elevated blood pressure has been confirmed on several occasions.

The workup of a child with severe hypertension requires careful evaluation for the presence of clinical findings that may represent either the primary cause of the elevated blood pressure or the secondary systemic effects of hypertension. Histories of frequent urinary tract infections, unexplained fevers, hematuria, dysuria, frequency, or edema all suggest renal disease. Previous umbilical artery catheterization increases the risk of renal artery stenosis or thrombosis. Ingestion of prescription, over-the-counter or illicit drugs, or rapid withdrawal of some antihypertensive medications, may support the

TABLE 33.1

BLOOD PRESSURE LEVELS (95TH AND 99TH PERCENTILES) FOR CHILDREN OF AVERAGE HEIGHT[a] (50TH PERCENTILE) AT SELECTED AGES

		Boys		Girls	
Age (yr)	BP percentile	SBP (mm Hg)	DBP (mm Hg)	SBP (mm Hg)	DBP (mm Hg)
1	95	103	56	104	58
	99	110	64	111	65
3	95	109	65	107	67
	99	116	73	114	74
5	95	112	72	110	72
	99	120	80	117	79
7	95	115	76	113	75
	99	122	84	120	82
10	95	119	80	119	78
	99	127	88	126	86
12	95	123	81	123	80
	99	131	89	130	88
14	95	128	82	126	82
	99	136	90	133	90
16	95	134	84	128	84
	99	141	92	135	91

[a]Children above or below the 50th percentile for height will have blood pressure ranges slightly above or below indicated values, respectively. For a more comprehensive listing, see *Pediatrics* 2004;114(2 suppl):555–576.
BP, blood pressure; SBP, systolic blood pressure; DBP, diastolic blood pressure.
Adapted from National High Blood Pressure Education Program Working Group on High Blood Pressure in Children and Adolescents. The fourth report on the diagnosis, evaluation, and treatment of high blood pressure in children and adolescents. *Pediatrics* 2004;114(2 suppl):555–576.

diagnosis of drug-related hypertension. A history of sweating, flushing, palpitations, fever, and weight loss may suggest a pheochromocytoma.

Physical examination should concentrate on identifying involved organ systems, paying particular attention to cardiovascular, renal, and central nervous systems. The cardiac examination should seek evidence of congestive heart failure (CHF) and pulmonary edema. Absent or decreased femoral pulses are suggestive of aortic coarctation. Abdominal examination may reveal the presence of a bruit or renal mass such as Wilms tumor, implicating a renovascular cause for the hypertension. Peripheral edema may suggest volume overload from renal or cardiac failure. Neurologic evaluation should include observation for sensorimotor symmetry and appropriate cerebellar function. Funduscopic examination for hypertensive changes such as hemorrhages, infarcts, and disc edema should be conducted, in addition to testing the pupillary light reflex and visual acuity.

Initial investigations for severe hypertension in the ED should be limited to the most basic of tests. Blood studies including a complete blood cell count, electrolytes, blood urea nitrogen, serum creatinine, and urinalysis are usually warranted. In addition, a urine culture should be considered in all girls and in boys with known renal pathologic conditions. A chest radiograph and electrocardiogram may help detect the presence of CHF or ventricular hypertrophy. If there are concerning findings on the initial cardiovascular examination, an echocardiogram may also be warranted. Additional studies are rarely part of the routine ED assessment of hypertension.

When the cause of hypertension is not readily apparent, a stepwise evaluation of the most common organ systems is indicated (Fig. 33.1), beginning with an evaluation for underlying renal disease, followed by consideration of cardiovascular and neurologic causes. A negative evaluation for an underlying cause of hypertension in the ED is compatible with, but not sufficient for, the diagnosis of essential hypertension. Follow-up is always indicated.

TABLE 33.2

COMMON CAUSES OF HYPERTENSION

Age group	Cause
Newborn infants	Renal artery thrombosis, renal artery stenosis, congenital renal malformations, coarctation of the aorta, bronchopulmonary dysplasia
Infancy–6 yrs	Renal parenchymal diseases[a], coarctation of the aorta, renal artery stenosis
6–10 yrs	Renal parenchymal diseases, renal artery stenosis, essential hypertension (including obesity)
Adolescence	Essential hypertension (including obesity), renal parenchymal diseases

[a]Includes renal structural and inflammatory lesions and tumors.
Adapted from the Task Force on Blood Pressure Control in Children. Report of the second task force on blood pressure control in children—1987. *Pediatrics* 1987;79:1–25.

TABLE 33.3

DIFFERENTIAL DIAGNOSIS OF HYPERTENSION

Anxiety	Clonidine withdrawal
Pain	Cocaine
Essential hypertension	Corticosteroids
Renal	Ephedrine
Obstructive uropathy, including kidney stones	Epinephrine
Renal parenchymal diseases	Heavy metal poisoning
Hemolytic uremic syndrome	Methylphenidate
Henoch–Schönlein purpura	Methysergide
Hypoplastic kidneys	Monoamine oxidase inhibitors
Lupus nephropathy	Oral contraceptives
Nephrotic syndrome	Phenylephrine
Polycystic kidney disease	Phencyclidine
Poststreptococcal glomerulonephritis	Phenylpropanolamine
Pyelonephritis	Pseudoephedrine
Reflux nephropathy	Reserpine
Renal trauma	**Endocrine**
Renal vascular disease	Congenital adrenal hyperplasia
Cardiovascular	Cushing syndrome
Bacterial endocarditis	Hyperaldosteronism
Coarctation of the aorta	Hyperparathyroidism
Vasculitis	Hyperthyroidism
Neurologic	Pheochromocytoma
Familial dysautonomia	**Tumors**
Guillain–Barré syndrome	Neuroblastoma
Increased intracranial pressure	Wilms tumor
Poliomyelitis	**Miscellaneous**
Drug induced/toxicologic	Acute intermittent porphyria
Anabolic steroids	Hypercalcemia
Anticholinergics	Hypernatremia
Amphetamines	Malignant hyperthermia

MANAGEMENT (SEE CHAPTER 108 RENAL AND ELECTROLYTE EMERGENCIES)

There is little consistency in the literature as to when treatment of hypertension should be initiated, particularly in the ED setting. According to the Fourth Report, immediate evaluation and treatment should be undertaken for patients with symptomatic stage 2 hypertension. However, some authors suggest that severe hypertension, even if asymptomatic, warrants acute treatment.

For children with symptomatic severe hypertension, treatment must be rapid but cautious. It is recommended that the blood pressure be reduced by no more than 25% in the first 6 to 8 hours. There is a compelling reason for a conservative approach. In long-standing hypertension, the range of blood pressure over which cerebrovascular autoregulation occurs shifts upward. As a result of prolonged hypertension, vascular endothelial inflammation and oxidative stress combine to make the vasculature less responsive to changes in blood pressure. If systemic blood pressure drops precipitously, cerebral perfusion may become dangerously low.

After initial stabilization, blood pressure may be lowered toward normal over the course of several days. This should take place in an intensive care unit, usually with intra-arterial blood pressure monitoring in place.

In addition to treating the elevation in blood pressure levels, the child with complications of hypertension may also require treatment of the specific complications. Attention should always be paid to managing the child's airway, breathing, and circulation. The child with seizures or CHF often requires the standard treatment of these problems in addition to antihypertensive therapy. However, when other complications are believed to be secondary to severe hypertension, treatment of the hypertension should take precedence.

SPECIFIC THERAPY

In a hypertensive emergency, adequate intravenous access should be secured immediately, and the patient should have cardiorespiratory and blood pressure monitoring. The intravenous route for medication administration is preferred for most hypertensive emergencies, as this allows for more accurate

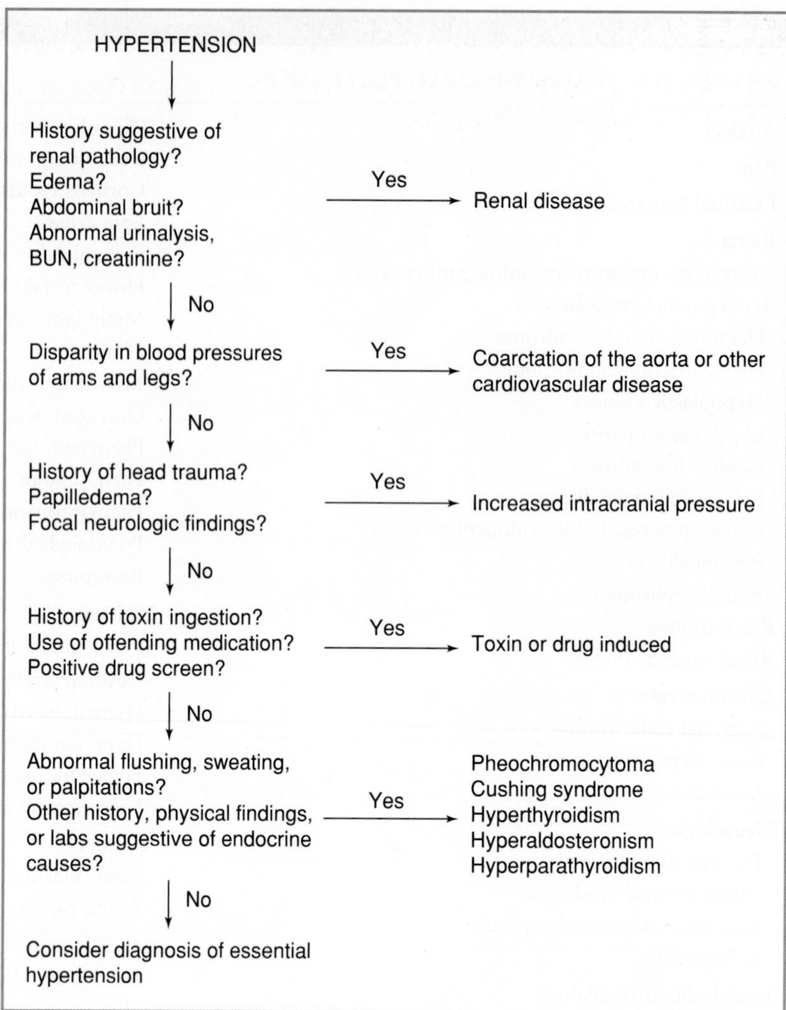

FIGURE 33.1 Diagnostic approach to the most common causes of acute, persistent hypertension in a previously healthy child. BUN, blood urea nitrogen.

titration of dose to response. Absorption and effect of medications given enterally may be less predictable, putting the patient at risk of relative hypotension. Management of hypertensive emergencies by continuous IV infusion of a short-acting titratable antihypertensive medication is ideal. The use of oral agents should be limited to hypertensive urgencies only.

Though there is insufficient randomized controlled trial data to recommend a specific drug protocol for hypertensive emergencies, the most commonly used agents for hypertensive emergencies remain labetalol, nicardipine, and sodium nitroprusside. Newer agents, such as clevidipine and fenoldopam, are gaining favor based on their kinetic and safety profiles. Specific medications (Table 33.4) should be chosen based on their availability, the physician's familiarity with the drug, and the underlying pathophysiology of the hypertensive process. The side effect profile of each medication and drug–drug interactions must be taken into account.

Intravenous Antihypertensive Medications

Labetalol

Labetalol is a combined α_1- and β-adrenergic blocking agent which has the ability to reduce peripheral vascular resistance with little effect on heart rate or cardiac output. It has a rapid onset of action (usually 5 to 10 minutes) and a plasma half-life of 3 to 5 hours when given intravenously. Because of its duration of action, labetalol can be more difficult to titrate to effect than other agents.

Labetalol may be administered by intermittent bolus dosing, or by a bolus dose followed by a continuous infusion (Table 33.4). Because of its β-blocking effects, it should not be used in patients with asthma, heart block, or CHF or for the treatment of hypertension in patients with pheochromocytoma or sympathomimetic drug overdose (e.g., cocaine; see Chapter 110 Toxicologic Emergencies), due to the potential for unopposed alpha effects.

Nicardipine

Nicardipine is a second-generation dihydropyridine calcium channel blocker that prevents vascular smooth muscle contraction, resulting in a reduction in peripheral vascular resistance without compromising cardiac output. Its onset of action within 1 to 2 minutes of administration and short elimination half-life make it relatively easy to titrate. Nicardipine is the preferred agent for the treatment of hypertensive emergencies at many institutions because of its safety profile, ability to produce a rapid effect, and low risk for causing hypotension. Recommended dosing is 1 to 3 μg/kg/min by continuous infusion. Hypotension, though uncommon, can be reversed by the administration of calcium. Nicardipine should be avoided in

TABLE 33.4

MOST COMMONLY USED ANTIHYPERTENSIVE AGENTS FOR THE TREATMENT OF HYPERTENSIVE URGENCIES AND EMERGENCIES IN CHILDREN[a,b]

Drug	Class	Route	Dose	Onset of action	Duration of action	Side effects/comments[c]
Labetalol	α_1- and β-Blocker	IV	Bolus dosing: 0.2–1 mg/kg (max 40 mg/dose) Infusion: 0.25–3 mg/kg/hr IV	5–10 min	2–4 hr	Contraindicated in asthma, heart failure, heart block, pheochromocytoma, cocaine toxicity; may mask symptoms of hypoglycemia
Nicardipine	Calcium channel blocker	IV	1–3 µg/kg/min	2–5 min	30–60 min	Risk of phlebitis at infusion site Reflex tachycardia May cause increased ICP
Sodium nitroprusside[d]	Direct vasodilator	IV	0.3–8 µg/kg/min	Seconds	During infusion only	Black box warning: Risk of cyanide/thiocyanate toxicity. May cause transient hypotension
Hydralazine[d]	Direct vasodilator	IV/IM	0.2–0.6 mg/kg/dose (max 20 mg)	10–30 min	4–12 hr	Commonly used in pregnancy May cause headaches, tachycardia, increased ICP, fluid retention
Esmolol	β_1-Blocker	IV	100–500 µg/kg/min	Seconds	10–20 min	May cause profound bradycardia Metabolism independent of hepatic or renal processes
Phentolamine[d]	α-Blocker	IV	0.05–0.1 mg/kg/dose (max 5 mg)	Seconds	15–30 min	Useful for catecholamine-induced hypertensive crisis
Fenoldopam[d]	Dopamine receptor agonist	IV	0.2–0.8 µg/kg/min	5–15 min	1–4 hr	Limited experience in children
Nifedipine	Calcium channel blocker	PO	0.25–0.5 mg/kg/dose (max 10 mg)	20–30 min	6 hr	Precipitous decrease in MAP associated with doses >0.25 mg/kg/dose Difficult to administer in exact doses May cause dizziness, flushing, rebound hypertension
Isradipine	Calcium channel blocker	PO	0.05–0.1 mg/kg/dose (max 5 mg)	30 min–2 hr	12 hr	Limited experience with pediatric use
Clonidine[d]	α_2-Receptor agonist	PO	0.05–0.1 mg/dose, may be repeated up to 0.8 mg of total dose	15–30 min	6–8 hr	Dry mouth, drowsiness

[a]Because several of these medications have not been extensively tested in children, existing pharmacokinetic data are frequently based on studies in adults.
[b]Dosing recommendations vary by source.
[c]See additional comments and cautions in text.
[d]Indicates drugs with Food and Drug Administration–approved pediatric labeling for use in hypertension.
IV, intravenous; ICP, intracranial pressure; IM, intramuscular; PO, by mouth; MAP, mean arterial pressure.

patients with increased intracranial pressure. Reflex tachycardia, usually clinically insignificant, and phlebitis are known adverse effects.

Sodium Nitroprusside

Nitroprusside is a powerful vasodilator, affecting both arteriolar and venous smooth muscle. Its onset is almost immediate, and its duration of action is extremely short, allowing for easy titration of the drug to the desired blood pressure. Because of its venous dilatory effects, nitroprusside reduces preload and often improves cardiac output in CHF. It may increase intracerebral blood flow, though this may be offset by a concomitant drop in systemic pressure. Because nitroprusside is metabolized to thiocyanate and cyanide, cyanide toxicity is a risk of its use, particularly for infusions lasting more than 24 to 48 hours or in those with liver or renal impairment. In such cases, thiocyanate levels should be monitored daily. Because of this known risk of toxicity, the FDA has added a black box warning to the labeling of the drug.

Nitroprusside is given as an intravenous infusion, starting at a dosage of 0.3 to 0.5 μg/kg/min and titrating upward as needed to 8 μg/kg/min. The average dosage required for the control of hypertension is approximately 3 μg/kg/min. Because nitroprusside has an extremely short half-life, blood pressure returns to pretreatment levels within 1 to 10 minutes of the cessation of the infusion.

Esmolol

Esmolol is an ultra–short-acting cardioselective β_1-blocker originally used in treatment of postoperative hypertension following repair of congenital heart disease. It has an onset of action of approximately 60 seconds and a duration of action of 10 to 20 minutes. It is usually administered by continuous infusion after an initial bolus dose. It is given as an initial bolus of 100 to 500 μg per kg followed by an infusion of 100 μg/kg/min, titrating to effect. Metabolism is independent of both hepatic and renal processes, making a good choice for use in patients with multiorgan failure. Although reported use in hypertensive children outside of the postoperative setting is limited, the drug certainly has potential for use in the ED setting. Because of its β-blocking effects, contraindications are similar to those of labetalol, and include second- and third-degree heart block, bradycardia, cardiac failure, and cardiogenic shock.

Hydralazine

Hydralazine is an arteriolar vasodilator that can be given intravenously, intramuscularly, and orally. Onset of action is in the order of 10 to 30 minutes when administered intravenously, with a duration ranging from 4 to 12 hours. Once the most commonly used agent for hypertension associated with pregnancy, it has largely been replaced by labetalol and nicardipine. Side effects include reflex tachycardia, fluid retention, facial flushing, and increased intracranial pressure. Hydralazine is given at a dose of 0.2 to 0.6 mg per kg intravenously or intramuscularly, or at a dose of 0.25 mg per kg orally to a maximum of 25 mg.

Phentolamine

Phentolamine is an α-adrenergic receptor antagonist whose use should be limited to treatment of hypertension associated with catecholamine-induced hypertensive crises, as seen with pheochromocytoma or sympathomimetic toxicity. Dosing recommendations vary widely. Some recommend 0.05 to 0.1 mg/kg/dose intravenously to a maximum of 5 mg, and others recommend a pediatric dose of 1 mg administered intravenously or intramuscularly, repeated as needed to achieve appropriate blood pressure control.

Enalaprilat

Enalaprilat is an angiotensin-converting enzyme inhibitor that can be useful in high renin states. It is contraindicated for use in patients with bilateral renal artery stenosis. Because of the high incidence of renovascular disease in the pediatric population, and limited pediatric experience with its use, caution must be exercised before using this agent for the treatment of severe hypertension in the ED. It should be administered at a dose of 0.05 to 0.1 mg per kg intravenously up to a maximum of 1.25 mg.

Newer Agents

Fenoldopam

Fenoldopam is a selective dopamine agonist causing vasodilation of the renal, coronary, cerebral, and splanchnic vasculature, resulting in a decrease in mean arterial pressure. The use of fenoldopam in pediatric patients has increased in recent years. Its use has been reported for controlled perioperative hypotension and in the intensive care setting when conventional therapy has failed.

Recent reports in children showed that although fenoldopam resulted in a decrease in blood pressure levels, this required higher doses than for adults and the decrease was less than that observed in adults. Peak effects are observed within 15 minutes, with steady-state serum levels achieved in 30 to 60 minutes. Initial infusion rates of 0.2 to 0.8 μg/kg/min are recommended. Side effects include reflex tachycardia, increased intracranial pressure, and increased intraocular pressure. Although pediatric experience with fenoldopam is limited, it appears to be a reasonable alternative when more conventional therapies fail.

Clevidipine

Clevidipine is an ultra–short-acting third-generation dihydropyridine calcium channel antagonist. It has high specificity for arteriolar smooth muscle, reducing peripheral resistance while increasing stroke volume and cardiac output. Its half-life is approximately 1 minute with more rapid onset and offset than even nicardipine, which eases titration, and is metabolized in plasma, independent of the liver or kidney. Combined, these characteristics make it a strong contender for the management of severe elevations in blood pressure levels in the ED. Clevidipine has not yet been approved for use in pediatric patients. Initial dosing recommendations in children suggest a starting dose of 0.5 to 1 μg/kg/min titrating upward.

Oral Antihypertensive Medications

Nifedipine

Short-acting nifedipine is a calcium channel blocker that decreases peripheral vascular resistance. Its use in children remains controversial, owing to the serious hypotensive side effects of the drug experienced in adults. However, similar exaggerated effects have not been clearly demonstrated in children.

Although previously administered sublingually, absorption is more predictable when the capsule is bitten and swallowed. Nifedipine is administered at a dose of 0.25 to 0.5 mg per kg up to a maximum of 10 mg. Onset of action is within 20 to 30 minutes; duration of action is approximately 6 hours. Precipitous decreases in mean arterial pressure (>25%) have been associated with doses exceeding 0.25 mg per kg.

Isradipine

A second-generation dihydropyridine calcium channel blocker, isradipine is another safe alternative for children with severe hypertension. Onset of action is usually 30 minutes to 2 hours,

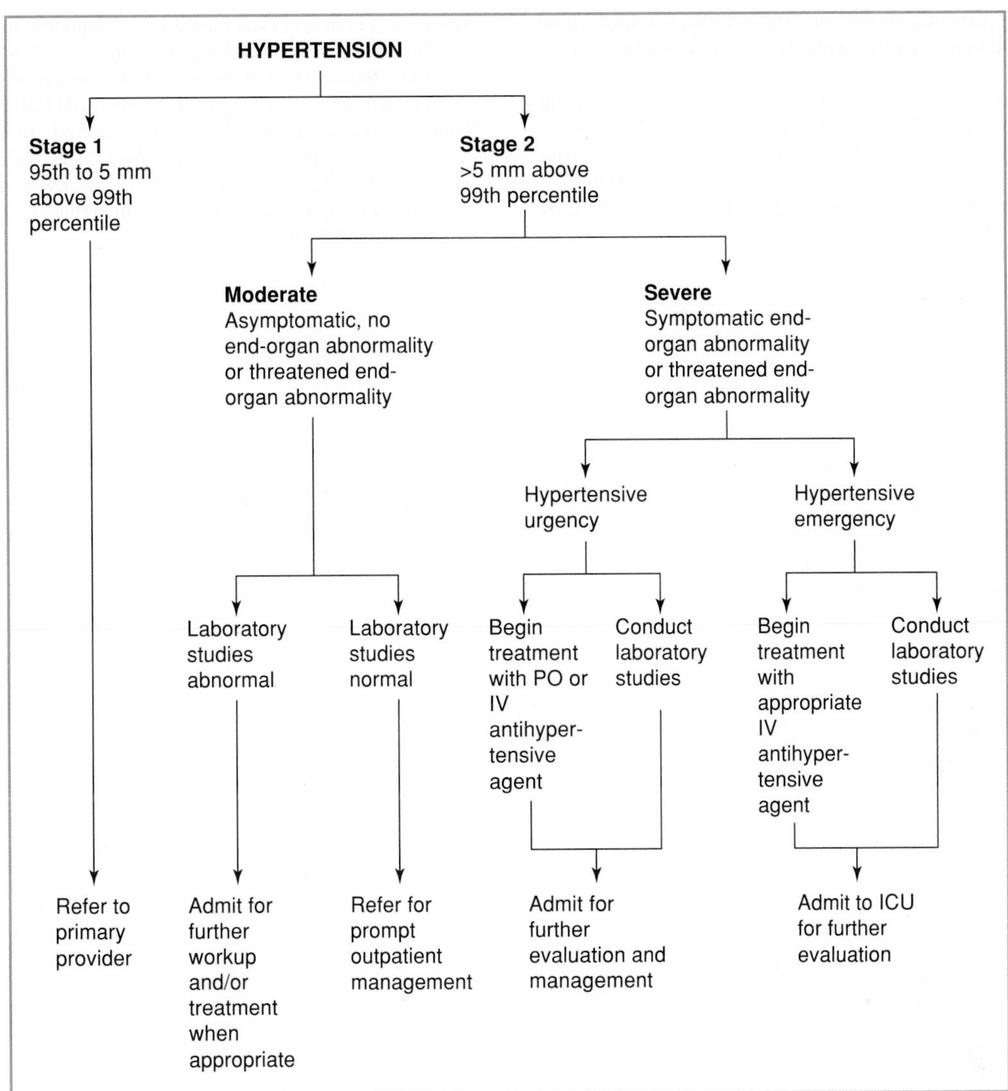

FIGURE 33.2 Approach to the initial emergency department triage and stabilization of the persistently hypertensive child. PO, oral; IV, intravenous; ICU, intensive care unit.

with a half-life of 3 to 8 hours. It has selective action on vascular smooth muscle, allowing it to be used in children with compromised myocardial function. Dosing ranges from 0.05 to 0.1 mg per kg per dose to a maximum of 5 mg, given two to four times daily.

Clonidine

Clonidine is an α_2-adrenergic agonist that works by reducing cerebral sympathetic output. Its onset of action is 15 to 30 minutes following administration. It is recommended by some for the management of hypertensive urgencies, although most studies have evaluated its use as a treatment of chronic primary hypertension in children older than 12 years.

SUMMARY

It is not unusual that a child presenting to the ED will have an elevation in blood pressure levels. In many cases, the blood pressure level will normalize with rest or acclimation to the environment. Occasionally, however, the elevation in blood pressure levels will be sustained. In children with asymptomatic mild hypertension and no target organ involvement, the emergency physician must ensure adequate follow-up. Moderate or severe hypertension that affects or threatens to affect end organs, in contrast, requires evaluation and initiation of treatment in the ED (Fig. 33.2). In severe or life-threatening cases, blood pressure reduction will often need to be instituted before the cause of the hypertension is known.

Suggested Readings and Key References

Flynn JT. Pediatric hypertension: recent trends and accomplishments, future challenges. *Am J Hypertens* 2008;21(6):605–612.

Flynn JT, Tullus K. Severe hypertension in children and adolescents: pathophysiology and treatment. *Pediatr Nephrol* 2009;24(6):1101–1112.

Hammer GB, Verghese ST, Drover DR, et al. Pharmacokinetics and pharmacodynamics of fenoldopam mesylate for blood pressure control in pediatric patients. *BMC Anesthesiol* 2008;8:6.

Heilpern K. Pathophysiology of hypertension. *Ann Emerg Med* 2008;51(3 suppl):S5–S6.

National High Blood Pressure Education Program Working Group on High Blood Pressure in Children and Adolescents. The fourth report on the diagnosis, evaluation, and treatment of high blood pressure in children and adolescents. *Pediatrics* 2004;114(2 suppl): 555–576.

Patel HP, Mitsnefes M. Advances in the pathogenesis and management of hypertensive crisis. *Curr Opin Pediatr* 2005;17(2):210–214.

Perez MI, Musini VM. Pharmacological interventions for hypertensive emergencies. *Cochrane Database Syst Rev* 2008;(1):CD003653.

Porto I. Hypertensive emergencies in children. *J Pediatr Health Care* 2000;14(6):312–317.

Sahney S. A review of calcium channel antagonists in the treatment of pediatric hypertension. *Paediatr Drugs* 2006;8(6):357–373.

Singh D, Akingbola O, Yosypiv I, et al. Emergency management of hypertension in children. *Int J Nephrol* 2012;2012:420247.

Tenney F, Sakarcan A. Nicardipine is a safe and effective agent in pediatric hypertensive emergencies. *Am J Kidney Dis* 2000;35(5):E20.

Yiu V, Orrbine E, Rosychuk RJ, et al. The safety and use of short-acting nifedipine in hospitalized hypertensive children. *Pediatr Nephrol* 2004;19(6):644–650.

CHAPTER 34 ■ IMMOBILE ARM

SARA A. SCHUTZMAN, MD AND GALINA LIPTON, MD

An infant or child brought for the evaluation of an "immobile arm" is not moving the limb because of pain or weakness. The evaluation is often a challenge because most of these children are preverbal; therefore, the history is second or third hand if available at all, patients are unable to report symptoms or pain location, and the physical examination is often difficult because of children's fear of strangers. These children can be considered as having an upper-extremity equivalent of "limp." By using historical information, physical findings, selective radiologic studies, and laboratory tests, children with this complaint can be diagnosed and managed.

DIFFERENTIAL DIAGNOSIS

Table 34.1 is a relatively comprehensive list of causes of decreased arm movement. Trauma is by far the most common cause of diminished arm use in children (Table 34.2). Although life- and limb-threatening causes (Table 34.3) are less common, clinicians should always have a high index of suspicion for these conditions in certain clinical scenarios.

Any injury from the clavicle to the fingertips can cause arm pain in children and can lead to decreased use of the limb. These injuries range from a simple contusion or sprain, to a fracture or dislocation with neurovascular compromise. Most young children with diminished arm use have radial head subluxation ("nursemaid's elbow"), fracture, or soft tissue injury. Radial head subluxation is by far the most common cause of arm disuse and is a common elbow injury that is unique to young children, typically those younger than 5 years (peak incidence age 2 to 3 years). The classic mechanism involves a sudden pull of the arm. However, oftentimes injuries are caused by other mechanisms including falling and twisting, and it is not uncommon to have no known history of trauma. The child with radial head subluxation typically holds the affected arm slightly flexed with the forearm pronated and without spontaneous arm movement. The child is usually not distressed unless the elbow is moved. Classically, there is no reproducible tenderness, warmth, or swelling (best evaluated with distracting the child).

With musculoskeletal injuries, the child may have an obvious abnormality, such as a deformity or ecchymosis, or more subtle findings of localized tenderness or decreased arm movement. Radiographs are useful for demonstrating most fractures or dislocations but may appear normal with Salter–Harris type I fractures and nursemaid's elbow, as well as with contusions and other minor soft tissue injuries (see also Chapter 119 Musculoskeletal Trauma).

Although one can often elicit a history of trauma, the diagnosis must be considered even in its absence because of unwitnessed events in preverbal children or, less commonly, intentional injuries inflicted by caregivers who are not forthcoming. In such cases, careful physical examination of the child often identifies other signs of inflicted trauma. In addition, inflicted fractures may have characteristic findings on radiographs. Identifying inflicted injuries is crucial to preventing further, potentially more serious injuries.

Children with hemophilia or other bleeding disorder may have hemarthrosis or hematoma with minimal trauma. The child will typically have a history of a bleeding disorder (although not with the first presentation) and may or may not have a history of trauma. The affected joint is swollen and tender with limited range of motion but there is typically no fever or other systemic symptoms.

Although much less common than trauma, infection may also cause decreased use of an arm. There may be a history of fever, and onset of arm disuse is often less abrupt than with trauma. The infection can be located at any point from the shoulder to finger and may be superficial (e.g., cellulitis, paronychia) or deep. Arthritis and osteomyelitis frequently have associated localized swelling, warmth, and tenderness; infected joints usually have limited, painful range of motion. With more severe infections, the child may be febrile and appear ill (especially if bacteremic). Laboratory findings may include elevated white blood cell count (WBC), elevated sedimentation rate (ESR), or elevated C-reactive protein (CRP) level, and blood culture results may yield the offending agent. Acutely, radiographs often are nondiagnostic; if arthritis or osteomyelitis is suspected, ultrasound, bone scintigraphy, or magnetic resonance imaging (MRI) should be considered (depending on the clinical scenario), with arthrocentesis or subperiosteal/bone aspiration as indicated (see Chapters 102 Infectious Disease Emergencies and 129 Musculoskeletal Emergencies). Congenital syphilis, although unusual, may present as pseudoparalysis in infants due to metaphysitis, periostitis, osteochondritis, or pathologic fracture, with bony changes evident on the radiograph (pseudoparalysis of Parrot).

In addition to bone or joint infections described above, one must keep in mind that soft tissue infections may also lead to decreased arm use. These include cellulitis and necrotizing fasciitis. Necrotizing soft tissue infections in children are most commonly caused by Group A Streptococcus, other agents include *Staphylococcus aureus* and anaerobic organisms. Predisposing factors include skin trauma (e.g., laceration, burn, surgery) and varicella, although skin may be intact. Children are usually febrile and the affected area is typically erythematous (without sharp borders), swollen, warm, shiny, and exquisitely tender, often with pain out of proportion to physical examination findings. WBC, CRP, and ESR are usually elevated. Compartment syndrome and complicating myonecrosis may occur and creatine phosphokinase (CPK) is often elevated.

Other inflammatory causes of arm pain include Lyme arthritis, other postinfectious arthritis, rheumatologic process (noninfectious arthritis), and myositis. In addition to a swollen, tender joint, children with these conditions may have

TABLE 34.1

DIFFERENTIAL DIAGNOSIS OF THE IMMOBILE ARM

Trauma
Fracture
Dislocation/subluxation
Hemarthrosis (hemophilia)
Soft tissue injury
Nerve injury
Splinter/hair tourniquet
Infection
Septic arthritis
Osteomyelitis
Soft tissue infection
Cellulitis
Fasciitis
Abscess
Lymphangitis
Paronychia/felon/tenosynovitis
Congenital syphilis
Tumor
Primary musculoskeletal
Bone
Cartilage
Soft tissue
Bone marrow infiltration
Leukemia
Neuroblastoma
Lymphoma
Inflammation
Arthritis
Juvenile idiopathic arthritis
Other collagen vascular
Postinfectious
Lyme
Myositis
Infarction
Hemoglobinopathy
Hand–foot syndrome (dactylitis)
Acute vasoocclusive crisis
Avascular necrosis
Avascular necrosis
Neurologic
Radiculopathy
Plexopathy
Neuropathy
Stroke
Todd's paralysis
Complex migraine
Traction
Pressure
Laceration
Injury
Miscellaneous
Complex regional pain syndrome (reflex sympathetic dystrophy)
Conversion disorder

TABLE 34.2

COMMON CAUSES OF DIMINISHED ARM USE

Newborns/infants
Clavicle fracture
Brachial plexus injury
Septic arthritis/osteomyelitis
Infants/preschool-aged children
Nursemaid's elbow
Fracture
Soft tissue injury

signs of systemic disease. These include multiple joint involvement, rash, fever, adenopathy, heart murmur, hematuria, or bloody stools. If the examination suggests an inflammatory arthritis but cannot exclude a septic process, then arthrocentesis is necessary for definitive diagnosis.

Tumors are a rare cause of diminished arm use. The tumors can be benign or malignant and of bone, cartilage, or muscle, or they may represent neoplastic infiltration of bone marrow (e.g., leukemia, neuroblastoma). Tumors are usually less acute in onset; cardinal symptoms may include pain and, perhaps, increasing limb or joint swelling, although the lesions may be asymptomatic. Occasionally, tumors lead to a pathologic fracture. Systemic complaints, including fever, malaise, and weight loss, may be present. Physical examination may reveal localized tenderness, joint swelling, or a mass of the soft tissue or bone. With leukemia or neuroblastoma, fever, abdominal mass, hepatosplenomegaly, or pathologic adenopathy may also be found. Plain radiographs are of obvious importance when tumor is considered; lesion location and radiologic appearance (density and peripheral margin) can be diagnostically significant. Complete blood cell count (CBC), CRP, and ESR are helpful in screening for possible infection or bone marrow neoplasm (see Chapter 106 Oncologic Emergencies).

Children with neurologic abnormalities will have diminished use of an arm because of weakness, with or without pain. An isolated monoplegia may be caused by a radiculopathy, plexopathy, or neuropathy that results from compression, inflammation, or injury. Trauma, particularly traction on the arm, is a common mechanism that leads to neurologic abnormalities (e.g., brachial plexus injury from birth); however, nontraumatic conditions may have an abrupt onset with no apparent antecedent illness. The child will have diminished arm movement, weakness, and may even experience pain; unlike the previously discussed causes of arm disuse, however,

TABLE 34.3

LIFE- AND LIMB-THREATENING CAUSES OF DIMINISHED ARM USE

Septic arthritis/osteomyelitis
Necrotizing cellulitis or fasciitis
Leukemia/other malignancy
Fracture with neurovascular compromise
Child abuse
Stroke

the pain (if present) is usually not reproducible with palpation and is not accompanied by swelling or redness. Reflexes may be diminished or absent. It is important to identify any associated neurologic abnormalities because facial or leg weakness may be subtle but would point to a lesion in the central nervous system.

Stroke is a rare cause of arm weakness in children and typically presents with an abrupt onset of hemiparesis (rather than isolated arm paresis). Children with sickle cell disease, structural heart disease, and coagulation disorders are at an increased risk for stroke. Although stroke may affect the arm more than the leg, suggesting a monoplegia, careful examination may reveal mild leg weakness, deep tendon reflex abnormalities, or extensor plantar response. Stroke may also have other associated neurologic signs such as headache, seizure, altered mental status, or speech difficulty.

There are several other neurologic conditions, which may lead to immobile arm. Todd's paralysis is a transient focal weakness that may occur after a seizure. The paralysis may be partial or complete. It is typically unilateral and although often a hemiparesis, it may be more prominent in one extremity. Complex migraine can be associated with focal motor deficits, usually hemiplegia. The evolution of symptoms is variable, but often includes scotomas, unilateral dysesthesia of the hand and mouth, and unilateral weakness (may involve only the arm and face, sparing the leg). These nonheadache symptoms may precede the headache by 30 to 60 minutes. Other features of migraine are often present and typically involve a headache, as well as nausea and vomiting. The neurologic symptoms typically last less than 24 hours. First episodes of hemiplegic migraine should only be diagnosed after acute stroke has been excluded by brain imaging.

Children with hemoglobinopathies (most commonly sickle cell disease) may present with decreased arm use because of stroke, or vasoocclusive crisis causing ischemia or infarction of bone marrow with acute bone pain. Long bones are commonly affected; however, young children frequently have involvement of the small bones of the hands and feet (dactylitis). Usually, no precipitating events are identified. The child experiences pain with localized tenderness and swelling of the involved areas; there may be associated warmth and erythema. Acutely, there are no bony abnormalities on radiographs. Because the "hand–foot syndrome" may be the first clinical manifestation of sickle cell disease, all children at risk for sickle cell disease with limb pain or swelling (or fever) must be screened for hemoglobinopathy if not tested previously. It is also particularly important to consider septic arthritis and osteomyelitis in children with sickle cell disease, as they are susceptible to infection, and the clinical findings may overlap with bone infarction, particularly if fever and leukocytosis are present (see Chapter 101 Hematologic Emergencies).

Several other much less common processes can cause decreased upper limb use. These include avascular necrosis of the humeral head or capitellum in otherwise healthy children, complex regional pain syndrome (reflex sympathetic dystrophy), and conversion disorder.

EVALUATION AND DECISION

The evaluation of the child who has diminished arm movement consists of a complete history and a thorough physical examination, with radiologic studies and laboratory tests when indicated. On the basis of these findings, appropriate management can be undertaken.

A history of any trauma should be ascertained. Details of the event may provide clues to the type of injury incurred; a fall onto an outstretched hand may cause a wrist, forearm, or elbow injury, whereas a sudden arm pull by a caregiver can cause dislocation or subluxation of the radial head ("nursemaid's elbow"). Of note is that some children with radial head subluxation may have a mechanism of injury other than a pull. If an immediate causative traumatic event is not elicited, the duration, course, and pattern of diminished arm use should be clarified. Fever, malaise, rash, or weight loss may give clues to a systemic illness. If the patient is an infant, it should be determined whether the arm disuse was from birth: a difficult delivery may lead to clavicular fractures or brachial plexus injuries. It should be remembered that infants do not always mount a febrile response to infection and may have only nonspecific symptoms of diminished feeding, increased sleeping, lethargy, or irritability. General medical history should include any history of inflammatory process, hemophilia, or sickle cell disease.

After a careful history, a physical examination should be performed. Fever should be noted and may be indicative of infection or, less likely, inflammatory or neoplastic process. Observation and inspection, sometimes from a distance, can provide information that might otherwise be unobtainable because many children cry when approached or touched by a stranger. The position of the arm should be noted. A child with nursemaid's elbow often holds the arm pronated and slightly flexed with obvious diminished movement, although often without apparent discomfort; a child with neurologic abnormality may hold the arm limply at the side of the body. Close inspection for areas of deformity, redness, swelling, or bruising should be done. Observation of the child's reach and grasp for an interesting object can provide information about the active range of motion and neurologic function. The clinician should palpate from clavicle to fingertips to identify areas of warmth, swelling, or tenderness (often best accomplished in the younger child while he or she is being distracted). Joints should be assessed for warmth, swelling, tenderness, and range of motion; however, if a history of trauma is present, manipulation can be deferred until an acute fracture has been excluded. Neurovascular integrity of the arm should be assessed carefully. A thorough general examination for rash, other joint abnormalities, hepatosplenomegaly, adenopathy, abnormal mass, and neurologic status should be performed, particularly for children without an obvious injury.

Plain radiographs are one of the most useful studies for evaluating children with diminished arm use. They may reveal a fracture or dislocation, joint effusion, or lytic bone lesion. If a discrete area of tenderness is identified, radiographs of that location, including the joint above and below, should be obtained. If the focus of pain is not apparent, it may be necessary to obtain radiographs of the entire limb from clavicle and shoulder to fingers.

A CBC may help in the diagnosis of infection, inflammation, malignancy, or hemoglobinopathy. Although nonspecific, an ESR or CRP may be useful in differentiating inflammatory or infectious processes from other causes.

Other tests helpful in selected cases include blood culture (if an infectious process is suspected), hemoglobin electrophoresis (if sickle cell disease is a possibility), bone scan, or MRI (for osteomyelitis, septic arthritis, or aseptic necrosis). If septic

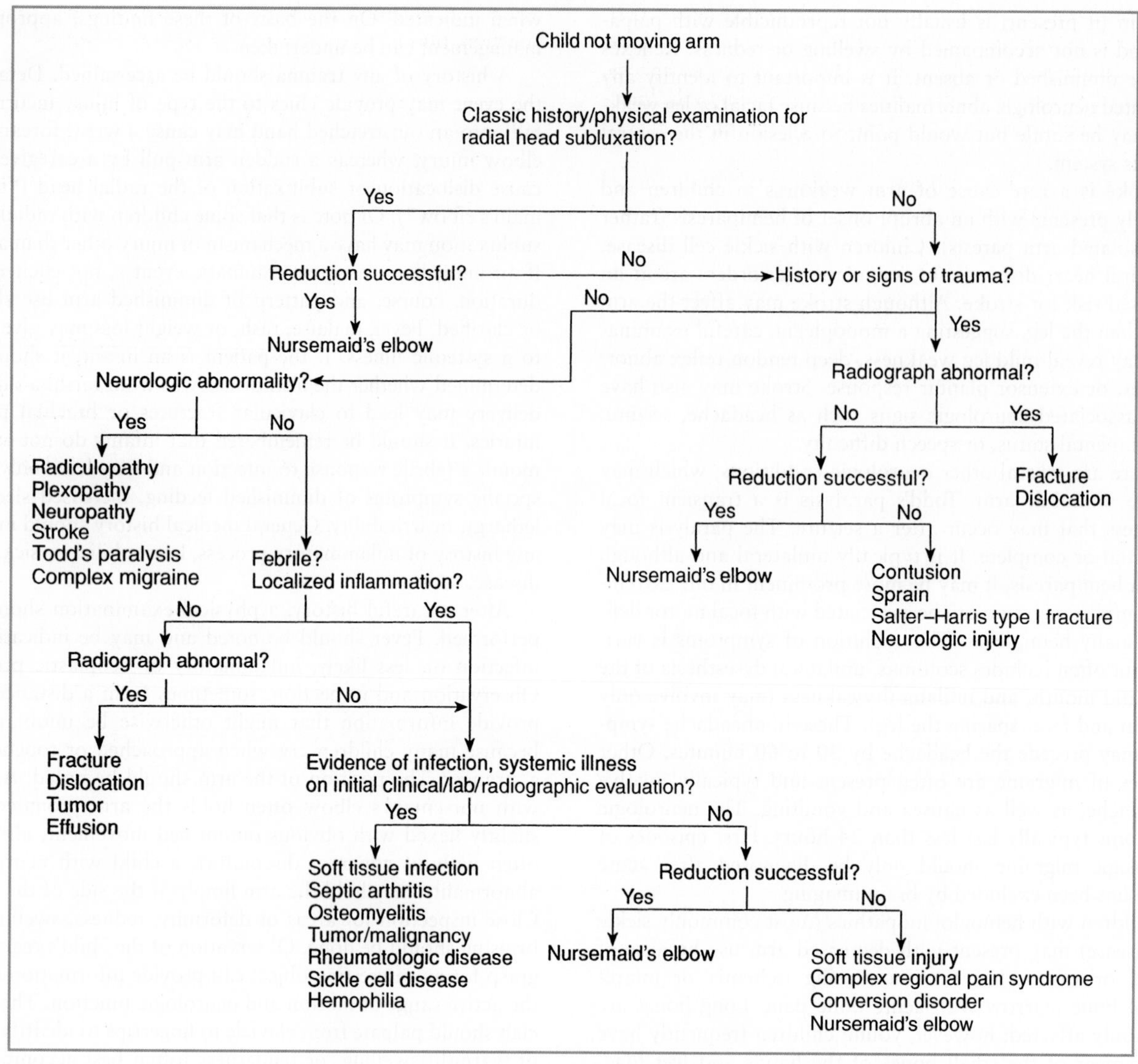

FIGURE 34.1 Approach to the child with diminished arm use.

arthritis or osteomyelitis is suspected, evaluation and treatment should proceed urgently. In the case of septic arthritis, arthrocentesis is imperative.

When a child is brought for the evaluation of diminished arm use, the physician should first determine whether this resulted from a specific traumatic event (Fig. 34.1). If the history is classic for radial head subluxation, the patient is holding the arm pronated and slightly flexed, there is no localized tenderness or swelling, and pain is elicited with slight pronation/supination, then the physician may attempt reduction (see Figure 129.11). If the child does not regain full use of the arm quickly, as in all other cases of trauma, radiographs should be obtained. In many cases, the radiographic studies provide the diagnosis (e.g., fracture, dislocation). Normal radiographs in the setting of acute trauma usually imply soft tissue injury and the patient should be treated symptomatically with close follow-up, provided that neurovascular integrity is established. If radiographs appear normal but the child has reproducible tenderness localized to the epiphyseal plate, then the patient should be presumptively treated for a Salter–Harris type I fracture. Occasionally, a child with a nursemaid's elbow may have an atypical history (e.g., "fell onto arm"); if radiographs exclude a fracture but the patient is holding the arm in a characteristic position, an attempt at reduction should be performed.

Children with neurologic abnormalities should be evaluated urgently to localize the site and cause of the impairment; the appropriate subspecialist (neurologist, neurosurgeon) should be involved.

If the child has no clear history of trauma but is afebrile with no obvious localized findings of infection, the limb should be evaluated radiographically. Abnormalities revealed might include fracture, dislocation, tumor, or effusion. If radiographs are normal in these children, one could consider obtaining a CBC, ESR, CRP, and blood culture, to evaluate for occult infectious or inflammatory processes. Hemoglobin electrophoresis should be considered for possible sickle cell disease in the appropriate clinical context, if prior screening has not been performed.

Children who are febrile, have signs of localized inflammation (e.g., warm, swollen joint), or have evidence of systemic illness should have a CBC and ESR, CRP, and blood culture tests in addition to radiographs. On the basis of specific findings, further evaluation might include arthrocentesis, bone scan, MRI, or rheumatologic tests. When the initial history, physical examination, laboratory tests, and radiographs localize the site and etiology of the pathology, the physician can begin specific management.

Some children with no history of trauma in whom a thorough initial evaluation is unrevealing will have a nursemaid's elbow. Therefore, an attempt at reduction is warranted in selected cases. Children with persistently diminished arm movement who are afebrile and nontoxic, with no localized findings, normal neurovascular function, and normal laboratory tests, likely have an occult soft tissue injury and can be managed as outpatients. A few of these children may have indolent pathologic processes or occult fractures; therefore, close follow-up must be ensured. These patients should be reevaluated every few days until normal arm use is regained or until evidence of a pathologic process develops. If arm disuse persists, a more extensive evaluation to diagnose or exclude occult fracture, infection, tumor, or inflammatory process is in order.

Suggested Readings and Key References

Aylor M, Anderson JM, Vanderford P, et al. Videos in clinical medicine. Reduction of pulled elbow. *N Engl J Med* 2014;371(21):e32. http://www.nejm.org/doi/full/10.1056/NEJMvcm1211809

Browner EA. Nursemaid's elbow (annular ligament displacement). *Pediatr Rev* 2013;34(8):366–367.

Carson S, Woolridge DP, Colletti J, et al. Pediatric upper extremity injuries. *Pediatr Clin North Am* 2006;53:41–67.

Eismann EA, Cosco ED, Wall EJ. Absence of radiographic abnormalities in nursemaid's elbow. *J Pediatr Orthop* 2014;34(4):426–431.

Fenichel GM. *Clinical pediatric neurology: a signs and symptoms approach*. 5th ed. Philadelphia, PA: Elsevier Saunders, 2005.

Rudloe TF, Schutzman S, Lee L, et al. No longer a "nursemaid's" elbow: mechanisms, caregivers, and prevention. *Pediatr Emerg Care* 2012; 28(8):771–774.

CHAPTER 35 ▪ INJURY: ANKLE

FRANCES TURCOTTE BENEDICT, MD, MPH AND ANGELA C. ANDERSON, MD, FAAP

Approximately 26% of sports-related injuries in school-aged children involve the ankle. It is often difficult for children to localize pain, therefore young children with ankle injuries may complain of pain anywhere from their mid-calf to their toes. Conversely, pathology in the lower leg and foot can cause referred pain to the ankle.

The ankle joint is composed of three bones: The tibia, the fibula, and the talus. The bony prominence of the distal fibula constitutes the lateral malleolus, whereas the prominence of the distal tibia forms the medial malleolus. The physes are located 1 to 2 fingerbreadths above the distal ends of the tibia and the fibula.

The ankle ligaments are attached to the epiphyses. The distal fibular physis is the most commonly injured growth plate in the lower extremities. It is second only to the distal radius in the incidence of physeal injuries.

Growth plates and bones are weaker than ligaments. Consequently, ankle trauma in preadolescent children is much more likely to cause fractures of the physis and the adjacent epiphysis and/or metaphysis than ligamentous injuries or sprains.

DIFFERENTIAL DIAGNOSIS

A number of traumatic injuries may cause ankle pain (Table 35.1). Although trauma is the most common cause of ankle pain in children, infectious, rheumatologic, inflammatory, neoplastic, and hematologic abnormalities also should be considered (Table 35.2) because trauma may occasionally merely exacerbate pain in children with underlying conditions. Again, keep in mind that a complaint of ankle pain may result from a lesion anywhere between the knee and the toe, particularly in preverbal children. The most common injuries vary according to age (Table 35.3).

ANKLE FRACTURES

Fractures of the ankle account for 5.5% of all fractures in pediatrics. The system used to classify ankle fractures in children differs from the one used in adults because of the presence of growth plates and the possible implications of physeal injuries. The Salter–Harris (S-H) classification is most commonly applied, as described in Chapter 119 Musculoskeletal Trauma.

Inversion ankle injuries in preadolescents most commonly cause a S-H type I fracture of the distal fibula (Fig. 35.1). Clinically, the patient presents with swelling about the lateral malleolus and tenderness at the distal fibular physis. Fractures confined to the physes may not be visible on radiographs. Consequently, routine radiographs may appear normal despite the presence of a fracture.

In severe inversion injuries, the distal fibular fracture described previously may be accompanied by a fracture of the medial malleolus (Fig. 35.2). This medial malleolus fracture is usually a S-H type III or IV fracture of the distal tibia. These patients will have tenderness at the medial malleolus and the distal fibular physis.

Fractures resulting from eversion of the ankle are usually a combination of a S-H type II fracture of the lateral tibia and a transverse fracture of the fibula (Fig. 35.3). The fibular fracture is relatively high (4 to 7 cm above the fibular physis). Therefore, it is important to examine the full length of the fibula in patients with ankle injuries.

Direct axial compression of the ankle is uncommon but can cause a S-H type V injury to the distal tibia.

External rotation injuries are responsible for lesions known as transitional fractures. Transitional fractures occur during adolescence when closure of the growth plates is beginning. Closure of the distal tibial physis starts centrally and then spreads medially, posteriorly, and finally laterally. The distal tibial physis closes before the distal fibular physis. As skeletal maturity (and physeal closure) progresses, the relative strengths of various parts of the tibia change. As a result, the same mechanism of injury may cause very different fracture patterns, depending on the age of the patient. The juvenile Tillaux fracture and the triplane fractures are examples of transitional fractures.

In the juvenile Tillaux fracture, a fragment of bone is torn off the lateral border of the tibia by the anterior tibiofibular ligament (Fig. 35.4). It is a S-H type III injury of the distal tibia. This fracture is seen almost exclusively in patients between the ages of 12 and 14 years. This is because the closure of the medial aspect of the distal tibial physis begins around 12 to 14 years of age, whereas the lateral aspect remains open and therefore less stable for approximately another 18 months. The greater the skeletal maturity of the patient, the more lateral the epiphyseal fracture line occurs.

Diagnosis of a juvenile Tillaux fracture may be difficult because routine radiographs may not show the fracture line well. If displacement is minimal, the only radiographic sign may be a slight widening of the lateral tibial physis or a faint vertical fracture line through the epiphysis on anteroposterior (AP) or oblique views. In some cases, the only finding may be local tenderness in the area of the lateral tibial physis. Multiple oblique views, or computed tomography (CT), may be needed to adequately delineate the extent of the fracture.

Growth arrest and angular deformity are rare because these fractures occur at the time of physeal closure. However, ankle joint arthritis may complicate the long-term outcome if the diagnosis is missed or if reduction is inadequate.

Triplanar fractures are characterized by a fracture line that runs in three planes: Coronal, sagittal, and transverse. Two types of triplane fractures have been described. The first is a three-fragment fracture (Fig. 35.5). The first fragment is the same as the one found in the juvenile Tillaux fracture—a fragment of the epiphysis torn off the anterolateral quadrant of the tibia. The second fragment is the remaining medial part

TABLE 35.1

DIFFERENTIAL DIAGNOSIS OF TRAUMATIC INJURIES THAT CAUSE ANKLE PAIN

Leg
Tibial fractures (toddler's fracture)
Fibular fractures
Contusions
Compartment syndrome of the calf
Ankle
Fractures
Distal tibial
Distal fibular
Physeal
Sprains
Contusions
Osteochondritis dissecans
Hemarthrosis
Foot
Fractures
Talar
Navicular
Fifth metatarsal (Jones or pseudo-Jones fracture)
Calcaneal
Sprains
Contusions

TABLE 35.2

DIFFERENTIAL DIAGNOSIS OF ANKLE PAIN

Trauma
Fractures
Sprains
Contusions
Osteochondritis dissecans
Hemarthrosis
Inflammatory
Tendonitis
Synovitis
Periostitis
Sever disease (calcaneal apophysitis)
Infectious
Osteomyelitis
Soft tissue abscess
Septic joint
Brodie abscess (subacute osteomyelitis of the distal tibia)
Rheumatologic
Juvenile idiopathic arthritis
Rheumatic fever
Reiter syndrome
Hematologic
Sickle cell disease (pain crisis)
Hemophilia (hemarthrosis)
Osteochondroses (avascular necrosis)
Kohler disease (navicular)
Freiberg disease (second metatarsal)
Tumors
Ewing sarcoma
Osteoid osteoma

of the epiphysis, which is attached to a posterior spike of the metaphyseal bone. The third fragment is the tibial shaft.

A two-fragment fracture has also been described. The first fragment is again the lateral tibial epiphysis, but it is attached to a posterior spike of the metaphyseal bone. The second fragment is the remaining medial epiphysis and is attached to the tibial shaft (Fig. 35.6).

On a radiograph, triplanar fractures have the appearance of a S-H type III fracture on the AP view and a S-H type II fracture on the lateral view. If only the AP view is obtained, it may be difficult to distinguish these fractures from the juvenile Tillaux fracture. The key to diagnosis is the posterior metaphyseal spike seen on the lateral film.

ANKLE SPRAINS

Ankle sprains in children or preadolescents are less common than fractures because the ligaments in this age group are much stronger than growth plates or even bone. If a ligamentous injury occurs in a child with an open growth plate, an associated avulsion fracture is almost always present. However, once skeletal maturity is reached, ankle sprains become the most common of sports injuries.

Inversion injuries cause 85% of ankle sprains. The most commonly injured structures are the lateral ligaments. Three lateral ligaments support the ankle joint: The anterior talofibular (ATFL), the calcaneofibular (CFL), and the posterior talofibular (PTFL) (Fig. 35.7). The ATFL is the weakest and most commonly injured of the three. The CFL is intermediate in strength and is rarely injured without an associated tear of the ATFL. The PTFL is the strongest and least injured of the lateral ligaments. Because its fibers run horizontally, only extreme dorsiflexion will stress this ligament. The peroneus brevis tendon also traverses the lateral aspect of the ankle

TABLE 35.3

COMMON INJURIES ASSOCIATED WITH ANKLE PAIN ACCORDING TO AGE

Toddler	Child	Adolescent
Spiral fracture of the tibia	Salter–Harris type I fracture of the distal fibula	Ankle sprain
Soft tissue contusion	Soft tissue contusion	Soft tissue contusion

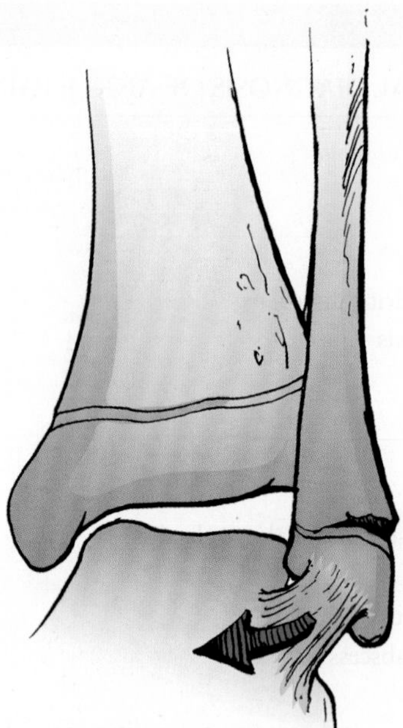

FIGURE 35.1 Inversion injury.

joint and can be injured by inversion stress. It inserts at the base of the fifth metatarsal.

Eversion injuries account for 15% of ankle sprains. The deltoid ligament, which supports the medial aspect of the ankle, is most commonly affected by this mechanism (Fig. 35.8). It is composed of deep and superficial fibers. Eversion may also cause disruption of the tibiofibular syndesmosis, which connects the distal tibia and the fibula.

Classification of Ankle Sprains

There are many systems of classification for ankle sprains. Table 35.4 provides guidelines that can be used in grading injuries to the lateral ligaments.

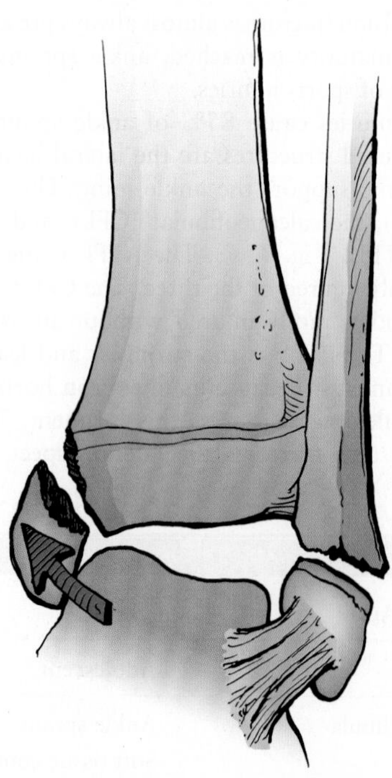

FIGURE 35.2 Severe inversion injury.

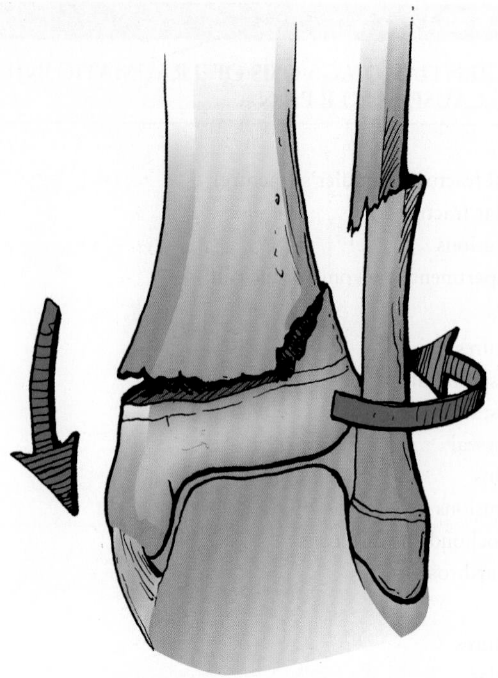

FIGURE 35.3 Eversion injury.

Injuries Associated with Ankle Sprains

Approximately 7% of ankle sprains are accompanied by osteochondral fractures of the talus. The medial dome is more commonly fractured than the lateral dome. Avulsions of the

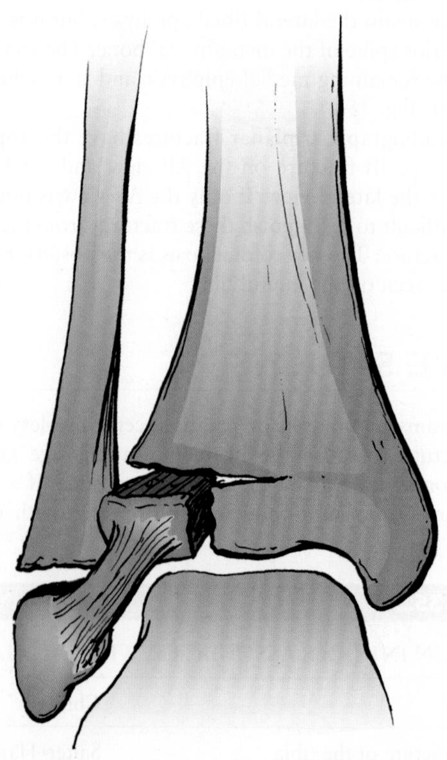

FIGURE 35.4 Juvenile Tillaux fracture or Salter–Harris type III fracture of the distal tibial physis; the medial part of the tibial physis is fused.

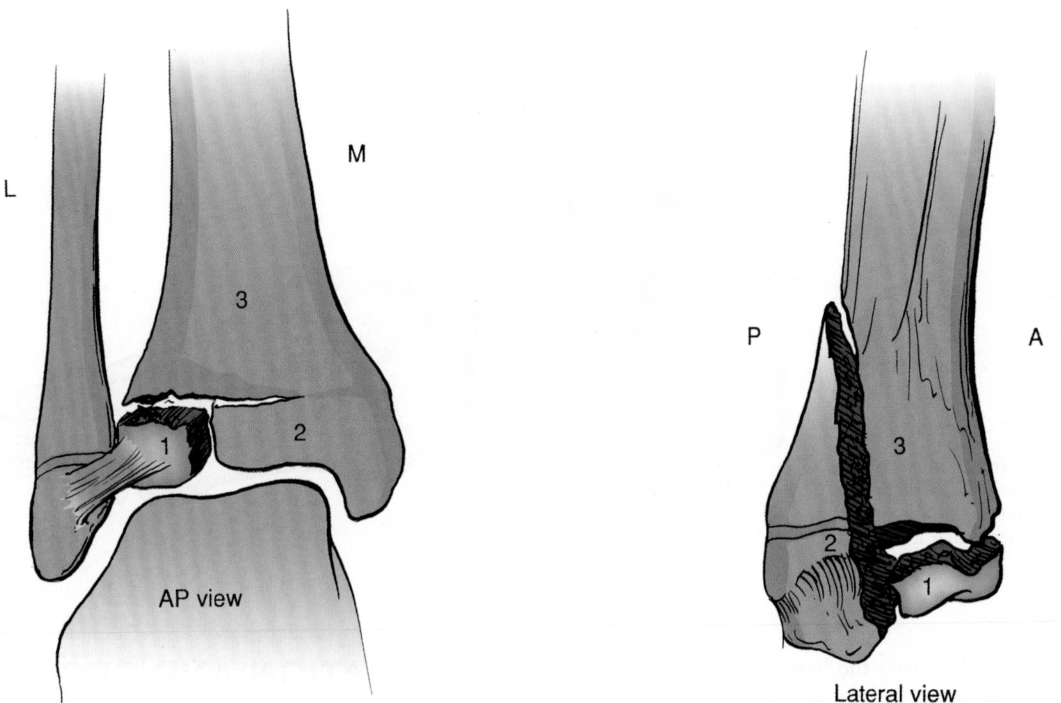

FIGURE 35.5 Anteroposterior and lateral views of three-fragment triplanar fracture. L, lateral; M, medial; P, posterior; A, anterior.

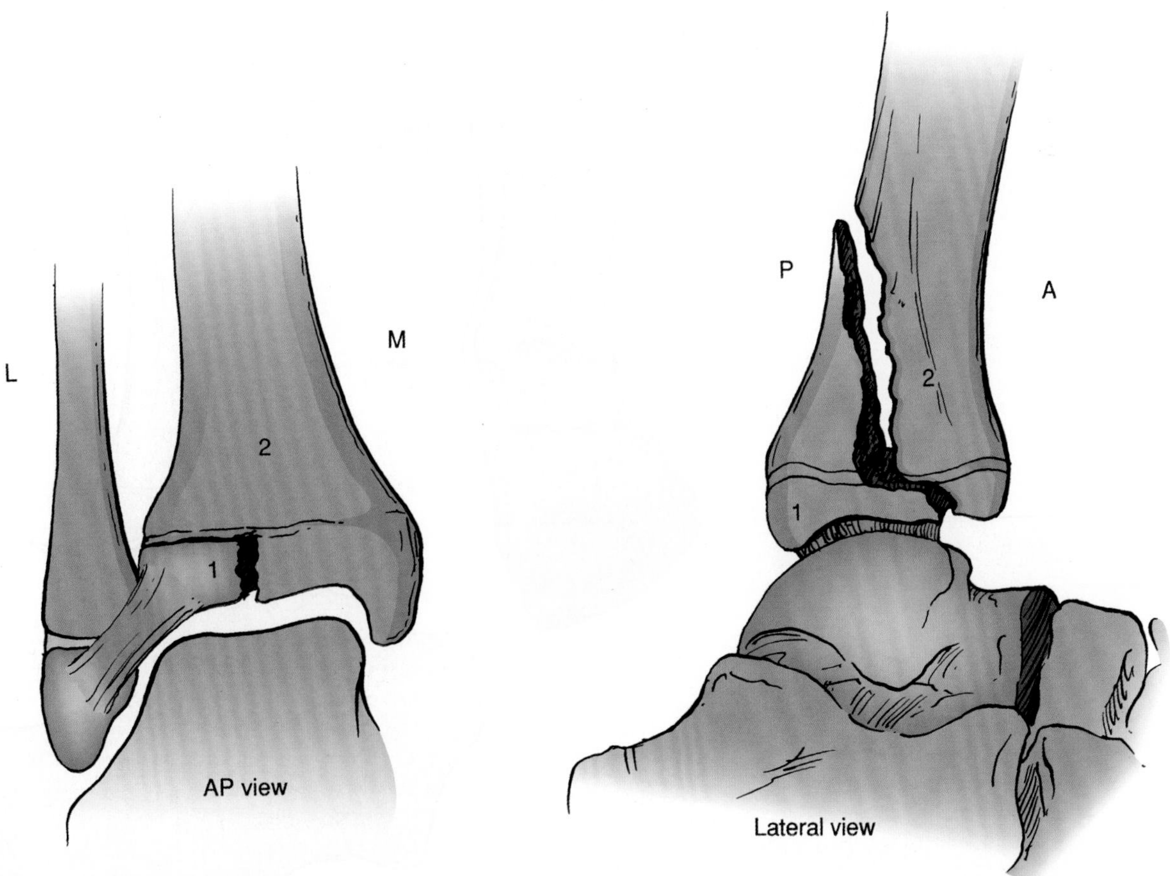

FIGURE 35.6 Anteroposterior and lateral views of two-fragment triplanar fracture. L, lateral; M, medial; P, posterior; A, anterior.

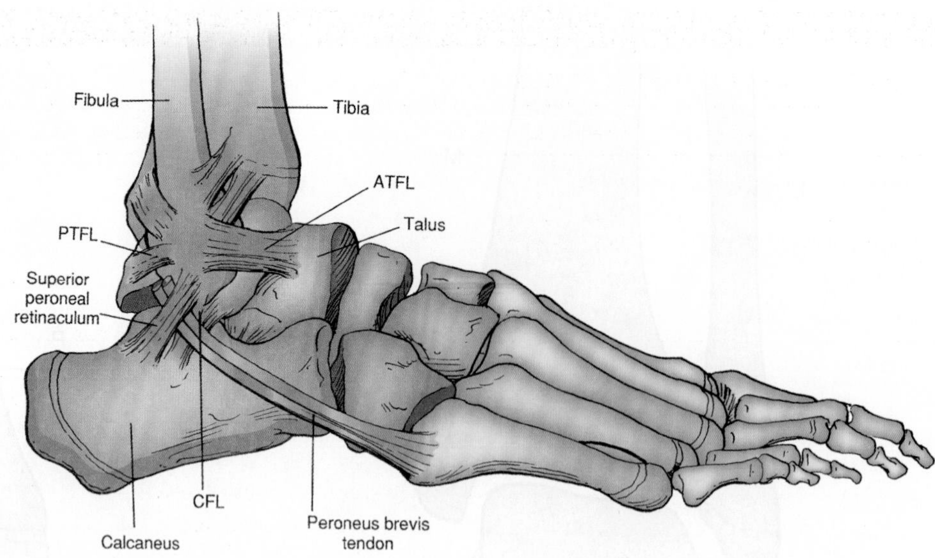

FIGURE 35.7 Lateral view of the ankle. ATFL, anterior talofibular ligament; PTFL, posterior talofibular ligament; CFL, calcaneofibular ligament.

peroneus brevis tendon from the base of the fifth metatarsal have been observed in up to 14% of patients with ankle ligament ruptures. If this injury occurs in children younger than 15 years, the avulsed fragment is usually an apophysis and is considered a S-H type I injury, often called a pseudo-Jones fracture. In older patients, the displaced portion represents a bony fragment from the metaphyseal–diaphyseal junction and is known as a Jones fracture.

EVALUATION AND DECISION

History

Trying to obtain a reliable history in ankle injuries can be difficult. Commonly, the description is: "I twisted it and it hurts." Nevertheless, the mechanism of injury, if obtainable, can provide a clue to the diagnosis. Other questions include

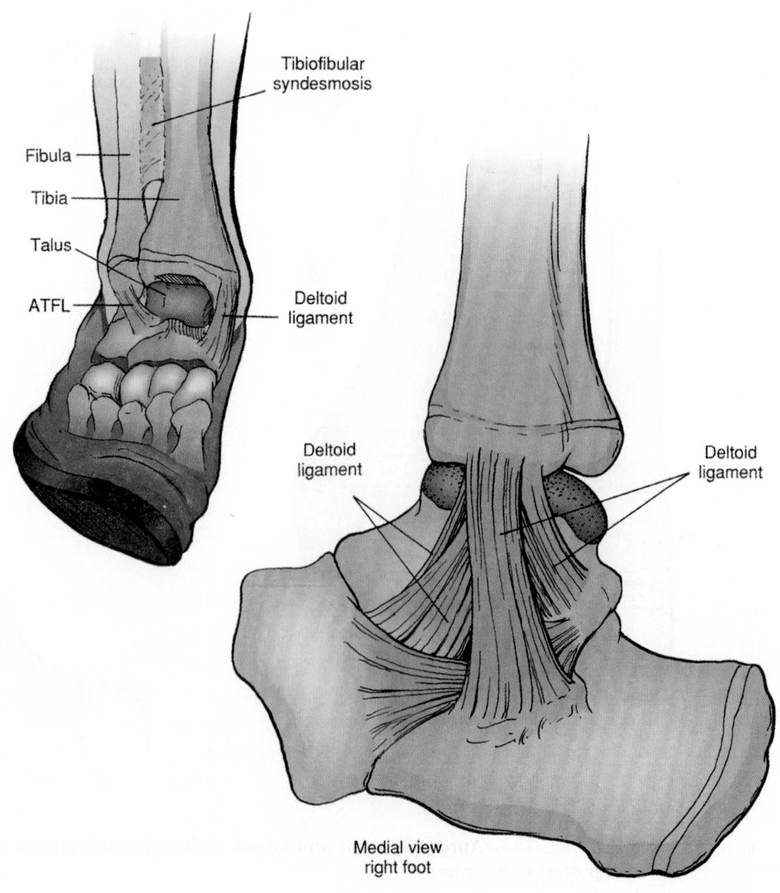

FIGURE 35.8 Ankle eversion injury. ATFL, anterior talofibular ligament.

TABLE 35.4

CLASSIFICATION OF ANKLE SPRAINS

	Grade I: Mild sprain	Grade II: Moderate sprain	Grade III: Severe sprain
Ligament injury	Minor	Near complete tear	Complete rupture
Swelling	Mild	Moderate	Severe
Tenderness	Mild, local	Moderate, diffuse	Marked
Functional loss	Minimal	Ambulates with difficulty	Inability to bear weight
Joint stability	Stable	No/mild instability	Unstable

the following: (i) When did the injury occur? (ii) Did swelling occur immediately or gradually? (iii) Is there a history of any previous injury to that limb? and (iv) Does the patient have a history of any other medical problems—osseous, neurologic, or muscular disease?

A history of fever, rash, or other joint involvement, in combination with a history of minimal or no trauma, suggests nontraumatic diagnoses such as septic joint, arthritis, or collagen vascular disease.

Physical Examination

General Inspection

Look for obvious deformities, open wounds, loss of anatomic landmarks, local swelling, and ecchymosis. If an obvious deformity is present, keep manipulation of the extremity to a minimum and assess neurovascular status promptly. Any break in the skin may communicate with the joint space or constitute an open fracture. The need for antibiotic coverage must be evaluated immediately.

Neurovascular Evaluation

Palpate the dorsalis pedis and posterior tibial arteries. Note skin temperature, color, and capillary refill. The absence of pulses or the presence of pallor requires immediate attention. A Doppler device may help identify pulses.

Vascular compromise is usually caused by a posterior dislocation. Traction reduction of the deformity should be attempted as rapidly as is feasible by performing the following steps: (i) Sedate the patient; (ii) apply longitudinal traction to the foot; (iii) if relocation is not accomplished in step (ii), apply longitudinal traction and pull the foot in a posterior to anterior direction; and (iv) immobilize the ankle and obtain radiographs. If the vascular status has not been compromised, continue with the examination and evaluate the nerves that cross the ankle. Test soft touch and pain sensation of the foot.

Bony Palpation

Trace all three bones of the ankle joint (tibia, fibula, and talus), searching for areas of point tenderness. It is very important to palpate the distal tibial and fibular physes because fractures in these areas may not be evident on radiographs. Any tenderness found along a physis should be considered a S-H type I fracture at the least, even if radiographic studies are negative. Also keep in mind that the only clue to a juvenile Tillaux fracture may be tenderness at the lateral tibial physis. Remember to palpate the fibula proximal to the ankle joint; external rotation and triplanar injuries may be associated with high fibular fractures.

Finally, examine the foot. This should include palpation of the dome of the talus. This is performed most easily with the foot in plantar flexion. Palpate the base of the fifth metatarsal. Tenderness here suggests an avulsion of the peroneus brevis tendon.

Once one area of point tenderness is found, continue to examine the entire joint. A single injury may cause many abnormalities.

Ligament Palpation

Palpate for tenderness along all three lateral ligaments, remembering that each one arises from the distal fibula. The ATFL can be further tested by inverting and plantar flexing the foot. This will increase pain if injury to this ligament is present. Swelling extending beyond an area of lateral ligament tenderness is highly suggestive of significant ligament injury.

Examine the superficial fibers of deltoid ligament on the medial aspect of the joint. The deep fibers are intra-articular and nonpalpable; therefore, rupture may be present without much medial tenderness. Isolated injuries to the deltoid ligament are rare because of the great strength of this ligament. If the deltoid ligament has been damaged, the tibiofibular syndesmosis is usually disrupted along with it.

Injuries to the tibiofibular syndesmosis may be explored by (i) squeezing the midshafts of the tibia and the fibula together, (ii) dorsiflexing and then externally rotating the foot while holding the tibia and the fibula stable, or (iii) forcefully dorsiflexing the ankle with the patient supine. Exacerbation of pain with these maneuvers suggests syndesmotic disruption.

Stability Testing

An attempt should be made to assess the stability of the ankle joint. However, stability testing in the immediate postinjury period may be limited significantly by pain, swelling, and/or muscle spasm. Several maneuvers are useful, but they are generally not performed if an ankle fracture is present.

- *Anterior drawer test*—The ATFL is the only structure that prevents forward subluxation of the talus. The anterior drawer test assesses the anterior stability of the ankle joint and the integrity of the ATFL (Fig. 35.9). The test result is positive if the foot can be pulled forward by more than 4 mm or if there is a significant difference in the degree of anterior movement in the injured ankle compared with the normal ankle.
- *Talar tilt test*—This test examines the lateral stability of the ankle joint. Firmly adducting the heel, looking for increased laxity compared with the noninjured joint (Fig. 35.9). Both the ATFL and CFL must be torn to cause gross lateral ankle instability.

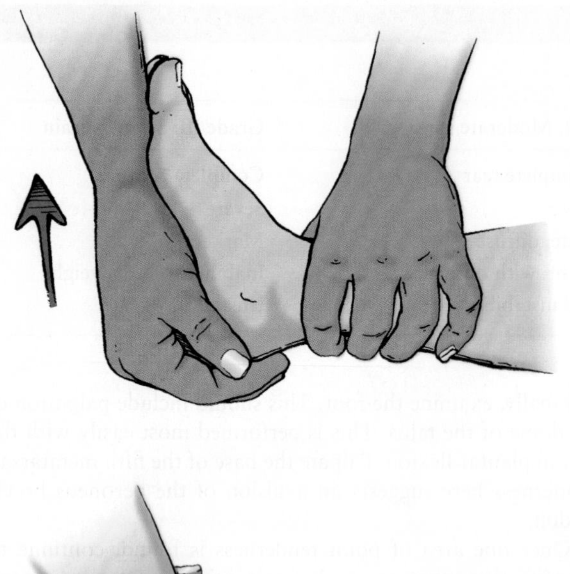

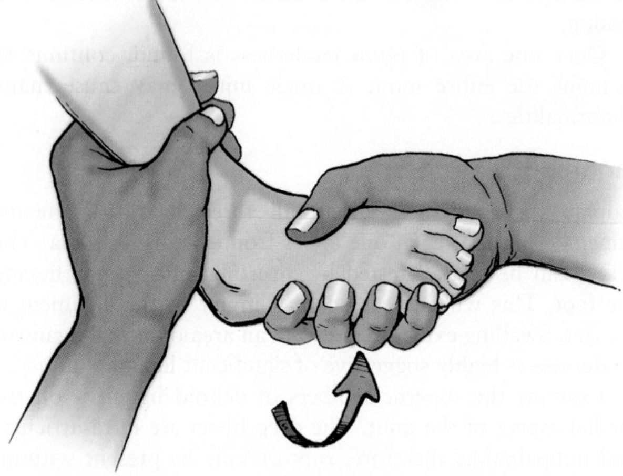

FIGURE 35.9 **Top:** The anterior drawer test is performed by placing the patient's heel in the palm of the examiner's hand with the ankle at a 90-degree angle to the long axis of the leg. The examiner gently, but firmly, moves the heel and foot forward (*arrow*). **Bottom:** In the talar tilt maneuver, the heel is firmly adducted (*arrow*) and assessed for increased laxity or instability compared with the noninjured side.

Radiographic Imaging

The Ottawa ankle rules (OAR) are used to predict radiographically evident ankle fractures in adults. The OAR maintain that ankle radiographs are required only if the patient has pain near the malleoli and one or both of the following: (i) Inability to bear weight immediately following the injury and in the emergency department (four steps) and (ii) bone tenderness at the posterior edge or tip of either malleolus. These rules are 100% sensitive in detecting clinically significant fractures in adults; pediatric studies caution the use of OARs to predict ankle fractures in children less than 6 years of age but in older children the OAR are 98.5% sensitive and reduce ankle radiography by 24.8%. The Low Risk Ankle Rule (LRAR) states that radiography may not be indicated to exclude a high-risk ankle injury (fracture of the foot, distal tibia and fibula proximal to the distal physis, tibiofibular syndesmosis injury, and ankle dislocations) if tenderness and swelling is isolated to the distal fibula and/or adjacent lateral ligaments distal to the tibial anterior joint line. Low-risk ankle injuries include lateral ankle sprains, nondisplaced S-H type I and II fractures of the distal fibula, and avulsion fractures of the distal fibula and lateral talus. One study found the LRAR to be 100% sensitive in children of ages 3 to 18 and reduced ankle radiography by 20%.

Radiographic evaluation of the ankle should include at least three views: AP, lateral, and mortise. If tenderness of the proximal fibula is noted, full-length views of the fibula are essential. Tenderness at the base of the fifth metatarsal mandates visualization of this area on the lateral film. If radiographic findings are questionable, consider obtaining comparison views of the noninjured ankle.

Note areas of soft tissue swelling. This may be the only clue to a S-H type I fracture of the distal fibula. Stress radiographs to evaluate growth plate injuries are rarely necessary and may cause further damage. Ultrasound may be a useful adjunct in identifying radiographic occult ankle fractures.

CT scan of the ankle is often necessary to fully evaluate triplane and juvenile Tillaux fractures. Magnetic resonance imaging (MRI) of ankle injuries is rarely performed during acute evaluation but may be useful in evaluating patients in whom one has a high clinical suspicion of injury despite normal radiographs. MRI may also delineate suspected tendon and ligament injuries in selected circumstances.

Approach

The approach (Fig. 35.10) to the evaluation and diagnosis of traumatic ankle injuries relies primarily on physical findings and the results of radiographic evaluation. Initially, pulses and sensation are assessed. Loss of pulses and/or sensation suggests a fracture/dislocation and the need for a rapid reduction; when available without delay, orthopedic consultation is advisable. After providing analgesia, immobilize the site to prevent further compromise, and obtain a radiograph. If neurovascular status is adequate and the general inspection reveals no obvious abnormalities, proceed with the rest of the physical examination as described previously.

Next, examine the area for open wounds. If present, apply a sterile saline dressing and immobilize the extremity before obtaining a radiograph. Consider administering intravenous antibiotics and tetanus prophylaxis.

If radiographic studies indicate a fracture or dislocation, provide treatment of the specific injury (see Chapter 119 Musculoskeletal Trauma). Administer analgesia as needed.

If no fracture is evident on the radiograph, but tenderness is elicited over a physis, the diagnosis of a S-H type I injury can be made and appropriate immobilization is performed (see Chapter 119 Musculoskeletal Trauma). One study demonstrated that approximately 18% of children with tenderness at the distal fibular physis and normal radiographs will develop new periosteal bone formation, thus implying the presence of an occult fracture. A negative radiographic result in the absence of bony tenderness suggests the diagnosis of contusion or ligamentous injury. A stable ankle in a patient who has pain with ligamentous stress or palpation characterizes a grade I sprain. A grade II sprain is more severe; instability is insignificant. Joint instability indicates a torn ligament and a grade III sprain.

TREATMENT

Fractures

Fracture reduction is usually accomplished by reversing the mechanism of injury. Closed reduction and a short leg cast are

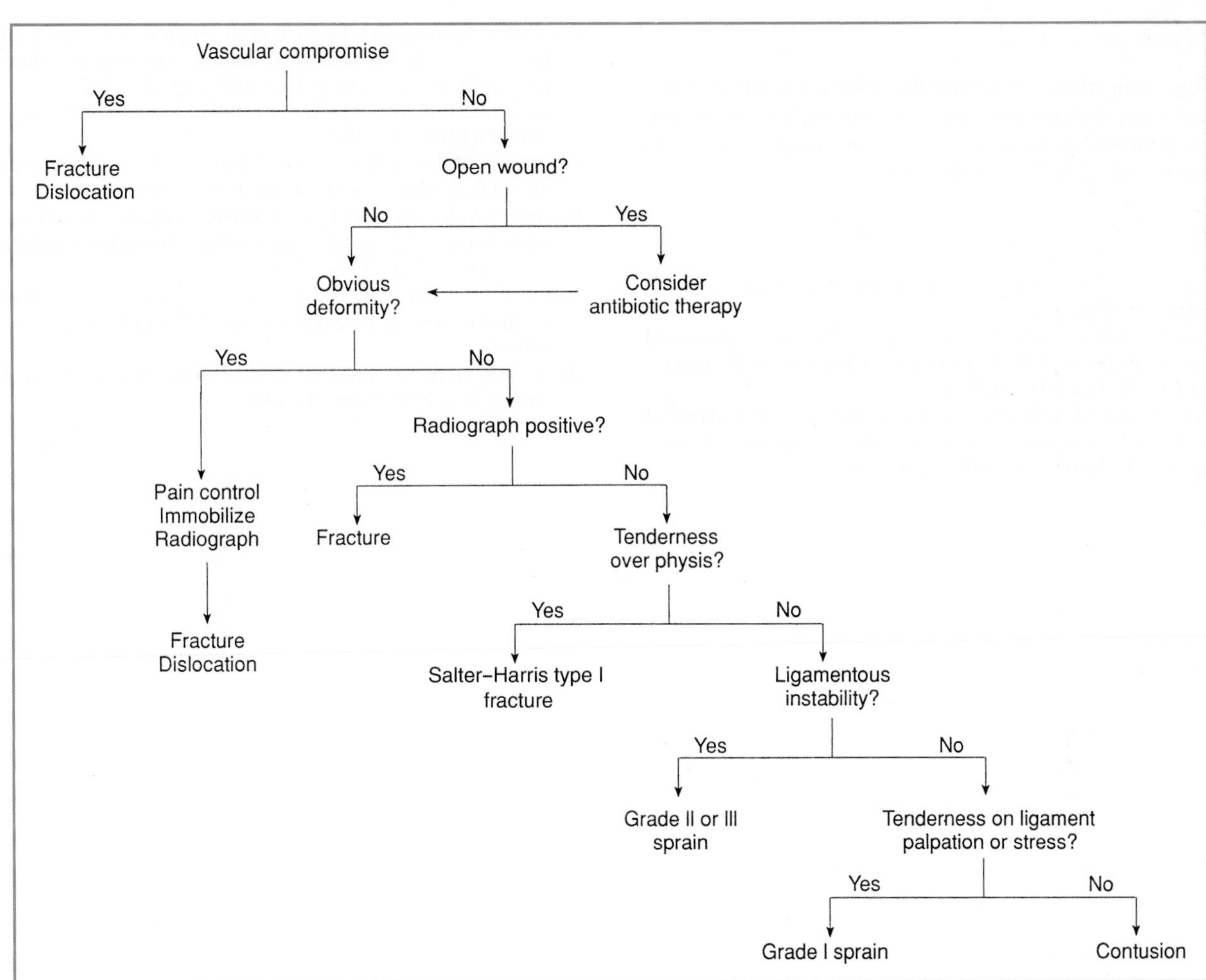

FIGURE 35.10 Evaluation and diagnosis of traumatic ankle injuries.

usually adequate for S-H type I and II fractures of the distal tibia and the fibula (see Chapter 119 Musculoskeletal Trauma). Some displacement can be accepted in younger patients because of their ability to remodel. Two studies have suggested that children with nondisplaced S-H type I fractures may benefit from less conservative therapy; those treated with crutches, a 5-day period of nonweight bearing, and the use of a removable ankle brace (e.g., an air-stirrup ankle brace or an elastic bandage) were able to return to normal activity sooner than those in whom short leg casts were used. Patients in these studies advanced their activities as tolerated. S-H type III and IV injuries involve the articular surface and are therefore less stable. They require anatomic realignment, frequently by open reduction. A long leg cast is commonly applied in any rotational injury.

Sprains

A common approach to the treatment of ankle sprains is described by the "RICE" (rest, ice, compression, elevation) mnemonic. It should be initiated within 36 hours of the injury.

- *Rest*—The patient is allowed to ambulate/exercise only if the activity does not cause pain or swelling during or within 24 hours. Otherwise, crutches and light weight bearing are recommended until ambulation without pain is possible.
- *Ice*—Apply ice directly to the ankle for 20 minutes, every 2 hours if possible, for the first 48 hours postinjury.
- *Compression*—The purpose of compression is to keep (and/or push) fluid out of the area of the ankle joint. This can be accomplished using an elastic bandage starting at the foot and wrapping proximally toward the ankle. For additional compression, any bulky padding can be applied to the malleoli and then secured with an elastic wrap. The combined application of an elastic wrap covered with an air-stirrup ankle brace may allow for an earlier return to normal function than either device used alone.
- *Elevation*—To help decrease or prevent swelling, elevate the ankle as often as possible.

Splinting

If swelling or pain is severe, apply a stirrup and/or posterior splint to the ankle (see Chapter 141 Procedures, Splinting section). Air splints can also be used; they allow dorsiflexion and plantar flexion while maintaining medial and lateral stability.

Rehabilitation

Plantar flexion and dorsiflexion exercises initiated as soon as possible, followed by toe raises and inversion/eversion exercises may shorten the period of disability considerably.

Orthopedic Referral

Absolute indications for orthopedic referral include (i) obvious deformity with growth plate involvement, (ii) neurovascular compromise, (iii) suspected syndesmotic injury, (iv) a grade III sprain, and (v) locking of the ankle.

Suggested Readings and Key References

Anderson S. Lower extremity injuries in youth sports. *Pediatr Clin North Am* 2002;49:627–641.

Beynnon BD, Renström PA, Haugh L, et al. Prospective, randomized clinical investigation of the treatment of first-time ankle sprains. *Am J Sports Med* 2006;34:1401.

Boutis K, Willan AR, Babyn P, et al. A randomized, controlled trial of a removable brace versus casting in children with low-risk ankle fractures. *Pediatrics* 2007;119:e1256–e1263.

Dowling S, Spooner CH, Liang Y, et al. Accuracy of Ottawa Ankle Rules to exclude fractures of the ankle and midfoot in children: a meta-analysis. *Acad Emerg Med* 2009;16(4):277–287.

Halstead ME. Pediatric ankle sprains and their imitators. *Pediatr Ann* 2014;43(12):e291–e296.

Lassiter TE, Malone TR, Garrett WE. Injury to the lateral ligaments of the ankle. *Orthop Clin North Am* 1989;20:629.

Malanga GA, Ramirez Del Toro JA. Common injuries of the foot and ankle in the child and adolescent athlete. *Phys Med Rehabil Clin North Am* 2008;19(2):347–371, ix.

Sankar WN, Chen J, Kay RM, et al. Incidence of occult fracture in children with acute ankle injuries. *J Pediatr Orthop* 2008;28: 500–501.

Wuerz TH, Gurd DP. Pediatric physeal ankle fracture. *J Am Acad Orthop Surg* 2013;21(4):234–244.

CHAPTER 36 ▪ INJURY: HEAD

SARA A. SCHUTZMAN, MD AND REBEKAH MANNIX, MD, MPH

PEDIATRIC HEAD TRAUMA

Head injuries in children are common, accounting for approximately 500,000 emergency department (ED) visits per year in the United States. Although the majority of these injuries are minor, head trauma causes significant pediatric morbidity and mortality. Trauma is the leading cause of death in children older than 1 year, and traumatic brain injury is the leading cause of death and disability caused by trauma in children, resulting in more than 2,000 deaths annually.

The most common mechanism of injury for pediatric head trauma is falls, followed by motor vehicle and pedestrian accidents and bicycle injuries; the majority of fatal injuries occur secondary to motor vehicle–related accidents. The mechanism of head injury varies with age; younger children are more likely to suffer falls or abuse, whereas older children are often injured in sporting or motor vehicle accidents (in addition to falls).

Many of the serious neurologic complications of head injury are evident soon after the traumatic event; however, some life-threatening injuries can appear initially as minor head trauma. To manage head injuries best, the physician must approach the child in a systematic manner to address all injuries (global resuscitation is the first priority of cerebral resuscitation), identify and treat any neurologic complications, and prevent ongoing cerebral insult.

PATHOPHYSIOLOGY

Neurologic injury following head trauma is related to the unique physiology and pathophysiology of the brain and the intracranial environment. The brain is a semisolid structure bathed in cerebrospinal fluid (CSF) and covered by the fine inner pia-arachnoid membrane and the outer thick fibrous layer of dura, all of which are encased in the skull, which is covered by the five-layered structure of the scalp. After infancy (when the skull sutures fuse), the cranial vault becomes a stiff and poorly compliant structure housing the brain. Because the intracranial volume is relatively fixed, any change in the volume of one of the intracranial components (blood, brain, and CSF) must occur at the expense of the others; if the other components do not decrease proportionally, intracranial pressure (ICP) will increase.

Brain injury occurs in two phases: primary and secondary. The primary injury is the mechanical damage sustained at the time of trauma and can be caused by direct impact of the brain against the internal calvarial structures, by bone or foreign bodies projected into the brain, and by shear forces delivered to the white matter tracts. Secondary brain injury is further neuronal damage sustained after the traumatic event to cells not initially injured. This results from numerous causes, including hypoxia, hypoperfusion, and metabolic derangements, and may also result from sequelae of the primary injury (e.g., cerebral edema, expanding intracranial mass) or be caused by extracranial injuries (e.g., hypotension from excessive blood loss, hypoxia from pulmonary contusion). The clinician's goal is to identify and treat any complications of primary brain injury in order to limit further neuronal damage by secondary brain injury.

One of the most common causes of secondary brain injury is cerebral ischemia resulting from impaired perfusion. Cerebral perfusion pressure is the difference between the mean arterial pressure of blood flowing to the brain and the ICP. In the healthy child, blood flow to the brain is maintained at a constant rate over a wide range of systemic blood pressures by means of autoregulatory changes in the cerebrovascular resistance so that the brain does not suffer ischemia or excessive blood flow during periods of relative hypotension or hypertension, respectively. With severe injuries, this autoregulatory control may be lost and the cerebral blood flow can become directly dependent on the cerebral perfusion pressure; with low mean arterial pressure or increased ICP, there will be inadequate blood flow and cerebral ischemia results. In addition to potential for causing decreased cerebral perfusion, increased ICP, if left unchecked, can lead to brain herniation and compression. This may be caused by a number of posttraumatic conditions, including cerebral edema and expanding intracranial mass.

Clinical symptoms of increased ICP or herniation include headache, vomiting, irritability, lethargy, visual disturbance, gait abnormalities, and weakness. Signs include depressed level of consciousness, abnormal vital signs (bradycardia, hypertension, respiratory irregularity), cranial nerve palsies, hemiparesis, and decerebrate posturing. The classic findings in transtentorial herniation are headache, decreasing level of consciousness followed by ipsilateral pupillary dilatation (cranial nerve III palsy), and contralateral hemiparesis or posturing. If the process continues unchecked, dilatation of the opposite pupil, alteration in respirations, and ultimately, bradycardia and arrest ensue (see Chapter 105 Neurologic Emergencies).

DIFFERENTIAL DIAGNOSIS

Head trauma may cause injuries of the scalp, skull, and intracranial contents. Although each is discussed here separately, the clinician must remember that these injuries may occur alone or in combination, and all potential injuries must be considered when dealing with one.

Scalp

The scalp consists of five layers of soft tissue that cover the skull; contusions and lacerations of this structure are common results of head trauma. The outermost layers of the scalp are skin and the subcutaneous tissue; edema and hemorrhage here may produce a mobile swelling. The third layer, the galea aponeurotica, is a strong membranous sheet that connects the frontal and occipital bellies of the occipitofrontalis muscle. The remaining two layers deep to the galea are the loose areolar tissue and pericranium. Subgaleal hematomas may result from more forceful blows as vessels in the fourth layer bleed and dissect the galea from the periosteum, or they may be signs of an underlying skull fracture. In subperiosteal hematomas, or cephalohematomas, the swelling is localized to the underlying cranial bone and most frequently occurs with birth trauma. Scalp lacerations may occur with or without underlying contusions or fractures and they often require suturing. Given the high vascularity of the scalp, these injuries can result in significant blood loss if not recognized and treated appropriately.

Skull

Skull fractures occurring in the calvarium, or bony skullcap, include frontal, parietal, temporal, and occipital fractures and may be linear, diastatic, depressed, comminuted, or compound. Fractures in the base of the skull are termed *basilar.* Most simple fractures require no intervention but are important in that they are a marker of significant impact to the head and are associated with at least a fivefold increased risk of intracranial injury (ICI).

Linear fractures account for 75% to 90% of skull fractures in children and often manifest with localized swelling and tenderness. Diastatic fractures are traumatic separations of cranial bones at a suture site or fractures that are widely split. A depressed skull fracture is present when the inner table of the skull is displaced by more than the thickness of the entire bone. These may be palpable and are diagnosed with tangential skull radiographs (SRs) or computed tomography (CT) scans. Compound fractures are those that communicate with lacerations.

Basilar skull fractures typically produce signs specific to their fracture location that lead to the diagnosis. Fractures of the petrous portion of the temporal bone may cause hemotympanum, hemorrhagic or CSF otorrhea, or Battle sign (bleeding into mastoid air cells with postauricular swelling and ecchymosis). Fracture of the anterior skull base may cause a dural laceration with subsequent drainage of CSF into paranasal sinuses and rhinorrhea. Anterior venous sinus drainage may cause blood leakage into the periorbital tissues (raccoon eyes). Given the location of basilar skull fractures, associated cranial nerve palsies may occur. There is a high incidence of associated ICI in children with basilar skull fracture, even in those with a Glasgow Coma Scale (GCS) score of 15 and normal neurologic examination results. Of note, not all basilar skull fractures are evident on CT; however, a patient with classic clinical signs should be considered to have this fracture even without demonstrable fracture on CT.

Intracranial Injury

Insults to intracranial contents include functional derangements without demonstrable lesions on CT scan (concussion, posttraumatic seizures), hemorrhage (cerebral contusion, epidural hematoma [EDH], subdural hematoma [SDH], subarachnoid hemorrhage, and intracerebral hemorrhage), and cerebral edema. Rarely, penetrating brain injuries occur in children. ICIs may also be classified as focal (e.g., contusions, hematomas, lacerations) or diffuse (e.g., diffuse axonal injury, with cerebral edema). Focal injuries are usually apparent on the initial CT scan, even if clinically asymptomatic. Diffuse injuries, in contrast, may not demonstrate striking abnormalities on early CT imaging, even if the patient manifests significant alteration in neurologic function.

Concussion

Concussion is typically a minor brain injury characterized by posttraumatic alteration in mental status that may or may not involve loss of consciousness (LOC). No consistent associated pathologic lesion has been identified on neuroimaging. The child may have a depressed level of consciousness, pallor, vomiting, amnesia, and confusion. The clinical picture often normalizes within several hours, however, in a small number of patients symptoms may persist for days or weeks. For more details please see Chapter 121 Neurotrauma.

Posttraumatic Seizure

Posttraumatic seizures can be divided temporally into immediate, early, and late, and they occur in 5% to 10% of children hospitalized for head trauma.

Immediate seizures occur within seconds of the trauma and may represent traumatic depolarization of the cortex. They usually are generalized and rarely recur.

Early seizures occur within 1 week of the trauma (the majority within 24 hours). Skull fractures, intracranial hemorrhage, and focal signs are associated with increased risk of early posttraumatic seizures; therefore, an early seizure should prompt investigation of these possibilities.

Late seizures occur more than 1 week after the traumatic event and may be attributed to scarring associated with local vascular compromise, distortion, and mechanical irritation of the brain. These seizures are more likely to occur in children with severe head injuries, dural lacerations, and intracranial hemorrhages. A substantial number of patients will have subsequent seizures.

Cerebral Contusion

Cerebral contusion is a bruising or crushing of brain and often results from blunt head trauma. The site of contusion may be a "coup" lesion, with the injured cerebral cortex directly beneath the site of impact (with or without skull fracture), or a "contrecoup" lesion, with damage opposite the site of impact; the contusion is demonstrable by CT scan. Children with cerebral contusion may have had LOC (not imperative), may show a depressed level of consciousness or symptoms of vomiting or headache, and may have focal neurologic signs or seizures.

Epidural Hematoma

EDH is a collection of blood between the skull and the dura. An overlying fracture is present in 60% to 80% of cases, and, depending on the location and vascular structure involved, the hemorrhage may be of arterial or venous origin; injury to the middle meningeal artery is frequently responsible for temporal EDH. The classic pattern of a "lucid interval" between initial

LOC and subsequent neurologic deterioration occurs only in a minority of children with EDH; furthermore, patients may occasionally develop EDH after relatively "minor" trauma with no history of LOC. Although many children present with marked lethargy, focal neurologic signs, or a clinical pattern consistent with temporal lobe herniation as the hematoma expands, some children may be alert with a nonfocal neurologic examination and may have symptoms only of headache or persistent vomiting; nevertheless, rapid deterioration can ensue.

Subdural Hematoma

SDHs occur as a result of bleeding between the dura and the arachnoid membranes covering the brain parenchyma. They may result from direct trauma or from shaking injuries and are typically due to tearing of the cortical bridging veins or due to bleeding from the cortex itself. SDHs may be bilateral, and frequently, there is an associated underlying brain injury. Skull fractures occur in only a minority of cases. Children with SDHs often have seizures, may present with evidence of acutely elevated ICP, or may have more nonspecific signs of vomiting, irritability, or low-grade fever. Physical examination often reveals an irritable or lethargic child, with a bulging fontanel in infants, who may or may not have neurologic abnormalities. CT scan commonly demonstrates crescent-shaped subdural collections.

Intracerebral Hematoma

Posttraumatic intracerebral hematomas are unusual in children. Blood within the parenchyma is usually the result of severe focal injury or penetrating trauma, usually manifests with severe neurologic compromise, and often portends a poor prognosis.

Subarachnoid Hemorrhage

Subarachnoid hemorrhage may occur following head trauma (including shaking injuries in infants) and may cause headache, neck stiffness, and lethargy in the child.

Diffuse Axonal Injury

Diffuse axonal injury is characterized by injury to the white matter tracts of the brain and is one of the most common causes of prolonged posttraumatic coma in children. The initial CT scan may be normal or may demonstrate multiple petechial hemorrhages in the deep white matter and central structures. The degree of microscopic injury is usually greater than that seen on diagnostic imaging, accounting for clinical symptoms that may be disproportionate to CT scan findings.

Cerebral Edema

Diffuse cerebral edema occurs frequently in children with severe head trauma. It appears to be a reactive phenomenon that occurs within hours of the traumatic event and is likely a final common manifestation of brain injury caused by a variety of pathophysiologic processes. The major effect of this swelling is potential for significant elevation of ICP. These children have a depressed level of consciousness and may have focal neurologic signs or symptoms of herniation.

Penetrating Injuries

Penetrating head injuries are uncommon in children and may be caused by bullets, teeth (e.g., dog bites), or other objects (e.g., dart, pencil, pellet) penetrating the skull. These injuries have obvious potential for extensive damage to the brain and intracranial vessels.

EVALUATION AND DECISION (SEE CHAPTER 89 HEAD TRAUMA)

The clinical spectrum of head injury in children varies from a small contusion of the scalp with no neurologic sequelae to severe ICI that causes death. The general approach is essentially the same as with any child who presents with trauma, paying particular attention to potential CNS damage. Following the ABCs (airway, breathing, and circulation) of resuscitation, the physician must systematically evaluate and stabilize the child with head trauma. The goals of management are to identify complications of the head trauma and to prevent secondary brain injury. Because some complications of head trauma may not manifest immediately, the assessment period includes the initial evaluation in the ED and a more extended observation period, either in the hospital or as an outpatient, as clinically indicated. Specific therapy will vary based on specific diagnosis in each case and may include supportive care and possible neurosurgical intervention. Although complications are more common in children with severe head injury, they also occur in children with apparently minor head trauma; thus, all patients merit some degree of scrutiny.

The immediate management of the child varies with the degree of compromise. A brief initial assessment is performed to determine immediate stability. In the older child, verbal response to a question often establishes the adequacy of the airway, ventilation, and cognitive function. If the child is unconscious or has unstable vital signs, immediate resuscitation is initiated to ensure a patent airway (with cervical spine immobilization), effective ventilation, and adequate tissue perfusion (see Chapter 4 Cardiopulmonary Resuscitation); efforts to decrease possible increased ICP may be indicated, depending on the degree of neurologic compromise (see Chapter 105 Neurologic Emergencies). The child with airway and hemodynamic stability and with only mild to moderate depression of mental status can undergo a more timely evaluation to identify subtle or occult abnormalities.

CLINICAL ASSESSMENT

History

The history should be obtained from the patient (if age and level of consciousness permit) and from any witnesses to determine the nature and severity of the impact and the prehospital course. Specifics of the traumatic event should include how, when, and where the trauma occurred, as well as details such as height of a fall, type of impact surface, and type and velocity of striking objects. Occurrence of LOC as well as duration should be determined. If the event was unwitnessed and the patient is amnestic, the clinician should assume that LOC occurred. Occurrence of seizure activity (including details of time of onset posttrauma, duration, and focality) and the child's level of alertness since the injury should be noted, as well as presence of vomiting, irritability, ataxia, and abnormal behavior—all signs of possible brain injury. Vomiting after a head injury is not uncommon; however, persistence for more than several hours may signal intracranial abnormalities. If the child is verbal, he or she should be questioned about the presence of headache or neck pain, amnesia, weakness, visual disturbances, or paresthesias. In many cases, elicited symptoms may be the only evidence of underlying CNS injury. In infants, symptoms of ICI may be subtle or absent; therefore, the clinician should pay particular attention to any alteration in behavior in this age group. Progression or resolution of any symptoms, neurologic signs, and level of consciousness since the traumatic episode must be defined clearly. One should also inquire about previous medical history and factors predisposing to head trauma (e.g., seizure disorder, gait disturbance, bleeding diathesis, alcohol abuse, or illicit drug use). When there are discrepancies in the history, when the history does not fit the physical findings, or when there is a skull fracture or ICI in a young child without a history of significant trauma, one should suspect nonaccidental injury.

Physical Examination

After a primary survey with appropriate resuscitation, a thorough physical examination should be performed, with special emphasis on the vital signs, head and neck, and neurologic examination. Bradycardia may be a sign of increased ICP; it is of particular concern when associated with hypertension, abnormal breathing pattern, depressed level of consciousness, or neurologic abnormality. Bradycardia may also be seen with spinal cord injuries caused by unopposed parasympathetic tone; in this case, it is often associated with hypotension, flaccidity, a sensory level, and absent deep tendon reflexes. Tachycardia may reflect hypovolemia (especially if associated with hypotension), hypoxia, or anxiety. Isolated head injuries rarely cause hypovolemia (except in infants with large subgaleal or intracranial hematomas); therefore, hypotension should alert the clinician to a possible extracranial or spinal cord injury.

The head should be inspected and palpated carefully for scalp swelling, lacerations, irregularities of the underlying bony structure, and fontanel fullness (in infants). Signs of basilar skull fracture (periorbital or postauricular hemorrhage in the absence of direct trauma, hemotympanum, CSF otorrhea, or rhinorrhea) and retinal abnormalities (hemorrhage or papilledema) should be noted. All children with depressed mental status or neck pain should have cervical spine immobilization maintained at least until its integrity has been confirmed radiographically; one should note cervical abrasions, deformity, or tenderness—findings that may indicate underlying cervical spine injuries.

Neurologic examination encompasses assessment of the child's mental status, as well as cranial nerve, motor, sensory, cerebellar, and reflex functions. Serial examinations are important in the child with head trauma to document improvement or deterioration. The GCS is a convenient way to quantify the level of consciousness and monitor neurologic progression. The GCS rates patient performance in three areas: eye opening, verbal ability, and motor ability. It also assesses the level of alertness, mentation, and major CNS pathways (Table 36.1); an individual's score may range from a low of 3 to a high of 15. The score has been modified for more age-appropriate behaviors in infants (Table 36.2). Although ICIs are more common in a child with a low GCS score, even a child with a GCS score of 15 may harbor potentially life-threatening complications of head trauma (e.g., EDH), especially if neurologic abnormalities are present. Further evaluation of mental status includes assessing orientation and memory. Subtle signs (irritability and high-pitched cry) may be indicative of underlying abnormalities in infants.

Cranial nerve function is assessed by checking for facial symmetry, corneal reflexes, presence of a gag reflex, full extraocular movements, pupillary size, and pupillary reactivity. In

TABLE 36.1

GLASGOW COMA SCALE SCORE

Activity	Best response	Score
Eye opening	Spontaneous	4
	To verbal stimuli	3
	To pain	2
	None	1
Verbal	Oriented	5
	Confused	4
	Inappropriate words	3
	Nonspecific sounds	2
	None	1
Motor	Normal spontaneous movements	6
	Localizes pain	5
	Withdraws to pain	4
	Abnormal flexion (decorticate rigidity)	3
	Abnormal extension (decerebrate rigidity)	2
	None	1

TABLE 36.2

MODIFIED COMA SCALE FOR INFANTS

Activity	Best response	Score
Eye opening	Spontaneous	4
	To speech	3
	To pain	2
	None	1
Verbal	Coos, babbles	5
	Irritable, cries	4
	Cries to pain	3
	Moans to pain	2
	None	1
Motor	Normal spontaneous movements	6
	Withdraws to touch	5
	Withdraws to pain	4
	Abnormal flexion (decorticate rigidity)	3
	Abnormal extension (decerebrate rigidity)	2
	None	1

the comatose patient or in the child with possible neck injury who is uncooperative, lateral gaze may be tested by caloric stimulation of the vestibular apparatus (but not the "doll's eye" maneuver) once tympanic membrane integrity has been established.

Examination of the motor system to evaluate both CNS and spinal cord function varies with age and level of consciousness. The alert patient should have individual muscle groups tested and gait evaluated. The child with a depressed level of consciousness may have motor responses elicited by noxious stimuli (e.g., sternal rub, nail bed pressure). Deep tendon reflexes and Babinski response should also be evaluated. Obviously, a complete physical examination with attention to possible thoracic, abdominal, pelvic, and extremity injuries should be performed.

Radiographic Investigation

Complications of head trauma may be identified with radiographic studies, which include plain radiographs of the skull and cervical spine and CT scan of the head; specific studies are indicated based on the child's history and physical findings. Although MRI is an additional imaging modality for the cranial contents, limited availability and prolonged study time limit its utility for evaluation of acute trauma at this time. All children with significant head trauma should be evaluated for associated cervical spine injuries. This evaluation will be clinical, with or without radiographic studies, based on the specific circumstances (see Chapter 120 Neck Trauma).

CT provides excellent images of the intracranial contents, and therefore, is the diagnostic modality of choice when intracranial pathology is suspected. CT imaging, however, has disadvantages, including exposure to ionizing radiation and the possible requirement for pharmacologic sedation, especially in younger patients. Ideally, CT imaging should be used selectively for patients at higher risk for ICI, limiting potentially unnecessary studies for those who are at low risk. Patients at intermediate risk can undergo CT versus observation based on the clinical scenario, provider experience, and parental preference.

Over the years, one of the most controversial issues in the management of head trauma has been the use of SRs. Since SRs give no direct information about ICI, their use has appropriately dwindled. However, they are useful for demonstrating skull fractures (one of the best predictors for ICI in infants and young children) and have the advantages of delivering lower doses of ionizing radiation, being more universally available, less costly, and not requiring sedation. Certainly, any child for whom there is significant concern for ICI should undergo CT imaging; however, there may still be a very small role for SRs in certain select circumstances when immediate CT is not warranted, yet significant chance of fracture exists to justify the test. Examples would include SRs as part of a skeletal survey, to evaluate for the location of a radiopaque foreign body, and in rare instances to screen for fracture in selected asymptomatic patients 3 to 12 months of age with concerning scalp hematoma or question of depression. Those with fractures identified on SR would need to have CT scans performed because they are at increased risk for associated ICI. In general, SRs should be performed only if they will be reviewed by a radiologist trained in their interpretation as they can be very challenging to interpret in young children, and the utility of the study depends on an accurate reading.

Approach

The goals of management are to define specific anatomic lesions (e.g., skull fracture and ICI) and to prevent secondary brain injury, while limiting unnecessary cranial irradiation. Pediatricians and emergency physicians will be the initial clinicians to evaluate and manage most children with head trauma. Neurosurgical consultation should be considered for all children with penetrating trauma, abnormal mental status or neurologic examination, skull fractures, and intracranial complications. The urgency of neurosurgical involvement varies with the acuity of the patient's clinical condition.

One approach to diagnosing complications of head trauma involves determining whether a penetrating injury has occurred. If so, brain or vascular injury is likely and emergent CT scanning and neurosurgical consultation are mandated in addition to stabilization.

If the head injury has resulted from blunt trauma, it must be determined whether an ICI is likely (Fig. 36.1). Since preverbal children may have differences in the presenting signs/symptoms of ICI compared to older children, the approach in evaluating for ICI should take age into account.

In children <2 years of age, high-risk historical features and physical findings include altered mental status, focal neurologic abnormality, signs of a skull fracture, a bulging fontanel, history of seizure, or concern for abuse. Children with any of these high-risk findings should be referred for emergent imaging. Special attention should be paid to infants <3 months of age who may present with a paucity of symptoms in the setting of ICI. Other historical or examination findings in children <2 years of age that suggest an increased risk of ICI include LOC ≥ 5 seconds, severe or unclear injury mechanism, caregiver concern, or persistent vomiting. Nonfrontal hematomas of greater concern include those that are temporoparietal, larger, and/or those that are present in younger children. While any of these factors may increase the risk of ICI, observation (versus emergent imaging) may be considered for children with only one finding (or two mild findings), based on the clinical scenario, provider experience, and parental preference. However, if emergent imaging is deferred, children should be observed in the ED for at least 4 to 6 hours after the injury for signs and symptoms of complications. These would include neurologic abnormalities, mental status depression, persistent vomiting, lethargy, or irritability. A CT scan should be obtained if these signs or symptoms develop. Abnormalities on CT might include intracranial hemorrhage or contusion, diffuse cerebral swelling, or skull fracture; if the CT scan is normal, then concussion or extracranial injury has likely occurred.

In children ≥2 years, high-risk clinical features include altered mental status, focal neurologic deficits, signs of a skull fracture, or seizures. Children with any of these features should be referred for emergent imaging. Additional findings concerning for increased risk of ICI include LOC, persistent vomiting, persistent/progressive or severe headache, or severe mechanism of injury. In children with one of these features (or two mild features), observation (versus emergent imaging) may be considered based on the clinical scenario, provider experience, and parental preference. If observation is initiated, the child should be observed for 4 to 6 hours for any signs of clinical deterioration, which would include neurologic abnormalities, mental status depression, persistent vomiting, or increasingly severe headache. A CT scan should be obtained

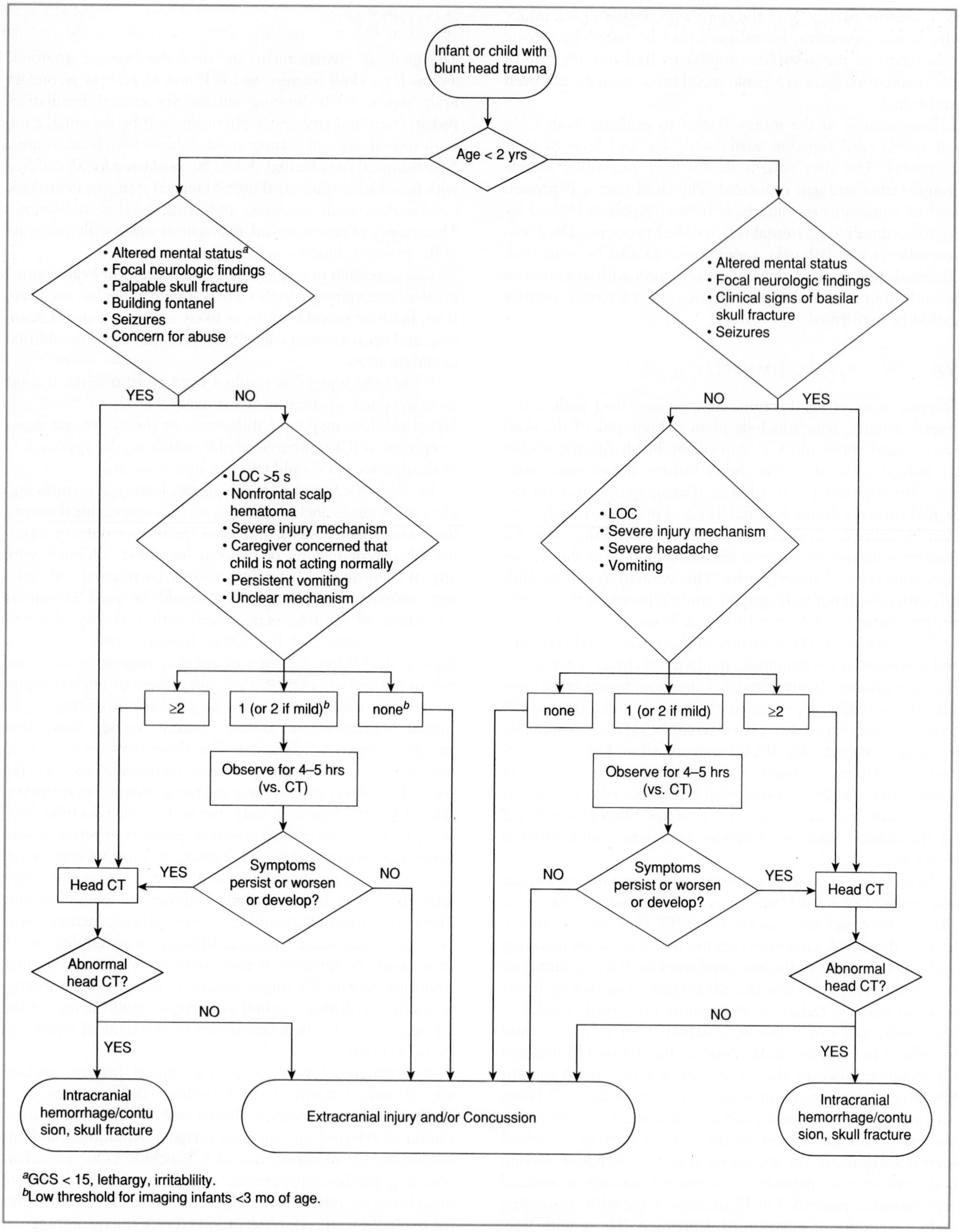

Infant or child with blunt head trauma

Age < 2 yrs

Age < 2 yrs:

- Altered mental status[a]
- Focal neurologic findings
- Palpable skull fracture
- Building fontanel
- Seizures
- Concern for abuse

YES → Head CT

NO →

- LOC >5 s
- Nonfrontal scalp hematoma
- Severe injury mechanism
- Caregiver concerned that child is not acting normally
- Persistent vomiting
- Unclear mechanism

≥2 → Head CT

1 (or 2 if mild)[b] → Observe for 4–5 hrs (vs. CT)

none[b] → Extracranial injury and/or Concussion

Symptoms persist or worsen or develop?

YES → Head CT

NO → Extracranial injury and/or Concussion

Abnormal head CT?

YES → Intracranial hemorrhage/contusion, skull fracture

NO → Extracranial injury and/or Concussion

Age ≥ 2 yrs:

- Altered mental status
- Focal neurologic findings
- Clinical signs of basilar skull fracture
- Seizures

YES → Head CT

NO →

- LOC
- Severe injury mechanism
- Severe headache
- Vomiting

none → Extracranial injury and/or Concussion

1 (or 2 if mild) → Observe for 4–5 hrs (vs. CT)

≥2 → Head CT

Symptoms persist or worsen or develop?

YES → Head CT

NO → Extracranial injury and/or Concussion

Abnormal head CT?

YES → Intracranial hemorrhage/contusion, skull fracture

NO → Extracranial injury and/or Concussion

[a]GCS < 15, lethargy, irritablility.
[b]Low threshold for imaging infants <3 mo of age.

FIGURE 36.1 Approach to the child with head trauma. CT, computed tomography; LOC, loss of consciousness; GCS, Glasgow Coma Scale.

TABLE 36.3

CRITERIA FOR DISCHARGE WITH HOME OBSERVATION

Traumatic force not life-threatening
Glasgow Coma Scale score of 15
Nonfocal neurologic examination
No significant symptoms
No history of prolonged loss of consciousness (or normal CT if it did occur)
No intracranial abnormalities on CT (if obtained)
Reliable caregivers who are able to return, if necessary
No suspicion of abuse or neglect

CT, computed tomography.

if these signs or symptoms develop. As previously stated, discrete abnormalities may be identified on CT scan, but if the scan is normal, then the child has suffered a concussion or extracranial injury. It is important to note that symptomatic children without evidence of ICI on CT scan may still suffer from persistent and/or debilitating symptoms that require admission or close outpatient follow-up.

Many children presenting to the ED after blunt head trauma will not require advanced imaging or observation. These remaining children, who sustained impact of minimal force, had no LOC, and are alert and asymptomatic with normal examinations, likely have only minor head trauma with or without extracranial injuries, including contusions and lacerations. Home observation is appropriate management for the majority of these patients. Rarely, intracranial complications develop in these children, causing symptoms hours after the traumatic event; therefore, the caregiver should be given a printed list of signs and symptoms (reviewed verbally by the clinician) indicative of increased ICP with instructions to check the child at regular intervals and to return to the ED if symptoms occur. Postconcussive counseling (especially with regard to return to sports), when indicated, should also be given. The caregivers must be reliable and able to return with the child if necessary, and there must be no suspicion of abuse or neglect—otherwise admission for observation in the hospital should be considered (Table 36.3).

Suggested Readings and Key References

Brenner D, Elliston CD, Hall EJ, et al. Estimated risks of radiation-induced fatal cancer from pediatric CT. *AJR Am J Roentgenol* 2001; 176(2):289–296.

Brenner DJ, Hall EJ. Computed tomography—an increasing source of radiation exposure. *N Engl J Med* 2007;357:2277–2284.

Committee on Quality Improvement, American Academy of Pediatrics. The management of minor closed head injury in children. *Pediatrics* 1999;104:1407–1415.

Dunning J, Daly JP, Lomas JP, et al. Derivation of the children's head injury algorithm for the prediction of important clinic events decision rule for head injury in children. *Arch Dis Child* 2006;91: 885–891.

Greenes DS, Schutzman SA. Clinical significance of scalp abnormalities in head-injured infants. *Pediatr Emerg Care* 2001;17:88–92.

Kuppermann N, Holmes JF, Dayan PS, et al. Identification of children at very low risk of clinically-important brain injuries after head trauma: a prospective cohort study. *Lancet* 2009;374:1160–1170.

Lyttle MD, Crowe L, Oakley E, et al. Comparing CATCH, CHALICE and PECARN clinical decision rules for paediatric head injuries. *Emerg Med J* 2012;29(10):785–794.

McCrory P, Meeuwisse W, Aubry M, et al. Consensus statement on concussion in sport—The 4th International Conference on Concussion in Sport Held in Zurich, November 2012. *Br J Sports Med* 2013;47(5):250–258.

Osmond MH, Klassen TP, Wells GA, et al. CATCH: a clinical decision rule for the use of computed tomography in children with minor head injury. *CMAJ* 2010;182:341–348.

Schunk JE, Schutzman SA. Pediatric head injury. *Pediatr Rev* 2012; 33(9):398–411.

Schutzman SA, Barnes P, Duhaime AC, et al. Evaluation and management of children younger than two years of age with apparently minor head trauma: proposed guidelines. *Pediatrics* 2001;107(5): 983–993.

CHAPTER 37 ▪ INJURY: KNEE

MARC N. BASKIN, MD AND CYNTHIA M. ADAMS, MD

Acute pain or injury to the knee is a common complaint in the emergency department (ED). Many injuries are minor and require only limited therapy; others, however, require consultation with an orthopedist, either in the ED or as outpatients after pain and inflammation subside. The emergency physician can provide appropriate therapy or determine the need for consultation, based on a comprehensive history, physical examination, and an appropriate radiographic evaluation.

DIFFERENTIAL DIAGNOSIS

The differential diagnosis of acute and chronic knee injuries is summarized in Table 37.1. The pertinent anatomy is illustrated in Figures 37.1 and 37.2.

Acute Injuries

Fractures

Preadolescents with open growth plates (physes) are especially susceptible to fractures. Since pediatric bone strength is less than pediatric ligament strength, an injury that would cause a ligamentous injury in adults may cause a Salter–Harris type physeal fracture in children. For bones around the knee, the epiphyses close by 17±1 years in females and by 18±1 years in males.

Fractures of the distal femoral epiphysis are classified by the Salter–Harris pattern (see Chapter 119 Musculoskeletal Trauma) and by the displacement of the epiphysis (usually lateral or medial). The injury usually follows significant trauma (e.g., being struck by a car and the knee hyperextended or during contact sports when sustaining a lateral hit with the foot fixed by cleats). Distal neurovascular status should be assessed because compromise of the popliteal artery occurs in 1% of cases and peroneal nerve injury occurs in 3% of cases.

Fractures of the proximal tibial epiphysis are rarer than those of the distal femoral epiphysis but are more likely to involve vascular compromise because of the proximity of the popliteal artery to the posterior aspect of the tibial epiphysis. With both fracture types, the patient will have severe pain, refusal to bear weight, extensive soft-tissue swelling, limited range of motion (ROM), and commonly, hemarthrosis. For both injuries, radiographs are usually diagnostic but may be normal if the injury is a nondisplaced Salter–Harris type I fracture. Although not necessary as part of ED evaluation, magnetic resonance imaging (MRI) may be needed when the physis is tender or a large effusion is present.

Acute traumatic avulsion of the tibial tuberosity is caused by acute stress on the knee's extensor mechanism. The quadriceps muscle group extends the knee by way of the patellar ligament. The patellar ligament inserts on the tibial tuberosity and may avulse it during sudden acceleration (e.g., beginning a jump) or deceleration (e.g., landing after a jump). The patient will have tenderness and swelling over the tibial tubercle and be unable to extend the knee fully (or perform a straight leg raise). A lateral radiograph is diagnostic.

Fractures of the patella are rare in younger children because the child's patella does not ossify until 3 to 6 years of age, leaving it with a thick cartilage layer that protects it from direct trauma. In addition, the soft tissue anchors of the patella are flexible which diffuses blunt forces. However, a direct impact on the patella into the distal femur can cause transverse or comminuted fractures. Much more common in children are avulsion fractures of the patella resulting from forceful contraction of the quadriceps. With patellar fractures, the patient's knee will be swollen, the patella tender, and knee extension painful. A radiograph is usually diagnostic although care must be taken not to miss small avulsion fragments including sleeve fractures which are unique to pediatrics (egg-shell–like bony fragment that dislocates with avulsed soft tissue). Bipartite patellas are a normal variant and may be confused with an acute fracture.

Osteochondral fractures are fractures of articular cartilage and underlying bone not associated with ligamentous attachments. These fractures often involve the femoral condyles or the patella. The injury may follow a direct blow to the knee, a twisting injury, or patellar dislocation. The patient will have severe pain, immediate swelling, and will hold the knee partially flexed. Hemarthrosis may be present. Knee radiographs need to include an intercondylar view because the fracture fragment may be in the intercondylar notch. Osteochondral fractures can be missed because only the small ossified portion of the osteochondral fragment is radiopaque. MRI may be necessary.

Analogous to an adolescent who ruptures the anterior cruciate ligament (ACL), patients 6 to 16 years old may sustain avulsion fractures of the tibial spine at the point where the ACL inserts. The tibial spine is incompletely ossified and may avulse before the ligament ruptures. The patient may have a hemarthrosis and will be unable to bear weight. If the patient tolerates an examination, the Lachman test (see Fig. 37.3) may be positive because the injury is similar mechanically to an ACL tear. AP, lateral, and intercondylar or tunnel-view radiographs will show the avulsed fragment. The visible ossified fragment may be small because the tibial spine is mostly radiolucent cartilage.

Dislocations

In a child, the knee joint itself rarely dislocates; usually, the distal femoral or proximal tibial epiphysis separates first. Dislocation occurs more frequently when the growth plates have closed and usually with trauma that involves significant force, such as a motor vehicle collision or contact sports. The knee will appear obviously deformed with the tibia or femoral condyles

TABLE 37.1

DIFFERENTIAL DIAGNOSIS OF THE INJURED KNEE

- Acute injuries
  - Fractures
    - Distal femoral epiphysis[a]
    - Proximal tibial epiphysis[a]
    - Tibial tubercle avulsion
    - Patella
    - Tibial spine avulsion
    - Osteochondral fractures
  - Soft-tissue injuries
    - Collateral ligament sprain[b] or tear
    - Anterior cruciate ligament sprain or tear
    - Posterior cruciate ligament sprain or tear
    - Meniscal tears
    - Quadriceps tendon rupture
    - Patellar tendon rupture
    - Hamstring strain[b]
  - Posttraumatic infections[a]
  - Dislocations and subluxations
    - Patellar[b]
    - Knee joint[a]
- Subacute injuries
  - Osgood–Schlatter's disease[b]
  - Patellofemoral dysfunction[b]
  - Patellar tendon tendinitis (jumper's knee)
  - Prepatellar bursitis
  - Osteochondritis dissecans (OCD)
  - Baker's cyst
  - Iliotibial (IT) band friction syndrome
- Other
  - Pathologic fractures[a]
  - Referred pain from hip disease
    - Slipped capital femoral epiphysis
    - Aseptic necrosis of the femoral head

[a]Life- or limb-threatening causes of the injured knee.
[b]Common causes of the injured knee.

abnormally prominent in an anterior or posterior dislocation, respectively. Disruption of the popliteal artery may occur with the dislocation, and the resulting hypoperfusion may be limb threatening. Posterior tibial and dorsalis pedis pulses and peroneal nerve function (sensation between the great and second toe and ankle dorsiflexion) must be documented. Radiographs will confirm the diagnosis.

Patellar dislocation occurs as the quadriceps muscles pull the patellar tendon to extend the knee, especially when the knee has a valgus stress or the extremity is suddenly abducted as when the leg slips laterally. If the vastus medialis fibers do not keep the patella in the intercondylar groove, the patella may dislocate laterally. This often recurrent injury rarely occurs from direct force. The patient may feel a popping sensation and will have intense pain and hold the knee flexed. The patella is displaced laterally, and the diagnosis is usually made based on history and examination. The dislocation may

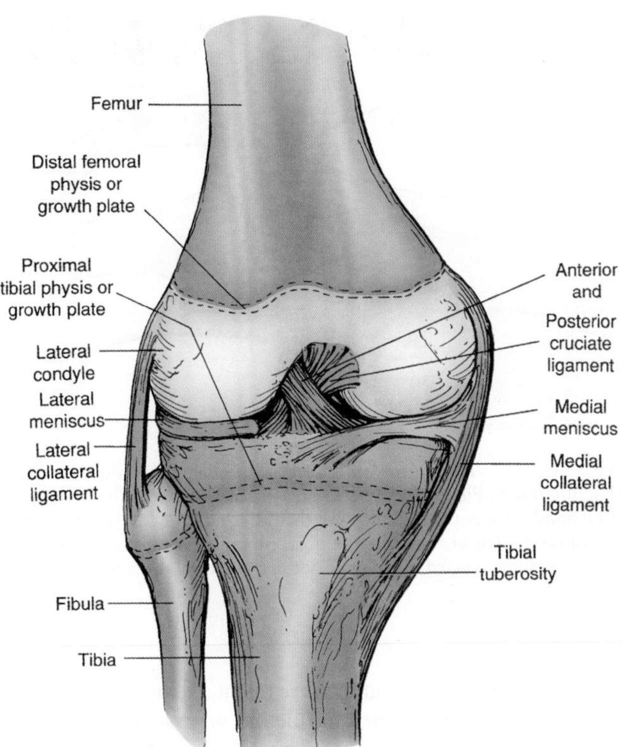

FIGURE 37.1 Anatomy of the knee—anterior view (patella removed).

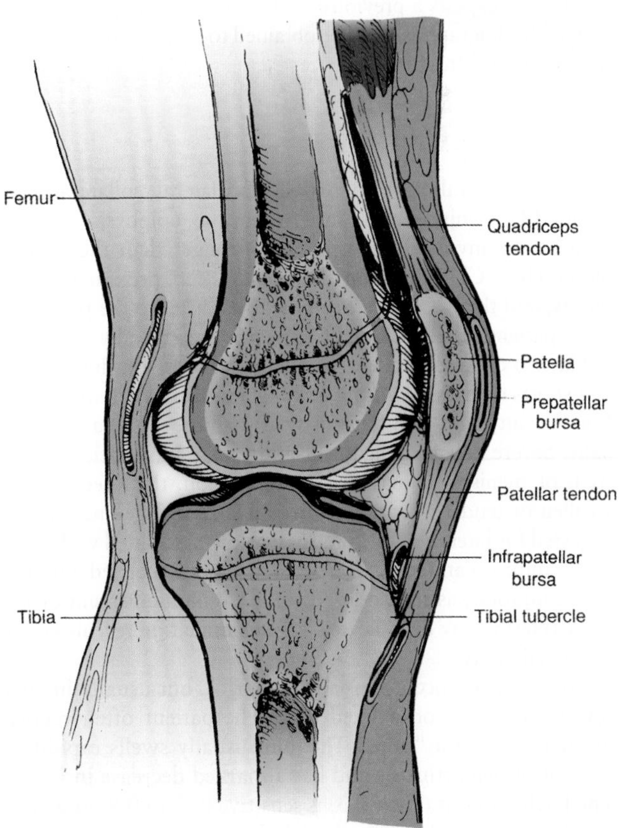

FIGURE 37.2 Anatomy of the knee—sagittal section.

SIGNS AND SYMPTOMS

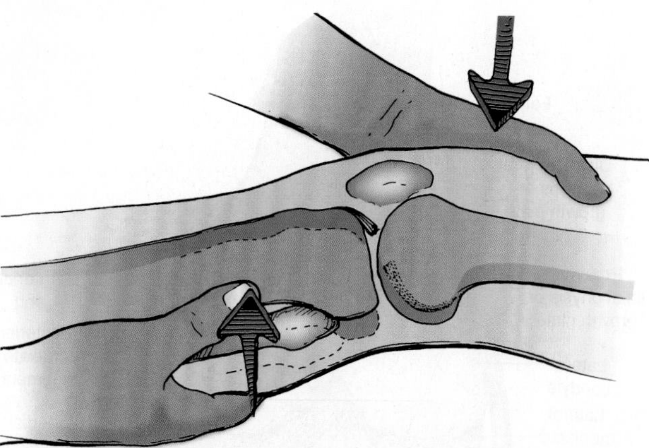

FIGURE 37.3 Testing for anterior cruciate ligament injury with the Lachman test. Flex the knee 20 to 30 degrees, support the thigh with one hand, and grasp the calf with the other hand. Move the tibia forward on the femur. Observe the tibial tubercle for movement and feel for excessive forward movement of the tibia in relation to the femur.

be reduced before radiographs are taken. Postreduction radiographs should be obtained to rule out an associated avulsion or osteochondral fracture of the patella.

If the history is consistent with dislocation but the patient is no longer in pain and has a normal examination, the patella may have subluxated or dislocated and self-reduced. A high-riding or laterally displaced patella may be observed. The patellar apprehension test can be performed by gently attempting to move the patella laterally. If the patient tightens the quadriceps, becomes apprehensive, or grabs the examiner's hand, this suggests a previously subluxated (or fully dislocated) patella. Radiographs should be obtained to look for an associated osteochondral fracture.

Soft-tissue Injuries

Medial collateral ligament (MCL) or lateral collateral ligament (LCL) injuries are rare when the epiphysis is open because the involved ligaments are stronger than the growth plate. The LCL inserts on the fibular head proximal to the physis, and the MCL inserts on the tibia distal to the physis. In older patients, the MCL or LCL may be damaged by a blow to the lateral or medial side of the knee, respectively, during contact sports or stressed during a skiing accident, when the athlete "catches an edge" and falls forward with the leg rotated externally. Severe collateral ligament injury may be associated with ACL or meniscal damage. On examination, the knee may be swollen or tender over the involved ligament. The knee should be tested for lateral laxity in full extension (associated with more severe injuries) and in 30 degrees of flexion (associated with less severe injuries), as shown in Figure 37.4. Non-emergent orthopedic referral may be indicated if the examination reveals lateral or medial laxity.

ACL injuries occur in many scenarios, but usually involve rotational forces on a fixed foot. The patient often reports the sensation of a "pop." The joint usually swells rapidly as a result of hemarthrosis and has a marked decrease in ROM. The Lachman test (Fig. 37.3) is sensitive (0.7 to 0.9) in detecting ACL injuries but may be falsely negative soon after the injury, when the knee is swollen and painful. Examining the

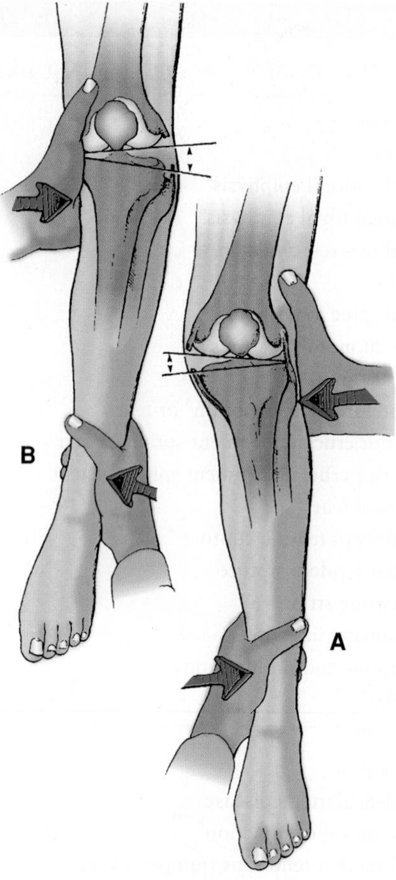

FIGURE 37.4 Testing for collateral ligament injury. Test the knee in full extension and in 30 degrees of flexion. To test for medial collateral ligament injury (**A**), hold and apply force to the medial side of the ankle with one hand and apply pressure over the fibular head with the other hand. To test for lateral collateral ligament injury (**B**), hold and apply force to the lateral side of the ankle with one hand and apply pressure just below the medial side of the knee with the other hand. If the knee "opens up" laterally or medially more than the uninjured knee, the collateral ligament is injured.

uninjured knee can be helpful for comparison. MRI and occasionally arthroscopy is often needed for definitive diagnosis. ACL injuries are rare before adolescence because in a child, the ACL's insertion point, the tibial spine, is incompletely ossified and more likely to be injured than the ligament. Radiographs may detect an epiphyseal fracture, tibial spine fracture, or an avulsed bone fragment due to associated MCL or LCL injury.

Posterior cruciate ligament injuries are extremely rare and usually result from direct force on the tibial tubercle, pushing the tibia posteriorly on the femur. The posterior drawer sign will be present in most cases (see Fig. 37.5).

The menisci are tough fibrocartilage pads that help distribute the body's weight over the femoral and tibial condyles. They can be injured when the knee is twisted during weight bearing. The patient, usually older than 12 years, may report a popping sensation and the feeling of the knee "giving out." Outside the acute period, the patient may report that the knee suddenly refuses to extend fully, "locking up," and then suddenly "unlocking." Joint-line tenderness is frequently present (sensitivity 0.7 to 0.8, specificity 0.2) but must be differentiated from the tenderness associated with collateral ligament

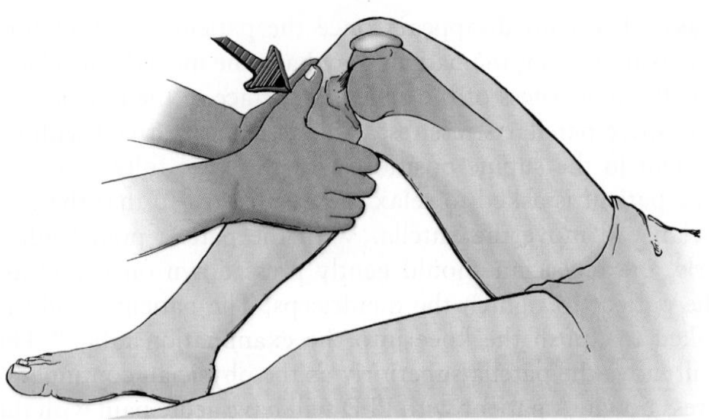

FIGURE 37.5 Testing for posterior cruciate ligament injury with the posterior drawer test. With the patient supine and the knee flexed to 90 degrees, sit on the patient's foot to stabilize it. Attempt to force the tibia posteriorly. Posterior movement greater on the injured side than on the uninjured side is abnormal and suggests a posterior cruciate ligament injury.

injuries. An effusion is commonly detected. Acutely, the injury may be difficult to diagnose because of diffuse pain and significantly reduced ROM, making the classic McMurray's sign difficult to elicit (see Fig. 37.6). The Apley compression test (see Fig. 37.7) requires less knee movement and may be easier

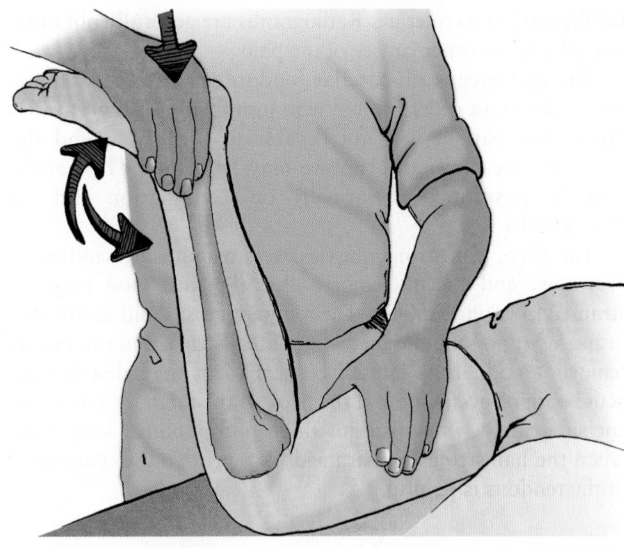

FIGURE 37.7 Testing for meniscal injury with the Apley compression test. With the patient prone and the knee flexed to 90 degrees, apply pressure to the heel while the tibia is rotated. If this produces pain that resolves when the tibia is distracted from the femur, a meniscal injury should be suspected.

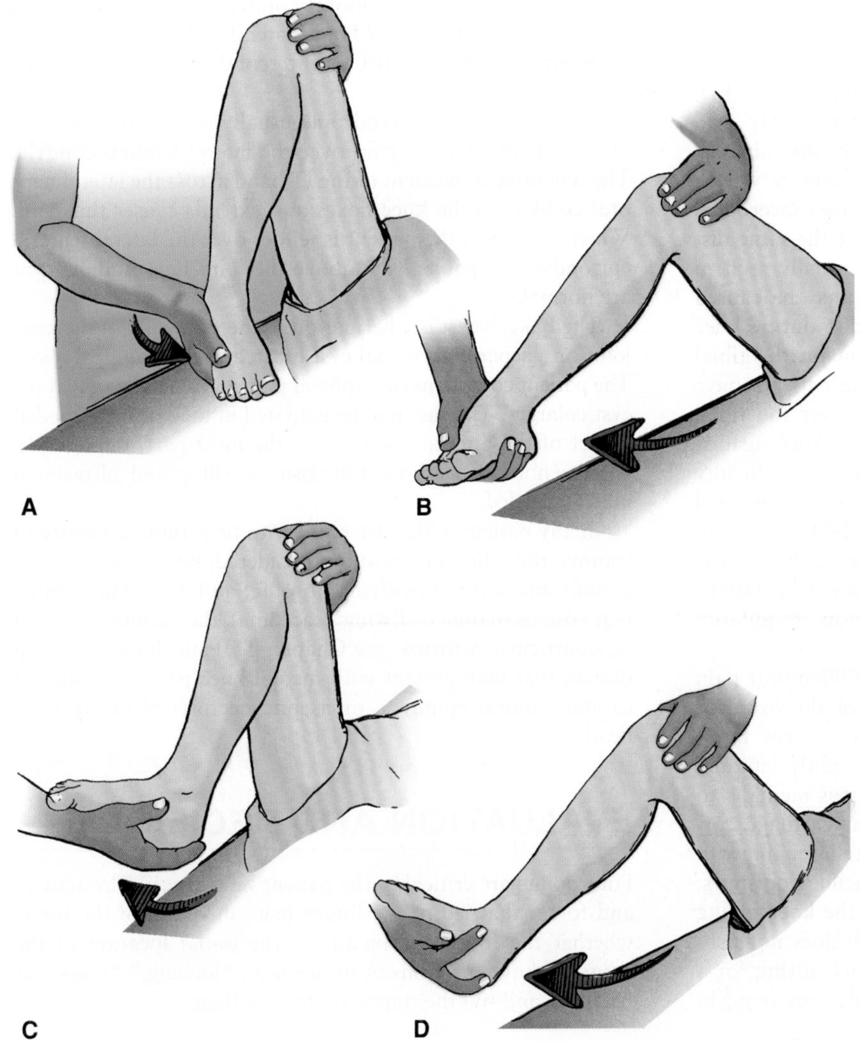

FIGURE 37.6 **A to D:** Testing for meniscal injury with the McMurray test. Grasp the patient's foot with one hand and place the other hand over the joint lines. Push on the lateral side of the knee to apply a valgus force. Start with the knee flexed and extend the knee while first internally rotating and then externally rotating the tibia. The injured meniscus may be felt as a painful click or snapping sensation as the knee is manipulated.

for the patient to tolerate. Radiographs are generally obtained to evaluate for other causes of the pain.

The quadriceps or patellar tendon can rupture acutely, especially in an older athlete who jumps or falls a great distance. The patient will not be able to actively extend the knee; the area over the rupture may be tender. The patella may be positioned abnormally on examination and on radiographs.

The three hamstring muscles (semitendinosus, semimembranosus, and biceps femoris) flex the knee and may be strained in young athletes. The semitendinosus and semimembranosus run along the medial popliteal space, and the biceps femoris tendon runs laterally. The patient may describe an acute pain or even a pop in the back of the thigh or may present subacutely with posterior thigh and popliteal knee pain when the hamstrings are strained by repetitive use. Palpation of the tendons is painful.

Posttraumatic Infection

Although not considered injuries, acute infections may present after a vague history of trauma. Physical findings of acute infection will be present. The most common disorders are septic arthritis, osteomyelitis, cellulitis, and septic prepatellar bursitis (see Chapters 102 Infectious Disease Emergencies and 129 Musculoskeletal Emergencies).

Subacute Injuries

Many subacute knee problems may present in the ED. Osgood–Schlatter's disease of the tibial tubercle may lead to similar symptoms as a traumatic avulsion of the tubercle; however, the symptoms have been noted for days or weeks. The symptoms of Osgood–Schlatter's disease are exacerbated by squatting or jumping, but they do not cause the same disability as an acute avulsion. The disease is usually seen in patients between 11 and 15 years of age. It may be caused by recurrent contractions of the patellar tendon during knee extension, traumatizing the tendon's insertion on the tibial tubercle during the child's growth spurt. The patients have localized tenderness and occasional swelling over the tibial tubercle. The patient will refuse to extend the knee against force (e.g., perform a deep-knee bend) and have difficulty going up or down stairs, although they may have a normal gait on a level surface. To eliminate the possibility of a neoplasm or a secondary avulsion if there is an acute change, the physician should obtain radiographs. In Osgood–Schlatter's disease, the radiographs will be normal or show irregularity of the tubercle.

Patellofemoral dysfunction (PFD) or patellofemoral pain syndrome may be caused by misalignment of the extensor mechanism of the knee. The vastus lateralis, vastus intermedius, and rectus femoris pull the patella slightly laterally and need to be balanced perfectly by the vastus medialis to keep the patella tracking across the articular cartilage correctly. The patient with PFD may have patellar pain with running and especially while going down inclines or stairs. The patient may also have the sensation of the knee giving out when descending, although an actual fall does not usually occur. The patient may describe pain when sitting for a prolonged time with the knee flexed at 90 degrees (e.g., in class). The pain disappears once the patient is ambulatory. On examination, the patient may have the medially displaced patella, tenderness of the articular surface of the patella, and a positive patellar stress test. This test is performed with the patient in the supine position with the knee fully extended. The patient is asked to relax the quadriceps so that the physician can move the patella. With the patella pulled inferiorly, the physician should gently press down on it and ask the patient to tighten the quadriceps. The patient should be asked to "push the knee into the examination table." This will move the patella superiorly as the physician continues to press down. A patient with PFD will have acute pain with this maneuver. Radiographs are normal.

Patellar tendonitis, or "jumper's knee," occurs in patients during their growth spurt, especially those involved in jumping (knee extension) sports. The knee is tender on the inferior pole of the patella and the adjacent patellar tendon, but not on the tibial tubercle; radiographs are generally normal.

Prepatellar bursitis occurs after acute or chronic trauma to this bursa, which overlies the patella. The patient will have swelling over the anterior aspect of the knee, especially over the patella. A septic bursitis may need to be ruled out by needle aspiration.

Osteochondritis dissecans (OCD) is the separation of a small portion of the femoral condyle with the overlying cartilage. The patient is usually an adolescent with a 1- to 4-week history of nonspecific knee pain. The physical examination may be normal, or the femoral condyle may be tender with the knee flexed. Because AP and lateral radiographs may not show the lesion, a tunnel or intercondylar view should be obtained.

Iliotibial (IT) band syndrome usually occurs in older runners who complain of pain over the lateral femoral condyle. The repetitive movement of the IT band across the lateral femoral condyle as the knee flexes and extends causes this pain. When examined, the patient is tender over the lateral femoral epicondyle, palpable 2 cm above the joint line. Radiographs are normal.

The Baker's cyst is a herniation of the synovium of the knee joint or a separate synovial cyst located in the popliteal fossa. The patient complains of popliteal pain and swelling only if the cyst enlarges. The sac may be palpated in the posterior medial aspect of the popliteal space. For the most part, radiographs will be normal or show soft-tissue swelling and ultrasound may be needed.

In any patient with knee pain, with or without a history of trauma, the following must be considered: Benign (e.g., osteochondroma and nonossifying fibroma) and malignant tumors (e.g., osteosarcoma or Ewing's sarcoma), the various causes of monoarticular arthritis (see Chapter 55 Pain: Joints) and hip disease that may present with medial knee pain (e.g., slipped capital femoral epiphysis or aseptic necrosis of the femoral head).

EVALUATION AND DECISION

Four points are critical in the patient's history: (i) The activity and forces that led to the injury (e.g., direction of the force, whether the foot was fixed); (ii) the initial location of the pain; (iii) any sensations or noises (e.g., "locking," "pops," or "tears"); and (iv) the timing of any swelling.

Most severe injuries (e.g., ACL, collateral ligament, or meniscal injuries) occur with high-velocity weight-bearing activities, especially running and making sharp cuts or being subjected to direct valgus or varus stress. Direct trauma to the front of the knee may cause posterior cruciate ligament injuries or patellar fractures, whereas lateral or medial forces may cause collateral or cruciate ligament damage or fractures.

Although the knee may "hurt all over" when seen in the ED, the patient may be able to localize the initial pain. Meniscal or collateral ligament injuries cause pain on the lateral or medial aspect of the knee, whereas ACL injuries hurt just inferior to the patella, and Osgood–Schlatter's disease is painful over the tibial tubercle.

Distinct popping noises or tearing sensations are reported in ACL injuries and patellar dislocation. Locking of the knee may be reported in meniscal injuries but not immediately after the injury. The sensation of the knee "giving out" may occur with meniscal injuries or PFD.

Swelling after acute injury should raise concern for significant pathology. Swelling within 2 hours strongly suggests hemarthrosis from an ACL injury, meniscal injury, or osteochondral fracture, while swelling within 24 hours has been associated with knee fractures.

The possibility of abuse in young children must always be considered, especially if the injury is unexplained, the history is implausible, or the delay in seeking medical care was unreasonable.

In subacute injuries, ask about hip or groin pain because the hip and knee share sensory nerves. Legg–Calvé–Perthes disease or a slipped capital femoral epiphysis may cause anterior thigh or knee pain. Patellar pain and the sensation of the knee giving way without actually falling when going down stairs or inclines suggest PFD.

Examination of the patient should include walking and standing to check for medially deviated "squinting" patellae. Inspect and palpate the knee in two positions, sitting relaxed with the knees at 90 degrees and supine. When sitting, inspect the knees for swelling and tenderness (e.g., swelling and tenderness over the tibial tubercle in Osgood–Schlatter's disease, or joint-line tenderness in meniscal injuries). With the patient supine, repeat inspection and palpation over the joint line, collateral ligaments, patella, proximal fibula, tibial tuberosity, and popliteal space. If the knee appears swollen, check for an effusion by milking any joint fluid centrally toward the patella. Normally, synovial fluid coats the patellar surface but does not separate the patella and femur. When fluid separates the two bones, a sharp pat on the patella results in the sensation of a tap as the two bones meet. If the joint contains a large amount of fluid, the patella will not touch the femur but will feel as if it is sitting on a cushion. Assess both active and passive ROM of the knee.

The physician should test for collateral and cruciate ligament damage, meniscal injuries, patellar subluxation, and PFD, using the appropriate maneuvers (Table 37.2).

A neurovascular exam should include palpation of the posterior tibial and dorsalis pedis pulses and testing of the peroneal nerve function. The deep peroneal nerve innervates the ankle dorsiflexors and the extensor hallucis longus, which can be tested by opposing dorsiflexion of the great toe. It also supplies sensation to the web space between the great and second toes.

Patients with knee symptoms should have a careful hip examination because patients with aseptic necrosis of the femoral head or a slipped capital femoral epiphysis may present with anterior thigh or knee pain.

TABLE 37.2

SUMMARY OF DIAGNOSTIC MANEUVERS FOR THE INJURED KNEE

Maneuver	Diagnosis
Collateral laxity test (Fig. 37.4)	Collateral ligament injury
Lachman test (Fig. 37.3)	Anterior cruciate ligament injury
Posterior drawer test (Fig. 37.5)	Posterior cruciate ligament injury
McMurray test (Fig. 37.6)	Meniscal injury
Apley compression test (Fig. 37.7)	Meniscal injury
Patellar apprehension test	Patellar subluxation
Patellar stress test	Patellofemoral pain syndrome

All patients with acute knee injuries should have AP and lateral radiographs, and if indicated, a patellar (or skyline view) radiograph. The Ottawa Knee Rules have demonstrated 100% sensitivity for knee fractures in large, prospective, multicentered adult trials. Studies in children are more limited but they also demonstrated a sensitivity of 100% (95% confidence interval = 95% to 100%) in a study involving 750 children of whom 70 had fractures. According to these rules, radiographs are required of children only if the patient has any of the following findings: (i) Isolated tenderness of the patella, (ii) tenderness of the head of the fibula, (iii) inability to flex to 90 degrees, (iv) inability to bear weight both immediately and in the ED (four steps) regardless of limping.

Figure 37.8 summarizes an approach to the child with an acutely injured knee. If the initial evaluation suggests vascular compromise, traction and reduction of the knee should be attempted and an emergent orthopedics consultation should be obtained. If the patella is obviously dislocated, it may be reduced before obtaining radiographs. If the patient's knee is too painful or swollen to allow a complete examination, and radiographs are negative, ligament or meniscal damage should be suspected. The patient should be instructed to use crutches and remain completely non–weight bearing until medical or surgical follow-up or until the patient improves. If radiographs demonstrate air in the joint, orthopedics should be consulted to assess for penetrating intra-articular injury. If there is a puncture wound or laceration near the knee joint, a saline load test should be performed to assess for penetrating intra-articular injury (Chapter 129 Musculoskeletal Emergencies).

Often, a patient may come to the ED with a history of trauma and knee pain that has been present for more than 2 or 3 days (see Fig. 37.9). In addition to the standard AP, lateral, and patellar views, a tunnel or intercondylar view should be taken to exclude fracture, tumor, and osteochondritis dissecans. If the initial knee and hip examinations do not suggest a diagnosis and no signs of infection exist, the diagnostic maneuvers in Table 37.2 should be completed. The patient may have a chronic collateral ligament, cruciate ligament, or meniscal injury and require an orthopedic referral.

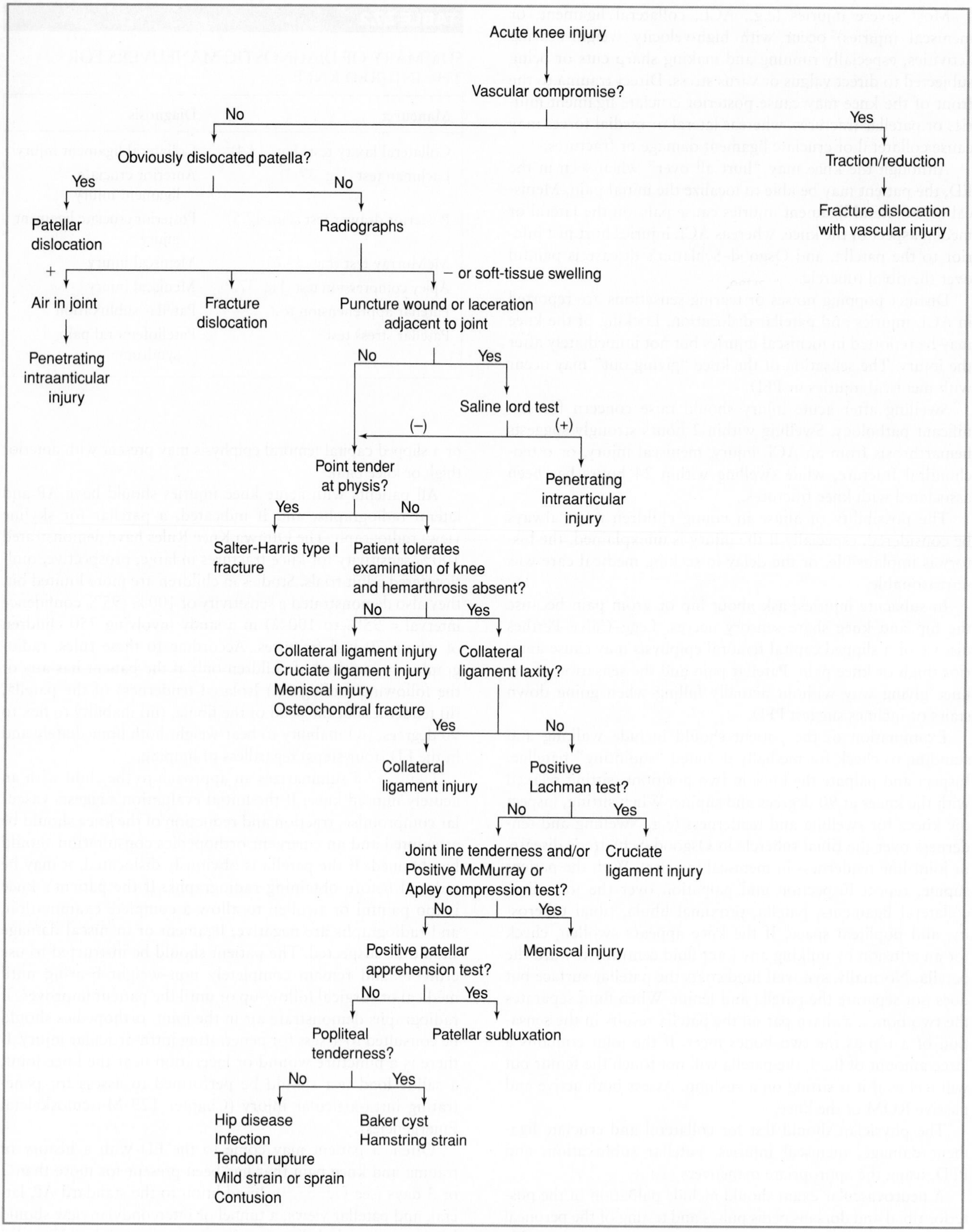

- Acute knee injury
  - Vascular compromise?
    - Yes → Traction/reduction → Fracture dislocation with vascular injury
    - No → Obviously dislocated patella?
      - Yes → Patellar dislocation
      - No → Radiographs
        - + → Air in joint → Penetrating intraanticular injury
        - Fracture dislocation
        - – or soft-tissue swelling → Puncture wound or laceration adjacent to joint
          - Yes → Saline lord test
            - (+) → Penetrating intraarticular injury
            - (–) → Point tender at physis?
          - No → Point tender at physis?
            - Yes → Salter-Harris type I fracture
            - No → Patient tolerates examination of knee and hemarthrosis absent?
              - No → Collateral ligament injury; Cruciate ligament injury; Meniscal injury; Osteochondral fracture
              - Yes → Collateral ligament laxity?
                - Yes → Collateral ligament injury
                - No → Positive Lachman test?
                  - Yes → Cruciate ligament injury
                  - No → Joint line tenderness and/or Positive McMurray or Apley compression test?
                    - Yes → Meniscal injury
                    - No → Positive patellar apprehension test?
                      - Yes → Patellar subluxation
                      - No → Popliteal tenderness?
                        - Yes → Baker cyst; Hamstring strain
                        - No → Hip disease; Infection; Tendon rupture; Mild strain or sprain; Contusion

FIGURE 37.8 Approach to the patient with an acute knee injury.

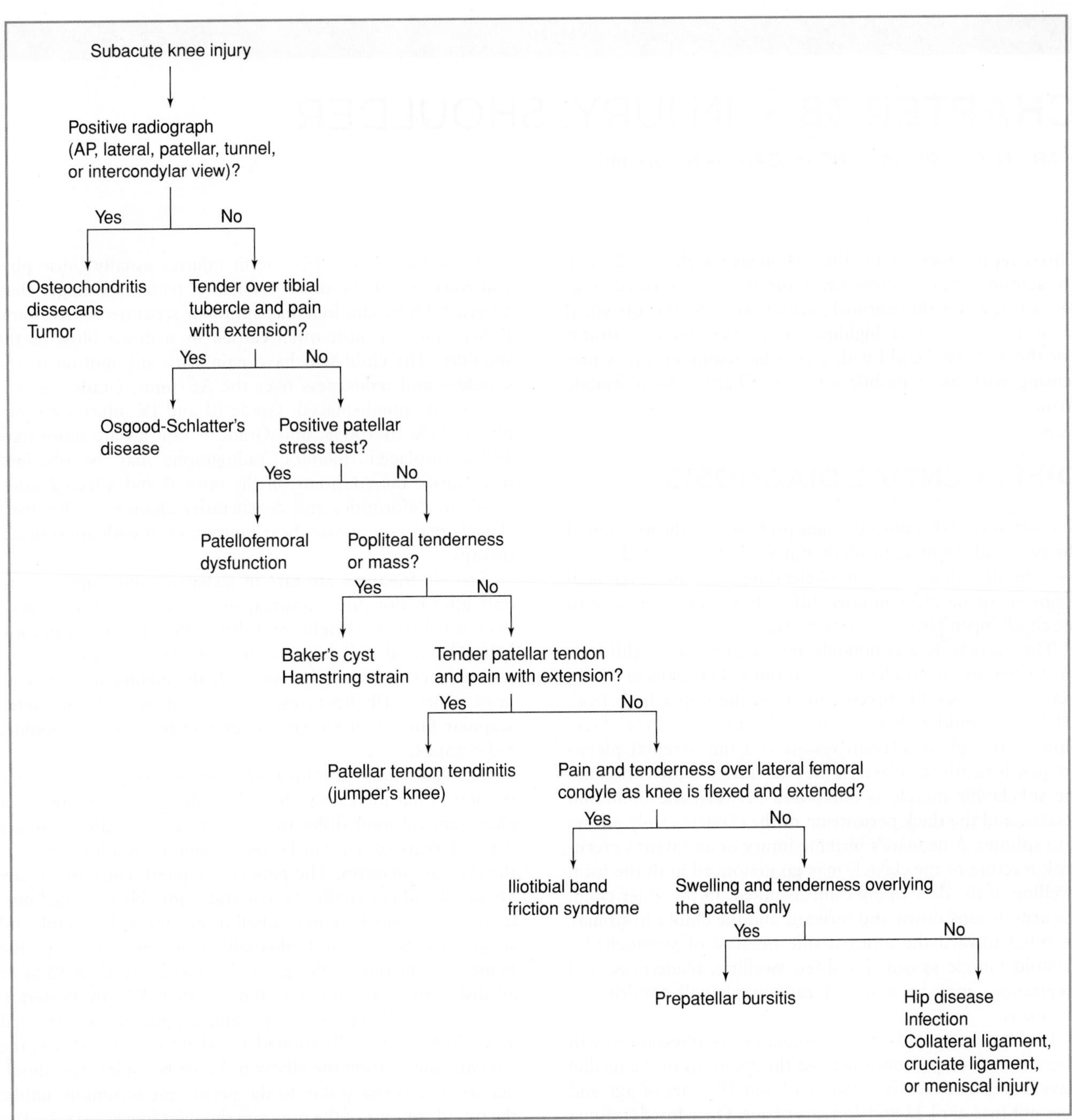

FIGURE 37.9 Approach to the patient with a subacute knee injury. AP, anteroposterior.

Suggested Readings and Key References

Bulloch B, Neto G, Plint A, et al. Validation of the Ottawa knee rules in children: a multicenter trial. *Ann Emerg Med* 2003;42: 48–55.

Cleland JA, Koppenhaver S. *Netter's Orthopaedic Clinical Examination: an evidence–based approach.* 2nd ed. Philadelphia, PA: Saunders Elsevier, 2011.

Micheli LJ, ed. *Encyclopedia of sports medicine.* Thousand Oaks, CA: SAGE Publications, 2011.

Micheli LJ, Kocher MS, eds. *The pediatric and adolescent knee.* Philadelphia, PA: Saunders Elsevier, 2006.

Micheli LJ, Purcell L, eds. *The adolescent athelete: a practical approach.* New York, NY: Springer Verlag, 2007.

Rockwood, Charles A. In: Beaty JH, Kasser JR, eds. *Rockwood and Wilkins' fractures in children.* 7th ed. Philadelphia, PA: Wolters Kluwer Lippincott Williams & Wilkins, 2010.

Solomon DH, Simel DL, Bates DW, et al. Does this patient have a torn meniscus or ligament of the knee? Value of the physical examination. *JAMA* 2001;286:1610–1620.

CHAPTER 38 ▪ INJURY: SHOULDER

MARC N. BASKIN, MD AND MEGAN HANNON, MD

This chapter focuses on the diagnosis of the child with an acutely injured shoulder. Injuries are described anatomically, from the sternoclavicular joint to the proximal humerus. Figure 38.1 highlights important bony anatomy. For the preverbal child with a possible shoulder injury presenting with an immobile arm, see Chapter 34 Immobile Arm.

DIFFERENTIAL DIAGNOSIS

The differential diagnosis depends primarily on the location of the pain and the mechanism of injury (Tables 38.1 and 38.2). As with all pediatric musculoskeletal injuries, the differential diagnosis of shoulder injuries differs from adults because of the child's open physes (growth plates).

The clavicle is a commonly fractured bone in children, most often in the middle or lateral third. The clavicle is subject to any medially directed force on the upper limb (e.g., a fall on shoulder) but is commonly fractured by a direct blow. Although subclavian vessels and the brachial plexus are just beneath the clavicle, they are rarely injured because the subclavius muscle is interposed between the bone and vessels, and the thick periosteum of the clavicle rarely allows it to splinter. A neonate's birthing injury or an infant's greenstick fracture of the clavicle may go unnoticed until the focal swelling of the developing callus is noted. In the older child, the arm droops down and forward and the child's head may be tilted toward the affected side because of sternocleidomastoid muscle spasm. Localized swelling, tenderness, and crepitations may be noted. A radiograph will confirm the diagnosis.

In children, medial clavicle trauma causes physeal (growth plate) fracture/separations because the epiphysis of the medial clavicle begins to ossify between 13 and 19 years of age and does not fuse until 22 and 25 years of age. Once fused, trauma in this location generally results in sternoclavicular joint dislocations. These injuries can be caused by direct trauma to the medial clavicle or by indirect trauma that forces the shoulder medially. Most dislocations are anterior, and the patient has swelling and tenderness over the sternoclavicular joint. If the dislocation is posterior, major vessels or trachea may be injured. The child may have dysphagia, hoarseness (laryngeal nerve), or difficulty breathing. Anteroposterior and superiorly projected lordotic radiographs comparing both clavicles may not visualize the injury and CT is usually necessary. Contrast is recommended to assess the great vessels as well as the bony anatomy.

Chronic clavicle pain or mild swelling 2 to 3 weeks after the initial injury may represent osteolysis. The distal clavicle may undergo bony resorption (osteolysis) of the pain even after minor injuries. Radiographs are diagnostic.

Acromioclavicular (AC) joint injuries usually cause physeal fractures of the distal clavicle in patients younger than 14 years. Older children may sprain or separate the AC joint. Either injury is most often caused by a direct blow to the shoulder. The child will have pain with any motion of the shoulder and tenderness over the AC joint. Grade I and II injuries are nondisplaced. Grade III and IV injuries are displaced 25% to 100%, and Grade V injuries are more than 100% displaced. Bilateral radiographs may be obtained to compare the AC joint on the normal and affected sides. Cosmetic deformities and degenerative changes of the distal clavicle may complicate these injuries, even with appropriate therapy.

Scapula fractures are rare in pediatrics and usually occur only after major direct trauma, such as a motor vehicle accident, a fall from a height, or a direct blow in American football. The child will have tenderness over the scapula. The patient often sustains other more life-threatening injuries (e.g., head injuries, rib fractures, or pneumothoraces). Dedicated scapular films improve yield over routine chest or shoulder radiographs.

The glenohumeral joint is shallow, allowing a wide range of motion but increasing the risk of dislocation. Shoulder or glenohumeral joint dislocations are rare in children younger than 12 years of age but become common in adolescence as the skeleton matures. The patient is injured when an already abducted and externally rotated arm is forcibly extended posteriorly (e.g., blocking in football or missing a slam dunk and striking the rim during basketball). This action leverages the humeral head out of the glenoid fossa. More than 95% of all dislocations are anterior, and less than 5% are posterior. The patient will be in severe pain, supporting the affected arm which is internally rotated and slightly abducted (i.e., the patient cannot bring the elbow to his or her side). The shoulder contour is sharp due to the prominent acromion, unlike the round contour of the opposite shoulder (see Fig. 38.2). The trauma can damage the axillary nerve or fracture the humeral head. Sensation over the lateral deltoid muscle (axillary nerve distribution), lateral proximal forearm (musculocutaneous nerve distribution), and distal pulses should be documented. Radiographs should always be obtained because a humeral head or clavicular fracture may mimic a shoulder dislocation. An AP, scapular "Y" view, and an axillary view are preferred to show the position of the dislocation and the presence of any fractures.

If the patient has a history consistent with dislocation but has more range of motion than expected and the radiograph is normal, the patient may have spontaneously reduced a dislocated shoulder or subluxated the glenohumeral joint and only sprained the ligaments overlying the glenoid fossa. An apprehension test may confirm the subluxation diagnosis (see Fig. 38.3).

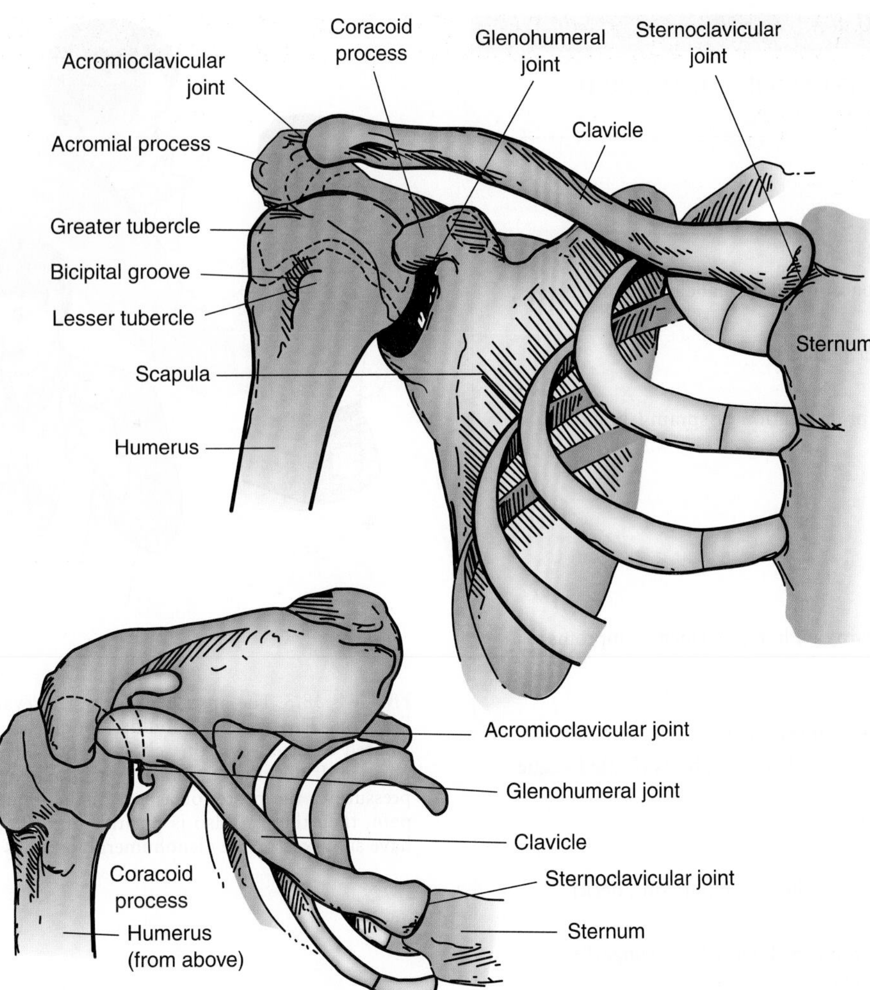

FIGURE 38.1 Anatomy of the shoulder.

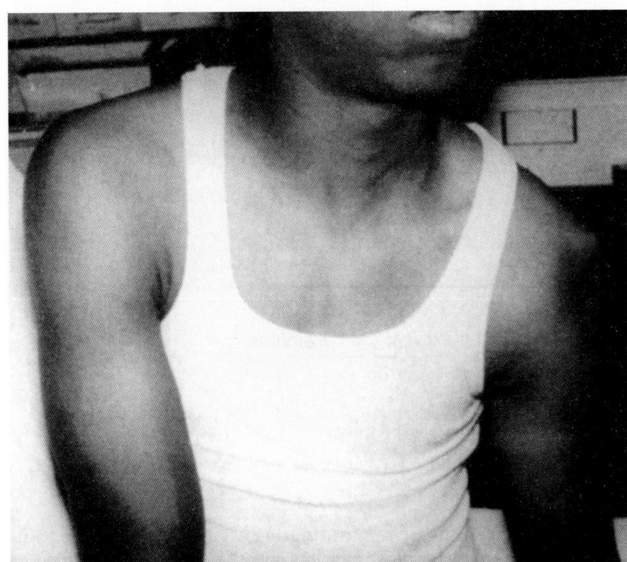

FIGURE 38.2 An older adolescent patient with left anterior glenohumeral joint dislocation. Notice the sharp contour of the shoulder, the fullness below the glenoid fossa, and the prominent acromion.

Actual tears of the rotator cuff are uncommon before 21 years of age. However, if the rotator cuff muscles are damaged or weak, the humeral head is displaced upward during overhead motion. This may impinge the tendon of the supraspinatus muscle and the subacromial bursa between the humeral head and the acromion or coracoid process. Impingement symptoms usually occur with repetitive overhead motions (e.g., throwing a ball). The pain is commonly notable over the deltoid area though it may be poorly localized. There are several tests for rotator cuff injuries but the painful arc test (see Fig. 38.4) has the best sensitivity and specificity. Plain radiographs are usually normal, and magnetic resonance imaging is necessary but does not need to be done emergently.

Before adolescence, proximal humerus fractures are usually transverse metaphyseal or Salter–Harris type I. The epiphysis closes between 16 and 18 years of age in males and about 1 year earlier in females. The injury occurs because of direct or indirect trauma (e.g., fall on an outstretched hand). The patient usually has mild swelling and local tenderness. AP and lateral radiographs can confirm the diagnosis, although they are less reliable in infants and children

TABLE 38.1

DIFFERENTIAL DIAGNOSIS OF THE INJURED SHOULDER

Sternoclavicular joint
Dislocation[a]
Sprain
Clavicle
Physeal fracture/separation of medial clavicle
Fracture
Contusion (shoulder pointer)
Osteolysis
Acromioclavicular joint dislocation or sprain (shoulder separation)
Scapula fracture
Glenohumeral joint
Dislocation
Subluxation
Labral tears
Rotator cuff tendinopathy with impingement symptoms
Rotator cuff tear
Humerus
Fracture of proximal humeral physis
Stress fracture of proximal humeral physis (Little League shoulder)
Biceps tendon tendonitis
Pathologic fracture[a]
Referred pain (from myocardium[a], diaphragm[a], neck)
Thoracic outlet syndrome[a]
Brachial plexus injury ("pinched nerve" or "stinger")

[a]Potentially life-threatening conditions.

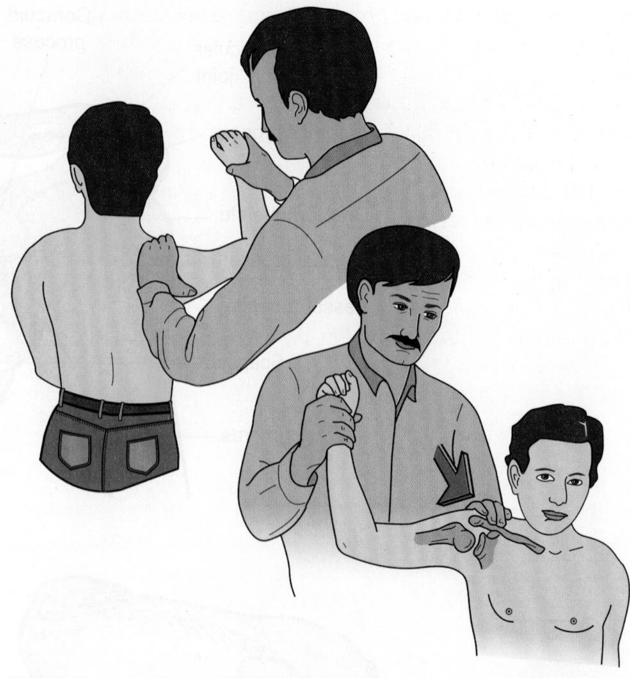

FIGURE 38.3 The apprehension test to evaluate for shoulder subluxation. The patient's shoulder should be abducted passively and rotated externally. If this elicits apprehension or pain, the test is positive. If not, the examiner then should apply anteriorly directed pressure to the posterior aspect of the humeral head. If this elicits pain, then the test also is positive and the patient's shoulder may have subluxed or the glenohumeral joint has some instability.

because the epiphysis is mainly cartilaginous. Even in older children, slight widening of the epiphysis may be difficult to appreciate, and comparison views of the uninjured side may be useful. If the child is tender over the physis and has normal radiographs, suspect a Salter–Harris I fracture. In infants <1 year of age strongly consider a skeletal survey and social work consultation due to risk of child abuse (see Chapter 95 Child Abuse/Assault).

TABLE 38.2

COMMON CAUSES OF THE INJURED SHOULDER

Clavicle fracture
Glenohumeral joint
Dislocation (shoulder dislocation)
Subluxation
Sprain
Humerus
Fracture of proximal humeral physis
Contusion

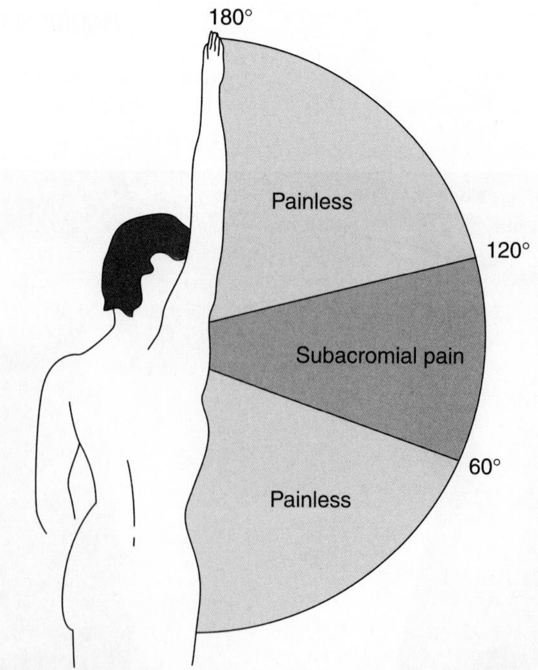

FIGURE 38.4 Painful arc test for rotator cuff injury. During the painful arc test the examiner moves the patients shoulder to full 180-degree abduction. If pain mainly occurs between 60 and 120 degrees, it is suggestive of rotator cuff injury. (Adapted from Shatzer M. *Physical medicine and rehabilitation pocketpedia*. 2nd ed. Philadelphia, PA: Lippincott Williams & Wilkins, 2012.)

Stress fractures of the proximal humeral epiphysis, or "Little League shoulder," are caused by repetitive internal rotation of an abducted, externally rotated shoulder during the throwing motion. The child, usually 11 to 16 years of age, has diffuse shoulder pain that worsens after throwing. The proximal humerus may be tender and radiographs may show widening of the proximal humeral physis. Radiographs of the contralateral humerus may be helpful.

In older patients, shoulder pain may be due to tendonitis of the long head of the biceps. This tendon is palpable as it runs through the bicipital groove just anterior and medial to the greater humeral tuberosity. The patient often has chronic pain and tenderness over the bicipital groove.

A painful shoulder or humeral fracture that follows minimal trauma may be caused by a benign or malignant tumor or by nonneoplastic bone lesions. Osteochondromas (exostoses) are outgrowths of benign cartilage from the bone adjacent to the epiphysis and present with a mass adjacent to a joint. Nonossifying fibromas also known as fibrous cortical defects are common asymptomatic lesions that may lead to pathologic fractures. Similarly, unicameral or "simple bone" cysts are benign fluid-filled cavities most commonly localized to the proximal humerus. They are usually asymptomatic until the bone fractures. Aneurysmal bone cysts are more expansile, blood channel–filled lesions that may cause pain and swelling. The malignant chondroblastoma is a rare tumor, but its most common location is the proximal humerus. The patient often has joint pain from an effusion associated with this tumor. Osteogenic sarcomas and Ewing sarcoma are more common but involve the humerus in only 10% of cases.

Shoulder pain may also be referred from the neck (e.g., cervical disc herniation), myocardium, or diaphragm (e.g., a splenic injury) after trauma to those areas.

Thoracic outlet syndrome results from compression of the lower roots of the brachial plexus (C8 to T1) or the axillary vein or artery, often in a pitcher, swimmer, or weight lifter. Patients may present with shoulder pain and associated numbness and paresthesias of the arm especially with repetitive overhead use of the arm. If thrombosis of the vein occurs, arm swelling, venous congestion, and distal cyanosis may occur. If the thrombus embolizes, the patient may have dyspnea and chest pain. The neurologic symptoms may be induced (Roos' test) by having the patient rapidly open and close their hands for 3 minutes with the arm abducted 90 degrees and the shoulder externally rotated (ask the patient to "signal for a touchdown"). The test is considered positive if it induces the patient's pain and paresthesias. A chest radiograph may identify a cervical rib. Ultrasonography is diagnostic of venous thrombosis.

Acute brachial plexus injuries ("pinched nerves" or "stingers") are common in high-impact sports. Most commonly, the shoulder is forcefully depressed and the head and neck tilted to the opposite side, stretching the brachial plexus (see Fig. 38.5). The patient has immediate arm weakness or paralysis, and paresthesias or numbness along a cervical dermatome, most commonly C5 and C6. C5 and C6 can be tested by assessing shoulder abduction (deltoid muscle and axillary nerve), external rotation (infraspinatus muscle and suprascapular nerve), and elbow flexion (biceps muscle and musculocutaneous nerve). The symptoms may resolve prior to the emergency department evaluation. Cervical spine injuries must be excluded.

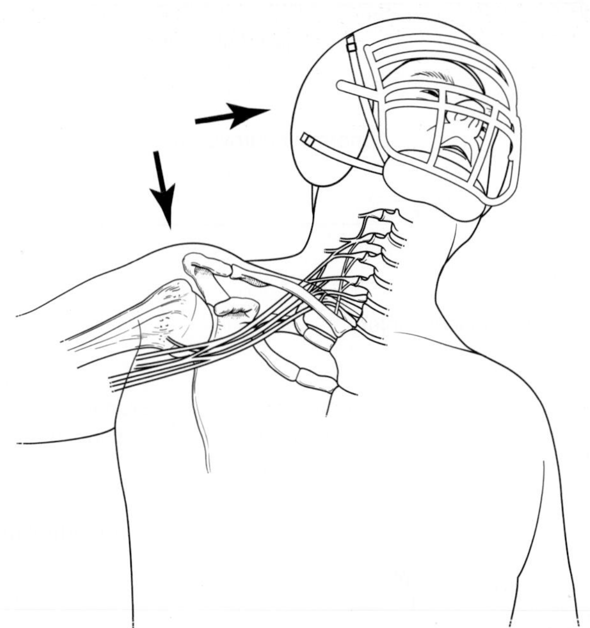

FIGURE 38.5 Burner/stinger syndrome. As in a football tackle, the shoulder is depressed while the head and neck and pushed away from the affected shoulder, resulting in a stinger. This same mechanism, combined with extension of the neck, may result in compression of the nerves on the contralateral shoulder, also resulting in a burner or stinger. (From Miniaci A. *Disorders of the shoulder: sports injuries*. Philadelphia, PA: Lippincott Williams & Wilkins, 2013.)

EVALUATION AND DECISION

Initially, the patient's neurovascular status is assessed and fracture stabilization provided, if necessary (see Fig. 38.6).

For an isolated shoulder injury, ask the patient to localize the pain as specifically as possible. Determine both the mechanism and the shoulder position during injury. If the pain is chronic, determine the position or motion that most exacerbates the pain. Ask the patient about any distal paresthesias, associated pain, and trauma (especially neck). Consider the possibility of abuse in young children, especially if the injury is unexplained, the history is implausible or inconsistent between caregivers, or the seeking of medical care was delayed unreasonably.

Observe the patient without clothes for positioning of the arm, swelling, deformity, or any asymmetry. Ask the patient to point with one finger to the most painful area. This observation period before the formal physical examination is especially important in a young, anxious child and helps prioritize the rest of the evaluation.

If the child seems anxious, examine the uninjured side first. Carefully palpate the entire shoulder from sternoclavicular joint to the shaft of the humerus. Swelling and tenderness at the sternoclavicular joint suggests a physeal separation or dislocation at this site. The clavicle is covered only by a thin platysma muscle, and a fracture is easily seen and palpated. Just lateral to the clavicle is the AC joint. Elevation of the clavicle above the acromion or tenderness of the articulation suggests AC joint separation or sprain. Just in front of the greater tuberosity of the humerus is the tendon of the long

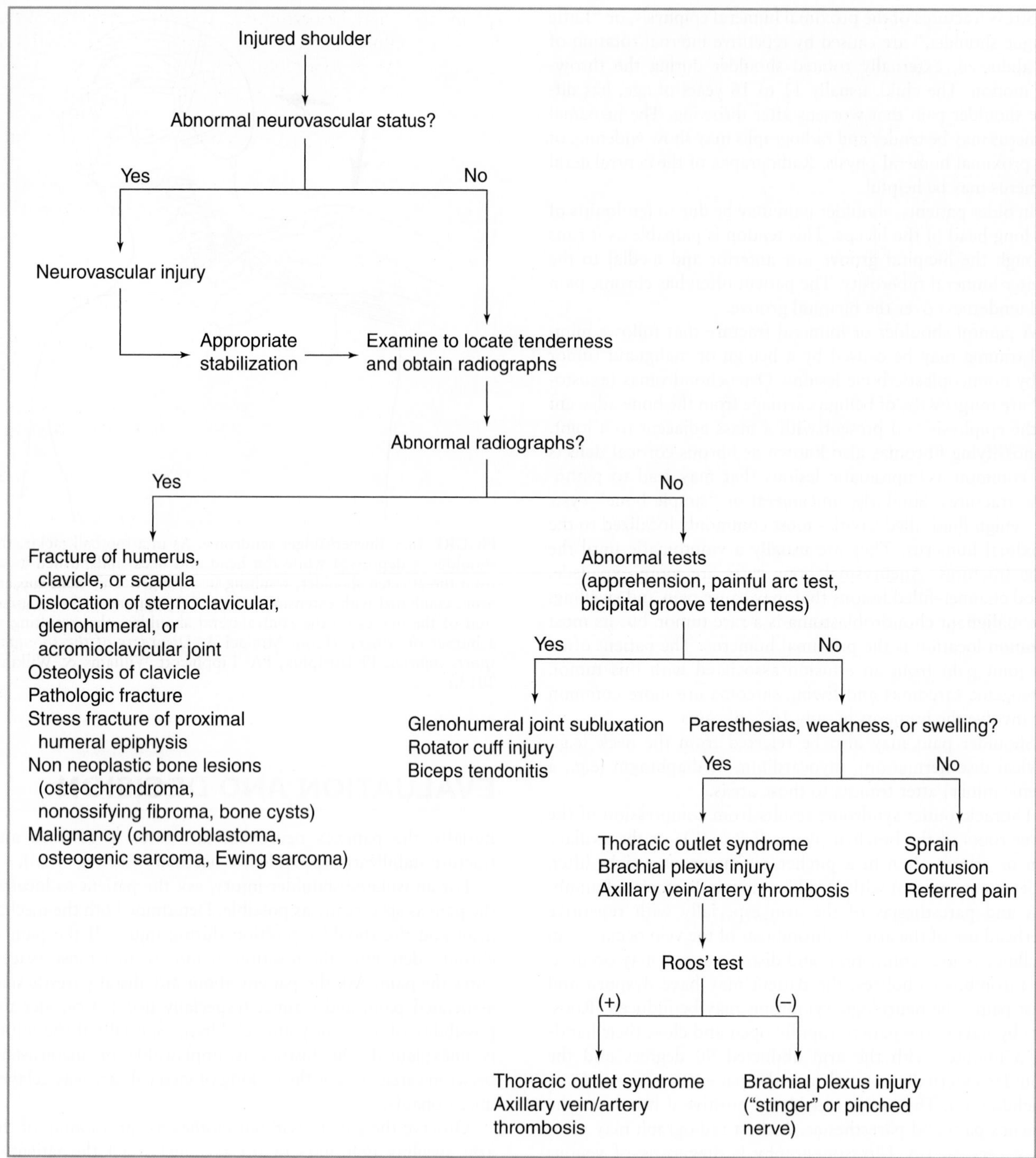

FIGURE 38.6 Approach to the patient with an injured shoulder.

head of the biceps within the bicipital groove. Pressure may produce exquisite tenderness in this area, so palpation should be gentle; if uncertainty about a finding of tenderness exists, a comparison with the examination of the uninjured side is helpful. Finally, the proximal humeral shaft and the scapula are palpated.

During the neurologic evaluation, it is important to test sensation over the deltoid muscle (to assess axillary nerve damage after shoulder dislocation) and over the lateral proximal forearm (to assess musculocutaneous nerve damage).

Next, examine the patient's active and passive range of motion (see Fig. 38.7). Internal and external rotation can be observed easily in a child by asking the patient to touch behind the neck (external rotation) and lower back to the inferior tip of the opposite scapula (internal rotation).

Once the pain has been localized, appropriate radiographs should be obtained. When indicated, additional

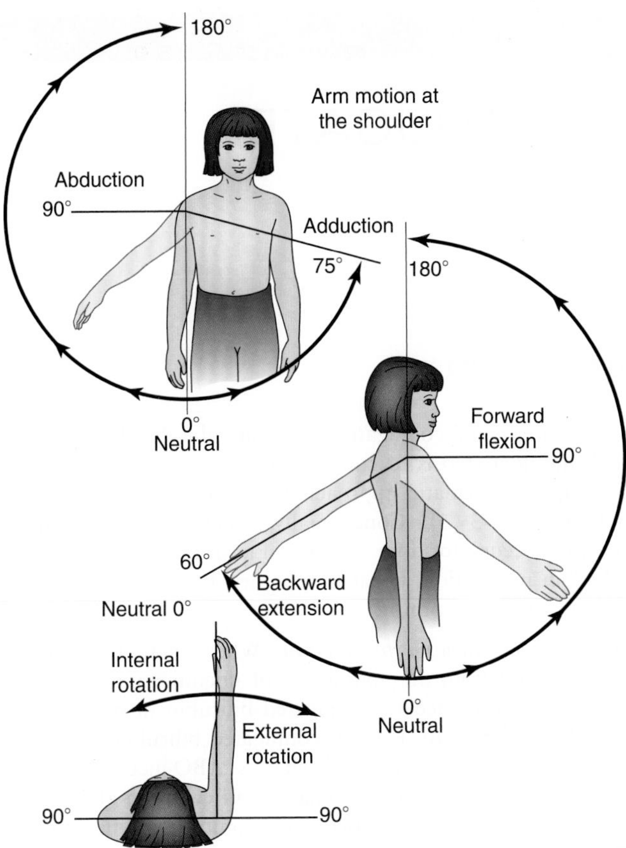

FIGURE 38.7 Range of motion of the shoulder joint.

specific tests may be performed: The apprehension test for shoulder subluxation and laxity (Fig. 38.4), painful arc (Fig. 38.3) test for rotator cuff injury.

If the patient has nonspecific pain with numbness, paresthesias, weakness, or diffuse swelling, Roos' test can be performed to distinguish between possible thoracic outlet syndrome and brachial plexus injury.

Patients with normal radiographs and negative maneuvers are most likely to have sprains or contusions, but occasionally, they may be experiencing referred pain.

Suggested Readings and Key References

Beaty JH, Kasser JR, eds. *Rockwood and Wilkins' fractures in children*. 7th ed. Philadelphia, PA: Lippincott Williams & Wilkins, 2010.

Dashe J, Roocroft JH, Bastrom TP, et al. Spectrum of shoulder injuries in skeletally immature patients. *Orthop Clin North Am* 2013;44:541–551.

Hermans J, Luime JJ, Meuffels DE, et al. Does this patient with shoulder pain have rotator cuff disease? The rational clinical examination systemic review. *JAMA* 2013;310(8):837–847.

Hoppenfeld S, Hutton R, Hugh T. *Physical examination of the spine and extremities*. Norwalk, CT: Appleton-Century-Crofts, 1976.

Irvin R, Iversen D, Roy S. *Sports medicine: prevention, assessment, management, and rehabilitation*. Boston, MA: Allyn & Bacon, 1998.

Micheli LJ, Purcell L, eds. *The adolescent athlete: a practical approach*. New York, NY: Springer, 2007.

Sarwark JF, ed. *Essentials of musculoskeletal care*. 4th ed. Rosemont, IL: American Academy of Orthopaedic Surgeons, 2010.

CHAPTER 39 ■ JAUNDICE: CONJUGATED HYPERBILIRUBINEMIA

ERIN B. HENKEL, MD AND SANJIV HARPAVAT, MD, PhD

INTRODUCTION

The pediatric emergency provider is typically confronted with the finding of hyperbilirubinemia in one of two situations: (1) a jaundiced child, or (2) an incidental finding during a laboratory evaluation. When conjugated hyperbilirubinemia is found, the challenge lies in determining if it is a sign of a life-threatening condition.

NORMAL BILIRUBIN PHYSIOLOGY

Senescent red blood cells release heme which is eventually converted to unconjugated bilirubin. Unconjugated bilirubin then binds to albumin and is transported to the liver. In the liver sinusoids, unconjugated bilirubin detaches from albumin and gains entry into the hepatocyte, where it is conjugated with glucuronide by the action of uridine diphosphate glucuronyl transferase. The soluble conjugated diglucuronide then is secreted out of the hepatocyte, across its canalicular membrane into the bile. Conjugated bilirubin, along with bile salts, phospholipids, cholesterol, and metabolites are the major constituents of bile. Bile flows through the intrahepatic biliary tree, into the extrahepatic bile ducts (including the common bile duct), and finally into the intestine at the ampulla of Vater. In the intestine, bacterial flora converts bilirubin to urobilinogen. Some urobilinogen is reabsorbed and taken up by the liver cells, only to be reexcreted into the bile. A small percentage of urobilinogen escapes into the systemic circulation and is excreted in the urine. The unabsorbed urobilinogen is excreted in the stool as fecal urobilinogen (see Chapter 40 Jaundice: Unconjugated Hyperbilirubinemia).

DEFINITION

The definition of conjugated hyperbilirubinemia is controversial. Some commonly used definitions are a conjugated bilirubin level higher than 2 mg/dL or a conjugated bilirubin that is more than 20% of the total bilirubin. Since these definitions are broad and frequently used in the absence of additional considerations, one risks missing significant liver diseases. A more sensitive definition is any conjugated bilirubin level above the laboratory's normal reference interval. Laboratory reference intervals are calculated using the 2.5th to 97.5th percentile of values in a population, that is, the middle 95% of values. This definition is very sensitive but less specific for liver disease. From the perspective of an emergency physician, following this definition will decrease the risk of missing diagnoses.

ETIOLOGIES

Once an elevated conjugated bilirubin value has been identified, the next step is to consider the causes that explain the finding. A systematic approach to making the diagnosis is helpful (Fig. 39.1). Conceptually, conjugated hyperbilirubinemia occurs for four reasons: Elevation from increased bilirubin production, hepatocyte injury, bilirubin transporter defects, or obstruction.

- *Increased bilirubin production:* When there is bilirubin overproduction, the abundance of unconjugated bilirubin must be converted to conjugated bilirubin in order for it to be excreted. As a result, conjugated bilirubin levels can rise. In newborns, red blood cell lysis, ABO incompatibility, G6PD, and cephalohematoma can all cause an abundance of unconjugated and subsequently conjugated bilirubin.
- *Hepatocyte injury:* Hepatocyte injury from any mechanism will cause the breakdown of the liver cell, which results in the release of conjugated bilirubin into the bloodstream. This occurs with liver failure, toxic injury, infections, and metabolic disorders.
- *Bilirubin transporter defects:* Transporter defects can be acquired in the setting of general liver injury. They can also be isolated, causing only conjugated hyperbilirubinemia without associated liver damage. In these situations, conjugated bilirubin is retained in the liver which can discolor the liver but does not cause direct toxicity. Other components of bile, such as toxic bile acids and metabolites, flow normally out of the liver and into the intestine. Dubin–Johnson syndrome is an example of a defect in conjugated bilirubin transporters.
- *Obstruction:* When the biliary tree becomes obstructed, liver damage results. The classic example is biliary atresia (BA), where bile salts backup into the liver and induce rapid fibrosis, cirrhosis, and eventual liver failure.

(See Table 39.1.)

HISTORY AND PHYSICAL EXAMINATION

The provider interviewing the patient and family with hyperbilirubinemia can often differentiate the cause and severity of the underlying issue with a thorough medical history and physical examination (Fig. 39.1). The following questions can help elucidate key points in differentiating the cause of conjugated hyperbilirubinemia:

1. Is this the first episode of jaundice? (to distinguish between an acute event or a chronic process)

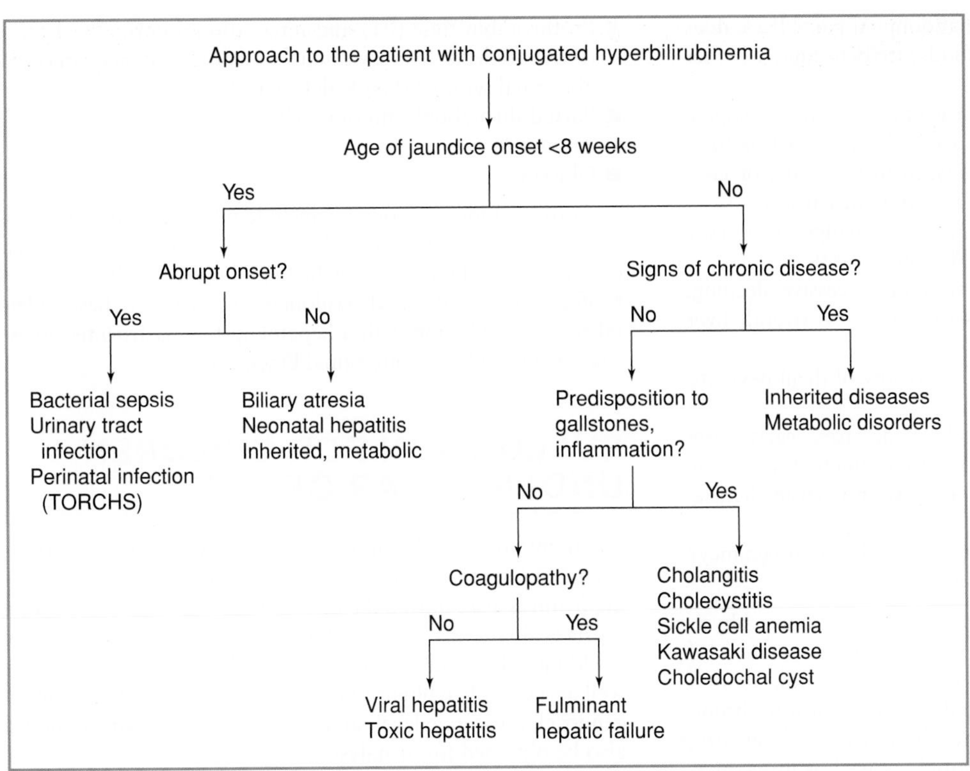

FIGURE 39.1 Approach to the patient with conjugated hyperbilirubinemia.

TABLE 39.1

CAUSES OF CONJUGATED HYPERBILIRUBINEMIA

Elevated production – Sickle hemoglobinopathies – ABO incompatibility – G6PD deficiency – Cephalohematoma **Hepatocyte injury** – Acute liver failure – Hepatotoxins: drugs such as acetaminophen – TORCHS and perinatal/congenital infections ■ Toxoplasmosis ■ Rubella ■ Cytomegalovirus ■ Varicella zoster ■ Herpes simplex virus ■ Coxsackievirus ■ Parvovirus B19 ■ Human immunodeficiency virus ■ Syphilis – Acquired infections ■ Sepsis ■ Urinary tract infection – Metabolic disorders ■ Galactosemia ■ Galactokinase deficiency ■ Hereditary fructose intolerance ■ α1-Antitrypsin deficiency – Cystic fibrosis – Autoimmune hepatitis	**Transporter problem** – Sepsis – Dubin–Johnson syndrome – Rotor syndrome – Hypopituitarism – Hypothyroidism – Cystic fibrosis – Idiopathic neonatal cholestasis or neonatal hepatitis syndrome – Progressive intrahepatic cholestasis types 1 and 2 (PFIC1, PFIC2) – Alagille syndrome – Wilson disease – Benign recurrent intrahepatic cholestasis (BRIC) **Obstruction** – Biliary atresia – Choledochal cyst – Cholelithiasis – Choledocholithiasis – Cholecystitis – Cholangitis – Pancreatic disease – Gallbladder hydrops ■ Kawasaki disease ■ Streptococcal infection ■ Staphylococcal infection – Inflammatory bowel disease ■ Ulcerative colitis ■ Crohn disease ■ Primary sclerosing cholangitis – Tumors of the liver and biliary tree

2. Are the stools acholic? Is there abdominal pain? If so, does the pain increase with certain foods? (to determine whether biliary obstruction is present)
3. Is fever, fatigue, emesis, or diarrhea present? (to investigate viral causes, including EBV, hepatitis A, and hepatitis B)
4. Are there any rashes, arthralgias, arthritic joints, or conjunctivitis? (to question about autoimmune causes)
5. Have there been any recent behavioral changes, especially in a teenager? (to evaluate for Wilson disease)
6. Is itching, bleeding, bruising, swelling, excessive sleeping, or mental status changes present? (to assess overall liver function)
7. What medications are taken, and are any of them new? (to identify potential hepatotoxins)
8. Is there a family history of liver diseases, early-onset emphysema, or iron overload? (to evaluate for genetic causes, such as Alagille syndrome, α_1-antitrypsin disease, or hemochromatosis)
9. (For infants) Were there any infections during pregnancy? Were the newborn screens normal?

It is also important to perform a meticulous physical examination, starting with the growth parameters of the child, including weight and height percentiles, as well as the growth curve. Central and distal perfusion should be assessed. While examining the abdomen, the liver size, contour, and texture should be noted, as well as an estimation of spleen size. The presence or absence of abdominal tenderness and the location should be identified in children with reliable examinations. The skin examination should include evaluation for bleeding, bruising, spider angiomas, caput medusa, excoriations or signs of pruritus, and palmar erythema. The neurologic examination should include mental status evaluation, as well as observation for dysarthrias, tremors, or rigidity.

EVALUATION

The most concerning etiologies for conjugated hyperbilirubinemia are the results of hepatocyte destruction or biliary obstruction. Identification of these conditions should be the focus of the evaluation in the emergency department. The first step is to obtain serum liver enzymes including:

- Aspartate aminotransferase (AST)
- Alanine aminotransferase (ALT)
- Gamma glutamyltransferase (GGT)
- Conjugated bilirubin
- Total bilirubin

If the liver studies above are normal except for a high conjugated bilirubin level, the clinician can be more reassured that hepatocyte damage or biliary obstruction is unlikely. However, in early stages of some liver diseases, conjugated bilirubin concentrations may rise before other signs of liver damage.

If there are abnormalities of the other liver enzymes, further investigation into hepatocyte injury or obstructive etiologies should be undertaken. A first step is to evaluate liver synthetic function, because abnormalities in liver function require admission and urgent evaluation by pediatric hepatology. Liver synthetic function is evaluated by measuring:

- Albumin (reflects liver synthetic function, but also reflects nutritional status and is a negative acute phase reactant)
- Prothrombin time (PT) and international normalized ratio (INR) (reflects liver synthetic function, but also may be abnormal with vitamin K deficiency)
- Partial thromboplastin time (PTT)
- Ammonia
- Glucose

Further studies to consider include infectious titers, thyroid studies, autoimmune antibodies, plasma amino acids, urine organic acids, PI phenotyping, hemoglobin electrophoresis, iron profile, sweat testing, and ceruloplasmin. These are best undertaken in consultation with a hepatologist or gastroenterologist (see Chapter 99 Gastrointestinal Emergencies).

EVALUATION FOR CHILDREN UNDER 1 YEAR OF AGE

For an infant under 2 months of age with conjugated hyperbilirubinemia, sepsis should always be considered. If any concerning features arise during the history or physical examination, a sepsis evaluation is warranted. Depending on the concern, this could include cultures blood, urine, and cerebrospinal fluid, as well as a complete blood cell, platelet count, blood urea nitrogen level, creatinine level, and blood sugar tests. Urine should also be obtained for urinalysis.

For these young infants, as well as children up to 12 months of age, state metabolic screens obtained during the newborn period should be reviewed. Additional studies of blood and urine that may be useful include protease inhibitor (PI) typing (for α_1-antitrypsin disease), TORCHS and hepatitis B virus serology, serum amino acids, thyroid function tests, red blood cell galactose 1-phosphate uridyltransferase activity, and urine examination for cytomegalovirus (CMV). Useful imaging includes chest radiograph to detect butterfly vertebrae characteristic of Alagille syndrome, and abdominal ultrasound to detect choledochal cysts. If BA is suspected, a more specialized evaluation is needed. Inpatient observation is appropriate in this age group because the diagnosis can rarely be established in the emergency department. Empiric therapy for sepsis or urinary infection is often warranted, pending culture results.

EVALUATION FOR CHILDREN OVER 1 YEAR OF AGE

In the evaluation of conjugated hyperbilirubinemia beyond infancy, it is necessary to know if there has been exposure to an infectious agent or a potential for sexual or vertical transmission of infections such as hepatitis or human immunodeficiency virus. Other risk factors for hepatitis (e.g., needle sticks, hemodialysis, transplant, transfusion of blood products, or factor use) need to be elicited. The physician should also ask about possible exposure to industrial toxins or foods previously implicated in hepatic injury (e.g., carbon tetrachloride, yellow phosphorus, tannic acid, alcohol, mushrooms of the *Amanita* species). The emergency physician must inquire about use of hepatotoxic medications including acetaminophen, salicylates, nonsteroidal anti-inflammatory drugs, iron salts, erythromycin, ceftriaxone, rifampin, nitrofurantoin, oxacillin, tetracycline, trimethoprim-sulfamethoxazole, ketoconazole, diphenylhydantoin, isoniazid, and chlorpromazine.

LIFE-THREATENING CAUSES NOT TO MISS

Congenital TORCHS Infections and Sepsis

One of the first signs of sepsis in a newborn could be conjugated hyperbilirubinemia, which may occur antecedent to more recognizable physical findings of sepsis or blood cultures becoming positive. Infants who have congenital infections may also have a low birth weight. They generally present in the immediate newborn period with cholestatic jaundice, irritability, jitteriness, and/or seizures. On examination, microcephaly, hepatomegaly, splenomegaly, and petechiae may be seen with the perinatal TORCHS complex. These include perinatal infections from toxoplasmosis, parvovirus B19, rubella, CMV, herpes simplex, varicella zoster, and syphilis. Jaundice may also be an early diagnostic sign of urinary tract infection (UTI) in the neonatal period. Gram-negative infections such as UTI and sepsis can lead to cholestasis as bile flow is sensitive to circulating endotoxins.

Biliary Atresia

Infants with BA present with a mild conjugated hyperbilirubinemia. They initially feed well and thrive. Their stools may be intermittently pigmented early in life and then become permanently without pigment usually by 4 to 6 weeks. The medical history and physical examination at presentation are generally reassuring, with the exception of jaundice and hepatomegaly. However, if these infants are not diagnosed early, they will have too much liver injury to be able to benefit from the Kasai portoenterostomy and will need liver transplantation for survival (see Chapter 99 Gastrointestinal Emergencies).

Evaluation for BA varies from institution to institution. Abdominal ultrasound is neither sensitive nor specific, though absence of gall bladder, irregular gall bladder walls, and polysplenia are findings that may be seen. The gold standard for diagnosis is an intraoperative cholangiogram to demonstrate obstruction of bile flow. Treatment includes the Kasai portoenterostomy to allow direct flow into the intestines, and has the highest success rate when performed earlier. Even if successful, 70% of children will continue to develop fibrosis, portal hypertension, and cirrhosis, and require liver transplantation.

Acute Liver Failure

Acute liver failure presents with both liver inflammation and dysfunction, and can be quite severe and rapidly progressive to shock and multi-organ failure. The most common etiologies are toxin-related (such as acetaminophen poisoning), infection, and idiopathic. Signs of acute failure include coagulopathy with elevated PT and PTT levels, and hepatic encephalopathy with an elevated ammonia level. Symptoms include vomiting, bruising, abdominal pain, jaundice, rash, and altered mental status. Common complications include gastrointestinal bleeding, electrolyte imbalances, renal failure, infection, and cerebral edema.

Aggressive therapy is needed as soon as acute liver failure is identified, and includes supportive care to maintain cardiac, cerebral, renal, and pulmonary function. N-acetylcysteine (NAC) should also be given in cases of acetaminophen toxicity. Procoagulation blood products are not necessarily recommended, because even though patients with acute liver failure have low levels of procoagulation factors (as measured by high INR), they maintain a balance because they also have low levels of anticoagulation factors which are seldom measured. Plasmapheresis, exchange transfusion, and hemodialysis may be necessary depending on the severity of the case. Mortality with acute liver failure can be 80% or higher; however, even with severe dysfunction, full recovery can occur. No reliable way currently exists to predict which patients presenting with acute liver failure will have a poor prognosis.

Metabolic Abnormalities

The metabolic and hepatic disorders have variable symptoms at onset. Infants with galactosemia, tyrosinemia, fatty acid oxidation disorders, and fructose intolerance can present with cholestasis and may appear ill in the emergency department due to metabolic derangement or secondary infection. Some cases present acutely; however, many children can have an antecedent history of failure to thrive, developmental delay, and inconstant jaundice. A family history of unexplained mortality in childhood or unexplained pulmonary, gastrointestinal, neurologic, or psychiatric disturbance in other family members may provoke diagnostic consideration.

Obstructive Etiologies: Gallstones, Cysts

Biliary calculi and acute inflammation of the gallbladder are less common causes of conjugated hyperbilirubinemia in the pediatric population except among patients with specific underlying conditions. For example, cholelithiasis may complicate any of the hemolytic anemias, particularly in patients with sickle hemoglobinopathies. Other risk factors for gallstones include obesity, Crohn disease, chronic parenteral nutrition, and cystic fibrosis. Cholecystitis may also accompany a variety of acute focal infections, such as pneumonia or peritonitis, and may occur in the course of bacterial sepsis. In less severe presentations of acute cholecystitis, fever, nausea, vomiting, abdominal distension, and right upper quadrant pain are prominent features.

Other causes of obstruction include choledochal cysts, which can present with triad of right upper quadrant abdominal mass, pain, and jaundice. Acute hydrops of the gall bladder, from Kawasaki disease or systemic streptococcal infection, can also appear with acute, painful right upper quadrant mass associated with jaundice. When cholelithiasis or other obstruction from stones or cysts is suspected, ultrasound of the right upper quadrant should be performed as it is highly sensitive and specific for stones in the gallbladder. Endoscopic retrograde cholangiopancreatography (ERCP) is more helpful to identify stones and abnormalities in the extrahepatic biliary tree and common bile duct. If a choledochal cyst is not seen by ultrasound but there is a high index of suspicion for this diagnosis, magnetic resonance cholangiopancreatography (MRCP) is the diagnostic test of choice.

Acetaminophen Toxicity

Acetaminophen toxicity is one of the most common unintentional and intentional overdoses seen in children and teenagers.

The acetaminophen metabolite *N*-acetyl-*p*-benzoquinoneimine (NAPQI) is responsible for hepatocyte injury by depleting glutathione, an antioxidant. Liver damage is more likely to occur with an ingested dose of 150 mg/kg or higher, or over 10 g total. In the first 8 hours after ingestion the patient can present with vague gastrointestinal symptoms such as nausea and vomiting, but generally will appear well for the first 24 hours. Liver enzymes will typically rise after 24 hours, and peak liver damage occurs between 24 and 48 hours after ingestion, manifesting with coagulopathy, encephalopathy, or hepatic failure and can progress to death. An acetaminophen level should be drawn at a minimum of 4 hours after ingestion, and the Rumack–Matthew nomogram can be used until 24 hours postingestion to determine toxicity.

Charcoal therapy is recommended only if the patient is seen within 1 hour of ingestion, is alert with stable vital signs, and is suspected to have ingested a toxic level of acetaminophen. NAC is given for a toxic level of acetaminophen in the blood based on the nomogram. NAC is a precursor to glutathione and helps the body to metabolize and excrete acetaminophen and NAPQI built up in the liver. Liver enzymes and coagulation studies should be followed serially for the first 24 hours after ingestion to monitor for progressive damage and need for further intervention.

Suggested Readings and Key References

Brumbaugh D, Mack C. Conjugated hyperbilirubinemia in children. *Pediatr Rev* 2012;33(7):291–302.

Gourley GR. Neonatal jaundice and disorders of bilirubin metabolism. In: Suchy FJ, Sokol RJ, Balistreri WF, eds. *Liver disease in children.* 3rd ed. New York, NY: Cambridge University Press, 2007.

Harb R, Thomas DW. Conjugated hyperbilirubinemia: screening and treatment in older infants and children. *Pediatr Rev* 2007;28(3):83–91.

CHAPTER 40 ▪ JAUNDICE: UNCONJUGATED HYPERBILIRUBINEMIA

DANA A. SCHINASI, MD

Jaundice is a yellowish discoloration of the skin, tissues, and bodily fluids that results from the deposition of unconjugated bilirubin pigment in the skin and mucous membranes. It is estimated that 60% to 80% of all term newborns develop jaundice. Hyperbilirubinemia refers to a serum bilirubin level greater than 5 mg per dL; unconjugated (indirect) hyperbilirubinemia is the most common form of jaundice encountered by emergency department (ED) practitioners. In conjugated (direct) hyperbilirubinemia, the conjugated fraction exceeds 2 mg per dL or is greater than 20% of the total serum bilirubin (TSB) (see Chapter 39 Jaundice: Conjugated Hyperbilirubinemia).

Clinicians must follow a systematic approach to distinguish between the physiologic and pathologic etiologies of unconjugated hyperbilirubinemia in order to promptly identify children in need of immediate intervention. The ultimate goal is to prevent the development of kernicterus—the permanent neurologic consequence of bilirubin deposition in brain tissue; the acute neurologic manifestations are known as acute bilirubin encephalopathy, the term recommended by the American Academy of Pediatrics (AAP).

PATHOPHYSIOLOGY

Bilirubin is the final product of heme degradation. Heme protoporphyrin is oxidized and subsequently reduced in macrophages to form unconjugated bilirubin, which is released into the plasma. At physiologic pH, bilirubin is insoluble in plasma and requires binding to albumin. When it exceeds the binding capacity of albumin, the unbound unconjugated bilirubin may cross the blood–brain barrier and deposit in the basal ganglia, causing acute bilirubin encephalopathy.

During normal physiologic conditions, the liver conjugates bilirubin by glucuronyl transferase and then excretes the conjugated form into bile. Most conjugated bilirubin is secreted through the bile into the small intestine, where bacterial enzymes degrade it to urobilinogen—90% is degraded and excreted in feces, while 10% is reabsorbed into the liver via enterohepatic circulation.

Newborn infants inherently possess multiple factors which contribute to the development of physiologic hyperbilirubinemia: increased red blood cell (RBC) volume, decreased RBC life span, immature hepatic uptake and conjugation, and increased enterohepatic circulation. Hyperbilirubinemia is considered pathologic when it is present in the first day of life, when the level exceeds the age-specific 95th percentile or has a concerning rate of rise (greater than 0.2 mg/dL/hr), when the conjugated fraction is high, or in the presence of concerning physical examination or laboratory findings.

DIFFERENTIAL DIAGNOSIS

The causes of unconjugated hyperbilirubinemia may be classified into three groups, based on mechanism of accumulation: excess bilirubin production, decreased bilirubin conjugation, impaired bilirubin excretion (Table 40.1).

Excess Bilirubin Production

The numerous causes of hemolysis may be categorized as intravascular or extravascular. Intravascular hemolysis may be further divided into intrinsic and extrinsic RBC defects. Inherited RBC enzyme deficiencies include glucose-6-phosphate dehydrogenase (G6PD) deficiency and pyruvate kinase deficiency. G6PD is common in children of African, Asian, and Mediterranean descent; patients with this disorder who are exposed to oxidant stress (e.g., fava beans, sulfa drugs) may present with acute rapid hemolysis (see Chapter 101 Hematologic Emergencies). Children with hemoglobinopathies, such as sickle cell disease and thalassemias, are prone to hemolysis. Congenital defects in the RBC membrane found in hereditary spherocytosis and hereditary elliptocytosis increase the fragility of the corpuscles, which predisposes patients to hemolytic episodes.

Maternal–fetal blood group incompatibility is critical to recognize early. When maternal antibodies are produced against fetal RBC antigens, the neonate can develop a Coombs positive isoimmune hemolytic anemia. ABO incompatibility generally occurs in infants with A or B blood groups whose mothers have type O blood group; maternal anti-A and anti-B antibodies are produced and can result in hemolysis with a positive direct Coombs test. Rh-negative mothers may become sensitized to an Rh-positive fetus during pregnancy and mount an antibody response during a subsequent pregnancy leading to Rh disease of the newborn. Administration of Rho (D) immune globulin (RhoGAM) to Rh-negative mothers who have not yet developed anti-Rh antibodies can prevent Rh isoimmunization. Infections such as sepsis, urinary tract infection (UTI), and malaria are also important causes of hemolysis. Other extrinsic causes of RBC destruction include the autoimmune, microangiopathic, and drug-induced hemolytic anemias.

Birth trauma, when associated with cephalohematoma, extensive bruising, or swallowed maternal blood, can result in hyperbilirubinemia. Intracranial, pulmonary, or other concealed hemorrhage can also lead to extravascular hemolysis. Similarly, polycythemia, caused by delayed clamping of the cord or maternal–fetal or fetal–fetal transfusion (in multiple gestations), increases the RBC mass and causes jaundice in neonates thereby increasing the risk for supraphysiologic

TABLE 40.1

CAUSES OF UNCONJUGATED HYPERBILIRUBINEMIA

Excess bilirubin production
Intravascular hemolysis
Intrinsic
Glucose-6-phosphate dehydrogenase deficiency, pyruvate kinase deficiency
Sickle cell disease, thalassemia
Hereditary spherocytosis, hereditary elliptocytosis
Extrinsic
Isoimmunization (ABO-incompatibility, Rh disease)
Infection
Hemolytic anemia (autoimmune, microangiopathic, drug-induced)
Extravascular hemolysis
Cephalohematoma
Swallowed blood during birth
Concealed hematoma (intracranial, pulmonary, intra-abdominal)
Polycythemia
Hypersplenism
Decreased bilirubin conjugation
Physiologic jaundice
Gilbert syndrome, Crigler–Najjar syndromes, Lucey–Driscoll syndrome
Galactosemia
Endocrine disorders (congenital hypothyroidism, infant of a diabetic mother)
Breast milk jaundice
Impaired bilirubin excretion
Breast-feeding jaundice
Bowel obstruction
Infection (sepsis, TORCH)
Toxin mediated

serum bilirubin. Various hypersplenic states, including splenic sequestration crisis in sickle cell disease, may result in anemia with accompanying hemolysis and hyperbilirubinemia.

Decreased Bilirubin Conjugation

Incomplete maturation of conjugation enzymes in the newborn infant's liver is the most common etiology of mild hyperbilirubinemia, with approximately 60% of neonates manifesting clinical signs of physiologic jaundice. Physiologic jaundice peaks between 3 and 5 days of life in the term infant, rarely exceeds 12 mg per dL, and requires no treatment.

Gilbert syndrome is a common cause of mild, intermittent, unconjugated hyperbilirubinemia that occurs in approximately 6% of the population. Patients with Gilbert syndrome have a partial deficiency of glucuronyl transferase. They generally present in late childhood with nonspecific abdominal pain, nausea, and mild jaundice in the setting of an intercurrent illness; there is no hepatosplenomegaly on physical examination and the remainder of liver function studies is normal. The serum bilirubin rarely exceeds 5 mg per dL in this benign cause of jaundice.

Crigler–Najjar syndrome is characterized by the absence or deficiency of the enzyme bilirubin glucuronyl transferase. Type I is the more severe form, manifests soon after birth, and is associated with high morbidity and mortality. Type II is milder, and is caused by an incomplete deficiency of the same enzyme; it typically presents in infancy or later in childhood. Lucey–Driscoll syndrome is a form of transient familial hyperbilirubinemia, and is caused by an inhibitor of glucuronyl transferase in the mother's serum; the syndrome resolves as the inhibitor is cleared from the neonate's blood.

Infants with galactosemia may exhibit an unconjugated hyperbilirubinemia during the first week of life, whereas older infants with galactosemia tend to have a conjugated hyperbilirubinemia (see Chapter 39 Jaundice: Conjugated Hyperbilirubinemia). Infants with galactosemia typically present with poor feeding, emesis, abdominal distention, failure to thrive, and hypoglycemia.

Unconjugated hyperbilirubinemia may be the only presenting sign of congenital hypothyroidism, preceding other manifestations by several weeks. The mechanism is thought to relate to reduced bile flow. Other signs include poor feeding, prolonged jaundice, constipation, and hypotonia. Infants of diabetic mothers are also at increased risk for jaundice, with as many as 19% developing nonphysiologic hyperbilirubinemia.

Breast milk jaundice occurs in 1% of newborns, and must be distinguished from breast-feeding jaundice (discussed below); it is associated with the breast milk itself and typically manifests after the fifth day of life. The underlying cause of breast milk jaundice is incompletely understood, but is likely hormonally mediated, and involves inhibition of bilirubin conjugation. Treatment requires temporary cessation of breast-feeding; however, the mother should be encouraged to express and store her breast milk during this time, and may resume breast-feeding when the neonatal bilirubin levels revert to normal.

Impaired Bilirubin Excretion

Exclusively breast-fed infants are at risk for exaggerated physiologic jaundice due to a relative caloric deprivation during the first few days of life. Decreased volume and frequency of feeds may result in a mild dehydration, as well as increased enterohepatic circulation. This is mitigated by increasing the frequency of feedings, improving latch and positioning, and occasionally by supplementing with formula in order to improve caloric intake.

Pyloric stenosis, duodenal atresia, malrotation with volvulus, meconium ileus, and Hirschsprung disease may present with jaundice along with other clinical signs of gastrointestinal (GI) obstruction. In neonates, obstruction can increase enterohepatic circulation resulting in unconjugated hyperbilirubinemia. Older children with jaundice in the setting of GI obstruction generally have a conjugated hyperbilirubinemia (see Chapter 39 Jaundice: Conjugated Hyperbilirubinemia).

Jaundice may be evident in cases of serious infection, such as sepsis and the congenital TORCH infections (Toxoplasmosis, Other [e.g., syphilis, parvovirus], Rubella, Cytomegalovirus, Herpes simplex virus). Bacterial endotoxins reduce bile flow, thereby impairing its excretion and leading to hyperbilirubinemia. Sepsis is exceedingly rare among well-appearing jaundiced neonates who have no additional signs or symptoms.

Intrauterine or breast milk exposure to certain drugs or toxins may also lead to impaired excretion of bilirubin in the neonate.

EVALUATION

Evaluation should always begin with a detailed history and physical examination. It is imperative to know the serum bilirubin level early in the course of evaluation. The need for additional studies—laboratory testing, imaging studies—is guided by the findings on history and physical examination.

History

Certain features of the birth history are critical in the evaluation of a neonate who presents with jaundice and concern for hyperbilirubinemia: gestational age, date and time of birth, birth weight, details of delivery (e.g., use of instrumentation such as forceps or vacuum), and maternal blood type and Rh status, as well as maternal exposure to infections such as syphilis. The history should also include a detailed feeding history, including type of milk and quantity, duration, and frequency of feeds. Urine output and character of stool should be elicited. Additionally, the presence or absence of other features that may indicate etiology (e.g., fever, emesis, lethargy) should be established. Exposures and previous bilirubin levels and the results of Coombs test should be reviewed, if applicable. Pertinent family history includes the presence of a first-degree relative with history of jaundice or anemia, and racial or ethnic origin associated with a hematologic disorder.

Physical Examination

The general appearance and vital signs of the patient will help guide the clinician as to the likelihood of a serious underlying condition such as bacterial sepsis. Hydration status should be ascertained. Hepatomegaly may indicate underlying liver dysfunction. Splenomegaly may be found in hypersplenic states or patients with hemolytic anemia. Neurologic examination should include evaluation for signs of acute bilirubin encephalopathy: hypotonia, irritability, retrocollis, opisthotonos, high-pitched cry, coma. Pallor may indicate concomitant anemia. Presence of a cephalohematoma or large areas of ecchymosis may suggest extravascular hemolysis as the cause of hyperbilirubinemia.

Clinical examination of jaundice involves close inspection of the sclera and skin under adequate light, applying gentle pressure with one finger to facilitate examination of color. In neonates, jaundice progresses in a cephalocaudal direction from the face to the trunk and extremities, and finally to the palms and soles. In neonates, visual assessment of jaundice has been found to correlate poorly with serum bilirubin measurement, with great interobserver variability noted.

Additional Studies

The total and fractionated (direct and indirect) serum bilirubin level should always be measured, as visual inspection alone is an unreliable indicator. Many times, these are the only laboratory studies indicated in the ED evaluation of a child who presents with jaundice; indication for other laboratory studies will be reviewed here. Occasionally, imaging studies are indicated in the evaluation of a child with jaundice or hyperbilirubinemia.

Laboratory Testing

Bilirubin Measurement. Transcutaneous measurements of bilirubin are correlated with serum bilirubin; however they are inaccurate at higher levels (greater than 12 to 15 mg per dL), and thus are best used as a screen. A TSB should always be obtained when therapeutic intervention is being considered.

Nearly all published data regarding the correlation of TSB levels to kernicterus or developmental outcome are based on capillary blood. Data on the relationship between capillary and venous sampling are conflicting. Capillary sampling is endorsed by the AAP; a confirmatory venous sample is not required. In neonates, it may be important to determine the rate of rise of TSB with serial measurements.

It is imperative to note that many clinical laboratories require the total and fractionated bilirubin to be ordered separately, as the total bilirubin reported on the hepatic function or comprehensive metabolic panels is unreliable in infants under 1 month of age. The ED clinician should be familiar with the accuracy of his or her laboratory assay in order to minimize error in the evaluation and management of neonates with suspected hyperbilirubinemia.

Other Laboratory Studies. If the TSB level is below 12 mg per dL, rises slowly, and resolves before 8 days of age, one can diagnose physiologic hyperbilirubinemia without further laboratory studies. When these conditions are not met, further testing is required to determine the etiology of elevated serum bilirubin.

A complete blood cell count should be obtained to evaluate for anemia. A peripheral blood smear should be examined microscopically for clues as to the etiology of the anemia: characteristic abnormal morphology, such as sickle cells, spherocytes, or elliptocytes, may be identified; helmet and fragmented cells are diagnostic of a microangiopathic hemolytic anemia; malarial ring forms may be apparent. The reticulocyte count may be elevated in the setting of hemolysis. Patients with anemia or hemolysis should also have a Coombs test performed to look for evidence of autoimmune hemolysis. In patients with a TSB level above threshold for exchange transfusion, a serum albumin should be obtained, and ratio of bilirubin to albumin should be calculated.

The child with fever, hypothermia, or ill appearance should be evaluated for serious bacterial infection, including blood, urine, and cerebrospinal fluid cultures as indicated. Serum electrolytes should be obtained in patients with clinical signs of dehydration, and those with a history of emesis excessive stool output. Hepatic function should be assessed in patients with hepatomegaly or in those with hyperbilirubinemia in the absence of anemia. Neonates with symptoms or newborn screen suggestive of congenital hypothyroidism should have a free T_4 level obtained.

Imaging Studies

If clinical signs of obstruction are present, the patient should undergo appropriate imaging studies such as abdominal radiographs, ultrasound, or upper GI series with contrast.

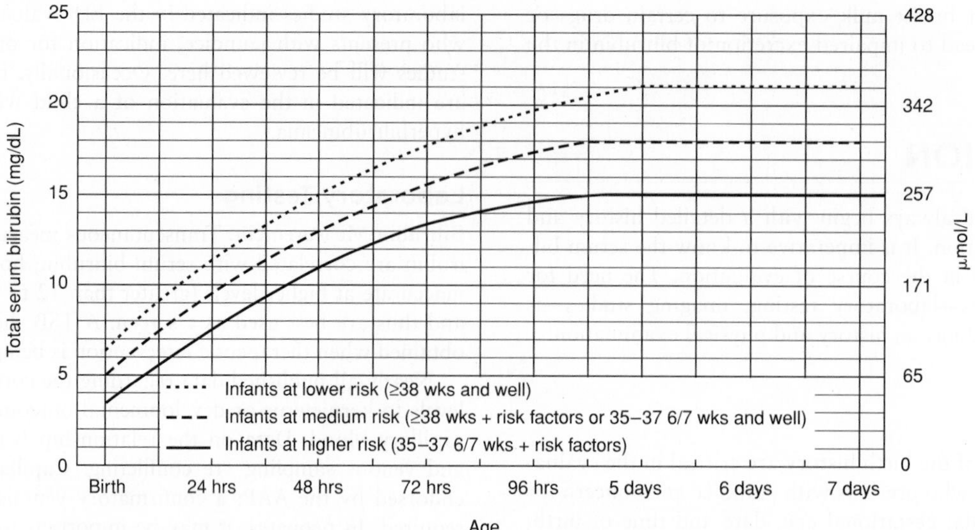

- Use total bilirubin. Do not subtract direct reacting or conjugated bilirubin.
- Risk factors—Isoimmune hemolytic disease. G6PD deficiency, asphyxia, significant lethargy, temperature instability, sepsis, acidosis, or albumin <3.0 g/dL (if measured).
- For well infants 35–37 6/7 wks can adjust TSB levels for intervention around the medium-risk line. It is an option to intervene at lower TSB levels for infants closer to 35 wks and at higher TSB levels for those closer to 37 6/7 wks.
- It is an option to provide conventional phototherapy in hospital or at home at TSB levels 2–3 mg/dL (35–50 μmol/L) below those shown but home phototherapy should not be used in any infant with risk factors.

FIGURE 40.1 Guidelines for phototherapy in hospitalized infants of 35 or more weeks of gestation. The guidelines refer to the use of intensive phototherapy, which should be used when the TSB exceeds the line indicated for each category. (Reprinted with permission from the American Academy of Pediatrics Subcommittee on Hyperbilirubinemia. Management of hyperbilirubinemia in the newborn infant 35 or more weeks of gestation. *Pediatrics* 2004;114(1):297–316. © 2004 by American Academy of Pediatrics.)

MANAGEMENT

The goal of neonatal hyperbilirubinemia management is to prevent neurotoxicity, acute bilirubin encephalopathy, and kernicterus. The jaundiced newborn needs to be kept well hydrated, and enteral feeding should be encouraged to promote bilirubin excretion. When bilirubin levels rise significantly, phototherapy and exchange transfusion may be indicated.

Phototherapy

Indications for phototherapy vary according to the age of the neonate; in the term neonate who develops jaundice and has no evidence of hemolysis, indications for phototherapy as recommended by the AAP Subcommittee on Hyperbilirubinemia are shown in Figure 40.1. When there is evidence of isoimmune hemolysis, phototherapy should be started immediately and a neonatologist should be consulted regardless of TSB level.

Phototherapy may be delivered by an overhead bank of lights or via a fiber optic light source in a blanket and should be initiated in the ED if an alternate site is not available quickly. The mechanism of phototherapy involves wavelengths of light that alter the unconjugated bilirubin in the skin, and convert it to less toxic, water-soluble photoisomers that may be excreted in the bile and urine without conjugation. TSB levels decline by 1 to 2 mg per dL within 4 to 6 hours using conventional phototherapy.

During phototherapy, the baby should be undressed to maximize the exposed surface area of the skin. The infant must wear an eye shield when using overhead lights in order to prevent retinal damage. Other risks of phototherapy include temperature instability, loose stools, and rash. Phototherapy is relatively contraindicated in patients with conjugated hyperbilirubinemia because it can cause a discoloration of the skin, or "bronze baby syndrome."

Exchange Transfusion

Exchange transfusion is the most rapid method for lowering serum bilirubin. Recommended TSB levels for exchange transfusion are based mainly on the goal of avoiding achievement of levels at which kernicterus has been reported. Indications for exchange transfusion as recommended by the AAP Subcommittee on Hyperbilirubinemia are shown in Figure 40.2.

Exchange transfusions should be performed in consultation with a neonatologist: fresh, irradiated, reconstituted whole blood is infused through an umbilical vein catheter while the neonate's blood is withdrawn through an umbilical artery catheter. During this procedure, the neonate's partially hemolyzed and antibody-coated RBCs are replaced with uncoated donor RBCs that lack the sensitizing antigen. Complications may impart significant morbidity, and include electrolyte disturbances, infection, and further hemolysis.

Hydration

Intravenous fluids are indicated for patients with clinical evidence of dehydration or shock. Jaundiced infants who are able to continue enteral hydration should be encouraged to do so, in order to diminish enterohepatic recirculation and promote bilirubin excretion. The interruption or discontinuation of breast-feeding should be discouraged, and is only appropriate

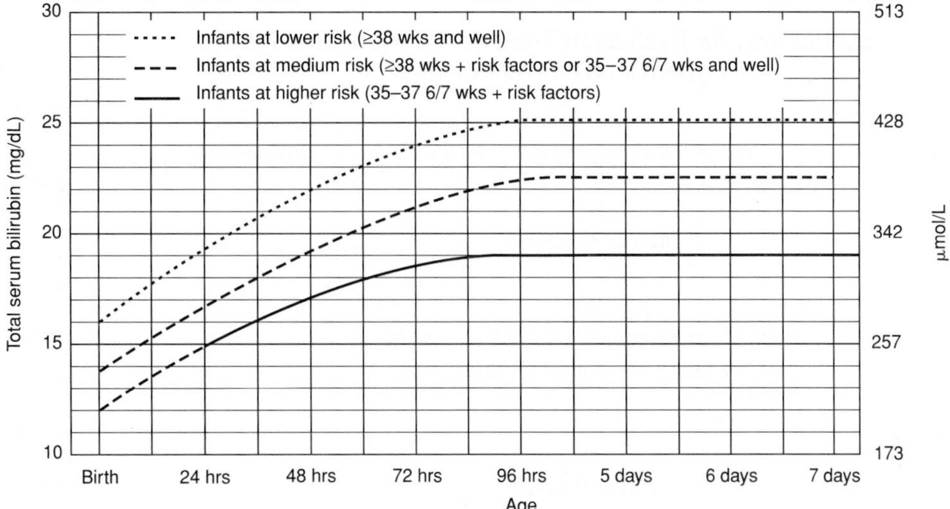

- The dashed lines for the first 24 hrs indicate uncertainty due to a wide range of clinical circumstances and a range of responses to phototherapy.
- Immediate exchange transfusion is recommended if infant shows signs of acute bilirubin encephalopathy (hypertonia, arching, retrocollis, opisthotonos, fever, high-pitched cry) or if TSB is ≥5 mg/dL (85 mol/L) above these lines.
- Risk factors—isoimmune hemolytic disease, (G6PD) deficiency, asphyxia, significant lethargy, temperature instability, sepsis, acidosis.
- Measure serum albumin and calculate B/A ratio (see AAP Subcommittee Guidelines).
- Use total bilirubin. Do not subtract direct reacting or conjugated bilirubin.
- If infant is well and 35–37 6/7 wks (median risk) can individualize TSB levels for exchange based on actual gestational age.

FIGURE 40.2 Guidelines for exchange transfusion in infants 35 or more weeks of gestation. Exchange transfusion is recommended if the TSB rises to these levels despite intensive phototherapy. Bilirubin/albumin (B/A) ratio can be used together with but not in lieu of the TSB level as an additional factor in determining the need for exchange transfusion. (Reprinted with permission from the American Academy of Pediatrics Subcommittee on Hyperbilirubinemia. Management of hyperbilirubinemia in the newborn infant 35 or more weeks of gestation. *Pediatrics* 2004;114(1):297–316. © 2004 by American Academy of Pediatrics.)

in certain settings (breast milk jaundice, exposure to toxins). Bottle-feeding expressed milk or supplementation of formula may be required in some instances. In an infant with poor oral intake and without contraindications, an oro- or nasogastric tube is an option to maintain enteral feedings.

Discharge

Neonates with presumed physiologic jaundice whose serum bilirubin levels fall below the threshold for intervention, are well-appearing, able to maintain adequate hydration, and have assurance of close follow-up, may be safely discharged from the ED.

The AAP recommends home phototherapy as an option for neonates whose TSB level does not cross the threshold for therapeutic intervention, but in whom the rate of rise may be concerning. Home phototherapy is not indicated for infants with TSB levels that are above phototherapy or exchange transfusion thresholds.

APPROACH

Clinical Pathway for Neonates

The main goal of the clinical pathway is to deliver consistent and efficient care to neonates born at greater than 35 weeks of gestational age presenting with jaundice or hyperbilirubinemia. The pathway emphasizes safe and consistent use of phototherapy, in order to prevent occurrences of acute bilirubin encephalopathy and kernicterus (Fig. 40.3). The pathway does not apply to infants with congenital medical or surgical conditions, those who are not normothermic, or who are known to have elevated serum bilirubin at time of ED presentation.

The bedside nurse is charged with initiating the clinical pathway, providing parents with basic education as to the goals of evaluation, and obtaining a total and fractionated serum bilirubin via heel stick (capillary blood). Once the sample is collected, the infant is placed on phototherapy. Logistically, by the time the history and physical examination are completed, the result of the TSB is available, allowing the clinician to rapidly make further diagnostic and therapeutic decisions. The pathway provides links to education modules for clinicians, discharge paper template that may be printed for patients, and the AAP Subcommittee on Hyperbilirubinemia manuscript.

Implementation of this clinical pathway has been shown to reduce time to phototherapy initiation, time to bilirubin measurement, and overall ED length of stay.

Beyond the Neonatal Period

For patients beyond the neonatal period, the approach is primarily directed at identification and treatment of the underlying cause. In some cases of severe hyperbilirubinemia, such as those caused by Crigler–Najjar syndrome type II and

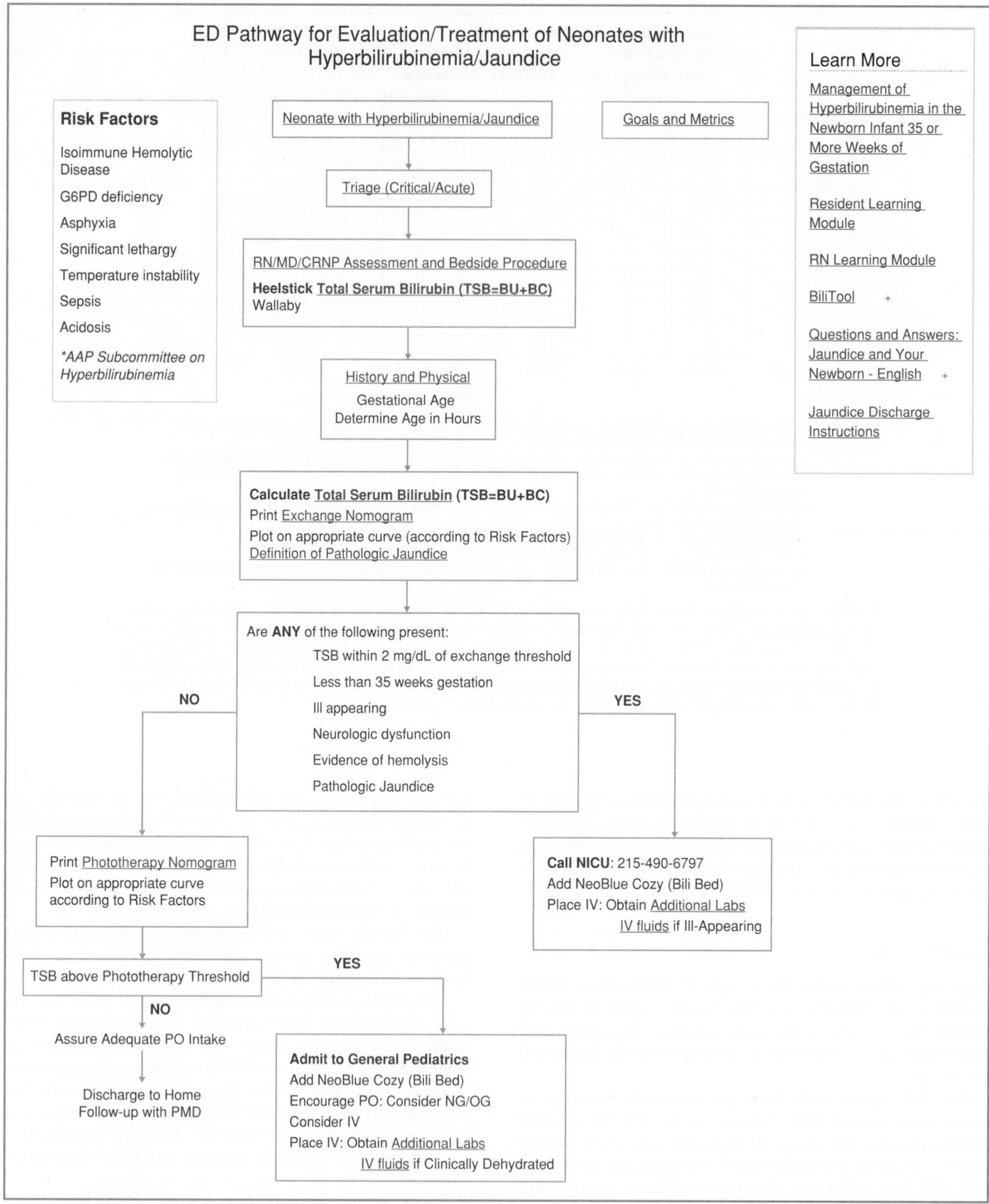

FIGURE 40.3 Clinical pathway for the evaluation and treatment of neonates with jaundice or suspected hyperbilirubinemia (http://www.chop.edu/professionals/clinical-pathways/ed-clinical-pathways.html). (© 2014 by The Children's Hospital of Philadelphia, all rights reserved.)

Lucey–Driscoll syndrome, phototherapy or phenobarbital may be indicated. If a patient appears acutely ill, the physician should proceed with the appropriate evaluation and treatment for sepsis. Among well-appearing patients, the presence or absence of anemia determines the likely diagnostic possibilities and appropriate studies. When unconjugated hyperbilirubinemia occurs without anemia, abnormal liver function tests will differentiate hepatic disease from inherited disorders of bilirubin metabolism. Anemic children should be evaluated for an underlying hemolytic process.

Suggested Readings and Key References

American Academy of Pediatrics Subcommittee on Hyperbilirubinemia. Management of hyperbilirubinemia in the newborn infant 35 or more weeks of gestation. *Pediatrics* 2004;114(1):297–316.

Ip S, Chung M, Kulig J, et al. An evidence-based review of important issues concerning neonatal hyperbilirubinemia. *Pediatrics* 2004; 114(1):e130–e153.

Maisels MJ, McDonagh AF. Phototherapy for neonatal jaundice. *N Engl J Med* 2008;358(9):920–928.

Moyer VA, Ahn C, Sneed S. Accuracy of clinical judgement in neonatal jaundice. *Arch Pediatr Adolesc Med* 2000;154:391–394.

Wolff M, Schinasi DA, Lavelle J, et al. Management of neonates with hyperbilirubinemia: improving timeliness of care using a clinical pathway. *Pediatrics* 2012;130(6):e1688–e1694.

CHAPTER 41 ■ LIMP

SUSANNE KOST, MD, FAAP, FACEP AND AMY D. THOMPSON, MD, FAAP, FACEP

Limping is a common complaint in the pediatric acute care setting. A *limp* is defined as an alteration in the normal walking pattern for the child's age. The average child begins to walk between 12 and 18 months of age with a broad-based gait, gradually maturing into a normal (adult) gait pattern by the age of 3 years. A normal gait cycle can be divided into two phases: Stance and swing. The stance phase, the time from the heel striking the ground to the toe leaving the ground, encompasses about 60% of the gait cycle. The swing phase involves a sequence of hip then knee flexion, followed by foot dorsiflexion and knee extension as the heel strikes the ground to begin the next cycle.

The causes of limping are numerous, ranging from trivial to life-threatening, but most children who limp do so as a result of pain, weakness, or deformity. Pain results in an antalgic gait pattern with a shortened stance phase. The most common causes of a painful limp are trauma and infection. Neuromuscular disease may cause either spasticity (e.g., toe-walking) or weakness, which results in a steppage gait to compensate for weak ankle dorsiflexion. Ataxia may be interpreted by parents as a limp. A Trendelenburg gait is characterized by the torso swinging back and forth to compensate for a pelvic tilt due to weak hip abductors or hip deformities. A vaulting gait may be seen in children with limb-length discrepancy or abnormal knee mobility. A stooped, shuffling gait is common in patients with pelvic or lower abdominal pain.

The evaluation of a child with a limp demands a thorough history and physical examination. A detailed history of the circumstances surrounding the limp should be obtained, with focus on the issues of trauma, pain, and associated fever or systemic illness. The physical examination must be complete because limping may originate from abnormalities in any portion of the lower extremity, nervous system, abdomen, or genitourinary tract. The location of the pain may not represent the source of the pathology, for example, hip pain may be referred to the knee area. Laboratory and imaging studies should be tailored to the findings in the history and physical examination, keeping in mind an appropriate age-based differential diagnosis.

DIFFERENTIAL DIAGNOSIS

The extensive differential diagnosis of the child with a limp may be approached from several angles: Disease category, location of pathology, or age of the child. Table 41.1 presents the differential diagnosis by disease category; Table 41.2 organizes the differential diagnosis by age and the location of pathology. This section reviews the differential diagnosis within the framework of an algorithmic approach (Fig. 41.1).

The most common cause of limping in all ages is trauma, either acute or repetitive microtrauma (stress fractures). Older children who limp as a result of trauma can generally describe the mechanism of injury and localize pain well. The toddler and preschool age groups, with their limited verbal ability and cooperation skills, often provide a diagnostic challenge. A common type of injury in this population (often not witnessed) is the aptly named "toddler's fracture," a nondisplaced spiral fracture of the tibial shaft that occurs as a result of torsion of the foot relative to the tibia. Occult fractures of the bones in the foot also occur in young children. Initial plain radiographic findings may be subtle, or at times nonexistent, but will become apparent in 1 to 2 weeks. Another fracture often lacking initial radiographic confirmation is a Salter–Harris type I fracture, which presents as tenderness over a physis after trauma to a joint area. Stress fractures may also lack overt radiographic findings. Common sites for overuse injury include the tibial tubercle (Osgood–Schlatter disease), the anterior tibia (shin splints), and the calcaneus at the insertion of the Achilles tendon (Sever disease). More information on the subject of fractures is found in Chapter 119 Musculoskeletal Trauma.

Trauma may also induce limping as a result of soft tissue injury. Although young children are more likely to sustain fractures than sprains and strains, the latter can occur. Joint swelling and pain out of proportion to the history of injury raises the possibility of a hemarthrosis as the initial presentation of a bleeding disorder (see Chapter 101 Hematologic Emergencies). Severe soft tissue pain and swelling in the setting of a contusion or crush injury suggests possible compartment syndrome. With compartment syndrome, pain is exacerbated by passive extension of the affected part; pallor and pulselessness are late findings. Severe pain of an entire limb out of proportion to the history of injury suggests complex regional pain syndrome. This entity is most common in young adolescent girls. It may be accompanied by mottling and coolness of the extremity, presumably as a result of abnormalities in the peripheral sympathetic nervous system.

A limp that is accompanied by a history of fever or recent systemic illness is likely to be infectious or inflammatory in origin. However, the absence of fever does not preclude the possibility of a bacterial bone or joint infection, and many infections are preceded by a history of minor trauma. Septic arthritis is the most serious infectious cause of joint pain and limp. It is more common in younger children and typically presents with a warm, swollen joint (although swelling in the hip is very difficult to detect clinically). Exquisite pain with attempts to flex or extend the joint is characteristic of septic arthritis, and the degree of pain with motion serves as a helpful clinical sign in distinguishing bacterial joint infection from inflammatory conditions. A common diagnostic challenge is differentiating septic arthritis from transient (or toxic) synovitis in a young child with fever, limp, and pain localized to the hip. Transient synovitis, a postinfectious reactive arthritis, follows a milder course. It is usually preceded by a recent viral respiratory or gastrointestinal illness. Acute-phase

TABLE 41.1

DIFFERENTIAL DIAGNOSIS OF LIMP BY DISEASE CATEGORY

Trauma or overuse	**Congenital**
Fracture	Vertical talus
Stress fracture	Tarsal coalition
Soft tissue injury	Other congenital limb abnormalities
Spondylolisthesis	Spinal dysraphism
Herniated nucleus pulposus	Inguinal hernia
Infectious	**Neurologic**
Septic arthritis	Muscular dystrophy
Osteomyelitis	Peripheral neuropathy
Lyme arthritis	Complex regional pain syndrome
Discitis	**Neoplasia**
Epidural abscess	Benign bone tumors
Appendicitis	Malignant bone tumors
Pelvic inflammatory disease	Leukemia
Deep cellulitis/abscess	Intra-abdominal tumors
Inflammatory	Sacral tumors
Transient synovitis	Spinal cord tumors
Reactive arthritis	**Metabolic**
Rheumatic disease	Rickets
Myositis	Hyperparathyroidism
Developmental or acquired	**Hematologic**
Developmental dysplasia of the hip	Sickle cell disease
Blount disease	Hemophilia
Limb-length discrepancy	
Torsional deformities	
Avascular necrosis	
Slipped capital femoral epiphysis	
Testicular torsion	

reactants may be elevated in both conditions, although usually less so in synovitis. A unilateral joint effusion, which is better visualized with ultrasound than plain films, may be present in both. Bilateral effusions are more suggestive of an inflammatory synovitis. Joint aspiration may be required for a definitive diagnosis because a septic hip is a surgical emergency requiring open drainage. Osteomyelitis is another potentially serious infectious cause of limp, although the presentation is typically more chronic than that of a septic joint. Osteomyelitis, which is also more common in younger children, presents with pain and occasionally warmth and swelling, usually over the metaphysis of a long bone. A reactive joint effusion may be present. Occasionally, osteomyelitis and septic arthritis will coexist. More detailed discussions of both septic joint and osteomyelitis are found in Chapters 102 Infectious Disease Emergencies and 129 Musculoskeletal Emergencies.

Rheumatic conditions that may result in limp are numerous. Many are accompanied by systemic symptoms and characteristic skin rashes. Examples include Henoch–Schönlein purpura, erythema multiforme, acute rheumatic fever, juvenile idiopathic arthritis (JIA), and systemic lupus erythematosus. Occasionally, limping from arthralgia will precede the development of the arthritis and systemic involvement. An approach to the child with joint pain is found in Chapter 55 Pain: Joints, and a detailed discussion of arthritis is found in Chapter 109 Rheumatologic Emergencies.

In the absence of obvious trauma, fever, or systemic symptoms, the next step in the approach to the differential diagnosis of a limp is to determine the focality of the findings and the degree of pain. Localized pain suggests repetitive microtrauma, bone tumor, or an acquired skeletal deformity. Repetitive microtrauma may be responsible for avascular necrosis of the foot bones in two locations: The tarsal navicular bone (Kohler disease) in younger children and the metatarsal heads (Freiberg disease) in adolescents. Both benign and malignant bone tumors may present with a painful limp. Benign lesions include bone cysts (unicameral or aneurysmal), fibrous dysplasia, and eosinophilic granulomas. Osteoid osteoma, caused by a painful nidus of vascular osteoid tissue, is another benign lesion unique to young people. The most common malignant pediatric bone tumors are osteogenic sarcoma and Ewing sarcoma. Bone tumor pain may be acute or chronic, with acute pain usually related to a pathologic fracture. Examples of acquired skeletal abnormalities causing painful limp include tarsal coalition and osteochondritis dissecans. Tarsal coalition occurs as a result of gradual calcification of a congenital cartilaginous bar between tarsal bones; it presents most commonly as a painful flatfoot in school-age children. Osteochondritis dissecans is related to osteonecrosis of the subchondral bone with separation of articular cartilage from underlying bony lesion; it most commonly affects the knees of adolescent boys.

Localized findings without pain suggest congenital or slowly developing acquired limb abnormalities. Three disorders of the hip fit into this category, each of which is characteristic of a specific age group. Developmental dysplasia of the hip includes a spectrum of abnormalities, ranging from mild dysplasia to frank dislocation. Most affected children with access to primary care are diagnosed with abnormal hip abduction on routine examination in infancy. Occasionally, the diagnosis will be missed, and the child then presents at the onset of walking with a painless short-leg limp, or waddling gait if bilateral, with weakness of the abductor musculature. Legg–Calvé–Perthes disease, an avascular necrosis of the capital femoral epiphysis, presents in young school-age children as an insidious limp with mild, activity-related pain. Slipped capital femoral epiphysis (SCFE) presents in young, typically obese adolescents with an externally rotated limp. The amount of pain experienced is related to the rate of displacement of the epiphysis, ranging from none to severe. Legg–Calvé–Perthes disease and SCFE are more common in boys. Other acquired skeletal deformities that may cause painless limp include limb-length inequality, Blount disease (with marked bowing of the proximal tibias), and torsional deformities. Baker cyst of the popliteal tendon may cause limping with minimal local discomfort.

Systemic bone or soft tissue involvement can lead to limping without localization of limb findings. A painful limp without localization or with migratory bone pain suggests a hematologic or oncologic cause, such as sickle cell disease or leukemia. Limping with bilateral leg pain localized to the muscles, especially the calves, suggests myositis. Benign acute childhood myositis is common during influenza epidemics. Recurrent diffuse aches after periods of vigorous activity, usually worse at night, suggest benign hypermobility syndrome or "growing pains." A painless, poorly localized limp may occur with metabolic bone disease (e.g., rickets).

TABLE 41.2

DIFFERENTIAL DIAGNOSIS OF LIMP BY AGE AND LOCATION OF PATHOLOGY

	Long bone	Skin/soft tissue	Any joint	Hip	Knee	Ankle/foot	Spine
Toddler	Fracture Toddler's Salter type I Periostitis Osteomyelitis Vasoocclusive crisis Congenital anomaly	Contusion Strain Foreign body Immunization Infection	Septic arthritis Reactive arthritis Rheumatic disease JIA Hemarthrosis	Transient synovitis DDH	Occult trauma Blount disease Referred hip pain	Poor shoe fit Occult trauma Vertical talus Kohler disease	Dysraphism Infection Tumor
School age	Fracture Salter type I Discrepant limb length Osteomyelitis Tumor Vasoocclusive crisis	Contusion Strain Myositis Growing pains Infection	Sprain Reactive arthritis Rheumatic disease EM, HSP, ARF, JIA Septic arthritis Lyme arthritis	Transient synovitis AVN	Baker cyst Referred hip pain	Poor shoe fit Salter type I fracture Tarsal coalition Kohler disease	Dysraphism Infection Tumor
Adolescent	Fracture Tumor Osteomyelitis Vasoocclusive crisis	Contusion Strain Tendonitis CRPS Infection	Sprain Reactive arthritis Rheumatic disease IBD, SLE, JIA Septic arthritis Gonococcal Lyme arthritis	SCFE	Osgood–Schlatter disease Osteochondritis dissecans Chondromalacia Baker cyst Referred hip pain	Poor shoe fit Salter type I fracture Bunion Freiberg disease Sever disease	Scoliosis Spondylolisthesis Herniated disc Infection Tumor

DDH, developmental dysplasia of the hip; JIA, juvenile idiopathic arthritis; AVN, avascular necrosis; EM, erythema multiforme; HSP, Henoch–Schönlein purpura; ARF, acute rheumatic fever; CRPS, complex regional pain syndrome; IBD, inflammatory bowel disease; SLE, systemic lupus erythematosus; SCFE, slipped capital femoral epiphysis.

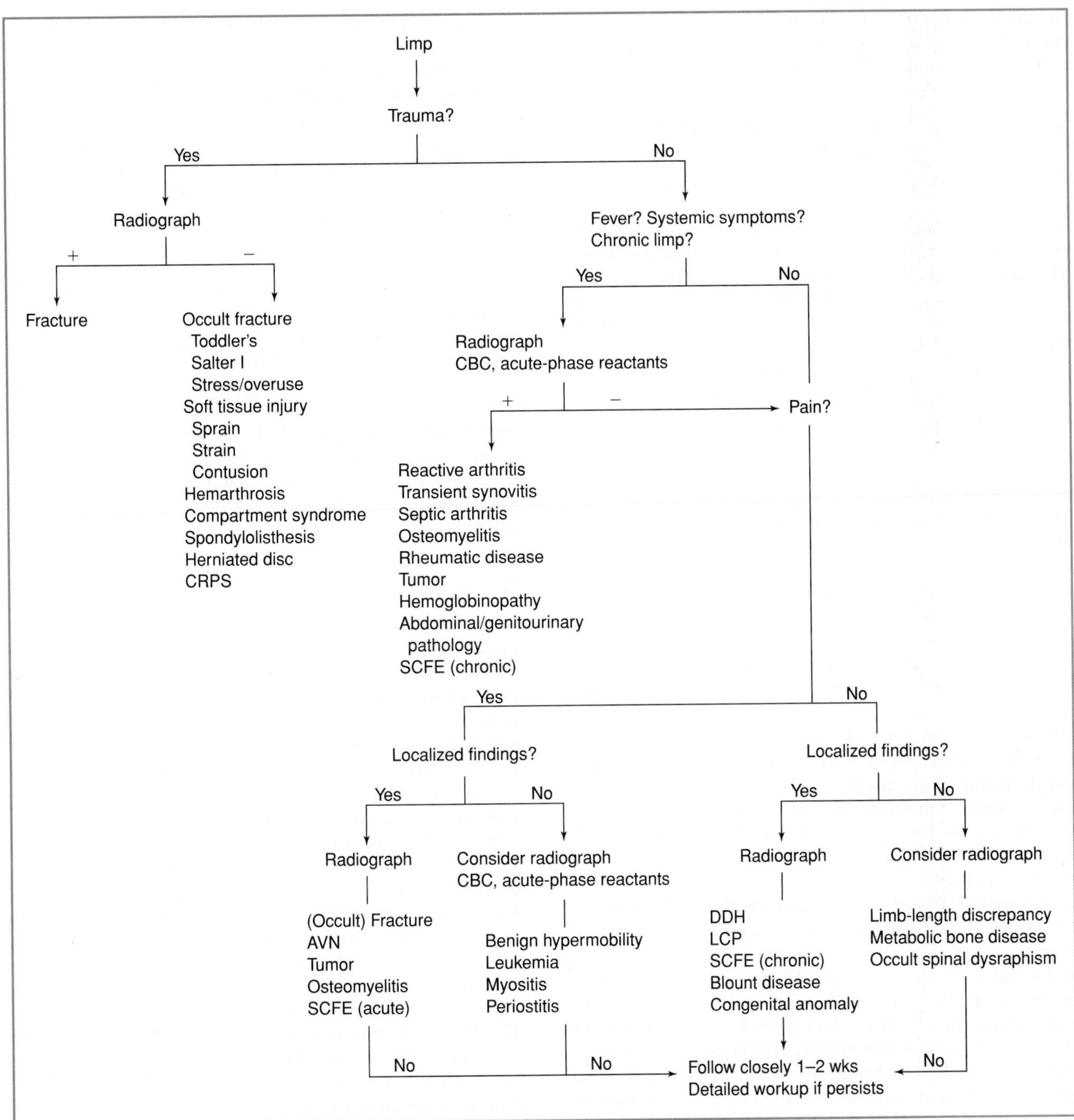

FIGURE 41.1 Algorithmic approach to the child with a limp. CRPS, complex regional pain syndrome; CBC, complete blood cell count; SCFE, slipped capital femoral epiphysis; AVN, avascular necrosis; DDH, developmental dysplasia of the hip; LCP, Legg–Calvé–Perthes disease.

Limping in the absence of localized limb findings may also suggest a nonlimb source such as the spine or the abdomen. Spinal problems that can cause leg pain, weakness, or limp include dysraphism, vertebral infection, spondylolisthesis, and herniated disc. Spinal dysraphism refers to a spectrum of abnormalities in the development of the spinal cord and vertebrae ranging from obvious (myelomeningocele) to occult (tethered cord). Associated neurologic and musculoskeletal findings, including pain, atrophy, high arches, and tight heel cords, may develop in early childhood. Vertebral infection typically presents with fever and back pain. Spondylolisthesis and herniated disc are rare in young children but may be seen in adolescents who complain of back pain or radicular pain. Limp may rarely present as an early symptom of a peripheral neuropathy, either hereditary (e.g., Charcot–Marie–Tooth disease) or acquired (Guillain–Barre syndrome, vitamin or medication related). Intra-abdominal pathology that can result in limp includes appendicitis, ovarian cyst, inflammatory bowel disease, pelvic or psoas abscess, and renal disease. Solid tumors, most commonly neuroblastoma, can cause limp through retroperitoneal irritation or extension into the spinal canal. Likewise, a sacral teratoma may affect the nerves of the cauda equina or sacral plexus. Testicular pain may present with limping in a boy who is reluctant or embarrassed to admit the true source of his discomfort.

EVALUATION AND DECISION

The conditions that lead to a presentation of limp range from mundane (poorly fitting shoes) to life-threatening (leukemia). The role of the pediatric acute care physician is to rule out the possibility of life- and limb-threatening pathologic conditions. The serious conditions include bacterial infection of the bone or joint space, malignancy, and disorders that threaten the blood supply to the bone, such as avascular necrosis and SCFE. Often, a definitive diagnosis will not be reached in the emergency department, and the patient will require follow-up with the primary care physician or specialist. Figure 41.1 provides an algorithmic approach to the child with a limp.

History

The history in a limping child should include information about the onset and duration of the limp, the family's perception of the origin of the problem, and associated symptoms such as pain, fever, and systemic illness. When pain is present, the physician should inquire about the location and severity. A history of trauma should be addressed, keeping in mind the inherent difficulty in obtaining an accurate trauma history in very young children. Conversely, obvious trauma in the absence of a consistent history raises the question of inflicted injury. In more chronic presentations, any cyclical or recurrent patterns should be noted. Stiffness and limp primarily in the morning suggest rheumatic disease, whereas evening symptoms suggest weakness or overuse injury. A history of joint or limb swelling should be investigated, with attention to the degree of swelling and any migratory or recurrent patterns.

The medical history should include birth and developmental history. Breech position is associated with developmental dysplasia of the hip, and mild cerebral palsy may present in childhood with abnormal gait. History of viral infections, streptococcal pharyngitis, medication use, and immunizations may provide clues to the cause of limping. A family history of rheumatic or autoimmune disease, neurologic disease, inflammatory bowel disease, hemoglobinopathy, or other bleeding disorders may help facilitate diagnosis. Finally, the review of systems should include questions about past trauma, infections, neoplasia, endocrine disease, metabolic disease, and congenital anomalies.

Physical Examination

The physical examination in a limping child should begin with observation of the child's gait. Ideally, the child should be observed walking in bare feet and wearing minimal clothing, preferably in a long hallway. The physician should attempt to observe the child unobtrusively to avoid gait changes caused by self-consciousness. The observer should note the symmetry of stride length, the proportion of the gait cycle spent in stance phase, hip abductor muscle strength (with weakness manifested by Trendelenburg or waddling gait), in-toeing or out-toeing, and joint flexibility. Muscle strength may be tested by asking the child to run, hop, and walk on toes and heels.

After observing the child in action, the physician should perform a complete examination with attention to the musculoskeletal and neurologic systems. The musculoskeletal examination begins with inspection of the limbs and feet for swelling or deformity. Supine positioning with the leg slightly flexed, abducted, and externally rotated at the hip is suggestive of fluid in the joint capsule. The spine should be inspected for curvature, both standing and bending forward, and the soles of feet and toes should be checked for foreign bodies and calluses. The bones, muscles, and joints should be palpated for areas of tenderness; range of motion of all joints should be checked; and limb lengths (from anterior-superior iliac spine to medial malleolus), as well as thigh and calf circumferences, should be measured for asymmetry. The neurologic examination should include inspection of the spine for lumbosacral hair or dimple (indicating possible spinal dysraphism), and testing of strength, sensation, and reflexes. The abdomen and external genitalia should be examined for tenderness or masses and the skin for rashes. A rectal examination may be indicated if sacral pathology is suspected. Finally, wear patterns on the child's shoes may provide clues to the nature and duration of the limp.

Laboratory and Imaging

Plain radiographs remain a mainstay of the workup of a limping child. They provide an excellent means of screening for fracture, effusion, lytic lesions, periosteal reaction, and avascular necrosis. In a child with an obvious focus of pain, the radiographs may be obtained with views specific to that area, noting that children with knee pain may have hip pathology. The need for comparative views (of the contralateral normal extremity) depends on the experience of the physician interpreting the films. Some radiographic findings can be subtle, and comparison with the opposite side may be helpful. Although the goal is to focus imaging on areas of greatest concern, in a young child or a child lacking obvious focus for the limp, anteroposterior and lateral views of both tibias should be ordered as an initial screen. If tibia/fibular films are negative, imaging of the pelvis, thigh, and foot may be considered. In children in whom hip pathology is suspected, anteroposterior and frog-leg lateral views of the pelvis are required. The frog-leg lateral view, obtained with the hips abducted and externally rotated, allows excellent visualization of the femoral heads. These radiographs should always include both hips to enable comparison of the femoral heads and width of the joint spaces. Radiographs of the spine are necessary if the child has neurologic signs or symptoms.

In children whose limp is associated with fever or systemic illness, laboratory studies, including a complete blood cell count, C-reactive protein level, and an erythrocyte sedimentation rate, are indicated. These studies serve as screens for infection, inflammation, malignancy, and hemoglobinopathy. While there is a clinically significant overlap in the erythrocyte sedimentation rate and white blood cell count in children with infectious and inflammatory arthritis, a C-reactive protein level of more than 2 mg per dL (20 mg per L) is more concerning for bacterial infection. A blood culture should be obtained in patients with concern for osteomyelitis, abscess or septic arthritis. Laboratory studies are also indicated in the absence of fever if the child has been limping for several days without evidence of trauma on plain films. While rheumatoid factor is typically negative in children with JIA, antinuclear antibody testing is frequently positive in patients with the polyarticular and pauciarticular onset forms of JIA. Low peripheral white blood cell counts (<4,000) and low to low-normal platelet counts (<150,000) in the setting of night-time limb pain suggest a diagnosis of leukemia rather than JIA. Children with evidence of infection or inflammation with a joint effusion may require arthrocentesis for definitive diagnosis. In areas of endemic Lyme disease, Lyme testing should be performed in a patient with monoarticular arthritis. A creatine phosphokinase level may be helpful if muscle inflammation is suspected.

When the initial history, physical examination, imaging, and laboratory evaluation indicate the cause of the limp, specific treatment can be initiated. Abnormalities in the initial workup without a definitive diagnosis should prompt further imaging or laboratory studies. Bone scintigraphy is more sensitive than plain radiographs for occult fracture, infection, avascular necrosis, and tumor; however, it is not specific for a given pathologic process. Computed tomography is an excellent imaging modality for cortical bone. It serves as a useful diagnostic adjunct in certain fractures, bony coalitions, and bone tumors. Ultrasound is the preferred modality for diagnosing hip effusions; it is also useful for guiding needle aspirations of the hip joint. Magnetic resonance imaging is useful in imaging the spinal cord, avascular necrosis, and bone marrow disease. Magnetic resonance imaging is becoming increasingly useful in the evaluation of infectious and oncologic musculoskeletal abnormalities as well, as an adjunct to bone scintigraphy or in place of it when the site of pathology is well localized.

If the initial workup in a limping child is completely normal, including screening radiographs and laboratory studies, the child may be followed closely as an outpatient. The child should be examined every few days until improvement is noted or a cause is determined. If the limp persists beyond 1 to 2 weeks without a diagnosis, further workup or consultation with a specialist is indicated.

Suggested Readings and Key References

Baron CM, Seekins J, Hernanz-Schulman M, et al. Utility of total lower extremity radiography investigation of nonweight bearing in the young child. *Pediatrics* 2008;121:e817–e820.

Jones OY, Spencer CH, Bowyer SL, et al. A multicenter case-control study on predictive factors distinguishing childhood leukemia from juvenile rheumatoid arthritis. *Pediatrics* 2006;117:e840–e844.

Levine MJ, McGuire KJ, McGowan KL, et al. Assessment of test characteristics of C-reactive protein for septic arthritis in children. *J Pediatr Orthop* 2003;23:373–377.

Milla SS, Coley BD, Karmazyn B, et al. ACR Appropriateness Criteria® limping child—ages 0 to 5 years. *J Am Coll Radiol* 2012; 9(8):545–553. Available at http://www.guideline.gov/content.aspx?id = 37914

Shavit I, Eidelman M, Galbraith R. Sonography of the hip-joint by the emergency physician: its role in the evaluation of children presenting with acute limp. *Pediatr Emerg Care* 2006;22:570–573.

Singhal R, Perry DC, Khan FN, et al. The use of CRP within a clinical prediction algorithm for the differentiation of septic arthritis and transient synovitis in children. *J Bone Joint Surg Br* 2011;93:1556–1561.

CHAPTER 42 ■ LYMPHADENOPATHY

KIYETTA H. ALADE, MD, RDMS, FAAP AND BETH M. D'AMICO, MD

Lymphadenopathy, defined as an enlargement of lymph nodes, is a frequent presenting sign in children. Most illnesses causing lymphadenopathy are common viral or bacterial infections that improve spontaneously or with an appropriate course of antimicrobial therapy. However, some serious illnesses, including malignancies, can present first as lymphadenopathy. Thus, a focused history, thorough physical examination, and knowledge of various causes of adenopathy are important in formulating an appropriate differential diagnosis.

MECHANISM OF LYMPHADENOPATHY

Enlargement of lymph nodes can be due to physiologic or pathologic causes. Most commonly, when lymph nodes perform their normal function, antigenic stimulation causes proliferation of lymphocytes, and nodes increase in size. This response is particularly active in children, who are frequently exposed to new antigens, thus accounting for the common observation of lymphadenopathy associated with pediatric infections. A second cause of lymph node enlargement occurs when bacteria or other pathogens that are present in lymphatic fluid stimulate an influx of inflammatory cells, local cytokine release, and symptoms of lymphadenitis. These include enlargement of the node, erythema, edema, and tenderness. A third cause of adenopathy is neoplastic disease, where malignant cells originate in or migrate to lymph nodes, infiltrating the node and causing enlargement. Last, in rare cases genetic storage diseases may lead to deposition of foreign material within the node.

A number of studies have described the presence of palpable lymph nodes in healthy infants and children. A seminal study of well infants and children up to 6 years of age reported more than half of the children had palpable nodes, most commonly in the cervical, occipital, and submandibular region. It is commonly accepted that lymph nodes in the cervical and axillary regions up to 1 cm in diameter, nodes in the inguinal region up to 1.5 cm in diameter, and nodes in the epitrochlear region up to 0.5 cm in diameter are considered normal in children.

DIFFERENTIAL DIAGNOSIS

As the differential diagnosis of lymphadenopathy is extensive, it is helpful to distinguish localized from generalized lymphadenopathy, and an acute from chronic time course. *Localized adenopathy* includes lymphadenopathy in a single region, and generally occurs in response to a focal infectious process. *Generalized lymphadenopathy* is defined as enlargement of more than two noncontiguous lymph node regions. The most common causes of generalized adenopathy are systemic infections, autoimmune diseases, and neoplastic processes. Lymphadenopathy of greater than 3 weeks duration is considered chronic.

The clinician caring for a child with lymphadenopathy will benefit from knowledge of the anatomic distribution of nodes in the area and their drainage patterns as described in Figures 42.1 and 42.2, as well as Table 42.1. The location of lymphadenopathy is often suggestive of a possible cause.

CAUSES OF LYMPHADENOPATHY BY REGION

Cervical

Enlargement of cervical lymph nodes is a common presenting sign in a variety of pediatric illnesses. In order to narrow the differential diagnosis, it is helpful to identify the time course of swelling (acute or chronic); history or presence of localized infections; occurrence of systemic symptoms; and specific location, symmetry, and characteristics of enlarged nodes. Cervical anatomy is complex, however nodes in the region can be classified generally as either superficial or deep. Superficial cervical nodes, palpated readily along the anterior and posterior borders of the sternocleidomastoid muscle, drain the shallow structures of the head and neck—particularly the oropharynx, external ear, and parotid. In contrast, deep cervical nodes, both superior and inferior, receive lymphatic drainage from a wider area of underlying structures of the head and neck, including the nasopharynx, tonsils and adenoids, larynx, and trachea. While there are numerous infectious and noninfectious causes of acute and chronic cervical lymphadenopathy, the most common etiologies in children are infectious (refer Chapter 102 Infectious Disease Emergencies).

By far, the most common cause of acute cervical adenopathy in children is reactive adenopathy associated with a viral upper respiratory tract infection. Superficial nodes are generally symmetrically enlarged, mobile, and minimally tender. Reactive adenopathy may persist for 2 to 3 weeks beyond the resolution of a viral illness. However, there should be no progression in the size or the extent of the adenopathy after resolution of symptoms of the virus.

Another common infectious cause of cervical lymph node enlargement, particularly in preschool-aged children, is lymphadenitis. Lymphadenitis occurs when an enlarged node becomes inflamed and tender over the course of a few days, as the result of a viral or bacterial infection. Viral adenitis is often associated with fever, conjunctivitis, pharyngitis, or other symptoms of an upper respiratory tract infection and causes acute bilateral swelling. Common causes are rhinovirus, adenovirus, enterovirus, influenza virus, respiratory syncytial virus, Epstein–Barr virus (EBV), and cytomegalovirus (CMV). Less commonly, herpes simplex, human herpes virus

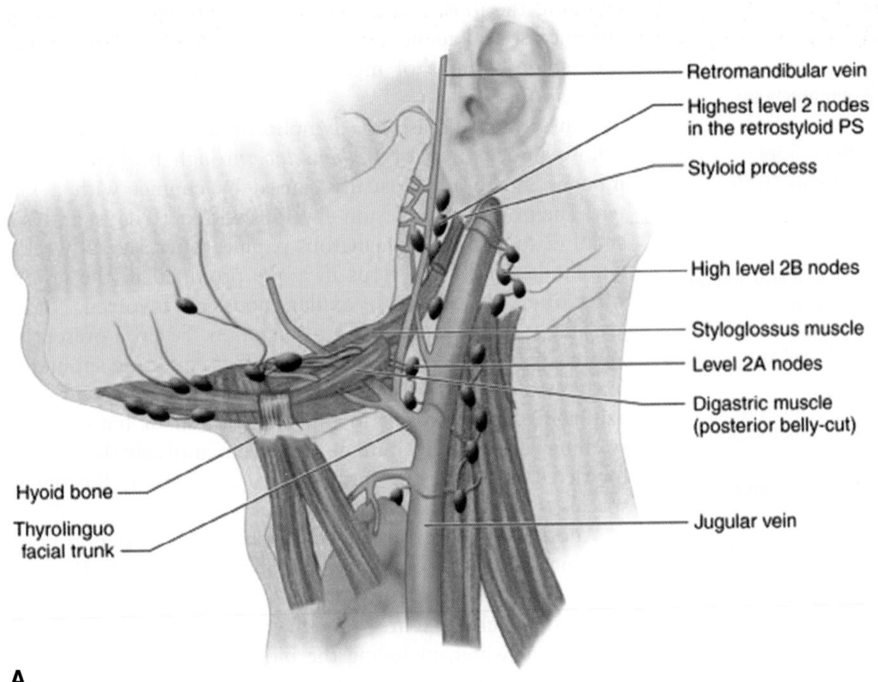

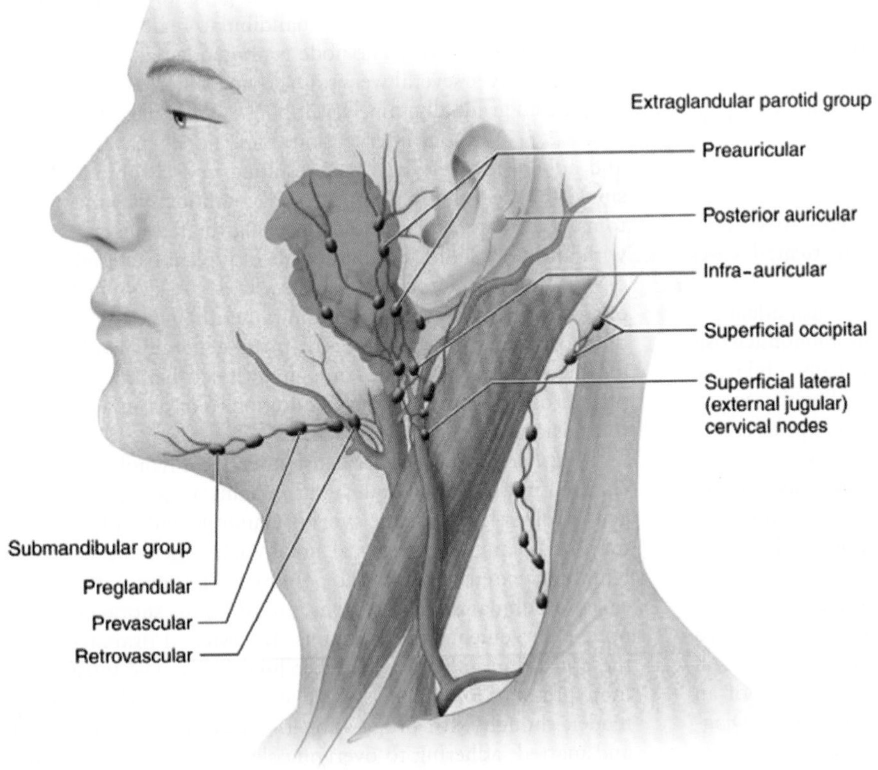

FIGURE 42.1 Lymph nodes of the head and neck. (From Mancuso AA. *Head and neck radiology*. Philadelphia, PA: Lippincott Williams & Wilkins, 2010.)

type 6 (roseola), or measles, mumps, or rubella are causative agents. In contrast, bacterial adenitis typically is unilateral and presents with the rapid onset of a firm, tender, and warm lymph node over 1 to 3 days. The overlying soft tissue becomes edematous and erythematous. Fever often accompanies the infection. If left untreated, the node may become suppurative, which is detectable on examination as fluctuance.

Acute bacterial adenitis is most often caused by group A β-hemolytic *Streptococcus* or *Staphylococcus aureus* (including methicillin-resistant *S. aureus* [MRSA]). Prompt initiation of oral antimicrobial therapy that empirically covers MRSA can prevent progression to a suppurative infection. However, patients who have failed to improve with oral antimicrobial therapy or those who present with signs of toxicity

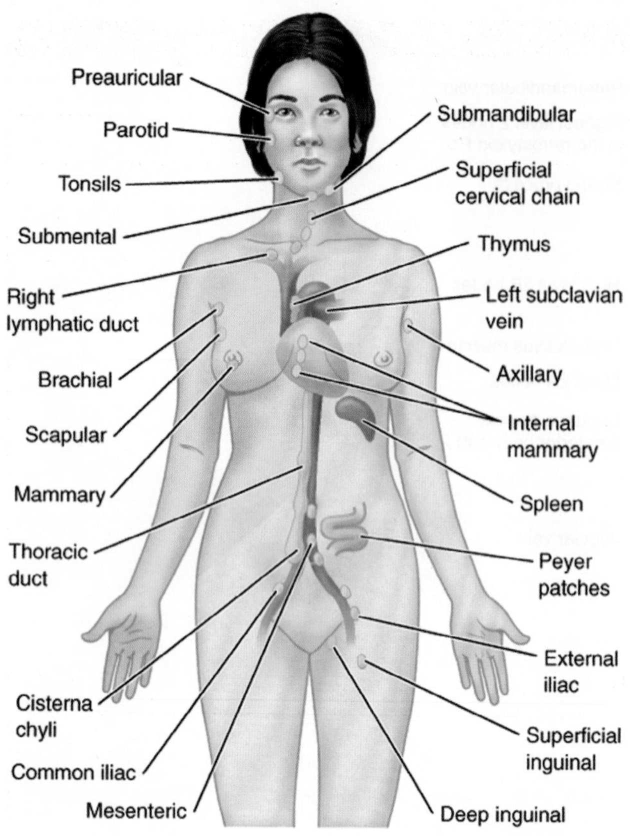

FIGURE 42.2 Lymph nodes of the body. (From Anderson MK. *Foundations of athletic training*. 5th ed. Philadelphia, PA: Lippincott Williams & Wilkins, 2012.)

require parenteral therapy. Drainage of the suppurative nodes is sometimes required, even in appropriately treated cases (Figs. 42.3 and 42.4).

A third commonly encountered cause of cervical adenopathy in children and adolescents is infectious mononucleosis caused by EBV, a herpes virus. EBV typically causes bilateral anterior and posterior cervical lymph node swelling that is tender to palpation. Nodes may be large and usually peak in size over the first week of illness, gradually subsiding over the next few weeks. The classic presentation of mononucleosis is a prodrome of malaise, headache, and elevated temperature prior to the development of an exudative pharyngitis, tender cervical adenopathy, and fever. Splenomegaly, abdominal pain, and anorexia may be present. Facial edema can accompany significant cervical adenopathy, presumably reflecting obstructed lymphatic drainage. Younger children with EBV infection may present less typically, with fever alone, symptoms of an upper respiratory infection, or abdominal complaints. Diagnosis of infectious mononucleosis can be made in adolescents with the detection of a positive heterophile–agglutinating antibody (e.g., monospot), however, the test may be falsely negative early in the disease course or in young children. Antibody titers directed to specific EBV antigens may be necessary to confirm the diagnosis. In addition, a complete blood count with differential (CBC/d) often shows a lymphocytosis with a large proportion of atypical lymphocytes.

In contrast to the acute cervical adenopathy seen with reactive lymphadenopathy, lymphadenitis, and infectious mononucleosis, there are a number of infectious agents that cause a more indolent course of cervical lymph node swelling. In children, the most common infections causing a subacute or chronic cervical adenopathy include *Bartonella henselae,* nontuberculous strains of mycobacterium, and *Mycobacterium tuberculosis.*

Cat-scratch disease is a lymphocutaneous syndrome that follows inoculation of *B. henselae* through broken skin or mucous membranes, usually caused by contact with a kitten. The primary skin lesion develops within 10 days, and is a small (2 to 5 mm) erythematous papule. After several weeks, lymphadenopathy develops in a site proximal to the lesion. Most often, the cervical or axillary nodes are involved. Nodes are single, large, and tender to palpation. Fever is present in approximately one-third of children. This condition spontaneously resolves within 1 to 3 months, though treatment with azithromycin will result in rapid resolution of lymph node swelling. The indirect immunofluorescent antibody (IFA) assay for detection of serum antibodies to antigens of *Bartonella* species is used for diagnosis of cat-scratch disease.

Another infectious cause of chronic cervical lymph node swelling is nontuberculous mycobacterium (NTM), also referred to as atypical mycobacterium. NTM is a group of acid-fast bacteria that are found in environmental sources such as soil and water, including the biofilm of home aquariums. Cervical lymphadenitis is the most common manifestation of NTM disease in childhood. Children younger than 5 years are affected. Lymph node involvement is generally unilateral, in the superficial cervical or submandibular region, and rarely larger than 3 to 4 cm. The node is nontender, and enlarges in size slowly over several weeks. Overlying skin may turn a deep purple and gradually thin, developing a paper-like appearance (Fig. 42.5). Without intervention, these nodes may suppurate and adhere to overlying skin, resulting in a chronic draining sinus. Infected children appear well, without systemic symptoms, and may have a history of being treated unsuccessfully with antibiotics aimed at pathogens of typical bacterial adenitis (group A *Streptococcus* or *S. aureus*). A clear history of exposure to NTM is the exception rather than the rule. Formal diagnosis is made by culture. Treatment generally involves surgical excision of the node, though antimicrobial therapy may play a role for some patients in addition to or as an alternative to excision.

M. tuberculosis is a rare cause of cervical lymphadenitis in children in the United States, but remains a significant pathogen in other parts of the world. Children with tuberculosis may be of any age. Cervical node enlargement occurs with lymphatic extension from the paratracheal nodes to the cervical and submandibular regions. In addition, supraclavicular node enlargement can be seen as the result of drainage from the apical lung pleura and upper lung fields. The most common presentation is an isolated enlarged node that is nontender, though with progression the node will become fixed and matted, adhering to overlying skin. In children with suspected tuberculous lymphadenitis, it is important to elicit any history of family members or close contacts with a diagnosis of tuberculosis, symptoms of active disease, or risk factors for acquisition (travel, homelessness, incarceration, human immunodeficiency virus [HIV] infection). Diagnosis is made by a combination of skin testing, chest radiograph, and if possible, culture data from the involved node. In addition, newly available serum interferon-γ–release assays (QuantiFERON-TB Gold In-Tube test or T-SPOT.TB test) detect interferon-γ generated by T cells in response to antigens found in *M. tuberculosis* and are available to aid in diagnosis. Treatment of

TABLE 42.1

CAUSES OF REGIONAL LYMPHADENOPATHY

Site	Drainage area	Common causes	Less common causes
Cervical	Head, neck, oropharynx	*Acute:* Viral URI Lymphadenitis (bacterial, viral) Pharyngitis Oropharyngeal infections EBV *Chronic:* EBV, CMV Cat-scratch disease Nontuberculous mycobacterium (NTM) lymphadenitis	*Acute:* Kawasaki disease *Chronic:* Malignancy (lymphoma, neuroblastoma, leukemia) Tularemia Toxoplasmosis Sarcoid Tuberculous lymphadenitis Histiocytosis (Langerhans cell histiocytosis, Rosai–Dorfman disease) Autoimmune lymphoproliferative syndrome (ALPS) Periodic fever, aphthous stomatitis, pharyngitis, cervical adenitis syndrome (PFAPA) Kikuchi–Fujimoto disease Kimura disease
Submental	Lower lip, gums, teeth, and floor of mouth	Dental caries/infections Gingivostomatitis	
Submandibular	Cheeks, buccal mucosa, lips, gums, teeth	Dental caries/infections Gingivostomatitis Chronically cracked/dry lips	
Anterior auricular (preauricular)	Anterior/temporal scalp, anterior ear canal, lateral conjunctiva, and eyelids	Conjunctivitis (viral/bacterial) Chlamydia conjunctivitis of neonate	Oculoglandular syndrome of cat-scratch disease, tularemia Rubella Parvovirus
Posterior auricular	Temporal and parietal scalp	Tinea capitis or other scalp infections	Roseola (HHV-6) Rubella
Occipital	Posterior scalp, neck	Pediculosis Tinea capitis Seborrheic dermatitis	Roseola (HHV-6) Rubella
Supraclavicular	Neck Right: mediastinum, lungs Left: upper abdomen	Malignancy (lymphoma or metastatic disease) Tuberculosis	
Axillary	Upper extremity, chest wall, upper abdominal wall, breast	Upper-extremity infections Reactive adenopathy after traumatic disruption in skin integrity Cat-scratch disease	Malignancy (leukemia, lymphoma) Rheumatologic disease of the hand/wrist Toxoplasmosis Rat-bite fever Tularemia
Epitrochlear	Ulnar side of hand, forearm	Local infection of hand	Rheumatologic disease of the hand/wrist Cat-scratch disease Sarcoid Tularemia Secondary syphilis
Inguinal	Scrotum/penis, vulva/vagina, perianal region, lower extremities, lower abdomen	Lower-extremity skin/soft tissue infections Perianal fissures or abscess Genital herpes Chlamydial/gonococcal infection	Syphilis Lymphogranuloma venereum Chancroid
Iliac	Lower extremities, abdominal viscera, urinary tract	Appendicitis UTI	Iliac adenitis

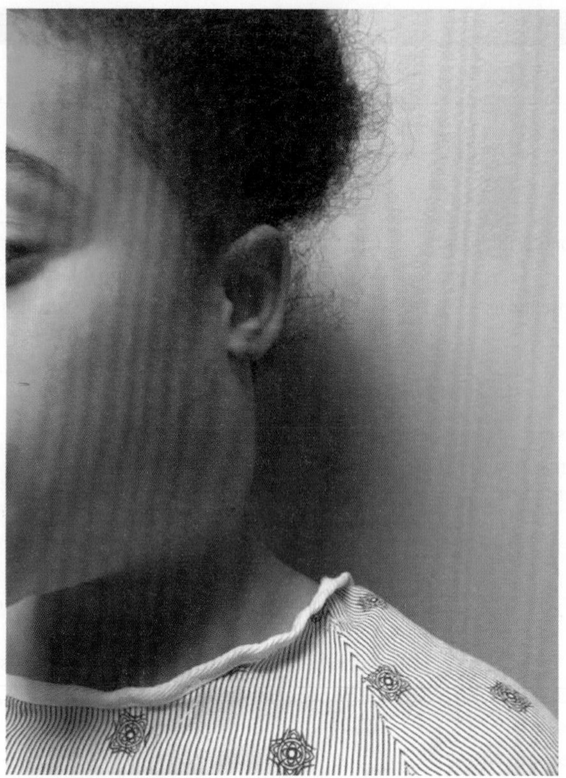

FIGURE 42.3 Child with lymphadenitis that progressed to lymph node abscess.

cervical lymphadenitis consists of antimycobacterial therapy, and should follow established recommendations, such as those from the Centers for Disease Control (CDC) (see Chapter 102 Infectious Disease Emergencies).

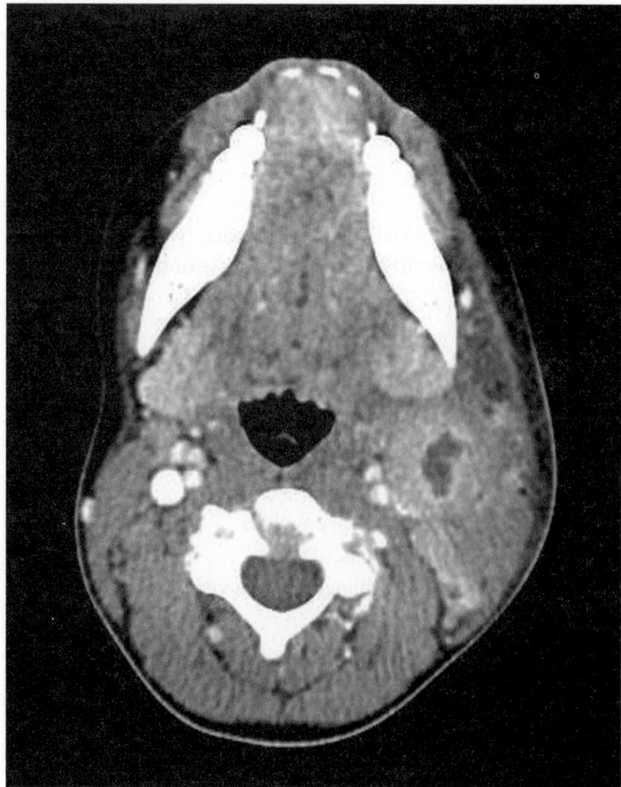

FIGURE 42.4 Computed tomography (CT) image of lymph node abscess.

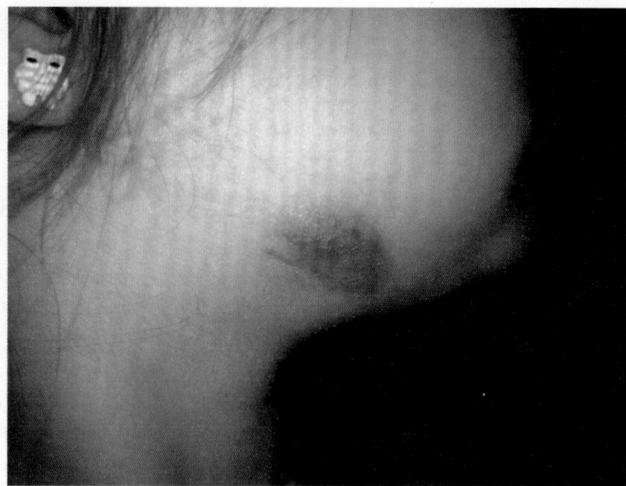

FIGURE 42.5 Child with nontuberculous mycobacterium (NTM) lymphadenitis.

There are several rare infectious causes of cervical lymphadenopathy that may be encountered in the pediatric emergency department. Tularemia, caused by infection with *Francisella tularensis,* occurs predominantly in the South Central United States (Arkansas, Oklahoma, Missouri, and Kansas). It occurs after contact with infected animals (rabbits, hamsters) or via tick or deerfly bites. The most common presentation in children is a febrile illness with tender cervical or occipital adenopathy that may become chronic. An associated papular or ulcerative lesion may be noted on the skin at the site of animal contact or insect bite. Diagnosis is made by detecting serum antibodies to *F. tularensis* and antimicrobial therapy with doxycycline or a fluoroquinolone is appropriate for mild illness. Toxoplasmosis, a parasitic infection caused by *Toxoplasma gondii,* is acquired via contact with oocytes in cat feces or consumption of undercooked pork or lamb containing cysts. Lymphadenopathy and fatigue are the most common symptoms of this self-limited illness, and adenopathy is discrete, nonsuppurative, and may persist for months in the cervical region. Serologic tests are the primary means of diagnosis.

In addition to infectious causes of cervical lymphadenopathy, there are numerous noninfectious etiologies that cause cervical node enlargement as a manifestation of systemic disease. Such noninfectious etiologies that may be encountered in pediatric patients include Kawasaki disease, malignancy, histiocytosis, lymphoproliferative disorders, and periodic fever syndromes.

An important cause of acute cervical adenopathy in young children is Kawasaki disease, or mucocutaneous lymph node syndrome (see Chapter 94 Cardiac Emergencies). Kawasaki disease usually affects children younger than 4 years of age and is rare after 8 years of age. Typical presentation of the disease is characterized by fever of at least 5 days duration, along with bilateral nonexudative conjunctivitis, changes to oral mucosa; peripheral extremity changes, a polymorphous rash, and cervical lymphadenopathy. The cervical lymphadenopathy in Kawasaki disease, seen in approximately 50% to 70% of patients, occurs during the early phase of the illness and may be unilateral or bilateral. The nodes are firm, mildly tender, and at least 1.5 cm in diameter. It is important to diagnose Kawasaki disease early because prompt treatment with intravenous immune globulin (IVIG) and aspirin can prevent coronary artery aneurysms, the most serious complication of this disease.

Various malignancies, including lymphoma and neuroblastoma may present with chronic cervical adenopathy. Lymph nodes in Hodgkin lymphoma are painless, with a rubbery and firm consistency, and located in the cervical, supraclavicular, or axillary regions. Palpation of such nodes in children, particularly when a history of nonspecific symptoms such as fatigue, anorexia, and weight loss are elicited, should lead to prompt evaluation with chest radiograph to evaluate for mediastinal masses. Neuroblastoma, most common in infants and children less than 2 years of age, is a neuroendocrine tumor arising in the adrenal glands, but can originate in the high thoracic and cervical sympathetic ganglia or metastasize to cervical and supraclavicular lymph nodes. Again, prompt imaging with chest radiograph, as well as abdominal imaging with computed tomography (CT) or magnetic resonance imaging (MRI) should be initiated in cases of suspected neuroblastoma.

Rare noninfectious causes of chronic cervical lymphadenopathy deserve consideration in the appropriate clinical context. Sarcoidosis is a multisystem granulomatous disorder that affects young adults, particularly African-Americans, causing systemic symptoms such as weight loss, cough, fatigue, and joint pain. Patients often have chronic bilateral cervical adenopathy, and chest radiograph in such patients may reveal hilar adenopathy, as well.

Autoimmune lymphoproliferative syndrome (ALPS), also known as Canale–Smith syndrome, is a genetic disorder of lymphocyte apoptosis leading to lymphadenopathy, splenomegaly, and pancytopenia. Children with ALPS present in the first year of life with massive cervical adenopathy and splenomegaly.

Histiocytic disorders, another uncommon group of diseases that cause prominent cervical adenopathy, occur when there is an overproduction of dendritic cells or macrophages which cause organ damage and tumor formation. Langerhans cell histiocytosis (LCH) affects children less than 3 years of age, causing lytic bone lesions and unilateral or bilateral soft and matted cervical lymphadenopathy. Sinus histiocytosis with massive lymphadenopathy (Rosai–Dorfman disease), presents in children as massively enlarged, nontender cervical lymphadenopathy, along with involvement of the nasal cavity, lytic bone lesions, pulmonary nodules, or rash.

Finally, the syndrome of periodic fever, aphthous stomatitis, pharyngitis, and cervical adenitis (PFAPA) is an autoinflammatory disease presenting in young children that cycles every 2 to 9 weeks. Children with PFAPA experience tender cervical lymphadenopathy with flares. There is no specific diagnostic test, and though corticosteroids and nonsteroidal anti-inflammatory drugs alleviate symptoms, the condition resolves spontaneously by 10 years of age.

Other Lymphadenopathy of the Head and Neck

Beyond cervical lymphadenopathy, acute localized adenopathy of the head and facial regions has a more narrow differential diagnosis, and the location of lymphadenopathy often suggests a cause, based on the location of focal infections and drainage patterns of nodes. Submandibular and submental nodes, draining the lips, buccal mucosa, and floor of the oropharynx, enlarge with infection within the oral cavity. This includes dental caries and abscesses, as well as gingivostomatitis. Herpetic gingivostomatitis generally affects the anterior tongue, buccal mucosa, or lips, while Coxsackievirus gingivostomatitis affects the posterior oropharynx, sparing the gingiva and lips, and causes characteristic lesions on palmar and plantar surfaces. Lymphadenopathy in the submandibular or submental regions on physical examination should prompt a careful oral and dental examination.

Preauricular nodes, located anterior to the ear, drain the conjunctiva and lateral eyelids. These nodes enlarge with eye or conjunctival infections, of which viral infections are a prominent cause. The combination of conjunctivitis and ipsilateral preauricular adenopathy is called oculoglandular syndrome, or Parinaud syndrome. Infections that can present as oculoglandular syndrome include adenovirus or chlamydial conjunctivitis in neonates. Rarely, cat-scratch disease and tularemia manifest as an oculoglandular syndrome.

Posterior auricular nodes, located behind the ear, and occipital nodes, found at the base of the scalp, commonly enlarge in response to scalp infections or chronic inflammation. Pediculosis (lice), tinea capitis, bacterial scalp infections, and inflammation from seborrheic dermatitis are all common causes of such node enlargement in children.

Axillary and Epitrochlear

Axillary adenopathy is commonly present with any infection or inflammation of the upper extremities. Most commonly, injuries to the hand, such as occur after falling or with puncture wounds or bites, may present with concomitant axillary adenopathy as a reactive response to disruption in skin integrity. Axillary adenopathy is also a common part of *B. henselae* infection (cat-scratch disease), as outlined previously as a cause of cervical adenopathy.

Epitrochlear adenopathy is significantly less common than axillary adenopathy in children, and any epitrochlear node greater than 0.5 cm is considered enlarged. Epitrochlear nodes may become inflamed after infections of the third, fourth, or fifth finger; medial portion of the hand; or ulnar portion of the forearm. Most commonly, these infections are caused by pyogenic bacteria (e.g., *Streptococcus pyogenes* or *S. aureus,* including MRSA), but depending on the inciting event, other pathogens may be responsible (e.g., *Streptobacillus moniliformis* and *Spirillum minus* in rat-bite fever or *F. tularensis* in tularemia). Rare causes of both axillary and epitrochlear adenopathy include rheumatologic disease of the hand or wrist and secondary syphilis.

Inguinal

Inguinal adenopathy most often results from lower-extremity skin or soft tissue infection. However, inguinal lymph nodes also drain tissues in the perianal region and unexplained adenopathy in this area should prompt examination for perirectal abscesses, fissures, or other inflammation. In addition, sexually transmitted diseases such as chlamydia or gonorrhea may cause inguinal adenopathy. Acute genital infection with herpes simplex virus-2 (HSV-2) often presents with tender inguinal adenopathy, occasionally as the only sign. Chancroid, lymphogranuloma venereum, and syphilis are rare causes of inguinal node swelling and tenderness. The presence of genital lesions, which may be either painful (as in herpes simplex virus or chancroid) or painless (as in syphilis), offers clues to these diagnoses. Therefore, careful history taking and physical examination are necessary to exclude these possibilities.

Iliac

Enlarged iliac nodes are palpable deeply over the inguinal ligament and become inflamed with lower-extremity infection, urinary tract infection, abdominal trauma, and appendicitis. Of note, iliac adenitis, which can present with fever, limp, and inability to fully extend the leg, may mimic the signs and symptoms of septic hip arthritis. Unlike in hip disease, however, hip motion is not limited on examination. Iliac adenitis may also be confused with appendicitis, but the pain initially occurs in the thigh and hip rather than in the periumbilical region or right lower quadrant.

GENERALIZED LYMPHADENOPATHY

Generalized lymphadenopathy, defined as enlargement of lymph nodes in two or more noncontiguous regions, can be a manifestation of both infectious and noninfectious systemic illnesses (Table 42.2). Akin to localized lymphadenopathy, generalized lymphadenopathy in children is most often caused by bacterial or viral infections. As an example, the high incidence of vomiting and abdominal pain in streptococcal pharyngitis has been attributed to abdominal lymph node swelling and inflammation, suggesting a more systemic pattern of adenopathy in streptococcal disease. More rare bacterial causes of generalized lymphadenopathy include the zoonotic infections brucellosis, leptospirosis, and tularemia. Brucellosis is acquired by exposure to cattle, sheep, goats, or unpasteurized milk or cheese and causes systemic symptoms including fever, night sweats, weight loss, arthralgias, and epididymoorchitis, as well as nonspecific examination findings including generalized lymphadenopathy and hepatosplenomegaly. Leptospirosis is most common in tropical climates, acquired via exposure to contaminated soil or water (particularly during swimming). Clinical manifestations are nonspecific, including fever, rigors, myalgias, headache, conjunctivitis, rash, hepatosplenomegaly, and lymphadenopathy. Brucellosis, leptospirosis, and tularemia (discussed previously) should be considered in the differential diagnosis of a child presenting with systemic symptoms, particularly fever, and physical examination findings of generalized lymphadenopathy if the appropriate exposure history is elicited.

Common viral causes of generalized adenopathy include EBV or CMV mononucleosis, and rubella and measles infections in parts of the world where these diseases are endemic. Though EBV mononucleosis classically causes fever, pharyngitis, and anterior and posterior cervical adenopathy; axillary and inguinal lymphadenopathy may also be presenting signs. In children with symptoms of infectious mononucleosis but a negative monospot and/or negative antibody titers to EBV antigens, CMV may be the cause. Rubella produces a prodrome of low-grade fever and lymphadenopathy (posterior cervical, postauricular, or generalized) followed by the development and rapid spread of a pink, maculopapular rash from face to the trunk and extremities. Measles (rubeola) produces a prodrome of fever, malaise, and anorexia followed by cough, conjunctivitis, coryza, and characteristic Koplik spots on the buccal mucosa. The exanthem of measles also has a cranial to caudal progression of a blanching, maculopapular rash, and lesions can become confluent. Children with severe measles may exhibit generalized lymphadenopathy and splenomegaly.

TABLE 42.2

CAUSES OF GENERALIZED LYMPHADENOPATHY

Systemic infection
Bacterial
Bacteremia
Group A streptococcus infection (pharyngitis, scarlet fever)
Brucellosis
Leptospirosis
Tularemia
Viral
Epstein–Barr virus
Cytomegalovirus
Human immunodeficiency virus
Adenovirus
Varicella
Rubella
Rubeola (measles)
Hepatitis B virus
Fungal
Histoplasmosis
Coccidioidomycosis
Blastomycosis
Parasitic
Toxoplasmosis
Malaria
Spirochete
Syphilis
Lyme disease
Autoimmune disease
Juvenile idiopathic arthritis
Systemic lupus erythematosus
Dermatomyositis
Serum sickness
Drug reaction with eosinophilia and systemic symptoms (DRESS)
Autoimmune hemolytic anemia
Chronic granulomatous disease (sarcoid)
Malignancy
Leukemia (acute lymphoblastic or acute myelogenous leukemia)
Non-Hodgkin lymphoma
Hodgkin lymphoma
Neuroblastoma
Histiocytosis
Hemophagocytic lymphohistiocytosis (HLH)
Langerhans cell histiocytosis (LCH)
Sinus histiocytosis with massive lymphadenopathy (Rosai–Dorfman disease)
Storage disease
Gaucher disease
Niemann–Pick disease
Miscellaneous
Autoimmune lymphoproliferative syndrome (ALPS)
Castleman disease
Hyperthyroidism

Last, HIV infection causes adenopathy in the cervical, axillary, and inguinal regions, particularly during the acute phase of infection. Nodes generally decrease in size after the first 1 to 2 weeks as the immune response to infection subsides, however a modest degree of adenopathy can persist. Children with unexplained recurrent or opportunistic infections, fevers, failure to thrive, hepatosplenomegaly, and generalized adenopathy should be evaluated for HIV infection.

Noninfectious systemic disease that also presents with generalized adenopathy includes inflammatory or autoimmune diseases, serum sickness, malignancy, histiocytosis, and genetic storage diseases. More than half of patients with systemic lupus erythematosus or systemic onset juvenile idiopathic arthritis manifest generalized adenopathy during the acute phase of illness. Nodes are typically soft, nontender, and located in the cervical, axillary, and inguinal regions.

Serum sickness is an immune complex–mediated hypersensitivity reaction to a number of drugs, with clinical manifestations including fever, rash, myalgias, and arthralgias. Symptoms begin 1 to 2 weeks after exposure to an inciting agent, and resolve spontaneously within weeks of discontinuation. Skin manifestations are variable, though typically urticarial and macular involving the lower trunk, groin, or axillary regions and spreading to the back, upper extremities, and hands. Lymphadenopathy may be noted with the rash, but may be seen without the rash and may be accompanied by splenomegaly. Table 42.3 lists drugs that have been implicated in serum sickness reactions.

Drug reaction with eosinophilia and systemic symptoms (DRESS) is a rare, potentially life-threatening drug-induced hypersensitivity reaction postulated to be caused by a drug-specific immune response and reactivation of herpes virus. Clinical manifestations include fever, diffuse morbilliform skin eruption, facial edema, hematologic abnormalities (eosinophilia, atypical lymphocytosis), lymphadenopathy, and visceral involvement (liver, kidney, lung, and/or bone marrow). The reaction begins 2 to 6 weeks after the initiation of the offending medication. The aromatic antiepileptic agents and the sulfonamides are the most frequent causes of this disorder (Table 42.3). Stopping the offending agent and avoiding similar cross-reacting drugs as well as supportive care are mainstay measures of treatment.

Neoplastic disease that causes generalized adenopathy may be primary to the lymph node, as in lymphoma or it may be caused by an invasion of the lymph node by extrinsic malignant cells, as in leukemia. Hodgkin lymphoma, discussed previously, results most often in cervical or supraclavicular adenopathy. In contrast, non-Hodgkin lymphoma presents with relatively rapid development (over weeks) of nontender, diffuse lymphadenopathy accompanied by abdominal pain, vomiting, facial swelling, or wheezing due to compression of surrounding structures in the mediastinum or abdomen. Children with acute leukemia often have generalized adenopathy, and nodes are firm or rubbery, nontender, and matted. These children usually appear ill, having other systemic signs, including fevers, weight loss, bony pain, bruising, petechiae, and hepatosplenomegaly with anemia and thrombocytopenia.

Histiocytic disorders, caused by the accumulation and infiltration of macrophages and dendritic cells in affected tissues, are a rare cause of generalized adenopathy. LCH and sinus histiocytosis (Rosai–Dorfman disease), discussed previously, cause cervical adenopathy; while hemophagocytic lymphohistiocytosis (HLH) is a potentially fatal disease in children less than age 4 that manifests with generalized adenopathy in one-third of patients. It presents as a febrile illness with adenopathy, cytopenias, coagulopathy, hepatitis, splenomegaly, and neurologic involvement. Characteristic laboratory findings include anemia, thrombocytopenia, and elevated liver enzymes, as well as extremely elevated ferritin levels and hypertriglyceridemia. Immune and cytokine studies, as well as genetic testing and bone marrow studies showing hemophagocytosis are used to establish the diagnosis.

Finally, rare causes of systemic adenopathy include lipid storage diseases, such as Gaucher and Niemann–Pick disease, which can cause diffuse adenopathy and are almost always associated with hepatosplenomegaly. Bone marrow biopsy, showing lipid-laden histiocytes, is diagnostic.

TABLE 42.3

DRUGS IMPLICATED IN SERUM SICKNESS AND DRUG REACTION WITH EOSINOPHILIA AND SYSTEMIC SYMPTOMS (DRESS)

Serum sickness
Common causes:
Antimicrobials: penicillin, trimethoprim–sulfamethoxazole, cefaclor
Uncommon causes:
Aspirin, indomethacin
Antimicrobials: ciprofloxacin, clarithromycin, itraconazole
Antiepileptics: carbamazepine
Captopril
Bupropion, fluoxetine
Heparin
Insulin
Iron-dextran
Barbiturates
DRESS
Antiepileptics: carbamazepine, lamotrigine, phenytoin
Antimicrobials: vancomycin, minocycline, dapsone, sulfamethoxazole
Sulfasalazine
Allopurinol

LIFE-THREATENING LYMPHADENOPATHY

In rare instances, lymphadenopathy can lead to a life-threatening condition. In children and adolescents affected by Hodgkin or non-Hodgkin lymphoma or metastatic neuroblastoma, bulky or rapidly enlarging mediastinal lymph nodes can cause compression of the superior vena cava (SVC) or the tracheobronchial tree. In SVC syndrome, lymph nodes that encircle the vena cava enlarge and cause obstruction to central venous blood flow. This obstruction leads to clinical manifestations including dilated chest and neck veins, facial swelling and plethora, and dyspnea. Progression may lead to headaches, confusion, and altered mental status as well as progressive respiratory distress. Children with bulky adenopathy of the mediastinal or paratracheal nodes may present solely with respiratory symptoms, including stridor or wheezing, caused by compression of the trachea or bronchi by enlarged lymph nodes. Emergency physicians who take care of children with suspected lymphoma must be aware of the acute risk of airway obstruction that may be exacerbated by changes in position (lying flat) or with sedation or anesthesia. In addition, when treating children with SVC syndrome, physicians must be careful to administer all intravenous therapy in the lower extremities, as poor circulation in the upper extremities and torso because of venous obstruction results in poor drug distribution and places the patient at increased risk of thrombus formation.

EVALUATION AND DECISION

The pediatric emergency physician who evaluates a child with lymphadenopathy is faced with an extensive differential diagnosis. However, a targeted history and thorough physical examination can help focus evaluation of the patient and will often lead to the correct diagnosis.

Historical data that need to be obtained include the time of onset, rate of growth, and presence of other symptoms. Local symptoms suggestive of infection are particularly relevant, including fever, conjunctivitis, otitis, pharyngitis, gingivostomatitis, or cellulitis, as these may correlate with acute regional lymphadenopathy. In well-appearing children, recent illnesses must be considered, particularly because reactive adenopathy may persist for 2 to 3 weeks after the resolution of a viral illness. During evaluation, it is important to note the presence of "red flag" constitutional symptoms, including prolonged fevers, weight loss, night sweats, arthralgias, rashes, and bruising or petechiae that may suggest underlying systemic pathology and prompt more aggressive evaluation.

Social history and ill contacts of children also provide important information in constructing a differential diagnosis. Ill contacts of children at school or in the home, particularly affected by viral respiratory infections, infectious mononucleosis, or group A streptococcus infections, should be noted. Inquiry about a child's close contacts with a diagnosis of tuberculosis, symptoms of active disease, travel, or risk factors for acquisition is imperative when considering tuberculous adenitis. Asking about pets (cats or fish tanks), residence (exposure to livestock), recent travel or outdoor activity (animal exposure and insect bites), and dietary patterns (consumption of unpasteurized milk or cheese, or undercooked meats) can provide key information in a given clinical context.

Finally, the clinician must ask about medication use and whether any prior treatment, such as antibiotic therapy, treatment with glucocorticoids, or attempted aspiration with cultures, has been initiated. For example, children with NTM adenitis or Kawasaki disease may present to the emergency department after a course of antistaphylococcal antibiotic therapy failed to reduce the size of the node. This information can often guide the physician to include or exclude certain diagnoses. The importance of avoiding glucocorticoids prior to making a definitive diagnosis of the cause of lymphadenopathy should be emphasized. Glucocorticoid treatment can mask or delay the histologic diagnosis of malignancy such as leukemia or lymphoma, and should not be given empirically to decrease node swelling.

The physical examination should include a careful measurement of the size of the enlarged nodes and documentation of the number of nodes involved to provide an adequate baseline for follow-up. Describing a node's consistency (soft, firm, rubbery, indurated, fluctuant), mobility (mobile or fixed), and degree of tenderness to palpation is essential. Skin changes around the node (erythematous and edematous, or violaceous and paper-thin) should be noted. Lymphadenopathy in any region should prompt examination of lymph nodes in all regions to assess for generalized involvement. Finally, a complete physical examination noting rashes, hepatosplenomegaly, joint swelling, or other abnormalities is critical.

In well-appearing children without systemic symptoms, further evaluation of acute localized lymphadenopathy is generally unnecessary. Children with symptoms of lymphadenitis (a unilateral node with erythema, edema, or tenderness) can be empirically treated with a 10- to 14-day course of antibiotics with MRSA coverage and reevaluated. Children without symptoms of an acute bacterial lymphadenitis can be observed over the same time course, provided they have no enlargement of the adenopathy and lack worrisome constitutional symptoms. Reactive adenopathy that occurs after a viral illness typically resolved within 2 to 3 weeks.

In children with localized adenopathy that persists past 2 to 4 weeks, ill-appearing children, and children with generalized lymphadenopathy, further evaluation should be performed, guided by the differential diagnosis that was formed based on history and physical examination. Any suspicion of malignancy warrants assessment with CBC with differential and peripheral blood smear examination, as well as chest radiograph to assess for mediastinal adenopathy. In addition, lactate dehydrogenase and uric acid may be elevated, indicating tissue damage and rapid cell turnover. Inflammatory markers, including C-reactive protein (CRP) and erythrocyte sedimentation rate (ESR) are nonspecific, but may be elevated in children with systemic inflammatory diseases and can be helpful in monitoring response to treatment. In children with nonspecific infectious symptoms, viral serologies (EBV, CMV, HIV) may be informative. As indicated by history and examination, serology for *B. henselae,* or tuberculin skin testing or serum testing for *M. tuberculosis* may be performed.

Various imaging modalities may aid in diagnosis of lymphadenopathy, including ultrasound (US), CT, and MRI. The type of diagnostic radiology necessary to evaluate lymphadenopathy depends on the location and chronicity of the lymph node(s). In efforts to limit radiation to doses as low as reasonably achievable (ALARA principle), US has proven to be a very effective, noninvasive, inexpensive, highly available, and nonradiating type of imaging to evaluate lymphadenopathy in children. US can distinguish between simple node enlargement and a suppurative lesion with higher sensitivity than CT. Color Doppler imaging can demonstrate increased blood flow to inflamed lymph nodes as well as a hypoechoic (dark) center in a suppurative node. Characteristics of the grouping of the lymph nodes can also aid the radiologist in narrowing the patient's differential diagnosis. CT may be preferred in the evaluation of lymphadenopathy when greater anatomic detail is desired, as in a preoperative radiologic evaluation or in the evaluation of deep cervical space neck infections. Contrast-enhanced CT is more sensitive than US for the diagnosis of an abscess but lacks specificity due to the similar radiologic appearance of frank pus and phlegmonous changes. MRI may provide these fine details without ionizing radiation, but the cost of imaging and need for sedation makes CT a more preferable and easily accessible modality when accessed from the emergency department.

Finally, in the course of evaluation of lymphadenopathy, the decision to perform a biopsy on an enlarged node remains a clinical one. In general, early node biopsy should be considered in children who are ill with systemic symptoms, persistent fever, or weight loss. Deep inferior cervical or supraclavicular adenopathy, with or without an abnormal chest film, is pursued aggressively with biopsy given the concern for malignancy, in particular lymphoma. Beyond this, in the face of an otherwise negative diagnostic workup, serial measurement over a period of weeks showing progressive or rapid enlargement of the affected node raises suspicion for malignant disease and biopsy should be strongly considered. Biopsy should also be considered if an enlarged node fails to regress in size after approximately 6 weeks of observation.

Suggested Readings and Key References

General References

Herzog LW. Prevalence of lymphadenopathy of the head and neck in infants in children. *Clin Pediatr* 1983;22(7):485–487.

Nield LS, Kamat D. Lymphadenopathy in children: when and how to evaluate. *Clin Pediatr* 2004;43:25–33.

Sahai S. Lymphadenopathy. *Pediatr Rev* 2013;34(5):216–227.

Twist CJ, Link MP. Assessment of lymphadenopathy in children. *Pediatr Clin North Am* 2002;49:1009–1025.

Bartonella Henselae Infection

English R. Cat-scratch disease. *Pediatr Rev* 2006;24(4):123–128.

Floren TA, Zaoutis TE, Zaoutis LB. Beyond cat scratch disease: widening spectrum of Bartonella henselae infection. *Pediatrics* 2008;121(5): e1413–e1425.

Massei F, Gori L, Macchia P, et al. The expanded spectrum of bartonellosis in children. *Infect Dis Clin North Am* 2005;19(3): 691–711.

Cervical Adenopathy

Gosche JR, Vick L. Acute, subacute, and chronic cervical lymphadenitis in children. *Semin Pediatr Surg* 2006;15(2):99–106.

Rajasekaran K, Krakovitz P. Enlarged neck lymph nodes in children. *Pediatr Clin North Am* 2013;60:923–936.

Imaging

Ludwig BJ, Wang J, Nadgir RN, et al. Imaging of cervical lymphadenopathy in children and young adults. *AJR Am J Roentgenol* 2012;199:1105–1113.

Restrepo R, Oneta J, Lopez K, et al. Head and neck lymph nodes in children: the spectrum from normal to abnormal. *Pediatr Radiol* 2009;39:836–846.

Mycobacterial Infections

Albright JT, Pranski SM. Nontuberculous mycobacterial infections of the head and neck. *Pediatr Clin North Am* 2003;50(2):503–514.

Cruz AT, Geltemeyer AM, Starke JR, et al. Comparing the tuberculin skin test and T-SPOT. TB blood test in children. *Pediatrics* 2011;127(1):e31–e38.

Marais BJ, Gie RP, Schaaf HS, et al. Childhood pulmonary tuberculosis: old wisdom and new challenges. *Am J Respir Crit Care Med* 2006;173(10):1078–1090.

Starke JR. Management of nontuberculous mycobacterial cervical adenitis. *Pediatr Infect Dis J* 2000;19(7):674–675.

Epstein–Barr Viral Infections

Luzuriaga K, Sullivan JL. Infectious mononucleosis. *N Engl J Med* 2010;362(21):1993–2000.

Kawasaki Disease

Bayers S, Shulman ST, Paller AS. Kawasaki disease. Part I: Diagnosis, clinical features and pathogenesis. *J Am Acad Dermatol* 2013;69(4): 501e2–501e11.

Bayers S, Shulman ST, Paller AS. Kawasaki disease. Part II Complications and treatment. *J Am Acad Dermatol* 2013;69(4):513e1–513e8.

Scuccimarri R. Kawasaki disease. *Pediatr Clin North Am* 2012;59: 425–445.

Son MB, Newburger JW. Kawasaki disease. *Pediatr Rev* 2013;34(4): 151–162.

Histiocytosis

Bhasin A, Tolan RW Jr. Hemophagocytic lymphohistiocytosis—a diagnostic dilemma: two cases and review. *Clin Pediatr (Phila)* 2013;52(4):297–301.

Drutz JE. Histiocytosis. *Pediatr Rev* 2011;32(5):218–219.

Risma K, Jordan MB. Hemophagocytic lymphohistiocytosis: updates and evolving concepts. *Curr Opin Pediatr* 2012;24(1):9–15.

Weitzman S, Jaffe R. Uncommon histiocytic disorders: the non-Langerhans cell histiocytoses. *Pediatr Blood Cancer* 2005;45(3): 256–264.

Windebank K, Nanduri V. Langerhans cell histiocytosis. *Arch Dis Child* 2009;94(11):904–908.

Other

Carroll MC, Yueng-Yue KA, Esterly NB, et al. Drug-induced hypersensitivity syndrome in pediatric patients. *Pediatrics* 2001;108(2): 485–492.

Shetty AK, Beaty MW, McGuirt WF Jr. Kimura's disease: a diagnostic challenge. *Pediatrics* 2002;110(3):e39.

Vigo G., Zulian F. Periodic fevers with aphthous stomatitis, pharyngitis, and adenitis (PFAPA). *Autoimmun Rev* 2012;12:52–55.

Yoo IH, Na H, Bae EY. Recurrent lymphadenopathy in children with Kikuchi-Fujimoto disease. *Eur J Pediatr* 2014;173(9):1193–1199.

CHAPTER 43 ▪ NECK MASS

CARLA M. PRUDEN, MD, MPH AND CONSTANCE M. MCANENEY, MD, MS

Neck masses are a common concern in the pediatric population. By definition, these include any visible swelling that disturbs the normal contour of the neck between the shoulder and the angle of the jaw. The patient's age and the location of the neck mass are important in determining the differential diagnosis. Four basic classifications of neck lesions are inflammatory, congenital, traumatic, and neoplastic. Inflammatory masses representing infectious changes in otherwise normal structures, such as lymphadenopathy and lymphadenitis, are the most common. Congenital anatomic defects of the neck including cystic hygromas, branchial cleft cysts, hemangiomas, thyroglossal duct cysts, and dermoids, may be minimally apparent, at birth, with progressive cyst formation over time. Traumatic hematomas surrounding vital structures may lead to significant distress. Malignant lesions of the head and neck are fairly uncommon, but must be ruled out, and often involve the lymphatic system. With multiple etiologies, an organized approach to the history and physical examination of the head and neck, including a working understanding of the embryology, is important to facilitate proper diagnosis and treatment.

Many factors, ranging from aesthetics to concern for malignancy may precipitate the initial emergency department (ED) visit. Direct compression of vital structures (airway, cardiovascular structures, or cervical spinal cord) can cause a principal threat to life. Rarely, systemic toxicity from progression of local infection or thyroid storm can cause uncompensated shock. In this chapter, recognition of masses that represent true emergencies will be addressed first (Table 43.1), followed by the approach to common, nonemergent lesions (Table 43.2). Table 43.3 lists causes of neck masses of children by location.

EVALUATION AND DECISION

Initial history and physical examination should rapidly assess immediate threats to airway, breathing, circulation, and neurologic status. Stridor, hoarseness, dysphagia, and drooling are ominous indications of airway compromise. Respiratory or cardiovascular compromise may manifest as mental status changes. Suspicion for traumatic injury warrants cervical spine immobilization. Table 43.1 lists disorders that constitute true emergencies because of local pressure on vital structures or because of systemic toxicity.

Child with Neck Mass and Respiratory Distress or Systemic Toxicity

Mechanism and duration of symptoms are crucial elements in the evaluation of a neck mass. Trauma from vehicular collisions, falls from heights, or sports injuries may cause hematoma formation near vital structures such as the carotid artery or trachea. If the trauma involves the cervical spine, a hematoma may occur over fractured vertebrae. Underlying coagulopathy can cause severe hemorrhage and compressive injury from hematoma, even with *mild* mechanisms of trauma. A high index of suspicion for bleeding disorders and nonaccidental trauma is necessary in these cases. Symptomatic arteriovenous fistulas may have a delayed presentation—up to weeks following the inciting neck trauma. Acute thoracic trauma or airway obstruction can cause increased transpulmonary pressure. The resulting air leak may dissect into the neck from the mediastinum or pleural spaces. Observation is warranted in a child presenting with crepitant neck swelling and tachypnea, as this may represent progression of a pneumomediastinum to pneumothorax. Allergic reactions ranging from local bee stings to anaphylaxis may precipitate an acute emergency if there is enough tissue edema to obstruct the trachea.

Local and regional infections may present with cervical lymphadenopathy, but can have more significant life-threatening aspects. Acute airway obstruction may result from viral or bacterial infections with associated tonsillar hypertrophy or laryngocele enlargement. Bacterial pharyngitis occasionally progresses to deep space neck infections including, retropharyngeal, lateral pharyngeal, and peritonsillar abscesses (PTAs). Lemierre syndrome, an uncommon parapharyngeal infection involving thrombophlebitis of the internal jugular vein with metastatic pulmonary abscesses, may manifest as respiratory distress and systemic toxicity in the adolescent with a history of pharyngitis. Dental infection that spreads to the floor of the mouth (Ludwig angina) and neck may cause neck masses and airway compression. Rarely, epiglottitis may present with associated cervical adenitis or the appearance of submandibular mass from ballooning of the hypopharynx. Concomitant dysphagia, drooling, and stridor would raise suspicion for these complications. Occasionally, branchial cleft cysts or cystic hygromas can become infected and progress to abscess formation or rarely to mediastinitis. More recently, children with human immunodeficiency virus (HIV) infection (see Chapter 102 Infectious Disease Emergencies) are reported to have parotitis or generalized lymphadenopathy (axillary, cervical, occipital), particularly visible in the neck as a presenting complaint. Children may have hyperthyroid symptoms when a neck mass represents thyromegaly. Similarly, patients with the mucocutaneous lymph node syndrome (Kawasaki disease) often have cervical lymphadenopathy and, on rare occasions, have active life-threatening vasculitis of the coronary vessels.

Although neck tumors generally grow outward, in children, they may become large enough to encroach on vital structures. Lymphoma, an uncommon but important cause of neck mass, is usually associated with painless enlargement (often of supraclavicular nodes) that occurs over several weeks in the older school-age child. Anterior mediastinal

TABLE 43.1

LIFE-THREATENING CAUSES OF NECK MASS

Hematoma secondary to trauma
- Cervical spine injury
- Vascular compromise or acute bleeding
- Late arteriovenous fistula

Subcutaneous emphysema with associated airway or pulmonary injury

Local hypersensitivity reaction (sting/bite) with airway edema

Airway compromise with epiglottitis, peritonsillar abscess, or infection of floor of mouth or retropharyngeal space (with adenopathy)

Bacteremia/sepsis associated with local infection of a cyst (cystic hygroma, thyroglossal, or branchial cleft cyst)

Non-Hodgkin lymphoma with mediastinal mass and airway compromise

Thyroid storm

Mucocutaneous lymph node syndrome with coronary vasculitis (Kawasaki disease)

Tumor—leukemia, lymphoma, rhabdomyosarcoma, histiocytosis X

Lemierre syndrome

node involvement creates airway collapse in the supine position secondary to tracheal compression. This may manifest as orthopnea. Cystic hygromas and hemangiomas occasionally enlarge sufficiently enough to interfere with feeding or to obstruct the airway. Other neoplasms, such as rhabdomyosarcoma, leukemia, neuroblastoma, and histiocytosis X, are life-threatening because of local invasion and metabolic and hematologic effects.

Child with Neck Mass and No Distress

Most children in the ED with a neck mass are not in distress; the leading diagnoses are reactive adenopathy or acute lymphadenitis from viral or bacterial infection. A common concern, however, is deciding which neck mass bears the diagnosis of malignancy and requires biopsy or further evaluation.

History

Age at presentation of the mass aids in narrowing the diagnosis. Congenital lesions often present in infancy, though not all masses are present within the first few months of life. A neck mass presenting at several weeks of life may represent

TABLE 43.2

COMMON CAUSES OF NECK MASS

Lymphadenopathy secondary to viral or bacterial infection

Cervical adenitis (bacterial)

Hematoma

Benign tumors—lipoma, keloid

Congenital cyst (squamous epithelial cysts)

TABLE 43.3

DIFFERENTIAL DIAGNOSIS OF NECK MASS BY ETIOLOGY

Congenital
- Squamous epithelial cyst (congenital or posttraumatic)
- Pilomatrixoma (Malherbe calcifying epithelioma)
- Hemangioma and cystic hygroma (lymphangioma)
- Branchial cleft cyst
- Thyroglossal duct cyst
- Laryngocele
- Dermoid cyst
- Cervical rib

Inflammatory
- Infection
  - Cervical adenitis—streptococcal, staphylococcal, fungal, mycobacterial, cat-scratch disease, tularemia
  - Adenopathy—secondary to local head and neck infection
  - Secondary to systemic "infection"—infectious mononucleosis, cytomegalovirus, toxoplasmosis, others
  - Retropharyngeal abscess
  - Focal myositis—inflammatory muscular pseudotumor
  - Lemierre syndrome
  - "Antigen" mediated
  - Local hypersensitivity reaction (sting/bite)
  - Serum sickness, autoimmune disease
  - Pseudolymphoma (secondary to phenytoin)
  - Mucocutaneous lymph node syndrome (Kawasaki disease)
  - Sarcoidosis
  - Caffey–Silverman syndrome

Trauma
- Hematoma
- Sternocleidomastoid tumor of infancy (fibromatosis colli)
- Subcutaneous emphysema
- Acute bleeding
- Arteriovenous fistula
- Foreign body
- Cervical spine fracture

Neoplasms
- Benign
  - Epidermoid
  - Lipoma, fibroma, neurofibroma
  - Keloid
  - Goiter (with or without thyroid hormone disturbance)
  - Osteochondroma
  - Teratoma (may be malignant)
  - "Normal" anatomy or variant
- Malignant
  - Lymphoma—Hodgkin disease, non-Hodgkin lymphoma
  - Leukemia
  - Other—rhabdomyosarcoma, neuroblastoma, histiocytosis X, nasopharyngeal squamous cell carcinoma, thyroid, or salivary gland tumor

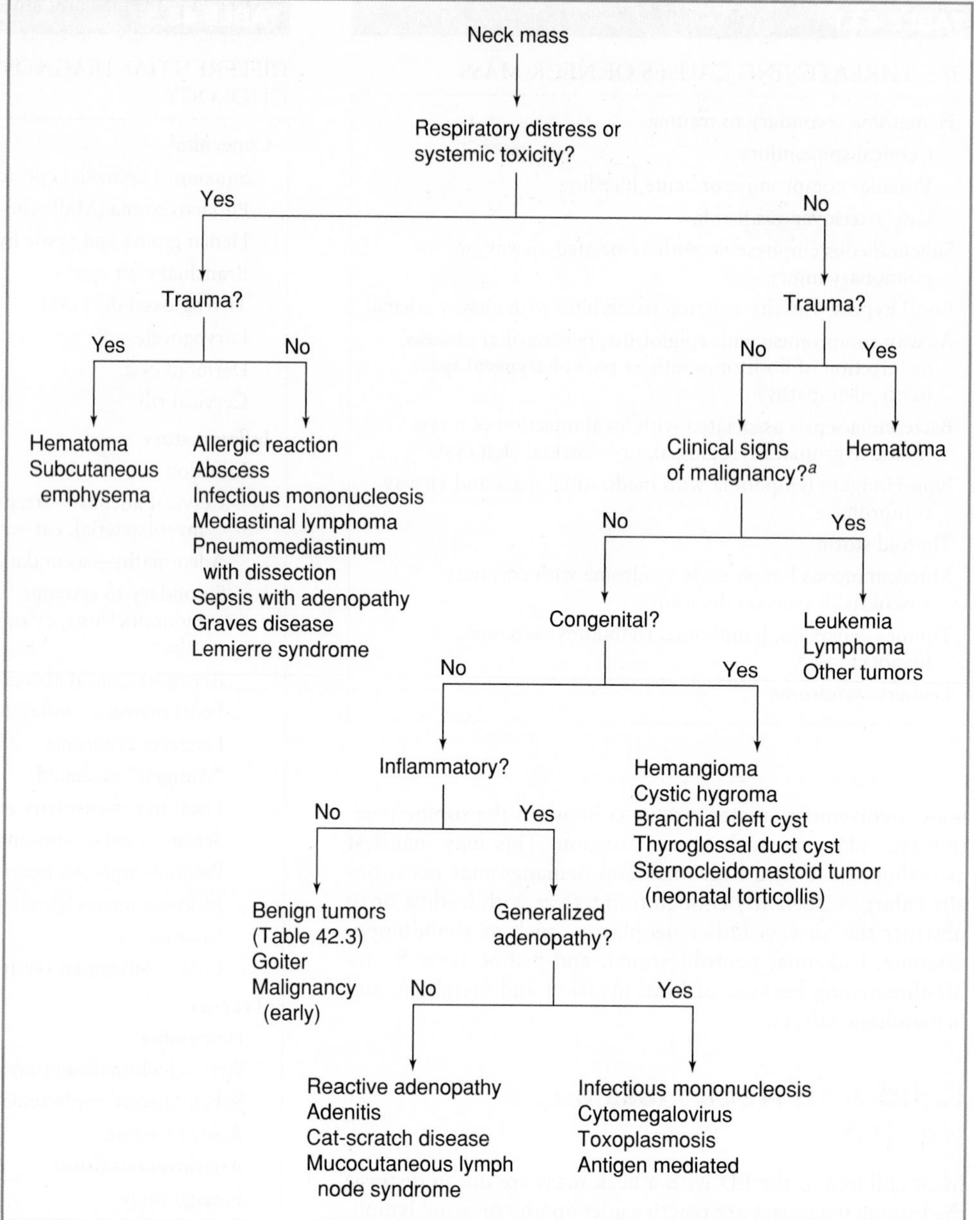

FIGURE 43.1 Evaluation of the child with a neck mass. [a]Malignancy: nontender, >3 cm diameter (and firm), enlarging mass of several weeks' duration, ulceration, location deep to superficial fascia or fixed to tissue, supraclavicular mass, systemic lymphadenopathy and bruising, superior vena cava syndrome.

birth trauma with hemorrhage into the sternocleidomastoid and resulting torticollis. Congenital cysts, however, may not come to attention until they have become recurrent secondary to repeated enlargement with infection or inflammation. A description of the mass, noting location, size and shape, is essential, as well as any changes in its nature over time. Recent trauma from animal scratches or bites can contribute to the differential diagnosis. Dimples, sinuses, drainage, and temporal exposure to known sick contacts may suggest infectious etiology.

In addition to establishing the duration of symptoms, it is important to ascertain the involvement of other organ systems. It is likewise important to elicit ENT and respiratory symptoms such as noisy breathing (wheezing or stridor), difficulty breathing, sore throat, and neck pain. History of fever, fatigue, weight loss, night sweats, or adenopathy elsewhere, can often suggest a diagnosis. Exposures to antibiotics or antiepileptic drugs may cause symptoms like serum sickness (fever, malaise, rash, arthralgias, nephritis) or pseudolymphoma, respectively (see Fig. 43.1).

Physical Examination

The child presenting with a neck mass should have a thorough head to toe examination, beginning with assessment for critical illness. It can be valuable to defer a meticulous neck evaluation until after completion of the remaining examination. Palpation will reveal the mass location, size, and shape. Presence of crepitation, thrill, bruit, fluctuance, or overlying skin changes should be noted. Normality of remaining structures should be ascertained to determine if additional lesions are present. Neck flexion and extension should be evaluated. Figure 43.2 diagrams common locations of neck mass. Inspection of the oral cavity should describe structures such as oral mucosa, dentition, Stensen duct (parotid gland), and other glands. Movement of the mass with swallowing or tongue protrusion is important to note. Completion of the

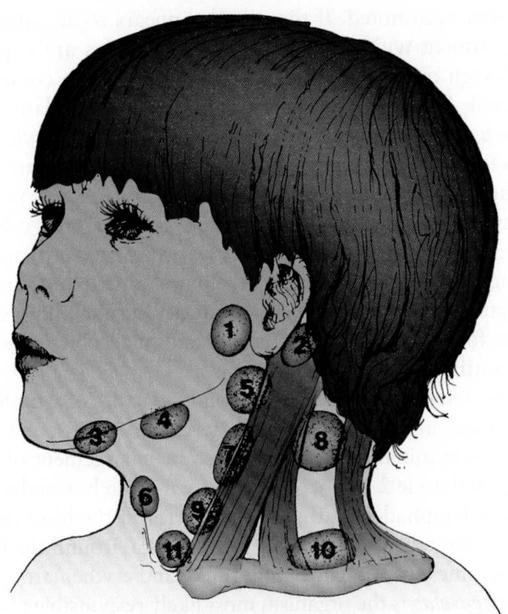

FIGURE 43.2 Differential diagnosis of neck mass by location. *Area 1. Parotid:* Cystic hygroma, hemangioma, lymphadenitis, parotitis, Sjögren and Caffey–Silverman syndrome, lymphoma. *Area 2. Postauricular:* Lymphadenitis, branchial cleft cyst (1st), squamous epithelial cyst. *Area 3. Submental:* Lymphadenitis, cystic hygroma, sialadenitis, tumor, cystic fibrosis. *Area 4. Submandibular:* Lymphadenitis, cystic hygroma, sialadenitis, tumor, cystic fibrosis. *Area 5. Jugulodigastric:* Lymphadenitis, squamous epithelial cyst, branchial cleft cyst (1st), parotid tumor, *normal*—transverse process C2, styloid process. *Area 6. Midline neck:* Lymphadenitis, thyroglossal duct cyst, dermoid, laryngocele, *normal*—hyoid, thyroid. *Area 7. Sternocleidomastoid (anterior):* Lymphadenitis, branchial cleft cyst (2nd, 3rd), pilomatrixoma, rare tumors. *Area 8. Spinal accessory:* Lymphadenitis, lymphoma, metastasis (from nasopharynx). *Area 9. Paratracheal:* Thyroid, parathyroid, esophageal diverticulum. *Area 10. Supraclavicular:* Cystic hygroma, lipoma, lymphoma, metastasis, *normal*—fat pad, pneumatocele of upper lobe. *Area 11. Suprasternal:* Thyroid, lipoma, dermoid, thymus, mediastinal mass. (From May M. Neck masses in children: diagnosis and treatment. *Pediatr Ann* 1976;5:517–535. Reprinted by permission.)

head examination should include assessment of the scalp, ears, sinuses, and nasopharynx.

Chest examination should pay special attention to auscultation. Extrathoracic compression of upper airway may only manifest as faint inspiratory stridor. Orthopnea or wheezing while supine may be an early sign of a mediastinal mass. Signs of systemic illness should be considered during completion of the examination. Signs of thyroid hormone excess (tachycardia, bounding pulses, systolic hypertension, exophthalmos) or deficiency may be associated with a goiter. Suspicion for malignancy increases with changes in the general appearance and color of the child, as with the presence of hepatosplenomegaly or an abdominal mass. Rashes, generalized lymphadenopathy, and fever may indicate an inflammatory or oncologic process. Failure to thrive or weight loss may also be found with multiple causes of infection or oncologic illness, including HIV disease, histiocytosis X, mycobacterial infections, and others. Finally, a close examination of the skin, not only observing the overlying skin but also noting any animal scratches or bites of the face and extremities, is imperative.

Details of chronicity, size, progression, and evidence of inflammation help distinguish between infection and neoplasm. Characteristics that may be associated with malignancy include masses that are firm and larger than 2 cm in diameter, nonpainful, progressively enlarging, ulcerating, deep to fascia or fixed to tissue, longer duration (weeks), or discovered in a newborn. These criteria are sensitive but not specific for cancer. Even with these characteristics, most lesions are benign congenital cysts or inflammatory masses. Although longer duration is concerning for malignancy, the duration the "node" is present is not reliable in discriminating benign from malignant.

DIFFERENTIAL DIAGNOSIS

Congenital Masses

Thyroglossal duct cysts are the most common congenital cyst of the neck, resulting from failure of embryologic thyroglossal duct obliteration prior to hyoid bone formation. Although 65% of these are found to be infrahyoid, they can develop anywhere in the *anterior triangle* (along the midline from the base of the tongue to the sternal notch). More than half are diagnosed in children before 10 years of age. Masses are classically soft, nontender, smooth, and may move cranially when the child swallows or protrudes the tongue. Thyroglossal duct cysts may be noticed initially after an upper respiratory infection (URI) or an episode of hemorrhage. When infected, they may be warm, erythematous, and drain externally. If drainage occurs by way of the foramen cecum, there may be an associated foul taste in the mouth. Antibiotics (for mouth and skin flora), warm compresses, and incision and drainage (if indicated) should be initiated for signs of infection. Complete excision is the treatment of choice after resolution of the acute infection.

Branchial cleft anomalies most commonly occur from defects in the development of the second branchial arch, giving rise to firm posterior triangle masses (along the anterior border of the sternocleidomastoid muscle near the angle of the mandible). Branchial cleft sinuses are painless and present with drainage at the junction of the middle and lower thirds of the sternocleidomastoid muscle. Blockage of the sinus tract may cause cysts which are usually fluctuant, mobile, and nontender. Infection of a cyst can cause pain and warmth, and may be precipitated by probing or injecting the tract. Consequently, incision and drainage should be avoided because it may result in fistula formation. Ultrasonography may be useful in identifying a thin-walled, anechoic, fluid-filled cyst. Treatment with antibiotics is necessary if the sinus or cyst is infected. Excision of the entire tract and cyst is important to prevent recurrence.

Cystic hygromas are lymphatic malformations occurring in the posterior triangle of the neck (superior to the clavicle and posterior to sternocleidomastoid). Many are identified at birth, and 90% present before a child's second birthday. These may be recognized only after injury or URI when "herniation" has occurred after crying, coughing, or other forceful Valsalva maneuvers. Though variable in size, these discrete lesions are compressible, mobile, nontender, and may transilluminate. Infection and airway compromise are rare, and additional signs would be as expected. Ultrasonography is useful in confirming its cystic nature. Chest radiograph is recommended to evaluate for extension into the mediastinum with resultant chylothorax or chylomediastinum. Computed tomography (CT) or magnetic resonance imaging (MRI) can determine the extent and involvement of surrounding structures. Spontaneous regression is rare; therefore, complete excision is the treatment of choice for small lesions. Larger lesions may need intralesional sclerotherapy.

Hemangiomas (including capillary, strawberry, and capillary-cavernous subtypes) are common head and neck lesions with a three to one female predominance. These are usually noticed during their period of rapid growth over the first year of life, but then involute over the next several years. Lesions are soft, mobile, nontender, and bluish or reddish with increased warmth. A thrill or bruit may be present, and capillary refill may be noted after palpation. Rare complications include thrombocytopenia from platelet consumption, disseminated intravascular coagulation, hemorrhage, airway obstruction, congestive heart failure, ulceration, infection, and necrosis. Lesions noted in the beard distribution, may be associated with glottic or subglottic hemangiomas, increasing the risk for airway compromise. Treatment for most hemangiomas is conservative and nonoperative because the issues are almost solely cosmetic and short term. Decisions about other treatments (corticosteroids, beta-blockers, laser treatment, intralesional sclerotherapy, and resection) are best reserved for the pediatric surgeon or vascular malformation subspecialist.

Neonatal torticollis, often caused by *fibromatosis colli* (also called sternocleidomastoid tumor), results from sternocleidomastoid fibrosis and shortening of the muscle. Presenting symptoms of torticollis occur in the first 3 weeks of life, with the infant holding his/her face and chin away from the affected side and the head tilted toward the fibrous mass. The mass is firm and seems attached to the muscle. Physical therapy, including massage, range-of-motion exercises, stretching exercises, and positional changes, is the preferred treatment. Facial and cranial asymmetry can develop without intervention. Surgical intervention is rarely needed.

Inflammatory Masses

Cervical lymphadenopathy is the most common reason for neck masses in children. Up to 90% of children between the ages of 4 and 8 years can have cervical adenopathy without obvious associated infection or systemic illness, though lymphadenopathy in newborns and young infants is rare and warrants investigation. Anterior cervical nodes drain the oropharynx and become enlarged with URIs, oral, and pharyngeal infections. Inflammation or infection of the scalp, and nasopharynx cause enlargement of posterior cervical nodes. Supraclavicular lymphadenopathy is considered pathologic and should be biopsied. Etiology for cervical adenopathy includes bacterial or viral infection (including rhinovirus, parainfluenza virus, respiratory syncytial virus, cytomegalovirus, and Epstein–Barr virus [EBV]) from local, regional, or systemic illness. With treatment of the underlying bacterial infection, cervical lymphadenopathy should resolve. Adenopathy secondary to viral infections is self-resolving, though duration of findings will vary by specific etiology.

Cervical lymphadenitis occurs when acute infection is present within the lymph node (see Chapters 102 Infectious Disease Emergencies and 126 ENT Emergencies). Commonly, one or more cervical lymph nodes become acutely enlarged, tender, warm, and erythematous after a URI, pharyngitis, tonsillitis, or otitis media. Systemic symptoms of fever and malaise may be present. Bacteria are the most common causes and include *Staphylococcus aureus* (possibly methicillin resistant) and group A β-hemolytic streptococci, although those caused by *Haemophilus influenzae,* anaerobic bacteria, and virus have also been noted. If the patient appears toxic, admission and treatment with intravenous (IV) antibiotics are appropriate, though most milder cases resolve with warm compresses and oral β-lactamase–resistant antibiotics. Clindamycin is effective against methicillin-resistant *S. aureus.* Knowledge of local resistance patterns is important when selecting antibiotic coverage. Without antibiotic treatment, infection may progress with nodal enlargement, suppuration, and regional cellulitis. Failure of outpatient management warrants further diagnostic investigation that may include serologies, ultrasound, fine needle aspiration, and incision and drainage. Purulent fluid should be sent for Gram stain and aerobic and anaerobic cultures to guide antibiotic management.

Cat-scratch disease is another common cause of lymph node enlargement in children. Typically, fever and malaise may have been present initially (30%), followed by enlargement of a single regional node 2 to 4 weeks after a cat scratch (usually a kitten). The lymphadenopathy can be cervical if the head or neck has been scratched (33% to 50%). The area around the lymph node becomes warm, tender, indurated, and erythematous. *Bartonella henselae* is the organism most likely responsible and needle aspiration may be both diagnostic and therapeutic. Surgical excision is unnecessary and can lead to formation of a draining sinus. Indirect immunofluorescent antibody assay for detection of serum antibodies to antigens of *Bartonella* organisms is useful in diagnosis. The indirect immunofluorescent antibody test is available in commercial laboratories, state public health department laboratories, and the Centers for Disease Control and Prevention. Polymerase chain reaction assays are available in some commercial and research laboratories. Generally, symptomatic treatment results in resolution over 2 to 4 months. Indications for antibiotic treatment include painful adenitis, systemic symptoms (hepatic or splenic involvement, endocarditis), or immunocompromise. Oral azithromycin, clarithromycin, rifampin, trimethoprim-sulfamethoxazole, and ciprofloxacin have all been shown to be effective. Azithromycin is the first-line antibiotic choice. Rifampin and a second drug (azithromycin or gentamicin) are suggested for those with hepatosplenic disease or prolonged fever. Parenteral ceftriaxone and gentamicin, with or without oral doxycycline, is suggested for those with culture negative endocarditis. Bartonella positive endocarditis is generally treated with doxycycline and gentamicin.

Mycobacterial infection of the cervical lymph nodes can be caused by the atypical strains of *Mycobacterium avium-intracellulare (MAI)* and *Mycobacterium scrofulaceum,* or less frequently, *Mycobacterium tuberculosis (M.tb).* The enlarged nodes of an atypical infection are generally submandibular in location, red, rubbery, and minimally tender to palpation. If systemic manifestations are present, an immune deficiency should be considered. In contrast, lymphadenopathy caused by *M.tb* more commonly involves supraclavicular nodes. Overlying skin may be pink to violaceous in color, and parchment-like in texture. Children with suspected mycobacterium infection should have a purified protein derivative (PPD) tuberculin skin test, and chest radiograph performed, though the PPD may be negative in atypical mycobacterium infections. A complete excisional biopsy may be necessary to identify and treat the organism definitively. Conversely, incision and drainage can result in a draining sinus. Treatment with clarithromycin with ethambutol or rifampin may be indicated in children with recurrent disease or incomplete excision. Treatment for *M.tb* lymphadenitis is the same as for pulmonary tuberculosis, with 6 to 9 months of antituberculosis chemotherapy.

Viral infections such as rhinovirus, parainfluenza virus, respiratory syncytial virus, cytomegalovirus, and EBV, may cause cervical lymphadenitis. A mononucleosis-like illness (most commonly from EBV) classically presents with large, hypertrophied tonsils, prominent posterior cervical nodes, in addition to diffuse lymphadenopathy. Fever, headache, malaise, and the presence of hepatosplenomegaly are frequently present. Generally, treatment for mononucleosis is supportive. Apparent exudative pharyngitis warrants evaluation for GAS, and should be treated with antibiotics if positive. Corticosteroids (prednisolone/prednisone at 1 mg/kg/day often prescribed short burst and then a taper) may be useful in patients with airway obstruction.

Kawasaki disease (*mucocutaneous lymph node syndrome;* see Chapter 109 Rheumatologic Emergencies) typically is described as presence of a single enlarged cervical lymph node (>1.5 cm diameter), nonexudative conjunctival injection, erythematous mouth, cracked lips, strawberry tongue, erythematous rash, induration of the palms of hands and soles of the feet, and fever of at least 5 days duration. Cervical lymphadenopathy is the least common of the presenting signs, however. The cause of this vasculitis is unknown. The peak incidence is 18 to 24 months, with the vast majority of the cases occurring in children younger than 4 years. Coronary artery aneurysm can be a long-term complication; thus, immunosuppressive therapy (IVIG) and aspirin should be started in consultation with a rheumatologist if it is suspected. An echocardiogram should be performed to rule out coronary artery aneurysms.

Retropharyngeal abscess (RPA), lateral pharyngeal abscess (LPA), and *peritonsillar abscess (PTA)* are potentially serious deep space neck infections that can present with neck mass, fever, dysphagia, sore throat, and pain with neck motion. RPAs are a result of infections of the nasopharynx, paranasal sinuses, or middle ear, and the paramedian lymph nodes that drain those areas. These infections commonly have associated pain with neck extension grater than neck flexion. Most cases of RPAs occur in children younger than 6 years. The usual pathogens are group A streptococcus, anaerobes, or *S. aureus.* PTAs and LPAs are associated with painful neck rotation, and are generally seen in school-aged children and adolescents, though they have similar microbial etiologies. Lateral neck films with appropriate positioning may reveal enlarged prevertebral space in cases of RPAs, though neck CT with contrast provides the most accurate imaging modality for evaluating deep space neck infections. Treatment includes monitoring for signs of airway compromise and IV antibiotic treatment using clindamycin, ampicillin/sulbactam, or cefazolin. Most children will need drainage, but IV antibiotics and observation may be sufficient for those determined to have retropharyngeal cellulitis.

Lemierre syndrome and *Ludwig angina* represent two additional deep space infections that can present with neck mass. *Lemierre syndrome* is an infection of the parapharyngeal space with septic thrombophlebitis of the internal jugular vein, leading to septic embolization to the lungs and/or central nervous system. It is generally seen in adolescents and adults. Sore throat, fever, fullness to one side of the neck, neck pain, trismus, dysphagia, dyspnea, and toxic appearance can be the presenting clinical signs and symptoms. The predominant pathogen is a gram-negative bacillus *Fusobacterium necrophorum,* though *S. aureus* can also cause a similar presentation. Anticoagulation is still controversial. *Ludwig angina* is an infection of the floor of the mouth via anaerobic oral flora following a dental procedure or trauma. It can present as submental swelling with toxicity, and elevation of the soft tissues can cause acute airway compromise. Treatment for either illness consists of either penicillin in combination with a β-lactamase inhibitor or a β-lactamase–resistant antibiotic in combination with a drug that is highly effective against anaerobes (clindamycin or metronidazole) for at least 6 weeks. Incision and drainage may be required when abscess is present.

Neoplasms

It is estimated that 80% to 90% of neck masses in children are benign, though differentiating between a benign and malignant lesion can be difficult. Presentation of neck neoplasm is usually a painless, firm, fixed cervical mass. Systemic symptoms may not be present. Duration and characteristics of the neck mass will lead to increased index of suspicion. Findings that would prompt further workup include: supraclavicular lymphadenopathy, a node larger than 2 cm in diameter, enlargement of a node for more than 2 weeks, no decrease in size of a lymph node after 4 to 6 weeks, lack of inflammation, firm or rubbery consistency, ulceration, failure to respond to antibiotics, and systemic symptoms. Neoplastic etiologies for neck mass in children include Hodgkin and non-Hodgkin lymphoma, rhabdomyosarcoma, neuroblastoma, thyroid carcinoma, nasopharyngeal carcinoma, and teratomas. If a malignancy is suspected, a complete blood count (CBC), chest radiograph, and selective CT or MRI should be obtained. Treatment is individualized according to specific tumor and extent of disease (see Chapter 106 Oncologic Emergencies).

GENERAL DIAGNOSTIC APPROACH

Clinical impression should guide decisions to obtain laboratory or imaging studies. In processes for which the risk of critical airway obstruction is impending, the utility of the arterial blood gas adds little initially, and the stress may lead to worsening of the obstruction. Oxygenation may be determined noninvasively by pulse oximetry. Soft tissue lateral neck films may be helpful to evaluate for intraoral, retropharyngeal, or airway infectious problems. In the child with respiratory distress, a chest radiograph is necessary to view the mediastinum, pleura, and lung for infection, tumor, pneumothorax, or pneumomediastinum. Cervical spine radiographs need to be obtained for trauma patients when instability or fracture of the cervical spine is suspected. Facial or mandibular films may be necessary to evaluate for some lower-face trauma or oral infections. When considering hematoma from trivial trauma and underlying coagulopathy, workup should include a CBC, prothrombin time, INR, and partial thromboplastin time.

For many of the common inflammatory conditions, no further workup is required. Of note, pharyngitis should prompt a rapid strep screen or throat culture, with consideration for heterophile antibody assay or, especially in the younger child, EBV-specific serologic tests to evaluate for infectious mononucleosis when confirmatory diagnosis is helpful. A white blood cell (WBC) count and differential can aid in diagnosing mono or oncologic processes. Serum thyroid hormone and thyroid-stimulating hormone levels may be warranted for suspected thyroid masses.

Ultrasound may be useful in defining a mass since lesions like cystic hygroma, lymphadenopathy, thyroglossal duct, and fibromatosis colli have fairly definitive patterns. Ultrasound may also help identify adenitis with abscess formation requiring drainage. Although not specific, the finding of calcification within a mass may suggest a teratoma or neuroblastoma. CT is often necessary to delineate deeper space infections. Lesional biopsy is required when the suspicion is high for malignancy.

DISPOSITION

In the ED, neck mass evaluation most often reveals benign adenopathy or adenitis requiring only systemic oral antibiotics and local care. Important to the approach to adenitis is the follow-up in several days to monitor clinical response and need for aspiration and drainage. When the mass is suspicious for tumor or congenital cyst, surgical consultation for biopsy or excision is indicated. Patients presenting with systemic toxicity, airway compromise, or severe local disease require hospitalization and initiation of definitive therapy.

Suggested Readings and Key References

Aciero SP, Waldhausen JH. Congenital cervical cysts, sinuses and fistulas. *Otolaryngol Clin North Am* 2007;40:161–176.

Ajulo P, Qayyum A, Brewis C, et al. Lemierre's syndrome: the link between a simple sore throat, sore neck and pleuritic chest pain. *Ann R Coll Surg Engl* 2005;87:303–305.

Al-Dajani N, Wootton SH. Cervical lymphadenitis, suppurative parotitis, thyroiditis, and infected cysts. *Infect Dis Clin North Am* 2007; 21(2):523–541.

Anne S, Teot LA, Mandell DL. Fine needle aspiration biopsy: role in diagnosis of pediatric head and neck masses. *Int J Pediatr Otorhinolaryngol* 2008;72:1547–1553.

Baddour LM, Wilson WR, Bayer AS, et al. Infective endocarditis: diagnosis, antimicrobial therapy, and management of complications: a statement for healthcare professionals from the committee on rheumatic fever, endocarditis, and Kawasaki disease, council on cardiovascular disease in the young, and the councils on clinical cardiology, stroke, and cardiovascular surgery and anesthesia, American Heart Association: endorsed by the Infectious Diseases Society of America. *Circulation* 2005;111:e394–e434.

Brown RL, Azizkhan RG. Pediatric head and neck lesions. *Pediatr Clin North Am* 1998;45:889–905.

Craig FW, Shunk JE. Retropharyngeal abscess in children: clinical perspective, utility of imaging, and current management. *Pediatrics* 2003;111:1394–1398.

Dulin MF, Kennard TP, Leach L, et al. Management of cervical lymphadenitis in children. *Am Fam Physician* 2008;78(9):1097–1098.

Eivazi B, Werner J. Extracranial vascular malformations (hemangiomas and vascular malformations) in children and adolescents-diagnosis, clinic, and therapy. *GMS Curr Top Otorhinolaryngol Head Neck Surg* 2014;13:doc02.

Green M(ed). The neck and lymphadenopathy. *Pediatric diagnosis.* 6th ed. Philadelphia, PA: Elsevier, 1998;61–65:398–403.

Long SS, Pickering LK, Prober CG. *Principles and practice of pediatric infectious diseases.* 4th ed. New York, NY: Churchill Livingstone, 2012.

Malik A, Odita J, Rodriguez J, et al. Pediatric neck masses: a pictorial review for practicing radiologists. *Curr Probl Diagn Radiol* 2002; 31:146–157.

Rajasekaran K, Krakovitz P. Enlarged neck lymph nodes in children. *Pediatr Clin North Am* 2013;60:923–936.

Tracy TF, Muratore CS. Management of common head and neck masses. *Semin Pediatr Surg* 2007;16(1):3–13.

Turkington JR, Paterson A, Sweeney LE, et al. Neck masses in children. *Br J Radiol* 2005;78:75–85.

Vieira F, Allen SM, Stocks RM, et al. Deep neck infection. *Otolaryngol Clin North Am* 2008;41:459–483.

CHAPTER 44 ■ NECK STIFFNESS

LEAH TZIMENATOS, MD, CHERYL VANCE, MD, AND NATHAN KUPPERMANN, MD, MPH

Neck stiffness is an important chief complaint in children evaluated in the emergency department. Commonly, neck stiffness is accompanied by neck pain. Certain clinical conditions, however, may lead a child to hold the neck in an abnormal posture (malposition) without neck pain. The underlying causes of neck stiffness or malposition in children range from relatively benign (e.g., muscle strain, cervical adenitis) to life-threatening (e.g., meningitis, fracture, or subluxation of the cervical spine).

Torticollis (meaning "twisted neck" from the Latin roots *tortus* and *collum*) is a subset of neck stiffness. With torticollis, the child holds the head tilted to one side and the chin rotated in the opposite direction, reflecting unilateral neck muscle contraction. This may result from various pathologic processes and may or may not be associated with neck pain. Torticollis is often congenital and/or muscular in origin. It can also be associated with acquired processes such as trauma, infectious or inflammatory illnesses, central nervous system neoplasms, drug reactions, and a variety of different syndromes.

This chapter reviews the differential diagnosis of neck stiffness including torticollis, both with and without neck pain, in children. Figure 44.1 offers an algorithmic approach to help distinguish potentially life-threatening from benign causes of neck stiffness, while providing a broad differential diagnosis.

DIFFERENTIAL DIAGNOSIS

Most patients presenting with neck stiffness are well appearing with benign, frequently self-limited conditions; however, the differential diagnosis of neck stiffness is broad and includes many potentially life-threatening causes, which must be considered and excluded when appropriate. A history of trauma, signs or symptoms of an infectious or inflammatory process, or evidence of spinal cord involvement may be helpful in identifying a number of specific diagnoses.

Table 44.1 lists most causes of neck stiffness in children, Table 44.2 lists the common causes, and Table 44.3 lists the life-threatening causes. The following descriptions categorize the causes of neck stiffness in children by underlying mechanism and severity.

Neck Stiffness Associated with Trauma

Potentially Life-threatening Causes

Neck trauma is a common cause of neck pain and stiffness (see Chapter 120 Neck Trauma). Fortunately, serious injuries to the cervical spine (fractures, subluxations, and spinal cord injuries) are uncommon, especially in children younger than 8 years. Because of a higher fulcrum of the cervical spine and relative weakness of the neck muscles compared to adults, these injuries generally occur in the upper cervical spine in younger children, as opposed to more widely across the cervical spine in older children and adolescents. Neck injuries in children most commonly result from high kinetic energy mechanisms, such as motor vehicle–related collisions, sports injuries, and falls.

Fractures of the Cervical Spine. Fractures of the cervical spine in children are very uncommon, occurring in 1% to 3% of hospitalized pediatric trauma patients. Although some children with fractures of the cervical spine are unresponsive at the time of evaluation, most are alert and verbal, limit their neck movement secondary to pain, and have no demonstrable neurologic deficits. At the minimum, the cervical spine should be immobilized and imaging of the cervical spine should be obtained on any child with an altered level of consciousness, pain or stiffness of the neck, any neurologic deficits, or distracting painful injuries after blunt trauma. Imaging should also be obtained in those who are unable to perceive pain (as a result of alcohol or drugs) or describe their symptoms. A large prospective study, the National Emergency X-Radiography Utilization Study (NEXUS), of blunt trauma victims identified five criteria (posterior midline cervical tenderness, altered alertness, distracting injury, intoxication, and focal neurologic signs) that identified all children with cervical spine injuries; however, there were few children younger than 9 years and none younger than 2 years with cervical spine injuries in that study. A multicenter attempt to retrospectively validate the NEXUS criteria among a different cohort of children (including those younger than 2 years) demonstrated a lower sensitivity, suggesting the need for refinement of these criteria before routine use in children. A more recent case-control study of 540 children with cervical spine injuries identified eight important risk factors: altered mental status, focal neurologic findings, neck pain, torticollis, substantial torso injury, conditions predisposing to cervical spine injury, diving, and high-risk motor vehicle collision mechanisms. Prospective refinement of risk factors, particularly in younger children, is necessary.

Subluxation of the Cervical Spine. Traumatic subluxations of the cervical spine are more common than fractures and are more likely to present more than 24 hours after injury. Subluxation may result from minor trauma (e.g., falls from low heights) but typically occurs after more severe trauma (see Chapter 120 Neck Trauma). The most common subluxation is rotary (or "rotatory") atlantoaxial subluxation. Clinically, rotary subluxation typically causes neck pain and torticollis without focal neurologic symptoms because the transverse ligament of the atlas remains intact and the spinal cord is not compromised. Sternocleidomastoid (SCM) spasm and neck tenderness are localized to the same side as the head rotation as the SCM attempts to "reduce" the deformity. This is in contrast to muscular torticollis, in which the spastic, tender SCM muscle is opposite to the direction of head rotation. In addition, in rotary subluxation, there is palpable deviation of the spinous process of C2 in the same direction as the head rotation. In

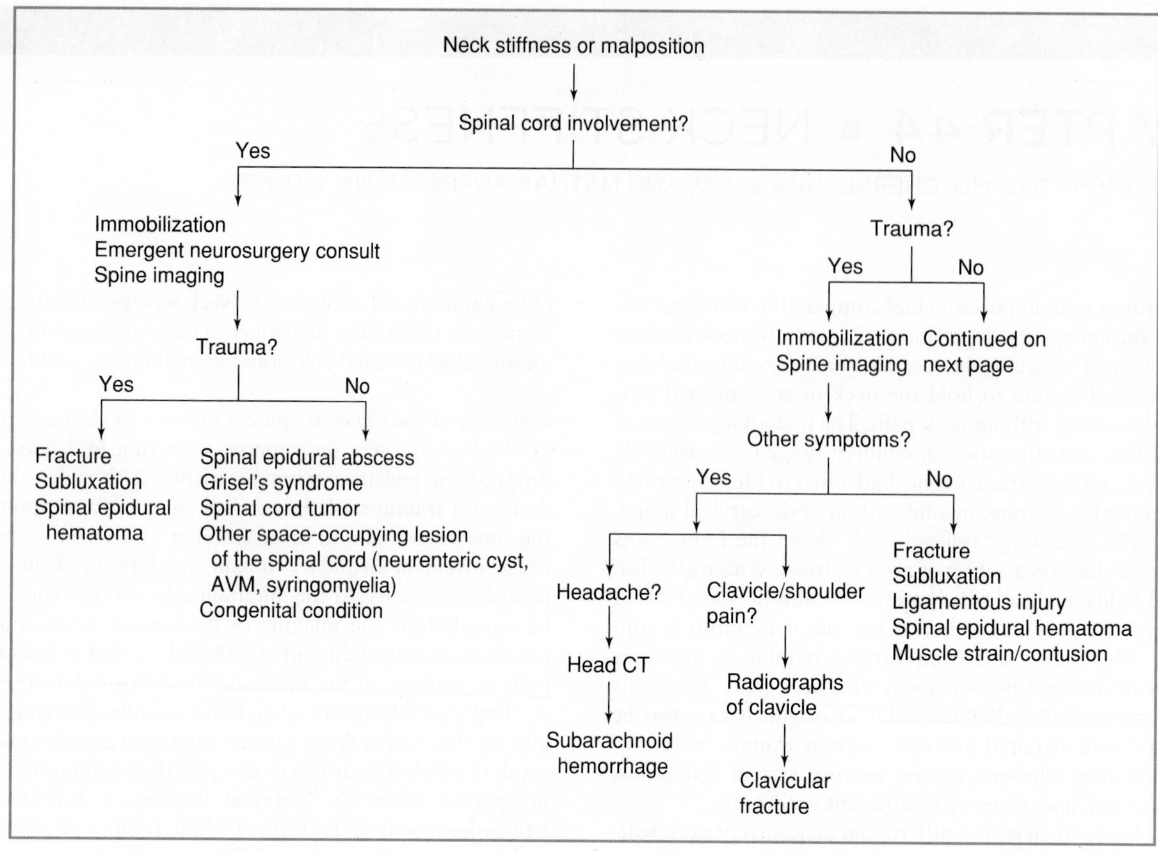

FIGURE 44.1 Approach to the child with stiff or malpositioned neck. Diagnostic studies included in this approach are intended to be *considerations* that may assist with making a diagnosis depending on the specific clinical scenario. C-spine XR, cervical spine radiograph; MRI, magnetic resonance imaging; ENT, ear, nose, and throat; AVM, arteriovenous malformation; CT, computed tomography; CBC, complete blood count; ESR, erythrocyte sedimentation rate; CRP, C-reactive protein; PPD, purified protein derivative; TB, tuberculosis; SCM, sternocleidomastoid; CXR, chest radiograph; US, ultrasound. *(continued)*

contrast, during normal neck rotation beyond 20 degrees, the spinous process of C2 deviates to the contralateral side.

Rotary atlantoaxial subluxation may be seen on plain radiographs. An anteroposterior open-mouth radiograph typically shows the rotation of C1 on C2, with the odontoid in an eccentric position relative to C1. However, definitive diagnosis is made by dynamic computed tomography (CT) scans of the neck showing a fixed rotation between C1 and C2 that fails to resolve with attempts to correct the torticollis. Most patients can be treated with a cervical collar and anti-inflammatory medications. Traction and immobilization may be necessary for more severe and/or long-standing rotary subluxation or if reduction is not achieved by conservative measures. Surgical intervention is rarely required.

Atlantoaxial subluxation with compromise of the spinal canal results when there is ligamentous laxity or rupture with resultant anterior movement of the atlas on the axis. Children with underlying conditions such as Down syndrome and Marfan syndrome are more susceptible to this due to laxity of the transverse ligament of the atlas. Radiographic findings may include a widened predental space and prevertebral soft tissue swelling. Treatment involves immobilization and cervical traction.

Epidural Hematomas of the Cervical Spine. Epidural hematomas of the cervical spine are uncommon but may occur even after apparently minor trauma. These may compress the spinal cord, leading to progressive neurologic symptoms and signs as well as neck stiffness or pain. Magnetic resonance imaging (MRI) of the spinal cord clearly demonstrates this injury. Emergent neurosurgical consultation and surgical decompression are indicated.

Subarachnoid Hemorrhage. Subarachnoid hemorrhage after trauma may lead to neck stiffness but is often accompanied by headache and/or other physical findings of head trauma. Rarely, subarachnoid hemorrhage may be due to nontraumatic causes such as aneurysm rupture.

Generally Non–life-threatening Causes

Traumatic Muscular Contusions of the Neck. Blunt trauma to the neck may result in neck pain as a result of muscular contusion and/or spasm. This is a diagnosis of exclusion and should not be entertained until a detailed physical examination and imaging of the cervical spine excludes more serious injuries. Treatment includes a soft cervical collar and analgesic medication.

Clavicular Fracture. Fracture of the clavicle in children is common and may cause torticollis because of SCM muscle spasm. This diagnosis is usually clear because pain, tenderness, and swelling are noted over the fracture site. The acute symptoms associated with clavicular fractures may occasionally mask an associated rotary atlantoaxial subluxation.

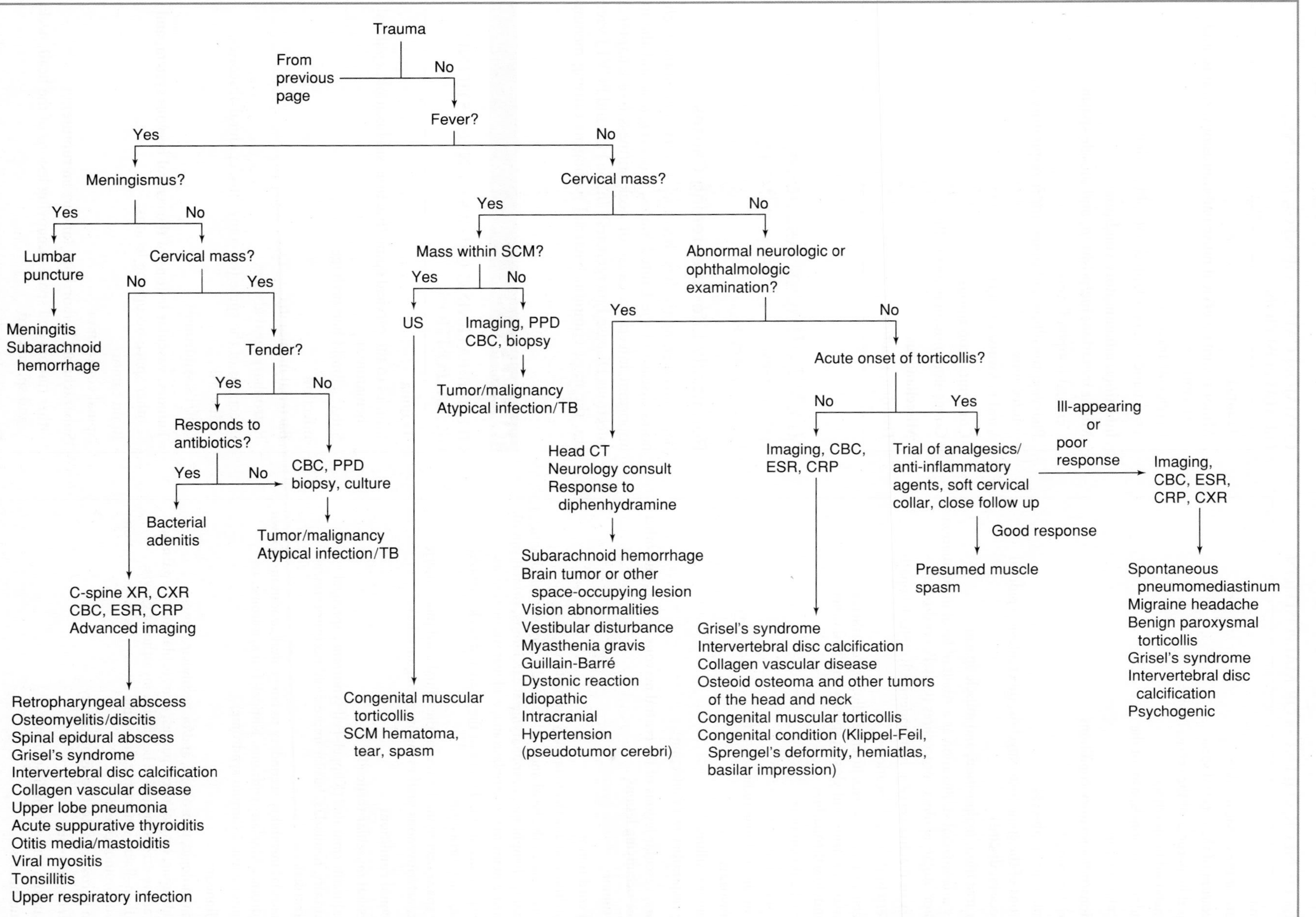

FIGURE 44.1 (*Continued*)

SIGNS AND SYMPTOMS

TABLE 44.1

CAUSES OF NECK STIFFNESS OR MALPOSITION

Trauma
Fracture of the cervical spine
Subluxation of the cervical spine
Epidural hematoma of the cervical spine
Subarachnoid hemorrhage
Muscular contusions/spasm of the neck
Clavicular fracture
Infectious/inflammatory conditions
Bacterial meningitis
Retropharyngeal abscess
Infections of the spine (osteomyelitis, tuberculosis, epidural abscesses, discitis)
Minor irritation, malposition, and muscle spasm
Rotary atlantoaxial subluxation as a result of local inflammation and/or otolaryngologic procedures (Grisel's syndrome)
Primary or reactive cervical lymphadenitis/lymphadenopathy
Intervertebral disc calcification
Collagen vascular diseases juvenile idiopathic arthritis, psoriatic arthritis, ankylosing spondylitis, and other spondyloarthropathies
Upper lobe pneumonia
Acute suppurative thyroiditis
Otitis media and mastoiditis
Viral myositis
Pharyngotonsillitis
Upper respiratory tract infection
Tumors, vascular lesions of the central nervous system, and other space-occupying lesions
Brain tumor
Spinal cord tumor
Subarachnoid hemorrhage (aneurysm rupture)
Other tumors of the head and neck (rhabdomyosarcoma, Ewing sarcoma, lymphoma, nasopharyngeal carcinoma, orbital tumor, acoustic neuroma, osteoblastoma, and metastatic tumors)
Other space-occupying lesions of the head and neck (Arnold–Chiari malformation)
Other space-occupying lesions of the spinal cord (neurenteric cyst, arteriovenous malformation, syringomyelia)
Congenital conditions
Congenital muscular torticollis
Skeletal malformations (Klippel–Feil syndrome, Sprengel deformity, hemiatlas, basilar impression, occipitocervical synostosis)
Atlantoaxial instability secondary to congenital conditions (Down syndrome, Marfan syndrome, Klippel–Feil syndrome, os odontoideum, Morquio syndrome)
Miscellaneous
Ophthalmologic, neurologic, and/or vestibular causes (strabismus, cranial nerve palsies, extraocular muscle palsies, refractive errors, migraine headache, myasthenia gravis, Guillain–Barré syndrome, idiopathic intracranial hypertension [pseudotumor cerebri])
Benign paroxysmal torticollis of infancy
Sandifer syndrome
Spontaneous pneumomediastinum
Spasmus nutans
Dystonic reaction
Psychogenic

TABLE 44.2

COMMON CAUSES OF NECK STIFFNESS OR MALPOSITION

Trauma
Minor trauma (cervical muscular contusions, strains, and spasm)
Clavicular fracture
Traumatic rotary atlantoaxial subluxation
Infectious/inflammatory conditions
Minor irritation, malposition, and muscle spasm
Cervical lymphadenitis
Pharyngotonsillitis and other upper respiratory tract infections
Viral myositis/myalgias
Congenital conditions
Congenital muscular torticollis
Miscellaneous
Dystonic reaction

Neck Stiffness Associated with Infectious/Inflammatory Conditions

Potentially Life-threatening Causes

Bacterial meningitis has become a very uncommon childhood disease in the United States, however, it is still the most important infectious cause of neck stiffness (see Chapter 102 Infectious Disease Emergencies). In the HiB and PCV13 vaccine era, the most common bacterial pathogens causing meningitis

TABLE 44.3

LIFE-THREATENING CAUSES OF NECK STIFFNESS OR MALPOSITION

Trauma
Injuries to the cervical spine (fracture, subluxation, epidural hematoma)
Subarachnoid hemorrhage
Infection
Bacterial meningitis
Retropharyngeal abscess
Infections of the spine (osteomyelitis, epidural abscesses, discitis)
Grisel's syndrome
Tumors, vascular lesions of the central nervous system, and other space-occupying lesions
Brain tumor
Spinal cord tumor
Subarachnoid hemorrhage (aneurysm rupture)
Other tumors and space-occupying lesions of the head, neck, and spinal cord
Congenital conditions
Atlantoaxial instability secondary to congenital conditions

after infancy are *Streptococcus pneumoniae* (including non–vaccine-type strains) and *Neisseria meningitidis.* Children with meningitis typically present with fever and headache with neck stiffness on physical examination. These findings may not be apparent in young infants or conditions with less inflammatory response (i.e., meningococcal meningitis). Torticollis has also been reported in patients with bacterial meningitis, although less commonly.

Retropharyngeal Abscess. There are several other important infectious processes for which neck stiffness and fever usually are the presenting signs. Retropharyngeal abscess is an infection that occupies the potential space between the posterior pharyngeal wall and the anterior border of the cervical vertebrae. Most commonly caused by *Staphylococcus aureus,* group A streptococcus, and oral anaerobes, these infections typically present with clinical toxicity, drooling, and sometimes stridor. Neck pain and/or stiffness are the presenting clinical findings in approximately two-thirds of these children. Limitation of neck extension and torticollis are particularly common. Lateral radiographs of the neck can be helpful in making the diagnosis and will reveal soft tissue swelling anterior to the upper cervical vertebral bodies. When radiographs are limited, however, due to inadequate neck extension or failure to obtain the image during inspiration, or when a positive finding of a widened prevertebral space is noted, CT imaging with contrast is required.

Infections of the Spine. Infectious processes involving the spine (osteomyelitis, epidural abscess, discitis) in children can involve the cervical region, although they occur most commonly in the thoracic and lumbar areas. Localized pain, fever, and elevation of inflammatory markers including erythrocyte sedimentation rate (ESR) and C-reactive protein generally accompany these infections.

Cervical vertebral osteomyelitis may lead to neck stiffness. Vertebral osteomyelitis is usually bacterial in origin (most commonly caused by *S. aureus*) but may be caused by mycobacteria as well. If the cervical spine is involved, radiographs of this area may reveal destruction of the vertebral body, local soft tissue swelling, or narrowing of the disc space. MRI is the imaging modality of choice and may reveal abnormalities of the spine before bony destruction is visible on plain radiography.

Although uncommon, spinal epidural abscesses are associated with significant morbidity and mortality. When these abscesses occur in the cervical region, severe neurologic deficits may occur, and emergent neurosurgical consultation is essential.

Discitis is uncommon in children; however, cases of cervical discitis have been reported. This disease is generally seen in children younger than 3 years of age. The most commonly identified microbiologic organism is *S. aureus,* although bacterial cultures are commonly negative and the cause has been debated. When evaluating for this condition, MRI is indicated.

Generally Non–life-threatening Causes

Torticollis Due to Minor Irritation, Malposition, and Muscle Spasm. Most well-appearing children with sudden onset of mild torticollis without a history of trauma, fever, or neurologic abnormalities do not have serious underlying pathology as a cause of their symptoms. Commonly, the patient awakens with mild neck pain and stiffness. On evaluation, there is no history of trauma, fever, preceding illness, pharyngotonsillitis, or any additional physical examination abnormality. The examination reveals a well-appearing child with mild torticollis, whose limitation of motion is primarily when he or she attempts correction of the malposition. Such muscular torticollis may be due to SCM spasm from awkward sleeping position or other mild irritation. In cases with this type of benign presentation, history, and examination, nothing more than careful clinical assessment, analgesic/anti-inflammatory medication, consideration of soft cervical collar, and close follow-up may be necessary.

Grisel's Syndrome. Rotary atlantoaxial subluxation uncommonly may occur as a result of inflammatory processes in the head and neck region (e.g., rheumatoid arthritis, systemic lupus erythematosus, tonsillitis, pharyngitis, otitis media, retropharyngeal abscess) or after otolaryngologic procedures (e.g., tonsillectomy, adenoidectomy). When due to such infectious or inflammatory conditions, the rotary subluxation is called Grisel's syndrome and is believed to occur as a result of ligamentous laxity. The subluxation may or may not be associated with displacement of the atlas, depending on the degree of involvement of the transverse ligament of the atlas. Most children with Grisel's syndrome have torticollis and neck pain, often localized to the ipsilateral SCM muscle. Fever and dysphagia are also common. The child's head is tilted to one side and rotated to the side opposite of the facet dislocation. As with rotary atlantoaxial subluxation from traumatic causes, radiographs may demonstrate the abnormality, but dynamic CT scan is diagnostic (see previous discussion). In the case of severe disease, or when there is evidence of spinal cord compression, neurosurgical consultation is necessary because cervical traction and immobilization are needed. Most commonly, however, the condition is mild and there is no anterior displacement. Grisel's syndrome often responds to analgesic medication, physical therapy, and a soft cervical collar. In addition to treating the subluxation, antibiotics to treat an underlying bacterial infection may be needed.

Cervical Lymphadenitis. Cervical lymphadenitis, either acute or chronic, is a common cause of neck pain and stiffness. The child with this condition typically has tender swelling over the lateral aspect of the neck, with or without fever. Most cases of cervical lymphadenitis are caused by *S. aureus* or group A streptococcus. Less commonly, Mycobacteria and other bacteria including *Bartonella henselae,* the cause of cat-scratch disease, may be responsible. Empirical antibiotics to treat the most common bacterial pathogens are usually sufficient therapy. A purified protein derivative (PPD) skin test to screen for tuberculosis should be performed if any risk factors are present.

Intervertebral Disc Calcification. Intervertebral disc calcification (IDC) is an uncommon, generally self-limited condition in which the nucleus pulposus of one or more intervertebral discs calcifies. Both the underlying cause of the condition and acute symptoms are unknown. Children typically present with 24 to 48 hours of neck pain associated with neck stiffness or torticollis; fever is often present as well. The ESR is usually elevated in IDC, and leukocytosis occurs in one-third of patients. Radiographs of the spine usually show the disc calcification, and CT scans help localize the calcification within the nucleus pulposus. The calcification resorbs spontaneously, and the disease is generally benign and self-limited, although disc protrusion and cord compression may uncommonly occur. One must distinguish infections of the spine and meningitis (see previous discussion) from IDC as symptoms and laboratory findings may overlap.

Collagen Vascular Disease. Collagen vascular disease (see Chapter 109 Rheumatologic Emergencies) may involve the cervical spine and lead to neck stiffness and/or pain. Children with juvenile idiopathic arthritis may have either insidious or acute onset of symptoms, which commonly include neck stiffness. Cervical involvement is a late finding in ankylosing spondylitis and other spondyloarthropathies. However, girls with psoriatic arthritis may have cervical involvement preceding sacroiliac and lumbar involvement.

Other Infectious/Inflammatory Conditions. Pharyngotonsillitis, upper respiratory tract infections, otitis media, and mastoiditis may be associated with neck pain. Torticollis may occasionally be seen with these conditions and may be accompanied by Grisel's syndrome as well. If neck pain is posterior in location and accompanied by fever, a lumbar puncture should be strongly considered to exclude meningitis. The diagnosis of viral myositis involving the neck can be made only after excluding the possibility of meningitis in a child with neck pain and fever. Upper lobe pneumonia may cause pain referred to the neck with or without associated stiffness. Although rare, acute suppurative thyroiditis may cause neck pain and stiffness and is associated with fever and a palpable, swollen thyroid gland.

Neck Stiffness Associated with Tumors, Vascular Lesions of the Central Nervous System, or Other Space-occupying Lesions

Potentially Life-threatening Causes

Space-occupying lesions of the brain and spinal cord may lead to neck stiffness, malposition, and/or pain. Even if the histology of these lesions is benign, they are potentially life-threatening because of the complications of intracranial pressure elevation and the potential for brain and spinal cord compression. Ruptured aneurysms may cause subarachnoid hemorrhage with associated neck stiffness.

Brain Tumors. Children with tumors of the posterior fossa, the most common location for pediatric brain tumors, may present with head tilt, neck stiffness, or torticollis. Posterior fossa tumors may cause many other symptoms and signs (e.g., vomiting, headache, ataxia, disturbances in vision including diplopia, papilledema, cranial nerve deficits, corticospinal or corticobulbar signs). Head tilt may result from attempts to compensate for diplopia. However, neck stiffness is believed to result from irritation of the accessory nerve by the cerebellar tonsils trapped in the occipital foramen or by tonsillar herniation.

Spinal Cord Tumors. Tumors of the spinal cord are uncommon in children and account for a small fraction of all central nervous system tumors. The most common spinal cord tumor is an astrocytoma. Typically, spinal cord tumors cause pain at the tumor site and neurologic defects (sensory and motor defects, impaired bowel and bladder function), but symptoms may be slow to develop, often leading to delays in diagnosis. Spinal cord tumors may also cause torticollis. Patients with these tumors may also hold their heads in a forward flexed position ("hanging head sign"). An MRI of the spine should be obtained on any child with symptoms and signs suggestive of a spinal cord tumor, and emergency neurosurgical consultation should be obtained.

Vascular Anomalies. Congenital berry aneurysms and acquired cerebral aneurysms may rupture spontaneously and result in life-threatening subarachnoid hemorrhages. These can present with abrupt onset of severe headache, meningismus, nausea and vomiting, photophobia, and possibly fever, thus mimicking meningitis.

Other Space-occupying Lesions of the Head and Neck. Head and neck tumors are uncommon in children, and diagnosis requires a high index of suspicion. Presenting signs and symptoms may include neck pain, stiffness, and/or torticollis. Rhabdomyosarcomas, Ewing sarcomas, and lymphomas account for most of the tumors of the neck but other tumors occurring in this region include nasopharyngeal carcinomas, orbital tumors, acoustic neuromas, osteoblastomas, and metastatic tumors. Arnold–Chiari malformations of the brain may also cause neck pain and stiffness.

Other Space-occupying Lesions of the Spinal Cord. Other uncommon space-occupying lesions of the cervical spine such as neurenteric cysts, arteriovenous malformations, spontaneous spinal epidural hematomas, and syringomyelia may also cause neck pain and stiffness, generally accompanied by neurologic findings. Early diagnosis by MRI is essential.

Generally Non–life-threatening Causes

Benign Tumors of the Head and Neck. Osteoid osteoma is a benign bone tumor that commonly affects older children and adolescents. Pain is the typical presenting symptom, often worse at night. If the osteoma is in the cervical spine, neck pain and/or stiffness result. Plain radiography is usually diagnostic, showing a well-demarcated radiolucent lesion surrounded by sclerotic bone. Treatment may be conservative medical management, radiofrequency ablation, or surgery. Eosinophilic granulomas and bone cysts are other rare, benign lesions of the spine that may cause neck pain and stiffness.

Congenital Causes of Neck Stiffness

Neck stiffness and/or torticollis from congenital abnormalities are usually not life-threatening. These congenital causes are usually muscular or skeletal in origin.

Congenital Muscular Torticollis. Congenital muscular torticollis is the most common cause of torticollis in infancy. The etiology is unclear but is believed to be related to birth trauma causing an injury to the SCM muscle with hematoma formation, followed by fibrous contracture of the muscle. Other theories suggest intrauterine malposition, infection, neurogenic causes, and intrauterine compartment syndrome of the SCM muscle. On examination, a palpable mass can often be detected in the inferior aspect of the SCM. The mass is generally not present at birth but appears in the neonatal period. The head is held in a characteristic position, with the patient's chin pointing away from the affected, contracted SCM muscle. Some degree of craniofacial asymmetry is commonly found in these patients, typically with contralateral flattening of the occiput and ipsilateral depression of the malar prominence. Ultrasound is the imaging modality of choice. Treatment is conservative with active positioning and manual stretching of the involved muscle. Surgical release of the SCM is required in approximately 5% of cases if the deformity persists for longer than 6 to 12 months.

Skeletal Malformations. Klippel–Feil syndrome is characterized by congenital fusion of a variable number of cervical vertebrae, which may result in atlantoaxial instability. The cause is unknown. It is often associated with many other bony abnormalities, and significant scoliosis develops in more than 50% of affected children. Limitation in range of motion of the neck is the most common physical sign. The classic triad also includes a low hairline and a short neck but is seen in fewer than half of patients.

Sprengel deformity is characterized by congenital failure of the scapula to descend to its correct position. The scapula rests in a high position relative to the neck and thorax. In its most severe form, the scapula may be connected by bone to the cervical spine and limit neck movement.

Hemiatlas is a malformation of the first cervical vertebra, which may cause severe, progressive torticollis. In time, the deformity becomes fixed; therefore, posterior fusion is recommended.

Basilar impression is a condition resulting from anomalies at the base of the skull and vertebrae, which lead to a short neck, headache, neck pain, and cranial nerve palsies due to compression of the cranial nerves. Many congenital conditions, including Klippel–Feil syndrome, achondroplasia, and neurofibromatosis, may cause basilar impression. Commonly associated with basilar impression is occipitocervical synostosis, a condition in which fibrous or bony connections between the base of the skull and the atlas cause neck pain, torticollis, high scapula, and several neurologic symptoms.

Atlantoaxial Instability. Several congenital conditions may be associated with atlantoaxial instability and may predispose the patient to cervical subluxation. In addition to Down, Marfan, and Klippel–Feil syndromes, these include other skeletal dysplasias and os odontoideum (aplasia or hypoplasia of the odontoid process of the axis). Children with these conditions should be screened for atlantoaxial instability. Morquio syndrome is a mucopolysaccharidosis resulting in flattening of the vertebrae and multiple skeletal dysplasias. In this syndrome, the odontoid is underdeveloped and may lead to atlantoaxial subluxation.

Miscellaneous Causes of Neck Stiffness

Head tilt, neck stiffness, and/or torticollis have been reported in other conditions, some of which are life-threatening and others generally benign.

Ophthalmologic, Neurologic, and/or Vestibular Causes. Head tilt or neck malposition may result from abnormalities of vision (strabismus, cranial nerve palsies, extraocular muscle palsies, refractive errors) or the vestibular apparatus. The child attempts to correct for the disturbance through changes in neck position. Careful ophthalmologic and neurologic examinations of the child with head tilt are necessary to exclude these possibilities. Torticollis has also been reported in patients with migraine headaches.

Myasthenia Gravis. Patients with myasthenia gravis may develop torticollis, although ptosis, impairment of extraocular muscular movement, and other cranial nerve palsies are generally earlier signs.

Guillain–Barré Syndrome. Neck stiffness has been reported in children with Guillain–Barré syndrome. Neck stiffness in this condition is seen in association with generalized motor weakness and areflexia.

Idiopathic Intracranial Hypertension (Pseudotumor Cerebri). Stiff neck and torticollis have also been reported in children with idiopathic intracranial hypertension, also known as pseudotumor cerebri. These neck symptoms may be the presenting signs of the condition, but more commonly patients present with headache, vomiting, and papilledema. Therefore, clinicians should inspect the optic discs of children with neck stiffness and/or torticollis. Lumbar puncture and removal of cerebrospinal fluid may quickly resolve the cervical symptoms and signs.

Benign Paroxysmal Torticollis of Infancy. Benign paroxysmal torticollis of infancy presents as recurrent episodes of head tilt sometimes accompanied by pallor, agitation, and vomiting. Typical onset is between 2 and 8 months of age, and the condition tends to remit by 2 to 3 years. Episodes subside spontaneously within a few hours or days. The etiology is unknown, and there is no effective treatment.

Sandifer Syndrome. Sandifer syndrome describes intermittent episodes of stiffening and torticollis related to gastroesophageal reflux. Children with this syndrome may have other symptoms associated with reflux including recurrent vomiting and failure to thrive.

Spontaneous Pneumomediastinum. Spontaneous pneumomediastinum may present with neck pain and torticollis. A history of severe coughing and/or retching is usually elicited. Crepitus is generally palpated along the neck.

Spasmus Nutans. Spasmus nutans is an acquired condition of childhood, characterized by nystagmus, head nodding, and torticollis. Children with these findings typically become symptomatic by 2 years. The condition is generally benign and self-limited. However, some children with the symptoms of spasmus nutans have underlying brain tumors. Therefore, imaging of the brain is necessary.

Dystonic Reaction. Certain drugs can cause acute dystonic reactions with torticollis. These most commonly include antipsychotic and antiemetic agents (e.g., haloperidol, prochlorperazine, and metoclopramide). Treatment with diphenhydramine may be diagnostic and therapeutic.

Psychogenic. Hysterical patients may present with torticollis. This diagnosis can be made only after excluding other causes.

EVALUATION AND DECISION

The evaluation of, and treatment plan for, neck stiffness is best organized around several important historical/clinical questions and physical examination findings: (i) Is there evidence of spinal cord involvement? (ii) Is there a history of trauma? (iii) Is there evidence of an infectious or inflammatory process (e.g., history or presence of fever)? (iv) Is a cervical mass present? (v) Are the symptoms acute or chronic?

The approach to the child with a stiff or malpositioned neck should focus initially on whether there is spinal cord involvement, as detailed in Figure 44.1. The diagnostic studies included in the figure represent suggested modalities for evaluation of children with those signs/symptoms. Decisions regarding specific diagnostic modalities will depend on each patient's individual presentation, history, and examination.

For any child with neck stiffness or pain, a history of weakness, paresthesias of the extremities, or abnormal bowel or bladder function should be sought. In addition, a complete ophthalmologic and neurologic examination should be performed, with the latter focusing on spinal cord function. Included in this examination should be an assessment of muscle strength, sensation, deep tendon reflexes, the Babinski reflex, and anal tone. Extra vigilance must be used if the patient is too young or incapacitated to provide an accurate history.

If *spinal cord involvement* is detected, immobilization, neurosurgical consultation, and imaging of the cervical spine are necessary. Conditions causing cervical spinal cord compromise may rapidly lead to permanent disability or death if not immediately addressed. If secondary to trauma, one should suspect cervical spine fracture, subluxation, or spinal epidural hematoma. In the setting of fever, a spinal epidural abscess should be considered. Atlantoaxial subluxation with instability secondary to otolaryngologic diseases or procedures should be considered in children with spinal cord involvement and consistent histories. Finally, spinal cord tumors and other space-occupying lesions should be considered if the development of symptoms is gradual and not associated with trauma or fever.

The next consideration is whether the neck stiffness is the result of an *acute traumatic event*. If acute trauma is the cause of the neck stiffness, the cervical spine should be properly immobilized (see Chapter 120 Neck Trauma) and imaging of the cervical spine obtained. Fractures and subluxations/dislocations will generally be identified on plain radiography of the cervical spine. Other modalities (e.g., flexion–extension views, CT, MRI) may be useful to detect ligamentous injury, rotary subluxation, or spinal epidural hematomas. In the setting of trauma, cervical muscle strain and/or contusion are diagnoses of exclusion. If other symptoms in addition to the neck stiffness are present, appropriate studies should be obtained. For example, the patient with neck stiffness and headache may have a subarachnoid hemorrhage for which a head CT scan would be indicated. The patient with clavicle fracture may have spasm of the SCM muscle and torticollis; however, tenderness is noted over the injured clavicle. Radiographs will confirm the diagnosis. Of note, rotary atlantoaxial subluxation may be associated with clavicle fracture.

Fever in the setting of neck stiffness suggests the presence of an infectious, inflammatory, or neoplastic process. Meningitis must be excluded either clinically or with a lumbar puncture (see Chapter 102 Infectious Disease Emergencies). On examination, meningismus should be sought. A lumbar puncture should be seriously considered in the presence of fever and neck stiffness of any type because meningitis may present with fever and atypical neck signs. Supporting findings include Brudzinski sign (flexion of the neck elicits flexion of the knee and hip) and Kernig sign (with the hip flexed, pain occurs with extension of the leg). Other conditions (e.g., subarachnoid hemorrhage) may also present with fever and meningismus, and a lumbar puncture is helpful in evaluating these conditions as well.

After meningitis has been excluded in the febrile patient with neck stiffness, the examination should focus on the *presence or absence of a cervical mass*. If a cervical mass is identified, a history of head or neck infections, contact with cats suggestive of *Bartonella*, or constitutional symptoms suggestive of malignancy should be elicited. If the cervical mass is tender and clinically consistent with lymph nodes, a trial of antibiotics directed at the most common bacterial pathogens may be all that is necessary. A PPD skin test should be placed to screen for tuberculosis if risk factors are present. If the cervical mass does not respond to an appropriate trial of antibiotics, cat-scratch disease, atypical mycobacterial infection, or malignancy may be the cause.

If no palpable cervical mass is present in the febrile child with neck pain and/or stiffness, a more in-depth evaluation may be necessary, based on the history and physical examination. Radiographic imaging of the neck may suggest retropharyngeal abscess in the child with drooling and neck stiffness, and stridor with more severe disease. Imaging of the cervical spine may detect atlantoaxial subluxation in the child with otolaryngologic disease or in the child who has recently had an otolaryngologic procedure. Additionally, advanced imaging (including CT, MRI, and nuclear medicine scans) may be useful in detecting other diseases involving the cervical spine, including vertebral osteomyelitis, discitis, IDC, spinal epidural abscess, and neck stiffness from collagen vascular disease. Although nonspecific, white blood cell count, ESR, or C-reactive protein levels will be elevated in most children with these conditions, as well as those with other infections of the head and neck (e.g., tonsillitis, mastoiditis). Finally, an upper lobe pneumonia identified on chest radiograph may be the cause of neck stiffness in the febrile child.

In the *afebrile* child with neck stiffness, a cervical *mass within the SCM* may be present. In an infant, this suggests congenital muscular torticollis, and neck ultrasound may be diagnostic. An SCM hematoma or tear may present with an SCM mass in an older child. If the cervical mass is not within the SCM, a malignancy or atypical infection may be the cause, and a complete blood cell count, PPD placement, and biopsy of the mass should be considered.

For the afebrile child with no cervical mass, an *abnormal neurologic or ophthalmologic examination* suggests a brain tumor, subarachnoid hemorrhage, other space-occupying lesions, or visual or vestibular disturbances causing the abnormal neck posture. At times, the patient does not have primary neck pain or stiffness but is attempting to correct these disturbances through changes in head position. In addition to careful neurologic and ophthalmologic examinations, a head CT or MRI scan may be necessary to evaluate for space-occupying lesions of the brain. Additionally, a lumbar puncture may be necessary to exclude subarachnoid hemorrhage, idiopathic intracranial hypertension, or Guillain–Barré syndrome. If myasthenia gravis is suspected, a neurologist should be consulted. Children with torticollis due to dystonic reactions after receiving neuroleptic or antiemetic medications will usually respond to intravenous diphenhydramine.

The child with neck stiffness without fever, cervical mass, or abnormal ophthalmologic or neurologic examination may have any of a number of conditions. *Timing of the symptoms* may be important in determining the appropriate evaluation. *Chronic symptoms* may suggest a congenital syndrome, collagen vascular disease, Sandifer syndrome, spasmus nutans, or a neoplastic process. Children with these conditions may also present with acute onset of symptoms. Some children with neck stiffness may have dysmorphic features, suggesting specific skeletal malformation syndromes. Radiographic imaging may help detect additional diagnoses such as osteoid osteoma or other benign tumors of the head and neck.

If symptom onset is *acute* and the patient *appears well,* muscle spasm may be the cause of torticollis. For the well-appearing child with sudden onset of mild torticollis without a history of trauma or fever and with a normal neurologic examination (e.g., the child who awakens with mild torticollis after sleeping in an unusual position), nothing more than careful clinical assessment, analgesic/anti-inflammatory medication, and close follow-up may be necessary. A soft cervical collar may provide comfort.

If the onset of torticollis is *acute* and the patient *does not respond to the above measures,* diagnoses may include benign paroxysmal torticollis in infants and migraine headache in older children. Pneumomediastinum may be seen on chest x-ray. Advanced imaging studies and laboratory evaluation may identify Grisel's syndrome and IDC, which may present with or without fever.

In conclusion, neck stiffness and/or malposition may indicate a wide array of medical and traumatic conditions, from life-threatening to relatively benign. A careful examination must be performed to exclude the presence of spinal cord involvement. Trauma and infection are the most important causes of neck stiffness in children, and a thorough history and physical examination will help guide the evaluation and decision making. Cervical spine fracture, subluxation/dislocation, and meningitis remain the most important diagnoses to exclude.

Suggested Readings and Key References

Beier A, Vachhrajani S, Bayerl S, et al. Rotatory subluxation: experience from the Hospital for Sick Children. *J Neurosurg Pediatr* 2012;9:144–148.

Cheng JC, Tang SP, Chen TM, et al. The clinical presentation and outcome of treatment of congenital muscular torticollis in infants—a study of 1,086 cases. *J Pediatr Surg* 2000;35:1091–1096.

Chi H, Lee YJ, Chiu NC, et al. Acute suppurative thyroiditis in children. *Pediatr Infect Dis J* 2002;21:384–387.

Cirak B, Ziegfeld S, Knight VM, et al. Spinal injuries in children. *J Pediatr Surg* 2004;39:607–612.

Cornejo VJ, Martinez-Lage JF, Piqueras C, et al. Inflammatory atlanto-axial subluxation (Grisel's syndrome) in children: clinical diagnosis and management. *Childs Nerv Syst* 2003;19:342–347.

Craig FW, Schunk JE. Retropharyngeal abscess in children: clinical presentation, utility of imaging, and current management. *Pediatrics* 2003;111:1394–1398.

Dai LY, Ye H, Qian QR. The natural history of cervical disc calcification in children. *J Bone Joint Surg Am* 2004;86:1467–1472.

Fąfara-Leś A, Kwiatkowski S, Maryńczak L, et al. Torticollis as a first sign of posterior fossa and cervical spinal cord tumors in children. *Childs Nerv Syst* 2014;30:425–430.

Fernandez M, Carrol CL, Baker CJ. Discitis and vertebral osteomyelitis in children: an 18-year review. *Pediatrics* 2000;105:1299–1304.

Leonard JR, Jaffe DM, Kuppermann N, et al. Cervical spine injury patterns in children. *Pediatrics* 2014;133(5):e1179–e1188.

Leonard J, Kuppermann N, Olsen C, et al. Factors associated with cervical spine injury in children after blunt trauma. *Ann Emerg Med* 2011;58:145–155.

Nigrovic LE, Kuppermann N, Malley R, et al. Children with bacterial meningitis presenting to the emergency department during the pneumococcal conjugate vaccine era. *Acad Emerg Med* 2008;15: 522–528.

Sans N, Faruch M, Lapègue F, et al. Infections of the spinal column–spondylodiscitis. *Diagn Interv Imaging* 2012;93:520–529.

Viccellio P, Simon H, Pressman BD, et al. A prospective multicenter study of cervical spine injury in children. *Pediatrics* 2001;108:e20.

Vitale MG, Goss JM, Matsumoto H, et al. Epidemiology of pediatric spinal cord injury in the United States years 1997 and 2000. *J Pediatr Orthop* 2006;26:745–749.

CHAPTER 45 ■ ODOR: UNUSUAL

ALISON ST. GERMAINE BRENT, MD

The human nose is able to discriminate approximately 4,000 odors! Occasionally, parents bring an infant or a child to the emergency department (ED) complaining of an unusual smell. Adolescents are more likely to note a new or an unusual odor themselves and present to the ED with specific complaints.

Olfaction is not a sense that most medical providers are trained to use, quantify, or describe. Before the development of sophisticated laboratory tests, clinicians relied heavily on the sense of smell and often made clinically perceptive diagnoses by aroma alone. Today, by incorporating the sense of smell into a clinical skill set, an astute provider can make a presumptive diagnosis of a metabolic disorder, intoxication, or infection and institute lifesaving therapy prior to laboratory confirmation.

PATHOPHYSIOLOGY

The olfactory area extends from the roof of the nasal cavity approximately 10 mm down the septum and superior turbinates bilaterally. The exact mechanism of stimulation of the olfactory receptors is unknown. Smell is more acute in the darkness and is believed to be linked to blood cortisol levels.

The unique odor emitted by a person is produced by a combination of body secretions and excretions, particularly those from the oropharynx, nasopharynx, and the respiratory tract, plus aromas from the skin and cutaneous lesions, urine, feces, and flatus. The most significant components of odor in healthy humans are the apocrine glands. These secretions are initially odorless, but bacterial breakdown that results in fatty acid production can cause an offensive odor. Body odor is altered by hygiene, metabolism, toxins, infections, and systemic disease.

When a child is unable to detect odor, anosmia should be considered. When a child complains of strange odors, especially if no one else is able to identify them, temporal lobe epilepsy should be contemplated.

DIFFERENTIAL DIAGNOSIS

A number of conditions, including metabolic disorders, intoxications, infections, dermatologic conditions, foreign bodies, various abnormalities of the body orifices, and a variety of systemic diseases, may result in noxious odor (Table 45.1).

Metabolic Disorders

The most common metabolic disorder with a characteristic odor is diabetic ketoacidosis (Table 45.2). The characteristic breath odor is described as sweet, fruity, or similar to nail polish remover. This distinctive aroma is caused by acetone from the breakdown of ketones bodies to ketoacids (acetone, acetoacetate, and betahydroxybutirate). It is important to note that any condition that results in a marked metabolic acidosis with ketosis will result in the characteristic sweet or fruity breath.

Inborn errors of metabolism that result in altered body, breath, or skin odors are unusual individually, but as a composite, they reflect a significant percentage of life-threatening illnesses of infancy (see Chapter 103 Metabolic Emergencies). Although definitive diagnosis depends on specific identification of serum and urine amino and organic acid levels, many such conditions are associated with a positive urine ferric chloride test, which when performed in the ED can yield presumptive diagnosis (Table 45.2).

Phenylketonuria is a disorder of amino acid metabolism associated with a deficiency of phenylalanine dehydroxylase and dihydropteridine reductase, which forces use of minor metabolic pathways of phenylalanine, resulting in the buildup of phenylacetic acid. It is the buildup of phenylacetic acid in sweat and urine that causes the characteristic aroma described as musty, mousy, horsey, wolf-like, barny, or stale sweaty locker-room towels. Clinical features of untreated phenylketonuria include white-blond hair, blue eyes, fair complexion, eczema, microcephaly, hypertonicity, seizures, and progressive mental deterioration. Although neonatal screening detects most of these cases, the observation of a characteristic odor in an infant should prompt immediate appropriate laboratory studies, which may include a urine ferric chloride test in the ED. Prompt diagnosis and dietary restriction of phenylalanine promote normal development.

Maple syrup urine disease is caused by a metabolic defect in the decarboxylation of the ketoacids of the branch-chain amino acids (leucine, isoleucine, and valine), which results in their accumulation in the blood. Sotolon (4,5-dimethyl-3-hydroxy-2[5H]-furanone), a metabolite of isoleucine in the urine, produces the characteristic odor described as maple syrup, caramel-like, malty, or boiled Chinese herbal medicine. Children with this disorder can have variable clinical manifestations, ranging from decreased appetite, vomiting, and ataxia, to progressive acidosis, seizures, coma, and death. Prompt diagnosis and limitation of dietary branched-chain amino acids promotes normal development.

Oasthouse urine disease, or methionine malabsorption syndrome, is caused by defective transport by the intestines and kidneys of methionine and, to a lesser extent, leucine, isoleucine, valine, tyrosine, and phenylalanine. The unabsorbed methionine in the gut is broken down by colonic bacteria to α-hydroxybutyric acid, which causes the distinctive odor, described as dried malt or hops (as in breweries), dried celery, or yeast. Clinical presentation includes fair hair and skin, hyperpnea, extensor spasms, fever, edema, and mental retardation. Successful treatment consists of a methionine-restricted diet.

The odor of sweaty feet syndrome, or isovaleric acidemia, is caused by a defect in the catabolism of leucine. The

TABLE 45.1

CLINICAL SOURCE AND CAUSE OF UNUSUAL ODORS

Urine		Body	
Metabolic diseases	**Metabolic disease odors**	**Toxins**	**Toxin odors**
Phenylketonuria	Mousy, musty, horsey, wolflike, barny	Marijuana (THC)	Sweet & sour
	Stale locker room towels	Nitrites, lacquer, ethanol, isopropyl alcohol, chloroform	Sweet, fruity
Maple syrup urine disease (branched-chain ketonuria)	Maple syrup, caramel, boiled Chinese herbal medicine	Paraldehyde, chloral hydrate	Pears
Oasthouse urine disease (methionine malabsorption)	Dried malt or hops (brewery), celery, years	Cyanide	Bitter almonds, peach pits
Odor of sweaty feet syndrome (isovaleric acidemia)	Sweaty feet or socks, ripe cheese	Cicutoxin	Carrots
Odor of cat's urine syndrome (biotin-responsive multiple carboxylase deficiency)	Male "Tomcat" urine	Disulfiram, mercaptan, hydrogen sulfide	Rotten eggs
Cystinuria	Rotten eggs	Zinc phosphide	Musty, fish, raw liver
Fish odor syndrome (trimethylaminuria)	Dead or rotting fish		
Odor of rancid butter syndrome (tyrosinemia)	Fishy, musty, rotten cabbage	Arsenic, phosphorous, dimethyl sulfoxide, thallium, tellurium, parathion, malathion, selenium	Garlic
Toxins	**Toxin odors**	Camphor, naphthalene, *p*-dichlorobenzene	Mothballs
Turpentine	Violets	Vacor	Peanuts
Infectious diseases	**Infectious disease odors**	O-Chlorobenzylidene, malononitrile	Pepper
Urinary tract infection	Ammonia	Ethchlorvynol	Aromatic, vinyl-like
Foreign body	**Foreign body odors**	Nitrobenzene	Shoe polish
Urethral foreign body	Foul, putrid	Methyl salicylate	Wintergreen
		Alcoholic beverages	Alcoholic beverages
		Metabolic diseases	**Metabolic disease odors**
		Phenylketonuria	Mousy, musty, horsey, wolflike, barny
		Odor of sweaty feet syndrome (isovaleric acidemia)	Cheesy, sweaty socks
		Infectious diseases	**Infectious disease odors**
		Typhoid fever	Freshly baked bread
		Yellow fever	Butcher shop
		Smallpox	Menagerie
		Scrofula	Stale beer
		Diphtheria	Sweet
		Rubella	Freshly plucked feathers
		Miliary fever	Rotten straw
		Omphalitis	Foul
		Miscellaneous diseases	**Miscellaneous disease odors**
		Scurvy	Putrid
		Gout	Fetid
		Pellagra	Sour or musty butter
		Psychiatric diseases	**Psychiatric disease odors**
		Schizophrenia	Pungent, heavy
		Antibiotics	**Antibiotic odors**
		Cephalosporin	Musty
		Penicillin	Ammonia
		Skin diseases	**Skin disease odors**
		Hidradenitis	Pungent
		Darier disease (keratosis follicularis)	Burned tissue
		Bromhidrosis	Pungent
		Ichthyosis, ulcers, necrosis, pemphigus	Foul, unpleasant
		Burns	Charred flesh
		Burns infected with *Pseudomonas aeruginosa*	Sweet, grapelike

(*continued*)

TABLE 45.1

CLINICAL SOURCE AND CAUSE OF UNUSUAL ODORS (*CONTINUED*)

Breath		Body fluids	
Toxins	**Toxin odors**	**Sputum**	**Sputum**
Amphetamines	Bad breath	*Infectious diseases*	*Infectious disease odors*
Cyanide	Bitter almonds	Bronchitis, empyema, abscess	Foul, putrid
Arsenic, phosphorus, tellurium, parathion, malathion	Garlic	**Vomitus**	**Vomitus**
		Infectious diseases	*Infectious disease odors*
		Peritonitis	Feculent
Iodine	Metallic	*Systemic diseases*	*Systemic disease odors*
Chloroform, lacquer, salicylate	Fruity, ripe apples	Gastrointestinal obstruction	Feculent
Chloral hydrate, paraldehyde	Pears	*Toxins*	*Toxin odors*
Methyl salicylate	Wintergreen	Arsenic, phosphorus	Garlic
Ethchlorvynol	Aromatic, vinyl-like	Turpentine	Violets
Camphor naphthalene, *p*-Dichlorobenzene	Mothballs	**Stool**	**Stool**
		Infectious diseases	*Infectious disease odors*
Hydrogen sulfide	Rotten eggs	*Shigella, Salmonella*	Rank
Infectious diseases	**Infectious disease odors**	Steatorrhea	Foul
Pharyngitis, tonsillitis, acute ulcerative gingivitis (Vincent angina, trench mouth), lung abscess, halitosis, dental abscess	Foul, putrid	*Systemic diseases*	*Systemic disease odors*
		Malabsorption, cystic fibrosis, celiac disease, chronic disease	Foul, vile
Diphtheria	Sweet grapes	*Toxins*	*Toxin odors*
Metabolic diseases	**Metabolic disease odors**	Arsenic	Garlic
DKA or any other condition that causes ketosis	Fruity or sweet	**General**	**General**
		Foreign body	*Foreign body odors*
Odor of sweaty feet syndrome (isovaleric acidemia)	Sweaty feet or socks, ripe cheese	Rectal foreign body	Foul, putrid
		Pus	**Pus**
Systemic diseases	**Systemic disease odors**	*Infectious diseases*	*Infectious disease odors*
Uremia	Fishy, ammonia	Gas gangrene	Sweet, rotten apples
Hepatic failure	Musty fish, raw liver, clover, feculent	Foreign body	Fetid, putrid
		Proteophylic bacteria	Feculent, ripe cheese
Gastrointestinal obstructions	Foul, feculent	Clostridium gas gangrene	Rotten apples
Foreign body	**Foreign body odors**	*Proteus*	Mousy
Nasal foreign body	Foul, putrid	Proteolytic bacteria	Overripe cheese
		Vaginal discharge	**Vaginal**
		Infectious diseases	*Infectious disease odors*
		Vaginitis, foreign body	Fishy, foul
		Systemic diseases	*Systemic disease odors*
		Malignancy	Fetid
		Foreign body	*Foreign body odors*
		Vaginal foreign body	Foul, putrid
		Ear discharge	**Ear discharge**
		Metabolic diseases	*Metabolic disease odors*
		Maple syrup urine disease	Maple syrup, caramel, boiled Chinese herbal medicine
		Infectious diseases	*Infectious disease odors*
		Pseudomonas	Foul
		Foreign body	*Foreign body odors*
		Otic foreign body	Foul, putrid

characteristic odor described as sweaty feet or socks or ripe cheese comes from the buildup of isovaleric acid. Clinically, children experience vomiting, dehydration, acidosis, and slowly progressive mental deterioration. Treatment includes restriction of leucine in the diet.

In the odor of cat's urine syndrome, the enzymatic defects are in the biotin-dependent enzymes β-methylcrotonyl-CoA carboxylase, pyruvate carboxylase, and propionyl-CoA carboxylase. The cause of the distinctive aroma of cat urine, referred to as male or "tomcat" urine, is unknown. Clinically,

TABLE 45.2

METABOLIC DISEASE ASSOCIATED WITH UNUSUAL ODORS

Disease	Odor	Odor source	Enzyme defect	Clinical features	Treatment	Rapid emergency department diagnosis
Diabetic ketoacidosis	Sweet or fruity	Breath	Lack of insulin or insulin activity	Polyuria, polydipsia, polyphagia, weight loss, coma, acidosis	Insulin administration	1 mL urine + 10% ferric chloride—red-brown color
Phenylketonuria	Musty, mousy, horsey, wolflike, barny stale locker room towels	Urine and body	Phenylalanine hydroxylase	Progressive mental retardation, eczema, decreased pigmentation, seizures, spasticity, white-blond hair, blue eyes, pyloric stenosis, microcephaly	Diet low in phenylalanine	1 mL urine + 10% ferric chloride—green color
Maple syrup urine disease (branched-chain ketonuria)	Maple syrup, caramel, boiled Chinese herbal medicine	Urine	Branched-chain ketoacid decarboxylase	Marked acidosis, seizures, vomiting, ataxia, decreased appetite, coma leading to death in first year or two of life or mental subnormality without acidosis or intermittent acidosis without mental retardation	Acutely ill: Start D10 ½ NS at 1.5 times maintenance to prevent catabolism. Diet low in branched-chain amino acid; protein restriction and/or thiamine in large doses	1 mL urine + 10% ferric chloride—blue, yellow, or blue-green color
Oasthouse urine disease (methionine malabsorption)	Dried malt or hops (brewery), celery, yeast	Urine	Defective transport of methionine, branched-chain amino acids, tyrosine, and phenylalanine	Mental retardation, spasticity, hyperpnea, fever, edema, fair hair and skin	Restrict methionine in diet	1 mL urine + 10% ferric chloride—purple or red-brown color
Odor of sweaty feet syndrome (isovaleric acidemia)	Sweaty feet or socks, ripe cheese	Urine, body, breath, all body fluids	Isovaleryl-CoA dehydrogenase	Recurrent bouts of acidosis, vomiting, dehydration, coma, aversion to protein foods, lethargy, hypotension	Acutely ill: Start D10 ½ NS at 1.5 times maintenance to prevent catabolism. Restrict leucine in diet	N/A
Odor of cat's urine syndrome (biotin-responsive multiple carboxylase deficiency)	Male or "tomcat" urine	Urine	β-Methylcrotonyl-CoA carboxylase, pyruvate carboxylase, propionyl-CoA carboxylase	Neurologic disorder resembling Werdnig–Hoffmann disease, ketoacidosis, failure to thrive	Leucine restriction Biotin administration	N/A
Fish odor syndrome (trimethylaminuria)	Dead or rotting fish	Urine	Deficiency in flavin monooxygenase 3	Stigmata of Turner syndrome, neutropenia, recurrent infections, anemia, splenomegaly	Dietary adjustments, hygiene	N/A
Cystinuria	Rotten egg	Urine	Inadequate reabsorption of (SLC 3A1 + SLC7A9)	Renal colic, hematuria, chronic backache, UTI	Hydration, urinary alkalinization	N/A
Odor of rancid butter syndrome (tyrosinosis)	Rancid butter, rotten cabbage, fishy, musty	Urine	Deficiency of fumarylacetoacetase succinylacetone	FTT, poor feeding, irritability, progressive neurologic deterioration, seizures, hepatic dysfunction, death	Dietary restriction phenylalanine and tyrosine	1 mL urine + 10% ferric chloride—transient blue-green color

N/A, not applicable.

children have failure to thrive, ketoacidosis, and neurologic symptoms similar to Werdnig–Hoffmann disease. Treatment consists of a low-leucine diet and the addition of biotin.

Fish odor syndrome, trimethylaminuria, results in the unmistakable odor of dead or rotting fish in the urine, breath, and sweat. This aroma is produced by a buildup of trimethylamine, caused by an inherited deficiency in flavin monooxygenase 3, the vital enzyme for the metabolism of trimethylamine. Clinical and laboratory presentation includes stigmata of Turner syndrome, history of recurrent pulmonary infections, a normal complement of chromosomes, neutropenia, and abnormal platelet function. While the disease itself is not life-threatening, it can be devastating from a psychosocial perspective and has been associated with suicide attempts, hence practitioners need to remain attentive to this often overlooked diagnosis. Unfortunately there is no cure or dietary adjustments that can reduce the excretion of trimethylamine and attention to body hygiene may be helpful adjuncts.

Tyrosinemia, the odor of rancid butter syndrome, is identified by a distinctive cabbage-like odor. This syndrome is caused by a deficiency of fumarylacetoacetase which results in the buildup of succinylacetone, the decarboxylation product of succinyl acetoacetate, a compound derived from the tyrosine catabolic intermediate fumarylacetoacetate. Clinical presentation may include failure to thrive, which may precede the appearance of more dramatic findings in tyrosinemia, including vomiting and diarrhea, which rapidly progressto bloody stool, lethargy, and jaundice, irritability, seizures, coma, progressive neurologic deterioration, and can result in early death secondary to infection and liver failure. In some cases, restriction of dietary phenylalanine and tyrosine has been helpful.

Cystinuria is caused by genetic mutations, resulting in inadequate reabsorption of cystine in the proximal of the kidney (SLC3A1 and SLC7A9). This causes an excessive concentration of this amino acid in the urine, which may precipitate out of the urine and form crystals or stones in the kidneys, ureters, or bladder. Patients with cystinuria usually present with renal colic, hematuria, chronic backache, and/or urinary tract infection. Since cystine is one of the sulfur-containing amino acids; the urine may have the characteristic odor of rotten eggs. The foundation of cystine stone prevention is adequate hydration and urinary alkalinization.

Toxicologic Considerations

Recognition of a characteristic odor is vital for rapid diagnosis and treatment of some potentially lethal ingestions prior to laboratory identification (Table 45.1) (see Chapter 110 Toxicologic Emergencies).

Due to the increased availability of both medical and recreational marijuana, medical care providers need to be vigilant to its impact on children. Marijuana refers to the dried leaves, flowers, stems, and seeds from the hemp plant Cannabis sativa, which contains the psychoactive chemical delta-9-tetrahydrocannabinol (THC), as well as other related compounds. This plant material can also be concentrated in a resin called hashish or a sticky black liquid called hash oil. Marijuana is usually smoked and has a pungent and distinctive, usually sweet-and-sour, odor that is easily recognized. Marijuana is also available as an edible, defined as a food item made with marijuana or infused with marijuana oils. Edibles are available in a wide variety of foods such as baked goods, sauces, candies (including animal or fruit-shaped gummies, lollipops, and chocolates) and as a beverage. The amount of THC can vary in edible marijuana products, especially in homemade marijuana edibles, making it harder to control how much THC is consumed.

After smoking or inhaling marijuana, the onset of symptoms is rapid (within 5 to 30 minutes), with the duration of effects for several hours. In contrast, after ingestion of marijuana edibles, the onset of symptoms is much slower (1 to 4 hours) with several hours duration. The most common overdose incidents in children occur with edibles and can have a more severe and prolonged effect because of the variable amounts of THC in edibles. Young children may mistake edible marijuana products for regular food and ingest it unknowingly. Small children are at higher risk based on their size and weight. Many young children who consume marijuana edibles require hospital admission due to the severity of their symptoms.

Salicylates are ubiquitous agents found in hundreds of over-the-counter (OTC) medications and in numerous prescription drugs, making salicylate toxicity an important cause of morbidity and mortality. Methyl salicylate (oil of wintergreen) or topically applied products may provide an early clue indicative of methyl salicylate poisoning by the pleasant minty smell of wintergreen. This can prompt the astute clinician to immediately institute lifesaving therapy.

A strong garlic odor is typical of arsenic, arsine gas, phosphorus, tellurium, parathion, malathion, selenium, dimethyl sulfoxide, and thallium. The odor of bitter almonds or peach pits is indicative of cyanide poisoning, in which the degree of excretion of the odor parallels toxicity (although the ability to detect this odor is genetically determined and may only be present in up to 40% of persons). Turpentine can be identified by the bouquet of violets. Diagnostic odors are found in several sedative-hypnotic medications that primarily have central nervous system manifestations. Ethchlorvynol (Placidyl) is a volatile agent that has an aromatic plastic or vinyl-like breath odor. Ingestion results in coma, hypothermia, respiratory depression, hypotension, and bradycardia. An overdose of chloral hydrate can result in central nervous system depression ranging from slurred speech, ataxia, and incoordination to deep coma, gastritis, and cardiac arrhythmias. It may be seen in children or as an intentional overdose in adults, and it imparts a fruity, pear-like scent. Disulfiram (Antabuse) gives the breath a rotten egg odor because of the sulfide metabolites.

Additional odors from toxins are listed in Table 45.1.

Infectious Diseases

Many microorganisms produce characteristic odors that suggest the diagnosis of their respective infectious diseases by olfaction alone (Table 45.1) (see also Clinical Pathway Chapter 92 UTI, Febrile). Omphalitis in the newborn can be life-threatening. It presents with a foul or putrid odor associated with a draining, erythematous umbilical area. Less common infections that have been historically associated with characteristic odors include typhoid's aroma of freshly baked bread, yellow fever's butcher shop smell, smallpox's menagerie odor, scrofula's odor of stale beer, diphtheria's sweet smell, and rubella's scent of freshly plucked feathers.

Medications also have distinguishing odors. Penicillins give off an ammoniacal scent, whereas cephalosporins are noted to have a musty odor. Topical benzoyl peroxide, applied in large quantities, emits a pungent, pervasive aroma.

Dermatologic Conditions

Many dermatologic diseases (Table 45.1) are associated with specific odors. Any cause of hyperhidrosis results in an offensive body odor. Hidradenitis has a characteristic pungent odor, whereas Darier disease (keratosis follicularis) is noted to have a pervasive aroma of burned tissue. An abscess or cellulitis is identified by the characteristic odors of the responsible microorganisms. In burn patients, there is the typical odor of charred flesh, which, when infected with *Pseudomonas aeruginosa,* takes on a characteristic sweet, grape-like odor.

Foreign Bodies

Foreign bodies are capable of producing a foul odor that results from secondary bacterial colonization or infection. Foreign body odors can be localized to a particular orifice, or they may pervade a patient's clothing, body, and surrounding environment. Foul-smelling, fetid, or feculent odors indicate anaerobic infections, whereas a sickly sweet odor is associated with *Escherichia coli,* and *Clostridia* is associated with a mousy odor.

Orifice Odors

Specific orifice odors can be diagnostic of infectious disease processes.

Oropharynx

A healthy mouth does not give off an offensive odor. Halitosis, or bad breath, is the result of a release of volatile sulfur compounds formed when the oral flora metabolizes amino acids from compounds in the saliva that adhere to the tongue, teeth, and gums. Halitosis is increased in states of diminished solid and liquid intake. Tonsillitis (see Chapters 69 Sore Throat and 102 Infectious Disease Emergencies) has an offensive odor, and group A β-hemolytic streptococcus gives off a characteristic "strep breath" smell. Dental abscesses (see Chapter 125 Dental Emergencies), gum or periodontal disease, and acute ulcerative gingivitis (Vincent angina, or trench mouth) are associated with a penetrating, offensive odor often described as metallic in nature. The oropharynx is also the portal of exit for deeper infections. Lung abscesses, empyema, bronchitis, and bronchiectasis result in foul breath and sputum. Nasal foreign bodies in toddlers are usually associated with an odor identified by parents as bad breath.

Nose

Nasal drainage can be clear and odorless or mucopurulent and odiferous. Nasal drainage and bleeding can reflect local infections, foreign bodies, irritations of the nasal passage, and sinus drainage.

Ear

Sterile inner ear fluid is odorless but gives off a rank smell when infected. Acute otitis externa is usually associated with a mucoid drainage, whereas chronic otitis externa produces a purulent, discolored drainage with a foul odor, usually caused by *P. aeruginosa* or *Staphylococcus aureus.*

Genitalia

Vaginal secretions are combinations of vulvar secretions from sebaceous, sweat, Bartholin and Skene glands, transudate through the vaginal wall, exfoliated cells, cervical mucus, endometrial and oviductal fluids, plus vaginal microorganisms and menstrual blood. These secretions are hormonally mediated and vary with the menstrual cycle. Odors are exacerbated by the presence of retained foreign bodies, including tampons and diaphragms.

Bacterial vaginosis (nonspecific vaginitis, *Gardnerella* vaginitis, *Corynebacterium* vaginitis, *Haemophilus* vaginitis, nonspecific vaginosis, and anaerobic vaginosis) is caused by an increase in anaerobic bacteria and a decrease in lactobacilli (see Chapter 100 Gynecology Emergencies). The anaerobic bacteria act synergistically with *Gardnerella vaginalis* to produce enzymes and aminopeptidases that degrade proteins, and decarboxylases that convert amino acids and other compounds to amines. The amines produce the characteristic "fishy" odor, which is best detected by alkalinization using 10% potassium hydroxide placed directly on a vaginal swab and smelling immediately. This odor also can be indicative of sexual abuse in children. Vaginal infection with *Trichomonas* often is associated with a fishy odor, whereas *Candida* vaginitis is notably free of odor.

A male counterpart, balanoposthitis, is associated with a urethral discharge that produces a fishy odor when alkalinized because of the same process and organisms as occur in bacterial vaginosis.

Urethral Meatus

A urinary tract infection caused by urea-splitting bacteria will emit an ammoniacal odor.

Rectum

Stool odors vary with diet, medications, and microbiologic flora. Various malabsorptive syndromes, such as sprue, cystic fibrosis (see Chapter 107 Pulmonary Emergencies), and Whipple disease, are associated with foul-smelling stool. The presence of blood in the stool has a distinctive pungent odor, as does pus. *Shigella* and *Salmonella* (see Chapter 102 Infectious Disease Emergencies) have distinctive rank odors.

Systemic Diseases

Several nutritional syndromes (Table 45.1), such as pellagra's stench of sour or musty butter and the putrid or fetid smell of scurvy and gout, have unique odors. Schizophrenia has a characteristic body odor described as heavy, unpleasant, and pungent. The odor-producing substance is *trans*-3-methyl-2-hexanoic acid, which is produced in the sweat. Uremic breath is produced by secondary and tertiary amines, dimethylamines, and trimethylamines that produce a fishy odor. Malignancy, especially when associated with an expanding external mass, bleeding, and necrosis, gives off a trenchant odor because of tissue and cellular breakdown plus gas formation. Hepatic failure gives an odor of "fetor hepaticus" (described as musty, rotten eggs, or garlic) and is noted in the breath or urine. In Crohn disease (see Chapter 99 Gastrointestinal Emergencies), the development of gastric fistulae is often heralded by a feculent odor.

A physiologic odor that often heralds the onset of puberty emanates from the underarms. This is usually the earliest sign of puberty and precedes all other physical changes. Age of onset is around 6 to 8 years and reflects the onset of adrenarche. Dehydroepiandrosterone sulfate is the androgen believed to be responsible for the pungent aroma of underarm body odor and can be measured for confirmation. Although the adrenal and hypothalamic–pituitary–gonadal axes are separate systems involved with the onset of puberty, they often become active nearly simultaneously.

EVALUATION AND DECISION

The evaluation of a child who presents to the ED should incorporate all the senses, including smell (Fig. 45.1). Both presence and absence of odors can be diagnostic. Each person has a unique odor, ranging from pleasant to offensive. Using the sense of smell should be done in stages; an initial evaluation of the prevailing odor of the examination room, followed by attention to overall body odor and identification of odors from individual orifices and body fluids. Body fluids such as ocular, ear, nasal, sinus tract, or umbilical drainage, vomitus, sputum, genital discharge, stool, ulcers, and superinfection of the dermis have unique identifiable odors.

Good or poor hygiene is readily detected in a closed examination room. When an unusual odor is detected, the history should include information about medications (topical, oral, or rectal), onset and duration of odor, methods used to alter odor, unusual drainage from body orifices, suspicion of foreign body, and fever.

In the evaluation of the significance of odors, attention must be paid to the child's age and developmental level. At birth, infant odors are a conglomeration of their own and their mother's physical environment. After birth, a well-cared-for, healthy infant should have a very pleasing scent and odorless breath. Offensive body odor in a newborn suggests an inborn error of metabolism, a localized infection such as omphalitis, or neglect. During infancy, inborn errors of metabolism (Table 45.3) are potentially life-threatening causes of unusual odor (Table 45.4). Infection localized to the umbilicus, omphalitis, produces a foul odor and is easily diagnosed on the basis of erythema, induration, and discharge. Other sources found in older children (foreign bodies, ingestions, and pharyngitis) are unusual in the infant.

TABLE 45.3

COMMON CAUSES OF UNUSUAL ODORS

Infants
Inborn errors of metabolism
Localized infections
Omphalitis
Neglect
Toddlers
Foreign bodies
Otic
Nasal
Vaginal
Urethral
Rectal
Localized infections
Stomatitis
Adolescents
Localized infections
Pharyngitis
Tonsillitis
Vaginitis
Toxins
Alcoholic beverages
Puberty

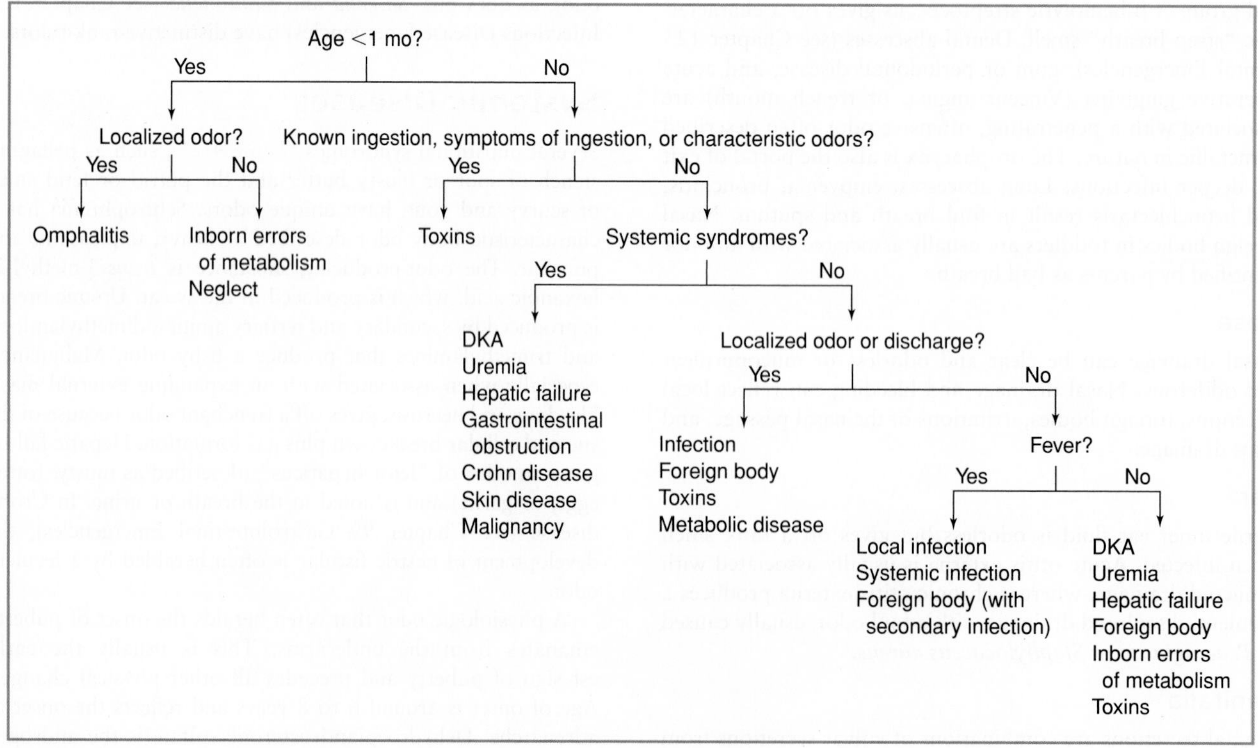

FIGURE 45.1 Evaluation and decision for unusual odors. DKA, diabetic ketoacidosis.

TABLE 45.4

LIFE-THREATENING CAUSES OF UNUSUAL ODOR

Metabolic disease
Inborn errors of metabolism
Diabetic ketoacidosis
Infectious diseases
Omphalitis
Diphtheria
Lung abscess
Toxins
Marijuana (THC)
Arsenic
Cyanide
Isopropyl alcohol
Methyl salicylate
Vacor
Systemic disease
Uremia
Liver failure
Gastrointestinal obstruction
Peritonitis

In an older child, the physician should determine a child's history and whether clinical signs of intoxication or chronic systemic diseases, such as diabetes, liver failure, or uremia, are present. The child with ketoacidosis usually appears dehydrated and manifests deep, rapid (Kussmaul) respirations; the breath may smell of ketones. Uremia develops in patients with renal failure who may have short stature, edema, hypertension, and a characteristic fishy odor of their breath. With liver failure, the patient may have jaundice, ascites, lethargy, or mental status changes, as well as breath and urine that emanate the odor of rotten eggs or garlic.

Body odors change with puberty through hormonally induced metabolic changes. The most significant change is the development of axillary odor related to apocrine secretions that are retained or spread by axillary hair. Normal quantities of sweat have a barely perceptible odor, whereas increasing quantities of sweat production cause increasingly noticeable and offensive odor.

Early on, the physician should determine the potential risk of ingestion of a toxic substance. In the adolescent, the risk of a significant ingestion increases and can be life-threatening (Table 45.4). Next, the physician should ascertain whether the odor emanates from a particular body orifice such as the ear, nose, pharynx, vagina, urethra, or rectum. Nasal foreign bodies are particularly common in children between the ages of 1 and 5 years. They may remain hidden for weeks, long beyond the child's memory of placing the object, and eventually, they produce a secondary infection that leads to a foul discharge. In some cases of foreign body, the odor may be so strong that it appears to be generalized. Thus, a careful examination of the various orifices, with particular attention to the nares, is advisable. The presence or absence of fever is another crucial variable in the evaluation of odor. Fever suggests an infectious cause, either systemic or localized. Pharyngitis and tonsillitis characteristically cause foul odor to the breath, much like a lung abscess. Occasionally, parents state that their child smells as if he or she had a "strep throat." Although foreign bodies occasionally produce obstruction and a secondary infection of severity sufficient enough to evoke a febrile response, in most cases, the inflammation is localized and the child is afebrile.

In the absence of a known history or obvious findings of chronic systemic disease, a visible foreign body, known ingestion, or fever, the clinician should perform a careful physical examination and a urinalysis. Diabetic ketoacidosis always causes glycosuria and ketonuria, but hepatic or renal failure may be less obvious. In addition, inborn errors of metabolism may first manifest well beyond the newborn period. Foreign bodies may defy routine attempts at visualization and, based on a high index of suspicion, may require endoscopy or imaging procedures. Persistence of an unusual odor or concern for chronic toxicity merits further laboratory evaluation. In cases in which an explanation of the odor is not uncovered, a follow-up evaluation in 2 to 3 days is prudent.

In patients who have died in the ED, a faint fecal odor is usually noted, feasibly related to the release of intestinal contents to the atmosphere. Unique identifiable odors detected at the time of death or autopsy can direct laboratory evaluation toward possible causes of death.

Suggested Readings and Key References

Chiang WK. Otolaryngologic principles. In: Goldfrank LR, Flomenbaum NE, Lewin NA, et al., eds. *Toxicologic emergencies*. 8th ed. Stanford, CT: Appleton & Lange, 2006:339–351.

Rezvani I. An approach to inborn errors of metabolism. In: Kliegman RM, Behrman RE, Jenson HB, et al., eds. *Textbook of pediatrics*. 18th ed. Philadelphia, PA: WB Saunders, 2007:527–567.

CHAPTER 46 ▪ OLIGOMENORRHEA

JEANNINE DEL PIZZO, MD, JENNIFER H. CHUANG, MD, MS, AND JAN PARADISE, MD

Oligomenorrhea, or infrequent menstrual bleeding, can usually be evaluated and managed in the outpatient setting. The pediatric emergency physician should be familiar with the common causes of oligomenorrhea as well as those presenting with true medical emergencies. This chapter will focus on how to evaluate a child presenting with oligomenorrhea, and when and where to refer.

DEFINITIONS

Although this chapter will focus on the approach to an adolescent with infrequent menstrual bleeding, the term "oligomenorrhea" is no longer used by the FIGO World Congress of Gynecology and Obstetrics nor by the American College of Obstetricians and Gynecologists. *For the pediatric emergency physician, oligomenorrhea* can be defined as an interval of more than 6 weeks between two menstrual periods. The newly accepted term of infrequent menstrual bleeding refers to one to two episodes of menstrual bleeding in a 90-day period. If menstrual cycles do not resume within 3 to 6 months, the term *secondary amenorrhea* is applied. Some patients with anovulatory menstrual cycles have oligomenorrhea punctuated by episodes of excessive bleeding. An approach to the evaluation of abnormal vaginal bleeding is presented in Chapter 75 Vaginal Bleeding.

This chapter will not specifically discuss primary amenorrhea—that is, failure to menstruate by a specified age, often 16 years. However, some disorders discussed here can also produce primary, as well as secondary amenorrhea and oligomenorrhea as part of an overall delay in pubertal development.

DIFFERENTIAL DIAGNOSIS

The differential diagnosis of oligomenorrhea is given in Table 46.1.

EVALUATION AND DECISION

History

The initial approach to any female complaining of oligomenorrhea should begin with history. It is essential to keep in mind that children and teenagers may not feel comfortable sharing certain information in front of their parents or caregivers. The emergency physician should plan on obtaining a history both with parents or caregivers present and with the patient alone. Some patients may feel comfortable discussing sexual information in front of parents and caregivers, however others will prefer to keep this information confidential.

Past medical history and current medications should be noted. A brief menstrual history should be obtained including onset of menstruation, timing of the last menstrual period, duration and frequency of typical menstruation cycles, number of pads or tampons used in a day, bleeding in between cycles, and the presence and size of clots passed. A patient should be asked if she engages in vaginal intercourse with males, if and which birth control methods are used, and if she is currently or has ever been pregnant. Patients should be asked if they have any recent weight loss or are restricting their caloric intake, increasing their physical activity, self-inducing vomiting, or using any medications (laxatives, diet pills, ipecac) for the purpose of weight loss.

Pertinent historical factors that can help exclude potentially dangerous causes of oligomenorrhea include any indicators of acute abdomen such as presence of abdominal pain, nausea, emesis, fever, or loss of appetite. Ascertain symptoms of increased intracranial pressure such as change in vision, neurologic symptoms, early morning emesis, or headache that is persistent, worsening, or waking the patient from sleep. Inquire about the presence of palpitations, tachycardia, sweating, weight loss, or agitation that may suggest hyperthyroidism. Conversely symptoms of hypothyroidism such as weight gain, cold intolerance, fatigue, and depressed mood should also be obtained.

Examination

Vital signs should be noted including the patient's height, weight, and body mass index (BMI). Tachycardia and hypotension may raise suspicion for ectopic pregnancy. Papilledema, blurred vision, cranial nerve VI palsy, visual field deficits, or other focal deficits may indicate increased intracranial pressure associated with pituitary tumors. Bradycardia and hypotension may suggest malnutrition due to caloric restriction, purging, or excessive energy expenditure. Note general appearance, mental status and perfusion, and perform a general examination. The patient should be observed for features such as overall body habitus, hirsutism, acanthosis nigricans, and acne. An abdominal examination should concentrate on the presence of peritoneal signs, a gravid uterus, or a palpable mass. Pubertal development including breasts and genitalia should be checked. If a history of galactorrhea is suspected, attempt to express fluid manually from the patient's breasts. The completed examination will separate the majority of patients who have no notable abnormalities from a minority with that point to a specific medical cause.

Pregnancy

Pregnancy is the first diagnosis to consider when evaluating an adolescent with one or several missed menstrual periods (Fig. 46.1). If the patient is not pregnant, evaluation can proceed at a more deliberate pace. Prompt diagnosis and referral

TABLE 46.1

DIFFERENTIAL DIAGNOSIS OF OLIGOMENORRHEA

I. Pregnancy and postpartum
  A. Intrauterine pregnancy
  B. Ectopic pregnancy
  C. Lactation
II. Iatrogenic
  A. Medications (see Table 46.3)
  B. Hormonal contraception
III. Endocrine
  A. Hyperandrogenism
    1. Polycystic ovarian syndrome
    2. Congenital adrenal hyperplasia
    3. Adrenocorticoid tumor
  B. Hypothalamic-pituitary axis disorders
    1. Caloric insufficiency
      a. Chronic illness
      b. Malabsorptive disorders
      c. Strenuous exercise
      d. Marked weight loss
      e. Anorexia nervosa
      f. Athletic triad
    2. Hyperprolactinemia
      a. Medications (see Iatrogenic)
      b. Pituitary tumor/other central nervous system tumors
  C. Ovarian disorders
    1. Ovarian failure
      a. Gonadal dysgenesis
      b. Alkylating antineoplastic agents
      c. Pelvic irradiation
      d. Autoimmune disease
    2. Hormone-secreting tumors
  D. Thyroid disorders
    1. Hypothyroidism
    2. Hyperthyroidism
IV. Miscellaneous
  A. Pseudocyesis
  B. Stress

are important; early and regular prenatal care is associated with reduced morbidity and mortality among pregnant teenagers and their offspring; early diagnosis also affords the pregnant adolescent time to consider all options including therapeutic abortion.

Early pregnancy is not always easy to recognize. Symptoms of fatigue, nausea, vomiting (not necessarily in the morning), urinary frequency, and breast growth or tenderness are common but by no means universal or specific. Some patients may report the result of a home pregnancy test. However, because of variability in the test's sensitivity for detecting urinary human chorionic gonadotropin (hCG), home pregnancy test kits commonly give falsely negative results. False-positive results can also occur, though rarely. Accordingly, the emergency physician should not rely solely on the reported result of a home pregnancy test to make or to exclude the diagnosis of pregnancy.

Qualitative urine and serum pregnancy tests performed in medical settings generally detect the β-subunit of hCG (β-hCG). The urine pregnancy test threshold is generally at β-hCG levels of ≥20 mIU per mL and will permit the detection of a normal pregnancy within about 10 days after conception and, in most but not all cases, by the time an expected menstrual period is missed. Serum β-hCG can be detected at lower levels though laboratories are variable regarding the level of detection (<1 vs. <5 mIU per mL). The emergency physician should know the detection level of the quantitative and qualitative β-hCG tests used by the local laboratory. Ectopic pregnancies often produce abnormally low levels of β-hCG compared to an intrauterine pregnancy of the same gestational age (see Chapter 75 Vaginal Bleeding). If a patient with one or several missed menstrual periods also complains of abdominal pain or abnormal vaginal bleeding, the diagnosis of *ectopic pregnancy* must be entertained (see Chapters 100 Gynecology Emergencies and 127 Genitourinary Emergencies). Although more than half of women with ectopic pregnancy have no risk factors, prior infections with chlamydia and gonorrhea, and pelvic inflammatory disease all increase the likelihood that a subsequent pregnancy will be ectopic.

Evaluation of Nonpregnant Patients

After pregnancy is excluded, the evaluation of an adolescent with oligomenorrhea can proceed at a deliberate pace (Fig. 46.1). During the first 2 years after menarche, it is not unusual for girls to have an occasional menstrual cycle that lasts less than 25 days or more than 40 days. After 3 years of menstruating, the typical menstrual cycle lasts 21 to 34 days for a majority of girls. As a rule, if an adolescent complains of only one or two prolonged menstrual cycles, is fewer than 2 years past menarche, and is not sexually active, further investigation in the emergency department (ED) is not warranted. However, the ED physician should be aware that, among adolescents who report oligomenorrhea at baseline (defined as an average cycle length of 42 to 180 days), the prognosis for developing regular cycles is guarded and may in fact be the earliest sign of a medical condition. After 3 years of follow-up, more than half will continue to have abnormally long cycles.

Adolescents with oligomenorrhea that has persisted for longer than 2 years after menarche or that involves three or more cycles longer than 42 days during the past year are candidates for further diagnostic evaluation, although ordinarily this ought to be accomplished in an outpatient setting rather than in an ED.

Postpartum

Breast-feeding is an obvious physiologic cause of prolactin secretion and oligomenorrhea.

Iatrogenic

Hyperprolactinemia causing oligomenorrhea and galactorrhea can have several etiologies: drugs (particularly antipsychotic agents), discontinuation of hormonal contraceptive agents, stimulation of the breasts, and excessive secretion of prolactin itself (e.g., primary hypothyroidism, pituitary adenoma). Drugs produce hyperprolactinemia by blocking pituitary

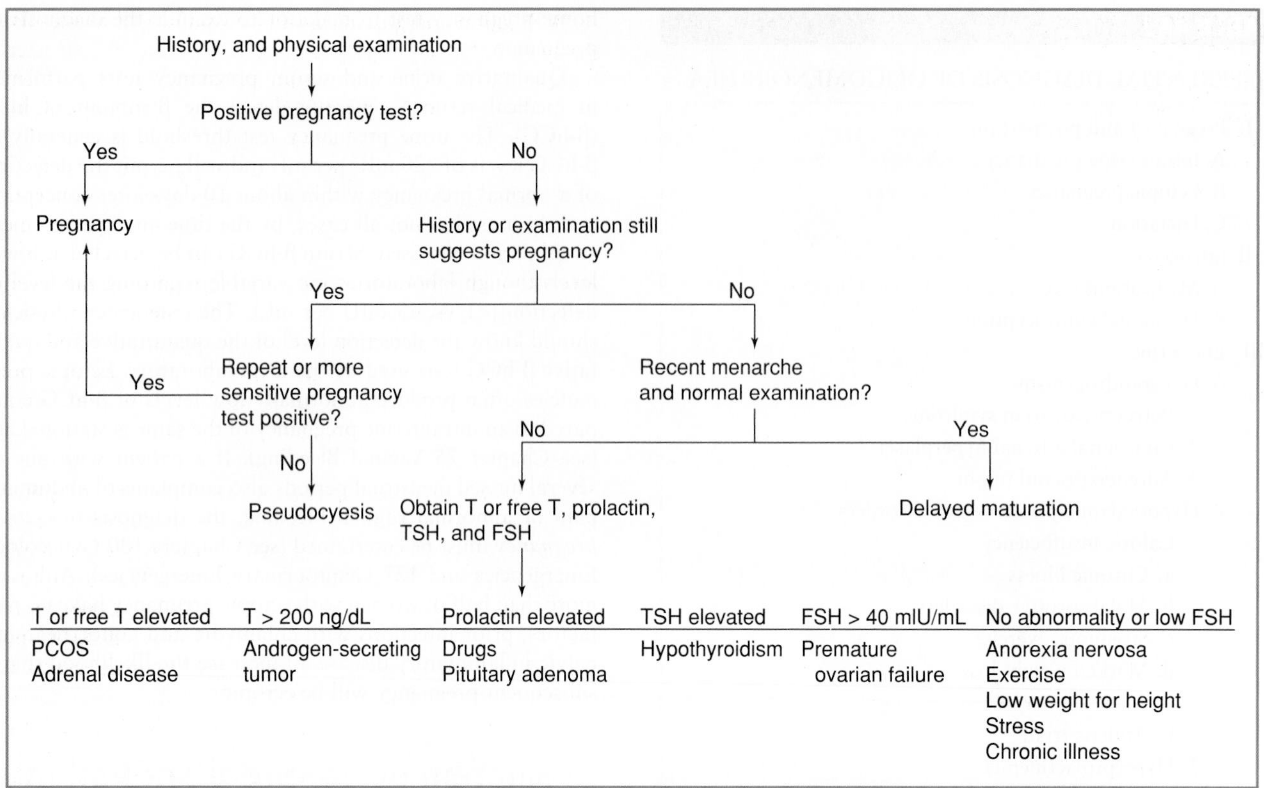

FIGURE 46.1 Strategy for initial diagnostic evaluation of the patient with oligomenorrhea. T, testosterone; TSH, thyroid-stimulating hormone; FSH, follicle-stimulating hormone; PCOS, polycystic ovary syndrome.

dopamine receptors or interfering in other ways with dopaminergic or serotoninergic central nervous system pathways.

A common cause for oligomenorrhea or amenorrhea is current or recent use of a hormonal contraceptive method. A parent may bring their child to a healthcare provider for complaint of oligomenorrhea; a confidential history may reveal that the patient is on a hormonal contraceptive method. Other diagnostic possibilities for oligomenorrheic patients with no abnormal physical findings include a wide variety of conditions. About half of women using contraceptive *medroxyprogesterone* injections for 12 months have amenorrhea; after 2 years of use, the proportion with amenorrhea is 68%. Amenorrhea also occurs in about 2% of menstrual cycles among patients taking combined hormonal contraceptives (pills, rings, patch). Some birth control pills are packaged for extended use, and the patient may only have withdrawal bleeding four times a year. However, amenorrhea persisting 12 months after the last injection of medroxyprogesterone or 6 months after birth control pills, ring, or patch have been stopped should be evaluated in the standard fashion.

Endocrine Abnormalities

Hyperandrogenism

Polycystic ovarian syndrome. Classically, hirsutism, obesity, ovarian enlargement, amenorrhea, or infertility constitutes the clinical features of *polycystic ovary syndrome* (PCOS, previously the Stein–Leventhal syndrome). Although hirsutism and obesity are classic features of PCOS, many adolescent patients with oligomenorrhea and the endocrinologic abnormalities of PCOS lack one or both of these signs. Patients with PCOS are a heterogeneous group with varying combinations of these features. An adolescent with PCOS may present to the ED with heavy abnormal uterine bleeding after several months of amenorrhea due to anovulatory cycles (see Chapter 75 Vaginal Bleeding). Few adolescents with clinical and biochemical evidence of PCOS have palpably enlarged ovaries, and their hyperandrogenism is typically mild. There are no distinct criteria for the diagnosis of PCOS in adolescents and currently, adolescents are diagnosed according to adult standards. Although several societies have published criteria guidelines for PCOS in adult women, the 2003 Rotterdam and the 2009 Androgen Excess Society's criteria are considered more applicable for adolescents. Table 46.2 provides both 2003 Rotterdam and 2009 Androgen Excess Society's criteria for the diagnosis of PCOS.

The pathophysiologic basis for PCOS is incompletely understood. However, the principal endocrinologic abnormalities involved are chronic anovulation, ovarian hyperandrogenism, and, in many affected patients, insulin resistance. Increased androgen production from the ovaries, adrenal glands, and peripheral conversion and high levels of free estrogen interferes with the hypothalamic-pituitary-ovarian feedback system, causing irregular menses.

The goals of treatment of adolescent patients with PCOS are to restore monthly menstrual cycles, to minimize hirsutism, to prevent the development of endometrial hyperplasia, and, it is hoped, to reduce the long-term risks of relative infertility, glucose intolerance, endometrial adenocarcinoma, and cardiovascular morbidity. Weight reduction can ameliorate the endocrinologic derangements and promote ovulation and regular menstruation in obese teens with PCOS, but few adolescents are able to achieve or to maintain substantial weight

TABLE 46.2

CRITERIA FOR THE DIAGNOSIS OF POLYCYSTIC OVARY SYNDROME

Rotterdam (2003) Requires two of three	Androgen Excess Society (2009)
1. Oligo- or anovulation 2. Clinical or biochemical signs of hyperandrogenism 3. Polycystic ovaries and exclusion of other etiologies	1. Hyperandrogenism: hirsutism and/or hyperandrogenemia 2. Ovarian dysfunction: oligo-anovulation and/or polycystic ovaries 3. Exclusion of other androgen excess or related disorders

Adapted from The Rotterdam ESHRE/ASRM-Sponsored PCOS Consensus Workshop Group. Revised 2003 consensus on diagnostic criteria and long-term health risks related to polycystic ovary syndrome. *Fertil Steril* 2004;81(1):19–25.
Adapted from Azziz R, Carmina E, Dewailly D, et al. The Androgen Excess and PCOS Society criteria for the polycystic ovary syndrome: the complete task force report. *Fertil Steril* 2009;91(2):456–488.

loss. The appropriate treatment of adolescents who do not desire pregnancy is a combined estrogen–progestin method—such as the pill, ring, or patch—to suppress ovarian or adrenal androgen production and to produce monthly menstrual bleeding. In adults, metformin has been used to treat PCOS by increasing peripheral tissue sensitivity to insulin. Spironolactone and other antiandrogenics have also been used in the treatment of PCOS. The practitioner should keep in mind that ovulatory cycles can potentially be restored with the use of metformin or antiandrogenics. Any adolescent who is sexually active with males should be counseled about contraceptive methods, regardless of whether she has PCOS or not.

Adrenal disorders. Nonclassic *congenital adrenal hyperplasia* is a rare cause of oligomenorrhea associated with hyperandrogenism. Though the patient may have signs of clitoromegaly on physical examination, it is usually indistinguishable clinically from PCOS and can be excluded by a normal 17-hydroxyprogesterone level in the morning during the follicular phase of the menstrual cycle. Other rare causes of oligomenorrhea, including *Cushing disease* and *ovarian and adrenal tumors,* should be suspected in patients with hirsutism accompanied by signs of glucocorticoid excess, or with rapidly developing, more severe virilization (male-pattern baldness, deepening of the voice, clitoromegaly), and in those with testosterone levels above 200 ng per dL.

Hypothalamic-Pituitary Axis Disorders

Caloric Insufficiency. Patients who have *insufficient caloric intake to meet energy expenditure* have an "energy drain" and commonly may experience oligomenorrhea or amenorrhea. There are various reasons why caloric intake may not be adequate: chronic diseases with increase metabolic rate, intestinal malabsorption problems, malnutrition and starvation due to unavailable food stores, or purposeful avoidance of food, such as in patients with eating disorders and in those who participate in high endurance sports or those that emphasize thinness.

Both leptin and ghrelin have been implicated as signals to the hypothalamic-pituitary system concerning overall energy balance. Regardless of the etiology of caloric insufficiency, the body's response is the same, shunting energy expenditure away from reproductive functions.

Accordingly, in assessing the nonpregnant adolescent with oligomenorrhea, one should inquire routinely about recent weight loss, chronic illness, behaviors characteristic of disordered eating, a restrictive eating pattern, and *strenuous exercise* (especially sports that put a premium on low body weight such as long-distance running, dance, and gymnastics). Many amenorrheic women who are athletes restrict their food intake; amenorrhea, disordered eating, and decreased bone mineral density together are termed "the female athletic triad."

Hyperprolactinemia. *Hyperprolactinemia* occurs in approximately 25% of adult women with secondary amenorrhea but is a much less common cause of oligomenorrhea in adolescents. Nevertheless, the possibility of hyperprolactinemia must be considered in all adolescents with oligomenorrhea because only 40% to 50% of hyperprolactinemic patients have spontaneous or expressible galactorrhea. Hyperprolactinemia can be a side effect of several commonly used medications (see Table 46.2). A pituitary adenoma is a rare, but important cause of hyperprolactinemia. In one retrospective review of teenagers with pituitary adenomas, over 50% of the females presented with either oligomenorrhea or secondary amenorrhea. Other central nervous system tumors should also be considered as a potential cause for hyperprolactinemia. The occasional patient with galactorrhea but with a normal prolactin level should be reevaluated periodically in an effort to identify a treatable cause of the problem.

Ovarian Disorders. Ovarian failure in adolescents may be caused by primary or acquired etiologies. Primary ovarian failure most commonly is due to gonadal dysgenesis from genetic causes, most commonly Turner syndrome. Secondary causes of premature ovarian failure include sequelae of chemotherapy, pelvic irradiation, or autoimmune disease. Ovarian tumors or other hormone-secreting tumors may result in ovarian failure. *Endometrial destruction* that results from overly vigorous curettage or pelvic tuberculosis is an exceedingly rare cause of oligomenorrhea.

Thyroid Disorders. *Hypothyroidism* and *hyperthyroidism* can both produce menstrual irregularities. The provider who sees a female patient presenting with either infrequent bleeding or excessive bleeding should have hypothyroidism and hyperthyroidism on the differential diagnosis.

Miscellaneous

Among adolescents who do not have overt signs of PCOS, hyperprolactinemia, or malnutrition, suppression of the hypothalamic-pituitary axis is the most common cause of oligomenorrhea that occurs more or persists for at least 2 years after menarche. Although oligomenorrhea in otherwise normal-appearing adolescents has historically been ascribed to psychosocial stressors (family disruption, moving, depression), many patients with apparently psychogenic menstrual irregularity prove on careful evaluation to have disordered eating patterns or nutritional deficits. It should be noted that diagnosis of stress as the cause of oligomenorrhea is one of exclusion.

Pseudocyesis is a rare cause of amenorrhea in women who believe they are pregnant and who exhibit many presumptive symptoms and signs of pregnancy, including nausea, vomiting, hyperpigmented areolae, galactorrhea, and abdominal distension. The diagnosis is made when a patient who insists that she is pregnant nevertheless has no true uterine enlargement, no demonstrable fetal parts or heart sounds, and a negative pregnancy test result. Psychiatric consultation should be obtained for such patients.

APPROACH TO DIAGNOSIS

Patients with oligomenorrhea but few other symptoms or signs of disease require laboratory evaluation to differentiate among the many potential causes of oligomenorrhea after pregnancy has been excluded. Figure 46.1 outlines a strategy for initial diagnostic evaluation. Determinations of serum levels of FSH, LH, testosterone and/or free testosterone, prolactin, and thyroid-stimulating hormone (TSH) are needed either to corroborate the suspected diagnosis or to categorize the patient whose history and physical examination have provided few diagnostic clues. Other laboratory tests should be performed as warranted by the clinical situation. The finding of a mildly elevated total or free testosterone level constitutes strong evidence for a diagnosis of PCOS. A total testosterone level of more than 200 ng per dL suggests an ovarian or adrenal tumor. An elevated prolactin level indicates a pituitary adenoma in patients who are not taking any of the drugs known to cause hyperprolactinemia and galactorrhea (Table 46.3). An elevated TSH level points to hypothyroidism either as the cause of oligomenorrhea or as a concomitant condition. FSH values of more than 40 mIU per mL confirm ovarian failure as the source of difficulty. If the laboratory evaluation discloses no abnormalities or only a low FSH level, the patient probably has one of the many conditions that cause hypothalamic-pituitary suppression. For definitive diagnosis, which may require additional laboratory testing, and for ongoing clinical management, all patients with oligomenorrhea should be referred to their primary care providers.

The administration of exogenous progestin is often used as an in vivo test of ovarian and endometrial function for oligomenorrheic patients. If the hypothalamic-pituitary axis is producing some gonadotropin, the ovaries are responding with some estradiol production, and the uterine endometrium is growing appropriately, then the addition of exogenous progestin (medroxyprogesterone acetate 10 mg per day for 7 days) will be followed by at least scanty menstrual bleeding within 7 days after the treatment is completed. This "withdrawal" flow, if it appears, provides the patient and her physician with tangible evidence of the basic integrity of these organs and the hypothalamic-pituitary-gonadal axis. For diagnosis in adolescents, however, laboratory investigation is much preferable to progestin administration. Keep in mind, however, that nearly all nonpregnant adolescents with oligomenorrhea will have a withdrawal bleed, and laboratory investigation may still be recommended. Appropriate follow-up at the primary care provider's office will be essential.

TABLE 46.3

PARTIAL LIST OF DRUGS THAT CAN CAUSE HYPERPROLACTINEMIA AND/OR GALACTORRHEA

1. *Antipsychotic and antidepressant agents*
   - Phenothiazines (e.g., chlorpromazine [Thorazine], clomipramine [Anafranil], fluphenazine [Prolixin], prochlorperazine [Compazine], thioridazine [Mellaril])
   - Haloperidol (Haldol)
   - Pimozide (Orap)
   - Risperidone (Risperdal)
   - Thiothixene (Navane)
2. *Drugs used to treat gastrointestinal disorders*
   - Cimetidine (Tagamet)
   - Metoclopramide (Reglan)
3. *Antihypertensive Agents*
   - Methyldopa (Aldomet)
   - Reserpine (Hydromox, Serpasil, others)
   - Verapamil (Calan, Isoptin)
4. *Opiates*
   - Codeine
   - Morphine

Suggested Readings and Key References

American Academy of Pediatrics, Committee on Adolescence, American College of Obstetricians and Gynecologists and Committee on Adolescent Health Care. Menstruation in girls and adolescents: using the menstrual cycle as a vital sign. *Pediatrics* 2006;118:2245–2250.

DiVasta AD, Emans SJ. Androgen abnormalities in the adolescent girl. In: Emans SJ, Laufer MR, Goldstein DP, eds. *Pediatric and adolescent gynecology*, 6th ed. Philadelphia, PA: Lippincott Williams & Wilkins, 2012:168–187.

Fraser IS, Critchley HO, Broder M, et al. The FIGO recommendations on terminologies and definitions for normal and abnormal uterine bleeding. *Semin Reprod Med* 2011;29(5):383–390.

Hillard PJ. Menstruation in adolescents: what's normal, what's not. *Ann N Y Acad Sci* 2008;1135:29–35.

O'Brien RF, Emans SJ. Polycystic ovary syndrome in adolescents. *J Pediatr Adolesc Gynecol* 2008;21:119–128.

Paradise JE. Evaluation of oligomenorrhea in adolescence. UpToDate Version 17.2. http://www.uptodate.com. Accessed October 13, 2009.

The American College of Obstetricians and Gynecologists. Practice bulletin: diagnosis of abnormal uterine bleeding in reproductive-aged women. *Obstet Gynecol* 2012;120(1):197–206.

Wiksten-Almstromer M, Hirschberg AL, Hagenfeldt K. Prospective follow-up of menstrual disorders in adolescence and prognostic factors. *Acta Obstet Gynecol Scand* 2008;87(11):1162–1168.

CHAPTER 47 ■ ORAL LESIONS

MARISSA A. HENDRICKSON, MD AND MARK G. ROBACK, MD

Children of all ages experience oral lesions, representing a wide range of illnesses. Lesions range from benign and self-resolving to indicative of life-threatening diseases. Many oral lesions, both congenital and acquired, are localized. However, lesions associated with systemic disease must also be considered (Fig. 47.1 and Table 47.1). Most often, patients with isolated complaints (e.g., a mouth sore or mass, drooling, pain, fever) are found to have common, self-limited conditions (Table 47.2). However, a complete history and physical examination is essential for all patients with oral lesions to rule out systemic and potentially life-threatening diseases (Table 47.3) that may present initially with isolated mouth findings.

PATHOPHYSIOLOGY

Oral lesions may result from localized or systemic pathophysiologic processes. Localized causes include congenital masses and cysts, infectious diseases, and oral tumors. Systemic illnesses with prominent oral involvement include a number of infectious, inflammatory, and toxin-mediated conditions. Given the broad spectrum of illnesses presenting with oral lesions, it is convenient to discuss individual causes under specific headings within the differential diagnosis. Several conditions with typical oral lesions exist that do not comfortably fit under any of these headings; these are discussed in the section on miscellaneous oral lesions.

DIFFERENTIAL DIAGNOSIS

Congenital Oral Lesions

Most oral lesions present at birth or in early infancy represent benign findings. Patients are largely asymptomatic, and the lesions resolve spontaneously.

Epstein pearls occur in more than 60% of newborns as small, white milia in the midline of the hard palate. These epithelial inclusion cysts are often found in clusters and resolve over the first few months of life. Epithelial pearls are similar to Epstein pearls and appear as shiny, small, white, self-limited lesions that occur on the gums.

Bohn nodules are also self-limited cysts that appear on the mandibular or maxillary dental ridges. Dental lamina cysts occur on the alveolar ridge of newborns and stem from trapped remnants of the dental lamina.

Natal teeth are prematurely erupted primary teeth present at birth; teeth erupting within the first month of life are termed neonatal teeth. These teeth are either supernumerary or true deciduous teeth and are usually found in the lower incisor region. Natal teeth may lead to ulcerations of the underside of the tongue, called Riga–Fede disease.

Patients with ankyloglossia may be referred to as "tongue tied" because of congenital shortening of the lingual frenum, which limits their ability to fully extend the tongue. Surgical correction is considered for patients when speech or feeding is affected.

Epulis is a congenital, fibrous, sarcomatous tumor that arises from the periosteum of the mandible or maxilla. The mass is firm and pedunculated and may regress spontaneously. Excision is required if the epulis interferes with feeding or breathing, or for cosmetic reasons.

Lymphangioma is a benign congenital tumor of lymphatic vessels that can appear on the tongue, lips, or buccal mucosa at birth or in early infancy. Hemangiomas are benign vascular malformations present at birth that may become more apparent as the patient grows. Oral hemangiomas are typically accompanied by vascular lesions internally and on the patient's skin.

White sponge nevus is an autosomal-dominant condition presenting with white, raised, folded-appearing tissue most commonly found on buccal mucosa. It may be mistaken for candidiasis.

Infectious Oral Lesions

Infectious oral lesions are most commonly viral in origin but may be caused by bacterial or fungal infections as well (see Chapter 102 Infectious Disease Emergencies).

Candidiasis, or thrush, is white plaque on the buccal mucosa, gingivae, and palate that cannot be removed with gentle scraping. Caused by *Candida albicans,* thrush is common in neonates and infants. Thrush outside of infancy should prompt consideration of the patient's immune status, as it is more common in patients infected with human immunodeficiency virus (HIV) or those who are otherwise immunosuppressed.

The typical lesions of herpes simplex virus (HSV) are groups of vesicles and erosions on erythematous bases in and around the mouth. Herpes gingivostomatitis, most commonly caused by HSV type 1 (HSV-1), represents primary infection and typically occurs in young children and infants. These patients have pain, fever, and drooling. Recurrent disease commonly manifests as herpes labialis or "cold sores." This consists of painful lesions that occur on the lips, most often the lower lip. Herpes labialis may be triggered by an acute febrile illness, sun exposure, or stress.

Hand, foot, and mouth disease is characterized by discrete shallow erosions in the mouth, especially on the soft palate, erythematous papulovesicular lesions on the hands and feet, and often high fevers. It is generally caused by enteroviruses, particularly coxsackievirus, and is self-limited. Herpangina is a similar infection, commonly caused by group A coxsackievirus. It is characterized by pharyngeal vesicles as well as fever, muscle aches, and malaise. Treatment in both cases is supportive, with antipyretics, topical and systemic analgesics, and attention to hydration.

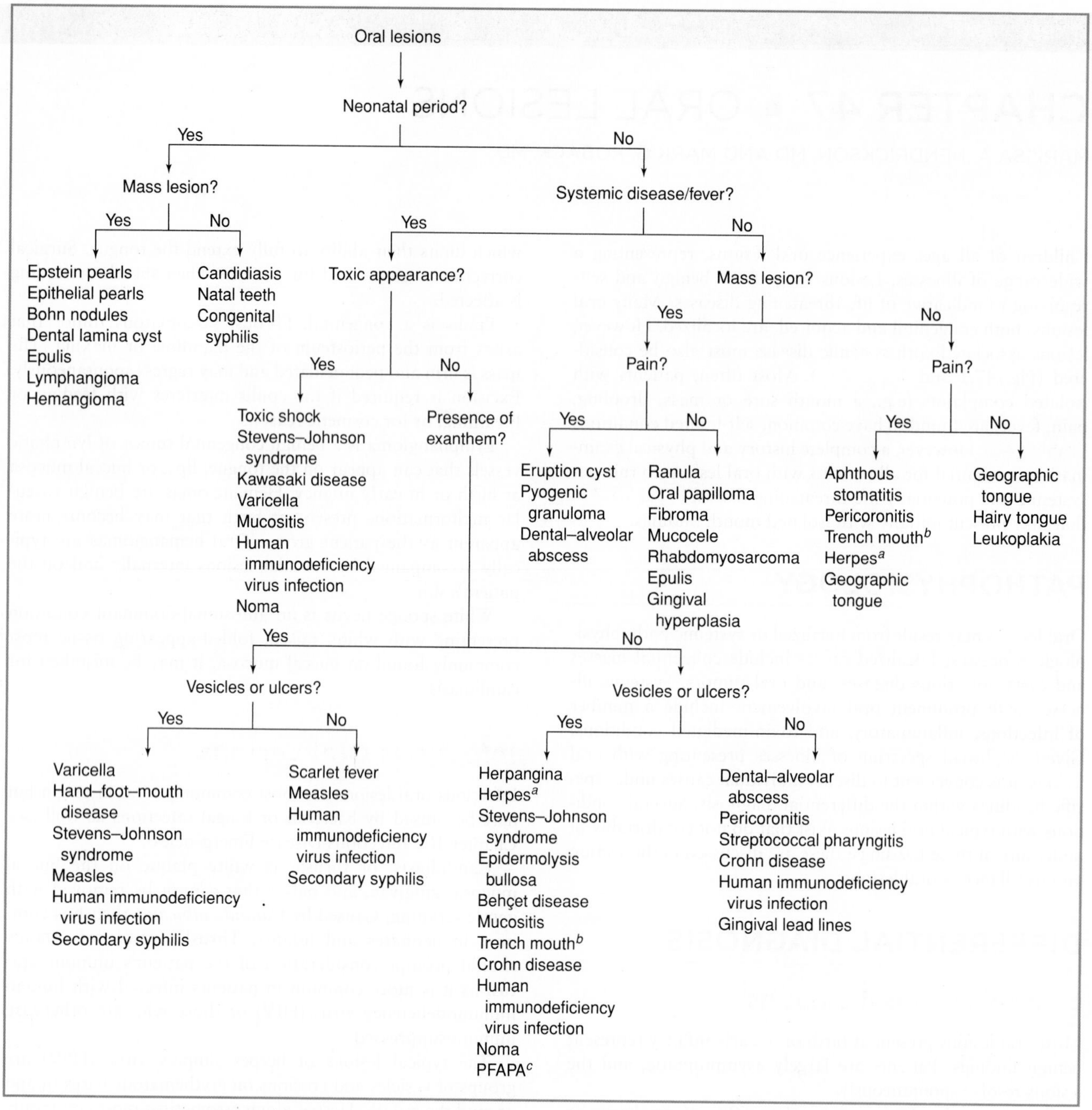

- Oral lesions → Neonatal period?
  - Yes → Mass lesion?
    - Yes: Epstein pearls; Epithelial pearls; Bohn nodules; Dental lamina cyst; Epulis; Lymphangioma; Hemangioma
    - No: Candidiasis; Natal teeth; Congenital syphilis
  - No → Systemic disease/fever?
    - Yes → Toxic appearance?
      - Yes: Toxic shock; Stevens–Johnson syndrome; Kawasaki disease; Varicella; Mucositis; Human immunodeficiency virus infection; Noma
      - No → Presence of exanthem?
        - Yes → Vesicles or ulcers?
          - Yes: Varicella; Hand–foot–mouth disease; Stevens–Johnson syndrome; Measles; Human immunodeficiency virus infection; Secondary syphilis
          - No: Scarlet fever; Measles; Human immunodeficiency virus infection; Secondary syphilis
        - No → Vesicles or ulcers?
          - Yes: Herpangina; Herpes[a]; Stevens–Johnson syndrome; Epidermolysis bullosa; Behçet disease; Mucositis; Trench mouth[b]; Crohn disease; Human immunodeficiency virus infection; Noma; PFAPA[c]
          - No: Dental–alveolar abscess; Pericoronitis; Streptococcal pharyngitis; Crohn disease; Human immunodeficiency virus infection; Gingival lead lines
    - No → Mass lesion?
      - Yes → Pain?
        - Yes: Eruption cyst; Pyogenic granuloma; Dental–alveolar abscess
        - No: Ranula; Oral papilloma; Fibroma; Mucocele; Rhabdomyosarcoma; Epulis; Gingival hyperplasia
      - No → Pain?
        - Yes: Aphthous stomatitis; Pericoronitis; Trench mouth[b]; Herpes[a]; Geographic tongue
        - No: Geographic tongue; Hairy tongue; Leukoplakia

FIGURE 47.1 Oral lesions. [a]Herpes gingivostomatitis or labialis. [b]Trench mouth, acute necrotizing ulcerative gingivitis. [c]PFAPA, *p*eriodic *f*ever, *a*phthous stomatitis, *p*haryngitis, and cervical *a*denitis syndrome.

Group A streptococcal pharyngitis can present with a characteristic "strawberry tongue," the result of hypertrophic red papillae on a thick white coat. Posterior pharyngeal findings include tonsillar hyperemia, hypertrophy, and exudate, as well as palatal petechiae (Fig. 47.2). If a "sandpaper" papular rash on a blanching erythematous base is present, most commonly on the trunk, the condition is termed scarlet fever.

Koplik spots are pinpoint white macules on markedly erythematous mucous membranes, occurring during the prodrome of measles, which includes cough, coryza, conjunctivitis, and fever. They generally resolve before the characteristic rash occurs.

Varicella lesions occurring in the mouth result in painful vesicles, which may become unroofed, on an erythematous base. Patients may be reluctant to swallow because of pain. Unless secondary bacterial infection occurs, these lesions are self-limited.

Oral lesions will be the initial presenting sign in approximately half of children with perinatally acquired HIV infection. Common lesions include oral candidiasis, parotid enlargement, herpes simplex vesicles or erosions, hairy leukoplakia, aphthous ulcers, linear gingival erythema, and necrotizing ulcerative gingivitis. Blue, purple, or red macules, papules, or nodules on the palate suggest oral Kaposi sarcoma, whereas diffuse swelling, discrete nodules, or ulcers of any oral mucosal surface may indicate non-Hodgkin lymphoma, although both are rare in children. Highly active antiviral therapy decreases the prevalence of oral lesions;

TABLE 47.1

DIFFERENTIAL DIAGNOSIS OF ORAL LESIONS

Congenital oral lesions	Tumorous oral lesions
Epstein pearls	Eruption cyst
Epithelial pearls	Oral papilloma
Bohn nodules	Fibroma
Dental lamina cysts	Mucocele
Natal teeth	Ranula
Ankyloglossia	Pyogenic granuloma
Epulis (gum boil)	Peripheral ossifying fibroma
Lymphangioma	Peripheral giant cell granuloma
Hemangioma	Melanotic neuroectodermal tumor of infancy
White sponge nevus	Rhabdomyosarcoma
Infectious oral lesions	**Oral lesions associated with systemic disease**
Candidiasis	Stevens–Johnson syndrome
Herpes simplex	Toxic shock syndrome
Gingivostomatitis—primary	Mucositis
Labialis—recurrent (cold sores)	Palatal mucormycosis
Hand–foot–mouth disease	Kawasaki disease
Herpangina	Crohn disease
Scarlet fever	Behçet syndrome
Streptococcal pharyngitis	Epidermolysis bullosa
Measles	Angular cheilitis
Varicella	**Miscellaneous oral lesions**
Human immunodeficiency virus infection	Aphthous stomatitis (including as part of PFAPA)
Dental–alveolar abscess	Geographic tongue
Pericoronitis	Gingival hyperplasia
Acute necrotizing ulcerative gingivitis (trench mouth)	Leukoplakia
Noma	Frictional keratosis
Syphilis	Linea alba
Acquired (secondary)	Peutz–Jeghers syndrome
Congenital	Melanotic nevi
Hairy tongue	

PFAPA, periodic fever, aphthous stomatitis, pharyngitis, and cervical adenitis.

increasing lesions may indicate low CD4 percentage and advancing disease.

The pain, erythema, and gingival swelling of dental–alveolar abscesses may be associated with loosening or extrusion of the associated tooth. Patients may also develop fever, significant lymphadenopathy, and facial cellulitis. Streptococci and anaerobes are common causes. Antibiotic therapy with penicillin or clindamycin is considered first-line therapy, though amoxicillin with or without clavulanate may be more palatable in suspension form. Antibiotics are secondary in importance to drainage of the abscess.

Pericoronitis is the local infection of the gingiva surrounding an erupting tooth. Although antibiotic therapy may be required, good oral hygiene is essential. Lymphadenopathy and facial swelling may accompany pericoronitis.

Acute necrotizing ulcerative gingivitis (ANUG), also called trench mouth or Vincent angina, is a spirochetal infection of the gingiva that occurs in adolescents. Patients report tender,

TABLE 47.2

COMMON CAUSES OF ORAL LESIONS

Candidiasis
Aphthous stomatitis
Herpes simplex
Gingivostomatitis—primary
Labialis—recurrent
Hand–foot–mouth disease
Herpangina

TABLE 47.3

LIFE-THREATENING CAUSES OF ORAL LESIONS

Stevens–Johnson syndrome
Kawasaki disease
Toxic shock syndrome
Human immunodeficiency virus infection
Noma (cancrum oris)

SIGNS AND SYMPTOMS

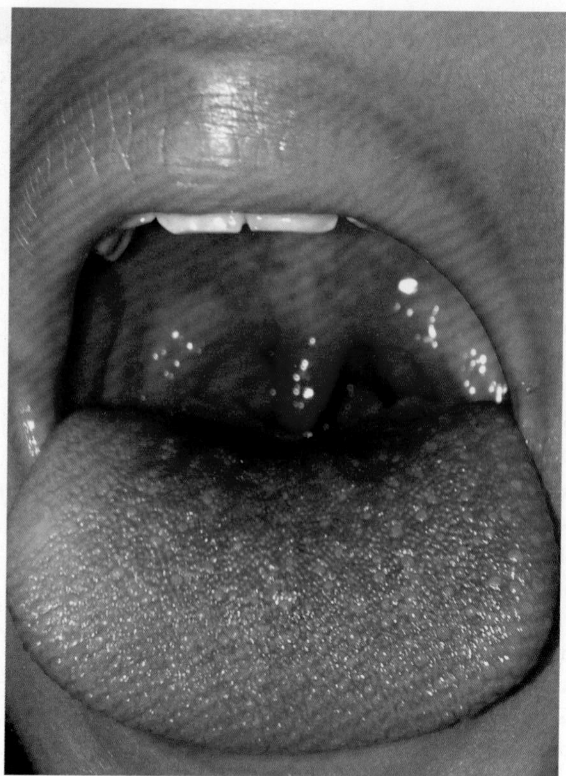

FIGURE 47.2 Palatal petechiae in streptococcal pharyngitis.

bleeding gums and fetid breath. Gums are hyperemic and appear "punched out" due to tissue loss between the teeth. Treatment involves attention to oral hygiene, mouth rinses with a dilute hydrogen peroxide solution, oral antibiotics, and in some cases debridement of necrotic tissue.

Noma, or cancrum oris, is a potentially fatal, gangrenous anaerobic infection of the oral cavity that may rapidly spread outward to involve large areas of the face. It typically begins as an oral mucosal ulcer or as ANUG, particularly after a bout of measles or other intercurrent illness in malnourished or immunocompromised patients. Currently, it is being recognized increasingly in HIV-infected and/or otherwise malnourished children in sub-Saharan Africa.

The oral lesions of congenital syphilis may not become obvious until several months of age. Erythematous papules can be seen in the mouth and other mucocutaneous sites. *Hutchinson teeth,* peg-shaped upper central incisors, present later in life. The secondary stage of acquired syphilis is characterized by patches of ulcers or raised lesions in the mouth and is seen in association with generalized rash, fever, malaise, and adenopathy.

Patients receiving long-term antibiotic therapy may develop elongation of filiform papillae of the dorsum of the tongue and a "hairy" appearance from fungal overgrowth called hairy tongue. Hairy leukoplakia of the lateral aspects of the tongue is found in HIV-infected patients in association with intraepithelial proliferation of Epstein–Barr virus infection.

Tumorous Oral Lesions

The vast majority of tumorous oral lesions in children are self-limited and benign in nature. Congenital oral lesions such as hemangioma, lymphangioma, and epulis have been considered previously.

Eruption cysts are associated with the eruption of teeth, appear on the alveolar ridge, and may contain blood.

Oral papillomas are finger-like extensions from the epithelium of the tongue, gums, lips, or buccal mucosa, commonly caused by human papilloma virus. They are typically benign, although a small percentage may become malignant.

A fibroma is a benign, smooth mass with a sessile base that frequently develops secondary to soft tissue injury from minor trauma. The tongue, lips, buccal mucosa, and palate are common sites for the development of fibromas.

Peripheral ossifying fibroma is a benign neoplasm found on the gingiva, likely arising from cells in the periodontal ligament and the periosteum. They appear as sessile nodules, and may be soft or firm. Recurrence after surgical resection is common. Peripheral giant cell granuloma is a similar lesion that may be found on the lingual or buccal aspect of the interdental papillae. Typical size is approximately 2 cm, and surgical excision and curettage is required.

Mucoceles are soft, well-demarcated masses that arise secondary to obstruction of salivary glands. Symptoms are minimal, but excision or marsupialization is typically required.

Ranula is a retention cyst or mucocele of the submaxillary or sublingual duct (Fig. 47.3). Ranulas are typically seen on the underside of the tongue or the floor of the mouth. Many of these lesions will resolve spontaneously, however persistence or repeated recurrence requires surgical resection.

Pyogenic granuloma represents granulation tissue that develops in response to an irritant such as trauma or a foreign body. Most commonly found on the gingiva, pyogenic granulomas are also found on the tongue, lips, and buccal mucosa. Treatment involves incision and drainage. Recurrence is common, especially when a foreign body is present.

Melanotic neuroectodermal tumor of infancy is a benign but rapidly growing osteolytic pigmented lesion, of neural crest

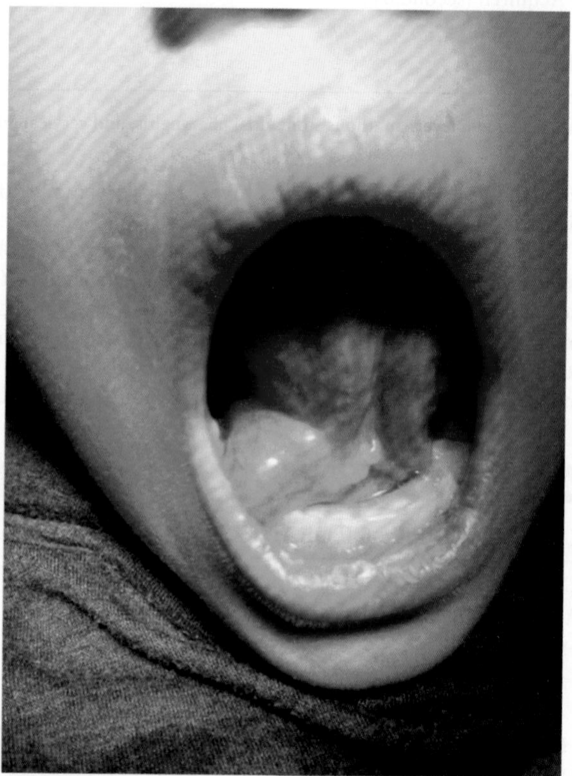

FIGURE 47.3 Ranula.

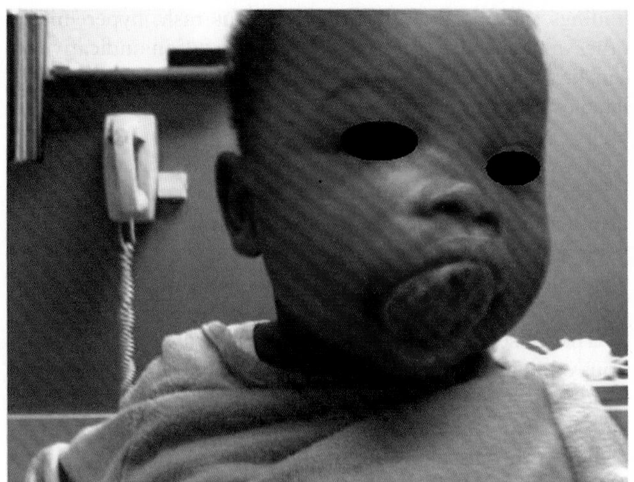

FIGURE 47.4 Melanotic neuroectodermal tumor of infancy.

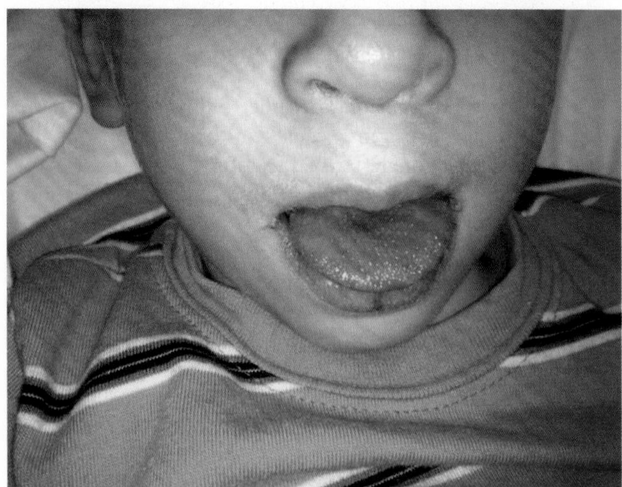

FIGURE 47.5 Strawberry tongue and cracked lips in Kawasaki disease.

origin, most commonly presenting between 1 and 6 months of age (Fig. 47.4). It appears as a blue or black lobulated sessile mass, often arising from the maxilla. Surgical treatment is usually curative.

Rhabdomyosarcoma is a rare malignant tumor that can present in the oral cavity. These lesions are typically ulcerative, fast growing, and may present with bleeding. Associated signs and symptoms are usually attributed to the mass lesion or obstructive sequelae. Other malignant oral tumors such as fibrosarcoma, carcinoma of the parotid, and osteosarcoma occur but are even rarer than rhabdomyosarcoma.

Oral Lesions Associated with Systemic Disease

Stevens–Johnson syndrome is a potentially life-threatening illness involving necrosis and detachment of the epidermis of skin and mucous membranes. It is most commonly triggered by medications, although infection may also be implicated. Oral lesions include erythema, erosions, scabs, and pseudomembranes often preceded by a prodrome of fever, malaise, and dysphagia. Removal of the offending medication is key, followed by intensive supportive care.

Toxic shock syndrome is a toxin-mediated disease that has oral manifestations including oropharyngeal erythema and strawberry tongue as well as systemic findings such as diffuse erythematous macular exanthem, hyperemic mucous membranes, fever, and shock. It is commonly caused by group A streptococci and by *Staphylococcus aureus* which may be associated with tampon use or nasal colonization. Patients may progress to septic shock.

Mucositis presents as ulcers, exudate, and pseudomembranes on the gingivae and buccal mucosa of patients with neutropenia often secondary to chemotherapy. Lesions are extremely painful, and the breath becomes fetid. Patients with hematologic malignancies or history of stem cell transplantation are at risk for the life-threatening fungal infection palatal mucormycosis, most commonly presenting as a black necrotic patch on the hard palate.

Kawasaki disease is a potentially life-threatening disorder that typically presents with an array of findings, including prolonged fever, rash, lymphadenopathy, nonpurulent conjunctivitis, and erythema or edema of the hands and feet. Oral changes include red, dry, cracked lips, erythematous oropharynx, and strawberry tongue (Fig. 47.5). Therapy is focused on prevention of coronary aneurysms.

The inflammatory lesions of Crohn disease may occur in any portion of the gastrointestinal tract. Oral lesions, seen most often in adolescents and young adults, include ulcers, polypoid papulous hyperplastic mucosa, and edema of the lips, gingiva, vestibular sulci, and buccal mucosa. Chronic, recurrent ulcers surrounded by erythema and gray exudate are found throughout the oral cavity in patients with Behçet syndrome. Genitourinary and skin lesions also occur. Behçet syndrome is rare, affecting older children and adolescents, usually boys.

More than 15 types of hereditary epidermolysis bullosa have been described. This rare, vesiculobullous condition affects mucous membranes and teeth, as well as the skin. Scarring may lead to restriction of mouth opening.

The painful cracking and erythema at the bilateral oral commissures of angular cheilitis may be due to nutritional deficiencies of riboflavin, folate, or iron, or due to infections, allergies, physical irritation, or bruxism. Treatment varies based on cause; antifungals may be helpful.

Miscellaneous Oral Lesions

Aphthous stomatitis is a painful, localized, self-limited ulceration of the oral epidermis of unknown cause. Lesions typically present as 5- to 10-mm ulcerations with a rim of erythema on the buccal mucosa, lips, and lateral aspect of the tongue. Patients are usually afebrile. Spontaneous resolution occurs in 7 to 10 days, but recurrence is common.

Less commonly, aphthous stomatitis also occurs with a constellation of symptoms seen in the syndrome of PFAPA (*p*eriodic *f*ever, *a*phthous stomatitis, *p*haryngitis, and cervical *a*denitis). Children with PFAPA are usually between 2 and 6 years of age, and experience episodes of 4 or 5 days of high fevers along with aphthous stomatitis, pharyngitis, and cervical adenitis recurring every 2 to 8 weeks. Although the episodes resolve spontaneously, there has been some reported benefit in symptom control with use of glucocorticoids, and tonsillectomy may prevent recurrence. Etiology is unknown, and there are no long-term effects.

Geographic tongue, or benign migratory glossitis, represents a benign inflammatory disorder that results in migratory smooth annular patches on the tongue. Although typically asymptomatic, patients may complain of pain. No treatment is required.

Traumatic tooth brushing or other habits leading to friction on the oral mucosa may cause white or gray lesions that may be smooth or rough, termed frictional keratosis. Lesions are most commonly found on the buccal mucosa and resolve with removal of the irritant.

Gingival hyperplasia seen in patients receiving long-term anticonvulsant therapy with phenytoin is irreversible. However, gingival overgrowth that occurs in association with the medications cyclosporine and nifedipine is reversible with discontinuation of the drugs. Poor dental hygiene appears to play a role in the cause. The gingivae undergo fibrous enlargement but are not inflamed or painful. Gingival fibromatosis is an inherited form of gingival hyperplasia.

Painless, leathery, white patches or plaques termed leukoplakia may develop in areas of long-term smokeless tobacco exposure. This is typically found on the mucosa of the buccal sulcus, and may result in dysplasia or carcinoma.

Linea alba is a sharply demarcated white line on the buccal mucosa opposite the plane of dental occlusion. It is a benign finding present in up to 5% of adolescents.

Areas of brown or black hyperpigmentation may be physiologic in patients with darker skin. Localized brown, blue, gray, or black macules or papules, most commonly on the hard palate, may represent melanotic nevi. These are often treated with excisional biopsy to rule out mucosal melanoma. The finding of multiple intraoral and perioral hyperpigmentations should prompt consideration of Peutz–Jeghers syndrome, an autosomal-dominant condition which requires referral to a gastroenterologist because of an increased risk of gastric malignancies.

EVALUATION AND DECISION

When evaluating patients with complaints of oral lesions, it is important to consider a myriad of associated signs and symptoms while taking a complete history and performing the physical examination. The patient's age, general health and appearance, presence of an exanthem or fever, and whether the lesions are painful must be considered. Once the presence of lesions is noted, they should be further characterized by color, type, and location and considered in the context of any additional physical findings.

Toxic-appearing patients require immediate evaluation for potentially life-threatening disease. Patients with Kawasaki disease or toxic shock syndrome (Table 47.3) have associated findings such as fever, diffuse cutaneous rash, hyperemia of other mucous membranes, or poor perfusion indicative of shock. However, Stevens–Johnson syndrome may cause isolated oral lesions initially and then rapidly progress to systemic involvement.

Once life-threatening causes have been considered, careful history and physical examination may lead to the diagnosis of other systemic diseases. Weight loss, abdominal pain, and diarrhea with or without blood loss suggest Crohn disease, whereas genital ulceration in an adolescent boy points to Behçet syndrome or secondary syphilis.

The presence of rash and fever makes disorders of infectious etiology more likely. Measles, varicella, scarlet fever, and hand–foot–mouth disease are generally diagnosed by history and physical examination alone. Laboratory evaluation might include a throat culture for streptococci and serologic testing for measles or HIV when these infections are suspected.

Infectious causes of oral lesions without exanthem may display obvious findings such as cachexia and alopecia in the neutropenic patient with mucositis, or they may be relatively localized to the oropharynx as in herpangina, herpes gingivostomatitis or labialis, and dental infections, which may or may not cause fever and lymphadenopathy.

Oral lesions without overt signs of systemic disease are mostly congenital or tumorous in nature. With the exception of candidiasis, lesions found in the newborn and during infancy are largely self-limited and most will resolve spontaneously. A few congenital lesions, including lymphangioma, hemangioma, and congenital epulis, may require intervention.

Children and adolescents experience an array of oral lesions not associated with signs of systemic disease that are typically further delineated by considering the type of lesion (i.e., mass, vesicle, ulcer) and whether they are painful. Most of these processes require little or no therapy, although rhabdomyosarcoma and other malignancies are obvious exceptions to this observation.

Suggested Readings and Key References

Bentley JM, Barankin B, Guenther LC. A review of common pediatric lip lesions: herpes simplex/recurrent herpes labialis, impetigo, mucoceles, and hemangiomas. *Clin Pediatr* 2003;42:475–482.

Esmeili T, Lozada-Nur F, Epstein J. Common benign oral soft tissue masses. *Dent Clin North Am* 2005;49:223–240.

Patel NJ, Sciubba J. Oral lesions in young children. *Pediatr Clin North Am* 2003;50:469–486.

Patton LL. Oral lesions associated with human immunodeficiency virus disease. *Dent Clin North Am* 2013;57:673–698.

Pinto A, Haberland CM, Baker S. Pediatric soft tissue oral lesions. *Dent Clin North Am* 2014;58:437–453.

CHAPTER 48 ■ PAIN: ABDOMEN

VINCENZO MANIACI, MD AND MARK I. NEUMAN, MD, MPH

Abdominal pain is a common complaint of children who seek care in the ED. Although most children with acute abdominal pain have self-limiting conditions, the presence of pain may herald a serious medical or surgical emergency. The diverse etiologies include acute surgical diseases (e.g., appendicitis, intussusception, strangulated hernia, trauma to solid or hollow organ), intra-abdominal nonsurgical ailments (e.g., gastroenteritis, urinary tract infection [UTI], gastric ulcer disease, gastroesophageal reflux disease), extra-abdominal conditions (e.g., pneumonia, pharyngitis, contusions of the abdominal musculature or soft tissue), systemic illnesses (e.g., "viral syndrome," leukemia, diabetic ketoacidosis, vasoocclusive crisis from sickle cell anemia), and, commonly, functional abdominal pain. Making a timely diagnosis of an acute abdomen, such as appendicitis or volvulus, early enough to reduce the rate of complications, particularly in infants and young children, often proves challenging.

PATHOPHYSIOLOGY

Abdominal pain can be stimulated by at least three neural pathways: visceral, somatic, and referred. Visceral pain generally is a dull, aching sensation caused by distention of a viscus that stimulates nerves locally and initiates an impulse that travels through autonomic afferent fibers to the spinal tract and central nervous system. The nerve fibers from different abdominal organs overlap and are bilateral, accounting for the lack of specificity to the discomfort. Children perceive the sensation of visceral pain generally in one of three areas: the epigastric, periumbilical, or suprapubic region. Somatic pain usually is well localized and intense (often sharp) in character. It is carried by somatic nerves in the parietal peritoneum, muscle, or skin unilaterally to the spinal cord level from T6 to L1. An intra-abdominal process will manifest somatic pain if the affected viscus introduces an inflammatory process that touches the innervated organ. Referred pain is felt at a location distant from the diseased organ and can be either a sharp, localized sensation or a vague ache. Afferent nerves from different sites, such as the parietal pleura of the lung and the abdominal wall, share pathways centrally. All three types of pain may be modified by the child's level of tolerance. Individual variation exists such that some children with an appendiceal abscess will appear to have minimal pain, whereas other children with a functional etiology of their abdominal pain will appear quite distressed.

A number of illnesses that present with abdominal pain including conditions such as tonsillitis with high fever, viral syndromes, and streptococcal pharyngitis cannot be readily explained neurophysiologically as the triggers of abdominal pain. Despite the appearance of localized abdominal pain, clinicians need to perform a thorough physical examination that should include the assessment of the oropharynx, lung, skin, and genitourinary system. The principal causes of abdominal pain in children and adolescents are summarized in Table 48.1. Table 48.2 highlights the life-threatening disorders.

DIFFERENTIAL DIAGNOSIS

Intra-abdominal injuries can be life-threatening (such as hemorrhage from solid organ laceration or fluid loss and infection from perforated hollow viscus) and rarely may occur after minor trauma. An accurate history may not always be provided and, thus, clinicians must specifically inquire about a history of trauma in a child presenting with acute abdominal pain. Typical mechanisms include motor vehicle crashes, falls, and child abuse (see Chapter 111 Abdominal Trauma).

Bowel obstruction may occur as a result of adhesions in a child with previous abdominal surgery. Malrotation with volvulus, and necrotizing enterocolitis, should be considered in neonates with bilious emesis. Intussusception typically occurs among children 2 months to 2 years of age. Colicky abdominal pain is a typical feature of intussusception. The presence of blood in the stool, or "currant jelly stool," is a relatively late finding among children with intussusception.

Among children of all ages, appendicitis can cause peritoneal irritation and focal tenderness. It occurs most commonly in children older than 5 years. The classic history of diffuse abdominal pain that later migrates to the right lower abdomen is not always elicited. The diagnosis of appendicitis in younger children can be more difficult and is often made later in the course of disease; as such, the rate of perforation in younger children is higher (see Clinical Pathway Chapter 83 Appendicitis (Suspected) and Chapter 124 Abdominal Emergencies for further information). Primary bacterial peritonitis is an uncommon cause of abdominal pain among children, but should be considered among children with nephrotic syndrome or liver failure.

Common conditions that are associated with acute abdominal pain include viral gastroenteritis, systemic viral illness, streptococcal pharyngitis, lobar pneumonia, and UTIs. Frequent causes of chronic or recurrent abdominal pain include colic (among young infants) and constipation. Other gastrointestinal (GI) conditions that may present with abdominal pain include inflammatory bowel disease (more often Chron's disease than ulcerative colitis), cholecystitis (more common among children with predisposing conditions such as hemolytic anemia or cystic fibrosis or among older adolescents), pancreatitis, dietary protein allergy (typically in infants), malabsorption, and intra-abdominal abscesses (most commonly observed in children with perforated appendicitis).

Incarcerated inguinal hernia is an extra-abdominal cause of abdominal pain that can be life-threatening. A careful genitourinary examination should be performed in all children with abdominal pain. Myocarditis and pericarditis are rare extra-abdominal causes of abdominal pain. Systemic life-threatening

TABLE 48.1

CAUSES OF ACUTE ABDOMINAL PAIN

<2 yrs	2–5 yrs	6–12 yrs	>12 yrs
Common			
Colic (age <3 mo)	Acute gastroenteritis	Acute gastroenteritis	Acute gastroenteritis
GERD	UTI	Trauma	Gastritis
	Trauma		
Acute gastroenteritis	Appendicitis	Appendicitis	Colitis
Viral syndromes	Pneumonia, asthma	UTI	GERD
	Sickle cell disease	Functional abdominal pain	Trauma
	"Viral syndromes"	Sickle cell disease	Constipation
	Constipation	Constipation	Appendicitis
		"Viral syndromes"	Pelvic inflammatory disease
			UTI
			Pneumonia, asthma
			"Viral syndromes"
			Dysmenorrhea
			Epididymitis
			Lactose intolerance
			Sickle cell disease
			Mittelschmerz
Less common			
Trauma (possible child abuse)	Meckel diverticulum (usually painless)	Pneumonia, asthma, cystic fibrosis	Ectopic pregnancy
Intussusception	Henoch–Schönlein purpura	Inflammatory bowel disease	Testicular torsion
		Peptic ulcer disease	Ovarian torsion
Incarcerated hernia	Toxin	Cholecystitis, pancreatic disease	Renal calculi
Sickle cell disease	Cystic fibrosis	Diabetes mellitus	Peptic ulcer disease
Milk protein allergy	Intussusception	Collagen vascular disease	Hepatitis
	Nephrotic syndrome	Testicular torsion	Cholecystitis or pancreatic disease
			Meconium ileus (cystic fibrosis)
			Collagen vascular disease
			Inflammatory bowel disease
			Toxin
Very uncommon or rare			
Appendicitis	Incarcerated hernia	Rheumatic fever	Rheumatic fever
Volvulus	Neoplasm	Toxin	Malignancy
Malignancy (e.g., Wilms tumor)		Renal calculi	Abdominal abscess
Toxin (heavy metal—Pb)	Rheumatic fever, myocarditis, pericarditis	Malignancy	
Malabsorptive syndromes	Hepatitis	Ovarian torsion	
	Inflammatory bowel disease	Meconium ileus (cystic fibrosis)	
	Choledochal cyst	Intussusception	
	Hemolytic anemia		
	Diabetes mellitus		
	Porphyria		

GERD, gastroesophageal reflux disease; UTI, urinary tract infection.
Modified from Liebman W, Thaler M. Pediatric considerations of abdominal pain and the acute abdomen. In: Sleisenger M, Fortran J, eds. *Gastrointestinal disease*. Philadelphia, PA: WB Saunders, 1978.

conditions that can be associated with abdominal pain include diabetic ketoacidosis and hemolytic uremic syndrome. Other extra-abdominal conditions in which abdominal pain is often present include the following: Henoch–Schönlein purpura (usually with a distinctive purpuric rash over the lower extremities and buttock), vasoocclusive crisis with sickle cell syndromes, testicular torsion, urolithiasis (typically with colicky pain and flank tenderness), and toxic ingestions (such as lead or iron).

Functional abdominal pain should be considered among children with recurrent abdominal pain, but should be a

TABLE 48.2

LIFE-THREATENING CAUSES OF ACUTE ABDOMINAL PAIN

<2 yrs	2–5 yrs	6–12 yrs	>12 yrs
Abdominal			
Malrotation/volvulus	Trauma	Trauma	Trauma
Intussusception	Intussusception	Appendicitis	Ectopic pregnancy
Trauma (possible child abuse)	Appendicitis	Megacolon (from inflammatory bowel disease)	Appendicitis
Severe gastroenteritis	Incarcerated hernia	Peptic ulcer disease (with perforation)	Intra-abdominal abscess secondary to pelvic inflammatory disease, cholecystitis, appendicitis, inflammatory bowel disease
Incarcerated hernia	Meckel diverticulum	Peritonitis (primary or secondary)	Peptic ulcer disease—bleeding or perforation
Hirschsprung disease	Obstruction secondary to prior abdominal surgery	Aortic aneurysm	Pancreatitis
Appendicitis Malignancy (e.g., Wilms tumor) Necrotizing enterocolitis	Peritonitis (i.e., primary, nephrosis)	Acute, fulminant hepatitis	Megacolon (from inflammatory bowel disease) Aortic aneurysm Acute fulminant hepatitis
Nonabdominal			
Heart disease (myocarditis, pericarditis)	Toxic overdose[a] Hemolytic uremic syndrome	Toxic overdose[a]	Collagen vascular disease
Metabolic acidosis due to inborn errors of metabolism	Diabetic ketoacidosis Sepsis	Sepsis	Diabetes mellitus (infection or ketoacidosis)
Toxic overdose Sepsis Hemolytic uremic syndrome	Myocarditis, pericarditis	Diabetic ketoacidosis Collagen vascular disease	Drug abuse/overdose

[a]Alcohol, amphetamines, aspirin, insecticide, iron, lead, phencyclidine, plants, etc.

diagnosis of exclusion. The pain rarely occurs during sleep and has no particular associations with eating, exercise, or other activities. The child typically has normal growth and development, and the abdominal examination is unremarkable; occasionally, mild midabdominal tenderness, without involuntary guarding, is elicited.

Among postmenarchal females, life-threatening conditions within the reproductive tract that can cause abdominal pain include pelvic inflammatory disease (PID) with tuboovarian abscess and ruptured ectopic pregnancy. Although intrauterine pregnancy may be associated with lower abdominal pain, ectopic pregnancy should always be considered.

EVALUATION AND DECISION

The first priority is the stabilization of the seriously ill or injured child. Attention to airway, breathing, and circulation is critical because cardiorespiratory disease and shock may present with abdominal pain as the major complaint and abdominal emergencies left untreated or with deterioration can lead to cardiorespiratory failure. The next priority is to identify the child who requires immediate or potential surgical intervention, whether for a traumatic injury, appendicitis, intussusception, or other congenital or acquired lesions. Third, an effort is directed to diagnose any of the medical illnesses from among a large group of acute and chronic abdominal and extra-abdominal inflammatory disorders that require emergency nonoperative management. Table 48.2 lists life-threatening causes of abdominal pain by age groups. Finally, the physician should consider those self-limiting or nonspecific causes of abdominal pain. The algorithm presented in this chapter for the approach to abdominal pain is shown in Figure 48.1.

Abdominal Pain in the Setting of Trauma

In the setting of major trauma, the physician should perform a rapid physical examination to distinguish superficial injury (e.g., soft tissue or muscle contusion) from significant intra-abdominal trauma (e.g., splenic hematoma or rupture, liver injury, or hollow viscus perforation) (see Chapter 111 Abdominal Trauma).

Children with localized and/or acute pain after blunt trauma may appear surprisingly well yet have significant solid organ or hollow viscus trauma. When significant intra-abdominal injury is suspected in a stable patient, an urgent computed tomography (CT) scan should be obtained to evaluate for solid organ injury. Lacerations of the liver and spleen are the most common intra-abdominal injuries seen in children. Bedside ultrasound (*f*ocused *a*ssessment with *s*onography in *t*rauma [FAST]) may be used to evaluate for hemoperitoneum. The sensitivity

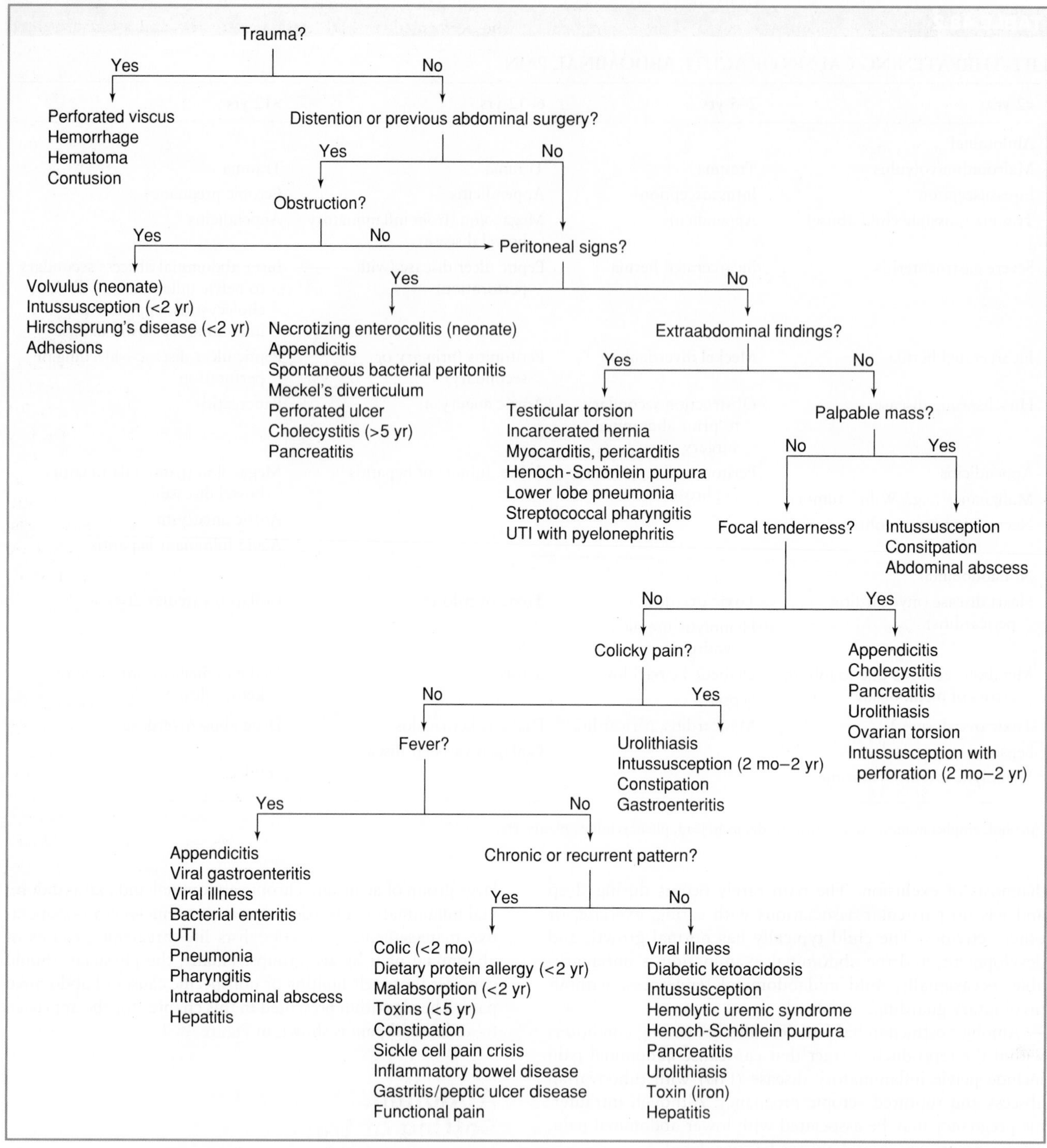

FIGURE 48.1 Acute abdominal pain (males and premenarchal females). UTI, urinary tract infection.

of ultrasound for the detection of solid organ injury is low, and some children with liver and splenic lacerations have minimal intra-abdominal fluid.

Considerations Among Children with Abdominal Distention or Prior Abdominal Surgery

A child who has had prior abdominal surgery presenting with abdominal pain and vomiting should have abdominal radiographs, including flat and upright views, obtained to evaluate for obstruction. Bowel obstruction may result from adhesions in this population. Ileus, manifesting clinically with distention and absent bowel sounds, often accompanies surgical conditions, such as volvulus and intussusception, but may also be observed among children with sepsis, infectious enterocolitis, or pneumonia. Obstruction may present with isolated vomiting. A low-grade fever suggests an inflammatory process, including peritonitis.

A patient with episodic colicky pain with interposed quiet intervals, even in the absence of a "currant jelly" stool, should raise suspicion for intussusception or midgut volvulus. An incarcerated hernia is a common cause of bowel obstruction in infants and young children. Inguinal hernias may incidentally incarcerate during acute illnesses in young, crying infants and may be a cause of abdominal obstruction. Signs of partial or complete obstruction with peritonitis indicate a perforated viscus from intussusception, volvulus, or, occasionally, appendicitis or Hirschsprung disease. An upper GI radiographic series should be performed if malrotation is suspected.

Abdominal Pain Associated with Peritoneal Signs

Rebound tenderness (including tenderness to percussion) or guarding suggests peritoneal inflammation. Children with peritonitis will often avoid motion and keep their hips flexed to relieve tension on the abdominal musculature. The abdomen may be distended, with decreased or absent bowel sounds. In neonates and young infants, abdominal tenderness, which is associated with peritoneal findings or abdominal distention with or without emesis, should raise suspicion for necrotizing enterocolitis. Systemic signs such as temperature instability, apnea, and lethargy may be present. The presentation of a child with appendicitis may vary widely, and the clinical signs and symptoms depend upon the stage of disease. Early in the course of illness children will most often complain of diffuse, nonspecific, periumbilical abdominal pain, nausea, and anorexia. As disease progresses, vomiting, fever, and migration of pain to the right lower abdomen are common findings. Ultrasound can be used to confirm the diagnosis of appendicitis, but the diagnosis cannot be excluded if the appendix is not well visualized, particularly early in the disease process. CT imaging has excellent test characteristics in the diagnosis of appendicitis; however, the risk of radiation must be considered. Various scoring systems, such as Alvarado Score and the Pediatric Appendicitis Score utilize various historical factors, physical examination findings, and laboratory results such as peripheral white blood cell count to risk stratify patients for imaging or surgery (see Chapter 124 Abdominal Emergencies).

Peritonitis in a child with nephrotic syndrome or liver failure may be due to spontaneous bacterial peritonitis. Pain localized to the epigastrium can be due to gastritis; however, the presence of peritonitis should raise suspicion for a perforated ulcer. Cholecystitis and pancreatitis may also produce peritonitis, with abdominal pain localized to the epigastrium or right upper abdomen. A child with Meckel diverticulum will usually present with painless rectal bleeding; however, abdominal pain may occur because of mucosal ulceration from ectopic gastric mucosa.

Extra-abdominal Conditions Associated with Acute Abdominal Pain

A thorough physical examination is required to exclude extra-abdominal conditions that can be associated with abdominal pain. On auscultation of the chest, localized, decreased, or tubular breath sounds or adventitious sounds (i.e., crackles) suggest pneumonia, not an uncommon cause of abdominal pain in the young febrile child. Children with "occult pneumonia" may have a normal respiratory rate and no detectable auscultatory findings on physical examination. Urinary symptoms may occur with pyelonephritis, and polydipsia with polyuria may suggest the onset of diabetes mellitus with abdominal pain from ketoacidosis.

In males, a complete genitourinary examination should be performed, as both testicular torsion and an incarcerated inguinal hernia can produce pain referred to the abdomen. Infectious mononucleosis and streptococcal pharyngitis may be associated with diffuse abdominal pain. The presence of tachycardia, a friction rub or gallop, or hepatosplenomegaly may suggest a cardiac etiology such as pericarditis or myocarditis. The diagnosis of Henoch–Schönlein purpura can be made if abdominal pain is associated with arthritis, along with a petechial or purpural rash of the lower extremities.

Palpable Mass

A palpable mass on the left side of the abdomen is sometimes appreciated in a child with constipation. The diagnosis of constipation should be made on clinical grounds, and radiography should be reserved for children in whom there is concern for obstruction or if the diagnosis is in doubt. A detailed history should include questions regarding the frequency of bowel movements, associated straining, and whether the stool is hard. In suspected constipation, a rectal examination may be helpful to confirm the presence of stool in the rectal vault (see Chapter 13 Constipation). A sausage-shaped mass in the right midabdomen is sometimes appreciated in children with intussusception. Less commonly, an abdominal abscess or neoplasm (commonly of renal origin) may be palpated.

Focal Tenderness

A child with a history of periumbilical pain that radiates to the right lower abdomen, fever, and vomiting should have high suspicion for the diagnosis of appendicitis. Typically, the child with appendicitis will have focal tenderness in the right lower quadrant; however, diffuse tenderness with involuntary guarding may be seen later in the course. The diagnosis of ovarian torsion should be considered in females with acute onset of lower abdominal pain and vomiting; less severe, but focal tenderness, can also be seen with a ruptured ovarian cyst. Epigastric tenderness may be observed in children with gastritis or pancreatitis. Right upper quadrant tenderness may be appreciated among children with hepatitis or cholecystitis. Jaundice or scleral icterus may be present. Pain or limitation of inspiration during palpation of the right upper quadrant (Murphy sign) may be elicited in patients with acute cholecystitis. Focal tenderness in the flank region suggests pyelonephritis or urolithiasis.

Colicky Pain

Intussusception should be considered in a child with colicky abdominal pain, particularly among children younger than 2 years of age. Among older children, a "lead" point for an intussusception should be considered (e.g., mesenteric adenitis, lymphoma, polyp, cystic fibrosis, anaphylactoid purpura). Abdominal radiographs may be useful in confirming obstruction or the presence of a mass; an air-contrast enema is indicated urgently if there is a high suspicion for intussusception. In low or moderate probability settings, an ultrasound is the standard imaging for diagnosis of intussusception. Flank tenderness and/or gross or microscopic hematuria may suggest urolithiasis. Gastroenteritis and constipation can be associated with colicky abdominal pain, but these diagnoses should be made after more serious conditions have been excluded.

Fever

Although most children with appendicitis will have peritoneal signs or focal tenderness, this diagnosis must be considered in any child with fever and abdominal pain. Children with gastroenteritis may have crampy abdominal pain and diarrhea. Although viral pathogens commonly cause gastroenteritis, the presence of fever, bloody stool, or severe abdominal pain may point to a bacterial etiology. A thorough physical examination should be performed to assess for extra-abdominal conditions such as pharyngitis, UTI, and pneumonia. Other conditions associated with abdominal pain and fever are shown in Figure 48.1.

Chronic or Recurrent Pattern

Chronic abdominal pain may occur as a result of many of the conditions listed in Table 48.1. Colic is a common cause of recurrent or chronic abdominal pain in infants younger than 3 months of age, but should only be considered if the pain is not accompanied by other findings or symptoms (see Chapter 15 Crying). Other causes of recurrent abdominal pain in infants must also be considered. These include gastroesophageal reflux, intussusception; malrotation with intermittent volvulus; mild-protein allergy; and various malabsorptive diseases such as cystic fibrosis, celiac disease, and lactase deficiency.

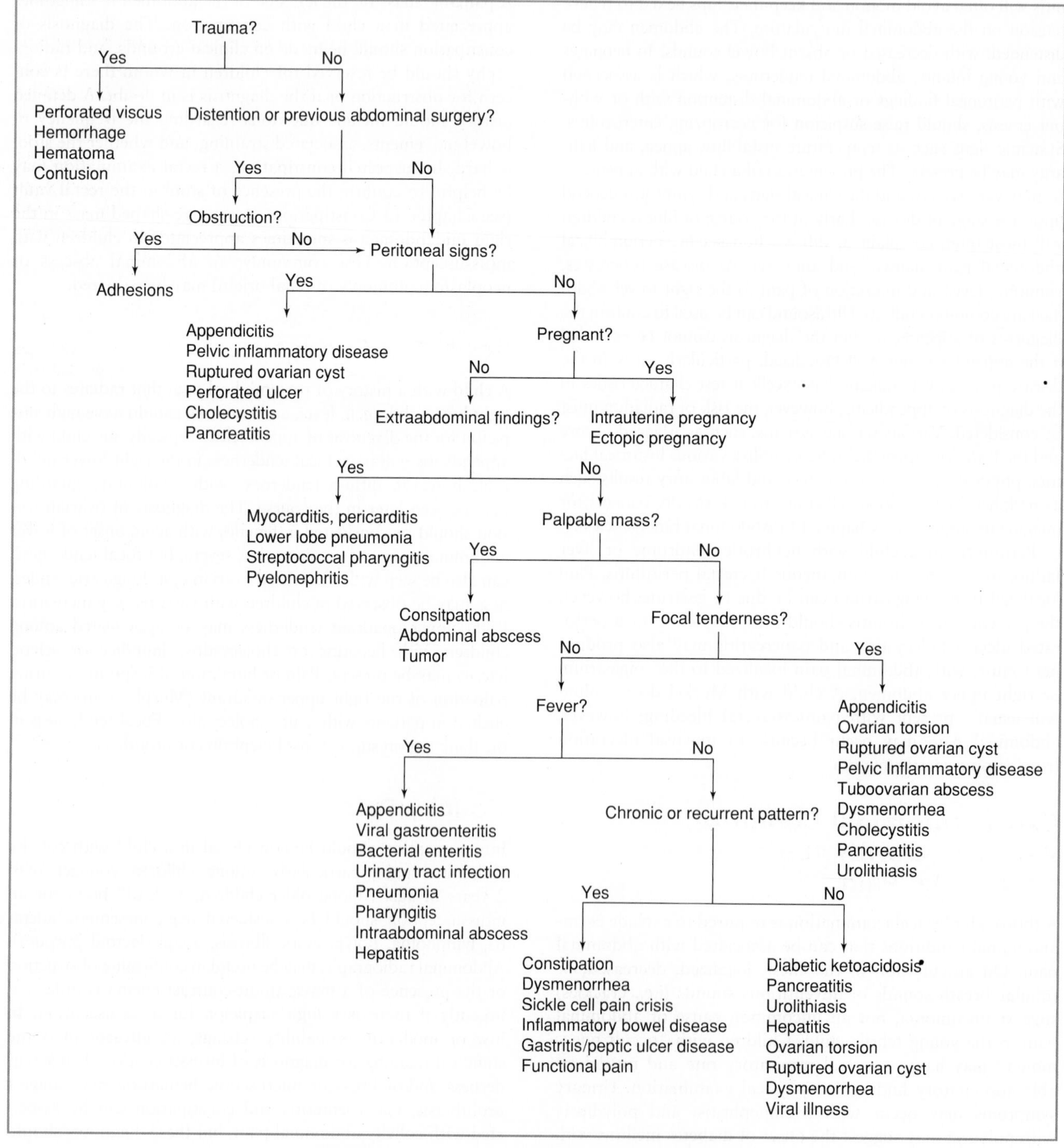

FIGURE 48.2 Acute abdominal pain (postmenarchal female).

Abdominal pain and pallor can occur rarely in a child with malignancy, as with bleeding into an abdominal Wilms tumor, hepatoma, or neuroblastoma. The presence of pallor and pain also raises the possibility of vasoocclusive crisis in a patient with sickle cell disease; splenic sequestration should also be considered. Jaundice may be observed in the child with hemolysis or with hepatitis. At times, an intra-abdominal vasculitis that causes pain may precede the rash of Henoch–Schönlein purpura or be a prominent finding with Kawasaki disease.

Chronic abdominal pain in the adolescents may be due to inflammatory bowel disease. In these children, inflammatory markers such as erythrocyte sedimentation rate and C-reactive protein levels are commonly elevated. In postpubertal females, dysmenorrhea, endometriosis, chronic PID, chronic UTI, or gallbladder disease can be associated with chronic or recurrent abdominal pain. Functional abdominal pain may be considered only after exclusion of other conditions; the presence of focal tenderness, rebound, guarding, or fever should prompt consideration of alternative diagnoses.

Additional Considerations in the Postpubertal Female with Acute Abdominal Pain

Among postpubertal females, pregnancy and complications of pregnancy must be considered (Fig. 48.2). A menstrual history and ascertainment of sexual activity are essential, and a urine β-hCG sample should be obtained in all females in whom pregnancy is a possibility.

The diagnosis of ectopic pregnancy must be considered among females with lower abdominal pain occurring within the first trimester of pregnancy (see Chapter 100 Gynecology Emergencies). Vaginal bleeding occurs in most patients with ectopic pregnancy but is not always present. A transvaginal or transabdominal ultrasound should be obtained. The diagnosis of ectopic pregnancy is not usually confirmed by ultrasound; however, the presence of an intrauterine gestational sac is reassuring and argues against the diagnosis of ectopic pregnancy. A quantitative serum β-hCG sample should be obtained; it may need to be repeated within 48 to 72 hours if the diagnosis remains uncertain. In addition, RhoD immune globulin (RhoGAM) should be administered to Rh-negative women. Although the diagnosis of ectopic pregnancy should be considered in all pregnant women, crampy lower abdominal pain is commonly reported among women with intrauterine pregnancy.

Rupture of an ovarian cyst is the most common cause of lower abdominal pain in postpubertal women; however, the diagnosis can be made only after the exclusion of more serious conditions. An ultrasound should be obtained if focal right or left lower abdominal tenderness is present on physical examination to evaluate for ovarian torsion and tuboovarian abscess. A pelvic examination is required in any sexually active female with abdominal pain. Cervical discharge or tenderness suggests the diagnosis of PID. Appropriate cultures and microscopic examinations for sexually transmitted diseases are indicated and presumptive antimicrobial treatment should be initiated.

Other, nongynecologic etiologies of abdominal pain, including appendicitis, must also be considered. Chronic or recurrent abdominal pain may be due to dysmenorrhea or endometriosis. Laparoscopy may be required to confirm the diagnosis.

SUMMARY

Abdominal pain is one of the most common complaints among children seeking care in the ED. An algorithmic approach to the child with acute abdominal pain should be performed, with a focus on traumatic and surgical conditions. Generation of a differential diagnosis should take into consideration the age of the child.

When evaluating a child with abdominal pain, the first priority should be the stabilization of the seriously ill or injured child. The next priority is to identify the child who requires immediate or potential surgical intervention, whether for a traumatic injury, appendicitis, intussusception, or other congenital conditions. Finally, a thorough examination should be conducted to determine the etiology of abdominal pain. Laboratory evaluations and radiographic studies may be used selectively to support or refute specific differential diagnoses generated by the history and physical examination.

Suggested Readings and Key References

Bachur RG, Dayan PS, Bajaj L, et al. The effect of abdominal pain duration on the accuracy of diagnostic imaging for pediatric appendicitis. *Ann Emerg Med* 2012;60:582–590.

Bundy DG, Byerley JS, Liles EA, et al. Does this child have appendicitis? *JAMA* 2007;298:438–451.

Collins BS, Thomas DW. Chronic abdominal pain. *Pediatr Rev* 2007; 28:323–331.

Fox JC, Boysen M, Gharahbaghian L, et al. Test characteristics of focused assessment of sonography for trauma for clinically significant abdominal free fluid in pediatric blunt abdominal trauma. *Acad Emerg Med* 2011;18:477–482.

Goldman RD, Carter S, Stephens D, et al. Prospective validation of the pediatric appendicitis score. *J Pediatr* 2008;153:278–282.

Kharbanda AB, Dudley NC, Bajaj L, et al. Validation and refinement of a prediction rule to identify children at low risk for acute appendicitis. *Arch Pediatr Adolesc Med* 2012;166:738–744.

Levy JA, Bachur RG. Bedside ultrasound in the pediatric emergency department. *Curr Opin Pediatr* 2008;20:235–242.

McOmber ME, Shulman RJ. Recurrent abdominal pain and irritable bowel syndrome in children. *Curr Opin Pediatr* 2007;19:581–585.

Neuman MI, Ruddy R. Approach to the child with acute abdominal pain. In: Rose BD, ed. *UpToDate*. Waltham, MA: UpToDate Inc, 2012.

Roskind CG, Ruzal-Shapiro CB, Dowd EK, et al. Test characteristics of the 3-view abdominal radiograph series in the diagnosis of intussusception. *Pediatr Emerg Care* 2007;23:785–789.

Scaife ER, Rollins MD, Barnhart DC, et al. The role of focused abdominal sonography for trauma (FAST) in pediatric trauma evaluation. *J Pediatr Surg* 2013;48:1377–1383.

Shaikh N, Morone NE, Lopez J, et al. Does this child have a urinary tract infection? *JAMA* 2007;298:2895–2904.

Weydert JA, Ball TM, Davis MF. Systematic review of treatments for recurrent abdominal pain. *Pediatrics* 2003;111:e1–e11.

CHAPTER 49 ▪ PAIN: BACK

KAREN S. FARBMAN, MD, MPH

Back pain is an uncommon presenting complaint in younger children and warrants careful attention, because it can be a sign of significant pathology. Back pain becomes a more common complaint in the teenage years. While benign musculoskeletal problems are more likely in adolescents, the differential remains broad and continues to deserve careful attention. The differential diagnosis for back pain and its evaluation is discussed here.

DIFFERENTIAL DIAGNOSIS

Trauma to the back is a common cause of back pain. The trauma may be an isolated direct force to the back or a more complex mechanism leading to multiple trauma (see Chapters 119 Musculoskeletal Trauma and 120 Neck Trauma). Vertebral compression fracture and spinal epidural hematoma are significant traumatic injuries. Trauma to the back can also occur as a result of repetitive stress injuries by the athlete or worker. Children, especially adolescents, can have muscular back strain from lifting. They can also have lumbar disc herniation, which is less common in children than in adults. In contrast, injury to the vertebral pars interarticularis is more common in children, especially adolescents. Spondylolysis is a stress fracture or separation at the pars, usually in the lower lumbar vertebrae. While some populations or those with certain conditions (e.g., Scheuermann kyphosis) are at increased risk for spondylolysis, it can occur in anyone, and typically occurs from repetitive hyperextension of the back. Athletes such as figure skaters and gymnasts are notorious for such hyperextension maneuvers. When there is bilateral spondylolysis at the same level, this can allow for slippage of the vertebral body anteriorly. This is known as spondylolisthesis.

A high index of suspicion for infectious etiologies of back pain in children is important, because these may present even without the classic signs of infection such as fever or elevated markers of inflammation. Discitis is more common in the young child, especially under age 5. Vertebral osteomyelitis is more common among adolescents. Sacroiliitis can have a bacterial source. Epidural abscess is a collection of pus located between the bony spine and the dura surrounding the cord. This is an infectious emergency that can compromise the spinal cord and must be diagnosed without delay. Those who abuse intravenous (IV) drugs are at increased risk for epidural abscess. There are other nonspinal sources of back pain with infectious etiologies, including pyelonephritis, and pyomyositis of the back muscles. Myalgias of the back can be the result of other infectious or postinfectious etiologies, especially influenza. Infections that can refer pain to the back include pneumonia, pelvic inflammatory disease, and abdominal pathology such as appendicitis, cholecystitis, and pancreatitis.

A host of neoplastic causes, both benign and malignant, may present with back pain. Osteoid osteoma is a benign tumor and is the most common tumor in children to present with back pain. Localized back pain can also result from primary bony malignancies including Ewing sarcoma, osteosarcoma, and osteoblastoma, as well as bony metastases from other sites. Other nonbony solid tumors can lead to regional pain, including neuroblastoma, Wilms tumor, and rhabdomyosarcoma. Leukemia, lymphoma, and other marrow infiltrative processes can also lead to back pain.

Inflammatory arthritis (collagen vascular diseases) may present with back pain in children. These include ankylosing spondylitis, arthritis associated with inflammatory bowel disease, reactive sacroiliitis, and psoriatic arthritis.

Finally, there are other causes of back pain that present with some frequency in children. Pulmonary disease, including pneumonia and pneumothorax, can present with thoracic back pain. Patients with sickle cell disease can have vasoocclusive crises of the spine, and are also at increased risk of infectious causes of back pain, especially osteomyelitis and sacroiliitis. Nephrolithiasis and obstruction along the urinary tract, such as UPJ obstruction, can cause severe back pain in children. Scheuermann kyphosis is anterior wedging in at least three adjacent vertebral bodies. Its etiology is unknown. It typically presents in the early teens with a fixed thoracolumbar kyphosis. Aortic aneurysm dissection is exceedingly rare in children, but should be considered in patients with Marfan syndrome or other connective tissue disorders who present with back pain. Psychogenic back pain is a diagnosis of exclusion (see Tables 49.1 and 49.2).

EVALUATION AND DECISION

History. Characterizing back pain is important. Pain that is constant, at night, or severe is especially worrisome. These characteristics might suggest neoplasm, infection, or nerve root compression. Musculoskeletal pain, in contrast, may be more dull or achy, and often more prominent after exercise or at the end of the day. Morning pain can be suggestive of collagen vascular disease. With discitis or other vertebral etiologies, there may be a history of the child preferring to be carried or refusing to bend forward. Nerve root pain can be intense, yet episodic. A lumbar herniated disc (unusual in children) often causes sciatic pain which radiates down the buttock and the back of the leg. While fever often suggests an infectious process, it can also be present with neoplastic or rheumatologic conditions which present with back pain.

Physical examination. Before commencing a detailed physical examination, one should first exclude any concern for unstable spinal injury. If symptoms or signs suggest neurologic deficits after trauma, the patient should remain immobilized

TABLE 49.1

CAUSES OF BACK PAIN

I. Traumatic, posttraumatic, or injury-related
   A. Compression fracture
   B. Muscle or ligamentous injury
   C. Spondylolysis
   D. Spondylolisthesis
   E. Disc herniation
   F. Spinal epidural hematoma
II. Infectious
   A. Spinal
      1. Discitis
      2. Vertebral osteomyelitis
      3. Spinal epidural abscess
   B. Nonspinal
      1. Pyelonephritis
      2. Pneumonia
      3. Sacroiliitis
      4. Pelvic Inflammatory Disease
      5. Pyomyositis
      6. Myalgias, typically viral
      7. Appendicitis
      8. Cholecystitis
      9. Pancreatitis
III. Reactive arthritis (collagen vascular disease)
   1. Ankylosing spondylitis
   2. Arthritis of IBD
   3. Reactive sacroiliitis
   4. Psoriatic arthritis
IV. Neoplastic
   1. Osteoid osteoma
   2. Leukemia
   3. Lymphoma
   4. Ewing sarcoma
   5. Osteogenic sarcoma
   6. Osteoblastoma
   7. Neuroblastoma
   8. Wilms tumor
V. Other
   1. Sickle cell disease
   2. Nephrolithiasis
   3. Urinary tract obstruction
   4. Scheuermann kyphosis
   5. Aortic dissection
   6. Psychogenic

TABLE 49.2

COMMON IMPORTANT CAUSES OF BACK PAIN IN CHILDREN

I. Traumatic
   A. Spondylolysis/spondylolisthesis
   B. Compression fracture
II. Infectious
   A. Pyelonephritis
   B. Pneumonia
   C. Vertebral osteomyelitis
   D. Discitis

and timely neurosurgical or orthopedic consultation should be sought. Otherwise, a comprehensive physical examination should ensue to better isolate the pain.

What is the appearance of the spine? Are any bruises noted over the back from injury? Is there kyphosis or lordosis? In spondylolysis there is excessive lumbar lordosis. With Scheuermann kyphosis there will be a fixed thoracic or lumbar kyphosis, unaffected by patient position. It is noteworthy that idiopathic scoliosis typically does not cause back pain, so scoliosis found on inspection of a child with back pain may suggest a concomitant finding.

Palpation of the spine can isolate areas of tenderness. With sacroiliitis, there is a positive FABERE or Patrick test. With this maneuver, while patient is supine, one knee is bent so that the ipsilateral ankle rests over the contralateral knee. Pushing down on the bent knee toward the examination table will produce pain at the ipsilateral, inflamed sacroiliac (SI) joint.

Ranging the back can ascertain pain with certain maneuvers. Discitis will have pain bending forward, as may certain spinal cord tumors. Children with spondylolysis may have pain with hyperextension of the back.

A detailed neurologic examination is also important. Do the muscles have good strength, bulk, and tone? Are the deep tendon reflexes present and strong? Is sensory function preserved, including light touch and prick? Is the child's gait normal or is there a limp? Does the patient have a positive straight leg raise (SLR) test suggesting radiculopathy, possibly secondary to disc herniation or spondylolisthesis?

Broader examination is also important. Is there tenderness to percussion along the flank suggesting lateral muscle strain, renal inflammation, or infection? Careful abdominal and pelvic examinations for referred causes of pain are necessary, along with dedicated hip and leg examinations.

Laboratory studies. Laboratory investigation is not routinely required, but rather directed by the history and physical examination. Urinalysis and urine culture are frequently obtained in the workup of back pain, especially with flank pain. When infection or arthritis is suspected, a CBC, C-reactive protein, ESR, and blood culture are typically sent. When neoplastic processes are considered, CBC, liver function, C-reactive protein, LDH, and uric acid may be helpful. If history and physical examination are suggestive, pancreatic enzymes or LFTs may be indicated.

Imaging. Plain film radiographs are the starting point for most conditions which need imaging. AP and lateral views of the spine will diagnose fractures, bony tumors, scoliosis, kyphosis, and lordosis. Oblique views can help diagnose a pars defect, although given low sensitivity more advanced imaging may be pursued at follow-up as needed. Chest radiographs are indicated if there is a suspicion for pneumonia (a relatively common cause of pediatric back pain) or to look for chest tumor and aortic size. CT scan is indicated for evaluation of acute, high force trauma to the back. Otherwise, MRI is often the study of choice to evaluate back pathology. It can increase yield of definitive diagnosis. The urgency of obtaining

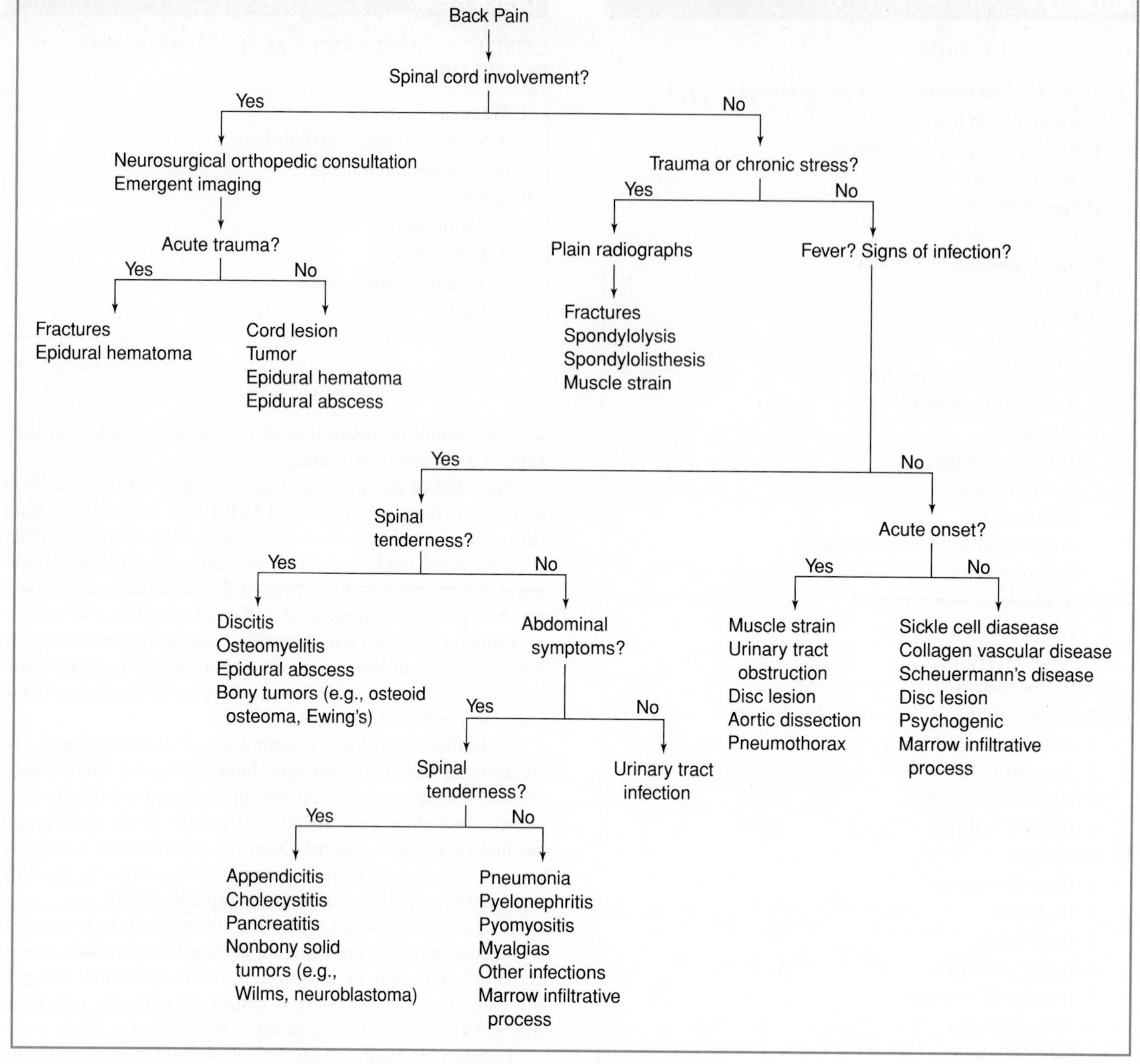

FIGURE 49.1 Back pain algorithm.

an MRI depends on the type and severity of symptoms, the presence of neurologic findings on examination, or concerning labs or plain film examination. MRI is very sensitive for spinal cord lesions, bony infection, discitis, and vertebral fractures, and does not incur radiation as does the CT scan.

Back pain in children deserves careful and comprehensive evaluation. Because back pain is a relatively uncommon chief complaint in pediatric emergency medicine, and because there is significant pathology within its differential diagnosis, close follow-up of patients presenting with back pain should be ensured (see Fig. 49.1).

Suggested Readings and Key References

Cruikshank M, Ramanan AV. Fifteen-minute consultation: a structured approach to the management of a child or adolescent with back pain. *Arch Dis Child Educ Pract Ed* 2014;99(6):202–207.

Jones GT, Macfarlane GJ. Epidemiology of low back pain in children and adolescents. *Arch Dis Child* 2005;90:312–316.

Purcell L, Micheli L. Low back pain in young athletes. *Sports Health* 2009;1(3):212–222.

Ramirez N, Flynn JM, Hill BW, et al. Evaluation of a systematic approach to pediatric back pain: the utility of magnetic resonance imaging. *J Pediatr Orthop* 2014;35(1):28-32.

CHAPTER 50 ■ PAIN: CHEST

ROBYN L. BYER, MD

The complaint of chest pain rarely represents a life-threatening emergency in children, in contrast to the same complaint in adults. Although heart disease is an uncommon source of chest pain in children, the fear of a cardiac origin for the pain may evoke anxiety in the child or in the parents. There are a wide variety of etiologies for chest pain including diseases of the respiratory, cardiac, gastrointestinal (GI), neurologic, psychiatric, and musculoskeletal systems; however, it is most commonly due to idiopathic noncardiac origins. Chest pain accounts for approximately 0.6% of all pediatric emergency room visits and affects boys and girls equally. Clinicians need to take a careful approach to the patient even in the pediatric setting. This chapter first briefly reviews the pathophysiology of chest pain, then outlines the differential diagnosis in children, and finally presents the evaluation, as appropriate in the emergency department (ED).

PATHOPHYSIOLOGY

To understand the possible origins of chest pain or discomfort, it is important to review how this sensation is transmitted. Musculoskeletal pain is produced by irritation of tissues and is transmitted through the sensory nerves. The stimulus is carried through the nerve in the dermatomal or intercostals distribution to the dorsal root ganglia, up the spinal afferents, and into the central nervous system (CNS). This local, peripheral sharp pain can also be produced by primary dorsal root irritation in the spine. Because of overlap of nerve distribution, pain may be sensed in locations distal to the irritation. For example, the third and fourth cervical nerves evoke pain as far caudally as the nipple line of the chest.

Tracheobronchial pain is transmitted by vagal afferents in the large bronchi and trachea to fibers in the cervical spinal column. Dull, aching, or sharp pain is felt in the anterior chest or neck. The irritation or sensation of cough is transmitted in a similar fashion. Pleural pain arises in the pain-sensitive parietal pleura and then travels through the intercostals nerves in the chest wall, giving rise to sharp, well-localized pain. The visceral pleura is insensitive to pain. The intercostal or phrenic nerves transmit diaphragmatic pain. Peripheral diaphragmatic irritation may cause local chest wall pain because of the intercostals innervation. Central diaphragmatic stimulation travels by the phrenic nerve, with the distribution of pain referred to the shoulder of the affected side.

The esophagus appears to be more pain sensitive in its proximal portion. Pain is transmitted by afferents to corresponding spinal segments, with resultant anterior chest or neck pain. The pericardium is innervated by portions of the phrenic, vagal, and recurrent laryngeal nerves, as well as by the esophageal plexus. This appears to give rise to various sensations, including chest or abdominal pain, dull pressure, and even referred angina-like pain.

Other mediastinal structures, such as the aorta, have pain fibers in the adventitia of the vessel wall. They transmit pain through the thoracic sympathetic chain to the spinal dorsal roots, giving rise to sharp, and variably localized chest pain. Cardiac pain probably is transmitted by a number of routes, including the thoracic sympathetic chain and the cardiac nerves through the cervical and stellate ganglia. It has been proposed that pain arises from abnormal ventricular wall movement and stimulation of the pericardial pain fibers. These routes account for the sensation of cardiac chest pain as pressure or crushing pain substernally or as sharp pain in the shoulder, neck, or arm.

DIFFERENTIAL DIAGNOSIS

A differential diagnosis of chest pain in children is included in Table 50.1. In the case of trauma, cardiac or pulmonary compromise may arise from direct injury to the heart, great vessels, or lung (see Chapter 123 Thoracic Trauma). Most chest pain in the nontraumatized child is caused by acute respiratory disease, musculoskeletal injury, anxiety, or inflammation (Table 50.2). Often, the physician does not make a causative diagnosis of the chest pain and calls it nonspecific or idiopathic in origin. Occasionally, this idiopathic chest pain may be unrecognized organic disease, such as gastroesophageal reflux disease. Chest pain in children usually occurs without associated cardiorespiratory signs or symptoms, often as an acute or chronic problem. By the time of the ED visit, frequently the pain has resolved. Although much less frequent, chest pain in association with cardiorespiratory distress demands immediate attention. Table 50.3 lists the life-threatening causes of chest pain by disease and mechanisms for decompensation. Chest pain in the dyspneic or cyanotic patient most often stems from a respiratory problem, such as pneumonia, asthma, pleurisy, or pneumothorax. Rarely does severe chest pain in an acutely ill child result from myocardial infarction (MI) due to aberrant coronary vessels, cocaine abuse, Kawasaki disease, hyperlipidemia, or other underlying cardiac diseases (aortic stenosis, an acute arrhythmia, or pericardial disease). Every individual evaluation must be started, however, with a broad differential diagnosis in mind to ensure proper diagnosis and management of the child with chest pain.

Although studies range in estimating a cardiac cause for chest pain in a pediatric patient, it is generally very low, <6%. The largest most recent study of pediatric patients with chest pain in a pediatric emergency setting found a cardiac cause for chest pain to be 0.6%. Major categories include arrhythmias, anatomic lesions, and acquired disorders such as myocarditis and pericarditis. Myocardial ischemia is very rare in pediatrics but can present with typical unrelenting substernal crushing chest pain with or without radiation to neck or arm, diaphoresis, nausea, dyspnea, and syncope. Patients are usually in

TABLE 50.1

CAUSES OF CHEST PAIN

I. Musculoskeletal/neural
- A. Muscle
  - Trauma—contusions, lacerations, strain
  - Infection—myositis
- B. Breast
  - Physiologic (fullness during menses or pregnancy)
  - Mastitis
  - Fibrocystic disease
  - Tumor (adenoma, other)
  - Gynecomastia
- C. Bone
  - Trauma—contusions, rib fractures
  - Osteitis, osteomyelitis
  - Costochondritis, Tietze syndrome
  - Tumor
  - Slipping rib syndrome
- D. Intercostal nerve
  - Neuritis—zoster, trauma
  - Toxin
- E. Dorsal root
  - Trauma
  - Radiculitis—viral, postviral
  - Spinal disease—scoliosis

II. Tracheobronchial (proximal bronchi)
- A. Foreign body
- B. Infection
  - Tracheitis
  - Bronchitis
  - Cystic fibrosis
- C. Asthma

III. Pulmonary/pleural/diaphragm
- A. Trauma—penetrating and blunt
- B. Pleurisy/pleurodynia—viral, mycobacterial
- C. Pneumonia
- D. Cystic fibrosis
- E. Pneumothorax, hemothorax, chylothorax
- F. Empyema
- G. Pneumomediastinum
- H. Malignancy/mediastinal mass
- I. Postpericardiotomy syndrome
- J. Pulmonary embolus/infarction
- K. Vasoocclusive crisis (sickle cell anemia)
- L. Tumor
- M. Subphrenic abscess/hepatic abscess
- N. Fitz-Hugh–Curtis syndrome

IV. Gastrointestinal
- A. Esophageal
  - Foreign body
  - Caustic ingestion
  - Gastroesophageal reflux/esophagitis
  - Esophageal spasms
  - Infection—*Candida*
  - Esophageal rupture/tear
- B. Hiatal hernia
- C. Gastritis/peptic ulcer disease
- D. Cholecystitis
- E. Pancreatitis

Cardiac (angina, pericardial, aortic)
- A. Angina—coronary insufficiency[a], anomalous vessels, pulmonary hypertension
- B. Hypertrophic cardiomyopathy
- C. Aortic stenosis, pulmonary stenosis
- D. Asymmetric septal hypertrophy
- E. Pericardial defects and effusions, pericarditis
- F. Acute arrhythmias[a]
- G. Myocarditis[a]
- H. Aortic aneurysm—idiopathic, syphilitic, Marfan syndrome
- I. Mitral valve prolapse

Central
- A. Psychiatric—anxiety, hyperventilation, conversion reaction, depression, phobia
- B. Idiopathic—Texidor's twinge (precordial catch)
- C. Other—visceral pain–associated disability syndrome

[a]Associated drug induced (especially cocaine).

TABLE 50.2

COMMON CAUSES OF CHEST PAIN

Common causes
Functional (anxiety/psychosomatic)
Musculoskeletal contusion/strain
Costochondritis/myositis
Cough or respiratory infections (bronchitis, pneumonia, pleurisy, upper respiratory infections)
Asthma
Gastroesophageal reflux
Idiopathic

distress and have physical examination abnormalities including pallor, diaphoresis, a gallop rhythm, a heart murmur, and decreased peripheral perfusion. Myocardial ischemia/infarction can occur as a result of a thrombosed coronary artery aneurysm. These aneurysms, which occur as a sequelae from Kawasaki disease, have both insufficient laminar flow and areas of stenosis that become obstructed via thrombosis leading to decreased myocardial perfusion. Case reports of myocardial ischemia without risk factors in adolescents have been attributed to vasospasm. Cocaine exposure can result in palpitations and coronary vasospasm leading to ischemia, MI, arrhythmias, or cardiomyopathy. Patients with cocaine toxicity are often anxious with confusion or combativeness and have significant tachycardia and hypertension. Other toxins have cardiac

TABLE 50.3

LIFE-THREATENING CAUSES OF CHEST PAIN

Category	Disease/injury	Decompensation
Traumatic	Rib fracture	Tension pneumothorax or shock from hemothorax
	Cardiac contusion	Arrhythmia or myocardial infarction
	Laceration—heart or great vessel	Shock
	Contusion—great vessels	Dissecting aneurysm/shock
	Pulmonary contusion	Adult respiratory distress syndrome
Cardiac	Congenital heart disease	Arrhythmia, shock, pulmonary hypertension
	Myocardial infarction (anomalous coronary artery, Kawasaki disease, cocaine toxicity)	Arrhythmia, cardiogenic shock
	Myocarditis	Arrhythmia, cardiogenic shock
	Pericarditis	Tamponade
	Rheumatic heart disease	Arrhythmia, congestive heart failure
	Aortic aneurysm	Rupture-shock, dissection
	Obstructive cardiac disease	Acute hypertension
Pulmonary	Pneumothorax (asthma, cystic fibrosis, spontaneous)	Tension pneumothorax, pulmonary hypertension, shock
	Hemothorax	Shock, hypoxemia
	Pulmonary infection or empyema	Pulmonary hypertension, sepsis
	Aspiration—foreign body	Acute airway obstruction, progressive pulmonary hypertension
	Acute asthma	Tension pneumothorax, pulmonary hypertension
	Pulmonary embolus	Pulmonary infarction, hypertension, cardiovascular collapse
	Pulmonary venoocclusive disease	Pulmonary hypertension
	Tumor (chest wall, chest, or mediastinum)	Airway compromise, progression of tumor
Miscellaneous	Drug ingestion/overdose (especially cocaine)	Arrhythmia, cardiomyopathy, shock
	Sickle cell crisis	Pulmonary infarction or hypertension
	Cholecystitis	Sepsis, peritonitis

effects. The herbal medications aconite, ephedra, and licorice have also been implicated as the cause of chest pain, congestive heart failure, arrhythmias, and MIs.

Anomalous coronary arteries which originate from the opposite sinus and traverse between the great vessels usually present with sudden death but can also cause chest pain with intense exercise. Pain is thought to be related to inadequate coronary perfusion via either compression of the great vessels, relative ostial stenosis, or both. The history is the key to this significant disease as the physical examination is usually normal.

Hypertrophic cardiomyopathy is the most common cardiac cause of sudden death, which is likely due to ventricular dysrhythmias, yet chest pain is not a common feature. This disease follows an autosomal dominant pattern of inheritance; however, spontaneous mutations may occur. Patients often have a systolic murmur which becomes more intense with standing or a Valsalva maneuver. Chest pain can also occur with severe obstruction from aortic stenosis which is likely to be discovered by the pathologic murmur on physical examination. The patient with chest pain that has onset with or worsening with exertion should be evaluated for these conditions.

Arrhythmias are not uncommon and children usually present with palpitations or a combination of chest pain and palpitations. Symptoms of heart pounding may occur with instantaneous initiation and termination whereas other children have been reported to abruptly stop an activity. Most arrhythmias are benign, such as premature atrial and ventricular contractions; however, children may present with signs of shock, congestive heart failure, or syncope secondary to supraventricular or ventricular tachycardia. Physical examination is often normal in the absence of active arrhythmias but long-term effects can lead to cardiomyopathy. Dilated cardiomyopathy presents with chest discomfort, fatigue, exercise intolerance, palpitations, and physical examination findings such as a gallop rhythm and a murmur secondary to mitral valve insufficiency.

Inflammatory conditions such as pericarditis and myocarditis can present with chest pain and systemic symptoms. Pericardial disease includes pericarditis, pericardial effusions, and cardiac tamponade. Pericarditis often presents with fever, a stabbing chest pain that improves with sitting up and leaning forward, respiratory distress, a friction rub, and distant heart sounds. Pericarditis and pericardial effusions can restrict outflow leading to neck vein distention and in severe cases of tamponade, pulsus paradoxus (see Chapter 94 Cardiac Emergencies). The presentation of myocarditis can be more subtle with mild chest pain and fatigue for several days followed by the development of fever, dyspnea, and worsening chest pain. The examination often shows tachycardia (or bradycardia when severe), orthostatic changes not improved by fluid resuscitation, pulsus paradoxus, and a gallop rhythm. Both pericarditis and myocarditis are usually associated with a preceding viral illness. Endocarditis is most often seen in children with a history of congenital heart disease but can present in those with no known predisposing condition. Patients are often ill appearing with a history of prolonged fever and may have signs of embolization. Other illnesses that can present with carditis include rheumatic heart disease and Kawasaki disease.

Chest pain associated with mitral valve prolapse is controversial. Studies have shown that mitral valve prolapse is not more common in those with chest pain than in the general population and other etiologies of the chest pain may exist in a patient with this condition. However, chest pain in patients with mitral valve prolapse may be secondary to papillary muscle or left ventricular endocardial ischemia. A midsystolic click and late systolic murmur should be found on physical examination. Pain secondary to mitral valve prolapse should be considered only when no other etiology may be found.

Patients with connective tissue disorders such as Marfan syndrome have the potential to develop aortic dilation, aortic dissection, and rupture. Symptoms of aortic dissection/rupture include generalized distress with unrelenting severe chest pain, decreased cardiac output, dyspnea, and often abdominal pain.

Children who present with chest pain days to months after cardiac surgery should be evaluated for signs of pericardial effusion known as postpericardiotomy syndrome. Patients with pulmonary hypertension may present with exercise intolerance, palpitations, and syncope. The resultant right ventricular dilatation may be found on physical examination as a narrowed second heart sound, hepatomegaly, and cyanosis if an ASD or VSD is present. Eisenmenger syndrome is severe pulmonary hypertension from an uncorrected congenital heart disease leading to cyanosis from right-to-left shunting of blood. Isolated anatomic abnormalities such as atrial septal defects have been known to present with chest pain and may or may not display the classic findings of a hyperactive precordium, widely split fixed second heart sounds, and both a systolic and diastolic murmur.

Unrecognized disease rarely causes isolated chest pain in a child who otherwise appears well, but the physician should consider drug exposure (e.g., cocaine; methamphetamine; nicotine; beta-agonist abuse; the triptans; combination of cold medications containing chlorpheniramine, dextromethorphan, and phenylpropanolamine; and herbal medications mentioned previously). Although cardiac conditions are infrequent, attention should be paid to diagnosing the rare patient with hypertrophic cardiomyopathy, angina, mitral valve prolapse, or early pericardial or myocardial inflammation (see Chapter 94 Cardiac Emergencies).

Pulmonary diseases are common and account for approximately 12% to 21% of chest pain cases. A first episode of reactive airway disease should be suspected when an associated night cough, history of wheezing, or family history of atopy is present. There is a high incidence of exercise-induced asthma which often presents with chest tightness, shortness of breath, and wheezing with exercise. These historical features are important as the physical examination may be completely normal during the ER visit. Infectious diseases of the respiratory tract are associated with fever, malaise, cough, and coryza, and may involve several family members simultaneously. Patients with pneumonia (see Chapter 107 Pulmonary Emergencies) often present with tachypnea and hypoxia in addition to fever and cough. Spontaneous (nontraumatic) pneumomediastinum and pneumothorax may occur in patients with reactive airway disease, cystic fibrosis, or as a result of barotrauma (i.e., Valsalva maneuver, forceful vomiting, or coughing). The pain of a pneumothorax is often unrelenting and pleuritic in nature. If the pneumothorax is moderate or large, then patients present with significant respiratory distress and decreased breath sounds on the affected side. Spontaneous (nontraumatic) pneumomediastinum is most often reported in male adolescents without underlying lung disease and those with asthma. It appears to occur with any activity that involves straining against a closed glottis. This is thought to cause a rise in intra-alveolar pressure and subsequently a rupture of the alveoli releasing air into the interstitial space. Air then dissects along facial planes of the hilum into the mediastinum and neck. Those with spontaneous pneumomediastinu m present with substernal chest pain which frequently radiates to the neck and is worse with deep inspiration and position changes, subcutaneous crepitus, Hamman sign (crunching heart sounds), dysphagia, and dysphonia. This diagnosis must be distinguished from pneumothorax, pericarditis, and esophageal perforation.

Pleural effusions can cause chest pain associated with decreased breath sounds and dullness to percussion on physical examination. Pleurodynia, often secondary to coxsackievirus B infection, causes sharp chest pain, fever, and a friction rub. Aspiration of a foreign body into the trachea or esophagus may occur without such history in a toddler or even in an older child, and approximately 50% of these children may complain of chest pain. Foreign bodies lodged in the airway often present with chest pain, cough, decreased breath sounds, and unilateral wheezing. However, auscultatory findings may be unimpressive despite a positive history.

Although pulmonary embolisms (see Chapter 107 Pulmonary Emergencies) are rare in children, they can present with pleuritic chest pain, cough, hypoxia, hemoptysis, dyspnea, respiratory distress, and the sense of impending doom. Usually this condition is associated with risk factors such as obesity, oral contraceptive use, pregnancy, collagen vascular disease, nephrotic syndrome, cigarette smoking, recent surgery, immobility, trauma (particularly spinal injury), a positive family history, a hypercoagulable condition (known or unknown), or prior cardiorespiratory problems. Finally, children with sickle cell disease can develop a vasoocclusive crises resulting in acute chest syndrome.

GI diseases account for approximately 4% to 7% of pediatric patients with chest pain. Diseases include gastroesophageal reflux, esophagitis, gastritis, ulcer disease, and rarely esophageal rupture or spasm. History is important in regard to symptom relationship to meals and body position. Pain of gastroesophageal reflux is typically described as burning, worse in the recumbent position, related to eating, and improved with antacid or hydrogen ion blocker therapy. The physical examination is usually normal or positive for epigastric tenderness. Foreign bodies in the GI tract can cause chest pain, drooling, dysphagia, and odynophagia. The history often uncovers this diagnosis and radiography may be helpful. Spontaneous esophageal perforation (Boerhaave syndrome) is secondary to transmitted increased pressure against a closed glottis most often seen with vomiting but also straining, coughing, defecation, seizure, childbirth, or forceful nose blowing. Presentation includes symptoms of chest pain, crepitus, pneumomediastinum, and hematemesis to hemorrhage and shock. Mackler triad includes vomiting, chest pain, and subcutaneous emphysema. There are case reports of adolescents diagnosed with diffuse esophageal spasm via motility testing after persistent chest pain. Intra-abdominal processes such as cholecystitis can present with postprandial pain and pain in the right upper quadrant.

Musculoskeletal causes of chest pain are common accounting for 15% to 56% of cases and are typically overuse injuries (muscle strain and inflamed tissue). Chest pain often occurs after physical activity and is reproducible by palpation and contraction of the muscle group on physical examination. Direct trauma may produce a contusion or rib fracture. Costochondritis is an inflammatory condition of the costochondral junctions which may be preceded by a respiratory illness and characteristically has reproducible pain on examination. The pain is described as sharp and exaggerated by physical activity or deep inspiration. Tietze syndrome is a benign inflammatory condition of unknown cause which results in isolated swelling of a costochondral junction. The inflamed area appears as a mass on the chest wall and results in chest pain that typically radiates to the shoulder or arm. This syndrome usually occurs in adults but has been reported in children and infants. When evaluating a chest wall mass the differential diagnosis should include osteomyelitis and tumors.

Slipping rib syndrome is a pain syndrome caused by hypermobility of the anterior aspect of the 8th to 10th ribs which do not directly attach to the sternum but instead are held together by fibrous tissue. It is thought that weakening of the fibrous tissue in the area allows the ribs to rub against the other irritating the intercostal nerve and referring pain to the chest wall and abdomen. Patients describe a popping or clicking sensation followed by pain which lasts several minutes. Pain is reproduced by hooking the lower ribs with the hand and pulling anteriorly.

A large group of children with chest pain will have no evidence of organic disease and no history of underlying cardiorespiratory disease or trauma. They may have a family history of chest pain and are able to identify a stressful situation that has precipitated the episode. Such children have psychogenic chest pain which represent approximately 5% to 17% of pediatric chest pain cases. Complaints of chest pain and other somatic aches often are chronic and other symptoms of psychiatric illness or hyperventilation may be present. Nonorganic chest pain may appear to cause respiratory distress in the hyperventilating teenager but close examination should distinguish this syndrome from serious problems (see Chapter 134 Behavioral and Psychiatric Emergencies).

Finally, idiopathic chest pain is a very common diagnosis of chest pain in pediatrics representing 23% to 45% of cases. The term is used to describe chest pain when no organic etiology and no psychological factors are present to explain the pain. It is typically described as occasional short episodes of sharp chest pain with or without exercise and no other associated symptoms. Physical examination is completely normal and pain is not reproducible. Precordial catch syndrome or "Texidor's twinge" is a relatively frequent cause of chest pain in healthy teenagers and young adults. It typically presents with an acute, sharp, well-localized pain (often in the left substernal region) that has a "split second" onset, is of short duration, worsened by deep inspiration, and usually occurs at rest or related to exercise. It is often relieved by position change (sitting up straight) which suggests that posture or ligamentous stretching of the supporting ligaments of the heart may have a role but the true etiology is unknown. The physical examination is normal without reproducible pain.

Other causes of chest pain include male adolescents with gynecomastia and female patients with fibrocystic breast disease. Rarely, chest pain, pressure, or shortness of breath, worse on supine position, will be associated with the presentation of a mediastinal mass.

EVALUATION AND DECISION

Child with Thoracic Trauma

The first step in evaluation of the child with chest pain is to perform a thorough history and physical examination. If the history is positive for a traumatic injury or there is any evidence of trauma to the chest (see Chapter 123 Thoracic Trauma), the patient requires rapid evaluation and may need immediate resuscitation as well (Fig. 50.1A). Correction of cardiac or respiratory insufficiency may diagnose and treat the cause of chest pain. Alveolar ventilation should be assessed for adequacy

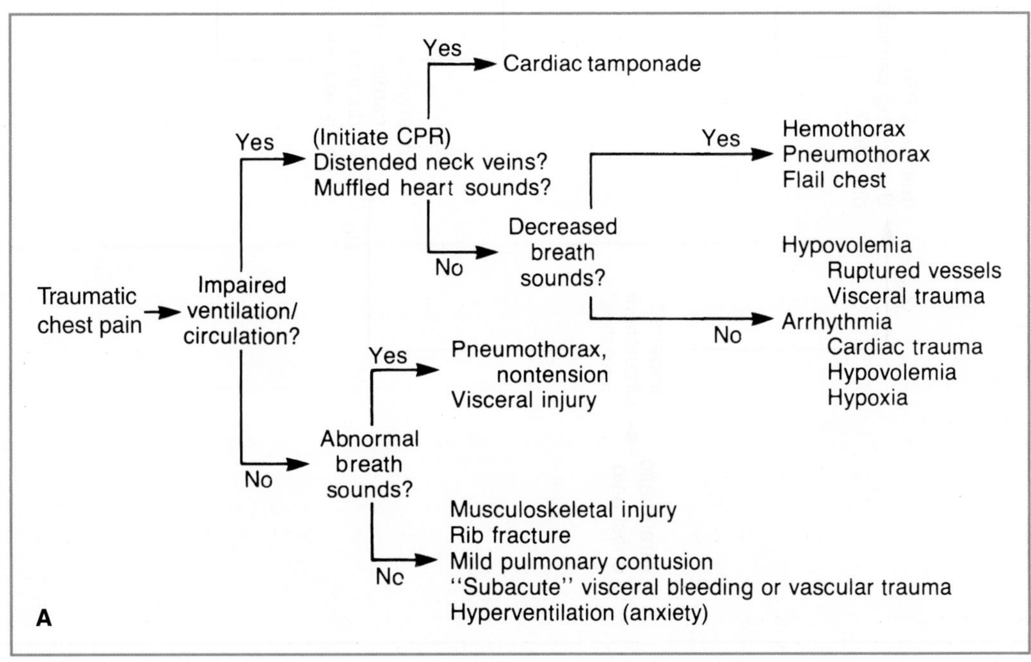

FIGURE 50.1 **A:** Diagnostic approach to traumatic chest pain. (*continued*)

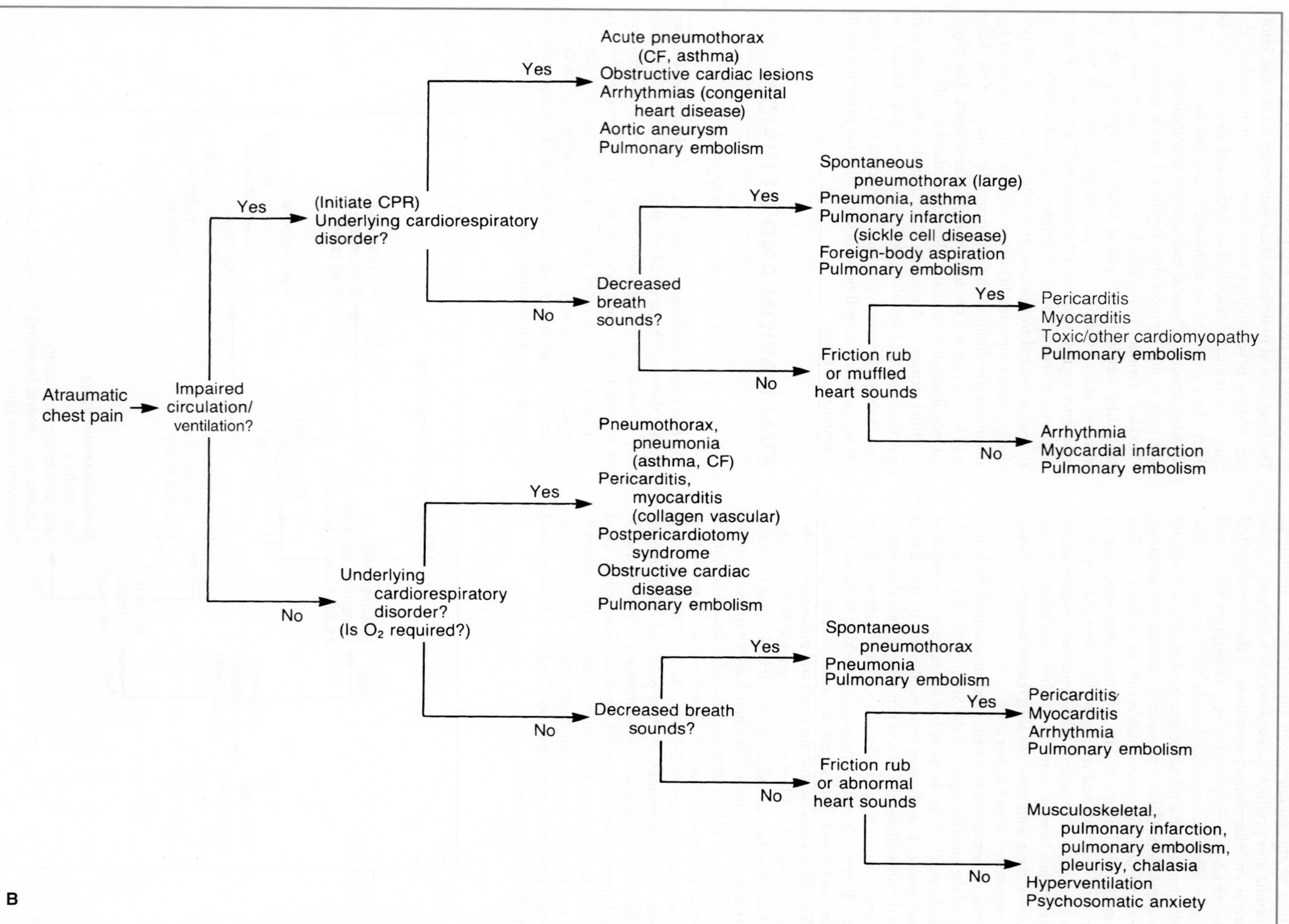

FIGURE 50.1 (*Continued*) **B:** Diagnostic approach to atraumatic chest pain. CPR, cardiopulmonary resuscitation; CF, cystic fibrosis.

and bilateral symmetry to distinguish acute respiratory failure from hemothorax or pneumothorax. In children with chest trauma, tachycardia with hypotension is generally caused by hypovolemia secondary to a hemothorax, hemopneumothorax, or vascular injury. Reduced cardiac output and perfusion, however, may also be secondary to a rhythm disturbance (from a myocardial contusion or tension pneumothorax) or cardiac tamponade (which causes muffling of the heart sounds and pulsus paradoxus). A discrepancy of the pulse or blood pressure between the extremities points to aortic diseases, such as traumatic avulsion or aneurysm. Ruptured esophagus and tracheobronchial disruption may result from rapid deceleration injuries and may present with chest pain, subcutaneous emphysema, respiratory distress, and hypotension.

Many children with thoracic injuries but no respiratory distress also complain of chest pain. Although a careful examination is mandatory in an effort to exclude significant intrathoracic trauma, the cause of the pain usually resides in the chest wall: contusions of the soft tissues or rib fractures. A history of significant trauma even in the absence of cardiovascular abnormality dictates that radiographs and an electrocardiogram (EKG) be obtained. Injury to the heart including myocardial contusions and acute rupture of cardiac structures can occur during rapid deceleration and compression-type injuries. Pulmonary injuries include contusions, pneumothoraces, and hemothoraces. These injuries may present with subtle physical examination findings. Patients have presented with chest pain following blunt trauma that was subsequently complicated by the development of posttraumatic ventricular septal defect and pseudoaneurysm.

Finally, the clinician should consider child abuse if rib fractures are seen in a young infant. In older children, a predisposing cause for fracture (i.e., bone cyst or tumor) should be sought.

Child with No Thoracic Trauma

As discussed above, the first step in evaluation of the child with chest pain is to perform a thorough history and physical examination assessing for cardiorespiratory instability. A thorough history including a complete review of symptoms, social history, and family history should be obtained. The description of chest pain should include quality, intensity, location, frequency, and duration as well as its relationship to exercise, food intake, position, or trauma. Chest pain relieved by leaning forward is consistent with pericarditis, while that which is worsened by reclining may represent pericarditis, gastroesophageal reflux, or hiatal hernia. The review of symptoms should be broad including systemic symptoms such as fever, fatigue, weight loss, diaphoresis, or intolerance to exercise; cardiac symptoms such as palpitations, heart racing, dizziness, or syncope; pulmonary symptoms such as dyspnea, cough, or wheezing; and GI symptoms such as vomiting, dysphagia, abnormal taste in the mouth, or abdominal pain. In general, chest pain that is acute in onset, described as crushing sternal pain with or without radiation to left arm or neck, awakens a patient at night or is associated with exertion, syncope, fever, fatigue, dyspnea, decreased exercise tolerance, or palpitations is concerning and demands a more extensive evaluation.

Next, the physician should inquire about a history suggestive of prior cardiorespiratory disease such as asthma, cystic fibrosis, congenital or structural heart conditions as well as high-risk past medical histories of collagen vascular disease, connective tissue disorders, hyperlipidemia, malignancy, thrombophilia, myopathies, Kawasaki disease, or a prolonged febrile illness. It is also important to determine if there is a family history of sudden death, hypercholesterolemia, cardiomyopathy, hyperlipidemia, pulmonary hypertension, hypercoagulability disorders, or early cardiovascular disease which could also place the patient at higher risk of a cardiopulmonary cause of the chest pain. Social history of drug use, cigarette use, and immobilization should be sought.

Children with respiratory illnesses, such as asthma or cystic fibrosis are at risk for pneumothorax, acute respiratory failure from mucous plugging or pneumonitis, and acute pulmonary hypertension. In the child with a history of cardiac arrhythmias (see Chapter 94 Cardiac Emergencies), congenital heart disease, cardiac surgery, or pericardial effusions, chest pain may signal an exacerbation of the underlying problem.

The social history should include recent stressors, cigarette, and drug use including prescription medications such as oral contraceptives, stimulants such as cocaine, and herbal medications. In addition, it may be helpful to determine the patient's perception of the pain and how it is affecting their life. Research has shown that approximately one-third of children with chest pain have missed school secondary to their symptoms and approximately half of children with chest pain associate this pain as a problem with their heart.

In the absence of prior cardiopulmonary disease or trauma, the approach must be directed toward unmasking evidence for any of the serious cardiorespiratory illnesses listed in Table 50.3. A thorough examination usually uncovers evidence of the cardiac and respiratory causes of chest pain. The clinician must carefully assess the vital signs looking for fever, tachycardia, bradycardia, tachypnea, bradypnea, hypertension, hypotension, and hypoxia. The patient may be well appearing with no apparent distress or ill appearing with significant distress. Concerning signs of the general appearance include cough, drooling, retractions, lethargy, pallor, or cyanosis. The physical examination in asthma shows a prolonged expiratory phase of respiration, variable degrees of chest hyperinflation, and wheezing accentuated by a forced expiratory effort. However, auscultatory findings, such as crackles or wheezing, may be minimal when obstructive pulmonary disease is moderately severe and a history of foreign body aspiration should also be sought with new-onset wheezing. Fever, hypoxia, tachypnea, decreased breath sounds, and/or crackles suggests pneumonia whereas dullness to percussion suggests effusion. Unilateral absent/decreased breathsounds are concerning for pneumothorax, pneumonia, foreign body aspiration, or a pulmonary embolism. Crepitus of the neck or chest wall is indicative of pneumomediastinum and/or pneumothorax. Tracheal deviation may be seen in severe cases of tension pneumothorax where patients are in obvious distress.

If breathsounds are equal, yet there is an abnormal heart sound, then a cardiac etiology is most likely. Pericardial disease can present with a friction rub, distant heart sounds, neck vein distention, hypotension, impaired circulation, pulses paradoxus, and chest pain worse in supine position and improved by leaning forward. Signs of myocarditis include persistent tachycardia and orthostasis, bradycardia, pulsus paradoxus, and a gallop rhythm. Physical examination findings such as dyspnea, crackles, wheezes, gallop rhythms, neck vein distention, and peripheral edema are seen in those with heart failure/cardiomyopathy. There is a wide range of clinical presentations of children with arrhythmias; they may be stable with irregular heart rates and rhythm or they can present in cardiovascular shock. Signs of MI include rate and rhythm disturbances, pallor, dyspnea, diaphoresis, as well as signs of heart failure.

Patients with a pulmonary embolism may present with a variety of physical findings depending on the degree of arterial obstruction and thus hemodynamic compromise (see Chapter 107 Pulmonary Emergencies). Tachypnea, tachycardia, decreased breathsounds, crackles, fever, a friction rub, an accentuated S2, unexplained cyanosis, pleural friction rub, and/or cardiovascular collapse.

In addition to the usual cardiac and pulmonary examination, one should search for "trigger points," where palpation of the chest wall reproduces the pain suggesting musculoskeletal inflammation. Reproduction of the pain by a "hooking maneuver" performed over the lower anterior ribs implicates the "slipping rib syndrome." Pain following a dermatome unilaterally suggests intercostal neuritis; children with zoster (shingles) may have pain preceding the development of rash.

When focal, peripheral pain is found without a "trigger point," the physician should consider pain referred from areas of sensory nerve overlap. A relationship of the pain to eating or swallowing suggests esophageal disease, and often, the physical examination may appear normal. Some of these patients will have a thin body habitus and/or cardiac findings of mitral valve prolapse.

Extrathoracic abnormalities, such as a rash or arthritis, may provide clues to collagen disorders (see Chapter 109 Rheumatologic Emergencies) or other systemic illness. Marfan syndrome should be suspected in the tall thin patient whose upper-extremity span exceeds his or her height and with overextensible fingers.

During the examination, it is useful to relate normal findings to the child and family because this reassurance often serves as the major "treatment" of self-limited or functional problems. Some families and patients are simply looking for reassurance that the chest pain is not cardiac in origin. Concerning physical examination findings such as fever, persistent tachycardia, persistent hypertension, hypotension, pathologic murmurs, a gallop rhythm, abnormal pulses, abnormal perfusion, hypoxia, and syncope warrant further investigation. Pulse oximetry is a quick and inexpensive screen that is helpful in determining the severity of any suspected pulmonary disease.

An EKG should be performed in most cases of chest pain if cardiac disease is a possibility. Studies have shown that most cases of cardiac-related chest pain can be picked up based on history, past medical history, concerning family history, physician examination, and an EKG. The EKG will be normal in almost all children with chest pain in which the physical examination is unremarkable. However, it may show signs of cardiac strain or ischemia with valvular heart disease, diseases of outflow obstruction, or ischemia. Acute cocaine exposure may present with classic signs of myocardial ischemia or myocardiopathy. A decreased QRS wave voltage and electrical alternans suggest the presence of a pericardial effusion in the child with muffled heart sounds. Decreased voltages, ST elevations, and T-wave abnormalities may also be seen in diseases such as myocarditis and pericarditis. Heart block and arrhythmias, such as atrial fibrillation and supraventricular tachycardia, can occur secondary to anatomic, ischemic, inflammatory, and drug-induced conditions. These electrical disturbances may be identified by careful evaluation of a rhythm strip. Finally, the S_1-Q_3-T_3 pattern may be seen on EKG evaluation in those with a pulmonary embolism.

Chest radiographs are not necessary for all patients who present with nontraumatic chest pain. They should be used selectively in patients in whom there is a clinical concern for a pulmonary or cardiac cause of the chest pain. One may consider obtaining a CXR in a patient with pulmonary symptoms such as cough or shortness of breath, unilateral chest pain, a concerning PMH, or abnormal physician examination findings such as abnormal breath sounds, unilateral breathsounds, a murmur, or abnormal vital signs such as tachypnea or tachycardia. The CXR may reveal findings consistent with asthma, pneumonitis, pleurisy, spontaneous pneumothorax, or mass. Foreign bodies ingested and lodged in the esophagus can be visualized if radiopaque (e.g., coins). In the cervical esophagus, they will lie flat and be fully visible in the posteroanterior view of the chest. A foreign body such as a coin in trachea typically appears "on end" on the posteroanterior view of the chest. Airway foreign-body aspiration most frequently manifests, however, by hyperinflation or atelectasis on radiographs because most tracheobronchial foreign bodies are not radiopaque. Inspiratory and expiratory films or decubitus chest radiographs may demonstrate focal hyperinflation (i.e., the lobe with an obstructed bronchus remains inflated in expiration or when placed on the dependent side on a decubitus film). Other characteristic radiographic changes include the wide mediastinum from an aortic aneurysm, abnormal cardiac silhouette related to a pericardial effusion or cardiomegaly, rib fractures, or bone changes of metabolic bone derangements. A calcified ring may be visualized in approximately one-third of patients with a history of Kawasaki disease. The presence of atelectasis may suggest mucous plugging or may be subtle evidence of pulmonary infarction from an embolus or a vasoocclusive crisis of sickle cell anemia. The presence of a wedge-shaped pulmonary infiltrate with an ipsilateral elevated hemidiaphragm is suggestive of a pulmonary embolism.

Studies other than chest radiographs and EKGs are rarely necessary. Laboratory studies (such as troponin) are typically not needed in the workup of most patients with chest pain. However, if there is clinical suspicion for cardiac abnormalities such as myocarditis, pericarditis, or acute MI based on history or an abnormal EKG, then selective use of a troponin assay is warranted. In general, myocarditis is often the cause of increased troponin as the diagnosis of acute MI is extremely low in children. Of note, troponin levels may be elevated in noncardiac disease states such as sepsis. B-type natriuretic peptide (BNP) can be useful in children with pre-existing heart disease or in those who are in congestive heart failure. Toxicologic screens are useful if the patient is considered at risk of drug abuse, particularly cocaine, or if the diagnosis remains unclear.

An elevated leukocyte count with a shift to the left may point toward infection as the cause of pain in patients with a systemic illness. Examination of a peripheral smear and a hemoglobin electrophoresis are indicated in the child suspected of having sickle cell disease as the cause of chest pain. In children with sickle cell disease, a CBC, reticulocyte count, and blood culture are indicated to assist in ascertaining acute chest syndrome or pneumonia, as well as the presence of acute anemia and its cause. If an intra-abdominal source for chest pain from diaphragmatic irritation is under consideration, a serum amylase may be obtained in the workup of pancreatitis. The evaluation of a possible right-sided subdiaphragmatic abscess would include liver function tests and further delineation by ultrasound or CT scan. Findings of low PaO_2, EKG abnormalities, and a positive D-dimer are suggestive of pulmonary embolism. This suspected diagnosis requires the performance of a helical CT scan for confirmation.

Esophageal causes of chest pain may often be diagnosed clinically in the ED with a trial of antacid therapy followed by H_2 antagonist or proton pump inhibitors. To confirm the findings of a hiatal hernia, esophagitis, or a radiolucent foreign body, a barium study or endoscopy may be required. The clinician may consider peak expiratory flow testing and/or therapeutic trial of bronchodilators when asthma is suspected as the cause of chest pain. Consultation with a pediatric cardiologist acutely for conditions such as myocarditis, pericarditis, acute MI, or significant findings on EKG may be necessary to assist with further workup and tests such as echocardiograms. The decision to obtain an urgent echocardiogram depends on the clinical suspicion for diseases such as myocarditis, pericarditis, pericardial effusion, or signs of congestive heart failure. Follow-up with a cardiologist may also be warranted for a concerning history such as exercise-induced chest pain, syncope and/or palpitations with chest pain, significant high-risk comorbidities/past medical history, significant family history (see discussion under "Child With No Thoracic Trauma") that places the child at high risk for cardiopulmonary disease, or EKG findings that require additional workup such as outpatient echocardiograms.

Not infrequently, the workup of chest pain including tests such as an EKG or chest radiographs is helpful in allaying parental fears of cardiac disease. However, the clinician should be aware that in some cases where a cardiac or respiratory condition is not suspected, ordering unnecessary tests may actually increase a patient's or parent's concern that true pathology exists. Definitive ongoing management requires referral to a primary care physician.

SUMMARY

Chest pain in children is a relatively uncommon sign of serious disease, but often has great importance to the patient or family. Most cases can be diagnosed by the emergency physician from the history and physical examination alone. Most all cardiac causes of chest pain can be diagnosed from the full history, physical examination, and EKG. Selective use of chest radiography and labs including troponin may be warranted in specific cases. The physician should always consider drug-induced chest pain (especially associated with cocaine) and other life-threatening conditions. Patients with a history of exercise-induced chest pain, palpitations and/or syncope, medical history of underlying cardiopulmonary condition, suspected Kawasaki disease, collagen vascular disease, connective tissue disorders, hyperlipidemia, malignancy, thrombophilia, myopathies, history of drug use, oral contraceptive and cigarette use, and family history of sudden death, early coronary artery disease, cardiomyopathy, hypercholesterolemia, hypercoagulability disorders, hyperlipidemia, and pulmonary hypertension appear to be at higher risk of cardiovascular disease. Psychogenic chest pain is a common occurrence and may be chronic or related to an acute stressful event. The possibility of cardiac disease needs to be addressed directly by the examining physician to alleviate fully the patient's (or family's) anxiety. The most common causes of organic chest pain are musculoskeletal (traumatic or inflammatory) and infectious disorders, usually self-limited or easily treated diseases. Occasionally, serious abdominal, pulmonary, or cardiac problems require immediate attention.

Suggested Readings and Key References

Angoff GH, Kane DA, Giddins N, et al. Regional implementation of pediatric cardiology chest pain guideline using SCAMP methodology. *Pediatrics* 2013;132:e1010–e1017.

Anwar S, Kavey RE. Pediatric chest pain: findings on exercise stress testing. *Clin Pediatr* 2012;51(7):659–662.

Asnes R, Santulli R, Bemborad J. Psychogenic chest pain in children. *Clin Pediatr* 1981;20(12):788–791.

Berezin S, Medow MS, Glassman MS, et al. Chest pain of gastrointestinal origin. *Arch Dis Child* 1998;63:1457–1460.

Brown JL, Hirsh DA, Mahle WT. Use of troponin as a screen for chest pain in the pediatric emergency department. *Pediatr Cardiol* 2012; 33:337–342.

Burns JC, Shike H, Gordon JB, et al. Sequelae of Kawasaki disease in adolescents and young adults. *J Am Coll Cardiol* 1996;28:253–257.

Cava JR, Sayger PL. Chest pain in children and adolescents. *Pediatr Clin North Am* 2004;51:1553–1568.

Chalumeau M, Le Clainche L, Sayeg N, et al. Spontaneous pnuemomediastinum in children. *Pediatr Pulmonol* 2001;31:67–75.

Christensen DD, Vincent RN, Campbell RM. Presentation of atrial septal defect in the pediatric population. *Pediatr Cardiol* 2005;26: 812–814.

Dekel B, Paret G, Szeinberg A, et al. Spontaneous pneumomediastinum in children: clinical and natural history. *Eur J Pediatr* 1996;155: 695–697.

Driscoll D, Glicklich L, Gallen N. Chest pain in children: a prospective study. *Pediatrics* 1976;57:648–651.

Drossner DM, Hirsh DA, Sturm JJ, et al. Cardiac disease in pediatric patients presenting to a pediatric ED with chest pain. *Am J Emerg Med* 2011;29:632–638.

Ernst E. Cardiovascular adverse effects of herbal medicines: a systematic review of the recent literature. *Can J Cardiol* 2003;19:818–827.

Friedman KG, Kane DA, Rathod RH, et al. Management of pediatric chest pain using a standardized assessment and management plan. *Pediatrics* 2011;128(2):239–245.

Frommelt PC, Frommelt MA, Tweddell JS, et al. Prospective echocardiographic diagnosis and surgical repair of anomalous origin of a coronary artery from the opposite sinus with an interarterial course. *J Am Coll Cardiol* 2003;42:148–154.

Gitter MJ, Goldsmith SR, Dunbar DN, et al. Cocaine and chest pain: clinical features and outcome of patients hospitalized to rule out myocardial infarction. *Ann Intern Med* 1991;115:277–282.

Glassman MS, Medow MS, Berezin S, et al. Spectrum of esophageal disorders in children with chest pain. *Dig Dis Sci* 1992;37(5):663–666.

Hayes D Jr. Chest pain. Hemothorax. *Clin Pediatr (Phila)* 2007;46(8): 746–747.

Hoerbelt R, Keunecke L, Grimm H, et al. The value of a noninvasive diagnostic approach to mediastinal masses. *Ann Thor Surg* 2003; 75:1086–1090.

Horton L, Mosee S, Brenner J. Use of the electrocardiogram in a pediatric emergency department. *Arch Pediatr Adolesc Med* 1994;148:184–188.

Hyman PE, Bursch B, Sood M, et al. Visceral pain-associated disability syndrome: a descriptive analysis. *J Pediatr Gastroenterol Nutr* 2002; 35:663–668.

Kane DA, Fulton DR, Saleeb S. Needles in hay: chest pain as the presenting symptom in children with serious underlying cardiac pathology. *Congenit Heart Dis* 2010;5:366–373.

Kocis KC. Chest pain in pediatrics. *Pediatr Cardiol* 1999;46(2):189–203.

Kundra M, Yousaf S, Maqbool S, et al. Boerhaave syndrome—unusual cause of chest pain. *Pediatr Emerg Care* 2007;23(7):489–491.

Kyle WB, Macicek SL, Lindle KA, et al. Limited utility of exercise stress tests in the evaluation of children with chest pain. *Congenit Heart Dis* 2012;7:455–459.

Lieberman A. Spontaneous pneumomediastinum in an adolescent patient. *J Adolesc Health Care* 1990;11:170–172.

Mahle WT, Cambell RM, Favaloro-Sabatier F. Myocardial infarction in adolescents. *Pediatrics* 2007;151:150–154.

Massin MM, Bourguignont A, Coremans C, et al. Chest pain in pediatric patients presenting to an emergency department or to a cardiac clinic. *Clin Pediatr* 2004;43:231–238.

Milov DE, Cynamon HA, Andres JM. Chest pain and dysphagia in adolescents caused by diffuse esophageal spasm. *J Pediatr Gastroenterol Nutr* 1989;9:450–453.

Mukamel M, Kornreich L, Horev G, et al. Tietze's syndrome in children and infants. *J Pediatr* 1997;131(5):774–775.

Neff J, Anderson M, Stephenson T, et al. Radiographs in the emergency department utilization criteria evaluation—pediatric chest pain. *Pediatr Emerg Care* 2012;28(5):451–454.

Perry T, Zha H, Oster ME, et al. Utility of a clinical support tool for outpatient evaluation of pediatric chest pain. *AMIA Annu Symp Proc* 2012;2012:726–733.

Rowe BH, Dulberg CS, Peterson RG, et al. Characteristics of children presenting with chest pain to a pediatric emergency department. *Can Med Assoc J* 1990;143(5):388–394.

Sabri MR, Ghavanini AA, Haghighat M, et al. Chest pain in children and adolescents: epigastric tenderness as a guide to reduce unnecessary work-up. *Pediatr Cardiol* 2003;24(1):3–5.

Saleeb SF, Li WY, Warren SZ, et al. Effectiveness of screening for life-threatening chest pain in children. *Pediatrics* 2011;128(5):e1062–e1068.

Selbst SM. Chest pain in children. *Pediatr Rev* 1997;18(5):169–173.

Selbst SM, Ruddy RM, Clark BJ, et al. Pediatric chest pain: a prospective study. *Pediatrics* 1988;82:319–323.

Selbst SM, Ruddy RM, Clark BJ, et al. Follow up of patients previously reported. *Clin Pediatr* 1990;29:374–377.

Taubman B, Vetter VL. Slipping rib syndrome as a cause of chest pain in children. *Clin Pediatr* 1996;35:403–405.

Tomita M, Suzuki N, Igarachi H, et al. Evidence against strong correlation between chest symptoms and ischemic coronary changes after subcutaneous sumatriptan injection. *Intern Med* 2002;41:622–625.

Walthen JE, Rewers AB, Yetman AT, et al. Accuracy of ECG interpretation in the pediatric emergency department. *Ann Emerg Med* 2005;46(6):507–511.

Woolf PK, Gewitz M, Berezin S, et al. Noncardiac chest pain in adolescents and children with mitral valve prolapse. *J Adolesc Health* 1991;12:247–250.

Yildirim A, Karakurt C, Karademir S, et al. Chest pain in children. *Int Pediatr* 2004;19(3):175–179.

Zavarus-Angelidou KA, Weinhouse E, Nelson DB. Review of 180 episodes of chest pain in 134 children. *Pediatr Emerg Care* 1992;8:189–193.

CHAPTER 51 ▪ PAIN: DYSPHAGIA

RAHUL KAILA, MD, RONALD A. FURNIVAL, MD, AND GEORGE A. WOODWARD, MD, MBA

The primary function of swallowing is the ingestion, preparation, and transport of nutrients to the digestive tract. Secondary functions of swallowing are the control of secretions, clearance of respiratory contaminants, protection of the upper airway, and equalization of pressure across the tympanic membrane through the eustachian tube. Dysphagia is defined as any difficulty or abnormality of swallowing. Dysphagia is not a specific disease entity but is a symptom of other, often clinically occult, conditions and may be life-threatening if respiration or nutrition is compromised. Odynophagia (pain on swallowing) or sialorrhea (drooling) may also be present in the dysphagic pediatric patient. Globus pharyngeus refers to the feeling of a lump in the throat. This chapter briefly presents the normal anatomy and physiology of swallowing, the differential diagnosis of disturbances of this process, and the evaluation and treatment of the pediatric patient with dysphagia.

PATHOPHYSIOLOGY

Swallowing begins in utero as early as the 10th to 14th week of gestation, playing an important role in gastrointestinal development and regulation of amniotic fluid volume. By the 34th week of gestation, this complex process, involving 26 muscles, 6 cranial nerves (V, VII, IX, X, XI, and XII), and cervical nerves C1 to C3, is functional, although incompletely coordinated with breathing. In the first few days after birth, each infant develops an individual pattern of sucking, swallowing, and breathing, usually with a 1:1 or 1:2 ratio of breaths per suckle, to prevent aspiration of material into the larynx. This stage of suckling, or suckle feeding, is primarily under medullary control, with minimal input from the cerebral cortex. A transitional period begins at 6 months of age, as the cortex gradually exerts more control over the pre-esophageal phase of swallowing, allowing for the introduction of solid foods. Swallowing in the esophageal region remains an autonomic process, with vagal sensorimotor control coordinating peristalsis of the upper striated and lower smooth muscle of the esophagus. By 3 years of age, the swallowing pattern is mature, although the pediatric patient, unlike the adult, may regress to a less mature stage if normal swallowing is disrupted.

To facilitate suckle feeding and breathing, the infant oropharynx is anatomically different from the adult, with a relatively larger tongue, smaller oral cavity, and more anterior and superior epiglottis and larynx. As the face and mandible grow, the oropharynx enlarges, creating more room for the eventual voluntary use of the tongue and dentition, and the larynx descends, eventually allowing for mouth breathing. Although breathing continues to cease during swallows, the older child depends less on close coordination between eating and breathing.

A normal swallow, using the suckling infant as an example, begins with rhythmic movement of the lips, tongue, and mandible. These parts function as a unit, creating negative intraoral pressure, while also compressing the nipple. The milk expressed from each suckle is stored in the posterior oral cavity until a larger fluid bolus is formed. As the tongue delivers the bolus to the pharynx, the nasopharynx is closed off by the posterior tongue and by elevation of the soft palate. The larynx elevates to a position under the tongue, closing the airway, as the epiglottis inclines to direct the bolus posterior. A pharyngeal wave of contraction sweeps the bolus toward the upper esophagus, where the cricopharyngeal sphincter relaxes, allowing passage into the esophagus. As the esophagus begins peristaltic contractions and the bolus moves past a relaxed lower esophageal sphincter into the stomach, the airway reopens, the cricopharyngeal sphincter constricts to close the upper esophagus, and respirations resume. Dysphagia can result from disruption of normal mechanisms at any stage of the swallowing process.

DIFFERENTIAL DIAGNOSIS

Acute dysphagia is one of the urgent symptoms needing immediate evaluation. While this may be an acute symptom in a healthy child, it may be a new or recurrent symptom in the increasing number of children surviving with chronic conditions. The incidence and prevalence of pediatric dysphagia is increasing, probably due to improved early medical and supportive care for prematurity and other conditions. The differential diagnosis for dysphagia is extensive and is commonly divided into pre-esophageal or esophageal disorders (Table 51.1). Pre-esophageal causes of dysphagia are further subdivided into anatomic categories, including nasopharyngeal, oropharyngeal, laryngeal, and generalized problems. Infectious and inflammatory disorders of either anatomic region may disrupt swallowing, whereas neuromuscular problems tend to be predominantly pre-esophageal, given the autonomic function of the esophagus. However, the esophagus can be affected by motility disorders intrinsic to smooth muscle. Finally, the differential diagnosis includes several systemic conditions that may affect the normal swallowing process. In a large case series of pediatric patients who underwent fiberoptic evaluation of swallowing function after presenting with dysphagia, 36% were found to have structural abnormalities of the aerodigestive tract or airway, 26% had neurologic diagnoses, 12% had gastrointestinal disorders, 8% had genetic syndromes, 5% had prematurity, 3% had cardiovascular anomalies, and 2% had metabolic issues.

In the adult patient, dysphagia most commonly results from a variety of neuromuscular disorders, whereas the pediatric patient more often has swallowing difficulty from congenital, infectious, inflammatory, or obstructive causes (Table 51.2). Dysphagia occurs in 85% of cerebral palsy patients, and is directly related to the severity of their overall neuromuscular

TABLE 51.1

DIFFERENTIAL DIAGNOSIS OF DYSPHAGIA

Pre-esophageal (nasopharynx, oropharynx, larynx)

- Mechanical/anatomic
  - Congenital syndromes
    - Pierre Robin
    - Treacher Collins
    - Crouzon's
    - Goldenhar's
    - Cornelia de Lange
  - Cysts (tongue, larynx, epiglottis)
  - Tumors (neuroblastoma)
  - Lymphangioma
  - Foreign-body aspiration
  - Traumatic (external, endotracheal intubation, endoscopy)
- Nasopharyngeal
  - Choanal stenosis/atresia
  - Nasal septum deflections
- Oropharyngeal
  - Cleft palate/lip
  - Submucosal cleft
  - Macroglossia
    - Down syndrome (trisomy 21)
    - Beckwith–Wiedemann syndrome
  - Micrognathia
  - Lip/teeth defects
  - Tongue/sublingual masses
    - Hemangioma
    - Lymphangioma
    - Lingual thyroid
    - Thyroglossal duct cyst
    - Branchial cleft cyst
  - Hypopharyngeal stenosis
  - Temporomandibular joint ankylosis
  - Pharyngeal diverticula (congenital/traumatic)
  - Adenoidal/tonsillar hypertrophy
- Laryngeal
  - Tracheostomy
  - Tracheoesophageal fistula
  - Cervical vertebral osteophytes
  - Airway obstruction
  - Laryngomalacia
- Inflammatory/infectious
  - Anaphylaxis
  - Tetanus
  - Rabies
  - Botulism (especially infant botulism)
  - Poliomyelitis
  - Angioneurotic edema
  - Sydenham chorea
  - Juvenile rheumatoid arthritis
  - Stevens–Johnson syndrome
- Nasopharyngeal
  - Nasal septal abscess
  - Sinusitis
- Oropharyngeal
  - Stomatitis (infectious, allergic)
  - Pharyngitis/tonsillitis/uvulitis
  - Retropharyngeal abscess
  - Peritonsillar abscess
  - Cervical adenitis
- Laryngeal
  - Epiglottitis
  - Diphtheria
  - Thyroiditis
- Neuromuscular
  - Prematurity
  - Hypoxic injury
  - Head trauma
  - Neurologic impairment
  - Cerebral palsy
  - Developmental delay
  - Meningitis
  - Cerebral abscess
  - Cerebral cortical atrophy/hypoplasia/agenesis
  - Arnold–Chiari malformation
  - Cerebrovascular disease
- Cranial nerve palsies (V, VII, IX–XII)
  - Palatal paralysis
  - Laryngeal paralysis
- Spinal cord impairment
  - Syringomyelia
  - Cricopharyngeal incoordination/spasm
- Moebius syndrome
- Myotonic muscular dystrophy
- Guillain–Barré syndrome
- Werdnig–Hoffman
- Myasthenia gravis
- Myotonic dystrophy
- Dermatomyositis
- Miscellaneous
  - Ingestions (neuroleptic-induced dystonic reaction)
  - Familial dysautonomia (Riley–Day syndrome)
  - Prader–Willi syndrome
  - Cerebrohepatorenal syndrome
  - Vitamin deficiencies (pellagra, scurvy)
  - Acrodynia
  - Infantile Gaucher disease
  - Psychiatric
  - Globus hystericus ("lump" in throat sensation)
  - Pseudodysphagia
  - Conversion reaction
  - Hyperphagia
  - Munchausen by proxy
- Respiratory distress

Esophageal causes of dysphagia

- Mechanical/anatomic
  - Tracheoesophageal fistula
  - Esophageal atresia/stenosis
  - Esophageal diverticula/duplication
  - Esophageal strictures
    - Congenital (webs, fibromuscular, tracheobronchial remnants)
    - Acquired (corrosive ingestion, esophagitis, postoperative)
  - Foreign-body ingestion
  - Thermal injury (burn from hot food/drink)
  - Esophageal tumors (hamartomas, leiomyoma, rhabdomyoma)
  - Esophageal polyps
  - External esophageal compression
  - Cardiovascular anomalies (aberrant right subclavian artery, vascular rings, double aortic arch)
  - Mediastinal tumors/infiltrations
  - Atopic thyroid
  - Diaphragmatic hernias
  - Paraesophageal hernia
  - Hiatal hernia
- Altered esophageal motility
  - Achalasia
  - Gastroesophageal reflux
  - Esophageal spasm
- Inflammatory/infectious
  - Eosinophilic esophagitis
  - Infectious esophagitis
  - Candida albicans
  - Herpes simplex
  - Cytomegalovirus
  - Human immunodeficiency virus
- Reflux esophagitis
- Allergic esophagitis
- Radiation injury
- Mediastinitis
- Esophageal perforation
- Crohn disease
- Chagas disease (Trypanosoma cruzi, a South American parasite)
- Miscellaneous
  - Connective tissue disease
    - Scleroderma
    - Systemic lupus erythematosus
    - Polymyositis
    - Dermatomyositis
    - Sjögren syndrome
    - Behçet disease
- Hyperkalemia, hypermagnesemia
- Muscular hypertrophy of esophagus
- Central nervous system tumors
- Demyelinating diseases
- Epidermolysis bullosa congenita
- Lesch–Nyhan syndrome
- Wilson disease
- Dyskeratosis congenita
- Opitz–Frias syndrome
- Lipidosis
- Myxedema
- Thyrotoxicosis
- Alcoholism
- Diabetes
- Amyloidosis
- Posttruncal vagotomy, antireflux surgery
- Subcutaneous emphysema

TABLE 51.2

COMMON CAUSES OF DYSPHAGIA

Newborn/infant
Prematurity
Tracheoesophageal fistula
Choanal stenosis/atresia
Birth trauma
Congenital abnormalities
Gastroesophageal reflux
Respiratory illness
Neurologic/neuromuscular disease
Infectious (botulism, candidiasis, herpetic esophagitis)
Inflammatory
Child
Foreign-body aspiration/ingestion
Caustic ingestion
Infectious
Ingestions (neuroleptic-induced dystonic reaction)
Neurologic impairment (cerebral palsy, mental retardation, head trauma)
Inflammatory

impairment. In the newborn or infant, swallowing may be disturbed as a result of prematurity, often associated with respiratory and neurologic disabilities. Gastroesophageal reflux is common in infants, although in a small percentage of patients, it may persist into childhood with reflux esophagitis. Eosinophilic esophagitis has recently been identified as an important cause of dysphagia, particularly in adolescents and young adults with environmental allergies, atopy, and food allergies. Ingestion or aspiration of a foreign body must always be considered in an infant or toddler who has either the acute or chronic onset of dysphagia (Fig. 51.1). Swallowing dysfunction is a common complication following pediatric head injury. In a review of 1,145 pediatric head injury patients, 68% of those with severe injury and 15% of those suffering moderate injury were found to have dysphagia requiring intervention. Postoperative dysphagia is also common after laryngotracheal reconstruction surgery or cardiovascular surgery. In a review of 2,255 children who had cardiovascular surgery, Sachdeva et al. found that 1.7% had vocal cord dysfunction associated with significant feeding problems and required prolonged gastrostomy feeding. These patients are predisposed to aspiration due to impaired airway protection.

TABLE 51.3

LIFE-THREATENING CAUSES OF DYSPHAGIA

Foreign-body aspiration/ingestion
Anaphylaxis
Tracheoesophageal fistula
Upper airway obstruction
Traumatic esophageal perforation
Epiglottitis
Retropharyngeal abscess
Botulism
Tetanus
Polio
Diphtheria
Central nervous system infection/abscess
Stevens–Johnson syndrome
Corrosive ingestion
Laryngeal paralysis

Life-threatening causes of dysphagia may involve airway compromise, serious local or systemic infection, and inflammatory disease (Table 51.3). The newborn may have a congenital anatomic abnormality, such as tracheoesophageal fistula, with aspiration of swallowed fluid into the lungs, or may have traumatic injury to the upper airway and esophagus from iatrogenic instrumentation in the delivery room. The older child may have a foreign body in the airway or esophagus, with the possibility

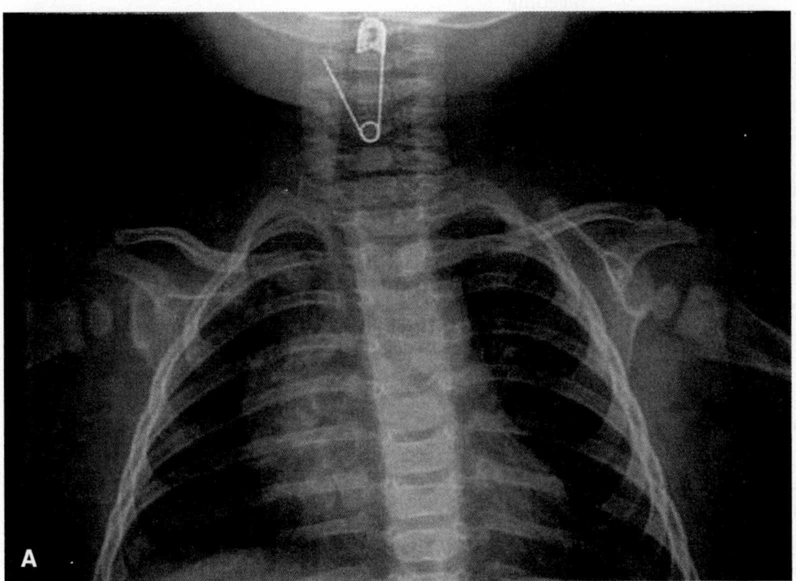

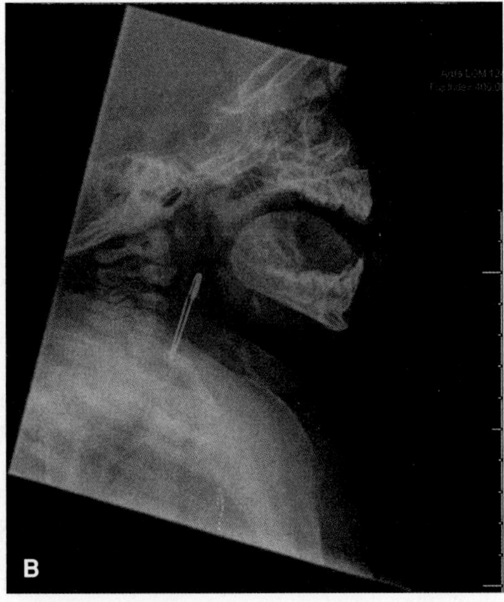

FIGURE 51.1 Six-month-old who came to the ED for choking episode and later abnormal breathing and drooling. AP (**A**) and lateral radiographs (**B**) of the neck showed open safety pin in the hypopharynx area.

of complete airway obstruction (see Chapter 3 Airway). Anaphylaxis or other allergic and infectious processes may present with dysphagia and can threaten airway integrity. These include epiglottitis, retropharyngeal abscess, Stevens–Johnson syndrome, and central nervous system infections.

EVALUATION AND DECISION

The evaluation of dysphagia in the pediatric patient begins with a detailed history, including pregnancy and delivery, family history, feeding history, growth and development, and a history of other illness (Table 51.4). An accurate and complete history should suggest the diagnosis in approximately 80% of patients. Prenatal polyhydramnios, maternal infection, maternal drug or medication use, bleeding disorders, thyroid dysfunction, toxemia, or irradiation may lead to or indicate swallowing problems in the newborn or infant. Association between decreased rate of fetal suckling and digestive tract obstruction or neurologic damage is well known. Maternal myasthenia gravis may also cause temporary feeding problems in the newborn.

A history of traumatic delivery may result in neurologic injury or laryngeal paralysis. Newborn intubation may be associated with trauma to the trachea, larynx, or esophagus, as well as hypoxic brain injury. A history of prematurity, developmental delay, failure to thrive, hypotonia, or associated congenital abnormalities may indicate a neuromuscular cause for dysphagia. The feeding history should include acute or chronic onset of symptoms, age at onset, weight loss, failure to thrive, and type and amount of food the child eats. Presence of fever, pain, respiratory symptoms, facial color, stridor, liquid or solid food intolerance, vomiting, regurgitation, drooling, voice change, position during feeding, and the timing of symptoms in relation to feedings should also be documented. For example, the infant with an upper airway obstruction may become fatigued or begin coughing and choking shortly after beginning to eat. Choking during feeding in an infant may be due to an underlying anatomic abnormality of the trachea, esophagus, or larynx. Congenital vascular lesions causing extrinsic compression of the esophagus may remain silent until the introduction of solid food, or may rarely manifest as dysphagia later in adulthood. Gastroesophageal reflux in infants may manifest as vomiting shortly after feeding or with a history of nighttime cough or emesis. Intrinsic lesions, from inflammation, tumor, or foreign body, may create problems with solid food but cause no difficulty with liquids. Infants with previously unrecognized neuromuscular disorders commonly present initially with dysphagia, particularly for liquids, drooling, prolonged feeding time, weak suckle, or nasal reflux of swallowed material. A history of fever may indicate aspiration pneumonia or other infectious or inflammatory causes of dysphagia. Determining whether symptoms are progressive or intermittent/nonprogressive can also be helpful.

The child with dysphagia should undergo a thorough general physical examination, initially focusing on the patient's cardiopulmonary status. Evidence of respiratory distress or cardiovascular compromise should be treated promptly in the appropriate manner, as outlined elsewhere in this text (see Chapters 3 Airway and 4 Cardiopulmonary Resuscitation). Assurance of a secure and stable airway should precede attempts to examine the oropharynx or to remove a foreign body (see Chapter 27 Foreign Body: Ingestion and Aspiration).

TABLE 51.4

IMPORTANT HISTORICAL FEATURES FOR DYSPHAGIA

- General
  - Age of onset
  - Acute/gradual onset
  - Weight gain
  - Growth and development
  - Constant, progressive, or intermittent
  - Pain (location/quality)
  - Fever
  - Ingestion history (neuroleptics, foreign bodies, or caustics)
  - Difficulty chewing
  - Difficulty swallowing
  - Change in voice quality
  - Altered swallowing sensation (lump, sticking, or foreign body)
  - Drooling/salivation
  - Solid/liquid intolerance
  - Cough/choking while feeding
  - Respiratory symptoms after feeding (stridor, wheezing, or apnea)
  - Vomiting (gastric contents) versus regurgitation (food without gastric contents, esophageal disorders)
  - Nasopharyngeal regurgitation
  - Gastroesophageal reflux
  - Peptic ulcer disease
  - Tobacco or alcohol usage
  - Recent esophageal or airway instrumentation
  - Arthritis, degenerative joint disease
  - Antibiotic use
  - Chemotherapy
  - Underlying illness, immunodeficiency
  - Newborn/infant
  - Prematurity
- Pregnancy history
  - Infections
  - Medications (especially antihypertensives)
  - Bleeding
  - Toxemia
  - Thyroid dysfunction
  - Polyhydramnios
  - Fetal irradiation
  - Food allergy
- Birth history
  - Birth trauma
  - Hypoxia
  - Endotracheal intubation or resuscitation
- Cough/gag/cyanosis/fatigue/stridor/irritability with feeding
- Feeding times greater than 30 min
- Respiratory distress associated with feeding
- Vomiting or regurgitation
- Level of alertness
- Weight gain or failure to thrive
- Nasal regurgitation
- Refusal to eat age-appropriate foods
- Recurrent pneumonias
- Family history of neuromuscular disease

In the stable dysphagic patient, evaluation of head size and shape, facial structure, mandibular development, tongue disproportion, and ear configuration may provide evidence of an underlying congenital abnormality, such as Pierre Robin, Treacher Collins, Crouzon, and Goldenhar syndromes. Evaluation of nasal airway patency in the infant can be determined by gently passing an 8F catheter through the nares into the stomach. If the catheter fails to pass easily, choanal stenosis, atresia, or esophageal obstruction must be considered. Inspection of the oral cavity, pharynx, and neck may reveal a cyst, mass, localized infection, or inflammatory cause for dysphagia. Cervical auscultation over the thyroid cartilage during feeding may note evidence of aspiration if upper airway breath sounds are abnormal or if the timing of breathing and swallowing is uncoordinated. The pulmonary examination may also detect signs of aspiration or respiratory compromise, including elevated respiratory rate, increased respiratory effort, stridor, stertor, rales, rhonchi, wheezing, or change in voice quality. Neurologic examination may reveal an altered level of arousal from an underlying brain injury or depressed sensorium from drugs or infection that may limit effective swallowing. Examination of the cranial nerves, particularly V, VII, IX, X, and XII, may reveal abnormalities from traumatic or surgical injury, tumor, or congenital disorder. Evaluation of muscle tone, strength, and reflexes in consideration of other neuromuscular causes of dysphagia completes the general physical examination.

Provided oral intake is not contraindicated by an expected procedure or intervention, observation of a typical feeding, given by a parent or primary caregiver, may help elucidate the cause of dysphagia. The manner of presentation of food to the patient, the consistency and amount given, patient position, duration of feeding, regurgitation (oral or nasal), agitation or behavior change, or the development of respiratory symptoms may further guide the diagnostic evaluation. Patients with upper airway obstruction may have an exacerbation of symptoms when attempting to drink. Patients with lesions such as tracheoesophageal fistula, vascular rings, or esophageal obstruction may begin coughing and choking soon after drinking without any initial difficulty. However, esophageal disorders such as extrinsic compression, strictures, tumors, or altered motility commonly are clinically silent and typically require use of radiographic or direct visual techniques for diagnosis.

Evaluation of the stable dysphagic patient may proceed on the basis of age and acute versus chronic onset of symptom development (Fig. 51.2). The neonate and young infant will require evaluation techniques and consideration of the age-related differential diagnoses outlined in Table 51.2, whereas the older child with an acute onset of dysphagia generally requires a more urgent approach. Witnessed or suspected foreign bodies, either ingested or aspirated, should be investigated with plain radiographs (or contrast studies if a radiolucent object is considered) and, if identified, emergently removed (see Chapter 27 Foreign Body: Ingestion and Aspiration). A history of neck trauma or caustic ingestion should lead to concern for aerodigestive tract abnormalities. These patients may present dramatically with neck pain, drooling, and evidence of facial or other trauma, but they may also have a subacute presentation (see Chapters 110 Toxicologic Emergencies, 114 ENT Trauma, and 120 Neck Trauma). Presence of fever or signs of systemic illness may result from potentially life-threatening infectious or inflammatory conditions (Table 51.3). Less severe problems (gingivostomatitis or thrush) may present with mouth lesions and can be managed on an outpatient basis after careful assessment of hydration status. Severe problems, including Stevens–Johnson syndrome, herpetic esophagitis, and diphtheria, may be discovered on examination and may require inpatient management.

Patients with a nonacute history of swallowing difficulty can be evaluated and managed as shown in Figure 51.2. The initial emphasis with these patients lies more in determination of nutritional status and development issues than in acute emergency department intervention, although prolonged feeding difficulty can develop into a life-threatening problem. Evaluation of these patients often involves a multidisciplinary approach. The child with obvious anatomic abnormalities, neurologic impairment, specific syndromes, or a tracheostomy may need referral to appropriate subspecialists after initial evaluation. The child without obvious anatomic or neurologic abnormality who has weight loss or failure to thrive may be evaluated as an outpatient.

Radiographic evaluation of the stable dysphagic patient usually begins with an examination of the airway and soft tissues of the neck, looking for evidence of a foreign body, mass, airway impingement, or other abnormality. A chest radiograph may suggest aspiration pneumonia, congenital heart disease, or mediastinal abnormality or, as in the patient with achalasia, demonstrate fluid levels within an enlarged esophagus. Helical computed tomography scan, echocardiography, or angiography may further identify problems suspected from initial studies.

A videofluoroscopic swallowing study (VFSS or modified barium swallow [BS]) is currently the gold standard for evaluating pre-esophageal disorders. This dynamic study may reveal evidence of aspiration, nasopharyngeal reflux, motility disorders, obstructions, masses, cricopharyngeal dysfunction, fistulas, inflammatory processes, or other causes of dysphagia. VFSS differs from the standard BS or upper gastrointestinal (UGI) series in that it does not use pure contrast, but instead uses food mixed with contrast in an attempt to simulate the normal feeding pattern as closely as possible. VFSS is less effective than a UGI series or BS at diagnosing gastroesophageal reflux or lower esophageal, gastric outlet, and small bowel abnormalities (Fig. 51.3), but it is superior in identifying pre-esophageal causes of dysphagia.

Fiberoptic endoscopic evaluation of swallowing (FEES) has also been used as the diagnostic and clinical tool for the pediatric dysphagia patient. With a nasopharyngeal approach under local anesthesia, FEES allows direct visualization of the swallowing process with the ability to document aspiration and functional pharyngeal or upper esophageal disorders. FEES may also be indicated for the suspected mass lesion, stricture, caustic ingestion, inflammatory lesion, or foreign body. FEES has been successfully used to initially screen dysphagia patients and to reevaluate swallowing function after feeding interventions to diet, position, presentation, and so on.

Other tests, such as a complete blood cell count and blood, urine or CSF cultures in the febrile patient, or blood gas for the patient with respiratory distress, may also be indicated. Cervical ultrasonography has been used to identify abnormalities with the tissues and function of the palate, tongue, and floor of the mouth; however, it is less useful than contrast studies for assessing airway problems and aspiration.

Treatment of dysphagia is dictated by the underlying diagnosis. Disorders with the potential to become life-threatening

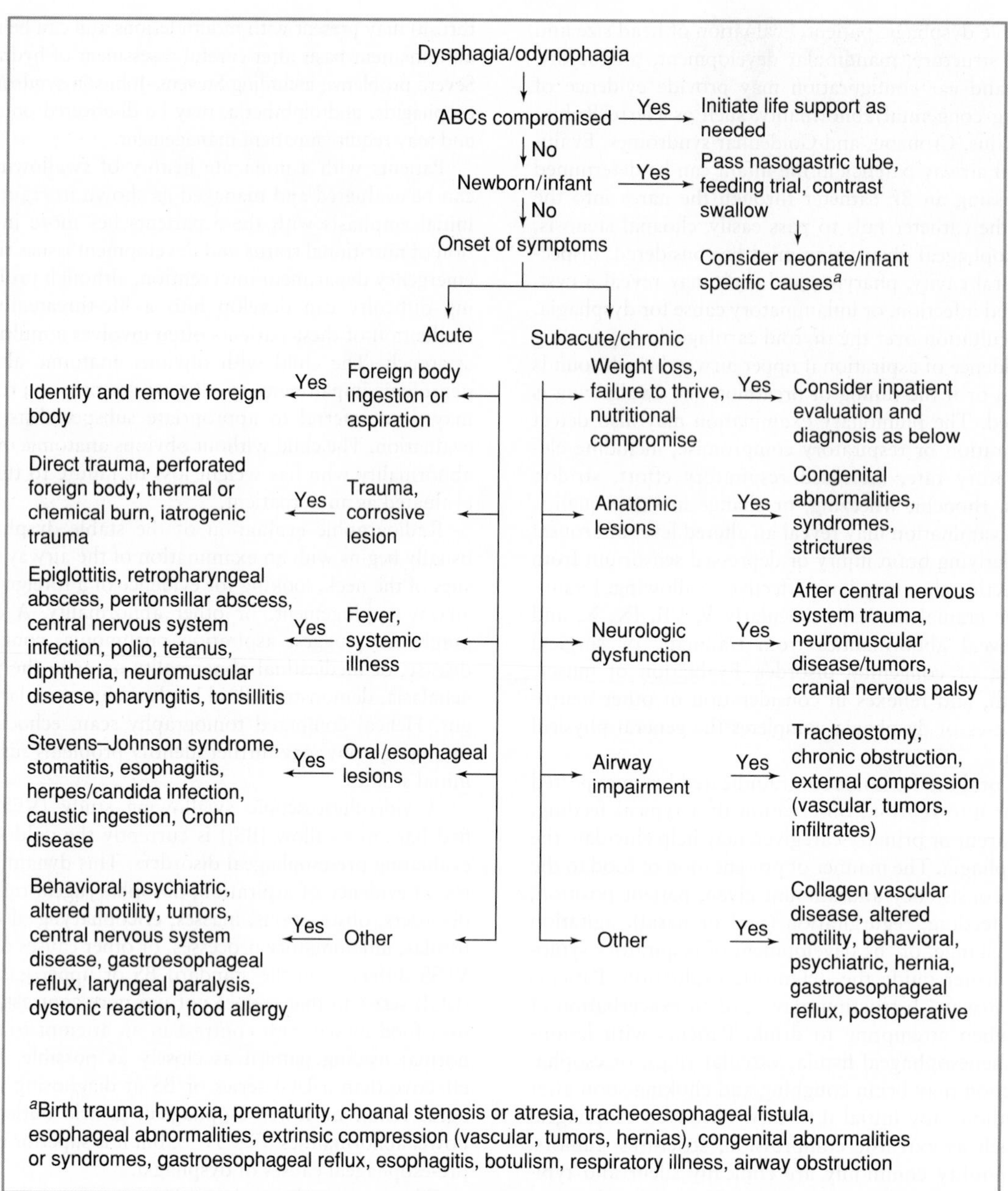

FIGURE 51.2 Evaluation scheme for the child with dysphagia or odynophagia. Radiographic and assessment options: neck, chest, abdomen, inspiratory/expiratory films, lateral decubitus films, fluoroscopy (including videofluoroscopy), contrast studies, ultrasonography, echocardiography, angiography, computed tomography, magnetic resonance imaging, esophageal manometry, laryngopharyngeal sensory testing, electromyography, endoscopy. Laboratory options: complete blood cell count, blood gas, cultures, toxin identifications, nutritional and electrolyte profile. Consultant options: pediatrics, general surgery, otolaryngology, gastroenterology, neurology, infectious disease, cardiology, pulmonology, rheumatology, oncology, nutrition, speech therapy, speech-language pathologist, occupational therapy. ABCs, airway, breathing, circulation.

should be treated in the hospital under the care of appropriate specialists. Chronic dysphagia with actual or potential aspiration should be identified. If nutrition has been severely compromised from chronic dysphagia, one should consider nasogastric, nasojejunal, or gastrostomy tube feedings. Many pediatric facilities have developed multidisciplinary feeding/swallowing teams to provide subspecialty expertise, while maintaining continuity and coordination of patient care. If such a specialty service is not available, involvement of appropriate individual specialists for the management of the patient with dysphagia is imperative as mentioned in Figure 51.2.

However, therapy for many disorders can be initiated on an outpatient basis. Gastroesophageal reflux and resultant esophagitis can often be successfully managed with small-volume thickened feeds and positioning. Several studies showed that gastroesophageal reflux is decreased in prone position rather than supine. Prone position is recommended only when the patient is awake and being observed as there is a higher risk of SIDS with sleeping prone in infants. Semi-supine positioning such as in a car seat or infant carrier is also not recommended as studies have shown more reflux in these position especially after feeding. Medical therapy consists of liquid antacids,

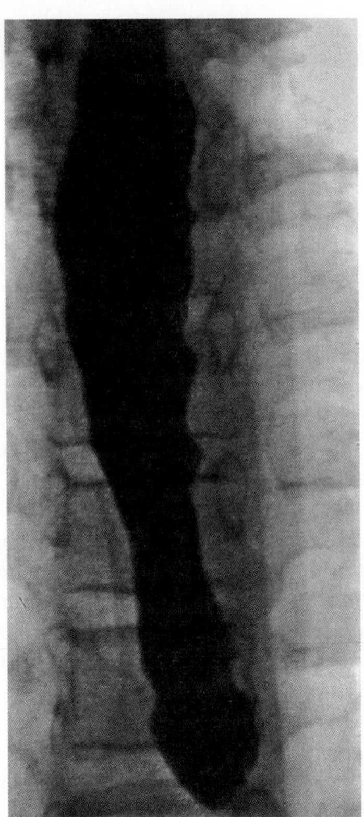

FIGURE 51.3 Upper gastrointestinal (UGI) series of a 14-year-old girl presenting with dysphagia. The UGI demonstrates a significantly dilated upper esophagus, with a functional spasmodic obstruction of the lower esophagus, characteristic of achalasia.

metoclopramide (should not be used long term due to risk of permanent dystonias), H_2-blockers, or proton pump inhibitors. Fishbein et al. found that gastroesophageal reflux disease overlapped with dysphagia, and swallowing dysfunction should be considered for persistently symptomatic patients already on appropriate reflux treatment, especially those with extreme prematurity, developmental delay, or who do not respond to antireflux medication. Children who have failed reflux therapy may also be candidates for an evaluation for eosinophilic esophagitis. Eosinophilic esophagitis is defined as vomiting and abdominal pain with solid dysphagia in children and esophageal impaction in postpubertal age. Treatment of eosinophilic esophagitis includes topical or oral steroids along with proton pump inhibitors. Mycostatin will be helpful in candidal esophagitis, whereas herpetic esophagitis often is self-limiting.

Pediatric dysphagia is an uncommon complaint in the pediatric emergency department but may be the presenting symptom for a wide variety of underlying clinical problems. The history and physical examination first must focus on potentially life-threatening causes and will often lead to a specific diagnosis. Causes of dysphagia not identified from the initial evaluation may require radiographic or subspecialty referral for further diagnostic and therapeutic management.

Suggested Readings and Key References

Benfer AK, SpPath B, Weir AK. Oropharyngeal dysphagia and gross motor skills in children with cerebral palsy. *Pediatrics* 2013;131:e1553.

Fishbein M, Branham C, Fraker C, et al. The incidence of oropharyngeal dysphagia in infants with GERD-like symptoms. *J Parenter Enteral Nutr* 2013;37:667–673.

Hartnick CJ, Hartley BE, Miller C, et al. Pediatric fiberoptic endoscopic evaluation of swallowing. *Ann Otol Rhinol Laryngol* 2000;109(11):996–999.

Morgan A, Ward E, Murdoch B, et al. Acute characteristics of pediatric dysphagia subsequent to traumatic brain injury: videofluoroscopic assessment. *J Head Trauma Rehabil* 2002;17(3):220–241.

Sachdeva R, Hussain E, Moss MM, et al. Vocal cord dysfunction and feeding difficulties after pediatric cardiovascular surgery. *J Pediatr* 2007;151(3):312–315, 315.e1–2.

CHAPTER 52 ■ PAIN: DYSURIA

JACQUELINE B. CORBOY, MD AND PATRICIA LOPEZ, MSN, CRNP

Many conditions of the genitourinary tract produce symptoms of pain or burning associated with urination, or *dysuria*. The sensation is produced by the muscular contraction of the bladder and the peristaltic activity of the urethra, both of which stimulate the pain fibers in the edematous and inflamed mucosa. Young children may complain of painful urination when they are instead experiencing related symptoms, such as pruritus. When a child is too young to verbalize his or her symptoms, parents may interpret various nonspecific statements or behaviors by their child as indicative of painful urination.

Dysuria is a commonly reported symptom associated with a number of infectious and noninfectious causes, but it usually stems from one of several common disorders of childhood and adolescence. Most children with dysuria as a chief complaint will have primary disorders of the genitourinary tract, and although patients with urethritis secondary to systemic illnesses may have dysuria as one of their many symptoms, it is only occasionally the principal reason for a visit to an emergency department (ED).

Most diseases causing dysuria are self-limited or easily treated; however, the rarely seen systemic causes of urethritis or the spread of some bacterial pathogens beyond the genitourinary tract may be life-threatening. A differential diagnosis of the many systemic, infectious, and noninfectious causes most commonly presenting as dysuria may be found in Table 52.1–52.4.

EVALUATION AND DECISION

The approach to the child with dysuria must be broad, and history will help determine the direction of the workup. A thorough investigation of possible causes should be conducted, including questions about trauma (both accidental and nonaccidental), and exposure to chemicals such as detergents, fabric softeners, perfumed soaps, bubble baths, and medications that have been reported to irritate the mucosal lining of the urethra or bladder. A negative history for injury may not be accurate, however, because most traumas are not recalled by young patients or, in the case of masturbation or abuse, may be denied. The detection of sexually transmitted infections (STIs), a common cause of dysuria in adolescents, may in turn be facilitated by obtaining a history about the nature and extent of sexual activity (Figs. 52.1 and 52.2).

A urethral or vaginal discharge suggests an infection of the genitalia: urethritis in the boy and urethritis or vulvovaginitis in the girl (see Table 52.3). *Neisseria gonorrhoeae* is an organism that commonly causes disease in this area. A Gram stain can be a helpful adjunct in determining the nature of the discharge. In prepubertal girls or boys of any age, the finding of gram-negative intracellular diplococci points to the diagnosis of gonorrhea. However, because nonpathogenic organisms that colonize the vagina after puberty have the same appearance as *N. gonorrhoeae* on Gram stain, additional testing is needed. The development of nucleic acid amplification tests (NAATs), which use ligase chain reaction (LCR) or polymerase chain reaction (PCR) technologies, allows first-catch urine (*not* clean-catch) to be tested for the presence of *Chlamydia trachomatis* and *N. gonorrhoeae* in a noninvasive manner. Where available, these provide an accurate screening tool for STIs without performing a cervical or male urethral swab culture. Self-collected vaginal swabs from adolescent female patients can also be used for testing and offer similar

TABLE 52.1

CAUSES OF DYSURIA: SYSTEMIC CONDITIONS

Disorder	Signs and symptoms	Physical examination
Stevens–Johnson syndrome (See Chapter 96 Dermatologic Urgencies and Emergencies)	Mucous membrane changes, conjunctivitis, oral ulcerations, urethritis	Genital ulcerations; target lesions
Reactive arthritis (Reiter syndrome)	Conjunctivitis, arthritis, urethritis; more common in males	No GU findings; joint pain (including heels, digits, and spine)
Crohn's disease (See Chapter 99 Gastrointestinal Emergencies)	Dysuria (often in setting of UTI); fistula formation (complication)	Perianal inflammation or perianal skin tags; may have associated fistulas or abscess
Bechet's syndrome	Recurrent oral ulcerations, ocular panuveitis, vasculitis, genital ulcerations (less common)	Genital ulcerations
Malignancy/tumor (See Chapter 106 Oncologic Emergencies)	Constitutional symptoms: fatigue, weight loss, and fever; genitourinary symptoms related to intra-abdominal mass	No GU findings; abdominal mass most common

TABLE 52.2

CAUSES OF DYSURIA: DERMATOLOGIC CONDITIONS

Disorder	Age	Signs and symptoms	Physical examination
Psoriasis	All	Pruritis	Sharply demarcated erythematous, thick, silver-scaled plaques of the scalp, elbows, and knees; may also involve nails, joints, axilla, and groin
Lichen sclerosis	Infants and young children (mostly female)	Dry, tender, and severely pruritic white plaques	Depigmentation in anogenital area (most common)

accuracy when compared with provider-obtained cervical specimens. In prepubertal patients, a urethral or vaginal culture may be required by local law enforcement agencies however NAAT results are accepted in most states. Postpubertal patients may be treated in the ED; treatment in young children should be based on symptoms and clinical findings after all needed testing has been collected for medical–legal documentation.

If no discharge is seen, urinalysis will identify the possibility of urinary tract infection (UTI) (see Chapter 92 UTI, Febrile). Clinical suspicion should remain high among those with a history of dysuria, prolonged fever, prior history

TABLE 52.3

CAUSES OF DYSURIA: LOCALIZED CONDITIONS (INFECTIOUS)

Disorder	Cause	Age	Signs and symptoms	Physical examination
Pyelonephritis (See Chapter 127 Genitourinary Emergencies)	*Escherichia coli*; other bacteria	All	Fever (often >38.5°C)	Flank tenderness
Cystitis	Viral (adenovirus) Bacterial: (*E. coli* and other organisms)	All	Suprapubic pain +/– fever (often low-grade fever)	Suprapubic tenderness
Urethritis, Bulbar urethritis (See Chapter 127 Genitourinary Emergencies)	*N. gonorrhoeae*; Chlamydia species; Herpes simplex; Mycoplasma and Ureaplasma	Adolescent males more common	Afebrile	Vesicles (HSV); urethral or discharge; prostatic tenderness (occasional)
Balanitis	Fungal (*Candida albicans*); Bacterial (*E. coli*, enterococci, *Staphylococcus aureus*, GABHS)	Infant males (most common)	Afebrile; genital itching, irritation, and pain; penile discharge, groin rash, excessive crying in infants	GU examination: erythema, edema, exudate, foul odor, scarring between glans and prepuce, and phimosis
Cervicitis (See Chapter 100 Gynecology Emergencies)	*N. gonorrhoeae*; Chlamydia species; Herpes simplex; Mycoplasma and Ureaplasma	Adolescent females	Purulent or mucopurulent vaginal discharge and/or vaginal bleeding; urinary frequency, vaginal irritation	Vaginal discharge; cervical motion tenderness
Pelvic inflammatory disease (See Chapter 100 Gynecology Emergencies)	*N. gonorrhoeae*; *C. trachomatis*	Adolescent females	Lower abdominal pain; vaginal bleed/discharge, fever, chills	Abdominal pain (greatest in lower quadrants) but may have RUQ pain, CMT, adnexal tenderness; vaginal discharge
Vulvitis/vulvovaginitis (See Chapter 100 Gynecology Emergencies)	Group A streptococcus; *C. albicans*	Prepubertal females	Vaginal discharge; afebrile	Erythema; cheese-like or mucoid discharge. Erythematous "satellite" lesions
Pinworms	*Enterobius vermicularis*	Infants, children, adolescents	Pruritis may be expressed as dysuria	Worms may be detected in the perianal area

SIGNS AND SYMPTOMS

TABLE 52.4

CAUSES OF DYSURIA—LOCALIZED (NONINFECTIOUS) AND MISCELLANEOUS

Disorder	Cause	Age	Signs and symptoms	Physical examination
Localized (Chemical)				
Chemical irritation	Detergents; fabric softeners; perfumed soaps; bubble baths	All	Afebrile	May have no physical findings; mild erythema; no discharge; no tenderness
Medications	Dopamine, cantharidin, ticarcillin, penicillin G, cyclophosphamide, ceftriaxone	All	Afebrile	Mild erythema; may have no physical findings
Recreational drugs	Ketamine (street); Jimson weed	Adolescents	Afebrile	Mild erythema; may have no physical findings
Localized (Trauma)				
Local injury	Straddle injury, blunt and penetrating trauma	All	Genital pain	Ecchymosis, laceration, erythema
Masturbation	NA	Adolescents	Genital pain	May have no physical findings
Sexual abuse (See Chapter 95 Child Abuse/Assault)	NA	All	Genital pain	Ecchymosis, laceration, discharge, erythema; may have no physical findings
Miscellaneous				
Hypercalciuria; uricosuria; urinary stones (See Chapter 108 Renal and Electrolyte Emergencies)	Congenital and acquired	All	Flank pain; hematuria;	Flank pain
Labial adhesions (See Chapter 100 Gynecology Emergencies)	Secondary to irritation/ inflammation, decreased estrogen	Prepubertal females (3 mo–6 y/o) peak 1–2 y/o	Asymptomatic (mostly); dysuria (from microtears)	Partial or complete adherence of labia minora
Imperforate hymen/anus	Congenital and acquired	Female	Cyclic abdominal or pelvic pain and hematocolpos; back pain, difficulties with urination	Marked distension of vagina; bluish discoloration of hymenal membrane
Urethral stricture (Congenital and acquired)	Congenital and acquired	All	Urinary retention	May have no physical findings
Dysfunctional voiding (Neurologic and nonneurologic)	Multifactorial; may be initially precipitated by UTI history	All	Urinary frequency, urgency	May have no physical findings

of UTI or abnormal urinary tract or presence of fever, and flank pain suggesting pyelonephritis. Urinalysis or urine dipstick evaluations may be performed as screening tools on the urine obtained. Clean catch urine is collected after thorough cleaning of the perineum or by urethral catheterization using sterile technique. A positive result on urine dipstick (moderate or large leukocyte esterase and/or positive nitrites) or the presence of pyuria on microscopic urine analysis (≥5 WBC/hpf AND bacteriuria) increases the likelihood of bacterial infection (urethritis, cystitis, or pyelonephritis); infection is confirmed by culture results meeting colony forming unit (CFU) criteria in the presence of a urinary pathogen. Inflammatory conditions, such as chemical urethritis, and nonbacterial infections may also evoke a leukocyte response. Empiric antibiotic therapy may be initiated based on urine dip or urinalysis results pending urine culture results.

In the young child with dysuria in the absence of pyuria, local trauma and chemical irritation are the most likely causes for the pain (see Table 52.4). In infants <6 months who empty their bladder frequently, it may be possible to miss pyuria, so the clinician may have a lower threshold for obtaining a urine culture. Most experts argue that the likelihood of infection is low in the absence of positive indicators on urine analysis, obviating the need for culture.

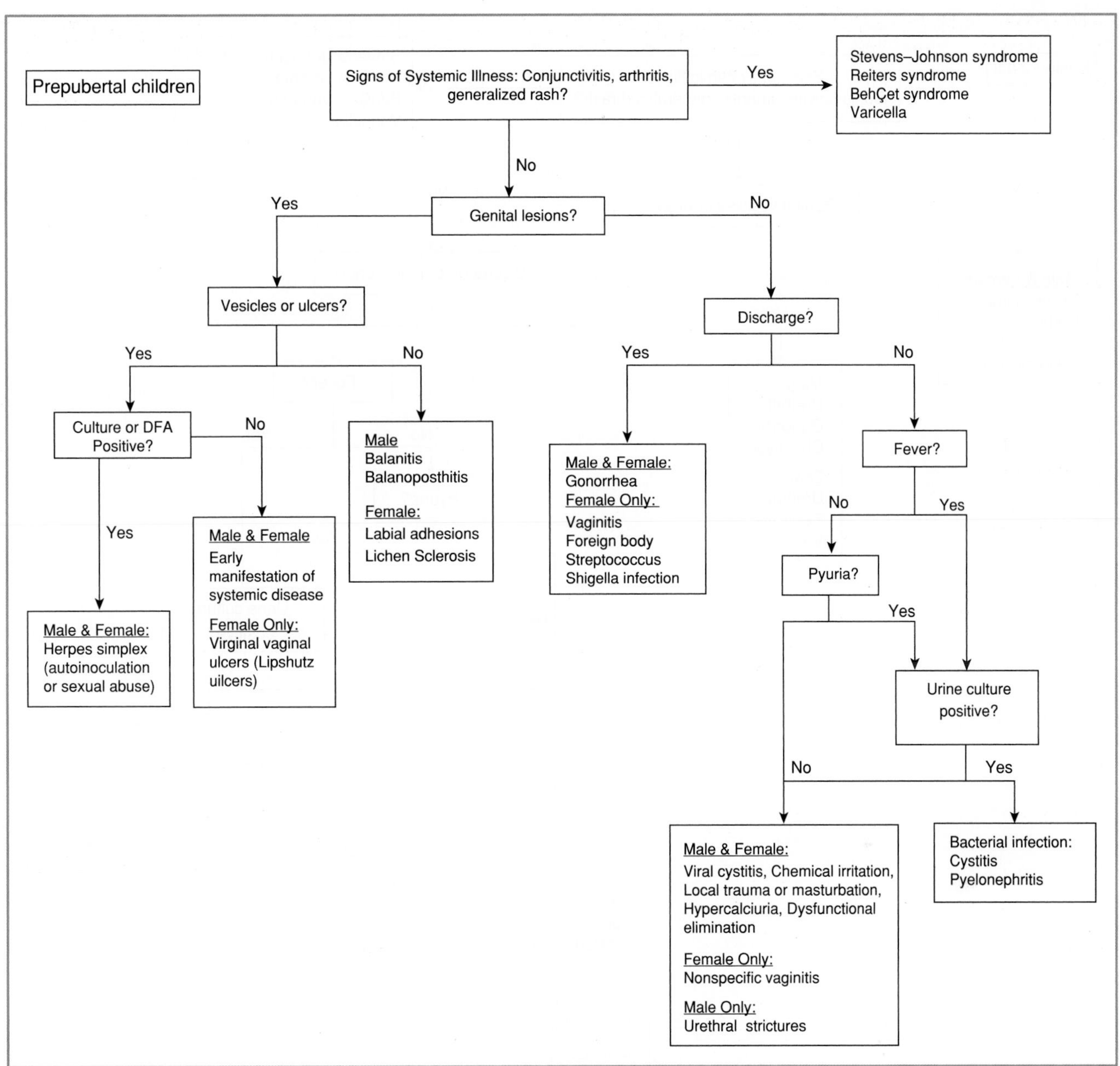

FIGURE 52.1 Prepubertal children pathway. (Adapted from Fleisher GR. *UpToDate: Evaluation of Dysuria in Children and Adolescents*. Updated May 08, 2013.)

Labial adhesions in prepubertal may be responsible for the painful urination (see Table 52.4). Since most girls with labial adhesions are asymptomatic, evaluation for infection or other cause for dysuria should be considered.

A few patients with a normal examination and negative cultures may complain persistently of dysuria. In this setting, dysfunctional voiding and idiopathic hypercalciuria represent potential diagnoses. If suspected, the diagnosis of hypercalciuria/uricosuria can be confirmed by measurement of calcium excretion in the urine. Another possible explanation in a female is that the patient is experiencing vaginal pruritus secondary to pinworms. Confirmation of this diagnosis requires either identification of the larvae or ova, or a response to a trial of mebendazole.

Last, the provider should give consideration to both sexual abuse and psychogenic dysuria. In most of these cases, further evaluation outside of the ED is needed.

SYMPTOMATIC MANAGEMENT

When a specific diagnosis has not been established and the provider is awaiting the results of cultures, therapy directed at the symptom of dysuria can provide some relief. Generally, dilute urine causes less irritation than concentrated urine, so a generous fluid intake is recommended. Warm water sitz baths may be helpful in the child with urethritis or vulvovaginitis. For the child older than 6 years, phenazopyridine (Pyridium)

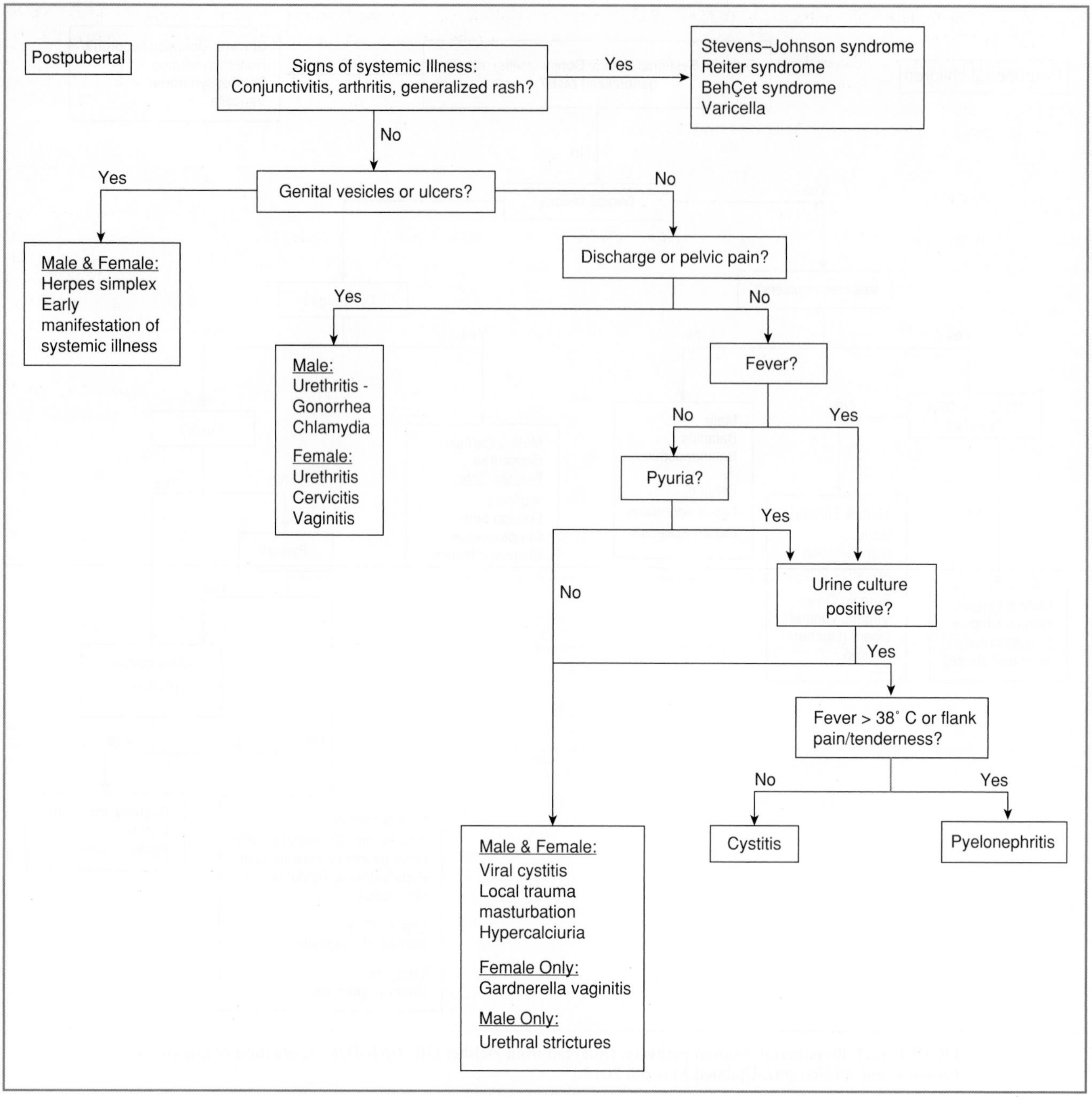

Postpubertal

Signs of systemic Illness: Conjunctivitis, arthritis, generalized rash?

Yes

Stevens–Johnson syndrome
Reiter syndrome
BehÇet syndrome
Varicella

No

Genital vesicles or ulcers?

Yes

Male & Female:
Herpes simplex
Early manifestation of systemic illness

No

Discharge or pelvic pain?

Yes

Male:
Urethritis - Gonorrhea
Chlamydia

Female:
Urethritis
Cervicitis
Vaginitis

No

Fever?

No

Pyuria?

Yes

Yes

Urine culture positive?

No

Yes

Fever > 38° C or flank pain/tenderness?

No

Cystitis

Yes

Pyelonephritis

Male & Female:
Viral cystitis
Local trauma
masturbation
Hypercalciuria

Female Only:
Gardnerella vaginitis

Male Only:
Urethral strictures

FIGURE 52.2 Postpubertal pathway. (Adapted from Fleisher GR. *UpToDate: Evaluation of Dysuria in Children and Adolescents*. Updated May 08, 2013.)

at a dosage of 12 mg/kg/day divided into three doses (daily maximum 600 mg per day), administered for up to 2 days, may be helpful as a urinary tract anesthetic.

Suggested Readings and Key References

Baraff LJ. Management of infants and young children with fever without source. *Pediatr Ann* 2008;37(10):673–679.

Benz MR, Stehr M, Kammer B, et al. Foreign body in the bladder mimicking nephritis. *Pediatr Nephrol* 2007;22(3):467–470.

Berwald N, Cheng S, Augenbraun M, et al. Self-administered vaginal swabs are a feasible alternative to physician-assisted cervical swabs for sexually transmitted infection screening in the emergency department. *Acad Emerg Med* 2009;16(4):360–363.

DeLago C, Deblinger E, Schroeder C, et al. Girls who disclose sexual abuse: urogenital symptoms and signs after genital contact. *Pediatrics* 2008;122(2):e281–e286.

Eberz B, Berghold A, Regauer S. High prevalence of concomitant anogenital lichen sclerosis and extragenital psoriasis in adult women. *Obstet Gynecol* 2008;111(5):1143–1147.

Etoubleau C, Reveret M, Brouet D, et al. Moving from bag to catheter for urine collection in non-toilet-trained children suspected of having urinary tract infection: a paired comparison of urine cultures. *J Pediatr* 2009;154(6):803–806.

Fang J, Husman C, DeSilva L, et al. Evaluation of self-collected vaginal swab, first void urine, and endocervical swab specimens for the detection of Chlamydia trachomatis and Neisseria gonorrhoeae in adolescent females. *J Pediatr Adolesc Gynecol* 2008;21(6): 355–360.

Farhat W, McLorie G. Urethral syndromes in children. *Pediatr Rev* 2001;22(1):17–21.

Fleisher G. Evaluation of dysuria in children and adolescents. Retrieved April 20, 2014 from www.uptodate.com.

Halachmi S, Toubi A, Meretyk S. Inflammation of the testis and epididymis in an otherwise healthy child: is it a true bacterial urinary tract infection? *J Pediatr Urol* 2006;2(4):386–389.

Johnson RE, Newhall WJ, Papp JR, et al. Screening tests to detect Chlamydia trachomatis and Neisseria gonorrhoeae infections—2002. *MMWR Recomm Rep* 2002;51(RR-15):1–38.

Omar HA. Management of labial adhesions in prepubertal girls. *J Pediatr Adolesc Gynecol* 2000;13(4):183–185.

Poindexter G, Morrell DS. Anogenital pruritus: lichen sclerosus in children. *Pediatr Ann* 2007;36(12):785–791.

Roberts KB; Subcommittee On Urinary Tract Infection, Steering Committee On Quality Improvement And Management. Urinary tract infection: clinical practice guideline for the diagnosis and management of the initial UTI in febrile infants and children 2 to 24 months. *Pediatrics* 2011;128(3):595–610.

Ruffolo C, Angriman I, Scarpa M, et al. Urologic complications in Crohn's disease: suspicion criteria. *Hepatogastroenterology* 2006; 53(69):357–360.

Santoro JD, Carroll VG, Steele RW. Diagnosis and management of urinary tract infections in neonates and young infants. *Clin Pediatr (Phila)* 2013;52(2):111–114.

Spitzer RF, Kives S, Caccia N, et al. Retrospective review of unintentional female genital trauma at a pediatric referral center. *Pediatr Emer Care* 2008;24(12):831–835.

Srinivasin A, Palmer LS. Genitourinary complications of epidermolysis bullosa. *Urology* 2007;70(1):179.e585–e586.

Srivastava T, Schwaderer A. Diagnosis and management of hypercalciuria in children. *Curr Opin Pediatr* 2009;21(2):214–219.

Suson KD, Mathews R. Evaluation of children with urinary tract infection–impact of the 2011 AAP guidelines on the diagnosis of vesicoureteral reflux using a historical series. *J Pediatr Urol* 2014; 10(1):182–185.

Yazici H. Behçet's syndrome: where do we stand? *Am J Med* 2002; 112(1):75–76.

CHAPTER 53 ■ PAIN: EARACHE

MARK D. JOFFE, MD

Ear pain or otalgia is a very common chief complaint in children seeking emergent or urgent care. In younger, preverbal children, ear pain is often inferred by parents from various child behaviors. While acute otitis media (AOM) may be the main parental concern, astute clinicians must consider a broader range of potential causes. Otalgia may result from diseases in all parts of the ear, and also from a variety of nonotogenic conditions. When ear pain is accompanied by neurologic signs and symptoms such as cranial nerve palsies, vertigo, or altered mental status, a more extensive evaluation is required.

DIFFERENTIAL DIAGNOSIS

Ear pain may be the presenting symptom of problems in external, middle, or inner ear (Fig. 53.1). Causes of external ear pain are often readily apparent. Trauma to the auricle is ascertained by history in most cases, and contusions, abrasions, hematomas, and lacerations are easily noted on physical examination. In younger children, and in particular in cases of inflicted injury, a history of ear trauma may be lacking. Swelling and/or bruising of the external ear, especially the medial aspect of the auricle, from forcible traction is a well-recognized manifestation of child abuse. Hematomas of the auricle are of particular concern because, interposed between the skin and underlying cartilage, the extravascular accumulation of blood disrupts the supply of nutrients to the cartilage. Necrosis of auricular cartilage leads to deformity and results in the characteristic "cauliflower ear." Pressure dressings on injured external ears may prevent the accumulation of significant auricular hematomas. Larger auricular hematomas may need to be drained.

The popularity of body piercing, and in particular multiple piercings of the ear, has increased the number of patients requiring treatment for complications. Infections of the ear lobe or of the cartilaginous portions of the auricle after piercing should be treated with topical and sometimes systemic antibiotics. While *Staphylococcus aureus* is the most frequent pathogen, cartilaginous infection with *Pseudomonas aeruginosa* is well described and requires specific treatment. Drainage, debridement, and treatment with fluoroquinolone antibiotics may be necessary. Preauricular cysts or sinuses may become infected. A small pit just anterior to the helix is noted in the center of the surrounding tender, red swelling.

Frostbite of the helix presents as a painful, pale ear that usually becomes hyperemic and swollen over time. Vesicles may develop in the latter stages. Rapid rewarming and analgesia are recommended. Most authorities discourage debridement of vesicular or hemorrhagic lesions.

Cerumen impaction may cause ear pain, especially after attempts to remove accumulations push the ear wax up against the tympanic membrane (TM). Removal of cerumen with a curette is best accomplished under direct visualization. Dry cerumen may be tightly adherent to the skin of the external canal which, when removed with a curette, causes abrasion and bleeding. Saline irrigation of the canal or instillation of peroxide-containing ear drops or docusate liquid can remove, soften, or detach adherent wax and is recommended prior to attempting to remove dry cerumen with a curette.

Children may have ear pain from foreign bodies placed in the ear. If the foreign body is difficult to remove or is close to the TM, removal under sedation by an otolaryngologist is advisable. Occasionally, live insects are noted in the external canal and their movement causes great pain and distress. Instillation of mineral oil will asphyxiate the insect prior to removal. Viscous lidocaine may have the added benefit of paralyzing the insect, reducing painful movements more quickly than mineral oil.

Shingles of the ear, or herpes zoster oticus, presents with painful or pruritic vesicles of the external auditory meatus and may also involve the TM. Although more common in adults, associated facial nerve palsy (Ramsay Hunt syndrome), hearing loss, or vertigo have been reported in children. Antiviral agents and systemic corticosteroids may be helpful in the early stages of this illness.

Labyrinthitis usually presents with vertigo that may be associated with nausea and vomiting, balance disturbance, and tinnitus. It is usually caused by a viral or bacterial infection of the inner ear, but may also be associated with middle ear infection and ear pain.

OTITIS EXTERNA

Otitis externa is a common problem during childhood, especially during summer when children are swimming and humidity is high. Cerumen is produced by glands in the external ear to coat the canal with a water-resistant, acidic, antibacterial substance that prevents maceration. Swimmers ear develops when water in the ear disrupts the protective cerumen layer. Attempts to remove water in the canal or to relieve pruritus may cause injury to the skin, creating portals of entry for bacteria in the external ear. Ear pain and sometimes visible ear discharge are the usual symptoms of otitis externa. Examination reveals an erythematous, swollen external canal filled with debris or purulence. Traction on the auricle causes pain with otitis externa, a finding that can help distinguish it from otitis media with perforation. Gentle removal of debris, instillation of topical antibiotics, and systemic analgesia are the usual treatment. When swelling is so severe that topical antibiotics may not reach the more proximal portion of the canal, a wick may be inserted to facilitate antibiotic entry. Systemic antibiotics are indicated if there is extensive cellulitis spreading beyond the external canal. Otitis externa is usually polymicrobial, but *S. aureus* and *P. aeruginosa* are important pathogens to cover, and polymyxin/neomycin or fluoroquinolone otic drops are the preferred treatment. Otitis externa with *P. aeruginosa*

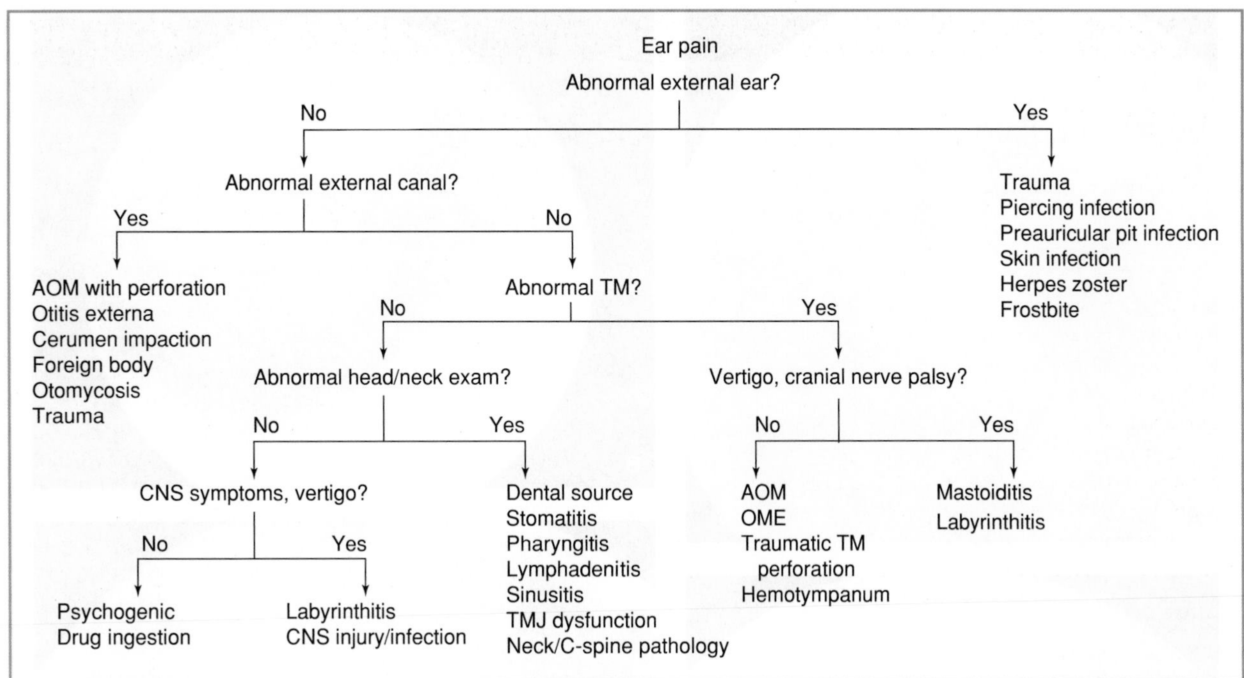

FIGURE 53.1 Ear pain algorithm. AOM, acute otitis media; CNS, central nervous system; TMJ, temporomandibular joint; OME, otitis media with effusion.

can be fulminant and necrotizing. Recalcitrant cases of otitis externa, especially if pruritus is a prominent symptom, may require evaluation for fungal disease (otomycoses) or deeper infection.

ACUTE OTITIS MEDIA

Otitis media is the most common illness prompting office visits and antimicrobial prescriptions in childhood, though both visits and prescriptions of OM have decreased. Clinical practice guidelines have encouraged a stricter diagnostic threshold for AOM, and immunization with PCV7 and influenza vaccines may have reduced the actual incidence of AOM.

AOM is defined as the rapid onset of signs and symptoms of inflammation in the middle ear. It is considered severe if there is moderate to severe otalgia or fever >39°C (102.2°F). Aside from ear pain, reported in only 50% to 60% of children with AOM, symptoms of AOM such as irritability, ear tugging, sleep disruption, and fever are nonspecific. Using strict but appropriate otoscopic criteria, a majority of children whose parent suspects AOM in fact have uncomplicated upper respiratory infection (URI).

Examination of the TM is one of the most difficult clinical skills to master. Agreement on AOM diagnosis between otolaryngologists, the gold standard, and pediatricians or family physicians is abysmal. Improved training in the diagnosis of AOM and careful physical examination is clearly warranted.

In younger children with respiratory symptoms, fever, or specific ear symptoms, adequate visualization of the TM is required. Despite the increasing pressure to manage and make a disposition for patients quickly, clinicians must take the time to accurately determine if AOM is present. Removal of cerumen with saline irrigation, peroxide-containing ear drops, docusate sodium syrup, and/or curettage will be a frequent procedure for clinicians caring for children. Immobilization of the uncooperative child and proper equipment must be available. The 2013 AAP/AAFP Clinical Practice Guideline eliminated the "Uncertain Diagnosis" category that was part of the 2004 guideline because the committee wanted to emphasize the necessity of proper, and in many cases time-consuming, assessment of the TM.

Bulging of the TM is the physical finding most specific for the presence of a bacterial pathogen in middle ear fluid (Fig. 53.2A–D). In children with acute symptoms, impaired TM mobility with pneumatic otoscopy and the presence of cloudy middle ear fluid are also strongly correlated with bacterial infection. A TM that appears hemorrhagic or strongly red is associated with AOM, but lesser degrees of redness are not useful diagnostically. Occasionally, examination of a child with AOM will reveal bullae on the TM. The organisms responsible for "bullous myringitis" are not significantly different from other cases of AOM and treatment should be similar. Children with AOM and TM perforation may present with purulent otorrhea that prevents adequate visualization of the TM. Otitis externa can usually be excluded on clinical grounds, so a diagnosis of AOM with perforation can be made.

Otitis media with effusion (OME) is a condition described by fluid in the middle ear cavity without signs and symptoms of acute inflammation. It may result from Eustachian tube obstruction or represent the aftermath of resolved AOM, but is not an acute bacterial infection.

Patients with ear pain from AOM should receive analgesic treatment because antibiotics do not generally provide symptomatic improvement for at least 24 hours. Acetaminophen or ibuprofen are effective analgesic treatments of AOM. Topical anesthetic–containing ear drops provide prompt, but short-lived pain relief. These oil-based preparations should not be administered if the TM has ruptured. Narcotic analgesia can be used for very severe pain, but should rarely be necessary.

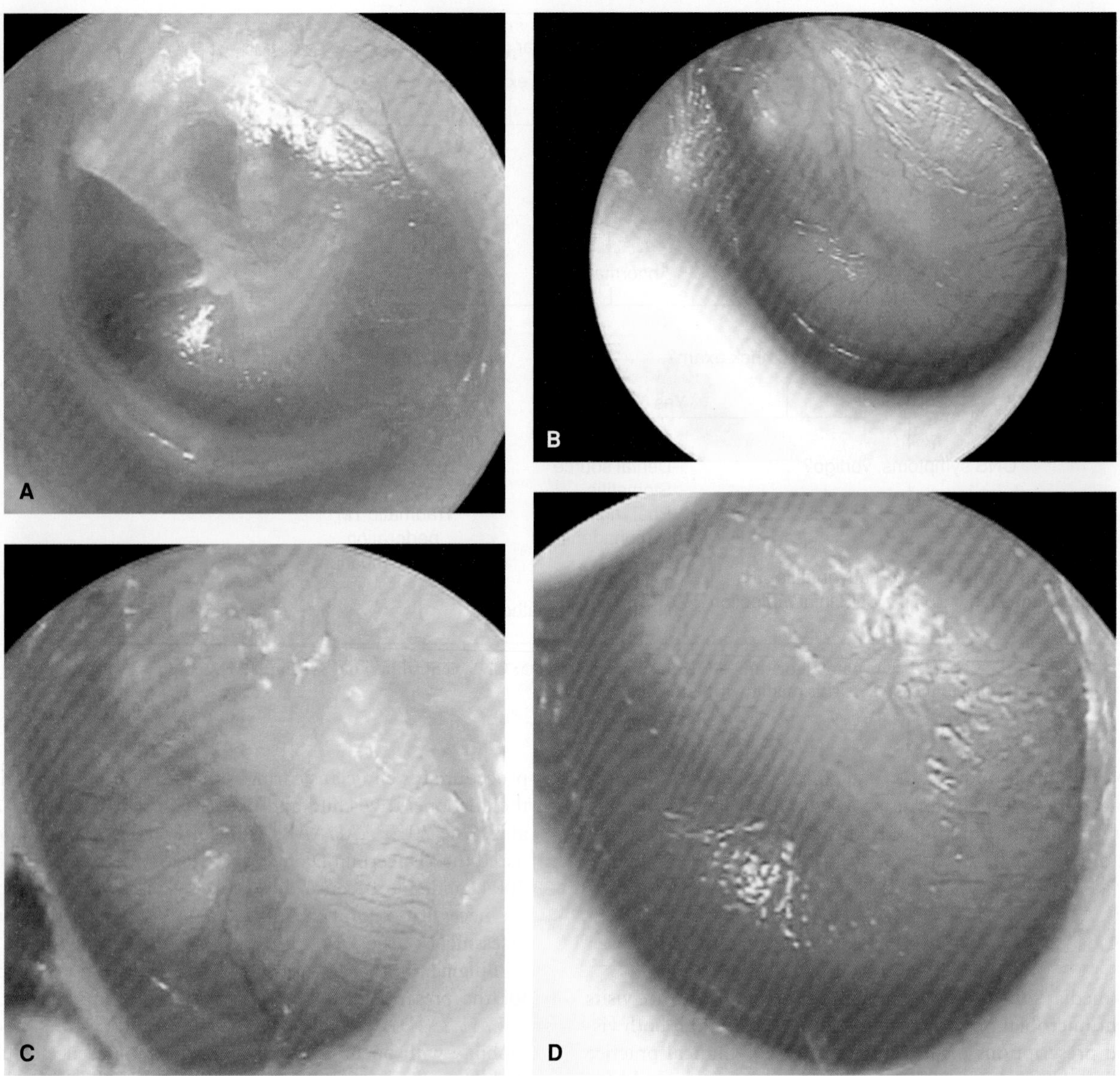

FIGURE 53.2 **A:** Normal tympanic membrane (TM). **B:** TM full/mild bulging (antibiotic treatment not indicated). **C:** TM with moderate bulging. **D:** TM with severe bulging.

Antibiotic treatment of AOM has been controversial due to the high spontaneous resolution rate of AOM in many studies. Using a more stringent diagnostic threshold for AOM, recent studies have documented a modest but statistically significant benefit of antibiotics for AOM. Antibiotic treatment is recommended for any child with AOM and severe symptoms, defined as moderate or severe otalgia, otalgia for greater than 48 hours or temperature >39°C (102.2°F). For children between 6 and 24 months of age, observation without antibiotics is an option if AOM is unilateral and symptoms are not severe. Observation is an option for patients >24 months of age with AOM without severe symptoms even if the AOM is bilateral. In all cases for which observation is the chosen option, the clinician must arrange for follow-up and the initiation of antibiotic therapy should the child worsen or if symptoms persist beyond 48 to 72 hours.

Most cases of AOM involve coinfection of a viral respiratory pathogen and bacteria. The Eustachian tube dysfunction caused by the viral URI leads to negative middle ear pressure, aspiration of contaminated upper airway secretions into the middle ear cavity, and subsequent development of acute bacterial infection. A viral prodrome followed by clinical worsening signals the onset of AOM. AOM may also develop secondary infection of ongoing middle ear fluid (OME).

Bacteria or bacterial DNA are found in middle ear fluid from almost all patients with properly diagnosed AOM. The predominant bacterial pathogens are nontypeable *Haemophilus influenzae, Streptococcus pneumoniae, Moraxella catarrhalis,* and occasionally *Streptococcus pyogenes.* Since the advent of immunization against *S. pneumonia, H. influenza* has become the most prevalent bacterial pathogen recovered from middle ear aspirates. While some *H. influenza* produce β-lactamase, the number of β-lactam–resistant strains is lower than previously thought. High-dose amoxicillin (80 to 90 mg/kg/day) achieves middle ear fluid concentrations that are greater than the minimum inhibitory concentrations of all penicillin-sensitive and intermediately resistant *S. pneumonia* serotypes, and many highly penicillin-resistant strains. Although all *M. catarrhalis* produce β-lactamase, most experts believe AOM from *M. catarrhalis* is mild, has a high spontaneous resolution

TABLE 53.1

ANTIBIOTIC TREATMENT OF AOM

First line	Treatment failure (after 48–72 hrs)
Amoxicillin 80–90 mg/kg/day in two doses	Amoxicillin-clavulanate 90 mg/kg/day amox in two doses
Amoxicillin-clavulanate 90 mg/kg/day amox in two doses	Ceftriaxone 50 mg IM or IV for 3 days
Penicillin allergy	**Alternative**
Cefdinir 14 mg/kg/day in one or two doses	Clindamycin 30–40 mg/kg/day in three doses plus third-generation cephalosporin
Cefpodoxime 10 mg/kg/day in two doses	Tympanocentesis and culture
Cefuroxime 30 mg/kg/day in two doses	
Ceftriaxone 50 mg IM or IV for 3 days	

rate and is without significant invasive potential, making coverage with a β-lactamase–resistant antibiotic unnecessary in the majority of cases.

High-dose amoxicillin (80 to 90 mg/kg/day in two divided doses) is the initial drug of choice for AOM provided the patient has not taken amoxicillin during the preceding 30 days, does not have concurrent conjunctivitis (*H. influenza* more likely), nor has a history of AOM treatment failure with amoxicillin (Table 53.1). Amoxicillin-clavulanate (80 to 90 mg/kg/day of amoxicillin, with 6.4 mg/kg/day of clavulanate in two divided doses) is recommended for antibiotic treatment failure, defined as worsening or persistent symptoms after 48 to 72 hours. Alternatives for treatment failure are ceftriaxone (50 mg IM or IV for 1 or 3 days) or clindamycin (30 to 40 mg/kg/day in three divided doses) plus a third-generation cephalosporin. Tympanocentesis and culture may be indicated after multiple antibiotic failures in persistently symptomatic patients.

Patients with a history of penicillin allergy may be treated with cefdinir (14 mg/kg/day in one or two divided doses), cefpodoxime (10 mg/kg/day in two divided doses), cefuroxime (30 mg/kg/day in two divided doses), or ceftriaxone (50 mg IM or IV for 1 or 3 days). These specific cephalosporins do not share similar side-chain structure with penicillin, ampicillin, or amoxicillin, and therefore do not pose an increased risk of allergic reaction in penicillin-allergic patients. Cephalosporins are not as effective as high-dose amoxicillin against *S. pneumonia* and should not be chosen as first-line therapy in patients who can take amoxicillin. Azithromycin and other macrolides have limited efficacy against *S. pneumoniae* and *H. influenza* and should not be used for the treatment of AOM.

A 10-day course of antibiotics is recommended for children less than 24 months of age with AOM. In patients with mild or moderate AOM who are over 24 months of age, a 7-day course of antibiotics is adequate. Evidence does not support routine 10- to 14-day follow-up for patients after treatment of AOM. A majority of children will have persistent middle ear fluid 2 weeks after the start of treatment, and almost half will still have fluid at 1 month. Children with persistent symptoms after treatment for AOM should follow-up with their primary care provider. Oral decongestants, intranasal decongestants, oral antihistamines, and steroid preparations are ineffective in the treatment of AOM and OME and should not be prescribed.

Persistent middle ear fluid without acute symptoms (OME) may be associated with a conductive hearing loss. Though the evidence for a long-term impact of mild and transient conductive hearing loss on otherwise normal children is weak, those in whom there is concern for developmental or cognitive delays should be followed more closely. Children with persistent middle ear effusion should not receive antibiotic prophylaxis. There is a modest, short-term benefit of antibiotic prophylaxis in reducing episodes of recurrent AOM. Antibiotic prophylaxis is not recommended for most children with recurrent AOM. Tympanostomy tube placement is a decision that is best made by primary care providers in consultation with otolaryngologists, and should be considered if a child has had three documented episodes of AOM within 6 months or four episodes within the preceding year.

OTORRHEA

Children with AOM and perforation improve more quickly when treated with oral antibiotic therapy rather than topical therapy. Many experts also recommend antibiotic ear drops in this setting, though there is little evidence for this dual therapy. Fluoroquinolone otic drops are safe in patients with perforated TMs. If the otorrhea is chronic, there is benefit from otic drops with a combination of fluoroquinolone and steroid. Patients with tympanostomy tubes who present with otorrhea without acute symptoms should be treated with ototopical antibiotic–steroid combination drops for 3 to 5 days, which is superior to oral antibiotics in resolving the otorrhea.

Complications of AOM are very rare considering the incidence of the disease. Mastoiditis can develop in children with AOM and may include osteitis and subperiosteal abscess formation. Patients with mastoiditis present with swelling behind the ear that displaces the auricle outward and downward. There is tenderness over the mastoid and the ipsilateral TM is usually abnormal in appearance. Intravenous antibiotic therapy is generally recommended and surgical drainage may be necessary in more severe cases. AOM with mastoiditis that involves the petrous portion of the temporal bone can cause cranial nerve palsies (Gradenigo syndrome). The trigeminal (V) and abducens (VI) nerves are most often affected with facial pain and diplopia as the presenting symptoms. The facial (VII) and acoustic (VIII) nerves can also be involved. The posterior and middle cranial fossae are adjacent to the middle ear and, on rare occasions, infection can spread to the central nervous system and cause meningitis, extradural abscess, subdural empyema, or brain abscess. Any child with AOM and cranial nerve palsy or signs of CNS infection should be evaluated with a CT or MRI to define the extent of the infection.

TRAUMATIC TM PERFORATION

The TM can be perforated by penetrating or blunt trauma to the external ear. Insertion of cotton swabs or other instruments to clean cerumen from the ear may lead to TM perforation. Blunt trauma from a punch or slap may create a positive pressure wave in the external canal that causes rupture of the TM. Proximity to an explosion, hyperbaric oxygen treatment, deep sea diving, or airplane travel may also rupture the TM. Ear pain is often severe but resolves with time. On examination, the perforation can usually be visualized, and pneumatic otoscopy will show no movement of the TM with positive or negative pressure. Most traumatic perforation will heal spontaneously, but patients with lesions over 20% of the diameter of the TM, acute hearing loss, vertigo, or cranial nerve deficits should be evaluated promptly by otolaryngology for possible surgical intervention. Head-injured children with basilar skull fractures may have cerebrospinal fluid otorrhea or hemotympanum on examination. With hemotympanum, the TM initially looks red from fresh bleeding with oxygenated blood. Over time the blood deoxygenates and appears dark purple behind the immobile ear drum. Basilar skull fractures are associated with many other signs and symptoms including facial nerve palsy, hearing loss, and vertigo. In general the management of the brain injury is the immediate priority.

REFERRED EAR PAIN

Patients may complain of ear pain when suffering from non-otogenic conditions. The sensory innervation of the auricle, external auditory canal, middle and inner ear involve cranial nerves V, VII, IX, and X. Dental infections, stomatitis, pharyngitis, sinusitis and in rare cases tumors of the head and neck may be associated with ear pain. The postauricular area is supplied by C2 and C3, and neck injuries, disc problems, arthritis may cause referred pain to that region. When no otic cause is found in children presenting with ear pain, clinicians should carefully evaluate the surrounding structures to identify other causes of the discomfort.

Suggested Readings and Key References

Conover K. Earache. *Emerg Med Clin North Am* 2013;31:413.

Ghanem T, Rasamny JK, Park SS. Rethinking auricular trauma. *Laryngoscope* 2005;115:1251.

Hoberman A, Paradise JL, Rockette HE, et al. Treatment of acute otitis media in children under 2 years of age. *N Engl J Med* 2011;364: 105–115.

Lieberthal AS, Carroll AE, Chonmaitree T, et al. Clinical practice guideline: the diagnosis and management of acute otitis media. *Pediatrics* 2013;131(3):e964–e999.

McCormick DP, Lim-Milia E, Saeed K, et al. Otitis media: can clinical findings predict bacterial or viral etiology? *Pediatr Infect Dis J* 2000; 19:256–258.

Pichichero ME. A review of evidence supporting the American Academy of Pediatrics recommendation for prescribing cephalosporin antibiotics for penicillin-allergic patients. *Pediatrics* 2005;115: 1048–1057.

Rosenfeld RM, Schwartz SR, Cannon CR, et al. Clinical practice guideline: acute otitis externa. *Otolaryngol Head Neck Surg* 2014; 150:S1–S24.

Spiro DM, Tay KY, Arnold DH, et al. Wait-and-see prescription for the treatment of acute otitis media: a randomized controlled trial. *JAMA* 2006;296:1235–1241.

CHAPTER 54 ■ PAIN: HEADACHE

CHRISTOPHER KING, MD, FACEP AND DENIS R. PAUZÉ, MD, FACEP

Headache is a common complaint of pediatric patients in the emergency department (ED). It is estimated that by the age of 15 years, up to 75% of children have experienced headaches, although most are cared for at home. Headache as an isolated complaint is a relatively unusual presentation in pediatric patients; it is more often one of a number of symptoms, such as fever, lethargy, sore throat, neck pain, and vomiting.

Like other challenging presentations, headache is seen with regularity and is often benign, but in a small subset of patients, it can portend a potentially life-threatening illness. Therefore, the primary responsibility of the emergency physician is to make the important discrimination between "bad" headaches and benign headaches. Fortunately, this differentiation can almost always be done successfully after a thorough history and physical examination, and when necessary, laboratory and radiographic tests. One notable exception to this rule, however, is brain tumor. Although most serious illnesses that cause headache (e.g., meningitis, encephalitis, ruptured vascular anomaly) will be readily classified in the "bad" category, the presence of a brain tumor may not be. The history can be subtle, and the examination is commonly unrevealing, often leading to a delay in diagnosis. Therefore, characteristics of headaches caused by a brain tumor are described in detail in this chapter. Above all, the key to proper management of such patients is ensuring appropriate follow-up care.

PATHOPHYSIOLOGY

For a headache to occur, there must be a noxious stimulus that affects one or more pain-sensitive structures. Injury to an area that is insensitive to pain, such as nonhemorrhagic stroke, may cause significant morbidity but will not manifest as headache. It is therefore useful to consider the sensory innervation of the head and neck. All extracranial structures are sensitive to pain. Thus, processes that affect the sinuses, oropharynx, scalp, or neck musculature often cause patients to complain of headache. In contrast, certain intracranial structures are sensitive to pain and others are not. For example, the brain, ependymal lining, choroid plexus, and much of the dura and pia-arachnoid over the hemispheres are insensitive to pain. Pathologic processes affecting these areas can cause headache, but only by impinging on adjacent pain-sensitive structures. The most pain-sensitive intracranial structures are the proximal portions of the large cerebral arteries at the base of the brain, the venous sinuses, and the large cerebral veins.

Various physiologic mechanisms come into play in causing headache. Painful stimuli can be broadly categorized as resulting from vascular effects, muscle contraction, inflammation, and traction/compression (Table 54.1). Examples of each of these types of headache etiology are described in the following discussion of differential diagnosis. It should be noted that visual problems are an unlikely cause of significant headaches in children. A child with persistent headaches that have previously been attributed to "eye strain" may, therefore, deserve a more careful evaluation.

Attempting to predict the neuroanatomic location of a pathologic process using only the site of headache described by a child is unreliable. In part, this is attributable to the unpredictable displacement of structures caused by a mass lesion. In addition, the extremely complex relationships of the various nerves involved in pain sensation of the head and neck lead to unexpected patterns of referred pain. Thus, a posterior fossa lesion can cause frontal or orbital pain, and supratentorial lesions may result in pain localized to the occiput or the back of the neck, for example.

DIFFERENTIAL DIAGNOSIS

A comprehensive discussion of the various causes of headache in pediatric patients is beyond the scope of this textbook. The conditions described here are those most likely to be seen in acute- and emergency-care settings (Table 54.2) and those with the greatest potential for imminent morbidity or mortality (Table 54.3). Fortunately, the majority of pediatric patients who present to the ED with headache have a benign condition. In a study of 432 children and teenagers evaluated in the ED for headache, Conicella et al. found that the most common etiologies were upper respiratory infection (19%), migraine (18.5%), posttraumatic headache (5.5%), and tension-type headache (4.6%). Anatomic abnormality (e.g., Chiari malformation), brain tumor, meningitis, idiopathic intracranial hypertension, and ventricular shunt failure were found in a total of 6% of patients.

Vascular

Headaches associated with vascular changes are believed to be caused primarily by vasodilation, although the exact mechanism has yet to be fully elucidated. One common example of this type of headache is migraine. Migraine headaches are typically chronic and remitting, with a characteristic pattern that is easily described by the patient or parents (see Chapter 105 Neurologic Emergencies). Often, a strong family history of migraines is present. For the emergency physician, the main issue with migraine patients is generally pain control, because the diagnosis is already known. However, a significant change in the quality, severity, or timing of headaches in these patients may represent a separate and potentially more serious problem. In such cases, the clinician should not be dissuaded by the existing diagnosis from pursuing an appropriate workup as indicated.

Headaches accompanying fever are also believed to be mediated by vascular effects. Because fever is such a common symptom, this is probably the most common cause of headaches in pediatric patients seen in the ED. Hypertension,

TABLE 54.1

PATHOPHYSIOLOGIC CLASSIFICATION OF HEADACHES

I. Vascular
  A. Febrile illness
  B. Migraine
  C. Systemic hypertension
  D. Hypoxia
  E. Caffeine withdrawal
II. Muscle contraction (tension)
III. Inflammation
  A. Intracranial infections
    1. Meningitis
    2. Encephalitis
    3. Brain abscess
  B. Pharyngitis
  C. Upper respiratory infection
  D. Dental infection
  E. Sinus infection
  F. Retroorbital cellulitis/abscess
IV. Traction/compression
  A. Brain tumor
  B. Intracranial hemorrhage
  C. Increased intracranial pressure
    1. Cerebral edema
    2. Hydrocephalus
    3. Idiopathic intracranial hypertension
  D. Brain abscess
  E. Lumbar puncture
  F. Arterial dissection
V. Posttraumatic
VI. Psychogenic

although rare, is another possible cause of vascular headaches in children. Renovascular disease leading to hypertension can in some instances be a life-threatening etiology. Additionally, children and teenagers may have an undiagnosed coarctation of the aorta leading to hypertension and associated headaches.

TABLE 54.2

COMMON CAUSES OF HEADACHE

Vascular
Febrile illness
Migraine
Inflammatory
Pharyngitis
Upper respiratory infection
Sinus infections
Dental infections
Muscle contraction
Tension-type headache
Posttraumatic
Psychogenic

TABLE 54.3

LIFE-THREATENING CAUSES OF HEADACHE

Vascular
Hypertension
Hypoxia
Coarctation of the aorta
Inflammatory
Meningitis
Encephalitis
Ventricular shunt infection
Traction/compression
Brain tumor
Intracranial hemorrhage
Hydrocephalus
Cerebral edema
Brain abscess
Arterial dissection
Ventricular shunt failure
Environmental
Carbon monoxide poisoning

Because of its rarity, this condition is easily misdiagnosed. Hypertension causes not only global changes in cerebral vasculature, but also possibly a component of increased intracranial pressure (ICP) that leads to headache.

Finally, hypoxia is a potent stimulus for cerebral vasodilation and can produce headaches on that basis. Therefore, children who experience a hypoxic insult (e.g., carbon monoxide poisoning) or those with disease states that predispose to hypoxia (e.g., cystic fibrosis, cyanotic heart disease) may present with headaches resulting from an acute process or an exacerbation of an underlying illness.

Muscle Contraction

Headaches can be caused by contraction of the scalp or neck muscles. This is the classic "tension" headache that is common in adults. These headaches usually occur when a patient has experienced prolonged mental or emotional stress or desk work with inadequate attention to ergonomic factors. This leads to recurrent episodes of muscle tension and/or spasm, which cause muscle soreness. The patient can often localize a specific site where the pain is felt, and the involved muscles may be tender to palpation. Although muscle contraction is an unlikely cause of headache in younger children, the stress of life during adolescence will often produce this type of headache. Onset is typically at the end of the day. A headache that is present on arising in the morning or that awakens a patient from sleep is an unusual manifestation of muscle contraction.

Inflammation

A wide variety of inflammatory conditions can result in headache, ranging from benign to potentially life-threatening entities. Children with bacterial meningitis or encephalitis may present with headache, although this is usually only one of a constellation of symptoms, such as fever, lethargy, neck pain, confusion, or coma. Headache is unlikely to be the sole complaint in these patients. However, an older child or adolescent with viral meningitis can present with a severe headache, mild, or sometimes no neck discomfort and no other signs of significant illness. Fortunately, viral meningitis is generally a benign process. Rare causes of inflammatory headache include retroorbital cellulitis or abscess and brain abscess. Focal findings on neurologic and/or ocular examination will normally provide clues to these unusual diagnoses.

Headaches can also be caused by inflammatory processes affecting other structures of the head and neck. For example, pediatric patients with pharyngitis caused by group A streptococcus will often complain of headaches. Indeed, the classic presentation for streptococcal pharyngitis in children is sore throat, fever, and headache, sometimes associated with abdominal pain. In a child who has difficulty localizing pain, otitis media and otitis externa can also present as headache. Pediatric patients with sinusitis will sometimes complain of facial or periorbital pain, although younger children may simply have a persistent nasal discharge. Dental abscess can be overlooked as a cause of headache because it is a relatively uncommon finding in children. Therefore, a careful examination of the teeth and gingiva should be performed for all pediatric patients with unexplained headaches. Finally, inflammation of the temporomandibular joint (TMJ) is a rare cause of unilateral headaches in children (TMJ syndrome). These patients typically report increased pain while chewing and have point tenderness over the mandibular condyle.

Traction/Compression

Headaches can be caused by mass effect from a pathologic lesion that produces traction and/or compression involving pain-sensitive structures of the head and neck. For the emergency physician, the most important conditions in this category are intracranial hemorrhage and brain tumor. An intracranial hemorrhage produces displacement of surrounding tissues and, in cases of more significant bleeding, increased ICP. In the pediatric population, this is most often the result of a severe head injury (see Chapter 121 Neurotrauma). However, in rare instances, a child can have a nontraumatic intracranial hemorrhage from a ruptured vascular anomaly (e.g., an arteriovenous malformation), which leads to bleeding into the brain parenchyma and ventricles. As with other vascular events, this type of hemorrhage is characterized by the abrupt onset of severe pain. In contrast, headaches resulting from a brain tumor typically have a more insidious onset. The child will often complain of progressively worsening headaches for several weeks or months. Additional symptoms, such as persistent vomiting or gait abnormalities, may also be present. Unfortunately, the physical examination can be normal during the early phase of the illness, and as mentioned previously, this commonly leads to a delayed diagnosis. Other processes that cause headache as a result of traction and compression include idiopathic intracranial hypertension, brain abscess, hydrocephalus, ventricular shunt failure, and persistent spinal fluid leak after lumbar puncture.

An unusual cause of headache in pediatric patients that deserves special mention because of its potentially life-threatening nature is arterial dissection. Patients may have a headache for hours or days before developing neurologic deficits caused by worsening vascular insufficiency and ultimately stroke. The classic presentation of vertebral artery dissection is neck pain and a severe occipital headache that occurs after minor (even trivial) trauma to the neck, followed by the onset of symptoms such as ataxia, nystagmus, and unilateral weakness. Although, as noted previously, nonhemorrhagic cerebral infarcts are not typically associated with headache, this is one important situation in which headache and ischemic stroke can coexist.

Psychogenic

Although less common than in adults, headaches of psychogenic origin are also seen in children. Possible causes include school avoidance behavior, malingering with secondary gain issues, and a true conversion disorder. These patients often have a history of chronic headaches that have been unresponsive to various treatment methods, and they may have undergone multiple tests without receiving a diagnosis. Parents of these children are usually worried and frustrated. Their reasoning in coming to the ED after an extensive prior workup is often simply to get another opinion. For the emergency physician, establishing definitively that a child's persistent headaches are the result of a psychogenic cause is generally impossible. Obviously, this should be considered a diagnosis of exclusion. However, if the history and physical examination do not suggest a more serious cause of headaches, the best management approach is to communicate genuine concern about the patient, attempt to allay some of the parental fears, and plan appropriate outpatient follow-up.

EVALUATION AND DECISION

As stated previously, the diagnosis for pediatric patients presenting with headache will be evident in all but a small minority of cases after a thorough history and physical examination. Laboratory tests and imaging modalities are rarely needed. Even if a definitive diagnosis cannot be established immediately, the identification of a potentially life-threatening cause of headaches will almost always be possible before the child leaves the ED. Concern about the possibility of a more serious cause warrants aggressive use of whatever diagnostic or therapeutic interventions are indicated, such as a computed tomography (CT) or magnetic resonance imaging (MRI) of the head, lumbar puncture, or intravenous antibiotics. Occasionally, a child with a suspected brain tumor will be appropriately discharged from the ED without undergoing any diagnostic tests. Such a disposition assumes that proper follow-up for such patients can be arranged and that MRI of the head will be performed shortly thereafter. An approach to the diagnostic evaluation of a child with headaches is outlined in Figure 54.1.

Clinical Assessment

History

Before proceeding to specific questions about headache symptoms, the clinician should inquire about the general health of the patient, particularly during the hours leading up to the current presentation. For example, the presence of a high fever, decreased activity, and poor oral intake are suggestive of a serious inflammatory cause such as meningitis. A patient with these same symptoms who also has an abrupt change in mental status may have encephalitis. If a child has been relatively well but has complained of headache associated with

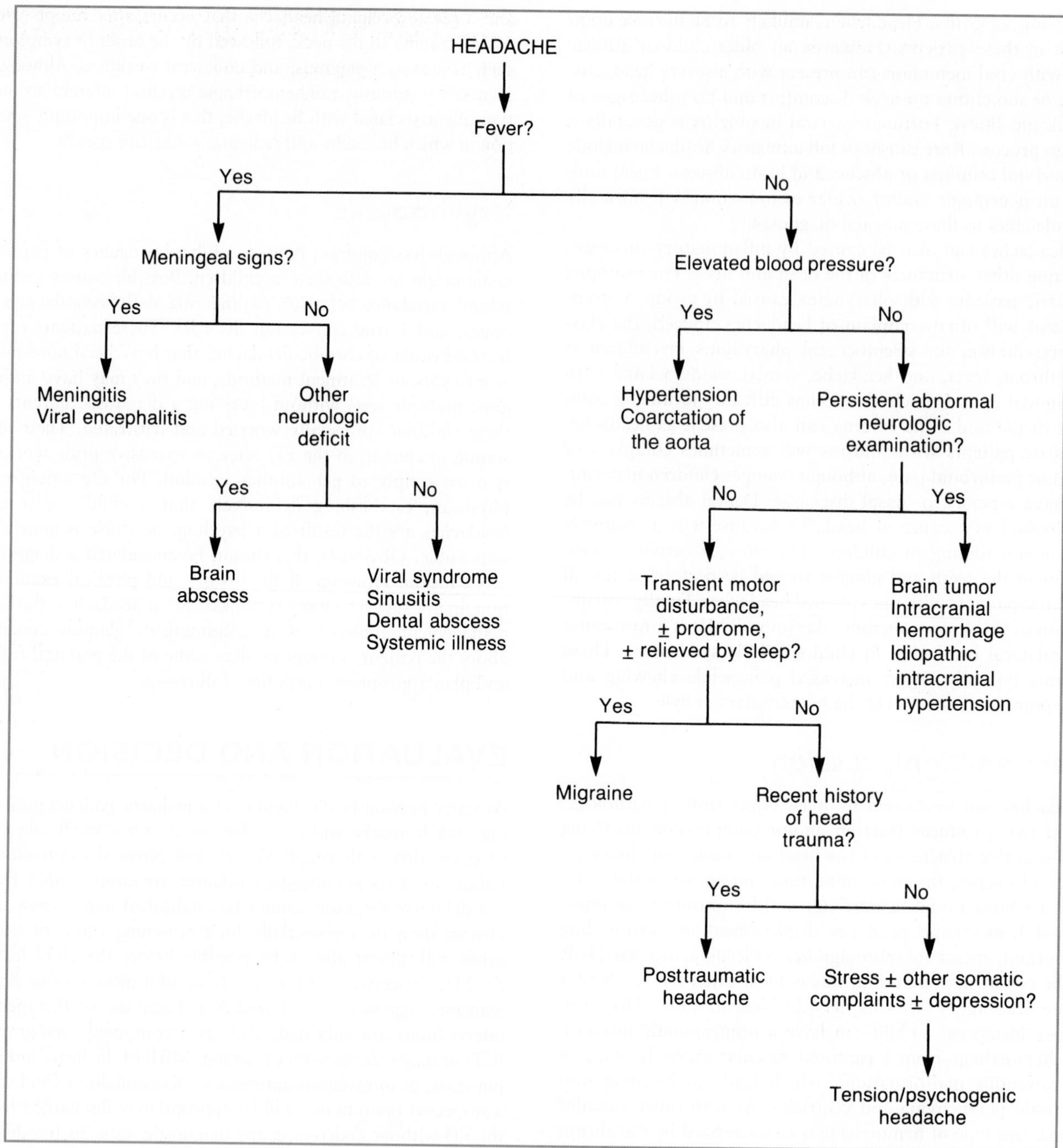

FIGURE 54.1 Approach to the diagnosis of headache.

persistent nasal discharge (especially if it is purulent), this may be caused by a sinusitis. A child with tooth pain, ear pain, or sore throat may also have a readily apparent reason for headaches.

After general health issues are covered, the clinician should then obtain a complete history regarding the headache itself. As with many illnesses, the cause of headaches can usually be diagnosed with a high degree of accuracy solely based on history; the physical examination is often merely confirmatory. One of the more important points to investigate is the mode of onset. A headache that starts abruptly and causes extreme pain may represent a vascular event such as a ruptured arteriovenous malformation, whereas a headache with a more gradual onset would be inconsistent with this diagnosis. It is sometimes useful to question the patient about the severity of the pain, although in younger children, this history may not always be reliable. A youngster who is smiling and playing with toys may nod "yes" in response to the question, "Is the pain very, very bad?" In such cases, the description of the severity of pain must obviously be correlated with the child's clinical appearance. Questions about the quality of pain (e.g., boring, throbbing) are often less useful in children.

The frequency and duration of headaches can also provide valuable clues about the origin of the pain. A child who complains of a constant headache for several days without respite (i.e., goes to sleep with it, wakes up with it) usually has a tension headache or, perhaps more likely, a psychogenic headache. In general, headaches that become progressively more frequent or prolonged should raise suspicion for a more serious underlying condition. Similarly, a child with headaches that have steadily worsened in severity over time warrants careful evaluation, again given the limitations of a child's description of pain. Parents can often help clarify such situations. For example, they may report that the child previously complained of headaches while continuing to play, but now the headaches cause the child to stop any activity, lie down, and start crying.

An important exception to the generally benign nature of headaches that are described as constant over prolonged periods is the rare patient who presents to the ED with undiagnosed idiopathic intracranial hypertension. Classically, an overweight female adolescent or young adult, these patients will often complain of severe, unrelenting headache that may gradually worsen over a period of several days. These patients are easily misdiagnosed as having such conditions as sinusitis or migraine or psychogenic headache. This presentation is especially significant if the patient also reports newly impaired vision, because this may be a sign of excessive pressure on the optic nerves, which, if untreated, can result in permanent blindness.

The time and circumstances of occurrence are also important historical points to ascertain. For example, headaches that are present when a child arises each morning or that awaken a child at night should raise suspicion about a possible brain tumor. In contrast, headaches that occur only later in the day are typically related to stress and result from muscle contraction. Vascular headaches are typically worsened by exertion. In addition, any precipitating events that consistently cause or exacerbate a headache should be identified. If an older child has a headache that is significantly worse when leaning down (e.g., to pick up something off the floor), this is most likely to be caused by sinusitis, although in rare cases, this history may be present in a child with a brain tumor.

The patient's past medical history and family history may contribute to the diagnosis. As mentioned previously, children with cystic fibrosis or congenital heart disease may have headaches caused by worsening hypoxia. Likewise, a patient with renal disease may develop headaches in response to an elevated blood pressure. Patients with neurofibromatosis, Down syndrome, a familial cancer, or previous therapy for leukemia are all at higher risk for developing brain tumors. For the child with a stable pattern of chronic, remitting headaches, the most important question regarding family history is whether anyone has had migraine headaches. It should be remembered, however, that many people use the term *migraine* rather broadly to refer to any type of severe headache. Therefore, the clinician may find it useful to describe typical migraine symptoms before questioning parents about this aspect of the history. Abrupt onset of headache and nausea in several members of one household (or headache and syncope in a child) may be the result of carbon monoxide poisoning.

Before leaving this subject, it is worth reemphasizing the importance of a thorough history in developing an appropriate clinical suspicion of a possible brain tumor. The time between onset of headaches and detection of abnormal physical findings is highly variable. Making a presumptive diagnosis of brain tumor as a likely cause of headaches during this early stage of the illness will, therefore, depend entirely on the history. In their classic article, Honig and Charney described several historical points that are characteristic of children with brain tumor headaches (Table 54.4). Although no single pathognomonic response on history unerringly establishes the diagnosis, eliciting one or more of these findings should certainly raise the level of concern that a child's headaches may be caused by a brain tumor.

TABLE 54.4

CHARACTERISTIC HISTORICAL FINDINGS OF BRAIN TUMOR HEADACHES IN CHILDREN

Nocturnal headache or pain on arising in the morning
Worsening over time (severity, frequency, and/or duration)
Associated with vomiting (although may also occur with migraine), especially if vomiting gets progressively worse
Behavioral changes
Polydipsia/polyuria (craniopharyngioma)
History of probable neurologic deficits (e.g., ataxia/incoordination/"clumsiness," blurred vision, or diplopia)

From Honig PJ, Charney EB. Children with brain tumor headaches: distinguishing features. *Am J Dis Child* 1982;136:121–141, with permission.

Physical Examination

Finding an abnormality on the physical examination of a child with headaches will be a relatively rare event. Nevertheless, a thorough examination should be performed in every case because identification of even a subtle finding (e.g., early papilledema) can significantly alter the course of evaluation and treatment. As with all children seen in the ED, the first step of the examination is to assess the patient's appearance. Does the child look sick or well? Does the child appear to be in severe pain, mild pain, or no pain at all? A child who appears ill may have a more serious underlying condition, such as meningitis or an intracranial hemorrhage, requiring a rapid examination and prompt initiation of treatment.

The vital signs should also be assessed, particularly the temperature and blood pressure. Although omitting the blood pressure is acceptable for many pediatric conditions, this is never acceptable for a patient with headaches. Significant hypertension, usually resulting from undiagnosed renal disease or an undiagnosed coarctation of the aorta, is a rare but potentially dangerous cause of headaches that can affect children of any age. For any patient with headache who complains of associated visual impairment, formal (age appropriate) visual acuity testing should be performed. Measuring basic growth parameters for a pediatric patient with headaches can also provide valuable information. Macrocephaly may be the result of hydrocephalus or a brain tumor, and short stature can be associated with a craniopharyngioma that causes impaired pituitary function.

The head and neck examination will sometimes reveal an obvious source of headache in a child. The scalp should be examined for evidence of head injury. Even when no history of trauma exists, the child may have had an unwitnessed event, or the history may be intentionally misleading with a victim of nonaccidental trauma. Tenderness of the scalp or neck muscles is often present with headaches resulting from stress and muscle contraction. Cranial auscultation may reveal a bruit in patients with arteriovenous malformation. The eyes should be examined to detect any abnormalities in pupillary responses or extraocular movements. A sluggish pupil may be caused by an expanding mass lesion that is compressing the third cranial nerve, and pain with extraocular movements may be elicited with a retroorbital cellulitis or abscess. The fundi should be carefully examined for signs of papilledema, which would suggest an elevated ICP. If necessary, a short-acting dilating eye drop such as tropicamide (Mydriacyl) can be administered to facilitate the examination. The clinician may find an otitis media or otitis externa. Streptococcal pharyngitis as a cause of headaches may be evident as swelling, erythema, and exudates of the tonsillar pillars. Facial tenderness and erythema are sometimes seen in children with maxillary or frontal sinusitis. The teeth and gingiva should be examined for evidence of inflammation or abscess. Nuchal rigidity can be a sign of meningitis, intracranial hemorrhage, or in rare cases, a brain tumor. If a child has a ventricular shunt, assessment of shunt function should be performed when appropriate (see Chapter 130 Neurosurgical Emergencies).

Examining the skin is also important for the child with headaches. Because the skin and central nervous system have a common embryologic origin, cutaneous lesions are sometimes seen with neurologic disorders. For example, a child with numerous hyperpigmented spots scattered over the body (café au lait spots) most likely has neurofibromatosis. This is a specific risk factor for brain tumors. Similarly, children with tuberous sclerosis will almost always have several small, hypopigmented spots (ash leaf spots) that are more apparent when viewed under a Wood ultraviolet lamp.

Every child with a complaint of headaches needs a complete neurologic examination. Any new focal finding suggests the presence of a focal lesion, such as a tumor, hemorrhage, or in rare cases, stroke. The findings of a large meta-analysis regarding the frequency of presenting complaints and physical findings of children with brain tumors are listed in Table 54.5 and those specifically for children under 4 years of age are listed in Table 54.6. Some children with migraine headaches develop focal neurologic abnormalities as part of their migraine syndrome (e.g., ophthalmoplegia), but parents can normally confirm that this is not a new problem. As mentioned previously, the mental status of a child with headaches must always be carefully assessed. A diminished level of consciousness may be the result of encephalitis, a large intracranial hemorrhage, or significantly elevated ICP. To the extent that the child can cooperate, cranial nerve function should also be evaluated. Cranial nerve abnormalities may result from an elevated ICP or direct compression by a mass lesion. Sensory and motor function should be examined, although here again the ability of a younger patient to cooperate may be limited. A reasonable evaluation can be accomplished by observing the child's gait while walking and/or running and by assessing the child's dexterity in performing age-appropriate activities, such as transferring a toy from hand to hand and tying shoelaces. Any evidence of abnormalities in gait or fine motor coordination warrants further investigation.

TABLE 54.5

FREQUENCY OF PRESENTING SIGNS AND SYMPTOMS IN CHILDREN WITH BRAIN TUMORS

Headache (33%)
Nausea and vomiting (32%)
Abnormal gait or coordination (27%)
Papilledema (13%)
Seizures (13%)
Squint (7%)
Change in behavior or school performance (7%)
Cranial nerve palsies (7%)

From Wilne S, Collier J, Kennedy C, et al. Presentation of childhood CNS tumours: a systematic review and meta-analysis. *Lancet Oncol* 2007;8: 685–695.

TABLE 54.6

FREQUENCY OF PRESENTING SIGNS AND SYMPTOMS IN CHILDREN UNDER 4 YEARS OF AGE WITH BRAIN TUMORS

Macrocephaly (41%)
Nausea and vomiting (30%)
Irritability (24%)
Lethargy (21%)
Abnormal gait and coordination (19%)
Weight loss (14%)
Bulging fontanelle (13%)
Seizures (10%)

From Wilne S, Collier J, Kennedy C, et al. Presentation of childhood CNS tumours: a systematic review and meta-analysis. *Lancet Oncol* 2007;8: 685–695.

Laboratory and Radiographic Testing

Most children presenting in an acute-care setting with headache as the chief complaint will not require any laboratory tests. The child with a possible serious infectious process causing headaches can require a variety of tests, including a complete blood cell count, blood cultures, and a lumbar puncture. Yet these patients are more likely to have other symptoms such as high fever and lethargy, rather than headache, as the primary complaint. When a lumbar puncture is necessary, it is important to remember that a head CT scan should be obtained first if the patient is suspected of having a lesion that could lead to subsequent cerebral herniation (e.g., a large intracranial mass or obstructive hydrocephalus). Signs suggestive of such a condition include focal neurologic deficits, papilledema, and mental status depression with unilateral pupillary dilation. This is generally considered a prudent practice despite the fact that considerable controversy exists about whether herniation is ever actually *caused* by a lumbar puncture, even if temporally related. For suspected idiopathic intracranial hypertension (i.e., a patient with papilledema who has a negative head CT), an opening pressure measurement should be obtained when the lumbar puncture is performed. Serum electrolytes, blood urea nitrogen, creatinine, and a urinalysis should be obtained for any child with headaches who is found to have an elevated blood pressure. The patient with a ventricular shunt who has fever and headaches will likely require a shunt tap by a neurosurgical consultant. Finally, a child with a suspected subarachnoid hemorrhage should undergo a lumbar puncture if the head CT scan is negative. This is necessary because a small hemorrhage may not be detected by CT, and in such cases, blood in the cerebrospinal fluid (CSF) is the only diagnostic finding. However, this is an uncommon situation in the pediatric population.

As with laboratory testing, few children with headaches who come to the ED will require an emergent imaging study. A child with a ventricular shunt may require a shunt series in addition to CT or MRI. Likewise, sinus radiographs are rarely indicated in pediatric patients because the diagnosis is almost always made on clinical grounds. Occasionally, a child with multiple episodes of an apparent sinus infection will require a CT scan of the sinuses, but this is normally done as an outpatient.

The two imaging modalities that are most widely used clinically to obtain detailed information about intracranial abnormalities are CT and MRI. Both tests have advantages and disadvantages. CT is more readily available on an emergent basis (many EDs have a dedicated scanner). Scanning time is also much shorter for CT, and the potentially unstable patient can be more easily observed. These characteristics make CT the test of choice to evaluate patients at risk for problems such as intracranial hemorrhage, cerebral edema, hydrocephalus, and herniation syndrome. Recent advances in MRI approaches have reduced the time needed for some MRI scans. For example, an MRI to evaluate VP shunt malfunction can now be performed in 3 to 5 minutes in some institutions. CT is especially useful for patients with head trauma.

CT does not offer the quality of image resolution provided by MRI. Smaller lesions, particularly those of the posterior fossa and brainstem, are more reliably detected by MRI. This is true even when the CT scan is performed using contrast material. Consequently, MRI is superior for children suspected of having a brain tumor who have a normal neurologic examination and no signs of elevated ICP. If these patients have a normal head CT scan in the ED, they will likely also require an outpatient MRI. Such duplication of testing is costly and usually unwarranted. While the use of MRI in the acute management of stroke has led to a substantial increase in overall scanning capacity, limited availability continues to be the main drawback of MRI. Even when the MRI is available, children may require deep sedation under the supervision of an anesthesiologist. This makes nonemergent MRI scans difficult to obtain from the ED even in large institutions. As discussed in the following, the emergency physician must take these and other factors into account in determining which, if any, imaging modality is indicated for a child with headaches.

Treatment and Disposition

Patients with headaches caused by a potentially life-threatening process (e.g., meningitis, encephalitis, ruptured vascular anomaly) require specific treatment approaches discussed elsewhere in this textbook. A patient with idiopathic intracranial hypertension may require drainage of CSF to reduce the ICP, which, in turn, often relieves the headache. Children with headaches that are presumptively diagnosed as benign can often be successfully treated with acetaminophen or ibuprofen. The various options available for treating pediatric migraine patients are described in Chapter 105 Neurologic Emergencies.

Although most children complaining of headache can be safely discharged from the ED with an appropriate follow-up plan, some will require admission to the hospital for further evaluation and treatment. For example, a child with headaches who is found to be significantly hypertensive must be admitted both for management of the blood pressure and investigation of the underlying cause. Any patient with idiopathic intracranial hypertension who also has decreased visual acuity requires emergent evaluation by an ophthalmologist and possibly a surgical procedure to relieve the pressure on the optic nerve. Patients with migraine who have intractable headache may also warrant admission to receive a more effective analgesic regimen. The child with a ventricular shunt who has severe headaches will usually require a shunt series, a CT scan of the head, and neurosurgical evaluation to assess the need for possible shunt revision. If neurosurgical consultation is not immediately available, the patient should be transported to an appropriate receiving facility.

A potentially confusing issue that the emergency physician will inevitably face is how to properly manage a child who is suspected of having a brain tumor. Should all these patients have a brain imaging study in the ED? As discussed previously, the resolution of even a contrast-enhanced head CT scan is inferior to MRI for detecting certain types of tumors. Also, a small but finite risk is associated with the administration of contrast material. However, obtaining a nonemergent MRI from the ED may not be an available option. What then is the appropriate diagnostic approach?

In general, a child with headaches who is suspected of having a brain tumor should undergo a head CT scan in the ED if there are any signs or symptoms of elevated ICP or mass effects. These include an altered mental status, visual changes, persistent vomiting, papilledema, or focal neurologic deficits. Because tumors that cause elevated ICP or mass effects are usually larger and more easily detectable, the reduction in image resolution with CT is less likely to result in missing an abnormality in such cases. Of note, if the CT scan is normal in a child with headache and new focal deficits on neurologic examination, it may be necessary to obtain an emergent MRI to exclude the diagnosis of stroke (e.g., arterial dissection), although this may simply represent the first presentation of a complex migraine syndrome.

But what about the child with a suspicious history (e.g., increasing frequency or duration of pain, headaches that awaken the child from sleep or occur every morning) who has a normal neurologic examination and no signs of elevated ICP? In most cases, if MRI is not available for a nonemergent scan from the ED, such patients can be safely discharged with an outpatient MRI scheduled shortly thereafter. In such cases, parents must be clearly instructed that any sign of deterioration, such as mental status changes or persistent vomiting, requires that the child be immediately returned to the ED for a reevaluation.

Suggested Readings and Key References

Brna PM, Dooley JM. Headaches in the pediatric population. *Semin Pediatr Neurol* 2006;13(4):222–230.

de Ribaupierre S, Rilliet B, Cotting J, et al. A 10-year experience in paediatric spontaneous cerebral hemorrhage: which children with headache need more than a clinical examination? *Swiss Med Wkly* 2008;138(5–6):59–69.

Hershey AD. Pediatric headache. *Pediatr Ann* 2005;34:426–429.

Honig PJ, Charney EB. Children with brain tumor headaches: distinguishing features. *Am J Dis Child* 1982;136:121–141.

Lanphear J, Sarnaik S. Presenting symptoms of pediatric brain tumors diagnosed in the emergency department. *Pediatr Emerg Care* 2014; 30(2):77–80.

Lateef TM, Grewal M, McClintock W, et al. Headache in young children in the emergency department: use of computed tomography. *Pediatrics* 2009;124:e12.

Lewis DW, Qureshi F. Acute headache in children and adolescents presenting to emergency department. *Headache* 2000;40:200–203.

Masi G, Favilla L, Millepiedi S, et al. Somatic symptoms in children and adolescents referred for emotional and behavioral disorders. *Psychiatry* 2000;63:140–149.

Mercille G, Ospina LH. Pediatric idiopathic intracranial hypertension: a review. *Pediatr Rev* 2007;28(11):e77–e86.

Metsähonkala L, Anttila P, Sillanpää M. Tension-type headache in children. *Cephalalgia* 1999;19(suppl 25):56.

Newton RW. Childhood headache. *Arch Dis Child Educ Pract Ed* 2008; 93:105–111.

Pavlakis SG, Frank Y, Chusid R. Hypertensive encephalopathy, reversible occipitoparietal encephalopathy, or reversible posterior leukoencephalopathy: three names for an old syndrome. *J Child Neurol* 1999;14:277–281.

Reulecke BC, Erker CG, Fiedler BJ, et al. Brain tumors in children: initial symptoms and their influence on the time span between symptom onset and diagnosis. *J Child Neurol* 2008;23: 178–183.

Rubin DH, Suecoff SA, Knupp KG. Headaches in children. *Pediatr Ann* 2006;35(5):345–353.

Sheridan DC, Meckler GD, Spiro DM, et al. Diagnostic testing and treatment of pediatric headache in the emergency department. *J Pediatr* 2013;163(6):1634–1637.

Walker DM, Teach SJ. Emergency department treatment of primary headaches in children and adolescents. *Curr Opin Pediatr* 2008; 20:248–254.

Wilne S, Collier J, Kennedy C, et al. Presentation of childhood CNS tumors: a systematic review and meta-analysis. *Lancet Oncol* 2007; 8:685–695.

CHAPTER 55 ■ PAIN: JOINTS

RICHARD J. SCARFONE, MD AND AARON CHEN, MD

Arthritis and arthralgia are common reasons for children to seek care in the emergency department (ED). Arthritis is joint inflammation marked by swelling, warmth, and limitation of motion; arthralgia is joint pain without inflammation. Establishing a diagnosis for the child with joint pain is challenging because the differential diagnosis is lengthy (Table 55.1), clinical and laboratory findings are rarely specific for a particular disease, and disease patterns for many of the etiologies are often highly variable among different patients. Among the most common causes of joint pain in children are infections, trauma, and postinfectious conditions (Table 55.2), whereas those most likely to be life-threatening are due to systemic disease and malignancy (Table 55.3). This chapter serves as a guide to the approach to the child with arthritis or arthralgia, with an emphasis on historical points and physical examination findings that can serve to narrow the diagnostic possibilities.

DIFFERENTIAL DIAGNOSIS

The initial differential diagnosis usually focuses on the most common or potentially serious etiologies (Tables 55.2 and 55.3). Children from 6 to 24 months of age have the highest incidence of nongonococcal bacterial (septic) arthritis, which results primarily from the hematogenous dissemination of an organism. The diagnosis of septic arthritis of the hip should not be delayed because pressure in the joint space will compromise the vascular supply to the femoral head, leading to necrosis (see Chapter 102 Infectious Disease Emergencies).

Osteomyelitis involving the distal end of long bones may manifest as arthralgia with or without objective signs of joint inflammation. Children with sickle cell anemia and Type 1 diabetes mellitus are at higher risk. Onset of symptoms is typically more indolent compared to septic arthritis.

In the first 10 days of illness, children with Kawasaki disease may have arthritis or arthralgia, often involving smaller joints in the hand. Beyond that time, involvement of larger joints of the lower extremities is more common. If an arthrocentesis is performed, the synovial fluid analysis resembles that seen with septic arthritis with 100,000 to 300,000 white blood cells (WBCs) per cubic millimeter (see Chapter 109 Rheumatologic Emergencies).

In the absence of a clear history of a tick bite, arthralgia secondary to early, localized Lyme disease may be a challenging diagnosis to establish because only about 40% to 70% of children have the characteristic erythema migrans rash, constitutional symptoms may be mild, and serologic tests will be normal in the early stages of disease. However, serologic testing will be confirmatory in patients with Lyme arthritis secondary to disseminated disease. Among those with monoarticular arthritis, it may be difficult to distinguish septic arthritis from arthritis associated with Lyme disease on clinical grounds alone, with or without analysis of synovial fluid. There are clinical features that favor the diagnosis of Lyme disease such as knee involvement, absence of recent fever, and lower inflammatory markers, but these characteristics may be shared with a subset of patients who have septic arthritis. Complicating this further is that synovial fluid analysis may not be definitive. There is a wide range of synovial WBC counts in children with Lyme disease and although median values are lower than those typically seen in patients with septic arthritis, there is considerable overlap. Given the difficulties of distinguishing Lyme disease from septic arthritis among children presenting with monoarticular arthritis, management of cases where suspicion for septic joint is significant may require an approach that includes analyzing synovial fluid and performing Lyme serology testing, especially if one practices in a region where Lyme disease is not endemic.

Transient (also called toxic) synovitis is a poorly understood inflammation of large joints, afflicting children 3 to 6 years of age. The diagnosis is typically made on clinical grounds, and this self-limited disease does not result in joint destruction. When the hip is involved, the challenge for clinicians is to distinguish transient synovitis from Lyme (in endemic areas) or septic arthritis.

Reactive, or postinfectious, arthritis is probably more common than septic arthritis. Arthritis following various enteric infections is not rare in children, and joint complaints after parvovirus B19 infection are seen among adolescents. *Chlamydia trachomatis* infection of the genitourinary tract should be considered in any sexually active adolescent with new-onset arthritis. With postinfectious arthritis, antimicrobial treatment does not modify the disease course.

Traumatic injuries to a joint may cause periarticular swelling or an effusion indicative of a hemarthrosis. In addition, ligamentous or tendon injuries will result in joint pain and impaired range of motion. Serum sickness and Henoch–Schönlein purpura (HSP) are marked by characteristic rashes.

EVALUATION AND DECISION

Figure 55.1 depicts an algorithm for the diagnostic approach to the child with joint pain. The evaluation should include inquiries about the specific joint(s) involved, symptom duration, and history of trauma, fever, rash, tick bites, sexual risk factors, intravenous drug use, and recent illnesses. The child's past medical and family histories should be reviewed. A family history of systemic lupus erythematosus (SLE), inflammatory bowel disease, or rheumatoid arthritis increases the child's risk for these diseases.

A comprehensive physical examination should be performed with particular attention paid to a search for rashes, heart murmurs, and abdominal abnormalities. Assessment of

TABLE 55.1

JOINT PAIN—DIFFERENTIAL DIAGNOSIS

Infection
Septic arthritis (bacterial)
Staphylococcus aureus
Streptococcus pneumoniae
Haemophilus influenza
Group B streptococci
Escherichia coli
Neisseria gonorrhea
Other infectious arthritis
Viral
Mycobacterial
Fungal
Osteomyelitis
Postinfectious
Viral: hepatitis B, parvovirus, Epstein–Barr virus, cytomegalovirus, varicella-zoster, herpesvirus 6, enterovirus, adenovirus
Bacterial: acute rheumatic fever, Lyme disease, chlamydia (Reiter syndrome), mycoplasma, shigella, campylobacter
Trauma/overuse
Contusion
Hemarthrosis
Fracture
Inflicted injury
Ligamentous sprain
Bursitis
Tendonitis
Slipped capital femoral epiphysis
Legg–Calvé–Perthes disease
Osteochondritis dissecans
Chondromalacia patellae
Osgood–Schlatter disease
Immune mediated/vasculitic
Juvenile idiopathic arthritis
Serum sickness
Kawasaki disease
Inflammatory bowel disease
Systemic lupus erythematosus
Henoch–Schönlein purpura
Other
Transient synovitis of the hip
Malignancy
Leukemia
Neuroblastoma
Bone tumor
Hemophilia

the affected joint(s) should determine if it is warm, swollen, or tender as well as its range of motion.

A complete blood count (CBC) and differential, C-reactive protein, and erythrocyte sedimentation rate (ESR) are indicated for the febrile child with signs of joint inflammation, especially in the absence of trauma. Blood cultures will have a low yield, but should be obtained in the febrile patient or when there is concern for bone or joint infection. Additional laboratory studies, such as an antistreptolysin-O titer or antinuclear antibody (ANA) test should be guided by the history and physical examination. Radiographs of the affected joint are particularly useful in the setting of trauma or acute monoarthritis without an obvious cause to evaluate for fractures and dislocations; the Ottawa knee rules can be used to guide the decision to obtain radiographs of the knee following injury. In a recent validation study in children aged 2 to 16 years of age, the rules were found to be 100% sensitive in detecting fractures while eliminating the need for about one-third of the radiographs, however there were a limited number of children below 5 years of age and caution must be used when applying these rules in younger children. Ultrasound is more sensitive than plain radiographs in detecting an effusion. In most febrile children with monoarthritis and a joint effusion, an arthrocentesis, usually ultrasound guided if involving the hip, is needed to assist in determining if septic arthritis is the etiology. Magnetic resonance imaging is most useful to detect subtle fractures not visualized on plain films and to help establish a diagnosis of osteomyelitis.

TABLE 55.2

COMMON CAUSES OF JOINT PAIN

Septic arthritis (bacterial)
Osteomyelitis
Kawasaki disease
Lyme disease
Transient synovitis
Postinfectious (reactive)
Traumatic
Serum sickness
Henoch–Schönlein purpura

Trauma

A key initial point in the history is whether trauma preceded the pain. A radiograph will detect fractures or a slipped capital femoral epiphysis (SCFE). Classically, an SCFE occurs in the obese adolescent with hip or knee pain (Chapters 119 Musculoskeletal Trauma and 129 Musculoskeletal Emergencies). Importantly, only about half of children will report preceding trauma and there may be bilateral disease in about one-third of children. Plain radiographs (including the frog-leg view of the hip)

TABLE 55.3

LIFE-THREATENING CAUSES OF JOINT PAIN

Acute rheumatic fever
Kawasaki disease
Malignancy
Leukemia
Neuroblastoma
Bone tumor

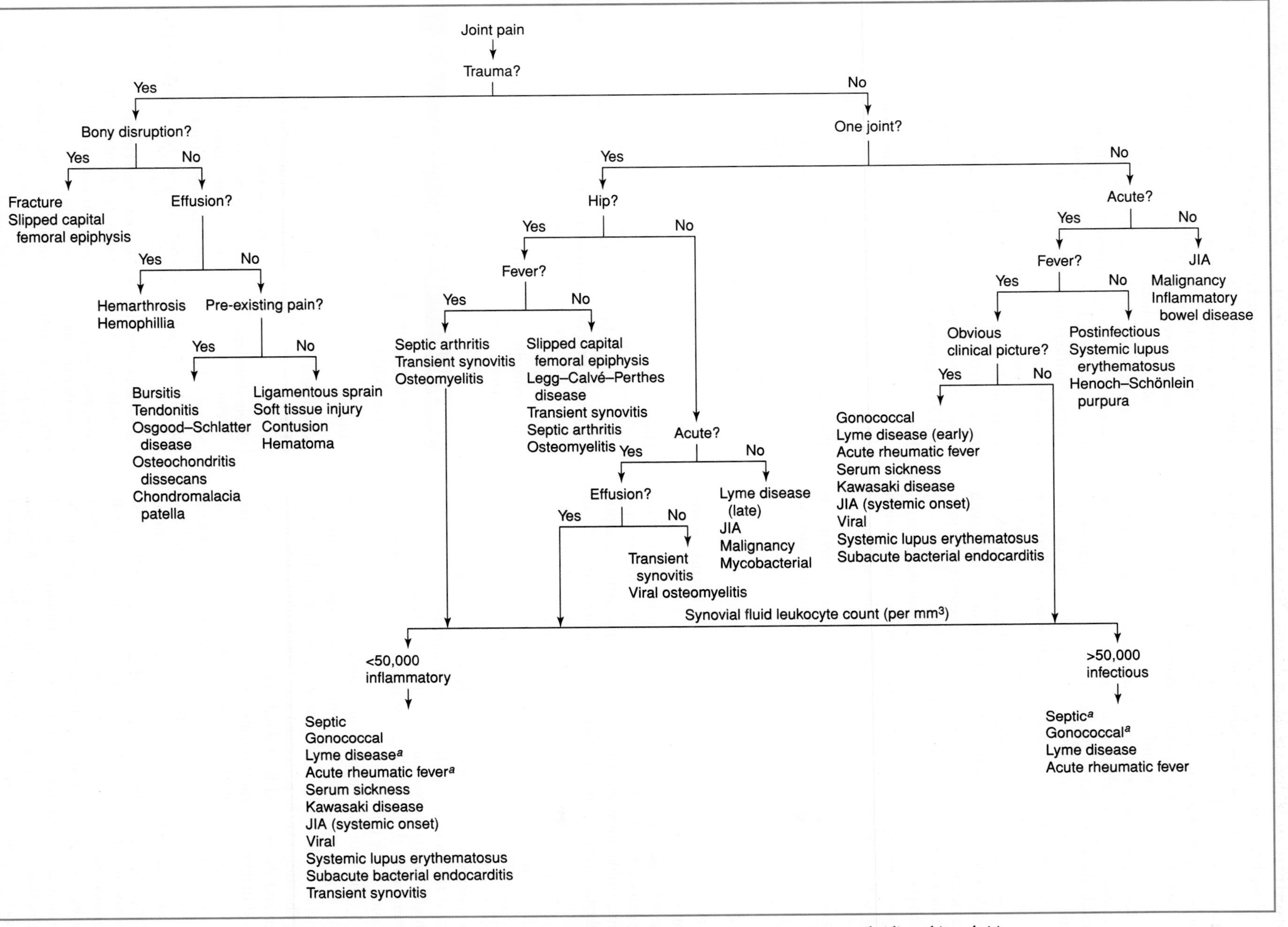

FIGURE 55.1 A diagnostic approach to joint pain. [a]Most likely leukocyte count. JIA, juvenile idiopathic arthritis.

showing a widened epiphysis and caudal displacement of the femoral head establish the diagnosis.

Metaphyseal corner ("bucket-handle") fractures resulting in joint pain are highly suggestive of inflicted injury. These typically occur in children of age 3 years or less and there may not be a clear history of trauma. These fractures result from traction or torsion forces such as occur when the arms or legs are pulled or swung violently.

Radiographs may also aid in determining whether swelling is caused by a joint effusion or is simply soft tissue swelling outside the joint space, a distinction that is often difficult to make on physical examination alone. In the setting of acute trauma and in the absence of fever, an effusion is indicative of a hemarthrosis and is rarely a diagnostic or therapeutic indication for performing an arthrocentesis. Clinicians must have a high index of suspicion for hemarthrosis in the child with hemophilia or other clotting disorder who presents with joint swelling, even without a clear history of trauma.

In the absence of an effusion, inquiries about the duration of symptoms should be made. Children with conditions such as bursitis, tendonitis, and Osgood–Schlatter disease typically have chronic, low-grade pain and may inadvertently come to medical attention after minor trauma. New-onset periarticular swelling and pain immediately after acute trauma suggests ligamentous or other soft tissue injury.

Monoarthritis

In the absence of trauma, monoarthritis of the hip may represent a true orthopedic emergency. Septic hips require operative drainage to prevent osteonecrosis and the most important prognostic factor is the length of delay in operative management. Unlike most other causes of fever and arthritis, septic arthritis involves only a single joint in more than 90% of affected children; 80% of these are hip, knee, or ankle infections. The absence of fever does not preclude the diagnosis; just 60% to 70% of children with septic arthritis are febrile at presentation. A child with septic arthritis of the hip will typically maintain external rotation of the hip, resist even the slightest range of motion and be unable to ambulate. In fact, if the child allows full range of motion, the diagnosis is highly unlikely. Neonates, on the other hand, will often present with thigh swelling, pseudoparalysis, and external rotation at the hip.

A child with acute onset of monoarthritis of the hip or any other large joint, marked by an effusion and severely restricted range of motion, with or without fever, needs an arthrocentesis. The study may be performed with bedside ultrasound guidance and the synovial fluid should be analyzed for cell count and differential, Gram stain, and culture. In two large series, about half of the children with septic arthritis of the hip had negative synovial fluid cultures. In these cases, children with synovial fluid WBC counts greater than 50,000 per mm^3 and positive blood cultures were presumed to have septic arthritis and managed accordingly. *Staphylococcus aureus* is the most common infecting agent for older children, whereas group B *Streptococcus* and gram-negative enteric organisms must also be considered in neonates. In recent years, clinicians are encountering a greater prevalence of community-associated methicillin-resistant *S. aureus* as a causative agent. *Kingella kingae,* a gram-negative coccobacillus, must be considered when evaluating a preschool-aged child, especially if the child has a chronic medical condition.

In contrast to septic arthritis, children with transient synovitis of the hip usually appear well, are afebrile, are often able to bear weight but have a limp, and allow almost complete range of motion of the affected joint. A prospective study of over 150 children presenting with an irritable hip found that just 2% of children had septic arthritis if each of these four risk factors were absent: Fever >38.5°C, refusal to bear weight, ESR >40 mm per hour, and WBC >12,000 cells per mm^3.

Often, based on clinical findings, a physician can make a diagnosis of transient synovitis without the need for laboratory testing or arthrocentesis. In more equivocal cases, inflammatory markers may be helpful and Lyme testing should be considered.

Inflammatory markers are usually elevated in patients with osteomyelitis, as well. In contrast to those with septic arthritis, children with osteomyelitis have a more subacute onset of pain, are less likely to be febrile, have focal bony tenderness, will have greater range of motion at the joint, and may not have signs of joint inflammation.

Legg–Calvé–Perthes disease, a condition of uncertain cause, occurs overwhelmingly in boys, with an onset between 4 and 8 years of age. The pain, which may be localized to the hip or referred to the thigh or knee, is insidious in onset. The aseptic or avascular necrosis of the femoral head will be manifest on plain radiographs as a small, osteopenic femoral head with a widened joint space although films obtained early in the clinical course may be normal.

Polyarthritis

Historical and physical examination findings help narrow the choices among the many causes of polyarthritis and fever (Tables 55.4 and 55.5). The ill-appearing adolescent with migratory arthritis, tenosynovitis involving the extensor tendons of the wrist or ankle, and scattered crops of vesiculopustules should be strongly suspected for gonococcal arthritis. This occurs three to five times more often in girls, often during menstruation. Of note, few patients report lower abdominal

TABLE 55.4

DISTINGUISHING CLINICAL FEATURES OF ETIOLOGIES OF POLYARTHRITIS

Disease	Clinical characteristics
Gonococcal	Adolescent, tenosynovitis, rash
Lyme	Tick bite, erythema migrans, endemic region, seasonality
Acute rheumatic fever	Recent streptococcal infection, extreme migratory pain, carditis
Serum sickness	Urticaria, angioedema
Kawasaki disease	Prolonged fever, rash, conjunctivitis, mouth changes
Subacute bacterial endocarditis	Congenital heart disease, fever, new murmur, splinter hemorrhages
Systemic lupus erythematosus	African-American female, skin or renal disease
Henoch–Schönlein purpura	Purpura below the waist, nephritis, abdominal pain, scrotal swelling
Inflammatory bowel disease	Abdominal pain, diarrhea, weight loss, anemia

TABLE 55.5

FEVER AND JOINT PAIN

Usually febrile at presentation
Septic arthritis (bacterial)
Osteomyelitis
Gonococcal
Acute rheumatic fever
Juvenile idiopathic arthritis (systemic onset subcategory)
Subacute bacterial endocarditis
Serum sickness
Kawasaki disease
May or may not be febrile at presentation
Leukemia
Mycobacterial
Postinfectious (reactive)
Lyme disease
Systemic lupus erythematosus
Inflammatory bowel disease

pain or vaginal discharge concurrently, and cultures of blood and synovial fluid are typically negative. The highest yield for establishing the diagnosis is by Gram stain of the skin lesions or by recovering the organism from the cervix, rectum, or throat.

Joint involvement with Lyme disease has two distinct patterns. In early localized or disseminated disease, the child may develop episodic migratory polyarthritis, affecting mainly large joints. However, more typically at this stage, the child has polyarthralgia without signs of joint inflammation. Weeks to months (mean 4 to 6 weeks) after the tick bite, half of untreated children develop a monoarthritis, usually of the knee. The joint is significantly swollen but only mildly painful, and patients are usually afebrile at this stage and without a history of trauma. A recent study of children in a Lyme-endemic area found that an absolute neutrophil count $<10 \times 10^3$ cells per mm^3 and an ESR <40 mm per hour helped distinguish Lyme arthritis from septic arthritis, although others have shown significant overlap in these labs across the two etiologies of arthritis.

Extremely painful, migratory joint inflammation involving multiple joints in a child with recent evidence of a group A streptococcal infection should raise the concern for acute rheumatic fever. Evidence of carditis, erythema marginatum, subcutaneous nodules, or a positive serology for antistreptococcal antibodies supports the diagnosis. The presence of diffuse urticaria and angioedema accompanying arthralgia or arthritis, especially 3 to 10 days after initiation of an antibiotic, helps distinguish serum sickness from other causes of polyarthritis and fever. Kawasaki disease is characterized by high and persistent fever, conjunctival injection without exudate, mouth and lip swelling and cracking, swelling and erythema of the hands and feet, a nonspecific rash, and lymphadenopathy. About 30% of patients will also develop arthritis or arthralgia, with about one-third of these having onset in the first 10 days of illness. Daily temperature spikes exceeding 40°C, especially if accompanied by a transient pink rash, suggest systemic-onset juvenile rheumatoid arthritis (JRA), one of the categories of juvenile idiopathic arthritis (JIA). A common viral-related arthritis is that caused by hepatitis B infection. The arthritis precedes the symptoms of hepatitis and resolves when the jaundice appears. Parvovirus B19 is the causative agent of erythema infectiosum; about 5% of affected children will complain of transient, bilateral joint swelling. Joint manifestations due to this virus can also occur in the absence of a rash causing a sudden onset of symmetric, self-limited polyarthritis, particularly in the hands. With subacute bacterial endocarditis, musculoskeletal symptoms are variable, ranging from asymptomatic joint effusions to frank arthritis of up to three joints. Pre-existing congenital heart disease, a prolonged fever, a new murmur, and splinter hemorrhages may all be clues to the diagnosis of this rare entity in children.

Postinfectious arthritis is one of the most common causes of acute polyarthritis without fever. One to 2 weeks after an illness (especially *C. trachomatis, Shigella,* or *Salmonella*) or urogenital infection (Reiter syndrome), a child may develop an asymmetric joint inflammation predominantly involving large joints of the lower extremities. The severity of the antecedent illness has little correlation with the arthritis. As with many of the diseases discussed to this point, SLE has a variable clinical presentation with regard to musculoskeletal involvement. In fact, no two patients have an identical pattern of immune complex formation or clinical disease expression. A symmetric polyarthritis involving peripheral joints of the hands or feet may be seen. However, small effusions of the knee are also common with active disease, and the arthritis may also be intermittent or migratory. Patients with this type of arthritis are usually afebrile, yet high fever may be a prominent finding. Further, although arthritis is one of several diagnostic criteria, it is uncommon for patients with SLE to present with isolated arthritis. Arthritis of the small joints, a positive test for ANA, and abnormalities of the skin, kidneys, lungs, or central nervous system should raise the clinician's suspicion for SLE.

HSP is rarely a diagnostic challenge thanks to the presence of petechiae and purpura in the characteristic below-the-waist distribution. Affected children may also have polyarthritis or arthralgia, colicky abdominal pain, and nephritis. As with the rash, periarticular swelling usually involves joints below the waist.

Chronic arthritis is less common than acute arthritis in children younger than age 16 years, with an incidence of 20 to 150 cases per 100,000. JIA is a newer term used to classify chronic childhood arthritis. This term describes children less than 16 years of age with joint inflammation for at least 6 weeks, in whom other causes have been eliminated, and encompasses all of the diseases referred to as JRA, as well as other causes of idiopathic arthritis. Subclassifications of disease are based on the patient's age at onset of symptoms, duration and pattern of arthritis, and presence or absence of systemic signs such as fever or rash. Tests for rheumatoid factor or ANA may assist in establishing a specific diagnosis. Since JIA has a highly variable presentation, it appears at many different points in the diagnostic algorithm. These are difficult diagnoses for ED physicians to establish based on a single patient encounter; children with chronic arthritis should be referred to a rheumatologist (see Chapter 109 Rheumatologic Emergencies).

In the absence of fever, chronic pain of one or more joints may also indicate malignancy. Specifically, leukemia or neuroblastoma can both present with true joint swelling, as can bony tumors. Pallor, adenopathy, weight loss, and other constitutional complaints, as well as anemia or cytopenias, would support this diagnosis.

A large joint oligoarthritis occurs as an extraintestinal complication of inflammatory bowel disease in about one-third of children, usually during times of active disease. Clues to the diagnosis include abdominal pain, hematochezia, anemia, and weight loss.

In summary, this review of joint pain in children should serve as a guide to the diagnostic evaluation. The clinician must choose from many different causes, each with variable and nonspecific characteristics. In addition, laboratory studies are rarely specific for a particular disease. However, by asking the appropriate questions, performing a careful physical examination, selectively obtaining adjunct studies, and developing pattern recognition skills, the clinician can follow the correct diagnostic path.

Suggested Readings and Key References

Bachur RG, Adams CM, Monuteaux MC. Evaluating the child with acute hip pain ("irritable hip") in a Lyme endemic region. *J Pediatr* 2015;166(2):407–411.

Caird MS, Flynn JM, Leung YL, et al. Factors distinguishing septic arthritis from transient synovitis of the hip in children. A prospective study. *J Bone Joint Surg Am* 2006;88:1251–1257.

Deanehan JK, Kimia AA, Tan Tanny SP, et al. Distinguishing Lyme from septic knee monoarthritis in Lyme-disease endemic areas. *Pediatrics* 2013;131:e695–e701.

Deanehan JK, Nigrovic PA, Milewski MD, et al. Synovial fluid findings in children with knee monoarthritis in Lyme disease endemic areas. *Pediatr Emerg Care* 2014;30:16–19.

Gough-Palmer A, McHugh K. Investigating hip pain in a well child. *BMJ* 2007;334:1216–1217.

Jones OY, Spencer CH, Bowyer SL, et al. A multicenter case-control study on predictive factors distinguishing childhood leukemia from juvenile rheumatoid arthritis. *Pediatrics* 2006;117:e840.

Kocher MS, Mandiga R, Zurakowski D, et al. Validation of a clinical prediction rule for the difference between septic arthritis and transient synovitis of the hip in children. *J Bone Joint Surg Am* 2004; 86:1629–1635.

Lehman TJA. Classification of juvenile arthritis. In: *UpToDate,* Rose BD, eds. UpToDate, Waltham, MA, 2014.

Nigrovic PA. Overview of hip pain in childhood. In: *UpToDate,* Rose BD, eds. UpToDate, Waltham, MA, 2015.

Thapa M, Vo JN, Sheills II WE. Ultrasound-guided musculoskeletal procedures in children. *Pediatr Radiol* 2013;43:S55–S60.

Thompson A, Mannix R, Bachur R. Acute pediatric monoarticular arthritis: distinguishing Lyme arthritis from other etiologies. *Pediatrics* 2009;123(3):959–965.

CHAPTER 56 ■ PAIN: SCROTAL

CATHERINE E. PERRON, MD AND STEVEN S. BIN, MD

Acute scrotal swelling or pain in a child is a potential surgical emergency requiring prompt evaluation. Although some causes of acute scrotal swelling are benign and require only observation and reassurance, other causes may lead to the rapid loss of a testis if diagnosis or treatment is delayed (testicular torsion). Many diagnoses in cases of scrotal pain are most reliably made clinically, differentiating by age, historical features relating to the evolution of pain and associated symptoms, and physical examination findings.

PATHOPHYSIOLOGY

An understanding of scrotal anatomy and development is important for rapid assessment. The structures contained in the scrotum include the testis; the epididymis; appendages of the testis; and the nerve, vascular, and lymphatic structures that constitute the spermatic cord and traverse the inguinal canal into the scrotum (Fig. 56.1). At 32 to 40 weeks' gestation, the testis descends through the inguinal canal from the abdomen to the scrotum. The testis descends within the process vaginalis, which is an outpouching of the peritoneal cavity. The abdominal portion of the process vaginalis then closes and the remaining portion, called the *tunica vaginalis,* is a potential space that encompasses the anterior two-thirds of the testicle. Within this space, fluids of various etiologies can collect. The testis, its related structures, and the layers of tissue that surround each testis in the scrotum may each relate to the pathology seen. Acute conditions of the scrotum may involve ischemia, inflammation, trauma, and tumor. These processes can alter blood flow to structures within the scrotum, making perfusion imaging modalities useful when correlated with clinical examination.

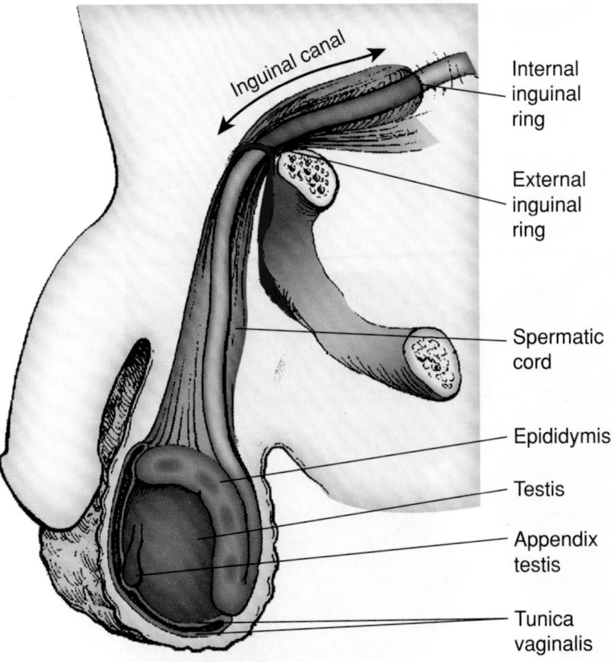

FIGURE 56.1 Anatomy of the scrotal contents.

DIFFERENTIAL DIAGNOSIS

Table 56.1 lists the principal causes of acute scrotal swelling, and Table 56.2 provides the most common diagnoses by age.

CAUSES OF PAINFUL SCROTAL SWELLING

Torsion of the Testis

Testicular torsion or twisting of the spermatic cord and its contents threatens the survival of the testis and is a true surgical emergency. Testicular torsion accounts for 10% to 15% of cases of acute scrotal pain and has two peaks in incidence; a small one in the newborn period, and a larger peak around puberty related to the increasing mass of the testis.

Torsion results from an inadequate fixation of the testis to the intrascrotal subcutaneous tissue (Fig. 56.2), resulting in the "bell-clapper" deformity. The testis, which hangs more

TABLE 56.1

CAUSES OF ACUTE SCROTAL SWELLING

Painful scrotal swelling
Torsion of testis
Torsion of appendage of testis
Epididymitis
Orchitis
Trauma—hematocele, hematoma, epididymitis, testicular rupture
Hernia—incarcerated
Tumor[a]—acute hemorrhage
Painless scrotal swelling
Hydrocele
Hernia
Varicocele
Spermatocele
Idiopathic scrotal edema
Henoch–Schönlein purpura[a] (can be painful)
Kawasaki disease[a] (can be painful)
Testis tumor[a]
Antenatal torsion of the testis

[a]Life-threatening causes.

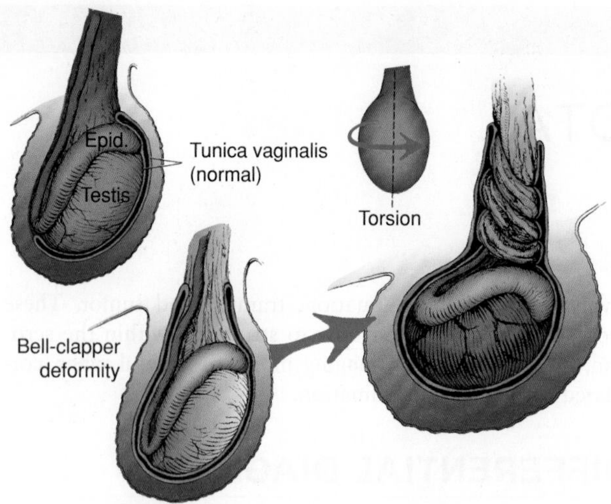

FIGURE 56.2 Torsion testis. Abnormality of testicular fixation—bell-clapper deformity—permits torsion of spermatic vessels with subsequent infarction of the gonad. Epid., epididymis.

freely within the tunica vaginalis in this deformity, may rotate, producing intravaginal torsion of the spermatic cord, venous engorgement of the testis, and subsequent arterial infarction (Fig. 56.3).

The sudden onset of severe scrotal pain and tenderness, often with radiation to the abdomen, and associated nausea and vomiting is typical. They may be associated with sports activity or mild testicular trauma that is perceived by the patient as the cause of pain. Prior episodes of similar pain that resolved may suggest intermittent torsion and spontaneous detorsion.

With torsion, the testis is acutely swollen, diffusely tender, and usually lies higher ("horizontal lie") in the scrotum than the contralateral testis. There may be overlying erythema of the scrotal skin. The cremasteric reflex (retraction of the testis with stroking of the inner thigh) is usually absent with testicular torsion, but may be present in early or incomplete torsion. The cremasteric reflex may be absent in some boys without torsion, usually less than 6 months of age. Since pain may be referred to the abdomen, genitalia should be examined carefully in every child who complains of abdominal pain. Urinalysis is usually negative.

The diagnosis of testicular torsion is made clinically when unilateral, acute scrotal pain presents with testicular changes, absent cremasteric reflex, and associated nausea or vomiting. Immediate surgical consultation for exploration and repair, without delay for imaging, is optimal. A clinical scoring system that takes into account the presence of nausea or vomiting (1 point), testicular swelling (2 points), hard testis on palpation (2 points), high riding testis (1 point), and absent cremasteric reflex (1 point) has been derived and validated. A score of ≥5 indicated testicular torsion with a sensitivity of 76%, specificity of 100%, and a positive predictive value of 100% (prevalence 15%). A score ≤2 excluded testicular torsion with a sensitivity of 100%, specificity of 87%, and negative predictive value of 100%.

Color Doppler ultrasound evaluates the size, shape, echogenicity, and perfusion of the testes and associated structures, and confirms the absence of torsion. In testicular torsion there is decreased or absent arterial blood flow within the affected testicle (Fig. 56.4). With high sensitivity (88.9%) and specificity (98.8%) and a low false-negative rate of 1%, ultrasound is the first-line imaging modality. False-positive scans occur when testicular flow appears decreased due to a large hydrocele, abscess, hematoma, or hernia. False-negative ultrasounds occur from spontaneous detorsion, partial or intermittent torsion, or late torsion when severe, overlying scrotal edema with increased vascularity obscures the underlying ischemic testis. Limitations of Doppler sonography exist in small, lower flow

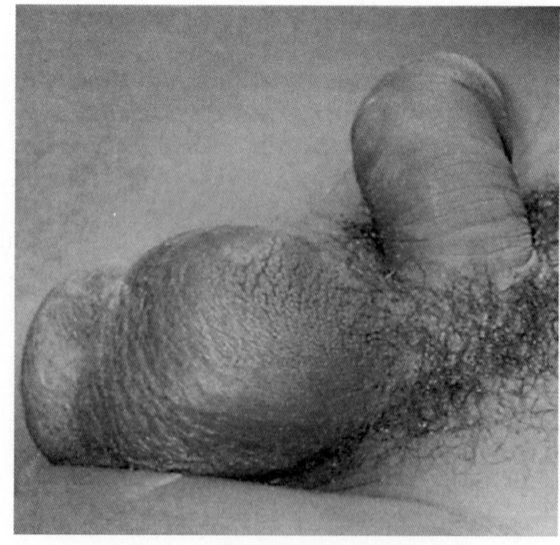

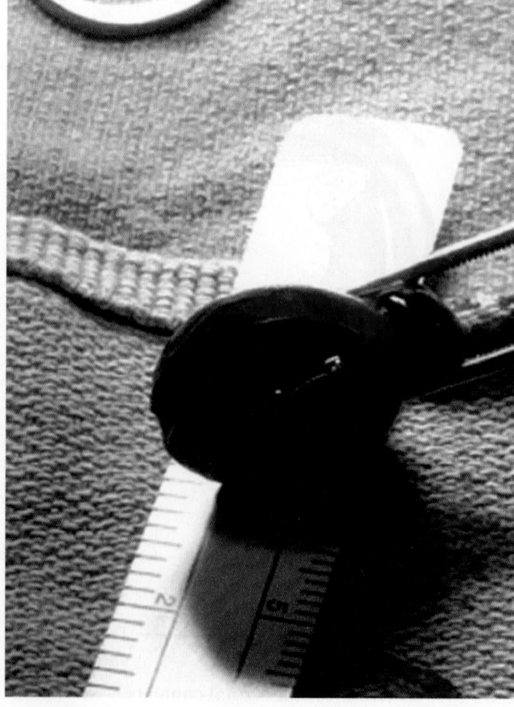

FIGURE 56.3 Torsion of testis. **A:** Swollen, diffusely tender testis high in the scrotum (from twisting of cord structures). **B:** Surgically exposed testis showing torsion of cord structures. Testis was infarcted and was removed.

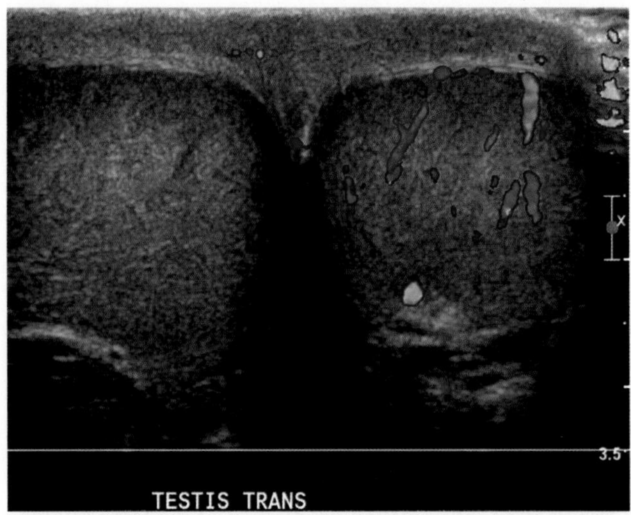

FIGURE 56.4 Torsion of testis. Ultrasound reveals enlarged right testicle and Doppler flow demonstrates no flow to necrotic testis.

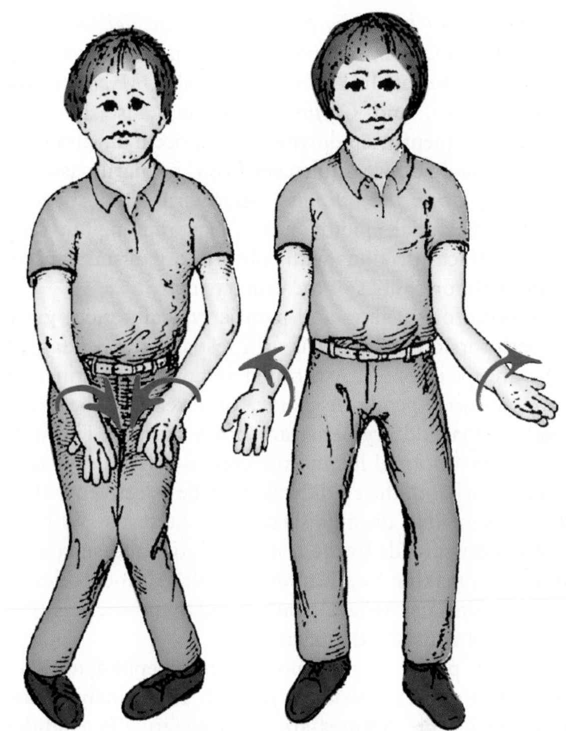

FIGURE 56.5 Torsion of testis. Because torsion typically occurs in a medial direction, manual detorsion should be attempted initially by rotating the testis outward toward the thigh.

prepubertal testes and due to operator-dependent nature of this test. Previously used nuclear perfusion scans are limited by associated time delay and radiation exposure. Again, imaging should not delay surgical consultation or treatment.

The treatment of testicular torsion is surgical exploration, detorsion, and fixation (orchiopexy) of the torsed and contralateral testis. A nonviable testis requires orchiectomy and fixation of the contralateral testis. If a testis has been twisted sufficiently to fully obstruct its blood supply for more than 6 to 12 hours, surgical detorsion is unlikely to salvage the gonad. Salvage rates are 90% to 100% within 6 hours of symptom onset, 50% beyond 12 hours, and 10% when beyond 24 hours. However, it is impossible to determine clinically whether the torsion has been partial or total, so regardless of the estimated duration of torsion immediate surgical intervention is required.

If a child is seen within a few hours of the onset of his torsion, before severe scrotal swelling has ensued, manual detorsion of the spermatic cord to restore blood supply to the testis can be considered. Ideally, this is undertaken by a physician experienced with the technique when surgery is not an immediate option. Sedation and analgesia should be administered. If available, a Doppler stethoscope reveals decreased arterial flow to the affected testis. Since torsion typically (in two-thirds of cases) occurs in a medial direction, detorsion should initially be carried out by rotating the testis outward toward the thigh (and may require more than one rotation (Fig. 56.5). Relief of pain and a lower position of the testis in the scrotum suggest a successful outcome. Doppler stethoscope or color Doppler ultrasound should be used to confirm the return of normal arterial pulsations to the testis. Orchiopexy of both the affected testis and the contralateral one, which is malfixed in more than 50% of cases, is still recommended.

Torsion of Testicular Appendage

Several vestigial embryologic remnants are attached to the testis or epididymis that may twist around their base, producing venous engorgement, and subsequent infarction. Appendage torsion is most common in boys of ages 7 to 12 years but can occur at any age. Mild to severe scrotal pain is the usual presenting feature. There can be associated nausea or vomiting, although less commonly than in testicular torsion (see Chapter 127 Genitourinary Emergencies).

If the child is seen early after the onset of pain, scrotal tenderness and swelling may be localized to the area of the twisted appendage, typically on the superior lateral aspect of the testis. It may be possible to have the patient point to the specific point of pain. If the site indicated is at the upper pole of the testis, a palpable, localized tender mass with the remainder of the testis being nontender, makes torsion of a testicular appendage likely. Although the classic "blue dot" sign of an infarcted appendage may be visualized through the scrotal skin, it often cannot be seen due to overlying edema. Later in the clinical course, increased scrotal tenderness and edema make differentiation from torsion of the testis difficult. The cremasteric reflex should be intact. Color Doppler ultrasound reveals normal or increased blood flow to the testis, and may demonstrate a low echogenicity structure with a central hypoechogenic area. Diagnostically, a surgical exploration may be required to be certain that torsion of the testis is not present.

The treatment of a torsed testicular or epididymal appendage is supportive with rest, support of the scrotum, and analgesic/anti-inflammatory medications. The pain usually resolves in 7 to 10 days. Rarely, removal of the torsed appendage occurs when there is severe or prolonged pain. Contralateral scrotal exploration is not indicated.

Epididymitis/Orchitis

Epididymitis is an infection or inflammation of the epididymis which occurs more frequently in sexually active adolescents and adults. In sexually active adolescents, it is most commonly associated with *Chlamydia trachomatis,* but *Neisseria gonorrhea, Escherichia coli, Mycobacterium,* and viruses are other important etiologies. In HIV-infected males, *Mycobacterium,* cytomegalovirus, and *Cryptococcus* must also be considered. Less frequently, epididymitis does occur in prepubertal and nonsexually active adolescent boys, primarily associated with *Mycoplasma pneumoniae,* enterovirus, and adenovirus infections. Bacterial epididymitis is uncommon, but related to urinary tract infections with coliform organisms caused by structural abnormalities of the urinary tract.

The onset of swelling and pain is typically more gradual than with torsion of the testis or a testicular appendage, but can be abrupt in onset. Associated symptoms of urinary frequency, dysuria, penile discharge, or fever may be present. Scrotal edema and erythema are often present. The testicle should have a normal lie and the cremasteric reflexes should be intact. Early on, the epididymis may be selectively enlarged and tender, readily distinguished from the testis. With time, inflammation spreads to the testis (orchitis) and surrounding scrotal wall, making localization difficult. Although elevation of the scrotum may relieve pain in epididymo-orchitis (Prehn sign) it is not considered a reliable.

Although pyuria is seen more often in epididymitis than in torsion, it is not consistently present. The urinalysis can be normal, and urine cultures are often negative in epididymitis, but are still recommended. The Centers for Disease Control and Prevention recommends a Gram stain and culture of urethral discharge or intraurethral swab, or nucleic acid amplification tests for *N. gonorrhea* and *C. trachomatis,* and a urinalysis and culture. Color Doppler sonography typically demonstrates an increase in size and blood flow to the testis and epididymis (Fig. 56.6).

Initial treatment for epididymitis includes analgesics, scrotal support, elevation, and bed rest. Antibiotic use depends on the suspected etiology. In sexually active adolescent males, in whom the most likely cause is chlamydia and gonorrhea, ceftriaxone (250 mg IM in single dose) plus doxycycline (100 mg PO twice a day for 10 days) is recommended. Due to increasing *N. gonorrhea* resistance, quinolones are not recommended for routine treatment. Patients allergic to cephalosporins and/or tetracyclines, or in whom enteric organisms are suspected, can be treated with fluoroquinolones such as ofloxacin or levofloxacin. Of note, doxycycline is not recommended for patients younger than 8 years of age, and fluoroquinolones are

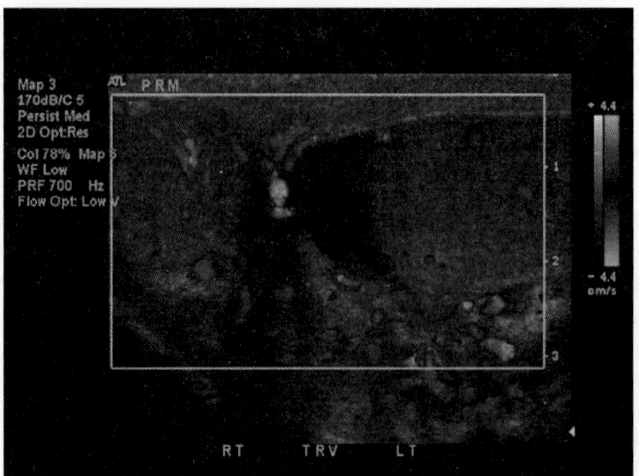

FIGURE 56.6 Epididymitis. Ultrasound image of enlarged epididymis seen on left side of image, testis on right. Color Doppler flow ultrasound reveals increased blood flow to inflamed epididymis.

not approved for use in patients younger than 18 years of age unless complicated urinary tract infection, or no other alternatives exist. In prepubertal boys epididymitis is often viral or idiopathic, but those with pyuria, positive urine cultures, or risk factors for urinary tract infection should be treated with antibiotic coverage for enteric organisms, such as trimethoprim-sulfamethoxazole or cephalexin. The patient should be warned that this process is frustratingly slow to resolve and discomfort and scrotal swelling will gradually subside over a few weeks.

At any age when epididymitis is associated with a urinary tract infection and in all prepubertal boys with bacterial epididymitis, referral for urologic follow-up to rule out a structural problem is recommended.

Orchitis

Orchitis is an inflammation or infection of the testis resulting from the extension of epididymitis, rarely as hematogenous spread of a systemic bacterial infection, or following certain viral infections, including mumps. Other viruses implicated include adenovirus, Epstein–Barr virus, coxsackievirus, parvovirus, and echoviruses. Fortunately, less common since the advent of vaccine against mumps and rare before puberty, orchitis occurs in about 18% of postpubertal boys with mumps parotitis. The onset of mumps orchitis occurs from 4 to 6 days after parotitis manifests. Rarely, it has been reported in the absence of parotitis. In 70% of cases, it is unilateral. It results in testicular atrophy, but not necessarily sterility, in 50% of affected testes. Treatment is supportive with analgesic/anti-inflammatory medications, rest, ice, and support of the scrotum.

Trauma/Hematocele

In children, most trauma to the scrotum results from a direct blow to the perineum or a straddle injury that compresses the testicle against the pubic bone. Penetrating injuries are less common, and the small size and greater mobility of the prepubertal testis make testicular injuries rare in this group (see Chapter 116 Genitourinary Trauma).

Scrotal trauma is a spectrum of injuries that ranges from minimal scrotal swelling to rupture of the testis with a tense, blood-filled scrotum (Fig. 56.7A). Scrotal ultrasound is useful in assessing the integrity of the testicle and the location of fluid within the scrotum (Fig. 56.7B). Urgent surgical evaluation should occur, unless the testis is clearly normal and without significant tenderness. Note that testicular torsion may present with a spurious history of trauma and a ruptured testis has the best salvage rate when surgically repaired.

An obvious ecchymosis of the scrotal wall after trauma suggests a hematocele, which is blood within the tunica vaginalis. Severe testicular injury can be associated with a hematocele, an intratesticular hematoma, or a laceration or rupture of the tunica albuginea which directly encases the testicle. Sonography can localize and identify blood, which is more echogenic than hydrocele fluid. Color Doppler ultrasound can also assess testicular blood flow. Scrotal exploration is indicated if testicular rupture or laceration is present, or in cases of large hematoceles, which heal more readily after surgical drainage. If the tunica albuginea can be determined to be intact, no surgical intervention is necessary.

If a scrotal laceration is present, it is essential that the testis and spermatic cord be evaluated for possible injury. This may

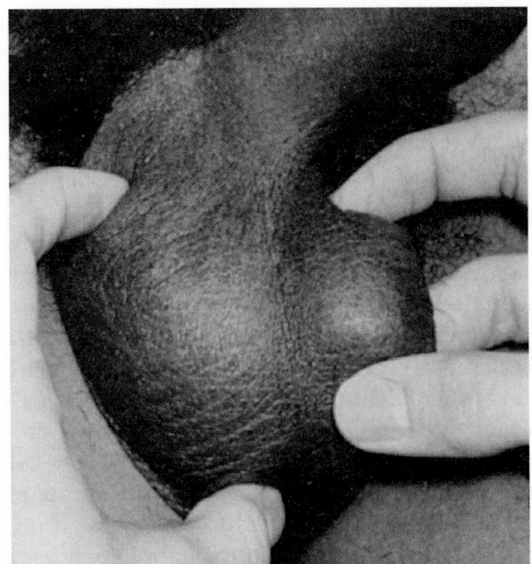

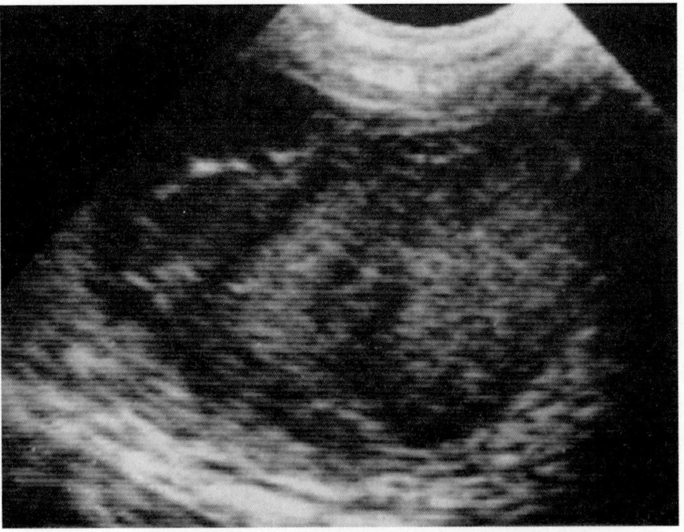

FIGURE 56.7 Rupture of testis. **A:** Testicular swelling and tenderness following kick to scrotum. **B:** Ultrasound examination of testis—central linear sonolucent area reflects site of testicular rupture. Surgical repair resulted in a well-preserved gonad.

require an examination under general anesthesia or an inguinal cord block with more severe injuries. For simple scrotal lacerations, careful hemostasis and closure of the laceration with chromic catgut is sufficient.

Traumatic epididymitis is local inflammation, resulting from blunt trauma to the scrotum, which usually evolves over a few days. Short-lived, acute pain associated with trauma is followed by a pain-free period after which pain returns. On examination, scrotal erythema, edema, and tenderness of the epididymis may be found. In this noninfectious variety of epididymitis, the urinalysis is negative. Sonography is helpful to rule out any more severe injury and will demonstrate hyperemia associated with the inflammation. Treatment is supportive.

Incarcerated Inguinal Hernia

Incarcerated inguinal hernias are herniations of bowel and omentum into the scrotum which present with pain and a scrotal mass. Their diagnosis and treatment are discussed in Chapters 29 Groin Masses and 127 Genitourinary Emergencies.

Henoch–Schönlein Purpura

Occasionally, a child may be seen with a petechial rash on the scrotum as the initial presentation of this systemic vasculitic syndrome, characterized by nonthrombocytopenic purpura, arthralgia, renal disease, abdominal pain, and gastrointestinal bleeding. More typically, the rash begins on the lower extremities or buttocks and later may involve the scrotum. If the associated swelling is not great, the cord structures and testes can be felt to be uninvolved and normal. In other cases with severe swelling, surgical exploration may be necessary to rule out testicular torsion, which rarely has been noted to coexist. When skin lesions are present, the diagnosis of Henoch–Schönlein purpura (HSP) must be suspected. Occasionally, an acutely painful scrotum is the dominant presenting symptom. Ultrasound may help rule out testicular torsion in these instances. For a more detailed discussion of HSP management, see Chapter 108 Renal and Electrolyte Emergencies.

Other Causes of a Painful Scrotum

Referred pain to the scrotum can present as acute scrotal pain without scrotal swelling, tenderness, or mass. The somatic nerves that innervate the scrotum are the genitofemoral, ilioinguinal, and posterior scrotal nerves. A retrocecal appendicitis is an uncommon, but important cause of referred pain. Other considerations may include urolithiasis, retroperitoneal processes like tumor, lumbar, or sacral nerve compression, or pain after hernia repair.

CAUSES OF PAINLESS SCROTAL SWELLING

Hydrocele

An accumulation of fluid within the tunica vaginalis that surrounds the testis—a hydrocele—is common in newborns; but also occurs with torsion of the testis or an appendage, epididymitis, trauma, or tumor. Examination of the underlying testis is required to exclude these conditions. If the testis can be felt to be normal and there is no abnormality of the overlying scrotal skin, it is a simple hydrocele. It represents fluid left in place after the processus vaginalis has closed. When the size of the hydrocele has no history of waxing or waning, it is considered a simple, noncommunicating hydrocele. Usually, the fluid is reabsorbed in the first 12 to 18 months of life.

If the hydrocele has a clear-cut history of changing in size (often with crying or exertion), particularly if it is associated with thickening of the cord structures as they are felt against the pubic tubercle (the silk-glove sign), then the processus vaginalis is patent and the diagnosis is a communicating hydrocele (Fig. 56.8). The processus vaginalis did not close spontaneously and may enlarge to permit the development of hernia. Surgical exploration and high ligation of the processus vaginalis with decompression of the hydrocele is appropriate treatment. Since a scrotal hernia may be confused with a hydrocele, aspiration should never be carried out in children, except by an experienced urologist.

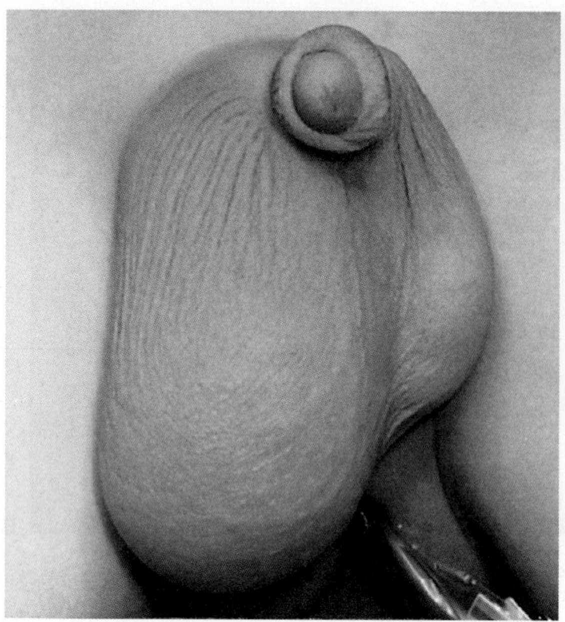

FIGURE 56.8 Hydrocele. Waxing and waning of size indicates a communicating hydrocele with a patent processus vaginalis, requiring surgical correction.

Occasionally, a hydrocele of the cord presents as a scrotal swelling just above the testis. Differentiation from an incarcerated hernia may be difficult and an ultrasound may be helpful. Surgical treatment like that for a hydrocele of the testis is appropriate.

Hernia

Although most inguinal hernias present in children with a mass in the groin, occasionally the hernia may extend and present as scrotal swelling. An incarcerated hernia may produce pain in some patients. The diagnosis and treatment of inguinal hernias are discussed in Chapter 124 Abdominal Emergencies.

Varicocele

A usually painless scrotal swelling, called a *varicocele,* is a collection of abnormally enlarged spermatic cord veins most commonly found on routine examination of asymptomatic boys ages 10 to 15 years. Most varicoceles occur on the left, representing spermatic vein incompetence caused by the left spermatic vein draining into the renal vein at a sharp angle, whereas the right spermatic vein drains into the inferior vena cava.

On occasion, a varicocele can present with mild pain or discomfort. The hemiscrotum appears full but overlying skin is normal. The testis and epididymis should be palpated to be normal. A mass of varicose veins described as "a bag of worms" can be appreciated above the testicle, which is more prominent when examined while standing. Doppler ultrasound demonstrates both normal flow to the testis and the collection of tortuous veins. Most varicoceles are asymptomatic and benign and just observed. Patients determined to have a varicocele, especially when they present with discomfort, should be referred for urologic follow-up. Some large varicoceles may require internal spermatic vein ligation or testicular vein embolization and effect testicular size and fertility. Inferior vena cava obstruction should be considered when the patient is prepubertal or if the varicocele is acute in onset, right sided, or remains unchanged in the supine position.

Spermatocele

Located above and posterior to the testicle in postpubertal boys, spermatoceles are sperm-containing cysts of the rete testes, ductuli efferentes, or epididymis. Multiple or bilateral spermatoceles may occur. On examination a small, nontender mass that transilluminates may be appreciated distinct from and posterior to the testicle. These masses must be differentiated from a hydrocele or tumor. Sonography may confirm the location and help distinguish a spermatocele from tumor. Referral to a urologist is indicated for the excision of large uncomfortable spermatoceles or for aspiration to differentiate a hydrocele from a spermatocele. Otherwise, no specific treatment is needed (see Chapter 127 Genitourinary Emergencies).

Idiopathic Scrotal Edema

Idiopathic scrotal edema is a rare entity that represents only 2% to 5% of acute scrotal swellings in otherwise normal children. Typically, a prepubertal child presents with the rapid onset of painless edema of the scrotal wall that may be bilateral and may extend up onto the abdomen. The skin of the scrotum may be erythematous. The child is usually afebrile, and urinalysis is negative. Through the edematous scrotum, the testes can be felt to be normal in size and nontender. This edema of the scrotal wall is of unknown origin, although it is believed to represent a form of angioneurotic edema. Other etiologies include insect bites, allergic reactions, cellulitis, and contact dermatitis. No specific therapy for idiopathic scrotal edema has been demonstrated to be effective. Bed rest and scrotal elevation may help. Children spontaneously begin to improve within 48 hours, regardless of treatment. Cellulitis, allergic reactions, and contact dermatitis should be appropriately treated. Occasionally, scrotal edema is seen secondary to diseases that cause generalized edema and/or ascites, such as nephrosis and cirrhosis.

Kawasaki Disease

Another vasculitis that can produce scrotal swelling and mild pain is Kawasaki disease, which has characteristic features, including fever, adenopathy, rash, conjunctivitis, and irritability. Although discussed in detail elsewhere (see Chapter 109 Rheumatologic Emergencies), it is important to note the association of scrotal swelling with this systemic disease to avoid unnecessary surgical explorations or delay in diagnosis of the underlying vasculitis.

Testis Tumor

Testicular or paratesticular tumors are rare in young children. However, in young males of ages 15 to 35 years, it is the most common solid tumor and represents 20% of cancers diagnosed in males. Testicular cancer usually presents as painless, unilateral, and firm to hard scrotal swellings discovered by the patient or physician on physical examination. Some patients report an achy feeling, and in rapid-growing tumors associated with hemorrhage or infarction, acute scrotal pain may be reported. Leukemic infiltration of the testis may present bilaterally. The mass does not transilluminate, but an associated reactive hydrocele may do so. In children younger than 2 years of age, the tumor usually is a yolk sac carcinoma, or teratoma, and after puberty, germinal cell tumors are seen. Evaluation involves an initial testicular ultrasound examination usually followed by surgical exploration and a possible radical inguinal orchiectomy.

Antenatal Torsion Testis (Newborn)

A newborn boy may present with a painless, smooth, testicular enlargement that is usually dark in color with minimal or no edema of the scrotum. This presentation occurs in 70% of newborn cases of torsion, represents prenatal, extravaginal torsion, whereby the entire testis and the tunica vaginalis twist together around the spermatic cord. The remaining cases of neonatal torsion occur postnatally during the first month of life, before fixation occurs. Salvage of the testis after neonatal torsion is rare and therefore management remains controversial. A recent survey of pediatric urologists indicate that most advocate for exploration of neonatal torsion through a scrotal incision with orchiopexy of the contralateral testicle, as most view neonatal torsion as a surgical emergency.

EVALUATION AND DECISION

Although this chapter is entitled scrotal pain, the most efficient approach to the differential diagnosis is through consideration of the important entities causing painful versus painless scrotal swelling. This approach is outlined in Figure 56.9. The specific causes of painful and painless scrotal swelling are discussed previously in this chapter (Table 56.1). As noted, some etiologies may cause either painful or painless scrotal swelling. No one aspect of the history or physical examination may be diagnostic, but collectively the clinical findings often suggest a diagnosis. Color Doppler ultrasonography is a helpful adjunct when the clinician is fully aware of the capabilities and limitations, and it is readily available so as not to delay necessary surgical intervention.

Initial Approach

As a first step in the evaluation of the child with a complaint of scrotal swelling or pain, the physician should determine whether the child is suffering from a generalized edematous state, such as the nephrotic syndrome. When the problem is localized to the scrotum, patients can be divided into those who have a painless swelling and those who are experiencing pain.

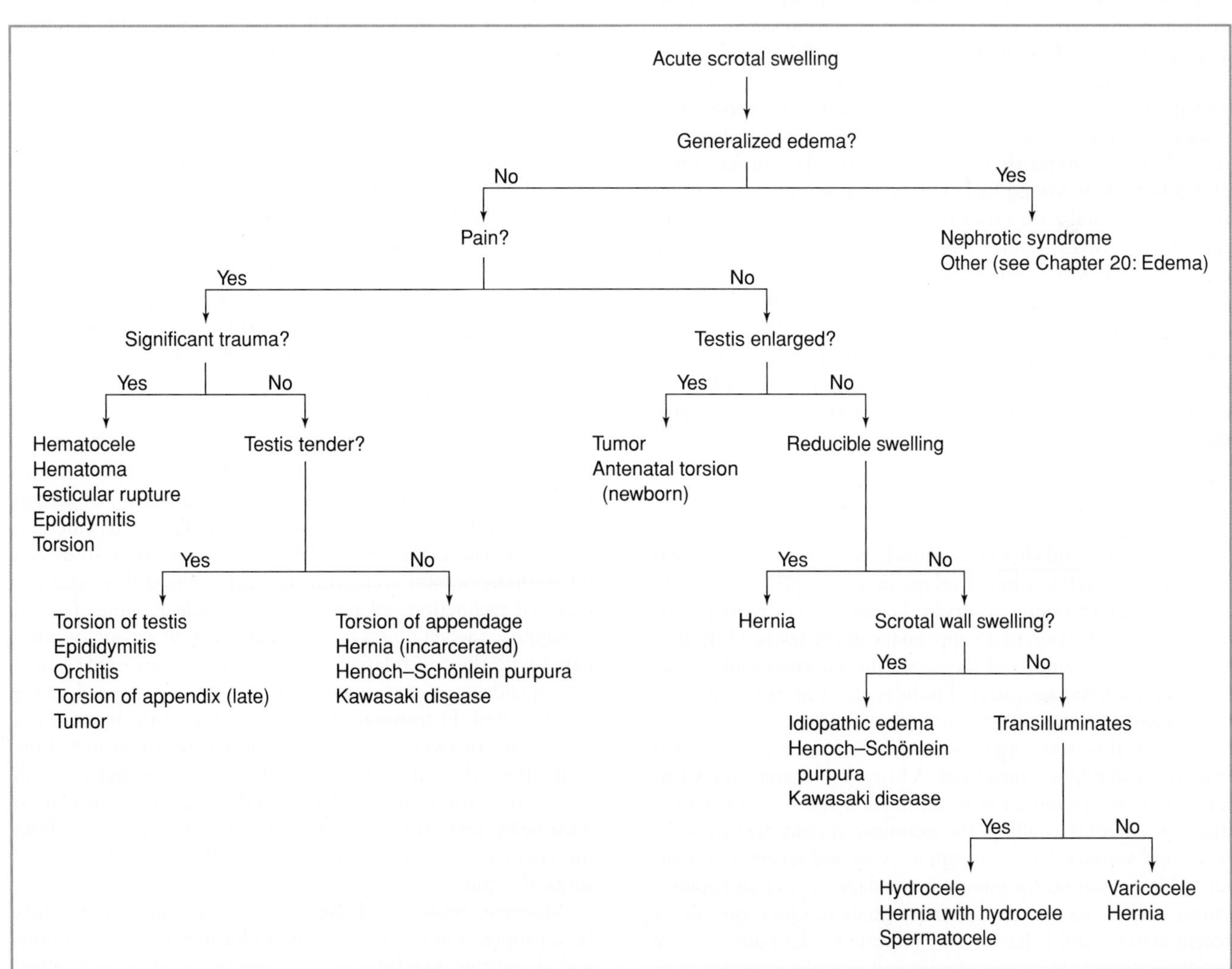

FIGURE 56.9 Diagnostic approach to acute scrotal swelling.

TABLE 56.2

COMMON CAUSES OF ACUTE SCROTAL SWELLING

Infancy
Hydrocele
Hernia
Childhood
Hernia
Torsion of the appendix testes
Torsion of the testes
Trauma
Adolescence
Epididymitis
Torsion of the appendix testes
Torsion of the testes
Trauma

In the immediate neonatal period, prenatal torsion may cause painless scrotal enlargement. In infancy, the most common causes of painless scrotal swelling (Table 56.2) are hernias and hydroceles; a hernia is often reducible. Beyond infancy, the physician must consider hernia, tumor, spermatocele, and varicocele when evaluating painless scrotal swelling determined to be within the scrotum. Kawasaki disease, HSP, and idiopathic scrotal edema involve the scrotal sac and cause swelling that is either painless or mildly painful.

Painful swelling may follow a well-documented injury, in which case the likely diagnoses are hematocele, hematoma, testicular rupture, and traumatic epididymitis. The physician should bear in mind that boys with testicular torsion often give a history of having had an incidental minor injury. Nontraumatic scrotal pain raises the suspicion of a testicular torsion, if the testis is tender. Unless the diagnosis of a systemic disorder (HSP, Kawasaki disease) is obvious, another structure such as an appendage is reliably determined to be the source of pain within the scrotum, the patient is an adolescent with the classic signs of epididymitis, or an incarcerated hernia is reduced, imaging via Doppler ultrasound is usually indicated. All patients in whom torsion is suspected require a surgical consultation.

History

The age of the child should be considered in evaluating scrotal pain and/or swelling, but overlaps in age at presentation do exist. Testicular torsion occurs in the newborn or early pubertal age range. Torsion of an appendage of the testis, HSP, idiopathic scrotal edema, and Kawasaki disease commonly occur in the prepubertal age group. Epididymitis is more common in adolescents but may occur in prepubertal boys.

Historical features regarding swelling, pain, and associated symptoms should be considered. A history of change in testicular or scrotal size should be determined. If there is pain associated with scrotal swelling, the examiner should determine its onset and severity. Pain is abrupt in onset and severe in testicular torsion, whereas the pain of appendage torsion and epididymitis may be less severe and more gradual. Questions about recent activity and behavior may indicate milder pain or more insidious course. The onset of pain and even the exact location of pain in children can be difficult to pinpoint because they may not initially localize sensation to the scrotum, but rather complain of lower abdominal pain. An embarrassed adolescent may not report scrotal pain early. Inquire about prior episodes of pain which may indicate intermittent torsion. Nausea and vomiting often accompany testicular torsion, and fever and symptoms of urinary tract infection may suggest epididymitis or other inflammatory diseases (vasculitides).

A history of trauma should always be addressed, recognizing the difference between significant trauma associated with severe acute pain and minor trauma to which the pain of torsion may mistakenly be attributed. Sexual activity history should be sought. A history of prior genitourinary surgeries may indicate a predisposition to urinary tract infections and epididymitis related to genitourinary abnormalities or prior instrumentation. Prior surgery for hernias, hydroceles, and undescended testis, unless associated with other genitourinary or anorectal abnormalities, does not suggest a predisposition to infection. In addition, torsion can occur despite prior scrotal surgeries believed to secure the testis.

Physical Examination

Initial observation of the patient's gait, resting position, and facial expression are helpful. Writhing or an especially quiet supine posture may indicate the degree of pain. Associated skin changes, presence and location of swelling, and the natural position (lie) of the testicle in the scrotum while standing should then be appreciated. Next note presence/absence of cremasteric reflexes and palpate the lower abdomen, inguinal canal, cord, and scrotal contents. Ask the patient to localize pain with one finger if possible. The unaffected hemiscrotum should be palpated first. Knowledge of the location and specific attempt at palpation of the appendix testis and epididymis is beneficial before palpation of the testis itself (Fig. 56.2). Use of a cotton-tipped swab to discretely localize tenderness in these areas may be helpful, and also less threatening to an uncomfortable patient. Appreciation of swelling, tenderness, and consistency should be noted for all intrascrotal structures. Transillumination may be helpful in some cases (Fig. 56.9).

Imaging Modalities

Color Doppler imaging with pulsed Doppler is the standard imaging modality as it provides both visualization of scrotal anatomy and intratesticular arterial blood flow determination and comparison. Widely available, this noninvasive study can differentiate scrotal wall from testicular blood flow and has replaced technetium-99 pertechnetate nuclear scans. Torsion is diagnosed when blood flow is diminished or absent, as compared with the contralateral testis. In cases of a torsed testicular appendage or epididymitis, blood flow is increased to the affected area. In trauma, ultrasound can localize blood, fluid collections, or swelling. The operator-dependent nature of the study, the technical challenges in the very young patient with small, low-flow testes, and the need for clinical correlation must be heeded. Any doubt in interpretation or concern about the adequacy of the signal should result in consideration of surgical exploration.

Magnetic resonance imaging of the scrotum has recently been proposed in cases of trauma to localize blood collections and determine the integrity of underlying structures when ultrasound is equivocal.

Suggested Readings and Key References

Baldisserotto M. Scrotal emergencies. *Pediatr Radiol* 2009;39:516–521.

Baker LA, Sigman D, Mathews RI, et al. An analysis of clinical outcomes using color Doppler testicular ultrasound for testicular torsion. *Pediatrics* 2000;105:604–607.

Barbosa JA, Tiseo BC, Barayan GA, et al. Development and initial validation of a scoring system to diagnose testicular torsion in children. *J Urol* 2013;189:1859–1864.

Broderick KM, Martin BG, Herndon CD, et al. The current state of surgical practice for neonatal torsion: a survey of pediatric urologists. *J Pediatr Urol* 2013;9(5):542–545.

Buckley JC, McAninch JW. Diagnosis and management of testicular ruptures. *Urol Clin North Am* 2006;33:111–116.

Garel L, Dubois J, Azzie G, et al. Preoperative manual detorsion of the spermatic cord with Doppler ultrasound monitoring in patients with intra-vaginal acute testicular torsion. *Pediatr Radiol* 2000;30:41–44.

Haecker FM, Hauri-Hohl A, von Schweinitz D. Acute epididymitis in children: a 4-year retrospective study. *Eur J Pediatr Surg* 2005;15: 180–186.

Karmazyn B, Steinberg R, Korneich L, et al. Clinical and sonographic criteria of acute scrotum in children: a retrospective study of 172 boys. *Pediatr Radiol* 2005;35:302–310.

Kim SH, Park S, Choi SH, et al. The efficacy of magnetic resonance for the diagnosis of testicular rupture: a prospective preliminary study. *J Trauma* 2009;66:239–242.

Leslie JA, Cain MP. Pediatric urologic emergencies and urgencies. *Pediatr Clin North Am* 2006;53:513–527.

Preston MA, Carnat T, Flood T, et al. Conservative management of adolescent varicoceles: a retrospective review. *Urology* 2008;72:77–80.

Santillanes G, Gausche-Hill M, Lewis RJ. Are antibiotics necessary for pediatric epididymitis? *Pediatr Emerg Care* 2011;27:174–178.

Schlamamon J, Ainoedhofer H, Schleef J, et al. Management of acute scrotum in children—the impact of Doppler ultrasound. *J Pediatr Surg* 2006;41:1377–1380.

Srinivasan A, Cinman N, Feber KM, et al. History and physical examination findings predictive of testicular torsion: an attempt to promote clinical diagnosis by housestaff. *J Pediatr Urol* 2011;7:470–474.

Workowski KA, Berman S; Center for Disease Control and Prevention. Sexually transmitted disease treatment guidelines, 2010. *MMWR Recomm Rep* 2010;59(RR-12):67–69.

CHAPTER 57 ■ PALLOR

SONAL N. SHAH, MD, MPH

Pallor, or the absence of skin coloration, is a relatively common problem in childhood. Throughout the world, the presence of pallor is often used as a screening tool to identify illness. The development of pallor can be acute and associated with a life-threatening illness, or it can be chronic and subtle, occasionally first noted by someone who sees the child infrequently. The onset of pallor can provoke anxiety for parents who are familiar with descriptions of the presentation of leukemia in childhood. In some instances, only reassurance may be needed, as in the case of a light complexioned or fair-skinned, nonanemic child. Even if there is a hematologic cause for the pallor, it is often a temporary condition readily amenable to therapy. However, pallor can portend a severe disease, and especially when acute in onset, can herald a true pediatric emergency for which rapid diagnosis and treatment are essential.

The degree of pallor depends on the concentration of hemoglobin in the blood and the distribution of blood in the blood vessels of the skin. Any condition that decreases the concentration of hemoglobin or alters the distribution of blood away from the body's surface may present as pallor. Clinically, pallor caused by anemia can usually be appreciated when the hemoglobin concentration is below 8 to 9 g per dL, although the complexion of the child and the rapidity of onset may influence this value.

DIFFERENTIAL DIAGNOSIS

The differential diagnosis for nonhematologic causes of pallor is outlined briefly in Table 57.1 and hematologic causes in Table 57.2. The concentration of hemoglobin in the blood can be lowered by three basic mechanisms: decreased erythrocyte or hemoglobin production, increased erythrocyte destruction, and blood loss. The most common causes of pallor and anemia seen in the emergency department (ED) are iron deficiency and blood loss (Table 57.3), but several less common diseases remain important considerations.

Decreased Production of Hemoglobin and Red Cells

Nutritional Anemias

Nutritional iron deficiency is the most common cause of decreased hemoglobin production in children. A peak in the prevalence of iron-deficiency anemia occurs between 12 and 24 months of age, when dietary iron content is often insufficient to meet the demands of a rapidly increasing red cell mass. Premature infants are more susceptible to developing iron-deficiency anemia because iron stores at birth are less than those found in term infants, whereas the growth (and therefore, expansion of the red cell mass) of the premature infant is often faster than that of term infants. The early exhaustion of iron stores in premature babies may result in pallor by 6 months of age, whereas in normal infants, signs of iron-deficiency anemia are uncommon before 10 to 12 months of age.

A thorough history and physical examination will provide important clues in the diagnosis of iron-deficiency anemia. History suggestive of a lack of iron in the diet may be readily apparent or may be recognized only after careful questioning, particularly regarding the daily consumption of cow's milk. The infant with severe iron deficiency is often irritable and very pale. A compensatory increase in cardiac output is seen, which, when coupled with conditions that increase systemic demands on the heart (such as fever), may provoke the development of congestive heart failure (see Chapter 94 Cardiac Emergencies).

Serum hemoglobin concentration may be as low as 2 g per dL in severe iron-deficiency anemia. Red blood cells are markedly microcytic and hypochromic, and wide variation in red cell size and shape is usually present. Although the percentage of reticulocytes may be elevated moderately, the absolute reticulocyte count is low.

The diagnosis of iron deficiency as the cause for an anemia can often be made on the basis of the history alone, and treatment is usually instituted before confirmatory laboratory studies are available. Free erythrocyte protoporphyrin, a precursor to mature hemoglobin, is increased in iron-deficiency anemia and readily assayed. It can be a useful measure when evaluating the severely anemic child in the ED. Measurements of serum iron and ferritin levels have too long of a turnaround time to be of much value in the emergency management of anemia, but are valuable confirmatory tests. The concentration of hemoglobin in the reticulocyte (CHr) is one of the indices reported with reticulocyte counts, and serves as a sensitive marker of response to iron therapy at outpatient follow-up.

Other nutritional anemias, such as vitamin B_{12} or folic acid deficiency, are uncommon in children in the United States. When present, these anemias are likely associated with particular conditions such as a grossly altered diet, extended hyperalimentation, intestinal resection, or chronic diarrhea. Affected infants usually present with failure to thrive and developmental delay. Older patients more commonly exhibit weight loss, constipation, and weakness. The diagnosis of vitamin B_{12} or folic acid deficiency may be suggested by the finding of anemia with megaloblastic features. Megaloblastic anemia is characterized by normochromic, macrocytic red blood cells, hypersegmented neutrophils, and an elevated serum level of lactic dehydrogenase. The diagnosis is confirmed by the finding of low serum levels of folic acid or vitamin B_{12} and the response to folic acid or vitamin B_{12} replacement therapy.

TABLE 57.1

PALLOR WITHOUT ANEMIA

Physiologic ("fair-skinned")
Shock: septic, hypovolemic, neurogenic, cardiogenic, anaphylactoid
Hypoglycemia and other metabolic derangements
Respiratory distress
Skin edema
Pheochromocytoma

Hypoplastic and Aplastic Anemia

Pallor is usually the first sign of aplastic or hypoplastic anemia. These anemias may be congenital or acquired. Congenital aplastic anemias are most commonly part of larger syndromes, with the two major syndromes recognized being Diamond–Blackfan and Fanconi anemia.

Diamond–Blackfan syndrome is a congenital hypoplastic anemia commonly detected in the first few months of life. The anemia can be severe at the time of diagnosis. The red cells are normocytic or macrocytic. The reticulocyte count is characteristically low. Associated congenital anomalies include microcephaly, cleft palate, web neck, and thumb irregularities. The diagnosis is made by examination of a bone marrow aspirate evidencing markedly reduced or absent erythrocyte precursors with normal marrow cellularity.

TABLE 57.3

RELATIVELY COMMON CAUSES OF PALLOR OR ANEMIA

Decreased erythrocyte or hemoglobin production
Iron deficiency
Transient erythroblastopenia of childhood
Increased erythrocyte destruction
Sickle cell syndromes
Autoimmune hemolytic anemia
G6PD deficiency
Blood loss

G6PD, glucose-6-phosphate dehydrogenase.

Fanconi anemia is an autosomal recessive condition that results in progressive bone marrow failure generally after 3 or 4 years of age. Fanconi anemia is characterized by a normochromic or macrocytic anemia as well as reductions in both white cell and platelet counts, in contradistinction to Diamond–Blackfan syndrome. Other phenotypic abnormalities associated with Fanconi anemia include hyperpigmentation or hypopigmentation, microcephaly, strabismus, small stature, mental retardation, and anomalies of the thumbs and radii. The diagnosis may be made in the proper clinical context by the presence of increased chromosomal breakage in lymphocytes cultured in the presence of DNA cross-linking agents.

TABLE 57.2

PALLOR WITH ANEMIA

I. Decreased erythrocyte or hemoglobin production
  A. Nutritional deficiencies
    1. Iron deficiency
    2. Folic acid and vitamin B_{12} deficiency or associated metabolic abnormalities
  B. Aplastic or hypoplastic anemias
    1. Diamond–Blackfan anemia
    2. Fanconi anemia
    3. Aplastic anemia[a]
    4. Transient erythroblastopenia of childhood
    5. Malignancy: leukemia, lymphoma, neuroblastoma[a]
  C. Abnormal heme and hemoglobin synthesis
    1. Anemia of chronic disease
    2. Lead poisoning[a]
    3. Sideroblastic anemias
    4. Thalassemias

II. Increased erythrocyte destruction
  A. Erythrocyte membrane defects: hereditary spherocytosis, elliptocytosis, stomatocytosis, pyknocytosis, paroxysmal nocturnal hemoglobinuria
  B. Erythrocyte enzyme defects
    1. Defects of hexose monophosphate shunt: G6PD deficiency most common
    2. Defects of Embden–Meyerhof pathway: pyruvate kinase deficiency most common
  C. Hemoglobinopathies
    1. Sickle cell syndromes[a]
    2. Unstable hemoglobins
  D. Immune hemolytic anemia
    1. Autoimmune hemolytic anemia[a]
    2. Isoimmune hemolytic anemia[a]
    3. Infection
      a. Viral: mononucleosis, influenzas, coxsackievirus, measles, varicella, cytomegalovirus
      b. Bacterial: *Escherichia coli, Pneumococcus, Streptococcus*, typhoid fever, *Mycoplasma*
    4. Drugs: antibiotics
    5. Inflammatory and collagen vascular disease
    6. Malignancy[a]
  E. Microangiopathic anemia
    1. Disseminated intravascular coagulation[a]
    2. Hemolytic uremic syndrome[a]
    3. Cavernous hemangioma

III. Blood Loss
  A. Severe trauma[a]
  B. Anatomic lesions
    1. Meckel diverticulum
    2. Peptic ulcer
    3. Idiopathic pulmonary hemosiderosis[a]

[a]Conditions that are known to present with acute, life-threatening anemia are or are associated with other serious abnormalities.
G6PD, glucose-6-phosphate dehydrogenase.

Acquired aplastic anemia can also present with severe pallor in children. The anemia is usually associated with granulocytopenia and thrombocytopenia. Acquired aplastic anemia is often idiopathic but has been associated with exposure to certain drugs and chemicals (e.g., chloramphenicol, felbamate, lindane, gold, benzene, and pesticides), radiation, and viral infections (especially hepatitis). The diagnosis is made by an examination of the bone marrow.

Transient erythroblastopenia of childhood (TEC) is a condition that is often associated with a recent viral illness and is characterized by moderate to severe anemia caused by diminished red cell production. The age at presentation can vary from infancy to 10 years, with a median of 18 to 26 months. The mean corpuscular volume (MCV) is usually normal at the time of diagnosis. The reticulocyte count is decreased, and a Coombs test is negative. The anemia of TEC may be associated with a normal or moderately decreased white cell count and a normal platelet count. Bone marrow examination shows an initial reduction or absence of erythrocytic precursors followed by erythroid hyperplasia during recovery. Transient erythroblastopenia that occurs in the first 6 months of life may be difficult to distinguish from Diamond–Blackfan anemia. Spontaneous recovery ultimately confirms the diagnosis of TEC.

Hypoplastic anemia can be the presenting symptom of childhood malignancies. The pallor can be severe, and although all three cell lines of the bone marrow are usually affected, anemia may be the only notable hematologic abnormality. The diagnosis can be suspected from the presence of other symptoms or findings, such as lymphadenopathy, bruising, limb pain, gum bleeding, or an abdominal mass.

Red cell aplasia may develop in patients with underlying hemolytic anemias such as hereditary spherocytosis or sickle cell disease (SCD), usually in association with parvovirus B19 infection. Decreased red cell production in the face of ongoing hemolysis causes an exacerbation of the anemia. The elevated reticulocyte count usually seen in hereditary hemolytic anemias falls to inappropriately low levels, often less than 1%. Although platelets and white cells are generally unaffected, they may be mildly decreased. Red cell transfusions are appropriate if the anemia is associated with cardiovascular compromise or if continuing reticulocytopenia indicates that the anemia is likely to become severe before the usual spontaneous recovery after 3 to 7 days. Patients with decreased erythrocyte production from a condition such as iron-deficiency anemia or human immunodeficiency virus (HIV) infection may also experience a transient aplastic crisis from parvovirus B19 infection. Hematologically normal children with underlying (though sometimes unrecognized) immunologic disorders may also develop parvovirus-induced anemia as a result of prolonged viremia.

Disorders of Heme and Globin Production

Pallor may be the presenting sign of nonnutritional disorders of hemoglobin synthesis, including the sideroblastic anemias and thalassemia syndromes. These disorders are characterized by a microcytic, hypochromic anemia with elevated reticulocyte counts.

Sideroblastic anemia results from a defect in the synthesis of heme in the red blood cell precursor; it may be inherited (sex linked) or acquired (often related to medication or toxin exposures). Iron use within the developing red cell is abnormal, accounting for the presence of diagnostic-ringed sideroblasts in the bone marrow. The serum iron and ferritin levels are often markedly elevated.

In the thalassemias, production of the globin portion of the hemoglobin molecule is impaired because of genetic defects in heme chain synthesis. Cooley anemia (β-thalassemia major) presents with severe pallor usually between 6 and 12 months of age, as fetal hemoglobin levels decline and the normal rise in adult hemoglobin (HbA) levels is compromised by a reduced or absent β-globin production. The anemia is the result of a unique combination of decreased hemoglobin synthesis and, as a result of imbalanced α and β globin chain production, accelerated red cell destruction. Consequently, erythropoietic hyperplasia of the bone marrow and extramedullary hematopoiesis occur. In severe β-thalassemia major, extramedullary hematopoiesis within craniofacial bones leads to a spectrum of characteristic facial features including prominence of frontal and parietal bones, depression of the nasal bridge, and protrusion of the upper teeth, resulting in the so-called "chipmunk facies." Bone marrow hyperplasia results in thinning of the cortex, widening of the medullary spaces, and osteoporosis. There is delayed skeletal maturation. This constellation of characteristic facies, bony abnormalities, presence of hepatosplenomegaly, and characteristic red cell morphology, including marked variation in red cell shape, usually makes this diagnosis readily apparent. Although β-thalassemia is often associated with Mediterranean ancestry, this disease and other thalassemias (e.g., E-β thalassemia, HbH disease) are also seen commonly in children of Southeast Asian, Indian, Pakistani, Arab, and Chinese ethnicity.

Lead poisoning affects heme synthesis, but significant anemia is unusual unless blood lead levels are markedly elevated. Iron deficiency is common in children with increased lead levels and usually accounts for the microcytic anemia found in these patients. If a concomitant hematologic disorder cannot be found in the anemic patient with plumbism, particular attention should be given to the possibility of severe lead intoxication.

Systemic Disease

Numerous disorders that are not primarily hematologic may be associated with pallor and anemia due to decreased production of hemoglobin or red cells. Occasionally, pallor is the only presenting finding of a serious systemic disorder. Chronic inflammatory diseases, such as juvenile idiopathic arthritis (JIA) and ulcerative colitis, are often accompanied by a normocytic or microcytic anemia related to impaired iron utilization by hematopoietic cells. The serum iron is reduced; however, low iron-binding capacity distinguishes this anemia of chronic inflammation from the anemia of iron deficiency. Similar clinical and laboratory findings may be associated with chronic infections such as HIV and subacute bacterial endocarditis. Other diseases in which anemia may be a prominent component include chronic renal disease, hyperthyroidism, and hypothyroidism. The anemia in these disorders is not severe enough to be considered a hematologic emergency unless complicated by other hematologic abnormalities. However, anemia may be the first clue to an underlying disease in which early treatment may improve the outcome substantially.

Increased Red Cell Destruction

The numerous conditions associated with shortened red cell survival can be congenital, as in the case of the hemoglobinopathies and membrane and enzyme defects. Acquired causes of shortened red cell survival include autoimmune hemolytic anemia, drug-associated hemolytic anemias, disseminated intravascular coagulation (DIC), and hemolytic uremic syndrome (HUS). The hemoglobin levels in these disorders can be normal, slightly depressed, or so low as to be life-threatening. The steady-state hemoglobin concentration is determined by a balance between the severity of the defect and the bone marrow's ability to respond to the presence of a shortened red cell survival. Compensation is achieved by an increase in erythrocyte production as is evident from the elevated reticulocyte count that is usually found in these conditions.

When the child with increased red cell destruction cannot compensate and make more red blood cells, this may result in a severe, life-threatening exacerbation of the underlying anemia (e.g., as is the case with acquired red cell aplasia from parvovirus B_{12} as discussed above). An aplastic crisis should be suspected in a patient with a known hemolytic anemia who develops increasing pallor and anemia associated with a reticulocyte count depressed in relation to its normally elevated baseline. The differential diagnosis of these underlying hemolytic conditions that result in red cell destruction is presented below.

Membrane Disorders

The degree of pallor associated with anemia caused by erythrocyte membrane abnormalities depends on the hemoglobin level. Hereditary spherocytosis, the most common of the membrane disorders, is usually characterized by well-compensated chronic hemolysis, which becomes clinically apparent only when the hemolysis is exacerbated by intercurrent infection. In rare instances, patients with hereditary spherocytosis may develop significant anemia, jaundice, and pallor in the newborn period. Moderate or severe anemia is less common in the other membrane disorders, such as hereditary elliptocytosis and hereditary stomatocytosis. The anemia of the erythrocyte membrane disorders is accompanied by reticulocytosis. A direct antiglobulin (Coombs) test will be negative. Red cell morphology usually permits the diagnosis to be made from the peripheral smear. A family history of anemia, splenomegaly, splenectomy, or cholecystectomy may be helpful as some of these disorders are inherited.

Infantile pyknocytosis is a hemolytic anemia seen during the first few months of life and is characterized by distorted and contracted erythrocytes and burr cells. The disorder may be associated with pallor and hyperbilirubinemia. Spontaneous recovery usually occurs by 6 months of age.

Enzyme Disorders

Erythrocyte enzymatic defects, such as pyruvate kinase deficiency and certain variants of glucose-6-phosphate dehydrogenase (G6PD) deficiency, may be associated with pallor due to increased red blood cell destruction. G6PD deficiency is the most common human enzyme defect to cause anemia, with predominance in people of Middle Eastern, South Asian, and African descent. This regional distribution is likely explained by the protection G6PD deficiency confers against malaria. In G6PD deficiency, pallor may be accentuated by acute hemolytic crises after exposure to oxidant stress (e.g., naphthalene-containing mothballs, antimalarials, sulfonamides, aspirin, methylene blue, or acidosis). Although alterations in red cell morphology are sometimes found in these enzyme disorders, assays of specific enzymes or substrates are required for definitive diagnosis.

Hemoglobinopathies

Pallor may result from the low hemoglobin level found in patients with sickle cell anemia and related hemoglobinopathies. Acute accentuation of pallor can result from an aplastic crisis, a complication of hemolytic disorders that is particularly common in sickle cell anemia. During an aplastic crisis, the normally elevated reticulocyte count may fall to zero, and the hemoglobin level may fall as low as 1 to 2 g per dL, resulting in severe pallor and signs of high-output cardiac failure.

The sequestration crisis of sickle cell anemia (HbSS) and related hemoglobin disorders (SC disease, S-β^0 thalassemia, S-β^+ thalassemia) is a true hematologic emergency. The presence of increased pallor and acute enlargement of the spleen in a patient with a sickling disorder should prompt immediate investigation of possible sequestration crisis. The condition results from pooling of red cells and plasma in the spleen resulting in sudden and severe anemia with associated hypovolemia. Emergent intervention is warranted as untreated cases may rapidly lead to death. Although this complication rarely occurs in children with homozygous SCD or S-β^0 thalassemia after the age of 5, sequestration crises may occur much later in children with sickling disorders such as SC disease or S-β^+ thalassemia, in which early splenic infarction is less common.

Immune Hemolytic Anemia

Pallor caused by autoimmmune hemolytic anemia is usually acute in onset and may be associated with severe anemia. Symptoms may include jaundice, dark urine, splenomegaly, and cardiovascular derangement. The presence of only moderate anemia (6 to 8 g per dL) at diagnosis should not detract from consideration of this disease as a hematologic emergency because brisk hemolysis may result in a sudden, additional fall in hemoglobin level. Autoimmune hemolytic anemia is usually, but not always, characterized by a positive direct antiglobulin (Coombs) test and an increased reticulocyte count. Spherocytes are commonly seen in the peripheral smear. Other causes of immune hemolytic anemia include infections, drug exposure, inflammatory diseases, and malignancies.

Microangiopathic Anemia

Alterations in the normal laminar flow of blood through the vascular system may cause increased red cell destruction. In DIC, abnormal fibrin deposition within small blood vessels results in mechanical injury to the erythrocytes. Thrombocytopenia and clotting abnormalities, which often herald the onset of DIC, may also contribute to the anemia via blood loss. The main diagnostic findings are red cell fragments in the peripheral blood smear, with platelet and clotting abnormalities typical of a consumptive coagulopathy (see Chapter 101 Hematologic Emergencies), and the clinical features of an underlying entity such as septic shock or extensive trauma, with which DIC is associated.

The increased red cell destruction in HUS and thrombotic thrombocytopenic purpura (TTP) is also caused by intravascular fibrin deposition. Thrombocytopenia and uremia may lower the hemoglobin concentration even further via blood loss, impaired red cell production, shortened red cell survival, and increased plasma volume. In some instances, anemia may be severe despite only mild uremia and absent thrombocytopenia, raising doubt about the diagnosis. In more typical cases, however, the diagnosis is readily apparent from the findings of oliguria, central nervous system abnormalities, increased blood urea nitrogen, thrombocytopenia, and abnormalities of red cell morphology on peripheral blood smear, including fragments and helmet cells.

Another form of microangiopathic anemia involves the proliferation of blood vessels within a cavernous hemangioma that may trap red cells or initiate a localized consumptive coagulopathy, causing erythrocyte destruction. Anemia in these cases is rarely severe unless the thrombocytopenia, which is more typical of the disorder, causes chronic blood loss.

Blood Loss

Pallor resulting from sudden, massive hemorrhage is commonly secondary to trauma; it is usually accompanied by signs of hypovolemic shock and evidence of injury. Patients may present in compensated or decompensated hypovolemic shock (see Chapter 5 Shock) and need to be emergently managed. Alternatively, the repeated loss of smaller amounts of blood over time may be associated with few findings other than pallor. The finding of iron-deficiency anemia despite normal dietary iron intake or iron supplementation may be a clue to the presence of chronic blood loss from the gastrointestinal (GI) tract or less commonly within the lungs or urinary tract.

EVALUATION AND DECISION

The initial assessment of the child with pallor should include an immediate determination of the severity of illness. Rapid evaluation and intervention is imperative for the severely ill child. In the presence of hypovolemic shock, immediate support of vascular volume is required. When high-output cardiac failure from severe anemia occurs, transfusion with small aliquots of packed red cells is necessary. After stabilization with initial therapeutic efforts, a thorough evaluation of the anemia can proceed.

If the child with pallor is not acutely ill, a deliberate search for the cause of pallor should be undertaken (Fig. 57.1). This may be accomplished by obtaining a thorough yet focused history, performing a detailed physical examination, and ordering appropriate laboratory investigations. The history should focus on several major components. First, particular attention should be paid to the time of onset of pallor. The slow development of pallor suggests diminished red cell production, as is found in bone marrow aplasia or iron deficiency. However, the acute onset of pallor is consistent with the brisk hemolysis of autoimmune hemolytic anemia, the splenic sequestration of SCD, or rapid blood loss.

After establishing the time course of the anemia, the history can be directed toward categories of anemia or specific diseases. A detailed dietary history, with particular attention to milk intake, is important in young children with suspected iron deficiency as excessive consumption of cow's milk often results in iron deficiency. Vitamin B_{12} deficiency may accompany strict vegetarian diets from which meat and egg products are excluded and may occur in breast-fed infants of vegetarian mothers or mothers with pernicious anemia. Nutritional folic acid deficiency is rare and can usually be readily deduced from the presence of severe dietary alterations and evidence of other vitamin deficiencies.

The family history helps in the diagnosis of hemoglobinopathies and inherited disorders of red cell membranes and enzymes. Because results of previous hemoglobin testing may have been explained inadequately or recalled inaccurately, a negative family history or newborn screening for hemoglobinopathies should not preclude evaluation of the patient's hemoglobin phenotype if a sickling disorder is suspected. The presence of a microcytic anemia unresponsive to iron in the parents suggests a thalassemic disorder. A history of splenomegaly, splenectomy, or cholecystectomy in family members may help identify a hemolytic disorder such as hereditary spherocytosis or pyruvate kinase deficiency.

Finally, a well-directed review of systems is essential in looking for systemic disorders such as chronic renal disease, hypothyroidism, or JIA. Pallor may be the presenting complaint in these and other disorders.

In the examination of the anemic patient, pulse and blood pressure (BP) should be measured to be sure hypovolemic shock and high-output cardiac failure are neither present nor imminent. If anemia or volume loss is mild, tachycardia may be present with a preserved BP. A systolic flow murmur is often heard if the hemoglobin level is below 8 g per dL. In the severely anemic patient, pallor of the skin and mucous membranes is usually readily apparent. When anemia is less severe or when the skin color is dark, pallor may be appreciated only in the nail beds, palmar surfaces, lips, and palpebral conjunctiva. Lymphadenopathy and splenomegaly may suggest a malignancy or an infectious disease such as mononucleosis. When splenomegaly occurs without lymphadenopathy, however, attention is drawn to hemolytic disorders such as hereditary spherocytosis and autoimmune hemolytic anemia or hemoglobinopathies (e.g., sickling disorders or thalassemia major). Scleral icterus may also be present in these disorders of shortened red cell survival. The finding of an unusually large and firm spleen in the absence of increasing scleral icterus suggests that red cells are being sequestered (e.g., splenic sequestration crisis of SCD, hypersplenism).

The skin in a patient with pallor should be examined for evidence of underlying disorders. The presence of hemangiomas might suggest microangiopathic anemia. If increased bruising or bleeding accompanies pallor, multiple blood elements are probably affected. The circulation time of platelets is short in comparison with that of red cells. Therefore, clinical findings of thrombocytopenia are often present by the time pallor develops in patients with acquired aplastic anemia, Fanconi anemia, and acute leukemia. Clinical evidence of thrombocytopenia may also suggest micorangiopathic anemia as described earlier. Sources of internal or external blood loss should be carefully sought. Chronic GI bleeding may escape detection until iron-deficiency anemia develops. Similarly, small pulmonary hemorrhages associated with idiopathic pulmonary hemosiderosis are often mistaken for other pulmonic processes until several recurrences of iron-deficiency

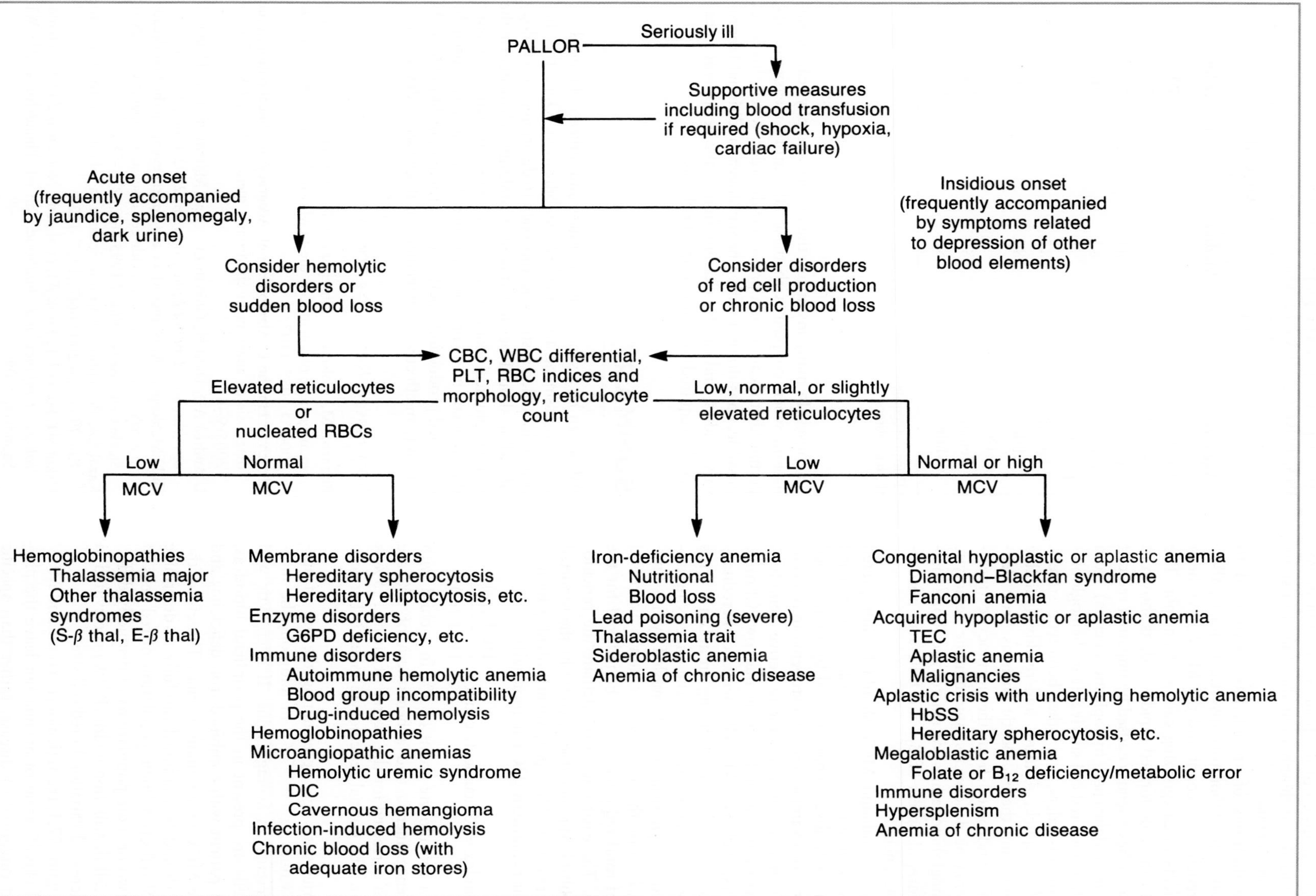

FIGURE 57.1 The diagnostic approach to pallor. CBC, complete blood cell; WBC, white blood cell; PLT, platelet; RBC, red blood cell; MCV, mean corpuscular volume; G6PD, glucose-6-phosphate dehydrogenase; DIC, disseminated intravascular coagulation; TEC, transient erythroblastopenia of childhood; HbSS, sickle cell anemia.

anemia suggest a hidden site of blood loss. Bony abnormalities associated with red cell disorders include frontal bossing from compensatory expansion of the bone marrow in hemolytic diseases and radial and thumb anomalies found in some patients with Fanconi anemia.

Numerous classifications of anemia have been used to assist the physician in the laboratory investigation of pallor. Historically, the reticulocyte count and the MCV have been helpful measurements in categorizing causes of anemia. The reticulocyte count can be performed rapidly and, as shown in Figure 57.1, distinguishes anemias caused by impaired red cell production (e.g., iron deficiency, hypoplastic anemia) from those caused by shortened red cell survival (e.g., hemoglobinopathies, membrane disorders, and other hemolytic states). The MCV provides a quick, accurate, and readily available method of distinguishing the microcytic anemias (iron deficiency, thalassemia syndromes) from the normocytic (membrane disorders, enzyme deficiencies, autoimmune hemolytic anemia, most hemoglobinopathies) or macrocytic (bone marrow/stem cell failure, disorders of B_{12} and folic acid absorption or metabolism) anemias.

The reticulocyte count and MCV should be interpreted with caution. As shown in Figure 57.1, disorders of shortened red cell survival are not always characterized by an increased reticulocyte count. For example, reticulocytopenia may occur in autoimmune hemolytic anemia, despite active hemolysis and increased erythropoiesis in the bone marrow. Chronic hemolytic disorders, such as sickle cell anemia or hereditary spherocytosis, may first be detected during an aplastic crisis when the reticulocyte count is low. Unless the underlying disorder is recognized, the physician may be misled by this finding. Furthermore, because the reticulocyte count is expressed as a percentage of total red cells, it must be indexed for the degree of anemia. The easiest way to calculate the reticulocyte index is to multiply the reticulocyte count by the reported hemoglobin or hematocrit (HCT pt [patient]) divided by normal hemoglobin or hematocrit (HCT nl [normal]):

$$\text{Reticulocyte index} = \text{Reticulocyte count} \times \frac{\text{HCT (pt)}}{\text{HCT (nl)}}$$

For example, a reticulocyte count of 5% in a child with severe iron-deficiency anemia and a hematocrit of 6% are not elevated when corrected for the degree of anemia (5% × 6%/33% = 0.9%). The normal reticulocyte index is between 1.0 and 2.0.

The MCV varies with age, necessitating the use of age-adjusted normal values (Table 57.4). In addition, the measured MCV represents an average value. If microcytic and macrocytic red cells are present in the peripheral blood as, for example, in a patient with combined iron deficiency and B_{12} deficiency, the MCV may remain normal. Therefore, the peripheral smear should be examined carefully to determine whether the MCV reflects a single population of red cells of uniform size, or two or more populations of distinctly different size. The red cell distribution width (RDW) is elevated in the presence of increased variation in red cell size.

As shown in Figure 57.1, the reticulocyte count and MCV help in the initial classification of anemia but leave the physician with broad categories of disease, rather than specific diagnoses. In many instances, the history and physical examination, when coupled with these laboratory measurements, permit identification of a particular disorder. When this is not possible, consultation with a hematologist, additional laboratory studies, and careful examination of the peripheral smear may be required to characterize the disease.

TABLE 57.4

AGE-RELATED VALUES FOR MEAN CORPUSCULAR VOLUME

	MCV (fL)	
Age (yrs)	Median	Lower limit[a]
0.5–2	77	70
2–5	79	73
5–9	81	75
9–12	83	76
12–14:		
Female	85	77
Male	84	76
14–18:		
Female	87	78
Male	86	77

[a]Third percentile.
fL, femtoliters.

SUMMARY

Pallor can be a sign of severe illness and indicate the need for rapid assessment and emergent stabilization. Once this has been initiated, a systematic approach to determine the etiology of pallor should be undertaken. Combining elements of the history, physical examination, and laboratory data will assist the clinician in identifying whether the anemia is caused by decreased production, increased destruction, or blood loss. As a result, an effective management strategy can be developed.

Suggested Readings and Key References

Bizzarro M, Colson E, Ehrenkranz R. Differential diagnosis and management of anemia in the newborn. *Pediatr Clin North Am* 2004;51:1087–1107.

Chalco JP, Huicho L, Alamo C, et al. Accuracy of clinical pallor in the diagnosis of anaemia in children: a meta-analysis. *BMC Pediatr* 2005;5:46.

D'Andrea AD, Dahl N, Guinan EC, et al. Marrow failure. *Hematology (Am Soc Hematol Educ Program)* 2002;1:58–72.

Gill FM, Sleeper LA, Weiner SJ, et al. Clinical events in the first decade in a cohort of infants with sickle cell disease. Cooperative Study of Sickle Cell Disease. *Blood* 1995;86(2):776–783.

Kazal LA. Prevention of iron deficiency in infants and toddlers. *Am Fam Physician* 2002;66(7):1217–1224.

Orkin SH, Fisher DE, Look AT, et al., eds. *Nathan and Oski's Hematology of infancy and childhood.* 7th ed. Philadelphia, PA: WB Saunders, 2009.

CHAPTER 58 ■ PALPITATIONS

JAMES F. WILEY II, MD, MPH AND STEVEN C. ROGERS, MD

Palpitations represent a disagreeable perception of the heartbeat by the patient. Descriptions commonly given include "pounding," "fluttering," "jumping in the chest," or a sensation of the heart "stopping." In children, most etiologies of palpitations are benign but can cause a great amount of anxiety. Pediatric patients demonstrate a high degree of variation in their sensitivity to changes in the heart rate (HR) or rhythm. A patient who actually has trivial cardiac events may express severe symptoms while children with a significant arrhythmia may remain asymptomatic. The challenge to the emergency physician is to determine which complaint can be managed in the emergency department (ED) and which merits further consideration by a cardiologist.

PATHOPHYSIOLOGY

The heart is innervated by the vagus nerve (cranial nerve X) and the sympathetic ganglion. Cardiovascular reflexes (e.g., vasovagal bradycardia) are transmitted by the vagus nerve. Pain sensation (e.g., related to myocardial ischemia) travels through afferent fibers associated with the sympathetic ganglia. In most patients, the sensation of the heartbeat is not felt. Children with documented arrhythmias, such as supraventricular tachycardia (SVT) and stable ventricular tachycardia (VT), may not complain of any symptoms. Even patients with heart murmurs audible to the unassisted ear can learn to ignore this obvious cue.

Patients with palpitations often relate an indirect perception of increased force of cardiac contraction, tachycardia, or irregular heartbeat. Increased force of the contraction is often detected when the patient is supine. At times, it may be described as a rushing or pounding in the ears, particularly when the ear is pressed against a pillow. Caffeine or alcohol consumption, illicit drug use, exercise, and emotional arousal can produce this same sensation. Patients with premature contractions and a compensatory pause may describe the feeling that their hearts "flip-flop" or "stop." Many patients with premature atrial or ventricular contractions notice the subsequent beat after the initial "short" beat because of the increased stroke volume ejected. Other patients may complain of a choking or full sensation in the neck. Jugular venous pulsation associated with right atrial contraction against a closed tricuspid valve (atrioventricular [AV] block with or without atrial tachycardia) can present in this way.

True cardiac arrhythmias arise from various mechanisms that are discussed in Chapter 94 Cardiac Emergencies.

DIFFERENTIAL DIAGNOSIS

Many conditions may produce palpitations (Table 58.1). Most children with palpitations do not have significant cardiac pathology (Table 58.2). However, many life-threatening conditions can come to medical attention because of abnormal cardiac sensation (Table 58.3). Wolff–Parkinson–White (WPW) syndrome and the prolonged QT syndrome are two potentially lethal diseases that may be diagnosed on a resting electrocardiogram (EKG). A patient with palpitations during exercise should also raise concern for hypertrophic cardiomyopathy, SVT, VT, or myocardial ischemia. In addition, palpitations in children with known congenital heart disease are frequently caused by a serious cardiac arrhythmia.

Diagnosis of noncardiac causes of life-threatening palpitations, including hypoxemia, hypoglycemia, hyperkalemia, and hypocalcemia, can be made by characteristic EKG changes, serum electrolyte determinations, rapid bedside glucose, and oxygen saturation measurements.

Hyperdynamic Cardiac Activity

Increased HR and contractility are physiologic responses to catecholamine release, like that which may occur with exercise, emotional arousal, hypoglycemia, and pheochromocytoma. Similarly, increased cardiac work accompanies conditions that increase the basal metabolic rate such as fever, anemia, and hyperthyroidism. Sympathomimetic and anticholinergic drugs are groups of commonly available substances that directly modulate the autonomic nervous system, causing tachycardia, hyperdynamic cardiac activity, and palpitations (Table 58.4).

Postural orthostatic tachycardia syndrome (POTS) describes a form of orthostatic intolerance characterized by chronic fatigue, tachycardia (more than 40 beats per minute over baseline or more than 120 or 130 beats per minute in patients 13 years of age and younger or 14 years of age and older, respectively) typically without hypotension upon standing. POTS is commonly seen in teenage girls and manifests as palpitations, dizziness, and tremulousness. The diagnosis may be made when no other serious cause for symptoms is found and the patient has replication of symptoms with head-up tilt table testing. Management consists of a multidisciplinary approach including family education, avoidance of precipitating factors (e.g., sudden posture changes, large meals, or vasodilating drugs), adequate water and salt intake, and regular exercise. Medications targeted at maintaining blood volume, avoiding vasodilation, or treating secondary symptoms are frequently required.

Sinus Bradycardia

Low basal metabolic rate associated with hypothyroidism may present with a slow HR and sinus rhythm. Similarly, in the absence of significant sympathetic nervous system input, the HR may be slow. This state may be responsible for the sinus bradycardia associated with sleep or with ingestion of drugs such as clonidine, sedative-hypnotics, or narcotics. Advanced physical training results in a highly efficient heart with high ventricular ejection fraction and sinus bradycardia.

TABLE 58.1

DIFFERENTIAL DIAGNOSIS OF PALPITATIONS

Hyperdynamic cardiac activity
Anemia
Anxiety/panic attacks/hyperventilation syndrome
Drug induced (Table 58.4)
Emotional/sexual arousal
Exercise
Fever
Hyperthyroidism
Hypoglycemia
Pheochromocytoma
Postural orthostatic tachycardia syndrome
Sinus bradycardia
Athleticism/advanced physical training (e.g., marathon runners)
Drug induced (Table 58.4)
Hypothyroidism
Sleep
True cardiac arrhythmias
Irregular rhythm or bradyarrhythmia
Complete heart block
Postoperative cardiac repair (especially ventriculoseptal defect, atrioventricular canal repairs)
Premature atrial contractions
Premature ventricular contractions
Sick sinus syndrome
Sinus arrhythmia/respiratory variation
Tachyarrhythmias (see Chapter 72 Tachycardia)

True Cardiac Arrhythmias

SVT represents the most common tachyarrhythmia of childhood and often presents with a chief complaint of palpitations. Possible underlying causes include drug exposure, congenital heart disease, and WPW syndrome (see Chapter 94 Cardiac Emergencies). Approximately 50% of children with SVT have no physical findings and no EKG abnormalities between episodes. In these patients, descriptions of abrupt onset and rapid termination of palpitations ("like a light switch") can often be elicited.

VT may also present with palpitations and may be associated with infections, drug exposure, or even exercise. Infections, especially viral myocarditis and acute rheumatic fever constitute some of the most common causes of acquired VT in children with normal cardiac anatomy. Similarly, ingestion of drugs that block fast sodium channels and/or potassium channels (e.g., tricyclic antidepressants, phenothiazines, and antiarrhythmic agents) is a preventable cause of torsades de pointes (polymorphic VT) and unstable VT in the otherwise normal child (Table 58.4). Palpitations associated with exercise may be caused by VT that occurs in conjunction with hypertrophic cardiomyopathy or myocardial ischemia (see Chapter 94 Cardiac Emergencies). Patients with the prolonged QT syndrome have a genetically determined predisposition to fatal VT or have an acquired long QT syndrome (LQTS) from drugs, hypokalemia, or hypomagnesemia. LQTS presents with palpitations, presyncope, syncope, cardiac arrest, and seizures (see Chapter 94 Cardiac Emergencies). Patients who have undergone ventriculotomy for tetralogy of Fallot comprise another group who are at high risk for VT as a result of the postoperative development of scarring in the right ventricular outflow tract. Finally, electrolyte disturbances, particularly hyperkalemia, hypocalcemia, and hypomagnesemia, may be causative in a child with palpitations and VT (see Chapter 108 Renal and Electrolyte Emergencies).

Premature atrial contractions produce the most common arrhythmia of childhood, with 50% of normal children experiencing at least one premature atrial contraction per day. Premature ventricular contractions (PVCs) also account for many reports of irregular heartbeat. Although this arrhythmia can herald serious underlying pathology, patients with an unremarkable history, normal physical examination, and unifocal PVCs that disappear with exercise do not require further evaluation. Patients with significant sinus or AV node dysfunction as a cause of an irregular or slow heartbeat often have a history of syncope or seizure, slow HR (25 to 50 beats per minute) on examination, a pulmonic flow murmur, or signs of congestive heart failure. Patients who have undergone intra-atrial repairs (D-transposition of the great arteries and atrial septal defect) are at highest risk for these potentially life-threatening arrhythmias.

TABLE 58.2

COMMON CAUSES OF PALPITATIONS

Exercise
Anxiety/hyperventilation syndrome
Emotional arousal
Drug induced (e.g., caffeine, over-the-counter sympathomimetic agents)
Supraventricular tachycardia
Premature atrial or ventricular contractions

TABLE 58.3

LIFE-THREATENING CAUSES OF PALPITATIONS

Cardiac
Wolff–Parkinson–White syndrome
Prolonged QT syndrome
Hypertrophic cardiomyopathy
Congenital heart disease/postoperative cardiac repair
Myocarditis/acute rheumatic fever
Mitral valve prolapse
Sick sinus syndrome
Complete heart block
Myocardial ischemia
Noncardiac
Hypoxemia
Hypoglycemia
Hyperkalemia
Hypocalcemia
Pheochromocytoma
Poisoning (Table 58.4)

TABLE 58.4

DRUGS THAT CAUSE PALPITATIONS/ARRHYTHMIAS

Sinus or supraventricular tachycardia
Albuterol
Amphetamines
Antidepressants
Antihistamines
Caffeine
Cocaine
Ephedra
Energy drinks
Ephedrine, pseudoephedrine
Hallucinogens (e.g., lysergic acid diethylamide [LSD] or phencyclidine [PCP])
Herbal stimulants
Marijuana
Methcathinones (bath salts) and khat (*Catha edulis* leaves, popular in Africa and the Middle East)
Phenothiazines
Synthetic cannabinoids (e.g., K2 or Spice)
Tobacco
Ventricular tachycardia or torsades de pointes
Amphetamines
Antiarrhythmic agents (e.g., quinidine, procainamide, mexiletine, flecainide, encainide)
Arsenic
Caffeine
Chloral hydrate
Chlorinated hydrocarbons
Chloroquine
Cocaine
Digoxin
Organophosphate pesticides
Phenothiazines
Tricyclic antidepressants
Bradycardia
Calcium channel blockers
Clonidine
Digoxin
Narcotics
Organophosphate pesticides
Sedative/hypnotic agents
β-Adrenergic blockers

EVALUATION AND DECISION

The ill-appearing child with palpitations requires rapid assessment for the presence of hypoxemia, shock, hypoglycemia, or an existing life-threatening arrhythmia. Further evaluation should include measurement of hemoglobin, serum glucose (Dextrostix), serum electrolytes, calcium, and pulse oximetry or arterial blood gas. The presence of heart disease should be assessed by a 12-lead EKG and rhythm strip, followed by continuous monitoring, frequent vital signs, and chest radiograph (Fig. 58.1). Specific arrhythmias should be treated as outlined in Chapter 94 Cardiac Emergencies.

The asymptomatic child with palpitations by history may also have an intermittent or continuing arrhythmia. Continuous cardiac monitoring and a resting 12-lead EKG performed while the patient is in the ED increase the likelihood that this abnormality will be detected. Patients with repeated episodes of palpitations may benefit from 24-hour ambulatory (Holter) or longer-term event monitoring, and warrant referral to a pediatric cardiologist. Any patient with a history of syncope, congenital heart disease, or particularly, postoperative or exercise-induced palpitations is at greater risk for having a true cardiac arrhythmia as the cause of his or her symptoms. Similarly, the presence of a short P-R interval with the typical delta wave morphology of WPW syndrome or a prolonged corrected Q-T interval (see Chapter 94 Cardiac Emergencies) indicates the need for evaluation and consultation by a pediatric cardiologist.

The presence or recent history of fever or an upper respiratory infection should prompt the emergency physician to look for signs and symptoms of myocarditis or acute rheumatic fever. Myocarditis describes inflammation of the muscle wall of the heart. Multiple organisms can cause this pathology, with the most common being viruses such as coxsackie, Epstein–Barr, and cytomegalovirus. Clinical features of myocarditis are fever, tachycardia out of proportion to activity or degree of fever, pallor, cyanosis, respiratory distress secondary to pulmonary edema, muffled heart sounds with gallop, and hepatomegaly caused by passive congestion of the liver. The EKG findings are nonspecific and include low-voltage QRS complexes (less than 5-mm total amplitude in limb leads), "pseudoinfarction" pattern with deep Q waves and poor R-wave progression in the precordial leads, AV conduction disturbances that range from P-R prolongation to complete AV dissociation, and tachyarrhythmias such as VT and SVT. A child with palpitations and clinical findings suggestive of myocarditis requires emergent supportive care (see Chapters 1 A General Approach to Ill and Injured Children and 5 Shock), echocardiography, and admission to a unit capable of intensive monitoring and rapid treatment of cardiac arrhythmias and hemodynamic instability.

Acute rheumatic fever follows pharyngeal streptococcal infection and is an inflammatory disease that targets the heart, vessels, joints, skin, and central nervous system (CNS). Diagnosis and management of acute rheumatic fever are discussed separately (see Chapter 94 Cardiac Emergencies).

A detailed history of recent medications or precipitating events may reveal the cause of palpitations in some patients. Ingestion of highly caffeinated beverages (including coffee, soft drinks, and energy drinks), cough and cold preparations, herbal preparations, dietary supplements, "health" drinks with herbal additives, use of illicit drugs, and a smoking history should be ascertained. The patient's emotional state before the onset of palpitations should be discussed to determine the likelihood of anxiety or emotional arousal as the cause of symptoms (see Chapter 134 Behavioral and Psychiatric Emergencies). The presence of diaphoresis, hypertension, and headache should encourage the assessment for pheochromocytoma, whereas widened pulse pressure and thyroid enlargement suggest hyperthyroidism (see Chapter 97 Endocrine Emergencies). Anemia may be the cause of symptoms in a patient with pallor (see Chapter 101 Hematologic Emergencies).

In some patients, an exact cause of palpitations cannot be determined at the time of ED evaluation. Patients with a single episode should have close follow-up arranged with their primary care physicians and should be instructed to return for further

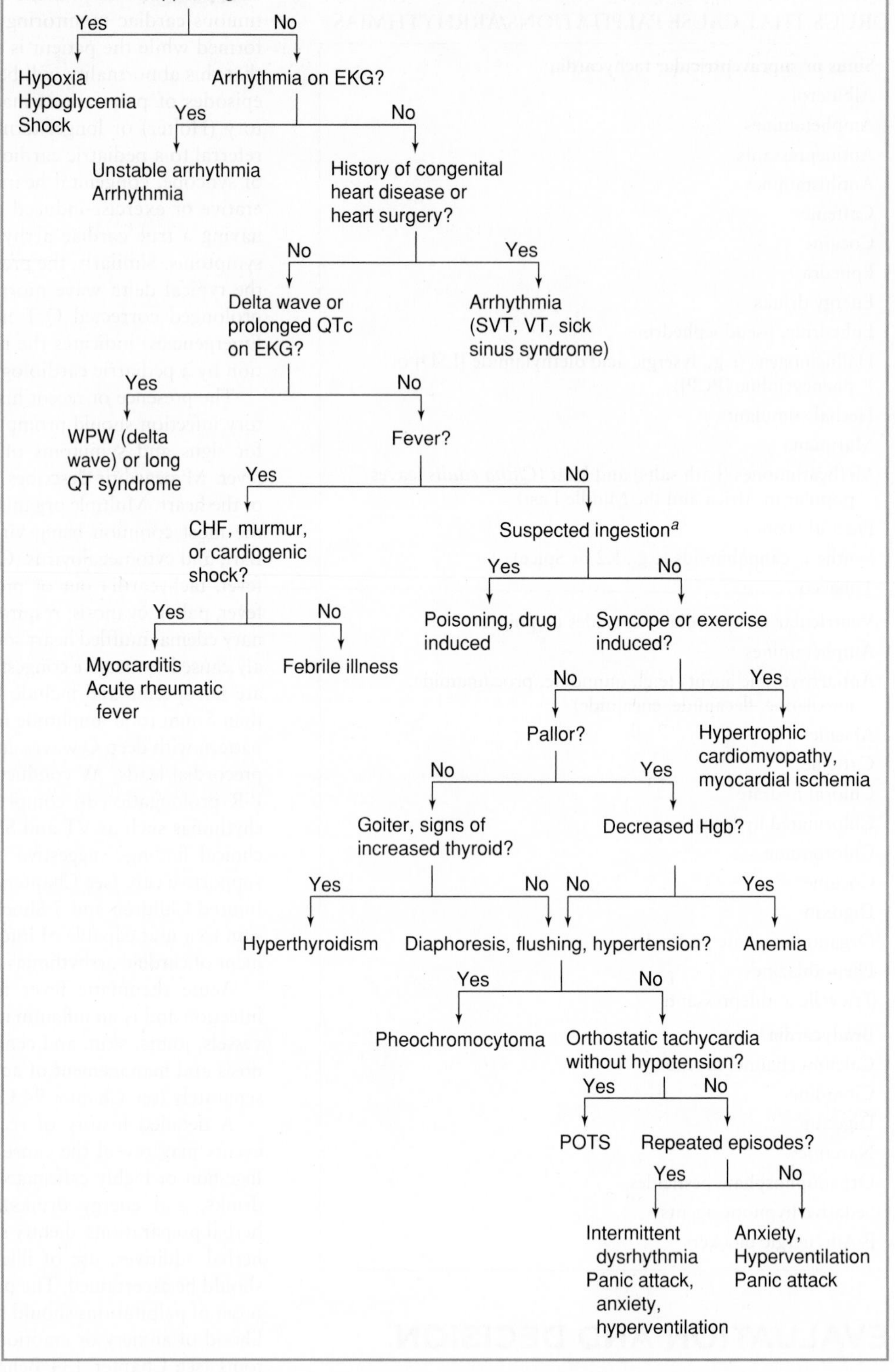

FIGURE 58.1 A diagnostic approach to palpitations. [a]Especially caffeine, diet supplements, herbal preparations, sympathomimetic medications, cocaine, or amphetamines. EKG, electrocardiogram; SVT, supraventricular tachycardia; VT, ventricular tachycardia; WPW, Wolff–Parkinson–White; CHF, congestive heart failure; Hgb, hemoglobin; POTS, postural orthostatic tachycardia syndrome.

evaluation if symptoms recur. Patients with multiple episodes of palpitations deserve further evaluation and consultation with a pediatric cardiologist.

Suggested Readings and Key References

Ginsburg GS, Riddle MA, Davies M. Somatic symptoms in children and adolescents with anxiety disorders. *J Am Acad Child Adolesc Psychiatry* 2006;45:1179–1187.

Kizilbash SJ, Ahrens SP, Bruce BK, et al. Adolescent fatigue, POTS, and recovery: a guide for clinicians. *Curr Probl Pediatr Adolesc Health Care* 2014;44:108–133.

Marzuillo P, Benettoni A, Germani C, et al. Acquired long QT syndrome: a focus for the general pediatrician. *Pediatr Emerg Care* 2014;30(4):257–261.

Rivera RF, Chambers P, Ceresnak SR. Evaluation of children with palpitations. *Clin Pediatr Emerg Med* 2011;12(4):278–288.

Sedaghat-Yazdi F, Koenig PR. The teenager with palpitations. *Pediatr Clin North Am* 2014;61(1):63–79.

CHAPTER 59 ■ POLYDIPSIA

KERRY CAPERELL, MD, MS AND RONALD I. PAUL, MD

Polydipsia, or excessive thirst, is an uncommon complaint in children. Although fluid consumption varies greatly among individuals, pathologic conditions exist when excessive drinking of fluids interferes with daily life or is accompanied by bizarre behavior, such as drinking from a toilet bowl. Polydipsia is routinely accompanied by urinary frequency (see Chapter 74 Urinary Frequency). Other accompanying symptoms depend on the underlying cause.

PATHOPHYSIOLOGY

The sensation of thirst and subsequent fluid intake is influenced by complex mechanisms that involve the hypothalamus, extracranial thirst receptors, and kidneys. As water is lost from the body, thirst centers in the hypothalamus are stimulated by an increase in serum osmolality. In response to signals from the hypothalamus, the pituitary gland releases an antidiuretic hormone, vasopressin, which causes reabsorption of water in the collecting ducts of the kidney. In addition to physiologic controls of thirst, cortical involvement and social conditioning also play a role and may be responsible for the wide variability in fluid consumption.

DIFFERENTIAL DIAGNOSIS

Diabetes mellitus (DM) is the single most common cause of polydipsia (Table 59.1). Additional prominent symptoms of DM include weight loss and polyuria. Other common causes of polydipsia include sickle cell anemia and diabetes insipidus (DI) (Table 59.2). In sickle cell anemia, chronic sickling of cells in the medulla of the kidney results in a limited ability to concentrate urine and mild polydipsia. In DI, a wide variety of lesions in the hypothalamus and neurohypophysis result in a deficiency of antidiuretic hormone. Inherited forms of nephrogenic DI may be autosomal dominant, autosomal recessive, or X-linked recessive. In instances in which the cause of DI cannot be readily determined, patients are diagnosed as idiopathic. These patients need frequent reevaluations because many are later diagnosed with intracranial tumors.

Less common metabolic and endocrine causes of polydipsia include electrolyte imbalances, catecholamine excess, and cystinosis. Primary renal causes of hyposthenuria include interstitial nephritis, renal tubular acidosis, medullary cystic disease (nephronophthisis), and obstructive uropathy. In nephrogenic DI, the renal tubule is unresponsive to antidiuretic hormone. Patients with nephrogenic DI usually have onset of symptoms in infancy and present with recurrent episodes of dehydration, fever, failure to thrive, and psychomotor retardation. Pharmacologic causes of polyuria and polydipsia include methylxanthines, amphotericin B, and diuretics. In addition, chronic lithium therapy may result in nephrogenic DI.

Primary polydipsia is diagnosed when the ingestion of water is in excess of that needed to maintain water balance. It can be caused by an inappropriate psychological thirst drive (psychogenic polydipsia or compulsive water drinking) or by hypothalamic damage that alters thirst but not antidiuretic hormone release (neurogenic polydipsia).

Most children with polydipsia have serious but nonacute problems. Potential life-threatening conditions may develop in certain circumstances (Table 59.3). Patients with DI or nephrogenic DI may develop severe dehydration if water is withheld for prolonged periods. Conversely, urgent management of hypernatremia is usually unnecessary if patients are able to drink and may be harmful if it is of chronic duration. Diabetic ketoacidosis may be an initial presentation of patients with DM, and can result in extreme electrolyte and acid–base imbalances. Patients with primary polydipsia who overload their kidneys' ability to excrete free water may present with hyponatremic seizures. Many of the brain lesions that cause DI can become life-threatening. Patients with severe brain injury often develop DI toward the end of life.

EVALUATION AND DECISION

When evaluating a child with polydipsia, the physician should seek information from the parent regarding the quantity and type of fluid taken each day and whether the child has used any unusual methods to satiate thirst. A history of nocturnal polydipsia and polyuria is helpful because most children with psychogenic polydipsia do not wake in the middle of the night for fluids. A medical history should include questions on growth and development, as well as past episodes of severe dehydration. Inquiries should be made about known causes of polydipsia such as sickle cell disease, DM, chronic kidney disorders, head trauma, and medications (Fig. 59.1). The physical examination should include a careful evaluation for known systemic and intracranial causes of DI, and particularly a full neurologic examination.

If the history and physical examination are not revealing, a urinalysis should be obtained. In almost all cases of polydipsia, the urine-specific gravity will be low (less than 1.010). A specific gravity greater than 1.020 usually represents appropriate thirst. If the urinalysis is abnormal, DM (glucosuria, possibly ketonuria, and pseudo-hypersthenuria), sickle cell disease (isosthenuric), or an intrinsic renal disorder (cellular elements and sediment) should be suspected. If the urinalysis is normal, electrolytes, calcium, and renal function tests may reveal conditions associated with electrolyte imbalances. Patients with poorly controlled DM, DI, or nephrogenic DI may have hypernatremia if they are examined when dehydrated. A hemoglobin electrophoresis may be needed to

TABLE 59.1

CAUSES OF POLYDIPSIA

Diabetes mellitus	Aneurysm
Electrolyte imbalances	Intraventricular hemorrhage
Hypercalcemia	Hereditary
Hypokalemia	Drugs
Bartter syndrome	Methylxanthines
Catecholamine excess	Amphotericin B
Pheochromocytoma	Diuretics
Neuroblastoma	Lithium
Ganglioneuroma	Renal causes
Cystinosis	Renal tubular acidosis
Diabetes insipidus (antidiuretic hormone deficient)	Nephrogenic diabetes insipidus
Craniopharyngioma	Sickle cell anemia
Pituitary adenoma	Interstitial nephritis
Langerhans cell histiocytosis	Obstructive uropathy
Head trauma	Primary polydipsia
Sarcoidosis	Psychogenic polydipsia
Leukemia	Neurogenic polydipsia
Infection	

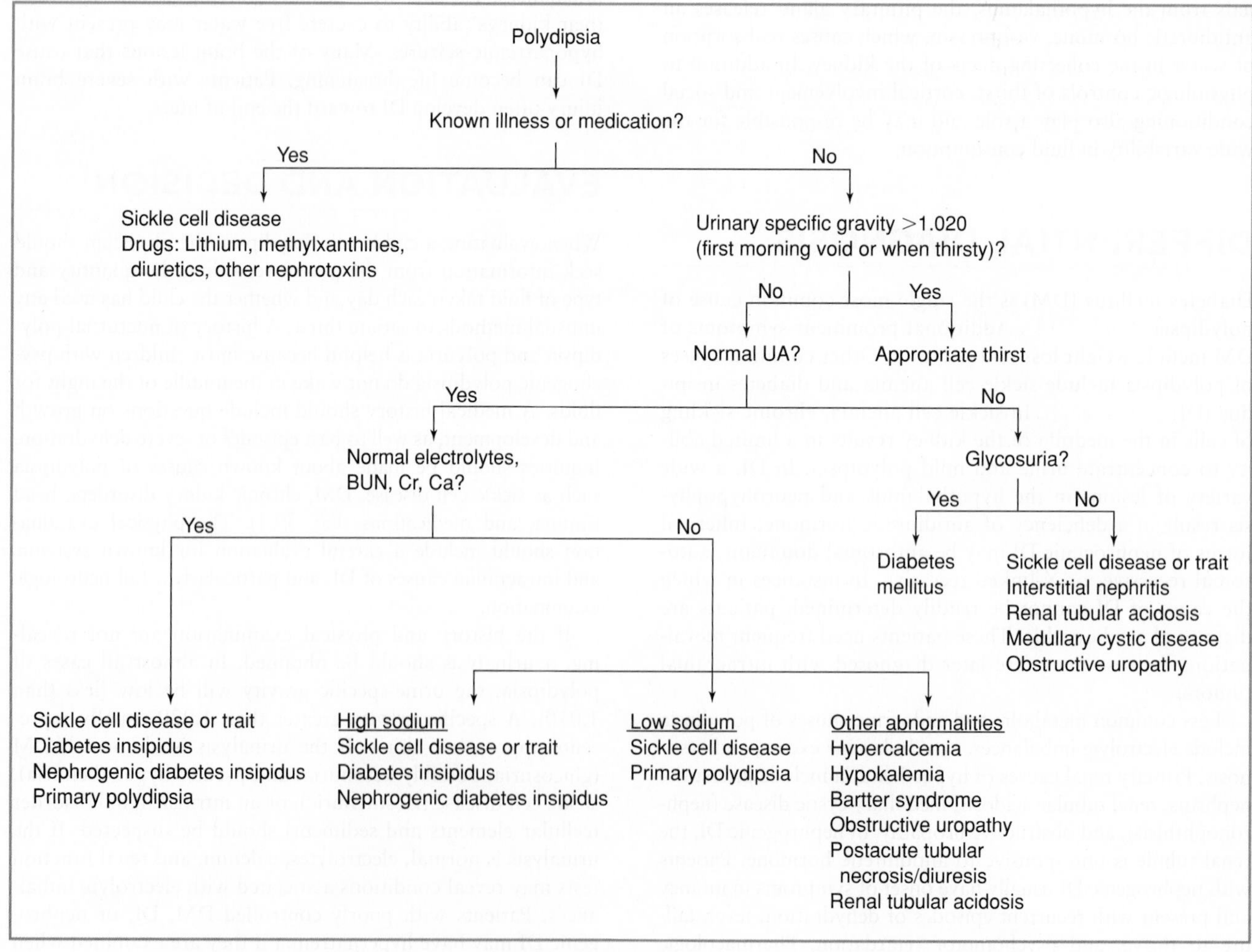

FIGURE 59.1 Diagnostic approach to a child with polydipsia. UA, urinalysis; BUN, blood urea nitrogen; Cr, creatinine; Ca, calcium.

TABLE 59.2

COMMON CAUSES OF POLYDIPSIA

Diabetes mellitus
Sickle cell anemia
Diabetes insipidus (antidiuretic hormone deficient)

TABLE 59.3

LIFE-THREATENING CAUSES OF POLYDIPSIA

Diabetes insipidus (antidiuretic hormone deficient)
Nephrogenic diabetes insipidus
Diabetes mellitus
Primary polydipsia

determine whether the patient has sickle cell disease. However, patients with sickle cell disease usually have the diagnosis confirmed before the development of tubular dysfunction and polydipsia. Because of the high resolution required to diagnose most intracranial causes, magnetic resonance imaging scan is usually necessary.

Patients suspected of having primary polydipsia, DI, and nephrogenic DI require further testing that can be dangerous. These tests should be performed in controlled settings and are usually inappropriate in the emergency department.

Patients with primary polydipsia should respond to a water deprivation test by increasing their urine specific gravity and osmolality. Patients with DI and nephrogenic DI should have rapid weight loss while continuing to excrete urine with a low specific gravity. They may become severely dehydrated if the weight loss is in excess of 3% to 5%. Constant observation should be maintained during the water deprivation test to ensure patients do not covertly consume water and to prevent severe dehydration. A trial of intranasal desmopressin (DDAVP) should distinguish between DI and nephrogenic DI because patients with antidiuretic hormone–deficient DI will respond to the exogenous hormone.

Unfortunately, even these tests are fraught with some inaccuracies. Patients with primary polydipsia who have chronic overhydration and diminished capacity to concentrate urine may have a blunted response to water deprivation. In addition, patients with DI and nephrogenic DI may produce hypertonic urine if the glomerular filtration rate is decreased as severe dehydration ensues. Radioimmunoassay for antidiuretic hormone can be helpful in confusing cases.

Suggested Readings and Key References

Bichet DG. Nephrogenic diabetes insipidus. *Adv Chronic Kidney Dis* 2006;13(2):96–104.

Cermeroglu AP, Buyukgebiz A. Psychogenic diabetes insipidus in toddlers with compulsive bottle-drinking: not a rare entity. *J Pediatr Endocrinol Metab* 2002;15(1):93–94.

De Buyst J, Massa G, Christophe C, et al. Clinical, hormonal, and imaging findings in 27 children with central diabetes insipidus. *Eur J Pediatr* 2007;166(1):43–49.

Di Iorgi N, Napoli F, Allegri A, et al. Diabetes insipidus—diagnosis and management. *Horm Res Paediatr* 2012;77:69–84.

Dundas B, Harris M, Narasimhan M. Psychogenic polydipsia review: etiology, differential, and treatment. *Curr Psychiatry Rep* 2007;9(3):236–241.

Rose S, Auble B. Endocrine changes after pediatric traumatic brain injury. *Pituitary* 2012;15(3):267–275.

CHAPTER 60 ▪ RASH: ATOPIC DERMATITIS, CONTACT DERMATITIS, SCABIES AND ERYTHRODERMA

PATRICK J. McMAHON, MD

DERMATITIS

Dermatitis is the general term used to describe an itchy, eczematous rash. In its acute form dermatitis is characterized by erythema, edema, exudation, scattered papules or vesicles, scaling, and crusting. Chronic dermatitis is characterized by lichenification (accentuated skin markings), hyperpigmentation, hypopigmentation, and excoriations. Diagnosis of the underlying cause of the dermatitis relies on patient history and physical examination findings, since histology is typically nonspecific. This chapter highlights common causes of dermatitis in children, including atopic dermatitis, nummular eczema, asteatotic eczema, dyshidrotic eczema, lichen simplex chronicus as well as contact dermatitis. In addition, this chapter includes discussions about scabies infestation and erythroderma.

Atopic Dermatitis

Atopic dermatitis is so far the most common cause of dermatitis in children (Table 60.1). It is a chronic and relapsing condition characterized by pruritic eczematous papules, patches, and plaques, and occurs in 10% to 20% of all children. There is often a personal or family history of allergic rhinitis, hay fever, or asthma. Most patients have the onset of symptoms before 6 months of age, with up to 90% developing symptoms by 5 years of age. Heat, stress, sweating, infection, and exposure to environmental (e.g., pet dander, pollen) and contact allergens (e.g., fragrances, soaps) may also precipitate flares.

The diagnosis is mainly based on typical history and physical examination findings, and the American Academy of Dermatology has developed criteria to summarize these features (Table 60.2). The broad differential diagnosis requires the exclusion of other skin conditions that present in a similar fashion such as seborrheic dermatitis, scabies, psoriasis, nutritional deficiencies (i.e., zinc), immune deficiencies, and cutaneous lymphoma. Importantly, while superficial bacterial infections, seborrheic dermatitis, and contact dermatitis may occur in isolation, they may also coexist in a patient with atopic dermatitis.

The typical distribution can vary by age. Infants have lesions on the cheeks, trunk, and extensor surfaces. Children show involvement of the hands, feet, and flexor areas, such as the antecubital and popliteal fossae, and the neck (Fig. 60.1). In adolescents and adults, flexor areas, hands, and feet are often involved. Xerosis (dry skin), ichthyosis vulgaris (inherited fish-like scaling of the extremities and hyperlinear palms), keratosis pilaris (follicularly based papules with cornified plugs in the upper hair follicles), infraorbital eyelid folds (Dennie–Morgan sign), pityriasis alba (scaly hypopigmented macules and patches on the cheeks), and follicular accentuation may be seen.

The main factors to assess when caring for patients with atopic dermatitis include pruritus, superinfection, and concomitant contact dermatitis. The pruritus of atopic dermatitis may be severe resulting in sleep disturbances in the child and caretakers as well as difficulty concentrating in school and work. The persistent itch-scratch cycle can also lead to severe excoriations in the skin. This damage to the skin barrier, along with inherent defects in the skin barrier and immunity that are associated with atopic dermatitis, makes patients particularly susceptible to superinfections with bacteria (*Staphylococcus aureus* or group A streptococcus), yeast (candida), and viral infections (herpes simplex, enterovirus, and molluscum contagiosum). The increased permeability of the skin barrier allows increased penetration of contact allergens that is felt to explain the increased incidence of contact dermatitis in this population (see below).

Management of atopic dermatitis includes minimizing triggers (irritants and allergens) with "gentle skin care" including an unscented soap, fragrance-free laundry detergent, hypoallergenic shampoo and conditioner, and regular application of thick unscented emollients immediately after bathing. Continual screening for new contactants is important since care providers may try new topical products in an effort to provide relief.

Screening for infection is critical in all patients with atopic dermatitis flares, including culturing active pustules for bacteria and obtaining a viral culture or polymerase chain reaction (PCR) sample from vesicles or erosions for herpes simplex virus, and in some cases, enterovirus. For localized areas, use of a topical antibiotic that covers gram-positive organisms is important. Empiric oral antibiotic or antiviral treatments may be needed in more involved cases. Dilute bleach baths have also been shown to be helpful in decreasing skin infections in atopic dermatitis and may help minimize flares.

Atopic dermatitis on the cheeks of infants is best managed by applying petrolatum-based ointments as a barrier prior to feeding and sleeping, avoidance of irritants (e.g., wet wipes, drool, food, pacifiers), and low- to midpotency topical corticosteroids as needed.

Topical corticosteroids are the mainstay of treatment for most patients with atopic dermatitis. One approach to minimize recurrences of *localized* atopic dermatitis after flares is to use topical corticosteroids twice daily during flares and then twice *weekly* for prevention. Alternatively, for more diffuse atopic dermatitis a more practical maintenance therapy may include twice daily use of a low-potency topical steroid

TABLE 60.1

DIFFERENTIAL DIAGNOSIS OF ECZEMATOUS RASH

Allergy
Atopic dermatitis
Allergic contact dermatitis
Autoeczematization
Drug reaction
Photoallergic reaction
Irritant
Irritant contact dermatitis
Lichen simplex chronicus
Nummular eczema
Asteatotic eczema
Dyshidrotic eczema (pompholyx)
Intertrigo
Frictional lichenoid dermatitis
Immunologic
Wiskott–Aldrich syndrome
Hyperimmunoglobulin E syndrome
Omenn syndrome
Severe combined immunodeficiency
Graft-versus-host disease
Agammaglobulinemia
Immune dysregulation, polyendocrinopathy, enteropathy, X-linked (IPEX)
Infectious
Seborrheic dermatitis
Dermatophyte infection
Scabies
Molluscum contagiosum
Pityriasis rosea
Human immunodeficiency virus
Oncologic
Histiocytosis (Letterer–Siwe)
Cutaneous T-cell lymphoma
Leukemia and lymphoma
Nutritional
Acrodermatitis enteropathica
Pellagra
Kwashiorkor
Other
Psoriasis
Erythroderma[a] (Table 60.4)
Netherton syndrome
Ichthyosis

[a]Potentially acute life-threatening condition.

compounded into a thick emollient (e.g., hydrocortisone 2.5% ointment mixed 1:1 with petrolatum). Referral to dermatology and/or allergy may be helpful to further manage moderate or severe atopic dermatitis. Particularly severe or persistent dermatitis should prompt consideration of an underlying systemic disorder associated with eczematous eruptions such as immunodeficiencies or nutritional deficiencies.

TABLE 60.2

AMERICAN ACADEMY OF DERMATOLOGY CONSENSUS CONFERENCE FEATURES OF ATOPIC DERMATITIS

Essential features (must be present)
Pruritus
Eczematous skin changes with chronic or recurring history, typical morphology, and distribution
■ Face, neck, extensor involvement in infants and children
■ Flexural lesions in any age group
■ Sparing of groin and axillary regions
Important features (seen in most cases, support the diagnosis)
Early age at diagnosis
Personal or family history of atopy
Immunoglobulin E reactivity
Associated features
Atypical vascular responses (e.g., facial pallor, white dermographism, delayed blanch response)
Keratosis pilaris/hyperlinear palms/ichthyosis/pityriasis alba
Ocular/periorbital changes
Other regional findings (e.g., perioral changes/periauricular lesions)
Perifollicular accentuation/lichenification/prurigo lesions

From Eichenfield LF, Tom WL, Chamlin SL, et al. Guidelines of care for the management of atopic dermatitis: section 1. Diagnosis and assessment of atopic dermatitis. *J Am Acad Dermatol* 2014;70(2):338–351.

Nummular Eczema

Nummular eczema presents as coin-shaped plaques that are erythematous and contain tiny vesicles, crusts, and at times, excoriations. Lesions occur on the extensor surfaces of the hands, arms, and legs (Fig. 60.2). They may be single or multiple and are often symmetric. Nummular eczema can be related to dry skin and atopy. Differential diagnosis includes dermatophyte infection, impetigo, and contact dermatitis (such as nickel in school chairs or desks).

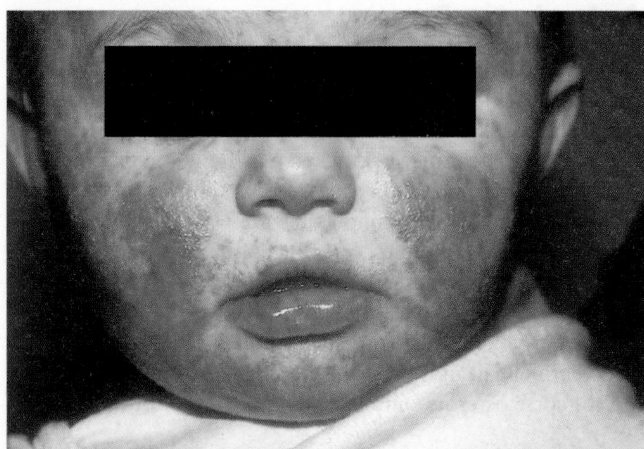

FIGURE 60.1 Infant with atopic dermatitis on the cheeks. (From Goodheart HP. *Goodheart's photoguide to common skin disorders.* Philadelphia, PA: Wolters Kluwer Health Lippincott Williams & Wilkins, 2009:52.)

SIGNS AND SYMPTOMS

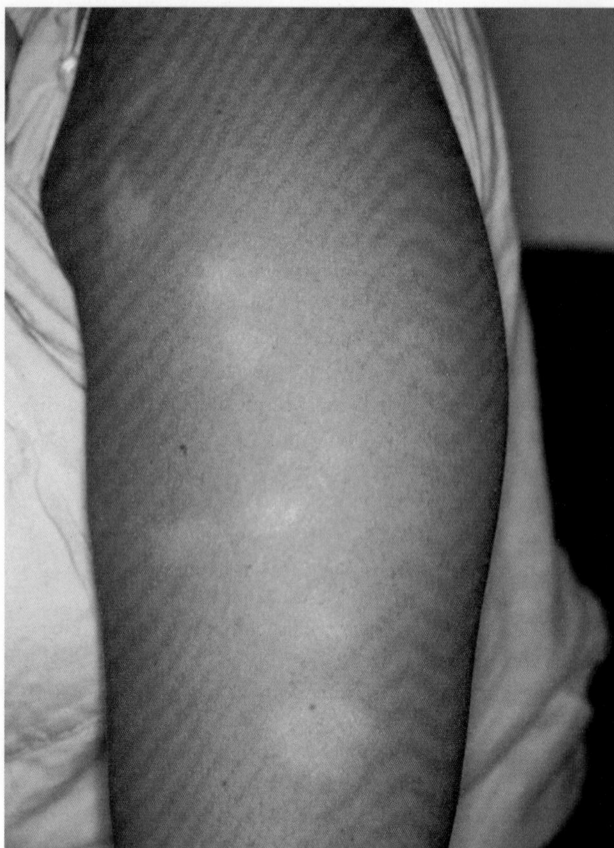

FIGURE 60.2 Nummular dermatitis. (From Lugo-Somolinos A, McKinley-Grant L, Goldsmith LA, et al. *VisualDx: essential dermatology in pigmented skin.* Philadelphia, PA: Lippincott Williams and Wilkins, 2011.)

Acute management of nummular eczema involves ruling out any coexistent superinfection with a bacterial culture from any eroded, crusted, pustular, or painful lesions along with potent topical steroids. Maintenance strategies include using daily petrolatum-based barrier ointments along with intermittent potent topical steroid use (e.g., twice weekly) for prevention.

Asteatotic Eczema

Asteatotic eczema, also called *winter eczema, xerotic eczema,* and *eczema craquele,* is a pruritic condition in which the skin is dry and cracked with red fissures and scale (Fig. 60.3). The skin has the appearance of cracked porcelain and patients may complain of burning and redness upon application of lotions or creams. The most common sites are the extensor surfaces. It tends to occur in adolescents during the winter and is associated with overbathing with drying soaps (often strongly scented body washes). Use of a gentle soap and petrolatum-based ointment or thick emollient applied twice daily is effective treatment in most cases. If needed, mid- to high-potency topical corticosteroid ointments could be used for flares.

Dyshidrotic Eczema

Dyshidrotic eczema, also called *pompholyx,* involves the hands and feet. There is sudden onset of pruritic, tiny, clustered, deep-seated vesicles that look like tapioca pearls (Fig. 60.4).

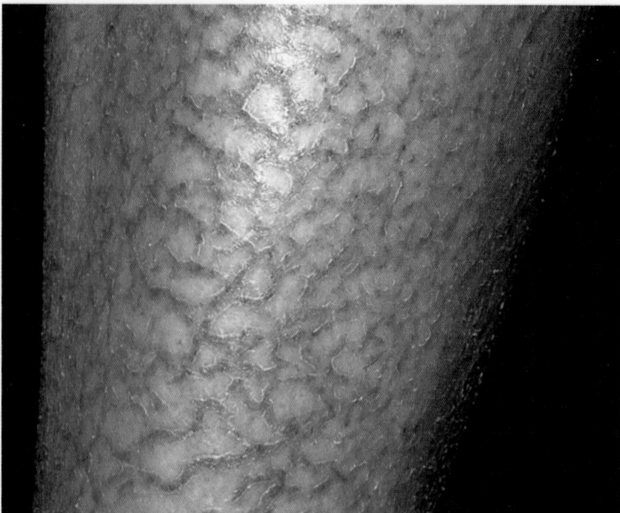

FIGURE 60.3 Asteatotic eczema. (From Goodheart HP. *Goodheart's photoguide of common skin disorders.* 2nd ed. Philadelphia, PA: Lippincott Williams & Wilkins, 2003.)

With time, scaling, lichenification, and painful fissures occur. Lesions appear on the palms, soles, and lateral digits. The process may be acute, chronic, or recurrent. It may be associated with hyperhidrosis and may also occur as a form of an Id reaction (autoeczematization) in the setting of a remote contact dermatitis or tinea capitis. Approximately 50% of patients have an atopic background. Acute presentations may be treated with thick emollients and potent topical corticosteroids, which can be applied under white cotton gloves nightly, if needed, to increase efficacy.

Lichen Simplex Chronicus

Lichen simplex chronicus refers to a chronic, localized lesion resulting from repeated rubbing and scratching. It has a predilection for the sites that are easily reached, such as the arms, legs, ankles, neck, and the anogenital area. It is rare in young children but fairly common in adolescents and adults. It may occur in a pre-existing area affected by dermatitis. Typical

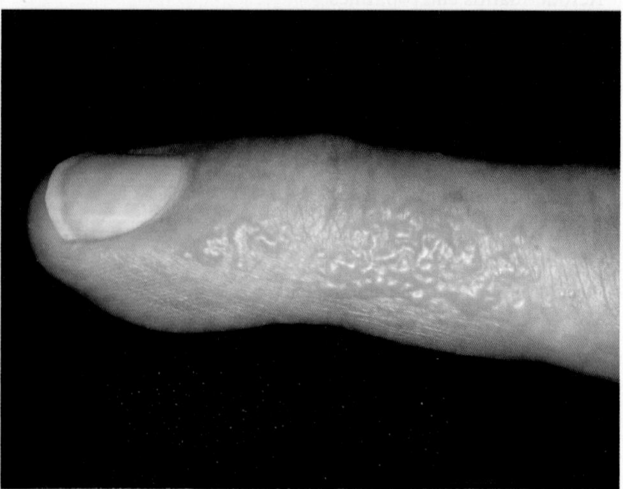

FIGURE 60.4 Dyshidrotic eczema. (From Craft N, Taylor E, Tumeh PC, et al. *VisualDx: essential adult dermatology.* Philadelphia, PA: Lippincott Williams & Wilkins, 2010.)

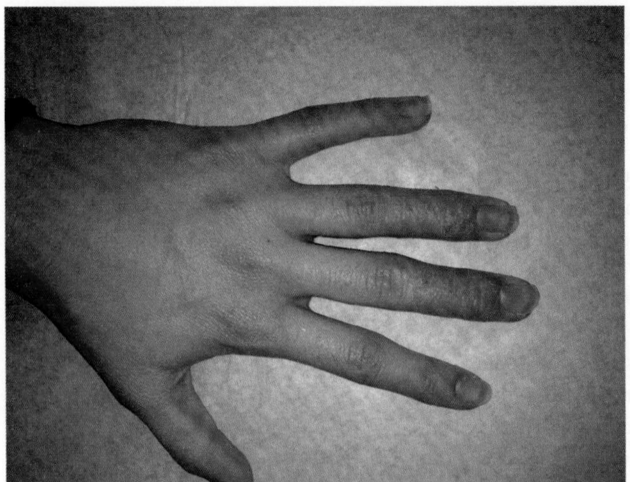

FIGURE 60.5 Contact dermatitis from a softball glove. Note the striking distribution of the dermatitis with a sharp cut-off on the third and fourth fingers corresponding to where the fingers contacted the inside of the glove.

lesions are single or multiple oval plaques from 5 to 15 cm in size. The skin is reddened and slightly edematous. Chronic lesions consist of well-demarcated areas of dry, thickened, scaly, hyperpigmented, or hypopigmented plaques. Intense pruritus is a hallmark and while topical corticosteroids can be effective, some lesions may respond best to occlusion with a corticosteroid-impregnated tape. Monitoring for signs of overuse including atrophy and striae is important while managing this chronic condition.

Contact Dermatitis

Contact dermatitis is an inflammatory reaction of the skin caused by an allergen (allergic contact dermatitis) or a primary irritant (irritant contact dermatitis). Acute eruptions have intense pruritus, severe erythema, edema, vesicles, and erosions with serous discharge and crusting (Fig. 60.5). A sharp demarcation between involved and unaffected skin along with a specific distribution may be a clue to this diagnosis. Subacute reactions have mild erythema, dry scale, less vesiculation, and mild thickening of the skin. Chronic exposures may result in lichenification, fissures, scales, excoriations, and hyperpigmentation. Itching, distribution, and the surface changes described above are key components that can help differentiate acute contact dermatitis from acute skin infections such as cellulitis.

Treatment of contact dermatitis includes avoidance of allergens or irritants and use of thick emollients and topical corticosteroids when needed. When oral corticosteroids are needed for severe or widespread contact dermatitis a longer treatment course with a slow taper over 14 days will decrease the risk for rebound dermatitis.

Allergic Contact Dermatitis

Allergic contact dermatitis is caused by a classic delayed T-cell–mediated hypersensitivity reaction (type IV). Repeated exposure causes an allergic sensitization. The eruption is delayed after the initial exposure for up to 7 to 10 days. Repeated exposures can cause the rapid appearance of an acute dermatitis

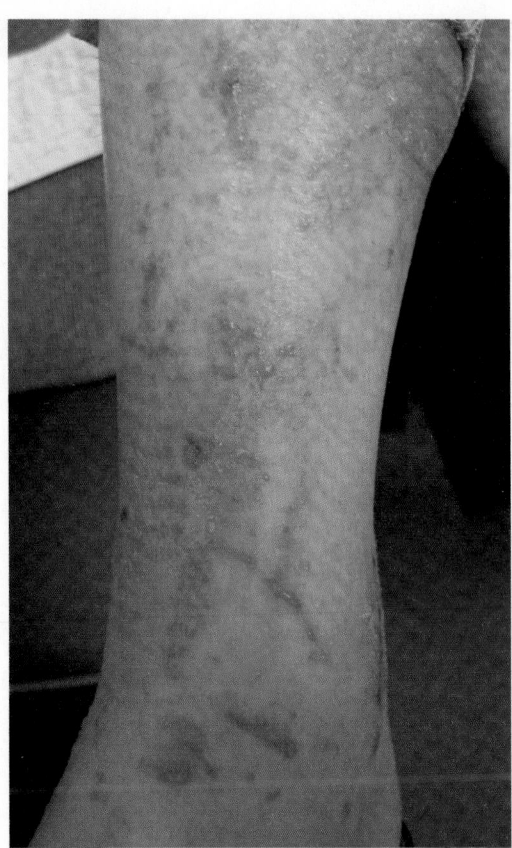

FIGURE 60.6 Allergic contact dermatitis caused by poison ivy. (From Stedman's Medical Dictionary. 28th ed. Philadelphia, PA: Lippincott Williams & Wilkins, 2005.)

(within 12 hours). Rhus dermatitis, caused by an oleoresin in the sap of poison ivy, poison oak, or poison sumac plants, is the most common cause of allergic contact dermatitis in the United States. Delayed exposure may occur because of contact with objects that have had contact with the plants (e.g., shoe laces, dogs). Typical presentation includes pruritus and erythema followed by development of papules, vesicles, and bullae, sometimes in a linear arrangement (Fig. 60.6). Burning of plants leads to aerosolization of the allergen, and may cause a widespread and severe outbreak on exposed skin surfaces including severe edema of the eyelids and lips in some cases. "Black dot poison ivy" can occur when a concentrated amount of the oleoresin gets deposited on the surface of the skin and oxidizes, creating a central black eschar surrounded by an acute dermatitis. This entity has been confused with a pigmented lesion or an insect bite. If possible, the black eschar should be removed by soaking or debridement to minimize spread of the resin. Other plants, flowers, pollens (especially ragweed), clothing, shoes, metals (e.g., nickel in jewelry), cosmetics, adhesive tape, and latex-containing products can also cause an allergic contact dermatitis. Nickel dermatitis occurs on earlobes as a result of nickel-containing earrings and on the abdomen due to pant buttons or belt buckles. Shoe dermatitis usually occurs on the dorsal surfaces of the feet, sparing interdigital spaces, in a symmetric manner.

Allergic contact dermatitis is rare in neonates because of their impaired ability to react to allergens. By 3 to 8 years of age, children react to allergens in a fashion similar to adults. The distribution, shape, pattern of the rash, and exposure history, may

TABLE 60.3

CAUSES OF CONTACT DERMATITIS

Allergen/irritant	Distribution
Poison ivy, oak, or sumac	Linear plaques with vesicles and crusting "Black dot poison ivy" (see above)
Nickel and cobalt	Lower abdomen (belt buckle, jean snaps); earlobe (earrings); preauricular and hands (cellphones)
Neomycin	Around wounds and abrasions
Nail polish (acrylates)	Eyelids
Fragrances (airborne)	Exposed surfaces including eyelids, face, upper chest, arms
Fragrances (in detergents)	Widespread under clothing
Dyes (in clothing)	Widespread under clothing
Disperse blue dye (in diapers)	Groin region in contact with blue dye
Car seat lining (irritant vs. allergic)	Occipital scalp, extensor elbows, posterior thighs, posterior lower legs
Mango peel	Perioral, hands
Wet wipes (methylisothiazolinone)	Perianal, groin, and perioral
Cocamidopropyl betaine (soaps and shampoos)	Widespread
Lanolin (found in emollients)	Widespread
Botanicals (found in many organic emollients)	Widespread
Rubber and leather (e.g., shoes)	Dorsal feet sparing, especially great toe. May affect soles.
Toilet seats (cleaning supplies)	Posterior thighs. May form ring including lateral and superior buttocks.
Sunscreens, fragrances (photoallergic contact dermatitis)	Photodistributed (face, chest, dorsal hands, and forearms)

elucidate the cause (Table 60.3). Newer contactants reported include blue dye in diapers and preservatives in wet wipes, which trigger an itchy diaper rash; toilet seat cleaning supplies triggering "*toilet seat dermatitis*" on the posterior thighs; and the vinyl lining of certain car seats which can cause "*car seat dermatitis*" on the outer elbows, posterior calves, and occipital scalp. Airborne processes (e.g., perfumes, body spray, spray deodorant) can trigger a rash on exposed surfaces, including eyelids, upper chest, distal arms, and legs. Photoallergic contact dermatitis occurs when an allergen is applied to the skin and exposed to the sun. Common agents implicated include phenothiazines, sulfonamides, thiazides, sunscreen components such as PABA, and some fragrances.

Irritant Contact Dermatitis

A primary irritant dermatitis is a nonallergic reaction of the skin caused by a single exposure or repeated contact with an irritating substance. Strong soaps and detergents, acidic juices, saliva, urine, stool contents, fiberglass particles, and bubble baths are common causes in children. *Lip licker's dermatitis* occurs as a result of excessive drooling, lip smacking, or lip licking, typically presenting as a sharply demarcated rash around the mouth. *Juvenile plantar dermatosis* is a form of irritant contact dermatitis resulting from exposure to wetness (e.g., sweat) and occlusive footwear without socks (e.g., flip-flops). This presents with extensive skin fissuring and glazed appearance of the planter surface of the foot. It may be treated with emollients, topical steroids, and breathable socks. *Frictional lichenoid dermatitis* is likely related to repeated rubbing and presents as shiny papules on the elbows, knees, and back of the hands, and occurs more frequently in individuals with atopic dermatitis. This condition is usually noted incidentally and is asymptomatic. Treatment of the above conditions includes minimizing contact with the primary irritants, frequent application of petroleum-based barrier ointments, and topical corticosteroids when needed.

Autoeczematization

Autoeczematization, or an Id reaction, occurs in the presence of an allergic contact dermatitis. The patient later develops a more extensive monomorphous papular eruption often accentuated on the extensor aspects of the elbows and knees as a result of autosensitization. A specialized form of this process is seen with dermatophyte infection—in particular, tinea capitis—and is called a *dermatophytid*. Dermatophytid reactions can be widespread on the head, neck, and body and are seen most commonly within the first week after initiating oral antifungal therapy for tinea capitis. Treatment of Id reactions includes removal or treatment of the inciting agent (allergen or tinea) and topical steroids for itching.

Scabies

The eruption of scabies is polymorphic, with papules, vesicles, nodules, excoriations, crusts, and eczematous plaques (Fig. 60.7). Only a small percentage of pediatric patients have the classically described linear tracts or burrows. *Norwegian or crusted scabies,* a severe form usually seen in immunosuppressed patients, is characterized by heavy crusting and hyperkeratosis. Infants may have similarly severe infestations, possibly related to a delay in diagnosis or use of topical steroids in a mistaken attempt to treat what was believed to be an atopic process.

Infants and young children have lesions accentuated on the axillae, diaper region, face, and scalp. The lesions may become generalized. Older children and adults tend to have involvement of the finger webs, flexural regions, breasts, and

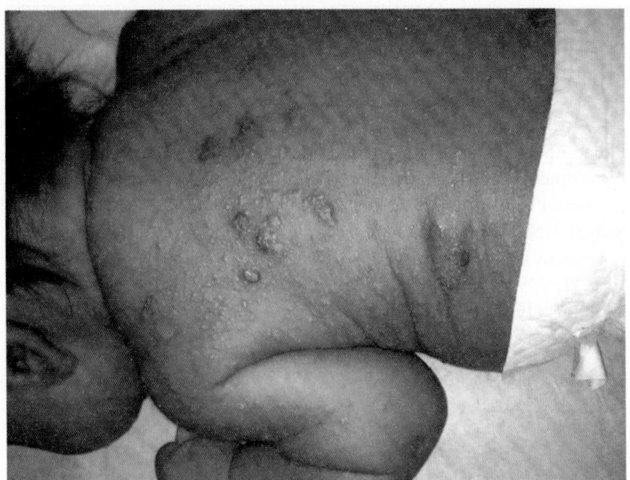

FIGURE 60.7 Scabies in an infant. Note the polymorphous appearance with widespread papules and clustered nodules with overlying scale and crust.

genital area. Diagnosis is confirmed by visualization of the mites, eggs, or fecal pellets from skin lesion scrapings. However, despite excellent specificity, a high false-negative rate exists. Diagnosis in the absence of confirmed mites is based on clinical features. Treatment consists of permethrin 5% cream applied overnight for the patient and any household contacts with a repeat treatment 1 week later. For infants over 8 weeks old it is recommended that the cream be applied to the head and neck as well as the body with careful attention to avoid the eyes, nose, and mouth. Bed linens and any fomites should be cleaned or wrapped in an airtight plastic bag for 1 week. Of note, the recommended treatment for infants under 8 weeks old is precipitated sulfur in petrolatum, however permethrin 5% cream has been used in this population without apparent major side effects.

Erythroderma

Erythroderma is a condition characterized by widespread erythema affecting >90% body surface area with (Fig. 60.8) or without overlying scale. Erythroderma may present acutely or subacutely and may be associated with fever, chills, or rigors. There are several possible triggers (Table 60.4) and erythroderma can be life-threatening if left untreated. In the acute phase, erythroderma can be complicated by temperature instability, electrolyte disturbances, fluid losses through the skin, high-output heart failure, pneumonia, and sepsis. Erythroderma may represent a severe form of a primary dermatologic condition (e.g., atopic dermatitis, psoriasis) or may be a sign of an underlying systemic disease (e.g., systemic drug reaction, staphylococcal-scalded skin syndrome, toxic shock syndrome).

Management of erythroderma includes identifying an underlying cause, supportive care, and often hospitalization. Blood work could include complete blood count with differential, comprehensive metabolic panel and more depending on the clinical scenario. Of note, a careful history should include screening for any high-risk medications that could trigger a systemic drug reaction, such as drug reaction with eosinophilia and systemic symptoms (DRESS) syndrome. DRESS present 10 to 14 days after starting a medication with a widespread morbilliform eruption that can progress to erythroderma within

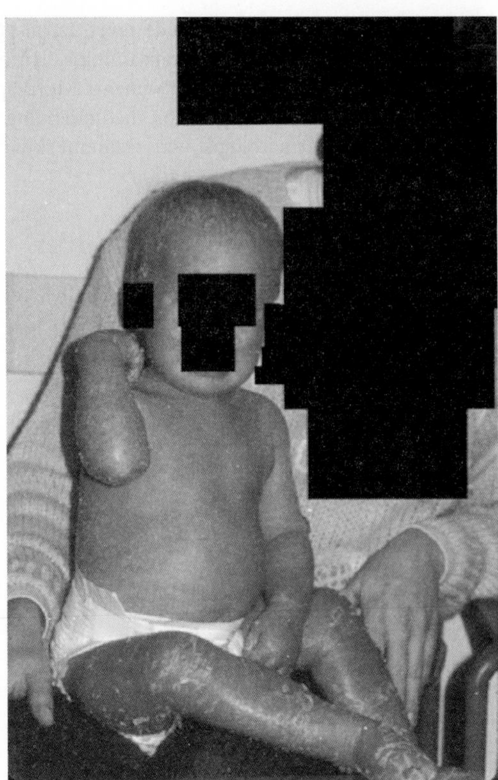

FIGURE 60.8 Erythroderma and scaling in an infant with immunodeficiency.

TABLE 60.4

CAUSES OF ERYTHRODERMA

Erythroderma with scale
Atopic dermatitis
Seborrheic dermatitis
Contact dermatitis
Psoriasis
Ichthyosis
Pityriasis rubra pilaris
Drug reactions (e.g., drug reaction with eosinophilia and systemic symptoms)
Immunodeficiencies (e.g., severe combined immunodeficiency)
Graft-versus-host disease
Cutaneous T-cell lymphoma
Kwashiorkor
Erythroderma without scale
Toxic shock syndrome
Staphylococcal-scalded skin syndrome (early)
Kawasaki disease (early accentuation in groin)
Erythroderma with blistering
Stevens–Johnson syndrome
Toxic epidermal necrolysis
Staphylococcal-scalded skin syndrome
Epidermolytic ichthyosis
Diffuse cutaneous mastocytosis/bullous mastocytosis
Pemphigus vulgaris or foliaceous

hours to days; additional features include fever, facial edema, eosinophilia, atypical lymphocytosis, transaminitis, lymphadenopathy, and rarely other visceral involvement. More specific treatment of erythroderma will depend on the underlying cause and consultation with a dermatologist with resultant skin biopsy may be needed to gather further information.

Suggested Readings and Key References

Admani S, Jacob SE. Allergic contact dermatitis in children: review of the past decade. *Curr Allergy Asthma Rep* 2014;14(4):421.

Krakowski AC, Eichenfield LF, Dohil MA. Management of atopic dermatitis in the pediatric population. *Pediatrics* 2008;122:812–824.

Noguera-Morel L, Hernández-Martín Á, Torrelo A. Cutaneous drug reactions in the pediatric population. *Pediatr Clin North Am* 2014; 61(2):403–426.

Paller AS, Simpson EL, Eichenfield LF, et al. Treatment strategies for atopic dermatitis: optimizing the available therapeutic options. *Semin Cutan Med Surg* 2012;31(3 suppl):S10–S17.

Sehgal VN, Srivastava G. Erythroderma/generalized exfoliative dermatitis in pediatric practice: an overview. *Int J Dermatol* 2006;45: 831–839.

Williams HC. Atopic dermatitis. *N Engl J Med* 2005;352:2314–2324.

CHAPTER 61 ■ RASH: BACTERIAL AND FUNGAL INFECTIONS

JAMES R. TREAT, MD

BACTERIAL INFECTIONS

Pustular Eruptions

Folliculitis

Folliculitis presents with pustules and red papules that are centered around hair follicles due to bacterial invasion of the follicle (Fig. 61.1). The infection is sometimes itchy but can be painful. When excoriated, the pustules may be unroofed and eroded, or crusted papules may predominate. Folliculitis can be widespread but is often concentrated in hair-bearing areas. Cultures of pustules prove the diagnosis, establish bacterial sensitivities, and guide therapy. Folliculitis is most commonly caused by *Staphylococcus aureus* (SA). Group A *Streptococcus* (GAS) causes folliculitis as well but may present with intermixed pustules, vesicles, and erosions.

Pseudomonas aeruginosa can survive in recirculated water and causes "hot tub" folliculitis. Pseudomonas infections from hot tubs or other recirculating water often present under the clothing where the bacteria get trapped. Therapy with antibacterial washes and topical antibiotics directed at *P. aeruginosa,* such as silver sulfadiazine, bacitracin/polymyxin B, gentamicin or neomycin, are often sufficient. For more widespread or symptomatic infections or those in immunocompromised hosts, systemic therapy with ciprofloxacin (off-label) should be considered.

Gram-negative folliculitis can be confused with acne; it can occur on the face and presents in adolescents with pustules, especially around the mouth. The differential diagnosis of bacterial folliculitis includes other nonbacterial causes of folliculitis such as *pityrosporum* yeast infections, especially on the upper trunk and neck of adolescents, or miliaria (heat rash) in patients who are sweating. Patients who are immunodeficient can have folliculitis due to gram-negative bacteria, disseminated yeast, and mold infections. Performing a swab culture of the pus expressed from an intact pustule establishes the diagnosis and guide therapy.

It is very important to recognize that vesicular eruption of herpes simplex virus (HSV) or varicella zoster virus (VZV) can also look pustular if the eruption has been present for a few days. Neutrophils infiltrate the vesicles and make them look pustular. Therefore, in neonates with pustular eruptions, and any child with recurrent localized areas of grouped pustules, HSV should be considered.

Disseminated *Gonococcal* Infections (See also Chapter 102 Infectious Disease Emergencies)

Localized genitourinary or oral infection with *Neisseria gonorrhoeae* can rarely disseminate to the skin, presenting with erythematous papules, petechiae, or vesicle-pustules on a hemorrhagic base. These cutaneous lesions usually develop on the trunk but may occur anywhere on the extremities. Disseminated *N. gonorrhoeae* should be considered in sexually active or sexually abused children, especially if the partner has a history of vaginal or penile discharge.

Diagnosis can be made by culture of vesiculopustular skin lesions, blood culture, or positive culture of oral or genital sites. Gram stains of pustules show gram-negative diplococci and can help support the clinical diagnosis, although *Neisseria meningitidis* may have the same appearance on Gram stain. Based on resistance patterns, recommended current therapy is ceftriaxone until clinical improvement is seen, at which point it can be changed to an oral antibiotic, such as cefixime, ciprofloxacin, ofloxacin, or levofloxacin, for a total of a 7-day course. Quinolones should not be used for infections in men who have intercourse with men or in those with a history of recent foreign travel or partners' travel, or infections acquired in other areas with increased resistance. Concomitant sexually transmitted diseases should be tested for and treated empirically.

Furunculosis

Furunculosis is an acute purulent abscess extending from the dermis into the subcutis. Furuncles manifest as painful red or purple fluctuant nodules with or without a pustule on top (Fig. 61.2). Furunculosis is most commonly caused by SA and can be methicillin sensitive or resistant (MRSA). Diagnosis is clinical but can be aided by ultrasound if it is unclear if there is fluctuance. Therapy is with incision and drainage and adding antibiotic coverage is controversial. The literature suggests antibiotics are not necessary for simple abscesses except in young children unless there is associated cellulitis, the lesion has failed incision and drainage previously, the patient is immunosuppressed or showing signs of sepsis, or the lesion is particularly difficult to drain. Cultures can be sent from the purulent drainage in order to confirm the diagnosis and measure the antibiotic sensitivities. Empiric therapy should be guided by local resistance patterns but is usually with clindamycin, trimethoprim-sulfamethoxazole, or doxycycline (if age appropriate) in order to cover for MRSA.

Recurrence of furunculosis is common. Reinfection from the patient's local environment can come from sources such as close contacts, pets, athletic equipment, or stuffed animals. Reinfection may occur because of reinoculation from the patient's own nares. Decolonization is challenging but nasal decolonization with intranasal mupirocin two times daily for 5 days for the patient and any close contacts can be effective. Four percent chlorhexidine washes or dilute sodium hypochlorite (¼ cup in 20 to 40 gallons of water for 15 minutes) baths can be used to decolonize the skin but caution in young children to assure they do not ingest or get the cleanser on the mucosa.

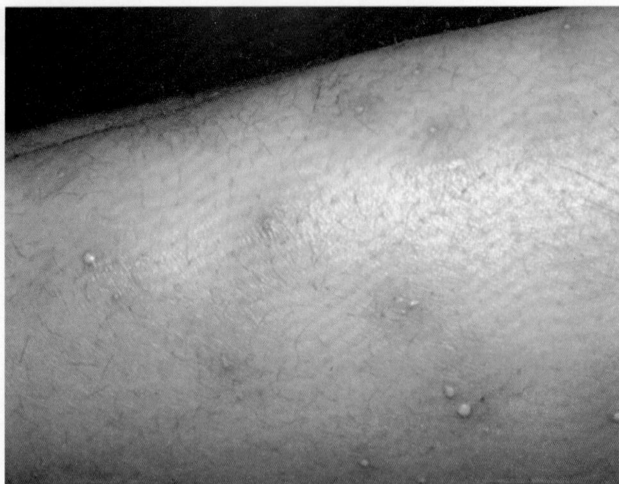

FIGURE 61.1 Folliculitis. (From Burkhart C, Morrell D, Goldsmith LA, et al. *Essential pediatric dermatology*. Philadelphia, PA: Lippincott Williams & Wilkins, 2009.)

Bullous Impetigo

Bullous impetigo is caused by a localized staphylococcal infection that produces an exfoliative toxin that cleaves the skin connection desmoglein 1 (DGS1). This allows fluid to build up within the epidermis and forms bullae (Fig. 61.3). When the bullae rupture, the roof of the bulla and the fluid dries to the skin giving the classic "honey-colored" crusting. SA colonization is most common in the nares and perianal areas and thus impetigo is more common on the face and perineum. Culture of the blister fluid will yield the pathogen and establish sensitivities for therapy. Localized bullous impetigo can often be treated with topical antibiotics such as mupirocin, bacitracin, or retapamulin. More widespread or severe infections or those in immunosuppressed hosts or neonates should be treated systemically.

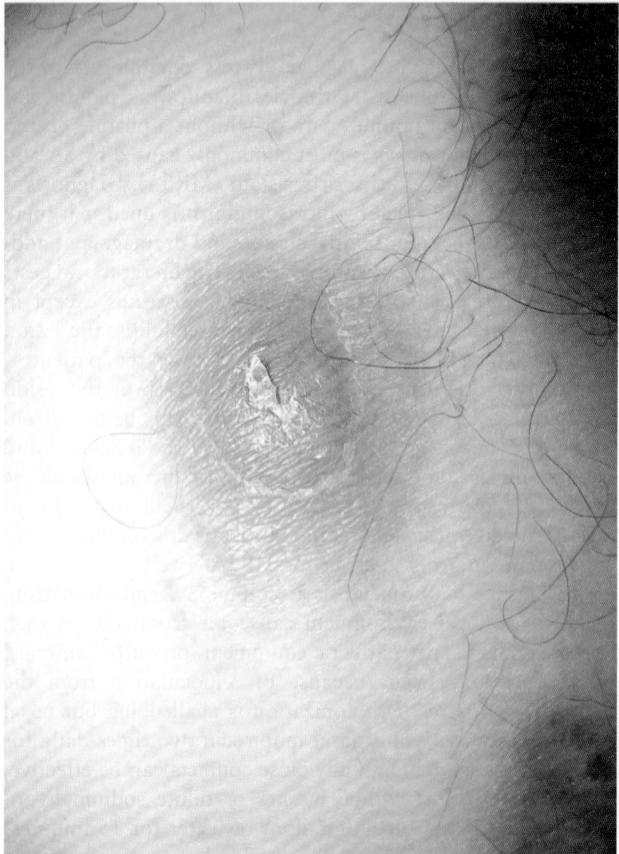

FIGURE 61.2 Furuncle. Note pustule with surrounding erythema and induration. (Image courtesy of Lee R. In: Elder DE, ed. *Lever's histopathology of the skin*. 11th ed. Philadelphia, PA: Wolters Kluwer, 2014.)

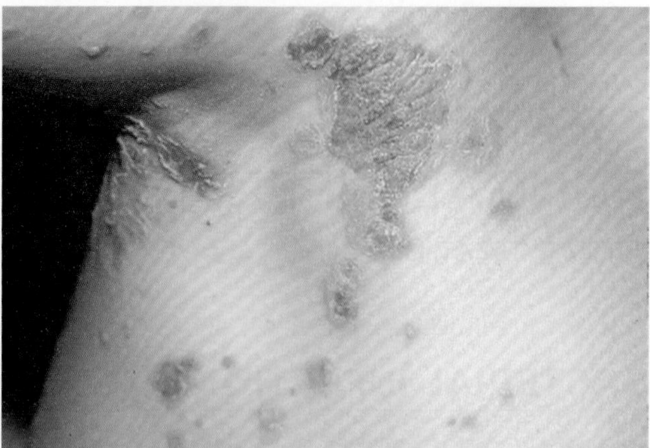

FIGURE 61.3 Bullous impetigo. (From Goodheart HP. *Goodheart's photoguide of common skin disorders*. 2nd ed. Philadelphia, PA: Lippincott Williams & Wilkins, 2003.)

Staphylococcal-Scalded Skin Syndrome

Staphylococcal-scalded skin syndrome (SSSS) is a severe infection resulting from dissemination of the exfoliative toxin produced by SA. SSSS is most common in children under 5 years of age and can present in neonates. The clinical appearance is diffuse redness that parents commonly liken to a sunburn. The skin then peels most characteristically around the mouth, nose, and eyes. Although the crusting and peeling is most prominent in these periorificial areas and can be exuberant, the actual conjunctiva and oral mucosa are not affected. Peeling is also typically prominent in the neck, axillary, and inguinal folds (Fig. 61.4). If the red skin is rubbed, a blister can often be induced (Nikolsky sign). The main clinical differential is Stevens–Johnson syndrome (SJS), which by definition must affect two mucous membranes. In the mucosa, desmoglein 3 is

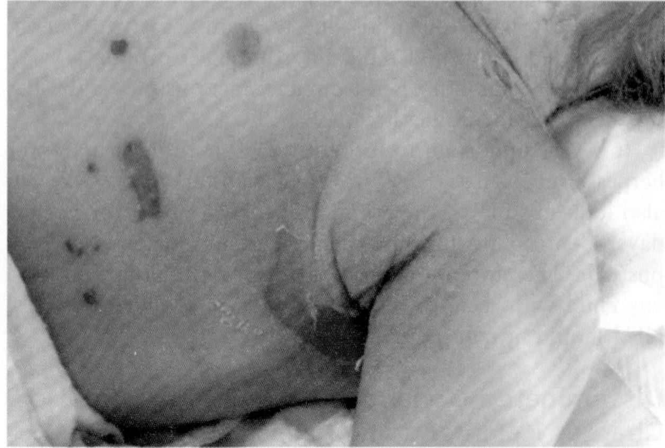

FIGURE 61.4 Staphylococcal-scalded skin syndrome. Note the scalded appearance of the skin under the ruptured bullae of the chest and axilla in this child with staphylococcal-scalded skin syndrome. (From Lippincott Nursing Assessment. February 2014. Philadelphia, PA: Wolters Kluwer, 2014.)

more important in keratinocyte cell–cell adhesion than DSG1. The exfoliative toxin only targets DSG1 and so the mucosa is spared in SSSS. Therefore, the most reliable way of differentiating SSSS from SJS is the lack of mucosal involvement in SSSS. Kawasaki can also cause peeling skin, especially on the hands and feet, but the peeling occurs at least 10 to 14 days after the initial febrile episode, while the exfoliation in SSSS occurs within the first few days of the onset of the illness.

The primary site of the staphylococcal infection is often unknown but recent surgeries (umbilical cord or circumcision in neonates) or other breaks in the skin should be evaluated and cultured. If no clear source of infection can be found, the nares and anus and most heavily crusted areas should be cultured in order to establish antibiotic sensitivities of the SA that is colonizing the child. Therapy for SSSS is with systemic antistaphylococcal antibiotics, typically oxacillin or other beta lactamase–resistant antibiotics. Clindamycin is often added because it inhibits bacterial ribosomal function, thus decreasing toxin formation. In critically ill patients vancomycin should be considered in case the infection is being caused by a resistant staphylococcal strain.

Ecthyma

Ecthyma is a skin infection with loss of the top layers of the skin caused by necrosis. The most common cause of ecthyma in children is GAS and typically presents with painful crusts and erosions (Fig. 61.5). Ecthyma gangrenosum is a term typically reserved for a pseudomonas infection that presents with a painful purple papule or nodule that quickly ulcerates with expanding redness. Pseudomonas ecthyma should not occur in normal hosts so if the diagnosis is made, the patient requires a workup as this can be a presentation of a malignancy or other immunosuppression. Other bacteria and opportunistic fungi may cause lesions of ecthyma in immunosuppressed children. Therefore, culture is vital to establish a diagnosis. Therapy should be guided by cultures but empiric broad-spectrum gram-positive and gram-negative coverage should be started immediately for suspected ecthyma gangrenosum in immunosuppressed patients. Consideration should also be given to starting an antifungal agent such as amphotericin and double-covering pseudomonas depending on the degree of immunosuppression and clinical appearance.

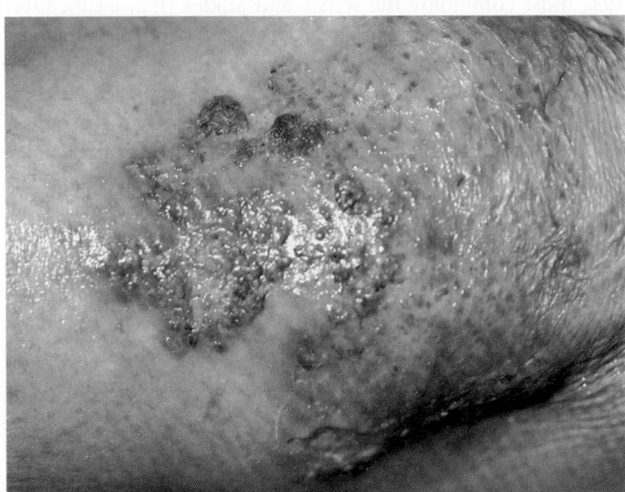

FIGURE 61.5 Ecthyma. Ecthyma with eroded, red papules with accompanying erosions and crust. (From Craft N, Fox LP, Goldsmith LA, et al. *Essential adult dermatology*. Philadelphia, PA: Lippincott Williams & Wilkins, 2010.)

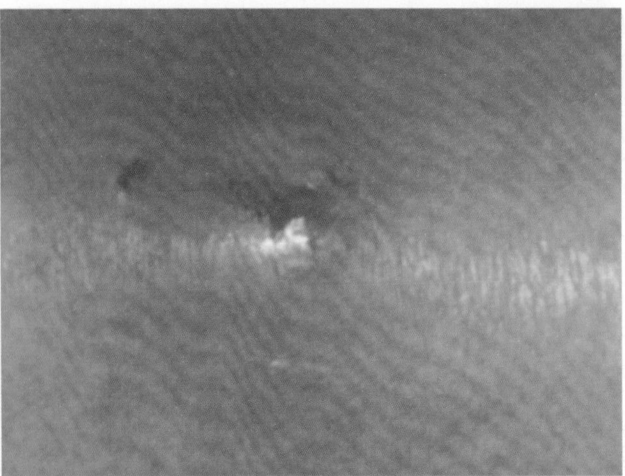

FIGURE 61.6 Erysipelas. (From Frontera WR. *FIMS sports medicine manual*. Philadelphia, PA: Lippincott Williams & Wilkins, 2011.)

Cellulitis

Cellulitis is the acute presentation of red, painful, swollen skin that is caused by a localized bacterial infection in the dermis and subcutaneous tissue. There may have been a break in the skin that leads to the infection but the infection then spreads underneath the skin. Because the infection is within the skin, it is difficult to culture the pathogen. Leading edge cultures have a low yield so most patients are treated empirically. Patients with disruption of the skin barrier (e.g., tinea pedis or atopic dermatitis) or lymphatic disruption (postsurgical or from a congenital lymphatic abnormality) have a higher risk of cellulitis. Erysipelas is a type of cellulitis that presents with swollen, red, painful edematous plaques due to infection of the superficial dermal lymphatics (Fig. 61.6). In erysipelas, there is often a step-off from affected edematous to normal skin. The differential diagnosis of cellulitis includes contact dermatitis. Contact dermatitis is often multifocal and itchy. Looking for linear areas of redness or vesiculation can help favor a contact allergy. Acute contact dermatitis of the face is often misdiagnosed as orbital or periorbital cellulitis. Usually contact dermatitis is less painful to touch, may have crusting overlying the rash, and fever and eye pain should be absent.

The most common causes for cellulitis are GAS and SA (erysipelas is only caused by GAS). *Vibrio vulnificus,* often due to exposure to infected oysters or salt water, is a rare cause of bullous, often purpuric cellulitis. Culture of blister fluid may yield the pathogen. Erysipeloid is a localized eruption of purple macules and patches often on the hands or other exposed areas caused by exposure to *Erysipelothrix rhusiopathiae,* often while handling raw chicken or fish (Fig. 61.7). Therapy of erysipeloid is with a first-generation cephalosporin such as cephalexin.

Secondary Infection of Inflamed Skin

Intertrigo describes inflamed, red skin folds that are a result of chronic irritation, yeast or bacteria. Streptococci or staphylococci can superinfect this inflamed skin and cause worsening pain, bright red erythema, and erosion in the skin fold. Intertrigo can be multifocal and common areas include the inguinal folds (in association with perianal streptococcal infection), or neck folds in infants where saliva is trapped

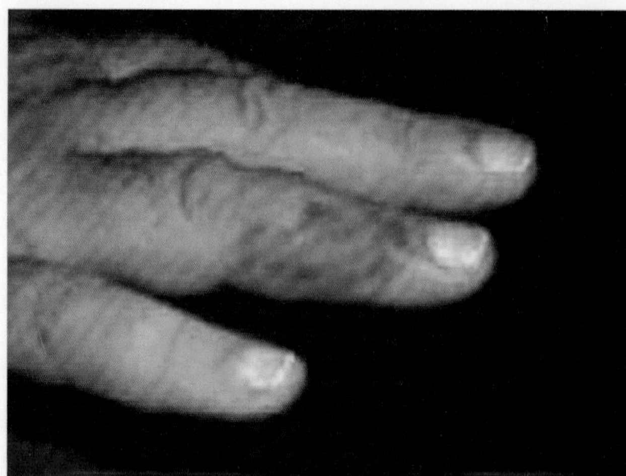

FIGURE 61.7 Erysipeloid. (From Betts RF, Chapman SW, Penn RL. *Reese and Betts' a practical approach to infectious diseases.* 5th ed. Philadelphia, PA: Lippincott Williams & Wilkins, 2002.)

(Fig. 61.8). Patients with atopic dermatitis are often colonized with SA and have downregulated innate immunity and so when scratched the skin can become readily infected. SA and GAS are the most common bacterial pathogens in superinfected atopic dermatitis. Clinically, there may be pustules or just honey-colored crusts and erosions.

Culture of the affected skin can yield the pathogen but caution is needed in interpreting these results as cultures will not differentiate colonization from true infection. Therapy with topical mupirocin or bacitracin is often effective for bacterial intertrigo but systemic antibiotics such as cephalexin or clindamycin can be used in more extensive cases.

OTHER PATHOGENS

Rocky Mountain Spotted Fever

Rocky Mountain spotted fever (RMSF), one of the most virulent infections identified in humans, is caused by *Rickettsia*

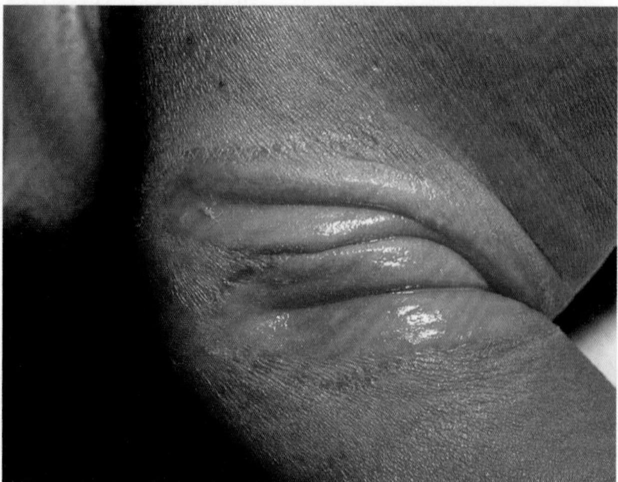

FIGURE 61.8 Intertrigo. PLEASE note, this is VERY likely a strep infection and not simple intertrigo. (From Burkhart C, Morrell D, Goldsmith LA, et al. *Essential pediatric dermatology.* Philadelphia, PA: Lippincott Williams & Wilkins, 2009.)

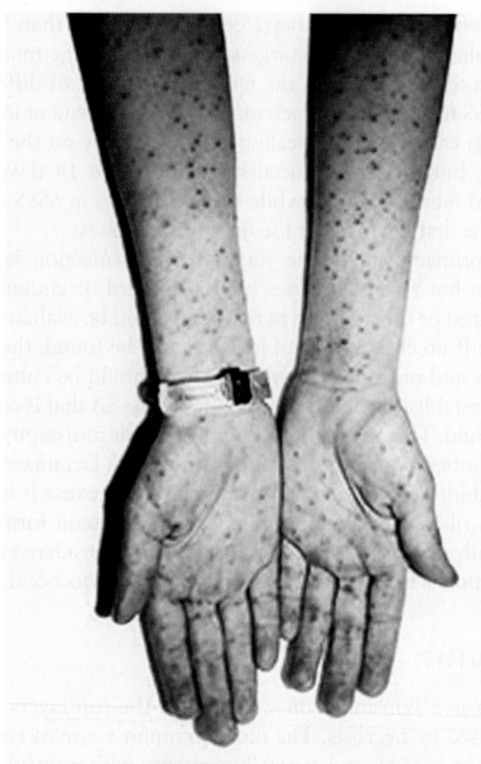

FIGURE 61.9 Rocky Mountain spotted fever. The rash starts on the wrists and ankles and spreads centripetally. (Courtesy of Sidney Sussman. In: Arndt KA, Hsu JT, Alam M, et al., eds. *Manual of dermatologic therapeutics.* 8th ed. Philadelphia, PA: Wolters Kluwer, 2014.)

rickettsii transmitted by the bite of a tick (see Chapters 96 Dermatologic Urgencies and Emergencies and 102 Infectious Disease Emergencies). Confirmed cases have been reported from all parts of the United States from varying tick vectors. RMSF is associated with a fatality rate of 5% with antimicrobial treatment and 13% to 40% without therapy. Patients who are treated with doxycycline by the fifth day of illness have the best survival.

The rash of RMSF begins on the third or fourth day of a febrile illness as a macular or papular eruption on the extremities, most commonly the wrists and ankles (Fig. 61.9). Over the next 2 days, the rash spreads typically to the palms and soles as well as centrally to involve the back, chest, and abdomen but still have an acral-predominant (arms, legs, palms, soles) distribution. Initially, the lesions are erythematous macules that then become more confluent and purpuric and can be papular. The severity of the rash is proportional to the severity of the disease.

All patients with RMSF have some degree of vasculitis that is the basis for many of the associated systemic symptoms. The patients are usually toxic appearing. Systemic signs and symptoms include fever, headache, myalgia, conjunctivitis, vomiting, seizures, myocarditis, heart failure, shock; periorbital, facial, or peripheral edema; and disseminated intravascular coagulation or purpura fulminans.

Most commonly, the diagnosis is based on clinical presentation with a history of potential tick exposure. The causative organism is not routinely cultured because of the danger to laboratory personnel. Diagnosis is best made by a serologic test such as indirect immunofluorescence antibody (IFA) assay.

Antibodies can be detected 7 to 10 days after onset of illness. Some reference laboratories are now offering polymerase chain reaction (PCR) testing. Thrombocytopenia, hyponatremia, and increased serum aminotransferase levels can develop as the disease progresses.

Doxycycline is the drug of choice for therapy in patients of all ages (despite its risk for potentially staining developing teeth) at a dose of 4 mg/kg/day in two divided doses (maximum of 100 mg bid), intravenously or orally. Chloramphenicol is a less optimal alternative and is not effective against ehrlichiosis, which can present similarly to RMSF. Therapy is continued until the patient is afebrile for at least 2 to 3 days (typically 7 to 10 days of antibiotic therapy).

Secondary Syphilis (See also Chapters 96 Dermatologic Urgencies and Emergencies and 102 Infectious Disease Emergencies)

Secondary syphilis is a widespread eruption that occurs due to dissemination of untreated primary syphilis. Manifestations of secondary syphilis usually occur 6 to 8 weeks after the appearance of the primary lesion, which is typically painless and so may have gone unnoticed. The rash of secondary syphilis is characterized by a generalized cutaneous eruption, usually composed of brownish, dull-red macules or papules that range in size from a few millimeters to 1 cm in diameter. They are generally discrete and symmetrically distributed, particularly over the trunk, where they follow the lines of cleavage in a pattern similar to pityriasis rosea. Papular lesions on the palms (Fig. 61.10) and soles, as well as the presence of systemic symptoms, such as general malaise, fever, headaches, sore throat, rhinorrhea, lacrimation, and generalized lymphadenopathy, help differentiate secondary syphilis. The exanthem extends rapidly and is usually pronounced and may be short lived or last months. One needs a high level of suspicion when viewing rashes in sexually active (or sexually abused) children to make the diagnosis of secondary syphilis.

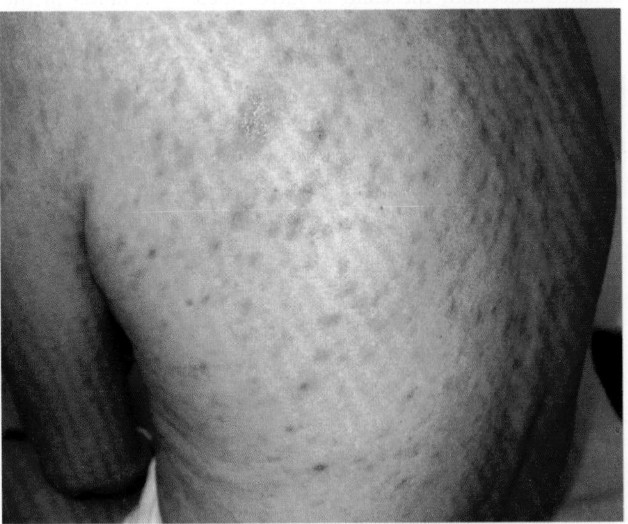

FIGURE 61.10 Secondary syphilis. (From Stedman's Medical Dictionary for the Health Professions and Nursing, Illustrated (Standard Edition). 6th ed. Philadelphia, PA: Lippincott Williams & Wilkins, 2007.)

Acquired syphilis is sexually contracted from direct contact with ulcerative lesions of the skin or mucous membranes of an infected individual. Diagnosis may be presumed after a positive nontreponemal test, such as the VDRL slide test, rapid plasma reagin test, or automated reagin test. Diagnosis should be confirmed by a treponemal test, such as the fluorescent treponemal antibody absorption test, the microhemagglutination test for *Treponema pallidum,* or the *T. pallidum* immobilization test. Penicillin is the treatment of choice unless contraindicated, in which case tetracycline, doxycycline, ceftriaxone, or erythromycin may be substituted. Length of therapy should be based on duration and stage of infection. Concomitant sexually transmitted diseases should be sought and treated empirically. HIV testing is recommended for patients with secondary syphilis.

FUNGAL INFECTIONS

Cutaneous fungal infections can be divided into a few clinical categories: dermatophytes, yeasts, deep fungal infections with cutaneous manifestations, and opportunistic fungal infections.

Dermatophytes (See also Chapter 96 Dermatologic Urgencies and Emergencies)

Dermatophytes are fungi that have a tropism for infecting skin, hair, and nails. The most common types are *Trichophyton* species, *Microsporum,* and *Epidermophyton* species. The specific types of infection are named for their body site of involvement because they can present differently based on location.

Tinea corporis presents with scaling patches that have a raised border (annular) (Fig. 61.11). Occasionally the fungi and resultant inflammation can cause blistering (bullous tinea). Tinea pedis can present with scaling around the base of the foot and often with extension in between the toes. Coincident onychomycosis is common and presents with toe nail thickening and subungual debris. Tinea manuum is the name for dermatophyte infection of the palms and is characterized by an extremely dry and sometimes fissured appearance that can mimic hand dermatitis. Often, patients with tinea manuum will have tinea pedis as well and present with both feet and one hand infected.

In North America, tinea capitis is most commonly caused by infection with *Trichophyton tonsurans* or *Microsporum canis.* Infection can manifest as scaling patches of alopecia, areas of distinct alopecia with broken hairs that manifest as "black dots" (Fig. 61.12), diffuse scaling with little alopecia, or an acute boggy plaque (kerion) (Fig. 61.13). Tinea capitis and other dermatophyte infections of hair-bearing areas (eyebrow, beard etc.) usually require systemic therapy since these are deeper infections of the hair shaft and follicle. Four to 8 weeks of griseofulvin (children over 2 years) or 2 to 6 weeks of terbinafine (children over 4 years) are commonly used therapies. In children under 2 years, oral fluconazole can be used, but topical therapy with an azole (e.g., clotrimazole) or an allylamine (e.g., terbinafine) may be effective if the hairs are fine.

Dermatophytes can be cultured by sending skin scrapings on a sterile tooth brush or in a sterile urine cup to the laboratory. Of note, some labs standardly perform a more broad fungal culture instead of a dermatophyte-specific culture.

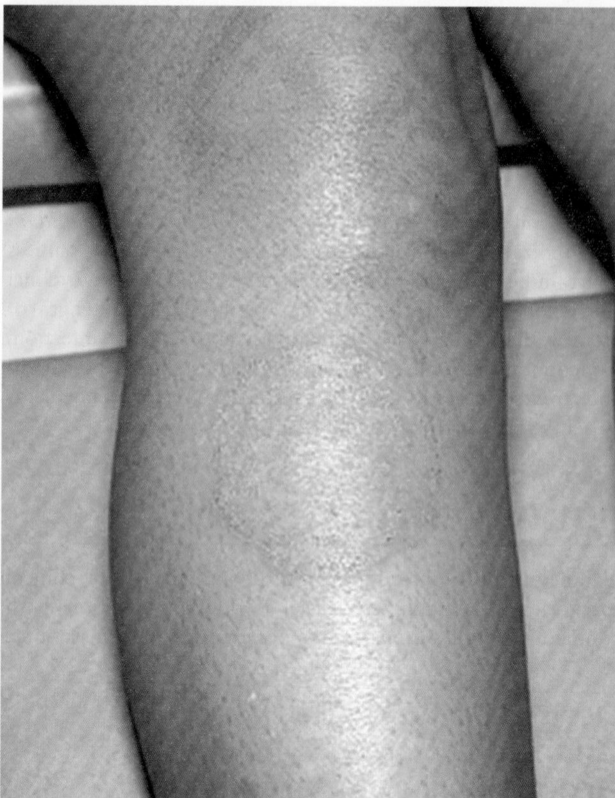

FIGURE 61.11 Tinea corporis (ringworm). Note the annular appearance, central clearing, and "active" scaly border that demonstrate hyphae on potassium hydroxide examination. (From Goodheart HP. *Goodheart's photoguide of common skin disorders*. 2nd ed. Philadelphia, PA: Lippincott Williams & Wilkins, 2003.)

Incidental, nonpathologic soil molds can grow on broader fungal cultures and the results must be interpreted with caution. Topical therapy for dermatophyte infections with azole agents such as clotrimazole or allylamines such as terbinafine is usually effective. In hair-bearing areas (scalp, beard, eyebrow) and nail infections, oral antifungals are usually needed to penetrate the hair follicle or nail. Tinea manuum and severe tinea pedis may also require oral antifungals due to the thickness of the stratum corneum.

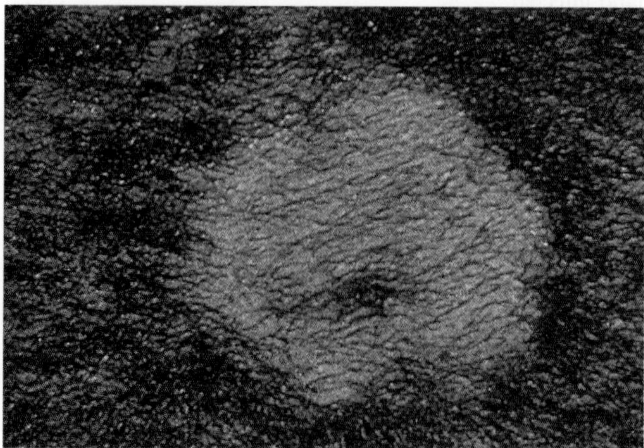

FIGURE 61.12 Tinea capitis. Alopecia with the "black dot" sign of broken hairs. (From Fleisher GR, Ludwig S, Baskin MN. *Atlas of pediatric emergency medicine*. Philadelphia, PA: Lippincott Williams & Wilkins, 2004.)

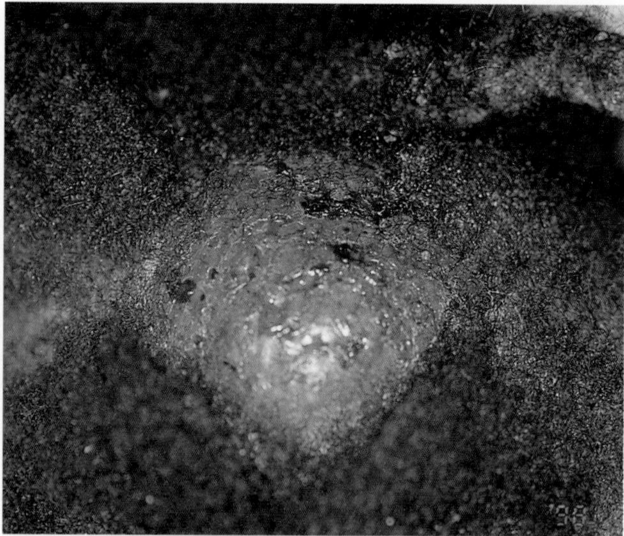

FIGURE 61.13 Tinea capitis with kerion. Note the boggy swelling from inflammation. (From Fleisher GR, Ludwig S, Baskin MN. *Atlas of pediatric emergency medicine*. Philadelphia, PA: Lippincott Williams & Wilkins, 2004.)

Candida Infections

Candida is a yeast that commonly superinfects inflamed, warm, moist skin. The typical clinical appearance is erythema in skin folds with pustules and peeling in the periphery (satellite pustules) (Fig. 61.14). Candidal infection of the oropharynx "thrush" presents with white papules and plaques that cannot be easily wiped off. Feeding may be painful. Thrush is common in young infants or after use of systemic antibiotics or steroids but in older children with no steroid or antibiotic exposure, it may be a marker of immunosuppression. Diagnosis is usually clinical but the white discharge can be cultured to prove the diagnosis. Therapy is with topical nystatin or clotrimazole troches (in older children) or oral fluconazole if severe.

Neonatal candida infections can be mild or severe depending on the age and weight of the child and the mode of infection. If there is premature rupture of membranes and an ascending candida infection, the child is surrounded by candida in the

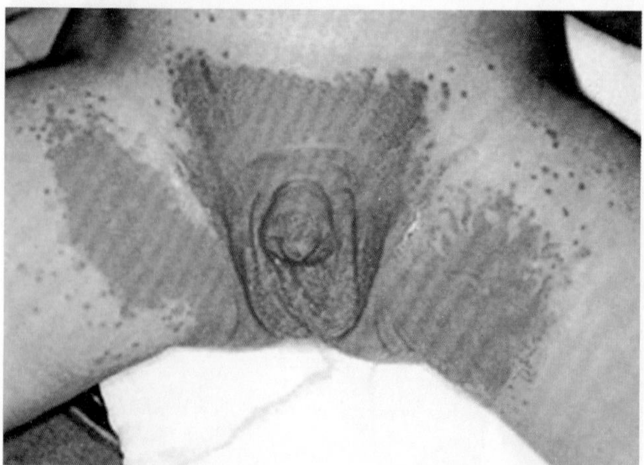

FIGURE 61.14 Candida infection. Note the intense confluent area of inflammation surrounded by discrete satellite lesions. (From Sauer GC, Hall JC. *Manual of skin diseases*. 7th ed. Philadelphia, PA: Lippincott-Raven, 1996.)

amniotic fluid. Infants may be born with broad redness that looks like a sunburn and then often develops superimposed pustules and then peels within a few days. This type of candida infection is severe and can be life-threatening, especially in children under 1,000 g. All children with congenital candidiasis should be evaluated for clinical signs of systemic infection and treated under the guidance of an infectious disease specialist. Those under 1,000 g should be treated systemically and evaluated for more widespread infection.

Localized candidal infections in healthy full-term infants often present in diaper, axillary, or other warm moist environments. In addition to therapy with topical antifungal agents, allowing the folds to dry is important to prevent reinfection.

Opportunistic Fungal Infections

There are some fungi and yeasts that should not grow in patients with normal immunity under normal circumstances. Therefore, infection with these opportunistic pathogens should warrant a workup for immunosuppression.

Fungi such as *Aspergillus* species, and molds such as *mucormycosis* (including *rhizopus* species), *fusarium* species, *alternaria*, and others can either cause infection by direct inoculation of the skin or by dissemination to the skin from a distant systemic infection in immunosuppressed patients. Infection through direct cutaneous inoculation presents with an eschar or deep purple nodule. The purple color is due to vascular invasion or infarction and can simulate a bruise. Infection is often at the site of trauma (including IV or surgical site). Localized infection with opportunistic fungi can also present as a pustular eruption if the fungus is present under occlusion such as tape or an armboard. It is vital to identify localized opportunistic fungal infections immediately to prevent dissemination. A biopsy with histopathologic evaluation and tissue culture can establish the diagnosis and fungal sensitivities. Since the cause of an erythematous or necrotic skin lesion in an immunosuppressed patient can be bacterial (gram negative or positive), viral, or fungal, a tissue Gram stain or frozen section from tissue biopsy can help make a rapid diagnosis. Patients with suspected opportunistic fungal infections should be treated with broad-spectrum antibiotics and antifungals under the guidance of an infectious disease specialist.

Deep Fungal Infections

Deep fungal infections are typically acquired as pulmonary infection through inhalation of the spores when the soil is disrupted and the spores are aerosolized. Cryptococcosis, histoplasmosis, blastomycosis, coccidioidomycosis, and paracoccidioidomycosis are common causes of deep fungal pulmonary infection in normal hosts in North America. This pulmonary infection can disseminate, or some of the spores can cause primary infection around the mouth. Primary infection is uncommon but presents with inflamed papules or nodules, often with crusting or erosion typically perioral, perinasal, or involving the oral mucosa. There also can be secondary reactive skin changes such as erythema nodosum (EN). EN is characterized by red, painful subcutaneous nodules, most specifically on the anterior shins. The nodules seem to be reactive and not truly infectious and there are many other causes of EN.

Deep fungal infections can also manifest as nodules or verrucous plaques when directly inoculated into the skin. Sporotrichosis often presents this way after direct inoculation of the fungus into the skin. The fungus *Sporothrix schenckii* lives on various plants and vegetation, including thorns (rose thorns), sphagnum moss, and carnations. Once inoculated into the skin, the fungus spreads along the lymphatic drainage (sporotrichoid pattern) up the affected arm or leg.

Diagnosis of cutaneous deep fungal infections is best proven with biopsy for histopathology and fungal culture. The specimen should also be sent for bacterial and mycobacterial culture since these can mimic deep fungal infections. Therapy is with systemic antifungals and should be guided by culture and infectious disease consultation depending on the specific fungus, extent of infection, and host factors such as immunosuppression.

Suggested Readings and Key References

Buckingham SC. Rocky Mountain spotted fever: a review for the pediatrician. *Pediatr Ann* 2002;31(3):163–168.

Demos M, McLeod MP, Nouri K. Recurrent furunculosis: a review of the literature. *Br J Dermatol* 2012;167(4):725–732.

Fritz SA, Camins BC, Eisenstein KA, et al. Effectiveness of measures to eradicate Staphylococcus aureus carriage in patients with community-associated skin and soft-tissue infections: a randomized trial. *Infect Control Hosp Epidemiol* 2011;32(9):872–880.

Hawkins DM, Smidt AC. Superficial fungal infections in children. *Pediatr Clin North Am* 2014;61(2):443–455.

Hussain S, Venepally M, Treat JR. Vesicles and pustules in the neonate. *Semin Perinatol* 2013;37(1):8–15.

Kress DW. Pediatric dermatology emergencies. *Curr Opin Pediatr* 2011;23(4):403–406.

Llera JL, Levy RC. Treatment of cutaneous abscess: a double-blind clinical study. *Ann Emerg Med* 1985;14(1):15–19.

Rivitti EA, Aoki V. Deep fungal infections in tropical countries. *Clin Dermatol* 1999;17(2):171–190.

CHAPTER 62 ■ RASH: VESICULOBULLOUS

MARISSA J. PERMAN, MD

Basic to all vesiculobullous (blistering) disorders is the disruption of cellular attachments. Blister formation, therefore, follows intracellular degeneration, intercellular edema (spongiosis), or damage to the anchoring structures associated with the basement membrane (hemidesmosomes, basal lamina, anchoring fibrils). The location of these changes can help the physician ascertain a specific diagnosis. When histologic information is not readily available or nondefinitive, however, the historical and clinical features of the case must be relied on. This chapter will discuss the following entities: infestations, mastocytosis, inherited blistering disorders, acquired autoimmune bullous disorders, friction blisters, and frostbite.

ACQUIRED BLISTERING ERUPTIONS

Infestations

Insect Bites

Insects generally bite exposed skin surfaces. Therefore, heaviest involvement occurs on the head, face, and extremities. Mosquito bites occur in the warm weather months, whereas flea (*Pulex irritans*) bites and bed bug (*Cimex lectularius*) bites occur throughout the year. Historical information includes contact with pets, recent camping trips, known exposure in close contacts, and involvement in outdoor activities. When blisters are present, the more characteristic urticarial papules are usually present in other locations, often clustered together or aligned linearly. This linear arrangement is often referred to as "breakfast, lunch, and dinner." The differential includes bullous impetigo which can easily be ruled out with a Gram stain or bacterial culture. In the case of bullous insect bites, the lesions should be negative for bacteria but can occasionally become secondarily infected.

If there is concern for flea bites, all pets should be evaluated by a professional. Bed bugs can be very difficult to locate but may be detected by turning on the lights in the middle of the night and inspecting along the mattress seams. Symptomatic treatment for insect bites includes mild to moderate potency topical corticosteroids and antihistamines such as diphenhydramine.

Scabies

While scabies in older children and adults most commonly presents as numerous ill-defined scaling, erythematous papules, interdigital scaling, and lesions in folds such as the umbilicus, groin, and axillae, infants and very young children can have vesiculobullous lesions on the palms (Fig. 62.1), soles, head, and face. It is important not to be misled by this distribution and appearance. Occasionally, the lesions can be nodular and often involve the genitals and axillae in young children. Generally, the parents or other close family contact are also infested and exhibit the typical appearance and pruritus of this disorder. First-line therapy for scabies includes permethrin cream (from the head down in infants, neck down in older children and adults) applied twice 1 week apart and washing all fomites in hot water followed by drying on high heat. Fomites not amenable to washing may be dry cleaned or placed in an air tight bag for several days. All close contacts should be treated. Ivermectin has also been used successfully.

Acropustulosis of Infancy

The appearance of pruritic vesicopustules in infants and young children on the palms and soles (Fig. 62.2), may also suggest acropustulosis of infancy. Vesicles often involve the lateral aspects of the fingers, palms, and soles. This condition was commonly misdiagnosed as dyshidrotic eczema in the past. Some speculate a relationship with antecedent scabies infestation in a subset of patients and may refer to this phenomenon as postscabetic pustulosis in this setting. Cyclic eruptions occur every 2 to 3 weeks, lasting 7 to 10 days. Spontaneous disappearance occurs at 2 to 3 years of age. Treatment with topical steroids may moderate some of the pruritus.

For a complete differential of acute vesiculobullous eruptions involving the palms and soles, see Table 62.1.

MASTOCYTOSIS

Cutaneous mast cell disease (mastocytosis or urticaria pigmentosa) may cause blistering in young children. Red-brown lesions that blister after stroking or trauma (Darier sign) indicate the release of histamine from mast cells. This collection may be isolated (mastocytoma) or generalized (urticaria pigmentosa or bullous mastocytosis). In addition to stroking, other triggers include mast cell destabilizers such as nonsteroidal anti-inflammatory drugs (NSAIDs), polymyxin B, some anesthetic medications (both topical and systemic), venom from bees or wasps, and narcotics. Additionally, extreme temperatures or sudden changes in temperature may also lead to mast cell destabilization and release of histamine. Refer to www.mastokids.org for more information about common mast cell degranulation triggers. Blistering of such lesions generally occurs in the first few years of life. After this time, only urticaria occurs.

The solitary lesion most often occurs on the arm near the wrist (Fig. 62.3) but can be located anywhere on the body. Lesions may be generalized and are often associated with more severe cutaneous disease or systemic mastocytosis. When a presumed pigmented lesion feels infiltrated, the physician

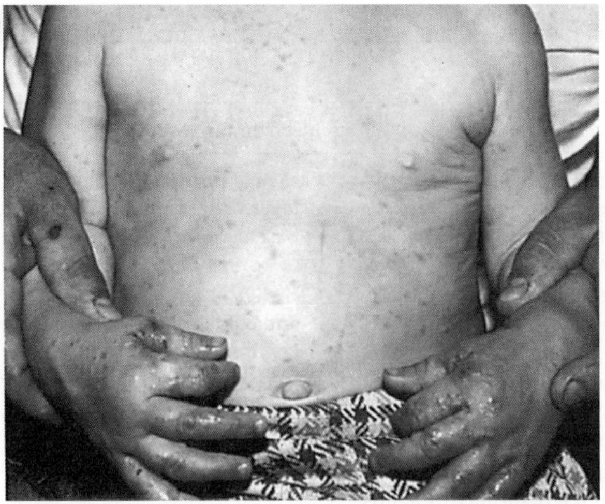

FIGURE 62.1 Blisters on hands of child infested with scabies.

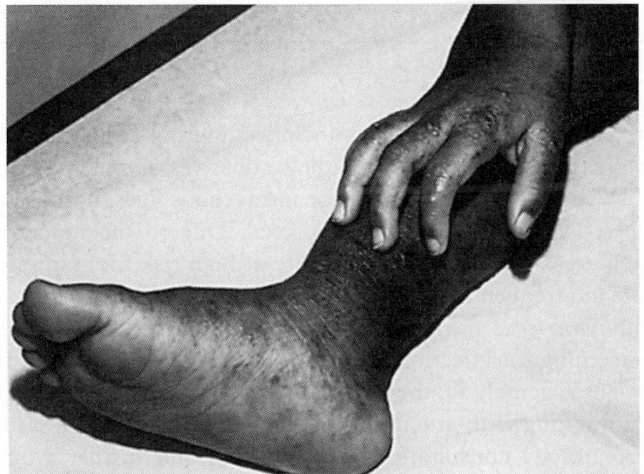

FIGURE 62.2 Note vesicles and pustules on child with acropustulosis of infancy.

TABLE 62.1

ACUTE VESICULOBULLOUS DISEASES INVOLVING PALMS AND SOLES

Child <3 yrs old
Scabies
Acropustulosis of infancy
Syphilis (transiently at birth)
Adolescent or older
Tinea pedis or manus
"Id" reaction
Epidermolysis bullosa of hands and feet
Any age
Drug reaction
Friction blisters or burns
Dyshidrotic eczema
Vasculitis (e.g., Henoch–Schönlein purpura)
Frostbite

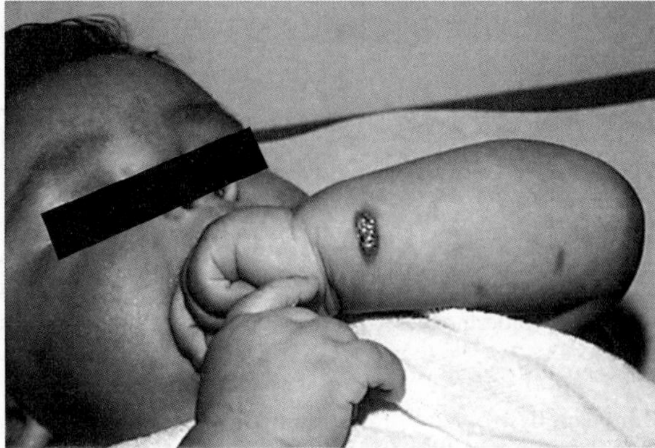

FIGURE 62.3 Infant with mastocytoma that has blistered because of trauma.

should think of mastocytosis—Darier sign will confirm the diagnosis. If asymptomatic and localized, active nonintervention is appropriate. For symptomatic disease, primary treatment is aimed at preventing histamine release with H1 and H2 antihistamines.

SIGNS AND SYMPTOMS

INHERITED BLISTERING DISEASES

Epidermolysis Bullosa

Epidermolysis bullosa (EB) is a group of inherited blistering disorders that tends to present in infancy or early in life with localized or widespread blistering at sites of friction. The cleavage plane leading to blistering is determined by specific mutations that lead to loss of function in the attachments between the epidermis and dermis. There are now over 30 subtypes of EB (Table 62.2), so for the purpose of this chapter, we will discuss general recognition of the condition.

The more severe subtypes of EB often present at or shortly after birth with large bulla and erosions at sites of friction or adhesion. They may affect all areas of the skin as well as the mucosa, particularly the oral mucosa, making early feedings a challenge due to pain. Patients may be born with large areas of absent skin known as congenital localized absence of skin (CLAS). Milia are also frequently seen at sites of blisters and erosions and may be present at birth. A hoarse cry may indicate airway involvement and is seen more commonly with junctional EB subtypes. Milder types may also present with localized blistering at birth, however some patients may not present until they are adolescents or adults. Certain types of EB simplex, for example, may not be diagnosed until the patients enter the army or other occupations where they are required to walk for long distances and subsequently develop blisters on their feet or use their hands in a repetitive motion leading to blistering on the palms. Patients may have other associated findings such as anonychia or dystrophic nails, and certain subtypes are associated with other systemic complications such as muscular dystrophy, pyloric atresia, or photosensitivity. Over time, severe subtypes may mitigate, and milder subtypes can become more severe. Mode of transmission varies depending on the subtype, therefore family history may be useful in making the diagnosis.

TABLE 62.2

EPIDERMOLYSIS BULLOSA SYNDROMES

Type	Typical inheritance	Clinical features	Electron microscope
Epidermolysis bullosa simplex	Autosomal dominant Autosomal recessive	Bullae present at birth, early infancy, or later in life; in areas of trauma; may improve in adolescence; rare mucous membrane involvement; nail involvement	Cleavage through the basal cell layer or suprabasal layer above basement membrane
Junctional epidermolysis bullosa	Autosomal recessive	Usually at birth; spontaneous bullae and large areas of erosion	Cleavage at junction of dermis and epidermis (above basement membrane)
Dominant dystrophic epidermolysis bullosa	Autosomal dominant	Early infancy and later; little or no involvement of hair and teeth; mucous membrane lesions and nail dystrophy	Dermal–epidermal separation beneath basement membrane
Recessive dystrophic epidermolysis bullosa	Autosomal recessive	Present at birth; widespread scarring and deformity with mitten deformity of hands; severe involvement of mucous membranes and nails	
Kindler syndrome	Autosomal recessive	Acral blistering; mottled pigmentation; photosensitivity: skin atrophy; involvement of mucous membranes	Cleavage at or near the dermal–epidermal junction

The differential diagnosis of EB in the newborn period includes infections such as herpes simplex virus (HSV) and bullous impetigo, and cultures should be obtained to rule out an infectious etiology. Epidermolytic ichthyosis, also known as bullous congenital ichthyosiform erythroderma, is a rare, autosomal dominant ichthyosis caused by mutations in keratins 1 and 10 found in the epidermis and presents with widespread superficial blistering and erythroderma in the neonatal period. The flexures, palms, and soles are most commonly involved, and mucosal surfaces are spared. With time, the skin develops thick, corrugated-like scale likely as compensation to the blistering.

Diagnosis is made by skin biopsy using immunofluorescence antigen mapping (IFM) and/or transmission electron microscopy (TEM) on newly induced blisters to detect the location of blistering and which cellular attachments are disrupted. However, more and more, genetic testing via mutation analysis is becoming first line as inducing new blisters can be challenging, especially in the newborn period. Additionally, mutation analysis allows for specific subclassification which is important for prognosis and genetic counseling.

In the emergency setting, the most important part of managing patients with possible or known EB is handling the patients with care. This includes limiting palpation only to areas of concern and avoiding adhesives as much as possible (this includes adhesives for intravenous lines, nasogastric tubes, electrocardiogram leads, etc.). Due to the numerous open areas of skin, EB patients are at high risk for skin infection and frequently become infected (as well as colonized) with *Staphylococcus aureus* and *Pseudomonas aeruginosa*. Areas concerning for infection should be cultured and treated. If the patient is acutely ill, they should be managed as needed in the acute setting with attention to skin as secondary. Once stable, dermatology consultation is warranted, and further wound care recommendations may be provided. For more information about EB, visit www.DEBRA.org.

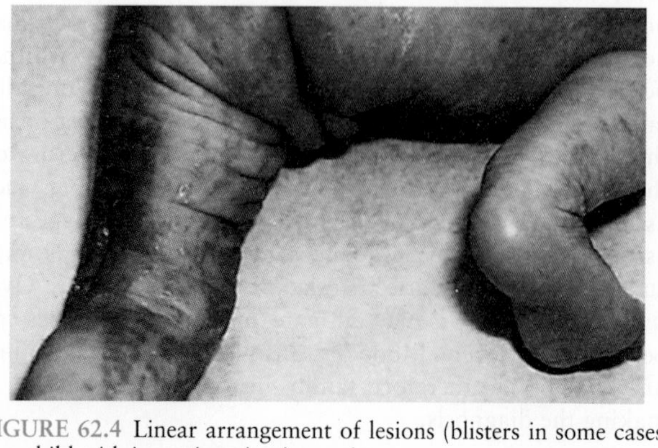

FIGURE 62.4 Linear arrangement of lesions (blisters in some cases) in a child with incontinentia pigmenti.

Incontinentia Pigmenti

Incontinentia pigmenti, a rare condition, occurs almost exclusively in females. Inflammatory vesicles and bullae erupt in crops in a linear or curvilinear distribution (especially on the extremities) for the first several weeks to months of life (Fig. 62.4). These affected areas then go on to a warty stage. Finally, swirl-like pigmentation occurs but not necessarily in the areas previously involved with warty or blistering lesions. During the vesiculobullous stage, peripheral eosinophilia occurs (18% to 50% eosinophils). These patients often have multisystem organ involvement and care must be coordinated with several subspecialists.

AUTOIMMUNE BULLOUS DISORDERS

Linear IgA Disease

Chronic bullous disease of childhood (CBDC), also known as linear immunoglobulin A (IgA) disease, may be seen in prepubertal children and is the most common acquired autoimmune blistering condition seen in childhood. It usually has an acute

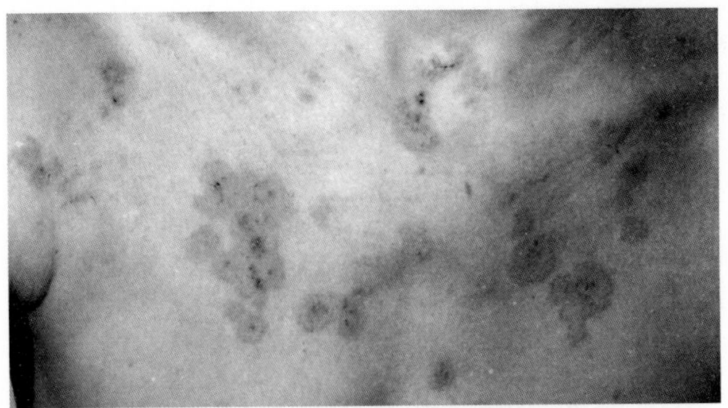

FIGURE 62.5 Chest of patient with chronic bullous dermatosis of childhood. Notice the resemblance to erythema multiforme.

onset with characteristic vesicles and bulla in an annular distribution often referred to as a "crown of jewels" or "string of pearls" (Fig. 62.5). Characteristic areas of involvement include the trunk, extremities, genital region, and face. The mucosa may be involved. Due to the acute onset and tense bulla, it may be initially misdiagnosed as bullous impetigo, but the recurrent nature and sterile bulla should suggest otherwise. Patients will often complain of pruritus. The lesions do not scar but may leave behind persistent hyperpigmentation at prior sites of blistering. The differential diagnosis includes bullous pemphigoid, dermatitis herpetiformis (DH), epidermolysis bullosa acquisita, and erythema multiforme.

Biopsy of a vesicle demonstrating a subepidermal blister with neutrophils along with direct immunofluorescence (DIF) of perilesional skin highlighting linear IgA staining at the basement membrane zone confirms the diagnosis. First-line therapy is dapsone. Other therapies include prednisone, sulfapyridine, colchicine, erythromycin, and topical steroids. The condition tends to spontaneously remit over months to years but occasionally can be chronic.

Bullous Pemphigoid

Bullous pemphigoid is a rare autoimmune blistering disorder that may develop as early as the newborn period and is due to autoantibodies to two hemidesmosal proteins, BP 230 and BP 180, which help to maintain dermal–epidermal attachment. Primary lesions include diffuse, large, tense, clear, or hemorrhagic bulla on a noninflammatory or erythematous base, although urticarial lesions occasionally predominate. Common locations include forearms, abdomen, thighs, genitals, palms, and soles. The striking acral involvement is more common in infancy and may help to distinguish clinically from other autoimmune blistering diseases. Mucosal involvement may be seen. Pruritus is common and may be severe.

Diagnosis is confirmed by biopsy of a vesicle demonstrating a subepidermal bulla with a predominantly eosinophilic infiltrate, and DIF from perilesional skin revealing linear deposition of immunoglobulin G (IgG) and C3. Enzyme-linked immunosorbent assay (ELISA) of BP 230 and 180 is commercially available as is indirect immunofluorescence testing for autoantibodies in the blood. BP may also be initially confused with bullous impetigo. The mainstay of treatment is oral corticosteroids, and the disease tends to last an average of 1 year for most patients.

DH presents as symmetric, intensely pruritic, crusted papules, papulovesicles, and urticarial plaques overlying extensor surfaces of the elbows and knees, posterior neck, scalp, and buttocks. Children with DH have gluten-sensitive enteropathy, however many are asymptomatic. Only about 10% of patients with a diagnosis of celiac disease will present with the classic eruption of DH.

Diagnosis is confirmed by biopsy of a papule or vesicle showing a predominately neutrophilic infiltrate focused at the tip of the dermal papillae. DIF reveals granular IgA deposition at the dermal papillae. Diagnosis may also be made by circulating serum IgA antibody to tissue transglutaminase in the blood. IgA levels should be checked as IgA deficiency may lead to a false-negative test. Additional diagnostic tests often included in a celiac panel include antiendomysial antibodies and antigliadin antibodies. Patients with DH should undergo endoscopy to assess for clinical evidence of gluten-sensitive enteropathy. Treatment includes dapsone, which leads to spontaneous remission of DH in 24 to 48 hours. A gluten-free diet is also recommended and may obviate the need for dapsone with strict adherence to a gluten-free diet.

For comparison of the above autoimmune bullous diseases, see Table 62.3.

TABLE 62.3

AUTOIMMUNE BULLOUS DISORDERS OF CHILDHOOD

	Bullous disease of childhood	Bullous pemphigoid	Dermatitis herpetiformis
Type of lesions	Large, tense, clear bullae; annular plaques with active vesicular borders	Large, tense bullae	Grouped papulovesicles, bullae, or urticarial lesions
Distribution	Scalp, lower trunk, genitals, buttocks, inner thighs	Trunk and flexor surfaces of extremities	Back, buttocks, scalp, extensor surface of extremities, often symmetric
Pruritus	None to severe	Mild	Intense
Mucous membrane involvement	Usually not	Yes	No
Duration	Months to years	Months to years	Months to years
Immunofluorescence	+ or –	+	+
	Linear IgA basement membrane (+ circulating IgA)	Linear IgG on basement membrane (+ circulating IgG)	Granular IgA at tips of dermal papilla of uninvolved perilesional skin
Treatment	Dapsone > Corticosteroids	Corticosteroids	Dapsone > Sulfapyridine

Systemic Lupus Erythematosus

Although not characteristic, widespread tense, bullous lesions can occur in systemic lupus erythematosus (SLE), usually in sun-exposed areas. Multisystem involvement suggests the diagnosis. Laboratory confirmation, which may include a skin biopsy and lupus band test, in conjunction with the complete clinical picture, is necessary for diagnosis.

OTHER BULLOUS ERUPTIONS THAT MAY BE CONFUSED WITH AUTOIMMUNE BLISTERING DISEASES

Many times, the appearance of a rash is so characteristic that a diagnosis becomes obvious. Such is the case with the conditions listed below, which are discussed in more detail in their respective chapters but are mentioned here for completeness when considering a vesiculobullous eruption.

Linear or geometric areas of vesiculation are the best clues to the presence of allergic contact dermatitis (see Chapter 60 Rash: Atopic Dermatitis, Contact Dermatitis, Scabies and Erythroderma). The shape of the dermatitis provides the information that helps identify the offending agent. A history of playing in a shrubbed area, camping, hiking, or being near burning leaves is helpful. Because children brush against poison ivy leaves, vesicles often are in a line and on exposed surfaces (e.g., the face, extremities). A round group of vesicles on the back of the wrist would point to contact sensitivity to nickel contained in the metal case of a wristwatch.

Dermatomal distribution of vesicles or bullae usually indicates the presence of herpes zoster. On rare occasions, in infants, the same dermatomal appearance may represent zosteriform herpes simplex infections. A positive Tzanck smear indicates the presence of the herpes virus. Viral cultures, rapid slide tests using monoclonal antibodies, or more recently, polymerase chain reaction tests are utilized to differentiate herpes simplex from herpes zoster (see Chapter 65 Rash: Papulosquamous Eruptions).

Target or iris lesions are pathognomonic of erythema multiforme. The lesion has a dusky center that may blister and has successive bright red bordering rings. At times, a doughnut-shaped blister occurs. This contrasts with annular urticaria, in which incompletely round (arcuate or polycyclic) wheals are observed and individual lesions typically resolve within less than 24 hours (see Chapter 60 Rash: Atopic Dermatitis, Contact Dermatitis, Scabies and Erythroderma). CBDC may be confused with erythema multiforme as discussed above.

Friction Blisters

Blisters usually occur in areas predisposed to trauma or friction such as on the heels after walking or playing sports or due to new, possibly poorly fitted, shoes. However, a persistent history may suggest EB, which may not always present in infancy in milder subtypes such as EB simplex as discussed above. See Table 62.2 for differentiation of the various types.

Occasionally, accidental burns or burns secondary to child abuse are seen. Abused children may have had cigarette burns or have had their feet dipped in scalding water.

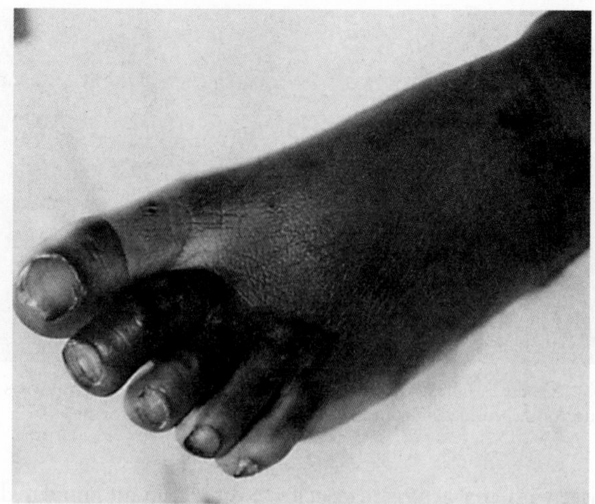

FIGURE 62.6 Frostbite. Child played in the snow for a prolonged period on a cold day wearing sneakers.

Frostbite

Fingers, toes, feet, nose, cheeks, and ears are affected by extreme cold. After exposed areas are damaged by the cold temperature, symptoms occur on rewarming. Erythema, swelling, and burning pain occur at first, followed by vesicles and bullae (at times hemorrhagic (Fig. 62.6)) within 24 to 48 hours. Prevention is most important with appropriate protection of these sites from extreme cold.

LABORATORY EVALUATION

If there is no clear idea about what caused the blister, the laboratory tests described next can be helpful.

Gram Stain

The Gram stain of fluid from an intact blister will be positive in impetigo and in a secondarily infected lesion. It will be negative, however, in all other conditions.

Tzanck Smear

Multinucleated giant cells will be present on a Tzanck smear of material scraped from the base of an intact, freshly opened vesicle caused by herpes simplex, herpes zoster, and varicella.

Rapid Slide Test for Direct Immunofluorescence

Fluorescent-tagged monoclonal antibody is applied to cells scraped from the blister base and can differentiate HSV-1, HSV-2, or varicella-zoster virus. Results can be available in 1 to 2 hours.

Bacterial or Viral Cultures

Cultures help confirm an etiologic diagnosis when Gram stain, Tzanck smears, and DIF are negative or indeterminate.

Polymerase Chain Reaction

An alternative or adjunct to traditional culture techniques, polymerase chain reaction techniques allow for amplification of DNA or RNA present within a specimen and rapid identification of the etiologic pathogen, including HSV, VZV, and enterovirus. The technique is useful even when the pathogen present is no longer viable.

Skin Biopsy

For perplexing cases undiagnosed by clinical and/or simple laboratory evaluation, dermatologic consultation and skin biopsy are required.

If the picture on histology is compatible with erythema multiforme, DIF should be considered. DIF will be negative in erythema multiforme but will be positive in bullous pemphigoid (linear IgG and C3 on the basement membrane), DH (granular IgA at tips of dermal papillae of uninvolved perilesional skin), and CBDC (linear IgA on the basement membrane). DIF can be negative in CBDC.

Indirect immunofluorescence can be performed to test for circulating antibodies. Circulating IgG is found in bullous pemphigoid; circulating IgA is found in CBDC.

CONCLUSION

Vesiculobullous diseases have a variety of presentations and several key features that may help to distinguish them from one another. While characteristic features in some make diagnosis straightforward, many of the blistering disorders require further diagnostic evaluation in order to confirm diagnosis. Treatment is aimed at the underlying pathogenesis.

Suggested Readings and Key References

Carr DR, Houshmand E, Heffernan MP. Approach to the acute, generalized, blistering patient. *Semin Cutan Med Surg* 2007;26:139–146.

Fine JD, Bruckner-Tuderman L, Eady RA, et al. Inherited epidermolysis bullosa: updated recommendations on diagnosis and classification. *J Am Acad Dermatol* 2014;70(6):1103–1126.

Fine JD, Mellerio JE. Extracutaneous manifestations and complications of inherited epidermolysis bullosa: part I. Epithelial associated tissues. *J Am Acad Dermatol* 2009;61(3):367–384; quiz 385–386.

Fine JD, Mellerio JE. Extracutaneous manifestations and complications of inherited epidermolysis bullosa: part II. Other organs. *J Am Acad Dermatol* 2009;61(3):387–402; quiz 403–404.

Kalil C, Fachinello FZ, Cignachi S, et al. Bullous dermatoses in childhood: part I. *Skinmed* 2007;6:73–78.

Kalil C, Fachinello FZ, Cignachi S, et al. Bullous dermatoses in childhood: part II. *Skinmed* 2007;6:128–134.

Lai-Cheong JE, McGrath JA. Kindler syndrome. *Dermatol Clin* 2010; 28(1):119–124.

Lara-Corrales I, Pope E. Autoimmune blistering diseases in children. *Semin Cutan Med Surg* 2010;29(2):85–91.

Mintz EM, Morel KD. Clinical features, diagnosis, and pathogenesis of chronic bullous disease of childhood. *Dermatol Clin* 2011;29(3): 459–462, ix.

Orion E, Marcos B, Davidovici B, et al. Itch and scratch: scabies and pediculosis. *Clin Dermatol* 2006;24:168–175.

Sansaricq F, Stein SL, Petronic-Rosic V. Autoimmune bullous diseases in childhood. *Clin Dermatol* 2012;30(1):114–127.

Steen CJ, Carbonaro PA, Schwartz RA. Arthropods in dermatology. *J Am Acad Dermatol* 2004;50:819–842.

Strong M, Johnstone PW. Interventions for treating scabies. *Cochrane Database Syst Rev* 2007;(3):CD000320.

Torrelo A, Alvarez-Twose I, Escribano L. Childhood mastocytosis. *Curr Opin Pediatr* 2012;24(4):480–486.

CHAPTER 63 ■ RASH: DRUG ERUPTIONS

MELINDA JEN, MD

DRUG ERUPTIONS

The spectrum of cutaneous drug eruptions ranges from the relatively benign, where the medication can be continued if essential, to the severe, where there can be significant morbidity and mortality. Thus, in cases of severe drug reactions, prompt and accurate diagnosis is critical and can be lifesaving. The primary morphology of the eruption helps guide the clinician to a diagnosis. Herein, we summarize the most salient features of the most common drug reactions, with a particular focus upon their primary morphologies.

URTICARIA

Urticaria (hives, wheals) consists of erythematous, edematous papules and plaques that can coalesce into larger polycyclic, arcuate, and annular plaques (Figs. 63.1 and 63.2). A key diagnostic feature is that individual lesions are transient, resolving within 24 hours, but with new lesions appearing elsewhere. As they resolve, purpuric macules secondary to capillary leak and hyperpigmentation may remain. Pruritus and angioedema, particularly of the eyelids, hands, and feet, are common.

Urticaria results from IgE degranulation of mast cells. Although the most common cause of urticaria is infection, medications can sometimes trigger urticaria. Urticaria typically appears within the first 2 weeks of starting the culprit medication. Cephalosporins, β-lactam antibiotics, sulfonamides, and anticonvulsants are common causes of drug-induced urticaria. Some medications, such as nonsteroidal anti-inflammatory drugs (NSAIDs), may cause urticaria through both immunologic and nonimmunologic pathways (via increased leukotriene synthesis).

Urticaria is often confused for erythema multiforme (EM). The key features differentiating urticaria from EM are morphology, individual lesion duration, symptomology, and distribution. Urticaria can be annular, polycyclic, and arcuate, but does not have the classic target appearance of EM. Additionally, urticaria does not vesiculate, while the central areas of EM lesions may be bullous. As noted above, individual lesions of urticaria last less than 24 hours, while lesions of EM are fixed and take several days to resolve. If symptomatic, urticaria is pruritic while EM may itch or burn. Urticaria can occur anywhere on the body, while EM typically first appears on the hands and feet before progressing centrally.

The treatment for drug-induced urticaria is withdrawal of the causative medication and treatment with both H1 and H2 blocking oral antihistamines for up to 4 to 8 weeks. For cases that persist despite maximum dosing of nonsedating H1 and H2 blocking antihistamines, oral steroids may be beneficial.

MORBILLIFORM

Morbilliform, or measles-like, describes an eruption characterized by both erythematous macules and papules (Fig. 63.3). The term "maculopapular" is often used to describe this eruption, but morbilliform is a more precise description. This is the most common type of drug rash. The eruption typically starts on the trunk before spreading to involve the extremities and face, though the mucous membranes are spared. The eruption can become diffuse and confluent. Pruritus may be present.

A morbilliform drug eruption typically appears 7 to 14 days after medication initiation, but in a previously sensitized patient it may appear within hours to days of reexposure. Antibiotics, in particular penicillins (Fig. 63.4), cephalosporins, and sulfonamides, as well as antiepileptics are common triggers.

A morbilliform drug eruption can be difficult to clinically distinguish from a viral exanthem. One unique example is that of the morbilliform eruption that may result from antibiotic administration, most commonly amoxicillin, during an Epstein–Barr virus (EBV) infection. Although early studies reported an incidence of 90% or more, a more recent study suggests that the true incidence is closer to 30%. This eruption, however, is not actually a drug hypersensitivity reaction (DHR), but rather is a viral exanthem.

Treatment involves a balance between the severity of the eruption and the importance of the causative medication. The rash is generally self-limited and will resolve within 7 to 14 days of stopping the medication. However, if the rash is mild and the medication is essential, then the medication can be continued with close monitoring. Morbilliform drug eruptions do not progress into more severe drug reactions, however, early on severe drug reactions may mimic a morbilliform drug eruption. Therefore, an uncomplicated morbilliform drug eruption must be distinguished from DHR, which has systemic involvement. If the eruption appears within the first 2 weeks of starting a medication, then it is more likely to be a morbilliform drug eruption. If the eruption is delayed by several weeks, then DHR is more likely. The presence of additional clinical features, such as facial edema and lymphadenopathy, and laboratory findings can also aid in distinguishing the two entities. If needed, topical steroids can help provide symptomatic relief of pruritus.

DRUG HYPERSENSITIVITY REACTION (DHR)/DRUG REACTION WITH EOSINOPHILIA AND SYSTEMIC SYMPTOMS (DRESS)

The cutaneous eruption of DHR, also known as drug reaction with eosinophilia and systemic symptoms (DRESS), is

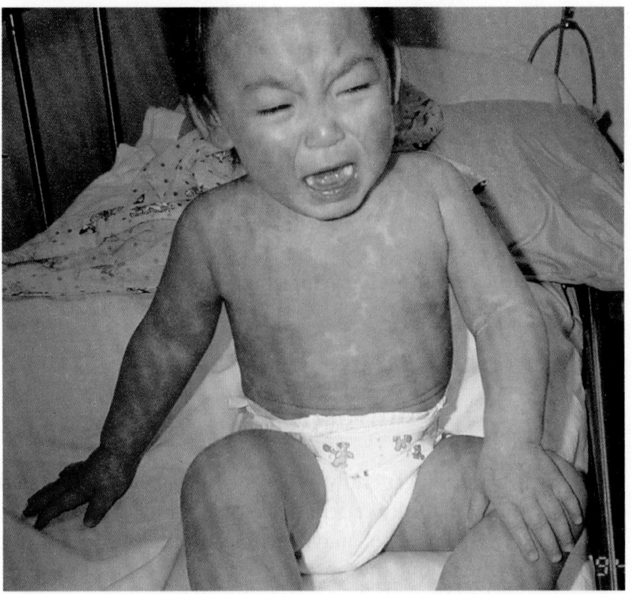

FIGURE 63.1 Widespread transient erythematous edematous papules and plaques. (From Fleisher GR, Ludwig S, Baskin MN. *Atlas of pediatric emergency medicine*. Philadelphia, PA: Lippincott Williams & Wilkins, 2004.)

a morbilliform eruption that starts on the face and spreads cephalocaudally. Additional clinical findings and systemic involvement distinguish DHR from a skin-limited morbilliform drug eruption. Facial edema is present in approximately 76%, fever in 90%, and lymphadenopathy in 54% of patients with DHR. In half of patients, there can be mild mucosal involvement, more commonly the oral mucosa. Systemic involvement commonly manifests with eosinophilia (95%) or atypical lymphocytosis (67%) on complete blood count. Liver involvement is seen in 75% of patients, and often presents as elevation of liver transaminases. In cases where patients have a prolonged clinical course or when they appear systemically ill, echocardiogram, renal function tests, and coagulation profiles should be checked for cardiac, renal, and severe hepatic involvement. Thyroid involvement is usually delayed in onset, so thyroid functions should be followed for 2 to 3 months after the DHR.

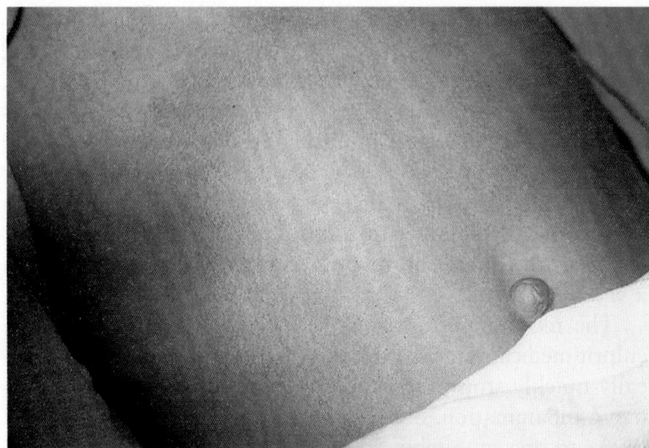

FIGURE 63.3 A morbilliform eruption presents with erythematous macules and papules on the trunk before spreading to the rest of the body. (Courtesy of George A. Datto, III, MD.)

DHR is a delayed-type hypersensitivity reaction that occurs 2 to 6 weeks, with an average of 22 days, after starting a medication. Antiepileptics (carbamazepine, phenytoin, phenobarbital, lamotrigine) are the most common cause of DHR. Other medications that commonly cause DHR are trimethoprim-sulfamethoxazole, minocycline, dapsone, sulfasalazine, and abacavir. There appears to be a genetic susceptibility for developing DHR to certain medications. For example, HLA-A*31:01 has been showed to be associated with an increased risk of DHR following exposure to carbamazepine in children. Other associations with DHR include human herpesvirus-6 (HHV6), in which reactivation has been detected in cases of DHR. Though the exact role of HHV6 in the pathogenesis of DHR is still unclear, some evidence suggests that HHV6 reactivation creates immune dysregulation that causes DHR, while others suggest that DHR-induced immune dysregulation allows for HHV6 reactivation.

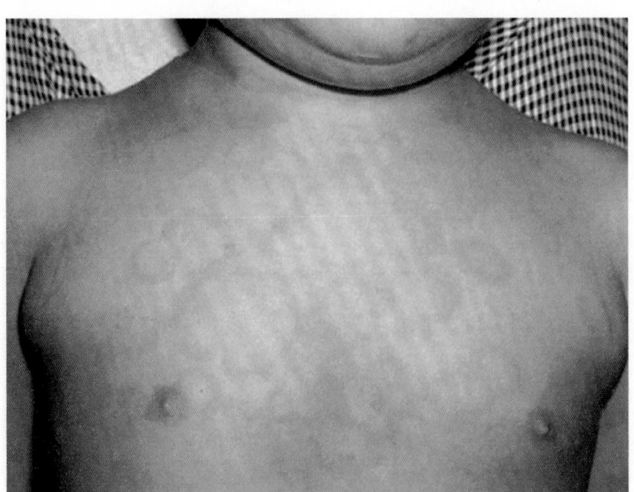

FIGURE 63.2 Urticaria often appears as annular or polycyclic plaques with central clearing or purpura. (From Burkhart C, Morrell D, Goldsmith LA, et al. *VisualDx: essential pediatric dermatology*. Philadelphia, PA: Lippincott Williams & Wilkins, 2009.)

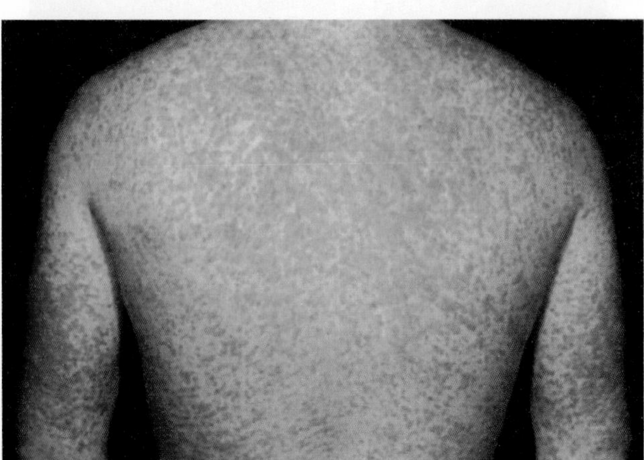

FIGURE 63.4 This morbilliform eruption presented several days after starting ampicillin therapy. (From Elder DE, Elenitsas R, Rubin AI, et al. *Atlas and synopsis of lever's histopathology of the skin*. 3rd ed. Philadelphia, PA: Lippincott Williams & Wilkins, 2012.)

The main differential diagnosis for DHR includes a cutaneous limited morbilliform drug eruption, Kawasaki disease, and viral exanthem. The presence of fever, facial edema, lymphadenopathy, and laboratory abnormalities distinguishes DHR from a cutaneous limited morbilliform eruption. The absence of conjunctivitis and mucous membrane involvement suggests DHR rather than Kawasaki disease. The initiation of a potential high-risk medication weeks before rash onset increases the likelihood that an eruption is DHR rather than a viral exanthem.

The most important treatment for DHR is stopping the culprit medication. Oral steroids of 1 to 2 mg/kg/day can typically quickly stop progression of the disease by treating systemic inflammation. Steroids should be tapered over several weeks to prevent a rebound of the reaction.

PUSTULAR

Acute generalized exanthematous pustulosis (AGEP) is a less commonly seen drug eruption in children. It presents with widespread erythema overlaid with numerous pinpoint, superficial, sterile pustules (Fig. 63.5). The pustules are fragile and easily ruptured, leaving superficial areas of desquamation over the background of erythema. The eruption frequently starts on the face or within skin folds before rapidly spreading to the rest of the body. Fever is usually present, while mucous membrane involvement is not seen.

AGEP presents within a few days of starting the triggering medication, usually an antibiotic. In one study, pristinamycin, aminopenicillins, and quinolones were the most common causes of AGEP, but cephalosporins, macrolides, clindamycin, tetracycline, and terbinafine are other causes.

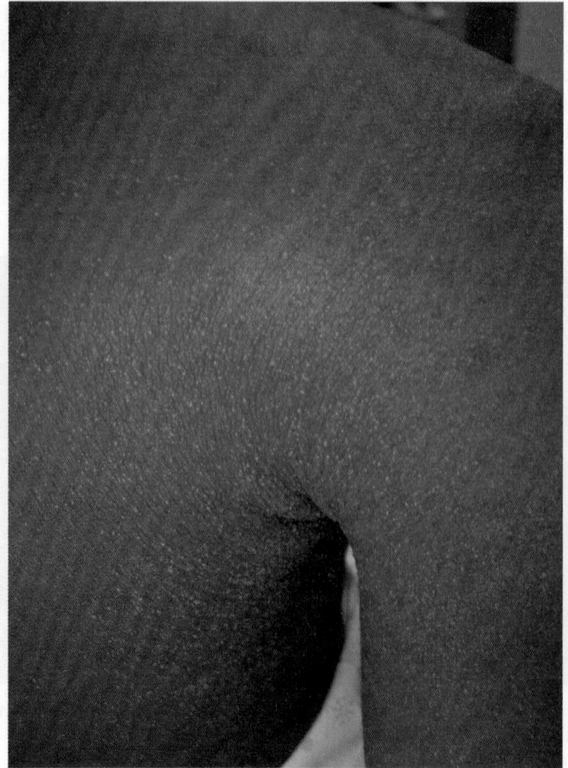

FIGURE 63.5 Innumerable superficial fragile pustules on a background of erythema. (Image provided by Stedman's.)

The differential diagnosis for AGEP includes DHR and pustular psoriasis. Careful inspection for pustules or for areas of desquamation, indicating ruptured pustules, in addition to laboratory evaluation, will help distinguish AGEP from DHR. Eliciting either a personal or family history of psoriasis or a history of a high-risk medication can help favor a diagnosis of either pustular psoriasis or AGEP, respectively.

AGEP generally resolves with desquamation within 4 to 10 days after stopping the drug. Topical steroids and oral antihistamines can provide symptomatic relief if needed.

VESICULOBULLOUS

Fixed Drug

Fixed drug eruption generally appears as a sharply demarcated erythematous to dusky, edematous oval or circular plaque (Fig. 63.6). The plaques may become bullous. Lesions can appear anywhere, but the lips, face, hands, feet, and genitals are commonly affected. They often leave hyperpigmentation that may take months to resolve. Although usually solitary, multiple or very large lesions may form in fixed drug eruption following repeated exposure to the triggering medication. The lesions can be pruritic, burning, or asymptomatic.

Initially, lesions appear within 2 weeks of starting a medication, but with repeated exposure, onset can occur in minutes to hours. Sulfonamides, particularly trimethoprim-sulfamethoxazole, are the most common causes of fixed drug eruption in children (Fig. 63.7), though NSAIDs and tetracycline are also frequent causes. Some foods and food additives have also been reported to cause fixed drug reactions.

Fixed drug eruption can often be confused for arthropod bites, urticaria, or EM. The history of recurrence in the exact same location with prominent postinflammatory hyperpigmentation is more suggestive of a fixed drug eruption rather than arthropod bites. Similarly, fixed drug eruption is typically not as pruritic as arthropod bites. As noted above, urticaria is transient, so individual lesions resolve within 24 hours, with any residual pigmentation or purpura resolving within days

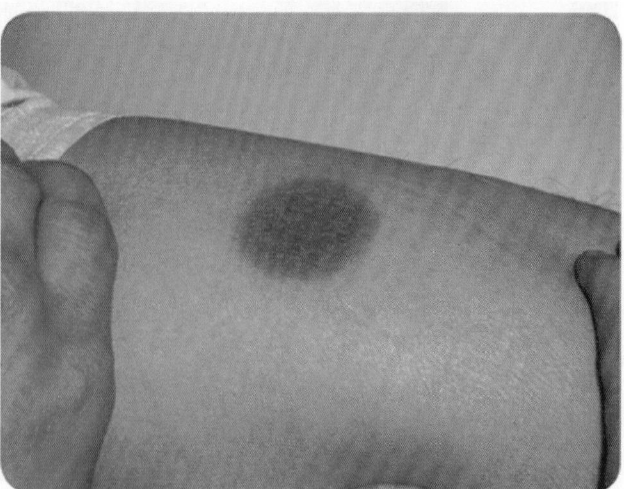

FIGURE 63.6 A characteristic well-demarcated erythematous circular plaque with a dusky center seen with a fixed drug eruption. (From Somolinos AL, Grant LM, Goldsmith LA, et al. *VisualDx: essential dermatology in pigmented skin*. Philadelphia, PA: Lippincott Williams & Wilkins, 2011.)

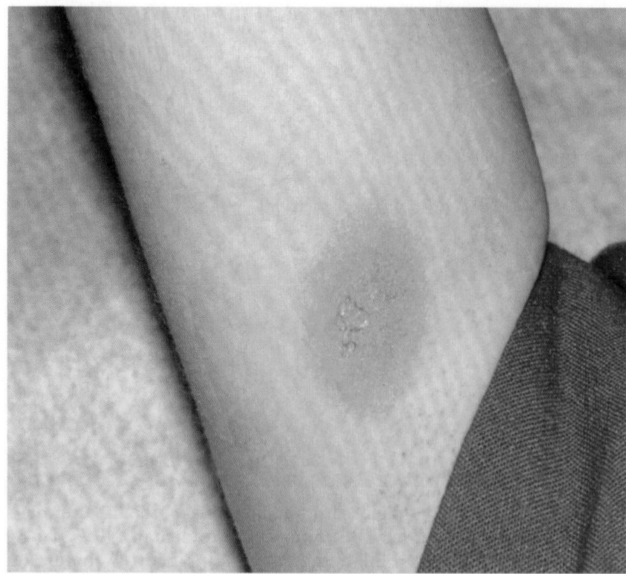

FIGURE 63.7 This erythematous oval plaque occurred at the identical site where it occurred the last time this patient was exposed to a sulfonamide antibiotic. (From Goodheart HP. *Goodheart's photoguide of common skin disorders.* 2nd ed. Philadelphia, PA: Lippincott Williams & Wilkins, 2003.)

rather than the months that fixed drug eruption hyperpigmentation may last. As compared to EM, the lesions of fixed drug eruption are larger, fewer, and in a different distribution.

Stopping and avoiding the causative medication allows for resolution of the fixed drug eruption and prevents recurrence. A fixed drug eruption does not progress to more severe drug eruptions, like DHR or Stevens–Johnson syndrome (SJS). If needed, a topical steroid can treat pruritus.

Erythema Multiforme

The lesions of EM have a classic target appearance, which appears as a well-defined round macule or papule with three distinct zones: two concentric rings around a dusky, bullous, or crusted center (Fig. 63.8A,B). The lesions are symmetrically distributed and favor the distal extremities, especially the upper extremities. Mucous membrane lesions can be seen in up to half of cases. Bullous lesions rupture easily, leaving swelling and crusting (Fig. 63.9). EM lesions are fixed, with individual lesions lasting approximately 7 days. Systemic symptoms of malaise, low-grade fever, myalgias, or arthralgias may be present.

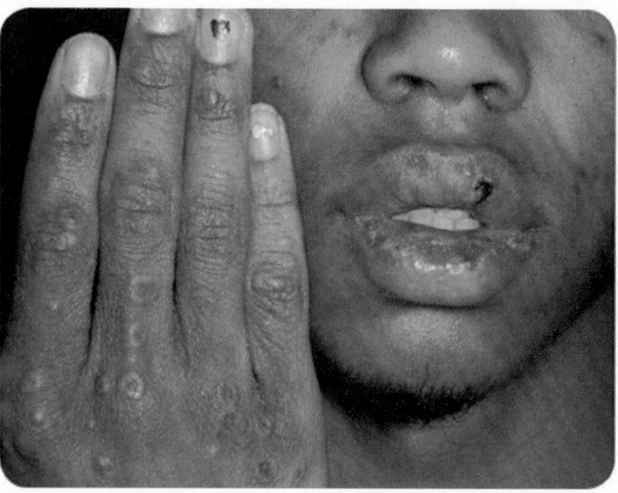

FIGURE 63.9 Erosions on the lips with target lesions on the hands. (From Somolinos AL, Grant LM, Goldsmith LA, et al. *VisualDx: essential dermatology in pigmented skin.* Philadelphia, PA: Lippincott Williams & Wilkins, 2011.)

EM is a hypersensitivity reaction most often secondary to an infectious trigger. EM has been associated with many infectious agents, including bacterial, viral, fungal, and parasitic infections. Herpes simplex virus 1 and 2 and Mycoplasma are the most common infectious triggers. Medications may be a cause of EM, most commonly sulfonamides, antiepileptic medications, and antibiotics.

EM is often confused for urticaria or SJS. EM can be distinguished from the transient and pruritic lesions of urticaria because of the classic target appearance of lesions that are

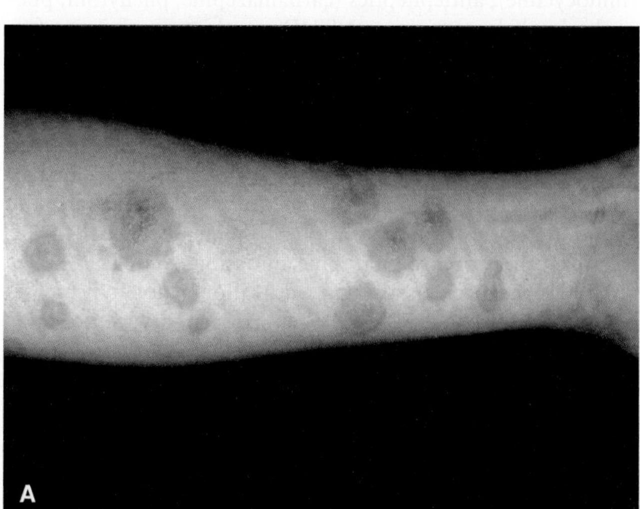

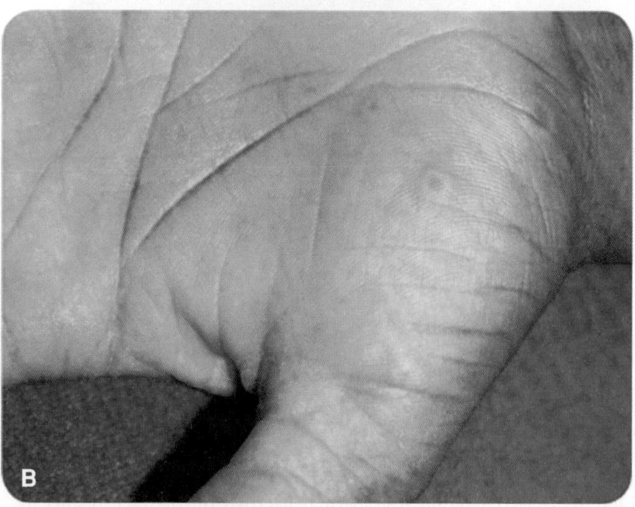

FIGURE 63.8 **A, B:** Classic target lesions seen in erythema multiforme with three distinct zones. (**A:** Reproduced with permission from Roche Laboratories. Sauer GC, Hall JC. *Manual of skin diseases.* 7th ed. Philadelphia, PA: Lippincott-Raven, 1996. **B:** From Somolinos AL, Grant LM, Goldsmith LA, et al. *VisualDx: essential dermatology in pigmented skin.* Philadelphia, PA: Lippincott Williams & Wilkins, 2011.)

fixed for several days. As discussed further below, SJS is a severe drug eruption that has lesions that are often confused for the targetoid lesions of EM, but they lack the characteristic three zones. Furthermore, in SJS two or more mucous membranes are typically involved with blisters, erosions, and crusting.

EM is a self-limited reaction resolving within 2 to 3 weeks. Because of its frequent association with herpes simplex virus, patients are often treated with acyclovir. If a medication trigger is suspected, then stopping the medication will help with resolution. Antihistamines can offer symptomatic relief.

Stevens–Johnson Syndrome/Toxic Epidermal Necrolysis

SJS and toxic epidermal necrolysis (TEN) are clinically similar, but exist in a spectrum distinguished by the degree of skin involvement. SJS involves <10% of body surface area; TEN involves >30% of body surface area; and 10% to 30% body surface area involvement is considered SJS/TEN overlap.

A prodrome of fever and constitutional symptoms (malaise, headache, sore throat, myalgias, arthralgias) sometimes precedes the onset of cutaneous lesions. Erythematous and purpuric macules start on the face and trunk and spread over hours to a few days to become more confluent and bullous. Tender erosions remain after the bullae rupture (Fig. 63.10). As the erythematous macules develop dusky centers indicating epidermal necrosis, they can have a targetoid appearance but lack the classic three zones seen in the target lesions of EM. Gentle lateral pressure to an area of macular erythema causes the epidermis to sheer off, known as the Nikolsky sign. Postinflammatory dyspigmentation is common.

Mucous membrane involvement can precede cutaneous involvement by 1 to 2 days. Two or more mucosal surfaces are usually involved, while any epithelial surface may be involved, including the eyes, lips (Fig. 63.11), tongue, buccal mucosa, nose, and genitalia. In severe cases, pulmonary and renal involvement has also been reported. Ocular manifestations include conjunctivitis with photophobia, keratitis, uveitis, or corneal ulcerations. Close ophthalmologic care is essential to prevent long-term complications, such as corneal neovascularization, symblepharon, and blindness. Bullae may not be obvious on mucous membranes, and often appear as a gray–white film that leaves erosions, ulcerations, and hemorrhagic crust. Mucosal involvement may lead to difficulty eating, drinking, dysuria, and pain with defecation. Ultimately, if scarring occurs, it can result in functional impairment from esophageal stenosis, urethral stenosis, vaginal stenosis, and anal strictures.

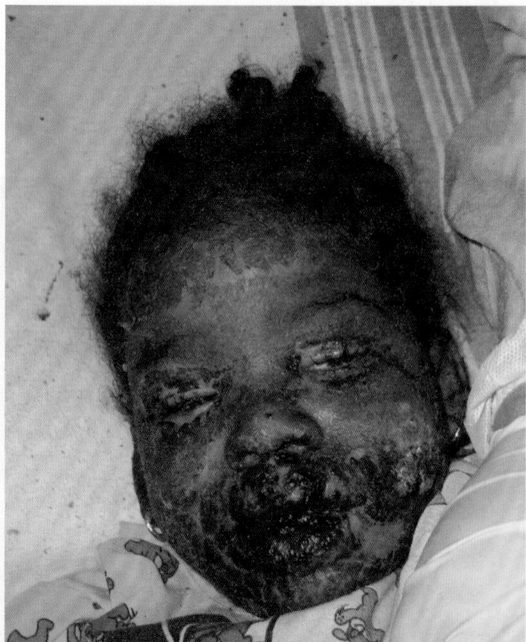

FIGURE 63.10 Confluent epidermal necrosis on the face results in diffuse desquamation and erosions. Note the involvement of the lips with hemorrhagic crust and erosions. (From Garg SJ. *Color atlas and synopsis of clinical ophthalmology—Wills Eye Institute—Uveitis*. Philadelphia, PA: Lippincott Williams & Wilkins, 2011.)

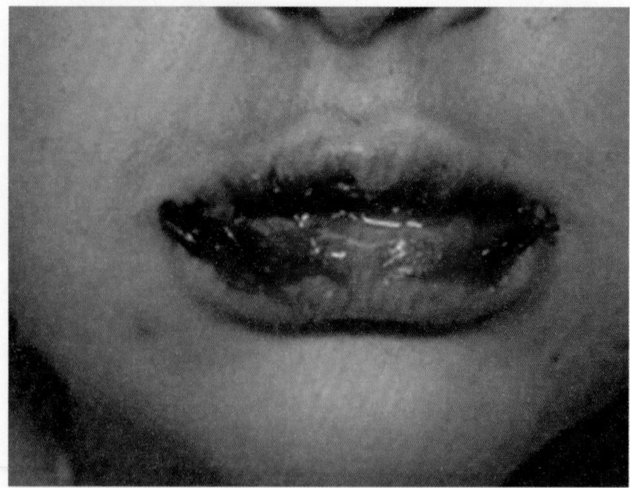

FIGURE 63.11 Hemorrhagic crust and erosions on the lip after desquamation. (From Onofrey BE, Skorin L, Holdeman NR. *Ocular therapeutics handbook*. Philadelphia, PA: Lippincott Williams & Wilkins, 2011.)

Drugs are the most common trigger for SJS, though a mucosal predominant form of SJS can be caused by mycoplasma infection. In contrast, medications are the exclusive cause of TEN. Antibiotics (trimethoprim-sulfamethoxazole, minocycline), antiepileptics (carbamazepine, phenytoin, phenobarbital, lamotrigine), NSAIDs, and nevirapine are frequent triggers for SJS/TEN. The first signs of SJS/TEN can present approximately 7 to 21 days after starting the medication. Similar to DHR, a genetic predisposition for SJS/TEN development may be present. Since the identification of the association between HLA-B*1502 and carbamazepine-induced SJS/TEN in patients of East Asian descent, the Food and Drug Administration recommends HLA-B*1502 testing prior to carbamazepine initiation. Similarly, HLA-B*5801 has been associated with allopurinol hypersensitivity and HLA-B*5701 has been associated with abacavir hypersensitivity.

The differential diagnosis for SJS/TEN includes EM, staphylococcal scalded skin syndrome (SSSS), and Kawasaki disease. As noted above, although SJS/TEN can have targetoid lesions, these are not the classic target lesions seen in EM. Additionally, SJS/TEN usually begins on the face and trunk, rather than the extremities as in EM. Likewise, although EM can have mucous membrane involvement, it does not involve two or more mucous membranes. SSSS affects the superficial epidermis, resulting in superficial desquamation rather than the full-thickness epidermal necrosis seen with SJS/TEN. SSSS also spares the oral mucosa, while SJS/TEN affects the oral mucosa. In contrast, Kawasaki disease often has a mucosal involvement, with conjunctivitis, strawberry tongue, and dry and cracked lips. However, the degree of involvement is not as severe as that seen in SJS/TEN, which may frequently consist of widespread erosions within the mouth and thick hemorrhagic crust on the lips.

Similar to other drug reactions, the most important step in managing SJS/TEN is stopping the causative medication. Wound care is critical to decrease the risk of complications, including infection and scarring. Petrolatum gauze or plain petrolatum should be liberally used in all affected areas, including the lips, genitals, and anus, to prevent scarring. Ophthalmology and urology should be consulted if there is suspected ocular or urethral involvement. The skin should be examined daily, and signs of infection should prompt aggressive treatment because the primary cause of mortality is infection. Mortality from SJS/TEN can be as high as 30%, with mortality increasing proportionally to the amount of body surface area involved. Pain management and nutritional support may need to be done parenterally since oral involvement may limit oral intake.

Regarding medical treatment, there is controversy and no consensus as to whether systemic steroids or intravenous immunoglobulins (IVIG) have benefit in this condition. Systemic steroids have generally fallen out of favor because of the increased risk of infection and delayed wound healing. IVIG is often used because it is thought to block apoptosis signaling pathways. When used, IVIG is given at 0.5 to 1 g/kg/day for 2 to 4 days to reach a total dose of 2 to 4 g per kg.

Suggested Readings and Key References

Urticaria

Peroni A, Colato C, Schena D, et al. Urticarial lesions: if not urticaria, what else? The differential diagnosis of urticaria: part I. Cutaneous diseases. *J Am Acad Dermatol* 2010;62:541–555.

Morbilliform

Amstutz U, Ross CJ, Castro-Pastrana LI, et al. HLA-A 31:01 and HLA-B 15:02 as genetic markers for carbamazepine hypersensitivity in children. *Clin Pharmacol Ther* 2013;94:142–149.

Chovel-Sella A, Ben Tov A, Lahav E, et al. Incidence of rash after amoxicillin treatment in children with infectious mononucleosis. *Pediatrics* 2013;131:e1424–e1427.

Ferrero NA, Pearson KC, Zedek DC, et al. Case report of drug rash with eosinophilia and systemic symptoms demonstrating human herpesvirus-6 reactivation. *Pediatr Dermatol* 2013;30:608–613.

Kardaun SH, Sekula P, Valeyrie-Allanore L, et al. Drug reaction with eosinophilia and systemic symptoms (DRESS): an original multisystem adverse drug reaction. Results from the prospective RegiSCAR study. *Br J Dermatol* 2013;169:1071–1080.

Acute Generalized Exanthematous Pustulosis

Sidoroff A, Dunant A, Viboud C, et al. Risk factors for acute generalized exanthematous pustulosis (AGEP)-results of a multinational case-control study (EuroSCAR). *Br J Dermatol* 2007;157: 989–996.

Stevens–Johnson Syndrome/toxic Epidermal Necrolysis

Chen P, Lin JJ, Lu CS, et al. Carbamazepine-induced toxic effects and HLA-B*1502 screening in Taiwan. *N Engl J Med* 2011;364: 1126–1133.

Ciralsky JB, Sippel KC, Gregory DG. Current ophthalmologic treatment strategies for acute and chronic Stevens-Johnson syndrome and toxic epidermal necrolysis. *Curr Opin Ophthalmol* 2013;24: 321–328.

Downey A, Jackson C, Harun N, et al. Toxic epidermal necrolysis: review of pathogenesis and management. *J Am Acad Dermatol* 2012; 66:995–1003.

Huang YC, Li YC, Chen TJ. The efficacy of intravenous immunoglobulin for the treatment of toxic epidermal necrolysis: a systematic review and meta-analysis. *Br J Dermatol* 2012;167:424–432.

Hung SI, Chung WH, Liou LB, et al. HLA-B*5801 allele as a genetic marker for severe cutaneous adverse reactions caused by allopurinol. *Proc Natl Acad Sci U S A* 2005;102:4134–4139.

Lee HY, Lim YL, Thirumoorthy T, et al. The role of intravenous immunoglobulin in toxic epidermal necrolysis: a retrospective analysis of 64 patients managed in a specialized centre. *Br J Dermatol* 2013;169: 1304–1309.

Mallal S, Nolan D, Witt C, et al. Association between presence of HLA-B*5701, HLA-DR7, and HLA-DQ3 and hypersensitivity to HIV-1 reverse-transcriptase inhibitor abacavir. *Lancet* 2002;359: 727–732.

Ravin KA, Rappaport LD, Zuckerbraun NS, et al. Mycoplasma pneumoniae and atypical Stevens-Johnson syndrome: a case series. *Pediatrics* 2007;119:e1002–e1005.

Sassolas B, Haddad C, Mockenhaupt M, et al. ALDEN, an algorithm for assessment of drug causality in Stevens-Johnson syndrome and toxic epidermal necrolysis: comparison with case-control analysis. *Clin Pharmacol Ther* 2010;88:60–68.

Wootton CI, Patel AN, Williams HC. In a patient with toxic epidermal necrolysis, does intravenous immunoglobulin improve survival compared with supportive care? *Arch Dermatol* 2011;147: 1437–1440.

CHAPTER 64 ■ RASH: NEONATAL

LESLIE CASTELO-SOCCIO, MD, PhD

Rashes are common in the neonatal period and can cause significant parental distress. The ability to distinguish worrisome rashes from those that are benign is of critical importance. To provide a schema for understanding rashes in the neonate, it can be helpful to divide the rashes into categories: pustules, vesicles, patches/plaques, birth marks/hamartomas, and dyspigmentation. Within these categories, there are sign and symptoms that push the clinician to be more or less concerned.

PUSTULAR (NEONATAL ACNE)

Pustular rashes in neonates are common and can be caused by inflammation (such as in erythema toxicum and transient neonatal melanosis) or infections (yeast, bacteria like *Staphylococcus aureus,* and, rarely, herpes virus [please see vesicular neonatal rashes below for full discussion of herpes simplex]). The goal of recognition is to spare healthy infants with benign pustular eruptions extensive workups and not to miss those with more serious pustular eruptions.

Erythema Toxicum Neonatorum

Erythema toxicum neonatorum (ETN) is usually evident within the first 48 hours of life. Characteristic lesions include erythema, wheals, papules, and pustules (Fig. 64.1). This transient rash resolves spontaneously without sequelae over the course of 1 to 2 weeks. Histologically, ETN shows an abundance of eosinophils. Etiology is unclear. One prospective study of 1,000 neonates suggested that risk factors include higher birth weight, greater gestational age, vaginal delivery, maternal age <30 years, and fewer than two previous pregnancies. Culture and Gram stain looking for eosinophils can help distinguish from bacterial infection. A similarly benign pustular eruption in neonates is transient neonatal pustular melanosis (TNPM), which is usually present at delivery. TNPM is characterized by small pustules (0.3 to 0.5 cm) on a nonerythematous base. These pustules rupture easily, and pigmented macules develop with surrounding collarettes of scales that may persist for weeks to months. The pustules are mostly located over the forehead, neck, and lower back, but occasionally, palms and soles may be involved (Fig. 64.2). No systemic manifestations have been reported.

Staphylococcal Pustulosis

If a neonate presents after 48 hours with new pustules, it is more likely to be caused by infection with staphylococcus or candida. Staphylococcal pustulosis is relatively common and can occur in the setting of infection of the umbilicus or circumcision site. Community-acquired *S. aureus* is common, so risk factors for acquiring staph in neonatal period include history of staph infection in close contacts. Simple bacterial swabs are the primary diagnostic tool. Pustules on the lower abdomen and in the diaper area are common. Few pustules, in an otherwise healthy neonate, can often be treated with oral and/or topical antibiotics. Providers should look for peeling in the folds of the skin and very red or hot skin because this can be a sign of staphylococcal scalded skin (Fig. 64.3).

Neonatal Candida

Congenital candidiasis usually presents within 12 hours of birth as redness on the affected area and then later with pustules with desquamation. *Candida albicans* and *Candida psiloparis* are the most common causes of neonatal candida infections. In full term healthy infants, congenital candida can often be treated topically and is usually a nonworrisome infection. In preterm infants, or other medically complex infants, candida can be invasive and can cause late-onset neonatal sepsis. Therefore, blood cultures, urine cultures, evaluation of the CSF, opthalmologic examination, echocardiogram, renal ultrasound, and systemic antifungal therapy are needed.

Moniliasis/Candidal Diaper Dermatitis

See Chapter 61 Rash: Bacterial and Fungal Infections. Moniliasis is the most characteristic of the diaper rashes (see below for a more detailed discussion of diaper dermatitis). The skin in the diaper area has clusters of erythematous papules and pustules that coalesce into an intensely red confluent rash with sharp borders (Fig. 64.4). Beyond these borders are satellite papules and pustules. At times, the infant has concomitant oral thrush. When the problem is chronic and recurrent, seeding from the gastrointestinal (GI) tract or from a mother with monilial vaginitis should be considered.

On rare occasions, an id reaction occurs. Besides the primary monilial diaper rash lies an antigenic dissemination with involvement of the intertriginous areas and scattered small patches or plaques of scaling erythema on other parts of the skin surface. Generally, *C. albicans* cannot be cultured from the plaques of the id reaction.

INFANTILE ACROPUSTULOSIS

Infantile acropustolosis is a recurrent, self-limited, vesiculopustular disorder affecting young children (Fig. 64.5). It presents with itchy, deep-seated pustules or vesicles on the palms and soles. Most cases occur after scabies infestation and this condition can wax and wane for years. Scraping for scabies mites should be performed and treatment initiated for scabies if mites are found. Therapy is midpotency topical steroids.

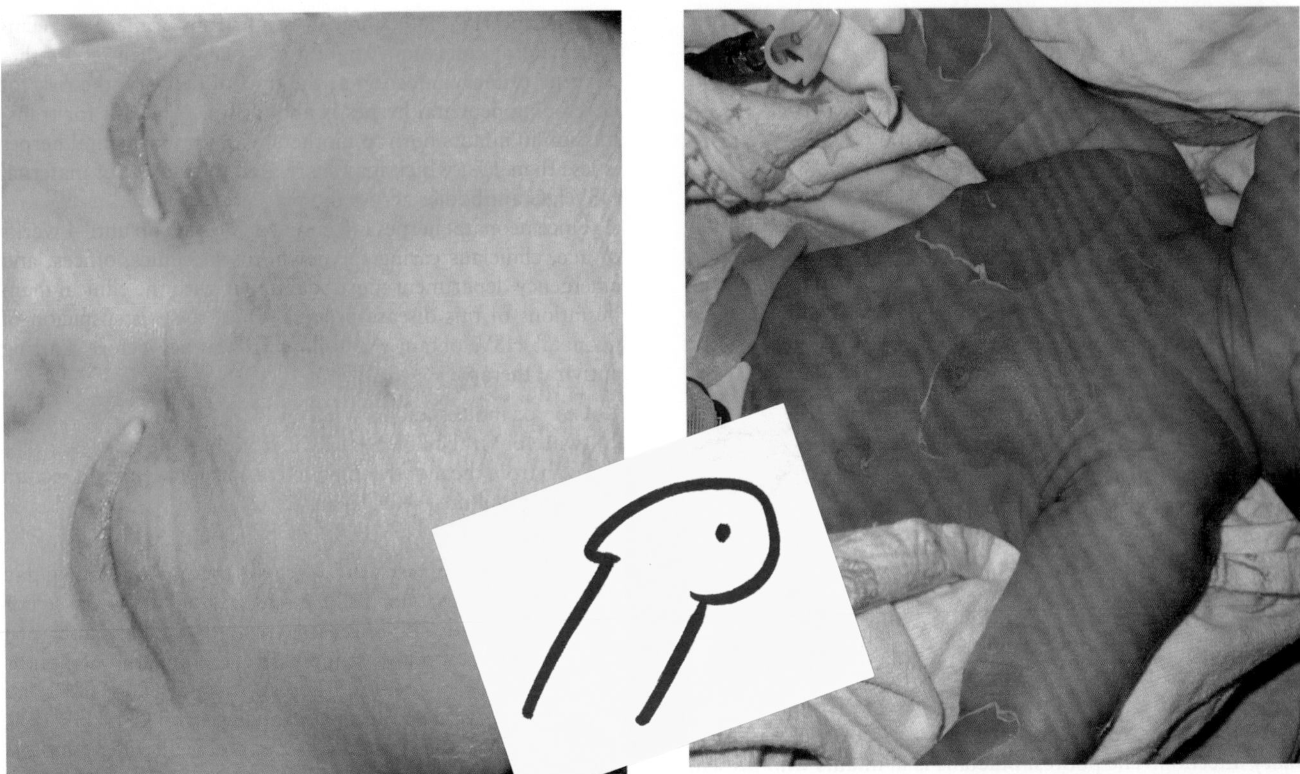

FIGURE 64.1 Infant with papules and pustules of erythema toxicum on the face.

FIGURE 64.3 Skin peeling on the trunk of infant with staphylococcal scalded skin syndrome.

VESICULAR ERUPTIONS

Neonatal herpes infection causes significant morbidity and mortality if not recognized and treated promptly (see Chapter 68 Septic Appearing Infant). Neonatal HSV can be acquired in utero (5%), in the peripartum period (85%) or in the postnatal period (10%). For the last two groupings, the extent of disease can be classified into the following categories: disseminated disease, central nervous system (CNS) disease, or skin, eye, and/or mouth (SEM) disease. A high index of suspicion is necessary in neonates presenting with vesicles or pustules, especially with a negative bacterial culture. About 40% of neonatal herpes is confined to the SEM. Most infections acquired during the peripartum period present between 9 and 11 days of life, though they can be seen earlier or later. Those infants with SEM disease are most easily diagnosed since they usually present with obvious vesicular lesions. HSV that develops in the skin usually begins as papules or vesicles that erode. Often erosions are the only visible lesions. They

FIGURE 64.2 Multiple collarets of scale on the leg of a newborn with TNPM.

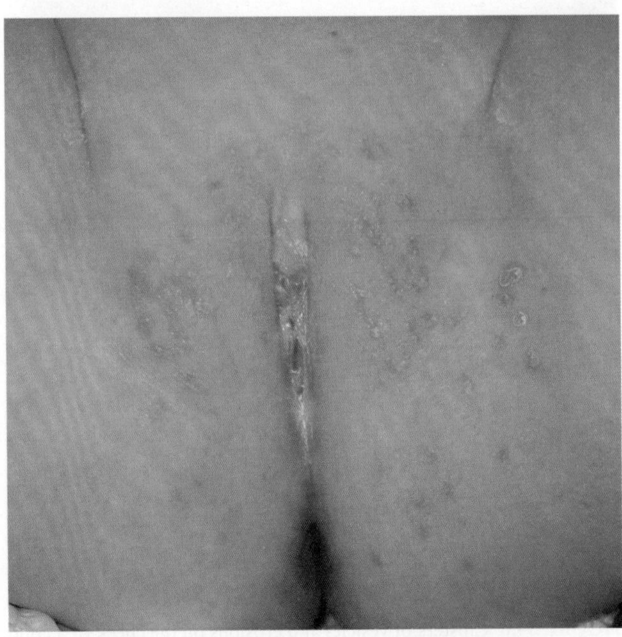

FIGURE 64.4 Infant with candidal diaper dermatitis.

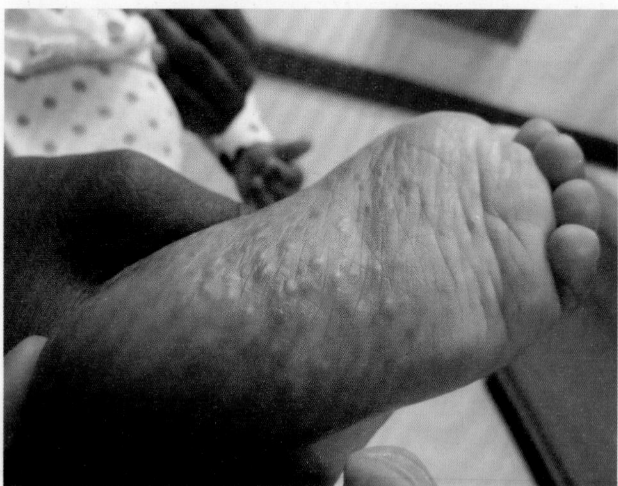

FIGURE 64.5 Acropustulosis of infancy.

usually have a red base and are 1 to 3 mm in diameter and can occur as a single unit or in clusters (Fig. 64.6). They appear anywhere on the body but are most commonly seen on the presenting parts such as the head in vertex presentation and buttocks in breach. Scalp probe sites can become sites of primary infection. The poorest outcome is in infants who present with widespread disease involving lungs, liver, adrenal gland, skin, eyes, and mouth. Infants presenting with disseminated herpes disease typically present with symptoms very similar to those associated with bacterial infection. Although the diagnosis may be easily confused, disseminated herpes disease may often be distinguishable from bacterial infection by the presence of vesicular lesions, neonatal hepatitis of unknown etiology, and DIC. Disseminated herpes infection may have a component of CNS involvement and the infant may therefore exhibit symptoms consistent with encephalitis or meningitis.

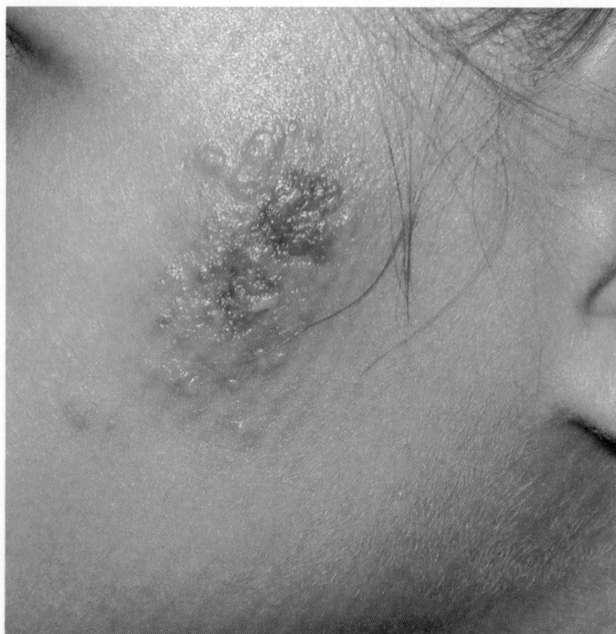

FIGURE 64.6 Clusters of vesicles and erosions on the cheek of a child with HSV.

Intrauterine HSV infection can result from primary or recurrent maternal infection. Highest risk occurs when the mother has true primary infection at the time of delivery; the risk for developing neonatal herpes is about 30%. The risk for transmission in infants born to mothers with known genital herpes is less than 1%, which may be related to transfer of maternal HSV IgG antibodies across the placenta.

Since neonatal herpes infection can be seen up until 4 weeks of age, clinicians caring for newborns in clinics, offices, and emergency department must be familiar with the clinical manifestations of this disease process. Once there is suspicion of neonatal HSV, obtain the following samples before starting antiviral therapy:

1. CSF for indices and HSV DNA PCR,
2. swab for viral culture +/– PCR from base of vesicles,
3. swab from the mouth, conjunctiva, nasopharynx and rectum for viral culture +/– PCR, and
4. whole blood for HSV DNA PCR.

Start empiric intravenous acyclovir therapy (60 mg/kg/day divided in 3 doses). For SEM disease, treat for 14 days. For disseminated and CNS diseases, treat for 21 days and then treat with oral acyclovir suppressive therapy for 6 months (900 mg/m^2/day divided in 3 doses). Also, for both CNS and disseminated diseases, repeat CSF analysis and CSF HSV PCR before stopping therapy and, if detectable in CSF, continue therapy until negative CSF PCR results. Dose of acyclovir should be weight-adjusted for the duration of therapy. Absolute neutrophil count should be monitored every 2 weeks for the first month and then monthly.

INCONTINENTIA PIGMENTI

Incontinentia pigmenti (IP) is a rare X-linked genodermatosis that affects mainly female neonates (see Chapter 62 Rash: Vesiculobullous). The first manifestation occurs in the early neonatal period and progresses through four stages: vesicular, verruciform, hyperpigmented, and hypopigmented. Clinical features also manifest themselves through changes in the teeth, eyes, hair, CNS, bone structures, skeletal musculature, and immune system. IP is often mistaken for an infectious process (Fig. 64.7). PCR and cultures of the vesicles yield negative

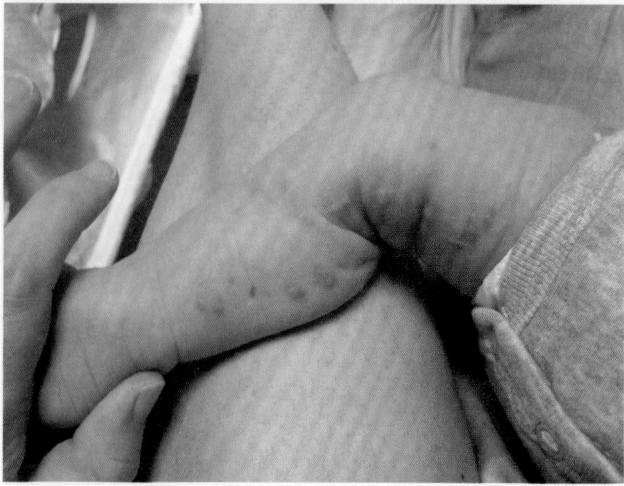

FIGURE 64.7 Linear vesicles in a newborn with the first stage of incontinentia pigmenti.

results. The clue to this diagnosis is that the vesicles usually occur on the arms and/or legs in a linear pattern that follows the lines of Blaschko. Genetic testing and/or a biopsy can help confirm the diagnosis. Rarely, boys that are XXY or have somatic mosaicism present with IP.

PATCHES AND PLAQUES

Annular Rashes

Neonatal lupus is an autoimmune disorder caused by the passive transfer of maternal autoantibodies, anti-Ro, anti-La, and, less commonly, anti-ribonucleoprotein (U1-RNP) (Fig. 64.8). The skin and heart are commonly affected, with the most serious complication being third-degree atrioventricular heart block (AVB), which results in fetal and neonatal mortality rates of 15% to 30%. Ten percent of patients experience thrombocytopenia, neutropenia, or anemia, which are usually transient. Neonatal lupus can present as annular, red, scaly patches, most commonly on the head and neck. Rash around the periorbital region should make suspicion very high (Fig. 64.9). Neonatal lupus can also manifest as scaly atrophic patches similar to discoid lupus. Mucosal erosions have been noted in some infants. The diagnosis also has implications for the mother and her future pregnancies. Women who have had a child with NLE have a 17% to 19% risk of having a child with neonatal lupus in subsequent pregnancies. Current recommendations suggest serial fetal weekly echocardiograms from 16 to 26 weeks of gestation, then every other week until 34 weeks. Up to 83% of mothers who have an infant diagnosed with NLE are asymptomatic at the time. However, approximately 50% of these mothers have or will subsequently develop an autoimmune disorder. Any annular erythematous rash in a newborn should be assumed to be NLE until definitively proven otherwise.

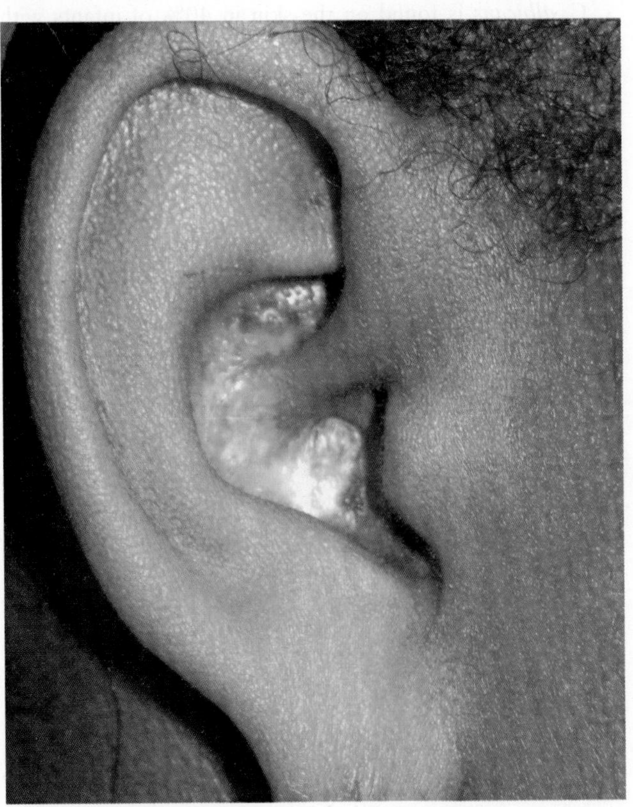

FIGURE 64.8 Infant with neonatal lupus.

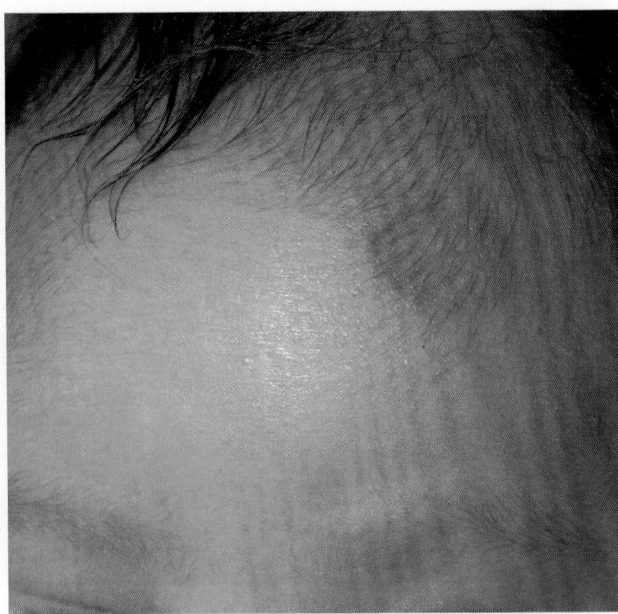

FIGURE 64.9 Annular red plaque near the eye of an infant with neonatal lupus.

Scaly Red Patches and Plaques

Dermatophyte Infections

Rarely, tinea has been reported in infants as young as a 2 to 3 weeks of life. Topical therapy is usually sufficient to treat tinea capitis or corporis in this group, and a dermatophyte screen can confirm the diagnosis. Please see Chapter 61 Rash: Bacterial and Fungal Infections for more details.

Atopic Dermatitis/Seborrheic Dermatitis

Neonates can present with scaly and greasy red patches as early as the first month of life. *Seborrheic dermatitis* is the term given to the salmon-colored patches with yellow, greasy scales occurring primarily in the so-called seborrheic areas (face, postauricular area, scalp, axilla, groin, and presternal area) (Fig. 64.10A,B). Seborrheic dermatitis is seen in infants or adolescents. Its onset occurs during the first 3 months. It may also reappear in adolescence. Often in the first months of life, atopic dermatitis and seborrheic dermatitis can overlap, leading to a head to toe pattern of redness and scale with accentuation on the scalp and face. For the seborrheic dermatitis component in the scalp, removing scales with a soft brush after application of an oil or petrolatum can be useful. Shampoos can be helpful for pure seborrheic dermatitis but will make atopic dermatitis worse because of increasing dryness. Low-potency topical steroids are usually sufficient to treat seborrheic dermatitis and atopic dermatitis. This should accompany gentle skin care, including use of moisturizing cleanser when bathing a few times a week and using moisturizers twice a day. A clue to the presence of atopic dermatitis is the waxing and waning of the rash (Fig. 64.11). Car-seat dermatitis (reaction to materials that line car seats) and other contact and irritant reactions (e.g., pacifiers) have been

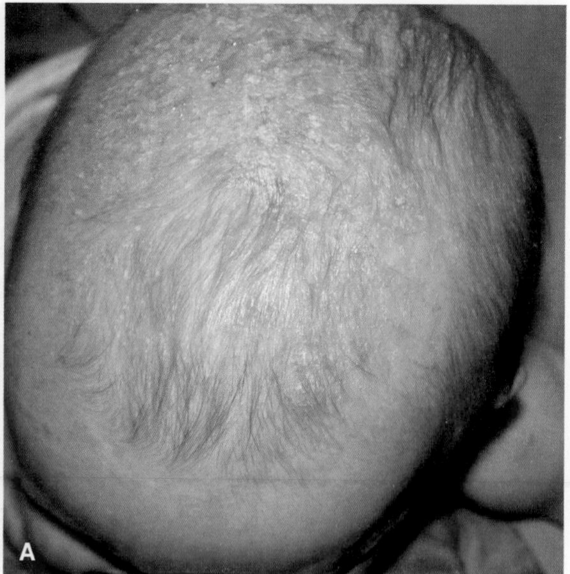

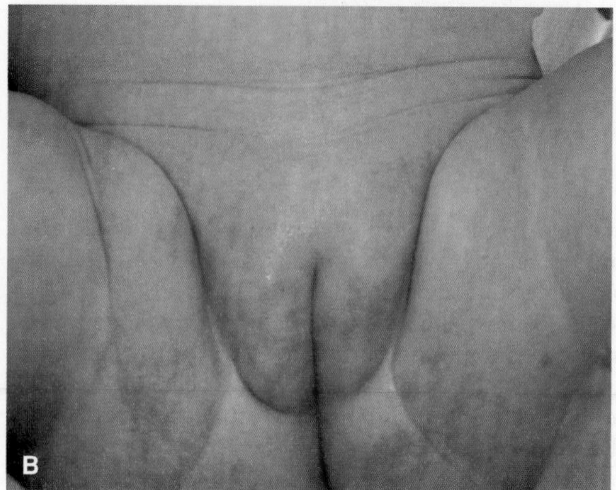

FIGURE 64.10 **A:** Infant with seborrheic dermatitis on scalp and face. **B:** Infant with seborrheic dermatitis in the diaper area.

reported in neonates as well. These typically present more suddenly and when the causative agent is removed the rash will resolve and not recur. Full discussion of atopic dermatitis can be found in Chapter 60 Rash: Atopic Dermatitis, Contact Dermatitis, Scabies and Erythroderma.

Diaper Dermatitis

Diaper dermatitis is a general term used to describe skin abnormalities beneath the diaper. The problem is common in children 2 years of age or younger who require the use of a diaper. It generally disappears after toilet training. The pathogenesis of the problem is multifactorial (Fig. 64.12) and not clearly defined. The possibilities include concentration of bacteria or fungi, action of organisms on urine, and moisture itself.

There is no conclusive evidence that bacteria play a major role in diaper dermatitis. However, bacterial overgrowth occurs with time on moist skin, and bacteria have been implicated in liberating ammonia from urine and raising urine pH. The rise in pH increases the activity of fecal proteases and lipases, which can damage skin. Bile salts can potentiate this damage.

C. albicans is found on the skin in 40% of infants with active diaper dermatitis within 72 hours of the appearance of

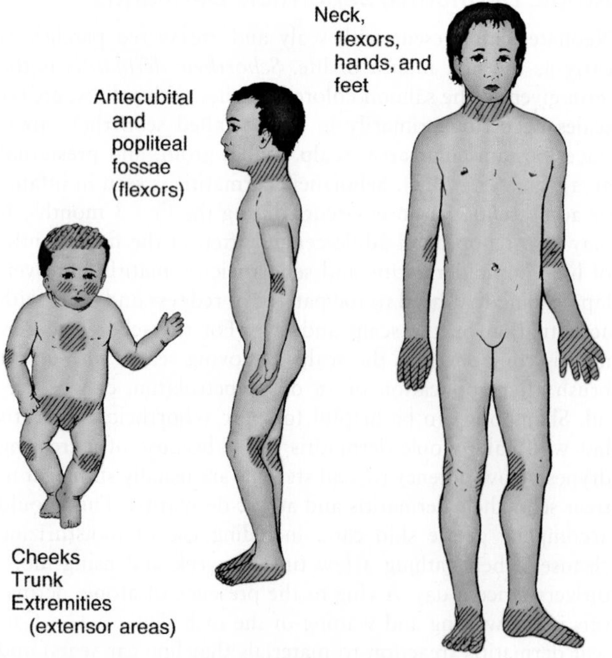

FIGURE 64.11 Distribution of atopic eczema at various ages.

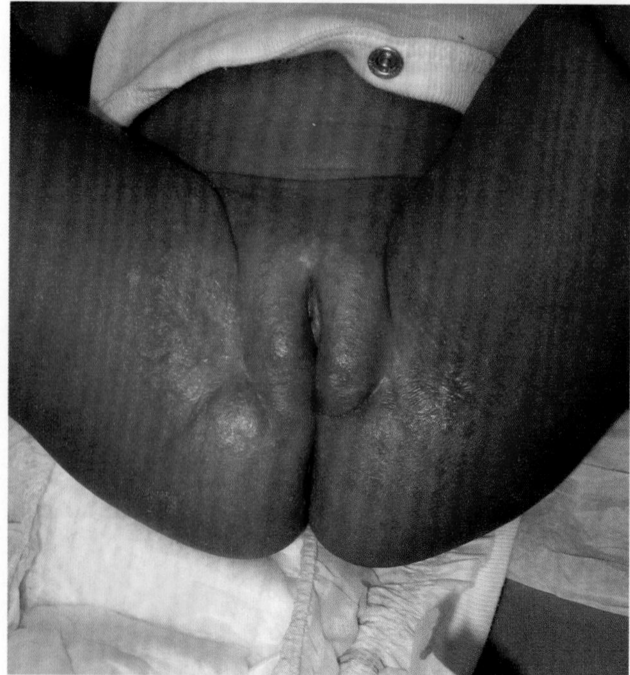

FIGURE 64.12 Infant with irritant/contact diaper dermatitis.

the rash. Because studies show that this organism is present in less than 10% of infants without diaper dermatitis, it may be playing a significant role. Sources of *C. albicans* include the GI tract and secondary implantation from a mother with candidal vaginitis.

If there is one major instigating factor, it is the effect of chronic exposure to moisture, which is critical to the development of diaper dermatitis. Chronic exposure of the skin to moisture, especially under occlusion by the diaper, leads to maceration and alteration of the epidermal barrier with overgrowth of bacteria (including group A β-hemolytic streptococci) and *C. albicans*. Traditional diaper creams and ointments create a moisture barrier and are usually recommended. These include petrolatum, silicone, and zinc oxide preparations.

Another consideration is the predisposition of certain individuals to react more easily and negatively to varying irritants. There are instances of true allergic contact dermatitis from baby wipes and dyes and fragrances found in diapers. Allergies to dyes usually occur at the waist band, the area that fits tightly around the leg, and in the center of the diaper, sparing the folds. If this is a concern, then switching to dye-free and fragrance-free diapers and using water or soft cloths with water instead of traditional disposable wipes may help. Generally, infants with an atopic or seborrheic predisposition are at greater risk for the development and persistence of diaper dermatitis. Differentiation of the various types of diaper dermatitis is difficult. Clues from the history and physical examination are necessary when characterizing the cause of this problem. The different types of diaper rashes include occlusion dermatitis, atopic dermatitis, seborrheic dermatitis, moniliasis, and mixed dermatitis. Acrodermatitis enteropathica, which is caused by zinc deficiency, psoriasis, and Langerhan cell histiocytosis, should also be considered in the differential diagnosis for diaper dermatitis that is persistent or does not respond to antifungals and anti-inflammatory medications.

Treatment is determined by the cause of the dermatitis. In general, proper skin care, which includes decreased frequency of washing, use of mild soaps, and use of barrier emollients, will help with any diaper dermatitis. With occlusive dermatitis, avoidance of tightly fitting diapers, plastic-covered paper diapers, and rubber pants is important. When atopic dermatitis is present, the use of topical steroids is necessary. It is important to avoid fluorinated or other potent steroids in the diaper area because occlusion by the diaper enhances the steroid effect and is more likely to produce skin atrophy and striae. The newer antifungal–steroid combinations should also be avoided for these same reasons. Therefore, 1% or 2.5% hydrocortisone cream or ointment no more than twice daily over a short period is recommended. Hydrocortisone (1% or 2.5%) is also effective for seborrheic diaper dermatitis and can be used intermittently. With monilial diaper dermatitis, the use of preparations such as econazole, miconazole, or nystatin twice daily is effective. If thrush is also present, oral nystatin suspension, 200,000 units (2 mL) four times a day for 7 days, is advisable. This medication will also be useful if the infant is seeding *C. albicans* from the GI tract onto the skin of the diaper area. Patients with id reactions, as described previously, require oral nystatin or econazole on the diaper and intertriginous areas and low-potency topical steroids applied to the plaques. Resolution usually takes 7 to 10 days. Secondarily infected dermatitis, such as bullous impetigo, should be treated with the appropriate systemic antibiotics or in some cases topical antibiotics.

Atrophic Patches

Aplasia Cutis

Aplasia cutis is a congenital defect that is characterized by localized absence of epidermis and dermis and, sometimes, subcutaneous fat. It generally occurs on the scalp (80% near the hair whorl) but can occur on any location of the body. Right after birth, aplasia cutis can appear as a scar or as a weeping, granulating oval or circular defect. Small defects are the most common but larger ones sometimes occur and may extend to the dura or meninges. Some lesions may present with an almost bullous appearance and when surrounded by dark hair or thicker hair (hair collar sign) may represent a form of neural tube defect. Patients with these lesions should undergo an MRI of the brain to look for underlying connection to the brain. Congenital absence of skin can also be seen with epidermolysis bullosa. Antithyroid drugs, most notably methimazole, have been implicated in some cases of aplasia cutis congenita.

Indurated Plaques

Subcutaneous Fat Necrosis

Subcutaneous fat necrosis is a skin change that leads to freely mobile nodules and plaques with or without redness. These can be asymptomatic or mildly tender. They usually appear within the first 6 weeks of life and are usually limited to areas of trauma or ischemia during delivery. Risk factors include high birth weight, prolonged labor, neuroprotective cooling, and other ischemia. The most common locations are the back, buttocks, and cheeks. Lesions resolve spontaneously in weeks to months. Mild atrophy of the skin may be noted after resolution. Complications include hyper- or hypocalcemia, lactic acidosis, high levels of ferritin, and transient thrombocytopenia; hypercalcemia is the most common. For extensive lesions, serum calcium, phosphorus, parathyroid hormone, and vitamin D levels should be monitored and patients should be observed closely for irritability, vomiting, anorexia, renal failure, or failure to thrive in the first 6 months. Pamidronate and low-calcium formula are used in severe cases. Corticosteroids have also been used to control hypercalcemia by interfering with the metabolism of vitamin D to the active 1,25-dihydroxyvitamin D. In most cases, reassurance is all that is needed.

Vascular Patches/Plaques and Hamartomas

Acute Hemorrhagic Edema of Infancy

Acute hemorrhagic edema of infancy is a distinctive, cutaneous small-vessel leukocytoclastic vasculitis of young children. Dark purple or pink in color, somewhat annular patches and plaques, without surface change, occur mostly on the face and extremities (Fig. 64.13). Infants otherwise look well and are usually afebrile or at most have a low-grade fever. Visceral involvement is uncommon, and spontaneous recovery usually occurs within 1 to 3 weeks without sequelae. The main differential diagnosis is Henoch–Schönlein purpura.

Hemangiomas

Hemangiomas of infancy (infantile hemangiomas) represent benign vascular tumors that are present in approximately 3%

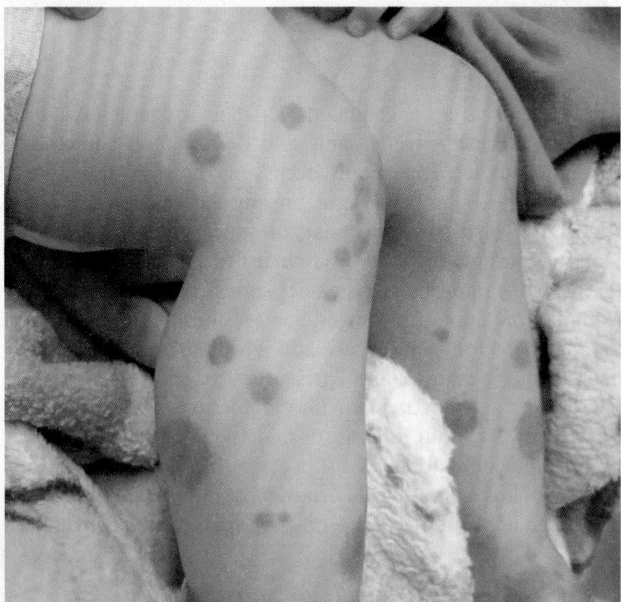

FIGURE 64.13 Infant with acute hemorrhagic edema of infancy.

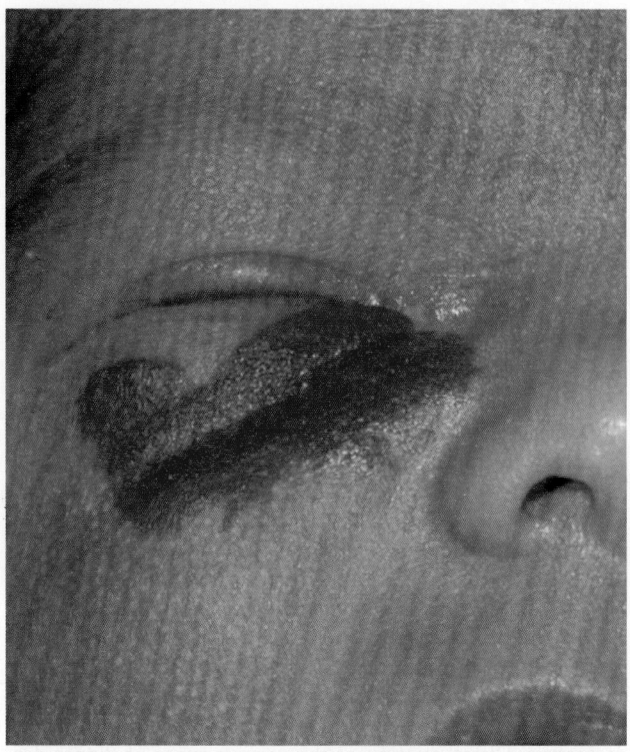

FIGURE 64.14 Infant with rapidly enlarging hemangioma of the eye.

of newborns and up to 10% of all infants. These are seen more frequently in premature and low–birth-weight infants and occur more commonly in girls than in boys. Superficial lesions possess a red color,resembling a strawberry or raspberry. Deep lesions appear soft, compressible, and often are faintly bluish. Mixed lesions may show features of both superficial and deep hemangiomas. These lesions typically undergo a proliferative phase during the first 4 to 6 months, plateau in growth during the second 6 months, and then begin a slow process of involution. Although most lesions generally involute with little to no complications given time, certain hemangiomas pose potential risks based on their anatomic location (see below). Beta-blockers, specifically systemic propranolol and topical timolol, are used to treat severe hemangiomas of infancy. Potential complications include bradycardia, hypotension, hypoglycemia, bronchospasm, and hypothermia; however, overall safety, even in young infants, has been good.

Rapidly enlarging hemangiomas near the eyes (Fig. 64.14) may result in amblyopia through obstruction of the visual axis (deprivation amblyopia) or because of the compression of the eyeball itself (strabismus or anisometropia) and require prompt intervention with systemic steroids or sometimes surgery. Hemangiomas in a "beard" distribution—around the mouth, preauricular areas, chin, or anterior neck—may indicate the presence of airway hemangiomas and warrant further evaluation by direct laryngobronchoscopy or radiologic imaging studies. Hemangiomas overlying the midline lower back may represent markers for spinal dysraphism or tethered cord syndrome and warrant imaging. Hemangiomas occurring in any area, but especially the oral or genital areas, may ulcerate and become secondarily infected, which may result in pain and permanent scarring. Treatment with topical or oral antibiotics, topical timolol with nonadherent dressings, can be helpful in managing these cases. Some may require treatment with a pulsed-dye laser. Finally, large, segmental facial hemangiomas have been associated with PHACE(S) syndrome, in which children suffer from *P*osterior fossa malformations; facial *H*emangiomas; *A*rterial anomalies, including coarctation of the aorta; structural *C*ardiac malformations; *E*ndocrinologic and structural *E*ye abnormalities; and midline *S*ternal defects or supraumbilical raphe. Intracranial vascular anomalies may predispose this subset of these children to an increased risk for stroke. The corollary in the pelvic region is called LUMBAR syndrome (lower body hemangioma and other cutaneous defects, urogenital anomalies, ulceration, myelopathy, bony deformities, anorectal malformations, arterial anomalies, and renal anomalies). These patients can also be at risk for arterial as well as other urogenital and bony abnormalities (Table 64.1).

Some vascular tumors, including kaposiform hemangioendotheliomas and tufted angiomas, may resemble hemangiomas. These unusual vascular tumors may undergo sudden

TABLE 64.1

COMPLICATIONS RELATED TO HEMANGIOMAS

Anatomic location	Associated complication
Periocular	Amblyopia
Beard area	Airway involvement
Midline prevertebral	Tethered cord syndrome; spinal dysraphism
Genital area	Ulceration
Large, facial lesion	PHACES (posterior fossa malformation; large facial hemangioma; arterial anomalies; coarctation of the aorta or other cardiac malformation; eye abnormalities; midline sternal defects)
Large pelvic area	LUMBAR (lower body hemangioma, urogenetial anomalies, ulceration, myelopathy, bony deformities, anorectal malformation, arterial anomalies, and renal anomalies)

swelling with resulting hemolytic anemia, thrombocytopenia, and congestive heart failure, resulting in a life-threatening syndrome known as *Kasabach–Merritt phenomenon.* Patients with this syndrome may require high doses of systemic corticosteroid or other chemotherapeutic interventions to control these complications.

DISORDERS OF PIGMENTATION

Brown Papules

Mastocytoma, Urticaria Pigmentosa

Parents of children with mastocytomas or lesions of urticaria pigmentosa generally describe a single yellow–tan–brown lesion that was present at or soon after birth (mastocytoma) or multiple pigmented papules that erupt during the first year of life (urticaria pigmentosa). One important clue is a history of these lesions becoming red (Fig. 64.15), hivelike, or blistered. The lesions may ooze and form crusts, much like impetigo; however, they do not respond to antibacterial preparations.

On physical examination, appearance is variable. The surface may have a peau d'orange appearance. Some papules are yellow and are easily mistaken for xanthomas. When they are tan to brown, they may be mistaken for raised moles. The key finding is a positive Darier sign, which is histamine-induced erythema, swelling, and urtication secondary to scratching and subsequent degranulation of mast cells.

When large amounts of these mediators are released, generalized flushing, persistent diarrhea, or hypotension may ensue. Children with these symptoms require therapy directed against histamine and prostaglandin D_2. Long acting H_1 blockers like cetirizine are often combined with long acting H_2 blockers like ranitidine. Shorter acting H_1 blockers, such as diphenhydramine and hydroxyzine, are sometimes used as rescue agents. NSAIDs are generally avoided in these patients because they are mast cell degranulators. There are limited data on the use of ibuprofen or indomethacin to inhibit prostaglandin synthesis but these are not first line therapy because often these make blistering worse. Children who suffer from persistent histamine-induced diarrhea may benefit from the addition of oral cromolyn sodium. An epinephrine pen should be provided for patients with systemic disease or extensive symptoms.

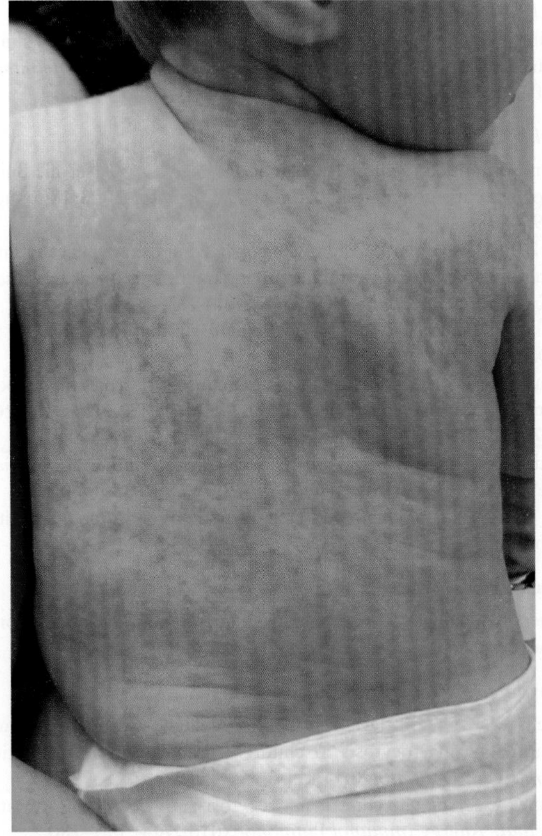

FIGURE 64.15 Infant with urticaria pigmentosa and positive Darier sign.

TABLE 64.2

COMMON ED MEDICATIONS AND PHYSICAL STIMULI TO BE AVOIDED IN PATIENTS WITH URTICARIA PIGMENTOSA

Medications	Physical stimuli
Alcohol	Rubbing of skin
Aspirin	Extreme water temperatures
Codeine	
Dextran	
Morphine/opiates	

Fortunately, with aging, the skin is no longer reactive, and most of the lesions disappear completely or leave only color change.

Table 64.2 lists medications and physical stimuli that cause mast cell degranulation and histamine and/or prostaglandin D_2 release. These agents should be avoided.

Hypopigmentation/Depigmentation

Pigmentary mosaicism exists when an individual is composed of two or more genetically different cell populations that lead to color variation; both hypo- and hyperpigmentation can occur within a Blaschkoid distribution. While small areas require reassurance, larger areas can be associated with neurologic, eye, cardiac, and skeletal anomalies. No definitive therapy exists.

A dominant form of partial albinism occurs in which localized areas of skin and hair are devoid of pigment. Ocular albinism is also seen. Two syndromes with albinism are Waardenberg syndrome (white forelock, heterochromia of the iris, and sensorineural hearing loss) and Chediak–Higashi syndrome (immunodeficiency and leukocytes with giant granules).

Loss of pigmentation can be a result of the absence of melanocytes as in vitiligo and halo nevi. Vitiligo is a symmetric, patchy loss of pigmentation. Hairs located in areas of vitiligo are often white. Vitiligo can be associated with alopecia areata, pernicious anemia, Addison disease, hypothyroidism, diabetes mellitus, hypoparathyroidism, and other endocrine disorders. Vitiligo, and some of the diseases associated with it, may be autoimmune disorders. Antibodies directed against melanocytes have been detected.

Suppression of melanocytic pigment production can cause loss of pigmentation, as in postinflammatory hypopigmentation. An example of this condition is the white patch of hypopigmentation and scaling often seen on the face, trunk,

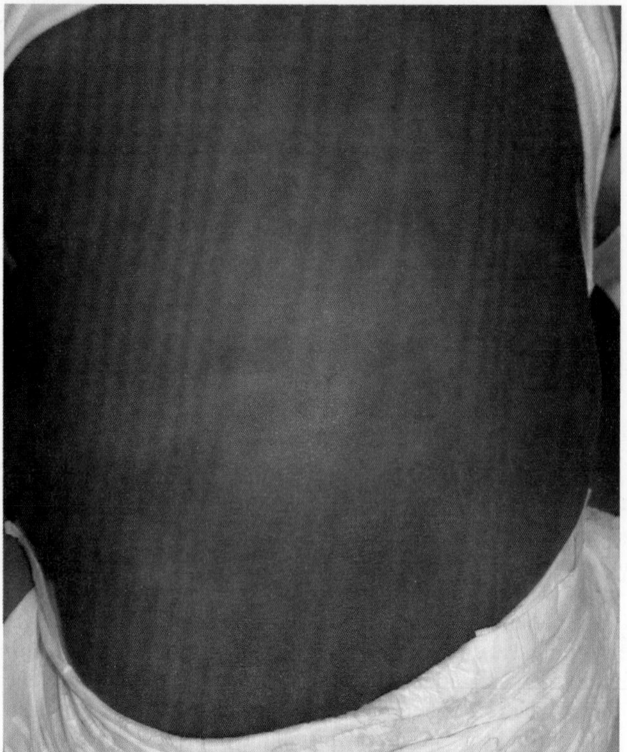

FIGURE 64.16 Dark blue patches on the buttocks and back of infant with dermal melanocytosis, formerly called Mongolian spots.

or extremities of children with atopic eczema. The ash-leaf macule is a flat, hypopigmented (whitish) spot that is present in more than 90% of patients with tuberous sclerosis. In patients with less skin pigment, they are more easily seen by shining a Wood lamp on the skin.

Hyperpigmentation

Diffuse hyperpigmentation is associated with Addison disease, acromegaly, and hemochromatosis.

Pigment deep in the dermis appears gray or blue at the surface of the skin. Mongolian blue spots, now called dermal melanocytes, are an example (Fig. 64.16). The Nevus of Ota is dermal pigment in the distribution of the ophthalmic branch of the fifth nerve; this pigmentation can also involve the sclera and palate.

Certain syndromes, including neurofibromatosis, are associated with pigmented skin lesions. Patients with this disease have café-au-lait spots, which are flat, nonpalpable, coffee-colored lesions of varying size and shape. When six or more lesions are present, greater than 0.5 cm in size, neurofibromatosis should be considered. The Peutz–Jeghers syndrome is a dominantly inherited condition that includes freckle-like lesions of the lips, nose, buccal mucosa, fingertips, and subungual areas associated with polyps in the small intestine, stomach, or colon. Melena and intussusception are the chief complications that may develop, usually in the second decade of life. McCune-Albright syndrome should be suspected when unilateral café-au-lait spots with irregular borders occur in the lumbosacral area. Included in this syndrome are bony abnormalities and precocious puberty. Children who have large, swirling areas of pigmentation following lines of Blaschko (lines representing planes of cutaneous embryogenesis) may have forms of cutaneous mosaicism as can be seen in linear and whorled nevoid hypermelanosis.

Spitz nevi are papules that can occur as a single papule or as a collection of papules. They can be pink, red, brown or black. They often occur on the face and extremities of children but can occur anywhere on the body. There is a lot of debate about these papules and most feel they are benign despite having histology that in the past was confused with melanomas. There are atypical variants of Spitz nevi and these require complete excision. True malignant melanoma is rare in children but can occur. They can arise *de novo* or within a congenital melanocytic nevus. Giant congenital melanocytic nevi have a high risk of malignant transformation, whereas small and medium have a much lower risk of transformation.

Suggested Readings and Key References

Pustules and Vesicles

Ehrenreich M, Tarlow MM, Godlewska-Janusz E, et al. Incontinentia pigmenti (Bloch-Sulzberger syndrome): a systemic disorder. *Cutis* 2007;79(5):355–362.

Ferrazzini G, Kaiser RR, Hirsig Cheng SK, et al. Microbiological aspects of diaper dermatitis. *Dermatology* 2003;206(2):136–141.

Fortunov RM, Hulten KG, Hammerman WA, et al. Evaluation and treatment of community-acquired Staphylococcus aureus infections in term and late-preterm previously healthy neonates. *Pediatrics* 2007;120(5):937–945.

Hundalani S, Pammi M. Invasive fungal infections in newborns and current management strategies. *Expert Rev Anti Infect Ther* 2013; 11(7):709–721.

Kimberlin DW. Neonatal herpes simplex infection. *Clin Microbiol Rev* 2004;17(1):1–13.

Paloni G, Berti I, Cutrone M. Acropustulosis of Infancy. *Arch Dis Child Fetal Neonatal Ed* 2013;98(4):F340.

Pinninti SG, Kimberlin DW. Management of neonatal herpes simplex virus infection and exposure. *Arch Dis Child Fetal Neontal Ed* 2014;99(3):F240–F244.

Patches and Plaques

Colon-Fontanez F, Fallon Friedlander S, Newbury R, et al. Bullous aplasia cutis congenital. *J Am Acad Dermatol* 2003;48(5 suppl): S95–S98.

Izmirly PM, Buyon JP, Saxena A. Neonatal Lupus: advances in understanding pathogenesis and identifying treatments of cardiac disease. *Curr Opin Rheumatol* 2012;24(5):466–472.

Klunk C, Domigues E, Wiss K. An update on diaper dermatitis. *Clin Dermatol* 2014;32(4):477–487.

Mitra S, Dove J, Somisetty SK. Subcutaneous fat necrosis in newborn - an unusual case and review of the literature. *Eur J Pediatr* 2011; 170(9):1107–1110.

Poindexter GB, Burkhart CN, Morrell DS. Therapies for pediatric seborrheic dermatitis. *Pediatr Ann* 2009;38(6):333–338.

Totri CR, Diaz L, Eichenfield LF. 2014 update on atopic dermatitis is children. *Curr Opin Pediatr* 2014;26(4):466–471.

Hamartomas

Püttgen KB. Diagnosis and management of infantile hemangiomas. *Pediatr Clin North Am* 2014;61(2):383–402.

Disorders of Pigmentation

Castells M, Metcalfe DD, Escribano L. Diagnosis and treatment of cutaneous mastocytosis in children: practical recommendations. *Am J Clin Dermatol* 2011;12(4):259–270.

Frieri M, Quershi M. Pediatric mastocytosis: a review of the literature. *Pediatr Allergy Immunol Pulmonol* 2013;26(4):175–180.

CHAPTER 65 ■ RASH: PAPULOSQUAMOUS ERUPTIONS

ALBERT C. YAN, MD, FAAP, FAAD

VIRAL SYNDROMES

Viruses are involved as the presumed cause or trigger for a variety of patterned skin disorders. Typically, these syn[illegible] arise either during the acute phase of the dise[illegible] Kaposi varicelliform eruption [KVE]), or as a reacti[illegible] enon as the viral infection resolves (as with papul[illegible] gloves-and-socks eruption [PPGS], unilateral lat[illegible] exanthem [ULE], and Gianotti–Crosti syndrome [G[illegible]

Kaposi Varicelliform Eruption

KVE is a collective term that indicates an acute, ofte[illegible] progressive, viral superinfection of an underlying inflammatory skin condition (Table 65.1). When herpes simplex virus, enterovirus, or vaccinia virus secondarily infects the skin in atopic dermatitis, the condition is referred to as eczema herpeticum (EH), eczema enteroviricum (coxsackium), or eczema vaccinatum, respectively. Less commonly, inflammatory diseases such as psoriasis, pityriasis rubra pilaris (PRP), or blistering skin diseases like pemphigus vulgaris, pemphigus foliaceus, keratosis follicularis (Darier disease), or benign familial pemphigus (Hailey–Hailey disease) can become superinfected, usually with herpes simplex virus and less commonly, varicella zoster virus.

The hallmarks of the condition are the acute onset and rapid progression of viral skin lesions. Initially localized vesicles or pustules will rapidly spread and later evolve into punched-out erosions (Fig. 65.1). These cutaneous findings characteristically occur at anatomic sites where the primary skin disease is either present or has previously been located, and help to differentiate KVE from a primary (first-episode) viral HSV or enteroviral outbreak.

KVE may be accompanied by fever, mucocutaneous involvement, malaise, and poor oral intake. Signs of bacterial superinfection with *Staphylococcus aureus* or *Streptococcus pyogenes* may be present. *S. pyogenes* by itself may cause superinfection in an atopic child that resembles eczema herpeticum, presenting with fever, cellulitis, and clusters of pustular skin lesions.

The decision to admit to hospital should be determined by the degree of toxicity. While patients may require in-hospital care for intravenous hydration or intravenous antibiotic therapy to address bacteremia, selected nontoxic patients with limited disease may be successfully and reasonably managed in the outpatient setting, as long as patients are followed closely and reconsidered for admission if they do not respond adequately or worsen clinically.

When a patient is suspected of having KVE, the initial history taking should identify the existence of an underlying primary skin disease history, its usual sites of anatomic involvement, and the suspected viral agent—herpes simplex, enterovirus, vaccinia, or varicella zoster.

Recomm[illegible] diagnostic studies include polymerase chain [illegible]say, direct fluorescent antibody testing, or [illegible]pes simplex virus, varicella zoster virus, and [illegible]viral PCR or culture. Vaccinia virus may be [illegible]ppropriate exposure context. Bacterial skin [illegible]ulture for bacteria may be obtained if a [illegible]on is suspected.

[illegible]erapy involves empiric antiviral treat[illegible]ainst herpes simplex, such as acyclovir or [illegible] antistaphylococcal *and* antistreptococ[illegible]erage may be considered if significant serous crusting is present, and especially if the child is febrile or ill appearing. The optimal agent depends on local antibiotic resistance patterns but will most likely include clindamycin, a first-generation cephalosporin such as cephalexin or cefazolin, a penicillinase-resistant agent such as oxacillin or nafcillin, or in more severe cases, vancomycin. If trimethoprim-sulfamethoxazole is used, it may need to be combined with another agent to provide adequate coverage for streptococci. Empiric antiviral therapy for eczema herpeticum reduces the length of hospital stay (LOS) when started promptly. In contrast, empiric systemic antibiotic therapy reduces LOS only when there is bacteremia.

Those patients with herpes simplex superinfection should be advised that reactivation of the virus may occur in between 15% and 50% within 6 to 12 months. Prompt antiviral treatment for any reactivation should be advised through their primary care clinician to avoid a recurrence of more widespread viral superinfection.

Papular-Purpuric Gloves-and-Socks Eruption

PPGS presents as an often painful petechial eruption concentrated on the palms and soles, but often extending proximally to involve the skin of the wrists, forearms, ankles, and lower legs in a so-called "gloves-and-socks" distribution (Fig. 65.2). The condition is triggered most commonly by infection with parvovirus B19, although other organisms have been linked to this condition, including cytomegalovirus, human herpesvirus 6 and 7, coxsackie B6, Epstein–Barr virus (EBV), hepatitis B virus, measles virus, *Arcanobacterium hemolyticum,* and *Mycoplasma pneumoniae.*

PPGS tends to affect young adults, typically during the spring and summer. Affected patients often have low-grade fevers along with painful, symmetrically distributed, petechial papules. There is often a sharp cutoff where the lesions stop. The oral mucosa may be affected. PPGS spontaneously resolves after approximately 1 to 3 weeks. However, it is important to

TABLE 65.1

KAPOSI VARICELLIFORM ERUPTION

Phenomenon	Primary skin disease	Superinfecting virus
Eczema herpeticum	Atopic dermatitis	Herpes simplex virus
Eczema enteroviricum (eczema coxsackium)	Atopic dermatitis	Enterovirus (coxsackie)
Eczema vaccinatum	Atopic dermatitis	Vaccinia virus
Pityriasis rubra pilaris herpeticum	Pityriasis rubra pilaris	Herpes simplex virus
Keratosis follicularis herpeticum	Darier disease (keratosis follicularis)	Herpes simplex virus
Pemphigus herpeticum	Pemphigus vulgaris, benign familial pemphigus (Hailey–Hailey)	Herpes simplex virus
Psoriasis herpeticum	Psoriasis	Varicella zoster virus

evaluate patients thoroughly in order to distinguish PPGS from more serious bleeding disorders, septicemias, or rickettsial disorders such as Rocky Mountain spotted fever. Rare associations have included coincident mononeuritis multiplex and red cell aplasia concurrent with PPGS attributed to the underlying parvovirus B19 infection.

Unilateral Laterothoracic Exanthem

ULE, also known as asymmetric periflexural exanthem, is a self-limited phenomenon attributed to a virus. It is thought to be viral because a viral prodrome may be associated, ULE occurs in community clusters, and patients generally do not experience recurrences. The condition is characterized by collections of blanchable pink macules, papules, and plaques originating in flexural creases such as the axillary, inguinal, or popliteal areas, which then extend unilaterally along the thorax and extremity (Fig. 65.3). Often, the eruption generalizes and becomes bilateral within several days. Symptoms may include mild itching.

While many viral exanthems resolve spontaneously within a week or so, ULE is longer lasting, and often takes approximately a month before it resolves. Recognition of the condition can allow the clinician to provide reassurance and an anticipated time course to the family regarding the natural history of the condition.

It is interesting to note that infection with molluscum contagiosum can trigger a ULE-like eruption. This reactive ULE-like phenomenon, however, is of often shorter duration and is typically responsive to topical steroid treatment, in contrast to ULE.

GIANOTTI–CROSTI SYNDROME (PAPULAR ACRODERMATITIS OF CHILDHOOD, PAPULOVESICULAR ACROLOCATED SYNDROME)

GCS is a self-limited reactive phenomenon clinically characterized by a blanchable papular and occasionally vesicular exanthem characteristically distributed on the cheeks of the face, the buttocks, as well as acral locations (arms and legs) (Fig. 65.4). These lesions exhibit variable pruritus. Early European and Japanese reports found an association between GCS and hepatitis B virus infection, but cases in the United States have been associated with other organisms, most notably EBV (Table 65.2).

Evaluation for a specific etiology is often not necessary unless the history or physical examination point to a specific etiology such as EBV or group A beta-hemolytic streptococcal infection, for which treatment may be necessary.

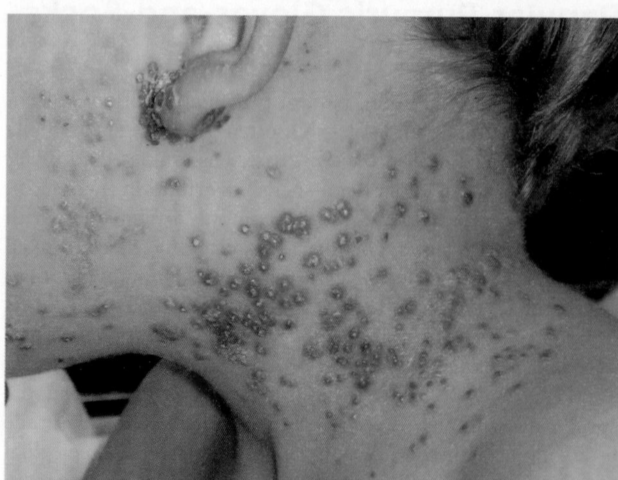

FIGURE 65.1 Kaposi varicelliform eruption. Note the crusted vesicles and pustules concentrated in areas where the pre-existing eczema has been active.

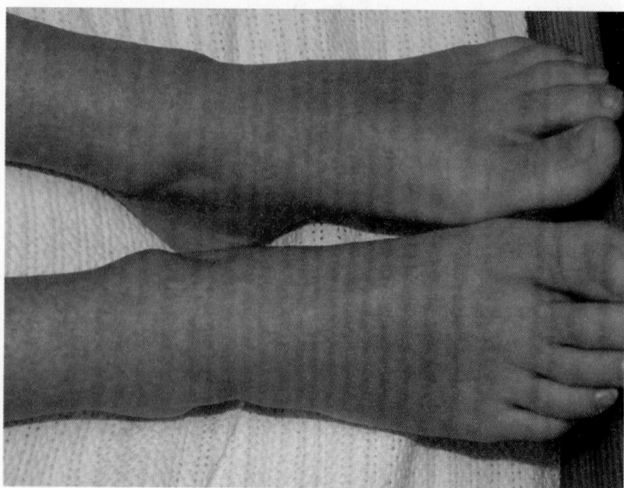

FIGURE 65.2 Papular-purpuric gloves and socks eruption caused by parvovirus B19. Note the multiple petechial papules on the ankles and feet which were also present on palms and forearms.

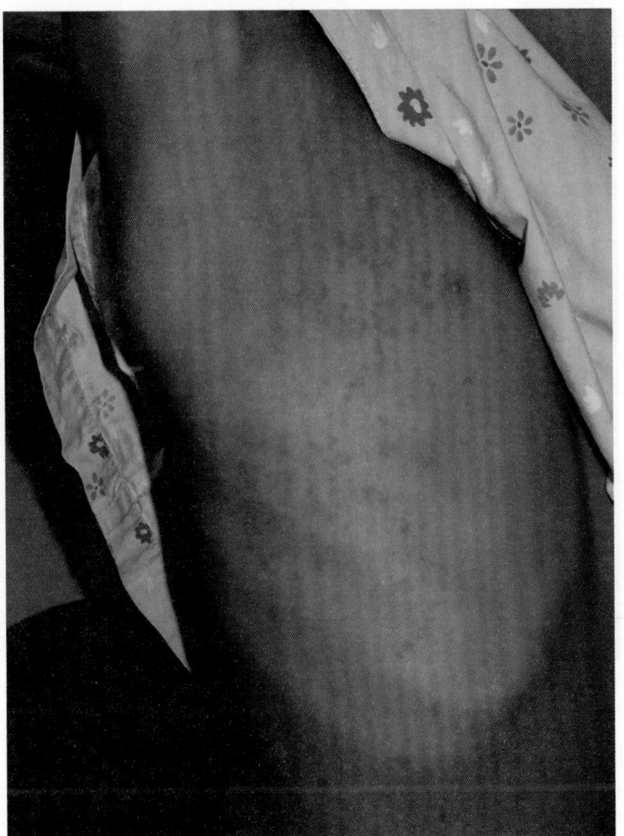

FIGURE 65.3 Unilateral laterothoracic exanthem characterized by a viral exanthem involving the right flank.

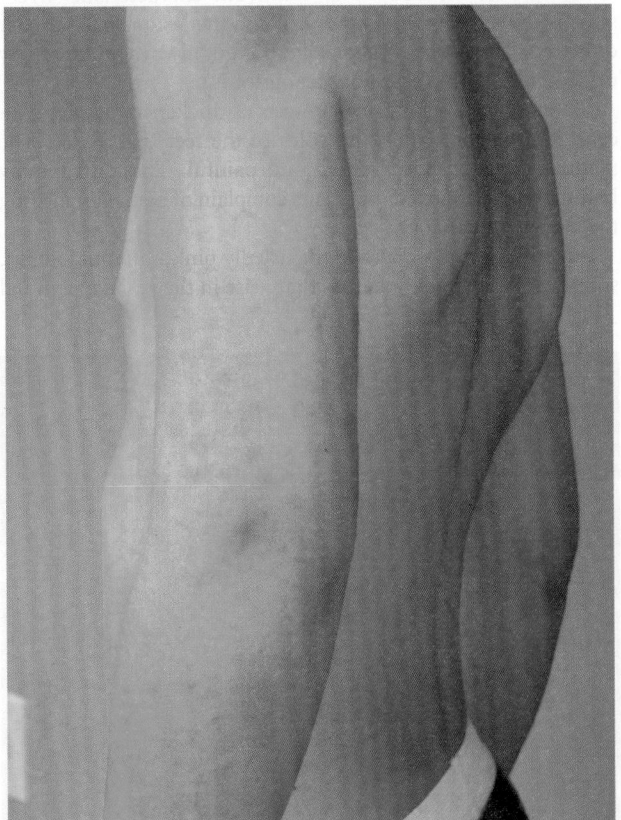

FIGURE 65.4 Gianotti–Crosti syndrome. Note the characteristic sparing of the distribution of this reactive process triggered by a viral syndrome.

TABLE 65.2

GIANOTTI–CROSTI SYNDROME: INFECTIOUS DISEASE ASSOCIATIONS

Viral	Epstein–Barr virus (most common), cytomegalovirus, enteroviruses, influenza and parainfluenza viruses, hepatitis viruses (B, C), herpes simplex virus, human herpes virus 6, human immunodeficiency virus, pox virus, respiratory syncytial virus, rotavirus
Bacterial	*Bartonella henselae, Borrelia burgdorferi, Neisseria meningitidis, Streptococcus pyogenes*
Other inflammatory triggers	Postimmunization (various)

Antihistamines may abate the pruritus symptoms although topical steroids have not been consistently beneficial in affected patients.

As with ULE, it is interesting to note that infection with molluscum contagiosum can trigger a GCS-like eruption. This reactive GCS-like phenomenon likewise, is of often shorter duration and is typically responsive to topical steroid treatment, in contrast to conventional GCS.

Papulosquamous Eruptions

Papulosquamous eruptions describe a set of skin conditions characterized by solid, elevated skin lesions (papules and plaques) that are associated with scaling. The prototypical skin condition is psoriasis; a variety of skin conditions can resemble psoriasis. These disorders can be differentiated on the basis of their morphology, configuration, distribution, and associated symptoms and signs.

The size of the lesions may be helpful for diagnosis. Tiny, flat-topped papular lesions may indicate lichen nitidus. Small drop-like papular lesions could suggest guttate psoriasis. Larger, oval, coin-sized plaques with peripheral scaling might point to pityriasis rosea (PR), secondary syphilis, lichen planus, or nummular eczema. Larger, confluent plaques would be more compatible with plaque-type psoriasis or PRP, or lichen planus.

The color of the lesions is often helpful in differentiating papulosquamous diseases. Salmon-colored erythema is typical of seborrheic dermatitis, while psoriasis is often a beefy red color. An orange-red color is characteristic of PRP, while purple with white striations is unique to lichen planus.

Configuration characterizes the local grouping of skin lesions. Koebnerization refers to the eruption of skin disease findings in a linear arrangement produced by scratching or incidental trauma (Fig. 65.5). When present, the clinician can focus on a more limited differential diagnosis because only certain skin conditions commonly produce the Koebner phenomenon: psoriasis, lichen planus, and lichen nitidus. That being said, linear lesions can be seen with allergic contact dermatitis and inoculation sites for warts or molluscum.

The distribution of skin lesions may also provide useful diagnostic clues. Plaque-type psoriasis favors the extensor surfaces of the extremities like the elbows and knees, as well as the scalp, ears, and intertriginous areas. While seborrheic

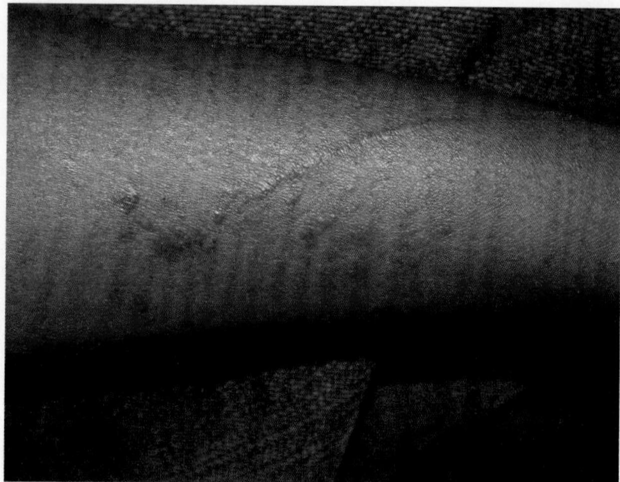

FIGURE 65.5 Note the linear purplish plaque consistent with koebnerization of lichen planus.

dermatitis also tends to involve intertriginous areas, it has a predilection for the perinasal areas, eyebrows, beard area, and external auditory canals. PR usually manifests predominantly on the torso, and skin lesions are characteristically distributed along skin cleavage lines producing the so-called "fir tree" or "pine tree" pattern on the back. Concomitant involvement of the diaper area, acral areas, and the face would raise the possibility of seborrheic dermatitis, acquired zinc deficiency, or acrodermatitis enteropathica.

Examination of the mucous membranes and skin appendages can provide corroborating evidence for a particular diagnosis. Geographic tongue may be a normal variant but is often a feature of psoriasis. Oral erosions or lacy white patterns in the mouth suggests lichen planus. Genital involvement is also a typical feature of psoriasis, lichen planus, lichen nitidus, and syphilis. Nail pitting is frequently seen in psoriasis, alopecia areata, and atopic dermatitis, but nails are generally normal in PRP despite its frequent resemblance to psoriasis.

The degree of pruritus is a helpful differentiating symptom for papulosquamous disorders. Many of the papulosquamous disorders are not particularly pruritic. When intense, itching would point to lichen planus or lichenoid drug eruptions (Table 65.3).

Psoriasis

Psoriasis is a relatively common, chronic papulosquamous disease that makes up approximately 4% of all skin disorders encountered in children. There is a predisposition for involvement of the scalp, perineum (particularly in infants), and the extensor surfaces of the body, particularly the elbows and knees. Psoriatic arthritis can occur in a minority of patients, but arthritis is more common among pediatric patients. One-third of adults with psoriasis experience onset of disease in childhood or adolescence. Among children with psoriasis, the majority develop the condition during adolescence although the condition arises in 12% before the age of 10 years.

Psoriasis occurs in several forms during childhood: plaque-type, guttate, palmoplantar, inverse, pustular, and erythrodermic. The most classic form is plaque-type psoriasis which is associated with thick, beefy red plaques with overlying silvery scales (Fig. 65.6) often in a symmetrical distribution on the extensor surfaces of the extremities, although other anatomic sites may be affected. When a scale is removed, pinpoint areas of bleeding may be revealed (Auspitz sign). Guttate psoriasis is one of the most common forms encountered in childhood manifesting as guttate (drop-like) erythematous scaly papules scattered over the body (Fig. 65.7). The characteristic silvery scale is only minimally expressed, and the lesions may appear quite red. This form is classically (but not always) preceded by or coincides with a streptococcal infection.

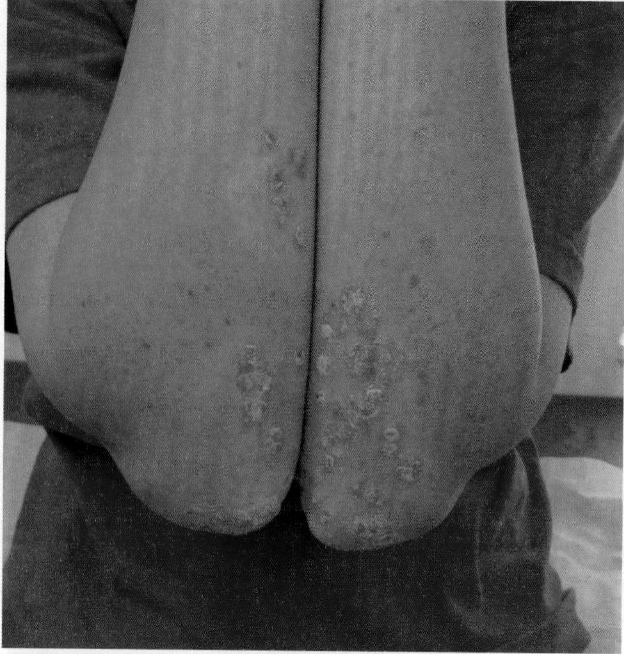

FIGURE 65.6 Classic plaque-type psoriasis tends to occur on extensor surfaces.

Palmoplantar psoriasis manifests as thickened plaques concentrated on the palms and soles of the feet (Fig. 65.8). The plaques may become fissured and painful. These areas may become so thickened that patients complain of pain with moving the fingers or walking.

Inverse psoriasis refers to the usually pink, salmon-colored, sometimes macerated plaques that arise in the axillae, inguinal

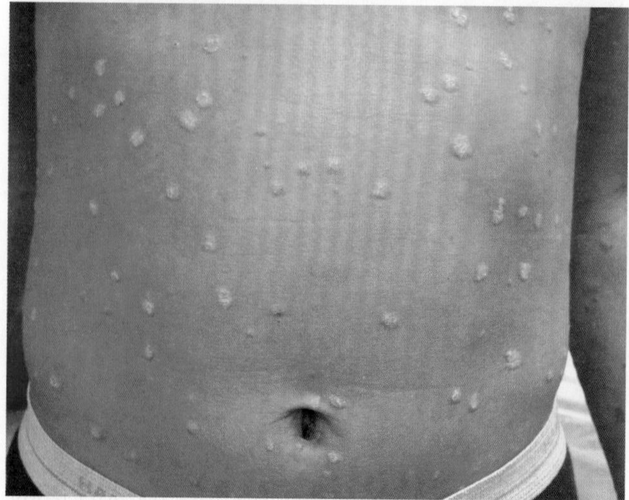

FIGURE 65.7 Small drop-like papules and plaques typical of guttate psoriasis.

TABLE 65.3

CLINICAL FEATURES OF PAPULOSQUAMOUS DISORDERS

Disorder	Morphology	Configuration	Distribution	Mucous membranes	Nails	Pruritus
Psoriasis	Beefy red plaques with overlying silvery scale	Papules, plaques; koebnerization can be seen	Scalp, ears, extensor surfaces, genital areas and buttocks; palms and soles	Geographic tongue	Pitting, "oil spot" onycholysis	Mild
Seborrheic dermatitis	Salmon-colored erythema and scaling	Patches and plaques	Scalp, eyebrows, perinasal, ears, intertriginous and genital areas in particular	Genital areas	Not typical	Minimal to mild
Pityriasis rosea	Oval scaly papules and plaques with collarettes of "trailing-edge" scale; first lesion may be larger "herald" patch or plaque	Papules and plaques	Torso and upper extremities; atypical forms involve palms and soles and legs	Not typical	Not typical	Minimal to mild
Pityriasis rubra pilaris	Orange-colored erythematous papules and plaques	Smaller papules coalescing into larger plaques with islands of sparing	Torso and extremities with palmoplantar keratoderma	Not typical	Not typical	Minimal to mild
Pityriasis lichenoides	Crusted papules (PLEVA) or scaly often hypopigmented patches and plaques (PLC)	Scattered lesions	Torso and extremities often with sparing of the face	Not typical	Not typical	Minimal to mild
Lichen nitidus	Flat-topped small white papules	Koebnerization often seen; lesions scattered	Torso, extremities, genital areas; face can be involved	Genital areas		Minimal to moderate
Lichen planus	Purplish, polygonal papules and plaques	Individual lesions may coalesce into larger plaques; koebnerization often seen	Torso, extremities; genital areas; face can be involved	Genital areas; oral white lesions and erosions can be seen	Not typical	Moderate to severe
Lichen striatus	Linear streaks of clustered pink papules and plaques, often discontinuous; lesions fade leaving behind hypopigmentation	Lesions follow lines of Blaschko	Most often extremities although face and torso have occasionally been involved	Not typical	Can cause nail dystrophy	Minimal to mild

areas, or on the genitalia and buttocks (Fig. 65.9). The gluteal crease is usually involved.

Erythrodermic psoriasis is less common and more severe. Onset may be abrupt or gradual, with a diffuse erythema and severe desquamation. In the growing child, there may be associated failure to thrive.

Pustular psoriasis is rarely seen in children and may arise suddenly. Patients may have other forms of psoriasis that then suddenly transition into pustular psoriasis flares, occasionally triggered by use of or withdrawal of systemic corticosteroid therapy. Various size sterile and superficial pustules develop on an erythrodermic background. Avoidance of systemic steroids may be prudent in patients with psoriasis since withdrawal can precipitate pustular flares of the disease.

Characteristically small, pitted lesions are seen on the nails in 25% to 50% of patients in all forms of the condition. Areas resembling tan-brown oil spots may appear as well within the nails.

Eighty percent of children have scalp involvement, and patients with early scalp psoriasis may be mistaken for having tinea capitis. In contrast to tinea capitis, most cases of psoriatic scalp involvement do not show frank hair loss or hair breakage, and scalp lymphadenopathy in psoriasis is uncommon.

A small proportion of patients develop arthritis between 9 and 12 years of age; some develop it before the onset of the skin eruption. The distal interphalangeal joints of the hands and feet are involved most often.

In the emergency department, patients with limited disease can be successfully managed with a course of topical corticosteroid until they can be referred back to their primary physician or dermatologist. Facial or genital areas may be treated with

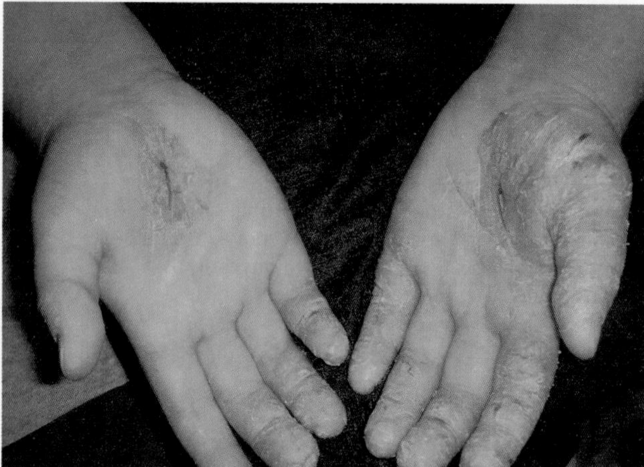

FIGURE 65.8 Palmar psoriasis.

a lower potency topical steroid such as hydrocortisone 1% or 2.5%, a vitamin D derivative topical (calcipotriene or calcitriol), or a topical calcineurin inhibitor such as pimecrolimus or tacrolimus. Body affected areas may be treated with a moderate potency topical steroid such as fluocinolone 0.025% or triamcinolone 0.1%. For the scalp, treatment with a steroid solution or oil-based compound is recommended, using a fluocinolone solution or oil, for example.

Previously diagnosed patients with psoriasis may be receiving other topical agents, including a variety of other more or less potent topical steroids, tar derivatives, topical vitamin A (tazarotene), topical vitamin D agents, emollients, and ultraviolet light. For severe cases, patients may be receiving treatment with systemic immunomodulating agents, including methotrexate, cyclosporine, acitretin, and a variety of biologic modifiers that address specific targets in T-cell physiology.

Patients with pustular or erythrodermic flares of their psoriasis may warrant admission in order to better control their disease, using more intensive wet wrap therapies with topical steroids or for initiation of systemic immunomodulating therapies. Patients with extensive skin involvement and skin barrier dysfunction may be at risk for hypothermia, skin infection, bacteremia, and electrolyte abnormalities, and should be evaluated accordingly. Older patients with psoriasis are also at risk for cardiovascular disease and lipid abnormalities such as hypertriglyceridemia and hypercholesterolemia.

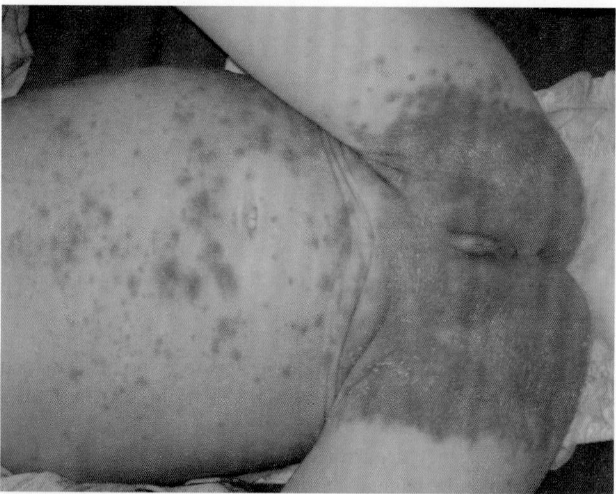

FIGURE 65.9 Inverse psoriasis. The classic diaper area or napkin psoriasis pattern is visible here.

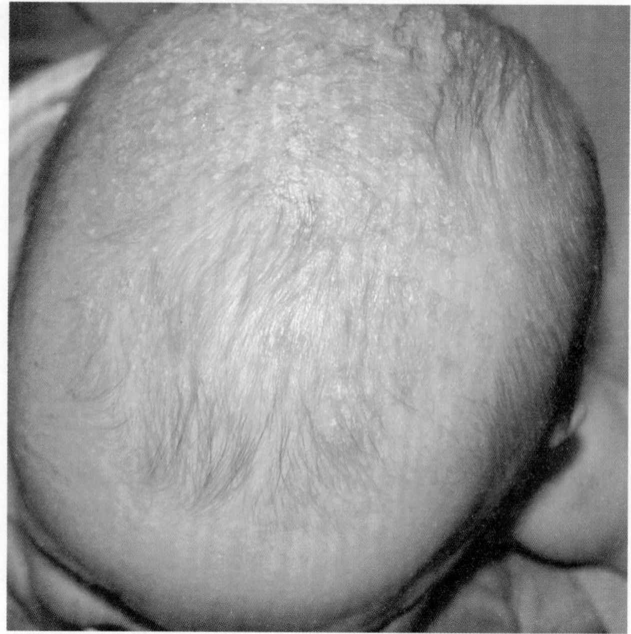

FIGURE 65.10 Infantile seborrheic dermatitis or "cradle cap."

Seborrheic Dermatitis

Seborrheic dermatitis is an inflammatory skin disorder characterized by salmon-colored erythema and greasy scale concentrated on areas rich in sebum production, including the scalp, eyebrows, ears, perinasal areas, beard areas, and less commonly, the midchest, axillary and inguinal areas (Fig. 65.10). Despite the intensity of the rash, pruritus is often mild or nonexistent.

Seborrheic dermatitis condition is most commonly seen in infants, adolescents, and adults. This is typically seen as an isolated phenomenon; however, it may occur as an overlap with psoriasis (the so-called sebopsoriasis phenomenon), atopic dermatitis (the so-called "sebotopic" or "atoporrheic" dermatitis); or arise in association with immunocompromised states, such as HIV, or Parkinson disease.

Scalp scaling is typically not associated with alopecia, which helps to differentiate it from tinea capitis. The scalp involvement often shows a faint, fine scaling in contrast to the more localized, thickly crusted cornflake-like scale encountered in Langerhans cell histiocytosis (LCH). An inflammatory reaction to local infection with Malassezia species has been demonstrated and may explain the efficacy of antifungal treatment of seborrheic dermatitis.

In cases where systemic findings are associated with seborrhea that is new-onset, chronic, or particularly severe, workup should include evaluation for HIV, immune deficiency, or LCH.

Treatment depends on the sites of involvement. For scalp involvement, an anti-inflammatory antifungal shampoo is appropriate: selenium sulfide, ketoconazole, or ciclopirox shampoos used daily for a week, and then maintained twice weekly is often sufficient. The facial involvement can be managed with once or twice daily use of a topical anti-inflammatory antifungal creams such as clotrimazole or ketoconazole cream prn. Occasionally, for more severe flares, brief courses of low-potency topical steroid (hydrocortisone 1% or 2.5%) or calcineurin inhibitor (pimecrolimus cream or tacrolimus ointment) can be applied twice daily for a week.

Parapsoriasis

Parapsoriasis is an inflammatory skin disorder characterized by scaly round, oval, or irregularly shaped papules and plaques (Fig. 65.11). The condition is typically divided on the basis of size into "small plaque" (SPP) and "large plaque" (LPP) types. The conditions are idiopathic. SPP is generally asymptomatic and viewed as a benign disorder that may spontaneously regress within months to years. LPP is often likewise benign, but may in a subset of cases (about 10%) represent a precursor to cutaneous T-cell lymphoma. The diagnosis is often made on the basis of excluding other entities such as PR, PRP, secondary syphilis, pityriasis lichenoides, or eczematous disorders. When the diagnosis is not clear, patients should undergo a skin biopsy to clarify the diagnosis. Treatment may involve use of topical corticosteroid or, for more severe cases, ultraviolet light phototherapy administered on an outpatient basis.

Pityriasis rosea

PR is a self-limited inflammatory skin disorder characterized by an initial larger herald patch or plaque, followed by the eruption of multiple smaller oval papules and plaques concentrated on the neck and torso areas. Individual lesions often show a collarette of scale (Fig. 65.12) and typically follow lines of cleavage in a so-called fir tree or Christmas tree pattern. The condition is most commonly seen among adolescents and adults. Younger patients and those with darker skin may show atypical features with greater involvement of palms and soles, or an inverse pattern with concentrated areas in the intertriginous folds.

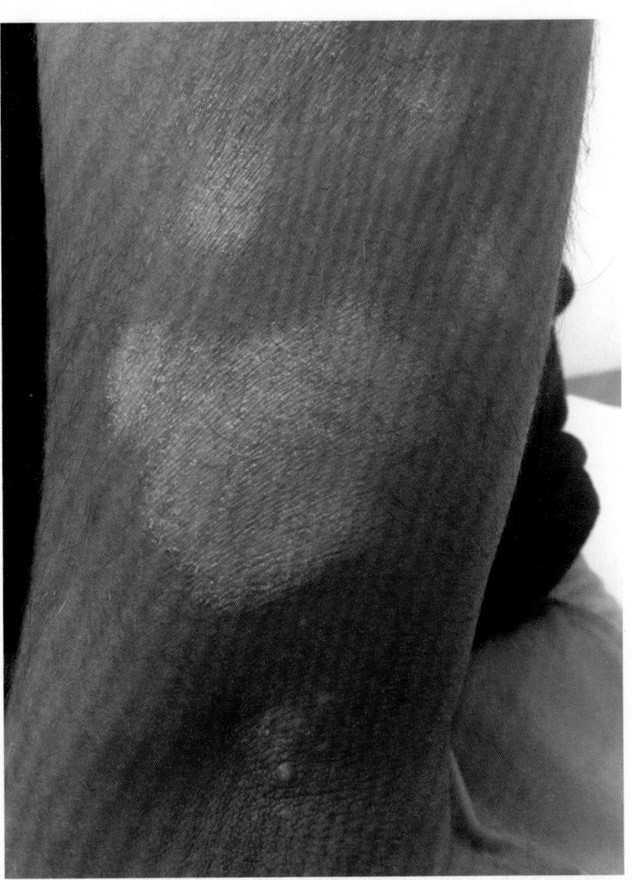

FIGURE 65.11 Parapsoriasis.

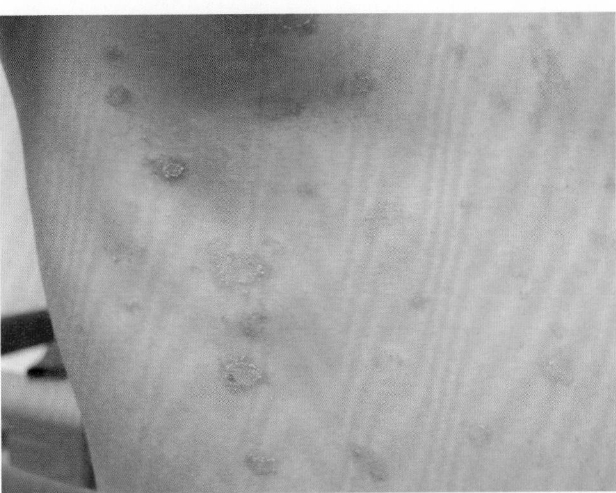

FIGURE 65.12 Pityriasis rosea with characteristic trailing edge scale within these oval papules and plaques.

PR is thought to be a reaction pattern to a preceding viral or other infectious process. Reactivation of latent human herpesvirus 6 or 7 (HHV 6,7) has been postulated as one potential mechanism. Given its clinical resemblance to secondary syphilis, adolescents and adults or those with risk factors for syphilis should be screened appropriately. Chronic cases of what looks like PR lasting longer than the typical 4 to 8 weeks should be evaluated for pityriasis lichenoides.

Since the condition is self-limited and often asymptomatic, reassurance and anticipatory guidance may be sufficient. For those who are symptomatic or desire a more rapid remission, treatment with oral acyclovir (to treat HHV6,7) or oral erythromycin (as a general anti-inflammatory agent) for 10 days may hasten resolution of the condition. Acyclovir appears to be more effective than erythromycin for this indication.

Pityriasis rubra pilaris

PRP is a chronic inflammatory skin condition typified by salmon-colored, orange-red follicular papules and larger plaques accompanied palmoplantar keratoderma. There are often characteristic islands of sparing (Fig. 65.13). It is most often confused with psoriasis, but PRP lesions lack the overlying silvery scale of psoriasis.

PRP is often idiopathic and sporadic in its occurrence. PRP can occur as a postinfectious process (most commonly streptococcal and occasionally HIV), as an adverse drug reaction, and in adults, as a paraneoplastic phenomenon associated with a variety of malignancies (adenocarcinoma, squamous cell carcinoma, laryngeal carcinoma, bronchogenic carcinoma, hepatocellular carcinoma). The condition has also been associated with CARD mutations and autosomal dominant inheritance (early-onset form).

Long-term treatments include use of emollients, topical corticosteroids, topical retinoids, vitamin D analogues, topical

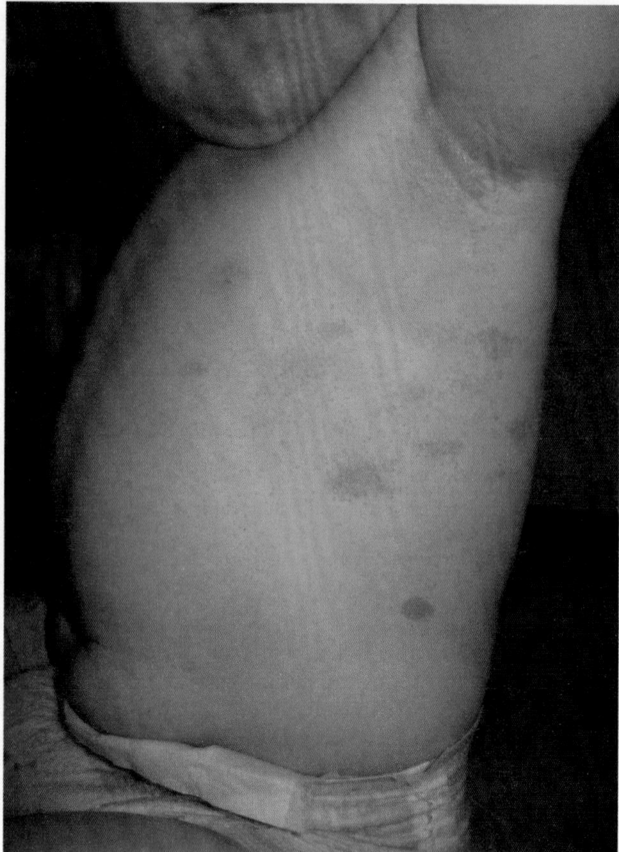

FIGURE 65.13 Pityriasis rubra pilaris. Note the orange or salmon-colored appearance of the papules.

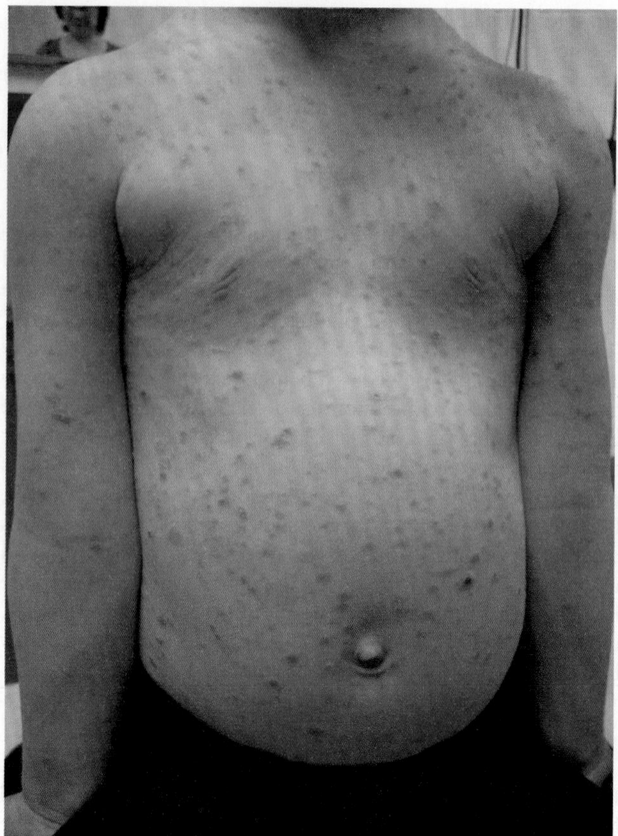

FIGURE 65.14 Crusted papules of pityriasis lichenoides et varioliformis acuta.

calcineurin inhibitors, and systemic agents such as phototherapy and biologic agents (infliximab, ustekinumab, etanercept, adalimumab).

In the emergency department, identification of an affected child should include evaluation for possible infectious triggers and treatment for any active infections. Referral to a dermatologist is recommended to institute longer-term treatment as needed.

Pityriasis lichenoides

Pityriasis lichenoides is a lymphocytic inflammatory skin condition that classically has been divided into the acute (pityriasis lichenoides et varioliformis acuta or PLEVA) form and the chronic (pityriasis lichenoides chronica) form. This distinction may be artificial as there are often overlapping features of both in an individual patient so the term pityriasis lichenoides is generally preferred. There is a rare and severe form known as febrile ulceronecrotic Mucha–Habermann (FUMH) syndrome.

Patients present with persistent crops of skin lesions that vary in appearance from crusted vesicles and papules (Fig. 65.14) to scaly patches and small plaques that may be hypopigmented in some cases (Fig. 65.15). These lesions are most often asymptomatic. There is often a predilection for sun-protected areas, and in summertime, areas exposed to sunlight often show fewer skin lesions. In FUMH syndrome, these lesions are often accompanied by fever and larger, often painful, ulcerated papules and plaques.

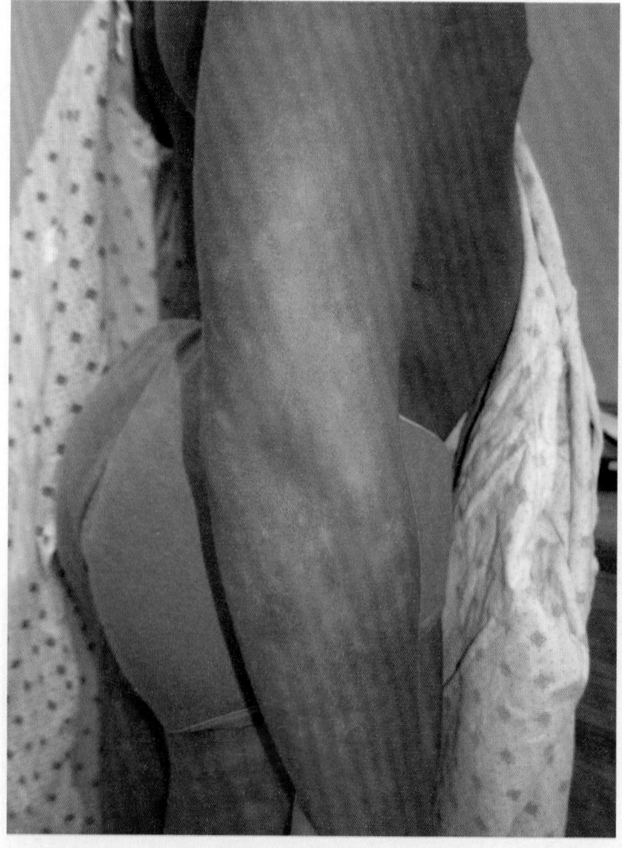

FIGURE 65.15 Scaly hypopigmented patches of pityriasis lichenoides chronica.

At times, the condition may be initially misdiagnosed as varicella, but PL patients are generally afebrile (except in FUMH), and the lesions of PL persist for months to years. At other times, the condition may resemble PR but PL will persist for months to years, differentiating it from PR. Infants who develop crusted papular eruptions that resemble PL should also be evaluated for the possibility of LCH.

While the diagnosis can sometimes be made on clinical grounds, consultation with a dermatologist for skin biopsy may be necessary to differentiate it from other conditions. Since the condition rarely represents a precursor to cutaneous T-cell lymphoma, periodic longer-term outpatient monitoring is advised.

Treatment for the condition typically involves an initial trial of macrolide derivatives such as erythromycin, and recalcitrant cases may be treated with ultraviolet light phototherapy. More severe cases, including those with FUMH, typically require systemic immunosuppressive therapy with agents such as methotrexate. Breaks from therapy can often be taken during the summer months when disease activity wanes from natural sunlight exposure. Long-term, the condition remits spontaneously over a period of several years.

Lichen nitidus

Lichen nitidus is a benign, self-limited condition characterized by crops of small, discrete flat-topped off-white papules scattered over the torso and extremities (Fig. 65.16), but which can involve the face and genitalia as well. Lesions often show characteristic groups of papules in a linear configuration demonstrating the phenomenon of koebnerization at sites of minor trauma. In contrast to follicular eczema, which is often pruritic, the skin findings are less often symptomatic. Treatment typically involves watchful waiting and reassurance, although some patients may respond to topical calcineurin inhibitors such as pimecrolimus cream or tacrolimus ointment.

Lichen planus

Lichen planus is often easily recognized by its intensely pruritic, purplish, often polygonal papules and plaques (Fig. 65.17). The condition can occur anywhere, but is usually seen involving the extremities. Areas may show koebnerization, with lesions appearing at sites of minor skin trauma. Affected patients should be asked about and examined for oral or genital involvement, which may or may not be symptomatic at these sites. On the mucous membranes, the condition has a lacy white appearance.

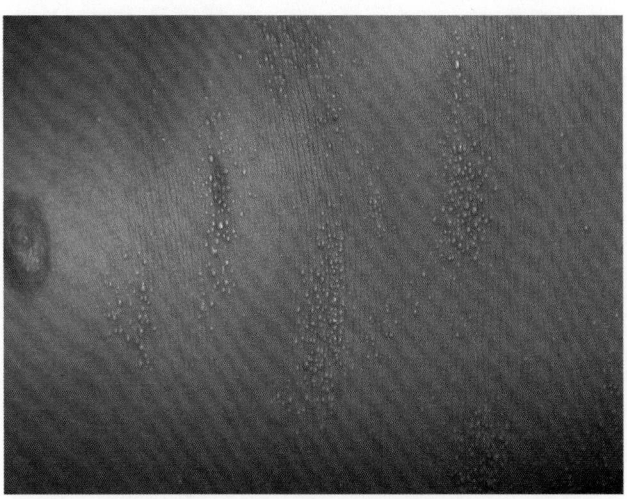

FIGURE 65.16 Lichen nitidus.

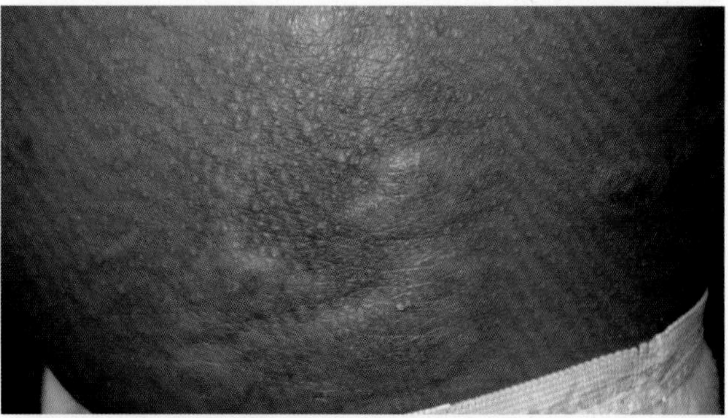

FIGURE 65.17 Lichen planus.

In adults, the condition may be associated with underlying hepatitis C infection, although children who present with lichen planus are generally otherwise healthy. Nonetheless, it is advisable to ask about any risk factors or family history of hepatitis C in affected patients.

Since patients with lichen planus are usually uncomfortably itchy, treatment is recommended. For the body affected areas of skin, topical therapy using moderate potency topical steroids such as fluocinolone 0.025% or triamcinolone 0.1% twice daily is suggested for 2 to 4 weeks to moderate the intense pruritus. For more widespread involvement seen in generalized lichen planus, or those with more severe oral or genital involvement which may be sore or painful, a course of oral corticosteroid therapy may be necessary. Since lichen planus is a chronic condition, consultation with a dermatologist is recommended.

Lichen striatus

Lichen striatus is a papulosquamous condition that most commonly presents as a single linear, scaly, and thickened plaque consisting of smaller pink papules, typically on an extremity. The lesion is often discontinuous and follows the curvilinear lines of Blaschko. After several months, the papular component fades, leaving behind hypopigmented areas in the same linear configuration (Fig. 65.18). Lichen striatus is most often seen in school-aged children. In contrast, inflammatory linear verrucous epidermal nevi (ILVEN) are often earlier in onset arising in infancy, and may be more widespread (Fig. 65.19).

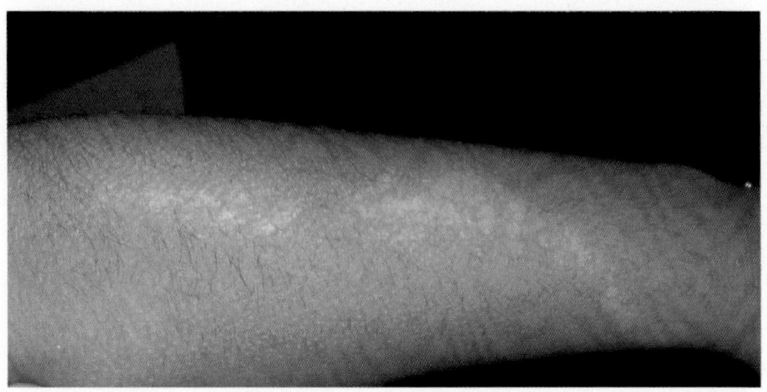

FIGURE 65.18 Lichen striatus.

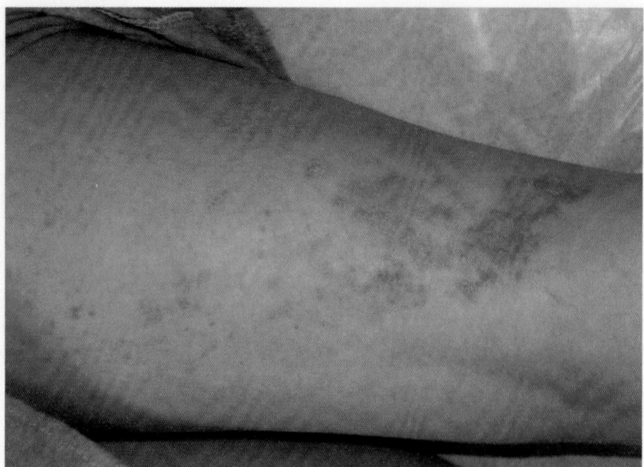

FIGURE 65.19 Inflammatory linear verrucous epidermal nevi (ILVEN). ILVEN is notable for its often larger collections of verrucous plaques with background inflammation.

Since lichen striatus resolves spontaneously in most typical cases, no treatment is necessary. In those with symptomatic pruritus, low-potency topical steroid use may be considered for intermittent use.

CONCLUSION

Viral syndromes and papulosquamous disorders are a highly heterogeneous group of skin disorders. While they share similar clinical characteristics with one another, an awareness of their distinguishing features and their natural histories will help in providing the patient a more accurate diagnosis, and direct appropriate therapy accordingly.

Suggested Readings and Key References

Aronson PL, Yan AC, Mittal MK, et al. Delayed acyclovir and outcomes of children hospitalized with eczema herpeticum. *Pediatrics* 2011;128(6):1161–1167.

Berger EM, Orlow SJ, Patel RR, et al. Experience with molluscum contagiosum and associated inflammatory reactions in a pediatric dermatology practice: the bump that rashes. *Arch Dermatol* 2012;148(11):1257–1264.

Ganguly S. A randomized, double-blind, placebo-controlled study of efficacy of oral acyclovir in the treatment of pityriasis rosea. *J Clin Diagn Res* 2014;8(5):YC01–YC04.

Harms M, Feldmann R, Saurat J-H. Papular-purpuric "gloves and socks" syndrome. *J Am Acad Dermatol* 1990;23:850–854.

Sugarman JL, Hersh AL, Okamura T, et al. Empiric antibiotics and outcomes of children hospitalized with eczema herpeticum. *Pediatr Dermatol* 2011;28(3):230–234.

CHAPTER 66 ■ RESPIRATORY DISTRESS

DEBRA L. WEINER, MD, PhD AND J. KATE DEANEHAN, MD, RDMS

Respiratory distress is one of the most common chief complaints of children seeking medical care. It accounts for nearly 10% of all pediatric emergency department visits and 20% of visits of children younger than 2 years. Twenty percent of patients admitted to the hospital and 30% of those admitted to intensive care units are admitted for respiratory distress. Primary respiratory processes account for approximately 5% of deaths in children younger than 15 years and 20% in infants. In addition, respiratory distress contributes substantially to deaths in patients with other primary processes. Respiratory arrest is one of the five leading causes of death in pediatric patients. Respiratory distress results from interruption of the respiratory or ventilatory pathway. Respiratory failure is caused by an inability to meet metabolic demands for oxygen (O_2) or by inadequate carbon dioxide (CO_2) elimination. Respiratory distress is usually reversible, but failure to treat the condition may result in cardiac arrest with long-term neurologic sequelae or death.

PATHOPHYSIOLOGY

The primary goals of respiration are to meet metabolic demands for O_2 and to eliminate CO_2. Secondary functions include acid–base buffering, host defense, and hormonal regulation. The upper airway or conducting zone, which includes the nose, nasopharynx, oropharynx, larynx, trachea, major bronchi, and terminal bronchioles, serves as a conduit for air movement. The lower airway, or respiratory zone, consists of respiratory bronchioles, alveolar ducts, sacs, alveoli and interstitium. Exchange of O_2 and CO_2 between the lungs and the blood occurs at the alveolocapillary membrane and depends on adequate and appropriately matched ventilation and perfusion.

Control of respiration is mediated by central and peripheral neural mechanisms. Respiration is an intrinsic brainstem function of the respiratory centers of the medulla. It is further influenced by the cerebellum, which alters respiration with postural change; by the hypothalamus, which controls respiration on a moment-to-moment basis; by the limbic system, which modulates respiration in response to emotion; and by the motor cerebral cortex, which controls volitional respiratory activity, including hyperventilation and hypoventilation and speech. Impulses are transmitted from the brain via the vagus and spinal nerves to the larynx, trachea, bronchi, bronchioles, and acini; the glossopharyngeal to the pharynx; the hypoglossal (CN XII) to the tongue; and the spinal accessory (CN XI) to accessory muscles. Cervical nerves (C2 to C4), the phrenic nerve (C3 to C5), and the intercostal nerves (T1 to T12), innervate accessory muscles, the respiratory diaphragm, and intercostal muscles, respectively.

Respiratory distress results from dysfunction or disruption of the respiratory tract and/or systems that control or modulate respiration.

Respiratory failure is the inability to meet the metabolic demand for O_2 (hypoxia) or the inability to eliminate CO_2 (hypercapnia). Criteria for defining respiratory failure vary widely; one set of criteria is presented in Table 66.1. Hypoxia can be categorized on the basis of mechanism. Arterial hypoxemia results from an inability to deliver adequate O_2 to the blood, most often, due to airway obstruction, central respiratory depression or impairment, neuromuscular or skeletal insufficiency, or restricted lung expansion. Other causes include low atmospheric PO_2 (e.g., high altitude), diffusion impairment (e.g., pulmonary edema, pulmonary fibrosis, acute respiratory distress syndrome, O_2 toxicity), anatomic or physiologic shunt (e.g., atelectasis, pneumonia, abnormal pulmonary blood flow), or increased metabolic demand (e.g., exercise, systemic illness). Anemic hypoxia is the result of the blood's inability to deliver adequate O_2 to tissues as a result of decreased hemoglobin oxygen-carrying capacity. It is caused by anemia (deficiency of red blood cells or of erythrocyte hemoglobin concentration) abnormal hemoglobin, carboxyhemoglobin, or methemoglobin. Hypokinetic, ischemic, or stagnant hypoxia also results in an inability of the blood to transport O_2 to the tissues. This type of hypoxia is caused by decreased blood flow to a localized area secondary to compromised cardiac output (e.g., cardiac failure), poor tissue perfusion (e.g., shock), sludging (e.g., polycythemia), or obstructed flow (e.g., vascular obstruction). Histotoxic hypoxia results from inability to metabolize O_2 at the tissue level as a result of inactivation of metabolic enzymes (e.g., by a chemical such as cyanide). Hypercapnia is caused by inadequate alveolar ventilation (e.g., central nervous system [CNS] depression, spinal cord injury, neuromuscular disease, diaphragmatic dysfunction), ventilation–perfusion imbalance with relative hypoventilation (e.g., restrictive airway disease, pulmonary embolism), or increased CO_2 production (e.g., metabolic/endocrine disturbance). Hypercapnia often contributes to respiratory failure as a result of hypoxemia and is less commonly the primary cause.

Infants are at an increased risk of respiratory distress compared with children and adults because of anatomic and physiologic differences (Table 66.2). These differences result in greater risk of airway obstruction, less efficient respiratory effort, limited respiratory reserve, and dysfunction of CNS respiratory control.

DIFFERENTIAL DIAGNOSIS

Establishing a diagnosis for respiratory distress in part depends on localizing the pathology to a particular organ system. Respiratory distress may result directly from a disturbance of the upper or lower respiratory system. It may also be caused by inability of the CNS or peripheral nervous system to interpret or process respiratory requirements, or of the

TABLE 66.1

CRITERIA FOR RESPIRATORY FAILURE[a]

Clinical	Laboratory
Tachypnea, bradypnea, apnea, irregular respirations	PaO_2 <60 mm Hg in 60% O_2[b]
Pulsus paradoxus >30 mm Hg	$Paco_2$ >60 mm Hg and rising
Decreased or absent breath sounds	pH <7.3
Stridor, wheeze, grunting	
Severe retractions and use of accessory muscles	
Cyanosis in 40% O_2[b]	
Depressed or heightened level of consciousness, decreased response to pain	
Weak to absent cough or gag reflex	
Poor muscle tone	

[a]Respiratory failure is likely if two clinical findings and one laboratory finding exist.
[b]Excluding cyanotic heart disease.

musculoskeletal system to perform the work of breathing. Alternatively, disease or dysfunction of other organ systems may indirectly result in respiratory disturbance by compromising respiratory system function or by stimulating compensatory respiratory mechanisms (Tables 66.3–66.5). Although respiratory effort can be immediately supported, treatment of the underlying cause is essential for definitive treatment of the respiratory distress.

Respiratory System

Respiratory distress may be caused by upper or lower airway obstruction or by disorders of the parenchyma or interstitium. Upper airway obstruction is common in infants and young children in part because of their airway anatomy and physiology (see Chapter 70 Stridor). The hallmark of complete upper airway obstruction is inability to phonate, that is, no speech, cry, or cough. Manifestations of upper airway obstruction may also include nasal flaring, stertor or snoring, gurgling, drooling, dysphagia, hoarseness, stridor, retractions, and paradoxical chest/abdominal wall movement. In neonates, common causes include nasal obstruction, upper airway anomalies (particularly laryngotracheomalacia), and congenital or postintubation subglottic stenosis. Common causes for upper airway obstruction in infants and children include croup, adenotonsillar hypertrophy, foreign body, retropharyngeal abscess, and tracheitis. Airway edema can be secondary to trauma, thermal or chemical burn, or anaphylaxis. *Epiglottitis,* although less common, is one of the most life-threatening causes of respiratory distress and is a true emergency. The incidence of epiglottitis has declined significantly since routine immunization against *Haemophilus influenzae* type b, the pathogen that once caused at least 75% of cases. Epiglottitis should be suspected in children who have abrupt onset of fever, dysphagia, drooling, muffled voice, labored respirations, and stridor. Children appear toxic and anxious and assume a sniffing position with protruding jaw and extended neck. These children are at risk of abrupt onset of respiratory arrest from obstruction. *Peritonsillar and retropharyngeal abscess* may present with symptoms similar

TABLE 66.2

ANATOMIC/PHYSIOLOGIC DIFFERENCES IN INFANT/CHILD AND ADULT AIRWAYS

Difference	Consequence
Nose: infants <4 mo preferential nose breathers	Nasal congestion may result in significant respiratory distress
Larynx: higher (C2–C3 vs. C6), softer, more elastic	More difficult to intubate
	Collapses more easily, particularly with fixed obstruction (i.e., Bernoulli principle—as the velocity of flow through a collapsible tube increases, the pressure that holds the tube open decreases)
Trachea: one-third diameter of adult at birth, shorter	Poiseuille law—resistance varies inversely with fourth power of the radius; 1-mm thickening decreases cross-sectional diameter by 20% in adult and by 80% in child
	More difficult to intubate/maintain proper depth
Alveoli: elastic fibers less well developed	Alveoli collapse more easily, results in ventilation–perfusion mismatch
Lungs: lower functional residual capacity	Reserve small, therefore limited protection when ventilation is interrupted, PaO_2 decreases more rapidly
Respiratory control apparatus: immature—reflexes that inhibit respiration, particularly Hering–Breuer reflex, which responds to stretch of lung, are very strong; central nervous system processing of information markedly affected by sleep state, cold, drugs, other metabolic derangements	Apnea or inability to respond appropriately to mechanical respiratory obstruction or increased metabolic demand
Chest wall: more compliant; intercostal muscles immature; ribs more horizontal; diaphragm flatter, fatigues; during rapid eye movement sleep, intercostal muscle movements become uncoordinated	Accessory muscle retractions Diaphragm does more work but is less effective

TABLE 66.3

CAUSES OF RESPIRATORY DISTRESS

Respiratory system	Spinal cord (congenital anomaly, tetanus, trauma)
Upper airway obstruction	Anterior horn (poliomyelitis, transverse myelitis, spinal muscular atrophy)
Nasopharynx (craniofacial anomalies, choanal atresia, nasal congestion, adenotonsillar hypertrophy, foreign body, trauma, mass)	**Peripheral nervous system**
Oropharynx (macroglossia, micrognathia, midface hypoplasia, tonsillitis, peritonsillar abscess, uvulitis Ludwig angina, trauma)	Peripheral motor nerve (phrenic nerve injury, Guillain–Barré syndrome, multiple sclerosis, tick paralysis, heavy metal or organophosphate toxicity, porphyria)
Larynx (epiglottitis, laryngomalacia, hemangioma, papilloma, webs, cysts, laryngoceles, laryngotracheal cleft, subglottic stenosis, croup, retropharyngeal abscess, tracheitis, anaphylaxis, angioneurotic edema, trauma, thermal or chemical burn, foreign body, vocal cord paralysis, laryngospasm, hypocalcemic tetany, mass)	Neuromuscular junction (myasthenia gravis, botulism, snake bite, organophosphate toxicity, antibiotics)
Trachea (tracheomalacia, stenosis, tracheoesophageal fistula, foreign body, mass)	Muscle (muscular/myotonic dystrophies, IEM, carnitine deficiency, polymyositis/dermatomyositis, fatigue)
Bronchi (bronchomalacia, stenosis, bronchogenic cyst, bronchitis, foreign body)	**Chest wall/intrathoracic**
Lower airway obstruction/acinar/interstitial disease	Air leak (pneumothorax, tension pneumothorax, pneumomediastinum, pneumopericardium)
Bronchioles (asthma, bronchiolitis, allergy, angioneurotic edema, bronchiectasis)	Space-occupying (esophageal foreign body, pleural effusion, empyema, chylothorax, hemothorax, anomalies great vessels, diaphragmatic hernia, cyst, mass)
Acini/interstitium	Boney and/or muscular deformity or dysfunction (congenital bone/muscle absence, spine deformity, pectus excavatum/carinatum, diaphragmatic hernia, contusion, rib fractures/flail chest, burn)
Disorders of lung maturity (transient tachypnea of newborn, respiratory distress syndrome, bronchopulmonary dysplasia, persistent fetal circulation, Wilson–Mikity syndrome)	**Cardiovascular**
Congenital malformation (congenital emphysema, cystic adenomatoid malformation, sequestration, pulmonary agenesis/aplasia/hypoplasia, pulmonary cyst)	Congenital (structural defect, arrhythmia)
Aspiration (meconium, foreign body, near drowning, gastroesophageal reflux, vomiting)	Acquired (cardiogenic shock, arrhythmia, valvular heart disease, myocarditis, myocardial ischemia or infarction, pericarditis, pericardial effusion, pericardial tamponade, aortic dissection or rupture, mass, coronary artery dilation/aneurysm, congestive heart failure)
Infection (pneumonia; bacterial, atypical bacteria, viral, chlamydial, pertussis, fungal, pneumocystis)	**Gastrointestinal**
Pulmonary collapse, (atelectasis), fluid (consolidation, edema, hemorrhage), mass	Distension/pain (necrotizing enterocolitis, mass, obstruction, perforation, laceration, hematoma, contusion, appendicitis, infection, inflammation, ascites)
Environmental/trauma (high-altitude pulmonary edema, thermal or chemical burn, smoke, carbon monoxide, biologic and chemical agents, hydrocarbon, drug-induced pulmonary fibrosis, bronchopulmonary traumatic disruption, pulmonary contusion)	**Metabolic/endocrine**
Central nervous system	Acidosis (exercise, fever, hypothermia, dehydration, sepsis, shock, IEM, liver disease, renal disease, diabetic ketoacidosis, salicylates)
Structural abnormality (agenesis, hydrocephalus, mass, arteriovascular malformation)	Hyperammonemia (IEM, liver failure)
Dysfunction/immaturity (apnea, hyperventilation/hypoventilation)	Serum chemistry disturbance (hyperkalemia/hypokalemia, hypercalcemia/hypocalcemia, hypophosphatemia, hypermagnesemia/hypomagnesemia)
Infection (meningitis, encephalitis, abscess)	Respiratory chain disturbance (cyanide, mitochondrial disorders)
Inherited or acquired degenerative disease	Endocrine (hyperglycemia/hypoglycemia, hyperthyroidism/hypothyroidism, hyperparathyroidism, adrenal hyperplasia)
Intoxication, central nervous system depression (alcohol, barbiturates, benzodiazepines, opiates, neurotoxins)	**Hematologic**
Seizure	Anemia, abnormal hemoglobin (inadequate erythrocyte numbers, decreased production, loss, hemoglobinopathy, methemoglobin, carboxyhemoglobin)
Trauma (birth asphyxia, hemorrhage)	Polycythemia

IEM, inborn error of metabolism.

to epiglottitis but are less likely to have stridor and the onset is more gradual. *Croup* or laryngotracheobronchitis is the most common cause of upper airway obstruction in children 3 months to 3 years of age. Croup causes subglottic narrowing and is characterized by a barky cough, inspiratory stridor, and hoarseness that are worse at night. Viral croup is most often caused by parainfluenza virus, frequently with several days of upper respiratory infection symptoms, which may or may not be accompanied by fever. Respiratory distress often occurs with wakening during the night in a child who was relatively

TABLE 66.4

MOST COMMON CAUSES OF RESPIRATORY DISTRESS

Neonates	Infants/children
Nasal obstruction	Croup
Congenital airway anomalies	Tracheitis
Transient tachypnea	Foreign body
Respiratory distress syndrome	Bronchiolitis
Meconium aspiration	Asthma
Pneumonia	Anaphylaxis
Sepsis	Pneumonia
Congenital heart disease	
Fever	
Sepsis	
Gastroenteritis/dehydration	

well before going to sleep. Children with croup-like symptoms that are recurrent or prolonged may have an underlying fixed or functional airway abnormality, most commonly subglottic stenosis or hemangioma. Children with chronic stridor, particularly those younger than 2 years, may also have an underlying congenital anomaly. *Tracheitis*, an infection of the trachea, may occur as a primary infection with abrupt onset, high fever similar to epiglottitis. More commonly, it presents as a secondary infection in a child with an initial croup-like illness but with a worsening clinical course. Although *tracheitis* is usually due to bacteria, most commonly streptococcus or staphylococcus, cases in which only viruses or no pathogen is identified are not uncommon. *Foreign-body aspiration*, which has a peak age of occurrence of 1 to 5 years, may cause obstruction of the upper or lower airway and is a leading cause of accidental death in toddlers. A history of abrupt onset of choking or gagging is suggestive. Drooling, dysphagia, and stridor suggest an upper airway foreign body, whereas unilateral wheeze, particularly first-time wheeze with acute onset, suggests lower airway position. Presentation, particularly with lower airway foreign body, may be delayed by days to weeks from time of aspiration.

Common causes of lower airway obstruction involve inflammation and bronchospasm and include asthma, allergy/anaphylaxis, and bronchiolitis. Wheeze, most often diffuse, is usually a predominant feature of these conditions (see Chapter 80 Wheezing). *Asthma* may be triggered by infection, exercise, environmental irritants, stress, and/or gastroesophageal reflux. Allergy, usually accompanied by coryza, congestion, mucosal edema, and/or rash, may be in response to environmental exposures, food, or medications. *Bronchiolitis* may be caused by respiratory syncytial virus as well as parainfluenza, influenza, adenovirus, metapneumovirus, and less commonly other viruses. It is the most common cause of lower respiratory illness in children

TABLE 66.5

MOST COMMON ACUTE LIFE-THREATENING CAUSES OF RESPIRATORY DISTRESS

Foreign body	Tension pneumothorax
Anaphylaxis	Pericardial tamponade
Epiglottitis	

younger than 2 years. These conditions cause airway obstruction by decreasing airway luminal area secondary to bronchospasm, edema, or thickening of the wall of the lumen. Lower airway obstruction is also caused by filling of the airway lumen by excessive secretions (e.g., from inflammation, infection, or toxin such as organophosphate) or aspirated fluids. External compression can also lead to a decrease in lumen (e.g., with emphysema and masses).

Disorders of the alveoli and interstitium involve pus or fluid collection, collapse, and structural or functional abnormality. Alveolar and interstitial disease is characterized by tachypnea, cough, grunting, crackles, rhonchi, wheeze, and decreased and/or asymmetric breath sounds with or without fever. In neonates, transient tachypnea of the newborn and meconium aspiration are common causes. *Pneumonia* is one of the most common causes of lower airway disease in children of all ages. Findings are more likely to be localized in the setting of bacterial pneumonia, whereas patients with viral and atypical pneumonias (e.g., *Mycoplasma* infection, *Chlamydia* infection, and pertussis) tend to have diffuse peribronchial, interstitial processes. Patients presenting during epidemics of severe respiratory illness secondary to coronavirus infections (e.g., SARS and MERS) also commonly have fever, chills, cough, and respiratory distress which can be life-threatening. Less commonly, aspiration, hemorrhage, and pulmonary edema cause fluid collection in the acini and interstitium. Atelectasis, or airway collapse, resulting from loss of air within the pulmonary parenchyma often occurs secondary to other processes, including pneumonia, particularly viral; bronchospasm; and inadequate lung expansion, most often resulting from pain, neuromuscular disease, or inactivity. Structural and/or functional abnormalities include bronchopulmonary dysplasia, respiratory distress syndrome, bronchiectasis (most commonly seen in cystic fibrosis), congenital or acquired emphysema, and pulmonary fibrosis (usually from radiation and chemotherapy).

Several biologic and chemical agents that are potential weapons of terrorism or warfare produce respiratory distress as their most predominant effect. These include the biologic agents inhalational anthrax, pneumonic plague, pneumonic tularemia, melioidosis; the toxins *Staphylococcus* enterotoxin B and ricin; and the chemical agents chlorine and phosgene (see Chapter 136 Biological and Chemical Terrorism). Respiratory findings include cyanosis, chest pain, cough, hemoptysis, dyspnea, tachypnea, stridor, rales, and/or wheeze. Chest radiographs may reveal infiltrates, pulmonary edema, pleural effusions, widened mediastinum, abscesses, and/or granulomas.

Nervous System

CNS disturbances may result in hypoventilation or hyperventilation, loss of protective airway reflexes, or airway obstruction from loss of pharyngeal tone. These conditions include CNS malformation, immaturity, infection, degenerative disease, seizures, mass, trauma, and intoxication. Focal neurologic deficits, visual disturbances, pupillary abnormalities, papilledema, abnormal muscle tone, and altered level of consciousness suggest CNS processes. Spinal cord trauma and anterior horn cell disease cause bulbar and respiratory muscle dysfunction, which results in airway obstruction and/or hypoventilation. Peripheral neuromuscular (i.e., peripheral nerve, neuromuscular junction, muscle) disorders result in muscle weakness or paralysis. Physical findings that suggest chest wall weakness may include hypotonia, hyporeflexia, muscle weakness, weak cry, hoarse voice, cough, gag, shallow or irregular respiratory pattern, and inability to lift the head or extremities (see Chapter 78 Weakness).

Chest Wall/Thoracic Cavity

Musculoskeletal deformity or disease involving the support structures of the chest may severely restrict lung expansion, limiting normal ventilatory efforts or attempts at compensatory ventilation for respiratory dysfunction and other systemic disturbances.

Intrathoracic conditions that may produce respiratory distress include air leak and space-occupying lesions, including fluid collections and masses. Air leak may be traumatic or spontaneous. Pneumothorax occurs when air enters the pleural space either by chest wall penetration (open pneumothorax) or by rupture of lung through the visceral pleura (closed pneumothorax) and causes collapse of the lung. With tension pneumothorax, air is able to enter but not egress. Pneumothorax often presents with nonspecific signs of respiratory distress, as well as ipsilateral chest wall hyperexpansion, decreased or absent breath sounds, and hyperresonance to percussion. Rarely, a patient will have bilateral pneumothoraces, in which case, the examination may be symmetric. With tension pneumothorax, there is also jugular venous distension (JVD) and deviation of the trachea and mediastinum away from the air leak. Tension pneumothorax decreases venous return and thus cardiac output. It is therefore life-threatening and must be relieved immediately by needle thoracostomy. Another space-occupying lesion is pleural effusion. Pleural effusion, which may be caused by infection, inflammation, ischemia, trauma, malignancy, major organ failure, drug hypersensitivity, or venous or lymphatic obstruction, is suggested on physical examination by decreased breath sounds and a pleural rub. Flail chest, caused by multiple rib fractures and resulting in inefficient expansion of the thorax is rare in children given the deformability of their immature bones. Absence of rib fractures does not preclude air leak, hemothorax, and/or pulmonary contusion. Mass lesions include congenital or traumatic diaphragmatic hernia, esophageal anomalies, benign or neoplastic masses, and vascular malformations (see Chapter 104 Neonatal Emergencies). Pectus that restricts lung expansion may also compromise ventilation.

Cardiovascular

Congenital and acquired heart disease may result in respiratory distress from decreased cardiac output, reduced O_2 saturation, and/or congestive heart failure (CHF). Compromised cardiac output, most commonly caused by congenital structural heart defects, cardiac arrhythmias, myocarditis or, pericarditis with effusion may result in insufficient tissue O_2 delivery to meet metabolic demands. *Pericardial tamponade* causes decreased cardiac output as a result of compromised cardiac filling. Classic physical examination findings of arterial hypotension, JVD, and distant heart sounds, referred to as Beck triad, are seen in fewer than one-third of patients. Pericardial tamponade may be caused by trauma, infection, inflammation, malignancy, or cardiac surgery. Acute tamponade may be immediately life-threatening and must be relieved expeditiously by pericardiocentesis. In children, congenital heart defects are the most common cause of CHF. Other cardiac causes of CHF include valvular heart disease, myocardial dysfunction, arrhythmias, ischemia, and infarction. Metabolic disturbances, sepsis, fluid overload, and severe anemia may also result in CHF. Pulmonary manifestations of CHF include tachypnea, increased work of breathing, dyspnea on exertion, orthopnea, perioral cyanosis, cough, wheeze, and bibasilar rales. Other manifestations include pallor, poor feeding, failure to thrive, fatigue, tiring with feeds, diaphoresis, edema, tachycardia, weak thready pulses, JVD, displaced point of maximum impulse, cardiac murmur, gallop, rub, cardiomegaly, and hepatosplenomegaly. Vascular causes of respiratory distress include pulmonary embolism, pulmonary hypertension, and pulmonary arteriovenous fistula (see Chapter 107 Pulmonary Emergencies).

Gastrointestinal

Abdominal obstruction, perforation of hollow viscous, laceration of solid organs, hematoma, contusion, appendicitis, infection, inflammation, ascites, or mass may result in impaired diaphragmatic excursion secondary to abdominal distension and/or pain. Prolonged shallow respiration may result in pulmonary hypoventilation. Gastroesophageal reflux or vomiting, particularly in children unable to protect their airway, may result in subglottic inflammation and/or pulmonary aspiration (see Chapter 99 Gastrointestinal Emergencies).

Metabolic and Endocrine Disturbances

Metabolic disturbances often manifest as compensatory alterations in respiratory status. Metabolic acidosis results in rapid, deep breathing. Hyperammonemia directly stimulates the respiratory center to produce tachypnea, which results in primary respiratory alkalosis with secondary metabolic acidosis. Disruption of O_2 metabolism is another cause for respiratory distress. Endocrine disturbances that cause alterations in metabolic rate or chemical imbalances also result in respiratory distress (see Chapters 97 Endocrine Emergencies).

Hematologic

Inadequate concentrations of hemoglobin, or hemoglobin with decreased oxygen-carrying capacity, result in deficient O_2 delivery to tissues. Polycythemia results in sludging of blood and therefore compromised O_2 delivery (see Chapter 101 Hematologic Emergencies).

EVALUATION AND DECISION

Triage and Stabilization

Every child with significant respiratory distress must be considered to be at potential risk of respiratory arrest. Airway patency, breathing, and circulation should be rapidly assessed and, if compromised, should be supported immediately before further evaluation (Table 66.6). Respiratory arrest can rapidly evolve into cardiac arrest if resuscitative interventions are not timely.

Cardiorespiratory status should be continuously monitored. A healthcare provider skilled in airway management

TABLE 66.6

LIFE-SAVING MANEUVERS TO RELIEVE RESPIRATORY DISTRESS

Maneuvers	Indications	Comments
Heimlich maneuver (abdominal thrusts) for age ≥1 yr	Relieve upper airway obstruction caused by foreign body	Contraindicated if conscious patient able to phonate
Back/chest blows for age <1 yr		Remove visible foreign body in the oropharynx, blind sweep contraindicated
Manual foreign-body extraction		
Head tilt/chin lift, jaw thrust	Relieve oropharyngeal obstruction	Head tilt/chin lift contraindicated if neck trauma
Nasopharyngeal airway	Relieve nasopharyngeal obstruction	Conscious or unconscious patient
		Contraindicated if bleeding diathesis, cerebrospinal fluid leak, nasal deformity
Oropharyngeal airway	Relieve obstruction by the tongue	Unconscious patient
Suction	Remove excess secretions, mucous plug	Nose, mouth, and, if intubated, trachea
Bag-valve-mask ventilation	Provide mechanical ventilation, deliver high-concentration oxygen	Self-inflating or anesthesia bag
Noninvasive positive pressure ventilation (CPAP, BiPAP)	Decreases work of breathing, increases oxygenation and ventilation	Contraindicated if decreased level of consciousness, apnea, increased secretions
Endotracheal intubation/assisted ventilation	Control ventilation for depressed central nervous system	Relatively contraindicated if severe midface trauma
	Absent pharyngeal reflexes	If epiglottitis, consider intubation in operating room
	Mechanical support for weak chest wall	
	Artificial airway for obstructed airway	Avoid intubation in severe asthma if possible
	Supplemental oxygen for damaged alveoli	
	Control intracranial pressure by hyperventilation	
	Provide tracheopulmonary toilet	
	Provide positive end-expiratory pressure to increase lung volume	
Needle cricothyroidotomy	Emergent artificial airway required to sustain life, upper airway obstruction cannot otherwise be relieved, tracheostomy cannot be immediately performed	Temporizing measure, tracheostomy to follow immediately
Tracheostomy	Emergent artificial airway required to sustain life, upper airway obstruction cannot be relieved by endotracheal intubation	Should be performed in operating room by experienced physician
Thoracentesis	Evacuation pneumothorax, tension pneumothorax, hemothorax, drainage pleural effusion, empyema	Pigtail or chest tube placement to follow immediately or performed instead
Thoracostomy	Evacuate, prevent reaccumulation pneumothorax, tension pneumothorax, hemothorax, effusion, empyema	Thoracentesis first if pigtail/chest tube cannot be placed immediately in life-threatening situation.
Pericardiocentesis	Relieve tamponade: effusion, hemopericardium, pneumopericardium	Improve cardiac output
		Requires ultrasound or ECHO guidance
Bronchoscopy	Foreign-body removal	Do not agitate the child before the procedure
		Esophagoscopy for esophageal foreign body

and resuscitation should remain with the patient at all times. Evaluation that is stepwise and focused is critical for determining the source and severity of respiratory distress. Anticipation and rapid aggressive management are essential for optimizing outcome. In the child who is alert and otherwise healthy, the position that he or she has naturally assumed is likely to be the one that minimizes respiratory distress and thus should be maintained. A child with significant respiratory distress should be allowed to remain with the parents and should not be agitated. Anxiety increases minute ventilation and adds significantly to the child's O_2 consumption. Any patient believed to have ventilatory compromise should be treated immediately with O_2 at the highest concentration available. Supplemental O_2 provides a small but often crucial margin of safety in ensuring adequate cerebral and myocardial oxygenation. In patients with decreased sensorium or neuromuscular disease, a position to optimize airway patency must be established. Airway devices or assisted ventilation may be necessary. For management of cardiorespiratory arrest, resuscitation efforts must be initiated immediately, as detailed in Chapters 1 A General Approach to Ill and Injured Children and 3 Airway.

History

A detailed history usually provides important clues to the cause of respiratory distress, but in a critically ill or injured child, comprehensive details should not be obtained at the expense of patient care. A brief history can be obtained while emergent treatment is initiated. Details can follow once the child is stabilized. Information obtained by history should include a description of respiratory and other symptoms, onset and duration of symptoms, possible precipitating factors including ill contacts, environmental exposures and recent travel, trauma, therapeutic interventions, history of previous similar symptoms, underlying medical conditions, particularly those that predispose to respiratory compromise, medications, allergies, and immunizations and family history of respiratory conditions.

Physical Examination

The physical examination should assess the degree of respiratory distress and should identify the site and likely cause of respiratory distress (Fig. 66.1A,B). Continuous cardiopulmonary monitoring and frequent assessment are important because respiratory status can change quickly. General appearance, level of consciousness, work of breathing, and vital signs, including respiratory rate and adequacy of oxygenation and ventilation give immediate information regarding the severity of respiratory distress and possible etiologies. Heightened level of consciousness, manifesting as restlessness, anxiety, or combativeness, is more likely an early sign of hypoxia, whereas diminished level of consciousness, manifesting as somnolence, lethargy, stupor, obtundation, or coma, tends to result from hypercarbia or severe hypoxia. The child's posture may provide clues regarding the source of the respiratory compromise. Children with upper airway obstruction tend to assume a sniffing position, an upright sitting posture with neck slightly flexed and head extended. For lower airway obstruction, a tripod position, in which the child is sitting up and leaning forward, may be preferred. Dysphagia and/or dooling are concerning for oropharyngeal or laryngeal obstruction. Pallor suggests possible anemia, structural heart disease, arrhythmia, sepsis, or hemorrhage. Peripheral cyanosis is caused by local vascular changes of the extremities that result in inadequate perfusion or vascular stasis.

Vital sign abnormalities provide important clues about the severity of illness and adequacy of compensatory mechanisms. Tachycardia is one of the early signs of respiratory compromise and is expected because of increased sympathetic tone due to respiratory distress. Bradycardia in a hypoxic child is a late and ominous sign that often signals impending cardiac arrest. Cardiac arrhythmias that compromise cardiac output may result in respiratory distress. Respiratory rate in children varies with age (Table 66.7). Tachypnea is a compensatory mechanism for hypoxia, hypercapnia, and acidosis, and it also occurs with pain, anxiety, and increased activity. Fever increases respiratory rate by 3 to 7 breaths per minute, per degree above normal, with increases as high as 11 breaths per minute in those <12 months of age. Although not specific for respiratory distress, tachypnea is one of the findings most consistently present with respiratory distress and is particularly pronounced with lower airway processes. Tachypnea may be the only manifestation of lower respiratory infection in children younger than 6 months. Bradypnea, or decreased respiratory rate, may reflect central respiratory depression, increased intracranial pressure, or fatigue of respiratory muscles. It is usually an ominous sign that heralds impending respiratory arrest. Blood pressure is often increased because of anxiety. Pulsus paradoxus, an exaggeration (more than 10 mm Hg) of the normal decrease in blood pressure during inspiration, correlates with degree of airway obstruction. Pulses paradoxus is also caused by compromised venous return because of forces on the pericardium that result in decreased cardiac output, particularly during forced inspiration. Hypotension in a child is a late and extremely worrisome finding. It suggests profound shock, significantly decreased cardiac output, and impending cardiorespiratory arrest. Oxygen saturation of >97% while awake is normal. Central cyanosis usually reflects at least 5 g/dL of unsaturated hemoglobin and an O_2 saturation of less than 90%. Peripheral cyanosis is not usually associated with a decrease in systemic O_2 saturation.

On inspection, in addition to respiratory rate, one should appreciate depth, rhythm, and symmetry of respirations; the use of accessory muscles; and perfusion. Rapid and shallow breathing may result from air trapping in obstructive lower airway disease. It may also result from chest pain, chest wall musculoskeletal dysfunction, or abdominal pain and/or distention. Kussmaul respirations (deep, regular, sighing breaths that may be rapid, slow, or normal in rate) are seen with metabolic acidosis, particularly diabetic ketoacidosis. Cheyne–Stokes respirations (respirations with increasing then decreasing depth alternating with periods of apnea) are seen with CNS immaturity in otherwise normal neonates and infants, particularly during sleep. In older children, this respiratory pattern is concerning for inadequate cerebral perfusion, brain injury, increased intracranial pressure, and central narcotic depression. Biot's, or ataxic, respirations (breaths of irregular depth interrupted irregularly by periods of apnea) suggest CNS infection, injury, or drug-induced depression. Asymmetric chest wall movement and/or expansion suggest unilateral chest wall or thoracic cavity pathology. Nasal flaring and supraclavicular, suprasternal, and subcostal retractions of accessory muscles of respiration usually reflect upper airway obstruction but may occur with lower processes (Table 66.8). Intercostal retractions are usually a sign of inadequate tidal volume as a result of lower airway disease. Head bobbing, more common in neonates and young infants, is another sign of accessory muscle use. Thoracoabdominal dissociation, also called respiratory alternans or see-saw respirations, in which the chest collapses on inspiration and the abdomen protrudes, is a common sign of respiratory muscle fatigue. Peripheral cyanosis should be distinguished from central cyanosis.

Palpation of the chest commonly reveals vibratory rhonchi over the large airways, which suggests fluid in the airway.

TABLE 66.7

NORMAL RESPIRATORY RATES

Age group	Respiratory rate (breaths/min)
Neonates	35–50
Older infants/toddlers	30–40
Elementary school-aged children	20–30
Older children/adolescents	12–20

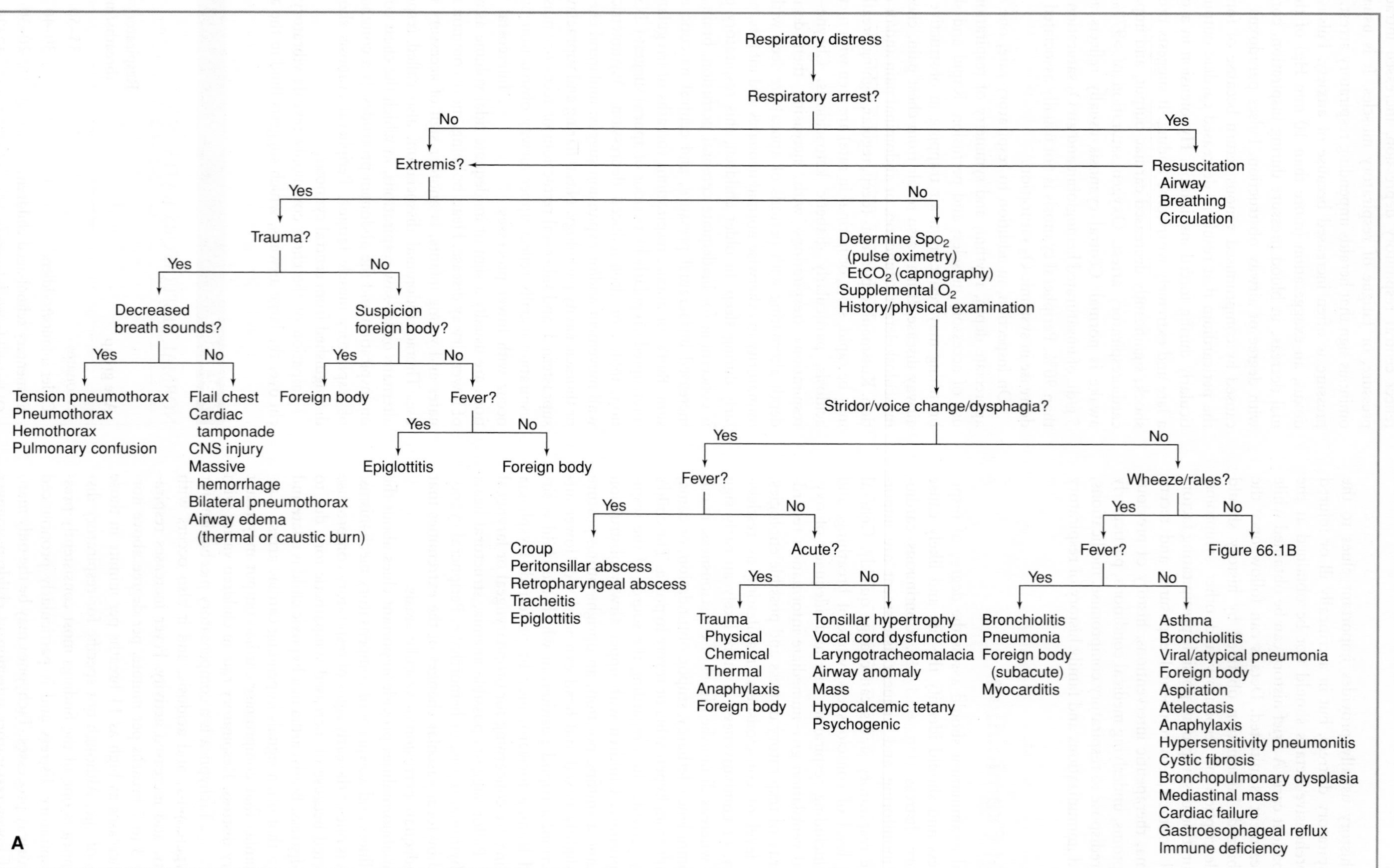

FIGURE 66.1 **A:** Approach to the child with respiratory distress. (*continued*)

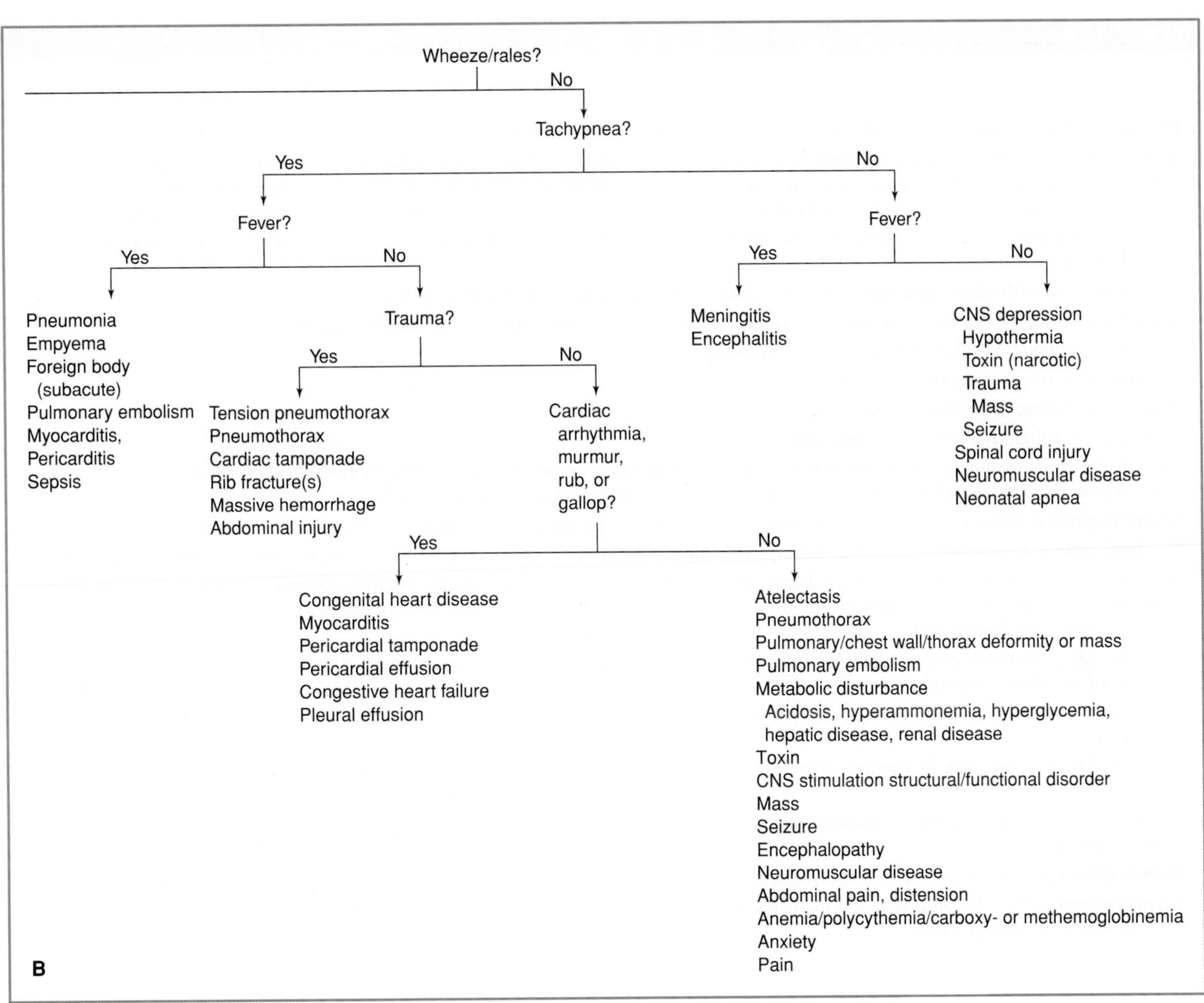

FIGURE 66.1 (*Continued*) **B:** Approach to the child with respiratory distress. SpO_2, percentage oxygen saturation; O_2, oxygen; $EtCO_2$, end-tidal carbon dioxide; CNS, central nervous system.

Increased tactile fremitus suggests bronchopulmonary consolidation or abscess, when decreased or absent, it suggests bronchial obstruction or space-occupying processes of the pleural cavity. Crepitus on palpation of the chest or neck may reveal subcutaneous emphysema caused by pneumothorax or pneumomediastinum.

Auscultation is particularly useful for localizing the site of respiratory distress (Table 66.8). Stertor, gurgle, dysphonia, aphonia, hoarseness, barky cough, and inspiratory stridor localize the respiratory distress to the upper airway. A lower airway cause is suggested by decreased or asymmetric breath sounds, changes in pitch of breath sounds, expiratory stridor, grunting, and/or adventitious sounds, including crackles, rhonchi, wheeze, rub, bronchophony, egophony, and whispered pectoriloquy. Transmission of breath sounds across the small pediatric chest may obscure focal findings, and upper airway sounds are often transmitted to lower airways. The ratio of inspiratory to expiratory phase of respiration, normally 1:1, can be useful in distinguishing an upper from lower respiratory tract cause of respiratory distress. Respiratory distress from upper airway disease usually results from difficulty of inward air movement. The inspiratory phase is often increased relative to the expiratory phase to a ratio between 1:1 and 2:1. Lower airway processes often impede outward air movement and may result in a prolonged expiratory phase with ratios of 1:3 to 1:4. Absence or disappearance of wheeze in a child with continued or worsening respiratory distress may represent severe obstruction and should not be considered reassuring but rather may herald impending respiratory arrest.

Percussion of the chest may reveal either hyperresonance, suggesting air trapping, or dullness, suggesting an area of consolidation, atelectasis, a mass in the lung or pleural space, or pleural fluid (Table 66.8). Air trapping is suggested by depressed position of the diaphragm. Diaphragmatic excursion can be accessed by measuring the difference between the level of dullness on percussion during full inspiration and full expiration. Poor diaphragmatic excursion may reflect diaphragmatic dysfunction.

The remainder of the physical examination should concentrate on the nervous, cardiac, gastrointestinal, renal, skin, metabolic/endocrine, and hematologic systems as potential source of respiratory distress.

TABLE 66.8

LOCALIZATION OF RESPIRATORY DISTRESS BY PHYSICAL EXAMINATION FINDINGS

Flaring: reflexive opening of nares during inspiration with airway obstruction

Retractions: accessory muscle use manifest as inward collapse of chest wall as a result of high negative intrathoracic pressure from increased respiratory effort; supraclavicular, suprasternal, and subcostal retractions usually reflect upper airway obstruction, intercostal retractions reflect lower airway obstruction or disease but may be seen with severe upper airway obstruction

Head bobbing: extension of head and neck during inhalation and flexion during exhalation, seen in neonates, young infants, reflects accessory muscle use

Stertor: snoring with nasal congestion, adenotonsillar hypertrophy, neuromuscular weakness

Gurgle: inspiratory and expiratory bubbling sounds caused by secretions oropharynx, trachea, large bronchi

Aphonia/dysphonia: vocal cord obstruction, dysfunction

Muffled voice: oropharyngeal obstruction

Hoarseness: laryngeal obstruction, dysfunction

Barky cough: subglottic, tracheal obstruction

Stridor: abnormal turbulence over airway obstruction; (i) inspiratory: quiet, high pitched from glottic, subglottic region; (ii) expiratory: loud, harsh from carina or below; and (iii) biphasic: loud, harsh from trachea

Grunt: expiration against a closed glottis to maintain expiratory lung volume with lower airway, gastrointestinal process

Tracheal deviation: shifting of trachea to nonaffected side of chest due to air, fluid space-occupying process on contralateral side

Wheeze: continuous, musical; (i) obstructed bronchi, bronchioles—polyphonic (variable pitched, regional differences) expiratory as in asthma; (ii) obstructed central airway—monophonic (low pitched, same in all lung fields) expiratory ± inspiratory as with tracheal foreign body, tracheomalacia

Crackles (rales): discontinuous, usually high-pitched, inspiratory; moist, from thin secretions in (i) bronchi, bronchioles (medium rales), or (ii) alveoli (fine rales)

Rhonchi (coarse rales): discontinuous, usually low-pitched, inspiratory; moist or dry, from exudate, edema, inflammation larger bronchi

Pericardial friction rub: saw-like sound, inspiratory, expiratory between sternum and apex of heart due to pericardial inflammation, fluid

Hamman crunch/sign: pericardial crackles synchronous with heart beat due to heart beating against pneumomediastinum, left-sided pneumothorax

Bronchophony, egophony, whispered pectoriloquy: alterations in voice sounds as a result of lobar pneumonia, pleural effusion

Tactile fremitus: vibration on percussion increased with consolidation, abscess, decreased/absent with bronchial obstruction, pleural cavity space-occupying lesion

Approach

The approach to the child with respiratory distress (Fig. 66.1A,B) begins with the assessment of airway patency and, oxygenation and ventilation. In arrest situations, appropriate resuscitation as per Pediatric Advanced Life Support guidelines, should be initiated immediately. Patients in extremis (Fig. 66.1A) also require emergent treatment for underlying conditions. In trauma patients, these most commonly include airway obstruction, tension pneumothorax, flail chest, or cardiac tamponade. Patients in extremis with no history of trauma require a very brief history and physical examination to determine etiology, most commonly foreign body, infection, or anaphylaxis.

For patients with mild to moderate respiratory distress, allow patients to assume and maintain a position that maximizes their respiratory function. Every effort should be made to avoid agitating the child as this may result in critical airway compromise and increased metabolic demand for O_2. The initial focus of the examination should be on the respiratory and cardiac systems. Assessment begins with the observation of patient position, general appearance, work of breathing, and respiratory sounds that can be appreciated without a stethoscope. This is followed by evaluation of oxygenation and ventilation, and auscultation to assess abnormal cardiopulmonary sounds. The remainder of the examination is performed when the child is sufficiently stable to tolerate the examination.

All patients with respiratory distress should have their oxygenation tested immediately by pulse oximetry. Capnography measures end-tidal carbon dioxide ($EtCO_2$) and CO_2 waveform as a rapid means of assessing ventilation and can help identify upper or lower airway obstruction.

Stridor, altered phonation, and/or dysphagia suggest partial airway obstruction. Children with abnormal auscultatory findings (i.e., wheeze, rales, rhonchi, and/or asymmetric breath sounds) and fever are likely to have pneumonia or bronchiolitis, whereas asthma, bronchiolitis, and foreign-body aspiration are common in afebrile patients.

Patients can be further categorized on the basis of tachypnea (Fig. 66.1B). Children with rapid respirations and fever may have pneumonia, even in the absence of rales; empyema, pulmonary embolism, and encephalitis are also important considerations. Tachypnea without fever points to trauma, cardiac disease, metabolic disturbances, toxic ingestions, or exposures.

Febrile children without tachypnea may have apnea or bradypnea as late manifestations of CNS infection. In afebrile patients, considerations include the myriad causes of CNS depression, spinal cord injury, neuromuscular disease, and neonatal apnea. Diagnostic tests should be used selectively

TABLE 66.9

DIAGNOSTIC STUDIES FOR EVALUATION OF RESPIRATORY DISTRESS

Test	Indications	Comments
Pulse oximetry	Respiratory distress, failure	Measures oxygen saturation Relative contraindication if agitation will worsen distress Not reliable if severe anemia No information about ventilation
Capnography	Respiratory distress, failure Confirm, monitor endotracheal tube placement, ventilatory failure Diagnose, differentiate upper, lower airway obstruction, monitor therapeutic interventions Monitor ventilation during sedation	Measures end-tidal CO_2 ($EtCO_2$), CO_2 waveform Can be used in intubated or nonintubated patients Approximates ABG $PaCO_2$ if cardiovascular status intact; $EtCO_2$ values 2–5 mm Hg $<PaCO_2$ Characteristic waveforms for apnea, hypoventilation, obstruction
ABG, VBG	Respiratory distress, failure, acidosis, carboxyhemoglobin, methemoglobin	Information about ventilation Most useful for lower airway process Relative contraindication if agitation will worsen distress ABG, VBG changes occur late and may not be seen until arrest (A-a) O_2 gradient increase suggests ventilation–perfusion mismatch
CBC count, blood cx, CSF analysis, cx, mono spot/EBV titers	Infection, allergy	Relative contraindication for lumbar puncture if agitation or positioning will worsen distress
Electrolytes, BUN, CR, glucose, Ca, PO_4, Mg, LFTs, ammonia, TFTs	Metabolic/endocrine disease, metabolic disturbance, disease Altered mental status Tetany	Calculate anion gap
PT/PTT	Bleeding/clotting disorder, pulmonary embolism	Negative D-dimer excludes PE in patients with low pretest probability for PE
D-dimer	Pulmonary embolism	
Toxicologic screen blood, urine	Ingestion/intoxication	Central nervous system depressants, neuromuscular blockade, electron transport chain poisons
Nasal, ocular, rectal swab: DFA, PCR, cx	Bronchiolitis, *Chlamydia* infection, pertussis, viral pneumonia	Neonates, infants
Sputum: stains, cx	Bacterial, TB, pneumocystis, fungal	Adolescents
TB skin test	TB	
Neck radiograph, AP/lateral	Tracheitis, abscess, foreign body	Not necessary for the diagnosis of croup Relative contraindication unstable airway Consider portable if unstable
Chest radiograph AP/lateral	Lower respiratory disease, atelectasis, foreign body, barotrauma, effusion, mass, chest wall trauma/deformity, cardiac process	
Forced expiratory or bilateral decubitus	Foreign body	Air trapping distal to foreign body
Unilateral decubitus	Distinguish effusion from infiltrate	Effusion layers
Abdominal radiograph, supine/prone, cross-table lateral, upright)	Abdominal mass, obstruction, perforation	
Fluoroscopy	Upper airway obstruction; structural or functional anatomic, foreign body, paralysis vocal cords, diaphragm	

(*continued*)

TABLE 66.9

DIAGNOSTIC STUDIES FOR EVALUATION OF RESPIRATORY DISTRESS (*CONTINUED*)

Test	Indications	Comments
Laryngoscopy/bronchoscopy	Upper or lower airway obstruction; structural or functional, foreign body	Esophagoscopy for esophageal processes
Head CT scan	Intracranial bleed, mass, hydrocephalus	
Chest CT scan	Intra/extrathoracic anomaly, mass, abscess, diaphragmatic hernia	
Abdomen CT scan	Obstruction, mass, appendicitis	
Pulmonary and cardiac US	Pleural or pericardial effusion, tamponade	
Electrocardiogram	Cardiac anomaly, failure, pericarditis	
ECHO	Structural, functional cardiac abnormality	
Thoracentesis, pericardiocentesis cytology, biochemical, cx	Infection, inflammation, oncologic process chest, heart, lymphatics	Also therapeutic Consider US guidance
Ventilation–perfusion scan	Pulmonary embolism (PE)	If concern PE, consider extremity US to evaluate for DVT
Barium swallow	Tracheoesophageal fistula, vascular ring, reflux	
Pulmonary function tests	Central or peripheral nervous system depression of chest wall function, respiratory system disease	Measures lung volume, flow, compliance
Electromyography	Central respiratory drive depressed, neuromuscular disease	Measures muscle activity generated by neural outflow from respiratory centers
Chest angiography	Vascular anomaly, PE	If concern PE, consider extremity US to evaluate for DVT

ABG, arterial blood gas; CBC count, complete blood cell count; cx, culture; CSF, cerebrospinal fluid; EBV, Epstein–Barr virus; BUN, blood urea nitrogen; CR, creatinine; Ca, calcium; PO_4, phosphate; Mg, magnesium; LFTs, liver function tests; TFTs, thyroid function tests; PT, prothrombin time; PTT, partial thromboplastin time; IFA, immunofluorescence assay; TB, tuberculosis; AP, anteroposterior; CT, computed tomography.

to evaluate for diagnoses suggested by history and physical examination (Table 66.9).

Rapid portable chest radiograph can be helpful in the determination of respiratory failure and impending failure, particularly because of lower airway processes, and may provide insights into its cause. Ultrasound can also be a useful adjunct to the physical examination and may help to both determine a diagnosis as well as to guide the management of a patient presenting with respiratory distress (Table 66.10). In the patient presenting with respiratory distress of unclear etiology, thoracic ultrasound can be used to evaluate for pneumonia, pleural effusion, and pneumothorax. Cardiac ultrasound can be used to detect a pericardial effusion and access cardiac function. For the novice ultrasonographer, these findings can then be confirmed with chest x-ray or ECHO respectively. In the trauma patient, thoracic ultrasound has been shown to be useful for the detection of hemothorax and pneumothorax. For complete details on thoracic and cardiac ultrasound technique and findings please refer to Chapter 142 Ultrasound.

Treatment

Regardless of the cause of respiratory distress, aggressive treatment must be initiated immediately to rapidly restore oxygenation and ventilation (Table 66.6). Airway patency, if inadequate, must be established. In the patient with decreased sensorium, positioning the airway by chin lift (contraindicated if neck injury is suspected) or jaw thrust may relieve soft tissue obstruction of the airway. The oral cavity should be cleared of secretions, vomitus, blood, and visible foreign matter. In the alert patient with suspected soft tissue obstruction of the airway, a nasopharyngeal airway may improve airway patency. In an unconscious patient, an oropharyngeal airway can be placed to relieve obstruction. Noninvasive positive pressure ventilation, in the form of CPAP of BiPAP may be trialed in select cooperative, hemodynamically stable, spontaneously breathing patients to decrease work of breathing and improve respiratory status and cardiac output. The child in whom airway patency and/or adequate ventilation and oxygenation cannot be established or maintained using noninvasive approaches, requires endotracheal intubation. Indications for endotracheal intubation directly related to respiratory distress include respiratory failure or impending failure, airway obstruction, inability to handle secretions, and risk of aspiration. Tension pneumo- or hemothorax, and/or pericardial fluid causing tamponade must be decompressed immediately. Ultrasound can be used to guide thoracentesis, thoracostomy, and pericardiocentesis. Placement of a nasogastric tube to decompress a distended abdomen often improves respiratory effort by allowing full expansion of the lungs. Correction of metabolic derangements and/or treatment of drug or toxin intoxication, may restore depressed respiratory drive and/or peripheral neuromuscular respiratory function.

TABLE 66.10

ULTRASOUND FOR EVALUATION AND TREATMENT OF RESPIRATORY DISTRESS[a]

Examination diagnosis	Probe, position	Key diagnostic findings	Therapeutic indications
Thoracic			
Pneumothorax	High-frequency probe Anteior chest midclavicular and anterior axillary line Marker to patient's head	Absence of lung sliding ("barcode sign" in M-mode) with lung point confirms pneumothorax Normal lung sliding ("seashore sign" in M-mode) with the presence of the comet tail artifact rules out pneumothorax	Thoracentesis, thoracotomy
Pleural effusion, hemothorax	Low-frequency probe RUQ, LUQ (FAST views) High- or low-frequency probe Anterior, lateral, and posterior lung zones Marker to patient's head	Anechoic fluid overlying the lung parenchyma, typically in the posterior/inferior region Fibrin strands, debris, loculations suggest empyema	Thoracentesis, thoracotomy
Pneumonia	High- or low-frequency probe Anterior, lateral, and posterior lung zones Marker to patient's head	Lung hepatization, air bronchograms (which can be also be seen with atelectasis)	
Cardiac			
Pericardial effusion	Low-frequency probe Subxiphoid, marker to patient's right Parasternal long, marker to patient's left hip	Anechoic fluid in the pericardial space between the pericardium and myocardium, tracks anterior to descending aorta in parasternal long view	Pericardiocentesis

[a]For details see Chapter 142 Ultrasound.

SUMMARY

Respiratory distress is one of the most common chief complaints of children seeking medical care. The causes of respiratory distress are numerous and varied. History and physical examination provides important clues that allow rapid localization of the site of impairment. The underlying cause must be identified and may be within the respiratory system or organ systems that control or impact respiration. Any disorder that causes respiratory distress may be life-threatening. Airway and ventilatory problems not only must be recognized but also must be anticipated and addressed aggressively. The underlying cause must also be treated. Patients must be monitored continuously and reassessed frequently. Airway, breathing, and circulation must be established and maintained. Diagnostic evaluation of body fluids, radiologic studies, direct visualization, and specialized tests of organ function must be performed prudently so that respiratory status is not further compromised.

Suggested Readings and Key References

Canducci F, Debiaggi M, Sampaolo M, et al. Two-year prospective study of single infections and co-infections by respiratory syncytial virus and viruses identified recently in infants with acute respiratory disease. *J Med Virol* 2008;80(4):716–723.

Cherry JD. Clinical practice. Croup. *N Engl J Med* 2008;358(4):384–391.

Dieckmann RA. Pediatric assessment. In: Gausche-Hill M, Fuchs S, Yamamoto L eds. *APLS: The pediatric emergency medicine resource.* Jones and Bartlett, Sudbury; 2010:2–37.

Durbin WJ, Stille C. Pneumonia. *Pediatr Rev* 2008;29:147–160.

Gadomski AM, Permutt T, Stanton B. Correcting respiratory rate for the presence of fever. *J Clin Epidemiol* 1994;47(9):1043–1049.

Hammer J. Acute respiratory failure in children. *Paediatr Respir Rev* 2013;14(2):64–69.

Kattwinkel J, Perlman JM, Aziz K, et al. Neonatal resuscitation: 2010 American Heart Association guidelines for cardiopulmonary resuscitation and emergency cardiovascular care. *Pediatrics* 2010;126(5):e1400–e1413.

King C, Henretig FM, King BR, et al., eds. *Textbook of pediatric emergency procedures.* 2nd ed. Baltimore, MD: Williams & Wilkins, 2007:85–251, 383–409, 823–901.

Kleinman ME, Chameides L, Schexnayder SM, et al. Pediatric advanced life support: 2010 American Heart Association guidelines for cardiopulmonary resuscitation and emergency cardiovascular care. *Pediatrics* 2010;126(5):e1361–e1399.

Krauss BS, Harakal T, Fleisher GR. The spectrum and frequency of illness presenting to a pediatric emergency department. *Pediatr Emerg Care* 1997;7(2);67–71.

Louie MC, Bradin S. Foreign body ingestion and aspiration. *Pediatr Rev* 2009;30:295–301.

Margolis P, Gadomski A. The rational clinical examination. Does this infant have pneumonia? *JAMA* 1998;279:308–313.

McIntosh K. Community-acquired pneumonia in children. *N Engl J Med* 2002;346(6):429–437.

Miller EK, Gebretsadik T, Carroll KN, et al. Viral etiologies of infant bronchiolitis, croup and upper respiratory illness during 4 consecutive years. *Pediatr Infect dis J* 2013;32(9):950–955.

O'Dempsey TJ, Laurence BE, Mcardle TF, et al. The effect of temperature reduction on respiratory rate in febrile illnesses. *Arch Dis Child* 1993;68(4):492–495.

Pfleger A, Eber E. Management of acute severe upper airway obstruction in children. *Paediatr Respir Rev* 2013;14(2):70–77.

Poets CF, Southall DP. Noninvasive monitoring of oxygenation in infants and children: practical considerations and areas of concern. *Pediatrics* 1994;93:737–746.

Rafei K, Lichenstein R. Airway infectious disease emergencies. *Pediatr Clin North Am* 2006;53:215–242.

Ralston SL, Lieberthal AS, Meissner HC, et al. Clinical practice guideline: the diagnosis, management, and prevention of bronchiolitis. *Pediatrics* 2014;134(5):e1474–e1502.

Shah S, Sharieff GQ. Pediatric respiratory infections. *Emerg Med Clin North Am* 2007;25:961–979.

Tibballs J, Watson T. Symptoms and signs differentiating croup and epiglottitis. *Paediatr Child Health* 2011;47(3):77–82.

Wald EL. Croup: common syndromes and therapy. *Pediatr Ann* 2010;39(1):15–21.

CHAPTER 67 ▪ SEIZURES

AMIR A. KIMIA, MD AND VINCENT W. CHIANG, MD

Seizure is the clinical expression of abnormal, excessive, synchronous discharges of neurons residing primarily in the cerebral cortex. This paroxysmal activity is intermittent and its duration may last from a few seconds to many hours. Seizures represent a neurologic emergency either due to the underlying trigger (bleed, infection) or due to potential of the neuronal death, the product of a prolonged seizure. Approximately 5% of children will have at least one seizure in the first 16 years of life. Physicians must have a fundamental knowledge of seizure classification (semiology), all aspects of seizure management (including initial stabilization), determination of cause (differential diagnosis), appropriate definitive treatment, and patient disposition.

BACKGROUND

A seizure is defined as a transient, involuntary alteration of consciousness, behavior, motor activity, sensation, and/or autonomic function caused by an excessive rate and hypersynchrony of discharges from a group of cerebral neurons. A convulsion is a seizure with prominent alterations of motor activity. Epilepsy, or seizure disorder, is a condition of susceptibility to recurrent seizures.

Seizures may be generalized or partial. *Generalized seizures* reflect involvement of both cerebral hemispheres. These may be convulsive or nonconvulsive. Consciousness may be impaired and this impairment may be the initial manifestation. Motor involvement is bilateral. Types of generalized seizures include absence (petit mal), myoclonic, tonic, clonic, atonic, and tonic–clonic (grand mal) seizures.

Partial (focal, local) seizures reflect initial involvement limited to one cerebral hemisphere. Partial seizures are further classified on the basis of whether consciousness is impaired. When consciousness is not impaired, the seizure is classified as a simple partial seizure. Simple partial seizures may have motor, somatosensory/sensory, autonomic, or psychic symptoms. When consciousness is impaired, the seizure is classified as a complex partial seizure. Both simple and complex partial seizures may evolve into generalized seizures (e.g., jacksonian march). It is important to recognize that generalized seizures with focal manifestations are also considered focal. These manifestations include lateral eye deviation, head tilt, postictal Todd paresis (or paralysis), or psychomotor seizures (also referred to as temporal lobe seizures).

Status epilepticus is a form of prolonged seizure. This is defined as seizures lasting more than 5 minutes or persistent, repetitive seizure activity without recovery of consciousness in between episodes. This is an operational definition of status that guides therapy because only 25% of pediatric seizures last longer than 5 minutes and the longer a seizure persists, the more difficult it becomes to control. If a child is seen in the ED with a reported/witnessed seizure that has resolved, a 30-minute cutoff is used to define status. This definition is used because 30 minutes is when the risk of permanent neuronal injury increases. Status epilepticus is the highest form of seizure emergency.

A postictal (decreased responsiveness) period usually follows a seizure. During this time, the patient may be confused, lethargic, fatigued, or irritable; also, headache, vomiting, and muscle soreness may occur. In general, the length of the postictal period is proportional to the length of the seizure. For brief seizures, there may be few or no postictal symptoms. Transient focal deficits (e.g., Todd paralysis) may occur during the postictal period, but one must first rule out a focal central nervous system (CNS) deficit.

PATHOPHYSIOLOGY

The underlying abnormality in all seizures is the hypersynchrony of neuronal discharges. Cerebral manifestations include increased blood flow, increased oxygen and glucose consumption, and increased carbon dioxide and lactic acid production. If a patient can maintain appropriate oxygenation and ventilation, the increase in cerebral blood flow is usually sufficient to meet the initial increased metabolic requirements of the brain. This will slow the rate of neuronal loss, which may still occur due to overstimulation. Brief seizures rarely produce any lasting effects. Multiple animal studies and a recent study in humans (FEBSTAT) indicate that 30 minutes of generalized convulsive status epilepticus increases the risk of permanent neuronal injury.

Systemic alterations may occur with seizures and result from a massive sympathetic discharge, leading to tachycardia, hypertension, and initially stress hyperglycemia. Failure of adequate ventilation, especially in patients in whom consciousness is impaired, can lead to hypoxia, hypercarbia, and respiratory acidosis. Patients with impaired consciousness may be unable to protect their airway and are at risk for aspiration. Prolonged skeletal muscle activity can lead to lactic acidosis, rhabdomyolysis, hyperkalemia, hyperthermia, and hypoglycemia.

DIFFERENTIAL DIAGNOSIS

It is important to remember that a seizure does not constitute a diagnosis but is merely a symptom of an underlying pathologic process that requires a thorough investigation (Table 67.1). Often, no underlying condition is identified, and the diagnosis of idiopathic epilepsy is made. However, it is important not to exclude potentially treatable causes prematurely. For instance, seizures that result from metabolic derangements (e.g., hyponatremia, hypoglycemia) are often refractory to anticonvulsant therapy until the abnormality is

TABLE 67.1

ETIOLOGY OF SEIZURES[a]

Infectious	Metabolic
Brain abscess	Hepatic failure
Encephalitis	Hypercarbia
Febrile (nonspecific)	Hyperosmolarity
Meningitis	Hypocalcemia
Parasites (central nervous system)	Hypoglycemia
Syphilis	Hypomagnesemia
Idiopathic	Hyponatremia
Subtherapeutic anticonvulsant level	Hypoxia
Withdrawal	Inborn errors of metabolism
Alcohol	Pyridoxine deficiency
Hypnotics	Uremia
Toxicologic	Vascular
Anticonvulsant	Cerebrovascular accident
Camphor	Hypertensive encephalopathy
Carbon monoxide	Oncologic
Cocaine	Primary brain tumor
Heavy metals (lead)	Metastatic disease
Hypoglycemic agents	Endocrine
Isoniazid	Addison disease
Lithium	Hyper/hypothyroidism
Methylxanthines	Obstetric
Pesticides (organophosphates)	Eclampsia
Phencyclidine	Traumatic
Sympathomimetics	Cerebral contusion
Tricyclic antidepressants	Diffuse axonal injury
Topical anesthetics	Intracranial hemorrhage
Degenerative cerebral disease	Congenital anomalies
Hypoxic ischemic injury	

[a]Bold type denotes most common causes. Given their nature, virtually all these etiologies are potentially life-threatening, except perhaps simple febrile seizures.

corrected. Therefore, rapid testing for glucose and sodium are recommended for pediatric status. Furthermore, every effort should be made to rule out a potentially life-threatening cause of seizures (e.g., intracranial injury or hemorrhage, meningitis, ingestions) before a less serious diagnosis is accepted.

Syncope, or the transient loss of consciousness that results from inadequate cerebral perfusion or substrate delivery, is the most common alternative diagnosis given to patients who present for the evaluation of a seizure episode (see Chapter 71 Syncope). Further complicating matters is the fact that a small percentage of patients with syncope exhibit some sort of convulsive movement. Although vasovagal episodes or orthostatic hypotension is the most common cause for syncope, it is important to evaluate these patients for potential underlying cardiac disease.

Psychogenic nonepileptic seizures (PNES) were formerly called "pseudoseizures." They are a movement disorder that resembles seizure activity, but have no corresponding abnormal brain electrical activity. PNES include a wide array of conditions ranging from conversion reaction to movement disorder and even parasomnias. When the event is psychogenic in nature, the movements can be quite startling, are typically bizarre and thrashing, and are often associated with a great deal of vocalization. There is usually no biting, incontinence, or injury associated with PNES. In contrast to seizures, PNES are rarely followed by a postictal period or postictal headache, and patients often possess a clear mental status after the event. PNES should also be suspected when the episodes are almost always witnessed or heard and never during sleep, rather than occurring randomly, and if the eyes are closed during the episodes (eyes are closed in less than 10% of actual seizures). In some cases, diagnosis may require long-term video and electroencephalographic (EEG) monitoring. Further complicating the issue is that PNES are most likely to occur in patients with an underlying seizure disorder (Table 67.2).

Breath-holding spells are common, affecting 4% to 5% of all children (see Chapter 134 Behavioral and Psychiatric Emergencies). They typically present between the ages of 6 and 18 months and rarely persist past 5 years of age. The two types of breath-holding spells—cyanotic and pallid—have common features, including a period of apnea and an alteration in the state of consciousness. Usually, some initiating event (e.g., pain, fear, agitation) triggers the episode. The diagnosis is based on the clinical findings, and the prognosis is excellent.

A variety of movement disorders can mimic seizures. Paroxysmal choreoathetosis is often associated with a positive family history for seizures and is exacerbated by intentional movement. Tic disorders can be manifested by twitching, blinking, head shaking, or other repetitive motions. These are usually suppressible and are not associated with any loss of consciousness. Shudder attacks are whole-body tremors similar to essential tremor in adults. Benign myoclonus of infancy can look like infantile spasms but is associated with a completely normal EEG.

Sleep disorders, such as somnambulism, night terrors (preschool-aged children), and narcolepsy (typically in adolescents) can often be diagnosed on the basis of the history

TABLE 67.2

DIFFERENTIAL DIAGNOSIS OF PAROXYSMAL EVENTS

Seizure disorders	Movement disorders
Psychogenic nonepileptic seizures	Paroxysmal choreoathetosis
(Pseudoseizures)	Tic disorders
Head trauma	Shudder attacks
Loss of consciousness	Benign myoclonus
Posttraumatic seizures	Psychiatric disorders
Syncope	Daydreaming
Hypovolemia	Attention-deficit hyperactivity disorder
Hypoxia	Panic attacks
Reduced cardiac output	Gastrointestinal disorder
Sleep disorders	Sandifer syndrome (gastroesophageal reflux)
Nightmares	Abdominal migraines
Night terrors	Cyclic vomiting
Narcolepsy	Breath-holding spells
Sleep apnea hypersomnia	Pallid
Somnambulism	Cyanotic
Apparent life-threatening event	Atypical migraines

alone (see Chapter 134 Behavioral and Psychiatric Emergencies). Infants with gastroesophageal reflux may exhibit torticollis or dystonic posturing (Sandifer syndrome). Atypical migraines and PNES are often diagnosed after other causes are excluded.

INITIAL STABILIZATION

This section will focus on patients with generalized convulsive status. The first priority in the seizing patient is to address airway, breathing, and circulation (the ABCs; see Chapter 1 A General Approach to Ill and Injured Children). An adequate airway is necessary to allow for effective ventilation and oxygenation. Patients with impaired consciousness are at risk for obstruction (the tongue, oral secretions, emesis), aspiration (loss of protective reflexes), and hypoventilation. Simple maneuvers such as the jaw thrust or suctioning of the oropharynx may improve the compromised airflow. The use of adjunctive airways (oral or nasopharyngeal) may also help maintain an adequate airway. In patients who are actively seizing, it may be difficult to insert these adjuncts and may cause injury if the intervention is forced. Furthermore, in patients for whom trauma is a possibility, these maneuvers must be undertaken with cervical spine (C-spine) immobilization. In patients in whom the airway remains unstable despite these actions, endotracheal intubation is warranted. When it is necessary to use a muscle relaxant to intubate a seizing patient, one should use the shortest-acting agent possible. The presence of motor activity may be the only clinical manifestation of seizure, and a long-acting muscle relaxant will mask the ongoing seizure activity. One should consider alternatives to succinylcholine in the setting of prolonged seizures because of the potential risk of hyperkalemia related to rhabdomyolysis.

The patient's circulatory status must also be closely monitored. Seizures generally cause a massive sympathetic discharge that result in hypertension and tachycardia. Continuous monitoring and intravenous (IV) access should be obtained. Blood samples, including rapid blood glucose testing, should be acquired at this time. Peripheral IV access, which is often difficult in the pediatric age group, may be nearly impossible in the actively seizing patient. Intraosseous and/or central venous access may be required in the patient with prolonged seizures.

Once the respiratory and circulatory functions have been assessed and maintained, efforts should be directed at stopping any ongoing seizure activity and making a diagnosis. As long as adequate ventilation and oxygenation are maintained, long-term sequelae are unlikely to result from a transient seizure. Consensus management suggests the initiation of anticonvulsant treatment of anyone who has been seizing for more than 5 minutes. This likely represents all patients who are brought to the ED actively seizing.

EVALUATION AND DECISION

History

As a result of the numerous potential causes of seizures, as well as the large number of events that can be mistaken for a seizure, a focused history is important. The parent or caregiver needs to carefully describe the episode and the preceding events. Was there a warning (aura) that the patient was about to have an event? Was there a loss of consciousness, tongue biting, or incontinence? Did the event involve the entire body or only a portion? How long did the event last? How did the patient act after the event was over? The clinician should take into account that the event characteristics may not be accurately perceived by a distressed parent. However, recently with smartphones and digital media being more common, parents may present a clip to the treating clinician, especially for recurring events.

In addition to the episode itself, the preceding events are also crucial. Was there a history of trauma, toxin exposure or ingestion, fever, or other systemic signs of illness (e.g., headache, ataxia, vomiting, diarrhea)? Does the child have an underlying seizure disorder, history of seizures, or other neurologic problems? Is the child taking any anticonvulsants? If yes, was there a recent change in dose, or were any medications started or stopped? Is there a chance that the patient could have a subtherapeutic level, for example, did the patient miss any doses? Other questions that should be asked include if there was any other significant medical history (including abnormal developmental history), any significant surgical history (including the placement of a ventricular shunt), family history of seizures, other medication use, and travel history to an endemic region (neurocysticercosis is one of the leading worldwide causes of seizures).

Physical Examination

With the history, a directed physical examination is performed to look for a possible cause of the seizure. Vital signs, including temperature, need to be obtained. An elevated temperature points to a potential infectious cause. The entire body needs to be examined for the evidence of trauma, either as a preceding cause or as a result of falling during the seizure episode. The skin should be examined for rashes or other congenital skin lesions. Dysmorphic features may be associated with other congenital CNS anomalies. Stigmata of underlying hepatic, renal, or endocrinologic disorders should also be noted.

The head should be carefully examined for swelling, deformity, or other signs of trauma. The presence of a ventricular shunt should be noted. The pupils are studied for shape, size, reactivity, and equality. The fundi are examined for the presence of retinal hemorrhages or papilledema. The tympanic membranes are examined for the presence of hemotympanum or for a source of potential infection. The mouth should be examined for the evidence of tongue biting.

The neck is assessed for meningeal irritation. If there is a history or other physical signs of trauma, neck immobilization should be maintained until the C-spine can be thoroughly examined. Examination of the chest, lungs, and abdomen is performed in the usual fashion. The extremities are examined for the evidence of trauma, especially as the result of falling during a seizure.

The neurologic examination may be limited by either ongoing seizure activity or a postictal state and may consist solely of the pupillary examination and an assessment of any asymmetric movements (focality). Any abnormal posturing (decerebrate or decorticate) should be noted and dealt with immediately, with emergent imaging and possibly neurosurgical intervention. During the postictal state, presence of a Todd paresis should be recorded.

If there is a question of a possible ingestion, the examination is also directed at uncovering a potential toxicologic syndrome (toxidrome) that may suggest a specific class of drugs or toxins that are responsible for the seizure (see Chapter 110 Toxicologic Emergencies). Important variables include temperature, heart rate, blood pressure, pupil size, sweating, flushing, and cyanosis.

As the patient recovers from the seizure episode, periodic reassessment is needed to assess for any underlying neurologic abnormalities.

DIAGNOSTIC APPROACH

Once it has been determined that a seizure may have taken place, the initial diagnostic evaluation (Fig. 67.1) starts with the history and physical examination. Laboratory, radiologic, and other neurodiagnostic testings (e.g., EEG) are other tools that can be a part of the seizure evaluation.

Patients with obvious trauma who are seizing should be treated per advanced trauma life support (ATLS) guidelines (see Chapter 2 Approach to the Injured Child), with close attention to possible intracranial injury (see Chapter 121 Neurotrauma).

Often, patients with a known seizure disorder will present to the ED actively seizing. Patients known or suspected to be taking anticonvulsants should have drug levels evaluated. A subtherapeutic anticonvulsant level is among the most common reasons for patients to present with seizures. At times a concurrent mild infectious process (URI, diarrhea) may have an effect on both seizure threshold and/or anticonvulsant absorption/metabolism.

Many different laboratory tests may reveal a cause for a seizure and, as a result, suggest a potential treatment. A rapid glucose reagent strip test should be performed with the initial blood sample. Hypoglycemia is a common problem that can often precipitate seizure activity. If hypoglycemia is documented or a rapid assessment is not available, treatment with 0.25 to 1 g per kg of dextrose is indicated. Normal glucose levels should not be used to exclude hypoglycemia as the seizure triggers, as secondary stress hyperglycemia may occur as the seizure progresses.

A *febrile seizure* is defined as a seizure caused by a fever, but this is a diagnosis of exclusion. Other infectious etiologies that present with a fever and can be the direct cause of a seizure (e.g., meningitis) must first be ruled out (see Chapters 26 Fever and 102 Infectious Disease Emergencies). Furthermore,

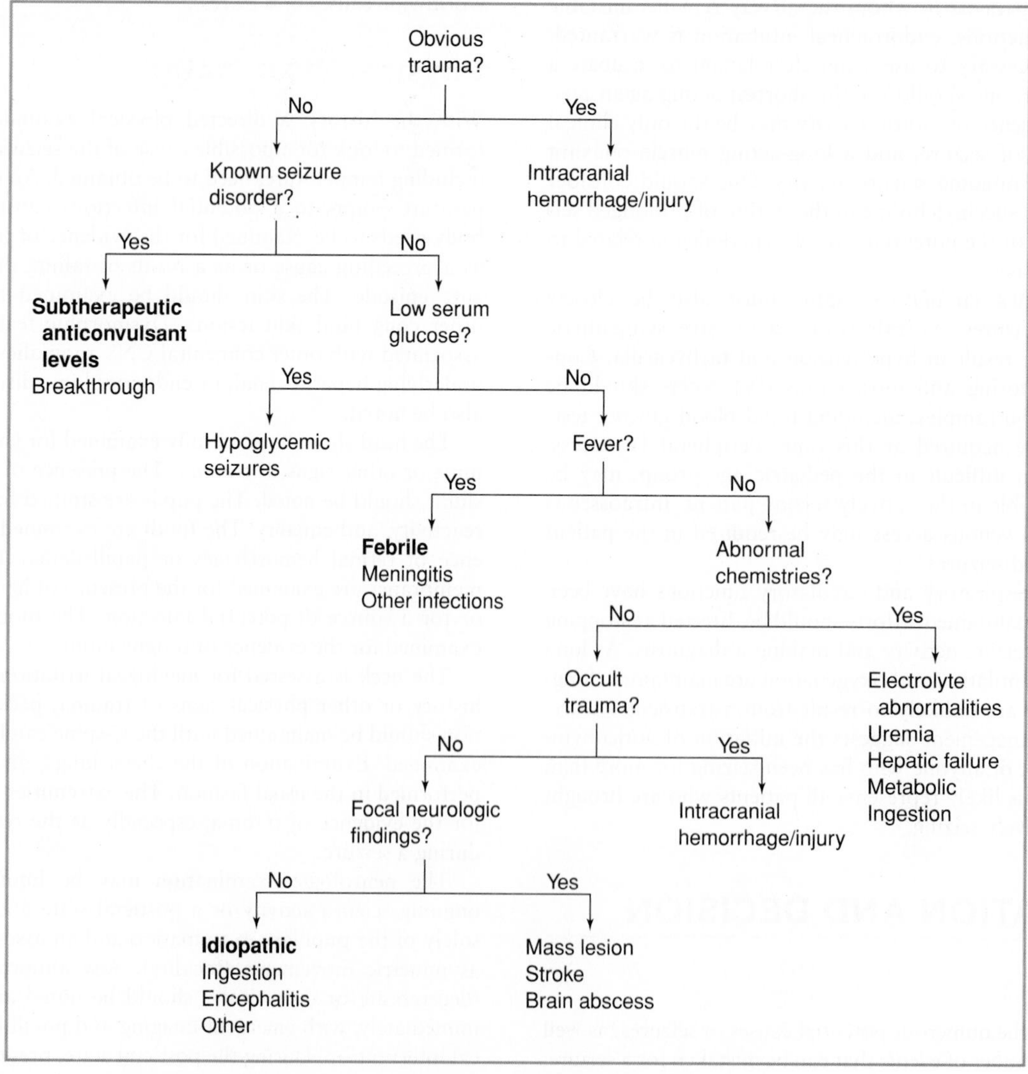

FIGURE 67.1 Diagnostic approach to seizures. The most common causes are in bold type.

infections not involving the CNS may still be the cause of the seizure through the elaboration of fever. Presence of fever or an elevated white blood cell (WBC) count may direct one to look for a potential infectious cause, yet stress response with peripheral leukocytosis occurs in up to a quarter of children with generalized seizures. Blood cultures should be limited to those patients at risk for bacteremia. Urinalysis and chest radiographs can also be used to confirm a source of infection.

A lumbar puncture (LP) with analysis of the cerebrospinal fluid (CSF) is the only way to make the diagnosis of meningitis and should be performed when meningitis is being considered. An elevated CSF protein, CSF pleocytosis, and a low CSF glucose level are all suggestive of CNS infection. CSF cultures, Gram stain, latex studies, and polymerase chain reaction may identify a specific agent. Ideally, CSF cultures should be obtained before antibiotic therapy is initiated. However, in the critically ill or unstable patient, antibiotics should not be withheld until an LP is performed. Furthermore, in cases in which a potential metabolic disease is being considered, CSF lactate, pyruvate, or amino acid level determinations can be used to diagnose a specific disorder. In these cases, it is often helpful to collect an extra tube of CSF to be frozen and used for later analysis. In any patient with signs of increased intracranial pressure, an LP should not be performed until head imaging can be done.

Electrolyte abnormalities may also cause seizures, with hyponatremia, hypocalcemia, and hypomagnesemia being the most common. Unfortunately, seizures caused by electrolyte derangements are often refractory to anticonvulsant therapy and patients will continue to seize until the underlying abnormality is corrected. In general, the routine screening for electrolyte abnormalities in a patient with brief seizure is of low value. Serum electrolytes should be measured in all patients with seizure with significant vomiting or diarrhea; patients with underlying renal, hepatic, neoplastic, or endocrinologic disease; patients who are taking medications that may lead to electrolyte disturbances; or patients who have seizures that are refractory to typical anticonvulsant management. One characteristic scenario involves hyponatremic seizures in infants, typically younger than 6 months, after prolonged feedings of dilute formula ("infantile water intoxication"). Other patients may be evaluated on a case-by-case basis. IV calcium, magnesium, and hypertonic (3%) sodium chloride should be used to treat the appropriate abnormal condition. In the case of hyponatremia, 3% sodium chloride should be infused rapidly until the seizure activity has been stopped; subsequent to seizure resolution, a slower rate of sodium correction should be used to avoid possible central pontine myelinolysis.

Rarely, other chemistries can be helpful in identifying specific organ dysfunction, either as a cause of the seizure activity or as an assessment of systemic injury. An elevated blood urea nitrogen or creatinine level suggests renal insufficiency (with associated findings such as hypertension and electrolyte disturbances) as a potential cause. Elevated liver function tests (transaminases or coagulation times) can be a reflection of hepatic failure. Metabolic acidosis or hyperammonemia can suggest an underlying metabolic disorder. In patients with prolonged seizures, an arterial or venous blood gas level can help in assessing adequacy of ventilation and a creatine kinase level can identify possible rhabdomyolysis.

Toxicologic screening can also be helpful in the seizing patient because certain ingestions are managed with specific antidotes or treatments. Typically, the clinical scenario is the young child with a possible accidental ingestion or the adolescent after a suicide attempt. In general, the toxicologic screen should be directed at agents known to cause seizures (Table 67.1) or those suggested by a clinical toxidrome.

Radiologic imaging of the patient with seizure generally consists of a computed tomography (CT) scan for emergent imaging or, preferably, a magnetic resonance imaging (MRI) study if the patient's condition allows. The following situations should be considered emergent: (i) a patient who has signs or symptoms of elevated ICP, (ii) a patient who has a focal seizure or a persistent focal neurologic deficit, (iii) a patient who has seizures in the setting of head trauma, (iv) a patient who has persistent seizure activity or status epilepticus, or (v) a patient who appears ill. Until C-spine injury is ruled out, it is important to maintain C-spine immobilization when head trauma is a concern. Patients with transient generalized seizures in whom a cause of the seizure activity is identified probably do not require any further head imaging studies. Patients with transient generalized seizures in whom no cause is identified and who appear clinically well can have their head imaging performed on a nonemergent basis in coordination with a pediatric neurologist.

In the past, because of easier availability and lack of a need for sedation for most patients, CT scans were most often the study of choice in the ED for a patient who presented with a seizure. However, given the recent heightened awareness of the risks of ionizing radiation associated with CT scans, patients who do not require emergent imaging may have an MRI study instead. An MRI study also has several other advantages; MRI is better at identifying underlying white matter abnormalities, disorders of brain architecture, lesions of the neurocutaneous syndromes, lesions in the posterior fossa and the brainstem, and small lesions.

EEG is an important diagnostic tool in the evaluation of seizure types, response to treatment, and prognosis. It is rarely indicated in the acute care setting.

EMERGENCY TREATMENT

Prolonged seizure activity is a true medical emergency. In one series, 88 of 239 patients who had convulsive status epilepticus for more than 1 hour had permanent neurologic sequelae. In the FEBSTAT study, 10% of children with febrile status epilepticus (30 minutes or longer) had MRI changes; half of these had permanent changes on follow-up MRI. Thus, following stabilization of the ABCs, further treatment is directed at stopping any seizure activity, as prolonged seizures are harder to control. Although certain causes of seizures may require a specific treatment, anticonvulsant therapy is initiated simultaneously during the evaluation of the seizing patient (Fig. 67.2). The approach to this subject is detailed in Chapter 105 Neurologic Emergencies, but some emergency treatment guidelines are reviewed here.

The benzodiazepines are the initial drug of choice for the treatment of seizures. Benzodiazepines work by blocking the GABA receptor, thus increasing the seizure threshold. Lorazepam (Ativan) has a rapid onset of action (less than 5 minutes) and should be given intravenously; intramuscular absorption is unreliably slow for the treatment of status epilepticus. The dose is 0.1 mg per kg, with a maximal dose of 4 mg and can be given over 1 to 2 minutes. Its anticonvulsant effects can last for several hours. It may be repeated at 5-minute intervals, but its effectiveness decreases with successive doses. The major side effects are

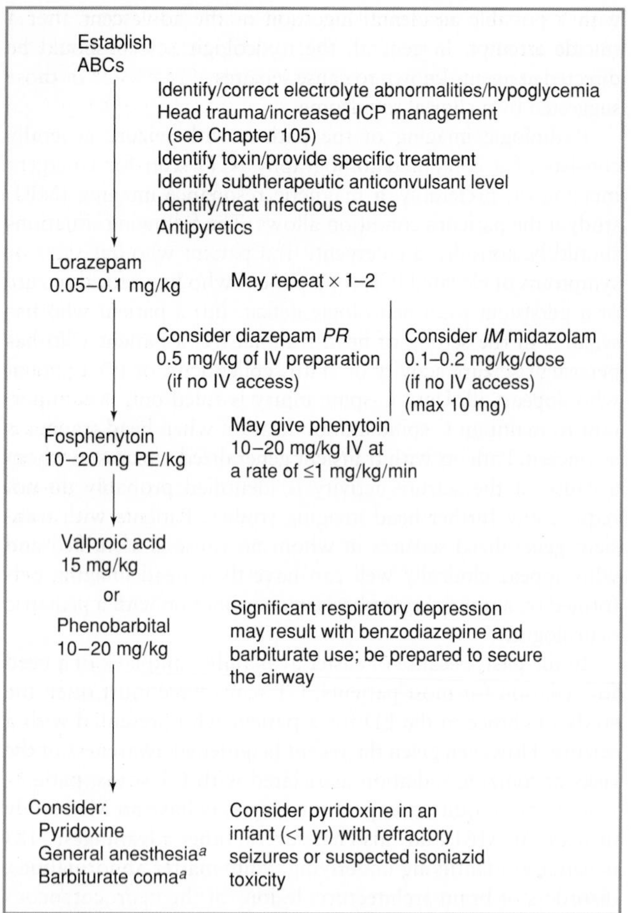

FIGURE 67.2 Management of status epilepticus. [a]Electroencephalogram monitoring and ICU setting required. ABCs, airway, breathing, circulation; ICP, intracranial pressure; PR, per rectum; IV, intravenous; IM, intramuscular; PE, phenytoin equivalent.

respiratory depression and sedation (dose-dependent), especially when combined with phenobarbital.

Diazepam (Valium) had been the standard initial treatment of seizures for many years before the development of the newer benzodiazepines. Diazepam is similar to lorazepam and is given in a dose of 0.2 mg per kg to a maximum of 8 to 10 mg. Diazepam has an advantage in that it can be given rectally, which is useful when a patient does not have IV access. A rectal gel is available in fixed doses of 5, 7.5, 10, 12.5, 15, 17.5, or 20 mg. The IV preparation of the drug may be used alternatively. Recommended rectal dosing for children up to 5 years of age is 0.5 mg per kg.

Midazolam can be given intramuscularly (0.2 mg/kg/dose; not to exceed a cumulative dose of 10 mg) and should be considered if there is delay in IV access. Midazolam has a theoretical advantage in that patients will return to baseline more quickly than with lorazepam or diazepam, thus allowing for better assessment of mental status and the need for CT scan and/or LP.

Phenytoin (Dilantin) is a second-line agent for the treatment of seizures. Phenytoin blocks sodium channels and thus acts by a different mechanism than the benzodiazepines. The dose is 10 to 20 mg per kg as an initial load. It has several limitations as compared with the benzodiazepines. First, peak CNS concentrations may not be reached until 10 to 30 minutes after its infusion is completed and, thus, it is much slower in onset. Furthermore, it must be administered slowly (no faster than 1 mg/kg/min, or 20 minutes for a dose of 20 mg per kg) because of concerns of cardiac conduction disturbances, which further lengthens its onset of action. It cannot be given in dextrose-containing solutions.

As a result of the limitations in the administration of phenytoin, fosphenytoin (Cerebyx) was created. It is a prodrug whose active metabolite is phenytoin. The drug is dosed as phenytoin equivalents (PEs), and the loading dose is 10 to 20 mg PE per kg. The advantages are that it can be given much more rapidly (up to 3 mg PE/kg/min, or 7 minutes for a dose of 20 mg PE per kg) and that it may be given in either normal saline or a 5% dextrose-containing solution or intramuscularly.

Phenobarbital (Luminal) is another second-line agent for the treatment of seizures. The loading dose is 10 to 20 mg per kg. Its advantage over phenytoin is that it can be given more rapidly (2 mg/kg/min, or 10 minutes for a dose of 20 mg per kg). Note that this is slower than fosphenytoin). However, it has an extremely long half-life (up to 120 hours) and a pronounced sedating effect. Furthermore, it can cause significant respiratory depression, especially when given after a benzodiazepine. One must be prepared to intubate a patient who has received both a benzodiazepine and a barbiturate for the treatment of seizures. It is important to remember that if a patient needs to be intubated, a muscle relaxant can mask the motor manifestation of seizure activity. The side effect profile of phenobarbital and the fact that it acts on GABA receptors (similar to the first line of benzodiazepines), make phenobarbital an inferior choice to the fast administered/fast acting fosphenytoin. Therefore, phenobarbital is now considered a third line agent.

Valproic acid (Depakene) is a commonly used antiepileptic agent and the IV preparation had been used in the past to rapidly attain therapeutic levels. Recently, there have been a few case series demonstrating its effectiveness in treating seizures in children who have been refractory to the first-line agents. As such, many now consider it a third-line agent for the treatment of status epilepticus. It is given intravenously at a dose of 15 to 40 mg per kg over 10 minutes. It is generally well tolerated and is less sedating than the barbiturates. IV levetiracetam (Keppra) has also been used for pediatric status, with a loading dose of 20 to 30 mg per kg given over 10 minutes.

Pyridoxine deficiency is an uncommon cause of seizures in newborns. One should consider its use primarily in patients younger than 3 months whose seizure activity is refractory to the other therapies (100 mg). Rarely, pyridoxine-dependent epilepsy may present in older patients, so some guidelines recommend its use in refractory status epilepticus in patients up to 18 months of age. Pyridoxine is also used in the treatment of isoniazid overdose (usual initial dose 70 mg per kg).

If all the described therapies fail, patients may require general anesthesia to abort the seizures. A variety of agents can be used, including inhalational anesthetics (e.g., halothane, isoflurane), large doses of short-acting barbiturates (e.g., pentobarbital 5 to 15 mg per kg load, then 1 mg/kg/hr starting dose), benzodiazepines (e.g., continuous infusion midazolam 0.2 mg per kg load, then 0.05 to 0.2 mg/kg/hr), or continuous infusion propofol (3 to 5 mg per kg load, then 1 to 15 mg/kg/hr).

The patient needs both to be intubated (if not already done) and to have continuous EEG monitoring in an intensive care unit. The level of anesthesia should be titrated to maintain either a flat-line or burst-suppression pattern on the EEG. The anesthesia can be then withdrawn slowly to see if any electrical seizure activity persists.

It is important to note that prior CNS insult or seizure disorder accounts for a high proportion of pediatric status epilepticus cases. Seizure management may be very complex and may involve multiple antiepileptic drugs; therefore, a seizure management plan should be developed as rapidly as possible in consultation with a pediatric neurologist.

SPECIAL CONSIDERATIONS

Febrile Seizures

Febrile seizures are the most common convulsive disorder in young children, occurring in 2% to 5% of the population. Most clinicians define a febrile seizure as a seizure occurring between 6 months and 5 years of age that is associated with a fever (temperature higher than 38°C [100.4°F]), but without the evidence of intracranial infection or other defined cause or neurologic disease. Some clinicians use 7 years as an upper age limit for febrile seizures, following the International League Against Epilepsy from 1993 defining the age cutoff of 1 month to 7 years.

Febrile seizures can be of any type, but most commonly, they are generalized tonic–clonic seizures. They are usually self-limited and last for only a few minutes. Febrile seizures are classified as simple when lasted less than 15 minutes, are generalized, and occur only once during a 24-hour period (two seizures within a time period of <30 minutes will be considered a single episode). In contrast, complex febrile seizures are prolonged, recur within 24 hours, or have focal manifestations. Simple febrile seizures (85%) are much more common. There is a family history of febrile seizures in an immediate family member in 25% to 40% of cases. Viral infections are frequently associated with febrile seizures, and human herpesvirus is a commonly identified agent.

After the first febrile seizure, approximately 33% of patients will have at least one recurrence and about 9% will have three or more episodes. The younger the patient is at first presentation, the greater the likelihood of recurrence. In addition, recurrences are more likely to recur in patients with lower temperatures on presentation of their first seizure (lower than 40°C) and shorter duration of fever before the seizure (less than 24 hours) and in patients with a family history of febrile seizures. Most recurrences (75%) will happen within 1 year. The exact risk of developing epilepsy after a febrile seizure is unknown, but most studies indicate that it is less than 5%. Risk factors for developing epilepsy after a febrile seizure include abnormal development before the episode, a family history of afebrile seizures, and a complex first febrile seizure; without any of these risk factors, the risk of developing epilepsy is approximately 1%, which is almost the same risk as in the general population.

The treatment of a patient who presents with a febrile seizure is nearly identical to that for other seizure types. The primary goal is the establishment of a clear airway; secondary efforts are then directed at the termination of the seizure and concurrent lowering of body temperature. However, because most febrile seizures are brief in duration, the typical patient who presents for the evaluation of a febrile seizure is no longer seizing upon arrival to the ED. In those instances, if the history is consistent with a simple febrile seizure, the patient has no stigmata of a CNS infection, and the patient's neurologic examination is completely normal (the patient may be postictal or slightly hyperreflexive), further evaluation for the cause of the seizure is unnecessary. As such, routine laboratory studies are not recommended for the patient with a simple febrile seizure. While seizure may be the first manifestation of meningitis, LP is only indicated for children in whom meningitis is clinically suspected and it is no longer recommended routinely. Similarly, routine neuroimaging or EEG screening is also not recommended for the patient with a first-time simple febrile seizure. However, the evaluation should focus on the possible cause of the fever. Outpatient EEG is recommended by some clinicians for patients with complex febrile seizure, in whom the risk of epilepsy is slightly higher.

A patient who has had a febrile seizure and is well appearing and back to baseline may be safely discharged to home. Parents should be reassured that febrile seizures are common and that most patients have no further episodes. They need to be cautioned that a recurrence may happen and should be given simple instructions on what to do should another seizure occur and indications for returning for evaluation. They can also be instructed on the proper use of antipyretics, even though studies have failed to demonstrate that this is effective in reducing the recurrence rate. Finally, any identified source of the fever should be properly treated.

Suggested Readings and Key References

Gaillard WD, Chiron C, Cross JH, et al. Guidelines for imaging infants and children with recent-onset epilepsy. *Epilepsia* 2009;50(9):2147–2153.

Hampers LC, Spina LA. Evaluation and management of pediatric febrile seizures in the emergency department. *Emerg Med Clin North Am* 2011;29(1):83–93.

Hirtz D, Ashwal S, Berg A, et al. Practice parameter: evaluating a first nonfebrile seizure in children: report of the quality standards subcommittee of the American Academy of Neurology, The Child Neurology Society, and The American Epilepsy Society. *Neurology* 2000;55(5):616–623.

Lewis DV, Shinnar S, Hesdorffer DC, et al.; FEBSTAT Study Team. Hippocampal sclerosis after febrile status epilepticus: the FEBSTAT study. *Ann Neurol* 2014;75(2):178–185.

Riviello JJ Jr, Ashwal S, Hirtz D, et al. Practice parameter: diagnostic assessment of the child with status epilepticus (an evidence-based review): report of the Quality Standards Subcommittee of the American Academy of Neurology and the Practice Committee of the Child Neurology Society. *Neurology* 2006;67(9):1542–1550.

CHAPTER 68 ■ SEPTIC APPEARING INFANT

STEVEN M. SELBST, MD AND BRENT D. ROGERS, MD

A young infant may be brought to the emergency department (ED) because he or she "just doesn't look right" to the parents. Inexperienced parents, whose first baby is just a few weeks old, will notice when their child is unusually sleepy, fussy, or not drinking well. To the physician in the ED, such an infant may appear quite ill with pallor, cyanosis, or ashen color. There may be notable irritability or lethargy, and fever or hypothermia may be present. The infant may be found to have tachypnea, tachycardia, or both. Hypotension or other signs of poor perfusion may also be apparent.

Generally, an ill-appearing infant will be immediately considered to have sepsis and managed reflexively. Although this is the correct approach in most cases, several other conditions can produce a septic-appearing infant.

This chapter establishes a differential diagnosis for infants in the first 2 months of life who appear ill. An approach to the evaluation and management of such an infant is discussed.

DIFFERENTIAL DIAGNOSIS

Numerous disorders (Table 68.1) may cause an infant to appear septic. The most common of these disorders (Table 68.2) include bacterial and viral infections. The remaining disorders demand diagnostic consideration because although uncommon, they are potentially life-threatening and treatable.

Sepsis

Sepsis should always be considered when the emergency physician is confronted with an ill-appearing infant (see Chapters 1 A General Approach to Ill and Injured Children, 5 Shock, and 102 Infectious Disease Emergencies). The signs and symptoms of sepsis may be subtle. The history may vary, and some infants are ill for several days whereas others deteriorate rapidly. Symptoms such as lethargy, irritability, diarrhea, vomiting, anorexia, or fever may be a manifestation of sepsis. Fever is generally an unreliable finding in the septic infant; many septic infants younger than 2 months will be hypothermic instead. (See Clinical Pathway Chapter 87 Fever in Infants.) On physical examination, a septic infant may be pale, ashen, or cyanotic. The skin is often cool and may be mottled because of poor perfusion. The infant may seem lethargic, obtunded, or irritable. There is often marked tachycardia, with the heart rate approaching 200 beats per minute, and tachypnea may be noted (respiratory rate more than 60 breaths per minute). If disseminated intravascular coagulopathy (DIC) has developed, scattered petechiae or purpura will be evident. A bulging or tense fontanel may be found if meningitis is present. If the infection has localized elsewhere, there may be otitis media, abdominal rigidity, joint swelling, tenderness in one extremity, or chest findings such as rales. Soft tissue infections from MRSA are becoming a more common cause of sepsis. Always examine the neonate for signs of omphalitis, an ascending infection originating in the umbilicus. Finally, if the disease process has progressed, the infant may develop shock and be hypotensive.

The laboratory is often helpful in suggesting a diagnosis of sepsis; however, definitive cultures require time for processing. Potential abnormal laboratory studies include a complete blood count (CBC) with a leukocytosis or leukopenia with left shift, a coagulation profile with evidence of DIC, and blood chemistries with hypoglycemia or metabolic acidosis. If localized infection is suspected, aspiration and Gram stain of urine, joint fluid, spinal fluid, or pus from the middle ear may reveal the offending organism. Similarly, a chest radiograph may show a lobar infiltrate if pneumonia is present. A Gram stain of a petechial scraping may also reveal the responsible organism.

Other Infectious Diseases

Overwhelming viral infections may cause a septic appearance, or systemic inflammatory response syndrome (SIRS) in the young infant (see Chapter 5 Shock). Approximately 25% of infants younger than 1 month with *enteroviral infections* develop a sepsis-like illness with high mortality. Respiratory distress and hemorrhagic manifestations, including gastrointestinal bleeding and bleeding into the skin, are commonly seen. Seizures, icterus, splenomegaly, congestive heart failure, and abdominal distention often occur. This infection is indistinguishable from bacterial sepsis, except that bacterial cultures are negative. Viral isolates from stool and cerebrospinal fluid (CSF) or enterovirus polymerase chain reaction (PCR) of the CSF may confirm the offending enterovirus.

Epidemics of *respiratory syncytial virus* (RSV) occur in the wintertime, and babies younger than 2 months may present with respiratory distress, cyanosis, or apnea. Those born prematurely or with previous respiratory or cardiac disorders are especially susceptible to apnea. Knowledge of illness in the community and a predominance of wheezing on chest examination may lead to the suspicion of RSV bronchiolitis. Still, some infants develop wheezing later in the course and, thus, the initial diagnosis in these septic-appearing infants is difficult. A rapid nasal wash test for RSV, if available, will be quickly diagnostic. Culture for RSV requires several days. A CBC may show a lymphocytosis, but because of stress, a left shift can also be found. Chest radiographs may show diffuse patchy infiltrates or lobar atelectasis (see Clinical Pathway Chapter 85 Bronchiolitis).

Another viral infection to consider is *herpes simplex*, which usually causes systemic symptoms and encephalitis at 7 to 21 days of life. Neonates present with fever, coma, apnea, fulminant hepatitis, pneumonitis, coagulopathy, and difficult to control seizures. History of maternal genital herpes should lead to suspicion of systemic herpes infection in the neonate, though in most cases the mother is completely asymptomatic. Focal neurologic signs and ocular findings, such as

TABLE 68.1

DIFFERENTIAL DIAGNOSIS OF THE SEPTIC-APPEARING INFANT

Infectious diseases
Bacterial sepsis[a]
Meningitis[a]
Urinary tract infection[a]
Viral infections—enterovirus, respiratory syncytial virus, herpes simplex[a]
Pertussis
Congenital syphilis
Omphalitis
Cardiac disease
Congenital heart disease[a]
Supraventricular tachycardia[a]
Myocardial infarction (most commonly aberrant left coronary artery)
Pericarditis
Myocarditis
Kawasaki disease
Endocrine disorders
Congenital adrenal hyperplasia
Metabolic disorders
Hyponatremia, hypernatremia[a]
Cystic fibrosis
Inborn errors of metabolism, galactosemia
Hypoglycemia[a]
Drugs/toxins—aspirin, carbon monoxide
Renal disorders
Posterior urethral valves
Hematologic disorders
Severe anemia[a]
Methemoglobinemia
Kernicterus
Gastrointestinal disorders
Gastroenteritis with dehydration[a]
Pyloric stenosis[a]
Intussusception
Necrotizing enterocolitis
Appendicitis
Volvulus
Incarcerated hernia[a]
Neurologic disease
Infant botulism
Shunt obstruction, infection[a]
Child abuse—intracranial hemorrhage[a]

[a]Indicates more common causes.

TABLE 68.2

MOST COMMON DISORDERS THAT MIMIC SEPSIS

Urinary tract infection	Congestive heart failure
Viremia	Gastroenteritis with dehydration

conjunctivitis or keratitis, may be noted. Strongly consider this infection if vesicular lesions are present on the skin, but they are present in only one-third to one-half of patients. Rapid diagnostic studies available include antigen detection tests and enzyme-linked immunosorbent assay (ELISA) antibody tests. The Tzanck preparation has low sensitivity and is not recommended as a rapid diagnostic test. Direct fluorescent antibody staining of vesicle scrapings is specific but less sensitive than culture. PCR is a sensitive method to detect the virus from CSF in infants suspected of herpes encephalitis and an electroencephalogram (EEG) or computed tomography (CT) scan may also be helpful to reveal abnormalities of the temporal lobe. The diagnosis is confirmed by culture of a skin vesicle, mouth, nasopharynx, eyes, urine, blood, CSF, stool, or rectum (see Clinical Pathway Chapter 87 Fever in Infants).

Pertussis is another infection to consider when evaluating a very ill infant. Apnea, seizures, and death have been reported in this age group. Parents may report respiratory distress, cough, poor feeding, and vomiting (often posttussive). History of exposure to pertussis may be lacking because the infant usually acquires the disease from older children or adults who have only symptoms of a common upper respiratory infection. Physical examination will distinguish the infection from sepsis if the infant has a paroxysmal cough. The characteristic inspiratory "whoop" after a coughing paroxysm (a hallmark in older patients) is uncommon in very young infants. Auscultation of the chest is usually normal; tachypnea and cyanosis may be present. Initial laboratory studies, abnormal in older children, may not be aberrant in young children with the condition. For instance, the classic CBC with a marked lymphocytosis is often absent in infants with pertussis and a chest radiograph may not show the typical "shaggy right heart border." Atelectasis or pneumonia may be present. PCR technique can reliably identify the condition from nasopharyngeal specimens and nasopharyngeal culture for *Bordetella pertussis* is confirmatory.

Infants with *congenital syphilis* may present in the first 4 weeks of life with extreme irritability, pallor, jaundice, hepatosplenomegaly, and edema. They may have pneumonia and often have painful limbs. Snuffles and skin lesions are common. Although these infants may appear ill on arrival in the ED, their histories reveal that they also have been chronically ill. Certainly consider the diagnosis if a history of maternal infection is obtained. Laboratory studies will be helpful in that radiographs of the infant's long bones may reveal diffuse periostitis of several bones, but a serologic test is needed to confirm the diagnosis.

Cardiac Diseases (See Chapter 94 Cardiac Emergencies)

In addition to infections, consider cardiac disease with a very ill infant. An infant with underlying *congenital heart disease* (CHD), such as ventriculoseptal defect, valvular insufficiency, valvular stenosis, hypoplastic left heart syndrome (HLHS), or coarctation of the aorta, may present with shock or congestive heart failure and clinical findings similar to those of an infant with sepsis. There may be tachycardia and tachypnea, as well as pallor, duskiness, or mottling of the skin. Cyanosis is not always present. There may also be sweating, decreased pulses, and hypotension caused by poor perfusion. A careful history and physical examination helps differentiate CHD with heart failure from sepsis. For instance, a chronic history of poor growth and poor feeding may suggest heart disease. The presence of a cardiac murmur may suggest a structural lesion, and a gallop rhythm, hepatomegaly, neck vein distention, and peripheral edema may lead one to consider primary cardiac pathology. Intercostal retractions and rales, rhonchi, or wheezing are nonspecific findings and may be present on chest examination in either heart failure or pneumonia. An infant with HLHS or coarctation of the aorta may present with shock toward the end of the first or second week of life as the patent ductus arteriosus (PDA) closes. A difference between upper- and lower-extremity blood pressures in a young baby suggests coarctation of the aorta, though pulse differences may not be detected if cardiac output is inadequate. Normal femoral pulses do not exclude a coarctation because the widened PDA provides flow to the descending aorta. Check the dorsalis pedis or tibialis posterior pulses; these are more sensitive for detecting coarctation or low cardiac output.

Further evaluation is essential in establishing cardiac disease as the cause of an infant's moribund condition. A chest radiograph often shows cardiac enlargement and may show pulmonary vascular engorgement or interstitial pulmonary edema rather than lobar infiltrates (as in pneumonia). The electrocardiogram (ECG) may reveal certain congenital heart lesions such as right-axis deviation with right atrial and ventricular enlargement in HLHS. The ECG may be nonspecific and an echocardiogram is usually required to define anatomy and confirm specific diagnoses. Finally, a CBC may be helpful in that the absence of leukocytosis and left shift may make sepsis a less likely consideration.

Rarely, an infant with anomalous or obstructed coronary arteries will develop myocardial infarction and appear septic initially. Such young infants may have colicky behavior, dyspnea, cyanosis, vomiting, pallor, and other signs of heart failure. However, these infants usually have cardiomegaly on chest radiograph. The ECG usually shows T-wave inversion and deep Q waves in leads I and AVL. Echocardiogram or cardiac catheterization is needed to confirm the diagnosis.

In addition to CHD, certain *arrhythmias* may cause an infant to appear ill. A young baby with *supraventricular tachycardia* (SVT) often presents with findings similar to those of a septic infant. This arrhythmia may be idiopathic (50%), associated with CHD (20%), or related to drugs, fever, or infection (20%). Young infants with SVT often go unrecognized at home for 2 days or more because they initially have only poor feeding, fussiness, and some rapid breathing. The infants will develop congestive heart failure as the condition goes untreated and may present with all the signs of sepsis, including shock. Fever can precipitate the arrhythmia, confusing the condition with sepsis, though a careful physical examination will make the diagnosis of SVT obvious. Particularly, the cardiac examination will reveal such extreme tachycardia in the infant that the heart rate cannot be counted, often exceeding 250 to 300 beats per minute. An ECG will show regular atrial and ventricular beats with 1:1 conduction, although P waves appear different than sinus P waves and may be difficult to see as they are often buried in the T waves. A chest radiograph may show cardiomegaly and pulmonary congestion.

Additional cardiac pathologies to consider include *pericarditis* and *myocarditis*. Pericarditis may be caused by bacterial organisms such as *Staphylococcus aureus;* myocarditis usually results from viral infections such as coxsackievirus B. These often are fulminant infections in infants and the baby will appear critically ill with fever and grunting respirations. A complete physical examination may help the physician distinguish these conditions from sepsis if signs of heart failure or unexplained tachycardia are present. Pericarditis may produce neck vein distention, distant heart sounds, and a friction rub if a significant pericardial effusion exists. Physical findings with myocarditis may include muffled heart sounds (because of ventricular dilatation), gallop, hepatosplenomegaly, and weak distal pulses with poor perfusion. A chest radiograph in a patient with pericarditis will show cardiomegaly and a suggestion of effusion. The ECG will show generalized T-wave inversion and low-voltage QRS complexes if pericardial fluid is present, and ST-T-wave abnormalities may be seen. The echocardiogram will confirm the presence or absence of a pericardial effusion and poor ventricular function in the case of viral myocarditis. The CBC will not distinguish these infections from sepsis because leukocytosis is common and a left shift may be present.

Kawasaki disease with associated coronary artery aneurysms is very rare in young infants and may present with cyanosis and shock. Usually, history reveals prolonged and unexplained fever, rash, and mucous membrane inflammation. The physical examination may distinguish this illness from sepsis if there is a diffuse, raised, erythematous rash or cracked red lips, swollen hands and feet, conjunctivitis, and cervical lymphadenopathy. Neonates with Kawasaki disease often have an atypical presentation and these classic features found in older infants and children may be absent in young babies. Routine laboratory studies may not differentiate this condition from sepsis either. A CBC may reveal leukocytosis and/or thrombocytosis. CSF usually shows a pleocytosis, with a lymphocytic predominance. Sterile pyuria is sometimes noted. In some cases of Kawasaki disease, findings consistent with myocardial ischemia or an arrhythmia may be noted on ECG. Normal findings or nonspecific abnormalities are more common. Coronary artery aneurysms may be discovered with an echocardiogram, making the diagnosis highly likely.

Endocrine Disorders (See Chapter 97 Endocrine Emergencies)

Certain endocrine disorders can also mimic sepsis. Infants with *congenital adrenal hyperplasia* (CAH) usually present in the first few weeks of life with a history of vomiting, lethargy, or irritability. Signs of marked dehydration may be present with tachycardia and possibly hypothermia. The recent history may be revealing in that such infants may have been poor feeders since birth and the symptoms may be progressive over a few days. The physical examination can be helpful in establishing the diagnosis in females if ambiguous genitalia are noted. The presence of marked hyponatremia with severe hyperkalemia on laboratory evaluation makes CAH a likely diagnosis. Other findings in this disorder include hypoglycemia, metabolic acidosis, and peaked T waves or arrhythmias on ECG. Elevated 17-hydroxyprogesterone and rennin, with decreased aldosterone and cortisol in the serum, confirm the diagnosis of CAH. Initiate treatment with hydrocortisone 100 mg per m^2 (or 2 mg per kg) intravenously as soon as the diagnosis is suspected. Hyperkalemia may result in sudden cardiac arrest; rapidly initiate protective measures with calcium, glucose, and insulin, and enhance elimination with kayexalate.

Metabolic Disorders

Various metabolic disorders can also present like sepsis. Prolonged diarrhea or vomiting can produce *hypoglycemia, dehydration, electrolyte disturbances,* and *acid–base abnormalities* such that an infant will appear quite ill. Young infants with diarrhea may develop marked hyponatremia caused by sodium losses or iatrogenic water intoxication. The latter occurs when well-meaning parents give excess free water to a young infant or improperly mix concentrated formula, leading to a rapid drop in serum sodium. Such infants may appear extremely lethargic, with slow respirations, hypothermia, and, possibly, seizures that are difficult to control. Likewise, dehydrated infants with *hypernatremia* may be lethargic or irritable, with muscle weakness, seizures, or coma. Infants with persistent vomiting may have hypochloremic alkalosis with hypokalemia, and may appear weak or have cardiac dysfunction (see Chapters 17 Dehydration and 108 Renal and Electrolyte Emergencies and Clinical Pathway Chapter 86 Dehydration).

A special cause of hyponatremic dehydration to consider is *cystic fibrosis* (see Chapter 107 Pulmonary Emergencies). The history in these cases may not be helpful initially, with vague symptoms including poor intake, poor growth, and increased lethargy. However, the parents may report that the infant usually gets very ill in hot weather and that the baby's skin tastes salty. The baby may have also had meconium plug syndrome (transient form of distal colonic obstruction secondary to inspissated meconium) or prolonged jaundice as a newborn. Pulmonary symptoms such as cough, tachypnea, or pneumonia may have been treated earlier in life. On examination, the dehydrated baby looks much like any other septic infant. However, laboratory tests showing profound hyponatremia that is not accounted for by gastrointestinal losses, suggest cystic fibrosis. A sweat test or DNA analysis will help confirm the diagnosis.

Rare inborn errors of metabolism, such as *inherited urea cycle disorders,* may produce vomiting in young infants, who will then present with lethargy, seizures, or coma resulting from metabolic acidosis, hyperammonemia, or hypoglycemia (see Chapter 103 Metabolic Emergencies). Galactosemia is due to a genetic defect in the metabolism of galactose and can cause a young infant to appear septic. Neonates with this enzyme deficiency present with vomiting, acidosis, failure to thrive, and jaundice when exposed to galactose. Some may have hypoglycemia and many will have liver dysfunction with a significant coagulopathy. Many develop urinary tract infections or sepsis due to gram-negative organisms. When considering metabolic conditions, it is essential to evaluate the CBC, electrolytes, bicarbonate, blood glucose, liver function (including coagulation studies), and plasma ammonia levels in young infants with significant symptoms of gastroenteritis, lethargy, or irritability. A urinalysis including ketones is also helpful. Collect extra plasma (2 mL) and urine (5 mL) for additional testing. Inquiry about neonatal screening is important; consider sending a follow-up blood filter paper specimen to the newborn screening laboratory. A rapid bedside test for blood sugar level is recommended for immediate recognition of hypoglycemia. *Hypoglycemia* also can be secondary to sepsis, certain drugs, or alcohol intoxication.

Another metabolic problem to consider is that of *toxins* (see Chapter 110 Toxicologic Emergencies). Young infants are incapable of accidental ingestions, but well-meaning parents may rarely cause salicylism in their attempts to aggressively treat fever with aspirin (despite current Reye syndrome warnings). Affected infants can then present with vomiting, hyperpnea, hyperpyrexia, convulsions, or coma. The history of medication given is crucial because the physical examination will not distinguish this ill baby from the infant with sepsis. The laboratory evaluation may lead to the suspicion of a metabolic problem because abnormalities of sodium, blood sugar, or acid–base balance are often found. Moreover, hypokalemia can be seen in salicylism, as well as abnormal liver function or renal function studies. An elevated salicylate level in the serum confirms the diagnosis of aspirin poisoning, but in chronic poisoning, the aspirin level may be relatively low despite a fatal course.

Carbon monoxide poisoning may present as an unknown intoxication when families are unaware of a defective heating system in the home. The young baby may have a history of sluggishness, poor feeding, and vomiting. A more careful history generally reveals that other family members are also ill with headache, syncope, or flu-like symptoms that improve after leaving the home environment. The classic "cherry red" skin color may be lacking, and physical examination may reveal only lethargy. Elevation of the carboxyhemoglobin level is diagnostic.

Renal Disorders (See Chapter 108 Renal and Electrolyte Emergencies)

A young infant may also appear extremely ill because of renal failure or dysplasia. Posterior urethral valves, especially in males, can cause bladder outlet obstruction resulting in renal failure. Approximately one-third of these cases is diagnosed by 1 week of age, but more than half go undetected for the first few months of life. The parents may give a history of vomiting, poor appetite, inadequate weight gain, or an abdomen that appears swollen. On physical examination, hypertension or an abdominal mass (hydronephrosis) may be detected, as well as urinary ascites. Laboratory tests will elucidate the diagnosis of posterior urethral valves even further, as suprapubic ultrasound may demonstrate the dilated posterior urethra and bladder. A voiding cystourethrogram will show a dilated posterior urethra, hypertrophy of the bladder neck, and trabeculated bladder. The serum creatinine and blood urea nitrogen levels may be markedly elevated. Urosepsis is a possible complication of posterior urethral valves.

Hematologic Disorders

It is important to consider hematologic disorders when confronted with a critically ill infant. Any infant with severe *anemia* caused by aplastic disease, hemolytic process, or blood loss can look quite ill (see Chapter 101 Hematologic Emergencies). Disorders of hemoglobin such as *methemoglobinemia* can also cause an infant to appear toxic. Although the chronic forms are uncommon inherited disorders of hemoglobin structure or enzyme deficiency, transient methemoglobinemia in infants is occasionally caused by environmental toxicity from oxidizing agents such as nitrates found in some specimens of well water or oxidant drugs (e.g., topical benzocaine in teething gels). This intoxication presents in very young infants with cyanosis, poor feeding, failure to thrive, vomiting, diarrhea, and lethargy. In other patients, the oxidant stress is less obvious, causing gastroenteritis and metabolic acidosis. Infants may present with severe diarrhea and metabolic acidosis. It is postulated that the infectious agent that causes the diarrhea or the secondary metabolic acidosis may produce an oxidant stress that leads to methemoglobin formation. On examination, these infants are lethargic, with hypothermia, tachycardia, tachypnea, and hypotension. They often appear mottled, cyanotic, or ashen. One key to the diagnosis of methemoglobinemia is that oxygen administration does not affect the cyanosis, although this may also occur with CHD with right-to-left shunt. Also, laboratory tests show a profound acidosis (pH 6.9 to 7.2), yet the Pa_{O_2} is normal despite the cyanosis. Leukocytosis and thrombocytosis are present, and prerenal azotemia may be noted. The blood itself may appear chocolate brown (most easily noted when a drop of blood on filter paper is waved in the air and compared with a normal control), and methemoglobin levels will be elevated up to 65% (normal 0% to 2%). Hemoglobin electrophoresis will be normal (except in rare cases of hemoglobin M), as is the glucose-6-phosphate dehydrogenase assay in most cases. With appropriate treatment, the methemoglobin level returns to normal. However, death can occur from methemoglobinemia in infants if not treated promptly.

When an infant presents to the ED appearing septic and with neurologic findings, consider *kernicterus,* or bilirubin encephalopathy (see Chapter 104 Neonatal Emergencies). This usually occurs in the first week of life in neonates with high levels of jaundice and the symptoms are due to the deposition of indirect bilirubin in the basal ganglia and brainstem nuclei. Premature infants are more susceptible to kernicterus, but the majority of infants who suffer are healthy, term infants who predominantly breast-feed. The clinical presentation early in the course is difficult to differentiate from sepsis, with lethargy and decreased feeding. As the illness progresses, the infant will develop respiratory distress and many neurologic signs, including decreased reflexes, a high-pitched cry, arching, opisthotonic posturing, twitching of the extremities, and convulsions. The neonate can even develop a bulging fontanel, making it difficult to differentiate from meningitis on clinical examination. Laboratory evaluation is crucial; obtain total and direct bilirubin counts, a CBC, blood typing, and Coombs. Kernicterus usually does not develop until the total bilirubin level has exceeded 25 to 30 mg per dL, but toxicity has occurred at levels as low as 20 mg per dL. Prompt phototherapy is indicated and most babies will require a double volume exchange transfusion to reduce bilirubin in the blood.

Gastrointestinal Disorders (See Chapter 99 Gastrointestinal Emergencies)

Gastrointestinal disorders can cause an infant to appear acutely ill. *Gastroenteritis,* even without electrolyte disturbances, can lead to profound dehydration. In a very young infant with little reserve, this can quickly result in lethargy and shock. Hypoglycemia is also common in young infants and can cause lethargy and coma. Bacterial infections such as *Salmonella* may cause sepsis in a young infant, and viral agents may mimic this. A history of bloody diarrhea suggests bacterial gastroenteritis. Stool cultures will diagnose infections, but a few days are needed for bacterial isolation and viral isolation takes even longer. A stool smear with polymorphonuclear leukocytes may indicate a bacterial infection and a CBC with many band forms despite a white blood cell (WBC) count in the normal range suggests *Shigella.* Fluid resuscitation may improve the infant's appearance and make dehydration the likely diagnosis. Regardless of laboratory studies and initial therapy, sepsis often cannot be ruled out in the ED.

There are several intra-abdominal surgical emergencies that mimic sepsis. The underlying pathophysiology is some combination of hypovolemia, electrolyte disturbances, hypoglycemia, and/or metabolic acidosis. Small bowel obstruction caused by *volvulus, intussusception,* or *incarcerated hernia* will generally present with bilious emesis and there may be bloody stools if there has been significant intestinal ischemia. Patients with intussusception may have a palpable mass. Abdominal distention may be present. Fluid requirements are significantly increased because of bowel wall edema. Plain films and contrast studies may be required to make a definitive diagnosis.

Pyloric stenosis causes severe vomiting in the young infant. This is most often seen in male infants 3 to 6 weeks old. An infant with pyloric stenosis may present to the ED afebrile, with significant dehydration and lethargy. A careful history reveals that increasingly projectile, nonbilious vomiting is the predominant feature of the illness, and there may be a positive family history for pyloric stenosis. The physical examination reveals the classic abdominal mass, or "olive," in less than half of the cases. Rarely, a peristaltic wave can be noted to pass over the epigastric area. Electrolytes typically show hypochloremia, hypokalemia, and alkalosis. Ultrasound of the upper gastrointestinal tract is used to confirm the diagnosis.

Several other unusual but important gastrointestinal disorders have to be considered in infants. *Necrotizing enterocolitis* (NEC) most often occurs in premature infants in the first few weeks of life, but can also occur in term infants, usually within the first 10 days of life. A history of an anoxic episode at birth or other neonatal stresses may suggest NEC. These infants are quite ill, with lethargy, irritability, anorexia, distended abdomen, and bloody stools. Radiographs of the abdomen may show pneumatosis cystoides intestinalis caused by gas in the intestinal wall. Neonatal *appendicitis* is another rare event, but several cases have been reported to closely mimic sepsis. The mortality for this disorder is close to 80%, and perforation worsens the prognosis. Rapid diagnosis is essential. The most common presenting signs include irritability, vomiting, and abdominal distention on examination. There may also be hypothermia, ashen color, and shock as the condition progresses, as well as edema of the right flank abdominal wall and possible erythema of the skin in that area. The WBC count may be elevated, with a left shift, and there may be a metabolic acidosis as well as DIC. Abdominal radiographs may show a paucity of gas in the right lower quadrant, evidence of free peritoneal fluid, or a right abdominal wall thickened by edema. Finally, consider rare diagnoses such as perforation caused by *trauma* from enemas or thermometers, and *Hirschsprung enterocolitis.*

Neurologic Diseases

Consider neurologic problems in the evaluation of a critically ill infant. An unusual process that produces a sepsis-like picture is *infant botulism* (see Chapter 102 Infectious Disease Emergencies). The symptoms of this illness are caused by neurotoxins elaborated by *Clostridium botulinum.* An infant with botulism often presents to the ED lethargic, with a weak cry, and possibly dehydrated. These infants are usually afebrile. A thorough history may help distinguish botulism from sepsis. The parents may note a more gradual progression with this illness that is preceded by constipation. The disease is associated with the ingestion of honey, breast-feeding, a recent change in feeding practices, a rural environment, and/or nearby construction. On physical examination, infants with botulism are notably hypotonic and hyporeflexic and may have increased secretions caused by bulbar muscle weakness. Infants with botulism differ from those with sepsis because they are generally well perfused with normal cardiovascular parameters. Also, the presence of a facial droop, ophthalmoplegia, and decreased gag reflex are consistent with botulism, whereas they remain unusual findings with a septic infant. The diagnosis of infant botulism is usually made by clinical findings; however, laboratory evaluation (normal WBC and negative cultures) helps rule out bacterial illness. A stool specimen that identifies toxins of *C. botulinum* is diagnostic, but requires considerable time for identification. Electromyography will show decreased muscle action potential with the "staircase" phenomenon in this disease, but this is rarely performed.

A young baby with a ventriculoperitoneal shunt in place because of hydrocephalus can develop serious complications that cause the baby to appear extremely ill (see Chapter 105 Neurologic Emergencies). *Shunt infection* could present with fever and irritability in a young infant. Abdominal pain or tenderness may be found on examination, as well as erythema or pus around the shunt itself. The definitive diagnosis is made by shunt aspiration under sterile conditions after ruling out other causes of fever such as meningitis. *Shunt obstruction* may result in increased intracranial pressure that causes a young infant to present with lethargy or poor feeding. On examination, the baby may have bradycardia, apnea, coma, opisthotonic posturing, bulging fontanel, or cranial nerve VI palsy. The shunt may be found to pump poorly. Radiographic evaluation of the shunt (shunt series) may be helpful if it shows a disconnection. Otherwise, a CT scan or MRI will demonstrate ventricle size and indicate the adequacy of shunt function.

Child Abuse

Intracranial hemorrhage that results from child abuse (see Chapter 95 Child Abuse/Assault) must be considered in the very ill infant. The absence of bruises on an infant does not rule out child abuse. Vigorous shaking of an infant or throwing the baby against a soft surface such as a mattress or sofa can produce subdural or subarachnoid hemorrhages. The history may or may not be helpful in establishing a diagnosis. A report that the infant was well and is now suddenly in critical condition raises suspicion of abuse. The parents may note that the child had respiratory distress at home; only a few admit to shaking the infant. On examination, the infant may appear gravely ill with apnea, bradycardia, hypothermia, bradypnea, or seizures. However, a careful physical examination suggests abuse rather than sepsis. Bruises may be present on the body, though more often, no external evidence of trauma is present. Consider that respiratory distress without stridor or lower airway sounds may be due to central nervous system dysfunction. The head circumference is often at or above the 90th percentile, and the fontanel may be full or bulging. Retinal hemorrhages are often found and strongly suggest intracranial hemorrhage from trauma. Some neurologic signs may be confused with meningitis, such as nuchal rigidity, irritability, coma, seizures, or posturing. The laboratory is helpful in confirming suspicions of intracranial bleeding. Although the CBC often shows a leukocytosis and thus is confusing, the spinal fluid from a shaken baby is usually bloody and fails to clear as the fluid is collected. A noncontrast CT scan or magnetic resonance imaging (MRI) usually demonstrates a small posterior, interhemispheric subdural hematoma. Such shaken babies have a high incidence of serious morbidity and mortality.

EVALUATION AND DECISION

Presume that any infant who is critically ill in the first few weeks of life may be septic. It is imperative to stabilize the baby rapidly (Fig. 68.1) because this life-threatening situation may respond to early treatment. Restore airway, breathing, and circulation and obtain vascular access. Unless another diagnosis is immediately obvious, it is best to give intravenous antibiotics while pursuing alternative diagnoses. If time permits, send cultures to the laboratory before giving antibiotics. Consider use of prostaglandins if cardiogenic shock after PDA closure is suspected.

Obtain a complete history including any previous medical problems such as known heart disease or failure to thrive. Determine the time of onset of symptoms, exposure to infection, medications given at home, and specific symptoms noted by the parents. Next, perform a careful physical examination because specific findings may lead to a diagnosis other than sepsis (Table 68.3). Follow with laboratory evaluation as indicated by findings on history and physical examination. Promptly obtain a rapid test for blood sugar as hypoglycemia may be life-threatening. For all sick infants obtain a blood culture and a urine culture, by a urethral catheter or suprapubic bladder tap. Perform a lumbar puncture unless physical findings point strongly to a diagnosis other than sepsis or the infant is too critically ill to tolerate the procedure. Bruising or bleeding with intravenous access attempts suggests the possibility of DIC and is a contraindication for lumbar puncture. A chest radiograph is also essential to look for pulmonary infection and to evaluate the heart size. Obtain a CBC as leukocytosis will add support to a suspicion of sepsis and also may be found in various other disorders including viral infections, myocarditis, pericarditis, intracranial bleeds, NEC, appendicitis, intussusception, and methemoglobinemia. For all sick infants, send studies to evaluate serum sodium, potassium, chloride, glucose, and bicarbonate level, as metabolic problems (disturbances in acid–base balance, electrolytes, blood sugar) can result from sepsis or be the primary problem that mimics sepsis. If hyponatremia is found, consider water intoxication, aspirin toxicity, cystic fibrosis, and CAH. If there is also a marked hyperkalemia, CAH is most likely. If there is hypochloremic alkalosis or alkalosis alone, then consider pyloric stenosis, aspirin toxicity, or gastroenteritis. Hypoglycemia may be secondary to poor glucose reserves in an ill infant or related to drug (aspirin) toxicity, inborn errors of metabolism, CAH, or methemoglobinemia. Confirm a low serum bicarbonate level with an arterial blood gas. The presence of acidosis could be due to poor perfusion caused by shock, as well as primary problems such as dehydration, drug toxicity, methemoglobinemia, appendicitis, CAH, and inborn errors of metabolism. If laboratory tests are not revealing for a specific disorder or the patient does not improve quickly as an inpatient receiving antibiotics, consider stool and CSF isolates for viruses.

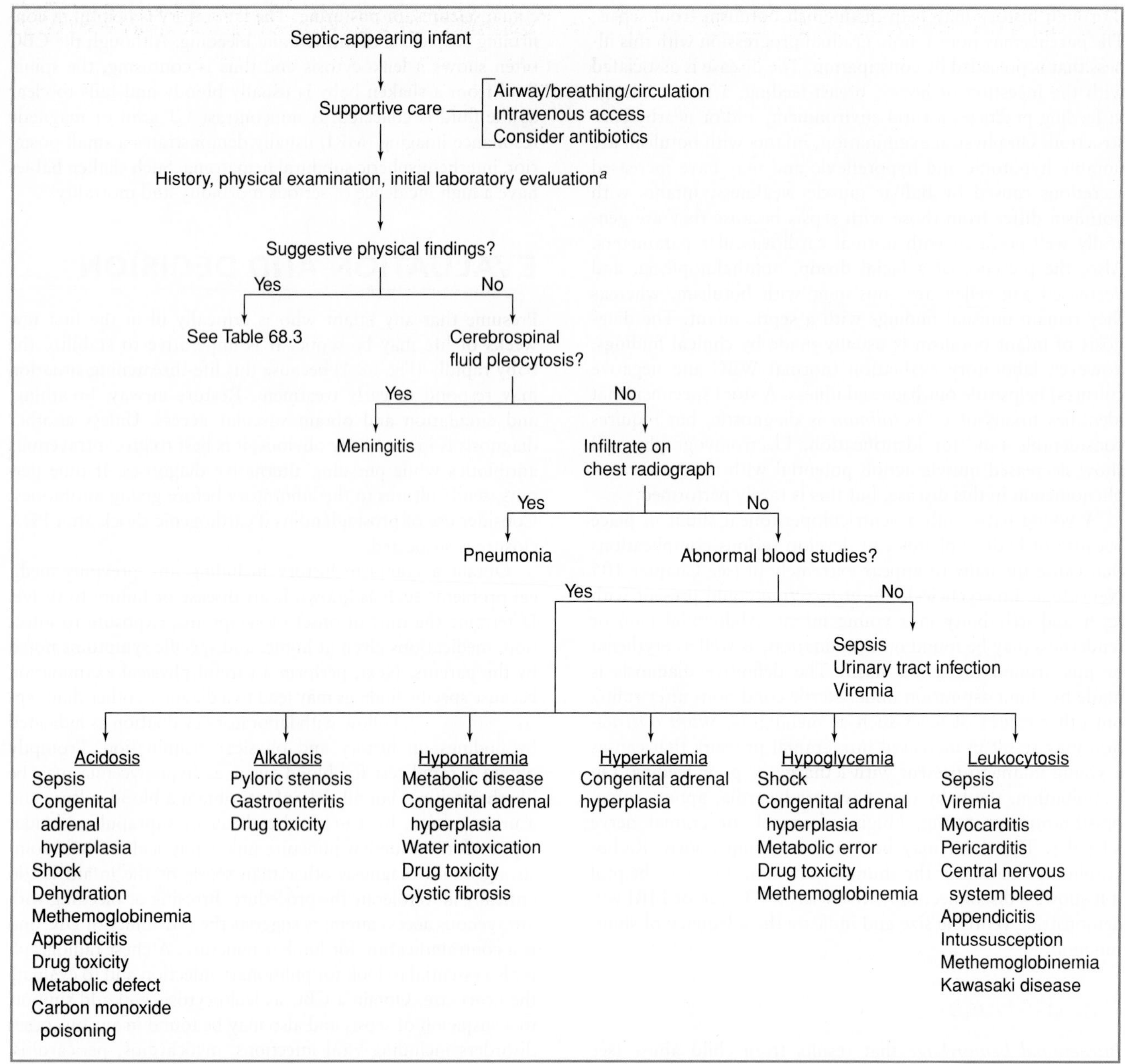

FIGURE 68.1 Initial approach to the septic-appearing child. [a]Initial laboratory evaluation: culture of blood, urine, usually cerebrospinal fluid, chest radiograph, complete blood cell count, urinalysis, electrolytes, glucose, bicarbonate, and may be arterial blood gas.

If the physical examination suggests a specific problem, it may be necessary to obtain additional tests (Table 68.3). An examination that reveals pallor, cyanosis, or cardiac abnormality (muffled heart sounds, murmur, unexplained tachycardia, or arrhythmia) raises concern for various cardiac disorders or methemoglobinemia. An ECG, arterial blood to measure Pa_{O_2}, and possibly an echocardiogram should then be obtained. Unusual neurologic findings, such as a bulging fontanel, warrant a lumbar puncture and previously mentioned blood studies to rule out meningitis. The presence of seizures should prompt a CT scan, EEG, and culture and treatment of herpes simplex. Retinal hemorrhages may suggest an intracranial bleed and, thus, a noncontrast CT scan, MRI, and lumbar puncture would be valuable studies. Likewise, abdominal distention, rigidity, mass, or bloody stools indicate a gastrointestinal emergency. In such cases, abdominal radiographs, ultrasound, or air-contrast studies are important diagnostic aids in addition to a sepsis workup.

If the physical examination reveals bruises or purpura, consider further evaluation for child abuse, coagulopathy, and sepsis. Long bone radiographs, coagulation profile (including platelet count), and Gram stain of the purpura may also be desirable. If vesicular lesions are seen on the skin, obtain a PCR and culture for herpes. If ambiguous genitalia are noted, send blood for 17-hydroxyprogesterone, renin, aldosterone, and cortisol levels to rule out CAH (see Chapter 97 Endocrine Emergencies). Finally, if wheezing is detected on chest examination, consider sending a nasopharyngeal swab for rapid detection of RSV or for the culture of RSV, and a chest radiograph.

TABLE 68.3

APPROACH TO THE SEPTIC-APPEARING INFANT WITH CHARACTERISTIC PHYSICAL FINDINGS

Physical findings	Diagnoses to consider	Specific tests
Cardiovascular abnormalities	Congenital heart disease	Echocardiogram, ECG
	Kawasaki disease	ECG, erythrocyte sedimentation rate
	Supraventricular tachycardia	ECG
	Myocarditis	Echocardiogram, ECG
	Myocardial infarction	ECG
	Methemoglobinemia	Pao_2 methemoglobin level
Neurologic abnormalities	Meningitis	Lumbar puncture
	Infant botulism	Stool for culture, ± electromyogram
	Child abuse	Long bone films, CT scan, or MRI
	Shunt malfunction	Shunt series, CT scan, or MRI
Skin abnormalities	Child abuse	Long bone films, CT scan, or MRI
	Coagulopathy	Coagulation profile
	Herpes simplex	PCR, electroencephalogram, CT scan, or MRI
Genitalia abnormalities	Congenital adrenal hyperplasia	Blood for 17-hydroxyprogesterone, renin, aldosterone, cortisol
Pulmonary abnormalities	Pertussis	PCR
	Pneumonia	Chest radiograph
	Bronchiolitis	Respiratory syncytial virus tests
	Metabolic acidosis	Arterial blood gas
Renal abnormalities (abdominal mass)	Posterior urethral valves	Abdominal, renal ultrasound, voiding cystourethrogram Blood urea nitrogen, creatinine

CT and MRI refer to intracranial imaging in this table.
ECG, electrocardiogram; CT, computed tomography; MRI, magnetic resonance imaging; PCR, polymerase chain reaction.

Suggested Readings and Key References

Sepsis

Brierley J, Carcillo JA, Choong K, et al. Clinical practice parameters for hemodynamic support of pediatric and neonatal septic shock: 2007 update from the American College of Critical Care Medicine. *Crit Care Med* 2009;37:666.

Polin RA; Committee on Fetus and Newborn. Management of neonates with suspected or proven early onset bacterial sepsis. *Pediatrics* 2012; 129:1006.

Stoll BJ, Hansen NI, Sánchez PJ, et al. Early onset neonatal sepsis: the burden of group B Streptococcal and *E. coli* disease continues. *Pediatrics* 2011;127:817.

Infectious Diseases

Caviness AC, Demmier GJ, Almendarez Y, et al. The prevalence of neonatal herpes simplex virus infection compared with serious bacterial illness in hospitalized neonates. *J Pediatr* 2008;153: 164–169.

Centers for Disease Control and Prevention (CDC). Congenital syphilis - United States, 2003–2008. *MMWR Morb Mortal Wkly Rep* 2010;59:413.

Guinto-Ocampo H, Bennett JE, Attia M. Predicting pertussis in infants. *Pediatr Emerg Care* 2008;24:16–20.

Khetsuriani N, LaMonte A, Oberste S, et al. Neonatal enterovirus infections reported to the national entervirus surveillance system in the United States, 1983–2003. *Pediatr Infect Dis J* 2006;25(10): 889–893.

Kowalzik F, Barbosa AP, Fernandes VR, et al. Prospective multinational study of pertussis infection in hospitalized infants and their household contacts. *Pediatr Infect Dis J* 2007;26:238.

Sawardekar KP. Changing spectrum of neonatal omphalitis. *Pediatr Infect Dis J* 2004;23:22.

Staat MA, Henrickson K, Elhefni H, et al. Prevalence of respiratory syncytial virus-associated lower respiratory infection and apnea in infants presenting to the emergency department. *Pediatr Infect Dis J* 2013;32:911.

Cardiac Diseases

Canter CE, Simpson KP. Diagnosis and treatment of myocarditis in children in the current era. *Circulation* 2014;129:115.

Dominguez SR, Friedman K, Seewald R, et al. Kawasaki disease in a pediatric intensive care unit: a case-control study. *Pediatrics* 2008; 122:e786–e790.

Weber MA, Ashworth MT, Malone M, et al. Clinicopathological features of paediatric deaths due to myocarditis: an autopsy series. *Arch Dis Child* 2008;93:594–598.

Endocrine Disorders

Speiser PW, Azziz R, Baskin LS, et al. Congenital adrenal hyperplasia due to steroid 21-hydroxylase deficiency: an Endocrine Society clinical practice guideline. *J Clin Endocrinol Metab* 2010;95: 4133.

Metabolic Disorders

Ballestero Y, Hernandez MI, Rojo P, et al. Hyponatremic dehydration as a presentation of cystic fibrosis. *Pediatr Emerg Care* 2006; 23:725–727.

Champion MP. An approach to the diagnosis of inherited metabolic disease. *Arch Dis Child Educ Pract Ed* 2010;95:40.

Ficicioglu C, Bearden D. Isolated neonatal seizures: when to suspect inborn errors of metabolism. *Pediatr Neurol* 2011;45:283.

Hematologic Disorders

Durracq MA, Daubert P, Osterhoudt K. A cyanotic toddler. *Pediatr Emerg Care* 2007;23:195–199.

Sgro M, Campbell D, Barozzino T, et al. Acute neurological findings in a national cohort of neonates with severe neonatal hyperbilirubinemia. *J Perinatol* 2011;31:392.

Gastrointestinal Disorders

Wang KS; Committee on Fetus and Newborn, American Academy of Pediatrics; Section on Surgery, American Academy of Pediatrics. Assessment and management of inguinal hernia in infants. *Pediatrics* 2012;130:768.

Neurologic Diseases

Long SS. Infant botulism and treatment with BIG-IV. *Pediatr Infect Dis J* 2007;26:261–262.

Risko W. Infant botulism. *Pediatr Rev* 2006;27:36–37.

Underwood K, Rubin S, Deakers T, et al. Infant botulism: a 30 year experience spanning the introduction of botulism immune globulin intravenous in the intensive care unit at Childrens Hospital Los Angeles. *Pediatrics* 2007;120:e1380–e1385.

CHAPTER 69 ▪ SORE THROAT

ANDREW M. FINE, MD, MPH AND GARY R. FLEISHER, MD

Sore throat refers to any painful sensation localized to the pharynx or the surrounding areas. Because children, particularly those of preschool age, cannot describe their symptoms as precisely as adults, the physician who evaluates a child with a sore throat must first define the exact nature of the complaint. Occasionally, young patients with dysphagia (see Chapter 51 Pain: Dysphagia), which results from disease in the area of the esophagus or with difficulty swallowing because of a neuromuscular disorder, will verbalize these feelings as a sore throat. Careful questioning usually suffices to distinguish between these complaints.

Although a sore throat is less likely to portend a life-threatening disorder than dysphagia or the inability to swallow, this complaint should not be dismissed without a thorough evaluation. Most children with sore throats have self-limiting or easily treated pharyngeal infections, but a few have serious disorders such as retropharyngeal or lateral pharyngeal abscesses. Even if the reason for the complaint of sore throat is believed to be an infectious pharyngitis, several different organisms may be responsible. Symptomatic therapy, antibiotics, anti-inflammatory drugs, or surgical intervention may be appropriate at times. Most children experience no adverse consequences from misdiagnosis and inappropriate therapy, but a few may develop local extension of infection or sepsis, chronically debilitating illnesses such as rheumatic fever, or life-threatening airway obstruction.

DIFFERENTIAL DIAGNOSIS

Infectious Pharyngitis

Infection is the most common cause of sore throat and is usually caused by respiratory viruses including adenoviruses, coxsackievirus A (various serotypes), influenza, or parainfluenza virus (see Chapter 102 Infectious Disease Emergencies and Tables 69.1–69.3). Several of the respiratory viruses produce easily identifiable syndromes, including hand–foot–mouth disease (coxsackievirus) and pharyngoconjunctival fever (adenovirus). These viral infections are closely followed in frequency by bacterial infections caused by group A streptococci (*Streptococcus pyogenes*). During streptococcal outbreaks, as many as 30% to 50% of episodes of pharyngitis may be caused by *S. pyogenes* in school-aged children. The only other common infectious agent in pharyngitis is the Epstein–Barr virus, which causes infectious mononucleosis. Although infectious mononucleosis is not often seen in children younger than 5 years (Fig. 69.1), it can occur even during these early years of life. More commonly, however, it affects the adolescent. An additional consideration in adolescents with an infectious mononucleosis-like syndrome is human immunodeficiency virus (HIV), which does not commonly cause significant pharyngeal inflammation.

Other organisms produce pharyngitis only rarely; these include *Neisseria gonorrhoeae, Corynebacterium diphtheriae, Francisella tularensis, Fusobacterium necrophorum,* and other bacteria. *N. gonorrhoeae* may cause inflammation and exudate but more often remains quiescent, being diagnosed only by culture. Diphtheria is a life-threatening but seldom encountered cause of infectious pharyngitis, characterized by a thick membrane and marked cervical adenopathy. Oropharyngeal tularemia is rare and should be entertained only in endemic areas among children who have an exudative pharyngitis that cannot be categorized by standard diagnostic testing and/or persists despite antibiotic therapy. Although unusual, mixed anaerobic infections should be considered in the ill-appearing adolescent with a severe pharyngitis because these organisms occasionally lead to sepsis (Lemierre disease). Other pathogens—group C and G streptococci, *Arcanobacterium haemolyticum, Mycoplasma pneumoniae,* and *Chlamydia pneumoniae*—have been implicated as agents of pharyngitis in adults, but in childhood, their roles remain unproved and their frequency is unknown. Of these, *A. haemolyticum* is the most frequent, having been isolated from 0.5% to 2.0% of adolescents with pharyngitis, often in association with a maculopapular rash.

Irritative Pharyngitis/Foreign Body

Drying of the pharynx may irritate the mucosa, leading to a complaint of sore throat. This condition occurs most commonly during the winter months, particularly after a night's sleep in a house with forced hot-air heating. Occasionally, a foreign object such as a fishbone or popcorn shell may become embedded in the pharynx.

Herpetic Stomatitis

Stomatitis caused by herpes simplex virus is usually confined to the anterior buccal mucosa but may extend to the anterior tonsillar pillars occasionally and involve the upper esophagus in immunocompetent patients on rare occasions (e-Fig. 69.1). Particularly, in these more extensive cases, the child may complain of a sore throat.

Peritonsillar Abscess

A peritonsillar abscess may complicate a previously diagnosed infectious pharyngitis or may be the initial source of a child's discomfort. This disease is most common in older children and adolescents. The diagnosis is evident from visual inspection, augmented occasionally by careful palpation. Trismus is common in these patients. These abscesses produce a bulge in the posterior aspect of the soft palate, deviate the uvula to the contralateral side of the pharynx, and have a fluctuant quality on palpation (e-Fig. 69.2).

TABLE 69.1

DIFFERENTIAL DIAGNOSIS OF SORE THROAT IN THE IMMUNOCOMPETENT HOST

Infectious pharyngitis
Respiratory viruses
Group A streptococci
Epstein–Barr virus (infectious mononucleosis)
Human immunodeficiency virus
Neisseria gonorrhoeae
Anaerobic bacteria
Group C and G streptococci
Arcanobacterium haemolyticum
Mycoplasma pneumoniae (unconfirmed)
Chlamydia pneumoniae (unconfirmed)
Francisella tularensis
Corynebacterium diphtheriae (diphtheria)
Other causes
Herpetic stomatitis
Irritative pharyngitis
Foreign body
Peritonsillar abscess
Retropharyngeal and lateral pharyngeal abscesses
Epiglottitis
Kawasaki disease
Stevens–Johnson syndrome
Chemical exposure
Psychogenic pain
Referred pain

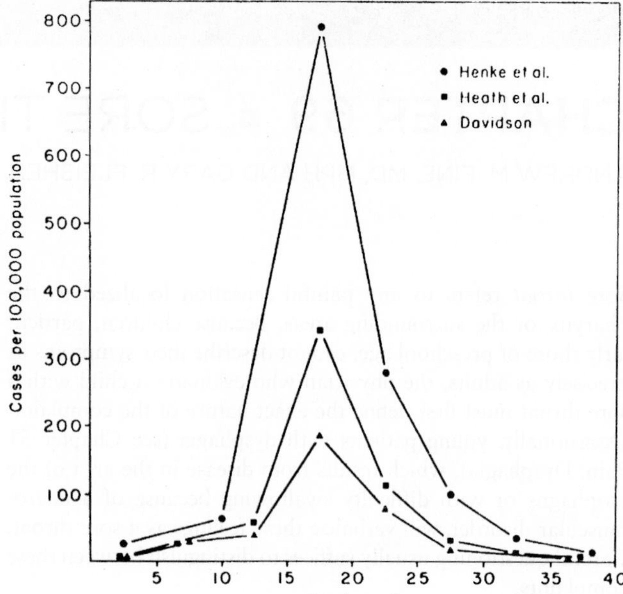

FIGURE 69.1 Incidence by age of infectious mononucleosis in three large studies.

Retropharyngeal and Lateral Pharyngeal Abscesses

Retropharyngeal abscess is an uncommon cause of sore throat, usually occurring in children younger than 4 years. Although most children with this disorder appear toxic and have respiratory distress, a few complain of sore throat and dysphagia without other manifestations early in the course. Occasional infants and young children may also manifest torticollis. A young child with a retropharyngeal abscess who presents with a high fever, toxic appearance, and torticollis is sometimes incorrectly thought to have meningitis. A soft tissue radiographic examination of the lateral neck demonstrates the lesion readily in most cases, whereas direct visualization is often impossible. Unfortunately, even limited flexion of the neck during the radiograph may cause a buckling of the retropharyngeal tissues that resembles a purulent collection. The physician must insist on a radiograph with the neck fully extended before hazarding an interpretation. If the diagnosis remains uncertain despite adequate radiographs, a computed tomography (CT) scan with contrast should be obtained.

Lateral pharyngeal abscesses manifest in a fashion similar to retropharyngeal infections but occur less often. High fever is a common symptom, and both trismus and swelling below the mandible may be seen. Lateral neck radiographs are often unrevealing. To confirm the diagnosis, a CT scan is appropriate.

Epiglottitis

The incidence of epiglottitis, a well-appreciated cause of life-threatening upper airway infection, has declined significantly since the introduction of vaccination against *Haemophilus influenzae* type b. This disease manifests with a toxic appearance, high fever, stridor, and drooling. In every reported series of cases, sore throat appears on the list of symptoms. Although this rarely may be the primary complaint in a child, other more striking findings almost always predominate. Epiglottitis should be excluded easily as a diagnosis in the patient with a sore throat who is without stridor and appears relatively well.

TABLE 69.2

COMMON CAUSES OF SORE THROAT

Infectious pharyngitis
Respiratory viruses
Group A streptococci
Epstein–Barr virus
Irritative pharyngitis
Forced hot air heating

TABLE 69.3

LIFE-THREATENING CAUSES OF SORE THROAT

Retropharyngeal and lateral pharyngeal abscesses
Epiglottitis
Tonsillar hypertrophy (severe) with infectious mononucleosis
Diphtheria
Peritonsillar abscess
Lemierre syndrome

Kawasaki Disease

Classic Kawasaki disease is characterized by several days of high fever along with at least four of the five following findings: (i) Bilateral bulbar conjunctivitis, (ii) oral mucous membrane changes, (iii) peripheral extremity changes (erythema and/or edema), (iv) polymorphous rash, and (v) cervical adenopathy (see Chapter 109 Rheumatologic Emergencies). The oral mucous membrane changes most commonly involve the lips, but occasionally pharyngitis may be a prominent feature. Other systemic inflammatory conditions (e.g., Behçet syndrome) may involve the pharynx as well.

Stevens–Johnson Syndrome

Stevens–Johnson syndrome, a disease of unknown etiology but presumed to be immune mediated, is characterized by vesicular and ulcerative lesions of the mucosa, including the pharynx, the genitalia, and the conjunctivae (e-Fig. 69.3A,B). In addition, children with this condition may have a diffuse rash, often characterized by target lesions or vesicles and bullae. Usually self-limited, an occasional case may lead to dehydration or progress to involve the pulmonary system.

Chemical Exposure

Certain ingestions, such as paraquat and various alkalis, may produce a chemical injury to the mucosa of the pharynx (see Chapter 110 Toxicologic Emergencies). Usually, these findings occur in the setting of a known ingestion and are accompanied by lesions of the oral mucosa.

Referred Pain

Occasionally, pain from the inflammation of extrapharyngeal structures is described as arising in the pharynx. Examples include dental abscesses, cervical adenitis, and, occasionally, otitis media.

Psychogenic Pharyngitis

Some children who complain of a sore throat have no organic explanation for their complaint after a thorough history and physical examination and a throat culture. In these cases, the physician should consider the possibility of anxiety, at times associated with frequent or difficult (globus hystericus) swallowing.

Pharyngitis in the Immunosuppressed Host

Immunosuppressed hosts may develop pharyngitis from any of the previously discussed causes. In addition, these patients exhibit a particular susceptibility to infections with fungal organisms such as *Candida albicans*.

EVALUATION AND DECISION

The history and physical examination should focus on findings seen with systemic illnesses causing pharyngitis and the appearance of the oral cavity. A medical history of an immunosuppressive disorder or missed immunizations raises the specter of unusual infections. A sudden onset is most characteristic of epiglottitis.

Fever, either historical or measured, points to an infection or, less commonly, Kawasaki disease. Toxicity and/or respiratory distress occur with infections leading to respiratory obstruction, such as peritonsillar, retropharyngeal, and lateral pharyngeal abscesses; epiglottitis; diphtheria; and infectious mononucleosis with severe tonsillar hypertrophy. Conjunctivitis suggests pharyngoconjunctival fever (adenovirus), Kawasaki disease, or Stevens–Johnson syndrome; generalized adenopathy occurs with infectious mononucleosis and HIV; and a rash is seen with scarlet fever (group A streptococci), Kawasaki disease, infectious mononucleosis, particularly after the administration of amoxicillin, and rarely with *A. hemolyticum* in adolescents.

The tendency of most clinicians is to assume that one of the common organisms is the cause of pharyngitis in the child with a sore throat. Before settling on infectious pharyngitis, however, the emergency physician should first at least briefly consider several more serious disorders (Fig. 69.2). Conditions that have immediate life-threatening potential include epiglottitis, retropharyngeal and lateral pharyngeal abscesses, peritonsillar abscess, severe tonsillar hypertrophy (usually as an exaggerated manifestation of infectious mononucleosis), and diphtheria. Generally, stridor and signs of respiratory distress accompany the complaint of sore throat in epiglottitis and retropharyngeal abscess. Drooling and voice changes are common

SIGNS AND SYMPTOMS

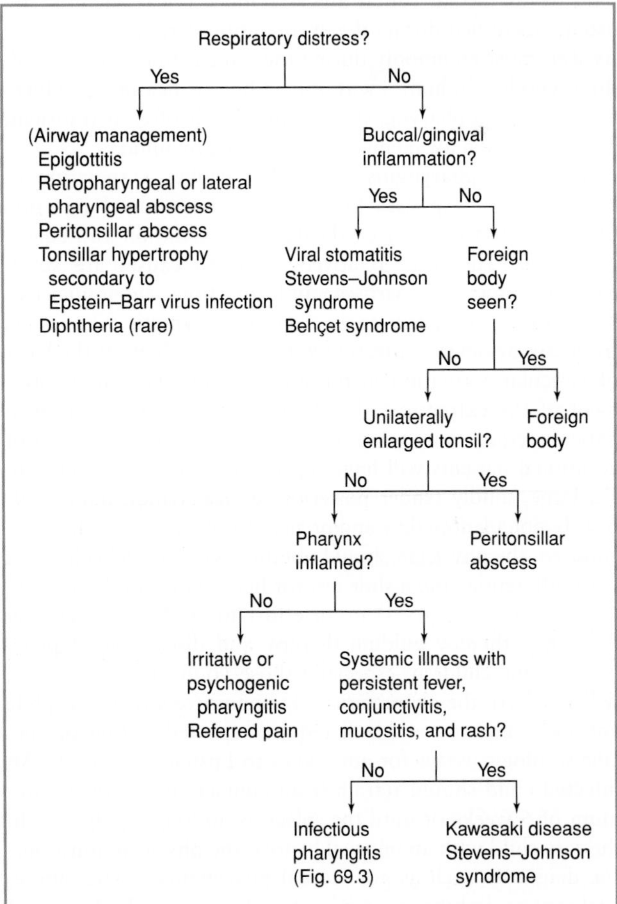

FIGURE 69.2 Diagnostic approach to the child with sore throat.

in children with these two conditions, as well as in patients with peritonsillar abscess and severe infectious tonsillar hypertrophy. In cases of epiglottitis or retropharyngeal abscess that are not clinically obvious, a lateral neck radiograph, obtained under appropriate supervision, is confirmatory. Peritonsillar abscess and tonsillar hypertrophy are diagnosed by visual examination of the pharynx. Diphtheria is rarely a consideration except in unimmunized children, particularly those from underdeveloped nations.

The next phase of the evaluation of the child with a complaint of sore throat hinges on a careful physical examination, particularly of the pharynx (Fig. 69.2). The appearance of vesicles on the buccal mucosa anterior to the tonsillar pillars points to a herpetic stomatitis or noninfectious syndromes such as Behçet or Stevens–Johnson syndrome (erythema multiforme). Uncommonly, a small, pointed foreign body, most commonly a fishbone, becomes lodged in the mucosal folds of the tonsils or pharynx; usually, the history suggests the diagnosis, but an unanticipated sighting may occur in the younger child. Significant asymmetry of the tonsils indicates a peritonsillar cellulitis or, if extensive, an abscess. Clinically, the diagnosis of an abscess is reserved for the tonsil that protrudes beyond the midline, causing the uvula to deviate to the uninvolved side. Kawasaki disease produces a systemic syndrome with a prolonged fever and other characteristic findings that are usually more prominent than the pharyngeal involvement.

The remaining organic diagnoses, once those already discussed have been eliminated by history, physical examination, and occasionally imaging, include referred pain, irritative pharyngitis, and infectious pharyngitis. Sources of referred pain (otitis media, dental abscess, and cervical adenitis) are usually identified during the examination. Irritative pharyngitis seen most commonly during the winter among older children who live in homes with forced hot-air heating, produces minimal or no pharyngeal inflammation. It often is transient, appearing upon awakening and resolving by midday.

Infectious pharyngitis (Fig. 69.3) evokes a spectrum of inflammatory responses that range from minimal injection of the mucosa to beefy erythema with exudation and edema formation. The three relatively common causes are streptococci, respiratory viruses, and infectious mononucleosis (Table 69.2). In a few cases, a viral pharyngitis that results from coxsackievirus infection will be self-evident on the basis of vesicular formation in the posterior pharynx or involvement of the extremities (hand–foot–mouth syndrome). Such patients require only symptomatic therapy. A small number of additional patients will have signs of infectious mononucleosis: large, mildly tender posterior cervical lymph nodes; diffuse lymphadenopathy; and/or hepatosplenomegaly. In these children, the physician should obtain a white blood cell count with differential and a slide test for heterophile antibody (e.g., "monospot," Fig. 69.4) in an effort to confirm the clinical diagnosis, thereby guiding therapy and discussion of prognosis. Some children, especially those younger than 5 years, will not have the characteristic lymphocytosis or heterophile antibody response and will require repeated testing or specific serologic assays for antibodies to Epstein–Barr virus. An infected child should refrain from contact sports for a minimum of 6 weeks or until the spleen is no longer palpable. In the rare child with an unusual history, the physician must pursue diagnoses such as gonococcal pharyngitis (sexual abuse, oral sex) or diphtheria (immigration from an underdeveloped nation, lack of immunization).

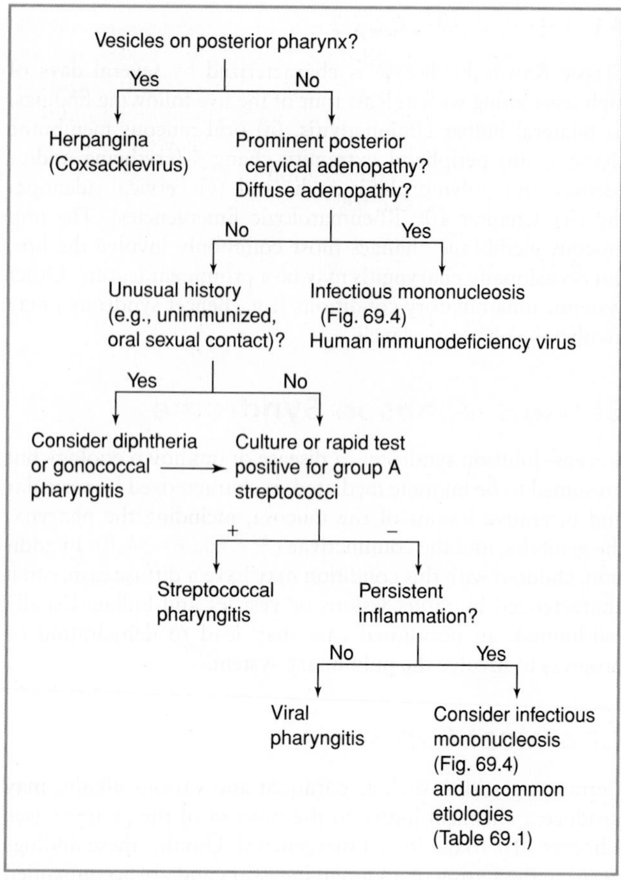

FIGURE 69.3 Diagnostic approach to infectious pharyngitis in the immunocompetent child.

Ultimately, most children will have a mildly to moderately inflamed pharynx but no specific etiologic diagnosis based solely on the history and physical examination. The local, recent incidence of group A streptococcal pharyngitis

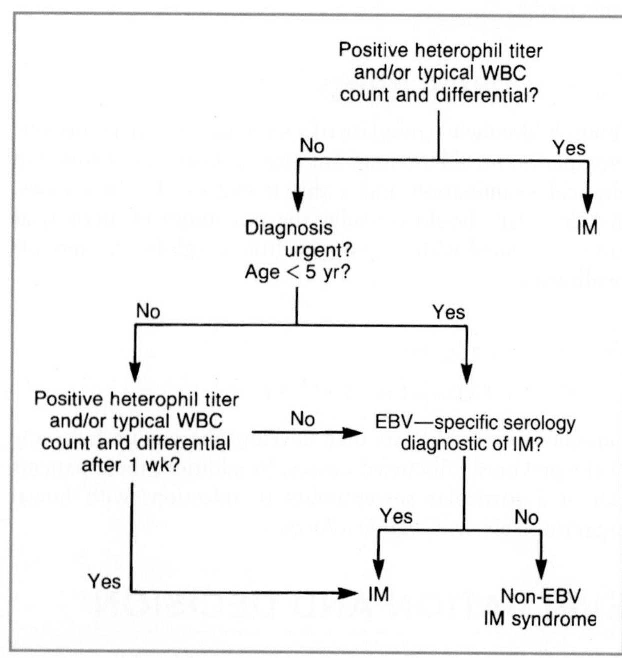

FIGURE 69.4 Diagnostic approach when findings are clinically suggestive for mononucleosis. WBC, white blood cell; IM, infectious mononucleosis; EBV, Epstein–Barr virus.

is an important predictor of strep throat among symptomatic patients. Integration of real-time biosurveillance data with the electronic health record has the potential to facilitate improved diagnosis of strep throat. Although certain symptoms and signs favor streptococcal infection, none is conclusive. Thus, obtaining a rapid test (latex agglutination or optical immunoassay) for group A streptococci, followed by a culture, if negative, is prudent. Rapid tests are most helpful when a positive result is obtained because specificity of the tests is high; however, a negative test result does not exclude streptococcal infection reliably, although some authorities would be satisfied with a negative optical immunoassay alone. With the more recent reported rise in the incidence of rheumatic fever, the accurate diagnosis of streptococcal pharyngitis assumes increasing importance. Generally, symptomatic therapy suffices in the patient with a negative rapid test, although the physician may elect to initiate therapy, usually with a penicillin (penicillin V or amoxicillin) but occasionally with a cephalosporin or macrolide, while awaiting the results of the throat culture in selected cases with highly suggestive clinical features. It is worth noting that the macrolides will not treat *Fusobacterium*, which rarely causes sore throat but is the primary pathogen in Lemierre syndrome.

Suggested Readings and Key References

Centor RM, Witherspoon JM, Dalton HP, et al. The diagnosis of strep throat in adults in the emergency room. *Med Decis Making* 1981;1:239–246.

Cornfeld D, Hubbard JP, Harris TN, et al. Epidemiologic studies of streptococcal infection in school children. *Am J Public Health Nations Health* 1961;51:242–249.

Craig FW, Schunk JE. Retropharyngeal abscess in children: clinical presentation, utility of imaging, and current management. *Pediatrics* 2003;111:1394–1398.

Davidson RJ. A survey of infectious mononucleosis in the North-East Regional Hospital Board area of Scotland, 1960–9. *J Hyg (Lond)* 1970;68(3):393–400.

Ebell MH, Smith MA, Barry HC, et al. The rational clinical examination. Does this patient have strep throat? *JAMA* 2000;284(22): 2912–2918.

Fine AM, Nizet V, Mandl KD. Improved diagnostic accuracy of group A streptococcal pharyngitis with use of real-time biosurveillance. *Ann Intern Med* 2011;155:345–352.

Fine AM, Nizet V, Mandl KD. Large-scale validation of the centor and mcisaac scores to predict group A streptococcal pharyngitis. *Arch Int Med* 2012;172(11):847–852.

Fine AM, Nizet V, Mandl KD. Participatory medicine: a home score for streptococcal pharyngitis enabled by real-time biosurveillance. *Ann Intern Med* 2013;159:577–583.

Fleisher GR, Lennette ET, Henle G, et al. Incidence of heterophil antibody responses in children with infectious mononucleosis. *J Pediatr* 1979;94:723–728.

Gerber MA, Baltimore RS, Eaton CB, et al. Prevention of rheumatic fever and diagnosis and treatment of acute Streptococcal pharyngitis: a scientific statement from the American Heart Association Rheumatic Fever, Endocarditis, and Kawasaki Disease Committee of the Council on Cardiovascular Disease in the Young, the Interdisciplinary Council on Functional Genomics and Translational Biology, and the Interdisciplinary Council on Quality of Care and Outcomes Research: endorsed by the American Academy of Pediatrics. *Circulation* 2009;119(11):1541–1551.

Gieseker KE, MacKenzie T, Roe MH, et al. Comparison of two rapid Streptococcus pyogenes diagnostic tests with a rigorous culture standard. *Pediatr Infect Dis J* 2002;21:922–927.

Goldenberg NA, Knapp-Clevenger R, Hayes T, et al. Lemierre's and Lemierre's like syndromes in children: survival and thromboembolic outcomes. *Pediatrics* 2005;116:e543–e548.

Heath CW, Brodsky AC, Potolsky AI. Infectious mononucleosis in a general population. *Am J Epidemiol* 1972;96(2):87–93.

Henke CD, Kurland LT, Elveback LR. Infectious mononucleosis in Rochester, Minnesota 1950 through 1969. *Am J Epidemiol* 1973; 98(6):483–490.

Kaltwasser G, Diego J, Welby-Sellenriek PL, et al. Polymerase chain reaction for Streptococcus pyogenes used to evaluate optical immunoassay for the detection of group A streptococci in children with pharyngitis. *Pediatr Infect Dis J* 1997;16:748–753.

Komaroff AL, Aronson MD, Pass TM, et al. Serologic evidence of chlamydial and mycoplasmal pharyngitis in adults. *Science* 1983; 222:927–929.

Lieu TA, Fleisher GR, Schwartz JS. Clinical evaluation of a latex agglutination test for streptococcal pharyngitis: performance and impact on treatment rates. *Pediatr Infect Dis J* 1988;7:847–854.

Lieu TA, Fleisher GR, Schwartz JS. Cost-effectiveness of rapid latex agglutination testing and throat culture for streptococcal pharyngitis. *Pediatrics* 1990;85:246–256.

MacKenzie A, Fuite LA, King J, et al. Incidence and pathogenicity of Arcanobacterium haemolyticum during a 2-year study in Ottawa. *Clin Infect Dis* 1995;21:177–181.

McIsaac WJ, Kellner JD, Aufricht P, et al. Empirical validation of guidelines for the management of pharyngitis in children and adults. *JAMA* 2004;291:1587–1595.

Shulman ST, Bisno AL, Clegg HW, et al. Clinical practice guideline for the diagnosis and management of group A streptococcal pharyngitis: 2012 update by the Infectious Diseases Society of America. *Clin Infect Dis* 2012;55(10):1279–1282.

Weisner PJ, Tronca E, Bonin P, et al. Clinical spectrum of pharyngeal gonococcal infection. *N Engl J Med* 1973;288:181–185.

Wessels MR. Clinical practice. Streptococcal pharyngitis. *N Engl J Med* 2011;364(7):648–655.

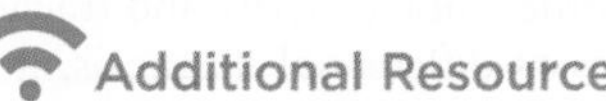

CHAPTER 70 ■ STRIDOR

ERIC C. HOPPA, MD AND HOLLY E. PERRY, MD

Stridor, although a relatively common occurrence, can be frightening to both children and parents. The presence of stridor necessitates a complete and careful evaluation to determine the cause of this worrisome and occasionally life-threatening symptom. This chapter presents the causes of stridor and provides the emergency practitioner with guidelines for initial evaluation and management.

PATHOPHYSIOLOGY

Stridor is a respiratory sound caused by turbulent airflow through a partially obstructed upper airway. Stridor can be inspiratory, expiratory, or biphasic depending on the level of airway obstruction. Inspiratory stridor occurs with obstruction of the extrathoracic trachea, biphasic stridor when the obstruction is at the level of the glottis or subglottis, and expiratory stridor when only the intrathoracic trachea is involved. The pitch of the stridor also varies with the location of the obstruction. Laryngeal and subglottic obstructions are associated with high-pitched stridor. In contrast, obstruction of the nares and nasopharynx results in a lower-pitched snoring or snorting sound called stertor. Because the passage of saliva and the flow of air are impeded in pharyngeal obstruction, these patients often have a gurgling quality of breathing. The relative length of inspiratory and expiratory phases may be helpful in localizing the airway obstruction. Laryngeal obstruction results in an increased inspiratory phase, whereas expiration tends to be prolonged in bronchial obstruction. Both inspiratory and expiratory phases are increased in patients with tracheal obstruction.

DIFFERENTIAL DIAGNOSIS

Stridor may occur in a wide variety of disease processes affecting the large airways from the level of the nares to the bronchi, but most often arises with disorders of the larynx and trachea (Table 70.1). For the purposes of differential diagnosis, it is helpful to categorize the common causes of stridor as acute or chronic in onset and to further divide acute onset into febrile and afebrile causes (Table 70.2). Life-threatening causes of stridor must be considered early during the evaluation process (Table 70.3).

Stridor with Acute Onset in the Febrile Child

Laryngotracheitis (croup) is by far the most common cause of stridor in the febrile child. Other diagnoses that should be considered include bacterial tracheitis, epiglottitis, and much less commonly retropharyngeal abscess or laryngeal diphtheria in the unimmunized child (see Chapter 102 Infectious Disease Emergencies). Though less common than croup, these diseases have a greater potential for life-threatening airway compromise.

Croup most commonly affects children between 7 and 36 months of age with peak incidence around 2 years of age but can be seen throughout childhood. Croup typically begins with symptoms of an upper respiratory tract infection and fever, usually ranging from 38° to 39°C (100.4° to 102.2°F). Within 12 to 48 hours, a barky, "seal-like" cough and inspiratory stridor are noted. The stridor is worsened when the child is agitated and often improves with nebulized racemic epinephrine. Supraclavicular and subcostal retractions may be present. Most children appear mildly to moderately ill, though the loud breathing and respiratory distress can be very alarming to family members.

Bacterial tracheitis has a varied presentation but can resemble croup. Patients tend to be older, appear more toxic, and may not improve as much as expected with nebulized racemic epinephrine. Dysphagia is common, and drooling may be present. The verbal child may complain of anterior neck pain or a painful cough.

Epiglottitis is an infection of the supraglottic structures. Historically, epiglottitis was most commonly caused by *Haemophilus influenzae type B*. Other causative pathogens include *Staphylococcus aureus, Streptococcus pneumoniae,* β-hemolytic streptococci, and viral agents (parainfluenza, HSV 1, and varicella). Noninfectious causes can include direct trauma and thermal injury. The incidence of epiglottis due to *H. influenzae* has plummeted to as low as 0.02 per 100,000 in Western countries following the introduction of the conjugate vaccine. Sporadic cases are seen in unimmunized children or vaccine failures. Patients with *H. influenzae* epiglottitis typically appear toxic with fever and drooling. Respiratory distress and a tripod stance (upright position, neck extended, and mouth open) are characteristic symptoms. Sudden airway compromise may occur and can be precipitated by the manipulation of the oropharynx.

In contrast, epiglottitis caused by pathogens other than *H. influenzae* has a more insidious onset, is more common in older children and adults, and is almost universally associated with dysphagia or sore throat. Importantly, the risk of airway compromise is less in this population. However, any child with suspected epiglottitis should be managed as if he or she has disease caused by *H. influenzae* with risk of imminent airway compromise.

A retropharyngeal abscess is an infrequent cause of stridor. Patients more commonly present with fever, limitation of neck movement, agitation, or lethargy. Physical examination may reveal midline fullness of the oropharynx.

Stridor with Acute Onset in the Afebrile Child

A foreign body in either the trachea or the esophagus may produce stridor. The majority of foreign body aspirations

TABLE 70.1

CAUSES OF STRIDOR BY ANATOMIC LOCATION

Nose and pharynx
Congenital anomalies
Lingual thyroid
Choanal atresia
Craniofacial anomalies (Apert and Down syndromes; Pierre Robin sequence)
Cysts (dermoid, thyroglossal)
Macroglossia (Beckwith syndrome)
Encephalocele
Inflammatory
Abscess (parapharyngeal, retropharyngeal, peritonsillar)
Allergic polyps
Adenotonsillar enlargement (acute infection, infectious mononucleosis)
Neoplasm (benign, malignant)
Adenotonsillar hyperplasia
Foreign body
Neurologic syndromes with poor tongue/pharyngeal muscle tone
Larynx
Congenital anomalies
Laryngomalacia
Web, cyst, laryngocele
Cartilage dystrophy
Subglottic stenosis
Cleft larynx
Inflammatory
Croup
Epiglottitis
Tracheitis
Anaphylaxis
Angioneurotic edema
Miscellaneous: tuberculosis, fungal infection, diphtheria, sarcoidosis
Vocal cord paralysis (multiple causes)
Psychogenic stridor (vocal cord dysfunction)
Neoplasm
Subglottic hemangioma
Laryngeal papilloma
Cystic hygroma (neck)
Malignant (e.g., rhabdomyosarcoma)
Laryngospasm (hypocalcemic tetany)
Trachea and bronchi
Congenital
Vascular anomalies
Webs, cysts
Tracheal stenosis
Tracheoesophageal fistula
Neoplasm
Tracheal
Compression by adjacent structure (thyroid, thymus, esophagus)
Foreign body (tracheal or esophageal)

TABLE 70.2

COMMON CAUSES OF STRIDOR

Acute, Febrile
Croup
Tracheitis
Epiglottitis
Acute, Afebrile
Foreign body
Caustic or thermal injury to airway
Spasmodic croup
Angioneurotic edema
Chronic
Laryngomalacia
Vascular anomalies
Adenotonsillar hyperplasia

occur in children under age 3 or in children with developmental delays. There may be a history of choking on food or a small object. Physical examination varies, depending on the location of the foreign body (see Chapter 27 Foreign Body: Ingestion and Aspiration).

Both ingestion and inhalation of caustic or thermally damaging substances may result in injury to the airway or hypopharynx (see Chapter 112 Burns). Symptoms of airway compromise may be delayed for as long as 6 hours. Blind finger sweeps have also been reported rarely to result in stridor. Other causes to consider include spasmodic croup, anaphylaxis, angioneurotic edema, and trauma.

Chronic Stridor

The differential diagnosis of chronic stridor varies by the age at onset. Stridor noted shortly after birth is most likely caused by an anatomical defect. This type of stridor tends to slowly worsen and is severe when the infant is crying or agitated. Laryngomalacia is the most common cause of congenital stridor accounting for up to 75% of chronic stridor in children younger than 1 year. Stridor associated with laryngomalacia is positional and may be relieved by placing the child in the prone position. It frequently disappears when the child cries.

TABLE 70.3

LIFE-THREATENING CAUSES OF STRIDOR

Usually febrile
Epiglottitis
Retropharyngeal abscess
Tracheitis
Usually afebrile
Foreign body
Anaphylaxis
Angioneurotic edema
Neck trauma
Neoplasm (compressing trachea)
Thermal or caustic injury

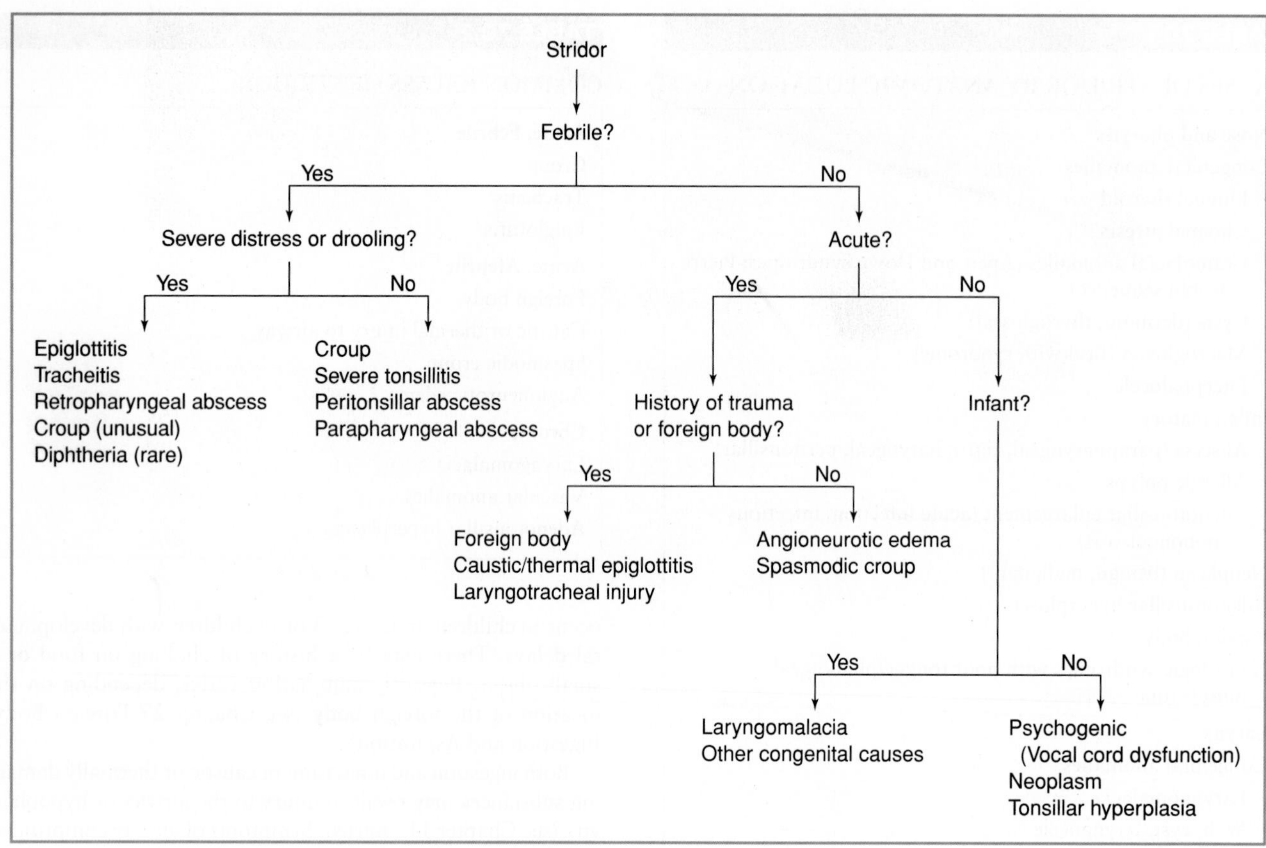

FIGURE 70.1 Diagnostic approach to stridor.

Other congenital causes of stridor include laryngeal webs, laryngeal diverticula, vocal cord paralysis, subglottic stenosis, tracheomalacia, and vascular anomalies such as a double aortic arch or a vascular sling. Stridor in infants has also been reported to be associated with gastroesophageal reflux, possibly related to associated laryngomalacia, or acutely secondary to partial laryngospasm.

Stridor in older children may be caused by papillomas or neoplastic processes. Patients with papillomas generally present between 2 and 4 years of age with complaints of hoarseness and stridor. Neoplastic processes causing tracheal compression can also lead to stridor in the older child.

Psychogenic or functional stridor (also called vocal cord dysfunction or paradoxical vocal cord movement) is an uncommon cause of stridor, and presents only in the older child. The diagnosis is three times more common in adolescent females than males. More than 50% of patients meet diagnostic criteria for a psychiatric disorder. This diagnosis can be challenging as many of these patients have asthma as a comorbid condition, and may present with apparent distress and poor aeration. Characteristically, stridor improves when the patient is unaware that he or she is being observed, and it may clear with cough. The diagnosis can be confirmed by nasopharyngoscopy in the symptomatic patient when the vocal cords are noted to be adducted during inspiration.

EVALUATION AND DECISION

The first priority is to ensure that the airway is adequate by assessing the level of consciousness, color, perfusion, air entry, breath sounds, and work of breathing, including respiratory rate, nasal flaring, and retractions. If possible, the child should be allowed to assume a position of comfort to minimize agitation and distress and maximize airway patency. Immediate resuscitative measures should be instituted as necessary (see Chapter 3 Airway). The child may then be evaluated systematically. In the child with acute onset of stridor, history should focus on associated symptoms such as fever, duration of illness, drooling, rhinorrhea, and history of choking or trauma (Fig. 70.1). Immunization status should be verified, particularly *H. influenzae* vaccination. In the case of a child with chronic stridor, important historical points include age at onset and progression of stridor, as well as ameliorating and aggravating factors.

Physical examination should include careful inspection of the nares and oropharynx, with particular attention to trismus, increased secretions or drooling, visible mass, and abnormal phonation. Of note, the examination and manipulation of the oropharynx of any child with suspected epiglottitis should be deferred until a secure airway can be established. Quality of the voice or cry should be noted as normal, hoarse (croup, vocal cord paralysis, papilloma), weak (neuromuscular disorder), or aphonic (laryngeal obstruction). Regional findings such as adenopathy, neck masses, meningismus, trauma, or bruising should also be sought. Position of comfort should be noted. Children with airway obstruction at or above the level of the larynx often hyperextend the neck and lean forward ("sniffing" position) in an effort to straighten the upper airway and maximize air entry. Finally, response to therapies, such as nebulized racemic epinephrine, should be noted.

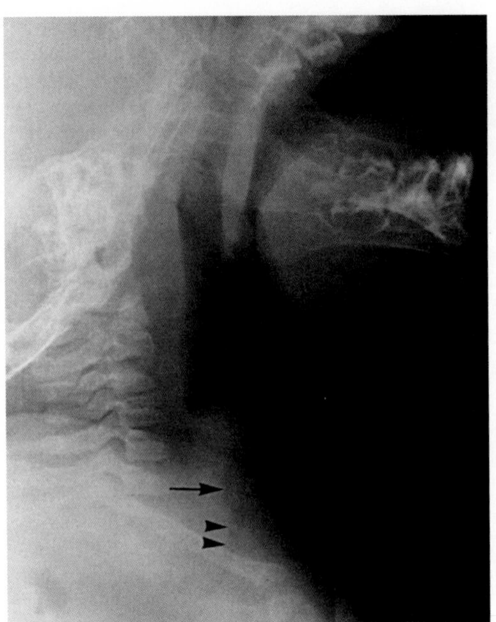

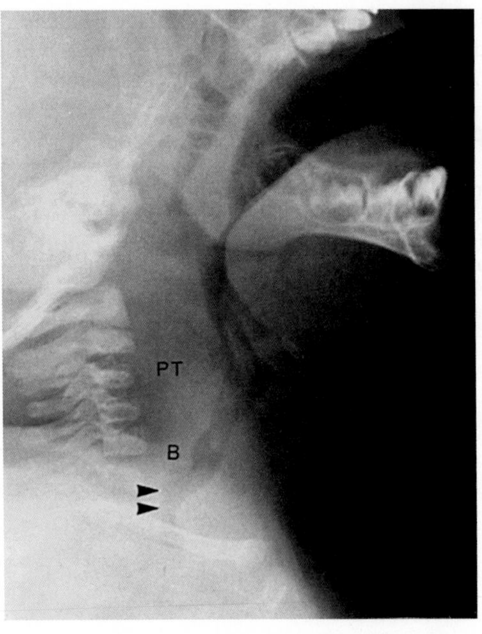

FIGURE 70.2 Inspiratory (**A**) and expiratory (**B**) lateral neck radiographs of a child with upper airway obstruction secondary to a granuloma (*arrow*) in the upper trachea. Note ballooning of the pharynx during inspiration (**A**) and narrowing of the trachea (*arrowheads*) below the level of obstruction. On expiration (**B**), note the normal pharyngeal lumen and dilation (*arrowheads*) of the trachea distal to the obstruction. The "bunching up" of the pharyngeal tissues (*PT*) and the buckling of the trachea (**B**) are normal findings on expiratory films.

Emergency management of the child with stridor depends on its severity and its likely cause. Oxygen, nebulized epinephrine, corticosteroids, laryngoscopy, intubation, and even emergency cricothyroidotomy or tracheostomy all have specific roles in the emergency department (ED) management of stridor, depending on its cause (see Chapters 114 ENT Trauma and 126 ENT Emergencies).

Febrile Child

In the febrile child with stridor, the onset is generally acute with croup being the most common cause. Other diagnostic possibilities to consider include bacterial tracheitis, epiglottitis, and much less likely retropharyngeal abscess. The child whose clinical picture is consistent with mild to moderate croup needs no further evaluation. History and physical examination alone are the most important diagnostic tools for croup. Radiographs are not necessary, in the evaluation of routine clinically diagnosed croup. However, anteroposterior and lateral neck radiographs should be obtained if the diagnosis of croup is in question or if the child does not respond to therapy as expected. If epiglottitis is strongly suspected, a lateral neck radiograph should only be obtained in stable and cooperative patients. Otherwise the child should have their airway secured by the most senior or skilled provider prior to other interventions, in the controlled setting of the operating room whenever possible.

Airway radiographs must be interpreted with care because they are affected by positioning, crying, swallowing, and the phase of respiration. To properly interpret the prevertebral space, the lateral neck radiograph must be taken with the patient's head extended and during inspiration. Normal tracheal buckling, which is seen during expiration in a young child, may be misinterpreted as tracheal mass lesion or deviation from an extrinsic mass (Fig. 70.2). Abnormal findings on a lateral neck radiograph include swollen epiglottis or aryepiglottic folds (epiglottitis), irregular tracheal borders or stranding across the trachea (tracheitis), and increased prevertebral width (retropharyngeal abscess) (e-Figs. 70.1 and 70.2). In children, the prevertebral space should be less than the width of the adjacent cervical vertebra. Radiographic findings consistent with croup are a narrowed subglottic area on anteroposterior view (the "steeple sign") and ballooning of the hypopharynx best appreciated on the lateral view.

Afebrile Child

In the afebrile child with acute onset of stridor, the duration of symptoms, the child's age, and the likelihood of foreign-body aspiration are all key elements to consider. Emergent otolaryngologic or surgical consultation should be obtained in a child with an evidence of airway obstruction if either aspirated foreign body or trauma is a likely cause of stridor. Stridor from anaphylaxis follows exposure to an allergen, and may be associated with vomiting, wheezing, facial or oral edema, urticaria, or hypotension. Angioneurotic edema, an autosomal-dominant trait, is characterized by rapid onset of swelling without discoloration, urticaria, or pain. Symptoms may occur in affected patients as young as 2 years of age but usually are not severe until adolescence. Symptoms may be precipitated by trauma, emotional stress, or menses. Determination of the C_1-esterase inhibitor level should be considered if angioneurotic edema is suspected.

A child with chronic stridor generally does not require an extensive evaluation in the ED unless significant respiratory distress is present. The infant with chronic stridor who is otherwise well should be referred to the private pediatrician or to an otolaryngologist. Once a neoplastic cause is deemed unlikely, the older child with chronic stridor should be referred to otolaryngology for evaluation, including nasopharyngoscopy and possible direct laryngoscopy for evaluation of the vocal cords.

Suggested Readings and Key References

Cherry JD. Croup. *N Engl J Med* 2008;358:384–391.

Craig FW, Schunk JE. Retropharyngeal abscess in children: clinical presentation, utility of imaging, and current management. *Pediatrics* 2003;111:1394–1398.

Guldfred LA, Lyhne D, Becker BC. Acute epiglottitis: epidemiology, clinical presentation, management and outcome. *J Laryngol Otol* 2008;122:818–823.

Hopkins A, Lahiri T, Salerno R, et al. Changing epidemiology of life-threatening upper airway infections: the reemergence of bacterial tracheitis. *Pediatrics* 2006;118:1418–1421.

Zoumalan R, Maddalozzo J, Holinger LD. Etiology of stridor in infants. *Ann Otol Rhinol Laryngol* 2007;116:329–334.

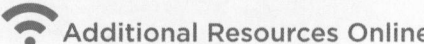

CHAPTER 71 ■ SYNCOPE

T. BRAM WELCH-HORAN, MD AND ROHIT P. SHENOI, MD

Syncope is a sudden, brief loss of consciousness and postural tone caused by transient global cerebral hypoperfusion and characterized by complete recovery. Presyncope is a feeling of impending sensory and postural changes without loss of consciousness. Syncope is a common condition in childhood, and in the United States accounts for about 1% of emergency department (ED) visits among children 7 to 18 years of age. The incidence peaks during the second decade of life. About 15% of children will have experienced syncope by the end of adolescence. Girls are more commonly affected than boys. The most common cause of syncope in children is vasovagal syncope, which is related to a loss of vasomotor tone and is generally benign. Occasionally, the etiology may be a life-threatening cardiac condition. The goal when evaluating a child who presents to the ED with syncope is to assess whether high-risk conditions are present or whether the symptoms can be attributed to a more benign etiology.

When normal individuals assume an upright position, cardiac output and cerebral arterial blood pressure (BP) are maintained by a combination of mechanical pumping activity of the skeletal muscles on venous return, the presence of one-way valves in the veins that facilitate venous return to the right atrium, arterial vasoconstriction caused by the baroreceptor reflex and cerebral blood flow autoregulation. If stroke volume is not maintained, then reflex sinus tachycardia develops. Vasovagal or neurocardiogenic syncope is believed to begin with excessive peripheral venous pooling that leads to a sudden decrease in peripheral venous return. This results in increased cardiac contractility and baroreceptor and left ventricular mechanoreceptor firing followed by an efferent response consisting of peripheral α-adrenergic withdrawal and enhanced parasympathetic tone. The hallmark is vasodilatation and bradycardia with hypotension. Sudden activation of a large number of mechanoreceptors in the bladder, rectum, esophagus, and lungs may also provoke such a response. In orthostatic hypotension, often due to fluid depletion, the compensatory responses and ensuing sinus tachycardia are not enough to maintain brain perfusion and syncope develops when the patient stands.

Syncope on exertion suggests a cardiac or cardiopulmonary cause such as obstruction to left or right ventricular outflow or pulmonary hypertension. In these conditions, cardiac output is unable to meet increased peripheral tissue needs. Failure to increase cardiac output sufficiently, together with a fall in peripheral resistance during exercise may lead to syncope on exertion. There are three main categories of syncope: autonomic (vasovagal or neurocardiogenic), cardiac, and others (Table 71.1).

AUTONOMIC (VASOVAGAL OR NEUROCARDIOGENIC) SYNCOPE

Autonomic syncope is the most common cause of syncope in children and adolescents, and accounts for almost 80% of cases. It belongs to a group of neurally mediated syncope conditions in which there is a brief inability of the autonomic nervous system to keep BP and sometimes heart rate at a level necessary to maintain cerebral perfusion and consciousness. Other conditions in this group include "situational" syncope which may occur after micturition, defecation, hair grooming, coughing, or sneezing. The precipitating causes for vasovagal syncope include prolonged standing, a crowded and poorly ventilated environment, brisk exercise in a warm environment, severe anxiety, perceived or real pain, and fear. There are three clinical types. In the first, there is marked hypotension (vasodepressor syncope). The second type is characterized by marked bradycardia (cardioinhibitory syncope) and in the third form there is a combination of hypotension and bradycardia. Some symptoms that herald a syncopal event include weakness, light-headedness, blurring of vision, diaphoresis, and nausea.

Breath-holding spells, a type of vasovagal syncope, occur in older infants and toddlers and may be triggered by anger, pain, or fear. There are two forms: cyanotic or pallid. In the cyanotic form, the child holds his or her breath, turns cyanotic, and then loses consciousness. In the pallid form, the loss of consciousness occurs before breath-holding. Occasionally the child may have associated tonic or clonic motor activity.

CARDIAC SYNCOPE

There are several cardiac conditions that can lead to syncope in children (Table 71.1). They account for 2% to 6% of pediatric syncope. The most important causes that may be associated with significant morbidity or death are discussed here.

Long QT Syndrome (LQTS)

This is an important cause of syncope and sudden cardiac death in children without structural heart disease. An abnormal ECG obtained when the patient is at rest is a key to the diagnosis. The upper limits of the corrected QT interval (QT_c) (using Bazett formula: $QT_c = (QT)/\sqrt{RR}$ interval) are <450 msec. There are congenital and acquired causes for a prolonged QT interval. The genetic arrhythmia syndromes consist of three subtypes: LQT1, LQT2, and LQT3. The disease occurs due to mutations in genes that encode for cardiac ion channels that are important in ventricular repolarization. Syncope in these patients is related to polymorphic ventricular tachycardia (torsades de pointes) and death is due to ventricular fibrillation. One form (LQT3) can also be associated with bradycardia and slow heart rates that may cause syncope. Most cases are associated with the autosomal dominant form of the syndrome (i.e., Romano–Ward syndrome), which shows variable penetrance. LQT1 is the most common form, and the triggers for syncope or sudden death in affected patients include emotional

TABLE 71.1

CAUSES OF PEDIATRIC SYNCOPE

Autonomic
Vasovagal[a]
Breath-holding spell[a]
Situational (micturition, defecation, hair grooming, coughing)
Cardiac[b]
Electrical disturbances[a]
Pre-excitation syndromes (Wolff–Parkinson–White syndrome)
Long QT syndromes (congenital and acquired)
Brugada syndrome
Polymorphic ventricular tachycardia
Bradycardia (complete heart block)
Structural heart disease
Hypertrophic obstructive cardiomyopathy
Ischemia (coronary artery anomalies, Kawasaki disease, and atherosclerotic disease)
Aortic valve stenosis
Dilated cardiomyopathy
Pulmonary hypertension
Myocarditis
Pericarditis
Postoperative cardiac repair
Others
Hypoglycemia[a]
Anaphylaxis[b]
Environmental
Heat syncope[b]
Orthostatic[a]
Dehydration or hemorrhage[b]
Toxins[a]
Carbon monoxide poisoning[b]
Inhalant abuse (volatile inhalants, nitrites)[b]
Hypoxia[b]
Drugs
Proarrhythmic agents (Class 1A and 1C antiarrhythmics), vasodilators, depressants
Conditions that mimic syncope
Seizures
Migraine
Conversion disorder[a]
Hyperventilation
Pseudoseizures
Intentional strangulation (e.g., "choking game")
Narcolepsy

[a]Common causes of syncope.
[b]Potentially life-threatening causes.

or physical stress such as diving and swimming. One form of LQT1, the Jervell and Lange-Nielsen syndrome, is autosomal recessive and associated with a high risk of sudden death and congenital deafness. In LQT2, syncope or sudden death can occur with stress or at rest. Events triggered by sudden loud noises, such as the ringing of an alarm clock, are virtually pathognomonic for this condition. Acquired causes for a prolonged QT_c interval include hypocalcemia, hypokalemia, hypomagnesemia, hypothyroidism, eating disorders, and the use of drugs that prolong QT interval (e.g., sotalol, haloperidol, methadone, and pentamidine).

It is crucial to obtain a full family history in patients suspected of having LQTS. Some clinical features such as QT morphologic characteristics, the response of the QT interval to exercise, triggers of arrhythmia, and response to therapies vary according to the disease-associated gene. In LQTS, recent and frequent syncopal episodes, QT_c prolongation >530 msec, and male gender between the ages of 10 and 12 years are predictive of risk for aborted cardiac arrest and sudden cardiac death during adolescence.

Brugada Syndrome

In this heritable disorder, there is an abnormality in the cardiac sodium channel which results in ST segment elevation in anterior precordial leads (V1 and V2) with a susceptibility to polymorphic ventricular tachycardia. The ECG pattern is diagnostic but may present only intermittently, and may change over time. If the arrhythmia degenerates to ventricular fibrillation, it may lead to sudden death; if it terminates, the patient may have only syncope.

Structural Heart Disease

Congenital heart conditions that interfere with cardiac output may result in syncope. Such structural problems include hypertrophic obstructive cardiomyopathy (HOCM), aortic valve stenosis, and coronary anomalies that cause cardiac ischemia. Functionally pulmonary hypertension may cause similar results. As with other cardiac causes of syncope, chest pain, dizziness, and dyspnea on exertion are concerning symptoms that should prompt further evaluation.

HOCM is a genetic disorder that affects the proteins of the cardiac sarcomere. In this condition the hypertrophied basal septum partially blocks the outflow of the left ventricle creating a functional obstruction. In addition, anterior motion of the mitral valve into the left ventricle during systole further compromises outflow. Patients present with dyspnea, exercise intolerance, angina, syncope, and sudden death.

Other Arrhythmias

Supraventricular tachycardia is the most common symptomatic pediatric tachyarrhythmia. Syncope results from compromised cardiac output. First-degree heart block may be an incidental finding in patients with syncope. However, second- and third-degree heart block need further investigation. Search for evidence of myocarditis, cardiomyopathy, or congenital heart disease when such arrhythmias are observed. Conduction disturbances are common after cardiac surgery. Patients who have undergone correction of tetralogy of Fallot, aortic stenosis, and transposition of the great arteries may be particularly prone to syncope. Ventricular arrhythmias may occur after repair of the ventricles in congenital heart disease. Rarely direct blunt trauma to the chest (commotio cordis) may cause ventricular arrhythmias leading to syncope or sudden death.

OTHER CONDITIONS AND THOSE THAT MIMIC SYNCOPE

There are several other conditions that may cause syncope. The most frequent of these are seizures and migraine. The rest are less frequent but still important conditions.

Hypoglycemia

Low blood sugar is usually associated with feelings of weakness, diaphoresis, light-headedness, and confusion that can mimic presyncope. Diagnosis is rapidly established by obtaining a blood glucose level.

Epilepsy

It may be difficult to differentiate an epileptic seizure from the seizures or posturing that may follow a brief but severe cerebral hypoxic event caused by vasovagal syncope. An important distinguishing feature is that in the latter, the patient usually displays a normal orientation after the syncopal event compared to the more prolonged postictal confusion and lethargy that usually follows a typical epileptic seizure. Nausea and sweating are also more common with syncope. Incontinence and fall-induced trauma may be observed in both conditions and are not discriminatory. A distant stare may precede an atonic seizure but is not typical of vasovagal syncope. The prodrome symptoms of vasovagal syncope differ from the aura that may precede a seizure in some patients. Prolonged clonic seizure activity after the patient is recumbent is not expected in a syncopal event.

Narcolepsy

Cataplexy, muscle weakness, and collapse in a patient with narcolepsy may mimic syncope. However, in these patients there are more likely to be disorders of the sleep–wake cycle, symptoms of daytime somnolence, and sometimes hallucinations.

Vertebrobasilar Migraine or Transient Ischemic Attacks

In such migraines, symptoms such as tinnitus, vertigo or other aura, and occipital headache may be observed. However, this constellation of symptoms is not specific. In vertebrobasilar migraine, as in vertebrobasilar arterial insufficiency causing transient ischemic attacks, loss of consciousness may be observed.

Psychogenic Causes of Syncope

Hyperventilation and conversion disorder can lead to syncopal events. These conditions are common in adolescence. Hyperventilation may occur as part of a panic disorder. Patients may complain of chest tightness, breathlessness, light-headedness, palpitations, and dizziness. Syncope-like symptoms due to conversion disorder occur in the presence of an audience and is not associated with injury. Episodes tend to last longer than the typical vasovagal syncope and are not posture dependent. Neurologic and autonomic manifestations are usually absent.

Orthostatic Intolerance

Syncope attributable to orthostatic hypotension occurs upon assuming an upright posture (i.e., orthostatis) due to a drop in BP. Symptoms of orthostatic hypotension consist of light-headedness, syncope or presyncope, vision changes, headaches, palpitations, tremulousness, and diaphoresis and are ameliorated by recumbent position. The causes include volume depletion (e.g., hemorrhage or dehydration), febrile illness, pregnancy, anemia, eating disorders, and use of medications such as diuretics, vasodilators, or calcium channel blockers. Symptoms typically abate upon treatment of the primary cause. In some patients, recurrent orthostatic symptoms may occur in the absence of true orthostatic hypotension, and may be associated with an excessive increase in heart rate during upright positioning. This condition is known as postural orthostatic tachycardia syndrome (POTS). It is diagnosed by orthostatic heart rate acceleration greater than 120 beats per minute or an absolute increase of 30 beats per minute or greater in the absence of significant orthostatic hypotension. There are two forms of POTS and both forms are observed more often in females than males. In the first and more common type, persistent tachycardia, associated with fatigue, exercise intolerance, and palpitations, is present while the patient assumes an upright position. This condition may occur after a viral illness, trauma, or surgery. The second or central form of POTS is often associated with migraines, tremor, and excessive sweating.

Dysautonomia

In rare cases, a child may exhibit an inadequate vasoconstriction in response to postural changes that would normally demand sympathetic nervous system activation. In such patients, the heart rate may not increase appropriately with standing, and BP may be labile, leading to syncope.

Drugs and Toxins

Medications that decrease cardiac output, such as barbiturates and tricyclic antidepressants, may cause syncope. Recreational drugs such as cocaine, alcohol, inhalants, and opiates may cause a loss of consciousness, though not true syncope. Carbon monoxide is an important environmental toxin to consider in applicable clinical scenarios.

CLINICAL EVALUATION

In children who present with syncope, the history usually offers key information to assist the clinician in making the diagnosis. However, objective findings are often absent, which can pose a challenge. An orderly approach in the evaluation of pediatric syncope is essential and consists of a meticulous history and physical examination, a 12-lead ECG, and the use of additional testing only in selected patients (Fig. 71.1). Extensive testing is usually unnecessary.

Determine the sequence of events leading up to the syncopal event and the position of the patient's body just before the syncope. It may be necessary to obtain information from eyewitnesses because the patient may not recollect the event. Search for precipitating factors, such as exercise, loud noise or a startle response, rapid postural changes, anxiety or

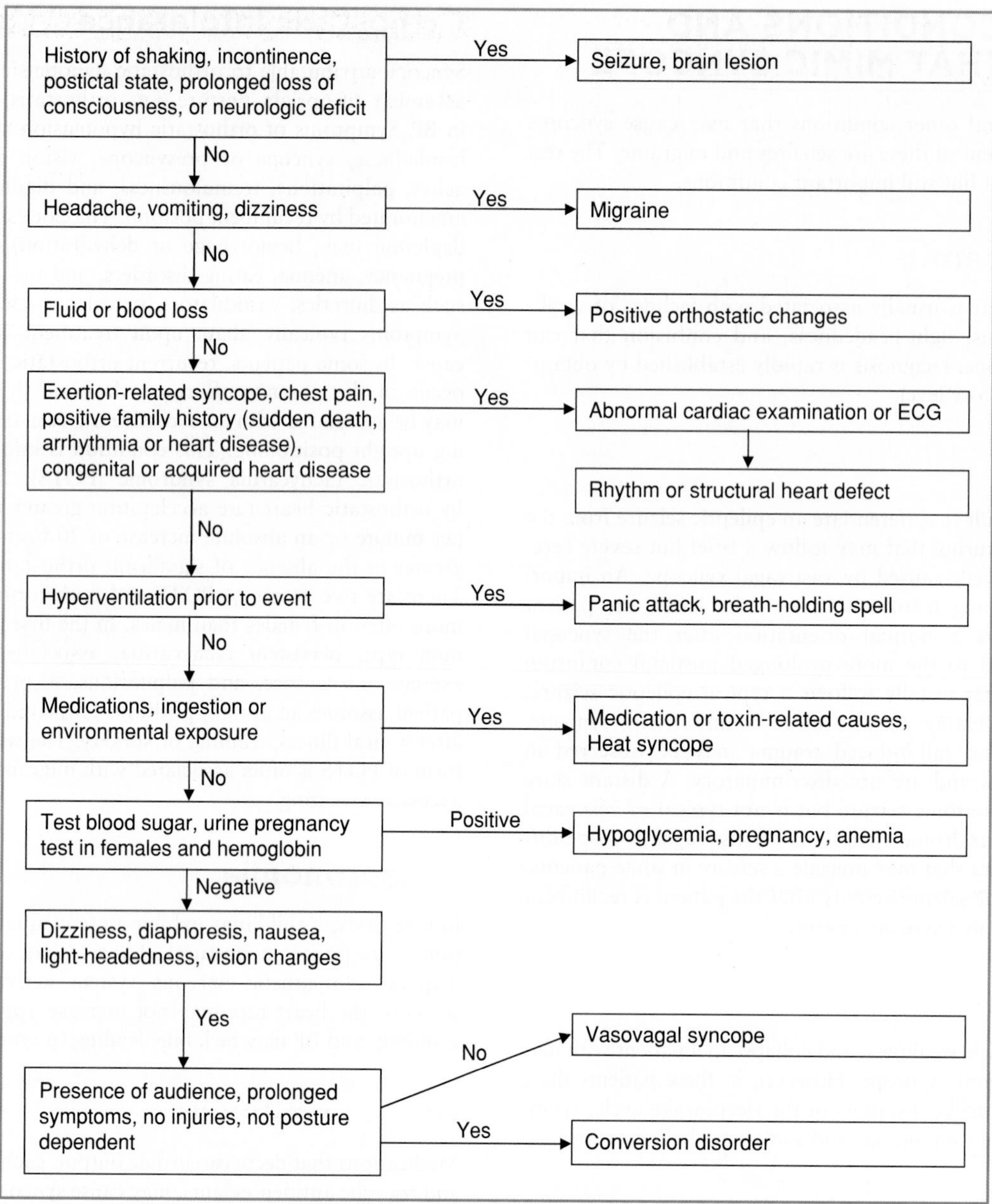

FIGURE 71.1 An approach to the diagnosis of pediatric syncope.

emotional stress, trauma, dehydration, and drug or medication intake. Exertion-related syncope suggests a cardiac cause. Sudden loud sounds or arousal may precipitate syncope in patients with long QT interval syndromes. In situational syncope, some specific activities such as stretching, arising suddenly from a recumbent position, swallowing, coughing, hair brushing, voiding, or defecation may be associated with loss of consciousness. Inquire about prodromal events such as pallor, light-headedness, sweating, vision changes, nausea, chest pain, palpitations, tinnitus, vertigo, diaphoresis, hyperventilation, or any aura. Sometimes a patient will anticipate a syncopal event and maneuver the body so as to avoid a sudden loss in postural tone. The presence of palpitations prior to the event may suggest a cardiac cause, but can also be seen in vasovagal syncope. Chest pain preceding syncope is almost never present in patients with primary electrical disorders of the heart but is more likely in patients with cardiomyopathies, congenital coronary artery abnormalities, or aortic disease (e.g., dissection or rupture associated with Marfan syndrome). With seizures, there may be posturing, clonic contractions or incontinence followed by postictal confusion, and the total time of the event is likely to be longer than that in a true syncope. Rarely, syncope may be severe enough to result in cardiopulmonary resuscitation, and any interventions by bystanders or emergency medical services should be discussed. Children and especially young athletes who have been outdoors for prolonged periods in warm weather may be at risk for dehydration and heat syncope. A history of drug ingestion (therapeutic or recreational use) should be elicited.

The *past medical history* may also provide information about the etiology for syncope. Patients may give a history of congenital heart disease, cardiac surgery or acquired conditions such as Kawasaki disease, rheumatic heart disease, myocarditis, or arrhythmia. Patients with seizure disorders, anemia, diabetes, or psychiatric conditions may also present with syncopal events. It is important to ask pubescent and adolescent girls about their menstrual history and the date of the last menstrual period, since pregnancy or dysfunctional uterine bleeding with resulting anemia may cause syncope. Adolescent patients with eating disorders may also present with syncope. Finally, ask about recent therapeutic or recreational drug use. Drugs that cause dehydration, heart rhythm disturbances, hypotension or mental status changes may be associated with syncope.

When inquiring about the *family history*, ask if there was a sudden death of any family member less than 50 years of age, any unexplained deaths, sudden infant death syndrome (SIDS), drowning, or motor vehicle crashes. Such events may occur in patients with LQTS or Brugada syndrome. Also ask for any family history of enlarged heart or heart rhythm problems, heart attack at age 50 or younger, pacemaker or implanted defibrillator, deafness at birth, hypercholesterolemia, Marfan syndrome, or unexplained fainting or seizures. A family history of vasovagal syncope may be present; genetic factors have been found to play a role in this disorder, though most cases follow complex patterns of inheritance and autosomal dominant inheritance, though possible, is rarely seen.

In most children with syncope, the *physical examination* is normal. The physical examination should focus on the vital signs, and the cardiac and neurologic examinations. Calculate the body mass index (BMI) in patients suspected with an eating disorder and inspect the patient for a Marfan disease body habitus. Check the patient for orthostatic changes as follows. Place the patient in the supine position for 2 minutes and then measure the BP and heart rate. Count the heart rate and respiratory rate for 1 minute. Next, make the patient stand for at least 1 minute and measure the BP and heart rate again. Observe for dizziness or light-headedness. If the patient is unable to stand, allow him or her to sit with the feet dangling for at least 2 minutes. The test is positive if the patient has any one of the following: systolic BP decreases >20 mm Hg; diastolic BP decreases >10 mm Hg or pulse increases >10 beats per minute; dizziness, syncope, or light-headedness. In the setting of hypovolemia, a positive test for orthostatic intolerance indicates a volume deficit of at least 10 to 15 mL/kg. The presence of orthostatic hypotension does not rule out other causes of syncope, particularly LQTS. During the cardiac examination, auscultate for the character of the heart sounds, abnormality in heart rhythm and the presence of a gallop, ejection clicks, rubs, or murmurs. Soft or muffled heart sounds may be heard with pericardial effusion. A loud second heart sound might point to pulmonary hypertension. Changing heart murmurs are observed in acute rheumatic carditis and a gallop may be auscultated in heart failure. Test the effect of maneuvers such as positional changes and holding the breath on the character of any heart murmur that is noted. The intensity of the ejection systolic murmur in HOCM decreases upon assuming a squatting position and increases with the Valsalva maneuver and upon standing. Search for signs of heart failure such as elevated jugular venous pressure, basilar lung crepitations, gallop, pathologic heart murmur, hepatomegaly, or edema. Finally, complete a full neurologic examination.

Electrocardiogram (ECG)

This is a very useful test in the diagnosis of cardiac causes of syncope and is recommended in all children who present with fainting or a similar event. Table 71.2 summarizes the ECG findings observed in important cardiac conditions that cause syncope. The 12-lead ECG provides information about both heart rhythm and atrioventricular (AV) conduction. Important findings include the delta wave signifying an accessory pathway and Wolff–Parkinson–White syndrome, a prolonged QT interval, high-grade ventricular ectopy, complete AV block, extremes of sinus, atrial, or junctional rates, and surface ECG changes specific for Brugada syndrome and increased QRS voltages with ST segment-T wave changes and deep Q waves in inferior and lateral leads in hypertrophic cardiomyopathy. Nonspecific ECG findings include moderate sinus arrhythmia, moderate sinus bradycardia, simple junctional rhythm, unifocal ventricular premature contractions, and right bundle branch block. Resting bradycardia may indicate drug ingestion, cardiac manifestation of eating disorders or central nervous system trauma, but can also be seen in healthy adolescents. Syncope is uncommon in patients with first- or second-degree heart block, but complete heart block can potentially lead to more serious symptoms. The combination of history, physical examination, and ECG allows identification of a cardiac cause of syncope in a majority of affected children, with reported sensitivity as high as 96%. Patients with clinical features or ECG findings suggestive of heart disease should be referred to a cardiologist.

TABLE 71.2

ECG FINDINGS IN IMPORTANT CARDIAC CAUSES OF PEDIATRIC SYNCOPE

Cause	ECG findings
Long QT syndrome	QT_c > 450 msec; morphology of QT segment and T wave may vary in different genetic subtypes
Brugada syndrome	Elevated ST segments in precordial leads V1 and V2. Coving seen in Type 1 syndrome; right bundle branch block
Wolff–Parkinson–White syndrome	Classic triad of delta wave, shortened PR interval, and widened QRS complex. There is a slurring in upstroke of R wave. Secondary ST-segment–T-wave changes are directed opposite to the major delta wave and QRS complex changes
Hypertrophic obstructive cardiomyopathy (HOCM)	The most frequent abnormalities found are large amplitude QRS complexes and associated ST-segment and T-wave changes consistent with left ventricular hypertrophy. Deep, narrow Q waves in leads II, III, aVF, V5, and V6 are most characteristic and specific findings of HOCM. Left atrial enlargement is also seen
Bradycardia	Second-degree and third-degree heart block

Other Tests

The patient should be placed on a continuous cardiac monitor to evaluate the heart rate and rhythm while in the ED. Routine use of screening blood tests in unselected pediatric patients with syncope will have a very poor diagnostic yield. Consider testing for hypoglycemia (via blood glucose), anemia (hemoglobin and hematocrit), pregnancy (urine pregnancy test), and recreational drugs (urine toxicology screen) in appropriate clinical scenarios. Check the serum chemistry in patients suspected to have electrolyte problems such as hypokalemia and hypocalcemia. Cardiac enzymes are not routinely recommended in pediatric patients with syncope. However, they may be necessary in an adolescent with chest pain or if the clinical evaluation suggests myocarditis or structural heart disease.

Echocardiography

The American Heart Association recommends the use of echocardiography only in patients with clinically suspected heart disease or exercise-induced syncope. In the absence of a history of exercise-induced syncope, positive family history, abnormal physical examination, or abnormal ECG, the echocardiogram does not contribute to the routine evaluation of pediatric syncope. However, the echocardiogram can identify underlying heart disease such as hypertrophic cardiomyopathy, aortic stenosis, or anomalous coronary arteries. It may suggest pulmonary hypertension if significant tricuspid regurgitation or right ventricular enlargement is present. Indications for an echocardiogram in a patient with syncope include known heart disease, pathologic murmur, evidence of chamber hypertrophy on ECG or chest radiograph, repolarization abnormalities with strain or ischemia, ventricular ectopy or concern for myocarditis, cardiomyopathy, or pulmonary hypertension.

Ambulatory ECG (Holter) monitoring may be useful if the screening ECG is normal but the history still suggests an arrhythmia as source of syncope, if there is exertional syncope, or if the relationship of a nonspecific ECG finding to symptoms is unclear. An *event recorder* is more practical because patients are able to keep the monitor for a month and use it at the time of their symptoms. The *stress test* may help in eliciting changes in QT intervals in patients with LQTS or arrhythmias in those with catecholaminergic polymorphic ventricular tachycardia but should be ordered by the cardiologist.

The *head-upright tilt table test (HUTT)* may be used to provoke a hypotensive episode that mimics the patient's symptoms. However, it has low sensitivity, and the results may not alter treatment. Some indications for use of this test are recurrent syncope or exertional syncope in which heart disease has been ruled out or recurrent syncopal episodes thought to be due to conversion disorder. *Implantable loop recorders* are small recording devices placed in a subcutaneous pocket and store retrospective ECG recording. They are used in patients with recurrent syncope in whom the diagnosis is uncertain despite conventional testing.

Neuroimaging is rarely required for a typical patient with syncope and the diagnostic yield is likely to be low. The only indication for neuroimaging is for a patient with focal neurologic deficits or persistently altered mental status in whom it is necessary to rule out significant intracranial injury or cerebrovascular accident. An *electroencephalogram (EEG)* may be performed on an outpatient basis if clinical features suggest a seizure and the patient has returned to a baseline neurologic status. However, it is important to remember that a normal EEG does not rule out epilepsy.

TREATMENT

Most children with syncope can be managed on an *outpatient* basis. Patients with vasovagal syncope and their families will need reassurance and education about the benign nature of the condition. They should be taught how to recognize prodromal symptoms. Maneuvers to prevent venous pooling (such as keeping the knees slightly bent when standing for a long time, isometric contraction of extremity muscles, toe raises, folding of the arms, and crossing of the legs) or even assuming a seated or supine position may help. Patients should be encouraged to increase their oral intake of water (up to 3 L per day in an adolescent), to add salty snacks to their diet, and to avoid consuming caffeinated beverages. If increased fluid and salt intake are not helpful, pharmacotherapy may be considered in patients with recurrent syncope. A variety of different medications have been tried in pediatric patients with recurrent syncope. Of these, midodrine, an α-adrenergic agonist, has shown some of the most beneficial results in reducing symptom recurrence with few side effects. Fludrocortisone, a mineralocorticoid, has also been used. However, recent studies have questioned its usefulness in preventing syncope and presyncope. Since depressive symptoms are common in these patients, management of depression may be beneficial. Also, selective serotonin reuptake inhibitors (SSRIs) may be useful in patients with coexisting anxiety or panic disorder.

The treatment of POTS requires education, hydration with clear, noncaffeinated beverages, increased salt intake, elevation of the head of the bed by 10 to 15 cm, and a gradual reconditioning exercise program spaced over 3 months.

Patients with recurrent symptoms who do not improve with conservative measures and pharmacotherapy and those with a suspected cardiac cause for syncope should be referred to a cardiologist for further management. Some situations may warrant hospital admission or observation of a child with syncope (Table 71.3), especially those involving persistent cardiovascular abnormalities or neurologic deficits.

For congenital LQTSs, the mainstay of therapy is the use of a long-acting beta blocker. Because syncope in these patients is adrenergically mediated, they are restricted from athletic activity. The use of an implantable cardioverter-defibrillator (ICD) is considered in a subgroup of patients felt to be at high risk for sudden death, such as those with symptoms before puberty, very long QT intervals (>500 msec), and those with recurrent syncope. The use of an ICD is also required in patients with hypertrophic cardiomyopathy and Brugada syndrome.

TABLE 71.3

CONDITIONS THAT MAY REQUIRE HOSPITALIZATION IN PEDIATRIC SYNCOPE

Abnormal cardiovascular examination and cardiovascular disease
Drug-related syncope
Attempted suicide
Neurologic
Persisting altered mental status
Focal neurologic deficits
Recurrent seizures
Recurrent hypoglycemia
Patients who require CPR
Orthostatic hypotension resistant to fluid therapy

CPR, cardiopulmonary resuscitation.

SUMMARY POINTS

Syncope is a common condition in children and is usually benign. Common causes for syncope include vasovagal syncope, breath-holding spells, and orthostatic intolerance. Life-threatening causes are usually cardiac in etiology. A comprehensive medical and family history, a thorough physical examination, and a 12-lead ECG will help identify most patients with life-threatening causes of syncope. Routine blood testing and imaging are unnecessary. Since recurrence is common, education and reassurance are important.

Suggested Readings and Key References

Goldenberg I, Moss AJ, Peterson DR, et al. Risk factors for aborted cardiac arrest and sudden cardiac death in children with the congenital long-QT syndrome. *Circulation* 2008;117: 2184–2191.

Grubb BP. Neurocardiogenic syncope. *N Eng J Med* 2005;352(10): 1004–1010.

Hobbs JB, Peterson DR, Moss AJ, et al. Risk of aborted cardiac arrest or sudden cardiac death during adolescence in the long-QT syndrome. *JAMA* 2006;296(10):1249–1254.

Morrow W, Berger S, Jenkins K, et al. Pediatric sudden cardiac arrest. *Pediatrics* 2012;129:e1094–e1102.

Pilcher TA, Saarel EV. A teenage fainter (dizziness, syncope, postural orthostatic tachycardia syndrome). *Pediatr Clin North Am* 2014;61(1):29–43.

Roden DM. Long-QT syndrome. *N Eng J Med* 2008;358:169–176.

Strickberger SA, Benson DW, Biaggioni I, et al. AHA/ACCF Scientific Statement on the evaluation of syncope. *Circulation* 2006;113: 316–327.

CHAPTER 72 ■ TACHYCARDIA

JAMES F. WILEY II, MD, MPH AND STEVEN C. ROGERS, MD

Fast heart rate or tachycardia is a common sign in children receiving emergency care. It may be noticed on initial evaluation by the emergency provider or may be raised as a concern by the caregiver who notes a rapid heart rate while holding the child or observes rapid jugular venous pulsations, increased apical heart rate, or pulse rate. The definition of tachycardia varies by age (callout to the table of normal vital signs in triage Chapter 73 Triage). In infants and young children, the higher resting heart rate, relative to older children, adolescents, and adults, reflects higher tissue oxygen utilization and metabolic rate. In most instances, the underlying cause for tachycardia in children is benign. However, children with a life-threatening etiology for their tachycardia require prompt recognition and treatment.

PATHOPHYSIOLOGY

Cardiac muscle has intrinsic automaticity that allows it to beat without any external stimulus. Resting heart rate typically reflects a balance of input from the vagus nerve (cranial nerve X) and the thoracic sympathetic ganglion (levels T1 to T4). Vagal stimulation results in slowing of the heart rate mediated by cholinergic receptors and has a greater impact on resting heart rate than on the sympathetic nervous system. Thus, medications with anticholinergic receptor effects (e.g., antihistamines, atropine) may cause tachycardia. Sympathetic stimulation results in increased heart rate and force of contraction primarily through the β_1-adrenergic receptors. These receptors may also be stimulated by circulating endogenous substances (e.g., epinephrine, increased carbon dioxide tension, hypoxemia) and by exogenous agents (e.g., sympathomimetic drugs).

Life-threatening cardiac tachyarrhythmias (e.g., supraventricular tachycardia [SVT], ventricular tachycardia) arise from various mechanisms that disrupt normal electrical conduction in the heart. The pathophysiology of these arrhythmias is discussed separately (see Chapter 94 Cardiac Emergencies).

DIFFERENTIAL DIAGNOSIS

Many conditions may produce tachycardia (Table 72.1). Most tachycardic children exhibit sinus tachycardia without significant cardiac pathology (Table 72.2). However, life-threatening conditions frequently come to medical attention because of fast heart rate and may reflect cardiac and noncardiac origins (Table 72.3).

Sinus Tachycardia

Fever, pain, and emotional arousal (e.g., crying, anxiety) are the most frequent causes of sinus tachycardia in children. Sympathetic stimulation from other conditions such as hypoxemia, hypoglycemia, hypercarbia, anemia, and excess circulating catecholamines (e.g., hyperthyroidism, pheochromocytoma) also increases SA node firing rate (Table 72.2). In addition, exogenous sympathomimetic or anticholinergic substances may cause sinus tachycardia. Over-the-counter medications that contain antihistamines or pseudoephedrine, "energy" drinks and diet pills that have high concentrations of caffeine, and commonly abused drugs (cocaine, amphetamines, methcathinones [e.g., bath salts], or synthetic cannabinoids [e.g., K2, Spice]) are frequently implicated (see Table 58.4).

Shock is a life-threatening cause of sinus tachycardia that requires rapid recognition and reversal to prevent permanent organ damage or death (see Chapter 5 Shock). Circulatory shock may result from intravascular volume loss, inadequate cardiac contractility, a marked drop in systemic vascular resistance, or a combination of these mechanisms. Physical findings help differentiate the different forms of shock (hypovolemic, cardiogenic, septic, and distributive) and identify the underlying cause.

Life-threatening Tachyarrhythmias

SVT represents the most common tachyarrhythmia of childhood (see Chapter 94 Cardiac Emergencies). The typical heart rate in infants with SVT exceeds 220 beats per minute, whereas older children usually have a heart rate in excess of 180 beats per minute. Infants and children with SVT demonstrate a spectrum of physical signs including no symptoms, palpitations, chest pain, tachypnea (often with feeding in infants), diaphoresis, and severe cardiogenic shock.

The most common form of SVT involves an accessory AV pathway. Additional etiologies include drug exposure, congenital heart disease, and Wolff–Parkinson–White syndrome. Sympathomimetics in cough and cold preparations are the most common drugs to incite SVT in children. Over-the-counter cough and cold preparations should not be used in children younger than 5 years of age. Unregulated dietary supplements such as ephedra (and its congeners, often advertised as "ephedra-free" products) and high-caffeine energy drinks also have the potential to precipitate SVT. Cardiac lesions associated with SVT include Ebstein anomaly, repaired dextrotransposition of the great arteries, and single-ventricle lesions status post-Fontan operation.

Ventricular tachycardia (monomorphic or polymorphic/torsades de pointes) and atrial flutter rarely occur in children (see Chapter 94 Cardiac Emergencies). Congenital heart disease, electrolyte disturbance (especially hyperkalemia, hypocalcemia, and hypomagnesemia), genetic predisposition (long QT syndromes), or poisoning accounts for most cases of ventricular tachycardia in children. Atrial flutter usually arises from an intra-atrial reentry circuit. Most children with atrial flutter have congenital heart disease. Although rare, atrial flutter

TABLE 72.1

DIFFERENTIAL DIAGNOSIS OF TACHYCARDIA

Sinus tachycardia
Fever
Crying
Pain
Hypoglycemia
Hypoxemia
Hypercarbia
Shock
Anemia
Poisoning (see Table 58.4)
Sepsis
Anaphylaxis
Hyperthyroidism
Pheochromocytoma
Drug induced (e.g., antihistamines, caffeine, dietary supplements)
Anxiety
Life-threatening cardiac tachyarrhythmias
Supraventricular tachycardia
Atrial flutter
Ventricular tachycardia (monomorphic and polymorphic/torsades de pointes)
Other cardiac causes
Myocarditis
Acute rheumatic fever
Kawasaki disease
Pericardial effusion with tamponade

carries a significant risk of sudden death if not controlled by medications or surgical intervention.

Other Cardiac Causes

Cardiac inflammation associated with viral myocarditis, acute rheumatic fever, or Kawasaki syndrome frequently presents with sinus tachycardia (see Chapter 94 Cardiac Emergencies). Patients with these conditions, especially myocarditis, are also at risk for life-threatening arrhythmias, myocardial ischemia, congestive heart failure, and/or cardiogenic shock. For patients with pericardial effusion, sinus tachycardia is a physiologic response to impaired cardiac outflow in order to maintain cardiac output

TABLE 72.2

COMMON CAUSES OF TACHYCARDIA

Fever
Pain
Crying
Anxiety
Anemia
Drug induced (e.g., caffeine, herbal medications, dietary supplements, illicit drugs)
Hypovolemic shock

TABLE 72.3

LIFE-THREATENING CAUSES OF TACHYCARDIA

Sinus tachycardia
Anaphylaxis
Hypoxia
Hypoglycemia
Sepsis
Shock
Pheochromocytoma
Poisoning (see Table 58.4)
Cardiac
Supraventricular tachycardia
Ventricular tachyarrhythmias
Atrial flutter
Other cardiac causes
Myocarditis
Pericardial effusion with tamponade

(see Chapter 94 Cardiac Emergencies). Pericardial effusion with tamponade may complicate pericarditis, blunt chest trauma, or recent cardiac surgery and results in decreased cardiac output with significant impairment of systemic circulation. In this setting, pericardiocentesis or surgical pericardiotomy is lifesaving (see Chapter 123 Thoracic Trauma).

EVALUATION AND DECISION

The child with tachycardia requires rapid assessment for the presence of hypoxia, hypoglycemia, an existing life-threatening arrhythmia, or shock (Fig. 72.1). Respiratory distress with cyanosis or low pulse oximetry (less than 90%) demands immediate provision of supplemental oxygen and further management of airway and breathing (see Chapters 3 Airway and 107 Pulmonary Emergencies). Hypoglycemia typically presents with altered mental status, diaphoresis, and/or hypertension and can be confirmed by measuring rapid blood glucose level. If an arrhythmia is suggested by an extremely rapid heart rate or a concerning tracing on the bedside cardiac monitor, a 12-lead electrocardiogram (EKG) and rhythm strip are necessary to confirm this impression and to guide further treatment (see Chapter 94 Cardiac Emergencies). Children with congenital heart disease or a family history of sudden death are at increased risk for a life-threatening tachyarrhythmia. Consultation with a pediatric cardiologist and emergent echocardiography are warranted. In patients with shock, additional history and physical findings help guide the clinician. Although the etiology may not be initially apparent, rapid treatment is imperative (see Fig. 5.3).

Children with fever and sinus tachycardia typically have a self-limited febrile illness. However, fever is also present in patients with cardiac pathology, including myocarditis, pericardial effusion, Kawasaki syndrome, and acute rheumatic fever, as well as in rare patients with thyroid storm. Myocarditis describes inflammation of the muscle wall of the heart. Clinical features of this disease are fever, tachycardia out of proportion to the activity or degree of fever, pallor, cyanosis, respiratory distress secondary to pulmonary edema, muffled

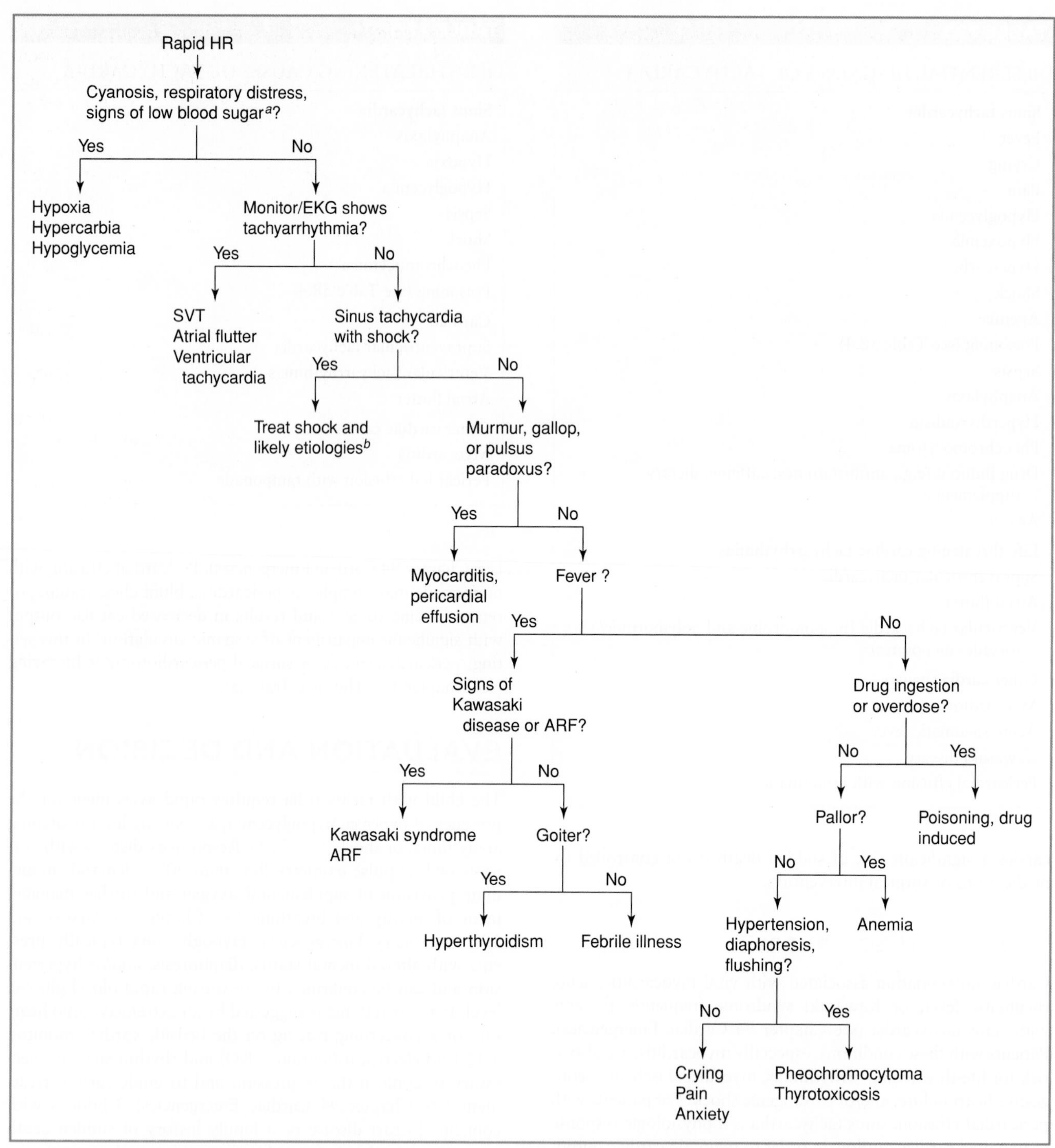

FIGURE 72.1 A diagnostic approach to tachycardia. [a]Altered mental status, diaphoresis, hypertension. [b]See Chapter 5, Shock. HR, heart rate; EKG, electrocardiogram; SVT, supraventricular tachycardia; ARF, acute rheumatic fever.

heart sounds with gallop, and hepatomegaly caused by passive congestion of the liver (see Chapter 94 Cardiac Emergencies). A child with tachycardia and clinical findings suggestive of myocarditis requires emergent supportive care (see Chapter 1 A General Approach to Ill and Injured Children), echocardiography, and admission to a unit capable of intensive monitoring and rapid treatment of cardiac arrhythmias and hemodynamic instability.

Pericardial effusion may occur after blunt chest trauma, viral infection, or as a component of inflammatory diseases such as systemic lupus erythematosus. Small effusions may be detected as a friction rub. Large effusions often cause cardiogenic shock and may lead to muffling of heart sounds and EKG changes, such as low-voltage or T-wave flattening with "strain" pattern in leads V1 through V6, but are nonspecific. Pericardial effusions are best identified using ultrasound. Patients with evidence of significant circulatory impairment should undergo a pericardial drainage procedure (e.g., placement of a pericardial catheter percutaneously under ultrasound guidance, pericardial window procedure).

Acute rheumatic fever follows pharyngeal streptococcal infection and is an inflammatory disease that targets the heart, vessels, joints, skin, and central nervous system (CNS). Diagnosis and management of acute rheumatic fever are discussed separately (see Chapter 94 Cardiac Emergencies). Clinical criteria for Kawasaki disease consist of prolonged high fever, conjunctivitis with perilimbic sparing, strawberry tongue, painful swelling of the hands and feet, rash, and lymphadenopathy. Early recognition and treatment of Kawasaki disease with intravenous γ-globulin is necessary to prevent the development of coronary artery aneurysms with potential for myocardial ischemia (see Chapter 109 Rheumatologic Emergencies).

Patients with thyroid storm may have marked sinus tachycardia, fever, goiter, and CNS stimulation (agitation, delirium, psychosis, seizures) accompanied by congestive heart failure (see Chapter 97 Endocrine Emergencies). Trauma, thyroid infection, thyroid surgery, and acute iodine load are frequent precipitants. Rapid recognition and institution of therapy to treat adrenergic symptoms (β-adrenergic blockers), block hormone synthesis (methimazole), prevent peripheral conversion of T4 to T3 (iodinated radiocontrast agents), and prevent thyroid hormone release (iodine) are necessary to prevent mortality.

Crying, pain, or anxiety is the most frequent cause of sinus tachycardia in afebrile children. Drug ingestion, poisoning, and anemia are important additional considerations (see Table 58.4). Rarely, sinus tachycardia may herald the presence of hyperthyroidism or pheochromocytoma, a catecholamine-secreting tumor that causes extreme hypertension, diaphoresis, and flushing (see Chapter 97 Endocrine Emergencies).

Suggested Readings and Key References

Doniger SJ, Sharieff GQ. Pediatric dysrhythmias. *Pediatr Clin North Am* 2006;53:85–105.

Manole MD, Saladino RA. Emergency department management of the pediatric patient with supraventricular tachycardia. *Pediatr Emerg Care* 2007;23(3):176–185.

Mazor S, Mazor R. Approach to the child with tachycardia. UpToDate. www.uptodate.com. Accessed on May 20, 2014.

Warrick BJ, Hill M, Hekman K, et al. A 9-state analysis of designer stimulant, "bath salt," hospital visits reported to poison control centers. *Ann Emerg Med* 2013;62:244–251.

Woods WA, McCulloch MA. Cardiovascular emergencies in the pediatric patient. *Emerg Med Clin North Am* 2005;23:1233–1249.

CHAPTER 73 ■ TRIAGE

DEBRA A. POTTS, MSN, RN, CPEN, CEN AND MARY KATE FUNARI, MSN, RN, CPEN

INTRODUCTION

Children are cared for in all emergency departments (EDs) from general EDs that see primarily adult patients to those general EDs with a separate pediatric section to pediatric EDs that exist within a pediatric institution. In the last two decades there has been a considerable increase in ED visits in the United States, a fourth of these visits by children. In 2010, there were 25.5-million ED visits for children less than 18 years of age. As the health burden on emergency services continues to rise it is critical to have a reliable method of triaging children presenting for services.

HISTORY OF TRIAGE

The term "triage" derived from the French word "trier," to sort, was first used back in the 18th century to document the severity of injury in warfare. Battlefield triage eventually made its way into the American medical system and in 1964 Wasserman et al. published the first use of civilian triage in EDs. Subsequently many institutions, federal agencies, and emergency medical systems have continued to study and refine triage systems in the United States.

CURRENT TRIAGE SYSTEMS

Pediatric triage requires rapid assessment of those presenting to the ED including determination of severity of illness or injury, assignment of acuity level, and anticipation of appropriate emergency care resources needed. With limited resources available, the goal of the triage process is "right patient, right provider, right care, right time," which demands a standardized approach. The American College of Emergency Physicians and the Emergency Nurses Association have recommended that EDs use a reliable and valid five-level triage system for prioritizing the care of children presenting to the ED. In 2010, the ACEP and ENA based on expert consensus of currently available evidence supported the adoption of a reliable, valid five-level triage system such as the Emergency Severity Index (ESI). Following the release of this position statement, the number of EDs using the five-level ESI triage system increased significantly.

Comprehensive triage has been the dominant model for assigning triage acuity in US EDs. Triage acuity systems have been based on the nurse's assessment of vital signs and physical examination along with subjective information including past medical history, medications, allergies, and history of the presenting complaint. These systems require the nurse to assign an acuity level by determining how acutely ill the patient is and how long they can wait to be seen by a provider.

The ESI is a five-level triage system developed by a group of emergency physicians and nurses in the late 1990s. The ESI is distinctive in its method of triage as it integrates both acuity and resource utilization. This system relies on nursing judgment for the more acutely ill patients (ESI levels 1 and 2), while asking nurses to assign lesser acuities (ESI levels 3 to 5) to the less acutely ill by predicting the number of resources such as diagnostic tests and procedures each patient will need in determining disposition. Triage nurses follow an algorithm for determining acuity (Fig. 73.1). The nurse answers specific questions for determining the more acutely ill at points A and B. Point B takes into consideration special high-risk conditions in pediatrics (Table 73.1). If the child is determined to be less acute, direction is given to what constitutes a resource and nurses are only required to estimate up to two resources (Table 73.2). Multiple studies of general ED populations have validated the ESI triage system with good interrater reliability and the ability to estimate ED resources when triage was performed by experienced and trained ED nurses.

The ESI has continually been validated and improved upon through research. ESI version 4 (2012 edition) was born out of the Pediatric ESI Research Consortium's large, multicenter study on pediatric triage and a comprehensive review of pediatric emergency courses and textbooks. Improvements to ESI included a designated chapter on pediatric triage and more pediatric triage case scenarios for educational use.

In 2009 the American Hospital Association reported that 57% of US hospitals were using the ESI triage system. Standardization of triage systems across the United States will allow for increased sharing of ED data and setting performance metrics for care. Establishing a standard for triage acuity assessment will further facilitate benchmarking, public health surveillance, and research.

The Center for Disease Control and Prevention National Center for Health Statistics reports national level data on ED visits. The report categorizes patients in five levels on how urgently they need to be seen by a provider and includes immediate (immediately), emergent (1 to 14 minutes), urgent (15 to 60 minutes), semi-urgent (1 to 2 hours), nonurgent (2 to 24 hours). While there is no research to support this classification it allows for sharing of national level data on acuity mix when patients present to the ED.

PEDIATRIC TRIAGE CONSIDERATIONS

The triage nurse needs a solid foundation of knowledge related to specific anatomic and physiologic issues that may put a child at risk, as well as age-dependent "red flags" that

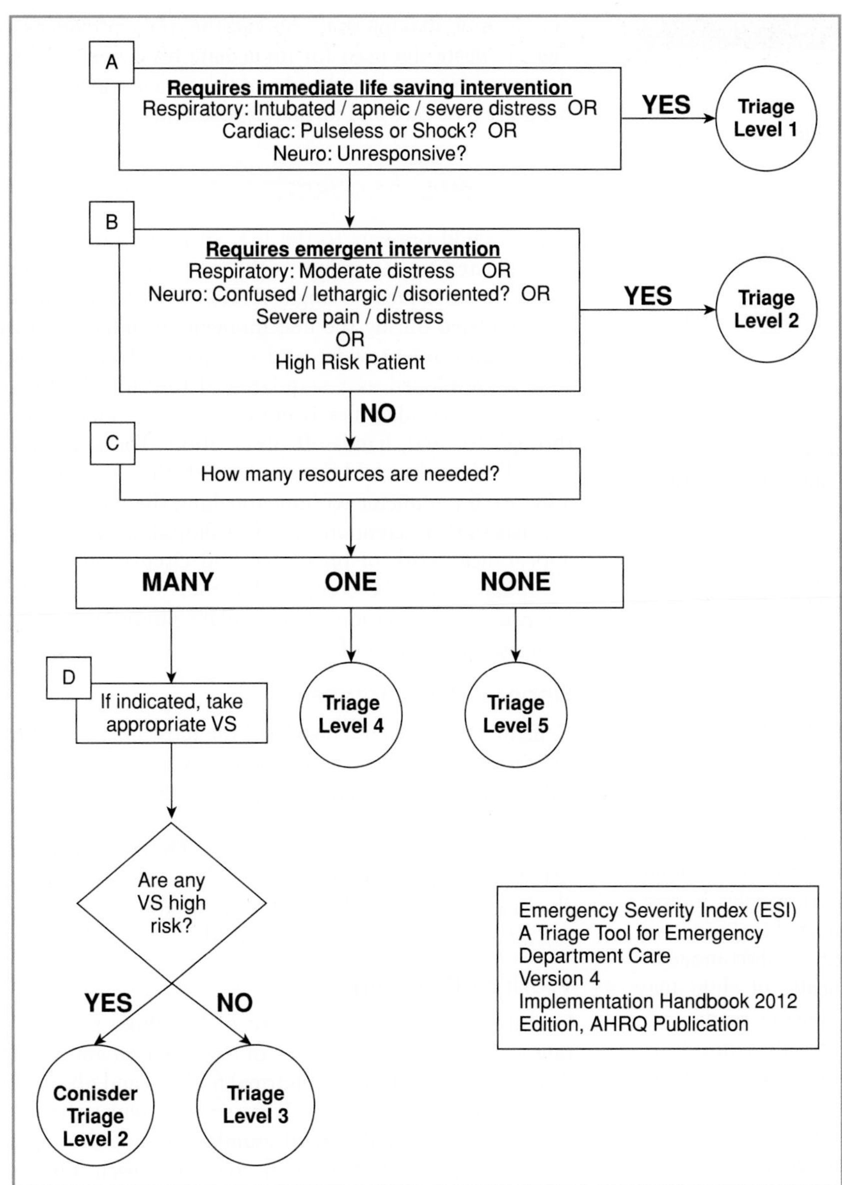

FIGURE 73.1 ESI triage algorithm.

TABLE 73.1

HIGH-RISK PATIENTS

• Hematology/oncology patient with fever	• Sickle cell patient with fever or pain
• Shunt patient with headache, nausea/vomiting, and/or fever	• Cardiac patient with change in normal saturation and/or increased need for O_2
• Diabetic with altered mental status, ± nausea/vomiting	• Infants ≤60 days with fever/hypothermia (temp ≤36°C or ≥38°C rectal by history or in ED)
• Bleeding disorder with significant trauma	• Eye injury with significant pain
• Ocular exposure	• Scrotal pain
• Posttonsillectomy and adenoidectomy bleed	• Apparent life-threatening event with history of cyanosis
• Suicidal ideation or attempt	• Ingestions (excluding foreign body)—consult ED physician for non–foreign-body ingestions
• Gastrostomy tube or gastrojejunal tube out and unable to place Foley in stoma in triage	• Cervical spine immobilized and on backboard
• Smoke inhalation/carbon monoxide exposure	• Abdominal trauma with significant abdominal pain
• Open fracture or altered neurovascular status with deformity	• Permanent tooth available for reimplantation
• Abdominal pain with peritoneal signs	

TABLE 73.2

TRIAGE RESOURCES

Aerosol treatments	Specialty consultation
IV or IM medications	IV fluids
Labs (blood, urine, cultures)	NG tube
X-rays	Simple procedure = 1 (Laceration or Foley)
ECG	Complex procedure = 2 (sedation)
CT or ultrasound	

must be considered during triage. The nurse should also be comfortable interacting with children of all ages. The following are key points when assessing a child:

1. Children have a larger body surface area than adults. This places them at risk for both heat and fluid loss.
2. Neonates have poor thermoregulation. They should not be undressed for any extended length of time as this cold stress causes increased metabolic demands resulting in potential physiologic decompensation.
3. Critically ill neonates/children can present with subtle signs such as hypothermia, poor feeding, and irritability.
4. Cardiac output is heart rate dependent in neonates and young children. Bradycardia or severe tachycardia can be very dangerous. Hypotension is a late finding.
5. Weight in kilograms is important in order to safely administer medications to children. Estimation of weights in critically ill children should be done with validated tools and estimated guesses by providers and caregivers are discouraged.
6. Children are portable. The most critically ill child may arrive being carried into your ED, you must be ready.
7. Caregivers' perception of illness is key. Providers must listen as caregivers know their children best and can explain when behavior is abnormal.
8. Triage nurses must be aware of risk factors for abuse. Anything that stresses a family puts children at risk such as lower socioeconomic levels, history of substance abuse, history of mental illness, and single caregiver households. Young children as well as children with chronic illness or disabilities are at increased risk. The nurse's knowledge of child development is very important when assessing injuries. The nurse needs to assess if the injuries can be explained knowing the current developmental level of the child.

Triage Process

As previously described, triage is fundamental in determining the severity of illness and immediate needs of a patient who presents to the ED. The pediatric triage process consists of a rapid initial assessment, primary survey, secondary survey, and triage decision. Ideally, triage should take no more than 3 to 5 minutes. Documentation of triage findings and interventions as well as reassessment of patients in the waiting room is also included in triage workflow. Care of pediatric patients requires a core understanding of developmental stages and their associated risk factors, injury and illness patterns, and physiologic compensatory mechanisms. As such, the triage process should be completed only by ED nurses experienced in pediatric patients who demonstrate sound assessment, clinical judgment, and decision-making skills. Should the triage provider's assessment indicate the need for immediate lifesaving intervention, the triage process should end and the patient moved to a treatment area for care and further assessment.

Pediatric Assessment Triangle

Once a child presents to the ED, an initial rapid assessment is conducted to determine "sick" or "not sick" utilizing the pediatric assessment triangle (PAT). This assessment should be completed during the first moments of interaction by any level healthcare provider and is separate from the primary survey. Developed as a standardized tool for children of all ages, the PAT identifies overall severity of illness or injury through focused, hands-off observation. The triage provider should allow the child to remain with their caregiver, evaluating each parameter without touching the patient. The PAT consists of three components of cardiopulmonary assessment: appearance, work of breathing, and circulation to the skin. Examination can be completed within 30 seconds, allowing for prompt recognition of immediate physiologic needs and their associated level of urgency.

General Appearance

General appearance is considered the most important factor in the assessment of a pediatric patient. While a child may meet "alert" criteria on the AVPU responsiveness scale, they can also display subtle signs of illness, injury, and deterioration through alterations in their general appearance. The mnemonic "tickles" (TICLS) should be utilized to identify deviations from normal characteristics through evaluation of tone, interactiveness, consolability, look/gaze, and speech/cry (Table 73.3).

Work of Breathing

In children, assessment of work of breathing provides accurate insight into the adequacy of oxygenation and ventilation through identification of abnormal findings and observation of compensatory mechanisms. The triage provider should listen from a distance for abnormal sounds including snoring, grunting, wheezing, and changes in voice or speech. Observation should include assessment of patient positioning, the presence and location of chest wall retractions, and nasal flaring.

Circulation to the Skin

Assessment of circulation to the skin reflects the integrity of vital organ perfusion. The child's skin should be exposed by the parent in a warm environment and visual examination performed, evaluating for pallor, mottling, cyanosis, and visible active bleeding.

TABLE 73.3

TICLS MNEMONIC

Tone	Moves spontaneously, sits or stands as age appropriate
Interactivity	Interacts with people, environment, objects
Consolability	Stops crying with comfort by caregiver
Look/gaze	Tracks objects, makes eye contact
Speech/cry	Age-appropriate speech or strong cry

Adapted from APLS: The Pediatric Emergency Medicine Resource, 5th Ed., 2012, American College of Emergency Physicians. Jones and Bartlett.

TABLE 73.4

TRIAGE "RED FLAGS"

Airway	Apnea, stridor, hoarse voice/cry, drooling, choking, gurgling, sniffing position, hypoxemia
Breathing	Increased work of breathing, retractions, grunting, nasal flaring, seesaw respirations, head bobbing, adventitious breath sounds, tripoding
Circulation	Tachycardia, bradycardia, hypotension, capillary refill >3 s or <1 s, decreased pulses, bounding pulses, cyanosis, mottling, uncontrolled bleeding
Disability	Altered level of consciousness, inconsolable crying, abnormal pupillary reaction, hypoglycemia
Exposure	Hypothermia, hyperthermia >105.1°F, rash (petechial, purpura), signs of abuse

Primary Survey

Once the overall urgency of care is determined through the PAT, the triage provider should complete a more detailed assessment of the patient's airway, breathing, circulation, disability, and exposure. This examination should be done in the specified order so that life-threatening findings are systematically identified and the patient immediately moved for appropriate intervention. As a general rule, any pediatric assessment should be completed from least invasive to most invasive to keep the child calm and allow for accurate assessment. Permit the child to remain as close as possible to their care provider, utilizing developmentally appropriate instruction and distraction to increase comfort, cooperation, and trust. Table 73.4 outlines the goals and "red flag" signs and symptoms of the primary survey.

Secondary Survey

The triage secondary survey centers on obtaining pertinent information about the patient's presentation to the ED and past medical history, with an additional focused physical assessment based on chief complaint. The patient's chief complaint is the subjective reason for visit provided by the patient or care provider. History taking in triage must be brief, with data obtained from the child's accompanying care provider, or the child if possible. Adolescents should be interviewed separately when presenting with mental health or sexual complaints. The secondary survey should also include an initial pain assessment utilizing developmentally appropriate scoring tools.

CIAMPEDS

The mnemonic CIAMPEDS provides a systematic approach to triage history taking. Information gathered helps the triage nurse determine potential triage interventions, isolation requirements, special needs, and triage acuity (Table 73.5).

TABLE 73.5

CIAMPEDS

C	**Chief complaint**
I	**Immunizations and isolation** *(assess need for)*
A	**Allergies** *(food, medications, dyes, latex, blood)*
M	**Medications** *(current)*
P	**Past medical history**
E	**Events surrounding the illness or injury**
D	**Diet and diapers** *(PO intake and urine output)*
S	**Symptoms associated with illness or injury**

Focused Physical and Pain Assessments

Comprehensive physical assessment is not warranted during the triage process as it prolongs the triage evaluation and delays definitive care. Once a chief complaint is determined, a focused physical assessment of the affected area(s) should be completed as abnormal findings often impact patient triage care and acuity. For instance, a distended, rigid abdomen or a decreased distal pulse in an injured extremity warrants expedited physician evaluation, and therefore, higher triage acuity. Pain assessment is incorporated into the triage secondary assessment to provide a baseline for the ED visit, and to assess for necessary triage intervention.

Vital Signs

Vital signs assessment during the triage process can provide key indicators as to the severity of illness and compensatory status of the pediatric patient. Table 73.6 depicts normal vital sign parameters by age as drawn from current existing literature. Pediatric vital signs should be assessed utilizing appropriately sized equipment to ensure accuracy in values. Blood pressure assessment should be based on nursing judgment as to patient need as it is not a critical factor in acuity assignment. As fever can impact acuity for numerous pediatric populations including neonates, immunocompromised and sickle cell patients, temperature should be evaluated during the triage process. Consistency, accuracy, and duration should determine the appropriate temperature assessment method. Higher acuity should be considered in patients with tachycardia without fever, or tachycardia outside expected range for fever (every degree Celsius rise in temperature should only show a 10% rise in heart rate). Pulse oximetry should be taken on patients who present with respiratory or cardiac complaints. If one vital sign parameter is abnormal, it is important to obtain a full set to determine appropriate acuity assignment.

TABLE 73.6

HIGH-RISK VITAL SIGNS

Age	Respiratory rate	Heart rate
<6 mo	>60	>180
6–12 mo	>50	>160
1–2 yrs	>40	>160
2–8 yrs	>30	>140
>8 yrs	>20	>100

Oxygen saturation <92%; capillary refill >2 seconds.

SIGNS AND SYMPTOMS

Triage Decision

Information gathered during the aforementioned aspects of the triage process is synthesized during this stage to provide appropriate triage interventions and assignment of acuity. The initiation of protocols in triage can help expedite patient care, improve ED flow, and positively impact patient/family satisfaction. Triage interventions are delineated by hospital and state protocols. Examples include administration of analgesia or antipyretics, initiation of NPO status or PO challenge, application of ice or basic splints, point of care testing, EKGs, simple wound care, x-ray orders, or clinical care pathways. Triage interventions should be agreed upon and clearly defined in departmental policy and procedure manuals. Isolation needs should also be addressed during this phase of triage if a patient is immunocompromised or suspected to have an infectious disease process. Once appropriate care is provided, the patient acuity should be assigned based upon the triage classification system utilized in the facility's ED. As previously mentioned, this acuity will determine the patient's priority and appropriate location of care.

Triage Documentation

Patient acuity, chief complaint, and pertinent subjective and objective data gathered during the triage process should be recorded in an organized fashion in the medical record, allowing for baseline patient information and triage decision-making factors to be shared with all necessary staff. Any triage care intervention should also be clearly charted. Additional documentation may be required per hospital or governmental standards. As safe pediatric care requires weight-based dosing, patients should have their weight obtained and recorded in kilograms.

Reassessment

With ever increasing ED crowding, patients often must wait to see a provider after triage is completed. Patients in the waiting room should be reassessed for progression of illness or injury and response to triage interventions. Individual departments should institute a reexamination plan based upon their available resources and patient flow, keeping in mind that assessment itself is strictly a nursing function, and cannot be delegated to unlicensed support staff.

EMTALA

To ensure appropriate access to emergency services, Congress passed the Emergency Medical Treatment and Active Labor Act (EMTALA) as part of the Consolidated Omnibus Budget Reconciliation Act (COBRA) in 1986. EMTALA requires all hospitals participating in Medicare programs to provide a medical screening examination (MSE) to each patient who presents to the facility requesting examination or treatment for an emergency medical condition (EMC) regardless of ability to pay, legal status, or citizenship. The MSE must be completed by a physician or qualified medical personnel (e.g., approved member of medical staff). An EMC is that which places the individual's health, organs, or bodily functions at serious risk. Once an EMC is identified, stabilizing treatment must be provided. If the facility is unequipped to appropriately stabilize, transfer to a higher level of care should occur with the patient, legal guardian, or power of attorney's consent. There are numerous directives which address discrimination, appropriate treatment area signage, insurance gathering, compliance reporting, and documentation standards. As such, participating hospitals should clearly address each EMTALA requirement in institutional policies and procedures. Triage nurses and emergency room medical staff should have a sound understanding of current EMTALA guidelines and institutional practices to ensure continued compliance.

TRENDS IN TRIAGE

Quality indicators including efficiency and effectiveness are often used in EDs. The overarching goal is to improve patient throughput while decreasing left-without-being-seen (LWBS) rates. Recognizing the need to improve throughput in pediatric EDs, the Child Health Corporation of America Emergency Department group set a national goal to decrease length of stay (LOS) in pediatric EDs by 25%. Outcome measures in ED LOS are segmented into door-provider, provider-decision, and decision to discharge or admit time. Some of the process measures suggested to expedite care in the ED include quick triage and registration and the use of a fast track area. Additionally, concepts including split flow, immediate bedding, and provider in triage have been implemented by some departments to help augment flow and ensure the appropriate resource and location for patients.

Split Flow

Designed to reduce wait times through immediate patient assessment, split flow expedites the care of the sickest patients while facilitating the flow of nonurgent patients who present to the ED. Patients are evaluated by a triage nurse during the initial registration process to determine their specific needs. They are then directed to an appropriate care location based upon their acuity and potential resource needs. This accelerates treatment and admission for acute patients, and decreases the LOS for those with nonurgent complaints. A shortened triage process can also be coupled with the split-flow concept to decrease intake times for less acute patients as well.

Immediate Bedding

Historically, the triage intake process occurs in a designated triage area, prior to patient bedding. To decrease time to provider, and improve the customer experience, the concept of immediate bedding has been applied in some EDs. Once a patient presents to the ED and completes their initial registration and screening process, a triage nurse directs them to their appropriate care area if a bed is available. In bypassing formal triage, unnecessary patient movement is decreased, and the provider and primary nurse are able to assess the patient at the bedside. The required elements of triage are then completed at the bedside, and appropriate care interventions initiated. Should no bed be available, normal triage processes in the waiting area would be followed.

Provider in Triage

Placement of a front-line provider in the triage intake area can help to expedite patient care and decrease LOS. Such providers can initiate care protocols and testing for those awaiting ED room placement, or could treat and discharge lower acuity patients from the waiting area itself. Level of care and interventions will depend upon the credentials of the provider (attending physician, nurse practitioner, or physician's assistant) and available team members and resources.

CONCLUSION

Children presenting to EDs bring unique challenges to the triage process. Utilizing a standardized approach, such as the validated AHRQ ESI triage tool, can improve the safe passage of the pediatric patient and family through triage. A pediatric triage nurse must be aware of the different patient–family care dynamics, communication challenges, developmental, physical, and environmental needs of children. A comprehensive triage orientation includes both didactic and hands-on review of pediatric considerations, the overall triage process, and accurate assignment of acuity. Additionally, a quality assurance and improvement program should monitor triage accuracy. Consideration should also be given to patient flow processes through triage to ensure "right patient, right provider, and right time." The triage nurse has a critical responsibility for quality and safety of the patient that begins at the time of patient entry to the ED. Triage nurses must have experience, and advanced assessment and critical thinking skills. Ideally, they are allotted time to participate in continuous quality improvement initiatives focused on the triage process.

Suggested Readings and Key References

American College of Emergency Physicians. Emergency Nurses Association. Joint Statement by the American College of Emergency Physicians (ACEP) and the Emergency Nurses Association (ENA): Triage Scale Standardization. Irving, TX: American College of Emergency Physicians; 2010.

Centers for Medicare and Medicaid Services. *Emergency medical treatment & labor act (EMTALA)*. CMS-1063F.

Chameides L, Sampson R, Schexnayder S, et al., eds. *Pediatric advance life support provider manual*. Dallas, TX: Amer Heart Association, 2011.

Dieckmann RA, Brownstein D, Gausche-Hill M. The pediatric assessment triangle: a novel approach for the rapid evaluation of children. *Pediatr Emerg Care* 2010;26(4):312–315.

Doyle SL, Kingsnorth J, Guzzetta C, et al. Outcomes of implementing rapid triage in the pediatric emergency department. *J Emerg Nurs* 2012;38:30–35.

ENA position statement. Holding, crowding, and patient flow. 2014. Available at https://www.ena.org/SiteCollectionDocuments/Position%20Statements/Holding.pdf

Fernades CB, Groth SJ, Johnson LA, et al. *A uniform triage scale in emergency medicine*. Dallas, TX: American College of Emergency Physicians, 1999.

Fernandes CM, Tanabe P, Gilboy N, et al. Five-level triage: a report from the ACEP/ENA five-level triage task force. *J Emerg Nurs* 2005; 31:39–50.

Fultz J, Sturt P, eds. Triage. In: *Mosby's emergency nursing reference*. 3rd ed. Missouri, MO: Elsevier Mosby; 2005:86–100.

Gilboy N, Tanabe P, Travers D. The emergency severity index version 4: changes to ESI level 1 and pediatric fever criteria. *J Emerg Nurs* 2005; 31:357–362.

Gilboy N, Tanabe P, Travers D, et al. Emergency severity index (ESI): a triage tool for emergency department care, version 4. *Implementation handbook 2012 Edition*. AHRQ Publication No. 12–0014. Rockville, MD. Agency for Healthcare Research and Quality, 2011.

Hohenhaus SM. Someone watching over me: observations in pediatric triage. *J Emerg Nurs* 2006;32:398–403.

Hohenhaus SM, Travers D, Mecham N. Pediatric triage: a review of emergency education literature. *J Emerg Nurs* 2008;34:308–313.

Iserson KV, Moskop JC. Triage in medicine, part I: concept, history, and types. *Ann Emerg Med* 2007;49(3):275–281.

Pitts SR, Niska RW, Xu J, et al. National hospital ambulatory medical care survey: 2006 emergency department summary. *Natl Health Stat Report* 2008;6(7):1–38.

Roberston-Steel I. Evolution of triage systems. *Emerg Med J* 2006; 23(2):154–155.

Tanabe P, Travers D, Gilboy N, et al. Refining emergency severity index triage criteria. *Acad Emerg Med* 2005;12:497–501.

Thomas DO, Bernardo LM, eds. Triage. In: *Core curriculum for pediatric emergency nursing*. 2nd ed. Emergency Nurse Association, 2009:71–76. Sudbury, Massachusetts: Jones and Bartlett.

Travers DA, Waller AE, Katznelson J, et al. Reliability and validity of the emergency severity index for pediatric triage. *Acad Emerg Med* 2009;16:843–849.

Wier LM, Yu H, Owens PL, et al. Overview of children in the emergency department. Healthcare Cost and Utilization Project 2013; statistical brief #157: 1–8.

CHAPTER 74 ■ URINARY FREQUENCY

ROBERT G. BOLTE, MD

Urinary frequency is a symptom of several commonly encountered clinical pediatric problems such as urinary tract infection (UTI), urethritis, vulvovaginitis, diabetes mellitus (DM), drug side effect (with caffeine, theophylline, and diuretics), or psychogenic stress. Moreover, urinary frequency may suggest underlying disease processes with life-threatening potential such as diabetic ketoacidosis, diabetes insipidus (DI), or congenital adrenal hyperplasia that require emergent diagnosis and management. Therefore, an organized approach in the emergency department (ED) evaluation of this symptom is important for any clinician providing acute care to children.

Urinary frequency (pollakiuria) is defined as an increase in the number of voids per day. It is a symptom distinct from polyuria (excretion of excessive amounts of urine). Although the two symptoms can be related, most children who present to the ED with frequency have a normal daily urine output, although the individual voids are frequent and small. Frequency is also distinct from *enuresis,* which is defined as inappropriate urination at an age when bladder control should be achieved.

PATHOPHYSIOLOGY

More than 90% of newborns void during the first day of life. Infants void between 6 and 30 times each day. Over the next 2 years, the number of voidings per day decreases by about half, whereas the volume of urine produced increases fourfold. Children between 3 and 5 years of ages average 8 to 14 voids per day. By 5 years of age, the number of voids decreases to 6 to 12 times per day. Adolescents average 4 to 6 voids per day. In the school-aged population, urinary frequency is usually defined as voiding more often than every 2 hours.

Normal bladder mucosa is both pressure and pain sensitive. An uncomfortable sensation is produced when urine volume approaches the age-dependent capacity of the bladder. Voiding is initiated by relaxation of the striated muscles of the urinary sphincter. There is an associated contraction of the smooth muscle of the bladder, resulting in bladder emptying. This mechanism is mediated by sacral nerves II to IV. Uncontrolled, "uninhibited" bladder contractions are the normal mechanism for infant and toddler voiding. Uninhibited (parasympathetic-mediated) bladder contractions do not normally occur after toilet training. By 5 years of age, 90% of children have achieved direct voluntary mastery of the voiding reflex and exhibit the adult pattern of urinary control.

Urinary frequency may be caused by reduced bladder capacity, polyuria, or psychological stress. The urinary volume per voiding will be low if frequency is related to reduced bladder capacity or psychological stress. Moreover, there will not be associated polydipsia. If frequency is secondary to polyuria, the urine volume per voiding will be normal or high, and there usually is associated polydipsia (see Chapter 59 Polydipsia).

A reduced bladder capacity may also be secondary to inflammation of the bladder, changes in the bladder wall induced by distal obstruction, or extrinsic masses pressing on the bladder. When the bladder is inflamed, its pain/pressure sensitivity threshold is markedly decreased, so less stimuli are necessary to initiate the urge to void.

Distal infravesical obstruction leads to bladder muscle hypertrophy because of the increased effort needed to empty the bladder. This hypertrophied muscle has a higher resting tone, so smaller than normal urine volumes are necessary to initiate the desire to void. A decrease in the size and force of the urinary stream and/or straining to urinate may be noted. Eventually, the bladder muscle fatigues and cannot empty the bladder effectively. This decompensated bladder has an increased residual urine volume with a resultant decrease in the functional bladder capacity. This large, hypotonic bladder contracts poorly, resulting in small, frequent voids.

Extrinsic extravesical masses that impinge on the bladder may cause frequency by mechanically interfering with normal bladder expansion. Extrinsic masses may also stimulate frequent voiding by causing an irritable focus in the bladder wall.

Normal pediatric values for urine output are useful in determining the presence of polyuria. The traditional definition of polyuria is a urinary output of more than 900 mL/m^2/day. An infant/toddler up to 2 years of age rarely exceeds 500 mL per day. Children 3 to 5 years of age void up to 700 mL per day. Children 5 to 8 years of age have an approximate maximum volume of 1,000 mL per day. Children 8 to 14 years of age void up to 1,400 mL per day. When polyuria is the cause of urinary frequency, the urine volume per void generally is more than 2 mL per kg.

Polyuria with dilute urine is classically associated with a decreased production of antidiuretic hormone or with impaired renal responsiveness to circulating antidiuretic hormone. Polyuria with dilute urine can also be seen when the stimulus for antidiuretic hormone release is absent (e.g., chronic water overloading). In all these situations, the specific gravity of urine seldom is greater than 1.005 and urine osmolality rarely exceeds 200 mOsm per kg. This contrasts with a normal urinary concentrating ability, which is confirmed by a specific gravity of greater than 1.020.

Polyuria with isotonic or slightly hypertonic urine occurs with an osmotic or solute diuresis. Unlike a water diuresis, there are increases in both urine flow rate and solute excretion. The urine osmolality is never lower than 300 mOsm per kg. However, the specific gravity of urine is variable, ranging from 1.010 when the solute is primarily electrolytes and urea (e.g., renal failure, administration of diuretics) to as high as 1.045 when the solute mass is large (e.g., DM, intravenous contrast agents).

Psychogenic/emotional stress may also induce urinary frequency. Cystometric studies have documented significant anxiety-related increases in intravesical pressure, usually accompanied by a desire to void.

DIFFERENTIAL DIAGNOSIS

A differential diagnosis of urinary frequency is outlined in Table 74.1. In-depth discussions of many of these subjects can be found in other chapters of this textbook (in particular, see Chapters 26 Fever, 33 Hypertension, 52 Pain: Dysuria, 59 Polydipsia, 88 Fever in Children, 92 UTI, Febrile, 97 Endocrine Emergencies, 100 Gynecology Emergencies, 108 Renal and Electrolyte Emergencies, 127 Genitourinary Emergencies, 134 Behavioral and Psychiatric Emergencies). The following discussion highlights selected topics in the differential diagnosis.

Frequency is often associated with UTIs; therefore, this diagnosis must always receive significant consideration in the differential, particularly in the febrile female patient younger than 2 years (see Chapters 26 Fever, 92 UTI, Febrile). Accurate diagnosis of pediatric UTI is important to ensure both appropriate initial treatment and follow-up evaluation.

The term *urethral syndrome* refers to an entity that can be seen in female adolescents, characterized by acute onset of frequency and dysuria with "insignificant" bacterial counts (less than 10^5 per mL). Pyuria is generally, but not absolutely, present. Vaginitis is a common cause of the urethral syndrome. *Chlamydia trachomatis* is also a relatively common etiology. The urethral syndrome can also occasionally be associated with *Neisseria gonorrhoeae*. There is evidence to support the causal relationship of low-level bacteriuria and symptomatic disease. Therefore, in the context of the urethral syndrome, after all other causes have been excluded, "significant" bacteriuria may be considered as 10^2 *Enterobacteriaceae* or more per mL.

Irritative vulvovaginitis (e.g., secondary to poor hygiene or bubble baths) is a relatively common cause of frequency, usually associated with dysuria but not with pyuria. Frequency may be secondary to urethral trauma secondary to straddle injuries, catheterization, masturbation, or sexual abuse. Pinworms (*Enterobius vermicularis*) may occasionally cause frequency in young females. Children with pinworm infestation may or may not present with perineal itching. Pyuria and dysuria are usually absent.

Frequency may be a presenting symptom of a pelvic mass pressing on the bladder, such as appendicitis, appendiceal abscess, or ovarian torsion. There is obvious potential for significant morbidity. Associated abdominal pain, by history and examination, should be present. Pyuria, microscopic hematuria, and proteinuria (but generally not bacteriuria) may also be present. Extrinsic compression from an abdominal tumor may also result in urinary frequency.

Frequency may be secondary to a partial distal urethral obstruction. The urinary stream in the male infant or child who presents with posterior urethral valves is usually nonforceful and nonsustained. Straining to urinate may also be noted. A lower abdominal mass (enlarged bladder) may be palpable.

A neurogenic bladder associated with a spinal cord lesion (e.g., tethered cord) may present with urinary frequency. There may be associated lumbosacral abnormalities (hairy patches, cutaneous dimples or tracts, lipoma, or bony irregularities). Decreased anal tone, as well as lower-extremity weakness or reflex abnormalities, may be noted. An enlarged bladder may be palpable.

TABLE 74.1

DIFFERENTIAL DIAGNOSIS OF URINARY FREQUENCY

Bladder/Urethra
Urinary tract infection (bacterial)[a]
Cystitis (viral)[a]
Cystitis (chemical)
Methicillin
Cyclophosphamide (Cytoxan)
Urethritis
Vulvovaginitis/balanitis (infectious, irritative/abusive, or foreign body)[a]
Meatal ulcerations/local trauma[a]
Urethral (frequency-dysuria) syndrome[a]
Pinworms (*Enterobius vermicularis*)
Urethral foreign body
Appendicitis/pelvic abscess, ovarian torsion, abdominal tumor[b]
Posterior urethral valves[b]
Neurogenic bladder (spinal cord lesion/injury)[b]
Constipation[a]
Pregnancy[a,b]
Uninhibited (unstable) bladder[a]
Mental retardation/behavioral disorders
Ectopic ureter
Renal
Osmotic diuresis
Diabetes mellitus[a,b]
Excess solute intake (inappropriately concentrated formula)[b]
Intravenous contrast agent
Intrinsic renal parenchymal disease[b]
Sickle cell anemia or trait[a]
Hypercalciuria[a]
Urinary calculi
Congenital adrenal hyperplasia (salt-losing form)[b]
Hypercalcemia
Chronic hypokalemia
Diabetes insipidus (nephrogenic)[b]
Diabetes insipidus (central)[b]
Head injury
Brain tumors (e.g., craniopharyngioma, optic nerve glioma)
Septo-optic dysplasia
Drugs[a]
Caffeine (caffeinated soft drinks, coffee, black teas, energy and chocolate drinks)
Theophylline
Ethanol
Lithium
Diuretics
Vitamin D
Psychogenic/Stress
Extraordinary urinary frequency syndrome[a]
Water intoxication[b]
Psychogenic water drinking
Munchausen syndrome by proxy

[a]Relatively common causes of frequency.
[b]Emergent/life-threatening causes of frequency.

SIGNS AND SYMPTOMS

It is well recognized that in children with urinary tract dysfunction, an association with constipation is often present. Large fecal masses may restrict maximal bladder capacity or directly produce symptoms of frequency by stimulating uninhibited bladder contractions. Resolution of the fecal accumulation decreases frequency symptoms.

Pregnancy should always be considered as a cause of frequent urination in the adolescent female. A lower abdominal mass may be palpable. To state the obvious, adolescent sexual histories are notoriously unreliable.

Uninhibited bladder contractions ("unstable bladder" syndrome) occur involuntarily in children who have failed to gain complete voluntary control over the voiding reflex. This appears to represent a delay in nervous system maturation. A child who attempts to maintain continence must constrict the voluntary urinary sphincter tightly. If the sphincter is relatively weak, urinary frequency associated with urgency and enuresis may result. Females may exhibit the so-called "curtsey" sign, so named because the child squats and attempts to prevent leakage by compressing the perineum with the heel of one foot. This maneuver will usually prevent major incontinence but generally small amounts of urine leakage occur. A history of recurrent UTIs is associated with the presence of this maneuver. If performed, a screening ultrasound examination would reveal normal (minimal) residual urine volumes. With maturity, spontaneous resolution of uninhibited contractions occurs in most cases. In children with significant mental retardation or behavioral disorders, the infantile pattern of spontaneous bladder contraction may persist. Unstable bladder syndrome may also develop in otherwise normal children who have undergone normal toilet training. If symptoms are persistent, a trial of extended-release oxybutynin, behavioral therapy, and/or biofeedback techniques after urologic consultation may be warranted.

Anatomic anomalies of the urogenital tract may result in a chronic leakage of urine. Ectopic ureter would be an example of such an anatomic defect.

Uncontrolled DM is a potentially life-threatening condition that can present with frequent urination. Polyuria results from a glucose-induced osmotic diuresis. At initial presentation, polydipsia, polyphagia, Kussmaul respirations, lethargy, and/or weight loss may also be noted.

In chronic renal failure and in certain diseases of the renal parenchyma (e.g., renal tubular acidosis, Fanconi syndrome, and Bartter syndrome), the renal tubules lose their ability to concentrate urine. This leads to polyuria and frequency with large volumes of relatively dilute urine. A concentration defect may also occur with sickle cell disease or trait and may be evident as early as 6 months of age.

Hypercalciuria has been reported as a significant noninfectious cause of the "frequency–dysuria syndrome" in pediatric patients. Onset of symptoms generally ranges from 2 to 14 years of age. Occasionally, hypercalciuria can present in early infancy, where irritability is a hallmark symptom. Symptoms often spontaneously resolve within 2 months. There may be a positive family history of calcium urolithiasis. Dysuria may or may not be present. Hematuria (generally microscopic) and/or crystalluria are often seen. However, the urinalysis may be normal. If the diagnosis is suspected and symptoms persist, studies of urinary calcium excretion and urologic consultation should be considered. A spot urinary calcium–creatinine ratio of 0.2 or more denotes hypercalciuria. Voiding dysfunction in the majority of patients with hypercalciuria responds to behavioral therapy and anticholinergics, with only a small minority of patients requiring treatment with thiazides.

The salt-losing form of congenital adrenal hyperplasia is a life-threatening, although a relatively rare, cause of frequency. Excessive urinary excretion of sodium leads to severe water loss and marked dehydration with associated hyperkalemia and hyponatremia. However, at initial presentation (usually in the first 2 months of life), urinary frequency as a symptom is generally not appreciated. Female infants may exhibit virilization of the external genitalia. Male infants may demonstrate increased pigmentation of the external genitalia and/or a relatively enlarged phallus.

DI is an uncommon, although life-threatening, cause of frequency in the ED. It is clinically characterized by polyuria (with resultant frequency) and polydipsia. It is caused by an inability of the kidneys to concentrate urine. This is related to a deficiency in the hypothalamic production of antidiuretic hormone (central DI) or a renal unresponsiveness to antidiuretic hormone (nephrogenic DI). Some causes of central DI (e.g., septooptic dysplasia) present in the neonatal period. However, most causes of central DI are acquired (e.g., head injury, brain tumors) and therefore can present at any age. The most common type of nephrogenic DI in childhood is the X-linked recessive type, which presents in males during early infancy. If fluids are not accessible or if the thirst sensation is impaired, hypernatremic dehydration develops. If DI is suspected, oral fluids should not be limited. The child should be admitted to the hospital for evaluation and treatment under strict medical supervision.

Drugs are a relatively common cause of frequency in childhood. Methylxanthines (caffeine, theophylline) and ethanol inhibit the production of antidiuretic hormone. In addition to caffeinated soft drinks, coffee, black teas, and energy drinks, chocolate drinks are potential sources of caffeine. Lithium, chronic hypokalemia, hypercalcemia, and vitamin D are also associated with urinary frequency, interfering with renal responsiveness to antidiuretic hormone. Diuretic agents may cause urinary frequency. These agents represent only a few of the many drugs that can cause urinary frequency as a side effect. Therefore, a detailed pharmacology history should be obtained in the child who presents with urinary frequency.

Frequency may result from polyuria secondary to water intoxication. Absence of nocturia and enuresis in the presence of polyuria would suggest an excessive fluid intake. The serum sodium and osmolality would generally be decreased. Psychogenic water drinking is an extremely unusual diagnosis in young children but may present in adolescence. Water intoxication secondary to Munchausen syndrome by proxy, an unusual presentation of abuse in the younger child, is also a consideration.

The "extraordinary urinary frequency syndrome" probably represents a relatively common cause of urinary frequency in pediatric primary care settings. Average age of onset is about 6 years (with a range of about 2 to 11 years). Daytime frequency occurs as often as every 5 minutes. Dysuria is not present. Nocturia is present in about half the cases but usually occurs only about one to two times per night. Polydipsia and polyuria are absent. The physical examination is normal. The urinalysis and serum electrolytes are also normal. A spot urinary calcium–creatinine ratio should be considered to exclude hypercalciuria. If the diagnosis of "extraordinary urinary frequency syndrome" is likely, reassurance and follow-up are indicated. Initial radiologic evaluation and pharmacologic therapy are generally unnecessary. Left untreated, frequent voiding often resolves spontaneously within about 2 months, although in some children, the duration of symptoms can be markedly longer. The etiology is unclear but often has a psychogenic component, with an apparent "trigger" (school problems, parental death, sibling illness, etc.) identifiable in about half the cases. More extensive urologic and possibly psychological evaluation is warranted if isolated urinary frequency persists for more than 2 months. After consultation, a trial of extended-release oxybutynin, behavior modification, and/or biofeedback techniques are therapeutic considerations.

As an isolated symptom, frequency would be an atypical presentation of pediatric sexual abuse. However, urinary frequency may be seen in association with pertinent history or physical findings (e.g., vulvovaginal venereal infection or genital trauma), which would be suggestive of sexual abuse.

EVALUATION AND DECISION

The primary role of the emergency physician in evaluating the child with urinary frequency is to exclude significant underlying pathology that may result in morbidity and to identify treatable conditions. When confronted with a child whose chief complaint is frequent urination, it should initially be determined whether the criteria for true urinary frequency have been met (see the "Pathophysiology" section above for age-related normal values). Additional history should then focus on symptoms related to the infection of the urinary tract. Are associated symptoms of dysuria, fever, or flank pain also present? Is there a history of UTIs? Questions specifically related to DM should also be included (polyuria, polydipsia, polyphagia, weight loss, family history). The presence or absence of nocturia and enuresis are also important historical points. The urine volume per voiding should be determined (large vs. small). Generally, the presence of polyuria (copious volumes of dilute urine) is obvious from the history. The onset and duration of the symptoms and the quality of the urinary stream should be documented.

In addition, other historical features may be pertinent. For example, are there symptoms to suggest central DI (polydipsia, nocturia, central nervous system abnormalities)? Is there a history of poor growth, suggesting renal disease? Is there a family history of sickle cell disease or trait? Is the child taking any medication or drug (including caffeinated beverages) associated with frequency? Is there a history of chronic constipation, vulvovaginal infection/trauma, or pruritus ani? Are there symptoms of abdominal pain, suggesting the possibility of acute appendicitis or appendiceal abscess? In young male patients, what is the quality of the urinary stream? In an adolescent female patient, when was her last menstrual period? Is there a family history of urolithiasis or renal disease?

A complete physical examination should be performed, including an accurate blood pressure measurement. The child's

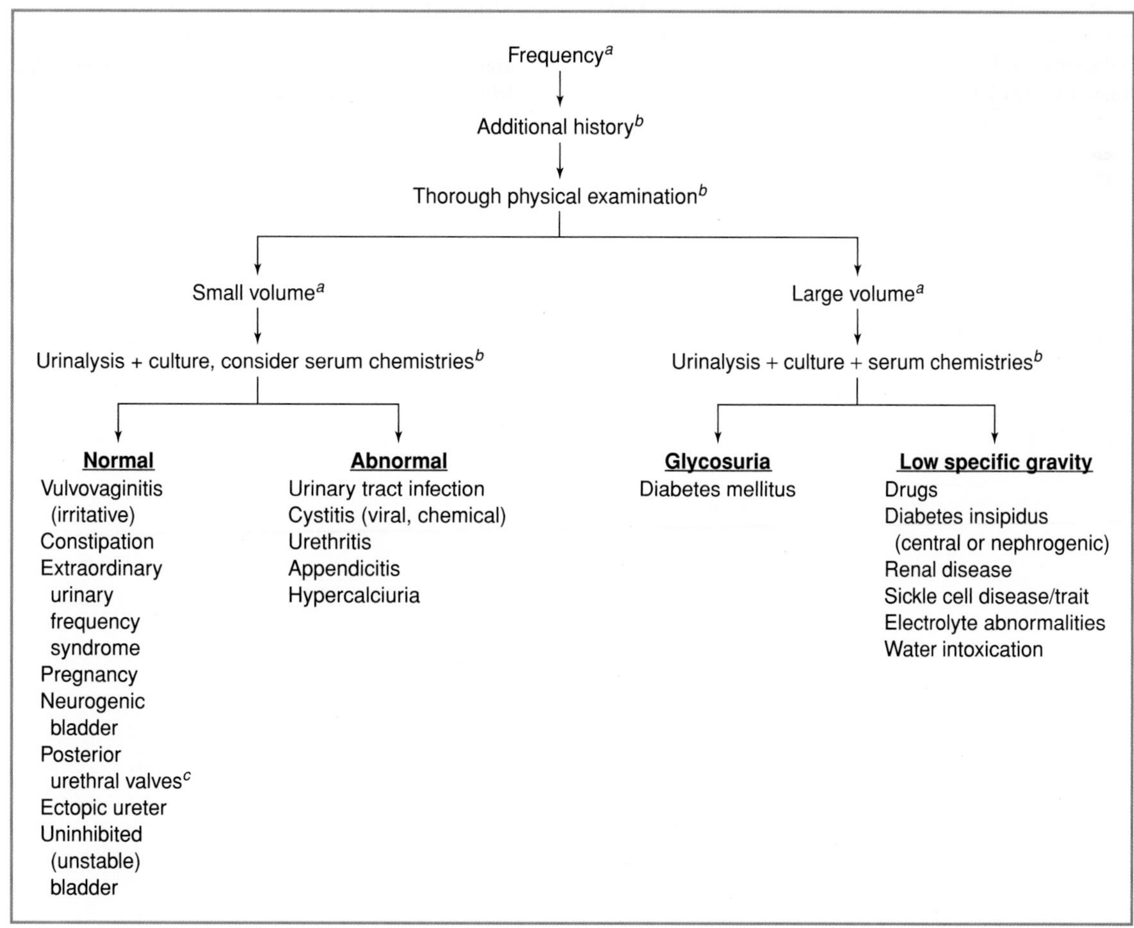

FIGURE 74.1 Evaluation of urinary frequency. [a]Refer to the "Pathophysiology" section for age-related normal values. [b]Refer to the "Evaluation and Decision" section. [c]Renal function tests may be abnormal.

growth parameters should be plotted, and the blood pressure should be compared with age-specific normal values to screen for hypertension (see Chapter 33 Hypertension). The abdomen should be palpated carefully for the presence of abdominal masses and/or tenderness. Percussion of the flanks should be performed. The lumbosacral area should be examined closely for anomalies (hairy patches, dimples, tracts, etc.). Special attention should be focused on the function of sacral nerves II to IV (anal wink and sphincter tone). Unless the diagnosis is readily apparent, a rectal examination should be performed, noting tone, tenderness, masses, and the quality and quantity of stool in the rectal vault. The external genitalia should always be thoroughly examined, meticulously searching for signs of infection, trauma, or anatomic abnormalities. Signs of virilization (in the female) or hyperpigmentation (in the male) should be evaluated. A thorough neurologic examination with careful attention to the retinal fundi and visual fields is warranted.

The laboratory evaluation is fairly straightforward. A urinalysis (including specific gravity) and urine culture should be performed as indicated by UA results. If a UTI is a significant differential consideration, then a catheterized specimen should be the standard in all children still wearing diapers. If a UTI is confirmed, additional elective radiologic evaluation should be considered. Glycosuria obviously suggests the diagnosis of DM.

If the diagnosis is not apparent at this point, serum chemistries (including electrolytes, glucose, blood urea nitrogen, creatinine, and calcium) should be obtained. A pregnancy test should be performed in the adolescent female patient. This workup is generally sufficient for those children who do not have both daytime and nighttime symptoms or anatomic and/or neurologic abnormalities.

In a child with progressive or worrisome urologic symptoms or signs (e.g., nocturia, persistent dysuria, poor urinary stream, straining to urinate, growth failure, hypertension, fixed low urinary specific gravity), urologic and/or nephrologic consultations are recommended. Additional studies may include a screening ultrasonogram of the urinary tract and abdomen, a voiding cystourethrogram, urinary calcium studies, and possible urodynamic investigation. If the presence of polyuria is in doubt, a 24-hour urine collection may be necessary to establish the diagnosis. If a neurogenic bladder (related to a spinal cord lesion such as a tethered cord) or a brain tumor is suspected, emergent radiologic evaluation with neurosurgical consultation is indicated.

A simplified schematic approach to the evaluation of the child with urinary frequency is outlined in Figure 74.1.

Suggested Readings and Key References

Bergmann M, Corigliano T, Ataia I, et al. Childhood extraordinary daytime urinary frequency—a case series and a systematic literature review. *Pediatr Nephrol* 2009;24:789–795.

Franco I. Functional bladder problems in children: pathophysiology, diagnosis, and treatment. *Pediatr Clin North Am* 2012;59(4):783–817.

Parekh DJ, Pope JC IV, Adams MC, et al. The role of hypercalciuria in a subgroup of dysfunctional voiding syndromes of childhood. *J Urol* 2000;164:1008–1010.

Shaikh N, Morone NE, Bost JE, et al. Prevalence of urinary tract infection in childhood: a meta-analysis. *Pediatr Infect Dis J* 2008;27:302–308.

Zorc JJ, Levine DA, Platt SL, et al.; Multicenter RSV-SBI Study Group of the Pediatric Emergency Medicine Collaborative Research Committee of the American Academy of Pediatrics. Clinical and demographic factors associated with urinary tract infection in young febrile infants. *Pediatrics* 2005;116:664–668.

CHAPTER 75 ■ VAGINAL BLEEDING

LAUREN E. ZINNS, MD, FAAP, JENNIFER H. CHUANG, MD, MS, JILL C. POSNER, MD, MSCE, MSEd, AND JAN PARADISE, MD

Vaginal bleeding is either a normal event or a sign of disease. Pathologic vaginal bleeding can indicate a local genital tract disorder, systemic endocrinologic or hematologic disease, or a complication of pregnancy. During childhood, vaginal bleeding is abnormal after the first few weeks of life until menarche. After menarche, abnormal vaginal bleeding must be differentiated from menstruation.

When evaluating patients with vaginal bleeding, it is important to distinguish between three types of bleeding: (1) Prepubertal bleeding, (2) bleeding in nonpregnant adolescent females, and (3) bleeding associated with pregnancy.

PREMENARCHAL VAGINAL BLEEDING

Evaluation and Decision

Important elements of the history include symptom onset, prior history of bleeding, associated abdominal pain, concern for foreign body, recent infections such as sore throat or diarrhea, rashes, masses, perineal skin changes, urinary and/or bowel symptoms and estrogen containing medications. When trauma is suspected, questions pertaining to the mechanism of injury and concerns for sexual abuse guide management (Fig. 75.1).

During the physical examination, the emergency clinician should note signs of hormonal stimulation (i.e., breast development, pubic hair growth, a dull pink vaginal mucosa, or physiologic leukorrhea), thyroid enlargement and skin findings such as petechiae, excessive bruising, or café-au-lait spots. Next, it is important to determine the source of bleeding. For the initial examination of the genitalia, an infant or child should be placed in frog-leg position with heels near the buttocks and while holding the legs flexed on the parent's lap or examining table (Fig. 75.2A). After inspecting the external genitalia, the physician gently grabs the middle of both labia majora and applies outward, downward traction to visualize the introitus and identify the source of bleeding. If the vaginal tissues cannot be visualized adequately, the knee-chest position is an alternative examination technique, which allows for relaxation of the abdominal musculature is an alternative examination technique (Fig. 75.2B). A vaginal speculum should *never* be used in a young, awake child.

As genital injuries can be associated with peritonitis and/or rectal perforation, a careful abdominal examination and consideration for rectal examination is warranted. Occasionally, a need for a more thorough examination under anesthesia by a pediatric surgeon, urologist or gynecologist is necessary.

Laboratory evaluation for prepubertal patients is based upon the most likely diagnoses.

Vulvar Bleeding

The vulva consists of several structures: the labia majora, labia minora, clitoris, and vaginal introitus. A premenarcheal girl with the complaint of vaginal bleeding whose vulva looks abnormal may have a vaginal disorder, vulvar disorder, or both.

Trauma

Most vaginal trauma results from a blunt straddle injury from a fall onto a hard surface causing abrasion, laceration, or a hematoma of the anterior genital tissues (labia, urethra, or clitoris). Penetrating trauma and sexual assault may damage the posterior tissues as well (hymen, vagina, rectum). Even a minor vulvar injury should alert the emergency physician to the possibility of concurrent, potentially serious vaginal, rectal, or abdominal injuries.

Vulvar lacerations do not often bleed excessively and usually do not require repair. However, resulting hematomas can extend widely through the tissue planes, forming large, painful masses that occasionally produce enough pressure to cause necrosis of the overlying vulvar skin. Pressure dressings and ice packs can aid with healing. Since minor periurethral injuries can produce urethral spasm and acute urinary retention, the injured child's ability to void should be assessed. Consider the possibility of sexual assault in every child with a genital injury.

Genital Warts

Similar to vulvar trauma, genital warts are recognized by inspection and can produce bleeding from minor trauma when they are located on the mucosal surface of the introitus. They appear as flesh-colored papules and are usually due to the human papilloma virus (HPV). In children younger than 2 years old, maternal-child transmission during vaginal birth is the most likely source. However, careful evaluation for sexual abuse in children >2 years old is indicated including screening for concurrent sexually transmitted infections and reporting to the State Child Protective Services Agency (see Chapter 95 Child Abuse/Assault). Topical podophyllin, used to treat warts, can produce systemic toxicity if absorbed in large amounts. A dermatologist or other knowledgeable clinician should be consulted to select an appropriate treatment for bleeding genital warts.

Vulvovaginitis

Vulvar inflammation can be seen in patients with bacterial or fungal vulvovaginitis (see also Chapter 76 Vaginal Discharge). Infections caused by *Shigella* species, group A hemolytic streptococci, *Staphylococcus epidermidis, Neisseria gonorrhoeae,* and *Candida albicans* produce vaginal bleeding or bloody discharge in a number of cases. Cultures to guide therapy can be collected by inserting a cotton swab in the vagina; avoid

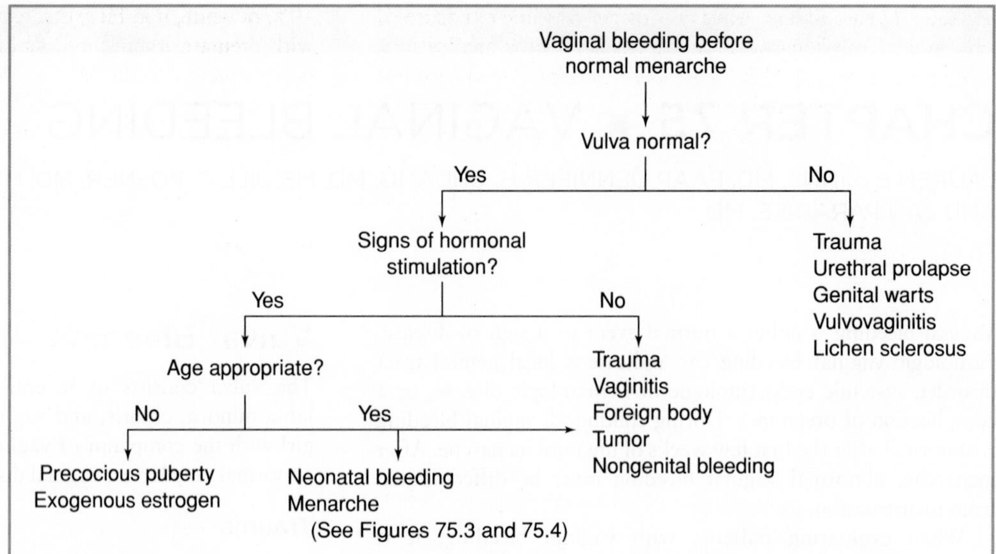

FIGURE 75.1 Diagnostic approach to vaginal bleeding before normal menarche.

contact with the hymenal tissues to reduce pain. *Enterobius vermicularis* (pinworm) infestations, though typically rectal, may also involve the vagina. Vigorous scratching may cause excoriation and resultant bleeding in the perineal area. Emergency physicians should recommend sitz baths, avoidance of bubble baths, thorough drying after bathing, and front-to-back wiping in all patients with vulvovaginitis. Occasionally, antibiotics or anthelmintics may be necessary depending on the organism isolated.

Lichen Sclerosis

Although bleeding per se is not common, ecchymoses, fissures, and telangiectasias are frequent clinical manifestations of lichen sclerosis, an uncommon, chronic, idiopathic skin disorder in children that most often affects the vulva. In this hyperestrogenic condition, white, flat-topped papules gradually coalesce to form atrophic plaques that involve the vulvar and perianal skin in a symmetric hourglass pattern. Topical treatment with corticosteroids or an immunomodulator is helpful in most cases. Consultation with a specialist is suggested for management of this uncommon disorder.

VAGINAL BLEEDING

Bleeding in the Neonate

During the first 2 weeks of life, hormonal fluctuations produce physiologic endometrial bleeding. Before female infants are born, high levels of placental estrogen from the mother stimulate growth of both the uterine endometrium and the breast tissue. As this hormonal support decreases after birth, some infants have an endometrial slough that results in a few days of light vaginal bleeding. The bleeding will stop spontaneously and requires no treatment except parental reassurance. A further workup is necessary if the bleeding persists after 3 weeks.

Bleeding in Young Children

Precocious Puberty

Precocious puberty is characterized by cyclic bleeding with or without associated breast development (thelarche), pubic hair growth (adrenarche), or accelerated linear growth in girls

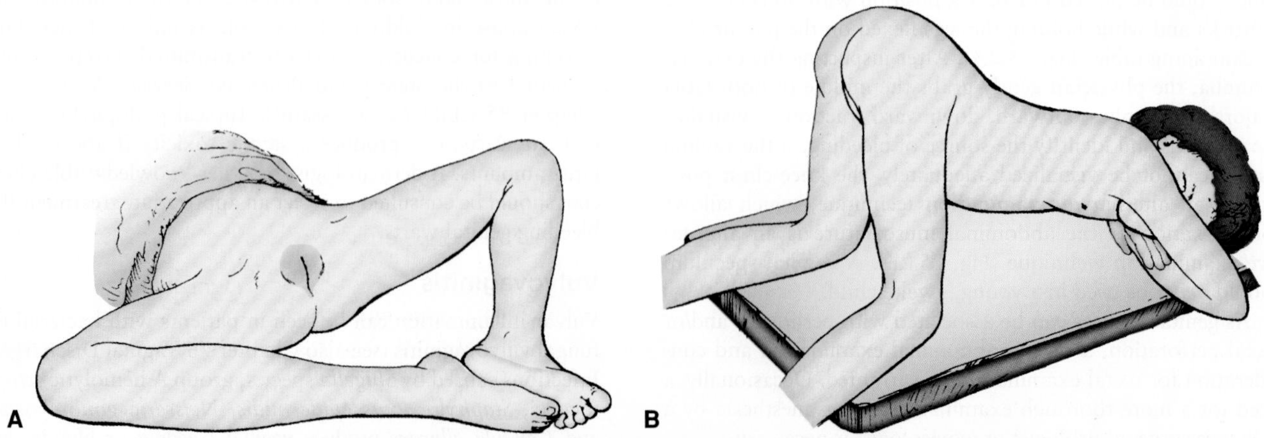

FIGURE 75.2 **A:** Girl in the frog-leg position for the examination of the external genitalia. **B:** Girl in the knee-chest position with exaggerated lordosis and relaxed abdominal muscles. The examiner can inspect the interior of her vagina by gently separating her buttocks and labia, using an otoscope without an attached speculum for illumination.

less than 8 years of age. Always consider possible exposure to exogenous feminizing hormones (e.g., creams or medications containing estrogen). Other considerations include ultrasound to identify an abdominal mass (endocrinologically active ovarian tumor or cyst affecting the gonads) and a careful examination to evaluate for central nervous system mass, symptoms/signs of hypothyroidism blood or coagulation disorders, or the presence of unilateral café-au-lait spots that may suggest McCune–Albright syndrome. The evaluation for precocious puberty is rarely emergent and best referred to a pediatrician and/or pediatric endocrinologist.

Foreign Body

Although a chronic, foul-smelling discharge is often considered the hallmark of a vaginal foreign body, many girls have intermittent vaginal bleeding or scant vaginal discharge. Direct inspection of the vaginal vault using the frog-leg or knee-chest position (Fig. 75.2B) usually reveals the foreign body easily. While the most common foreign body—toilet paper—is not radiopaque, pelvic ultrasound may be useful when toy parts, crayons, or coins are suspected. If a foreign body is strongly suspected but cannot be seen, vaginal irrigation often successfully flushes out the foreign body. Instill normal saline via gravity using a Foley catheter and a 50-mL syringe with the plunger discarded. Application of 2% viscous lidocaine to the introital tissues reduces discomfort and the majority of children tolerate the procedure well. A rectal examination may provide further information. An examination under procedural sedation or general anesthesia with a pediatric gynecologic specialist is sometimes necessary to ensure that a retained foreign body is removed to prevent complications such as fistula formation and vaginal stenosis.

Infections

About half of all patients with *Shigella* vaginitis have bleeding that may be more noticeable than vaginal discharge. Most patients do not have concurrent diarrhea. Vaginal infections with group A streptococci, *N. gonorrhoeae,* and *C. albicans* also cause bleeding in some cases. A vaginal culture will provide the diagnosis and guide the selection of appropriate therapy. The manifestations and treatment of vaginal infections in children are discussed in more detail in Chapters 76 Vaginal Discharge and 100 Gynecology Emergencies.

Tumors

Malignant tumors, such as endodermal sinus tumors and rhabdomyosarcomas including sarcoma botryoides are a rare cause of vaginal bleeding in young females. Sarcoma botryoides present as a polypoid, "grape-like" mass protruding from the introitus and often has metastasized to the lungs, pericardium, liver, kidney, and bones when initially diagnosed. Peak incidence is 2 years of age but can present between 1 and 5 years old. Pelvic ultrasound aids in making this diagnosis. A pediatric gynecologist and oncologist should be consulted immediately because treatment requires surgical excision, chemotherapy, and radiation therapy after a tissue biopsy.

Vascular Anomalies

Vascular anomalies, such as malformations or tumors, may cause vaginal bleeding in young children. Infantile hemangiomas are the most common vascular tumor, occurring in up to 10% of white, non-Hispanic females. They are often associated with prematurity and infants of mothers with multiple gestation, advanced maternal age, placenta previa, or preeclampsia. They typically present in the first weeks of life and tend to regress spontaneously. Infrequently, they may lead to ulceration and bleeding. Treatment with corticosteroids, laser therapy, and possible excision may be necessary.

Idiopathic

Occasionally, a prepubertal patient with a history of vaginal bleeding has no abnormalities and no bleeding at the time of the examination. The patient's urine and stool should be checked for blood and close follow-up with the pediatrician or a gynecologic specialist may be warranted.

Urethral Bleeding

Urethral prolapse (see Chapter 100 Gynecology Emergencies) is a common cause of apparent vaginal bleeding. Urethral prolapse more commonly affects school-aged African-American children. The etiology remains unknown. Factors contributing to urethral prolapse include estrogen deficiency, trauma, urinary tract infection, weak pelvic floor muscles, and increased intra-abdominal pressure associated with chronic cough or constipation. Some patients with urethral prolapse complain of dysuria or urinary frequency but most have painless bleeding as their only symptom. Prolapse is diagnosed by its characteristic nontender, soft, doughnut-shaped mass anterior to the vaginal introitus. The ring of protruding urethral mucosa is swollen and dark red with a central dimple that indicates the meatus. When the child is supine, the prolapse is often large enough to cover the vaginal introitus and appears to protrude from the vagina. Bleeding comes from the ischemic mucosa. Urethral prolapse is sometimes mistaken for a urethral cyst or polyp, which may lead to vaginal bleeding; these lesions do not surround the entire urethral orifice symmetrically. If the diagnosis of urethral prolapse is in doubt, one may safely catheterize the bladder through the prolapse to obtain urine. Most patients will improve with the use of sitz baths and topical estrogen creams applied twice daily. In rare circumstances where the patient has difficulty voiding or if estrogen therapy fails, referral for surgical evaluation and possible excision of the prolapsed tissue is necessary.

ABNORMAL BLEEDING AFTER MENARCHE

When an adolescent girl presents with a chief complaint of irregular menses, the ED physicians must first differentiate between normal and abnormal bleeding. In most cases, a comprehensive history and physical examination, along with minimal ancillary testing, will uncover the etiology and guide management. An understanding of the menstrual cycle and its hormones is key to treating the most common cause of adolescent uterine bleeding, anovulatory cycles.

Normal Menstrual Cycle

Menstrual patterns during the first 2 years after menarche vary. The normal menstrual cycle averages 28 days but varies

TABLE 75.1

DIFFERENTIAL DIAGNOSIS OF VAGINAL BLEEDING

I. At any time
  A. Trauma
  B. Tumor
II. Before normal menarche
  A. Hormonal
    1. Neonatal bleeding
    2. Exogenous estrogen
    3. Precocious puberty
  B. Nonhormonal
    1. Urethral prolapse
    2. Genital warts
    3. Lichen sclerosus
    4. Infectious vaginitis
    5. Foreign body
III. After menarche
  A. Bleeding diathesis
  B. Pelvic infection
  C. Endocrinologic problem
    1. Midcycle spotting
    2. Dysfunctional uterine bleeding
      a. Hormonal contraception
      b. Axis immaturity
      c. Polycystic ovary syndrome
      d. Hypothyroidism
      e. Ovarian cyst
  D. Ectopic pregnancy
  E. Spontaneous abortion
  F. Placenta previa
  G. Abruptio placentae

from 21 to 35 days. Ninety-five percent of young adolescents' menstrual periods last between 2 and 8 days; duration of 8 days or more is abnormal. An occasional interval of less than 21 days from the first day of one menstrual period to the first day of the next is normal for teenagers, but several short cycles in a row are abnormal. Typical bleeding requires adolescents to change a pad or tampon 4 to 5 times daily without resultant anemia.

During puberty, the hypothalamic–pituitary–ovarian axis regulates menstruation. The pituitary allows for menarche and the development of secondary sexual characteristics. During the early teenage years, the menstrual cycles may be irregular due to immaturity of the hypothalamic–pituitary–ovarian axis. Occasionally, an adolescent girl is brought to the emergency department (ED) by her parents to confirm their belief that she is having her first menstrual period. About 65% of girls are in sexual maturity stage 4 (Tanner stage 4) for breast development when menarche occurs (Table 75.1). Of the remaining girls, about 25% are in breast development stage 3 and 10% are in stage 5. If the adolescent's chronologic age and degree of pubertal development are consistent with this expected pattern of maturation, no further evaluation is necessary.

The normal menstrual cycle is divided into three phases based on the physiologic processes occurring in the ovary and uterus. The ovarian cycle consists of the follicular phase, ovulation, and luteal phase, whereas the uterine cycle is divided into menstruation, proliferative phase, and secretory phase. By convention, the cycle is counted in days beginning with the first day of bleeding. During the follicular phase, ovarian follicles are stimulated by the release of pituitary follicle stimulating hormone (FSH), one or two of the follicles become dominant and the nondominant follicles atrophy. The predominant hormone during the follicular phase is estrogen, which is secreted in increasing amounts, and induces proliferation within the uterine lining. Approximately midcycle, there is a surge in secretion of luteinizing hormone (LH) from the pituitary stimulating ovulation, the release of an egg from the dominant follicle. In the absence of fertilization, the ovum becomes the corpus luteum and secretes large amounts of progesterone. Progesterone counteracts the estrogen effects on the endometrium, inhibiting its proliferation and producing glandular changes to prepare the lining for implantation of a fertilized ovum. Estrogen and progesterone exert a negative feedback on FSH and LH secretion and these levels subsequently decrease. In the absence of implantation, the corpus luteum involutes, progesterone and estrogen levels fall, the endometrium involutes, and menstruation ensues, starting the cycle over again.

Terminology

Abnormal bleeding may be characterized as *menorrhagia,* defined as bleeding that occurs at regular intervals but lasts more than 7 consecutive days or in excess of 80 mL. *Metrorrhagia* is defined as bleeding that occurs at irregular intervals. *Menometrorrhagia* denotes heavy and irregular bleeding. It should be noted that the American College of Obstetrics and Gynecology has recommended abandonment of these terms. Moreover, the term *abnormal uterine bleeding* (AUB) in an adolescent should replace *dysfunctional uterine bleeding* (DUB).

BLEEDING IN THE NONPREGNANT ADOLESCENT PATIENT

Evaluation and Decision in the Nonpregnant Adolescent

A comprehensive history and physical examination, along with minimal ancillary testing, usually points to an etiology to guide management (see Fig. 75.3). The detailed history includes a review of the patient's menstrual history including age at menarche, usual cycle duration, a relative estimate of usual blood loss, and how the current symptoms may differ from baseline. Heavy bleeding from the first period may indicate an underlying bleeding disorder, most commonly von Willebrand disease. Abdominal cramping, a response to progesterone secreted in the luteal phase, indicates that ovulation has occurred. The presence of dysmenorrhea argues against a diagnosis of anovulatory bleeding. Other pertinent historical details include the presence or absence of trauma, fainting, dizziness, fever, easy bruising, and excessive bleeding at other sites. Postural dizziness and other signs of anemia can be elicited. Questions regarding sexual activity, the possibility of pregnancy, sexual abuse, and/or sexually

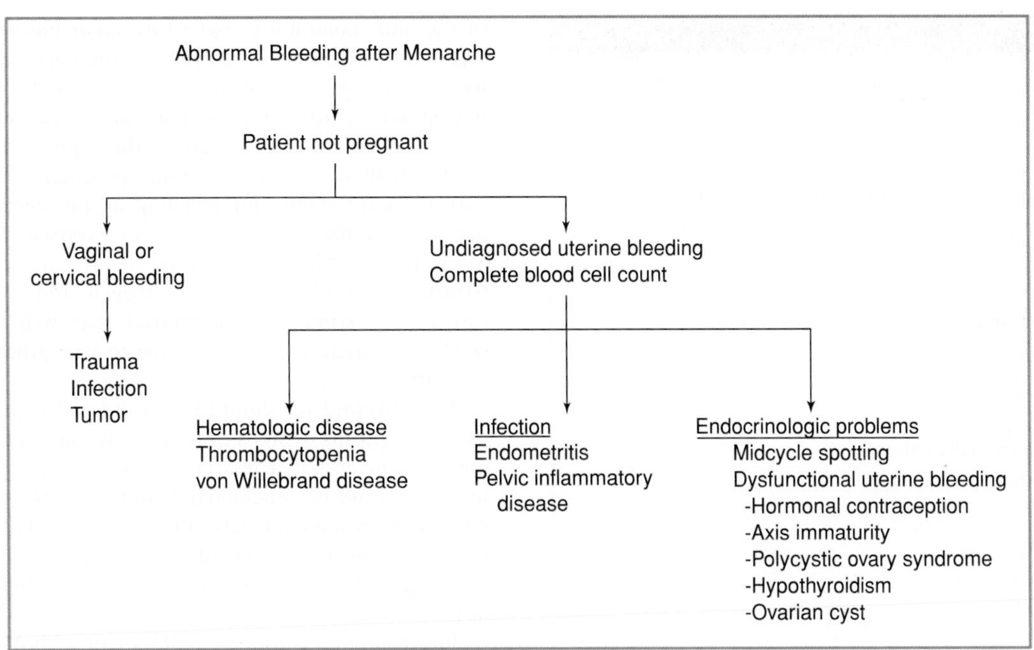

FIGURE 75.3 Diagnostic approach to abnormal uterine bleeding after menarche—nonpregnant patients.

transmitted infection should be asked with the teen alone. An opportunity for private conversation between a teen and her physician without parent(s) is a routine and necessary part of the adolescent medical evaluation regardless of chief complaint.

The physical examination helps the clinician determine the severity of blood loss in order to narrow the differential diagnosis. The ED physician begins with an assessment of vital signs and the patient's hemodynamic status. Tachycardia, hypotension, orthostatic changes, and/or signs of anemia may indicate more significant blood loss. The mucous membranes, conjunctiva, and palms of the hands/feet should be assessed for pallor. The skin should be examined for signs of androgen excess such as acne, hirsutism, or acanthosis nigricans as well as purpura or petechiae to suggest an underlying bleeding disorder. The thyroid should be palpated for nodules or enlargement. Heart rate and the presence of a soft systolic flow murmur should be noted during the cardiac examination. Additional emphasis should be placed on the abdominal examination—palpating for a uterine fundus, suprapubic and/or lower quadrant tenderness. Particular attention should be placed on pelvic examination, which consists of visualizing the external genitalia, performing the bimanual examination, and using a speculum to visualize the vaginal vault and cervix. Visualization of the external genitalia allows the clinician to verify the origin of the bleeding, assign Tanner pubertal staging, and assess for signs of virilization, trauma or discharge. For adolescents with more significant blood loss, anemia, or concerns for sexually transmitted infection, the examination then includes a bimanual examination to assess for the presence of a vaginal foreign body or mass and to determine cervical motion and/or adnexal tenderness. The speculum examination may be reserved for girls who have significant, on-going blood loss. Otherwise, this procedure, perceived as relatively invasive by many teens, may not be necessary to collect cervical specimens, especially since newer methods of STI testing (such as urine or self-collected vaginal swabs) are available.

Since the risks associated with missed diagnosis of pregnancy are high, universal pregnancy testing is necessary for all adolescent girls presenting with abnormal bleeding. Often teens do not feel comfortable disclosing their sexual history. Uterine bleeding in the pregnant patient is an obstetric emergency. A complete blood count (CBC) with differential is indicated for teens presenting with heavy bleeding because estimates of blood loss are typically inaccurate. Given the prevalence of sexually transmitted infection in this age group, screening for *Chlamydia trachomatis* and *N. gonorrhoeae* via urine nucleic acid amplification testing is recommended. Further evaluation for bleeding disorders and/or endocrine causes is indicated based on clinical suspicion. Coagulation studies such as PT/PTT, fibrinogen, von Willebrand assay (includes von Willebrand factor antigen, ristocetin cofactor assay, and factor VIII), and bleeding time may be helpful in patients with heavy cyclical bleeding from menarche and those with more severe degree of anemia (hemoglobin less than 10 mg/dL). Von Willebrand studies, however, may be misleadingly normal range during acute bleeding or in the presence of estrogen. Endocrine studies may be considered including TSH, prolactin, DHEAS, testosterone profile, androstenedione, and 17-hydroxyprogesterone. Consultation with adolescent, hematology, and endocrine specialists can be considered when indicated.

Causes of Uterine Bleeding in the Adolescent Patient

The differential diagnosis of abnormal genital bleeding is broad, and one must consider all the diagnostic possibilities during the evaluation. For the vast majority of adolescents evaluated in the ED for excessive bleeding, the most common causes are anovulation and sexually transmitted infection. It is crucial to evaluate for pregnancy-related conditions early in all postpubertal girls with bleeding, even if sexual activity is denied. Vaginal bleeding may be the result of accidental injury

TABLE 75.2

DIFFERENTIAL DIAGNOSIS OF ADOLESCENT ABNORMAL UTERINE BLEEDING

Anovulation
Hypothalamic–pituitary–adrenal axis immaturity
Polycystic ovarian disease
Hormonal contraceptives
Pregnancy
Threatened, spontaneous or missed abortion
Placenta previa, acretia
Ectopic pregnancy
Infection
Cervicitis (especially chlamydial)
Pelvic inflammatory disease
Trauma
Laceration
Sexual abuse
Foreign body
Hematologic
Von Willebrand disease, platelet dysfunction
Thrombocytopenia
Coagulation defects, factor deficiencies
Endocrine
Polycystic ovarian syndrome
Thyroid disorders
Adrenal disorders
Hyperprolactinemia

or trauma from either a consensual or abusive relationship. A foreign body such as a retained tampon or an intrauterine device may cause abnormal bleeding. Rare causes include hematologic disorders, thyroid or adrenal disease, or central nervous system neoplasm such as a prolactinoma. Structural abnormalities of the reproductive tract such as uterine fibroids or polyps are highly unusual causes in the adolescent age group (see Table 75.2).

Endocrine: Endocrinologic phenomena—whether physiologic, pharmacologic, or pathologic—are the most common causes of AUB in nonpregnant adolescents. During physiologically normal menstrual cycles, the occasional adolescent has spotty bleeding for 24 hours or less in association with the transient decline in estrogen level that occurs at midcycle. The unilateral pain of mittelschmerz can accompany this brief bleeding episode.

Hormonal contraception is a common, pharmacologic cause of irregular menstrual bleeding. Of women who use birth control pills containing 35 μg or less of estrogen, 5% to 10% will have breakthrough intermenstrual spotting or bleeding, especially during the first 3 months of contraceptive pill use. Breakthrough bleeding is also a common side effect of progestin-only contraceptive pills, injectable medroxyprogesterone, and long-acting progestin implants. Many patients using birth control pills experience estrogen withdrawal bleeding if they forget to take one or several pills.

Physiologic anovulatory cycles are frequent, especially in the first 2 years after menarche, stemming from immaturity of the hypothalamic–pituitary–ovarian axis. The physiology of anovulatory cycles deserves special mention as it is one of the most common causes of irregular bleeding in adolescents. In the absence of ovulation, the corpus luteum never forms, and estrogen continues to act on the endometrium unopposed by progesterone. The lining becomes increasingly thicker and eventually outgrows the supporting capabilities of the stroma. Punctate areas of endometrial shedding give way to more significant bleeding as the deeper layers are affected and the spiral arterioles are exposed. The treatment of AUB from physiologic anovulation requires the administration of both exogenous estrogen and progesterone—estrogen to stimulate endometrial regrowth in the excessively thin areas and progesterone to strengthen the stromal support.

Hypothyroidism should be considered if the patient has other symptoms or signs of thyroid dysfunction. A functioning ovarian cyst is a less common cause of vaginal bleeding but should be considered especially in the teenager with AUB and an adnexal mass or tenderness. Polycystic ovarian syndrome is considered in adolescents with abnormal bleeding and stigmata of androgen excess (hirsutism, acne, obesity).

Infection: In the nonpregnant patient with AUB, infectious causes such as cervicitis or pelvic inflammatory disease should be considered, especially if there is pelvic pain or tenderness. Abnormal bleeding occurs in nearly one-third of patients with pelvic inflammatory disease, generally as a result of endometritis. Sexually transmitted infections and pelvic inflammatory disease are discussed in detail in Chapter 100 Gynecology Emergencies. Every sexually active patient with abnormal vaginal bleeding should be screened for *N. gonorrhoeae* and *C. trachomatis* genital tract infections. Bleeding genital warts should not be treated with topical podophyllin because toxic amounts of the resin can be absorbed systemically (see Chapter 100 Gynecology Emergencies).

Trauma: The evaluation and management of victims of sexual assault are discussed in detail in Chapter 95 Child Abuse/Assault. Hymenal tears produced by coitus rarely require treatment beyond reassurance. More significant trauma may occur necessitating a careful physical examination. Retained foreign body such as a tampon or condom can cause vaginal bleeding. Evaluation via bimanual examination, speculum examination, or ultrasound may be helpful. Malignant genital tract tumors are a rare cause of vaginal bleeding during adolescence.

Hematologic: Hematolgoic causes of AUB are relatively rare. The most common hematologic cause of excessive menstrual bleeding is thrombocytopenia (caused by, e.g., idiopathic thrombocytopenic purpura, hematologic malignancy, or chemotherapeutic agents). Clotting factor disorders produce heavy bleeding much less frequently than does thrombocytopenia, but von Willebrand disease should be considered in the differential diagnosis, especially when heavy bleeding has been present since menarche.

Treatment Options

The treatment for adolescents with AUB depends on the underlying cause and the severity of the bleeding. AUB is categorized as mild, moderate, or severe based on the measured hemoglobin level. Mild bleeding (hemoglobin >12 mg/dL) can be managed by close monitoring via the teen's maintenance of a menstrual calendar and careful follow-up. All patients with anemia should receive iron replacement, typically ferrous

TABLE 75.3

CONTRAINDICATIONS TO ESTROGEN THERAPY

Migraine with aura
Acute VTE or history of VTE
Inherited prothrombotic disorders
Lupus with positive or unknown antiphospholipid antibodies
Hypertension (SBP >160 mm Hg or DBP >100 mm Hg)
Current and history of certain heart conditions
Certain liver diseases
Postpartum (<21 days)
Stroke
Current diagnosis of breast cancer

For a complete list of contraindications see the CDC's US Medical Eligibility Criteria for Contraceptive Use.

sulfate 325 mg orally three times daily. The treatment goals of more moderate (hemoglobin 10 to 12 mg/dL) or severe (hemoglobin <10 mg/dL) AUB is to stop the bleeding and prevent or reverse anemia. The mainstay of therapy is monophasic oral contraceptive pill (OCP), as long as there are no contraindications to estrogen therapy (see Table 75.3). The OCP selected should contain 30- to 35-μg ethinyl estradiol pill, ideally with an androgenic progestin such as norgestrel or levonorgestrel. If the patient is acutely bleeding but is hemodynamically stable, a 50-μg ethinyl estradiol pill with 0.5 mg norgestrel may be used. If there is no active bleeding, OCPs are initiated one pill daily for 6 months. If there is active, ongoing bleeding, then an OCP taper is in order: one pill every 6 hours for 4 days, then one pill every 8 hours for 3 days, then twice daily for 14 days, then daily thereafter. For patients with contraindications to estrogen therapy, if there is no acute bleeding, norethindrone 0.35 mg daily is administered in place of a combined OCP. If there is active bleeding and contraindications to estrogen, the treatment is medroxyprogesterone acetate 10 mg every 6 hours until bleeding stops, and then the medroxyprogesterone may be tapered gradually (four times a day for 4 days, three times a day for 3 days, and then twice a day for 2 weeks). Norethindrone (5 to 10 mg daily until bleeding stops then taper) may also be used as a progestin-only alternative, though at high doses norethindrone may be peripherally converted ethinyl estradiol. In the rare cases of hemodynamic instability, intravenous administration of conjugated estrogens 25 mg IV every 6 hours inpatient can be considered with transition to OCPs once bleeding has stopped. Antiemetics are recommended as needed for patients receiving combined oral contraceptives more than once daily due to associated nausea with the medications. Iron supplementation of 65 mg of elemental iron twice daily should be prescribed and a stool softener should be considered. Consider hospitalization for adolescents with severe, ongoing blood loss, orthostatic hypotension or other symptoms of anemia, and/or hemoglobin less than 8 g per dL.

BLEEDING IN THE PREGNANT PATIENT

The emergency physician should consider complication of pregnancy in any adolescent that presents with vaginal bleeding (Fig. 75.4). A β-hCG test should be performed in

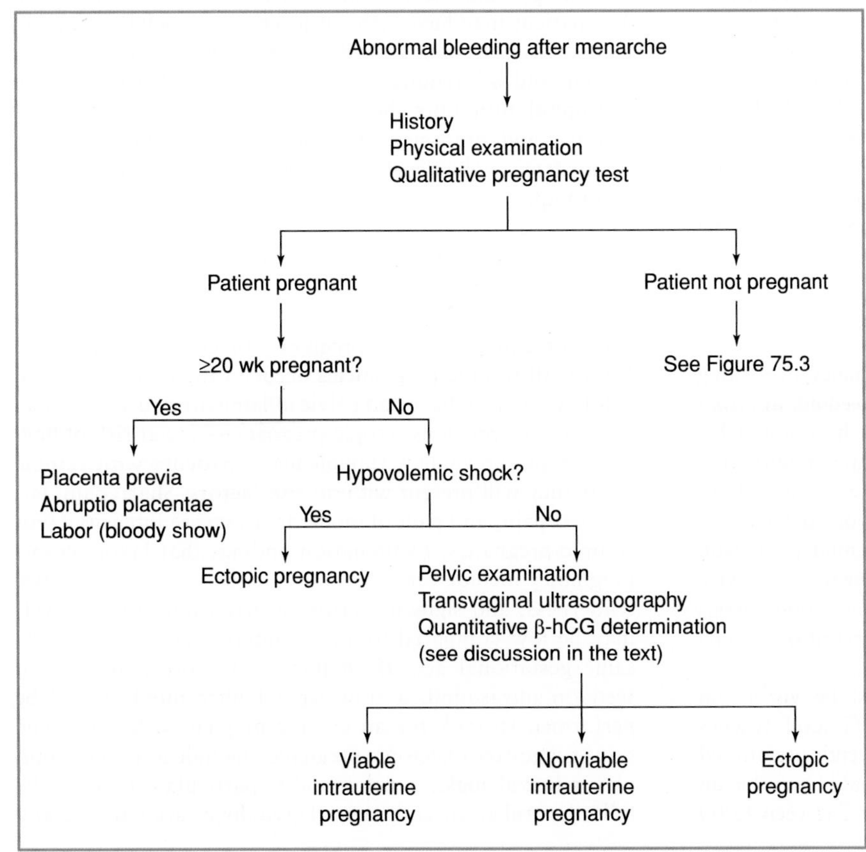

FIGURE 75.4 Diagnostic approach to abnormal uterine bleeding after menarche—pregnant patients. β-hCG, β-human chorionic gonadotropin.

all adolescent females with vaginal bleeding, regardless of whether the patient believes that she is pregnant or whether she has reported sexual activity. A pregnancy test should be obtained even if the patient with an episode of abnormal bleeding says she has had regular menstrual periods because approximately 25% of patients with ectopic pregnancies do not report having missed a menstrual period, and recollection of menstrual history dates may not be reliable. The emergency physician should obtain the social history from the patient in a confidential setting, separate from the parent. Although the patient may not disclose a history of sexual activity, there is often a hesitancy to share an intimate report of her life with a healthcare provider she is meeting in the ED for the first time. Oftentimes, the patient may fear disclosure regarding sexual activity to her parent in the emergency room setting. The patient may not also be forthcoming with the information if she has been a victim of sexual abuse or sexual violence. Adolescents tend to present to a healthcare provider with concerns of pregnancy much later than women in their 20s and 30s. In addition to the above disclosure concerns, an adolescent may be less knowledgeable about recognizing early signs of pregnancy such as nausea, breast tenderness, or fatigue. Menstrual cycles are often irregular among adolescents, so the patient may not also notice a missed period.

The urine pregnancy test usually detects at β-hCG levels of ≥20 mIU/mL and will permit the detection of a normal pregnancy within about 10 days after conception. Serum β-hCG can be detected at lower levels though laboratories are variable regarding levels of detection (<1 vs. <5 mIU/mL). Ectopic pregnancies often produce abnormally low levels of β-hCG compared to an intrauterine pregnancy of the same gestational age (see Chapter 127 Genitourinary Emergencies). If the β-hCG is positive or if there is clinical suspicion of pregnancy, a pelvic ultrasound should be performed to evaluate whether the pregnancy is intrauterine or ectopic. Early intrauterine pregnancies and ectopic pregnancies are best visualized by transvaginal ultrasound, though the clinician may want to perform a speculum examination to assess if the cervical os is open before obtaining a transvaginal ultrasound. If available at the institution, an obstetrician should evaluate any adolescent with bleeding during pregnancy.

Bleeding During Early Pregnancy

Among adults in the first trimester of pregnancy presenting to an ED with abdominal pain or vaginal bleeding, approximately 60% have normal pregnancies, 30% have nonviable intrauterine pregnancies, and 10% have ectopic pregnancies. In a pregnant patient with abdominal pain or vaginal bleeding in the first trimester, symptoms that favor an intrauterine pregnancy (rather than ectopic) include mild pain, pain located in the midline, and uterine size greater than 8 weeks. On examination, the diagnosis of incomplete spontaneous abortion is straightforward if the internal cervical os is open or tissue fragments are visible.

A normal intrauterine pregnancy should be visible on transabdominal ultrasound when the β-hCG level reaches about 6,000 mIU per mL at the sixth or seventh gestational week (4 to 5 weeks after conception) and should be visible on transvaginal ultrasound when the level reaches between 1,000 to 2,000 mIU per mL at approximately the fifth week of gestation (3 weeks after conception), though visibility on the ultrasound is also operator dependent. It should be remembered that β-hCG levels for any given gestational age are higher in twin pregnancies.

Failure to visualize a gestational sac on transvaginal ultrasound in a patient whose β-hCG level exceeds 3,000 mIU per mL strongly suggests a nonviable pregnancy. Among patients with vaginal bleeding, no intrauterine gestational sac on transvaginal sonography, and a β-hCG level of 2,000 mIU per mL or higher, about 40% will miscarry, about 55% have ectopic pregnancies, and only about 5% have normal intrauterine pregnancies. The likelihood of ectopic pregnancy is increased in symptomatic patients whose β-hCG levels are less than 1,500 mIU per mL. Spontaneous abortion includes threatened, incomplete, complete, septic, and missed abortions. During a threatened abortion, the patient has experienced vaginal bleeding but the cervical os remains closed. In the case of a threatened abortion, the pregnancy may still be viable and requires close follow-up by an obstetrician. Incomplete, complete, and missed abortions occur when a spontaneous miscarriage is occurring or has already occurred. The obstetrician or emergency physician may need to complete the evacuation of the products of conception in the case of an incomplete abortion. During management for spontaneous abortion, the patient will need close follow-up from an obstetrician and may require admission to the hospital. In a normal pregnancy, between days 5 and 42 after conception and above an initial level of 100 mIU per mL, the β-hCG level doubles approximately every 2 days. A decline in β-hCG levels on serial measurement or an increase of less than 66% in 48 hours suggests a nonviable fetus.

Septic abortion may complicate an intrauterine infection from a spontaneous abortion or from an induced abortion. The patient may have signs of fever, severe pelvic pain, and leukocytosis. Retained products of conception may still be present and will require surgical evacuation. Broad spectrum parenteral antibiotics should be initiated to cover for gram-positive and gram-negative bacteria. Infections may also occur from polymicrobial organisms, anaerobic bacteria, and fungi.

Bleeding During an Ectopic Pregnancy

An ectopic pregnancy is a pregnancy that is not intrauterine. Nearly all ectopic pregnancies occur in the fallopian tubes. Adolescents who have had pelvic inflammatory disease, tubal surgeries, or previous ectopic pregnancies are at risk of having ectopic pregnancy, though many patients with ectopic pregnancy will present with no risk factors. Sharp pain, lateralized pain, and pain of moderate to severe intensity favor ectopic pregnancy. Examination findings that favor ectopic pregnancy include cervical motion tenderness, lateral pelvic tenderness, and signs of peritoneal irritation. β-hCG levels may be low compared to an intrauterine pregnancy of the same gestational age. If an intrauterine pregnancy is not seen on ultrasound, a transvaginal ultrasound should be performed to look for an ectopic pregnancy. Sonographic signs suggestive of ectopic pregnancy include a solid or complex adnexal mass, a pelvic mass, particulate fluid in the fallopian tube, an endometrial pseudogestational sac, and cul-de-sac fluid that is either moderate to large in volume or echogenic. Occasionally, obtaining a serum progesterone concentration may be helpful; serum progesterone levels are usually higher in intrauterine pregnancies than in ectopic and nonviable pregnancies. However, the utility of the serum progesterone level is limited when β-hCG and ultrasound are available. If an ectopic pregnancy is diagnosed, an ob/gyn or other appropriate surgical service should be called to manage the patient. The mainstay of treatment is surgery, though early ectopic pregnancies may be managed medically with the administration of methotrexate. Patients who present with ruptured ectopic pregnancy must be monitored closely for signs of hemodynamic instability, sepsis, and shock.

Bleeding During Late Pregnancy

If the patient is 20 weeks pregnant or more by history or abdominal examination, potential causes of bleeding that must be identified urgently are placenta previa (placenta close to or overlying cervical os), abruptio placentae (premature separation of the placenta), uterine rupture, and vasa previa (fetal vessels traversing closely to cervical os). An obstetrician should be consulted at the earliest opportunity regarding further ED management of the pregnant patient with second- or third-trimester bleeding.

Digital vaginal examination in a female in late pregnancy presenting with vaginal bleeding should initially be avoided because uncontrollable hemorrhage may be provoked in a patient with placenta previa. Vital signs, physical examination, and laboratory studies should be obtained to evaluate for hemodynamic instability. A transabdominal ultrasound should be performed to assess for the location of the placenta. A transvaginal ultrasound may also need to be performed to better visualize the placenta location in relation to the cervical os. The fetal heart rate should be monitored, and a large-bore intravenous catheter should be inserted. Initial laboratory evaluation should include determinations of the blood type and antibody screen, hematocrit, platelet count, fibrinogen level, and coagulation studies to screen for disseminated intravascular coagulation, which may be present in moderate and severe abruption.

Bleeding with Shock

If the patient with vaginal bleeding is in the first or early second trimester of pregnancy and has shock or early signs of cardiovascular instability (pallor, perspiration, vomiting), ruptured ectopic pregnancy or septic abortion must be ruled out. Because of the urgency of the situation, treatment of shock and diagnostic measures should be undertaken simultaneously. Pelvic examination is performed and obstetric consultation should be obtained rapidly. Emergency surgery may be necessary for critically ill patients with ectopic pregnancy. Fluid resuscitation and antibiotics should be administered for patients with suspected septic abortion.

If the patient is ≥20 weeks of gestation, hypovolemic shock should be suspected from placenta previa, abruption placenta, uterine rupture, or vasa previa. Appropriate measures should be taken to provide volume resuscitation, and obstetrics must evaluate urgently.

Suggested Readings and Key References

General

Boyle C, McCann J, Miyamoto S, et al. Comparison of examination methods used in the evaluation of prepubertal and pubertal female genitalia: a descriptive study. *Child Abuse Negl* 2008;32:229–243.

Vaginal Bleeding During Childhood

Daniels RV, McCuskey C. Abnormal vaginal bleeding in the nonpregnant patient. *Emerg Med Clin North Am* 2003;21:751–772.

Guthrie B. Vaginal bleeding in the prepubescent child. *Clin Ped Emerg Med* 2009;10:14–19.

Hill NC, Oppenheimer LW, Morton KE. The aetiology of vaginal bleeding in children: a 20-year review. *Br J Obstet Gynaecol* 1989;96:467–470.

Kondamudi NP, Gupta A, Watkins A, et al. Prepubertal girl with vaginal bleeding. *J Emerg Med* 2014;46(6):769–771.

Lacy J, Brennand E, Ornstei M, et al. Vaginal laceration from a high-pressure water jet in a prepubescent girl. *Pediatr Emerg Care* 2007;23:112–114.

Paradise JE, Willis ED. Probability of vaginal foreign body in girls with genital complaints. *Am J Dis Child* 1985;139:472–476.

Poindexter G, Morrell DS. Anogenital pruritus: lichen sclerosus in children. *Pediatr Ann* 2007;36:785–791.

Scheidler MG, Shultz BL, Schall L, et al. Mechanisms of blunt perineal injury in female pediatric patients. *J Pediatr Surg* 2000;35:1317–1319.

Striegel AM, Myers JB, Sorenson MD, et al. Vaginal discharge and bleeding in girls younger than 6 years. *J Urol* 2006;176:2632–2635.

Sugar NF, Feldman KW. Perineal impalements in children: distinguishing accident from abuse. *Pediatr Emerg Care* 2007;23:605–616.

Tsanadis G, Avgoustatos F, Sotiriadis A, et al. Isolated menses: a benign, self-limited process. *J Obstet Gynaecol* 2002;22(3):323.

Valerie E, Gilchrist F, Frischer J, et al. Diagnosis and treatment of urethral prolapse in children. *Urology* 1999;54:1082–1084.

Vaginal Bleeding During Pregnancy

Barnhart KT, Casanova B, Sammel MD, et al. Prediction of location of a symptomatic early gestation based solely on clinical presentation. *Obstet Gynecol* 2008;112:1319–1326.

Cox JE. Teen pregnancy. In: Emans SJ, Laufer MR, eds. *Pediatric and adolescent gynecology*. 6th ed. Philadelphia, PA: Lippincott Williams & Wilkins, 2012:474–486.

Dart R, Ramanujam P, Dart L. Progesterone as a predictor of ectopic pregnancy when the ultrasound is indeterminate. *Am J Emerg Med* 2002;20:575–579.

Doubilet PM, Benson CB, Bourne T, et al. Diagnostic criteria for nonviable pregnancy early in the first trimester. *N Engl J Med* 2013;369(15):1443–1451.

Kohn MA, Kerr K, Malkevich D, et al. Beta-chorionic gonadotropin levels and the likelihood of ectopic pregnancy in emergency department patients with abdominal pain or vaginal bleeding. *Acad Emerg Med* 2003;10:119–126.

Norwitz ER, Park JS. Overview of the etiology and evaluation of vaginal bleeding in pregnant women. UpToDate Online Version 14.0. http://www.uptodate.com/contents/overview-of-the-etiology-and-evaluation-of-vaginal-bleeding-in-pregnant-women?source=search_result&search=bleeding+in+pregnancy&selectedTitle=1~150. Accessed 2014.

Sinha P, Kuruba N. Ante-partum haemorrhage: an update. *J Obstet Gynecol* 2008;28:377–381.

http://www.acr.org/~/media/ACR/Documents/AppCriteria/Diagnostic/FirstTrimesterBleeding.pdf. Accessed on August 10, 2014.

SIGNS AND SYMPTOMS

Vaginal Bleeding in the Nonpregnant Adolescent

Bennett AR, Gray SH. What to do when she's bleeding through: the recognition, evaluation, and management of abnormal uterine bleeding in adolescents. *Curr Opin Pediatr* 2014;26:414–419.

DeVore GR, Owens O, Kase N. Use of intravenous premarin in the treatment of dysfunctional uterine bleeding-a double-blind randomized control study. *Obstet Gynecol* 1982;59:285–291.

Hillard PJA. Menstruation in adolescents: what's normal, what's not. *Ann N Y Acad Sci* 2008;1135:29–35.

James A, Matchar DB, Myers ER. Testing for von Willebrand disease in women with menorrhagia: a systematic review. *Obstet Gynecol* 2004;104:381–388.

Seravalli V, Linari S, Peruzzi E, et al. Prevalence of hemostatic disorders in adolescents with abnormal uterine bleeding. *J Pediatr Adoles Gynecol* 2013;26:285–289.

Strickland JL, Wall JW. Abnormal uterine bleeding in adolescents. *Obstet Gynecol Clin North Am* 2003;30:321–335.

CHAPTER 76 ■ VAGINAL DISCHARGE

JENNIFER H. CHUANG, MD, MS AND KAREN J. DIPASQUALE, DO, MPH

Vaginal discharge among children and adolescents is a common complaint, and the differential diagnosis can be very broad. Discharge may be physiologic as a normal part of development, or it may be infectious and require further testing and treatment. Physiologic leukorrhea, a clear or whitish discharge is caused by circulating estrogen that stimulates the vaginal epithelium. This can be seen in newborns up to 3 weeks of age, the discharge resolves spontaneously as the effects of maternal estrogen wane. It also occurs before menarche, due to an increase in circulating estrogen levels.

Vaginal discharge beyond the newborn period and prior to puberty is an abnormal finding. Appropriate treatment is guided by history, physical examination, laboratory testing, and imaging if needed. The possibility of sexual abuse must always be considered in any girl presenting with vaginal complaints.

Postpubertal females presenting with vaginal discharge usually have a specific cause, including sexually transmitted infections, candidiasis, bacterial vaginosis, or physiologic leukorrhea (see Chapter 100 Gynecology Emergencies).

EVALUATION OF VAGINAL DISCHARGE IN THE PREPUBERTAL CHILD

Differential Diagnosis

The etiology of vaginal discharge in the prepubertal child differs from that of the adolescent (Figure 76.1). Normal vaginal flora in this age group may contain *Staphylococcus epidermidis, Streptococcus viridans,* diphtheroids, mixed anaerobes, enterococci, lactobacillus, and *Escherichia coli.* Lack of estrogen in the prepubertal child results in thinner, atrophic labia and an alkaline pH, making the vaginal mucosa more susceptible to irritation and infections. This is potentiated by the higher prevalence of poor local hygiene, the close proximity to the rectum, more frequent use of bubble baths and other harsh soaps, the use of tight, nonabsorbent clothing, and exploratory behaviors with insertion of foreign bodies in this age group.

Vaginitis is the most common gynecologic problem in prepubertal girls, and the differential diagnosis can be quite extensive (Table 76.1). In addition to vaginal discharge, other symptoms can include dysuria, itching, soreness, erythema, and bleeding.

Nonspecific vaginitis occurs in 25% to 75% of girls presenting with symptoms of vaginal discharge. In these cases, no specific pathogen is isolated. The etiology is most likely the result of poor perineal hygiene or mechanical or chemical irritation. Symptoms resolve within 2 to 3 weeks with vaginitis treatment.

Children with infection caused by respiratory and enteric pathogens often present with a purulent, bloody, or mucoid discharge. The most common respiratory pathogen associated with this infection is *Streptococcus pyogenes*. A recent history of sore throat is often obtained. Other bacteria found less commonly include *Staphylococcus aureus,* nontypable *Haemophilus influenzae, Streptococcus pneumoniae, Neisseria meningitides,* and *Moraxella catarrhalis.* Enteric pathogens that may or may not be associated with diarrhea include *Shigella flexneri* and *Yersinia enterocolitica.*

The possibility of sexual abuse must always be considered in a child who presents with vaginal complaints. Sexually transmitted infections in this age group most commonly result from sexual abuse and include *Neisseria gonorrhoeae, Chlamydia trachomatis, Trichomonas vaginalis,* human papilloma virus, and herpes simplex virus.

N. gonorrhoeae infection causes a purulent vaginal discharge. *C. trachomatis* may produce a scant, mucoid discharge, but is often asymptomatic. Chlamydia may be transmitted perinatally and may persist for several months until 3 years of age. However, the possibility of sexual abuse must be thoroughly investigated as it is more common. *T. vaginalis* infection beyond the newborn period is transmitted through sexual contact. Vaginal discharge and other vaginal symptoms are often mistakenly diagnosed as candidal infections in prepubertal girls. In contrast to the postpubertal adolescent, candidal infection in the prepubertal child typically causes perineal dermatitis rather than vaginal discharge and vulvar inflammation. Candidal vulvovaginitis infections are not common in the prepubertal child, and if present, most often occur in those children who are immunosuppressed or who have had recent antibiotic treatment.

Foreign bodies in the vagina usually present with a foul-smelling discharge and/or bleeding. Other presenting symptoms may include dysuria and vaginal, pelvic, or abdominal pain. The most common items retained are toilet paper, hair accessories, toys, and paper clips, although any object that is small enough to pass through the introitus has the potential to be an intravaginal foreign body.

An ectopic ureter, which can originate from a duplex collecting system or from a dysplastic kidney, and can insert into or near the vagina, can cause chronic symptoms of vulvar irritation, wetness, and a purulent discharge in prepubertal girls. A history of chronic vaginal discharge and recurrent urinary tract infections should increase the examiner's index of suspicion for this diagnosis.

Other causes of vaginal complaints in the prepubertal child include cervical polyps and tumors, systemic illnesses such as Kawasaki disease and Crohn's, certain infectious diseases including scarlet fever and some viral illnesses, parasitic diseases such as pinworms, and skin diseases such as atopic dermatitis, contact dermatitis, and lichen sclerosis.

TABLE 76.1

DIFFERENTIAL DIAGNOSIS OF VAGINITIS IN THE PREPUBERTAL CHILD

Associated with vaginal discharge
Nonspecific vaginitis
Specific etiology
Respiratory and enteric flora
Streptococcus pyogenes
Staphylococcus aureus
Nontypable *Haemophilus influenzae*
Streptococcus pneumoniae
Neisseria meningitides
Moraxella catarrhalis
Shigella flexneri
Yersinia enterocolitica
Sexually transmitted infections
Neisseria gonorrhoeae
Chlamydia trachomatis
Trichomonas vaginalis
Foreign body
Congenital abnormalities
Ectopic ureter
Urethral prolapse
Other vulvovaginal complaints that may not have associated discharge
Sexually transmitted infections
Herpes simplex
Condyloma acuminata
Pinworms and other helminths
Tumors, polyps
Trauma
Systemic illnesses
Kawasaki disease
Crohn disease
Scarlet fever
Viral infections
Skin conditions
Atopic dermatitis
Contact dermatitis
Lichen sclerosis

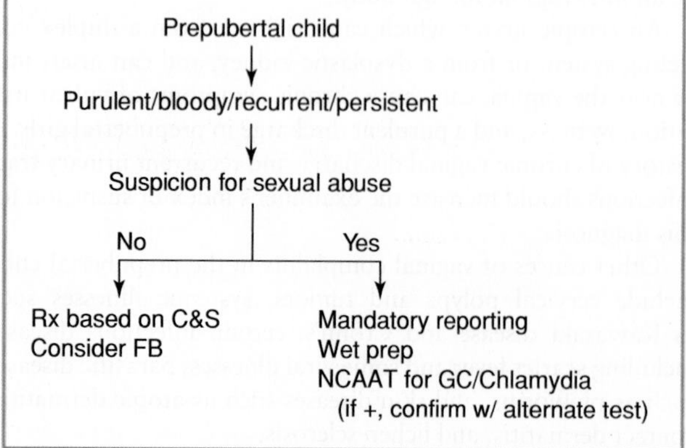

FIGURE 76.1 Diagnostic approach to vaginal discharge.

Examination

In the prepubertal patient, examination should begin with a general physical examination. Examination of the external genitalia is often best accomplished by having the infant or child lie supine in the frog-leg position. The child's parent can assist by placing the child on his or her lap or between the parent's legs on the examining table. The examination should include inspection of the perineal area, vulva, and vaginal introitus. Specimen testing can be obtained by either using a cotton-tipped swab moistened with sterile nonbacteriostatic saline. Specimens may also be obtained with a small feeding tube or urinary catheter attached to a syringe containing non-bacteriostatic saline. A small amount of saline can be instilled into the vaginal opening and then aspirated into the syringe to obtain the specimen. This method can also be used as a means of flushing out a retained foreign body.

Diagnostic Testing and Treatment

In the majority of prepubertal girls who present with vaginal discharge, no specific etiology can be found. Treatment of nonspecific vaginitis includes practicing good perineal hygiene and removing any mechanical and chemical sources of irritation.

Nonspecific Vaginitis Treatment

- Avoid bubble baths and harsh soaps
- Bathe daily for 10 to 15 minutes in warm water
- Supervise children under 5 years and assist with toilet hygiene, including front to back wiping
- Allow for air circulation with sleepwear; nightgowns are preferred over pajama bottoms
- Wear cotton underpants
- Avoid the use of fabric softeners and other dryer additives
- Launder clothing with hypoallergenic detergents
- Avoid tight-fitting clothes
- Change into dry clothing as soon as possible after swimming
- Protect the vulvar skin with a barrier ointment, such as A&D or zinc oxide

Antibiotic treatment for infectious causes of vaginal discharge should be guided by clinical index of suspicion, vaginal culture, and sensitivities (see Chapter 100 Gynecology Emergencies).

If sexual abuse is suspected, testing for sexually transmitted diseases should be performed. Urine or vaginal testing using nucleic acid amplification tests (NAATs) is a reliable alternative to culture in initial testing for either *C. trachomatis or N. gonorrhoeae* genital infection in prepubertal children (with high sensitivity and specificity). Be familiar with local requirements for forensic evidence as some states still require culture confirmation. Diagnosis of Trichomonas infection is confirmed by obtaining a vaginal specimen for rapid antigen detection.

Vaginal irrigation often successfully flushes out retained intravaginal foreign bodies. Apply topical lidocaine jelly to the hymen, insert a small feeding tube or urinary catheter without touching the hymenal rim and irrigate with warm saline. Palpation and removal of small round objects can also be accomplished by a digital rectal examination by palpation and application of gentle outward pressure. In rare cases, if the patient is unable to cooperate for the procedure or the foreign body is sharp or too large, the examination under sedation or general anesthesia by a gynecologist or pediatric surgeon may be required. If a foreign body is suspected but not visualized, a plain radiograph of the pelvis may be helpful in providing information as to the identity, size, and shape of an intravaginal foreign body, although in most cases the foreign body is not radioopaque. The diagnosis of ectopic ureter is confirmed by imaging with ultrasound and IVP. Treatment is surgical.

EVALUATION OF VAGINAL DISCHARGE IN THE ADOLESCENT

Differential Diagnosis

Vaginal discharge may be due to physiologic leukorrhea, candidal vulvovaginitis, bacterial vaginosis, or may be a presenting symptom of cervicitis from a sexually transmitted infection from *N. gonorrhoeae, C. trachomatis,* or *T. vaginalis.* Sexually transmitted infections are covered in further detail in Chapter 100 Gynecology Emergencies.

A sexually active adolescent presenting with a vaginal discharge may have a sexually transmitted infection caused by Chlamydia, gonorrhea, or another nongonococcal bacteria. Because of biologic, behavioral, and epidemiologic factors among adolescents, the risk of acquiring a sexually transmitted infection is quite high. Keeping in mind that an adolescent may not be initially forthcoming in her history regarding sexual activity, the possibility of sexually transmitted infection must always be considered.

Bacterial vaginosis occurs as a result of a disruption in the normal vaginal flora, leading to absence of the hydrogen peroxide–producing lactobacillus as well as an overgrowth of *Gardnerella vaginalis* and anaerobic bacteria. Although most common among females who have had vaginal intercourse, bacterial vaginosis may also be found in women who have sex with women, females who have received oral sex, and females who have never engaged in sexual activity.

Cervicitis is commonly caused by *C. trachomatis* or *N. gonorrhoeae,* but may also be caused by *Mycoplasma genitalium, Ureaplasma urealyticum,* and other bacteria that are sexually transmitted but not commonly identified in laboratory tests. The adolescent female may present with a yellow, white, or green discharge. She may also complain of prolonged menses, intermenstrual bleeding, or pain with intercourse (dyspareunia). However, the majority of adolescents with Chlamydia or gonorrhea may be asymptomatic. The untreated or reinfected patient may develop pelvic inflammatory disease, which may leave her at risk for future fertility problems.

A malodorous, often bloody vaginal discharge in adolescent females may also be the result of a retained foreign body. The most commonly found foreign body is a forgotten retained tampon.

Examination

Evaluation of the adolescent begins by visual inspection of the external genitalia to examine for signs of folliculitis, herpetic ulcers, candidal vulvovaginitis, clitoromegaly, and signs of excoriation. Speculum examination may be omitted in nonsexually active females who are presenting with signs of physiologic leukorrhea with scant discharge. A speculum examination followed by a bimanual examination may be necessary to evaluate sexually active females with vaginal discharge accompanied by foul odor, irregular bleeding, pelvic pain, or dyspareunia.

The postpubertal patient with candidal vulvovaginitis typically complains of a white, thick, curd-like discharge and intense itching. Signs of vulvar inflammation, such as edema, redness, and excoriation are often present. *T. vaginalis* causes a copious white, yellow, or green discharge that may be malodorous. Bacterial vaginosis causes a gray, white, or yellow discharge with a malodorous "fishy" odor.

The need for a bimanual examination with or without a speculum examination should be carefully considered in adolescents with vaginal symptoms if there is concern for upper genital tract disease, foreign body, mass, or nonmenstrual source of bleeding (see Chapter 100 Gynecology Emergencies).

Diagnostic Testing and Treatment

Diagnostic Testing

Bedside testing of the vaginal discharge for pH, wet mount microscopy with saline and 10% KOH may assist in identifying etiologies. Vaginal pH (from the fornix) and wet mount microscopy for clue cells support the diagnosis of bacterial vaginosis. Rapid antigen tests for trichomonas offer higher sensitivity than KOH wet mount and are available widely. Urine for NAAT for gonorrhea and Chlamydia can be obtained from the patient, specimens can also be obtained by endocervical collection or self-collected vaginal swabs.

Candidal vulvovaginitis is a clinical diagnosis, if tested pH is normal and KOH wet mount may reveal hyphae or pseudohyphae. Vaginitis caused by Trichomonas is associated with vaginal pH >4.5 and saline wet mount preparation slide may reveal flagellated motile trichomonads. Rapid trichomonal antigen tests performed on vaginal discharge offer a higher sensitivity for diagnosis of infection so are replacing bedside testing. Bacterial vaginosis is characterized by vaginal pH >4.5, the presence of a fishy odor (enhanced by the addition of KOH wet mount), and the presence of clue cells on saline wet mount (epithelial cells present stippled with Gardnerella) (see Table 76.2). Presence of three of the four Amstel criteria are used to make the diagnosis (Table 76.2).

TABLE 76.2

AMSEL CRITERIA FOR DIAGNOSIS OF BACTERIAL VAGINOSIS

1. Homogenous discharge that adheres to the vaginal walls
2. pH ≥4.5
3. Positive "whiff test" (a fishy odor noted before or after the addition of one drop of 10% KOH to a sample of the discharge)
4. Presence of clue cells (comprising at least 20% of the cells)

TABLE 76.3

TREATMENT OF INFECTIOUS CAUSES OF VAGINITIS AND VAGINAL DISCHARGE

Recommended regimens for the treatment of candidal vulvovaginitis	**Recommended regimens for the treatment of *Trichomonas vaginalis***
Over-the-counter intravaginal agents:	**Metronidazole** 2 g orally in a single dose
Butoconazole 2% cream 5 g intravaginally for 3 days	**Tinidazole** 2 g orally in a single dose
Clotrimazole 1% cream 5 g intravaginally for 7–14 days	**Recommended regimens for the treatment of *Chlamydia trachomatis***
Clotrimazole 2% cream 5 g intravaginally for 3 days	**Azithromycin** 1 g orally in a single dose
Miconazole 2% cream 5 g intravaginally for 7 days	**Doxycycline** 100 mg orally twice a day for 7 days
Miconazole 4% cream 5 g intravaginally for 3 days	**Recommended regimens for the treatment of *Neisseria gonorrhoeae***
Miconazole 100 mg vaginal suppository, one suppository for 7 days	**Ceftriaxone** 250 mg IM in a single dose
Miconazole 200 mg vaginal suppository, one suppository for 3 days	PLUS
Miconazole 1,200 mg vaginal suppository, one suppository for 1 day	**Azithromycin** 1 g orally in a single dose
Tioconazole 6.5% ointment 5 g intravaginally in a single application	OR
Prescription intravaginal agents:	**Doxycycline** 100 mg orally twice a day for 7 days
Butoconazole 2% cream (single-dose bioadhesive product), 5 g intravaginally for 1 day	**Recommended regimen for outpatient treatment of pelvic inflammatory disease**
Nystatin 100,000-unit vaginal tablet, one tablet for 14 days	**Ceftriaxone** 250 mg IM in a single dose
Terconazole 0.4% cream 5 g intravaginally for 7 days	PLUS
Terconazole 0.8% cream 5 g intravaginally for 3 days	**Doxycycline** 100 mg orally twice a day for 14 days
Terconazole 80 mg vaginal suppository, one suppository for 3 days	WITH or WITHOUT
Oral agent:	**Metronidazole** 500 mg orally twice a day for 14 days
Fluconazole 150 mg oral tablet, one tablet in single dose	**Recommended regimen for inpatient treatment of pelvic inflammatory disease**
Recommended regimens for the treatment of bacterial vaginosis	**Cefotetan** 2 g IV every 12 hrs
Metronidazole 500 mg orally twice a day for 7 days[a]	OR
Metronidazole gel 0.75%, one full applicator (5 g) intravaginally, once a day for 5 days	**Cefoxitin** 2 g IV every 6 hrs
Clindamycin cream 2%, one full applicator (5 g) intravaginally at bedtime for 7 days	PLUS
	Doxycycline 100 mg orally or IV every 12 hrs

[a]Consuming alcohol should be avoided during treatment and for 24 hrs thereafter.

Microscopy from a cervical specimen in patients with cervicitis may reveal greater than 10 white blood cells per high power field. NAATs for *C. trachomatis* and *N. gonorrhoeae* from urine, endocervical swab collection, or self-collected vaginal swab will identify infection. Keep in mind that a patient who was recently treated for a positive NAAT may continue to have a false-positive test for up to 3 weeks.

Treatment

Physiologic leukorrhea does not require treatment. Candidiasis and bacterial vaginosis should be treated with appropriate antimicrobials, and the patient counseled regarding good hygiene including avoidance of harsh soaps, tight-fitting clothes, and douching. Suspected sexually transmitted infection should be treated accordingly, even before receiving the results of laboratory tests (Table 76.3). Treatment of a retained foreign body is removal of the foreign body. Follow-up of the adolescent patient to assure resolution of symptoms and compliance with treatment course is recommended. Patient partners within the preceding 2 months should be referred testing and treatment. Pelvic rest is recommended for 7 days after the completion of treatment of the sexually transmitted infection. Patients treated for pelvic inflammatory disease should have follow-up at 72 hours as worsening symptoms may indicate need for inpatient admission (Table 76.4).

TABLE 76.4

CRITERIA FOR ADMISSION TO THE HOSPITAL FOR PELVIC INFLAMMATORY DISEASE

- Surgical emergency cannot be excluded
- Pregnancy
- Failed clinical improvement on appropriate PO antibiotics
- Poor compliance or inability to tolerate PO outpatient regimen
- Presence of severe illness, nausea and vomiting, or high fever
- Suspected/confirmed tuboovarian abscess

Suggested Readings and Key References

Amsel R, Totten PA, Spiegel CA, et al. Nonspecific vaginitis: diagnostic criteria and microbial and epidemiologic associations. *Am J Med* 1983;74(1):14–22.

Bazella C, Greenfield M. Vaginal discharge and odor. In: Adams Hillard P, ed. *Practical pediatric and adolescent gynecology.* 1st ed. Cleveland, OH: John Wiley & Sons Ltd, 2013:14–17.

Emans SJ. Vulvovaginal problems in the prepubertal child. In: Emans SJ, Laufer MR, Goldstein DP, eds. *Pediatric and adolescent gynecology.* 6th ed. Philadelphia, PA: Lippincott Williams & Wilkins, 2012:42–59.

Emans SJ, Woods ER. Vulvovaginal complaints in the adolescent. In: Emans SJ, Laufer MR, Goldstein DP, eds. *Pediatric and adolescent gynecology.* 6th ed. Philadelphia, PA: Lippincott Williams & Wilkins, 2012:305–324.

Joishy M, Ashtekar CS, Jain A, et al. Do we need to treat vulvovaginitis in prepubertal girls? *BMJ* 2005;330(7484):186–188.

Lara-Torre E. The physical examination in pediatric and adolescent patients. *Clin Obstet Gynecol* 2008;51(2):205–213.

Neinstein LS, Gordon CM, Rosen DS, et al. Vaginitis and vaginosis. In: Hwang Ly, Shafer MB, eds. *Adolescent health care: a practical guide.* 5th ed. Philadelphia, PA: Lippincott Williams & Wilkins, 2008:723–732.

Someshwar J, Lufti R, Nield LS. The missing "Bratz" doll: a case of vaginal foreign body. *Pediatr Emerg Care* 2007;23(12):897–898.

Stricker T, Navratil F, Sennhauser F. Vulvovaginitis in prepubertal girls. *Arch Dis Child* 2003;88(4):324–326.

Sweet RL, Gibbs RS. *Atlas of infectious diseases of the female genital tract.* Philadelphia, PA: Lippincott Williams & Wilkins, 2005.

Workowski KA, Berman S; Centers for Disease Control and Prevention. Sexually transmitted diseases treatment guidelines, 2010. *MMWR* 2010;59(No. RR-12):40–67.

CHAPTER 77 ▪ VOMITING

MARIDETH C. RUS, MD AND CARA B. DOUGHTY, MD, Med

Vomiting is the forceful oral expulsion of gastric contents associated with contracture of the abdominal and chest wall musculature. Vomiting may be caused by a number of problems in diverse organ systems. Vomiting is extremely common in the pediatric emergency department (ED), and usually represents a transient response to a self-limited infectious, chemical, or psychological insult. However, vomiting may also be the primary presentation of significant gastrointestinal, infectious, neurologic, or metabolic disorders requiring immediate evaluation and treatment to prevent morbidity and mortality. Thus, an orderly approach to diagnosis is crucial.

Vomiting is a complex act with multiple phases: pre-ejection, retching, and ejection phases. Gastric relaxation and retroperistalsis occur in the first phase, followed by rhythmic contractions of chest and abdominal wall muscles against a closed glottis in the retching phase. In the ejection phase, contraction of the abdominal muscles combines with relaxation of the esophageal sphincter to result in ejection. "Projectile" vomiting should be concerning as a sign of gastric outlet obstruction such as pyloric stenosis.

Recent therapeutic advances arise from an evolving understanding of neurotransmitter activity in the central nervous system (CNS), GI tract, and other sites. Serotonin (5-hydroxytryptamine) receptors are prevalent in the CNS and gut and participate in the induction of emesis. Use of serotonin receptor antagonists (such as ondansetron) has proven to be successful in decreasing or preventing emesis associated with many chemotherapeutic and radiotherapeutic cancer treatments, in emetogenic poisonings, and in children with viral gastroenteritis. Increasing evidence shows that ondansetron use in pediatric patients with viral gastroenteritis is safe, effective in reducing emesis, and unlikely to mask underlying pathology in appropriately selected patients.

A related complaint, often heard in the ED, is that of young infants who "spit up." This refers to the nonforceful reflux of milk into the mouth, which often accompanies eructation. Such nonforceful regurgitation of gastric or esophageal contents is most often physiologic and of little consequence, although it occasionally represents a significant disturbance in esophageal function with clinical consequences for the infant.

It is convenient to attempt to organize the many diverse causes of regurgitation and vomiting into age-related categories (Table 77.1). Although there is considerable overlap, the most common and serious entities can be easily organized into such groupings.

EVALUATION AND DECISION

General Approach

Given the myriad causes of vomiting an orderly approach to the differential diagnosis of this symptom is critical. Three clinical features should guide initial evaluation and management: The child's *age*, evidence of *obstruction,* and signs or symptoms of *extra-abdominal disease.* Other important considerations include *appearance* of the vomitus, *overall degree of illness* (including the presence and severity of dehydration or electrolyte imbalance), and *associated GI symptoms.*

History

The history should focus on the key elements noted above. The patient's age is often significant because certain critical entities (especially those that cause intestinal obstruction) are seen predominantly in neonates, older infants, or children beyond the first year of life. Evidence of obstruction, including abdominal pain, obstipation, nausea, distention, and increasing abdominal girth, is sought in addition to vomiting. Associated GI symptoms may include diarrhea and anorexia. The suspicion of significant extra-abdominal organ system disease is raised by *neurologic symptoms* such as severe headache, stiff neck, blurred vision or diplopia, clumsiness, personality or school performance change, or persistent lethargy or irritability; by *genitourinary symptoms* such as flank pain, dysuria, urgency and frequency, hematuria, or amenorrhea; by *infectious complaints* such as fever, sore throat, or rash; or by *respiratory complaints* such as cough, increased work of breathing, or chest pain (Tables 77.2 and 77.3). Other associated GI symptoms may include diarrhea, anorexia, flatulence, and frequent eructation with reflux.

The appearance of the vomitus (by history and inspection when a specimen is available) is often helpful in establishing the site of pathology. Undigested food or milk should suggest reflux from the esophagus or stomach caused by lesions such as esophageal atresia (in the neonate), gastroesophageal reflux (GER), or pyloric stenosis. Bilious vomitus suggests obstruction distal to the ampulla of Vater, although it may occasionally be seen with forceful prolonged vomiting of any cause when the pylorus is relaxed. Fecal material in the vomitus is seen with obstruction of the lower gastrointestinal tract. "Coffee-grounds" emesis suggests blood that has been exposed to gastric acid. Hematemesis usually reflects a bleeding site in the upper GI tract; its evaluation is detailed in Chapter 28 Gastrointestinal Bleeding.

Physical Examination

The physical examination should begin by evaluating the overall degree of toxicity. Are there signs of sepsis or poor perfusion? Is there the inconsolable irritability of meningitis? Are there signs of severe dehydration or concern for symptomatic hypoglycemia? Does the child exhibit the bent-over posture, apprehensive look, and pained avoidance of unnecessary movement typical of peritoneal irritation in appendicitis? Next, attention is directed to the abdominal examination. Are there signs of obstruction such as ill-defined tenderness, distention,

TABLE 77.1

VOMITING AND REGURGITATION: PRINCIPAL CAUSES BY USUAL AGE OF ONSET AND ETIOLOGY

Newborn (birth to 2 wks)

- Normal variations
- Gastroesophageal reflux (± hiatal hernia)
- Esophageal stenosis, atresia
- Infantile achalasia
- Obstructive intestinal anomalies
  - Intestinal stenosis, atresia
  - Malrotation of bowel (± midgut volvulus)
  - Meconium ileus (cystic fibrosis)
  - Meconium plug
  - Hirschsprung disease
  - Imperforate anus
  - Enteric duplications
- Other gastrointestinal causes
  - Necrotizing enterocolitis
  - Milk protein intolerance
  - Lactobezoar
  - Gastrointestinal perforation with secondary peritonitis
- Neurologic
  - Intracranial bleeding (Subdural hematoma)
  - Hydrocephalus
  - Cerebral edema
  - Kernicterus
- Renal
  - Obstructive uropathy
  - Renal insufficiency/uremia
- Infectious
  - Meningitis
  - Urinary tract infection
  - Sepsis
- Metabolic
  - Inborn errors of urea cycle; amino acid, organic acid, and carbohydrate metabolism (phenylketonuria, galactosemia)
  - Congenital adrenal hyperplasia

Older infant (2 wks to 12 mo)

- Normal variations
- Gastroesophageal reflux
- Acquired esophageal disorders (corrosive esophagitis ± stricture, foreign bodies, retroesophageal abscess)
- Rumination
- Gastrointestinal obstruction
  - Bezoars, foreign bodies
  - Pyloric stenosis
  - Malrotation (with or without volvulus)
  - Enteric duplications
  - Meckel diverticulum (complications)
  - Intussusception
  - Ascariasis
  - Incarcerated hernia
  - Hirschsprung disease
- Other gastrointestinal causes
  - Gastroenteritis
  - Celiac disease
  - Peritonitis
  - Paralytic ileus
- Neurologic
  - Brain tumors
  - Other intracranial mass lesions
  - Cerebral edema
  - Hydrocephalus
- Renal
  - Obstructive uropathy
  - Renal insufficiency
- Infectious
  - Meningitis
  - Sepsis
  - Urinary tract infection
  - Pertussis
  - Hepatitis
- Metabolic
  - Metabolic acidosis (inborn errors of amino acid and organic acid metabolism, renal tubular acidosis)
  - Galactosemia
  - Hereditary fructose intolerance
  - Adrenal insufficiency
- Drug overdose
  - Aspirin
  - Theophylline
  - Digoxin
- Respiratory (posttussive)
  - Reactive airways disease
  - Respiratory infection
  - Foreign body (FB)

Older child (older than 12 mo)

- Gastrointestinal obstruction
  - Acquired esophageal strictures
  - Foreign bodies, bezoars
  - Peptic ulcer disease
  - Posttraumatic intramural hematoma
  - Malrotation (with or without volvulus)
  - Meckel diverticulum (complications)
  - Meconium ileus equivalent (cystic fibrosis)
  - Ascariasis
  - Incarcerated hernia
  - Adhesions (postsurgical, peritonitis)
  - Intussusception
  - Hirschsprung disease
  - Superior mesenteric artery syndrome
- Other gastrointestinal causes
  - Gastroenteritis, gastritis, duodenitis
  - Gastroesophageal reflux
  - Appendicitis
  - Peptic ulcer disease
  - Pancreatitis
  - Peritonitis
  - Paralytic ileus
  - Crohn disease
- Neurologic
  - Intracranial mass lesions (brain tumors, other)
  - Cerebral edema
  - Migraine
  - Motion sickness
  - Concussion
  - Seizures
- Renal
  - Obstructive uropathy
  - Renal insufficiency/uremia
  - Renal tubular acidosis
- Infectious
  - Meningitis
  - Urinary tract infection
  - Hepatitis
  - Upper respiratory infection (postnasal drip)
- Metabolic
  - Diabetic ketoacidosis
  - Reye syndrome
  - Adrenal insufficiency
  - Inborn error of metabolism (urea cycle or fatty acid oxidation defect; acute, intermittent porphyria)
- Toxins and drugs
  - Aspirin
  - Ipecac
  - Digoxin
  - Iron
  - Lead (chronic)
- Respiratory (posttussive)
  - Asthma exacerbation
  - Infectious respiratory disease (pneumonia, bronchiolitis)
  - Foreign body
- Other
  - Pregnancy
  - Cyclic vomiting

TABLE 77.2

LIFE-THREATENING CAUSES OF VOMITING

Newborn (birth to 2 wks)
Anatomic anomalies—esophageal stenosis/atresia; intestinal obstructions (Table 77.1), especially malrotation and volvulus; Hirschsprung disease
Other gastrointestinal (GI) causes
Necrotizing enterocolitis
Peritonitis
Neurologic—kernicterus, mass lesions, hydrocephalus
Renal—obstructive anomalies, uremia
Infectious—sepsis, meningitis
Metabolism—inborn errors, especially congenital adrenal hyperplasia
Older infant (2 wks to 12 mo)
Intestinal obstruction (Table 77.1), especially pyloric stenosis, intussusception, incarcerated hernia, malrotation with volvulus
Other GI causes, especially gastroenteritis (with dehydration)
Neurologic—mass lesions, hydrocephalus
Renal—obstruction, uremia
Infectious—sepsis, meningitis, pertussis
Metabolic—inborn errors of metabolism
Toxins, drugs
Older child (older than 12 mo)
GI obstruction, especially intussusception (Table 77.1)
Other GI causes, especially appendicitis, peptic ulcer disease
Neurologic—mass lesions
Renal—uremia
Infectious—meningitis, sepsis
Metabolic—diabetic ketoacidosis, adrenal insufficiency, inborn errors of metabolism
Toxins, drugs

high-pitched bowel sounds (or absent sounds in ileus), or visible peristalsis? A complete physical examination must include a search for signs of neurologic, infectious, toxic/metabolic, and genitourinary causes, as well as an evaluation of hydration status (see Chapter 17 Dehydration).

The diverse nature of causes for vomiting makes a routine laboratory or radiologic screen impossible. The history and physical examination must guide the approach in individual patients. Certain well-defined clinical pictures demand urgent radiologic workup. For example, abdominal pain and bilious vomiting in an infant requires supine and upright plain films, as well as a limited upper GI series for evaluation of congenital obstructive anomalies such as malrotation. A child with paroxysms of colicky abdominal pain and grossly bloody stools requires immediate ultrasound for rapid diagnosis of intussusception, or in clear-cut cases should proceed directly to an air-contrast enema for both diagnosis and reduction of the intussusception. Other situations require no imaging studies (e.g., a typical case of viral gastroenteritis). In many cases, cultures or serum chemical analyses are essential for making a diagnosis (e.g., meningitis, aspirin toxicity, urinary tract infection [UTI], pregnancy) or for guiding management (e.g., degree of metabolic derangement in severe dehydration, pyloric stenosis, diabetic ketoacidosis). For most straightforward, common illnesses (e.g., gastroenteritis, respiratory infections with posttussive emesis), laboratory investigation is unwarranted.

TABLE 77.3

COMMON CAUSES OF VOMITING

Newborn (birth to 2 wks)
Normal variations ("spitting up")
Gastroesophageal reflux
Gastrointestinal (GI) obstruction—congenital anomalies
Necrotizing enterocolitis (premature birth)
Infectious—meningitis, sepsis
Older infant (2 wks to 12 mo)
Normal variations
Gastroesophageal reflux
Gastrointestinal (GI) obstruction—especially pyloric stenosis, intussusception, incarcerated hernia
Gastroenteritis
Infectious—sepsis, meningitis, urinary tract infection
Posttussive—reactive airways disease, respiratory infections, foreign body
Drug overdose
Older child (older than 12 mo)
GI obstruction—incarcerated hernia, intussusception
Other GI causes—gastroenteritis, gastroesophageal reflux, appendicitis
Infectious—meningitis, urinary tract infection
Posttussive—asthma, respiratory infections, foreign body
Metabolic—diabetic ketoacidosis
Concussion
Toxins/drugs
Pregnancy

APPROACH TO CHILDREN BY AGE GROUPS

With these introductory concepts in mind, we can approach the differential diagnosis of the principal causes of vomiting on

TABLE 77.4

SIGNS AND SYMPTOMS ASSOCIATED WITH SIGNIFICANT UNDERLYING CAUSES OF VOMITING

Bilious emesis—concerning for obstruction distal to the ampulla of Vater
Headache, especially early morning—concerning for increased intracranial pressure
Hematemesis—concerning for esophagitis, gastritis, or peptic ulcer disease
Hematochezia/melena—may suggest mucosal GI disease such as inflammatory bowel disease (IBD)
Weight loss or poor weight gain—consider chronic illness such as celiac disease, IBD, metabolic disorders
Severe dehydration—concerning for electrolyte imbalance, warrants exclusion of underlying conditions such as obstruction

an age-related basis. An algorithm for such an approach that uses the key clinical features previously outlined is illustrated in Figure 77.1.

Neonates

A careful history should focus on the perinatal history, onset and duration of vomiting, nature of the vomitus, associated GI symptoms, and the presence of symptoms referable to other organ systems. Onset of vomiting in the first days of life should always prompt evaluation for one of the common *congenital GI anomalies* that cause obstruction, such as esophageal or intestinal atresia or web, malrotation, meconium ileus, or Hirschsprung disease. If the vomiting is bilious, bright yellow, or green, an urgent surgical consultation is required. In most cases, a serious and possibly life-threatening mechanical obstruction may be the cause of bilious vomiting. All neonates in whom the possibility of GI obstruction is entertained must have immediate flat and upright abdominal films and an upper GI series. Other clinical features, such as toxicity, dehydration, and lethargy, attest to the length of time of the obstruction and its severity. Except for some cases of malrotation, most neonates with a congenital basis for their bowel obstruction will present during their initial nursery stay; only rarely will the first presentation be in the ED. In those rare cases where an intestinal atresia presents to the ED in the first few days of life, infants will have vomiting since birth, evidence of obstruction with abdominal distention and bilious emesis, and plain abdominal films may show findings such as the "double bubble" of duodenal atresia. Correction of dehydration and metabolic abnormalities, nasogastric decompression, and surgical consultation are the most immediate ED interventions. Neonates or infants with malrotation and volvulus may present with abdominal pain (crying, drawing up their knees, poor feeding), with evidence of obstruction (bilious emesis), or an acute abdomen (abdominal distention or rigidity). Malrotation is confirmed by the abnormal radiographic location of the duodenal–jejunal junction (upper GI series) and/or the cecum (contrast enema). Immediate fluid resuscitation, GI decompression, and surgical consultation are indicated.

Infants with Hirschsprung disease most commonly present with delayed passage of meconium in the nursery, but may also present later with a distended abdomen and bilious vomiting. Children with delayed diagnosis may also present with Hirschsprung-associated enterocolitis, with foul-smelling diarrhea, fever, and abdominal distention, or progress to life-threatening toxic megacolon. Prompt recognition and treatment of electrolyte imbalance, antibiotics, and surgical consultation are essential.

Other serious causes of neonatal vomiting that may present to the ED include *infection,* such as meningitis, sepsis, pyelonephritis, omphalitis, or necrotizing enterocolitis (it should be noted that such serious infections may not be accompanied by fever in the neonate); *increased intracranial pressure* (ICP) related to cerebral edema, subdural hematoma, or hydrocephalus; *metabolic acidosis* or *hyperammonemia* caused by the inborn errors of amino acid and organic acid metabolism; and *renal insufficiency* or *obstruction.* Such infants usually appear ill, with associated lethargy and irritability. In some cases, findings such as fever, a full fontanel, a diminished urinary stream, an abdominal mass, or respiratory signs will suggest the underlying cause. Any ill-appearing neonate with vomiting, with or without evidence of intestinal obstruction, requires hospitalization and prompt, broad evaluation for sepsis and neurologic, renal, and metabolic disease.

Commonly, however, a young infant in the first 2 to 4 weeks of life who appears entirely well is brought to the ED with the complaint of persistent vomiting. The birth history and perinatal course are unremarkable. The baby is vigorous, has gained weight appropriately (5 to 7 oz per week after the first week of life), and has a normal physical examination. Usually, a close description of the "vomiting" (or a trial feeding in the ED) reveals the problem to be *physiologic regurgitation* or *reflux.* This is a common and usually insignificant problem, representing normal variation in the developmental maturation of the lower esophageal sphincter (LES). GER in infants is discussed further below.

Older Infants

Older infants presenting with vomiting must also be evaluated for signs of obstruction, however the causes of obstruction in this age group differ from those in the neonate. Although malrotation with volvulus must continue to be considered, other causes of obstruction in this age group include hypertrophic pyloric stenosis (HPS), intussusception, enteric duplication cysts, incarcerated hernia, and complications of Meckel diverticulum. Causes of intestinal obstruction most often diagnosed in the neonatal period, such as Hirschsprung disease, may also present at this age, though less commonly. The various causes of intestinal obstruction must be considered in the vomiting infant before nonobstructive causes are considered in order to make a timely diagnosis and initiate treatment.

HPS most commonly presents between 3 and 6 weeks of age. It is caused when thickening of the pyloric muscle leads to gastric outlet obstruction. Infants present with nonbilious emesis, during or shortly after feeds, which is often described as projectile. Emesis tends to worsen in frequency and severity over days to weeks. In the past, diagnosis was made by clinical history and palpation of the hypertrophied pyloric muscle, or "olive" in the abdomen. Infants often presented with dehydration and electrolyte abnormalities caused by repeated vomiting, typically a hypokalemic, hypochloremic metabolic alkalosis. However, with earlier presentation and diagnosis, fewer patients have an olive palpated at diagnosis, and the majority do not have the classic electrolyte derangements at presentation.

HPS should be suspected in the young infant presenting with progressively worsening nonbilious emesis, and can be diagnosed using ultrasound. A hypertrophied pylorus with muscle wall thickness of 4 mm or greater and length of 15 mm or greater with no passage of gastric contents into the small intestine confirms the diagnosis. Treatment is surgical, with laparoscopic pyloromyotomy. Prior to surgery, the patient should be well hydrated and any electrolyte abnormalities should be corrected.

Intussusception occurs when one portion of the bowel telescopes into its distal segment, commonly the terminal ileum into the cecum. The peak incidence for intussusception is between 3 months and 3 years of age, although it remains one of the most common causes of obstruction up to 6 years of age. Patients typically present with intermittent episodes of abdominal pain, during which they may cry or pull up the legs. Children may be lethargic between episodes, and infants may present only with lethargy and without the classic episodes of pain. Bilious emesis and blood-tinged "currant jelly"

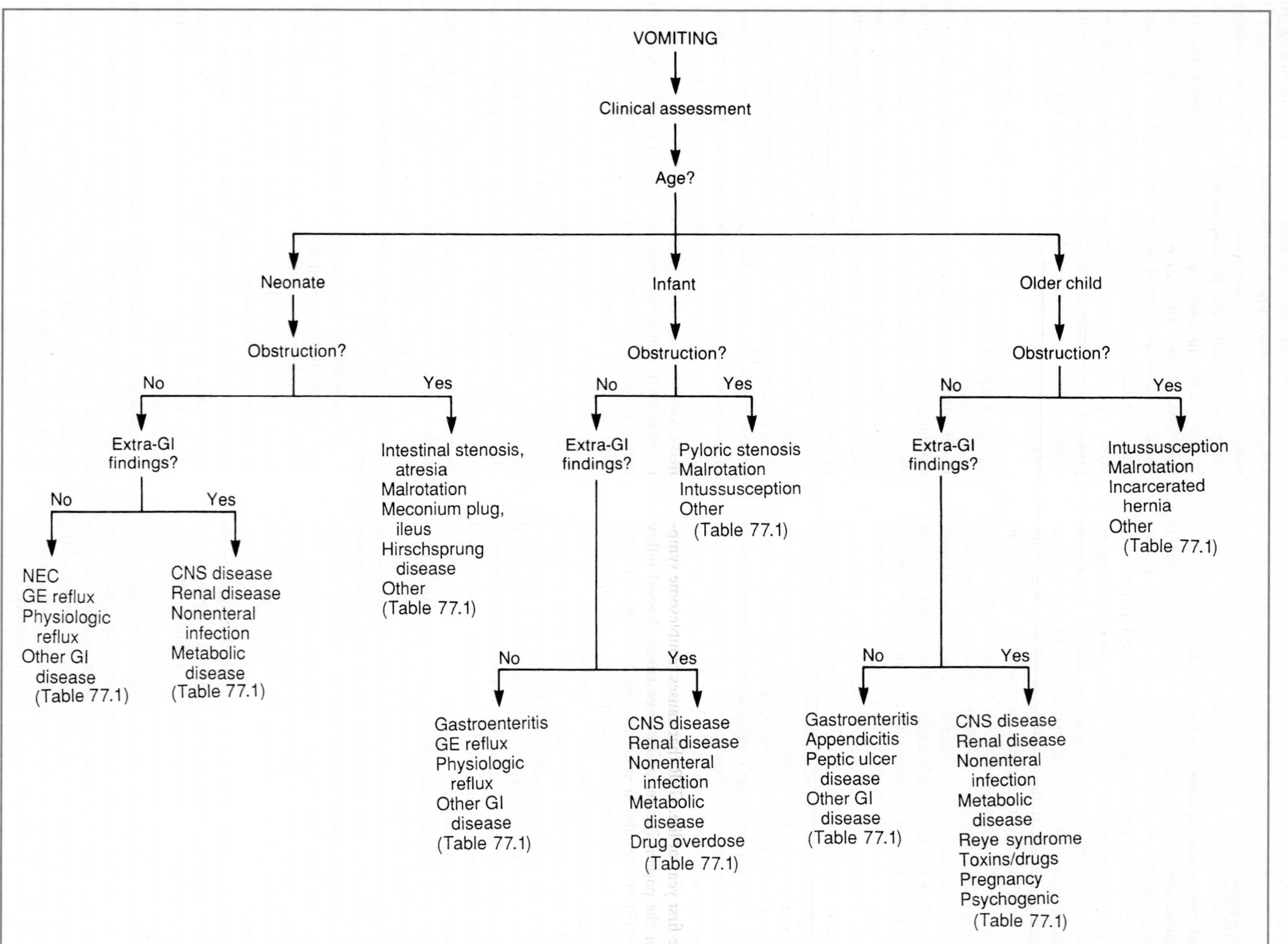

FIGURE 77.1 Differential diagnosis of vomiting. GI, gastrointestinal; NEC, necrotizing enterocolitis; GE, gastroesophageal; CNS, central nervous system.

stools may be seen. However, the classic triad of abdominal pain, vomiting, and bloody stools is seen in less than a quarter of children with intussusception, so a high level of clinical suspicion must be maintained when any of these symptoms are present (refer Chapter 48 Pain: Abdomen).

Less common causes of obstruction should also be considered in infants presenting to the ED with vomiting. A thorough clinical examination should be performed to evaluate for signs of incarcerated inguinal or umbilical hernias. Meckel diverticulum, which results from incomplete obliteration of the omphalomesenteric duct, is the most common congenital anomaly of the GI tract in children. While the majority of patients are asymptomatic, children can occasionally present with obstruction. Enteric duplication cysts can also lead to intestinal obstruction or can act as lead points for intussusception.

While the clinician must first rule out obstructive causes of vomiting in infants, nonobstructive causes are more common than obstructive causes. Nonobstructive causes of vomiting in this age group include GI, infectious, neurologic, renal, and metabolic disorders.

GER is a common cause of emesis in this age group. GER results when relaxation of the LES allows retrograde passage of gastric contents. Infants with GER may present with repeated episodes of emesis of stomach contents usually within 30 minutes of feeding. Emesis is generally nonbloody and nonbilious, and is fairly constant over time. Most infants will have some degree of GER or "spitting up," with a peak at age 4 months (up to 67% of infants) and gradually tapering over the first year of life. GER that causes troublesome symptoms for the patient is referred to as gastroesophageal reflux disease (GERD). Troublesome symptoms that suggest GERD include poor weight gain, vomiting associated with irritability or refusal to feed, arching of the back during feeding, and respiratory symptoms such as cough or wheezing related to reflux. For infants who present with reflux but without any of these troublesome symptoms, there is generally no need for any further diagnostic testing or for medical management. Nonpharmacologic treatments suffice for the vast majority of infants with reflux. Upper GI contrast radiography and esophageal pH probes are the most commonly used tests in the diagnosis and evaluation of GERD, but are almost never indicated in the PED for reflux evaluation.

Management of both GER and GERD should include lifestyle modifications. These modifications can include both positioning and feeding changes. Positioning the infant in a completely upright or left lateral position after feeds has been shown to decrease total number of reflux episodes, while little change has been demonstrated when infants are placed in a semi-supine position after feeds. Feeding changes may include avoiding overfeeding, diet changes, and avoiding feeding in the supine or semi-supine position. As milk–protein allergy can mimic GERD, a trial of eliminating milk and eggs from the diet of mothers of breast-fed infants or a trial of hydrolyzed protein formula in formula-fed infants may be warranted. Medications should be reserved for infants with continued worrisome symptoms of GERD after trials of feeding modifications, with the two classes of medications most commonly used in infants being histamine-2 receptor antagonists (H2RAs) and proton pump inhibitors (PPIs). PPIs may be preferable to H2RAs as a fairly rapid tachyphylaxis can develop after initiation of treatment with H2RAs. It is important to stress to parents that these medications will reduce acid exposure in children with GERD, but that they will not decrease the amount of reflux itself. There has been a shift away from acid-suppression therapy because of lack of efficacy and possible adverse effects.

Viral gastroenteritis is another common cause of vomiting in infants. The infant will generally present with diarrhea as well, although they may present without diarrhea or early in the disease course before diarrhea has developed. It is crucial to assess hydration of infants presenting with gastroenteritis and to ensure adequate oral intake, particularly in those infants who also have diarrhea as this age group is at much higher risk of dehydration than older children.

Vomiting in infants may also be caused by pathology of organ systems outside the digestive system and should be considered in the infant presenting with vomiting. These include infectious, neurologic, renal, and metabolic causes. Infections outside the GI tract can present with vomiting in infants. One of the most common infections to cause vomiting outside of the GI tract is UTI. UTIs are a common source of fever in children, particularly in infants. Clinical symptoms are often nonspecific in infants, but may include vomiting in as many as one-third of infants with UTI, poor feeding, or malodorous urine. Infants with pneumonia may also present with fever and vomiting, along with tachypnea, cough, or increased work of breathing. Any respiratory illness causing cough, including bronchiolitis, pneumonia, and pertussis, can be associated with posttussive emesis in this age group.

Neurologic causes of vomiting in infants include CNS infections such as meningitis, hydrocephalus, intracranial mass, and intracranial hemorrhage. Signs and symptoms of increased ICP in infants may include vomiting in addition to lethargy, irritability, bulging anterior fontanel, seizures, or focal neurologic findings.

Other causes of vomiting outside the GI tract include renal and metabolic causes. Infants with renal tubular acidosis (RTA) may present with vomiting, growth failure, and recurrent episodes of dehydration. Children with renal failure may also present with vomiting. Vomiting can be an early symptom of many of the inborn errors of metabolism, including urea cycle disorders and organic acidemias. Infants with inborn errors of metabolism may present with vomiting, lethargy, and poor feeding, and this diagnosis should be kept in the differential diagnosis of infants presenting with recurrent vomiting. Infants with congenital adrenal hyperplasia may present with vomiting, growth failure, and lethargy. They may appear critically ill with a similar appearance to those with sepsis, and may have electrolyte abnormalities including hyponatremia and hyperkalemia.

Infant rumination syndrome is a rare syndrome characterized by voluntary regurgitation of gastric contents into the mouth. The Rome III criteria were developed by gastroenterologists to guide practitioners in the diagnosis of functional gastrointestinal disorders, and include criteria for the diagnosis of infant rumination syndrome. All of the following criteria must be met for at least 3 months to make the diagnosis: (1) Repetitive contraction of the abdominal muscles, diaphragm, and tongue, (2) regurgitation of gastric contents into the mouth, which is either expectorated, rechewed, or reswallowed, and (3) three or more of the following, (a) onset between 3 and 8 months of age, (b) does not respond to management for GERD or to anticholinergics, formula changes, or gastrostomy tube feedings, (c) unaccompanied by signs of nausea or distress, or (d) does not occur during sleep or when the infant is interacting with individuals in the environment. Rumination syndrome is thought to result from dysfunction of the parent–child interaction, and treatment should focus on improving this interaction.

Older Child

In the older child, several of the obstructive causes of vomiting can continue to occur, although less commonly than in infancy. Children in this age group may present with malrotation and volvulus, intussusception, incarcerated hernia, or enteric duplication cysts. Children with a history of abdominal surgery may present with bowel obstruction caused by adhesions. Signs of obstruction in this age group include vomiting (particularly bilious), abdominal distention, and pain.

Nonobstructive causes of vomiting continue to be more common than obstructive causes of vomiting in older children. GI causes such as appendicitis, peptic ulcer disease, and gastroenteritis can lead to vomiting, as well as several extra-abdominal causes. Appendicitis can present with vomiting in children, along with other symptoms including abdominal pain, anorexia, and fever. Often, pain will begin in the periumbilical region and then shift to the right lower quadrant, and pain may be increased with coughing or hopping (refer clinical pathway Chapters 83 Appendicitis (Suspected) and 124 Abdominal Emergencies).

Other nonobstructive causes of vomiting in older children related to the digestive system include pancreatitis, cholelithiasis and cholecystitis, gastritis, and peptic ulcer disease. Children with pancreatitis may present with vomiting and severe pain and tenderness in the epigastric region. Children with cholelithiasis may present with vomiting and pain in the right upper quadrant, with symptoms worsening particularly after eating fatty foods, while those with cholecystitis may present with similar symptoms with the addition of fever. Peptic ulcer disease may also present with vomiting, as well as abdominal pain worst in the epigastric region and hematemesis in severe cases.

Acute gastroenteritis (AGE) is the most common cause of vomiting in this age group. AGE is an infection characterized by diarrhea, often accompanied by vomiting and is a common reason for children to present to the ED. Fever may or may not be present. The degree of dehydration will help to determine how to manage the child. Several scales exist to assess the severity of dehydration (mild, moderate, or severe) in children with AGE based on physical examination, including criteria from the World Health Organization (WHO), the Gorelick scale, and the Clinical Dehydration Scale (CDS). Laboratory studies may also be helpful in children with signs of severe dehydration, with serum bicarbonate level having been shown to correlate with dehydration in several studies, but are rarely indicated in children with mild or moderate dehydration (see Chapter 17 Dehydration). Intravenous fluids are generally recommended for the treatment of severe dehydration, and admission to the hospital may be indicated in these children, particularly if ongoing losses exceed intake. However, oral rehydration should be attempted prior to intravenous rehydration in children with mild or moderate dehydration. Ondansetron may be helpful in children prior to attempting oral rehydration in vomiting patients. It is important that parents realize that rehydration in the ED is only the first phase of treatment of dehydration, with the second and third phases being replacement of ongoing losses and continuation of normal feeding. Education on how to replace ongoing fluid losses after discharge from the ED should be provided. Symptoms will generally improve over a few days to a week. While most cases of AGE are caused by viral infection, bacterial and parasite infections can also cause gastroenteritis, and clinicians must be alert to signs and symptoms that suggest more evaluation is warranted. Blood in the stool may be a sign of bacterial infection, and stool cultures can be sent if a bacterial infection is suspected. Symptoms that persist beyond the usual timeframe for viral infections may suggest a parasitic infection, particularly in children with a history of recent travel or consumption of fresh water from streams or ponds, with the diagnosis being confirmed by sending stool studies for ova and parasite inspection.

Neurologic causes continue to be an important consideration in the differential diagnosis of vomiting in older children. Increased ICP in this age group may present with vomiting and headaches. Older children may complain of progressively worsening headaches over a period of weeks to months, with headache worst in the morning. They may also have nighttime headaches that wake them from sleep. Vomiting with headaches, particularly if it is occurring regularly and most frequently in the morning, is a worrisome sign. Migraine headaches may also be associated with vomiting, but in this case headaches are often acute, with associated symptoms such as photophobia and phonophobia. It is important to obtain a thorough history and perform a full examination, including neurologic, as well as to examine the fundus for papilledema in children presenting with headaches and vomiting, to determine which children require urgent neuroimaging.

Renal causes remain in the differential diagnosis in this age group, and include renal failure and nephrolithiasis. Diabetic ketoacidosis may present with frequent vomiting in addition to headaches, tachypnea, and altered mental status. Ingestions of medications or toxins, either accidental or intentional, may also lead to vomiting.

Cyclic vomiting syndrome (CVS) is characterized by recurrent episodes of severe vomiting in children. Patients are generally otherwise healthy, and are asymptomatic between the stereotypical episodes. Vomiting and nausea are acute in onset and last for hours to days. Associated symptoms may include headaches, photophobia, abdominal pain, and anorexia. There is a strong association between CVS and migraine headaches, with many patients suffering from CVS having a family history of migraine headaches. Diagnosis can initially be challenging, and may not be suspected until a pattern of recurrent episodes has been established. The Rome III diagnostic criteria may be used when CVS is considered in a child. These criteria include (1) two or more periods of intense nausea and unremitting vomiting or retching lasting hours to days and (2) return to usual state of health lasting weeks to months. Treatment includes lifestyle modifications and medications. Lifestyle modifications include avoiding triggers (similar to those known to trigger migraine headaches), such as fasting, chocolate, caffeine, and sleep deprivation. Medications can be divided into those for acute symptoms and those used for prophylaxis. Nausea and vomiting in acute episodes can be relieved with ondansetron, and intravenous fluids are frequently necessary. Depending on the severity of the episode, sedatives such as chlorpromazine, diphenhydramine, or lorazepam may be considered. When CVS episodes occur frequently, prophylaxis can be provided with tricyclic antidepressants including cyproheptadine in children of age 5 years and under, or amitriptyline for children over the age of 5 years.

Propranolol has also been used for prophylaxis, and can be used in both younger and older children.

Symptomatic relief of vomiting can be provided with antiemetic medication, providing significant benefit for oral rehydration attempts. In the past, many antiemetics were used with caution due to the possibility of dangerous adverse effects in children, including extrapyramidal symptoms. However, ondansetron has emerged as an antiemetic with a low side effect profile. Studies have shown that use of ondansetron does not mask symptoms of dangerous causes of vomiting, such as obstruction. Although most commonly used to decrease nausea and vomiting in gastroenteritis, ondansetron has been used by practitioners for vomiting caused by a variety of conditions, including concussion, pneumonia, and appendicitis.

Suggested Readings and Key References

General

Granado-Villar D, Cunill-De Sautu B, Granados A, et al. Acute gastroenteritis. *Pediatr Rev* 2012;33:487–496.

Louie JP. Essential diagnosis of abdominal emergencies in the first year of life. *Emerg Med Clin N Am* 2007;25:1009–1040.

McCollough M, Sharieff GQ. Abdominal pain in children [review]. *Pediatr Clin North Am* 2006;53(1):107–137.

Parashette KR, Croffie J. Vomiting. *Pediatr Rev* 2013;34(7):307–321.

Malrotation

McVay M, Kokoska ER, Jackson RJ, et al. The changing spectrum of intestinal malrotation: diagnosis and management. *Am J Surg* 2007;194:712–719.

Nagdeve NG, Qureshi AM, Bhingare PD, et al. Malrotation beyond infancy. *J Pediatr Surg* 2012;47:2026–2032.

Strousse PJ. Malrotation [review]. *Semin Roentgenol* 2008;43(1):7–14.

Hirschsprung Disease

Haricharan RN, Georgeson KE. Hirschsprung disease. *Semin Pediatr Surg* 2008;17:266–275.

Stensrud KJ, Emblem R, Bjornland K. Late diagnosis of Hirschsprung diease-patient characteristics and results. *J Pediatr Surg* 2012;47:1874–1879.

Gastroesophageal Reflux Disease

Blanco F, Davenport KP, Kane TD. Pediatric gastroesophageal reflux disease. *Surg Clin N Am* 2012;92:541–558.

Lightdale JR, Gremse DA; Section on Gastroenterology, Hepatology, and Nutrition. Gastroesophageal reflux: management guidance for the pediatrician. *Pediatrics* 2013;131:e1684.

Loots C, Kritas S, wan Wijk M, et al. A randomized trial of body positioning and medical therapy for infantile Gastroesophageal reflux symptoms. *J Pediatr Gastroenterol Nutr* 2014;59(2):237–243.

Rosen R. Gastroesophageal reflux in infants: more than just a phenomenon. *JAMA Pediatr* 2014;168(1):83–89.

Pyloric Stenosis

Glatstein M, Carbell G, Boddu SK, et al. The changing clinical presentation of hypertrophic pyloric stenosis: the experience of a large, tertiary care pediatric hospital. *Clin Pediatr* 2011;50(3):192–195.

Ranells JD, Carver JD, Kirby RS. Infantile hypertrophic pyloric stenosis: epidemiology, genetics and clinical update. *Adv Pediatr* 2011;58:195–206.

Intussusception

Applegate KE. Intussusception in children: imaging choices. *Semin Roentgenol* 2008;43(1):15–21.

Fike FB, Mortellaro VE, Holcomb GW, et al. Predictors of failed enema reduction in childhood intussusception. *J Pediatr Surg* 2012;47:925–927.

Waseem M, Rosenberg HK. Intussusception. *Pediatr Emerg Care* 2008;24(11):793–800.

Rumination Syndrome

Hyman PE, Milla PJ, Benninga MA, et al. Childhood functional gastrointestinal disorders: neonate/toddler. *Gastroenterology* 2006;130:1519–1526.

Appendicitis

Aspelund G, Fingeret A, Gross E, et al. Ultrasonography/MRI versus CT for diagnosing appendicitis. *Pediatrics* 2014;133:586–593.

Goldman RD, Carter S, Stephens D, et al. Prospective validation of the pediatric appendicitis score. *J Pediatr* 2008;253:278–282.

Mandeville K, Pottker T, Bulloch B, et al. Using appendicitis scores in the pediatric ED. *Am J Emerg Med* 2011;29:972–977.

Pepper VK, Stanfill AB, Pearl RH. Diagnosis and management of pediatric appendicitis, intussusception, and Meckel diverticulum. *Surg Clin N Am* 2012;92:505–526.

Cyclic Vomiting Syndrome

Li BU, Lefevre F, Chelimsky GG, et al. North American Society for Pediatric Gastroenterology, Hepatology, and Nutrition consensus statement on the diagnosis and management of cyclic vomiting syndrome. *J Pediatr Gastroenterol Nutr* 2008;47:379–393.

Rasquin A, Di Lorenzo C, Forbes D, et al. Childhood functional gastrointestinal disorders: child/adolescent. *Gastroenterology* 2006;130:1527–1537.

Imaging

Hryhorczuk AL, Lee EY. Imaging evaluation of bowel obstruction in children: updates in imaging techniques and review of imaging findings. *Semin Roentgenol* 2012;47:159–170.

Ng L, Marin JR. Pediatric emergency ultrasound. *Ultrasound Clin* 2014;9:199–210.

Reid JR. Practical imaging approach to bowel obstruction in neonates: a review and update. *Semin Roentgenol* 2012;47:21–31.

Gastroenteritis and Ondansetron

Colletti JE, Brown KM, Sharieff GQ, et al. The management of children with gastroenteritis and dehydration in the emergency department. *J Emerg Med* 2010;38(5):686–698.

Fedorowicz Z, Jagannath VA, Carter B. Antiemetics for reducing vomiting related to acute gastroenteritis in children and adolescents. *Cochrane Database Syst Rev* 2011;(9):CD005506.

Freedman SB, Ali S, Oleszczuk M, et al. Treatment of acute gastroenteritis in children: an overview of systematic reviews of interventions commonly used in developed countries. *Evid Based Child Health* 2013;8:1123–1137.

Sturm JR, Hirsh DA, Schweickert A, et al. Ondansetron use in the pediatric emergency department and effects on hospitalization and return rates: are we missing alternative diagnoses? *Ann Emerg Med* 2010;55:415–422.

CHAPTER 78 ■ WEAKNESS

NICHOLAS TSAROUHAS, MD AND CHRISTOPHER F. VALENTE, MD

Weakness is defined as an inability to generate normal voluntary force in a muscle or normal voluntary torque about a joint. Although often associated, *hypotonia* is not always synonymous with weakness. Neurologists define hypotonia as decreased resistance to "passive" motion. Not all hypotonic patients are weak; for example, a patient with Down syndrome may have normal strength yet have decreased tone.

PATHOPHYSIOLOGY

Weakness is a reflection of a disease process that may involve any component of the motor neuron unit. These diseases are classically categorized as upper or lower motor unit disorders (Table 78.1). Upper motor neuron disease affects structures extending from the motor strip of the cerebral cortex, through the corticospinal tracts of the spinal cord, to (but not including) the anterior horn cell. Although upper motor neuron disease is generally characterized by increased deep tendon reflexes (DTRs) and spasticity, early in the clinical course there may be flaccid paralysis. Lower motor neuron disease may involve the anterior horn cell, the peripheral nerves, the *neuromuscular junction* (NMJ), or the muscle fibers. In general, lower motor neuron disease is associated with fasciculations, muscle atrophy, hypotonia, and hyporeflexia, and may ultimately lead to flaccid paralysis.

DIFFERENTIAL DIAGNOSIS

The *cerebral cortex* can be damaged by *cerebrovascular accidents* (CVAs), which include *cerebral infarctions* and *cerebral hemorrhages*. CVAs, while rare (2.1 to 13.1 per 100,000 children per year), cause some of the most catastrophic cases of weakness (Table 78.2). These children usually present with sudden, unilateral, or asymmetric weakness.

Cerebral hemorrhage is usually due to a *ruptured arteriovenous malformation* (AVM), but may also be caused by a *ruptured aneurysm*. Most AVMs are asymptomatic until rupture, but some children do complain of periodic "migraine-like" headaches. *Brain tumor hemorrhage* may also present acutely as weakness, severe headache, and vomiting.

Cerebral infarctions usually occur in the setting of predisposing factors, which include sickle cell disease, homocystinuria, structural arterial disease (e.g., moyamoya), hypercoagulable states (e.g., antithrombin III, protein C and S deficiencies, and factor V Leiden mutations). Other more common hypercoagulable states include pregnancy, malignancy, infections, and severe dehydration. Recent studies have shown increased risk associated with hypertension, diabetes, obesity, and hypercholesterolemia in younger teenage populations. Substance abuse with tobacco, alcohol, cocaine, and amphetamines have also been associated with cerebral infarction. Atherosclerosis and atrial fibrillation, common culprits in adult stroke, remain rare causes of stroke in children. *Embolic* causes that should be considered in pediatric patients include children with congenital heart disease, mitral valve prolapse, or a history of rheumatic fever.

Transient ischemic attacks (TIAs) often present with resolving weakness. TIAs are defined as transient neurologic deficits referable to a cerebral artery territory in a child whose cranial magnetic resonance imaging (MRI) shows no acute ischemia, but whose history/workup suggests cerebrovascular disease. Transient focal deficits are common after a seizure and are called *Todd postictal paralysis*. Deficits usually resolve within minutes to hours after a seizure has ended, but one study demonstrated a mean symptom duration of 15 hours and persistence of up to 36 hours. In this same study, 8/14 patients with Todd postictal paralysis had an underlying CNS lesion.

Because a Todd paralysis resolves with time, if the patient is not improving (regaining function) in 30 to 45 minutes, the differential diagnosis should be broadened to ensure a cerebrovascular event or mass lesion is not the cause of the focal weakness. Cranial imaging is crucial in cases of prolonged postictal paralysis, especially if the mental status remains impaired, or if other focal deficits persist. The reference standard study is MRI. However, access to MRI may be limited or may not be immediately practical or safe (e.g., need for deep sedation). Consequently, a computed tomography (CT) scan of the head is often the initial study of choice. The head CT is most useful to rule out acute bleeds and large mass lesions. In some cases, a CT angiogram is necessary to identify vascular lesions or anomalies.

Traumatic injuries may seriously damage or compress the spinal cord. *Spinal cord concussion* is defined as a transitory disturbance in spinal cord function caused by a direct blow to the back. Symptoms may include flaccid paraplegia or quadriplegia, a sensory level at the site of injury, loss of tendon reflexes, and urinary retention. Recovery usually begins within a few hours and is usually complete within a week. *Spinal epidural hematoma* may cause spinal cord compression as the hematoma expands. Emergent spinal MRI scanning is indicated when an epidural hematoma is suspected. Other traumatic injuries include vertebral body compression fractures, dislocations, and spinal cord transections.

Another serious cause of spinal cord compression is *epidural abscess,* which is usually caused by hematogenous spread of bacteria, most commonly *Staphylococcus aureus,* or by direct spread from an adjacent carbuncle or vertebral osteomyelitis. This is a rare (0.2 to 1.2 per 10,000 hospital admissions), but potentially devastating disease entity often unidentified until progression to severe neurologic sequelae. Patients commonly present with fever and back pain, but may also have headache, vomiting, stiff neck, and bowel and bladder dysfunction. Point tenderness may be elicited over the affected area. The diagnosis is confirmed by MRI, which helps also

TABLE 78.1

DIFFERENTIAL DIAGNOSIS OF WEAKNESS

UPPER MOTOR UNIT DISORDERS	LOWER MOTOR UNIT DISORDERS
Cerebral cortex	**Anterior horn cell**
Cerebrovascular infarction	Poliomyelitis
Cerebrovascular hemorrhage	Postasthmatic amyotrophy
■ Ruptured arteriovenous malformation	Spinal muscular atrophy
■ Ruptured aneurysm	Amyotrophic lateral sclerosis
Brain tumor hemorrhage	**Peripheral nerve**
Cerebral embolism	Guillain–Barré syndrome
Transient ischemic attack	Erb/Klumpke palsy
Todd postictal paralysis	Heavy metal poisoning
Amyotrophic lateral sclerosis	Pharmacologic medicines
Spinal cord	Marine toxins
Trauma	Acute intermittent porphyria
■ Cord concussion	**Neuromuscular junction**
■ Epidural hematoma	Botulism
■ Fracture	Myasthenia gravis
■ Dislocation	Tick paralysis
■ Transection	Organophosphates
Epidural abscess	Neuromuscular blockers
Discitis	Snake envenomations
Spinal cord tumor	**Muscle**
Transverse myelitis	Muscular dystrophy
Anatomic	Myotonic dystrophy
■ Atlantoaxial dislocations	Dermatomyositis
■ Chiari malformations	Infectious
■ Tethered spinal cord	■ Pyomyositis
Amyotrophic lateral sclerosis	■ Viral myositis
Miscellaneous disorders	■ Trichinosis
Congenital hypothyroidism	Metabolic abnormalities
Benign congenital hypotonia	Periodic paralysis
Alternating hemiplegia	Rhabdomyolysis/myoglobinuria
Acute hemiplegic migraine	Inborn errors of metabolism
Critical illness neuromuscular disease	Endocrine disorders
Conversion disorder/malingering	Steroid myopathy

TABLE 78.2

LIFE-THREATENING CAUSES OF WEAKNESS

Cerebrovascular accident
Brain tumor hemorrhage/edema
Epidural hemorrhage/abscess:
Cord compression (tumor/trauma)
Heavy metal/organophosphate poisoning
Myoglobinuria/rhabdomyolysis
Guillain–Barré syndrome
Myasthenia gravis
Botulism
Tick paralysis

to distinguish the abscess from a *vertebral discitis.* Similarly, spinal cord tumors are another important cause of spinal cord compression.

Transverse myelitis is an acute demyelinating disorder of the spinal cord. It is frequently attributed to a preceding viral infection, but may be immune mediated. It presents as an acute episode of fever and back pain at the level of cord involvement. The hallmark of transverse myelitis is the demarcation of the lesion by a sensory loss below a spinal cord level (usually thoracic). Leg paresthesias and weakness evolve rapidly over the course of 2 days. Asymmetric leg weakness is common. Tendon reflexes may be increased or reduced. Bowel and bladder continence are often lost. Urgent MRI of the spine is required to exclude cord compression.

Anatomic anomalies of the spine and spinal cord associated with weakness also include the *atlantoaxial dislocations* associated with Klippel–Feil and Down syndrome. Patients with *Chiari malformations/myelomeningoceles* also have weakness (as well as other deficits). In the growing child, a *tethered spinal cord* may cause weakness and neurologic deficits, as the tether causes the spinal cord to stretch. Clumsiness may be the presenting symptom of leg weakness. Bladder control problems are also common.

Juvenile amyotrophic lateral sclerosis (ALS) is a rare hereditary disorder involving upper and lower motor neurons. Similar to "adult" ALS, or Lou Gehrig disease, it causes spasticity and muscular atrophy. The course is progressive and is ultimately fatal.

Anterior horn cell disease affects the most proximal component of the lower motor neuron unit. Because these diseases affect the motor neurons, sensory function is normal. Reflexes are generally lost early in the course of the disease. Ultimately, muscle atrophy and fasciculations develop. Cranial nerve nuclei are often affected as well.

Poliomyelitis is the classic example of an anterior horn cell disease, but it has been largely eradicated by immunization. In 2014, anterior horn cell disease emerged in association with enterovirus D68. A peculiar entity that mimics poliomyelitis is idiopathic *postasthmatic amyotrophy,* or Hopkins syndrome. It presents as a sudden onset of weakness, generally 1 to 2 weeks after an acute asthma attack. Like polio, prognosis is poor, with all patients left with some degree of permanent paralysis.

The three pediatric types of *spinal muscular atrophy* (SMA) comprise a group of autosomal recessive genetic disorders in which the anterior horn cells in the spinal cord and motor nuclei of the brainstem are progressively lost. There is widespread muscle denervation and atrophy. The weakness is usually symmetric, progressive, and proximal, and presents anytime from birth to adulthood. Later in the disease course, tongue fasciculations and diminished DTRs may occur. Importantly, intellect and cardiac, sensory, and sphincter functions are preserved.

Spinal muscular atrophy I (acute infantile SMA, or Werdnig–Hoffman disease) is the most severe form of SMA. The weakness and severe generalized hypotonia begin before 6 months of age. These patients can never sit alone. Death often occurs by 4 years of age, usually from overwhelming pneumonia. *Spinal muscular atrophy II* (chronic infantile SMA) usually has its onset of weakness between 6 and 18 months. These patients can sit alone, but can never walk. In this "intermediate" SMA, survival to adulthood is expected. *Spinal muscular atrophy III* (mild juvenile SMA, or Kugelberg–Welander disease) usually presents with weakness after 18 months. These patients can walk without support.

Neuropathies (primary disorders of the axon or its myelin sheath) usually present as progressive symmetric distal weakness. Weakness and sensory loss may move in a "glove and stocking" fashion. Tendon reflexes are usually lost early. Dysesthesias ("pins and needles" or burning sensations) usually occur in acquired conditions.

Guillain–Barré syndrome (GBS), or acute inflammatory demyelinating polyradiculopathy (AIDP), is the classic acquired immunologic neuropathic disorder. It is the most common cause of acute motor paralysis in children. GBS occurs when activated immune mechanisms, induced by an antecedent viral infection, trigger inflammation and demyelination (see Chapter 105 Neurologic Emergencies). Many viruses have been implicated, including adenovirus, Epstein–Barr virus, cytomegalovirus, human immunodeficiency virus, varicella-zoster virus, measles virus, *Rubulavirus* (mumps), and vaccinia virus. *Mycoplasma pneumoniae* and *Campylobacter jejuni* infections, as well as some vaccines (i.e., swine flu 1976), have also been implicated.

The most common complaint is weakness, but patients also present with leg and back pain, and in younger children, an abnormal gait. The symptoms may progress for days to weeks. The weakness is usually symmetric and may be ascending or descending. There is often a sensory loss, as well as loss of position and vibratory sense. DTRs are diminished or absent in the weak muscles. Bowel and bladder incontinence, autonomic dysfunction (hypotension), and cardiac dysrhythmias also occur.

Respiratory paralysis occurs in 20% to 30%. Cranial nerve involvement is seen in 30% to 40% of patients, usually manifested by facial weakness or ocular paresis. The *Miller Fisher* variant of GBS includes the triad of ataxia, areflexia, and ophthalmoplegia.

Required clinical criteria for diagnosis include a progressive motor weakness of more than one limb, and areflexia. Examination of the cerebrospinal fluid demonstrates an elevated protein without pleocytosis (albuminocytologic dissociation). Important diseases to consider in the differential diagnosis include acute cerebellar ataxia, transverse myelitis, toxic neuropathy, tick paralysis, botulism, myasthenia gravis (MG), and acute viral myositis. A chronic form of GBS, chronic inflammatory demyelinating polyneuropathy (CIDP), also exists. The course of CIDP varies widely and ranges from complete spontaneous recovery to frequent relapses with gradually declining function. Therapies for both GBS and CIDP include steroids, IVIG, plasmapheresis, and physiotherapy.

Birth trauma may produce traction injuries to the nerve roots causing a restricted pattern of focal weakness. *Erb palsy,* a proximal (C5/C6) brachial plexus palsy, is the most common brachial plexus injury. These infants assume the "waiter's tip" posture: arm adducted, humerus internally rotated, elbow extended, forearm pronated, wrist flexed. *Klumpke palsy,* an injury to the lower trunk (C8/T1) of the plexus, is much rarer. This typically manifests as an infant holding the arm in supination with the elbow flexed and wrist extended. Fortunately, most birth-related traction injuries of the brachial plexus result in only a self-limited neuropraxia from stretching of the nerves, with resolution of symptoms by 6 months of age. More extensive brachial plexus injuries can be associated with Horner syndrome (ptosis, miosis, anhidrosis) due to injury of the stellate ganglion. Avulsions or ruptures of the nerves usually result in more permanent weakness. Flaccid weakness of the arms and legs may result from excessive traction on the spinal cord during a difficult delivery.

Heavy metals, such as lead, mercury, arsenic, and thallium, are known neuropathic toxins. Lead, in particular, may cause a distal motor weakness with foot and wrist drop. Drug-induced neuropathies occur with drugs of abuse, as well as pharmacologic medicines. Several antimicrobials (isoniazid, nitrofurantoin, and zidovudine), as well as antineoplastics (vincristine, vinblastine, cytosine arabinoside, and cisplatin), are known to cause paresthesias and muscle weakness.

The seas also harbor deadly neurotoxins. Ciguatera and paralytic shellfish poisoning are caused when toxin-elaborating dinoflagellates are ingested by fish or shellfish, which are then eaten by unsuspecting humans. Cone snail stings, blue-ringed octopus bites, sea snake bites, and puffer fish ingestion may also result in life-threatening paralysis. On land, the *Crotalidae* (pit vipers) and *Elapidae* (coral snakes) families of snakes in the United States are responsible for nearly 8,000 envenomations each year. Pit viper bites initially cause localized pain, erythema, edema, and even tissue necrosis, but then severe multiorgan systemic symptoms, including weakness, may develop. Coral snakes, on the other hand, have a paucity of local signs associated with their bites, but then weakness and severe neurotoxicity ensue. A respiratory paralysis results from the toxin's presynaptic neuromuscular blockade; this ultimately proves fatal in 10 to 20 human cases per year.

Acute intermittent porphyria is an autosomal dominant inborn error of metabolism that usually presents after puberty (women > men) with neurovisceral attacks causing severe abdominal pain, nausea, vomiting, tachycardia, hypertension, and, in some cases, central and peripheral neuropathies. Motor weakness is more common than sensory symptoms, and the proximal muscles are more affected than the distal musculature. Autonomic dysfunction and mental status changes also occur. Medications (griseofulvin, barbiturates, sulfonamides, and estrogens) as well as stress, infections, and alcohol have been implicated as triggers.

Diseases of the NMJ can be recognized by their cranial nerve abnormalities and autonomic dysfunction. Importantly, sensory function is unaffected. In botulism, *Clostridium botulinum,* a gram-positive anaerobe, produces several potent neurotoxins that prevent presynaptic release of acetylcholine, resulting in descending flaccid paralysis. Preformed toxin may be ingested from improperly home-canned foods or any incompletely cooked food. Botulinum spores are also found in the soils of some areas of the United States, particularly in eastern Pennsylvania and California. There are three distinct clinical presentations of natural disease: infant botulism, classic botulism, and wound botulism (see Chapter 105 Neurologic Emergencies). In addition, the potential use of botulinum toxin as a weapon of bioterrorism has been described (see Chapter 136 Biological and Chemical Terrorism).

Infant botulism is one of the more common causes of generalized weakness seen in young infants (Table 78.3). The bacterial spores are ingested, and then they germinate and colonize in the intestinal tract, leading to *in vivo* toxin production. Infant botulism has been linked to ingestion of honey, which has a high rate of contamination by the spores. The spores are also found naturally in soil; consequently, areas in which disturbed soil is found, such as construction sites and rural farming areas, also have been associated with disease. Peak incidence is between 2 and 3 months of age, but it may be seen in infants up to 9 months old. Infant botulism commonly

TABLE 78.3

CAUSES OF WEAKNESS IN INFANTS

Infant botulism
Congenital hypothyroidism
Inborn errors of metabolism
Benign congenital hypotonia
Transient/familial myasthenia
Congenital muscular dystrophy/myopathies
Spinal muscular atrophy
Chiari malformation/myelomeningocele
Tethered cord
Erb palsy

presents with a history of constipation, lethargy, and feeding difficulties. On physical examination, the infants are hypotonic with generalized muscle weakness and a noticeably weak cry. There may be reduced facial expressions, pooling of oral secretions, a decreased gag reflex, ptosis, and dilated pupils that respond poorly to light. A progressive bulbar and descending skeletal muscle weakness ensues, with loss of tendon reflexes over the next several days. Sensory examination is normal. While this subacute presentation is most common, a "sepsis-like" or catastrophic presentation is also possible. Importantly, constipation, lethargy, weak cry, and hypotonia are much more commonly caused by *congenital hypothyroidism,* which lacks the more dramatic bulbar symptoms and progressive paralysis that occur later in the course of infant botulism.

Classic botulism, which is usually seen in older children and adults, is caused by eating food contaminated by the preformed botulinum exotoxin. Even tiny amounts of toxin can produce severe paralysis. Symptoms develop 12 to 36 hours after ingestion of the toxin. These may include nausea and vomiting, followed by blurred vision, diplopia, ptosis, photophobia, and then dysphagia and dysarthria from sequential involvement of cranial nerves. A descending skeletal muscle paralysis follows in many patients—without any sensory involvement.

In *wound botulism,* a wound is contaminated with soil containing the spores of *C. botulinum*. Subsequent production of botulinum toxin results in muscle weakness and bulbar dysfunction 4 to 14 days after the wound has been infected. The severe muscular spasms of generalized *tetanus* ("lockjaw"), caused by *Clostridium tetani,* are in contrast to the muscle weakness of botulism. Wound botulism presents similarly to classic botulism, except that no gastrointestinal symptoms are associated.

A less common disorder of the NMJ is juvenile *myasthenia gravis,* which occurs as a result of an antibody-mediated autoimmune reaction against the postsynaptic acetylcholine receptors in skeletal muscle. The sine qua non of MG is muscle weakness provoked by activity and relieved by rest. There is weakness and fatigability of ocular, bulbar, and extremity striated muscles. Most patients present with ptosis. Sensory examination and DTRs are normal.

Ten percent to 15% of babies born to mothers with MG develop *transient neonatal myasthenia,* which is caused by a transient impairment of neuromuscular transmission secondary to the passive transfer of antibodies versus acetylcholine receptors. These babies may present with weak suck or cry, ptosis, dysphagia, generalized weakness, or respiratory distress in the first few hours or days of life. The condition usually resolves in the first few weeks, but occasionally the symptoms may take months to disappear.

Familial infantile myasthenia, or congenital myasthenia, should not be confused with transient neonatal myasthenia. Familial infantile myasthenia is not autoimmune, and these infants are not born to mothers with MG. Children with this type of myasthenia also exhibit respiratory muscle weakness, feeding difficulties, ptosis, hypotonia, and limb fatigability.

Paralyzing toxins may also be introduced by human–animal interactions, a dramatic example being *tick paralysis.* This is a toxin-mediated paralysis transmitted from the bite of one of several species of ticks in North America. The dog tick, *Dermacentor variabilis,* and the Rocky Mountain wood tick, *Dermacentor andersoni,* among others, elaborate a salivary gland toxin that most likely acts at the NMJ to induce a rapid, profound, generalized, flaccid weakness. The tick exposure often precedes the paralysis by 5 to 10 days. Although patients may complain of paresthesias, the sensory examination is usually normal. DTRs are absent or decreased, thus mimicking GBS. Removal of the tick results in dramatic resolution of symptoms.

Organophosphates, which are used in commercial insecticides, inhibit acetylcholinesterases at the NMJ. This leads to the prolonged attachment of acetylcholine at the postsynaptic receptor. Severe muscle cramps and life-threatening weakness ensues. Similarly, children treated with neuromuscular blockers for long periods of time may have exaggerated weakness and remain flaccid for days or weeks after the drugs are discontinued.

Myopathies are primary disorders of muscle fibers. Proximal weakness is the usual presenting feature, and sensory function is normal. *Muscular dystrophy* (MD) is a progressive inherited myopathy caused by defects in structural muscle proteins. These defects result in muscle degeneration and loss of strength. In the two main MDs, Duchenne and Becker, there is a reduction of the structural protein dystrophin. Although MD primarily affects striated skeletal muscle, striated cardiac muscle may also be involved. Four criteria must be met to diagnose MD: a primary myopathy (not neurogenic), genetic cause, progressive course, and myofiber degeneration.

Duchenne muscular dystrophy (DMD) is an X-linked recessive disorder that presents before the age of 5 years as gait disturbance, frequent falling, waddling gait (hip girdle weakness), and difficulty rising from the floor. The classic examination finding is the Gower sign, whereby the hands and arms are used to push up off the floor, and then "walked" up the thighs to straighten into the erect position. Boys with DMD often have low normal intellectual ability. Proximal muscles are weaker than the distal muscles. These children have large, rubbery, hypertrophic calf muscles without tenderness. DTRs are present early, but disappear later. Sensory examination is normal. The diagnosis is supported by a creatine kinase (CK) elevation that may range from 10 to 10,000 times normal, and is confirmed by muscle biopsy. Death occurs from progressive respiratory insufficiency or infection, dysrhythmia secondary to cardiomyopathy, or congestive heart failure. *Becker muscular dystrophy* is also an X-linked recessive MD, but is less severe, with a later presentation, intact IQ, preservation of ambulation, rare cardiac involvement, and favorable survivability.

Myotonic dystrophy is an autosomal-dominant, multisystem disorder that presents from infancy to adolescence with myotonia and distal muscle weakness. Its classic feature, myotonia, is defined as a disturbance in muscle relaxation after contraction. It causes an inability to quickly relax a contracted muscle or release an object. Unlike MG, this myotonia is worsened by rest. A characteristic facial weakness, the "Cheshire cat smile," is an inability for a child to relax a smile.

Dermatomyositis is a systemic angiopathy that is manifested by intravascular occlusion and infarction in muscles, connective tissue, skin, the gastrointestinal tract, and small nerves (see Chapter 109 Rheumatologic Emergencies). It is caused by antibody or immune complex–mediated immune response against a vascular endothelial component. Patients commonly present with fever, anorexia, and fatigue, followed by rash, and then the myositis. The classic "heliotrope" rash is a violaceous discoloration and edema of periorbital and malar areas. Over time, the rash spreads to the extensor surfaces of the joints. Papular, erythematous, scaly lesions over the knuckles are referred to as the "Gottron sign." Arthralgias and cardiac complications are common. *Polymyositis,* a similar disorder, is rare in children.

Infectious processes of the muscle may also present with weakness. *Pyomyositis* is caused by multifocal abscesses associated with a bacterial infection of the muscle. Causative agents include *S. aureus,* streptococci, *Escherichia coli, Yersinia,* and *Legionella* species. Although most common in immunocompromised patients, it can also occur in normal hosts. Clinical presentation includes muscle pain, tenderness, and fever.

Viral myositis is one of the more common causes of acute weakness seen in children (Table 78.4) and commonly follows influenza or other viral respiratory illness. Several days of prodromal constitutional symptoms lead to severe symmetric muscle pain and generalized weakness. On examination, the muscles are exquisitely tender to palpation. *Myoglobinuria* (positive urinary "dipstick" for heme, in the absence of red blood cells) and *rhabdomyolysis* (markedly elevated serum CK) sometimes complicate viral myositis. Viral myositis resolves with rest, adequate hydration, and analgesics. Rhabdomyolysis and myoglobinuria may also occur from excessive physical exertion, prolonged seizures, toxic exposures, and envenomations. Along with weakness and muscle tenderness, patients present with the characteristic dark or tea-colored urine of myoglobinuria, which may lead to renal insufficiency or failure. Uremia itself may also lead to muscle weakness.

Trichinosis is the most common parasitic disease of skeletal muscle. It occurs when *Trichinella spiralis* is ingested in inadequately cooked meat (usually pork). Most patients are asymptomatic, but some develop constitutional symptoms (fever, headache, abdominal pain, and diarrhea) along with myalgias and generalized weakness. Cysticercosis and toxoplasmosis may have similar presentations.

Myopathies may also be caused by various metabolic abnormalities. Hyponatremia, hypocalcemia, and hypochloremia are frequently associated with weakness. High, low, or normal potassium levels have been described with distinct familial syndromes that present with weakness. These autosomal-dominant *periodic paralysis syndromes* may present from infancy to adolescence. Attacks of weakness may be precipitated by rest, shortly after exercise. Mild attacks last for less than an hour, whereas severe attacks can cause flaccid paralysis for many hours. During attacks, the serum potassium is high or low, and electrocardiogram changes sometimes occur.

Inborn errors of metabolism, such as defects in glycogen metabolism (acid maltase deficiency, or Pompe disease), and disorders of lipid or mitochondrial metabolism may also cause weakness. Hyperthyroidism/hypothyroidism, hyperparathyroidism/hypoparathyroidism, and hyperadrenalism/hypoadrenalism are just a few of the endocrinologic causes of myopathies. Even exogenous steroid use has been implicated in myopathies. Corticosteroids are sometimes associated with a usually mild, proximal, "steroid myopathy" 4 to 14 days after therapy is started.

Critical illness neuromuscular disease is the term given to patients who develop acute weakness or paralysis during the course of a life-threatening disease. Risk factors include sepsis or multisystem organ failure, treatment with steroids or neuromuscular blocking agents, and even hyperglycemia. While incompletely understood, neuromuscular structural changes, consisting of axonal nerve degeneration, myosin loss, and muscle necrosis, lead to electrical inexcitability of nerves and muscles. This may manifest as a polyneuropathy, or as an acute myopathy, and is perhaps an underappreciated cause of some patients' inability to wean from mechanical ventilation.

Several disorders are difficult to place using conventional neuroanatomic and pathophysiologic classifications. *Benign congenital hypotonia* is the term given to an infant with generalized hypotonia, but without major weakness. Biopsy, electromyogram, and all other studies are normal. Most children spontaneously improve. Alternating hemiplegia and acute hemiplegic migraine are poorly understood disorders that present with acute onset hemiplegia. Acute hemiplegic migraine may be associated with CVAs later in life.

Finally, patients with weakness caused by a conversion disorder demonstrate a deficit in voluntary motor function without physiologic basis. Most prevalent in adolescent females, patients with conversion disorders have a striking lack of concern for their impairments. They may complain of severe pain without concomitant sympathetic signs. Their examination is often illogical both anatomically and physiologically. Patients with a "paralyzed leg" who are suspected to have a conversion disorder should have normal DTRs. They should also be tested for the presence of the "Hoover sign." With the patient supine, the patient is asked to raise the "paralyzed" leg. The contralateral (unaffected) leg should push down on the bed (on top of the examiner's hand) to strain to raise the weak "paralyzed" leg. A positive "Hoover sign" demonstrates no volitional effort on the patient's behalf to actually try to raise the leg. This may indicate malingering.

In summary, there is a wide range of diagnostic possibilities for the child presenting with weakness. Although the neuroanatomic classification system followed above is most helpful pathophysiologically, an easy-to-remember mnemonic, which represents the major disease processes categorized by type of pathologic injury, might also be useful to the clinician. This mnemonic is VITAMINS (Table 78.5), with *V* representing *v*ascular events; *I* *i*nfectious, *i*mmunologic, and *i*nflammatory diseases; *T* *t*rauma and *t*oxins; *A* *a*natomic conditions; *M* *m*yopathies and

TABLE 78.4

COMMON CAUSES OF ACUTE WEAKNESS IN CHILDREN

Viral myositis
Guillain–Barré syndrome
Medications/toxins
Tumors
Seizures

TABLE 78.5

"VITAMINS" MNEMONIC FOR THE DIFFERENTIAL DIAGNOSIS OF WEAKNESS

Vascular events	**Anatomic conditions**
Cerebral infarction	Atlantoaxial dislocation
Arteriovenous malformation	Chiari malformation/myelomeningocele
Infectious diseases	Tethered spinal cord
Botulism	**Myopathies**
Epidural abscess	Muscular dystrophy
Pyomyositis	Spinal muscular atrophy
Transverse myelitis	Myotonic dystrophy
Poliomyelitis	**Metabolic disturbances**
Viral myositis	Congenital hypothyroidism
Trichinosis	Periodic paralysis
Immunologic diseases	Myoglobinuria/rhabdomyolysis
Guillain–Barré syndrome	Acute intermittent porphyria
Myasthenia gravis	Acid maltase deficiency
Transient neonatal myasthenia	**Idiopathic (and miscellaneous) disorders**
Inflammatory diseases	Benign congenital hypotonia
Dermatomyositis	Hemiplegic migraine
Polymyositis	Postasthmatic amyotrophy
Trauma	Critical illness neuromuscular disease
Spinal cord concussion	Conversion
Spinal epidural hematoma	Malingering
Fracture, dislocation, transection	**Neuropathies**
Birth trauma	Juvenile amyotrophic lateral sclerosis
Toxins	Familial infantile myasthenia
Pharmacologic	**Neoplasia**
Tick paralysis	Brain tumors
Heavy metals	Spinal cord tumors
Marine toxins	**Seizures**
Snake envenomations	

*m*etabolic disturbances; *I* *i*diopathic disorders; *N* *n*europathies and *n*eoplasia; and *S* seizures.

EVALUATION AND DECISION

The acuity and severity of weakness onset are critical features in guiding one's diagnostic approach (Fig. 78.1). A history of a severe or sudden deterioration (Fig. 78.2) should lead one to consider catastrophic processes such as cerebral infarctions, ruptured AVMs, or hemorrhaging brain tumors. After appropriate stabilization, emergent imaging (CT/MRI) and subspecialty consultation (neurology/neurosurgery) is mandatory. Patients with transient, less fulminant presentations may be experiencing a TIA or Todd postictal paralysis. Importantly, a conversion disorder may present as an acute, apparent "paralysis." Clues include recent psychosocial stressors, unrelated chronic medical conditions, and underlying psychiatric histories. It is important to remember that these patients are not fabricating their symptoms or malingering, but subconsciously attempting to resolve some internal conflict, with the resulting physical manifestations.

A history of trauma is commonly associated with minor concussions of the spinal cord, but more severe edema and hematomas may rapidly lead to paralysis. Similarly, vertebral column fracture/dislocations may also be devastating. Birth

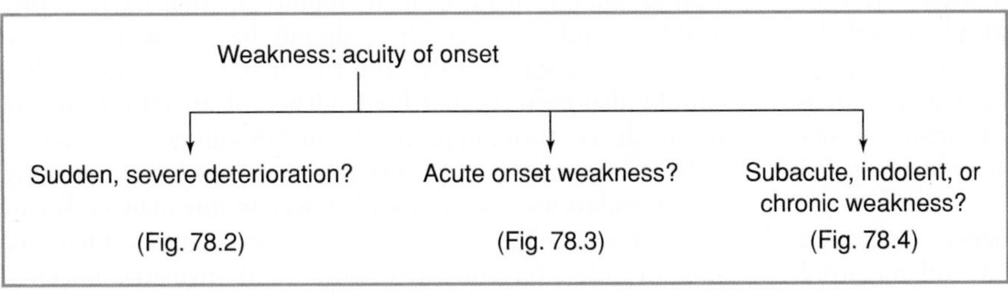

FIGURE 78.1 Diagnostic approach to weakness.

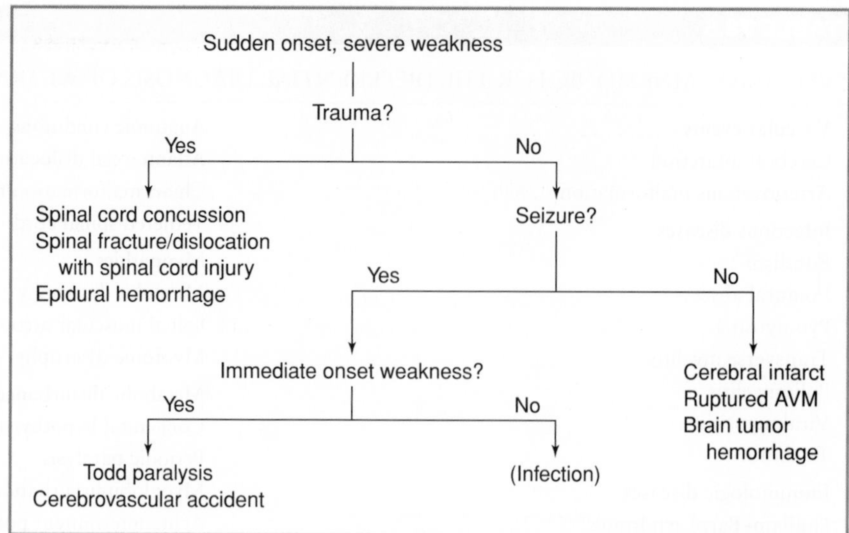

FIGURE 78.2 Approach to sudden onset of severe weakness. AVM, arteriovenous malformation.

trauma is usually obvious and may present with findings ranging from subtle limb weakness (Erb palsy) to complete quadriplegia from a spinal column distraction injury. Other conditions are manifested by less sudden, but still relatively acute onset, over hours to days (Fig. 78.3). Constipation and feeding difficulties, followed over a day or two by facial and extremity weakness in an infant strongly implicate infant botulism. A recent tick bite coupled with an acute progression of paralysis makes tick paralysis the likely diagnosis. A descending paralysis in a patient with a skin wound could be a case of wound botulism, whereas ingestion of improperly prepared or undercooked foods would suggest classic botulism or trichinosis. Fish ingestion with concomitant vomiting and other gastrointestinal symptoms might implicate ciguatera or paralytic shellfish poisoning.

A thorough history of medication use or toxin exposure is always important. Many pharmacologic medications have weakness and paresthesias as an adverse effect. Certain drugs can trigger an attack of acute intermittent porphyria. Drugs of abuse, as well as heavy metals, are associated with both weakness and mental status changes. A mild steroid myopathy is quite common, whereas a rare postasthmatic amyotrophy has been described in asthmatics irrespective of steroid use. Critical illness neuromuscular disease may occur in the context of steroid use, but should be considered in all severely ill children who require intensive care.

Patients who develop delayed onset of weakness after a prolonged seizure might have rhabdomyolysis with resultant myoglobinuria. Rhabdomyolysis (CK levels greater than 5 times normal, or greater than 1,000 IU/L) may also occur after viral syndromes, strenuous physical activity, heat stroke, cocaine abuse, sympathomimetic overdoses, neuroleptic malignant syndrome, and serotonin syndrome. These patients may have a history of dark or tea-colored urine.

Weakness that is worse after activity (and better with rest) should suggest MG. Patients with hypokalemic/hyperkalemic periodic paralysis, however, have their attacks initiated by rest shortly after exercise. Similarly, the weakness of myotonic dystrophy is worsened by rest. Patients with autoimmune disorders are more prone to myasthenic syndromes and dermatomyositis.

A history (or recent history) of fever suggests infectious (abscess, pyomyositis, viral myositis) and inflammatory (dermatomyositis) disorders. Headache is usually associated with viral processes such as myositis, but may also herald an AVM, an acute hemiplegic migraine, or brain tumor (the latter, especially if associated with emesis upon awakening or cranial nerve palsies). Back pain is common with GBS, an epidural abscess, and transverse myelitis. Abdominal pain should prompt consideration of food poisoning, such as botulism, but is also characteristic of acute intermittent porphyria.

A subacute, indolent, and/or chronic course of muscle weakness (Fig. 78.4) suggests neuropathies and myopathies. This weakness is almost always first noticed in the legs because parents will report clumsiness or gait disturbance as their initial concern. Furthermore, many neuromuscular disorders affect the legs before the arms. Although the history commonly revolves around the child's ability to walk, run, play, and climb stairs, questions should also be directed toward activities of daily living such as hair combing, buttoning, coloring, and writing.

Following the development of an appropriate differential diagnosis via a comprehensive history, the physical examination can further establish the likely diagnosis. Because weakness may cause respiratory insufficiency, one should first evaluate the effectiveness of aeration and oxygenation. Altered mental status may portend acute intracranial emergency such as stroke, hemorrhage, or CNS infection. Severe headache along with bradycardia and hypertension suggests increased intracranial pressure. Trauma patients require adequate cervical spine immobilization to prevent further injury.

Once triage for true neurologic emergencies is complete, the examination should continue by observing the child's activity. Infants should be observed for gaze tracking and maintenance, head control, global tone, and strength of suck. Strength and tone can be assessed by holding the infant vertically and allowing them to bear weight on the legs, as well as pulling them up from supine position by the arms. Toddlers and older children should be assessed for their ability to sit, stand, walk, and run. The muscles themselves should also be inspected for evidence of atrophy from disuse or denervation, hypertrophy or "doughiness" caused by MD, failure to relax appropriately as in myotonic dystrophy, or fasciculations common with lower motor neuron disease such as SMA. Tenderness to palpation suggests inflammation or infection consistent with viral myositis, bacterial

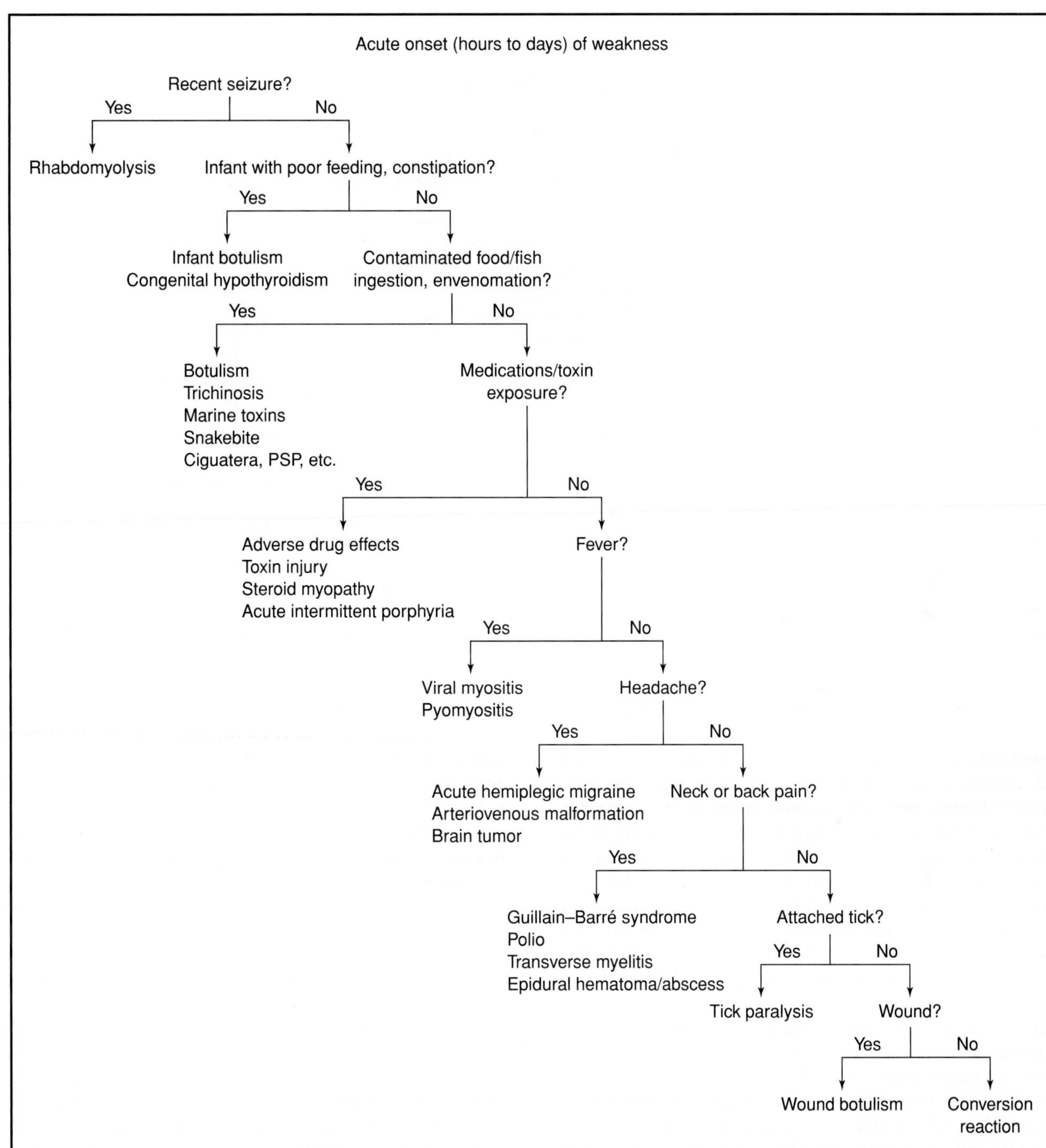

FIGURE 78.3 Approach to acute onset of weakness. PSP, paralytic shellfish poisoning.

pyomyositis, or dermatomyositis. Focal tenderness of the back may be a clue toward diagnosis of an epidural abscess or transverse myelitis.

Muscle strength of all the major muscle groups should be carefully assessed and documented (Table 78.6). "Give" weakness, whereby the patient resists passive motion up to a certain point and then suddenly loses strength is not physiologic and is usually the product of perceived pain or fatigue or frank malingering. When performance on muscle strength testing is suspect, stealthy observation during simple functional tasks such as the patient walking to the bathroom may prove valuable.

Toe walking and heel walking assess for gastrocnemius muscle and anterior compartment muscle weakness, respectively. The classic "Gower sign" of MD denotes proximal pelvic weakness as the child adopts the prone position before standing, and uses the hands to "walk" up the thighs. To test the arm muscles, have the child suspend himself above the floor in the "push-up" position. In general, myopathies such as MD present with proximal greater than distal muscle weakness, in contradistinction to neuropathies where the opposite is usually true. Proximal muscle weakness is also characteristic of viral myositis, rhabdomyolysis, dermatomyositis, acute intermittent porphyria, and anterior cord syndrome. Although

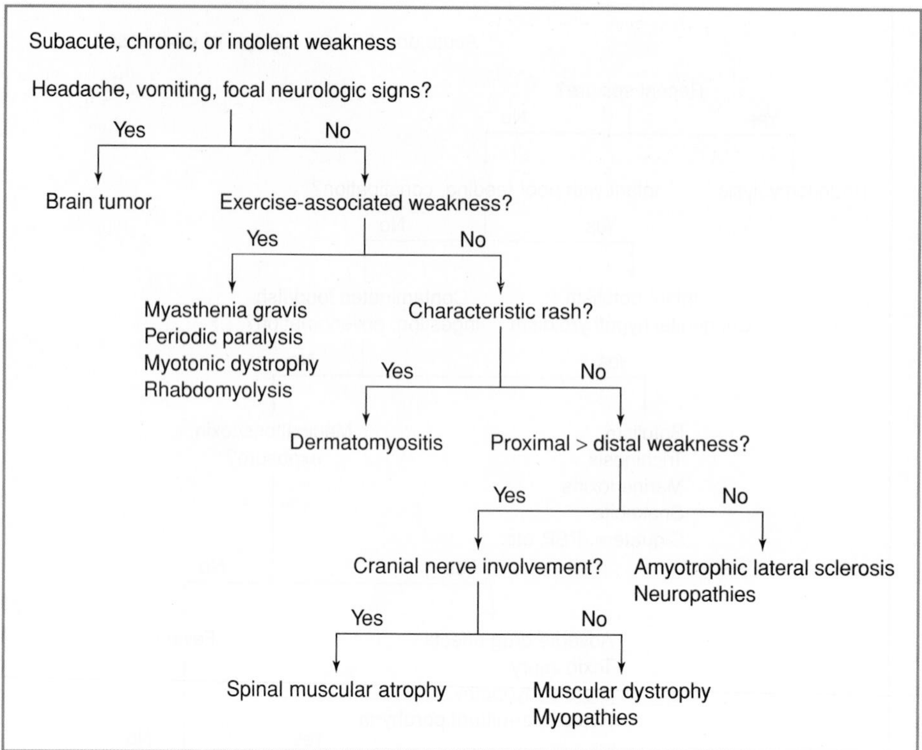

FIGURE 78.4 Approach to subacute, indolent, or chronic weakness.

most disorders have symmetric muscle weakness (GBS, MD, SMA, botulism), some diseases are commonly associated with asymmetric muscle weakness (transverse myelitis, polio, other CNS lesions, complex migraines). Regional weakness with a nearby feeding tick cements the diagnosis of tick paralysis. A novel bedside measure of bulbar muscle fatigue has been dubbed the "slurp" test. Children are given a 4-oz cup of water with a flex straw and are encouraged to drink the water as quickly as possible until the "slurping" sound at the end. This test, which has been used in children with MG, has been shown to be valuable for identifying patients with bulbar muscle compromise and for monitoring these children during times of decompensation.

After the general motor examination, the neurologic examination continues with the assessment of the cranial nerves. Diseases where cranial nerve involvement is most notable include GBS (Miller Fisher variant with ophthalmoplegia), SMA, MG, and infant botulism. Ptosis is common to both MG and infant botulism, while multiple prominent cranial nerve palsies are most often seen with infant botulism. In general, sensory deficits suggest spinal cord dysfunction or peripheral neuropathies, in contrast to NMJ disorders and myopathies. Sensory involvement is usually seen in GBS and transverse myelitis, whereas MG, MD, SMA, and botulism usually spare the senses. The DTRs are diminished in GBS, MD, botulism, and tick paralysis, whereas the DTRs are normal in MG.

Cerebellar function may be tested using heel-to-toe walk, finger-to-nose, and Romberg testing (patient stands with feet together and eyes closed; a test is positive test when the patient cannot maintain truncal stability). Ataxia, dysmetria, or positive Romberg indicate cerebellar mass, infection, inflammation, or demyelination. Specifically, a positive Romberg uncovers vestibular or proprioceptive system pathology otherwise compensated for by visual input.

The rest of the physical examination also yields important clues. While meningismus is often suggestive of infectious meningitis, it may be present with intracranial hemorrhage, abscess, or even polio. An abnormal cardiac examination may be present in GBS, MD, dermatomyositis, periodic paralysis, uremia, and acid maltase deficiency (Pompe disease). The characteristic heliotrope rash is the hallmark of dermatomyositis. Finally, when the examination is illogical or does not correspond to anatomic or physiologic principles, one should consider a conversion disorder or malingering.

In conclusion, weakness can be a vexing presenting complaint. The differential diagnosis is extensive and the disease processes complex. Although Figure 78.1 outlines a diagnostic approach, therapeutics should precede diagnostics when the patient is in existing or impending crisis. Patients with acute neurologic, respiratory, or circulatory compromise must be stabilized first. Once the patient is stable, a careful history and physical examination will narrow the differential diagnosis. Furthermore, select diagnostic laboratory and imaging studies may often assist in the search for the definitive diagnosis. Finally, subspecialty consultation and inpatient hospitalization are often indicated for these challenging patients.

TABLE 78.6

GRADING SCALE OF MUSCLE WEAKNESS

0	No movement
1	Trace movement
2	Movement in a horizontal plane but not against gravity
3	Movement against gravity but not against resistance
4	Weak strength against resistance
5	Full strength against resistance

Suggested Readings and Key References

Caramant L, Diadori P. The neurologic examination. In: Maria BL, ed. *Current management in child neurology.* 2nd ed. BC Dekker Inc., 2002.

Sander HW, Hedley-White ET. Case records of the Massachusetts General Hospital. Weekly clinicopathological exercises. Case 6-2003. A nine-year-old girl with progressive weakness and areflexia. *N Engl J Med* 2003;348(8):735–743.

Sanger TD, Chen D, Delgado MR, et al. Taskforce on Childhood Motor Disorders. Definition and classification of negative motor signs in childhood. *Pediatrics* 2006;118(5):2159–2167.

Shellhaas RA, Smith SE, O'Tool E, et al. Mimics of childhood stroke: characteristics of a prospective cohort. *Pediatrics* 2006;118(2): 704–709.

Tabarki B, Coffiniéres A, Van Den Bergh P, et al. Critical illness neuromuscular disease: clinical, electrophysiological, and prognostic aspects. *Arch Dis Child* 2002;86(2):103–107.

CHAPTER 79 ■ WEIGHT LOSS

SHABANA YUSUF, MD AND PAMELA J. BAILEY, MD

INTRODUCTION

Unexplained weight loss in a child is always concerning for parents and may prompt a visit to the emergency department. The differential diagnosis of weight loss is vast and the emergency physician must have a methodical approach to its evaluation so that children with potentially life-threatening causes of weight loss can be promptly identified and treated. Most causes of weight loss in children are not immediate threats to life but still require thoughtful evaluation, appropriate referral, and good follow-up.

PATHOPHYSIOLOGY

The major determinants of body weight are water and the organic fuels, carbohydrates, protein, and fat. Normal body weight is maintained by a balanced intake of water, protein, carbohydrates, and fats. Weight loss occurs when the daily energy balance becomes negative for one of these components. By far, the most common cause of acute (less than 2 weeks) weight loss in children of any age is loss of water, usually associated with an acute infectious illness. In addition, most infectious illnesses in children are associated with anorexia and increased short-term metabolic demand. Chronic weight loss (occurring over more than 2 weeks) results when there is persistent insufficient intake and retention of protein and energy to meet cellular metabolic demands and tissue synthesis. Causes of chronic weight loss include decreased energy intake, normal energy intake with increased metabolic requirement, and normal energy intake in the face of malabsorption or impaired use.

Understanding the basic physiologic abnormalities that cause weight loss in children provides a general framework which allows the emergency physician to generate a very broad differential diagnosis (Table 79.1). These physiologic categories apply to children of all ages. The child's age, severity and duration of the weight loss, specific symptoms and physical examination findings, as well as the judicious use of laboratory and radiographic studies help narrow the differential diagnosis into a more manageable list.

It is particularly important to recognize potentially life-threatening causes of weight loss in children in the emergency department (Table 79.2).

EVALUATION AND DECISION

General Approach

A thorough history and physical examination are key components in the evaluation of the patient with weight loss. Consideration of the child's age and the severity and duration of the weight loss, along with the presence of other systemic symptoms and specific physical examination findings, refines the extensive differential diagnosis. Many diagnoses are exclusive to specific age groups. For the emergency physician, severity is an important consideration because sudden losses are more suggestive of life-threatening disorders that require prompt recognition and treatment. Acute weight loss is most often caused by anorexia, poor fluid and energy intake, increased losses, and increased metabolic need in association with an intercurrent illness. Weight loss is a sensitive indicator for dehydration and commonly occurs in the presence of any significant febrile illness. In this setting, the history includes an estimation of intake, losses, and increased need for fluid and energy intake. The types of losses (e.g., urine, stool, or emesis) may pinpoint the location of the pathology. Inborn errors of metabolism usually present as sepsis-like picture either in neonatal or infancy (see Chapter 103 Metabolic Emergencies). Patients can also present as hepatic and cardiac failure. Others may demonstrate a picture of chronic developmental and neurologic sequelae.

Chronic weight loss results from a combination of factors including anorexia, poor utilization or malabsorption, and increased requirements, as well as health consequences imposed by the underlying disease state. When considering the cause of chronic weight loss, broad categories exist, including loss (i) secondary to a medical cause (underlying infection, absorptive defect, inflammatory, or neoplastic disease); (ii) related to a psychosocial or psychiatric cause; or (iii) resulting as a consequence of both problems. Once again, the importance of a thorough history and physical examination cannot be overemphasized. A complete review of systems, in search of fever, night sweats, arthritis, abdominal pain, and/or diarrhea, dermatitis, and other constitutional symptoms, helps the physician reach the diagnosis (Table 79.3).

A complete and careful physical examination with weight, height for age, weight for height, vital signs, state of hydration, and findings suggestive of specific disease states (e.g., anomalies of the face, general appearance, hygiene, pallor, jaundice, murmur, and/or cyanosis, clubbing, lymphadenopathy, dermatitis, hyperpigmentation, abdominal mass and/or tenderness, oral ulcers, anal skin tags, arthritis, neurologic abnormalities) provide useful clues. The shape of the head is important and points to various syndromes. Nutritional inspection includes an evaluation of body fat, muscle mass, hair, skin, and nails. Physical signs associated with vitamin deficiencies are nonspecific and occur late in the course of malnutrition. Dysmorphic features should be noted and a thorough neurologic examination should be performed. Infants should be observed nursing or being bottle-fed, with attention to any gagging, choking, reflux, or respiratory distress. The assessment of the airway might be necessary to initiate a safe feeding plan.

The essential components of the physical examination include measurement of weight, recumbent length in babies younger than 2 years, standing height in children older than

TABLE 79.1

PHYSIOLOGIC ABNORMALITIES CAUSING WEIGHT LOSS

Decreased calorie intake	Increased caloric requirements
■ Inadequate or improperly prepared food/formula ■ Mechanical feeding difficulties ■ Diseases causing vomiting ■ Diseases causing anorexia ■ Psychological or behavioral problems	■ Chronic or recurrent infection ■ Malignancies ■ Congenital heart disease ■ Chronic respiratory disease ■ Renal insufficiency
Decreased calorie absorption/utilization	**Increased caloric expenditure**
■ Gastrointestinal malabsorption ■ Pancreatic insufficiency ■ Liver disease, short gut ■ Chronic inflammatory bowel disease ■ Vitamin or mineral deficiencies ■ Genetic/chromosomal abnormalities ■ Inborn errors of metabolism, diabetes	■ Hyperthyroidism ■ Chronic heart and lung disease ■ Exercise ■ Chronic infection ■ Malignancies ■ Immunodeficiency ■ Trauma/burns, sepsis

2 years, and head circumferences in those younger than 3 years. Use of growth charts to evaluate the child's weight and height relative to each other and previous values is important. Anthropometric measurements may be helpful in sorting out adequacy of growth of children consistently less than 5% after the ED evaluation. Looking at growth parameters over time is extremely helpful, although usually unavailable in the ED; a consistent fall in a downward direction requires a diligent search for an underlying chronic illness.

The severity of malnutrition can be defined further by using the actual weight expressed as a percentage of the ideal weight for the patient's actual height. Mild protein-energy malnutrition exists when the actual weight is 80% to 90% of the ideal body weight for actual height, moderate when 70% to 80%, and categorized as severe when 60% to 70%. The degree of malnutrition is important when considering the refeeding regimen and decision making regarding the patient's disposition.

Routine laboratory tests should not be performed unless indicated by history and physical examination. If history and physical examination are normal, a trial of adequate nutrition should be attempted. If the child does not gain weight despite these measures, further testing may be considered.

TABLE 79.2

LIFE-THREATENING CAUSES OF WEIGHT LOSS

Infants	Children and adolescents
Inborn error of metabolism	Diabetes mellitus
Congenital adrenal hyperplasia	Addison disease
Congenital heart disease	Acute dehydration
Congenital immune deficiencies	Eating disorders
Acute dehydration	

TABLE 79.3

HISTORY FOR WEIGHT LOSS

Birth history
Birth weight
Fetal factors
TORCHES
Congenital anomalies
Extended neonatal intensive care unit stay
Drugs, alcohol, and smoking
Dietary history
Type of feeding, types of food consumed, feeding techniques, feeding schedule
Intake
Output
Past medical history
Recent illness
Chronic medical conditions
Hospitalizations
Surgery
Developmental history
Gestational and perinatal history, prematurity, developmental milestones
Family history
Parental height, medical conditions in the family, inherited diseases, history of developmental delay, psychological history
Growth chart
Social history
Care givers, socioeconomic status, major life events, history of child protective services involvement
Review of systems

Normal Determinants of Growth

Infants should regain their birth weight by 10 to 14 days of age. A normal infant gains an average of 25 to 30 g per day for the first 3 months of life, 20 g per day in the third to sixth months, and 12 g per day in the second half of the first year. The growth in infancy is largely nutrition based. There is a transition from primarily nutrition-based growth in infancy to growth hormone–dependent growth during childhood and growth/sex hormone growth during adolescence.

The growth of a child depends on genetic, environmental, and constitutional factors. Environmental factors include prenatal factors, maternal, placental factors, and infections during pregnancy. Approximately 25% of infants shift to a lower percentile in the first 2 years of life and follow that percentile based on their genetic predisposition; these infants should not be diagnosed with weight loss or failure to thrive. These include constitutional growth delay, familial short stature, and intrauterine growth retardation. Children with constitutional failure have normal history and physical but delayed bone age.

They are usually normal at birth but cross percentiles before 2 years of age. They are often referred to as "late bloomers."

DIFFERENTIAL DIAGNOSIS BY AGE

A few life-threatening diseases associated with weight loss must be separated from conditions that carry no immediate risk (Table 79.2). Severe dehydration in the presence of gastroenteritis or other acute illness may be life-threatening in any age group (see Chapter 17 Dehydration).

Infants and Preadolescents

In young infants and older children, the patients can be divided into three diagnostic categories:

1. Organic etiology (18%) of patients which includes gastrointestinal, neurologic, pulmonary, cardiovascular, endocrine, and metabolic causes.
2. Nonorganic (58%) includes feeding problems, constitutional growth delay, genetic short stature, and social problems.
3. Undetermined etiology where no definitive diagnosis is established. Multiple mechanisms may come into play for a given case of weight loss.

The single most common cause of acute weight loss in all age groups is dehydration that occurs in conjunction with an acute infectious illness. The most common cause of chronic weight loss or failure to gain weight in the first 3 years of life is undernutrition. As a child ages, the probability increases that the cause of chronic weight loss is due to an underlying medical or psychiatric illness rather than under nutrition. In some instances, an exact diagnosis is not made at the time of the ED visit, but a workup may be initiated and an appropriate referral should be made (Table 79.4).

In young infants, several disease states need to be considered in the differential diagnosis (Table 79.5). When evaluating the infant with weight loss or inadequate weight gain, the physician should include the perinatal history and the onset and character of the symptoms. The presence of vomiting and acute weight loss in an otherwise well baby with a good appetite suggests gastroesophageal reflux or pyloric stenosis. Poor sucking or swallowing and delayed development suggests neurologic or neuromuscular disease. Vomiting and anorexia, altered mental status, seizures, and characteristic body fluid odors point to metabolic disease. Kidney failure, renal tubular acidosis, and liver disease also may cause anorexia, vomiting, and poor growth. Frequent infections, dermatitis, and diarrhea are associated with immune-deficiency syndromes. The infant who tires or becomes diaphoretic with feedings may have congenital heart or pulmonary disease. The presence of malodorous and loose stools suggests primary malabsorption or cystic fibrosis. Blood-streaked, water-loss stools may be related to milk protein allergy or infectious (especially bacterial) enteritis.

Toddlers and preadolescents may present with life-threatening diseases that are associated with weight loss (e.g., adrenal crisis, diabetes mellitus with ketoacidosis, severe dehydration, and eating disorders). Children with Addison disease have gradual onset of fatigue and weakness, anorexia, weight loss, and low blood pressure. If the diagnosis is not made, adrenal crisis may occur, leading to circulatory failure, which may be rapidly fatal. Hyperpigmentation (particularly around the genitalia, nipples, axilla, and umbilicus) provides a clue to the diagnosis. Ketoacidosis is the initial manifestation in many children with diabetes; these children often give a history of weight loss in the presence of polyphagia, polydipsia, and polyuria (see Chapter 97 Endocrine Emergencies).

TABLE 79.4

LABORATORY TESTS FOR INFANTS AND PREADOLESCENTS

Type of study
Hematologic: Complete blood cell count, ESR, coagulation studies, iron profile
Chemistry: Serum glucose, electrolytes, BUN, creatinine, calcium, phosphate, liver function tests, ammonia, lactate, CRP
Urine: Analysis, VMA, amino acids, organic acids, reducing substances
Imaging: Chest x-ray, echocardiogram, upper GI, bone age, renal ultrasound
Endocrine: Thyroid function tests, growth hormone screening, cortisol
Serologic: Immunologic studies, chromosomes, serum amino acids
Stool studies: Stool culture, stool for fat and trypsin
Miscellaneous: Sweat test, EKG

TABLE 79.5

CAUSES OF WEIGHT LOSS IN INFANTS AND CHILDREN

Infectious	Chronic infections, HIV, tuberculosis
Genetic and congenital	Various syndromes, e.g., Smith–Lemli–Opitz syndrome
Metabolic	Aminoacidopathies, inborn errors of metabolism
Cardiac	Congenital and acquired heart disease
Hepatic	Biliary atresia, hepatitis, cirrhosis
Pulmonary	Bronchopulmonary dysplasia, chronic hypoxemia, cystic fibrosis
Renal	Renal tubular acidosis, chronic renal disease, recurrent UTIs
Endocrine	Hyperthyroidism, hyperaldosteronism, diabetes
Hematologic	Malignancies
Gastrointestinal	Reflux, TE fistula, obstruction, malrotation, orofacial disorders, IBD, celiac disease
Neurologic	Intracranial lesions, chronic neurologic disorders
Psychosocial	Apathy, abnormal interaction between infant and caregiver, neglect, hyper vigilance

Adolescents

Just as in younger children, inflammatory and infectious processes, malignancies, and endocrinopathies are all important

TABLE 79.6

PHYSICAL EXAMINATION AND LABORATORY ABNORMALITIES IN ANOREXIA NERVOSA

Physical examination	Laboratory abnormalities
Hypothermia	Pancytopenia
Bradycardia	Hypoglycemia
Hypotension	Hypokalemia
Emaciation	Elevated BUN
Acrocyanosis	Elevated cholesterol
Dry skin	Hypoalbuminemia
Lanugo	Mild transaminase elevations
Thinning hair	
Peripheral edema	
Breast atrophy	
Hypercarotenemia	

causes of weight loss and growth failure in adolescence. Adolescents also are prone to experiencing bio-psychosocial causes of significant, unexplained weight loss.

Eating disorders are now among the most common chronic diseases in teenagers, especially for girls. The lifetime prevalence of anorexia nervosa and bulimia nervosa in females ranges from 0.5% to 3.7% and 1.1% to 4.2%, respectively (see Chapter 46 Oligomenorrhea). Even if the weight loss does not meet strict diagnostic criteria for an eating disorder, adolescents who participate in sports may follow unhealthy weight-control practices to seek advantage in their athletic activities, including food restriction, vomiting, over exercise, diet pills, stimulants, insulin, nicotine, and voluntary dehydration.

Anorexia nervosa should be suspected when the adolescent is unwilling or unable to maintain body weight over a minimally normal weight for age and height and when attitudes and behaviors about eating or body image are distorted. The history may reveal infrequent or absent menses, compulsive exercising, refusal to eat in front of others, or ritualistic eating practices such as cutting their food into very small pieces. These behaviors are practiced in secret, and are often denied. Physical examination findings and laboratory abnormalities commonly found in children with anorexia nervosa are listed in Table 79.6. Early in calorie malnutrition, initial laboratory tests are usually normal.

Hypochloremic hypokalemic metabolic alkalosis suggests vomiting, bulimia, or diuretic abuse. Metabolic acidosis suggests surreptitious laxative use. Initial magnesium, calcium, and phosphorus can be normal but fall to life-threatening low levels during refeeding. Patients noted to have low thyroid hormone in the setting of an eating disorder should not receive thyroid replacement without consultation. An EKG may reveal nonspecific ST and T wave abnormalities, widened QT_c, and a right-axis deviation because of the emaciated body habitus.

Disposition

Most children with mild to moderate weight loss can be discharged safely from the ED and referred back to their pediatrician for management. Hospitalization is indicated in any child who is suspected to have sustained trauma or been abused and may be indicated in those with physical findings consistent with severe malnutrition, hypothermia, bradycardia, or hypotension. Severe malnutrition requires inpatient management as refeeding requires careful monitoring of electrolytes. Subspecialty consultations with social work, nutrition, cardiology, gastroenterology, or endocrinology may be necessary and are readily available if the child is hospitalized. Management of these children requires a multidisciplinary approach. Nutrition is a central component of well-being in the growing child, and malnutrition carries significant morbidity and mortality. Thus, persons who care for children need to have an understanding of normal growth and must develop an approach for the evaluation and treatment of growth failure.

SUMMARY

Weight loss in a child requires a careful evaluation. Infants are more likely to have psychosocial growth failure. Older children and adolescents are more likely to have an organic cause. Acute weight loss is most often associated with an acute intercurrent illness and these children will regain their weight spontaneously as their illness resolves. Chronic weight loss is more often related to less common diseases with a much broader differential diagnosis. It is very important to understand normal growth and have an organized approach for the evaluation and management of weight loss.

Suggested Readings and Key References

American Academy of Pediatrics, Committee on Adolescence. Identifying and treating eating disorders. *Pediatrics* 2003;111(1):204–211.

American Academy of Pediatrics Committee on Sports Medicine and Fitness. Promotion of health weight-control practices in young athletes. *Pediatrics* 2005;116(6):1557–1564.

Cole SZ, Lanham JS, Mai MC. Failure to thrive: an update. *Am Fam Phys* 2011;83(7):829–834.

Ficicioglu C, Haack K. Failure to thrive: when to suspect inborn errors of metabolism. *Pediatrics* 2009;124(3):972–979.

Jolley CD. Failure to thrive. *Curr Probl Pediatr Adolesc Health Care* 2003;33:183–206.

Kreipe RE, Birnford SA. Eating disorders in adolescents and young adults. *Med Clin North Amer* 2000;84(4):1027–1049.

Krugman SD. Failure to thrive. *Am Fam Phys* 2003;68(5):879–884.

Powers PS, Santana CA. Eating disorders: a guide for the primary care physician. *Prim Care* 2002;29(1):81–98.

Shah MD. Failure to thrive in children. *J Clin Gastroenterol* 2002; 35(5):371–374.

Sigman GS. Eating disorders in children and adolescents. *Pediatr Clin North Am* 2003;50:1139–1177.

Wright CM. Identification and management of failure to thrive: a community perspective. *Arch Dis Child* 2000;82:5–9.

SIGNS AND SYMPTOMS

CHAPTER 80 ■ WHEEZING

DANICA B. LIBERMAN, MD, MPH AND VINCENT J. WANG, MD, MHA

Wheezes are whistling or musical adventitious sounds that are the hallmark of lower airway constriction and/or obstruction. Whereas rales or crackles are discontinuous or intermittent popping noises, wheezes are continuous sounds most frequently heard during expiration. The most common diseases causing wheezing in children are bronchiolitis and asthma, but the differential diagnosis is broad, and the causes are multifactorial. An episode of wheezing may occur at least once in 20% of infants younger than 1 year of age, and in almost 50% of children younger than 6 years of age, but fewer than 15% of children will develop asthma. This chapter presents an organized approach to the diagnosis of conditions associated with wheezing in children beyond the newborn period.

PATHOPHYSIOLOGY

Obstruction to air flow is the common denominator in all conditions that produce wheezing. Wheezing usually results from obstruction of the intrathoracic lower airways (bronchioles) and less commonly by narrowing of the trachea or bronchi. Obstruction of the lower airway passages may be anatomic or physiologic and is the result of intrinsic airway narrowing or extrinsic airway compression. Intrinsic airway narrowing may be caused by bronchial or bronchiolar constriction, inflammation, and/or intraluminal airway blockage. It may also be caused by a combination of these factors simultaneously, as in asthma. When wheezing is audible during the inspiration and expiration phases of respiration, wheezing is more likely to be caused by extrinsic airway compression. In contrast, when wheezing is predominantly expiratory, intrinsic airway narrowing is more likely to be the cause.

DIFFERENTIAL DIAGNOSIS

Table 80.1 lists the life-threatening causes of wheezing, and Table 80.2 outlines the relative prevalence of conditions that may present acutely with wheezing, categorized by age.

Common Conditions

Bronchiolitis is an acute viral infection of the lower respiratory tract caused predominantly by respiratory syncytial virus (RSV). Other causes include rhinovirus, parainfluenza virus, adenovirus, influenza virus, coronavirus, and human metapneumovirus. Occurring primarily in epidemics between November and April, bronchiolitis affects children younger than 2 years of age. Proliferation of cells and submucosal edema lead to obstruction of the bronchioles. Rhinorrhea and a low-grade fever typically accompany a prominent staccato-like cough and a variable degree of respiratory distress. The concurrence of respiratory symptoms in other family members is common. Degree of severity is multifactorial, with factors such as parental smoking, prematurity, congenital heart disease, and reactive airway disease contributing to the individual patient's response to the viral infection.

Asthma is a chronic inflammatory disorder of the airways, characterized clinically by *recurrent* exacerbations involving symptoms of coughing and/or wheezing. Acute asthma attacks are usually triggered by respiratory infections, allergens, exercise, and irritants, such as cigarette smoke or particulate air pollution. Patients with asthma have a higher incidence of associated atopic diseases, which include allergic rhinitis and conjunctivitis, and atopic dermatitis. Immediate family members are also more likely to be affected by asthma and atopic disease. Although many hesitate to make the diagnosis of asthma in a child younger than 2 years of age, many asthmatics have their first episode of wheezing before this age. However, 60% of those who wheeze before 3 years of age will not wheeze by school age. In addition, it is unknown if bronchiolitis predisposes patients to develop asthma, or if the response to bronchiolitis is different for a patient who is predisposed to developing asthma.

Less Common Conditions

Other infectious causes of wheezing include viral or bacterial pneumonia. Most cases are preceded by several days of upper respiratory tract symptoms and fever. Physical examination will usually reveal tachypnea, retractions, rales, and/or wheezes. Auscultatory findings are often localized rather than diffuse. As with bronchiolitis, the most common causes of pneumonia are viral. Bacterial causes include *Streptococcus pneumoniae, Mycoplasma pneumoniae, Chlamydia pneumoniae,* group A *Streptococcus,* and *Staphylococcus aureus. S. pneumoniae* has been the most common bacterial agent, but the incidence has decreased since the widespread utilization of the conjugate pneumococcal vaccine.

Pulmonary aspiration is a less common cause of wheezing that occurs in several fairly characteristic clinical circumstances. In otherwise healthy children, the abrupt onset of respiratory distress, associated with an episode of coughing, choking, or gagging, suggests the pulmonary aspiration of a foreign object (see Chapter 27 Foreign Body: Ingestion and Aspiration). Foreign-body aspiration is typically seen in toddlers, although older infants may aspirate solid food particles or small objects placed within their reach. Rarely, an older child may also aspirate food particles or other objects. The aspiration of a small object or food substance may not be witnessed, and thus, may go unrecognized for weeks or months until persistent lower respiratory symptoms trigger a search for an underlying cause. In these circumstances, persistent cough, wheezing, and sometimes recurrent fever is associated with an area of consolidation and/or collapse on radiograph. These symptoms fail to resolve despite seemingly appropriate medical therapy.

TABLE 80.1

LIFE-THREATENING CAUSES OF WHEEZING

Asthma
Bronchiolitis
Foreign-body aspiration
Pulmonary hemorrhage
Mediastinal tumor
Congestive heart failure
Chemical pneumonitis
Anaphylaxis

Recurrent aspiration of food or gastric contents is usually seen in infants younger than 1 year of age, or in older patients with severe intellectual disability or neuromuscular disease. Disordered swallowing and gastroesophageal (GE) reflux typically contribute in varying degrees to the recurrent aspiration that occurs in these patients. Repeated aspiration is also seen in children with tracheostomies and in children with structural anomalies of the tracheolaryngeal complex or an H-type tracheoesophageal fistula, which are rare. Patients with chronic recurrent aspiration may develop wheezing and respiratory distress in the absence of a well-defined episode of choking or severe coughing because many such patients have depressed cough reflexes or experience "microaspiration." Fever often accompanies pulmonary aspiration, reflecting associated chemical inflammation or infection of the tracheobronchial tree.

Wheezing attributable to anaphylaxis is also of sudden onset and may be accompanied by one or more other clinical findings that include urticaria, angioedema, stridor, hypotension, abdominal pain, vomiting, and diarrhea. When wheezing is the only finding, anaphylaxis may be suspected when the onset of respiratory difficulty is associated with Hymenoptera envenomation, medication or food ingestion, or another allergic precipitant. Wheezing in this context typically responds promptly to epinephrine administration and/or to bronchodilator therapy.

The development of chronic respiratory problems in the neonatal period, due to complications such as prematurity, assisted ventilator support, and oxygen dependence, all lead to a common condition referred to as chronic lung disease (CLD). This condition is the childhood equivalent of chronic obstructive pulmonary disease and represents a pathophysiologic continuum that includes varying degrees of structural damage and airway inflammation. Although gradual improvement in lung function occurs during infancy and early childhood, bronchial hyperactivity and recurrent episodes of wheezing may persist until later in childhood.

Transient wheezing may also occur with smoking and air pollutant exposures. It is important to note, that 90% of cigarette smokers start before the age of 21 years. Wheezing and bronchiolitis have also been associated with passive smoke exposure. Air pollution containing particulate matter less than or equal to 10 microns in diameter, which is small enough to travel into the distal airways, nitrogen dioxide, nitrogen oxide, and carbon monoxide have been associated with wheezing, and can exacerbate other causes of wheezing.

Rare Conditions

Cardiovascular abnormalities are one of many uncommon causes of wheezing in children. Small airway edema in the setting of congestive heart failure or airway impingement by enlarged cardiovascular structures is the usual pathophysiologic mechanism. Most cardiac conditions are associated with other abnormal physical findings, including cyanosis,

TABLE 80.2

CLINICAL CLASSIFICATION OF WHEEZING: AGE AT DIAGNOSIS AND DISEASE PREVALENCE

Disease prevalence	<1 yr	1–3 yr	>3 yr
Common	Bronchiolitis	Bronchiolitis Asthma	Asthma
Less common	Pneumonia Pulmonary aspiration GE reflux CLD Swallowing disorders	Pneumonia Pulmonary aspiration Anaphylaxis CLD	Pneumonia Anaphylaxis CLD Smoking/air pollution
Rare	Congenital heart disease Tracheobronchomalacia Cystic fibrosis Immunodeficiency Tracheoesphageal fistula Cystic malformations of lung Primary ciliary dyskinesia Vascular rings/slings Congenital lobar emphysema	Immunodeficiency Mediastinal lymphadenopathy Congenital heart disease Cystic fibrosis Sarcoidosis GE reflux Bronchiectasis Pulmonary edema Parasitic infections	Psychogenic wheezing (vocal cord dysfunction) Mediastinal lymphadenopathy Cystic fibrosis Immunodeficiency Tuberculosis Sarcoidosis Bronchiectasis Pulmonary edema Pulmonary aspiration Parasitic and fungal infections

GE, gastroesophageal; CLD, chronic lung disease.

SIGNS AND SYMPTOMS

murmurs, abnormal pulses, poor perfusion, or signs consistent with congestive heart failure. Though abnormal cardiac physical findings are generally absent in patients with a vascular ring or sling, these structural abnormalities may cause wheezing and dysphagia due to esophageal compression; and a right-sided aortic arch is often noted on chest radiograph.

While pulmonary disease, including wheezing, is the hallmark of cystic fibrosis (CF), individuals with CF (see Chapter 107 Pulmonary Emergencies) will often also exhibit steatorrhea and failure to thrive because of pancreatic insufficiency and malabsorption. Similar to CF, patients with primary ciliary dyskinesia also develop repeated respiratory tract infections, sinusitis, and otitis media, often in association with situs inversus viscerum and bronchiectasis (Kartagener's syndrome).

Wheezing may result from pulmonary edema, which may be caused by congenital or acquired heart disease with congestive heart failure. However, pulmonary edema may also be caused by other disease processes, such as pneumonia, acute respiratory distress syndrome, and hypoalbuminemic states, such as nephrotic syndrome and liver failure. Hydrocarbon aspiration, leading to a chemical pneumonitis, may also cause pulmonary edema.

An adolescent patient may present with moderate to severe respiratory distress that is unresponsive to beta agonist therapy. Consideration should be given to precipitating factors and the diagnosis of psychogenic wheezing (also called vocal cord dysfunction). These patients may generate wheezing noises in their larynx.

Children with cell-mediated or humoral immune deficiency syndromes often present with recurrent wheezing and bacterial pulmonary infections; and can have opportunistic infections or repeated extrapulmonary infections, including meningitis, otitis media, otitis externa, furunculosis, and mucocutaneous candidiasis.

Other uncommon causes of wheezing include extrinsic tracheobronchial compression by an enlarged lymph node or tumor (see Chapter 106 Oncologic Emergencies). Mediastinal or hilar lymph node enlargement may be the result of malignancy, sarcoidosis, or a mycobacterial or fungal infection. Mediastinal tumors that are most likely to produce pulmonary symptomatology include lymphoma, neuroblastoma, pheochromocytoma, ganglioneuroma, thymoma, teratoma, or thyroid carcinoma; however, any malignancy can metastasize to the lungs and cause extrinsic compression of the airways.

Among the rarest causes of wheezing in children are congenital structural anomalies of the respiratory tract, including bronchogenic cysts, cystic malformations of the lung, congenital lobar emphysema, intrinsic stenosis, and webs. Respiratory symptoms typically begin in the neonatal period or early infancy. The predominant clinical features are determined by the site of abnormality within the tracheobronchial tree. Stridor and a croupy cough are typical of laryngotracheal constriction, whereas wheezing and recurrent pneumonia are more characteristic of bronchial narrowing. Respiratory findings generally worsen with intercurrent respiratory infection and may accentuate with crying and activity. Some diagnoses are discovered only when persistence of symptoms necessitates imaging studies.

Bronchiectasis is the term used to describe irreversible bronchial dilatation, and is the common end result of various disease processes. The most common cause is cystic fibrosis, but bronchiectasis may also be caused by primary ciliary dyskinesia, immunodeficiency disorders, congenital anatomical abnormalities, and infection. Cough is prominent and accompanied by purulent sputum production.

Even though the diagnosis of bronchitis is more commonly associated with adult patients, children may develop a nonspecific bronchial inflammation associated with various viral agents. The pathophysiology is similar to bronchiolitis and may be preceded by upper respiratory symptoms. Cough is usually prominent and may be followed by wheezing.

Other rare conditions are listed in Table 80.2.

EVALUATION

History

Thorough history-taking is the key to arriving at an accurate diagnosis in a child with wheezing. In particular, consideration of the age at onset, course and pattern of illness, and associated clinical features provide a useful framework for approaching a differential diagnosis (Figs. 80.1 and 80.2).

In patients with respiratory distress, it may be necessary to perform a focused history pertaining to life-threatening causes of wheezing (Table 80.1). Such a battery of questions may include the following: (i) How acutely did the symptoms present? (ii) Was the patient choking or did he or she become cyanotic? (iii) Has this occurred before? (iv) Are there concurrent upper respiratory symptoms? (v) Does the patient have a history of cardiac disease or failure to thrive? (vi) Does anyone in the family have asthma? Table 80.3 reviews salient features of common disorders that cause wheezing.

The onset of wheezing in the neonatal period is associated with congenital structural airway anomalies; although a history of prematurity, mechanical ventilation, and oxygen dependence is more suggestive of CLD. The *first episode* of wheezing in an otherwise healthy infant in association with respiratory symptoms suggests bronchiolitis, especially if the episode occurs in the winter months. Recurrent episodes of wheezing precipitated by respiratory infections and a variety of other triggers are the hallmark of asthma. However, recurrent wheezing beginning in infancy, or "difficult to control asthma" at any age, should lead to a consideration of other less common diagnoses, such as CF, GE reflux, recurrent pulmonary aspiration, a retained airway foreign body, and immune deficiency. Persistent wheezing at any age suggests mechanical airway obstruction from a variety of causes, including congenital airway narrowing, pulmonary foreign body, and compression by a mediastinal tumor. Sudden onset of wheezing is characteristic of pulmonary aspiration or anaphylaxis.

As indicated previously, the diagnosis of a chronic wheezing disorder, such as asthma, relies on the identification of recurrent episodes of obstructive lower airway disease. It is often useful to ask if the child has ever had "breathing problems," or has ever been treated with a "breathing medicine." In a large longitudinal study, major risk factors for asthma included eczema or a parental history of asthma, and minor risk factors included wheezing between viral illnesses, nonviral rhinitis, and eosinophilia. Cough, as a salient feature in patients with obstructive lower airway disease, cannot be overemphasized (see Chapter 14 Cough). In fact, in patients with cough variant asthma, recurrent dry cough may be the predominant presenting clinical feature and wheezing may be absent despite careful lung auscultation.

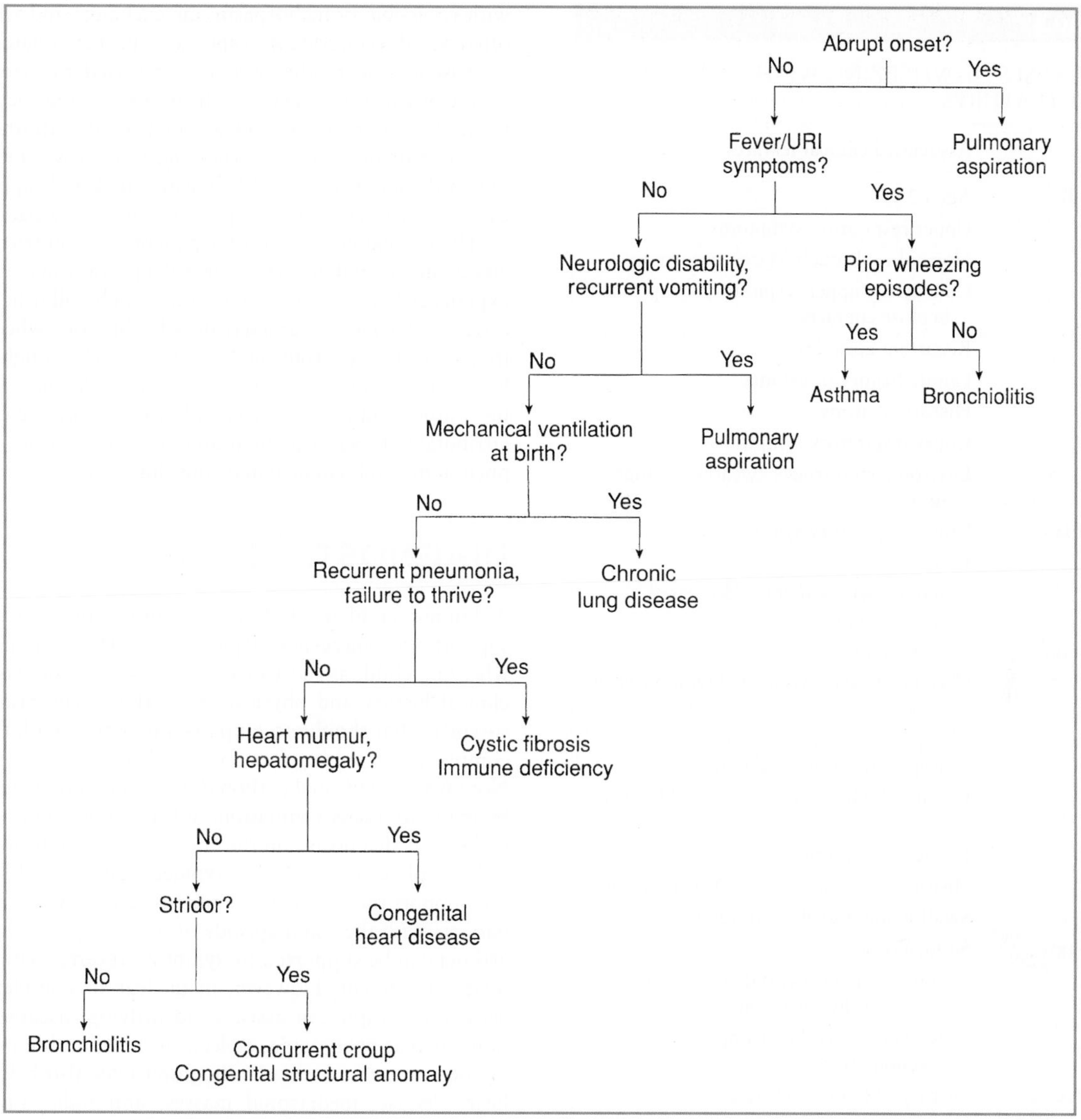

Abrupt onset?
No
Yes
Fever/URI symptoms?
Pulmonary aspiration
No
Yes
Neurologic disability, recurrent vomiting?
Prior wheezing episodes?
Yes
No
Asthma
Bronchiolitis
No
Yes
Mechanical ventilation at birth?
Pulmonary aspiration
No
Yes
Recurrent pneumonia, failure to thrive?
Chronic lung disease
No
Yes
Heart murmur, hepatomegaly?
Cystic fibrosis
Immune deficiency
No
Yes
Stridor?
Congenital heart disease
No
Yes
Bronchiolitis
Concurrent croup
Congenital structural anomaly

FIGURE 80.1 Approach to wheezing in children younger than 1 year. URI, upper respiratory infection.

Abrupt onset?
No
Yes
Fever/URI symptoms?
Uriticaria, stridor?
No
Yes
No
Yes
Recurrent pneumonia?
Asthma
Bronchiolitis
Pneumonia
Foreign-body aspiration
Anaphylaxis
No
Yes
Asthma
Cystic fibrosis
Immune deficiency
Foreign body

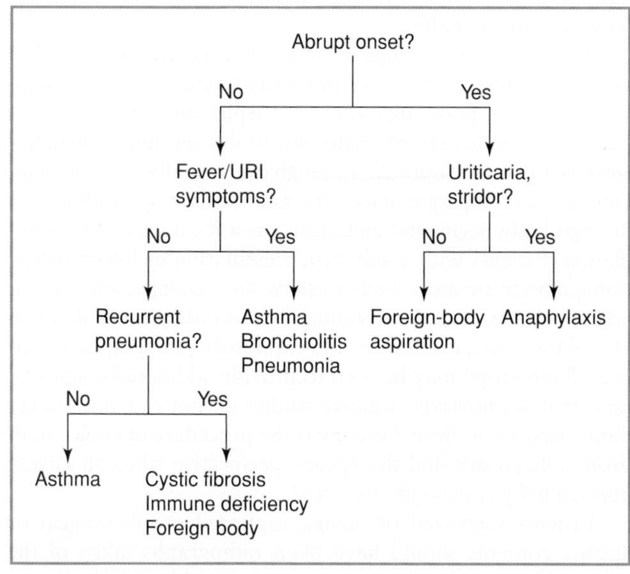

FIGURE 80.2 Approach to wheezing in children 1 year or older. URI, upper respiratory infection.

Physical Examination

Wheezing must be distinguished from other causes of "noisy breathing" in children, including the stridor of upper airway obstruction (see Chapter 70 Stridor), the stertor of nasal congestion, and audible rhonchi. Because of the dynamic flexibility of airway structures, these clinical features of airway obstruction vary in accordance with the respiratory phase. Accordingly, upper airway collapse and stridor are typically worse on inspiration, whereas lower airway narrowing and wheezing are accentuated on expiration. Moreover, sounds originating in the upper airway passages (e.g., stridor, stertor) are transmitted with uniform quality and intensity across both lung fields. In contrast, wheezes tend to be polyphonic in pitch and distributed somewhat unevenly in intensity and location due to inevitable variation in airway narrowing that occurs. Importantly, wheezes consistently limited to a single lung field suggest a localized obstructive process, such as a foreign body, pneumonia, or an extrinsic mass lesion.

The intensity of wheezes and their pitch and duration are a function of the degree of airway narrowing and the velocity of

TABLE 80.3

MAJOR CAUSES OF WHEEZING WITH ASSOCIATED CLINICAL FEATURES

Causes	Associated clinical features
Bronchiolitis	Age <2 yr
	Upper respiratory symptoms
	November through March occurrence
	Concurrent upper respiratory symptoms in close contacts
Asthma	Recurrent episodes
	Family history of asthma
	History of atopy
	Upper respiratory symptoms
	Environmental trigger (weather change, etc.)
Pneumonia	Upper respiratory symptoms
	Fever
	Unilateral wheezing/rales/decreased breath sounds
Foreign-body aspiration	Age >6 months
	Choking episode associated with onset of symptoms
	Abrupt onset or prolonged symptoms despite appropriate therapy
	Unilateral wheezing or decreased breath sounds
	Intellectual disability
	History of tracheal surgery/tracheostomy
	Swallowing disorder, GE reflux
Anaphylaxis	Sudden onset
	Accompanying urticaria, angioedema, stridor, or hypotension
	New exposure or Hymenoptera envenomation
Congestive heart failure/cardiac disease	History of failure to thrive
	Heart murmur, hepatomegaly, poor perfusion
	Cardiomegaly
Cystic fibrosis	History of failure to thrive
	Recurrent respiratory tract infections
	Steatorrhea

Adapted from Martinati LC, Boner AL. Clinical diagnosis of wheezing in early childhood. *Allergy* 1995;50:701–710.

airflow at the site(s) of obstruction. In patients with minimal airway obstruction, wheezing may be difficult to detect. When such instances are suspected, forced exhalation may reveal low-pitched wheezes limited to the end of expiration. Subtle wheezes can be accentuated further by combining forced exhalation with simultaneous manual compression applied by the examiner in the anteroposterior dimension of the chest (so-called "squeezing the wheeze"). As airway narrowing and minute ventilation increase, wheezes become louder and higher pitched. However, when airway obstruction becomes more severe, airflow and wheezes will diminish proportionately. A "quiet chest" in the face of significant respiratory distress may indicate impending respiratory failure. Conversely, in patients with reversible bronchospasm, air exchange and wheezes are often noted to increase in response to bronchodilator therapy.

Auscultation of the neck may be used to determine the source of wheezing. Wheezing heard only in the chest, and not the neck, is more likely to be associated with intrathoracic airway obstruction, whereas wheezing heard over the neck, but not in the chest, is more likely associated with upper airway causes of wheezing, such as psychogenic wheezing.

The clinical evaluation of a patient with obstructive lower airway disease will invariably reveal a prominent cough. To the experienced clinician or parent, this cough will usually be perceived as having a characteristic whistling or "wheezy" quality that is distinct from the "seal-like" barky cough of croup. Physical examination of the wheezing child may also reveal inspiratory and expiratory crackles, which are far more often attributable to subsegmental atelectasis than to an associated pneumonia and parenchymal consolidation.

DIAGNOSTIC TESTS

A limited number of diagnostic modalities are needed to support the emergency department (ED) evaluation of the wheezing child, as most diagnoses can be made based on the clinical history and physical exam alone. The primary measurement that should accompany any patient with respiratory complaints is pulse oximetry, which measures oxygenation. Noninvasive end-tidal carbon dioxide measurements may also be made to assess ventilation. When bronchiolitis or asthma is the clear diagnosis and the course is uncomplicated, a chest radiograph can usually be avoided. The available data do not support the utility of obtaining a chest radiograph for all patients with their first episode of wheezing. The diagnosis of asthma can be supported by symptom reversal with bronchodilator treatment. However, in unclear or complex cases, a chest radiograph can assist in identifying disease complications such as pneumonia, atelectasis, pneumothorax, or pneumomediastinum. A chest radiograph may also help diagnose heart disease, mediastinal masses, and radiopaque foreign bodies of the airway and esophagus. Varying degrees of hyperaeration, bronchiolar thickening, and subsegmental atelectasis are the most common radiographic findings in patients with bronchiolitis or asthma.

An immediate and aggressive workup is always justified in patients suspected of having an airway foreign body (see Chapter 27 Foreign Body: Ingestion and Aspiration) on the basis of acute and sudden symptomatology. In this setting, chest radiographs are usually normal, although occasionally they can demonstrate a radiopaque object, the faint outline of a radiolucent foreign body, segmental atelectasis, or a focal area of hyperinflation. Patients with a subacute presentation of lower airway foreign body are more likely to show focal collapse and consolidation that is evident on standard chest radiographs. Bilateral decubitus views, inspiratory and expiratory radiographs, or airway fluoroscopy may be used to provide additional diagnostic information, however negative studies do not rule out foreign body aspiration. Bronchoscopy is the procedure of choice both from a diagnostic and therapeutic perspective when an airway foreign body is strongly suspected.

Patients suspected of having aspirated oropharyngeal or gastric contents should have plain radiographs taken of the chest. Nonspecific findings consistent with lower airway obstruction generally precede the appearance of infiltrates.

Patients believed to have recurring episodes of pulmonary aspiration should have further testing at a subsequent time to identify swallowing dysfunction, GE reflux, or actual tracheobronchial soiling. Such inpatient or outpatient tests might include a swallow study, esophageal pH monitoring, esophageal endoscopy and biopsy, or radionuclide scintigraphy. Flexible bronchoscopy may be required to diagnose patients with a tracheoesophageal fistula.

The diagnosis of CLD is established on the basis of chronic respiratory symptoms superimposed on a background of neonatal lung disease. Nevertheless, a chest radiograph characteristically shows hyperexpansion and streaky or patchy infiltrates, punctuated by areas of alternating local hyperaeration and atelectasis. Comparison to previous radiographs is often helpful in distinguishing chronic changes from acute processes.

Newborn screening should identify most children with CF, but screening is dependent on the state standards, and the test does not have 100% sensitivity. Thus, infants with recurrent wheezing, particularly in combination with failure to thrive and chronic diarrhea should be referred for sweat chloride or DNA testing.

A patient suspected of having congenital or acquired heart disease should have an electrocardiogram and a chest radiograph performed in the ED. Definitive diagnosis generally requires echocardiography. A barium swallow, computed tomography scan, or magnetic resonance imaging are usually sufficient to diagnose the presence of a vascular ring or sling, although computed tomography angiography or magnetic resonance angiography may be necessary for exact anatomic definition.

APPROACH

The evaluation of a wheezing child begins with an immediate assessment of the degree of respiratory distress and consideration of the need for general supportive measures. Patients with impending respiratory failure should be managed aggressively, as outlined in Chapter 1 A General Approach to Ill and Injured Children, and in Chapter 66 Respiratory Distress. Clinical features suggestive of impending respiratory failure include severe respiratory distress, agitation or lethargy, dusky mucous membranes, signs of autonomic excess (tachycardia, diaphoresis, peripheral vasoconstriction), poor air movement on lung auscultation, pulse oximetry reading of less than 90%, and elevated noninvasive end-tidal carbon dioxide measurements. Blood gas analysis may also aid in recognizing and monitoring the progression of respiratory failure.

Supplemental oxygen should be offered promptly to any patient with respiratory distress and adjusted to maintain a pulse oximeter reading of 93% or greater. Higher altitude medical centers may accept lower pulse oximetry readings. In otherwise healthy children with no feeding difficulty or respiratory distress, recent American Academy of Pediatrics recommendations suggest that a pulse oximeter reading of 90% or greater is acceptable for patients with bronchiolitis. Patients suspected of having reversible bronchospasm should be given an inhaled bronchodilator, such as albuterol, while proceeding with further evaluation and management.

Expeditious management is essential in patients with poor baseline pulmonary function because they can develop respiratory failure quickly. Such patients include children with significant CLD and advanced cases of progressive chronic lung disorders such as CF. Moreover, in patients with chronic respiratory insufficiency, careful titration of inspired oxygen concentration is important to avoid respiratory drive suppression.

CHILDREN YOUNGER THAN 1-YEAR OLD

An algorithm for elucidating the cause of wheezing in the child younger than 1-year old is presented in Figure 80.1. It is important to note that age cutoffs are not absolute. The abrupt onset of wheezing, often immediately preceded by an episode of choking, gagging, or vomiting, is highly suggestive of pulmonary aspiration of a foreign body. If wheezing is subacute in presentation and accompanied or preceded by fever or respiratory symptoms, bronchiolitis or asthma should be considered. Most infants who present with a first episode of wheezing have bronchiolitis. A similar complex of physical findings in an older infant with a history of bronchiolitis or wheezing and clear improvement after bronchodilator administration is characteristic of asthma.

The remaining disorders are often found in infants who have overt evidence of chronic or severe underlying illness and who typically present with recurrent or persistent episodes of wheezing and respiratory distress. Pulmonary aspiration of gastric contents may occur in infants and children with neurologic disability, as well as the occasional otherwise healthy child or adolescent. A report of mechanical ventilation at birth and/or a prolonged neonatal intensive care unit admission may be a clue to CLD. Recurrent pneumonia, failure to thrive, and steatorrhea are characteristic of infants with CF, whereas pneumonia in association with repeated extrapulmonary infection is suggestive of an immune deficiency. A heart murmur and other clinical findings consistent with congestive heart failure are indicative of congenital heart disease and pulmonary edema. Wheezing accompanied by stridor commonly indicates the coexistence of viral croup but may reflect intrinsic congenital airway narrowing, such as tracheobronchomalacia or extrinsic compression by a mediastinal mass. In the absence of any of the clinical clues listed, the first episode of wheezing in an otherwise healthy child, especially when it occurs during the winter months, is most likely to represent bronchiolitis.

CHILD 1 YEAR OR OLDER

After 1 year of age, congenital diagnoses in children become less prominent, and the diagnoses may be organized as described in Table 80.2. As with those under 1 year old, it is important to note that overlap occurs between age groups. After age 2 years, symptoms are most likely attributable to asthma, but rare conditions can occur at any age. Figure 80.2 outlines an algorithmic approach to the more common causes of wheezing in the child who is older than 1 year. The sudden onset of respiratory distress and wheezing associated with an episode of choking and coughing is likely to indicate foreign-body aspiration, particularly in a toddler who has been eating or playing with a small object. An abrupt onset of wheezing may also accompany stridor, urticaria, and hypotension in the child with an anaphylactic reaction. When symptoms present subacutely, associated cough and rhinorrhea suggest the diagnosis of bronchiolitis in the toddler 1 to 2 years of age. Most recurrent episodes of wheezing represent asthma, and 80% of children with asthma will develop symptoms before the age of five years. Typically, asthma exacerbations are precipitated by a concurrent respiratory infection, weather change, exercise, or allergic trigger, and the patient should clinically improve with bronchodilator administration. Less commonly, recurrent episodes may represent an exacerbation of CLD, whereas nonrecurrent episodes may be caused by pneumonia or bronchitis.

Wheezing and recurrent pneumonia in multiple pulmonary segments are characteristic of patients with defects in host defense mechanisms, such as CF, an immunodeficiency, or primary ciliary dyskinesia. When older children are diagnosed with these disorders, there is usually a history of lower respiratory illness that began in infancy, as well as other signs and symptoms suggestive of chronic disease. Repeated pneumonia in the same pulmonary segment in an otherwise healthy child that begins in late infancy or in early childhood is likely to represent a previously unrecognized bronchial foreign body or external compression of the local airway. In the absence of any of the clinical clues previously listed, the first episode of wheezing in an otherwise healthy child is most likely to represent asthma.

It is imperative that *all* patients with wheezing receive outpatient follow-up with their primary care provider or, in some instances, with a specialist. With few exceptions, follow-up evaluation should take place within a day to a week of the ED visit.

Suggested Readings and Key References

American Academy of Pediatrics, Subcommittee on Diagnosis and Management of Bronchiolitis. Diagnosis and management of bronchiolitis. *Pediatrics* 2006;118(4):1774–1793.

Ducharme FM, Tse SM, Chauhan B. Diagnosis, management, and prognosis of preschool wheeze. *Lancet* 2014;383:1593–1604.

Edwards DK. The child who wheezes. In: Hilton SW, Edwards DK, eds. *Practical pediatric radiology,* 3rd ed. Philadelphia, PA: Saunders, 2006.

Martinati LC, Boner AL. Clinical diagnosis of wheezing in early childhood. *Allergy* 1995;50:701–710.

Nagler J, Krauss B. Capnographic monitoring in respiratory emergencies. *Clin Ped Emerg Med* 2009;10:82–89.

Taussig LM, Wright AL, Holberg CJ, et al. Tucson children's respiratory study: 1980 to present. *J Allergy Clin Immunol* 2003;111(4):661–675.

Weinberger M, Abu-Hasan M. Pseudo-asthma: when cough, wheezing, and dyspnea are not asthma. *Pediatrics* 2007;120(4):855–864.

Wilmott RW, Boat TF, Bush A, et al., eds. *Kendig and Chernick's disorders of the respiratory tract in children,* 8th ed. Philadelphia, PA: Saunders, 2012.

Zorc JJ, Hall BC. Bronchiolitis: recent evidence on diagnosis and management. *Pediatrics* 2010;125:342–349.

SECTION III
Clinical Pathways

CHAPTER 81 ■ INTRODUCTION TO CLINICAL PATHWAYS

JANE LAVELLE, MD, JOSEPH ZORC, MD, MSCE, AND AILEEN SCHAST, PhD

BACKGROUND

Medical professionals must increase focus on providing healthcare with high value—that which provides the best outcomes achieved with the least cost. Over the past several decades, variation in clinical care has been recognized as a core problem in achieving high value care. Variation results from a number of causes including: 1. Clinical uncertainty: high quality evidence is available to the guide the care of patients only 10% to 20% of the time; 2. Growth in medical knowledge: the exponential growth in new knowledge of clinical medicine has made it impossible for a single provider to assimilate and apply this information to current practice; 3. The growing complexity of patient conditions and treatments which requires strong team collaboration, and, finally; 4. Misaligned financial incentives for providers that allows reimbursement for unnecessary testing, procedures and treatments. Healthcare utilization across different geographic regions has been documented to show wide variation. This variation cannot be explained by illness, best practice evidence or well-informed patient preferences. Variation has also been documented across all types of providers, and within an individual provider's practice, confirming that some portion of variation comes from individual provider preference. Finally, as research enters the mainstream, translation to the bedside is often left to clinician judgment, applied inconsistently, often without measurement.

QUALITY IMPROVEMENT THEORY

Quality improvement theory provides powerful tools to increase value in healthcare through standardization of healthcare processes and promotion of strong clinician teamwork. Principles of process improvement, coupled with organizational/behavioral psychology and the scientific method form the basis of quality improvement theory. It directs the management's focus onto processes and systems rather than individual clinicians, and it provides a set of principles by which teams of clinicians can measure and document the best patient outcomes at the lowest necessary cost.

Healthcare delivery is a process—a series of linked steps designed to achieve a certain outcome. The healthcare system is a series of processes interacting together. Through designing process interventions, testing change, and measuring outcomes, quality improvement theories can be applied to healthcare in meaningful ways.

APPROACH TO CLINICAL PATHWAY DEVELOPMENT

The clinical pathways presented in this chapter represent examples of a multidisciplinary effort over the last decade to standardize processes for a given chief complaint or clinical condition to improve care in our emergency department (ED). Each pathway provides a road map or mental model for all members of the ED clinician team. As this shared model is incorporated into culture, communication, teamwork and quality improve, and unnecessary variation and costs decrease. There are many others available at http://www.chop.edu/professionals/clinical-pathways/.

A clinical pathway provides a standard, detailed process of care for patients with a particular chief complaint or clinical problem. It results from multidisciplinary work by front line clinicians who possess the fundamental knowledge around that particular care process. Existing evidence, guidelines, and expert consensus are translated into a practical tool that can be utilized during bedside care. The pathways live in a web-based format and are accompanied by an electronic order set and other tools bringing decision support to the clinical team, making it easier for them to do what is recommended.

To develop a pathway, clinical leaders and frontline clinicians first select a high priority condition, one in which there is known practice variation, substantial existing evidence or guidelines, concerns for safety/quality issues and importantly, a will for change. A multidisciplinary clinician group is formed with representation from all relevant stakeholders and led by a strong clinical champion/s best represented by a physician and nurse team. Important additional team members include an improvement advisor and a data analyst who can facilitate the process and steer the project to completion. This team, meets to review the current process and gather patient data, safety events, and information form clinicians. They work together to review existing evidence, generate expert consensus, and develop an algorithm that defines the steps in the processes of care. Supplementary guidance is provided via hyperlinks to specific decision nodes on the algorithm. The algorithm/flow chart becomes the foundation for the care process; the shared mental model promoting strong teamwork and effective team communication.

The pathway must reflect the flow of work, so the team must consider staffing, training and education, supplies, physical layout, educational materials and clinical decision support. The pathway is then shared with stakeholders to recruit support and to incorporate important feedback. As much of this work is based on expert consensus due to lack of evidence, it is imperative to have stakeholder agreement. The pathway, including the algorithm, hyperlinks, supporting evidence, important policies/procedures and websites is then posted on the internet for easy access to all clinicians. Each pathway has an accompanying electronic order set with built-in decision support, including pre-checked selections that highlight recommended tests and medications and doses appropriate for the particular clinical problem. These tools make it easy for the clinician to provide the care recommended in the pathway, but do not prevent the provider from making different choices if necessitated by the patient's unique presentation.

MEASURING IMPROVEMENT

The pathway provides the basis for consistent practice based on scientific information and peer consensus. This consistency facilitated the ability to measure both the care delivery processes and patient outcomes. Clinicians can then apply the scientific method to systematically improve care. Credible data is required to inform the team, so an adequate data system must be put into place. This requires a significant commitment and investment for needed resources from the organization.

The Pathway Team then decides on a few key measures to follow during implementation and improvement. Aims, which detail how much improvement is to be made by a targeted date are documented. The team designs iterative Plan-Do-Study-Act (PDSA) cycles to test whether changes made in the care delivery process result in improvements. At weekly huddles, the team meets to review the most recent data and design the next test of change. This process continues until the aim is achieved. Monitoring of the process continues to ensure that the change has taken hold. Statistical Process Control Charts (SPC) are an ideal way to track the process, separating deviation arising from differences in patient presentation (appropriate, common or random variation) and those arising from external practice patterns (inappropriate, special or assignable cause). The goal is to eliminate unnecessary variation across clinicians over time and to retain variation that arises from important individual patient differences.

Through our efforts over the past 10 years, we have found this work to be rewarding; it engages clinicians to be curious about their current practices. Additionally, sharing what we have learned with our colleagues has sparked interest in pathways-based quality improvement at our own institution as well as at hospitals around the world.

Suggested Readings and Key References

James BC. Implementing practice guidelines through clinical quality improvement. *Front Health Serv Manage* 1993;10(1):2–37.

Langley GJ, Moen RD, Nolan TW, et al. *The Improvement Guide: A Practical Approach to Enhancing Organization Performance,* 2nd edition. California: Jossey-Bossey, 2009.

Provost LP, Murray SK. *The Health Care Data Guide: Learning form Data Improvement.* California: Jossey-Bossey, 2011.

CHAPTER 82 ■ ABDOMINAL PAIN IN POSTPUBERTAL GIRLS

CYNTHIA J. MOLLEN, MD, MSCE, MARY SCHUCKER, RN, BSN, MSN, CRNP, AND NAOMI LOVE, RN, BSN, CPEN

BACKGROUND (EPIDEMIOLOGY, EVIDENCE)

Abdominal pain is a frequent chief complaint in the pediatric emergency department (ED). National data noted 8,137,774 visits to the ED for abdominal pain between 2006 and 2009; 70% of these visits were by females, and over 70% of visits were by adolescent patients. The differential diagnosis for these patients is broad; even once narrowed by age and gender, the provider must consider a long list of potential diagnoses, including gynecologic causes such as pelvic inflammatory disease (PID), ovarian cyst rupture, or ovarian torsion; pain from pregnancy or complications of pregnancy, such as ectopic; and others, such as appendicitis, pyelonephritis, nephrolithiasis, constipation, or trauma.

Of note, an estimated one in eight sexually active adolescent girls develop PID before reaching 20 years of age, and patients with PID are at risk of serious acute and chronic complications such as tubo-ovarian abscesses, infertility, and chronic pelvic pain. The diagnosis of PID can be difficult to make, however, as the clinical presentation may mimic other pelvic and abdominal processes. In order to assist clinicians with these complex diagnostic decisions, the Centers for Disease Control and Prevention has developed standardized guidelines for the diagnosis and treatment of PID; although comprehensive, these guidelines are lengthy and can be difficult to navigate.

Despite evidence-based national guidelines, the prevalence and the risk of complications from PID, multiple studies have demonstrated that the ED treatment of patients with PID is less than ideal. For example, an analysis of data from the National Hospital Ambulatory Medical Care Survey (NHAMCS) from 1992 to 1997 identified 351 records for adolescents diagnosed with a sexually transmitted infection, representing 1.2 million adolescent visits. Of patients diagnosed with PID, only 35% were treated in accordance with the CDC guidelines. Similarly, a telephone survey–based study of 51 ED pediatricians found that management of adolescent girls with PID was often less aggressive than that recommended by the CDC; particularly regarding admission criteria and ensuring adequate follow-up.

With respect to pregnancy testing, although almost 800,000 adolescents give birth each year, a recent study of national data found that only 20% of adolescent females underwent pregnancy testing during their ED visit; of patients with complaints potentially related to pregnancy, the number rose to only 44.5%. Even if a positive pregnancy test is unrelated to the presenting symptoms, identifying pregnancy early allows for initiation of pregnancy precautions and prenatal care if childbirth is desired, earlier detection of life-threatening complications such as ectopic pregnancy, opportunity for consideration of options such as therapeutic abortion or adoption, and increased time for counseling, regardless of the patient's ultimate choice.

Given the potential for significant sequelae from some diagnoses if not rapidly identified, the chief complaint of lower abdominal pain in the postpubertal female provides an excellent opportunity for pathway development. The identification and management of these diagnoses requires a streamlined, multidisciplinary approach, with the entire care team aware of issues around testing, confidentiality, and appropriate treatment.

PATHWAY GOALS AND MEASUREMENTS

Goals

- Increased assessment of pregnancy status in adolescent females
- Improved timeliness of care
- Improved adherence to recommended antibiotic regimens for the treatment of PID
- Improved follow-up

Specific Goals

- Assure β-hCG testing in all patients ≥13 years old presenting with abdominal pain who have not been tested within the last 72 hours
- Use the CDC recommended antibiotic regimens in all patients diagnosed with PID

Measurements

- Percent pregnancy tests in female patients ≥13 years old with chief complaint of abdominal pain
- Time from arrival to MD evaluation, time from MD evaluation to order entry, and time from arrival to ultrasound, if indicated
- Review of specific antibiotics prescribed for patients diagnosed with PID
- Documented follow-up after implementation of electronic order built in EMR discharge set

Algorithm and Key Hyperlinks

- See Figure 82.1
- http://www.chop.edu/clinical-pathway/lower-abdominal-painclinical-pathway-post-pubertal-girls

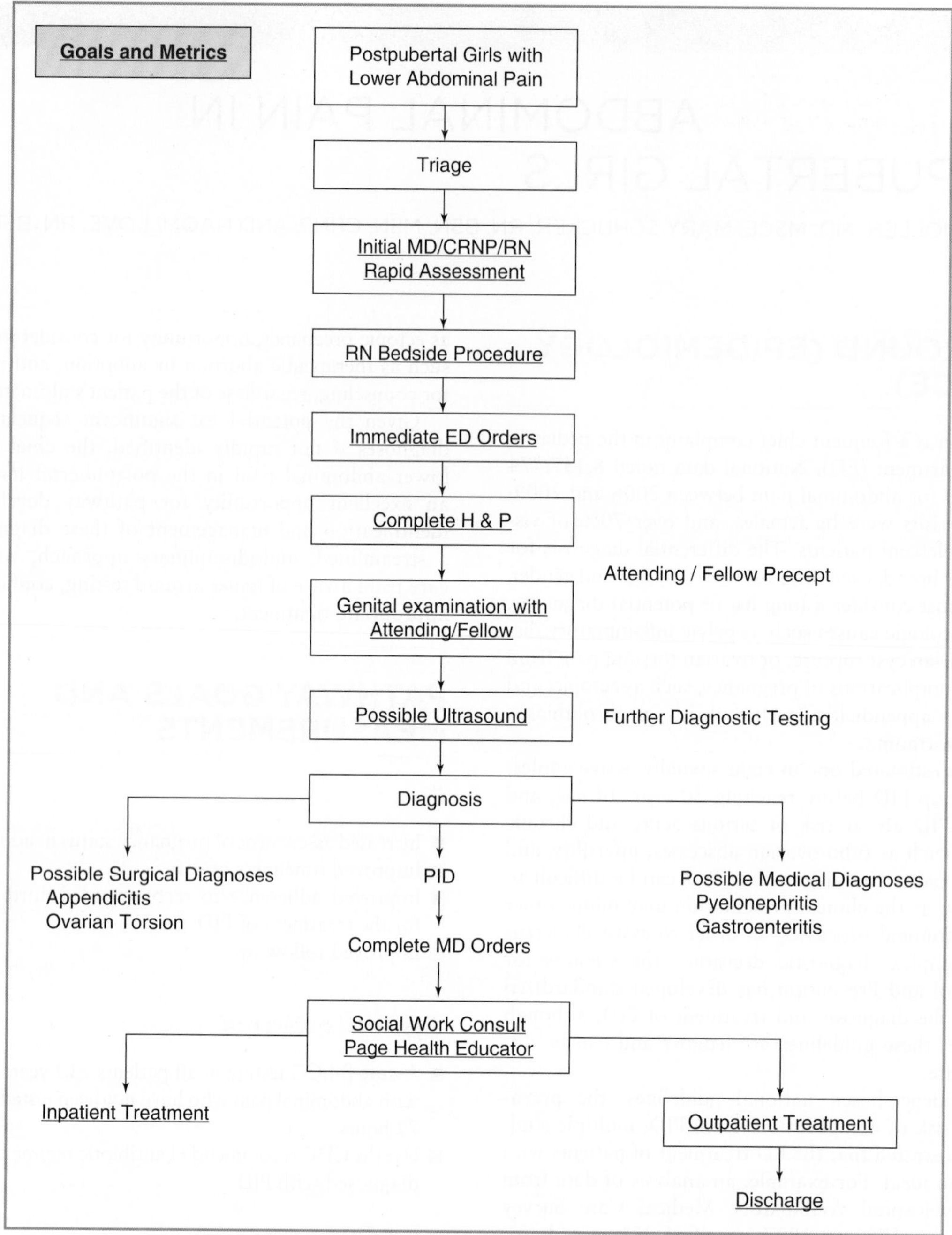

FIGURE 82.1 Pathway for the evaluation and treatment of postpubertal female with lower abdominal pain. *Pathway Authors: C. Mollen, MD, Monika Goyal, MD, J. Lavelle, MD, M. Schucker, CRNP.*

PATIENT POPULATION/ STRATIFYING PATIENT RISKS

This pathway is intended for all postpubertal female patients presenting with abdominal pain without vaginal bleeding. While the goals of the pathway focus on pregnancy testing and PID treatment, this pathway can be used for all adolescent patients with abdominal pain, as the initial assessment is appropriate for patients who ultimately are found to have alternative diagnoses, such as appendicitis, gastroenteritis, or constipation. The clinician can refer to additional pathways as the differential diagnosis narrows.

Of note, this pathway is for higher acuity patients triaged as ESI level 3 or higher, as it is presumed that these patients are likely to require intravenous fluids and laboratory evaluation, regardless of their ultimate diagnosis. However, this pathway can be utilized to assist the clinician in determining necessary testing and treatment for less acutely ill patients diagnosed with PID.

Finally, an important early decision point for patients being treated using this pathway is determining the clinician's concern for ovarian torsion as a potential diagnosis. In these patients, a pelvic ultrasound is necessary in an urgent fashion, and if transabdominal ultrasounds are the test of choice in the institution

TABLE 82.1

INDICATIONS FOR ULTRASOUND

Indications for ultrasound	Severe pain Significant focality to pain Palpable mass on PE Uncertain diagnosis Elevated inflammatory markers

Consider retrograde filling of the bladder, refer to the Bladder Filling Procedure.

(rather than transvaginal ultrasounds), the patient must have a full bladder. Therefore, the pathway recommends rapid assessment by the care team to determine need for an ultrasound, and subsequent serum β-hCG testing while refraining from urine studies until after the ultrasound (see Tables 82.1 and 82.2).

CLINICAL DECISION SUPPORT

Electronic Order Set

The Electronic Order Set assists in the coordination of standardized, evidence-based care and encourages communication among team members. If designed properly, it facilitates care and ultimately improves timeliness of care, as the physician/care provider can place the correct orders quickly and the nurse can then initiate care without delay, encouraging collaborative care between the nurse and physician or other care provider (see Table 82.3).

Other Electronic Tools

Additional electronic hyperlinks include a discharge order set with specific reminders around follow-up, obtaining patient information for providing confidential test results after the ED visit, as well as a link to the CDC STI treatment guidelines. Hyperlinks on the pathway include social work evaluation and evaluation by a health educator, who can provide confidential sexual health risk reduction counseling and testing for HIV.

TABLE 82.3

LABORATORY STUDIES

Urine	HCG (if not serum) Aptima for chlamydia and GC if evaluating for STIs Point of care urine dip Consider urine culture based on dip results and clinical scenario
Blood	HCG (if not urine) CBC CRP ESR BMP Amylase, Lipase as clinically indicated RPR hepatitis B and C serology, HIV PCR as clinically indicated (e.g., RPR in patients diagnosed with PID; Hepatitis B and C if clinical evidence of hepatitis; HIV PCR in sexually active patients if not recently tested—consider plan for result notification)
Vaginal swab	Rapid trichomonas antigen test Gram stain (not culture)
Lesion swab	HSV PCR

Communication/Team Work

The team communication goal is to recognize that all adolescent females presenting with abdominal pain need pregnancy assessment; the method of testing (serum vs. urine) is determined by the clinicians' concern for severity of illness. Ovarian torsion and pregnancy-related complications require rapid evaluation and treatment.

The ED workup proceeds after team evaluation of the patient. If the patient is unable to be assessed in a team manner (attending/frontline clinician/nurse) then the patient's nurse can initiate the pathway after brief discussion with the ordering clinician.

The treating frontline clinician discusses testing with the patient/guardian, keeping in mind issues around confidentiality,

TABLE 82.2

CRITERIA FOR THE DIAGNOSIS OF PELVIC INFLAMMATORY DISEASE

Minimum criteria	Elaborate criteria[a]	Most specific criteria
Uterine/adnexal tenderness or	Oral temperature >38.3°C	Ultrasound showing thickened fluid-filled tubes with or without free pelvic fluid or tubo-ovarian complex
Cervical motion tenderness	Abnormal cervical or vaginal mucopurulent discharge Presence of WBCs on Gram stain of vaginal secretions Elevated ESR Elevated CRP Laboratory documentation of GC Chlamydial infection	Laparoscopic findings

2015 CDC STD Treatment Guidelines.
[a]Improves specificity, not necessary to initiate treatment.

TABLE 82.4

INDICATIONS FOR ADMISSION

Indications for admission	
Indications for admission	Age <15 yrs Immunodeficiency TOA Failed outpatient treatment Vomiting Severe disease Concern for compliance, follow-up Uncertain diagnosis Significantly elevated inflammatory markers

and documents an accurate phone number in the EMR to reach the guardian and/or patient to discuss test results and follow-up care. Provider/patient discussions regarding confidentiality (e.g., the patient may give permission for a parent or guardian to be given test results) should be documented in the medical record, to assist with follow-up (see Chapter 100 Gynecology Emergencies).

Given the potential for poor follow-up in these patients, the risk of potential sequelae from PID, and the need to provide test results for STI testing after the ED visit, a systematic follow-up system must exist. The ED pediatric nurse practitioner reviews laboratory results and calls patients to assess follow-up needs and progression of symptoms. The order set includes an electronic follow-up note, and a link on the pathway reminds clinicians about the 72-hour time recommended time frame for a follow-up appointment, and reminds the clinician to obtain a specific phone number from the patient.

Nurse Specific Education

A key component of nursing care is considering the next step in care/potential for changes in clinical status. Nurses recognize the need for an immediate ultrasound and subsequent potential for a full bladder prior to ultrasound. Additionally, the bedside nurse considers the npo status and need for analgesia, and talks with the teen about the possible need for bimanual examination. If a full bladder is required for ultrasound and time is of the essence, the bedside nurse prepares for retrograde bladder filling. Finally, as with all patients, the nurse is a vital team partner for ensuring the patient and family are kept up to date around the care plan and results of the evaluation.

TABLE 82.5

INPATIENT TREATMENT FOR PID

Regimen A	Cefoxitin 2 g IV q6h *plus* • Doxycycline 100 mg po BID • Add Flagyl if TOA is present
Regimen B	Clindamycin 900 mg IV q8h *plus* • Gentamicin 2 mg/kg IV, then 1.5 mg/kg q8h

TABLE 82.6

OUTPATIENT TREATMENT FOR PID (*BOTH DRUGS ARE REQUIRED*)

Drug	Dose
Ceftriaxone	250 mg IM or IV
Doxycycline	100 mg po BID for 14 days

Quality Measurement

Specific measures of quality for this pathway include assessment of pregnancy testing, review of antibiotic choices, timeliness of care, and provision of analgesia.

Next Steps

The pathway team will work to educate care providers about the need for pregnancy testing in all patients, with the potential of increased serum testing (rather than urine testing) in order to serve the dual purpose of reducing time to ultrasound and overall length of stay. Additionally, the team will work to improve follow-up for patients diagnosed with PID, with consideration of adopting technology such as text messaging, for example. This requires the team to develop a process for standardized follow-up, working with colleagues in adolescent medicine. Once the new process is refined, the pathway is updated, and another aspect of the pathway is addressed additional information. See Tables 82.4, 82.5, and 82.6 for additional information.

Suggested Readings and Key References

Beckmann KR, Melzer-Lange MD, Gorelick MH. Emergency department management of sexually transmitted infections in US adolescents: results from the national hospital ambulatory medical care survey. *Ann Emerg Med* 2004;43(3):333–338.

Benaim J, Pulaski M, Coupey SM. Adolescent girls and pelvic inflammatory disease: experience and practices of emergency department pediatricians. *Arch Pediatr Adolesc Med* 1998;152(5):449–454.

Centers for Disease Control and Prevention. Sexually transmitted diseases treatment guidelines. *MMWR Recomm Rep* 2015;64:1–140. Available at: http://www.cdc.gov/std/tg2015/default.htm. Aaccessed July 30, 2015.

Centers for Disease Control and Prevention. Update to CDC's sexually transmitted diseases treatment guidelines, 2010: oral cephalosporins no longer a recommended treatment for gonococcal infections. *MMWR Morb Mortal Wkly Rep* 2012;61(31):590–594.

Goyal M, Hersh A, Luan X, et al. Frequency of pregnancy testing among adolescent emergency department visits. *Acad Emerg Med* 2013;20(8):816–821.

Johnson TJ, Weaver MD, Borrero S, et al. Association of race and ethnicity with management of abdominal pain in the emergency department. *Pediatrics* 2013;132(4):e851–e858.

Kane BG, Degutis LC, Sayward HK, et al. Compliance with the Centers for Disease Control and Prevention recommendations for the diagnosis and treatment of sexually transmitted diseases. *Acad Emerg Med* 2004;11(4):371–377.

Tarr ME, Gilliam ML. Sexually transmitted infections in adolescent women. *Clin Obstet Gynecol* 2008;51(2):306–318.

CHAPTER 83 ■ APPENDICITIS (SUSPECTED)

MANOJ K. MITTAL, MD, MRCP(UK), DOLORES H. ALBERT, BSN, RN, CPEN, KATELYN N. YOUNG, RN, MSN, CPEN, JOY L. COLLINS, MD, FAAP, AND JANE LAVELLE, MD

BACKGROUND (EPIDEMIOLOGY, EVIDENCE)

Appendicitis is the most common surgical emergency in children leading to more than 70,000 pediatric appendectomies annually in the United States. The diagnosis can be challenging, with a substantial proportion misdiagnosed if based on clinical features and laboratory tests alone. Negative appendectomy and perforation rates remain high, indicating a need to reevaluate the diagnostic assessment for this condition. Over the last decade, computed tomography (CT) has been heavily relied on in the evaluation of children with possible appendicitis to improve diagnostic accuracy. However, because of increasing concern over the long-term malignancy risk related to CT-associated ionizing radiation in children, its routine use is being reappraised. Standardizing the approach to patients with suspected appendicitis has been shown to reduce variability, thus promoting the delivery of efficient, safe, and cost effective health care. Clinical prediction rules are used to stratify patients based on their risk for having appendicitis, thus allowing for tailored management. There is increasing use of ultrasound (US) as the primary imaging modality. The US has been shown to accurately confirm or exclude appendicitis in cases where the appendix is clearly identified. When appendix is not identified, however, other clinical approaches should be considered; these include repeat clinical assessment; laboratory testing including a potential future role for biomarkers; admission for repeat clinical examinations and repeat US; and/or focused right lower quadrant CT or magnetic resonance imaging, or discharge home with close follow-up.

Appendicitis may also serve as a model disease for examining healthcare disparities in children given its acute nature, high prevalence, and known adverse outcomes associated with appendiceal perforation. Higher rates of appendiceal perforation have been found in patients with decreased healthcare access such as in minorities, patients on Medicaid, and in Hispanics with limited English proficiency.

PATHWAY GOALS AND MEASUREMENT

Goals

The goals for this pathway include the following:

- Use of US as first-line imaging modality for all patients to avoid unnecessary radiation exposure
- Standardized US radiology reports to facilitate clinician decision making
- Standardized order sets for laboratory studies to assist frontline clinicians in initiating timely workups
- Expectation for timely communication with the surgical team guided by the clinical certainty of diagnosis at different stages of the evaluation process
- Expectation for timely fluid and pain management
- Standard antibiotic regimen based on regional susceptibility data

Measurement

- US, CT utilization
- Time to OR from ED arrival
- Use of appropriate antibiotics
- Pain management
- Negative appendectomy rate
- Perforation rate
- Revisit rate, diagnosis at revisit
- "Missed" diagnosis
- Equity-related criteria: assessing the above criteria across different racial, ethnic, and insurance groupings

Algorithm and Key Hyperlinks

- See Figure 83.1
- http://www.chop.edu/clinical-pathway/suspected-appendicitis clinical-pathway

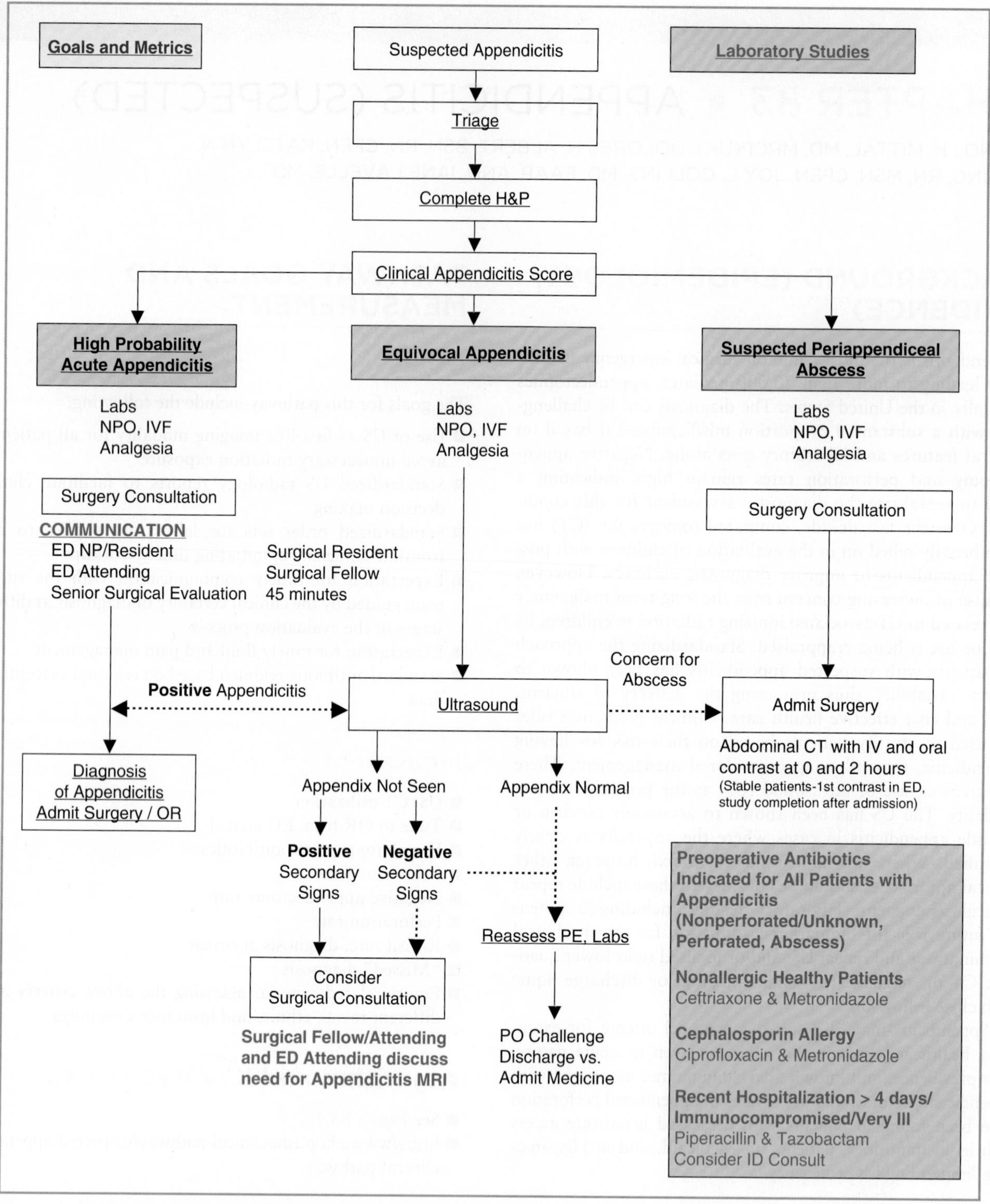

FIGURE 83.1 Pathway for the evaluation of children with suspected appendicitis. *Pathway Authors: Lavelle, MD, J. Collins, MD, C. Jacobstein, MD, M. Mittal, MD, M. Joffe, MD, J. Zorc, MD, M. Nance, MD, K. Darge, MD, K. Young, RN, D. Albert, RN.*

Patient Population/Stratifying Patient Risk

TABLE 83.1

PATIENT POPULATION/STRATIFYING PATIENT RISK

High probability acute appendicitis	Symptoms less than 48 hrs Migration of pain from periumbilical region to RLQ Anorexia, nausea, vomiting Pain preceding vomiting Pain with movement (cough, car ride, jumping on right foot) RLQ tenderness with or without rebound
Equivocal acute appendicitis	Presenting with focal abdominal tenderness (usually right sided) with some of the features of high probability acute appendicitis
Suspected periappendiceal abscess	Systemic toxicity Fever Prolonged symptoms >48–72 hrs Urinary and/or rectal urgency Palpable RLQ mass WBC, ANC, CRP consistent with marked inflammation

Clinical Appendicitis Score

TABLE 83.2

CLINICAL APPENDICITIS SCORE

Pediatric Appendicitis Score Low Risk <4; High Risk ≥7		Alvarado/Mantrels Score Low Risk <4; High Risk ≥7	
Nausea/vomiting	1		1
Anorexia	1		1
Migration of pain to RLQ	1		1
Fever	1	Temperature ≥37.3°C	1
Cough/percussion/hopping tenderness	2	Rebound tenderness	1
RLQ tenderness	2		2
Leukocytosis (WBC >10,000)	1		2
Neutrophilia (ANC >7,500)	1		1

Experienced physician's clinical impression is comparable to these scores.

Electronic Order Set

Laboratory studies recommended for all patients are preselected in the electronic order set to assist the frontline ordering clinician. There are additional recommendations for radiographic studies, as well as standard recommendations for IVF, pain medications, and antibiotic therapy. See Table 83.3.

TABLE 83.3

LABORATORY STUDIES

All patients	CBC with ANC, CRP
As clinically indicated	CMP Lipase, amylase Urine HCG Urine for GC, Chlamydia LCR Vaginal swab for Trichomonas
Ill patients	Blood culture Coagulation studies Lactate Type and screen

NOTE: Type and screen is not indicated for routine appendectomy.

Radiology Studies

TABLE 83.4

RADIOLOGY STUDIES

Initial imaging	All US abdomen RLQ—appendicitis only Females US pelvis with Doppler
Secondary imaging	MR abdomen W/O contrast CT abdomen and pelvis, IV contrast only

Standardized Radiology Reporting

Radiologists include the following descriptions in their reports, to assure that clinicians interpret the impressions in the same manner to aid in reducing the need for additional diagnostic studies:

- Appendix seen and normal
- Appendicitis
- Appendix not seen, secondary signs present
- Appendix not seen, no secondary signs

Communication/Teamwork

The communication plan aims at triaging high-risk patients for senior surgical consultation to expedite time to definitive care and further reduce unnecessary imaging. Conversely, ED workup proceeds for the patients with equivocal signs and symptoms in an effort to reduce unnecessary surgical consultation, as patients with reassuring US and ANC/CRP results can often be reassessed and safely discharged with good follow-up.

RN Specific Education

The RN champion education focuses on timely and ongoing fluid resuscitation, pain assessment and treatment, and antibiotics.

TABLE 83.5

QUALITY IMPROVEMENT DATA: IMAGING UTILIZATION FOR PATIENTS WITH SUSPECTED APPENDICITIS

Imaging utilization	No imaging 2.2% US only 85% US + CT 11.8%

Quality Measurement

Over a 1-year period, the electronic order set for appendicitis was used in approximately 20% of children presenting with a chief complaint of abdominal pain. Of this cohort, 50% had the diagnosis of appendicitis, representing 10% of all children with the chief complaint of abdominal pain. See Table 83.5.

Next Steps

Use data to inform the pathway team on new opportunities for improvement. Use clinical decision support to further improve care processes.

Suggested Readings and Key References

Anderson M, Collins E. Analgesia with acute abdominal pain and diagnostic accuracy. *Arch Dis Child* 2008;93(11):995–997.

Bachur RG, Dayan PS, Bajaj L, et al.; Pediatric Emergency Medicine Collaborative Research Committee of the American Academy of Pediatrics. The effect of abdominal pain duration on the accuracy of diagnostic imaging for pediatric appendicitis. *Ann Emerg Med* 2012;60(5):582–590.

Ebell MH, Shinholser J. What are the most critically useful cutoffs for the Alvarado and Pediatric Appendicitis Scores? A systematic review. *Ann Emerg Med* 2014;64(4):365–372.

Goldin AB, Khanna P, Thapa M, et al. Revised ultrasound criteria for appendicitis in children improve diagnostic accuracy. *Pediatr Radiol* 2011;41(8):993–999.

Grim PF. Emergency medicine physicians' and pediatricians' use of computed tomography in the evaluation of pediatric patients with abdominal pain without trauma in a community hospital. *Clin Pediatr (Phila)* 2014;53(5):486–489.

Hatcher-Ross K. Sensitivity and specificity of the pediatric appendicitis score. *J Pediatr* 2009;154(2):308.

Kharbanda AB. Appendicitis: do clinical scores matter? *Ann Emerg Med* 2014;64(4):373–375.

Kharbanda AB, Dudley NC, Bajaj L, et al.; Pediatric Emergency Medicine Collaborative Research Committee of the American Academy of Pediatrics. Validation and refinement of a prediction rule to identify children at low risk for pediatric appendicitis. *Arch Pediatr Adolesc Med* 2012;166(8):738–744.

Kharbanda AB, Taylor GA, Fishman SJ, et al. A clinical decision rule to identify children at low risk for appendicitis. *Pediatrics* 2005;116(3):709–716.

Leeuwenburgh MM, Jensch S, Gratama JW, et al.; OPTIMAP study group. MRI features associated with acute appendicitis. *Eur Radiol* 2014;24(1):214–222.

Ohle R, O'Reilly F, O'Brien KK, et al. The Alvarado Score for predicting acute appendicitis: a systemic review. *BMC Med* 2011;9:139.

Russell WS, Schuh AM, Hill JG, et al. Clinical practice guidelines for pediatric appendicitis evaluation can decrease computed tomography utilization while maintaining diagnostic accuracy. *Pediatr Emerg Care* 2013;29(5):568–573.

Samuel M. Pediatric appendicitis score. *J Pediatr Surg* 2002;37(6):877–881.

Saucier A, Huang EY, Emeremni CA, et al. Prospective evaluation of a clinical pathway for suspected appendicitis. *Pediatrics* 2014;133(1):e88–e95.

Schneider C, Kharbanda A, Bachur R. Evaluating appendicitis scoring systems using a prospective pediatric cohort. *Ann Emerg Med* 2007;49(6):778–784.

Wagner JM, McKinney WP, Carpenter JL. Does this patient have appendicitis? *JAMA* 1996;276(19):1589–1594.

CHAPTER 84 ■ ASTHMA

JOSEPH ZORC, MD, MSCE, ANN MARIE REARDON, MSN, CRNP, AND WARREN FRANKENBERGER, PhD, RN, CCNS

BACKGROUND EPIDEMIOLOGY, EVIDENCE

Asthma is the most common chronic childhood illness and a leading cause for emergency department (ED) visits and hospitalizations. In recent decades, rising rates of asthma prevalence and hospitalizations have led to a focus on improving the quality of care, including guidelines published by the National Heart, Lung, and Blood Institute (NHLBI) and international organizations. Asthma emergency visits vary seasonally, coinciding with common triggers including respiratory viruses and environmental allergens. In peak periods, typically in the fall months after children return to school, asthma visits occur in epidemic fashion and can overwhelm ED and hospital resources. Adequate preparation and system organization are key to managing the predictable seasonal surge of asthma.

Unlike many pediatric illnesses, there is a strong evidence base for treatment of asthma in the ED drawn from clinical trials, systematic reviews, and comparative effectiveness research. The NHLBI Guideline algorithm stresses rapid assessment and categorization of asthma severity in the ED, leading to early treatment with inhaled bronchodilators and oral corticosteroids. Severity assessment in children relies on a multifaceted clinical assessment, as acutely ill children are often unable to perform lung function tests used as a standard approach in adults. Diagnostic tests, such as chest radiographs and arterial blood gases, are not required for most patients. Recommended therapies that have been shown to improve outcomes in severe asthma exacerbations include high-dose beta-agonist and anticholinergic bronchodilators and systemic corticosteroids. Timeliness is a key principle for treatment of acute asthma, as the mechanism of action of this combined treatment regimen takes several hours to reach peak effect. Recent studies have found a reduction in hospitalization rate when the time from arrival to the administration of oral corticosteroids was decreased by methods such as administration in triage.

Despite this strong evidence base, deficiencies in the quality of asthma care for children in EDs are well documented. Benchmarking studies have found wide variation in oral corticosteroid and chest radiograph rates across EDs in the United States, including children's hospitals. Of broader concern are the deficiencies in long-term preventive primary care that have been observed for populations of children seeking care in EDs. The NHLBI Guidelines recognize the importance of ED providers assessing these deficiencies and connecting patients with appropriate resources for long-term care.

As with any challenging problem, a concerted team approach is the key to successful asthma care in the ED. This is particularly the case for asthma, given the multidisciplinary nature of treatment, which typically includes physicians, midlevel providers, nurses, and respiratory therapists. Communication and a clear understanding of the steps of the algorithm and doses of medication are key to improving timeliness and eliminating errors. An initial team assessment at the bedside sets the direction for care on the pathway, with timed reassessments. Assessment of long-term needs of the child, such as access to preventive primary care, triggers in the home environment, prescription of controller medications when appropriate, and use of asthma devices, is also best accomplished by a collaborative approach. Regular review of performance on asthma treatment goals and feedback to the quality team working on improving care can drive system changes.

PATHWAY GOALS AND MEASUREMENTS

Goals

The goals for this pathway include the following:

- Increase the use of effective, evidence-based treatments for acute asthma including bronchodilators and systemic corticosteroids based on an initial severity assessment.
- Improve timeliness of care by improving team-based care and encouraging a coordinated assessment.

- Identify long-term asthma preventive care issues for children seen in the ED including smoking, triggers, and access to controller medications.

Measurement

- Decreased time to beta-agonist and corticosteroid therapy for moderate and severe patients
- Decreased ED length of stay (disposition within 2 hours of start of treatment)
- Increased rate of corticosteroid administration for moderate and severe patients
- Decreased hospitalization rate
- Decreased chest radiograph rate
- Increased initiation of asthma controller therapy at ED discharge
- Reduction in prescribing errors

Algorithm and Key Hyperlinks

See Figure 84.1 (http://www.chop.edu/clinical-pathway/asthma-clinical-pathway)

PATIENT POPULATION/ STRATIFYING PATIENT RISKS

Quality Measurement

Population

Patients presenting to the ED with asthma (defined as prior diagnosis of asthma or history of two prior wheezing episodes), age >12 months, and acute wheezing and respiratory distress. See Table 84.1.

TABLE 84.1

QUALITY MEASUREMENT

Corticosteroid administration	Achievable benchmark: 80% of all asthma patients (Knapp et al., PEC 2010)
Arrival to corticosteroid administration	80% of triage level ½ patients administered within 1 hr of arrival
Chest x-ray rate	Achievable benchmark: 17% of all asthma patients (Knapp et al., PEC 2010)
ED length of stay	Follow monthly
ED admission rate	Follow monthly
Revisit 72 hrs w/ admission	Follow monthly, balancing measure

Next Steps

Utilizing a rapid improvement cycle framework (which emphasizes small tests of changes), the QI team will provide focused interventions. Potential areas for intervention include decreasing time to steroids by changes in the logistics of care, such as providing corticosteroids at triage and changing the type of steroid to dexamethasone, which has been shown to be better tolerated and requires a shorter course at discharge. Use data to further define areas for process improvement. Improve methods of screening for long-term asthma preventive issues and implement systems for education, identification of high-risk patients, and linkage to primary care resources.

CHILD WITH ASTHMA AND RESPIRATORY COMPLAINT

Asthma Definition for Pathway

- Acute trouble breathing and/or wheezing
- Age >12 months
- Prior diagnosis of asthma or history of two significant wheezing episodes

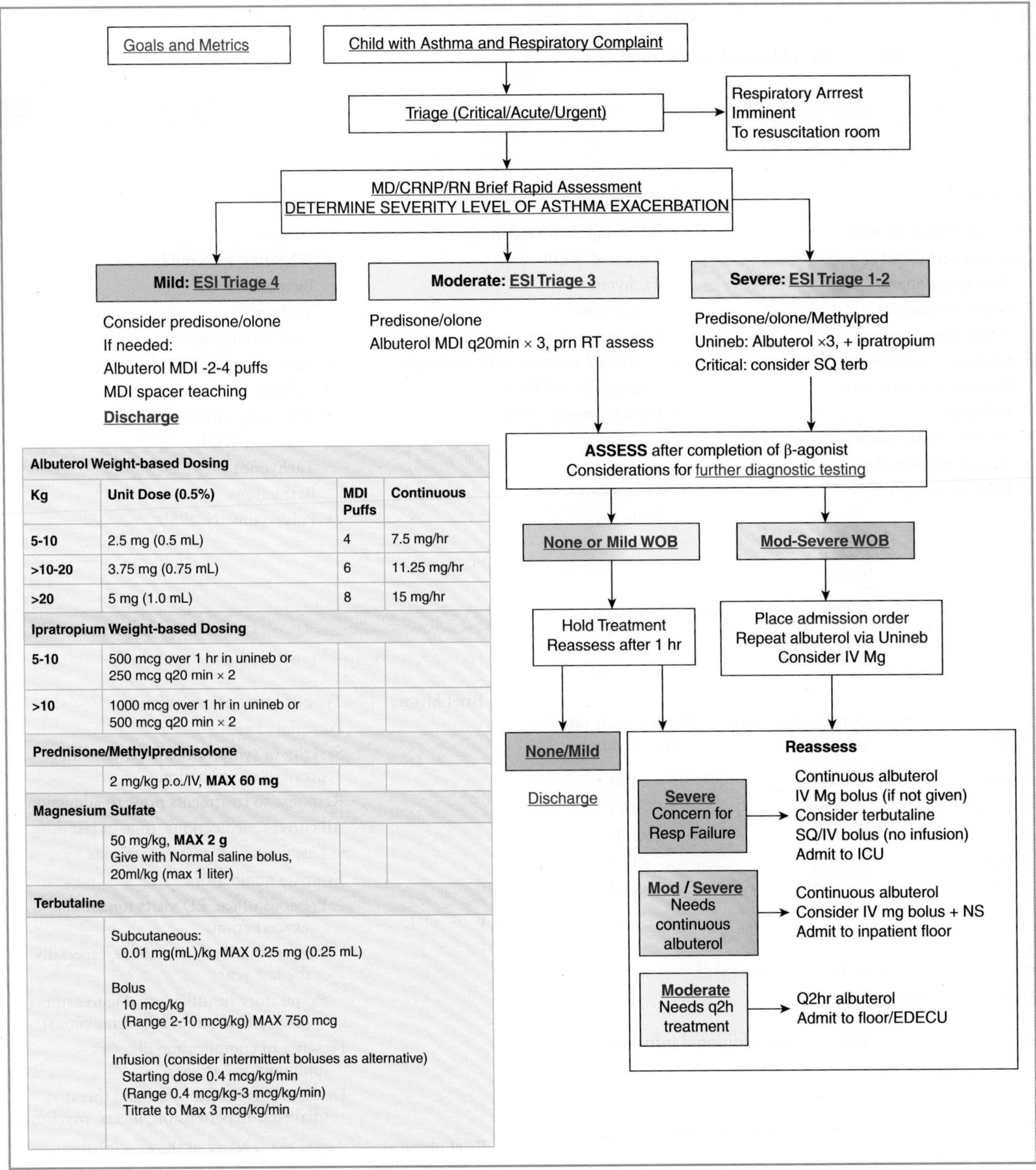

Albuterol Weight-based Dosing			
Kg	**Unit Dose (0.5%)**	**MDI Puffs**	**Continuous**
5-10	2.5 mg (0.5 mL)	4	7.5 mg/hr
>10-20	3.75 mg (0.75 mL)	6	11.25 mg/hr
>20	5 mg (1.0 mL)	8	15 mg/hr
Ipratropium Weight-based Dosing			
5-10	500 mcg over 1 hr in unineb or 250 mcg q20 min × 2		
>10	1000 mcg over 1 hr in unineb or 500 mcg q20 min × 2		
Prednisone/Methylprednisolone			
	2 mg/kg p.o./IV, **MAX 60 mg**		
Magnesium Sulfate			
	50 mg/kg, **MAX 2 g** Give with Normal saline bolus, 20ml/kg (max 1 liter)		
Terbutaline			
	Subcutaneous: 0.01 mg(mL)/kg MAX 0.25 mg (0.25 mL) Bolus 10 mcg/kg (Range 2-10 mcg/kg) MAX 750 mcg Infusion (consider intermittent boluses as alternative) Starting dose 0.4 mcg/kg/min (Range 0.4 mcg/kg-3 mcg/kg/min) Titrate to Max 3 mcg/kg/min		

FIGURE 84.1 ED pathway for the evaluation and treatment of children with asthma. *Pathway Authors: J. Zorc, MD; R. Scarfone, MD; A. Reardon, CRNP; N. Stroebel, CRNP; W. Frankenberger, RN; L. Tyler, RT; D. Simpkins, RT; R. Abaya, MD; E. Delgado, MD; E. Brill, RN.*

Triage (Critical/Acute/Urgent)

See Tables 84.2 and 84.3 for additional information.

TABLE 84.2

RESPIRATORY DISTRESS

1—critical	2—acute	3–4 urgent
• Severe wheezing with: Severe tachypnea Bradypnea/apnea Severe retractions Nasal flaring Grunting respirations Decreased muscle tone Lethargy • Absent breath sounds • Agonal respirations • Pulse oximetry <92%	• Wheezing with moderate: Increased WOB Tachypnea Retractions Intermittent grunt • Decreased aeration with moderate Tachypnea and WOB • Pulse oximetry <95%	**3—urgent** • Wheezing with mild: Increased WOB Tachypnea Mild retractions • Pulse oximetry ≥95% **4—urgent** • Wheezing with minimal: Increased WOB Tachypnea Retractions • Pulse oximetry ≥95%

TABLE 84.3

GUIDE TO BREATHING AND HEART RATES IN AWAKE CHILDREN

Age	Normal respiratory rate (per minute)	Normal heart rate (per minute)
<2 mo	<60	<160
2–12 mo	<50	<160
1–2 yrs	<40	<120
2–5 yrs	<40	<110
6–8 yrs	<30	<110

MD/CRNP/RN Brief Rapid Assessment

See Tables 84.4, 84.5 and 84.6 for additional information.

TABLE 84.4

MD/CRNP/RN BRIEF RAPID ASSESSMENT

Brief history	Time of onset of exacerbation Potential causes Severity of symptoms compared with previous exacerbation Response to treatments prior to admission All current medications, time of last dose Last course of systemic steroids Estimate number of: Previous office, ED visits for asthma exacerbations Hospitalizations for asthma, especially in the last year Respiratory insufficiency due to asthma (LOC, intubation, ICU admissions) Presence of complicating illnesses (pulmonary, cardiac) Diseases aggravated by steroid therapy (diabetes, hypertension, ulcers, psychosis)
Brief physical examination	Assess the severity of the exacerbation VS, pulse oximetry Level of alertness Hydration status Presence of cyanosis, pallor Respiratory distress Wheezing, decreased aeration Identify complications: Pneumonia Pneumothorax Pneumomediastinum Rule out upper airway obstruction (croup, foreign body, etc.)

TABLE 84.5

ASTHMA ASSESSMENT—KEY POINTS

Variability	Asthmatic children show acute airway obstruction differently depending on many factors including age and baseline lung function. One set of criteria cannot define asthma severity accurately across this wide spectrum of disease. Assignment of acute asthma severity is based on an **overall integrated assessment** of available signs, symptoms, and (if able) lung function.
Spirometry/peak flow	Pulmonary function tests are objective measures to directly assess airway obstruction. Valid measurement requires **good effort** by the patient and should be interpreted based on **baseline lung function** (when available) or a **value predicted by height.**
PASS	Pediatric Asthma Severity Score (range 0–6, see below) includes key examination elements (**wheezing, work of breathing, prolongation of expiration**) that correlate with the overall assessment to follow trends over time.
Pulse oximetry	Assessment for hypoxemia is important, as it may not be apparent on physical examination. It most often reflects **ventilation–perfusion mismatch** due to mucus plugging or bronchospasm which may not correlate with asthma severity. This effect may be temporarily worsened by bronchodilator therapy. Decisions about oxygen therapy should be based on overall saturation trends. Continuous pulse oximetry should be withdrawn as patients improve.

TABLE 84.6

DETERMINE SEVERITY LEVEL OF ASTHMA EXACERBATION

	Mild	Moderate	Severe	Respiratory arrest imminent
Key examination elements (PASS)				
Wheezing	**None or mild (0)** None or end of expiration only	**Moderate (1)** Throughout expiration	**Severe (2)** Inspiratory/expiratory or absent due to poor air exchange	Diminished due to poor air exchange
Work of breathing	**None or mild (0)** Normal or minimal retractions	**Moderate (1)** Intercostal retractions	**Severe (2)** Suprasternal retractions, abdominal breathing	Tiring, inability to maintain work of breathing
Prolonged expiration	**None or mild (0)** Normal or minimally prolonged	**Moderate (1)**	**Severe (2)**	Severely prolonged
Other examination elements				
Breath sounds/aeration	Normal	Decreased at bases	Widespread decrease	Absent/minimal
Symptoms				
Breathlessness	With activity or agitation	While at rest For infants: Soft or shorter cry Difficulty feeding Prefers sitting	While at rest For infants: Stops feeding Sits upright	
Talks in	Sentences	Phrases	Words	
Alertness	Alert	May be agitated	Agitated	Drowsy, confused
Measurements				
Pulse oximetry	>94%	Variable	Variable	Variable
PEF (% predicted by height)	>70%	40–69%	<40%	

FURTHER DIAGNOSTIC TESTING

Chest x-ray

Routine chest imaging is NOT recommended.

Consider if the patient has persistence of any of the following:

- Severe symptoms
- Significant hypoxemia
- Marked asymmetry on lung examination

Viral Testing

Routine viral testing is NOT recommended.

Consider if:

- Suspected influenza infection if patient meets criteria for treatment
- See Table 84.7.

RN/MD DISCHARGE INSTRUCTIONS

Before Discharge from ED

- Family should review controlling asthma video
- Prescribe oral steroids for 4 days if indicated
- Consider initiating controller medication if persistent symptoms present by history
- Review educational material on asthma and device sheets
- Review dosing of new and home medications
- Schedule follow-up appointment with primary care physician as soon as possible
- Review signs that would require a return to the ED

Inpatient

- Patient followed by a subspecialty service should be admitted to that service (pulmonary, allergy/immunology)
- Continue q2h nebulized treatments versus continuous albuterol nebulization
- Assess respiratory examination hourly while in the ED

TABLE 84.7

DIAGNOSTIC TESTING

Good response	Incomplete response	Poor response
Patient has **mild** symptoms: Pulse oximetry >94% Mild tachypnea Normal mental status Minimal ↑ WOB Good aeration End expiratory wheeze PEF >70%	Patient continues with **moderate** symptoms: Pulse oximetry 91–95% Moderate tachypnea Mildly anxious Moderate ↑ WOB Fair-good aeration Loud expiratory wheeze PEF 50–80% Continue q2h albuterol puffs or nebulizations (weight based) Consider continuous albuterol nebulization Assess need for additional therapies (see poor response)	Patient continues with SEVERE symptoms: Pulse oximetry <91% Severe tachypnea Anxious Severe ↑ WOB Poor aeration Inspiratory, expiratory wheezing Place IV, send basic metabolic panel Continuous albuterol nebulization IV magnesium sulfate 50 mg/kg, maximum of 2 g IV terbutaline Bolus infusion 2–10 μg/kg Infusion 0.08–0.4 μg/kg/min (maximum 6 μg/kg/min)

Suggested Readings and Key References

Bhogal SK, McGillivray D, Bourbeau J, et al. Early administration of systemic corticosteroids reduces hospital admission rates for children with moderate and severe asthma exacerbation. *Ann Emerg Med* 2012;60:84–91.

Global Strategy for Asthma Management and Prevention, Global Initiative for Asthma (GINA). 2014. Available at: http://www.ginasthma.org/.

Knapp JF, Hall M, Sharma V. Benchmarks for the emergency department care of children with asthma, bronchiolitis, and croup. *Pediatr Emerg Care* 2010;26:364–369.

National Asthma Education and Prevention Program. *Expert panel report 3: Guidelines for the diagnosis and management of asthma. National Institutes of Health Pub. # 08–5846*. Bethesda, MD, 2007. Available at: http://www.nhlbi.nih.gov/guidelines/asthma/asthmafullrpt.pdf.

Scarfone RJ, Zorc JJ, Capraro GA. Patient self-management of acute asthma: adherence to national guidelines a decade later. *Pediatrics* 2001;108:1332–1338.

Zemek R, Plint A, Osmond MH, et al. Triage nurse initiation of corticosteroids in pediatric asthma is associated with improved emergency department efficiency. *Pediatrics* 2012;129:671–680.

CHAPTER 85 ■ BRONCHIOLITIS

SHANNA R. DOOLEY, BSN, RN, CPEN, BONNIE RODIO, RN, BSN, CEN, CPHQ, LISA TYLER, MS, RRT-NPS, CPFT, AND JOSEPH ZORC, MD, MSCE

BACKGROUND EPIDEMIOLOGY, EVIDENCE

Bronchiolitis is a common pediatric illness caused by infection of the lower respiratory tract with respiratory syncytial virus (RSV), rhinovirus, metapneumovirus, or other pathogens. About a third of children acquire bronchiolitis in the first 2 years of life, and it is the leading cause of hospitalization for infants in the United States. Rising hospitalization rates and costs due to bronchiolitis over recent decades have led to a focus on improving the quality of care, including guidelines published by the American Academy of Pediatrics.

Bronchiolitis visits peak during the winter respiratory viral epidemic and can consume high amounts of ED and hospital resources. Although inevitable, the severity and specific timing of RSV season vary each year, which is a challenge for planning. Another important concern is the potential for spread of nosocomial infection to high-risk children, such as premature infants and children with immunodeficiency or cardiac disease. Finally, assessment of infants with bronchiolitis is somewhat challenging, as status can change rapidly due to clearance of secretions from the airways or response to treatments such as suctioning. Although many bronchiolitis scores have been developed for research and clinical care, no single widely accepted approach exists to define a standard clinical assessment.

A key concern as a team develops a plan of care for bronchiolitis is the high degree of variation that researchers have observed across hospitals in the ordering of tests and treatments. As discussed in the AAP Guideline, diagnostic tests such as viral testing and chest radiographs are used widely in some settings without clear evidence that they assist in diagnosis or management decisions, beyond what is gained from a simple history and physical examination. Similarly, use of treatments such as bronchodilators and corticosteroids varies widely across settings, although clinical trials have not found benefit in children with typical bronchiolitis. Use of unnecessary tests and treatments increases costs, delays care, and introduces the potential for harm due to adverse effects. A successful bronchiolitis pathway needs to focus on a standard clinical assessment with clear indications for additional tests and treatments.

The bronchiolitis pathway presented here is based on an initial assessment of severity and classification as mild, moderate, or severe. Repeated reassessments and clear documentation are important to note change in clinical status and response to treatment. Standard supportive care such as suctioning is encouraged. We have embedded lists of indications and reminders about appropriate use of chest radiographs and viral testing in the pathway and associated order set. Regular review of performance and feedback from the quality team was successful in reducing use of chest radiographs in low-acuity patients as shown in Figure 85.2.

PATHWAY GOALS AND MEASUREMENT

Goals

Encourage clinical diagnosis of bronchiolitis

Decrease use of tests and treatments without strong evidence base for benefit

- Chest radiograph
- Viral testing
- Albuterol use
- Continuous oxygen monitoring in mild patients
- Antibiotic use

Decrease ED length of stay, admission rate, revisit rate
Decrease hospital length of stay, readmit rate
Improve parental satisfaction

Metrics

General

- ED length of stay
- ED admission rate
- ED revisit rate

Testing

- Viral testing rate
- Chest radiograph rate

Treatment

- Albuterol trial use
- Racemic epinephrine use
- Steroid use
- Antibiotic use

Volume/cost
Use of order set

Algorithm and Key Hyperlinks

See Figure 85.1 (http://www.chop.edu/clinical-pathway/bronchiolitis-emergent-evaluation-and-treatment-clinical-pathway).

Quality Measurement

Population

This pathway should be used for healthy patients <2 years of age presenting to the ED with a clinical presentation consistent with the diagnosis of bronchiolitis including the following:

- Viral URI and cough, with signs of lower respiratory tract infection
- Work of breathing

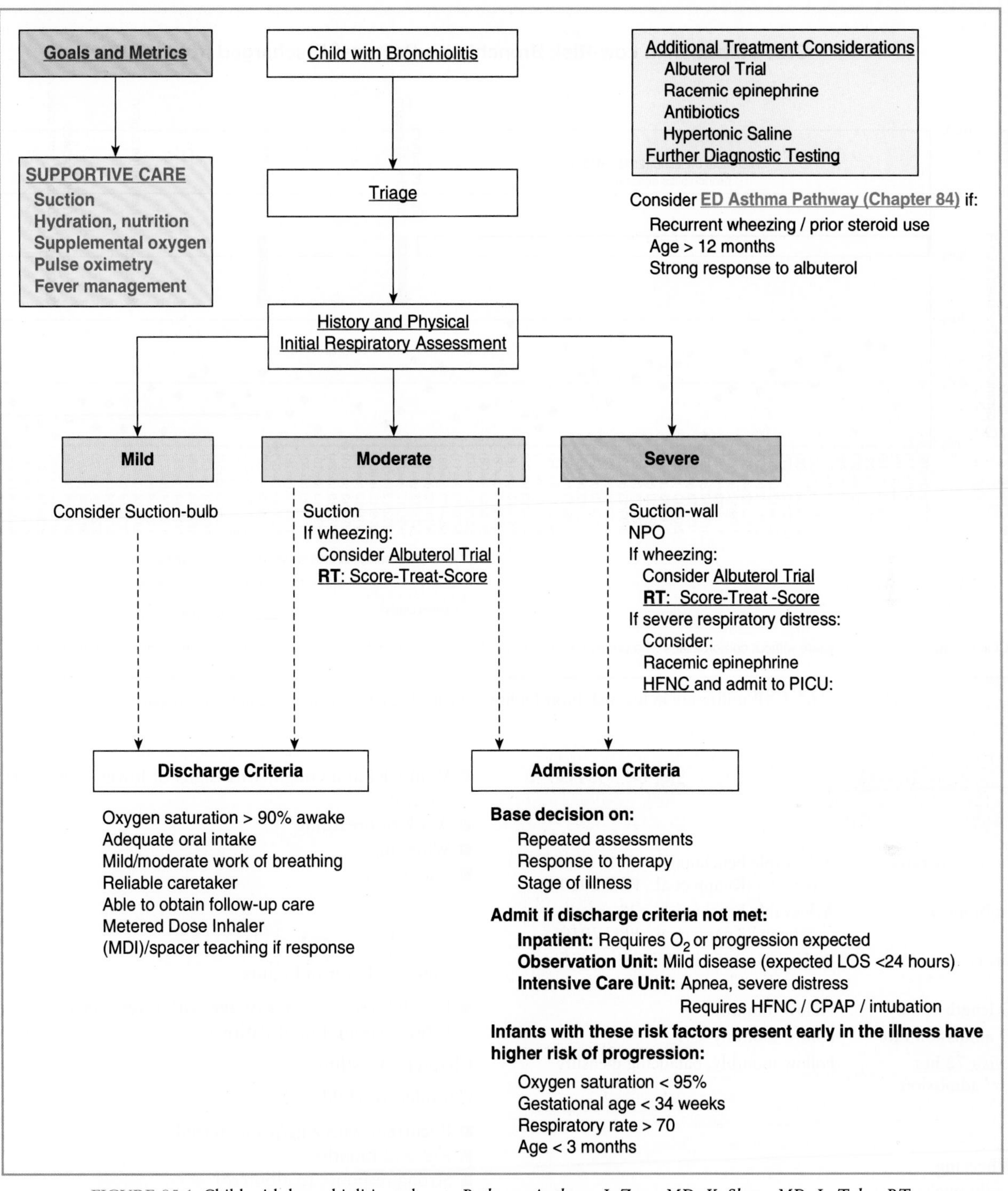

FIGURE 85.1 Child with bronchiolitis pathway. *Pathway Authors: J. Zorc, MD; K. Shaw, MD; L. Tyler, RT; B. Rodio, RN; S. Dooley, RN.*

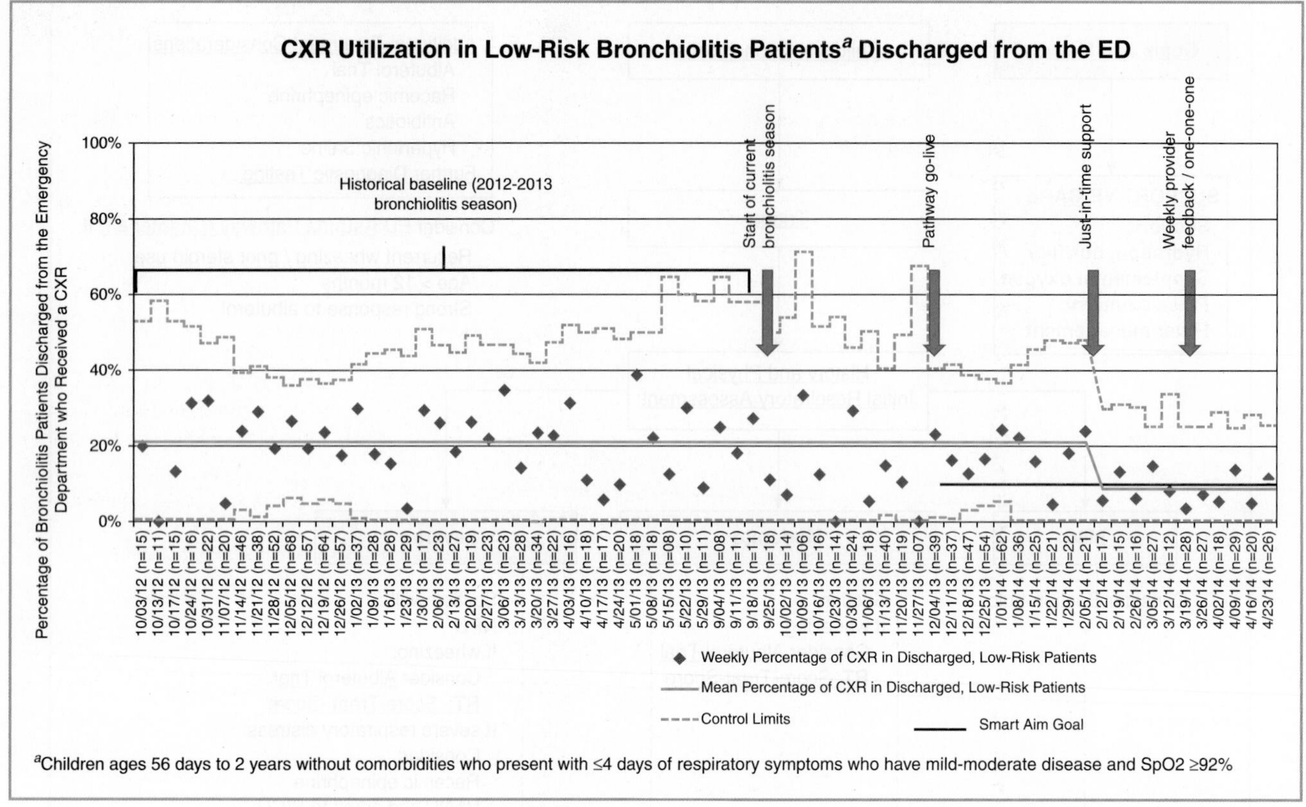

FIGURE 85.2 CXR utilization in low-risk bronchiolitis patients discharged from the emergency department.

TABLE 85.1

QUALITY MEASUREMENT

Chest x-ray rate	Achievable benchmark: <17% of all patients (Knapp et al., PEC 2010)
Antibiotic use	Achievable benchmark: <2% of all patients (Knapp et al., PEC 2010)
Corticosteroid use	Reduce to <10% in children with first episode of bronchiolitis
ED length of stay	Follow monthly
ED admission rate	Follow monthly
Revisit 72 hrs w/ admission	Follow monthly, balancing measure

- Wheezing
- Tachypnea
- See Figure 85.2 and Table 85.1

Next Steps

Use data to further define areas for process improvement. Consider using decision support in the electronic health record to further guide use of treatment and testing.

CHILD WITH BRONCHIOLITIS

This pathway should be used for healthy patients <2 years of age with the clinical presentation consistent with the diagnosis of bronchiolitis including:

- Viral URI and cough, with signs of lower respiratory tract infection
- Work of breathing
- Wheezing
- Tachypnea

Associated Pathways:

Chapter 87 Fever in Infants

- For children ≤56 days of age with fever ≥38°C, refer to the Febrile Young Infant Pathway

Chapter 84 Asthma

Consider for children if:

- Recurrent wheezing/prior steroid use
- Age >12 months
- Strong response to albuterol

Exclusion Criteria

- Known asthma
- Cardiac disease
- Airway defects
- Immunodeficiency
- Significant lung disease (on baseline meds or O_2)
- Complex, chronic medical condition

Initial Respiratory Assessment: Key Points

See Table 85.2 for additional information.

TABLE 85.2

INITIAL RESPIRATORY ASSESSMENT: KEY POINTS

Variability	The **physical exam findings vary** from minute to minute based on physiology and response to treatment as well as the child's position, level of alertness, and cooperation.
Physical examination	Assessment is ideally done with the **child upright, awake after suctioning the upper airway,** as nasal congestion may transmit to the lungs and simulate wheezing. A reliable assessment often **requires repeated examinations** over the course of the ED visit.
Progression of illness	Symptoms tend to **worsen over the first 3–5 days of illness** and then gradually resolve over the following weeks. Assessment of the stage of illness and potential progression is an important factor in the disposition decision.
Pulse oximetry	Hypoxemia is due to **ventilation–perfusion mismatch** from mucus plugging of the airways.
	Bronchodilator therapy can worsen this effect temporarily.
	Pulse oximetry is important, as mild hypoxemia may not be apparent on physical examination. However, changes can be transient, the decisions to initiate oxygen should be based on **repeated observation of pulse oximetry <90%** after routine measures such as positioning and suctioning.
	Mild hypoxemia (<95%) is a predictor of potential progression to severe disease requiring hospitalization, particularly if the child is in the early stages of the illness.
Apnea	Apnea is a concern in young and premature infants. Factors predicting very low risk of apnea include the following:
	Age >4 wks for full term or 48 wks postconception for preterm (<37 wks' gestation)
	Absence of prior history of apneic episode before presentation

Baseline Assessment and Pathway Status Determination

The highest rating in any category dictates the patient's current assessment. Key elements including respiratory rate, work of breathing, and mental status can be used to assess trend overtime. See Table 85.3.

TABLE 85.3

BASELINE ASSESSMENT

		Mild (0)	Moderate (1)	Severe (2)
RR	<3 mo	30–60	61–80	>80
	3–<12 mo	25–50	51–70	>70
	1–2 yrs	20–40	41–60	>60
WOB		None or mild	Intercostal retractions	Nasal flaring, grunting, head bobbing
Mental status		Baseline	Fussy or anxious	Lethargic or inconsolable
Oxygen requirement		None	<1.5 L	>1.5 L
Suctioning		Bulb	Wall/bulb	Wall
Breath sounds		Clear	Crackles, wheezing	Diminished breath sounds or significant crackles, wheezing
Cough		Absent or mild	Moderate	Severe

ALBUTEROL TRIAL/RT: SCORE-TREAT-SCORE

Pretreatment

- Suction nares per nursing standard
- Assess, document intervention score on bronchiolitis flow sheet
- Pulse oximetry
- Albuterol trial X1 treatment with nebulizer

Posttreatment

- Assess, document intervention score on bronchiolitis flow sheet
- See Table 85.4 for Albuterol Dosing
- Use the Respiratory Intervention Score (RIS) in Table 85.5 to assess children after each intervention.

CLINICAL PATHWAYS

TABLE 85.4

ALBUTEROL DOSING

Weight (kg)	Intermittent nebulization (0.5% solution [5 mg/mL])	MDI (90 µg/puff)
<5	1.25 mg (0.25 mL)	Per physician's discretion
≥5	2.5 mg (0.5 mL)	2–4 puffs

NOTE: Albuterol should NOT be continued if the patient does not respond to test dose.
If responsive to albuterol test dose, may continue:
MDI every 2–4 hrs
Intermittent nebulization every 2–6 hrs

TABLE 85.5

RESPIRATORY INTERVENTION SCORE (RIS)

		Mild (0)	Moderate (1)	Severe (2)
RR	<3 mo	30–60	61–80	>80
	3–<12 mo	25–50	51–70	>70
	1–2 yrs	20–40	41–60	>60
WOB		None or mild	Intercostal retractions	Nasal flaring, grunting, head bobbing
Mental status		Baseline	Fussy or anxious	Lethargic or inconsolable

Supportive Care

Supportive care is the primary treatment for infants with bronchiolitis (Table 85.6).

TABLE 85.6

SUPPORTIVE CARE FOR INFANTS WITH BRONCHIOLITIS

Suction	• Decreases work of breathing by clearing secretions • May improve feeding • Bulb suction is preferred, especially in infants with low intervention score • Wall suctioning is reserved for infants with respiratory distress requiring admission • Perform Respiratory Intervention Score before and after
Hydration nutrition	• Consider NG feeds if: Poor oral intake Moderate respiratory distress Choking with feeds • NPO and IVF if: Severe respiratory distress Concern for worsening of respiratory status
Monitoring respiratory status	• Use Respiratory Intervention Score (RIS) • Frequency depends on level of the pathway
Pulse oximetry	• Severe RIS Continuous pulse oximetry is indicated • Moderate RIS Intermittent pulse oximetry (continuous monitoring is not required) • Mild RIS Spot check pulse oximetry with regular assessments **Note:** Continuous monitoring has been correlated with longer hospital LOS
Supplemental O_2	• Consider if O_2 saturation is consistently: 90% while awake for >20 s after suction, position 88% while asleep for >20 s after suction, position • Brief desaturations (<20 s) less than 90% in a sleeping infant do not routinely require supplemental oxygen • Begin O_2 wean when saturations are >90%

ADDITIONAL TREATMENT CONSIDERATIONS

May be considered in infants with significant respiratory distress that is not alleviated sufficiently by supportive care interventions (Table 85.7).

TABLE 85.7

ADDITIONAL TREATMENT CONSIDERATIONS

Albuterol	Albuterol should **not** be continued if the patient does not respond to test dose. If responsive to albuterol test dose, may continue: MDI every 2–4 hrs Intermittent nebulization every 2–6 hrs
Racemic epinephrine	α- and β-adrenergic agonist ***Consider*** use in patients with increasing severe respiratory distress Requires MD order/bedside assessment for administration
High flow nasal cannula (HFNC)	Provides warmed, humidified air with adjustable oxygen concentration Reduces WOB Refer to high-frequency protocol
Antibiotics	Do **not** prescribe antibiotics without evidence of bacterial infection: Bacterial superinfections are uncommon in this age group. Prescribe antibiotics only when there is a specific secondary infection Associated pathways *Febrile UTI pathway, OM, PNA* *ED Febrile Infant Pathway*

FURTHER DIAGNOSTIC TESTING

See Table 85.8 for additional information.

TABLE 85.8

DIAGNOSTIC TESTING FOR CHILDREN WITH BRONCHIOLITIS

Chest x-ray	X-rays are **not** routinely recommended *Consider if:* • Clinical picture is not consistent with typical bronchiolitis • Clinical course suggests super infection • New fever late in the disease process • Severe disease/toxic appearance with a lack of upper respiratory symptoms
Viral RRP	Viral testing is not routinely recommended *Consider testing if:* • The diagnosis is in question • Prolonged fever • Local epidemiology indicates significant flu activity • When there is a high clinical suspicion of flu and ■ The child is being seen within the window when antivirals will be effective (for patients to be discharged) ■ The child is being admitted
Pertussis PCR	Pertussis testing is not routinely recommended *Consider if:* • History of apnea and prolonged cough • Known exposure • Unimmunized or only partially immunized • Significant pertussis activity in the community

Suggested Readings and Key References

Knapp JF, Hall M, Sharma V. Benchmarks for the emergency department care of children with asthma, bronchiolitis, and croup. *Pediatr Emerg Care* 2010;26:364–369.

Shay DK, Holman RC, Newman RD, et al. Bronchiolitis-associated hospitalizations among US children, 1980–1996. *JAMA* 1999; 282(15):1440–1446.

Subcommittee on Diagnosis and Management of Bronchiolitis. Clinical practice guideline: the diagnosis, management, and prevention of bronchiolitis. *Pediatrics* 2014;134(5):1474–1502. Available at: www.pediatrics.org/cgi/doi/10.1542/peds.2014-2742.

CHAPTER 86 ■ DEHYDRATION

MERCEDES M. BLACKSTONE, MD, PHILIP SPANDORFER, MD, MSCE, AND MARK D. JOFFE, MD

BACKGROUND (EPIDEMIOLOGY, EVIDENCE)

Acute gastroenteritis continues to be a leading cause of morbidity in both the developed and developing worlds, disproportionately affecting young children. Among children 1 to 5 years of age, diarrhea and dehydration is responsible for up to 10% of all hospitalizations and 3.7-million physician visits per year. Though the majority of these infections are viral, bacterial gastroenteritis and food-borne illnesses add to this enormous toll. Even for those not ill enough to require hospitalization, this affliction continues to be a tremendous burden on the healthcare system in terms of ED and clinic visits and on families in terms of days missed from work and school.

Research has shown that oral rehydration therapy (ORT) is a safe and effective way to rehydrate most children with dehydration secondary to gastroenteritis and it is advocated by the AAP and the CDC. In children with vomiting, a single oral dose of ondansetron given in the ED has been shown to decrease episodes of vomiting and increase the success of ORT, thereby reducing hospital admissions.

Patients who require intravenous hydration, either because they have severe dehydration or because they fail ORT, may benefit from obtaining some dextrose in their fluids in addition to normal saline. Dextrose-containing fluids help to reverse ketosis, which likely contributes to nausea and poor appetite. Studies suggest that patients who receive more dextrose in the ED reduce their ketone levels and may be less likely to require return visits with admission. As such, this pathway advocates a second bolus of 20 cc/kg of D_5NS given over an hour after the initial traditional NS bolus is given in the subset of patients with significant dehydration and ketosis (defined as having ketones on urinalysis or an anion gap >15).

PATHWAY GOALS AND MEASUREMENTS

Goals

The goals for this pathway include the following:

- Make ORT the standard of care for children with mild and moderate dehydration
- Timely administration of ondansetron in appropriate patients
- Safely and rapidly IV rehydrate children who fail ORT
- Educate families about how to keep children hydrated during an illness
- Rapidly administer dextrose-containing fluids in dehydrated, ketotic children to reverse ketosis
- Reduce unnecessary laboratory testing in mild to moderately dehydrated patients

Measurements

- Time to initiation of ORT, ondansetron
- Number of patients who fail ORT and require IVFs
- Admission rate—ORT versus IVF group, group who received antiemetic, group who received dextrose-containing IVFs
- Revisit rate/revisits with admission

Algorithm and Key Hyperlinks

- See Figure 86.1 (http://www.chop.edu/clinical-pathway/gastroenteritis-and-dehydration-clinical-pathway)
- http://www.healthychildren.org/English/health-issues/conditions/abdominal/Pages/Diarrhea.aspx
- http://www.cdc.gov/mmwr/preview/mmwrhtml/rr5216a1.htm

PATIENT POPULATION/ STRATIFYING PATIENT RISKS

This pathway is to be used for the treatment of children with gastroenteritis and associated dehydration. It is important to assess the child for surgical, neurologic, and metabolic conditions before using this treatment pathway. ORT may also be used for other causes of dehydration, for example, fever, pharyngitis, stomatitis, postoperative conditions. This pathway is not intended for children with significant underlying disease or for infants under 1 month of age.

Children who have vomiting or diarrhea but who are not dehydrated or have only mild dehydration, do not need to be rehydrated in the ED. These patients and families will benefit from education about use of ORT at home. Similarly, we encounter a great many children who are not drinking well for a variety of reasons but who do not have significant ongoing losses or an existing fluid deficit. Some of these children deserve a "po trial" in the ED but do not necessarily require true ORT, which refers to specific small volumes of specific rehydrating fluids.

Many dehydration scales have been proposed in order to help clinicians assess the degree of dehydration based on the

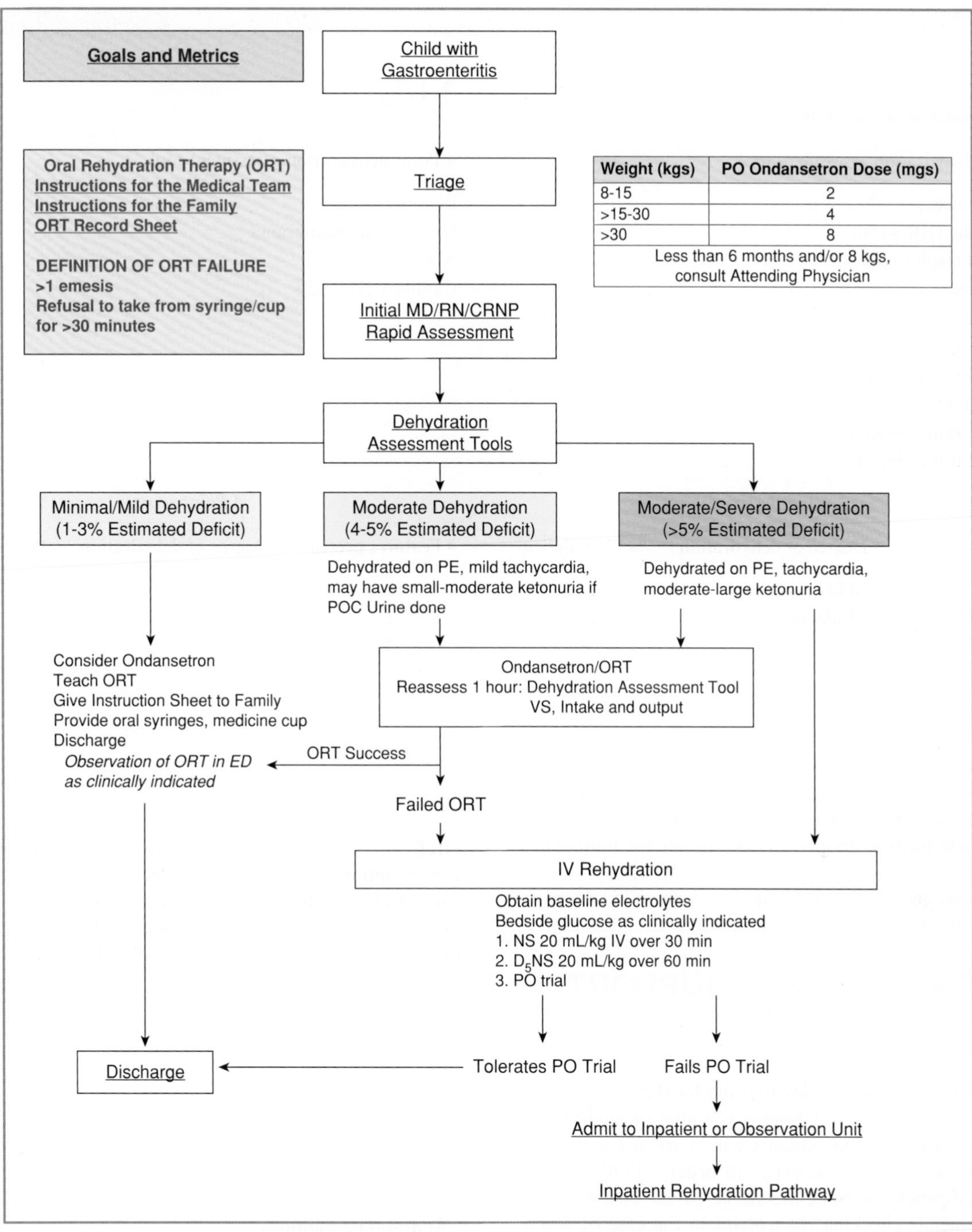

Weight (kgs)	PO Ondansetron Dose (mgs)
8-15	2
>15-30	4
>30	8
Less than 6 months and/or 8 kgs, consult Attending Physician	

FIGURE 86.1 Algorithm for the treatment of children with gastroenteritis and dehydration. *Pathway Authors: M. Joffe, MD; M. Blackstone, MD; J. Lavelle, MD; T. Crowley, RN; D. Hoser-Glatts, RN.*

CLINICAL PATHWAYS

TABLE 86.1

DEHYDRATION ASSESSMENT TOOLS

Dehydration assessment tools					
10 Point dehydration assessment tool			**4 Point dehydration assessment tool**		
Ill appearance Tachycardia (HR >150) Abnormal respirations Sunken eyes Absent tears Dry mucous membranes Abnormal radial pulse Capillary refill >2 s Decreased skin elasticity Decreased urine output			Ill appearance Dry mucous membranes Absent tears Capillary refill >2 s		
10 Point score			**4 Point score**		
# Features present	**Degree of dehydration**	**% Fluid deficit**	**# Features present**	**Degree of dehydration**	**% Fluid deficit**
<3	Mild	1–3	1	Mild	1–3
≥3 and <7	Moderate	4–6	2	Moderate	4–6
≥7	Severe	>6	3–4	Severe	>6

physical examination, but the most accurate method is to calculate the change in weight from baseline. In the ED setting, baseline weight is often unknown so we use the following assessment tools in an attempt to estimate the fluid deficit (Table 86.1).

See sections on "triage" and "rapid assessment" in the pathway for additional help distinguishing dehydration severity.

CLINICAL DECISION SUPPORT

Electronic Order Set

The electronic order set includes an order for the bedside nurse to initiate the pathway. No laboratory studies or medications are prechecked since many patients will be treated with ORT alone. There are options, however, to order a POC glucose, POC urine dipstick, or basic metabolic panel. This pathway only recommends checking electrolytes in the case of severe dehydration or failed ORT when an IV is being placed. A POC glucose should also be checked, however, in any patient who appears somnolent or lethargic. The electronic order set also includes commonly administered IVFs and rounded, weight-based doses of ondansetron. There is an option for an abdominal film for patients with isolated emesis where there is a concern for obstruction.

Other Electronic Tools

The pathway also provides links to the electronic tools shown here that can be printed out to make the ORT process go more smoothly. These include "Instructions for the Medical Team," "Instructions for the Family," and an "ORT Record Sheet." Hyperlinks are also provided in the pathway to assist in admission and discharge criteria.

ORT Instructions for the Medical Team

ORT works via the sodium glucose cotransport mechanism, which optimizes intestinal absorption of water. Utilizing the correct electrolyte solution is critical for its success. Adding juice to the solutions alters the sodium to glucose concentration and diminishes the efficacy of ORT (see Tables 86.2, 86.3, and 86.4).

TABLE 86.2

ORT SOLUTIONS

Appropriate solutions	
• Pedialyte	
• Gatorade ½ strength with saltine crackers in older patients	
Total volume to be given over 3–4 hrs	
Mild/moderate dehydration	50 mL/kg
Moderate/severe dehydration	100 mL/kg
Ongoing losses	
• 5–10 mL/kg for each diarrheal stool	
• 2 mL/kg for each emesis	
Aliquot volume to be given every 5 min	
Mild/moderate dehydration	1 mL/kg
Moderate/severe dehydration	2 mL/kg
Double the aliquot volume as tolerated after the first 30 min	
Maximum aliquot volume is 30 mL	

TABLE 86.3

ORAL REHYDRATION THERAPY INSTRUCTIONS FOR FAMILIES

Oral Rehydration Therapy (ORT) is a treatment we use for dehydrated patients.

- A small amount of liquid (1–2 mL/kg of the child's body weight) is administered every 5 min with a syringe or small cup over 3–4 hrs. If the ORT is going well, we may ask you to continue it at home after a couple of hours of observation in the ED. To treat your child today, we will start with _____ mL every 5 min.
- Pedialyte is the best fluid choice for young children. Older children may refuse this, so ½ strength Gatorade with saltine crackers is substituted. These fluids have the most favorable ratio of glucose and sodium, which helps the intestines to reabsorb water.
- Although your child may want more, it is important to give the fluid slowly. This allows the stomach to absorb the liquid and helps prevent vomiting. Please watch the clock and give only the recommended amount every 5 min.
- Your child may refuse the fluid initially, but with a few feeds it often gets much easier and the child begins to take the fluids.
- If your child vomits, let your nurse know. If it is only a small amount, we will continue ORT. If it is a large amount, we may need to stop and place an IV.
- If your child repeatedly refuses the feeds or is passing frequent, large-volume stools, we may need to place an IV.

TABLE 86.4

ORAL REHYDRATION RECORD SHEET

Patient Sticker:		**Preweight:______** **Postweight:______**	
Time	**Amount of fluid taken (mL)**	**Emesis (# times)**	**Diarrhea (# times)**

Communication/Teamwork

For this patient population, communication focuses on ensuring that we have the correct patient cohort and early recognition of dehydration with prompt initiation of therapy. The majority of patients require only ORT, often with the addition of ondansetron. Severely dehydrated patients or those with altered mental status need an immediate dextrose checked and placement of an IV. In both cases, our nurses can initiate this therapy after a brief discussion with a front line provider and an order to initiate the pathway. Once patients are on the pathway, we rely on good communication from our nursing colleagues in terms of how the rehydration is progressing and whether we need to consider additional therapies or steps toward disposition. Good communication with families is also essential. We provide them with education on ORT to empower them both in the ED and at home.

Nurse-specific Education

Nursing-specific education has focused on physical examination findings in dehydration, normal ranges for pediatric vital signs, and importance of ORT for mild and moderate dehydration. Nurses are taught how to initiate ORT and how to educate families about it. They monitor intake and output for these patients. They are knowledgeable about the natural course of infectious diseases leading to dehydration so that they can counsel patients effectively at discharge about how to advance diet and when to return to the ED. Nurses provide syringes and medicine cups for families so they can easily continue ORT at home.

Quality Measurement

Although we have only limited quality improvement data from our own institution, randomized trials have demonstrated that ORT is as effective as IV fluids for moderately dehydrated patients with gastroenteritis in the ED. They have also shown that a single dose of ondansetron administered in the ED can reduce ED length of stay, episodes of emesis, and need for IVFs and immediate hospital admission. More recently, however, a large multicenter study showed that despite a considerable increase in ondansetron usage, use of IVFs and hospitalization rates did not improve. This is likely due to a failure of knowledge translation since ondansetron is likely not being given to the right patients at the right time. This highlights the need for pathways such as this one to be applied to the appropriate patient population and for interventions to be carefully considered and optimally timed.

Next Steps

Potential next steps would include careful tracking of clinical time points to ensure that ORT (and ondansetron when appropriate) is being promptly initiated and looking at how many patients are converted to IVFs. Admission rates and return visits with admission before and after the recent implementation of dextrose-containing IVFs in the resuscitation phase should be studied.

Suggested Readings and Key References

Colletti JE, Brown KM, Sharieff GQ, et al.; ACEP Pediatric Emergency Medicine Committee. The management of children with gastroenteritis and dehydration in the pediatric emergency department. *J Emerg Med* 2010;38(5):686–698.

Fedorowicz Z, Jagannath VA, Carter B. Antiemetics for reducing vomiting related to acute gastroenteritis in children and adolescents. *Cochrane Database Syst Rev* 2011;(9):CD005506.

Freedman SB, Adler M, Seshadri R, et al. Oral ondansetron for gastroenteritis in a pediatric emergency department. *N Engl J Med* 2006; 354(16):1698–1705.

Freedman SB, Hall M, Shah SS, et al. Impact of increasing ondansetron use on clinical outcomes in children with gastroenteritis. *JAMA Pediatr* 2014;168(4):321–329.

Gorelick MH, Shaw KN, Murphy KO. Validity and reliability of clinical signs in the diagnosis of dehydration in children. *Pediatrics* 1997; 99(5):E6.

Hartling L, Bellemare S, Wiebe N, et al. Oral versus intravenous rehydration for treating dehydration due to gastroenteritis in children. *Cochrane Database Syst Rev* 2006;(3):CD004390.

Keren R. Ondansetron for acute gastroenteritis: a failure of knowledge translation. *JAMA Pediatr* 2014;168(4):308–309.

Levy JA, Bachur RG. Intravenous dextrose during outpatient rehydration in pediatric gastroenteritis. *Acad Emerg Med* 2007;14(4): 324–330.

Roslund G, Hepps TS, McQuillen KK. The role of oral ondansetron in children with vomiting as a result of acute gastritis/gastroenteritis who have failed oral rehydration therapy: a randomized controlled trial. *Ann Emerg Med* 2008;52(1):22–29.

Spandorfer PR, Alessandrini EA, Joffe MD, et al. Oral versus intravenous rehydration of moderately dehydrated children: a randomized, controlled trial. *Pediatrics* 2005;115(2):295–301.

CHAPTER 87 ■ FEVER IN INFANTS

RICHARD J. SCARFONE, MD, PAYAL K. GALA, MD, AND MARY KATE FUNARI, MSN, RN, CPEN

BACKGROUND (EPIDEMIOLOGY, EVIDENCE)

Febrile young infants (FYIs) are at higher risk for serious bacterial infection (SBI) compared to older children. Published data indicate that 8% to 12% of FYIs have an SBI, most commonly pyelonephritis. To provide high-value care, clinicians who are evaluating FYIs in the ED must be appropriately vigilant in assessing for SBI while trying to minimize the inherent risks of overtesting and overtreating including obtaining false-positive cultures, unnecessary hospitalizations, increased costs, increased lengths of stay in the ED, and parental anxiety.

To date, there is not a universally accepted evaluation and treatment strategy for this population. Rather, most clinicians follow hospital-specific guidelines that vary widely among medical institutions. For example, there is variation in practice for several fundamental clinical decision points including the age below which a lumber puncture (LP) should be performed routinely, the clinical scenarios in which herpes simplex virus (HSV) screening and/or empiric therapy should be initiated, and whether or not an LP is necessary for FYI with pyuria. A review of the literature helps to provide guidance and serves as the basis for the recommendations here. Huppler et al. published a 25-year review of 22 studies assessing the performance of low-risk criteria for SBI among this cohort. Just two neonates <4 weeks old had bacterial meningitis. None of 29- to 56-day old infants who otherwise met low-risk criteria had bacterial meningitis suggesting that an LP may be safely omitted in this setting. On the other hand, about one-third of neonates with HSV infection do not have skin vesicles and in a significant proportion of cases, their mothers have asymptomatic herpes infections at delivery. Thus, maternal history and physical examination of the neonate alone may miss the diagnosis; this supports a conservative approach for HSV screening among those likely to be at highest risk. Schnadower et al. reported that among 1,895 infants 29 to 60 days old with fever and pyelonephritis, 5 had concomitant bacterial meningitis. This rate, while low, is higher than that reported for FYI without pyelonephritis leaving individual clinicians to determine the utility of routinely performing an LP among FYI found to have pyuria. For questions such as the ones raised here, instituting a clinical pathway based on supporting evidence in the literature can help standardize care for this population of patients.

PATHWAY GOALS AND MEASUREMENTS

Goals

The goals for this pathway are as follows:

- Standardize the care of FYI who do not have clearly identifiable sources of illness
- Streamline the ED evaluation of FYI
  - Obtain all necessary studies to evaluate for possible SBI
  - Omit unnecessary testing that is not likely to yield a diagnosis
  - Define appropriate candidates for HSV screening and the appropriate screening tests
  - Define when it is cost-effective to perform enteroviral testing of cerebrospinal fluid (CSF)
- Improve timeliness of key points of care of FYI including times from ED arrival to:
  - MD evaluation
  - Urinary catheterization to screen for UTI
  - Peripheral intravenous (PIV) line placement and serologic tests
  - LP (if indicated)
  - Chest radiograph (if indicated)
  - Antibiotics (if indicated)
- Standardize order sets for laboratory studies to assist front-line clinicians, including RNs in initiating timely workups
- Reexamine the practice of routinely performing an LP in all febrile infants 29 to 56 days old; for those who meet low-risk criteria, assess utility of LP

Measurement

- Time from ED arrival to MD evaluation, urinary catheterization, PIV placement, serologic testing, LP, appropriate antibiotics
- Use of acyclovir empirically among FYI at risk for HSV infection
- Use of order set for laboratory studies and antibiotics
- Proportion of patients with SBI
- Admission rates
- ED length of stay
- Proportion of FYI 29 to 56 days old who have LP performed
- Low-risk infants 29 to 56 days old who are discharged home:
  - Rates of successful phone follow-up after ED discharge
  - Outcomes at time of follow-up
  - ED revisit rates within 72 hrs
  - Outcomes at time of revisit
- Negative predictive value of low-risk criteria for excluding bacterial meningitis among 29- to 56-day-old cohort
- Proportion of patients who are high risk and are ultimately diagnosed with bacterial meningitis
- Cost analysis
  - Costs of laboratory testing and procedures

Algorithm and Key Hyperlinks

- See Figure 87.1 (http://www.chop.edu/clinical-pathway/febrile-young-infants-0–56-days-old-clinical-pathway)

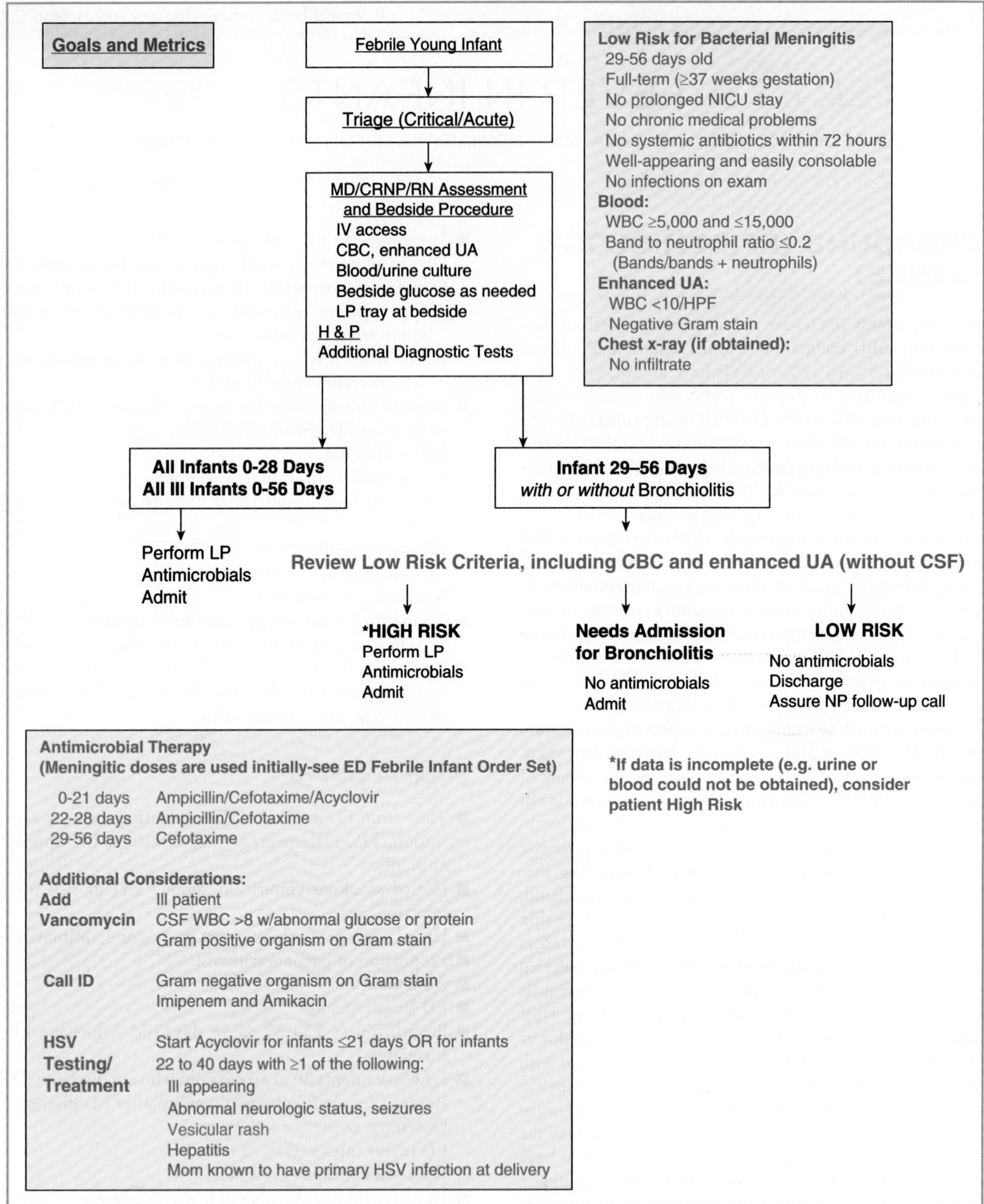

FIGURE 87.1 Algorithm for the evaluation and treatment of febrile young infants (0 to 56 days). *Pathway Authors: R. Scarfone, MD; P. Gala, MD; A. Murray, MD; MK Funari, RN; J. Lavelle, MD; L. Bell, MD.*

TABLE 87.1

RISK OF BACTERIAL MENINGITIS

Low-risk bacterial meningitis	**History and physical examination:** 29–56 days old Full-term (≥37 wks' gestation) No prolonged NICU stay No chronic medical problems No systemic antibiotics within 72 hrs prior to arrival Well appearing and easily consolable No infections on examination **Blood:** Peripheral WBC ≥5,000 and ≤15,000 Band to neutrophil ratio <0.2 (bands/bands + neutrophils) **Enhanced urinalysis:** WBC <10/HPF Negative Gram stain **Chest x-ray (if obtained):** No infiltrate
High-risk bacterial meningitis	**Does not meet low-risk criteria including:** Ill appearing Abnormal mental status Abnormal perfusion Hypothermia Specific bacterial infection diagnosed on examination (omphalitis, mastitis, cellulitis, etc.)

PATIENT POPULATION/ STRATIFYING PATIENT RISK

Patient Population

All FYIs 0 to 56 days old should be treated based on pathway criteria and recommendations.

Stratifying Patient Risk

- Febrile neonates <29 days old are at high risk for SBI. It is difficult to accurately judge a neonate's degree of illness and bacterial infections more easily spread from the initial focus of infection in this population. As such, it is recommended that every FYI <29 days old have a complete evaluation for SBI including blood, urine, and CSF cultures, be treated empirically with broad-spectrum antibiotics, and be hospitalized while awaiting culture results.
- If the FYI is 29 to 56 days old, utilize clinical and laboratory criteria to stratify patients into low- and high-risk categories for SBI:
  - A CBC and blood culture is recommended
  - Urine should be obtained by catheterization and sent for enhanced urinalysis (UA) and culture
  - Chest radiographs should be obtained only for those with signs or symptoms of respiratory illness
  - An LP may be omitted in low-risk infants with normal CBC and UA
  - An LP should be performed for any infant who fails to meet *all* low-risk criteria
  - CSF results are *not* used to stratify risk
- An infant's risk for HSV must be assessed. HSV risk factors include the following:
  - <21 days old
  - Ill appearance
  - Abnormal neurologic status or seizure
  - Vesicular rash
  - Hepatitis
  - Mom known to have primary HSV disease
- A conservative approach would be to evaluate for HSV infection in any infant with any one of these risk factors. A less conservative approach would be to not routinely evaluate all those <21 days old, if no other risk factors are present.
- Blood and CSF should both be obtained for HSV PCR testing.
- If skin vesicles are present, they should be unroofed and the fluid sent for HSV PCR testing. See Table 87.1.

CLINICAL DECISION SUPPORT

The electronic order set includes an order for the bedside nurse to initiate the pathway. Laboratory studies recommended for all patients are preselected to assist the clinician. There are additional recommendations for laboratory studies as indicated for specific populations; for example, enterovirus testing for summer months, HSV testing for neonates less than 21 days old. There are also standard recommendations for antibiotic therapy categorized by each age group as seen in the pathway algorithm.

Communication/Teamwork

Prompt care of the FYI is dependent on strong communication amongst all members of the ED and inpatient care team, as well as the patient's family. The communication plan aims at early identification of the FYI that meets pathway initiation criteria and subsequent timely workup and disposition. Triage and bedside nurses should immediately notify ordering clinicians of a FYI's presenting history and physical examination for appropriate order set placement. Since the medical care of the FYI involves multiple invasive procedures in rapid succession, family education is paramount to help alleviate anxiety during this potentially stressful time. Throughout the ED visit, the status of procedures, laboratory results, and changes in severity of illness should be conveyed to all members of the team to ensure consistency and timeliness of care. Should a FYI be discharged from the ED, detailed follow-up practices for both families and outpatient providers must be in place for continued patient safety.

Nurse-Specific Education

ED nursing staff must receive pathway-specific education to ensure safe, consistent, and quality team care. Education should include initiation criteria, risk for infection, family education, timing of procedures and antibiotics, and anticipatory guidance for worsening severity of illness. Basics of neonatal care including thermoregulation and glucose needs should also be reviewed as the FYI may have periods of prolonged exposure during examinations and procedures and may also have decreased feeding during their illness. The ED RN should adhere to existing hospital policies concerning straight catheterization, IV placement, laboratory draws, and medication administration.

Upon identifying a FYI, the nurse should collaborate with providers for appropriate order placement. Care for the unstable infant should be tailored to the patient's immediate needs. To facilitate timely interventions, the nurse and/or physician provider should educate the family on the overall plan for their ED stay. Since the FYI is a high-risk patient, each should be placed on a centralized continuous monitor per facility guidelines. For stable patients, procedural priority should be given to obtaining urine and blood specimens. It is encouraged that urine specimens are obtained prior to IV placement/laboratory testing since FYIs often void when upset. It is often challenging to obtain IV access in ill, dehydrated FYI; placement of hot packs or use of transillumination devices or bedside ultrasound may assist in successful IV placement. ED nursing and technician staff should receive hands on training on appropriate methods for holding and supporting the infant during an LP. Safety considerations include vital signs monitoring since bradycardia, desaturation and apnea may occur. The LP should be deferred in any infant who is compromised in this manner during the procedure. Nursing should be reminded to hold antibiotics/antivirals until all cultures are obtained, unless instructed otherwise by the treating physician. For patients who can be discharged, nurses should provide appropriate anticipatory guidance for care and follow-up, as well as emphasize the importance of frequent hand washing.

Next Steps

The medical care of the FYI has evolved over time, reflecting the publication of studies attempting to answer key patient management questions. Clinicians must continue to monitor the publication of additional data that will fine-tune decision making in the future. Similarly, in recent decades there has been a shift in the pathogens likely to cause SBI among young infants. There has been a notable decline in the incidence of Group B streptococcal disease; gram-negative organisms are now the most common SBI encountered by these patients. Thus, clinicians must also monitor shifting patterns of etiology in order to make proper judgments regarding presumptive antibiotic use.

Suggested Readings and Key References

Baker MD, Bell LM. Unpredictability of serious bacterial illness in febrile infants from birth to 1 month of age. *Arch Pediatr Adolesc Med* 1999;153:508–511.

Baker MD, Bell LM, Avner JR. Outpatient management without antibiotics of fever in selected infants. *New Engl J Med* 1993;329: 1437–1441.

Baker CJ, Byington CL, Polin RA; Committee on Infectious Diseases, Committee on Fetus and Newborn. Policy statement- Recommendations for the prevention of perinatal group B streptococcal disease. *Pediatrics* 2011;128:611–616.

Baskin MN, O'Rourke EJ, Fleischer GR. Outpatient treatment of febrile infants 28 to 89 with intramuscular administration of ceftriaxone. *J Pediatr* 1992;120:22–27.

Bramson RT, Meyer TL, Silbiger ML, et al. The futility of the chest radiography in the febrile infant without respiratory symptoms. *Pediatrics* 1993;92(4):524–526.

Byington CL, Kendrick J, Sheng X. Normative cerebrospinal fluid profiles in febrile infants. *J Pediatr* 2011;158:130–134.

Byington CL, Reynolds CC, Korgenski K, et al. Costs and infant outcomes after implementation of a care process model for febrile infants. *Pediatrics* 2012;130:e16–e24.

Greenhow TL, Hung YY, Herz AM. Changing epidemiology of bacteremia in infants aged 1 week to 3 months. *Pediatrics* 2012;129: e590.

Huppler AR, Eickhoff JC, Wald ER. Performance of low-risk criteria in the evaluation of young infants with fever: review of the literature. *Pediatrics* 2010;125:228–233.

Kimberlin DW. When should you initiate acyclovir therapy in a neonate? *J Pediatr* 2008;153:155–156.

Kimberlin DW, Baley J; Committee on infectious diseases, Committee on fetus and newborn. Guidance on management of asymptomatic neonates born to women with active genital herpes lesions. *Pediatrics* 2013;131:e635–e646.

Pantell RH, Newman TB, Bernzweig J, et al. Management and outcomes of care of fever in early infancy. *JAMA* 2004;291:1203–1212.

Ralston S, Hill V, Waters A. Occult serious bacterial infection in infants younger than 60 to 90 days with bronchiolitis. *Arch Pediatr Adolesc Med* 2011;165:951–956.

Schnadower D, Kuppermann N, Macias CG. Febrile infants with urinary tract infections at very low risk for adverse events and bacteremia. *Pediatrics* 2010;126:1074–1083.

Shah SS, Volk J, Mohamad Z, et al. Herpes simplex virus testing and hospital length of stay in neonates and young infants. *J Pediatr* 2010;156:738–743.

Zorc JJ, Levine DA, Platt SL, et al. Clinical and demographic factors associated with urinary tract infection in young febrile infants. *Pediatrics* 2005;116:644–648.

CHAPTER 88 ■ FEVER IN CHILDREN

KERI A. COHN, MD, MPH, DTM&H, FRAN BALAMUTH, MD, PhD, MSCE, RONALD F. MARCHESE, MD, PhD, ELIZABETH R. ALPERN, MD, MSCE, AND FRED M. HENRETIG, MD

BACKGROUND (EPIDEMIOLOGY, EVIDENCE)

Fever is among the most common causes for parents to seek care for their children in an emergency department. The importance of fever lies in its role as a physiologic expression of disease. The care of a febrile child focuses on discovering the cause of the fever and treating the underlying illness. Height and duration of fever, associated signs and symptoms, exposures, and host factors are all essential clues to the proper evaluation of the febrile patient. The changing epidemiology of infectious agents, especially in an era of new vaccines and antibiotic resistance, complicates the approach to medical evaluation and treatment. Combining expert consensus and evidence-based medicine in an algorithmic approach may prevent unnecessary medical testing and antibiotic treatment, while identifying those patients who warrant further evaluation. Time spent on educating parents about supportive care during an acute febrile viral illness may minimize return visits and assuage concern, while providing clear indications for when to seek care for further evaluation. Additionally, patients at higher risk for severe infections or conditions can be identified promptly, and their management aggressively pursued in order to optimize patient care and outcome.

PATHWAY GOALS AND MEASUREMENTS

Goals

- Identify patients with fever who are at increased risk for infection requiring antimicrobials or supportive medical intervention.
- Early identification, evaluation, and management of patients with high-risk factors or severe signs and symptoms of disease.
- Adequate review of discharge instructions with patients and families including indications for return to medical care and review of supportive care including hydration and antipyretics.

Measurements

- Appropriate antibiotic choice and use
- Decrease in ancillary testing for patients with viral acute respiratory tract infection
- Time to antibiotics, appropriateness of antibiotic choice in high-risk patients
- Increased documented use of appropriate discharge instructions to families including indications for return to medical care, and review of supportive care including hydration and antipyretics

Algorithm and Key Hyperlinks

See Figure 88.1.

ALGORITHM AND RELATED CHAPTERS

Signs and Symptoms
- Dehydration: Chapter 17
- Fever: Chapter 26
- Lymphadenopathy: Chapter 42
- Neck Stiffness: Chapter 44
- Oral Lesions: Chapter 47
- Pain: Earache: Chapter 53
- Rash: Bacterial and Fungal Infections: Chapter 61
- Rash: Vesiculobullous: Chapter 62
- Rash: Papulosquamous Eruptions: Chapter 65
- Respiratory Distress: Chapter 66
- Septic Appearing Infant: Chapter 68
- Sore Throat: Chapter 69
- Stridor: Chapter 70
- Tachycardia: Chapter 72
- Triage: Chapter 73

Clinical Pathways
- Pneumonia, Community-Acquired: Chapter 90
- UTI, Febrile: Chapter 92
- Bronchiolitis: Chapter 85
- Fever in Infants: Chapter 87
- Shock: Chapter 91

Medical Emergencies
- Dermatologic Urgencies and Emergencies: Chapter 96
- Infectious Disease Emergencies: Chapter 102
- Pulmonary Emergencies: Chapter 107
- Rheumatologic Emergencies: Chapter 109

Surgical Emergencies
- Abdominal Emergencies: Chapter 124
- Dental Emergencies: Chapter 125
- ENT Emergencies: Chapter 126

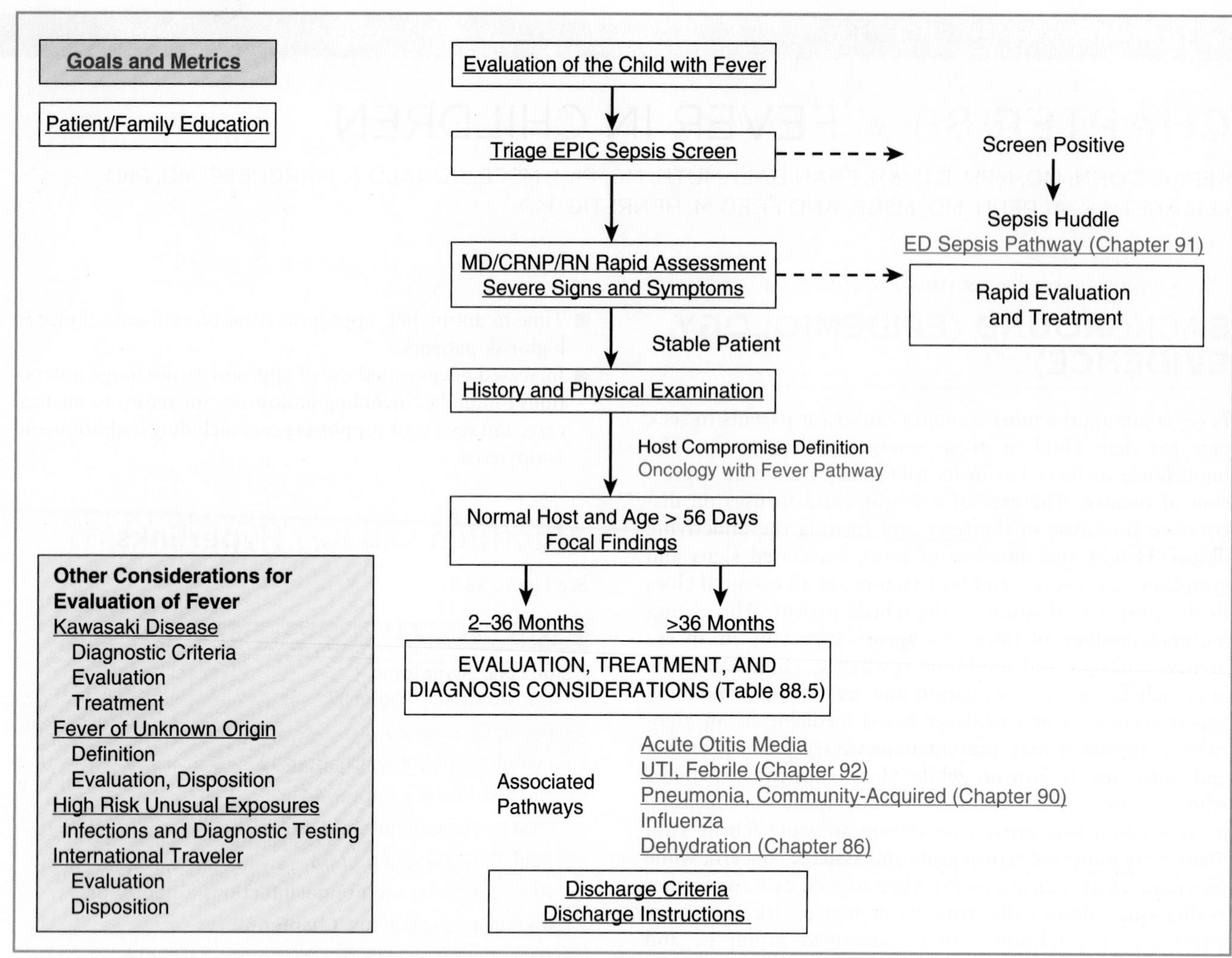

FIGURE 88.1 Pathway for the evaluation of the child with fever.

PATIENT POPULATION/ STRATIFYING PATIENT RISKS

For more information please see *Tables 88.1 through 88.6.*

TABLE 88.1

DEFINITION OF FEVER

Fever defined for specific age groups or children with particular risk factors	
Infants ≤56 days of age	≥38.0°C (100.4°F)
Children >56 days of age	≥38.5°C (101.3°F)
Patients with underlying immunocompromised state	≥38.5°C once ≥38.0°C three times within 24-hr period (1 hr apart)
Fever of unknown origin	≥38.3°C (101°F) in patients with fever >8 days
Rectal	Most closely approximates core body temperature Use this route in infants ≤56 days of age
Oral	Acceptable for school-age children with appropriate developmental abilities
Temporal artery	May underestimate high temperatures, overestimate low ones

Temperature should be taken in child in resting state, unbundled from heavy outer clothing or blankets.
History of tactile temperatures without measured fever in ED may prompt repeated reassessment depending on underlying patient risk factors.

TABLE 88.2

SEVERE SIGNS AND SYMPTOMS OF LIFE-THREATENING INFECTIONS

Prior to performing a full history and examination, it is important to consider and identify signs and symptoms of life-threatening infections.	
Meningitis/encephalitis	Altered sensorium, convulsion, meningismus, or focal neurologic deficits *Of note, <1 yr with meningitis often do not have meningismus, but they may instead have irritability, anorexia, lethargy, vomiting, or bulging fontanel
Epiglottitis, severe croup, retropharyngeal abscess	Stridor, excessive drooling, and tripod positioning
Severe pneumonia, myocarditis or sepsis syndrome	Dyspnea and/or tachypnea, cyanosis or pallor, tachycardia, and hypotension, +/– altered mental status
Meningococcemia, Rocky Mountain spotted fever, other sepsis syndrome (or toxic shock syndrome)	Hemorrhagic rash (or erythroderma), especially with toxic appearance, poor perfusion
Necrotizing fasciitis	Severe muscle tenderness, overlying skin changes, poor perfusion
Rapid response considerations	If severe signs or symptoms are present: Provide emergent stabilization of airway, breathing, and circulation Anticipate need for airway subspecialist or operating room airway placement Rapid initiation of IV access and fluids, laboratory studies, radiographic testing, and empiric antibiotics Seizure control as indicated Surgical subspecialty consultation as required by condition Consider infectious disease consultation for specific antimicrobial recommendations Consider appropriate dosing of antimicrobials to allow for crossing blood–brain barrier for patients at risk for meningitis

TABLE 88.3

HISTORY AND PHYSICAL EXAMINATION

History		
General history of present illness	Onset, duration, method of temperature taking, height of fever and diurnal variations	
	Associated signs and symptoms	
	Medications (including antipyretics and antibiotics)	
	Presence of ill contacts, travel history, and pet or insect exposures	
	Prior evaluation and treatments during this illness	
Past medical history	Recurrent febrile illnesses	
	Presence of any diseases or drug regimens that would compromise normal host defenses	
	Sickle cell anemia	
	Asplenia (functional, congenital, or surgical)	
	Malignancy (noting particularly chemotherapeutic or radiation treatments)	
	Human immunodeficiency virus (HIV)	
	Renal disease	
	Prolonged steroid or other immune-modulating agent use	
	Indwelling catheters or other internal foreign material	
	Immunization status	
Physical examination		**Diagnosis to consider**
General	Alertness, responsiveness	
	Work of breathing, color, feeding activity	
	Gross motor functions	
	Presence of "paradoxical irritability"	
HEENT	Eyelid swelling, erythema, tenderness	*Periorbital, orbital cellulitis*
	Conjunctival erythema, discharge +/– rhinorrhea, nasal mucosal inflammation (i.e., +/– URI)	*Conjunctivitis, viral syndrome*
	Tympanic membrane redness, bulging, decreased mobility, loss of landmarks and light reflex, air–fluid level behind, or purulent drainage from a perforation	*Otitis media*
	Rhinorrhea, nasal mucosal inflammation	*Viral upper respiratory infection (URI)*
	URI symptoms persisting ≥10 days or severe onset of fever >39°C and purulent nasal discharge for at least 3 consecutive days	*Acute bacterial sinusitis*
	Barky cough, +/– URI findings, stridor as illness progresses	*Croup*
	Oropharyngeal erythema, exudate, tonsillar hypertrophy, peritonsillar swelling	*Acute pharyngitis (viral or streptococcal), tonsillitis, peritonsillar abscess*
	Oral ulcers, gingival inflammation	*Stomatitis*
	Dental caries, tenderness, gingival inflammation	*Tooth abscess*
	Parotid swelling, tenderness	*Parotitis*
Neck	Tender swollen cervical lymph nodes	*Adenitis*
	Cervical spinous process tenderness	*Osteomyelitis, discitis*
	Meningismus	*Meningitis*
Chest	Wheezing, tachypnea, and fever in infants	*Bronchiolitis*
	Tachypnea, fever, nasal flaring, retractions; rales	*Pneumonia*
	Evidence of consolidation or pleural effusion	
	Wheezing, tachypnea, disproportionate tachycardia, +/– mild hypotension, or other signs of poor perfusion	*Myocarditis*
	(+/– abnormal CXR and electrocardiogram)	

TABLE 88.3

HISTORY AND PHYSICAL EXAMINATION (*CONTINUED*)

Abdomen	Pain or tenderness Vomiting, and/or diarrhea	*Viral gastroenteritis, early hepatitis, or pancreatitis*
	Pain, tenderness (severe, particularly predominant right lower quadrant tenderness and peritoneal signs)	*Appendicitis peritonitis/ intra-abdominal abscess from other sources*
	In children, fever with abdominal pain may also represent	*Lower lobe pneumonia, streptococcal pharyngitis, or urinary tract infection (UTI)*
	Suprapubic or costovertebral angle tenderness (however, young children may manifest only fever)	*UTI*
	Adolescent girls with pelvic or abdominal pain and fever	*Pelvic inflammatory disease, UTI*
Musculoskeletal	Joint swelling, effusion, tenderness, limited range of motion	*Septic arthritis, Lyme disease*
	Bony tenderness, abnormal posture, or limp	*Osteomyelitis, discitis, etc.*
	Severe muscle tenderness, poor perfusion	*Myositis, pyomyositis, compensated shock*
Neurologic	Bulging fontanel (infants) and altered sensorium, convulsion, meningismus, or focal neurologic deficits (older children)	*Meningitis, encephalitis*
Skin	Characteristic febrile exanthems	*Varicella, rubeola, scarlet fever, and Coxsackievirus*
	Fever and petechiae Petechiae only above the nipple line, normal white blood cell (WBC) count and coagulation studies, and well appearance make invasive disease less likely Ill appearance, laboratory abnormality, or progressive petechial rash requires full evaluation, empiric antibiotics	*Meningococcemia, other bacteremic disease, Rocky Mountain spotted fever, viral infection or streptococcal pharyngitis*
	Diffuse erythroderma, especially with multiorgan dysfunction and/or hemodynamic instability	Toxic shock syndrome, other toxin-mediated illness

TABLE 88.4

HOST COMPROMISE

Definition	Patients ≤56 days of age Recent surgery Presence of internal foreign material (surgical instrumentation/patches; central lines, shunts) Primary immunodeficiency Secondary (acquired immunodeficiency) • HIV/AIDS • Long-term corticosteroids (daily or alternate day corticosteroids for ≥14 days) • Neutropenia (from underlying malignancy, chemotherapy, effects of other drugs) • Malignant neoplasm • Stem cell or solid organ transplantation • Asplenia or functional asplenia (e.g., sickle cell disease) • Chronic renal disease • Receiving immune system altering medications including chemotherapy, anti metabolic, biologic immune modulation, or radiation therapy (high-risk patients would include oncologic, rheumatologic, IBD patients) • Children who have a disease (e.g., systemic lupus erythematosus) that, in itself, is considered to suppress the immune response

TABLE 88.5

EVALUATION, TREATMENT, AND DIAGNOSIS CONSIDERATIONS

2–36 mo	Consider UTI (*see UTI Pathway chapter*) Consider obtaining a blood culture and CBC in unimmunized or not fully immunized patient Consider pneumonia if >3–4 days of fever in setting of respiratory symptoms, hypoxia, tachypnea If ≥1 yr of age, may consider acute bacterial sinusitis if fever ≥39°C for at least 3 days and purulent nasal discharge Consider diagnosis of Kawasaki disease if fever ≥5 days (including fever alone if <6 mo) Fever of unknown origin if >8 days of fever without a source Influenza or other seasonal or locally endemic infection to consider
>36 mo	Consider acute bacterial sinusitis if fever ≥39°C for at least 3 days and purulent nasal discharge Consider *Kawasaki disease* if fever ≥5 days Consider sinusitis if persistent and not improving nasal discharge ≥10 days Fever of unknown origin if ≥8 days of fever without a source Influenza or other seasonal or locally endemic infection to consider

TABLE 88.6

ED PLAN, DISCHARGE CRITERIA, DISCHARGE INSTRUCTIONS

ED plan	Consider the following during the ED visit prior to discharge: Period of observation PO challenge Antipyretic medications Repeat vital signs Consider evaluation for viral myocarditis for persistent tachycardia after resolution of fever and dehydration
Discharge criteria	Nontoxic appearing Normal vital signs (resolution of fever not necessary for discharge) Tolerating PO and able to keep up with losses Parental understanding of follow-up instructions and reasons to return to the ED Access to good outpatient follow-up
Discharge instructions	**Take the time to review discharge instructions with family, including:** Likely etiology of fever Minimize "fever phobia" Emphasize monitoring for signs and symptoms of serious disease Emphasize need for increased oral hydration Emphasize need for comfort in setting of febrile illness: • Keep child lightly dressed to avoid environmental elevation in temperature • Goal of antipyretics—comfort, *not for* normalizing temperature Acetaminophen and ibuprofen both safe and effective in appropriate doses, review dosing with parent Avoid aspirin and alcohol baths **Reasons to return to immediate medical attention:** Inability to take adequate oral hydration, no urination >8 hrs, other signs of dehydration Lethargy or inconsolable crying/irritability Stiff neck Development of purple/reddish spots on the skin (petechiae/purpura) Difficulty breathing that does not improve with cleaning out the nose Inability to swallow and is drooling Seizure or convulsion **Return to Medical evaluation if:** Increased or new pain Continued fever for ≥48 hrs without other concerning symptoms Continued other symptoms that are not improving after 48–72 hrs from discharge You have any other concerns

CLINICAL DECISION SUPPORT

Electronic Order Set

As noted above, there are several pathways that address management of the febrile child. Each of these have an accompanying order set with preselected testing recommendations as well as clinical decision support regarding appropriate antibiotic selection and duration, including recommendations for PCN/cephalosporin drug allergy.

RN Specific Education

Nursing education has focused on use of protocol orders for antipyretics and reassessing vital signs. Additionally, RNs can assess need for point-of-care urine testing and place a urine bag on children who are not yet toilet trained, can institute ORT for patients with dehydration and provide nasal suctioning to patients with bronchiolitis. Additionally, the bedside RN can provide education about the causes of fever in children, discuss the use of antipyretics, the normal physiologic responses of children to fever, and concerning signs and symptoms.

Quality Measurement

The emergency department team has worked with the antibiotic stewardship program to develop standard antibiotic recommendations with the goal of using the narrowest spectrum and least expensive antibiotics for the given clinical condition. The pathway guidance and the electronic order set have resulted in improved adherence to antibiotic recommendations for pneumonia, UTI, and otitis media.

Suggested Readings and Key References

El-Radhi AS, Barry W. Thermometry in paediatric practice. *Arch Dis Child* 2006;91(4):351–356.

Finnell SM, Carroll AE, Downs SM; Subcommittee on Urinary Tract Infection. Technical report—Diagnosis and management of an initial UTI in febrile infants and young children. *Pediatrics* 2011; 128(3):e749–e770.

Ishimine P. Risk stratification and management of the febrile young child. *Emerg Med Clin North Am* 2013;31(3):601–626.

Joffe MD, Alpern ER. Occult pneumococcal bacteremia: a review. *Pediatr Emerg Care* 2010;26(6):448–454.

Newburger JW, Takahashi M, Gerber MA, et al.; Committee on Rheumatic Fever, Endocarditis, and Kawasaki Disease, Council on Cardiovascular Disease in the Young, American Heart Association. Diagnosis, treatment, and long-term management of Kawasaki disease: a statement for health professionals from the Committee on Rheumatic Fever, Endocarditis, and Kawasaki Disease, Council on Cardiovascular Disease in the Young, American Heart Association. *Pediatrics* 2004;114(6):1708–1733.

Schwartz MD. Fever in the returning travelers, part II: a methodological approach to initial management. *Wilderness Environ Med* 2003;14:120–130.

Wald ER, Applegate KE, Bordley C, et al.; American Academy of Pediatrics. Clinical practice guideline for the diagnosis and management of acute bacterial sinusitis in children aged 1 to 18 years. *Pediatrics* 2013;132(1):e262–e280.

CHAPTER 89 ■ HEAD TRAUMA

MARK R. ZONFRILLO, MD, MSCE AND SHARON TOPF, RN, BSN, CPEN

BACKGROUND (EPIDEMIOLOGY, EVIDENCE)

One of the leading causes of death and disability in children worldwide is traumatic brain injury (TBI). For children 18 years and younger in the United States, TBI accounts for more than 6,000 deaths, 60,000 hospital admissions, and 600,000 emergency department visits annually. Emergency department visits for TBI have increased in recent years, which is likely a direct result of increased awareness and recognition of mild TBI and concussion. While head computed tomography (CT) is the standard of care to diagnose intracranial hemorrhage and skull fractures following head injury, there has been a movement to avoid unnecessary testing and radiation exposure, particularly in pediatric patients. Prediction rules provide helpful decision-making guidance for emergency physicians, and can decrease testing, promoting cost-effectiveness.

One of the most commonly used set of rules for head injury in children were derived and validated in over 42,000 patients and can accurately predict children with acute head trauma who are at very low risk for a clinically important intracranial injury and who do not require a head CT. These two sets of rules, one for children less than 2 years old and one for children 2 years and older, are based on specific criteria accounting for injury mechanism, and presenting signs and symptoms. Additional studies based on the same cohort have focused on the risk of injury for isolated signs and symptoms, and in certain patient populations with pre-existing conditions which have provided additional guidance on which patients are at low risk for intracranial injury. For children who do not meet the prediction rule criteria, there are certain situations that represent higher risks of injury and for which a CT should be considered. Conversely, observation in the emergency department may be useful to avoid head CTs for children who do not meet all criteria but are still at lower risk. Children who are determined to be low risk typically do not require hospitalization for ongoing neurologic observation beyond their time in the emergency department.

It may be feasible to integrate these head trauma prediction rules into the electronic health record and facilitate risk determination while still maintaining an efficient clinical workflow. These rules may be robustly applied in a shared decision-making process with clinicians and parents of children with head trauma in order to maximize safety and efficient health-care utilization, and avoid unnecessary testing fueled by parental anxiety or preference.

The overall goal of the head trauma pathway is to standardize patient evaluation and management following acute head trauma through rapid identification of potentially serious intracranial injury, minimization of unnecessary head CT use, and reduction of time to ultimate disposition through a joint clinician–guardian decision-making process.

PATHWAY GOALS AND MEASUREMENTS

Goals

The goals for this pathway include the following:

- Standardize patient evaluation following acute head trauma.
- Minimize the inappropriate use of head CT.
- Rapidly identify potentially serious intracranial injury.
- Reduce time to ultimate disposition.
- Promote shared decision making between the ED clinicians and the patient/family.
- Educate patient/family with concussion discharge instructions and schedule appropriate follow-up.
- Always consider occult nonaccidental injury in children <2 years of age.
- Provide a structured mental model for the ED clinicians and a common platform for communication and collaboration.

Measurement

- Head CT utilization by ED clinician.

Algorithm and Key Hyperlinks

www.chop.edu/clinical-pathway/acute-head-trauma-clinical-pathway

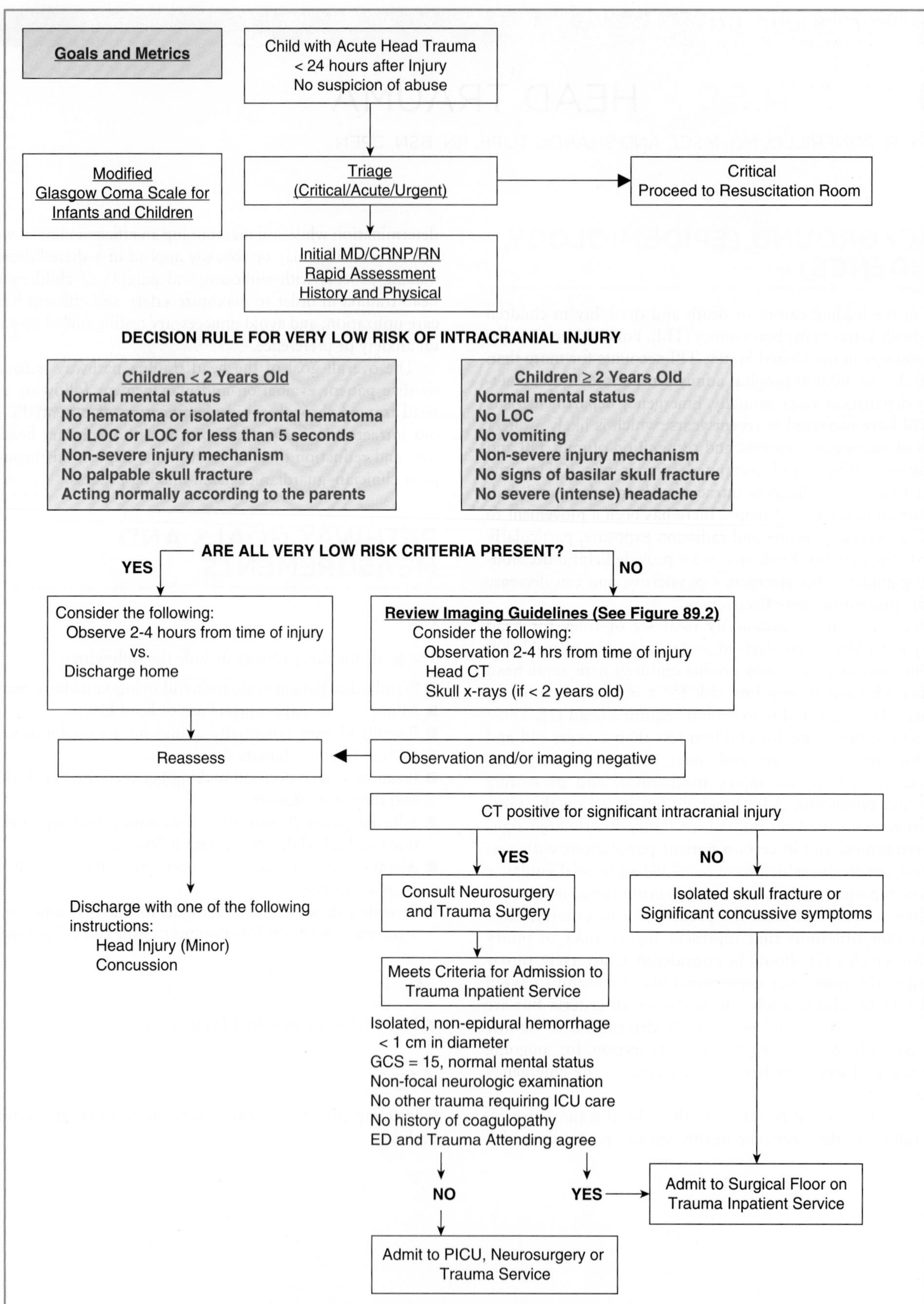

FIGURE 89.1 Algorithm for the evaluation and treatment of children with acute head trauma.

Patient Population/Stratifying Patient Risks

This pathway should be used to guide the care of healthy children with history of head injury in the preceding 24 hours in which there is a very low suspicion of nonaccidental trauma (see Chapter 95 Child Abuse/Assault). Patients with underlying medical conditions that predispose them to intracranial bleeding are excluded; these include but are not limited to existing intracranial pathology such as hydrocephalus, VP shunt, existing neurologic abnormalities that interfere with adequate neurologic assessment, or existing coagulopathy.

Clinical Decision Support

Immediate access to Decision Rule for Very Low Risk of Intracranial Injury by the clinician at the point of care.

TABLE 89.1

HEAD TRAUMA DECISION RULES FOR CHILDREN <2 YEARS OLD

Very low risk of intracranial injury if all of the following are present:	
Normal mental status	Altered mental status is defined as: GCS < 15 Agitation Somnolence Slow responses when developmentally appropriate Repetitive questioning
No hematoma or isolated frontal hematoma	
No LOC or LOC <5 s	
Nonsevere injury mechanism	Severe defined as any of the following: Motor vehicle crash with: Patient ejection Death of another passenger Rollover Pedestrian or bicyclist without helmet struck by a motorized vehicle Falls of >3 ft Head struck by a high-impact object
No palpable skull fracture	
Acting normally according to the parents	

TABLE 89.2

HEAD TRAUMA DECISION RULES FOR CHILDREN ≥2 YEARS OLD

Very low risk of intracranial injury if all of the following are present:	
Normal mental status	Altered mental status is defined as: GCS < 15 Agitation Somnolence Slow responses Repetitive questioning
No LOC	
No vomiting	
Nonsevere injury mechanism	Severe defined as any of the following: Motor vehicle crash with: Patient ejection Death of another passenger Rollover Pedestrian or bicyclist without helmet struck by a motorized vehicle Falls of >5 ft Head struck by a high-impact object
No signs of basilar skull fracture	
No severe headache	

TABLE 89.3

REASSESS AND DISCHARGE

Consider discharge if:
Mental status, neurologic examination is normal
Vomiting subsides, patient can tolerate oral fluids
Headache improved after analgesia
No other injuries requiring further intervention
No social, caretaker concerns

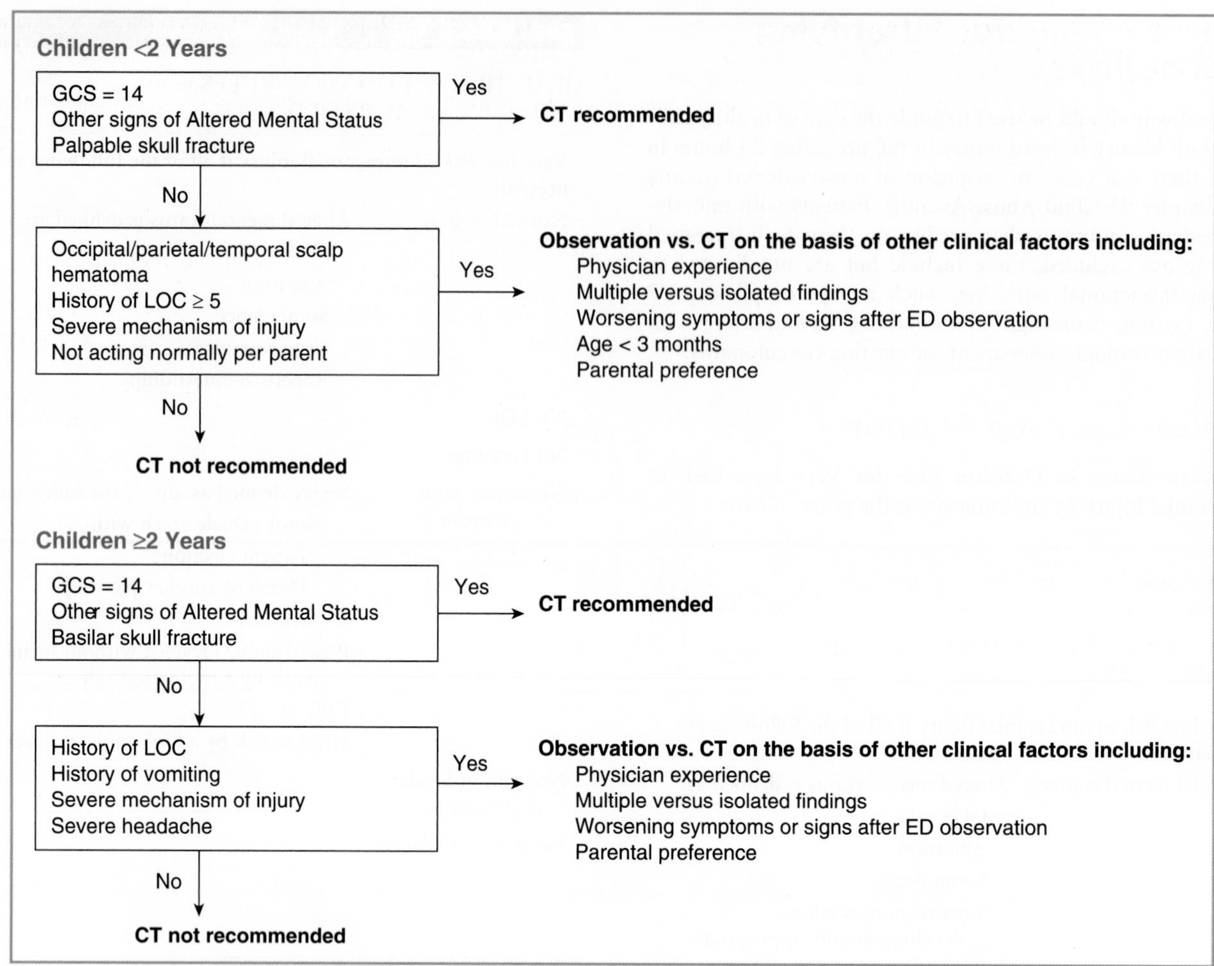

FIGURE 89.2 Imaging algorithm. (From Kupperman N, Holmes JF, Dayan PS, et al. Identification of children at very low risk of clinically important brain injuries after head trauma: a prospective cohort study. *Lancet* 2009; 374:1160–1170.)

Communication/Teamwork

The communication plan aims at standardizing the assessment and treatment of acute head trauma patients to reduce unnecessary imaging and radiation exposure. Clear and defined decision rules are listed to accurately identify children with very low risk of clinically significant TBI. It is important that the clinician team including the ED attending, resident physicians, nurse practitioners, and consultants share the same information with the patient and the family.

Nurse-specific Education

- Hourly GCS, vital signs, neurologic checks, cardiorespiratory monitor
- Initial trauma score
- Pain score/assessment
- Cervical spine immobilization
- NPO status for possible sedation
- Medications: analgesia, antiemetics, IV fluids
- MD notification for concerns about patient appearance or parental concerns
- Concussion/minor head injury discharge teaching for families

QUALITY MEASUREMENT

- Population: Patients presenting to the ED, with acute head trauma <24 hours after injury with no suspicion of abuse.
- Outcomes:
  Head CT utilization
  Time from arrival to head CT
  Percent of CTs requiring sedation
  Revisits at 72 hours

Next Steps

Current EMRs provide an opportunity to provide clinician-specific metrics to guide clinical decision making in the future, such as CT utilization by ESI triage level and patient age. Additionally, data from the pathway cohort can further inform the pathway team on opportunities for improvement, such as efforts to reduce emergency department visits by appropriate follow-up for concussion care.

Suggested Readings and Key References

Centers for Disease Control and Prevention, National Center for Injury Prevention and Control. Traumatic brain injury in the United States: emergency department visits, hospitalizations, and deaths 2002–2006. Available at: http://www.cdc.gov/traumaticbraininjury/pdf/blue_book.pdf. Accessed October 1, 2013.

Dayan PS, Holmes JF, Atabaki S, et al. Association of traumatic brain injuries with vomiting in children with blunt head trauma. *Ann Emerg Med* 2014;63(6):657–665.

Dayan PS, Holmes JF, Schutzman S, et al. Risk of traumatic brain injuries in children younger than 24 months with isolated scalp hematomas. *Ann Emerg Med* 2014;64(2):153–162.

Hess EP, Wyatt KD, Kharbanda AB, et al. Effectiveness of the head CT choice decision aid in parents of children with minor head trauma: study protocol for a multicenter randomized trial. *Trials* 2014;15:253.

Holmes JF, Borgialli DA, Nadel FM, et al. Do children with blunt head trauma and normal cranial computed tomography scan results require hospitalization for neurologic observation? *Ann Emerg Med* 2011;58(4):315–322.

Kuppermann N, Holmes JF, Dayan PS, et al. Identification of children at very low risk of clinically-important brain injuries after head trauma: a prospective cohort study. *Lancet* 2009;374(9696):1160–1170.

Lee LK, Dayan PS, Gerardi MJ, et al. Intracranial hemorrhage after blunt head trauma in children with bleeding disorders. *J Pediatr* 2011;158(6):1003–1008 e1–e2.

Lee LK, Monroe D, Bachman MC, et al. Isolated loss of consciousness in children with minor blunt head trauma. *JAMA Pediatr* 2014;168(9):837–843.

Marin JR, Weaver MD, Yealy DM, et al. Trends in visits for traumatic brain injury to emergency departments in the United States. *JAMA* 2014;311(18):1917–1919.

Natale JE, Joseph JG, Rogers AJ, et al. Cranial computed tomography use among children with minor blunt head trauma: association with race/ethnicity. *Arch Pediatr Adolesc Med* 2012;166(8): 732–737.

Nigrovic LE, Lee LK, Hoyle J, et al. Prevalence of clinically important traumatic brain injuries in children with minor blunt head trauma and isolated severe injury mechanisms. *Arch Pediatr Adolesc Med* 2012;166(4):356–361.

Nigrovic LE, Lillis K, Atabaki SM, et al. The prevalence of traumatic brain injuries after minor blunt head trauma in children with ventricular shunts. *Ann Emerg Med* 2013;61(4):389–393.

Nigrovic LE, Schunk JE, Foerster A, et al. The effect of observation on cranial computed tomography utilization for children after blunt head trauma. *Pediatrics* 2011;127(6):1067–1073.

Sheehan B, Nigrovic LE, Dayan PS, et al. Informing the design of clinical decision support services for evaluation of children with minor blunt head trauma in the emergency department: a sociotechnical analysis. *J Biomed Inform* 2013;46(5):905–913.

Stiell IG, Bennett C. Implementation of clinical decision rules in the emergency department. *Acad Emerg Med* 2007;14(11): 955–959.

CHAPTER 90 ■ PNEUMONIA, COMMUNITY-ACQUIRED

JEFFREY SEIDEN, MD AND JAMES M. CALLAHAN, MD

BACKGROUND (EPIDEMIOLOGY, EVIDENCE)

Globally, pneumonia is the leading cause of mortality in children under 5 years of age, accounting for nearly 20% of all such deaths. In the United States, community-acquired pneumonia (CAP) is the most common serious bacterial infection in childhood, accounting for approximately 3 million outpatient visits per year. Further, CAP is one of the most common reasons for inpatient hospitalizations; for every 100,000 children under 19 years of age, 200 will be hospitalized with CAP. Despite the frequency with which physicians encounter CAP in the emergency department (ED), there exists a tremendous degree of practice variation with respect to the diagnosis, management, and disposition for children with suspected CAP. Even when adjusting for level of severity, rates of inpatient admission for pneumonia vary from 19% to 69% among freestanding US children's hospitals. Similar variability exists in the rates of ED resource utilization, such as diagnostic imaging and laboratory evaluation, as well as in the use of antimicrobial agents. As a result, efforts to standardize care and optimize outcomes are essential. Development and implementation of clinical pathways are an effective method for increasing the value of healthcare.

There are two main areas that warrant special attention in the development of a clinical pathway for CAP: diagnostic testing and antibiotic treatment. A wide variability has been described in the use of radiographic imaging, blood tests, and viral studies among inpatients with CAP in freestanding children's hospitals in the United States. Increased diagnostic testing was associated with increased hospital length of stay, but had no effect on other outcomes, such as hospital readmission after discharge. In addition, increased testing has been associated with a higher frequency of broad-spectrum antibiotic usage. Despite solid evidence that broad-spectrum antibiotics, including cephalosporins and macrolides, provide little benefit over penicillins in the treatment of CAP, they continue to be prescribed quite frequently. The majority of children admitted to the hospital for the treatment of CAP are actually treated in community hospitals and children's hospitals within larger hospitals. In one retrospective cohort study, a similar variability in diagnostic testing has been shown to exist in these settings. There was decreased variability in the choice of antibiotic regimen in these settings but unfortunately more than 75% of patients in this review of an administrative database were inappropriately treated with a third-generation cephalosporin as part of their regimen and 10% were treated with macrolides alone, which frequently do not provide adequate coverage for the organisms which most often cause CAP in children. Creating evidence-based, consensus guidelines to standardize the approach to CAP aims to minimize unnecessary diagnostic testing, prevent the unnecessary use of broad-spectrum antibiotics, and ensure the best possible outcomes for children presenting with suspected CAP. The Pediatric Infectious Diseases Society (PIDS) and Infectious Disease Society of America (IDSA) have issued clinical guidelines that may be used to guide the development of local guidelines in 2011. Quality improvement efforts, in particular rapid tests of change using plan-do-study-act cycles, have been shown to be an effective way to produce a rapid increase in compliance with such guidelines. A web-based pathway allows ready access to evidence and expert consensus to the clinicians at the point of care to provide support to clinical decision making for all team members.

PATHWAY GOALS AND MEASUREMENT

Goals

- Increase the use of amoxicillin as first-line antibiotic therapy in children with CAP.
- Reduce the use of diagnostic tests that provide little information to guide management decisions.
- Minimize treatment failures and need for revisit/readmission to primary care provider, ED, or hospital.

Measurement

- The proportion of children with CAP if treated with antibiotics, treatment with amoxicillin.
- The proportion of children with CAP who have the following tests performed: erythrocyte sedimentation rate (ESR), C-reactive protein (CRP), rapid respiratory panel (RRP), mycoplasma PCR, and/or blood culture.
- The proportion of children with CAP who require another visit to primary care provider, ED, or hospital with diagnosis of pneumonia and antibiotic prescription within 14 days.

ALGORITHM AND KEY HYPERLINKS

http://www.chop.edu/clinical-pathway/community-acquired-pneumonia-clinical-pathway see Tables (90.1-90.3) and Figure 90.1.

PATHWAY AUTHORS

J. Gerber, MD, PhD; T. Metjian, PharmD; M. Siddharth, MD; D. Davis, MD, MSCE; T. Florin, MD; J. Zorc, MD; T. Blinman, MD; D. Mong, MD; X. Bateman, CRNP; E. Pete Devon, MD; R. Keren, MD, MPH; L. Bell, MD; L. Utidjian, MD; E. Moxey, RN, MPH

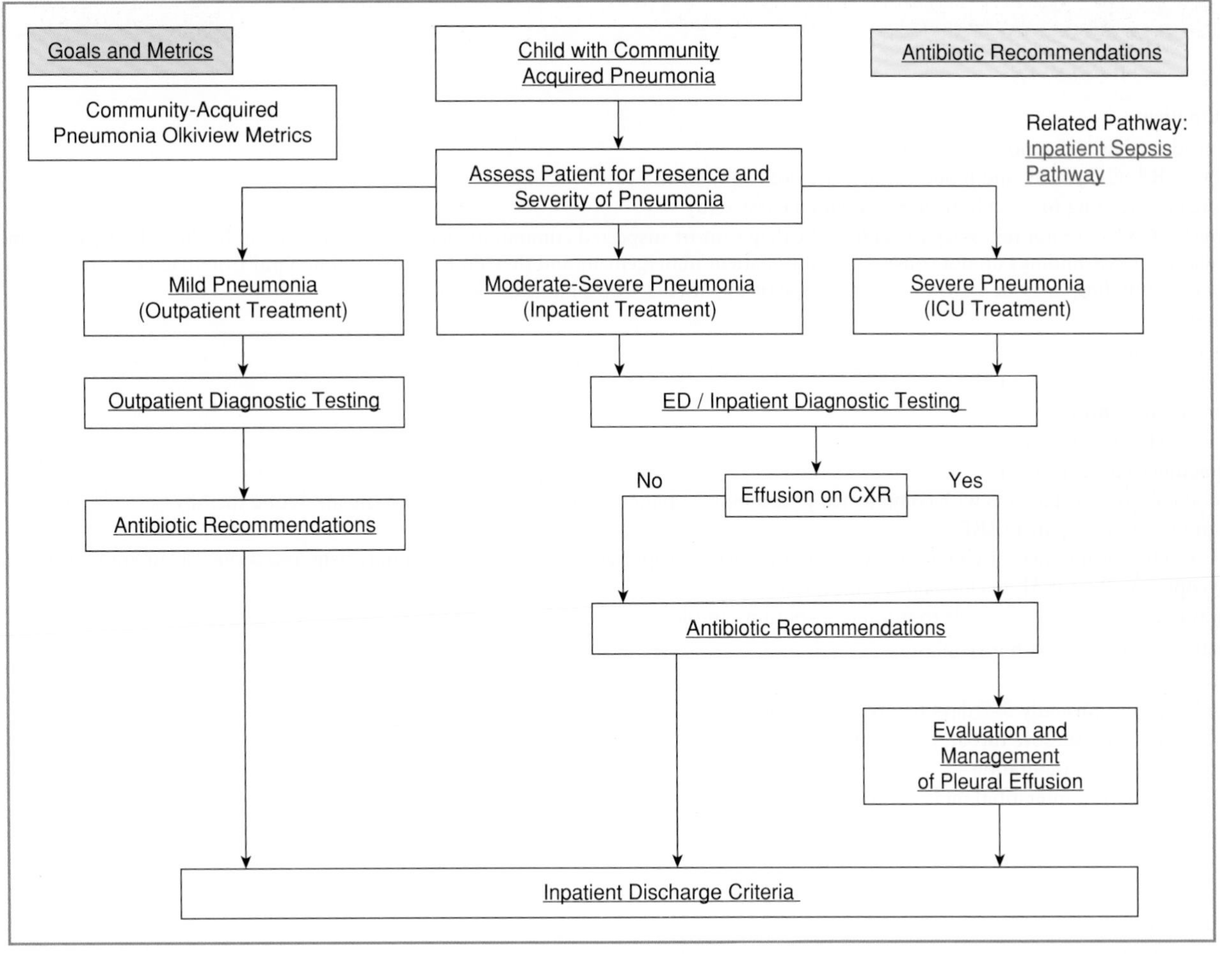

FIGURE 90.1 Algorithm for the evaluation and treatment of child with community-acquired pneumonia (CAP).

TABLE 90.1

PATIENT POPULATION/STRATIFYING PATIENT RISK

Mild pneumonia Outpatient treatment	**Moderate–severe pneumonia Inpatient treatment**	**Severe pneumonia ICU treatment**
Age >3 mo Absence of: Retractions Grunting Nasal flaring Apnea Pulse oximetry >90% in room air Nontoxic appearance Ability to tolerate oral medications and fluids Adequate observation/follow-up care	Any of the below: Age <3 mo Moderate–severe dyspnea Retractions Grunting Nasal flaring Apnea Pulse oximetry <90% in room air Alteration in mental status Moderate to large parapneumonic effusion Concern for inadequate outpatient care/observation/follow-up Dehydration, vomiting, or inability to take oral medication Clinical concern for inpatient-level observation/care Failure of initial outpatient treatment	Any of the below: Need for mechanical ventilator support with artificial airway New or increased CPAP or BiPAP support Apnea, inadequate ventilation, severe respiratory distress Hypoxemia despite significant support defined as: Pulse oximetry <92% on 40% high-flow nasal cannula or 50% face mask Inability to transition from 100% nonrebreather mask Systemic signs of inadequate perfusion (change in mental status, hemodynamic instability) Parapneumonic effusion requiring emergent drainage Clinical concern for impending respiratory failure

TABLE 90.2

DIAGNOSTIC TESTING

Outpatient

Consider CXR if diagnosis is uncertain

CBC, CRP, ESR, RRP, and blood cultures are *not* routinely indicated

Note on screening for occult pneumonia with a chest x-ray

Routine CXRs are not necessary to confirm the diagnosis of suspected community-acquired pneumonia in healthy children with mild disease. CXR findings do not consistently alter patient management and they do not differentiate viral from bacterial etiology. Typical findings may be absent in early disease or in patients with significant dehydration.

Inpatient

Recommended

CXR, CBC with differential

Not recommended

ESR, CRP, procalcitonin

Sometimes recommended

Blood culture: For patients with complicated pneumonia or patients worsening on appropriate antibiotic therapy

Rapid respiratory panel (RRP)

Consider for inpatient if viral etiology, such as influenza suspected as sole cause which may help assess the role of antiviral therapy

Mycoplasma PCR if *M. pneumoniae* is suspected

Sputum culture in children able to produce a sputum sample

Features associated with mycoplasma

Age >5 yrs

Insidious onset; usually 5–7 days before presentation

Headache, malaise, sore throat, prominent cough

Diffuse rales on auscultation

Diffuse, bilateral, interstitial infiltrates on x-ray

TABLE 90.3

ANTIBIOTIC RECOMMENDATIONS FOR CHILDREN WITH CAP

	First-line therapy[a]	Beta-lactam allergy[b]	Duration of therapy/comments
Mild pneumonia outpatient	Amoxicillin: 90 mg/kg/day, divided BID-TID Max: 1 g/dose	Clindamycin PO: 30 mg/kg/day divided TID Max: 1.8 g/day OR Levofloxacin (PO) ≥6 mo and <5 yrs 20 mg/kg/day divided q12h ≥5 yrs 10 mg/kg/day, once daily Max: 500 mg	Duration: 7 days Target pathogen: *S. pneumoniae* High-dose amoxicillin against most *S. pneumonia* Clindamycin active against ~90% Levofloxacin active against >95% Oral cephalosporins inferior to high-dose amoxicillin for *S. pneumonia* Azithromycin resistance in up to 40% of *S. pneumoniae*
Moderate pneumonia inpatient	Ampicillin 300 mg/kg/day divided every 6 hrs Max: 2 g/dose	Clindamycin IV 40 mg/kg/day Divided every 8 hrs Max: 2.7 g/day Clindamycin PO 30 mg/kg/day Divided TID Max 1.8 g/day	Duration: 7 days, or at least 48 hrs from resolution of fever and tachypnea (whichever is longer) including oral/outpatient therapy Target pathogen: *S. pneumonia* High-dose amoxicillin against most *S. pneumonia* Ceftriaxone for treatment failure[c] with outpatient amoxicillin

TABLE 90.3

ANTIBIOTIC RECOMMENDATIONS FOR CHILDREN WITH CAP (*CONTINUED*)

	First-line therapy[a]	Beta-lactam allergy[b]	Duration of therapy/comments
		OR Levofloxacin IV/PO ≥6 mo and <5 yrs 20 mg/kg/day divided q12h ≥5 yrs 10 mg/kg/day, once daily Max: 500 mg	
Complicated pneumonia[d] inpatient	Clindamycin IV 40 mg/kg/day Divided every 8 hrs Max: 2.7 g/day Clindamycin PO 30 mg/kg/day Divided TID Max 1.8 g/day AND Ceftriaxone 100 mg/kg every 24 hrs Max: 2 g/dose	Clindamycin IV 40 mg/kg/day Divided every 8 hrs Max: 2.7 g/day Clindamycin PO 30 mg/kg/day Divided TID Max 1.8 g/day AND Levofloxacin IV/PO ≥6 mo and <5 yrs 20 mg/kg/day divided q12h ≥5 yrs 10 mg/kg/day, once daily Max: 500 mg	Duration: 7 days from drainage of effusions. If not amenable to drainage, 7 days from afebrile. Please consult Infectious Disease team for pneumonia with mod–large effusion or empyema. Target pathogens: *S. pneumonia* *S. pyogenes* *S. aureus* Clindamycin for suspected CA-MRSA active ~85% of MRSA (CA and HA)
Severe pneumonia inpatient (ICU)	Vancomycin 15 mg/kg/dose Divided every 6 hrs Max: 500 mg/dose AND Ceftriaxone 100 mg/kg every 24 hrs Max: 2 g/dose	Vancomycin 15 mg/kg/dose Divided every 6 hrs Max: 500 mg/dose AND Levofloxacin IV/PO ≥6 mo and <5 yrs 20 mg/kg/day divided q12h ≥5 yrs 10 mg/kg/day, once daily Max: 500 mg	Duration 7 days from afebrile. Please consult Infectious Disease team for pneumonia with mod–large effusion or empyema Target pathogens: *S. pneumonia* *S. pyogenes* *S. Aureus* Vancomycin for suspected CA-MRSA in severe or life-threatening conditions

[a]For **typical,** presumed bacterial community-acquired pneumonia.
Atypical pneumonia (often characterized by nonlobar, patchy, or interstitial pattern on CXR; insidious onset; low grade of fever, malaise, H/A, cough; minimal auscultatory findings relative to CXR) is often caused by respiratory viruses, but may be caused by atypical bacterial pathogens including *Mycoplasma pneumoniae*. Most atypical pneumonia is mild and self-limited; however, for disease requiring hospitalization, consider PCR testing for respiratory viruses and *M. pneumoniae*. Drugs for confirmed *M. pneumoniae* infection, or for presumed infection in the presence of severe disease, include **azithromycin:** 10 mg/kg on day 1, single dose (max: 500 mg/day), followed by 5 mg/kg/day, once daily, days 2 to 5 (max: 250 mg/day) **OR Levofloxacin** (as above).
[b]Defined by urticaria or anaphylaxis.
[c]After >48 hrs of therapy with high-dose amoxicillin in a patient who was tolerating the outpatient PO regimen.
[d]Includes pneumonia with moderate–large parapneumonic effusion.

ASSOCIATED PATHWAYS

http://www.chop.edu/clinical-pathway/severe-sepsis-clinical-pathway-infants-28-days-age-and-children

This pathway is to be used for healthy children >56 days through 18 years of age with suspected/proven CAP managed in the outpatient, ED, inpatient, or intensive care setting. Children with immunodeficiency, chronic lung disease (excluding asthma), tracheostomy, or concern for aspiration or hospital-acquired pneumonia are excluded from these recommendations.

CLINICAL DECISION SUPPORT

The electronic order set includes recommendations for appropriate radiographic studies, laboratory studies, intravenous fluids, and antibiotic therapies to blend standard recommendations for evaluation and treatment into the flow of work while making it easier for the clinician to do the right thing.

COMMUNICATION/TEAMWORK

The effectiveness of this pathway is dependent at least in part on good communication between community (primary care) providers, emergency physicians, and physicians providing care for children with CAP in an inpatient setting. Practitioners across the entire healthcare system have to be familiar with the most common causes of CAP in various age groups and prevailing patterns of antimicrobial sensitivity testing. In addition, there should be agreement about what, if any, diagnostic testing is required among patients with differing severity of symptoms and in different practice settings. The PIDS and IDSA Guidelines provide evidence-based recommendations that should be the basis of these communications. These recommendations serve to minimize diagnostic testing which does not contribute to clinical decision making, and to begin treatment with the narrowest spectrum antibiotic that will treat the majority of patients with CAP. The web-based pathway provides a platform for communication across the institution around this clinical diagnosis.

NURSE-SPECIFIC EDUCATION

Nursing education should include a familiarity with risk factors and findings in patients more likely to have severe disease including young age, moderate to severe dyspnea or signs of respiratory distress, significant hypoxemia, presence of dehydration or inability to tolerate oral fluid intake and/or oral medications, and alterations in mental status. In the presence of such findings, nurses should be prepared to obtain IV access and laboratory studies and look for direction regarding whether the patient should be kept NPO. Education should also be provided regarding the appropriateness of narrow-spectrum antibiotic treatment for the majority of patients with CAP so that appropriate education can be provided to parents and other caregivers. This allows for standard communication within the clinical team as well as with the patients and their families.

QUALITY MEASUREMENT

The CAP pathway was implemented at The Children's Hospital of Philadelphia in October 2012 across the outpatient, ED, and inpatient settings. ED metrics that have been monitored since then include antibiotic selection, diagnostic testing performed, length of stay, cost of care, and return visits to the ED. Since pathway implementation, the rate of prescribing of amoxicillin or use of intravenous ampicillin has increased from a baseline rate in the month before pathway implemented of 61% to rates as high as 91% on a monthly basis. Overall, mean rates of narrow-spectrum antibiotic prescribing have remained at about 72%. Blood cultures are obtained in fewer patients who do not have severe disease, cost of care provided has decreased and return visits remain very rare (<1% in most months). It has been shown that rapid cycle improvement QI methodology can lead to marked increases in compliance with published guidelines for the evaluation and management of CAP.

NEXT STEPS

The next steps in development of this pathway are to utilize the data gathered to inform the pathway team on opportunities for improvement. For example, if the data demonstrate an increased rate of revisits/readmissions among certain subgroups of patients, the team may need to alter the definitions of pneumonia severity to reflect these newly discovered risk factors. Other areas for possible performance improvement may include the timeliness of antibiotic therapy for patients diagnosed with CAP.

Suggested Readings and Key References

Ambroggio L, Thomson J, Kurowski EM, et al. Quality improvement methods increase appropriate antibiotic prescribing for childhood pneumonia. *Pediatrics* 2011;131:e1623–e1631.

Bourgeois FT, Monuteaux MC, Stack AM, et al. Variation in emergency department admission rates in US children's hospitals. *Pediatrics* 2014;134(3):539–545.

Bradley JS, Byington CL, Shah SS, et al. The management of community-acquired pneumonia in infants and children older than 3 months of age: clinical practice guidelines by the Pediatric Infectious Diseases Society and the Infectious Diseases Society of America. *Clin Infect Dis* 2011;53:e25–e76.

Brogan TV, Hall M, Williams DJ, et al. Variability in processes of care and outcomes among children hospitalized with community-acquired pneumonia. *Pediatr Infect Dis J* 2012;31(10):1036–1041.

Kronman MP, Hersh AL, Feng R, et al. Ambulatory visit rates and antibiotic prescribing for children with pneumonia, 1994–2007. *Pediatrics* 2011;127(3):411–418.

Lee GE, Lorch SA, Sheffler-Collins S, et al. National hospitalization trends for pediatric pneumonia and associated complications. *Pediatrics* 2010;126(2):204–213.

Leyenaar JK, Lagu T, Shieh M, et al. Variation in resource utilization for the management of uncomplicated community-acquired pneumonia across community and children's hospitals. *J Pediatr* 2014;165(3):585–591.

Wardlaw T, Salama P, Johansson EW, et al. Pneumonia: the leading killer of children. *Lancet* 2006;368(9541):1048–1050.

CHAPTER 91 ▪ SHOCK

FRAN BALAMUTH, MD, PhD, MSCE, DEBRA A. POTTS, MSN, RN, CPEN, CEN, MARY KATE FUNARI, MSN, RN, CPEN AND JANE LAVELLE, MD

BACKGROUND (EPIDEMIOLOGY, EVIDENCE)

Pediatric sepsis syndrome is a leading source of morbidity, mortality, and healthcare costs in infants and children in the United States. In the United States, there are approximately 21,000 cases of severe sepsis requiring hospitalization annually with estimated mortality estimates from 5% to 20%. Timely antimicrobial therapy and fluid resuscitation is essential in the treatment of severe sepsis and septic shock. The Surviving Sepsis Campaign recommends antibiotic administration within 1 hour of recognition of septic shock, as well as prompt fluid resuscitation in both adults and children. In addition, timely sepsis care has been identified as a quality metric. Several pediatric institutions have successfully implemented protocol-based sepsis care and have demonstrated associated improvements in the timeliness of care delivery. These improvements have been associated with improved ICU and hospital length of stay. Recognizing which patient requires these intensive severe sepsis therapies remains a challenge. Ideally, sepsis recognition tools should be built with high sensitivity such that no patients with sepsis are missed, they should also have high specificity to avoid unnecessary antibiotic use and resource utilization. Because of the time-sensitive nature of sepsis interventions, implementing pediatric sepsis protocols in the emergency department settings requires strong teamwork and strong interdisciplinary collaboration.

PATHWAY GOALS AND MEASUREMENTS

Goals

- Improved identification of patients with severe sepsis
- Timely antibiotic therapy
- Timely fluid resuscitation
- Decrease patients in whom sepsis is diagnosed within 24 hours of admission

Measurements

- Time to fluid management (40 mL per kg, 60 mL per kg)
- Time to first appropriate antibiotics, percent in <1 hour
- Multisystem organ failure at 0, 24, 48 hours

Algorithm and Key Hyperlinks

- See Figure 91.1 (http://www.chop.edu/clinical-pathway/severe-sepsis-clinical-pathway-infants-28-days-age-and-children)
- See Tables 91.1 and 91.2

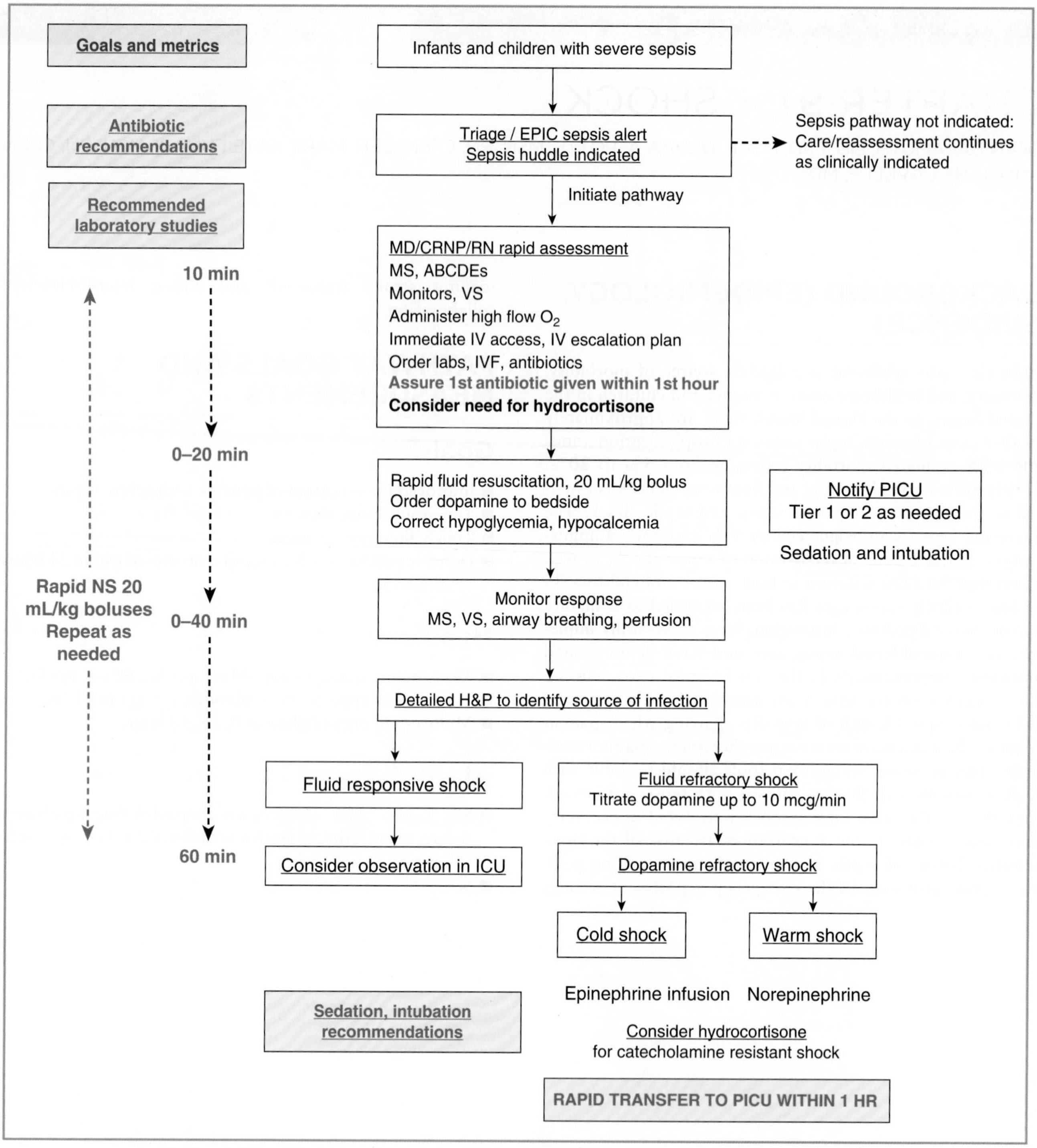

Goals and metrics

Antibiotic recommendations

Recommended laboratory studies

Infants and children with severe sepsis

Triage / EPIC sepsis alert
Sepsis huddle indicated

Sepsis pathway not indicated: Care/reassessment continues as clinically indicated

Initiate pathway

10 min

MD/CRNP/RN rapid assessment
MS, ABCDEs
Monitors, VS
Administer high flow O_2
Immediate IV access, IV escalation plan
Order labs, IVF, antibiotics
Assure 1st antibiotic given within 1st hour
Consider need for hydrocortisone

0–20 min

Rapid fluid resuscitation, 20 mL/kg bolus
Order dopamine to bedside
Correct hypoglycemia, hypocalcemia

Notify PICU
Tier 1 or 2 as needed

Sedation and intubation

Rapid NS 20 mL/kg boluses Repeat as needed

0–40 min

Monitor response
MS, VS, airway breathing, perfusion

Detailed H&P to identify source of infection

Fluid responsive shock

Fluid refractory shock
Titrate dopamine up to 10 mcg/min

60 min

Consider observation in ICU

Dopamine refractory shock

Cold shock

Warm shock

Epinephrine infusion

Norepinephrine

Sedation, intubation recommendations

Consider hydrocortisone
for catecholamine resistant shock

RAPID TRANSFER TO PICU WITHIN 1 HR

FIGURE 91.1 Pathway for evaluation and treatment of infants >28 days of age and children with severe sepsis. *Pathway Authors: F Balamuth, MD; MK Funari, RN; H Scott, MD; E Alpern, MD; D Davis, MD; M Mittal, MD; C Jacobstein, MD; J Gerber, MD; T Metjian, PharmD; J Lavelle, MD.*

TABLE 91.1

PATIENT POPULATION/STRATIFYING PATIENT RISKS

Use the following criteria to identify children with history, symptoms suggestive of infection and inadequate tissue perfusion:	
Temperature abnormality	Fever >38.5°C or <36°C
Heart rate abnormality	See table below
Plus one of the following:	
Mental status abnormality	Anxiety, restlessness, agitation, irritability, inappropriate crying Drowsiness, confusion, lethargy, obtundation
Perfusion abnormality	Cool extremities, capillary refill >3 s, diminished pulses, mottling or Flushed, warm extremities, bounding pulses, flash capillary refill
High risk conditions	<56 days of age Central line presence BMT or solid organ transplants Malignancy Immune compromised, suppression Asplenia, sickle cell disease Immunosuppressive therapy Static encephalopathy Petechial, purpuric rash Erythroderma

TABLE 91.2

VITAL SIGN TARGETS

Age	Tachycardia[a]	RR[a]	Systolic BP Hypotension	Systolic BP 50th percentile
1 mo–1 yr	>180	>34	<75	85–95
>1–5 yrs	>140	>22	<74	88–95
>5–12 yrs	>130	>18	<83	96–106
>12–18 yrs	>120	>14	<90	108–118

Remember, heart rate is affected by pain, anxiety, medications, and hydration status.
[a]>95th percentile.

CLINICAL DECISION SUPPORT

Sepsis Screening Tools

The use of screening tools for sepsis or SIRS aids the clinician team in early identification of at-risk patients. Tools should include history of fever/hypothermia or concern for infection, abnormal vital signs, mental status and perfusion, as well as presence of any high-risk conditions. A positive screen prompts immediate clinician team assessment to determine if pathway activation is required. While paper can be used to complete this screen, many EHRs support clinical decision alerts which also provides for immediate data retrieval to provide timely feedback to clinicians.

Electronic Order Set

The electronic order sets specific to the emergency care of pediatric sepsis patients include prechecked laboratory studies; additional orders for care are selected by the clinician and include IV placement and fluid resuscitation orders, recommended antibiotics for different patient populations, stress steroid dosing, vasopressor infusions, recommended RSI medications, blood bank and imaging orders. The organized order set makes it easier for the clinician to rapidly enter orders for the care that is needed. (See Figure 91.2, Table 91.3, and Table 91.4)

TABLE 91.3

FLUID RESUSCITATION AND VASOPRESSORS

Fluid resuscitation	First hour Rapid warmed NS 20 mL/kg boluses every 5 min Reassess, repeat boluses to improve perfusion Begin dopamine if poor response to fluids (40 mL/kg)
Rapid fluid infusion techniques	Push–pull technique (<50 kg) 30-mL syringe Macrodrip set up with three-way stopcock T-connector Pressure bag (≥50 kg) Rapid infuser (≥50 kg) Set up for patients ≥50 kg
Volume	20 mL/kg NS boluses up to ≥60 mL/kg Continue rapid volume infusion as needed following clinical parameters Use warmed NS when possible
Dopamine	Order dopamine infusion to bedside Begin at 5 mcg/kg/min as clinically indicated
Other considerations	Order D_5NS fluids to run at maintenance to provide adequate glucose Order FFP if INR, PT/PTT abnormal Order PRBC if Hgb <10 mg/dL Order platelets for platelet count <50,000

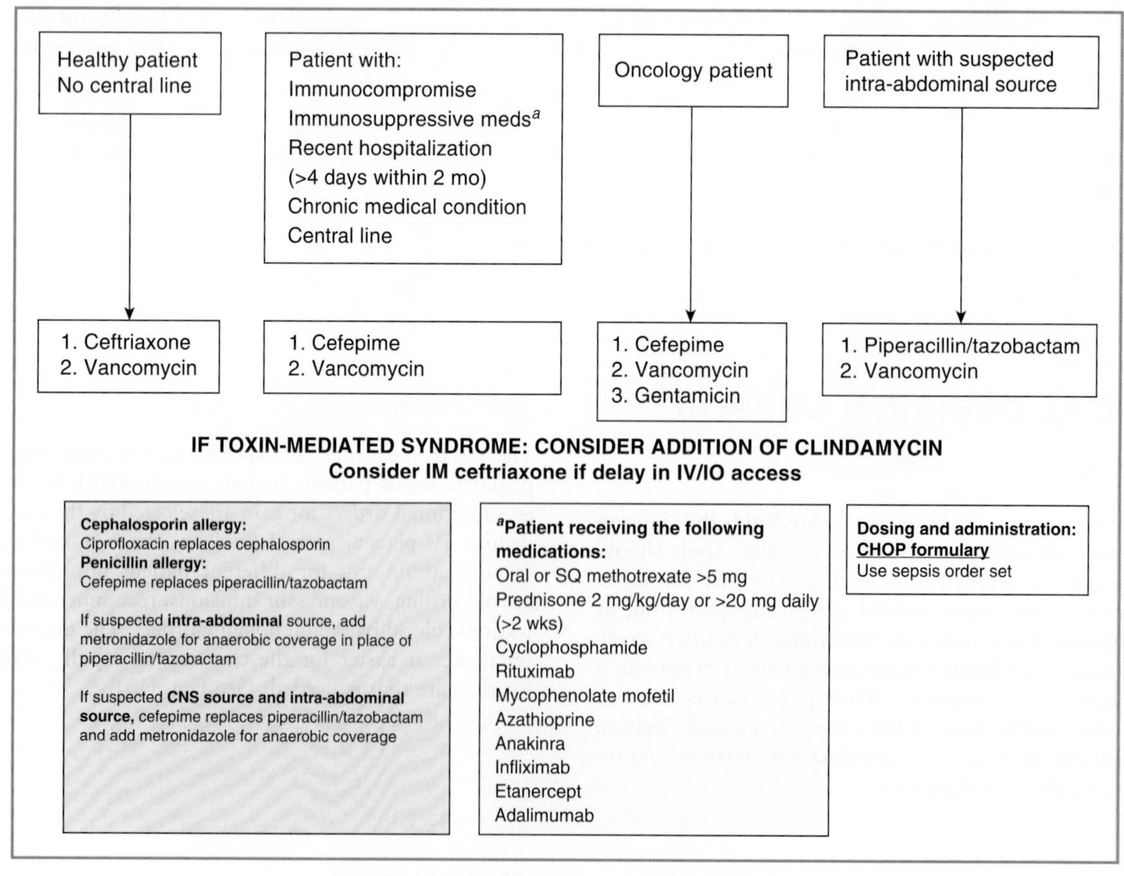

FIGURE 91.2 Antibiotics by patient characteristics.

TABLE 91.4

REFRACTORY SHOCK DEFINITION AND PRESSORS

Fluid refractory shock	NS >40–60 mL/kg administered without adequate clinical response
	Start, increase dopamine (5–10 mcg/kg/min)
	Consider central venous line
	Continue fluid boluses until perfusion improves or signs of fluid overload develop
Dopamine refractory shock	Shock state persists despite NS >60 mL/kg and
	Dopamine at 10 mcg/kg/min
Cold shock	Evidence of vasoconstriction on physical examination
	Capillary refill >3 s
	Diminished peripheral pulses
	Mottled, cool extremities
	Begin epinephrine
Warm shock	Evidence of vasodilatation on physical examination
	Brisk capillary refill
	Bounding peripheral pulses
	Warm, flushed extremities
	Wide pulse pressure
	Begin norepinephrine

Communication/Teamwork

Triage and bedside nurses must recognize patients at high risk for sepsis and alert frontline clinicians. Prompt bedside evaluation (sepsis huddle) then ensues with the entire care team. As many invasive procedures and resuscitative interventions are completed in quick succession, additional nursing or support staff needs are identified at the start of care. Verbalization of treatment priorities is helpful as competing tasks can delay optimum time to therapy. For example, a clear plan for IV escalation and communication to the attending is key. Response to therapy, changes in severity of illness and the status of procedures, laboratory work and antibiotics are frequently monitored and documented by the care team to ensure appropriate escalation of care and admission. Development of a standardized response can promote consistency, efficiency, and safe care in this patient population. (See Tables 91.5 and 91.6)

Nurse-specific Education

The nursing staff receives comprehensive education to ensure safe passage of the septic child through the ED. Prior to education on the pathway itself, didactic and interactive learning about pediatric sepsis including basic pathophysiology, physical examination findings of warm and cold shock, laboratory values, appropriate interventions and complications should be completed. Additionally, high-risk vital signs and hypotension should be reviewed. Focus should be on early identification, team collaboration, and recognition of worsening severity of illness.

TABLE 91.5

IV ESCALATION PLAN

Minutes	Access procedure
0–5	First peripheral IV with largest gauge possible
	Consider IO immediately in severely ill patients
5–10	2nd peripheral attempt
	Consider US-guided peripheral IV
	Consider EJ (US guided)
	Notify vascular access specialist (IV team)
10–15	If still no access
	EZ-IO
	EJ (consider US guided)
	Central line (consider US guided) or
	Call PICU to assist at bedside
	Consider chief surgical fellow as additional resource

TABLE 91.6

RN REASSESSMENT

RN documentation	
q15min	HR, RR, BP
	Oxygen saturation
q30min	Mental status
	Respiratory effort
	Capillary refill
	Quality of pulses
	Skin temperature
q60min	Temperature
	I/O

After initial education is complete, pathway-specific education is incorporated. Initial nursing actions should be discussed with attention to timing of procedures. Difficult IV access algorithms should be reviewed for appropriate escalation of care. Goal antibiotic and fluid administration times are key, with emphasis placed on concurrent administration, IV push of antibiotics, and use of push–pull, pressure bag or rapid infuser for rapid resuscitation. Additional patient safety considerations include continued monitoring for change in patient status and trending of resuscitation measures.

Quality Measurement

Consistent with prior published data, since implementation of this pathway, time to antibiotics and IV fluid resuscitation has improved. Example statistical process control charts for median time to initial IV antibiotic and for proportion of patients receiving initial IV antibiotic within 60 minutes are shown in Figure 91.3. Hospital and ICU length of stay has also decreased as number of patients with sepsis diagnosed within 24 hours of hospital admission.

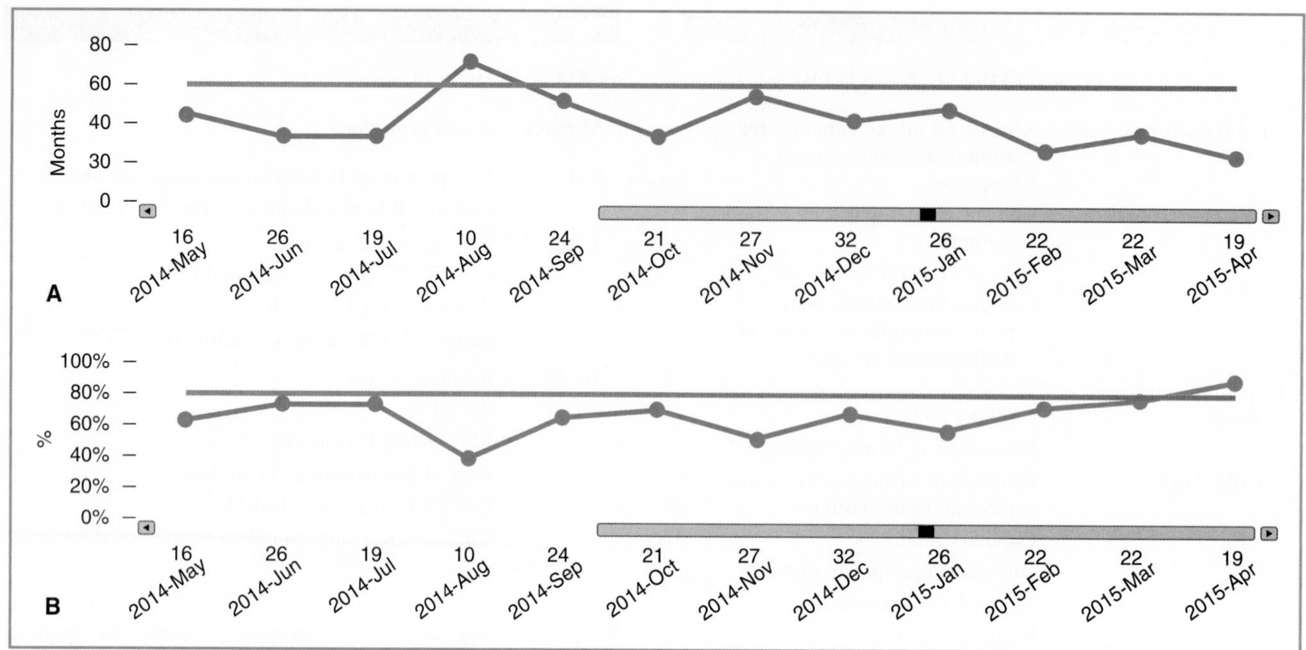

FIGURE 91.3 **A:** Median minutes from sepsis recognition to initial IV antibiotic administration. **B:** Proportion of patients receiving initial IV antibiotics within 60 minutes of sepsis recognition.

Next Steps

Next steps include continued efforts to improve timeliness of antibiotic and fluid administration, tracking of patient level morbidity outcomes such as organ dysfunction, and continued improvement in sepsis recognition in the ED to decrease patients diagnosed with sepsis within the first 24 hours following ED visit.

Suggested Readings and Key References

Balamuth F, Weiss SL, Neuman MI, et al. Pediatric severe sepsis in US children's hospitals. *Pediatr Crit Care Med* 2014;15(9):798–805.

Carcillo JA, Davis AL, Zaritsky A. Role of early fluid resuscitation in pediatric septic shock. *JAMA* 1991;266(9):1242–1245.

Cruz AT, Perry AM, Williams EA, et al. Implementation of goal-directed therapy for children with suspected sepsis in the emergency department. *Pediatrics* 2011;127(3):e758–e766.

Cruz AT, Williams EA, Graf JM, et al. Test characteristics of an automated age- and temperature-adjusted tachycardia alert in pediatric septic shock. *Pediatr Emerg Care* 2012;28(9):889–894.

Dellinger RP, Levy MM, Rhodes A, et al; Surviving Sepsis Campaign Guidelines Committee including the Pediatric Subgroup. Surviving sepsis campaign: international guidelines for management of severe sepsis and septic shock: 2012. *Crit Care Med* 2013;41(2):580–637.

Goldstein B, Giroir B, Randolph A; International Consensus Conference on Pediatric Sepsis. International pediatric sepsis consensus conference: definitions for sepsis and organ dysfunction in pediatrics. *Pediatr Crit Care Med* 2005;6(1):2–8.

Goldstein B, Giroir B, Randolph A. Reply: values for systolic blood pressure. *Pediatr Crit Care Med* 2005;6(4):500–501.

Hartman ME, Linde-Zwirble WT, Angus DC, et al. Trends in the epidemiology of pediatric severe sepsis. *Pediatr Crit Care Med* 2013; 14(7):686–693.

Larsen GY, Mecham N, Greenberg R. An emergency department septic shock protocol and care guideline for children initiated at triage. *Pediatrics* 2011;127(6):e1585–e1592.

Odetola FO, Gebremariam A, Freed GL. Patient and hospital correlates of clinical outcomes and resource utilization in severe pediatric sepsis. *Pediatrics* 2007;119(3):487–494.

Paul R, Melendez E, Stack A, et al. Improving adherence to PALS septic shock guidelines. *Pediatrics* 2014;133(5):e1358–e1366.

Paul R, Neuman MI, Monuteaux MC, et al. Adherence to PALS sepsis guidelines and hospital length of stay. *Pediatrics* 2012;130(2): e273–e280.

Scott HF, Donoghue AJ, Gaieski DF, et al. The utility of early lactate testing in undifferentiated pediatric systemic inflammatory response syndrome. *Acad Emerg Med* 2012;19(11):1276–1280.

Weiss SL, Fitzgerald JC, Balamuth F, et al. Delayed antimicrobial therapy increases mortality and organ dysfunction duration in pediatric sepsis. *Crit Care Med* 2014;42(11):2409–2417.

CHAPTER 92 ■ UTI, FEBRILE

KATHY SHAW, MD, MSCE, MERCEDES M. BLACKSTONE, MD, PATRICIA LOPEZ, MSN, CRNP, AND CHRISTINE ROPER, BSN, RN

BACKGROUND (EPIDEMIOLOGY, EVIDENCE)

Acute pyelonephritis is currently the most common serious bacterial infection in childhood yet is difficult to detect on history or physical examination as symptoms are nonspecific. In the nonverbal infant or young child in diapers, fever is the primary finding. Although the risk of sepsis is small outside the neonatal period, it is not zero, with estimates as high as 3% in febrile infants 2 to 24 months. Early detection and treatment with antibiotics relieves symptoms and halts progression of disease as measured by nuclear renal scans done at time of diagnosis and improvement in inflammatory markers. There remains uncertainty in the relationship between childhood UTI and risk of end-stage renal failure based on current data, but there is general agreement that timely diagnosis and treatment of UTI in febrile infants is important.

Clinicians should be selective in screening young febrile children for UTI to avoid the consequences of false-positive tests, unnecessary catheterization, treatment, and imaging. Empiric treatment should be based upon results of the initial urine screen results. An understanding of specific risk factors for UTI in individual young febrile children helps the clinician to reduce unnecessary testing.

The 2011 guidelines from the American Academy of Pediatrics support using predictive models to rationally determine which young febrile children should be tested, using evidence-based predictors including height and duration of fever, sex, race, other potential sources for the infant's fever, and circumcision status. This clinical pathway uses the predictive model by Gorelick and Shaw to help the clinician determine the pretest probability of UTI for a given child and whether screening is indicated. This selective approach allows one to avoid undesirable extremes—indiscriminately obtaining urine on all febrile children resulting in increased cost at little additional benefit, or the overly restrictive approach of not screening until the child presents with fever for 4 to 5 days.

Screening for UTI can be painful, time-consuming, and costly. This pathway describes a two-step approach to screening febrile children 6 to 24 months of age. Initially, a urine bag is placed to obtain urine for screening. A point-of-care (POC) urine dipstick is performed on children meeting specific criteria. If the urine screen is positive, urethral catheterization is performed to obtain sterile urine for culture. Urine specimens obtained via bag should not be sent for culture due to high contamination rates. Evidence supports the use of the urine dipstick; it performs as well as a standard urinalysis at less cost and yields a more timely result. Using specific values of moderate (2+) or large leukocyte esterase (3+) *or* presence of nitrites as threshold for obtaining a culture reduces the catheterization and false-positive rates. This two-step screening process allowed for a decrease in catheterization rates from 70% to <30% for screening in febrile children without increasing our ED length of stay.

PATHWAY GOALS AND MEASUREMENT

Goal

The goals of this clinical pathway are to standardize the following:

- Recommendations for screening for UTI in febrile children
- Urine collection and testing methods
  - Decrease number of unnecessary invasive catheterizations
  - Ensure bag specimens are not sent for culture
- Indications and antibiotic recommendations for empiric treatment

Measurements

- Febrile children <2 years of age are appropriately screened for UTI
- POC testing by urine dipstick is performed, not laboratory urinalysis
- Urine obtained for culture by correct method per age and toilet-training status
- Appropriate empiric treatment based on UA results with correct antibiotic

Algorithm and Key Hyperlinks

See Figure 92.1 (http://www.chop.edu/clinical-pathway/febrile-uti-clinicalpathway)

Associated Pathways

- Chapter 91 Shock (http://www.chop.edu/clinical-pathway/severe-sepsis-clinicalpathway-infants-28-days-age-and-children)
- Chapter 82 Abdominal Pain in Postpubertal Girls (http://www.chop.edu/clinical-pathway/lower-abdominalpain-clinical-pathway-post-pubertal-girls)

PATIENT POPULATIONS/ STRATIFYING PATIENT RISKS

This pathway provides recommendations for the screening of infants >56 days and children through 18 years of age, with fever >38°C for possible UTI. These recommendations should not be used for patients with known urinary tract abnormality, neurogenic bladder, immunodeficiency, or recent GU surgery.

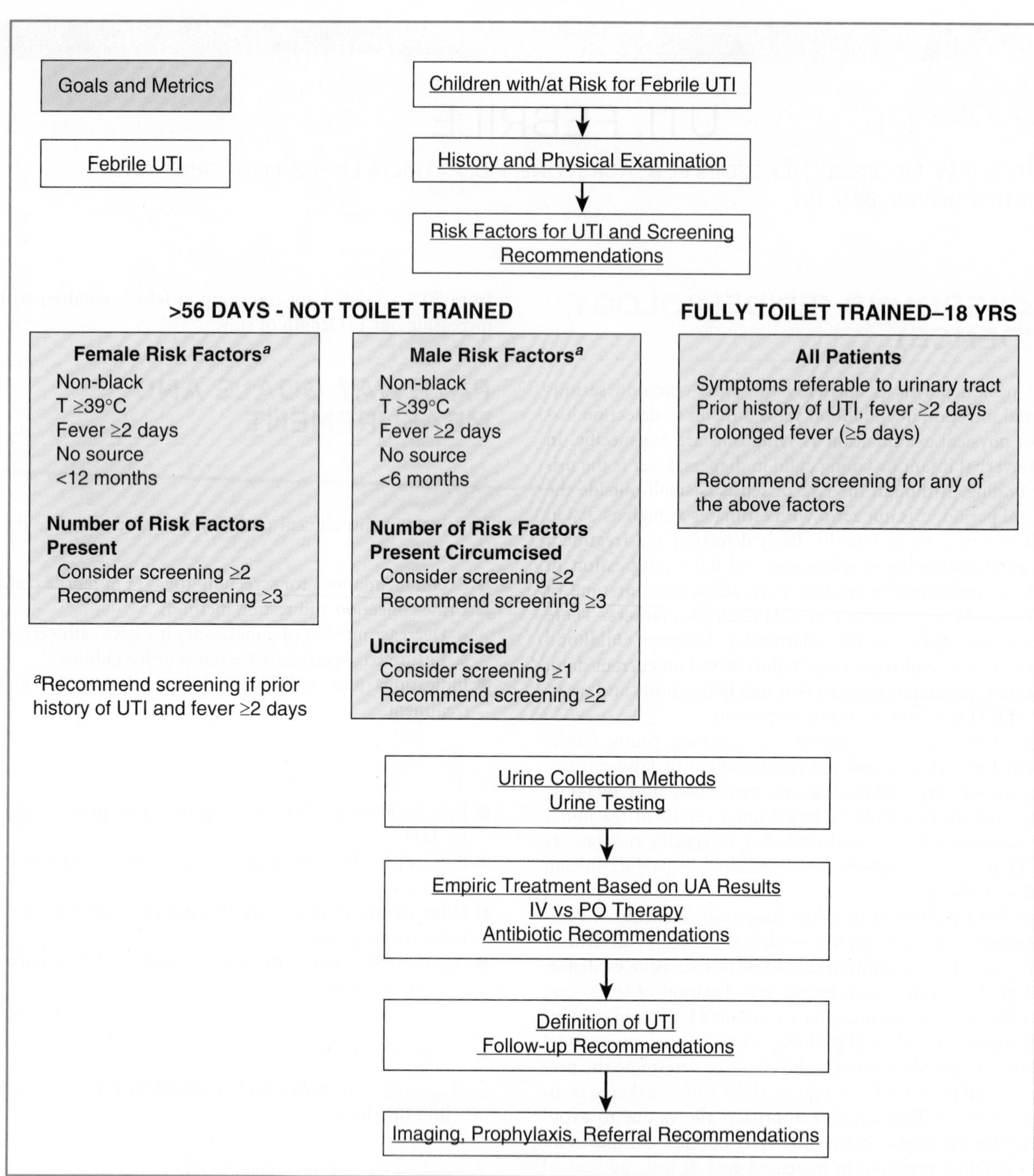

FIGURE 92.1 Pathway for the evaluation and treatment of children with febrile UTI. *Pathway Authors: K. Shaw, MD; N. Plachter, CRNP; J. Lavelle, MD; T. Kolon, MD; M. Carr, MD; R. Keren, MD; R. Patel, MD; M. Dunne, MD; J. Kim, MD; J. Gerber, MD; M. Pradhan, MD; K. Ota, MD; C. Jacobstein, MD; K. McGowan, PhD; T. Metjian, PharmD.*

Prospective epidemiologic studies have identified risk factors for UTI which can help stratify risk in febrile young children. Consider the following risk factors for young febrile children >56 days of age who are not yet toilet trained:

- White race
- Fever ≥39°C
- Fever for ≥2 days
- No other source of infection
- Young age (<12 months for females, <6 months for males)

To maximize sensitivity and specificity, the pathway recommends the following approach:

- Screening should be considered if two risk factors are present and it is recommended if ≥3 are present.
- Since uncircumcised males have an increased risk of infection especially in the first year of life, screening should be considered if one risk factor is present and recommended if two to three are present.

Identifying a definite source of infection is challenging. Children with unequivocal sources for their fever such as

TABLE 92.1

URINE COLLECTION METHODS

Patients who are not fully toilet trained	
Bagged urine specimens	Can be used for screening UA in >6 mo of age NEVER use for culture If UA positive, obtain a catheterized specimen for culture
Catheterization	Optimal method to obtain urine for culture in children who are not fully toilet trained
Suprapubic tap	Requires US guidance May be useful in children when catheterization fails, for example, uncircumcised, abnormal urethra or fused labia
Patients who are fully toilet trained	
Clean catch	Fully toilet trained defined as no daytime accidents, no pull-ups at night/dry, and no history of constipation

pneumonia, cellulitis, etc. or recognizable clinical syndromes such as roseola or Kawasaki rarely require screening. For those with nonspecific viral syndromes, the clinician is left to decide whether or not that constitutes the source of the current fever. (See Table 92.1)

URINE TESTING

- Dipstick should be performed within 1 hour.
- Dipstick is the preferred screening method and is as good as a formal UA when done correctly.
- Do not send a urinalysis if the dipstick is negative.
- All specimens obtained by catheterization or suprapubic tap should be sent for culture.
- If Dipstick or UA from clean catch is negative, a urine culture should NOT be sent.

Cleansing the Perineum

Baby wipes are the preferred method of reducing contamination with clean-catch or urine bag specimens.

Supervision of cleansing and midstream clean catch may help reduce contamination rates that are reported to be as high as 50% in young children (2 to 6 years old).

Urine Test Results

See Table 92.2 for additional information.

TABLE 92.2

EMPIRIC ANTIBIOTIC TREATMENT BASED ON URINALYSIS RESULTS

Use the following criteria to empirically treat for UTI:	
Dipstick	Positive nitrite *OR* LE 2+/3+
Standard UA	>5 WBC/hpf AND bacteria

TABLE 92.3

EMPIRIC ANTIBIOTIC RECOMMENDATIONS

	First line	Beta-lactam allergy	Duration/ comments
Outpatient	Cephalexin	Trimethoprim-sulfamethoxazole Sulfa allergy: ciprofloxacin	<6 mo 10 days ≥6 mo 7 days
Inpatient	Ampicillin *plus* gentamicin	Gentamicin alone	Gentamicin levels are not necessary unless treatment >48 hrs

Uncircumcised Males with Phimosis

Consider treatment with betamethasone 0.05% cream twice daily for 4 weeks or refer to Urology.

EMPIRIC ANTIBIOTIC RECOMMENDATIONS

- Consider initial IV treatment if <6 months of age, moderate/severe dehydration, inability to tolerate PO fluids, antibiotics or concern for follow-up.
- If previous UTI, review organism sensitivities.
- If patient is on prophylaxis, do not use the same antibiotic for treatment.
- See Table 92.3

The diagnosis of UTI requires an abnormal urine test *and* growth of a urinary pathogen. (See Tables 92.4 and 92.5)

ALL urine cultures need careful follow-up.

Patients Treated Empirically

- Check urine culture results.
- If positive, review sensitivities, change antibiotic as needed, assure response to therapy within 48 hours.
- Educate family about follow-up for future febrile illnesses.
- If negative, discontinue antibiotics, inform family that child did not have UTI.

TABLE 92.4

DEFINITION OF UTI

Specimen	Definite cfu/mL	Possible cfu/mL
Catheterization	>50,000	>10,000
Clean catch	>100,000	>50,000

TABLE 92.5

COMMON URINARY TRACT PATHOGENS AND CONTAMINANTS

Urine pathogens		Common contaminants
E. coli, *Proteus* sp.	*Klebsiella* sp.	*Lactobacillus* sp.
Enterococcus sp.	*Enterobacter* sp.	*Corynebacterium* sp.
Pseudomonas sp.	Group B streptococci	Coagulase-negative staphylococci
Serratia sp.	*Staphylococcus aureus*	Alpha-hemolytic streptococci
Corynebacterium urealyticum		

Positive Urine Cultures

- Review sensitivities.
- Assure appropriate antibiotic therapy and response to treatment within 48 hours.
- Educate family about follow-up for future febrile illnesses.

Negative Urine Cultures

Inform family that the patient did not have a UTI.

CLINICAL DECISION SUPPORT

The electronic UTI order set includes a preselected POC urine dip order. If there is a positive urine dip (moderate or large leukocytes and/or positive nitrites), a urine culture is ordered.

First-line empiric antibiotic recommendations are based on medication allergies and prior organisms and sensitivities among those with prior UTIs and local prevalence. Routine laboratory testing, including blood culture, CBC, CRP, and BMP are not recommended unless there are other concerns (i.e., urosepsis).

Follow-Up Recommendations

A process for review of culture results and patient follow-up is key (Table 92.6). For those started on empiric therapy, it is important to inform the family of negative urine culture results and discontinue antibiotics. For this circumstance, an electronic order is placed to notify the nurse practitioner so the family can be notified even if the culture results are negative. At the time of follow-up, the urine test results, the organism, colony count, and sensitivities are reviewed to make recommendations regarding treatment. If the diagnosis of UTI is made, the need for follow-up is reinforced with their primary care provider for further management.

Communication/Teamwork

Informed clinical providers who work as a team and communicate well are essential for prompt screening of febrile children for urinary tract infection and subsequent timely patient disposition. Identification of patients meeting screening criteria should occur at the earliest possible point of patient contact to expedite care in the ED. As such, the bedside RN may

TABLE 92.6

PATIENT FOLLOW-UP BASED ON URINE TEST AND URINE CULTURE RESULTS

UA results	Culture results	Recommendation	Follow-up
UA meets criteria for empiric treatment	Cfu criteria met with pathogen	Check sensitivities, treat 7–10 days	RBUS
	Cfu criteria not met but pathogen present	Check sensitivities, treat 7–10 days	RBUS
	Contaminant or negative	Stop treatment	
UA positive but does not meet empiric treatment criteria	Cfu criteria met with pathogen	Check sensitivities, treat 7–10 days	RBUS
	Cfu criteria not met but pathogen present	Check patient Febrile, check sensitivities, treat 7–10 days Afebrile, no treatment	RBUS
UA negative	Cfu criteria met with pathogen or Cfu criteria not met but pathogen present	Check patient Febrile, repeat specimen Afebrile, no treatment (Asymptomatic bacteriuria)	
	Contaminant	No treatment	

initiate specimen retrieval procedures prior to MD evaluation. Nursing and frontline clinicians then partner to determine need for urine test and culture. If unable to obtain urine in a timely manner, the need for additional interventions or alternative screening methods are discussed by the team.

Nurse-Specific Education

ED nurses should be educated on febrile UTI pathway inclusion criteria and applicable interventions. Nurses must identify patients >56 days of age with symptoms concerning for a UTI and initiate age and developmentally indicated screening techniques as described in the pathway. Pertinent patient–family education and appropriate urine collection materials must be provided to maintain specimen integrity and comprehensive care. Urethral catheterization is the recommended method for urine collection for children less than 6 months of age, while initial urine collection by placing a urine bag is appropriate for older, non–toilet-trained children. Parents are encouraged to participate in their child's care by offering the patient oral fluids and are given the call bell to alert the nurse when urine is present in the bag so the sample can be collected and tested in a timely manner. They also need to be alerted to the fact that a urine catheterization will be indicated for culture if the urine screen is positive. For toilet-trained children and teenagers a clean-catch sample is collected after explaining how to utilize the hospital-approved cleansing agent to clean the perineum and then collecting a midstream urine sample in the provided sterile container. The ED RN should adhere to hospital-specific procedural standards for urine collection via catheterization and clean catch. When utilizing a urine bag for screening, nurses should position patients to thoroughly clean the perineum with hospital-approved cleansing agent and utilize a no-sting barrier to ensure adequate bag adhesion, preventing specimen loss and contamination. For patients who can be discharged, nurses should provide appropriate anticipatory guidance for care and follow-up, as well as preventative techniques.

Quality Measurement

The ED team conducted a continuous quality-improvement project between October 18, 2013 and March 8, 2014 with the aim of reducing catheterization rates by first screening with a urine bag. Data showed a marked and steady reduction of catheterization rate from a baseline of 70% (2,759/3,943) to 24% (43/179) over a 4-month period with no change in the revisit rate, no missed UTIs in the subset followed in our healthcare system, no urine cultures inappropriately sent from bagged specimens, or increased ED length of stay (296 minutes for patients screened with bag vs. 321 minutes for those screened with catheterization). An unintended positive effect was an increase in POC testing (47% vs. 65%). During this time, more than 350 children have been safely spared a catheterization. Initial screening by means of urine bag placement was shown to successfully reduce unnecessary catheterization in febrile infants without increasing ED LOS or decreasing screening or detection of febrile UTI in this high-risk group. We intentionally excluded infants less than 6 months of age as no screening test is 100% accurate, and this group is at higher risk for both UTI and its morbidity.

Next Steps

The ED physician must set expectations if the diagnosis of UTI is confirmed by the culture results. At present, only a renal bladder ultrasound is indicated for most patients with first-time uncomplicated acute pyelonephritis. Next steps include adherence to recommended empiric treatment recommendations as well as to potentially decrease unnecessary radiographic screening studies.

Suggested Readings and Key References

Al-Orifi F, McGillivray D, Tange S, et al. Urine culture from bag specimens in young children: are the risks too high? *J Pediatr* 2000; 137:221–226.

American Academy of Pediatrics Subcommittee on Urinary Tract Infection, Steering Committee on Quality Improvement and Management, Roberts KB. Urinary tract infection: clinical practice guideline for the diagnosis and management of the initial UTI in febrile infants and children 2 to 24 months. *Pediatrics* 2011;128(3): 595–610.

Gorelick MH, Hoberman A, Kearney D, et al. Validation of a decision rule identifying febrile young girls at high risk for urinary tract infection. *Pediatr Emerg Care* 2003;19(3):162–164.

Gorelick MH, Shaw KN. Clinical decision rule to identify febrile young girls at risk for urinary tract infection. *Arch Pediatr Adolesc Med* 2000;154(4):386–390.

Hoberman A, Chao HP, Keller DM, et al. Prevalence of urinary tract infection in febrile infants. *J Pediatr* 1993;123(1):17–23.

Hoberman A, Wald ER, Hickey RW, et al. Oral versus initial intravenous therapy for urinary tract infections in young febrile children. *Pediatrics* 1999;104(1 pt 1):79–86.

Montini G, Tullus K, Hewitt I. Febrile urinary tract infections in children. *N Engl J Med* 2011;365:239–250.

Round J, Fitzgerald AC, Hulme C, et al. Urinary tract infections in children and the risk of ESRF. *Acta Peadiatr* 2012;101:278–282.

Shaikh N, Morone NE, Lopez J, et al. Does this child have a urinary tract infection? *JAMA* 2007;298(24):2895–2904.

Shaw KN. Call for a rational approach for testing for urinary tract infection as a source of fever in infants. *Ann Emerg Med* 2013; 61(5):566–568.

Shaw KN, Gorelick M, McGowan KL, et al. Prevalence of urinary tract infection in febrile young children in the emergency department. *Pediatrics* 1998;102(2):e16. Available at: www.pediatrics.org/cgi/content/full/102/2/e16.

Shaw KN, McGowan KL, Gorelick MH, et al. Screening for urinary tract infection in infants in the emergency department: which test is best? *Pediatrics* 1998;101(6):E1.

CHAPTER 93 ■ ALLERGIC EMERGENCIES

MICHELLE D. STEVENSON, MD, MS, FAAP AND RICHARD M. RUDDY, MD

GOALS OF EMERGENCY THERAPY

- Rapid treatment with epinephrine (intramuscularly, lateral thigh) is imperative in anaphylaxis to reverse shock and respiratory distress.
- Hereditary angioedema management should include rapid, controlled airway management in cases of laryngeal edema, with prompt administration of C_1-esterase inhibitor concentrate (or alternative therapy) to reduce the risk of morbidity and mortality due to acute attacks.
- The goals of treatment of serum sickness include removal of antigen exposure (if known), control of painful arthralgias and pruritis through nonsteroidal anti-inflammatory drugs (NSAIDs) and antihistamines, and appropriate monitoring for organ dysfunction (particularly renal involvement).
- Although there is a paucity of comparative effectiveness data in children, intranasal corticosteroids are often considered to be a first-line agent in symptom management for allergic rhinitis. Oral nonsedating antihistamines and oral montelukast are common alternative therapies.

RELATED CHAPTERS

Signs and Symptoms
- Edema: Chapter 20
- Eye: Red Eye: Chapter 22
- Rash: Papulosquamous Eruptions: Chapter 65
- Sore Throat: Chapter 69
- Stridor: Chapter 70
- Wheezing: Chapter 80

Clinical Pathways
- Shock: Chapter 91

Medical Emergencies
- Dermatologic Urgencies and Emergencies: Chapter 96
- Pulmonary Emergencies: Chapter 107

ANAPHYLAXIS

Goals of Treatment

Early recognition, aggressive support of respiratory and circulatory compromise, and immediate treatment with intramuscular epinephrine in the lateral thigh are essential goals in the evaluation and treatment of anaphylaxis.

CLINICAL PEARLS AND PITFALLS

- Anaphylaxis is a life-threatening emergency which is not rare.
- Stridor, hoarseness, respiratory distress, and hypotension require rapid intervention.
- Delayed administration of intramuscular epinephrine is associated with an increased risk of morbidity and mortality.
- Most, but not all children with anaphylaxis will experience skin manifestations such as urticaria, which may be transient or masked by medications.
- Hypotension or shock may be present, but absence of circulatory compromise does not exclude the diagnosis of anaphylaxis, especially in children.
- Diphenhydramine and corticosteroids are not considered first line, but rather adjunctive therapy in the management of anaphylaxis due to lack of data regarding efficacy.

Current Evidence

Anaphylaxis is a potentially life-threatening manifestation of immediate hypersensitivity. The severity of these reactions varies from mild urticaria to shock and death. Anaphylaxis most commonly involves the pulmonary, circulatory, cutaneous, gastrointestinal (GI), and central neurologic systems.

The classic anaphylactic response is an IgE-mediated reaction that occurs after reexposure to an antigen to which the patient has previously been sensitized. The term *anaphylactoid reaction* is sometimes used to refer to a clinically similar syndrome that is not IgE mediated and does not necessarily require previous exposure to the inciting agent. It has become a common practice to use *anaphylaxis* to describe the clinical syndrome, regardless of the responsible mechanism. Although the mortality rate for children <18 years is low (estimated at 0.1 per million population), anaphylaxis causes approximately 20,000 emergency department (ED) visits per year in the United States across all age groups.

Any route of exposure, including parenteral, oral, or inhalation, has been associated with anaphylaxis. Food allergens represent the most common inciting agents among children in the United States with exposure most often occurring outside medical facilities. Other common triggers include hymenoptera

TABLE 93.1

COMMON CAUSES OF ANAPHYLAXIS

Insect venom
Hymenoptera
Fire ants
Drugs
Antibiotics—penicillin, cephalosporins, sulfonamides
Anesthesia-related drugs—lidocaine, neuromuscular blocking agents
Aspirin
Radiocontrast media
Foods
Peanuts
Cashews
Other tree nuts
Milk
Seafood—shellfish
Grains
Fruit
Blood products
Immunotherapy
Allergen extracts
Other
Latex
Idiopathic

stings, drugs, immunotherapy, radiocontrast media, and blood products (Table 93.1). The causative agent for anaphylaxis goes undetected in a significant proportion of cases.

Certain conditions are known to increase the risk of severe or fatal anaphylaxis. Systemic mastocytosis is a risk factor for severe anaphylaxis due to hymenoptera stings and venom subcutaneous immunotherapy. Peanut, cashew, and other tree nut triggers, especially when consumed outside the home environment, represent an important risk factor. Adolescents appear to be at the greatest risk for death, possibly due to risk-taking behavior. Asthma is also a worrisome historical feature in patients presenting with anaphylaxis, as is a delay in epinephrine administration. Most patients with a fatal reaction to a food have a history of an allergy to the specific food allergen trigger, but the severity of prior reactions may have been quite different.

During IgE-mediated anaphylaxis, IgE binds to high-affinity receptors on mast cells and basophils. The resultant sudden release of numerous mediators is presumed to be responsible for the pathophysiologic features of anaphylaxis (bronchospasm, increased vascular permeability, and altered systemic and pulmonary vascular smooth muscle tone). The most notable of these mediators is histamine, but others that have been implicated include prostaglandin D2, leukotrienes, anaphylatoxins (C3, C4a, C5a), platelet-activating factor (PAF), heparin, tryptase, and chymase. Levels of serum PAF, a proinflammatory phospholipid, are often elevated in patients with anaphylaxis and correlate with symptom severity.

Certain agents can stimulate the release of mediators directly by an unknown mechanism that does not involve IgE or complement. Agents capable of direct stimulation include hyperosmolar solutions such as mannitol and radiocontrast media. Other causes of apparent anaphylaxis have less clear mechanisms. These include reactions after the ingestion of aspirin and other NSAIDs and exercise-induced anaphylaxis in which vigorous exercise, often preceded by an allergenic food such as wheat or shellfish, is the trigger.

Clinical Considerations

Clinical Recognition

The time between exposure to the inciting agent and onset of symptoms can vary from minutes to hours, although epidemiologic data suggest that most children will experience symptoms within 30 minutes. Guidelines from multiple national and international allergy societies state that anaphylaxis is highly likely under any of the following circumstances: (1) Sudden onset of skin (e.g., urticaria, periorbital erythema, pruritus, flushing) and/or mucous membrane (e.g., oral/uvula swelling) changes in combination with either (a) acute respiratory symptoms (e.g., wheezing, stridor, or hypoxia) or (b) hypotension or signs of end-organ dysfunction (e.g., fainting/incontinence); (2) sudden involvement of at least two body organ systems after exposure to a likely allergen or trigger for that patient (skin/mucosa, GI, respiratory tract, central nervous system [CNS], or circulatory system); or (3) age-specific hypotension (or >30% decline in systolic blood pressure) after exposure to a known allergen.

Skin manifestations usually emerge first but may be absent. GI symptoms are relatively common and include nausea, vomiting, diarrhea, and crampy abdominal pain. Swelling of the lips or tongue can potentially impair swallowing and ventilation. An immediate life-threatening feature of anaphylaxis is upper airway obstruction that results from edema of the larynx, epiglottis, and other surrounding structures. Airway involvement may manifest either as subtle discomfort or pruritus of the throat, or as obvious stridor and respiratory distress. Anaphylaxis can also cause lower airway disease secondary to bronchospasm. This leads to findings similar to acute asthma, such as a sense of chest tightness, cough, dyspnea, wheezing, and retractions.

Another potential life-threatening feature of anaphylaxis is cardiovascular collapse and hypotensive shock. Arrhythmias and electrocardiographic evidence of myocardial ischemia may also be seen. These features are less commonly seen in anaphylaxis among children compared to adults. CNS involvement can include dizziness, syncope, seizures, and an altered level of consciousness.

Triage Considerations

Because evaluation and management of anaphylaxis is time sensitive, rapid identification and triage of patients presenting with signs and symptoms concerning for anaphylaxis is critical to minimize morbidity and mortality. Vital signs, pulse oximetry, and cardiopulmonary status should be immediately assessed upon arrival to the ED in children presenting with a possible "allergic reaction." After ensuring a patent airway, supplemental oxygen should be administered if respiratory compromise is present or anaphylaxis is highly likely. Patients with circulatory compromise should be placed in the Trendelenburg position. Potential triggers should be immediately removed. Standardized protocols and immediate assembly of rescue or resuscitation teams can assist with appropriate, rapid management of affected patients. Cardiopulmonary resuscitation may be necessary in severe cases. Change in voice, difficulty in swallowing, dyspnea, and a sense of impending doom are characteristics of potentially serious anaphylaxis.

Clinical Assessment

After a rapid cardiopulmonary assessment and appropriate interventions have been initiated (see Fig. 93.1 and Management section), a more detailed assessment should be performed. The history should be directed toward determining the nature and severity of the reaction, the rapidity with which symptoms evolved, the management prior to arrival, and the evidence of ongoing progression.

Attempts should also be made to determine the offending agent. The history should focus on the 1- to 2-hour period

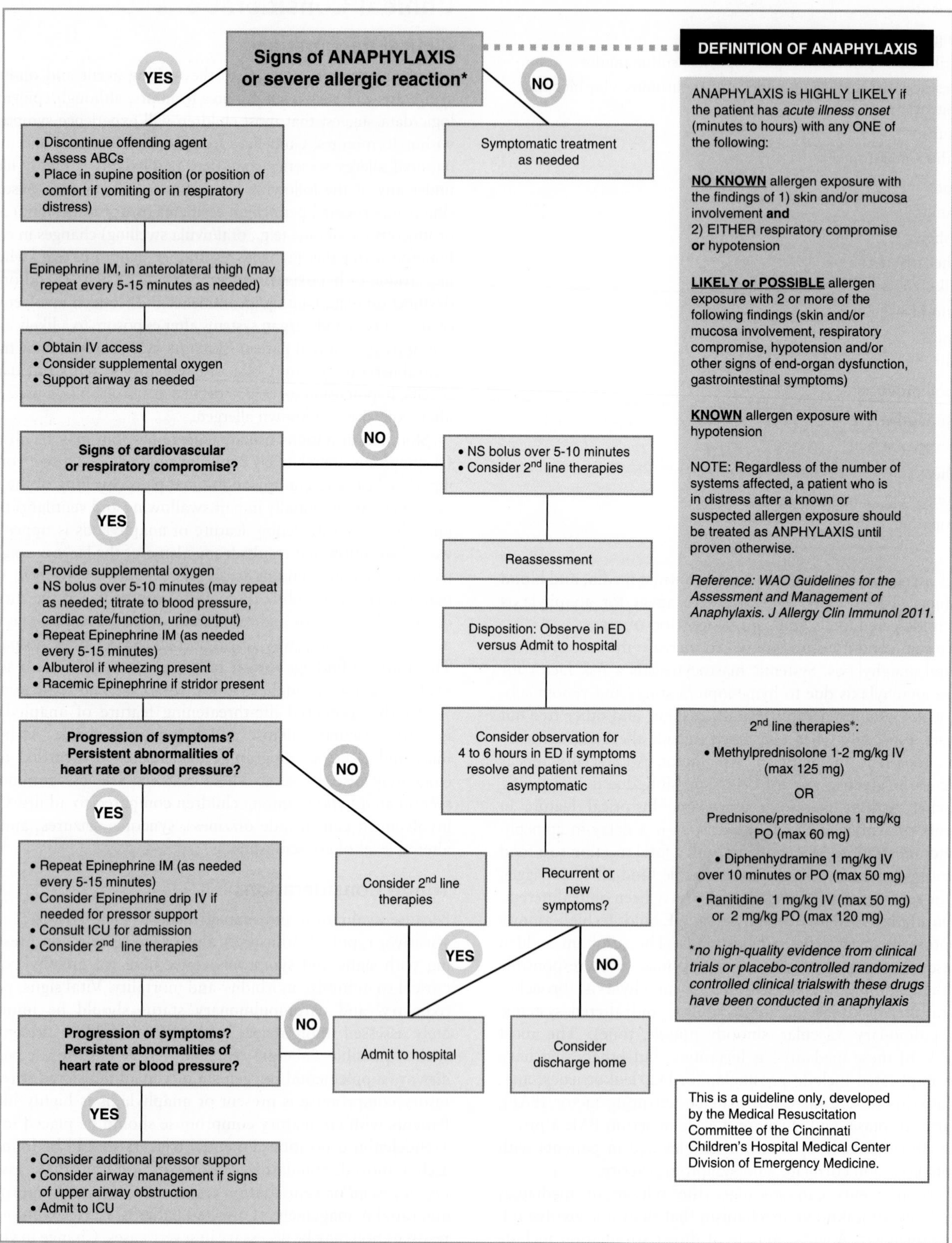

FIGURE 93.1 Anaphylaxis pathway. (From the guidelines established by the Medical Resuscitation Committee of the Cincinnati Children's Hospital Medical Center Division of Emergency Medicine.)

before the onset of symptoms. While there may be history of an obvious sting or drug exposure, the association of anaphylactic reactions with food is often confusing. Although patients often identify a particular food as the cause, a more detailed history may implicate something else in the meal. For example, it is common to associate reactions with chocolate whereas the nuts in many chocolate preparations generally are the offending agents. Many patients will not have a prior history of reaction to the ingested trigger.

Factors that may place the child at increased risk for a severe reaction should also be ascertained. These include a personal history of asthma or atopic disease or a previous allergic reaction. Although not commonly used in children, certain medications such as β-blockers, calcium channel blockers, and angiotensin-converting enzyme inhibitors may make anaphylaxis more severe or difficult to manage. Nonsteroid anti-inflammatory medications, ethanol ingestion, and concurrent respiratory illness may also exacerbate symptoms of anaphylaxis.

Anaphylaxis remains a diagnosis based upon clinical assessment. Although serum tryptase can be measured and may assist with the diagnosis of anaphylaxis in reactions in some cases, its suboptimal sensitivity and specificity, particularly in food-associated anaphylaxis, does not support routine use of this biomarker for confirmatory testing. Levels should only be considered if the diagnosis is uncertain, and appropriate follow-up of results can be assured. PAF measurements appear to have limited potential utility due to the transient nature of its elevation.

Management

Management of a life-threatening anaphylactic reaction requires simultaneous evaluation and management of the airway, breathing, and circulation, as well as the immediate administration of intramuscular epinephrine, preferably within 5 minutes. Any known trigger (e.g., intravenous medication) should be discontinued or removed promptly.

Epinephrine, the first-line drug for anaphylaxis, should be administered as soon as possible. There is no absolute contraindication for its use in anaphylaxis. Intramuscular epinephrine is indicated when anaphylaxis is highly likely or strongly suspected. It should be considered for any patient who experiences an isolated cutaneous reaction (e.g., urticaria, flushing) who also has risk factors for fatal anaphylaxis, or who has a history of a near-fatal episode, particularly when a known trigger is present. The recommendation to administer it sooner, rather than later, in the course of anaphylaxis comes from the increased likelihood of a fatal reaction among patients who receive delayed administration of epinephrine.

As an α-adrenergic agonist, epinephrine promotes vasoconstriction, which increases blood pressure and decreases capillary leakage. As a β-adrenergic agonist, it relaxes bronchial smooth muscle, increases cardiac rate and contractility, and inhibits further mediator release. Epinephrine should be administered via intramuscular injection to the thigh as a 1:1,000 solution (1 mg per mL), at a dose of 0.01 mg per kg (maximum 0.5 mL in adults, 0.3 mL in children). At some centers, pharmacy or ED storage of epinephrine 1:1,000 is not maintained, so sites have kept EPIPEN Jr (0.15 mg) and EPIPEN (0.3 mg) in the departments for convenience and safety, administering the full amount if <15 kg or >15 kg respectively. Epinephrine doses may be repeated every 5 to 15 minutes for persistent or recurrent symptoms. There is clear evidence that absorption is more rapid and peak plasma levels are greater when epinephrine is administered via the intramuscular route compared to subcutaneously.

If the patient is hypotensive or significantly hypoperfused, or if multiple intramuscular doses are ineffective, epinephrine should be administered intravenously or through an interosseous needle as a 1:10,000 solution, at a dose of 0.01 mg per kg (maximum 0.1 mL per kg) slowly *over 1 to 2 minutes.* In severe cases, this may need to be followed by a continuous epinephrine infusion of 0.1 μg/kg/min, which can be titrated to effect up to a maximum dose of 1 μg/kg/min. Inhaled epinephrine does not achieve adequate plasma levels and should not be substituted for the intramuscular dose during initial therapy for anaphylaxis. Ventricular arrhythmias, pulmonary edema, and hypertensive crises may be seen with epinephrine overdose.

Maintenance of the Airway

The physician should administer maximal supplemental oxygen, with bag-valve-mask ventilation when indicated, to assist ventilation. If there is complete airway obstruction, preparation for immediate endotracheal intubation should parallel the rapid administration of epinephrine, which can mitigate or ease the airway management. If intubation is unsuccessful, cricothyrotomy (in an older child) or percutaneous transtracheal ventilation (younger child) offers a lifesaving alternative to bypassing upper airway edema causing obstruction.

Maintenance of the Circulation

Hypotensive patients should be placed in the Trendelenburg position, and a rapid bolus of 20 mL per kg of a crystalloid solution of normal saline should be administered and repeated as necessary. Decreased plasma volume from fluid leak and profound vasodilation with resultant increases in intravascular capacity may result in the need for large amounts of fluid. If hypotension persists after epinephrine administration, normal saline boluses, and positioning, a continuous infusion of epinephrine should be started as previously described. Other vasopressors may be considered for refractory anaphylaxis, and anticholinergics and glucagon may be beneficial in patients taking a β-adrenergic blocking medication.

Other Therapy

Recent systematic reviews have revealed a striking paucity of studies that examine adjunctive therapies such as antihistamines or glucocorticoids in the management of anaphylaxis. Based on evidence surrounding the treatment of asthma, it is reasonable to treat bronchospasm associated with anaphylaxis with inhaled β_2-agonists such as albuterol and systemic glucocorticoids.

Glucocorticoids do not take effect during the initial resuscitative phase of anaphylaxis. Their role in preventing biphasic reactions is unclear, but glucocorticoids are frequently recommended because of known efficacy for other allergic diseases. They can be administered as methylprednisolone 1 to 2 mg per kg IV (maximum 125 mg) or, for mild symptoms, prednisone 0.5 to 1 mg per kg by mouth (maximum 60 mg). Children who have received steroids within the last several months, who have underlying asthma, or who are experiencing severe reactions should receive IV corticosteroids. Stress-dose hydrocortisone should be considered for those with life-threatening anaphylaxis.

Despite a paucity of evidence to directly support their use in anaphylaxis, the H_1-receptor antihistamines such as diphenhydramine (1 to 1.25 mg per kg intramuscularly or intravenously; maximum 50 mg) may still be used to alleviate itching and mucocutaneous symptoms. In stable patients, some providers prefer the oral route of administration.

The role of H_2-blocking antihistamines such as cimetidine (5 mg per kg; maximum 300 mg) or ranitidine (1 to 2 mg per kg; maximum 50 mg) in addition to H_1-blocking antihistamines in anaphylaxis has not been studied with methodologic rigor in children. Guidelines highlight the prioritization of epinephrine over these second-line agents, and many no longer recommend routine administration of these medications, alluding to the need for higher-quality data. In summary, glucocorticoids and H_1 and H_2 antihistamines should be considered second-line therapy since there is little role in the acute treatment of cardiovascular compromise.

Disposition

The recommended period of observation after anaphylaxis should be individualized and based upon severity, risk factors, and access to care. An observation period of 4 to 6 hours may be appropriate for patients with mild to moderate episodes that resolve promptly with therapy. Patients with severe reactions that involve upper airway obstruction or shock generally should be monitored for a minimum of 8 to 24 hours. The incidence of biphasic reactions varies across the literature but approaches 20% in some studies and can occur up to 72 hours after initial symptoms. Children with a history of asthma appear to be at increased risk for delayed, biphasic, and severe reactions and may also require prolonged monitoring. In addition, a longer period of observation may be indicated for patients in whom the allergen could continue to be absorbed, those with a slower onset of symptoms, or those with a history of biphasic reactions.

Discharge Considerations

Adjunctive therapy initiated in the ED is often continued for 48 to 72 hours, although there is a lack of evidence to support this practice. Follow-up with the child's primary care physician within that time frame is also advised. Referral to an allergist is indicated in most cases for further evaluation and testing.

Strategies to avoid exposure to the offending agent should be discussed and emphasized. Formal action plans may be helpful. All children with a history of anaphylaxis, especially those with asthma or a reaction to peanuts or tree nuts, should be instructed to carry a preloaded syringe of epinephrine to be used in emergencies and wear a medic alert tag. The chosen epinephrine dose should be nearest to 0.01 mg/kg/dose, typically 0.3 or 0.15 mg, and may be rounded up for patients at higher risk of a severe reaction. In children weighing less than 10 kg, dosing may be more appropriately achieved via syringe administration of a predetermined dose of 1:1,000 epinephrine at 0.01 mg/kg/dose.

It has been shown that practical demonstrations at the time of prescription of an epinephrine autoinjector dramatically increase the likelihood of effective administration. Because several different types of autoinjectors have been approved by the Food and Drug Administration (FDA), it may be prudent for patients to also review use of the autoinjector prior to leaving the pharmacy. Multiple online resources for education of parents of children with sensitization to allergens are available, some of which have been validated through federal funding and are available free of charge (http://www.cofargroup.org/).

Following an episode of anaphylaxis, approximately 30% of children have a second episode within 7 years. Children with atopic dermatitis, a documented sensitivity to food allergens, or a history of urticaria/angioedema appear to be at increased risk for recurrence.

HEREDITARY ANGIOEDEMA

CLINICAL PEARLS AND PITFALLS

- Hereditary angioedema is a rare but life-threatening disorder triggered by direct mechanical friction or trauma.
- The diagnosis should be considered for patients with recurrent angioedema without urticaria, abdominal pain/vomiting, or laryngeal edema, especially with a positive family history.
- Acute attacks of abdominal pain, facial swelling, or laryngeal swelling can be life-threatening.
- Recently approved C_1-esterase inhibitor concentrate and plasma kallikrein inhibitor should be strongly considered in the management of acute attacks of hereditary angioedema.

Current Evidence

Pathophysiology

Hereditary angioedema is caused by a deficiency of C_1-inhibitor function. It is a rare episodic disorder and can be the result of either low levels of the protein (type I) or poor functionality (type II), causing recurrent episodes of vascular permeability. Because of the autosomal-dominant inheritance pattern, many children with the disorder have a positive family history. However, 20% to 25% of cases are due to spontaneous mutations. Onset is most common in school age children (8 to 12 years). Patients may present with subcutaneous angioedema (involving circumscribed areas of edema of the skin, most commonly the extremities, without erythema or pruritis), abdominal attacks (severe pain, distention, and vomiting), or laryngeal edema (life-threatening hoarseness, stridor, and voice changes). Lack of C_1-esterase inhibitor results in activation of the kallikrein–kinin system, with resultant release of bradykinin, which causes vasodilation and increased vascular permeability.

Triggers

A number of triggers for angioedema have been established. Episodes of angioedema may be triggered by direct mechanical friction or trauma. Affected children should therefore avoid contact sports. Viral infections can also be an etiology and therefore exposures (i.e., early daycare) should be limited when possible. Puberty often worsens acute episode frequency and duration. Stress, dental manipulation, estrogens, and angiotensin-converting enzyme inhibitors can also serve as the inciting agents of edema.

Goals of Treatment

The goals of treatment of hereditary angioedema include rapid, controlled airway management in cases of laryngeal edema, with prompt administration of C_1-esterase inhibitor concentrate (or alternative therapy) to reduce the risk of morbidity and mortality due to acute attacks.

Clinical Considerations

Clinical Recognition

Diagnosis of hereditary angioedema early in life is critical but often delayed. A complete history and physical examination, with special attention to the airway, posterior pharynx, and abdomen, should be performed. Occasionally, abdominal ultrasonography is useful in discriminating angioedema from a surgical process. Findings include hyperemia of the bowel wall, and often ascites. Patients may report a prodrome of paresthesias at the location where edema will arise, with the self-limited episodes lasting from 2 to 4 days.

Laboratory Assessment

The diagnosis is suspected from C4 levels that are usually low because of increased conversion of C4 to C1, while C3 is normal. Functional and antigenic C_1-inhibitor levels should be determined but may be falsely low in infants younger than 2 years.

Management

Airway management and monitoring, fluid resuscitation, and pain control are important during initial management. Intubation should be strongly considered in the presence of an inability to swallow, voice changes, or dyspnea. Because of the potential for landmark distortion and an acute increase in edema, direct laryngoscopy is best performed in a controlled setting where a definitive surgical airway can be achieved when required. Unfortunately, corticosteroids and antihistamines are usually ineffective in the management of hereditary angioedema. Epinephrine (nebulized or intramuscular) may transiently improve symptoms, although it is most commonly ineffective.

There have been a limited number of young children enrolled in individual trials evaluating efficacy of therapies for hereditary angioedema. However, many international guidelines recommend treatment of children with acute attacks of angioedema given the risk of morbidity and the available safety data. *Human C_1-esterase inhibitor concentrate* has approval by the FDA for routine prophylaxis in adolescents and adults (Cinryze, 1,000 units every 3 to 4 days) and in the management of acute attacks. C_1-esterase inhibitor concentrate can be administered immediately parenterally (20 units per kg up to 1,000 units [Berinert], or 50 units per kg up to 4,200 units of the recombinant product [Ruconest]) to patients presenting with laryngeal edema or symptoms of an acute abdominal process. This treatment generally begins to alleviate symptoms within 30 to 60 minutes. Repetitive doses are sometimes required. Hospitalization is often necessary in the course of severe laryngeal or abdominal attacks. With appropriate training, patients can be prescribed C_1-esterase inhibitor concentrate (Berinert) for home self-administration, provided that epinephrine is available in case of hypersensitivity. Patients who self-administer C_1-esterase inhibitor concentrate for laryngeal attacks should be advised to seek immediate medical treatment due to the risk of airway obstruction. Education remains critical in assisting patients with long-term management.

Other relative new therapies include the plasma kallikrein inhibitor ecallantide (Kalbitor, 30 mg as three 10 mg subcutaneous injections for patients age ≥12 years) and the bradykinin B_2-receptor antagonist icatibant (Firazyr, 30 mg subcutaneously, patients ≥18 years).

SERUM SICKNESS

CLINICAL PEARLS AND PITFALLS

- True serum-sickness reactions are becoming less common due to decreased utilization of medications derived from heterologous serum.
- Serum sickness-like reactions which are characterized by fever, urticarial or vasculitic-appearing rash, and arthralgias, are more common in young children, often due to exposure to an antibiotic or other medication in the prior 7 to 14 days.
- Renal involvement should be excluded.
- Most children with serum sickness-like reactions can be managed with supportive care (NSAIDs, antihistamines, and oral corticosteroids for severe/protracted cases).

Current Evidence

Background

Serum sickness is an immune complex–mediated disease. It was first described in 1905 in patients who had received heterologous antisera, which, at that time, was used routinely to treat various infectious diseases. The use of therapeutic agents obtained from heterologous serum has decreased dramatically. These preparations are currently found in antithymocyte globulins used to prevent organ transplant rejection and in antitoxins for the management of clostridia infections, diphtheria, tetanus, and specific arachnid, snake, and scorpion envenomations. Today, the most common cause of serum sickness is exposure to medication, usually described as a serum sickness–like reaction.

Currently, the medications implicated most frequently in serum sickness–like reactions include the penicillins, sulfonamides, cephalosporins, streptomycin, hydantoins, griseofulvin, bupropion, fluoxetine, and thiouracil. Because these drugs are all low–molecular-weight substances, they cannot act as antigens directly but must bind to proteins, usually through their metabolites. This makes it difficult to substantiate sensitization. Chimeric human-murine monoclonal antibodies such as infliximab (used to treat psoriasis and inflammatory bowel disease) and rituximab (used to treat autoimmune disorders and lymphomas), and the humanized anti-IgE antibody omalizumab (used to treat allergic disorders and asthma) can also induce serum sickness. Less commonly, exposures to various chemical, infectious agents, or autologous antigens result in a serum sickness–like illness.

Pathophysiology

In the classical serum-sickness model, exposure to a foreign serum protein causes characteristic symptoms 7 to 10 days later. During the initial period after exposure to the foreign protein, there is a period of antigen excess. Antibodies develop after approximately 6 to 10 days causing antibody-antigen complexes to form. These immune complexes deposit in the tissues and may also activate complement. Symptoms often develop when soluble immune complexes are being cleared by the body. These immune complexes can activate the classical complement pathway. Complement activation generates the anaphylactic toxins C3a and C5a, which then increase vascular permeability, cause histamine release, and produce bronchospasm. In addition, this leads to inflammation around deposits of complexes in various tissues.

Clearance of immune complexes depends on their size and the effectiveness of the reticuloendothelial system. The most vulnerable organs to injury include the kidneys and the vascular system.

Goals of Treatment

The goals of treatment of serum sickness include removal of antigen exposure (if known), control of painful arthralgias and pruritis (through NSAIDs and antihistamines), and appropriate monitoring for organ dysfunction (particularly renal involvement).

Clinical Considerations

Clinical Recognition

The severity of serum sickness and the specific clinical manifestations vary widely. The reaction is characterized by fever, malaise, and a rash that is most commonly urticarial but may also appear as a maculopapular or vasculitic eruption. Other manifestations include arthralgias or arthritis, lymphadenopathy, angioedema, and nephritis. Other less common problems include abdominal pain, carditis, anemia, and neuritis. In serum sickness–like reactions, signs are generally limited to fever, pruritis, urticaria/rash, and arthralgias. Serum sickness is usually self-limited and typically resolves within 1 to 2 weeks with or without therapy.

Characteristically, the onset of symptoms occurs 7 to 14 days after the primary exposure. If there has been prior sensitization, however, reexposure can result in onset within a few days.

The history should be directed toward identifying the offending agent and determining the extent and severity of the symptoms. The physician should review possible exposures up to 14 days before symptoms to ascertain a possible cause for the process. Because a secondary exposure can produce a more rapid onset of symptoms (1 to 4 days), inquiries about this interval and about previous exposures may also be revealing.

In addition, the history should elicit information about the extent of systemic illness and the involvement of specific organ systems. It is important to determine the time course and nature of the rash; the degree of joint pain, swelling, or warmth; and evidence of renal involvement such as hematuria, edema, and reduced urine output. In light of the potential for involvement of other organ systems, a complete review of systems is indicated.

The physical examination serves to determine the severity and extent of involvement of the reaction. A general inspection will help ascertain how ill and uncomfortable the child is. Most children with serum sickness–like reactions will not appear toxic. Examination of the skin may reveal a maculopapular eruption, urticaria, or palpable purpura of a cutaneous vasculitis. Painful angioedema is commonly present. Generalized lymphadenopathy often occurs. In more severe reactions, the joints show erythema, warmth, and effusion. Wheezes may be appreciated on auscultation of the lungs, and a pericardial friction rub may be audible if pericarditis is present. The liver and the spleen often enlarge. Rarely, neurologic deficits occur secondary to a vasculitis of the CNS.

Laboratory Assessment

The selection of laboratory studies should be determined by the severity of the reaction, the evidence of specific organ system involvement, and the degree of diagnostic uncertainty. For most patients, a urinalysis to look for the evidence of renal involvement is all that is required. A list of other studies that may be indicated for individual patients with immune complex–mediated disease is outlined in Table 93.2.

TABLE 93.2

POSSIBLE LABORATORY EVALUATION OF SERUM SICKNESS[a]

Blood tests
Erythrocyte sedimentation rate
Complete blood cell count with differential
CH_5O, C3, C4
Blood urea nitrogen, creatinine
Antinuclear antibody
Rheumatoid factor
Hepatic enzymes
Hepatitis B screen
Heterophile antibody
Immune complex assay
Other laboratory tests
Urinalysis
Electrocardiogram
Stool heme test
Computed tomography scan

[a]Laboratory evaluation should be tailored for each individual patient as noted in the text.

The erythrocyte sedimentation rate may be elevated. CBC with differential counts may reveal leukopenia or leukocytosis. The C3, C4, and CH_5O may decrease because of complement activation. Any of the tests for circulating immune complexes (e.g., cryoglobulins) may be elevated. Stool testing for blood should be considered for patients with abdominal pain or other symptoms involving the GI tract. If carditis is suspected, a screening electrocardiogram and chest radiograph should be obtained; an echocardiogram may also be considered. Severe headache or focal neurologic deficits are indications for neuroimaging, usually a computed tomography scan. Serum sickness–like reactions will not be accompanied by hypocomplementemia or renal dysfunction.

Management

The treatment of serum sickness is based on the extent and severity of the disease. Keeping in mind that the reaction is usually self-limited, the goal is to provide symptomatic relief and to monitor for complications. If possible, the offending antigen should be eliminated.

Pharmacologic management usually involves one or more of the following: antihistamines, NSAIDs, and corticosteroids. Pruritus, rash, and angioedema can be managed with an antihistamine such as diphenhydramine (5 mg/kg/24 hrs divided every 6 hours) or hydroxyzine (2 mg/kg/24 hrs divided every 6 to 8 hours, with a maximum of 200 mg per 24 hours). Although experience in the treatment of serum sickness is limited, the use of second-generation, nonsedating antihistamines may also be considered (Table 93.3). Mild joint involvement and/or fever often improve with the use of an NSAID such as ibuprofen (5 to 10 mg/kg/dose every 6 to 8 hours up to a

TABLE 93.3

TREATMENT OF ALLERGIC RHINITIS AND CONJUNCTIVITIS (SYSTEMIC, TOPICAL NASAL, AND TOPICAL OPHTHALMIC)

Medication	Dose	Comments
Oral antihistamines		
Loratadine		Available over the counter
10-mg tab or 10-mg/10-mL syrup	5 mg daily	Age 2–5 yrs
	10 mg daily	Age ≥6 yrs
Desloratadine		
0.5-mg/mL syrup, 2.5-mg or 5-mg dispersible tablets or 5-mg tablets	1 mg daily	Age 6–11 mo
	1.25 mg daily	Age 12 mo–5 yrs
	2.5 mg daily	Age 6–11 yrs
	5 mg daily	Age ≥12 yrs
Fexofenadine		Available over the counter
30-mg/5-mL suspension, 30-mg dispersible tablets, 30-mg tablets, 60-mg tabs/caps, 180-mg tabs	30 mg bid	Age 2–11 yrs
	60 mg bid	Age ≥12 yrs
	180 mg daily	Age ≥12 yrs
Cetirizine		Available over the counter
5-mg tabs, 10-mg tabs	2.5 mg daily	Age 6–11 mo
5-mg/5-mL syrup	2.5 mg daily or 2.5 mg bid	Age 1–5 yrs
	5–10 mg daily	Age 6–11 and ≥12 yrs
Levocetirizine		
2.5 mg/5 mL, 5-mg tabs	1.25 mg daily	Age 6 mo–5 yrs
	2.5 mg daily	Age 6–11 yrs
	5 mg daily	Age ≥12 yrs
Topical corticosteroids		
Beclomethasone (aqueous: 42 μg/spray)	1–2 sprays each nostril bid	Age ≥6 yrs
Budesonide (32 μg/actuation)	1–2 sprays each nostril daily	Age 6–11 yrs
	2–4 sprays each nostril daily	Age ≥12 yrs
Fluticasone propionate (50 μg/spray)	1–2 sprays each nostril daily	Age ≥4 yrs, available over the counter
Triamcinolone (55 μg/spray)	1 spray each nostril daily	Age 2–5 yrs
	1–2 spray each nostril daily	Age ≥6 yrs
Flunisolide (25 μg/spray)	2 sprays each nostril bid	Age 6–14 yrs
	2 sprays each nostril bid-tid	Age ≥15 yrs
Mometasone furoate (50 μg/spray)	1 spray each nostril daily	Age 2–11 yrs
	2 sprays each nostril daily	Age ≥12 yrs
Other therapy		
Cromolyn sodium (5.2 mg/spray, mast-cell stabilizer)	1 spray each nostril q4–8h	Age ≥2 yrs, available over the counter
Azelastine (137 μg/spray, antihistamine)	1 spray each nostril bid	Age 5–11 yrs
	1–2 sprays each nostril bid	Age ≥12 yrs
Ipratropium bromide (0.03%, 21 μg/spray)	2–3 sprays each nostril bid-tid	Age ≥6 yrs
Montelukast sodium		
4-mg granules	4-mg po daily	Age 6 mo–5 yrs
4- and 5-mg chewable	5-mg po daily	Age 6–14 yrs
10-mg tab	10-mg po daily	Age ≥15 yrs

bid, twice a day; tid, three times a day; po, by mouth.

maximum 2.4 g per 24 hours). In more severe disease or after failure to respond to these measures, a burst of corticosteroids may be prescribed at a dose of 1 to 2 mg/kg/day of prednisone (maximum 60 to 80 mg per day) for 7 to 10 days, followed by a taper for 2 weeks. In life-threatening serum sickness with significant circulating immune complexes, plasmapheresis may play a role, but this procedure has not been used extensively for the treatment of this disease. Most children with serum sickness can be managed as outpatients, with close follow-up by their primary care physicians and long-term avoidance of the offending agent. Children with more severe involvement or refractory symptoms may benefit from hospitalization, particularly if the diagnosis is in question.

ALLERGIC RHINITIS AND CONJUNCTIVITIS

CLINICAL PEARLS AND PITFALLS

- Allergic rhinitis is a common cause of morbidity and direct healthcare costs in children.
- Although there is a paucity of comparative effectiveness data in children, intranasal corticosteroids are often considered to be a first-line agent in symptom management. Oral nonsedating antihistamines and oral montelukast are common alternative therapies.

Current Evidence

Background

Allergic rhinitis is the most common manifestation of atopic disease, resulting in significant direct and indirect healthcare costs. Peak incidence occurs in the pediatric age group, affecting up to 40% of children and adolescents. Although not a life-threatening problem, allergic rhinitis can have a significant, often underestimated, negative impact on the quality of life of affected children. Severe nasal symptoms have been directly linked to poor school performance. The morbidity of allergic rhinitis results from the direct manifestations of the disease and from associated complications such as sinusitis, acute asthma, sleep disturbances, dysosmia, and the consequences of chronic mouth breathing.

Pathophysiology and Classification

Allergic rhinitis is caused by an IgE-mediated hypersensitivity response of the nasal mucosa to foreign allergens. Following sensitization to a foreign antigen, reexposure triggers an immediate hypersensitivity reaction. This early response is characterized by the activation of mast cells and the release of preformed mediators such as histamine, prostaglandins, and leukotrienes. These mediators cause vasodilation, mucosal edema, mucus secretion, stimulation of itch receptors, and reduction in the threshold for sneezing.

Historically, allergic rhinitis has been categorized as seasonal or perennial. *Seasonal* allergic rhinitis is most commonly caused by exposure to tree pollens (early spring), grass pollens (late spring and early summer), and ragweed or other weed pollens (late summer and fall). Allergens responsible for *perennial* allergic rhinitis include animal dander, house dust mites, and mold spores. Updated duration-based terminology established by the World Health Organization includes *intermittent* (<4 days per week or for <4 weeks per year) and *persistent* (>4 days per week and >4 weeks per year) allergic rhinitis. These terms were chosen because not all patients with sensitivity to typical perennial allergens exhibit constant symptoms and because year-round pollens may be found in many parts of the world. It is important to recognize that food allergens do not typically cause isolated allergic rhinitis.

Goals of Treatment

Goals of emergency management of allergic rhinitis include acute symptomatic relief of nasal obstruction and secretions, and eye irritation and pruritus. Referral to the primary care physician and/or allergist for chronic management is warranted in most cases.

Clinical Considerations

Clinical Recognition

The classic symptoms of allergic rhinitis include nasal congestion, paroxysmal sneezing, pruritus of the nose and eyes, and watery, profuse rhinorrhea. Other complaints may include noisy breathing, snoring, repeated throat clearing or cough, itching of the palate and throat, "popping" of the ears, and ocular complaints such as redness, itching, and tearing.

The physical examination is variable but may reveal the "gaping" look of a mouth breather, dark discoloration of skin on the infraorbital ridge caused by venous congestion (allergic shiners), and a transverse external nasal wrinkle secondary to chronic rubbing of the nose (allergic salute). Intranasal findings are variable. The mucosa is often edematous and may appear pale or violaceous. The nasal secretions may be clear, mucoid, or opaque.

Management

There are several approaches to the management of allergic rhinitis, although high-quality evidence for most pharmacologic interventions in children is limited. Options include the identification and avoidance of environmental allergens and irritants, oral antihistamine drugs, topical decongestants, topical anti-inflammatory agents (cromolyn and/or corticosteroids), and immunotherapy.

Recognizing that long-term therapy must be highly individualized, the emergency physician will generally limit interventions to those that safely provide rapid, symptomatic relief and then refer the child to the primary care physician for long-term evaluation of allergic triggers and associated therapy. Data in adults suggest that adequate treatment of allergic rhinitis in asthmatic patients can significantly reduce healthcare utilization due to bronchospasm. In this important subgroup, parents should be reminded during the ED visit to seek appropriate chronic management of allergic rhinitis.

Topical corticosteroids are considered first-line therapy for chronic allergic rhinitis but may require as long as 2 weeks to achieve maximal relief. Rapid relief can generally be achieved through use of a nonsedating antihistamine (Table 93.3). First-generation antihistamines (such as chlorpheniramine, brompheniramine) are no longer recommended as first-line therapy because of the over-the-counter availability of many generic formulations of second-generation antihistamines with a better side-effect profile. Antihistamines acutely reduce the rhinorrhea, pruritus, and sneezing associated with allergic rhinitis. Combination oral antihistamine-decongestant preparations are available for children ≥12 years and adults, but are primarily appropriate for short intervals for rescue therapy. Topical antihistamines such as azelastine can also provide symptomatic relief to children and adults with intermittent allergic rhinitis, but may have a bitter aftertaste and are considered second-line therapy. Other nonpharmacologic measures such as saline nasal rinses may also provide some symptomatic relief.

There is some evidence supporting the role of montelukast in the management of persistent allergic rhinitis in preschool children, seasonal allergic rhinitis in older children and adolescents, and in the management of allergic rhinitis in patients with asthma who already take inhaled corticosteroids. Although there is little evidence to support allergen avoidance for indoor allergens, it is logical to limit exposures when possible in patients with significant allergic rhinoconjunctivitis, especially during pollen seasons. Children with significant ocular symptoms may also benefit from local ophthalmic treatment (see Table 131.2). While there is a paucity of evidence to guide pharmacologic treatment of allergic rhinitis in children, there is at least a moderate level of evidence supporting subcutaneous immunotherapy in the chronic management of allergic rhinitis in children and adults. Sublingual immunotherapy and omalizumab are other important chronic therapies under investigation.

Suggested Readings and Key References

Anaphylaxis

Brown SG, Stone SF, Fatovich DM, et al. Anaphylaxis: clinical patterns, mediator release, and severity. *J Allergy Clin Immunol* 2013; 132(5):1141–1149.e5.

Campbell RL, Li JT, Nicklas RA, et al. Emergency department diagnosis and treatment of anaphylaxis: a practice parameter. *Ann Allergy Asthma Immunol* 2014;113:599–608.

Dhami S, Panesar SS, Roberts G, et al. Management of anaphylaxis: a systematic review. *Allergy* 2014;69(2):168–175.

Ma L, Danoff TM, Borish L. Case fatality and population mortality associated with anaphylaxis in the United States. *J Allergy Clin Immunol* 2014;133(4):1075–1083.

Simons FE, Ardusso LR, Bilo MB, et al. World Allergy Organization anaphylaxis guidelines: summary. *J Allergy Clin Immunol* 2011; 127(3):587–593.e1–22.

Simons FE, Ardusso LR, Dimov V, et al. World Allergy Organization anaphylaxis guidelines: 2013 update of the evidence base. *Int Arch Allergy Immunol* 2013;162(3):193–204.

Hereditary Angioedema

Bork K. An evidence based therapeutic approach to hereditary and acquired angioedema. *Curr Opin Allergy Clin Immunol* 2014; 14(4):354–362.

Bowen T, Cicardi M, Farkas H, et al. 2010 International consensus algorithm for the diagnosis, therapy and management of hereditary angioedema. *Allergy Asthma Clin Immunol* 2010;6(1):24.

Craig TJ, Levy RJ, Wasserman RL, et al. Efficacy of human C1 esterase inhibitor concentrate compared with placebo in acute hereditary angioedema attacks. *J Allergy Clin Immunol* 2009;124(4): 801–808.

Zuraw BL, Banerji A, Bernstein JA, et al. US Hereditary Angioedema Association Medical Advisory Board 2013 recommendations for the management of hereditary angioedema due to C1 inhibitor deficiency. *J Allergy Clin Immunol* 2013;1(5):458–467.

Serum Sickness

Segal AR, Doherty KM, Leggott J, et al. Cutaneous reactions to drugs in children. *Pediatrics* 2007;120(4):e1082–e1096.

Shah KN, Honig PJ, Yan AC. "Urticaria multiforme": a case series and review of acute annular urticarial hypersensitivity syndromes in children. *Pediatrics* 2007;119(5):e1177–e1183.

Tamburro JE, Esterly NB. Hypersensitivity syndromes. *Adolesc Med* 2001;12(2):vii, 323–341.

Allergic Rhinitis

Al Sayyad JJ, Fedorowicz Z, Alhashimi D, et al. Topical nasal steroids for intermittent and persistent allergic rhinitis in children. *Cochrane Database Syst Rev* 2007;(1):CD003163.

Bousquet J, Khaltaev N, Cruz AA, et al. Allergic Rhinitis and its Impact on Asthma (ARIA) 2008 update (in collaboration with the World Health Organization, GA(2)LEN and AllerGen). *Allergy* 2008;63(suppl 86):8–160.

Brozek JL, Bousquet J, Baena-Cagnani CE, et al. Allergic Rhinitis and its Impact on Asthma (ARIA) guidelines: 2010 revision. *J Allergy Clin Immunol* 2010;126(3):466–476.

Glacy J, Putnam K, Godfrey S, et al. *Treatments for seasonal allergic rhinitis.* Rockville, MD: Agency for Healthcare Research and Quality (US); 2013. Available from http://www.ncbi.nlm.nih.gov/books/NBK153714/

Lin SY, Erekosima N, Suarez-Cuervo C, et al. *Allergen-specific immunotherapy for the treatment of allergic rhinoconjunctivitis and/or asthma: comparative effectiveness review.* Rockville, MD: Agency for Healthcare Research and Quality (US); 2013. Available at http://www.ncbi.nlm.nih.gov/books/NBK133240/

CHAPTER 94 ■ CARDIAC EMERGENCIES

CASANDRA QUIÑONES, MD AND BETH BUBOLZ, MD

GOALS OF EMERGENCY THERAPY

Pediatric cardiac emergencies are caused by a wide variety of pathophysiologic states and so have a variety of presentations. Cardiac emergencies may be due to congenital heart disease (CHD), arrhythmias, acute heart failure syndromes (AHFS), trauma, and sequelae of treatment. The common denominator in cardiac emergencies is that cardiac output is compromised. The challenge for emergency medicine (EM) providers is to identify cardiac emergencies promptly even when the chief complaint is not cardiac in nature. With the proper mental model for interpreting the patient's signs and symptoms, the provider can determine the correct approach to these complex patients. The clinician must consider heart disease when evaluating common symptoms such as feeding difficulty, abdominal pain, wheezing, or respiratory distress and can make the correct diagnosis if the proper framework for interpreting signs and symptoms is applied.

If the provider understands framework, an exhaustive knowledge of every anatomic variation of CHD is not necessary. Instead, the EM provider can recognize cardiac disease by the presenting symptoms and the patient may be assessed rapidly and accurately and restoration of adequate cardiac output can be started.

KEY POINTS

- CHD should be a consideration in any neonate presenting with acute decompensation in the first 2 months of life.
- CHD often presents with cyanosis or shock in the first 2 weeks of life, coinciding with closure of the ductus arteriosus (DA).
- CHD often presents with pulmonary over circulation and poor feeding around 2 months of life coinciding with fall in pulmonary vascular resistance (PVR).
- Pediatric patients with AHFS often present with nonspecific, noncardiac complaints many times before the correct diagnosis is made.
- Incessant tachycardia may lead to heart failure at any age.
- Children with implanted cardiac devices may present with complications of implantation or device failure.

RELATED CHAPTERS

Resuscitation and Stabilization

- Cardiopulmonary Resuscitation: Chapter 4

Medical Emergencies

- Neonatal Emergencies: Chapter 104

Signs and Symptoms

- Coma: Chapter 12
- Cyanosis: Chapter 16
- Dizziness and Vertigo: Chapter 19
- Fever: Chapter 26
- Heart Murmurs: Chapter 31
- Pain: Chest: Chapter 50
- Pain: Joints: Chapter 55
- Rash: Bacterial and Fungal Infections: Chapter 61
- Respiratory Distress: Chapter 66
- Seizures: Chapter 67
- Septic Appearing Infant: Chapter 68
- Syncope: Chapter 71
- Tachycardia: Chapter 72
- Weight Loss: Chapter 79
- Wheezing: Chapter 80

CONGENITAL HEART DISEASE

Goals of Treatment

The goals of treatment are the rapid recognition, stabilization, and restoration of cardiac output in patients who present with undiagnosed congenital or acquired heart disease as well as the stabilization of a child with an underlying heart condition who presents with an emergent noncardiac condition.

CLINICAL PEARLS AND PITFALL

- Recognition of the most common presentation patterns for patients with CHD will guide appropriate therapy.
- CHD should be a consideration in any neonate presenting with acute decompensation.
- Evaluate femoral pulse in all newborns and infants to detect coarctation of the aorta.
- Palliation or incomplete repair of a congenital heart defect in an infant is a red flag for a patient who may not tolerate other stressors.
- Pediatric patients with cardiac disease often present with nonspecific symptoms involving the gastrointestinal or pulmonary systems.
- Endotracheal intubation and mechanical ventilation can significantly decrease cardiac demands.

Current Evidence

Congenital heart malformations are the most common types of birth defects, affecting nearly 1% or approximately

TABLE 94.1

GLOSSARY OF CONGENITAL HEART DEFECTS

Structural congenital heart defect	Definition
Left coronary artery anomalies	Anomalous Left main Coronary Artery arises from the Pulmonary Artery rather than the aortic root (ALCAPA) Desaturated blood with low coronary perfusion pressure compromises blood flow as PVR drops in the newborn This and other variations of the coronaries may present as sudden death or CHF
Aortic Regurgitation (AR)	Diastolic regurgitation of blood from the aorta back into the left ventricle
Aortic Stenosis (AS)	Three types: subvalvar, valvar, and supravalvar Subtotal narrowing/obstruction of the left ventricular outflow at or near the aortic valve
Aortopulmonary window	Defect between the aorta and pulmonary artery Pulmonary overcirculation and left-sided volume overload
Atrial Septal Defect (ASD)	A communication between the right and left atria Usually asymptomatic Causes right-sided volume overload
Atrioventricular Septal Defect (AVSD)	Incomplete fusion of the embryonic endocardial cushions resulting in defects of the lower atrial septum (primum ASD), inlet ventricular septum, and atrioventricular valves, in isolation or combination
Bicuspid Aortic Valve (BAV)	Aortic valve composed of two cusps, or three cusps with two commissures yielding two effective cusps
Congenital Mitral Stenosis	Mitral valve leaflets are thickened and/or fused, producing a narrowed opening from the left atrium to the left ventricle, may be associated with an abnormal papillary muscle (parachute MV)
Coarctation of the Aorta (CoA)	A discrete narrowing of the distal segment of the aortic arch, typically just distal to the left subclavian artery at the point of ductal insertion
Cor triatriatum	The pulmonary veins join in a confluence that is not completely incorporated into the left atrium
Double-Outlet Right Ventricle (DORV)	The majority of the semilunar valve orifices of both great arteries arise from the morphologic right ventricle Variable presenting physiology depending on great vessel and VSD anatomy
Ebstein anomaly	The tricuspid valve is displaced downward with resultant "atrialization" of a portion of the right ventricle The proximal part of the right ventricle is thin-walled and continuous with the right atrium and thus the functional right ventricle is small
Hypoplastic left heart syndrome (HLHS)	Syndrome in which the mitral valve, left ventricle, ascending aorta, and/or aortic arch are underdeveloped Cardiac output travels from the right ventricle via the main pulmonary artery to the lungs Systemic flow is blood shunted via the ductus arteriosus to the descending aorta Often the ascending aorta fills retrograde from the ductus arteriosus Blood returns to the right atrium where it is mixed with pulmonary venous return shunting from left atrium to right atrium via an ASD
Mitral valve regurgitation (MR)	Systolic regurgitation of blood from the left ventricle into the left atria
Mitral valve prolapse (MVP)	Mitral valve prolapses into the left atrium after it closes, during systole
Patent Ductus Arteriosus (PDA)	The ductus arteriosus, which connects the pulmonary artery and the aorta in the fetus, remains open after birth rather than closing within 15 hours and sealing around 3 wks to become ligamentum arteriosum
Pulmonary atresia	Pulmonary valve does not develop at all
Pulmonary Stenosis (PS)	Narrowing near or at the pulmonary valve
Pulmonary vein stenosis	Defined as subtotal obstruction of one or more pulmonary veins
Single ventricle	Univentricular heart due to a variety or anatomic defects Some examples are hypoplastic left heart, tricuspid atresia, unbalanced AV septal defect, double inlet right ventricle (some cases), double inlet LV, etc. Any lesion with an underdeveloped LV or RV may be considered a single ventricle Blood flow from the two atria is directed through the left and/or right AV valves into a single ventricular chamber
Tetralogy of Fallot (TOF)	Lesion composed of: large nonrestrictive VSD, right ventricular outflow tract obstruction from pulmonic stenosis, aorta overriding the ventricular septal defect, and right ventricular hypertrophy Right and left ventricular pressures are equal because of nonrestrictive VSD so the amount of right ventricular outflow tract obstruction determines pulmonary blood flow and cyanosis

(*continued*)

TABLE 94.1

GLOSSARY OF CONGENITAL HEART DEFECTS (*CONTINUED*)

Structural congenital heart defect	Definition
D-Transposition of the Great Arteries (D-TGA)	Aorta and the pulmonary artery are transposed in relation to the ventricular septum, with the aorta arising from the right ventricle and the main pulmonary artery arising from the left ventricle
L-Transposition of the Great Arteries (L-TGA or ventricular inversion)	The anatomic LV receives blood from the right atrium and pumps to the pulmonary artery, the anatomic RV receives blood from the left atrium and pumps to the aorta. Physiology is defined by associated defects Often develop AV block spontaneously
Truncus arteriosus	Single great artery departing the heart that gives rise to aorta, pulmonary arteries, and coronary arteries. Associated VSD is always present Systemic and pulmonary pressures are equal causing early pulmonary hypertension
Tricuspid Atresia	Hypoplastic RV due to tricuspid atresia No communication between the right atrium and the right ventricle All RA blood flows to the LA and then to the LV PDA required for pulmonary perfusion
Total Anomalous Pulmonary Venous Return (TAPVR)	None of the four pulmonary veins drain into left atrium thus all pulmonary veins terminate in a systemic vein or the right atrium Four forms depending on where pulmonary veins drain: supracardiac (most common), cardiac, intracardiac, and mixed
Ventricular Septal Defect (VSD)	Septum dividing right and left ventricle has a hole or defect

40,000 live births per year in the United States. Nearly half of the deaths from CHD occur in the first year of life. Recent data reveals that 15% of CHD is associated with chromosomal abnormalities. Twenty-nine percent of CHD is associated with other major noncardiac malformations. This is a complex patient population who often seek medical care in the ED.

All forms of CHD occur along a spectrum. For example, tetralogy of Fallot (TOF) may range from pulmonary atresia to very mild pulmonary stenosis, or absent pulmonary valve (no stenosis). Therefore, presentation of TOF can range from fulminant cyanosis and shock to mild cyanosis to congestive heart failure (CHF). It is not necessary to know the exact anatomical defect at the time of presentation but rather focus on the cardiac physiology. Anatomical details will be defined by an echocardiogram, but that full information is not necessary for recognition of common patterns of presentation and stabilization in the emergency department (ED).

Clinical Considerations

Clinical Recognition

Many times when an infant or child presents to the ED, the diagnosis is not immediately evident and management is initiated without complete certainty of the underlying pathology. This is especially true with CHD. However, a framework can be used to assist in forming a differential diagnosis, instituting therapy, and communicating with the pediatric cardiologist. This approach encourages the provider to categorize patients into groups according to their presenting vital signs and predominant symptoms.

Presentation of CHD often occurs at the time of transition from fetal to postnatal circulation. The adaptation to extrauterine life involves closure of three shunts: The DA, patent foramen ovale in the atrial septum, and ductus venosus. Pulmonary vascular resistance (PVR) drops dramatically with the first breath and continues to diminish significantly over the next 2 months. It follows that closure of the DA and fall in PVR may cause infants with cardiac malformations to become symptomatic.

Structural CHD can be divided into four major categories. Each of the four categories has typical presenting symptoms due to the underlying hemodynamics. The key to diagnosis is associating presenting symptoms and physical findings with each of the major categories of CHD. The four categories of structural CHD are: (1) Ductal dependent lesions that require a patent ductus arteriosus (PDA) for pulmonary blood flow (PBF); (2) ductal dependent lesions that require a PDA for systemic blood flow; (3) shunt lesions with right-to-left flow; and (4) shunt lesions with left-to-right flow (Tables 94.1 and 94.2).

Categorization of a patient into one of these four groups requires knowing the patient's age, weight, vital signs, and physical examination findings, which all may be gathered quickly. This simplified method of understanding heart disease can help the provider identify and treat emergencies due to CHD (Table 94.3 and e-Table 94.1).

Ductal Dependent Lesions

After birth, circulating prostaglandins decrease and the DA naturally closes. Cardiac defects, which depend on ductal patency for stable circulation, will present at this time, typically within the first 2 weeks of life. Either pulmonary or systemic blood flow may be dependent on a PDA. These lesions have very different presentations, which can be recognized by the astute clinician.

Ductal Dependent Pulmonary Blood Flow

Cardiac defects in which the pulmonary outflow tract is atretic depend completely on patency of the DA for survival. When the ductus closes, these patients become extremely hypoxic and present with severe cyanosis and shock. Defects such as critical pulmonary stenosis, pulmonary atresia with intact ventricular septum, and severe TOF, present in this dramatic fashion.

Less severe forms of ductal dependency for PBF present with varying degrees of cyanosis at the time this vessel closes. The degree of cyanosis is determined by the amount of blood flow to the lungs. These infants feed and grow well initially, have normal respiratory rate and effort, and normal vital signs. Defects such as TOF and some forms of tricuspid atresia and double outlet right ventricle (DORV) present in this fashion.

Ductal Dependent Systemic Blood Flow

Patients with severe left ventricular outflow tract obstructive (LVOTO) lesions depend on blood flow from the pulmonary artery via the DA to supply the descending aorta. By definition, this is a right-to-left shunt that causes desaturated blood to be circulated systemically, and it is necessary to provide systemic blood flow. Cyanosis is usually mild. Early symptoms include mild tachypnea or cyanosis, which can quickly progress to cardiogenic shock when the ductus closes. Cardiovascular collapse may be the first indication that there is a heart defect. Resulting acidosis and pressure loading of the ventricle accelerate decompensation and end-organ failure rapidly follows. LVOTO lesions such as hypoplastic left heart syndrome (HLHS), critical aortic stenosis, and severe coarctation of the aorta present in this fashion.

Shunt Lesions

Left-to-right Shunts

Left-to-right shunt lesions allow oxygenated blood to pass from the systemic circulation to the pulmonary circulation. The amount of flow is determined by the size of the defect and the relative PVR compared to systemic vascular resistance (SVR). If the PVR is high or if the defect is small, left-to-right shunting is limited and the patient is relatively asymptomatic. As PVR drops, left-to-right shunting increases causing increased PBF, which results in pulmonary over circulation. Over circulation of the lungs presents as tachypnea, sinus tachycardia, poor feeding, sweating with feeds, and failure to thrive, which may be mistaken for a respiratory illness. Typical examples of left-to-right shunt lesions include ventricular septal defect (VSD) and PDA.

Patients with left-to-right shunts usually present between 6 and 8 weeks of life. They present with tachypnea (not cyanosis) and have a history of poor feeding and/or weight gain. They may also have started out life feeding well and asymptomatic, but their feeding has worsened as their PVR dropped and pulmonary over circulation increased. On physical examination, the provider may or may not appreciate a murmur. A large, nonrestrictive VSD will not produce a murmur at all, since left ventricle (LV) and right ventricle (RV) pressures are equal. Small VSDs produce louder murmurs due to the pressure gradient from LV to RV. The murmur of a small VSD may become louder as PVR falls. Hepatomegaly is a prominent feature in large left-to-right shunts.

Right-to-left Shunts

Right-to-left shunts include defects that allow deoxygenated blood to pass from the right side of the heart into the systemic circulation resulting in cyanosis. Defects such as TOF are examples of this group. The physiology of TOF is defined by the large, nonrestrictive VSD and pulmonary stenosis even though TOF is described anatomically as pulmonary stenosis, a large nonrestrictive VSD, overriding aorta and right ventricular hypertrophy. The stenotic pulmonary outflow tract offers higher resistance to blood flow than SVR and blood preferentially shunts right-to-left through the VSD. The degree of pulmonary stenosis determines the volume of right-to-left shunting and thus the degree of cyanosis. The murmur is determined by the degree of pulmonary stenosis, not the VSD. These infants present with normal feeding, weight gain, and vital signs but they are cyanotic. Dehydration may worsen cyanosis.

Right-to-left and Left-to-right Shunts (Total Mixing Lesions)

Total mixing lesions such as atrioventricular septal defects (AVSDs) may present with mild cyanosis and pulmonary overcirculation. These patients have right-to-left *and* left-to-right shunting causing both cyanosis and pulmonary over circulation. Presentation will also be affected by associated defects such as pulmonary stenosis, unbalanced ventricles (one ventricle larger than the other), and so forth. If either of these associated defects is present with AVSD, they will present as a ductal dependent lesion, rather than as pulmonary over circulation.

Triage. Age, vital signs, weight, color, and respiratory status will indicate acuity of most congenital heart lesions (Table 94.3).

Initial Assessment/H&P. Newborn infants with significant congenital heart malformations may be completely asymptomatic until the DA closes or PVR drops. Large population studies have shown that screening newborns using pulse oximetry combined with physical examination prior to hospital discharge can detect up to 82.8% of all cardiac defects. The most likely defects to be missed in the newborn nursery are left ventricular (LV) obstructive lesions. This is important because the infant who is discharged from the nursery with undetected CHD, is at increased risk for mortality and morbidity.

In the ED, history should focus on age at presentation, feeding patterns, weight gain, breathing patterns, and color changes. When the patient presents in shock, cardiac and noncardiac diagnoses must be considered. Cardiac lesions that present with shock include those dependent on the DA for systemic blood flow (LV obstructive lesions) or severe ductal dependent right ventricular outflow tract obstruction

TABLE 94.2

CONGENITAL HEART DISEASE: INITIAL DIAGNOSIS

Structural congenital heart lesions	Age	Cyanosis	Murmur	Unique PE findings	CXR	EKG
Ventricular Septal Defect (VSD)	2 mo	No	II/VI–V/VI harsh holosystolic murmur LLSB Smaller the VSD the louder the murmur; Very large VSDs have no murmur	Tachypnea Poor weight gain after 6–8 wks of life	Cardiomegaly Increased pulmonary vascular markings	LAH LVH
Patent Ductus Arteriosus (PDA)	2–6 wks	Not usually (Cyanosis in lower extremities only, with pulmonary hypertension)	1–4/6 Continuous machinery-like left infraclavicular area	Bounding peripheral pulses Wide pulse pressure	Normal Cardiomegaly + increased pulmonary vascular markings	Mild: normal Moderate-large: sinus tachycardia, atrial fibrillation, LVH, LAE
Pulmonary Stenosis (PS)	PPS-newborn Critical PS-birth Not critical-childhood	Critical PS—Yes Not Critical—No	Systolic ejection murmur at the LUSB that radiates to the back Valvar PS + click PPS is benign murmur of newborn (I-II/VI)	Not critical—asymptomatic with murmur	Critical PS—Paucity of blood flow to lung fields	RVH Possible P-Pulmonale
Tetralogy of Fallot (TOF)	Birth to 2 wks (ductal closure) Depends on degree of PS	Yes (proportional to pulmonary stenosis)	Systolic thrill lower and middle left sternal border, loud single S2, aortic ejection click, loud grade 3–5/6 SEM in middle–lower sternal border	Tet Spell—agitated (See text for management)	Boot shaped heart Normal heart size Decreased pulmonary vascular markings	RAD RVH (RBBB post op)
Aortic Stenosis (AS) (subvalvar, valvar, and supravalvar)	Birth, Subaortic stenosis may develop later	No	II–IV/VI rough/harsh SEM at right upper intercostal space or left intercostal space with radiation to neck Aortic valve stenosis + Click	Supravalvar associated with William syndrome	Cardiomegaly LVH	Severe: LVH with strain pattern
Aortic Regurgitation (AR)	Adolescence to adulthood	No	High pitched diastolic decrescendo murmur heard best at LLSB	Secondary to procedure on aortic valve (i.e., AS s/p valvuloplasty)	Cardiomegaly	LAE/LVE
Bicuspid Aortic Valve (BAV)	Young adult	No	SEM + ejection click	Most common congenital heart defect Risk for stenosis later in life	Normal	Normal

Atrial Septal Defect (ASD)	Any time after 1 yr	No	Pulmonary flow murmur, widely split and fixed S2 II–III/VI SEM upper left sternal border with mid diastolic rumble	Asymptomatic Rarely, develop PHN, more often in association with trisomy 21 Late SSS and atrial arrhythmias	Cardiomegaly (RVE) with increased pulmonary vascular markings	RAD RVH RBBB, IRBBB RAE Crotchetage III
Coarctation of the Aorta (CoA)	2 wks (ductal closure) Later in childhood	No	Grade II–III/VI SEM ULSB	Weak pulses Brachial–femoral delay in pulses, decreased pulses in lower extremities Infancy—CHF, shock Child—asymptomatic murmur, nosebleeds, HTN Adult—asymptomatic, hypertension	Shock (no blood flow to lower body when PDA closes) Cardiomegaly Pulmonary edema Rib notching “3 sign” (older children) Hypertension	RVH RBBB
D-Transposition of the Great Arteries (TGA)	Birth	Yes-severe	None Loud, single S2	Profound cyanosis	Normal to minimally enlarged heart Narrow superior mediastinum (involuted thymus) “Egg-on-a-string”	RAD RVH
Atrioventricular Septal Defect (AVSD)	6–8 wks	Yes If unrepaired—Eisenmenger syndrome	Systolic thrill Holosystolic AV valve regurgitant murmur Loud Split S2	Hyperactive precordium, Commonly with trisomy 21	Increased pulmonary vascular markings Cardiomegaly	Superior QRS axis RVH RBBB LVH Prolonged PR
Malposition/ Heterotaxy			Depends on associated defects		Right-sided heart Inversion of abdominal organs may also be seen	
Mitral valve regurgitation (MR)	Depends on degree	No	Systolic regurgitant murmur over the apex, possible diastolic inflow murmur if severe		LA or LV enlargement depending or severity	Usually normal
Mitral valve prolapse (MVP)	Depends on degree	No	Mid systolic click Possible systolic regurgitant murmur that gets louder with standing if MR present	Associated with connective tissue disorders (Marfan syndrome)	Depends on associated findings (MVR, aortic root dilation in Marfan)	Usually normal

(*continued*)

TABLE 94.2

CONGENITAL HEART DISEASE: INITIAL DIAGNOSIS (*CONTINUED*)

Structural congenital heart lesions	Age	Cyanosis	Murmur	Unique PE findings	CXR	EKG
Mitral stenosis	Depends on degree, associated symptoms and congenital vs. acquired	No	Diastolic inflow murmur	Possible syncope with exercise		Possible LA enlargement
Cor triatriatum	1–3 yrs old or Asymptomatic until adulthood	No	Soft, blowing systolic murmur		Pulmonary venous congestion	RVH
Pulmonary vein stenosis	Neonatal	No	None		Reticular pattern of PV obstruction in lung fields	
Hypoplastic Left heart syndrome (HLHS)	Birth to ductal closure	Yes	Single S_2 heart sound SEM Examination may be normal	Diminished pulses Shock	Cardiomegaly Pulmonary edema	Nonspecific RAE May show RVH Peaked T waves
Pulmonary atresia	Birth	Yes	Single S_2 heart sound		Normal	Decreased right-sided forces Relative LAD
Double-Outlet Right Ventricle (DORV)	Birth to ductal closure to 2 months	Varies with associated lesions	DORV presentation may vary from TOF like physiology to D-TGA physiology, depending on arrangement of PA, degree of PS, and proximity to VSD			
Single ventricle	Birth—ductal closure	Yes	Varies with associated lesions	Includes tricuspid atresia, HLHS, unbalanced AVSD, some DILV, DORV, etc.		
Tricuspid atresia	Birth—ductal closure	Yes	Single S2 VSD and PDA murmurs	Cyanosis	Normal OR Small heart size	RAH LAH LVH
Ebstein anomaly	Prenatal to adulthood Depends on severity	Yes	Mid systolic click	Cyanosis CHF	Massive cardiomegaly ("wall-to-wall") Decreased pulmonary vascularity	RAH, RBBB Pre-excitation + LBBB Low voltage right-sided QRS First-degree AV block

Truncus Arteriosus	Birth	Mild	Loud regurgitant systolic murmur at LSB Systolic ejection click at apex/LSB Single heart sound	Cyanosis CHF Accentuated and bounding pulses	Cardiomegaly Pulmonary vascular congestion Interstitial edema Right-sided aortic arch	Normal OR RVH LVH
Total Anomalous Pulmonary Venous Return (TAPVR)	Obstructed TAPVR = birth Unobstructed = later	mild to moderate	None	CHF Shock	Cardiomegaly (if no pulmonary venous obstruction) Increased pulmonary vascular markings Supracardiac—"snowman" or "figure eight" (>4 mo)	RAD RVH RAE
Aortopulmonary window	2 mo	No	Accentuated S2, narrow split prominent ejection click in pulmonic area loud SEM LUSB or machinery like (similar to PDA) Bounding pulses when PVR drops	CHF Tachypnea		
Anomalous Left Coronary Artery from the Pulmonary Artery (ALCAPA)	10 wks	No	Mitral regurgitation may occur due to LV enlargement CHF findings	Fussy, irritable, wheezing, poor feeding, grey color skin, hepatomegaly	Cardiomegaly Pulmonary edema	MI: deep, wide Q waves, inverted T waves, ST segment changes in precordial leads
Vascular ring/sling	Birth to adulthood	No	None	Asymptomatic Signs tracheal compression Signs of esophageal compression	Normal	Normal
Cardiac tumor	Varies with size and location	None	Varies with size and location; any outflow or regurgitant murmur vs. normal	Varies with size and location; CHF vs. obstructive symptoms vs. arrhythmia vs. sudden cardiac death	Varies with size and location	Varies with size and location

RAD, right axis deviation; LVH, left ventricular hypertrophy; RVH, right ventricular hypertrophy; LAE, left atrial enlargement; RAE, right atrial enlargement; SSS, sick sinus syndrome; PVR, pulmonary vascular resistance; PDA, patent ductus arteriosus; PPS, peripheral pulmonary stenosis; RUSB, right upper sternal border; LUSB, left upper sternal border; LSB, left sternal border; VSD, ventricular septal defect; LA, left atrium; RA, right atrium; LV, left ventricular; RV, right ventricular; HTN, hypertension; CHF, congestive heart failure; PS, pulmonary stenosis; SEM, systolic ejection murmur.

TABLE 94.3

AGE AND VITAL SIGNS OF INFANTS WITH CYANOSIS OR CHF/PULMONARY OVER CIRCULATION

	Cyanosis	CHF/Pulmonary over circulation
Age	2 wks	2 mo
Weight gain	Normal	Poor after 6–8 wks
Oxygen saturation	<95%	>95%
RR	Normal	>50/min
HR	Normal	Slightly high
BP	Normal	Normal or arm HTN or leg lower than arm

CHF, Congestive heart failure; RR. respiratory rate; HR, heart rate; BP, blood pressure; HTN, hypertension

(RVOTO). In addition, identifying a genetic syndrome may shed light on likely cardiac diagnoses (Table 94.4).

Management/Diagnostic Testing of an Infant in Shock, Suspected Ductal Dependent Lesion. While immediate attention to airway, breathing, circulation, and high-quality CPR are first steps in the management of a patient in shock, initiation of prostaglandin (PGE_1) to re-establish ductal patency is a lifesaving therapy. The dose of PGE_1 is 0.05 to 0.1 mcg/kg/min via intravenous (IV) or intraosseus (IO) line. Side effects of PGE_1 include hypotension, apnea, fever, and rash. Titrate PGE_1 until femoral pulses are palpable or oxygen saturations improve. Effect should be seen within 30 minutes.

Endotracheal intubation and mechanical ventilation decrease the work of breathing by reducing cardiac demands and guard against apnea caused by PGE_1. Epinephrine and other drugs for resuscitation should be drawn up and ready for administration during endotracheal intubation, since there is a high likelihood of cardiac arrest during this procedure. Once the airway is secured, aim to maintain oxygen saturations at approximately 75%. Over ventilation and hyperoxygenation may cause systemic blood pressure to drop significantly since oxygen is a potent pulmonary vasodilator. Pulmonary vasodilation drops the PVR, thereby increasing shunting of systemic blood flow into the lungs, and thus causing systemic hypotension. If the blood pressure falls, check for over ventilation or oxygen saturations above 75% to 85%. If possible, lower saturations to control PBF and restore systemic BP.

Chest x-ray (CXR) is useful to assess heart size and pulmonary circulation or pulmonary venous congestion. It also shows the cardiac silhouette, thoracic and abdominal situs, and aortic arch sidedness. Cardiac rhythm should be monitored. EM physicians trained in emergency ultrasound may assess cardiac function. Electrocardiogram (EKG) with rhythm strip is the gold standard for arrhythmia diagnosis, and may also offer clues in structural heart disease. Refer to Table 94.2 for typical presenting signs and symptoms, CXR, and EKG findings on initial evaluation of suspected CHD. Table 94.5 outlines common issues in patients after cardiac surgery.

Laboratory evaluation should include venous or arterial blood gas (ABG), electrolytes, blood urea nitrogen (BUN),

TABLE 94.4

GENETIC CONDITIONS AND TYPICALLY ASSOCIATED CHD

Alagille syndrome	PPS, TOF ±PA, ASD, VSD, coarctation of aorta
CHARGE syndrome	TOF, aortic arch anomalies
Cornelia de Lange	VSD, ASD, PS, HCM
DiGeorge Syndrome	Truncus arteriosus, complex TOF
Deletion 1p36 syndrome	Ebstein anomaly, Noncompaction left ventricle, dilated cardiomyopathy, TOF/PA, PDA
Deletion 4p syndrome (Wolf–Hirschhorn syndrome)	Pulmonic stenosis, ASD, VSD
Trisomy 21 (Down syndrome)	AVSD, VSD (all types), ASD (secundum type), PDA, TOF
Holt–Oram syndrome, TBX5 gene	ASD and possible VSD
Noonan syndrome	HCM, PS with dysplastic pulmonary valve, partial AVSD, coarctation of aorta
Goldenhar syndrome	TOF
Jacobsen syndrome	HLHS, VSD
Marfan syndrome	Aortic root dilation, mitral valve prolapse
Partial trisomy 9	HLHS
Smith–Lemli–Opitz	HLHS, secundum ASD, VSD, AVSD, TAPVR
Tetrasomy 22p (Cat Eye syndrome)	TAPVR, PAPVR
Trisomy 13	Conotruncal: DORV, TOF, Common AVSD, ASD, VSD, PDA, polyvalvar dysplasia
Trisomy 18	VSD, TOF, DORV, AVSD, polyvalvar dysplasia, bicuspid aortic valve
Turner syndrome 45,XO	Coarctation of aorta, bicuspid aortic valve, AS, mitral valve anomalies, MVP, HLHS
Williams–Beuren syndrome	PS, supravalvar AS
Williams syndrome	Supravalvar AS, abnormal origin of coronary arteries, PS, PPS
Deletion 7p	ASD, VSD

CHD, congenital heart disease; PPS, peripheral pulmonary stenosis; TOF, tetralogy of Fallot; PA, pulmonary atresia; ASD, atrial septal defect; VSD, ventricular septal defect; PDA, patent ductus arteriosus; AVSD, atrioventricular septal defect; HCM, hypertrophic cardiomyopathy; HLHS, hypoplastic left heart syndrome; TAPVR, total anomalous pulmonary venous return; PAPVR, partial anomalous pulmonary venous return; DORV, double outlet right ventricle; MVP, mitral valve prolapse; PS, pulmonary stenosis; AS, aortic stenosis

TABLE 94.5

CONGENITAL HEART DISEASE REPAIRS: PEARLS AND PITFALLS

Repair	Type	Use/lesions	Description	Pearls and pitfalls
Blalock–Taussig Shunt (modified) (mBTS)	Palliative	Cyanotic lesions and decreased PBF: HLHS, TOF, RVOTO, Pulmonary atresia	Gortex graft from subclavian artery to ipsilateral PA creates a left-to-right aortopulmonary shunt Original BTS involved diverting subclavian artery directly to the PA	Ideal oxygen saturations ~75% Assess for shunt murmur to establish patency Beware of PHTN, dehydration, systemic hypotension Treat obstructed shunt with IV fluid bolus, Heparin and emergency surgery
Norwood stage I	Palliative	HLHS/Single ventricle	Performed at birth. Patient with HLHS and aortic atresia. Hypoplastic aorta is reconstructed using MPA. mBTS central or Sano (ventricle to PA) shunt for pulmonary blood flow. See mBTS above	Avoid 100% oxygen and overventilation, which lead to pulmonary overcirculation at the expense of the systemic circulation. Mortality rate is ~15% due to vagal events, arrhythmia, ischemia, CHF, mBTS malfunction. Place NG tube with caution
Norwood stage II (Bidirectional Glenn Shunt)	Palliative	Single ventricle, ex: HLHS, unbalanced AVSD, Tricuspid atresia, etc.	Performed at age 3–6 mo. Anastomosis of the superior vena cava to pulmonary artery (cavopulmonary shunt) See bidirectional Glenn Shunt BTS is taken down at this stage	Flow from the SVC to PA depends on low PA pressures. Oxygen sats typically 70–80% Avoid PHTN, hypoxia, acidosis, and positive pressure ventilation, hypovolemia Treat with O_2 and preload/fluids
Fontan	Final palliation	HLHS, or any lesion with a single ventricle	Performed at age 2 yrs to adulthood. SVC and IVC surgically connected to the PA. Pulmonary venous return to the single ventricle, ventricular outflow through the neoaorta to the body	No murmur with good hemodynamics but possible loud, single S2. AV valve regurgitation or AS murmur indicate poor hemodynamics Risk for CHF, chylous effusions, arrhythmias, and protein losing enteropathy from GI tract
Rastelli Procedure	Final repair	Pulmonary atresia or TOF with large conal branch coronary	RV to PA conduit	Often develop pulmonary insufficiency requiring conduit replacement in adulthood if symptomatic
Pulmonary Artery Banding	Palliative	"Swiss cheese" septum, i.e. multiple muscular VSD's, some single ventricle anatomy, i.e., unbalanced AVSD	Performed in newborn to limit pulmonary blood flow until definitive repair	Too tight will present cyanotic and too loose present in CHF
Arterial switch	Final repair	D-TGA	Transposed aorta and pulmonary artery are surgically switched, coronary arteries are re-implanted	Usually presents at birth to 2 wks. Sequelae include coronary artery insufficiency and aortic or pulmonic valve insufficiency
Mustard or Senning	Final palliation	D-TGA surgical repair used prior to arterial switch operation	Baffle from IVC and SVC to the tricuspid valve & baffle from pulmonary veins to the mitral valve	Not used after 1990s. Prone to tachycardia and bradycardia. Anatomic RV is systemic ventricle and often develops CHF
ASD closure	Final repair	Secundum ASD	Surgical stitch, patch or catheter device closure	Amplatzer occluder device commonly used for transvenous closure in cath laboratory

(continued)

TABLE 94.5

CONGENITAL HEART DISEASE REPAIRS: PEARLS AND PITFALLS (*CONTINUED*)

Repair	Type	Use/lesions	Description	Pearls and pitfalls
VSD closure	Final repair	VSD	Surgical patch or (rarely) catheter device closure	Residual defects and post op complete heart block are main complications
PDA ligation	Final repair	Hemodynamically significant PDA	Surgical ligation or coil closure in the cath laboratory	Echo pre-op to rule out any ductal dependent lesions
Coarctation of aorta anastomosis	Final repair	End–to-end or extended end-to-end anastomosis	Narrowed segment removed with end-to-end or oblique anastomosis	End-to-end may re-stenosis, always check arm–leg blood pressures
Ross procedure	Final repair	Aortic valve stenosis	Aortic valve is removed and replaced with patient's own pulmonary valve (autograft). Donor pulmonary homograft (human cadaver) valve is put into the pulmonary position. Coronary arteries are reimplanted	Autograft allows for growth of aortic valve, relatively high failure rate. Pulmonary homograft often develops pulmonary insufficiency Prone to coronary insufficiency
Tetralogy of Fallot	Palliation or final repair	Initial surgery may be mBTS followed by full repair	mBTS used in critical PS, PAtr. These lesions are ductal dependent. Less severe TOF may be fully repaired at 6–9 mo of life	mBTS risks and risk of Tet spells in unrepaired infants Later may have atrial or ventricular arrhythmias and free pulmonary insufficiency
Valve replacement	Final repair	For stenosis, regurgitation	Prosthetic vs. homograft	Risk for bleeding if anticoagulated (prosthetic), valve malfunction/ insufficiency Listen for metallic click to evaluate valve on physical examination
Heart transplantation	Palliation	CHF, myocarditis, severe congenital heart defects	Removal of native heart and replacement with donor heart	Rejection always a concern, CHF, coronary artery disease may develop, nonadherence, bradycardia and sensitivity to adenosine
Damus–Kaye–Stancel	Palliation	Used to bypass LVOTO in single ventricle lesions	Bypass AS or sub AS in complex lesions. May be part of initial palliation in Norwood I operation	Bypasses aortic stenosis (AS), but AS murmur still present

PBF, pulmonary blood flow; HLHS, hypoplastic left heart syndrome; TOF, tetralogy of Fallot; RVOTO, right ventricular outflow tract obstruction; PAtr, pulmonary atresia; PA, pulmonary artery; VSD, ventricular septal defect; ASD, atrial septal defect; D-TGA, dextro-transposition of the great arteries; LVOTO, left ventricular outflow tract obstruction; PHTN, pulmonary hypertension; IVC, inferior vena cava; SVC, superior vena cava; CHF, congestive heart failure; AS, aortic stenosis; AV, atrioventricular.

creatinine (Cr), ionized calcium, magnesium, glucose, complete blood count (CBC), liver function tests (LFTs), and coagulation studies. Blood tests reflect end-organ damage of the liver and kidneys.

Judicious fluid resuscitation based on clinical presentation may be employed. If the patient is anemic and cyanotic, red blood cell infusion may be used to expand intravascular volume. A urinary catheter should be inserted for fluid management. Initiate inotropic support as needed with dopamine 5 to 10 mcg/kg/min. Other inotropes to consider include epinephrine, norepinephrine, and milrinone.

As soon as cardiac pathology is suspected, consult cardiology. Consult cardiac surgery early if extracorporeal membrane oxygenation (ECMO) or surgical intervention is anticipated.

Management/Diagnostic Testing of an Infant with Cyanosis and Suspected Ductal Dependent Lesion. The presentation of cyanosis due to ductal dependent lesions is variable as ductal dependent lesions exist along a wide spectrum. If cyanosis is the predominant symptom, first administer 100% oxygen. Oxygen supplementation will not improve cyanosis due to cardiac causes but pulmonary causes should respond. Oxygen administration may be diagnostic as well as therapeutic in the stable patient. The hyperoxia test can help differentiate cardiac from pulmonary disease. After receiving 100% oxygen for 10 minutes, an ABG is tested. If the PO_2 is greater than 150 mm Hg, it is normal. PO_2 less than 100 mm Hg suggests cardiac etiology. Pulse oximetry should not be used for the hyperoxia test.

Treatment of cardiac cyanosis is the re-establishment of PBF by opening the DA using PGE_1 (0.05 to 1 mcg/kg/min) as discussed above. Endotracheal intubation and mechanical ventilation will protect the infant from apnea, a common side effect of PGE_1.

A hypercyanotic spell (Tet spell) is a cyanotic emergency, which may result in altered mental status, loss of consciousness, or death. Events are typified by hyperpnea, tachypnea, and agitation. It occurs when a patient with TOF or similar lesion involving RVOTO, experiences an event in which the muscular infundibular portion of the RVOT becomes diminishingly small, preventing blood flow to the lungs. All blood is then shunted right-to-left across the nonrestrictive VSD. The pulmonary stenosis murmur disappears. Extreme cyanosis ensues.

Treatment of a hypercyanotic event follows a stepwise progression. Initially, bring the knees to the chest, allowing the parent to comfort the patient in this position. Monitor closely. Knee to chest position in infants, or squatting in older children, increases SVR and decreases right-to-left shunting. Administer 100% oxygen. If the spell persists, morphine (0.1 mg/kg IM or IV) can be used to calm agitation. Normal saline bolus (5 to 10 mL/kg) ensures adequate preload and may be repeated if the patient is dehydrated. If these steps are not successful a continuous intravenous (IV) infusion of phenylephrine, an alpha agonist (0.5 to 5 mcg/kg/min), may be titrated to increase SVR. Propranolol, a beta-blocker, may be used to decrease heart rate and promote ventricular filling, but care should be exercised when administering this drug as hypotension may occur. If the spell still is not broken, general anesthesia and emergent surgery for placement of a systemic–pulmonary shunt or full repair is the next step. Ketamine 1 to 2 mg/kg IM or IV is an excellent drug for sedation for endotracheal intubation or other procedures.

After stabilization the patient should be admitted to an intensive care unit skilled in cardiac care. Chronic oral beta blocker therapy may be initiated in an attempt to decrease RVOT infundibular reactivity and thus prevent further spells. Definitive care is surgical repair or palliation with an aortopulmonary shunt.

Management/Diagnostic Testing of Infant Presenting with Left-to-right Shut and Pulmonary Overcirculation. Diuretic therapy is the mainstay of acute treatment for pulmonary overcirculation due to left-to-right shunt lesions. When used with afterload reduction the symptoms of overcirculation may be mitigated until the time of surgical repair. Hospital admission may be necessary for initiation of medical therapy, treatment of concurrent infections, or surgery if medical management is not effective. IV fluids and oxygen should be avoided in these patients, as either intervention will worsen pulmonary overcirculation.

Clinical Indications for Discharge or Admission. Any child newly diagnosed with hemodynamically significant CHD should be admitted to the hospital. Consultation with a pediatric cardiologist can guide this decision. Very ill patients such as those requiring a PGE_1 infusion, should be admitted to an intensive care unit skilled in the care of sick neonates with heart disease. The safest mode of transport is with a skilled pediatric transport team.

Congenital Heart Disease: Postoperative and Other Considerations. For a reference on congenital heart defects, surgical repairs, common complications, and sequelae, see Table 94.5.

Some guiding principles will help EM providers navigate the specifics of a patient with CHD whose diagnosis is known. Red flags in CHD include age less than 2 months, especially with palliated or unrepaired defects, poor cardiac function, single ventricle anatomy, and arrhythmias. Special consideration should also be given to infants or older children with respiratory illness, especially respiratory syncytial virus, with palliative surgery or infants with pulmonary overcirculation.

Aortopulmonary shunts (modified Blalock–Taussig (BT), central shunts, etc.) may be larger or smaller than optimal, causing problematic over or under circulation of the lungs. The size of the shunts can be judged by oxygen saturation. Patients with excessive shunt flow will present with high saturations (>95%) and pulmonary edema. Patients with inadequate shunt flow due to shunt malfunction or decreased systemic blood pressure, or a small shunt present with cyanosis (saturations <75%).

A patient with *BT shunt obstruction* will present with cyanosis that may progress to cardiac arrest. History of CHD, worsening cyanosis, and lack of a shunt murmur raise the suspicion for shunt obstruction. Risk factors include shunt size <4 mm, very young age at the time of shunt placement, and low weight. The obstruction may be due to thrombus formation, often in the setting of dehydration or may be due to kinking of the shunt. No shunt murmur is audible on auscultation of the right or left infraclavicular area.

Treatment of shunt stenosis or clotting is administration of an IV normal saline bolus, heparin, and emergent surgical consultation. Shunt obstruction can be confirmed with an echocardiogram. Endotracheal intubation may be needed. Pressors may be used to augment systemic blood pressure to perfuse the shunt. Consider pulmonary hypertensive crisis in the differential diagnosis of a patient who presents with cyanosis and no shunt murmur. Pulmonary hypertensive crisis is treated with hyperventilation, oxygen, correction of acidosis, and sedation. Ketamine is a good choice for sedation if needed in these patients.

Infants who have undergone the first stage (Norwood Stage I) palliation for single ventricle are at high risk for sudden cardiac death (SCD). About 15% of these infants will die before the second palliative operation. Respiratory or other intercurrent noncardiac illnesses are very concerning and may be fatal. Nasogastric tubes should be placed with caution to avoid significant vagal stimulation. Coronary blood flow may be compromised in some patients, leading to acute heart failure and/or ventricular arrhythmias. Management of these patients in the ED should be expedited and cardiology consultation should be obtained prior to discharge. Caution should be used even when the infant is well appearing.

Postpericardiotomy syndrome (PPS) is a postsurgical syndrome of fever, pericardial and pleural inflammatory response, with effusions and malaise. It usually occurs one to several weeks after open-heart surgery, cardiac catheterization, or transvenous device implantation. The etiology is thought to be an autoimmune reaction. If pericardial fluid accumulates rapidly, it may present as cardiac tamponade.

If PPS is suspected, evaluate for leukocytosis and eosinophilia on CBC. Echocardiogram can detect pericardial fluid and assess for tamponade. PPS is treated with salicylates and pericardiocentesis if needed. Steroids are indicated if salicylates are not effective or the effusion is large.

Pleural effusions may be seen acutely after discharge from the hospital following any type of congenital heart surgery. Chylous or serous effusions may be chronic following Fontan procedure (caval pulmonary anastomosis) due to increased central venous pressures (lymphatic congestion).

Postoperative cardiac patients may present to the ED with wound infection, sepsis, endocarditis, and/or mediastinitis. Sepsis presents with fever or florid septic shock and occurs in 2.6% of patients after cardiac surgery. The usual pathogens are group A beta-hemolytic *Streptococcus, Escherichia coli, Listeria monocytogenes, Staphylococcus aureus,* and *Pseudomonas aeruginosa.* Endocarditis presents with nonspecific symptoms of fever, poor feeding, and malaise. High-risk situations for endocarditis include the presence of an abnormal aortic valve, residual VSD, TOF, and extensive repairs involving foreign material such as prosthetic valves. Atrial septal defects and right-sided defects are at lower risk for endocarditis. A new murmur may develop from dehiscence of a patch/conduit or turbulent flow caused by vegetations. Common pathogens implicated in endocarditis include *Staphylococcus aureus, Streptococcus pyogenes,* and *Streptococcus viridans* (Chapter 102 Infectious Disease Emergencies).

Mediastinitis is a serious postoperative complication that presents with local erythema, pain, induration, fluctuance, and purulent drainage from the sternotomy incision. This local infection may cause wound dehiscence and sternal instability. The most common pathogen causing mediastinitis is *Staphylococcus aureus.* Approximately 50% of patients with mediastinitis will have concurrent bacteremia.

When an infection is suspected, CBC, erythrocyte sedimentation rate (ESR), urinalysis, urine culture, and blood cultures should be obtained. Concern for sepsis, endocarditis, or mediastinitis warrants prompt treatment with empiric broad-spectrum IV antibiotics although cultures should be obtained from the wound or blood before antibiotics if the patient is stable. Judicious fluid resuscitation for septic shock depends on the heart disease. Give aliquots of 10 mL/kg crystalloid for fluid resuscitation in patients with poor ventricular function, volume overload, or significant AV valve regurgitation. Reassess frequently for signs of CHF. In all surgical complications, cardiothoracic surgery and cardiology should be consulted.

Cardiac Transplantation. Pediatric heart transplant patients presenting to the ED require special consideration. The ED physician must be well versed on common problems encountered in this group of patients. Concerns following transplant include rejection, infection, nonadherence, cardiac allograft vasculopathy (CAV), and issues arising from long-term immunosuppression.

Rejection, infection, and CAV may all present in a similar fashion. Pediatric transplant patients with these conditions present with subtle complaints including tachycardia, tachypnea, lethargy, irritability, abdominal pain, nausea, vomiting, and/or poor feeding. Abdominal pain is frequently endorsed in pediatric patients with rejection or symptomatic CAV. Atypical chest pain may also be a sign of CAV and of rejection (chest pain can occur as some patients partially reinnervate over time). Low-grade fever, malaise, and heart failure symptoms may also be present. Arrhythmias and conduction disturbances may be a sign of rejection or coronary artery vasculopathy. Physical signs may include jugular venous distension, hepatomegaly, new murmur, and a gallop.

Infections are a threat to the immunocompromised transplant patient. Prophylaxis against fungal (nystatin), CMV (ganciclovir, especially in CMV + donor), and protozoal (TMP–SMX) infections is used after transplant. In the first month following transplant, the greatest risk of infection is bacterial or fungal. In the second month, CMV and other viruses pose the greatest threat.

Long-term immunosuppression increases the transplant recipient's risk for posttransplant lymphoproliferative disorder/malignancy, hypertension, and renal failure. In the adolescent age group, nonadherence is a leading cause of late rejection and death. Adherence to the medical regimen should be asked of all adolescent patients presenting to the ED. The transplanted patient should be carefully evaluated with these issues in mind when presenting to the ED for any reason.

Following a careful physical examination, B-type natriuretic peptide (BNP), chemistry, CBC, blood cultures, viral studies, CXR, EKG, and echocardiogram may aid diagnosis and treatment. Prompt consultation with the cardiac transplant service is recommended when these patients present to the ED.

For more information on complications specific to particular lesions or complications specific to particular procedures/surgical repairs refer to Table 94.6.

Adults with Congenital Heart Disease

As a result of advances in diagnosis and surgical management, most patients born today with CHD survive into adulthood. There are an estimated 1 million adults living with CHD in the United States of America. These patients require specialized care provided by cardiologists trained in this field. Commonly encountered complications in adults with congenital heart disease (ACHD) include poor cardiac function and atrial arrhythmias. Similar to children with CHD, history should elicit information about diagnosis, baseline cardiac function, concurrent medical history, medication, and previous problems encountered.

Intraatrial reentrant tachycardia (IART) is a variation of atrial flutter where the reentrant circuit is caused by scarring in the atrium from previous surgeries. Often the rate of IART is relatively slow and the amplitude of the P waves is low, making this arrhythmia hard to detect. The heart rate in IART may be 80 to 86 BPM and may look like sinus rhythm. Patients with single ventricle palliation typically do not tolerate any nonsinus rhythm, even if its rate is controlled. Adenosine blocks AV conduction transiently but usually does not terminate tachycardia. Due to the low amplitude of the P waves, continuation of IART during adenosine administration is often missed. Synchronized cardioversion is typically the treatment of choice.

Sudden death can be a complication after repair of CHD. Risk increases with increasing age of the patient, complexity of the repair, and with poor ventricular function. Long term, the highest risk lesions include TOF, aortic stenosis, transposition of the great arteries, coarctation of the aorta, AVSD, pulmonary stenosis, and anomalies that undergo the Fontan procedure. Repaired VSD and PDA ligation are low risk procedures with respect to SCD.

ARRHYTHMIC EMERGENCIES

Goal of Treatment

The primary goal of treatment in a cardiac arrhythmic emergency is rapid recognition and correction of unstable arrhythmias while simultaneously documenting the rhythm on EKG. A secondary goal is to identify patients with subtle signs of aborted SCD.

TABLE 94.6

LESION SPECIFIC COMPLICATIONS

Congenital heart lesion	Complication	Details	Presentation	Treatment
Coarctation of the aorta	Arch obstruction/restenosis Aortic dissection Aortic aneurysm	Restenosis is more likely if balloon angioplasty of the coarctation was performed Aortic dissection at coarctation site with or without aneurysm	Hypertension; Arm–leg blood pressure discrepancy	Cardiology consultation; resuscitation as needed
TOF	Atrial and ventricular arrhythmias Asymptomatic RBBB on EKG	Normal to have PS murmur with Pulmonary insufficiency	Fatigue and free pulmonary insufficiency	May require RVOT conduit replacement
ASD (Catheter Device Closure)	Device may erode through atrium; possibly into the esophagus (rare). Device may impinge on AV Node	Usually w/ large device/large defect and small patient	Shock, tamponade bradycardia—usually noted at procedure	Stabilization and emergent surgery
ASD (Surgical repair)	PPS SSS AFlut	PPS—early post op complication SSS and AFlut—late	Fever, pericardial effusion, tamponade Symptomatic Bradycardia Palpitations	NSAIDs, drainage Pacemaker (SSS) Catheter ablation or medication (AFlut)
D-TGA	Coronary artery insufficiency LV outflow obstruction and aortic or pulmonary valvar insufficiency	Coronary artery problems usually early postop complication Valvar issues arise later	Exertional chest pain or syncope Possible new murmur	Cardiology consultation
VSD	Asymptomatic RBBB Complete heart block CHB Residual VSDs	CHB early postop, rarely late Challenging defect closure if multiple muscular VSDs ("Swiss cheese septum")	Syncope with late onset CHB Pulmonary over circulation with residual VSDs	Medical management; Consider device closure in cath laboratory PA banding to limit PBF
AV Septal Defect	Bradycardia-SSS, mitral valve insufficiency	Cleft in left side of the AV valve often a source of insufficiency	CHF	Medical management or reoperation

TOF, tetralogy of Fallot; PS, pulmonary stenosis; RVOT, right ventricular outflow tract; RBBB, right bundle branch block; EKG, electrocardiogram; ASD, atrial septal defect; PPS post pericardiotomy syndrome; SSS, sick sinus syndrome; AFlut, atrial flutter; D-TGA, D-transposition of the great arteries; LV, left ventricle; CHB, complete heart block; VSD, ventricular septal defect; PA, pulmonary artery; PBF, pulmonary blood flow; AV, atrio-ventricular; CHF, congestive heart failure.

CLINICAL PEARLS AND PITFALLS

- Any incessant tachycardia can cause CHF and diminished LV function.
- In dilated cardiomyopathy (DCM), it may be difficult to discern which came first: tachycardia or DCM.
- Arrhythmias are not well tolerated in the setting of structural heart disease, especially single ventricle or in those who have undergone palliative repairs.
- Arrhythmias are not well tolerated in patients with poor LV function.
- Adenosine may be diagnostic as well as therapeutic.
- Never give adenosine in a wide complex irregular rhythm.
- In heart transplant patients, use adenosine with extreme caution at one-third to half the normal recommended dosage. Be prepared to pace in the event of asystole.
- Ventricular tachycardia (VT) may look narrow in infants.
- Long QT syndrome (LQTS) presents more frequently with sudden death as the first symptom in pediatrics than in adults.

Current Evidence

Arrhythmias may occur in healthy individuals as well as in those with heart disease. They may be congenital or acquired, fast or slow, and anywhere on the spectrum from benign to fatal. Recent advances have improved rhythm management, particularly of tachyarrhythmias, in the pediatric population. Cardiac catheter ablation can cure most tachyarrhythmias and is safe in young patients. Implantable pacemakers and defibrillators are small enough to be used in infants and children. Many diseases that predispose patients to sudden cardiac death (SCD) may be identified by genetic markers, facilitating primary preventive therapy.

Clinical Considerations

Clinical Recognition

Patients with either bradycardia or tachycardia may present with signs of decreased cardiac output including fatigue, dizziness, syncope, and sudden death. Presentation depends on how fast or slow the rhythm is, the age of the patient at presentation, how long the patient has been in the abnormal rhythm, and co-existing conditions such as structural heart disease.

Infants with dysrhythmias may present with increased crying, poor color, decreased responsiveness, poor feeding, vomiting, wheezing, or tachypnea. Abnormal heart rates may be picked up on routine well child visit and subsequently referred to the ED. There may be a history of tachycardia in utero or earlier in life.

Older children and adolescents with tachycardia often state their heart is "beeping" fast. In addition, they endorse dizziness, palpitations, fatigue, or sudden onset/offset of symptoms. Stomach pain, combativeness, or vomiting may be signs of poor cardiac output due to dysrhythmias. Some patients with incessant tachycardia may be asymptomatic and have the abnormality discovered incidentally.

Rarely do older children or adolescents with bradycardia endorse the feeling of the heart beating too slowly. Rather, they present with irritability, pallor, combativeness, fatigue, or syncope.

Triage. Any patient presenting with a heart rate that is out of the normal range for age and clinical situation should have full vital signs and perfusion checked. The emergency physician should evaluate any symptomatic patient giving special consideration to patients with a cardiac history, pacemaker or implantable cardioverter–defibrillator (ICD), syncope, or history of arrhythmias.

Initial Assessment/H&P. The history should focus on the presence of red flags including previous tachycardia, current medications and adherence to medical therapy, prior response to adenosine, length of symptoms, prior heart operation/catheterization/EP procedure, or presence of a pacemaker or ICD. Tachycardia in patients with underlying cardiac dysfunction should raise concern, even if the patient looks well. Infants, patients with heart transplant, single ventricle or palliated heart disease, and adults with CHD should also raise the provider's index of concern. The focus of the initial examination is to assess the hemodynamic status using heart rate, perfusion, level of consciousness, tachypnea, and hepatomegaly or other signs of CHF. Printing prior EKGs performed when the patient was in sinus rhythm or in episodes of tachycardia may be very helpful in analyzing an arrhythmia. Review of a prior episode of tachycardia on EKG, likewise is helpful. Often, treatment that was effective in prior episodes will be effective again; so if time allows, obtain this information from the medical record or the family.

Management/Diagnostic Testing of Tachycardia. The gold standard for arrhythmia diagnosis is a 12 or 15 lead EKG. Using the EKG, the rhythm may be classified into narrow or wide, and regular or irregular. The mechanism can be discerned from the rate and the P wave relationship to the QRS. Extremely regular tachycardia suggests a re-entrant circuit as the mechanism. Any irregularity of the rate or rhythm may reveal the mechanism of the arrhythmia and therefore these irregularities should be recorded on an EKG for scrutiny after the patient is stabilized.

When a patient presents to the ED with tachycardia a standard approach should be taken. First, assess hemodynamics and determine if the patient is stable or unstable. An unstable patient should rapidly be prepared for cardioversion or defibrillation according to Pediatric Advanced Life Support (PALS) guidelines. A simple rhythm strip should be recorded through the external defibrillator. If the patient is pulseless, high-quality CPR should be initiated, airway and IV access should be secured. Unstable nonsinus tachycardia should be cardioverted or defibrillated. Synchronization should be employed in all rhythms except ventricular fibrillation (VF) to prevent the shock from being delivered at a vulnerable time on the T wave, potentially inducing VF. If tachycardia persists, the shock should be repeated with higher energy according to PALS guidelines (see Chapter 4 Cardiopulmonary Resuscitation). After delivery of the shock, CPR should resume immediately. One provider should check the rhythm strip while another team member re-assesses the patient. If the rhythm has converted to normal sinus rhythm and the patient is stable, obtain an EKG, and assess for CHF. The patient should constantly be monitored for any deterioration in condition or change in rhythm. Inotropes are arrhythmogenic, so if necessary they should be initiated with care. Consult cardiology and admit to an intensive care unit skilled in care of dysrhythmias.

If the patient is stable, obtain an EKG with long rhythm strip to determine whether the QRS is narrow or wide and whether the rhythm is regular or irregular. That information drives subsequent actions.

Narrow Complex, Irregular Tachycardia. An irregularly, irregular, narrow QRS rhythm, is almost always atrial fibrillation (or less commonly, atrial flutter/intraatrial reentrant tachycardia with variable conduction). These rhythms will respond to synchronized cardioversion (0.5 to 1 J/kg), or medication for rate control. Due to the risk of stroke, one should avoid cardioversion in a patient who has been in atrial fibrillation for 48 hours or more, or who is unable to tell when tachycardia started. Either beta-blockers or calcium channel blockers may be used (but not in combination) to control rate until the patient is fully assessed for a possible clot in the left atrium. Calcium channel blockers are not given to patients less than 2 years of age. Amiodarone or sotalol are commonly used for chronic control atrial fibrillation and when used acutely may cause conversion to sinus rhythm.

Wide Complex, Irregular Tachycardia. A wide rhythm, which is irregularly irregular may be VT or atrial fibrillation with Wolff–Parkinson–White (WPW) and will require cardioversion/defibrillation. Assess for hemodynamic stability and proceed according to the PALS algorithms. WPW with atrial fibrillation should be cardioverted, just as for atrial fibrillation without WPW. Do not give adenosine to any patient with a wide complex *irregular* rhythm (see adenosine below).

Narrow Complex, Regular Tachycardia. Evaluation of a relatively stable patient with narrow complex tachycardia, includes asking the patient to perform a vagal maneuver *while recording the rhythm*. An external defibrillator/pacer should be available. The vagal technique chosen should be appropriate for the age of the patient. In infants, knee to chest position, rectal stimulation with a thermometer, or the diving reflex may be used. To elicit the diving reflex in an infant, gently place a slurry of ice and water in a plastic bag over the nose and eyes of the patient for no more than 35 seconds. Older children and adolescents may perform knee to chest, hold their breath, immerse their face in cold water, or bear down. If vagal maneuvers are unsuccessful in converting tachycardia to sinus rhythm, IV access should be obtained for administration of adenosine.

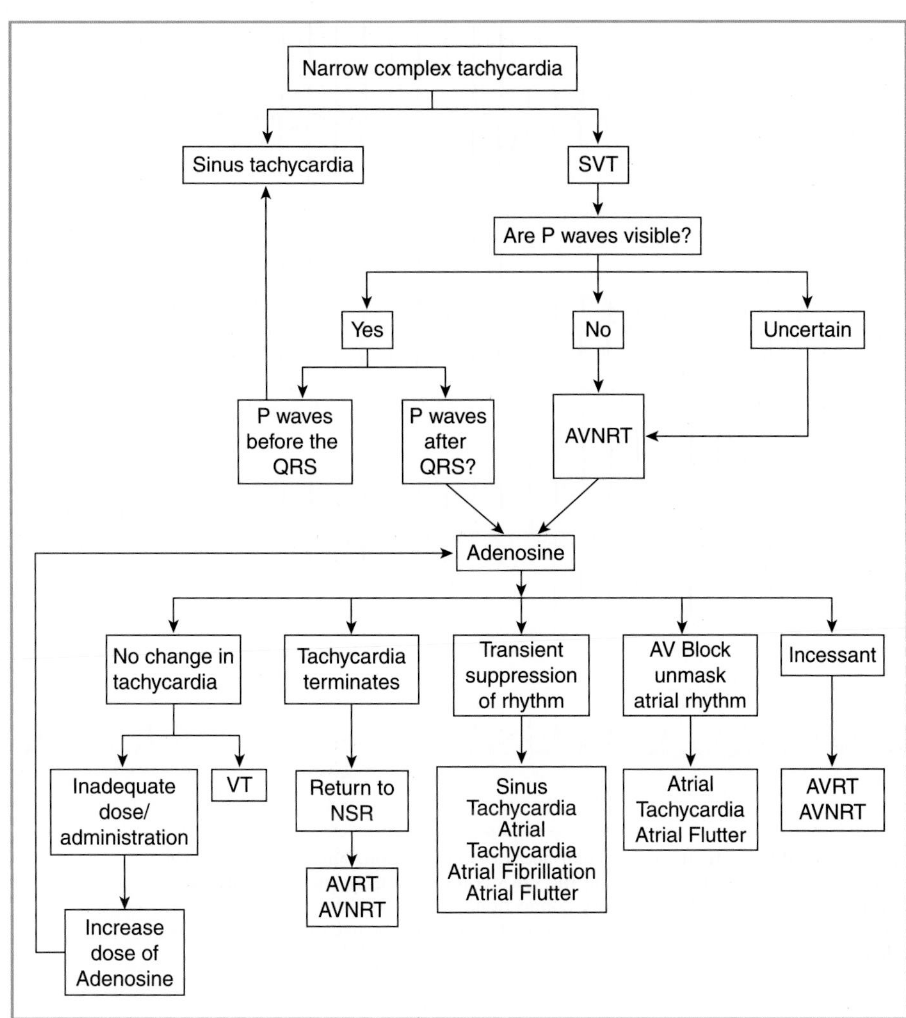

FIGURE 94.1 Narrow complex tachycardia and adenosine response. SVT, supraventricular tachycardia; AVNRT, atrioventricular nodal reentrant tachycardia; AV, atrioventricular; VT, ventricular tachycardia; NSR, normal sinus rhythm; AVRT, atrioventricular reentrant tachycardia.

Adenosine is the drug of choice in regular, narrow complex tachycardia. It is an amino acid that is rapidly metabolized by erythrocytes and the endothelium, giving it a half-life of about 9 seconds. Therefore, adenosine must be delivered via a large-bore IV placed as close to the heart as possible, followed by rapid or simultaneous flush of 10 mL normal saline to ensure that the medication reaches the heart before it is metabolized. The starting dose of adenosine is 0.1 mg/kg IV, followed by 0.2 mg/kg IV as needed three times. In patients weighing more than 50 kg, give 6 mg IV followed by 12 mg IV. One-third to one-half of the normal adenosine dose should be used when given to heart transplant recipients. Adenosine has reportedly been effective when administered through an IO line but results are inconsistent.

Adenosine briefly blocks conduction in the atrioventricular (AV) node causing disruption of any tachycardia circuit that depends on AV nodal conduction for perpetuation of the tachycardia. Interpretation of the adenosine's effect on conduction cannot be analyzed on the bedside monitor screens, so it is important to record a rhythm strip during adenosine administration as well as during vagal maneuvers. Once adenosine has been administered, assess the EKG for adequate response of AV or VA dissociation from the adenosine. Note signs of AV dissociation, tachycardia termination, slowing or irregularity of the rhythm. The mechanism of tachycardia is often revealed with initiation or termination of the rhythm.

Administration of adenosine will result in one of three possible outcomes: It may have no effect on the rhythm; it may terminate tachycardia resulting in sinus rhythm; or it may reveal atrial flutter waves or atrial tachycardia during transient blocking of the AV node. Tachycardia will resume after adenosine is metabolized (Fig. 94.1).

In the first case, when adenosine has no effect on the rhythm, it is either because the dose was too low, it was metabolized before it reached the heart, or the rhythm is VT. The dose should be doubled and properly administered. The higher dose may be given twice. If the rhythm is determined to be VT, follow the management of wide complex arrhythmias below.

In the second case, when adenosine successfully terminates tachycardia, next steps include recording the EKG in sinus rhythm and monitoring on telemetry until admission, transfer, or cardiology consultation. If adenosine is successful in terminating tachycardia but it recurs, adenosine may be given again. Another option is to administer a longer-acting drug and then repeat conversion with adenosine.

The third case is when adenosine administration reveals atrial flutter or atrial tachycardia. One common pitfall is the assumption that the tachycardia briefly stopped and then restarted in response to adenosine, when in reality adenosine simply unmasked the rhythm by blocking AV conduction to the ventricles thus making the atrial flutter waves obvious. To avoid this pitfall, look for flutter waves or atrial

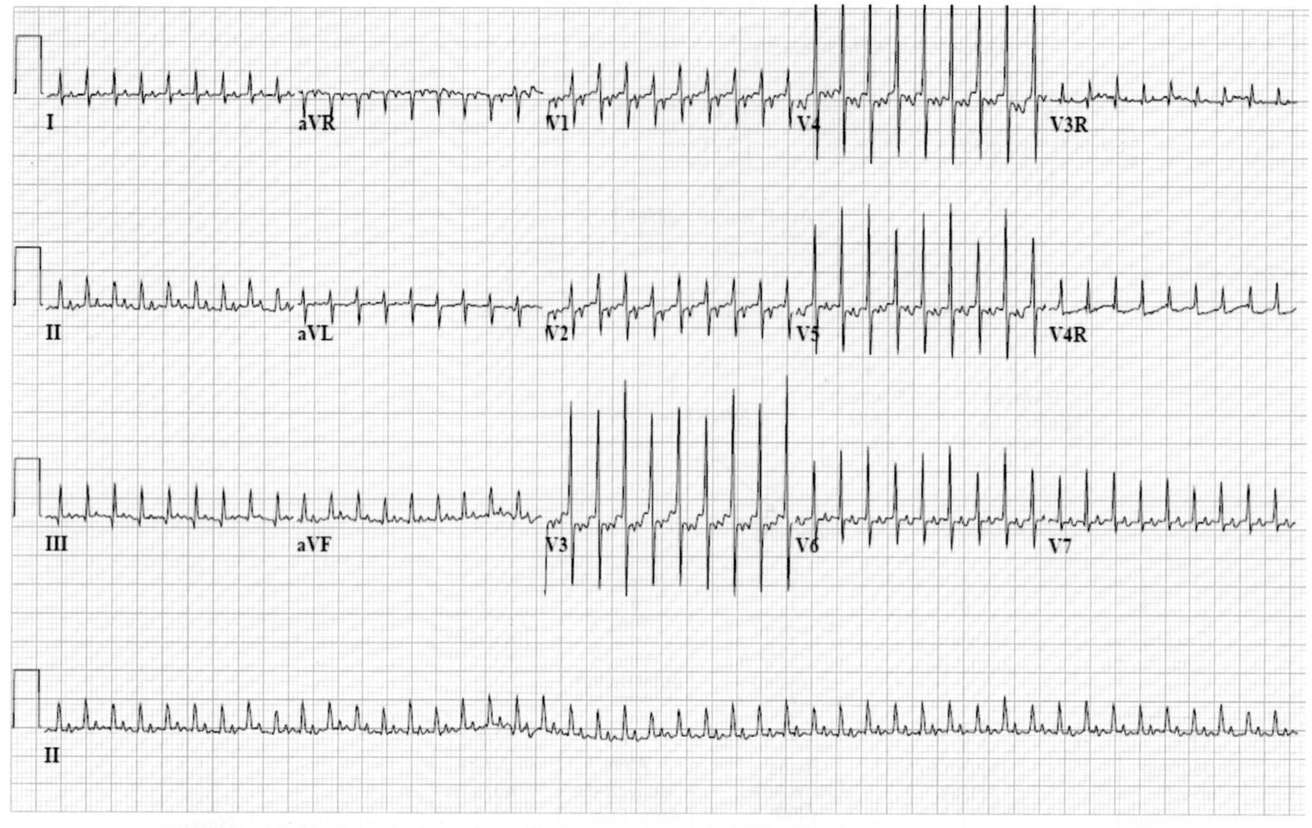

FIGURE 94.2 Supraventricular tachycardia due to atrioventricular accessory connection. This is SVT at nearly 300 BPM. Retrograde P waves are seen immediately following the QRS complex suggesting atrioventricular reentrant tachycardia mediated by an atrioventricular accessory connection, such as Wolff–Parkinson–White. Ventricular pre-excitation is not seen in tachycardia, but rather in sinus rhythm. This tachycardia should break with valsalva maneuvers or adenosine.

tachycardia P waves during the time of slowing/AV node inhibition (Figs. 94.2–94.5).

If adenosine successfully converts SVT to sinus rhythm, but the tachycardia recurs, electrical cardioversion offers no advantage over redosing adenosine. In this case, a longer-acting medication is needed. If the patient is on chronic antiarrhythmic therapy, consider giving this medication. Useful IV medications include procainamide, esmolol, or amiodarone. Oral beta-blockers, sotalol, or flecainide may be used. Calcium channel blockers should not be used in patients less than 2 years of age, in combination with beta-blockers, or with poor ventricular function. Cardiology consultation is advised. If adenosine fails to convert tachycardia at all, electrical cardioversion is indicated.

Although adenosine is generally a benign drug, it can have adverse side effects. When administering adenosine the provider should be prepared for defibrillation, external pacing, or airway management.

Adenosine is absolutely contraindicated in patients with WPW syndrome presenting in atrial fibrillation (i.e., wide complex, irregular rhythm). Blocking the AV node may then cause atrial fibrillation to be conducted rapidly to the ventricle via the accessory connection leading to VF and possibly death.

Adenosine is relatively contraindicated in heart transplant recipients due to prolonged sinus pauses in the transplanted heart, which is denervated from the autonomic nervous system. Besides prolonged asystole, the heart is vulnerable to malignant escape rhythms. Starting with one-third the recommended dose, and increasing if necessary may mitigate the effect of adenosine on the transplanted heart. Finally, there are rare reports of adenosine causing bronchospasm in asthmatics.

Wide Complex Regular Tachycardia. A wide complex regular tachycardia may be VT, SVT with aberrancy, antidromic WPW, or sinus tachycardia with aberrancy/bundle branch block. A quick history including symptoms, previous tachycardia, baseline EKG, and any cardiac surgery or CHD will guide treatment. The EKG and rhythm strip should be scrutinized to identify P waves and establish the mechanism of tachycardia. Assess for hemodynamic stability and proceed according to the PALS algorithms. Adenosine may be given with continuous rhythm strip recording in a nonsinus regular tachycardia. Cardiology should be consulted early to guide therapy.

While VT in adults is commonly due to ischemia secondary to coronary artery disease, in children, ischemic VT is usually due to congenital coronary anomalies or postoperative complications. Nonischemic VT may be due to scars in postoperative CHD, ion channelopathies (LQTS, catecholaminergic polymorphic ventricular tachycardia [CPVT] or Brugada syndrome), cardiomyopathies (myocarditis, DCM, HCM, and arrhythmogenic right ventricular dysplasia [ARVD]), cardiac tumors, or drugs. Idiopathic VF is diagnosed after cardiac arrest when no cause for VF is identified in spite of a complete workup.

There are two types of monomorphic VT commonly encountered in the normal heart. One is VT arising from the RVOT (LBBB, inferior axis) and the other is Belhassen VT a

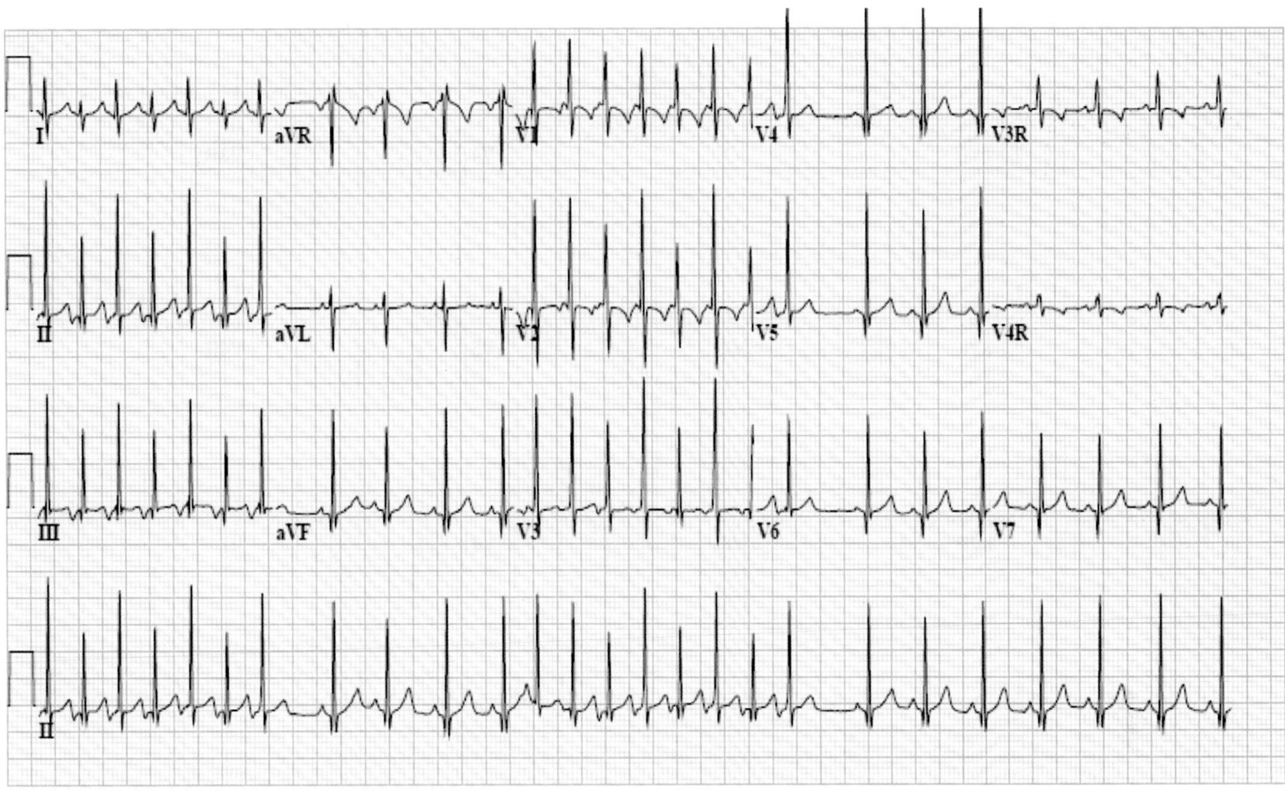

FIGURE 94.3 Supraventricular tachycardia due to an atrial ectopic focus. This shows runs of SVT at a rate of 200 BPM. The P waves precede the QRS complex, but do not have the morphology of sinus P waves, suggesting tachycardia mediated by an ectopic atrial focus. The rhythm is alternating atrial tachycardia (SVT) and sinus rhythm on this EKG, suggesting an incessant tachycardia. This rhythm will not be terminated by adenosine and may be associated with dilated cardiomyopathy.

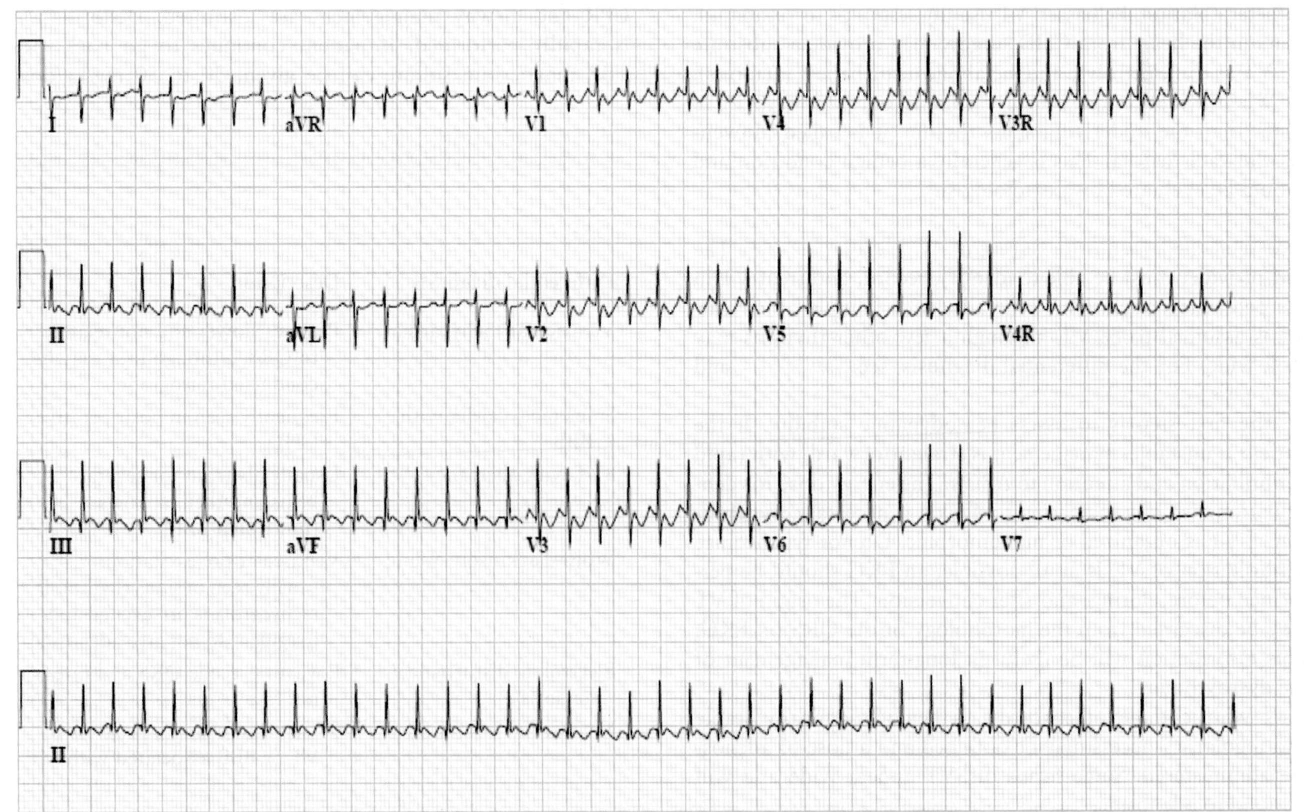

FIGURE 94.4 Narrow complex tachycardia due to atrial flutter: This shows atrial flutter at 240 BPM. Flutter waves are subtle, but may be discerned in a 2:1 ratio to QRS complexes especially in lead V1 through V4 and in the right sided chest leads V3R and V4R.

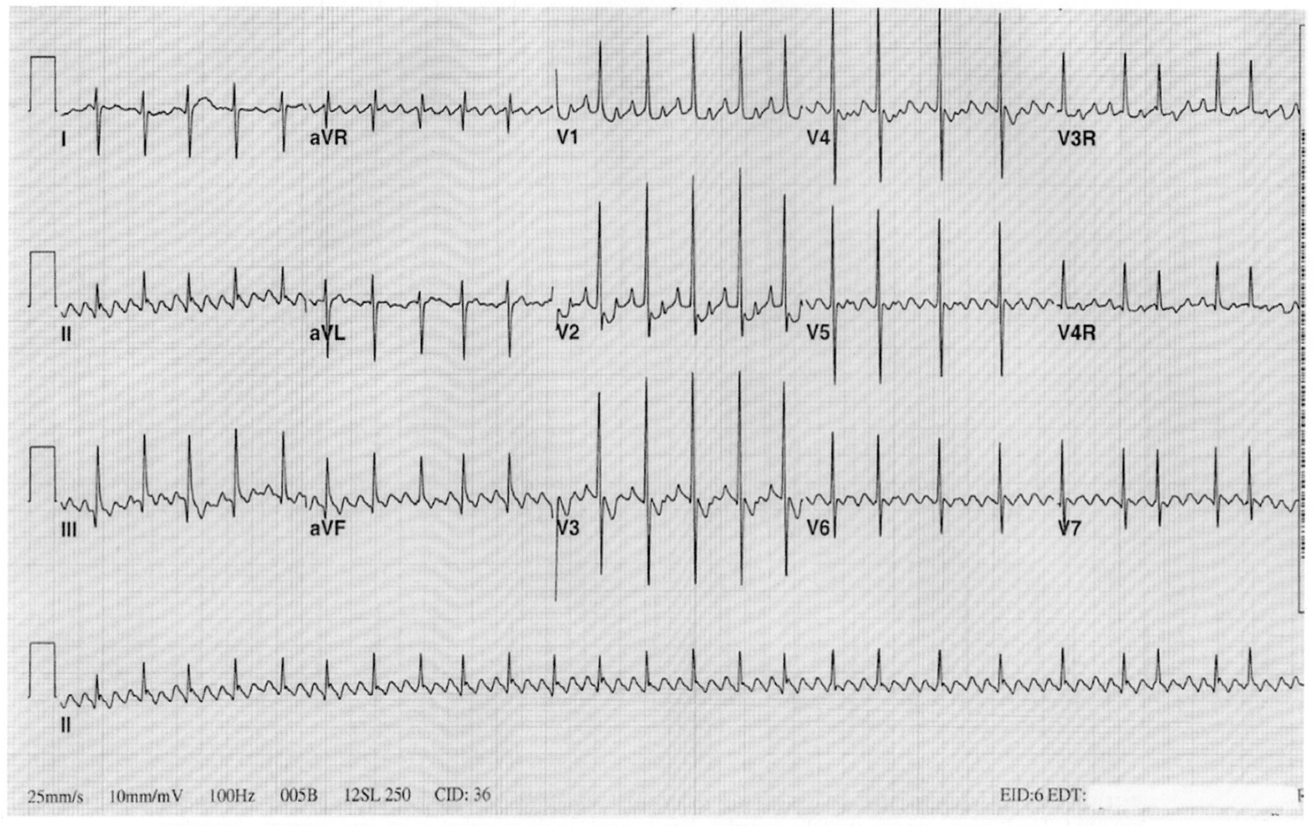

FIGURE 94.5 Atrial flutter with 3:1 and 4:1 atrioventricular block. If AV conduction occurs in a 1:1 or 1:2 ratio (as in Fig. 94.4) adenosine may make flutter waves more visible as seen here.

left fascicular tachycardia (RBBB and left axis). Both are relatively benign and may be treated with medication or cured by catheter ablation. Belhassen VT usually responds to verapamil. Scars in the heart from CHD surgery may provide a substrate for VT as can electrolyte and metabolic disturbances (acidosis).

When wide complex tachycardia is only 15% to 20% faster than the underlying sinus rhythm, it is called idioventricular tachycardia. This is generally a benign condition and should be evaluated by a cardiologist.

Management/Diagnostic Testing of Wide Complex VT. The EM provider must be able to identify, record, and treat VT in the pediatric population. Generally, wide complex tachycardia is assumed to be VT, although a few other rhythms may look wide. For the differential diagnosis, see Table 94.7 and Figure 94.6.

The first step is to assess hemodynamic stability. If the patient is unstable, management is straightforward, with rapid defibrillation and attention to ABC's. The energy dose for defibrillation is 2 J/kg increasing to 4 J/kg, if necessary. Synchronize if VT is organized or monomorphic. Do not synchronize defibrillation of VF. If at all possible, an EKG should be performed before, during, and after conversion. The origin of VT may be discerned from the morphology of the QRS on EKG. This information will be useful in long-term management of the dysrhythmia.

If wide complex tachycardia is hemodynamically stable and regular, IV access may be obtained and a dose of adenosine administered. Some forms of SVT appear wide and will respond to adenosine.

Conversely, some VT in children is relatively narrow. See Figures 94.7 and 94.8.

Management/Diagnostic Testing of Channelopathies. Long QT presents as syncope due to torsades de pointes (TdP). CPR and airway management are instituted. Defibrillation is rapidly performed. If patient continues to go back into TdP, magnesium sulfate can be given, 30 to 50 mg/kg/dose

TABLE 94.7

DIFFERENTIAL DIAGNOSIS FOR WIDE COMPLEX TACHYCARDIA

Differential diagnosis	Description
Ventricular tachycardia	P waves slower and not related to QRS, although they may be conducted retrograde
Sinus tachycardia with BBB	Frequently seen in postoperative CHD
SVT with aberrancy	Usually aberrant for several beats and then narrows (functional BBB)
Wolff–Parkinson–White	Ventricular pre-excitation: usually seen in sinus rhythm. If tachycardia is pre-excited and irregular, do not give adenosine
Electrolyte disturbance/acidosis	P waves precede QRS and rate is not fast
Myocardial infarction	ST segment changes progress to VT or BBB associated with MI

BBB, bundle branch block; CHD, congenital heart disease; SVT, supraventricular tachycardia; VT, ventricular tachycardia; MI, myocardial infarction.

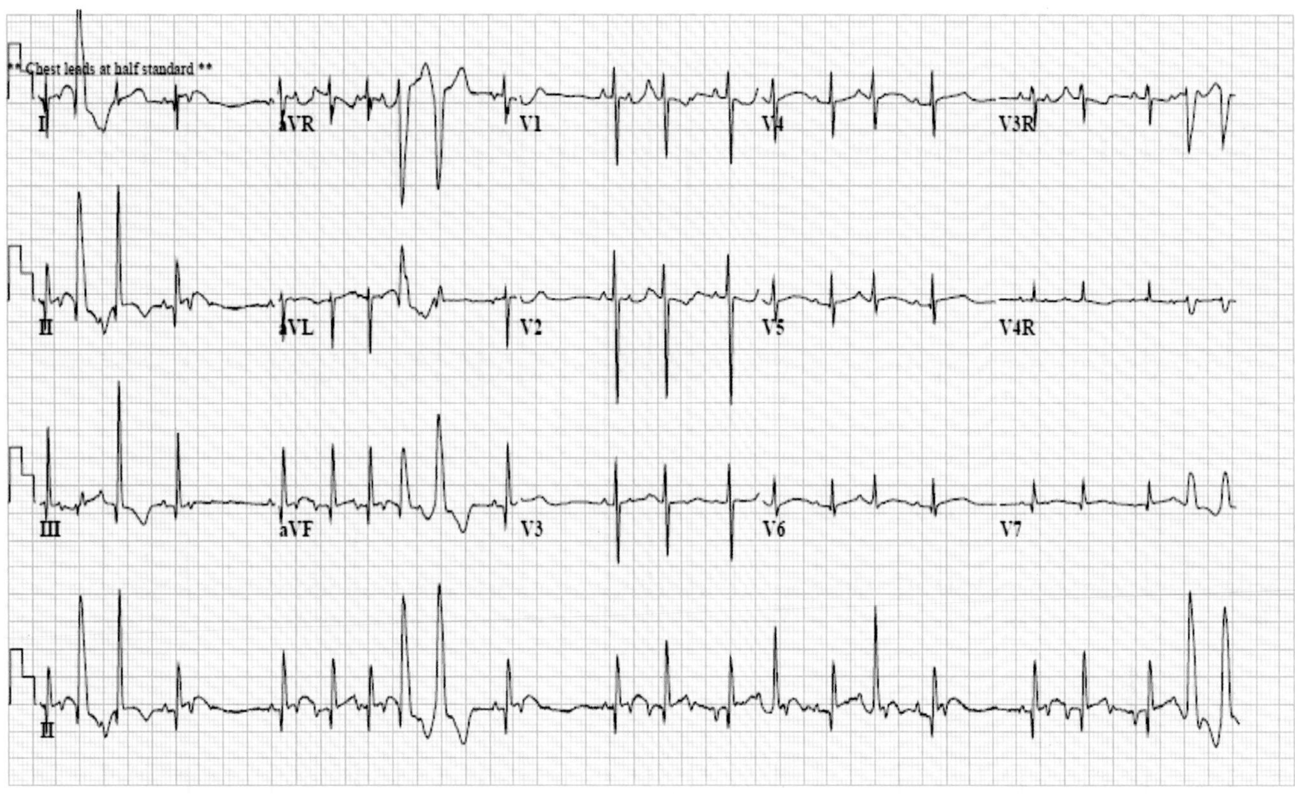

FIGURE 94.6 Supraventricular tachycardia with aberrancy. It is one example of SVT, which may be confused with ventricular tachycardia. It is distinguished from ventricular ectopy by the P wave preceding each wide complex.

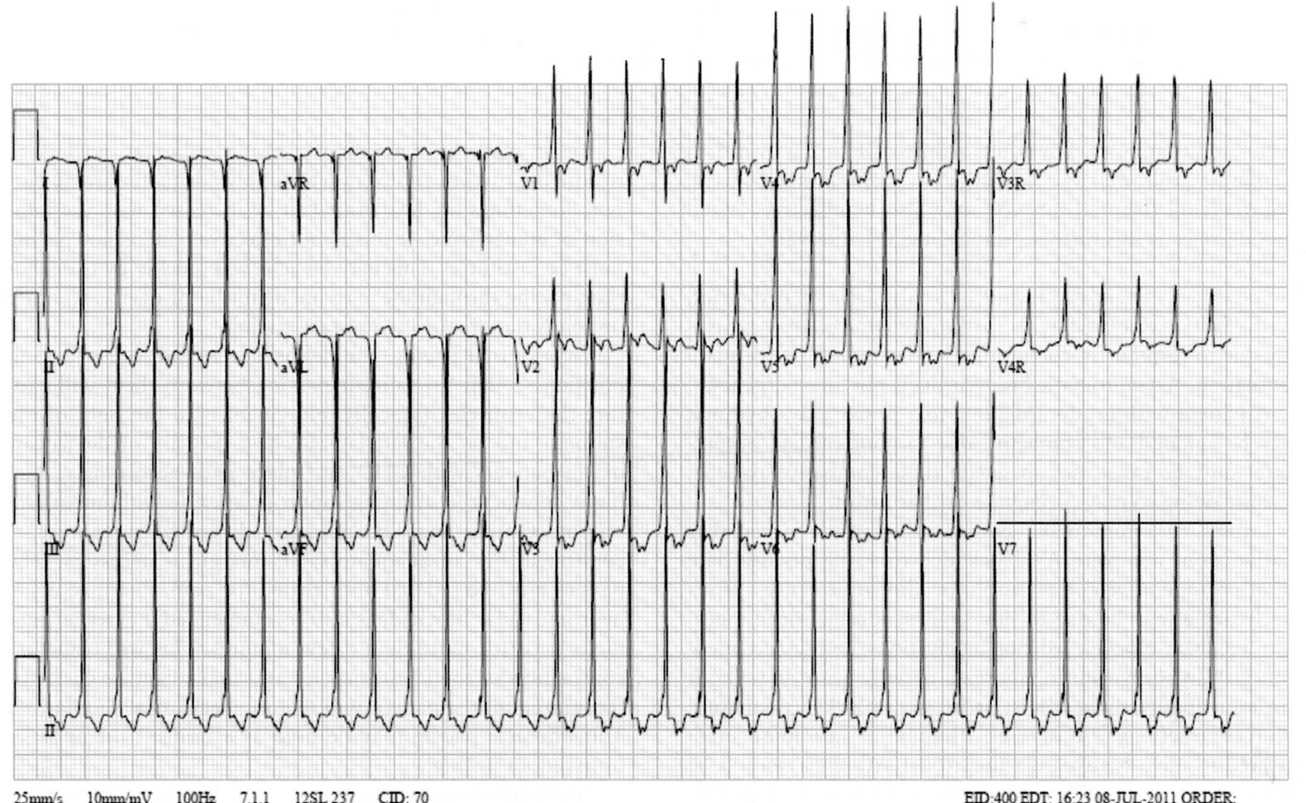

FIGURE 94.7 Ventricular tachycardia. This is a “narrow QRS tachycardia” at 200 BPM recorded in an infant. Retrograde P waves are visible in the ST segment, suggesting possible SVT, although the QRS axis is not normal. In the pediatric age group, it is common to have normal retrograde conduction via the AV node.

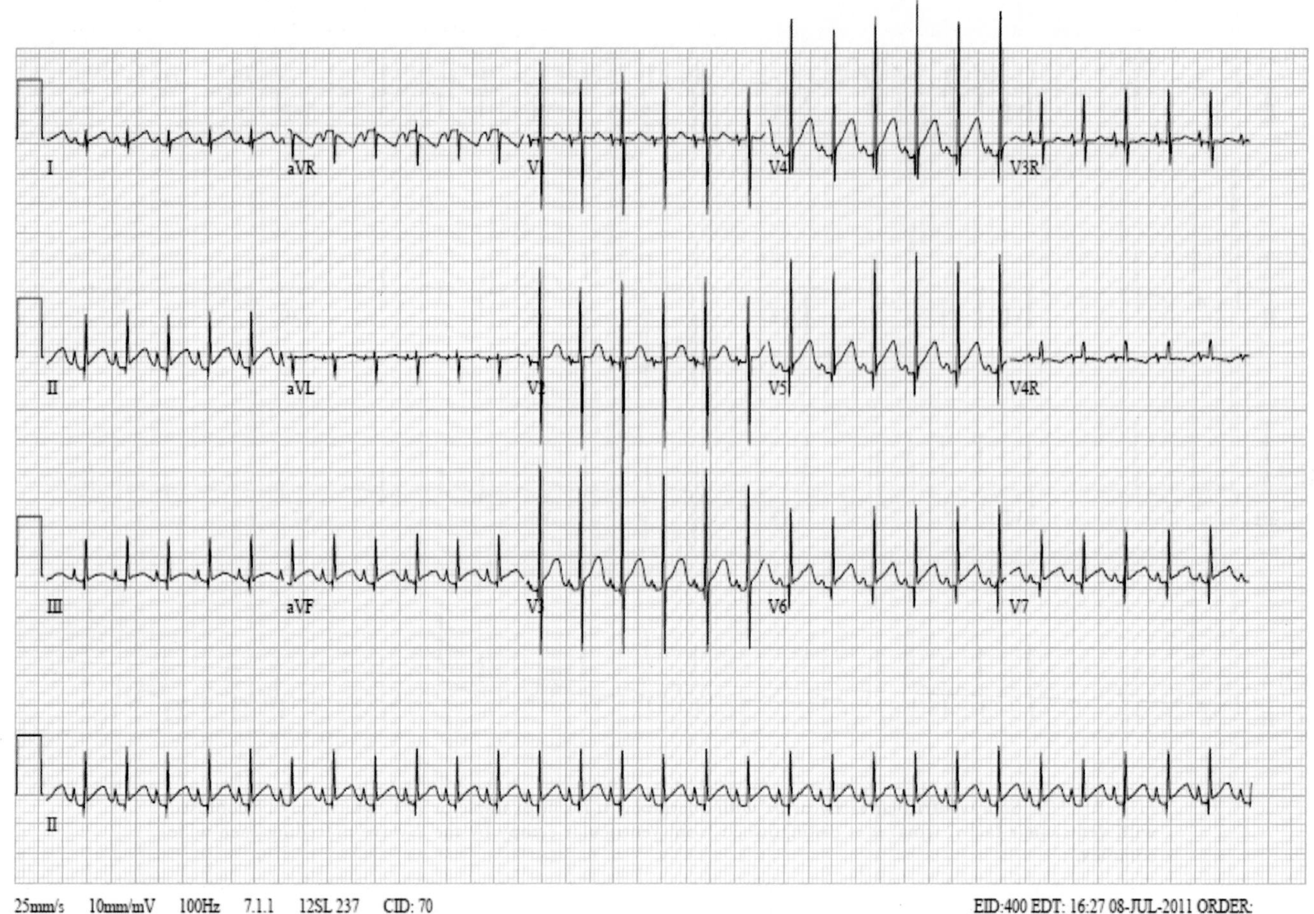

FIGURE 94.8 Sinus rhythm. This is sinus rhythm after synchronized cardioversion of the rhythm shown in Figure 94.7. This illustrates the relatively narrow appearance of VT in infants and young children. Consider VT when a "narrow QRS tachycardia" does not convert with adenosine.

over 5 to 20 minutes. For adults a dose of 1 to 2 g over 5 to 20 minutes, followed by a drip of 0.5 to 1 g/hour may be used. Isoproterenol (Isuprel) infusion may also be effective. Avoid amiodarone, as this further prolongs the QT interval.

Management/Diagnostic Testing of Bradycardia. In pediatrics, bradycardia associated with cardiovascular collapse is usually due to respiratory compromise and responds to adequate ventilation. Asymptomatic bradycardia is not an emergency.

A patient with bradycardia due to a primary dysrhythmia may be agitated and combative due to poor cardiac output. Care must be taken not to sedate these combative patients because doing so may precipitate cardiac arrest.

Causes of symptomatic bradycardia include pacemaker malfunction, complete AV block due to Lyme disease, late onset postoperative complication, or idiopathic causes. Sinus bradycardia may be due to sick sinus syndrome, drug ingestion (i.e., beta-blocker, sedating medications, and seizure medications), hypothyroidism, anorexia nervosa with or without cardiomyopathy, myocarditis, or frequent blocked premature atrial contractions (PACs) (Figs. 94.9 and 94.10). Infants discovered to have bradycardia due to 2:1 AV block should be assumed to have LQTS until proven otherwise by a pediatric electrophysiologist. EKG and long rhythm strip should be obtained. These patients should be monitored on telemetry in case TdP develops.

In all cases of symptomatic bradycardia the goal is to restore the rhythm and/or rate to supply adequate cardiac output. Sometimes the heart rate can be increased with the infusion of epinephrine. If this is not effective, emergency pacing must be instituted. This may be achieved quickly by transthoracic pacing through the external defibrillator device. Another option is transvenous temporary pacing.

For external pacing, the defibrillation pads are placed in position so that the current passing between them will capture the ventricle. Typically, placement is to the right of the sternum and on the left lateral chest. Beware of dextrocardia in patients with CHD and place pads accordingly. Pacing is commenced at an age appropriate rate with maximum output. Output may be adjusted down when capture is confirmed, but an adequate safety margin is necessary. The patient must be sedated and treated for pain. Pharmacologic neuromuscular blockade is also recommended if external pacing is used for more than a few minutes. This will eliminate contraction of the chest muscles and make capture easier to recognize, but the patient will require mechanical ventilation. Transthoracic pacing may be used as a bridge to temporary transvenous pacing.

For transvenous pacing, access to the RV via the right internal jugular, subclavian, or femoral vein is obtained. Placement is best achieved in the catheterization laboratory under fluoroscopic guidance. In the ED catheter position is documented

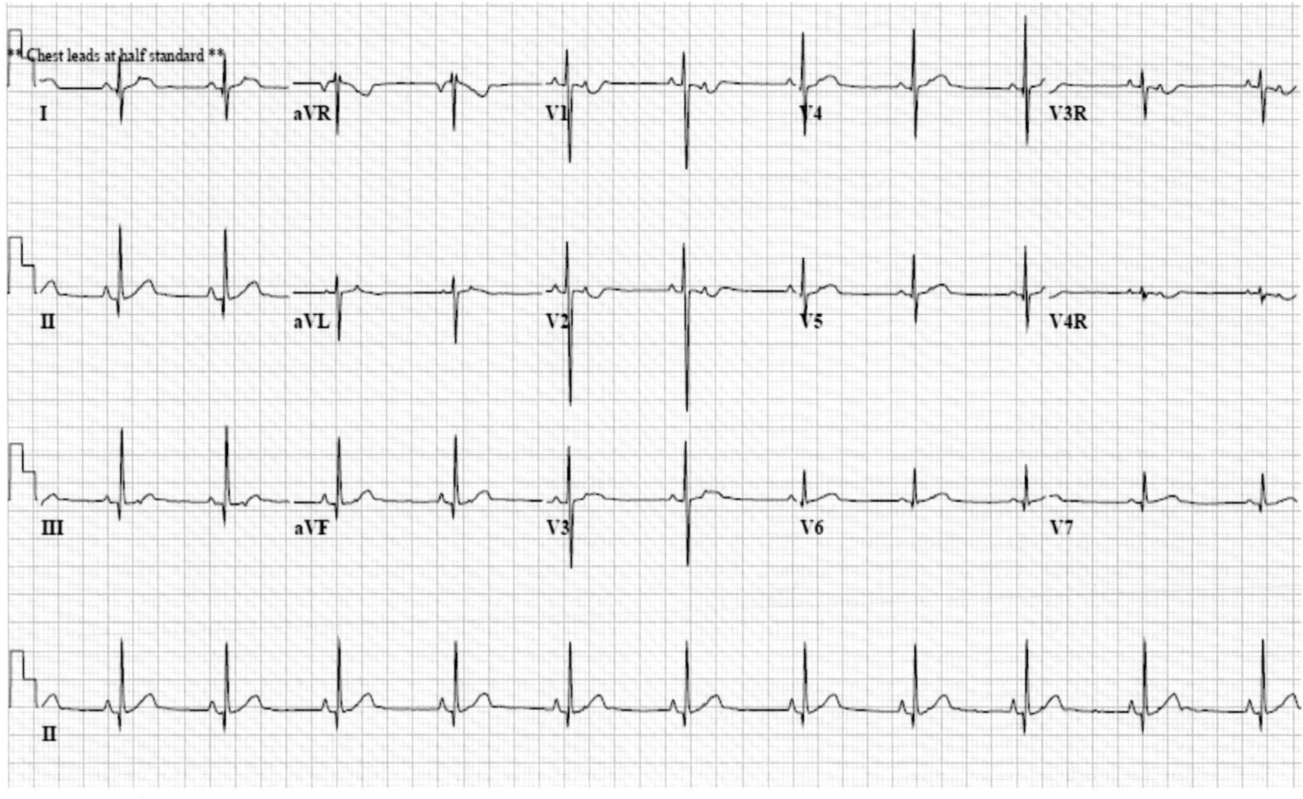

FIGURE 94.9 Bradycardia due to blocked premature atrial contractions.

and confirmed with a CXR. The pacing catheter is advanced to the RV and connected to an external pacemaker. This temporary pacemaker is programmed to maximum output at an appropriate rate. Capture is confirmed by palpating a pulse. The catheter should be secured with a sterile dressing. Risks of perforation, dislodgement, and infection increase in smaller patients. Pediatric cardiology and/or electrophysiology should be consulted early.

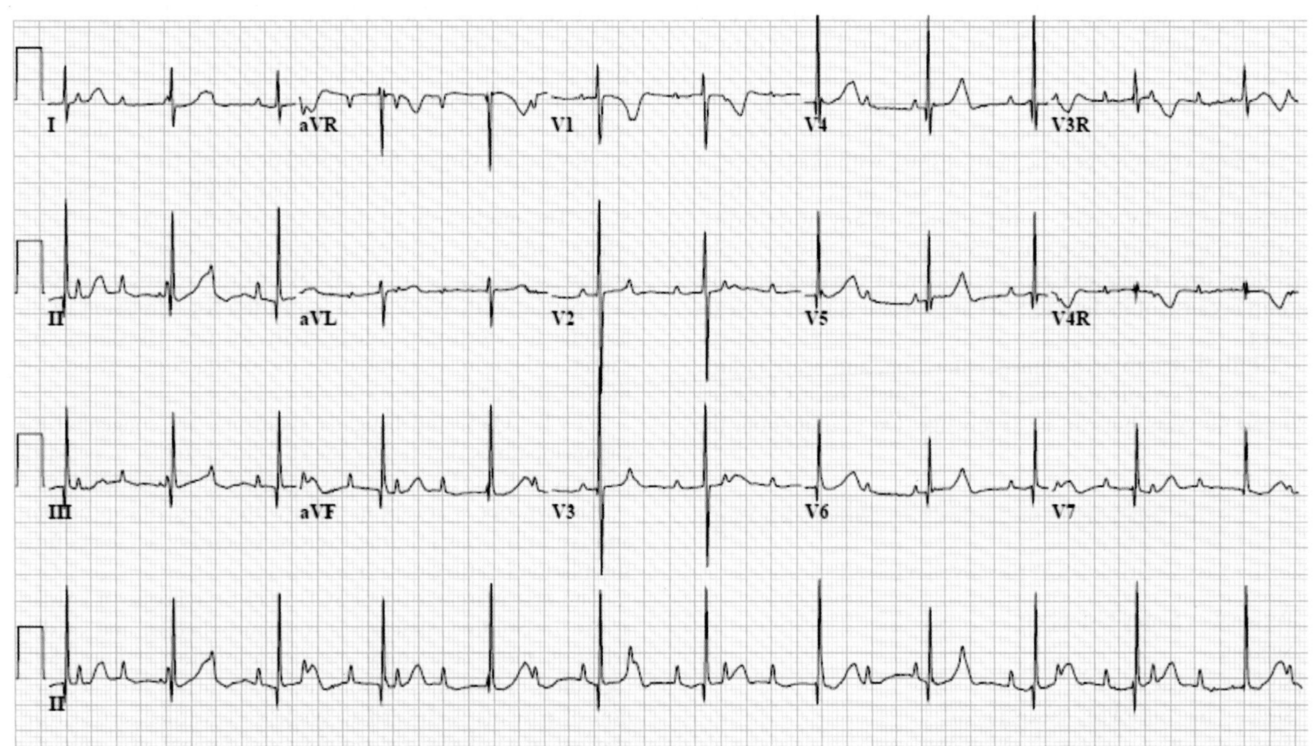

FIGURE 94.10 Bradycardia due to complete heart block. Note there is no association between P waves and QRS complexes.

SUDDEN CARDIAC DEATH

CLINICAL PEARLS AND PITFALLS

- Screen for SCD with a thorough personal and family history in all syncope patients.
- Knowledge of the cardiac causes of sudden death can guide resuscitation, stabilization, and laboratory investigation.
- Consider SCD in patients presenting with syncope without prodrome and that occurs around the time of exercise.

SCD is death occurring within 24 hours of onset of symptoms. The incidence of SCD in infants, children, and adolescents is 1.3 to 8.5 per 100,000 patient-years. Hypertrophic cardiomyopathy (HCM) is the most frequent cause of SCD in people under 35 years of age. Other common causes of SCD in the young include congenital coronary artery anomalies, disorders of the ventricular myocardium (myocarditis, dilated cardiomyopathies, and ARVD), aortic rupture and arrhythmias (including channelopathies) make up the balance.

In adults with CHD, SCD increases with increasing age, increasing complexity of CHD, and poor ventricular function. Arrhythmias are not tolerated well in these patients.

SCD is often is heralded by syncope. For detection of syncope that is more likely to be high risk, obtain a thorough history of the patient's and family's prior experience with similar episodes, syncope, heart disease, sudden death younger than 50 years old, drowning, and/or single motor vehicle accidents. Some syncope has been misdiagnosed as seizure. Carefully inquire about each incident of syncope that the patient has experienced. Also, obtain an EKG for all patients presenting with syncope (Table 94.8). Restrict from exercise and refer to cardiology if the episode was around the time of exertion. Admit to the hospital on a monitored bed if patient received CPR.

HCM is a genetic disease involving 1,400 mutations in 11 or more genes encoding proteins of the cardiac sarcomere. It is the most common genetic heart disease with prevalence of 1:500. It manifests as increased LV wall thickness without dilation of the LV cavity in the absence of any other explanation (i.e., obstruction, hypertension, etc.). Hypertrophy develops over time, and gains attention in the pediatric age group because of its link to SCD in people less than 35 years of age.

Death is due to arrhythmias, infarction, and heart failure. The onset of symptomatic heart failure usually occurs between 20 and 40 years but can be at any age. On examination, the EM provider should appreciate a LVOTO murmur at the left sternal border or apex that is louder with standing or valsalva and becomes softer when supine. EKG is almost always abnormal and may show LV hypertrophy, ST and T wave changes, deep Q waves, or lack of R waves in the lateral precordial leads. Echocardiogram is diagnostic. CXR is remarkable for cardiomegaly and a globular shaped cardiac silhouette.

TABLE 94.8

SUDDEN CARDIAC DEATH/SYNCOPE 5 S's

Personal or family history of:
Syncope
Sudden cardiac death
Seizures (uncontrolled, unexplained)
"Swimming" (i.e., unexplained drowning)
Single car accidents (unexplained)

Patients with HCM can develop atrial fibrillation, SVT, and VT. These rhythms are not well tolerated and even SVT can degenerate to cause SCD. Syncope, near syncope, palpitations, exercise intolerance, and chest pain are all ominous signs in HCM. At times, the first symptom may be SCD. The typical murmur or family history should be sought in all other patients presenting with these signs or symptoms to assure that HCM is not overlooked. Cardiology should be consulted when HCM is suspected or new symptoms are discovered.

Anomalous Coronary Arteries can also lead to SCD. The most common variation is origin of the anomalous left coronary artery from the pulmonary artery (ALCAPA) but other variations exist. Syncope and sudden death may be the presenting symptoms. Patients may be asymptomatic until exertion when flow to the coronaries is impaired leading to ischemia, arrhythmia, or sudden death. Bland White Garland Syndrome refers to presentation of ALCAPA in an infant around 10 weeks of age. When the PVR drops significantly around this age, the anomalous LCA is not perfused and ischemia causes the infant to cry with feeds, develop cardiac wheezing, and respiratory distress. CHF and SCD may ensue. Although 10 weeks is the classic age of presentation, these patients may be asymptomatic until later in childhood or adolescence. At the later age, presentation is with chest pain, syncope, or SCD.

Clinical assessment should include EKG and echocardiogram in a laboratory skilled in imaging coronary arteries. Chest radiograph can be helpful. Treat with supplemental oxygen, sedation, and analgesia for chest pain. Patients with syncope concerning for cardiac etiology, should have consultation with a cardiologist. Diagnosing any child with ALCAPA requires a high index of suspicion. Consult cardiology and cardiovascular surgery for surgical definitive treatment.

About 0.1% of all patients with WPW will experience SCD. The mechanism of death starts with atrial fibrillation, which leads to VF if the atrial fibrillation is conducted rapidly via the accessory pathway (WPW) to the ventricle. Syncope in a patient with WPW is an indication for admission to the hospital for electrophysiology study for risk assessment and catheter ablation. Generally, the use of digoxin is avoided in these patients.

CPVT, LQTS, and Brugada syndrome are congenital ion channelopathies that render the rhythm unstable. In pediatric patients with LQTS, the first symptom may be sudden death.

The syncope is abrupt in onset with a negligible prodrome and typically occurs during exercise or during acute auditory stimulation (alarm clock) (Fig. 94.11).

The first presentation of SCD may be syncope or cardiac arrest. In children, syncope is frequently benign and cardiac arrest is most commonly due to respiratory failure. Still, regardless of how uncommon, the goal remains early recognition of patients with cardiac syncope or cardiac arrest from aborted SCD. Early recognition will impact not only the patient, but potentially prevent morbidity and mortality in close relatives by commencing a screening evaluation.

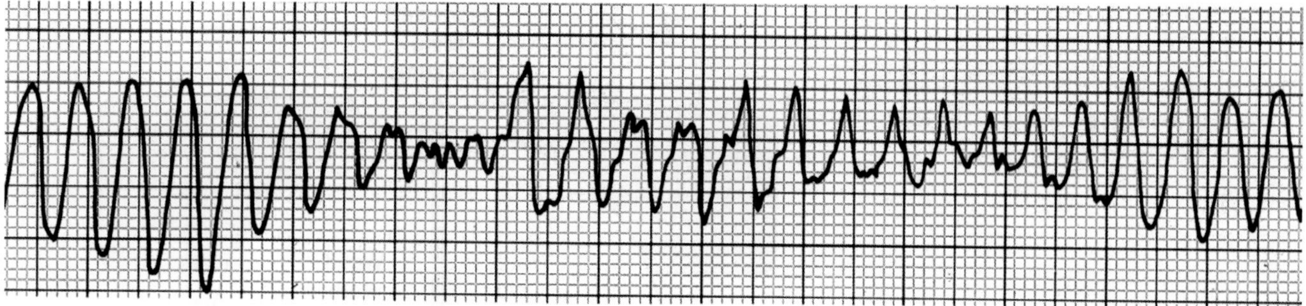

FIGURE 94.11 Torsades de pointes is the rhythm leading to sudden cardiac death in long QT syndrome.

ACUTE HEART FAILURE SYNDROMES

CLINICAL PEARLS AND PITFALLS

- In the pediatric population, CHF is most commonly due to CHD.
- Initiation of diuretic therapy promptly in the emergency department has been shown to decrease length of stay in adults presenting to the ED with worsening CHF.

Current Evidence

AHFS include new onset heart failure or decompensation of chronic heart failure. In the pediatric population, AHFS is most commonly the sequelae of CHD. Still, AHFS can also develop in the setting of many inherited and acquired conditions (Table 94.9).

Goal of Treatment

The goal is to identify patients in CHF early in order to initiate diuretic and other therapy in the Emergency Department.

Clinical Considerations

Clinical Recognition

CHF in pediatrics is notoriously difficult to diagnose because patients present with a wide variety of signs and symptoms that are seen in common or benign pediatric ailments. Despite much effort, there is still no reliable, simple way to recognize this condition. A high index of suspicion is essential in making the diagnosis. In the neonate, common manifestations include tachypnea, tachycardia, hepatomegaly, cardiomegaly, rales, rhonchi, and feeding difficulties. CHF can masquerade as bronchiolitis or asthma by presenting with respiratory insufficiency, increased work of breathing, or dyspnea. It may mimic gastroenteritis, hepatitis, or renal failure with volume overload. Older children may present with symptoms similar to adults such as dyspnea on exertion, exercise intolerance, and/or syncope, peripheral or facial edema, pleural effusions, ascites or hepatomegaly. In the ED, the diagnosis of CHF should be considered when patients thought to be dehydrated do not respond as expected to fluid bolus or patients with wheezing do not respond to beta agonists. Consider CHF early in patients who have presented with CHF before or in patients with CHD.

TABLE 94.9

ETIOLOGIES OF ACUTE HEART FAILURE SYNDROMES IN CHILDREN

Cardiomyopathies	Myocarditis, mitochondrial disorders, storage diseases, metabolic disorders, nutritional deficiencies
High output states	Severe anemia, thyrotoxicosis, AV malformation
Cardiovascular disease	Hypertension, cardiac tumors, congenital heart disease, coronary artery insufficiency
Infectious diseases	Septicemia
Medications	Chemotherapy

Initial Assessment/H&P. A history assessing for CHF should consist of an inquiry into viral illnesses, family history of cardiomyopathy, existing or repaired CHD, prior heart failure, heart transplantation, presence of comorbid conditions including rheumatic heart disease, hypothyroidism, Kawasaki disease (KD), or cancer receiving anthracyclines for chemotherapy. One should inquire about antecedent viral syndromes as seen with myocarditis, check pulses for coarctation of the aorta, and auscultate for murmurs or tachycardia.

Diagnostic and laboratory testing provide supportive evidence for the diagnosis of CHF. CXR should be obtained to assess for cardiomegaly and increased pulmonary vascular markings. Obtain a CBC to assess for anemia. EKG is useful to evaluate for arrhythmia or changes consistent with myocarditis or cardiac ischemia. BNP aids in differentiating AHFS from lung disease and can be trended after initiation of treatment. Although echocardiogram is the definitive test to assess cardiac function, bedside emergency ultrasound has been increasingly used in pediatric EM to evaluate LV systolic function. Additional evaluation is case dependent and geared toward suspected etiologies (i.e., thyroid function, metabolic evaluation, etc.).

Management. The priority is to restore hemodynamic stability. To initiate proper therapy AHFS should be categorized (Fig. 94.12). Diuretics are the mainstay of management of CHF with volume overload. Administration of diuretics should not be delayed in these patients. Inotropic therapy, such as dopamine, epinephrine, norepinephrine, milrinone, or dobutamine may be necessary in patients with poor perfusion. Milrinone therapy may be instituted if blood pressure is adequate. Dopamine at 5 to 20 μg/kg/min is appropriate in patients with poor perfusion. Epinephrine and norepinephrine support

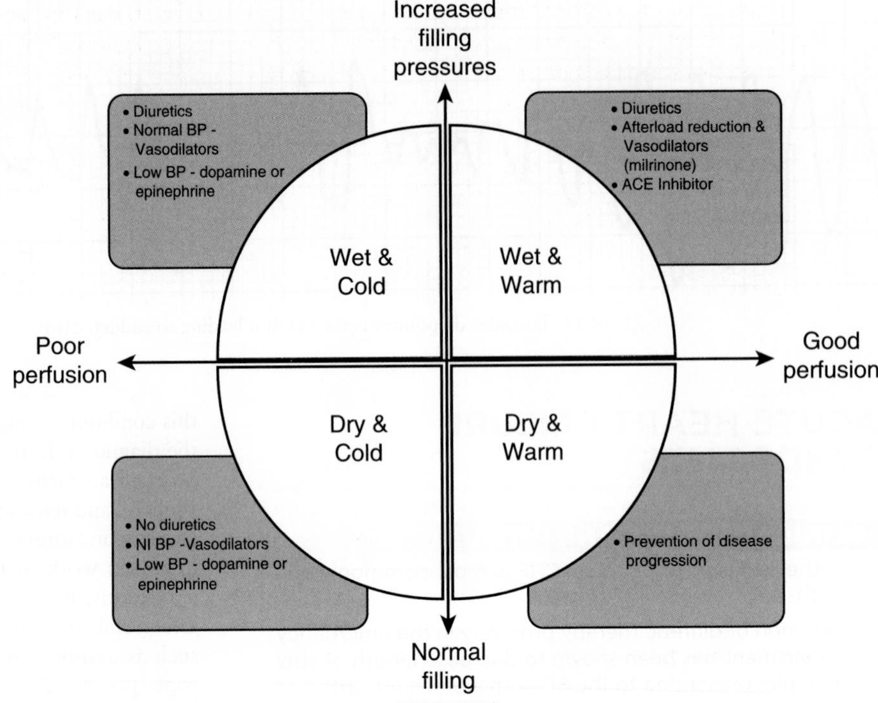

FIGURE 94.12 Acute heart failure syndromes: Assessment and management. BP, blood pressure; ACE, angiotensin converting enzyme.

blood pressure. Milrinone or dobutamine are used in pulmonary hypertension. Digoxin has fallen out of favor because of time needed to reach therapeutic levels and narrow therapeutic window and availability of better drugs now. Afterload reduction therapy is beneficial in some cases. Patients should be admitted and monitored in a critical care unit with continuous telemetry. It is very important to record any arrhythmia that occurs in the EC. Cardiology should be consulted early.

ACQUIRED HEART DISEASE

Goals of Treatment

The goal of the EM provider includes the early recognition of acquired pediatric heart disease. Even with a high index of suspicion, it is challenging to make these diagnoses since symptoms can be very nonspecific. This section gives an overview of common acquired heart disease in pediatrics to facilitate early recognition. Diseases reviewed include cardiomyopathies (hypertrophic, dilated, and restrictive), myocarditis, pericarditis/tamponade and endocarditis, acute rheumatic fever (ARF), KD, and cardiac trauma.

CLINICAL PEARLS AND PITFALLS

- Myocarditis presents with nonspecific symptoms that mimic common pediatric ailments.
- The most common sign of myocarditis is unexplained tachycardia.
- Infective endocarditis is most common in children with structural heart disease.
- KD is the most common form of acquired heart disease in children in industrialized nations.
- KD and incomplete KD are risk factors for the development of coronary artery aneurysms (CAA).

CARDIOMYOPATHIES

HCM is a genetic disease in which cardiac hypertrophy and symptoms develop over time. In this sense it is an acquired cardiomyopathy. Please see the section on SCD earlier in this chapter for more discussion (Table 94.10).

DCM is the end result of various disease processes. While the majority of DCM in pediatrics is idiopathic, some cases are familial or due to inborn errors of metabolism (mitochondrial disorders, Barth syndrome, carnitine deficiency). In older children the most commonly identified causes are myocarditis and neuromuscular disease (Duchenne and Becker muscular dystrophy). LVOTO obstructive lesions and incessant tachycardia may also produce DCM, which is often reversible when the obstruction or tachycardia is corrected. KD, rheumatic fever, and Lyme disease are also recognizable causes of DCM. Some patients who have received anthracyclines for chemotherapy will develop DCM.

TABLE 94.10

ETIOLOGIES OF HYPERTROPHIC CARDIOMYOPATHY

Autoimmune disease	
Nutritional deficiencies	Selenium, carnitine, thiamine
Endocrine dysfunction	GH deficiency, thyroid disease, hypocalcemia, diabetes mellitus, pheochromocytoma
Infiltrative diseases	Glycogen storage disease, hemochromatosis, amyloidosis
Toxins	Cobalt, lead
Drugs	Alcohol, sympathomimetics, anthracyclines
Other	Chronic tachycardia, muscular dystrophies

The incidence of DCM in children younger than 18 years old is 0.57 cases per 100,000 per year. A higher incidence has been noted in boys, Blacks compared to Whites, and infants less than 1 year old. DCM may lead to CHF and is the most common reason for cardiac transplantation in the pediatric population. Patients with familial or idiopathic DCM that are older than 6 years of age, or have CHF at diagnosis are at highest risk for heart transplantation.

DCM presents with shortness of breath and exercise intolerance. Young children have vague symptoms such as tachypnea, dyspnea, irritability, and poor feeding. Symptoms usually are insidious except in acute viral myocarditis. Physical examination may reveal signs of CHF and a mitral regurgitation murmur or S3 gallop. EKG usually shows sinus tachycardia, LVH, and nonspecific ST and T wave changes. Incessant tachyarrhythmias such as SVT and VT are poorly tolerated in patients with DCM and should thus be treated aggressively. The goal of treatment of DCM in the emergency department is early identification of CHF and supportive care. ECMO can be a bridge to recovery or transplant and cardiac surgery should be involved early. For management of CHF, see Section on "Acute Heart Failure Syndromes."

Restrictive Cardiomyopathy (RCM) is due to increased stiffness of the myocardium leading to a rise in ventricular filling pressures. RCM is the least common type of cardiomyopathy, although patients with HCM and end-stage DCM may develop restrictive physiology. RCM is commonly idiopathic or familial with predominately autosomal dominant inheritance. Other causes of RCM are rheumatologic (sarcoidosis, scleroderma), infectious (parasitic), infiltrative (glycogen storage disease, hemochromatosis, amyloidosis), carcinoid, nutrition, and drugs. A gallop and loud P2 may be appreciated on cardiac examination. The EKG commonly has abnormal right or left atrial enlargement, ST depression, and ST–T wave abnormalities. Cardiomegaly and pulmonary venous congestion will be noted on CXR. ECHO is diagnostic for RCM. These patients require adequate preload.

Unclassified cardiomyopathies such as *Left Ventricular Noncompaction (LVNC)* are now being recognized. In LVNC the heart has prominent LV trabeculae and deep intertrabecular recesses. LVNC occurs independent of or in conjunction with CHD such as Ebstein anomaly, complex heart disease, or neuromuscular disease. LVNC may be transient in neonates.

MYOCARDITIS

Myocarditis is an acute, nonischemic, inflammatory disorder of the myocardium usually with preserved LV size (as opposed to DCM which has LV dilation and reduced ejection fraction). Myocarditis is primarily caused by viral infections but it also may occur due to autoimmune, pharmacologic, toxic, and vasculitic processes. The most common viral causes are enterovirus (Coxsackie B, echovirus) and adenovirus. There may be a history of preceding or concurrent viral upper respiratory tract infection or gastroenteritis 10 to 14 days before. A high index of suspicion is essential for early recognition of myocarditis as it may present subtly and go unrecognized by clinicians. Most children with myocarditis are *not* diagnosed on initial presentation, but require multiple visits to a medical provider before this elusive diagnosis is suspected. The challenge lies in the vague and nonspecific nature of the presentation. Presenting symptoms are common and nonspecific: Fever, lethargy, poor feeding, vomiting, diaphoresis, and pallor. Signs and symptoms can be easily mistaken for common illnesses such as bronchiolitis, sepsis, or dehydration. Older children may exhibit fatigue, dyspnea, chest pain (>10 years old), abdominal pain from hepatic congestion in CHF, or arrhythmias. Myocarditis can be classified into three categories: Acute, fulminant, and chronic. In some cases, myocarditis may resolve spontaneously. In others, recognition may be delayed until the disease has progressed or even worse after sudden death and identification on postmortem or autopsy. In fulminant disease, the patients present in extremis with cardiogenic shock. Physical examination should focus on signs or respiratory distress, tachypnea, abnormal lung examination, and hepatomegaly. Myocarditis is a clinical diagnosis, but supportive information can be obtained from additional testing. The classic EKG in myocarditis shows sinus tachycardia, low-voltage QRS complexes, and inverted or low-voltage T waves. In myocarditis, cardiac death is a result of dysrhythmias/conduction disease such as VT, atrial fibrillation, supraventricular tachycardia, or complete AV block. Myocarditis may present with CHF or VT. CXR shows cardiomegaly and pulmonary edema. Cardiac enzymes (troponin, creatinine kinase-MB fraction, BNP) may be elevated to help diagnose heart failure as a result of myocarditis from heart failure as a result of DCM or anomalous left coronary arising from the pulmonary artery (ALCAPA). ECHO can establish cardiac function. The gold standard for diagnosis remains endomyocardial biopsy (EB). Cardiac MRI identifies areas of myocardial inflammation and can even be used to increase the sensitivity of EB.

Management consists of addressing ABCs, treating CHF and arrhythmias, and/or stabilizing those patients presenting in cardiogenic shock. The goal should be rapid stabilization and cardiology consultation. Transfer to institution that offers ECMO, ventricular assist device (VAD) implantation, and/or heart transplant capabilities is ideal and can be life saving. Transfer should be via PALS transport team.

PERICARDITIS

Pericarditis is inflammation of pericardium. In infancy, viral disease (Coxsackie, echovirus, adenovirus, influenza) is most common etiology. Bacterial causes include *Staphylococcus aureus, Streptococcus pneumoniae, Haemophilus influenzae, Neisseria meningitis,* and tuberculosis. Other important causes are PPS (discussed above) and ARF. The pericardial space, between visceral serous and parietal serous pericardium, normally contains less than 20 to 30 mL of serous fluid for lubrication. If fluid accumulates gradually, a large amount may be tolerated, but rapid accumulation often leads to cardiac tamponade. In this condition ventricular filling is impaired, leading to decreased stroke volume and hypotension. See section on cardiac tamponade.

Acute pericarditis is usually preceded by an illness. Obtain history of any antecedent upper respiratory tract infection, pneumonia, empyema, osteomyelitis, pyelonephritis, or tonsillitis. The typical presenting complaint is chest pain as a result of pericardial inflammation. Pericarditis is the second most commonly identified cardiac cause of chest pain after musculoskeletal pain in the pediatric population. The pain may be precordial or substernal in location and is typically described as squeezing, sharp, or dull with worsening in the supine position. Severity of symptoms depends on the rate of accumulation of fluid and health of the myocardium. Pericarditis becomes a medical emergency when the fluid causes cardiac tamponade.

On examination, evaluate for a pericardial friction rub, which is pathognomonic for pericarditis. A rub will not be present in large effusions; therefore, the absence of a rub does not rule out pericarditis. Pericarditis is the most frequent cause of ST elevation in children. Accordingly, an EKG showing low-voltage QRS complexes and diffuse ST segment elevations will support the diagnosis of pericarditis. Slurring of the PR interval is also a sign of pericardial inflammation. ST segment elevations will normalize later in the disease and T waves may flatten or invert. CXR in pericarditis classically reveals cardiomegaly, although heart size may be normal. Management and treatment in a patient with suspected pericarditis involves early recognition. ECHO demonstrates the presence and size of an effusion as well as any evidence of tamponade physiology. Depending on whether the effusion causes hemodynamic compromise or not, treatment includes nonsteroidal antiinflammatory drugs (NSAIDs), steroids, emergent percutaneous drainage, or surgical drainage with creation of a pericardial window.

CARDIAC TAMPONADE

Cardiac tamponade is the accumulation of fluid or some other substance (blood, chyle, air, pus) in the pericardial space that compresses the heart and thus impairs diastolic function resulting in decreased stroke volume and hypotension. Cardiac tamponade can be a complication of malignancies, cardiac tumors, uremia, bacterial/viral infections, rheumatologic conditions, autoimmune disorders, blunt/penetrating trauma, myocardial perforation after central venous catheterization, cardiac perforation from ASD occluder devices, ECMO, or positive pressure ventilation (PPV).

Patients with cardiac tamponade typically present with dyspnea, cough, anorexia, and/or vomiting. The physical examination is notable for tachycardia, tachypnea, and poor peripheral pulses. Beck triad of distant heart sounds, JVD, and hypotension is more commonly seen in adults. EKG demonstrates electrical alternans in 10% to 15% of patients or decreased voltages. CXR may have straightening of the left heart border or a progressively enlarging globular heart as the fluid accumulates. Pathognomonic findings on echocardiogram are pericardial effusion causing diastolic collapse of the right atrium and ventricle. Cardiac tamponade is a true medical emergency that requires immediate attention. Indications for pericardiocentesis include low cardiac output, hypotension, suspected bacterial pericarditis, pericardial effusion in an immunocompromised host, or for diagnosis. Pericardial fluid (if obtained) should be sent for cell count, glucose, protein, Gram stain, acid-fast bacilli stain, bacterial culture, viral culture, fungal culture, and microscopic analysis. For the procedure, select sedation and analgesia that will result in minimal respiratory depression. PPV can decrease cardiac output, so use with caution. Intravascular volume expansion is indicated in hypotensive patients. Avoid diuretics in these patients. Consult cardiology or surgery early for percutaneous or surgical drainage.

BACTERIAL ENDOCARDITIS

Endocarditis is an infection of the endocardium of the heart usually involving the heart valves. Endocarditis occurs most commonly in the pediatric population in association with CHD where it causes significant morbidity and mortality. Insidious and acute onset CHF can be a complication of infective endocarditis and can impact prognosis. High-risk conditions include prosthetic valves, previous history of endocarditis, complex cyanotic heart disease, residual shunts (jet lesions), and indwelling central venous catheters or devices. Patients with endocarditis may present with fulminant disease and sepsis, but often have a more indolent presentation with fever, chills, malaise, and myalgias. Carefully evaluate each CHD patient for new murmur and examine the teeth for decay or infection. Vascular and immunologic phenomena associated with endocarditis including Janeway lesions and Osler nodes may or may not be seen. Echocardiogram and blood cultures prior to antibiotics are essential for the diagnosis and management of bacterial endocarditis. Consult cardiology for admission. Cardiac surgery may be needed if endocarditis involves large vegetations in danger of embolization or significant valve insufficiency or perivalvar abscess. Treatment in the ED includes empiric antibiotics in the critically ill child with suspected endocarditis adequate to cover MRSA and Gram-negative organisms (e.g., vancomycin and cefotaxime) (see Chapter 102 Infectious Disease Emergencies).

ACUTE RHEUMATIC FEVER

In ARF, Group A streptococcus (GAS) causes acute inflammation in the multiple organs of the body including the heart. The degree to which the heart is affected and the course of the illness are variable. In the emergency department, a high suspicion and detection of patients with GAS provides the best chance of preventing the cardiac sequelae of ARF. EKG may show prolonged PR interval.

KAWASAKI DISEASE

Kawasaki disease (KD) is the most common generalized systemic vasculitis and the most common form of acquired heart disease in children in the United States. The heart can be affected in both the acute and chronic phase. KD typically affects infants and young children less than 5 years old. It is rare under the age of 4 months or in adults. These patients often present to the emergency department with fever, rash, and irritability. They have a hyperdynamic precordium, sinus tachycardia, rub, gallop, or murmur. They may exhibit signs of depressed myocardial function, myocarditis, or pericarditis during the acute phase. Coronary artery aneurysms (CAA) or ectasia occur in 25% of untreated children with KD. Children with incomplete features of KD are at increased risk of developing CAA due to delays in making the diagnosis resulting in delays in therapy. CAA typically develop in the second to third weeks of illness with coronary stenosis developing later. Although myocardial infarction is rare, affecting <3% of patients within 1 year of onset; myocardial infarction, sudden death, and ischemic heart disease may occur. KD should be considered in any child with 5 days of fever. Workup includes complete blood count, C-reactive protein level, erythrocyte sedimentation rate, liver function tests and urinalysis and urine culture. These tests will provide supporting evidence for the diagnosis as well as prognostic indicators. Thrombocytopenia is a risk factor for development of CAA. Electrocardiogram typically has sinus tachycardia and nonspecific ST and T changes. An echocardiogram is needed in the future to evaluate the coronary arteries, but if there is concern about the cardiac function early echocardiogram in the emergency department should be obtained.

Recognition and treatment within 10 days of the onset of fever lowers the risk of developing CAA. Treatment is intravenous immunoglobulin (IVIG) 2 g/kg, and high-dose aspirin 80 to 100 mg/kg/day every 6 hours for anti-inflammatory effect. See Chapter 102 Infectious Disease Emergencies for full discussion of KD.

MYOCARDIAL INFARCTION

Myocardial ischemia occurs when myocardial oxygen demand is not met and may lead to infarction. Myocardial infarctions are rare in children, yet the diagnosis should be considered in young patients with any condition that affects the coronary arteries (i.e., CHD or KD) or chest pain with exertion. Symptoms of ischemic chest pain include exertional pain, dyspnea, diaphoresis, and syncope. Pain is typically described as substernal pressure or burning, may radiate to neck or arm, and may even be short lived, lasting only 2 to 10 hours. Considerations when evaluating for causes of acute MI in the pediatric population should include coronary artery pathology: anomalous coronary arteries, KD with coronary involvement, surgery involving the coronary arteries or aortic root (coronary artery reimplantation in the arterial switch operation for D-TGA, aortic root replacement [Ross procedure]), mismatch between supply and demand (HCM, severe aortic stenosis, tachycardia with limited coronary blood flow), or severe hypoxia. Physical examination and EKG are often normal by the time the patient reaches the ED. If EKG is indicative of an MI, treatment follows Advanced Cardiac Life Support (ACLS) guidelines: oxygen, morphine, nitroglycerine, and monitoring. Cardiology should be consulted immediately or transfer to a facility capable of pediatric cardiac catheterization and coronary artery intervention should be initiated

A special case is the infant presenting with anomalous left coronary artery arising from the pulmonary artery (ALCAPA). These infants typically present around 10 weeks of age with crying with feeds, grey color, wheezing, tachypnea, or even loss of consciousness. They may be treated for gastroesophageal reflux or reactive airway disease. A high index of suspicion is necessary to make this diagnosis. Workup includes EKG and CXR, and blood work. Treatment may include diuretics, endotracheal intubation, cardiac inotropic support, and admission to a cardiac intensive care unit. Definitive treatment is surgery.

CARDIAC TRAUMA

Goals of Treatment

The focus in the emergency department is prompt recognition of cardiac trauma using a systematic approach and intervening quickly with any stabilizing interventions necessary (Chapter 123 Thoracic Trauma).

CLINICAL PEARLS AND PITFALLS

- Cardiac trauma can be blunt, penetrating, or electrical.
- Blunt trauma is the most common cause of cardiac trauma in pediatrics.
- Commotio cordis is a fatal ventricular rhythm experienced with chest trauma by a projectile such as a hockey puck or baseball in children.

Current Evidence

Much of the data available on cardiac trauma is from the adult population. Few data exist on children with traumatic injuries to the heart.

Clinical Considerations

Clinical Recognition

The key to recognition of cardiac trauma in children is a high level of suspicion in any child with injury to neck, axilla, chest, upper abdomen, or back.

Triage Considerations. Pediatric trauma patients should be evaluated immediately upon arrival to the emergency department. Ideally, the patient should be transported from the scene to a Level I pediatric trauma center or transferred to such facility promptly after stabilization.

Clinical Assessment. Children who have suffered a trauma should have a full primary and secondary survey immediately upon arrival. All garments should be removed and the chest closely examined. Diagnostic studies will vary depending on the nature and severity of the injury.

Management. Address ABCs: Airway, oxygenation, volume resuscitation, bleeding control. Perform necessary procedures when indicated. Patient with cardiac tamponade should undergo immediate pericardiocentesis. Penetrating cardiac injury often times requires emergent thoracotomy.

Blunt

Blunt cardiac trauma is typically sustained in MVC, but can be from any blunt force including blow to the chest, falls, acceleration–deceleration, compression in a crush injury, or a blast injury. The risk for rupture is greater if compression occurs when chambers are maximally filled (end diastole). Blunt cardiac trauma can cause injury to pericardium (pericardial contusion, pericardial rupture), myocardium (myocardial contusion, myocardial rupture, septal disruption, ventricular aneurysm), or great vessels. Commotio cordis causes SCD from blunt cardiac trauma. In a crush injury, patients are at risk of myocardial rupture if compression occurs at the time of maximal chamber filling. Blunt trauma can also result in pericardial tamponade.

Penetrating

The EM physician should assume cardiac injury with any penetrating injury to the chest, neck, axilla, back, or upper abdomen. Gunshot and stab wounds account for the majority of penetrating injury to the heart. Gunshots cause rapid exsanguination from extensive tissue destruction as a result of the bullet's kinetic energy. Stab wounds are more likely than gunshot to lead to cardiac tamponade.

Electrical

Electrical injury to the heart can occur from man-made electricity or lightning. Death is secondary to dysrhythmias. If a child sustains electrical injury, obtain an EKG and manage dysrhythmias per PALS protocol. Death is most commonly a result of VF. If a patient is asymptomatic with a normal EKG, no further cardiac evaluation is warranted.

EVALUATION OF THE PATIENT WITH A CARDIAC DEVICE

Goals of Treatment

The focus of the EM physician is to recognize and anticipate device-related malfunctions and complications in patients presenting to the emergency department.

CLINICAL PEARLS AND PITFALLS

- Atrial septal defect occluder devices may, on rare occasions, present with erosion through the heart and hemorrhagic shock.
- Initial history should identify pacemaker-dependent patients.
- Patients with a malfunctioning ICD that cannot deliver lifesaving therapy should be admitted to the hospital on telemetry in a unit that can respond rapidly to a potentially lethal rhythm.
- Complications involving pacemakers and ICDs occur more frequently around the time of implant.

Current Evidence

Pacemakers and ICD are small enough to be used routinely in pediatric patients for treatment of bradycardia or life-threatening tachyarrhythmias, respectively. ASD occlude devices are replacing surgical closure. Many other devices may be safely employed to close defects, vessels, replace valves, and maintain cardiac output.

Clinical Considerations

Pacemakers

Pacemakers are implanted for rate support in bradycardia. The most frequent indication in pediatrics is AV block, but symptomatic sinus bradycardia is also an indication. Patients may have single-chamber (atrial or ventricular) pacemakers or dual-chamber pacemakers that sense and pace both chambers.

Device failure may present with collapse, syncope, or the less dramatic symptom of fatigue. If the patient presents with extremis, temporary pacing or epinephrine for positive chronotropy may be necessary. History should reveal if the patient is pacemaker dependent, the type of pacemaker implanted, the date of implant, and the low rate programming or settings. Patients are issued an identification card at the time of device implant, which records information, including type of device and manufacturer, and name of the cardiologist. The initial evaluation of the pacing system should include an EKG and rhythm strip with and without magnet application, review of a comparison EKG and CXR, and review of a comparison film for lead placement.

The basics of troubleshooting a pacemaker include evaluation of the lead and the device itself. The lead is the most vulnerable part of the pacing system. Lead fractures/damage, dislodgements, poor connections, high pacing capture thresholds, or infection may cause pacemaker noncapture. Mechanical lead dislodgment or poor connections most frequently occur early after implant and result in inconsistent or noncapture, heart rate below the programmed rate, or an irregular heart rate. The lead fractures occur later after implant. One common site for lead fracture (or crush injury) is between the clavicle and the first rib. The lead is also vulnerable in trauma or hyperextension of the arm. CXR (two views) may reveal these lead problems. If the leads are intact, the battery may be the underlying issue. Battery failure is generally not without warning, although electromagnetic interference may cause problems.

If the pacing wires and battery are intact, device programming should be evaluated. Irregularities, such as over or under sensing of the rhythm, may be corrected by adjusting the pacemaker settings. Consultation with a pediatric cardiologist trained in pacemaker programming is required. It is not adequate to have a representative from the pacemaker manufacturer download the device information if a cardiologist is not available to interpret that information and guide therapy.

Pacemaker infections are usually seen within weeks of implant and may involve a stitch, the pacemaker pocket, or the entire pacing system. Presenting symptoms are similar to that of local wound infection or endocarditis. Blood cultures, EKG, and echocardiogram should be obtained. Consultation with the implanting physician for management is recommended. Noncapture may be a risk of an infected pacemaker and the ED physician should be prepared to give rate support. Infections as well as some medications may lead to high pacing thresholds.

ICD

ICDs are implanted to rescue the patient from potentially fatal VT or fibrillation by delivering high-energy shock to the heart. Most ICDs can also function as pacemakers. Devices may be implanted for primary prevention (high-risk conditions before symptoms develop) or secondary prevention (after aborted SCD).

Malfunction of the ICD leaves the patient vulnerable to SCD. Just as with pacemakers, ICD malfunction may be due to lead or battery failure and/or over or under sensing of the rhythm. Patients may receive appropriate or inappropriate shocks. The patient may even experience a phantom shock (the perception of a shock in the absence of a discharge from the device). This may be discerned by accessing information recorded by the device. In addition, inadequate energy delivery to convert the rhythm to sinus rhythm can be a serious malfunction. Evaluation of an ICD should include a history, EKG, two-view CXR, device interrogation, and electrophysiology consultation. Representatives from the device manufacturers are available to download information from the devices and can provide relevant information about safety and function recalls on the device. A cardiologist trained in the management of ICDs should be consulted. Malfunctions that cannot be reprogrammed for proper function in the ED should be admitted for telemetry monitoring and definitive plans for correction. If the device delivered a shock appropriately, consult cardiology for further management.

Ventricular Assist Devices

Ventricular assist devices (VADs) are mechanical pumps that take over the function of one or both ventricles. They serve as a bridge to transplantation and are being used increasingly as

TABLE 94.11

OTHER CARDIAC DEVICES

Cardiac device	Key points	
Stents	*Indication:*	Stent opens stenotic or hypoplastic vessel (i.e., pulmonary artery, coarctation of aorta with late postoperative restenosis)
Trans-catheter valves	*Indication:*	Replacement of insufficient pulmonary or aortic valves
ASD occluder	*Indication:*	Closure of atrial septal defect
	Complications:	Erosion through heart, atrioventricular block
	Treatment:	Emergent surgical repair, pacing
Ductal occluder	*Indication:*	Occlude PDAs and other aortopulmonary collaterals
	Complications:	Embolization, usually during procedure
	Treatment:	Catheter or surgical retrieval

techniques improve and smaller devices are available. Patients may be discharged home with these devices in place and therefore may present from home to the ED with these devices. VADs generate cardiac output, but not with pulsatile flow; therefore, a pulse will not be palpable. Immediate consultation with cardiac surgeon is imperative when these patients present to ED. Complications of VADs include stroke, bleeding, and infection.

Extracorporeal Membrane Oxygenation (ECMO)

ECMO is used to support circulation in reversible conditions or as a bridge to definitive therapy (transplant, ventricular function recovery, etc.). Consider the use of ECMO early and include cardiothoracic surgery in the decision-making process as soon as possible.

Information on other cardiac devices that may be encountered in the emergency department are discussed in Table 94.11.

Suggested Readings and Key References

Cardiac Emergencies

Congenital Heart Disease

Aronson PL, Chen J. The neonate after cardiac surgery: What do you need to worry about in the emergency department? *Clin Pediatr Emerg Med* 2011;12(4):313–322.

Brown K. The infant with undiagnosed cardiac disease in the emergency department. *Clin Pediatr Emerg Med* 2005;6(4):200–206.

Dolbec K, Mick NW. Congenital heart disease. *Emerg Med Clin North Am* 2011;29:811–827.

Hartman RJ, Rasmussen SA, Botto LD. The contribution of chromosomal abnormalities to congenital heart defects: a population-based study. *Pediatr Cardiol* 2011;32(8):1147–1157.

Hoffman JL, Kaplan S. The incidence of congenital heart disease. *J Am Coll Cardiol* 2002;39(12):1890–1900.

Lee C, Mason LJ. Pediatric cardiac emergencies. *Anesthesiol Clin North America* 2001;19(2):287–308.

Mahle WT, Newburger JW, Matherne GP, et al. Role of pulse oximetry in examining newborns for congenital heart disease: a scientific statement from the AHA and AAP. *Pediatrics* 2009;124:823–836.

Miller A, Riehle-Colarusso T. Congenital heart defects and major structural noncardiac anomalies, Atlanta, Georgia, 1968 to 2005. *J Pediatr* 2011;159(1):70–78.

Oster ME, Lee KA, Honein MA, et al. Temporal trends in survival among infants with critical congenital heart defects. *Pediatrics* 2013; 131(5):e1502–e1508.

Oyen N, Poulsen G, Boyd HA, et al. Recurrence of congenital heart defects in families. *Circulation* 2009;120;295–301.

Reller MD, Strickland MJ, Riehle-Colarusso T, et al. Prevalence of congenital heart defects in Atlanta, 1998–2005. *J Pediatr* 2008; 153:807–813.

Rudolph AM. The changes in the circulation after birth: their importance in congenital heart disease. *Circulation* 1970;41:343–359.

Savitsky E, Alejos J, Votey S. Emergency department presentations of pediatric congenital heart disease. *J Emerg Med* 2003;24(3):239–245.

Shaddy R, Parisi F. Pediatric Heart Transplantation. In: Allen HD, Driscoll DJ, Shaddy R E, eds. *Moss and Adams' heart disease in infants, children, and adolescents including the fetus and young adult.* 8th ed. Philadelphia, PA: Lippincott Williams and Wilkins, 2013: 1384–1400.

Tsai W, Klein BL. The postoperative cardiac patient. *Clin Pediatr Emerg Med* 2005;216–221.

Tuo G, Marasini M, Brunelli C, et al. Incidence and clinical relevance of primary congenital anomalies of the coronary arteries in children and adults. *Cardiol Young* 2013;23:381–386.

Woods WA, McCulloch MA. Cardiovascular emergencies in the pediatric patient. *Emerg Med Clin North Am* 2005;23:1233–1249.

Yee L. Cardiac emergencies in the first year of life. *Emerg Med Clin North Am* 2007;25:981–1008.

Arrhythmic Emergencies

Cannon BC, Snyder CS. Disorders of Cardiac Rhythm and Conduction. In: Allen HD, Driscoll DJ, Shaddy RE, et al. eds. *Moss and Adams' heart disease in infants, children, and adolescents including the fetus and young adult.* 8th ed. Philadelphia, PA: Lippincott Williams and Wilkins, 2013:441–472.

Hazinski MF, Smason R, Schexnayder S. 2010 Handbook of emergency cardiovascular care for healthcare providers. *American Heart Association* 2012, 72–79.

Sinz E, Navarro K. Advanced Cardiovascular Life Support Provider Manual. *American Heart Association* 2011:59–73, 104–127.

Taylor S. Temporary pacing in children. In: Gillette PC, Ziegler VL, eds. *Pediatric cardiac pacing.* Futuro Publishing Co, 1996:115–148.

Sudden Cardiac Death (SCD)

Maron BJ, Maron MS. Hypertrophic cardiomyopathy. *Lancet* 2013; 381(9862):242–255.

Maron BJ, Haas TS, Murphy CJ, et al. Incidence and causes of sudden death in U.S. college athletes. *J Am Coll Cardiol* 2014;63(16): 1636–1643.

Omar HR, Camporesi EM, Sprenker C, et al. The use of isoproterenol and phenytoin to reverse torsade de pointes. *Am J Emerg Med* 2014; 32(6):683.e5–683.e7.

Silka MJ, Bar-Cohen Y. A contemporary assessment of the risk for sudden cardiac death in patients with congenital heart disease. *Pediatr Cardiol* 2012;33:452–460.

Walsh E. Sudden death in adult congenital heart disease: risk stratification in 2014. *Heart Rhythm* 2014;11(10):1735–1742. [Epub ahead of print].

CHF

Cohen S, Springer C, Avital A, et al. Amino-terminal pro-brain-type natriuretic peptide: heart or lung disease in pediatric respiratory distress? *Pediatrics* 2005;115(5):1347–1350.

Costello JM, Almodovar MC. Emergency care for infants and children with acute cardiac disease. *Clinical Pediatric Emergency Medicine* 2007;8(3):145–155.

Durani Y, Giordano K, Goudie BW. Myocarditis and pericarditis in children. *Pediatr Clin North Am* 2010;57(6):1281–1303.

Faris R, Flather MD, Purcell H, et al. Diuretics for heart failure. *Cochrane Database of Syst Rev* 2006;25(1). Art. No.: CD003838. DOI: 10.1002/14651858.CD003838.pub2.

Macicek SM, Macias CG, Jefferies JL, et al. Acute heart failure syndromes in the pediatric emergency department. *Pediatrics* 2009; 124(5):e898–e904.

Acquired Heart Disease

Baddour LM, Wilson WR, Bayer AS, et al. Infective endocarditis: diagnosis, antimicrobial therapy, and management of complications: a statement for healthcare professionals from the committee on rheumatic fever, endocarditis, and Kawasaki disease, council on cardiovascular disease in the young, and the councils on clinical cardiology, stroke, and cardiovascular surgery and anesthesia, American heart association: endorsed by infectious disease society of America. *Circulation* 2005;111:e394–e434.

Chang YJ, Chao HC, Hsia SH, et al. Myocarditis presenting as gastritis in children. *Pediatr Emerg Care* 2006;22(6):439–440.

Cramm KJ, Cattaneo RA, Schremmer RD, et al. An infant with tachypnea. *Pediatr Emerg Care* 2006;22(11):728–731.

Durani Y, Giordano K, Goudie BW. Myocarditis and pericarditis in children. *Pediatr Clin North Am* 2010;57(6):1281–1303.

Elliot P, Anderson B, Arbustini E, et al. Classification of the cardiomyopathies: a position statement from the European society of cardiology working group on myocardial and pericardial diseases. *Eur Heart J* 2008;29:270–276.

Gewitz M, Taubert KA. Infective endocarditis and prevention. In: Allen HD, Driscoll DJ, Shaddy RE, et al., eds. *Moss and Adams' heart disease in infants, children, and adolescents including the fetus and young adult.* 8th ed. Philadelphia, PA: Lippincott Williams and Wilkins, 2013:1363–1376.

Towbin JA, Lowe AM, Colan SD, et al. Incidence, causes, and outcomes of dilated cardiomyopathy in children. *JAMA* 2006;296(15): 1867–1876.

Zaidi AN, Daniels CJ. Myocardial ischemia. In: Allen HD, Driscoll DJ, Shaddy RE, et al., eds. *Moss and Adams' heart disease in infants, children, and adolescents including the fetus and young adult.* 8th ed. Philadelphia, PA: Lippincott Williams and Wilkins, 2013:1377–1383.

Cardiac Trauma

Smith GA, Feltes TF. Cardiac trauma. In: Allen HD, Driscoll DJ, Shaddy RE, et al., eds. *Moss and Adams' heart disease in infants, children, and adolescents including the fetus and young adult.* 8th ed. Philadelphia, PA: Lippincott Williams and Wilkins, 2013:552–559.

Pacemakers, Defibrillators, and Other Implanted Cardiac Devices

Berul CI, Van Hare GF, Kertesz NJ, et al. Results of a multicenter retrospective implantable cardioverter-defibrillator registry of pediatric and congenital heart disease patients. *J Am Coll Cardio* 2008; 51:1685–1691.

Chessa M, Carminati M, Butera G, et al. Early and late complications associated with transcatheter occlusion of secundum atrial septal defect. *J Am Coll Cardiol* 2002;39(6):1061–1065.

Fraser CD, Jaquiss RD, Rosenthal DN, et al. Prospective trial of a pediatric ventricular assist device. *N Engl J Med* 2012;367(6): 532–541.

Kaszala K. Evaluation troubleshooting and management of pacing system functions. In: Ellenbogen K, Kaszala K, eds. *Cardiac pacing and ICD's.* 6th ed. Blackwell and Wiley, 2014:272–275.

Sharma MS, Webber SA, Morell VO, et al. Ventricular assist device support in children and adolescents as a bridge to heart transplantation. *Ann Thorac Surg* 2006;82(3):926–932.

Sharma MS, Webber SA, Morell VO, et al. Ventricular assist device support in children and adolescents with heart failure: the Children's Medical Center of Dallas experience. *Artif Organs* 2012; 36(7):635–639.

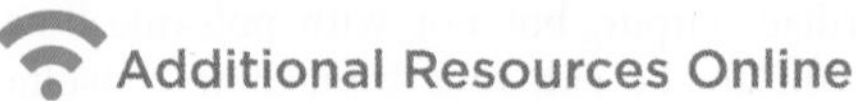

CHAPTER 95 ▪ CHILD ABUSE/ASSAULT

JOANNE N. WOOD, MD, MSHP, JAMES M. CALLAHAN, MD, AND CINDY W. CHRISTIAN, MD

GOALS OF EMERGENCY CARE

Prompt recognition and evaluation of injuries resulting from physical abuse is important to allow for (1) appropriate treatment of the presenting injury, (2) identification of occult injuries including fractures, traumatic brain injury (TBI), or intra-abdominal injury that may require medical intervention, and (3) protection of the child and possibly other children from further injury. Distinguishing abusive injuries from accidental injuries in the ED, however, can be challenging especially in young, preverbal children due to the potential unreliability of caregiver histories and limitations of physical examination in this population. Thus, providers should consider the possibility of physical abuse in young children with injuries without a clear accidental etiology. In children with injuries suspicious for abuse, a thorough evaluation including history and physical examination should be performed once the patient is medically stabilized (Tables 95.1–95.3). Depending on the age of the child, radiologic and laboratory testing for occult injuries may be indicated as victims of physical abuse presenting with minor injuries may have more serious clinically occult injuries (Table 95.4). A report to child protective services (CPS) must be made if the provider has reasonable suspicion that the child may be a victim of abuse. Physicians and nurses are mandated reporters of child abuse in all states; in many states, other healthcare workers are also mandated reporters. Emergency department providers should be familiar with the mandatory child abuse reporting laws governing the area in which they practice. Failure to recognize, evaluate, and report cases of physical abuse can result in children suffering complications from injuries undiagnosed at the time of presentation, and keeps children vulnerable to future abuse that can lead to additional injuries and death.

KEY POINTS

- Physical abuse is common; over 120,000 children are substantiated as victims of physical abuse each year in the United States.
- Abuse should be considered in the differential diagnosis of injuries without obvious accidental etiologies.
- Children <1 year old are at the highest risk of serious and fatal abuse.
- Victims of physical abuse may present with misleading histories.
- Young victims of abuse frequently have occult injuries including fractures, TBI, and intra-abdominal injuries not detected on history or physical examination.
- Medical providers are mandated to make a report to CPS if there is a reasonable suspicion for abuse.

RELATED CHAPTERS

Resuscitation and Stabilization
- Approach to the Injured Child: Chapter 2

Signs and Symptoms
- Coma: Chapter 12
- Crying: Chapter 15
- Seizures: Chapter 67

Medical, Surgical, and Trauma Emergencies
- Abdominal Trauma: Chapter 111
- Burns: Chapter 112
- Dental Trauma: Chapter 113
- ENT Trauma: Chapter 114
- Musculoskeletal Trauma: Chapter 119
- Neurotrauma: Chapter 121
- Thoracic Trauma: Chapter 123
- Sexual Assault: Child and Adolescent: Chapter 135

INJURIES FROM PHYSICAL ABUSE: GENERAL

Clinical Considerations

Clinical Recognition

Children of all ages may present to the emergency department with abusive injuries, but infants are at the greatest risk of sustaining severe or fatal injuries. Victims of physical abuse may present with injuries to any body system, but cutaneous injuries and fractures are the most common injuries for which victims of physical abuse are brought for care. TBI is also common among young victims of physical abuse and is the leading cause of morbidity and mortality in this population. Intra-abdominal injuries are rare but are the second leading cause of morbidity and mortality from physical abuse.

Triage Considerations

The triage of children with suspected abusive injuries is similar to children with accidental injuries and is dependent on the severity and type of the injury. The severity of the child's clinical condition may be underestimated initially because the history provided at triage is often false or incomplete.

Clinical Assessment

The initial clinical assessment of a child with possible abusive injuries does not differ from the approach for a child with similar accidental injuries. After the child is stabilized, further evaluation is necessary to determine the level of concern for abuse and guide next steps in ensuring the safety of the child. Distinguishing abusive injuries from accidental injuries in the

TABLE 95.1

FINDINGS IN THE HISTORY THAT MAY BE SUGGESTIVE OF PHYSICAL ABUSE

- No history of trauma provided to explain the injury
- History is inconsistent with the injury
- History is inconsistent with the developmental age of the child
- History changes with time
- History of sibling or home resuscitative efforts causing injuries
- Conflicting histories provided from different caregivers
- Unexplained or unexpected delay in seeking care

ED can be difficult as there are few single injuries pathognomonic for abuse and overlap exists in the spectrum of injuries resulting from accidental and abusive trauma. Findings on history and physical examination, however, can help to identify cases concerning for abuse that warrant further evaluation (Tables 95.1 and 95.2). A thorough history including history of trauma, developmental history, past medical history, and social history should be performed. A complete physical examination including review of vital signs, thorough skin examination, and neurologic examination, should be performed in addition to the assessment of the presenting injury. If available, photodocumentation with a size standard or ruler should be performed for cutaneous findings (Table 95.5).

TABLE 95.2

DIFFERENTIAL DIAGNOSIS OF CUTANEOUS FINDINGS SUSPICIOUS FOR PHYSICAL ABUSE[a]

Disease	Key features
Differential diagnosis of bruises	
Abusive bruises[b]	• Bruises in young, nonmobile infants without verifiable history of trauma • Bruises over soft tissue areas on the ear, neck, face, abdomen, buttock, back, hands, feet, genitals • Patterned bruises, clusters of bruises • Loop marks
Accidental bruises[b]	• History of accidental trauma matching bruise location/pattern • Often over bony prominences • Common in ambulatory children
Dermal melanesia	• Blue-gray macules that do not appear red or inflamed • Less distinct borders than bruises • Do not change in color or size over days to weeks • May fade during childhood
Phototoxicity: psoralens	• Exposure to psoralens in citrus fruit or other plants • Erythematous, purple or hyperpigmented lesions, erosions, and blisters following exposure to sunlight
Photoallergy: bergamot	• Exposure to bergamot in perfume or other liquids • Blisters and hyperpigmented lesions following exposure to sunlight
Henoch–Schönlein purpura (HSP)	• Palpable purpura typically located on the buttocks and extensor surface of the extremities in children of 2 to 7 years old. May be associated with arthritis, abdominal pain, elevated ESR, and thrombocytosis
Hemangioma	• Superficial hemangiomas: Purple/red telangiectatic macules and papules • Deep hemangiomas: Poorly defined bluish nodules • Grow rapidly for first 6 months of life, then grow slowly until 12 to 18 months, followed by involution
Cao gio (coin rolling)	• Linear petechiae or purpura on torso • History of rubbing back or chest with a coin or other object as part of a folk health remedy
Erythema multiforme	• ± preceding viral illness • Fixed annular, macular papular lesions on palms, soles, and extensor surfaces of extremities that develop concentric zones of color change with central crusting or blistering
Idiopathic thrombocytopenic purpura	• Acute onset with bruising and petechiae • Low platelet count • Usually self-limited
Coagulopathies (congenital and acquired)	• ± history of easy bruising, epistaxis, gingival bleeds, menorrhagia bleeding, bleeding into joints or muscles, excessive bleeding following circumcision, surgical procedures or trauma in patient or family • Laboratory tests (CBC, PT, INR, aPTT, VWF antigen, VWF activity, Factors VIII and IX) and/or consultation with a hematologist should be considered if there is suspicion for coagulopathy
Differential diagnosis of burns	
Abusive scald burn[b]	• Cigarette burns (0.5 to 1.0 cm, clearly demarcated, round burn that forms a scar with a hypopigmented center) • Patterned burns with inadequate history • Immersion burns with stocking, glove pattern • Multiple distinct areas of burns • Burns involving the perineum or genitals in children <2 years old

TABLE 95.2

DIFFERENTIAL DIAGNOSIS OF CUTANEOUS FINDINGS SUSPICIOUS FOR PHYSICAL ABUSE[a] (*CONTINUED*)

Disease	Key features
Abusive contact burn[b]	• Often clearly demarcated and patterned • Multiple burns • May be located on trunks, extremities, and dorsum of hands
Accidental scald burn[b]	• History of hot liquid spill or flowing hot water that matches burn location/pattern • Irregular margins • May involve head/face, neck, trunk, upper body • If involves lower extremities typically asymmetric distribution • Usually does not involve perineum/genital region in young children
Accidental contact burn[b]	• Burn in location consistent with child accidentally touching hot item • Blurred margins/not clearly demarcated • Single burn
Bullous impetigo	• Honey crusted lesions that vary in size and may spread
Phototoxicity/ photoallergy	• See description in bruise section above
Senna-containing laxative blistering dermatitis	• Ingestion of senna-containing laxative • Diamond-shaped lesion on buttock with linear borders that line up with diaper edge • Sparing of perianal tissue and gluteal cleft

[a]Includes some but not all of the medical conditions that can mimic cutaneous injuries from abuse. Evaluation for additional conditions may be indicated in some cases.
[b]The pattern and distribution of bruises and burns can help in identifying lesions associated with an increased likelihood of abuse, but are not diagnostic for abuse and must be interpreted within the context of the history, physical examination, and results of laboratory and radiographic evaluation.

TABLE 95.3

DIFFERENTIAL DIAGNOSIS OF FRACTURES SUSPICIOUS FOR PHYSICAL ABUSE[a]

Disease	Key features
Abusive fractures[b]	• Fracture in a nonmobile infant <12 months old without verifiable history of trauma • Femoral fracture or humeral fracture in young, nonambulatory child • Rib fractures in child <3 years old • Classic metaphyseal lesions (CML) • Multiple fractures
Accidental fractures[b]	• Child ≥18 months old • History of accidental trauma mechanism that matches fracture type • Distal buckle fracture of radius/ulna or tibia/fibula in ambulatory child • Femoral fracture in ambulatory child • Supracondylar humeral fracture with history of fall
Infantile cortical hyperostosis (Caffey disease)	• Infant <6 months old • Cortical thickening of mandible, clavicle, and long bones • Associated soft tissue swelling and irritability
Osteogenesis imperfect (OI)	• Features vary depending on the type but may include the following: triangular facies, blue sclera, limb deformities, hyperextensible joints, hearing loss, macrocephaly, hernias, short stature, teeth abnormalities, scoliosis, kyphosis, and demineralized or Wormian bones on radiography • Genetic testing, and/or collagen analysis can aid in diagnosis
Osteopenia	• History of risk factors for osteopenia including prematurity, immobility, or chronic disease • Demineralization on radiographs
Rickets	• Laboratory abnormalities including low 25-hydroxy vitamin D level, elevated alkaline phosphatase level, elevated PTH • Radiologic findings of bone demineralization, widened metaphyses, and cupping and fraying of the metaphyses and costochondral junctions

[a]Includes some but not all of the medical conditions that can mimic abusive fractures. Evaluation for additional conditions may be indicated in some cases.
[b]Specific types of fractures are associated with an increased likelihood of abuse but are not diagnostic for abuse and must be interpreted within the context of the history, physical examination, and results of laboratory and radiographic evaluation.

TABLE 95.4

LABORATORY AND RADIOLOGIC TESTS FOR EVALUATION OF OCCULT INJURIES IN CASES OF SUSPECTED PHYSICAL ABUSE

Test	Indications
Abdominal trauma laboratory tests	
• ALT, AST, amylase, lipase, urine analysis	• Consider in suspected victims of physical abuse of any age to screen for occult abdominal trauma
Abdominal imaging	
• Abdominal CT with intravenous contrast	• Obtain in children with clinical concern for abdominal trauma based on history, physical examination, or laboratory findings
Head imaging	
• CT for acutely symptomatic children • MRI for asymptomatic children Note: CT may be more readily available but MRI may be more sensitive for subtle injuries and provide more detailed information.	• Obtain in children with suspected intracranial injury • Obtain in neurologically asymptomatic suspected victims of abuse <2 years old with any of the following high risk criteria: 1. Age <6 months 2. Rib fractures 3. Multiple fractures 4. Facial injury • Consider in neurologically asymptomatic suspected victims of abuse <2 years old who do not meet high risk criteria
Cervical spine imaging	
• CT or MRI	• Obtain in children with suspected spinal injury based on history or physical examination • Obtain in children with suspected abusive head trauma
Skeletal imaging	
• Skeletal survey	• Obtain in ALL children <2 years old with injuries suspicious for physical abuse to screen for occult fractures • Consider in children of 2 to 3 years with severe abusive injuries to screen for occult fractures • Repeat in 2 weeks in high-risk cases

If results of the history and physical examination suggest that an injury is suspicious for abuse, laboratory and/or radiologic studies to screen for occult injuries may be indicated based on the age of the child (Table 95.4). Testing for diseases that may mimic abusive injuries or predispose a child to sustain injuries with minimal accidental trauma such as bleeding disorders in children with unexplained bruising or osteogenesis imperfecta in the children with multiple fractures should be considered as well (Tables 95.2 and 95.3). Although screening tests for some of these disorders may be able to be obtained in the emergency department, it may be necessary to refer patients to appropriate specialists for further testing (e.g., referral to a hematologist for specialized testing for bleeding disorders if a platelet count and basic coagulation profile testing is normal or to a geneticist if there is a concern for osteogenesis imperfecta).

Management

With few exceptions, the initial management of patients with abusive injuries does not differ from the management of children with accidental injuries. Severely injured children should be stabilized prior to the evaluation for suspected abuse being performed. If based on the history, physical examination, and laboratory and radiographic evaluation, the ED provider has a reasonable suspicion to suspect physical abuse; a report to CPS must be made and should be discussed with the caregivers. Children with injuries from physical abuse can be discharged from the ED if the following conditions have been met: (1) Injuries do not require further inpatient management, (2) medical evaluation including evaluation for occult injuries is complete, and (3) a safe discharge environment has been identified; this requires collaboration with the local child welfare agency. If these conditions have not been met, hospital admission may be advisable.

Once the medical provider makes a report, the CPS agency will make a determination as to whether there is sufficient information to suggest that an investigation for suspected child abuse is warranted. If the report is "screened in" for investigation, a CPS caseworker will initiate an investigation which may include but is not limited to speaking with the family, child, medical providers, and other contacts as well as performing a home assessment. After making the report, the medical provider should cooperate with the CPS investigation and provide the relevant medical information. The Health Insurance Portability and Accountability Act (HIPAA) rules allow for medical providers who have made a mandatory report of suspected child maltreatment to share information with CPS without legal guardian authorization. During the investigation, the CPS caseworker will also assess the family's strengths and needs, and when appropriate provide services to support the family. If there is an immediate concern for the safety of the child in the home environment, the child may be discharged from the hospital to foster care, a relative's home, or a shelter while the investigation is being conducted, but

TABLE 95.5

PHOTODOCUMENTATION TIPS

- **Do** take photos of any injury visible on physical examination.
- **Do** take an initial photograph of the patient's identification bracelet.
- **Do** photograph each injury separately.
- **Do** take a photograph of the injury at a distance, followed by a close-up photograph.
- **Do NOT** take only close-up photos without wider angle photos of each injury. Remember that what appears obvious to you in the room with the patient may not be identifiable to you months or years later.
- **Do** review your photographs to be sure that both the injury and body part are identifiable to a provider who has not seen the patient in person.
- **Do** use a size standard or ruler in close-up photographs.

Camera settings and information

- Try photographing bruises with and without direct lighting and with and without flash, to see which conditions show bruising the best. Each case will be different, so some experimentation may be necessary to determine which lighting conditions are best.
- To obtain close-up photos, move the camera closer rather than using the built-in zoom feature.
- Photograph against a neutral background, like the sheets.
- Center the injury in the middle of the frame.

only a minority of children reported to CPS enter out-of-home placement.

If based on the results of the investigation the CPS worker determines that there is sufficient evidence to conclude that the child was abused, the case will be substantiated or founded. The CPS agency may initiate child protection or child dependency hearings in juvenile court if deemed necessary for the child's protection. Depending on the severity of the maltreatment and perceived risk for future maltreatment, the CPS agency may determine that the child is safe to remain in their home with voluntary or mandated services for the family. In cases of severe abuse or high risk, the child may be placed in a foster home, relative's home, or shelter.

CUTANEOUS MANIFESTATIONS OF ABUSE: BRUISES, BURNS, AND BITES

Goals of Treatment

Most cases of abusive bruising do not require medical intervention. Prompt recognition and evaluation of abusive bruising is important, however, to allow for (1) identification of occult injuries including fractures, TBI, or abdominal trauma that may require medical intervention, and (2) protection of the child from further injury. In cases of extensive bruising with muscle breakdown, monitoring for and treatment of rhabdomyolysis and renal failure may be necessary. Abusive burns and bite marks should be medically managed as clinically indicated based on the type and severity of the injury with the addition of the need to evaluate for and treat any additional occult injuries (Table 95.4) and make a report to CPS.

CLINICAL PEARLS AND PITFALLS

- Skin is the most commonly injured body organ in physical abuse.
- Accidental bruising is very uncommon in young non-mobile infants.
- Bruises may be the only external sign of injury in abuse victims with serious internal injuries.
- Bleeding disorders and other medical diseases should be considered in the differential diagnosis of cutaneous findings suspicious for abuse.
- The majority of burns in children result from accidental trauma.
- A high percentage of genital/perineal scald burns in children <2 years old are abusive.

Current Evidence

Cutaneous injury, and bruising in particular, is the most common injury identified in young victims of physical abuse. Cutaneous injuries such as bruising can be the only outward sign of more serious abusive injuries including fractures and abusive head trauma (AHT). Abusive bruising is a frequent precursor to more serious forms of physical abuse including AHT.

Clinical Considerations

Clinical Recognition

Bruises. The age and developmental stage of the child as well as the distribution and pattern of injuries can help to distinguish abusive from accidental bruises (Table 95.2). Young nonmobile infants infrequently sustain accidental bruises during routine daily activities. Therefore, *any* unexplained bruising in a nonmobile infant should raise consideration of possible abuse. As children become more mobile the frequency of accidental bruising increases. Among mobile children, most accidental bruises are located over bony prominences including the forehead, shins, and knees. Accidental trauma is less likely to cause bruises over soft tissue areas on the face, abdomen, buttock, back, arms, hands, and feet; bruising in these locations should prompt consideration of abuse. Patterned bruises, bruises occurring in clusters, and multiple bruises of uniform shape should raise suspicion for possible abuse. The mnemonic "TEN 4" can assist clinicians in identifying the following bruise patterns suspicious for abuse: Bruising of the torso, ear, or neck in a child ≤4 years old, or bruising in any location in a child <4 months old. Although, these features can help in identifying bruises associated with an increased likelihood of abuse, they are not diagnostic for abuse. Bruises, as with other injuries, must be interpreted within the context of the medical and social history, physical examination, and results of laboratory and/or radiographic evaluation. During the evaluation of suspected abusive bruising, providers should also consider the possibility of dermatologic conditions, hematologic and oncologic diseases, connective tissue disorders, vasculitis, and folk remedies that increase risk of bruising or cause lesions that can be mistaken for bruises (Table 95.2). Bruises, whether accidental or abusive, cannot be accurately aged based on their appearance.

Bites. Victims of physical abuse may present with areas of bruising, abrasions, lacerations, and avulsions from human bite marks. Human bite marks are typically ovoid or elliptical in shape and may have an area of central bruising. Bite marks should be photographed with and without a scale and, if acute, they should be swabbed for forensic evidence using a cotton swab moistened with sterile water. The size and pattern may be helpful in distinguishing between child and adult bite marks; an intercanine distance of greater than 3 cm is suggestive of an adult bite mark.

Burns. Although the majority of burns in children are due to accidental injury, the proportion of burns due to abuse is not well documented; it is estimated that between 1% and 35% of children admitted to burn units are victims of abuse. The mean age of children with abusive burns is between 2

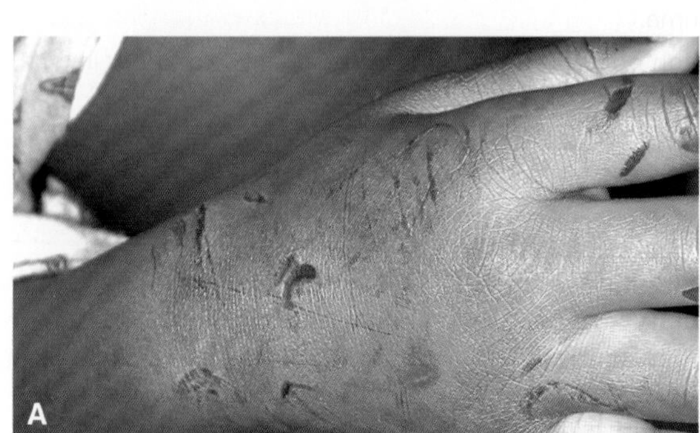

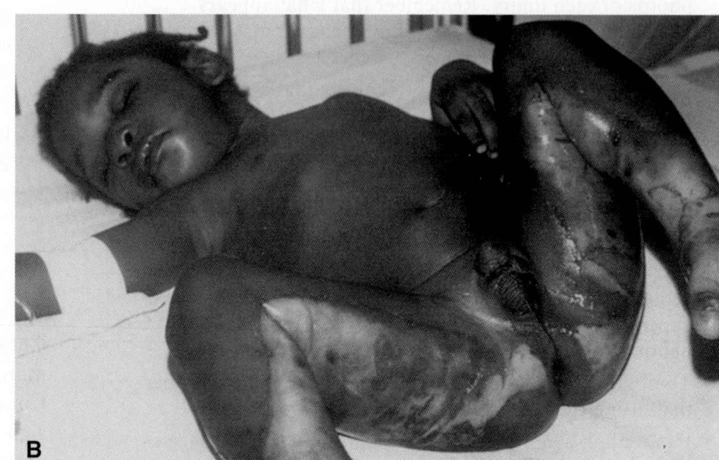

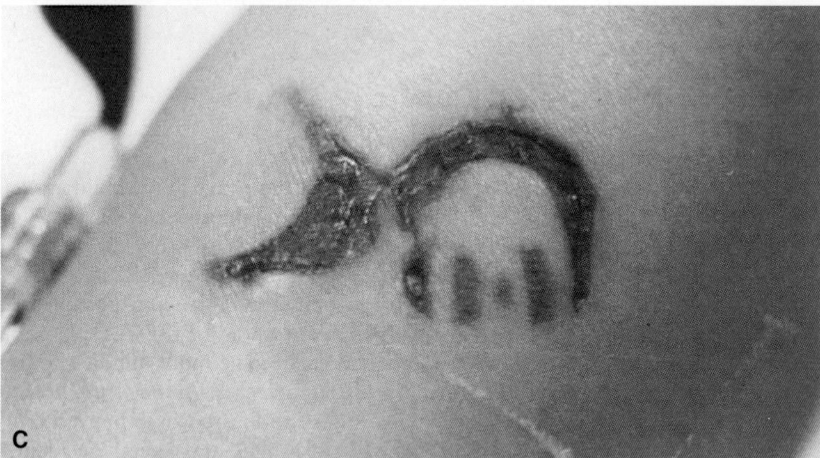

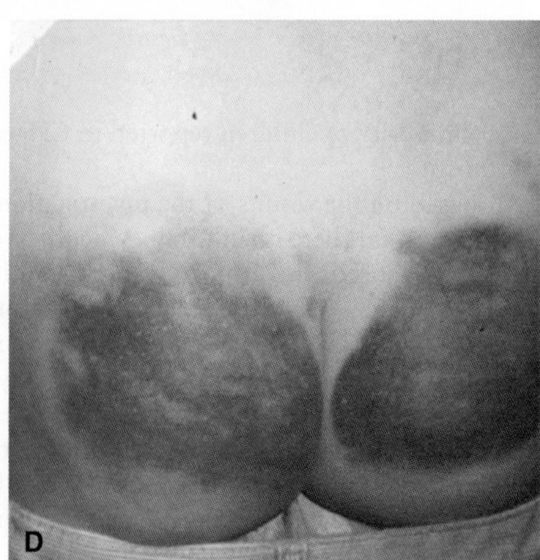

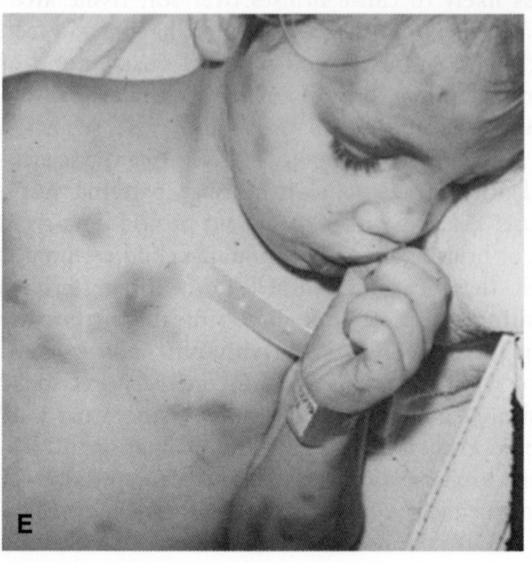

FIGURE 95.1 Cutaneous manifestations of child abuse. **A:** Multiple patterned scars including loop-shaped marks. **B:** Hot water burn in an immersion pattern. **C:** Pattern burn from cigarette lighter. **D:** Buttock bruises as a cause of myoglobinuria. **E:** Multiple bruises in a central pattern.

and 4 years old, higher than for other types of abusive injuries. As with other injuries, the pattern and distribution of burns may help to distinguish abusive from accidental injuries although there can be overlap between the two etiologies (Table 95.2). Scald burns are the most common type of burn seen in children. Scald burns of the buttocks and/or perineum from immersion in hot tap water should raise concern for abuse. Intentional scalds are more likely than accidental scald burns to have clear upper margins and a symmetric distribution. The identification of additional unexplained injuries on physical examination or radiologic studies can also help to distinguish abusive from accidental scald burns. Contact burns, the second most common type of burn in children, can also occur from accidental and abusive etiologies. Findings suggestive of abuse in cases of contact burns include the presence of clearly demarcated circular cigarette burns or other clearly demarcated patterned burns, multiple burns, or a history not consistent with the burn pattern. The pattern and distribution of the burn can help in identifying burns associated with an increased likelihood of abuse, but they are not diagnostic for abuse and must be interpreted within the context of the history, physical examination, laboratory, and/or radiographic evaluation results. In addition to accidental burns, dermatologic and infectious conditions should be considered in the differential diagnosis of lesions concerning for abusive burns (Table 95.2, Fig. 95.1).

OROPHARYNGEAL INJURIES FROM ABUSE

Goals of Treatment

Severe and life-threatening oropharyngeal abusive injuries including pharyngeal lacerations can occur and should be medically managed the same as similar accidental injuries. Most abusive oropharyngeal injuries, however, are mild, with bruises, abrasions, and lacerations being most common and will heal without medical intervention. Prompt identification and evaluation of inflicted oropharyngeal injuries is important in order to allow for identification of occult injuries (Table 95.4) and protection of the child from further injury.

CLINICAL PEARLS AND PITFALLS

- The oropharynx should be examined carefully in suspected victims of abuse for injuries including fractured or avulsed teeth; frenum tears; as well as bruises; burns; and lacerations of the lips, tongue, palate, pharynx, or retropharynx.
- Injuries to the oral cavity may be overlooked by physicians who do not routinely examine the structures within the mouth.
- Injuries within the ear, nose, or throat, should arouse suspicion of abuse, especially in infants and young children. When recurrent, these injuries are almost always inflicted.
- Tears to the frena in young infants should raise a suspicion of abuse; these injuries are sometimes disregarded, only to have the infant return with additional injury.

Current Evidence

Abusive injuries to the oropharynx may be the result of blunt or penetrating trauma. The majority of injuries are mild, although these injuries are often associated with more severe internal injuries.

Clinical Considerations

Clinical Recognition

Trauma to the mouth may cause contusions or lacerations of the upper or lower lip. Blows directed at the child's mouth may result in the oral tissues coming into forceful contact with the child's teeth, resulting in "bite marks" of the inner lip from the child's own teeth. Bruising or laceration at the corners of the lips also can result from the use of a gag to silence a child.

Most abusive injuries to the tongue are a result of the child biting the tongue inadvertently. A blow to the jaw can trap the tongue between upper and lower teeth. These injuries usually involve the lateral or anterior surfaces of the tongue and resemble jagged indentations seen with any bite mark in soft tissue. If the bite involves posterior areas of the tongue, the marks may appear more like crushed tissue rather than showing definite bite marks.

In young infants, intraoral injuries including frenum tears and pharyngeal perforations should always raise the possibility of abuse. Injury is often related to forced feeding, leading to mild to severe contusions of the lips and gingivae as well as lacerations of the labial frenum or perforation of the posterior pharynx. Although accidental frenum tears are common in the 8- to 18-month old who is learning to walk, similar injuries in young infants and in older, more stable children should raise a suspicion of abuse. Along with lacerations cause by forced feeding, other forms of abusive trauma can tear these tissues. Blows to the face can displace the lip far enough to stretch the lip's attachment tissue beyond its elastic limit, lacerating the frenum. Invasive trauma that introduces a hard or sharp object into the mouth also can lacerate these areas. Frenum tears will usually heal on their own, although can require sutures if the wound is large or the alveolar bone is exposed.

Abuse-related injuries to teeth can include movement of the teeth within the socket, fracture, or loss of the tooth, typically from blows to the face. Teeth can be moved anteriorly or posteriorly, intruded into or avulsed from the socket, or moved mesially or distally if adjacent teeth are not in tight contact. Teeth can also be fractured. This can happen with accidental injuries as well as from abuse. Traumatic tooth avulsion requires immediate dental consultation. The tooth must be kept moist in isotonic saline solution or milk. The chances for successful reimplantation are best if the procedure is accomplished within 30 minutes of the avulsion.

Trauma that affects teeth also is likely to affect the surrounding gingivae. In addition, trauma from an object striking the child can produce contusions or lacerations of the gingivae without visible trauma to adjacent teeth. Radiographic examination is necessary in cases of gingival trauma to properly diagnose any damage to adjacent teeth or alveolar bone.

Pharyngeal and cervical esophageal perforations due to child abuse are uncommon but well described, and are typically caused by penetrating trauma to the child's mouth. Pharyngeal or esophageal lacerations introduce air, oral secretions, and bacteria into the soft tissues of the neck and mediastinum, with potentially life-threatening sequelae. Children with perforating injuries may present with fever, drooling, respiratory distress, erythematous cervical swelling, dysphagia, dysphonia, subcutaneous emphysema, or pneumomediastinum. Abused children may also have foreign bodies forced into their mouth and adjoining structures, leading to respiratory distress or asphyxiation.

ABUSIVE FRACTURES

Goals of Treatment

The acute medical management of abusive fractures does not differ from the management of accidental fractures. Once the patient is stabilized evaluation for occult injuries including occult fractures and TBI should be performed depending on

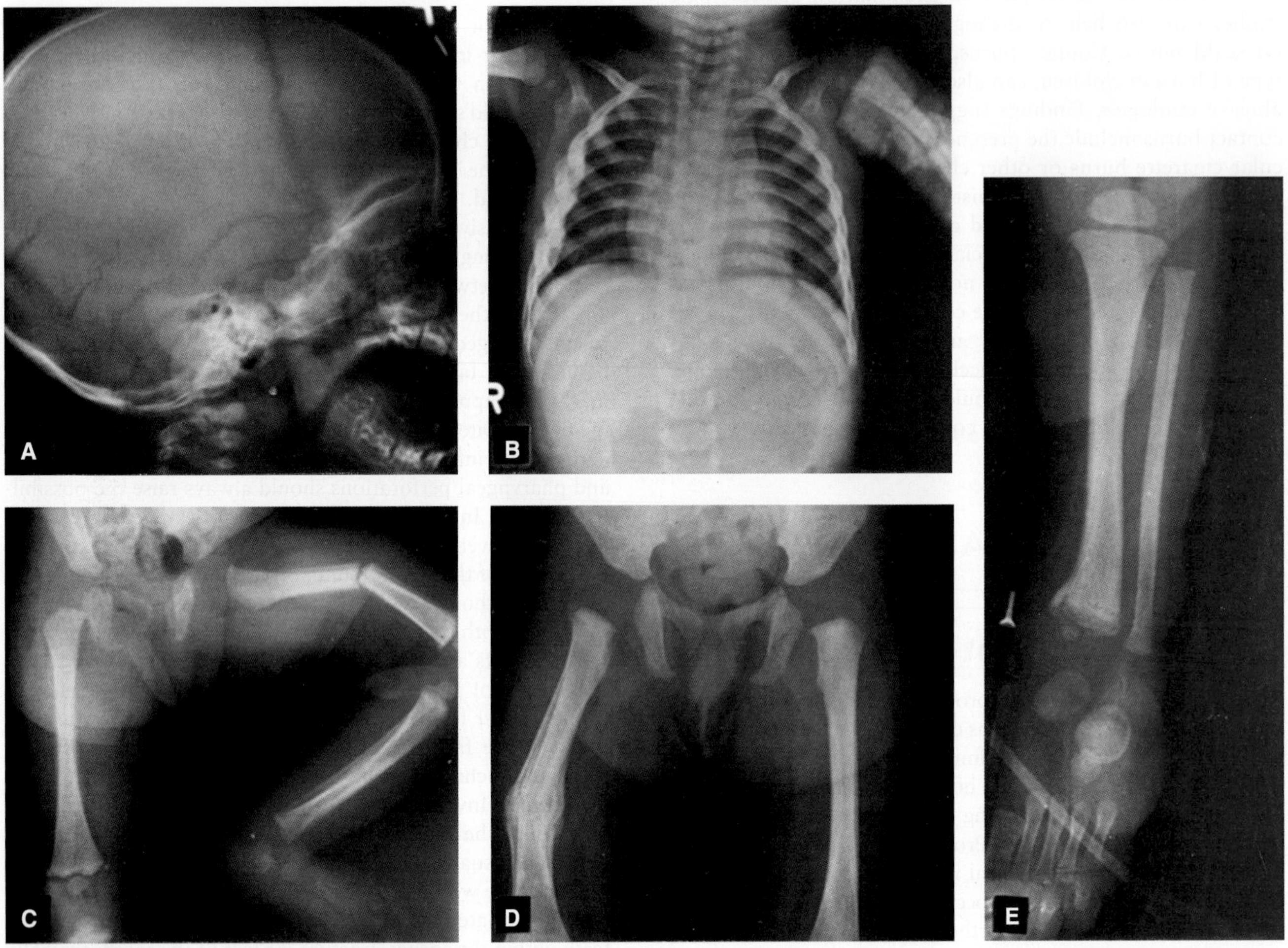

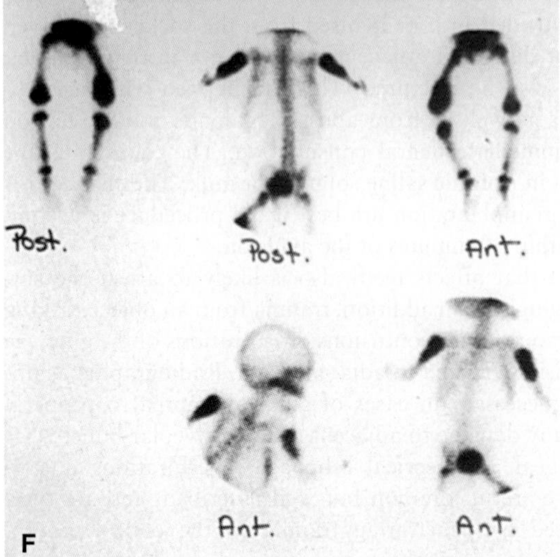

FIGURE 95.2 Abusive fractures. **A:** Multiple skull fractures in an infant. **B:** Left humerus fracture and multiple old healing rib fractures. **C:** Left femur fracture and metaphyseal chip avulsion fractures of the right distal femur. **D:** Healing fracture of the right femur with callus formation and new periosteal bone formation. **E:** "Bucket-handle" deformity of healing distal tibial metaphyseal fracture. **F:** Bone scans showing multiple areas of increased uptake caused by trauma. Some of these areas appeared normal on the original radiographs. Ant., anterior; Post., posterior.

the age of the child (Table 95.4) and a report should be made to CPS to ensure the safety of the child.

CLINICAL PEARLS AND PITFALLS

- Fractures are a common abusive injury and a common accidental injury in young children.
- Rib fractures and metaphyseal fractures have a high specificity for physical abuse.
- Occult injuries including additional fractures and TBI are common among young children presenting with abusive fracture(s).
- Physical abuse is the most common cause of multiple fractures in infants and young children, but underlying bone disorders may present with multiple fractures or bony lesions that may be mistaken for fractures.

Current Evidence

Fractures are one of the most common injuries for which victims of child abuse will present for medical care (Fig. 95.2). Approximately 1 in 5 children under the age of 12 months and 1 in 15 children 12 to 23 months old with a fracture will be diagnosed with physical abuse.

Clinical Considerations

Clinical Recognition

The age and developmental stage of the child as well as the location and type of fracture can help to distinguish abusive from accidental fractures. Abusive fractures most commonly are identified in young children, especially infants less than 12 months old, and are uncommon in children over 36 months. Rib fractures have one of the highest specificities for physical abuse, with 60% to 100% of non-MVC related, nonpathologic rib fractures attributed to abuse in children under the age of 36 months. Approximately half of femur fractures and 40% of humerus fractures in children less than 18 months are attributed to abuse while the vast majority of these fractures in children greater than 18 months are attributed to accidental trauma. Abuse is the most common etiology identified in children with classic metaphyseal fractures and in children presenting with multiple fracture sites. Children with genetic or metabolic bone disease can present with fractures and multiple fractures. Thus, history, physical, and radiologic images should always be reviewed for any signs of an underlying bone disease and if present, further evaluation and consultation with specialists should be considered (Table 95.3).

ABUSIVE HEAD TRAUMA

Goals of Treatment

Children presenting with AHT should be medically managed the same as children with accidental head injury with the recognition that the history provided can be false or incomplete and underestimate the severity of the injury. Once the patient is stabilized evaluation for retinal hemorrhages and evaluation for occult injuries including occult fractures should be performed (Table 95.4). As in all cases in which there is a reasonable suspicion for abuse, a report should be made to CPS to ensure the safety of the child.

CLINICAL PEARLS AND PITFALLS

- TBI is the leading cause of morbidity and mortality from physical abuse.
- AHT peaks at around age 8 to 12 weeks, and is most common in infants.
- Infants with AHT may present with nonspecific symptoms (i.e., fussiness, emesis) and no outward signs of trauma.
- Infants with AHT may not have any signs or symptoms of neurologic injury.
- Occult injuries, including fractures, are common among young children with AHT.

Current Evidence

AHT is the leading cause of morbidity and mortality from child physical abuse. Given the limitations of the history and physical examination in identifying AHT, the diagnosis can be easily missed resulting in children suffering complications from untreated injuries and being subjected to ongoing abuse. Among young infants with identified AHT, prior visits to medical providers with signs and symptoms of abusive injuries that were not recognized are common. Thus, clinicians should have a low index for suspicion when evaluating young infants with clinical symptoms that may be suggestive of head injury. Clinically occult AHT is common (as high as 30%) among neurologically asymptomatic infants presenting with noncranial abusive injuries such as multiple fractures or facial bruising. Thus, evaluation for occult AHT may be indicated in children with suspected abusive injuries depending on the child's age and presenting injuries (Table 95.4).

Clinical Considerations

Clinical Recognition

The majority of victims of AHT are less than 1 year old but toddlers and older children may sustain AHT. The clinical presentations of cases of AHT vary widely; some children present with obvious physical examination findings of head trauma and severe neurologic manifestations including seizures, coma, and apnea while other children may present with only nonspecific symptoms such as emesis or fussiness and no external signs of trauma. Rarely a history of inflicted trauma is provided; in most cases a history of accidental trauma or no history of trauma is provided. Although rare, severe and even fatal head injuries can occur from accidental household trauma and should be distinguished from AHT. The age, developmental stage of the child, presenting history, as well as the type and pattern of TBI and presence or absence of associated injuries such as noncranial fractures and retinal hemorrhages can help to distinguish AHT from accidental head trauma.

All infants and children with suspected AHT should have neuroimaging with a CT and/or MRI (Fig. 95.3). CT may be more readily available than MRI and is sensitive in identifying

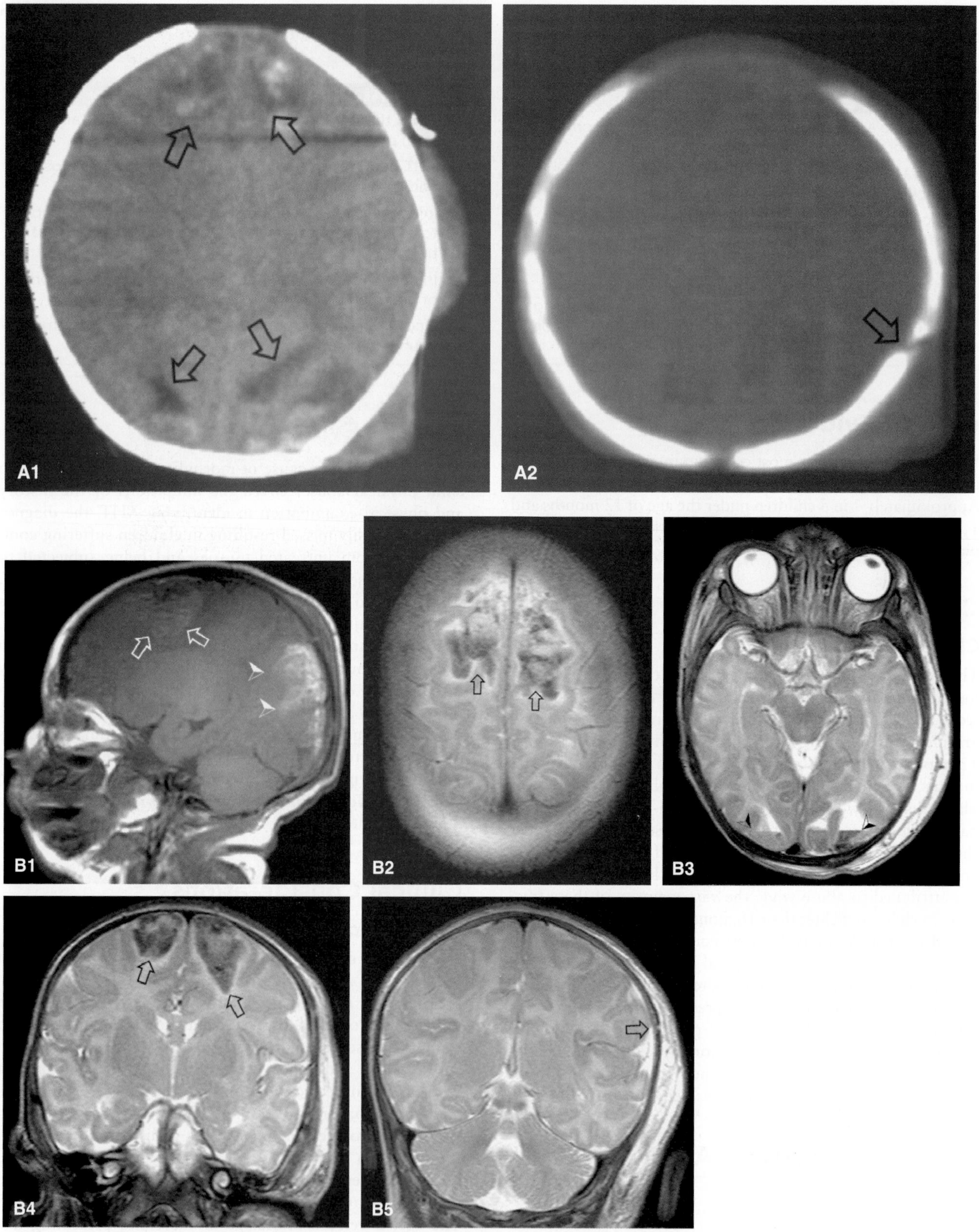

FIGURE 95.3 Radiographic Imaging of Abusive Head Trauma. **A:** Six-week-old infant examined by computed tomography (CT) without contrast. **A1:** Axial CT shows focal areas of increased and decreased density in the anterior and posterior parasagittal regions (*arrows*). Scalp swelling is present on the left. **A2:** Axial bone window shows fracture of the right parietal bone (*arrow*). **B:** Six-week-old infant examined by magnetic resonance imaging (MRI) studies. Same patient as A1. **B1:** Sagittal T1WI shows both an older clot with methemoglobin as high signal intensity in the parieto-occipital region (*arrowheads*) and a more recent clot as deoxyhemoglobin in the frontal region (*arrows*). **B2:** Axial T2WI shows the frontal parasagittal hemorrhagic areas of injury (*arrows*). **B3:** Axial T2WI shows the posterior, parieto-occipital older areas of injury as areas of bleeding with blood fluid levels (*arrowheads*). **B4:** Coronal T2WI through the frontal region shows bilateral parasagittal hemorrhagic changes (*arrows*). **B5:** Coronal T2WI at the site of fracture (*arrow*) shows overlying scalp swelling and bleeding.

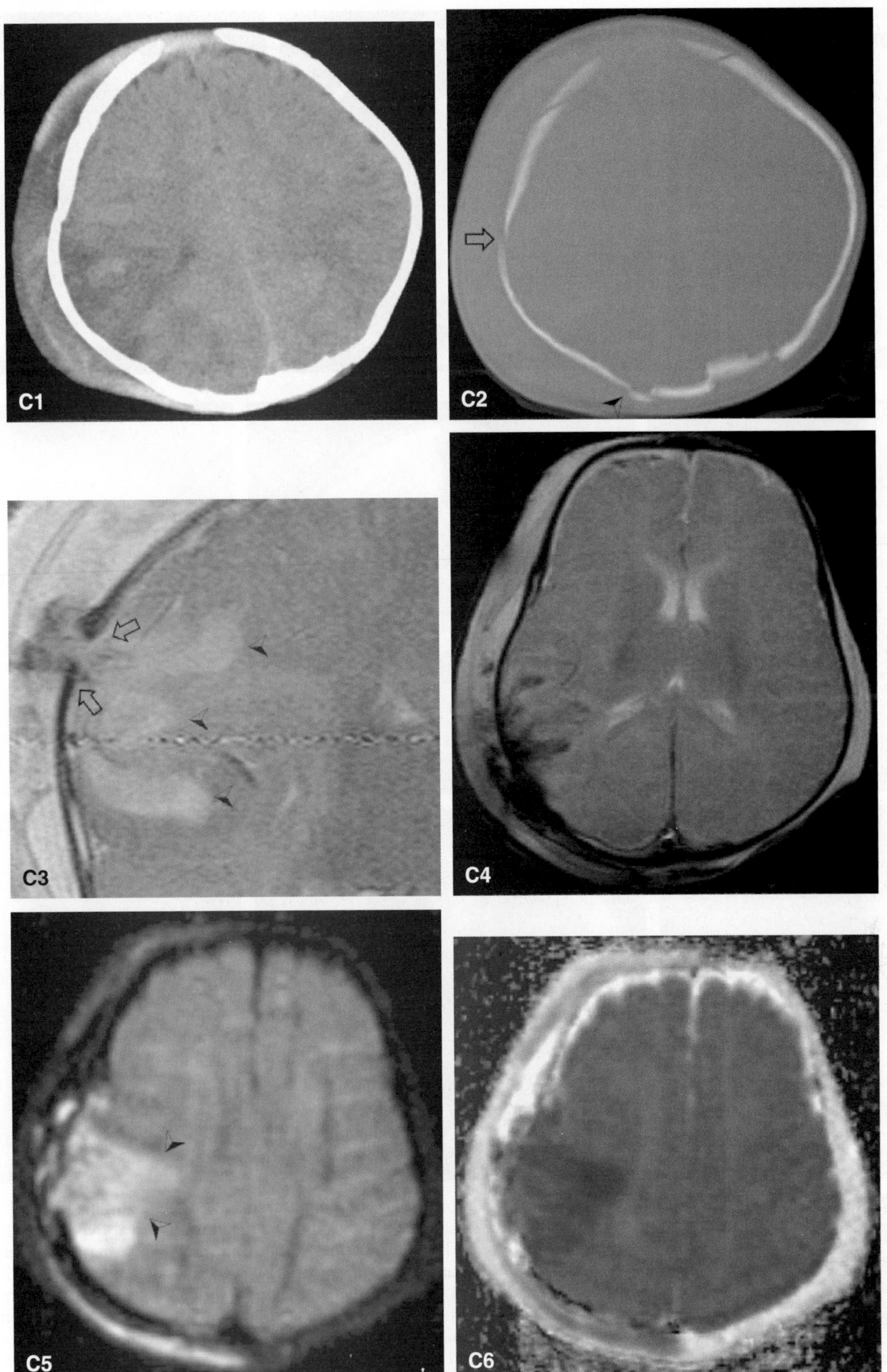

FIGURE 95.3 (*Continued*) **C:** Five-month-old male infant examined by CT and MRI on the day of admission. Parts C1 and C2, axial CTs without contrast; parts C3 to C6, MRI images. **C1:** Axial CT, brain windows, shows hemorrhage within the soft tissues of the scalp; underlying hypodensity and hyperdensity within the brain in the right parietal region consistent with contusional change. **C2:** Axial bone window at the same level as C1 shows a fracture of the right parietal bone (*arrow*) and an additional area of fracture posteriorly at the lambdoid suture (*arrowhead*). **C3:** Coronal T2WI demonstrates separation of the bone at the site of fracture (*arrow*) and underlying brain swelling involving the cortex, consistent with contusion (*arrowheads*). Abnormality is present at the site of the fracture in the extracalvarial soft tissues, consistent with hemorrhage and/or herniation of brain tissue through the fracture. **C4:** Axial two-dimensional FLASH susceptibility gradient echo scan demonstrates extensive intraparenchymal and soft-tissue scalp areas of signal loss consistent with bleeding. **C5:** Axial diffusion imaging through the site of contusion shows restricted motion of water consistent with cytotoxic edema (*arrowheads*). **C6:** Axial apparent diffusion coefficient (ADC) map at the site of the restricted motion of water shows hypointensity consistent with cytotoxic edema. (*continued*)

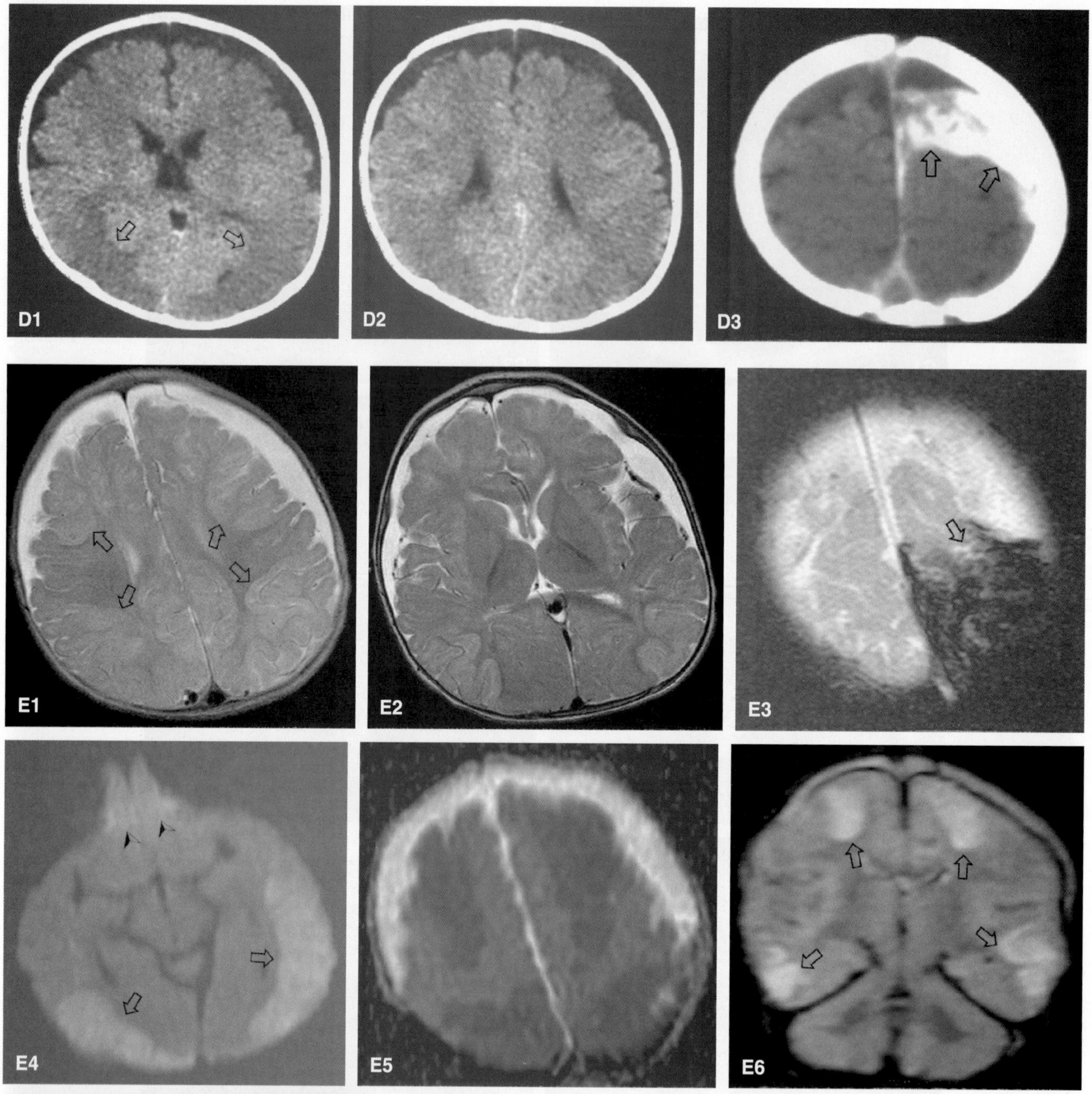

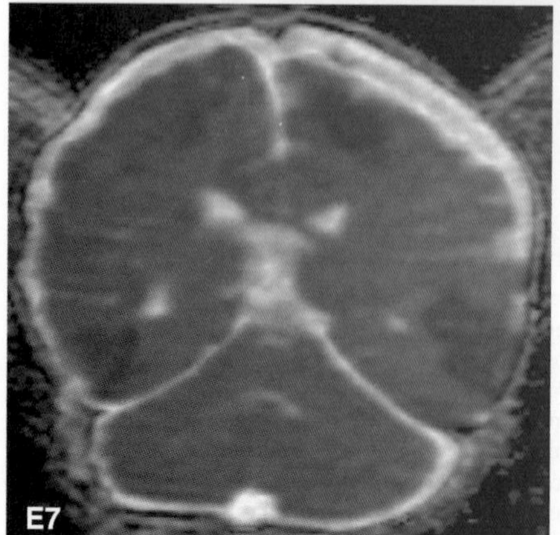

FIGURE 95.3 (*Continued*) **D:** Four-month-old male infant examined by CT on the day of presentation (noncontrast study). **D1:** Axial image shows bilateral hypodense fluid collection surrounding the frontal lobes. The temporo-occipital gray–white matter shows loss of definition bilaterally (*arrows*) consistent with injury. **D2:** Axial CT at a higher level in the brain shows the same findings as in A. **D3:** Still higher axial CT shows extensive subdural hemorrhage on the left side covering the frontal lobe (*arrows*) and extending into the midline along the falx cerebri. **E:** Four-month-old male infant (same as D) examined on the day of presentation. **E1:** Axial T2WI shows bilateral subdural fluid collection surrounding the frontal lobes. There is abnormal subtle increased T2 signal intensity in the cortex both anteriorly and posteriorly within the brain (*arrows*). There is sparing of the rolandic region. **E2:** Axial T2WI at a lower level shows the same findings. **E3:** Axial T2WI gradient echo susceptibility scan shows extensive area of hemorrhage in the subdural space overlying the left parietal region (*arrow*). **E4:** Axial diffusion weighted image shows bilateral temporo-occipital areas of restricted diffusion consistent with cytotoxic edema (*arrows*). Note anteriorly in the region of the gyrus rectus that there is also bilateral cytotoxic edema (*arrowheads*). **E5:** Axial ADC map at a higher level in the brain shows the hypointense signal in the bilateral parasagittal watershed region frontally, consistent with cytotoxic edema, as well as posteriorly in the bilateral parietal region. **E6:** Coronal diffusion weighted image shows bilateral parasagittal posterior frontal areas of cytotoxic edema and bilateral temporal watershed areas (*arrows*). **E7:** Coronal ADC map of these injuries shows hypointense signal at the site of cytotoxic edema. (All images courtesy of Robert A. Zimmerman, MD.)

scalp swelling, skull fractures, and acute hemorrhage. MRI is the preferred modality for assessing cerebral hypoxia and ischemia and can provide detailed information about subtle or old injuries. Thus, MRI is recommended for evaluation of intracranial injury in neurologically asymptomatic infants presenting with noncranial injuries. MRI should also be performed in children with abnormal CT findings. Imaging in victims of AHT may reveal scalp swelling, skull fracture, subdural hemorrhage, subarachnoid hemorrhage, parenchymal hemorrhage and contusions, cerebral hypoxia, ischemia, or diffuse axonal injury. Epidural hemorrhages and isolated skull fractures without associated intracranial hemorrhage can be seen in cases of abuse but are more common in accidental injuries. All infants and children with suspected AHT should undergo a fundoscopic examination but this does not have to occur in the emergency department setting. Retinal hemorrhages are common in cases of AHT. Retinal hemorrhages can also be seen in cases of accidental head trauma but are uncommon. The severity and pattern of retinal hemorrhages can help to distinguish cases of AHT from accidental head trauma.

Evaluation for underlying medical diseases including coagulopathies and metabolic disorders such as Glutaric Aciduria type 1 that may increase a child's risk of intracranial bleeding should be considered, especially in children presenting with isolated intracranial hemorrhage and no additional injuries.

ABUSIVE ABDOMINAL TRAUMA

Goals of Treatment

Severe and life-threatening intra-abdominal injuries to solid organs and hollow viscous organs, can occur in cases of physical abuse and should be medically managed the same as similar accidental injuries. Once the patient is medically stable a thorough evaluation including radiologic testing for occult injuries is indicated in order to allow for identification of occult injuries (Table 95.4). Victims of abuse may have clinically occult intra-abdominal injuries; thus evaluation for abdominal trauma should be performed in children presenting with nonabdominal injuries suspicious for abuse. In all cases in which there is a reasonable suspicion for abuse, a report should be made to CPS to ensure the safety of the child.

CLINICAL PEARLS AND PITFALLS

- Abdominal trauma is the second leading cause of mortality in victims of physical abuse.
- Children may sustain serious internal abdominal injuries without abdominal wall bruising or other external signs of injury.

Current Evidence

Abdominal trauma is an uncommon form of child physical abuse but is associated with a high mortality rate; thus prompt identification and treatment is important. Liver and splenic injuries are most common but pancreatic, renal, duodenal/jejunal, adrenal, mesenteric, and vascular injuries can also occur. Diagnosing abusive abdominal trauma in the ED can be challenging due to its rarity. In addition the presence of a misleading history and lack of external abdominal bruising in many cases, can add to the challenge in making a timely diagnosis.

Clinical Considerations

Children with abusive abdominal trauma are typically older than children with AHT and abusive fractures, with a mean age of 2 to 4 years, but tend to be younger than victims of accidental abdominal trauma. Children with abdominal injuries from abuse may present with a misleading history of accidental trauma or may present with no history of trauma and have nonspecific symptoms such as emesis, lethargy, or shock. Physical examination reveals abdominal bruising in less than 50% of cases. Abdominal tenderness and peritoneal signs may or may not be present. Elevated liver and pancreatic enzymes can be useful in identifying children with abdominal trauma and should be performed in cases of suspected acute physical abuse even in the absence of findings on examination suggestive of abdominal injury. Abdominal imaging with intravenous contrast-enhancing CT scan should be performed if abusive abdominal trauma is suspected based on history, physical examination, or screening laboratory studies.

Hollow viscous injuries are identified more frequently in victims of abuse than in children with accidental trauma, but solid organ injuries are the most commonly seen injury in both victims of abuse and accidental injury. The presence of both solid organ injury and hollow viscous injury is rare in accidental trauma and should raise consideration for abuse.

Suggested Readings and Key References

General Physical Abuse/Assault

American College of Radiology. ACR-SPR practice parameter for skeletal surveys in children. "Diagnostic Radiology" Radiography Practice Parameters and Technical Standards. Res. 54-2011, Amended 2014. Available at: http://www.acr.org/~/media/ACR/Documents/PGTS/guidelines/Skeletal_Surveys.pdf. Accessed 8/4/2015.

Christian CW, Committee On Child A, Neglect. The evaluation of suspected child physical abuse. *Pediatrics* 2015;135:e1337–e1354.

Duffy SO, Squires J, Fromkin JB, et al. Use of skeletal surveys to evaluate for physical abuse: analysis of 703 consecutive skeletal surveys. *Pediatrics* 2011;127(1):e47–e52.

Flaherty EG, Thompson R, Litrownik AJ, et al. Effect of early childhood adversity on child health. *Arch Pediatr Adolesc Med* 2006; 160(12):1232–1238.

Section on Radiology, American Academy of Pediatrics. Diagnostic imaging of child abuse. *Pediatrics* 2009;123(5):1430–1435.

Sheets LK, Leach ME, Koszewski IJ, et al. Sentinel injuries in infants evaluated for child physical abuse. *Pediatrics* 2013;131(4):701–707.

U.S. Department of Health and Human Services. Administration for children and families, administration on children, youth and families, children's bureau. *Child Maltreatment* 2011. 2012; http://www.acf.hhs.gov/programs/cb/research-data-technology/statistics-research/child-maltreatment. Accessed 8/26/13.

Abusive Cutaneous Injuries

Feldman KW. The bruised premobile infant: should you evaluate further? *Pediatr Emerg Care* 2009;25(1):37–39.

Greenbaum AR, Donne J, Wilson D, et al. Intentional burn injury: an evidence-based, clinical and forensic review. *Burns* 2004;30(7):628–642.

Kemp AM, Maguire SA, Nuttall D, et al. Bruising in children who are assessed for suspected physical abuse. *Arch Dis Child* 2014;99(2): 108–113.

Maguire S, Mann M. Systematic reviews of bruising in relation to child abuse—what have we learnt: an overview of review updates. *Evid Based Child Health* 2013;8(2):255–263.

Pierce MC, Kaczor K, Aldridge S, et al. Bruising characteristics discriminating physical child abuse from accidental trauma. *Pediatrics* 2010;125(1):67–74.

Sugar NF, Taylor JA, Feldman KW. Bruises in infants and toddlers: those who don't cruise rarely bruise. Puget sound pediatric research network. *Arch Pediatr Adolesc Med* 1999;153(4):399–403.

Abusive Oropharyngeal Injuries

Kellogg N, American Academy of Pediatrics Committee on Child Abuse and Neglect. Oral and dental aspects of child abuse and neglect. *Pediatrics* 2005;116(6):1565–1568.

Abusive Fractures

Leventhal JM, Martin KD, Asnes AG. Incidence of fractures attributable to abuse in young hospitalized children: results from analysis of a United States database. *Pediatrics* 2008;122(3):599–604.

Maguire S, Cowley L, Mann M, et al. What does the recent literature add to the identification and investigation of fractures in child abuse: an overview of review updates 2005–2013. *Evidence-Based Child Health: A Cochrane Review Journal* 2013;8(5):2044–2057.

Ravichandiran N, Schuh S, Bejuk M, et al. Delayed identification of pediatric abuse-related fractures. *Pediatrics* 2010;125(1):60–66.

Taitz J, Moran K, O'Meara M. Long bone fractures in children under 3 years of age: is abuse being missed in Emergency Department presentations? *J Paediatr Child Health* 2004;40(4):170–174.

Wood JN, Fakeye O, Mondestin V, et al. Prevalence of abuse among young children with femur fractures: a systematic review. *BMC Pediatr* 2014;14:169.

Abusive Head Trauma

Christian CW, Block R. Committee on Child Abuse and Neglect; American Academy of Pediatrics.Abusive head trauma in infants and children. *Pediatrics* 2009;123(5):1409–1411.

Jenny C, Hymel KP, Ritzen A, et al. Analysis of missed cases of abusive head trauma. *JAMA* 1999;281(7):621–626.

Maguire SA, Kemp AM, Lumb RC, et al. Estimating the probability of abusive head trauma: a pooled analysis. *Pediatrics* 2011;128(3):e550–e564.

Maguire SA, Watts PO, Shaw AD, et al. Retinal hemorrhages and related findings in abusive and non-abusive head trauma: a systematic review. *Eye (Lond)* 2013;27(1):28–36.

Rubin DM, Christian CW, Bilaniuk LT, et al. Occult head injury in high-risk abused children. *Pediatrics* 2003;111(6):1382–1386.

Abusive Abdominal Trauma

Lindberg D, Makoroff K, Harper N, et al. Utility of hepatic transaminases to recognize abuse in children. *Pediatrics* 2009;124(2):509–516.

Maguire SA, Upadhyaya M, Evans A, et al. A systematic review of abusive visceral injuries in childhood—their range and recognition. *Child Abuse Negl* 2013;37(7):430–435.

Trokel M, DiScala C, Terrin NC, et al. Blunt abdominal injury in the young pediatric patient: child abuse and patient outcomes. *Child Maltreat* 2004;9(1):111–117.

Wood J, Rubin DM, Nance ML, et al. Distinguishing inflicted versus accidental abdominal injuries in young children. *J Trauma* 2005;59(5):1203–1208.

CHAPTER 96 ■ DERMATOLOGIC URGENCIES AND EMERGENCIES

LESLIE CASTELO-SOCCIO, MD, PhD

GOALS OF EMERGENCY CARE

The goals in treating dermatologic conditions are to recognize signs of systemic illness and complications such as secondary infection.

KEY POINTS

- The ability to describe a rash precisely and accurately will dramatically improve the likelihood of a correct diagnosis.
- Key features of the history include duration of the rash (acute or chronic), initial distribution, extent of spread (generalized or localized), ill contacts (including sexual partners), and any associated systemic symptoms, including fever.
- Key features of the physical examination include a careful systematic inspection of all mucocutaneous surfaces, with special attention paid to involvement of the oropharynx, palms and soles, extensor or flexor surfaces, scalp, and trunk.

RELATED CHAPTERS

Signs and Symptoms

- Rashes: Chapters 61 to 65

Medical, Surgical, and Trauma Emergencies

- Infectious Disease Emergencies: Chapter 102
- Rheumatologic Emergencies: Chapter 109

Clinicians are often confronted with a skin rash or skin lesion. An accurate diagnosis depends on a systematic approach that requires assessing the skin carefully and knowing dermatology, terminology, morphology, and differential diagnoses. Although not always diagnostic, morphology and configuration of cutaneous lesions are important parts of categorizing and making a differential diagnosis. Terminology is an important part of this process. Descriptors can be divided into primary and secondary. Primary descriptors include macules (flat <10 mm), papules (raised <10 mm), patches (flat <10 mm), plaques (raised >10 mm), nodules (solid lesion 0.5 to 2 cm), pustules (elevation with white material), abscesses (elevated lesion >10 mm with purulent material), wheals (elevated lesion with local transient edema), vesicles (elevated lesion <10 mm containing fluid), and bullae (elevated lesion >10 mm containing fluid). Secondary descriptors include crust, scale, fissuring, erosions, ulceration, umbilication, excoriation, atrophy, lichenification, and scar. In addition to these descriptions it is also important to understand the distribution of the rash or lesion. Distribution characteristics include localized, blaschkoid (following lines of embryologic development), widespread, and photodistributed (predilection for sun-exposed areas). Characterizing a rash or lesion using these descriptors narrows the differential diagnosis significantly. The following sections of this chapter will divide skin changes by their primary descriptor and then will provide a framework for adding secondary characteristics to improve diagnosis.

PAPULES

Papules can be quite varied and the following algorithm is used to help practitioners diagnose varying papular lesions (Fig. 96.1).

Papules with a Characteristic Appearance

Many conditions can be diagnosed on sight. For example, the experienced eye can easily distinguish milia from molluscum contagiosum (MC) and warts from the uncommon xanthoma. Several clues make the process of separating these entities from one another easier such as color, distribution, and patient characteristics. Skin biopsy is a valuable tool available to the dermatologist and may be required to differentiate many of the entities discussed here.

Milia

Milia are 1- to 2-mm firm, white papules. They are produced by retention of keratinous and sebaceous material in follicular openings. Newborns often have milia on their face. They frequently disappear by the age of 1 month. Milia can also arise from skin trauma, and can be seen in scars after burns and in healed wounds in patients with blistering disorders like epidermolysis bullosa. Persistent milia may be a manifestation of the oral–facial–digital syndrome, hereditary hypotrichosis (Marie Unna type), and certain rare ectodermal dysplasias (Basan's syndrome). Because lesions that are not associated with syndromes disappear spontaneously, no therapy is indicated.

Molluscum Contagiosum

The lesion, produced by the common poxvirus, is a papule with a white center (Fig. 96.2). It occurs at any age during childhood. It is more common in swimmers and wrestlers. Patients with atopic eczema are especially susceptible. Most

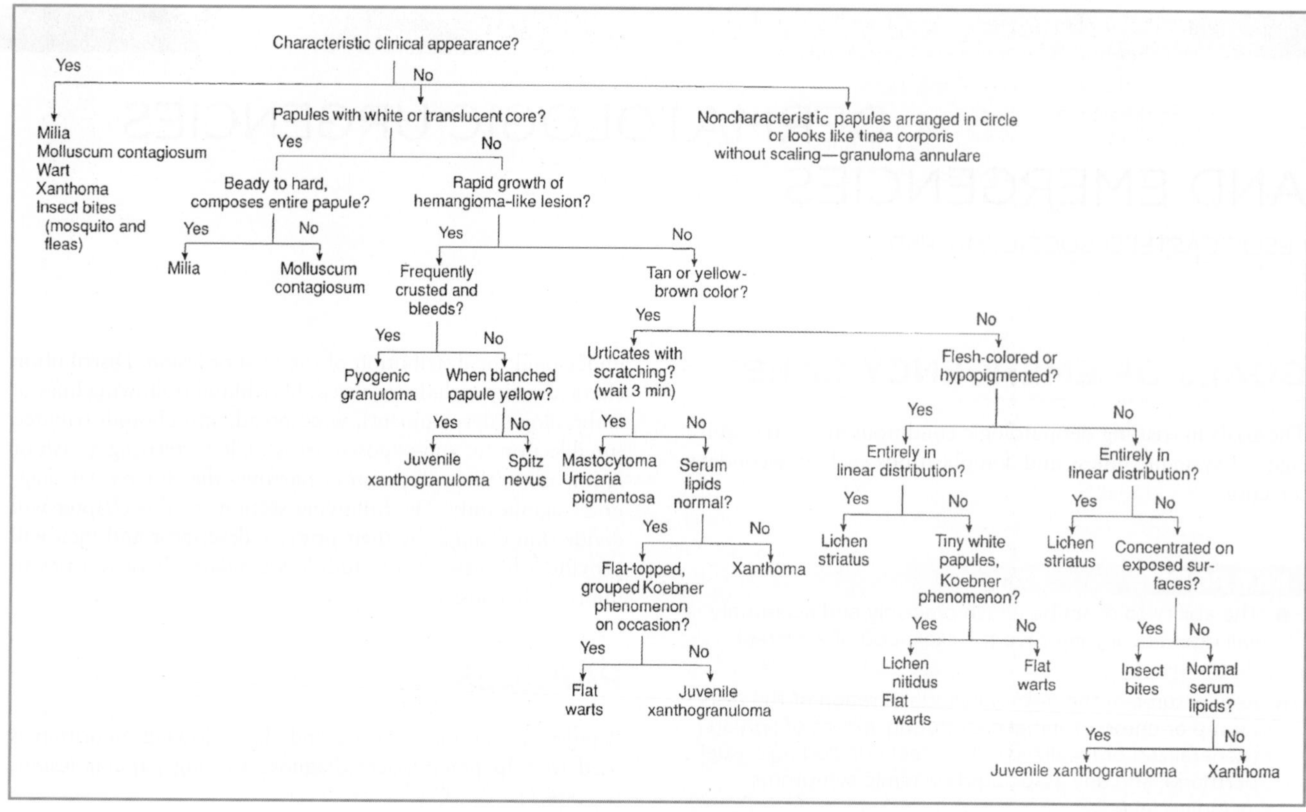

FIGURE 96.1 Approach to diagnosis of papular lesions.

lesions resolve in 6 to 9 months, but some may persist for more than 3 years. Spread is by autoinoculation.

Lesions can be single or numerous and favor intertriginous areas such as the groin. They are usually 2 to 5 mm in diameter, but several can coalesce and form a lesion 1.5 cm in diameter. They may become inflamed, which sometimes herald spontaneous disappearance. Often when inflamed they look "infected" but culture is usually negative. At times, an eczematous reaction occurs around some lesions.

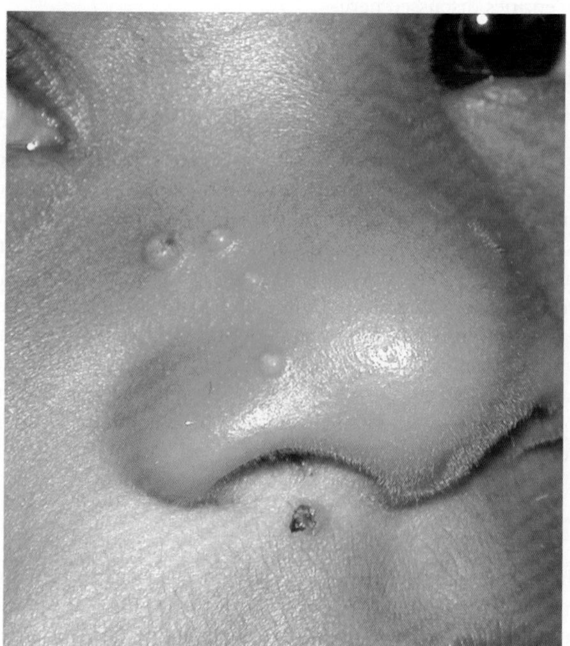

FIGURE 96.2 Child with lesion of molluscum.

Since spontaneous resolution is common, treatment, if elected, should be gentle. Removal of the white core will cure the lesion. This treatment can be performed by applying a local anesthetic cream (e.g., EMLA or LMX-4) under occlusion to the lesion 1 to 2 hours before treatment. This procedure will anesthetize the area and allow the physician to prick the skin open over the core with a 26-gauge needle, and squeeze the core out with a comedone extractor. Multiple light touches with liquid nitrogen can also be effective. With widespread lesions, nonpainful procedures are preferable as multiple painful treatments will cause great fear in the patient and make future visits to a physician difficult for the family. Application of 0.1% tretinoin cream one to two times daily may induce enough inflammation to hasten the host's immune response or cause extrusion of the central core but caution should be observed since tretinoin may exacerbate secondary eczematization around molluscum lesions. A dilute formulation of cantharidin, a natural toxin derived from the blister beetle, can be used successfully to treat molluscum. Cantharidin can be applied to individual molluscum lesions for 1 to 4 hours and then washed off. The medication is generally painless when applied but may result in subsequent blistering of treated areas and should be avoided on the face or genital areas.

Warts

Warts affect 7% to 10% of the population and are one of the most common dermatologic problems encountered in pediatrics. The peak incidence is during adolescence. Sixty-five percent of common warts disappear spontaneously within

2 years, and 40% of plantar warts disappear within 6 months in prepubertal children. However, immunosuppressed patients may experience extensive spread of the lesions.

The common wart resembles a tiny cauliflower. Lesions disrupt the natural skin lines and may also manifest with small black dots, representing thrombosed capillaries. The shape of the wart varies with its location on the skin. They may be long and slender (filiform) on the face and neck or flat (verruca plana) on the face, arms, and knees. When located on the soles, they are called *plantar warts,* and when in the anogenital area, they are referred to as *condyloma acuminata.*

The tendency for recurrence of warts makes the treatment of this condition frustrating. Because most warts disappear spontaneously with time, procedures that are least traumatic for the child should be attempted first. The simple, nontraumatic method of airtight occlusion with plain adhesive tape or duct tape for 1 month has been shown to be successful on many occasions. Topical application of 17% salicylic acid in flexible collodion (Duofilm) or duct/occlusive tape is good for home use. Plantar warts can be treated with 40% salicylic acid. When simple methods are unsuccessful, touching the warts with liquid nitrogen or volatile cryogens such as dimethyl ether, propane, or isobutane (Verruca Freeze) for 10 to 30 seconds or surgical removal can be attempted on a 2- to 4-week schedule until the lesions clear completely. Both procedures are painful.

Anogenital warts can be treated with topical preparations such as podophyllotoxin gel (Condylox) or imiquimod cream (Aldara). Podophyllotoxin gel is applied on the condylomata three consecutive nights each week while imiquimod is used every other night three times weekly. Both agents may be used for up to 3 months or so or until the warts clear. Topical cidofovir in 1% or 3% preparation can also be used for warts and molluscum. Child abuse should be considered in any child with genital warts but keep in mind that maternal transmission can occur during delivery.

Xanthomas

Papules, plaques, nodules, and tumors that contain lipid are called *xanthomas.* These lesions can appear on any skin surface and are often associated with disturbances of lipoprotein metabolism.

Insect Bites

Mosquitoes are probably the most common cause of insect bites in children, followed closely by fleas (Fig. 96.3) and bed bugs. Mosquito bites are generally limited to the warm months of the year. In contrast, fleabites, which predominate from spring to fall, can also occur during the winter months as a result of cats, dogs, and rodent who live indoors.

The distribution of lesions is a valuable clue in making the diagnosis of mosquito or fleabites. Insect bites generally involve the exposed surfaces of the head, face, and extremities. The lesions are usually urticarial wheals that occur in groups or along a line on which the insect was crawling. Some lesions may manifest a central punctum. On occasion, both mosquito bites and fleabites can cause blistering lesions. These lesions are not caused by secondary infection but rather by an immune response to the bite. Certainly, excoriation with resulting secondary infection with *Staphylococcus aureus* or *Group A streptococci* can complicate a simple bite.

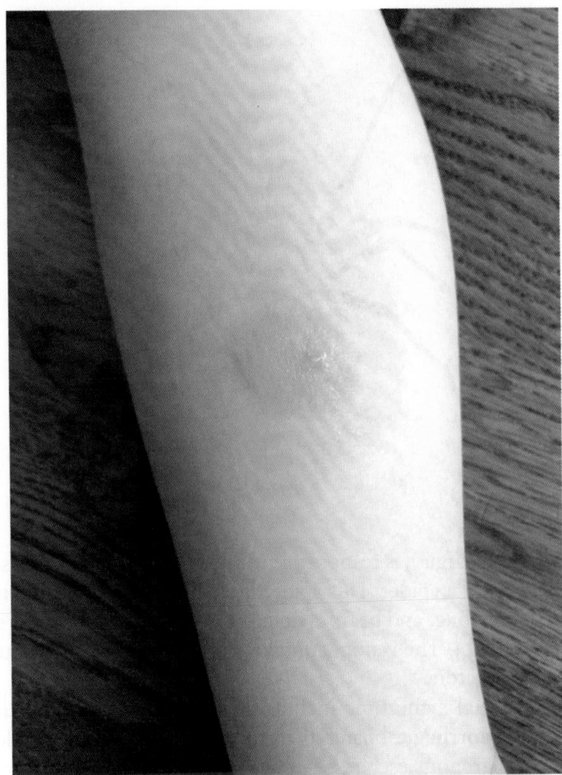

FIGURE 96.3 Insect bite in a child.

Unfortunately, no specific treatment exists for insect bites. Antihistamines, calamine lotion, or topical steroids have a limited or temporary effect. Prevention through the prophylactic use of insect repellents and protective clothing offers the best solution. Obviously, elimination of the biting insects by treatment of the homes with insecticides or treatment of the infested animals is important. For additional information about insect bites, see Chapter 62 Rash: Vesiculobullous.

Tick Bites

Tick bites usually cause only local reactions. Erythema migrans is the characteristic rash of Lyme disease and looks like large bull's eye; the rash does generally appear 7 to 10 days post tick exposure but the range is 3 to 30 days. Rarely, tick bites are associated with significant systemic illness, including Rocky Mountain spotted fever (RMSF), tick paralysis, and Lyme meningitis.

When ticks are removed, it is important not to leave fragments of the mouthparts in the skin or to introduce body fluids containing infectious organisms. Various methods have been recommended for removal of ticks from the skin. The safest method is to use a blunt-curved forceps, tweezers, or fingers protected by rubber gloves. The tick is grasped close to the skin surface and pulled upward with a steady even force. The tick should not be squeezed, crushed, or punctured. If mouthparts are left in the skin, they should be removed.

Spider Bites

Loxosceles reclusa, or the brown recluse spider (Fig. 96.4), found most commonly in the south central United States (from southeastern Nebraska through Texas, east through southern

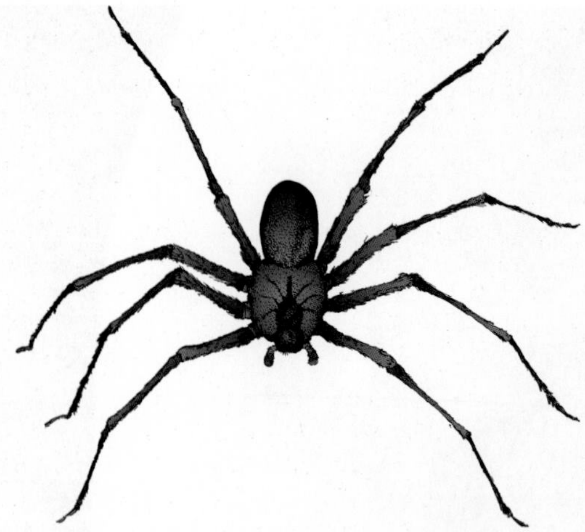

FIGURE 96.4 Spider recluse.

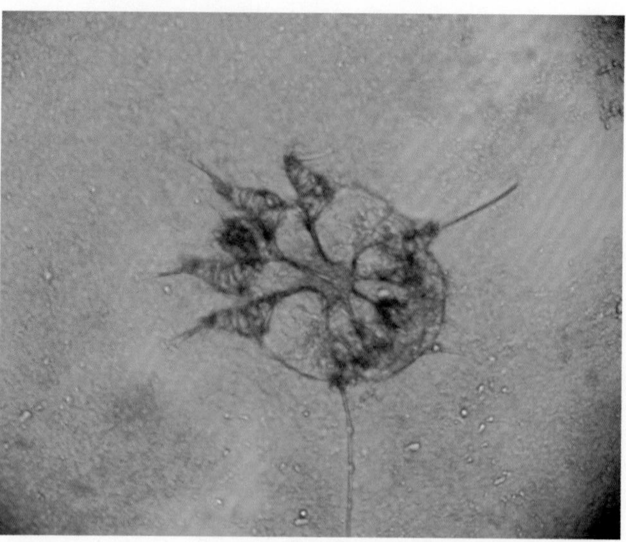

FIGURE 96.5 Scabies mite.

Ohio and Georgia), is responsible for most skin reactions caused by the bite of a spider. This spider is small, the body being only 8 to 10 mm long, and bears a violin-shaped band over the dorsal cephalothorax. The venom contains necrotizing, hemolytic, and spreading factors.

The initial symptoms include mild stinging and/or pruritus. A hemorrhagic blister then appears, which can develop into a gangrenous eschar. Severe bites can cause a generalized erythematous macular eruption, nausea, vomiting, chills, malaise, muscle aches, and hemolysis. Treatment includes tetanus prophylaxis, the use of dapsone in selected cases where there is apparent necrosis (but never in patients with G6PD deficiency), and surgical removal of the necrotic area to prevent spread of the toxin. Antibiotics are indicated if there are signs of secondary infection. Some authors recommend corticosteroids if the patient presents within 12 hours of a bite but the efficacy of this approach is unproven. An antivenom exists if there are systemic signs.

Scabies Infestation

Please see Chapter 62 Rash: Vesiculobullous for more details. The cardinal symptom of any infestation with scabies is pruritus. Two clues should be considered when attempting to make this diagnosis: (i) Distribution (red papules with concentration on the hands, feet, and folds of the body, especially the finger webs and genital areas) and (ii) involvement of other family members. It is important not only to ask other family members if they have pruritus but also to examine their skin. In contrast to adults, infants may develop blisters and exhibit lesions on the head and face.

The diagnosis is made by scraping involved skin and looking for mites under the 10× microscope objective (Fig. 96.5). Once an infestation occurs, it usually takes 1 month for sensitization and pruritus to develop.

Louse Infestation

Three forms of lice infest humans: (i) The head louse, (ii) the body louse, and (iii) the pubic or crab louse (Fig. 96.6). The major louse infestation in children involves the scalp and causes pruritus. The female attaches her eggs to the hair shaft. The egg then hatches, leaving behind numerous nits that

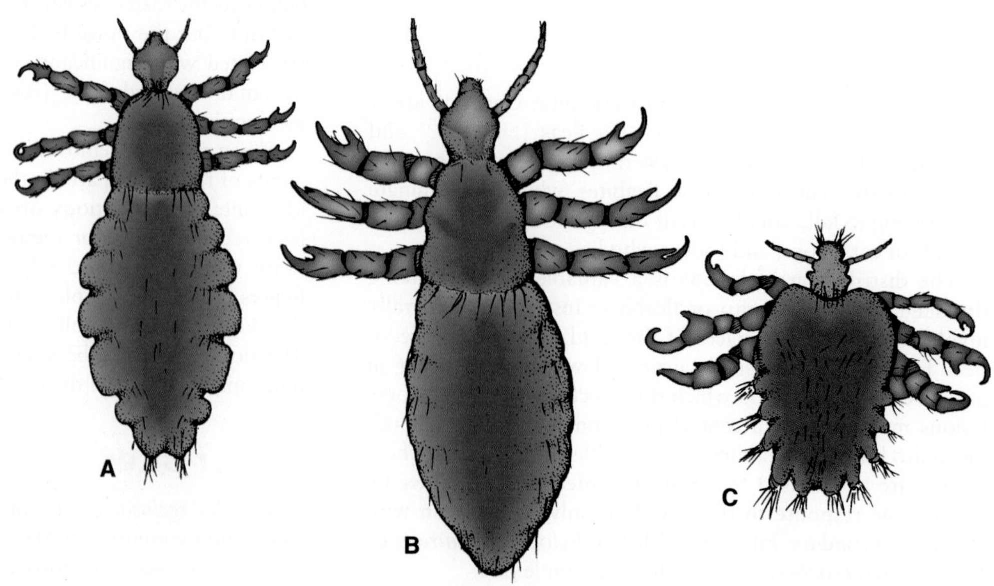

FIGURE 96.6 Louse.

resemble dandruff. Secondary infection can occur from vigorous scratching. Body lice generally reside in the seams of clothing and lay their eggs there. They go to the body to feed, particularly the interscapular, shoulder, and waist areas. Red pruritic puncta that become papular and wheal-like then occur. Pubic lice occur in the genital area, lower abdomen, axillae, and eyelashes. Transmission is usually venereal. Blue macules (maculae caeruleae) that are 3 to 15 mm in diameter can be seen on the thighs, abdomen, or thorax of infested persons. These macules are secondary to bites.

Because the body louse resides in clothing, therapy consists mainly of disinfecting the clothing with steam under pressure. Pediculosis capitis is usually effectively treated with 1% permethrin or pyrethrin creme rinse though resistance to this medication is not uncommon. The patient's hair should be shampooed, rinsed, and toweled dry. Enough medication to saturate the hair and scalp is applied. The medication is washed out after 10 minutes. Additionally benzyl alcohol–containing products (Ulesfia) and topical ivermectin (SKLICE) products can also be used. Patients with resistant disease may also respond to topical petrolatum applied to hair and scalp nightly for 1 week as a lice suffocant or trimethoprim-sulfamethoxazole given orally for 5 to 7 days, which kills the symbiotic parasite present in the GI tract of head lice. Pediculosis pubis is best treated with the same permethrin or pyrethrin preparations used for head lice. Any nits are removed with a fine-toothed comb. The safest treatment for lice in the eyelashes is the application of Vaseline twice daily for 8 days. The lice stick to the Vaseline, cannot feed, and die. Another treatment alternative is physostigmine ophthalmic ointment, although it may carry more significant toxicity.

Vascular Papules and Nodules

Vascular papules and nodules can be congenital or acquired. Those in infants generally fall in the category of benign with hemangiomas being most common. Other vascular nodules including kaposiform hemangioendotheliomas and sarcomas should be considered for vascular papules or nodules that feel firm or do not follow the natural history of infantile or congenital hemangiomas. See further discussion in Chapter 64 Rash: Neonatal. Acquired lesions include Spitz nevi and pyogenic granulomas.

Spitz nevus. Spitz nevi appear suddenly between 2 and 13 years of age. Preferred sites of growth include the cheek (15%), shoulder, and upper extremities (Fig. 96.7). The lesion has a pink to red surface because of numerous dilated blood vessels. Pressure produces blanching of this pink to red color. The lesions can reach a size of 1.5 cm in diameter but are completely benign. Pigmented Spitz nevi, another variant of Spitz nevi, often appear black in the skin rather than pink-red, and their appearance is often worrisome for malignant melanoma. Because the histologic appearance of these lesions can be confused easily with a malignant melanoma, an experienced histopathologist should interpret the findings. Most clinicians still recommend that Spitz nevi be removed surgically.

Pyogenic granulomas. Pyogenic granulomas (Fig. 96.8) are bright red to reddish-brown or blue-black pedunculated, vascular papules/nodules ranging from 0.5 to 2 cm in size that develop rapidly at the site of an injury, such as a cut, scratch, insect bite, or burn. Pyogenic granulomas occur commonly in children and young adults, usually on the fingers, face, hands, and forearms.

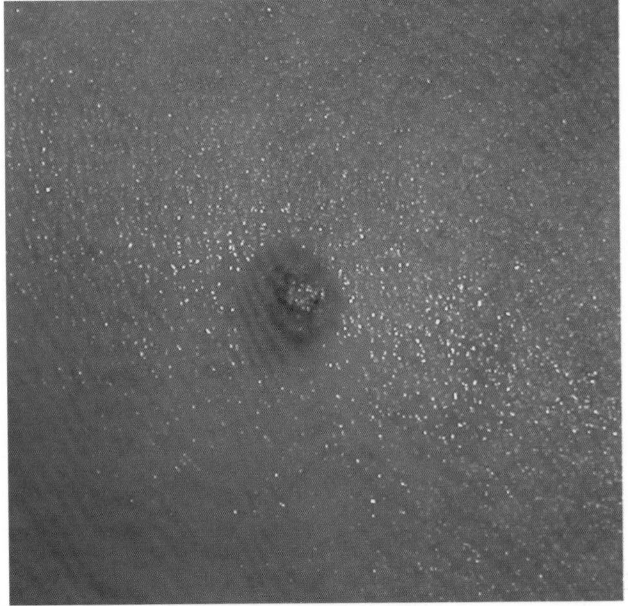

FIGURE 96.7 Spitz nevus.

They bleed easily. Generally, they are asymptomatic. Because spontaneous disappearance is rare, the lesions must be removed by curettage, excision, electrosurgery, cryosurgery, laser surgery, or some combination of these various modalities. Management of acute bleeding may include chemical (e.g., aluminum chloride or silver nitrate though silver nitrate can leave a tattoo) or electrical cautery, placement of constrictive sutures, or full-thickness excision and suturing.

Yellow, Tan, or Brown Papules

Many papules are yellow tan or brown. The yellow, tan, and brown papules include the lesions seen in urticaria pigmentosa (see Chapter 64 Rash: Neonatal), flat warts, xanthomas, insect bites, juvenile xanthogranulomas as well as melanocytic nevi.

One way to differentiate the various papules from one another is to scratch them. If hiving of a scratched lesion (Darier

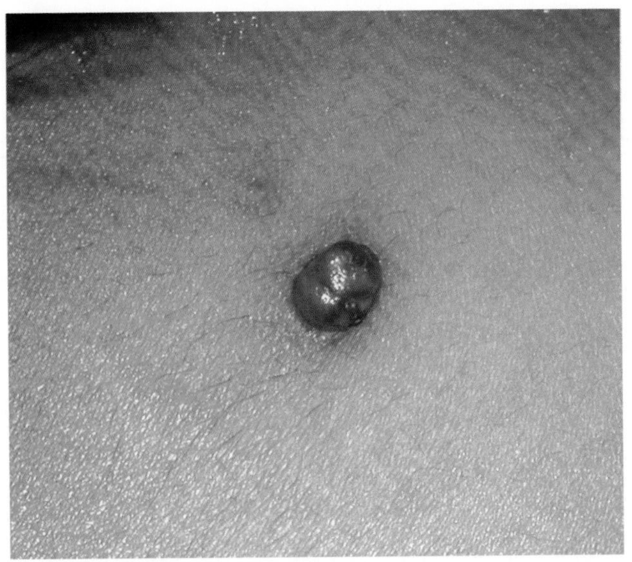

FIGURE 96.8 Pyogenic granuloma.

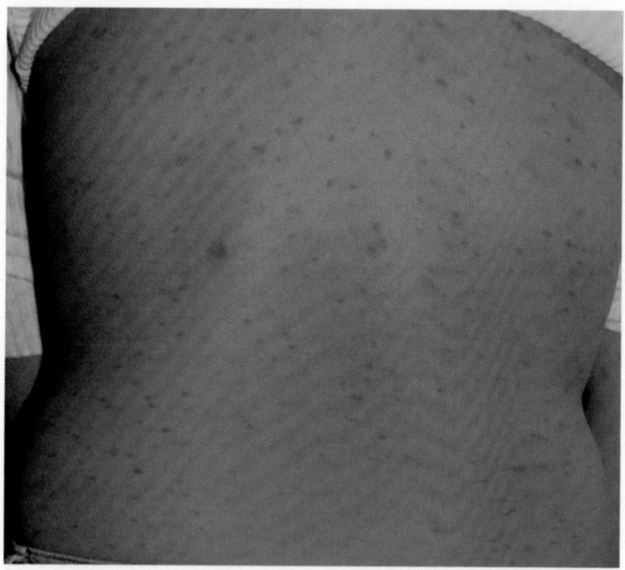

FIGURE 96.9 Urticaria pigmentosa with Darier sign.

sign) occurs within a short period of time (3 to 5 minutes), the lesion contains mast cells (i.e., a mastocytoma or urticaria pigmentosa) (Fig. 96.9). Make sure to scratch normal skin to rule out the presence of dermatographism. The latter condition will produce a false-positive Darier sign. When no urtication occurs, a biopsy may be helpful. Flat warts tend to be grouped, are flat topped, and can be autoinoculated in scratch lines (pseudo-Koebner phenomenon). Lesions characteristic for JXGs are not flat topped, tend to be singular in number (or when multiple are scattered about), and do not demonstrate the Koebner phenomenon (recapitulation of the eruption in traumatized areas) (Fig. 96.10). JXG lesions may also look like xanthomas. Unlike xanthomas, however, abnormal lipid levels do not occur with JXGs.

Mastocytoma, Urticaria Pigmentosa

These are red/brown papules that urticate. For additional information please see Chapter 64 Rash: Neonatal.

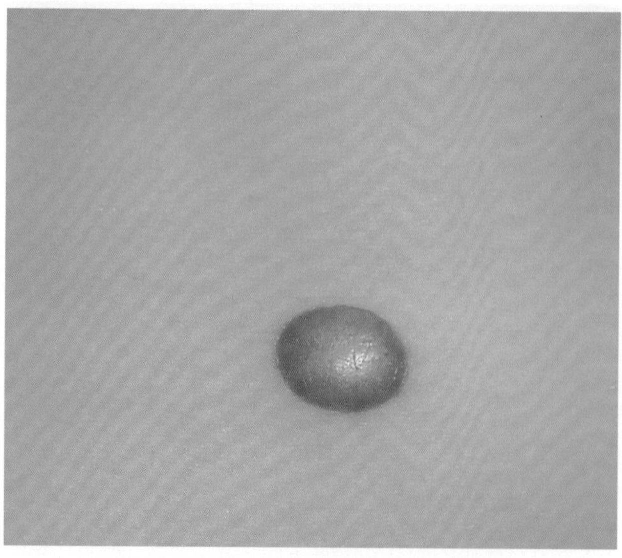

FIGURE 96.10 Juvenile xanthogranuloma (JXG).

Juvenile Xanthogranulomas

Juvenile xanthogranuloma. JXGs can be confused with urticaria pigmentosa or xanthomas. Numerous yellow or reddish-brown papules appear on the face and upper trunk in the first year of life. The number of lesions may increase until the child is 18 months to 2 years of age. Serum lipid levels are normal, and the Darier sign (urtication after scratching) is negative. The lesions often disappear spontaneously after 2 years of age; therefore, intervention is generally unnecessary. When JXGs are multiple, particularly on the head and neck, evaluation of the eyes for intraocular JXGs is recommended because of their potential for visual impairment. The presence of JXGs in a young child with neurofibromatosis (type 1) has been a marker associated with an increased risk of juvenile myelomonocytic leukemia.

Flesh-colored Papules

Many entities may present as flesh-colored papules. Here we will highlight lichen striatus and lichen nitidus. When the papules are arranged linearly, streaming down an extremity or across the face or neck, lichen striatus should be considered. If the papules are not arranged linearly but are tiny pinpoint, flesh-colored papules, lichen nitidus should be considered, especially if a Koebner phenomenon is present. Flat warts may be flesh colored as well.

Lichen Striatus

Lichen striatus is an asymptomatic eruption of unknown cause. The flat-topped papules are arranged linearly and may be confluent. Lesions may occur in a wide band but remain characteristically linear or more accurately curvilinear patterns corresponding to lines of Blaschko. The lesions are flesh colored to erythematous in Caucasians and hypopigmented in African Americans. The eruption follows the long axis of an extremity (Fig. 96.11) or may involve any other part of the skin surface (especially the face). Because the eruption resolves spontaneously within 2 years, no treatment is necessary.

Lichen Nitidus

Lichen nitidus is characterized by tiny, pinpoint, flat-topped, flesh-colored papules (Fig. 96.12). The papules are often grouped and are found in scratch lines (i.e., the Koebner phenomenon). Although any skin surface may be involved, the trunk and genitalia are common sites. The lesions are often asymptomatic but may occasionally itch. The lesions persist for variable periods and generally do not respond to therapy.

If this algorithm for papules has not helped in making a diagnosis, a consultant should be called. Many entities can be difficult to differentiate.

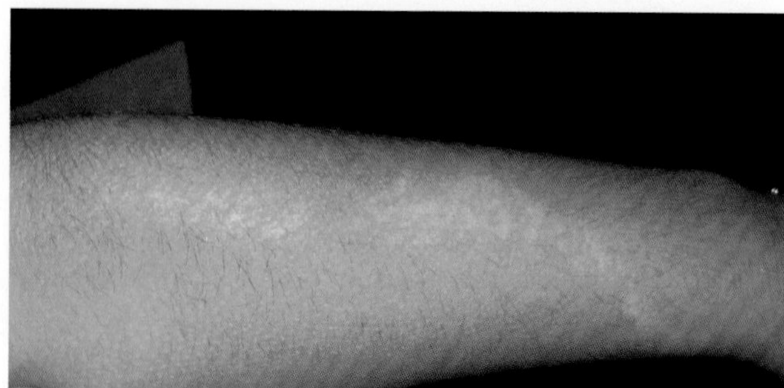

FIGURE 96.11 Lichen striatus.

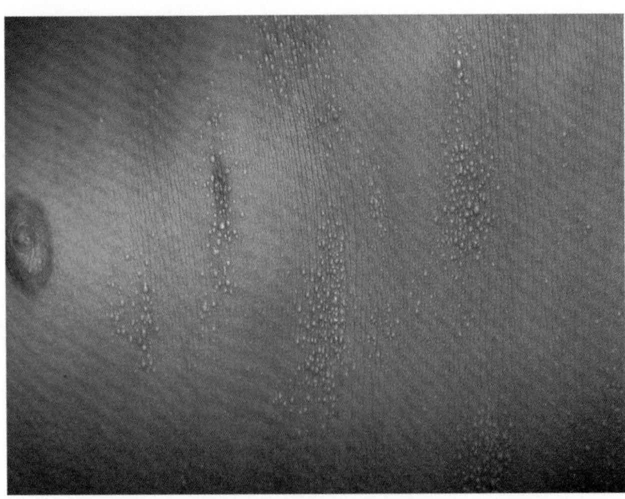

FIGURE 96.12 Lichen nitidus.

PLAQUES

Annular Plaques

Granuloma Annulare

Granuloma annulare is believed to be an idiosyncratic response to trauma and looks to many like tinea corporis ("ringworm") without the scale. This skin change may begin as a flesh-colored or violaceous papule that clears centrally as the margins advance, or it may appear as a group of papules arranged in a ring-like configuration (Fig. 96.13). The central portion of the lesion is often dusky or hyperpigmented. The key point on physical examination is the lack of scaling. This physical finding distinguishes granuloma annulare from tinea corporis and cannot be stressed enough. The border is firm on palpation, unlike tinea corporis. The rings can be 5 cm in diameter or larger.

A potassium hydroxide test would be definitive in ruling out tinea corporis. It would be difficult to obtain scales from a granuloma annulare lesion using this procedure. It is important to diagnose this entity correctly because one can reassure parents that three-fourths of lesions clear spontaneously within a 2-year period. Recurrences are common until children outgrow this tendency.

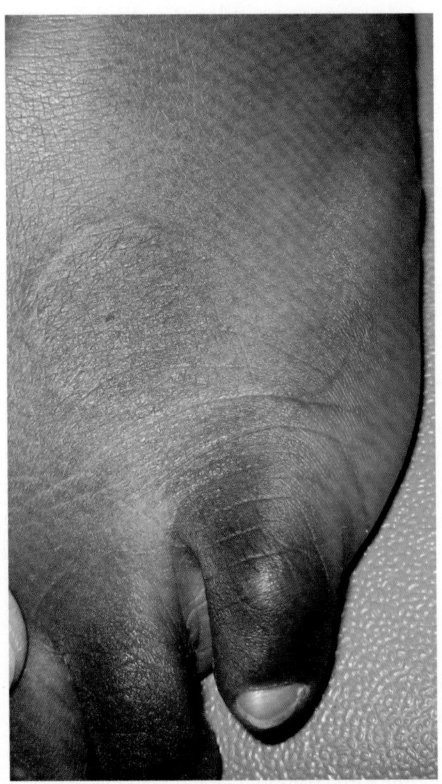

FIGURE 96.13 Granuloma annulare.

Lupus

Neonatal lupus and systemic lupus can sometimes be composed of annular plaques. Lupus has a varied appearance depending on type and whether it is skin limited or systemic. For more discussion please see Chapter 64 Rash: Neonatal for discussion of neonatal lupus and Chapter 62 Rash: Vesiculobullous for discussion of bullous lupus.

NODULES

Nodules in the skin can be difficult to diagnose and many require a skin biopsy. There are a few inflammatory conditions of the skin that are characteristically nodules and should not be missed.

Panniculitis

Erythema Nodosum

Erythema nodosum seems to be a hypersensitivity reaction leading to inflammation of the subcutaneous fat and may be related to infection (streptococci, tuberculosis, coccidioidomycosis, histoplasmosis), inflammatory bowel disease, sarcoidosis, and medications (e.g., oral contraceptives). The exact immunologic mechanism has not been clarified. The entity occurs predominantly in adolescents during the spring and fall. Women are affected more often than men.

The lesions of erythema nodosum appear as deep, tender, erythematous nodules, or plaques on the extensor surfaces of the extremities. The sedimentation rate is generally elevated and usually returns to normal with disappearance of the eruption, unless an underlying disease is present. The reaction usually lasts 3 to 6 weeks. Treatment should be directed toward the cause when and if established; otherwise, it is symptomatic (nonsteroidal anti-inflammatory drugs and antihistamines). Hospitalization is unnecessary. Corticosteroids should not be used, except in severe cases after an underlying infection has been ruled out.

Cold Panniculitis

Cold panniculitis is caused by cold injury to fat. During the cold of winter, infants and some older children develop red, indurated nodules and plaques on exposed skin, especially on the face. The subcutaneous fat in infants and some children solidifies more readily at a higher temperature than that of an adult because of the relatively greater concentration of saturated fats. Infants who hold ice chips or popsicles in their mouths are also susceptible to this phenomenon. The lesions gradually soften and return to normal over 1 or more weeks. Treatment is unnecessary.

GENERALIZED MACULES AND PAPULES/MORBILLIFORM ERUPTIONS

Morbilliform rashes are common in pediatric practice, and children often present to the emergency department (ED) for their evaluation and treatment. Morbilliform or "measle-like" eruptions are often described as maculopapular rashes.

The causes of morbilliform eruptions rashes are diverse (Table 96.1) and range from benign to life-threatening (Table 96.2). Common causes include viral exanthems and drug reactions. The diagnostic approach to these disorders is based on the presence or absence of fever, characteristic clinical appearance, location, chronicity, and medication history. Some of these conditions have very characteristic clinical appearances (Table 96.3); however, manifestations of these illnesses can be sufficiently variable that a proportion of the cases are difficult to diagnose.

EVALUATION AND DECISION

In approaching a child with an exanthem, the initial steps are to take a history and to fully examine all cutaneous surfaces.

TABLE 96.1

RASHES COMPOSED OF MACULES AND PAPULES: ETIOLOGIC CLASSIFICATION

Infectious	*Fungal*
Viral	Pityriasis versicolor
Roseola infantum	*Other infections*
Rubeola	Rocky Mountain spotted fever
Rubella	Ehrlichiosis
Erythema infectiosum (fifth disease)	Mycoplasma (15% of cases)
Varicella (early manifestations before bullae)	*Etiology uncertain but thought to be viral*
Epstein–Barr virus (10–15% of cases have macular or maculopapular rash)	Pityriasis rosea
Molluscum contagiosum (papules)	Kawasaki disease
Dengue	Papular acrodermatitis
"Nonspecific" viral	**Noninfectious**
Enterovirus	*Bites and infestations*
Echovirus	Insect bites
Coxsackievirus	Scabies
Adenovirus	*Miscellaneous*
Bacterial	Drug reaction
Scarlet fever	Allergic contact dermatitis
Syphilis	Irritant contact dermatitis
Disseminated gonorrhea	Papular urticaria
	Erythema multiforme
	Guttate psoriasis
	Pityriasis lichenoides
	Lichen nitidus

TABLE 96.2

POTENTIALLY LIFE-THREATENING ILLNESSES ASSOCIATED WITH DIFFUSE MORBILLIFORM ERUPTION

Rocky Mountain spotted fever
Kawasaki disease
Erythema multiforme
Dengue fever
Rubeola
Ehrlichiosis
Drug Reaction with Eosinophilia and Systemic Symptoms (DRESS)

The most important historical features include the duration of the rash (acute or chronic), initial distribution, extent of spread (generalized or localized), ill contacts (including sexual partners), and any associated systemic symptoms, including fever. The physical examination should include a careful systematic inspection of all mucocutaneous surfaces, with special attention paid to involvement of the oropharynx, palms and soles, extensor or flexor surfaces, scalp, and trunk.

For patients with widespread rash who appear particularly ill, the potential diagnoses of drug hypersensitivity reaction, viral and bacterial illness should be considered. Figure 96.12 may help with an approach to morbilliform/mixed macular and papular eruptions.

For patients who do not appear ill, certain exanthems will have distinctive patterns that will immediately strike the examiner and make the diagnosis readily apparent. Erythema multiforme (EM), rubella, coxsackievirus infections (Fig. 96.14), erythema infectiosum (Fig. 96.15A,B), scarlet fever, varicella, MC (Fig. 96.16), tinea versicolor (Fig. 96.17), pityriasis rosea (Fig. 96.18), and roseola all have recognizable clinical appearances. Many of these illnesses have characteristic distributions or associated signs and symptoms that aid in their diagnoses. If the pattern of the rash does not evoke immediate recognition from the examiner, a more methodical approach is indicated, as outlined in Figure 96.19.

TABLE 96.3

GENERALIZED RASHES THAT OFTEN HAVE CHARACTERISTIC CLINICAL APPEARANCES

Rubeola
Erythema infectiosum (fifth disease)
Hand–foot–mouth disease (coxsackievirus A16)
Molluscum contagiosum
Scarlet fever
Pityriasis versicolor
Pityriasis rosea
Roseola infantum
Insect bites
Erythema multiforme
Stevens–Johnson syndrome
Drug reaction with eosinophilia and systemic symptoms

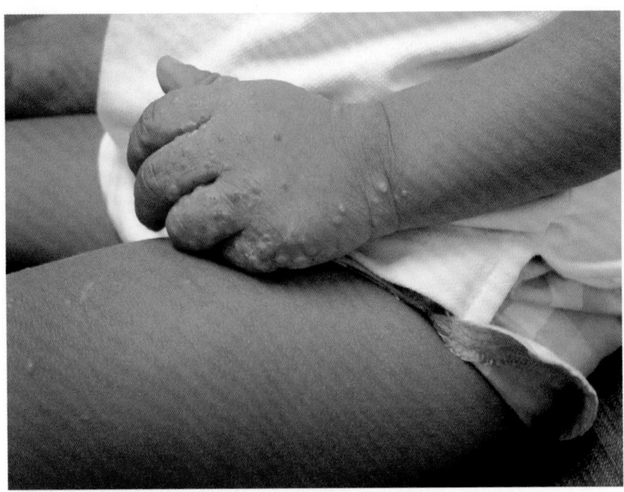

FIGURE 96.14 Coxsackie virus/enterovirus.

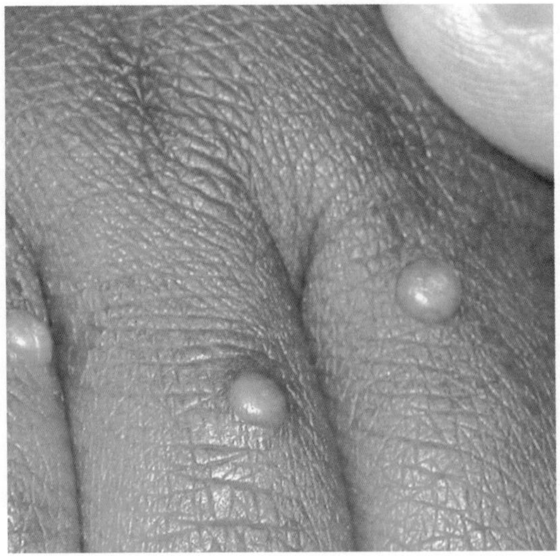

FIGURE 96.16 Molluscum contagiosum.

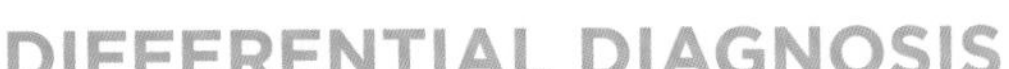

DIFFERENTIAL DIAGNOSIS

Presence of Fever

The potentially life-threatening rashes (Table 96.2) are all acute illnesses most commonly associated with fever and significant systemic symptoms. EM and rubeola have recognizable clinical appearances, whereas Kawasaki disease (KWD), RMSF, and dengue fever require a high level of clinical suspicion. Drug hypersensitivity reactions can often cause fevers.

Potentially Life-threatening Illnesses

Drug Hypersensitivity Reactions

Please see Chapter 63 Rash: Drug Eruptions for a full discussion of drug reactions. The spectrum of cutaneous drug eruptions ranges from the relatively benign to the severe. Morphology of the eruption as well as suspected drug causing the eruption helps establish when clinicians should worry about morbidity and mortality. Morphologies range from urticarial to morbilliform (sometimes called maculopapular) to pustular and vesiculobullous. Many drug hypersensitivity reactions are associated with fever.

Kawasaki Disease (see Chapter 109 Rheumatologic Emergencies)

KWD can present with a wide variety of rashes, including morbilliform and urticarial. Conjunctivitis, when present, is unique in that it is nonexudative with limbal sparing. Other dermatologic manifestations include red cracked lips, strawberry tongue, and erythematous oropharynx, and erythema, swelling, and/or induration of peripheral extremities.

The most commonly associated rash is a generalized exanthem with raised erythematous plaques; however, the rash may also present with an erythematous maculopapular, morbilliform, scarlatiniform, or erythema marginatum–like pattern. Peeling in the diaper/groin area is also frequently observed early. The exanthem may be fleeting or persist for 2 to 3 days. During the later stages of the acute phase, periungual desquamation and peeling of the palms, soles, or perineal area develop.

Measles (Rubeola)

Measles was one of the most common viral exanthems before the measles vaccine. It is now on the rise again because of increased opting out of vaccinations for children. The incubation period is 10 to 14 days after direct contact with droplets from an infected person. In its classic form, measles has a

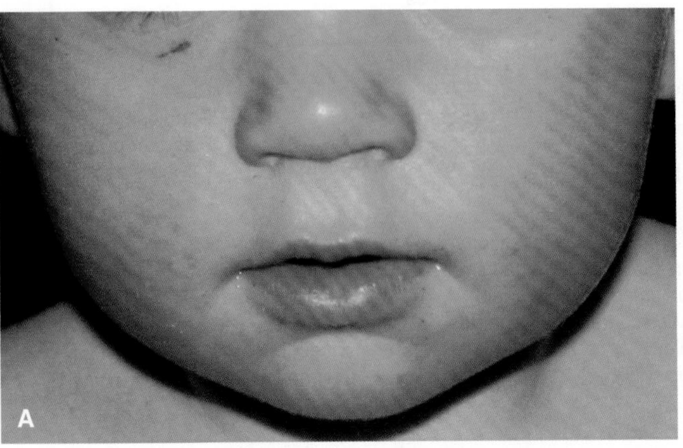

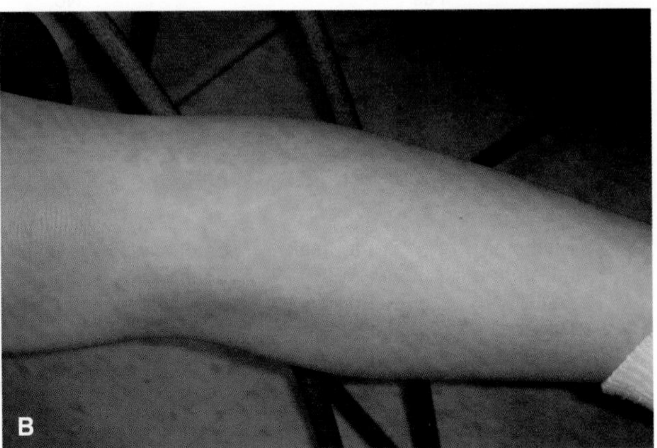

FIGURE 96.15 **A:** Erythema infectiosum—slapped cheeks. **B:** Erythema infectiosum—exanthema.

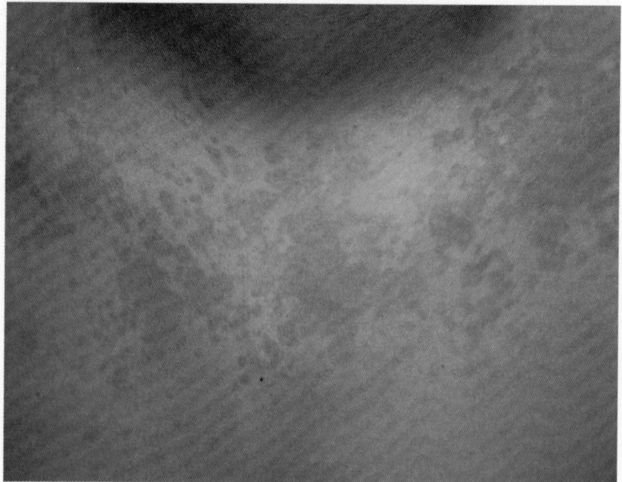

FIGURE 96.17 Tinea versicolor.

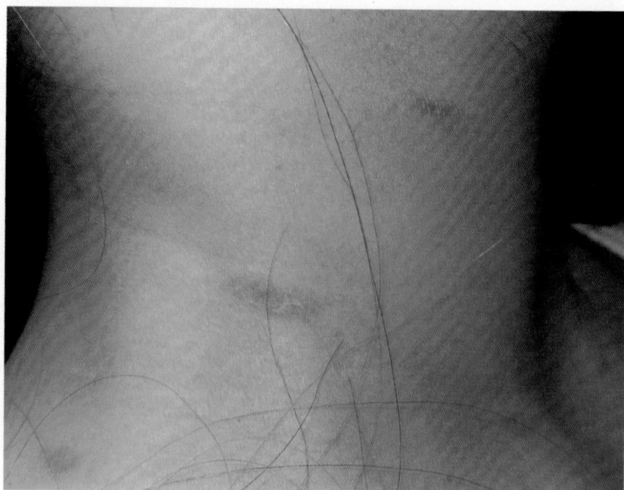

FIGURE 96.18 Pityriasis rosea.

highly characteristic natural history. Two to 3 days after the onset of the prodromal symptoms of cough, coryza, conjunctivitis, and fever, Koplik spots occur in the mouth, followed 12 to 24 hours later by the cutaneous exanthem. Most typically, Koplik spots appear as pinpoint white lesions on a red base on the buccal mucosa adjacent to the molars; however, they may be seen on any of the mucosal surfaces of the oral cavity except the tongue.

The measles exanthem begins on the head as reddish maculopapules and spreads caudally during the next 4 to 5 days. Within 1 to 2 days of its appearance, the discrete maculopapular lesions coalesce to produce the confluent phase of the rash. Hence, within 2 to 3 days of onset, the rash on the face becomes confluent, whereas the rash on the lower extremities still consists of individual maculopapules. Modified measles occurs in children who have received serum immunoglobulin after exposure to measles. Measles may still occur, but the incubation period may be delayed up to 21 days. The symptoms, although following the usual progression, will be milder. A faint rash and mild febrile illness may occur 7 to 10 days after immunization with the live attenuated measles vaccine.

Rocky Mountain Spotted Fever

RMSF is caused by *Rickettsia rickettsii* transmitted by the bite of a tick (see Chapter 61 Rash: Bacterial and Fungal Infections). Although initially confined to the Rocky Mountain States

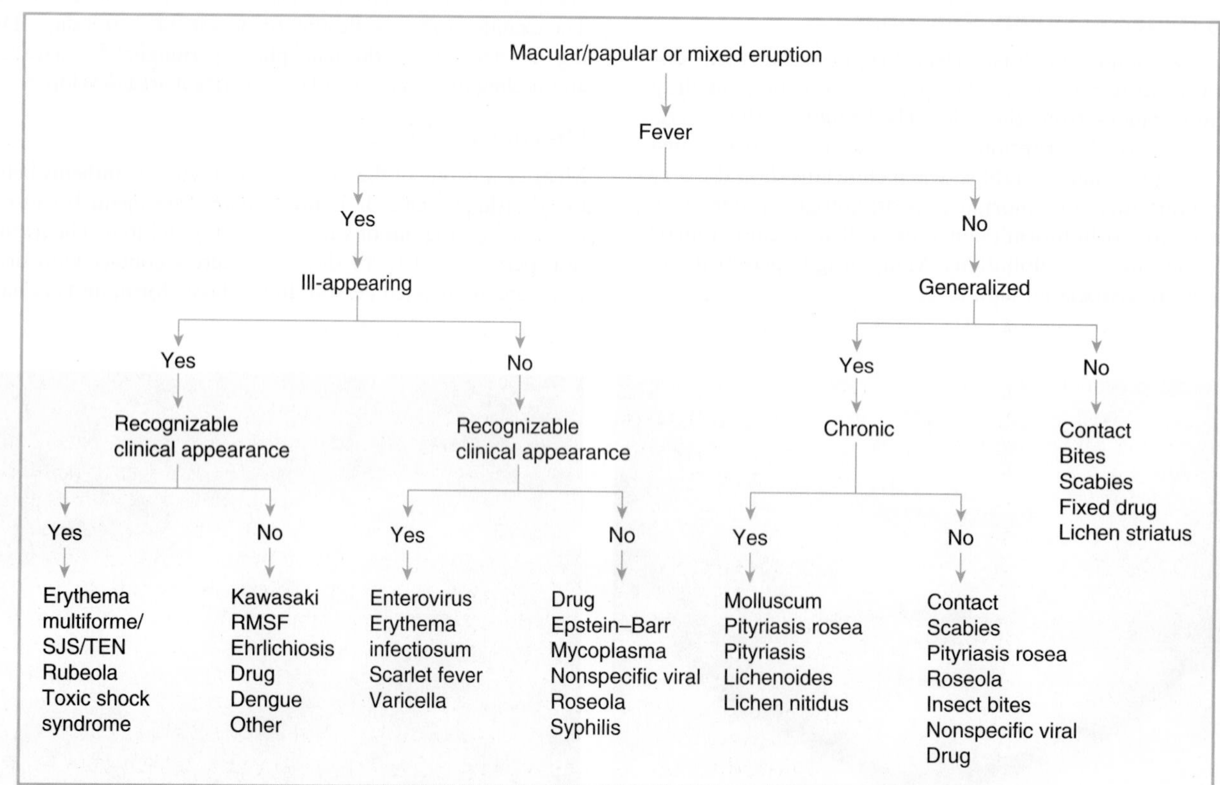

FIGURE 96.19 Schematic approach to morbilliform or mixed macular and papular eruptions.

(hence, its name), confirmed cases have been reported from all parts of the United States with varying tick vectors. The primary determinants in patient outcome are early diagnosis and treatment. The best outcomes are associated with the initiation of doxycycline therapy by day five of illness.

The rash of RMSF begins on the third or fourth day of a febrile illness as a morbilliform eruption on the extremities, most commonly the wrists and ankles. Over the next 2 days, the rash becomes generalized by spreading centrally to involve the back, chest, and abdomen. Initially, the rash consists of erythematous macules that blanch on pressure; they then become more confluent and purpuric. Notably, the hemorrhagic lesions predominate in the peripheral distribution, involving the palms of the hands and the soles of the feet. The severity of the rash is proportional to the severity of the disease.

All patients with RMSF have some degree of vasculitis that is the basis for many of the associated systemic symptoms. An overall toxic appearance is common. Systemic signs and symptoms include fever, headache, myalgia, conjunctivitis, vomiting, seizures, myocarditis, heart failure, shock; periorbital, facial, or peripheral edema; and disseminated intravascular coagulation or purpura fulminans.

Diagnosis is best made by polymerase chain reaction (PCR) testing. Thrombocytopenia, hyponatremia, and increased aminotransferases usually develop as the disease process progresses but antibiotics should hopefully have been started prior to the development of these findings.

Doxycycline is the drug of choice for therapy in patients of all ages, despite its risk for potentially staining developing teeth at a dose of 4 mg/kg/day in two divided doses (maximum of 100 mg two times a day), intravenously or orally.

Ehrlichiosis

Ehrlichiosis is another tick-borne disease with increasing prevalence that is most common during the warmer months when ticks are most prevalent. Nomenclature has undergone multiple changes. Currently, disease in the United States is due to three distinct obligate intracellular bacteria: *Ehrlichiosis chaffeensis* (human monocytic ehrlichiosis or HME), *Anaplasma phagocytophilum* agent (human granulocytic anaplasmosis or HGA), or *Ehrlichia ewingii* (*E. ewingii* ehrlichiosis). Infections with any of these bacteria cause an illness very similar to RMSF. Rash is a less consistent feature of ehrlichiosis but when present may be macular, morbilliform, or petechial and is more commonly seen in pediatric patients infected with *E. chaffeensis*. Unlike RMSF, rash may occur anywhere on the body and is less commonly seen on the palms and/or soles. Vasculitis is less prominent, and leukopenia, anemia, and hepatitis are more common in ehrlichiosis than in RMSF.

As for RMSF, doxycycline is the drug of choice for therapy in patients of all ages and at the same dose (see above). Therapy is continued until the patient is afebrile for at least 2 to 3 days and for a minimum total course of 5 to 10 days. Clinical improvement is usually apparent within 3 days, and if not, an alternative diagnosis should be sought. Disease may be more severe or even fatal in untreated patients. Early initiation of therapy minimizes morbidity and mortality.

Dengue Fever

Dengue fever is caused by four dengue viruses transmitted by Aedes mosquitos and is seen in tropical and subtropical areas of almost all continents (including areas of Puerto Rico and the Caribbean basin and now in Florida). Many cases are asymptomatic. In symptomatic cases, initial constitutional symptoms include sudden onset of high fever, severe headache, myalgia, arthralgia, and abdominal pain. During the course of fever that lasts 2 to 7 days, back and leg pain may be severe, hence, the disease's nickname "breakbone" fever. The development of a hemorrhagic vasculitis, most common in patients younger than 15 years, leads to the more concerning subtype called dengue hemorrhagic fever. The term dengue shock syndrome is used in even more severe cases when increased vascular permeability leads to shock. Encephalopathy, hepatitis, myocardiopathy, intestinal bleeding, and pneumonia are other complications.

Two distinct rashes may be seen, which coincide with the disease's biphasic fever pattern. The first rash is a generalized, transient, macular rash that blanches under pressure and is seen within the first 24 to 48 hours of the onset of systemic symptoms. The second rash coincides with or occurs 1 to 2 days after defervescence and is a generalized morbilliform sparing the palms and soles.

Diagnosis is based on clinical suspicion and potential exposure based on the virus's geographic distribution. Serologic testing is available as is viral isolation and measurement of serum immunoglobulin antibodies in paired serum specimens obtained 4 weeks apart. Treatment is supportive, and may require aggressive fluid management and pain control. Intravenous immunoglobulin and/or plasma exchange may be of benefit in severe cases.

Causes of Other Widespread Rashes Associated with Fever

Non–life-threatening illnesses associated with fever and widespread rash include coxsackievirus infections, erythema infectiosum, scarlet fever, and early varicella. Harder to diagnose are rashes associated with Epstein–Barr virus, *Mycoplasma* infections, roseola infantum, disseminated gonorrhea, secondary syphilis. Also consider primary and secondary reaction such as the amoxicillin rash that occurs in the setting of Epstein–Barr virus infection.

Erythema Infectiosum (Fifth Disease)

Erythema infectiosum is a benign disease caused by parvovirus B19, the same virus that can cause aplastic crises in patients with sickle cell anemia. For the normal, nongravid host, fifth disease is usually of no consequence, with the only systemic symptom being fever in 15% to 30% of cases. On the face is a characteristic, intensely erythematous, "slapped cheek" rash, often with a relative circumoral pallor (Fig. 96.15A). In addition, a symmetric red lace-like rash is seen on the arms and then trunk, buttocks, and thighs, which may be pruritic (Fig. 96.15B). In its acute phase, the rash usually lasts only for a few days but can wax and wane in intensity with environmental changes (e.g., exposure to heat or sunlight) for weeks and sometimes months. In a small subset of patients, parvovirus B19 causes the atypical papular purpuric gloves and socks syndrome (PPGSS) with a typically painful purpuric exanthem limited to the hands and feet. Immunocompromised children or those with hemolytic anemias can develop red cell aplasia and symptoms associated with a chronic anemia.

Diagnosis is usually made on a clinical basis alone but may be confirmed in an immunocompetent host by measuring parvovirus B19–specific IgM antibody. PCR is the best modality for diagnosis in an immunocompromised host. No specific therapy is necessary in immunocompetent hosts. For a chronic infection in an immunodeficient patient, IVIG therapy should be considered. Because parvovirus is associated with fetal anemia, congestive heart failure and hydrops-exposed pregnant women should be referred to their physicians to discuss possible parvovirus antibody testing.

Scarlet Fever

Scarlet fever is caused by phage-infected *Group A Streptococcus* that makes an erythrogenic toxin. This disease is still seen with regularity but does not appear to be any more serious than Group A streptococcal infection without rash. Scarlet fever is most commonly associated with streptococcal pharyngitis but may occur in association with pyoderma or an infected wound.

The diagnosis of scarlet fever can be made clinically in a child with signs and symptoms of pharyngitis who has a fine, raised, generalized morbilliform rash. The skin has a coarse or sandpapery feel on palpation. Typically, there is sparing of the circumoral area, leading to circumoral pallor. There is usually a bright erythema of the tongue and hypertrophy of the papillae, leading to the term *strawberry tongue*. Pastia's lines, bright red, orange, or even hemorrhagic lines, can occasionally be seen in the axillae or antecubital fossa. The rash generally lasts 3 to 5 days, followed by brownish discoloration and peeling of the skin as small flakes to entire casts of the digits. A rapid streptococcal test or throat culture should be sent to confirm infection.

Epstein–Barr Virus

Between 5% and 15% of patients with Epstein–Barr viral infection, otherwise known as infectious mononucleosis, will have an erythematous maculopapular eruption. Infection in young children is usually asymptomatic or so mild that diagnosis is not sought. Older patients between 15 and 25 years of age are more likely to present for evaluation. Fifty percent to 100% of patients with infectious mononucleosis develop a maculopapular rash after receiving concurrent ampicillin or amoxicillin-containing antibiotics—most commonly for an incorrect diagnosis of streptococcal pharyngitis.

The illness begins insidiously with headache, malaise, and fever, followed by sore throat, membranous tonsillitis, and lymphadenopathy. Splenomegaly is common. The exanthem occurs within 4 to 6 days as a macular or maculopapular morbilliform eruption most prominent on the trunk and proximal extremities. An enanthem consisting of discrete petechiae at the junction of the hard and soft palate occurs in approximately 25% of patients. A small subset of patients develops more serious disease, often involving the central nervous system.

Diagnosis is often presumed clinically but may be supported by an absolute increase in atypical lymphocytes or a positive heterophile antibody (monospot) test (obtained after the first week of symptoms), or may be confirmed by serology. The heterophile antibody test is less sensitive in children younger than 4 years of age. The illness is most commonly self-limited, requiring no therapy, but due to the frequency of associated splenomegaly, affected children should not be allowed to participate in contact sports until fully recovered and the spleen is no longer palpable. Amoxicillin should be avoided for any concurrent infections. Corticosteroids may be considered for patients with particularly severe tonsillitis.

Mycoplasma Infections

Infections with *Mycoplasma pneumoniae* may cause morbilliform rashes in up to 15% of cases. The classic clinical presentation is of a child with malaise, low-grade fever, and prominent cough. The cough is initially nonproductive but may become productive, particularly in older children, and may persist for 3 to 4 weeks. Physical examination may reveal bilateral rales.

Diagnosis is suggested by mycoplasma PCR of the sputum or by IgM or IgG titers of the blood. Erythromycin, clarithromycin, or azithromycin are the treatment of choice.

Mycoplasma can also induce Stevens–Johnson syndrome (see Chapter 63 Rash: Drug Eruptions). The rash here is characterized by hemorrhagic lips and mucosal involvement with fewer bullous lesions on the rest of the skin.

Roseola Infantum

Roseola infantum, also called *exanthem subitum* or *sixth disease,* is attributed to primary infection with human herpes virus (HHV)-6. The illness is characterized by the onset of a maculopapular rash that appears following a 3- to 4-day febrile illness. The fever is characteristically high. The rash is widely disseminated, appearing as discrete, small, pinkish macules that rarely coalesce, beginning on the trunk and then extending peripherally. The rash may last for hours to days. The occurrence of the rash within 24 hours of defervescence rather than the morphologic appearance of the rash leads to the correct diagnosis. The rash can appear very similar to that seen in measles, but the child with roseola appears well and no longer febrile. Diagnosis is made clinically and care is supportive.

Disseminated Neisseria Gonorrhea

Disseminated *Neisseria gonorrhoeae* should be considered in sexually active or potentially abused children, especially if associated with a history of vaginal or penile discharge. A distinct minority of patients develop disseminated gonorrhea infection through hematogenous spread. Disseminated gonorrhea may cause a range of cutaneous lesions, including small erythematous papules, petechiae, or vesicle-pustules on a hemorrhagic base. These cutaneous lesions usually develop on the trunk but may occur anywhere on the extremities.

An etiologic diagnosis can be established by demonstration of the organism on Gram stain of the skin lesion, positive blood culture, or positive culture of oral or genital sites. Based on resistance patterns, recommended current therapy is ceftriaxone 50 mg/kg/day (maximum 1 g per day) until clinical improvement is seen, at which point it can be changed to an oral antibiotic, such as cefixime, ciprofloxacin, ofloxacin, or levofloxacin, for a total of a 7-day course. Quinolones should not be used for infections in men who have intercourse with men or in those with a history of recent foreign travel or partners' travel, or infections acquired in other areas with increased resistance. Concomitant sexually transmitted diseases should be sought and treated.

Secondary Syphilis

One needs a high level of suspicion when viewing rashes in sexually active (or potentially abused) children to make the diagnosis of secondary syphilis, caused by the spirochete *Treponema pallidum*. Manifestations of secondary syphilis

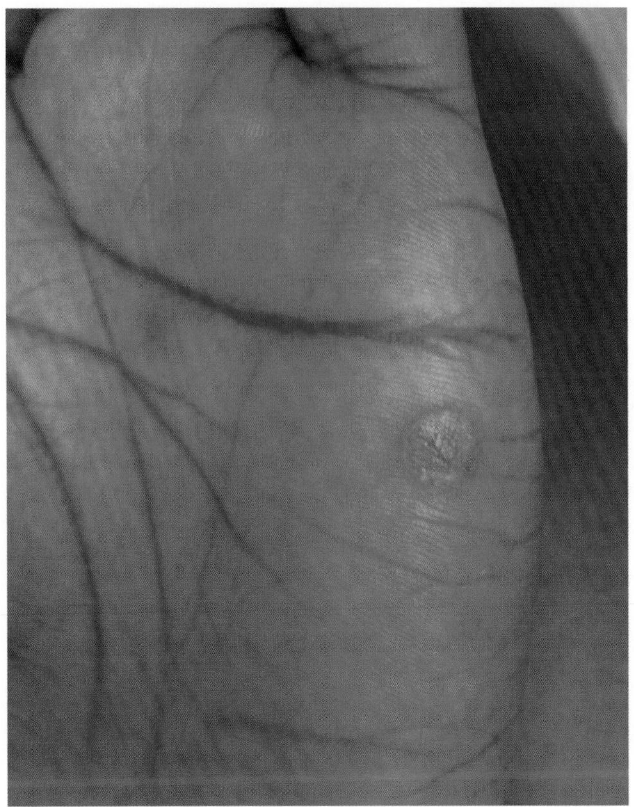

FIGURE 96.20 Secondary syphilis.

usually occur 6 to 8 weeks after the appearance of the primary lesion, which may have gone unnoticed. The exanthem extends rapidly and is usually pronounced.

The rash of secondary syphilis is characterized by a generalized cutaneous eruption, usually composed of brownish, dull-red macules or papules that range in size from a few millimeters to 1 cm in diameter (Fig. 96.20). They are generally discrete and symmetrically distributed, particularly over the trunk, where they follow the lines of cleavage in a pattern similar to pityriasis rosea. Papular lesions on the palms and soles, as well as the presence of systemic symptoms, such as general malaise, fever, headaches, sore throat, rhinorrhea, lacrimation, and generalized lymphadenopathy, help differentiate secondary syphilis.

Acquired syphilis is sexually contracted from direct contact with ulcerative lesions of the skin or mucous membranes of an infected individual. Diagnosis may be presumed after a positive nontreponemal test, such as the VDRL slide test, rapid plasma reagin (RPR) test, or the automated reagin test. Diagnosis should be confirmed by a treponemal test, such as the fluorescent treponemal antibody absorption test, the microhemagglutination test for *T. pallidum,* or the *T. pallidum* immobilization test. Definitive diagnosis may also be made by identifying spirochetes by microscopic dark-field examination or direct fluorescent antibody tests of lesion exudate or tissue. Penicillin is the treatment of choice unless contraindicated, in which case tetracycline, doxycycline, ceftriaxone, or erythromycin may be substituted. Length of therapy should be based on duration and stage of infection. Concomitant sexually transmitted diseases should be sought and treated empirically. HIV testing is recommended for patients with secondary syphilis.

Nonspecific Viral Exanthems

Many times, a specific diagnosis cannot be made even after considering such factors as exposure history, history of preceding illness, description of eruption, time and site of onset, character of initial lesion, progression, distribution patterns, and occurrence of mucosal lesions. This should not be surprising, given the large number of viruses that can be associated with macular or morbilliform eruptions. In particular, enteroviruses and adenoviruses can cause a macular or morbilliform eruption. In fact, enterovirus 71 is now known to be the cause of a subset of cases of hand–foot–mouth disease. There is little to distinguish the rash caused by one of these viruses from that of another, based on the location and morphology, with the exception of those viral infections previously discussed. One usually arrives at the diagnosis of nonspecific viral exanthem in a child in whom other diagnoses have been excluded and who may have signs of associated illness or systemic features such as fever. If specific diagnosis is required, it can be determined by viral isolation and/or a rise in diagnostic titer.

Generalized Eruptions without Fever

Many generalized eruptions are not associated with fever. Many are fairly easily recognizable such as psoriasis, contact dermatitis, pityriasis rosea.

Guttate Psoriasis and Pityriasis Rosea

Please see Chapter 65 Rash: Papulosquamous Eruptions for full discussion of papulosquamous skin rashes.

Rubella

Rubella is rarely seen in the postvaccine era in the United States. In a classic case of rubella, the rash, similar to measles, begins on the head and spreads caudally. The progression occurs over 2 to 3 days, and typically, the rash is entirely gone by the fourth day. The rash always remains macular and never becomes confluent, which is an important distinguishing characteristic. One-third of all rubella virus infections is clinically silent (i.e., they have no exanthem). The rash of rubella may show extensive variation in location, progression, and duration, at times disappearing within 12 hours or being localized to one part of an extremity without any progression.

Unlike measles, in which systemic toxicity and fever are the rule, fever is uncommon. Associated symptoms and complaints in rubella include joint pain and adenopathy (most commonly suboccipital, postauricular, and cervical). Arthralgia that occurs with a viral exanthem is highly characteristic for rubella. Diagnosis is based on clinical presentation, and treatment is supportive.

Vesicles/Bullae

Enterovirus Infections

Enterovirus infection can not only cause morbilliform exanthems but can also cause vesicles and blisters. The classic exanthem of coxsackievirus A16 infection, also appropriately called *hand–foot–mouth disease,* is common and easily recognized. Infections may occur in epidemics, most commonly in the late summer or early fall. Multiple infected members within a household are common.

Coxsackievirus A16 infection begins with a prodrome of low-grade fever, anorexia, mouth pain, and malaise, followed within 1 to 2 days by an oral enanthem and then shortly thereafter by red macules and papules. The oral lesions begin as small red macules, most often located on the palate, uvula, and anterior tonsillar pillar, which evolve into small vesicles that ulcerate and heal over a 1- to 6-day period. The exanthem develops into small crescent or football-shaped vesicles on an erythematous base (Fig. 96.14). These vesicles, which may be pruritic or mildly tender, are usually located on the dorsal and lateral aspects of fingers, hands, and feet but may develop on the buttocks, arms, legs, and face. The lesions improve over 2 to 7 days.

The other types of coxsackievirus cause similar or even indistinguishable exanthems, which may more commonly involve the face, trunk, and proximal extremities. Often, children with these exanthems will be diagnosed with nonspecific viral infections. Other symptoms attributed to coxsackie virus infection include aseptic meningitis and less commonly myopericarditis, pleuritis, encephalitis, or paralysis. Severe and/or persistent infections may be seen in immunocompromised hosts.

Diagnosis is usually made clinically, although the virus can be detected by PCR directly from the vesicles or from the stool. The virus is commonly shed for weeks from stool. Coxsackievirus infections are usually self-limiting, so no specific treatment is necessary. IVIG with high antibody titer may be considered for immunocompromised patients or in life-threatening neonatal infections. Coxsackie virus also frequently infects eczema prone areas and in this case is called eczema coxsackium (similar to eczema herpeticum).

Varicella (Chickenpox)

Although varicella is an easily recognizable vesiculobullous eruption, on occasion, the earliest phase can be confusing. The initial skin manifestations of varicella virus infection are small, red macules. Some of the lesions remain as macules, but most progress to papules and then the characteristic umbilicated, tear-shaped vesicles. The earliest lesions appear on the chest and spread centrifugally, but there are many exceptions to the pattern of spread. Mucosal lesions can be seen but are usually not a prominent feature. Occasionally, a child with mild chickenpox may have only a few scattered macules with only one or two progressing to the more typical vesicular lesions. Of children receiving varicella vaccine, 7% to 8% may develop a mild maculopapular or varicelliform rash within 1 month of vaccination.

Other Bullae/Vesicles

Blisters can be related to bug bites, contact allergy, friction, drug reaction, vasculitis, primary genetic disease of the skin, and fluid overload. A full discussion of blisters can be found in Chapter 62 Rash: Vesiculobullous. Chapter 65 Rash: Papulosquamous Eruptions, covers HSV and Chapter 60 Rash: Atopic Dermatitis, Contact Dermatitis, Scabies and Erythroderma, covers eczema herpeticum.

Localized Eruptions without Fever

Contact dermatitis, insect bites, papular acrodermatitis, and scabies usually present in a localized distribution; however, all may appear as a more generalized eruption in extensive cases.

Contact Dermatitis

Contact dermatitis may be caused either by a primary exposure to an irritant or by an acquired delayed hypersensitivity response to a sensitizing substance. A sharp demarcation commonly exists between the involved and uninvolved skin areas. Affected skin is erythematous with variable numbers and combinations of macules, papules, vesicles, and/or bullae.

Diagnosis depends on obtaining a thorough history of exposure and the presence of a characteristic localized pattern of rash. Treatment for both types of these dermatitides includes eliminating exposure to offending irritants, providing topical or systemic antipruritic agents, and for more severe cases, providing topical or systemic steroids. Please see Chapter 60 Rash: Atopic Dermatitis, Contact Dermatitis, Scabies and Erythroderma for additional information.

Insect Bites

Virtually all children experience insect bites. Mosquitoes, fleas, and bedbugs are the most common offenders. Diagnosis depends on the season, the climate, exposure to animals, and distribution and appearance of the lesions. Care is aimed at minimizing discomfort with topical or systemic antihistamines and/or topical steroids.

Papular Acrodermatitis (Gianotti–Crosti Syndrome)

Papular acrodermatitis is an eruption of unclear cause that has been associated with hepatitis B, EBV, and other viral infections in young children. In the pediatric population, 85% are younger than 3 years. The eruption may follow a low-grade fever or mild upper respiratory symptoms.

The eruption consists of flesh-colored papules that occur anywhere on the body but often concentrate on the extensor surfaces of the arms, legs, and buttock. Lesions are particularly prominent over the elbows and knees. The rash usually lasts 2 to 8 weeks and then disappears. No treatment is needed for the cutaneous eruption; however, a subset of patients with cutaneous lesions develops generalized lymphadenopathy and hepatosplenomegaly. These children should be evaluated for hepatitis and follow-up in 2 weeks is recommended for patients with only cutaneous involvement to exclude hepatitis.

Scabies

Scabies is discussed in Chapter 65 Rash: Papulosquamous Eruptions.

Chronic Eruptions without Fever

Chronic eruptions are defined as those that are usually present for a minimum of 2 weeks.

Atopic Dermatitis

Although the eruption may have a variable appearance (erythema, edema, papules, vesicles, serous discharge, and crusting), its constant feature is pruritus. The eruption often has a characteristic distribution, depending on age, and often occurs in allergic (atopic) individuals or those with a family history of allergies (e.g., hay fever, asthma, allergic rhinitis, food allergies, eosinophilic gastroenteritis). Please see full discussion in Chapter 60 Rash: Atopic Dermatitis, Contact Dermatitis, Scabies and Erythroderma.

Pityriasis Lichenoides

Pityriasis lichenoides is a relatively rare disorder of unknown cause that can appear in childhood and young adulthood. There are two forms: acute and chronic. The acute disease is characterized by a macular, papular, or papulovesicular rash that is often distributed most heavily on the trunk and upper arms. The lesions occur in successive crops, rapidly evolving into vesicular, necrotic, and even purpuric lesions, which may leave pock-like scars. Resolution occurs spontaneously but may take several weeks to months and recurrences may occur. Parents may describe these recurrences as "he keeps getting the chickenpox." The more chronic form may evolve from the acute form or may arise de novo and often lasts for several years. There is no established therapy though light therapy, topical steroids, erythromycin, and tetracyclines have all been used.

Tinea

Dermatophyte infections usually last longer than 2 weeks. A full discussion can be found in Chapter 61 Rash: Bacterial and Fungal Infections. In short, tinea corporis is characterized by one or more sharply circumscribed scaly patches. The center of the circular patch generally clears as the leading edge spreads out. The leading edge may be composed of papules, vesicles, or pustules. The lesions are most commonly confused with nummular eczema. The diagnosis can be made by scraping the active outer rim of papules and examining the scales with a potassium hydroxide (KOH) preparation under the microscope. These lesions do not fluoresce under the Wood light. Treatment with topical antifungal agents such as clotrimazole, miconazole, econazole, terbinafine, and butenafine produces clearing in 7 to 10 days. Therapy should be maintained for at least 2 weeks. If improvement does not occur, treatment with griseofulvin (15 to 20 mg/kg/day in two divided doses) will usually resolve the problem.

Tinea Capitis

Although tinea capitis is commonly caused by *Microsporum* species and *Trichophyton tonsurans,* the two forms have different clinical appearances. The *Microsporum* species generally causes round patches of scaling alopecia (Fig. 96.21). Illumination of a lesion with a Wood lamp gives a blue-green

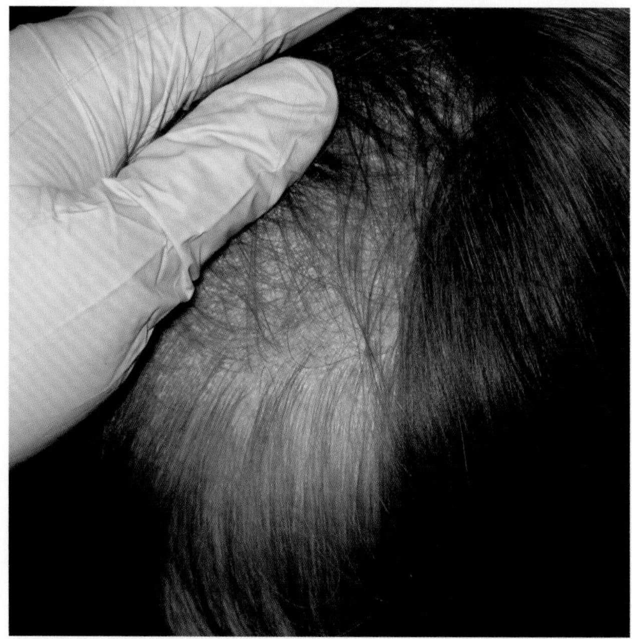

FIGURE 96.21 Tinea capitis with round patches of scaling alopecia.

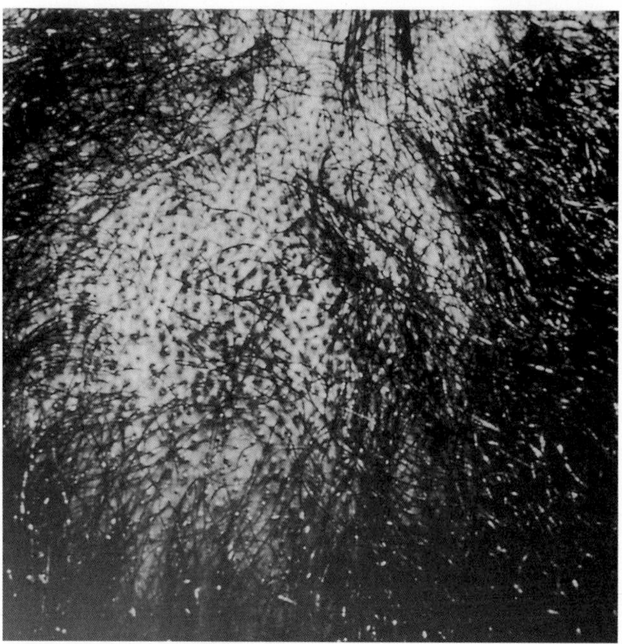

FIGURE 96.22 Black dot tinea capitis.

fluorescence. Kerion formation can occur as a swollen, boggy abscess. The *Trichophyton* species usually causes scattered alopecia with seborrheic-like scaling, not always oval or rounded; the alopecia is irregular in outline with indistinct margins. Normal hairs grow within the patches of alopecia. At times, the hairs break off at the surface of the scalp, leaving a "black dot" appearance (Fig. 96.22). Diffuse scaling may simulate dandruff, and although minimal hair loss is present, it is not perceived. Wood light examination of lesions caused by *Trichophyton* species does not produce fluorescence. The organism can cause a folliculitis, suppuration, and kerion formation (Fig. 96.23). Diagnosis is made by culturing the affected scalp area. The clinician should consider the presence of tinea capitis when a nonresponsive seborrheic or atopic dermatitis of the scalp is present, black dots are seen, or increased scaling follows the use of topical steroids. If a kerion is present, the swelling (allergic reaction to the fungus) can be controlled by a combination of griseofulvin and prednisone.

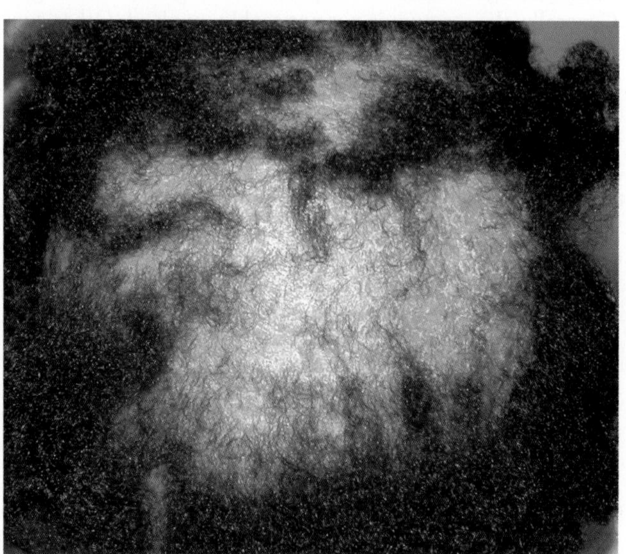

FIGURE 96.23 Inflammation characteristic of a kerion.

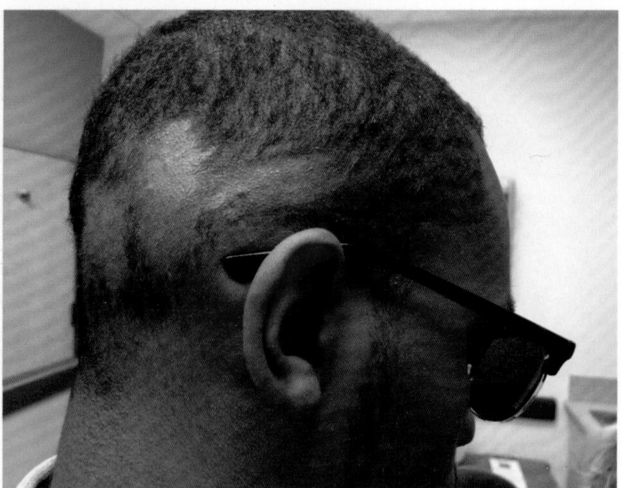

FIGURE 96.24 Nonscarring alopecia on the scalp of a child characteristic of alopecia areata.

In the differential diagnosis of patchy hair loss, as is seen in tinea capitis, the clinician should consider alopecia areata (Fig. 96.24). However, with alopecia areata, no inflammation or scaling of the scalp occurs. *Trichotillomania* (also *trichotillosis*), the term given to the habit children develop of rubbing, twirling, or playing with their hair to the point that the hair breaks and is lost in irregular sometimes geometric patches, should also be considered. Hairs are characteristically of different length within the affected area, indicating breakage at different times. In addition, there is no scaling or inflammation typically seen. Traction alopecia occurs with certain hairstyles. Hair is lost at the margins of the hairline with the ponytail style or frequent use of tight hair styles. At times, papules or pustules occur where the skin has been disrupted by the traction. Infants who are left on their backs for long periods may lose hair at the occiput from the constant friction in that area.

Tinea Cruris

Tinea cruris begins as a small, red, scaling rash in the groin that spreads peripherally and clears centrally. The edges are sharply marginated and scalloped, extending down the thighs. Generally, the scrotum is not noticeably involved. Other conditions to consider are seborrheic dermatitis (which usually can be differentiated by involvement of other areas of the body such as the ears, scalp, and eyelids), intertrigo (generally secondary to friction and maceration), contact dermatitis, candidiasis (which usually involves the inner thigh and causes the scrotum to appear bright red), and erythrasma (which will fluoresce under Woods lamp). The clinician should always check the feet to ensure there is no fungal involvement in that area as well. In general, this condition affects only postpubertal children. Diagnosis is made by KOH preparation. Nonspecific measures for treatment include loose-fitting clothing, reducing the amount of perspiration. Clotrimazole, miconazole, tolnaftate, and econazole are useful as topical antifungal agents. Rarely, oral griseofulvin may be needed in severe cases.

Tinea Pedis

Tinea pedis is generally caused by *Trichophyton rubrum* or *Trichophyton mentagrophytes.* It occurs most commonly in postpubertal children. The cracking and peeling of the skin suggestive of tinea pedis in prepubertal children more often indicates the presence of atopic eczema or hyperhidrosis. KOH preparation will demonstrate hyphae, especially when samples are taken from between the fourth and fifth interspaces of the toes. Clinically, the skin has a dry, white, hazy appearance and is often pruritic. When secondary bacterial infection is present, an odor occurs. At times, an inflammatory lesion (caused by *T. mentagrophytes*) causes blistering. The presence of an id reaction indicates dissemination of antigen to other parts of the body, especially the hands.

The differential diagnosis of tinea pedis includes simple maceration, contact dermatitis, and atopic eczema. Treatment consists of drying the feet thoroughly after washing; wearing dry, clean socks; avoiding caffeine-containing foods to decrease sweating; keeping shoes off as much as possible; and walking barefoot or in sandals. Topical antifungal agents and/or oral griseofulvin are used to treat this condition.

Tinea Versicolor

Tinea versicolor refers to a superficial infection of the skin caused by *Malassezia,* which produces color changes of the skin, hypopigmentation, hyperpigmentation, and sometimes a salmon-colored redness (Figs. 96.17 and 96.25). Wood light examination usually shows yellowish-brown fluorescence. Because moisture promotes growth of the organism, exacerbations occur in warm weather or in athletes who sweat excessively. The infection is difficult to eradicate and recurs frequently. A KOH preparation shows short, stubby hyphae and large clusters of spores, often referred to as "spaghetti and meatballs."

Treatment consists of lathering the entire body with selenium sulfide shampoo (2.5% concentration) or ketoconazole shampoo after wetting the skin surface in a shower. The lather is left on for 5 to 10 minutes and is then showered off. This procedure is carried out daily during the first week, with decreasing frequency over the ensuing weeks. Maintenance therapy once weekly throughout the summer or warmer seasons is advisable because of the high incidence of recurrence. Localized areas of involvement can be treated with topical antifungal agents (e.g., econazole, ketoconazole topically). Adolescents can be treated with 400 mg of ketoconazole given as a single oral dose and then 200 mg at monthly intervals during the warm summer months or during a sports season when the patient sweats frequently. Because tinea versicolor

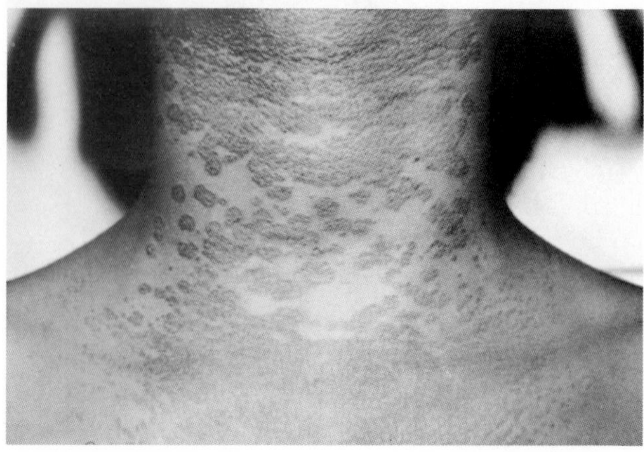

FIGURE 96.25 Scaly white patches consistent with tinea versicolor.

tends to be a recurrent problem, retreatment in subsequent years may be necessary.

PAPULOSQUAMOUS ERUPTIONS/SCALY RED PATCHES AND PLAQUES

Papulosquamous eruptions are discussed in Chapter 65 Rash: Papulosquamous Eruptions. These are conditions that are a mixture of papules or plaques with scale. They are often red but can be more pink or purple in color as in lichen planus.

Conditions that Lack Pruritus

Parapsoriasis

Parapsoriasis is an uncommon pediatric skin condition. When it occurs, however, the course is chronic and, on rare occasions, may progress to cutaneous lymphoma. The appearance of this eruption is easily mistaken for nummular eczema, psoriasis, tinea corporis, or a lichenoid change. Small oval scaling, erythematous (Fig. 96.26) to yellow-brown macules are concentrated on the trunk. The skin lesions are asymptomatic, and the patient feels healthy.

Treatment is unnecessary because the disease is asymptomatic. Topical steroids may be helpful but may not entirely clear the skin changes. The eruption clears spontaneously after varying periods.

Pityriasis Rosea

For more information about pityriasis rosea, see Chapter 65 Rash: Papulosquamous Eruptions. This is a harmless skin condition that generally occurs in preadolescents to adults and contains scaly pink or red plaques often in a "Christmas tree" distribution on the back (Fig. 96.18). There are atypical variants that are more papular and scaly and include the head and neck. One should consider secondary syphilis in the differential of pityriasis rosea (Fig. 96.20). Guttate psoriasis should also be included in the differential.

Secondary Syphilis

Please see previous discussion in this chapter.

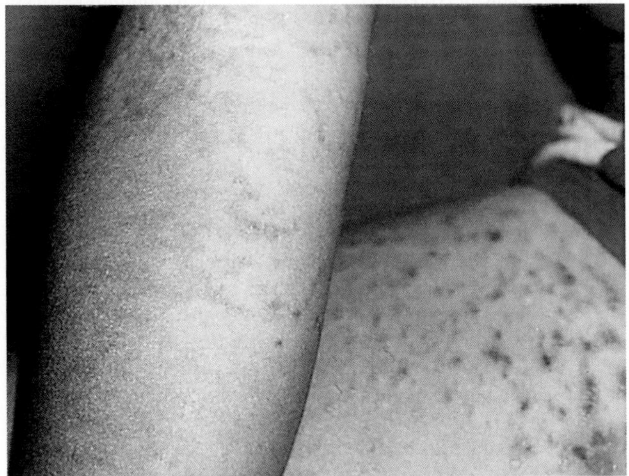

FIGURE 96.26 Digitate scaly red patches consistent with parapsoriasis.

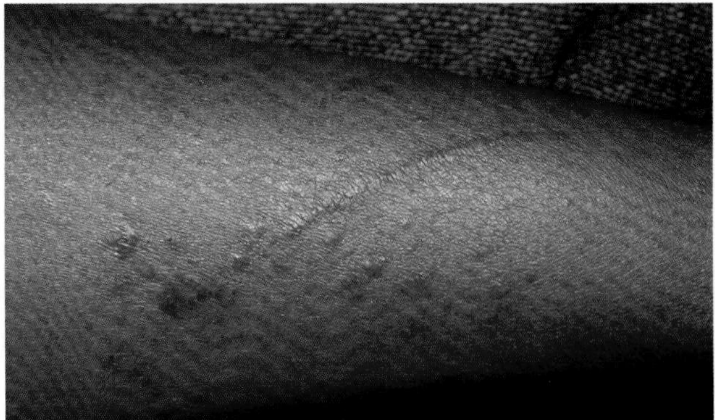

FIGURE 96.27 Purple polygonal papules consistent with lichen planus.

Pruritic Papulosquamous Disorders

Lichen Planus

Lichen planus is seen occasionally in pediatric patients as a chronic, pruritic, reddish-blue (violaceous) to purplish eruption. Two percent to 3% of cases occur in patients younger than 20 years of age.

The eruption generally involves the flexors of the wrist, forearms, and legs, especially the dorsum of the foot and ankles. The highly pruritic lesions appear as small, violaceous, shiny, flat-topped, polygonal papules (Fig. 96.27). These qualities may be recalled with the alliterative mnemonic of the five *p*'s: *p*ruritic, *p*urplish, *p*lanar, *p*olygonal, *p*apules. Some add a sixth *p* indicating a predilection for so-called "private" areas such as penis or vulva. The surface of these papules may have white cross-hatching, called Wickham striae. Lesions may occur in sites of trauma or injury (Koebner phenomenon). The scalp may be involved, often resulting in a scarring alopecia, called lichen planopilaris. It is important to examine the buccal mucous membranes and the genital areas for a reticulated or lace-like pattern of white papules or streaks. This finding is characteristic for lichen planus. The nails are often pitted, dystrophic, or ridged (pterygium nails). The lesions in lichen planus can be vesicular or bullous. Hypertrophic and linear lesions occur but are less common. Persistent, severe, postinflammatory hyperpigmentation is common in African Americans. In two-thirds of patients, the lesions clear within 8 to 15 months. The cause of the disorder is unknown. Topical therapy with steroids can be helpful, and treatment with oral steroids may be necessary for extremely symptomatic patients. For chronic cases, ultraviolet light phototherapy can be an effective adjunct to therapy.

Seborrheic Dermatitis

For more information about seborrheic dermatitis, see Chapter 64 Rash: Neonatal. This is a red eruption with greasy scale that is seen in neonates and then in adolescence and adulthood.

Pityriasis Rubra Pilaris

Pityriasis rubra pilaris (PRP) is characterized by follicular papules and yellow-orange skin that surrounds islands of normal skin. Of patients with PRP, 30% are children.

The onset of the disease is gradual, beginning in the scalp and spreading to involve the face and ears. Acuminate follicular papules with keratotic plugs occur on the back of the fingers, side of the neck, and extensors of the extremities. The skin is generally salmon colored and scaly. As the eruption progresses, it surrounds islands of normal skin. Yellow thickening of the palms and soles is characteristic. In contrast to psoriasis, nail pitting is rarely ever observed in PRP. Three subtypes have been described: The familial form has its onset in infancy and childhood, a localized type is found in 60% of cases, and the acquired form occurs in persons older than 15 years. The cause of this disease is unknown, although it is a disorder of keratinization. The condition responds to vitamin A and its derivatives.

Psoriasis

Psoriasis occurs in three forms during childhood: guttate, erythrodermic, and pustular. Any or all of these types may develop with silvery scales into the chronic, plaque-type psoriasis. For a more detailed discussion please see Chapter 65 Rash: Papulosquamous Eruptions.

VASCULAR LESIONS

Pyogenic Granulomas

Pyogenic granulomas (Fig. 96.8) are vascular nodules that develop rapidly at the site of an injury, such as a cut, scratch, insect bite, or burn. Clinically, the lesions are bright red to reddish-brown or blue-black. The vascular nodules are pedunculated, ranging from 0.5 to 2 cm in size. Their surfaces are glistening, or raspberry-like, often becoming eroded and crusted. They bleed easily. Removal by curettage, excision, or laser is advisable because few spontaneous resolve. Acute bleeding may be managed by cautery, by constriction with a suture, or by excision.

Hemangioma

Hemangiomas, including PHACE and LUMBAR syndromes, are detailed in Chapter 64 Rash: Neonatal.

URTICARIA/WHEALS

Urticaria is often encountered in the pediatric population, occurring in 2% to 3% of all children. In most cases, no cause is identified. A small number of cases are caused by allergic reactions from the ingestion of drugs or foods (e.g., nuts, eggs, shellfish, strawberries). Urticaria also follows viral (e.g., Epstein–Barr virus, hepatitis), bacterial (streptococcal), or parasitic infections. Physical factors, including dermographism, cholinergic stimulation (induced by heat, exercise, and emotional tension), cold (acquired and familial), and solar exposure, can induce urticaria. Finally, urticaria may be caused by factors producing a vasculitis or other autoimmune phenomena (particularly thyroid diseases) and substances causing degranulation of mast cells (e.g., radiocontrast material). Episodes of urticaria that last less than 6 weeks are termed *transient* or *acute*. The most common causes of urticaria are infection, insect bites, drugs, and foods. Chronic urticaria is defined as that which lasts for more than 6 weeks. No cause is found in 90% of children. These cases include the physical urticarias or urticarial vasculitis. The lesion itself follows vasodilation and leakage of fluid and red blood cells from involved vessels. The vascular damage can be caused by mediators such as histamine complement and immune complexes. IgE can attach to and cause degranulation of mast cells in sensitized individuals, with resulting histamine release. Urticarias are usually acute and transient but at times become chronic and recurrent.

Clinical Manifestations

The typical urticarial lesions are familiar to all physicians. They can be localized or generalized (involving the entire body). At times, the lesions are giant with serpiginous borders. Individual wheals rarely last more than 12 to 24 hours. Most commonly, the lesions appear in one area for 20 minutes to 3 hours, disappear, and then reappear in another location. The total duration of an episode is usually 24 to 48 hours; however, the course can last 3 to 6 weeks. In young children, urticaria may have an annular or polycyclic (coalescent annular) or arcuate (partially annular) appearance and may be associated with edema of the hands or feet. Because this is frequently confused with EM (which manifest with more fixed, targetoid lesions), this annular urticarial hypersensitivity has sometimes been referred to as *urticaria multiforme*.

Management

Acute relief can be accomplished by oral diphenhydramine 1 mg per kg (max 50 mg). Oral antihistamines are useful for maintenance therapy for transient urticaria. H1 antihistamines for 4 to 6 weeks are usually effective for controlling urticaria. Many recommend combinations of H1 and H2 antihistamines, but there is currently insufficient evidence to support this as a routine practice. Shorter-acting agents like hydroxyzine can be used for breakthrough.

Suggested Readings and Key References

General

Eichenfield LF, Esterly NB, Frieden IJ. *Textbook of neonatal dermatology.* Philadelphia, PA: Elsevier Health Sciences, 2014.

Goldsmith LA, Katz SI, Gilchrest B, et al. *Fitzpatrick's dermatology in general medicine.* 8th ed. New York, NY: McGraw-Hill, 2012.

Goldsmith L, Papier A. *VisualDx: essential pediatric dermatology.* Visual Dx: The Modern Library of Visual Medicine, 2009.

Harper J, Oranje A, Prose N. *Textbook of pediatric dermatology.* Oxford, England: Blackwell Science, 2012.

James WD, Berger TG, Elston D. *Andrews' diseases of the skin.* 11th ed. Philadelphia, PA: WB Saunders, 2011.

Paller AS, Mancini AJ. *Hurwitz clinical pediatric dermatology.* 4th ed. Philadelphia, PA: WB Saunders, 2011.

Schachner LA, Hansen RC. *Pediatric dermatology.* 4th ed. New York, NY: Churchill Livingstone, 2011.

Treat JR. *Curbside consultation in pediatric dermatology.* 1st ed. Slack Inc., 2012.

Atopic Dermatitis

Flohr C, Mann J. New insights into the epidemiology of childhood atopic dermatitis. *Allergy* 2014;69(1):3–16.

Lio PA, Lee M, LeBovidge J, et al. Clinical management of atopic dermatitis: practical highlight and updates from the atopic dermatitis practice parameter 2012. *J Allergy Clin Immunol Pract* 2014;2(4): 361–369.

Mathes EF, Oza V, Frieden IJ, et al. "Eczema coxsackium" and unusual cutaneous findings in an enterovirus outbreak. *Pediatrics* 2013;132(1):e149–e157.

Sanders JE, Garcia SE. Pediatric herpes simplex virus infections: an evidence-based approach to treatment. *Pediatr Emerg Med Pract* 2014;11(1):1–19.

Torti CR, Diaz L, Eichenfield LF. 2014 update on atopic dermatitis in children. *Curr Opin Pediatr* 2014;25(4):466–471.

Allergic Contact Dermatitis

Adami S, Jacob SE. Allergic contact dermatitis in children: review of the past decade. *Curr Allergy Asthma Rep* 2014;14(4):421.

Epstein WL. Topical prevention of poison ivy/oak dermatitis. *Arch Dermatol* 1989;125:499–501.

Diaper Dermatitis

Berg RW, Buckingham KW, Stewart RL. Etiologic factors in diaper dermatitis: the role of urine. *Pediatr Dermatol* 1986;3:102–106.

Blume-Peytavi U, Hauser M, Lünnemann L, et al. Prevention of diaper dermatitis in infants-a literature review. *Pediatr Dermatol* 2014; 31(4):413–429.

Honig PJ, Gribetz B, Leyden JL, et al. Amoxicillin and diaper dermatitis. *J Am Acad Dermatol* 1988;19:275–279.

Shin HL. Diagnosis and management of diaper dermatitis. *Pediatr Clin North Am* 2014;61(2):367–382.

Drug Reactions

Dodiuk-Gad RP, Laws PM, Shear NH. Epidemiology of severe drug hypersensitivity. *Semin Ctan Med Surg* 2014;33(1):2–9.

Kirchhof MG, Miliszewski MA, Sikora S, et al. Retrospective review of Stevens-Johnson syndrome/toxic epidermal necrolysis treatment comparing intravenous immunoglobulin with cyclosporine. *J Am Acad Dermatol* 2014;71(5):941–947.

Mathur AN, Mathes EF. Urticaria mimickers in children. *Dermatol Ther* 2013;25(6):467–475.

Mockenhaupt M. Stevens-Johnson syndrome and toxic epidermal necrolysis: clinical patterns, diagnostic considerations, etiology and therapeutic management. *Semin Cutan Med Surg* 2014;33(1): 10–16.

Schawartz RA, McDonough PH, Lee BW. Toxic epidermal necrolysis: Part II. Prognosis, sequelae, diagnosis, differential diagnosis, prevention and treatment. *J Am Acad Dermatol* 2013;69(2):187.

Wong S, Koh M. PD33—Drug Reaction and Eosinophilia with systemic symptoms (DRESS): a 10 year review in a pediatric population. *Clin Transl Allergy* 2014;4(suppl 3rd Pediatric Allergy and Asthma Meeting):P33.

Staphylococcal Scalded Skin Syndrome

Braunstein I, Wanat KA, Abuabara K, et al. Antibiotic sensitivity and resistance patterns in pediatric staphylococcal scalded skin syndrome. *Pediatr Dermatol* 2014;31(3):305–308.

Stanley JR, Amagai M. Pemphigus, bullous impetigo and the staphylococcal scaled skin syndrome. *N Engl J Med* 2006;355:1800–1810.

Bites and Infestations

Fuller LC. Epidemiology of scabies. *Curr Opin Infect Dis* 2013;26(2): 123–126.

Howard R, Frieden IJ. Papular urticaria in children. *Pediatr Dermatol* 1996;13:246–249.

Jucket G. Arthropod bites. *Am Fam Physician* 2013;88(12):841–847.

Mounsey KE, McCarthy JS. Treatment and control of scabies. *Curr Opin Infect Dis* 2013;26(2):133–139.

Paller AS. Scabies in infants and small children. *Semin Dermatol* 1993; 12:3–8.

Shmidt E, Levitt J. Dermatologic infestations. *Int J Dermatol* 2012; 51(2):131.

Fungal Infections

Hawkins DM, Smidt AC. Superficial fungal infections in children. *Pediatr Clin North Am* 2014;61(2):443–455.

Honig PJ, Caputo GL, Leyden JJ, et al. Microbiology of kerions. *J Pediatr* 1993;123:422.

Honig PJ, Caputo GL, Leyden JJ, et al. Treatment of kerions. *Pediatr Dermatol* 1994;11:69.

Jensen RH, Arendrup MC. Molecular diagnosis of dermatophyte infections. *Curr Opin Infect Dis* 2012;25(2):126–134.

Hemangiomas

Iacobas I, Burrows PE, Frieden IJ, et al. LUMBAR: association between cutaneous infantile hemangiomas of the lower body and regional congenital anomalies. *J Pediatr* 2010;157(5):795–801.

Johnson EF, Smidt AC. Not just a diaper rash: LUMBAR syndrome. *J Pediatr* 2014;164(1):208–209.

Metry DW, Dowd CF, Barkovich AJ, et al. The many faces of PHACE syndrome. *J Pediatr* 2001;139:117–123.

Metry DW, Hebert AA. Benign cutaneous vascular tumors of infancy: when to worry, what to do. *Arch Dermatol* 2000;136:905–914.

Urticaria

Berstein JA, Lang DM, Khan DA, et al. The diagnosis and management of acute and chronic urticarial: 2014 update. *J Allergy Clin Immunol* 2014;133(5):1270–1277.

Ghosh S, Kanwar AJ, Kaur A. Urticaria in children. *Pediatr Dermatol* 1993;10:107.

Zuberbier T, Aberer W, Asero R, et al. The EAAC1/GA(2) LEN/EDF/ WAO Guideline for the definition, classification, diagnosis and management of urticarial: the 2013 revision and update. *Allergy* 2014;69(7):868–887.

Warts and Molluscum

Brown J, Janniger CK, Schwartz RA, et al. Childhood molluscum contagiosum. *Int J Dermatol* 2006;45:93–99.

Kwok CS, Gibbs S, Bennett C, et al. Topical treatments for cutaneous warts. *Cochrane Database Syst Rev* 2012;9:CD001781.

Olsen JR, Gallacher J, Piguet V, et al. Epidemiology of molluscum contagiosum in children: a systemic review. *Fam Pract* 2014;31(2): 130–136.

Smolinski KN, Yan AC. How and when to treat molluscum contagiosum and warts in children. *Pediatr Ann* 2005;34:211–221.

Congenital Herpes Simplex

Antaya RJ, Robinson DM. Blisters and pustules in the newborn. *Pediatr Ann* 2010;39(10):171–179.

Berardi A, Lugli L, Rossi C, et al. Neonatal herpes simplex virus. *J Matern Fetal Neonatal Med* 2011;24(suppl 1):88–90.

Brown ZA, Selke S, Zeh J, et al. The acquisition of herpes simplex virus during pregnancy. *N Engl J Med* 1997;337:509–515.

Brown ZA, Vontver LA, Benedetti J, et al. Effects on infants of a first episode of genital herpes during pregnancy. *N Engl J Med* 1987;317: 1246–1251.

Kimberlin DW. Herpes simplex virus infections in neonates and early childhood. *Semin Pediatr Infect Dis* 2005;16:271–281.

Kimberlin DW, Lin CY, Jacobs RF, et al. Natural history of neonatal herpes simplex virus infections in the acyclovir era. *Pediatrics* 2001; 108:223–229.

Kimberlin DW, Lin CY, Jacobs RF, et al. Safety and efficacy of high-dose intravenous acyclovir in the management of neonatal herpes simplex virus infections. *Pediatrics* 2001;108:230–238.

Pityriasis Rosea

Chuh AA, Dofitasa BL, Comisel GG, et al. Interventions for pityriasis rosea. *Cochrane Database Syst Rev* 2007;2:CD005068.

Drago F, Broccolo F, Rebora A. Pityriasis rosea: an update with a critical appraisal of its possible herpesviral etiology. *J Am Acad Dermatol* 2009;61(2):303–318.

Drago F, Rebora A. Treatments for pityriasis rosea. *Skin Therapy Lett* 2009;14(3):6–7.

Hartley AH. Pityriasis rosea. *Pediatr Rev* 1999;20:266–269.

CHAPTER 97 ■ ENDOCRINE EMERGENCIES

MICHAEL S.D. AGUS, MD AND KATE DORNEY, MD

KEY POINTS

DKA/Hyperglycemia

- 1% of children with diabetic ketoacidosis will develop cerebral edema
- Risk factors for cerebral edema include elevated blood urea nitrogen, low Pco_2, treatment with bicarbonate, failure of serum Na to rise steadily with correction of hyperglycemia, age <3 years, new-onset diabetes
- Hyperglycemia in ED setting can result from numerous triggers including intercurrent illness or trauma in patient with known DM, new-onset DM, other illnesses associated with hyperglycemia, spurious sample, medication effect

Hypoglycemia

- Prompt recognition of hypoglycemia is important to avoid adverse outcomes
- Hypoglycemia in absence of ketones is consistent with hyperinsulinism or fatty acid oxidation enzyme deficiencies

Hypopituitarism

- The acute presentation of hypopituitarism is most likely to occur when the child is stressed by injury, illness, or fasting
- Children with hypopituitarism are prone to hypoglycemia
- Hypopituitarism is associated with intracranial developmental anomalies or lesions

Adrenal Insufficiency/Congenital Adrenal Hyperplasia

- Cortisol and aldosterone replacement in patients with adrenal insufficiency under stress conditions is imperative
- ED presentations include addisonian crisis, ambiguous genitalia, acute salt-wasting crisis, and precocious puberty
- Patients with acute salt-wasting crisis must be recognized and treated immediately with fluid resuscitation, stress dose hydrocortisone, careful monitoring of electrolytes

Pheochromocytoma

- Often presents with headache, palpitations, sweating; but also nervousness, tremulousness, fatigue, chest/abdominal pain, and flushing
- Most associated with hypertension although can be paroxysmal; alpha blockade is antihypertensive of choice, avoid pure beta blockade as can lead to severe hypertension

Diabetes Insipidus

- Inability of kidneys to concentrate urine resulting in polyuria/polydipsia
- Hypertonic dehydration if thirst is not intact or access to fluids is restricted; if occurs abruptly, patient at risk for central pontine myelinolysis
- Consider in patients with increased urine excretion, enuresis, and increased thirst
- Management is similar to hypernatremic dehydration with initial reexpansion of intravascular volume, then repletion of maintenance over 48 hours

Syndrome of Inappropriate Antidiuretic Hormone Secretion

- Associated with bacterial meningitis (50%), positive pressure ventilation (20%), Rocky Mountain spotted fever (70%), and numerous other illnesses
- For severe lethargy, seizure, or coma administer 3% saline emergently (3 mL per kg every 10 to 20 minutes as needed), consider furosemide, initiate antiepileptic drugs if indicated, and treat underlying cause

Hyperparathyroidism

- Uncommon in children
- Family history is important as hyperparathyroidism is associated with MEN I, II and being an infant born to a mother with hypoparathyroidism
- Demineralization and bone resorption seen on x-ray

Hypoparathyroidism

- Rare in children but tends to be associated with familial autoimmune syndromes, immunologic deficiencies, or iatrogenic etiologies

Rickets

- Rickets is caused by inadequate dietary intake of vitamin D; incidence is decreasing as increased awareness and increased supplementation in food
- Failure of calcification affects those parts of the skeleton that are growing most rapidly or that are under stress; a clinical diagnosis that is confirmed by radiology

Thyroid Storm

- Thyroid storm is the fulminant intensification of hyperthyroid state
- Precipitated by intercurrent infection, trauma, or after subtotal thyroidectomy with an inadequately prepared patient
- Presence of high fever (often to 105.8°F [41°C]) is primary distinguishing feature of Thyroid Storm from hyperthyroid
- Marked increase in cardiac workload may result in high-output heart failure and hypotension and pulmonary edema rather than classic hypertension

Neonatal Thyrotoxicosis

- Neonatal thyrotoxicosis is a life-threatening condition found in 1% to 5% of infants born to mothers with history of hyperthyroidism; mother's thyroid disease does not have to be active during pregnancy

Congenital Hypothyroidism

- Increased incidence of ED visits for congenital hypothyroidism now that infants are being routinely screened at birth
- Untreated disease may result in impairment of neurologic development

See Table 97.1.

TABLE 97.1

SUMMARY OF CLINICAL FEATURES, INVESTIGATIONS, AND INITIAL TREATMENT OF PEDIATRIC ENDOCRINE EMERGENCIES

Condition	Major clinical features	Urgent investigations	Initial treatment
Diabetic ketoacidosis	Polyuria, polydipsia, dehydration, ketotic breath, hyperpnea, nausea, vomiting, abdominal pain, coma	Blood glucose, pH	0.9% saline 10 mL/kg in first 1–2 hrs IV; insulin infusion 0.1 Unit/kg/hr; later, may need KAcetate 10–60 mEq/L and KPhos 10–20 mEq/L
Hypoglycemia	*Older child:* hunger, sweatiness, dizziness, convulsions, coma *Neonate:* apnea, hypotonia, hypothermia, irritability, tremor, convulsions	Blood glucose Serum for growth hormone, cortisol, insulin; first voided urine for organic acids and toxin screen	25% dextrose 1–2 mL/kg IV bolus or 10% dextrose 5–10 mg/kg/min IV infusion, glucagon 0.5–1 mg IM stat (if hyperinsulinism)
Congenital adrenal hyperplasia	Ambiguous genitalia in females; poor feeding, weight loss, irritability, vomiting, dehydration	Plasma sodium, potassium, glucose, 17-hydroxyprogesterone; karyotype and pelvic ultrasound	0.9% saline 20 mL/kg in first hour IV; hydrocortisone 25 mg IV stat (neonatal dose)
Adrenal insufficiency	Nausea, vomiting, abdominal pain, weakness, malaise, hypotension, dehydration, hyperpigmentation	Plasma sodium, potassium, glucose, cortisol, and ACTH (for retrospective confirmation of diagnosis)	Hydrocortisone 100 mg IV stat; 10% dextrose in 0.9% saline 20 mL/kg in first hour
Hypercalcemia (hyperparathyroidism)	Headache, irritability, anorexia, constipation, polyuria, polydipsia, dehydration, hypertension	Plasma calcium, phosphate	0.9% saline at two to three times maintenance rate; furosemide 1 mg/kg
Hypocalcemia (hypoparathyroidism)	Cramps, carpopedal spasms, paresthesias, lethargy, apathy, convulsions, hypotension	Plasma calcium, phosphate, alkaline phosphatase	10% calcium gluconate 1 mL/kg IV over 15 min
Diabetes insipidus	Polyuria, polydipsia, dehydration, irritability, fever, drowsiness, coma	Paired plasma and urine osmolality and sodium	*Central:* IV fluids at two-thirds maintenance rate plus replete deficit over 48 hrs; Pitressin 1–10 mU/kg/hr IV *Nephrogenic:* IV fluids at urine output plus replete deficit over 48 hrs
Syndrome of inappropriate antidiuretic hormone secretion	Anorexia, headache, nausea, vomiting, irritability, seizures, coma	Paired plasma and urine osmolality and sodium	*Seizures:* 3% saline at 1–3 mL/kg IV; furosemide 1 mg/kg IV stat; benzodiazepines *Otherwise:* fluid restriction
Thyroid storm	Goiter, exophthalmos, high fever, tachycardia, congestive cardiac failure, delirium, stupor	Free T_4, TSH	Propranolol 10 µg/kg IV over 15 min; Lugol iodine 9–15 drops/day orally; methimazole 20–30 mg q6–12h (initially); tepid sponging
Neonatal thyrotoxicosis	Goiter, failure to gain weight, irritability, tachycardia, congestive cardiac failure	Free T_4, TSH	Propranolol 1 mg/kg tid orally; potassium iodide two drops bid orally; methimazole 0.5–0.7 mg/kg/day divided tid orally
Congenital hypothyroidism	Asymptomatic: hypothermia, hypoactivity, poor feeding, constipation, prolonged jaundice, large posterior fontanel	Free T_4, TSH	L-thyroxine 10–15 µg/kg/day orally
Hypopituitarism	See features listed for adrenal insufficiency and hypoglycemia		

IV, intravenous; IM, intramuscular; ACTH, adrenocorticotropic hormone; TSH, thyroid-stimulating hormone; tid, three times daily; bid, twice per day.

DIABETIC KETOACIDOSIS

Goals of Treatment

To identify patients with DKA and initiate treatment per algorithm.
To recognize patients with cerebral edema (1%) and intervene with appropriate treatment.

CLINICAL PEARLS AND PITFALLS

- Clinically significant cerebral edema is the most serious immediate risk to the child, occurring in 1% of cases, and it remains so during the first 24 hours of therapy, despite the more apparent issues of hypovolemia and acidosis.
- The treatment for symptomatic cerebral edema is mannitol and/or 3% saline.
- Avoid bicarbonate administration.

Current Evidence

Insulin deficiency initially leads to hyperglycemia that, once above the renal threshold of 180 mg per dL, leads to polyuria due to an osmotic diuresis. Without vigorous oral repletion at home, the child quickly becomes hypovolemic, prompting a stress response and elevations of the counterregulatory hormones glucagon, cortisol, growth hormone, and catecholamines. These hormonal changes produce significant insulin resistance and stimulate glycogenolysis and gluconeogenesis that worsens the hyperglycemia, hypovolemia, and stress response. In this insulin-deficient state, adipose tissue is broken down in large quantities into free fatty acids, subsequently converted into ketoacids in the liver. Ketoacids readily dissociate in the blood to produce free hydrogen ions, and metabolic acidosis ensues. This reaction is partially compensated for by a respiratory alkalosis (hyperventilation), with a resultant lowering of Pco_2 and plasma bicarbonate (HCO_3^-).

Intracellular potassium is depleted because of transcellular shifts of this ion brought about by the exchange of potassium with excess free hydrogen ions and extracellular dehydration. Protein catabolism secondary to insulin deficiency causes a negative nitrogen balance and results in additional efflux of potassium from cells. The potassium is then lost in the urine during the osmotic diuresis. Volume depletion causes secondary hyperaldosteronism, which further promotes urinary potassium excretion. Thus, total body depletion of potassium occurs, although the plasma potassium concentration may not reflect the loss at the time of presentation.

Clinical Considerations

Clinical Recognition

In cases of new-onset diabetes, the child usually has a history of polyuria and polydipsia for a few days or weeks before the acute decompensation. Significant weight loss often occurs despite a vigorous appetite. Vomiting is common once the child has ketoacidosis; these further losses plus the inability to compensate for polyuria contribute to the hypovolemia.

In children known to have diabetes, the prodrome may be less than 24 hours and precipitated by an intercurrent illness, inappropriate sick day management, or omission of insulin doses.

Triage

On physical examination, particular attention should be paid to the degree of dehydration, including skin turgor and dryness of mucous membranes. Urine output is not a reliable sign of hydration status. In severe cases, the child may exhibit signs of compensated shock, including a thready pulse and cold extremities, and rarely, as uncompensated shock with hypotension. The smell of ketones on the breath and the presence of hyperpneic (Kussmaul) respirations reflect the ketoacidosis. The patient's consciousness level, which may range from full alertness to deep coma, should be noted.

Initial Assessment/H&P

Patients may complain of nausea, vomiting, and abdominal pain, and the parents may have noticed increasing listlessness. Less than 2% of children are in coma at the time of hospital admission, although a higher percentage has an altered state of consciousness. The history and physical examination usually suggest the diagnosis; however, particularly in the patient with new-onset diabetes, presenting clinical features can be misdiagnosed, especially in the infant or young child. For example, abdominal pain may be misinterpreted as appendicitis; hyperpnea may be mistaken as a sign of pneumonia or asthma; and polyuria may be incorrectly diagnosed as a urinary tract infection. Enuresis, polydipsia, and irritability are sometimes wrongly categorized as behavioral problems. The child may have exquisite abdominal tenderness with guarding and rigidity, which can mimic an acute abdomen. The ears, throat, chest, and urine should be examined because infection is often a precipitating factor. Careful attention should be paid to the skin examination because there have been several case reports of fasciitis copresenting with DKA. The presence of hyperpigmentation (acanthosis nigricans) on the posterior neck is a sign of long-standing insulin resistance and should alert the clinician to the possibility of non–insulin-dependent diabetes.

Management/Diagnostic Testing

Diagnostic laboratory findings include plasma glucose greater than 200 mg per dL (commonly 400 to 800 mg per dL), the presence of glucose and ketones in the urine, and acidosis (venous pH less than 7.3 and serum bicarbonate less than 15 mEq per L). Additionally, high or normal plasma potassium, and slightly elevated blood urea nitrogen are common. Occasionally, DKA can occur with normoglycemia when persistent vomiting and decreased intake of carbohydrates are accompanied by continued administration of insulin or when patients have kept themselves particularly well hydrated with non–glucose-containing fluids. The measured serum sodium is usually low or in the low to normal range. In the setting of hyperglycemia, the measured sodium will be lowered; a commonly used estimate for correction is a decrease of 2 mEq/L Na for every 100 mg per dL elevation in glucose above normal. Leukocytosis with a left shift may be noted but does not necessarily signify an underlying infection. Hyperglycemia in the absence of acidosis should cause the clinician to consider additional possibilities (see Hyperglycemia section).

For the severely dehydrated child, initial treatment is directed toward expansion of intravascular volume and administration of insulin. Subsequent treatment is directed at the normalization of the remaining abnormal biochemical parameters. Medical intervention carries significant risks of hypokalemia and cerebral edema (Tables 97.2 and 97.3).

TABLE 97.2

PRINCIPLES OF MANAGEMENT OF DIABETIC KETOACIDOSIS

Life-threatening complications

Cerebral edema

Cardiovascular collapse

Profound metabolic acidosis

Hyperkalemia

Hypokalemia

Hypophosphatemia

Areas of management decisions

- *Fluids.* Treat hypovolemia with crystalloid extracellular fluid expander. Use normal saline (0.9%) and infuse 10 mL/kg in the first 1–2 hrs. (Avoid hypotonic solutions initially because they are inefficient volume expanders and may contribute to cerebral edema.) Continue infusion at this rate until perfusion is improved and urine output is reestablished. After first 1–2 hrs, start half-normal saline—use greater tonicity, up to normal saline, if the initial serum sodium is less than 135 mmol/L or if the serum sodium falls with therapy. Total fluid administration in first 48 hrs should rarely exceed one and one-half to two times maintenance.
- *Alkali.* Avoid bicarbonate therapy in DKA. Only consider if arterial pH <6.9 and impaired cardiac contractility and vascular tone, or if patient has life-threatening hyperkalemia.
- *Potassium.* Start potassium therapy with administration of insulin. Starting concentration in fluid should be 40 mEq/L as a combination of potassium acetate and potassium phosphate. If the patient is hypokalemic (<4 mmol/L), a higher concentration of potassium, 60–80 mEq/L, may be necessary. Administer high concentrations of potassium only with electrocardiographic monitoring. If hyperkalemic (>6 mmol/L), decrease the concentration to 0–20 mEq/L.
- *Insulin.* Should be given as a continuous IV infusion (0.1 Unit/kg/hr).
- *Glucose.* Add 5% glucose to solutions when plasma glucose is approximately 300 mg/dL. Continue adding glucose up to 12.5% in a peripheral IV in order to keep plasma glucose in target range of 200–300 mg/dL.
- *Phosphate.* Add one-half of potassium in IVF as potassium phosphate up to 20 mEq/L, unless severe hypophosphatemia (PO_4 <2 mmol/L).

Monitoring

- *Clinical monitoring.* Blood pressure, pulse, respirations, neurologic status, and fluid intake and output. Continuous noninvasive $ETCO_2$ monitoring, if available.
- *Laboratory monitoring.* Obtain initial glucose, electrolytes, blood gases, and blood urea nitrogen. Measure blood glucose every hour initially as guide to insulin dosage. Repeat electrolytes and pH measurements two to four times hourly as necessary, every hour if severe abnormalities.
- *Use flow sheet.*

DKA, diabetic ketoacidosis; IV, intravenous; IVF, intravenous fluids; $ETCO_2$, end-tidal CO_2.

TABLE 97.3

RISK FACTORS FOR CEREBRAL EDEMA IN DIABETIC KETOACIDOSIS

Elevated blood urea nitrogen

Low PCO_2

Treatment with bicarbonate

Failure of measured serum [Na^+] to rise steadily with correction of hyperglycemia

Age <3 yrs

New-onset diabetes

Fluid and Electrolyte Replacement

Fluid replacement should be instituted promptly. In the first 1 to 2 hours, if hypovolemia is apparent, 10 mL per kg isotonic (0.9%) crystalloid (either normal saline or lactated Ringer's) should be infused intravenously to establish an adequate intravascular volume and improve tissue perfusion. Normal saline is generally preferred for initial resuscitation given that DKA patients already have a degree of lactic acidosis, however, lactated Ringer's has the benefit of a reduced chloride load. A small head-to-head trial showed no significant differences between the two fluids. Repeat bolus if the pulse rate and capillary refill rate do not improve, but rarely is more than 20 mL per kg required in the first hour. The goal of this initial rehydration therapy is not euvolemia but adequate perfusion of end organs, often best judged by monitoring mentation, capillary refill, and heart rate.

Once adequate intravascular volume is established, the fluid deficit should be replaced over the next 48 hours. During the first 4 to 6 hours of this period isotonic fluids should be used with appropriate additional electrolyte supplementation as detailed below. The total body water deficit may be estimated based on a clinical estimate of dehydration, or intravenous (IV) fluid may be administered at a rate between one and one-half and two times maintenance fluid requirements (see Chapters 17 Dehydration and 108 Renal and Electrolyte Emergencies). Urine output should be monitored and ongoing urinary losses in excess of 5 mL/kg/hr (osmotic diuresis) should also be replaced.

The Na^+ deficit typically approximates 10 mEq per kg body weight and Na^+ maintenance is 3 mEq per 100 mL of maintenance fluid. From a practical point of view, half-normal (0.45%) saline can be started after the initial 4- to 6-hour period of isotonic fluids. The measured serum sodium should rise with initiation of therapy. If the initial serum sodium is less than 136 mEq per L, or if the serum sodium falls with therapy, the IV fluid should be changed to a more concentrated sodium stock, and the patient should be watched particularly closely. Serum sodium failing to rise with therapy has been identified as a risk factor for cerebral edema. Correcting the serum sodium for the degree of hyperglycemia may be useful in following the patient's total body sodium status:

$$\text{Corrected } [Na^+] = \text{measured } [Na^+] + [2 \times (\text{measured plasma glucose} - 100)/100].$$

All children with DKA are total-body potassium depleted (5 mEq per kg body weight); therefore, potassium replacement is an important part of therapy. If the initial serum [K^+] is 3 to 4.5 mEq per L, 40 mEq per L of potassium is added to the infusion after vascular competency has been established and the child has urinated. If the serum [K^+] is 4.6 to 5.0 mEq per L, only 20 mEq per L of potassium should be added, and if the [K^+] is above 5.0 mEq per L, potassium should be withheld in the initial fluids. Generally, K^+ is provided as potassium acetate (or chloride) and potassium phosphate in equal amounts. If the initial serum [K^+] is less than 4 mEq per L, potassium replacement should be initiated promptly; if less than 3 mEq per L, IVF concentrations of K^+ of 60 mEq per L or greater may be necessary. With the higher concentrations of potassium, the phosphate component must be adjusted not to exceed the maximum rate. If the K^+ initial concentration is low, monitoring via an electrocardiogram (EKG) is indicated.

Phosphate depletion is almost universal in patients with DKA; however, the clinical significance of this reaction remains uncertain. As noted earlier, half of the K^+ replacement is with potassium phosphate, up to a maximum of 20 mEq potassium phosphate per liter except in the rare situation of severe hypophosphatemia (serum phosphate less than 2 mEq per L). Infusion of excess phosphate results in hypocalcemia, which may be complicated by tetanic seizures.

Bicarbonate Therapy

In retrospective reviews of patients with DKA who developed significant cerebral edema, bicarbonate administration was identified as a significant risk factor (Table 97.3). This may be because the sickest patients are the ones most likely to have received bicarbonate therapy; however, without further clarification of the pathophysiology, bicarbonate therapy is reserved for patients with both severe acidosis (pH <6.9) and secondary hemodynamic compromise that is unresponsive to inotropic agents.

A theoretical mechanism for the complications observed with bicarbonate therapy is the development of a paradoxical acidosis of the central nervous system (CNS) and resultant cerebral depression. Paradoxical acidosis occurs because administered HCO_3^- combines with excess H^+ ions in the bloodstream to form H_2O and CO_2. Because the blood–brain barrier is relatively more permeable to CO_2 than to HCO_3^-, CO_2 accumulates in the CNS, resulting in further exacerbation of acidosis in this compartment, while acidosis is being corrected systemically.

Insulin and Glucose

Regular insulin is used for the treatment of ketoacidosis, but it should not be administered until the initial isotonic fluids have been administered for 1 hour. Insulin is initially necessary to stop ongoing ketone body production, the primary cause of the acidosis. Insulin should be started after 1 hour of initial fluid expansion to steadily correct the acidosis and may be either infused intravenously or, if necessary, injected intramuscularly at hourly intervals. Subcutaneous injections of insulin should be avoided because of the uncertainties of absorption in a dehydrated patient. The starting dose of insulin for continuous infusion is 0.1 Unit/kg/hr, infused by a regulated pump. Failure of the glucose to decrease in response to insulin suggests improper insulin preparation, inadequate hydration, or serious underlying disease (e.g., appendicitis or fasciitis with resultant significant increases in counterregulatory hormones). It is unnecessary and possibly detrimental to give an initial bolus of insulin. The dose for the hourly intramuscular (IM) injection, used if IV access cannot be obtained, is 0.1 Unit/kg/hr.

Once the blood glucose approaches 300 mg per dL, dextrose should be added to the IV fluids. As long as the child remains acidotic, insulin infusion should never be stopped; instead, the amount of dextrose in the IV infusion should be increased in stepwise fashion up to a concentration of 12.5 g per dL to maintain the blood glucose between 200 and 300 mg per dL. If the blood glucose continues to drop, the rate of IV fluid administration should be increased to twice maintenance. If the blood glucose still cannot be maintained, the insulin infusion should be decreased by increments of 0.025 Unit/kg/hr.

When the child is able to eat and the anion gap has closed (normal = 10 to 12), IV infusion of insulin can be discontinued. If hourly IM injections are used, they should be continued until the blood glucose is less than 300 mg per dL and acidosis is correcting. Because IV insulin is metabolized rapidly, subcutaneous insulin must be given 30 minutes prior to the discontinuation of the infusion. The initial dose of subcutaneous insulin should be calculated, with consultation by a pediatric endocrinologist, based on a daily dose of 0.75 Unit/kg/day in the prepubertal child up to 1.0 Unit/kg/day in the pubertal child and beyond. The total daily dose must be divided into long-acting and short-acting insulins.

Cerebral Edema

Despite several investigations of the causes and risk factors for clinically significant cerebral edema in patients with DKA, and subsequent modifications in therapy, the incidence of the complication has not changed significantly during the past 20 years and remains at approximately 1%. Table 97.3 lists the leading risk factors published in more recent years. Clinical signs and symptoms of significant cerebral edema include abnormal motor or verbal response to pain, decorticate or decerebrate posturing, new cranial nerve palsy, and abnormal respiratory pattern. Other concerning signs are decrease or fluctuation in level of consciousness (e.g., Glasgow Coma Scale), age-inappropriate incontinence, vomiting, headache, and heart rate deceleration.

If these signs are noted by the physician at the bedside, a clinical diagnosis of cerebral edema must be made and treatment initiated without any diagnostic imaging. The patient should receive mannitol 1 g per kg IV over 10 minutes. There is some evidence that mannitol is the preferred first-line agent, but that hypertonic saline (3%) may be an appropriate second-line agent; however, only a large retrospective study and case series data are currently available.

Endotracheal intubation should be rarely considered, primarily if the patient's mental status does not assure a safe airway, and secondarily if the patient is not able to maintain a respiratory alkalosis to partially compensate for the metabolic acidosis. Noninvasive ventilation may also be considered in order to support the patient's efforts to achieve a respiratory alkalosis. If intubated, the patient should be initially hyperventilated to the P_{CO_2} he/she was maintaining prior to the neurologic decompensation (generally 10 to 20 mm Hg in the presence of severe ketoacidosis); this can be gradually reduced over several hours as the acidosis resolves and the cerebral edema is treated.

Only after the patient is fully stabilized should a confirmatory computed tomography of the head be considered, unless a diagnosis of intracerebral hemorrhage or thrombosis is strongly suspected.

Clinical Indications for Discharge or Admission

Close monitoring is mandatory, and a well-organized flowsheet ensures all parameters are being observed. Admission to an intensive care unit or specialized intermediate care unit should be considered if the patient is younger than 1 year of age, has a Glasgow Coma Scale score of less than 12, has a venous pH below 7.1, has an initial measured [Na^+] of more than 145 mEq per L, or has an initial [K^+] of less than 3 mEq per L.

The patient should be maintained on continuous cardiorespiratory monitoring with hourly assessments of blood pressure and level of consciousness until the patient's trajectory of illness has been clearly established. Careful neurologic examination, with particular attention to arousability and pupillary reactivity, should be performed frequently. The fluid input and output must be reviewed hourly to ensure appropriate rehydration is occurring. The IV fluids should be checked frequently so that pump failure or fluid leakage into the subcutaneous tissues can be corrected quickly. In the severely ill child, an EKG should be performed in the setting of hyperkalemia or hypokalemia. The plasma glucose should be measured hourly until the blood glucose is stable and less than 300 mg per dL, and as long as the child is on an insulin infusion. Glucose measurement may be less frequent once the patient has been changed to subcutaneous insulin. Serum [K^+] needs to be measured every 2 to 4 hours until the acidosis and hyperglycemia are normalized, or more frequently if hypokalemia is encountered or bicarbonate therapy is used. Calcium, phosphate, and magnesium should be assessed initially and followed every 2 to 4 hours, more frequently if any are being actively replaced. With the advent of point-of-care ketone measurements, it may be advisable to follow serum ketone concentration every 2 to 4 hours, although continuous noninvasive capnography with nasal cannula end-tidal CO_2 ($ETCO_2$) or transcutaneous CO_2 monitoring is also useful in tracking the degree of acidosis over time. Venous pH may be obtained to follow resolution of the acidosis if the above monitoring options are not available. Arterial sampling is not necessary for metabolic monitoring, and central venous access is rarely necessary.

When the child is better hydrated and the acidosis resolves, mental alertness will improve and symptoms of nausea, vomiting, and abdominal pain should remit. If they do not resolve, an abdominal disorder should be considered. Some patients complain of blurred vision, which is caused by lens distortion resulting from fluid shifts of rehydration and correction of hyperglycemia—this should resolve within 24 hours of conclusion of therapy. When the anion gap has closed, most patients are able to tolerate oral fluids, at which point rehydration can be continued orally *ad libitum*.

MILD KETOACIDOSIS/ HYPERGLYCEMIA

Goals of Treatment

To identify patients with hyperglycemia and/or mild ketoacidosis and initiate treatment per algorithm.

To create a sick day plan for patients able to orally rehydrate, create sick day plan for them upon discharge with close follow-up with their diabetes specialist.

CLINICAL PEARLS AND PITFALLS

- Fasting laboratory plasma glucose of greater than 126 mg per dL or a random glucose greater than 200 mg per dL on two separate occasions is diagnostic of diabetes in an otherwise healthy person. This definition was developed by specialists in adult diabetes and may not be completely applicable to the pediatric population.
- Hyperglycemia in ED setting can result from numerous triggers including intercurrent illness or trauma in patient with known DM, new-onset DM, other illnesses associated with hyperglycemia, spurious blood sample, and medication effect.
- For purposes of definition, a patient with hyperglycemia does not have DKA if venous pH is greater than 7.3 and serum bicarbonate is greater than 15 mEq per L.

Current Evidence

As noted in the previous section on diabetes and the following section on hypoglycemia, glucose homeostasis reflects the balance between glucose input (from gut absorption, hepatic glycogen breakdown, or gluconeogenesis) and disposal (via storage or oxidation). With the exception of gut absorption, this process is largely regulated by insulin, although counterregulatory hormones also have a significant effect. Furthermore, tissue factors and medication also impact the insulin effect.

Clinical Considerations

Clinical Recognition

Plasma glucose concentrations in the 200 to 300 mg per dL range rarely result in symptoms. This level of hyperglycemia may be accompanied by intermittent increased frequency of urination; however, parents are rarely aware of their child's frequency of urination once the child is toilet trained unless the frequency becomes disruptive (e.g., nocturia or "accidents" at school). Children and adolescents have no sense of what is the normal frequency of urination, so they rarely complain unless the frequent urination is accompanied by dysuria. Higher levels of glucose (greater than 300 mg per dL) may be associated with subtle clinical findings, such as blurring of vision or dryness of oral membranes. Significant hyperglycemia may occur without significant symptoms and can be tolerated for a prolonged period without clinical signs.

Triage

Generally these patients are asymptomatic and very well appearing. Care must be taken to distinguish from patients with more severe diabetic ketoacidosis and possible cerebral edema.

Initial Assessment/H&P

In the ED, hyperglycemia is likely to be seen in several different situations. First, the child may be known to have diabetes and present with an intercurrent illness or traumatic injury. Both illness and injury result in increased counterregulatory hormones, which may lead to relative insulin resistance and hyperglycemia. The second presentation is the child for whom diabetes is suspected because of classical symptoms of polyuria, polydipsia, and polyphagia accompanied by weight loss. Almost half of children with new-onset diabetes mellitus present to their pediatrician or to the ED in this way. Third, some medical conditions are associated with persistent hyperglycemia, such as recurrent urinary tract infections and vaginal yeast infections. Furthermore, type 2 diabetes is increasingly being reported in minority adolescents; in many, hyperpigmentation of the posterior neck and axilla (acanthosis nigricans) may be noted. Fourth, a laboratory panel obtained for some other reason (e.g., abdominal pain) may reveal hyperglycemia.

If a child is severely ill and has concomitant hyperglycemia, close attention should be paid to the underlying illness. Severity of hyperglycemia in the setting of critical illness is correlated with mortality, and it can be thought of as a general index of severity of illness in this nondiabetes setting.

Management/Diagnostic Testing

Children who are mildly dehydrated (5%) with slight acidosis will benefit from an IV fluid bolus (10 to 20 mL per kg of isotonic crystalloid); furthermore, this bolus may be given while awaiting laboratory test results.

Insulin therapy can be initiated subcutaneously, at a total daily dose of 0.25 to 0.5 Unit/kg/day for the prepubertal child and 0.5 to 0.75 Unit/kg/day for the adolescent. There are two general regimens for dividing this total daily dose. In the conventional regimen, two-thirds of the total daily dose is administered in the morning, and one-third before dinner; two-thirds of the morning dose and evening dose should be as an intermediate-duration insulin (NPH, Lente), the remaining one-third of the total daily dose is rapid-acting insulin (lispro, aspart). Using the basal-bolus approach, one-half of the total daily dose is administered as insulin glargine or detemir, two 24-hour–acting analogs, and rapid-acting insulin (lispro, aspart) is dosed as a combination of coverage for ingested carbohydrates and as a correction for the degree of hyperglycemia above a chosen target—these initial dosages should be calculated along with the help of a consulting diabetes specialist.

Hyperglycemia associated with critical illness should be managed in the context of the underlying illness. Specific therapy for hyperglycemia should generally not be initiated in the ED, but can wait until the patient arrives in the ICU.

Clinical Indications for Discharge or Admission

Some children with new-onset diabetes may also have hyperglycemia without ketoacidosis or with only mild acidosis. Generally, these patients are hospitalized for 24 to 48 hours to allow time to educate the family and stabilize the insulin dosage. Children with known diabetes often develop hyperglycemia and ketosis without significant acidosis (venous pH greater than 7.3 or bicarbonate greater than 15 mEq per L) during the course of intercurrent illness, especially gastroenteritis, or secondary to omission of insulin doses. Once the laboratory results are available, the physician must decide whether to hospitalize the child, continue treatment in the ED, or send the child home. Several factors must be considered before sending a child home.

1. Is the child fully conscious and alert?
2. Can the child drink and retain oral fluids?
3. Can home glucose monitoring be done and are all related supplies available in the home?
4. Can ketones be measured at home, either in the urine with chemical test strips or in the serum with a point-of-care blood measurement device?
5. Will the child have competent supervision at home?
6. Does the family have access to both a telephone and transportation?
7. Is there a clinician available with whom the family can communicate by telephone?
8. Is the family comfortable with managing the mild acidosis at home?

If these questions can be answered in the affirmative, the child may be sent home. Recommendations should be made to the family regarding fluid intake, insulin administration, and monitoring. Specific recommendations may vary with the age of the child and the experience of the family, but the following scheme may be helpful. Oral intake should be about the same as would be given intravenously to resolve the deficit and provide maintenance (e.g., the 10-year-old child [30 kg] would normally receive a 300-mL bolus followed by 100 to 140 mL per hour, for a total of up to 1 L during the first 6 hours intravenously if he/she was hospitalized; therefore, the physician should suggest that the family try to get in 150 to 180 mL of liquid every hour for the next 6 hours). It is best if this liquid is taken in as sips. Supplements of short-acting insulin will be required in addition to the patient's usual long-acting doses. In the ED, two decisions will need to be made regarding insulin.

- First, how much short-acting insulin (lispro or regular) should be given to the child before discharge? One way to dose additional insulin is using the 5–10% to 10–15% rule.
  - If blood glucose is 250 to 400 mg per dL without urinary ketones, 5% of the child's usual total daily dose will suffice.
  - If blood glucose is more than 400 mg per dL without ketones, or is 250 to 400 mg per dL with moderate or large ketones, 10% of the daily dose will be needed.
  - If blood glucose is more than 400 mg per dL and ketones are moderate or large, the child will need 15% of the daily dose and admission to the hospital should be reconsidered.
- Second, how much insulin should be given at home and with what frequency? Once home, the preceding 5–10% to 10–15% rule is generally applicable and should be given every 4 hours, based on blood glucose and blood or urinary ketones. The family can begin using this algorithm once the child is able to return to a normal intake. For any child to be safely discharged home, however, he or she must be able to maintain adequate oral intake and have frequent contact with a clinician who is comfortable managing pediatric diabetes. Finally, hourly monitoring of blood glucose, urine output, and ketones is recommended with the expectation that the blood glucose should decline, the urine output should fall, and the ketones should begin to clear.

Failure to respond to these simple measures, whether in the ED or at home, should lead to a consultation with the child's endocrinologist. If oral fluids must be restricted and the child is hyperglycemic (e.g., a child with traumatic injury requiring surgery), IV fluids without glucose should be used and glucose should be monitored frequently. As blood glucose concentration reaches 200 mg per dL, dextrose should be added to the IV fluid to maintain target blood glucose of 150 to 250 mg per dL. Additional supplemental insulin may be required, depending on when the child last received insulin and the response to simple hydration. Note, if hyperglycemia is a coincidental finding, the diagnosis requires thoughtful consideration. How traumatic was the blood draw? How upset was the child? What medications or IV fluids were given to the child just before the phlebotomy? What was the child drinking while waiting to see the physician? Are the symptoms in any way related to the hyperglycemia? How sick is the child? The sicker the child is, the less likely it is that hyperglycemia is reflective of diabetes. Three simple evaluations are helpful in determining whether the hyperglycemia is circumstantial or suggestive of diabetes. Brief hyperglycemia resulting from a stress response to phlebotomy or secondary to oral intake rarely results in significant glucosuria; therefore, a urine dip for glucose is often helpful. Second, in the absence of ongoing stress or input, glucose tends to fall over time. A point-of-care glucose is rarely stressful. Therefore, repeating a glucose measurement by fingerstick 1 to 2 hours after the original sample was sent is useful in separating disease from nondisease. Third, hyperglycemia secondary to these factors is usually mild (150 to 250 mg per dL). More significant hyperglycemia should raise the suspicion of diabetes, glucose intolerance, or an underlying medical illness that is producing a significant counterregulatory response.

HYPOGLYCEMIA

Goal of Treatment

To recognize hypoglycemia, initiate a diagnostic laboratory evaluation, and begin corrective treatment immediately if exhibiting any symptoms.

CLINICAL PEARLS AND PITFALLS

- Hypoglycemia in absence of ketones is consistent with hyperinsulinism or fatty acid oxidation enzyme deficiencies.
- Every acutely ill child with an altered level of consciousness should have a rapid bedside glucose determined.
- Treat severe hypoglycemia with rapid IV administration of 0.25 g dextrose per kg body weight.

TABLE 97.4

CAUSES OF CHILDHOOD HYPOGLYCEMIA

Decreased availability of glucose
Decreased intake—fasting, malnutrition, illness
Decreased absorption—acute diarrhea
Inadequate glycogen reserves—defects in enzymes of glycogen synthetic pathways
Ineffective glycogenolysis—defects in enzymes of glycogenolytic pathways
Inability to mobilize glycogen—glucagon deficiency
Ineffective gluconeogenesis—defects in enzymes of gluconeogenic pathway
Increased use of glucose
Hyperinsulinism—islet cell adenoma or hyperplasia, ingestion of oral hypoglycemic agents, insulin therapy
Large tumors—Wilms tumor, neuroblastoma
Diminished availability of alternative fuels
Decreased or absent fat stores
Inability to oxidize fats—enzymatic defects in fatty acid oxidation
Unknown or complex mechanisms
Sepsis/shock
Reye syndrome
Salicylate ingestion
Ethanol ingestion
Adrenal insufficiency
Hypothyroidism
Hypopituitarism

Current Evidence

Hypoglycemia is generally defined as plasma glucose of less than 50 mg per dL, regardless of whether symptoms are present. A differential diagnosis of hypoglycemia, as it may present in the ED, is provided in Table 97.4. Hypoglycemia may be secondary to insulin therapy for diabetes. Excluding this category, almost all hypoglycemia in children occurs during periods of decreased or absent oral intake, often coupled with increased energy demand (e.g., viral gastroenteritis with fever). Postprandial hypoglycemia is unusual in children, except in those who have had prior gastrointestinal surgery. A few select poisonings can produce hypoglycemia. Because glucose is necessary for cellular energy production in most human tissues, the maintenance of an adequate blood glucose concentration is important for normal function. The plasma glucose reflects a dynamic balance among glucose input from dietary sources, glycogenolysis and gluconeogenesis, and glucose use by muscle, heart, adipose tissue, brain, and blood elements. The liver plays a unique role in glucose homeostasis because it stores glucose as glycogen. With fasting, this glycogen is degraded to glucose, which is released into the bloodstream. In addition, the liver synthesizes new glucose from glycerol, lactate, and certain amino acids. During fasting, lipolysis occurs and the resultant fatty acids are used for the production of both energy and ketones (acetoacetate and β-hydroxybutyrate) by the liver. The energy generated from the metabolism of fatty acids is essential to sustain maximal rates of gluconeogenesis and ureagenesis in the liver. The ketones are an important auxiliary fuel for most tissues, including the brain. Muscle contains significant quantities of glycogen and protein. Under fasting conditions, the glycogen is degraded and used endogenously but is not released as free glucose into the bloodstream. Certain amino acids, particularly alanine and glycine, are released from the muscle and subsequently used by the liver for gluconeogenesis. Muscle derives an increasing proportion of its energy requirement from fatty acids as fasting proceeds. Brain tissue is highly dependent on glucose for its energy requirements. Under certain circumstances, it can extract a limited proportion of its energy requirement from other substrates (e.g., glycerol, ketones, lactate), although this process requires a period of adaptation and does not obviate the need for a constant supply of glucose. Insulin is the primary hormone that regulates the blood glucose level. Insulin stimulates the uptake of glucose and amino acids into skeletal, cardiac, and adipose tissue and promotes glycogen and protein synthesis. It inhibits lipolysis and glycogenolysis. The net effect of insulin action is to accelerate the removal of glucose and gluconeogenic substrates from the bloodstream. Opposing or modulating the effects of insulin are cortisol, glucagon, epinephrine, and growth hormone. The effects of these hormones include inhibition of glucose uptake by muscle, mobilization of amino acids for gluconeogenesis, activation of lipolysis, inhibition of insulin secretion, and induction of gluconeogenic enzymes. The net effect is to increase the availability of gluconeogenic substrates to the liver, and to increase the accessibility and use of nonglucose fuels by other tissues.

Clinical Considerations

Clinical Recognition

The acutely ill child warrants a glucose determination if the level of consciousness is altered because hypoglycemia may accompany an illness that interferes with oral intake. The symptoms and signs of hypoglycemia are nonspecific and are often overlooked, especially in the infant and young child. Any child presenting with a seizure, other than a breakthrough seizure with known epilepsy, or unconsciousness should have a plasma glucose determination.

Triage

Children with known diabetes who appear ill need a rapid bedside glucose for possibility of hypoglycemia or hyperglycemia. All children with acute alterations in consciousness, including those with dehydration and fussy or lethargic young infants, should have a point-of-care glucose measurement.

Initial Assessment/H&P

Because hypoglycemia in children occurs after a period of fasting, a careful chronology of dietary intake during the preceding 24 hours should be obtained, as well as a history either of poor fasting tolerance (irritable upon awakening until feeding), or of fasting avoidance (sleeps with bottle in crib). The possibility of a toxic ingestion should be considered because ethanol, β-blockers, and oral hypoglycemic agents are in common use. Family history should be explored for evidence of an undiagnosed metabolic disorder.

The clinical findings of hypoglycemia reflect both the decreased availability of glucose to the CNS and the adrenergic stimulation caused by decreasing or low blood glucose. Adrenergic symptoms and signs include palpitations, anxiety, tremulousness, hunger, and sweating. Irritability, headache, fatigue, confusion, seizure, and unconsciousness are neuroglycopenic symptoms. Any combination of these symptoms should lead to a consideration of hypoglycemia.

Management/Diagnostic Testing

If hypoglycemia is suspected, blood should be drawn before treatment, if at all possible. An extra tube (3 mL serum) should be obtained and refrigerated until the laboratory glucose is known. Rapid screening should be performed using a bedside glucose meter while awaiting definitive laboratory results. In some clinical laboratories, blood glucose can be emergently obtained with heparinized "whole" blood samples along with blood gases. Therapy should be instituted if this screen is suggestive of hypoglycemia. This method may lead to some overtreatment because of error of bedside devices; however, treatment holds minimal risk. It is preferable to overtreat than to allow a child to remain hypoglycemic until definitive laboratory results are available. If the laboratory glucose confirms that the blood glucose was less than 50 mg per dL, the reserved serum can be used for chemical (β-hydroxybutyrate, acetoacetate, amino acid profile, acylcarnitine profile), toxicologic, and hormonal (insulin, growth hormone, cortisol) studies, and may provide the correct diagnosis without extensive additional testing. If adequate blood is obtained before correction, other metabolites to be considered are glucagon, C-peptide, lactate, and pyruvate. If blood is obtained with 15 minutes of glucose administration, it may still be helpful, although possibly not diagnostic. The first voided urine after the hypoglycemic episode should be saved for toxicologic, organic acid evaluation, and acylglycine profile. In the ED, the urine should also be tested immediately for ketones. With hypoglycemia, ketones should be present. Failure to find moderate or large ketone concentrations in the presence of hypoglycemia strongly suggests either that fats are not being mobilized from adipose tissue, as might occur in hyperinsulinism, or that fat cannot be used for ketone body formation, as might occur in enzymatic defects in fatty acid oxidation (e.g., medium chain acyl dehydrogenase [MCAD] deficiency, and many other metabolic defects—see Chapter 103 Metabolic Emergencies). Both the urine and the serum results will be useful in determining the underlying cause of hypoglycemia.

The preferred treatment for hypoglycemia is rapid IV administration of 0.25 g of dextrose per kg body weight (2.5 mL per kg of 10% dextrose, 1.0 mL per kg of 25% dextrose). The plasma glucose should then be maintained by an infusion of dextrose at a rate of 6 to 8 mg/kg/min. Generally, this goal can be accomplished by providing 10% dextrose at one and one-half times maintenance rates. While waiting for vascular access, mucosal and enteral routes should be considered if can be done safely. Glucagon (0.03 mg per kg up to a maximum of 1 mg intramuscularly) may be used to treat hypoglycemia that is known to be caused by hyperinsulinism but is not indicated as part of the routine therapy of hypoglycemia. Glucocorticoids should not be used because they have minimal acute benefit and may delay identification of the cause of hypoglycemia.

The adequacy of therapy should be evaluated both chemically and clinically. The plasma glucose should be monitored frequently and consistently until a stable level higher than 70 mg per dL is attained on more than one measurement. Adrenergic symptoms should resolve quickly. The resolution of CNS symptoms may be prolonged, particularly if the child was initially seizing or unconscious. Seizures that do not respond to correction of hypoglycemia should be managed with appropriate anticonvulsants (see Chapters 67 Seizures and 105 Neurologic Emergencies). The mild acidosis (pH 7.25 to 7.35) usually seen in hypoglycemia will correct without specific intervention. Marked acidosis (pH <7.10) suggests shock or serious underlying disease and should be managed appropriately (see Chapter 5 Shock).

Clinical Indications for Discharge or Admission

Any child with documented hypoglycemia not secondary to insulin therapy, or due to another known entity, should be considered for hospitalization for careful monitoring and diagnostic testing. Exceptions to hospitalization might include children with significant dehydration in the setting of a gastroenteritis illness where symptoms are improving or controlled after proper rehydration in the ED. If being considered for discharge, these children will need repeat blood glucose measurements off IV infusions for several hours prior to discharge.

HYPOPITUITARISM

Goal of Treatment

The goal of treatment in those with known hypopituitarism includes the replacement of essential hormones especially during times of stress such as illness or injury.

CLINICAL PEARLS AND PITFALLS

- The acute presentation of hypopituitarism is most likely to occur when the child is stressed by injury, illness, or fasting.
- Children with midline neurologic defects are at risk for hypopituitarism.
- Children with hypopituitarism are prone to hypoglycemia.
- Hypopituitarism is associated with intracranial lesions.
- Cortisol replacement in patients with adrenal insufficiency under stress conditions is imperative.

Current Evidence

The term *hypopituitarism* generally applies to any condition in which more than a single pituitary hormone is deficient. This condition may include deficiencies resulting from a lack of hypothalamic-releasing factors, as well as deficiencies of anterior and posterior pituitary hormones. Diabetes insipidus (DI), the lack of antidiuretic hormone (ADH), may occur alone or in association with other hormonal defects and is discussed in a subsequent section. Adrenocorticotropic hormone (ACTH) primarily affects adrenal glucocorticoid production; generally, it does not affect mineralocorticoid synthesis, which is primarily regulated by the renin–angiotensin system. A deficiency of ACTH production manifests as cortisol deficiency. Because cortisol plays a role as an insulin counterregulatory hormone, a lack of either ACTH or cortisol may result in hypoglycemia during stress or a prolonged fast. Because the only identified role for thyroid-stimulating hormone (TSH) is the stimulation of thyroid hormone production, a deficiency of TSH is most likely to manifest as hypothyroidism. Luteinizing hormone (LH) and follicle-stimulating hormone (FSH) are involved in gonadal maturation, as well as the regulation of gonadal functions. LH and FSH play an important role in testicular descent and penile growth in the male fetus, as well as affecting the onset of puberty in all adolescents. The circulating levels of these two pituitary hormones are low in children and have no significant role before onset of puberty. Prolactin is primarily involved in the maintenance of lactation and is of minimal significance in childhood under normal conditions. Growth hormone is a principal regulator of linear growth and an important insulin counterregulatory hormone. The absence of growth hormone may be associated with hypoglycemia, particularly in infants and young children during a prolonged fast.

Clinical Considerations

Clinical Recognition

The symptoms and signs of hypopituitarism depend on the deficient hormones. The acute presentation of hypopituitarism is most likely to occur when the child is stressed by injury, illness, or fasting. The presentation may involve either an unusually rapid decompensation, reflecting the role of cortisol in adaptation to stress, or as hypoglycemia, mirroring the role of both cortisol and growth hormone in opposing the effects of insulin.

Triage

Children with known hypopituitarism are at risk for severe decompensation during illness or other forms of stress. Children who are normally on replacement therapy should be assessed for compliance and tolerance of medications. Special attention should be given to abnormal vital signs and mental status.

Initial Assessment/H&P

Patients with known hypopituitarism who present to the ED are at risk for decompensation thus it is important to carefully assess for injury, illness, or fasting state that may precede crisis. A history of vomiting or noncompliance with taking medications, particularly steroids, should be elicited. Questions related to what and how much the patient has been eating and drinking are important. Urine output and fluid status (weight trend if known) are helpful in determining total body water status. Physical examination should focus on addressing vital sign abnormalities and assessment of mental status, hydration state, perfusion as well as a focused assessment of the patient's presenting problem. Understanding which specific hormone deficits the presenting patient has will help guide further history, physical, and the treatment.

Cortisol deficiency can present insidiously with fatigue, vomiting, and failure to thrive. Consider it specifically in patients with unexplained hypoglycemia and/or hyponatremia. Cortisol deficiency can also present more acutely, as in patients who have fluid and pressor refractory hypotension (see Acute Adrenal Insufficiency section for more information).

Patients with thyroid hormone deficiency as a result of hypopituitarism will often have general complaints of fatigue, cold intolerance, constipation, weight gain, and hair thinning/loss. Children often have delayed growth. Infants can have hypotonia, hypothermia, and significant constipation (see Congenital Hypothyroidism section).

Patient with DI have extreme thirst and polydipsia as well as polyuria. Consider in patients who have a history of polydipsia, however, appear volume depleted on examination (see Diabetes Insipidus section).

Isolated growth hormone deficiency is most likely to present with poor linear growth, although occasionally an infant or young child will present with hypoglycemia.

In the older child, no specific symptoms or signs indicate a lack of LH and FSH. An association between a lack of these hormones and anosmia has been noted (Kallmann syndrome). In the adolescent, a deficiency of LH and FSH may be evidenced as pubertal delay. In the neonatal male, hypopituitarism may be accompanied not only by hypoglycemia, but also by micropenis (less than 2 cm, stretched length). This condition illustrates the role of LH and FSH in stimulating testicular function in utero.

No specific signs or symptoms have been associated with a deficiency of prolactin in childhood. Significant liver dysfunction in the neonatal period may be associated with congenital hypopituitarism. Hypopituitarism is seen with various midline structural anomalies, including optic nerve hypoplasia, cleft palate, absence of the septum pellucidum, and spina bifida. In the older child, intracranial mass lesions, particularly with craniopharyngioma and other pituitary abnormalities, may cause hypopituitarism. The presence of visual field abnormalities may aid in localizing the site of the lesion. A history of severe head trauma, surgery for CNS tumors, or CNS irradiation should increase the suspicion of hypopituitarism.

Management/Diagnostic Testing

The child with hypopituitarism may require any or all the following therapies. Adequate cortisol replacement is an absolute necessity in children with known or suspected secondary adrenal insufficiency (ACTH deficiency) during a time of physiologic stress. Cortisol replacement under stress conditions (e.g., trauma, fever) should be the equivalent of 50 mg of hydrocortisone/m^2/day (hydrocortisone IV infusion 12.5 mg per m^2 every 6 hours; hydrocortisone continuous IV infusion at 50 mg/m^2/day; cortisone 50 mg per m^2 intramuscularly every 24 hours). A child with hypopituitarism presenting in extremis or with severe electrolyte abnormalities should immediately receive an initial rescue dose of hydrocortisone of 50 mg per m^2. When a surface area calculation cannot be immediately done, a dose of 1 to 2 mg per kg should be administered. In general, all cases of adrenal insufficiency should be treated with hydrocortisone because it is the only pharmacologic glucocorticoid that stimulates both the glucocorticoid receptor and the mineralocorticoid receptor. If a patient is known to have hypopituitarism, other steroids may be used in equipotent doses and the mineralocorticoid production can be assumed to be normal because it does not involve the pituitary. Because both cortisol and growth hormone are insulin counterregulatory hormones, children with hypopituitarism are prone to hypoglycemia. If enteral intake is interrupted for prolonged periods, glucose should be supplied intravenously. Blood glucose should be monitored to ascertain the adequacy of therapy. Both adrenal insufficiency and DI can lead to fluid and electrolyte abnormalities; therefore, electrolytes should be determined at presentation and followed closely. Changes in IV therapy should be based on serum electrolytes. Judicious use of 1-desamino-8-d-arginine vasopressin (DDAVP) may be helpful in managing DI, as outlined subsequently; however, this treatment is usually unnecessary at the time of acute presentation.

Although both thyroid hormone and sex hormone(s) may need to be replaced, this treatment is not required in the ED. Growth hormone replacement therapy is generally not indicated in the ED setting in the absence of hypoglycemia. Administration of growth hormone to critically ill adults has been shown to increase mortality, apparently as a result of hyperglycemia and increased incidence of sepsis, so it should generally be withheld in the critically ill patient.

Because hypopituitarism often results from intracranial lesions, the demonstration of a pituitary or a hypothalamic mass, or a history of a significant cranial insult, should lead to a diligent search for hormonal deficits. Similarly, documented pituitary deficits should lead to a thorough radiologic investigation of the cranial cavity.

Clinical Indications for Discharge or Admission

Diagnostic testing and therapeutic management of hypopituitarism is generally conducted as an outpatient. General clinical indications ought to guide the decision to admit or discharge to outpatient follow-up, including stability of serum electrolytes and ability to tolerate medications and fluids.

TABLE 97.5

COMMON CAUSES OF ACUTE ADRENAL INSUFFICIENCY IN CHILDREN

Primary adrenal insufficiency
Adrenoleukodystrophy (X-linked)
Congenital adrenal hyperplasia
Autoimmunity
Tuberculosis
Meningococcal septicemia
Adrenal hemorrhage
Secondary adrenal insufficiency
Suppression of adrenocorticotropic hormone by pharmacologic doses of glucocorticoid administration
Pituitary or hypothalamic tumors
Central nervous system surgery or irradiation
Structural abnormalities (septooptic dysplasia)
Congenital hypopituitarism

ACUTE ADRENAL INSUFFICIENCY

See Table 97.5.

Goal of Treatment

To stabilize hemodynamics and correct electrolytes.

CLINICAL PEARLS AND PITFALLS

- Adrenal insufficiency may present with nonspecific symptoms such as fatigue, weight loss, and abnormal electrolytes.
- Children with chronic steroid use are at risk for life-threatening adrenal insufficiency with intercurrent infection or after trauma or surgery.

Current Evidence

Acute adrenal insufficiency occurs when the adrenal cortex fails to produce enough glucocorticoid and mineralocorticoid in response to stress. Because the production of corticosteroids by the adrenal cortex is under pituitary and hypothalamic control, adrenal insufficiency can result from either an adrenal (primary) or hypothalamic–pituitary (secondary) disorder. Specific adrenal problems resulting in adrenal insufficiency include inborn errors of hormonal biosynthesis (discussed in the Congenital Adrenal Hyperplasia section), autoimmune destructive processes, X-linked adrenoleukodystrophy, and adrenal hemorrhage. Hypothalamic–pituitary causes include CNS tumors, trauma, and radiation therapy for a variety of neoplastic disorders. Exogenous administration of glucocorticoids also suppresses the adrenal–pituitary axis, an effect that often lasts well beyond the cessation of corticosteroid therapy.

Glucocorticoids are essential for withstanding stress; therefore, adrenal insufficiency is most likely to be manifested during an intercurrent infection or after trauma. Mineralocorticoids, especially aldosterone, play an important role in salt and water homeostasis by promoting salt reabsorption in the distal renal tubules and collecting ducts. Mineralocorticoid production is primarily regulated by the renin–angiotensin system; thus, adrenal insufficiency resulting from hypothalamic–pituitary causes is rarely associated with a lack of aldosterone. However, aldosterone deficiency is a common feature in primary adrenal insufficiency. Because of the nature of the pituitary–adrenal axis, primary adrenal insufficiency is accompanied by significantly elevated ACTH levels.

Clinical Considerations

Clinical Recognition

Adrenal insufficiency is generally recognized in patients with general fatigue associated with weight loss and abnormal electrolytes or more acutely in critically ill patients who decompensate after a minor prodrome and do not respond to early interventions.

Triage

In children with known adrenal insufficiency, early assessments should focus on vital signs and mental status.

Initial Assessment/H&P

Children with a primary adrenal defect are more likely to have had a gradual onset of symptoms, such as general malaise, anorexia, fatigue, and weight loss. Salt craving and postural hypotension may also have been noted. Waterhouse–Friderichsen syndrome, or acute adrenal infarction, should be considered in a patient with fulminant sepsis and hypotension unresponsive to vasopressors or inotropes, especially if due to meningococcemia. A child with secondary adrenal insufficiency is more likely to have a history of neurosurgical procedures, head trauma, CNS pathology, or chronic disease necessitating the prolonged use of glucocorticoids.

Findings on physical examination are more likely to be characteristic of the precipitating illness or trauma rather than specifically suggestive of adrenal insufficiency. Although a lack of glucocorticoid and aldosterone can be associated with hypotension and dehydration, a better clue to the possibility of adrenal insufficiency is inappropriately rapid decompensation in the face of metabolic stress. Hyperpigmentation may be present in primary adrenal insufficiency, especially of long duration. Red hair and peripheral eosinophilia may be noted in Addison disease or autoimmune destruction of the adrenals.

Management/Diagnostic Testing

Biochemical evidence suggestive of adrenal insufficiency includes hyponatremia, hyperkalemia, hypoglycemia, and hemoconcentration. Metabolic acidosis and hypercalcemia may be present. The definitive diagnosis depends on the demonstration of an inappropriately low level of cortisol in the serum. Blood should be obtained for the measurement of both cortisol and ACTH at baseline if the diagnosis is suspected, but should not delay the administration of hydrocortisone if the patient is critically ill. For stable children, cortisol measurement can be measured 60 minutes after IV or IM administration of 0.25 mg of a synthetic ACTH preparation (i.e., cosyntropin). Although practice varies across institutions, we recommend using an ACTH dose that is weight based for those under 10 kg of 0.015 mg per kg. Results are unlikely to be available on an emergency basis.

Treatment of adrenal crisis with shock is based upon rapid volume expansion and the administration of glucocorticoids. Immediate management consists of 50 to 100 mg per m^2 of hydrocortisone intravenously. In the absence of a body surface area calculation, hydrocortisone can be given as 1 to 2 mg per kg in critical illness. Subsequent management is hydrocortisone 50 mg/m^2/24 hrs given intravenously continuously or divided every 6 hours. Volume expansion is accomplished with normal saline (20 to 60 mL per kg) in the first hour, followed by fluids appropriate for maintenance and replacement. Additional Na^+ may be needed in primary adrenal insufficiency because of ongoing urinary Na^+ losses. These fluids should contain 10% dextrose and should not contain potassium until the serum potassium is within the normal range.

Mineralocorticoid therapy is rarely important in the acute phase, provided fluid therapy is adequate; however, patients with primary adrenal insufficiency may need replacement with a mineralocorticoid for long-term management. Hydrocortisone acts at the mineralocorticoid receptor when dosed at stress levels of 50 mg/m^2/day. Subsequent long-term therapy can be accomplished with fludrocortisone. Specific therapy directed toward correction of the hyperkalemia is rarely required unless cardiac EKG changes (peaked T wave, prolonged QRS duration) or arrhythmias are present. Hypoglycemia is remedied by the use of dextrose and by the hyperglycemic effects of glucocorticoids. The precipitating factor, such as infection, also requires appropriate therapy.

Improvement in peripheral circulation and blood pressure should occur quickly with therapy. Dramatic improvement often occurs in all parameters within hours after the first dose of glucocorticoid. Because adrenal crisis is commonly brought on by another stress such as infection, the symptoms of malaise, anorexia, and lethargy may take longer to resolve.

Clinical Indications for Discharge or Admission

Once instituted, high-dose glucocorticoid therapy should be continued for 48 hours, and adequate hydration should be maintained either orally or intravenously. The patient known to be at risk for adrenal insufficiency should wear an identifying bracelet to alert ED personnel to this possibility.

CONGENITAL ADRENAL HYPERPLASIA

Goal of Treatment

To rapidly initiate treatment for acute salt-wasting crisis and adrenal insufficiency.

CLINICAL PEARLS AND PITFALLS

- ED presentations include ambiguous genitalia, acute salt-wasting crisis, and precocious puberty.
- Patients with acute salt-wasting crisis must be recognized and treated immediately with fluid resuscitation, glucocorticoids, careful monitoring of electrolytes.
- Administer emergency glucocorticoid therapy (50 mg per m^2) to patients with known AI/congenital adrenal hyperplasia (CAH) with fever (T >101.3°F [38.5°C]), emesis/diarrhea, fracture, altered mental status, or shock.

Current Evidence

Inborn errors of adrenal steroid biosynthesis are grouped under the term *congenital adrenal hyperplasia* (CAH). Two major modes of presentation occur in early infancy and require prompt diagnosis and treatment: acute salt-losing crisis and ambiguous genitalia (Table 97.6). CAH may also present in children as precocious virilization. This form of CAH warrants investigation, but it does not require emergency management. The most common form of CAH presenting in infancy is 21-hydroxylase deficiency, which is recessively inherited and accounts for 90% of all cases. Clinically apparent salt wasting develops in approximately two-thirds of affected patients. In the United States, the incidence of 21-hydroxylase deficiency is approximately 1 in 15,000 live births. The enzymes 21-hydroxylase, 11β-hydroxylase, 3β-hydroxysteroid dehydrogenase, and 20,22-desmolase are involved in the production of both cortisol and aldosterone (Fig. 97.1 and Table 97.6). Because the hypothalamic–pituitary axis is under feedback control by cortisol, the lack of production of this hormone caused by the enzyme deficiency results in a significant increase in ACTH. In turn, ACTH stimulates the adrenal to increase steroid hormone production. Because cortisol synthesis is impaired, the precursors of cortisol accumulate significantly. The symptoms and signs characteristic of each enzymatic deficiency reflect either the absence of cortisol or aldosterone or the accumulation of their precursors.

Impairment of mineralocorticoid synthesis by 21-hydroxylase, 3β-hydroxysteroid dehydrogenase, and 20,22-desmolase deficiency can result in salt wasting. Although 11β-hydroxylase deficiency also blocks aldosterone production, the immediate precursor to the block, desoxycorticosterone, has potent mineralocorticoid activity. Thus, instead of developing salt loss, patients with this enzyme defect often develop hypertension during childhood.

Androgenic compounds accumulate in 21-hydroxylase and 11β-hydroxylase deficiencies. Females with these defects are virilized in utero and are born with ambiguous genitalia; therefore, females are often identified in the newborn period. Some female infants are so virilized that they are mistaken as males with bilateral cryptorchidism. Males have normal genital development; therefore, the diagnosis is generally missed until they present with salt-wasting crisis during infancy or with evidence of precocious puberty during childhood.

Deficiency of 3β-hydroxysteroid dehydrogenase leads to underproduction of testosterone. Boys with this deficiency are undervirilized because only weak androgens are produced, whereas girls are mildly virilized because of these weak androgens. Lack of cortisol renders the patient more susceptible to hypoglycemia and reduces the tolerance to severe stress, such as dehydration.

Clinical Considerations

Clinical Recognition

CAH may manifest at birth with the discovery of ambiguous genitalia, between 2 and 5 weeks of age when the baby presents with acute salt-losing crisis, or during childhood with the onset of precocious puberty. The affected child may come to the ED for any of these reasons. Although many US states now screen newborns for CAH, the results may not be available for 3 to 4 weeks and the acute salt-losing crisis may occur before this time. Furthermore, the report of an abnormal test result may precipitate a visit to the ED: Unless the child is ill, consultation with a pediatric endocrinologist is highly recommended before initiating therapy. Salt wasting is present shortly after birth, but acute crisis usually does not occur until the second week of life.

Triage

Consider CAH as etiology of ill-appearing neonate; recognize importance of quickly visualizing genitalia and obtaining point-of-care blood glucose.

Initial Assessment/H&P

The appearance of symptoms of salt-wasting crisis can be insidious, with a history of poor feeding, lack of weight gain, lethargy, irritability, and vomiting. The nonspecific symptoms may lead to consideration of diagnoses other than CAH and delay initiation of treatment.

Examination of the child should include the vital signs and an assessment of the degree of dehydration. In severe cases,

TABLE 97.6

CLINICAL AND LABORATORY FEATURES OF VARIOUS FORMS OF CONGENITAL ADRENAL HYPERPLASIA

	Clinical features				
	Newborn with sexual ambiguity				
Enzyme deficiency	Female	Male	Salt wasting	Hypertension	Postnatal virilization
21-Hydroxylase					
Nonsalt wasting	Y	N	N	N	Y
Salt wasting	Y	N	Y	N	Y
11β-Hydroxylase	Y	N	N	Y	Y
3β-Hydroxysteroid dehydrogenase	Y	Y	Y	N	N
17α-Hydroxylase	N	Y	N	Y	N
Cholesterol desmolase	N	Y	Y	N	N
18-Hydroxylase	N	N	Y	N	N
17β-Hydroxysteroid dehydrogenase	N	Y	—	—	Y

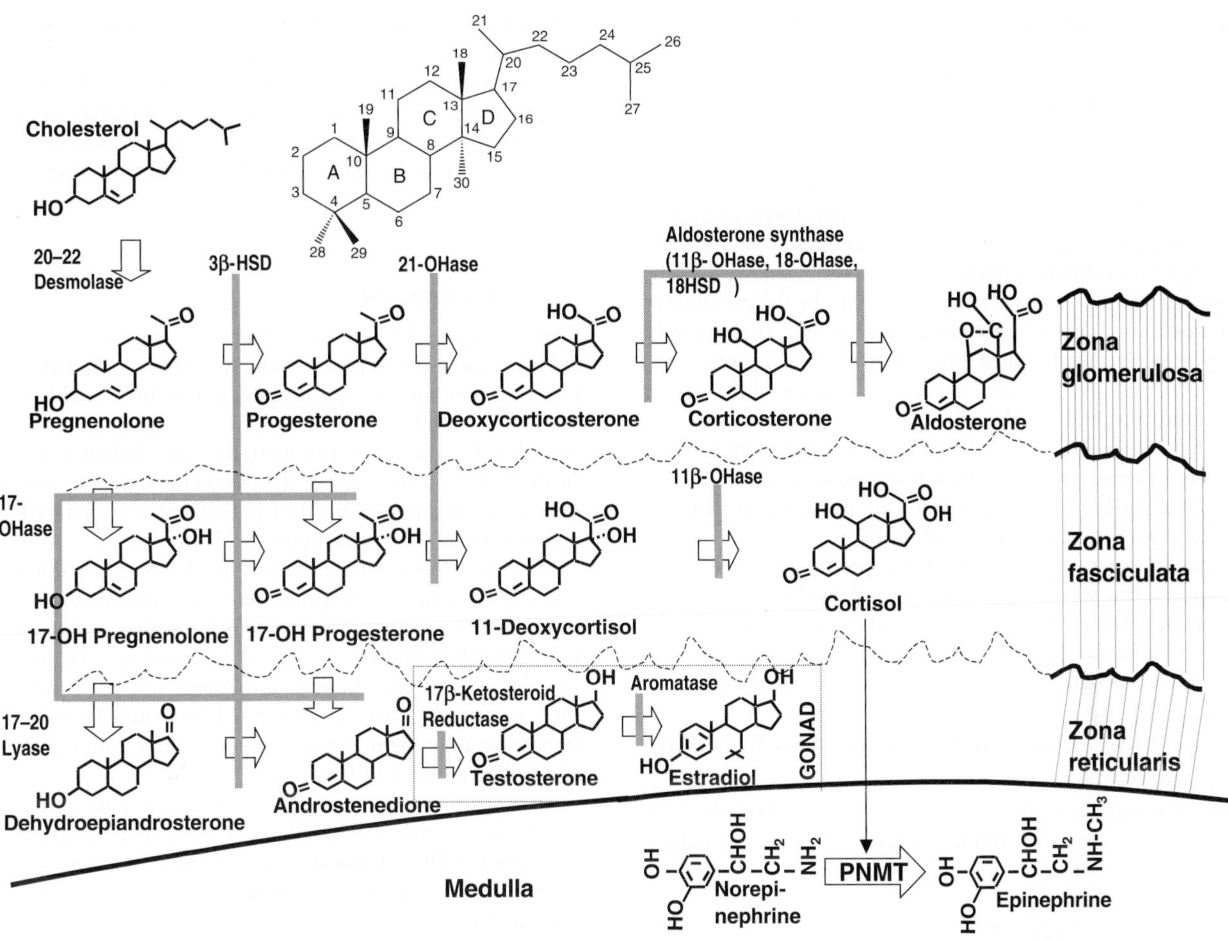

FIGURE 97.1 Adrenal steroid hormone biosynthesis. The pathways for the synthesis of adrenal steroid hormones (adrenal cortex) and catecholamines (adrenal medulla) are arranged from left to right. Synthesis of all compounds originates from cholesterol in the mitochondria of the adrenal cortex. Subsequent conversions are shown with enzyme names located next to *open arrows,* and *gray lines* indicating enzymatic blocks in the various forms of congenital adrenal hyperplasia (CAH). Mineralocorticoids (aldosterone) are produced in the zona glomerulosa, glucocorticoids (cortisol) in the zona fasciculata, and androgens (testosterone) and estrogens (estradiol) in the zona reticularis. Cortically produced cortisol is required for full induction of the medullary conversion of norepinephrine to epinephrine. (Courtesy of Joseph Majzoub, MD, Children's Hospital Boston.)

there may be shock and metabolic acidosis. The genitalia should be examined carefully because the degree of ambiguity of the genitalia varies considerably. Virilized females may have an enlarged clitoris and fusion of the labial folds. An undervirilized male may have a small phallus and/or hypospadias. The presence of gonads in the inguinal canals or labioscrotal fold is suggestive of a male karyotype. Hyperpigmentation of the labioscrotal folds and the nipples is occasionally present in the neonatal period; however, it is rarely prominent enough to alert the examiner to the possibility of CAH.

Management/Diagnostic Testing

In the ED, the most urgent investigations are plasma electrolytes and blood glucose. The combination of hyperkalemia and hyponatremia is often the first clue to the diagnosis of CAH, especially in males. The plasma potassium is elevated, but in the presence of vomiting and diarrhea, the rise may be blunted. Potassium levels between 6 and 12 mEq per L are occasionally encountered, and can paradoxically be seen without any clinical cardiac dysfunction or EKG changes. The plasma bicarbonate level is usually low, reflecting the metabolic acidosis that results from the retention of hydrogen ions in exchange for sodium loss. The blood glucose is usually normal; however, hypoglycemia may occur secondary to the lack of cortisol and the reduced caloric intake during the acute illness. Serum should be drawn for determination of an adrenal steroid profile to include cortisol, 17-hydroxyprogesterone, dehydroepiandrosterone, androstenedione, testosterone, and if possible, ACTH. Ideally, blood should be obtained for these tests before the administration of hydrocortisone. For the child in crisis, the diagnosis must be based on physical findings and electrolyte abnormalities, and treatment must be instituted before the definitive results of the adrenal steroid profile are available.

Emergency glucocorticoid therapy, delivered at the stress dose of hydrocortisone 50 mg/m^2/day should be administered to any patient with known CAH or other form of adrenal insufficiency in the setting of temperature above 38.5°C, emesis and/or diarrhea, bony fracture of any type, or in the setting of altered mental status or shock. If the patient appears ill, an initial dose of hydrocortisone 50 mg per m^2 may be given either intramuscularly or intravenously, followed by that dose divided in four and given every 6 hours. If the patient is not ill appearing and is tolerating oral fluids and medications, his/her usual daily dose may be tripled and given in three equal parts daily, or hydrocortisone 50 mg/m^2/day may be given orally in three equal parts daily if the home dose cannot be readily established.

Correction of Hyperkalemia, Hypoglycemia, and Acidosis

- Infants with CAH tolerate hyperkalemia far better than do other children and adults, with potassium levels as high as 12 mEq per L reported without clinical signs. Volume restoration with normal saline is the major and, usually, the only measure needed to lower the potassium. In the presence of arrhythmias, IV 10% calcium gluconate 1 mL per kg can be given for its membrane-stabilizing properties. Therapy with glucose and insulin is contraindicated because of the danger of precipitating hypoglycemia.
- If hypoglycemia is found at the time of presentation, it should be treated acutely by the administration of dextrose (0.25 g per kg) intravenously and by the subsequent inclusion of 10% dextrose in the infusate.
- Acidosis generally does not require specific treatment; however, the low serum bicarbonate may take days to fully correct. Bicarbonate therapy is reserved for patients with both severe acidosis (pH <6.9) and secondary hemodynamic compromise that is unresponsive to inotropic agents.

Clinical Indications for Discharge or Admission

Hemodynamic instability, inability to tolerate oral medications or maintain hydration, significant electrolyte or acid/base abnormalities, and refractory hypoglycemia are indications for admission.

PHEOCHROMOCYTOMA

Goal of Treatment

To recognize the presentation of pheochromocytoma and to control hypertension.

CLINICAL PEARLS AND PITFALLS

- Pheochromocytoma presents with episodic headache, palpitations, sweating; but also nervousness, tremulousness, fatigue, chest/abdominal pain, and flushing.
- Associated hypertension can be paroxysmal; alpha blockade is antihypertensive of choice, pure beta blockade as a treatment for hypertension should be avoided as it can precipitate severe hypertension.

Current Evidence

Pheochromocytomas are functional tumors that arise in chromaffin tissues. In most children, these tumors are in the adrenal medulla, but they may be found in aberrant tissue along the sympathetic chain. Less than 5% of all pheochromocytomas occur in children. They are twice as common in males as in females, with the incidence of malignancy estimated to be 2% to 4%. Most information on pheochromocytoma is derived from adult studies, especially regarding signs and symptoms. Few detailed studies are available on children.

Catecholamines are low–molecular-weight substances produced in the CNS, the sympathetic nerves, the adrenal medulla, and the extra-adrenal chromaffin cells. Catecholamines affect metabolic processes in most tissues of the body and have many effects, including accelerated heart rate, increased myocardial contraction, and changes in peripheral vascular resistance. Excessive production of catecholamines by a pheochromocytoma results in intensification of the normal physiologic effects.

Clinical Considerations

Clinical Recognition

The detection of a pheochromocytoma requires expert clinical awareness. Most patients are symptomatic, but the symptoms are episodic, nonspecific and, in the child, are likely to be attributed to other disease entities. The symptoms and signs are related to the excess production of catecholamines and can be explained on the basis of the pharmacologic effects of these substances. Up to one-third of pheochromocytomas are associated with familial syndromes.

The most common symptoms are headache, palpitations, and excessive or inappropriate sweating. The headache, characteristically, is pounding and may be severe and associated with altered mental status. The palpitations may be accompanied by tachycardia. Almost all patients will have one of the three symptoms listed, and most will have at least two. Other symptoms may include nervousness, tremor, fatigue, chest or abdominal pains, and flushing.

Because the hypertension may be continuous or paroxysmal, frequent and repeated blood pressure determinations may be necessary. Hypertension is most likely to be found when the patient is symptomatic. A hypertensive patient who is asymptomatic is unlikely to have a pheochromocytoma.

Triage

The most useful screening tool for pheochromocytoma is the blood pressure cuff because most pheochromocytomas are associated with hypertension.

Initial Assessment/H&P

Paroxysmal symptoms and hypertension should lead to consideration of this diagnosis. The diagnosis of a pheochromocytoma should also be considered in patients with malignant hypertension, in those who fail to respond or respond inappropriately to antihypertensive medications, and in those who develop hypertension during the induction of anesthesia or during surgery. Incidence of pheochromocytomas is increased among patients with neurofibromatosis and with the multiple endocrine neoplasia syndrome types II and III.

Management/Diagnostic Testing

Documentation of excess catecholamine in either the urine or serum confirms the diagnosis of pheochromocytoma. The most readily available and widely used test for this purpose remains the measurement of urinary catecholamines or their metabolites (3-methoxy-4-hydroxymandelic acid and total metanephrines) in a 24-hour urine collection accompanied by a patient symptom log. The finding of significant elevations of these substances is adequate confirmatory data. Some false-negative results may occur using urinary catecholamines. When the degree of suspicion is high, repeated specimens may be needed. Plasma metanephrine concentration has now been shown to be a superior screening and confirmatory test, however, and ought to be employed where available.

Once the diagnosis is confirmed, anatomic localization is necessary using either computed tomography or nuclear magnetic resonance imaging. Occasionally, arteriography with selective sampling for epinephrine production is necessary for localization. Cure is by the surgical removal of the tumor.

The focus of ED management should be on controlling hypertension and hypertensive crisis that may occur before the surgical procedure. α-Adrenergic blocking agents are useful in controlling hypertension and in minimizing blood pressure fluctuations during the surgical procedure. Preferred drugs for controlling hypertension are phenoxybenzamine (Dibenzyline) and prazosin (Minipress). Dosage schedules and quantity must be tailored to the individual for adequate control of hypertension. Hypertensive crisis may be appropriately managed with IV phentolamine (Regitine 1 mg IV for children; 5 mg IV for adolescents) or sodium nitroprusside (0.5 to 8.0 μg/kg/min). Beta blockade must be avoided because it may lead to unopposed alpha action on the part of secreted catecholamines and resultant severe hypertension.

Clinical Indications for Discharge or Admission

Admission is warranted if there is strong clinical consideration of pheochromocytoma due to paroxysmal hypertension; especially preoperatively so that blood pressure control can be adequately attained.

DIABETES INSIPIDUS

Goal of Treatment

In DI, the goal of treatment is to rapidly restore the intravascular volume needed to stabilize the patient and then replace remaining deficit over 48 hours.

CLINICAL PEARLS AND PITFALLS

- Hypertonic dehydration occurs if thirst is not intact or access to fluids is restricted.
- Children may present with severe dehydration despite a history of normal urine output.
- The degree of dehydration may be underestimated due to the patient's hyperosmolar state, a patient is at risk for central pontine myelinolysis if DI causes very rapid dehydration.

Current Evidence

DI is caused by an inability of the kidneys to concentrate urine and is characterized clinically by polyuria and polydipsia. Either a deficiency of ADH secretion from the hypothalamus and posterior pituitary gland or renal unresponsiveness to ADH can cause this disease (Table 97.7).

Most causes of central DI in children are acquired and can present at any age. In contrast, the most common cause of nephrogenic DI in children is X-linked recessive and manifests in males during early infancy. Renal lesions associated with nephrogenic DI can present in later childhood.

ADH is synthesized in the supraoptic and paraventricular nuclei of the hypothalamus. It is transported along nerve axons to the posterior pituitary gland, where it is stored, generally bound to its carrier protein neurophysin II. ADH is released in response to increased plasma osmolality, hypernatremia, and decreased right atrial pressure secondary to hypovolemia. The distal convoluted tubules and the collecting ducts of the kidneys respond to ADH by inserting a water channel (aquaporin) into the luminal membrane of the collecting duct and allowing water reabsorption along the medullary concentration gradient. Lack of ADH (central DI) can result from a wide variety of hypothalamic and pituitary lesions (Table 97.7).

In nephrogenic DI, ADH levels are normal or elevated because the defect resides in the renal collecting tubules, which are resistant to the action of ADH. In either case, failure of water reabsorption results in polyuria. A normal thirst mechanism contributes toward fluid balance by promoting adequate fluid intake; however, if this balance is not achieved, hypertonic dehydration ensues. If a hyperosmolar state develops abruptly, it may lead to dehydration of neural tissues, which can cause serious neurologic sequelae or result in death. The pons is particularly sensitive to this effect resulting in central pontine myelinolysis.

TABLE 97.7

CAUSES OF DIABETES INSIPIDUS IN CHILDREN

Causes
Antidiuretic hormone deficiency
Head injury
Meningitis
Idiopathic
Suprasellar tumors and their treatment by surgery and/or radiotherapy
Craniopharyngioma
Optic nerve glioma
Dysgerminoma
Septooptic dysplasia
Association with midline cleft palate
Familial (dominant or sex-linked recessive)
Wolfram syndrome (diabetes insipidus, diabetes mellitus, optic atrophy, deafness)
Histiocytosis X (Hand–Schuller–Christian disease)
Nephrogenic diabetes insipidus
Sex-linked recessive
Renal disease
Polycystic kidneys
Hydronephrosis
Chronic pyelonephritis
Hypercalcemia
Hypokalemia
Toxins:
Demeclocycline
Lithium
Sickle cell disease
Idiopathic

Clinical Considerations

Clinical Recognition

Urine excretion is increased in both volume and frequency in the child with DI. This condition may manifest as enuresis in the younger child. Provided the thirst mechanism is intact and fluids are accessible, the child can compensate for the water loss by drinking excessively. If fluids are not available or if fluid intake is interrupted because of an illness, dehydration rapidly ensues. The patient will present with signs of dehydration despite the apparent "normal" urine output. With severe dehydration, the child may have signs of altered mental status.

Triage

Recognize the dehydrated child and consider DI in the setting of dilute urine output with hypovolemia. Children with known DI will decompensate if noncompliant with medication or any illness.

Initial Assessment/H&P

A history may be elicited of the child's awakening in the middle of the night to drink. In the young infant who is not provided with adequate fluids and consequently is chronically dehydrated, the child may fail to thrive or may have a history of intermittent low-grade fevers due to intermittent hypernatremia. However, if the cries of the infant are interpreted as hunger rather than thirst, the infant with DI may be obese.

Physical examination may be normal, or signs of dehydration, such as dryness of mucous membranes, decreased skin turgor, sunken eyes, and in an infant, a depressed anterior fontanel, may be present. Because of the hyperosmolarity, the degree of dehydration may be underestimated on physical examination. Hypothalamic or pituitary lesions can lead to other endocrine abnormalities such as secondary hypothyroidism and growth failure. A craniopharyngioma or optic nerve glioma may affect the visual fields or cause raised intracranial pressure, which is indicated by papilledema.

Management/Diagnostic Testing

DI is diagnosed by demonstrating that the kidneys fail to concentrate urine when fluid intake is restricted. This condition can be difficult to prove in children. Criteria for the diagnosis of DI may be met by finding an elevated serum osmolality (greater than 300 mOsm per L) and an elevated serum [Na^+] (greater than 145 mEq per L) in the presence of dilute urine (osmolality less than 600 mOsm per L). Blood glucose and serum creatinine levels are normal.

In many cases, the diagnosis can be ruled out by the demonstration of appropriately concentrated urine and normal serum osmolality on specimens obtained upon awakening. The definitive diagnosis is made by a formal water deprivation test. This test is performed electively in cases in which the diagnosis is uncertain and should never be performed if the child is already dehydrated. The measurement of ADH by radioimmunoassay is available but generally is not useful in the diagnosis of DI.

In most cases, a diagnosis of DI is not known at the time of presentation; therefore, the acute management is directed toward correction of the dehydration and the hyperosmolar state. The treatment of DI is similar to that described for hypernatremic dehydration (see Chapter 17 Dehydration), with the notable addition that the fluid required for the replacement of urinary fluid losses will be far greater. In fact, the high urinary output, despite significant dehydration, often provides the first and most convincing evidence for DI.

If the child is hypotensive or if the serum [Na^+] is greater than 160 mEq per L, initial volume expansion is necessary, using 20 mL per kg normal saline during the first hour or more rapidly, if needed. Once an adequate intravascular volume has been achieved, further fluid replacement is accomplished slowly because overly rapid volume correction can cause cerebral edema, seizures, and death.

If the child is not hypotensive, or once the hypotension and perfusion have been corrected, free water replacement is done over 48 hours. Calculations of appropriate fluids must include maintenance requirements, replacement needs, and ongoing urinary losses (see Chapter 17 Dehydration).

If DI is strongly suspected on the basis of discrepant serum and urine osmolality, DDAVP (10 μg intranasally or 0.2 to 0.4 μg per kg subcutaneously) may be a useful adjunct to IV fluid therapy. If DDAVP is not available or cannot be used for some reason, other antidiuretic agents are available. Aqueous Pitressin may be administered as a continuous IV infusion starting at 1 mU/kg/hr and slowly (every 5 to 10 minutes) increasing the rate (maximum 10 mU/kg/hr) to decrease urine output to less than 2 mL/kg/hr.

DDAVP and Pitressin act rapidly to promote tubular resorption of free H_2O; clinically, this response is apparent as decreased urinary output with increased osmolality within 15 minutes of administration. Once the patient has responded, however, extreme care must be used in subsequent fluid management because the patient can no longer excrete excess water. Therefore, baseline IV fluid administration must be maintained at 1 L per m^2 of body surface area per day (or roughly two-thirds maintenance fluids) using a low sodium infusate, such as 5% dextrose with one-fourth normal saline (0.23%), in addition to the fluid designed to replete the initial estimated free water deficit over 48 hours.

Failure to respond to either form of ADH suggests the possibility of tubular unresponsiveness to ADH (nephrogenic DI); however, more commonly, failure to respond results from improper administration of the medication or use of DDAVP that has lost its potency. Because of these factors, if cessation of diuresis is not noted within 2 hours of administration of the first dose, a second dose from a different bottle of DDAVP should be tried. The use of an ADH agonist generally simplifies management by reducing the quantity of fluid that must be infused; however, careful monitoring of input and output remains essential. Children who fail to respond to DDAVP are likely to have nephrogenic DI and must be acutely managed with fluid therapy alone. Hypercalcemia and renal failure are the most common causes of nephrogenic DI. Paradoxically, the thiazide diuretics have proven to be useful in the chronic control of nephrogenic DI.

The child should be closely observed for changes in level of consciousness, pulse rate, and blood pressure. Fluid input and output should be meticulously monitored. Serum osmolality and [Na^+] should be determined every 1 to 2 hours until the rate of their decline can be determined. Urine osmolality should be measured every 1 to 2 hours to determine the responsiveness of the renal tubule to DDAVP. Because large volumes of dextrose-containing fluids are used, the blood glucose should also be followed closely. If the blood glucose exceeds 160 mg per dL, the concentration of dextrose in the infusate should be decreased.

Clinical Indications for Discharge or Admission

Clinically significant electrolyte derangements or the inability to maintain hydration status are indications for admission in well-appearing child. Children with intact thirst mechanism who are able to tolerate PO can be discharged with plan for close outpatient follow-up.

SYNDROME OF INAPPROPRIATE ANTIDIURETIC HORMONE SECRETION

Goals of Treatment

The goals of treatment in a child with syndrome of inappropriate antidiuretic hormone (SIADH) are to raise the serum sodium and improve the neurologic status of the patient; secondarily, causes of SIADH should be identified.

CLINICAL PEARLS AND PITFALLS

- Most patients are asymptomatic from SIADH until the serum sodium <125 mEq per L.
- SIADH is associated with bacterial meningitis (50%), positive pressure ventilation (20%), Rocky Mountain spotted fever (70%), and numerous causes of moderate and severe illness.
- For severe lethargy, seizure, or coma administer 3% saline emergently (3 mL per kg every 10 to 20 minutes as needed) and consider Lasix with a normal saline infusion.

For asymptomatic or mildly symptomatic patients, treat with rigorous fluid restriction and consider a vasopressin receptor antagonist if recurrent.

Current Evidence

Excessive secretion of ADH accompanying normal or low plasma osmolality or $[Na^+]$ is inappropriate because it further depresses the plasma osmolality and $[Na^+]$. The overall incidence of the SIADH secretion in childhood is unknown, but it is common in certain disease states. Normal ADH secretion is stimulated by hypertonicity of the fluid surrounding the hypothalamic osmoreceptors, volume receptors in the right atrium, and ill-defined nervous impulses from higher cortical centers. Disorders of the CNS (Table 97.8) may cause excessive ADH secretion by producing either a local disturbance of the hypothalamic osmoreceptors or some undetermined nervous stimuli. Many intrathoracic conditions are associated with SIADH, probably due to the vestigial ability of the lung to produce ADH. Physical and emotional stress, severe pain, and nausea are also potent stimuli of ADH secretion. Excessive secretion of ADH leads to water retention by the collecting tubules of the kidneys, a mechanism mediated by insertion of water channels into the luminal membrane of the collecting duct and allowing water reabsorption along the medullary concentration gradient. The retained water expands the intravascular compartment, dilutes all plasma constituents, and lowers the plasma osmolality.

TABLE 97.8

SOME CAUSES OF SYNDROME OF INAPPROPRIATE ANTIDIURETIC HORMONE SECRETION IN CHILDREN

Disorders of central nervous system
Infection (meningitis, encephalitis)
Trauma, postneurosurgery
Hypoxic insults, especially in the perinatal period
Brain tumor
Intraventricular hemorrhage
Guillain–Barré syndrome
Psychosis
Intrathoracic disorders
Infection (tuberculosis, pneumonia, empyema)
Positive pressure ventilation
Asthma
Cystic fibrosis
Pneumothorax
Patent ductus arteriosus ligation
Miscellaneous
Pain (e.g., after abdominal surgery)
Nausea
Severe hypothyroidism
Tumors (e.g., neuroblastoma)
Drug induced
Increased antidiuretic hormone secretion
Vincristine
Cyclophosphamide
Carbamazepine
Adenine arabinoside
Phenothiazines
Morphine
Potentiation of antidiuretic hormone effect
Acetaminophen
Indomethacin

Clinical Considerations

Clinical Recognition

Most patients with SIADH are asymptomatic until the plasma $[Na^+]$ falls to less than 125 mEq per L. Associated with the low serum sodium, children may be weak, have altered mental status, or have seizures. Patients may have mild signs of hypervolemia.

Triage

Assess mental status and neurologic examination, treat for precipitating conditions.

Initial Assessment/H&P

- Symptoms associated with hyponatremia range from anorexia, headache, nausea, vomiting, irritability, disorientation, and weakness to seizures and coma, leading potentially to death.
- Absence of edema and dehydration are usual and significant clinical findings.

Management/Diagnostic Testing

Laboratory investigations for diagnostic purposes must include concomitant serum and urine samples (Table 97.9).

TABLE 97.9

CRITERIA FOR DIAGNOSIS OF SYNDROME OF INAPPROPRIATE ANTIDIURETIC HORMONE SECRETION

Hyponatremia, reduced serum osmolality
Urine osmolality inappropriately elevated (a urine osmolality <100 mOsm/kg usually excludes the diagnosis)
Urinary Na^+ concentration that is excessive in comparison to the degree of hyponatremia (usually >18 mmol/L)
Normal renal, adrenal, and thyroid function
Absence of volume depletion (euvolemic to hypervolemic state)

Hyponatremia, hypoosmolality (serum), and low blood urea nitrogen will be present. In contrast, the urinary osmolality and [Na^+] are inappropriately elevated for the hypotonicity of the serum. Due to the euvolemic or hypervolemic state, aldosterone is suppressed and urine potassium will be low. Radioimmunoassay for ADH is now available and has been helpful in defining this syndrome; however, the results of this test are unlikely to be available on an emergency basis.

The underlying cause of the syndrome should be investigated according to the physician's clinical judgment. Hyperlipidemia may falsely lower laboratory measurement of [Na^+], leading to a factitious hyponatremia. Hyperglycemia and hypoproteinemia, however, lead to true hyponatremia. Renal salt wasting, secondary to adrenal insufficiency, should be accompanied by hyperkalemia and dehydration. Cerebral salt wasting may have laboratory parameters similar to SIADH but is characterized by hypovolemia and a high urine output as long as renal perfusion remains intact. The urine osmolality in water intoxication states is usually low compared with that found in SIADH.

Severely Symptomatic Children

- Patients with a persistent seizure attributable to severe hyponatremia and those who are severely lethargic or comatose need urgent treatment with hypertonic (3%) saline by fusing small amounts of 3% saline in the range of 3 mL per kg every 10 to 20 minutes until symptoms remit. One milliliter per kilogram of 3% saline should raise the serum [Na^+] by approximately 1 mEq per L. Since the administration of 3% is high-risk therapy, it should only be given in the quantity needed to treat the adverse clinical finding (e.g., altered mental status, seizure). A single dose of furosemide (1 mg per kg) also can be administered intravenously. Close monitoring of fluid balance, plasma and urinary sodium, potassium, and osmolality is essential.
- Seizures should be treated concomitantly with a standard emergency anticonvulsant protocol (see Chapters 67 Seizures and 105 Neurologic Emergencies). Of note, phenytoin (Dilantin) or fosphenytoin (Cerebyx) intravenously (5 to 10 mg per kg) inhibits ADH release and may be helpful in the patient with seizures secondary to CNS causes of SIADH.
- The underlying cause of SIADH, such as meningitis or pneumonia, should be treated when possible; successful treatment is usually accompanied by remission of inappropriate water retention.

Asymptomatic or Mildly Symptomatic Children

- Asymptomatic or mildly symptomatic children are best treated by rigorous fluid restriction. Fluid input should be sharply limited, often below insensible loss, until the [Na^+] and osmolality begin to rise (800 cc per m^2). If the initial [Na^+] is less than 125 mEq per L, all fluids must be withheld.
- Frequent measurements of plasma electrolytes, glucose, and osmolality, as well as close monitoring of fluid input and output, are essential. As the serum [Na^+] rises and urine osmolality falls, the rate of fluid administration can be gradually increased.
- The child with chronic or recurrent episodes of SIADH may require treatment with a drug in the "vaptan" class, which block vasopressin binding to its receptor. Pediatric dosing parameters have not yet been formally established. Consultation with a pediatric endocrinologist should be conducted to guide dosing.

Clinical Indications for Discharge or Admission

Admission is indicated for children who are symptomatic, or are newly diagnosed with hyponatremia until a reassuring trajectory has been established.

HYPERPARATHYROIDISM

Goal of Treatment

The major ED treatment goal is to address clinical effects of severe hypercalcemia and hypophosphatemia while trying to correct these electrolytes.

CLINICAL PEARLS AND PITFALLS

- Consider the diagnosis of hyperparathyroidism in a critically ill infant who presents with hypercalcemia.
- May present in adolescence with nonspecific symptoms including nausea and constipation. The patient will have hypercalcemia.
- Family history is important as hyperparathyroidism is associated with MEN I, II and being an infant born to a mother with hypoparathyroidism.

Current Evidence

The parathyroid glands are derived from the third and fourth pharyngeal pouch and are usually embedded in the posterior aspect of the thyroid gland. Occasionally, a gland may be found in the anterior mediastinum. Parathyroid hormone (PTH) is the primary hormone produced by the parathyroid glands. PTH is synthesized and released constitutively; its secretion is stimulated by low, and suppressed by high, serum ionized calcium concentration. Prolonged hypocalcemia, most commonly in the setting of renal failure, may lead to hypertrophy of the parathyroid glands and secondary hyperparathyroidism. PTH acts on the kidney to decrease the excretion of calcium, magnesium, and hydrogen, while increasing the excretion of phosphate, sodium, and bicarbonate. Many of the effects are mediated by cyclic adenosine monophosphate (cAMP), and an increased quantity of cAMP is present in the urine of patients with hyperparathyroidism. PTH also increases the formation of 1,25-dihydroxyvitamin D in the kidneys. PTH may increase intestinal absorption of calcium, although this effect is primarily mediated by 1,25-$(OH)_2$D. Both PTH and 1,25-$(OH)_2$D affect bone mineralization. PTH acts on bone to increase the release of calcium by increasing the number and activity of the osteoclasts, whereas vitamin D decreases calcium use in bone formation by decreasing the number of osteoblasts. The net effect of the actions of PTH and vitamin D is to increase serum calcium by decreasing renal calcium excretion, decreasing new bone formation, increasing bone resorption, and increasing intestinal absorption of calcium.

Clinical Considerations

Clinical Recognition

Hyperparathyroidism has two common presentations in children. The first presentation is the critically ill infant who is found to have severe hypercalcemia during the course of diagnostic investigations. The serum calcium level may be extremely high. The second presentation is a child in the early to midteens with nonspecific symptoms including nausea, constipation, unexplained weight loss, personality changes, and headaches. Diffuse bone pain or renal colic may be reported, although these symptoms are less common in children than in adults.

Triage

Consider hyperparathyroidism as a potential diagnosis in the critically ill neonate.

Initial Assessment/H&P

The physical findings of hypercalcemia are hypotonia, weakness, listlessness, anorexia, constipation, and vomiting, and in the neonate, respiratory distress and apnea. There may be hypertension, shortened QTc interval on EKG, polyuria (due to renal unresponsiveness to ADH), and rarely, encephalopathy with seizures. A palpable mass may occasionally be located in the parathyroid region. Certain characteristic features have been associated with idiopathic hypercalcemia in infancy, including hypertelorism, broad forehead, epicanthal folds, prominent upper lip, an underdeveloped nasal bridge, and a small mandible. Not surprisingly, these same features have been noted in infants with hyperparathyroidism. A family history may be helpful because hyperparathyroidism has been associated with both multiple endocrine neoplasia types I and II, which are inherited as autosomal-dominant conditions. Hyperparathyroidism may also occur in infants of hypoparathyroid mothers.

Management/Diagnostic Testing

Radiologic findings consistent with hyperparathyroidism include evidence of demineralization and bone resorption (Figs. 97.2 and 97.3). Osteitis fibrosa cystica, although highly suggestive of the diagnosis, is unusual in children. Hypercalcemia is usually present but may be subtle or intermittent in mild cases. The serum inorganic phosphate level is usually low but may be normal, especially in patients with decreased renal function. Mild hyperchloremic acidosis may be present. Alkaline phosphatase level and urinary hydroxyproline excretion may be elevated secondary to increased osteoclast activity. Because PTH causes a significant increase in cAMP in the kidney tubule, the presence of excess cAMP in the urine is strongly suggestive of excess PTH production. The determination of PTH levels is critical for diagnostic purposes,

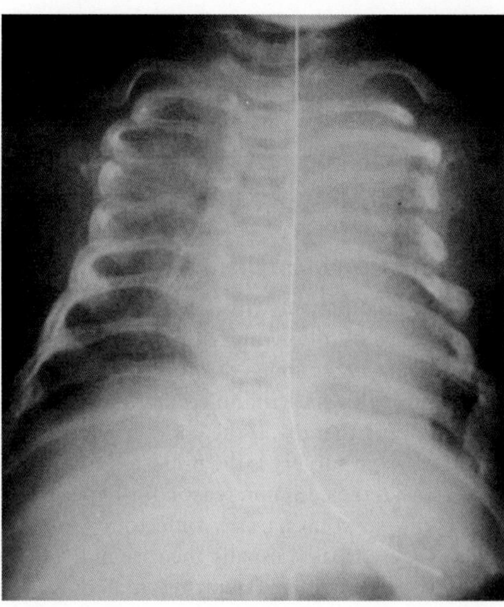

FIGURE 97.2 Primary hyperparathyroidism in a 3-day-old girl. Roentgenogram of the chest shows profound demineralization of the skeleton with loss of a well-defined cortical margin. Cystic changes in rib and subperiosteal bone resorption in humerus are seen. (Courtesy of Soroosh Mahboubi, MD, The Children's Hospital of Philadelphia.)

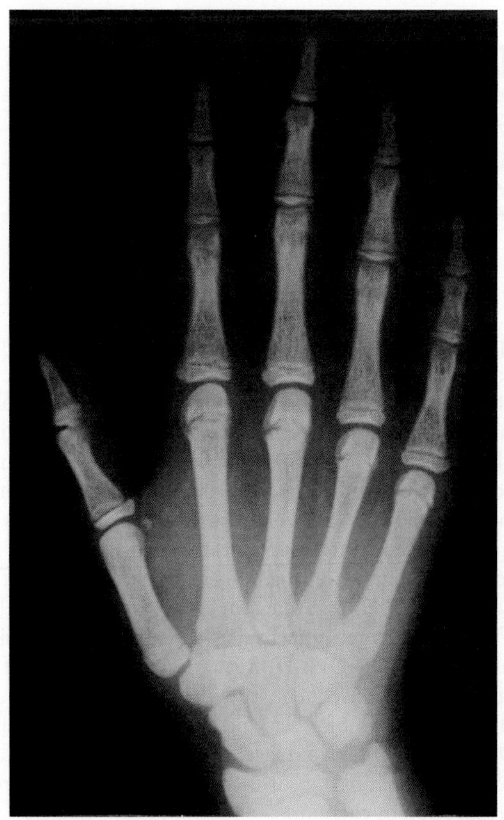

FIGURE 97.3 Secondary hyperparathyroidism in a 12-year-old girl with chronic pyelonephritis. There is moderate subperiosteal erosion on the radial side of the middle phalanges; note a lacy appearance of the periosteum and small-tuft erosion. Subperiosteal bone resorption is the most significant radiologic finding in hyperparathyroidism; subperiosteal bone resorption and tuft erosion are seen in both primary and secondary hyperparathyroidism. (Courtesy of Soroosh Mahboubi, MD, The Children's Hospital of Philadelphia.)

and elevated levels of PTH, when the patient is hypercalcemic, are a definitive laboratory finding. Acute management of hyperparathyroidism is essentially the same as management of hypercalcemia (see Chapter 108 Renal and Electrolyte Emergencies). The specific management of hyperparathyroidism depends on the level of calcium and on the presence of signs and symptoms.

Clinical Indications for Discharge or Admission

In the asymptomatic patient with serum calcium of less than 12 mg per dL, careful follow-up with close attention to both bone mass and renal function is recommended. Young infants with feeding difficulty or irritability may need low calcium formula and diuretic therapy. If the child is persistently hypercalcemic, parathyroid surgery is the preferred treatment. In the case of hyperplasia, the common reason for hyperparathyroidism in the infant, subtotal parathyroidectomy is indicated. If an adenoma is present, as is usually the case in the older child, simple removal of the involved parathyroid gland is adequate.

HYPOPARATHYROIDISM

Goal of Treatment

Treatment goals for children with hypoparathyroidism include addressing the clinical effects of hypocalcemia and to initiate treatment with vitamin D and calcium.

CLINICAL PEARLS AND PITFALLS

- Presents with signs and symptoms of hypocalcemia.
- Hypocalcemic seizures may be difficult to control.
- Calcium infusions must be done slowly to avoid life-threatening arrhythmias.

Current Evidence

Hypoparathyroidism can occur sporadically or be part of a familial syndrome consisting of combinations of several autoimmune diseases (e.g., Addison disease, diabetes mellitus, lymphocytic thyroiditis, pernicious anemia, ovarian failure). It is also associated with thymic aplasia and severe immunologic deficiencies (DiGeorge syndrome). A transient form of hypoparathyroidism, lasting for as long as 1 year, has been reported in some infants. Hypoparathyroidism may also result from damage incurred during thyroid surgery or irradiation.

The lack of PTH, regardless of cause, has several deleterious effects on calcium homeostasis. Because PTH has significant effects on 1,25-$(OH)_2D_3$ formation, the absence of PTH is magnified by a consequent reduction in 1,25-$(OH)_2D_3$. The net effect of the lack of PTH (and decreased quantity of vitamin D) is a declining serum level of calcium, primarily caused by decreased intestinal absorption of calcium and decreased renal resorption of calcium.

Clinical Considerations

Clinical Recognition

The predominant historical features and clinical manifestations of hypoparathyroidism are the same as those of hypocalcemia. Presenting complaints are often related to paresthesias and tetany that result from hypocalcemia. General complaints such as bone pain, headaches, fatigue, and insomnia are also common. Physical examination findings are generally nonspecific aside from tetany, when present, or the ability to elicit the Chvostek or Trousseau sign. Labs abnormalities include elevated phosphorous, low calcium, low calcitriol, and low PTH (see Chapter 108 Renal and Electrolyte Emergencies).

Triage

Hypocalcemia should be considered in a child who has neurologic irritability or myoclonus.

Initial Assessment/H&P

Unique historical information that may suggest the diagnosis of hypoparathyroidism includes other family members with autoimmune endocrine disease, recurrent episodes of serious infection in the affected child, and previous thyroid manipulations. Most symptoms and signs of hypoparathyroidism are the same as those related to hypocalcemia. The particular symptoms and signs found depend on the age at disease onset, the chronicity of the disease, and the presence of other autoimmune or syndromic phenomena.

Papilledema without hemorrhage may be seen during the initial examination and tends to resolve within several days after the initiation of therapy. Lenticular cataracts are common in hypoparathyroidism and are associated with long-standing hypocalcemia of any cause. Psychiatric and neurologic disorders occur in association with hypoparathyroidism. Subnormal intelligence occurs in about 20% of children with the idiopathic form of hypoparathyroidism and the severity correlates closely with the period of untreated hypocalcemia.

Dry, scaly skin is a common finding, as is patchy alopecia. Psoriasis or mucocutaneous candidiasis may be found on occasion. Unusually brittle fingernails and hair are often found. Hypoplasia of tooth enamel may be seen if hypoparathyroidism was present at the time of dental development. Intestinal malabsorption and steatorrhea have been reported in association with hypoparathyroidism.

Management/Diagnostic Testing

In most cases, the diagnosis of hypoparathyroidism is first considered when low serum calcium is found. If an elevated phosphate accompanies low calcium, low or normal serum alkaline phosphate, and normal blood urea nitrogen, hypoparathyroidism is a likely possibility. Finding a low or nonmeasurable level of PTH in the presence of hypocalcemia and hyperphosphatemia makes the definitive diagnosis. Because PTH increases cAMP levels in the urine, the excreted amount of cAMP in the urine is low in patients with hypoparathyroidism and rises briskly with the administration of exogenous PTH. The presence of antibodies in other endocrine tissues or organs may help in delineating the cause of the hypoparathyroidism.

The acute management of hypoparathyroidism is essentially the management of the hypocalcemia (see Chapter 108 Renal and Electrolyte Emergencies). Long-term management consists of treatment with vitamin D, usually with one of its more active analogs—1,25-$(OH)_2D_3$ at 0.01 to 0.05 μg/kg/day. Supplemental oral calcium is almost always necessary. The goals of long-term therapy are to maintain the serum calcium in the lower range of normal and to avoid both vitamin D toxicity and hypercalcemia. Preparations of PTH are not available for the long-term management of hypoparathyroidism.

Clinical Indications for Discharge or Admission

Asymptomatic patients may be treated as outpatients with close follow-up.

RICKETS

Goals of Treatment

To initiate vitamin D (and potentially calcium treatment) to normalize serum phosphate and effect positive changes on radiographs.

To avoid a potentially dangerous drop in calcium with initiation of treatment.

CLINICAL PEARLS AND PITFALLS

- Caused by inadequate dietary intake of vitamin D; incidence is decreasing as increased awareness and increased supplementation in food.
- Failure of calcification affects those parts of the skeleton that are growing most rapidly or that are under stress; a clinical diagnosis that is confirmed by radiology.
  - Premature infants are at increased risk for the development of rickets.
  - Significant hypocalcemia is unusual in rickets.

Current Evidence

Incidence of rickets is falling given increased supplementation of diets however is still seen among certain ethnic groups, premature infants, children with severe malabsorption problems, and patients with serious renal disease. Rickets is caused by the failure of mineralization of bone matrix in growing bone resulting from a lack of vitamin D. Consequently, unmineralized cartilage is excessive, and bone is soft. In addition to inadequate intake of vitamin D, the other causes of rickets are inability to form the active metabolite of vitamin D, excess phosphate excretion, and excess accumulation of acid.

Vitamin D may be obtained from dietary sources (especially animal fat) or synthesized from cholesterol via a complex pathway requiring the interaction of the precursor molecule with sunlight. Further hydroxylation of vitamin D in the liver (25-hydroxylation) and kidney (1-alpha-hydroxylation) leads to the formation of the active metabolite 1,25-dihydroxyvitamin D. Therefore, failure to form 1,25-$(OH)_2D_3$ may result from inadequate intake of vitamin D or insufficient exposure to sunlight. This is a particular problem among ethnic groups that eat small quantities of animal meat and that are extensively clothed when outdoors. Because vitamin D is fat soluble, any problem leading to prolonged fat malabsorption can result in rickets. Diseases affecting kidney or liver function may also lead to inadequate production of 1,25-$(OH)_2D_3$. An inherited deficiency of the 1-alpha-hydroxylase in the kidney (vitamin D–dependency rickets) is known. Certain drugs, such as phenobarbital and phenytoin, affect liver metabolism of vitamin D and can lead to rickets. Premature infants are particularly prone to vitamin D deficiency because of their minimal stores of vitamin D and their limited capacity for vitamin D synthesis.

Phosphate is a critical component of bone formation. Excess excretion of phosphate may lead to clinical rickets. Conditions that lead to excess phosphate excretion include primary hyperphosphaturia, Lowe syndrome, and Fanconi syndrome. Vitamin D–resistant rickets is a misnomer because the primary defect is in the renal tubular resorption of phosphate and not a resistance to vitamin D. Both an X-linked recessive and an autosomal-dominant form of phosphate wasting are known.

Rickets may also occur in conditions leading to chronic acidosis because bone is resorbed to buffer the acid load. This condition is seen in patients with distal renal tubular acidosis and may be partially responsible for the rachitic changes associated with Fanconi syndrome.

Clinical Considerations

Clinical Recognition

Children with rickets may come to medical attention because of specific physical abnormalities (bowed legs), limb pain and swelling, seizures, failure to thrive (renal tubular acidosis), biochemical abnormalities (hypocalcemia), radiographic findings (broadened, frayed metaphysis), or during the evaluation of a fracture.

Triage

Rickets should be considered in patients with nonspecific bony complaints.

Initial Assessment/H&P

A thorough social and dietary history is helpful in delineating the probable cause of the rickets and in sparing the patient an extensive and expensive evaluation. A family history may be useful in identifying the 1-hydroxylase deficiency or renal phosphate wasting. If the child has previously been treated with vitamin D, the reported response to that treatment may be helpful in identifying the likely site of defect.

The clinical findings in rickets may vary considerably, depending on the underlying disorder, the duration of the problem, and the child's age. Most features are related to skeletal deformity, skeletal pain, slippage of epiphyses, bony fractures, and growth disturbances. Muscular weakness, hypotonia, and lethargy are often noted.

Failure of calcification affects those parts of the skeleton that are growing most rapidly or that are under stress. For example, the skull grows rapidly in the perinatal period; therefore, craniotabes is a manifestation of congenital rickets. However, the upper limbs and rib cage grow rapidly during the first year of life, and abnormalities at these sites are more common at this age (i.e., rachitic rosary, flaring of the wrist). Bowing of the legs is unlikely to be noted until the child is ambulatory. Dental eruption may be delayed, and enamel defects are common.

Management/Diagnostic Testing

Radiography is the optimal way to confirm the clinical diagnosis of rickets because the radiologic features reflect the histopathology. Characteristic findings include widening and irregularity of the epiphyseal plates, cupped metaphyses, fractures, and bowing of the weight-bearing limbs (Figs. 97.4 and 97.5).

The clinical laboratory is often helpful in correctly identifying the cause of rickets. Frank hypocalcemia (<7 mg per dL) is unusual in rickets. Calcium levels in the 7 to 9 mg per dL

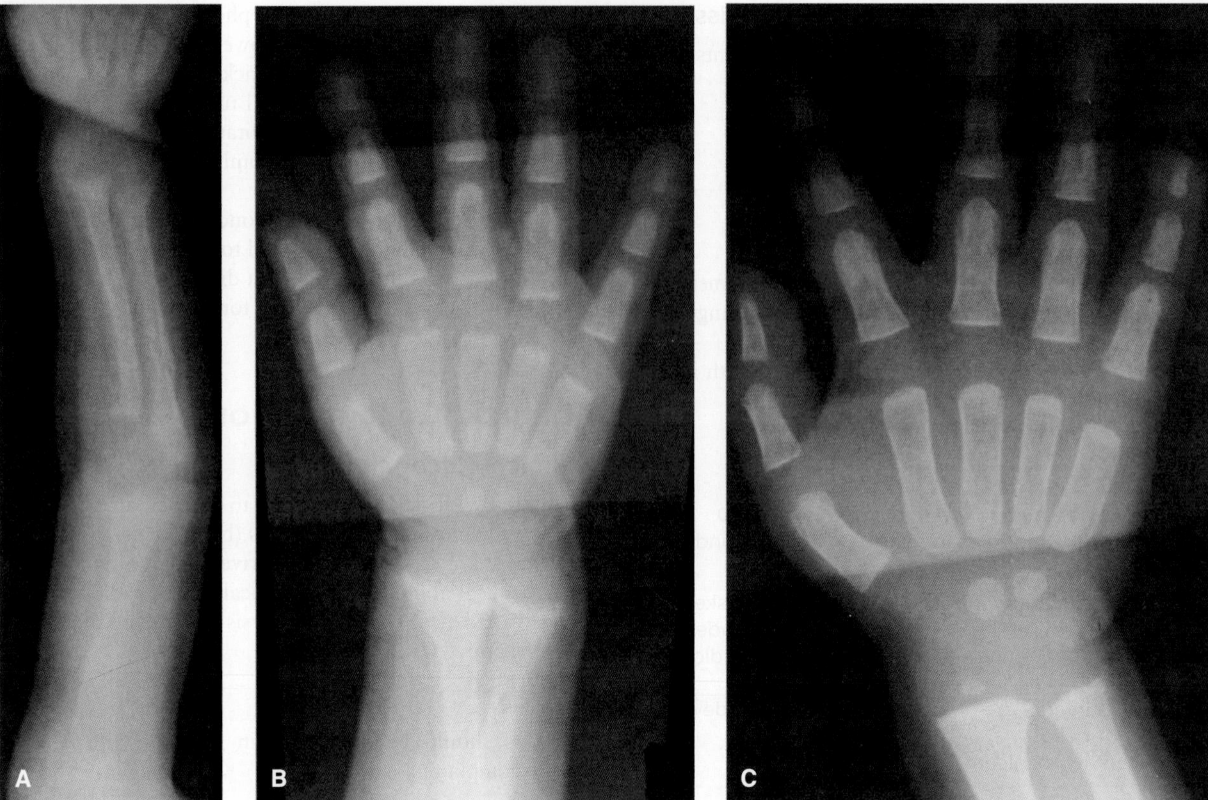

FIGURE 97.4 Rickets in an 11-month-old boy, breast-fed since birth. **A:** Roentgenogram of the upper extremity shows profound demineralization of the skeleton, with frayed, irregular cupping of the end of the metaphysis and poorly defined cortex. Note retardation of skeletal maturation. **B:** Same patient with some healing 4 weeks after supplemental vitamin D. Severe rachitic changes are noticeable. Periosteal cloaking, both of the metacarpals and of the radius and ulna, is evidence of healing. **C:** Complete healing of the rickets 8 months after treatment. Note the reappearance of the provisional zone of calcification. (Courtesy of Soroosh Mahboubi, MD, The Children's Hospital of Philadelphia.)

range are common and warrant careful attention because the initiation of vitamin D treatment increases bony deposition of calcium and may lead to a fall in serum calcium. Phosphate levels are often low. An amino aciduria is often present and may lead to some confusion of simple vitamin D deficiency

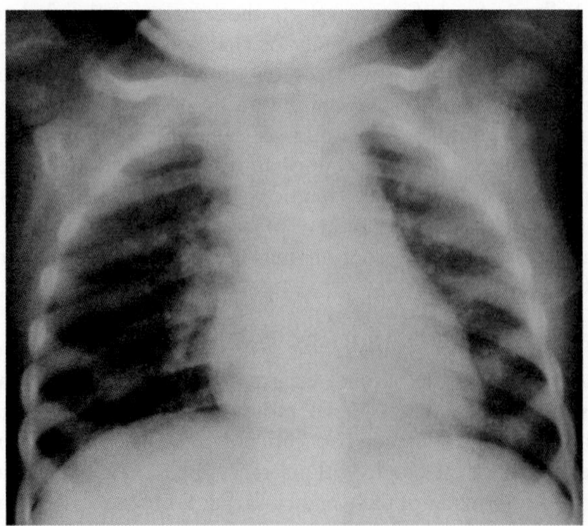

FIGURE 97.5 Rickets in an 11-month-old boy, breast-fed since birth. Roentgenogram of the chest shows demineralization of the skeleton with cupping of the distal end of ribs and humerus. (Courtesy of Soroosh Mahboubi, MD, The Children's Hospital of Philadelphia.)

with Fanconi syndrome. Alkaline phosphatase levels are significantly increased, reflecting extremely active bony metabolism. Although PTH levels are elevated, the results of this test are unlikely to be available at the time initial clinical decisions are made. Chronic acidosis, liver disease, and renal disease should be ruled out.

Treatment depends on the nature of the underlying disease. The response to treatment may be helpful in differentiating simple dietary vitamin D deficiency from more complex causes of rickets.

In the absence of chronic disease, dietary rickets may be adequately treated with daily doses of 1,200 to 1,600 IU of vitamin D (ergocalciferol) until healing occurs. Alternatively, a single high IM dose to replenish stores may be administered as ergocalciferol 50,000 to 100,000 IU. Serum phosphate usually returns to normal within 1 to 2 weeks, and radiographic improvement is generally apparent by 2 weeks. Once healing is complete, the child should continue to be treated with 400 IU per day to prevent recurrence.

If the initial serum calcium is borderline low or low, supplemental calcium should be initiated 48 hours before the institution of vitamin D, especially in the young child. Otherwise, the institution of vitamin D may cause a further decrease in serum calcium and elicit frank hypocalcemia. This presentation may occur naturally if the vitamin D–deficient patient has relatively low serum calcium concentration and then has prolonged exposure to the sun. This may lead to abrupt increases in vitamin D, ultimately leading to a rapid increase in bone recalcification (hungry bone syndrome) and severe hypocalcemia with possible seizures. This syndrome is seasonally termed "spring fits."

Clinical Indications for Discharge or Admission

Children with symptomatic hypocalcemia or with initial serum calcium of less than 7 mg per dL on presentation warrant hospitalization and frequent calcium determinations. Failure to respond to vitamin D treatment suggests that the child has a more complex cause of rickets, and consultation with a pediatric nephrologist or endocrinologist is recommended.

THYROID STORM

Goals of Treatment

After recognizing thyroid storm, the goals of emergency treatment are to control the metabolic rate and reduce cardiac workload.

CLINICAL PEARLS AND PITFALLS

- Thyroid storm is precipitated by intercurrent infection, trauma, or after subtotal thyroidectomy with an inadequately prepared patient.
- The presence of high fever (often to 105.8°F [41°C]) is the primary distinguishing feature of thyroid storm from a simple hyperthyroid state.
- A marked increase in cardiac workload may result in high-output heart failure and hypotension and pulmonary edema rather than classic hypertension.

Current Evidence

In thyroid storm, thyroid hormone is suddenly released into the circulation, which results in the uncoupling of oxidative phosphorylation and/or increased lipolysis, both of which contribute to excessive thermogenesis. Insensible fluid loss increases as a result of increased metabolism and sweating. Tachycardia is caused by both the hyperthermia and the direct action of thyroid hormones on the cardiac conduction system. Widened pulse pressure occurs as the result of increased cardiac contractility and decreased peripheral resistance. The mortality rate in adults may be as high as 20%; similar data are not available for children.

Clinical Considerations

Clinical Recognition

Almost all cases of thyroid storm occur in patients with known hyperthyroidism, although occasionally, a patient will present initially with thyroid storm.

Triage

Consider thyroid storm in patients with known hyperthyroidism who presents with fever, tachycardia, and systolic hypertension; these patients should receive expedited evaluation and treatment should be initiated quickly.

Initial Assessment/H&P

Most patients will have clinical findings characteristic of hyperthyroidism, including goiter (more than 95%), exophthalmos, tachycardia, bounding pulses, and systolic hypertension. Diastolic hypotension, tremulousness, restlessness, mania, delirium, or frankly psychotic behavior may be present. A primary feature that distinguishes thyroid storm from uncomplicated hyperthyroidism is the presence of high fever, often as high as 41°C (105.8°F). The marked increase in cardiac workload may result in high-output cardiac failure, in which case hypotension and pulmonary edema may be seen, rather than more classic hypertension.

Management/Diagnostic Testing

Thyroid studies including serum-free thyroxine (T_4), free triiodothyronine (T_3), and TSH should be obtained. Many clinical laboratories can now perform free T_4 assays on an emergency basis, alternatively total T_4 or total T_3 are adequate indices along with T_3-binding resin uptake; however, in many cases, therapy must be initiated on the basis of clinical evidence. Furthermore, the T_4 and T_3 values seen in thyroid storm overlap with those found in frank hyperthyroidism without storm. Serum electrolytes should be obtained but are unlikely to reveal any characteristic abnormalities, except for evidence of modest dehydration. Chest radiograph and EKG are helpful in evaluating and following cardiac status as treatment is initiated.

Initial treatment is directed toward lowering the metabolic rate and reducing the cardiac workload. Subsequent treatment is directed toward controlling thyroid hormone production.

Because many of the hypermetabolic effects of hyperthyroidism are mediated by the adrenergic system, a β-adrenergic antagonist (propranolol starting at 10 μg per kg intravenously over 10 to 15 minutes; or an esmolol infusion may be initiated with a loading dose of 500 μg/kg/min over 1 minute with maximal infusion doses of 50 to 250 μg/kg/min) is useful in the acute management of thyroid storm. Maintenance dosing of propranolol is 2 mg/kg/day divided every 6 hours in neonates and 10 to 40 mg every 6 hours in older children. EKG monitoring for heart rate and arrhythmias is recommended.

Because the metabolic rate is increased about 10% for every degree of body temperature higher than 36.5°C (97.7°F), lowering body temperature is an effective means of reducing the metabolic rate in the patient with thyrotoxicosis. Tepid sponging, use of a cooling blanket, and administration of acetaminophen can accomplish this task. Aspirin should not be used because it is a potential uncoupler of oxidative phosphorylation that may exacerbate the hypermetabolic state.

Treatment of the hyperthyroidism in thyroid storm is accomplished by the use of iodide and an inhibitor of iodine oxidation in the thyroid gland such as methimazole 0.5 to 0.7 mg/kg/day divided into three oral doses, which blocks iodine's ability to combine with tyrosine to form thyroxine and triiodothyronine (T_3); of note neither medication inactivates circulating T_4 and T_3. Propylthiouracil was a first-line agent, but, due to its association with pediatric liver failure, it has now become contraindicated in children. Iodide rapidly terminates thyroid hormone release; however, this effect is overcome after 3 to 5 days of iodide therapy. Iodide also decreases the vascularity of the thyroidal arterial supply and can be particularly useful as a preoperative agent. Lugol iodide (or SSKI) 3 to

5 drops once every 8 hours orally or sodium iodide 125 to 250 mg per day intravenously over 24 hours is the usual mode of iodide therapy. While iodide can reduce thyroid hormone secretion within 24 hours, methimazole's effects are minimally useful in acute management because the reduction in thyroid levels may take several days.

Adequate hydration is essential for effective treatment of thyroid storm. The estimate of fluid replacement should include a consideration of the significant increase in fluid requirements caused by fever and an accelerated metabolic rate. Glucocorticoids are useful in the acute presentation because they appear to inhibit thyroid hormone release from the thyroid and decrease the peripheral conversion of T_4 to T_3. Dexamethasone (0.2 mg per kg) or hydrocortisone (5 mg per kg) can be given parenterally during the acute phase.

Intercurrent infection may be the precipitating factor, thus it should be searched for and treated appropriately. Broad-spectrum antibiotics should be considered while awaiting the results of cultures, as there is a known association between thyrotoxicosis and pneumococcal bacteremia. Improvement should be seen within a few hours after the initiation of treatment with propranolol, especially in terms of cardiovascular status.

Clinical Indications for Discharge or Admission

All patients in thyroid storm should be admitted. Full recovery and adequate control of the underlying thyroid disease take several days to achieve. For the patient presenting with thyroid storm, serious consideration should be given to permanent treatment of the hyperthyroidism, either by surgery or radioiodide ablation.

NEONATAL THYROTOXICOSIS

Goals of Treatment

The goals of treatment are to control metabolic rate and reduce cardiac workload.

CLINICAL PEARLS AND PITFALLS

- Neonatal hyperthyroidism is a life-threatening condition found in 1% to 5% of infants born to mothers with history of hyperthyroidism.
- Infants of mothers with thyroid disease can have hyperthyroidism even if the mother's thyroid condition is not active during pregnancy or well controlled.

Current Evidence

Neonatal thyrotoxicosis may not be correctly diagnosed in the newborn nursery and may be discovered only when the child presents in extremis in the ED. It is caused by excessive thyroid hormone produced by the neonatal thyroid that has been stimulated by maternal thyroid-stimulating antibodies present in the immunoglobulin G (IgG) fraction that have crossed the placenta. TSH, T_4, and T_3 do not cross the placenta in significant quantities. In most cases, the disease is self-limiting, and hyperthyroidism remits within about 6 weeks. Occasionally, the disease may run a protracted course and arise in the absence of maternal thyroid-stimulating antibodies.

Clinical Considerations

Clinical Recognition

The diagnosis should be considered in neonates with maternal history of hyperthyroidism; especially if they are presenting with tachycardia, failure to thrive, or congestive heart failure.

Triage

Assess for signs/symptoms of congestive heart failure.

Initial Assessment/H&P

The child usually presents with a history of failure to gain weight despite a ravenous appetite. The child may also be irritable and have tachycardia, as well as signs of congestive heart failure. The physical examination is usually remarkable for a goiter and exophthalmos, acknowledging that a goiter may be difficult to appreciate in a small infant with a short neck.

Management/Diagnostic Testing

Laboratory investigations should include estimations of serum total and free T_4 and T_3, and serum TSH. Increased concentration of T_4 in the presence of suppressed TSH levels is consistent with the diagnosis. If the mother is taking antithyroid medication, thyroid function tests on the infant may be unreliable in the first days of life because of suppression of the fetal thyroid by transplacental passage of maternal antithyroid medication. When tested, the bone age may be advanced.

In most cases, treatment must be initiated on the basis of historical and clinical findings. For an infant who has an elevated level of T_4 but who has few, if any, symptoms or signs, consultation with a pediatric endocrinologist is strongly recommended. Total T_4 levels in all infants tend to be higher than those in older children because of increased thyroid-binding globulin (TBG) induced by maternal estrogen that crosses the placenta. Also, an elevated total thyroxine may be seen with defects that alter the binding of T_4 to TBG or the end-organ sensitivity to T_4.

Treatment is identical to that outlined for thyroid storm in older children. The duration of treatment is uncertain and should be based on serial thyroid function tests, especially TSH. It is anticipated that treatment need be continued only for 6 to 8 weeks in most cases because the causative agent is a subclass of IgG molecules with a serum half-life of about 2 weeks.

Clinical Indications for Discharge or Admission

Consider admission for symptomatic children.

CONGENITAL HYPOTHYROIDISM

Goal of Treatment

The major goal of treatment is to address acute clinical manifestations of hypothyroidism, confirm the diagnosis, and plan replacement therapy.

CLINICAL PEARLS AND PITFALLS

- Congenital hypothyroidism should be considered in infants with significant constipation, prolonged jaundice, hypotonia, or hypothermia.

Current Evidence

The incidence of congenital hypothyroidism is 1 in 3,500 live births. Emergency physicians should be knowledgeable about congenital hypothyroidism so they can appropriately educate parents and initiate therapy. Acquired hypothyroidism rarely results in urgent clinical problems that lead to ED visits.

The causes of congenital hypothyroidism are numerous; most cases (90%) are permanent. About 20% of patients have ectopic glands, and another 50% have hypoplastic or aplastic thyroid glands. Other causes are less common and include dyshormonogenesis, maternal ingestion of antithyroid medication, hypothalamic–pituitary disorders, and defects in thyroglobulin metabolism. The dyshormonogenic disorders are inherited as autosomal-recessive conditions. Congenital thyroid deficiency may result in impaired neurologic development if not treated before 1 month of age.

Clinical Considerations

Clinical Recognition

Clinical symptoms and signs of congenital hypothyroidism may be subtle and nonspecific, especially during the first month of life.

Triage

Patients are generally well appearing and at minimal risk for decompensating.

Initial Assessment/H&P

Severely affected infants may be relatively large at birth, have a large posterior fontanel, manifest hypothermia and hypoactivity, feed poorly, tend to become constipated, and have prolonged jaundice. An enlarged tongue, coarse facies, and a hoarse cry may also be noted but are unusual in the first weeks of life. An umbilical hernia may be present. If treatment is not started, the physical characteristics become more prominent as the child grows older.

Management/Diagnostic Testing

Thyroid function tests beyond the first 2 days of life are most useful diagnostically. The TSH level is elevated in primary hypothyroidism, and the total and free T_4 levels are low or normal for age. A thyroid ultrasound or scan (^{123}I) may be helpful in identifying the particular type of primary hypothyroidism, but treatment should not be delayed to obtain this study. A low total T_4 level in the absence of elevated TSH level may result from a deficiency of TBG, a pituitary deficiency of TSH, or prematurity.

In term infants, treatment with l-thyroxine, 10 to 15 µg/kg/day should be instituted as soon as the relevant diagnostic tests are performed. In premature infants, 8 µg/kg/day can be administered. This dosage can be adjusted to maintain a TSH value that is normal for age; on appropriate replacement, the TSH will normalize within 4 weeks. Total T_4 and free T_4 concentrations should be maintained in the upper half of the normal range for age. Both undertreatment and overtreatment must be avoided.

Clinical Indications for Discharge or Admission

Generally, treatment is as outpatient. Careful follow-up on a monthly basis during the first several months, preferably by a physician who is accustomed to dealing with congenital hypothyroidism, is strongly recommended.

Suggested Readings and Key References

Diabetic Ketoacidosis

American Diabetes Association. Diagnosis and classification of diabetes mellitus. *Diabetes Care* 2004;27:S5–S10.

Butkiewicz EK, Liebson CL, Obrien PC, et al. Insulin therapy for diabetic ketoacidosis: bolus injection versus continuous insulin infusion. *Diabetes Care* 1995;18:1187–1190.

Butler AM, Talbot NB. Metabolic studies in diabetic coma. *Trans Assoc Am Physicians* 1947;60:102–109.

DeCourcey DD, Steil G, Wypij D, et al. Increasing use of hypertonic saline over mannitol in the treatment of symptomatic cerebral edema in pediatric diabetic ketoacidosis: an 11 year retrospective analysis of mortality. *Pediatr Crit Care Med* 2013;14:694–700.

Edge JA, Hawkins MM, Winter DL, et al. The risk and outcome of cerebral oedema developing during diabetic ketoacidosis. *Arch Dis Child* 2001;85:16–22.

Ghetti S, Lee JK, Sims CE, et al. Diabetic ketoacidosis and memory dysfunction in children with type 1 diabetes. *J Pediatr* 2010;156:109–114.

Glaser N, Barnett P, McCaslin I, et al. Risk factors for cerebral edema in children with diabetic ketoacidosis. The Pediatric Emergency Medicine Collaborative Research Committee of the American Academy of Pediatrics. *N Engl J Med* 2001;344:264–269.

Jacobson AD, Hauser ST, Willett J, et al. Consequences of irregular versus continuous follow-up in children and adolescents with insulin dependent diabetes mellitus. *J Pediatr* 1997;131:727–733.

Klekamp J, Churchwell KB. Diabetic ketoacidosis in children: initial clinical assessment and treatment. *Pediatr Ann* 1996;25:387–393.

Krane EJ, Rockoff MA, Wallman JK, et al. Subclinical brain swelling in children during treatment of diabetic ketoacidosis. *N Engl J Med* 1985;312:1147–1150.

Lindsey R, Bolte RG. The use of insulin bolus in low-dose insulin infusion for pediatric diabetic ketoacidosis. *Pediatr Emerg Care* 1989;5:77–79.

Morris AD, Boyle DI, McMahon AG, et al. Adherence to insulin treatment, glycaemic control and ketoacidosis in insulin dependent diabetes mellitus. *Lancet* 1997;350:1505–1510.

Muir AB, Quisling RG, Yang MC, et al. Cerebral edema in childhood diabetic ketoacidosis: natural history, radiographic findings, and early identification. *Diabetes Care* 2004;27:1541–1546.

Puttha R, Cooke D, Subbarayan A, et al. Low dose (0.05 units/kg/h) is comparable with standard dose (0.1 units/kg/h) intravenous insulin infusion for the initial treatment of diabetic ketoacidosis in children with type 1 diabetes-an observational study. *Pediatr Diabetes* 2010;11:12–17.

Thompson CJ, Cummings F, Chalmers J, et al. Abnormal insulin treatment behavior: a major cause of ketoacidosis in the young adult. *Diabet Med* 1995;12:429–432.

Wolfsdorf JI, Allgrove J, Craig ME, et al. ISPAD Clinical Practice Consensus Guidelines 2014. Diabetic ketoacidosis and hyperglycemic hyperosmolar state. *Pediatr Diabetes* 2014;15(suppl 20):154–179.

Hypoglycemia

Aynsley-Green A. Hypoglycemia in infants and children. *Clin Endocr Metab* 1982;11:159–193.

Cornblath M, Schwartz R. *Disorders of carbohydrate metabolism in infancy.* Cambridge: Blackwell Publications, 1991.

Haymond MW. Hypoglycemia in infants and children. *Endocrinol Metab Clin North Am* 1989;18:211–252.

LaFranchi S. Hypoglycemia of infancy and childhood. *Pediatr Clin North Am* 1987;34:961–982.

Pagliara AS, Karl IE, Haymond M, et al. Hypoglycemia in infancy and childhood. Parts I and II. *J Pediatr* 1973;82:365–379, 558–577.

Stanley CA. Advances in diagnosis and treatment of hyperinsulinism in infants and children. *J Clin Endocrinol Metab* 2002;87:4857–4859.

Wolfsdorf JI, Weinstein DA. Glycogen storage diseases. *Rev Endocr Metab Disord* 2003;4:95–102.

Hypopituitarism

DeVile CJ, Stanhope R. Hydrocortisone replacement therapy in children and adolescents with hypopituitarism. *Clin Endocrinol* 1997;47:37–41.

Geffner ME. Hypopituitarism in childhood. *Cancer Control* 2002;9:212–222.

Lovinger RD, Kaplan SL, Grumbach MM. Congenital hypopituitarism associated with neonatal hypoglycemia and microphallus: four cases secondary to hypothalamic hormone deficiencies. *J Pediatr* 1975;87:1171–1181.

Rogol AD. Hypopituitarism. *Curr Ther Endocrinol Metabol* 1994;5:26–29.

Stahnke N, Koehn H. Replacement therapy in hypothalamus-pituitary insufficiency: management in the adolescent. *Horm Res* 1990;4 (suppl 33):38–44.

Willnow S, Kiess W, Butenandt O, et al. Endocrine disorders in septo-optic dysplasia: evaluation and follow-up of 18 patients. *Eur J Pediatr* 1996;155:179–184.

Acute Adrenal Insufficiency

August GP. Treatment of adrenocortical insufficiency. *Pediatr Rev* 1997;18:59–62.

Dorin RI, Qualls CR, Crapo LM. Diagnosis of adrenal insufficiency. *Ann Intern Med* 2003;139:194–204.

Lipiner-Friedman D, Sprung CL, Laterre PF, et al. Adrenal function in sepsis: the retrospective Corticus cohort study. *Crit Care Med* 2007;35:1012–1018.

New MI. Replacement doses of glucocorticoids. *J Pediatr* 1991;119:161.

Perry R, Kecha O, Paquette J, et al. Primary adrenal insufficiency in children: twenty years experience at the Sainte-Justine Hospital, Montreal. *J Clin Endocrinol Metab* 2005;90:3243–3250.

Urban MD, Kogut MD. Adrenocortical insufficiency in the child. *Curr Ther Endocrinol Metab* 1994;5:131–135.

Congenital Adrenal Hyperplasia

Cutler GG Jr, Laue L. Congenital adrenal hyperplasia due to 21-hydroxylase deficiency. *N Engl J Med* 1990;323:1906–1913.

Joint LWPES/ESPE CAH Working Group. Consensus statement on 21-hydroxylase deficiency from the Lawson Wilkins Pediatric Endocrine Society and the European Society for Paediatric Endocrinology. *J Clin Endocrinol Metab* 2002;87:4048–4053.

Levine LS. Congenital adrenal hyperplasia. *Pediatr Rev* 2000;21:159–170.

Miller WL. Congenital adrenal hyperplasia. *Endocrinol Metab Clin North Am* 1991;20:721–749.

Newfield RS, New MI. 21-hydroxylase deficiency. *Ann NY Acad Sci* 1997;816:219–229.

Pang S. Congenital adrenal hyperplasia. *Endocrinol Metab Clin North Am* 1997;26:853–891.

Speiser PW, Azziz R, Baskin LS, et al. Congenital adrenal hyperplasia due to steroid 21-hydroxylase deficiency: an Endocrine Society clinical practice guideline. *J Clin Endocrinol Metab* 2010;95:4133–4160.

Pheochromocytoma

Bravo EL, Tagle R. Pheochromocytoma: state-of-the-art and future prospects. *Endocr Rev* 2003;24:539–553.

Caty MG, Coran AG, Geagen M, et al. Current diagnosis and treatment of pheochromocytoma in children. *Arch Surg* 1990;125:978–981.

Ein SH, Pullerits J, Crighton R, et al. Pediatric pheochromocytoma: a 36-year review. *Pediatr Surg Int* 1997;12:595–598.

Fonkalsrud EW. Pheochromocytoma in childhood. *Prog Pediatr Surg* 1991;26:103–111.

Lenders JW, Keiser HR, Goldstein DS, et al. Plasma metanephrines in the diagnosis of pheochromocytoma. *Ann Intern Med* 1995;123:101–109.

Werbel SS, Ober KP. Pheochromocytoma: update on diagnosis, localization and management. *Med Clin North Am* 1995;79:131–153.

Diabetes Insipidus

Buonocore CM, Robinson AG. The diagnosis and management of diabetes insipidus during medical emergencies. *Endocrinol Metab Clin North Am* 1993;22:411–413.

Harris AS. Clinical experience with desmopressin: efficacy and safety in central diabetes insipidus and other conditions. *J Pediatr* 1989;144:711–718.

Knoers N, Monnens LA. Nephrogenic diabetes insipidus: clinical symptoms, pathogenesis, genetics and treatment. *Pediatr Nephrol* 1992;6:476–482.

Lee YJ, Huang FY, Shen EY, et al. Neurogenic diabetes insipidus in children with hypoxic encephalopathy: six new cases and a review of the literature. *Eur J Pediatr* 1996;155:245–248.

Ober KP. Endocrine crisis: diabetes insipidus. *Crit Care Clin* 1991;7:109–125.

Oiso Y, Robertson GL, Nørgaard JP, et al. Clinical review: treatment of neurohypophyseal diabetes insipidus. *J Clin Endocrinol Metab* 2013;98:3958–3967.

Schrier RW, Cadnapaphornchai MA. Renal aquaporin water channels: from molecules to human disease. *Progr Biophys Molec Biol* 2003;81:117–131.

Seckl JR, Dunger DB. Diabetes insipidus: current treatment recommendations. *Drugs* 1992;44:216–224.

Syndrome of Inappropriate Antidiuretic Hormone Secretion

DeFronzo RA, Goldberg M, Agus ZS. Normal diluting capacity in hyponatremic patients. Reset osmostat or a variant of the syndrome of inappropriate antidiuretic hormone secretion. *Ann Intern Med* 1976;84:538–542.

Ganong CA, Kappy MS. Cerebral salt wasting in children: the need for recognition and treatment. *Am J Dis Child* 1993;147:167–169.

Kaplan SL, Feigin RD. Syndromes of inappropriate secretion of antidiuretic hormone in children. *Adv Pediatr* 1980;27:247–274.

Kappy MS, Ganong CA. Cerebral salt wasting in children: the role of atrial natriuretic factor. *Adv Pediatr* 1996;43:271–308.

Palmer BF. Hyponatremia in patients with central nervous system disease: SIADH versus CSW. *Trends Endocrinol Metab* 2003;14:182–187.

Schrier RW, Gross P, Gheorghiade M, et al. Tolvaptan, a selective oral vasopressin V2-receptor antagonist, for hyponatremia. *N Engl J Med* 2006;355:2099–2112.

Hyperparathyroidism

Lawson ML, Miller SF, Ellis G, et al. Primary hyperparathyroidism in a paediatric hospital. *Q J Med* 1996;89:921–932.

Marcocci C, Bollerslev J, Khan AA, et al. Medical management of primary hyperparathyroidism: proceedings of the fourth International Workshop on the Management of Asymptomatic Primary Hyperparathyroidism. *J Clin Endocrinol Metab* 2014;99:3607–3618.

Matsuo M, Okita K, Takemine H, et al. Neonatal primary hyperparathyroidism in familial hypocalciuric hypercalcemia. *Am J Dis Child* 1982;136:728–731.

Moe SM, Drueke TB. Management of secondary hyperparathyroidism: the importance and the challenge of controlling parathyroid hormone levels without elevating calcium, phosphorus, and calcium-phosphorus product. *Am J Nephrol* 2003;23:369–379.

Ross AJ, Cooper A, Attie MF, et al. Primary hyperparathyroidism in infancy. *J Pediatr Surg* 1986;21:493–499.

Hypoparathyroidism

Rosen JF, Fleischman AR, Finberg L, et al. 1,25-Dihydroxycholecalciferol: its use in the long-term management of idiopathic hypoparathyroidism in children. *J Clin Endocrinol Metab* 1977;45:457–468.

Taylor SC, Morris G, Wilson D, et al. Hypoparathyroidism and 22q11 deletion syndrome. *Arch Dis Child* 2003;88:520–522.

Winter WE, Silverstein JH, Maclaren NK, et al. Autosomal-dominant hypoparathyroidism with variable, age-dependent severity. *J Pediatr* 1983;103:387–390.

Rickets

Chesney RW, Mazess RB, Rose P, et al. Long-term influence of calcitriol and supplemental phosphate in X-linked hypophosphatemic rickets. *Pediatrics* 1983;71:559–567.

Dwyer JT, Dietz WH, Hass G, et al. Risk of nutritional rickets among vegetarian children. *Am J Dis Child* 1979;133:134–140.

Lovinger RD. Rickets. *Pediatrics* 1980;66:359–365.

Mughal Z. Rickets in childhood. *Semin Musculoskelet Radiol* 2002;6:183–190.

Rajakumar K. Vitamin D, cod-liver oil, sunlight, and rickets: a historical perspective. *Pediatrics* 2003;112:e132–e135.

Thacher TD, Fischer PR, Pettifor JM. Vitamin D treatment in calcium-deficiency rickets: a randomised controlled trial. *Arch Dis Child* 2014; 99:807–811.

Wharton B, Bishop N. Rickets. *Lancet* 2003;362:1389–1400.

Thyroid Storm

Bahn Chair RS, Burch HB, Cooper DS, et al. Hyperthyroidism and other causes of thyrotoxicosis: management guidelines of the American Thyroid Association and American Association of Clinical Endocrinologists. *Thyroid* 2011;21:593–646.

Foley TP Jr. Thyrotoxicosis in childhood. *Pediatr Ann* 1992;21:43–49.

Foley TP Jr, Charron M. Radioiodine treatment of juvenile Graves' disease. *Exp Clin Endocrinol Diabetes* 1997;105(suppl 4):61–65.

Hung W. Graves' disease in children. *Curr Ther Endocrinol Metab* 1997; 6:77– 81.

Rivkees SA, Mattison DR. Ending propylthiouracil-induced liver failure in children. *New Engl J Med* 2009;360:1574–1575.

Segni M, Gorman CA. The aftermath of childhood hyperthyroidism. *J Pediatr Endocrinol Metab* 2001;14(suppl 5):1277–1282.

Neonatal Thyrotoxicosis

De Groot L, Abalovich M, Alexander EK, et al. Management of thyroid dysfunction during pregnancy and postpartum: an Endocrine Society clinical practice guideline. *J Clin Endocrinol Metab* 2012;97:2543–2565.

Dirmikis SM, Munro DS. Placental transmission of thyroid-stimulating immunoglobulins. *Br Med J* 1975;2:665–666.

Foley TP Jr. Maternally transferred thyroid disease in the infant: recognition and treatment. *Adv Exp Med Biol* 1991;299:209–226.

Levy-Shraga Y, Tamir-Hostovsky L, Boyko V, et al. Follow-up of newborns of mothers with Graves' disease. *Thyroid* 2014;24:1032–1039.

Singer J. Neonatal thyrotoxicosis. *J Pediatr* 1977;91:749–750.

Congenital Hypothyroidism

Barsano CP, DeGroot LJ. Dyshormonogenetic goitre. *Clin Endocrinol Metab* 1979;8:145–165.

Bongers-Schokking JJ, Resing WC, de Rijke YB, et al. Cognitive development in congenital hypothyroidism: is overtreatment a greater threat than undertreatment? *J Clin Endocrinol Metab* 2013;98:4499–4506.

Burrow GN, Dussault JH. *Neonatal thyroid screening.* New York, NY: Raven, 1980.

Grüters A, Krude H. Detection and treatment of congenital hypothyroidism. *Nat Rev Endocrinol* 2012;8:104–113.

Lazarus JH, Bestwick JP, Channon S, et al. Antenatal thyroid screening and childhood cognitive function. *N Engl J Med* 2012;366:493–501.

Léger J, Olivieri A, Donaldson M, et al. European Society for Paediatric Endocrinology consensus guidelines on screening, diagnosis, and management of congenital hypothyroidism. *J Clin Endocrinol Metab* 2014;99:363–384.

CHAPTER 98 ■ ENVIRONMENTAL EMERGENCIES, RADIOLOGICAL EMERGENCIES, BITES AND STINGS

DESIREE M. SEEYAVE, MBBS AND KATHLEEN M. BROWN, MD

RELATED CHAPTERS

Resuscitation and Stabilization
- Airway: Chapter 3
- Cardiopulmonary Resuscitation: Chapter 4
- Shock: Chapter 5
- Pain: Abdomen: Chapter 48

Signs and Symptoms
- Seizures: Chapter 67

Clinical Pathways
- Shock: Chapter 91

Medical, Surgical, and Trauma Emergencies
- Cardiac Emergencies: Chapter 94
- Renal and Electrolyte Emergencies: Chapter 108
- Burns: Chapter 112

DROWNING

Goals of Treatment

Treatment of submersion injuries aims to resuscitate and stabilize those who need it, and prevent further pulmonary and neurologic deterioration.

CLINICAL PEARLS AND PITFALLS

- Outcome of submersion victims depends on duration of submersion, degree of pulmonary damage by aspiration, and effectiveness of initial resuscitative measures.
- Supplemental O_2 should be given to all victims of submersion, regardless of neurologic or pulmonary function on presentation.

Current Evidence

Drowning is defined as water submersion with resultant asphyxiation and death within 24 hours; *near drowning* implies that resuscitation has extended survival beyond 24 hours. Each term is further classified according to whether aspiration has occurred.

Drowning affects all age groups and males two to three times more often than females. Individuals with epilepsy have a 15- to 19-fold higher risk of drowning when compared to the general population. It is the major cause of death following water-related natural disasters such as Hurricane Katrina.

Drowning is the second leading cause of injury death in children 1 to 14 years of age. Older infants and toddlers are disproportionately represented in these accidents, with lower survival rates. They are vulnerable to immersion in household buckets, baths, hot tubs, swimming pools, and other bodies of water near their homes. Young teenagers are also at greater risk because adult supervision decreases and impulsive behavior increases. However, coexisting trauma, drug or alcohol use, and suicidal intent must be considered in each case.

Fresh water aspirated into the lungs is rapidly taken up into the circulation, resulting in a transient rise in circulating blood volume and hemodilution. Salt-water aspiration causes decreased intravascular volume and hemoconcentration. Occasionally massive hemolysis may occur. Electrolyte abnormalities that occur after massive aspiration in laboratory animals rarely achieve clinical significance in human victims.

Even small (1 to 3 mL per kg) quantities of fresh water cause disruption of surfactant, a rise in surface tension in the lungs, and alveolar instability. Capillary and alveolar membrane damage allows fluid to leak into the alveoli, with subsequent pulmonary edema. Aspiration of salt water (osmolality greater than normal saline) does not denature surfactant but creates an osmotic gradient for fluid to accumulate in the lungs, which dilutes surfactant.

Both fresh- and salt-water aspiration decrease pulmonary compliance, increase airway resistance and pulmonary artery pressure, and diminish pulmonary flow. As nonventilated alveoli are perfused, an intrapulmonary shunt develops, leading to a drastic fall in partial pressure of arterial oxygen (PaO_2). Tissue hypoxia then leads to severe metabolic acidosis. The victim is usually able to correct a rise in partial pressure of arterial carbon dioxide ($PaCO_2$). Aspiration of bacteria, gastric contents, and foreign materials may cause additional trauma to the lungs.

Hypoxemia results in loss of consciousness. If anoxia ensues, irreversible central nervous system (CNS) damage begins after 4 to 6 minutes. Fear or cold may trigger the diving reflex (commonly encountered in infancy), which shunts blood to the brain and heart primarily and affords several minutes of additional perfusion. Cold water is relatively protective of the CNS, but probably only if immersion hypothermia develops very rapidly or before compromise of oxygenation. Hypothermia is more rapid in the victim who is younger (because of greater surface area:volume ratio) or is struggling in or swallowing icy water. If laryngospasm or aspiration occurs before a fall in core body temperature and cerebral metabolic rate, protection is probably minimal.

Cardiovascular effects are primarily those expected with myocardial ischemia, severe systemic acidosis, hypothermia, and intravascular volume changes. After aspiration of fresh water, the transient rise in intravascular volume later contributes to problems of cerebral and pulmonary edema.

Clinical Recognition

In the first moments after rescue, the appearance of the child who has nearly drowned may range from apparently normal to apparently dead. Body temperature is often low, even in warm water. Respiratory efforts may be absent, irregular, or labored, with pallor or cyanosis, retractions, grunting, and cough productive of pink, frothy material. The lungs may be clear, or there may be rales, rhonchi, and wheezing. Infection may develop as a consequence of aspirated mouth flora or organisms in stagnant water, but this is not usually important in the first 24 hours.

Respiratory function may improve spontaneously or deteriorate rapidly as pulmonary edema and small airway dysfunction worsen. Deterioration may also occur slowly over 12 to 24 hours. Intense peripheral vasoconstriction and myocardial depression may produce apparent or actual pulselessness.

The child may be alert and normal or have any level of CNS compromise. Superficial evidence of head trauma may be noted if the submersion episode was a secondary event. Head CT most typically shows diffuse loss of gray–white differentiation and/or bilateral basal ganglia edema/infarction.

Triage Considerations

Outcome depends on the duration of submersion, the degree of pulmonary damage by aspiration, and effectiveness of initial resuscitative measures. Most children are salvageable, and all should receive the benefit of excellent cardiopulmonary resuscitation without delay at the scene. They should all be given 100% oxygen, even if rescued with spontaneous ventilation and minimal or no neurologic dysfunction, to minimize the risk of progressive hypoxemia and acidosis with secondary myocardial and cerebral damage. Physical examination is notoriously insensitive to hypoxemia; a seriously hypoxemic child may be alert and talking. Once the child has arrived at an emergency facility (and cardiovascular stability is achieved), pulmonary and neurologic assessment should guide further treatment.

Initial Assessment

Initial assessment should focus on signs of neurologic, respiratory, and hemodynamic compromise. One prospective study devised a prediction rule for children submerged in nonicy water who presented to the emergency department (ED) in a comatose state: Lack of pupillary light reflex, male gender, and hyperglycemia were variables used to predict unfavorable outcome (vegetative state or death). A retrospective study of children presenting to the ED after warm-water submersion suggested that hemodynamic, rather than neurologic, status was more highly predictive of poor neurologic outcome.

More recent studies indicate that patients with asystole on arrival in the ED have uniformly poor neurologic outcomes. The emergency physician may reasonably discontinue resuscitative efforts after consideration on a case-by-case basis.

Management and Diagnostic Testing

Effective therapy of drowning depends on the reversal of hypoxemia and metabolic acidosis. The pulmonary status is assessed initially with a chest radiograph (Fig. 98.1) and with measurement of arterial oxygen saturation ($Sa{O_2}$) and arterial blood gas (ABG), as in Figure 98.2. If oxygenation is normal on breathing room air, the child can be assumed to have suffered drowning without aspiration. Observation for 6 to 24 hours with repeat $Sa{O_2}$ or ABG determination should be sufficient to assess the possibility of late deterioration in gas exchange.

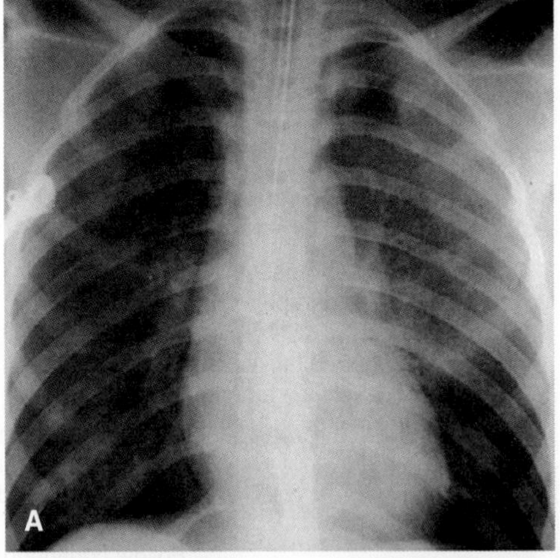

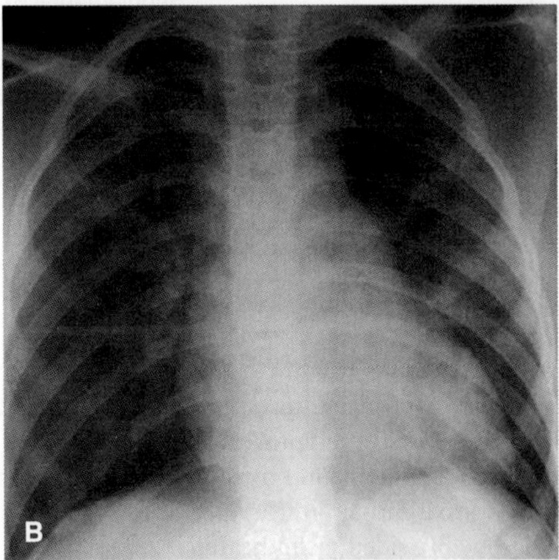

FIGURE 98.1 Drowning in a 4-month-old girl. **A:** There is bilateral disseminated alveolar pattern, more on the left than on the right, consistent with the pulmonary edema of drowning. This change may be the result of neurologic pulmonary edema rather than aspirated water. **B:** Two days later, the patient has been extubated and there is marked improvement in appearance of pulmonary edema secondary to drowning. (Courtesy of Soroosh Mahboubi, MD.)

Other initial laboratory evaluation should include complete blood cell count (CBC), electrolytes, and urinalysis. Patients with abnormalities of gas exchange with normal chest radiographs can usually be managed with supplemental oxygen and pulmonary physiotherapy. Noninvasive ventilatory support, such as high-flow humidified nasal cannula oxygen or CPAP, may be beneficial. Any change in mental status or increase in respiratory distress may reflect arterial hypoxemia and should also prompt a repeat ABG determination. Continuous $Sa{O_2}$ or serial $Pa{O_2}$ measurements will guide the physician to continue conservative treatment or to intensify ventilatory support.

Patients with obvious respiratory distress, hypoxemia ($Sa{O_2}$ less than 90% or $Pa{O_2}$ less than 60 on 60% inspired oxygen), and extensive pulmonary edema or infiltration generally require more vigorous treatment. All should be monitored

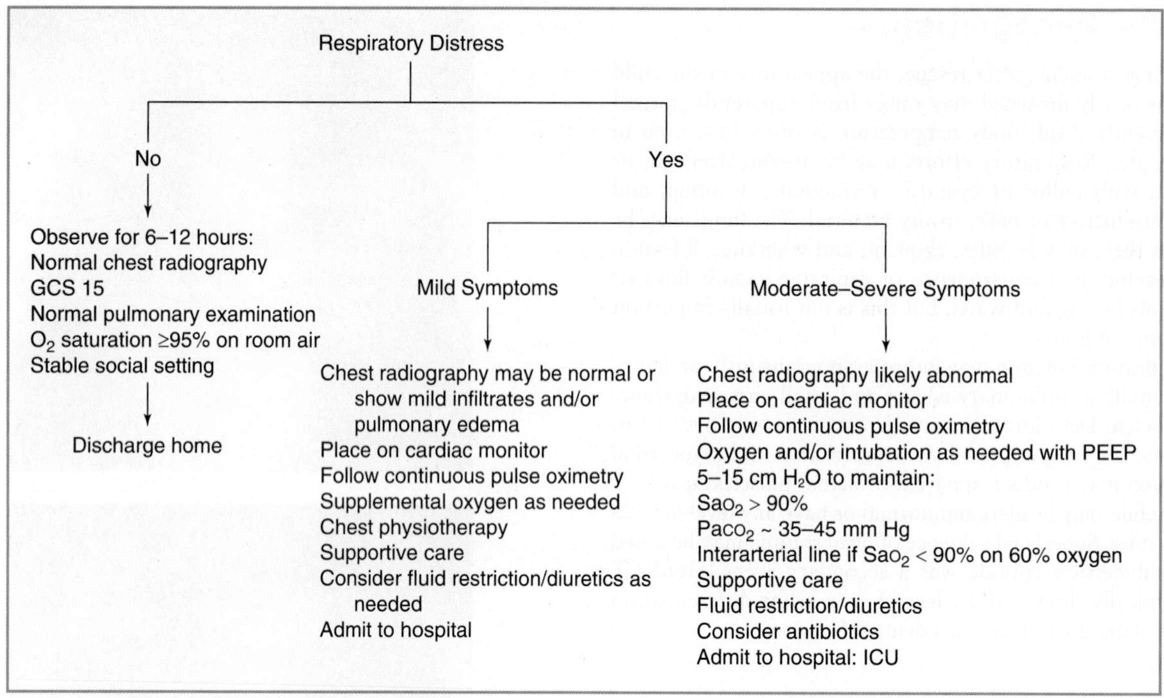

FIGURE 98.2 Algorithm for pulmonary assessment for drowning.

for heart rate, cardiac rhythm, respiratory rate, and blood pressure (BP). Most will require frequent blood gas analysis and may be more easily monitored through arterial cannulation. Intubation, supplemental oxygen, and mechanical ventilation with positive end-expiratory pressure (PEEP; 5 to 15 cm H_2O) should be provided, as indicated.

Once BP is stabilized, fluid restriction (to approximately one-half the maintenance rate) and diuretic therapy (e.g., furosemide 0.5 to 1 mg per kg intravenously, usual maximum 20 mg per dose) may improve gas exchange. In the setting of extensive pulmonary damage, pulmonary and cardiovascular components of the disease are intimately entwined. Optimum management requires monitoring of blood gases and systemic arterial pressure.

Patients who have experienced significant hypoxemia and are not able to be aroused, can be further divided into three subcategories according to neurologic findings: (i) Those with decorticate response to pain and Cheyne–Stokes breathing, (ii) those with decerebrate response to pain and central hyperventilation, and (iii) those who are flaccid with fixed, dilated pupils and apneustic breathing or apnea. Again, reversal of hypoxemia and acidosis is critical, as well as fluid resuscitation and avoidance of hyperglycemia. Avoiding hypercapnia and resultant cerebral hyperemia is generally accepted, but hyperventilation, barbiturate coma, and other measures initially believed to provide cerebral protection and prevent or treat elevated intracranial pressure have not been helpful in these patients.

Hypothermia does appear to have some protective effect. Extreme hypothermia should be corrected to at least 32°C (89.6°F) to achieve hemodynamic stability and to minimize the risk of infection. The child should then be allowed to rewarm passively. Although data in humans are limited, animal studies suggest that maintenance of mild brain hypothermia may minimize reperfusion injury. Hyperthermia, a common result of active rewarming, should be avoided.

There is no benefit to prophylactic antibiotics, which should be reserved for strongly suspected or proven bacterial infection. Exceptions are when grossly contaminated water is aspirated or when maximal ventilatory support is required to provide any margin for survival. Bronchoalveolar lavage and steroids have no demonstrated benefit.

Renal function, normal electrolytes, and an adequate hemoglobin level (more than 10 g per 100 mL) should be maintained. If significant hemoglobinuria exists, diuresis is required.

Indications for Discharge or Admission

The patient's clinical condition in the ED dictates further management and may provide prognostic clues. Patients may be assigned to one of three groups: alert, blunted, or comatose (Table 98.1). Patients in the first group should be observed in the ED (as above). If they maintain normal oxygenation and normal work of breathing they can be discharged to home. Patients in the second group should be admitted for careful monitoring.

Patients in the third group have experienced severe CNS asphyxia. The prognosis for this group includes a much greater risk of death or severe anoxic/ischemic encephalopathy. Risk increases with depth of coma on presentation. Patients in the third subdivision (flaccid with fixed, dilated pupils) rarely survive intact regardless of treatment, although coexistent hypothermia has provided some remarkable exceptions.

SMOKE INHALATION

Goals of Treatment

The goals of emergency care include early intubation (if there are signs of airway compromise), stabilization of respiratory

TABLE 98.1

NEUROLOGIC ASSESSMENT AFTER DROWNING

Group	Description	Treatment
A (alert)	Alert Fully conscious	Observe
B (blunted)	Obtunded but arousable Purposeful response to pain Normal respiratory pattern	Prevent further hypoxic damage Monitor clinical neurologic status Therapy as required for pulmonary and cardiovascular stability Normalize temperature
C (comatose)	Comatose, not arousable Abnormal response to pain Abnormal respiratory pattern	Prevent further hypoxic damage Therapy as required for pulmonary and cardiovascular stability Maintain normocapnia or mild hyperventilation Monitor core temperature Warm to 32°C (89.6°F), then allow passive warming to 37°C (98.6°F) Avoid hyperthermia
C.1	(Decorticate) Flexion response to pain Cheyne–Stokes respiration	
C.2	(Decerebrate) Extension response to pain Central hyperventilation	Monitor temperature
C.3	(Flaccid) No response to pain Apnea or cluster breathing	Consider withdrawal of support if no protection from hypothermia

and cardiovascular status, and maintenance of fluid and electrolyte balance. One must recognize concomitant carbon monoxide or cyanide poisoning or other inhalants that contribute to morbidity.

CLINICAL PEARLS AND PITFALLS

- Early intubation should be done with any evidence of airway burns or edema.
- Severe smoke inhalation can occur without cutaneous burns.
- Respiratory status, and not evidence of airway burns or labs, should guide treatment.

Current Evidence

Respiratory complications of smoke inhalation rank with carbon monoxide poisoning as a major cause of early death from fire. Although serious cutaneous injury may occur in the absence of pulmonary involvement, inhalation injury dramatically increases the morbidity and mortality associated with any given percent body surface area burn.

The severity of carbon monoxide inhalation and respiratory problems is related to the duration of exposure, the occurrence in a closed space (more likely in very young or elderly victims), the nature of materials involved, and the presence of products of incomplete combustion. Severe hypovolemic shock, massive tissue destruction, extensive fluid resuscitation, and infection further complicate direct inhalational trauma.

The relatively low heat capacity of dry air and the excellent heat exchange properties of the nasopharynx usually limit direct thermal injury to the upper airway. Dry air above 160°C (320°F) has little effect on the lower airway. The greater heat capacity of steam increases the risk of lower airway damage. In addition, continuing combustion of soot particles carried deeply into the lung may exacerbate thermal injury.

Chemical injury may occur at any level of the respiratory tract. Oxides of sulfur and nitrogen combine with lung water to form corrosive acids. Incomplete combustion of any carbon-containing material, such as wood, may produce carbon monoxide. Combustion of cotton or plastic generates aldehydes that cause protein denaturation and cellular damage. Burning polyurethane may produce cyanide gas. Fire retardants that contain phosphorus may actually produce phosgene gas. The upper airway filters most soot particles, but those carried into the lung may adsorb various substances and cause reflex bronchospasm to further extend chemical damage.

Immediate effects of smoke inhalation on the lower airway include loss of ciliary action, mucosal edema, bronchiolitis, alveolar epithelial damage, and impaired gas exchange, particularly oxygenation. Areas of atelectasis or air trapping, and loss of surfactant activity, worsen ventilation–perfusion mismatch and hypoxemia. Hours later, sloughing of tracheobronchial mucosa and mucopurulent membrane formation increases the degree of obstruction, poor gas exchange, and likelihood of infection. Beyond the first 24 hours, pulmonary pathology that results from smoke inhalation is largely indistinguishable from adult respiratory distress syndrome, which arises from other insults. Children who die from smoke inhalation may sustain serious respiratory damage in the absence of cutaneous injury.

Clinical Recognition

A history of exposure in a closed space should heighten concern for smoke inhalation. Need for CPR at the site implies significant carbon monoxide poisoning and/or hypoxia secondary to decreased ambient oxygen concentration or severe respiratory disease. The physician should also consider the types of material involved to determine the risk of poisoning from carbon monoxide or other toxins.

Physical examination that reveals facial burns, singed nasal hairs, pharyngeal soot, or carbonaceous sputum justifies a presumption of smoke inhalation. Any sign of neurologic dysfunction, including irritability or depression, should be presumed related to tissue hypoxia until proven otherwise. Signs of respiratory dysfunction, including tachypnea, cough, hoarseness, stridor, decreased breath sounds, wheezing, rhonchi, or rales may be detected on presentation or may be delayed for 12 to 24 hours, depending on the severity of the insult.

Auscultatory findings often precede chest radiograph abnormalities by 12 to 24 hours. Radiographic changes may include diffuse interstitial infiltration or local areas of atelectasis and edema (Fig. 98.3). Acute respiratory failure may occur at any point. ABG analysis provides the ultimate assessment of effective respiratory function. Bronchoscopy can document the extent of inhalation injury and help remove debris but may worsen airway edema. In general, it is respiratory function, not the appearance of lesions, that guides supportive care; therefore, most patients can be treated effectively without bronchoscopy.

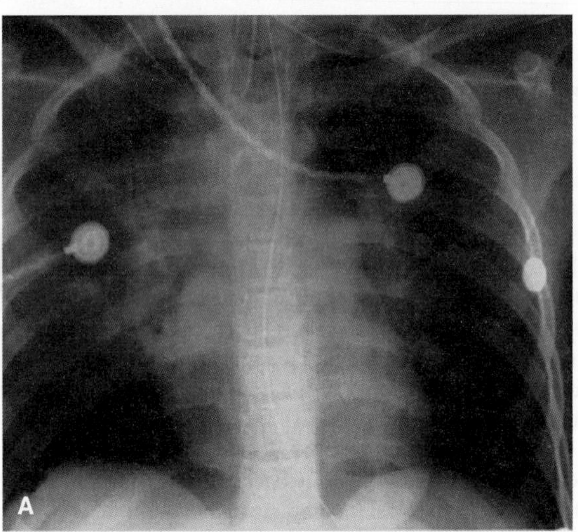

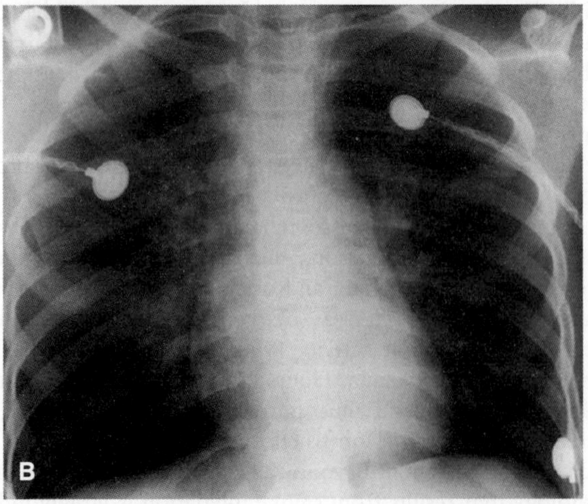

FIGURE 98.3 Smoke inhalation in a 9-year-old girl. **A:** There is bilateral central alveolar process consistent with acute smoke inhalation. **B:** A day later, the patient has been extubated and there is marked improvement in the appearance of pulmonary edema. (Courtesy of Soroosh Mahboubi, MD.)

Triage Considerations

Initial assessment and resuscitation at the scene should proceed according to the principles outlined in Chapter 1 A General Approach to Ill and Injured Children. Because of the likelihood of carbon monoxide exposure and the difficulty of assessing hypoxemia clinically, all victims should receive the maximum concentration of inspired oxygen possible in transport and in the ED until further evaluation is complete (Table 98.2).

Clinical Assessment

In the ED, assessment of airway and respiratory functions must proceed simultaneously with cardiovascular stabilization. Thermal injury to the nose, mouth, or face, or compromise of

TABLE 98.2

MANAGEMENT OF SMOKE INHALATION

Initial management
Remove from contaminated environment
Cardiopulmonary resuscitation as needed
Provide 100% supplemental oxygen
Insure patent airway
Laboratory determinations
Arterial blood gas analysis
Carboxyhemoglobin level, troponin
Chest radiograph
Monitor
Heart rate, electrocardiogram, respiratory rate, blood pressure, SaO_2
Consider central venous pressure
Consider pulmonary artery catheterization
Fluids
5% dextrose in normal saline at maintenance rates or less to maintain urine output at 0.5–1.0/mL/kg/hr
Volume expansion in presence of cutaneous burns; normal saline, lactated Ringer solution, or 5% albumin
Respiratory management
Intubation for:
1. Upper airway obstruction
2. PaO_2 <60 mm Hg on 60% oxygen
3. Central nervous system depression with loss of cough and gag reflexes. Continuous positive airway pressure 5–15 cm H_2O for PaO_2 <60 mm Hg on 60% oxygen
Intermittent mandatory ventilation for:
1. Hypoxia unresponsive to continuous positive airway pressure or
2. $PaCO_2$ >50 mm Hg
Humidification of inspired gases
Meticulous pulmonary toilette
Consider inhaled bronchodilators

the upper airway (stridor, hoarseness, barking cough, retractions, delayed inspiration, or difficulty handling secretions) indicates the need for direct laryngoscopy. The presence of significant pharyngeal, supraglottic, or glottic edema mandates elective endotracheal intubation. Worsening edema over 24 hours may lead to respiratory arrest and a difficult emergency intubation through a distorted airway, and thus early endotracheal intubation is indicated. Elective tracheostomy may be considered if placing or securing the endotracheal tube will further traumatize an edematous airway or severe facial burns. However, in the presence of extensive cutaneous burns, tracheostomy dramatically increases the risk of systemic and pulmonary infection.

Management and Diagnostic Studies

The details of burn therapy are elaborated in Chapter 112 Burns but, in general, the goals are stabilization of cardiovascular function without fluid overload and compromise of gas exchange. Pulse rate and BP should guide administration of fluid volume. Maintenance of urine output of at least 0.5 mL/kg/hr should provide adequate tissue perfusion. Careful monitoring of renal and cardiovascular systems may prevent or minimize acute pulmonary edema and delayed pulmonary dysfunction secondary to late fluid mobilization and infection.

Oxygen saturation and serial blood gas determinations should be obtained to guide oxygen supplementation and to assess adequacy of ventilation. Intubation is indicated if adequate oxygenation ($Sa{O_2}$ greater than 90% or $Pa{O_2}$ greater than 60 mm Hg) cannot be maintained with an inspired oxygen concentration of 40% to 60%, if $Pa{CO_2}$ rises above 50 mm Hg, or if the work of breathing appears unsustainable. Spontaneous ventilation with continuous positive airway pressure causes less cardiovascular interference; this patient should receive humidified gas mixtures and be encouraged to take deep breaths and cough frequently. If there is severe CNS depression or severe pulmonary parenchymal damage, mechanical ventilation with PEEP will likely be necessary. Maximally humidified oxygen should be delivered by mask or artificial airway to prevent inspissation of debris and occlusion of the airway. If intubation is necessary, meticulous pulmonary toilette is essential, with frequent suctioning to remove edema fluid, mucus, and sloughed epithelium that may otherwise occlude the endotracheal tube.

High-frequency percussive ventilation (hi-fi) is superior to conventional mechanical ventilation in reducing work of breathing. There is also evidence that extracorporeal membrane oxygenation (ECMO) may be useful in severely burned children.

After the first few hours, diuretic therapy (furosemide 0.5 to 1 mg per kg intravenously), within the limits of cardiovascular stability, may also improve oxygenation and pulmonary compliance, leading to more effective ventilation. Chemical and particulate irritation of upper airway receptors may cause reflex bronchoconstriction and contribute to lower airway obstruction. Bronchodilators such as nebulized albuterol may help reverse bronchospasm, but relief depends mostly on removal of secretions and debris from the respiratory tree.

Studies have not demonstrated a role for steroids or prophylactic antibiotics. When steroids are used, there is evidence that sodium and fluid retention increase, healing is delayed, and bacterial clearance from the lung is decreased.

One study in children has demonstrated some benefit to aerosolized heparin and N-acetylcysteine in decreasing the incidence of atelectasis, reintubation, and overall mortality. Whole-body hypothermia has been shown to be effective in controlling bronchoalveolar damage in animal models.

Indications for Discharge or Admission

Determination of disposition from the ED will depend on the history and clinical status. Patients with significant respiratory distress or decreased neurologic status should be admitted to an intensive care unit (ICU). Patients who appear well on presentation to the ED but have a significant history of exposure or physical evidence of significant smoke inhalation should be monitored closely for at least 6 hours for signs of respiratory distress or significant cough.

CARBON MONOXIDE POISONING

Goals of Treatment

The goals of treatment are immediate removal from the source of contamination, provision of 100% oxygen to foster elimination, and treatment/prevention of tissue hypoxia, metabolic acidosis, and cerebral edema.

CLINICAL PEARL AND PITFALLS

- Carbon monoxide poisoning may occur in spaces with improper ventilation, even with doors and windows open.
- The classically described "cherry red" skin color is unreliable in diagnosis.
- $Pa{O_2}$ and pulse oximetry arterial saturation ($Sa{O_2}$) are likely to be normal in carbon monoxide intoxication.

Current Evidence

Unintentional carbon monoxide poisoning claims approximately 500 lives per year in the United States and is largely responsible for early deaths related to fire. Exposure may occur in a variety of other settings unrelated to accidental fires, including incomplete combustion of any carbon-containing fuel (i.e., propane-powered forklifts), improperly vented wood- or coal-burning stoves, and automobile exhaust in garages, even with doors and windows open. Passengers may be poisoned in vehicles or boats with open backs, or with faulty or blocked exhaust systems.

In the normal person, carboxyhemoglobin levels are less than 1%. In smokers, levels of 5% to 10% are common. Inhaled carbon monoxide has two important effects that cause tissue hypoxia: (i) It binds to hemoglobin with an affinity 200 to 300 times greater than that of oxygen, and (ii) it shifts the oxyhemoglobin dissociation curve to the left and changes the shape from sigmoidal to hyperbolic (Fig. 98.4). The first effect decreases oxygen content of the blood, whereas the second causes oxygen release at lower-than-normal tissue oxygen levels. Other endogenous (anemia) and exogenous (high altitude, or displacement of ambient oxygen during fires) factors contribute further to hypoxia. Although oxygen content of the

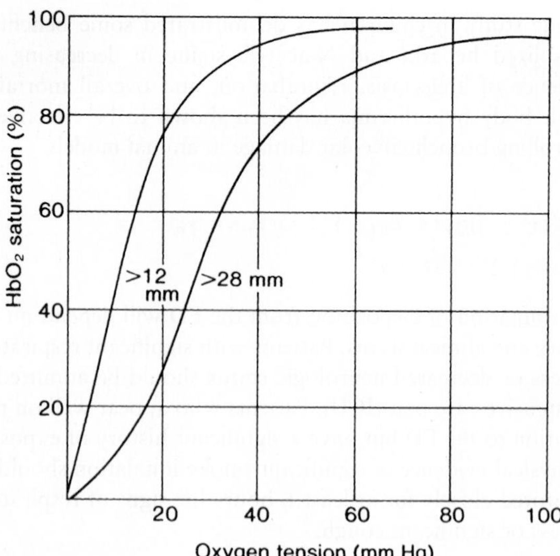

FIGURE 98.4 Carbon monoxide shifts the oxyhemoglobin dissociation curve to the left and changes its shape, making the unloading of oxygen in the tissues more difficult and provides an inadequate diffusion gradient. (*Left curve, P_{50}* >12 mm; *right curve, P_{50}* >28 mm.)

blood is low, the PaO_2 remains normal. Because carotid body receptors respond to PaO_2, respiration may not be stimulated until late, when metabolic acidosis activates other centers. Tissue hypoxia increases cerebral blood flow, cerebrospinal fluid pressure, and cerebral capillary permeability, which predispose the patient to cerebral edema.

Carbon monoxide interacts with several other cellular proteins, including cytochrome oxidase. It appears to interfere with oxidative energy production and may generate free radicals, which exacerbate CNS dysfunction. Neuronal necrosis, as well as apoptosis, is seen in animal models in the frontal cortex, globus pallidus, and cerebellum, likely contributing to delayed cognitive effects such as deficits in learning, memory, and dementia. Carbon monoxide also binds to myoglobin; individuals, particularly with pre-existing coronary disease, may develop cardiac ischemia and/or dysrhythmias.

Clinical Recognition

History provides the most valuable clue to diagnosis. Carbon monoxide poisoning should be suspected in all fire victims and considered in children exposed to other hazards noted earlier. Presence or absence of the classically described "cherry red" skin color is of no diagnostic value. In fact, patients with thermal injury may appear red, whereas those with vasoconstriction may be quite pale. Both color and respiratory rate may be deceptive and may lead the physician away from recognition of severe tissue hypoxia. PaO_2 and arterial saturation as determined by pulse oximetry (SaO_2) are likely to be normal in carbon monoxide intoxication; low values reflect coexistent pulmonary dysfunction.

Triage Considerations

Most important is removal of the victim from the contaminated environment. Resuscitation should proceed according to general principles. As soon as possible, the patient suspected of suffering carbon monoxide poisoning should be provided 100% oxygen to hasten elimination.

Clinical Assessment

Determination of blood levels of carboxyhemoglobin may help aid in diagnosis and prognosis. Spectrophotometric methods are most widely used clinically. Venous blood may be used because of the high affinity of carbon monoxide for hemoglobin, but an arterial sample provides more precise information about acid–base balance and adequacy of ventilation. The level of hemoglobin should also be determined.

Levels of carboxyhemoglobin as low as 5% in nonsmokers may impair judgment and fine motor skills. Mild intoxication (20% carboxyhemoglobin) produces headache, mild dyspnea, visual changes, and confusion. Moderate poisoning (20% to 40%) produces drowsiness, faintness, nausea and vomiting, tachycardia, dulled sensation, and decreased awareness of danger. At lower levels, these symptoms are noted only with exertion, but as the fraction approaches 40%, they are present at rest. Between 40% and 60%, weakness, incoordination, and loss of recent memory occur, and cardiovascular and neurologic collapse is imminent. Above 60%, coma, convulsions, and death are almost certain. Although carboxyhemoglobin levels and symptoms tend to follow the pattern just described, individual patients may be more or less symptomatic than predicted. An important caveat is that blood carboxyhemoglobin levels will fall rapidly with time and may not reflect cellular dysfunction, especially in high-demand tissues of the heart and CNS.

Patients with severe poisoning are vulnerable to pressure trauma to skin, subcutaneous tissue, and muscle, especially at sites that support body weight or that are pinned under fallen objects. The history may suggest which sites are most vulnerable, and pain is an early symptom. Muscle breakdown and myoglobin deposition in renal tubular cells may precipitate acute renal failure.

A syndrome of delayed neuropsychologic sequelae (DNS) has been described in patients after exposure to carboxyhemoglobin. These patients develop neurologic symptoms acutely, appear to recover with treatment, and then exhibit a broad spectrum of neurologic and psychiatric abnormalities days to weeks after the exposure. Studies of DNS, many of which are methodologically flawed, have elucidated neither an exact mechanism nor a consensus on prevention and treatment.

Management and Diagnostic Studies

After removal from the contaminated environment, 100% oxygen should be administered (Table 98.3). If the patient is breathing spontaneously, this can be accomplished with a nonrebreathing face mask. The half-life of carboxyhemoglobin is approximately 4 hours in a patient breathing room air at sea level and approximately 1 hour if pure oxygen is inspired. The half-life is further reduced to less than 30 minutes if the patient has access to hyperbaric oxygen (HBO) at 2 to 3 atmospheres of pressure. There is no widespread agreement on indications for HBO, and transfer to a hyperbaric chamber should not jeopardize cardiopulmonary stabilization. However, HBO administration may have effects beyond the mere reduction in carboxyhemoglobin half-life. Some studies in adults suggest a role for HBO in reducing the incidence of mortality and DNS, but there are no studies in children addressing its effectiveness. Early consultation with a poison control center or an HBO facility should be considered while the patient is receiving 100% oxygen (Table 98.4).

TABLE 98.3

MANAGEMENT OF CARBON MONOXIDE POISONING

Initial management
Remove from contaminated environment
Cardiopulmonary resuscitation as needed
Provide 100% supplemental oxygen
Laboratory determinations
Arterial blood gas analysis
Carboxyhemoglobin level, troponin
Complete blood cell count, electrolytes
Urinalysis for myoglobin
Monitoring
Heart rate, electrocardiogram, respiratory rate, blood pressure
Treatment
Correct anemia Hgb <10 g/dL
Continue supplemental oxygen until carboxyhemoglobin ≤5%
Decrease oxygen consumption with bed rest, avoid producing anxiety
Maintain urine output >1 mL/kg/hr
Consider hyperbaric oxygen

Severe metabolic acidosis in the context of normal carboxyhemoglobin and methemoglobin should suggest the possibility of coexistent cyanide poisoning in patients involved in closed-space fires (especially where nitrogen-containing synthetic materials have burned). Cyanide has high mortality but a short half-life (approximately 1 hour), so empiric cyanide levels on patients who have survived the scene are not recommended generally unless confirmation is needed. If cyanide poisoning is strongly suspected in an early presenting patient, the cyanide antidote kit (formerly known as the Lilly kit) may be considered. This two-step kit must be used with caution because the nitrite-containing first step induces methemoglobinemia. In case of doubt, the thiosulfate-containing second step, which is able to scavenge cyanide without significant additional toxicity, may be given alone. Anemia (hemoglobin less than 10 g per 100 mL) must be corrected to maximize oxygen-carrying capacity. Hydroxocobalamin (a synthetic form of vitamin B_{12}) was approved by the FDA in 2006 for use in cyanide poisoning. Its mechanism of action is that the hydroxyl group of the vitamin binds to free cyanide, forming the nontoxic cyanocobalamin. The dose is 70 mg per kg (max 5 g) given over 15 minutes, with a repeat dose if necessary. The minimal side effects of hydroxocobalamin make this an attractive alternative to the traditional nitrite therapy.

TABLE 98.4

CONSIDERATIONS FOR HYPERBARIC OXYGEN THERAPY[a]

Neurologic symptoms or signs (syncope, seizure, coma) either on presentation or that persist despite normobaric oxygen
Signs of cardiac ischemia or metabolic acidosis
Pregnancy

[a]Consider early consultation with a poison control center or HBO facility.

If myoglobinemia or myoglobinuria is present, vigorous hydration and diuresis with furosemide (1 mg per kg intravenously) and/or mannitol (0.25 to 1 g per kg intravenously) with close attention to urine output may preserve renal function. If hydration and diuresis are ineffective, renal failure should be considered and fluids restricted accordingly (see Chapter 108 Renal and Electrolyte Emergencies).

Indications for Discharge or Admission

Determination of disposition from the ED will depend on the history and clinical status. Patients with significant respiratory distress or decreased neurologic status should be admitted to an ICU. Patients who appear well on presentation to the ED but have a significant history (loss of consciousness at the scene) or elevated CO levels should be admitted for monitoring for other sequelae of smoke inhalation.

ENVIRONMENTAL AND EXERTIONAL HEAT ILLNESS

Goals of Treatment

Treatment of heat stroke involves rapid reversal of hyperpyrexia, cardiovascular support, and correction of electrolyte imbalances.

CLINICAL PEARLS AND PITFALLS

- Heat cramps may mimic an acute abdomen.
- Heat stroke is differentiated from heat exhaustion by the presence of circulatory failure and/or severe CNS dysfunction.
- Active cooling may be achieved effectively using evaporation with fans after spraying with cool water.

Current Evidence

Environmental and exertional heat illness occurs with excessive heat generation and storage. These conditions arise when high ambient temperature prevents heat dissipation by radiation or convection, and humidity limits cooling by sweat evaporation. The spectrum of illness is broad, including heat cramps, heat exhaustion, and heat stroke; the latter is an acute medical emergency with significant associated morbidity and mortality.

The elderly are most vulnerable (more than 80% of cases occur in people older than 50 years), but heat illness is also significant among healthy young people. Of the weather-related deaths noted previously for which the age of the decedent was recorded, 164 (4%) occurred in children younger than 15 years. Children with increased risk include those with cystic fibrosis or congenital absence of sweat glands, children receiving medications that cause oligohidrosis, infants left in automobiles on hot days, and young athletes. Heat stroke remains the third most common cause (after head injury and cardiac disorders) of exercise-related mortality among U.S. high school athletes, despite the fact that survival following acute heat stroke has improved over the last century from an estimated 20% to more than 90%.

Heat-sensitive centers of the posterior hypothalamus control sympathetic tone. This tone regulates vasoconstriction of arterioles and subcutaneous arteriovenous anastomoses, which, in turn, controls heat conduction from the body core to the skin. Flow through these areas may represent 0% to 30% of total cardiac output. High flow provides efficient heat transfer from the body core to the skin, which is an effective radiator. Low flow to the skin prevents radiation and allows only inefficient diffusion through the insulating skin and subcutaneous tissues. When body temperature rises, blood in the preoptic area of the anterior hypothalamus is warmer than optimal. Impulses from this area increase and are conducted through autonomic pathways to the spinal cord and then, through cholinergic fibers to the sweat glands, where sweat is released. Exercise and certain emotional states release circulating epinephrine and norepinephrine to increase sweat production.

Clinical Recognition

Three types of heat illnesses are recognized and represent different physiologic disturbances (Table 98.5). Heat cramps refer to the sudden onset of brief, intermittent, and excruciating cramps in muscles after they have been subjected to severe work stress. Cramps tend to occur after the work is done, on relaxing, or on taking a cool shower. Occasionally, abdominal muscle cramps may simulate an acute abdomen. The usual victim is highly conditioned and acclimatized. Typically, these individuals can produce sweat in large quantities and provide themselves with adequate fluid replacement but inadequate salt replacement. Electrolyte depletion is probably the cause of cramps.

Most spasms last less than a minute, but some persist for several minutes, during which a rock-hard mass may be palpated in the affected muscle. Cramps often occur in clusters. Rapid voluntary contraction of a muscle, contact with cold air or water, or passive extension of a flexed limb may reproduce a cramp. Laboratory investigation reveals hyponatremia and hypochloremia and virtually absent urine sodium. The blood urea nitrogen (BUN) level is usually normal but may be mildly elevated.

Heat exhaustion is less clearly demarcated from heat stroke than are heat cramps. In most cases, water depletion predominates because individuals who live and work in a hot environment do not always voluntarily replace their total water deficit. Progressive lethargy, intense thirst, and inability to

TABLE 98.5

CHARACTERISTICS OF HEAT ILLNESS

Illness	Who	When	Characteristic	Laboratory
Heat cramp	Highly conditioned Highly acclimatized Adequate water replacement Inadequate salt replacement	After severe work stress Usually when relaxing Triggered by cold	Excruciating cramps in affected muscle occurring in clusters (may simulate acute abdomen)	↓ Serum Na^+Cl^- ↓↓ Urine Na^+ BUN nl or slightly ↑
Heat exhaustion A. Predominant water depletion	Generally unacclimatized Working in hot environment Inadequate water replacement	During periods of hot weather After physical exertion	T ≤39°C (102.2°F) Progressive lethargy Thirst Inability to work or play Headache Vomiting CNS dysfunction ↓ BP ↑ HR	Na, Cl ↑ Hct ↑ Urine-specific gravity ↑
B. Predominant salt depletion	Unacclimatized Inadequate salt replacement Cystic fibrosis	During periods of hot weather After physical exertion	T ≥39°C (102.2°F) Weakness, fatigue Headache GI symptoms exertion Prominent Muscle cramp ↑ HR Orthostatic hypotension	Na ↓ Hct ↑ Urine Na ↓↓
Heat stroke	Extremes of age Overdressed infants Infants in closed cars Extreme exertion (young athletes) Drug use (e.g., phenothiazines)	During heat waves After excessive exertion	T ≥41°C (105.8°F) Hot skin Circulatory collapse Severe CNS dysfunction Rhabdomyolysis Renal failure	Na, Cl nl or ↑ CPK ↑ Ca ↓

BUN, blood urea nitrogen; nl, normal; T, temperature; CNS, central nervous system; BP, blood pressure; HR, heart rate; Hct, hematocrit; GI, gastrointestinal; CPK, creatinine phosphokinase.

work or play progress to headache, vomiting, CNS dysfunction (including hyperventilation, paresthesias, agitation, incoordination, or actual psychosis), hypotension, and tachycardia. Hemoconcentration, hypernatremia, hyperchloremia, and urinary concentration are typical. Body temperature may rise but rarely to higher than 39°C (102.2°F). If unattended, heat exhaustion may progress to frank heat stroke.

Heat exhaustion may also occur secondary to predominant salt depletion. As in heat cramps, water losses are replaced but without adequate electrolyte supplementation. Symptoms include profound weakness and fatigue, frontal headache, anorexia, nausea, vomiting, diarrhea, and severe muscle cramps. Tachycardia and orthostatic hypotension may be noted.

Hyponatremia, hemoconcentration, and significantly diminished urine sodium are consistent findings. Children with cystic fibrosis, particularly those who are young and unable to meet increased salt requirements, are at risk for electrolyte depletion because salt losses in their sweat apparently do not respond to acclimatization and aldosterone stimulation of the sweat gland.

Heat stroke (Table 98.5) is a life-threatening emergency. Classic signs are hyperpyrexia (41°C [105.8°F] or higher); hot, dry skin that is pink or ashen, depending on the circulatory state; and severe CNS dysfunction. Often sweating ceases before the onset of heat stroke.

The onset of the CNS disturbance may be abrupt, with sudden loss of consciousness. Often, however, premonitory signs and symptoms exist. These include a sense of impending doom, headache, dizziness, weakness, confusion, euphoria, gait disturbance, and combativeness. Posturing, incontinence, seizures, hemiparesis, and pupillary changes may occur. Any level of coma may be noted. Cerebrospinal fluid findings are usually normal. The extent of damage to the CNS is related to the time and extent of hyperpyrexia and to the adequacy of circulation. In severe cases, coma may persist even after the body temperature is lowered.

Patients able to maintain cardiac output adequate to meet the enormously elevated circulatory demand are most likely to survive. Initially, the pulse is rapid and full, with an increased pulse pressure. Total peripheral vascular resistance falls as a result of vasodilation in the skin and muscle beds, and splanchnic flow diminishes. If hyperpyrexia is not corrected, ashen cyanosis and a thin, rapid pulse herald a falling cardiac output. The cause may be either direct thermal damage to the myocardium or significant pulmonary hypertension with secondary right ventricular failure. Even after body temperature is returned to normal, cardiac output remains elevated and peripheral vascular resistance remains low for several hours, resembling the compensatory hyperemia after ischemia noted in posttrauma, postshock, and postseptic states. Persistently circulating vasoactive substances probably account for this phenomenon.

Severe dehydration is not a necessary component of heat stroke but may play a role if prolonged sweating has occurred. Electrolyte abnormalities may occur, especially in the unacclimatized victim, if NaCl has not been replaced. In acclimatized persons, NaCl is conserved but often at the expense of a severe potassium deficit. Polyuria is sometimes noted, often vasopressin resistant and possibly related to hypokalemia. Acute tubular necrosis may be seen in as many as 35% of cases and probably reflects combined thermal, ischemic, and circulating pigment damage. Hypoglycemia may also be noted.

Nontraumatic rhabdomyolysis and acute renal failure have been described as consequences of various insults, including hyperthermia and strenuous exercise in unconditioned persons. Clinically, there may or may not be musculoskeletal pain, tenderness, swelling, or weakness. Laboratory evidence includes elevated serum creatinine phosphokinase (CPK) (300 to 120,000 units) and urinalysis that is orthotolidine (Hematest)-positive without red blood cells and shows red-gold granular casts. Typically, serum potassium and creatinine levels rise rapidly relative to BUN. An initial hypocalcemia, possibly a consequence of deposition into damaged muscle, progresses to hypercalcemia during the diuretic phase a few days to 2 weeks later.

Management and Diagnostic Studies

Heat Cramps

Most cases of heat cramps are mild and do not require specific therapy except for rest and increased oral salt intake. In severe cases with prolonged or frequent cramps, IV infusion of normal saline is effective. Approximately 5 to 10 mL per kg over 15 to 20 minutes should be adequate to relieve cramping. Oral intake of fluids and salted foods can then complete restoration of salt and water balance.

Heat exhaustion

Heat exhaustion as a result of predominant water depletion is treated with rehydration and rest in a cooled or well-ventilated place. If the child is able to eat, he or she should be encouraged to drink cool liquids and be allowed unrestricted dietary sodium. If weakness or impaired consciousness precludes oral correction, IV fluids are given as in any hypernatremic dehydration.

Heat exhaustion caused by predominant salt depletion also requires rest in a cool environment. Alert, reasonably strong children can be given relatively salty drinks, such as tomato juice, and should be encouraged to salt solid foods. Hypotonic fluids (e.g., water, Kool-Aid) should be avoided until salt repletion has begun. Patients with CNS symptoms or gastrointestinal (GI) dysfunction may be rehydrated with IV isotonic saline or Ringer lactate. Initial rapid administration of 20 mL per kg over 20 minutes should improve intravascular volume with return of BP and pulse toward normal. Further correction of salt and water stores should be achieved over 12 to 24 hours. In especially severe cases with intractable seizures or muscle cramps, hypertonic saline solutions may be used. The initial dose of 3% saline solution is 5 mL per kg by IV over 15 minutes for seizures, more slowly over 30 to 60 minutes for cramping. An additional 5 mL per kg should be infused over the next 4 to 6 hours.

Heat Stroke

Treatment centers on two priorities: (i) Immediate elimination of hyperpyrexia and (ii) support of the cardiovascular system (Table 98.6). Clothing should be removed and patients should be cooled actively. They should be transported to an emergency facility in open or air-conditioned vehicles. Ice packs may be placed at the neck, groin, and axilla. Although immersion in ice water may be a more efficient means of lowering body temperature, it may complicate other support and monitoring. Among the most efficient but invasive and rarely used methods is iced peritoneal lavage. Iced peritoneal lavage is contraindicated in the pregnant patient and those with a

TABLE 98.6

MANAGEMENT OF HEAT STROKE

Initial management
Remove clothing
Begin active cooling
Transport to cool environment
Cardiovascular support
Laboratory determinations
Complete blood cell count, PT/PTT
Electrolytes, BUN, creatinine, CPK, Ca, P
Urinalysis, including myoglobin
Arterial blood gas
Monitoring
Temperature
Heart rate, electrocardiogram, blood pressure
Peripheral pulses and perfusion
Urine output
Central nervous system function
Treatment
Active cooling
Fluids
Maintenance: 5% dextrose in normal saline at maintenance rates
Resuscitation: ≤20 mg/kg lactated Ringer's or 0.9% sodium chloride
Additional fluids as determined by electrolytes, output, and hemodynamic status
Inotropic support
Dobutamine 5–20 mcg/kg/min or
Diuresis for myoglobinuria
Maintain urine output >1 mL/kg/hr
Consider furosemide 1 mg/kg
Consider mannitol 0.25–1 g/kg

PT, prothrombin time; PTT, partial thromboplastin time; BUN, blood urea nitrogen; CPK, creatine phosphokinase.

history of abdominal surgery. In addition, a canine model of heat stroke suggested that an evaporative technique in which fans blew room air over subjects sprayed with 15°C (59°F) tap water was equally efficient. Temperature should be monitored continuously with a rectal probe, and active cooling should be discontinued when rectal temperature falls to approximately 38.5°C (101.3°F). Sedation and paralysis of the patient can greatly augment the cooling process.

The severity of the patient's presentation determines the degree of cardiovascular support. If the skin is flushed and BP adequate, lowering body temperature with close attention to heart rate and BP may be sufficient. Although severe dehydration and electrolyte disturbances are uncommon, these should be assessed and corrected if necessary. Fluids cooled to 4°C (39.2°F) hasten temperature correction but may precipitate arrhythmias on contact with an already stressed myocardium. Adult patients rarely have required more than 20 mL per kg over the first 4 hours, but determinations of electrolytes, hematocrit, and urine output, and clinical assessment of central vascular volume should guide precise titration of fluids and electrolytes.

Inotropic support may be required after a fluid challenge (see Chapter 5 Shock). Dobutamine is probably most appropriate: Its β-agonist properties increase myocardial contractility and maintain peripheral vasodilation. Isoproterenol has been used successfully in the past but may cause myocardial oxygen consumption to exceed oxygen delivery. Additional fluid resuscitation may be necessary with the initiation of either dobutamine or isoproterenol to fill the effectively increased vascular space. Normal saline or albumin should be given to maintain the arterial BP in the normal range. Dopamine may also be effective, infused at rates compatible with inotropic support without vasoconstriction (i.e., 5 to 15 mcg/kg/min). In cases of extreme hemodynamic instability, extracorporeal circulation may provide both circulatory support and a means of rapid temperature correction. Agents with α-agonist characteristics (epinephrine and norepinephrine) are not recommended for initial management; they cause peripheral vasoconstriction, interfere with heat dissipation, and may compromise hepatic and renal flow further. Atropine and other anticholinergic drugs that inhibit sweating should be avoided.

Renal function should be monitored carefully, especially in patients who have been hypotensive or in whom vigorous exercise precipitated heat stroke. In general, BUN, creatinine, electrolytes, calcium, and urinalysis for protein and myoglobin should be obtained. Once the patient's vascular volume has been restored and arterial pressure normalized, hourly urine output should be monitored. If urine output is inadequate (less than 0.5 mL/kg/hr) in the face of normovolemia and adequate cardiac output, furosemide (0.5 to 1 mg per kg by IV) and/or mannitol (0.25 to 1 g per kg by IV) should be given. If the response is poor, acute renal failure should be suspected, and fluids should be restricted accordingly. Rapidly rising BUN or potassium should prompt consideration of early dialysis.

Indications for Admission and Discharge

Patients with heat cramps can generally be discharged for the ED after resolution of symptoms. Children with heat exhaustion may require admission for ongoing fluid and electrolyte replacement and serial testing. Children with heat stroke require admission to the ICU. Patients with ashen skin, tachycardia, and hypotension demonstrate cardiac output insufficient to meet circulatory demand and are in imminent danger of death. Monitoring of the electrocardiogram (ECG) and arterial BP (with an indwelling arterial line) should determine support.

ACCIDENTAL HYPOTHERMIA

Goals of Treatment

The goals of treatment include general supportive measures, cardiopulmonary resuscitation, and rewarming.

CLINICAL PEARLS AND PITFALLS

- A high index of suspicion is needed to recognize hypothermia.
- Hypothermia can mimic death, hence rewarming must be done before pronouncing death.

Current Evidence

Hypothermia was responsible for nearly 14,000 deaths in the United States from 1979 to 1998. Neonates, with large surface:volume ratios and small amounts of subcutaneous fat, conserve heat poorly and are unable to produce heat by shivering. Therefore, minor deviations in the thermal environment may produce hypothermia in neonates. The capacity for nonshivering thermogenesis—primarily metabolism of brown fat—is intact, but oxygen consumption is significantly increased. This may result in metabolic acidosis, hypoglycemia, and hypocalcemia. Adolescents are psychologically less likely to conserve energy and to take preventive or corrective measures, thus increasing their risk of hypothermia. Physical disability, especially immobilizing conditions, and drug or alcohol ingestion increase risk at any age. Healthy young people who work or play to exhaustion in a cold environment are also at risk. The rising popularity of cold weather sports is producing more cases of accidental hypothermia. However, environmental conditions need not be extreme, and the diagnosis should be considered even in temperate climates.

When core temperature begins to fall to less than 37°C (98.6°F), physiologic mechanisms that produce and conserve heat are activated. Cooled blood stimulates the hypothalamus to increase muscle tone and metabolism (oxidative phosphorylation and high-energy phosphate production) and to augment heat production by 50% during nonshivering thermogenesis. When muscle tone reaches a critical level, shivering begins, and heat production increases two to four times basal levels.

Although the surface temperature of the body, especially of the extremities, may drop to nearly the environmental temperature, several mechanisms work to conserve heat and to protect blood and core structures from ambient air temperature, humidity, and wind. Sweating is abolished, decreasing heat loss by evaporation (unless there is external moisture), whereas vasoconstriction of cutaneous and subcutaneous vessels reduce losses further. Piloerection, which in many animal species traps an insulating layer of air next to the skin, occurs but is ineffective in humans.

Once homeostatic mechanisms fail and core temperature falls, predictable physiologic changes take place. If shivering does not occur, basal metabolic rate decreases steadily, reaching 50% of normal at 28°C (82.4°F). As a result, oxygen consumption and carbon dioxide production decline. The oxygen–hemoglobin dissociation curve shifts to the left.

Although respiratory depression occurs late, impaired mental status and cold-induced bronchorrhea predispose the patient to airway obstruction and aspiration. Acid–base balance follows no predictable pattern. Respiratory acidosis occurs, but tissue hypoxia, increased lactic acid production, and decreased lactate clearance by the liver produce metabolic acidosis.

Decreased heart rate contributes primarily to a drop in cardiac output. Peripheral vasoconstriction and an early increase in central vascular volume cause a transient rise in BP, which later falls to become clinically significant at less than 25°C (77°F). A variety of cardiac conduction abnormalities arise, including decreased sinus rate, T-wave inversion, prolongation of ECG intervals, and the appearance of pathognomonic J waves (Fig. 98.5), which may provide the first clue to the diagnosis. Atrial fibrillation may occur at temperatures less than 33°C (91.4°F) but is usually not hemodynamically significant.

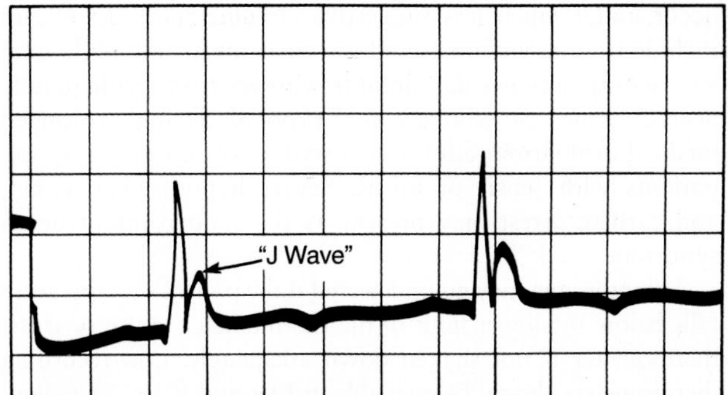

FIGURE 98.5 J wave (Osborn wave), pathognomonic of hypothermia. Rounded contour distinguishes it from an RSR′. It may also be confused with a T wave with a short Q-T interval. (Reprinted from Welton D, Mattox K, Miller R, et al. Treatment of profound hypothermia. *JAMA* 1978;240:2291–2292, with permission.)

At less than 28°C (82.4°F), myocardial irritability increases dramatically, and ventricular fibrillation becomes likely.

Cold-induced vasoconstriction and elevated central blood volume and pressure contribute to a diuresis, which subsequently diminishes intravascular volume. At lower temperatures, tubular dysfunction allows salt and water loss. Acidosis causes potassium to shift from cells to the urine, where it is eliminated. Increased capillary permeability results in loss of fluid into the extracellular space.

Hematologic abnormalities may also occur. Plasma loss causes an increased hematocrit level, whereas splenic sequestration may be responsible for a fall in white blood cell and platelet counts. Disseminated intravascular coagulation is sometimes seen.

CNS abnormalities are progressive. Each fall of 1°C produces a 6% to 7% decline in cerebral blood flow. Plasma loss increases blood viscosity, which further contributes to impaired cerebral microcirculation and mentation. Peripheral nerve conduction slows, and deep tendon reflexes decrease. Pupils dilate and react sluggishly, if at all, at less than 30°C (86°F). The electroencephalogram deteriorates progressively with falling temperature, from high-voltage slow waves, to burst suppression patterns, to electrical silence at 20°C (68°F).

GI motility decreases at less than 34°C (93.2°F). The liver's capacity for detoxification or conjugation of drugs and products of metabolism is poor. Insulin release abates, and serum glucose rises. Frank pancreatic necrosis may also occur, producing clinical evidence of pancreatitis.

Clinical Recognition

Elevated body temperature is a routine concern for most physicians, especially pediatricians. However, hypothermia, defined as core temperature at or less than 35°C (95°F), is often overlooked. Reduced body temperature may be a consequence or cause of many disorders but is diagnosed only if healthcare providers maintain a high index of suspicion. Special thermometers may be required to detect hypothermia.

Triage Considerations

A history of sudden immersion in icy water or prolonged exposure to low environmental temperatures provides the obvious clue, but significantly low core temperatures may occur under much less suggestive circumstances. Examples include trauma victims found unconscious or immobile on a wet, windy, summer day; infants who are from inadequately heated homes or who are left exposed during prolonged medical evaluation; adolescents with anorexia nervosa; and patients with sepsis or burns. Severe hypothermia, coma, and cardiac arrest may present as the sudden infant death syndrome.

Hypothermia may go undetected if the patient's temperature falls below the lower limit of the thermometer in use or if the thermometer is not shaken down adequately. Low-recording thermometers should be available in EDs and ICUs. This diagnosis should be kept in mind for any patient with a suggestive history or coma of uncertain cause.

Initial Assessment

Physical examination reveals a pale or cyanotic patient. At mild levels of hypothermia, mental status may be normal, but CNS function is progressively impaired with falling temperature until frank coma occurs at approximately 27°C (80.6°F). BP also falls steadily at less than 33°C (91.4°F) and may be undetectable. Heart rate slows gradually unless atrial or ventricular fibrillation occurs. Intense peripheral vasoconstriction and bradycardia may render the pulse unapparent or absent. At less than 32°C (89.6°F), shivering ceases, but muscle rigidity may mimic rigor mortis. Pupils may be dilated and may not react. Deep tendon reflexes are depressed or absent. Evidence of head trauma or other injury, drug ingestion, and frostbite should be sought (Figs. 98.6 and 98.7).

Severe hypothermia mimics death. However, the significant decrease in oxygen consumption may allow life to be sustained for long periods, even after cessation of cardiac function. Signs usually associated with certain death (i.e., dilated pupils or rigor mortis) have little prognostic value. If the patient's history suggests that hypothermia is the primary event and not a consequence of death, resuscitation should be attempted and death redefined as failure to revive with rewarming.

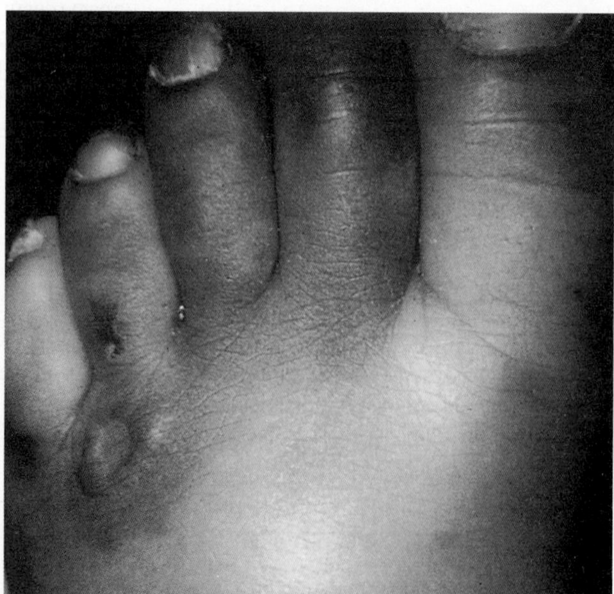

FIGURE 98.6 Frostbite of toes. Note the line of demarcation and ulcerative lesion.

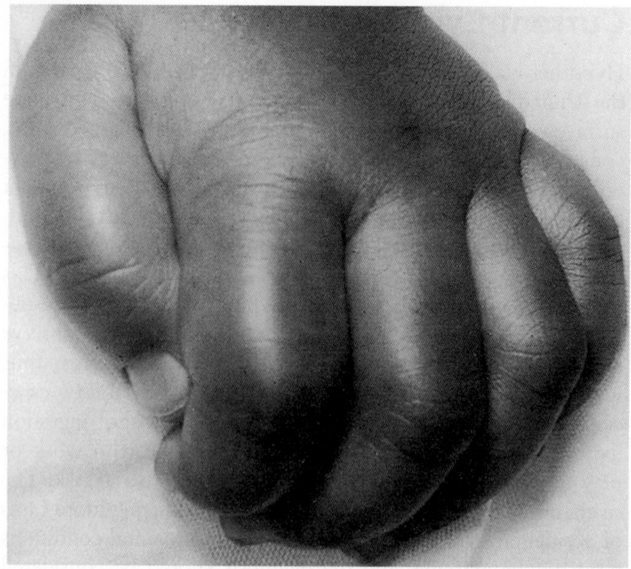

FIGURE 98.7 Swollen fingers of a child with cold exposure.

Initial laboratory tests should include CBC, platelet count, clotting studies, electrolytes, BUN and creatinine, glucose, serum amylase, and ABGs corrected for temperature (Table 98.7). Urine should be sent for drug screening.

Management and Diagnostic Studies

Therapy for hypothermia can be divided into two parts: general supportive measures and specific rewarming techniques (Table 98.8). Once hypothermia is diagnosed, temperature must be monitored continuously as treatment progresses.

All patients should be given supplemental oxygen. Patients with profuse secretions, respiratory depression, or impaired mental status should be intubated and mechanically ventilated. Intubation should be performed as gently as possible to minimize the risk of arrhythmias.

A decreased metabolic rate produces less carbon dioxide, and usual minute ventilation would produce respiratory alkalosis, increasing the risk of dangerous arrhythmias. Therefore, ventilation should begin at approximately one-half the normal minute ventilation.

Assessment of acid–base status and ventilation in the hypothermic patient is the subject of considerable confusion. Blood gas machines heat the patient's blood sample to 37°C (98.6°F) before measuring pH and gas partial pressures (thus providing theoretical values if the patient were 37°C [98.6°F]). If the patient's actual temperature is provided with the sample, the

TABLE 98.7

EFFECT OF BODY TEMPERATURE ON ARTERIAL BLOOD GASES MEASURED AT 37°C (98.6°F)

	For each elevation of 1°C	For each depression of 1°C
pH	–0.015	+0.015
Pa_{CO_2} (mm Hg)	+4.4%	–4.4%
Pa_{O_2} (mm Hg)	+7.2%	–7.2%

TABLE 98.8

MANAGEMENT OF HYPOTHERMIA

Initial management
Provide supplemental oxygen
Cardiopulmonary resuscitation for asystole, ventricular fibrillation, or any nonperfusing rhythm (use Echo to distinguish PEA from perfusing rhythm if pulses are not palpable)
Laboratory determinations
Arterial blood gas analysis corrected for temperature
Complete blood cell count, platelet count
Prothrombin time, partial thromboplastin time
Electrolytes, blood urea nitrogen, creatinine
Glucose, amylase
Urine drug screen
Monitoring
Heart rate, electrocardiogram, respiratory rate, blood pressure
Temperature
Consider central venous pressure
Treatment
Correct hypoxemia, hypercarbia
Correct hypokalemia
Correct hypoglycemia, 25% dextrose 1 g/kg IV
Tolerate hyperglycemia
Temperature
≥32°C (89.6°F): passive rewarming or simple external rewarming
<32°C (89.6°F) (acute): external or core rewarming
<32°C (89.6°F) (chronic): core rewarming
Fluid replacement
(acute) 5% dextrose in normal saline at maintenance rates
(chronic) normal saline, 5% albumin, and/or fresh frozen plasma to maintain blood pressure

machine can correct the values according to the nomogram of Kelman and Nunn. (Table 98.7 shows one set of guidelines for appropriate correction.) However, it is important to understand two concepts. The first is the ectothermic principle, which relies on the following aspect of physiology: Dissociation of ions and partial pressures of gases are decreased in cooled blood. In hypothermia, therefore, neutral pH is higher, whereas "normal" PCO_2 is lower than is encountered at 37°C (98.6°F). For example, hypoventilation of the hypothermic patient with a pH of 7.5 would actually induce an undesirable respiratory acidosis. A second, more practical concept is that if the patient's blood volume is restored and oxygenation maintained, acidosis will be corrected spontaneously as the patient is warmed.

Heart rate and rhythm should be monitored continuously and the patient handled gently to avoid precipitation of life-threatening arrhythmias in an irritable myocardium. Sinus bradycardia, atrial flutter, and atrial fibrillation are common but rarely of hemodynamic significance. Spontaneous reversion to sinus rhythm is the rule when temperature is corrected. It may be difficult to detect pulses in the hypothermic patient; therefore, it is important to provide chest compressions until pulseless electrical activity has been ruled out by echocardiography or arterial BP monitoring. Ventricular fibrillation may occur spontaneously or with trivial stimulation, especially at temperatures less than 28° to 29°C (82.4° to 84.2°F). Electrical defibrillation is warranted but frequently is ineffective until core temperature rises. Closed chest massage should be initiated and maintained until the temperature is higher than 30°C (86°F), when defibrillation is more likely to be effective. Drug therapy is rarely effective and fraught with hazards associated with decreased hepatic and renal metabolism.

Fluid replacement is essential. Relatively little plasma loss occurs in acute hypothermia but losses may be great in hypothermia of longer duration. Normal saline or lactated Ringer solution, warmed to about 43°C (109.4°F) in a blood-warming coil, is appropriate initially. Electrolyte determinations should guide further replacement. If clotting abnormalities occur, fresh-frozen plasma (10 mL per kg) is a useful choice for volume expansion (see Chapter 101 Hematologic Emergencies). As temperature rises and peripheral vasoconstriction diminishes, hypovolemia is expected. Fluid volume should be sufficient to maintain an adequate arterial BP.

Hypoglycemia, if present, is treated with glucose (0.5 to 1 g per kg by IV). Hyperglycemia, which may result from impaired insulin release in the hypothermic pancreas, should be tolerated to avoid severe hypoglycemia with rewarming.

A number of rewarming strategies exist (Fig. 98.8). Passive rewarming implies removal of the patient from a cold environment and use of blankets to maximize the effect of basal heat production. For patients with mild hypothermia (temperature higher than 32°C [89.6°F]), this may be adequate. As shown in the algorithm, the adequacy of perfusion and the degree of hypothermia are the major factors in the selection of rewarming strategies. For patients with an adequate pulse, passive rewarming is used as the initial strategy if the temperature is greater than 32°C and active core rewarming if the temperature is less than 32°C. Those with poor perfusion require active rewarming with a temperature greater than 32°C and ECMO, if available, with temperature less than 32°C.

Active rewarming is divided into external and core rewarming techniques. Electric blankets, hot-water bottles, overhead warmers, and thermal mattresses are simple, easily available sources of external heat. Immersion in warm-water baths is also possible but complicates monitoring or response to arrhythmias. These methods, however, cause early warming of the skin and extremities with peripheral vasodilation and shunting of cold, acidemic blood to the core. This causes the well-known phenomenon of "afterdrop" of core temperature. Severe hypotension may also occur in chronic cases as vasodilation increases the effective vascular space. External rewarming techniques limited to the head and trunk may minimize vasodilation and afterdrop. In acute hypothermia, active external rewarming is appropriate, but there is some evidence that in chronic cases (more than 24 hours), mortality is higher if active external rewarming is used instead of simple passive techniques.

Core rewarming techniques are almost certainly more rapid and less likely to be associated with afterdrop, dangerous arrhythmias, or significant hypotension. These methods are especially valuable in the setting of severe chronic hypothermia (temperature less than 32°C [89.6°F]), where fluid shifts are most likely to occur. A nonshivering human model

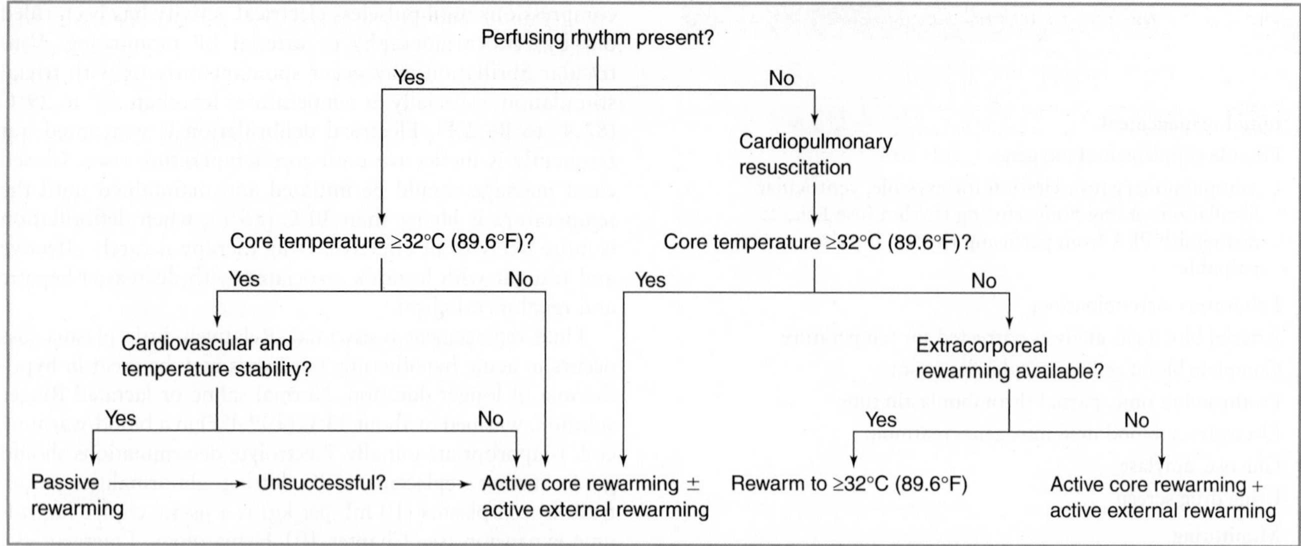

FIGURE 98.8 Algorithm for rewarming. (Adapted from Danzl DF, Pozos RS. Accidental hypothermia. *N Engl J Med* 1994;331(26):1756–1760.)

of severe hypothermia indicated that inhalation rewarming offered no rewarming advantage, whereas forced air warming (approximately 200 W) allowed a 6- to 10-fold increase in rewarming rate over controls. A canine study of experimental hypothermia found that heated aerosol inhalation alone contributed less heat than endogenous metabolism, but peritoneal lavage and pleural lavage had similar effect on rewarming (6°C/hr/m^2). In humans, peritoneal dialysis with dialysate warmed to 43°C (109.4°F) is effective and requires only equipment routinely available in most hospitals. Gastric or colonic irrigation has also been advocated, but placement of the intragastric balloon may precipitate dysrhythmias. Hemodialysis, extracorporeal blood rewarming, and mediastinal irrigation are effective but require mobilization of sophisticated equipment and personnel. Thus, new endovascular warming catheters, introduced after cannulization of the femoral vein and advancement to the inferior vena cava, use closed-loop circuitry to maintain the patient's temperature. In one case report, a woman's temperature increased by 2.8°C per hour, with a temperature of 37°C (98.6°F) achieved after 5 hours.

Indications for Admission and Discharge

In patients with mild temperature depression (greater than 32°C [89.6°F]), external rewarming techniques and supportive care based on vital signs, ABGs, and metabolic parameters such as glucose and calcium levels, should result in prompt recovery. Patients with mild hypothermia due to environmental exposure who improve with passive rewarming may be discharged after observation in the ED. However, it should be noted that other causes of hypothermia should be ruled out prior to discharge.

Children who present with a temperature less than 32°C (89.6°F), and especially those in whom hypothermia developed over 24 hours or more, require meticulous attention to continuously changing vital signs and metabolic needs. More elaborate core rewarming techniques are appropriate.

FROST BITE INJURY

CLINICAL PEARLS AND PITFALLS

- Care should be taken not to rub or apply pressure to the affected areas.
- Rewarming is painful and analgesics should be provided.

Clinical Recognition

Frostbite is injury or destruction of the skin and its underlying tissue. It may result from extended exposure to freezing temperatures; the most typical body parts affected include the fingers, toes, ears, and nose. The clinical presentation can range from superficial areas of pallor and edema to more severe hemorrhagic blisters and necrosis. Treatment can be described in three phases. The initial prethaw period, usually performed by prehospital personnel, involves getting the patient out of the cold environment and then removing wet clothing. Soft padding should be applied to protect the affected area; care must be taken not to rub any of these tissues as this may cause further damage. The second phase, the actual rewarming process, will take place over the next 15 to 30 minutes with the affected area being immersed in water that is preheated to 40° to 42°C. Because rewarming is quite painful, IV analgesics will likely be required. The third phase, the postthaw period, involves careful wound management and application of loose, sterile dressings. Digits are typically separated with cotton, and extremities are splinted. Tetanus prophylaxis is warranted. Prophylactic antibiotic use is controversial; however, coverage for staphylococci, streptococci, and pseudomonas should be considered if there is any indication of infection.

HIGH-ALTITUDE ILLNESS

Goals of Treatment

Early recognition and treatment can lead to complete recovery. Severe illness needs to be treated with cardiopulmonary resuscitation and descent to prevent pulmonary edema and cerebral edema.

CLINICAL PEARLS AND PITFALLS

- The four major illnesses seen with altitude include high-altitude headache (HAH), acute mountain sickness (AMS), high-altitude cerebral edema (HACE), and high-altitude pulmonary edema (HAPE).
- Treatment for HAH or mild AMS includes acetazolamide, analgesics, hydration, and antiemetics.
- For more severe AMS or HACE, oxygen, hyperbaric therapy, and dexamethasone are indicated.

Current Evidence

Physiologic changes accompanying altitude may be attributed to hypobaric hypoxia. As altitude increases, barometric pressure decreases, with a subsequent reduction in the partial pressure of oxygen. Temperature also has an inverse relationship to altitude, with hypothermia compounding these hypoxic effects. The individual's response to hypoxia is to increase ventilation, which raises alveolar oxygen while reducing alveolar carbon dioxide simultaneously. Hypocapnia produces an alkalosis that, in turn, will serve as a "check and balance" for the body by limiting further increases in the respiratory rate. The pH returns to neutral as the kidneys excrete bicarbonate in response to this alkalosis. Acetazolamide (Diamox) is used to inhibit carbonic anhydrase to create a metabolic acidosis that allows the ventilatory rate to remain high and to maintain better oxygenation.

Clinical Recognition

The four major illnesses seen with altitude include HAH, AMS, HACE, and HAPE. Headache is typically the initial symptom upon climbing to higher altitudes; it may occur alone as in HAH or progress to AMS. AMS is defined as having a headache in the setting of at least one of four other symptoms: nausea/vomiting, fatigue, difficulty sleeping, and dizziness. Vasogenic edema is believed to explain the pathophysiology underlying AMS, with clinical progression to encephalopathy occurring as cerebral edema, or HACE, worsens. HAPE is the most common cause of death when exposed to high altitudes; younger individuals appear to be the most susceptible, especially children with upper respiratory symptoms. Pulmonary vascular leak leads to elevated pulmonary artery pressures.

Triage and Initial Assessment

The recognition of altitude illness depends mainly on a compatible history of exposure to high altitude. Children may be exposed to higher altitudes through participation in sporting events, family vacations, and school activities. One source defines high altitude as 1,500 to 3,500 m (4,921 to 11,483 ft), very high altitude as 3,500 to 5,500 m (11,483 to 18,045 ft), and extreme altitude as greater than 5,500 m (18,045 ft).

Initial Assessment

The diagnosis of altitude illness in children can be challenging, especially in the preverbal age group. Factors that affect whether an individual gets sick include the altitude itself, rate of ascent, the altitude where sleeping occurs routinely, and the individual's physiology. Information regarding any potential genetic basis of high-altitude illness is limited, with no specific genetic polymorphisms identified to date. However, from an anatomical perspective, those who are able to tolerate brain swelling (i.e., the elderly whose brain size diminishes with age, or infants with their immature sutures and open fontanelles) are less susceptible to altitude illnesses. A recent study from Switzerland finds a prevalence of AMS in both healthy children and adolescents of 37.5%; fortunately, the symptoms were relatively mild and responded to supportive care without the need for descent.

Management and Diagnostic Studies

Treatment for HAH and mild AMS includes stopping the ascent and acclimatizing at the current altitude; acetazolamide given early will hasten this process. Analgesics, hydration, and antiemetics are also given for supportive care. Once AMS worsens, low-flow oxygen should be given in conjunction with acetazolamide and/or dexamethasone, and either HBO therapy with a portable compartment or immediate descent should occur. Therapy should be more aggressive if HACE ensues, with dexamethasone administered in addition to oxygen, HBO, and immediate descent or evacuation. The addition of the calcium-channel blocker nifedipine will reduce pulmonary vascular pressures in patients with HAPE. Exertion should be limited, oxygen provided, and either HBO or immediate descent arranged.

Prevention

Prevention efforts may minimize an individual's chance of developing altitude illness. For example, different formulas exist regarding ideal ascent rates (i.e., above 3,000 m [9,842 ft], sleeping elevations should not exceed the previous day by more than 300 to 500 m and rest should occur every 3 days), following the mantra of "climb high, sleep low." If physically fit individuals follow such climbing guidelines, prophylaxis with acetazolamide is not typically required. However, because of the ease of getting to high elevations via car or airplane, individuals who ascend quickly, and/or have significant underlying diseases (hepatic, renal, or cardiopulmonary dysfunction in particular) may warrant acetazolamide prophylaxis. Most sources recommend using 250 mg twice daily, with pediatric dosing extrapolated from acetazolamide dosing for edema at 5 to 10 mg/kg/dose every 6 hours, not to exceed 1 g per day. Care should be taken in the individual with a sulfa allergy because acetazolamide contains a sulfa moiety; while the incidence of cross-reactivity is low at 7% to 10% in patients with a self-reported sulfa allergy, anaphylaxis has been reported and thus use of dexamethasone may be more prudent in these cases.

ELECTRICAL INJURIES

Goals of Treatment

The goals of emergency therapy are stabilization of cardiopulmonary status, treatment of external injuries, and assessment for potential internal injuries.

CLINICAL PEARLS AND PITFALLS

- Children who have sustained minor household electrical injuries and are asymptomatic usually do not require laboratory evaluation, cardiac evaluation, or hospitalization.
- In more severe injuries, entry and exit wounds and arc burns are poor predictors of internal damage. Tissue that appears viable initially may become ischemic over several days.

Current Evidence

The spectrum of electrical injury is enormous, ranging from low-voltage household accidents to million-volt lightning strikes (Table 98.9). Appropriate management requires an understanding of the basic physical aspects of electricity, the physiologic responses to injury, and the potential for immediate and delayed damage. Lightning that strikes individuals carries a 30% risk of mortality and claims approximately 100 lives annually in the United States. The death rate is highest among children ranging from 15 to 19 years of age. Harnessed electrical power is responsible for approximately 700 deaths per year, of which 10% are children. Household electrical cords are the major cause of electrocution in children 12 years of age and younger. High-tension electrical injuries dominate in older children who climb on trees, buildings, or utility structures. Tasers and stun guns, which are high-voltage, low-current stimulators, cause pain due to involuntary muscle contractions.

The severity of electrical injury depends on six factors: (i) The resistance of skin, mucosa, and internal structures; (ii) the type of current (alternating or direct); (iii) the frequency of the current; (iv) the intensity; (v) the duration of contact; and (vi) the pathway taken by the current. Precise separation of the effect of these factors, which are interrelated, is impossible. Together, they produce either heat or current, and a variety of injuries result.

Resistance is a major factor determining the amount of current flow through tissue. Tissue injury is inversely related to resistance. Dry skin provides resistance of approximately 40,000 ohms, whereas thick, callused palms may provide up to 1×10^6 ohms. Thin, moist, or soiled skin lowers resistance to the 300- to 1,000-ohm range. The highly vascular, moist oral mucosa has even lower resistance.

TABLE 98.9

LIGHTNING VERSUS HIGH-VOLTAGE ELECTRICAL INJURY

Factor	Lightning	High voltage
Duration	Brief	Prolonged
Energy level	100,000,000 V 200,000 A	Much lower
Type of current	Direct	Usually alternating
Shock wave	Present	Absent
Cardiac	Asystole	Ventricular fibrillation
Burns	Superficial, minor	Deep, frequently obscured
Renal failures	Rare	Common secondary to myoglobinuria
Fasciotomy and amputation	Rare	Common, early, extensive

The type of current is another important determinant of injury. Alternating current (AC) at low voltage is able to induce tetanic muscle contraction and is, therefore, more dangerous than direct current (DC). Normal household 60-Hz current changes direction 120 times per second, a frequency that induces an indefinite refractory state at neuromuscular junctions. The resultant muscle contractions prevent the victim from releasing his grip ("locking-on"), thus extending the duration of contact. Higher-frequency commercial currents are less likely to induce such a state and may be less harmful.

DC is used in medical settings for cardiac defibrillation, countershock, and pacing. Currents as low as 1 mA may trigger ventricular fibrillation, and high currents may damage the heart and conducting tissues directly. Lightning is another example of DC, discharged in a single, massive bolt that lasts 1/10,000 to 1/1,000 second. The brevity of exposure makes deep thermal injury unlikely.

In general, high-voltage injury is more dangerous than low-voltage injury. A higher voltage is more likely to cause "locking-on" and associated deep tissue injury, although its tendency to throw victims from the source of current may mitigate this effect. The possibility of head and cervical spine injuries must be considered in these cases. The value of the current, or amperage, is of even greater importance than the voltage. Flow as low as 1 to 10 mA may be perceived as a tingling sensation. Progressively higher flows may paralyze muscles and ventilation, precipitate ventricular fibrillation, and cause deep tissue burns.

Clinical Recognition

Electrical injury may produce a variety of clinical sequelae, ranging from local damage to widespread multisystem disturbances. Victims of the most severe accidents are commonly pulseless, apneic, and unresponsive. Current that passes directly through the heart may induce ventricular fibrillation. Brainstem (medullary) paralysis or tetanic contractions of thoracic muscles may result in cardiopulmonary collapse. Lightning injury is capable of inducing asystole, from which the heart may recover spontaneously, but the accompanying respiratory failure is commonly prolonged. Unless ventilation is initiated promptly, hypoxia leads to secondary ventricular fibrillation and death.

Other cardiac disorders, including arrhythmias and conduction defects, are common among survivors. Supraventricular tachycardia, atrial and ventricular extrasystoles, right bundle branch block, and complete heart block are most common. Complaints of crushing or stabbing precordial pain may accompany nonspecific ST-T wave changes. Some patients sustain myocardial damage or even ventricular wall perforation. Despite evidence of important cardiac injuries, patients without secondary hypoxic-ischemic injury usually regain good myocardial function.

Nervous system injury is also common and may involve the brain, spinal cord, peripheral motor and sensory nerves, and sympathetic fibers. Loss of consciousness, seizures, amnesia, disorientation, deafness, visual disturbances, sensory deficits, hemiplegia, and quadriparesis occur acutely but may be transient. Vascular damage may produce subdural, epidural, or intraventricular hemorrhage.

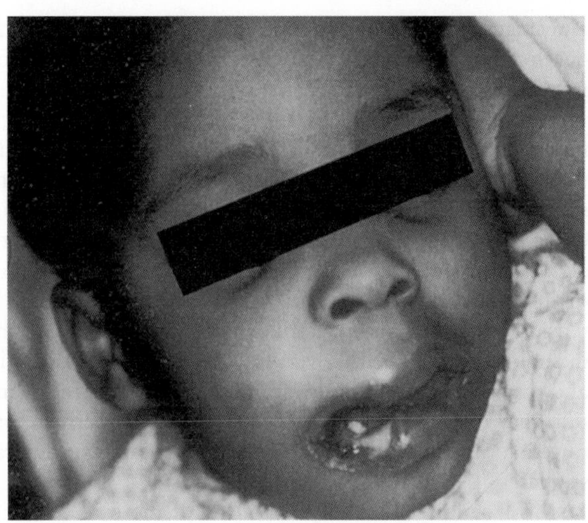
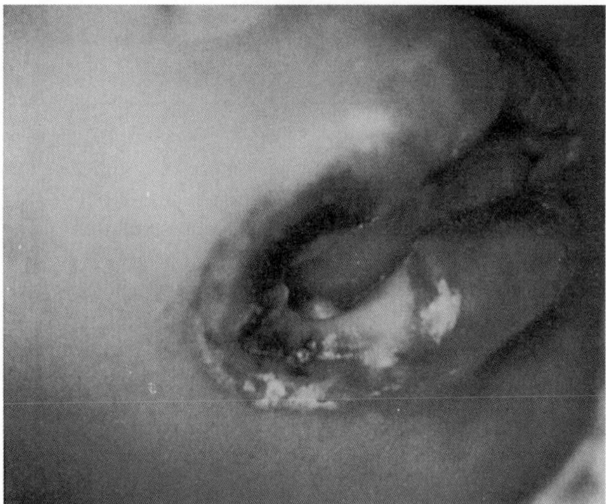

FIGURE 98.9 Patient with electrical burns to the corner of the mouth after biting on an electrical cord. (Courtesy of Evaline Alessandrini, MD.)

Additional problems develop within hours to days after injury. The syndrome of inappropriate antidiuretic hormone secretion may precipitate cerebral edema. Electroencephalograms reveal diffuse slowing, epileptiform discharges, or burst suppression patterns, but these may not have prognostic significance. Spinal cord dysfunction more often results in motor than sensory deficit. Peripheral neuropathies with patchy distribution may reflect direct thermal injury, vascular compromise, or current flow itself. A variety of autonomic disturbances may resolve spontaneously or persist as reflex sympathetic dystrophy.

Ocular damage is common, particularly after lightning strikes. Direct thermal or electrical injury, intensive light, and confusion contribute to the presentation. Findings include corneal lesions, hyphema, uveitis, iridocyclitis, and vitreous hemorrhage. Choroidal rupture, retinal detachment, and chorioretinitis occur less often. Autonomic disturbances in a lightning victim may cause fixed dilated pupils, which should not serve as a criterion for brain death without extensive investigation of other neurologic and ocular functions. Cataracts and optic atrophy are possible late developments.

Electrical injury may induce direct or indirect complications in other organ systems. Tetanic contractions may cause joint dislocations and fractures, especially of the upper-extremity long bones and vertebrae. Fractures of the skull and other long bones may occur when high-tension shock throws the victim from the site of contact. Early cardiopulmonary insufficiency, as well as direct renal effects, may cripple renal function. Damaged muscle releases myoglobin and CPK. As in crush injuries, myoglobin may induce renal tubular damage and kidney failure. Pleural damage may cause large effusions, whereas primary lung injury or aspiration of gastric contents may lead to pneumonitis. Gastric dilation, ileus, diffuse GI hemorrhage, and visceral perforation may occur immediately or later.

In addition to burns at the site of primary contact, burns are common where current has jumped across flexed joints. Such burns are most common on the volar surface of the forearm and across the elbow and axilla. Arcing current may also ignite clothing and produce thermal burns. Entry and exit wounds and arc burns are poor predictors of internal damage. Tissue that appears viable initially may become edematous and then ischemic or frankly gangrenous over several days. Diminished peripheral pulses may provide immediate evidence of vascular damage, but strong pulses do not guarantee vascular integrity. Blood flow falls to a minimum at about 36 hours, but current or thermal damage may lead to vasospasm, delayed thrombosis, ischemic necrosis, or aneurysm formation and hemorrhage weeks after the injury. Viable major arteries near occluded nutrient arteries may account for apparently adequate circulation and uneven destruction of surrounding tissues.

Young children are vulnerable to orofacial burns, especially of the lips (Fig. 98.9). These full-thickness burns of the upper and lower lips and oral commissure usually involve mucosa, submucosa, muscles, nerves, and blood vessels. The lesion usually has a pale, painless, well-demarcated, depressed center with surrounding pale gray tissue and erythematous border. After a few hours, the wound margin extends and marked edema occurs. Drooling is common. The eschar separates in 2 to 3 weeks and bleeding may occur at this time; granulation tissue gradually fills the wound. Scarring may produce lip eversion, microstomia, and loss of function. Damage to facial or even carotid arteries may result in delayed hemorrhage. Devitalization of deciduous and secondary teeth may occur.

Inadequately debrided burned or gangrenous tissue provides a medium for serious infection. Staphylococcal, pseudomonal, and clostridial species are common pathogens in the extremities. Streptococci and oral anaerobic organisms may infect mouth wounds.

Management and Diagnostic Studies

The first step in emergency management (Table 98.10) is to separate the victim from the current source. The rescuer must be well insulated to avoid becoming an additional casualty. If the current cannot be shut off, wires can be cut with a wood-handled ax or appropriately insulated wire cutters.

Any victim in cardiopulmonary arrest should be resuscitated promptly following the guidelines discussed in Chapters 2 Approach to the Injured Child, 3 Airway, and 4 Cardiopulmonary Resuscitation. Prolonged efforts to restore adequate cardiopulmonary and cerebral function, especially in the lightning victim, may be appropriate in the context of bizarre neurologic

TABLE 98.10

MANAGEMENT OF ELECTRICAL INJURIES

Initial management
Remove from source of current
Cardiopulmonary resuscitation as needed
Provide mechanical ventilation until spontaneous ventilation is adequate
Immobilize neck and spine
Clinical assessment
Neurologic examination
Peripheral pulses and perfusion
Oral burns/edema
Chest wall injury
Abdominal distention
Eye or ear trauma
Cutaneous burns or bruises
Laboratory determinations
Complete blood cell count
Blood urea nitrogen, creatinine, urinalysis including myoglobin
Electrolytes
Troponin
Electrocardiogram (ECG)
Consider skull, spine, chest, long bone radiographs
Consider computed tomography scan of brain
Consider electroencephalogram
Monitoring
Heart rate, ECG, respiratory rate, blood pressure
Management
Maintenance fluids: 5% dextrose in normal saline
Volume expansion in presence of thermal burns or extensive deep tissue injury: 0.9% sodium chloride, lactated Ringer solution, or 5% albumin
Fluid restriction for central nervous system injury
Maintain urine output >1 mL/kg/hr
Treat arrhythmias
Treat seizures
Tetanus toxoid; consider penicillin/other antibiotics
Consider general, oral, or plastic surgical consultation

phenomena that inhibit ventilatory efforts, consciousness, or pupillary function. The patient who fails to respond to resuscitative efforts over hours to days and meets standard brain death criteria can be pronounced dead.

Any patient who sustains electrical injury deserves a comprehensive physical examination. Bleeding or edema from orofacial burns may compromise the upper airway. The head, particularly eyes, and neck should be examined carefully for evidence of trauma. The skin should be examined carefully for burns and bruises. Limbs should be evaluated for pulses, perfusion, and motor and sensory function, as well as for soft tissue swelling or evidence of fractures. Burns and deep tissue injury may progress over hours to days, so repeated examination and monitoring are important.

Neurologic evaluation is especially important in all but the most minor, localized peripheral injuries. Level of consciousness and mental status should be assessed according to the child's developmental level. Evaluations of cranial nerve, cerebellar, motor, and sensory function are essential.

Children who have sustained minor household electrical injuries and are asymptomatic usually do not require laboratory evaluation, cardiac evaluation, or hospitalization. In one series, investigators were unable to assess the clinical significance of loss of consciousness, tetany, wet skin, or current flow across the heart, and recommended cardiac monitoring if any of these factors were present. If the history is one of a high-tension injury or lightning strike, laboratory evaluation should include ECG, CBC, CPK (with fractionation), BUN, creatinine, and urinalysis, including urine myoglobin. Physical examination that reveals evidence of bruises, bony tenderness, or distorted long bones should prompt appropriate radiographic studies.

Most children who sustain burns of the oral commissure (usually after biting an electrical cord) do not require extensive evaluation or admission. In cases of severe orofacial burns, use of an artificial airway should be considered before progressive edema leads to catastrophe. Mechanical ventilation may be necessary to overcome CNS depression or primary lung involvement.

Patients with persistent coma and loss of protective airway reflexes should be intubated to avoid aspiration. Good oxygenation and ventilation adequate to maintain a normal pH and $Paco_2$ of 35 to 40 mm Hg must be ensured. Seizure activity should be treated (see Chapter 67 Seizures).

The neck and back should be immobilized if the patient was thrown from the site of injury. If the mechanism of injury was severe, a cervical collar should be maintained in place despite normal cervical spine radiographs. If a child fails to regain consciousness within a short time or shows signs of neurologic deterioration, a computed tomography scan will help exclude intracranial hemorrhage.

Cardiopulmonary support is nonspecific. Most patients resume circulatory stability unless severe hypoxia and ischemia have weakened the myocardium. Arrhythmias should be treated along usual lines (see Chapter 94 Cardiac Emergencies).

Patients struck by lightning require only maintenance fluids. Patients with ordinary thermal burns should be treated according to standard recommendations (see Chapter 112 Burns), although body surface area calculations may seriously underestimate fluid requirements. Extensive vascular and deep tissue destruction may lead to extensive fluid sequestration. Isotonic fluid should be given in amounts to maintain normal pulse and BP. In all cases, fluids should be given with attention to possible CNS complications.

Cerebral edema may develop over hours to days after injury, especially after a lightning strike. If the child's neurologic status fails to improve or deteriorates, intracranial pressure monitoring and treatment may be necessary. Serum and urine electrolytes and osmolality should be followed closely to recognize promptly the syndrome of inappropriate antidiuretic hormone secretion.

Myoglobin in the urine is consistent with muscle breakdown and sets the stage for renal failure. Hydration and brisk diuresis with furosemide and/or mannitol may prevent renal damage but must be undertaken with caution if there is coexistent CNS injury. Extensive muscle damage after lightning injury is uncommon, however, and major CNS injury is common. Treatment should proceed with these relative risks in mind until definitive information is available.

Most burns associated with lightning injury are superficial. Although they may become more apparent after several hours, most remain first- or second-degree burns. Minor burns on the extremities can be treated with antibiotic ointment and should be allowed to slough and heal. Oral and plastic surgeons should evaluate children who sustain oral burns. In most cases, similar conservative management is recommended, but a removable stent may be necessary to minimize scarring.

High-voltage injuries commonly require aggressive treatment. Fasciotomy may be necessary to restore adequate circulation to an injured extremity. The approach to debridement of wounds is controversial, but repeated examinations are considered most useful for detecting nonviable tissue. Approximately 30% of survivors of high-tension injuries ultimately require amputation of some part of an extremity.

The risk of infection in patients with deep tissue injury is high. Any patient not clearly immunized against tetanus should be given tetanus toxoid. Prophylactic antibiotics have been recommended for oral injuries, but in general, antimicrobial therapy should be reserved for proven or strongly suspected infection.

Indications for Discharge and Admission

Any patient who has sustained cardiopulmonary arrest, loss of consciousness, or deep tissue injury should be admitted to the hospital for evaluation and treatment. Heart rate, respiratory rate, and BP should be monitored regularly. Doppler evaluation may be helpful in cases of vasospasm, which may complicate assessment of BP and subsequent fluid management. True hypotension may require pressor support and ICU care.

INJURIES INVOLVING RADIATION

Goals of Treatment

The emergency physician should be aware of the basic principles and management of radiation incidents in order to recognize when it happens, know procedures for decontamination of victims, alleviate public fears and psychological trauma about potential incidents, and prevent mismanagement of potential victims. Frequent training and drills are essential to ensure that the ED staff has the knowledge, procedural skills, and supplies to deal with possible victims exposed to radiation accidents. The goals of treatment are to decontaminate the patient without contaminating healthcare providers and to recognize early signs of radiation injury.

CLINICAL PEARLS AND PITFALLS

- No survivable radiation injury requires immediate life-saving treatment, hence medical staff should focus their attention on injury-related life-threatening conditions.
- The greatest risk of whole-body radiation exposure occurs 3 to 4 weeks later when bone marrow depression reaches its nadir.
- Risk of contamination of ED staff is usually minimal.
- Emergency preparedness for radiation injuries is crucial to managing these incidents and preventing widespread panic among staff and the public.

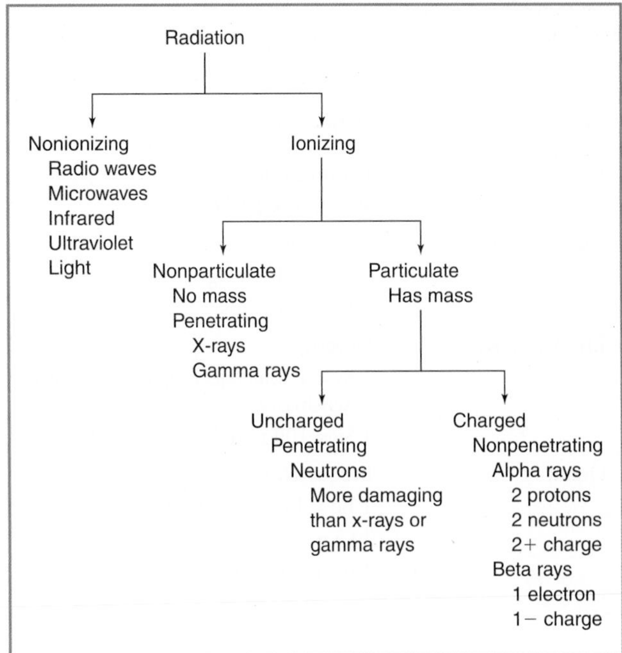

FIGURE 98.10 Types of radiation.

Current Evidence

Types of Radiation

Radiation is a very general term used to describe energy that is emitted from a source (Fig. 98.10). *Ionizing radiation,* for example, x-rays, deposits a large amount of energy in a small volume of tissue; energy is sufficient to strip electrons from atoms. *Nonionizing radiation,* for example, visible light and infrared, is less energetic and of longer wavelength, and primarily deposits heat in tissue.

Ionizing radiation can be further subdivided into types of radiation that have no associated mass (*nonparticulate*) and those that have mass (*particulate*). X-rays and gamma rays are nonparticulate types of radiation and can penetrate deeply into the body and affect radiation-sensitive tissues, for example, bone marrow and the lining of the GI tract. X-rays are emitted by excited electrons, whereas gamma rays are emitted by excited or unstable nuclei (radioisotopes or radionuclides). Once x-rays or gamma rays have been emitted, they are indistinguishable.

Particulate radiation can be further divided into charged and uncharged particles. Neutrons, a type of particulate radiation that has no electrical charge, can penetrate the body to depths similar to x-rays and gamma rays. Because neutrons deposit their energy in a more concentrated area, they cause more biologic damage than x-rays or gamma rays.

Alpha particles have a 2+ electrical charge and a large mass (two protons and two neutrons). Beta particles have a single negative charge and a small mass (one electron). Charged particles do not penetrate the body very well. Because of their larger mass and charge, alpha rays cannot penetrate even the dead layers of skin. ^{239}Pu, an alpha emitter, is a biologic hazard only when it is inhaled, ingested, or otherwise introduced into the body. Beta particles ("beta rays") are more penetrating and in high doses can severely damage the skin. Beta rays cannot damage the deep radiation-sensitive organs in the body unless the radioactive source is incorporated into the body. At

TABLE 98.11

INTERNATIONAL RADIATION UNITS

Metric	Definition
Exposure	Roentgen, R R = 2.58×10^{-4} C/kg air
Absorbed dose	Gray, Gy 1 Gy = 1 Joule/kg 1 Gy = 100 rads
Effective dose	Sievert, Sv 1 Sv = 1 Joule/kg, weighted for tissue sensitivity 1 Sv = 100 rems
Quantity	Becquerel, Bq 1 Bq = 1 disintegration/s 1 Ci = 3.7×10^{10} Bq 1 mCi = 37 MBq

TABLE 98.12

COMMON RADIATION DOSES

Sources	Effective dose
Roundtrip intercontinental air flight	20–30 μSv
Chest radiograph	50–100 μSv
Living in brick house	0.20 μSv/yr
Natural radiation	3 mSv/yr
Angiography	10 mSv
Abdominal computed tomographic scan	10–30 mSv

the Chernobyl nuclear plant accident in Russia, some of the firefighters had severe skin damage due to intense beta particle exposure, which contributed to their deaths.

The words "radiation" and "radioactive" are often confused. An atom that is unstable spontaneously gives off energy as radiation and is therefore radioactive. In contrast, an x-ray machine cannot spontaneously give off radiation: An external power source is needed. Therefore, an x-ray machine is not radioactive. A patient who has been exposed to radiation does not become radioactive. Patients emit radiation only if they have radioactive atoms on them (external contamination) or within them (internal contamination).

Amounts of Radiation

Geiger counters can measure amounts of radiation far below levels that have a measurable biologic effect. They are inexpensive and readily available in the nuclear medicine department at most hospitals. Because a Geiger counter can detect and quantify the radiation exposure rate immediately, detecting and managing a radiation hazard may be easier than detecting and managing biologic or chemical hazards.

Radiation exposure is commonly measured in three different units in the United States: roentgen, rad, and rem. However, new international units are being used by regulatory and professional organizations (Table 98.11). The roentgen (R) is a measure of radiation exposure in air. Absorbed dose in an organ is measured in grays (Gy); 1 Gy is equal to 100 rads. Effective dose, in sieverts (Sv), is a measure of overall risk to an individual when the irradiation is weighted for the sensitivity of each organ to late effects of radiation. One sievert is equal to 100 rems. Quantity of radioactivity is measured by becquerels (Bq), defined as 1 atomic disintegration per second. The former unit, the curie (Ci), is equal to 3.7×10^{10} Bq, and 1 mCi is equal to 37 MBq.

We are exposed to about 3 mSv of radiation each year from natural sources. During a 70-year lifetime, a person's total radiation exposure from natural sources will be more than 200 mSv, with no measurable biologic effect of radiation. Typical radiation exposures encountered during life and in medicine are listed in Table 98.12.

The hazard posed by a radionuclide depends on its quantity, decay scheme, the energies of its emissions, its half-life, and length of exposure. For example, a radionuclide that decays by emitting only alpha particles is not a hazard if kept outside the body, since alpha particles cannot penetrate even the dead layers of the skin. However, some radionuclides (e.g., ^{131}I) that are readily absorbed by the body and/or are concentrated by an organ can be a hazard in small amounts.

Although the radiation doses to personnel involved in the care of a victim contaminated by radioactive material are likely to be very small, simple protective measures should be employed to minimize the doses. There are three methods of protection from radiation exposure: minimizing *time* of exposure, maximizing *distance* from the material to the extent practical, and using *shielding* as appropriate (Fig. 98.11). The amount of exposure received is directly proportional to the time spent near the source of radiation. Distance is the most practical and effective method of reducing radiation exposure because the

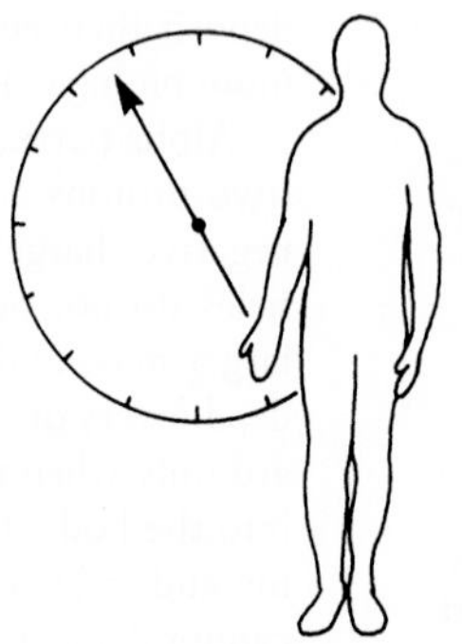
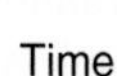

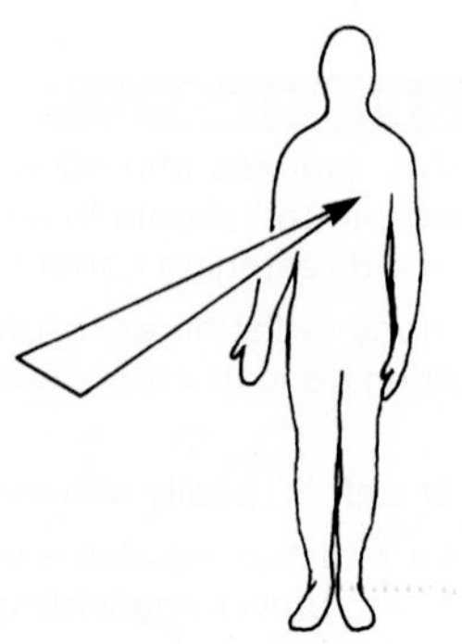

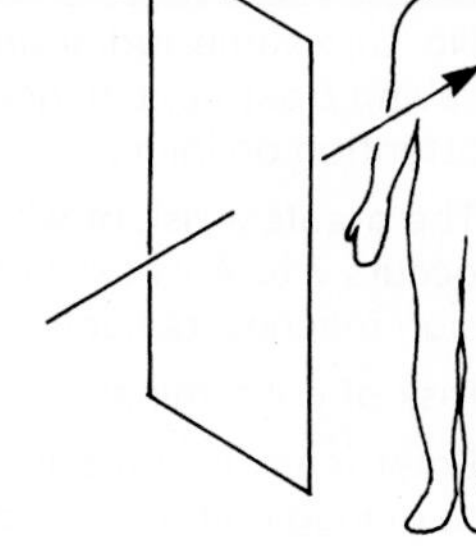

FIGURE 98.11 Three methods of reducing radiation exposure.

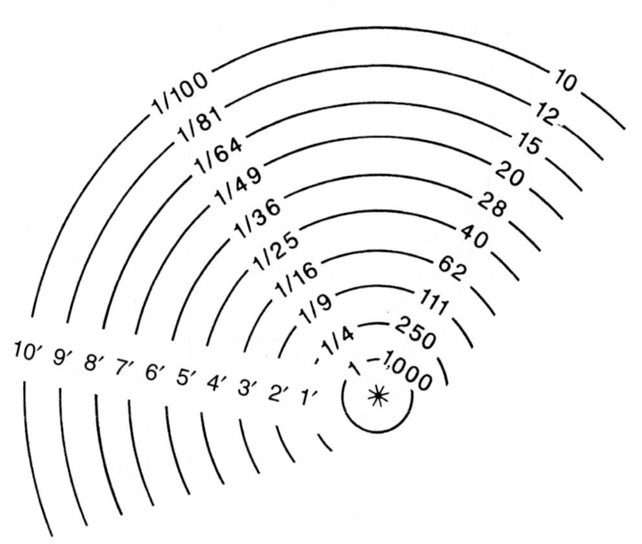

FIGURE 98.12 The effect of distance on radiation exposure from a point source of radiation.

dose decreases by the square of the distance (Fig. 98.12). This is known as the inverse square law. The lead aprons used in radiology departments, where the radiation comes from low-energy scattered radiation, are not generally useful in radiation event management. Lead aprons do not provide very effective protection against the higher-energy radionuclide emissions likely to be encountered with radioactive contamination.

Recognition

Radiation exposures can be recognized by understanding three questions: (i) Who is likely to be affected by a radiation exposure or accident? (ii) What are the likely sources of radiation? and (iii) What are the likely injuries? The people most likely to be involved in a radiation exposure event are individuals whose work involves radiation. Other individuals who may be exposed to radiation include members of the general public who inadvertently come into contact with a radiation hazard, for example, the population surrounding the Chernobyl powerplant, those who are intentionally poisoned, and patients who have undergone medical procedures (e.g., fluoroscopy or radiation therapy). To cause a significant radiation injury, an intense radiation source is needed. The four major types of possible intense radiation sources are listed in Table 98.13. Because of their various physical properties, different sources are likely to cause different types of radiation injuries.

There are three major types of radiation injuries (Table 98.14): perceived, exposure, and contamination. The first and by far the most common injury is the perceived radiation injury, due to public misconceptions and fear. The psychological stress caused by misdiagnosis can be significant. Healthcare workers educated about radiation risks should be able to anticipate and mitigate these concerns. The second major type of radiation injury is exposure to radiation. Because these patients do not have radioactive dirt on or in them, they are not radioactive and can be treated without any additional precautions on the part of healthcare workers. Two types of injury from radiation exposure are possible—whole body and local injury. A high dose of penetrating radiation over a short period of time to a large portion of the body (i.e., whole-body radiation) causes the acute radiation syndrome. Large doses of radiation over a short period of time to a small portion of the body cause a local radiation injury. Analogous medical situations would be whole-body radiation as conditioning for bone

TABLE 98.14

TYPES OF RADIATION INJURIES

Perceived
Exposure
Whole body
Local
Contamination
External
Internal
Metal fragment
Hot particle
Terrorist event

TABLE 98.13

INTENSE RADIATION SOURCES

Type of source	Examples	Likely injuries
Sealed	Industrial radiography Brachytherapy Some radiation therapy machines Industrial sterilizers	Contamination unlikely Local radiation injury with small source Whole-body exposure with large source
Unsealed	Medical radionuclides (e.g., ^{131}I, ^{32}P) Accidental release by a reactor Radium dial painters	External and internal contamination likely
Radiation devices	Cyclotron Linear accelerator Fluoroscopy unit	Local radiation injury likely
Uncontrolled fission	Nuclear reactor Uranium enrichment Weapons production	Large whole-body doses likely On- and off-site contamination possible for nuclear reactors

TABLE 98.15

DOSE-EFFECT RELATIONSHIP AFTER ACUTE WHOLE-BODY RADIATION EXPOSURE

Whole-body absorbed dose (Sv)	Comments
0.1	Asymptomatic (minimal detectable dose using cytogenetics)
0.5	Asymptomatic (minor depression of white blood cell and platelets)
1	Nausea and vomiting in approximately 15% of patients within 2 days of exposure
2	Nausea and vomiting in most patients
4	Nausea, vomiting, and diarrhea within 48 hrs; severe hematologic depression; 50% mortality without medical treatment
6	100% mortality within 30 days without medical treatment; 50% mortality with medical treatment
7	Gastrointestinal syndrome; survival unlikely; death in 2–3 wks
50	Neurovascular syndrome; death in 24–72 hrs

marrow transplantation and localized radiation therapy for breast cancer. The signs and symptoms of the acute radiation syndrome (Table 98.15) begin to appear after whole-body radiation doses of approximately 1 Gy. Organs with rapidly dividing cells such as bone marrow and GI tract lining are the most susceptible to radiation damage. The amount of damage that occurs is dependent both on the dose and on the dose rate, for example, a dose of 1 Gy per minute would probably cause symptoms but 1 Gy at a dose rate of 10 mGy per day for 100 days would likely be asymptomatic. Doses of about 4 to 6 Gy may be lethal in approximately 50% of people if they do not receive medical treatment. With maximum medical treatment, the dose of radiation that will kill 50% of people may be as high as 6.5 to 7 Gy.

The acute radiation syndrome consists of three distinct phases (Table 98.16): prodromal, latent, and manifest illness. The *prodromal* phase begins minutes to hours after the radiation

TABLE 98.16

ACUTE RADIATION SYNDROME—SIGNS AND SYMPTOMS

Prodromal (0–2[a])	Latent (2–20[a])	Manifest illness (21–60[a])
Fatigue	Asymptomatic	Bone marrow depression
Nausea and vomiting		Sepsis
Diarrhea		Bleeding
Headache		Diarrhea
Dizziness		
Decreased lymphocyte count		

[a]Days after exposure.

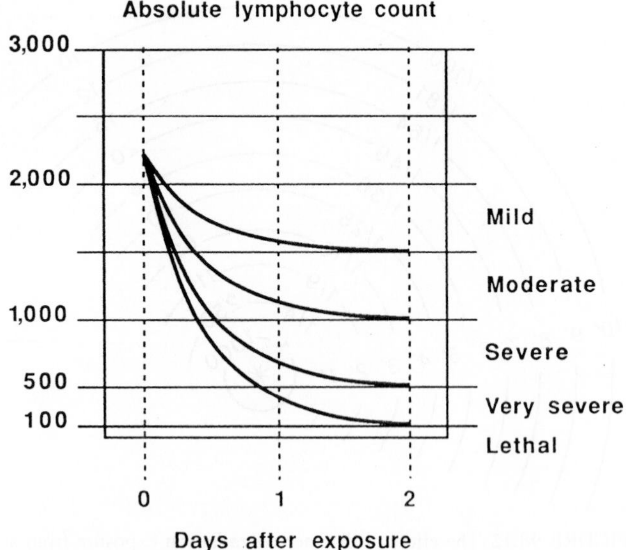

FIGURE 98.13 Effect of whole-body radiation on lymphocytes in the first 2 days after exposure.

exposure, lasts for 2 to 3 days, and common symptoms are nausea, vomiting, diarrhea, fatigue, and/or headache. The prodromal phase is followed by the *latent* phase, in which the patient is relatively asymptomatic and generally lasts days or weeks after the exposure. The *manifest illness* phase poses the greatest risk for infection and bleeding due to bone marrow suppression and GI epithelial damage. As the radiation dose increases, the duration of the prodromal phase increases and the length of the latent phase decreases.

With doses of 2 to 4 Gy, the primary effect of whole-body radiation is to depress the bone marrow. Although the absolute lymphocyte count (Fig. 98.13) decreases rapidly within the first 24 hours, there is no need for specific medical treatment. The patient will be at greatest risk 3 to 4 weeks after the radiation exposure when the white blood cell and platelet counts reach a nadir (Fig. 98.14). At this time, the patient is vulnerable to death from infection and bleeding. If the patient can be supported during this period of vulnerability and if the bone marrow is not irreversibly damaged, a recovery phase ensues.

The GI syndrome occurs from absorbed doses of more than approximately 7 Gy. During the prodromal phase there is prompt onset of severe nausea, vomiting, and diarrhea. There is a latent period of approximately 1 week and then recurrence of GI symptoms, sepsis, electrolyte imbalance, and likely death. The patient is susceptible to infection due to lack of granulocytes and because pathogens can readily enter the body across the damaged GI tract lining.

At dose levels of more than 50 Gy, the cardiovascular/CNS syndrome predominates. There is almost immediate nausea, vomiting, prostration, hypotension, ataxia, and convulsions. The permeability of blood vessels increases and there is brain edema and hypotension caused by the difficulty of maintaining a normal intravascular space. Death usually occurs within 1 to 4 days.

Estimating the whole-body radiation dose may be difficult, especially when complicated by injuries that are not due to radiation. The signs and symptoms during the prodromal period are quite nonspecific except for a rapidly decreasing lymphocyte count. Nausea and vomiting are sensitive but

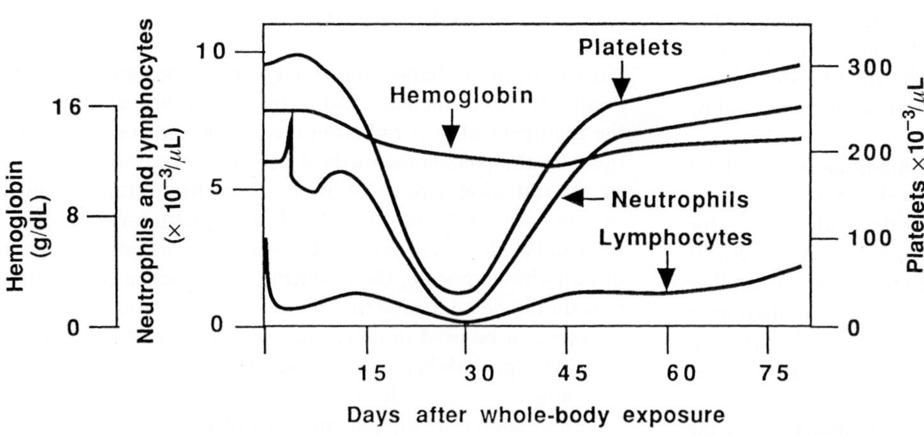

FIGURE 98.14 Effect of whole-body radiation on blood cell counts in the days after exposure.

nonspecific symptoms. Patients who do not have nausea and vomiting are unlikely to have been exposed to a radiation dose that is large enough to cause acute radiation syndrome. However, individuals may have nausea and vomiting for reasons other than exposure to radiation. The whole-body radiation dose from radiation accidents is rarely uniform. The nonuniform nature of the radiation dose makes it more difficult to predict the biologic effects of the exposure. Chromosome analysis (cytogenetic dosimetry) may be helpful in estimating the radiation dose, but the results may not be available for about 1 week.

The second type of radiation exposure that can occur involves a large radiation dose to a small part of the body. Large doses can be tolerated if only a small part of the body is exposed. Local radiation injuries may cause bone marrow depression if accompanied by a significant whole-body radiation dose. These injuries are rarely life-threatening, but they are difficult to manage because they often cause a slowly progressive injury that takes months to years to fully evolve. The injury develops slowly because the radiation causes progressive fibrosis of the blood vessels, which, in turn, causes tissue necrosis. The ultimate extent of the injury may not be appreciated initially. Healing following amputation or reconstructive surgery is poor because of deficient blood supply.

The hand is the most common site for localized irradiation injuries. The next most common sites are the thighs and buttocks because individuals are likely to put things that they find into their pockets. A patient who has undergone a fluoroscopic procedure would have local radiation injury to the skin overlying the region imaged. For example, the radiation source is typically positioned posterior to a patient undergoing a cardiac catheterization and therefore a radiation burn would be on the back. Most industrial radiography sources deliver an extremely high dose on direct contact with the skin. In contrast, analytical x-ray crystallography machines, which emit x-rays of much lower energy than the photons of ^{192}Ir, are not likely to cause deep blood vessel injury.

Local radiation injuries can be readily differentiated from thermal burns. The effects of a thermal burn appear immediately. If a patient presenting with a burn-like injury does not know the cause or time of the injury, a local radiation injury should be suspected. Table 98.17 lists the dose-related findings expected after a local radiation exposure.

If erythema is seen within the first 48 hours, ulceration will probably occur. The erythema may come in waves that appear, disappear, and then reappear. With transepidermal injury, blister formation may occur at 1 to 2 weeks with doses in the range of 100 Gy and at 3 weeks after dose levels of 30 to 50 Gy. Treatment is required to prevent infection and to relieve pain. Skin grafting, especially musculocutaneous flaps, may be appropriate if the radiation exposure was localized and superficial. Progressive gangrene, due to the obliterative changes in the small vessels, will occur if the radiation exposure is large and involves deep structures. Under these circumstances, amputation may be necessary.

Contamination

Contamination represents the third major type of radiation injury. Contamination occurs when radioactive dirt or liquid remains on the patient (external contamination) or, when inhaled or ingested, inside the patient (internal contamination). Contamination is the only type of radiation injury that requires the medical staff to take any radiation-related precautions. There is little danger to the medical staff when caring for a contaminated person once they are in the hospital; however, medical personnel who respond to the accident site may be exposed to large, potentially life-threatening doses of radiation. For these rescue workers, 0.5 Gy is the voluntary limit suggested by the National Council on Radiation Protection and Measurements (NCRP) for lifesaving activities.

External contamination. External contamination rarely is a significant medical problem. To prevent additional radiation exposure to the patient, medical staff, and the public, external contamination should be removed and dispersal of radioactive materials should be prevented. The goal of treatment of any contaminated patient is to keep radiation exposures "as low as reasonably achievable." This is called the ALARA

TABLE 98.17

APPROXIMATE ABSORBED DOSE TO PRODUCE SKIN CHANGES

Absorbed dose (Gy)	Findings
3	Threshold for erythema (100 keV diagnostic x-rays)
6	Threshold for erythema (10 MeV therapeutic x-rays)
15	Moist desquamation
20	Skin ulceration with slow healing
>30	Gangrenous changes

principle and requires advance planning, specific supplies, and appropriate protective clothing. Preventing the dispersal of radioactive materials is accomplished by treating the patient in a single location, controlling access to that location, and by using standard contact precautions.

Internal contamination. Internal contamination can be a serious problem because it is difficult to eliminate some long-lived radioactive materials from within the body. Death due to radiation from internal contamination is rare. A few deaths have been caused by medical misadministrations. A familiar example of intentional, nonlethal internal contamination is the bone scan performed in a nuclear medicine department. Treatment of hyperthyroidism with ^{131}I also is, in a sense, planned internal contamination.

Metal fragment. Another source of contamination is the radioactive metallic fragment, which can be intensely radioactive. These could, in principle, be found if a "dirty bomb" were constructed with a radioactive metal source such as ^{192}Ir. Radioactive metal fragments can be embedded in the patient's skin and should never be touched with fingers. Tongs or forceps will increase the distance between the radioactive metal fragment and the fingers and thus greatly reduce any radiation dose to the healthcare worker.

Hot particles. "Hot" particles are microscopic particles that can be highly radioactive. Typically, they contain ^{60}Co or fission products and might be found on a nuclear reactor worker after a reactor accident. These particles can be difficult to localize and remove, and may give a large radiation dose to a small volume of tissues. If the particle is trapped under a nail or is in the fold of the skin, routine washings may not dislodge it. The particle can sometimes be localized by using a thick piece of lead. If the lead is placed between the particle and the radiation detector, the exposure rate should decrease substantially. Once the particle is localized, it can usually be removed by using simple mechanical means. Rarely, a punch biopsy of the skin may be necessary.

Terrorist events. Nuclear materials may be used intentionally in a terrorist event. An intact sealed source could be placed in a populated area, generating whole-body exposures but no contamination. A conventional explosive combined with radioactive materials, the so-called "dirty bomb," could be employed to disseminate radioactive materials over a local or wide area. Victims of such an attack would likely have radiation exposure as well as injuries from the explosion itself. An attack on a research or commercial power reactor could produce a large-scale dispersion of nuclear material; victims could be exposed to whole-body and localized radiation, as well as internal and external contamination. Transported nuclear materials such as radiopharmaceuticals or radioactive waste could be the subject of a terrorist attack. The effects would vary depending on whether the containers were breached—intact containers would produce only external exposures, whereas destruction of the containers and dispersal of their contents could also lead to contamination. A "dud" nuclear weapon that does not undergo a nuclear reaction would still disperse radioactive materials by the associated conventional explosion, leading to contamination in addition to effects from the conventional explosion itself. A nuclear weapon effectively detonated by a terrorist group might be relatively small scale but still capable of widespread damage, including thermal and blast effects from the denotation along with contamination and exposure of affected persons and equipment.

Triage Considerations

No survivable radiation injury requires immediate lifesaving treatment; hence medical staff should focus their attention on the treatment of non–radiation-related life-threatening conditions. In the past, some medical personnel were so distracted by the radiation aspects of an accident that routine medical care was delayed. Once stabilized, the radiation-related injuries can be addressed. Because there is no immediate treatment of radiation exposure, the problem of radioactive contamination should be addressed first. In most circumstances, a Geiger counter can be used to determine the presence of contamination. The probability of contamination can be assessed by obtaining an accurate description of the accident and the likely radiation source. If the patient is a radiation worker, finding his or her radiation badge and performing a "reenactment" of the accident may be critical for dose estimation.

Management and Diagnostic Studies

Internal Contamination

Treatment of internal contamination is most effective if initiated promptly. The requirement for prompt treatment is a dilemma for the physician as it is difficult to determine if internal contamination is present until the external contamination has been removed. Moistened cotton Q-tips can be used to perform nasal swabs. If these show radioactivity, inhalation of radioactive materials is possible. The nature of the accident may provide clues to the possibility of internal contamination (e.g., a fire with smoke leading to the inhalation of radioactive particles). The most effective treatment requires knowledge of the radionuclide involved and its chemical form. This information is usually not immediately available. Fortunately, there are simple general treatment measures that can be effectively instituted before the magnitude of the internal contamination is fully known.

If given soon after exposure, stable iodine is effective for preventing the uptake of radioactive iodine by the thyroid gland. Prompt administration of stable iodine should be considered if there is a possibility of external contamination, or ingestion or inhalation of radioactive iodine (Table 98.18). Because radioactive iodine is volatile, it is likely to be inhaled. If a contaminated child were brought to the ED after an accident with a radiopharmaceutical truck carrying radioactive iodine, administration of stable iodine would be appropriate. If further investigation revealed no radioactive iodine, little harm would have been done by having administered the stable iodine. A single dose of oral iodine is highly unlikely to cause any adverse reactions, even in persons who have serious reactions to iodinated contrast agents or seafood.

TABLE 98.18

DOSE OF STABLE IODINE (SSKI) BY AGE

Age	Dose (po) (mg)
<1 mo	16
1 mo–3 yrs	32
3–18 yrs	65
>18 yrs	130

After a nuclear reactor accident that results in the release of a large amount of radioactive iodine, three steps can be taken to minimize the adverse effects on the public. First, the public should be sheltered or evacuated to prevent further exposure via fallout or gaseous materials. Second, potassium iodide (KI) may be administered if available. However, it is important to note that many of the nuclear reactors in the United States do not house radioactive iodine, making KI useless. Third, the food supply can be monitored carefully to prevent further ingestion of radioactive iodine or other radionuclides. If a reactor accident occurs that involves contamination of the public, understandable concern by members of the public will ensue. If this happens, emergency medical facilities should try to preserve their valuable resources for patients who need lifesaving medical treatment. Plans must be made to refer uninjured persons and persons with minor injuries to other facilities. Hospitals should not become decontamination centers.

Several simple steps can be taken to treat internal contamination nonspecifically. The goals of treatment are to prevent the absorption of the radionuclide and to enhance its excretion. Safe techniques that prevent the absorption of radionuclides include the administration of activated charcoal and alginate-containing antacids. Enhanced excretion can be achieved by hydration and administration of a purgative. Specific treatment of internal contamination depends on the radionuclide, its chemical and physical forms, and the route of internal contamination. Recommendations for many specific treatments can be found in the NCRP Report 161, titled *Management of Persons Contaminated with Radionuclides*. This report should be available in every hospital ED and can be downloaded for free from the NCRP website (http://www.ncrponline.org) (Fig. 98.15). This report was updated

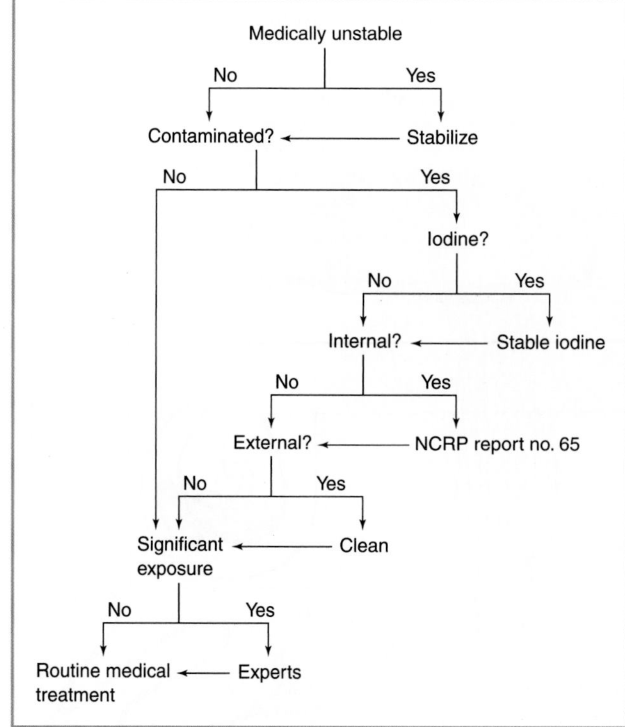

FIGURE 98.15 Treatment of radiation injuries. NCRP, National Council on Radiation Protection and Measurements.

in 2012. Initiation of treatments that entail some risk to the patient (e.g., pulmonary lavage, intravenous chelating agents) should be undertaken only after consultation with experts; the benefits of the treatment should be significantly greater than the risks. The most effective treatment of internal contamination is preventing the internal contamination in the first place.

External Contamination

External contamination is treated in the same way as contamination by other hazardous chemical or biologic agents. Personnel should wear gloves, a gown, shoe covers, and a mask, which keeps them clean and makes cleanup easier. The garments do not decrease the exposure to penetrating radiation. If available, film badges or other devices to measure radiation exposure should be worn by hospital staff in close contact with the patient.

If external contamination is widespread, it may be helpful to cover the floor. If only a small area of contamination is present, spread can be prevented by simply wrapping the contaminated area until it can be cleaned. Because it is much easier to detect radioactive contamination than chemical or biologic hazards, cleanup following a radiation accident will be much more effective.

External contamination is rarely a significant medical problem but decontamination requires preplanning. The patient should be admitted through a separate entrance of the ED. If this is not possible, the patient can be placed on a clean stretcher outside the ED and wrapped in a cloth (not plastic) sheet and then transported to the desired area of the hospital. Access to the treatment area should be controlled.

Removal of the patient's clothing will eliminate up to 90% of the external contamination (Table 98.19). Contaminated articles should be placed in labeled plastic bags. Residual contamination is likely to be on the hands, face, hair, and wounds. These should be washed with lukewarm water and soap. Cleaning the skin with damp washcloths is better than cleaning with running water. The radioactive dirt on the damp washcloth can be contained by placing the cloth in a plastic bag. Radioactive dirt in wash water is much more difficult to control but, when necessary in the course of patient care, may be discharged to the sewer system by flushing. Shaving should not be performed because this may make small cuts and increase absorption through the skin. Excessive rubbing of the skin may also increase transdermal uptake.

TABLE 98.19

DECONTAMINATION

Remove clothes	Cover clean wounds to prevent contamination
Wash with a damp cloth	Prevent external and tepid water contamination from becoming internal
Pay special attention to skin folds and fingernails	Do not abrade the skin

TABLE 98.20

APPROPRIATE LABORATORY TESTS FOR PATIENTS INVOLVED IN A SIGNIFICANT RADIATION ACCIDENT

In the emergency department
Complete blood cell count; repeat every 6 hrs for 24 hrs
Nasal swabs
Collect all excreta
Later
Cytogenetics
Sperm count
Eye examination (baseline for cataracts)
Human leukocyte antigen typing

Open uncontaminated wounds should be covered to prevent them from becoming contaminated. Contaminated wounds should be cleaned like any other dirty wound. All samples from the patient should be saved and labeled if there is any question about the identity of the radionuclides.

A Geiger counter should be used to monitor and document the progress of the decontamination efforts. If contamination persists, the source may be fixed to the skin or may be internal. Radiation experts should be consulted before performing more aggressive decontamination. Some residual contamination may be acceptable.

Exposure

Other than symptomatic measures, there is no immediate treatment to reverse whole-body or local radiation exposure. Medically significant whole-body radiation exposure is unlikely if the patient does not have nausea and vomiting. Serial CBCs are also helpful in excluding the diagnosis of a recent large whole-body exposure to radiation (Table 98.20). In the absence of other major trauma, the absolute lymphocyte count will rapidly fall in patients who have been exposed to a large radiation dose. If a patient has been exposed to a large dose of radiation, there is little in the way of specific medical treatment in the ED. The threat to the patient's life will occur within days to weeks after the exposure.

The diagnosis of a local radiation injury requires vigilance. The physician should consider the possibility of a local radiation injury whenever there is an unexplained painless "burn" blister, ulceration, or necrosis of the skin. A CBC to exclude an accompanying whole-body exposure is indicated. The prognosis of a local radiation injury depends on the dose. The dose can be estimated only by having a qualified physicist reconstruct the accident that led to the exposure.

BITES AND STINGS

Goals of Treatment

General care should include relief of pain and itching, tetanus prophylaxis, antibiotics if needed, and emotional support. Animals must be identified as venomous or not. The emergency physician must determine whether the bite or sting is symptomatic or not, and clinical observation may be the only means of determining this.

CLINICAL PEARLS AND PITFALLS

- Knowledge of common animals in your location of practice is essential in identification and/or treatment of potential victims.
- Shock can occur even with seemingly minor local injury because of the systemic effects of toxins.
- Consider tetanus prophylaxis in all victims of bites or stings.
- Wound closure may be delayed when there is a high risk of infection.

MARINE INVERTEBRATES

Phylum Coelenterata (Cnidaria)

The phylum is divided into three large classes: the Hydrozoa (hydras, Portuguese man-of-war), Scyphozoa (true jellyfish), and Anthozoa (soft corals, stone corals, anemones). They have tentacles with specialized organelles called nematocysts, which are used for entangling, penetrating, anchoring, and poisoning prey (Fig. 98.16). When the tentacles touch an object, the nematocysts fire, releasing toxin-coated, barbed threads. The severity of envenomation is related to venom toxicity, number of nematocysts discharged, and general condition of the victim. Stings from sessile forms are generally not as severe as stings from free-floating forms. Jellyfish venoms affect autonomic nervous systems via several mechanisms. Paralysis and CNS effects appear to be related primarily to toxic proteins and peptides. Burning pain and urticaria are secondary to the release of various mediators of inflammation, including serotonin, histamine, or histamine-releasing agents in the venom.

Class Hydrozoa

Feathered hydroid (*Pennaria tiarella*) is found from Maine to Florida and along the Texas coast just below the low-tide line.

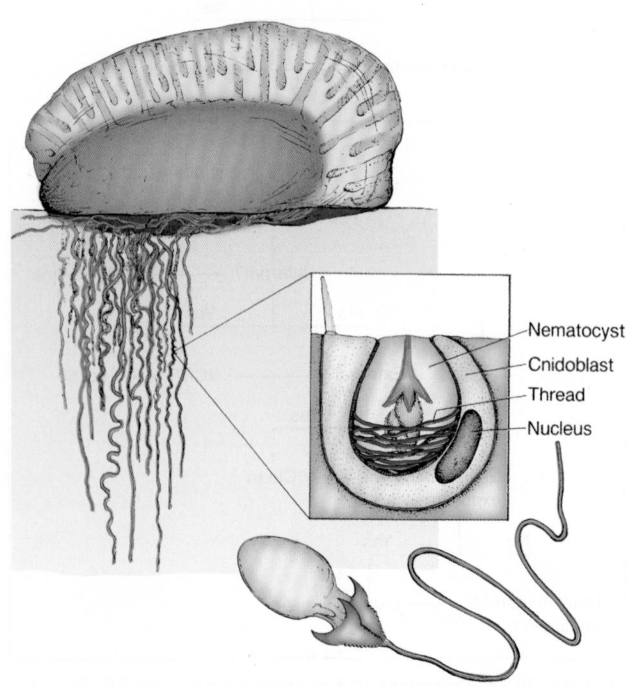

FIGURE 98.16 Marine invertebrate causing human sting.

They attach to solid objects, including pilings and floats. They cause a mild sting that may be treated with local care.

Portuguese man-of-war (*Physalia physalis*) is a hydrozoan colony, although it is commonly erroneously considered a jellyfish. The float can be up to 30 cm in length, with tentacles hanging from the float that may reach more than 75 ft long and contain about 750,000 nematocysts each. This pelagic animal is often driven ashore by storms along the Atlantic coast.

Tentacles on the skin should be fairly easy to recognize as the cause of symptoms. Releasing one of the most powerful marine toxins, the nematocysts of the Portuguese man-of-war may discharge even when it is dead and washed up on the beach. Because of the length and transparency of the tentacles in the water, swimmers are often stung without seeing the animal.

The toxin contains polypeptides and degradative enzymes. Local effects include pain and irritation. Systemic reactions include headache, myalgias, fever, abdominal rigidity, arthralgias, nausea and vomiting, pallor, respiratory distress, hemolysis, renal failure, and coma. Death may occur if the area stung is extensive in relation to the size of the victim.

The unexploded nematocysts are inactivated with topical application for 30 minutes with vinegar (3% acetic acid), a slurry of baking soda, or meat tenderizer (papain). Papain should not be left on for more than 15 minutes. Vinegar is generally the best disarming agent; however, for Portuguese man-of-war, vinegar has been shown to be ineffective and may activate the nematocysts. The area should be washed with seawater or normal saline. The affected limbs should be immobilized. There is no antivenin available for *Physalia* or the scyphozoans, with the exception of the sea wasp, *Chironex fleckeri,* of Australia. Shock may require cardiorespiratory support. General supportive measures for systemic reactions include oral antihistamines, oral corticosteroids, and opiates for pain. Muscle spasms have been treated with 10% solution of calcium gluconate 0.1 mL per kg (10 mg per kg) given intravenously, although the efficacy is controversial. Local dermatitis should be treated with a topical corticosteroid cream.

Class Scyphozoa

The common purple jellyfish (*Pelagia noctiluca*) is only mildly toxic. Local skin irritation is the major clinical manifestation. Sea nettle (*Chrysaora quinquecirrha*) is a common jellyfish found along the Atlantic coast. Clinical manifestations are the same as those for purple jellyfish. Lion's mane (*Cyanea capillata*) is a highly toxic creature that can reach a width of 244 cm, with tentacles as long as 61 cm. The animal is found along both coasts. Contact with the tentacles produces severe burning. Prolonged exposure causes muscle cramps and respiratory failure. Treatment of scyphozoan stings is the same as above for hydrozoan stings.

Class Anthozoa

The anemones found within United States tidal zones are only mildly toxic. Coral cuts and stings can be a problem for swimmers off the Florida coast. The stinging ability of stony corals is minor; coral cuts can be severe due to a combination of lacerations, nematocyst venom, foreign debris in the wound, and secondary bacterial infection. The clinical picture is one of stinging sensation followed by wheal formation and itching. If the wound is untreated, an ulcer with an erythematous base may form within a few days. Cellulitis, lymphangitis, fever, and malaise commonly occur.

Treatment consists of cleaning the wound and irrigation with copious amounts of saline, removal of foreign particles, and debridement. Marine bacteria that can inoculate wounds are generally heterotrophic, motile, and facultatively anaerobic, gram-negative rods. Organisms include *Vibrio* species, *Erysipelothrix rhusiopathiae,* and *Mycobacterium marinum.* Wounds should be left open. Broad-spectrum antibiotic therapy, particularly tetracycline, at a dosage of 40 mg/kg/day in four divided doses, has been advocated but should not be used routinely in children younger than 8 years. For children younger than 8 years, cephalexin (50 mg/kg/day in four divided doses) or trimethoprim-sulfamethoxazole (10 mg TMP/kg/day divided in two doses) should be used.

Phylum Echinodermata

Phylum Echinodermata includes starfish, sea urchins, and sea cucumbers. Of the three classes, only the *Echinoidea,* the sea urchins, have clinical relevance for US children. The long-spined urchins (e.g., Diadema) are dangerous to handle. They do not appear to possess venom like tropical urchins, but the spines, composed of calcium carbonate, easily pierce the skin, wet suits, and sneakers and can lodge deep in the flesh. Most injuries occur during wading in shallow water.

Penetration of skin by spines is accompanied by intense pain followed by redness, swelling, and aching. Complications include tattooing of the skin, joint arthritis, secondary infection, and granuloma formation.

Management. All spines should be removed as completely as possible using local anesthetic if needed. Any spines not reachable will be absorbed in time. Soaking in warm water may be helpful for pain. Systemic antistaphylococcal antibiotics should be used if infection develops.

MARINE VERTEBRATES

Stingrays

Current evidence. Stingrays are the most important group of venomous fishes, accounting for an estimated 1,000 attacks per year in North America. Stingrays are bottom feeders that bury themselves in sand or mud of bays, shoal lagoons, and river mouths. They are found along the Atlantic, Pacific, and Gulf coasts and range from several inches in diameter to more than 14 ft in length. Six different species are represented in North American waters. Envenomations usually occur when an unsuspecting swimmer steps on the back of the animal and causes it to hurl its barbed tail upward into the victim as a reflex defense response. Most injuries are confined to the lower extremities, although wounds to the chest and abdomen have been reported.

The venom apparatus consists of a serrated, retropointed, dentinal caudal spine located on the dorsum of the tail. Spines vary in length, depending on the size of the ray, but may reach a length of 122 cm in some species. The spine is encased in an integumentary sheath that contains specialized secretory cells that hold the venom. When the stingray's barb strikes the victim, it easily penetrates the skin, rupturing the integumentary sheath over the spine and causing the venom to pass along the ventrolateral grooves of the barb, into the wound. The barb is retropointed, so the wound it produces is a combination of puncture and laceration. Wounds may vary in length from 3.5 to 15 cm. Life-threatening puncture wounds may occur that require immediate resuscitation. The venom is a heat-labile toxin that depresses medullary respiratory centers, interferes with the cardiac conduction system, and produces severe local pain.

The sting is followed immediately by pain, which spreads from the site of injury during the next 30 minutes and peaks within 90 minutes. Syncope, weakness, nausea, and anxiety are common complaints due to effects of the venom and the vagal response to the pain. Vomiting, diarrhea, sweating, and muscle fasciculations of the affected extremity may also occur. Generalized cramps, paresthesias, hypotension, arrhythmias, and death may occur. The wound often has a jagged edge that bleeds profusely, and the wound edges may be discolored. Discoloration may extend several centimeters from the wound within hours after injury and may subsequently necrose if untreated. Often, parts of the stingray's integumentary sheath contaminate the wound.

Treatment is aimed at treating shock, direct pressure to control bleeding, preventing complications of the venom, alleviating pain, and preventing secondary infection. At the scene, the wound should be irrigated with cold saltwater as this can remove much of the venom. Remnants of the integumentary sheath should be removed if it can be seen in the wound. The extremity should be placed in hot water (40° to 45°C [104° to 113°F]) for 30 to 90 minutes. After soaking, the wound should be reexplored, debrided again if necessary, and closed. Pain relief is best achieved with morphine. Tetanus prophylaxis should be considered, but antibiotics are reserved for wounds that become secondarily infected.

Sharks

Shark attacks may be preceded by one or more "bumps," which may cause extensive abrasions from the rough denticles of the shark's skin. Two types of bite wounds are described: tangential injury and a definitive bite. Tangential injury, caused by the slashing movement of the open mouth as the shark makes a close pass, causes severe lacerations, incised wounds, and loss of tissue. Definitive bite wounds cause lacerations, loss of soft tissue, amputations, and comminuted fractures. Most injuries involve only one or two bites and are confined to the extremities.

Hypovolemic shock is the immediate threat to life in shark attacks. Bleeding should be controlled at the scene with direct compression, and intravascular volume should be replaced with crystalloid until blood products are available. The victim should be kept warm and given oxygen when being transported to an ED. Wounds should not be explored in the field. Tetanus toxoid and tetanus immune globulin therapies should be considered, and prophylactic antibiotics with a third-generation cephalosporin or trimethoprim-sulfamethoxazole is suggested.

Scorpaenidae

The 80 species found in the Scorpaenidae family include the zebra fish, scorpion fish proper, and stonefish. In California, the sculpin is commonly involved. Scorpaenidae are generally found in shallow water, around reefs, kelp beds, or coral. They are nonmigratory, slow swimming, and often buried in sand. The venom apparatus consists of a number of dorsal, anal, and pelvic spines covered by integumentary sheaths containing venom glands that lie within anterolateral grooves. The venoms are unstable, heat-labile compounds. Most often envenomation occurs when the fish are handled during fishing excursions.

Severe pain at the site of the wound is the first and primary clinical sign for all species. The wound and surrounding area becomes ischemic and then cyanotic. Paresthesia and paralysis of the extremity may occur. Other clinical signs include nausea, vomiting, hypotension, tachypnea proceeding to apnea, and myocardial ischemia with electrocardiographic changes.

Treatment involves irrigating the wound with sterile saline. The injured extremity is then immersed in very hot water (40° to 45°C [104° to 113°F]) for 30 to 60 minutes or until the agonizing pain is completely relieved. Pain relief is best achieved with morphine 0.1 mg per kg IV, IM, or SC. The patient should be monitored carefully for cardiotoxic effects and respiratory depression. Antivenin is available only for the stings of the stonefish of Australia.

Catfish

The catfish is a popular food and sport fish found in many lakes and rivers throughout the United States. The venom apparatus consists of a number of spines located in the dorsal and pectoral fins. The integumentary sheaths covering the spines contain venom glands. The venoms are unstable, heat-labile compounds.

Injuries can be a combination of puncture wounds and lacerations, foreign-body reactions, and the effects of venom. The spines may become imbedded in flesh, causing soft tissue swelling, infection, or foreign-body reaction. The venom produces a local inflammatory response with local intense pain, edema, hemorrhage, and tissue necrosis.

Treatment involves irrigating the wound with sterile saline. The injured extremity is then immersed in hot water (40° to 45°C [104° to 113°F]) for 30 to 60 minutes or until pain is relieved. Pain relief is best achieved with morphine. The wound should be explored, spines removed and debrided if needed. Systemic antibiotics to cover gram-negative organisms are recommended. Wounds may be closed by using a delayed primary closure.

TERRESTRIAL INVERTEBRATES

Phylum Arthropoda

The arthropods make up the largest phylum in the animal kingdom. All arthropods have an exoskeleton with jointed appendages. The phylum is divided into two subphyla: the Chelicerata, which includes scorpions, spiders, ticks, and mites, and the Mandibulata, which includes insects.

Scorpions

There are 650 known scorpion species (class Arachnida), but only a limited number are dangerous to humans. In the Southwest United States, *Centruroides sculpturatus* is the potentially lethal inhabitant. Although *C. sculpturatus* and *Centruroides exilicauda* have been considered separate species in the past, more recent taxonomic classification treats the two as one species. It has two pinching claws anteriorly and a tail or pseudoabdomen that ends in a telson (Fig. 98.17), that houses a pair of poison glands and a stinger. The animals are

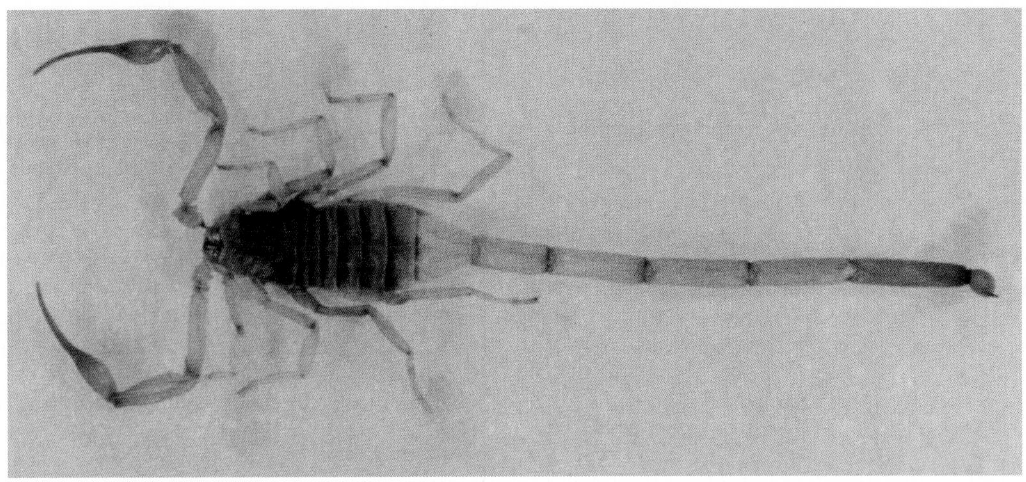

FIGURE 98.17 *Centruroides exilicauda* (sculpturatus). (Courtesy of F. E. Russell.)

nocturnal; during the day, they seek shelter under stones and debris. They often crawl into sleeping bags and unoccupied clothing. In one report, 80% of stings occurred in children younger than 10 years.

The scorpion produces a neurotoxin and a local cytotoxin. The general neurotoxicity is excitatory, affecting the autonomic and skeletal neuromuscular system. Common symptoms include local pain, restlessness, hyperactivity, roving eye movements, and respiratory distress. Other associated signs may include convulsions, drooling, wheezing, hyperthermia, cyanosis, GI hemorrhage, and respiratory failure. Death may result from respiratory paralysis, pulmonary edema, or shock. The diagnosis may be difficult because history of a sting may not be forthcoming. There is no laboratory test for confirmation of envenomation.

Treatment begins with general supportive care. Cryotherapy of the site of sting has been advocated to reduce swelling and local induration. An antivenin had been developed and used in Arizona; however, the production ended in 2001. Since the last vials expired, an increase in ICU admissions has been reported. Calcium gluconate (0.1 mL per kg [10 mg per kg] of the 10% solution) has been given intravenously to reduce muscular contractions and associated pain, but benefit has not been proved. Sedative anticonvulsants, in particular, phenobarbital (5 to 10 mg per kg) or benzodiazepines (midazolam 0.05 to 0.1 mg per kg) intravenously are used to treat persistent hyperactivity, convulsions, and/or agitation. A continuous infusion of midazolam may optimize treatment in extreme cases (start at 0.1 mg/kg/hr and titrate to relief of symptoms). Corticosteroids and antihistamines have little, if any, proven benefit.

Spiders

Current evidence. There are more than 100,000 species of spiders (class Arachnida). Most spiders are shy creatures, will not bite unless provoked, have mild venom and fangs that are too short and fragile to penetrate human skin. Only two species in the United States are dangerous: the brown recluse and the black widow spiders.

Loxoscelism (Bite of the Brown Recluse Spider). **Current evidence.** Three species of Loxosceles have caused envenomation, primarily in the southern and midwestern states, but can be found throughout the continental United States. They are small (1 to 1.5 cm in length) with a brown violin-shaped mark on the dorsum of the cephalothorax. They are found outdoors but will establish nests indoors, especially in closets. As its name implies, the most common species, *Loxosceles reclusa,* is shy and will only attack when provoked. The venom is cytotoxic and also contains a factor similar to hyaluronidase.

Clinical recognition. The bite is usually innocuous and may initially go unnoticed. The spectrum of reaction ranges from minor local reaction to severe necrotic arachnidism (Fig. 98.18). The local reaction consists of mild to moderate pain 2 to 8 hours after the bite, with erythema and a central blister or pustule. Within 24 hours, there is subcutaneous discoloration that spreads over 3 to 4 days, reaching a size of 10 to 15 cm. At this time, the pustule drains, producing an ulcerated "crater." Scar formation is rare if there is no evidence of necrosis within 72 hours of the bite. Systemic reaction is most common in small children, and occurs within 24 to 48 hours. Symptoms include fever, chills, malaise, weakness, nausea, vomiting, joint pain, morbilliform eruption with petechiae, intravascular hemolysis, hematuria, and renal failure.

Management. Treatment varies with the clinical stage of the bite. There is no specific serologic, biochemical, or histologic test to diagnose envenomation accurately. Many of

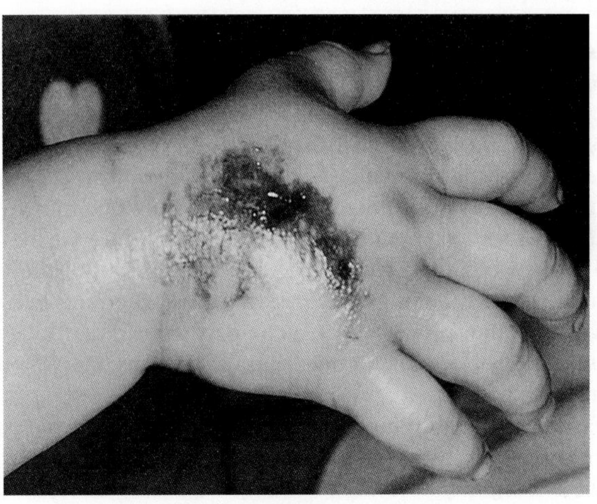

FIGURE 98.18 Spider bite necrotizing.

TABLE 98.21

SPIDERS KNOWN TO CAUSE NECROTIC LESIONS

Genus name	Common name	Geographic distribution
Argiope	Golden orb weaver	Throughout North America (individual species more restrictive)
Cheiracanthium	Running spider	Throughout United States
Loxosceles	Brown recluse	Kansas and Missouri to Texas West to California
Lycosa	Wolf spider	Throughout United States
Phidippus	Black jumping spider	Atlantic Coast to Rocky Mountains

the presumed bites outside the endemic range are caused by other spiders (Table 98.21) or other conditions. Pediatric conditions that have been misdiagnosed as brown recluse bites include infections with staphylococci or streptococci, herpes simplex, herpes zoster, erythema multiforme, Lyme disease, fungal infection, pyoderma gangrenosum, chemical burn, poison ivy/oak, and localized vasculitis. Unless the spider is brought for identification, definitive diagnosis cannot be made. Table 98.21 lists the spiders found in the United States, known to cause necrotic lesions. An algorithm for management of suspected bites is shown in Figure 98.19. Serious complications are rare in adults. Most victims will heal with supportive care. Occasionally surgical excision and skin grafting are required.

Studies have found no significant alteration of necrosis from the venom by steroids, heparin, dapsone, or HBO. Current recommendations are to limit the use of dapsone to adults with proven brown recluse bites. Dapsone should not be used in children due to the risk of methemoglobinemia. Antivenom is not yet commercially available. For systemic manifestations, vigorous supportive care is needed. Most deaths are caused by hemolysis and respiratory failure. A CBC and platelet count for evidence of hemolysis are needed, as well as monitoring of hemoglobin, urine sediment, BUN, and creatinine levels for evidence of hemolysis and renal failure.

Latrodectism (Bite of the Black Widow Spider). **Current evidence.** The bite of *Latrodectus mactans* is the leading cause of death from spider bites in the United States. The spider is shiny black, with a brilliant red hourglass marking on the abdomen of mature females. It may be present on the male, but the male is not a threat because it is only one-fourth the size of the female, and its fangs are unable to penetrate human skin. The webs are usually found in corners or out-of-the-way places. The female is not aggressive unless guarding her egg sac or provoked. The venom, a complex protein that includes a neurotoxin, stimulates myoneural junctions, nerves, and nerve endings.

Clinical recognition. Bites are seldom mistaken if the child is old enough to describe the spider. There is generalized pain and rigidity of muscles 1 to 8 hours after the bite. No local symptoms are associated with the bite itself. The pain is

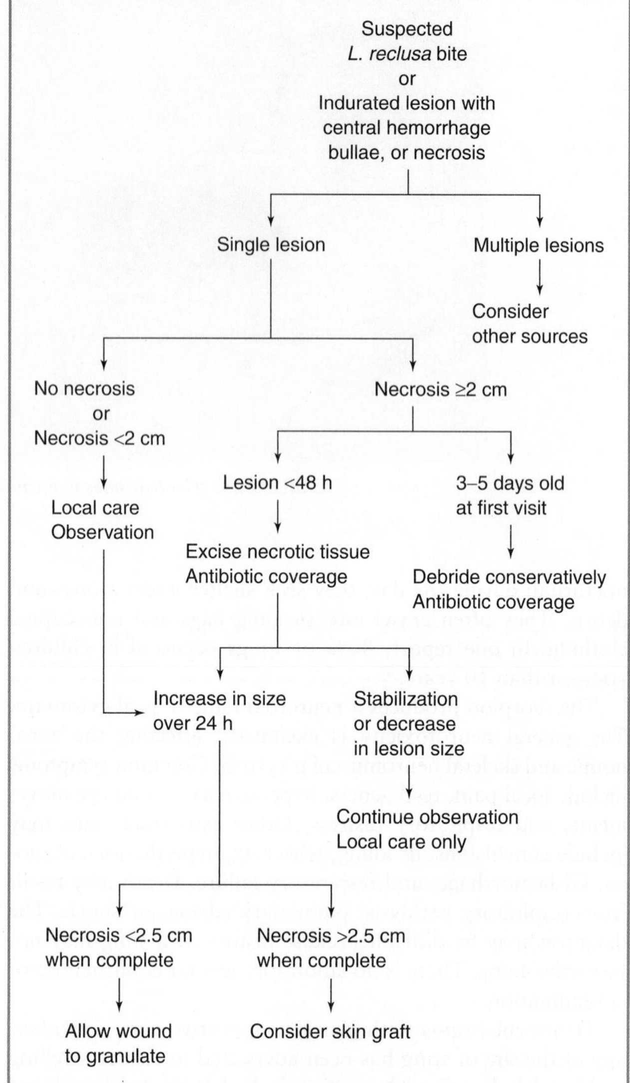

FIGURE 98.19 Management of suspected brown recluse spider bite.

cramping and felt in the abdomen, flanks, thighs, and chest. Nausea and vomiting are often reported in children. Respiratory distress, chills, urinary retention, and priapism can occur. There is a 4% to 5% mortality rate, with death resulting from cardiovascular collapse. The mortality rate in young children may be as high as 50%.

Management. A child who has severe pain and muscle rigidity after a spider bite should be considered a Latrodectus bite victim. A clinical grading scale has been developed by Clark (Table 98.22). Treatment with Latrodectus antivenin (Lyovac, Merck, Sharp & Dohme) should be instituted as soon as a bite is confirmed in children who weigh less than 40 kg; the usual dose is 2.5 mL (one vial). Antivenin should be administered by following the package insert and after skin testing to determine the risk of hypersensitivity to horse serum. For children who weigh more than 40 kg, it is not as urgent to institute antivenin treatment, but indications for its use include patients who are younger than 16 years, who have respiratory difficulty, or who have significant hypertension (grades II and III). Antivenin is usually effective within 30 minutes and may be repeated once within 2 hours if symptoms return. Serum sickness is a possible side effect. Because

TABLE 98.22

GRADING SCALE FOR *LATRODECTUS* ENVENOMATION

Grade	Symptoms
1	Asymptomatic Local pain at bite site Normal vital signs
2	Muscular pain—localized Diaphoresis—localized Normal vital signs
3	Muscular pain—generalized Abnormal vital signs Nausea, vomiting Headaches Diaphoresis

the dosage is low, however, serum sickness is uncommon, with a rate lower than those reported for other types of antivenom. Calcium gluconate 10% solution was given in the past to control leg and abdominal cramps. Recent series found calcium gluconate effective in only 4% of cases. Methocarbamol (Robaxin) appears to be even less efficacious than calcium gluconate. Muscle relaxants such as diazepam have also been advocated, but they are variably effective and the effects are short lived. Analgesia may be achieved with opiates.

Tarantulas and Others. Tarantulas do not bite unless provoked. The venom is mild, and envenomation is not a problem. The wolf spider (*Lycosa* species) and the jumping spider (*Phidippus* species) have also been implicated in bites. They also have mild venom that causes only local reactions. Bites from all three of these spiders should be treated with local wound care.

Tick Paralysis

Current evidence. Ticks are responsible for transmitting a variety of infectious agents, including spirochetes, viruses, rickettsiae, bacteria, and protozoa. Examples of tick-borne illness, which are discussed in Chapter 102 Infectious Disease Emergencies, include Rocky Mountain spotted fever, Lyme disease, tularemia, ehrlichiosis, babesiosis, relapsing fever, and Colorado tick fever. Tick paralysis is associated with the bite of the wood tick, *Dermacentor andersoni;* the dog tick, *Dermacantor variabilis;* and the deer tick, *Ixodes scapularis.* The gravid engorged tick releases a neurotoxin that can produce cerebellar dysfunction or an ascending weakness. The mechanism of action of the toxin is not well understood.

Clinical assessment. Following tick attachment, there is a latent period of 4 to 7 days, followed by symptoms of restlessness, irritability, and ascending flaccid paralysis. Respiratory paralysis and death may follow if the tick is not detected. Laboratory data, including cerebrospinal fluid, are usually normal, but lymphocytic pleocytosis has been reported.

Management. Management is based on general supportive care and a diligent search for the tick. Ticks should be removed using blunt forceps or tweezers. The tick should be grasped as close to the skin surface as possible and pulled upward with a steady even pressure. A twisting or jerking motion may cause the mouthparts to break off. Do not squeeze or crush the body of the tick because this may introduce infective agents. After the tick is removed, the bite site should be cleaned. Once the tick is removed, the paralysis is reversible without apparent sequelae.

Centipedes and Millipedes

Centipedes (class Myriapoda order Chilopoda) are venomous, biting with jaws that act like stinging pincers. Bites can be extremely painful; however, the toxin is relatively innocuous, causing only local reaction. Treatment consists of injection of local anesthetic at the wound site and local wound care.

American millipedes (order Diplopoda) are generally harmless.

Insects

The insects (class Insecta) constitute the largest number of animal species. Hymenoptera is the most important order of the class and includes bees, wasps, hornets, yellow jackets, and ants (Fig. 98.20). Hymenoptera are responsible for 50% of human deaths from venomous bites and stings. A variety of toxic reactions are seen but the most common is allergic. Ants are discussed separately due to differences in venom composition and rate of systemic reactions.

Bee, Hornet, Yellow Jacket, Wasp. **Clinical recognition.** Clinically, the stings of bees and wasps differ because the barbed stinger of the bee remains in the victim's skin, whereas the wasp may sting multiple times. The venoms of the bee, hornet, yellow jacket, and wasp contain protein antigens that can elicit an immunoglobulin E antibody response. Venoms contain various biogenic amines, phospholipase, phosphatase, and hyaluronidase. Because of the similarity of the venoms, cross-reactivity can occur. Local reaction to a sting results in pain, erythema, and swelling.

Triage: Systemic allergic reactions may be grouped by severity.

- Group I consists of urticaria, generalized erythema, malaise.
- Group II includes angioedema or two or more of the following: chest or throat tightness, nausea, vomiting, and dizziness.
- Group III consists of dyspnea, wheezing, or stridor and two or more of the following: dysphagia, dysarthria, hoarseness, weakness, confusion, feeling of impending disaster.
- Group IV consists of life-threatening systemic reactions, including hypotension, and shock. Anaphylactic reactions secondary to insect stings occur in 0.5% to 5% of the population.
  - The barbed honeybee stinger with venom sac is avulsed and often remains in the victim's skin; it must be removed if seen. Delays in removal are likely to increase the dose of venom received. The method of removal of the stinger is irrelevant (scraping vs. pulling vs. squeezing).

Management. Treatment of stings is based on the severity of the allergic reaction. Local reactions can be treated with cold compresses at the site of sting.

- Group I reactions are treated with a second-generation antihistamine (loratidine, cetirizine).
- Group II and Group III reactions are treated with epinephrine 1:1,000 solution 0.01 mL per kg (maximum 0.3 mL) IM followed by antihistamines orally. Oral steroids (prednisone/prednisolone 2 mg/kg/day) are recommended. These children should be observed in the hospital for 24 hours.

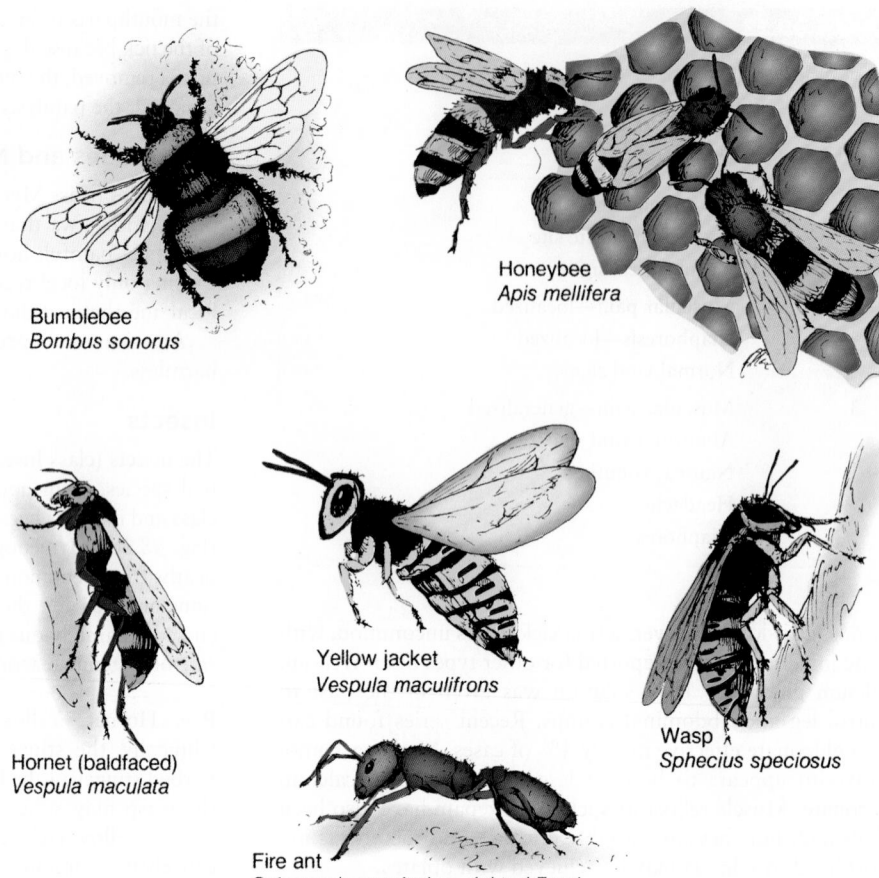

FIGURE 98.20 Hymenoptera capable of causing allergic reactions.

- Group IV reactions may require intubation if upper airway obstruction is present. Hypotension should be treated with a fluid bolus of saline or lactated Ringer solution 10 to 20 mL per kg given over 20 to 30 minutes. IV epinephrine (1:10,000) should be considered if hypotension fails to respond to IM epinephrine and fluid bolus. Hydrocortisone (2 mg per kg) may be given intravenously for 4 days. All children in this group should be admitted to an ICU.

Children who have had a group II, III, or IV reaction should be followed by an allergist for hyposensitization. Parents of these children should keep an insect sting emergency kit. The EpiPen and EpiPen Jr are spring-loaded autoinjectors triggered by placing pressure on the thigh with the instrument. The pens inject 0.3 or 0.15 mg (EpiPen and EpiPen Jr, respectively) of epinephrine. The pens are used as first aid in the field by the parent or guardian and are not meant to substitute for prompt definitive treatment at a medical facility. Parents should receive information regarding the use of epinephrine autoinjectors and avoidance of situations and behaviors that would attract stinging insects.

Fire Ants. **Current evidence.** Fire ants (*Solenopsis richteri* and *Solenopsis invicta*) cause bites and envenomations in the South and increasing in the North. The venom is an alkaloid with a direct toxic effect on mast cell membranes. There is no cross-reactivity with other members of the Hymenoptera species.

Clinical recognition. The fire ant bites with well-developed jaws and then uses its head as a pivot to inflict multiple stings. There is immediate wheal and flare at the site. The local reaction varies from 1 to 2 mm, up to 10 cm, depending on the amount of venom injected. Within 4 hours, a superficial vesicle appears. After 8 to 10 hours, the fluid in the vesicle changes from clear to cloudy (pustule), and the vesicle becomes umbilicated. After 24 hours, the lesion is surrounded by a painful erythematous area that persists for 3 to 10 days. Edema, induration, and pruritus at the site occur in up to 50% of patients. Occasionally, systemic reactions occur as with other Hymenoptera.

Management. Treatment is symptomatic. Local care includes ice and frequent cleansing to prevent secondary infection. Topical steroids, antibacterial medications, and antihistamines do not appear to be efficacious in prevention of pustule formation. Antihistamines are useful for pruritus. Systemic reactions are rare and should be treated similarly to other Hymenoptera reactions.

TERRESTRIAL VERTEBRATES

Venomous Reptiles

Goals of Emergency Care

Venomous substances are secreted by 15% of the United States' 120 snake species. An estimated 8,000 people are bitten annually by poisonous snakes in the United States. Emergency care is directed at providing timely antivenin therapy and expedient supportive medical care, and has dramatically reduced mortality and morbidity from poisonous snakebites. Only 10 to 15 deaths are reported per year, but the morbidity in limb dysfunction and other complications, although unknown, is undoubtedly much

TABLE 98.23

POISONOUS SNAKES INDIGENOUS TO THE UNITED STATES

Family	Genus	Species	Common name
Crotalidae			Pit vipers
	Crotalus		Rattlesnakes
		C. adamanteus	Eastern diamondback
		C. atrox	Western diamondback
		C. horridus	Timber rattlesnake
		C. viridis	Western rattlesnake
		C. v. viridis	Prairie rattlesnake
		C. v. helleri	Southern Pacific rattlesnake
		C. v. oreganus	Northern Pacific rattlesnake
		C. v. abyssus	Grand Canyon rattlesnake
		C. v. lutosus	Great Basin rattlesnake
		C. cerastes	Sidewinder
		C. ruber	Red diamond rattlesnake
		C. mitchellii	Speckled rattlesnake
		C. lepidus	Rock rattlesnake
		C. tiaris	Tiger rattlesnake
		C. willardi	Ridge-nosed rattlesnake
		C. scutulatus	Mojave rattlesnake
		C. molossus	Black-tailed rattlesnake
		C. pricei	Twin-spotted rattlesnake
	Sistrurus		
		S. catenatus	Massasauga rattlesnake
		S. miliarius	Pygmy rattlesnake
	Agkistrodon		
		A. piscivorus	Water moccasin
		A. contortrix	Copperhead
Elapidae		*Micruroides euryxanthus*	Sonovan (Arizona) coral snake
		Micrurus fulvius	Eastern coral snake

higher. With appropriate therapy, most long-term morbidity can be prevented.

CLINICAL PEARLS AND PITFALLS

- Identification of the snake may not be possible, but snakebite victims should be treated based on clinical symptoms.
- Extraction of venom is not usually helpful.

Current Evidence

The pediatric population, especially males, ages 5 to 19 years, accounts for a disproportionately large number of snakebite victims. The highest incidence occurs in the Southeast and Southwest, between April and October, although venomous snakebites occur at least sporadically in most states. Approximately 25% of bites are in patients younger than 17 years.

The poisonous snakes indigenous to the United States are members of the Crotalidae (pit viper) or Elapidae families (Table 98.23). The rattlesnake, water moccasin, and copperhead are pit vipers and are responsible for 99% of venomous snakebites. The coral snake is the only member of the Elapidae family in this country and, along with imported exotic snakes, accounts for the remaining 1% of serious snakebites.

Pit Vipers

The pit vipers have several characteristic features that distinguish them from nonvenomous snakes (Fig. 98.21): (i) Two pits with heat-sensitive organs that assist these poor-visioned reptiles to localize their prey are located on each side of the head, between the eye and nostril; (ii) the pupils are elliptical and vertically oriented; (iii) two curved fangs or hollow maxillary teeth are folded posteriorly against the palate and advance forward when the pit viper strikes; (iv) the head is relatively more triangular; and (v) the scutes, or scales, on the ventral portion caudad to the anal plate continue in a single row, whereas nonpoisonous snakes have a cleft, or double row.

The rattlesnake (*Crotalus*) is distributed widely throughout most of the United States and is the culprit in approximately 60% of all pit viper attacks. Several species are notably more menacing and toxic to humans. The large and gold diamondbacks (*Crotalus adamanteus* and *Crotalus atrox*) often stand their ground when approached by humans and inflict most lethal snakebites in North America. The pygmy rattler and massasauga are considered rattlesnakes because, in common

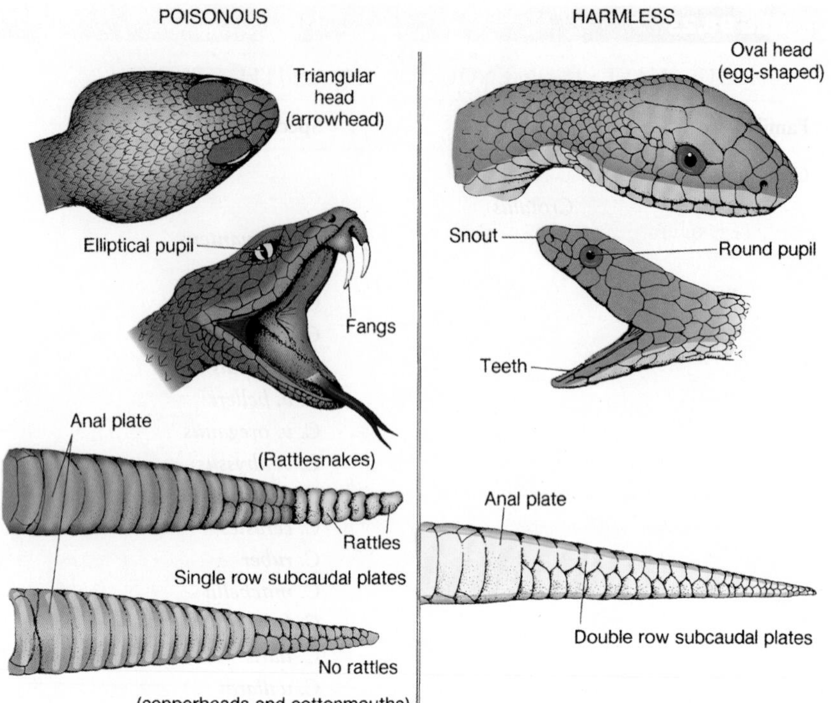

FIGURE 98.21 Comparison of poisonous and nonpoisonous snakes.

with *Crotalus* species, they possess a "rattler" on their tail. However, these two relatively small snakes are members of the genus *Sistrurus*, and their bites are not as toxic as those of true rattlesnakes.

The copperhead (*Agkistrodon contortrix*) is a common poisonous snake that lives in the Southeast and much of the Northeast, extending westward as far as Texas and Nebraska. This snake accounts for approximately 30% of venomous snakebites but, luckily, is seldom a serious threat to life or limb. Emergency physicians must become familiar with the particular species in their areas.

Coral Snakes

The relatively passive coral snake is responsible for only 10 to 15 snakebite cases per year in the United States. It is a member of the Elapidae family, and unlike pit vipers, it has round pupils, a blunt head, ventral caudal scutes, and lacks pits. Unlike the nonpoisonous snakes, the coral snake has two small maxillary fangs.

The snout of the coral snake is always black and is followed by a yellow ring and subsequent black band. Red and black bands then alternate down the approximately 2-ft length of the coral snake, with narrow yellow rings bordering the red band (Fig. 98.22). The nonvenomous king snake is often confused with the coral; it has red bands directly bordered by black bands. The yellow rings in this snake are within the black bands. The adage about coral snakes holds true.

Red on yellow, kill a fellow.
Red on black, venom lack.

There are two species of coral snakes: the eastern (*Micrurus fulvius*) and the Arizonan (*Micruroides euryxanthus*). *M. fulvius* is responsible for most human envenomations and is found in most states east of the Mississippi, with the exception of the Northeast. *M. euryxanthus* is indigenous only to Arizona and New Mexico.

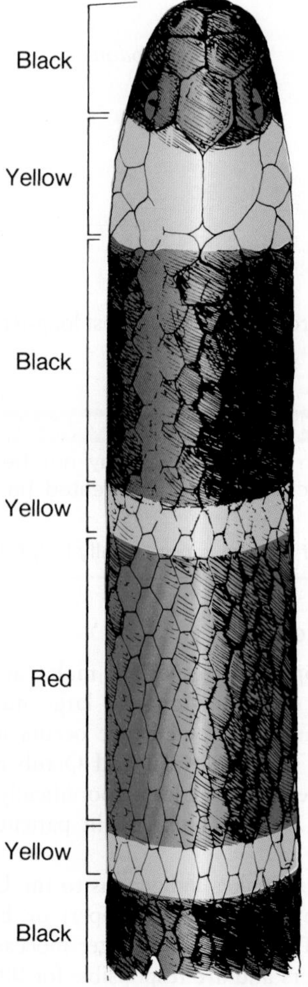

FIGURE 98.22 Coral snake.

Clinical Considerations

Snakebite envenomation is a complex poisoning because of the combination of the effects of venoms and the human and snake variables that influence venom toxicity. Venoms are mixtures of potent enzymes, primarily proteinases, and low-molecular-weight peptides that possess extensive pathophysiologic properties. A crotalid venom often has a combination of necrotizing, hemotoxic, neurotoxic, nephrotoxic, and/or cardiotoxic substances. Many venoms induce increased endothelial permeability and venous pooling, creating intravascular depletion. A transient hemoconcentration may be present during this plasma "leak." Hemotoxic effects induce hemolysis, fibrinogen proteolysis, and thrombocytopenia, which, along with activation of plasminogen, can lead to a bleeding diathesis in severe envenomation. Respiratory failure may occur because of pulmonary edema or a shock state.

Human factors that influence toxicity to snakebites include the victim's size and general health and wound characteristics. A small child is more susceptible to a given volume of venom than a larger person and unfortunately, young children are commonly bitten more than once. Fang penetration of a vessel or subfascial compartment ensures a more rapid absorption and serious systemic effects. Likewise, a bite on the head, neck, or trunk (3% of snakebites) hastens systemic absorption.

Snake variables include the snake's size, the amount of venom injected, and the potency of the particular species' venom. Conditions that facilitate venom secretion (e.g., long, healthy fangs or full stores of venom) add to the toxicity of the bite. An angered and hungry rattlesnake unloads more venom than a recently satiated and surprised rattlesnake.

Clinical Recognition

Pit viper. A *Crotalus* envenomation causes intense local pain and burning within a couple of minutes. Victims of a significant rattlesnake bite often complain within minutes of perioral numbness, extending to the scalp and periphery, with a metallic taste in the mouth. Local ecchymoses and vesicles usually appear within the first few hours, and hemorrhagic blebs are often present by 24 hours. Lymphadenitis and lymph node enlargement may also become apparent. Without appropriate therapy, there may be progression to necrosis that may extend throughout the bitten extremity. Secondary infection is a risk as the snake's oral flora includes gram-negative bacteria. Table 98.24 summarizes local characteristics of pit viper bites.

Patients may have nausea, vomiting, weakness, chills, sweating, syncope, and other more ominous symptoms of systemic venom absorption. A copperhead or pygmy rattlesnake envenomation produces less local symptoms, and systemic consequences are often minimal or nonexistent unless a small child, multiple bites, or larger than average snake is involved. The water moccasin's effects are more variable.

TABLE 98.24

LOCAL SIGNS OF PIT VIPER ENVENOMATION

Pain	Ecchymosis
Edema	Vesicles
Erythema	Hemorrhagic blebs

TABLE 98.25

SYSTEMIC SIGNS OF CROTALID (PIT VIPER) ENVENOMATION

General
Anxiety, diaphoresis, pallor, unresponsiveness
Cardiovascular
Tachycardia, decreased capillary perfusion, hypotension, shock
Pulmonary
Pulmonary edema, respiratory failure
Renal
Oliguria, hemoglobinuria, hematuria
Neuromuscular
Fasciculations, weakness, paralysis, convulsions
Hematologic
Bleeding diathesis

There is a relative lack of serious pain or swelling with the Mojave rattler bite, although, as in other *Crotalus* bites, the patient may complain of paresthesia in the affected extremity. Within several hours, these patients may develop neuromuscular symptoms such as diplopia, difficulty in swallowing, lethargy, nausea, and progressive weakness from the large portion of neurotoxin in this species.

The wound should be inspected for fang punctures, and if two are present, the distance between them should be noted. An interfang distance of less than 8 mm suggests a small snake; 8 to 12 mm, a medium snake; and more than 12 mm, a larger snake. Fang wounds by small snakes such as the pygmy rattler may be extremely subtle; in larger crotalid snakebites, the fang marks may be hidden within hemorrhagic blebs and edema. Occasionally, only one puncture or two scratches will be present, but both wounds may be potentially venomous. Ten percent to 20% of known rattlesnake strikes do not inject venom. Other causes of puncture wounds such as rat bites and thorn wounds must also be kept in mind. Nonpoisonous snakes sometimes leave an imprint of their two rows of teeth, but the wounds should lack fang puncture marks.

The dramatic signs of crotalid envenomation are derived primarily from the victim's hypovolemic state, hemorrhagic tendencies, and neuromuscular dysfunction. Table 98.25 outlines the more notable physical signs.

Coral snake. Coral snakes leave unimpressive local signs but can neurologically cripple their prey. The bite may have one or two punctures, at most 7 to 8 mm apart, and other small teeth marks. Local wound and, eventually, extremity paresthesia and weakness may be reported. Over several hours, generalized malaise and nausea, fasciculations, and weakness develop insidiously. There may be diplopia with difficulty talking or swallowing. Physical examination reveals bulbar dysfunction and generalized weakness. Respiratory failure may ensue.

Triage

Pit viper. The airway, breathing, and circulation of the patient must be addressed before attending to the snakebite (Fig. 98.23). The first priority of prehospital care of the snakebite victim is rapid transport to a medical facility. All activities in the field must be tempered by the fact that time is of the essence.

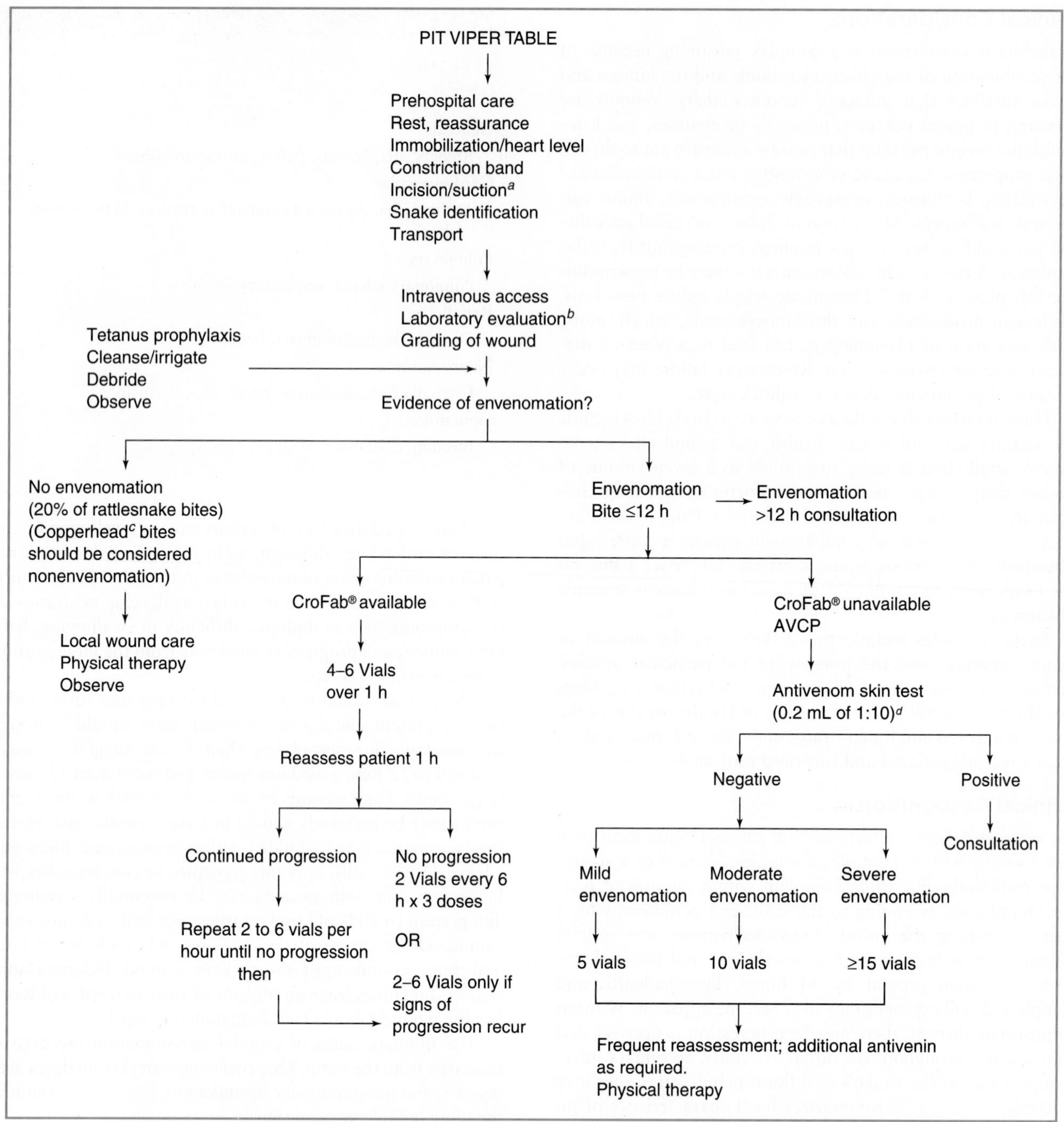

FIGURE 98.23 Management of pit viper bite. [a]Perform within 5 to 10 minutes of bite; continue suction for 30 to 60 minutes. [b]Complete blood cell count, platelet count, prothrombin time, partial thromboplastin time, urinalysis, type and hold; in moderate or severe cases, add fibrinogen, arterial blood gases, electrolytes, blood urea nitrogen, and creatinine. [c]Seldom need antivenin; exceptions with large snakes and small children. [d]1:100 dilution if allergy history; saline control; resuscitation medications at hand; antivenin seldom indicated if greater than 12 to 24 hours since bite.

It is important to approach the patient with reassurance and to place him or her at rest. The affected extremity should be stripped of any constricting jewelry or clothing and immobilized in a position of function below the level of the heart. The patient should be kept warm and not allowed anything by mouth.

Tourniquets, inadvertently tightened for prolonged full vascular occlusion, have created more problems than they have solved and therefore cannot be recommended for prehospital care. In experienced hands, however, a constriction band that obstructs lymph and venous flow can be valuable when a long transport is anticipated (longer than 30 to 60 minutes). The band should be at least 2 cm wide and placed 5 to 10 cm proximal to the wound (proximal to the nearest joint if the wound is nearby). The constriction should be loose enough to admit a finger and preserve good distal arterial pulses. Vigilant observation for adequate perfusion is necessary because of progressive edema; the constriction band should be shifted to remain proximal to the swelling. To be effective, the band must be applied initially within 1 hour of the pit viper bite. It may be removed when antivenin therapy is started.

TABLE 98.26

GRADING OF CROTALID (PIT VIPER) SNAKEBITES

	Mild	Moderate	Severe
Local	Fang mark Intense pain Edema Erythema Ecchymosis ± Vesicles Within 10–15 cm of bite	All local signs extend beyond wound site	Entire extremity involvement
Systemic	None Anxiety related	Nausea/vomiting Weakness/fainting Perioral, scalp paresthesias Metallic taste Pallor Tachycardia Mild hypotension Fasciculations	As in moderate Hypotension Shock Bleeding diathesis Respiratory distress
Laboratory	No abnormalities	Hemoconcentration Thrombocytopenia Hypofibrinogenemia	Significant anemia Prolonged clotting time Metabolic acidosis

Incision and suction (extractors) of the pit viper wound is no longer advised. The usefulness of extractors can be supported only if applied within minutes of the bite and even then recovery of venom is variable in a laboratory setting. No animal studies have shown an increase in survival.

In the rare situation in which skilled personnel and supplies are at the scene and a long transport is expected, it is reasonable to allow one or two attempts at IV access. Many authorities also suggest capturing or killing the snake for later verification, but again, prudence dictates that time not be wasted and that an inexperienced person not risk the bite of an agitated snake. If the snake arrives in the ED, treat it with respect—decapitated snakes can bite reflexively for up to 1 hour.

Management

If the history and physical examination on arrival in the ED are consistent with a venomous snakebite, immediate laboratory evaluation and IV access are indicated. A CBC, coagulation studies, platelet count, urinalysis, and blood crossmatching should be obtained, as blood may be difficult to crossmatch after massive hemolysis. In moderate or severe poisoning, analyses of serum electrolytes, BUN, creatinine, fibrinogen, and ABG levels are also indicated. Hemolysis, anemia, thrombocytopenia, hypofibrinogenemia, prolonged bleeding times, and metabolic acidosis all may be seen in severe poisoning. Repeat the laboratory studies every 6 hours to ensure no significant changes occur.

Therapy will be based on the clinician's overall grading of venom toxicity. Local and systemic manifestations, as well as laboratory findings, weigh heavily in this judgment. The clinical pattern may change as the venom's effects unfold and frequent reassessment is crucial. The physician should measure and record the circumference of the injured extremity at the leading point of edema and 10 cm proximal to this level every 30 minutes for 6 hours, then at least every 4 hours for a total of 24 hours. Table 98.26 is derived from a grading system suggested by the Scientific Review Subcommittee of the American Association of Poison Control Centers.

Any prehospital care (e.g., extremity immobilization) should be rechecked. If an occluding tourniquet is inappropriately present, the physician should place a more proximal constriction band and then cautiously remove the tourniquet, being prepared to respond therapeutically to a systemic release of venom.

The older antivenom (Crotalidae) polyvalent (AVCP; Wyeth-Ayerst Pharmaceuticals) is no longer available; it was derived from horse serum and was highly antigenic. The newer antivenom was licensed in 2000 and is a polyclonal, polyvalent Fab affinity purified (FabAV; CroFab Prothenics, Inc.) product derived from sheep. It has less adverse reactions than seen with AVCP. The antivenom is effective for rattlesnake and water moccasin envenomations. Mojave rattlesnake venom was used in the development of FabAV; therefore, its efficacy may be better in bites from this species. Copperhead venom was not used in either AVCP or FabAV. The need for antivenin in cases of copperhead envenomation has been questioned in patients without significant systemic effects or severe swelling and pain. For maximal venom binding, the antivenin should be given within 4 hours of the snake strike. The benefits of antivenin administration after 12 hours are questionable for either antivenin. Their use is generally not indicated after 24 hours (an exception may be continued coagulopathy). The dosage regimen for FabAV is different than AVCP. Unbound Fab may be cleared before venom emerges from tissue deposits. For this reason, FabAV is given either on a fixed schedule or on a sliding scale. Relative contraindications for use include known hypersensitivity to papain, papaya, latex, or FabAV.

For patients receiving FabAV, an initial dose of four to six vials is given over 1 hour. Skin testing is not needed for FabAV. Each vial is reconstituted with 10 mL of sterile water and then the total dose is mixed in 250 mL of normal saline. The infusion should be started slowly, at a rate of 25 to 50 mL per hour for 10 minutes, while observing for allergic reaction. The rate should be increased so the 250 mL is given over 1 hour. If mild allergic manifestations develop, the infusion should be stopped and diphenhydramine (1 to 2 mg per kg IV) given. Once the allergic symptoms have resolved, a minimum of 5 minutes should pass, then the infusion should be restarted at a slower rate. Reactions have been associated with faster infusion rates. Initial dosage from FabAV (CroFab) is given irrespective of degree of envenomation. Subsequent doses are based on signs of progression. The patient should be reassessed after the initial dose. If there is progression of envenomation, then the initial dose should be repeated. If there is no progression, two different schedules are suggested. One choice is to give two vials every 6 hours for three doses. The other regimen is to give two to six vials only if signs of envenomation progression recur. All patients should be reassessed every 2 to 5 days after discharge.

Wound care includes irrigation, cleansing, a loose dressing, and tetanus prophylaxis. The affected extremity should be maintained just below the level of the heart and in a position of function. Cotton padding can be used between swollen digits, and analgesics if needed. Current studies question the need for prophylactic antibiotics. Surgical excision of the wound, routine fasciotomy, and application of ice are contraindicated. Excision of the wound does not remove significant venom after 30 minutes, and cryotherapy has been associated with increased extremity necrosis and amputations. Fasciotomy should be reserved for the rare case of a true compartmental syndrome. Necrosis is usually the result of the proteolytic enzymes or inappropriate therapy and is not caused by compartmental pressure. Superficial debridement will be required at 3 to 6 days; one possible wound care regimen suggested at this stage includes local oxygen, aluminum acetate (1:20 solution) soaks, and triple dye. Physical therapy is beneficial during the healing phase.

Supportive care focuses on correction of the intravascular depletion that results from increased venous capacitance, interstitial third spacing, and hemorrhagic losses. There should be two IV lines for antivenin therapy and volume replacement. Shock usually develops between 6 and 24 hours after the snakebite but may present within the first hour in severe envenomation. Central vascular monitoring and accurate urine output measurements are desirable for optimal therapy. Normal saline or lactated Ringer solution (20 mL per kg over 1 hour), followed by fresh whole blood or other blood components, often corrects the hypovolemia (see Chapter 5 Shock). Vasopressors are usually needed only transiently in the more severe cases. A bleeding diathesis is best managed with fresh whole blood, or blood component therapy, primarily packed cells (10 mL per kg), and fresh-frozen plasma (10 mL per kg). With life-threatening bleeding, platelets (0.2 units per kg) and a more concentrated fibrinogen source (cryoprecipitate—dose one bag per 5 kg body weight) should also be considered. Abnormal clotting parameters, including fibrinogen and platelet and blood counts, should be reevaluated every 4 to 6 hours. Respiratory and renal support may also be required.

The rate of serum sickness with FabAV (CroFab) is much lower than that seen with older products. Signs of serum sickness include rashes, arthralgias, edema, malaise, lymphadenopathy, fever, and/or GI symptoms that evolve over several days. Prednisone (2 mg/kg/day, maximum 80 mg) until symptoms abate (and then a tapering schedule) has been used with success in most cases. Diphenhydramine (5 mg/kg/day in four divided doses, max 50 mg per dose) is often given as an adjunct.

Coral snake. When coral snake wounds are present or the history or specimen is consistent with an Eastern coral snakebite, antivenin for *M. fulvius* (Wyeth) is administered before development of further symptoms. The antivenin's access is restricted in the United States (contact http://www.Wyeth.com for information). This is also an equine serum and requires preliminary skin testing (see package insert). The initial recommended dosage is three to five vials by IV; an additional three to five vials may be given as needed for signs of venom toxicity. There is no antivenin available for the Arizona coral snake (*M. euryxanthus*). Supportive care should provide a satisfactory outcome in these cases. Constriction bands, suction and drainage, and other local measures do not retard coral snake venom absorption, and hence, are not indicated.

Exotic snakes. The clinician confronted with an exotic snakebite or a clinician inexperienced in snakebites should consult a local medical herpetologist, poison control center, or the American Association of Zoologic Parks and Aquariums and the American Association of Poison Control Centers. These centers keep an up-to-date database of exotic antivenoms. Access to this information is available at 800-222-1222. Report all illegally possessed reptiles to the police or to the appropriate fish and game agency.

MAMMALIAN BITES

Goals of Treatment

Treatment aims to decrease the overall morbidity of mammalian bites in terms of infectious complications, cosmesis, disability, psychological trauma, and medical expenses.

CLINICAL PEARLS AND PITFALLS

- Cat and human bites have a high infectious complication rate.
- Wound closure can be delayed when there is a high risk of infection.
- Local wound care is more important than prophylactic antibiotics in prevention of infection.

Current Evidence

At least 1 to 2 million people are bitten each year, and about 1% of ED visits are prompted by bite wounds. Dog bites account for the overwhelming majority (80% to 90%) of mammalian bites. An estimated 4.5 million dog bites occur in the United States annually, with approximately 885,000 people seeking medical care. The most common dog attack involves a 5- to 14-year-old boy close to home and a large-breed or mixed-breed canine. The dog's owner can be identified 85% to 90% of the time; in fact, in 15% to 30% of cases, the dog belongs to the victim's family. Usually, the dog has been provoked, although most often unintentionally. Animal jealousy has been implicated in unprovoked biting of infants and accounts for about 10 fatal cases each year in the United States.

Other mammalian bites are perpetrated by cats (5% to 10%), rodents (2% to 3%), humans (2% to 3%), and other wild or domesticated animals. Human and cat bites both have high infectious complication rates.

Clinical Considerations

Anatomic wound characteristics and the microbiologic inoculum of the offending species determine the pathologic consequences of the bite.

Many dog bites cause crush injuries with infection-prone devitalized tissue, a result of the enormous pressures (200 to 400 lb/square inch) dogs can generate in their bites. Overall only 5% to 10% of dog bites become infected, probably because the resulting lacerations and abrasions are so accessible to good wound hygiene. The feline bite is a deep puncture wound that is difficult to irrigate or cleanse, hence its high infection rate (up to 50% in some series). The penetration of tendons, vessels, facial compartments, and bones also increases the risk of infection. The hand offers all these anatomic components in a relatively small cross-sectional area, hence its increased risk of infection, regardless of the biting species.

Aerobic and anaerobic bacteria indigenous to mammalian oral flora are inoculated into the wound during biting. The most commonly isolated bacteria in infected cat and dog bite wounds are *Staphylococcus aureus* and *Pasteurella* species, a gram-negative rod. In one series, *Pasteurella multocida* and *Pasteurella canis* were found in 50% and 80% of infected dog and cat wounds, respectively. Other more common bacteria have also been isolated: streptococci, coagulase-negative staphylococci, *S. aureus,* and enteric bacteria. Anaerobic bacteria are usually recovered (not alone but only in mixed cultures with aerobes).

Human bite infections are mixed bacterial infections, with *Streptococcus viridans* or *S. aureus* being the predominant organism. Anaerobic bacteria, especially *Bacteroides* and *Peptostreptococcus* species, are commonly cultured. The more serious morbidity in infected human bites of the hand has been correlated with *S. aureus* isolation and, more recently, with *Eikenella corrodens,* a facultative anaerobe.

Finally, the multiple systemic diseases that may be transmitted by mammalian bites need to be considered.

Clinical Assessment

Mammalian bite wounds cause a spectrum of tissue injuries from trivial to life-threatening. Scratches, abrasions, contusions, punctures, lacerations, and their complications are commonly seen in the ED. The complications usually involve secondary infections or damage to structures that underlie the bite.

Dog bites are insignificant lesions in at least half of the cases that come to medical attention, 5% to 10% warrant suturing and 2% require hospital admission. Approximately 33% of dog bites involve the upper extremity, 33% involve the lower extremities, and 20% involve the head and neck area. The remainder of bites involves multiple areas. Other than bites on the hand, the rate of secondary infection in dog bites given good local care approximates that of nonbite wounds.

Young children suffer more serious canine injuries. The dog strikes the head and neck in 60% to 70% of victims younger than 5 years and in 50% of those younger than 10 years. On rare occasions, life-threatening injuries occur, including depressed skull fractures, intracranial lesions, major vascular injury, visceral penetration, and chest trauma. Death is usually secondary to acute hemorrhagic shock.

Cat bites are located in the upper extremities in two-thirds of cases and are usually puncture wounds rather than lacerations or contusions. *P. multocida* infections characteristically present within 12 to 24 hours of the injury and rapidly display erythema, significant swelling, and intense pain. Local infections from other organisms usually present 24 to 72 hours after the bite in a less fulminant manner. Viridans streptococcal infections are occasional exceptions to this generalization and may resemble a *P. multocida* clinical course.

Cat scratches also commonly occur in the periorbital region, and may involve corneal abrasions. Cat-scratch disease, an uncommon complication of these injuries, is characterized by a papule at the scratch site and a subsequent regional lymphadenitis. The primary lesion is typically a crusted, erythematous papule, 2 to 6 mm in diameter that develops 3 to 10 days after the scratch. A tender regional lymphadenopathy occurs 2 weeks after the primary lesion. Malaise and fever are associated symptoms in approximately 25% of patients. Rarely, encephalopathy, exanthem, atypical pneumonia, and parotid swelling may occur. The disease is self-limiting, with resolution of the symptoms within 2 to 3 months. *Bartonella henselae* is the causative organism. An indirect fluorescent antibody test to Bartonella is useful in the diagnosis and is available through the Centers for Disease Control and Prevention. Polymerase chain reaction assays are available in some commercial labs.

Human bites in older children and adolescents are most commonly incurred when a clenched fist strikes the teeth of an adversary. The wound overlies the metacarpal–phalangeal joint, with bacterial penetration into the relatively avascular fascial layers. Hand infections, usually present with mild swelling over the dorsum of the hand 1 to 2 days after injury. If there is pain with active or passive finger motion, a more serious deep compartmental infection or tendonitis should be suspected. Osteomyelitis occasionally occurs in hand infections. In younger children, human bites are more often on the face or trunk than on the hands. Often, a playmate inflicts the wound, but child abuse must always be considered. Systemic diseases that may be spread by human bites include hepatitis B and syphilis.

Rodent bites usually occur in disadvantaged socioeconomic groups or among laboratory workers and have a relatively low incidence of secondary infection (10%). Ratbite fever is a rare disease that may present after a 1- to 3-week incubation period with chills, fever, malaise, headache, and a maculopapular or petechial rash. There are two forms: Haverhill fever (*Streptobacillus moniliformis*) and Sodoku (*Spirillum minus*), both of which are responsive to IV penicillin.

Another uncommon bacterium for which lagomorphs, particularly rabbits, are hosts is *Francisella tularensis*. Tularemia is usually spread to humans by rabbit bites, although contact with or ingestion of contaminated animals or insect vectors is sufficient for transmission. Ulceroglandular tularemia is the most common form of the disease, and gentamicin, ciprofloxacin, or doxycycline is the agent of first choice in its treatment. Streptomycin may be used but is no longer readily available in the United States.

Serious infections from multiple bacteria, including osteomyelitis, sepsis, endocarditis, and meningitis, have been reported as complications of mammalian bite wounds. The risk of rabies or tetanus always must be considered in animal bites.

Management

Meticulous and prompt local care of the bite wound is the most important factor in satisfactory healing and prevention of infection. The wound should be forcefully irrigated with a minimum of 200 mL normal saline. A 19-gauge needle or catheter attached to a 30-mL syringe will supply sufficient pressure for wound decontamination and will decrease the infection rate by 20-fold. Stronger irrigant antiseptics—povidone-iodine, 20% hexachlorophene, alcohols, or hydrogen peroxide—may damage wound surfaces and delay healing. Soaking in various preparations has not proved helpful in reducing infections.

Most open lacerations from mammalian bites can be sutured if local care is provided within several hours of the injury and good surgical technique is used. Facial wounds often mandate primary closure for cosmetic reasons and, overall, are low infection risks because of the good vascular supply. In fact, one study demonstrated a lower infection rate in sutured dog bite wounds than in those left open. Other more recent studies support the low infection rate in selected sutured bite wounds. The exceptions to suturing are minor hand wounds and other high-risk bites. In large hand wounds, hemorrhage should be carefully controlled. We suggest closing the subcutaneous dead space in these wounds with a minimal amount of absorbable suture material. Cutaneous sutures can be placed after 3 to 5 days if there is no evidence of infection.

Extremities with extensive wounds should be immobilized in a position of function and kept elevated as much as possible. This is especially true of hand wounds, which should have bulky mitten dressings and be supported by an arm sling. All significant wounds should be rechecked in follow-up in 24 to 48 hours.

The following wounds may be considered at high risk for infection: puncture wounds, minor hand or foot wounds, wounds given initial care after 12 hours, cat or human bites, and wounds in immunosuppressed patients. As a rule, these wounds should not be sutured. The use of prophylactic antibiotics is controversial. Suggested indications for antibiotics include the following:

- Human and cat bites through dermis
- Bites closed prematurely
- Bites more than 8 hours old with significant crush injury or edema
- Potential damage to bones, joints, or tendons
- Bites to hands and feet
- Patients with increased risk of infection
- Signs of infection within 24 hours

No single antibiotic is ideal for all the most common organisms involved in infected mammalian bite wounds. Amoxicillin-clavulanic acid (Augmentin) (30 to 50 mg/kg/day) is effective for *P. multocida,* Streptococcus, and anaerobes, as well as in providing methicillin-susceptible *S. aureus* (MSSA) coverage. Combination therapy with phenoxymethyl penicillin (penicillin VK) and cephalexin or dicloxacillin has been suggested by some authorities. An extended-spectrum cephalosporin or trimethoprim-sulfamethoxazole PLUS clindamycin is an alternative for the penicillin-allergic patient. The initial dose of antibiotic should be given in the ED and continued for the next 3 to 5 days. It must be emphasized that local care ultimately prevents infection more effectively than prophylactic antibiotics. Studies indicate that prophylactic oral antibiotics for low-risk dog bite wounds are not indicated because the differences in the rate of infection are not significant and the cost–benefit ratio is not worth the risk of allergic reaction.

Moderate to severe hand infections or other wounds that involve deep structures usually require debridement and exploration under general anesthesia. Aerobic and anaerobic culture swabs should sample the depth of the wound; or, in cases of cellulitis, the specimen can be collected by needle aspiration of the leading edge of erythema. While awaiting cultures, a Gram stain is often helpful in differentiating the probability of staphylococci or streptococci from *P. multocida.*

Parenteral antibiotics and admission to the hospital are indicated if the child has systemic symptoms or has wounds with potential functional or cosmetic morbidity. The choice of parenteral antibiotics should be governed by the same factors considered in selection of prophylactic antibiotics and then modified by culture results.

Tetanus immunization status should be checked in every injury that violates the epidermis, regardless of the cause. Recommendations for tetanus immunoglobulin and immunization are noted elsewhere (see Chapter 102 Infectious Disease Emergencies).

Concern for rabies is the factor that prompts many patients to seek medical care. Although the incidence of rabies in the United States (one to five cases per year) is extremely low, the physician must always assess the possibility of rabies exposure and promptly initiate prophylaxis when indicated. Dogs and cats account for only 5% of animal rabies in the United States. The history should include the apparent health of the animal and any provocation for attack. Wild carnivores and bats should generally be regarded as rabid; rodents (rats, mice, squirrels) and lagomorphs (rabbits) can usually be considered no risk. Exposure to bats by a sleeping or very young child even without bite or scratch should warrant serious consideration of prophylaxis. Rabies prophylaxis is not indicated in bites by a healthy dog or cat with a known owner, assuming the animal's health does not deteriorate over the following 10 to 14 days. Bites by strays and other domesticated mammals should be considered individually and with consultation of the local health department. Scratches, abrasions, and animal saliva contact with the victim's mucous membranes are capable of rabies spread.

If postexposure antirabies immunization is indicated both passive antibody (RIG, rabies immune globulin, human) and vaccine (HDCV, human diploid cell rabies vaccine) should be given (see also Chapter 102 Infectious Disease Emergencies). Immunization with RIG is administered only once, in a dose of 20 IU per kg. Half the dose, or as much as possible, is infiltrated locally around the wound and the remainder is given intramuscularly. The HDCV immunization should be administered intramuscularly in the opposite deltoid (vastus lateralis in infants) from RIG on days 0, 3, 7, 14, and 28 for a total of five doses, each 1.0 mL.

Suggested Readings and Key References

Drowning

Baum CR. Environmental emergencies: weighing the ounce of prevention. *Clin Pediatr Emerg Med* 2003;4:121–126.

Bell GS, Gaitatzis A, Bell CL, et al. Drowning in people with epilepsy: how great is the risk? *Neurology* 2008;71:578–582.

Brenner RA; Committee on Injury, Violence, and Poison Prevention, American Academy of Pediatrics. Technical report: prevention of drowning in infants, children, and adolescents. *Pediatrics* 2003;12: 440–445.

Causey AL, Tilelli JA, Swanson ME. Predicting discharge in uncomplicated near-drowning. *Am J Emerg Med* 2000;18:9–11.

Modell JH. Drowning. *N Engl J Med* 1993;328:253–256.

Zuckerman GB, Conway EE. Drowning and near drowning: a pediatric epidemic. *Pediatr Ann* 2000;29:360–366.

Smoke Inhalation

Committee on Injury and Poison Prevention, American Academy of Pediatrics. Reducing the number of deaths and injuries from residential fires. *Pediatrics* 2000;5:1355–1357.

Palmieri TL, Warner P, Mlcak RP, et al. Inhalation injury in children: a 10 year experience at Shriners Hospitals for children. *J Burn Care Res* 2009;30:206–208.

Pierre EJ, Zwischengerger JB, Angel C, et al. Extracorporeal membrane oxygenation in the treatment of respiratory failure in pediatric patients with burns. *J Burn Care Rehabil* 1998;19:131–134.

Carbon Monoxide Poisoning

Chambers CA, Hopkins RO, Weaver LK, et al. Cognitive and affective outcomes of more severe as compared to less severe carbon monoxide poisoning. *Brain Inj* 2008;22:387–395.

Cho CH, Chiu NC, Ho CS, et al. Carbon monoxide poisoning in children. *Pediatr Neonatol* 2008;49:121–125.

Chou KJ, Fisher JL, Silver EJ. Characteristics and outcome of children with carbon monoxide poisoning with and without smoke exposure referred for hyperbaric oxygen therapy. *Pediatr Emerg Care* 2000; 6:151–155.

Geller R, Barthold C, Saiers JA, et al. Pediatric cyanide poisoning: causes, manifestations, management, and unmet needs. *Pediatrics* 2006;118:2146–2158.

Martin JD, Osterhoudt KC, Thom SR. Recognition and management of carbon monoxide poisoning in children. *Clin Pediatr Emerg Med* 2000;1:244–250.

Weaver LK. Clinical practice. Carbon monoxide poisoning. *N Engl J Med* 2009;360:1217–1225.

Environmental and Exertional Heat Illness

Hadad E, Rav-Acha M, Heled Y, et al. Heat stroke: a review of cooling methods. *Sports Med* 2004;34:501–511.

Martin TJ, Martin JS. Special issues and concerns for the high school- and college-aged athletes. *Pediatr Clin North Am* 2002;49:533–552.

Accidental Hypothermia

Danzl DF, Pozos RS. Accidental hypothermia. *N Engl J Med* 1994; 331:1756–1760.

Hughes A, Riou P, Day C. Full neurological recovery from profound (18.0 degrees C) acute accidental hypothermia: successful resuscitation using active invasive rewarming techniques. *Emerg Med J* 2007;24:511–512.

Laniewics M, Lyn-Kew K, Silbergleit R. Rapid endovascular warming for profound hypothermia. *Ann Emerg Med* 2008;51:160–163.

Ulrich SA, Rathlev NK. Hypothermia and localized cold injuries. *Emerg Med Clin North Am* 2004;22:281–298.

High-altitude Illness

Basnyat B, Murdoch DR. High-altitude illness. *Lancet* 2003;361: 1967–1974.

Bloch JC, Duplain H, Rimoldi SF, et al. Prevalence and time course of acute mountain sickness in older children and adolescents after rapid ascent to 3450 meters. *Pediatrics* 2009;123:1–5.

Hackett PC, Roach RC. High-altitude medicine. *N Engl J Med* 2001;345:107–114.

Kriemler S, Kohler M, Zehnder M, et al. Successful treatment of severe mountain sickness and excessive pulmonary hypertension treated with dexamethasone in a prepubertal girl. *High Alt Med Biol* 2006; 7:256–261.

Electrical Injuries

Centers for Disease Control and Prevention. Lightning-associated deaths—United States, 1980–1995. *MMWR Morbid Mortal Wkly Rep* 1998;47:391–394.

Garcia CT, Smith GA, Cohen DM, et al. Electrical injuries in a pediatric emergency department. *Ann Emerg Med* 1995;26:604–608.

Jumbelic MI. Forensic perspectives of electrical and lightning injuries. *Semin Neurol* 1995;5:342–350.

Kleinschmidt-DeMasters BK. Neuropathology of lightning-strike injuries. *Semin Neurol* 1995;5:323–328.

Rabban JT, Blair JA, Rosen CL, et al. Mechanisms of pediatric electrical injuries. *Arch Pediatr Adolesc Med* 1997;51:696–700.

Radiation

American College of Radiology. *Disaster preparedness for radiology professionals: response to radiological terrorism.* Reston, VA: American College of Radiology, 2006.

Armed Forces Radiobiology Research Institute (AFRRI). *Medical management of radiological casualties.* 2nd ed. Bethesda, MD: AFRRI, 2003.

Gusev IA, Guskova AK, Mettler FA, eds. *Medical management of radiation accidents.* 2nd ed. Boca Raton, FL: CRC Press, 2001.

Mettler FA Jr, Voelz GL. Major radiation exposure—what to expect and how to respond. *N Engl J Med* 2002;345:1554–1561.

National Council on Radiation Protection and Measurements (NCRP). *Management of terrorist events involving radioactive material (NCRP Report No. 138).* Bethesda, MD: NCRP, 2001.

National Council on Radiation Protection and Measurements (NCRP). *Management of persons contaminated with radionuclides (NCRP Report No. 161).* Bethesda, MD: NCRP, 2012.

Ricks RC, Berger ME, O'Hara FM Jr, eds. *The medical basis for radiation—accident preparedness: the clinical care of victims.* Boca Raton, FL: Parthenon-CRC Press, 2002.

Bites and Stings

Auerbach PS. Marine envenomation. *N Engl J Med* 1991;325:486–493.

Bailey PM, Little M, Jelinek GA, et al. Jellyfish envenoming syndromes: unknown toxic mechanisms and unproven therapies. *Med J Aust* 2003;178:34–37.

Campbell RL, Li JT, Nicklas RA, et al.; Members of the Joint Task Force, Practice Parameter Workgroup. Emergency department diagnosis and treatment of anaphylaxis: a practice parameter. *Ann Allergy Asthma Immunol* 2014;113(6):599–608.

Halstead BW. *Poisonous and venomous marine animals of the world.* Princeton, NJ: Darwin Press, 1978.

Halstead BW, Vinci JM. Venomous fish stings. *Clin Dermatol* 1991;5: 29–35.

McGoldrick J, Marx JA. Marine envenomations, I: vertebrates. *J Emerg Med* 1991;9:497–502.

McGoldrick J, Marx JA. Marine envenomations, II: invertebrates. *J Emerg Med* 1992;10:71–77.

Singletary EM, Rochman AS, Bodmer JC, et al. Envenomations. *Med Clin North Am* 2005;89:1195–1224.

Echinodermata

Burnett JW, Burnett MG. Sea urchins. *Cutis* 1999;64:21–22.

Stingrays

Bitseff EL, Garoni WJ, Hardison CD, et al. The management of stingray injuries of the extremities. *South Med J* 1970;63: 417–418.

Evans RJ, Davies RS. Stingray injury. *J Accid Emerg Med* 1996;13: 224–225.

Fenner PJ, Williamson JA, Skinner RA. Fatal and non-fatal stingray envenomation. *Med J Aust* 1989;151(11/12):621–625.

Scorpaenidae

Bonnet MS. The toxicology of Trachinus vipera: the lesser weeverfish. *Br Homeopath J* 2000;89:84–88.

Catfish

Baack BR, Kucan JO, Zook EG, et al. Hand infections secondary to catfish spines: case reports and literature review. *J Trauma* 1991;31: 1432–1436.

Arthropoda

Bentur Y, Taitelman U, Aloufy A. Evaluation of scorpion stings: the poison center perspective. *Vet Human Toxicol* 2003;45(2):108–111.

Berg RA, Tarantino MD. Envenomation by the scorpion Centruroides exilicauda (C. sculpturatus): severe and unusual manifestations. *Pediatrics* 1991;87:930–933.

Brown SG, Blackman KE, Stenlake V, et al. Insect sting anaphylaxis; prospective evaluation of treatment with intravenous adrenaline and volume resuscitation. *Emerg Med J* 2004;21:149–154.

Clark RF, Wethern-Kestner S, Vance MV, et al. Clinical presentation and treatment of black widow spider envenomation: a review of 163 cases. *Ann Emerg Med* 1992;21:782–787.

Freeman TM. Hypersensitivity to hymenoptera stings. *N Engl J Med* 2004;351:1978–1984.

Gendron BP. Loxosceles reclusa envenomation. *Am J Emerg Med* 1990; 8:51–54.

Jerrard DA. ED management of insect stings. *Am J Emerg Med* 1996; 14:429–433.

LoVecchio F, McBride C. Scorpion envenomations in young children in Central Arizona. *J Toxicol Clin Toxicol* 2003;41:937–940.

Rees R, Campbell D, Rieger E, et al. The diagnosis and treatment of brown recluse spider bites. *Ann Emerg Med* 1991;16:945–949.

Saucier JR. Arachnid envenomation. *Emerg Med Clin North Am* 2004; 22:405–422.

Sicherer SH, Simons ER; Section on Allergy & Immunology. Self-injectable epinephrine for first-aid management of anaphylaxis. *Pediatrics* 2007;119:638–646.

Volcheck GW. Hymenoptera (Apid and Vespid) allergy: update in diagnosis and management. *Curr Allergy Asthma Rep* 2002;2:46–50.

Venomous Reptiles

Alberts MB, Shalit M, LoGalbo F. Suction for venomous snakebite: a study of "mock venom" extraction in a human model. *Ann Emerg Med* 2004;43:181–186.

Behm MO, Kearns GL, Offerman S, et al. Crotaline FAB antivenom for treatment of children with rattlesnake envenomation. *Pediatrics* 2003;112:1458–1459.

Bond GR. Controversies in the treatment of pediatric victims of Crotalidae snake envenomation. *Clin Pediatr Emerg Med* 2001;2: 192–202.

Dart RC, McNally J. Efficacy, safety, and use of snake antivenoms in the United States. *Ann Emerg Med* 2001;37:181–188.

Gold BS, Dart RC, Barish RA. Bites of venomous snakes. *N Engl J Med* 2002;347(5):347–356.

McKinney PE. Out-of-hospital and interhospital management of crotaline snakebite. *Ann Emerg Med* 2001;37:168–174.

Pizon AF, Riley BD, LoVecchio F, et al. Safety and efficacy of Crotalidae polyvalent immune Fab in pediatric crotaline envenomations. *Acad Emerg Med* 2007;14:373–376.

Schmidt JM. Antivenom therapy for snake bites in children: is there evidence? *Curr Opin Pediatr* 2005;17:234–238.

Trinh HH, Hack JB. Use of CroFab antivenin in the management of a very young pediatric copperhead envenomation. *J Emerg Med* 2005;29:159–162.

Mammalian Bites

Aghababian RV, Conte JE Jr. Mammalian bite wounds. *Ann Emerg Med* 1980;9:79–83.

Ball V, Younggren BN. Emergency management of difficult wounds: part I. *Emerg Med Clin North Am* 2007;25:101–121.

Morgan M, Palmer J. Dog bites. *BMJ* 2007;334:413–417.

Rupprecht CE, Gibbons CE. Prophylaxis against rabies. *N Engl J Med* 2004;351:2626–2635.

CHAPTER 99 ■ GASTROINTESTINAL EMERGENCIES

ERIC A. RUSSELL, MD, BRUNO P. CHUMPITAZI, MD, MPH, AND CORRIE E. CHUMPITAZI, MD

GOALS OF EMERGENCY CARE

Abdominal complaints are among the most common reasons for a child to present to the emergency department. While the majority of these complaints are not life-threatening, the emergency provider must be able to recognize the most serious diagnoses and initiate appropriate therapy. The goal for the ED physician is to identify and stabilize gastrointestinal (GI) emergencies early in their course. This includes the recognition of hemodynamic instability or impending instability secondary to infection, bleeding, organ dysfunction, or ischemia. This can be aided by the identification of patients at high risk for life-threatening emergencies such as those with a history of abdominal surgery, organ transplantation, biliary manipulation, immunodeficiency, or primary hepatic, pancreatic, oncologic, or renal disease.

RELATED CHAPTERS

Signs and Symptoms

- Abdominal Distension: Chapter 7
- Constipation: Chapter 13
- Diarrhea: Chapter 18
- Gastrointestinal Bleeding: Chapter 28
- Jaundice: Conjugated Hyperbilirubinemia: Chapter 39
- Jaundice: Unconjugated Hyperbilirubinemia: Chapter 40
- Pain: Abdomen: Chapter 48
- Vomiting: Chapter 77

Clinical Pathways

- Abdominal Pain in Postpubertal Girls: Chapter 82
- Appendicitis (Suspected): Chapter 83

Medical, Surgical, and Trauma Emergencies

- Infectious Disease Emergencies: Chapter 102
- Oncologic Emergencies: Chapter 106
- Renal and Electrolyte Emergencies: Chapter 108
- Abdominal Trauma: Chapter 111
- Abdominal Emergencies: Chapter 124
- Thoracic Emergencies: Chapter 132
- Transplantation Emergencies: Chapter 133

KEY POINTS

- Abdominal pain may be a presenting sign of systemic disease.
- Brisk bleeding is uncommon but can rapidly become life-threatening.
- GI bleeding may be a sign of bowel ischemia.
- Previous hepatic or biliary surgery places a patient at high risk for cholecystitis and ascending cholangitis.
- Hepatic encephalopathy is not universally seen in patients with acute liver failure (ALF), but when identified, may be a life-threatening finding of ALF.

GASTROINTESTINAL BLEEDING

Goals of Treatment

GI bleeding is a common and occasionally life-threatening condition in infants and children. An orderly approach to this problem is essential (see Chapter 28 Gastrointestinal Bleeding). Significant GI bleeding places a patient at risk of circulatory collapse. The goal for the ED physician is to address life-threatening GI bleeding by stopping the ongoing losses and replacing intravascular volume. Addressing ongoing bleeding will require a team of professionals, including the emergency physician, surgeon, and/or gastroenterologist. Addressing potential circulatory compromise achieves two principal objectives: Oxygen carrying capacity is improved through administration of blood products and the perfusion pressure to vital organs is preserved via blood product and intravenous (IV) fluid administration.

The vast majority of patients with either upper or lower GI bleeding will not have experienced significant blood loss. These patients can be managed successfully with judicious laboratory investigation, supportive care, and follow-up with a primary care provider or an appropriate subspecialist.

Upper Gastrointestinal Bleeding

Esophageal Varices

Goals of Treatment. The initial goals of therapy of suspected variceal hemorrhage are identical to those of massive upper GI bleeding from any source. Volume resuscitation to maintain adequate perfusion and oxygen carrying capacity is necessary, but overexpansion of the intravascular volume should be avoided because it may contribute to rebleeding. Patients with actively bleeding esophageal varices (EV) may also have liver dysfunction and, as a result, early therapy should also correct existing coagulopathies.

Current Evidence. Upper GI bleeding from EV is a major cause of morbidity and mortality in patients with underlying

CLINICAL PEARLS AND PITFALLS

- Patients with varices are likely to have portal hypertension, and therefore are at risk for ascites, spontaneous bacterial peritonitis, bleeding, and splenomegaly with associated thrombocytopenia and leukopenia.
- Overexpansion of intravascular volume may contribute to rebleeding.
- Patients with portal hypertension are also at risk for bleeding from congestive gastritis.
- Coagulation abnormalities in the setting of active bleeding should be managed aggressively with IV vitamin K, fresh frozen plasma (FFP), and platelets. Coagulation abnormalities without active bleeding do not require FFP or platelets.
- Prophylactic antibiotics are part of initial pharmacologic management. Bleeding varices may be the initial sign of sepsis in patients with liver disease.
- Octreotide is part of initial pharmacologic management with severe active bleeding due to portal hypertension.

liver disease and portal hypertension. Causes of EV can be seen in Table 99.1. Varices that develop as a result of portal hypertension are a type of portal-systemic collateral, which develop secondary to the abnormally elevated pressure within the portal system and can form in any area where veins draining the portal venous system are in close approximation to veins draining into the caval system (i.e., submucosa of the esophagus, submucosa of the rectum, and anterior abdominal wall). Patients with EV often have underlying portal hypertension, and their varices may develop over a few months or after many years. Patients with portal hypertension are also at risk of GI bleeding from congestive or hemorrhagic gastritis.

EV are very common in patients with certain types of high-risk underlying liver disease, particularly biliary atresia (BA) and portal vein thrombosis where EV have been reported to be present in as many as 70% of patients. Patients are at increased risk for EV if they have splenomegaly, thrombocytopenia, or hypoalbuminemia. In addition to primary liver disease, patients with congestive heart failure are known to be at high risk for EV. These factors should be taken into account when evaluating a patient with a history of an upper GI bleed or when counseling families for their risk of upper GI bleed.

Clinical Considerations

Clinical Recognition. Patients with EV may have occult bleeding, but more commonly, the bleeding is brisk. Patients will have hematemesis, hematochezia, and/or melena. The possibility of bleeding EV should be considered in any patient with a history of jaundice (beyond the newborn period), hepatitis, ascites, chronic right-sided heart failure, portal vein thrombosis, pulmonary hypertension, omphalitis, umbilical vein catheterization, or one of the hepatic parenchymal diseases noted in Table 99.1.

Triage Considerations. While it is common that bleeding will have stopped prior to arrival in the ED, patients with EV have the potential for significant blood loss. Close attention should be given to tachycardia as an early indicator of hemodynamic compromise and patients should be triaged accordingly. Patients with significant upper GI bleeding may also be at risk for airway compromise.

Clinical Assessment. One should have a high suspicion of EV in any patient presenting with an upper GI bleed and any of the risk factors listed above. One can also evaluate for the stigmata of portal hypertension, such as jaundice, ascites, rectal hemorrhoids, and hepatosplenomegaly (Table 99.2). Other signs or symptoms of right-sided heart failure would also place a patient at higher risk. Given the risk for sudden and life-threatening bleeding, assessing this risk is essential.

In patients with severe upper GI bleeding from EV, two large-bore IVs should be started immediately (Fig. 99.1). An nasogastric (NG) tube should be placed to evaluate for ongoing bleeding and to remove blood from the stomach, which may act as an irritant and potentially worsen hepatic encephalopathy. Variceal bleeding is not a contraindication for passing an NG tube. Immediate laboratory studies should include

TABLE 99.1

CAUSES OF PORTAL HYPERTENSION AND ESOPHAGEAL VARICES

Location of lesion	Example	
Prehepatic	• Portal vein thrombosis • Portal vein obstruction (i.e., malignancy) • Splenic vein obstruction	• Increased portal or splenic blood flow • Portal vein sclerosis/venopathy (i.e., schistosomiasis, HIV, cystic fibrosis)
Intrahepatic	• Cirrhosis from biliary atresia, primary sclerosing cholangitis, cystic fibrosis, α_1-antitrypsin deficiency, chronic hepatitis B/C, autoimmune hepatitis, chronic alcohol use	• Schistosomiasis • Idiopathic portal hypertension • Congenital hepatic fibrosis • Nonalcoholic fatty liver disease
Posthepatic	• Budd–Chiari syndrome: thrombosis or exterior compression (i.e., malignancy) • Inferior vena cava obstruction • Constrictive pericarditis	• Congestive heart failure • Venoocclusive disease

TABLE 99.2

SIGNS AND SYMPTOMS OF PORTAL HYPERTENSION

System	Physical examination findings	Clinical complications
CNS	Altered mental status	Hepatic encephalopathy
Hematologic	Splenomegaly Petechiae/purpura Ecchymosis Pallor	Thrombocytopenia Leukopenia Anemia
Circulatory	Bounding pulses Systolic flow murmur Warm extremities Abdominal distention/ascites Peripheral vasodilation/ palmar erythema Edema Venous hum over collateral vessels	Hypotension Ascites Hepatorenal syndrome Hepatopulmonary syndrome Portopulmonary hypertension
GI	Hepatomegaly Splenomegaly Nausea/vomiting Melena/hematochezia Hematemesis Abdominal pain/fever Dilated abdominal vasculature Abdominal distention/pain Jaundice Fetor hepaticus (rare in children) Spider angiomas	Gastroesophageal varices Recta varices Congestive/ hemorrhagic gastritis Ascites Spontaneous bacterial peritonitis
Pulmonary	Dyspnea Hypoxemia Digital clubbing Cyanosis	Hepatopulmonary syndrome Portopulmonary hypertension
Renal	Edema Abdominal distention/ascites	Hepatorenal syndrome Hypervolemia

type and crossmatch, complete blood cell (CBC) count, platelet count, prothrombin time (PT), and partial thromboplastin time (PTT). Additional laboratory studies may be indicated on the basis of the differential diagnosis of the most likely cause of the patient's bleeding. Arterial blood gases should also be followed when severe blood loss is associated with shock. The hematocrit is an unreliable initial index of acute blood loss because it may be normal or only slightly decreased and not accurately reflect the actual value in a rapid bleed.

Transfusion of blood products may be necessary to maintain adequate end-organ perfusion with severe GI bleeding. The volume of blood products that should be administered as

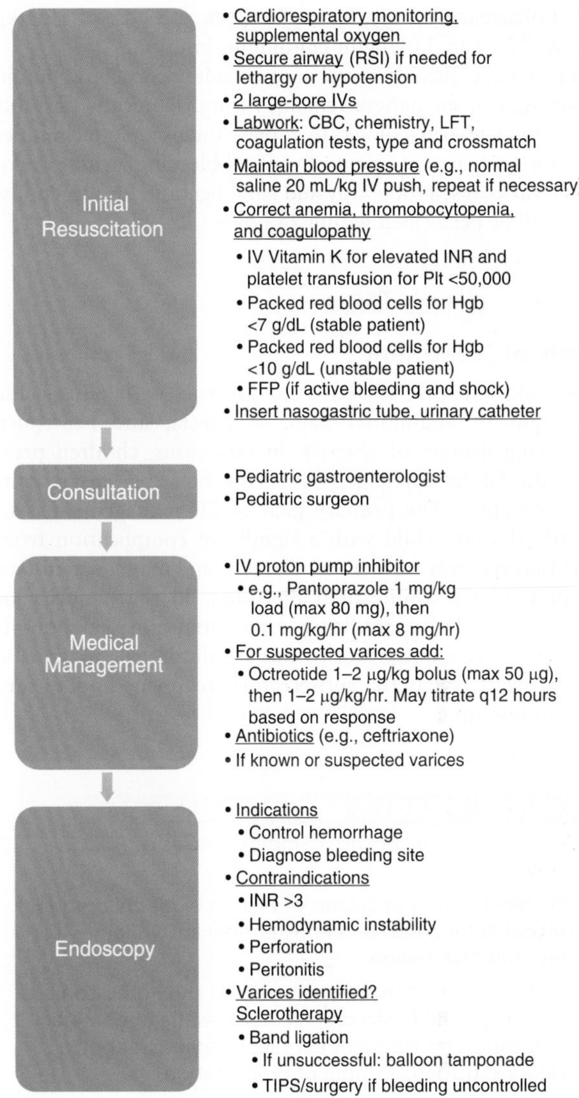

FIGURE 99.1 Emergency management of severe UGI bleeding. The management involves a multidisciplinary approach from resuscitation, to consultation, to medications, to endoscopy if indicated.

well as the timing of those transfusions is controversial. Current recommendations generally target a hemoglobin transfusion goal of 7 to 8 g/dL. Excessive blood administration, especially in the setting of non–life-threatening bleeding, should be avoided, as it is known to contribute to rebleeding. Coagulation abnormalities should be managed aggressively only if there is active bleeding, as transfusion of blood products may lead to volume overload. In patients who are not actively bleeding, the ED physician should not attempt to correct a coagulopathy as a patient's PT and INR can be very difficult to correct and are not reliable indicators of bleeding risk in those with underlying liver disease. It is also important to note that bleeding varices may be the initial sign of sepsis in patients who have cirrhosis. Prophylactic broad-spectrum antibiotics, after appropriate cultures are obtained, are recommended in the setting of a significant esophageal bleed.

Therapies for acute variceal hemorrhage include both pharmacologic and endoscopic therapy. Multiple pharmacologic agents have been studied, including vasopressin, somatostatin, and octreotide. Octreotide has been found to be the most effective with the best side effect profile and is the preferred initial pharmacotherapy. It may be given at a dose of 1 μg/kg followed by 1 to 5 μg/kg/hr continuous infusion.

Emergency flexible esophagogastroduodenoscopy should be arranged if the patient remains hemodynamically unstable after initial pharmacologic therapies. Endoscopic techniques used for acute management of variceal bleeding include endoscopic variceal sclerotherapy and band ligation. Ideally, endoscopy will be performed within 24 hours (Fig. 99.1).

Peptic Ulcer Disease

Goals of Treatment

Peptic ulcer disease (PUD) often presents with nonspecific symptoms of abdominal pain, dyspepsia, and heartburn to varying degrees of severity. In rare cases, children present with GI hemorrhage, GI perforation, or gastric outlet obstruction. The primary goal of ED management is to identify the rare child with a significant complication from PUD that requires further stabilization and management (see Chapter 28 Gastrointestinal Bleeding). In the majority of cases, once PUD is identified as a potential cause of abdominal pain, it is appropriate to initiate outpatient diagnostic testing, start a gastric antisecretory regimen, and ensure close follow-up.

CLINICAL PEARLS AND PITFALLS

- Stress-related ulcers are common causes of PUD in early infancy.
- The most common causes of PUD in older children are *Helicobacter pylori* and nonsteroidal anti-inflammatory drug (NSAID) usage.
- Gastric outlet obstruction from PUD should be considered in the child with chronic nonspecific abdominal symptoms and frequent nonbilious emesis of both liquids and solids at time of presentation.
- Proton pump inhibitors (PPIs), if discontinued abruptly, may result in rebound hypersecretion and exacerbation of symptoms.

Clinical Evidence

While the term PUD describes a group of disorders which involves changes to the mucosal lining of the upper GI tract (esophagus, stomach, and duodenum), this section will focus on diseases of the stomach and duodenum. PUD has various levels of severity with the most common causes of ulcers in stomach and duodenum being *H. pylori* infection followed by NSAIDs. Less common etiologies include stress-induced gastropathy, portal gastropathy, caustic ingestion, inflammatory bowel disease (IBD), and eosinophilic gastritis.

Ulcer disease occurs when there is an imbalance between cytotoxic factors, (e.g., acid, pepsin, NSAIDs, *H. pylori*) and cytoprotective factors, including the secretion of mucus and bicarbonate by superficial epithelial and mucous cells in the upper GI tract. Local blood flow, delayed gastric emptying, duodenal reflux, and other factors have been suggested as important factors in the development of gastric ulceration, but the exact pathogenesis of the condition remains unclear.

The role of the bacterium *H. pylori* in the etiology of ulcer disease in children has been investigated. *H. pylori* produces a localized inflammatory reaction that contributes to epithelial damage either by direct toxic effect or via immunopathologic means. *H. pylori* infection usually occurs in childhood with earlier acquisition and higher prevalence noted in developing countries. There are higher prevalence rates among family members and institutionalized populations, suggesting person-to-person transmission via either an oral route or a fecal-to-oral route. A family history of ulcer disease is typically present in 50% or more of children with duodenal ulcers.

Clinical Considerations

Clinical Recognition. Symptoms of PUD vary with the patient's age. Stress ulcers account for 80% of peptic disease in early infancy, and often present as medical emergencies. Infants may present either with nonspecific feeding difficulties and vomiting, or with upper GI bleeding or perforation. Nonspecific signs and symptoms predominate among older infants and preschool-aged children, with boys and girls affected equally. Preschool-aged children often complain of poorly localized abdominal pain, vomiting, or GI hemorrhage, which can manifest as either hematemesis or melena. Among teenagers with ulcer disease, a male predominance is seen, with boys outnumbering girls nearly 4:1. Older children and adolescents generally present with abdominal pain, which is classically described as waxing and waning, sharp or gnawing, and localized to the epigastrium. It may awaken the child at night or in the early hours of the morning. Other historical clues include a family history of ulcer disease and the presence of predisposing factors such as smoking or regular use of NSAIDs.

Initial Assessment/H&P. History should focus on the presence of hematemesis and whether melanotic stools have been passed. Physical examination may reveal orthostasis, pallor, as well as abdominal tenderness, which is poorly localized in young children, but localized to the epigastrium or to the right of the midline in older children and adolescents. Stool should be tested for occult blood. The remainder of the physical examination should include an oral examination looking for dental enamel erosion, which would suggest chronic gastroesophageal reflux (GER) or recurrent emesis, and an examination of the lungs for wheezing, which also might suggest bronchospasm due to or exacerbated by reflux. Weight loss may be noted.

Management/Diagnostic Testing. A CBC and fecal occult blood test are good screening tests when one is considering the possibility of significant PUD. If physical examination findings reveal significant abdominal tenderness with guarding or rebound tenderness, plain radiographs of the abdomen including an upright view should be obtained to evaluate for perforation or secondary bowel obstruction. IV access should be obtained in all patients who have significant emesis, dehydration, weight loss, or concerning abdominal examination findings. An initial bolus of normal saline (20 mL per kg) should be given and vital signs monitored frequently, with additional boluses given as needed to achieve hemodynamic stability.

An upper GI series is not recommended for the routine evaluation of PUD given its relatively poor sensitivity. However, it may be useful in diagnosing children with gastric outlet obstruction secondary to PUD. Noninvasive *H. pylori* testing using either fecal antigen testing and/or C13 urea breath test should be undertaken in all patients for whom an obvious cause of secondary gastric or duodenal ulceration (e.g., NSAIDs, stress, sepsis, or burns) does not exist. Practice guidelines by the North American Society for Pediatric Gastroenterology, Hepatology, and Nutrition (NASPGHAN) recommend initial diagnostic *H. pylori* testing with positive histopathology on EGD plus a positive rapid urease test or a positive culture. Tissue culturing of the organism may assist in the determination of appropriate antibiotic therapy, particularly in communities where antibiotic resistance is high. Serologic tests based on the detection of antibodies (IgG, IgA) against *H. pylori* in serum, whole blood, urine, and saliva are not reliable for use in the clinical setting.

A number of approaches are available for the treatment of PUD. Therapies can be categorized as those that neutralize acid (i.e., antacids), block acid secretion, are cytoprotective, or are anti-infective. Antacids are a low-cost, safe, primarily short-term means of treating PUD in children. They can be prescribed for patients of any age. Adverse effects of antacids are related to the metal ion present in the preparation: Magnesium-containing products may cause diarrhea, whereas aluminum-containing products may cause constipation. Some products are available as a combination of the two to minimize these effects. The usual dosage for children is 0.5 mL per kg, given 1 hour after eating and before going to the bed. Patients with food-related or nocturnal abdominal pain without associated signs of serious illness can be started on empirical therapy with antacids, and followed by a primary care physician.

H_2-receptor antagonists (e.g., ranitidine or famotidine) are used to block acid secretion and treat ulcer disease. Alternatively PPIs (e.g., omeprazole or lansoprazole) can be used and are more effective at decreasing gastric acid secretion than H_2-receptor antagonists. PPIs should be used in patients with anemia or who have moderate to severe PUD. Potential short-term adverse effects with PPI usage include headache, abdominal pain, diarrhea, nausea, and vomiting. When initiating therapy, follow-up is important, as is providing a sufficient quantity so that the child can take the medication until the outpatient visit has occurred.

Sucralfate (40 to 80 mg/kg/day by mouth every 6 hours) is an aluminum salt that insulates the gastric mucosa from further damage by acid, pepsin, or bile. It is recommended to be given on an empty stomach 1 hour before meals and at bedtime, and not given at the same time as other medications given its ability to bind them.

Current protocols for first-line therapy for *H. pylori* include a PPI plus two antibiotics (choosing two of the following: amoxicillin, clarithromycin, or metronidazole for 10 to 14 days). Compliance is an important consideration because it is a major determinant of the success of treatment. Antibiotic susceptibility testing for clarithromycin is recommended before initial clarithromycin-based triple therapy in areas/populations with a known high resistance rate (>20%) as this will adversely affect eradication rates.

Mallory–Weiss Tears/Prolapse Gastropathy

Mallory–Weiss tears are mucosal lacerations of the distal esophagus and proximal stomach induced by forceful retching. Patients typically present with a recent history of repeated vomiting prior to onset of the hematemesis and less frequently, with pain from the tear. While the amount of blood can vary, Mallory–Weiss tears usually are self-limited and do not require any medical or surgical intervention. Upper GI bleeding after retching or vomiting may also be due to prolapse gastropathy, when the stomach prolapses through the lower esophageal sphincter causing mucosal injury. Management is generally conservative with antiemetic therapy, PPI, and observation.

Lower GI Bleeding

Inflammatory Bowel Disease

Goals of Treatment. The goals of emergency therapy include initial supportive care and the identification of any IBD complication. These complications may include perforation, intra-abdominal or perirectal abscess, toxic megacolon, severe anemia, electrolyte imbalances, superinfection, and dehydration. In severe cases initial supportive care may include rehydration, addressing electrolyte abnormalities, and packed red blood cell transfusions. Diagnostic tests to assess the presence and/or severity of the disease include laboratory markers, stool testing, and radiologic imaging. Communication with gastroenterologists and, when needed, surgeons helps to ensure efficient and directed care.

CLINICAL PEARLS AND PITFALLS

- Lower GI bleeding in a child with IBD should not immediately be attributed to a flare of the chronic underlying disease as these children often receive immunosuppressive therapies and are at high risk for infections (e.g., *Clostridium difficile*).
- In an ill-appearing child with Crohn's disease and fever, the clinician should consider intra-abdominal abscess and perforation in the differential diagnosis.
- Children with IBD may have extraintestinal manifestations including arthralgia, arthritis, muscle diseases, erythema nodosum, and ocular manifestations such as uveitis.
- Narcotic and anticholinergic usage should be avoided when possible in children with IBD colitis to avoid toxic megacolon.
- Pancreatitis should be considered with acute worsening of abdominal pain in children with IBD, particularly those on thiopurine (e.g., azathioprine or 6-MP) therapy.

Current Evidence. IBD is primarily used to describe two chronic lifelong intestinal disorders: (i) Ulcerative colitis (UC), characterized by inflammation and ulceration confined to the colonic mucosa; and (ii) Crohn's disease, manifested by transmural inflammation that may affect any segment of the GI tract. The incidence of IBD, particularly of Crohn's disease, has been increasing in children and adults with an estimated 1.17 million Americans having IBD. The etiology of IBD is unclear but is thought to result from a confluence of host genetic makeup and environmental factors. One of the most important risk factors is a family history of the disease.

IBD likely results from the inappropriate and ongoing activation of the GI mucosal immune system driven by the presence of normal bacterial flora. Growth failure is common in children with IBD. The cause of growth failure in patients with IBD is multifactorial, but inadequate nutrient intake is most likely the final common pathway. Malabsorption, especially with small bowel involvement of the disease, may also occur and micronutrient deficiencies may result in part from the area of intestine affected (e.g., duodenal inflammation is associated with iron deficiency). Hematochezia, protein-losing enteropathy, and increased fecal losses of cellular constituents result from chronic inflammation and damage to the intestinal mucosa. The cause of diarrhea is also multifactorial, resulting from extensive mucosal dysfunction, bile acid malabsorption in terminal ileal disease, bacterial overgrowth secondary to strictures and disordered motility, and protein exudation from inflamed surfaces. Extraintestinal manifestations of the disease are often partially the result of a breakdown in the normal barrier and immunoregulatory functions of the GI tract as a result of chronic inflammation.

Clinical Considerations

Clinical Recognition. Clinical manifestations of IBD can be varied and related to either GI inflammation or the development of either GI tract or extraintestinal complications. Many clinical features are common to both UC and Crohn's disease, including diarrhea, GI blood and protein loss, abdominal pain, fever, anemia, weight loss, and growth failure. Children with UC are more likely to present with rectal bleeding, diarrhea, and tenesmus. In contrast, children with Crohn's disease are more likely to present with chronic abdominal pain, weight loss, and failure to thrive. Perianal disease, including fissures, skin tags, fistulae, and abscesses, occurs in 15% of children with Crohn's disease but not in UC. Perianal disease may precede the appearance of the intestinal manifestations of Crohn's disease by several years. Extraintestinal manifestations involving the joints (arthritis), skin (erythema nodosum), eyes (uveitis), and liver (chronic hepatitis or sclerosing cholangitis) are seen with both disorders, although they are generally more common with Crohn's disease.

Abdominal pain and diarrhea with or without occult blood are the most common symptoms at presentation. The pain is often colicky and occurs soon before or during bowel movements in UC. In Crohn's disease, given possible ileal involvement, the abdominal pain may localize to the right lower quadrant. The abdominal examination may elicit guarding and rebound tenderness prompting consideration of acute appendicitis in the differential diagnosis. Eliciting a history of chronic symptoms and identification of inflammation of other portions of intestine beyond the appendix alone during the evaluation may aid in differentiating IBD from appendicitis.

IBD occasionally causes massive upper or lower GI bleeding due to intestinal mucosal breakdown and potential involvement of blood vessels underneath. Rarely, due to the ability of Crohn's disease to cause fibrostenosing inflammation, children may present with complete intestinal obstruction. Partial obstruction from significant intraluminal narrowing from stricturing disease, often in the ileum, is more common. Children with Crohn's disease may develop intra-abdominal abscesses or fistulas due to the transmural nature of the inflammation.

The presence of significant abdominal distention, accompanied by diminished or absent bowel sounds, should raise the suspicion of actual or impending perforation, even in the absence of severe pain. Perforation may occur even after minor abdominal trauma and must be ruled out when patients with known IBD complain of abdominal pain after trauma.

In addition the development of massive colonic distention, termed toxic megacolon, is a rare complication of both UC and Crohn's disease. Toxic megacolon represents a life-threatening emergency that has a reported mortality rate of as high as 25%. Although rare in children, up to half of the cases occur with the first attack of IBD; another 40% are seen in patients receiving high-dose steroid therapy for fulminant colitis. Toxic megacolon almost always involves the transverse colon. The pathophysiology is believed to be an extension of the inflammatory process through all layers of the bowel wall, with resulting microperforation, localized ileus, and loss of colonic tone. The result is imminent major perforation, peritonitis, and overwhelming sepsis. Antecedent barium enema, opiates, or anticholinergics may all precipitate toxic megacolon. Clinical features include (i) a rapidly worsening clinical course usually associated with fever, malaise, and even lethargy; (ii) abdominal distention and tenderness usually developing over a few hours or days; (iii) a temperature of 38.5°C (101.3°F) or higher and a neutrophilic leukocytosis; and (iv) an abdominal radiograph showing distention of the transverse colon of more than 5 to 7 cm. In a recent case-control study of children with toxic megacolon, fever, tachycardia, dehydration, and electrolyte abnormalities were significantly more common than in age-matched controls with UC without toxic megacolon. The differential diagnosis of acute fulminant colitis includes acute bacterial enteritis, amebic dysentery, ischemic bowel disease, and radiation colitis.

Other potential clinical manifestations of IBD related to extraintestinal complications include thrombosis of cerebral, retinal, or peripheral vessels that may lead to coma, seizures, or focal visual or motor deficits; gallstone cholecystitis; renal calculi leading to hematuria; and pancreatitis. Pancreatitis, in particular, should be considered in an IBD patient on thiopurine maintenance therapy.

Triage. Children with initial presentations of significant GI hemorrhage, toxicity from toxic megacolon, severe dehydration or perforation will be triaged rapidly with standard triage protocols. Children with known IBD presenting with symptoms of a flare (e.g., abdominal pain and diarrhea) with a fever should be evaluated more promptly. The differential includes infectious etiology (e.g., *C. difficile*), toxic megacolon, or intra-abdominal abscess (more so in Crohn's disease). *C. difficile* in particular has become a significant clinical challenge in children with IBD with increased amounts of colonization and infection being reported. Children with signs of orthostasis, dehydration, significant abdominal pain, or active lower GI bleeding may also need to be evaluated promptly.

Initial Assessment/H&P. The initial medical history should be detailed, including family history, for any potential new diagnoses of IBD. Physical examination should include ophthalmic, skin, joint, and perianal evaluation in addition to a comprehensive abdominal examination. In those with an established diagnosis of IBD, medication compliance and identification of medications used for the disease should be completed, particularly those which are immunosuppressive (e.g., steroids). The H&P should also be directed to identify other potential etiologies associated with painful rectal bleeding including intussusception, Henoch–Schönlein purpura (HSP), and hemolytic uremic syndrome (HUS).

Management/Diagnostic Testing. Abdominal radiography, including an upright view, is indicated in cases of suspected partial or full obstruction, toxic megacolon, or perforation. Abdominal ultrasound is the preferred initial modality to evaluate for an abscess, and has a sensitivity approaching 90% and specificity approaching 100% to identify bowel inflammation. Computed tomographic (CT) imaging should be used sparingly and only if urgent information related to inflammation or a possible extraenteric complication is needed, as children with IBD have been identified as having moderately increased exposure to radiation over the course of their chronic disease. MRI enterography has gained favor for a nonradiation method when further delineation beyond ultrasound is desired and may be completed once the child is admitted or in the outpatient setting.

LABORATORY TESTING. Laboratory evaluation should include a CBC with differential, chemistry panel (chem 10, especially in those with chronic diarrhea or vomiting), liver panel (albumin, protein, aminotransferases, bilirubin), erythrocyte sedimentation rate (ESR), C-reactive protein, amylase, and lipase. ESR is elevated in up to 80% of patients with newly diagnosed Crohn's disease and in 60% of those with newly diagnosed UC. It may also be used to assess the efficacy of therapies in those with previously diagnosed IBD. A blood type and crossmatch is indicated in cases of suspected or confirmed severe anemia. Stool testing for *C. difficile,* stool culture, as well as ova and parasites should be obtained. Increasingly, fecal calprotectin, a protein produced by neutrophils, is being used to help diagnose IBD and monitor the severity of inflammation in those with established disease.

MANAGEMENT. Management is guided by the history, physical, and diagnostic testing. The role of the ED physician is to provide supportive care while ensuring a significant medical complication (e.g., significant dehydration, electrolyte imbalance, severe anemia, superinfection) or potential complication requiring surgical intervention (e.g., toxic megacolon, intra-abdominal or perirectal abscess, perforation) is identified and addressed if present.

Initial supportive medical care includes rehydration with crystalloid per established protocols. Blood transfusions may be required in those with severe anemia. If toxic megacolon or perforation is suspected, arrangements should be made for admission to an intensive care unit (ICU) and for surgical consultation. An NG tube should be placed. Patients should be started on aggressive doses of broad-spectrum antibiotics such as piperacillin/tazobactam. Suitable alternative therapies may include ampicillin/sulbactam, or cefoxitin in combination with gentamicin.

Management of significant GI bleeding should be performed as described in Chapter 28 Gastrointestinal Bleeding. Emergency management of suspected intestinal obstruction includes gastric decompression with NG drainage and IV rehydration, initially with normal saline. Prompt surgical consultation is required in cases of perforation or toxic megacolon. Concomitant consultation by a pediatric gastroenterologist and surgeon may be indicated with identification of an intra-abdominal or perirectal abscess, fistulizing disease, and partial or complete obstruction to coordinate care during an admission.

Clinical Indications for Discharge or Admission

- The diagnosis of IBD is based on a combination of clinical, pathologic, and radiologic data. In those cases where a medical or surgical emergency is not identified, and diagnostic testing has been completed or started (e.g., stool infectious workup), then discharge of a child with suspected IBD with close follow-up by a pediatric gastroenterologist is appropriate. Further diagnostic studies such as esophagogastroduodenoscopy, colonoscopy, or GI contrast studies can be arranged on an outpatient basis. The initiation of therapies such as corticosteroids, aminosalicylic acid compounds (e.g., mesalamine), immunomodulators (e.g., 6-mercaptopurine), or biologics (e.g., infliximab) can started on an outpatient basis, often after confirmation of the diagnosis.
- Psychosocial factors such as concern for possible negligence by the child's guardians, poor history of follow-up, or significant abdominal pain which cannot be managed at home, may also result in hospital admission. Patients with known IBD who are deemed to have mild to moderate flares may only require adjustments of their IBD maintenance regimen and can be discharged from the ED with close follow-up with their gastroenterologist.
- Severe anemia requiring red blood cell transfusion, failure to maintain adequate hydration, electrolyte imbalances requiring rehydration and replacement, and severe failure to thrive are indications for supportive care and admission. Those children with suspected IBD or known IBD in whom a significant medical or surgical manifestation has occurred should be admitted to the appropriate care setting. Children with suspected severe colitis and frequent bloody bowel movements but with normal hemoglobin values should be considered for admission if close follow-up cannot be arranged.
- Children with known IBD with a significant flare may be admitted for modification of existing therapies or initiation of new therapies in consultation with the child's gastroenterologist. There is increasing use of biologics (e.g., infliximab) in children with IBD early in their course in conjunction with immunomodulators (e.g., azathioprine, mercaptopurine) which will translate to ED physicians seeing more children with established IBD on strong immunosuppressive therapies.

Dietary Protein Gastrointestinal Disorders

Goals of Treatment

The initial goals of therapy for dietary protein GI disorders are to identify the suspected protein and remove it from the diet. In the vast majority of cases reassurance, making a dietary change recommendation, and ensuring close follow-up is all that is needed.

CLINICAL PEARLS AND PITFALLS

- Lower GI bleeding in an otherwise healthy-appearing infant is most often dietary protein–induced proctocolitis. Complete resolution of bleeding after an effective dietary change may take several weeks.
- Infants with dietary protein disorders may present with vomiting, diarrhea, and/or shock. Food protein–induced enterocolitis syndrome (FPIES) should be of particular consideration when a child presents with one, or especially, multiple episodes of shock.
- Esophageal food impaction may be the first presentation of a child with eosinophilic esophagitis (EE). The diagnosis of EE should be considered in a child with multiple food impactions without a known anatomic contributor.
- Laboratory and stool testing available to the ED physician is not sensitive in these dietary protein disorders but may include peripheral eosinophilia on a CBC with differential. Stool specimens may also demonstrate elevated eosinophils when testing for fecal leukocytes.

Current Evidence

Food allergy affects nearly 8% of children. Dietary proteins may induce significant bowel injury via both IgE and non–IgE-based immunologic mechanisms. Children may present with GER, dysphagia, colic, abdominal pain, and/or constipation. The symptoms correlate with the portion of GI tract affected (e.g., dysphagia is seen in EE). These allergic diseases begin at different ages with FPIES and allergic proctitis affecting primarily infants while EE more typically is seen in early childhood and later. The symptoms resolve after the offending protein(s) are eliminated from the diet.

Clinical Considerations

Clinical Recognition. The typical presentation of milk-protein sensitivity (allergic) colitis is that of acute onset of blood-streaked, mucoid stool in an otherwise well-appearing infant often younger than 3 months. Blood loss is typically limited, so infants do not appear acutely ill or dehydrated. They are afebrile, and weight gain has typically been normal since birth. In contrast, children with FPIES may present with significant vomiting, diarrhea, and dehydration resulting in shock. Children with EE often have other chronic symptoms which mimic GER but are more likely to present to the ED acutely in the case of food impaction.

Initial Assessment/H&P. Dietary history including any recent changes in the child's diet or, in the case of breast-feeding infants the mother's diet, should be noted. A past medical history of asthma, eczema, or rhinitis may be helpful in older children. A strong family history of atopy or food allergy may be found. With infants with rectal bleeding, external anal fissures can be ruled out by careful physical examination. Identification of eczema may support the diagnosis.

Management/Diagnostic Testing. Infants with allergic proctocolitis are rarely hemodynamically unstable or seriously ill; therefore, initial ED management is focused on making a presumptive diagnosis based on history and physical examination, initiating appropriate dietary therapy (e.g., partially hydrolyzed formula), and arranging adequate follow-up with the patient's primary care physician or a pediatric gastroenterologist. One might consider obtaining CBC count with white blood cell (WBC) differential to assess the hemoglobin level and check for eosinophilia in cases which are severe, refractory, or where there is concern for anemia. Examination of stool for blood, fecal leukocytes, bacterial culture should be performed on infants who have proven refractory to dietary therapy or if there is a known exposure. *C. difficile* may also be considered though infants may be colonized with this organism. Infants who have milk-protein sensitivity colitis will characteristically have leukocytes seen on fecal smear and eosinophils may also be present. In cases of suspected food impaction, a two-view CXR is often obtained but often does not identify the nonradiopaque food item.

Treatment consists of identifying and eliminating the offending protein from the diet. There is generally improvement in symptoms within 72 hours of the dietary change, though complete resolution may take weeks. Guaiac-positive stools may also persist for several weeks.

Mothers of breast-feeding infants may be asked to eliminate milk protein or other suspected culprit proteins from their diet, but breast-feeding can often be continued. Infants receiving cow's milk-based or soy protein formulas should be changed to a formula containing casein hydrolysate as the protein source. Nutramigen, Pregestimil, and Alimentum are currently available in the United States. Occasionally, in patients with severe allergic colitis or FPIES, an amino acid–based elemental formula, such as Neocate or Elecare, is recommended.

Children with EE presenting with food impaction require removal of the impaction by either gastroenterology, surgery, or ENT, depending on institutional protocol.

Clinical Indications for Discharge or Admission. Most children can be safely discharged from the emergency department. Parents should be counseled that infants who respond to dietary elimination should not be challenged with a milk- or soy-based formula until 1 year of age. Allergic symptoms may also change with age, such as the development of vomiting and diarrhea in addition to GI bleeding. Infants with evidence of persistent gross bleeding 2 weeks following formula change require further evaluation and potential consideration for a more intensive dietary change or workup for an alternative diagnosis.

Children with vital sign instability, significant failure to thrive, failure to gain weight on amino acid–based formulas, or significant anemia should be considered for admission and more extensive evaluation.

Additional Causes of Gastrointestinal Bleeding

Hemolytic Uremic Syndrome

HUS is a disorder characterized by the triad of acute microangiopathic hemolytic anemia, thrombocytopenia, and oliguric renal failure (see Chapter 108 Renal and Electrolyte Emergencies). The disease is heralded by a prodrome of intestinal symptoms, typically with abdominal cramps and diarrhea. While initially nonbloody, 70% of patients experience hemorrhagic colitis within 1 to 2 days. Fever (30%)

and vomiting (30% to 60%) are also commonly seen. Acute infectious gastroenteritis or colitis secondary to infection with *Escherichia coli* O157:H7 is responsible for 70% of cases of HUS in North America and Western Europe. Acute renal failure occurs in 55% to 70% of patients.

All children with HUS require admission to the hospital. Laboratory studies should be obtained, including a CBC count, platelet count, PT, PTT, electrolytes, blood urea nitrogen (BUN), and creatinine. IV access needs to be secured for the correction of dehydration and the potential administration of blood products. The GI manifestations of HUS usually resolve without sequelae or the need for antibiotic treatment of the initial intestinal infection.

Henoch–Schönlein Purpura

HSP is a systemic vasculitis that may cause edema and hemorrhage in the intestinal wall. Peak age of onset is between 3 and 7 years and the male to female ratio is 2:1. The presentation consists of the onset of a purpuric rash, typically confined to the buttocks and lower extremities, followed by arthralgias, angioedema, and diffuse abdominal pain. GI symptoms may precede the usual cutaneous symptoms and include abdominal pain (60% to 70%), occult bleeding (50%), gross bleeding (30%), massive hemorrhage (5% to 10%), and intussusception (3%). All children with suspected HSP and GI symptoms should have a stool guaiac test performed, as well as a urinalysis to monitor for the onset of renal involvement (nephritis). Children with HSP limited to the involvement of the skin and joints can often be managed as outpatients. However, severe abdominal pain or GI hemorrhage is an indication for admission.

Gastrointestinal Vascular Malformations

GI vascular malformations, including hemangiomas, angiodysplasia, Dieulafoy lesions, and arteriovenous malformations (AVMs), are rare causes of GI bleeding in children and are most often seen as a part of congenital syndromes such as Klippel–Trenaunay–Weber syndrome. Diffuse visceral hemangiomatosis is rare, often fatal, and is always associated with cutaneous vascular lesions. GI hemangiomatosis should be suspected in any child with unexplained anemia and a syndrome of cutaneous hemangiomas.

Intestinal AVMs are rare in the pediatric age group, may occur both as solitary and as multiple AVMs, and are typically part of a congenital syndrome (e.g., Osler–Weber–Rendu disease). Many GI vascular malformations, particularly cavernous hemangiomas and AVMs, can be detected using CT scans with IV contrast. Intestinal angiography or tagged red blood cell scans are often used to identify the source of bleeding during an acute hemorrhage. ED management of patients with GI bleeding from vascular malformations is the same as for any patient with potentially significant blood loss. After initial stabilization, referral to an appropriate subspecialty consultation for final diagnosis and definitive treatment is warranted.

Foreign Bodies

Swallowed foreign bodies can cause significant trauma and GI bleeding. Eighty percent to 90% of ingested foreign bodies are able to pass without intervention, even those with sharp edges (Fig. 99.2). Approximately 10% to 20% must be removed endoscopically, and only approximately 1% requires surgery. Removal by endoscopy is indicated if significant bleeding occurs or if the foreign body is retained in the esophagus. Consideration for endoscopic and/or surgical removal should be made if the foreign body is causing symptoms (e.g., obstruction), involves multiple magnets, or is greater than 5 cm in length (see Chapter 27 Foreign Body: Ingestion and Aspiration).

PANCREATITIS

Goals of Treatment

Pancreatitis can be difficult to diagnose in children and is often overlooked as it is uncommon and no specific pathognomonic symptoms are associated with the condition. The goal of ED management is to make an early diagnosis, recognize any potential causative factors, and address any complications that may already be present at the time of presentation. Once identified, the goals of medical treatment include suppression of pancreatic secretion, relief of pain, and treatment of early complications such as hypovolemia, hypocalcemia, respiratory distress, and potential infection.

CLINICAL PEARLS AND PITFALLS

- Pancreatitis should be considered in any child with acute or chronic epigastric abdominal pain, vomiting, or ascites of unknown origin. Approximately 30% to 40% of cases are associated with an infectious agent or after blunt trauma.
- Mild trauma from small pointed objects, such as sticks, handlebars, or fence posts, may transmit injury directly to the organ.
- Secondary complications may be present at the time of the initial ED visit and can contribute greatly to morbidity and mortality.
- Serum amylase and lipase levels may not correlate with severity of disease.

Current Evidence

Pancreatitis in children is uncommon, however the incidence is increasing. In infants and toddlers, pancreatitis is most commonly associated with multisystem disease such as HUS or pulmonary disease. In older children and adolescents, the most common cause of pancreatitis remains unknown or "idiopathic" followed closely by trauma and structural disease. Many patients who were previously labeled idiopathic have been found to have genetic abnormalities such as a cystic fibrosis transmembrane regulator (CFTR) mutation. Table 99.3 lists the causes of pancreatitis. Regardless of the initiating event, acute pancreatitis results in the activation of the numerous pancreatic enzymes, including proteolytic enzymes, lipase, amylase, elastase, and phospholipase A, which causes autodigestion of the gland. The process may be focal or diffuse. Mild disease, or *acute edematous pancreatitis,* is by far the most common form seen in children, is usually self-limited, and associated with complete recovery. *Necrotic* or *hemorrhagic pancreatitis,* occurs when the autodigestive process intensifies with increased inflammation, fat necrosis, and hemorrhagic changes. It is associated with significant morbidity and mortality, with the mortality rate

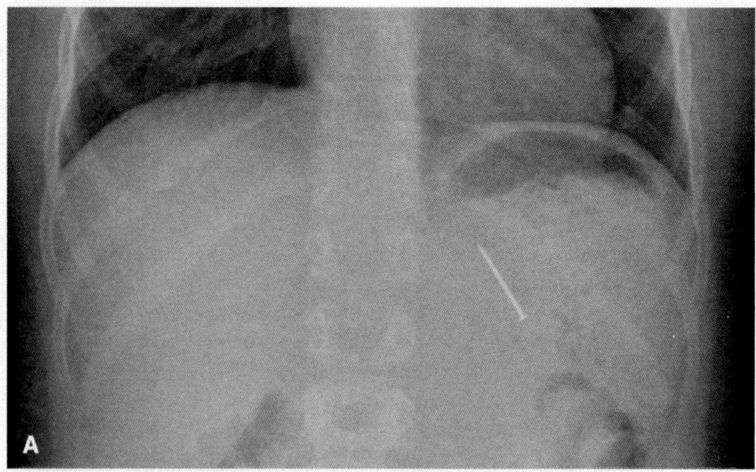

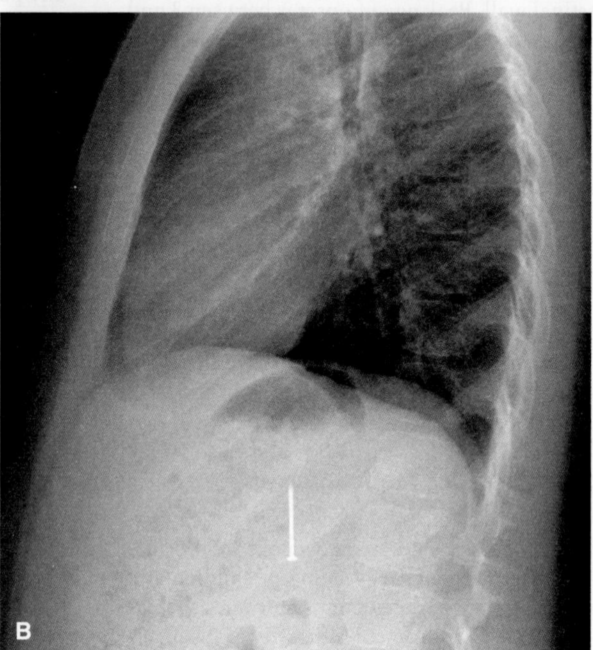

FIGURE 99.2 **A, B:** Gastric foreign body. A 9-year-old female accidentally ingested a 2.7-cm nail when hanging stockings and was holding nail in her mouth.

approaching 10%. Complications from severe pancreatitis include pseudocyst formation, necrosis, secondary bacterial infections, acute respiratory distress syndrome, shock, multiorgan system failure, and death. Early in the disease it is difficult to predict which patients are at risk for severe disease and a poor prognosis. There are several well-validated scoring systems in adults, including the Modified Glasgow score, Ranson criteria, and APACHE II, however they have been shown to be poor predictors of outcome in children.

Clinical Considerations

Clinical Recognition

The majority of children with acute pancreatitis initially present with nonspecific signs and symptoms. Abdominal pain (87%) and vomiting (64%) are the most common presenting symptoms. The character of the abdominal pain may range from tolerable distress to severe incapacitating pain. Classically, the pain is constant and localized to the epigastrium and may radiate to the back (left or right scapula) or to the right or left upper quadrants. The pain is classically described as knifelike in quality and is aggravated when the patient lies supine. Vomiting may be severe and protracted. Fever, abdominal distention, and jaundice may also be present. In cases of severe necrotic pancreatitis, patients may complain of dizziness or present with hypotension and shock. Mental status changes including psychosis and coma are common in necrotic pancreatitis.

Triage Considerations

Most patients with pancreatitis present with nonspecific signs and symptoms and are hemodynamically stable. A minority of patients, especially those with necrotic or hemorrhagic disease may present in shock or jaundice. These patients require immediate recognition and appropriate stabilization.

Clinical Assessment

The abdomen may be distended but is usually not rigid, and the patient may prefer sitting or lying on their side with knees flexed. There may be mild to moderate voluntary guarding in

TABLE 99.3

CAUSES OF ACUTE PANCREATITIS IN CHILDREN

Trauma: blunt, penetrating, surgical
Infectious: mumps, coxsackievirus B infection, hemolytic *Streptococcus* infection, *Salmonella* infection, hepatitis A and B
Obstructive: cholelithiasis, ascaris infection, congenital duodenal stenosis, duplications, tumor, choledochal cyst
Drugs: steroids, chlorothiazides, salicylazosulfapyridine, azathioprine, alcohol, valproic acid, tetracyclines, borates, oral contraceptives
Systemic: systemic lupus erythematosus, periarteritis nodosa, malnutrition, peptic ulcer, uremia
Endocrine: hyperparathyroidism
Metabolic: hypercholesterolemia, cystic fibrosis, vitamin A and D deficiency
Hereditary
Idiopathic

the epigastrium. A palpable epigastric mass suggests pseudocyst. Ascites is rare. Bowel sounds may be decreased or absent. Associated physical findings may include signs of parotitis, mild hepatosplenomegaly, epigastric mass, pleural effusions, and mild icterus. Although rare, rebound tenderness or a rigid abdomen is a poor prognostic sign. Similarly, a bluish discoloration around the umbilicus (Cullen sign) or flanks (Grey Turner sign) is rare in children but portends a poor prognosis and suggests a diagnosis of hemorrhagic pancreatitis. Signs of overt hemodynamic instability are rarely evident at initial presentation. It is particularly important to evaluate patients for clinical signs of hypocalcemia (Trousseau and Chvostek signs). Jaundice may suggest distal biliary obstruction.

Two easily attainable laboratory tests are used to diagnose pancreatitis: serum amylase and lipase. The combination of clinical symptoms and an elevation of the level of one or both of these enzymes, particularly if >3 times the upper limit of normal, strongly point to pancreatitis. There is some evidence to suggest that serum lipase may be a more sensitive marker for pancreatitis. A recent study of 320 patients with acute pancreatitis found that 18.8% of patients with acute pancreatitis did not have an elevated amylase on their initial ED visit, whereas only 2.9% of patients did not have an elevated serum lipase. It has been taught that amylase is more rapidly cleared whereas an elevated lipase may remain elevated for days after the acute onset of disease. While this is frequently true, it is not a reliable finding.

Elevated serum amylase and lipase levels are not pathognomonic for pancreatitis. Many clinical situations, including penetrating or perforated ulcer, intestinal obstruction or infarction, IBD, pneumonia, hepatitis, liver trauma, acute biliary tract disease, salpingitis, salivary adenitis, renal failure, diabetic ketoacidosis, and benign macroamylasemia can cause an amylase elevation. Serum lipase levels may be elevated with a perforated peptic ulcer or bone fracture with pulmonary fat embolism and remain elevated for up to 14 days after the onset of acute pancreatitis.

Ultrasound is a useful adjunctive test for the diagnosis of pancreatitis, as it can assess pancreatic size, contour, and the presence of calcifications or pseudocyst formation. Ultrasound should be considered in all cases of suspected pancreatitis, especially to evaluate for an obstructive etiology such as gallstones. Abdominal CT scan, magnetic resonance pancreatography, and endoscopic retrograde cholangiopancreatography (ERCP) are being used more often to assess the severity of pancreatitis and pseudocyst formation and to determine possible causes of pancreatitis. ERCP has the additional advantage of providing the option for therapeutic maneuvers such as stone removal or sphincterotomy.

Management

While not common, patients may present with hypotension and shock. IV fluids should be started immediately, and the patient's oral intake should be discontinued. Once the acute shock episode is resolved, IV fluids should be administered at 1.5 times the maintenance rate. Vital signs and urine output should be monitored frequently. Continuous NG suction should be started to prevent the delivery of gastric acid into the duodenum, which in turn diminishes hormonal stimulation of the pancreas. NG suction also relieves pain and prevents development of ileus. The use of anticholinergic or H_2-receptor antagonists to reduce gastric secretion is controversial and is not recommended in the initial management of patients. A crucial part of management is the treatment of abdominal pain. There is no strong evidence regarding the choice of pharmacologic agent for pain control.

Laboratory studies that should be performed in the ED in patients with severe disease should include amylase, lipase, CBC count, electrolytes, BUN, calcium, glucose, AST, ALT, bilirubin (direct and indirect), alkaline phosphatase, serum gamma-glutamyltransferase (GGT), triglyceride, PT, and PTT. A chest radiograph should be obtained and evaluated for pleural effusion, interstitial pneumonic infiltrates, and basilar atelectasis. A flat and upright abdominal radiograph can assist in evaluating for perforation, ascites, and pancreatic calcifications. An abdominal ultrasound should be performed.

Antibiotics are not routinely indicated in the initial management of pancreatitis; however, infection is very common with necrotizing pancreatitis and is associated with morbidity and mortality. Pancreatic abscess or superinfection should be considered if the patients present with fever and in those cases, broad-spectrum antibiotic coverage is indicated. Surgical consultation is indicated if active intraperitoneal bleeding, suspected abscess, biliary duct obstruction, or traumatic transection is suspected.

Clinical Indications for Admission

All patients with acute pancreatitis should be admitted to the hospital. The decision to admit to the ICU should be based on hemodynamic status and concern for complications.

BILIARY TRACT DISEASE

Biliary Atresia

Goals of Treatment

BA is uncommon, but is associated with very high morbidity and mortality. Excellent evidence suggests that a delay in diagnosis and subsequent treatment will have a significant negative impact. The goal of an ED physician is to suspect BA and facilitate its diagnosis and subsequent definitive surgical care to improve patient outcomes. In a patient who has undergone surgical correction, an ED physician must recognize that the patient is at high risk for ascending cholangitis and progression of their underlying disease leading to cirrhosis, portal hypertension, and ultimately liver failure requiring transplant.

CLINICAL PEARLS AND PITFALLS

- Liver and biliary tract diseases should be considered in any patient >1 week of age with persistent jaundice.
- BA should be considered in any young infant with even minimal conjugated hyperbilirubinemia (greater than normal) regardless of the ratio to unconjugated bilirubin.
- Patients with acholic stools should be investigated for biliary disease.
- Cholangitis is the most common complication after a hepatoportoenterostomy (Kasai) procedure.

Current Evidence

The incidence of BA varies based on geography, occurring most commonly in East Asia with an incidence of 1 in 5,000 births in Taiwan and 1 in 10,000 to 15,000 births in the United States. It is the leading cause of liver transplant and death from liver failure in children. There is no universal screening tool at present, although some countries have had success with stool color cards as a public health measure to help families identify acholic stools (Fig. 99.2). The cause of BA remains unknown. There are several subtypes of BA, but the end result in all patients is that there is an inflammatory process that destroys both intrahepatic and extrahepatic biliary tracts and leads to complete biliary obstruction, liver damage, progressive liver cirrhosis, and if untreated, death before age 2 to 3 years. Treatment is surgical, which restores biliary flow via a hepatoportoenterostomy. There is strong evidence that early diagnosis and surgical correction of BA improves both long-term morbidity and mortality. Patients who received surgical correction prior to 60 days of life had a 10-year survival rate of 73%, whereas patients who received surgery after 90 days of life had a 10-year survival rate of 11%. Unfortunately, the mean age for surgical correction in the United States is 65.5 days of life, which has not improved in the past 20 years. Up to 20% of patients have other congenital abnormalities. The most common co-occurring congenital abnormalities are splenic malformations (polysplenia), situs inversus, and other vascular abnormalities. Patients are also at risk for congenital cardiac defects and intestinal malrotation.

Clinical Considerations

Clinical Recognition. Patients with BA are generally well appearing on initial presentation. A clinician must have a high index of suspicion for patients with persistent jaundice. There are many causes of jaundice in a newborn (see Chapters 39 Jaundice: Conjugated Hyperbilirubinemia and 40 Jaundice: Unconjugated Hyperbilirubinemia). In general, 15% of newborns are jaundiced at 2 weeks of age and 2% to 6% at 4 weeks of age. Persistent jaundice beyond 2 weeks of age should be evaluated for possible BA with a measurement of serum conjugated bilirubin.

Triage Considerations. In most patients, there are no specific triage considerations for patients with BA as they are typically well appearing. While uncommon, if a patient presents after the newborn period with jaundice, it is possible that they could already have advanced liver disease, portal hypertension, and splenomegaly.

Clinical Assessment. Patients are typically well appearing and present with persistent jaundice. Acholic stools, dark brown urine, and failure to thrive may also be present. On examination, there may not be any physical findings other than skin discoloration and icterus, yet splenomegaly may be present if a patient has developed portal hypertension. Dysmorphic features may be identified that likely suggest another disorder, such as Alagille syndrome (AS) (see section below).

Initial laboratory evaluation of any patient with persistent jaundice should include a serum conjugated bilirubin level. If the newborn has a conjugated hyperbilirubinemia, BA should be suspected and high on the differential. Other laboratory abnormalities may demonstrate a cholestatic disease process with an elevation in liver function enzymes (AST, ALT), serum GGT, and alkaline phosphatase. Synthetic liver function is generally normal early in the course of the disease, and most patients are not hypoalbuminemic or coagulopathic.

Ultrasound is an important initial step in evaluation of a patient with possible BA. Findings may include hepatomegaly, an absent or atretic gallbladder, or the "triangular cord sign" which is a hyperechoic area that results from a fibrous hepatic duct. This finding is operator dependent and has reported sensitivities of 49% to 80%, but if found may be 98% specific. Bile duct dilation is never present. If inconclusive, additional diagnostic testing may be performed in consultation with Gastroenterology and Surgery to differentiate BA from other cholestatic disease processes.

In patients who have already been diagnosed and undergone surgical repair, the most common complication is cholangitis, occurring in up to 55% of patients in the first 2 years after surgery. Many patients also develop portal hypertension (see section on portal hypertension), hepatic malignancy, or hepatopulmonary syndrome which results in increased pulmonary vascular blood flow and hypoxia. Patients may also present with worsening cirrhosis and liver failure as a result of progression of their underlying disease.

Management. The most important role for the emergency physician in managing a patient with BA is early identification of the disorder. Once the diagnosis is made, management is primarily surgical. In patients with a conjugated hyperbilirubinemia, ED providers should further evaluate for cholestasis (total and fractionated bilirubin, GGT, alkaline phosphatase), aminotransferase elevation (AST, ALT), and liver function (albumin, PT/INR, PTT) (see Figure 39.1 for further information on the workup of Conjugated Hyperbilirubinemia). Patients should also receive an abdominal ultrasound with Doppler to assess for other anatomic causes as well as obstruction and chest x-ray to assess for possible vertebral body changes or rib cage changes suggestive of Alagille's. The patient should be urgently referred to Gastroenterology and Pediatric Surgery.

Cholelithiasis/Cholecystitis

Gallstones or cholelithiasis occasionally occur in adolescents. Often the condition remains asymptomatic until a complication develops, such as cholecystitis. It is primarily seen in patients with hemolytic anemias (pigment stones) such as sickle cell disease and hereditary spherocytosis, however it becoming increasingly common in otherwise healthy children, likely as a result of childhood obesity and diabetes. Other risk factors for developing gallstones includes the use of total parenteral nutrition (TPN), systemic infection, antibiotic use, biliary anatomic abnormalities, cystic fibrosis, increased estrogen, and family history. While not nearly as common in adults, children do account for 4% of all cholecystectomies, and two-thirds are female.

Biliary colic results from acute transient obstruction of the cystic duct or common bile duct by gallstone(s). Cholecystitis is an aseptic inflammatory process that develops as a reaction to chemical injury triggered by obstruction to the cystic duct by a gallstone. Cholangitis results from secondary bacterial infection by enteric organisms in the face of biliary tract obstruction or after surgical manipulation of the biliary tract. Acute cholangitis may be mild and superficial, producing only short-lived symptoms, or it may be severe, causing suppurative cholangitis with septic shock and formation of hepatic abscesses.

The pain of biliary colic is acute in onset, often follows a meal, and is usually localized to the epigastrium or right upper quadrant. Some children localize the pain to the periumbilical area. In contrast to the colicky pain of intestinal or ureteral origin, biliary colic does not worsen in relatively short cyclic paroxysms or bursts but instead is characterized by its sustained, intense quality. Unlike pancreatitis, the patient tends to move about restlessly and the pain is not improved by changes in position. In addition, referred pain is common, particularly to the dorsal lumbar back near the tip of the right scapula. Nausea and vomiting are commonly associated with biliary colic but are not severe and protracted as seen with pancreatitis. Mild jaundice occurs in 25% of patients. An attack of acute cholecystitis begins with biliary colic, which increases progressively in severity or duration. Pain lasting longer than 4 hours suggests cholecystitis and the temperature is usually mildly elevated. As the inflammation worsens, the pain changes character, becoming more generalized in the upper abdomen and increased by deep respiration and jarring motions.

In contrast, acute cholangitis should be suspected in the patient who has right upper quadrant abdominal pain, shaking chills with spiking fever, and jaundice (Charcot triad). These patients usually have a history of abdominal surgery. A dangerous aspect of this disorder is that overwhelming sepsis can develop rapidly. Listlessness and shock are characteristic of advanced or severe cholangitis and usually reflect gram-negative septicemia. Cholangitis can evolve rapidly before the development of significant jaundice. Clinically apparent jaundice may be absent even in postsurgical BA patients.

Laboratory tests are typically nonspecific in cholecystitis. A CBC and blood smear may show evidence of hemolysis. The leukocyte count averages 12,000 to 15,000 per mm^3 with a neutrophilic leukocytosis. Elevated leukocyte counts raise concern for cholangitis. The level of serum bilirubin may be elevated but rarely exceeds 4 mg per dL. Higher values are more compatible with either complete common bile duct obstruction or cholangitis. The levels of serum transaminases (ALT and AST) and alkaline phosphatase may be mildly elevated but are often normal. Marked elevation in the levels of transaminases may occur with acute, complete common duct obstruction. Serum amylase levels may be mildly elevated without other evidence of pancreatitis.

The general management for the ED physician includes discontinuation of oral intake, support with IV fluids, pain control, and surgical consultation. If acute cholangitis is suspected, antibiotics should be given empirically, with coverage directed toward enteric organisms. Blood cultures should be drawn prior to antibiotic administration.

Alagille Syndrome

AS is another cause of cholestasis in a newborn or infant, and is secondary to bile duct paucity. As such, it can be easily confused with BA. AS is a progressive disorder. Infants with AS may not have biliary paucity if their biopsy is performed before 6 months of life. In contrast, 90% of infants over 6 months of age will demonstrate biliary paucity on biopsy. The majority (95%) of patients less than 1 year of age will demonstrate cholestasis on laboratory evaluation, while their synthetic function is typically intact. Hepatomegaly under 1 year of age is common. Over months to years, however, patients' hepatic disease tends to worsen as the biliary tract deteriorates. With time, 10% to 50% of patients who initially present in infancy will develop severe portal hypertension, cirrhosis, or liver failure and 20% to 50% will require liver transplant.

In addition to cholestasis and hepatic disease, AS is associated with cardiac, renal, facial, and musculoskeletal abnormalities (Table 99.4). More recently, a particular genetic mutation (Jagged1) has been associated with AS, and aids in the diagnosis. On physical examination, ED providers may see syndromic facies, jaundice, excoriations secondary to extreme pruritus, hepatosplenomegaly, stigmata of portal hypertension (Table 99.2), xanthomas, heart murmur, or sequelae of congenital heart disease, such as cyanosis. In addition to cholestatic disease, congenital heart disease is the most common abnormality seen in AS, and is the highest cause of mortality in infancy. It may be seen in as many as 90% of patients with AS. The most common types of congenital heart disease include pulmonic valve stenosis, tetralogy of Fallot, pulmonary atresia, truncus arteriosus, ASD and VSD. The mortality rates of patients with tetralogy of Fallot and AS are higher than patients without AS. Intracranial bleeding is also common in patients with AS and is a major cause of mortality. Renal disorders are very common in AS, occurring in about 40% to 50% of patients. These include, but are not limited to, renal artery stenosis, solitary kidney, dysplastic kidneys, renal tubular acidosis, and juvenile nephronophthisis.

There are multiple reasons for an infant to present with cholestasis, and for the ED physician treating a patient with, or suspected of AS, it is important to understand the high potential for additional congenital abnormalities in addition to liver disease. While phenotypes and congenital abnormalities can vary greatly, it is the comorbidities that are

TABLE 99.4

CHARACTERISTICS OF ALAGILLE SYNDROME

Classic Alagille syndrome criteria

1. Bile duct paucity plus
2. 3 of 5 major criteria:
   - "Alagille Facies"
   - Cholestasis (conjugated hyperbilirubinemia)
   - Congenital heart disease
   - Vertebral anomalies
   - Ocular anomalies

Additional clinical characteristics

Hepatic: chronic cholestasis, portal hypertension, liver fibrosis, liver cirrhosis, liver failure, hepatocellular carcinoma

Cardiac: tetralogy of Fallot, pulmonic valve stenosis, pulmonary atresia, truncus arteriosus, aortic stenosis, ASD and VSD

Ocular: posterior embryotoxon, Axenfeld anomaly, Rieger anomaly, congenital macular dystrophy, cataracts, exotropia, strabismus, retinal fundus hypopigmentation

Vertebral: butterfly vertebrae, shortened digits, spina bifida occulta, fusion of adjacent vertebrae, rickets, osteopenia/osteoporosis, pathologic fractures

Facial features: prominent forehead, macrocephaly, hypertelorism, deep set eyes, upslanting palpebral fissures, depressed nasal bridge, sinus abnormalities, large ears

Renal: renal tubular acidosis, renal insufficiency, small/ectopic/horseshoe/single kidneys, renal cysts

Vascular: stroke, intracranial bleeding, cerebral artery anomalies, vascular malformations, moyamoya syndrome, renal artery stenosis

Endocrine: pancreatic exocrine insufficiency, insulin-dependent diabetes mellitus, hypogonadism

Gastrointestinal: malabsorption, failure to thrive, malrotation, microcolon, atresia

Other: growth retardation, mental retardation, learning difficulties

the likely cause for morbidity and mortality in the infancy period.

LIVER DISEASE

Acute Liver Failure

Goal of Treatment

ALF in children occurs when the vital synthetic functions of the liver fail (coagulopathy) in the setting of known hepatic injury in the absence of known chronic liver disease. ALF can be associated with hypoglycemia, hyperbilirubinemia, hypoproteinemia, and possible encephalopathy. Liver failure can develop acutely, or it may be chronically progressive. ALF is a clinical syndrome due to a myriad of etiologies including infections (e.g., viral hepatitis) and metabolic diseases (e.g., Wilson disease). Clinical presentation can be quite variable. The goal of the ED physician is early recognition of ALF in the setting of nonspecific signs and symptoms. In patients with recognized liver failure, the ED physician should address acute and common complications such as electrolyte imbalances, hypoglycemia, and encephalopathy. In addition, patients are often coagulopathic, which should be corrected in the setting of active bleeding. If there is no active bleeding, correction of a coagulopathy should be weighed against the risk of volume overload. Finally, patients with ALF are at very high risk for infection and should be treated aggressively if one is suspected.

CLINICAL PEARLS AND PITFALLS

- Childhood ALF may be diagnosed in the setting of coagulopathy, evidence of hepatic injury, and in the absence of chronic liver disease.
- Children with ALF may not present with hepatic encephalopathy or asterixis.
- Hypoglycemia is a common complication of ALF.
- Coagulopathies are difficult to correct and aggressive attempts at correction may lead to volume overload.
- Renal function should be monitored closely.
- Patients with ALF are at high risk for infectious complications and should be treated aggressively if infection is suspected.

Current Evidence

ALF in children can be secondary to a variety of causes, however all result in the progression of irreversible hepatocyte injury. In children younger than 1 year of age, ALF most commonly occurs in the setting of a metabolic disease such as urea cycle disorders, galactosemia, type I tyrosinemia, or an underlying mitochondrial disorder (see Chapter 103 Metabolic Emergencies). Other causes include viral hepatitis such as herpes simplex or enterovirus and medications such as acetaminophen. In children older than 1 year of age, the etiology is not determined in half of all cases (Table 99.5). In identified cases, pharmaceutical agents such as acetaminophen or antiepileptic drugs are the most common causes. Importantly, prolonged and inappropriate acetaminophen dosing is likely an important contributor to ALF in children, however it is much more difficult to assess with current testing mechanisms, which more accurately assesses for acute toxicity (see Chapter 110 Toxicologic Emergencies). Metabolism of acetaminophen is known to be quite variable, and there are likely patients who are slow metabolizers that may increase their risk of ALF with prolonged use, even when correct weight-based dosing is given. Other causes include autoimmune hepatitis and infections such as viral hepatitis. Herbal drugs have also been known to cause ALF. In developing countries, viral hepatitis is by far the most common etiology of ALF in all age groups of children.

The development of hepatic encephalopathy is not seen in children as frequently as in adults, but when seen, is more common in patients with non–acetaminophen-induced ALF. The Pediatric Acute Liver Failure Study Group evaluated children with ALF in North America and Europe and found that on presentation 57% of nonacetaminophen and 40% of acetaminophen groups had clinical evidence of HE.

Clinical Considerations

Clinical Recognition. Patients often do not exhibit serious clinical features of ALF. Patients may present with nonspecific

TABLE 99.5

ETIOLOGY OF ACUTE LIVER FAILURE BY AGE GROUP

Less than 1 yr (%)	>1 yr (%)
Metabolic[a] (42)	Unknown (47)
Neonatal hemochromatosis (16)	Viral hepatitis
	Non-A and non-B (27)
Undetermined (16)	Hepatitis A (10)
Viral hepatitis (15)	Hepatitis B (4)
Other (10)	Drug induced[b] (10)
	Other (2)

[a]Type 1 tyrosinemia, mitochondrial, urea cycle disorder, galactosemia, fructose intolerance.
[b]Acetaminophen, amanita, isoniazid, valproic acid.
This table was adapted from Cochran JB, Losek JD. Acute liver failure in children. *Ped Emerg Care* 2007;23:129–135.

prodromal symptoms or in septic shock. Often children present with multisystem disease or sepsis, making the diagnosis of primary ALF challenging. Adult definitions, which rely on HE, are often not reliable in children.

Triage Considerations. Many patients simply present with nonspecific prodromal symptoms such as fatigue, nausea, and vomiting. Others may present in shock with multisystem organ failure. As with any life-threatening condition, patients should be triaged and treated accordingly.

Clinical Assessment. Patients may initially complain of fatigue, nausea, vomiting, fever, and diffuse abdominal pain. Occasionally, right upper quadrant pain is severe. Commonly, a history of a prodromal viral illness can be elicited. The presence of jaundice usually initiates the first visit to the physician. As liver failure progresses, patients become more jaundiced and lethargic, and may report easy bruising or bleeding. History should include any infectious and medication exposures including prescription and nonprescription medications and herbal and other alternative remedies. ED physicians should be cognizant of chronic acetaminophen exposure in addition to acute toxicity. Family history should be assessed for Wilson disease, α_1 antitrypsin deficiency, autoimmune conditions, infant deaths, metabolic or mitochondria disorders, or liver failure of unknown etiology.

Physical examination findings may include small size, poor nutritional status, jaundice, bruising, or petechiae. Hepatomegaly is common and some patients may have splenomegaly. Findings associated with chronic liver disease and portal hypertension would suggest an alternative diagnosis. Encephalopathy is graded on a scale from I to IV from drowsiness, poor concentration, and irritability to aggressive behavior or unresponsiveness. Those with severe encephalopathy can develop cerebral edema and increased intracranial pressure (ICP). Cerebral edema is a major cause of death in patients with liver failure and requires aggressive supportive management.

Because it may be difficult to diagnose patients clinically, biochemical evidence of liver failure is necessary. PT is a helpful measure of synthetic function. Other laboratory markers suggestive of severe liver failure include evidence of increasing cholestasis manifested by a rising serum bilirubin level, hypoalbuminemia, and hypoglycemia.

It is also important to monitor serum transaminase levels. Falling transaminase levels usually indicate resolving liver disease, though in the setting of increasing jaundice and coagulopathy, this trend may indicate excessive hepatocyte loss rather than hepatocyte recovery. Serum fibrinogen is usually decreased in patients with liver failure. In cases in which the patient has splenomegaly, thrombocytopenia and leukocytopenia may be present.

Hypoglycemia almost always accompanies ALF because the liver is the primary organ for gluconeogenesis and glycogen storage is often depleted. This may complicate the signs of encephalopathy. Hepatorenal syndrome occurs in approximately 75% of patients who reach severe encephalopathy. The cause of hepatorenal syndrome is unclear; however, the result is oliguria in the presence of near-normal intravascular pressures. Metabolic acidosis occurs in approximately 30% of patients who have liver failure, and the risk of sepsis is increased secondary to the patient's compromised immune function.

Management. All patients suspected of having liver failure should undergo a complete physical examination, including a thorough and serial neurologic evaluation. Laboratory testing should include serum glucose, transaminases, total and direct bilirubin, albumin, PT, GGT, CBC count with differential, electrolytes, blood culture, and fibrinogen.

Infection can be both the cause and complication of ALF and is a major cause of morbidity and mortality. Infection may be the cause of death in up to 20% of patients. Patients with ALF may not present with an elevated WBC count and fever, so the ED clinician should have a very low threshold for empiric broad-spectrum antibiotics.

Patients with hypoglycemia should receive IV fluids with 10% dextrose, with additional dextrose boluses as necessary, and should undergo frequent blood glucose monitoring (every 1 hour) until their blood glucose level stabilizes. Metabolic acidosis should be corrected; however, correction of hyponatremia should be gradual in patients with ascites.

Patients who have a life-threatening coagulopathy should be given IV vitamin K (2.5 mg in infants; 5 mg in older children and adolescents). In the case of non–life-threatening coagulopathy, vitamin K should be given subcutaneously because of the risk of infusion reactions. A repeat PT should be performed 6 to 8 hours after administration. An uncorrectable PT is suggestive of severe hepatocyte damage. Clinicians should be cautious about aggressive management of coagulopathies in patients without active bleeding, as this may quickly lead to difficulties with patient volume status without significant improvement in the patient's coagulopathy. Recombinant Factor VII may help correct a coagulopathy without the need for significant volume, however the data of its efficacy in children is lacking. In addition, there is a decrease in both procoagulant and anticoagulant factors, so an elevated PT and INR may not accurately reflect a patient's risk of bleeding. Patients also often exhibit thrombocytopenia secondary to decreased production and increased consumption. Platelet dysfunction is also seen in liver failure.

Therapeutic management of ascites should occur only in the face of respiratory distress or renal failure. In these cases, IV 25% albumin (1 g per kg) followed by IV furosemide can be used. Otherwise, the introduction of a diuretic (e.g., spironolactone) to achieve a slow, gradual change in ascites is all that is initially required. Aggressive diuresis may precipitate or worsen hepatorenal syndrome.

Patients with encephalopathy should be frequently monitored for changes in neurologic function. Bowel therapy with lactulose is a common therapy directed at hyperammonemia. Patients with HE should also have medications reviewed for any medication that may worsen their mental status. Blood within the GI tract, if present, provides a high protein load and may also worsen HE. Patients should also be monitored for signs of elevated ICP. Cerebral edema is a major cause of mortality. Invasive monitoring, however, has not been shown to improve outcome and can be difficult in the setting of intractable coagulopathies. Patients should be monitored in an intensive care setting and neurosurgical consultation is necessary.

Additional medical treatments include steroids, N-acetylcysteine, and plasmapheresis. Steroids have been shown to be beneficial in the setting of adrenal insufficiency, autoimmune hepatitis, or with medication reactions. Steroids should not be used nonspecifically with other general causes of ALF. Acetaminophen toxicity should be treated aggressively with N-acetylcysteine (see Chapter 110 Toxicologic Emergencies). N-acetylcysteine may have some benefit in certain groups of patients with non–acetaminophen-induced liver failure, however evidence is lacking for its broad use in all cases of ALF. Plasmapheresis has been used to perform the detoxification functions of the liver, however evidence of its benefit on patient outcome is lacking. Finally, if medical management has failed, patients may require liver transplant. Ten percent to 15% of pediatric liver transplants in the United States are secondary to ALF (see Chapter 133 Transplantation Emergencies).

Portal Hypertension

Portal hypertension is a clinical syndrome caused by either increased or restricted blood flow within the portal vasculature leading to a splenomegaly and the development of portosystemic blood vessel collaterals as blood is shunted to the systemic vasculature. The disease becomes clinically significant when effects of this elevation in pressure or collateral vessels become evident. Most patients present with splenomegaly, however some will also present with GI bleeding or ascites. The management of these complications is important for the ED provider as they may be life-threatening.

Portal hypertension most commonly occurs when there is an obstruction to normal portal blood flow. The lesion may be prehepatic (i.e., portal vein thrombosis or splenic vein obstruction), intrahepatic (i.e., cirrhosis from BA, α_1-antitrypsin deficiency, or cystic fibrosis), or posthepatic (i.e., hepatic vein thrombosis or tumor). Prehepatic disease in children is most commonly due to portal vein thrombosis from omphalitis, but may also be related to sepsis, severe dehydration, or prothrombotic conditions. Globally, schistosomiasis is a leading cause of portal hypertension due to intrahepatic parasitic disease causing inflammation, fibrosis, and obstruction. (See Table 99.1 for additional causes of portal hypertension in children.) Portal hypertension is typically a clinical diagnosis through recognition of the signs and symptoms of portal hypertension, such as the development of ascites, GI bleeding, identification of varices without active bleeding, or splenomegaly. Additional diagnostic testing such as ultrasound, liver biopsy, or measurement of the portal pressure gradient would, of course, supplement any new diagnosis.

The effects of portal hypertension are systemic, and complications can affect every organ system (Table 99.2). The most common complication, with high morbidity and mortality, is GI hemorrhage from the development of portosystemic varices (i.e., gastric or EV), or congestive or hemorrhagic gastritis. (Variceal bleeding is discussed in the Gastrointestinal Bleeding section of this chapter.) Effects on the circulatory system are complex and multifactorial, but ultimately result in an increased cardiac output, hypervolemia, decreased systemic vascular resistance, and hypotension. This is largely due to an overall decrease in venous and splanchnic arterial tone, retention of sodium and free water, and subsequent increase in circulatory volume and venous return. The increase in venous return and decreased peripheral resistance (mediated by a variety of vasoactive factors such as nitric oxide) result in an overall increase in cardiac output. These changes in circulatory physiology contribute to additional complications such as ascites, hepatorenal, and hepatopulmonary syndrome.

Ascites results from an imbalance in the oncotic and hydrostatic pressures within the abdominal vasculature. Hydrostatic pressure is increased secondary to the increased pressure within the draining splanchnic and portal system, as well as the increased circulating blood volume from factors discussed above. In addition, there may be a decrease in oncotic pressure as the liver's synthetic function deteriorates. Treatment for ascites may include fluid restriction, diuretic therapy, and albumin administration; however, one must be cognizant of the patient's functional intravascular volume status. Patients with portal hypertension are at high risk of infectious complications, such as spontaneous bacterial peritonitis in patients with ascites. Indeed, an underlying infection is often the cause for a sudden clinical deterioration.

Hematologic complications are generally, but not completely, related to splenomegaly, and patients may present with thrombocytopenia, leukopenia, and anemia. Coagulopathies are often present, but are secondary to the underlying liver disease and liver failure, as opposed to the portal hypertension itself. When the patient is not actively bleeding, these hematologic abnormalities should not be treated aggressively as treatment may result in hypervolemia and place a patient at higher risk for GI bleeding. A provider should not attempt to correct thrombocytopenia and anemia to normal levels. Active and life-threatening bleeding should be treated more aggressively with blood products. The management of GI bleeding and transfusion parameters are discussed in the GI bleeding section of this chapter.

Pulmonary complications include hepatopulmonary syndrome and portopulmonary hypertension. Hepatopulmonary syndrome occurs when there is an increase in the levels of vasoactive agents, causing pulmonary vasodilation and subsequent ventilation–perfusion mismatch. There is also likely a degree of venous–arterial shunting within the pulmonary vasculature. Both can result in hypoxemia. Portopulmonary hypertension may also occur and likely results from vascular remodeling and endothelial cell dysfunction. Ultimately, significant pulmonary hypertension may result in right-sided heart failure.

Renal complications are secondary to the changes in circulatory physiology described above and may result in hepatorenal syndrome.

Ultimately, portal hypertension is a chronic and complex problem that requires a multidisciplinary team to manage. Emergency management is directly related to the presenting complications. The emergency provider must be familiar with the complex pathophysiology in patients with advanced portal hypertension as it directly affects the emergency management of conditions that may carry significant morbidity and mortality.

Acute Viral Hepatitis

Goals of Emergency Therapy

The initial evaluation of a patient with abnormal liver biochemical and function tests (LFTs) includes obtaining a history to identify potential risk factors for liver disease and performing a physical examination to look for clues to the etiology and for signs of chronic liver disease. Subsequent testing is determined based on the information gathered from the history and physical examination as well as the pattern of LFT abnormalities. The goal of emergency care is to determine if the patient is at risk for fulminant liver failure.

CLINICAL PEARLS AND PITFALLS

- A high index of suspicion is required to detect patients with viral hepatitis as the aminotransferase elevation may be very mild in children.
- A history of immigration or adoption from high prevalence countries or family/personal history of high-risk exposures should prompt screening for hepatitis B virus (HBV) and hepatitis C virus (HCV), even if liver transaminases are only mildly elevated.
- Hepatitis A virus (HAV) IgM suggests current or recent hepatitis A infection in the setting of HAV total antibody positivity. Treatment is supportive.
- HBV is 100-fold more infectious than human immunodeficiency virus (HIV). A positive anti-HBs (surface antibody) are present. All HBsAg- and HBcAb-positive patients merit confirmatory HBV DNA.
- Infants at risk for vertical HCV transmission should not be tested until 18 months of age as maternal HCV antibody can circulate for over 1 year. If positive, confirm with HCV ribonucleic acid (RNA) quantitative polymerase chain reaction (PCR) and refer to Hepatology.

Current Evidence

The existing alphabet of viral hepatitis is now up to G, excluding F, with new variants awaiting discovery. HAV, the cause of "infectious" or epidemic hepatitis, is a RNA virus transmitted by the fecal–oral route. Hepatitis A is the second most common vaccine preventable infection in travelers and has an incubation period of 28 days (range 15 to 50). Peak infectivity occurs during the 2-week period before onset of jaundice or elevation of liver enzymes, when concentration of virus in stool is highest. Highly effective vaccines exist for its prevention for travelers over 12 months of age. The vaccine is sufficient for most patients; however, an immunoglobulin is an option for high-risk individuals, such as patients under 12 months of age or patients with an underlying liver disease traveling to an endemic area. On a worldwide scale, fewer than 5% of cases are clinically recognized. HAV is a rare cause of fulminant hepatitis. No chronic carrier state exists. The virus is maintained in the human population through person-to-person transmission, and there is no evidence of maternal to neonate transmission. About 30% of the United States shows evidence of past infection. Immunization of children (1 to 18 years of age) consists of two or three doses of the vaccine. Adults need a booster dose 6 to 12 months following the initial dose of vaccine. The vaccine is thought to be effective for 15 to 20 years or more. Because Hepatitis A vaccine is inactivated, no special precautions need to be taken when vaccinating immunocompromised persons.

HBV is endemic in the human population. Although predominantly transmitted by the parenteral route or sexual contact, the high incidence of infection in family contacts suggests that the virus may also spread by saliva or breast milk. The ability of HBV to produce a chronic carrier state in the DNA in 5% to 10% of infected subjects allows maintenance of an infectious pool without serial transmission. Children who contract HBV at birth have a 30% chance of dying from a liver-related cause. HBV vaccine provides protection against hepatitis B for 15 years and possibly much longer. Currently, the Center for Disease Control and Prevention recommends that all newborns and individuals up to 18 years of age be vaccinated. Three injections over a 6- to 12-month period are required to provide full protection.

HCV accounts for about 95% of hepatitis infections in recipients of blood transfusion and 50% of cases of sporadic non-A, non-B hepatitis. Most of these patients will progress to chronic hepatitis, and about 20% will develop cirrhosis. Maternally acquired antibodies can persist in an infant, so patients should not be tested for perinatally acquired disease until after the infant is 18 months of age.

HDV requires hepatitis B helper functions for the propagation in hepatocytes and may occur either simultaneously with hepatitis B infection (coinfection) or as superinfection in chronic hepatitis B carriers. Clinically, the effect of HDV appears to worsen the course of HBV. Hepatitis E is an enterically transmitted virus responsible for large epidemics of acute hepatitis in Asia, the Middle East, and parts of Africa. Mortality as high as 10% is reported worldwide in pregnant women. Hepatitis G virus (HGV) is known to infect humans but has not been definitively shown to cause disease. A variety of nonhepatotropic viruses that cause systemic disease are known to cause a number of systemic viral infections that may cause hepatitis, the most common of which are Epstein–Barr virus (EBV) and cytomegalovirus (CMV).

Clinical Considerations

Clinical Recognition. The majority of patients who are diagnosed with hepatitis present with nonspecific symptoms and clinically may appear jaundiced. Symptoms may include nausea, vomiting and anorexia, or may include flu-like symptoms of cough, pharyngitis, rhinorrhea, headache, or myalgias. A history of immigration or adoption from high prevalence countries, such as those from Eastern Europe, Asia, Sub-Saharan Africa, Northern South America, or family/personal history of high-risk exposures, such as IV drug use, multiple sexual partners, unregulated tattoo parlors, should prompt screening HBV and HCV even if liver transaminases are only mildly elevated.

Triage. The basic tenets of contact transmission apply, thus encourage patients and providers to wash hands after using the bathroom and before fixing food or eating.

Initial Assessment/H&P. Most childhood cases of acute hepatitis produce minimal symptoms, are anicteric, and, unless suspected by palpation of tender hepatomegaly, are usually confused with a GI flu–like illness. Clinical hepatitis classically consists of a 5- to 7-day prodrome of variable constitutional symptoms (low-grade fever, anorexia, nausea, vomiting, malaise, fatigue, and epigastric or right upper quadrant abdominal pain), followed by acute onset of scleral icterus, jaundice, and passage of dark urine. Pruritus and diarrhea are rare. Physical examination after the onset of jaundice may reveal tender hepatomegaly. Mild splenomegaly is present in 25% to 50% of patients. HBV patients may also present with extrahepatic signs and symptoms such as arthralgia, arthritis, or papular acrodermatitis (on face, buttocks, and extensor surfaces of arms and legs). The rash may be associated with lymphadenopathy and fever (Gianotti–Crosti syndrome), and has been reported with several viruses although HBV is the most common. Onset of the icteric phase of acute hepatitis most commonly is temporarily associated with improvement in the constitutional symptoms. In up to 15% of cases, severe fatigue, anorexia, nausea, and vomiting persist. The icteric period usually lasts 1 to 4 weeks. Occasionally, the jaundice is prolonged for 4 to 6 weeks, with increasing pruritus at 2 to 3 weeks. A number of infectious agents may mimic a viral hepatitis-like illness. The most common are EBV (infectious mononucleosis) and CMV. Both agents rarely produce clinical jaundice, and high fever and diffuse adenopathy are more characteristic. Less common agents include herpes, adenovirus, coxsackievirus, rheovirus, echovirus, rubella, arbovirus, leptospirosis, toxoplasmosis, and tuberculosis.

Management/Diagnostic Testing. Most causes of hepatocellular injury are associated with an AST elevation that is lower than that of ALT. An AST to ALT ratio of 2:1 or greater is suggestive of alcoholic liver disease, particularly in the setting of an elevated GGT, although much more common in the adult population. The following laboratory tests should be performed in all cases of suspected viral hepatitis: serum transaminases (AST and ALT), alkaline phosphatase, serum GGT, total and direct bilirubin, CBC, PT, electrolytes, BUN, glucose, total protein, albumin, and globulin. AST and ALT are the best indicators of ongoing hepatocellular injury, although it is important to note that in those with chronic and advanced disease, ALT and AST may be normal or only mildly elevated despite significant damage and fibrosis. Alkaline phosphatase levels are usually less than two times the upper limit of normal for age. Levels greater than three times normal should raise suspicions of EBV or CMV hepatitis or biliary tract disease. Hepatitis classically produces direct fractions of serum bilirubin in excess of 30% of total, indicating definite liver disease. Hyperbilirubinemia may be present in the absence of scleral icterus or jaundice because these signs usually cannot be appreciated until levels of total bilirubin exceed 3 to 4 mg per dL. Serum bilirubin levels peak 5 to 7 days after the onset of jaundice.

Serum albumin and globulin are usually within normal levels. Decreased albumin or increased globulin levels should suggest an acute flare of chronic liver disease. Serum ceruloplasmin levels should be drawn in all patients older than 5 years who have suspected hepatitis to evaluate for Wilson disease. Figure 99.3 contrasts the sequence of clinical, biochemical, and serologic events in typical HAV and HBV infection. The serodiagnosis of acute hepatitis is best approached

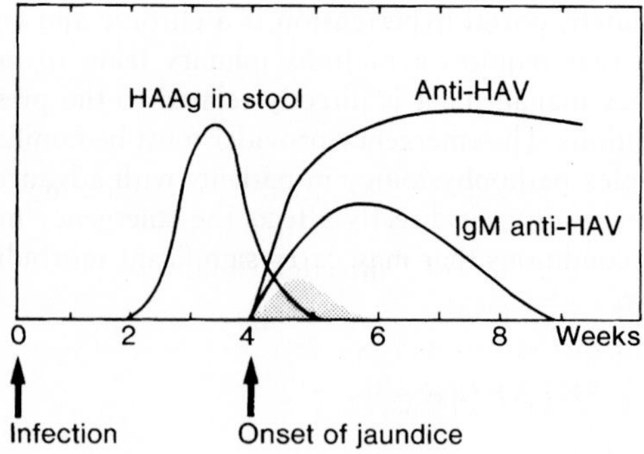

FIGURE 99.3 Serologic changes in hepatitis A. HAAg, hepatitis-associated antigen; HAV, hepatitis A virus.

by first testing for anti-HAV IgM, HB surface antigen, HB e antigen, HB serum DNA (quantitative), anti-HB core Ab, anti-HCV, hepatitis C serum PCR (quantitative), anti-CMV, and EBV serology. The finding of serum IgM anti-HAV is diagnostic of acute HAV infection because the antibody is present at the time of clinical symptoms. A positive HB surface antigen suggests the diagnosis of HBV in a symptomatic patient. A positive HB e antigen or anti-HB core Ab is helpful in the rare patient who rapidly clears HB surface antigen from the serum. It is also important to note that in long-term HB surface antigen carriers who have HDV superinfection, the suppression of HBV replication may lead to a transient absence of HBV markers in the serum; unless HDV markers in the serum are sought, the diagnosis may be missed. Anti-HCV does not appear in the patient's circulation until 1 to 3 months after the onset of acute illness, and in rare cases, detectable levels may not be demonstrated for up to 1 year. Thus, unless the acute presentation is actually a flare of chronic HCV, serodiagnosis of an HCV infection (Hep C PCR) will await long-term follow-up.

No specific treatment of acute viral hepatitis is available. Most patients can be managed at home. No restrictions in diet or ambulation are necessary. The traditional recommendations of a low-fat, high carbohydrate diet and bed rest are now recognized to have no effect on the symptoms or duration of the disease. Parents should be told that anorexia and fatigue are common symptoms. Small, frequent feedings may be helpful. Hepatotoxic drugs should be strictly avoided. The key for both the patient and other household contacts is personal hygiene. Infants and children should avoid contact with the patient even after they have received immunoprophylaxis. In HAV, shedding of the virus may occur for up to 2 weeks after the onset of jaundice. Patients should be kept at home during this time. After this, they may return to school. Indications for hospitalization of a patient who has acute hepatitis include (i) dehydration secondary to anorexia and vomiting, (ii) bilirubin levels more than 20 mg per dL, (iii) abnormal PT, (iv) WBC count more than 25,000 per mm^3, or (v) levels of transaminases more than 3,000 units per L.

Patients who have acute hepatitis and who are hospitalized should be isolated. Follow-up studies of all patients with acute hepatitis should be performed to document biochemical resolution. Follow-up serology may also establish a specific cause in cases of apparent non-A, non-B hepatitis (fourfold increase in CMV serology, development of anti-HCV). Reevaluation of patients with HBV is especially important either to ensure clearance of HB surface antigen or to recognize the development of the HB surface antigen carrier state.

Postexposure Prophylaxis

Hepatitis A

The mean incubation period for HAV infection is about 4 weeks (range, 15 to 50 days). Conventional immune serum globulin (ISG; 0.02 mL per kg IM) confers passive protection against clinical HAV infection if given within 2 weeks of exposure and protects for up to 3 months. Seventy-five percent of this group will develop detectable levels of anti-HAV IgM, suggesting passive–active immunity. Postexposure immunoprophylaxis is suggested for household and close personal contacts, institutionalized contacts, newborns of HAV-infected mothers, those exposed to an infected food handler and contacts within a day care facility. Schoolroom exposure of an isolated case and routine play contacts do not require ISG. However, a second case within a class is an indication for immunoprophylaxis of the rest of the class. Serologic testing of close contacts is not recommended, as it adds to unnecessary cost and potential treatment delay. Importantly, current guidelines recommend pre-exposure prophylaxis via routine HAV immunization for all children. Recently, studies have shown that immunizing patients postexposure with the hepatitis A vaccine is as effective as providing immune globulin.

Hepatitis B

Prophylactic treatment to prevent infection after exposure to HBV should be considered in individuals who do not have documented immunity from the HBV vaccine in the following ED situations: (i) Sexual exposure to the HBV surface antigen–positive patient, (ii) inadvertent percutaneous or permucosal exposure to HBV surface antigen–positive blood, (iii) household exposure of an infant younger than 12 months to a primary caregiver who has acute HBV. Before treatment in the first two situations, testing for susceptibility is recommended if it does not delay treatment beyond 14 days postexposure. Breast-feeding of an infant by a HBV surface antigen–positive mother poses no additional risk if the infant has received HBV and HB immunoglobulin. Testing for anti-HBV core Ab is the most efficient prescreening procedure. HBV is 100-fold more infectious than HIV. Do not dismiss a positive anti-HBsAg (surface antigen) as postvaccination response if risk factors present as it can be a marker of chronic infection. All HBsAg- and HBcAb-positive patients merit confirmatory HBV DNA confirmation. All susceptible persons should receive a single dose of hepatitis B immunoglobulin (0.06 mL per kg) intramuscularly and hepatitis B vaccine in recommended doses.

MISCELLANEOUS ABDOMINAL EMERGENCIES

Gastroesophageal Reflux Disease

Gastroesophageal reflux disease is one of the most common abdominal complaints seen in pediatrics. The NASPGHAN defines GER as the physiologic passage of gastric contents into the esophagus and gastroesophageal reflux disease (GERD) as reflux associated with troublesome symptoms or complications. GER is reported in ⅔ of otherwise healthy infants and complications from GERD account for a significant number of ED visits annually. GER complications or complaints can be esophageal or extraesophageal. Esophageal complaints include vomiting, poor weight gain, esophagitis, abdominal pain, or retrosternal pain. Extraesophageal complaints include cough, recurrent pneumonia, laryngitis, dental erosions, and wheezing in infancy. There is no strong evidence, however, to suggest that treating GERD will improve reactive airway disease or recurrent pneumonia. The degree to which GER contributes to any extraesophageal complaint can be difficult to associate. Importantly, there are certain "red flag" complaints that are not associated with GERD and should raise concerns for an alternative diagnosis (Table 99.7). There are certain populations that seem to be at higher risk for developing complications of GER, including those patients with severe neurologic impairment, Cornelia de Lange syndrome, underlying severe pulmonary disease (cystic fibrosis, bronchopulmonary dysplasia), premature infants, repaired esophageal achalasia or atresia, and patients with lung transplants. GERD may also contribute to Apparent Life-Threatening Events (ALTE), however the prevalence of this relationship is not clear. GERD complaints also vary by age group. GERD in infants seems to peak at around 50% by 4 months of age, whereas only 5% to 10% of patients have clinically significant GERD at 1 year. In general, GERD is a clinical diagnosis and no additional testing is necessary; however, additional diagnostic testing modalities include pH and impedance probe monitoring and endoscopy.

The (NASPGHAN) guidelines for the management of GERD recommend multiple options including lifestyle changes and pharmaceuticals. Lifestyle changes for infants include changing formulas (e.g., partially hydrolyzed trial), changing the mother's diet if the patient is breast-fed, decreased volume and more frequent feedings, frequent burping, and keeping the patient in a more upright position during and after feeding. Those with a milk protein allergy may benefit from more aggressive lifestyle changes. In breast-fed infants, GERD is typically not so severe that breast-feeding should be discontinued, especially with lifestyle changes. (See section on Dietary Protein Gastrointestinal Disorders for a more complete discussion.) Caregivers may also

TABLE 99.6

SIGNS AND SYMPTOMS OF GERD BY AGE

Infants <1 yr of age	Children >1 yr of age
Recurrent vomiting/regurgitation	Abdominal pain
Recurrent regurgitation without vomiting	Recurrent vomiting
Poor weight gain	Chest pain
Irritability	Heartburn
Back arching	Chronic cough
Sleep interruption	Sleep interruption
Cough	Burping
Choking/gagging	Food refusal
Food refusal	
Dystonic posturing (Sandifer syndrome)	
Apparent life-threatening event	

Adapted from Lightdale JR, Gremse DA. Gastroesophageal reflux: management guidance for the pediatrician. *Pediatrics* 2013;131(5): e1684–e1695.

TABLE 99.7

RED FLAG SIGNS AND SYMPTOMS IN CHILD WITH VOMITING

Significant weight loss	Fever
Bilious emesis	Lethargy
GI bleeding	Hepatosplenomegaly
Forceful vomiting	Macro- or microcephaly
Failure to thrive	Seizure
Constipation/diarrhea	Hyper- or hypotonia
Recurrent pneumonia	Abdominal pain/distention
Onset after 6 mo of age	Apparent life-threatening event

Adapted from Lightdale JR, Gremse DA. Gastroesophageal reflux: management guidance for the pediatrician. *Pediatrics* 2013;131(5): e1684–e1695.

choose to trial thickening agents, which have shown to decrease the height of esophageal reflux and frequency of regurgitation. An example of thickening would be to add one teaspoon of thickening cereal to 1 oz of formula. It is important to know that there is an association between thickening agents and necrotizing enterocolitis in preterm infants. The Food and Drug Administration does not recommend thickening agents in infants born before 37 weeks' gestation, those who are hospitalized, or those who were hospitalized within the past 30 days. Prone positioning has also been found to improve symptoms, however this benefit is outweighed by the increased risk of Sudden Infant Death Syndrome. Similarly, positioning a patient on his or her side is also not recommended. In older children and adolescents, lifestyle change includes cessation of alcohol and tobacco, dietary modifications (decrease in caffeine, chocolate, and spicy foods), weight loss, and position changes. Position changes include sleeping with the head of the bed elevated and in the left lateral decubitus position.

The principal medication therapies for GERD are histamine-2 receptor antagonists (H2RAs) and PPIs. Both have been shown to increase gastric pH. H2RAs antacid effect lasts for approximately 6 hours. PPIs effect is longer, but not well defined due to metabolism variability. PPIs also decrease intragastric volumes. Despite their efficacy at increasing gastric pH, studies have not demonstrated beneficial effect of PPIs over placebo in infants with symptoms of GERD. In fact, one study found increased side effects without significant benefit in infants with suspected GERD treated with PPIs versus placebo. In children greater than 1 year of age, both have been shown to improve symptoms of GERD and esophagitis, with PPIs being more effective than H2RAs. Despite their apparent benign nature, both medications have side effects including nausea, diarrhea, headaches, and constipation. The use of both H2RAs and PPIs may also be associated with an increased risk for community-acquired pneumonia, gastroenteritis, candidemia, and necrotizing enterocolitis in preterm infants. The chronic use of antacids in pediatrics is not currently recommended under the guidelines and like any new medication, emergency patients should be referred to their pediatrician for chronic management.

Celiac Disease

Celiac disease (also known as celiac sprue and gluten-sensitive enteropathy) is an immune-mediated enteropathy triggered by the ingestion of gluten-containing grains such as wheat, rye, and barley in genetically susceptible persons. The vast majority of patients with celiac disease carry either the human leukocyte antigen (HLA)-DQ2 or HLA-DQ8 haplotype; however, many unaffected people may also carry the alleles. More recent prevalence data generated on large, population-based samples of subjects from the United States and Europe indicate that the disease is far more common than originally thought. Data suggest that it occurs in nearly 1% of the US population. Among at-risk groups such as first- or second-degree relatives or symptomatic patients, the prevalence varied from 1 in 56 to 1 in 22. Celiac disease is also associated with other conditions and syndromes such as type I diabetes mellitus, IgA deficiency, autoimmune thyroiditis, Down syndrome, Turner syndrome, and Williams syndrome. Celiac disease presents with a diverse spectrum of disease presentations and the age-related variability in manifestations require emergency physicians to maintain a high degree of suspicion for the disorder when evaluating patients with a variety of complaints.

In patients with the genetic predisposition for celiac disease, exposure to gluten triggers an autoimmune reaction resulting in

TABLE 99.8

SEROLOGIC CHANGES IN HEPATITIS

Test	Antigen/antibody	Interpretation
HBsAg	Hepatitis B surface antigen	Detection of acute or chronic infection. Not present after vaccine.
Anti-HBs	Antibody to HBsAg	Resolved infection with HBV or immunocompetent vaccinated.
HBeAg	Hepatitis B e antigen	Detects HBV infection with increased risk of transmission.
Anti-HBe	Antibody to HBeAg	Detects HBV infection with decreased risk of transmission.
Anti-HBc	Antibody to HBV core antigen	Detects acute, resolved, or chronic HBV infection. Not present after immunization.
IgM anti-HBc	IgM antibody to HBV core antigen	Identifies acute or recent HBV infection (within past 6 mo).
HBV DNA by PCR	Amplified HBV DNA	Detects virus in blood or liver tissues. Indicates ongoing infection.
HCAb	Hepatitis C antibody	Detects Chronic HCV infection, if positive confirm with HCV RNA quantitative PCR.

From http://www.cdc.gov/hepatitis/hbv/pdfs/serologicchartv8.pdf http://www.cdc.gov/hepatitis/hcv/pdfs/hcv_graph.pdf

crypt hyperplasia, epithelial lymphocytosis, increased plasma cells, and villous atrophy. There is undisputed evidence regarding the role of gluten as the triggering agent. In the continued presence of gluten, celiac disease is self-perpetuating. Clinically, patients may present with malabsorption and failure to thrive. Other common GI symptoms include diarrhea, constipation, anorexia, and recurrent abdominal pain. Non-GI symptoms have also been appreciated with Celiac disease, such as anemia, joint pain, arthritis, chronic fatigue, irritability, and other behavioral changes. Celiac disease should also be considered in patients with dermatitis herpetiformis, dental enamel hypoplasia, short stature, delayed puberty, osteopenia, and iron deficiency anemia that are unresponsive to oral iron supplementation. These nonspecific signs and symptoms in part explain the observation that the average time from onset of symptoms to diagnosis in US children is typically several years. It is likely that ED physicians frequently come in contact with patients with undiagnosed celiac disease who present with nonspecific abdominal or systemic complaints.

Initial testing for celiac disease should be via the measurement of IgA antibody to human recombinant tissue transglutaminase (anti-TTG). The measurement of serum IgA levels aids in the diagnosis as some children have significant IgA deficiency, thus decreasing the usefulness of IgA anti-TTG. Intestinal biopsy may also be helpful, but is out of the scope of ED practice and this review. The only effective treatment of celiac disease is the complete avoidance of gluten-containing grains. Early diagnosis of the disease and dietary elimination of gluten are currently the only ways to avoid complications of the disease that may manifest in adulthood, including intestinal lymphoma and diabetes mellitus. A gluten-free diet should result in the resolution of GI symptoms and non-GI symptoms including improved growth and bone mineralization. Poor adherence to a gluten-free diet is often responsible for a lack of symptom resolution or recurrence of symptoms and may be assessed through repeat IgA anti-TTG testing.

Mesenteric Lymphadenitis

Mesenteric lymphadenitis (ML) or mesenteric adenitis is typically used to refer to an inflammatory process involving abdominal lymph nodes. This inflammatory process is thought to contribute to patients' abdominal pain, especially when no other abdominal pathology is identified. Given that enlarged lymph nodes are so frequently identified in symptomatic and asymptomatic patients, it can be difficult to determine the clinical significance of an enlarged abdominal lymph node.

ML is likely a common and important cause of both acute and recurrent abdominal pain in children. Enlarged lymph nodes can be associated with other intra-abdominal inflammatory processes such as appendicitis, however when seen as an isolated finding it is likely often due to viral infections. It is also associated with particular bacterial infections (see Chapters 42 Lymphadenopathy and 102 Infectious Disease Emergencies). Frequently the enlarged lymph nodes are seen in the right lower quadrant, and may mimic appendicitis. Multiple studies have attempted to evaluate the incidence and significance of enlarged mesenteric lymph nodes in children but the results have been inconclusive. All that can be said is that enlarged abdominal lymph nodes are commonly seen in pediatrics, and the diagnosis of ML should probably be reserved for those patients with lymph nodes greater than 10 mm and no other identifiable pathology.

Reye Syndrome

Reye syndrome is a distinct, reversible syndrome occurring after an antecedent viral infection, characterized by severe noninflammatory encephalopathy and fatty degeneration of the liver. Once the link between antecedent aspirin exposure and the onset of Reye syndrome was established, the incidence has declined to about two cases per year. Isolated case reports continue to be described, indicating the need to continue to consider Reye syndrome when evaluating patients with the typical clinical presentation. Most of the clinical features of Reye syndrome, including lactic acidosis, elevated fatty acids, nitrogen wasting, hyperammonemia, cellular fat accumulation, and cytotoxic cerebral edema, may be explained in the context of primary mitochondrial damage.

A biphasic clinical history is remarkably constant. First, the child has a history of a recent, usually febrile, illness that is waning or has resolved. Approximately 90% of the children have an antecedent upper respiratory tract infection. Varicella virus or influenza B infections have been most associated. The abrupt onset of protracted vomiting usually starts within 1 week following the prodromal illness. The vomiting is unresponsive either to restriction of oral intake or to antiemetic therapy.

Coincident with the onset of vomiting (or shortly thereafter), signs of encephalopathy appear. At first, encephalopathy may be manifested by unusual quietness or disinterest. However, a rapid sequential progression to irritability, combativeness, confusion, disorientation, delirium, stupor, and coma may occur. Seizures are a late sign in older children but may occur during early stages of encephalopathy in infancy (usually secondary to hypoglycemia).

In the ED, patients are usually afebrile. Tachycardia and hyperventilation commonly occur. At the initial presentation, only 50% of patients have hepatomegaly. The liver usually increases in size during the first 24 to 48 hours after the diagnosis is made. The absence of jaundice and scleral icterus is characteristic and is the major mitigating clinical sign against hepatic encephalopathy secondary to acute fulminant hepatitis. Despite evidence of encephalopathy, no focal neurologic signs or signs of meningeal irritation are apparent.

The hallmark of the acute encephalopathy of Reye syndrome is the associated evidence of liver abnormality. The levels of transaminases (ALT and AST) and blood ammonia are almost always elevated at the time of the onset of protracted vomiting. The range of transaminase elevation is highly variable and has not been shown to correlate well with severity of the disease. Ammonia levels more than 300 g per L have been shown to be an indicator of a poor prognosis. The PT is elevated by more than 50% in at least one-half of the patients, although clinical bleeding is rare and evidence of disseminated intravascular coagulation is absent. The level of serum bilirubin rarely exceeds 2 mg per dL. Hypoglycemia is rare, except in children who present in coma and in infants younger than 1 year, in whom the incidence is reported to be as high as 70% to 80%. Azotemia and ketonuria are common, secondary to starvation and dehydration from vomiting and poor oral intake. Patients most often have a mixed respiratory alkalosis and mild metabolic acidosis. The metabolic acidosis correlates with the level of ammonia elevation and reflects the degree of mitochondrial dysfunction.

Once the diagnosis is made, immediate plans to admit the child to an ICU should be made, because the progression of the encephalopathy may be rapid, resulting in increased morbidity and mortality.

Increased ICP secondary to cerebral edema is the major factor contributing to morbidity and mortality. With the ability to monitor ICP, numerous different invasive therapies have been introduced in an attempt to rapidly reduce and control cerebral edema. However, none of these therapies, including hyperventilation and muscle paralysis using neuromuscular-blocking drugs, hyperosmolar agents, high-dose barbiturates, exchange transfusions, or hypothermia, have been clearly proven to protect the brain from progressive ischemic insult. Ultimately, the management of Reye syndrome is supportive because no specific curative therapy is currently available.

Finally, it is important to note that there are multiple diseases secondary to inborn errors of metabolism (mostly mitochondrial) that present in a very similar fashion to Reye syndrome. Given the rarity of Reye syndrome, any child who is suspected of having Reye syndrome should have a thorough metabolic evaluation.

Suggested Readings and Key References

Overview

Thompson DA, Eitel D, Fernandes CM, et al. Coded chief complaints–automated analysis of free-text complaints. *Acad Emerg Med* 2006; 13(7):774–782.

Gastrointestinal Bleeding

Alarcon T, Jose Martinez-Gomez M, Urruzuno P. Helicobacter pylori in pediatrics. *Helicobacter* 2013;18(suppl 1):52–57.

Ertem D. Clinical practice: Helicobacter pylori infection in childhood. *Eur J Pediatr* 2013;172(11):1427–1434.

Hernandez C, Serrano C, Einisman H, et al. Peptic ulcer disease in Helicobacter pylori-infected children: clinical findings and mucosal immune response. *J Pediatr Gastroenterol Nutr* 2014;59(6):773–778.

Koletzko S, Jones NL, Goodman KJ, et al. Evidence-based guidelines from ESPGHAN and NASPGHAN for Helicobacter pylori infection in children. *J Pediatr Gastroenterol Nutr* 2011;53(2):230–243.

Oderda G, Mura S, Valori A, et al. Idiopathic peptic ulcers in children. *J Pediatr Gastroenterol Nutr* 2009;48(3):268–270.

Reid-Adam J. Henoch-schönlein purpura. *Pediatr Rev* 2014;35(10): 447–449.

Esophageal Varices

Fagundes ED, Ferreira AR, Roquete ML, et al. Clinical and laboratory predictors of esophageal varices in children and adolescents with portal hypertension syndrome. *J Pediatr Gastroenterol Nutr* 2008; 46(2):178–183.

Lykavieris P, Gautheir F, Hadchouel P, et al. Risk of gastrointestinal bleeding during adolescence and early adulthood in children with portal vein obstruction. *J Pediatr* 2000;136(6):805–808.

Shneider BL, Bosch J, de Franchis R, et al; Expert panel of the Children's Hospital of Pittsburgh of UPMC. Portal hypertension in children: expert pediatric opinion on the report of the Baveno v Consensus Workshop on Methodology of Diagnosis and Therapy in Portal Hypertension. *Pediatr Transplant* 2012;16(5):426–437.

Villanueva C, Colomo A, Bosch A, et al. Transfusion strategies for acute upper gastrointestinal bleeding. *N Engl J Med* 2013;368(1): 11–21.

Inflammatory Bowel Disease

Church PC, Guan J, Walters TD, et al. Infliximab maintains durable response and facilitates catch-up growth in luminal pediatric Crohn's disease. *Inflamm Bowel Dis* 2014;20(7):1177–1186.

Dambha F, Tanner J, Carroll N. Diagnostic imaging in Crohn's disease: what is the new gold standard? *Best Pract Res Clin Gastroenterol* 2014;28(3):421–436.

Dulai PS, Thompson KD, Blunt HB, et al. Risks of serious infection or lymphoma with anti-tumor necrosis factor therapy for pediatric inflammatory bowel disease: a systematic review. *Clin Gastroenterol Hepatol* 2014;12(9):1443–1451.

Hashash JG, Binion DG. Managing Clostridium difficile in inflammatory bowel disease (IBD). *Curr Gastroenterol Rep* 2014;16(7):393.

Hoffenberg EJ, Park KT, Dykes DM, et al. Appropriateness of emergency department use in pediatric inflammatory bowel disease: a quality improvement opportunity. *J Pediatr Gastroenterol Nutr* 2014;59(3):324–326.

Huang M, Rose E. Pediatric inflammatory bowel disease in the emergency department: managing flares and long-term complications. *Pediatr Emerg Med Pract* 2014;11(7):1–16.

Kappelman MD, Moore KR, Allen JK, et al. Recent trends in the prevalence of Crohn's disease and ulcerative colitis in a commercially insured US population. *Dig Dis Sci* 2013;58(2):519–525.

Kostakis ID, Cholidou KG, Vaiopoulos AG, et al. Fecal calprotectin in pediatric inflammatory bowel disease: a systematic review. *Dig Dis Sci* 2013;58(2):309–319.

Lee SS, Kim AY, Yang SK, et al. Crohn disease of the small bowel: comparison of CT enterography, MR enterography, and small-bowel follow-through as diagnostic techniques. *Radiology* 2009;251(3):751–761.

Palmer L, Herfarth H, Porter CQ, et al. Diagnostic ionizing radiation exposure in a population-based sample of children with inflammatory bowel diseases. *Am J Gastroenterol* 2009;104(11):2816–2823.

Rabizadeh S, Dubinsky M. Update in pediatric inflammatory bowel disease. *Rheum Dis Clin North Am* 2013;39(4):789–799.

Walters TD, Kim MO, Denson LA, et al; PRO-KIIDS Research Group. Increased effectiveness of early therapy with anti-tumor necrosis factor-alpha vs an immunomodulator in children with Crohn's disease. *Gastroenterology* 2014;146(2):383–391.

Dietary Protein Gastrointestinal Disorders

Guibas GV, Tsabouri S, Makris M, et al. Food protein-induced enterocolitis syndrome: pitfalls in the diagnosis. *Pediatr Allergy Immunol* 2014;25(7):622–629.

Ludman S, Harmon M, Whiting D, et al. Clinical presentation and referral characteristics of food protein-induced enterocolitis syndrome in the United Kingdom. *Ann Allergy Asthma Immunol* 2014;113(3): 290–294.

Machida HM, Catto Smith AG, Gall DG, et al. Allergic colitis in infancy: clinical and pathologic aspects. *J Pediatr Gastroenterol Nutr* 1994;19(1):22–26.

Maloney J, Nowak-Wegrzyn A. Educational clinical case series for pediatric allergy and immunology: allergic proctocolitis, food protein-induced enterocolitis syndrome and allergic eosinophilic gastroenteritis with protein-losing gastroenteropathy as manifestations of non-IgE-mediated cow's milk allergy. *Pediatr Allergy Immunol* 2007;18(4):360–367.

Wolfe JL, Aceves SS. Gastrointestinal manifestations of food allergies. *Pediatr Clin North Am* 2011;58(2):389–405.

Hemolytic Uremic Syndrome

Noris M, Remuzzi G. Hemolytic uremic syndrome. *J Am Soc Nephrol* 2005;16(4):1035–1050.

GI Vascular Malformations

Lee YT, Walmsley RS, Leong RW, et al. Dieulafoy's lesion. *Gastrointest Endosc* 2003;58(2):236–243.

Lilje C, Greiner P, Riede UN, et al. Dieulafoy lesion in a one year old child. *J Pediatr Surg* 2004;39(1):133–134.

Acute Pancreatitis

Benifla M, Weizman Z. Acute pancreatitis in childhood: analysis of literature data. *J Clin Gastroenterol* 2003;37(2):169–172.

Isenmann R, Runzi M, Kron M, et al; German Antibiotics in Severe Acute Pancreatitis Study Group. Prophylactic antibiotic treatment in patients with predicted severe acute pancreatitis: a placebo-controlled, double-blind trial. *Gastroenterology* 2004;126(4):997–1004.

Jackson WD. Pancreatitis: etiology, diagnosis, and management. *Curr Opin Pediatr* 2001;13(5):447–451.

Kandula L, Lowe ME. Etiology and outcome of acute pancreatitis in infants and toddlers. *J Pediatr* 2008;152(1):106–110.

Smith RC, Southwell-Keely J, Chesher D. Should serum pancreatic lipase replace serum amylase as a biomarker of acute pancreatitis? *ANZ J Surg* 2005;75(6):399–404.

Biliary Atresia

Goldman M, Pranikoff T. Biliary disease in children. *Curr Gastroenterol Rep* 2011;13(2):193–201.

Hartley JL, Davenport M, Kelly D. Biliary atresia. *Lancet* 2009; 374(9702):1704–1713.

Harvapavat S, Finegold MJ, Karpen SJ. Patients with biliary atresia have elevated direct/conjugated bilirubin levels shortly after birth. *Pediatrics* 2011;128(6):e1428–e1433.

Hsiao CH, Chang MH, Chen HL, et al; Taiwan Infant Stool Color Card Study Group. Universal screening for biliary atresia using an infant stool color card in Taiwan. *Hepatology* 2008;47(4): 1233–1240.

Petersen C. Pathogenesis and treatment opportunities for biliary atresia. *Clin Liver Dis* 2006;10(1):73–88.

Raval MV, Dzakovic A, Bentrem DJ, et al. Trends in age for hepatoportoenterostomy in the United States. *Surgery* 2010;148(4):785–791.

Cholelithiasis/Cholecystitis

Goldman M, Pranikoff T. Biliary disease in children. *Curr Gastroenterol Rep* 2011;13(2):193–201.

Poffenberger CM, Gausche-Hill M, Ngai S, et al. Cholelithiasis and its complications in children and adolescents: update and case. *Pediatr Emerg Care* 2012;28(1):68–76.

Walker SK, Maki AC, Cannon RM, et al. Etiology and incidence of pediatric gallbladder disease. *Surgery* 2013;154(4):927–931.

Alagille Syndrome

Goldman M, Pranikoff T. Biliary disease in children. *Curr Gastroenterol Rep* 2011;13(2):193–201.

Piccoli DA, Spinner NB. Alagille syndrome and the Jagged1 gene. *Semin Liver Dis* 2001;21(4):525–534.

Turnpenny PD, Ellard S. Alagille syndrome: pathogenesis, diagnosis, and management. *Eur J Hum Genet* 2012;20(3):251–257.

Acute Liver Failure

Cochran JB, Losek JD. Acute liver failure in children. *Pediatr Emerg Care* 2007;23(2):129–135.

Squires RH Jr. Acute liver failure in children. *Semin Liver Dis* 2008; 28(2):153–166.

Squires RH, Dhawan A, Alonso E, et al. Intravenous N-acetylcysteine in pediatric patients with nonacetaminophen acute liver failure: a placebo-controlled clinical trial. *Hepatology* 2013;57(4):1542–1549.

Squires RH Jr, Shneider BL, Bucuvalas J, et al. Acute liver failure in children: the first 348 patients in the pediatric acute liver failure study group. *J Pediatr* 2006;148(5):652–658.

Portal Hypertension

Bosch J, Berzigotti A, Garcia-Pagan JC, et al. The management of portal hypertension: rational basis, available treatments, and future options. *J Hepatol* 2008;48(suppl 1):S68–S92.

Gugig R, Rosenthal P. Management of portal hypertension in children. *World J Gastroenterol* 2012;18(11):1176–1184.

Ling SC. Portal hypertension in children. *Clin Liver Dis* 2012;1(5): 139–142.

Shneider BL, Bosch J, de Franchis R, et al; Expert panel of the Children's Hospital of Pittsburgh of UPMC. Portal hypertension in children: expert pediatric opinion on the report of the Baveno V Consensus Workshop on Methodology of Diagnosis and Therapy in Portal Hypertension. *Pediatr Transplant* 2012;16(5):426–437.

Viral Hepatitis

Alter MJ. Prevention of spread of hepatitis C. *Hepatology* 2002;36(5 suppl 1):S93–S98.

Broderick AL, Jonas MM. Hepatitis B in children. *Semin Liver Dis* 2003;23(1):S59–S68.

Mack CL, Gonzalez-Peralta RP, Gupta N, et al; North American Society for Pediatric Gastroenterology, Hepatology, and Nutrition. NASPGHAN practice guidelines: diagnosis and management of hepatitis C infection in infants, children, and adolescents. *J Pediatr Gastroenterol Nutr* 2012;54(6):838–855.

NIH consensus statement on management of hepatitis C: 2002. *NIH Consens State Sci Statements* 2002;19(3):1–46.

Pratt DS, Kaplan MM. Evaluation of abnormal liver-enzyme results in asymptomatic patients. *N Engl J Med* 2000;342(17):1266–1271.

Sokal EM, Bortolotti F. Update on prevention and treatment of viral hepatitis in children. *Curr Opin Pediatr* 1999;11(5):384–389.

Gastroesophageal Reflux Disease

Vandenplas Y, Rudolph CD, Di Lorenza C, et al. Pediatric gastroesophageal reflux clinical practice guidelines: joint recommendations of the North American Society for Pediatric Gastroenterology, Hepatology, and Nutrition (NASPGHAN) and the European Society for Pediatric Gastroenterology, Hepatology and Nutrition (ESPGHAN). *J Pediatr Gastroenterol Nutr* 2009;49(4):498–547.

Lightdale JR, Gremse DA. Gastroesophageal reflux: management guidance for the pediatrician. *Pediatrics* 2013;131(5):e1684–e1695.

Deal L, Gold BD, Gremse DA, et al. Age-speciic questionnaires distinguish GERD symptom frequency and severity in infants and young children: development and initial validation. *J Pediatr Gastroenterol Nutr* 2005;41(2):178–185.

Celiac Disease

Fasano A. Celiac disease–how to handle a clinical chameleon. *N Engl J Med* 2003;348(25):2568–2570.

Fasano A, Berti I, Gerarduzzi T, et al. Prevalence of celiac disease in at-risk and not-at-risk groups in the United States: a large multicenter study. *Arch Intern Med* 2003;163(3):286–292.

Green PH, Cellier C. Celiac disease. *N Engl J Med* 2007;357(17):1731–1743.

Hill ID, Dirks MH, Liptak GS, et al; North American Society for Pediatric Gastroenterology, Hepatology and Nutrition. Guideline for the diagnosis and treatment of celiac disease in children: recommendations of the North American Society for Pediatric Gastroenterology, Hepatology and Nutrition. *J Pediatr Gastroenterol Nutr* 2005;40(1):1–19.

Mesenteric Lymphadenitis

Carty HML. Paediatric emergencies: non-traumatic abdominal emergencies. *Eur Radiol* 2002;12(12):2835–2848.

Simanovsky N, Hiller N. Importance of sonographic detection of enlarged abdominal lymph nodes in children. *J Ultrasound Med* 2007;26(5):581–584.

Vayner N, Coret A, Polliack G, et al. Mesenteric lymphadenopathy in children examined by US for chronic and/or recurrent abdominal pain. *Pediatr Radiol* 2003;33:864–867.

Reye Syndrome

Bhutta AT, Van Savell H, Schexnayder SM. Reye's syndrome: down but not out. *South Med J* 2003;96(1):43–45.

da Silveira EB, Young K, Rodriguez M, et al. Reye's syndrome in a 17 year-old male: is this disease really disappearing? *Dig Dis Sci* 2002;47(9):1959–1961.

Glasgow JF, Middleton B. Reye syndrome—insights on causation and prognosis. *Arch Dis Child* 2001;85(5):351–353.

McGovern MC, Glasgow JF, Stewart MC. Lesson of the week: Reye's syndrome and aspirin: lest we forget. *BMJ* 2001;322(7302):1591–1592.

Schrör K. Aspirin and Reye syndrome: a review of the evidence. *Pediatr Drugs* 2007;9(3):195–204.

CHAPTER 100 ■ GYNECOLOGY EMERGENCIES

MARGARET WOLFF, MD, JENNIFER H. CHUANG, MD, MS, AND CYNTHIA J. MOLLEN, MD, MSCE

GOALS OF EMERGENCY CARE

Pediatric gynecologic complaints are common and there is often considerable anxiety surrounding these complaints. The goals of evaluation are to identify life-threatening etiologies, such as ruptured ectopic pregnancy, to ensure appropriate diagnosis and treatment of other etiologies, such as infection and disorders of menstruation, and to ensure appropriate follow-up care with subspecialists or the primary care physician.

KEY POINTS

- Pregnancy should be considered in all adolescent patients presenting to the emergency department.
- Patients with severe abnormal uterine bleeding should be quickly assessed for hemodynamic instability.
- Pelvic inflammatory disease can lead to long-term pain and dysfunction if inadequately treated.

RELATED CHAPTERS

Signs and Symptoms
- Breast Lesions: Chapter 11
- Groin Masses: Chapter 29
- Oligomenorrhea: Chapter 46
- Vaginal Bleeding: Chapter 75
- Vaginal Discharge: Chapter 76

Clinical Pathways
- Abdominal Pain in Postpubertal Girls: Chapter 82
- http://www.chop.edu/clinical-pathway/lower-abdominal-pain-clinical-pathway-post-pubertal-girls

Medical, Surgical, and Trauma Emergencies
- Infectious Disease Emergencies: Chapter 102
- Genitourinary Trauma: Chapter 116
- Genitourinary Emergencies: Chapter 127
- Behavioral and Psychiatric Emergencies: Chapter 134
- Sexual Assault: Child and Adolescent: Chapter 135

PREGNANCY

Goals of Treatment

- Consideration of pregnancy and pregnancy-related complications on the differential diagnosis for adolescent females
- Rapid stabilization of unstable patients
- Identification of appropriate resources to ensure adequate treatment and follow-up
- Attention to consent and confidentiality issues

CLINICAL PEARLS AND PITFALLS

The symptoms of pregnancy in teenagers are variable. It should be considered in the differential diagnosis for almost every chief complaint of the postpubertal adolescent girl. Additionally, physicians should remember to include the possibility of pregnancy in teens with chronic illness. One study of sexual behaviors in adolescents with chronic illness or disability indicates that teenagers with chronic conditions are as sexually active as their otherwise healthy counterparts, regardless of the visibility of the chronic condition. Furthermore, contraception may be less effective in teenagers with chronic illness for multiple reasons.

Confidentiality and Legal Issues

Confidentiality should be maintained throughout the visit to encourage autonomy, protect privacy, promote necessary medical follow-up, and guard the teen from any physical harm or humiliation that may result from disclosing pregnancy status to family members. The results of the test are best initially shared with the adolescent alone. At this time, the practitioner has the opportunity to encourage the teen to share the information with a trusted adult friend who can offer support and assistance to the teen in necessary follow-up. The teen may choose to share this information with those that have accompanied her to the emergency department (ED) or her partner, or may want to contact another adult. A nonjudgmental and compassionate approach will assist the teen in choosing the option that suits her life situation best because she is the one who will be most affected by that choice. However, there are certain situations in which disclosure is required, regardless of the teen's wishes. Every state has enacted mandated reporter statutes that include suspected physical or sexual abuse and suicidal or homicidal ideation; some states include pregnancy in women younger than 13 years old in the definition of abuse.

Current Evidence

According to the Youth Risk Behavior Survey, about 47% of high school students have ever been sexually active; of those who are currently sexually active, 59% report condom use and 19% report birth control use during their last sexual encounter. Twenty percent of sexually active teenagers become pregnant yearly, accounting for approximately 620,000 pregnancies to young women ages 15 to 19 years in 2010. Of these, just over half (approximately 368,000) resulted in live births. With respect to intention to become pregnant, approximately 75% of 15 to 19 year olds who give birth report their pregnancy was unplanned; others, however, report a positive attitude about becoming pregnant.

Clinical Considerations

Clinical Recognition

Although pediatric ED visits for pregnancy account for less than 1% of all visits, the rate of visits to pediatric EDs by pregnant teenagers is increasing. In addition, of nonpregnant teens seeking care in the ED, pregnancy risk may be high due to high rates of sexual activity and lack of contraceptive use. Causey et al. retrospectively compared adolescents presenting to a general emergency department (GED) who were diagnosed with pregnancy with those in whom the diagnosis was not made during an ED visit who subsequently went on to have a child. They found that 43% presented during the first trimester, 25% in the second trimester, and 33% in the third trimester. Of the 100 patients in whom the diagnosis was not made, one-third of these patients had complaints that were suspicious for pregnancy.

The most common presenting complaint associated with early pregnancy is a missed or abnormal menstrual period. However, the menstrual history is particularly unreliable in teenage women secondary to anovulatory cycles. Other symptoms commonly associated with pregnancy include fatigue, dizziness, breast tenderness, weight gain, nausea, and morning sickness. Many adolescents report nonspecific complaints related to the gastrointestinal or genitourinary tracts. Less commonly, the presenting symptom is associated with complications of early pregnancy, including vaginal bleeding, hyperemesis, hypertension, headache, hyperglycemia, vaginal discharge, or dysuria.

Clinical Assessment

It is important to consider performing a pregnancy test in peri- and postmenarchal teenage women. A recent study of national data found that only 20% of adolescent females underwent pregnancy testing during their ED visit; of patients with complaints potentially related to pregnancy, the number rose to only 44.5%. Even if a positive pregnancy test is unrelated to the presenting symptoms, there are several advantages to the patient in identifying pregnancy as early as possible. These include earlier initiation of pregnancy precautions and prenatal care if childbirth is desired, earlier detection of life-threatening complications such as ectopic pregnancy, opportunity for consideration of options such as therapeutic abortion or adoption, and increased time for counseling, regardless of the patient's ultimate choice. If the pregnancy test is negative and pregnancy is suspected, repeat testing should be done in 1 week.

In the ED, it is imperative to recognize those patients who are immediately at risk for life-threatening complications, and require acute resuscitation and emergent evaluation by a surgical subspecialist. Pregnant patients who present with vaginal bleeding, with or without abdominal pain, represent a high-risk group. First-trimester vaginal bleeding occurs in 20% to 25% of patients. Common etiologies include ectopic pregnancy, spontaneous and incomplete abortion, missed or threatened abortion, sexually transmitted infections, and trauma. The initial laboratory workup should always include a complete blood count, both to assess the amount of blood loss and to provide a baseline if bleeding continues. A urinalysis can detect the presence of white blood cells, bacteria, glucose, or protein. Other laboratory screening tests that are rarely indicated during an ED evaluation include Papanicolaou smear, syphilis serology, HIV testing, rubella serology, and hepatitis B serology. If unknown, Rh determination is indicated if there is uterine bleeding. It is important to note that Rh-negative teens with pregnancies greater than 8 weeks' gestation should receive Rh immunoglobulin if there is risk of fetal or placental blood loss.

Ectopic pregnancy is the leading cause of maternal mortality in the United States during the first half of pregnancy; therefore, timely recognition and treatment is imperative. The prevalence of ectopic pregnancy among women presenting to an ED with first-trimester bleeding and/or pain ranges from 6% to 16%. Although the overall incidence of ectopic pregnancy in teenagers is low, this group has the highest mortality rate, largely due to a tendency to delay seeking care. Risk factors for ectopic pregnancy include prior ectopic pregnancy, tubal abnormalities, prior upper genital tract infection, and assisted reproduction.

The diagnosis of ectopic pregnancy must be considered in any patient with vaginal bleeding and/or abdominal pain. Patients can present with a wide spectrum of symptoms, including abnormal vaginal bleeding; intermittent crampy, lower abdominal pain; or acute abdominal pain associated with shock (with or without vaginal blood loss). Fortunately, with the development of sensitive urine pregnancy tests, most patients with ectopic pregnancy present before rupture has occurred.

Spontaneous abortion is another cause of vaginal bleeding in the pregnant teenager, which can be septic, threatened (or missed), inevitable, or complete. Spontaneous miscarriage is very common in early pregnancy; up to one-half of all fertilized ova that implant into the endometrium are lost. Most spontaneous abortions occur during the first trimester, although a small number occur after 20 weeks' gestation. Vaginal bleeding can indicate threatened abortion, when the patient's external cervical os is closed, or an inevitable abortion, when the external os is open. If products of conception are found in the vaginal vault of a patient with an inevitable abortion, the abortion is incomplete.

Management

Pregnancy. Once the diagnosis of pregnancy has been determined, goals of the ED evaluation may include (i) dating the pregnancy, (ii) recognizing symptoms that require immediate referral for obstetric or gynecologic evaluation, (iii) identifying and treating presenting and potential nonsurgical complications, (iv) assessing chronic medical conditions, (v) providing appropriate counseling, and (vi) securing appropriate and timely follow-up. These goals can be tailored to specific settings, depending on consultant availability and access to close follow-up for the patient. In the ED setting, it is optimal to ensure scheduled follow-up in 2 to 3 days with the teen's primary care provider or an adolescent medicine specialist, where counseling about options can occur in a less rushed, less chaotic environment. It is also important to review the patient's medical insurance and link him or her to eligible coverage/resources. The need to arrange close follow-up and to facilitate connection to care following the ED visit should not be underestimated.

For patients diagnosed with pregnancy, the approach may include subspecialty consultation, quantitative serum β-hCG levels, serum progesterone levels, abdominal and/or transvaginal ultrasound, depending on the practice setting, as well as close follow-up. In a normal singleton pregnancy, serial serum β-hCG levels should increase by 67% every 48 hours during the first month of pregnancy. Levels that do not rise or rise more slowly than expected are indicative of an abnormal pregnancy (usually an ectopic pregnancy or a pregnancy that is destined to spontaneously abort). Serum progesterone levels may play some role in the diagnosis of normal versus abnormal pregnancy. A progesterone level greater than 25 ng per dL is seen in 95% of normal pregnancies; a level less than 5 ng per dL suggests an abnormal pregnancy. Ultrasound is used to visualize the uterine cavity to assess for the presence of a gestational sac. When the β-hCG level reaches the discriminatory zone (a level that varies based on local transvaginal ultrasound expertise), a gestational sac should be visible within the uterus. If no sac is seen, the pregnancy is presumed to be ectopic.

For patients diagnosed with ectopic pregnancy, conservative medical management may be appropriate in adolescents who are stable, have no evidence of any bleeding, have a hemoglobin of greater than 8 g per dL and a gestational sac less than 4 cm, who are not immunocompromised, and do not have a bleeding diathesis, or liver, or renal disease, providing that close follow-up can be secured. As many as 83% of patients meeting these criteria may experience spontaneous abortion and resorption.

Although less common, those presenting with an acutely ruptured ectopic pregnancy have an immediate life-threatening condition. These patients usually have a history of abnormal vaginal bleeding and intermittent pelvic pain. On physical examination, vital signs may reflect compensated or uncompensated shock, the abdomen is tender, the uterus is tender and may be slightly enlarged, and an adnexal mass may or may not be palpated after rupture has occurred. These patients require immediate subspecialty consultation with either gynecology or pediatric surgery, depending on the care setting. They should have continuous vital sign monitoring, fluid resuscitation with normal saline, and packed red blood cells as needed. Serial hemoglobin determination, coagulation profile, Rh screening, and type and cross are important components of the laboratory evaluation. Emergency surgical evaluation is the treatment of choice. Ultrasound is contraindicated in the unstable patient and may delay surgical intervention.

Finally, the possibility that sexual abuse may exist in teens concerned about pregnancy and/or diagnosed with pregnancy in the ED needs to be considered and explored. Healthcare providers are mandated to report significant concern for sexual abuse in all patients younger than 18 years of age. It is also important to assess safety issues and screen these teens for depression, substance abuse, and suicide risk. Usually, a multidisciplinary approach is required to ensure that the patient is safe, as well as able to obtain appropriate counseling and medical follow-up.

Delivery. Patients presenting to the ED in active labor should be transferred to the obstetrical unit as soon as possible. However, even in a PED, patients have presented when the newborn is crowning, making transfer impossible. Fortunately, the majority of deliveries occur spontaneously, and the primary role of the clinician is to control the process. However, a subspecialist should be called to the ED to deliver the newborn whenever possible.

VAGINITIS

Goals of Treatment

The goals of treatment are to identify the offending agent and either eliminate it or treat with antimicrobials as indicated.

CLINICAL PEARLS AND PITFALLS

- Vaginitis can be caused by infectious agents, foreign bodies, or irritants.
- In prepubertal girls, vaginitis presents as vaginal discharge, bleeding, or both.
- In pubertal girls, vaginitis presents as discomfort or a change in the character of vaginal discharge.

Current Evidence

Vaginitis, or inflammation of the vagina, can be produced by chemical and mechanical irritants, foreign bodies, and a variety of infectious agents including viruses, chlamydial species, bacteria, fungi, protozoa, and helminths. At least half of all symptomatic premenarcheal girls with vaginal discharge visible on physical examination will prove to have specific vaginal infections that warrant antimicrobial treatment. During childhood, vaginitis is characterized by the presence of vaginal discharge, bleeding, or both. After puberty has begun, girls normally have an asymptomatic vaginal discharge; vaginitis is then indicated by the discomfort it produces or by a change in the character of the discharge. The etiology, clinical manifestations, diagnosis, and treatment of common vaginal infections are presented in this chapter. For a review of the differential diagnosis of vaginal bleeding and discharge, see Chapters 75 Vaginal Bleeding and 76 Vaginal Discharge. Table 100.1 summarizes the treatment of common vaginal infections.

At least half of all symptomatic premenarcheal girls with vaginal discharge visible on physical examination will prove to have specific vaginal infections that warrant antimicrobial treatment. Among prepubertal girls in the United States, *Neisseria gonorrhoeae* causes the greatest number of these specific infections. Less common offenders include *Shigella* species, *Streptococcus pyogenes,* and in infants and after puberty has begun, *Trichomonas vaginalis.* Although staphylococci and *Haemophilus influenzae* usually colonize the lower genital tract without producing symptoms, they are associated with vaginal discharge in only a small proportion of patients. *Candida albicans* is the most common vaginal pathogen among both pubertal (but premenarcheal) and postmenarcheal girls.

The relative prevalence of vaginal infections in a population of postmenarcheal adolescents depends primarily on how many of them are sexually active. Bacterial vaginosis is found commonly and nearly exclusively among sexually active adolescents. Diabetes mellitus, pregnancy, immunodeficiency, and the use of broad-spectrum antibiotics and corticosteroids predispose patients to developing *Candida* vulvovaginitis, but the infection is most often seen in patients who lack any of these risk factors. Trichomoniasis is transmitted vertically or by sexual contact. Up to one-third of patients with trichomoniasis have concurrent gonorrhea, but there is no increased rate of infection with *Chlamydia trachomatis.*

TRICHOMONAL VAGINITIS

Clinical Considerations

Clinical Recognition

A small proportion of vaginally delivered female neonates acquire trichomonal vaginitis from their infected mothers. Infants harboring only a few trichomonads may never develop

TABLE 100.1

TREATMENT OF VAGINITIS

Infection	Drug	Dose, route
Bacterial vaginosis	Metronidazole	500 mg orally bid for 7 days
	Metronidazole gel 0.75%	One full applicator vaginally daily for 5 days
	Clindamycin 300 mg	One orally twice daily for 7 days
Vulvovaginal	Intravaginal agents	
candidiasis	Butoconazole 2% cream[a]	5 g intravaginally for 3 days
	Butoconazole 2% cream (butoconazole 1-sustained release)	Singe intravaginal application
	Clotrimazole 1% cream[a]	5 g intravaginally for 7–14 days
	Clotrimazole 100 mg vaginal tablet	One vaginally daily for 7 days
		2 tablets vaginally for 3 days
	Miconazole 2% cream[a]	5 g intravaginally for 7 days
	Miconazole 100 mg vaginal suppository[a]	One vaginally daily for 7 days
	Miconazole 200 mg vaginal suppository[a]	One vaginally daily for 3 days
	Miconazole 1,200 mg vaginally suppository[a]	Once vaginally
		One vaginally daily for 14 days
	Tioconazole 6.5% ointment[a]	5 g intravaginally daily for 7 days
	Terconazole 0.4% cream	5 g intravaginally daily for 7 days
	Terconazole 0.8% cream	5 g intravaginally daily for 3 days
	Terconazole 80 mg vaginal suppository	One vaginally daily for 3 days
	Oral agent: fluconazole 150 mg	Once orally
Trichomoniasis	Metronidazole	2 g orally as single dose
	Tinidazole	2 g orally as single dose

[a]Over-the-counter preparations.
Adapted from Workowski KA, Bolan GA; Centers for Disease Control and Prevention. Sexually transmitted diseases treatment guidelines, 2015. *MMWR Recomm Rep* 2015;64(RR-3):1–137.

clinical disease, but the remainder will have a thin whitish or yellowish vaginal discharge that appears within 10 days after birth and may persist for several months if untreated. Infected babies may be fussy but are otherwise well.

The classic vaginal discharge of trichomonal vaginitis after puberty is pruritic, frothy, and yellowish. However, many infected women do not complain of excessive discharge and the discharge may be scant or nondescript. A "strawberry cervix" with multiple punctate areas of hemorrhage is pathognomonic for trichomoniasis but is visible without colposcopy in only about 2% of infected patients.

Clinical Assessment

For patients of all ages, the diagnosis can be made if characteristically motile, flagellated trichomonads are seen in a saline suspension of discharge examined microscopically within about 15 minutes after the specimen has been obtained (Fig. 100.1). If a longer delay occurs, the organisms will gradually lose their mobility and normal shape, making them more difficult to identify. The sensitivity rate for wet mount examinations is 50% to 60%. Cultures from a specialized parasite medium have a sensitivity of 85% to 95%, but results are delayed. Newer diagnostic methods, such as nucleic acid amplification testing (NAAT), can be performed with a patient collected vaginal swab and have a sensitivity rate of greater than 95%.

Management

Metronidazole is effective for the treatment of vaginal trichomoniasis. The dosage for infants is 15 mg/kg/day orally in two to three divided doses for 7 days. Recommended treatment of adolescents includes metronidazole 2 g orally in a single dose or tinidazole 2 g orally in a single dose. Because trichomoniasis is a sexually transmitted disease, the adolescent patient's partner(s) must also be referred for treatment.

Nausea and an unpleasant taste are common side effects of nitroimidazoles. Alcohol should be avoided during treatment and 24 to 72 hours after treatment to prevent the occurrence of more severe abdominal pain, vomiting, flushing, and headache (disulfiram reaction). Patients should continue to abstain from alcohol for 24 hours after completion of metronidazole and 72 hours after completion of tinidazole. Recent data indicate that metronidazole is not a teratogen, but many clinicians prefer to postpone treatment of pregnant patients until the second trimester. Intravaginal clotrimazole (two intravaginal tablets at bedtime for 7 days) can provide symptomatic relief for pregnant patients but will cure only 10% to 20%.

SHIGELLA VAGINITIS

Clinical Considerations

Clinical Recognition

Shigella flexneri, Shigella sonnei, Shigella boydii, and *Shigella dysenteriae* can produce vaginal infections in infants and children but do not appear to cause genital disease after puberty. The vaginitis is characterized by a white to yellow discharge that is bloody in three-fourths of cases. Associated pruritus

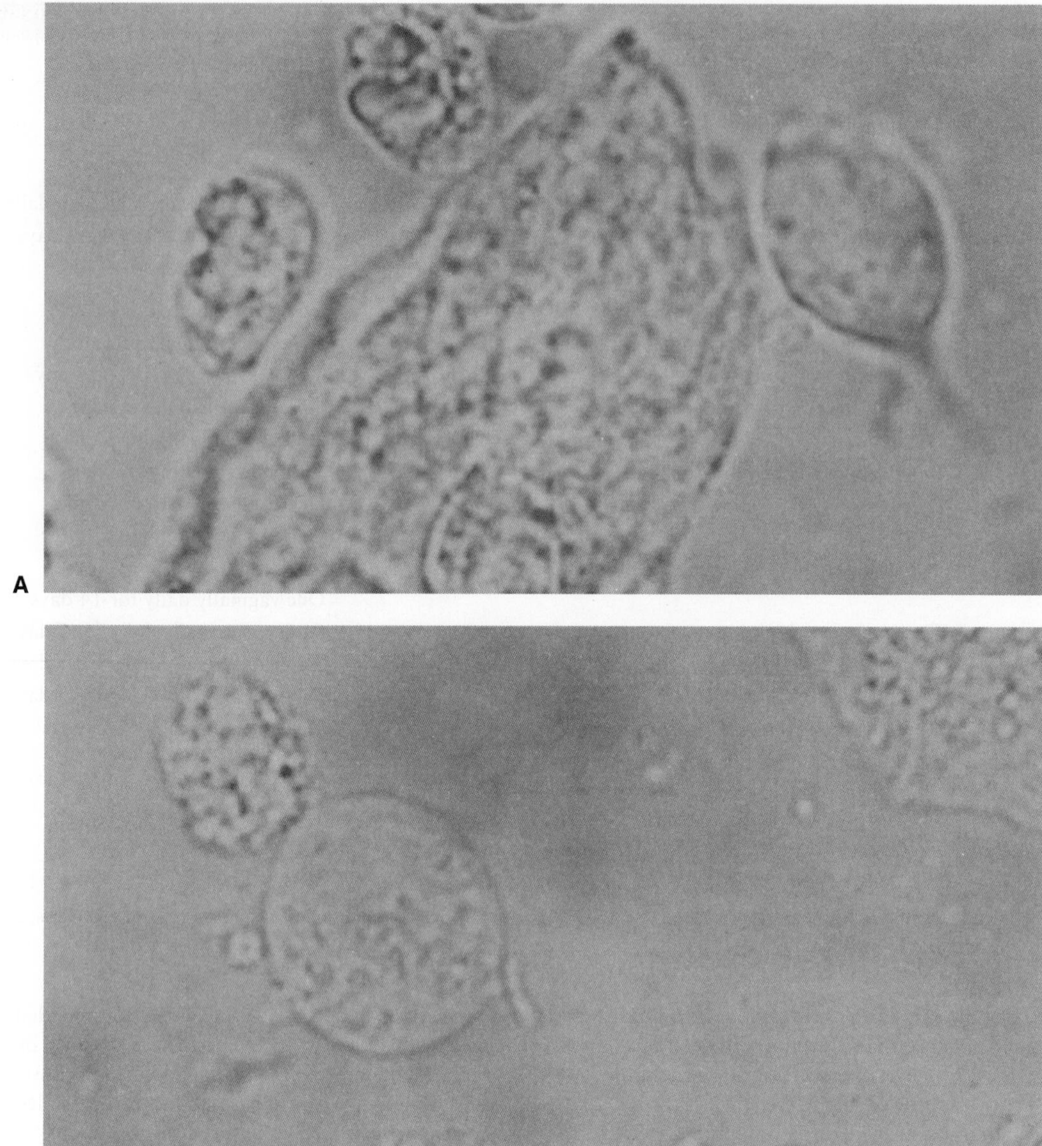

FIGURE 100.1 **A:** Trichomonad in the vaginal discharge of a 17-year-old patient with gonococcal pelvic inflammatory disease. The flagellated protozoan is elliptical and somewhat larger than the adjacent polymorphonuclear leukocytes (×225 magnification). **B:** After suspension in saline solution for microscopy, trichomonads gradually become swollen and immobile. This balloon-shaped trichomonad is barely recognizable (×225 magnification).

and dysuria are uncommon. One-third of patients have diarrhea that precedes, accompanies, or follows the vaginal discharge. On inspection, the vulvar mucosa is often inflamed or ulcerated.

Clinical Assessment

The diagnosis is established by culture of a specimen of vaginal discharge. Rectal cultures are positive for *Shigella* species in some cases.

Management

Patients with *Shigella* vaginitis should be treated with oral antibiotics chosen on the basis of sensitivity testing. If the antibiotic sensitivity is unknown, trimethoprim-sulfamethoxazole (8 mg/kg/day orally of trimethoprim in two divided doses for 5 days) should be used.

STREPTOCOCCAL VAGINITIS

Clinical Considerations

Clinical Recognition

S. pyogenes can be identified in cultures of vaginal specimens taken from about 14% of prepubertal girls with scarlet fever. Most of these vaginal infections produce either no symptoms or minor discomfort, but a few patients develop outright vaginitis with a purulent discharge. Streptococcal vaginitis can accompany or follow symptomatic pharyngitis and causes genital pain or pruritus which can mimic candidal or gonococcal vaginitis.

Clinical Assessment

A swab of the patient's discharge should be cultured to verify the clinical diagnosis. Testing for other potential etiologies, such as gonococcal infection, should be considered on a case-by-case basis.

Management

As for any other infection with group A β-hemolytic streptococci, penicillin is the preferred antibiotic. Intramuscular benzathine penicillin G is an alternative if poor compliance with oral treatment is anticipated. For some patients who are allergic to penicillin, a 10-day course of a narrow-spectrum (first-generation) oral cephalosporin is indicated. However, as many as 5% to 10% of penicillin-allergic people also are allergic to cephalosporins. Patients with immediate or type I hypersensitivity to penicillin should not be treated with a cephalosporin; in these patients, oral clindamycin (20 mg/kg/day in three divided doses; maximum, 1.8 g/day) for 10 days is an acceptable alternative. Additionally, an oral macrolide or azalide (such as erythromycin, clarithromycin, or azithromycin) is also acceptable for patients allergic to penicillin. Therapy for 10 days is indicated **except** for azithromycin (12 mg/kg/day; maximum, 500 mg on day 1, then 6 mg/kg/day; maximum, 250 mg per day), which is given on days 2 through 5.

CANDIDAL VAGINITIS

Clinical Considerations

Clinical Recognition

Candidal vaginitis is one of the most common causes of vaginitis in pubertal adolescents. *C. albicans* frequently colonizes the vagina after the onset of puberty when estrogen stimulates local increases in glycogen stores and acidity that both appear to enhance its growth. If the ecologic balance of the vagina is changed by inhibition of the normal bacterial flora, impaired host immunity, or an increase in the availability of nutrients (broad-spectrum antibiotics, immunodeficiency states, corticosteroids, diabetes mellitus, pregnancy), the resulting proliferation of *Candida* may produce symptoms. However, most patients with candidiasis have no identifiable predisposing risk factors. Because of the importance of estrogen in promoting fungal growth, candidal vulvovaginitis is rare among prepubertal girls.

Clinical Assessment

The most common clinical manifestation of vulvovaginal candidiasis is vulvar pruritus. In severe infections, vulvar edema and erythema can occur. "External" dysuria is produced when urine comes in contact with the inflamed vulva. Vaginal discharge is variable in quantity and appearance. In severe cases, the vaginal vault is red, dry, and has a whitish, watery, or curd-like discharge that may be relatively scanty. Patients with mild disease may have only intermittent itching and an unimpressive discharge.

The diagnosis can be made with the presence of *C. albicans* on wet mount, Gram stain, or culture of vaginal discharge in a patient with vaginitis symptoms; however, candidiasis is most often a clinical diagnosis—testing can be limited to patients who are not responding to appropriate therapy or if an alternative diagnosis is being considered. Microscopic examination of a sample of vaginal discharge suspended in 10% potassium hydroxide solution to clear the field of cellular debris can provide a rapid diagnosis of candidiasis if hyphae are seen. However, in as many as 50% of cases, wet mounts are falsely negative. Gram-stained smears of discharge are somewhat more sensitive because hyphae and yeast cells are Gram-positive and easily visible. Symptomatic women with negative wet mounts and Gram stains should have a culture performed if possible or should receive empiric therapy. From these considerations, it is apparent that, although the presence of *C. albicans* can be confirmed by laboratory tests, the diagnosis and subsequent treatment of this infection should be guided by the presence or absence of clinical disease. It is important to remember that candidal vaginitis does not exclude sexually transmitted infections.

Management

Topical imidazoles will promptly cure 80% to 90% of patients with candidal infections. Most are available without prescription. The creams are packaged with intravaginal applicators, but many premenarcheal and virginal girls can be treated adequately and more comfortably by applying cream to the vulva alone. Effective, nonprescription, short-course treatments of patients with mild to moderate candidal vulvovaginitis include butoconazole 2% cream (5 g at bedtime for three nights), clotrimazole 2% cream (5 g intravaginally at bedtime for three nights), miconazole 200-mg suppositories (one suppository at bedtime for three nights), and tioconazole 6.5% ointment (one full applicator as a single dose). For patients with severe discomfort, one of the 5- or 7-day formulations of a topical agent is likely to be more effective. Creams and suppositories in this regimen are oil-based and might weaken latex condoms and diaphragms. Patients should be referred to condom product labeling for more information. Fluconazole, 150-mg oral tablet in a single dose, cures candidal vulvovaginitis as effectively as the topical preparations, and many patients prefer oral to topical treatment. However, the potential for promoting fungal resistance and the risks, albeit low, of systemic toxicity and allergy are important disadvantages of oral antifungal agents.

BACTERIAL VAGINOSIS

Clinical Considerations

Clinical Recognition

Bacterial vaginosis is a syndrome characterized clinically by the presence of three of the following four signs: (i) a homogeneous, white adherent vaginal discharge; (ii) vaginal pH above 4.5; (iii) a fishy, amine-like odor released when 10% potassium hydroxide solution is added to a sample of the discharge; and (iv) the presence of clue cells (Amsel criteria). The syndrome occurs when lactobacilli that normally predominate in the genital tract are displaced by an overgrowth of mixed flora, including *Gardnerella vaginalis, Mobiluncus* species, other anaerobes, and *Mycoplasma hominis*. What accounts for this change in the vaginal microflora is not understood. The high prevalence of the syndrome in sexually active women and in women attending STI clinics suggests that a wide range

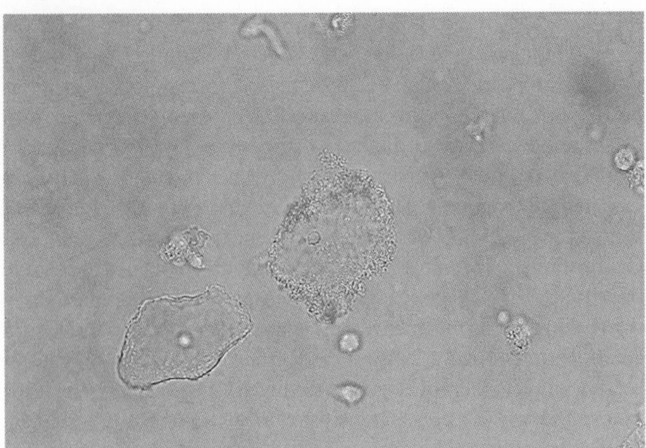

FIGURE 100.2 A clue cell. The vaginal epithelial cell on the right has shaggy borders obscured by coccobacilli (×100 magnification).

of epidemiologic and microbiologic factors may contribute to its pathogenesis.

Clinical Assessment

The symptoms of bacterial vaginosis—malodor and discharge—are not distinctive and can resemble those of trichomonal infection. A complaint of dysuria or pruritus goes against the diagnosis. As many as half of women who have signs of vaginosis are asymptomatic. The vaginal discharge is moderate or copious, grayish-white, and homogeneous. On examination, the vulva, vagina, and cervix are not inflamed, but concomitant infection with trichomonas or gonococci can complicate this picture.

Compared with the composite Amsel criteria, the use of single tests (e.g., pH, clue cells, or whiff test alone) produces lower positive and negative predictive values for the diagnosis of bacterial vaginosis. When a wet mount of vaginal discharge is examined, clue cells can be seen which are epithelial cells that are studded with large numbers of small bacteria giving them a granular appearance with shaggy borders (Fig. 100.2). The ratio of epithelial cells to polymorphonuclear leukocytes in the discharge is 1 or higher. Lactobacilli (long rods) are sparse. Gram stain can be used to confirm the presence of clue cells and the scarcity of long Gram-positive rods (lactobacilli). Because 35% to 55% of women without bacterial vaginosis have positive cultures for *G. vaginalis,* culture is not a useful diagnostic test. In addition, a rapid, antigen-based test has been developed to assess for bacterial vaginosis using a vaginal swab sample, similar to the rapid antigen test for *T. vaginalis.* This test has improved sensitivity and specificity over Gram stain. Trichomonal infection is the major diagnostic alternative for patients suspected of having bacterial vaginosis.

Management

The standard treatment of bacterial vaginosis is oral metronidazole, 500 mg twice daily for 7 days. Treatment of patients' sexual partners does not reduce the recurrence rate and is not recommended. Common side effects of metronidazole include GI upset, headache, and a metallic taste. Patients should abstain from alcohol during treatment and for 24 hours after treatment with metronidazole to avoid the disulfiram reaction. Metronidazole in standard doses is not a human teratogen; however, some clinicians prefer to postpone treatment of pregnant women until the second trimester. Intravaginal clindamycin cream (2%, 5 g) and metronidazole gel (0.75%, 5 g) are alternative treatment options for nonpregnant women. Oral clindamycin (300 mg twice a day for 7 days) is an alternative treatment regimen for pregnant patients with bacterial vaginosis.

NONSPECIFIC VAGINITIS

Clinical Considerations

Clinical Recognition

The term *nonspecific vaginitis,* referring to a disorder of prepubertal girls, encompasses a variety of genitourinary symptoms and signs that are sometimes caused by poor perineal hygiene but that in other cases have no readily identifiable cause. Genital discomfort, discharge, itchiness, and dysuria are relatively common childhood complaints. In a reported series of premenarcheal girls with vaginitis who have been systematically evaluated, between 25% and 75% are ultimately categorized as having nonspecific vaginitis. The diagnosis should not be made until other entities have been excluded.

Clinical Assessment

When a prepubertal girl with vaginitis symptoms has either a normal vulva and vagina or only mild vulvar inflammation on physical examination, a specific vaginal infection is unlikely, and other possible explanations for the complaint—smegma, pinworms, urinary tract infection, a local chemical irritant, or sexual abuse, for example—should be sought with appropriate questions and laboratory tests. (It should be noted that commercially available bubble bath is not often the culprit.) If, however, a vaginal discharge is present on physical examination, the specific vaginal infections discussed in this chapter are diagnostic possibilities and cultures or other specific testing should be obtained.

Management

General measures to promote cleanliness and comfort should be initiated for the girl with nonspecific vaginitis. Daily soaking in a bath of warm water, either plain or with some baking soda added, gentle perineal cleaning with a soft washcloth, and the use of cotton underwear can be recommended. The girl should be taught to wipe toilet paper anteroposteriorly. Using these suggestions, most girls with perineal irritation will show improvement within 2 weeks. The remaining patients should be reevaluated to exclude any specific but previously unrecognized disorder. If none is found, these girls may benefit from a brief course of topical estrogen cream (a small amount dabbed onto the vulva nightly for 2 to 4 weeks) to stimulate thickening of the vaginal mucosa so that it is more resistant to local irritation. Parents should be cautioned that estrogen cream is capable of producing breast growth if it is used for a prolonged period of time.

CERVICITIS

Goals of Treatment

To identify the causative agent and treat with antibiotics or removal of offending agent as appropriate. Patients should also be screened for other sexually transmitted infections, evaluated for pelvic inflammatory disease (PID), and counseled on safe sexual practices.

CLINICAL PEARLS AND PITFALLS

- The most common etiology of acute cervicitis is infectious.
- Cervicitis may be diagnosed incidentally in asymptomatic women.
- Sexually active women with cervicitis should be treated empirically for gonorrhea and chlamydia while test results are pending.

Current Evidence

Cervicitis, or inflammation of the cervix, can be acute or chronic in nature. The etiology of acute cervicitis is most often infectious, with *N. gonorrhoeae* and *C. trachomatis* being the most common offenders. Many of the cases of acute cervicitis will not have a specific infectious etiology identified. Other etiologies of acute cervicitis include mechanical irritation (e.g., tampon, intrauterine device, sexual intercourse) and chemical irritation (e.g., contraceptive cream, douche). Chronic cervicitis is more often due to a noninfectious etiology. If untreated, infections can ascend the genitourinary tract and cause PID which may lead to infertility, chronic pelvic pain, and increased risk of ectopic pregnancy. In addition, cervical infections can be transmitted to sexual partners and increases the risk of acquiring HIV infections if exposed.

Clinical Considerations

Clinical Recognition

Patients with cervicitis may be asymptomatic. Symptomatic patients with cervicitis present with variable and nonspecific symptoms including purulent vaginal discharge, intermenstrual bleeding, postcoital bleeding, and dyspareunia. Less frequently, patients will present with urinary symptoms such as dysuria and urinary frequency due to a concomitant urethral infection. Patients with isolated cervicitis are unlikely to have fever or significant pain. The presence of these should signal other conditions such as PID or a herpes simplex virus infection (HSV).

Clinical Assessment

On physical examination, patients with acute cervicitis will have purulent (or mucopurulent) discharge from the cervix on speculum examination. The clinician may also notice that the cervix tends to bleed easily after minor trauma from a swab used during the examination due to cervical friability. Testing for etiology is essential as it is difficult to determine based on examination findings alone. There are, however, several characteristic findings that may aid the diagnosis. Edema in the zone of ectopy may suggest gonorrhea or chlamydia; ulcerations or vesicles are characteristic of HSV; and punctate hemorrhages are seen in *T. vaginalis*. As many adolescent patients, particularly those in the ED setting, can be assessed without a speculum examination, the diagnosis can be made based on the clinical picture. After determining the patient has cervicitis based on physical examination findings of cervical discharge or endocervical friability, or based on vaginal discharge in a patient at risk for a sexually transmitted disease, testing should be performed for gonorrhea, chlamydia, bacterial vaginosis, and trichomoniasis. Testing for gonorrhea and chlamydia can be performed with NAAT using urine, a vaginal sample, or an endocervical sample (least preferred, and not necessary if the speculum examination is not indicated). Trichomonas can also be detected using NAAT. Testing for bacterial vaginosis generally requires wet prep and vaginal pH testing (see bacterial vaginitis discussion). It is important to remember the diagnosis of one sexually transmitted infection does not exclude other infections. In addition to laboratory tests, the clinician should perform a bimanual examination to assess for concurrent PID.

Management

Patients with acute cervicitis should receive empiric therapy for gonorrhea and chlamydia while awaiting test results. This can be treated with ceftriaxone (250 mg intramuscularly or intravenously; lidocaine hydrochloride can be used as diluent to decrease discomfort) and azithromycin (1 g orally), or doxycycline (100 mg orally twice a day for 7 days). Treatment of Trichomonas, bacterial vaginosis, and herpes simplex virus (HSV) are discussed in the corresponding sections. Patients should be counseled to abstain from sexual activities for 7 days following treatment.

PELVIC INFLAMMATORY DISEASE

Goals of Treatment

The goals of treatment of PID are early recognition, initiation of appropriate antimicrobial treatment, and detection of complications.

CLINICAL PEARLS AND PITFALLS

- One in eight sexually active adolescent girls will develop PID.
- PID can lead to chronic pelvic pain, ectopic pregnancy, and infertility.
- Acute presentation of PID is variable and patients may be well-appearing despite serious consequences of untreated disease.

Current Evidence

PID is a polymicrobial inflammatory condition of the female upper genital tract caused by an ascending sexually transmitted infection that variably involves the endometrium, fallopian tubes, ovaries, adjacent structures, and pelvic peritoneum. An estimated one in eight sexually active adolescent girls develop PID before reaching 20 years of age. Young age, a large number of sexual partners, and nonbarrier contraceptive methods are risk factors for infection with *N. gonorrhoeae* and *C. trachomatis,* the microorganisms responsible for initiating most cases of acute PID. Other risk factors include cigarette smoking, recent douching, bacterial vaginosis, previous gynecologic surgery, and HIV infection. Patients with PID are at risk of serious acute and chronic complications such as tuboovarian abscesses, infertility, and chronic pelvic pain. It has been estimated that 20% of women with PID will have chronic pelvic pain. Half of all ectopic pregnancies are thought to be the result of tubal damage produced by PID. Women with a history of PID have a 10-fold risk of infertility with repeated bouts substantially increasing the likelihood of infertility.

Clinical Considerations

Clinical Recognition

Although the constellation of symptoms and signs associated with PID—abdominal pain, irregular uterine bleeding, abnormal vaginal discharge, and lower abdominal and pelvic tenderness—is well known, no single symptom or sign or a combination of symptoms and signs is both sensitive and specific. Clinical findings that improve the specificity of the diagnosis of PID (i.e., increase the likelihood that the diagnosis is correct) do so only at the expense of sensitivity (i.e., exclude patients who do in fact have PID). Criteria for the diagnosis of PID suggested by the CDC are shown in Table 100.2. Because the diagnosis of PID is imprecise, and the potential for damage to the reproductive health of the patient is great, providers should maintain a low threshold for the diagnosis of PID.

TABLE 100.2

DIAGNOSTIC CRITERIA FOR PELVIC INFLAMMATORY DISEASE

Minimum criteria	Sexually active patient with pelvic or lower abdominal pain, no cause other than PID identified, *and* one of the following: Cervical motion tenderness *or* Uterine tenderness *or* Adnexal tenderness
Additional criteria	These findings enhance the specificity of the minimum criteria and support a diagnosis of PID: Oral temperature >101°F (>38.3°C) Abnormal cervical or vaginal mucopurulent discharge Abundant numbers of white blood cell on saline microscopy of vaginal secretions Erythrocyte sedimentation rate >15 mm/hr Elevated C-reactive protein Documented gonococcal or chlamydial cervical infection
Specific criteria	These findings offer a definitive diagnosis of PID Endometrial biopsy with histopathologic evidence of endometritis Laparoscopic abnormalities consistent with PID Transvaginal sonography or magnetic resonance imaging techniques showing thickened, fluid-filled tubes or tuboovarian complex, or Doppler studies showing tubal hyperemia

PID, pelvic inflammatory disease.
Adapted from Workowski KA, Berman S; Centers for Disease Control and Prevention. Sexually transmitted diseases treatment guidelines, 2010. *MMWR Recomm Rep* 2010;59(RR-12):1–110.

Triage Considerations

The majority of patients with PID will be stable. However, patients presenting with an ill appearance or peritonitis require prompt treatment and surgical consultation. These findings may suggest a complication such as a perforated tuboovarian abscess.

Clinical Assessment

The emergency physician should focus on identifying patients with relatively mild illness; the CDC encourages clinicians to err on the side of providing rather than withholding antibiotic treatment. Additionally, the EM practitioner should identify women with relatively severe illness, through additional diagnostics, focusing on the consideration of major competing diagnoses. Many patients with PID will have negative cultures, which does not exclude the diagnosis, as PID is a polymicrobial clinical syndrome rather than a specific bacterial infection.

An important pathophysiologic irony is the observation that tubal occlusion is associated more often with a relatively unimpressive clinical presentation of PID (i.e., long duration of symptoms, no signs of peritonitis, normal peripheral leukocyte count) than with a "hot" clinical disease (i.e., short duration of symptoms, fever, peritoneal signs, leukocytosis). Similarly, chlamydial PID is associated with both a longer duration of pain at patient presentation and a higher risk of infertility than is gonococcal PID. Thus, if the diagnosis of PID is allowed to depend substantially on patients' appearance—as either "well" or "sick"—clinicians may be tempted to reject the diagnosis of PID and to withhold antibiotic treatment of those patients at highest risk of subsequent ectopic pregnancy and infertility (Fig. 100.3).

A complication of PID that warrants prompt diagnosis is ruptured tuboovarian abscess. About 15% of tuboovarian abscesses rupture spontaneously. The symptoms and signs of a ruptured abscess may be mild if only a small amount of pus has leaked out, but the usual clinical picture includes peritonitis

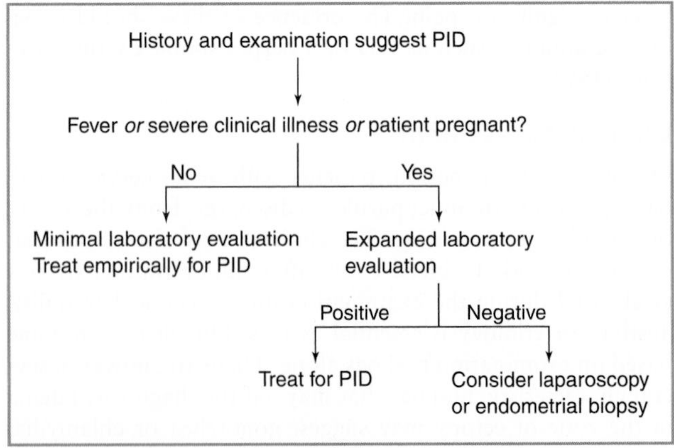

FIGURE 100.3 Strategy for diagnosis of pelvic inflammatory disease (PID). Minimal laboratory evaluation should include tests for gonococcal and chlamydial cervicitis. Expanded laboratory investigation may include, in addition to the minimal evaluation, complete blood cell count, C-reactive protein or erythrocyte sedimentation rate, and pelvic or transvaginal ultrasonography. (Adapted from Kahn JG, Walker CK, Washington AE, et al. Diagnosing pelvic inflammatory disease. A comprehensive analysis and considerations for developing a new model. *JAMA* 1991;266:2594–2604.)

and shock. A pelvic mass is palpable in less than one-half the cases. Prompt surgical intervention can be lifesaving.

Perihepatitis (Fitz-Hugh–Curtis syndrome), consisting of right upper quadrant pain and tenderness produced by inflammation of the liver capsule in association with PID, occurs in 4% to 30% of cases of PID and is more likely to occur with gonococcal infection and more severe diseases. On transvaginal ultrasonography, about one-third of patients with PID will have visible fallopian tubes and about one-fifth will have a demonstrable tuboovarian abscess (Fig. 100.4).

Laparoscopy confirms the diagnosis of PID in only about 60% of patients who are suspected, either by gynecologists or by primary care physicians, on clinical grounds of having the disease. Conditions most often mistaken for PID are acute appendicitis, endometriosis, hemorrhagic and nonhemorrhagic ovarian cysts, and ectopic pregnancy. In up to 25% of women judged clinically to have PID, no abnormality can be identified laparoscopically.

Finally, the emergency physician must consider the possibility of pregnancy in adolescents with presumed PID. Ascending genital tract infection is rare during pregnancy. As a result, alternative diagnoses to PID, including ectopic pregnancy, should be considered. Hospitalization is recommended for all pregnant patients with PID.

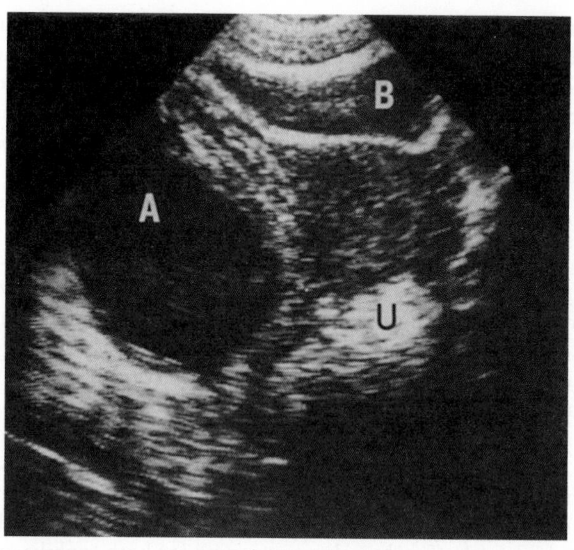

FIGURE 100.4 Transverse real-time sonogram of the pelvis of a 15-year-old patient with gonococcal salpingitis, demonstrating a 6- × 8-cm right tuboovarian abscess (A) containing a fluid–debris level. U, uterus; B, bladder.

Management

The 2015 CDC guidelines for the treatment of PID are summarized in Table 100.3. The antibiotics listed were selected for their effectiveness in combination against *N. gonorrhoeae, C. trachomatis,* and the aerobes and anaerobes responsible for polymicrobial PID. Hospitalization is recommended for any patient with PID whose diagnosis is uncertain, particularly if ectopic pregnancy or appendicitis seems likely; for patients

TABLE 100.3

TREATMENT REGIMENS FOR PELVIC INFLAMMATORY DISEASE

	Initial therapy	Subsequent therapy	Comments
Regimen A			
Extended parenteral treatment	Cefotetan 2 g IV every 12 hrs *or* Cefoxitin 2 g IV every 6 hrs *with* Doxycycline 100 mg po or IV every 12 hrs	Doxycycline 100 mg po bid to complete 14 days of therapy	Oral doxycycline is preferred to avoid infusion pain Parenteral treatment may be stopped 24 hrs after clinical improvement
Regimen B[a]			
Extended parenteral treatment	Clindamycin 900 mg IV every 8 hrs *with* Gentamicin 2 mg/kg and then 1.5 mg/kg IV or IM every 8 hr (single daily dosing may be substituted)	Doxycycline 100 mg po bid *or* Clindamycin 450 mg po qid to complete 14 days of therapy	Clindamycin is preferred for oral treatment of tuboovarian abscess Parenteral treatment may be stopped 24 hrs after clinical improvement
Regimen C			
Combined parenteral/oral treatment	Ceftriaxone 250 mg IM *PLUS* Azithromycin 1 g orally in a single dose or doxycycline 100 mg orally twice daily for 7 days[a] *or* Cefoxitin 2 mg IM with probenecid 1 g po	Doxycycline 100 mg po bid for 14 days	Ceftriaxone has better coverage than cefoxitin against *Neisseria gonorrhoeae* Adding metronidazole (500 mg orally twice a day for 14 days) will treat the bacterial vaginosis associated with many cases of PID and will enhance anaerobic coverage

[a]Fluoroquinolones are no longer recommended for the treatment of gonococcal infections.
IV, intravenous; IM, intramuscular; bid, twice a day; qid, four times daily.
Adapted from Workowski KA, Bolan GA; Centers for Disease Control and Prevention. Sexually transmitted diseases treatment guidelines, 2015. *MMWR Recomm Rep* 2015;64(RR-3):1–137; Centers for Disease Control and Prevention (CDC). Update to CDC's Sexually transmitted diseases treatment guidelines, 2010: oral cephalosporins no longer a recommended treatment for gonococcal infections. *MMWR Morb Mortal Wkly Rep* 2012;61(31):590–594.

with severe clinical illness, including those with fever or suspected pelvic abscess; and for patients who are either immunodeficient or pregnant. Parenteral treatment is recommended for patients likely to fail a course of oral antibiotics because of either poor compliance or vomiting and for those whose illnesses have not responded to prior oral antibiotics.

The follow-up of outpatients should include a return visit after about 3 days of treatment. The average duration of symptoms among women with gonococcal salpingitis treated with oral antibiotics is 3 to 4 days; the corresponding interval for nongonococcal salpingitis is 4 to 6 days. A poor response to therapy should alert the physician to the possibilities of inadequate compliance, abscess formation, or an alternative diagnosis.

Follow-up for all patients should include reexamination at the end of antibiotic therapy to check for residual pelvic tenderness and adnexal masses. All patients with gonococcal and chlamydial infections should be counseled about the HIV infection and offered serologic screening for both syphilis and HIV infection.

The importance of identifying and treating sexual partners of women with PID cannot be overemphasized. About 25% of such men have asymptomatic urethritis and are unlikely to seek treatment on their own. If these men are not treated, they become part of the reservoir of undetected carriers of STIs. The success of various patient referral strategies conducted by public healthcare personnel to achieve treatment of partners ranges from 29% to 59%. The success rate of patient-initiated partner treatment is unknown in the adolescent population, although several small studies in adult women suggest this strategy may reduce the rate of reinfection. The legal and policy landscape around expedited partner therapy is complicated and constantly changing; the CDC maintains an up-to-date website in order to assist clinicians who wish to provide this treatment to patients (http://www.cdc.gov/std/ept/legal/default.htm). All sexual partners with contact with a patient with PID (or any STI) within the prior 2 months should be treated.

ADNEXAL TORSION

Goals of Treatment

The primary goals for the emergency physician are consideration of ovarian torsion on the differential diagnosis of female patients with abdominal pain, rapid assessment with ultrasonography to make the diagnosis, and rapid referral to an appropriate specialist for surgical intervention.

CLINICAL PEARLS AND PITFALLS

- Ovarian torsion is a difficult diagnosis to make, given the lack of specific or sensitive historical or physical examination factors.
- The diagnosis of ovarian torsion can be made in prepubertal girls, although postmenarchal patients account for the majority of diagnoses.
- Enlargement of the ovary is the most common finding on ultrasound; Doppler findings can be inconsistent due to the dual blood supply of the ovary, so demonstration of blood flow should not definitively rule out ovarian torsion.

Current Evidence

Adnexal torsion is a rare diagnosis with an estimated incidence of 4.9 per 100,000 in women less than 20 years of age. Pediatric patients are the minority of cases of adnexal torsion; large pediatric centers report 0.3 to 3.5 cases annually. With respect to treatment, many surgeons are moving away from oophorectomy and instead treat patients with detorsion and conservative measures. This is due in part to the rarity of malignancies as a cause of torsion in pediatric patients, and in part to increasing evidence of the rarity of complications and good clinical outcomes. Of note, multiple studies have indicated that the intraoperative appearance of the ovary does not predict permanent damage or long-term sequelae of torsion.

Clinical Considerations

Clinical Recognition

Adnexal torsion can be a difficult diagnosis to make, given that the clinical picture can overlap with other, more common, abdominal diagnosis, such as appendicitis. Most patients with adnexal torsion will present with acute onset of lower abdominal or pelvic pain; the location of the pain can vary in younger children, as the ovaries can be located higher in the abdomen than in adult women, but symptoms are almost universally unilateral. Additional symptoms may include nausea, vomiting, fever, and symptoms referable to the urinary tract. Many patients report constant pain, although the pain can be intermittent.

Clinical Assessment

Female patients presenting with acute onset of abdominal pain should be assessed with a complete history and physical examination, which can start to narrow the broad differential diagnosis. Because studies suggest that right-sided adnexal torsion is more common than left-sided, many patients will need to be evaluated concurrently for adnexal torsion and appendicitis. Additional diagnoses to consider include nephrolithiasis, mesenteric adenitis, intussusception (in the younger patient), and urinary tract infection, to name several. A recent retrospective chart review of 82 cases of adnexal torsion found that most patients presented with 24 hours of severe, intermittent pain, and commonly reported nausea, vomiting, and abdominal tenderness on examination. This larger study was consistent with findings from smaller, previous studies. Similarly, a retrospective study of 94 patients found that the presence of intermittent pain and nonradiating pain were statistically associated with the diagnosis of torsion. While laboratory studies can assist in the diagnosis of other entities causing abdominal pain, when there is high suspicion for adnexal torsion a pelvic ultrasound is the first study of choice. While a wide spectrum of morphologic changes have been reported on ultrasound, the majority of patients will have a unilaterally enlarged ovary. As noted above, the presence of arterial blood flow does not rule out the diagnosis of adnexal torsion. However, the absence of Doppler flow is highly suggestive of torsion. While computed tomography can demonstrate findings consistent with adnexal torsion, it is used most commonly when alternative diagnoses are suspected. Similarly, while magnetic resonance imaging can diagnosis torsion, the logistical difficulty of obtaining the study in many centers, combined with the high cost and potential delay in diagnosis, limit its utility for this diagnosis.

Management

As with all patients with potential surgical diagnoses, patients with suspected adnexal torsion should remain npo with intravenous fluids. Pain management with opioids may be needed. When the diagnosis of adnexal torsion is confirmed, the patient should be assessed immediately by a surgeon. Most patients will undergo conservative management and detorsion rather than oophorectomy. The duration of symptoms has not been shown to correlate with ovarian salvage.

DISEASES THAT PRODUCE EXTERNAL GENITOURINARY LESIONS

CLINICAL PEARLS AND PITFALLS

- HSV may not present with classic symptoms making laboratory testing essential.
- Primary HSV infections are typically characterized by more lesions and greater systemic involvement.
- Human papillomavirus (HPV) affects the majority of young women in some populations.

Herpes Simplex Virus Infection

HSV can cause disease of the skin, mucus membranes including genitalia, eyes, liver, lung, and the central nervous system. Genital lesions can be caused by either serotype of HSV (HSV-1 or HSV-2). Patients may present with any of the three disease states of HSV: primary, nonprimary first episode, and recurrent. A patient with HSV infection without pre-existing antibodies to HSV-1 or HSV-2 has primary HSV infection. Nonprimary HSV infection refers to a patient who develops a genital infection with HSV-1 who has pre-existing antibodies to HSV-2 or vice versa. Recurrent infections occur when there is reactivation of HSV and the lesions are the same serotype as the serum antibodies. Patients with primary infections tend to have significant systemic and local signs and symptoms, though some patients may be asymptomatic or have mild symptoms. When present, systemic symptoms include fever, myalgias, and malaise. Local symptoms include painful lesions that may also be pruritic, dysuria, and tender lymphadenopathy. Lesions tend to last 2 to 3 weeks. Rarely, patients with severe primary infection may present with acute urinary retention due to lumbosacral radiculopathy. Nonprimary first infections tend to be less severe with fewer lesions. Recurrent infections are typically less severe than primary infections with a shorter duration of symptoms (mean duration 10 days) and may be preceded by a prodrome of tingling or pain in the legs, buttocks, or genitalia. Local symptoms are more common than systemic symptoms in recurrent disease.

Patients will classically present with painful, shallow, tender ulcers that may contain a vesicular component. In addition, some patients may have systemic symptoms as noted above. Other etiologies of genital ulcerations include syphilis which tends to be a painless ulcer and chancroid which tends to be a deep, purulent ulcer with very tender lymphadenopathy. Diagnosis of HSV made by history and physical examination alone may be inaccurate; therefore diagnosis should be confirmed by laboratory testing. Testing options include viral culture, polymerase chain reaction (PCR), and direct fluorescent antibody (DFA). Viral culture is the least sensitive of the available methods and requires several days prior to diagnosis, making this option less desirable if alternate methods are available. If viral culture is performed, the culture should be obtained by unroofing an active genital lesion and sampling the vesicular fluid. PCR and DFA are more sensitive methods and PCR testing is the test of choice for cerebrospinal fluid testing. Tzanck testing is insensitive and difficult to interpret and should not be relied upon for the diagnosis of HSV.

TABLE 100.4

TREATMENT REGIMENS FOR HERPES SIMPLEX VIRUS INFECTIONS

Primary infection	Suppressive	Recurrent infection
Acyclovir 400 mg po tid for 7–10 days OR Acyclovir 200 mg po five times daily for 7–10 days OR Famciclovir 250 mg po tid for 7–10 days OR Valacyclovir 1 g po bid for 7–10 days	Acyclovir 400 mg po bid OR Famiciclovir 250 mg po bid OR Valacyclovir 500 mg po once a day OR Valacyclovir 1 g po once a day	Acyclovir 400 mg po tid for 5 days OR Acyclovir 800 mg po bid for 5 days OR Acyclovir 800 mg po tid for 2 days OR Famciclovir 1000 mg po bid for 1 day OR Valacyclovir 500 mg po bid for 3 days OR Valacyclovir 1 g po once daily for 5 days

Adapted from Workowski KA, Bolan GA; Centers for Disease Control and Prevention. Sexually transmitted diseases treatment guidelines, 2015. *MMWR Recomm Rep* 2015;64(RR-3):1–137.

Primary HSV can cause prolonged and significant pain and discomfort. Therefore, all patients with primary infection should receive antiviral therapy (Table 100.4) to reduce symptom severity and shorten disease course. Recurrences are common with HSV infections, making suppressive therapy desirable to some patients and have the added benefit of decreasing partner transmission. Alternatively, some patients may prefer episodic therapy for recurrent episodes. Antivirals are most effective when started within 72 hours of symptom onset. Management should also include symptomatic relief of pain, dysuria, and systemic symptoms. Sitz baths may be effective for patients with dysuria due to painful lesions.

HPV

HPV affects a large number of young women with the prevalence approaching 60% in some populations of young women in the United States. There are over 100 types of HPV that affect different sites of the body. The types affecting the anogenital region can cause genital warts (condyloma acuminatum) or squamous intraepithelial lesions which can lead to carcinoma of the vagina, vulva, cervix, and anus in women. Patients presenting with anogenital warts will have variable symptoms depending on the location, size, and number of lesions present. If warts are small in size and number, patients will often be asymptomatic. Patients that are symptomatic may experience burning, tenderness, pruritus, or pain. Occasionally, large mass-like warts will form that can interfere with defecation or intercourse.

Condylomata acuminata consists of pink- or skin-colored lesions that may be small, flat papules or large and papilliform. Physical examination is usually sufficient for diagnosis, but lesions should be distinguished from the flat and velvety lesions seen in secondary syphilis. In some patients, further evaluation with speculum examination or anoscopy will be necessary to determine the extent of involvement. If diagnosis remains uncertain after visual inspection or if a patient is immunocompromised, a biopsy can be obtained to confirm the diagnosis.

Management depends on location, size, and number of lesions as well as patient preference. Spontaneous regression of anogenital lesions is possible, but patients often prefer to have the lesions treated to hasten removal and should be referred to gynecology or adolescent medicine to facilitate this. Lesions can be removed by physical destruction, immunologic therapy, and surgical therapy. However, many lesions recur regardless of method of removal employed. Patients with anogenital warts should also be counseled about the potential presence of squamous intraepithelial lesions and need for screening. An HPV vaccine exists, recommended as a 3-shot series over a 6-month period for all young adolescents ages 11 or 12 years. According to the CDC, young women can receive the vaccine through age 26 years; young men are eligible through age 21 years, with special populations (immunocompromised, men who have sex with men) eligible through 26 years old.

DISORDERS OF MENSTRUATION

Dysmenorrhea

Goals of Treatment

To provide appropriate pain relief to adolescents experiencing severe cramping from dysmenorrhea.

CLINICAL PEARLS AND PITFALLS

- Nonsteroidal anti-inflammatory drugs (NSAIDs) are usually effective first-line treatment for primary dysmenorrhea and are most effective when started at the first sign of cramping or menstrual bleeding.
- If a patient's pain persists despite appropriate use of NSAIDs, hormonal management usually ameliorates symptoms of primary dysmenorrhea.
- Suspect secondary dysmenorrhea due to endometriosis or other pelvic pathology if the patient's pain does not improve after the use of NSAIDs and a hormonal method for 3 to 6 months.

Background

Pelvic pain related to menses is a common complaint in the ED. The adolescent may experience dysmenorrhea (pain with menses) when she begins ovulatory cycles—typically 1 to 3 years after menarche. In the majority of cases, the pain is caused by primary dysmenorrhea (in the absence of any pelvic pathology). Pain that does not respond appropriately to treatment for primary dysmenorrhea may be secondary to endometriosis, reproductive tract anomalies, or other pelvic pathology.

Current Evidence

It is believed that the production of prostaglandins, particularly PGF2α and PGE_2, plays a central role in the discomfort of dysmenorrhea. These prostaglandins can account for uterine contractions, nausea, and diarrhea that are often associated with menstrual cramps. NSAIDs are typically the first-line treatments for dysmenorrhea to alleviate symptoms. NSAIDs act to inhibit the cyclooxygenase pathway, thereby ultimately hindering prostaglandin synthesis.

Clinical Assessment

A detailed menstrual history is important to obtain from the patient complaining of severe menstrual cramps. Information about the timing of her first period (menarche), regularity of her cycles, duration of menstrual flow, and the amount of blood flow per period are important to know. The practitioner should ask about accompanying signs such as nausea, vomiting, dizziness, or diarrhea. Knowing whether the cramps keep the patient home from school gives a clue that the adolescent's ability to function well is affected by the dysmenorrhea. Asking about which medications have been attempted for alleviation of symptoms is important, as symptoms are usually better controlled with NSAIDs than with acetaminophen.

A physical examination for dysmenorrhea does not routinely include a pelvic examination unless the provider is concerned about an imperforate hymen, adnexal masses, or a sexually transmitted infection. For patients with a history of sexual activity and presenting with pelvic pain, a bimanual examination should be performed to evaluate for PID. Findings of cervical motion tenderness, adnexal tenderness, or uterine tenderness would be consistent with a clinical presentation of PID. Patients who are sexually active should be tested for chlamydia and gonorrhea, as they may present with pelvic pain or with irregular or heavy vaginal bleeding. Endometriosis may also have findings of adnexal, uterine, or rectovaginal tenderness or nodularity on bimanual or rectal examination. If pelvic anatomy should be further explored, ultrasonography or MRI are options to consider. Pelvic ultrasound is an appropriate initial imaging study to evaluate uterine and ovarian anatomy. An MRI may be a better modality to evaluate vaginal and bladder lesions. Intraperitoneal lesions, however, are difficult to visualize on imaging studies.

Management

NSAIDs are first-line medications for most adolescents with dysmenorrhea and have both analgesic and anti-inflammatory effects. The NSAIDs block cyclooxygenase, thus inhibiting production of prostaglandins from arachidonic acid. The patient should be counseled that the NSAIDs are most effective when started 1 to 2 days prior to onset of menstrual bleeding. If the patient is unable to predict the onset of her period, then she should be advised to start the NSAIDs at the first signs of cramping or bleeding. Naproxen (500 mg PO q12h) and ibuprofen (600 to 800 mg PO q6h) are effective NSAIDs to use for dysmenorrhea; failure to respond to one NSAID does not preclude use of another. NSAIDs should be avoided in patients with ulcers, gastrointestinal bleeding, renal disease, or clotting disorders.

In patients where NSAIDs are contraindicated, tramadol may be used, as it is a centrally acting analgesic agent that binds to μ-opioid receptors and inhibits the reuptake of norepinephrine and serotonin. Tramadol is prescribed as 50 to

100 mg by mouth every 6 hours, not to exceed 400 mg per day. Use tramadol with caution in patients with a history of seizures. Drug dependence is also possible in patients taking tramadol.

Patients whose pain is not alleviated by NSAIDs should be offered a hormonal method to treat the dysmenorrhea. Combined oral contraceptive pills (OCPs) with estrogen and progestin formulations are widely used to treat dysmenorrhea by suppressing ovulation, reducing the amount of endometrial growth, and reducing the amount of endometrial tissue available for prostaglandin production. Patients who continue to have significant pain during the week of placebo pills may be considered for an extended cycle regimen (e.g., prescribing a 91-day pack rather than the standard 28-day pack). The combined contraceptive transdermal patch (Ortho Evra) or vaginal ring (NuvaRing) delivers similar results as OCPs. Any patient who is sexually active should be counseled to consider beginning a hormonal method of birth control as well. Before initiating any therapy containing estrogen, the patient should be assessed for any contraindication to estrogen (described in detail under Abnormal Uterine Bleeding section).

Patients in whom estrogen is contraindicated or not preferable may respond well to progestin-only medications. The injectable depot medroxyprogesterone (Depo-Provera) is particularly effective in suppressing ovulation and alleviating pain from dysmenorrhea and can be administered every 12 weeks. Implantable subdermal progestin (Nexplanon) and progestin-releasing intrauterine devices (Mirena) may also be longer-acting alternatives to treat dysmenorrhea. Most patients with primary dysmenorrhea will respond to NSAIDs and hormonal medication to alleviate symptoms within 3 months. Patients whose menstrual-associated pain continue to be severe despite 6 months of NSAIDs and hormonal management should be assessed for dysmenorrhea secondary to endometriosis or other pelvic pathology. A laparoscopy may be performed to evaluate for endometriosis.

ABNORMAL UTERINE BLEEDING

Goals of Treatment

The goal for the ED physician is to reduce the patient's vaginal bleeding in a prompt yet safe manner.

CLINICAL PEARLS AND PITFALLS

- The physician should assess for signs for hemodynamic instability including checking orthostatic vital signs and hemoglobin.
- The differential diagnosis for abnormal uterine bleeding (AUB) should also include von Willebrand disease and other coagulation disorders.
- Assess whether there are any contraindications for administering the patient an estrogen containing therapy.

Background

AUB refers to irregular, prolonged, or excessive menstrual bleeding unrelated to pregnancy. The term AUB has replaced the previous terminology of dysfunctional uterine bleeding. The majority of adolescents who present to the ED with AUB will have bleeding related to anovulatory cycles. Normal menstrual cycles in an adolescent may range from 21 to 45 days, though the adult menstrual cycle is generally 21 to 35 days. Regular ovulatory cycles may not occur until about 2 years after menarche, and the majority of AUB within 18 months of menarche are due to anovulatory cycles. Bleeding that persists beyond 9 days, recurs at intervals of fewer than 21 days, soaks greater than one pad per hour, produces large clumps of clots, causes anemia, or creates hemodynamic instability, warrants attention.

The normal ovulatory menstrual cycle is divided into an initial follicular and a subsequent luteal phase. The parallel phases of endometrial development are termed, respectively, proliferative and secretory. At the start of the ovulatory cycle, pituitary follicle–stimulating hormone (FSH) promotes the growth of ovarian follicles. The follicles produce estradiol which stimulates the proliferation of endometrial stroma and glands and induces a midcycle surge of luteinizing hormone (LH), which triggers ovulation. Ovulation typically occurs 14 days prior to the onset of menses, and the ovarian follicle forms a corpus luteum that secretes progesterone and estradiol; subsequently the levels of FSH and LH gradually decline. The progesterone produced by the corpus luteum promotes growth of the endometrial secretory glands and spiral blood vessels, though it also limits the ultimate thickness of the endometrium. As the corpus luteum degenerates, circulating levels of estrogen and progesterone fall which lead to endometrial necrosis and menstrual sloughing.

The majority of adolescents who present with AUB experience intervals of anovulation. Without ovulation, there is no progesterone secreted by the corpus luteum to promote structural integrity of the endometrium. Estrogen levels secreted by the ovarian follicles may fluctuate, including secreting large amounts that cause greater endometrial proliferation and thus heavy vaginal bleeding.

Clinical Manifestations

History, physical, and laboratory tests help the clinician guide the severity of the patient's vaginal bleeding. Bleeding that has been occurring for 8 days or more, at intervals more frequently than every 21 days, bleeding greater than 80 mL per menstrual period, or bleeding large clots that are at least quarter sized, should be evaluated by a healthcare provider for AUB. Unlike bleeding during an ovulatory cycle, AUB from anovulatory cycles tends to be painless and without significant cramps. Pertinent history should also include whether the patient is pregnant, has been sexually active, or has any underlying platelet or bleeding disorder (e.g., thrombocytopenia, von Willebrand disease).

The physical examination starts with the measurement of the patient's vital signs, including checking for orthostatic changes in the pulse and blood pressure. Pallor and symptomatic orthostasis are concerning for significant anemia. Petechiae, bruising, and mucosal bleeding may indicate a bleeding disorder. Signs of polycystic ovarian syndrome include hirsutism, acne, obesity, and acanthosis nigricans (an indication of insulin resistance). The clinician may choose to perform a speculum examination to note for the presence of bleeding from the cervical os, an incomplete abortion, cervicitis, or a retained foreign body. A bimanual examination may be performed to assess for uterine tenderness and adnexal masses. If necessary, rectoabdominal palpation can be substituted for the standard bimanual examination.

A complete blood count should be ordered to assess the hemoglobin, hematocrit, and platelet count. A reticulocyte count may be helpful as an indicator of bone marrow response to the blood loss. Screen sexually active adolescents with a pregnancy test as well as a vaginal swab or urine collection for a NAAT for *N. gonorrhoeae* and *C. trachomatis*. Be aware that many adolescents may not be forthcoming about their sexual history, and if the clinician has an index of suspicion that the patient may have been sexually active consider sending the tests.

Coagulation disorders—such as von Willebrand disease, thrombocytopenia, or platelet dysfunction—should be considered in adolescents who present with heavy bleeding at menarche or who bleed heavily with each menses. Coagulation studies to send in addition to a complete blood count include prothrombin time, partial thromboplastin time, fibrinogen, and a von Willebrand panel—consisting of von Willebrand factor, ristocetin cofactor activity, and factor VIII activity. The von Willebrand panel should be drawn prior to the administration or 7 days after discontinuing any hormonal medications, particularly those containing estrogen, as the estrogen may raise the von Willebrand factor into normal range. Bleeding may also be related to the use of medications such as anticoagulants or platelet inhibitors. TSH should also be sent, as hyperthyroidism and hypothyroidism may cause menstrual irregularities. An evaluation for polycystic ovarian syndrome may include laboratory studies for FSH, LH, DHEAS, free and total testosterone, and androstenedione, though these results will not be available to the emergency physician but useful to the patient's outpatient provider. If there are concerns for a prolactinoma, including signs of visual field deficits, a prolactin level may be sent. Adolescents with androgenic signs and clitoromegaly may be evaluated for congenital adrenal hyperplasia by sending 17-hydroxyprogesterone.

Management

For patients with brisk hemorrhage or hemodynamic instability, hospitalization and prompt volume resuscitation are necessary as well as possible blood transfusion. Control of the bleeding is usually accomplished with hormonal treatment, commonly using a combined estrogen and progestin approach (Table 100.5). Estrogen is used to stop the bleeding and support the endometrium. A progesterone agent must be administered simultaneously or soon after the administration of estrogen to produce a more stabilized secretory endometrium. Any of the OCPs with 0.03 mg to 0.05 mg of ethinyl estradiol and a progestin provides a convenient means of administering the two hormones together. Commonly used pills include ethinyl estradiol 0.03 mg/norgestrel 0.3 mg or ethinyl estradiol 0.05 mg/norgestrel 0.5 mg. For brisk bleeding, one tablet may be given up to four times a day until the bleeding stops. The medication may then be gradually tapered as long as the bleeding remains ceased (e.g., one tablet three times a day for 3 days, then one tablet two times a day for 3 days, then one tablet a day). Nausea is a common side effect of estrogen and can be treated symptomatically with antiemetics. If the emergency physician is discharging the patient home, provide two prescriptions to the patient: the first prescription with the above taper regimen with instructions to skip the placebo week in

TABLE 100.5

MANAGEMENT OF ABNORMAL UTERINE BLEEDING

Mild (Hgb >12 mg/dL)	May monitor as an outpatient Offer OCPs or progestin-only pills
Moderate (Hgb 10–12 mg/dL)	Ethinyl estradiol 0.03 mg/norgestrel 0.3 mg OCP every 6 hrs until bleeding stops. Then pills may be tapered if the bleeding has not resumed to three pills a day for 3 days, two pills a day for 3 days, then one pill daily If estrogen is contraindicated, then may use medroxyprogesterone 10 mg or norethindrone acetate 5–10 mg up to four times a day. May give four times a day for 4 days, then taper to three times a day for 3 days, then two times a day for 2 wks. Follow-up will be needed by her outpatient provider Iron 65 mg/day and consider a stool softener Antiemetics as needed Follow-up as outpatient with primary care provider, adolescent medicine, gynecologist, or hematology
Severe (Hgb <10 mg/dL)	Assess for hemodynamic instability Volume resuscitation and consider blood transfusion If bleeding is severe and poorly controlled, consider conjugated estrogen (Premarin) 25 mg IV every 4 hrs for 2–3 doses Otherwise, most patients respond to ethinyl estradiol 0.05 mg/norgestrel 0.5 mg OCP every 6 hrs until bleeding stops. Then pills may be tapered if the bleeding has not resumed to three pills a day for 3 days, two pills a day for 3 days, then one pill daily If estrogen is contraindicated, then may use medroxyprogesterone 10 mg or norethindrone acetate 5–10 mg up to four times a day. May give four times a day for 4 days, then taper to three times a day for 3 days, then two times a day for 2 wks. Follow-up will be needed by her outpatient provider Antiemetics as needed Iron 65 mg/day and consider a stool softener Rarely, curettage if hormonal therapy fails

the pill pack; the second prescription to take one tablet daily after finishing the pill pack from the first prescription. The diagnoses should be included on the prescriptions, as many insurance companies will not initially approve of dispensing more than one pill pack per month.

Patients with severe bleeding, hemodynamic instability, and hemoglobin <10 g per dL should be considered for hospital admission. Refill the intravascular space with isotonic fluids and evaluate need for potential blood transfusion. For acute severe hemorrhage, conjugated estrogen (Premarin) 25 mg IV every 4 hours for two or three doses may be given. Keep in mind, however, that conjugated estrogen has a higher risk of thromboembolism than the combined oral contraceptives. A combined estrogen and progestin pill is still administered within 24 to 48 hours after starting conjugated estrogen for stabilization of the endometrium by progestin. Patients whose bleeding does not significantly improve after one to two doses of conjugated estrogen should be reevaluated for an alternate cause of bleeding (e.g., bleeding diatheses, anatomic abnormality).

Before starting any estrogen containing therapy, assess the patient for any contraindications to estrogen (Table 100.6). Absolute contraindications include a history of migraine with aura, deep venous thromboembolism or pulmonary embolism, inherited prothrombotic disorders, systemic lupus erythematosus with positive or unknown antiphospholipid antibodies, hypertension (SBP >160 mm Hg or DBP >100 mm Hg), certain heart conditions (ischemic heart disease, complicated valvular heart disease, peripartum cardiomyopathy), certain liver conditions (hepatocellular adenoma, liver malignancy, severe cirrhosis), postpartum <21 days, stroke, current diagnosis of breast cancer, or history of complicated solid organ transplant. For a full list see the United States Medical Eligibility Criteria for Contraceptive Use at http://www.cdc.gov/reproductivehealth/unintendedpregnancy/usmec.htm.

If estrogen is contraindicated or not tolerated, progestin-only regimens may be used but the resulting hemostasis is less prompt and less predictable. Medroxyprogesterone and norethindrone acetate are progestin-only pill options that may be used. Medroxyprogesterone 10 mg or norethindrone acetate 5 to 10 mg may be given orally up to four times a day. A typical taper may begin as four times a day for 4 days. If the bleeding stops, then the taper may continue as three times a day for 3 days, and then twice a day for 2 weeks. The patient's outpatient provider may continue to taper the progestin pill to one tablet daily and gradually discontinue the medication. The clinician should keep in mind that norethindrone at high doses converts peripherally to ethinyl estradiol. Other medication options that are available—though not typically administered in an ED setting—include depot medroxyprogesterone, tranexamic acid, and levonorgestrel-releasing intrauterine system (Mirena IUS). Consultation to adolescent medicine, hematology, or gynecology may be warranted.

For the patient who has developed anemia from ongoing vaginal bleeding, it is important to provide iron supplementation to rebuild iron stores. Because iron and estrogen may cause gastrointestinal discomfort, some practitioners delay administration of the first dose of iron until the estrogen is tapered to a lower dosage. It is important for the patient to have follow-up with her outpatient primary care doctor, adolescent medicine specialist, or gynecologist for long-term control of AUB and irregular menses.

TABLE 100.6

CONTRAINDICATIONS TO THE USE OF ESTROGEN CONTAINING MEDICATIONS

History of migraine with aura
History of venous thromboembolism (deep venous thromboembolism, pulmonary embolism, stroke)
Inherited prothrombotic disorders
Systemic lupus erythematosus with positive or unknown antiphospholipid antibodies
Hypertension (SBP >160 mm Hg or DBP >100 mm Hg)
Certain heart conditions (ischemic heart disease, complicated valvular disease, peripartum cardiomyopathy)
Certain liver conditions (hepatocellular adenoma, liver malignancy, severe cirrhosis)
Postpartum <21 days
Current diagnosis of breast cancer
History of complicated solid organ transplant

Adapted from Centers for Disease Control and Prevention. United States Medical Eligibility Criteria Contraceptive Use, 2010. *MMWR Recomm Rep* 2010;59(RR–4):1–85; For a full list see the United States Medical Eligibility Criteria for Contraceptive Use at http://www.cdc.gov/reproductivehealth/unintendedpregnancy/usmec.htm

CLINICAL PEARLS AND PITFALLS

- Patients may present with vaginal bleeding or concern for trauma.
- Lichen sclerosis will cause permanent scarring and sexual dysfunction if untreated.

LICHEN SCLEROSIS

Lichen sclerosis is an uncommon, chronic, idiopathic skin disorder that most often affects the vulva. In this condition, white, flat-topped papules gradually coalesce to form atrophic plaques that involve the vulvar and perianal skin in a symmetric hourglass pattern around the vulvar and perianal areas. Patients may present with vulvar pruritus or pain or bleeding from the affected tissue. Findings may also be misinterpreted as trauma causing parents to bring their child in for concern of possible sexual abuse.

Diagnosis in children can usually be made by visual inspection. In addition to the white, hourglass appearance of the affected skin, ecchymoses, fissures, and telangiectasias are frequently present (Fig. 100.5).

Lichen sclerosis can lead to loss of the normal labia and architecture of the vulva causing long-term sexual dysfunction if not treated. Therefore, goals of treatment are proper identification and initiation of treatment to prevent long-term effects. Treatment is with topical, high-potency corticosteroids (clobetasol 0.05% ointment) applied to the affected area twice daily for 2 weeks. Patients should be reexamined at 2 weeks to assess for response. Patients usually require 6 to 12 weeks of treatment with topical steroids until symptoms and visible findings have resolved. After this point, the topical steroid should be tapered to avoid rebound that can be seen with abrupt cessation. Immunomodulators are an alternative to topical steroids.

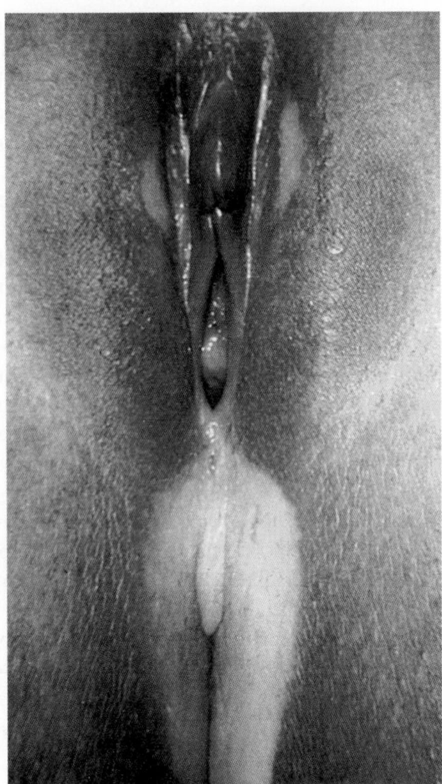

FIGURE 100.5 Figure-of-eight pattern of vulvar and perianal hypopigmentation in a 10-year-old girl with lichen sclerosus.

CONGENITAL VAGINAL OBSTRUCTION

CLINICAL PEARLS AND PITFALLS

- Vaginal outlet anomalies should be considered in infants presenting with an abdominal mass or in adolescents with abdominal pain, particularly if the patient has normal pubertal development without the onset of expected menarche.
- Vaginal outlet obstruction can cause acute urinary retention in any age female.
- A complete physical examination can easily diagnose imperforate hymen.

An obstructed vagina will eventually accumulate fluid, causing distention and, eventually, symptoms. Anatomic vaginal obstructions present most often during adolescence, when menstrual blood fills the vagina, producing hematocolpos or hematometrocolpos. There are multiple case reports of vaginal obstruction presenting in the neonatal period (incidence of approximately 0.006%), when vaginal distension is caused by mucus secreted as a result of stimulation by maternal hormones. This condition is called hydrometrocolpos.

The two most common anomalies that lead to vaginal outlet obstruction are imperforate hymen (approximately 0.1% of term female neonates) and transverse vaginal septum (sometimes called vaginal atresia; 1 in 30,000 to 84,000 women). These malformations are probably produced between the 16th and 20th weeks' gestation if the developing vaginal plate fails to perforate at its junction with either the fused paramesonephric (müllerian) ducts proximally or the urogenital sinus caudally. Unlike patients with a transverse vaginal septum or imperforate hymen, patients with complete agenesis of the vagina (Rokitansky–Küster–Hauser syndrome) have rudimentary uteri or none at all, so hydrocolpos does not occur.

Although vaginal obstruction should be properly identified during the initial examination of the newborn female, infants with hydrocolpos often go unrecognized until days or weeks later when they develop the three hallmarks of this condition: (i) a lower abdominal mass, (ii) difficulty with urination, and (iii) a visible bulging membrane at the introitus. In more severe cases, infants may also have constipation, hydronephrosis, edema of the lower extremities, and hypoventilation. A complete physical examination should immediately indicate the proper diagnosis. In adolescence, a female with congenital vaginal obstruction will usually present with either primary amenorrhea or lower abdominal pain; this condition should be suspected in patients with normal pubertal development without expected menarche. As the hematocolpos grows, it will finally interfere with urination, causing urgency, frequency, or dysuria. Although the differential diagnosis for a patient with amenorrhea and a lower abdominal mass on physical examination includes pregnancy or tumors, the characteristic appearance of the introitus covered by a bluish bulging membrane is diagnostic of hematocolpos with imperforate hymen. Patients with a high transverse vaginal septum will be more difficult to diagnose because the introitus will appear normal. However, palpation of the vagina will demonstrate obstruction, and the cervix will not be palpable.

The emergency physician should also consider the diagnosis of congenital vaginal obstruction in patients with acute urinary retention. Due to chronic intrinsic pressure, patients can have variable degrees of hydroureter or hydronephrosis; rarely, infants will present with respiratory insufficiency or inferior vena caval obstruction because of the large mass. While imperforate hymen is usually an isolated anomaly, other types of obstruction, chiefly transverse vaginal septum, are regularly associated with renal malformations, including hypoplastic or single kidneys, and duplicated or ectopic collecting systems; presence of additional anomalies should be considered when this condition is diagnosed.

Patients with congenital vaginal obstruction need surgical treatment; surgery should be planned urgently for adolescents but can be performed electively for asymptomatic infants and children.

LABIAL ADHESIONS

CLINICAL PEARLS AND PITFALLS

- Labial adhesions are a common, usually asymptomatic disorder of childhood.
- Treatment is not necessary in asymptomatic cases.
- Manual separation of adhesions should be avoided.

Labial adhesions are a common disorder of childhood, occurring in approximately 0.6% to 3% of prepubertal girls. Labial adhesions are not a congenital disorder; rather, they are classically thought to occur due to a lack of estrogen combined with irritation, due to poor hygiene or diaper rash, for example. However, more recent studies suggest that there may be etiologic factors other than estrogen insufficiency. Most labial adhesions are asymptomatic and are noted by a parent at home

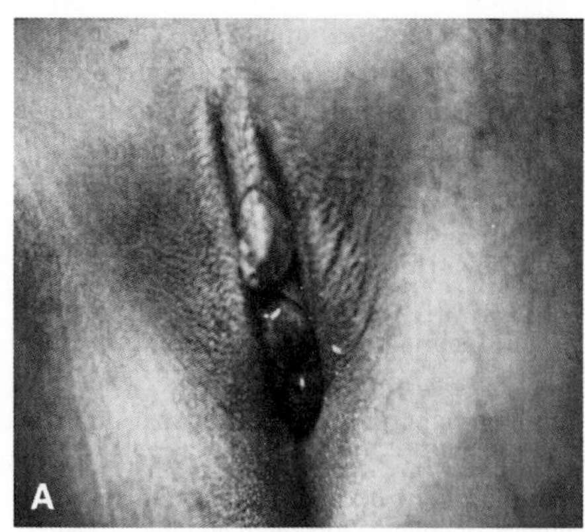

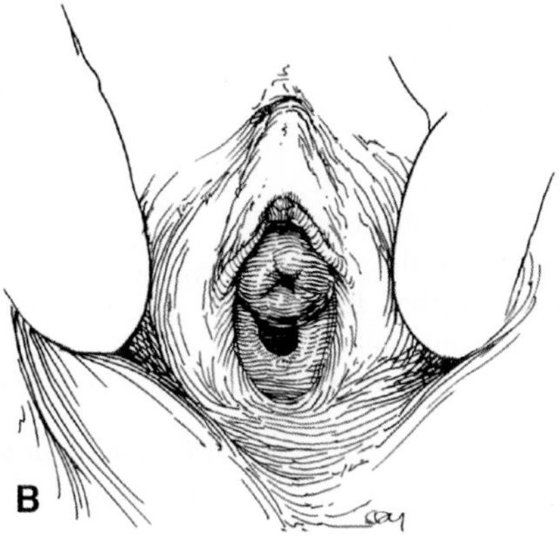

FIGURE 100.6 **A:** Urethral prolapse in a 6-year-old girl with "vaginal" bleeding. The vaginal orifice cannot be seen. **B:** The smooth doughnut shape and central lumen are characteristic features of a urethral prolapse, which if large or swollen, often conceals the vagina below it.

or a physician during the child's routine physical examination. The classic physical examination finding is a flat plane of tissue marked by a central vertical line of adhesion that obstructs the view of the introitus. Even when adhesions appear to have closed the vulva completely, a pinpoint opening usually remains that permits urination.

Some patients with labial adhesions present with symptoms such as dysuria, frequency, or refusal to void that may be a result of either the mechanical obstruction or concurrent urinary tract infection. Whether associated urinary tract infections are a cause or an effect of adhesions is unclear. For girls with urinary tract infections, urine cultures should be performed and appropriate medical follow-up provided. Because vaginal infection is not associated with adhesions, vaginal cultures are not indicated except in patients who have concurrent vaginal discharge.

Treatment is not indicated for asymptomatic girls with labial adhesions because the condition spontaneously resolves early in puberty as a result of increasing endogenous estrogen. Some parents, however, prefer that their children be treated. Of girls with labial adhesions, up to 90% (published success rates range from 16% (one study) to 50% to 88%) can be treated successfully with a small amount of estrogen cream (Premarin or Dienestrol) dabbed onto the adhesions at once or twice a day for 2 to 4 weeks. Potential side effects include skin hypopigmentation and breast budding; more serious complications, such as vaginal bleeding or precocious puberty, are theoretical concerns. More recently, some authors have investigated treatment with topical betamethasone (0.05%), with some success. Labial adhesions should never be manually separated. The procedure is painful and usually results in recurrence when the irritated, newly separated labia readhere. Even with medical treatment recurrence rates vary from 15% to 40%, so care after separation is important. Proper hygiene is recommended, as well as daily application of a bland emollient such as petroleum jelly.

URETHRAL PROLAPSE

CLINICAL PEARLS AND PITFALLS

- The peak age for urethral prolapse in prepubertal children is 5 to 8 years.
- The majority of children with urethral prolapse present with vaginal bleeding.
- A doughnut-shaped protrusion from the vulva is found in urethral prolapse.
- Prompt attention is needed to correct the prolapse to avoid tissue necrosis.

Urethral prolapse is the protrusion of the distal urethral mucosa outward through its meatus, with a cleavage plane between the longitudinal and circular-oblique smooth-muscle layers of the urethra. Most prolapses happen spontaneously, but some episodes are noted to have occurred following a sudden or recurrent increase in intra-abdominal pressure (coughing, seizure, straining with constipation, lifting heavy objects). The prolapsed segment is constricted at the meatus and venous blood flow is impaired, so the involved tissue becomes swollen, edematous, and dark red or purplish. If the urethral prolapse is not corrected, the tissue can become thrombosed and necrotic.

About half of affected females are prepubertal children, while the majority of the remainder are postmenopausal women. Most urethral prolapses during childhood occur between the ages of 2 and 10 years, with the peak at 5 to 8 years of age. The majority of prepubertal children with urethral prolapse are African-Americans.

Clinical Manifestations

Vaginal bleeding or spotting is the chief complaint of 90% of children with significant urethral prolapses. The bleeding is painless, occasionally misinterpreted as hematuria or menstruation, and is sometimes accompanied by urinary frequency or dysuria. On examination of the child's perineum, a red or purplish, soft, doughnut-shaped mass is seen (Fig. 100.6). Most prolapses are not tender and measure 1 to 2 cm in diameter. By retracting the labia majora posterolaterally, the examiner can often demonstrate that the mass is separate from and anterior to the vaginal introitus; this process may be difficult if the prolapse is large. A small central dimple in the mass indicates the urethral lumen, though the dimple can be missed if lighting is inadequate, bleeding is active, or mucosal edema is significant. In most cases, the appearance of the prolapse is diagnostic. However, if the diagnosis is in doubt, sterile straight catheterization of the bladder through the mass can be performed to demonstrate the anatomic relationships safely and rapidly. Urinalysis may show red blood cells and urine cultures are routinely sterile, though these tests may not be clinically indicated if the child otherwise looks well. Urethral polyps, prolapsed ureterocele, sarcoma botryoides, and urethral carcinoma may be included in the differential diagnosis, but they are rare in children and lack the characteristically annular appearance of a urethral prolapse.

Management

For the symptomatic patient with a small segment of prolapsed mucosa that is not necrotic, warm moist compresses or sitz baths, combined with a 2-week course of topical estrogen cream, may be prescribed. Most patients treated in this way have improved within 10 to 14 days and remained normal thereafter, thus avoiding surgery. Patients with dark-red or necrotic mucosa should be treated surgically within several days by reduction of the prolapse and/or excision of necrotic tissue. After the diagnosis is confirmed by cystoscopy, the prolapse is excised and the cut edges are sutured together. It is also important for the practitioner to address any precipitant related to the prolapse such as chronic constipation or other Valsalva-related intra-abdominal strain.

Suggested Readings and Key References

Pregnancy

Chernick L, Kharbanda O, Santelli J, et al. Identifying adolescent females at high risk of pregnancy in a pediatric emergency department. *J Adolesc Health* 2013;51:171–178.

Goyal M, Hersh A, Luan X, et al. Frequency of pregnancy testing among adolescent emergency department visits. *Acad Emerg Med* 2013;20:816–821.

Kann L, Kinchen S, Shanklin SL, et al.; Centers for Disease Control and Prevention. Youth risk behavior surveillance—United States, 2013. *MMWR Surveill Summ* 2014;63:24–29.

Lau M, Lin H, Flores G. Pleased to be pregnant? Positive pregnancy attitudes among sexually active adolescent females in the United States. *J Pediatr Adolesc Gynecol* 2014;27:210–215.

Timm NL, McAneney C, Alpern E, et al. Is pediatric emergency department utilization by pregnant adolescents on the rise? *Pediatr Emerg Care* 2012;28:307–309.

Vaginitis

Hellberg D, Nilsson S, Mårdh PA. The diagnosis of bacterial vaginosis and vaginal flora changes. *Arch Gynecol Obstet* 2001;265: 11–15.

Nyirjesy P, Sobel JD. Vulvovaginal candidiasis. *Obstet Gynecol Clin North Am* 2003;30:671–684.

Tasker GL, Wojnarowska F. Lichen sclerosus. *Clin Exp Dermatol* 2003;28:128–133.

Workowski KA, Berman S; Centers for Disease Control and Prevention. Sexually transmitted diseases treatment guidelines, 2010. *MMWR Recomm Rep* 2010;59(RR–12):1–110. http://www.cdc.gov/mmwr/preview/mmwrhtml/rr5912a1.htm. Accessed on June 14, 2014.

Cervicitis

Centers for Disease Control and Prevention. Screening tests to detect Chlamydia trachomatis and Neisseria gonorrhoeae infections–2002. *MMWR Recomm Rep* 2002;51(RR-15):1–38.

Centers for Disease Control and Prevention. Recommendations for the laboratory-based detection of Chlamydia trachomatis and Neisseria gonorrhoeae—2014. *MMWR Recomm Rep* 2014; 63(No. RR-2):1–19.

Johnson LF, Lewis DA. The effect of genital tract infections on HIV-1 shedding in the genital tract: a systematic review and meta-analysis. *Sex Transm Dis* 2008;35:946–959.

Workowski KA, Bolan GA; Centers for Disease Control and Prevention. Sexually transmitted diseases treatment guidelines, 2015. *MMWR Recomm Rep* 2015;64(RR-3):1–137. http://www.cdc.gov/std/tg2015/default.htm. Accessed on July 30, 2015.

Pelvic Inflammatory Disease

Banikarim C, Chacko MR. Pelvic inflammatory disease in adolescents. *Adolesc Med Clin* 2004;15(2):273–285.

Beckmann KR, Melzer-Lange MD, Gorelick MH. Emergency department management of sexually transmitted infections in US adolescents: results from the National Hospital Ambulatory Medical Care Survey. *Ann Emerg Med* 2004;43(3):333–338.

Centers for Disease Control and Prevention (CDC). Update to CDC's Sexually transmitted diseases treatment guidelines, 2010: oral cephalosporins no longer a recommended treatment for gonococcal infections. *MMWR Morb Mortal Wkly Rep* 2012;61(31):590–594.

Workowski KA, Bolan GA; Centers for Disease Control and Prevention. Sexually transmitted diseases treatment guidelines, 2015. *MMWR Recomm Rep* 2015:64(RR-3):1–137. http://www.cdc.gov/std/tg2015/default.htm. Accessed on July 30, 2015.

Adnexal Torsion

Applebaum H, Abraham C, Choi-Rosen J, et al. Key clinical predictors in the early diagnosis of adnexal torsion in children. *J Pediatr Adolesc Gynecol* 2013;26:167–170.

Gerscovich EO, Corwin MT, Sekhon S, et al. Sonographic appearance of adnexal torsion, correlation with other imaging modalities, and clinical history. *Ultrasound Q* 2014;30:49–55.

Rossi BV, Ference EH, Zurakowski D, et al. The clinical presentation and surgical management of adnexal torsion in the pediatric and adolescent population. *J Pediatr Adolesc Gynecol* 2012;25:109–113.

Schmitt ER, Ngai SS, Gausche-Hill M, et al. Twist and shout! Pediatric ovarian torsion clinical update and case discussion. *Pediatr Emerg Care* 2013;29:518–523.

HSV

Eberhardt O, Küker W, Dichgans J, et al. HSV-2 sacral radiculitis (Elsberg syndrome). *Neurology* 2004;63(4):758–759.

Gupta R, Warren T, Wald A. Genital herpes. *Lancet* 2007;370(9605): 2127–2137.

Workowski KA, Bolan GA; Centers for Disease Control and Prevention. Sexually transmitted diseases treatment guidelines, 2015. *MMWR Recomm Rep* 2015;64(RR-3):1–137. http://www.cdc.gov/std/tg2015/default.htm. Accessed on July 30, 2015.

HPV

Diaz ML. Human papilloma virus: prevention and treatment. *Obstet Gynecol Clin North Am* 2008;35(2):199–217.

Dunne EF, Unger ER, Sternberg M, et al. Prevalence of HPV infection among females in the United States. *JAMA* 2007;297(8):813–819.

Tarkowski TA, Koumans EH, Sawyer M, et al. Epidemiology of human papillomavirus infection and abnormal cytologic test results in an urban adolescent population. *J Infect Dis* 2004;189(1): 46–50.

Dysmenorrhea

Harel Z. Dysmenorrhea in adolescents and young adults: an update on pharmacological treatments and management strategies. *Expert Opin Pharmacother* 2012;13(15):2157–2170.

Laufer MR. Gynecologic pain: dysmenorrhea, acute and chronic pelvic pain, endometriosis, and premenstrual syndrome. In: Emans SJ, Laufer MR, Goldstein DP, eds. *Pediatric and Adolescent Gynecology.* 6th ed. Philadelphia, PA: Lippincott Williams & Wilkins, 2012:238–271.

Abnormal Uterine Bleeding

Centers for Disease Control and Prevention (CDC). United States Medical Eligibility Criteria for Contraceptive Use, 2010. *MMWR Recomm Rep* 2010;59(RR–4):1–85. http://www.cdc.gov/reproductivehealth/unintendedpregnancy/usmec.htm. Accessed on Dec 20, 2014.

Gray SH, Emans SJ. Abnormal vaginal bleeding in the adolescent. In: Emans SJ, Laufer MR, Goldstein DP, eds. *Pediatric and Adolescent Gynecology.* 6th ed. Philadelphia, PA: Lippincott Williams & Wilkins, 2012:159–167.

Congenital Vaginal Obstruction

Ameh EA, Mshelbwala PM, Ameh N. Congenital vaginal obstruction in neonates and infants: recognition and management. *J Pediatr Adolesc Gynecol* 2011;24:74–78.

Ero lu E, Yip M, Oktar T, et al. How should we treat prepubertal labial adhesions? Retrospective comparison of topical treatments: estrogen only, betamethasone only, and combination estrogen and betamethasone. *J Pediatr Adolesc Gynecol* 2011;24:389–391.

Shaked O, Tepper R, Klein Z, et al. Hydrometrocolpos—diagnostic and therapeutic dilemmas. *J Pediatr Adolesc Gynecol* 2008;21:317–321.

Urethral Prolapse

Emans SJ. Vulvovaginal problems in the prepubertal child. In: Emans SJ, Laufer MR, Goldstein DP, eds. *Pediatric and Adolescent Gynecology.* 6th ed. Philadelphia, PA: Lippincott Williams & Wilkins, 2012:42–59.

Rome ES. Vulvovaginitis and other common vulvar disorders in children. *Endocr Dev* 2012;22:72–83.

Van Eyk N, Allen L, Giesbrecht E, et al. Pediatric vulvovaginal disorders: a diagnostic approach and review of the literature. *J Obstet Gynaecol Can* 2009;31(9):850–862.

CHAPTER 101 ■ HEMATOLOGIC EMERGENCIES

STACY E. CROTEAU, MD, MMS, ERIC W. FLEEGLER, MD, MPH, AND MARISA BRETT-FLEEGLER, MD

GOALS OF EMERGENCY THERAPY

The management of pediatric hematologic emergencies is directed toward immediate stabilization of the acutely ill patient to prevent morbidity and mortality related to severe anemia, infection, bleeding, and thrombosis. Patients at risk for infection and sepsis, such as neutropenic or asplenic patients, require prompt attention; quality metrics focus on time to initiation of antibiotic therapy for these patients. Simultaneously, significant hematologic findings of unknown etiology require thorough evaluation, especially where necessary therapies may obscure the underlying diagnosis or impede later diagnostic testing.

Hematologic emergencies arise in children who have been previously well, who have known blood disorders, or who have systemic disease. Initial measures of support, diagnosis, and treatment are based on general principles that often do not require a definitive diagnosis to initiate management.

RELATED CHAPTERS

Resuscitation and Stabilization
- Approach to the Injured Child: Chapter 2
- Shock: Chapter 5

Signs and Symptoms
- Gastrointestinal Bleeding: Chapter 28
- Pain: Abdomen: Chapter 48
- Pallor: Chapter 57
- Tachycardia: Chapter 72

Clinical Pathways
- Shock: Chapter 91

Medical Emergencies
- Gastrointestinal Emergencies: Chapter 99
- Oncologic Emergencies: Chapter 106

Trauma
- Abdominal Trauma: Chapter 111
- Thoracic Trauma: Chapter 123

Surgical Emergencies
- Abdominal Emergencies: Chapter 124
- Thoracic Emergencies: Chapter 132

KEY POINTS

- Hemoglobin levels may be normal in acute blood loss.
- The decision to transfuse red blood cells (pRBCs) should be based on etiology, severity, and chronicity of the anemia as well as on clinical symptoms and end-organ perfusion rather than hemoglobin values.
- Patients with sickle cell disease require prompt evaluation for complications including stroke, acute chest syndrome, splenic sequestration, infection, vasoocclusive episodes, and priapism.
- Prompt evaluation and treatment of neutropenic patients is essential to decrease morbidity and mortality associated with infection. Appropriate cultures should be obtained but should not delay empiric antibiotic treatment. Disposition should be based on the underlying etiology of the neutropenia and clinical presentation.
- Increasingly, the management of immune thrombocytopenia (ITP) is guided by bleeding symptoms rather than platelet count.
- Platelet disorders and von Willebrand disease (vWD) typically result in mucosal-type bleeding whereas hemophilia causes hemarthrosis and deep muscle bleeds. Drugs that interfere with platelet function (e.g., aspirin, nonsteroidal anti-inflammatory agents) should be avoided in patients with hemostatic defects.

ANEMIA

Goals of Treatment

Severe anemia requires rapid evaluation and treatment to prevent hypoxia, congestive heart failure, end-organ damage, and death. When the etiology of the anemia is not immediately apparent, management focuses simultaneously on diagnostic and therapeutic interventions. Many management strategies for the anemic child are similar regardless of etiology, but special considerations are necessary in the setting of a destructive red cell process.

CLINICAL PEARLS AND PITFALLS

- The stabilization of the severely anemic child is guided by the clinical presentation more than by laboratory values. In chronic blood loss, low hemoglobin levels may be relatively well tolerated due to compensatory mechanisms and should not be the sole indication for transfusion.
- The acuity or chronicity of a clinical condition will impact the clinical status and thereby affect management. Prompt transfusions and isotonic fluid resuscitation needed for acute blood loss may be detrimental in chronically anemic patients.
- Transfusion risks versus benefits must be considered based on the clinical situation.

TABLE 101.1

CLASSIFICATION OF ANEMIA BY RED BLOOD CELL SIZE

Macrocytic (MCV >100)
- Megaloblastic anemia: folic acid or vitamin B_{12} deficiency
- Liver disease (target cells)
- Reticulocytosis
- Hypothyroidism
- Myelodysplastic syndrome
- Antiretrovirals, e.g., AZT

Microcytic (MCV <80)
- Iron deficiency
- Thalassemia
- Anemia of chronic disease
- Sideroblastic anemia
- Lead poisoning

Normocytic (MCV 80–100)
- Low reticulocyte count
- Iron deficiency (especially early)
- Anemia of chronic disease
- Chronic renal disease (low erythropoietin)
- Hypothyroidism, adrenal insufficiency, or hypopituitarism
- Primary bone marrow disorder
- Aplastic anemia
- Malignancy, e.g., leukemia, metastases
- Myelodysplastic syndromes
- Infection, e.g., parvovirus B19 (causes red cell hypoplasia or aplastic anemia)
- Blood loss
- Hemolysis

Adapted from Zeiger Roni F, McGraw-Hill's Diagnosaurus 4.0: http://accessmedicine.mhmedical.com/diagnosaurus.aspx

Current Evidence

Anemia in the pediatric patient ranges from an incidental finding in an asymptomatic patient to acute or chronic processes presenting in a critically ill patient. The classification of causes of anemia according to (i) blood loss, (ii) increased RBC destruction, and (iii) decreased RBC production provides a framework for the evaluation of the anemic child.

Alternatively, comparing the MCV level with age appropriate normal values allows for classification of anemia as macrocytic, normocytic, or microcytic (see Table 101.1). A reticulocyte count indicates the reactivity of the marrow, and elevated levels are often found in blood loss and hemolysis. Decreased levels of serum haptoglobin, elevated lactate dehydrogenase, and increased unconjugated bilirubin along with the presence of heme in the urine suggest hemolysis.

BLOOD LOSS

CLINICAL PEARLS AND PITFALLS

- In acute hemorrhage, measured hemoglobin changes may lag behind blood loss, and normal values should not provide reassurance against clinically significant blood loss.

Clinical Considerations

Clinical Recognition

Anemia due to blood loss occurs from a variety of causes (Fig. 101.1). Overall, these conditions are divided into traumatic or atraumatic bleeding. The possibility of occult nonaccidental trauma must always be considered, particularly in younger children. Gastrointestinal hemorrhage is the most common cause of atraumatic blood loss, but postsurgical (e.g., posttonsillectomy hemorrhage), renal, gynecologic, and other etiologies may also present. In some cases, an anatomic lesion or process may combine with a congenital or acquired coagulopathy to precipitate significant anemia. For example, adolescent girls with unrecognized von Willebrand disease (vWD) may present with anemia due to both acute and chronic blood loss during menses.

Assessment for anemia should be considered in any patient with pallor, jaundice, or unexplained tachycardia. Asymptomatic chronic anemia may be detected as an incidental finding that requires further evaluation.

Triage

In the patient with known or suspected anemia due to blood loss, hypotension, hypoxia, or evidence of end-organ dysfunction is a medical emergency and warrants immediate intervention to prevent progression to cardiopulmonary collapse. Patients with both acute and chronic blood loss may become unstable. The chronicity of symptoms should not reassure the clinician, as it may be the exhaustion of physiologic compensatory mechanisms that prompts the patient to present to medical attention.

Initial Assessment

Initial assessment of a patient presenting with anemia secondary to blood loss includes a focused history targeted at potential etiology and symptoms of compromise related to anemia/hypoxia. In suspected blood loss, the clinician must assess for evidence of trauma including nonaccidental injury, postprocedure bleeding, symptoms of upper or lower gastrointestinal bleeding, medication use that could precipitate gastrointestinal bleeding, reports of epistaxis, hematuria or menorrhagia, and any concern for complications of pregnancy or hemorrhagic ovarian cyst. History related to symptomatic anemia should include fatigue, exercise intolerance, syncope, orthostasis, chest pain or dyspnea, decreased urine output, and any change in mental status.

Assessment of hemodynamic parameters to identify signs of impending cardiopulmonary collapse (e.g., hypotension, hypoxia, and severe tachycardia) is critical. Physical examination should assess for location of blood loss and signs of systemic illness that may cause anemia. Signs of end-organ dysfunction, such as change in mental status, congestive heart failure, or renal insufficiency should be noted. In the trauma patient, bleeding may be evident or occult, as in the case of femoral, pelvic, or abdominal (including both intra- and retroperitoneal) hemorrhage. These may be hemodynamically significant but not immediately obvious. The presence of trauma itself may be subtle in nonaccidental injury. Look for evidence of gastrointestinal or gynecologic bleeding when the bleeding etiology is unclear.

Management/Diagnostic Testing

Laboratory testing for patients with suspected blood loss includes complete blood count (CBC), reticulocyte count,

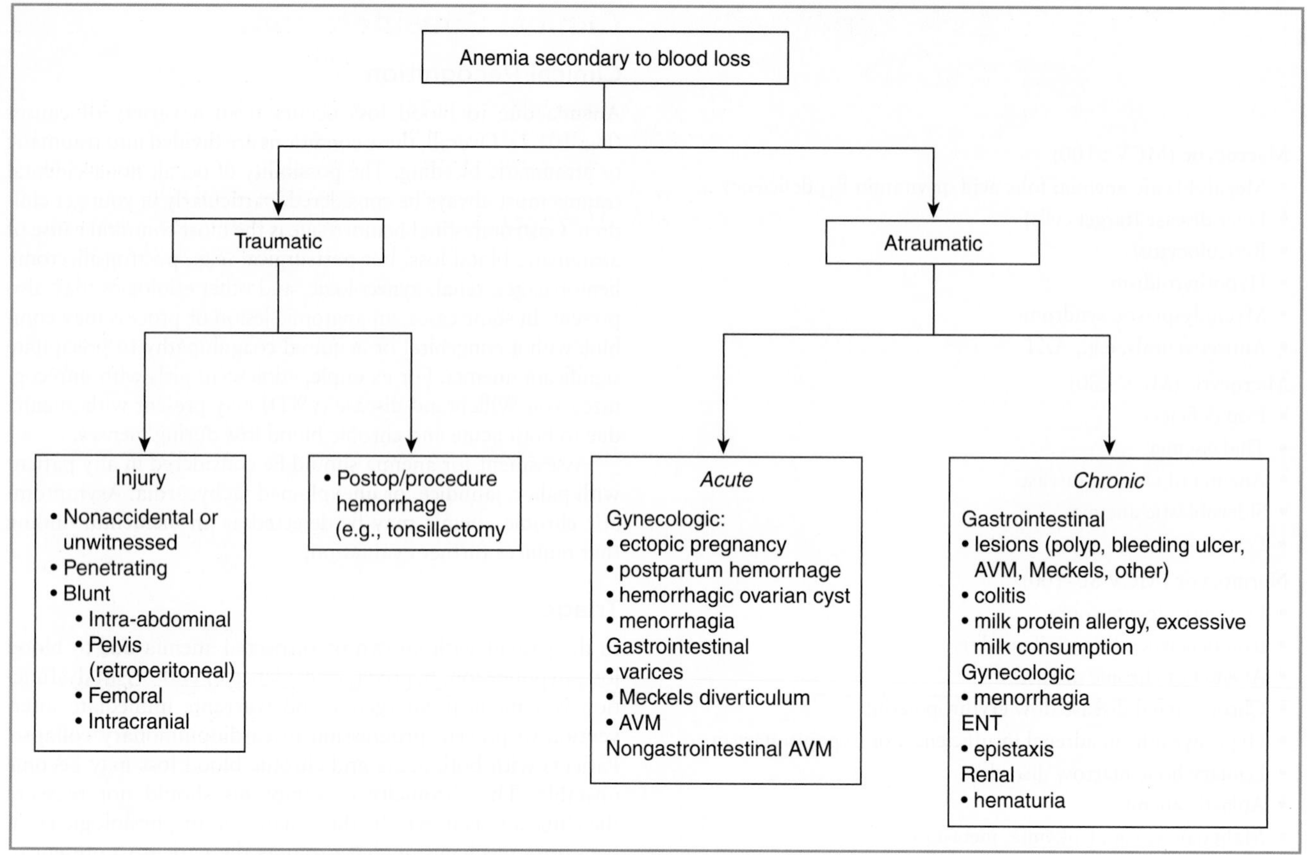

FIGURE 101.1 Causes of blood loss.

coagulation studies and a type and screen, or type and cross if transfusion is anticipated. If the etiology of the anemia is unclear, obtain stool guaiac for occult blood, hemolysis labs, and other studies as outlined below (see section on Hemolytic Anemia). Send a pregnancy test if clinically indicated.

Management

Initial management steps for all patients include immediate vascular access, cardiorespiratory monitoring, and administration of oxygen, regardless of oxygen saturation to maximize oxygen-carrying capacity of the existing RBC mass and plasma. Unstable patients require multiple sites of vascular access. Peripheral intravenous (IV) catheters are typically more useful than central lines for rapid volume resuscitation; intraosseous access may also be used. If transfusion is anticipated, the blood bank should be notified promptly.

Trauma patients (see Chapter 2 Approach to the Injured Child) require a multidisciplinary team to complete primary, secondary, and tertiary surveys. Occult blood loss as discussed above should be considered in all trauma patients. The use of ultrasound and FAST (focused assessment with sonography in trauma) may be helpful in assessing for intra-abdominal hemorrhage in the multisystem trauma patient (see Chapter 142 Ultrasound). Management is simultaneously directed at immediate hemodynamic stabilization and plans to control blood loss through surgical and catheter-guided embolization strategies as indicated. Patients in uncompensated shock (hypotension, signs of end-organ dysfunction) require rapid fluid resuscitation. Initial crystalloid boluses of 20 ml/kg should be given via pressure bags, rapid infusers, or other means of rapid fluid administration. Patients with uncompensated shock due to hemorrhage despite fluid resuscitation require transfusion (see Table 101.2). While some patients may need immediate transfusion, crystalloid fluids are typically available more quickly and should be used until O-negative blood is available. Hemoglobin changes typically lag behind acute blood loss and are not a useful guide to initial management. Patients with isolated tachycardia but no other signs of end-organ dysfunction such as altered mental status, decreased urine output, or poor perfusion (compensated shock) should be managed based on the severity of the tachycardia, anticipated trajectory of the blood loss, and the need for embolization or operative management. Failure to respond to initial crystalloid resuscitation in these patients may be an indication for transfusion. Traumatic hemorrhage may result in coagulopathy that could worsen bleeding. Trauma patients requiring massive transfusion will need additional blood product support with platelets and fresh-frozen plasma (see Table 101.2) and careful monitoring for electrolyte derangements associated with these treatments. Patients with atraumatic acute blood loss are resuscitated based on the presence of uncompensated shock, on the ability to achieve hemostasis, and the need for procedural intervention. In the stable patient with chronic blood loss, IV fluids should be used with caution, if at all, due to the potential for hemodilution. The decision to transfuse in these cases is based on symptoms, the trajectory of the blood loss, and ability to reverse the inciting cause. Pediatric data are limited, but transfusion in adult patients with hemoglobin >7 g per dL has not improved outcomes. Patients with a hemoglobin below 5 to 6 g per dL frequently require transfusion.

TABLE 101.2

BLOOD PRODUCTS AND DRUGS TO MANAGE BLEEDING

Product/drug	Indication(s)	Dose	Pearls
Packed red blood cells (pRBCs)	Anemia	Volume of packed RBCs = ([desired hemoglobin – current hemoglobin] × pts blood volume)/hemoglobin of packed RBCs Estimated blood volume (mL) = weight (kg) × 70 mL/kg Estimated hemoglobin of unit of packed RBCs = 19–25 g/dL	• Desired Hb level dictated by clinical situation • 10 mL/kg of pRBCs should raise the Hb about 2 g/dL • Rate of transfusion is dictated by clinical presentation and differs for acute versus chronic etiologies of anemia
Platelets	Thrombocytopenia with bleeding Platelet function defects	One unit per 5–10 kg (~50–60 mL/unit), ≥5.5 × 10^{10} platelets/unit OR One apheresis unit (~200 mL), ≥3 × 10^{11} platelets/unit	• Use with caution/clear clinical need for patients with ITP, DIC, TTP, HIT • Random donor units are a pooled donor source. An apheresis unit is from a single donor • One unit of random donor platelets should increase count by 5,000–10,000/µL in average adult • One apheresis unit should increase count by 30,000–50,000/µL in average adult
Fresh-frozen plasma (FFP)	Bleeding associated with abnormal coagulation panel Factor deficiency replacement Reversal of Vitamin K antagonist Massive transfusion requirement	10–20 mL/kg/dose (~200–250 mL/unit)	• Contains all plasma clotting factors, but with variable concentrations
Cryoprecipitate (Cryo)	Bleeding associated with deficiency of fibrinogen, FVIII, FXIII, or vWF	1–2 units for every 10 kg of body weight	• Contains fibrinogen, FVIII, FXIII, and vWF
Recombinant factor products	Factor 8 products: treatment or prophylaxis of FVIII deficiency Factor 9 products: treatment or prophylaxis of FIX deficiency Factor 7 (rFVIIa): treatment or prophylaxis of FVII deficiency or treatment or prophylaxis for FVIII or FIX patients with inhibitors	Factor VIII: (number of units = desired level (%) × weight of patient [kg] × 0.5) Factor IX: (number of units = desired level (%) × weight of patient [kg]) Factor VII: Replacement: 15–30 mcg/kg q4–6 hrs FVIII or FIX inhibitors: 90 mcg/kg q2hr, space as clinically tolerated	• Plasma-derived factor replacement products also available
Antihemophilic factor/vWF complex	Von Willebrand disease (vWD)	Dosing based on vWF:RCo units/kg	
Prothrombin complex concentrates	Bleeding with deficiency of FII, FVII, FIX, FX or familial vitamin K deficiency or reversal of vitamin K antagonist	Consult hematologist, dose for factor replacement based on specific factor deficiency and target level Dose for reversal depends on specific product and predose INR	• Contraindicated in DIC, HIT, or known hypersensitivity
DDAVP (desmopressin)	Type I vWD or mild hemophilia A (if patients known to respond)	IV formulation—0.3 mcg/kg in 50 mL NS by IV infusion over 30 min (max dose 20 mcg) Nasal spray formulation stimate (desmopressin acetate) 1.5 mg/mL—metered dose pump delivers 0.1 mL (150 mcg) per actuation for patients ≥50 kg—2 sprays (1/nostril); <50 kg—1 spray	• Causes release of vWF and FVIII from endothelial cells • Can exacerbate the thrombocytopenia seen with type 2B vWD • Side effects: facial flushing, headache, and, rarely, hypertension, hypotension, and water retention, hyponatremic seizures have occurred

(continued)

TABLE 101.2

BLOOD PRODUCTS AND DRUGS TO MANAGE BLEEDING (*CONTINUED*)

Product/drug	Indication(s)	Dose	Pearls
Aminocaproic acid (amicar)	Mucocutaneous bleeding	Aminocaproic acid (pediatric): 50–100 mg/kg loading dose then 50 mg/kg q6hr (usual max: 2 g/dose) not to exceed 12 g/day. Aminocaproic acid (adult): 5 g loading (PO or IV) then 2–5 g q6h, titrated by patient need.	• Contraindicated in DIC. Avoid use with upper urinary tract bleeding (hematuria), can lead to intrarenal obstruction.
Tranexamic acid	Mucocutaneous bleeding Menorrhagia	Tranexamic acid: 1,300 mg PO or 10 mg/kg IV TID (dose reduction for creatinine >1.4) Formulation: 650 mg tabs or IV solution	• Avoid use with upper urinary tract bleeding (hematuria), can lead to intrarenal obstruction.

In patients with chronic blood loss, evidence of insufficient end-organ perfusion is an indication for transfusion; however, overly rapid or voluminous transfusion can lead to circulatory overload and collapse. For severe anemia with a tenuous hemodynamic status, exchange transfusion may be necessary to safely and efficiently correct the anemia. Specific treatment strategies may be available for some conditions, such as use of estrogen for menorrhagia.

The need for transfusion in a patient with anemia should be carefully considered, given the low but real associated risks of transmission of infectious agents and transfusion reaction. As a practical guide to rapid decision-making, a volume of 10- to 15-ml packed red blood cells (pRBCs) per kg may be given for acute blood loss, with the infusion rate varying from rapid to over 4 hours, depending on the degree of patient instability and rate of ongoing blood loss. In contrast, for severe, chronic anemia, 5-ml pRBCs per kg over 4 hours may be necessary to avoid circulatory overload.

Clinical Indications for Discharge or Admission

In stable patients with anemia, without physiologic compromise, discharge may be considered if the etiology of the condition is known, not expected to progress or accelerate, and close and reliable follow-up is available.

HEMOLYTIC ANEMIA

CLINICAL PEARLS AND PITFALLS

- Promptly evaluate patients with acute onset of pallor and jaundice for hemolytic anemia.
- Autoimmune hemolytic anemia (AIHA) can be life-threatening, especially in cases of severe anemia and reticulocytopenia.
- Early consultation with hematology and the blood bank helps to optimize patient management and to provide sufficient time for compatibility testing if transfusion is needed.
- With evidence of hemolysis, transfusion indications include symptomatic anemia or low presenting hemoglobin (<5 to 6 g per dL in children, <6 to 7 g per dL in adolescents).
- Avoid excessive crystalloid fluid resuscitation in severely anemic patients with hemolytic process.

Current Evidence

The premature destruction of RBCs in circulation (hemolytic anemia) is most commonly due to intrinsic defects of erythrocytes (membranopathies, enzymopathies, or hemoglobinopathies) in pediatric patients; however, extrinsic or extracorpuscular factors such as antibodies, environmental stresses, infection, or microangiopathic damage may also cause hemolysis. The severity of anemia can range from mild to life-threatening and is often influenced by the underlying mechanism. For example, erythrocyte membrane disorders (hereditary spherocytosis, hereditary elliptocytosis, hereditary stomatocytosis) and metabolic abnormalities (glucose-6-phosphate dehydrogenase [G6PD] deficiency, pyruvate kinase deficiency) do not usually cause severe anemia and rarely constitute a life-threatening emergency. AIHA, on the other hand, may present with a precipitously falling hemoglobin level in a child who appears critically ill with signs of congestive heart failure. Reported mortality rates for pediatric patients with hemolytic anemia range from 4% to 10%. Fortunately, this is a rare condition in children.

Goals of Treatment

Successful treatment of hemolytic anemia requires stabilization of the hemoglobin level and maintenance of sufficient oxygen-carrying capacity and cardiac output. Clinical outcomes depend on early recognition and intervention for uncompensated anemia.

Clinical Considerations

Clinical Recognition

Hemolytic anemia arises in all age groups. The typical presenting features include pallor, jaundice, and dark urine. Other symptoms include fatigue, malaise, dizziness, fever, and abdominal or back pain. Symptoms often develop suddenly, and in cases of rapid hemolysis, the presenting hemoglobin level may be as low as 3 to 4 g per dL. Some patients follow an indolent course presenting with symptoms evolving over days or weeks. Any unexplained low hemoglobin level, typically accompanied by a reticulocytosis, should prompt consideration of a hemolytic anemia.

Triage

Children with hemolytic anemia often present in a relatively compensated state; however, their clinical status can deteriorate rapidly. Severe, uncontrolled hemolytic anemia can be fatal with patients succumbing to insufficient oxygen-carrying capacity and cardiovascular collapse. Ongoing assessment of cardiovascular and neurologic status is crucial during the diagnostic evaluation and until the rate of hemolysis is controlled. Alert the hematology service and blood bank to patients with suspected hemolytic anemia early in the evaluation process.

Initial Assessment/H&P

The history should focus on systemic complaints relevant to anemia and hemolysis such as fatigue, light-headedness or near-syncope, fussiness/irritability in young children, and dyspnea. Probe for symptoms of a systemic autoimmune process, an immunologic disorder, and malignancy as these can be associated with AIHA. Elicit any personal or family history of an intrinsic RBC defect or AIHA. Attention to recent exposures including symptoms suggestive of a recent or concurrent viral illness, toxins (e.g., naphthalene-containing mothballs), and medications can also provide clues about possible triggers (Table 101.3). Typical examination findings for patients with hemolytic anemia include jaundice/icterus, pallor, tachycardia in some cases accompanied by murmur from a high output cardiac state, and mild hepatosplenomegaly. Other findings such as lymphadenopathy or massive hepatosplenomegaly may suggest underlying infection or malignancy. The presence of jugular venous distention, significant hepatosplenomegaly, gallop rhythm, respiratory distress, hypotension, or poor perfusion heralds imminent cardiovascular collapse.

Diagnostic Testing

A basic approach to the evaluation of hemolytic anemia is presented in Figure 101.2. The initial laboratory evaluation should include a CBC and differential, peripheral blood smear, reticulocyte count, blood type and antibody screen (indirect antibody test, formerly known as an indirect Coombs test), direct antiglobulin test (DAT, formerly called a direct Coombs test), haptoglobin, serum electrolytes, BUN/Cr, and bilirubin level. The goal is to identify a hemolytic anemia, prepare for transfusion in case the hemoglobin is critically low or falling rapidly, and narrow the differential of the causative mechanism. Reticulocytosis is present in most cases but can be absent or delayed in up to 10% of patients. Consideration of hemolytic anemia should not be eliminated based solely on a low reticulocyte count. Distinguishing between an immune- and a non–immune-mediated hemolytic anemia is an essential first step as this dictates therapy. The DAT uses broad-spectrum Coombs serum (IgG, IgM, and complement) to detect the presence of antibodies on erythrocytes and is usually positive in AIHA. A positive DAT prompts additional testing by the blood bank to further characterize the antibody. Acute hemolysis is most commonly associated with a warm (37°C)-reactive IgG antibody with or without complement (C3). This type of hemolysis is usually extravascular, occurring in the spleen. IgM-mediated cold agglutinin disease is less common in children than in adults, but can occur following mycoplasma (anti-I) or infectious mononucleosis (anti-i). These antibodies bind to RBCs in the cold and characteristically cause intravascular hemolysis as complement is bound and activated at warmer temperatures. Cold-reactive IgG antibodies (Donath–Landsteiner test) cause paroxysmal cold hemoglobinuria (PCH), which in children frequently follows a viral infection. A negative DAT does not definitively exclude an immune-mediated process. Rarely, IgA or warm reactive-IgM antibodies may be present but not detected by the Coombs reagent. Additionally, in rare cases, the causative warm-IgG antibodies are below the level of detection. When there is a high degree of suspicion for an immune-mediated process despite a negative DAT, specialized assays are required for antibody detection.

Examination of the peripheral blood smear is helpful in diagnosing subsets of nonimmune hemolytic anemia especially in the acute care setting when the results of disease-specific

TABLE 101.3

EXTRACORPUSCULAR CAUSES OF HEMOLYTIC ANEMIA

Infections
- Mycoplasma
- Epstein–Barr virus (EBV)
- Cytomegalovirus (CMV)
- Parvovirus
- Human herpes virus 6 (HHV-6)
- HIV

Toxins
- Naphthalene (mothballs) (in children with G6PD deficiency)
- Copper (Wilson disease)
- Lead

Medications (abbreviated list)
- Penicillin family
- Quinidine
- Hydrochlorothiazide
- Rifampin
- Sulfonamides
- Isoniazid
- Alpha-methyldopa
- Interferon-α
- IVIg

Autoimmune disorders
- Systemic lupus erythematosus
- Evans syndrome
- Thyroiditis
- Rheumatic disease

Immunologic disorders
- Common variable immunodeficiency (CVID)
- Autoimmune lymphoproliferative syndrome (ALPS)

Malignancies
- Lymphoma

Mechanical fragmentation
- Heart valve homografts or synthetic prostheses
- Uncorrected valvular disease
- Hemolytic-uremic syndrome (HUS)
- Thrombotic thrombocytopenic purpura (TTP)
- Collagen vascular disease
- Bone marrow transplantation associated microangiopathy

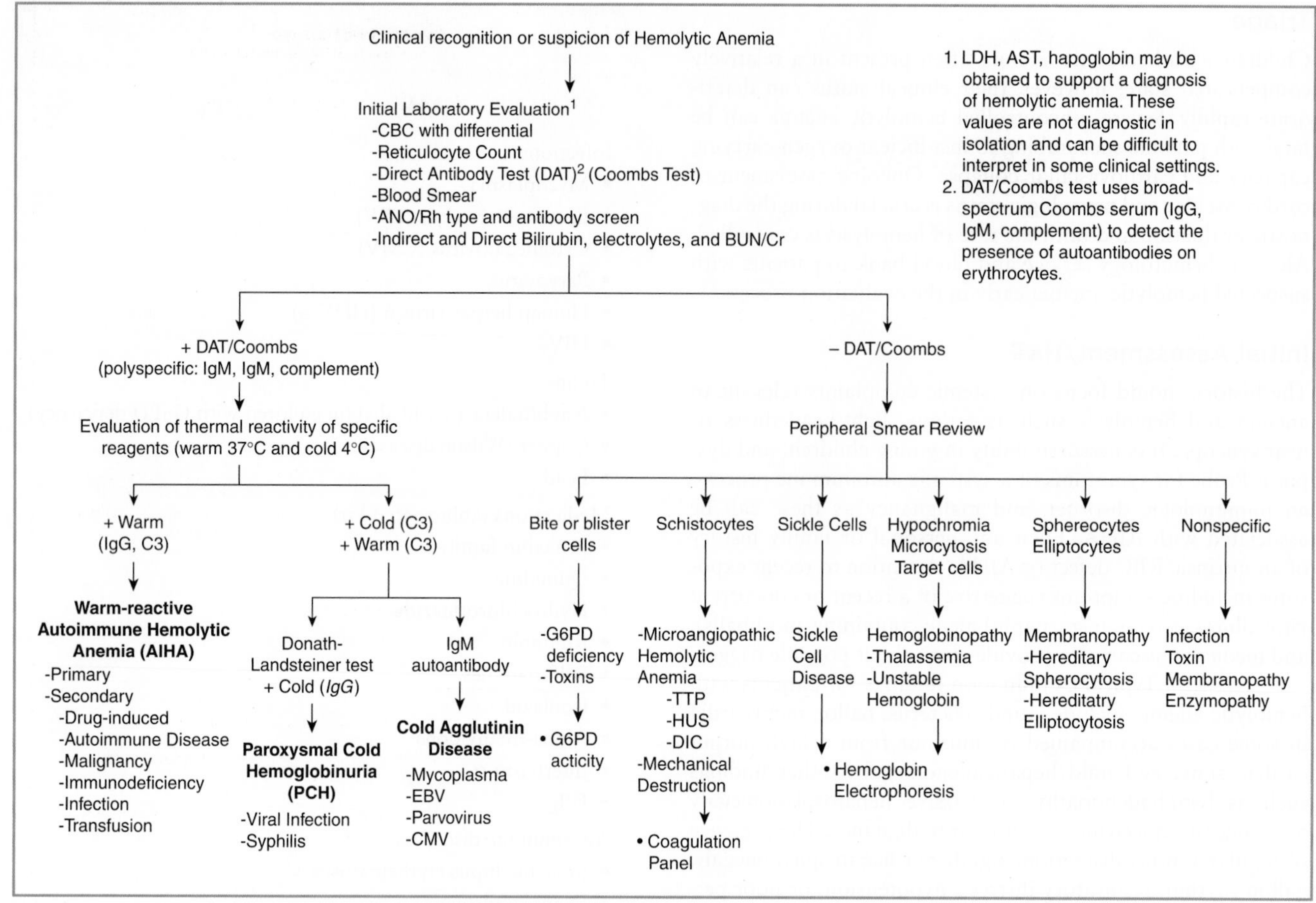

FIGURE 101.2 Approach to evaluation of hemolytic anemia.

testing such as osmotic fragility, hemoglobin electrophoresis, or G6PD activity will not be available. Certain patterns of red cell morphology can support a diagnosis of hemoglobinopathy or enzymopathy. The presence of RBC fragments (schistocytes) on the peripheral smear suggests mechanical damage to the erythrocyte. If the diagnosis is uncertain, a pretransfusion blood sample should be saved for additional testing such as the measurement of specific enzyme levels or hemoglobin electrophoresis. The diagnosis of microangiopathic processes such as hemolytic uremic syndrome (HUS) and thrombotic thrombocytopenic purpura (TTP) is important and should be considered in patients with diarrhea, and in the presence of acute kidney injury, thrombocytopenia, and fever and neurologic changes. Disseminated intravascular coagulation (DIC) occurs in the context of systemic illness, including sepsis, trauma, or malignancy. If considering any microangiopathic process, evaluation should also include a coagulation panel.

Management

AIHA. Prompt initiation of therapy for AIHA is necessary to stabilize the rate of hemolysis. Hospitalization for careful observation and treatment is usually necessary; the hemoglobin level may continue to fall precipitously despite initial therapy. Patients with symptomatic or severe anemia (hemoglobin <5 to 6 g per dL in children, <6 to 7 g per dL in adolescents) should receive a pRBC transfusion. Hemolytic transfusion reactions are a potential hazard. Transfuse an initial 5 to 10 mL of blood slowly to test for a significant hemolytic transfusion reaction associated with the selected aliquot of blood. If the patient does not manifest signs or symptoms of acute worsening during the initial infusion, increase the transfusion rate. Ultimately, the transfusion rate must exceed the rate of ongoing hemolysis. Careful monitoring of hemoglobin levels is important, with a stable hemoglobin goal of 6–8 g per dL.

The management strategy differs for those with a warm-reactive antibody versus those with a cold-reactive antibody as highlighted in Figure 101.3. Hemolysis and erythrocyte clearance in the setting of a warm-reactive antibody is generally extravascular, taking place in the spleen. These patients typically respond to corticosteroid therapy, but may also benefit from concomitant IVIG or splenectomy in more dire circumstances. Cold-reactive AIHA is intravascular hemolysis, dominated by complement activation and with limited response to corticosteroids or splenectomy. These patients should be kept warm (i.e., avoid cold exposure), and they may benefit from plasmapheresis in severe cases. In the setting of intravascular hemolysis, accumulation of circulating free hemoglobin and cellular contents can be toxic to the renal tubular system. Careful fluid management to ensure adequate renal clearance without excessive dilution of the red cells is imperative.

Nonimmune Hemolytic Anemia. Most etiologies of nonimmune hemolytic anemia require observation and supportive care, including removal of the offending agent and prevention of renal damage due to significant hemolysis (see Table 101.3). Infectious agents that may induce hemolytic anemia include malaria, other protozoa, and a wide variety of gram-positive and gram-negative organisms that require identification and

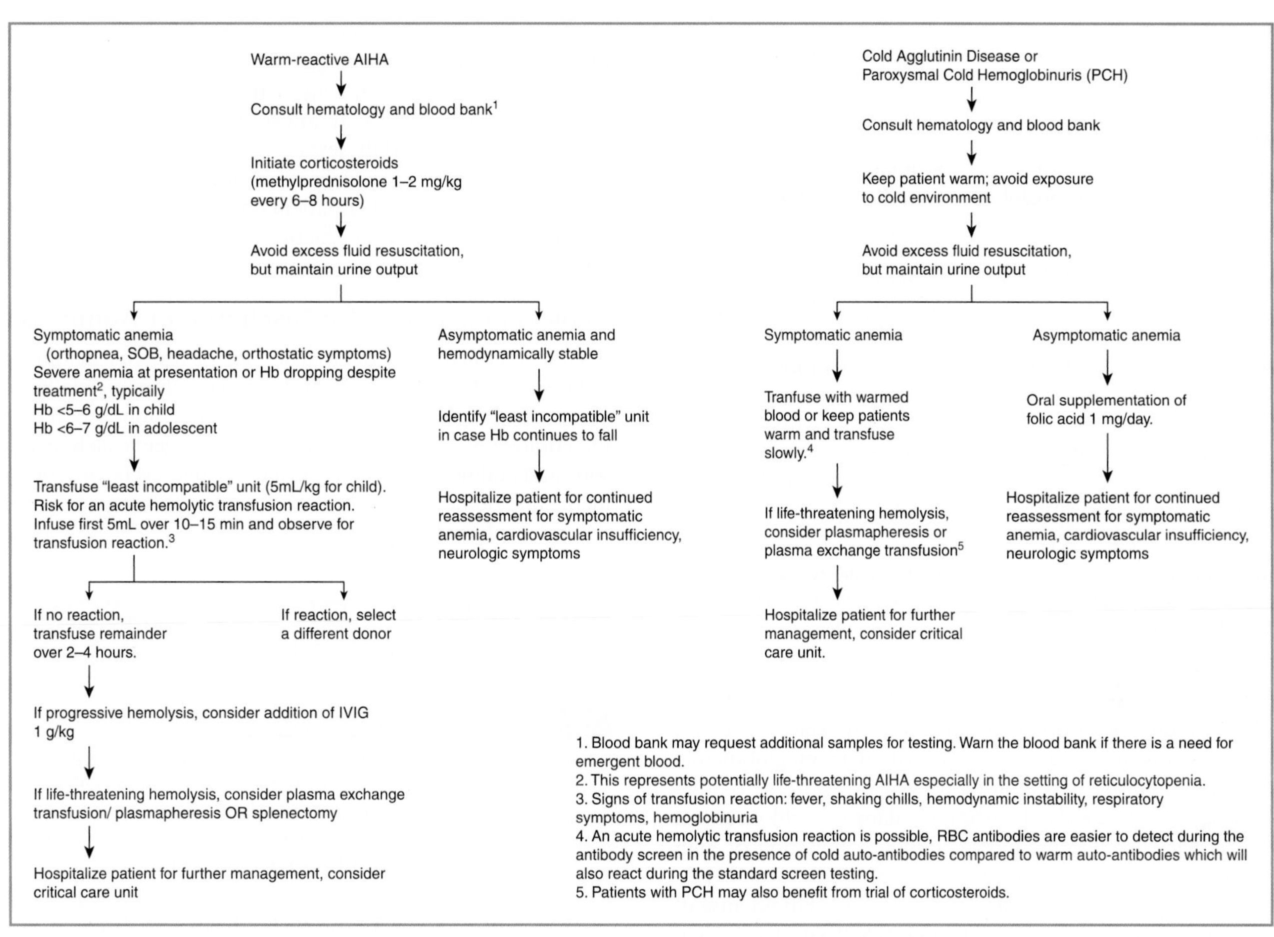

FIGURE 101.3 Management of autoimmune hemolytic anemia.

prompt treatment. When hemolysis is a result of small vessel disease, treatment of the underlying disorder (e.g., collagen vascular disease) or primarily affected organs (e.g., renal failure in hemolytic-uremic syndrome) is the first priority. The prompt institution of plasma exchange for TTP can be lifesaving.

Clinical Indications for Discharge or Admission

Hospitalize patients with severe or symptomatic anemia or an unclear clinical trajectory for close clinical monitoring and treatment. Frequently a critical care setting is appropriate for these patients. Consider outpatient management in patients with a clear or well-established underlying diagnosis and mild anemia with short interval follow-up for monitoring and ongoing management.

METHEMOGLOBINEMIA

Goals of Treatment

Methemoglobin (MHb) is the end product of a number of mechanisms (toxic exposure, dietary trigger, acidosis, genetic abnormality) that oxidize the iron associated with a heme group from the ferrous (Fe^{2+}) to ferric state (Fe^{3+}) rendering it unable to reversibly bind oxygen. In high quantities, insufficient gas exchange may be incompatible with life. The primary goal of treatment is to remove the causative agent, provide supportive care to optimize end-organ oxygenation, and allow time for reduction of MHb back to hemoglobin. In symptomatic and life-threatening situations, therapeutic intervention can hasten the reduction process.

CLINICAL PEARLS AND PITFALLS

- Suspect MHb when a cyanotic patient has a normal arterial PO_2, and pulse oximetry (generally in the mid-80s) is significantly lower than the oxygen saturation reported on arterial blood gas.
- MHb levels are reported as percent of total hemoglobin; therefore, patients with anemia will manifest more symptoms at lower levels of MHb.
- Methylene blue administration for methemoglobinemia is contraindicated in patients with G6PD.

Clinical Considerations

Methemoglobinemia is an uncommon cause of cyanosis in infants and children, but can cause significant morbidity and even death. Oxidant stress under physiologic conditions produces MHb that is reduced back to hemoglobin by cellular mechanisms. In normal individuals, MHb exists in a steady state of about 1% of total hemoglobin; this may be higher in those chronically exposed to tobacco smoke. Congenital forms of methemoglobinemia present in the neonatal period or early infancy and result from defects in or absence of the endogenous reductase systems. Defects in globin chains (α- or β-chain) can also alter the oxidation state of the heme iron

TABLE 101.4

SYMPTOMS ASSOCIATED WITH MHb LEVELS

Methemoglobin concentration (g/dL)	% total hemoglobin	Symptoms (assuming Hb 15 g/dL)
<1.5	<10	None
1.5–3	10–20	Cyanosis
3–4.5	20–30	Anxiety, lightheadedness, headache, tachycardia
4.5–7.5	30–50	Fatigue, confusion, dizziness, tachypnea, increased tachycardia
7.5–10.5	50–70	Coma, seizures, arrhythmias, acidosis
>10.5	>70	Death

Reprinted with permission from Wright RO, Lewander WJ, Woolf AD. Methemoglobinemia: etiology, pharmacology, and clinical management. *Ann Emerg Med* 1999;34:646–656.

resulting in cyanosis. Termed M hemoglobins, they are inherited in an autosomal dominant fashion and typically do not require treatment. Acquired forms of methemoglobinemia are more common. Ingestion or topical exposure to oxidizing drugs or chemicals (benzocaine, dapsone, chloroquine, nitrates, paraquat) occurs most commonly. Ingestion of high levels of nitrates, such as through well water, can cause MHb. Systemic acidosis in infants may also result in MHb because of the relative immaturity of NADH-dependent enzyme system early in life.

Clinical Recognition

Consider the diagnosis of methemoglobinemia when cyanosis occurs in the absence of cardiac or pulmonary disease and does not improve with oxygen therapy. Symptoms depend on the actual concentration of MHb (see Table 101.4). At low levels, patients may present with cyanosis only. As the level rises, symptoms of headache, fatigue, anxiety, and lightheadedness develop. A MHb level greater than 30% is considered life-threatening, and these patients may exhibit altered mental status, dyspnea, tachypnea, tachycardia, seizures, respiratory depression, and arrhythmia. Coma may occur at MHb levels above 50%.

Management/Diagnostic Testing

The treatment of methemoglobinemia depends on the clinical severity. In all cases, attempt to identify and remove the causative oxidant stress. If symptoms are mild after oxidant exposure, therapy may be unnecessary. RBCs with normal metabolism will reduce the MHb in several hours. In general, treat patients with MHb level >20% with 1 to 2 mg per kg of methylene blue as a 1% solution in saline infused intravenously over 5 minutes. Administer a second dose if symptoms are still present 1 hour later. Patients with a significant concurrent medical condition, especially cardiopulmonary conditions, should be considered for treatment at MHb levels starting at 10%. Methylene blue is an oxidant at high dosages, so total dosage should not exceed 7 mg per kg to avoid paradoxical methemoglobinemia.

Use methylene blue with extreme caution in patients with G6PD due to the risk of hemolytic anemia. The mechanism of action of methylene blue relies on NADPH. These patients may not produce sufficient quantities of NADPH to respond to this therapy; however, some patients have partial enzyme activity. Methylene blue at lower doses (0.3 to 0.5 mg/kg/dose) may lower MHb levels without causing significant hemolytic anemia. The addition of ascorbic acid 5 to 8 mg/kg/day may benefit G6PD patients. Consider exchange transfusion in patients who fail methylene blue treatment or have absent G6PD activity.

Clinical Indications for Discharge or Admission

Even if treatment with methylene blue or ascorbic acid in the ED is successful, admit any child with symptomatic methemoglobinemia to the hospital for close observation, especially if the etiology is unknown. Some oxidizing agents such as dapsone and aniline have been reported to cause cyclic or rebound methemoglobinemia. Consultation with toxicology or poison control is advised.

INEFFECTIVE OR DECREASED RED BLOOD CELL PRODUCTION

CLINICAL PEARLS AND PITFALLS

- Decreased RBC production may be due to congenital abnormalities (Diamond–Blackfan anemia [DBA]), marrow infiltrative processes (malignancy, fibrosis, lysosomal storage disease), or acquired insults (viral suppression, toxins, nutritional deficiency).
- β-Thalassemia major usually presents only after 2 to 3 months of age with the switch from γ- to β-globin chain production; it may present with severe anemia causing a hematologic emergency.
- Iron replacement therapy for iron-deficiency anemia consists of 3 to 6 mg/kg/day of elemental iron given orally as ferrous sulfate at night on an empty stomach (and ideally with ascorbic acid) as a single daily dose. IV or SQ formulations do not provide an advantage in the absence of malabsorption.
- The goal of transfusion for chronic, severe anemia is relief of symptoms, not restoration of a normal hemoglobin level. If transfusion is necessary, provide small aliquots of RBCs (5 mL per kg) slowly with close monitoring and consideration of furosemide administration.

Current Evidence

Thalassemia

The thalassemias are mutations or deletions of the globin genes that result in reduced or loss of production of α- or β-globin chains, the building blocks of hemoglobin. Hemoglobin A (normal adult hemoglobin $\alpha 2\beta 2$) begins rising just prior to birth as the body switches production from γ- to β-globin chains, and increases steadily over the first year of life to become the predominant hemoglobin.

The β-thalassemia gene mutations occur most commonly in populations living in regions bordering the Mediterranean, North Africa, the Middle East, Central and Southeast Asia, and India. In β-thalassemia, reduced (β^+) or no (β^0) β-globin chains are produced. β-Thalassemia major phenotype results from β^0/β^0 or β^0/β^+, intermedia phenotype from β^+/β^+, and carrier state from β/β^+.

In the first year of life, infants with β-thalassemia major usually develop a sallow complexion, increased fatigue, and poor weight gain and linear growth. Physical examination shows pallor, icterus, and enlargement of the liver and spleen. In thalassemia major, the hemoglobin level may decrease to 3 or 4 g per dL, and the mean corpuscular volume is low. The RBCs are hypochromic and microcytic, with striking variation in size and shape; nucleated RBCs are present on the peripheral smear. Children and adolescents with thalassemia intermedia have a moderate anemia, with hemoglobin levels usually between 7 and 10 g per dL. Hemoglobin electrophoresis is used to make the initial diagnosis of β-thalassemia, although in many cases index of suspicion is high due to family history. Hemoglobin electrophoresis may also reveal other mutant β-chains such as hemoglobin E or C. Independently, these hemoglobins may not cause a significant clinical phenotype; however, in combination with a β^0 or β^+ mutation, patients may have a β-thalassemia major or intermedia phenotype.

Patients with β-thalassemia major require lifelong transfusion or bone marrow transplantation. They may present to the emergency department with symptoms of severe anemia prior to initial diagnosis or later in life due to toxicity related to iron overload (often due to poor compliance with iron chelation therapy). The β-thalassemia intermedia phenotype is variable, but patients typically only need transfusions for acute exacerbations of their anemia during illness, pregnancy, or perioperatively. Patients who carry one-mutated β-gene are asymptomatic but their red cells are microcytic (low MCV) and a mild anemia may be evident.

The α-thalassemia gene mutations occur most commonly in populations living in Mediterranean countries, northern Africa, the Middle East, India, and Southeast Asia. Loss of one or two of the four α-globin genes is clinically trivial and manifests as a silent carrier or α-thalassemia trait, respectively. Loss of three α-globin genes causes hemoglobin H disease, usually associated with a moderate anemia and chronic hemolysis. Loss of all four α-globin genes results in production of Hemoglobin Barts (γ_4) and hydrops fetalis (stillborn or death soon after birth). Hemoglobin electrophoresis does not aid the diagnosis of α-thalassemia trait but can identify Hemoglobin H. Hemoglobin Barts can be detected on newborn screen.

Congenital and Acquired Aplastic/Hypoplastic Anemia

The differential diagnosis of aplastic and hypoplastic anemias is discussed in Chapter 57 Pallor. DBA and transient erythroblastopenia of childhood (TEC) are the more common causes of pure RBC aplasia in early childhood. In DBA, the level of RBC adenosine deaminase (ADA) is frequently elevated, and blood samples for this test should be obtained before transfusion. TEC typically presents in previously healthy children from infancy to toddlerhood with severe anemia and reticulocytopenia but otherwise normal blood counts. For patients with a hypoplastic anemia suggestive of TEC, a bone marrow aspirate may be helpful in predicting the course of the disease during the next few days and, in particular, the likelihood that pRBC transfusions will be required. For example, if a patient with TEC has a hemoglobin level of 4 g per dL, low reticulocyte count, and few RBC precursors on bone marrow evaluation, a further decrease in the hemoglobin concentration should be anticipated and pRBC transfusions will almost certainly be required. However, if the bone marrow aspirate shows numerous erythrocyte precursors progressing through all levels of erythrocyte maturation, a peripheral reticulocytosis can be expected within 24 hours and RBC transfusions may be unnecessary.

Nutrition Deficiencies and Excess

Nutritional anemias in children constitute more of a public health problem than a hematologic emergency; however, in some cases the hemoglobin level may be very low at the time of diagnosis. Some of the most common micro-nutrients related to anemia include deficiencies of iron, B_{12}, folate, zinc, vitamin C, and excess of copper. Of these, iron-deficiency anemia is the most common in the pediatric population.

Severe iron deficiency occurs mainly in toddlers due to excess cow's milk consumption (more than 1 quart [32 fl oz or ~1 L] daily). Adolescent girls make up another group at high risk for iron deficiency because a diet normally marginal in iron content becomes inadequate in the face of menstrual blood losses. The presenting complaints in severe iron-deficiency anemia include pallor, lethargy, irritability, or poor exercise tolerance. Iron replacement therapy consists of 3 to 6 mg/kg/day of elemental iron given orally as ferrous sulfate at night on an empty stomach (and ideally with ascorbic acid) as a single daily dose. The hematologic response to parenterally administered iron is no faster than the response to orally administered iron for patients with intact gastrointestinal absorption. Historically, intravenously administered iron has been associated with anaphylaxis, but such reactions are rare with modern preparations.

Vitamin B_{12} and folate deficiency result in megaloblastic macrocytic anemia. Infants exclusively breast-fed by a vegetarian mother may develop vitamin B_{12} deficiency. In folic acid deficiency caused by impaired folate absorption, nonhematologic symptoms such as diarrhea, slowed development, or altered mental status and coma may be more prominent than the symptoms of anemia. When considering replacement of folic acid or vitamin B_{12}, traditional replacement doses of 1 mg of folic acid and 100 mcg of vitamin B_{12} daily are undoubtedly excessive, but their common use reflects the safety and concentrations of the available compounds. The administration of supplemental iron, vitamin B_{12}, or folic acid should not be considered a substitute for adequate dietary intake when nutritional deficiency is recognized. Unlike most hematologic emergencies, the rapid improvement after treatment of these disorders may reduce the likelihood of further visits despite attempts to ensure adequate follow-up care. Therefore, a strong effort to restructure the diet should begin at the time of the initial contact.

Clinical Considerations

Clinical Recognition

Patients with congenital and acquired disorders of effective RBC production may be detected incidentally, with mild symptoms such as pallor, fatigue or malaise, or due to severe symptoms such as cardiopulmonary compromise. Some viral infections, such as parvovirus, may precipitate an anemic crisis in a previously stable patient with a chronic process due to suppression of erythropoiesis. A mild anemia due to chronic disease may be the presentation of a child with systemic illness. Age of onset helps to guide differential diagnosis. While acquired etiologies can arise at any age, congenital forms of aplastic anemia and thalassemia major typically present during infancy or early childhood.

Initial Assessment/H&P

History should include a thorough review of systems including general complaints of fatigue or decreased exercised tolerance, dietary history, family history and ethnic origin, and menstrual history where appropriate. Physical examination should assess for lymphadenopathy, organomegaly, and signs of bleeding.

Diagnostic Testing

Laboratory testing should include a CBC, reticulocyte count, review of peripheral blood smear, type and cross, reticulocyte hemoglobin (CHr), indirect antibody test (i.e., indirect Coombs test), and DAT (i.e., Coombs test), total and direct bilirubin, ferritin, plasma iron, total iron binding capacity (TIBC), chemistry panel, urinalysis, and a stool examination for occult blood. Additional testing including hemoglobin electrophoresis, micronutrient levels, ADA activity, genetic testing for congenital aplastic anemias may also be appropriate and should be guided by consultation with a hematologist. Often these subspecialized tests are not interpretable in the weeks following a transfusion, so communication with hematology prior to transfusion is preferable if clinical situation permits.

Management

The decision regarding transfusion of pRBCs depends on the etiology and severity of the anemia. Replacement of nutrient deficiencies and elimination of toxin exposures is necessary (see Table 101.5). If the hemoglobin level is mildly decreased from baseline levels and the patient has no evidence of cardiovascular compromise, transfusion may be unnecessary. However, transfusion should be considered in any patient with cardiovascular compromise, or borderline cardiovascular symptoms in the setting of expected ongoing losses. The goal of transfusion should be relief of symptoms, not restoration of a normal hemoglobin level. If transfusion is necessary, provide small aliquots of pRBCs (5 mL per kg) slowly. The administration of a rapid-acting diuretic (furosemide 1 mg/kg/dose, maximum 20 mg per dose) may diminish the risk of fluid overload.

For patients requiring recurrent or chronic transfusions or patients who may be candidates for bone marrow transplantation, blood bank measures to provide CMV-negative products and reduce the likelihood of alloimmunization by leukoreduction of pRBC units or extended RBC antigen typing are beneficial. First-degree relatives should *not* be chosen as blood donors to avoid allosensitization to family minor HLA antigens.

SICKLE CELL DISEASE

Goals of Treatment

Patients with sickle cell disorders suffer from three broad categories of complications: vascular occlusion, infection, and end-organ damage. Immediate recognition and early management of these complications can prevent hospitalizations, decrease the need for significant interventions such as exchange transfusions, and avoid long-term morbidity and death.

CLINICAL PEARLS AND PITFALLS

- Sickle cell patients require aggressive pain control when they present with a vasoocclusive episode. Management includes IV fluids to improve vascular flow, nonsteroidal anti-inflammatory drugs (NSAIDs), and administration of narcotics.
- Acute chest syndrome presents as fever, respiratory symptoms (increased work of breathing, hypoxia, or chest pain), and a new infiltrate on CXR. Acute chest syndrome can evolve rapidly to become life-threatening.
- Patients with sickle cell disease have a 300-fold higher risk of stroke compared with other children. New neurologic findings should prompt emergent hematology consultation, plans for exchange transfusion, and head imaging.
- Patients are functionally asplenic and at increased risk of severe bacterial infections. Fever >101.5°F/38.5°C necessitates blood culture (other cultures as clinically indicated) and empiric coverage with a broad-spectrum antibiotic such as ceftriaxone.
- Splenic sequestration results from pooling of blood within the spleen and can lead to hypovolemic shock necessitating transfusion. Most presentations are in children <3 years old; however, later presentations can occur in patients with HbSC or Hb Sickle β-thalassemia.

TABLE 101.5

TREATMENT OF ANEMIA

Cause	Treatment
Iron deficiency	Iron supplementation and increase dietary intake
Vitamin B_{12} and folic acid deficiency	Cobalamin and folate supplements
Lead poisoning	Remove child from site of exposure; intestinal irrigation if radiographs demonstrate retained lead particles; chelation therapy if severe; iron and folate supplementation
Hemolytic anemia	Supportive care with iron and folate supplementation and cessation of possible causative medications; autoimmune: steroids or Intravenous immunoglobulin (IVIG), plasmapheresis; transfusions if clinically unstable
Anemia of chronic disease	Treat underlying disease process
Aplastic anemia	Bone marrow transplant
Thalassemia	Chronic transfusions, iron chelation for prevention of iron overload and close monitoring for end-organ effects of iron toxicity; bone marrow transplant
Transient erythroblastopenia of childhood	Supportive, self-resolving; transfusion only in the case of clinical decompensation
Diamond–Blackfan anemia	Steroids; if unresponsive, bone marrow transplant; supportive care with transfusions
Gastrointestinal losses	Supportive, acid blocker; endoscopy to identify source of bleeding; octreotide infusion and transfusion if severe
Menstrual losses	Supportive, estrogen therapy, tranexamic acid, and transfusion if severe

Clinical Considerations

Clinical Recognition

Patients with sickle cell disease require prompt evaluation for complications including stroke, vasoocclusive episodes, acute chest syndrome, splenic sequestration, infection, and priapism. Consider the diagnosis of sickle cell disease in genetically susceptible children with unexplained pain or swelling (especially of the hands or feet), pneumonia, meningitis, sepsis, neurologic abnormalities, splenomegaly, or anemia. Recognition of sickle cell disease is key to appropriate intervention. Definitive testing to diagnose sickling disorders, hemoglobin electrophoresis, is not usually performed in the ED.

Triage

Immediately evaluate any sickle cell patient with fever, concern for stroke, acute chest syndrome, splenic sequestration, or priapism.

Vasoocclusive Pain Episodes

Initial Assessment/H&P

Vasoocclusive pain episodes are responsible for nearly 90% of all emergency department visits and 70% of hospitalizations related to sickle cell disease. Pain may be severe and debilitating for patients. Many patients live their entire lives with some degree of baseline pain. Cold exposure and dehydration trigger increased sickling. Joint pain presents a diagnostic challenge because vasoocclusive pain and the symptoms of trauma and infection (septic arthritis and osteomyelitis) present similarly and the physical examination findings, laboratory tests, and imaging features are often nonspecific. For a given patient, pain that is typical and/or at a recurrent location supports a vasoocclusive etiology. Dactylitis (infarction of the metacarpals, metatarsals, and phalanges) usually results in swelling of the hands and feet and is a common presentation in children 6 months to 2 years of age. Pain usually resolves after several days, but swelling may persist for 1 to 2 weeks.

Management/Diagnostic Testing

No definitive test exists for diagnosing a vasoocclusive episode. Hydration and prompt pain management are key (see Table 101.6). Improving intravascular volume with a normal saline bolus of 10 to 20 mL per kg followed by fluids at 1 to 1.5 times maintenance, depending on patient's hydration status, can help improve distal blood flow. Overly aggressive fluid management should be avoided due to the risk of hemodilution in the setting of anemia or cardiac strain in a patient with known or suspected underlying cardiac dysfunction. Concurrently, initiate a pain control regimen with the use of NSAIDs, such as ketorolac or ibuprofen, and narcotics. Frequent and appropriately dosed narcotics are essential, keeping in mind that patients with regular home use of oral narcotics may have a degree of tolerance. Timely and efficient use of pain control early in the crisis decreases hospital admission rates and length of stay. Patients can frequently identify the medications that best treat their pain. In some circumstances, oral, intranasal, or intramuscular administration of opiates is appropriate when IV access is not available. Consider patient/nurse-controlled analgesia (PCAs) and admission for those patients with inadequate analgesia after 2 to 3 doses of parental narcotics. Transdermal and subcutaneous administration of opioids can provide adjunctive therapy. Hesitancy in using parenteral narcotics may result in inadequate pain relief, mounting anxiety, and a loss of trust between physician and patient. This is a particularly common occurrence when the patient has repeated visits to the ED and physicians are suspicious of the stated degree of discomfort. Monitoring patients' self-reported pain scales at regular intervals will help determine the effectiveness of pain management.

Consider alternative diagnoses when pain fails to respond to appropriate treatment. If septic arthritis is strongly suspected, perform an arthrocentesis. Gram stain and culture are important in guiding management since the cell count and differential may be similar in septic arthritis and infarction. Bone biopsy may help diagnose osteomyelitis. *Staphylococcus aureus* is the most common cause of osteomyelitis; however *Salmonella* and other gram-negative organisms (including *Escherichia coli*) are more common in sickle cell patients than the general population.

Patient disposition depends on initial response. Consider discharge home on a standing NSAID and narcotic regimen for those patients who have significant improvement or complete resolution of pain. Instruct patients to decrease frequency of pain medication use over 48 to 72 hours in consultation with hematologist or PCP.

Visceral Pain Crises and Hepatobiliary Disease

Initial Assessment/H&P

Infarction of abdominal organs may produce symptoms similar to other nonhematologic disease processes. In the child with sickle cell disease and right upper quadrant abdominal pain, the differential diagnosis includes liver infarction from sickling in the vascular beds, cholelithiasis secondary to calculi due to chronic hemolysis, hepatitis from infectious causes, pancreatitis, peptic ulcer disease, and biliary obstruction. Common surgical problems such as appendicitis may be difficult to assess and laboratory values may not differentiate visceral vasoocclusive crisis from other problems.

Management/Diagnostic Testing

If the patient describes pain as typical in location and quality to a vasoocclusive crisis, begin fluids, provide analgesia, and observe the patient for improvement. Elevated aspartate aminotransferase (AST) and hyperbilirubinemia may be present in infarction as well as biliary disease. Abdominal ultrasound can assess the anatomy of the liver, gall bladder, and biliary tree.

Cholelithiasis is the most common hepatic and biliary tract complication in children with sickle cell disease, with an incidence of 12% in 2- to 5-year olds and approximately 40% by the age of 15 to 18 years. Patients can present with acute right upper quadrant pain and tenderness, hyperbilirubinemia, and elevated liver enzyme levels. Typically, surgery is delayed until acute inflammation has subsided to reduce the risk of complications. The optimal treatment includes elective laparoscopic cholecystectomy after adequate preparation for surgery (transfusions).

Rarely acute intrahepatic sickling or viral hepatitis can result in a similar clinical presentation with massive hyperbilirubinemia and elevated enzyme levels. Fulminant hepatic failure with hepatic encephalopathy and shock can also occur as a rare, often fatal, syndrome that may be amenable to exchange transfusion.

TABLE 101.6

SICKLE CELL ANEMIA: COMPLICATIONS AND MANAGEMENT

Complication	Clinical features	Management	Comments
Vasoocclusive episode	1. Joint or bone pain 2. Joint swelling (e.g., dactylitis) 3. Abdominal pain (may mimic acute abdomen)	1. Mild or moderate pain • Oral or IV hydration (bolus 10–20 ml/kg then 1–1½ times maintenance volume) • Analgesia ■ Oral medications such as oxycodone may be sufficient for some patients ■ IV (intermittent) doses of morphine, fentanyl, or hydromorphone ■ NSAIDs • Consider admission if ■ pain worsens ■ inadequate oral fluid intake ■ repeat emergency department visits 2. Severe pain • IV bolus 10–20 ml/kg followed by hydration at 1–1½ times maintenance volume • Analgesia ■ IV (intermittent) doses of morphine, fentanyl, or hydromorphone ■ PCA (early) ■ NSAIDs (ketorolac) • Admit unless pain markedly reduced and patient tolerates oral fluids	IV fluid can be D5 normal saline or ½ normal saline solution NSAID may be ibuprofen or ketorolac and should continue after discharge until pain resolves If delayed or difficult IV access, intranasal fentanyl may be considered for initial therapy Patient-controlled analgesia (PCA) may include a continuous infusion of opioid If using fentanyl patient may require PCA due to short duration of action
Priapism	1. Prolonged erection lasting more than 3 hrs 2. Pain 3. May experience difficulty urinating	1. Oral or IV hydration (10–20 ml/kg bolus, then 1–1½ times maintenance) 2. Oral pseudoephedrine 3. Analgesia as needed to control pain 4. Consult with urology, if no relief within 3 hrs.	Urology may consider early aspiration of the corpora
Splenic sequestration	1. Left upper quadrant pain 2. Pallor 3. Lethargy 4. Splenomegaly 5. May have altered vital signs (tachycardia, hypotension) 6. Worsened anemia with elevated reticulocytes and mild to moderate thrombocytopenia	1. Immediate volume replacement • IV fluids • Simple red blood cell transfusion 2. Admission to hospital 3. Splenectomy in refractory patients	Onset of symptoms is often sudden Usually occurs before age 5 but may develop later in patients with hemoglobin SC disease
Acute chest syndrome	1. Chest pain 2. Oxygen saturation below patient's baseline 3. Symptoms of respiratory distress 4. New finding on chest radiograph 5. Fever often present	1. Antibiotic therapy • Third-generation cephalosporin; if allergy to cephalosporins consider quinolones (e.g., levofloxacin), azithromycin, or clindamycin. • Macrolide 2. Consideration of red blood cell transfusion for patients with respiratory distress • Simple transfusion if hemoglobin <10 g/dL • Exchange transfusion if hemoglobin ≥10 g/dL	Therapy with steroids not usually needed unless patient has a history of asthma and signs of an asthma exacerbation

TABLE 101.6

SICKLE CELL ANEMIA: COMPLICATIONS AND MANAGEMENT (CONTINUED)

Complication	Clinical features	Management	Comments
Ischemic or hemorrhagic stroke	1. Focal neurologic deficits • Focal weakness • Dysarthria • Aphasia 2. Increased ICP • Severe headache • Vomiting • Bradycardia 3. Seizure 4. Impaired mental status/coma 5. Nuchal rigidity (hemorrhagic stroke)	1. Immediate CT 2. If stroke present, initiate exchange transfusion. Simple transfusion maybe used as a bridge while exchange is being setup if hemoglobin <10 g/dL 3. MRI if within 2–4 hrs of symptoms 4. 1.5–2X-volume exchange transfusion 5. Angiography to target management	Ischemic strokes may be more subtle than hemorrhagic strokes
Hemolytic anemia crisis	1. Fatigue 2. Pallor 3. Scleral icterus 4. Jaundice 5. Tachycardia 6. Headache 7. Fall in the hematocrit from baseline 8. Elevated reticulocyte count 9. Elevated bilirubin	1. Usually self-limited, routine supportive care 2. Transfusion of pRBCs if severe symptoms (altered mental status, impaired oxygen delivery, significant tachycardia)	Transfusions usually not required
Aplastic anemia crisis	1. Fatigue 2. Pallor 3. Tachycardia 4. Absence of jaundice 5. Altered mental status (severe anemia) 6. Headache 7. Dyspnea 8. Fall in the hematocrit from baseline 9. Low reticulocyte count 10. Absence of acute hemolysis	1. Usually self-limited, routine supportive care 2. Transfusion of pRBCs if severe symptoms (altered mental status, impaired oxygen delivery, significant tachycardia)	Small transfusions often sufficient to support oxygen delivery while awaiting bone marrow recovery Often parvo B19 related though other infections as well
Bacteremia/ sepsis	1. Fever 2. Hypotension 3. Lethargy 4. Tachycardia	1. Cultures of blood, and if indicated, urine and spinal fluid. 2. Prompt antibiotic administration (don't delay if culture difficult to obtain). Third-generation cephalosporin, vancomycin. If allergy to cephalosporins consider quinolones (e.g., levofloxacin), azithromycin, or clindamycin. 3. IV fluids 4. Simple or exchange transfusion for sepsis, acidosis, or hypoxia 5. Admission	High risk for infection with *Streptococcus pneumoniae, Haemophilus influenzae, Salmonella, Staphylococcus aureus, Escherichia coli* Can rapidly deteriorate

Priapism

Initial Assessment

Priapism is a painful vasoocclusive crisis causing a tender and engorged penis that may persist for hours. Urination may be difficult.

Management/Diagnostic Testing

Treatment is similar to other painful crises with management directed at hydration and analgesia. A number of systemic therapies can also be utilized. Pseudoephedrine can be given orally, while terbutaline delivery is either oral or subcutaneous. Terbutaline has been studied for the treatment of priapism in nonsickle cell disease patients and has some demonstrated efficacy in the sickle cell disease group. Consider early consultation with a pediatric hematologist and urologist.

Infection/Sepsis

Initial Assessment

Sickle cell patients have a higher risk of bacterial infection than the general population due to functional asplenia, low serum immunoglobulin levels, and abnormal opsonization and complement activation. The risk is highest for serious infections with encapsulated bacteria such as *Streptococcus pneumoniae, Haemophilus influenzae,* and *Salmonella* species, as well as *S. aureus* and *E. coli.* Sepsis, meningitis, pneumonia, osteomyelitis, abscesses, and septic arthritis are all possible. The use of oral penicillin prophylaxis until age 5 and vaccination for *H. influenzae* and *S. pneumoniae* have decreased the rate of serious bacterial infection from 3–5% to 0.8%; however, infection remains a meaningful concern in the setting of an acutely ill, febrile patient with sickle cell anemia. In one recent retrospective study at a tertiary care center, the bacteremia rate in 1,118 acutely febrile patients with sickle cell was 0.8%; the nine cases of bacteremia included 4 cases of *Salmonella,* 2 *S. pneumoniae,* 2 *E. coli,* and 1 *S. aureus.*

Management/Diagnostic Testing

In the emergency department, a toxic-appearing child with sickle cell disease requires careful and immediate evaluation, monitoring, fluid resuscitation, and antibiotics. Obtain cultures of blood, and, if indicated, urine and spinal fluid. Do not delay antibiotic administration due to difficulty obtaining labs or performing procedures. Include a type and cross. In regions with endemic resistant *S. pneumoniae* strains, use vancomycin in addition to a third-generation cephalosporin. As in other patients with reduced or absent splenic function, clinical deterioration may be extremely rapid. The patient who arrives alert to the ED may become moribund and hypotensive within 30 minutes. In the ill patient with sepsis, acidosis, or hypoxia, provide simple or exchange transfusions to decrease massive sickling, which can cause secondary organ damage. Mortality from bacteremia may approach 20% to 30%.

Have a high level of suspicion for meningitis in the young, irritable child with sickle cell disease and unexplained fever. Perform a lumbar puncture on toxic children and anyone with signs or symptoms of meningitis. Use the same antibiotic therapy for meningitis as recommended for hematologically normal children with meningitis. Simple or exchange transfusion to lower the percentage of sickle hemoglobin may reduce the risk of intracerebral sickling in areas of brain swelling that can lead to infarction. When hemoglobin S is less than 30% of the total hemoglobin, sickling is unlikely, and decisions regarding fluid management can be directed by the central nervous system findings as opposed to the need to ameliorate sickling.

The nontoxic, febrile child (temperature >38.5°C) with sickle cell disease requires a thorough history and physical examination. Detailed history should focus on length, duration, and height of fever, and the presence of associated symptoms such as cough, respiratory distress, and abdominal pain. Elicit immunization status and compliance with prophylactic antibiotics. Without a clear source of infection, laboratory assessment should include a CBC with a reticulocyte count and blood culture. Other evaluations, if the history or physical examination suggest, should include a chest x-ray, urinalysis with culture, cerebrospinal fluid analysis, and type and cross, especially if history suggests splenic sequestration, acute chest syndrome, or significant neurologic symptoms. Administer antibiotics promptly, prior to knowledge of laboratory results. Typically, prescribe ceftriaxone (50 mg per kg up to 2,000 mg) for broad-spectrum antibiotic coverage lasting 24 hours while cultures are pending; outpatient management is appropriate in stable patients without early concerns for developing complications and who have reliable caretakers with the means to return if necessary. Consider levofloxacin, azithromycin, or clindamycin in patients allergic to cephalosporins and depending on local sensitivities.

Acute Chest Syndrome

Initial Assessment

Acute chest syndrome is a life-threatening complication of sickle cell disease indicative of pneumonia, pulmonary infarction or both. Lifetime risk of acute chest syndrome is 48% and causes 25% of sickle cell disease–related deaths. The patient usually presents with fever, tachypnea, chest pain, rales, and hypoxia. In a dehydrated patient, the initial physical examination findings may be minimal.

Management/Diagnostic Testing

Any sickle cell patient who presents with chest pain requires immediate assessment, monitoring, and treatment including: IV access, fluids, oxygen administration, laboratory testing including: CBC with reticulocyte count, type and screen, blood culture, and chest x-ray (see Table 101.6). Consider any infiltrate to be within the spectrum of acute chest syndrome and treat with antibiotics including ampicillin or a third-generation cephalosporin such as ceftriaxone and atypical coverage with a macrolide. Add vancomycin in the severely ill patient. All patients with acute chest syndrome require admission for further management. Monitor closely patients with chest pain without radiographic findings or hypoxia and encourage incentive spirometry, as splinting puts them at risk for the development of acute chest syndrome.

Consider simple transfusion in the presence of severe anemia (hemoglobin <6 to 7 g per dL) and simple or exchange transfusion for hypoxia or radiologic or clinical evidence of severe or rapidly progressive disease. The distinction between pneumonia and an acute chest/vasoocclusive crisis can be difficult, making aggressive management prudent. Euvolemia is the goal of fluid resuscitation in acute chest, as pulmonary edema can worsen respiratory distress and hypovolemia can increase sickling. Therapy with corticosteroids is controversial. Although some studies show short-term benefit, significant complications can occur and therefore routine use of steroids has not been adopted. Patients with the comorbidity of asthma may require steroids as part of their acute management; however, a taper rather than the standard 5-day course is necessary.

Stroke

Initial Assessment

The combined incidence of ischemic and hemorrhagic stroke is nearly 300-fold higher in patients with sickle cell disease compared with all children. Eleven percent of all sickle cell anemia patients will suffer a stroke, with occurrence at a median age of 20 years. Fatalities with ischemic strokes are less likely than with hemorrhagic stroke; however, neurologic sequelae are common with both. Typical presenting symptoms and signs for ischemic stroke include focal weakness, dysarthria, aphasia, and seizure. Hemorrhagic strokes present with evidence of increased intracranial pressure including severe headache, vomiting, impaired mental status, bradycardia, nuchal rigidity, coma, focal neurologic deficits, and seizure. Risk factors include young age, low baseline hemoglobin concentration, and high leukocyte count. Historical risk factors include previous stroke, moya moya, cerebral aneurysms, acute chest syndrome, acute hypertension, hypertransfusion, and recent corticosteroid use. Cerebral aneurysms occur with increased frequency in patients with sickle cell disease. The origin of this complication, which is usually detected in teenagers or adults, remains obscure but may relate to local vessel damage. The severe morbidity and high mortality associated with ruptured cerebral aneurysms require careful evaluation of patients with sickle cell disease and headaches or other neurologic findings (vertigo, syncope, nystagmus, ptosis, meningismus, or photophobia). Unfortunately, the aneurysm often escapes detection until after major, and often fatal, subarachnoid or intracerebral bleeding.

Management/Diagnostic Testing

Use CT for initial evaluation of sickle cell patients with concern for stroke. MRI can assist in early diagnosis in ischemic strokes (within 2 to 4 hours of symptoms) that may not be apparent on CT. A 1.5 to 2X volume exchange transfusion should begin immediately for ischemic strokes. This reduces the likelihood of further intravascular sickling and may prevent extension of cortical damage. MRA should be performed in patients with identified intracranial hemorrhage to guide further diagnosis and management. If an accessible aneurysm is identified and bleeding persists, surgical or interventional radiology intervention should follow radiologic confirmation.

Anemia

Initial Assessment/H&P

The baseline anemia of a patient with sickle cell disease may worsen acutely due to acute hemolysis triggered by a viral or bacterial infection or by an aplastic crisis usually in the setting of infection with parvovirus B19 halting RBC production for 2 to 4 days. In both cases, patients will present with fatigue, pallor (or jaundice if hemolysis), and tachycardia.

Management/Diagnostic Testing

Laboratory studies will demonstrate a fall in the hemoglobin from baseline. Patients with a hemolytic crisis will typically have scleral icterus, jaundice, and a reticulocytosis. Both hemolytic and aplastic crises are usually self-limited; once the infection clears, the patient recovers. Patients with severe symptoms such as altered mental status, impaired oxygen delivery, and significant tachycardia should receive a transfusion of pRBCs. Transfusion volume should be calculated to target the patient's baseline hemoglobin level and not exceed 10 to 11 g per dL.

Splenic Sequestration

Initial Assessment/H&P

Splenic sequestration, a potentially life-threatening event, usually presents in children younger than 5 years of age before the spleen has completely fibrosed. The lifetime risk is 20%. It may be the first presenting symptom of sickle cell disease in children less than 2 years. Patients with HbSC and sickle β-thalassemia have less splenic fibrosis and may experience splenic sequestration at any age. During sequestration, the spleen becomes acutely engorged in some cases with a significant portion of the blood volume. Patients will present with acute onset of left upper quadrant abdominal pain, progressive pallor, increasing tachycardia, and lethargy over several hours. The spleen is palpable and may be tender. A prominent reticulocytosis is usually present. Hypotension and cardiovascular collapse can occur with a 10% to 15% mortality rate.

Management/Diagnostic Testing

The mainstay of treatment is replenishment of the intravascular volume for patients in hypovolemic shock. Resuscitation with crystalloid is used to stabilize perfusion emergently. However, aggressive crystalloid use can compromise tissue oxygenation due to dilutional worsening of anemia. Transfuse pRBCs for patients in shock (5 to 10 mL per kg, begin carefully with 2 to 3 mL per kg). Since RBCs will be released from the spleen as the sequestration reverses, do not overcorrect the hemoglobin (return it to patient's baseline) with initial transfusion to avoid complications of circulatory overload and erythrocytosis. Reversal of shock and a rising hemoglobin signals improvement of a sequestration crisis. The spleen becomes less firm and smaller over the course of days. For milder cases, admission for serial splenic examinations and establishing trend of hemoglobin is appropriate.

Papillary Necrosis

Initial Assessment/H&P

Papillary necrosis in the kidneys causes hematuria that is usually sudden and painless and often persistent. A history of recent trauma, streptococcal infection, or recurrent urinary tract infection should alert the physician to other causes of hematuria. Similarly, hypertension suggests the presence of nephritis rather than simple vasoocclusion.

Management/Diagnostic Testing

Laboratory evaluation should include CBC, reticulocyte count, type and cross, BUN/Cr and urinalysis. In papillary necrosis, microscopic examination of the urine shows numerous RBCs but RBC casts are rarely seen. Pyuria and proteinuria in excess of what might be attributed to the blood in the urine are not found in papillary necrosis and may indicate nephritis. Renal ultrasound may be obtained to confirm the diagnosis and evaluate for alternative etiologies for the hematuria. Admission to the hospital is often required for IV hydration. In severe hematuria, significant anemia may necessitate RBC transfusion. Simple or exchange transfusion may also shorten the course of ongoing hematuria. The lifetime risk of renal failure is 11%.

Avascular Necrosis

Sickle cell disease is the most common cause of pediatric femoral head avascular necrosis. This complication is even more common in patients with HbSC disease. The lifetime risk of avascular necrosis is 21%. Risk factors include a high baseline hematocrit and a clinical history of frequent or severe painful crises.

Management/Diagnostic Testing

Treatment options are limited. Bed rest and core decompression are the initial approaches. Total hip replacement may become necessary.

Transfusions

Patients with sickle cell disease may receive many transfusions throughout their lives and are at risk for developing alloantibodies. Perform extended RBC antigen testing before their first transfusion; their primary hematologist usually performs this during routine outpatient monitoring. Alloantibodies make future cross-matching more challenging and increase the risk of a hemolytic transfusion reaction. The volume of simple transfusion should be calculated to avoid raising the patient's hemoglobin level above 10 to 11 g per dL. Exchange transfusion may be needed in some clinical settings, as discussed in the complication sections above; this procedure requires adequate large bore IV access, or central venous access, and often requires a plasmapheresis machine. Infants may be exchange transfused with simple syringes, but this too should occur in consultation with a hematologist. If sophisticated blood banking services are not available, consider transferring the patient to such a center.

Clinical Indications for Discharge or Admission

Admit patients for IV analgesics if their pain is inadequately managed with an oral pain regimen. Additionally, admit patients who are unable to maintain adequate oral intake and are at risk of dehydration. Ill-appearing patients or those with clinical concern for acute chest syndrome, sepsis, splenic sequestration, or stroke require hospitalization and potentially intensive care management. Consider hospitalization for febrile patients who are well appearing but are younger than 6 months, under-immunized, if there is a concern for the reliability of follow-up, and in those with more than 5% (absolute) drop in hematocrit below baseline, or a Hb <6 g per dL. Febrile nontoxic patients with sickle cell disease may be discharged following blood cultures and antibiotic administration if they are able to follow-up within 24 hours.

NEUTROPENIA

Goals of Treatment

Prompt evaluation and treatment of neutropenic patients is essential to decreasing morbidity and mortality associated with infection. Cultures should be obtained but should not delay empiric antibiotic treatment. Numerous quality improvement initiatives in pediatric emergency medicine have shown improvement in time to initiation of antibiotic therapy in patient populations known to be at risk of neutropenia.

CLINICAL PEARLS AND PITFALLS

- Neutropenia is defined as an absolute neutrophil count (ANC) less than 1,500 per μL, with severe neutropenia <500 per μL.
- Severe neutropenia increases the risk for serious infection due to increased susceptibility to bacterial and fungal infections, but not typically to viral or parasitic infections.
- Risk of serious infection in neutropenic patients varies depending on the etiology of the neutropenia and patient comorbidities.
- Incidental neutropenia identified in a previously healthy child likely represents viral suppression.

Current Evidence

Neutrophils are an essential component of host defense against invasive organisms including bacteria and fungi. Neutropenia or defects in neutrophil function can result in clinically significant immunocompromise.

Clinical Considerations

Asymptomatic neutropenia has multiple etiologies and diagnostic evaluation can occur as an outpatient. Antibiotic administration to febrile neutropenic patients should occur promptly while awaiting culture results. Neutropenic states associated with repeated, severe infections require an aggressive attempt to identify a causative organism. Obtain blood and urine cultures, along with appropriate cultures from identified sources of infection (e.g., skin abscess, cellulitis). Examine cerebrospinal fluid when CNS infection is suspected.

Clinical Recognition

There are a wide range of causes of neutropenia in children. Etiologies of neutropenia can be divided into congenital or acquired. Congenital forms of neutropenia such as severe congenital neutropenia and cyclic neutropenia arise from specific genetic mutations. Several syndromes including myelokathexis/WHIM syndrome, Shwachman–Diamond syndrome, and Chédiak–Higashi syndrome are also associated with neutropenia. Acquired forms arise from infections, drugs, or autoimmunity (see Table 101.7). Immune-mediated conditions are caused by neutrophil-specific antibodies. These include neonatal alloimmune neutropenia, a severe but self-limited neutropenia secondary to transplacental maternal antibodies, and primary autoimmune neutropenia. Idiopathic neutropenia occurs without evidence of congenital, immune, or cyclic neutropenia.

Triage

The most important triage consideration is to identify febrile neutropenic patients, and among those to recognize ill-appearing children who require aggressive management. Early administration of broad-spectrum IV antibiotics should be a primary focus.

Initial Assessment/H&P

Attention to frequency, site, and severity of prior infections is critical. Ascertain the height of fever, other constitutional symptoms, the presence of oral inflammation, and history of other infections. Family history may help diagnose cyclic neutropenia. Detailing exposure to medications and toxins

TABLE 101.7

CAUSES OF NEUTROPENIA AND DISORDERS OF NEUTROPHIL FUNCTION IN CHILDREN

Inherited neutropenia
Severe congenital neutropenia, includes autosomal dominant (neutrophil elastase mutation), autosomal recessive Kostmann disease
Cyclic neutropenia
Dyskeratosis congenita
Shwachman–Diamond syndrome
Congenital neutropenia associated with pigmentation and or immune disorders—Chédiak–Higashi syndrome, Griscelli syndrome, Hermansky–Pudlak syndrome
Reticular dysgenesis, myelokathexis/WHIM syndrome
Other neutropenias—Metaphyseal chondrodysplasia or cartilage-hair hypoplasia, Barth syndrome, glycogen storage type 1b, Gauchers disease, Niemann–Pick disease
Acquired neutropenias
Drugs and chemical toxins
Anticonvulsant: carbamazepine, valproate
Antimicrobial: sulfonamides, penicillins, trimethoprim/sulfamethoxazole, quinine
Antipsychotic: clozapine, olanzapine, phenothiazines
Antirheumatic: Gold, levamisole, penicillamine
Antithyroid: methimazole, propylthiouracil
Other: aminopyrine, deferiprone, rituximab, levamisole-adulterated cocaine, phenothiazines, thiouracil
Dose dependent myeloid suppression, cytotoxic drugs, antimetabolites
Iatrogenic causes (radiotherapy, radioactive treatments)
Infection (bacterial, viral, rickettsial, protozoal)—usually transient
Bacterial: Brucella, parathyphoid, tuberculosis, tularemia, typhoid
Viral: CMV, EBV, HIV, influenza, parvovirus B19, Hepatitis A, B, RSV, rubella, measles, varicella
Rickettsial: *Anaplasma phagocytophilum,* other rickettsia
Protozoan: *Plasmodium vivax, Plasmodium falciparum*
Bone marrow infiltration or failure (leukemia, aplastic anemia, hypogammaglobulinemia, hemophagocytic lymphohistiocytosis)
Nutritional deficiencies (starvation; anorexia nervosa; vitamin B_{12}, folate, zinc, and copper deficiencies)
Immune neutropenias (collagen vascular diseases, Felty syndrome, neonatal isoimmune neutropenia, autoimmune neutropenia including chronic benign neutropenia of childhood)
Disorders of neutrophil function
Abnormal adhesion (leukocyte adhesion deficiency)
Abnormal chemotaxis (hyperimmunoglobulin E syndrome)
Abnormal opsonization and ingestion (complement deficiency, leukocyte adhesion deficiency)
Abnormal degranulation (Chédiak–Higashi syndrome)
Abnormal oxidative metabolism (chronic granulomatous disease, myeloperoxidase deficiency)
Acquired disorders of phagocytic dysfunction (malnutrition, malignancies, severe burns)

including herbal or "natural" remedies may reveal a cause of acquired disease. Congenital neutropenia usually presents in infancy with severe or recurrent bacterial or fungal infections typically of the skin, mucosa, or lungs. Explore the family history for recurrent infections or deaths in early childhood that might suggest a congenital neutropenia.

On physical examination, evidence of mouth ulcers, gingival, periodontal, or dental issues may indicate neutropenia. Acute abdominal pain and fever should raise concerns about neutropenic colitis (also known as typhlitis) and sepsis. Examine the perirectal and anal area for cellulitis. In the absence of neutrophils, the degree of induration may lead clinicians to underestimate the severity of infection.

Management/Diagnostic Testing

Management of neutropenic patients depends on the degree and etiology of the neutropenia (see Table 101.7). Neutropenic oncology patients are a special category (see Chapter 106 Oncologic Emergencies). Febrile neutropenic patients require CBC and blood cultures. For ill-appearing febrile patients and febrile neutropenic patients with poor marrow function (congenital neutropenias and bone marrow failure syndromes), treat with broad-spectrum IV antibiotic therapy that includes antibiotics effective against skin and gastrointestinal flora, and anaerobic coverage if abdominal pain is present. An example initial regimen may include ceftriaxone, vancomycin, and metronidazole. For persistent fever (>4 days), empiric antifungal coverage should be considered. Febrile neutropenic patients with normal marrow function (autoimmune-mediated neutropenias) who are well appearing with reassuring vital signs are often managed as outpatients following a dose of ceftriaxone.

Neutropenia is occasionally discovered during an evaluation for fever. In most of these instances both the fever and neutropenia result from a viral illness. Serious secondary

TABLE 101.8

BUCHANAN AND ADIX BLEEDING SEVERITY FOR CHILDREN WITH ITP

Overall bleeding severity		
Score	**Description**	
0	None	Definitely no new hemorrhage of any kind
1	Minor	Few petechiae (≤100 total) and/or ≤5 small bruises (≤3 cm diameter)
2	Mild	Many petechiae (>100 total) and/or >5 large bruises (>3 cm diameter); no/minimal mucosal bleeding
3	Moderate	Overt mucosal bleeding (epistaxis, gum bleeding, oropharyngeal blood blisters, menorrhagia, gastrointestinal bleeding, etc.) that does not require immediate medical attention or intervention
4	Severe	Mucosal bleeding or suspected internal hemorrhage (in the brain, lung, muscle, joint, etc) that requires immediate medical attention or intervention
5	Life-threatening	Documented intracranial hemorrhage or life-threatening or fatal hemorrhage in any site

Reproduced with permission from Buchanan GR, Adix L. Grading of hemorrhage in children with idiopathic thrombocytopenic purpura. *J Pediatr* 2002;141:683–688.

bacterial infections are unlikely with mild to moderate neutropenia; however, because the neutropenia usually cannot be attributed with certainty to a viral illness, other causes of neutropenia should be considered including the use of drugs associated with neutropenia (see Table 101.7), as well as other underlying disorders. Genetic testing for congenital neutropenias should be pursued in infants, usually at follow-up with a pediatric hematologist. Consider underlying disorders such as malignancies or nutritional disturbances (folate and vitamin B_{12}). If no etiology is identified and neutropenia persists on repeat follow-up testing, additional evaluation should be performed in consultation with a pediatric hematologist. Work up for patients with unexplained neutropenia should include CBC with differential and peripheral smear review, nutritional studies (such as folate and vitamin B_{12}), and may include antineutrophil antibodies, bone marrow aspiration and biopsy (if neutropenia is persistent and without clear etiology), serum immunoglobulins, and virology screen. Patients with some forms of chronic neutropenia may be treated with granulocyte colony stimulating factor (G-CSF), especially in the setting of recurrent infections. Neonatal alloimmune neutropenia may be treated with IVIG and eventually resolves as the maternal antibody titer wanes.

Clinical Indications for Discharge or Admission

In the afebrile patient, clinical status is more important than the ANC. For well-appearing patients with good marrow function, outpatient management is reasonable. If the ANC is greater than 500 per μL, manage the child as one would a nonneutropenic patient. An ill-appearing child or a child with poor marrow function requires inpatient management for empiric IV antibiotics and clinical monitoring.

DISORDERS OF NEUTROPHIL FUNCTION

Numerous disorders of neutrophil function tend to have normal or elevated neutrophil counts; however, these conditions can be associated with serious infections. Evaluate and treat patients with abnormal neutrophil function based on the specific cause and the history of serious infection. For example, chronic granulomatous disease (CGD) has characteristic features including the site of infection (liver, bones, GI tract) and specific causative organisms that require directed therapy (*Aspergillus* species, *Pseudomonas cepacia, Serratia marcescens*). Guidelines for the management of febrile illnesses are generally similar to those for the management of patients with neutropenia.

PLATELET DISORDERS

Goals of Treatment

The management of platelet disorders is targeted at preventing and managing hemorrhage, notably intracranial hemorrhage or bleeding causing hemodynamic compromise. In most cases, bleeding dictates the need for platelet transfusion or other therapy, rather than the platelet count. Patients often manifest different degrees of bleeding at a given platelet count, especially across different causative mechanisms.

IMMUNE THROMBOCYTOPENIA

CLINICAL PEARLS AND PITFALLS

- Bleeding stigmata due to decreased platelet number are variable but mucosal bleeding and petechiae are most typical.
- Significant spontaneous bleeding is uncommon above platelet counts of 20,000 per μL.
- For thrombocytopenia with minimal or no bleeding symptoms, observation is typically appropriate.
- Parents and clinicians must be vigilant for signs or symptoms of intracranial hemorrhage.

Current Evidence

ITP, formerly known as idiopathic thrombocytopenic purpura, is the most commonly encountered cause of severely low platelets in children. This isolated thrombocytopenia arises due to immunologic destruction without a known precipitant in the case of primary ITP, or in association with autoimmune disorders, viral processes or drugs in the case of secondary ITP. Serious bleeding is rare (<2%). This low frequency is particularly remarkable because the disease is most common in children between the ages of 1 and 4 years, who have the expected developmental predilection toward minor trauma.

ITP may be newly diagnosed, persistent (3 to 12 months) or chronic (>12 months). For the diagnosis and management of persistent or chronic ITP, hematology consultation is advised. Anemia is uncommon but hemorrhagic manifestations can result in moderate or severe anemia. Adolescents with ITP may develop significant anemia due to heavy menstrual bleeding. Evans syndrome, immune destruction of two or more blood cell lines, can be an alternative explanation for anemia with ITP. The life-threatening complication of ITP is intracranial hemorrhage. Consider intracranial hemorrhage in any patient with ITP with symptoms of intracranial injury (change in mental status, vomiting, neurologic abnormality) even in the absence of a clear history of head trauma, as the precipitating event can be quite minor. The relationship between platelet count and bleeding symptoms is not precise. Intracranial hemorrhage is fortunately rare, but patients are at highest risk when platelet counts are less than <10,000 per µL. Other severe hemorrhage can occur from the nasal mucosa, gastrointestinal tract, or other internal sites.

Clinical Considerations

Clinical Recognition

The classic presentation of the child with ITP is a well-appearing child with unexplained ecchymoses and petechiae that may be accompanied by gingival bleeding, epistaxis, and hematuria. Any child with unexplained bleeding warrants evaluation for thrombocytopenia, followed by evaluation for its etiology. The peak incidence of childhood ITP is children 2 to 6 years old. There may be a history of a recent immunization or antecedent viral illness. In children less than 1 year of age consider a possible underlying immunodeficiency. In adolescent patients, there is a higher prevalence of concurrent autoimmune disorders. ITP is a diagnosis of exclusion; atypical features warrant evaluation for other etiologies.

Triage

A child with petechiae and fever, even if well appearing, should be assumed to have an infectious process and to be at risk for systemic inflammatory response syndrome (SIRS) until proven otherwise and managed accordingly. Initial triage for afebrile patients includes evaluation for evidence of hemodynamic instability, related to associated hemorrhage and anemia, and neurologic changes concerning for intracranial hemorrhage. A localized bruising pattern is atypical for ITP should prompt consideration of nonaccidental injury.

Initial Assessment/H&P

The history of the present illness in suspected ITP should focus on any history of bleeding or bruising. Questions about nosebleeds or gingival bleeding with teeth brushing can be helpful. Less commonly, patients will report blood in urine or stool. Postmenarchal patients should be queried about menorrhagia. Evaluate any recent medication use that could affect platelet function. Review of systems should include evaluation for fever, fatigue, anorexia, weight loss, bone or joint pain, or other clues to an underlying systemic process. Although often limited in pediatric patients, a history of prior surgical procedures including circumcision, tonsillectomy and adenoidectomy, or dental procedures (extractions), are important to assess response to hemostatic challenges that may prompt suspicion of a congenital bleeding disorder. Family history should include questions regarding hematologic and immunologic processes. The physical examination should focus first on vital signs. In the hemodynamically stable patient, perform a thorough physical examination, with particular attention to evidence of mucosal bleeding (epistaxis, gingival bleeding, oropharyngeal hematomas, positive stool guaiac), tachycardia (a clue to possible underlying anemia), hepatosplenomegaly (may suggestive a consumptive process), lymphadenopathy (suggestive of an infectious or malignant process), and a dermatologic examination for evidence of petechiae, purpura, or ecchymoses. Children with ITP generally have a normal physical examination except for petechial rash, ecchymoses, and other signs of bleeding.

Management/Diagnostic Testing

Initial Evaluation and Diagnosis. The diagnosis of ITP should be considered in all patients with isolated thrombocytopenia with a platelet count less than 100,000 per µL. Initial lab tests include CBC, reticulocyte count, blood smear for review, type and screen for all patients. Direct antibody test (Coombs), coagulation panel, uric acid, blood cultures, and other tests should be performed based on clinical presentation. Atypical features should prompt consideration of other diagnoses and further evaluation.

The well-appearing child with a normal physical examination, isolated thrombocytopenia, characteristic findings on peripheral blood smear, an unremarkable personal and family history, and absence of history or examination findings suggestive of an alternate diagnosis may be diagnosed with ITP. Although some controversy exists, bone marrow biopsy and aspiration is generally unnecessary in children older than 12 months with a typical presentation. Any historical or physical examination features raising concern for an oncologic process should prompt bone marrow evaluation before the initiation treatment. If a patient with acute leukemia is mistakenly diagnosed as having ITP and treated with steroids, the correct diagnosis of leukemia may be delayed and long-term outcome could be adversely affected.

Treatment

Increasingly, the management of ITP is guided by bleeding symptoms rather than the platelet count. Management of an acute episode for a patient with persistent or chronic ITP should be based on past successful therapy and in conjunction with the primary hematologist. There is practice heterogeneity for when and how to treat pediatric patients with acute ITP. Here we provide an approach based on the recent American Society of Hematology guidelines. Many patients with acute ITP with absent or mild bleeding may be managed with observation. Indications for pharmacologic intervention include moderate bleeding symptoms (see Table 101.8), inability to keep patients safe from significant head trauma, or the need for surgery. Most, though not all, of these patients will have platelet counts below 30,000 per µL. For patients with moderate–severe bleeding symptoms, several initial medications and dosing regimens are cited in the literature. Table 101.9 presents a few examples of regimens used. IVIG and steroids are the two most common first-line treatments. Anti-D is relatively contraindicated if hematocrit is low due to bleeding or if there is evidence of autoimmune hemolysis, and now carries an FDA black box warning due to risk of severe hemolysis. For life-threatening bleeding, which is fortunately rare in this population, platelet transfusion and in some cases emergent splenectomy are required in addition to initiating pharmacotherapy.

TABLE 101.9

TREATMENT REGIMENS FOR ACUTE ITP

	Treatment		
	Corticosteroids	IVIG	Rh_o(D) immune globulin (WinRho)
Treatment regimen	Prednisone or prednisolone 2 mg/kg BID × 5 days OR 2 mg/kg/day × 10 days Max dose: 40 mg BID	1 g/kg IV × 1–2 doses	50 mcg/kg IV initial dose, subsequent doses based on response and hemoglobin level
Benefits	• Enteral • Outpatient therapy • Inexpensive	• Fastest rise of platelet count • Steroid sparing	• Short infusion time • Steroid sparing
Risks/side effects	• Emotional instability • Hyperphagia • Hyperactivity • If diagnosis incorrect potential to partially treat ALL	• Hypersensitivity reaction • Severe headache • Aseptic meningitis • Fever/chills • Immune mediated • Hemolysis • Long infusion time • Expensive	• Only for Rh+ patients • Black box warning: life-threatening acute/subacute immune-mediated intravascular hemolysis • Fever/chills

Avoid drugs that interfere with platelet function such as aspirin and NSAIDs, as well as activities that increase the risk of head injury.

Adjuvant therapies to control bleeding for the patient with ITP, as outlined in Table 101.2, may be of use until specific ITP treatments are effective. Nasal packing and topical phenylephrine are useful for persistent epistaxis. Excessive menstrual bleeding may require hormonal therapy. Antifibrinolytics such as aminocaproic acid may be useful in decreasing mucocutaneous bleeding. Intractable symptoms warrant hematology consultation for consideration of second-line or extraordinary measures.

Management of Head Trauma

Intracranial hemorrhage in the setting of ITP is rare, but it is also the major cause of mortality in ITP and therefore requires immediate recognition and intervention. Figure 101.4 provides an algorithm for managing head trauma in the setting of ITP. No universally accepted guideline for the evaluation and management of head trauma in ITP patients exists. Carefully consider each case and manage in conjunction with hematology.

Clinical Indications for Discharge or Admission

Many patients with ITP can be managed on an outpatient basis. Consider age, developmental level, parental comfort, and distance from the hospital when identifying patients who are safe for discharge with close outpatient follow-up.

OTHER DISORDERS ASSOCIATED WITH THROMBOCYTOPENIA

Neonatal Thrombocytopenia

Thrombocytopenia can arise in neonates from a number of different etiologies: immune mediated, perinatal asphyxia, inherited thrombocytopenias, drug/medication toxicity, and infection. Careful assessment of the clinical status of the neonate as well as the timing of the thrombocytopenia can help narrow the differential diagnosis. The two most common immune-mediated causes are neonatal alloimmune thrombocytopenia (NAIT) and autoimmune neonatal thrombocytopenia.

NAIT can emerge in an otherwise healthy neonate and can lead to significant morbidity and mortality if unrecognized. NAIT develops when a fetus expresses a paternally inherited antigen on its platelets that the mother does not. Maternal exposure to these fetal platelets generates an IgG antibody that can cross the placenta and cause destruction of fetal platelets and megakaryocytes. This can occur with a first pregnancy and often more severely with subsequent pregnancies. When recognized, it is an indication for future high-risk obstetrical care. Severe thrombocytopenia leads to increased risk of intracranial hemorrhage. Maintaining the platelet count greater than 30,000 per μL during the first week of life and greater than 20,000 per μL subsequently is appropriate in nonbleeding infants. Greater than 50,000 per μL is the goal in the setting of bleeding. Random donor platelet transfusion may be ineffective if those platelets carry the offending antigen, so monitor platelet counts after transfusion. If available, platelet products negative for the causative antigen or maternal platelets may be more effective. IVIG administration may also help to boost the platelet count. Consider corticosteroids for neonates who are refractory to therapy with bleeding symptoms.

Autoimmune neonatal thrombocytopenia can occur in infants whose mothers have primary ITP or ITP secondary to an autoimmune condition such as SLE. This condition tends to result in less severe thrombocytopenia compared to NAIT. Fortunately, significant bleeding episodes such as intracranial hemorrhage are rare. Monitor the platelet count and provide therapy for neonates with platelet counts less than 30 to 50 × 10^3 per μL. Survival of donor platelets (platelet transfusion) is

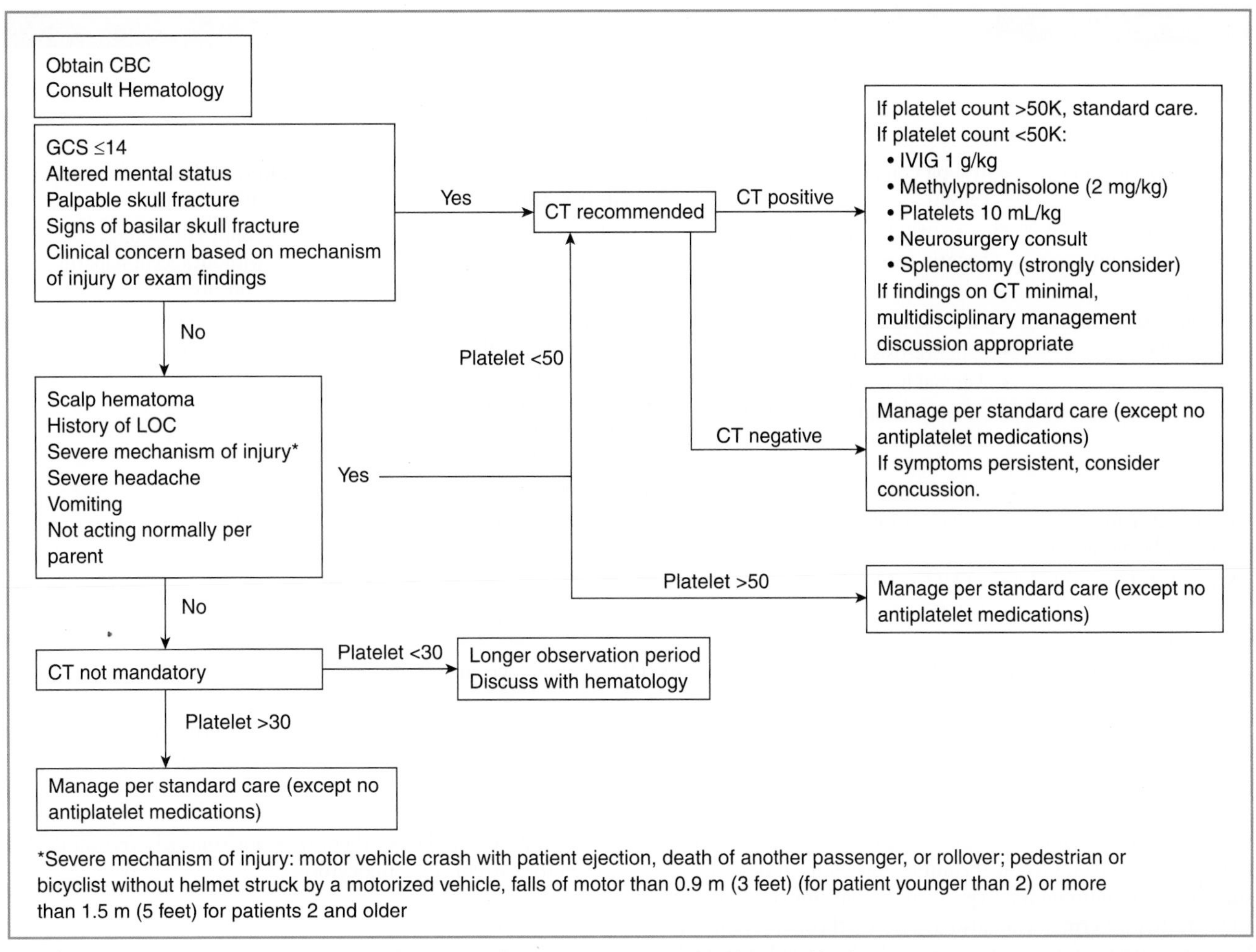

FIGURE 101.4 ITP with head trauma or concern for CNS bleed.

significantly shortened due to the presence of antibody. Treatment with IVIG improves the platelet count in most patients. Both NAIT and maternal autoantibody–mediated neonatal thrombocytopenia are self-limited as the maternal IgG antibody wanes over the course of weeks to months.

Heparin-induced Thrombocytopenia

Children treated with heparin are at risk for developing heparin-induced thrombocytopenia (HIT). The incidence has increased over recent years likely due to increased recognition of this entity in pediatric patients. In the right clinical context, HIT is an important diagnosis to consider because it is associated with an increased risk of thrombosis and can threaten life and limb if undiagnosed. The degree of thrombocytopenia, timing of the fall in platelet count relative to heparin exposure, presence of thrombosis, and other potential causes of thrombocytopenia are all important considerations when risk stratifying for the likelihood of HIT. Table 101.10 presents a scheme for estimating a patient's pretest probability of HIT.

Most commonly HIT develops due to formation of an IgG antibody that recognizes an antigen formed by the complex of heparin and platelet factor 4 (PF4), a protein secreted by activated platelets. The antibody mediates destruction of platelets resulting in thrombocytopenia. HIT more frequently develops in the setting of unfractionated heparin (UFH) use but can also emerge in patients receiving low–molecular-weight heparin (e.g., enoxaparin). The typical pattern for HIT is the downtrending of the patient's platelet count 5 to 10 days following the initiation of heparin therapy. The platelet count may fall to 50% of baseline values for the patient, but generally the nadir is mild to moderate with median counts reported in the 50 to 60 × 10^3 per μL range. If the patient has had a recent exposure to heparin and had circulating antibodies present at the time of heparin reinitiation, the platelet count may fall in the first 24 hours. If HIT is strongly suspected, discontinue heparin therapy immediately and use an alternate anticoagulant in consultation with a hematologist. Alternative treatment options include direct thrombin inhibitors such as argatroban and bivalirudin, but studies are currently limited in pediatric patients.

Nonimmune Thrombocytopenia

Nonimmune etiologies of thrombocytopenia are less common but important to consider particularly in mild to moderate thrombocytopenia. Platelet production can be affected by intrinsic defects or absence of megakaryocytes (platelet progenitors), suppression mediated by infection, medications, toxins, or marrow replacement by malignant cells such as leukemia or a metastatic solid tumor. Platelet destruction can

TABLE 101.10

4T's SCORE FOR HIT PRETEST PROBABILITY

	2	1	0
Thrombocytopenia	>50% plt count fall and nadir ≥20K cells/μL	30–50% plt count fall to nadir 10–19K cells/μL	<30% plt count fall or nadir ≤10K cells/μL
Timing of fall in platelet count	Onset 5–10 days or <1 day (if heparin exposure within 30 days)	>10 days or timing unclear or <1 day with recent heparin 31–100 days	Plt count fall <4 days (without recent heparin exposure)
Thrombosis or other sequelae	• New thrombosis • Skin necrosis at injection site • Adrenal hemorrhage • Anaphylactoid reaction to IV heparin bolus	• Progressive or recurrent thrombosis on therapeutic anticoagulation • Erythematous skin lesion at injection site • Suspected but not confirmed thrombosis	None
Other cause for thrombocytopenia	No other cause evident	Possible other cause evident	Probable/definite other cause present

Score 0–3: Low probability of HIT (<5%). Testing not advised.

Score 4–5: Intermediate probability of HIT (10–30%). Consider sending screening test (HIT antibody screen); discuss with hematology

Score 6–8: High probability of HIT (20–>80%). Send both tests (HIT antibody screen and the serotonin release assay).

Modified from Warkentin TE, Linkins LA. Nonnecrotizing heparin-induced skin lesions and the 4T's score. *J Thromb Haemost* 2010;8:1483–1485.

arise in the setting of microangiopathic coagulopathies such as DIC, TTP, or HUS. Occult thrombus, mechanical destruction such as cardiopulmonary bypass, and environmental stresses such as hypothermia can also result in thrombocytopenia. Platelet sequestration is most commonly due to splenomegaly. Pseudothrombocytopenia (laboratory artifact when platelets clump in a specimen) is also a consideration in an otherwise healthy individual with isolated and unexpected thrombocytopenia.

Severe thrombocytopenia in the setting of a nonimmune process puts a patient at greater risk of bleeding than ITP. Patients usually respond well to platelet transfusions. Transfusions should be reserved for severe or persistent bleeding or for significant trauma. Many affected patients have chronic disorders and require repeated transfusions. The excessive use of platelet transfusions, whether prepared from multiple, single, or HLA-matched donors, may contribute to the formation of antiplatelet antibodies. Such antibodies make subsequent transfusions challenging since platelets are often quickly destroyed by these alloantibodies leading to a minimal or short-lived increase in the platelet count. Use single-donor transfusions (apheresis units) and leukocyte-depleted blood products whenever possible for this patient population to decrease the risk of alloimmunization.

THROMBOCYTOSIS

Goals of Treatment

Treatment for thrombocytosis is typically unnecessary in the pediatric population. Unlike primary thrombocytosis, secondary or reactive thrombocytosis has not been associated with a significant increased risk of thrombotic or hemorrhagic complications and empiric antiplatelet therapy is not routinely recommended even for extreme thrombocytosis.

Clinical Considerations

Clinical Recognition

Thrombocytosis is defined as a platelet count greater than 450×10^3 per μL. Primary thrombocytosis is rare in the pediatric population. Hereditary or familial forms have been associated with mutations in genes that encode thrombopoietin and the thrombopoietin receptors, and transmit in an autosomal dominant fashion. Clonal forms of thrombocytosis result from myeloproliferative syndromes, though these are extremely rare in children. The pathophysiology and natural history of primary thrombocytosis has been predominantly explored in the adult population. Evidence of increased risk of thrombotic and hemorrhagic events has been reported in children but to a lesser degree than observed in adults. Risk assessment and stratification tools have not been validated in pediatrics. The degree of thrombocytosis can range from mild (>450×10^3 per μL) to extreme (>$1{,}500 \times 10^3$ per μL) regardless of a primary or secondary etiology. Secondary thrombocytosis is common and occurs in the setting of infection, inflammation, other physiologic stress (Table 101.11).

Clinical Assessment/Diagnostic Testing

Thrombocytosis is usually an incidental finding. Spurious causes of thrombocytosis such as cell fragments or microorganisms should be excluded by reviewing a peripheral blood smear. Initial evaluation should focus on identifying an inciting cause. In the absence of symptoms, laboratory evidence of acute inflammation such as C-reactive protein, von Willebrand

TABLE 101.11

ETIOLOGIES OF REACTIVE THROMBOCYTOSIS

Acute infectious disease
Chronic infection (tuberculosis, hepatitis, osteomyelitis)
Autoimmune/inflammatory disease
• Inflammatory bowel disease (IBD)
• Kawasaki disease
• Ankylosing spondylitis
• Rheumatoid arthritis
Medication effect
• Glucocorticoids
• Epinephrine
• Low-molecular-weight heparin
• Vincristine
Malignancy
Tissue damage
• Postprocedure
• Thermal burns
• Trauma
Asplenia or functional asplenia
Iron deficiency
Hemolytic anemia
Acute blood loss
Inflammation
Exercise
Rebound following thrombocytopenia

factor (vWF), fibrinogen, and proinflammatory cytokines (IL-6) may suggest an underlying inflammatory state. The presence of Howell–Jolly bodies on peripheral blood film may suggest an asplenic or functionally asplenic state.

Management

Patients with asymptomatic thrombocytosis do not require emergency medical therapy to lower their platelet count; however, they may require treatment directed at the underlying cause of their thrombocytosis. Patients should follow-up with their primary care provider to ensure platelet count normalization; the platelet count may remain elevated for weeks to months. Consultation with a pediatric hematologist is advised if thrombocytosis persists beyond this timeframe. The use of antiplatelet (aspirin) or cytoreductive agents (hydroxyurea, anagrelide) should only be started in consultation with a pediatric hematologist. Evidence for their use and the optimal agent for a given clinical situation are limited in children due to the rarity of this diagnosis. An individualized treatment plan for patients with additional thrombotic risk factors is appropriate.

DISORDERS OF HEMOSTASIS

Goals of Treatment

Achieving hemostasis in the setting of spontaneous or traumatic bleeding is paramount. Additionally, taking appropriate pre-emptive steps prior to procedural intervention for patients with ongoing or potential hemorrhage is critical.

CLINICAL PEARLS AND PITFALLS

- Factor replacement is the primary goal in any hemophilia patient with suspected or known bleeding.
- Measured levels of factor VIII and factor IX typically predict clinical severity; however, levels for other factor deficiencies including VII and XI do not reliably correlate with bleeding phenotype.

Current Evidence

The most common inherited bleeding disorders are vWD, factor VIII deficiency (hemophilia A), and factor IX deficiency (hemophilia B). These bleeding disorders are reviewed in more detail in the following sections. Other rare inherited disorders include isolated defects or deficiencies in specific factor proteins which contribute to the initiation of clot formation such as factor II, factor V, factor VII, factor X, factor XI, proteins responsible for clot stabilization such as factor XIII, and proteins which counter the fibrinolytic pathway such as plasminogen activator inhibitor type-1 (PAI-1). Each of these deficiencies has a clinically variable phenotype. This combined with their rarity has hindered the development of clinical practice guidelines for rare bleeding disorders. Once a diagnosis is made, therapeutic decisions must be tailored to the individual patient based on bleeding severity and location. Acquired defects of hemostasis are uncommon in the pediatric population, but consider these disorders in the setting of acute onset of an unexpected bleeding episode in the absence of any personal or family history of bleeding. Among the more common acquired causes are DIC, which can arise in the setting of sepsis or severe trauma, uremia and drug-induced platelet dysfunction, and decreased factor synthesis due to liver disease and cholestasis.

Clinical Considerations

Clinical Recognition

Severe congenital disorders of hemostasis typically present during infancy. Mild and moderate disorders may go undetected until later childhood or even adulthood when patients sustain a challenge that exceeds the capability of their hemostatic system, such as major surgery or trauma, invasive dental procedure or extraction, or menarche. Emergency physicians may encounter patients who are referred for an abnormal coagulation laboratory result obtained by a primary care physician, often because of an expressed concern for bleeding or easy bruising, or because of a family history of a bleeding disorder. Consider underlying coagulation disorders in patients who return with postoperative and traumatic bleeding that seems out of proportion to the clinical situation. Infants may present to the ED with prolonged bleeding from the site of circumcision or the umbilical stump. Older children may present with a pattern of mucosal bleeding including epistaxis or menorrhagia, or with deep muscle or joint bleeds, usually trauma associated.

Triage

If a child presents with active bleeding, initial assessment should focus on the site and severity of hemorrhage and prioritize therapeutic interventions to achieve hemostasis. Evidence of hemodynamic compromise should prompt rapid resuscitation efforts to reestablish circulating volume. Consider the need for prompt surgical involvement if clinically indicated.

Clinical Assessment

A detailed history of the patient's prior bleeding events and a thorough family history is necessary to determine the level of concern for an underlying bleeding disorder. Pertinent history includes:

- Are bleeding episodes related to mild–moderate trauma or procedures or do they occur spontaneously?
- Is the bleeding typically a mucocutaneous pattern (epistaxis, oral bleeding, petechiae, easy bruising, GI bleeding, or menorrhagia)?
- Is there bleeding into the deep muscles or joints?
- Is there a history of poor wound healing?
- Are bleeding episodes more likely to occur hours versus days after a procedure or injury?

Additionally, family history of responses to hemostatic challenges may suggest an inherited defect of hemostasis. Mucocutaneous bleeding is usually associated with defects of primary hemostasis such as platelet count (see section on thrombocytopenia above) or dysfunction, or vWD. Bleeding into deep muscles or joints, especially when spontaneous, is characteristic of hemophilia. Poor wound healing or delayed bleeding following a procedure has been described with factor XI, factor XIII, and PAI-1 deficiencies. A physical examination should focus on findings of active or recent bleeding including a careful HEENT and dermatologic examination.

Diagnostic Testing

The initial screening laboratories to investigate for hemostatic abnormalities should include: CBC, examination of the peripheral blood smear, prothrombin time (PT), and activated partial thromboplastin time (aPTT), thrombin time (TT), and fibrinogen. Save blood for additional assays of specific factors. An approach to initial interpretation of these tests is presented in Figure 101.5. The CBC reveals the platelet count, aids in recognition of associated anemia resulting from bleeding, and reveals white blood cell count abnormalities that may suggest underlying sepsis or malignancy. Review of a peripheral blood smear enables verification of the platelet count and also allows for visualization of platelet morphology, such as the presence of normal granulation necessary for platelet function. Other elements seen on the peripheral smear may also yield clues to the underlying diagnosis such as RBC fragments seen with microangiopathic coagulopathy or peripheral blasts suggestive of an underlying hematologic malignancy. The PT evaluates factors II, V, VII, X and fibrinogen, while aPTT evaluates factors II, V, VIII, IX, X, XI and fibrinogen. These initial tests can

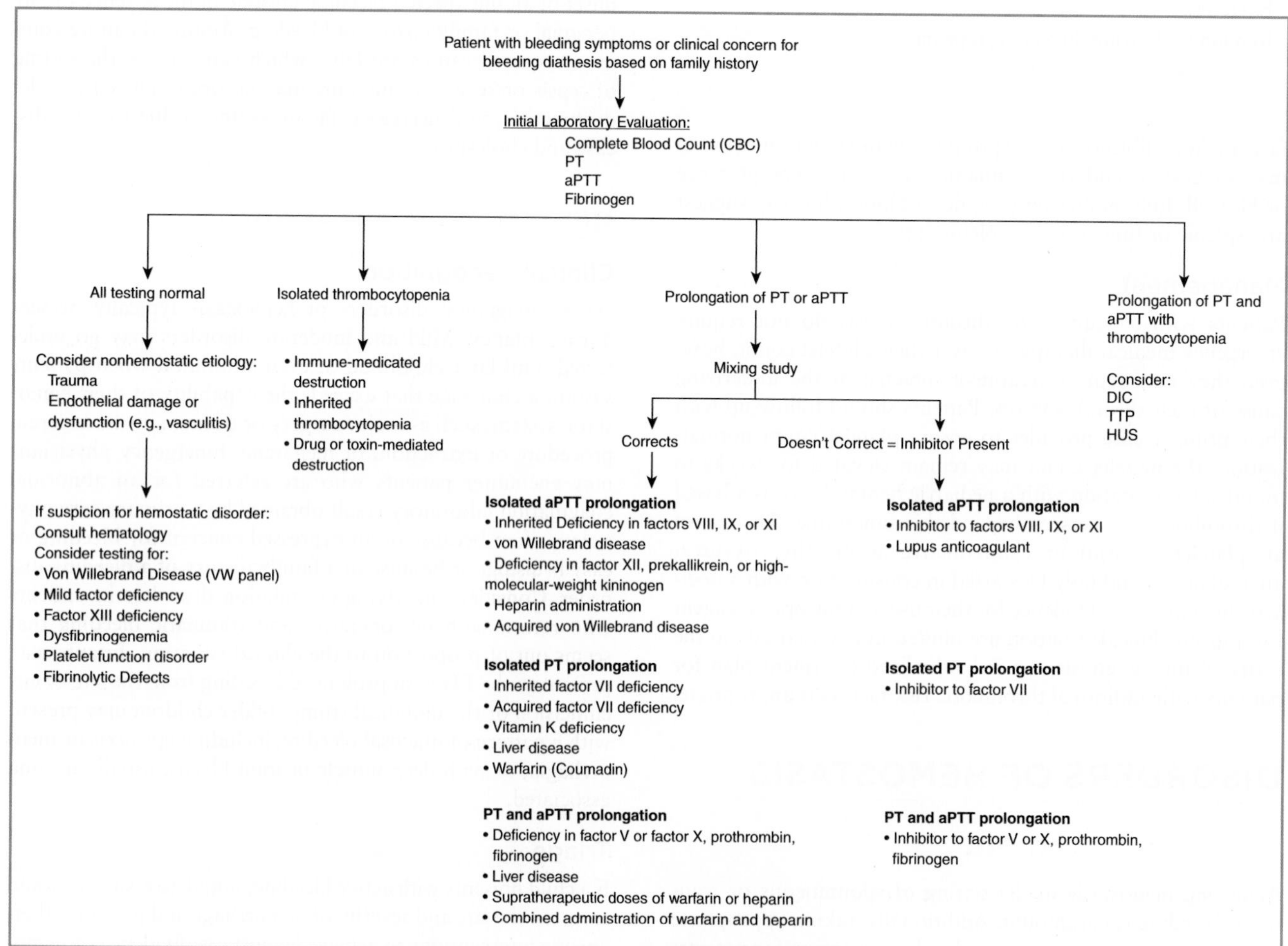

FIGURE 101.5 Approach to diagnosis of a bleeding disorder.

help emergency physicians narrow the differential diagnosis, but more extensive evaluation is usually needed to make a final diagnosis. Such tests may include a von Willebrand panel, assays for specific factor levels, inhibitor assays, platelet function (aggregometry) studies; these tests are almost never available in real time for clinical use in an emergency department. Fortunately, initial steps in management are not hindered by the lack of a precise diagnosis. It is important to note that proper collection of the blood sample for these specialized coagulation studies is paramount for accurate results. Samples that are drawn through heparinized indwelling catheters, over shaken, or not promptly processed often yield erroneous results.

Management

Establishment of a specific hemostatic disorder diagnosis should not take precedence over the timely management of a serious bleeding episode. Where applicable, use local measures such as pressure dressings and nasal packing, as well as other adjuncts such as estrogen in the case of menorrhagia. Agents useful for achieving hemostasis are reviewed in Table 101.2. Specific management strategies for treating vWD and Hemophilia A and B are detailed below.

Rare Inherited Coagulation Factor Deficiencies

There are no clinical practice guidelines for managing the rare, inherited coagulation factor deficiencies, in part because of small patient numbers and in part due to the clinical heterogeneity of these disorders. For patients with known deficiencies, implementation of their bleeding management plan or consultation with their hematologist is advised. For severe bleeding episodes, major trauma or an emergent operative procedure, replacement of the missing factor protein is generally advised. For factors VII and XIII, recombinant products are available; plasma-derived protein concentrates are also available for these factors and for factor XI. Cryoprecipitate contains concentrated quantities of factor XIII, fibrinogen, factor VIII, and vWF. Fresh-frozen plasma may be used for any factor deficiencies; however, large volumes of product are often required to achieve hemostatic levels. If patients have primarily mucosal bleeding, antifibrinolytic therapies may provide sufficient hemostasis.

Disseminated Intravascular Coagulopathy (DIC)

Treatment of the inciting disease process is critical. Therapy to correct the coagulopathy is appropriate in an actively bleeding patient; however, it provides only a temporary solution. Infusion of platelets, fresh-frozen plasma, and cryoprecipitate (Table 101.2) may be trialed to improve hemostasis; however, replacement therapy should not be continued without clinical benefit. The role of heparin therapy for DIC remains controversial and should only be initiated in consultation with a hematologist. The use of agents such as antithrombin, rFVIIa, and direct thrombin inhibitors has been reported in the adult literature, but there are presently no data to support their use in the pediatric population with DIC.

Other Acquired Disorders of Hemostasis

As discussed above, acquired disorders of hemostasis include liver disease, vitamin K deficiency, and development of inhibitors to vWF or other coagulation factor proteins, often in the setting of an autoimmune condition. Patients with chronic liver disease and vitamin K deficiency may benefit from vitamin K supplementation. When patients have bleeding, replacement of factor deficiencies and platelets, if low, may be useful. Patients with renal failure require optimal management of their uremia and may benefit from platelet transfusion, cryoprecipitate, and DDAVP in the right clinical setting. For patients who develop inhibitors to coagulation factors (acquired hemophilia), management is complex and should involve a hematologist.

Clinical Indications for Discharge or Admission

Patients with uncontrolled bleeding or with clinical concern for bleeding risk should be admitted for ongoing inpatient management and diagnostic evaluation if necessary. If a bleeding disorder is suspected on the basis of initial laboratories or patient or family history, but the child is not actively bleeding, additional evaluation may occur in the outpatient setting with a hematology consultation.

HEMOPHILIA

Goals of Treatment

Early identification of bleeding in hemophilia patients is crucial for treating life-threatening bleeds and preventing the long-term sequelae of recurrent joint bleeding.

CLINICAL PEARLS AND PITFALLS

- Drugs that interfere with platelet function (e.g., aspirin, NSAIDs) should not be given to patients with hemophilia.

Current Evidence

Hemophilia A (factor VIII deficiency) and Hemophilia B (factor IX deficiency) are X-linked disorders of hemostasis. Hemophilia A accounts for roughly 85% of cases (incidence ~1:5,000 males), and Hemophilia B for the remaining 15% (incidence ~1:30,000 males). The bleeding phenotype can usually be predicted from the level of factor coagulant activity. If factor activity is less than 1% (severe hemophilia), bleeding episodes can occur spontaneously. Patients with moderate hemophilia (factor level between 1% and <5%) and mild hemophilia (factor level between 5% and 50%) typically do not have spontaneous hemorrhage but may have severe bleeds related to trauma and procedures. Increasingly, children and young adults are started on prophylactic administration of factor replacement to reduce the frequency of spontaneous bleeding, with regular infusions scheduled to maintain through factor levels above 1% or as needed to support their baseline activity level.

Clinical Considerations

Clinical Recognition

The most common bleeding events for hemophilia patients include hemarthrosis (joint bleed), muscle bleed, and subcutaneous bleed. These episodes may be spontaneous or associated with trauma. Patients with hemophilia usually know when they have a spontaneous bleed prior to any clinical findings. Signs of early hemarthrosis include a sensation of bubbling or tingling within the joint, joint discomfort that may accompany mild edema, or slight reduction in range of motion. As an untreated or inadequately treated bleed progresses, swelling, erythema, warmth, difficulty bearing weight and limited range of motion will become evident. Bleeds within a muscle may present similarly, however, tenderness and edema will localize to a muscle. Ecchymosis may or may not be present. Distinguishing between hip hemorrhage and an iliopsoas bleed may be difficult but is clinically very important since retroperitoneal bleeds can become life-threatening. An iliopsoas bleed will produce severe pain with hip flexion and extension but minimal pain with hip rotation. Iliopsoas bleeds may cause compression of the lateral femoral nerve resulting in numbness. Hip bleeds, on the other hand, produce severe pain with hip rotation and mild pain with flexion or extension.

A patient's disease severity should also inform a clinician's level of clinical concern. For example, after mild head trauma, the patient with severe hemophilia is at greater risk of developing intracranial bleeding than the patient with mild hemophilia and must be evaluated and managed more aggressively. On the other hand, if a patient with mild hemophilia presents with extensive hemorrhage, there should be a heightened suspicion for significant trauma and possible associated injury to internal organs.

Neutralizing antibodies (inhibitors) against factors occur in 20% to 30% of children with factor VIII deficiency and 3% to 5% of patients with factor IX deficiency. Inhibitor development is influenced by the severity of hemophilia, age, genetics, number of prior factor infusions, and the pattern of exposure to factor replacement products. Inhibitors do not change the typical sites, or frequency or severity of bleeding, but they make timely and adequate control of bleeding more challenging. Inhibitors are measured in Bethesda units (BU) where one BU equals the amount of inhibitor in 1 mL of plasma that destroys 50% of factor VIII or IX. High-titer inhibitors are considered greater than 10 BU. Immune tolerance or desensitization protocols are available to attempt to eliminate the inhibitor. The recognition of a newly developed inhibitor occurs when response to previously effective therapy is insufficient or may be detected on routine outpatient monitoring. Patients with moderate hemophilia may have increased bleeding frequency and an inadequate response to treatment with an inhibitor. A real-time inhibitor level measurement will not be available during the initial management of an emergent bleed. When an inhibitor is suspected, measurement of aPTT or a mixing study may be supportive. In the presence of a high-titer inhibitor, a level of factor activity adequate to normalize the aPTT (20% to 40% factor VIII) is rarely achieved with standard doses of factor replacement and aPTT is not correctable mixing the patient's plasma with normal plasma.

Triage

Bleeding emergencies in hemophilia patients should be promptly identified and treated. Infusion of factor replacement prior to completing radiologic evaluation is appropriate to avoid unnecessary delays in the treatment. Life- and limb-threatening bleeds in hemophilia patients include intracranial hemorrhage, iliopsoas bleeds, gastrointestinal bleeds, and compartment syndrome. Additionally, children with hemophilia will present with the same surgical emergencies that affect children with normal hemostasis and will require prompt administration of factor. Early hematology consultation is warranted for any patient with hemophilia anticipated to need operative or procedural intervention.

Management/Diagnostic Testing

The primary treatment for hemophilia is infusion of factor VIII or factor IX concentrate. Factor concentrate is manufactured as a lyophilized (freeze-dried) powder from either recombinant-DNA derived factor protein or plasma-derived protein that has been treated to attenuate possible viral contaminants from donors. The management of the patients with hemophilia is dictated by type and severity of bleed (see Table 101.12). In general, goal hemostatic factor levels for mild–moderate bleeding are 35% to 50% and for severe/life-threatening bleeding or surgical procedures are 100%.

The aPTT may be normal when the factor VIII or IX level is as low as 20% to 30% depending on the assay method used. Measurement of the factor coagulant level is needed to assess the adequacy of response to treatment when levels above 30% are desired. Although the aPTT need not be measured after routine treatment of minor hemorrhages, it can be useful in demonstrating a response to factor replacement in the setting of major hemorrhage or prior to operative management. If a minor bleed fails to respond to conventional dosing, a pre- and posttreatment factor level should be measured to be certain that the desired level is being achieved. Consider the possibility of a newly developed inhibitor in this setting.

CNS Bleed/Head Injury. All major head injuries require evaluation by a physician and immediate treatment with a goal of correction to 100% factor activity level. For patients with minor trauma without any symptoms or external evidence of injury, or the child with mild hemophilia, replacement therapy may not be required. Any child with moderate or severe hemophilia needs careful attention to the type of trauma and bleeding history for the physician to decide whether to use replacement therapy.

A CT scan of the head is indicated for patients with hemophilia if there is any sign of trauma (hematoma), history of falling down stairs or from crib/changing table, hitting the head on a hard surface or corner, altered mental status, vomiting, or focal neurologic changes. There should be a low threshold to perform a CT scan on patients with prior history of head bleed even if the mechanism of injury seems minor. Children with seemingly insignificant trauma may develop the first obvious signs of intracranial bleeding several days later when concern has diminished. For patients with mild to moderate hemophilia, imaging is indicated for any clinical features concerning for neurologic injury such as lethargy, vomiting, or focal neurologic changes. For children with indeterminate presentations (e.g., mild mechanism of injury and normal neurologic examination), consideration of imaging versus observation is based on the severity of the hemophilia combined with usual management strategies for pediatric head trauma. If the trauma is mild (a light bump on the forehead), patients may be observed at home for the usual signs of intracranial hemorrhage or increased intracranial pressure. Ruling out intracranial hemorrhage does not exclude the possibility of a concussion. Persistent symptoms after an intracranial bleed has been excluded warrant follow-up with the patient's primary provider and specialists as indicated.

TABLE 101.12

TREATMENT GUIDANCE FOR BLEEDING IN HEMOPHILIA

Type of hemorrhage	Factor replacement guidance	Additional management
• Life-threatening hemorrhage • Severe head injury • CNS bleed or nerve compression • Major trauma • Throat/Neck swelling • Intra-abdominal/GI bleed	100% factor correction; may consider continuous factor infusion depending on injury (FVIII) or q12h dosing (FIX)	Appropriate intensive care Head imaging Additional imaging studies
Major bleed/procedure • Hemarthrosis • Iliopsoas or thigh bleed • Compartment syndrome (forearm/calf) • Periodontal surgery • Major surgery	50–100% initial factor correction and will likely need repeated doses	Rest, ice, compression, elevation No weight bearing Non-NSAID pain control Measurements may be helpful to check for enlargement
Minor bleed/procedure • Expanding SQ bleed • Muscle • Fracture • Tooth extraction/filling • Mild/moderate trauma • Sutures	25–50% factor correction, may need repeated doses Fractures require factor replacement at least until swelling subsides (at least 2 days and generally 5–7 days)	Rest, ice, compression, elevation No weight bearing Non-NSAID pain control Measurements may be helpful to check for enlargement
Minimal bleeding • Epistaxis • Subcutaneous bleed • Mouth/tongue laceration • Abrasions/lacerations (no sutures)	Factor replacement typically not needed	Hold pressure/cold compress. Consider antifibrinolytic agent Measurement of bruise may be helpful to check for enlargement
Hematuria (painless/nontraumatic)	Factor replacement only if fails all conservative measures	Increase fluid intake PO/IV Exclude infectious etiology Bed rest Steroids (0.5–1 mg/kg/day) × 3 days if persists after 24 hrs of increased hydration Antifibrinolytic medications contraindicated

Emergent or Major Surgery. The indications for surgery are similar to those for children without coagulation disorders, provided an appropriate correction of clotting abnormalities has been achieved. When the need for surgery has been definitively established, correction up to 100% should be given and the aPTT should be measured to ensure its normalization.

Throat or Neck Swelling. For bleeds of the neck muscles, careful evaluation of airway patency is essential. Pressure on the airway from a subcutaneous bleed of the neck may become life-threatening, requiring steps to ensure airway patency such as endotracheal intubation, in addition to correction of the factor level to 100%. Complete airway obstruction may also result from extensive bleeding in the tongue. Early anticipation of the need to secure the airway is essential in these presentations.

Compartment Syndrome. If there is concern for nerve compression or vascular insufficiency in a child with a muscle or soft tissue bleed immediate correction is important. Compartment syndrome is a limb-threatening event. Imaging of the affected area and consultation with orthopedics is necessary.

Iliopsoas or Thigh Hemorrhage. Retroperitoneal bleeds can be life-threatening and may present with lower abdominal pain. A mass is sometimes palpable deep in the pelvis, and sensation in the distribution of the femoral nerve may be diminished. Loss of the psoas shadow may be seen on an abdominal radiograph, and a hematoma may be demonstrated by ultrasonography. The hemoglobin level should be measured initially and, if bleeding persists, at regular intervals thereafter.

Hematuria. When the child with hemophilia develops hematuria or flank tenderness after trauma, a more aggressive approach to diagnosis and treatment is required. Perform ultrasonography, CT, MRI, or IV pyelography as soon as possible to look for subcapsular or intrarenal bleeding or an obstructive clot at the pelvic–ureteral junction. To prevent parenchymal damage and deterioration of renal function, administer replacement therapy to achieve a level of 70% to 100% immediately. Atraumatic, painless hematuria generally does not require replacement therapy.

Management of Patients with Inhibitors. The treatment of bleeding episodes in the child with hemophilia and antibodies against the missing or diminished factor is challenging and should be managed in conjunction with a hematologist. Options for treatment depend on the clinical scenario and inhibitor titer. Possible therapies include: massive doses (100 to 200 units per kg) or continuous infusion of factor product, aPCCs (activated prothrombin complex concentrates such as FEIBA ["Factor Eight Inhibitor Bypassing Agent"], or rFVIIa [NovoSeven]). Hemophilia B patients with inhibitors are at risk of severe allergic reaction/anaphylaxis when receiving factor; FEIBA is contraindicated in this setting because it contains factor IX. Factor IX inhibitor complexes can precipitate and eventually cause nephrotic syndrome. Exchange transfusion followed by infusion of factor IX concentrate may be useful if the hemorrhage is severe or life-threatening.

Clinical Indications for Discharge or Admission

Severe, life-threatening bleeding events require monitoring for CNS or airway complications. Hemarthrosis may require hospitalization for immobilization and elevation of limb, pain control, or serial examinations. Minor or moderate bleeds including some hemarthroses and superficial muscle bleeds can usually be managed on an outpatient basis.

VON WILLEBRAND DISEASE

CLINICAL PEARLS AND PITFALLS

- DDAVP is a good therapeutic option for patients with Type 1 disease who have previously demonstrated response to a DDAVP challenge.
- DDAVP is generally ineffective for those with Type 2 and Type 3 disease and can exacerbate symptoms in patients with Type 2B disease by accelerating platelet clearance.
- Patients with Type 3 vWD typically manifest a clinical phenotype similar to patients with severe hemophilia.

Current Evidence

vWD is the most common inherited bleeding disorder affecting about 1% of the population; however, only a small fraction of patients manifest bleeding symptoms. vWF plays a key role in coagulation by facilitating platelet aggregation and adhesion and serving as a carrier molecule for factor VIII. There are three main types of vWD: Type 1 is a deficiency of vWF, Type 2 subtypes are functional defects associated with vWF, and Type 3 is an absence of vWF. The vast majority of patients with vWD have Type 1, inherited in an autosomal dominant pattern with variable expressivity and penetrance.

Clinical Considerations

Clinical Recognition

The sites of bleeding in vWD (Types 1 and 2) resemble the mucocutaneous bleeding found in patients with platelet disorders such as bruising, epistaxis, oral bleeding, and menorrhagia. Joint and deep muscle bleeding is unusual except in cases of children affected by Type 3 vWD. Since the most common type of vWD is a dominant mutation, family history is often positive for bleeding symptoms, however, even within a family the degree of symptomatology can be variable. Type 3 vWD is rare and inherited in an autosomal recessive fashion; clinical symptoms resemble severe hemophilia.

Diagnostic Testing

Patients with vWD will typically have a normal initial coagulation screen, except for Type 3 patients who have a prolonged aPTT. The diagnosis of vWD requires a special coagulation study which examines vWF antigen level (vWF:Ag), its function, often ristocetin induced platelet agglutination (vWF:RCo), and factor VIII (FVIII:C), the protein that it carries in plasma. The normal level for each of these components is greater than 50%. The lower limit of normal and how to define vWD has been controversial, but it is presently generally accepted that levels <30% constitute vWD and levels between 30% and 50% are designated as "low von Willebrand." Part of the challenge arises because vWF level is influenced by blood type (e.g., lower with blood type O) and disease states such as acute illness and hypothyroidism. It can be elevated by estrogen levels and exercise. Some patients with low von Willebrand will manifest a bleeding phenotype and may require treatment for menorrhagia or prophylaxis prior to dental procedures while others will be asymptomatic despite hemostatic challenges. A diagnosis of a Type 2 subtype is often suggested by a ristocetin cofactor to antigen ratio of less than 0.6. Additional testing to evaluate von Willebrand multimers and ristocetin-induced platelet aggregation (RIPA) may be necessary to make a diagnosis but is outside of the scope of testing typically sent from the emergency department.

Management

Most patients with vWD only require episodic management at the time of a bleeding episode or planned procedure. For most mild bleeding events including epistaxis, gingival bleeding, or menorrhagia, antifibrinolytic therapy with aminocaproic acid or tranexamic acid is appropriate (see Table 101.2). Patients with menorrhagia may benefit from estrogen therapy. DDAVP (desmopressin) is another staple of therapy for patients with type 1 vWD who respond. DDAVP stimulates the secretion of vWF from endothelial cells and can transiently result in a sufficient increase to facilitate hemostasis and may be used for bleeding symptoms or prior to a procedure. Common side effects include facial flushing, tachycardia, and headache. Careful attention to fluid management is necessary to avoid severe hyponatremia. For children with vWD who do not respond to DDAVP, treatment with plasma-derived factor VIII concentrates containing vWF is indicated. Recombinant vWF products are not yet available in the United States but are available in other parts of the world. Dosing is based on the ristocetin cofactor activity. For minor bleeding episodes, raising the vWF:RCo level above 50% should provide adequate hemostasis. For more serious bleeding or for the prevention of surgical bleeding, an initial dose calculated to raise the vWF:RCo to 100%, followed by repeat dosing every 12 hours, is recommended.

HYPERCOAGULABILITY

Goals of Treatment

The primary goal of thrombus treatment is to halt progression of abnormal coagulation and to prevent or minimize morbidity due to restricted perfusion. In cases of inherited deficiencies of a natural anticoagulant such as protein C, protein S, or antithrombin protein, replacement with fresh-frozen plasma or protein-specific concentrate is needed to replete the missing protein prior to initiation of anticoagulation. Evaluation of an underlying thrombophilia (predisposition to abnormal clot formation) may be warranted for some patients; however, this investigation should not delay initial management. Except for the rare deficiencies of anticoagulant factors noted above, the underlying genetic risk factors do not alter the initial approach to anticoagulation.

CLINICAL PEARLS AND PITFALLS

- The most frequent risk factor for thrombosis in children is the presence of a central venous catheter.
- Levels of anticoagulant factors must be interpreted with care (and in consultation with hematology) as normal levels are age dependent and can be affected by acute thrombosis or use of warfarin.

Current Evidence

Recognition of thrombotic events in pediatric patients has increased over recent years due to increased awareness and expanded critical care capabilities. The majority of thrombotic events in children occur in the setting of identifiable, acquired risk factors: presence of a central venous catheter, medications (L-asparaginase, corticosteroids, estrogen-containing oral contraceptive pills), tumors, inflammatory conditions (inflammatory bowel disease, vasculitis, antiphospholipid syndrome, autoimmune disorders), prolonged immobilization, obesity, and anatomic variants (Paget–Schroetter syndrome, May–Thurner syndrome). Inherited risk factors play an important, but less common role in pediatric thrombosis. In decreasing order of frequency the following laboratory findings have been associated with an increased risk of thrombophilia: Factor V Leiden, prothrombin gene mutation G20210A, protein C deficiency, protein S deficiency, antithrombin deficiency.

These inherited (or *de novo*) mutations disrupt the normal balance of procoagulant and anticoagulant proteins in favor of thrombus formation. These mutations confer an increased risk of thrombosis in the heterozygous state but are even more severe in the homozygous state. Factor V Leiden results from a point mutation of the factor V gene that renders it resistant to activated protein C, and thus factor V remains active and drives thrombin formation. Likewise insufficient amounts of the natural anticoagulant factors (protein C, protein S, antithrombin) or excess prothrombin permit unchecked propagation of the coagulation cascade. Heterozygosity for Factor V Leiden is found in 3% to 6% of the Caucasian population in the United States, but it is rare in those of African or Asian descent. It carries a two- to sevenfold increased relative risk of venous thromboembolism compared with normal individuals, whereas the relative risk for homozygotes is 80-fold. Homozygous protein C deficiency may cause widespread thrombosis in the neonatal period leading to purpura fulminans (hemorrhagic skin necrosis) and cerebral thrombosis.

Clinical Considerations

Clinical Recognition

Thrombosis may manifest as deep venous thrombosis (DVT), pulmonary embolus (Chapter 107 Pulmonary Emergencies), stroke or sinus venous thrombosis (Chapter 126 ENT Emergencies). History should attempt to identify underlying risk factors. Carefully review the family history for the occurrence of venous thrombosis or pulmonary embolus, stroke, myocardial infarction, and recurrent miscarriages. Patients with homozygous protein C, protein S, or antithrombin typically have a severe clinical presentation in infancy with purpura fulminans. In the heterozygous state patients may present later in life with unprovoked thrombosis.

Management/Diagnostic Testing

Clinical features of purpura fulminans in an infant not explained by infection should prompt consideration for homozygous protein C, protein S, or antithrombin deficiency. Administer FFP (10 to 20 mL per kg q6 to 8 hours) to patients while awaiting the evaluation of these protein levels. As noted above, levels of these anticoagulants can be difficult to interpret in infancy and in the setting of acute thrombosis, so levels drawn from the patient's parents may be more informative. For other patients, initiation of treatment should be managed as described below and a workup for underlying risk factors, including protein levels, can be pursued at a later point. Consult hematology to tailor the evaluation based on the presentation, as well as personal and family thrombotic history. Prior to starting anticoagulation therapy, document the patient's platelet count, PT, aPTT, renal function, and hepatic function since these values may be affected by the anticoagulant.

For non–life- or limb-threatening thrombosis start therapeutic enoxaparin (LMWH) at a dose of 1 mg per kg SQ q12 hours (max initial dose 40 mg BID). The antifactor Xa assay is used to monitor treatment with LMWH, 4 hours after the second or third dose. In general, the therapeutic goal is an antifactor Xa level of 0.5 to 1 unit per mL. Infants up to 2 months of age need a higher starting dose of 1.5 to 2 mg per kg SQ q12 hours in order to reach the same goal anti-Xa level. For patients with complex medical issues, renal insufficiency or increased risk of bleeding, an individualized anticoagulation plan in consultation with hematology may be appropriate. Alternatively, IV UFH can be used. Treatment with UFH is usually initiated with a bolus injection of 50 to 75 units per kg followed by a constant infusion of 20 units/kg/hour for children older than 1 year and 28 units/kg/hour for neonates and infants. Adjust the UFH dose according to readily available nomograms (Table 101.13). Anticoagulation with LMWH is equal in safety and efficacy to UFH; however, a therapeutic level can often be more quickly achieved with LMWH. UFH has the advantage of a short half-life, so its effects are more easily reversible in the setting of a bleed or need for a procedure.

When venous or arterial thrombosis is extensive or occludes blood flow, threatening a patient's life or the integrity of a limb or vital organ, infusion of a thrombolytic agent can result in the dissolution of the thrombus and re-establishment

TABLE 101.13

SYSTEMIC HEPARIN ADMINISTRATION AND ADJUSTMENT

1. Loading dose: heparin 50–75 units/kg IV over 10 min
2. Initial maintenance dose: 20 units/kg/hr
3. Adjust heparin to maintain aPTT 55–85 sec as follows:

aPTT (seconds)	Bolus (Units/kg)	Hold (minutes)	Rate change (%)	Repeat aPTT
<50	50	0	+10%	4 hrs
50–59	0	0	+10%	4 hrs
60–85	0	0	0	Next day
86–95	0	0	–10%	4 hrs
96–120	0	30	–10%	4 hrs
>120	0	60	–15%	4 hrs

4. Obtain blood for aPTT 4 hrs after administration of the heparin loading dose and 4 hrs after every change in the infusion rate.
5. When aPTT values are therapeutic continue monitoring with daily CBC and aPTT.

Reproduced with permission from Andrew M, Marzinotto V, Massicotte P, et al. Heparin therapy in pediatric patients: a prospective cohort study. *Pediatr Res* 1994;35:78–83.

of blood flow. Thrombolytic agents such as tissue plasminogen activator (tPA), streptokinase, and urokinase have been used extensively in adult practice for decades, but tPA is the agent of choice in pediatric patients. For maximum effectiveness in the appropriate clinical setting, tPA is given as soon as possible after the symptoms begin and the extent of vascular occlusion is documented. Therapy can be administered systemically or directed to the distal end of the thrombosis by catheter placement. Most clinicians use 0.1 to 0.5 mg/kg/hour, but total dose and infusion duration are individualized. Unanswered questions regarding thrombolysis in children include whether concomitant heparin infusion is safe, how long therapy can be safely administered, and how to best evaluate the degree of thrombolysis. The thrombolytic state is monitored by increases in PT and aPTT, reduction in the fibrinogen concentration, and rise in the concentration of fibrin degradation products or D-dimer. The major risk of thrombolytic therapy is bleeding; therefore, thrombolysis is contraindicated in patients who have had recent abdominal or brain surgery.

Clinical Indications for Discharge or Admission

For patients with uncomplicated DVT, outpatient management is possible if the resources to teach the patient/family how to administer LMWH are available and short-interval follow-up with hematology is assured. For patients requiring UFH infusion or with PE or stroke, inpatient management is appropriate.

TRANSFUSION REACTIONS

Clinical Recognition

Reactions to transfused blood products may be acute (during or within 24 hours of transfusion) or delayed (days to weeks posttransfusion). The most feared, but fortunately now uncommon transfusion reaction, is an acute hemolytic transfusion reaction. This type of reaction occurs due to the presence of a complement-fixing RBC antibody that causes rapid and often severe intravascular hemolysis. The patient will have a newly positive DAT (Coombs). The uncommon occurrence of this problem is, in large part, a tribute to careful blood banking practices and close attention to the administration of the properly identified RBC product to the correct recipient thereby avoiding infusion of ABO incompatible red cells. The release of proinflammatory cytokines as a result of complement activation gives rise to the characteristic symptoms of apprehension, fever, chills, abdominal or flank pain, chest tightness, and hypotension as well as activation of the coagulation cascade potentially manifesting as DIC. Other potentially life-threatening transfusion reactions include: Transfusion-related acute lung injury (TRALI), transfusion-associated circulatory overload (TACO), anaphylactic transfusion reaction, and septic transfusion reaction (see Table 101.14). TRALI is defined as acute lung injury with hypoxemia (PaO_2/FiO_2 ≤300 or room air O_2 saturation <90%) that occurs within 6 hours of a transfusion in a patient without prior risk factors for acute lung injury. Respiratory symptoms can be severe and may progress to respiratory failure in some cases. While symptoms typically resolve within 48 to 72 hours, the associated mortality is about 10%. TACO should be considered prior to transfusion in patients at risk for circulatory volume overload such as patients with chronic anemia or those with compromised cardiac function. Delayed hemolytic transfusion reactions can occur days to weeks after a RBCs transfusion. These reactions may be due to formation of an antibody in response to a newly encountered RBC antigen or an amnestic response of an antibody that originally developed in response to a previous transfusion but was undetectable at the time of the most recent cross-match. The rate of RBC destruction is usually slower with a delayed hemolytic transfusion reaction than with an acute hemolytic reaction, so patients may have symptoms of anemia and hyperbilirubinemia, but not shock and renal insult.

Management

In the event of a suspected transfusion reaction, the transfusion should be stopped immediately. The blood bank should

TABLE 101.14

TRANSFUSION REACTIONS

Transfusion reaction	Signs and symptoms	Reaction mechanism	Evaluation	Management
Potentially life-threatening				
Acute Hemolytic	Fever, chills, rigors, hypotension, shock, dyspnea, DIC, hemoglobinemia, hemoglobinuria	Complement-fixing RBC antibody (e.g., ABO incompatibility)	• Blood samples for evaluation of DAT (Coombs), hemoglobin, free hemoglobin, BUN, Cr, coagulation panel • Blood samples (patient and transfused unit) to blood bank for repeat serologic testing • Urine sample to evaluate for hemoglobinuria	• Stop transfusion • Supportive care to manage cardiorespiratory distress and coagulopathy, if present
Anaphylactic	Fever, chills, dyspnea, wheeze, rash	Antibody to IgA, haptoglobin, or C4	• Evaluate patient for IgA deficiency	• Stop transfusion • Epinephrine • Corticosteriods • Diphenhydramine • Cardio-respiratory support
Transfusion associated acute lung injury (TRALI)	Fever, chills, respiratory distress, hypoxia, pulmonary edema, hypotension	Donor antibody to HLA or granulocyte-specific antigen	• Exclude acute hemolytic reaction and bacterial contamination • Test for HLA or granulocyte-specific antibody in donor plasma	• Supportive care
Transfusion associated circulatory overload (TACO)	Respiratory distress, headache, hypertension, pulmonary edema, congestive heart failure	Circulatory volume overload		• Stop transfusion • Supportive care • Diuretics
Septic	Fever, chills, rigors, shock	Bacterial contamination of transfused product	• Exclude acute hemolytic reaction and TRALI • Blood cultures	• Stop transfusion • Parenteral antibiotics
Not typically life-threatening				
Febrile Nonhemolytic	Fever, chills	Antibody to transfused platelets, plasma proteins, or passenger WBCs	• Exclude acute hemolytic reaction, bacterial contamination, and TRALI • Diagnosis of exclusion	• Stop/hold transfusion • Antipyretics
Allergic	Pruritus, urticaria, flushing	Antibody to plasma proteins		• Stop transfusion • Administer antihistamines • If reaction mild and resolves completely in 30 min, may restart transfusion
Delayed hemolytic	Fever, weakness, pallor, malaise	Primary immunization or anamnestic response	• Hemoglobin, DAT (Coombs), bilirubin, BUN, Cr, coagulation panel	• Supportive care

be alerted to the concern for a possible transfusion reaction. Supportive care to ensure adequate respiratory support and end-organ perfusion is essential. Evaluation and management considerations by reaction type are highlighted in Table 101.14. The name, identification number, and blood type of the patient should be compared with those on the unit of blood to ensure that the blood was given to the patient for whom it was intended. Laboratories to evaluate for hemolysis, coagulopathy, and renal function should be sent to exclude the possibility of a hemolytic reaction. Specifically, these include the following labs: hemolysis (DAT, indirect antiglobulin test, hemoglobin, plasma/free hemoglobin, bilirubin, LDH, evaluation for hemoglobinuria), renal function (BUN, creatinine), and coagulation (PT, aPTT, fibrinogen, platelet count). Additionally, an aliquot of the unit should be returned to the blood bank for confirmation of the original compatibility testing and labeling. For patients with severe acute hemolysis, aggressive fluid resuscitation, sometimes including diuretic therapy is needed to maintain urine output and minimize the toxic effects of free hemoglobin on the renal tubules. While nonhemolytic and febrile transfusion reactions are more common, they may be difficult to distinguish from the more dangerous hemolytic reaction prior to laboratory evaluation.

Suggested Readings and Key References

Anemia

Bansal D, Oberoi S, Marwaha RK, et al. Approach to a child with bleeding in the emergency room. *Indian J Pediatr* 2013;80:411–420.

Hayward CP, Moffat KA. Laboratory testing for bleeding disorders: strategic uses of high and low-yield tests. *Int J Lab Hematol* 2013; 35:322–333.

Jackson J, Carpenter S, Anderst J. Challenges in the evaluation for possible abuse: presentations of congenital bleeding disorders in childhood. *Child Abuse Negl* 2012;36:127–134.

Blood Loss

Carson JL, Grossman BJ, Kleinman S, et al.; Clinical Transfusion Medicine Committee of the AABB. Red blood cell transfusion: a clinical practice guideline from the AABB*. *Ann Intern Med* 2012; 157:49–58.

Janz TG, Johnson RL, Rubenstein SD. Anemia in the emergency department: evaluation and treatment. *Emerg Med Pract* 2013; 15:1–15; quiz 15–16.

Tyrrell CT, Bateman ST. Critically ill children: to transfuse or not to transfuse packed red blood cells, that is the question. *Pediatr Crit Care Med* 2012;13:204–209.

Villanueva C, Colomo A, Bosch A, et al. Transfusion strategies for acute upper gastrointestinal bleeding. *N Engl J Med* 2013;368: 11–21.

Hemolytic Anemia

Aladjidi N, Leverger G, Leblanc T, et al.; Centre de Reference National des Cytopenies Auto-immunes de, l'Enfant (CEREVANCE). New insights into childhood autoimmune hemolytic anemia: a French national observational study of 265 children. *Haematologica* 2011; 96:655–663.

Dhaliwal G, Cornett PA, Tierney LM Jr. Hemolytic anemia. *Am Fam Physician* 2004;69:2599–2606.

Petz LD. A physician's guide to transfusion in autoimmune haemolytic anaemia. *Br J Haematol* 2004;124:712–716.

Methemoglobinemia

Cortazzo JA, Lichtman AD. Methemoglobinemia: a review and recommendations for management. *J Cardiothorac Vasc Anesth* 2014; 28:1055–1059.

Wright RO, Lewander WJ, Woolf AD. Methemoglobinemia: etiology, pharmacology, and clinical management. *Ann Emerg Med* 1999; 34:646–656.

Sickle Cell Disease

Baskin MN, Goh XL, Heeney MM, et al. Bacteremia risk and outpatient management of febrile patients with sickle cell disease. *Pediatrics* 2013;131:1035–1041.

Field JJ, DeBaun MR. Asthma and sickle cell disease: two distinct diseases or part of the same process? *Hematology Am Soc Hematol Educ Program* 2009:45–53.

Ogunlesi F, Heeney MM, Koumbourlis AC. Systemic corticosteroids in acute chest syndrome: friend or foe? *Paediatr Respir Rev* 2014;15:24–27.

Quinn CT. Sickle cell disease in childhood: from newborn screening through transition to adult medical care. *Pediatr Clin North Am* 2013;60:1363–1381.

Rees DC, Williams TN, Gladwin MT. Sickle-cell disease. *Lancet* 2010; 376:2018–2031.

Venkataraman A, Adams RJ. Neurologic complications of sickle cell disease. *Handb Clin Neurol* 2014;120:1015–1025.

Neutropenia

Boxer LA, Newburger PE. A molecular classification of congenital neutropenia syndromes. *Pediatr Blood Cancer* 2007;49:609–614.

Dokal I, Vulliamy T. Inherited aplastic anaemias/bone marrow failure syndromes. *Blood Rev* 2008;22:141–153.

Newburger PE, Dale DC. Evaluation and management of patients with isolated neutropenia. *Semin Hematol* 2013;50:198–206.

Immune Thrombocytopenia

Buchanan GR, Adix L. Grading of hemorrhage in children with idiopathic thrombocytopenic purpura. *J Pediatr* 2002;141:683–688.

Labarque V, Van Geet C. Clinical practice: immune thrombocytopenia in paediatrics. *Eur J Pediatr* 2014;173:163–172.

Neunert CE, Buchanan GR, Imbach P, et al.; Intercontinental Childhood ITP Study Group Registry II Participants. Severe hemorrhage in children with newly diagnosed immune thrombocytopenic purpura. *Blood* 2008;112:4003–4008.

Neunert C, Lim W, Crowther M, et al.; American Society of Hematology. The American Society of Hematology 2011 evidence-based practice guideline for immune thrombocytopenia. *Blood* 2011;117: 4190–4207.

Other Disorders Associated With Thrombocytopenia

Balduini CL, Pecci A, Noris P. Diagnosis and management of inherited thrombocytopenias. *Semin Thromb Hemost* 2013;39:161–171.

Bertrand G, Kaplan C. How do we treat fetal and neonatal alloimmune thrombocytopenia? *Transfusion* 2014;54:1698–1703.

Warkentin TE, Linkins LA. Non-necrotizing heparin-induced skin lesions and the 4T's score. *J Thromb Haemost* 2010;8:1483–1485.

Thrombocytosis

Bleeker JS, Hogan WJ. Thrombocytosis: diagnostic evaluation, thrombotic risk stratification, and risk-based management strategies. *Thrombosis* 2011:1–16.

Fu R, Zhang L, Yang R. Paediatric essential thrombocythaemia: clinical and molecular features, diagnosis and treatment. *Br J Haematol* 2013;163:295–302.

Schafer AI. Thrombocytosis and thrombocythemia. *Blood Rev* 2001; 15:159–166.

Teofili L, Larocca LM. Advances in understanding the pathogenesis of familial thrombocythaemia. *Br J Haematol* 2011;152:701–712.

Disorders of Hemostasis

Chitlur M. Challenges in the laboratory analyses of bleeding disorders. *Thromb Res* 2012;130:1–6.

Lee LK, Dayan PS, Gerardi MJ, et al.; Traumatic Brain Injury Study Group for the Pediatric Emergency Care Applied Research Network (PECARN). Intracranial hemorrhage after blunt head trauma in children with bleeding disorders. *J Pediatr* 2011;158:1003–1008.e1–e2.

Nichols WL, Hultin MB, James AH, et al. von Willebrand disease (VWD): evidence-based diagnosis and management guidelines, the National Heart, Lung, and Blood Institute (NHLBI) Expert Panel report (USA). *Haemophilia* 2008;14:171–232.

Sarnaik A, Kamat D, Kannikeswaran N. Diagnosis and management of bleeding disorder in a child. *Clin Pediatr (Phila)* 2010;49:422–431.

Singleton T, Kruse-Jarres R, Leissinger C. Emergency department care for patients with hemophilia and von Willebrand disease. *J Emerg Med* 2010;39:158–165.

Hypercoaguability

Andrew M, Marzinotto V, Massicotte P, et al. Heparin therapy in pediatric patients: a prospective cohort study. *Pediatr Res* 1994;35:78–83.

Kenet G, Nowak-Gottl U. Venous thromboembolism in neonates and children. *Best Pract Res Clin Haematol* 2012;25:333–344.

Monagle P, Chan AK, Goldenberg NA, et al.; American College of Chest Physicians. Antithrombotic therapy in neonates and children: Antithrombotic Therapy and Prevention of Thrombosis, 9th ed: American College of Chest Physicians Evidence-Based Clinical Practice Guidelines. *Chest* 2012;141:e737S–e801S.

Raffini L. Thrombophilia in children: who to test, how, when, and why? *Hematology Am Soc Hematol Educ Program* 2008;228–235.

Roach ES, Golomb MR, Adams R, et al.; American Heart Association Stroke Council, Council on Cardiovascular Disease in the Young. Management of stroke in infants and children: a scientific statement from a Special Writing Group of the American Heart Association Stroke Council and the Council on Cardiovascular Disease in the Young. *Stroke* 2008;39:2644–2691.

Yang JY, Chan AK. Pediatric thrombophilia. *Pediatr Clin North Am* 2013;60:1443–1462.

Transfusion Reactions

Osterman JL, Arora S. Blood product transfusions and reactions. *Emerg Med Clin North Am* 2014;32:727–738.

CHAPTER 102 ■ INFECTIOUS DISEASE EMERGENCIES

NICOLAUS W.S. GLOMB, MD, MPH AND ANDREA T. CRUZ, MD, MPH

GOALS OF EMERGENCY CARE

Fever is one of the most common presenting complaints for children seen in the emergency department (ED). ED physicians face the challenge of differentiating potentially life-, limb-, or sensory-threatening causes of infection from the vast majority of children with febrile illnesses that will spontaneously resolve without intervention. For infectious disease (ID) emergencies, the clinical evaluation should focus upon prompt recognition of potentially serious conditions. Evidence-based diagnostic strategies can facilitate care and avoid unnecessary evaluations of otherwise well-appearing children.

RELATED CHAPTERS

Signs and Symptoms
- Diarrhea: Chapter 18
- Fever: Chapter 26
- Lymphadenopathy: Chapter 42
- Neck Mass: Chapter 43
- Oral Lesions: Chapter 47
- Septic Appearing Infant: Chapter 68
- Sore Throat: Chapter 69
- Tachycardia: Chapter 72

Clinical Pathways
- Fever in Infants: Chapter 87
- Fever in Children: Chapter 88
- Pneumonia, Community-Acquired: Chapter 90
- Shock: Chapter 91
- UTI, Febrile: Chapter 92

Medical, Surgical, and Trauma Emergencies
- Cardiac Emergencies: Chapter 94
- Gastrointestinal Emergencies: Chapter 99
- Gynecology Emergencies: Chapter 100
- Oncologic Emergencies: Chapter 106

BACTEREMIA AND SEPSIS

CLINICAL PEARLS AND PITFALLS

- It can be difficult to differentiate among children with uncomplicated viral infections and occult bacteremia.
- With reduction in vaccine-preventable diseases, most positive blood cultures are false positive with contaminants.
- Evidence-based guidelines can optimize management in the young febrile child.

Current Evidence

The epidemiology of pediatric bacteremia has changed dramatically over the last three decades due to widespread use of the pneumococcal conjugate and *Haemophilus influenzae* type B (Hib) vaccines. The most common isolates now causing bacteremia are listed in Table 102.1. While rates of pneumococcal bacteremia have declined in the postpneumococcal conjugate vaccine era, *Streptococcus pneumoniae* still comprises most cases of bacteremia, along with *Staphylococcus aureus, Salmonella,* group A streptococcus (GAS), and meningococcus; group B streptococcus (GBS) and Gram-negative rods remain the most common causes of bacteremia and sepsis in neonates and young infants. In some studies, contaminants are up to sevenfold more common than true pathogens. As a consequence, use of evidence-based algorithms in the approach to the febrile child (Chapters 87 Fever in Infants and 88 Fever in Children) can reduce unnecessary evaluation and optimize treatment of the non–toxic-appearing child.

Goals of Treatment

The goals of treatment are to recognize which children may be at higher risk for bacteremia than the general pediatric population (e.g., asplenic children, children with central venous catheters [CVC], neutropenic children) and to be cognizant of the most common organisms causing bacteremia seen in a given region. Thus, knowledge of local antibiotic resistance patterns is critical for the ED physician.

Clinical Considerations

Clinical recognition: Children at highest risk for bacteremia are under 2 years of age. For meningococcus, biphasic peaks occur: one during infancy and a second during adolescence. Thus, algorithms for fever management focus heavily upon young children due to higher incidence at this age and because the signs of occult bacteremia are difficult to discern. In many tertiary care centers, the children at highest risk for bacteremia and sepsis are children with indwelling CVC, neutropenia, or short gut. These children may have baseline tachycardia from anemia, making triage recognition more problematic.

Triage considerations: Recognition of abnormal vital signs (e.g., tachycardia, hypothermia) and signs of poor perfusion are critical for rapid initiation of resuscitation in the ED. Given the variation in normal vital sign ranges through the pediatric age spectrum, recognition can be facilitated if alerts are built into electronic health records.

Clinical assessment: Several studies have attempted to stratify the risk of bacteremia and other serious bacterial infections in febrile children. Table 102.2 describes clinical and laboratory predictors of occult bacteremia in young children.

TABLE 102.1

MOST COMMON CAUSES OF PEDIATRIC OCCULT BACTEREMIA IN THE POSTPNEUMOCOCCAL CONJUGATE VACCINE ERA

				Pathogen (% of total isolates)					
Authors	Year[a]	Age	# of positive cultures	*S. pneumoniae* (%)	*E. coli* species (%)	Group B streptococcus (%)	*S. aureus* (%)	Other (%)	Contaminant: pathogen ratio
Benito-Fernández, et al.	2010	3–36 mo	22/3088 (0.7%)	82	0	0	0	18	N/A
Laupland, et al.[b]	2009	<18 yrs	N/A	47	18	0.4	26	9	N/A
Rudinsky, et al.	2009	<24 mo	5/690 (0.7%)	20	20	20	0	40	6.8:1
Wilkinson, et al.	2009	3–36 mo	26/8408 (0.3%)	65	8	0	0	27	6.1:1
Carstairs, et al.	2007	<36 mo	15/1428 (1.1%)	87[c]	0	0	0	13	2.9:1
Sard, et al.	2006	1–36 mo	21/2971 (0.7%)	62	5	19	0	14	4:1
Stoll, et al.	2004	2–36 mo	3/329 (1%)	100	0	0	0	0	1.3:1

[a]Year of publication.
[b]Reported bacteremia that was considered community acquired; data from administrative database, and clinical variables could not be assessed. As such, all bacteremia reported may not have been "occult."
[c]All in unimmunized children.

TABLE 102.2

CLINICAL AND LABORATORY PREDICTORS OF SERIOUS BACTERIAL INFECTION

Predictor	Author	Year[a]	Age range	Finding
Fever duration	Bressan, et al.	2010	<1 mo	ANC and CRP were more predictive of SBI in children febrile for at least 12 hrs; both performed better than WBC in predicting SBI
Fever magnitude	Trautner, et al.	2006	<18 yrs	In children with fever ≥106°F, approximately 20% each had SBI and documented viral infections
	Stanley, et al.	2005	<3 mo	In infants with fever ≥104°F, one-third had SBI
WBC	De, et al.	2014	<5 yrs	WBC had a sensitivity of 47% and specificity of 76% for SBI
	Brauner, et al.	2010	3–36 mo	39% with extreme leukocytosis had SBI, primarily pneumonia
	Shah, et al.	2005	2–24 mo	Extreme leukocytosis (WBC ≥25,000/mm) had rates of bacteremia similar to those with WBC 15,000–24,999/mm)
	Lee, et al.	2001	3–36 mo	Cost-effectiveness analysis indicated that blood cultures should only be sent if WBC ≥15,000/mm in the post-PCV era
	Jaffe and Fleisher	1991	3–36 mo	WBC (>10,000/mm) performed better than temperature as an indicator of bacteremia (sensitivity 92%; false-positive rate 57%)
ANC	De, et al.	2014	<5 yrs	ANC had a sensitivity of 41% and specificity of 78% for SBI
Bandemia	Kuppermann and Walton	1999	0–24 mo	Absolute band count or band: neutrophil ratio did not help identify SBI after adjusting for age, temperature, clinical appearance, and ANC
CRP or procalcitonin	Mahajan, et al.	2014	0–36 mo	Procalcitonin was more sensitive for SBI than traditional screening tests
	Yo, et al.	2012	7 days–3 yrs	Meta-analysis showed procalcitonin was more sensitive for SBI (83%) than WBC (58%) or CRP (74%)
	Andreola, et al.	2007	7 days–36 mo	PCT and CRP are more accurate markers of SBI than WBC and ANC
	Pulliam, et al.	2001	1–36 mo	CRP is a better predictor of bacteremia and SBI than the WBC or ANC

[a]Year of publication; classic articles on SBI were included, but articles published in the post-PCV era were emphasized.
ANC, absolute neutrophil count; CRP, C-reactive protein; SBI, serious bacterial infection; WBC, white blood count; PCV, pneumococcal conjugate vaccine.

Management: Empiric antibiotic management depends upon knowledge of the most common causes of bacteremia in a community. While there has been a decline in pneumococcal isolates causing occult bacteremia, there have been increases in the rates of penicillin- and cephalosporin-resistant pneumococcal isolates. As such, if there is concern for invasive pneumococcal disease, initiating treatment with vancomycin and a third-generation cephalosporin (cefotaxime or ceftriaxone) would be appropriate. In the event that the isolate is cephalosporin susceptible, a cephalosporin would be a much more effective bactericidal drug than vancomycin. However, if resistance to a cephalosporin is present, then the child is receiving a drug to which the isolate retains susceptibility. This regimen would also provide coverage for the most common other causes of bacteremia and sepsis in immunocompetent children outside the neonatal period. If staphylococcal disease is suspected, children could receive nafcillin as well; in the event that they have methicillin-susceptible *S. aureus* (MSSA), nafcillin is far more bactericidal than vancomycin. In immunocompromised hosts, the causes of bacteremia are more diverse, and antipseudomonal coverage should be considered *a priori.* In addition, these children may also be at higher risk for antibiotic-resistant organisms from prior antibiotic exposure(s). Reviewing prior culture data to evaluate for a history of infection with drug-resistant organisms can help optimize ED-based management. Empiric coverage with vancomycin and an antipseudomonal beta-lactam (e.g., ceftazidime, piperacillin/tazobactam, or ticarcillin/clavulanate) may be considered.

OTHER SYSTEMIC INFECTIOUS EMERGENCIES

Goals of Treatment

The goals of treatment are to rapidly identify children at risk for some less common pathogens that can result in fulminant infection and to plan an empiric treatment course while awaiting diagnostic testing.

CLINICAL PEARLS AND PITFALLS

- If rickettsial disease is suspected based upon epidemiologic risk factors and clinical presentation, doxycycline should be started immediately.
- Doxycycline is the treatment of choice for the most deadly rickettsial disease in the United States, Rocky Mountain spotted fever (RMSF); this is true for all age groups.
- The "classic" triad for RMSF of fever, headache, and a rash is present in approximately 60% of cases.
- Babesiosis presents with symptoms similar to malaria, but in a child who lacks a travel history to a malaria-endemic region.
- Asplenic patients are at highest risk for babesiosis complications.

Toxic Shock Syndrome

Toxic shock syndrome (TSS) is characterized by severe, prolonged shock and is caused by toxins produced by *S. aureus* or GAS. TSS presents with the sudden onset of high fever, vomiting, and watery diarrhea. Pharyngitis, headache, and myalgias may also occur, and oliguria rapidly develops. Within 48 hours, the disease progresses to hypotensive shock. The patient has a fever, usually 39° to 41°C (102.2° to 105.8°F); a diffuse, erythematous maculopapular rash; and hyperemia of the mucous membranes. In almost one-half of cases of streptococcal TSS, no portal of entry is identified, or only minor, nonpenetrating skin trauma is identified in retrospect. The Centers for Disease Control and Prevention (CDC) definitions of TSS are described in e-Table 102.1. Laboratory findings include leukocytosis with a left shift, thrombocytopenia, transaminitis, elevated creatinine, elevated creatinine kinase, myoglobinuria, and coagulopathy. Complications can include acute respiratory distress syndrome (seen in over one-half of patients), acute kidney injury occurs in almost all children (creatinine elevation precedes hypotension), and disseminated intravascular coagulation. The initial diagnosis is clinical. The following laboratory tests should be obtained from all children suspected of having TSS: CBC, platelet count, PT, PTT, D-dimer, electrolytes, blood urea nitrogen (BUN), creatinine, AST, alanine aminotransferase (ALT), and creatinine kinase. Cultures of the blood, urine, stool, throat, and vagina serve to isolate *S. aureus* and to rule out other infectious causes of shock. A lumbar puncture (LP) is often required to exclude bacterial meningitis. The management of TSS is the same as that for shock caused by other organisms (see Chapter 91 Shock). Broad-spectrum antibiotics (vancomycin and ceftriaxone) are indicated for patients who are hemodynamically unstable, while those who are less ill may have treatment limited to an antistaphylococcal agent. Many authorities recommend the addition of clindamycin, which inhibits the toxin.

Rickettsial Diseases

The most severe endemic rickettsial disease in the United States is RMSF, caused by *Rickettsia rickettsii.* Transmitted by dog and wood ticks, RMSF is found in the southeastern United States and most cases present during the spring and summer months. Fever, headache, and a rash are considered the characteristic triad of RMSF, but are found in only 60% of cases. The rash begins as a maculopapular rash on the wrist and ankles and progresses centrally, later becoming petechial. Laboratory findings include thrombocytopenia, hyponatremia, and transaminitis. Multisystem involvement is seen with this systemic vasculitic condition, and the high mortality rate (up to 80% in untreated patients) usually is attributable to disseminated intravascular coagulation and shock. As a consequence, treatment with doxycycline should begin immediately if RMSF is suspected, without awaiting confirmatory diagnostics (acute and convalescent serologies). Doxycycline use has been shown to decrease morbidity and mortality over the second-line drug, chloramphenicol, and doxycycline also treats ehrlichiosis, which can present with symptoms similar to RMSF. Doxycycline is the preferred treatment for RMSF in children of all ages, unless a child has a severe doxycycline allergy.

Babesiosis

Babesiosis is caused by *Babesia microti,* an intraerythrocytic parasite whose symptoms mimic those of malaria in persons who lack a travel history to a malarial-endemic region. Babesiosis is seen in the northeastern and upper Midwestern United States; it is transmitted by the same *Ixodes* ticks that transmit Lyme disease and has also been transmitted via blood transfusion. Symptoms include fever and influenza-like illness; signs can be minimal, but in more severe cases, tachypnea, hypotension, icterus, and mild hepatosplenomegaly can be seen. Disease can be severe in asplenic patients, who have very high parasite burdens. The diagnosis is made by thick and thin blood smears demonstrating the organism's classic Maltese cross form within erythrocytes. Treatment is clindamycin and quinine for 7 to 10 days. Exchange transfusion may be needed for patients with parasitemia above 10%.

CNS INFECTIOUS EMERGENCIES

Meningitis, Bacterial

CLINICAL PEARLS AND PITFALLS

- The most common causes of meningitis in the first month of life are GBS and Gram-negative rods; beyond the first month of life, the most common etiologies are pneumococcus and meningococcus.
- The "classic" signs and symptoms of meningitis, including nuchal rigidity, are insensitive in infancy.
- The Gram stain of the cerebrospinal fluid (CSF) should be used to broaden, but not to narrow, empiric antibiotic selection.
- Empiric antibiotic therapy should comprise bactericidal agents that cross the blood–brain barrier. For neonates, ampicillin and either cefotaxime or ceftriaxone can be used. For infants and older children, vancomycin (for enhanced pneumococcal coverage) and either cefotaxime or ceftriaxone (for meningococcal coverage) should be utilized.
- In neonates and young infants with a CSF pleocytosis, addition of acyclovir (20 mg/kg every 8 hours) is reasonable until herpes simplex virus (HSV) is excluded.

Current Evidence

The most common causes of bacterial meningitis by age are listed in Table 102.3. In the first month of life, *Escherichia coli* and GBS are usually isolated; *Listeria monocytogenes,* a Gram-positive rod, accounts for 1% to 3% of the cases. Between 30 and 60 days of age, GBS continues to be recovered frequently, followed by *S. pneumoniae* and *Neisseria meningitidis;* Hib occurs rarely. After the first 2 months of life, *S. pneumoniae* and *N. meningitidis* cause the majority of meningeal infections; *Haemophilus influenzae* remains a consideration primarily among children not immunized with conjugated Hib vaccine. *Salmonella,* an uncommon etiologic agent in the United States, should be suspected in the first few months of life if meningitis occurs in association with gastroenteritis. The incidence of acute bacterial meningitis has declined in the last three decades due to widespread use of the Hib and polyvalent pneumococcal conjugate vaccines.

Goals of Treatment

The goal of treatment is the rapid recognition and treatment of bacterial meningitis to decrease a child's risk of neurologic sequelae. The clinical team should consider neuroimaging prior to LP in the immunocompromised child or the child with focal neurologic deficits. Clinical outcomes include time to appropriate parenteral antibiotics, CSF sterility at 24 to 48 hours, and neurologic outcome.

TABLE 102.3

ETIOLOGIES OF ACUTE BACTERIAL MENINGITIS CHILDREN OUTSIDE THE NEONATAL PERIOD

	Age			
Pathogen	**30–90 days (%)**	**3 mo–<3 yrs (%)**	**3–<10 yrs (%)**	**10–18 yrs (%)**
S. pneumoniae	14	45	47	21
N. meningitidis	12	34	32	55
Group B *Streptococcus*	39	11	5	8
Gram-negative rods	32	9	3	8
Other bacteria	3	1	13	8

From Nigrovic, Kuppermann M, Malley R; Bacterial Meningitis Study Group of the Pediatric Emergency Medicine Collaborative Research Committee of the American Academy of Pediatrics. Children with bacterial meningitis presenting to the emergency department during the pneumococcal conjugate vaccine era. *Acad Emerg Med* 2008;15:522–528.

Clinical Considerations

Clinical recognition: The most common signs and symptoms of bacterial meningitis are listed in Table 102.4. Before 2 to 3 months of age, the history is usually that of irritability, an altered sleep pattern, vomiting, and decreased oral intake. In particular, paradoxical irritability points to the diagnosis of meningitis. Irritability in the infant without inflammation of the meninges is generally alleviated by maternal fondling; however, in the child with meningitis, any handling, even directed toward soothing the infant, may increase irritability by its effect on the inflamed meninges. The amount of time spent sleeping may either increase because of obtundation or decrease from irritability. Bulging of the fontanelle, an almost certain sign of meningitis in the febrile, ill-appearing infant, is a late finding. Vomiting is a sensitive but nonspecific feature of infantile meningitis.

TABLE 102.4

SIGNS AND SYMPTOMS OF MENINGITIS

		Signs	
Age	**Symptoms**	**Early**	**Late**
0–3 mo	Paradoxical irritability	Lethargy	Bulging fontanelle
	Alerted sleep pattern	Irritability	Shock
	Vomiting	Fever	
	Lethargy	Hypothermia (<1 mo)	
4–24 mo	Irritability	Fever	Nuchal rigidity
	Altered sleep pattern	Irritability	Coma
	Lethargy		Shock
>2 yrs	Headache	Fever	Coma
	Neck pain	Nuchal rigidity	Shock
	Lethargy	Irritability	

As the child ages past 3 months, the symptoms gradually become more specific for involvement of the central nervous system (CNS). A change in the level of activity is almost always noticeable. However, it is only in the child older than 2 years that meningitis manifests reliably with complaints of headache, neck stiffness, and photophobia.

The physical examination in the young infant rarely provides specific corroboration, even when the history suggests meningitis. Fever may be absent in these children, despite the presence of bacterial infection. Any child younger than 2 to 3 months who is brought to the ED with a documented temperature of ≥100.4°F should be considered at risk for meningitis. The physical signs are sufficiently elusive that many experts caution that one should not rely exclusively on the examination to rule out meningeal infection. In several studies, 5% to 10% of these young infants had meningitis (although mostly aseptic), despite being judged clinically well by experienced clinicians.

After 2 to 3 months of age, increasing, but not absolute, reliance can be placed on the physical findings; fever is typically noted. Specific evidence of meningeal irritation is often present, including nuchal rigidity and, less often, Kernig (pain with extension of the leg on a flexed femur) and Brudzinski (involuntary lifting of the legs when the head is raised while the child is lying supine) signs. When an LP fails to confirm the diagnosis of meningitis, despite the presence of meningeal signs, other conditions must be pursued that can mimic the findings on physical examination. Conditions capable of producing the findings typical of meningismus (irritation of the meninges without pleocytosis in the CSF) include severe pharyngitis, retropharyngeal abscess (RTA), cervical adenitis, arthritis or osteomyelitis of the cervical spine, upper lobe pneumonia, subarachnoid hemorrhage, pyelonephritis, and tetanus.

Seizures are a presenting complaint for 20% of children with bacterial meningitis. Many of these are focal, recurrent, or prolonged seizures. Most clinicians advise that children younger than 6 months with a first-time febrile seizure should routinely have LP performed to discern the presence of CNS infection, unless there are specific contraindications or an alternative diagnosis is readily apparent. Febrile seizures are reviewed in Chapters 26 Fever and 67 Seizures.

Triage considerations: Children with fever and altered mental status or neck pain should be evaluated promptly for meningitis. Associated tachycardia and hypotension can be seen in children with meningitis who are in compensated or uncompensated shock, respectively. If meningococcus is suspected, providers should wear simple face masks and utilize droplet precautions.

Clinical assessment: Initial considerations in the management of children with bacterial meningitis are listed in Table 102.5. Confirmation of meningitis is by sampling of the CSF. The most common CSF parameters associated with various causes of meningitis are summarized in Table 102.6. The CSF Gram stain will be positive for an organism in approximately two-thirds (40% to 90%) of cases of bacterial meningitis and the results of Gram stain should be used to add additional antimicrobial therapy when appropriate. It is generally prudent to await culture confirmation before antibiotic coverage is narrowed. In certain patients, computed tomography (CT) should be considered prior to LP. These criteria are not as well defined for pediatric patients, but in adult patients, they include immunocompromised state; history of focal CNS disease; presence of papilledema; and focal neurologic deficit.

Seizures occur in 20% of children with bacterial meningitis and, occasionally, in those with viral infections of the CNS, such as meningoencephalitis due to HSV. One should always be suspicious of derangement of the glucose or sodium as a cause of convulsive activity. However, most seizures are caused by irritation of the brain from the infectious process. They are controlled using routine antiepileptic agents. Subdural effusion and, less often, empyema occur in 20% to 40% of young children with meningitis but usually appear later in the course.

Management: The optimal antibiotics for empiric treatment of acute bacterial meningitis would offer coverage for the most common pathogens, be bactericidal, and cross the blood–brain barrier. Treatment options for meningitis in normal hosts are described in Table 102.7. Treatment of tuberculosis meningitis and HSV meningitis is described elsewhere. Evaluation and treatment of meningitis in immunocompromised hosts (e.g., human immunodeficiency virus [HIV]-infected children) should be undertaken with consultation with an ID specialist. Consideration should be given to admitting children with suspected bacterial meningitis to an intensive care unit setting for close initial monitoring. Standard precautions are indicated for most causes of bacterial meningitis, except for meningococcus (droplet precautions) and tuberculosis meningitis (airborne precautions). Electrolyte imbalances seen in bacterial meningitis and their treatment are discussed in Chapter 108 Renal and Electrolyte Emergencies.

TABLE 102.5

IMMEDIATE MANAGEMENT STEPS FOR CHILDREN WITH SUSPECTED OR CONFIRMED BACTERIAL MENINGITIS

Immediate evaluation	Initiate hemodynamic monitoring and support
	Achieve venous access; use cardiorespiratory monitors
	Ensure adequate ventilation and cardiac function
Laboratory evaluation	CSF for cell count and differential; Gram stain and culture; glucose; protein
	Consider holding CSF in the laboratory for enteroviral or HSV PCR, AFB culture, cryptococcal, or arboviral studies
	CBC, blood culture, electrolytes, serum glucose, BUN and creatinine, prothrombin time and partial thromboplastin time
Medications	Fluid resuscitation for septic shock, if present
	If *Mycobacterium tuberculosis* or *H. influenzae* type b is the suspected cause of meningitis, consider dexamethasone (0.15 mg/kg) before or with the first dose of antibiotics
	Antibiotics (see Table 102.7)
	Glucose (if serum glucose <50 mg/dL) 0.25–1 g/kg
	Treat acidosis and coagulopathy, if present.

CSF, cerebrospinal fluid; HSV, herpes simplex virus; PCR, polymerase chain reaction; AFB, acid-fast bacilli; CBC, complete blood count.

TABLE 102.6

USUAL RANGES FOR CEREBROSPINAL FLUID PARAMETERS

	Neonate, normal parameters	Child, normal parameters	Bacterial meningitis	TB meningitis	Lyme meningitis[a]	Viral meningitis
WBC (per mm^3)	<30	<10	200–20,000	10–500	10–500	10–1,000
Protein (mg/dL)	<170	<40	>100	80–400	40–150	40–100
Glucose (mg/dL)	>30	>40	<30	<40	>40	>30

[a]One predictive model for Lyme meningitis utilized CSF monocytic predominance, duration of headache, and presence of cranial neuropathy and had a 100% positive predictive value (Garro AC, Rutman M, Simonsen K, et al. Prospective validation of a clinical prediction model for Lyme meningitis in children. *Pediatrics* 2009;123:e829). Another study found that children were at low-risk for Lyme meningitis when the "rule of 7s" were met: headache for <7 days; <70% CSF monocytes, and the absence of seventh cranial nerve or other palsies (Cohn KA, Thompson AD, Shah SS, et al. Validation of a clinical prediction rule to distinguish Lyme meningitis from aseptic meningitis. *Pediatrics* 2012;129(1):e46–e53).
TB, tuberculosis; WBC, white blood count.

Herpes Simplex Virus, Neonatal

CLINICAL PEARLS AND PITFALLS

- Most mothers of infants with HSV infection do not provide a history of HSV, as primary infection can be asymptomatic and vesicular lesions deep in the female genitourinary tract cannot be visualized by the mothers. Thus, a "negative" maternal history of herpes does not rule out herpes in an infant.
- HSV has substantial overlap with bacterial causes of sepsis and meningitis.
- The three main forms of neonatal disease are skin, eye, and mouth (SEM) disease, CNS disease, and disseminated disease.
- HSV should be considered in the differential diagnosis of any febrile neonate with a CSF pleocytosis and in infants with elevated hepatic transaminases or coagulopathy.
- Early recognition of HSV disease and prompt initiation of acyclovir can decrease the substantial morbidity and mortality in infants.

Current Evidence

HSV has three major manifestations in the neonatal period. HSV genital lesions will be described in the section on sexually transmitted infections (STIs). It is estimated that 45% of adults in the United States are seropositive for HSV-1 and 16% for HSV-2. Both viruses can cause oral or genitourinary infection, but approximately 75% of neonatal HSV disease is caused by HSV-2. Neonatal HSV is thought to complicate 1 in 3,200 deliveries, resulting in approximately 1,500 cases per year in the United States. Risk factors for transmission to neonates include primary maternal infection; vaginal delivery; prolonged rupture of membranes; HSV-2; and use of fetal scalp electrodes. The risk of neonatal HSV is highest during the primary infection in the mother, as viremia is often higher than with recurrent infections, and an effective immune response has yet to be mounted. However, 75% of mothers of HSV-infected neonates did not report a history of herpes, as primary infection can be asymptomatic. As such, the lack of maternal history of HSV should not provide false reassurance to the PEM clinician.

TABLE 102.7

EMPIRIC ANTIBIOTIC THERAPY FOR SUSPECTED ACUTE BACTERIAL MENINGITIS

Age	Most common pathogens	Empiric antibiotics
<1 mo	Group B streptococcus (*S. agalactiae*), *E. coli*, *Listeria monocytogenes*, *Klebsiella* species	Ampicillin (50 mg/kg every 8 hrs in the first week of life; 50 mg/kg every 6 hrs on days 8–28) *and* Cefotaxime (50 mg/kg every 8 hrs in the first week of life; 50 mg/kg every 6 hrs on days 8–28)
1–23 mo	*Streptococcus pneumoniae*, *Neisseria meningitidis*, group B streptococcus, *E. coli*, *H. influenzae* type b	Vancomycin (15 mg/kg every 6 hrs) *and* Cefotaxime (75 mg/kg every 6 hrs, maximum 2 g/dose) or ceftriaxone (50 mg/kg every 12 hrs, maximum 2 g/dose)
≥24 mo	*N. meningitidis*, *S. pneumoniae*	Vancomycin (15 mg/kg every 6 hrs) *and* Cefotaxime (75 mg/kg every 6 hrs, maximum 2 g/dose) or ceftriaxone (50 mg/kg every 12 hrs, maximum 2 g/dose)

From Tunkel AR, Hartman BJ, Kaplan SL, et al. Practice guidelines for the management of bacterial meningitis. *Clin Infect Dis* 2004;39:1267–1284.

TABLE 102.8

MANIFESTATIONS OF NEONATAL HERPES SIMPLEX VIRUS INFECTION[a]

Type	%	Age (days)	Symptoms	% with vesicles	% with CNS disease	Mortality/Neurologic sequelae[a]
Skin, eye, mouth	45	10–12	Vesicular rash on erythematous base; consider in any child with a suspected pustule where the Gram stain is negative for bacteria	80–100	—	0%/100%
Central nervous system (CNS)	30	16–19	Fever, focal or generalized seizures, bulging fontanelle, temperature instability	60–70	100%	4%/70%
Disseminated	25	10–12	CNS findings (above), respiratory distress or failure, hepatic failure with coagulopathy, adrenal insufficiency, hemorrhagic pneumonitis	80	65–70%	29%/20%

[a]Sequelae in children who did not receive herpes antiviral suppressive therapy after completion of acyclovir.
From Pinninti, et al. Neonatal herpes simplex virus infections. *Infect Dis Clin N Am* 2013;60:351–365.

Goals of Treatment

The goal of treatment of neonatal HSV is the rapid recognition and initiation of acyclovir promptly. Clinical outcomes include time to antiviral therapy and neurologic sequelae.

Clinical Considerations

Clinical recognition: There are three manifestations of HSV in the neonatal period: SEM disease, seen in approximately 45% of cases; CNS disease, seen in 30%; and disseminated disease, seen in 25%. The most common clinical and laboratory presentations are described in Table 102.8. In utero infection rarely is seen (1 in 300,000 deliveries) and children are symptomatic at birth with cutaneous, ophthalmologic, and neurologic findings. There is substantial overlap between the three most common disease entities, as many children with vesicles have more invasive disease, and many children with disseminated disease have CNS involvement. Children with isolated SEM disease have the best prognosis, with few reported cases of death or neurologic sequelae. While the mortality rate for CNS disease is low, most children have neurologic sequelae. In contrast to older patients, in whom HSV has a tropism for the temporal lobes, neonatal CNS HSV infection often involves multiple portions of the brain. Children with disseminated disease present septic, and require multiorgan system support, as they often have severe synthetic hepatic dysfunction resulting in coagulopathy and can develop HSV pneumonitis, which is often hemorrhagic. Adrenal involvement is common; as such, the provider should consider hydrocortisone for children with suspected HSV disease. The most severe disease typically occurs in children who never develop a vesicular rash, as the diagnosis often is delayed in these children. As such, the absence of a rash should not lead the clinician to eliminate HSV from the differential diagnosis.

Triage considerations: Febrile and hypothermic neonates should be evaluated promptly for HSV in addition to bacterial infections. The clinician's index of suspicion for HSV should be increased in the following circumstances: vesicles; seizures or abnormal neurologic examination; CSF pleocytosis; or evidence of hepatic dysfunction, including coagulopathy.

Clinical assessment: The diagnosis is confirmed by isolation of HSV via culture or polymerase chain reaction (PCR). Surface cultures should be obtained from the conjunctivae, nose, mouth, and anus, in addition to cultures being obtained from vesicles. In the latter instance, the swabs should be rubbed against the base of the vesicle, as opposed to aspirating fluid from the vesicle itself. HSV PCR of the CSF is more sensitive (90% to 100%) than viral culture of the CSF, but the sensitivity is lower early in the disease process. As such, a negative HSV CSF PCR does not rule out CNS involvement. If the index of suspicion for HSV disease is high, it is reasonable to repeat PCR testing prior to stopping therapy. PCR (qualitative or quantitative) can also be obtained from the blood; this is of particular utility in children who are coagulopathic or have other clinical features which make LP difficult. HSV serologies are not useful in the acute setting. In addition to routine laboratory evaluation and cultures, ALT, prothrombin time, and partial thromboplastin time should be obtained. Obtaining a serum glucose is also useful, as hepatic dysfunction can result in an inability to mobilize glycogen stores and result in hypoglycemia.

Management: Neonates with suspected HSV should receive parenteral acyclovir (20 mg per kg every 8 hours). Children in whom ocular disease is present should be promptly evaluated by an ophthalmologist and receive topical antiviral therapy, such as 1% trifluridine (one drop every 6 hours) to the affected eye(s), in addition to parenteral acyclovir. Neonates, especially those with disseminated disease, are likely to require blood products and fresh frozen plasma to treat coagulopathy. Many of the considerations noted in the section on bacterial meningitis also are applicable for HSV meningoencephalitis. Standard and contact precautions (if vesicles are present) should be used for children with suspected HSV disease.

Meningitis, Aseptic

Both infectious and noninfectious processes can produce aseptic meningitis (Table 102.9). The most common cause is viral meningitis. In Lyme-endemic regions, clinicians should

TABLE 102.9

CAUSES OF ASEPTIC MENINGITIS

Viral	Enteroviral Herpes simplex virus Arboviral Lymphocytic choriomeningitis virus Mumps Other viral infections
Bacterial	Early or partially treated bacterial meningitis Parameningeal infection *Mycobacterium tuberculosis* *Borrelia burgdorferi* (Lyme disease) Rickettsial diseases *Bartonella henselae* (cat scratch) *Leptospirosis* *Treponema pallidum* (syphilis) Mycoplasma
Fungal	*Cryptococcus* Histoplasmosis *Candida*
Parasitic	*Naegleria* Toxoplasmosis *Taenia solium* (neurocysticercosis) Malaria Trichinosis
Noninfectious	Neoplasia Kawasaki disease Hemorrhage Collage vascular diseases Hypersensitivity reactions Heavy metal poisoning Sarcoidosis

also suspect *Borrelia burgdorferi* as a cause of aseptic meningitis. The signs and symptoms of aseptic meningitis mimic those of acute bacterial meningitis, but alterations in level of consciousness or focal neurologic deficits are rarer than in bacterial meningitis. Initial laboratory evaluation should parallel that described for bacterial meningitis. Enteroviral PCR should be sent on the initial CSF. Ill-appearing children or infants in the first 1 to 2 months of life should have HSV PCR on the CSF and serum sent as well (see HSV meningoencephalitis section) and acyclovir (20 mg per kg every 8 hours for children 0 to 3 months; 15 mg per kg every 8 hours for children >3 months of age) should be initiated. Most patients need no further tests, but in atypical situations, consideration should always be given to nonviral causes that may mandate additional diagnostic steps or specific therapy. If tuberculosis is suspected based on family contacts, a low CSF glucose with lymphocytic predominance, or pulmonary findings, then a Mantoux tuberculin skin test (TST) and chest radiograph are useful for confirmation. In endemic areas, serologic studies for Lyme disease and antibiotic therapy may be indicated based upon the exposure history and time of year. A CT scan provides essential information about patients with symptoms or signs of parameningeal infection, HSV encephalitis, or CNS tumors and hemorrhages. Immunosuppressed patients develop infections with a wide variety of unusual bacteria, fungi, and parasites that can be identified in many cases with appropriate examination and culture of the CSF (e.g., India ink and acid-fast stains, cryptococcal antigen testing, fungal and mycobacterial cultures).

Because the CSF findings in aseptic meningitis overlap those in bacterial infections, hospital admission is usually warranted until the CSF culture results are available. However, the experienced clinician may choose to follow the older child as an outpatient if the family is reliable and nonviral causes (e.g., Lyme disease, tuberculosis, cryptococcosis) are clinically unlikely. To guide clinicians, the Bacterial Meningitis Score has been derived and validated to identify children at very low risk (negative predictive value 99.7%) for bacterial meningitis. Low-risk features are negative CSF Gram stain; CSF absolute neutrophil count (ANC) <1,000 cells/μL, CSF protein <80 mg per dL, peripheral ANC <10,000 cells per mm^3, and no seizures at or prior to presentation. Additionally, a positive rapid enteroviral PCR may support outpatient management if available and the patient is clinically well.

Encephalitis and Meningoencephalitis

Encephalitis is an inflammation of the brain that can occur with or without associated meningeal irritation; the former is termed meningoencephalitis, but the terms will be used interchangeably in this section. The clinical manifestations can overlap with those of meningitis. The etiologies most commonly associated with encephalitis are listed in e-Table 102.2; however, an etiology is found in only a small fraction of children and adults with encephalitis. In circumstances where etiologies are found, almost 70% are viral (most commonly enterovirus, followed by HSV and Epstein–Barr virus [EBV]) and approximately 20% are bacterial. In the last two decades, it has been recognized that several arboviruses endemic in the United States can cause encephalitis. These viruses, which include West Nile, St. Louis, La Crosse, and the equine encephalitides, are termed arboviruses because they are arthropod-borne viruses, not because they share phylogenetic characteristics. The clinical manifestations include altered consciousness or behavioral changes, seizures, hemiparesis, or ataxia, often with nausea and vomiting. Fever is not uniformly present. Postinfectious cases can have associated demyelination in the absence of acute signs of infection; most cases of brainstem encephalitis are postinfectious. The differential diagnosis of encephalitis includes ingestion, metabolic disorders, structural lesions (masses, bleeds, emboli), acute demyelinating encephalomyelitis (ADEM), and autoimmune encephalitis (NMDAR). One diagnostic approach to the child with suspected encephalitis is listed in Table 102.10, realizing that repeated history taking may be necessary to elucidate all exposures a child may have had. Children with encephalitis should be started on acyclovir (20 mg per kg every 8 hours) pending HSV PCR, as this is one of the few treatable causes of encephalitis. If a CSF pleocytosis exists, empiric initiation of parenteral antibiotics (e.g., vancomycin [15 mg per kg every 6 hours] and cefotaxime [75 mg per kg every 6 hours; maximum: 2 g per dose]) is reasonable pending bacterial culture

TABLE 102.10

EVALUATION OF A CHILD WITH SUSPECTED ENCEPHALITIS OR MENINGOENCEPHALITIS

All suspected cases	
CSF	Cell count and differential, protein/glucose, bacterial culture, HSV PCR, enteroviral PCR
	Consider holding CSF in the laboratory for additional diagnostic studies (see below)
Serum	CBC, chemistries, blood cultures, EBV/CMV serologies, HIV, HSV PCR, *Bartonella* serologies, *Mycoplasma* serologies
Other	Enteroviral PCR (respiratory, stool), PCR of respiratory specimens
Specific risk factor or features	
Tuberculosis risk factors	Should be suspected in any child with CSF pleocytosis and a high CSF protein and/or low CSF glucose: chest radiograph (abnormal in approximately 90% of children with tuberculosis meningitis; tuberculin skin test; interferon gamma release assay; gastric aspirate or sputum for acid-fast culture; CSF PCR for *Mycobacterium tuberculosis*
Immunocompromised	Acid-fast culture for tuberculosis, cryptococcal antigen (serum, CSF), human herpesvirus 6 and 7, JC virus, Toxoplasma serum IgG; cultures for *Listeria monocytogenes,* VZV PCR, histoplasmosis serologies/urinary antigen
Sexually active	RPR/VDRL for syphilis
Summer/fall	West Nile IgM (CSF, serum), Arboviral panel (CSF, serum), and serologies for other geographically appropriate arboviruses (e.g., St. Louis, La Crosse, and the equine encephalitides)
	Serologies for *Rickettsia rickettsii* (Rocky Mountain spotted fever) and ehrlichiosis as well as *Borrelia burgdorferi* (Lyme disease) if in the appropriate geographic region
Winter	Influenza PCR
Raw or unpasteurized food products	*Toxoplasma* IgG, serologies for *Coxiella,* culture for *Listeria monocytogenes,* evaluation for *Gnanthostoma* if history of travel to Southeast Asia or Latin America
Animal exposures	Rabies (bites from unimmunized dogs/cats or contact with bats or wild carnivores), *Bartonella* (cat scratches or bites from cat fleas), LCMV (exposure to rodent urine or feces)
Ticks	Serologies or PCR for *Rickettsia rickettsii, Ehrlichia chaffeensis, Anaplasma, Borrelia burgdorferi*
Insect contact	Serologies for equine encephalitides, St. Louis encephalitis, Japanese encephalitis, West Nile virus, La Crosse virus and smear for malaria (if appropriate travel histories) for mosquito contact; *Bartonella bacilliformis* serologies (sandflies); trypanosomiasis serologies (tsetse flies)
Swimming in brackish or stagnant water	Wet mount for *Naegleria fowleri*
Travel history	Serologies for fungal infections endemic in certain regions; consider early consultation with an infectious diseases specialist. Infections more common outside industrialized nations are discussed in the section on Infections in Returned Travelers
Vesicular rash	PCR of lesion for HSV, VZV
Diarrhea and seizure	Stool for bacterial culture (*Shigella, E. coli*) and for rotavirus PCR
CSF eosinophilia	*Baylisascaris* (raccoon roundworm) serologies

CSF, cerebrospinal fluid; HSV, herpes simplex virus; PCR, polymerase chain reaction; CBC, complete blood count; EBV, Epstein–Barr virus; CMV, cytomegalovirus; HIV, human immunodeficiency virus; VZV, varicella zoster virus; RPR, rapid plasma reagin; VDRL, venereal disease research laboratory; LCMV, lymphocytic choriomeningitis virus.
From Tunkel AR, Glaser CA, Bloch KC, et al. The management of encephalitis: clinical practice guidelines by the Infectious Diseases Society of America. *Clin Infect Dis* 2008;47:303–327.

results. Consideration should be given to admission of these patients to intensive care unit settings for closer monitoring given concerns for changes in the ability to protect the airway, increased intracranial pressure, or electrolyte imbalances. Standard precautions are recommended for most forms of encephalitis.

Other CNS Infections

Goals of Treatment

The goal is to rapidly identify infections which may result in intracranial extension, and to recognize that the empiric antibiotic selection in these cases must include antibiotics that are both bactericidal and achieve adequate CNS penetrance.

CLINICAL PEARLS AND PITFALLS

- The most common comorbidity in children with brain abscesses is congenital heart disease.
- Staphylococci and streptococci are the most common organisms isolated.
- One common regimen to treat suspected CNS invasion from contiguous structures is the combination of vancomycin, ceftriaxone or cefotaxime, and metronidazole, all at meningitic doses.

Brain Abscesses

Brain abscesses can result from contiguous spread from head and neck infections (e.g., mastoiditis, sinusitis, odontogenic) or from direct seeding from septic emboli, most commonly in children with congenital heart disease. The latter remains the most common risk factor for pediatric brain abscesses. The most common organisms are streptococci (aerobic and anaerobic streptococci, GAS, and pneumococcus) and *S. aureus,* followed by fungal (primarily *Aspergillus*) and Enterobacteriaceae. Early symptoms are nonspecific and can include fever, malaise, vomiting, and headache. The most common signs are focal neurologic deficits, papilledema, meningeal signs, hemiparesis, and ataxia, although symptoms will vary by abscess location (cerebral hemisphere is the most common location) and size. Mental status changes are late signs with ominous prognoses. LP rarely yields an organism, and blood cultures infrequently are positive. ED-based diagnosis can be made by contrast CT of the brain, although magnetic resonance imaging (MRI) will better delineate brainstem and cerebellar abscesses. Early neurosurgical intervention is critical. Empiric antibiotics should be broad-spectrum antibiotics with CNS penetrance covering staphylococci, streptococci, and anaerobes. One regimen would be vancomycin, cefotaxime, and metronidazole, all at meningitic doses. Standard precautions should be used.

Sinusitis

Sinusitis is an inflammation of the paranasal sinuses. While the ethmoid and maxillary sinuses are present at birth, the frontal and sphenoid sinuses do not develop until children are school aged. The most common etiologies mimic those causing acute otitis media and include pneumococcus, nontypeable *H. influenzae, Moraxella,* and GAS. The most common signs and symptoms of acute sinusitis are listed in e-Table 102.3. Children with chronic sinusitis can have milder, more indolent symptoms, such as cough that is often worse when the child is supine and rhinorrhea; pyrexia is less common in this group of children, and physical examination often is normal. The diagnostic criteria are summarized in e-Table 102.4. Complications of sinusitis include orbital cellulitis, brain abscess, epidural or subdural empyema, and cavernous sinus thrombosis.

Most sinusitis is managed solely with medical therapy in the outpatient setting. Amoxicillin (80 to 90 mg/kg/day) remains the mainstay of therapy; a 10-day course is recommended for most cases of uncomplicated acute sinusitis. Two- to 3-week courses may be needed for chronic sinusitis or for immunocompromised or chronically ill children with acute sinusitis. Inpatient therapy should be considered for toxic-appearing children, those with facial swelling, or children with suspected or confirmed intracranial extension. The AAP recommendations for sinusitis treatment are summarized in e-Table 102.5. Standard precautions should be used.

Mastoiditis

Mastoiditis, an infection of the mastoid air cells, is a rare complication of acute otitis media. The most common organism is pneumococcus, followed by *S. aureus,* GAS, and *Pseudomonas;* historically, Hib has also been implicated. The most common signs are fever, ear proptosis, and postauricular redness, pain, and swelling; the tympanic membrane is usually erythematous and bulging. Complications can include intracranial extension of the abscess, damage to the facial nerve, labyrinthitis, bacteremia, and osteomyelitis. The diagnosis is confirmed by CT of the temporal bone. Tympanocentesis cultures reflect etiology of mastoiditis in approximately 50% of cases. Treatment is a combination of medical and surgical management. Empiric antibiotics should target streptococci and staphylococci. In regions where MRSA and penicillin-resistant pneumococci are common, a reasonable regimen would include vancomycin and a third-generation cephalosporin. Standard precautions should be used.

Orbital Cellulitis

Orbital cellulitis is an infection posterior to the orbital septum caused primarily by *S. aureus,* streptococci, pneumococcus, and nontypeable *H. influenzae.* The most common signs are fever, proptosis, limited ocular range of motion, pain with eye motion, chemosis, and an afferent pupillary defect. Blood cultures should be obtained; LP should be considered for young infants and for children with signs of meningitis. Contrasted CT of the orbit and brain confirms the diagnosis and allows for evaluation for intracranial extension, which would alter antibiotic management. Many children with uncomplicated orbital cellulitis are managed medically; however, early consultation with surgical subspecialists would be advised. Empiric antibiotic selection should cover the same organisms as for mastoiditis; if intracranial extension is not evident on CT, substitution of vancomycin for clindamycin can ease the transition of a child from parental to an entirely oral regimen after clinical improvement even if an isolate is not recovered. Indications for operative management include intracranial extension, visual loss, or optic nerve dysfunction. Standard precautions should be used.

Botulism

Botulism is a neurotoxic disorder caused by *Clostridium botulinum* that causes a descending flaccid paralysis. The most common pediatric manifestation is infantile botulism, most common in children under 6 months of age, caused by ingestion of spores; botulism is the reason that honey is not recommended for infants. Affected infants have decreased movement, bulbar nerve palsies, expression-less facies, loss of head control, and descending hypotonia. Diagnosis is confirmed by isolation of toxin or spores from stool. The mainstay of treatment is supportive therapy; intubation may be necessary. Infants with botulism should immediately receive botulism immune globulin (BabyBIG) intravenously. Antibiotics are not indicated for infantile botulism, and aminoglycosides may worsen the toxin's paralytic effects. Older patients with wound botulism after penetrating or crush trauma should receive penicillin or metronidazole after receiving an equine-derived Heptavalent Botulinum Antitoxin (HBAT). Standard precautions should be used.

Tetanus

Tetanus is caused by another neurotoxin in the Clostridium family, *Clostridium tetani.* Spores are ubiquitous in the environment and can contaminate wounds of unimmunized or underimmunized persons. Neonatal tetanus is most common in developing nations where infants are unprotected because of the lack of maternal immunity. Local tetanus refers to muscle spasms in areas contiguous to the wound, and can result in generalized tetanus (lockjaw), with trismus, risus sardonicus, and generalized muscle spasming. The differential diagnosis includes hypocalcemia and drug reactions. Tetanus is a clinical diagnosis; culture yield is poor. Treatment is tetanus immune globulin (TIG), with some infiltrated around the wound and the rest administered intramuscularly. Metronidazole (preferred) or penicillin for 10 to 14 days also is needed. The recommendations for ED management of tetanus prophylaxis are described in Table 102.11. It is important that the ED

TABLE 102.11

TETANUS PROPHYLAXIS FOR PATIENTS WITH WOUNDS OR BITES

	Clean, minor wounds		Contaminated, crush, burn, frostbite, projectile, or puncture wounds	
Scenario	Vaccine	TIG	Vaccine	TIG
<3 tetanus vaccines or tetanus vaccine history unavailable	Yes	No	Yes	Yes
≥3 tetanus vaccines	No if <10 yrs after last tetanus vaccine	No	No if <5 yrs after last tetanus vaccine	No
	Yes if ≥10 yrs since last tetanus vaccine	No	Yes if ≥5 yrs since last tetanus vaccine	No

DTaP is used for children <7 yrs of age; Tdap is for children ≥7 yrs old who have not received Tdap before; Td is for children ≥7 yrs old who have already received Tdap.
TIG, tetanus immune globulin.

physician asks about tetanus vaccination, as opposed to assuming that children are up-to-date on this immunization; a recent national surveillance study found that only 82% of toddlers were appropriately immunized against tetanus. Standard precautions should be used.

NECK INFECTIOUS EMERGENCIES

Cervical Lymphadenitis

CLINICAL PEARLS AND PITFALLS

- The most common organisms causing cervical lymphadenitis are staphylococci and streptococci. However, thorough travel and exposure histories should be taken to evaluate for less common etiologies.
- Signs of inflammation also can help differentiate among the causes of localized infectious lymphadenopathy. Nontender adenopathy should lead the clinician away from most pyogenic causes, and should increase the index of suspicion for viral upper respiratory infections (URIs) or mycobacterial disease, depending upon the duration of illness.

Current Evidence

Cervical lymphadenitis is a bacterial infection of the lymph nodes in the neck. This condition must be distinguished from lymphadenopathy, an enlargement of one or more lymph nodes that occurs with viral infections, or as a reaction to bacterial disease in structures that drain to the nodes. The most common etiologies are listed in e-Table 102.6 (see also Chapter 42 Lymphadenopathy).

Goals of Treatment

Clinical outcomes for children with lymphadenitis include limiting the use of CT among patients with uncomplicated bacterial lymphadenitis.

Clinical Considerations

Clinical recognition: The child with cervical lymphadenitis is usually noted to have swelling in the neck. If sufficiently old, he or she will complain of pain. Fever occurs only occasionally, more often in children younger than 1 year. The infected node may vary in size from 2 cm to more than 10 cm. Initially, it has a firm consistency, but fluctuance develops in about 25% of the infected nodes. The skin overlying the node becomes erythematous, and there may be associated edema. Children with nontuberculous mycobacterial infections may have nontender adenopathy with violaceous discoloration of the overlying skin.

Triage considerations: Children with lymphadenitis should be promptly assessed for deep neck infections and for infections that may affect the airway. Lymphadenitis should be considered in the differential diagnosis of a child with a painful neck mass. Associated toxic appearance or pain out of proportion to the examination may imply a deeper extension of the infection and demand emergent treatment and surgical consultation.

Clinical assessment: The WBC count is usually normal but may be elevated in the younger, febrile child. Aspiration of the node often identifies the organism by both Gram stain and culture, even if fluctuance is not appreciated. Children with infections from *Mycobacterium tuberculosis* usually react to the TST and may have findings compatible with tuberculosis seen on chest radiograph. Complications of bacterial adenitis are unusual. Organisms such as *S. aureus* and group A streptococci (GAS) can spread locally if unchecked. A draining sinus tract may develop in untreated children with atypical mycobacterial adenitis. Recurrence of infection suggests a local anatomic abnormality (e.g., branchial cleft cyst or thyroglossal duct cyst) or immunocompromising conditions such as chronic granulomatous disease.

Management: If the node is fluctuant, aspiration provides useful etiologic information and speeds the rate of resolution. Children who fail to respond to empiric antibiotic therapy and children with tuberculosis risk factors who present with adenitis should have a TST placed. Children with cervical adenitis who are otherwise healthy should receive an antibiotic effective against *S. aureus* and the GAS. While clindamycin (10 mg/kg/dose three times daily; maximum: 600 mg per dose) has activity against both pathogens, trimethoprim-sulfamethoxazole (TMP-SMZ) will not offer GAS coverage. The decision about which oral antibiotic to select depends on the level of methicillin-resistant *S. aureus* (MRSA) in a community.

Indications for inpatient admission and parenteral antibiotics include: toxic appearance; young age (<3 months); immunocompromised host; suspicion of deeper neck extension; development of a draining sinus track; or failure to improve with outpatient oral antibiotic therapy. For these children, clindamycin (10 to 13 mg per kg every 8 hours; maximum: 600 mg per dose) or vancomycin (15 mg per kg every 8 hours; maximum: 2 g per dose) offers alternatives in the face of penicillin and/or cephalosporin allergy or in geographic areas where coverage for MRSA must be considered. Standard precautions should be used unless children have draining lesions (in which case contact precautions should be used) or if children are suspected of having tuberculosis lymphadenitis (in which case airborne precautions should be used until pulmonary involvement is excluded).

Other Neck Infectious Emergencies

Lemierre's Syndrome

Lemierre's syndrome refers to a deep neck abscess with a contiguous septic thrombophlebitis of the internal jugular and septic pulmonary emboli. The most common cause historically has been *Fusobacterium necrophorum;* in recent years, *S. aureus* has been the most common etiology. Examination is notable for a tender cord in the lateral neck and dyspnea is common as the number of septic pulmonary emboli increases. The diagnosis can be made by CT neck with contrast-showing flow voids in the jugular; apical cuts through the lungs on neck CT may show the embolic lesions. Children with suspected Lemierre's should receive broad-spectrum antibiotics covering both MRSA and anaerobes (e.g., vancomycin plus metronidazole).

Cat-scratch Disease

Cat-scratch disease, caused by *Bartonella henselae,* is caused by cat scratches or cats licking abraded skin or from the bite of infected cat fleas. These most commonly occur to the upper extremities and result in tender, fluctuant axillary or epitrochlear lymphadenitis, but cervical adenopathy can be seen if scratches or bites occur to the face. In some pediatric series, *Bartonella* and EBV are the most common causes of fever of unknown origin. Diagnosis is based on history (cat, especially kitten, exposure), examination (slowly healing papule at inoculation site), and serologies. While most lesions will resolve in 1 to 2 months, antibiotics may decrease symptom duration. Optimal antibiotics are unclear; rifampin, azithromycin, TMP-SMZ, and fluoroquinolones have all been utilized. Standard precautions should be used.

RESPIRATORY TRACT INFECTIOUS EMERGENCIES

Upper Respiratory Tract Infectious Emergencies

Goals of Treatment

Infections in the neck can rapidly enter other tissue planes that can result in spread to contiguous structures, including compromising the airway or neck vasculature. Clinicians need to be cognizant that while most upper airway infections are relatively benign (e.g., pharyngitis), some can progress from benign etiologies to life-threatening complications (e.g., Lemierre's syndrome). The clinical manifestations, diagnosis, and treatment of upper respiratory tract infections are summarized in Table 102.12.

CLINICAL PEARLS AND PITFALLS

- Many clinical entities can be differentiated on the basis of the child's age, history, and oropharyngeal examination.
- Airway instrumentation in a child with suspected epiglottitis should be performed in the more controlled environment of the operating room.
- Many upper airway infections are caused by streptococcal and staphylococcal species, simplifying empiric ED antibiotic selection.

Epiglottitis

Epiglottitis is characterized by fever, drooling, dysphagia, and inspiratory stridor in a toxic-appearing child who is not hoarse and does not have a barky cough. The illness is rapidly progressive over hours and is most common in children 1 to 8 years of age. The most common organism historically was Hib, but now *S. pneumoniae, Streptococcus pyogenes,* and *S. aureus* comprise many of the cases. Soft tissue lateral neck radiographs can show an enlarged epiglottis ("thumbprint sign"), and visualization demonstrates a swollen, erythematous epiglottis. However, instrumentation is best performed in the operative setting to prevent airway compromise. Immediate involvement of otolaryngology and broad-spectrum antibiotics (e.g., vancomycin and cefotaxime) and attempting to keep the child calm are the mainstays of ED management. Standard precautions should be used.

Retropharyngeal Abscess

RTAs are characterized by nuchal rigidity or torticollis, difficulty swallowing, drooling, stridor, and fever. Anterior bulging of the posterior pharynx can be difficult to appreciate. Children with RTAs usually are preschool aged, and GAS and *S. aureus* are the most common organisms. A soft tissue lateral neck radiograph can suggest the diagnosis if there is increased prevertebral space; however, a contrast CT neck is better to delineate the anatomy prior to operative intervention. Empiric antibiotics should target streptococci and staphylococci (e.g., clindamycin). Standard precautions should be used.

Peritonsillar Abscess

Peritonsillar abscesses (PTAs) are characterized by unilateral swelling of the tonsils, change in caliber of the voice, trismus, unilateral odynophagia, displacement of the uvula toward the unaffected side, and fever. PTAs are most common in adolescents, and GAS and *S. aureus* are the most common organisms. The diagnosis is clinical, although in some cases ultrasound can be used to aid the diagnosis and CT may be useful to evaluate for deeper extension of the abscess. Empiric antibiotics should target streptococci and staphylococci (e.g., clindamycin). Standard precautions should be used.

Ludwig Angina

Ludwig angina is a rapidly progressive cellulitis of the floor of the mouth. This can be a complication of dental abscesses, especially of the mandibular molars. Children with Ludwig angina develop fever, halitosis, odynophagia, submandibular lymphadenopathy, and induration to the floor of the mouth. The

TABLE 102.12

PRESENTATION OF AIRWAY AND NECK INFECTIONS

Site	Age (yrs)	Symptoms	Diagnosis	Organisms	Empiric treatment[a]
Epiglottitis	1–8	Fever, drooling, dysphagia, inspiratory stridor	Lateral neck radiograph with "thumbprint" sign	GAS, *S. aureus*, pneumococcus, Hib in the unvaccinated	Vancomycin and a third-generation cephalosporin
Diphtheria	All	Gray pseudomembrane over nose or larynx; swelling to neck soft tissues ("bull neck"), fever, dyspnea; can see myocarditis, arrhythmias, and cranial nerve palsies	Clinical diagnosis; inform laboratory if suspect diphtheria, as it has unique culture requirements	*C. diphtheriae*	Equine antitoxin (from CDC in the United States) + penicillin or erythromycin to eradicate organism
Retropharyngeal	<5	Fever, torticollis, odynophagia, stridor, drooling. Physical examination is insensitive for detecting the anterior bulging of the posterior pharynx	Lateral neck radiograph may demonstrate increased prevertebral space; CT neck often needed to guide surgical management	GAS, *S. aureus*	Clindamycin (offers coverage for both GAS and *S. aureus*)
Peritonsillar	Adolescent	Fever, unilateral odynophagia, trismus, change in quality of the voice; examination reveals unilateral tonsillar swelling	Clinical. CT neck may be indicated if deeper extension of the abscess is suspected	GAS, *S. aureus*	Clindamycin (offers coverage for both GAS and *S. aureus*)
Lemierre's	All	Tender cord in lateral neck (internal jugular), pain out of proportion to examination, dyspnea	CT neck with contrast; apical slices through the chest may demonstrate septic pulmonary emboli. Blood cultures	*S. aureus*, anaerobes	Vancomycin and metronidazole
Ludwig angina	All	Fever, halitosis, odynophagia, tender regional adenopathy, and a brawny appearance to the floor of the mouth	Clinical. CT neck may be indicated to determine the extent of the infection	Anaerobes	Broad-spectrum antibiotics (e.g., vancomycin and piperacillin/tazobactam)

[a]Empiric treatment should be based upon antibiotic susceptibility patterns in the community and any available prior culture results for the child.
GAS, Group A streptococcus; Hib, *Haemophilus influenzae* type b; CDC, Centers for Disease Control and Prevention; CT, computed tomography.

most feared complication is airway obstruction, but infection into multiple neck planes can result from Ludwig's. Anaerobes, including microaerophilic (nonpneumococcal, non-group A) streptococcal species, are most commonly isolated. Diagnosis is clinical, but imaging by CT can help evaluate the extent of infection. Antibiotics should not be held pending imaging or other diagnostic evaluation. Surgical consultation and admission to a critical care unit are necessary with strong consideration for early endotracheal intubation. Broad-spectrum coverage for aerobes and anaerobes (e.g., clindamycin, piperacillin/tazobactam) should be considered for this fulminant infection. Standard precautions should be used.

Pharyngitis

GAS accounts for 15% to 36% of exudative pharyngitis cases in children and adolescents; the majority of the remaining etiologies are viral. Throat swabs should be obtained from both tonsillar pillars and swabs that first touch the tongue should be discarded, as saliva can result in false-negative rapid streptococcal assay results. Rapid streptococcal assays show variable sensitivity based on the experience of the person collecting the specimen. Reported sensitivities range from 60% to 99%; as such, throat cultures should be sent for all children in whom rapid streptococcal assays are negative. The treatment of choice is amoxicillin or penicillin. There are good data behind the use of a single-daily dose of amoxicillin (50 mg per kg daily, maximum: 1 g per day) for 10 days. For children with difficulty swallowing or in whom nonadherence is a concern, a single intramuscular dose of penicillin should be considered (penicillin G benzathine [Bicillin] ≤27 kg: 600,000 units; >27 kg: 1.2 million units). Regimens for penicillin-allergic patients include cephalosporins and macrolides. There are no data suggesting that the use of cephalosporins decreases the risk of relapse or leads to symptoms resolution faster than more narrow-spectrum antibiotics. Amoxicillin-clavulanate offers no advantages over amoxicillin or penicillin, as there

TABLE 102.13

MOST COMMON CAUSES OF PNEUMONIA BY AGE

Age	Viral	Pyogenic bacteria	Other
<3 wks	CMV RSV hMPV HSV Rubella	Group B streptococcus (*S. agalactiae*) Gram-negative enterics (*E. coli, Klebsiella*) *S. pneumoniae* *S. aureus,* especially in hospitalized neonates	*Bordetella pertussis* *Chlamydia trachomatis* *Mycobacterium hominis* *Treponema pallidum* (syphilis) *Ureaplasma urealyticum*
3 wks–3 mo	RSV hMPV Parainfluenza Adenovirus Influenza	*S. pneumoniae* *S. aureus* *H. influenzae* (nontypeable)	*Bordetella pertussis* *Chlamydia trachomatis*
3 mo–5 yrs	RSV hMPV Parainfluenza Adenovirus Influenza	*S. pneumoniae* *S. pyogenes* (group A streptococcus) *S. aureus*	*Mycoplasma pneumoniae* *Chlamydophila pneumoniae* *Mycobacterium tuberculosis*
5–18 yrs	hMPV Influenza Adenovirus	*S. pneumoniae* *S. pyogenes* (group A streptococcus) *S. aureus*	*Mycoplasma pneumoniae* *Chlamydophila pneumoniae* *Mycobacterium tuberculosis*

CMV, cytomegalovirus; RSV, respiratory syncytial virus; hMPV, human metapneumovirus; HSV, herpes simplex virus.

have been no GAS isolates found to be resistant to beta-lactams. Approximately 5% of U.S. GAS isolates are resistant to macrolides and 20% to 25% to clindamycin. Standard precautions should be used.

LOWER RESPIRATORY TRACT INFECTIOUS EMERGENCIES

Lower respiratory tract infections are one of the most common causes of death in children less than 5 years of age in developing nations. The morbidity of these infections in industrialized nations remains high. The following section will review the diagnosis and management of pneumonia and other common lower respiratory tract infections. Tuberculosis is covered separately later in this chapter in the section on infection in returned travelers, reflecting the epidemiology of this disease in industrialized nations.

Pneumonia

CLINICAL PEARLS AND PITFALLS

- The most common causes of community-acquired pneumonia are viral infections.
- Beyond the neonatal period, the most common bacterial cause is pneumococcus.
- Less common, but more severe bacterial causes of pneumonia include *S. aureus* and GAS.
- While chest radiography can be useful to evaluate for complications of pneumonia, such as empyema or lung abscess, radiographic appearance alone is not useful for differentiating viral from bacterial etiologies.

Current Evidence

The most common causes of pneumonia in different age groups are listed in Table 102.13. Among the bacteria, *S. pneumoniae* predominates at every age beyond the newborn period. Hib formerly ranked second to pneumococcus in children 2 months to 3 years of age but now occurs rarely in countries utilizing the conjugate Hib vaccine. *S. aureus* causes a severe, rapidly progressive but uncommon pneumonia in young children; 60% of these infections occur in the first year of life. GAS is also uncommon but may also be severe, *N. meningitidis* has been described rarely, and anaerobic bacteria play a role primarily following aspiration.

Goals of Treatment

Early recognition of children with respiratory distress and findings consistent with bacterial pneumonia is ideal. The clinical team should be cognizant of indications for imaging other than chest radiographs, as well as what radiographic patterns may be more consistent with certain pathogens. Clinical outcomes for patients with pneumonia include appropriate antibiotic utilization and indications for admission for treatment.

Clinical Considerations

Clinical recognition: Bacterial pneumonia generally has an abrupt onset with fever, often accompanied by chills. A cough is a common but nonspecific complaint. Younger children may have decreased activity level or appetite. Pleuritic chest pain may be seen. The most common examination finding other than pyrexia is tachypnea. The observation of the child at rest before the examination often provides the key to the diagnosis of pneumonia. A hasty effort at auscultation that disturbs the quiet infant obscures this finding. Grunting respirations in a young child should arouse a strong suspicion of pneumonia.

TABLE 102.14

MANAGEMENT OF UNCOMPLICATED COMMUNITY-ACQUIRED PNEUMONIA IN PREVIOUSLY HEALTHY CHILDREN[a]

Age	Outpatient	Inpatient[b]	Other considerations
Neonates	N/A	Ampicillin + third-generation cephalosporin	Consider empiric influenza antiviral therapy in children with moderate–severe pneumonia during influenza season, even if rapid influenza diagnostic test results are negative (these tests are insufficiently sensitive to guide empiric therapy)
Infants	Amoxicillin	Ampicillin	
Preschool aged	Amoxicillin[c]	Ampicillin	
School aged	Amoxicillin + macrolide	Ampicillin + macrolide	
Adolescents	Amoxicillin + macrolide	Ampicillin + macrolide	

[a]Based upon the 2011 Infectious Diseases Society of America and the Pediatric Infectious Diseases Society guidelines for the management of community-acquired pneumonia in children: *Clin Infect Dis* 2011;53(7):e25. Management for children with complicated pneumonia (e.g., empyema, lung abscess) is discussed elsewhere. Unimmunized children should have a third-generation cephalosporin added to ampicillin, for coverage of *H. influenzae* type B.
[b]Vancomycin or clindamycin should be added if there is clinical, laboratory, or radiographic reason to suspect staphylococcal pneumonia; critically ill children should be treated with broad-spectrum antibiotics for pneumonia (e.g., vancomycin and cefotaxime), given that rates of resistant pneumococci are increasing in many industrialized nations.
[c]The guidelines state that antimicrobial therapy is not required routinely for preschool-aged children with community-acquired pneumonia, as the great majority will have a viral etiology.
N/A, not applicable.

Localized findings, more often seen in the child older than 1 year, include inspiratory rales, decreased breath sounds (sometimes the only abnormality), and less often, dullness to percussion. Patients with lower lobe pneumonia may present with abdominal pain; occasionally, the abdominal findings in pulmonary infections mimic appendicitis. With upper lobe pneumonia, the pain may radiate to the neck, causing meningismus; the diagnosis of pneumonia must, therefore, be considered in the child with nuchal rigidity and normal CSF.

Triage considerations: Children with fever and respiratory distress should be evaluated for pneumonia, despite the recognition that only a minority of febrile infants and children with respiratory distress will harbor a bacterial pathogen. Some children with pneumonia will require supplemental oxygen, more advanced airway support, and/or fluid resuscitation.

Clinical assessment: The diagnosis often is made by chest radiograph, which can be falsely negative in dehydrated or neutropenic children. While there are no pathognomonic findings to differentiate viral from bacterial pneumonia, certain patterns in radiographic findings are of use to the PEM clinician. A lobar consolidation is assumed to be of bacterial origin, needing treatment with antibiotics, whereas a minimal, diffuse interstitial infiltrate in a previously healthy toddler suggests a viral infection that can be managed with symptomatic therapy or, in an adolescent, *Mycoplasma pneumoniae,* calling for treatment with erythromycin or azithromycin. Bilateral involvement, pleural effusion, and pneumatoceles point to more severe disease.

Further laboratory studies are obtained only on specific indications. A WBC count may be helpful in differentiating viral from bacterial disease or in assessing the likelihood of bacteremia in the young child. The rate of occult pneumonia in children with leukocytosis >20,000 per mm^3 remains 10% to 15% in the postpneumococcal conjugate vaccine era. An elevated C-reactive protein (CRP) correlates with the bacteremia and lobar infiltrates more closely than the WBC count but is rarely needed. A blood culture is helpful when positive.

The most common complication of pneumonia is dehydration due to decreased intake and increased insensible losses; this is particularly true for young children. Rarely, extensive pulmonary involvement compromises ventilation, leading to respiratory failure. ABGs should be considered for any child with significant respiratory distress or transcutaneous oxygen saturation below 90%. The most common causes of parapneumonic effusions are pneumococcus and staphylococcus. Bacteremia may result in additional foci of infection, including meningitis, pericarditis, epiglottitis, and septic arthritis.

Management: The PEM physician should consider whether or not the child is a candidate for outpatient therapy (e-Table 102.7). Professional societies have formulated consensus guidelines on which children can be classified as moderate or severe pneumonia and may benefit from intensive care unit care (e-Table 102.8). Empiric antibiotic management is reviewed in Table 102.14. Immunocompromised children should receive broad-spectrum antibiotics, including pseudomonal coverage. The management of children with complicated pneumonia is described elsewhere in the sections on empyema and lung abscess. Standard precautions should be utilized for children with suspected community-acquired pneumonia.

Other Respiratory Tract Infectious Emergencies

Tracheitis

Bacterial tracheitis is predominantly caused by *S. aureus* in the post-Hib vaccine era. It can mimic the presentation of epiglottitis (see above) with a rapid course. While children present with fever and stridor, they are more toxic appearing than children with croup and are in more respiratory distress. Radiographs may reveal tracheal narrowing and direct laryngoscopy may demonstrate a pseudomembrane. The first step in management is to secure the airway; the emergency medicine physician should anticipate that intubation may be difficult; if anesthesiologist or otolaryngology support is available at a facility, consideration should be given to having them at the bedside prior to intubation being attempted. Broad-spectrum antibiotics (e.g., vancomycin and ceftriaxone) should be started and the child should be admitted to an intensive care unit. Standard precautions should be used.

Empyema

Empyemas are purulent pleural effusions that can complicate pneumonia. Empyemas are most commonly seen with *S. aureus* and pneumococcal pneumonia and increasing incidence rates of staphylococcal pneumonia have been seen in the post-Prevnar era. Gram-negative pathogens should be suspected in immunocompromised hosts, neonates, and patients with indwelling chest tubes. The most common symptoms are fever, shortness of breath, and pleuritic chest pain. The most common examination finding is tachypnea; auscultation can reveal rales or decreased breath sound. Pleural friction rubs are rarely heard in young children. Chest radiography demonstrates blunting of the costophrenic angle. A decubitus or cross-table lateral radiograph can be performed to see if the fluid is free-flowing. Ultrasonography can be very useful to determine if sufficient fluid is present for thoracentesis; for older children, a decubitus fluid layer at least 1 cm thick is considered sufficient to attempt thoracentesis. CT allows for better differentiation between an empyema and lung abscess. Thoracentesis for pleural fluid can be sent for cell count and differential, lactate dehydrogenase (LDH), protein, glucose, and pH in addition to Gram stain and cultures. Cultures that should be obtained include aerobic, anaerobic, and acid-fast cultures. Adenosine deaminase (ADA) should be sent from the pleural fluid if tuberculosis is suspected. The pleural fluid parameters that help differentiate causes of pleural effusion are reviewed in e-Table 102.9. Some children with empyema will need video-assisted thoracoscopic surgery with debridement; this has been shown to decrease hospital length of stay and fever duration. Empiric antibiotic therapy should target pneumococcus, *S. aureus,* and GAS. For mildly ill patients, ampicillin and azithromycin treatment for community-acquired pneumonia may be appropriate. For children with risk for staphylococcal disease (e.g., history of staphylococcal disease, presence of pneumatocele), combination therapy with clindamycin and a third-generation cephalosporin is reasonable. Critically ill children should be treated with vancomycin and a third-generation cephalosporin. Anaerobic coverage should be considered for neonates, immunocompromised hosts, associated neck infections (especially with jugular thrombophlebitis), and patients with indwelling chest tubes. Standard precautions are recommended for children with empyema unless tuberculosis is suspected (in which case, airborne precautions should be used) or unless the child has draining skin lesions (in which case contact precautions should be utilized).

Lung Abscess

Most lung abscesses are polymicrobial and caused by aspiration of oral flora, especially in patients with underlying neurologic disorders. The predominant anaerobes are *Bacteroides, Peptostreptococcus,* and *Prevotella.* Anaerobes, *S. aureus,* pneumococcus, and nontypeable *H. influenzae* are the most common pathogens identified in otherwise healthy children. Fungal pathogens and *Pseudomonas* should be considered in immunocompromised children. *M. tuberculosis* will be discussed separately in the section on travel medicine. The most common symptoms are fever, cough, shortness of breath, and chest pain. Symptoms have often been present for up to 2 to 3 weeks before the child is recognized to have a lung abscess; as a consequence, weight loss is seen in some children, whereas it is an uncommon occurrence for children with community-acquired pneumonia. Auscultation of the lungs is often nonfocal, particularly in young children. The diagnosis usually is made by chest radiograph, which can show a thin- or thick-walled cavity with an air–fluid level. Intrathoracic adenopathy can be found in more subacute causes of lung abscess (e.g., tuberculosis, fungal). CT can be of use if operative intervention is planned to better delineate the anatomy. Leukocytosis with a neutrophilic predominance is common; blood cultures are positive in 10% to 15% of cases. Gram stain of the sputum is rarely useful unless the abscess has ruptured into a bronchus and is communicating with the airway. Percutaneous aspiration or bronchoscopy is more sensitive in yielding a microbiologic diagnosis. Empiric antibiotic coverage should target *S. aureus,* pneumococcus, and anaerobes. Clindamycin and cefotaxime is one such regimen, with the advantage that it can be readily converted from a parenteral regimen to oral equivalents. However, for toxic-appearing children, or in regions where cephalosporin-resistant pneumococci or clindamycin-resistant staphylococci are commonly seen, vancomycin should be included in the initial regimen. Standard precautions should be used for patients with lung abscesses unless tuberculosis is suspected (in which case, airborne precautions should be implemented).

Pertussis

Pertussis (whooping cough) is caused by *Bordetella pertussis* or *Bordetella parapertussis* (the latter being the cause of kennel cough in dogs). A similar clinical syndrome can be caused by adenovirus or *Chlamydia trachomatis* in infants. There are three clinical stages. The first symptoms are indistinguishable from a viral URI. This catarrhal phase, characterized by a mild cough, conjunctivitis, and coryza, lasts for 1 to 2 weeks. An increasingly severe cough heralds the onset of the second stage (paroxysmal), which continues for 2 to 4 weeks. After a prolonged spasm of coughing often involving 10 or more coughs in succession, the sudden inflow of air produces the characteristic whoop (young infants lack the ability to generate sufficient negative inspiratory pressure and may, therefore, not whoop). During episodes, children can appear to choke, become cyanotic, and appear anxious. Posttussive emesis is common. When not coughing, the child has a remarkably normal history and physical examination, except for an occasional subconjunctival hemorrhage. Young infants can exhibit apnea unrelated to coughing paroxysms. During the third stage (convalescent), the intensity of the cough wanes. At times, pertussis may present as a chronic cough without other signs of infection. The fatality rate for pertussis is approximately 1% for patients in the first month of life and 0.3% for those between age 2 and 12 months. Complications often occur during the paroxysmal stage. The most immediately life-threatening complication is complete obstruction of the airway by a mucous plug, leading to respiratory arrest. Secondary bacterial pneumonia occurs in 25% of children with pertussis and accounts for 90% of the fatalities. Seizures are seen in 3%, and encephalitis in 1%. Sudden increases in intrathoracic pressure can cause intracranial hemorrhages, rupture of the diaphragm, and rectal prolapse.

The white blood count often is elevated, at times with a leukemoid reaction (the latter more common in infants over 6 months of age) and a lymphocytic predominance. Chest radiographs often are normal. The diagnosis is by PCR of nasopharyngeal secretions. Early treatment can reduce symptoms and shorten the clinical course although it is unclear if antibiotics influence course during paroxysmal phase (does still reduce transmission); however, it is important to start antibiotic treatment when pertussis is suspected and prior to confirmatory testing. The preferred treatment is azithromycin (10 mg per kg on the first day, followed by 5 mg per kg on days 2 to 5). Erythromycin (40 mg/kg/day divided every 6 to 8 hours × 14 days, maximum dose: 2 g per day) can also be utilized, though the more frequent dosing interval (every 6 to 8 hours) and longer treatment duration may be associated with reduced adherence. Household and close contacts (even if fully immunized) require chemoprophylaxis with either azithromycin (10 mg per kg daily for 5 days, maximum dose: 500 mg) or erythromycin (same regimen as treatment dose). Contacts who are not fully immunized should also receive a booster dose of the vaccine (DTaP for children <7 years of age, TDaP for children 7 years and above). Receipt of the acellular pertussis vaccine does not obviate the need for postexposure prophylaxis (PEP) for healthcare workers, so strict use of droplet precautions (gloves, mask) is needed for any provider caring for a child with suspected pertussis.

CARDIAC INFECTIOUS EMERGENCIES

Kawasaki Disease

See also:
Chapter 94 Cardiac Emergencies
Chapter 109 Rheumatologic Emergencies

CLINICAL PEARLS AND PITFALLS

- Kawasaki disease (KD) is the most common form of acquired heart disease in children in industrialized nations.
- KD is a clinical diagnosis in a child with fever to 102°F for at least 5 days who has four of five additional symptoms: oral mucosal changes; rash; nonpurulent conjunctivitis; extremity changes; and cervical lymphadenopathy.
- Incomplete KD, where children do not meet all the diagnostic criteria, is more common in young infants, and is a risk factor for the development of coronary artery aneurysms (CAAs).

Current Evidence

KD is a vasculitic condition of unknown etiology that can cause CAAs or ectasia in up to 25% of untreated children. It is the most common form of acquired heart disease in American children. While first described in Japanese children, it occurs in children of all races and ethnicities and is most common in infants and preschool-aged children.

Goals of Treatment

The goal of treatment is to recognize and initiate treatment in children with KD before the 10th day of symptoms, as delayed treatment increases the risk of CAA development.

Clinical Considerations

Clinical recognition: The symptoms of KD are summarized in Table 102.15. Incomplete KD, in which a child does not meet all diagnostic criteria, is more common in infants and rates of CAA are higher in children with incomplete KD. It is important that clinicians ask all caregivers of children with fever of at least 5 days duration about KD symptoms. Not all symptoms may be present at the time of ED presentation. The differential diagnosis of KD is extensive and includes viral infections (especially adenovirus, but can also include EBV, cytomegalovirus [CMV]), scarlet fever, staphylococcal-scalded skin syndrome, TSS, rickettsial diseases (e.g., RMSF), leptospirosis, drug hypersensitivity reactions, and some rheumatologic conditions.

Triage considerations: Children with KD can be intravascularly depleted from insensible losses from several days of high fever. Fluid resuscitation may be needed in the ED. If there is concern for cardiac function based upon examination (e.g., murmur, hepatomegaly), fluid resuscitation should proceed cautiously and early cardiac imaging (or a baseline electrocardiogram) should be obtained.

Clinical assessment: Supporting laboratory criteria are described in Table 102.24.

Management: The treatment for KD is intravenous immunoglobulin (IVIG) at 2 g per kg as a single dose given over 10 to 12 hours. In addition, children should be started on high-dose aspirin (80 to 100 mg/kg/day divided every 6 hours). An echocardiogram should be ordered. A clinician's threshold for treating should be lower as a child approaches day 10 of fever than it is at day 5. Standard precautions should be used.

Other Cardiac Infectious Emergencies

Goals of Treatment

ED recognition of new cardiac infections is poor, especially in the child without pre-existing structural heart disease. For example, most children with myocarditis are missed at the time of initial ED presentation. Recognition of children at risk for endocarditis, as well as the most common manifestations of myocarditis and pericarditis, can prevent the ED physician from inadvertently worsening cardiac function from rapid fluid resuscitation.

CLINICAL PEARLS AND PITFALLS

- Infective endocarditis is most common in children with structural heart disease, but increased rates of *S. aureus* endocarditis in children with normal heart valves have recently been described.
- The most common sign of myocarditis is unexplained tachycardia.
- The chest radiograph in a child with pericarditis and a large pericardial effusion may be normal.
- Bedside ultrasound can provide rapid assessment for pericardial effusion and contractility.

Endocarditis

Endocarditis is an infection of cardiac valves most commonly caused by *S. aureus*, viridans streptococci, the so-called HACEK organisms (*Haemophilus noninfluenzae* species, *Actinobacillus*

TABLE 102.15

CLINICAL AND LABORATORY FINDINGS IN KAWASAKI DISEASE

Feature		Details	Frequency	Caveats
Clinical (need fever + four of five other clinical criteria)	Fever ≥5 days	At least 102°F/38.8°C daily; KD cannot be diagnosed in the absence of fever	100%	Can diagnose KD after 4 days if a child meets all clinical criteria
	Oral mucosal changes	Erythema, cracking, or bleeding of lips; strawberry tongue, erythema of oral mucosa	95–98%	Ulcerative or exudative lesions are not consistent with KD
	Conjunctival injection	Bulbar conjunctival injection with perilimbic sparing	90–95%	Purulent conjunctivitis is not consistent with KD
	Rash	Polymorphous, late desquamation	90–95%	Rash can have any appearance except bullous or vesicular
	Extremity changes	Firm, tender or painless induration to hands and/or feet; periungal desquamation occurs 1–3 wks after fever onset	80–90%	1–2 mo later, can see Beau lines on nails
	Cervical adenopathy	At least one node needs to be ≥1.5 cm in diameter; nodes usually in anterior cervical chain, unilateral, and nontender or minimally tender	70–80%	The least common finding in KD
Laboratory	WBC	Often >15,000 cells/μL	50%	Predominance of neutrophils and bands
	Hemoglobin	Normocytic anemia is common	Common	Anemia requiring intervention is rare
	Platelets	Thrombocytosis common (usually >450,000/mm^3 after the 7th day of illness); peaks in 3rd week	Very common	Thrombocytopenia is a risk factor for coronary artery aneurysms
	ESR/CRP	Acutely elevated (ESR ≥40 mm/hr, CRP ≥3 mg/dL); usually normalize by 6–8 wks	Almost 100%	ESR will be falsely elevated after IVIG
	AST/ALT	Transaminitis with AST/ALT in low 100s U/L	40%	GGT elevated in 67%
	Bilirubin	Hyperbilirubinemia; no evidence of synthetic hepatic dysfunction	10%	Indirect hyperbilirubinemia
	Albumin	Hypoalbuminemia ≤3 g/dL	Common	Hypoalbuminemia worsens with increased symptom duration
	Urinalysis	Sterile pyuria (≥10 WBC/HPF)	3–5%	Likely due to urethritis, as suprapubic aspirates show no pyuria
	CSF WBC	Sterile pleocytosis seen in 50% of KD children who receive a lumbar puncture; normal protein and glucose	50%	Monocytic predominance

KD, Kawasaki disease; WBC, white blood count; ESR, erythrocyte sedimentation rate; CRP, C-reactive protein; IVIG, intravenous immunoglobulin; AST, aspartate aminotransferase; ALT, alanine aminotransferase; GGT, gammaglutamyl transpeptidase; HPF, high-power field.

actinomycetemcomitans, Cardiobacterium hominis, Eikenella corrodens, and *Kingella kingae*), and *Coxiella* (Q-fever). Endocarditis is more common in children with existing structural heart disease. The most common symptoms are fever, chills, fatigue, myalgias, and examination and laboratory findings may include evidence of embolic phenomenon (pulmonary infarcts, intracranial or subconjunctival hemorrhages), Janeway lesions (nontender hemorrhagic macules on palms/soles), immunologic phenomenon (glomerulonephritis, Osler nodes [red, tender raised lesions on palms/soles], or Roth spots [white-centered retinal hemorrhages]). The diagnosis is based on the modified Duke criteria, which combine major criteria (blood culture positivity with an organism known to cause endocarditis; echocardiogram findings) with minor criteria, which include predisposing structural heart disease, fever, and embolic or immunologic phenomenon. ED-based diagnosis involves obtaining several large-volume blood cultures before antibiotics are initiated to optimize culture yield. The laboratory should be instructed to hold the blood cultures for several weeks, as some of the organisms causing endocarditis are fastidious and require long periods to grow. Empiric management in the critically ill child with suspected endocarditis should cover MRSA and Gram-negative organisms (e.g., vancomycin and cefotaxime). Standard precautions should be used.

Myocarditis

Myocarditis is a variably painful inflammation of the myocardium primarily caused by viral infections, most commonly enteroviruses, but parvovirus, influenza, parainfluenza, and adenovirus, and other viruses can also cause myocarditis. In children with a consistent travel history, Chagas disease (*Trypanosoma cruzi*) and parasitic infections can also cause myocarditis. Myocarditis has been found in 15% to 20% of sudden infant death syndrome victims and the same proportion of adolescents who suffer from sudden cardiac death. Early symptoms mimic the nonspecific findings of viral infections; the most common symptoms are shortness of breath, vomiting, poor feeding, rhinorrhea, and fever. Chest pain is more commonly verbalized by older children. The most common examination findings are tachypnea, hepatomegaly, fever, and crackles. Findings may become more obvious after a child receives fluid boluses, emphasizing the importance of serial examinations between fluid boluses. EKGs are abnormal in over 90% of patients; the most common EKG findings are sinus tachycardia, low-voltage QRS complexes, and T-wave inversion. Chest radiographs are abnormal in 60% to 90% of children, most commonly showing cardiomegaly and pulmonary edema. Laboratory evaluation should include troponin, creatine kinase MB, B-type natriuretic peptide (BNP), and early cardiology intervention should be sought. Standard precautions should be used.

Pericarditis is caused by a more heterogeneous group of pathogens (enterovirus being the primary viral etiology, while pneumococcus, meningococcus, *S. aureus,* and tuberculosis are among the more common bacterial causes). Rheumatologic disorders, uremia, pancreatitis, and other noninfectious etiologies can also result in pericardial inflammation. Symptoms are nonspecific and include fever, cough, shortness of breath, abdominal pain, and vomiting. Chest pain is an early finding and is worst over the precordium, may radiate to the left shoulder, is worse when supine, and better when the child is sitting upright or leaning forward. Examination findings include a pericardial friction rub, muffled heart tones, tachycardia, jugular venous distension (JVD), and narrowed pulse pressures. Pulsus paradoxus, where the systolic blood pressure decreases by >10 mm Hg with inspiration, is concerning for tamponade physiology. Beck triad is pathognomonic for tamponade: JVD, muffled heart sounds, and hypotension. EKGs are abnormal in >90%. Diffuse ST elevation is seen first, followed by ST depression and PR decrease, then normalization of intervals with T-wave inversions. As the pericardial effusion increases, QRS voltages are dampened and there may be evidence of electrical alternans. The chest radiograph often is normal in pericarditis, as it is estimated that an effusion has to be at least 250 mL (adult) before being apparent on plain radiograph. Early cardiology intervention and echocardiogram is critical. Nonsteroidal anti-inflammatory drugs are the mainstay of pericarditis treatment. Children with tamponade physiology may require pericardiocentesis. Standard precautions should be used.

GASTROINTESTINAL INFECTIOUS EMERGENCIES

Gastroenteritis is an inflammation of the alimentary tract that, in its acute form, is overwhelmingly infectious in origin. Viruses are the organisms most commonly found in children with diarrhea in the United States and can be isolated from approximately 30% of patients. In 10% of patients, bacteria are recovered, including *Salmonella, Shigella, Campylobacter, Yersinia,* and pathogenic *E. coli; Aeromonas hydrophila* and *Vibrio* species, such as *Plesiomonas shigelloides,* are occasional pathogens. *Clostridium difficile,* which elaborates a toxin, may cause colitis, particularly after the use of antibiotics. Parasitic infestations rarely lead to diarrhea in developed countries. *Giardia lamblia* and *Cryptosporidium* should be considered, particularly in outbreaks in daycare centers, and *Entamoeba histolytica,* among immigrants or travelers from tropical areas; cryptosporidiosis also commonly affects patients with HIV. These topics are covered later in this chapter, in the sections on travel medicine and HIV, respectively. Current diagnostic techniques are unable to identify an etiologic agent in most of the remaining episodes.

Viral hepatitis is covered in Chapter 99 Gastrointestinal Emergencies. Bacterial infections of the liver and bacterial cholangitis, almost exclusively abscesses, are rare in otherwise healthy children; more commonly, they complicate either an anatomic malformation (e.g., biliary atresia) or affect neonates or immunocompromised hosts.

Because calculi in the bile ducts rarely occur before adolescence, cholecystitis occurs much less often in children than in adults. Occasionally, episodes are seen in teenagers or children predisposed to stone formation, as in the chronic hemolytic anemias. Less commonly, salmonellosis, leptospirosis, or KD produces acalculous cholecystitis. These diseases are discussed elsewhere in this chapter.

In childhood, peritonitis almost invariably reflects an intra-abdominal catastrophe that requires surgical intervention. However, the accumulation of ascitic fluid in children with diseases such as nephrosis and cirrhosis allows the development of a primary infection of the peritoneum.

Gastroenteritis—Viral

The most common etiologies of acute gastroenteritis (AGE) in the United States are viral, most commonly noroviruses and rotavirus, which comprise almost 40% of viral AGE in the United States. Rotavirus has been on a major decline since the introduction of routine vaccination. Please also see Chapter 18 Diarrhea. Adenovirus, sapovirus, astrovirus, parechovirus, and bocavirus comprise an additional 30% of cases in preschool-aged children. Most causes of viral gastroenteritis are self-limited in healthy children; however, young children can shed viruses in feces for weeks to months after acute infection, contributing to secondary spread in the community. The most common symptoms are diarrhea and/or vomiting, crampy abdominal pain, and fever. Signs on examination may include pyrexia, tachycardia, and hyperactive bowel sounds. Hematochezia and high fever in the older child may suggest a bacterial etiology, as would a history of international travel to a developing nation. No laboratory studies are indicated in uncomplicated gastroenteritis in the previously healthy child with mild dehydration. Stools WBC or stool lactoferrin is more indicative of a bacterial pathogen.

Gastroenteritis—Bacterial

Five bacterial pathogens commonly produce gastroenteritis: *Salmonella, Shigella, Yersinia, Campylobacter,* and pathogenic *E. coli* (*Campylobacter,* typhoid fever, and pathogenic *E. coli* are discussed in the travel medicine section of this chapter).

Together, these organisms cause approximately 10% of the diarrheal illnesses seen in children coming to the ED. In underdeveloped countries and occasionally in the United States, *Vibrio* species must also be considered. In addition, *A. hydrophila* has been associated occasionally with diarrheal illnesses in children. *C. difficile* causes toxin-associated colitis, particularly in patients who receive antibiotics.

Salmonella, Shigella, Yersinia, and *Campylobacter* do not normally inhabit the alimentary tract. Thus, recovery of one of these organisms suffices for the diagnosis of gastroenteritis. *E. coli,* however, is part of the normal bowel flora, only occasionally assuming a pathogenic role. Serotyping is useful for detecting *E. coli* O157:H7, which along with related strains is capable of inducing hemolytic uremic syndrome (HUS), but identification of other disease-producing strains is not readily available to the clinician.

Hemolytic Uremic Syndrome

Shiga toxin-producing *E. coli* (STEC) can cause HUS and colitis. The most common serotype causing HUS in the United States is *E. coli* O157:H7, but *Shigella, Campylobacter,* and pneumococcus have also been associated with HUS. The pathogen is spread via fecal–oral transmission, and recent cases have been linked to contaminated fruits and vegetables, undercooked beef, and use of community pools. While HUS is rare, the morbidity and mortality are substantial and the disease can be difficult to diagnose in the early stages. Children present with bloody diarrhea, hematuria, oliguria, and altered mental status 5 to 10 days after exposure. Laboratory findings include elevated BUN and creatinine, thrombocytopenia, and anemia. The CDC case definition specifies that anemia must be accompanied by microangiopathic changes (e.g., schistocytes, burr cells, or helmet cells on peripheral smear), and that renal involvement may consist of hematuria, proteinuria, and elevated creatinine (≥1 mg per dL in children <13 years of age and ≥1.5 mg per dL in older children). Thrombocytopenia, not part of the case definition, is an early finding and may resolve within a week. Atypical HUS is associated with certain genetic anomalies of complement activation, is associated with multiorgan system involvement (myocardial infarction, hepatitis, pancreatitis), more severe renal disease, and worse prognosis than typical infectious HUS. Treatment historically has been supportive. Antibiotic use in children with *E. coli* O157:H7 colitis was thought to increase risk of progression to HUS, but meta-analyses have not borne out this association; they also did not show that antibiotic use was beneficial. Use of antimotility agents is discouraged. Early hydration during the diarrheal phase may have benefit. Early involvement of nephrology and admission is essential, as some children will progress to severe anemia and renal failure requiring careful management of fluids, electrolytes, and potentially dialysis. Platelet transfusion should only be performed for life-threatening bleeding. Eculizumab, a monoclonal antibody that decreases complement system activation, has been used in atypical HUS, severe HUS, and to prevent relapses. Standard and contact precautions should be used for children with HUS.

Nontyphi *Salmonella*

Nontyphoidal *Salmonella* serotypes are spread via consumption of infected animal products (e.g., poultry, dairy, eggs); non-human mammals, reptiles, amphibians, and birds serve as reservoirs (typhoid fever is discussed in the travel medicine section of this chapter). These are one of the most common food-borne pathogens reported in the United States, estimated to cause 1.2 million illnesses annually. The following patients are at higher risk for nontyphi salmonellosis: children younger than 4 years of age; the elderly; sickle cell disease patients or patients with functional or anatomic asplenia; HIV-infected persons; and immunosuppressed or immunocompromised persons. *Salmonella* can cause asymptomatic carriage, mild to severe gastroenteritis, and extraintestinal disease (osteomyelitis, CNS disease). Bacteremia can be seen in children with *Salmonella* gastroenteritis, and up to 10% will develop focal extraintestinal infections. The organism can be cultured from blood, stool, or CSF. Scenarios under which children with nontyphi *Salmonella* require treatment are reviewed in e-Table 102.10. Increasing rates of amoxicillin, TMP-SMZ, and fluoroquinolone resistance have been reported in Asia. Azithromycin remains a viable option for children with uncomplicated salmonellosis. Contact precautions should be used for incontinent children. Of note, preschool-aged children can excrete the organism in the stool for weeks to months after initial infection.

Shigella

Shigellosis is caused by several species in the *Shigella* genus; the most common species in the United States are *Shigella sonnei* and *Shigella flexneri.* These are Gram-negative rods spread via fecal–oral transmission. Risk factors for infection include daycare attendees and their caregivers; international travel, especially to Africa and Asia; HIV-infected patients with CD4+ cell counts <200 per mm^3; and men who have sex with men. It is estimated that over 500,000 cases of shigellosis occur in the United States annually. *Shigella* can cause asymptomatic infections, mild disease (watery stools in the absence of constitutional symptoms), dysentery, or extraintestinal manifestations. Dysentery is characterized by fever and abdominal pain which precede the diarrhea. Stools may contain mucus and blood. A *Shigella* infection may produce CNS irritation or seizures because of the release of toxin before the onset of diarrhea; as such, shigellosis must be on the differential of a child with meningismus without a CSF pleocytosis.

Bandemia, even in the absence of leukocytosis, in a child with dysentery should increase the provider's suspicion for shigellosis. *Shigella* grows readily in standard stool cultures; fecal leukocytes often are present. While treatment may not be indicated for mild shigellosis, it has been shown to decrease shedding of the organism in stool (potentially preventing secondary spread) and decreasing diarrheal duration. Treatment is recommended for patients with bacteremia or other severe disease, for dysentery, and for immunocompromised children. Amoxicillin and TMP-SMZ resistance is common, and oral cephalosporins are not useful for treating shigellosis. Parenteral macrolides or cephalosporins are recommended for empiric therapy of shigellosis if antibiotic susceptibilities are not available. While fluoroquinolones are beneficial, they are not recommended for children. Resistance to macrolides and fluoroquinolones has been reported in several U.S. outbreaks. Antidiarrheals are not recommended. Malnourished children should also receive vitamin A (200,000 IU as a single dose) and zinc (10 to 20 mg daily for 10 to 14 days). Contact precautions are recommended.

Antibiotic-associated Colitis

While many children receiving antibiotics develop diarrhea, *C. difficile* infection is rare in children. However, it has increased twofold between the mid-1990s and the mid-2000s in hospitalized children in the United States. *C. difficile* is a Gram-positive, toxin-producing anaerobic rod that is the causative agent of pseudomembranous colitis. The most common antibiotics associated with *C. difficile* in children reflect antibiotics most commonly used in the outpatient setting: penicillins, cephalosporins, clindamycin, and macrolides. Other risk factors include use of feeding tubes, proton pump inhibitors, immunocompromised, and recent hospitalization.

Colitis with *C. difficile* varies widely in severity. Typically, profuse watery or mucoid diarrhea begins after several days of antibiotic therapy. Many older children complain of crampy abdominal pain. On examination, the usual findings include fever and diffuse abdominal tenderness. Often, the WBC count rises above 15,000 per mm^3. The stool may be guaiac-positive or frankly bloody; leukocytes (by stool microscopy or by measuring stool lactoferrin) are found in approximately 50% of patients. An etiologic diagnosis requires the identification of *C. difficile* toxin in the stool; recovery of the organism on culture is suggestive but not sufficient. The diagnosis is more difficult in children less than 2 years of age, who can have asymptomatic intestinal colonization by toxogenic *C. difficile.* If *C. difficile* colitis goes unrecognized and untreated, complications, including toxic megacolon, perforation, and peritonitis, may develop. Case fatality rates as high as 10% to 20% were described before the introduction of specific treatments.

Treatment of asymptomatic carriers is not recommended. Mild cases without fever or other systemic signs of infection may resolve with discontinuation of the inciting antibiotic(s) and supportive care. Treatment of moderate to severe infection, defined as pyrexia, voluminous diarrhea, dehydration, colitis, or leukocytosis, warrants systemic therapy.

Oral metronidazole (30 mg/kg/day in four divided doses; maximum: 2 g per day) is the first-line choice for initial treatment of mild/moderate disease and for treatment of the first relapse. Oral vancomycin (40 mg/kg/day in four divided doses; maximum: 500 mg to 2 g per day) or vancomycin administered per rectum (500 mg in 100 mL of 0.9% normal saline administered four times daily with 30 to 60 minutes retention through clamping of catheter) combined with intravenous metronidazole is recommended for severe disease, for patient with ileus, and for patients who do not respond to metronidazole monotherapy. Treatment should continue at least 10 days. Relapses are seen in up to one-quarter of children after therapy is discontinued. Antidiarrheal agents should be avoided. Contact precautions should be used. Alcohol-based hand hygiene products do not kill spores; instead, providers should wash their hands with soap and water.

Intra-abdominal Abscesses

The most common cause of intra-abdominal abscesses in childhood will be from perforated appendicitis. Blood cultures rarely are positive unless the child is immunocompromised or toxic-appearing. These infections are polymicrobial, and cultures often grow a combination of Gram-negative enterics and anaerobes. As such, broad-spectrum antimicrobial coverage should be offered. The Infectious Disease Society of America has published guidelines for empiric therapy for children with complicated intra-abdominal infections. Monotherapy has been found to be equivalent in terms of outcomes to combination therapy. Single-agent regimens include ticarcillin-clavulanate, piperacillin-tazobactam, and carbapenems (meropenem, imipenem-cilastin, and ertapenem) for children with community-acquired infections. Recommended multidrug regimens include a third-generation cephalosporin with metronidazole; metronidazole or clindamycin with an aminoglycoside, with or without ampicillin.

GENITOURINARY INFECTIOUS EMERGENCIES

Urinary tract infections (UTIs) and renal abscesses are discussed in this section. The diagnosis and management of children with pelvic inflammatory disease are covered in Chapter 100 Gynecology Emergencies.

Urinary Tract Infections

CLINICAL PEARLS AND PITFALLS

- The most common pathogen causing UTIs is *E. coli;* in many regions, over 50% of *E. coli* isolates from the urinary tract are resistant to amoxicillin and/or TMP-SMZ.
- UTIs are on the differential diagnosis of fever of unknown origin and of failure to thrive in infants.
- Most children outside the neonatal period who have UTIs can be managed in the outpatient setting.
- Isolation of *S. aureus* from a urinary culture should prompt evaluation for a renal abscess.

Current Evidence

Infections occur along the urinary tract from the tip of the urethra to the renal parenchyma. Clinical syndromes that may accompany infections include urethritis, cystitis, and pyelonephritis. *Bacteriuria* refers to the presence of bacteria in the urine, arising from any site in the urinary tract, with or without symptoms. Significant bacteriuria describes the presence of bacteria in sufficient quantity such that infection is more likely than contamination or colonization. Significant bacteriuria may be asymptomatic, and the clinical syndromes mentioned previously may occur in the absence of infection. Because cystitis and pyelonephritis may coexist or be difficult to distinguish clinically and share a similar etiology, they are discussed together, using the common term *UTI*.

The predominant pathogen isolated in UTIs is *E. coli,* which is recovered in 90% of cases. Next in frequency are other members of the Enterobacteriaceae family, including *Enterobacter* and *Klebsiella.* Among the Gram-positive organisms, enterococci are seen at all ages, staphylococcal species (*Staphylococcus saprophyticus*) occur most often in adolescents, and group B streptococci are recovered primarily in infants and during pregnancy. *P. aeruginosa, C. albicans,* and a number of other bacteria and fungi infect patients with immunocompromise, anatomic obstruction, or indwelling catheters. Cystitis may be caused, in addition, by adenoviruses. *S. aureus* is not a common pathogen unless there is bacteremia, urinary tract abnormality, or indwelling hardware.

The frequency of infections of the urinary tract varies by age, gender, and race (e-Table 102.11). Overall, infections occur commonly in neonates, decrease in frequency during childhood, and then rise in incidence after puberty in sexually active females. Males are more commonly infected than females in the first 6 months of life, in part because of a higher incidence of congenital urinary tract anomalies, but they rarely acquire infections beyond this period unless uncircumcised and even these infections are uncommon beyond a year of age. Females have a rather high incidence of symptomatic infection between 6 months and 2 years of age and of asymptomatic bacteriuria throughout childhood. Children with UTIs have a higher incidence of genitourinary anomalies than the general population, although in most infections, no anatomic or functional abnormalities are identified.

Goals of Treatment

Treatment begins with the recognition of which children are at risk for UTIs. The clinical team should consider prior culture results and regional antibiotic susceptibility patterns for children with urinalyses consistent with UTIs.

Clinical Considerations

Clinical recognition: The manifestations of UTIs vary with age, being particularly nonspecific in infancy. In neonates, a septic appearance or fever is often the only finding. UTIs in infants may also cause vomiting, diarrhea, and irritability. Beyond 2 to 3 years of age, symptoms more often localize to the urinary tract. Differentiation between upper and lower tract disease in children, as compared to adults, is not feasible for the clinician. In most cases, children who are febrile (greater than or equal to 38.5°C [101.3°F]) should be assumed to have pyelonephritis. However, some patients will have typical syndromes that localize disease to the upper or lower tract. Typically, children with cystitis appear relatively well and complain of dysuria and suprapubic pain. On examination, they have a lower-grade fever and tenderness on the suprapubic area. In contrast, patients with pyelonephritis may be toxic and usually have additional symptoms, including vomiting and flank pain. The physician is often able to elicit tenderness to percussion in the costovertebral area, either unilaterally or bilaterally.

Triage considerations: Young children (girls <2 years of age, circumcised boys <6 months of age, uncircumcised boys <12 months of age), children with a history of UTIs, and children with known anatomic anomalies that would predispose to UTIs should be evaluated for UTIs if they present with fever without localizing source and/or dysuria. Tachycardia may be the first sign of urosepsis.

Clinical assessment: The diagnosis of UTI usually is based on urinalysis in the ED. The performance characteristics of various aspects of the urinalysis are reviewed in Table 102.16. Either spun or unspun urine may be studied through the microscope, with or without the aid of a Gram stain. Urine culture should be obtained in any child in whom a UTI is suspected, as some young infants will not develop pyuria in response to a UTI and the urinalysis may be falsely negative. Urine cultures are documented in terms of colony counts (Table 102.17).

Bacteremia accompanies UTIs primarily during the first 12 months of life. In the very young infant, bacteremia may be present in the absence of fever and should be suspected in any child during the first year of life with a temperature ≥102.2°F. Indications for a CBC count and blood culture with a suspected UTI include (i) signs of clinical toxicity (extreme tachycardia, low blood pressure, shaking chills); (ii) age

TABLE 102.16

PERFORMANCE CHARACTERISTICS OF URINALYSIS VARIABLES

Test	Sensitivity (range), %	Specificity (range), %
Leukocyte esterase	83 (67–94)	78 (64–92)
Nitrite	53 (15–82)	98 (90–100)
Either leukocyte esterase or nitrite positive	93 (90–100)	72 (58–91)
Microscopy (WBC/HPF)	73 (32–100)	81 (45–98)
Microscopy (bacteria)	81 (16–99)	83 (11–100)
Leukocyte esterase, nitrite, or microscopy positive	99.8 (99–100)	70 (60–92)

WBC, white blood count; HPF, high-power field.
From The Subcommittee on Urinary Tract Infection. Urinary tract infection: clinical practice guideline for the diagnosis and management of the initial UTI in febrile infants and children 2 to 24 months. *Pediatrics* 2011;128:595.

TABLE 102.17

CRITERIA FOR THE DIAGNOSIS OF A URINARY TRACT INFECTION BY CULTURE

Source	Colony count (pure culture)	Probability of infection
Suprapubic aspiration	Gram-negative rods: any	99%
	Gram-positive cocci ≥1,000	99%
Transurethral catheterization	≥100,000	95%
	10,000–100,000	Infection likely
	1,000–10,000	Suspicious: repeat
	≤1,000	Infection unlikely
	≥10,000	Infection likely
Clean void: boy	≥10,000	Infection likely
Clean void: girl	three specimens ≥100,000	95%
	two specimens ≥100,000	90%
	one specimen ≥100,000	80%
	50,000–100,000	Suspicious; repeat
	10,000–50,000	Symptomatic: suspicious; repeat
	10,000–50,000	Asymptomatic: infection unlikely
	<10,000	Infection unlikely

Adapted from The Subcommittee on Urinary Tract Infection. Urinary tract infection: clinical practice guideline for the diagnosis and management of the initial UTI in febrile infants and children 2 to 24 months. *Pediatrics* 2011;128:595.

younger than 3 months; and (iii) age 3 months to 1 year and temperature greater than or equal to 39°C (102.2°F). Children with dehydration or likely pyelonephritis (as opposed to cystitis) require measurement of electrolytes, BUN, and creatinine.

Management: Most patients are candidates for oral therapy. Indications for parenteral antibiotics include toxicity; young age (<2 months); refusal to drink or vomiting; immunocompromised; anatomic factors that may cause an obstruction to urinary flow; or culture-positivity for a pathogen known to be resistant to oral antibiotics (e.g., extended spectrum beta-lactamase [ESBL]-producing *Klebsiella* or *E. coli* isolates). It is critical that providers are cognizant of antibiotic resistance patterns in their area. If urine culture results are already available, the most narrow spectrum antibiotic providing coverage should be selected. If the child is in an area where many *E. coli* isolates are resistant to ampicillin and/or TMP-SMZ, empiric therapy with a latter generation cephalosporin is reasonable. For children requiring parenteral antibiotics, a third-generation cephalosporin often is used. It is recommended that a 7- to 14-day course of antibiotics be prescribed, as these have been shown to be superior to shorter (1 to 3 day) courses for children. Standard precautions are indicated for children with UTIs.

Renal Abscesses

Renal abscesses can occur as either a complication of pyelonephritis, where they typically are caused by Gram-negative rods, or from hematogenous seeding from systemic bacteremia, in which case *S. aureus* is the most common etiology. Risk factors for renal abscesses due to pyelonephritis include anatomic obstruction (e.g., nephrolithiasis) or vesicoureteral reflux. These abscesses can occur in either the renal cortex or medulla. Risk factors for hematogenous spread include endocarditis or intravenous drug use; in some instances, children have had a preceding minor skin infection, with transient bacteremia seeding the kidneys. These abscesses primarily are found in the renal cortex. Symptoms include fever, malaise, back or abdominal pain, and weight loss. The absence of dysuria does not exclude a renal abscess. Costovertebral angle tenderness is found in a majority of adults, but is less sensitive in children.

Laboratory findings include leukocytosis with a left shift and elevated erythrocyte sedimentation rate (ESR) and CRP. Patients whose abscesses connect with the collecting system may have urinalyses demonstrating pyuria, proteinuria, and bacteriuria. For patients whose abscesses are due to hematogenous spread, initial urinalyses can be normal, but the organism will grow in culture. Renal abscesses should always be suspected in a child with a presumed *S. aureus* UTI. Ultrasound often cannot distinguish a purulent collection from a hematoma, whereas a contrasted CT can help determine the extent of disease. Medical management alone is usually sufficient for renal abscesses less than 5 cm in diameter, whereas percutaneous drainage in addition to antibiotics is needed for larger abscesses. Broad-spectrum antibiotics covering both Gram-negative organisms (pseudomonal coverage should be considered for immunocompromised hosts or persons who previously have had pseudomonal UTIs) and *S. aureus* should be started pending culture results. Improvement is followed clinically (fever curve) and through laboratory parameters (normalization of white count and inflammatory markers). Standard precautions are indicated.

SKIN AND SOFT TISSUE INFECTIOUS EMERGENCIES

The major infections of the skin, soft tissues, and bones include impetigo, cutaneous abscesses, cellulitis and superficial abscesses, fasciitis, septic arthritis, and osteomyelitis. Additionally, mastitis and omphalitis occur in the neonate. Among the disorders in this group, impetigo and cellulitis are both common complaints in the ED. Although children with bone and joint infections are seen infrequently, the differential diagnosis of several common complaints (e.g., fever, limp) often includes these conditions. Thus, the emergency clinician who cares for children should be familiar with such infections, particularly because a prolonged delay in the institution of therapy can result in appreciable morbidity.

Impetigo

Impetigo is a superficial pustular infection of the epidermis. In contrast, ecthyma involves the dermis. Bullous impetigo is characterized by lesions greater than 1 cm in diameter. GAS is the most common cause of impetigo, while *S. aureus* is the most common cause of bullous impetigo, but can also cause nonbullous impetigo. Impetigo is predominantly a disease of the preschool-aged child, and is more common during summer months. Children typically lack systemic signs and symptoms of infection. Skin findings include honey-crusted or bullous lesions with minimal surrounding erythema or induration; regional adenopathy is not common. Routine laboratory evaluation is unnecessary in the well appearing, previously healthy child. Complications may include cellulitis and glomerulonephritis if the child is infected with a nephritogenic strain. The risk of renal disease is not decreased by treatment of local infection. Mupirocin can eradicate most cases of impetigo, especially if the disease is limited in distribution, and may decrease selection for antibiotic resistance. Systemic therapy may be indicated for bullous impetigo or if use of topical antibiotics is impractical due to extent of disease. Oral treatment options include cephalexin, or clindamycin. TMP-SMZ offers coverage for the vast majority of staphylococcal isolates (both MRSA and MSSA), but does not cover GAS. Knowledge of the rates of MRSA in your area can help optimize empiric antibiotic therapy. Contact precautions should be used.

Cellulitis

Cellulitis is an infection of the skin and subcutaneous tissues. A related disease is erysipelas, which involves the more superficial skin layers. Erysipelas lesions are beefy red, raised above the skin surface, and have very well-demarcated borders; the most common cause is GAS. The most common causes of cellulitis by location and exposure type are listed in e-Table 102.12. Clinical manifestations include erythema, edema, warmth, and pain; only 10% to 20% develop fever. Regional adenopathy is common. Blood cultures rarely are positive in well-appearing immunocompetent hosts, except in children with pneumococcal, *H. influenzae,* or group B streptococcal disease. However, these children are usually not well appearing. Needle aspirates from the center of the cellulitic region are positive in between 5% and 40% of cases, with punch biopsies having a higher culture yield. Bedside ultrasound may allow the clinician to differentiate abscesses from cellulitis. Treatment should be directed at *S. aureus* and GAS, with empiric selection guided by the local prevalence of MRSA and past cultures. While most children with cellulitis can be managed in the outpatient setting, initial parenteral therapy should be considered in the following cases: immunocompromised; toxic-appearance; rapidly progressive lesions; crepitance or violaceous skin discoloration; pain out of proportion to examination; facial cellulitis; or circumferential cellulitis. Standard precautions should be used unless draining lesions exist, in which case contact precautions should be implemented.

Mastitis, Neonatal

Mastitis is an infection of breast tissue; in neonates, it is most commonly seen in the first 3 weeks of life and is more common in girls and in term infants. The most common etiology is *S. aureus,* but GBS, *E. coli,* and *Salmonella* can also cause neonatal mastitis. Infants present with unilateral painful erythema and induration of the breast bud. Fever may be absent even in bacteremic children. Blood cultures usually are negative; cultures of purulent drainage often are positive. Empiric antibiotic coverage should include nafcillin (for coverage of GAS, GBS) and gentamicin and vancomycin if the child lives in an area with high MRSA prevalence. Incision and drainage is advisable in the case of local fluctuance, with careful attention to avoiding injury to the developing breast bud, which is already at risk of damage from the infectious process and may lead to cosmetic issues of the breast first noted at adolescence. Standard precautions should be used unless draining lesions exist, in which case contact precautions should be implemented.

Omphalitis

Omphalitis is an infection of the umbilical stump and surrounding tissues. The most common pathogens are *S. aureus* and GAS; GBS (*Streptococcus agalactiae*) and Gram-negative enterics can also cause omphalitis. The incidence has decreased in industrialized countries because of triple dye placed on the stump immediately after delivery; omphalitis usually is seen in the first 14 days of life. It is more common in premature infants and in infants with complicated deliveries. The first symptoms are purulent, foul-smelling drainage and later erythema around the stump (ultimately, many children have erythema that completely encircles the stump). Later manifestations include lethargy, fever or hypothermia, and irritability; late examination findings include erythema and induration of the anterior abdominal wall. Minimal drainage or noncircumferential erythema is not sufficient to diagnose omphalitis, as some drainage from the umbilical stump is common in the absence of infection. Evaluation for bacteremia and other systemic disease is necessary; Gram stain and cultures from umbilical drainage should be sent. Empiric antibiotic coverage should include nafcillin (for coverage of GAS, GBS) and gentamicin and vancomycin if the child lives in an area with high MRSA prevalence. Standard precautions should be used unless draining lesions exist, in which case contact precautions should be implemented.

Septic Arthritis

CLINICAL PEARLS AND PITFALLS

- Children with septic arthritis present with joint pain (and refusal to walk, if the affected joint is in the lower extremities) and decreased range of motion.
- Laboratory findings supportive of the diagnosis of septic arthritis include elevated inflammatory markers.
- The definitive diagnosis is made via arthrocentesis and culture. Cell count parameters allow the clinician to help differentiate between inflammatory and infectious etiologies.
- Empiric therapy for septic arthritis outside the neonatal period should target *S. aureus,* the most common cause of septic arthritis.
- In Lyme-endemic regions, *B. burgdorferi* can also cause arthritis, though the children with Lyme arthritis typically have less fulminant courses than with pyogenic arthritis.

Current Evidence

Septic arthritis is a bacterial infection of the joint space. The etiologies vary by age. In the neonatal period and early infancy, GBS and *S. aureus* are the predominant pathogens, with Gram-negative bacilli and *Candida* seen sporadically, especially in hospitalized infants. Beyond this time period, *S. aureus* overwhelmingly is the most common pathogen causing septic arthritis. Pneumococcus, GAS, gonococcus, and *K. kingae* also are associated with septic arthritis in children. *Salmonella* can be seen in children with hemoglobinopathies. *Brucella* septic arthritis can be associated with consumption of unpasteurized milk products and has a predilection for the sacroiliac joint. Hib is a rare cause of septic arthritis in the modern era. Lyme arthritis and tuberculosis arthritis are discussed elsewhere.

Goals of Treatment

The goal of treatment is to rapidly identify children with septic arthritis so that prompt arthrocentesis can be performed and antibiotics administered. Clinical outcomes include orthopedic sequelae (e.g., chondrolysis, osteonecrosis) and differentiation of septic arthritis from other orthopedic complaints of childhood.

Clinical Considerations

Clinical recognition: The most common manifestation is limp, as 90% of children with septic arthritis have monoarticular involvement of a lower extremity joint. In the child who is limping or refusing to ambulate, occasionally it will be difficult to determine a focal lesion after manipulation of the lower extremity joints and palpation of the long bones. Clinicians should be sure to evaluate the sole of the foot for foreign bodies and also to palpate over the sacroiliac joint to assess for tenderness. Pain may be referred to other areas (e.g., hip septic arthritis presenting as knee pain). The child with a septic hip often lies quite still with the leg abducted and in external rotation. Fever is present in almost two-thirds of children with septic arthritis, but can be absent in adolescents with gonococcal infections or in neonates. An erythematous swelling may surround a superficial joint that is infected. Although a temperature difference exists between the affected and unaffected sites, it can be difficult to discern in the febrile child. Inflammation within the joint distends the capsule and produces pain with movement. If a child allows the physician to manipulate an extremity through a full range of motion, septic arthritis is unlikely.

Triage considerations: Any child with fever and a limp or other joint complaint should be promptly evaluated for septic arthritis. The most urgent of locations is septic arthritis of the hip, as this can result in compromised vascular flow to the femoral capitis. Associated tachycardia and/or hypotension can imply sepsis and would require fluid resuscitation.

Clinical assessment: Septic arthritis is diagnosed via aspiration and culture of joint fluid. Arthrocentesis is not only diagnostic, it is therapeutic; many children report decreased pain after synovial fluid is aspirated. As such, early consultation with orthopedic surgery is critical. Most children with pyogenic septic arthritis have synovial fluid white blood cell count (WBC) of >50,000 cells per mm^3 and a neutrophilic predominance. However, cell counts may be lower with *Brucella* or tuberculosis arthritis and may exceed 50,000 cells per mm^3 with some noninfectious causes of arthritis, such as juvenile idiopathic arthritis. A Gram stain should be sent, as some organisms may be seen in the synovial fluid and not grown in culture, even in children without antibiotic pretreatment, as synovial fluid has some bacteriostatic properties. Approximately 50% of children with septic arthritis will have positive synovial fluid cultures. Culture yield is enhanced for certain pathogens with appropriate specimen handling. If *Kingella* is suspected, synovial fluid should be injected into a blood culture bottle to increase yield. If *Brucella* is suspected, the laboratory should be notified so that the cultures can be kept far beyond the usual protocol, as it often takes weeks for this organism to grow. Acid-fast cultures and *M. tuberculosis* PCR should be sent in immunocompromised hosts or children with epidemiologic risk factors for tuberculosis. Fungal, anaerobic, and acid-fast cultures (the latter for nontuberculous mycobacteria) should be obtained in children with penetrating trauma, as these infections often are polymicrobial and can be caused by a broad spectrum of pathogens.

Ancillary laboratory evaluation should include a blood culture, complete blood count, ESR, and CRP. The ESR and CRP are the most consistent abnormal laboratory studies and can be used to monitor response to therapy. Radiographic studies (e.g., MRI) can be used to evaluate for contiguous osteomyelitis. This is particularly common in the first year of life, because at this time, the metaphysis is located within the joint capsule. Recognition of osteomyelitis in association with septic arthritis is an important consideration when determining the duration of therapy.

Clinical algorithms have been developed for septic arthritis. The best known is the Kocher criteria for septic arthritis of the hip. The risk factors assessed were nonweight bearing on the affected side, ESR >40 mm per hour, fever, and WBC >12,000 per mm^3. When all four criteria are met, there is a 99% chance that the child has septic arthritis. However, the negative predictive value is not as robust; 40% of cases with only 2/4 criteria have a septic joint.

Management: Prompt surgical intervention is typically advocated for septic arthritis of the hip. All children with suspected septic arthritis should be admitted to the hospital for parenteral antibiotics. Antistaphylococcal coverage should be initiated in children of any age with suspected septic arthritis. The selection of vancomycin over clindamycin depends upon local antibiotic susceptibility patterns and any prior culture results available for the child. Coverage should be expanded beyond staphylococcal coverage if the Gram stain demonstrates organisms other than Gram-positive cocci in clusters, if gonococcal arthritis is suspected based upon history or cultures from nonjoint sites (e.g., oropharynx, rectum), or in immunocompromised children or children whose arthritis is due to penetrating trauma to the joint. In neonates and young infants, ampicillin and a third-generation cephalosporin should be added to augment coverage for GBS and Gram-negative rods. Standard precautions should be used unless draining lesions exist, in which case contact precautions should be implemented.

Lyme Disease Arthritis

A common cause of septic arthritis in Lyme-endemic regions (northeastern, mid-Atlantic, and Great Lakes states in the United States) is *B. burgdorferi.* Lyme arthritis is a monoarticular or pauciarticular (affecting 2 to 4 joints) arthritis that most often affects the large joints, especially the knees, which are involved in over 90% of cases. After the knee, the shoulder, ankle, and elbow are the most commonly affected joints. It affects approximately 7% of children with Lyme disease. The symptoms mimic those of septic arthritis caused by pyogenic organisms (acute bacterial septic arthritis). There are some features that can enable the provider to differentiate the two entities (e-Table 102.13). One clinical prediction rule derived and validated in a Lyme-endemic region showed that children were at low risk for septic arthritis if the ANC was <10,000 per mm^3 and the ESR was <40 mm per hour. Serologic tests are insensitive in the first month after Lyme infection, but are always positive when arthritis exists. Tiered screening, beginning with an enzyme immunoassay (EIA) or immunofluorescent antibody (IFA) assay, with confirmation of positive results by a Western blot, is recommended. Two-step screening is needed because false positives on EIA or IFA can occur due to other spirochete infections, varicella, EBV, and some collagen vascular disorders. Lyme serologies should not be sent in children who have not lived in or traveled to Lyme-endemic regions, as any positive results in these children are far more likely to represent false positives. The treatment of initial and recurrent arthritis due to Lyme disease is summarized in e-Table 102.14. Macrolides are less effective than other antibiotics, and as such are recommended only for patients who cannot tolerate cephalosporins, penicillins, or tetracyclines. Standard precautions are used for children with suspected Lyme disease.

Osteomyelitis

CLINICAL PEARLS AND PITFALLS

- Children with osteomyelitis usually present with fever and focal bone pain. Range of motion may be limited by pain, and findings can thus mimic septic arthritis.
- The most common cause of osteomyelitis is *S. aureus*.
- Blood cultures are positive in approximately 50% of children, as such, bone biopsy should be attempted. Under optimal circumstances, the biopsy would occur prior to the child receiving antibiotics, if the child is nontoxic and immunocompetent.

Current Evidence

Osteomyelitis is a bacterial infection of the bone. In 90% of cases, only one bone (most commonly in the lower extremity) is involved. The upper extremity is involved in approximately 25% of cases. The most common cause, across all age groups, is *S. aureus*. There is substantial overlap between the organisms causing septic arthritis and those causing osteomyelitis. *P. aeruginosa* may infect the bones of the foot after a puncture wound. In children with sickle cell hemoglobinopathies, *Salmonella* species account for almost half the cases of osteomyelitis. Unusual pathogens may be recovered from immunocompromised children.

Goals of Treatment

The goal of treatment is the prompt recognition of osteomyelitis in the febrile child with bone pain. The clinical team should consider advanced imaging by MRI to evaluate for contiguous infections.

Clinical Considerations

Clinical recognition: As the most common bones involved are the femur and tibia, limp is a common presentation. The multiplicity of bones that may be involved leads to a wide spectrum of chief complaints. Vertebral osteomyelitis manifests as backache, torticollis, or stiff neck, and involvement of the mandible causes painful mastication. Infection of the pelvis is particularly elusive and may masquerade as appendicitis, septic hip, neoplasm, or UTI. Infants with osteomyelitis localize the symptoms less well than older children. Initially, irritability may be the only complaint.

Fever is seen in 70% to 80% of children with osteomyelitis. The infant with a long bone infection often manifests pseudoparalysis, an unwillingness to move the extremity. Movement may also be decreased in the older child, but to a lesser degree. Point tenderness is seen commonly in osteomyelitis; however, it is nonspecific, as it is found in other conditions, such as trauma, may be difficult to discern in the struggling infant, and does not always occur early in the course of the infection. Percussion of a bone at a point remote from the site of an osteomyelitis may elicit pain in the area of infection. When purulent material ruptures through the cortex, diffuse local erythema and edema appear. This finding occurs often in infants, but late in the course, and is confined primarily to children in the first 3 years of life (before the cortex thickens sufficiently to contain the inflammatory exudate).

Triage considerations: Any child with fever and a focal bone pain should be evaluated for osteomyelitis. Associated tachycardia and/or hypotension can imply sepsis and would require fluid resuscitation.

Clinical assessment: Bone biopsy cultures are positive in approximately 60% of children with acute hematogenous osteomyelitis, and blood cultures are positive in 50% of cases. The ESR and CRP are the most consistent abnormal laboratory studies and can be used to monitor response to therapy. Plain radiographs of the affected extremity should be obtained, although they are often normal early in the disease course. Within 3 to 10 days, some radiographic anomalies become evident: Muscle edema will obliterate the lucent planes separating muscle groups. Visualization of bony destruction requires loss of over 40% of the bony matrix, and is a finding uncommon prior to 10 to 14 days. MRI is used to evaluate for drainable fluid collections (e.g., subperiosteal abscess or pyomyositis), and the most common finding on MRI in children with osteomyelitis is bone marrow edema. In the era of MRSA, many centers have noted that some children with osteomyelitis have infected deep venous thromboses (DVTs) in the adjacent blood vessels. MRI also allows for evaluation of DVTs (which appear as flow voids). Recognition of DVTs is important, as it could alter antibiotic therapy (e.g., make it more likely to select a bactericidal antibiotic as opposed to a bacteriostatic drug) and would prompt anticoagulation.

Management: In contrast to septic arthritis, well-appearing children with suspected osteomyelitis do not require immediate parenteral antibiotic therapy. If a child has age-appropriate vital signs, is previously healthy, and there is a low likelihood of osteomyelitis, blood cultures and an MRI can be obtained while the child is observed off of antibiotics. As blood cultures will be positive in only one-half of children, identification of an organism from bone biopsy is critical. The clinician should contact orthopedic surgery (or interventional radiology) early about culturing the infected bone prior to initiation of antibiotics in these patients. However, if the child were to change clinically, or in the toxic-appearing or immunocompromised child, antibiotics should not be withheld. Empiric therapy should target *S. aureus*. The selection of vancomycin over clindamycin depends upon local antibiotic susceptibility patterns and any prior culture results available for the child. Nafcillin is a more bactericidal drug for MSSA than vancomycin or clindamycin and change to a beta-lactam antibiotic (nafcillin or cefazolin) should occur if the child is known to have MSSA. Coverage should be expanded beyond staphylococcal coverage in immunocompromised children, children in whom other pathogens have been cultured in the past, and for septic children. Standard precautions should be used.

Necrotizing Fasciitis

Fasciitis is cellulitis extending to deeper tissues, such as fascia and muscle, but not to bones or joints. The most common causes in the modern era are GAS and *S. aureus*. Widespread use of the varicella vaccine has decreased the incidence of necrotizing fasciitis, where GAS could complicate varicella infection. The family may report that the lesion is rapidly progressive. Fasciitis can be differentiated from cellulitis by pain out of proportion to examination findings and more systemic signs; toxic appearance, high fever, tachycardia, and hypotension are more common. In some cases of anaerobic fasciitis, subcutaneous crepitance may be noted. Patients generally have a leukocytosis with a neutrophilic predominance, and blood cultures (aerobic and anaerobic) should be obtained, as bacteremia is present in a majority of cases. Fasciitis is a medical and surgical emergency. Debridement is needed in many instances to prevent spread to adjacent tissues. Antimicrobial therapy should be targeted toward GAS, *S. aureus*, and anaerobes, especially with fasciitis of the head and neck (or any area with evidence of gas production in the tissues). Multidrug empiric therapy with penicillin (which is more bactericidal for GAS than clindamycin or vancomycin), clindamycin (for anaerobic coverage), and vancomycin (for MRSA) should be initiated. Contact precautions should be used.

TABLE 102.18

GEOGRAPHIC DISTRIBUTION OF INFECTIOUS AGENTS

Region	Pathogens
Africa, sub-Saharan	African tick-bite fever, amebiasis, anthrax, *Brucella,* Chikungunya, cholera, cutaneous larval migrans, cysticercosis, dengue, *Echinococcus,* filariasis, hemorrhagic fever viruses, hepatitis A, B, and C, leishmaniasis (visceral), malaria, meningococcus, onchocerciasis, plague, polio, rabies, schistosomiasis, tetanus, trypanosomiasis, tuberculosis, typhoid and nontyphi *Salmonella,* yellow fever
Africa, Northern and Middle East	Anthrax, *Brucella, Echinococcus,* filariasis, leishmaniasis (cutaneous, visceral), malaria, onchocerciasis, rickettsial disease, tuberculosis
Asia and Indian subcontinent	Amebiasis, Angiostrongyliasis, anthrax, *Brucella,* Chikungunya, cutaneous larval migrans, cysticercosis, dengue, *Echinococcus,* filariasis, hepatitis A, B, and C, Japanese encephalitis, leishmaniasis (visceral), malaria, melioidosis, plague, rabies, schistosomiasis, tetanus, tick-borne encephalitis, tuberculosis, typhoid
Caribbean	Cholera, cutaneous larva migrans, dengue, diphtheria, filariasis, leishmaniasis (cutaneous), malaria, melioidosis, typhoid, nontyphi *Salmonella,* tuberculosis
Central/South America	Amebiasis, anthrax, *Brucella, Campylobacter,* Chagas disease, cholera, cutaneous larva migrans, cysticercosis, *Echinococcus,* filariasis, hepatitis A and B, hemorrhagic fever viruses, leishmaniasis (visceral cutaneous), leptospirosis, malaria, melioidosis, onchocerciasis, plague, rabies, *Strongyloides,* tetanus, typhoid and nontyphi *Salmonella,* yellow fever, tuberculosis
Europe, Eastern	Anthrax, *Brucella,* diphtheria, *Echinococcus,* hepatitis B and C, polio, tick-borne encephalitis
Europe, Western	*Brucella,* leishmaniasis (visceral), Lyme disease, meningococcus, tick-borne encephalitis
Mediterranean	*Brucella, Echinococcus,* hepatitis A, B, and C, rickettsial disease

INFECTIONS IN RETURNED TRAVELERS

Introduction

Over the last 20 years, there has been an enhancement of medical provider networks designed to improve surveillance and medical care for international travelers. More than 80% of U.S. citizens visiting pretravel clinics are traveling to resource-poor countries, with Africa being the most commonly visited region. Approximately 29 million residents of the United States traveled internationally in 2013, with approximately 8% reporting travel-associated illnesses. While most are mild, self-limited conditions, such as traveler's diarrhea, a proportion of these individuals will present to the ED after returning home. Pediatric travelers may be classified into several groups: children returning from international travel; children returning from visiting friends and relatives (VFRs) in the child or parents' country of origin; international adoptees; and recently emigrated children. These groups may have distinct risk factors for infection and certain groups (VFRs) historically have been at higher risk for travel-associated infections because their families infrequently seek medical attention prior to international travel.

It is critical for the emergency medicine provider to ask families not only about locations to which the child has traveled (Table 102.18 for infections common in specific regions), but what regions (e.g., urban vs. rural) the child visited and what activities were undertaken. Knowing when a child returned home can help narrow the differential diagnosis using the incubation period for certain pathogens. The incubation period and symptoms of most common diseases in the returned traveler are summarized in Table 102.19, and the diagnosis and treatment of these diseases are presented in Table 102.20. These diseases are categorized in one of three ways: diseases endemic in both industrialized and developing nations; vaccine-preventable illnesses more common internationally; and diseases endemic only outside industrialized nations.

In the next section, six major diseases or syndromes will be reviewed: malaria, tuberculosis, typhoid, dengue, chikungunya, and diarrheal diseases. Other IDs will then be organized based on the primary organ system involved. HIV will be covered at the end of this chapter.

Malaria

CLINICAL PEARLS AND PITFALLS

- Persons returning to their native countries (VFRs) are at particular risk for malaria, since many fail to take the necessary precautions either to avoid insect exposure or to take prophylaxis.
- Malaria should be considered in the differential diagnosis of any febrile child who has returned from a malaria-endemic region in the preceding month; one negative blood smear should not lead the PEM provider to rule out malaria.
- Chloroquine resistance is widespread, and this drug should not be used as empiric therapy for the ill child with suspected malaria.

Current Evidence

Malaria is the most important parasitic disease of man with prevalence estimated to be approximately 300 to 500 million with over 2 million deaths each year, most of whom are children. The majority of morbidity and mortality is due to *Plasmodium falciparum.* Malaria is endemic throughout tropical regions worldwide; in 2013, 104 countries were malaria-endemic, and over 3 billion persons were at risk of malaria.

TABLE 102.19

EPIDEMIOLOGY, HISTORICAL, AND CLINICAL FINDINGS IN COMMON INFECTIONS IN RETURNED TRAVELERS

Disease	Region	Incubation period (days)	Historical features	Symptoms
Amebiasis (*Entamoeba histolytica*)	Latin America, southern Asia, western/southern Africa	14–28, but can remain latent for years	Fecal–oral: contaminated water sources or history of eating uncooked or contaminated fruits or vegetables, poor personal hygiene	Acute colitis: fever, chills and bloody or mucoid diarrhea Mild: abdominal discomfort with diarrhea (containing blood or mucus), weight loss Liver abscess: fever, cough, right upper quadrant pain, referred shoulder pain (more common in adults)
Babesiosis (*Babesia microti*)	Northeast, upper Midwest	7–28	Tick-borne disease more common in warmer months (May–October); ticks need to feed for 48 hrs to effectively transmit disease; some cases also reported after blood transfusion	Fever, nonspecific flu-like symptoms, nonproductive cough, jaundice, and hemolytic anemia *Illness is much more severe in asplenic patients and other immunocompromised hosts*
Brucellosis (*Brucella abortus*)	Europe, Africa, Middle East, central America, India, central and South America, and Mexico	5–60	Contact through breaks in skin with animal tissue, blood, urine, aborted fetuses and placentas; ingestion of raw milk or dairy products from infected animals	Continued, intermittent, or irregular fever of variable duration, headache, weakness, profuse sweating, chills, arthralgia, joint pain, and weight loss
Campylobacter (*C. jejuni*)	Worldwide; one of most common bacterial causes of diarrhea in the United States	2–5	Consumption of undercooked meat (particularly poultry) and other contaminated food and water; contact with infected animals (particularly kittens or puppies) or infants	Diarrhea (frequently bloody), abdominal pain, malaise, fever, nausea, and/or vomiting; 1/1,000 develop Guillian–Barré; smaller percentage develop reactive arthritis or iritis
Chagas (*Trypanosoma cruzi*)	Central and South America	7–21	History of exposure to or bitten by cone-nosed or kissing bugs	Acute: Fever, lymphadenopathy, malaise and hepatosplenomegaly generally occur in children; chagoma (inflammatory response at site of infection) may last for up to 8 wks; unilateral bipalpebral edema (Romana sign) is seen in a minority of cases Chronic: irreversible myocardial damage, arrhythmias and major EKG abnormalities, and development of intestinal complications of megaesophagus and megacolon
Chikungunya (togavirus)	Africa, Southeast Asia, India, Sri Lanka, and the Philippines	1–12	*Aedes* mosquito; diagnosis made by excluding other diseases found in the same region	High fever, headache, lymphadenopathy, leukopenia, arthralgia or arthritis (symmetrical, multiple joints affected) lasting days to months, rash (erythematous, petechial, erythroderma, or desquamation; often lasts 2–3 days and does not spare palms or soles); seizures and neurologic complications more common in children

(*continued*)

TABLE 102.19

EPIDEMIOLOGY, HISTORICAL, AND CLINICAL FINDINGS IN COMMON INFECTIONS IN RETURNED TRAVELERS (*CONTINUED*)

Disease	Region	Incubation period (days)	Historical features	Symptoms
Cholera (*Vibrio cholera*)	Most cases in Africa, Indian subcontinent, Southeast Asia; outbreaks common after disasters (Haiti)	2–5	Consumption of contaminated water or food (especially seafood), poor hygiene and sanitation, and crowded living conditions (urban slums, refugee camps)	Most infections asymptomatic or with mild gastroenteritis; severe cases with sudden onset painless watery (rice-water) diarrhea, nausea, profuse vomiting; potential to develop severe dehydration, hypovolemic shock, acidosis, circulatory collapse, hypoglycemia, renal failure and death
Cryptosporidium	Worldwide	1–12	Fecal–oral infection of the parasite including person–person, animal–person, waterborne and foodborne transmission	Diarrhea (may be profuse and watery), preceded by anorexia and vomiting in children; cramping abdominal pain
Cutaneous larval migrans (hookworm)	Southern United States, sub-Saharan Africa, south and Southeast Asia, and Latin America	1–28	Infection via skin (foot, abdomen, buttock) coming in contact with damp contaminated soil	Erythematous, pruritic papule at the site of entry, which becomes elevated and vesicular; larvae tunnel under skin leaving serpiginous tracks; risk of secondary infections due to extreme itching
Dengue	Asia, Africa, Caribbean, South and central America In the United States, cases reported in Florida, South Texas	3–14	Bite of infected mosquitoes (*Aedes aegypti*—a day- and night-feeding mosquito)	Stage 1: Sudden onset, fever for 2–7 days, intense headache, retroorbital pain, myalgia, arthralgia, anorexia, nausea, vomiting, and transient ash; minor bleeding in some patients Stage 2: Dengue hemorrhagic fever symptoms: acute onset of severe fever, hemorrhagic diathesis, abnormal blood clotting, increased vascular permeability leading to hypovolemic shock, pleural effusions Stage 3: recover phase starting 2–3 days after Stage 2; may see pruritic maculopapular rash
Diphtheria (*Corynebacterium diphtheriae*)	Southeast Asia, Central Africa, Middle East	2–5	Human-to-human contact with a carrier or patient with the disease; contact with clothing that had been soiled with cutaneous lesions of infected people; raw milk	Asymmetric grey-white membrane with surrounding inflammation typically involving the mucous membranes of the upper respiratory tract; lymphadenopathy in some cases leading to severe swelling of the neck creating a "bull neck" appearance; cutaneous lesions with some infections
E. coli 0157:H7	Worldwide; most US cases in the southwestern, western, and northeastern states	3–9	Linked to undercooked beef and vegetables	Watery diarrhea that becomes bloody after 1–5 days; severe abdominal pain, usually afebrile. Hemolytic uremic syndrome (HUS)
Filariasis	Latin America, Africa, Asia, and the Pacific Islands	6–12 mo for *W. bancrofti* 3–6 mo for *Brugia species*	Bite of mosquito infected with one of three different forms of filariasis causing infection of the lymphatic system	Acute, recurrent lymphadenitis, high fever; hydrocele, chyluria, lymphedema, elephantiasis of extremities and genital region; tropical pulmonary eosinophilic syndrome, manifested by paroxysmal nocturnal asthma, chronic interstitial lung disease, recurrent low-grade fever, profound eosinophilia
Giardia	Worldwide	3–25	Fecal–oral transmission, anal intercourse, ingestion of contaminated water	Acute self-limited diarrhea; chronic diarrhea, steatorrhea, abdominal cramping, bloating, frequent loose and pale greasy stools, fatigue, malabsorption and weight loss

Hantavirus	Southwest; other foci in Brazil, Argentina, Chile, Pacific coast	3–30	Patients with history exposure to field rodents (presumed via aerosol transmission from rodent urine and feces), especially inside homes	Hemorrhagic fever with renal syndrome: acute onset of fever, lower back pain, varying degrees of hemorrhagic manifestations and renal involvement; five clinical phases including febrile, hypotensive, oliguria, diuretic, and convalescent Hantavirus pulmonary syndrome: fever, myalgia, gastrointestinal complaints followed by abrupt onset of acute respiratory distress and hypotension, leading to respiratory failure, shock and possible death
Hemorrhagic fever viruses other than dengue (e.g., Ebola, Marburg)	Ebola: central/west Africa Marburg: west Africa Lassa: west Africa Also seen in South America (e.g., Argentinean, Bolivian, Venezuelan hemorrhagic fever)	2–21	Animal exposure: bats (Marburg), rodents (Lassa, South American hemorrhagic fevers); exposure to blood products (Ebola)	Fever, myalgia, headache, vomiting, diarrhea, abdominal or chest pain, mental status changes; rash begins around day 5 (usually on trunk), progressing from erythema to petechiae as disseminated intravascular coagulation evolves
Leishmaniasis (*Leishmania* species, protozoa)	90% of cases in Bangladesh, Brazil, Ethiopia, India, Nepal, and Sudan, but endemic in 70 countries	7–60 Weeks–months for cutaneous; months–years for visceral and mucosal	Transmitted by bite of infected female phlebotomine sandflies; domestic and stray dogs as reservoirs	Cutaneous: macule formation (single or multiple) developing into a painless papule (most common on face, extremities), then ulcer formation with some lesions spontaneously healing within weeks to months; some disseminate to include mucosal lesions and may become locally destructive Visceral (Kala-Azar): fever, weight loss, hepatosplenomegaly Mucosal: ulcerative lesions near nose and mouth, very locally destructive and disfiguring
Leptospirosis (Spirochetes, several pathogenic species)	Worldwide distribution, higher incidence in tropical climates	2–28	Contact of the skin (especially if abraded) or mucous membranes with moist soil or vegetation contaminated with urine of infected animals, with contaminated waters (flooding, swimming, occupational) with urine, fluids or tissues of infected animals; occasionally through drinking or ingestion of food or water contaminated with urine of infected animals (often rats) or inhalation of droplet aerosols of contaminated fluids	Mild, influenza-like illness, retroorbital pain, vomiting; Weil syndrome: characterized by jaundice, renal failure, hemorrhage, myocarditis with arrhythmias; meningitis or meningoencephalitis; and pulmonary hemorrhage with respiratory failure

(*continued*)

TABLE 102.19

EPIDEMIOLOGY, HISTORICAL, AND CLINICAL FINDINGS IN COMMON INFECTIONS IN RETURNED TRAVELERS (*CONTINUED*)

Disease	Region	Incubation period (days)	Historical features	Symptoms
Malaria (*Plasmodium* species, most importantly *P. falciparum*)	Central and northern South America, sub-Saharan Africa, Southeast Asia and Indian subcontinent	7–30	Vector *Anopheles* mosquitoes (feed at dusk and night) Ask about specific regions of travel (compare to CDC website) and ask if child received malaria prophylaxis during the trip	Fever, vomiting, headache, abdominal pain, malaise, jaundice; hepatosplenomegaly *Fever in children returning from malaria-endemic areas should be considered malaria until proven otherwise*
Measles	Worldwide	7–18	Unimmunized patients that come in contact with airborne droplets of infected individuals	Prodromal fever, cough, coryza, conjunctivitis, Koplik spots; red blotchy rash develops on days 3–7 beginning on the face then progress caudally; by the time the rash is seen on the feet, it has typically disappeared from the face
Mumps	Worldwide	16–18	Unimmunized patients come in to contact with airborne droplets or via direct contact with saliva of infected individuals	Fever, tenderness of one or more salivary glands (usually the parotid); tender regional adenitis; orchitis (usually unilateral); sensorineural hearing loss
Cysticercosis (*Taenia solium*)	Central and South America, sub-Saharan Africa, Indian subcontinent, and Southeast Asia	Months–years	Pork consumption; vegetarians and persons not eating pork can inquire infection from fecal–oral contamination with eggs from carriers	Seizures from neurocysticercosis (lesions average 1–2 cm in diameter); visual loss if ophthalmic involvement; massive cysts; burden in muscles can present as pseudohypertrophy
Polio	Afghanistan, India, Nigeria, and Pakistan	7–14	Human-to-human spread in unvaccinated patients mainly through fecal–oral route	Fever, malaise, headache, nausea and vomiting in 10% of patients; acute onset of flaccid paralysis seen in <1% of patients
Rabies	Worldwide	21–56	Patient with a history of exposure to virus-laden saliva from a rabid animal introduced through a bite, scratch, or contact with a mucosal surface (e.g., for bats)	Onset consists of apprehension, fever, headache, malaise, and parasthesia at site of animal bite; excitability, aero- and/or hydrophobia with spasms of the swallowing muscles commonly follow; delirium; convulsions; progressive viral encephalitis that is nearly always fatal
Salmonella typhi (*S. enterica* serotype typhi)	Higher case rates in Indian subcontinent; also seen in Asia, sub-Saharan Africa, western South America	10–20	Ingestion of food or water contaminated with feces and urine of patients and carriers; ask if received oral typhoid vaccine (the intramuscular typhoid vaccine offers poor protection)	Sustained fever, significant headache, anorexia, malaise, relative bradycardia, constipation and abdominal discomfort, mild cough, splenomegaly; erythematous blanchable rose spots on the trunk in 25% of patients; late onset of diarrhea (nonbloody); convulsions (more common in preschool-aged children); possible death secondary to toxemia, myocarditis, intestinal hemorrhage or perforation
Salmonella, nontyphi	Worldwide Most common bacterial cause of food-borne infections in the United States	12–36 hrs	Contaminated foods, including undercooked eggs, raw milk/milk products, contaminated water, meat/meat products, poultry/poultry products, and contaminated products	Sudden onset of headache, fever, abdominal pain, diarrhea (may be bloody), nausea and sometimes vomiting; reactive arthritis and iritis occur in a small percentage as postinfectious phenomenon

Schistosomiasis	85% of cases in Africa; others in Middle East, Southeast Asia	14–42 (acute form), months–years (chronic form)	Patients wading, bathing or swimming in freshwater containing the infected snail vectors	*S. mansoni* and *S. japonicum* typically give rise to hepatic and intestinal symptoms including hepatosplenomegaly, diarrhea, and abdominal pain; *S. haematobium* can give rise to urinary tract manifestations including dysuria, urinary frequency, and hematuria; acute onset of Katayama fever weeks after infection: fever, abdominal pain, hepatosplenomegaly, diarrhea, eosinophilia
Shigella (*Shigella flexneri, sonnei*)	Worldwide	1–3	Fecal–oral transmission from a symptomatic patient or asymptomatic carrier; ingestion of contaminated food or water as well as from person-to-person transmission; associated with daycare attendance	Small volume loose stool (may contain blood and mucous), fever, nausea, vomiting, cramps; reactive arthritis and iritis occur in a small percentage as postinfectious phenomenon
Strongyloides (*Strongyloides stercoralis*, a nematode)	Endemic in Latin America, Southeast Asia, sub-Saharan Africa	14–21	Infective larvae develop in feces or moist soil contaminated with feces and penetrate human skin entering the venous circulation	Abdominal pain, diarrhea, and urticarial, nausea, vomiting, weakness, constipation; transient dermatitis with initial infection (serpiginous urticarial rash most often involving perianal region and torso); cough, rales, pneumonitis when involves the lungs *Immunocompromised hosts are at risk for hyperinfection, characterized by a high number of worms (especially in the lungs), or by worms in ectopic sites (e.g. brain), or both*
Tick-borne diseases, Rickettsial	Worldwide	3–14	Ticks need to feed for several hours prior to transmission; more common in warm weather months	Fever, rash, headache (while the classic triad for Rocky Mountain spotted fever, is seen in only 60% of children), myalgias
Tuberculosis (*Mycobacterium tuberculosis*)	Worldwide, but 90% of burden is in developing nations Over 50% of cases in US from New York, California, Texas, Florida	14–70 Weeks–months (shorter incubation in infants and immunocompromised children)	Ask about tuberculosis contacts; exposure to bacteria in airborne, aerosolized droplets produced by patients with pulmonary or high respiratory tract TB; persons at risk for TB: homeless, incarcerated, HIV positive, previously treated for TB	Fever, weight loss, malaise, cough. Night sweats and hemoptysis rare in young children. Most common site of extrapulmonary diseases are extrathoracic lymphadenopathy and meningitis
Yellow fever (Flavivirus)	Central and South America, Central Asia	3–16	Transmitted to humans via the bite of infective *Aedes* spp. mosquitoes (feeding morning and evening)	Most patients asymptomatic Most common symptoms: sudden onset of fever, chills, headache, backache, myalgias, nausea and vomiting; minority of patients (15%) will continue to develop hemorrhagic symptoms including epistaxis, gingival bleeding, hematemesis, melana, and multiorgan system failure

TABLE 102.20

DIAGNOSIS AND TREATMENT OF COMMON INFECTIONS IN RETURNED TRAVELERS

Disease	ED-based testing	Definitive diagnosis	Treatment
Amebiasis	Stool (better for colitis) or serum (better for hepatic abscess) antigen detection Serology (better for hepatic abscess) Ancillary: leukocytosis, anemia, elevated ALT; abdominal imaging to help differentiate from pyogenic abscesses, *Echinococcus,* and malignancy	Microscopy to detect eggs in stool or antigen detection (stool, serum) or serology	Noninvasive or asymptomatic disease: paromomycin (termed a luminal agent) Colitis: metronidazole Amebic abscess: metronidazole + paromomycin or another luminal agent
Babesiosis	Thick and thin smears with Giemsa/Wright staining Anemia, low haptoglobin, elevated lactate dehydrogenase, and reticulocyte count; thrombocytopenia common	Visualization of trophozoites (Maltese cross) Antibody detection by indirect immunofluorescence assays	Mild–moderate: atovaquone + azithromycin or clindamycin + quinine for 7–10 days If parasitemia >10% (especially in asplenic patients), significant anemia, or hepatorenal or pulmonary compromise, exchange transfusion should be considered
Brucella	Serology (acute and convalescent titers) Lab should be notified that Brucella is suspected as cultures require an incubation of 4 wks minimum	Serology	Trimethoprim-sulfamethoxazole and rifampin for at least 4–6 wks Addition of an aminoglycoside should be added for the first 14 days in case of suspected meningitis, endocarditis, and osteomyelitis
Campylobacter	Stool culture	Stool culture	Fluid resuscitation Azithromycin or erythromycin × 3–5 days
Chagas	Giemsa Staining or direct wet mount Serology testing available by CDC for chronic cases	Giemsa staining	Benznidazole for 30–90 days or Nifurtimox for 90–120 days
Chikungunya	Usually a clinical diagnosis: fever + severe arthralgia/arthritis + travel to or residence in endemic area within 15 days of symptom onset + virologic evidence	PCR is preferred in early stages Serology: IgM usually detectable in 2–7 days (lasts <3–4 mo)	Supportive, nonsteroidal anti-inflammatories Small series have noted possible benefit of ribavirin and chloroquine, but these have not been validated in large trials
Cholera	Stool culture with use of salt-containing media (TBS) Ancillary: may see hypoglycemia, hypokalemia, and other electrolyte disturbances secondary to dehydration	Stool culture	Fluid resuscitation Antibiotics (fluoroquinolones, tetracyclines) reduce disease severity and duration- important to prevent secondary spread
Cryptosporidium	Stool culture for oocysts (use of formalin ethyl acetate stool concentration method is recommended and at least three stool specimens collected on separate days are required because shedding can be intermittent	Stool culture for oocysts	Most do not require therapy Nitazoxanide oral suspension
Cutaneous larval migrans	Clinical diagnosis	Clinical diagnosis	Thiabendazole 500 mg four times a day for 5 days

Dengue	PCR is best modality for all stages Ancillary: Stage 1: Thrombocytopenia, leukopenia, elevated hepatic transaminases Stage 2: DIC, hypoalbuminemia, severe thrombocytopenia Stage 3: No specific laboratory findings	Stage 1: PCR or ELISA Stage 2: PCR Serologic tests cross-react with other flaviviral infections or flaviviral vaccines (e.g., yellow fever, Japanese encephalitis virus)	Supportive care, fluid resuscitation
Diphtheria	Clinical diagnosis confirmed by nasopharyngeal or cutaneous lesion cultures (positive cultures should be sent to CDC)	Nasopharyngeal or cutaneous lesion cultures	IV equine antitoxin Erythromycin (oral or parenteral) Penicillin G IM or IV for 14 days
E. coli (0157:H7)	Conventional Stool culture	Stool culture	Supportive care
Filariasis	Microscopic detection of microfilaria on blood smears obtained at night PCR and immunologic testing also available	Microscopic detection of microfilaria on blood smears obtained at night	Microfilaria of *W. bancrofti:* Diethylcarbamazine citrate (DEC) 2 mg/kg × 1 dose, or 50 mg DEC to children <12 yrs old × 1 dose
Giardia	Stool culture (sensitivity is higher for diarrheal stool specimens) PCR	Stool culture (sensitivity is higher for diarrheal stool specimens)	Metronidazole 5–7 days
Hantavirus	Serology, PCR Ancillary: thrombocytopenia, metabolic acidosis, elevated creatinine, elevated hepatic transaminases Culture not recommended due to risk to laboratory personnel	Serology (should be sent to CDC)	Supportive care
Hemorrhagic fever viruses (other than dengue)	Serology Ancillary: thrombocytopenia, disseminated intravascular coagulation	Serology (subject to cross-reaction with other arboviruses in the same class)	Supportive Lassa: ribavirin highly effective if given before day 7 of illness
Hepatitis viruses	Serology testing	Serology testing	Acute hepatitis A and B: supportive Chronic hepatitis C: Interferon or peginterferon-alpha Peginterferon-alpha in combination with ribavirin
Leishmaniasis	Direct visualization of protozoa from bone marrow aspirate Serology if other diagnostic tests unavailable Ancillary for visceral form: marrow suppression, elevated hepatic transaminases, hypoalbuminemia, hypergammaglobulinemia	Visualization of protozoa from bone marrow or splenic aspiration Serology not useful for cutaneous form	Consultation with CDC should be performed Standard treatment involves pentavalent antimonials and sodium stibogluconate; amphotericin has also been used

(continued)

TABLE 102.20

DIAGNOSIS AND TREATMENT OF COMMON INFECTIONS IN RETURNED TRAVELERS (*CONTINUED*)

Disease	ED-based testing	Definitive diagnosis	Treatment
Leptospirosis	PCR, culture, or immunohistochemical staining (culture is sensitive and slow) Ancillary: can see lymphocytic cerebrospinal fluid pleocytosis with elevated protein and opening pressure; elevated hepatic transaminases and bilirubin; urinalysis showing pyuria, proteinuria, and hematuria; elevated creatinine, creatine kinase, and amylase	PCR is sensitive and continues to be positive even after initiation of therapy Serology (microscopic agglutination test (MAT) If sending blood cultures, need to notify laboratory to hold culture for 2–4 mo	Penicillin or ampicillin for severe disease Doxycycline or amoxicillin for mild disease, and doxycycline also recommended for prophylaxis Need to monitor for Jarisch–Herxheimer reaction with initiation of therapy
Malaria	Thick, thin smear Anemia, thrombocytopenia, hypoglycemia, metabolic acidosis, elevated creatinine, bilirubin, and serum transaminases. Obtain type and screen and G6PD level (need to know status before treating with primaquine for the hypnozoite form seen in *P. vivax and ovale*) If strongly suspect malaria, do not withhold treatment if initial smears negative, simply repeat smears in 12–24 hrs In a malaria-endemic region, low-grade parasitemia may not explain all a child's symptoms	Thick smear: quantify level of parasitemia Thin smear: allows for speciation; presence of >1 ring form in a erythrocyte suggests *P. falciparum,* the species responsible for most deaths globally	Check CDC site for regions where parasites retain chloroquine susceptibility *P. falciparum:* Atovaquone/Proguanil (Malarone) × 3 days or Artemether-lumefantrine (Coartem) × 3 days or Quinine + (clindamycin or doxycycline) × 7 days or Mefloquine (Larium) × 2 doses Severe/complicated malaria: quinine + clindamycin × 7 days; exchange transfusion considered for cerebral malaria and high-grade parasitemia For *vivax/ovale:* atovaquone. Proguanil + primaquine
Measles	Serology for IgM antibody	Serology for IgM antibody	Supportive treatment Vitamin A once daily for 2 days associated with decreased morbidity and mortality (WHO recommendation)
Mumps	Clinical diagnosis PCR and serology testing	PCR and serology testing	Supportive treatment
Neurocysticercosis	CSF serology, characteristic neuroimaging: hypodense cysts with well-defined edges; can see edema as parasites die Ancillary: CSF eosinophilia	Serology in CSF (serum serology cross-reacts with *Echinococcus*)	Utility of treatment if cysts is controversial and can be associated with acute inflammation Use of albendazole or praziquantel with steroids can be used
Polio	Culture of throat or stool (obtain two or more for enterovirus isolation obtained at least 24 hrs apart)	Culture of throat or stool	Supportive
Rabies	Serology Ancillary tests of minimal value, except to exclude other causes of meningoencephalitis	Serology Visualization of Negri bodies on cerebellar or nape of neck biopsies	Supportive care, but prognosis dismal once symptoms develop

Salmonella typhi	Stool culture for gastroenteritis Bone marrow culture or blood culture for those with enteric fever	Stool culture	Supportive if asymptomatic or uncomplicated (noninvasive) gastroenteritis Ampicillin, amoxicillin, or trimethoprim-sulfamethoxazole for susceptible strains For invasive disease, empiric treatment with expanded spectrum cephalosporin, azithromycin, or a fluoroquinolone
Salmonella, nontyphi	Conventional stool culture	Stool culture	Ceftriaxone or azithromycin if need treatment; bacteremic, <3 mo old, immunocompromised host (including children with hemoglobinopathies)
Schistosomiasis	Identification of eggs in stool (*S. mansoni* or *japonicum*) or urine (*S. hematobium*) Eosinophilia	Identification of eggs Serology does not differentiate acute and chronic infection	Praziquantel (most effective against adult worms, not immature stages, so retreatment after 3–4 mo often needed)
Shigella	Conventional stool culture Ancillary: leukocytosis with bandemia is common	Stool culture	Fluid resuscitation Azithromycin or Ceftriaxone daily for 3 days
Strongyloides	Stool to detect larvae (often need to obtain multiple stool samples)	Visualization of larvae in stool	Ivermectin is treatment of choice by WHO Also used: mebendazole Watch for anaphylaxis during treatment of hyperinfected patients
Tuberculosis	Respiratory specimen (expectorated sputum, induced sputum, or gastric aspirate) for acid-fast culture; additional cultures if extrapulmonary TB is suspected Ancillary: tuberculin skin test, interferon gamma release assay (IGRA), chest radiograph; check for HIV	Most children will have negative cultures, and diagnosis is made on basis of (1) consistent clinical and radiographic findings, (2) epidemiologic link to a source case, (3) immunologic evidence of TB (skin test, IGRA), and exclusion of other diagnoses	Azithromycin or ceftriaxone daily for 3 days Multidrug therapy (isoniazid, rifampin, pyrazinamide, ethambutol) administered via directly observed therapy Consultation with specialists in pediatric TB is warranted given infrequency of diagnosis in children in the United States
Yellow fever	Serology Ancillary: thrombocytopenia, elevated PT, PTT, hyperbilirubinemia, prolonged elevation of hepatic transaminases	Serology Patients who received yellow fever vaccine can have an elevated IgM for several years; cross-reaction with other flaviviruses can be seen	Supportive Avoid nonsteroidal anti-inflammatories

CDC, Centers for Disease Control and Prevention; PCR, polymerase chain reaction; ELISA, enzyme-linked immunosorbent assay; CSF, cerebrospinal fluid; EKG, electrocardiogram; TB, tuberculosis; HIV, human immunodeficiency virus; DIC, disseminated intravascular coagulation; G6PD, glucose-6-phosphate dehydrogenase; WHO, World Health Organization.

The most common species worldwide are *Plasmodium vivax,* prevalent on the Indian subcontinent and in central America, and *P. falciparum,* prevalent in Africa and in Papua New Guinea. High-risk regions include sub-Saharan Africa, Papua New Guinea, the Solomon Islands and Vanuatu.

Approximately 40% of the reported cases of malaria in the United States are from foreign travelers. Infections with *P. falciparum* can progress rapidly, some fatally, and must be considered in the differential diagnosis in all febrile children who have recently visited an endemic region. Approximately 90% of *P. falciparum* infections are acquired in sub-Saharan Africa, and up to 90% of travelers who are infected begin to have symptoms within 1 month after their return. In contrast to *P. falciparum* infections, travelers infected with *P. vivax* and *Plasmodium ovale* may show symptoms several months to years after exposure. Seventy percent of *P. vivax* infections are acquired in Asia or Latin America.

Chloroquine-sensitive malaria exists in central America as well as the Caribbean and limited parts of South America. There are regions that have developed chloroquine and mefloquine (Lariam) resistance, specifically in Southeast Asia. It is vital for the clinician to ask about not only if malaria prophylaxis was taken but also the medication and how it was administered. Both chloroquine and mefloquine kill the parasite only in the hematogenous phase; it is thus vital to take these medications for 4 weeks upon leaving the endemic region. Early termination of these medications could result in malaria even in someone who was "taking prophylaxis."

Goals of Treatment

The goal of treatment is for the clinician to rapidly recognize that the febrile child returning from a malaria-endemic region should be evaluated for plasmodial infection and that empiric antimalarial therapy, even in the absence of a positive blood smear, should be initiated for the toxic-appearing child.

Clinical Considerations

Clinical recognition: The most common symptoms of malaria are fever, malaise, headache, myalgia, vomiting, and diarrhea. Signs include pyrexia, tachycardia, tachypnea, dehydration, pallor, splenomegaly, and icterus. While the frequency and spectrum of complications differ among the plasmodial species (e-Table 102.15), signs and symptoms cannot differentiate between species. The malaria species and degree of parasitemia will affect the types and degree of symptoms that are displayed. Severe malaria is defined as shock, acidosis, hypoglycemia, end-organ involvement (e.g., CNS, renal), and/or parasitemia exceeding 5% of erythrocytes.

Triage considerations: Given the constellation of symptoms, malaria should be considered in all febrile travelers almost regardless of their clinical presentation.

Clinical assessment: The blood smear is considered the diagnostic reference standard. Both thick and thin smears should be obtained. Thick smears allow for a much larger volume of blood to be examined and thus for the detection of smaller numbers of parasites (leading to increased sensitivity), while the thin smear will allow for the identification of the species and the percentage of affected red blood cells. If the initial blood films are negative for malaria and the disease is still clinically suspected, examination of the thick and thin smears should be repeated at least once within 12 to 24 hours after the initial evaluation. One negative blood smear should not cause the clinician to exclude malaria from the differential diagnosis. In malaria-endemic areas, many children have low-level parasitemia. It is therefore important to consider other pathogens when children are found to have low-grade parasitemia on blood smear. Thrombocytopenia without leukocytosis is a characteristic feature of malaria, as is splenomegaly. Rapid assays for malaria are also available. In laboratories where personnel may be less familiar with performing blood smears, these rapid assays may be far superior to blood smears.

Management: Malaria is a reportable disease to the U.S. CDC. Empiric treatment should be decided upon in consultation with an ID specialist. Most children with malaria treated in the United States are admitted for treatment. Empiric therapy is based upon the disease severity, the species, and data regarding drug resistance in different geographic regions. Children with severe malaria should be admitted to an intensive care unit for monitoring and because some children will require exchange transfusion (if parasitemia exceeds 10% or there is evidence of cerebral or renal involvement). These children should receive parenteral therapy (clindamycin with either quinine or quinidine; artesunate is a newer parenteral regimen). Blood smears should be repeated after therapy is initiated to evaluate response to therapy and need for additional interventions. Primaquine is needed to kill the dormant phase seen in *P. vivax* and *P. ovale* infections. Prior to use of primaquine, patients need to be screened for glucose-6-phosphate dehydrogenase (G6PD) deficiency (primaquine can cause hemolytic anemia in patients with G6PD); women of childbearing age also need to be screened for pregnancy (primaquine is a potential teratogen). Both chloroquine and quinidine are available in intravenous preparations from the CDC. Standard precautions are used for patients with malaria.

Tuberculosis

CLINICAL PEARLS AND PITFALLS

- Intrathoracic tuberculosis (pulmonary parenchymal disease, intrathoracic lymphadenopathy, and pleural disease) and peripheral lymphadenopathy account for over 90% of all cases of childhood tuberculosis.
- Most children with tuberculosis have negative acid-fast sputum smears and cultures; the diagnosis is instead based on a triad of findings: a positive TST or TB blood test (interferon gamma release assays [IGRAs]); compatible radiographic and clinical findings; and contact with a person known to have tuberculosis disease.
- Preadolescent children with pulmonary tuberculosis without cavitary findings on radiography rarely are contagious; however, providers should utilize airborne precautions because in many instances, the child is brought to the ED by the person from whom they acquired tuberculosis, and that adult is by definition contagious.

Current Evidence

The most common sites of infection are intrathoracic (pulmonary parenchymal, intrathoracic adenopathy, and/or pleural effusions) and peripheral lymphadenopathy. Together, these account for over 90% of all childhood TB cases. Meningeal tuberculosis comprises 1% to 2% of all childhood TB cases, and is most common in children in the first 2 years of life.

Latent tuberculosis infection (LTBI) is defined as a positive TST (e-Table 102.16) in a child who lacks TB symptoms and has a normal chest radiograph and physical examination.

While LTBI will rarely be an ED-based diagnosis, clinicians may see children with LTBI for nontuberculosis concerns or for medication adverse events. Children with LTBI are not contagious and have no specific infection control considerations. As most tuberculosis medications are hepatically metabolized, the clinician should be aware of potential hepatotoxicity if a child receiving tuberculosis medication presents with abdominal pain, vomiting, anorexia, or icterus. Isoniazid (INH) can also cause peripheral neuropathy and can cause benzodiazepine-refractory seizures in cases of overdose (the antidote is pyridoxine, administered as a gram-to-gram dose based on the estimates of the INH dose ingested).

Goals of Treatment

The goal of treatment is to recognize which children with pulmonary, meningeal, or lymphadenitis may have tuberculosis as opposed to other diagnoses.

Clinical Considerations

Clinical recognition: Tuberculosis disease (e-Table 102.17) should be included in the differential diagnosis of children with fever of unknown origin; pneumonia refractory to therapy for community-acquired pneumonia; cavitary pneumonia/lung abscesses; hilar or mediastinal adenopathy; miliary pattern on chest radiograph; free-flowing pleural effusions with or without consolidation; chronic nontender adenopathy; chronic otorrhea or chronic otitis media; and meningitis with an elevated CSF protein. Children with pulmonary tuberculosis often have chest radiographs that look far worse than the child. Weight loss in combination with pneumonia should lead the provider to broaden the differential diagnosis outside of the usual pathogens causing community-acquired pneumonia. TB meningitis has an insidious onset, and in the early stages, children may have fever and constitutional symptoms alone. Unexplained protracted vomiting (due to increased intracranial pressure) often is identified only in retrospect. Given the nonspecific initial symptoms and the rarity of the diagnosis in industrialized nations, many children with TB meningitis have had multiple healthcare encounters prior to diagnosis.

Triage considerations: While prepubertal children with noncavitary chest radiographs rarely are contagious, the person bringing the child to medical attention may be the person who transmitted tuberculosis to the child. As such, airborne precautions should be used more to protect healthcare workers and other patients from the caregivers, as opposed to from the patient him/herself.

Clinical assessment: The diagnosis of tuberculosis in a child infrequently is made based upon microbiologic confirmation. Acid-fast cultures of respiratory secretions are positive in a minority of children; the highest culture yield occurs in children with peripheral lymphadenopathy or skeletal disease. Instead, children usually are diagnosed based on a triad of findings: epidemiologic links to a person with known or suspected tuberculosis disease; a positive TST or IGRA; and compatible clinical or radiographic findings. A chest radiograph should be performed in all children in whom TB is suspected. The majority of children with extrapulmonary disease (especially those with meningitis) will have abnormal chest radiographs. CT of the brain should be obtained in children with suspected TB meningitis, as hydrocephalus and tuberculomas (mass-occupying lesions) may be present and hydrocephaly may require shunting. All infants in whom TB disease is suspected should undergo LP for routine studies, acid-fast culture, and *M. tuberculosis* PCR. While TSTs are helpful when positive, a negative test does not rule out TB. All children in whom TB disease is suspected should be screened for HIV and have a baseline CBC and hepatic transaminases performed.

Management: Initiation of multidrug tuberculosis therapy should be performed in conjunction with ID specialists. The management of children with drug-resistant tuberculosis is outside the scope of this chapter. Airborne precautions should be used.

Typhoid

CLINICAL PEARLS

- Typhoid fever is caused by the bacteria *Salmonella enterica* serotype typhi. It is a human pathogen transmitted via the fecal–oral route and can cause local (diarrheal) or invasive disease (bacteremia, meningitis, bowel perforation, osteomyelitis). For many children fever alone is the only presenting symptom.
- Typhoid fever is more common in the pediatric and immunocompromised hosts of any age and should be suspected in any febrile child who has returned from Asia, Africa, or Latin America in the preceding month.

Current Evidence

Typhoid fever is endemic in sub-Saharan Africa, the Indian subcontinent, Southeast Asia, East Asia, the Middle East, and central and South America with an estimated incidence of 22 million per year. It is most prevalent in impoverished areas where sanitary conditions are poor. Approximately 300 returned travelers to the United States are diagnosed with typhoid fever every year. In the United States, 67% of imported cases were from South Central Asia, 10% from Southeast Asia, and 10% from sub-Saharan Africa. Increasing rates of antibiotic resistance to cephalosporins, fluoroquinolones, and macrolides have been seen in recent years. In Southeast Asia, reduced susceptibility to fluoroquinolones has complicated empiric therapy.

***Goals of treatment*:** The goal of treatment is the rapid recognition that fever in a returned traveler could represent typhoid fever, and for the PEM clinician to be cognizant of drug-resistance patterns globally that may impact empiric antibiotic selection.

Clinical Considerations

Clinical recognition: Many patients infected with *S. enterica* subtype typhi are either asymptomatic or have mild symptoms; 60% to 90% do not seek medical attention or are treated on in the outpatient setting. Patients with typhoid fever have an insidious onset of fever and development of symptoms over a period of 5 to 21 days after the ingestion of contaminated food or water. A majority of patients develop anorexia, abdominal pain, chills, in addition to malaise, tender splenomegaly, marked headache, relative bradycardia (given the degree of pyrexia), and a nonproductive cough in the early stages. Approximately 25% of Caucasian patients will develop painless, erythematous, blanchable, subcentimeter, maculopapular "rose spots" on the trunk. Constipation is more common than diarrhea in young children. The severity of illness is influenced by the particular strain virulence, quantity of inoculum, the age of the patient, duration of illness before initiation of treatment, and current vaccination status. Complications of severe disease include shock, meningitis, pneumonia (primary *Salmonella* pneumonia or secondary bacterial infection), gastrointestinal perforation, or hemorrhage. Chronic carriers play an important role in the transmission of the disease; they typically excrete a large number of organisms yet have a high level of immunity.

Triage considerations: Clinicians should consider typhoid fever in patients with abdominal pain, fever, and chills, and with recent travel to developing nations.

Clinical assessment: Diagnosis is made by blood culture. Stool cultures are positive in approximately 30% of bacteremic patients. Bone marrow cultures may be useful because they remain positive long after treatment has been initiated and are more sensitive than blood culture. Serology is not recommended as it often cross-reacts with other *Salmonella* serotypes.

Management: Empiric management of children with suspected typhoid is reviewed in e-Table 102.18. Historically, fluoroquinolones have been the treatment of choice. However, the recent evolution and recognition of multidrug-resistant *Salmonella* isolates has complicated empiric therapy. In general, fluoroquinolones should not be first-line therapy if typhoid fever in patient from South Asia or other regions where there is a known increase in resistance to fluoroquinolones. In some sub-Saharan African nations, up to 40% of *Salmonella* isolates are resistant to latter generation cephalosporins. In patients with severe systemic illness, such as typhoid-associated shock or encephalopathy, dexamethasone (3 mg per kg followed by 1 mg per kg every 6 hours for 48 hours), should be considered. The chronic carrier state can be eradicated by 4 weeks of oral fluoroquinolones. Contact and standard precautions should be used for providers caring for children with suspected typhoid fever.

Dengue

CLINICAL PEARLS AND PITFALLS

- Dengue is the most prevalent mosquito-transmitted viral illness and should be considered in the differential diagnosis of any febrile patient presenting in the ED within 2 weeks of return from a tropical or subtropical region.
- Clinical manifestations include self-limited dengue fever to life-threatening dengue hemorrhagic fever with shock syndrome.
- Treatment is with supportive care and fluid resuscitation, including blood transfusion.

Current Evidence

Dengue is transmitted by the *Aedes aegypti* mosquitoes, which are most active during the day, but can bite at any time of day or night. The disease is endemic to central and South America, sub-Saharan Africa, the Indian subcontinent, and Southeast Asia. Concurrently, there has been a broadening of the geographic distribution of the disease. In the last decade, outbreaks have been reported in Texas, Florida, and Hawaii, and the mosquito vector already is widespread throughout the southern United States. The worldwide incidence has been increasing in the past several decades due to a number of factors including population growth, overcrowded urban living with poor sanitation, increasingly mobile/transient population and therefore increased mobility of the mosquitoes, virus and infected individuals, and lack of effective mosquito control. Each year there are an estimated 50 to 100 million dengue infections, with >500,000 cases of dengue hemorrhagic fever, and >20,000 deaths, primarily in children.

Goals of Treatment

The goal of dengue management is to identify which children are at risk for dengue based on travel history and for the PEM clinician to be aware that rapid fluid shifts after fluid resuscitation can lead to volume overload.

Clinical Considerations

Clinical recognition: The differential diagnosis includes febrile illness with similar clinical manifestations such as influenza, enteroviral infection, measles, and rubella. The diagnosis is typically a clinical one when treating patients with recent travel to dengue endemic regions. Only 50% of patients infected with dengue develop symptoms. Clinical manifestations range from self-limited dengue fever to dengue hemorrhagic with shock syndrome. Symptoms typically develop within 3 to 14 days after the bite of an infected mosquito; the risk of severe disease is much higher in sequential infections. In 2009, the World Health Organization (WHO) published revised dengue case definitions (e-Table 102.19). Three distinct phases exist. The first is the febrile phase. Here, children develop pyrexia (or hyperpyrexia), vomiting, joint pain. Some develop a transient maculopapular rash, lasting approximately 3 to 7 days. Most patients do not progress to the next phase and improve without intervention. Phase 2 is called the critical or capillary leak phase and consists of clinical or radiographic evidence of serositis, ascites, or pulmonary edema. Children in phase 2 are at risk for developing hypotension and uncompensated shock. Patients may be refractory to fluid resuscitation and may develop abdominal pain, persistent emesis, tender hepatomegaly, mucosal bleeding, and altered mentation. Phase 3 (the convalescence or reabsorption phase) begins approximately 2 to 3 days after the initiation of phase 2. Patients typically experience both clinical and laboratory rapid improvement as the body reabsorbs extravasated plasma and fluid. Some patients develop a pruritic vasculitic rash that may desquamate during resolution of the illness (2 to 3 weeks).

Triage considerations: Dengue should be considered in every patient seen in the ED presenting with fever and recent return (<2 weeks) from tropical or subtropical regions.

Clinical assessment: Dengue is predominantly a clinical diagnosis. Definitive diagnosis is via PCR or ELISA; IgM antibodies are detectable by day 4 to 5 after fever onset. Children with suspected dengue should get the following laboratory evaluation: complete blood count (to evaluate for leukopenia, anemia, and thrombocytopenia), BUN and creatinine to evaluate for acute kidney injury, type and screen, hepatic transaminases, prothrombin time, and partial thromboplastin time to evaluate for disseminated intravascular coagulation.

Management: Treatment of dengue is supportive including fever control, and fluid resuscitation and red blood cell transfusion. There appears to be no indication for platelet transfusion; the consumptive coagulopathy seen in dengue appears to be refractory to transfusions. There are no antivirals that are of use in dengue. There are some small, nonrandomized trials of corticosteroids for dengue shock syndrome that have shown some possible benefit, but more data are lacking. Standard precautions are recommended.

Chikungunya

CLINICAL PEARLS AND PITFALLS

- Chikungunya is endemic in Africa, the Indian subcontinent, and Southeast Asia.
- Clinical manifestations mimic dengue and include fever and bilateral polyarthralgia. Hemorrhagic manifestations are more common in children. Most recover fully over a period of weeks, but approximately 5% to 10% experience chronic joint symptoms.

Current Evidence

The main vectors for chikungunya are the *A. aegypti* and *Aedes albopictus* mosquitoes, which also transmit dengue. Chikungunya is found throughout Africa, India, China, and Southeast Asia, but cases in travelers returning to North America, the Caribbean, France, and Italy have been reported. In late 2013, the first transmission in the western hemisphere was reported in St. Martin and other French territories in the Caribbean. As the incubation period is relatively short, it is most common in travelers who have recently returned from endemic regions.

Goals of Treatment

As with other travel-related infections, it is important for the clinician to recognize that some imported infections will present similarly to infections endemic in the United States (e.g., influenza virus). Asking about recent travel will help broaden the differential diagnosis.

Clinical Considerations

Clinical recognition: The incubation period is 2 to 12 days and the first symptom is often rapid-onset arthralgia of multiple joints. Subsequently, patients develop myalgia, high fever, generalized lymphadenopathy, and conjunctivitis. Initial symptoms usually resolve over 2 to 3 days and are followed by the development of a maculopapular rash in about 50% of patients. Fever may recur and some develop hemorrhagic manifestations (more common in children).

Triage Considerations

Clinical assessment: Chikungunya mimics dengue in symptomatology and geographic distribution. One of the distinguishing features between the two is that the arthralgia in Chikungunya is polyarticular, something rarely seen with dengue. Chikungunya is more likely to present with lymphopenia than dengue, while dengue is more likely to result in neutropenia. Thrombocytopenia can be found with both diseases although severe thrombocytopenia is more common in dengue. Fluid resuscitation may be needed due to dehydration from reduced intake and increased insensible losses. Most children recover fully over a period of weeks but approximately 5% to 10% experience chronic joint symptoms. Severe complications include meningoencephalitis, cardiopulmonary compromise, acute renal failure, and death; these are more common in patients with comorbidities and the elderly. The primary diagnostic tool used is serology. ELISA tests identify IgM (1 to 12 days after infection) and IgG (2 weeks postinfection) antibodies. Viral culture and molecular techniques are used primarily for research purposes.

Management: Treatment is supportive. Repeat episodes are more likely to be severe. Nonsteroidal anti-inflammatories or corticosteroids may help to relive arthralgia. Standard isolation precautions should be used. The risk of human infection may be reduced by utilization of insect repellant (no more than 30% DEET recommended for children >2 months), wearing long pants and long sleeve shirts, and staying in screened or air-conditioned dwellings during peak feeding times (dusk to dawn). Standard precautions are recommended.

Diarrheal Diseases

CLINICAL PEARLS

- Diarrheal disease is a significant cause of morbidity and mortality worldwide.
- Diarrhea is often accompanied by other clinical signs and symptoms including vomiting, dehydration, fever, and electrolyte abnormalities.
- There exist more than 40 different enteropathogens that can cause gastroenteritis and is neither possible nor necessary to arrive at an etiologic diagnosis in all cases.

Current Evidence

Many children who travel to developing countries develop diarrhea. Most episodes of traveler's diarrhea resolve during or shortly after the travel. Five percent to 10% of travelers report diarrhea that lasts for 2 weeks or longer and 1% to 3% have diarrhea that lasts 4 weeks or longer. In the majority of cases, the etiologic agent of traveler's diarrhea cannot be isolated. However, among cases in which a pathogen is isolated, 50% to 75% are identified within 2 weeks of developing symptoms. As the duration of the diarrhea increases (typically greater than 2 weeks), the likelihood of identifying a specific bacterial cause decreases; in contrast, the likelihood of identification of a parasitic cause increases. The most commonly identified parasitic infections include *G. lamblia, Cryptosporidium parvum, E. histolytica,* and *Cyclospora cayetanensis,* although these are detected in less than one-third of travelers with chronic diarrhea and in only 1% to 5% of travelers with acute diarrhea. Infected children are predominantly asymptomatic, but bloody or nonbloody diarrhea, hepatobiliary symptoms, and failure to thrive may occur.

Viral hepatitis should be considered when evaluating a child with nonspecific gastrointestinal symptoms, particularly when jaundice is present. Hepatitis A is prevalent in both developed and developing nations and is acquired through contaminated food and water. Hepatitis A is usually asymptomatic or manifests as mild symptoms in young children. Hepatitis E must be considered because it is a common etiology of acute hepatitis in developing countries. Although rarely presenting acutely, hepatitis B and C are common in the developing world and should be considered in any adolescent or young adult who is sexually active or has had a tattoo or body piercing while traveling.

There are several common noninfectious causes of chronic diarrhea in travelers including tropical sprue, postinfectious disaccharidase deficiency, and irritable bowel syndrome. Tropical sprue is characterized by acute or chronic diarrhea, weight loss, and malabsorption of nutrients. It occurs in residents of or visitors to the tropics and subtropics; the cause is unknown. e-Table 102.20 reviews the differences between inflammatory and noninflammatory diarrhea. Importantly, a diarrheal illness that develops more than 1 month after travel is not likely due to travel exposure.

Goals of Treatment

The goal is for the clinician to know in which children bacterial or protozoal pathogens would be a more likely etiology for diarrheal disease, and, therefore, which children would be more likely to benefit from antibiotic therapy.

Clinical Considerations

Clinical recognition: Invasive or inflammatory enteropathy (e.g., dysentery) should be suspected in persons with bloody diarrhea, fever, or leukocytes detected in the mucous portion of the stool. Invasive enteropathy has a fairly abrupt onset (over a period of hours generally) and may be complicated by metastatic infections, reactive arthropathy, or, in the case of infection with *Campylobacter jejuni,* Guillain–Barré syndrome. Amoebic dysentery, caused by *E. histolytica* among other amoebae, often presents slowly over the course of days and may be complicated by hepatic abscess formation.

Triage considerations: Early recognition of the dehydrated child, or of the child with possible electrolyte disturbances, is essential. While most children with mild or moderate dehydration will respond to oral volume resuscitation, parenteral resuscitation will be needed for the severely dehydrated child.

Clinical assessment: Returning travelers with diarrhea should have stool samples cultured for enteric pathogens and examined microscopically for ova and parasites if there is evidence of an invasive enteropathy, if the diarrhea is persistent, if the diarrhea is unresponsive to empirical therapy, or if the infected person is immunocompromised. Assays for the detection of *C. difficile* toxins may also be indicated. The routine microbiologic techniques oftentimes cannot detect many of the bacteria associated with persistent diarrhea. The sensitivity of a single stool specimen for the detection of ova and parasites varies, depending on the parasite, but it rarely exceeds 80%. The likelihood of identifying a parasite may be increased by examining additional stool samples (three samples obtained on separate occasions increase the sensitivity to more than 90%).

Management: In many cases of persistent diarrhea, no causative agent can be identified. In these cases, some experts recommend empiric antimicrobial therapy such as a fluoroquinolone or a macrolide for suspected bacterial enteritis. Metronidazole (or a related agent) is recommended for presumed giardiasis, since *G. lamblia* is the most commonly identified intestinal parasite in travelers. Multiple courses of antimicrobial agents should be avoided. For travelers whose diarrhea persists, endoscopic examination and biopsy should be considered to exclude entities such as tropical sprue and inflammatory bowel disease. Contact precautions are recommended.

SYSTEMIC INFECTIONS IN THE RETURNED TRAVELER

There are several treatable infections that may affect travelers who have systemic manifestations, including hemorrhage. These include meningococcemia, malaria, leptospirosis, and rickettsial infections. There are a handful of viral infections (in addition to dengue and yellow fever) that are also associated with fever and hemorrhage; these, however, are rarely acquired by travelers. Viral hemorrhagic fevers (such as Lassa fever and Ebola fever) need to be considered in travelers who present with fever and hemorrhage; these diseases also have important infection control and public health concerns. Epidemiologic clues include history of visits to rural areas or recent contact with ill persons in areas where the viral hemorrhagic fevers are endemic. Most patients with viral hemorrhagic fevers note the onset of fever within 3 weeks after exposure to infected persons, contaminated water, or infected insects/vectors.

There is currently no specific treatment available for the viral hemorrhagic fevers. Supportive care with special attention to careful fluid and electrolyte management is indicated. Endothelial dysfunction makes hydration challenging; pulmonary edema occurs rapidly with intravenous hydration. To prevent agitation, analgesia and sedation may be useful.

Yellow Fever

Yellow fever is a tropical zoonotic infection caused by a flavivirus transmitted from non-human primates to humans by mosquitoes of the *Aedes* (in Africa) and *Haemagogus* (in Latin America) genera. Following a 3- to 6-day incubation period, patients develop an influenza-like illness with fever, chills, headache, photophobia, back pain, and myalgias lasting approximately 4 days, followed by spontaneous resolution in almost 80% of patients. The remaining 15% to 20% of patients then develop fever, abdominal pain, vomiting, and jaundice. Oliguria and hemorrhagic findings can be seen. Laboratory findings include leukopenia, thrombocytopenia, transaminitis, disseminated intravascular coagulation, and proteinuria. Most patients experience remission of symptoms after an initial 3- to 4-day period. Patients who continue to have symptoms or develop biphasic illness can progress to multiorgan system dysfunction; in these cases, mortality rates range from 20% to 50%. Treatment is supportive, often in an intensive care unit setting. A live-attenuated vaccine is available for children older than 6 to 9 months and is required for entry into some Latin American and sub-Saharan African nations. Standard precautions are recommended.

Leptospirosis

Leptospirosis is caused by *Leptospira interrogans,* a spirochete transmitted in the urine or placental tissue of rodents and other infected non-human animals. As organisms can remain viable under moist conditions (soil or water) for months, the infection can also be spread via contact with bodies of water or after persons have been in regions where flooding has occurred. Humans become infected via entry of leptospires through mucosal surfaces or skin abrasions. While it has a global distribution, it is more common in tropical and subtropical regions. Most cases are mild or asymptomatic. Severe cases typically are bimodal, with an initial septicemic phase and a second immune phase. The septicemic phase can be icteric (Weil syndrome) or anicteric and is characterized by an influenza-like illness lasting less than 1 week. Following this, a subset of patients will develop headache, nuchal rigidity, rash (sometimes petechial), hepatomegaly, and conjunctival suffusion. Renal involvement may consist of pyuria, hematuria, proteinuria, or acute kidney injury. The most severe form is Weil syndrome, characterized by icterus and hepatorenal syndrome; it carries a 5% to 10% mortality rate. The diagnosis is based upon acute and convalescent serologies. Parenteral penicillin is the treatment of choice. Clinicians should be aware of Jarisch–Herxheimer reactions (acute febrile illness, myalgia, headache lasting less than 1 day) after initiation of therapy as the spirochetes die. Doxycycline can be used in older patients with milder disease. Contact precautions are recommended.

Tick-borne Diseases

Rickettsial diseases in the returned traveler may include *Rickettsia africae* (African tick typhus), *Rickettsia conorii* (causing varying clinical syndromes in different geographic regions, and called by a number of names: Boutonneuse fever; or Mediterranean, Israeli, Kenyan, or Indian tick typhus), and *Orientia tsutsugamushi* (scrub or bush typhus in Japan and Russia). These are all arthropod transmitted from game and cattle ticks, dog ticks, and mites ("chiggers"), respectively. Symptoms are similar to endemic rickettsial diseases: fever, headaches, myalgia, and rashes. A painless eschar can sometimes be found at the site of the bite. Risk factors include hiking, camping, or traveling on safari in grassy or scrubby regions. Examination findings may include localized lymphadenopathy and a petechial or nonpetechial rash (African tick typhus typically presents without rash, or with a few macular or vesicular lesions). Laboratory findings include leukopenia and thrombocytopenia. The diagnosis is usually clinical and treatment with doxycycline should not await confirmatory serologies or PCR-based diagnostics. Standard precautions are recommended.

Plague

Plague is caused by a Gram-negative coccobacillus, *Yersinia pestis,* which is a zoonotic infection of rodents and fleas. It can be transmitted by respiratory droplet from person-to-person. Plague cases are consistently recorded throughout several countries in Africa, Asia, and the Americas with a vast majority of these cases occurring in Africa. In the United States, the main risk factor is contact with prairie dogs, and it is most common in the upper Midwestern states. The most common form is bubonic plague, characterized by an initial brief prodrome of fever, anorexia, and headache followed by the development of tender regional adenopathy (often in the inguinal area after flea bites to the lower extremities). These nodes develop a reddish discoloration and proceed to necrosis. More severe forms include pneumonic and septicemic plague. Most patients have a rapidly progressive course characterized by fever; initial symptoms mimic influenza. If untreated, pneumonic and septicemic plague is almost uniformly fatal and bubonic plague has a mortality rate approaching 50%. The proximate causes of death are disseminated intravascular coagulation, respiratory failure, and renal failure. The diagnosis is made by culture; Gram stain demonstrates a bipolar appearance to the bacillus that appears like a safety pin with clustering of the stain at the poles with relative central clearing. The treatment of choice is an aminoglycoside. Alternative agents include fluoroquinolones or chloramphenicol for plague meningitis, tetracyclines, or doxycycline. Cephalosporins are not recommended. TMP-SMZ is not recommended as monotherapy. The disease must be reported to public health authorities. Droplet precautions should be used for patients with pneumonic plague.

CENTRAL/PERIPHERAL NERVOUS SYSTEM

There are numerous processes that may cause fever and neurologic manifestations; however, special consideration should be given to specific etiologies in the returning traveler. Malaria, tuberculosis, typhoid fever, rickettsial infections, leptospirosis, poliomyelitis, rabies, and the viral encephalitides (including Japanese encephalitis, West Nile encephalitis, and tick-borne encephalitis) are possible infections that affect the CNS. Travelers to the "meningitis belt" regions in Africa (during the months of December to June) and those who travel to the Arab world around the time of the annual pilgrimage to Mecca for the Hajj are at increased risk for developing meningococcal meningitis. CNS involvement with eosinophilia should also raise the possibility of coccidioidomycosis and angiostrongyliasis (the latter caused by the rat lungworm *Angiostrongylus cantonensis*).

Neurocysticercosis

Cysticercosis is caused by the pork tapeworm, *Taenia solium,* commonly found throughout central and South America, South Asia, and China. Human cysticercosis is acquired via fecal–oral transmission by ingestion of tapeworm eggs from a human tapeworm carrier or by autoinfection. The incubation period may be several years. Morbidity is almost entirely due to infection of the CNS; most commonly, seizures (partial seizures with or without secondary generalization) due to larval cysts in the brain parenchyma serving as a seizure focus. Other manifestations can include gait dysfunction from cerebellar involvement, ocular disease with visual loss, or encephalitis. One study in Chicago found that neurocysticercosis was a common cause of new-onset afebrile seizures in Latino children. Subcutaneous cysts are primarily only of cosmetic significance and produce painless palpable nodules.

The diagnosis is made primarily via CT scanning or MRI demonstrating calcified, hypodense or ring-enhancing larval cysts. Antibody assays detecting IgG to *T. solium* in the CSF and serum are the confirmatory diagnostic tests available via the CDC and multiple commercial laboratories. Serum serologies are more sensitive than CSF serologies.

Neurocysticercosis treatment has to be individualized on the basis of the number and viability of cysts present on neuroimaging and where they are located. Calcified, or nonviable cysts, only require symptomatic treatment and anticonvulsant therapy in children with seizures. Parenchymal cysts without enhancement typically respond to antihelminthic treatment: either praziquantel (100 mg/kg/day PO in three doses × 1 day, then 50 mg/kg/day in 3 doses × 29 days) or albendazole (15 mg/kg/day, max 800 mg, in two doses for 8 to 30 days). Albendazole is better tolerated than praziquantel, is indicated for children of all ages, and does not interact with most antiepileptic medications. Studies have demonstrated that a shorter 8-day course of albendazole is of equivalent efficacy compared to the prior recommended 30-day course. One large meta-analysis found that antihelminthic treatment was associated with decreased seizure frequency and more rapid radiographic resolution of granulomas that form around cysts. Coadministration of corticosteroids for the initial 2 to 3 days of treatment is recommended if extensive CNS involvement is suspected, but is not associated with improved neurologic outcomes. Clinicians should be aware that patients may have paradoxical worsening during therapy, as most of the CNS effects of neurocysticercosis are immune mediated and often worsen as the host inflammatory response is activated. Anticonvulsant therapy is recommended until resolution of neurologic symptoms and patient has been seizure free for 1 to 2 years. Surgical excision is generally recommended for intraventricular and ocular cysts. Standard precautions should be observed.

Rabies

Rabies is an almost uniformly fatal zoonotic infection caused by a rhabdovirus. While most commonly spread to humans from dogs internationally (more than 95% of cases occur in Africa and Asia), the majority of US cases are caused by exposure to bats and wild carnivores (raccoons, skunks, foxes, coyotes). Among domesticated animals, cats are reported as rabid three times more commonly than dogs. The incubation period is longer for bites on the distal extremities than on the trunk or face. The two major clinical syndromes are furious and paralytic rabies; each lasts approximately 2 to 10 days. Furious rabies consists of hyperesthesia at the bite site, agitation, confusion, hallucinations, aerophobia, and hydrophobia; in the absence of an exposure history, early symptoms can be difficult to differentiate from psychiatric illness. Paralytic rabies (approximately 30% of all cases) begins with paresis of the muscles surrounding the bite site and progress to generalized paralysis. This form often is underreported. There are a few case reports of rabies survivors (protocol available at www.mcw.edu/rabies), but treatment generally is supportive; contact precautions should be used. Pre-exposure prophylaxis with the rabies vaccine is recommended for veterinarians and others at risk for bites from wild or domesticated animals. PEP indications are summarized in e-Table 102.21 and include both the rabies vaccine and receipt of rabies immunoglobulin (RIG).

Polio/Acute Flaccid Paralysis

Polio is caused by three enteroviral serotypes and is transmitted via the fecal–oral route. There is no non-human reservoir; most cases are transmitted during summer months, and it primarily affects children less than 5 years of age. It can result from administration of the oral polio vaccine, a live-attenuated vaccine no longer utilized in the United States. As of 2014, only three countries were classified as polio endemic by the WHO: Afghanistan, Nigeria, and Pakistan. Approximately 400 cases were reported in 2013. Seventy percent of infections are asymptomatic, and almost one-quarter of cases have mild disease, characterized by low-grade fever and upper respiratory tract symptoms. Acute flaccid paralysis is seen in 1% of cases as a result of motor neuron disease. The paralysis is asymmetric, flaccid, and associated with areflexia. Leg paralysis is most common; of paralyzed patients, 5% to 10% develop paralysis of cranial nerves or respiratory muscles. The diagnosis is clinical, with culture or PCR of stool or pharyngeal swabs serving as confirmatory tests. Treatment is supportive. Contact precautions are recommended.

African Trypanosomiasis

African trypanosomiasis ("African sleeping sickness") is a protozoal infection transmitted through the bite of the tsetse fly. Wild animals serve as the reservoir for *Trypanosoma brucei rhodesiense* (East African trypanosomiasis), whereas humans are the most important reservoir for *Trypanosoma brucei gambiense* (West African trypanosomiasis). Clinical manifestations vary by subspecies. An erythematous swelling or chancre at the site of the fly bite, intermittent high fevers, retrobulbar headache, posterior cervical adenopathy (Winterbottom sign), myalgia, and myocarditis can be preceded by the meningoencephalitis. Chronic meningoencephalitis is associated with behavioral changes, delusions, and the somnolence that result in the illness name. Laboratory findings include anemia, thrombocytopenia, transaminitis, and, rarely, disseminated intravascular coagulation. During the acute phase, trypomastigotes are often detectable on blood smears of buffy coats or aspirates of lymph nodes. Serologies are not available for East African trypanosomiasis. Early treatment is essential because the prognosis is poor once CNS involvement has occurred. In the absence of CNS disease, pentamidine is used for West African and suramin for East African trypanosomiasis. CNS involvement requires use of eflornithine for West African and melarsoprol for East African trypanosomiasis. Drugs for trypanosomiasis are difficult to obtain in the United States and care should be coordinated via the CDC Drug Service: (404) 639-3670. Standard precautions are recommended.

CARDIAC INFECTIONS

Chagas Disease

Chagas disease, an infection caused by the protozoan parasite *T. cruzi*, is seen in Mexico and central and South America. The parasite is transmitted through feces of infected triatomine insects (kissing bugs) after a blood meal. The global prevalence is 8 to 10 million. The common initial presentation is a painless red nodule known as a chagoma that develops at the site of initial inoculation. Most develop low-grade fever, generalized lymphadenopathy, and malaise. Rare acute presentations include myocarditis, hepatosplenomegaly, edema, and meningoencephalitis. While most cases resolve over 1 to 3 months, in approximately 20% of patients, serious sequelae such as dilated cardiomyopathy, megaesophagus, and megacolon may occur years to decades after the initial infection. Cardiac manifestations include pericardial effusion which can lead to tamponade physiology, left ventricular aneurysms, abnormal diastolic function, contractile anomalies, and characteristic EKG findings (right bundle branch block, left anterior block, AV block, sinus bradycardia, and ST segment, T- and Q-wave abnormalities). Mortality is due to ventricular arrhythmias, complete heart block, congestive heart failure, or emboli. Diagnosis is made via Giemsa staining of blood specimens or by direct wet mount prep. Serologies, available via the CDC, are used to diagnose chronic Chagas. Treatment is with antitrypanosomal medications such as benznidazole (for 30 to 90 days) or nifurtimox (for 90 to 120 days). Travelers should avoid contact with the triatomine bug by utilizing insecticide and bed netting and avoiding habitation in buildings constructed of mud, palm thatch, or adobe brick. Standard precautions are recommended.

RESPIRATORY TRACT INFECTIONS

The most common respiratory infections in returned travelers will be simple viral infections. However, knowledge of the region of travel can alert clinicians to either common viruses with different seasonality in other hemispheres (e.g., influenza virus in the middle of the calendar year in subequatorial nations) or for pathogens more common in other settings. The latter includes tuberculosis (described earlier in the chapter), some vaccine-preventable diseases more common in developing nations (e.g., diphtheria), and emerging infections, such as the coronaviruses causing Severe Acute Respiratory Syndrome (SARS) and Middle Eastern Respiratory Syndrome (MERS), which were first reported in Asia and the Middle East, respectively.

Coronaviruses (SARS, MERS)

Coronaviruses are common causes of mild upper respiratory tract infections, and are known to cause lower respiratory tract disease, primarily in young or immunocompromised children. In 2002, SARS caused a febrile illness associated with ARDS and a mortality rate that exceeded 50% in older adults. Disease severity was milder in young children. Laboratory findings included leukopenia, elevated LDH, and elevated creatinine kinase. In 2012, MERS was first described in a Saudi Arabian man who died of ARDS. Symptoms include fever, chills, myalgias, and a minority of patients develop diarrhea. Acute kidney injury and multiorgan failure can be seen. In May 2014, the first MERS imported case was reported, and within 2 weeks the first case transmitted within the United States was reported from Illinois. Treatment is supportive. Contact and droplet precautions should be used.

Diphtheria

Diphtheria, a bacterial infection caused by an exotoxin-producing Gram-positive bacillus, *Corynebacterium diphtheriae,* remains an important disease in resource-poor countries and has experienced resurgence in recent years in Russia, Haiti, and other countries. Diphtheria is spread via contact with respiratory secretions (airborne, droplet, or direct contact) or skin lesions. Infection may lead to an asymptomatic carrier state, respiratory disease, or cutaneous disease. Faucial (nasopharyngeal) diphtheria is the most common form of the disease and is characterized by the gradual onset of a moderate fever, malaise, and pharyngitis in 80% with a gray-white pseudomembrane usually covering one or both tonsils. There is usually a characteristic odor present. Extensive membranous pharyngitis may ensue, causing significant swelling of the tonsils, uvula, anterior neck, and regional lymph nodes causing a "bull neck" appearance. Stridor can be seen with laryngeal involvement. Fever, if present at all, usually is low grade. Severe complications are seen in approximately 10% of patients and include myocarditis with arrhythmias or heart failure, or neuritis of the palatal, bulbar, or skeletal muscles. Baseline EKGs should be obtained in a patient with suspected diphtheria. Cutaneous diphtheria is now more common than nasopharyngeal disease in the West, with recent resurgence seen in homeless persons in the United States. Chronic, painless nonhealing scaly rashes with well-demarcated borders or ulcers with a grey membrane appearance characterize skin involvement.

The diagnosis is made clinically and confirmed by culture. The laboratory should be notified that diphtheria is suspected, as the organism has specific culture requirements (cysteine-tellurite blood agar or modified Tinsdale agar). Treatment involves administration of IV equine antitoxin and antibiotics. Antibiotic treatment with erythromycin (oral or parenteral) or penicillin G IM or IV for 14 days will stop toxin production and prevent dissemination. Cutaneous lesions should be thoroughly washed with soap and water and treated with antimicrobial treatment as discussed above. Household contacts and providers, irrespective of their immunization status, should receive nasopharyngeal cultures and be offered PEP with either oral erythromycin or intramuscular penicillin G. Persons receiving PEP also should be offered a booster dose of a diphtheria-containing vaccine. Droplet precautions are recommended for all patients and carriers with pharyngeal diphtheria until nasopharyngeal cultures collected 24 hours after completing antimicrobial treatment are negative.

Hantavirus

Hantaviruses are members of the Bunyaviridae family and are spread by infected rodents. Two different syndromes have been reported: hemorrhagic fever with renal syndrome (HFRS) and Hantavirus cardiopulmonary syndrome. The clinical features of HFRS include fever, hemorrhage, hypotension, and renal failure. The clinical features of Hantavirus cardiopulmonary syndrome consist of a 2- to 8-day prodrome, and a febrile phase associated with diffuse interstitial edema with respiratory compromise developing within 72 hours. Patients may develop chills, headaches, vomiting, myalgia, and diarrhea. Symptoms typically seen with upper respiratory tract infections are notably absent, except for cough. Laboratory findings include a neutrophilic leukocytosis with bandemia, thrombocytopenia, and increased hemoglobin. Renal manifestations include proteinuria and hematuria. The diagnosis is serologic. Treatment is supportive. Mortality rates approaching 40% have been reported for Hantavirus cardiopulmonary syndrome, whereas death from HFRS is rare. Standard precautions are recommended; it has not been associated with healthcare transmission or person-to-person infection.

Lymphadenopathy

The differential diagnosis for lymphadenopathy in the returned traveler is broad, and should include both pathogens endemic to the region of travel as well as infectious agents with a global distribution. Most returned travelers with infectious adenopathy will have viral etiologies, similar to the epidemiology in children who have not traveled. However, there are some systemic diseases for which the initial manifestations may be lymphadenopathy or lymphadenitis. These are summarized below. Filarial diseases, which cause lymphedema, are discussed separately later in the chapter.

Measles

Measles is caused by a paramyxovirus that is transmitted by droplet and airborne routes. It is one of the most contagious infections of humans. While rare in the United States in immunized children, approximately 1 million children per year develop measles globally, with an estimated 120,000 deaths, primarily in children less than 5 years of age who live in tropical regions. Transmission is directly from respiratory secretions and cases are infectious only during the early stages of illness. Children present with fever, upper respiratory tract symptoms, nonpurulent conjunctivitis, and an erythematous blanchable rash that begins on the head and moves in a cephalocaudal manner. The presentation can mimic that of Kawasaki disease. Oral lesions (Koplik spots) are transient and not seen in all children. Acute complications include pneumonitis and meningoencephalitis, and the dreaded delayed complication is subacute sclerosing panencephalitis, associated with irreversible neurocognitive decline years after the initial infection. The diagnosis is primarily clinical, with confirmatory serologies available. Treatment is supportive. In developing nations, the use of vitamin A daily for 2 days has been associated with reductions in morbidity and mortality. Any child with suspected measles should be placed in a negative-pressure room and airborne precautions taken by providers.

Mumps

Mumps is caused by a paramyxovirus transmitted by infected respiratory tract secretions. Humans are the only known natural host. Mumps occurs worldwide (peaking in the winter), although there has been a significant reduction in the number of cases since the introduction of the mumps vaccine in the United States in 1977. In 2013, fewer than 450 cases were reported in the United States. Approximately 20% are asymptomatic. The incubation period is approximately 2 weeks; children then develop a nonspecific prodrome of myalgia, low-grade fever, and headache. Subsequently, there is a swelling of the salivary glands (primarily parotid glands). However, multiorgan involvement (epididymitis, prostatitis, oophoritis, mastitis, myocarditis, hearing impairment, hepatitis, pancreatitis, thyroiditis, and arthritis) can be seen. Diagnosis is made clinically, with confirmatory laboratory PCR and serology testing available. Treatment is supportive. The infectious period is from 3 days prior to onset of symptoms to the 4th day of active disease. Standard and droplet precautions are recommended.

Brucella

Brucellosis is a systemic infection caused by the bacteria in the genus *Brucella,* small Gram-negative aerobic bacilli. Brucella is a zoonotic infection of livestock that is most common in the Mediterranean region, Indian subcontinent, and Latin America. *Brucella* can be transmitted via inhalation of aerosols, mucosal or skin contact, or ingestion of unpasteurized dairy products, raw meat, liver, or bone marrow. Symptoms include fever, night sweats, malaise, anorexia, headache, abdominal pain, and myalgia. Complications include meningitis, arthritis, osteomyelitis, and endocarditis. Diagnosis is made by isolation of the organism from the blood and acute and convalescent titers; the laboratory should be instructed that *Brucella* is suspected, as cultures need to be incubated for a minimum of 4 weeks. Treatment of children consists of TMP-SMZ and rifampin for at least 4 to 6 weeks. Adolescent and adult patients are preferably treated with either doxycycline or TMP-SMZ and rifampin; an aminoglycoside should be added for the first 14 days of therapy in cases of suspected meningitis, endocarditis, and osteomyelitis. Rifampin monotherapy is not recommended for concern for selecting for antibiotic resistance. Standard precautions can be used.

GASTROINTESTINAL/ GENITOURINARY

Amebiasis

Amebiasis, caused by the parasite *E. histolytica,* is responsible for approximately 70,000 deaths per year globally; it is estimated that 8 to 10 million persons are infected. The disease is most common in tropical regions. Amebiasis is transmitted via fecal–oral contact with amebic cysts; humans are the only reservoir. High-risk groups include foreign travelers, migrant workers, immunocompromised individuals, children in daycare centers, and prisoners. Less than 20% of persons who consume infected cysts develop symptoms. The spectrum of infection ranges from asymptomatic carriers to intestinal amebiasis, hepatic abscesses, or amebomas. Intestinal amebiasis typically has an insidious onset consisting of weight loss, abdominal pain, and initially nonbloody progressing to dysentery. Fever is rare. Complications include intestinal ulcers, fulminant colitis, and perforation. Hepatic amebic abscesses present clinically as fever, cough, tachypnea, hepatomegaly, and right upper quadrant pain with referred shoulder pain (the latter is more common in adults). Liver abscesses are the most common extraintestinal form of amebiasis. Rupture of the abscess with peritoneal seeding can be fatal. While drainage may be adjunctive to medical therapy, percutaneous drainage under controlled circumstances is optimal to prevent peritoneal seeding. Other extraintestinal manifestations are rare, but may include pericardial, pleuropulmonary, cerebral, genitourinary, and cutaneous amebiasis. Amebomas are annular lesions of cecum or colon that can mimic cancer or pyogenic abscesses. These usually can be managed medically.

Diagnosis is made via visualization of cysts in stool (for colitis) or serum antigen testing (for hepatic abscesses). CT can help identify extraintestinal manifestations. Ancillary testing may reveal leukocytosis, anemia, or transaminitis. Treatment of asymptomatic carriers is with diloxanide furoate (20 mg/kg/day in three divided doses [maximum: 500 mg per dose] for 10 days) or paromomycin (25 to 35 mg/kg/day in three divided doses for 7 days). Treatment of colitis is with metronidazole (35 to 50 mg/kg/day divided into three doses for 7 to 10 days; maximum: 750 mg per dose). Treatment of liver abscesses, ameboma, or moderate/severe intestinal amebiasis is a metronidazole and paromomycin. Contact precautions are recommended.

Giardia

Giardiasis is caused by *Giardia intestinalis,* a protozoan spread by fecal–oral transmission. While humans are the primary reservoir, domesticated and wild animals can also be infected. Most U.S. outbreaks have been associated with contaminated drinking water, daycare facilities, and food handlers. One-half to three-quarters of infections are asymptomatic. Symptoms include malodorous watery, nonbloody diarrhea, flatulence, abdominal pain, and weight loss. Anemia may be noted. Children with humoral immunodeficiencies can develop chronic symptomatic infection. The diagnosis is based on EIA or direct fluorescent antibody (DFA) assays, which have sensitivity and specificity far superior to identification of organisms in the stool. Treatment is not needed for self-limited infections in normal hosts, and treatment of asymptomatic carriers is not recommended unless they live in the home with an immunocompromised person. For patients requiring treatment, metronidazole (5 mg per kg every 8 hours [maximum: 250 mg per dose for 5 to 7 days]), tinidazole (single dose, licensed for children 3 years of age and older: 50 mg per kg [maximum: 2 g]), or nitazoxanide (3-day course for children 1 year of age and older: 1 to 3 years: 100 mg twice daily, 4 to 11 years: 200 mg twice daily, ≥12 years: 500 mg twice daily) are options. Standard and contact precautions should be used for incontinent children.

Cryptosporidium

Cryptosporidiosis is caused by *C. parvum* and *C. hominis,* protozoal species spread by fecal–oral transmission. Humans, cattle, and other animals are reservoir species. In the United States, almost 750,000 cases occur annually, so a travel history is not a prerequisite for infection. Risk factors include swallowing contaminated water, hiking and drinking unfiltered water, daycare attendees, workers, and the families of children who attend day care, and travelers. Asymptomatic infection can be seen. Most patients will develop low-grade fever, watery, nonbloody diarrhea with crampy abdominal pain, vomiting, and weight loss. Symptoms last 1 to 2 weeks, although more severe and chronic symptoms can be seen in HIV-infected patients and other immunocompromised hosts. In addition, immunocompromised children can develop extraintestinal manifestations: biliary tract and pneumonitis. DFA and EIAs are more sensitive than detection of oocytes in stool. Self-limited illness in immunocompetent hosts usually does not require treatment. Nitazoxanide is approved for children 1 year of age and older (3-day course for children 1 year of age and older: 1 to 3 years: 100 mg twice daily, 4 to 11 years: 200 mg twice daily, ≥12 years: 500 mg twice daily). Longer treatment courses may be needed in HIV-infected children and other immunocompromised hosts. Standard and contact precautions should be used for the incontinent child.

Gram-negative Enterics: Vibrio, *E. coli,* Campylobacter

Several Gram-negative enteric pathogens are more common in developing nations than in industrialized countries. These include *Vibrio cholera,* enterotoxigenic, enteropathic, enteroinvasive, and enteroaggregative *E. coli,* and *Campylobacter* (e-Table 102.22). Cholera is characterized by painless watery diarrhea, and persons most at risk are those with low gastric acidity. It can be easily spread in congregate settings, and is a major cause of diarrhea in camps for displaced persons. The character of diarrhea varies based on *E. coli* type, and some types produce a Shiga-like toxin. *Campylobacter* is also a cause of dysentery (bloody stools with fecal leukocytes) in the United States, but is more common internationally. In addition to the acute symptoms (which are more severe in immunocompromised hosts), patients with *Campylobacter* can also have postinfectious sequelae with Guillain–Barré syndrome including the Miller Fisher variant. All three pathogens can be cultured on routine stool culture media. The mainstay of therapy is rehydration. Adjunctive antibiotic treatment is recommended to decrease symptom duration, decrease fecal shedding, and decrease secondary transmission. Standard and contact precautions are recommended.

Schistosomiasis

Schistosomiasis is caused by mammalian blood trematodes (flukes) in the *Schistosoma* genus. Freshwater snails transmit the infection through penetration of intact skin. Schistosomiasis is endemic in more than 75 countries worldwide including in Africa, the Middle East, China, Southeast Asia, Brazil, Venezuela, and the Caribbean. Adult worms can live as long as 30 years, causing disease decades after patients have left an endemic area. The clinical manifestations of the most common syndromes caused by schistosomes are summarized in e-Table 102.23. The severity of chronic illness is associated with worm burden. Those with low to moderate burden may never develop significant illness, while those with significant worm burden may develop mucoid bloody diarrhea and tender hepatomegaly. Severe infection with the intestinal form of the disease may result in development of portal hypertension, ascites, esophageal varices, and hematemesis. The drug of choice is praziquantel (dosing varies depending on the species) and the treatment must be repeated approximately 1 to 2 months later due to failure of the medication to kill developing worms. Schistosomal dermatitis (swimmer's itch) does not require therapy. Standard precautions exist for isolation of infected patients.

Soil Helminthic Infections

A number of helminthic infections cause human disease. Most are transmitted through the fecal–oral route, though in some cases helminths can penetrate intact skin. The most common helminthic infections are *Enterobius vermicularis* (pinworms), *Trichuris trichiura* (whipworm), *Ascaris lumbricoides* (roundworm), *Ancylostoma* (hookworm), cutaneous larva migrans (CLM) (sandworm), and *Strongyloides.* Most infected individuals are asymptomatic. Clinical manifestations are strongly related to the intensity of the infection and worm burden. Some infections result in anemia or impaired growth and cognition. Diagnosis is usually made via visualization of larvae in the stool. The clinical manifestations, diagnosis, and treatment are summarized in e-Table 102.24. Most can be treated with either albendazole or mebendazole; albendazole is typically more tolerable for patients in terms of taste and side effects. The albendazole dose is 400 mg for both children and adults. A single-dose regimen is the recommended treatment for *Ancylostoma, Ascaris,* and *Enterobius,* whereas *Trichuris* requires a 3-day course and *Strongyloides* a 7-day course with twice-daily dosing.

SKIN/SOFT TISSUE INFECTIONS

Dermatologic conditions are common among persons who have recently traveled (Table 102.21). Urticaria are common, and can be caused by *Strongyloides stercoralis,* scabies, schistosomiasis, onchocerciasis, or insect bites. Insect bites (such as bedbugs and fleas) are the most common cutaneous finding in the returning traveler. The most common cause of ulcers

TABLE 102.21

DERMATOLOGIC CONDITIONS SEEN IN RETURNING TRAVELERS

Morphology	Disease	Region	Manifestations
Burrows	Botfly (myiasis)	Central/South America	Botfly embryo penetrates hair follicle and develops into a boil-like pocket
	Burrowing flea (tungiasis)	Caribbean, Latin America, Africa, Indian subcontinent	After impregnation, female flea burrows under skin, releasing eggs from boil-like orifice
Eschar	*S. aureus*, group A streptococcus	Global	Shallow, painful, purulent lesions that are secondarily infected by pyogenic bacteria
	Rickettsial diseases	Africa, Asia	Subcentimeter painless lesion at the site of the tick bite
Ulcers	Buruli ulcer disease (*Mycobacterium ulcerans*)	Americas, Africa, Asia, eastern Mediterranean	Painless progressive ulcers with cotton appearance and surrounding skin hyperpigmentation
	Leishmaniasis	Latin America (*espundia*) Central Asia	Papules which become nodules then shallow painless ulcers with raised borders. Granulomatous inflammation can be destructive; most common on the face
	Sporotrichosis (*Sporothrix schenckii)*	Tropical/subtropical regions in western hemisphere	Ulcerative, papular, or nodular lesions at site of minor trauma, usually from contact with soil. Can spread in a lymphatic pattern
Urticarial	Cutaneous larva migrans	Caribbean, Africa, Asia, Latin America, southeastern United States	Migrating intensely pruritic serpiginous tracks most common on buttocks and feet
	Onchocerca volvulus (river blindness)	Sub-Saharan Africa	Pruritic rash after contact with blackfly larvae
	Sea anemone larvae (*Edwardsiella lineata*), jellyfish larvae (*Linuche unguiculata*)	Caribbean, Latin America, Philippines, Southeast Asia	Pruritic papular rash caused by larvae entrapped under the bathing suit
	Scabies (*Sarcoptes scabiei*)	Worldwide	Pruritic erythematous eruption most common in webspaces of digits and along areas where clothing fits tightly; in infants, diffuse rash can be seen
	Schistosomiasis—Katayama fever	Sub-Saharan Africa	High fever, urticaria, eosinophilia weeks after contact with freshwater in endemic areas
	Schistosoma—swimmer's itch (freshwater), digger's itch (saltwater)	Sub-Saharan Africa	Pruritic rash after skin is penetrated by schistosomal cercaria

is pyoderma, caused by streptococci and staphylococci, but can also be caused by cutaneous leishmaniasis. Eschars may be seen in rickettsial disorders such as Mediterranean spotted fever, scrub typhus, and African tick typhus. Burrowing lesions can be caused by botflies (myiasis) and fleas (tungiasis).

Leishmaniasis

Leishmaniasis is a parasitic disease caused by the protozoan flagellates of *Leishmania* genus that are transmitted to humans through the bite of the phlebotomine sandfly. The annual incidence is 1.5 to 2 million. The disease is found worldwide in tropical zones in the Americas, Africa, South America, southern Europe, and Asia. There are three major clinical manifestations including cutaneous, mucosal, and visceral forms. Immunosuppression is a risk factor for the visceral form. More than 90% of visceral leishmaniasis cases occur in the Middle East, where as 90% of mucosal leishmaniasis cases occur in Peru, Brazil, and Bolivia. Cutaneous leishmaniasis is more widely distributed and occurs in central America, northern South America, northern Africa, the Middle East, and scattered portions of southern Europe. Cutaneous infection presents as painless skin lesions localized to exposed parts of the body that are accessible to sandflies (e.g., extremities, face). The incubation period is approximately 1 month. The skin lesions initially present as erythematous papules, which evolve into nodules and then to shallow volcano-like ulcerative lesions that are locally destructive and have associated localized lymphadenopathy. Mucosal infection may occur simultaneously or months to years after a cutaneous lesion heals. Parasites may extend into the nasopharyngeal mucosa and cause nasal congestion. The infection may continue to spread to the buccal mucosa and laryngeal membrane. Advanced stages of the disease can involve severe tissue necrosis and disfigurement. The incubation period for visceral leishmaniasis is 2 to 6 months and the onset of symptoms may be acute or chronic. In sudden onset cases, patients develop a persistent high fever, anorexia, a protuberant abdomen, and wasting of the limbs. Painless splenomegaly is an early finding; while hepatomegaly is less common, icterus is a marker of poor prognosis.

Laboratory findings include anemia, thrombocytopenia, hypoalbuminemia, and hypergammaglobulinemia. Untreated visceral infection is nearly always fatal. Diagnosis of the cutaneous form is through identification of leishmanial organisms via Wright or Giemsa stain of tissue samples. Visceral disease is diagnosed via bone marrow (iliac crest in children), spleen, or less commonly, liver aspirations. Treatment is always indicated for the mucosal and visceral cases. The drug of choice for visceral and mucosal disease is liposomal amphotericin B. Sodium stibogluconate, an antimonial, has also been used in the treatment of leishmaniasis, but has multiple potential adverse events including cardiotoxicity (EKG changes findings include ST-elevation or depression, T-wave inversion, and QT-interval prolongation), hepatitis, pancreatitis, nephrotoxicity with proteinuria, phlebitis, myelosuppression, and optic atrophy. Treatment of localized cutaneous disease depends on the type and characteristics of the lesion. Those that are rapidly self-healing can remain untreated. Systemic treatment is recommended for large or multiple cutaneous lesions. Diffuse cutaneous disease is resistant to treatment. Expert consultation is available through the CDC Division of Parasitic Diseases and Malaria: (770) 488-7775 or (770) 488-7100. Standard isolation precautions are recommended.

Cutaneous Larva Migrans

CLM is caused by the larval form of canine and feline hookworms (*Ancylostoma* species), found in fecal material in soil or sand. These nematodes can penetrate intact skin; infection is most common in tropical regions, especially on beaches. While most common in travelers returning from the Caribbean, Latin America, Asia, and Africa, the infection is also seen in the southeastern United States. Patients present with itchy papules at the entry site with a migratory, raised, erythematous, serpiginous pattern as the larvae migrate. The feet and buttocks most commonly are affected. The parasites enter the bloodstream and have a maturation phase in the lungs. With a large inoculation, eosinophilic pneumonitis (Löeffler syndrome) can be seen. Eosinophilia can also be seen with invasive enteritis, but is not a feature of isolated CLM. The diagnosis is clinical; biopsy is not recommended, but pathology may demonstrate an eosinophilic infiltrate. Serologies and EIAs are not commercially available. While usually a self-limited disease, albendazole or mebendazole can be used for treatment. Patients with substantial eosinophilia should be monitored for manifestations of mast cell degranulation after treatment, and some may require corticosteroids along with antiparasitic therapy.

Filariasis

Filariases are mosquito-borne infections caused by the nematodes (roundworms) *Wuchereria bancrofti, Brugia malayi,* or *Brugia timori* (e-Table 102.25). The incubation period ranges from 3 to 12 months depending on the species. *W. bancrofti's* clinical manifestations include acute adenolymphangitis (ADL), hydrocele, lymphedema, elephantiasis, chyluria, and tropical pulmonary eosinophilia (TPE). ADL is characterized by malaise, fever, chills, and enlarged painful lymph nodes, usually in the lower limb. Hydrocele (unilaterally or bilateral) is the most common chronic manifestation of *W. bancrofti.* Chronic lymphedema may progress to elephantiasis and typically involves the lower extremities. Edema usually becomes nonpitting with skin thickening and loss of skin elasticity. Secondary bacterial and fungal infections are common. Chyluria is seen when dilated lymphatics rupture and drain into the urinary excretory system. It is typically recurrent and lasts for days to weeks. TPE is the result of immune hyperresponsiveness to microfilaria in the lung. Patients with TPE typically present with nocturnal coughing and wheezing and extreme eosinophilia (counts >3,000 cells per mm^3). If left untreated, TPE may progress to chronic interstitial fibrosis and permanent lung damage. Brugian filariasis (caused by both *B. malayi* and *B. timori*) is very similar to Bancroftian filariasis, except that hydroceles, genital manifestations, and chyluria are less common, and that the elephantiasis is usually limited to the lower legs in Brugian filariasis.

Lymphatic filariasis may be diagnosed via microscopic detection of microfilaria on blood smears obtained at night. In addition, adult worms or microfilaria may be detected with skin biopsy, and ultrasonography can sometimes be used to detect adult worms. Nocturnal microfilaria of *W. bancrofti* and *B. malayi* may be provoked to enter the bloodstream during the day with a one-time dose of diethylcarbamazine citrate (DEC). Blood examination should be performed 30 to 60 minutes after administration of DEC. PCR and immunologic testing are also available. The drug of choice for lymphatic filariasis is DEC (2 mg/kg/dose three times daily after food for 12 days; there is no maximum adult dose). Ivermectin (150 μg per kg; there is no maximum adult dose) is effective against the microfilaria of *W. bancrofti* but has no effect on the adult worm. Consequently, combination therapy with DEC-ivermectin or ivermectin-albendazole is needed for suppression of microfilaremia. TPE is treated with DEC for 12 to 21 days. Appropriate and prompt treatment of secondary infections is crucial. Standard precautions exist for isolation of patients with lymphatic filariasis and there is no human-to-human transmission of microfilaria and adult worms with the exception of transfusion with infected blood.

Onchocerciasis (river blindness) is caused by *Onchocerca volvulus* and transmitted by *Simulium* blackflies. Approximately 18 million people worldwide are infected, over 500,000 have severe visual disability. Clinical manifestations may be dermatologic or ocular. Skin manifestations present as a pruritic rash with multiple papules that may resolve spontaneously or continue to spread. Painless, firm, mobile granulomas may develop in subcutaneous tissue, but rarely cause morbidity. Ocular lesions involve both the anterior and posterior segments. Anterior segment lesions result from an acute inflammatory reaction around microfilariae and are reversible with therapy. Posterior segment lesions involve the optic nerve and chorioretinitis and may result in blindness. Diagnosis can be made clinically or via the Mazzotti test which involves the administration of DEC by mouth and observing for intense pruritus and skin rash 1 to 24 hours later. Laboratory confirmation may be sought via PCR or microscopic examination of skin snips for microfilariae. The diagnosis is primarily clinical, as microfilariae may not be present in patients with lymphedema. Treatment is with ivermectin in a single dose of 150 μg per kg (there is no maximum adult dose). Standard precautions should be used.

SEXUALLY TRANSMITTED INFECTIONS

STIs are the most commonly reported infections in the United States and represent an important pediatric problem, particularly during infancy or adolescence. This chapter focuses on HIV, syphilis, HSV outside the neonatal period, and neonatal chlamydia and gonorrheal infections and nongenital gonorrheal infections. STIs causing pelvic inflammatory disease and cervicitis are covered elsewhere (Chapter 100 Gynecology Emergencies) and management of STIs in the abused child is discussed in Chapter 95 Child Abuse/Assault. In these children, the most common pathogens are *Trichomonas, C. trachomatis,* and *Neisseria gonorrhea,* and one study in sexually abused girls found that 8% of girls had one or more STIs. As many adolescents with one STI can be infected with more than one pathogen, identification of one STI should prompt diagnostic evaluation for others. The manifestations, diagnosis, and treatment of common STIs are described in Table 102.22.

Chlamydia, Neonatal

C. trachomatis can cause a number of syndromes in infants: conjunctivitis, trachoma, and pneumonia. Chlamydia is the most common STI in the United States, and adolescent females comprise the most at-risk group. Vertical transmission occurs in up to 50% of infants born to infected mothers. Chlamydia conjunctivitis is characterized by a serous, slightly purulent eye discharge that can be first noticed within 5 days to several weeks after delivery. There is conjunctival injection and lid edema. The drainage typically lasts 1 to 2 weeks. Approximately 30% of children with neonatal chlamydia conjunctivitis also will have chlamydial pneumonia. Chlamydia conjunctivitis and trachoma are not prevented by erythromycin that is given in the immediate newborn period to prevent ophthalmia neonatorum (see below). Trachoma is a sequela of chronic chlamydial eye infection and is characterized by corneal neovascularization which can result in blindness. While rare in the United States, trachoma is the leading infectious cause of blindness globally, estimated to impact up to 80 million persons. *C. trachomatis* pneumonia occurs most commonly from 2 weeks to 5 months after birth and is characterized by an afebrile illness with repetitive, paroxysmal cough similar to pertussis. In contrast to pertussis, leukemoid reactions are rare, but eosinophilia can be seen. Upper respiratory tract symptoms are common from chlamydial colonization of the nasopharynx.

Radiographic findings may include hyperinflation and patchy interstitial infiltrates. The diagnosis is made on the basis of IgM, culture, complement fixation, or microimmunofluorescent assays. Of note, complement fixation does not differentiate between chlamydia species. DFA testing is the only FDA-approved test for the detection of *C. trachomatis* from nasopharyngeal specimens. The treatment of chlamydia conjunctivitis is 14 days of erythromycin, whereas chlamydia pneumonia can be treated with either 14 days of erythromycin or 5 days of azithromycin. Despite the association between use of erythromycin in neonates and the development of pyloric stenosis, erythromycin remains the treatment of choice. Even with erythromycin therapy, cure is achieved in only 80% of cases; consequently, retesting after treatment is necessary to see if the child requires a second antibiotic course. The treatment of trachoma is topical erythromycin twice daily for 2 months; however, given poor adherence, the WHO recommends a single dose of azithromycin (20 mg per kg, maximum dose: 1 g). In contrast, topical therapy for chlamydia conjunctivitis is not recommended. Standard precautions are recommended.

Gonorrhea, Neonatal

The most common site of neonatal gonorrheal infection is the eye (ophthalmia neonatorum). While rare in the United States due to neonatal ocular prophylaxis, it may occur if prophylaxis does not occur (e.g., children born in nonhospital facilities) for children born to mothers with gonococcal chorioamnionitis. Infants present within the first week of life (most commonly between days 2 and 5 of life) with a hyperpurulent conjunctivitis. The diagnosis can be made by a Gram stain of the exudate, which demonstrates Gram-negative diplococci. Blood cultures should be sent, as gonorrheal infections can involve the meninges, joints, skin/soft tissue (e.g., from scalp electrodes), and bacteremia.

Prompt treatment and ophthalmologic evaluation are necessary to avoid the recognized complications of corneal ulceration and iridocyclitis. The treatment for ophthalmia neonatorum is a single dose (25 to 50 mg per kg, maximum 125 mg) of ceftriaxone, administered intravenously or intramuscularly. This is also the recommended treatment for asymptomatic infants born to mothers with untreated gonorrhea. Antibiotic eye ointment is not adequate as monotherapy and not beneficial when the child is receiving systemic therapy. For disseminated disease, 7 to 14 days of intravenous cefotaxime or ceftriaxone are recommended. Empiric treatment for chlamydia should be considered. Standard precautions are recommended.

Gonorrhea, Disseminated

Disseminated gonococcal disease is rare, estimated to occur in 1% to 3% of all untreated cases. The most common extragenital sites include skin and joints (arthritis–dermatitis syndrome). The rash is polymorphous, but often maculopapular or pustular painful lesions more commonly found on the extremities than the trunk; they may involve the palms and soles. The rash may have a hemorrhagic component. Joint complaints include a migratory polyarthralgia of the knees, ankles, elbows, and wrists. Tenosynovitis most commonly affects the wrist and ankles. Septic joints, most commonly at the knee, can also be seen and are clinically indistinguishable from streptococcal and staphylococcal septic arthritis; this is most common after the rash has disappeared. Gonococcal pharyngitis can be a complication of oral sex and can present with odynophagia, fever, and an exudative pharyngitis. Other manifestations include endocarditis (more common in males and in patients with collagen vascular diseases; the aortic valve is most commonly involved) and meningitis, though both are rare.

The diagnosis can be made by culturing all mucosal surfaces (cervix, rectum, and pharynx) and obtaining blood cultures and joint aspirate cultures. Nucleic acid amplification tests on urine can also increase culture yield. The treatment for extragenital gonorrhea outside the neonatal period is a third-generation cephalosporin administered for 7 days for arthritis–dermatitis and for 28 days for meningitis and endocarditis.

TABLE 102.22

CLINICAL PRESENTATION, DIAGNOSIS, AND TREATMENT OF COMMON SEXUALLY TRANSMITTED INFECTIONS

Infection	Presentation	Diagnosis[a]	Treatment
Chlamydia, congenital[b]	Conjunctivitis: ocular edema and discharge developing days to weeks after birth; less purulent than gonorrheal conjunctivitis Pneumonia: afebrile staccato cough in infants 2–19 wks of age	Culture *PCR-based tests not approved for chlamydial conjunctivitis or pneumonia* CXR; hyperinflation; infiltrates (no characteristic pattern)	Erythromycin 50 mg/kg/day in four divided doses for 14 days Conjunctivitis cannot be treated with topical therapy alone Up to 20% of children may require retreatment
Gonorrhea, neonatal[b]	Ocular: hyperpurulent conjunctivitis that can result in permanent vision loss Scalp abscess: associated with fetal scalp monitoring Disseminated: arthritis, bacteremia, meningitis (see row below)	Culture	Conjunctivitis: ceftriaxone 50 mg/kg × one (maximum dose: 125 mg) IM Arthritis/dermatitis: ceftriaxone 50 mg/kg/day (maximum dose: 1 g/day) IV or IM for 7 days Should also be treated with erythromycin for *Chlamydia*
Gonorrhea, disseminated	Arthritis: monoarticular Dermatitis: polymorphic lesions which can appear as pustules, abscesses, or ecthyma Genitourinary: purulent urethritis (with dysuria and apparently sterile pyuria), proctitis, or epididymitis	Culture PCR on urine, endocervical or vaginal swabs, or male urethral swabs *PCR-based tests not approved for pharyngeal or rectal swabs due to cross-reaction with nongonococcal neisserial species and should not be used for children in whom sexual assault/abuse is suspected*	Arthritis/dermatitis: • 45 kg: ceftriaxone 50 mg/kg/day (maximum dose: 1 g/day) IV or IM daily for 7 days • ≥45 kg: ceftriaxone 1 g IV daily for 7 days Conjunctivitis: ceftriaxone 1 g IM once Epididymitis, urethritis: ceftriaxone 250 mg IM once Meningitis or endocarditis: • 45 kg: ceftriaxone 50 mg/kg/day (maximum dose: 2 g/day) IV or IM q12h for 10–14 days for meningitis, 28 days for endocarditis • ≥45 kg: ceftriaxone 1–2 g IV q12h for 10–14 days for meningitis, 28 days for endocarditis Should also be treated empirically for *Chlamydia* with azithromycin 1 g PO once
HSV, acquired[c]	Orolabial: multiple vesicles that appear indistinguishable from herpangina, but are not limited to the posterior tonsillar pillars; instead, they can be found throughout the mouth, on the tongue, and lips Anogenital: painful vesicles or ulcers with fever, influenza-like illness, pruritus, dysuria, and tender inguinal adenopathy	Culture, PCR	Acyclovir; alternatives include valacyclovir and famciclovir Topical antiviral therapy is not recommended for orolabial or anogenital disease
HIV	See e-Tables 102.26, 102.31	ELISA, PCR	Combination antiretroviral therapy
Syphilis, congenital	See e-Table 102.32	e-Table 102.32	See e-Table 102.33
Syphilis, acquired	See e-Table 102.34	Nontreponemal tests (VDRL, RPR) for screening; treponemal tests (FTA-ABS, MHA-TP, TP-PA) for confirmation	See Table e-102.33

[a]All patients with one sexually transmitted infection (STI) should be screened for other STIs.
[b]Culture should be obtained for children in whom sexual assault/abuse is suspected.
[c]Neonatal HSV disease is discussed earlier in the chapter.
PCR, polymerase chain reaction; IM, intramuscular; IV, intravenous; PO, by mouth; HSV, herpes simplex virus; HIV, human immunodeficiency virus; ELISA, enzyme-linked immunosorbent assay; VDRL, venereal disease research laboratory; RPR, rapid plasma reagin; FTA-ABS, fluorescent treponemal antibody absorption; MHA-TP, microhemagglutination test for antibodies to *Treponema pallidum;* TP-PA, *Treponema pallidum* particle agglutination.

Children should also be empirically treated for *Chlamydia*. Standard precautions are recommended.

Herpes Simplex Virus, Nonneonatal

HSV in the neonatal period is discussed earlier in the chapter. The most common sites of infection are the anogenital region and the oropharynx; while the former is most commonly caused by HSV-2 and the latter by HSV-1, both HSV-1 and HSV-2 can cause infection in either location. HSV can also cause skin infection in abraded skin, as is seen with herpes gladiatorum (in wrestlers) and in herpetic whitlow on the digits. It was estimated that in 2007, over 23,000 patients visited the ED for herpetic gingivostomatitis. HSV-1 seroprevalence is approximately 25% in children in early elementary school and increases to over 30% by early adolescence. In contrast, HSV-2 seroprevalence was 1.4% among teenagers from 2005 to 2008. Only a minority of patients who are seropositive for HSV-2 report having symptoms compatible with genital HSV infection.

The most common symptoms are vesicles on an erythematous base. However, as the vesicles are friable, unroofed painful ulcers may instead be noted on examination. Painful regional adenopathy is common, especially with the primary infection. The virus grows readily in standard viral culture. HSV identified from genital lesions should be typed; while HSV-1 can be autoinoculated into the genital region from oral infection, sexual abuse needs to be considered in prepubertal children with genital HSV-2. PCR assays are also commercially available. Type-specific antibodies do not enable differentiation of orolabial and anogenital infections and are plagued with both false-negative (in early infection) and false-positive results.

Antiviral therapy is recommended for patients with initial and recurrent genital HSV infection to shorten symptom duration and decrease viral shedding. There are fewer data on the utility of antiviral therapy for mucocutaneous HSV in immunocompetent hosts. Acyclovir remains the first-line therapy (20 mg per kg every 6 hours [maximum: 800 mg per dose] for young children and 400 mg three times daily for postpubertal patients) for 7 to 10 days. An alternative regimen for older patients who can swallow pills is valacyclovir (1 g twice daily for 7 to 10 days), which may increase adherence given the less frequent dosing interval. Topical acyclovir is not recommended for herpes labialis or gingivostomatitis. Contact precautions are recommended for children with mucocutaneous HSV.

Human Immunodeficiency Virus

CLINICAL PEARLS AND PITFALLS

- Acute HIV infection presents as a mononucleosis-type illness; serologies often are negative, and the diagnosis is contingent upon PCR.
- Knowledge of the child's CD4+ cell count can allow the clinician to determine which opportunistic infections (OIs) are most likely.
- Antiretroviral therapy has a host of potential adverse events, as well as multiple potential drug interactions that can result in toxicity.

Current Evidence

It is estimated that there are approximately 11,000 children living with HIV in the United States and 3.3 million globally.

TABLE 102.23

APPROXIMATE RISK OF HUMAN IMMUNODEFICIENCY VIRUS ACQUISITION AFTER A SINGLE EXPOSURE LISTED BY SOURCE

Exposure	Risk of infection (per 10,000)
Transfusion with positive blood unit	950
Intravenous drug use	67
Percutaneous exposure (needlestick)	30
Receptive penile–anal intercourse	50
Insertive penile–anal intercourse	10
Receptive penile–vaginal intercourse	10
Insertive penile–vaginal intercourse	5
Receptive oral sex	1
Insertive oral sex	0.5

While HIV acquired vertically from mothers to infants has declined in recent years (approximately 150 cases of perinatal infection are reported annually in the United States), increasing case rates have been reported in adolescents. Twenty-six percent of persons living with HIV in 2010 were infected when they were between 13 and 24 years of age, and the incidence in this age group was 24 per 100,000. While most adolescent females acquire infection via heterosexual contact (80% vs. 20% from injection drug use), most adolescent males acquire HIV via male-to-male sexual contact (75% vs. 13% from injection drug use, and the remainder from heterosexual contact). The risk of HIV transmission from different routes is summarized in Table 102.23. It is estimated that approximately 20% of HIV-infected persons are unaware of their HIV status. HIV-infected children may present to the ED for a number of reasons: acute HIV infection, OIs (children in whom the diagnosis of HIV may or may not have been established), and with complications of antiretroviral therapy.

Goals of Treatment

The goal of treatment is to rapidly identify the most serious causes of infection in the HIV-infected child, as well as to understand what infections should lead you to consider HIV testing in a child who currently does not carry the diagnosis of HIV.

Clinical Considerations

Clinical recognition: Initial ED recognition of children with known HIV infection should include categorizing children as likely OIs (e-Tables 102.26 and 102.27) based on their CD4+ cell count, infections caused by pathogens which also infect normal hosts, and drug toxicities from their antiretroviral regimen or from prophylactic antibiotics or antiviral medications (e-Table 102.28 reviews antiretroviral medications, and e-Table 102.29 reviews adverse events). ED clinicians should also be cognizant of the presentations of acute HIV infection (Table 102.24) in adolescents and of the presentations of OIs in as-yet undiagnosed children with perinatally acquired HIV infection (e-Table 102.30), most of whom will become symptomatic during infancy.

TABLE 102.24

CLINICAL MANIFESTATIONS AND DIAGNOSIS OF ACUTE HIV INFECTION

Symptoms	Signs	Laboratory findings
Fever	Pyrexia	HIV PCR
Pharyngitis	Generalized lymphadenopathy	ELISA, Western blot often initially negative, convert to positive by 2–4 mo
Rash	Maculopapular rash	Leukopenia
Myalgias	Mucocutaneous ulcerations	Thrombocytopenia
Headache	Hepatomegaly	
Nausea, vomiting	Splenomegaly	
Diarrhea	Neurologic symptoms: aseptic meningitis, meningoencephalitis, neuropathy, radiculopathy, facial nerve palsy, Guillian–Barré syndrome, psychosis	

HIV, human immunodeficiency virus; PCR, polymerase chain reaction; ELISA, enzyme-linked immunosorbent assay.

Triage considerations: HIV-infected children should be roomed as rapidly as possible to prevent them from acquiring a nosocomial infection while in the ED. Triage assessment should include obtaining pulse oximetry, as indolent hypoxemia may be the first sign of early *Pneumocystis jirovecii* pneumonia (PCP). Triage personnel need to be cognizant that HIV-infected children are at risk for overwhelming bacterial and viral sepsis, similar to other immunocompromised children.

Clinical assessment: The most common clinical presentations of HIV-infected children and one diagnostic approach are reviewed in e-Table 102.31. The first branch point in decision making for the febrile HIV-infected child is whether or not they are ill appearing. Most infections, even in HIV-infected children will be caused by common pathogens also seen in immunocompetent children. However, it is important that providers realize that the rates of bacteremia are higher in HIV-infected children than in their immunocompetent peers. It appears that serious bacterial, viral, or OIs are relatively uncommon among well-appearing HIV-positive children who present to the ED with fever.

HIV-positive patients with fever who appears ill should be treated like other ill-appearing, febrile children because they are likely to be infected with the same types of organisms that infect immunocompetent children. An LP is indicated for those with meningismus, change in mental status, or an underlying abnormal mental status makes assessment difficult; the clinician should consider obtaining a CT of the brain prior to LP to evaluate for a mass-occupying lesion. If a child is believed to be so unstable that LP is not safe, it can be delayed. In either case, the child should be started on parenteral broad-spectrum antimicrobials. Ceftriaxone (100 mg/kg/day divided every 12 hours) is an appropriate choice because it covers the organisms that most commonly cause sepsis in children. In young children, because of the possibility of PCP presenting with fever and ill appearance, TMP-SMZ (5 mg/kg/dose of trimethoprim every 6 hours) should be considered if there are respiratory symptoms, with or without a positive chest radiograph. Treatment for suspected PCP should not be delayed because of concern of interfering with the diagnostic workup. Fungal infections, with the exception of oral thrush, are uncommon in HIV-infected children. However, candidal sepsis should be considered in hospitalized patients who do not improve with antibiotics.

Chronic fever is common in HIV-infected children and has a broad differential diagnosis. The major focus of such an evaluation in the ED is to rule out acute bacterial infection. A careful history and physical examination should be followed by a CBC, urinalysis, chest and sinus films, and blood, urine, and stool cultures. Recurrent otitis media is commonly seen, and some children may have recurrent parotitis or sinusitis. If no source is recognized on examination and the initial testing is negative, more unusual infections need to be considered. Tuberculosis, although common among HIV-infected adults, is uncommon in children but may be more likely among adolescents. *Mycobacterium avium* complex may cause chronic fevers in HIV-infected children. This pathogen is often associated with anemia secondary to bone marrow infiltration and can be cultured from blood, stool, and bone marrow. Numerous viruses can cause chronic infections associated with fever in these children. EBV and CMV are among the more common, with CMV often presenting with chronic hepatitis and bloody diarrhea. It may also cause pneumonia and retinitis. A blood buffy coat specimen can be sent for quantitative CMV-antigen detection. Most HIV-positive children with fever of unknown origin are hospitalized to facilitate the diagnostic process. The possibility of drug fever must also be considered.

Two OIs warrant special attention: PCP and lymphoid interstitial pneumonitis (LIP). PCP is caused by a fungal pathogen and is the most common initial manifestation of HIV in the perinatally infected infant. The infant or child typically is febrile, with marked tachypnea, wheezing, rhonchi, and diminished breath sounds. Rales are not usually part of the PCP picture, and cough may be absent. When coughing is present, it is typically dry and nonproductive. Over hours to days, the patient develops hypoxia and increased respiratory distress. Initial ED evaluation should include beginning supplemental oxygen, obtaining pulse oximetry, an arterial blood gas, a chest radiograph, and serum LDH levels. Radiographs may show a diffuse interstitial ("ground glass") pattern, but infants may develop patchy infiltrates or complete opacification of the lung fields. The diagnosis often requires bronchoscopy with specimens sent for silver stains. However, if the ED physician suspects PCP, it is appropriate to start IV TMP-SMZ at a dosage of 20 mg/kg/day of TMP divided every 6 hours. The child should be hospitalized for close observation and further evaluation as needed. In general, patients with PCP do not respond rapidly to antibiotic therapy. Patients intolerant of TMP-SMZ can be treated with pentamidine (4 mg/kg/day as a single daily dose) or atovaquone, but these should be considered second-line agents. Corticosteroid therapy in children with severe PCP improves survival and is generally recommended for patients with Pao_2 less than 70 mm Hg or an alveolar–arterial gradient of greater than 35 mm Hg. Standard precautions are indicated.

LIP is a lymphoid hyperplastic condition associated with both HIV and EBV infections. LIP results in a slowly progressive hypoxemic condition in children outside infancy. The most common symptoms are chronic cough, mild tachypnea, generalized adenopathy, marked hypoxemia, and digital clubbing. Chest radiography reveals an interstitial nodular pattern, and bronchiectasis can be seen on high-resolution CT of the chest. The diagnosis is confirmed via biopsy. Fever is an unusual manifestation of LIP and should prompt evaluation for secondary pyogenic bacterial infections. Therapy may be with antiretroviral therapy; in acute respiratory compromise, empiric corticosteroid therapy may be warranted. If the Pao_2 is less than 65 mm Hg, LIP is treated with 1 to 2 mg/kg/day of prednisone (maximum: 60 mg per day) for 2 to 4 weeks and subsequently tapered to maintain the Pao_2 above 70 mm Hg. If the patient is febrile, tuberculosis or MAI must be ruled out before beginning steroid therapy.

Management: Whenever a child with HIV infection presents with high-grade fever (temperature higher than 39°C or 102.2°F), a complete blood cell count (CBC) with differential and blood culture is recommended. If the child is still in diapers, a urine sample should be obtained for analysis and culture. Older children who are toilet trained usually complain of dysuria or frequency if they have a UTI. If the child has any respiratory signs or symptoms, including isolated tachypnea, or if the CBC has an elevated leukocyte count with a shift to left, regardless of the presence of respiratory signs, pulse oximetry and a chest radiograph should be ordered. The WBC count is best evaluated in relation to baseline counts because many HIV-infected children have some degree of leukopenia. If it is known that the child is not leukopenic or the baseline is not available, a WBC count of 15,000 per mm^3 or more should be considered suggestive of bacterial infection. If the child appears well and the evaluation has not revealed a source for the fever that requires hospitalization, the child may be sent home (if the child's caregiver can be easily contacted and has the means to return if necessary) with instructions to return if symptoms worsen or if the patient develops lethargy or will not take adequate amounts of fluids. Clinicians can choose to offer empiric antibiotics (e.g., ceftriaxone) for children being considered for outpatient care. A follow-up evaluation by telephone or a revisit to the child's regular provider or the ED should be scheduled for the next day.

PEP: Providers may be asked by families about PEP after children are exposed to HIV via contact with blood or other body fluids, after contact with discarded needles in a nonhealthcare setting, or after sexual assault. The risk after specific exposures is reviewed in Table 102.23. It is important for families to realize that risk of drug-associated adverse events, estimated to cause treatment cessation in over one-third of HIV-infected patients, is substantially higher than the risk of transmission. PEP is not recommended for needlesticks from discarded needles, nor is it suggested that needles are sent for testing for HIV. Consultation with a local HIV specialist is recommended prior to the PEM provider initiating prophylaxis.

Syphilis, Congenital

Congenital syphilis has an incidence of 10 per 100,000 live births in the United States. While cases have declined over the last two decades, risk factors for a child being born with congenital syphilis include birth in Southern states and birth to African-American mothers. Clinical findings early in congenital syphilis can range from very profound (stillbirth) to initially asymptomatic. The rate and the severity of infection correlate with the staging in the mother. Women with untreated early syphilis are estimated to have a 40% rate of spontaneous abortion. The rate of transmission to the fetus is very high in maternal secondary syphilis but decreases for mothers with latent or tertiary syphilis. The most common symptoms and the diagnostic criteria for congenital syphilis are summarized in e-Table 102.32. Other findings include diffuse bilateral pneumonia (pneumonia alba), chorioretinitis, nephritis, and testicular masses. Late findings of congenital syphilis include dental changes (Hutchinson teeth—small hypoplastic teeth with enamel anomalies; mulberry molars—maldevelopment of the cusps), other bony changes (frontal bossing, prominent mandible, shortened maxilla, saddle nose, saber shins), swelling of the sternoclavicular joint (Higouménakis sign), sensorineural hearing loss, and interstitial keratitis. Any infant whose mother has inadequately treated syphilis, or the infant with any symptoms consistent with congenital syphilis and positive serologic tests for syphilis, should be managed as a presumptive case.

The treatment of choice for syphilis and the only accepted regimen for pregnant women is penicillin. Treatment recommendations are summarized in e-Table 102.33. Treatment for nonpregnant adolescents and adults who are penicillin-allergic is doxycycline 100 mg twice daily for 14 days for primary, secondary, or early latent syphilis and for 4 weeks for late latent or latent syphilis of unknown duration. Contact precautions should be used for infants with congenital syphilis, as nasal secretions and dermatologic manifestations are heavily laden with spirochetes.

Syphilis, Acquired

Acquired syphilis is stratified into stages based on clinical manifestations and serologic findings. The clinical and laboratory findings present at different stages are summarized in e-Table 102.34, and the treatment recommendations by stage are reviewed in e-Table 102.33. One cause of confusion relates to serologic testing for syphilis. Two broad categories of tests exist. The first test developed were nontreponemal tests, which measure primarily IgG. These include the rapid plasma reagin (RPR) and the venereal disease research laboratory (VDRL); the former is a serum test, the latter performed on CSF. These tests have the advantage of being inexpensive (optimal for screening tests) and decreasing in response to therapy, allowing for serial monitoring. These tests have disadvantages including false-positive results, which have been best described in patients with anticardiolipin antibody, autoimmune disease, HIV infection, and pregnancy; and false-negative results in some patients with secondary syphilis and in many patients with late-stage syphilis. The second class is treponemal tests. These include the FTA-ABS (fluorescent treponemal antibody absorption), MHA-TP (microhemagglutination test for antibodies to *Treponema pallidum),* and the TP-PA (*Treponema pallidum* particle agglutination). These tests are confirmatory assays when nontreponemal tests are positive, and also are useful in the diagnosis of late stages of syphilis. They are as sensitive as nontreponemal tests for late disease, and are much more specific. These tests cannot be used to monitor response to therapy, as they do not revert to negative with therapy. All patients with syphilis should be screened for HIV and other STIs. Contact precautions should be used for any syphilis patient with open lesions or secretions.

Suggested Readings and Key References

Infectious Disease Emergencies

Systemic Infections (Bacteremia & Shock, Rickettsial Diseases, Babesiosis)

Andreola B, Bressan S, Callegaro S, et al. Procalcitonin and C-reactive protein as diagnostic markers of severe bacterial infections in febrile infants and children in the emergency department. *Pediatr Infect Dis J* 2007;26(8):672–677.

Benito-Fernandez J, Mintegi S, Pocheville-Gurutezeta I, et al. Pneumococcal bacteremia in febrile infants presenting to the emergency department 8 years after the introduction of the pneumococcal conjugate vaccine in the Basque Country of Spain. *Pediatr Infect Dis J* 2010;29(12):1142–1144.

Brauner M, Goldman M, Kozer E. Extreme leukocytosis and the risk of serious bacterial infection in febrile children. *Arch Dis Child* 2010;95(3):209–212.

Bressan S, Andreola B, Cattelan F, et al. Predicting severe bacterial infections in well-appearing febrile neonates: laboratory markers' accuracy and duration of fever. *Pediatr Infect Dis J* 2010;29(3): 227–232.

Carstairs KL, Tanen DA, Johnson AS, et al. Pneumococcal bacteremia in febrile infants presenting to the emergency department before and after the introduction of the heptavalent pneumococcal vaccine. *Ann Emerg Med* 2007;49(6):772–777.

De S, Williams GJ, Hayen A, et al. Value of white cell count in predicting serious bacterial infection in febrile children under 5 years of age. *Arch Dis Child* 2014;99(6):493–499.

Graham J, Stockley K, Goldman RD. Tick-borne illnesses: a CME update. *Pediatr Emerg Care* 2011;27(2):141–147.

Jaffe DM, Fleisher GR. Temperature and total white blood count as indicators of bacteremia. *Pediatrics* 1991;87(5):670–674.

Kuppermann N, Walton EA. Immature neutrophils in the blood smears of young febrile children. *Arch Pediatr Adolesc Med* 1999; 153(3):261–266.

Laupland KB, Gregson DB, Vanderkooi OG, et al. The changing burden of pediatric bloodstream infections in Calgary, Canada, 2000–2006. *Pediatr Infect Dis J* 2009;28(2):114–117.

Lee GM, Fleisher GR, Harper MB. Management of febrile children in the age of the conjugate pneumococcal vaccine: a cost-effectiveness analysis. *Pediatrics* 2001;108(4):835–844.

Mahajan P, Grzybowski M, Chen X, et al. Procalcitonin as a marker of serious bacterial infections in febrile children younger than 3 years old. *Acad Emerg Med* 2014;21(2):171–179.

Mistry RD, Wedin T, Balamuth F, et al. Emergency department epidemiology of pneumococcal bacteremia in children since the institution of widespread PCV7 vaccination. *J Emerg Med* 2013;45(6): 813–820.

Pulliam PN, Attia MW, Cronan KM. C-reactive protein in febrile children 1 to 36 months of age with clinically undetectable serious bacterial infection. *Pediatrics* 2001;108(6):1275–1279.

Rudinsky SL, Carstairs KL, Reardon JM, et al. Serious bacterial infections in febrile infants in the post-pneumococcal conjugate vaccine era. *Acad Emerg Med* 2009;16(7):585–590.

Sard B, Bailey MC, Vinci R. An analysis of pediatric blood cultures in the postpneumococcal conjugate vaccine era in a community hospital emergency department. *Pediatr Emerg Care* 2006;22(5): 295–300.

Shah SS, Shofer FS, Seidel JS, et al. Significance of extreme leukocytosis in the evaluation of febrile children. *Pediatr Infect Dis J* 2005;24(7):627–630.

Simonsen KA, Harwell JI, Lainwala S. Clinical presentation and treatment of transfusion-associated babesiosis in premature infants. *Pediatrics* 2011;128(4):e1019–e1024.

Stanley R, Pagon Z, Bachur R. Hyperpyrexia in infants younger than 3 months. *Pediatr Emerg Care* 2005;21(5):291–294.

Stoll ML, Rubin LG. Incidence of occult bacteremia among highly febrile young children in the era of the pneumococcal conjugate vaccine. *JAMA Pediatr* 2004;158(7):671–675.

Trautner BW, Caviness AC, Gerlacher GR, et al. Prospective evaluation of the risk of serious bacterial infection in children who present to the emergency department with hyperpyrexia (temperature of 106 degrees F or higher). *Pediatrics* 2006;118(1):34–40.

Wilkinson M, Bulloch B, Smith M. Prevalence of occult bacteremia in children aged 3 to 36 months presenting to the emergency department with fever in the post pneumococcal conjugate vaccine era. *Acad Emerg Med* 2009;16(3):220–225.

Woods CR. Rocky Mountain spotted fever in children. *Pediatr Clin North Am* 2013;60:455–470.

Yo CH, Hsieh PS, Lee SH, et al. Comparison of the test characteristics of procalcitonin to C-reactive protein and leukocytosis for the detection of serious bacterial infections in children presenting with fever without source: a systematic review and meta-analysis. *Ann Emerg Med* 2012;60(5):591–600.

Central Nervous System Infections (Meningitis, Encephalitis, Brain Abscesses, Botulism, Tetanus)

Centers for Disease Control and Prevention. National, state, and local area vaccination coverage among children aged 19–35 months – United States, 2012. *MMWR Morb Mortal Wkly Rep* 2013;62(36): 733–740.

Cohn KA, Thompson AD, Shah SS, et al. Validation of a clinical prediction rule to distinguish Lyme meningitis from aseptic meningitis. *Pediatrics* 2012;129(1):e46–e53.

Garro AC, Rutman M, Simonsen K, et al. Prospective validation of a clinical prediction model for Lyme meningitis in children. *Pediatrics* 2009;123(5):e829–e834.

Goodkin HP, Harper MB, Pomeroy SL. Intracerebral abscesses in children: historical trends at Children's Hospital Boston. *Pediatrics* 2004;113(6):1765–1770.

Halgrimson WR, Chan KH, Abzug MJ, et al. Incidence of acute mastoiditis in Colorado children in the pneumococcal conjugate vaccine era. *Pediatr Infect Dis J* 2014;33(5):453–457.

Hardasmalani MD, Saber M. Yield of diagnostic studies in children presenting with complex febrile seizures. *Pediatr Emerg Care* 2012;28(8):789–791.

Kaplan SL, Barson WJ, Lin PL, et al. Early trends for invasive pneumococcal infections in children after the introduction of the 13-valent pneumococcal conjugate vaccine. *Pediatr Infect Dis J* 2013;32(3):203–207.

Nigrovic LE, Kuppermann N, Malley R, et al. Children with bacterial meningitis presenting to the emergency department during the pneumococcal conjugate vaccine era. *Acad Emerg Med* 2008; 15(6):522–528.

Pifko E, Price A, Sterner S. Infant botulism and indications for administration of botulism immune globulin. *Pediatr Emerg Care* 2014;30(2):120–124.

Pinninti SG, Kimberlin DW. Neonatal herpes simplex virus infections. *Pediatr Clin North Am* 2013;60(2):351–365.

Seltz LB, Smith J, Durairaj VD, et al. Microbiology and antibiotic management of orbital cellulitis. *Pediatrics* 2011;127(3):e566–e572.

Subcommittee on Febrile Seizures of the American Academy of Pediatrics. Neurodiagnostic evaluation of the child with a simple febrile seizure. *Pediatrics* 2011;127(2):389–394.

Tunkel AR, Glaser CA, Bloch KC, et al. The management of encephalitis: clinical practice guidelines by the Infectious Diseases Society of America. *Clin Infect Dis* 2008;47(3):303–327.

Tunkel AR, Hartman BJ, Kaplan SL, et al. Practice guidelines for the management of bacterial meningitis. *Clin Infect Dis* 2004;39(9): 1267–1284.

Upper and Lower Respiratory Tract Infections

Bradley JS, Byington CL, Shah SS, et al. The management of community-acquired pneumonia in infants and children older than 3 months of age: clinical practice guidelines by the Pediatric Infectious Diseases Society and the Infectious Diseases Society of America. *Clin Infect Dis* 2011;53(7):e25–e76.

Fine AM, Nizet V, Mandl KD. Large-scale validation of the Centor and McIsaac scores to predict group A streptococcal pharyngitis. *Arch Intern Med* 2012;172(11):847–852.

Murphy CG, van de Pol AC, Harper MB, et al. Clinical predictors of occult pneumonia in the febrile child. *Acad Emerg Med* 2007;14(3):243–249.

Rutman MS, Bachur R, Harper MB. Radiographic pneumonia in young, highly febrile children with leukocytosis before and after universal conjugate pneumococcal vaccination. *Pediatr Emerg Care* 2009;25(1):1–7.

Van Driel ML, De Sutter AI, Keber N, et al. Different antibiotic treatments for group A streptococcal pharyngitis. *Cochrane Database Syst Rev* 2013;4:CD004406.

Wald ER, Applegate KE, Bordley C, et al. Clinical practice guideline for the diagnosis and management of acute bacterial sinusitis in children aged 1 to 18 years. *Pediatrics* 2013;132(1):e262–e280.

Cardiac Infections

Baddour LM, Wilson WR, Bayer AS, et al. Infective endocarditis: diagnosis, antimicrobial therapy, and management of complications: a statement for healthcare professionals from the Committee on Rheumatic Fever, Endocarditis, and Kawasaki Disease, Council on Cardiovascular Disease in the Young, and the Councils on Clinical Cardiology, Stroke, and Cardiovascular Surgery and Anesthesia, American Heart Association: endorsed by the Infectious Diseases Society of America. *Circulation* 2005;111(23):e3940434.

Durani Y, Giordano K, Goudie BW. Myocarditis and pericarditis in children. *Pediatr Clin North Am* 2010;57(6):1281–1303.

Newburger JW, Takahasi M, Gerber MA, et al. Diagnosis, treatment, and long-term management of Kawasaki Disease: a statement for health professionals from the Committee on Rheumatic Fever, Endocarditis, and Kawasaki Disease, Council on Cardiovascular Disease in the Young, American Heart Association. *Circulation* 2004;110(17):2747–2771.

Gastrointestinal Infections

Belingheri M, Possenti I, Tel F, et al. Cryptic activity of atypical hemolytic uremic syndrome and eculizumab treatment. *Pediatrics* 2014;133(6):e1769–e1771.

Centers for Disease Control and Prevention. Foodborne diseases active surveillance network (FoodNet). Available online at: http://www.cdc.gov/foodnet/surveillance.html. Accessed May 23, 2014.

Chhabra P, Payne DC, Szilagyi PG, et al. Etiology of viral gastroenteritis in children <5 years of age in the United States, 2008–2009. *J Infect Dis* 2013;208(5):790–800.

Freedman SB, DeGroot JM, Parkin PC. Successful discharge of children with gastroenteritis requiring intravenous rehydration. *J Emerg Med* 2014;46(1):9–20.

Heiman KE, Karlsson M, Grass J, et al. Notes from the field: shigella with decreased susceptibility to azithromycin among men who have sex with men – United States, 2002–2013. *MMWR Morb Mortal Wkly Rep* 2014;63(6):132–133.

Safdar N, Said A, Gangon RE, et al. Risk of hemolytic uremic syndrome after antibiotic treatment of Escherichia coli O157:H7 enteritis: a meta-analysis. *JAMA* 2002;288(8):996–1001.

Solomkin JS, Mazuski JE, Bradley JS, et al. Diagnosis and management of complicated intra-abdominal infection in adults and children: guidelines by the Surgical Infection Society and the Infectious Diseases Society of America. *Clin Infect Dis* 2010;50(2):133–164.

Szajewska H, Guarino A, Hojsak I, et al. Use of probiotics for management of acute gastroenteritis: a position paper by the ESPGHAN Working Group for Probiotics and Prebiotics. *J Pediatr Gastroenterol Nutr* 2014;58(4):531–539.

Wendt JM, Cohen JA, Mu Y, et al. Clostridium difficile infection among children across diverse US geographic locations. *Pediatrics* 2014;133(4):651–658.

Genitourinary Infections

Bachur R, Harper M. Reliability of the urinalysis for predicting urinary tract infections in young febrile children. *Arch Pediatr Adolesc Med* 2001;155(1):60–65.

The Subcommittee on Urinary Tract Infection. Urinary tract infection: clinical practice guideline for the diagnosis and management of the initial UTI in febrile infants and children 2 to 24 months. *Pediatrics* 2011;128(3):595–610.

Skin and Soft Tissue Infections

Denehan JK, Kimia AA, Tan Tanny SP, et al. Distinguishing Lyme from septic knee monoarthritis in Lyme Disease-endemic areas. *Pediatrics* 2013;131(3):e695–e701.

Wormser GP, Dattwyler RJ, Shapiro ED, et al. The clinical assessment, treatment, and prevention of Lyme disease, human granulocytic anaplasmosis, and babesiosis: clinical practice guidelines by the Infectious Diseases Society of America. *Clin Infect Dis* 2006;43(9): 1089–1134.

Travel Medicine

General Travel Medicine Articles

Alirol E, Getaz L, Stoll B, et al. Urbanisation and infectious diseases in a globalised world. *Lancet Infect Dis* 2011;11(2):131–141.

Flores-Figueroa J, Okhuysen PC, von Sonnenburg F, et al. Patterns of illness in travelers visiting Mexico and Central America: the GeoSentinel experience. *Clin Infect Dis* 2011;53(6):523–531.

Harvey K, Esposito DH, Han P, et al. Surveillance for travel-related diseases–GeoSentinel Surveillance System, United States, 1997–2011. *MMWR Surveill Summ* 2013;62:1–23.

Kotlyar S, Rice BT. Fever in the returning traveler. *Emerg Med Clin North Am* 2013;31(4):927–944.

Lozano R, Nghavi M, Foreman K, et al. Global and regional mortality from 235 causes of death for 20 age groups in 1990 and 2010: a systematic analysis for the Global Burden of Disease Study 2010. *Lancet* 2012;380(9859):2095–2128.

Mangili A, Gendreau MA. Transmission of infectious diseases during commercial air travel. *Lancet* 2005;365(9463):989–996.

Spira AM. Assessment of travellers who return home ill. *Lancet* 2003;361(9367):1459–1469.

Malaria

Freedman DO. Clinical practice; malaria prevention in short-term travelers. *N Engl J Med* 2008;359(6):603–612.

White NJ, Pukrittayakamee S, Hein TT, et al. Malaria. *Lancet* 2014;383(9918):723–735.

World Health Organization. *World Malaria Report 2013*. Geneva, 2014. Available online at: http://www.who.int/malaria/publications/world_malaria_report_2013/wmr2013_no_profiles.pdf?ua=1. Accessed June 5, 2014.

Tuberculosis

Centers for Disease Control and Prevention. Trends in tuberculosis – United States, 2013. *MMWR Morb Mortal Wkly Rep* 2014;63(11):229–233.

Centers for Disease Control and Prevention, American Thoracic Society, and Infectious Diseases Society of America. Treatment of tuberculosis. *MMWR* 2003;52(RR-11):1–74.

Perez-Velez CM, Marais BJ. Tuberculosis in children. *N Engl J Med* 2012;367(4):348–361.

World Health Organization. Global tuberculosis report 2013. Geneva: WHO, 2013. Available online at: http://www.who.int/tb/publications/global_report/en./ Accessed May 16, 2014.

Typhoid

Beeching NJ, Parry CM. Outpatient treatment of patients with enteric fever. *Lancet Infect Dis* 2011;11(6):419–421.

Buckle GC, Walker CL, Black RE. Typhoid fever and paratyphoid fever: systematic review to estimate global morbidity and mortality for 2010. *J Glob Health* 2012;2(1):010401.

Dengue

Hung NT. Fluid management for dengue in children. *Paediatr Int Child Health* 2012;32(suppl 1):39–42.

Huy NT, Van Giang T, Thuy DH. Factors associated with dengue shock syndrome: a systematic review and meta-analysis. *PLoS Negl Trop Dis* 2013;7(9):e2412.

Murray NE, Quam MB, Wilder-Smith A. Epidemiology of dengue: past, present, and future prospects. *Clin Epidemiol* 2013;5:299–309.

Simmons CP, Farrar JJ, Nguyen VV, et al. Dengue. *N Engl J Med* 2012;366(15):1423–1432.

World Health Organization. Dengue: guidelines for diagnosis, treatment, prevention, and control. Geneva: 2009. Available online at: http://www.who.int/tdr/publications/documents/dengue-diagnosis.pdf. Accessed June 6, 2014.

Chikungunya

Burt FJ, Rolph MS, Rullie NE, et al. Chikungunya: a re-emerging virus. *Lancet* 2012;379(9816):662–671.

Gibney KB, Fischer M, Prince HE, et al. Chikungunya fever in the United States: a fifteen year review of cases. *Clin Infect Dis* 2011; 52(5):e121–e126.

Staples JE, Breiman RF, Powers AM. Chikungunya fever: an epidemiological review of a re-emerging infectious disease. *Clin Infect Dis* 2009;49(6):942–948.

Diarrheal Diseases

Kollaritsch H, Paulke-Korinek M, Wiedermann U. Travelers' diarrhea. *Infect Dis Clin North Am* 2012;26(3):691–706.

Central/Peripheral Nervous System Infections

Otte WM, Singla M, Sander JW, et al. Drug therapy for solitary cysticercus granuloma: a systematic review and meta-analysis. *Neurology* 2013;80(2):152–162.

Rosenfeld EA, Byrd SE, Shulman ST. Neurocysticercosis among children in Chicago. *Clin Infect Dis* 1996;23(2):262–268.

Sotelo J, del Brutto OH, Penagos P, et al. Comparison of therapeutic regimen of anticysticercal drugs for parenchymal brain cysticercosis. *J Neurol* 1990;237(2):67–72.

Cardiac Infections

Lescure FX, Le Loup G, Freiliij H, et al. Chagas disease: changes in knowledge and management. *Lancet Infect Dis* 2010;10(8):556–570.

Martins-Melo FR, Lima MD, Ramos AN Jr, et al. Prevalence of Chagas disease in pregnant women and congenital transmission of Trypanosoma cruzi in Brazil: a systematic review and meta-analysis. *Trop Med Int Health* 2014;19(8):943–957.

Respiratory Tract Infections

Al-Abdallat MM, Payne DC, Alqasrawi S, et al. Hospital-associated outbreak of Middle East Respiratory Syndrome Coronavirus: a serologic, epidemiologic, and clinical description. *Clin Infect Dis* 2014;59(9):1225–1233.

Bialek SR, Allen D, Alvarado-Ramy F, et al. First confirmed cases of Middle East Respiratory Syndrome Coronavirus (MERS-CoV) infection in the United States. Updated information on the epidemiology of MERS-CoV infection, and guidance for the public, clinicians, and public health authorities–May 2014. *MMWR Morb Mortal Wkly Rep* 2014;63(19):431–436.

Farizo KM, Strebel PM, Chen RT, et al. Fatal respiratory disease due to Corynebacterium diphtheria: case report and review of guidelines for management, investigation, and control. *Clin Infect Dis* 1993;16(1):59–68.

Hartline J, Mierek C, Knutson T, et al. Hantavirus infection in North America: a clinical review. *Am J Emerg Med* 2013;31(6):978–982.

Stockman LJ, Massoudi MS, Helfand R, et al. Severe acute respiratory syndrome in children. *Pediatr Infect Dis J* 2007;26(1):68–74.

Vapalahti O, Mustonen J, Lundkvist A, et al. Hantavirus infections in Europe. *Lancet Infect Dis* 2003;3(10):653–661.

Gastrointestinal/Genitourinary

Barzilay EJ, Schaad N, Magloire R, et al. Cholera surveillance during the Haiti epidemic – the first 2 years. *N Eng J Med* 2013;368(7): 599–609.

Colley DG, Bustinduy AL, Secor WE, et al. Human schistosomiasis. *Lancet* 2014;383(9936):2253–2264.

Greenwood Z, Black J, Weld L, et al. Gastrointestinal infection among international travelers globally. *J Travel Med* 2008;15(4):221–228.

Harris JB, LaRocque RC, Qadri F, et al. Cholera. *Lancet* 2012; 379(9835):2466–2476.

Stanley SL Jr. Amoebiasis. *Lancet* 2003;361(9362):1025–1034.

Skin/Soft Tissue Infections

Huekelbach J, Wilcke T, Meier A, et al. A longitudinal study on cutaneous larval migrans in an impoverished Brazilian township. *Travel Med Infect Dis* 2003;1(4):213–218.

Knopp S, Steinmann P, Hatz C, et al. Nematode infections: filariasis. *Infect Dis Clin North Am* 2012;26(2):359–381.

Schwartz E, Hatz C, Blum J. New world cutaneous leishmaniasis in travelers. *Lancet Infect Dis* 2006;6(6):342–349.

Van Griensven J, Diro E. Visceral leishmaniasis. *Infect Dis Clin North Am* 2012;26(2):309–322.

Sexually Transmitted Infections

Centers for Disease Control and Prevention. Congenital syphilis – United States, 2003–2008. *MMWR Morb Mortal Wkly Rep* 2010; 59(14):413–417.

Centers for Disease Control and Prevention. Seroprevalence of herpes simplex virus type 2 among persons aged 14–49 years – United States, 2005–2008. *MMWR Morb Mortal Wkly Rep* 2010;59(15): 456–459.

Centers for Disease Control and Prevention. Sexually transmitted diseases treatment guide, 2010. *MMWR Morb Mortal Wkly Rep* 2010;59:1–109.

Centers for Disease Control and Prevention. HIV surveillance report: estimated HIV incidence in the United States, 2007–2010. CDC, 2011. Available online at: http://www.cdc.gov/hiv/pdf/statistics_hssr_vol_17_no_4.pdf. Accessed May 29, 2014.

Centers for Disease Control and Prevention. Revised surveillance case definition for HIV infection – United States, 2014. *MMWR Recomm Rep* 2014;63(3):1–11.

Elangovan S, Karimbux NY, Srinivasan S, et al. Hospital-based emergency department visits with herpetic gingivostomatitis in the United States. *Oral Surg Oral Med Oral Pathol Oral Radiol* 2012;113(4):505–511.

Girardet RG, Lahoti S, Howard LA, et al. Epidemiology of sexually transmitted infections in suspected child victims of sexual assault. *Pediatrics* 2009;134(1):79–86.

Saloojee H, Velaphi S, Goga Y, et al. The prevention and management of congenital syphilis: an overview and recommendations. *Bull World Health Organ* 2004;82(6):424–430.

Xu F, Lee FK, Morrow RA, et al. Seroprevalence of herpes simplex virus type 1 in children in the United States. *J Pediatr* 2007;151(4): 374–377.

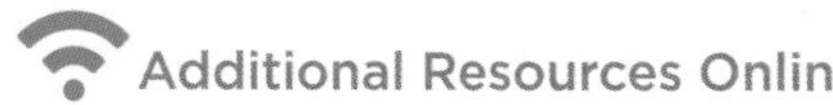

CHAPTER 103 ▪ METABOLIC EMERGENCIES

DEBRA L. WEINER, MD, PhD

GOALS OF EMERGENCY THERAPY

Recognition and understanding of inborn errors of metabolism (IEMs) in the acutely ill child in the emergency department (ED) is critical for appropriate, and possibly lifesaving, management. Individually, metabolic diseases are rare, but collectively are common with over 5,000 identified. In the United States, the incidence is approximately 1 in every 1,000 to 1,500 newborns. Goals of emergency care are to recognize the possibility of IEM in the differential diagnosis of acutely ill, previously undiagnosed patients, and to identify, treat, and prevent acute metabolic derangements in patients with suspected or known IEMs, including the asymptomatic neonate with a positive newborn screening (NBS).

KEY POINTS

- IEMs usually manifest in the neonatal period or infancy but can present at any age, even during adulthood.
- Clinical manifestations vary from those of acute life-threatening decompensation to subacute progressive degenerative disease.
- Newborn screening varies by state, results may not be available in the first days to weeks of life, and false negatives and false positives occur.
- ED care does not require an extensive knowledge of individual metabolic diseases or biochemical pathways, but rather an understanding of the pathophysiology of categories of IEMs.
- History, physical examination, and routine laboratory tests provide clues regarding when IEM should be considered. Most important in making the diagnosis of metabolic disease is a high index of suspicion.
- Successful emergency treatment of suspected and known IEMs depends on prompt institution of therapy to correct and prevent further metabolic derangement and is critical to prevent acute and long-term morbidity and mortality.
- Specialists with expertise in inborn errors of metabolism should be consulted to guide diagnosis and management, and consideration should be given to consultation even if this requires referral outside of your facility.

UNKNOWN SUSPECTED IEM

Goals of Treatment

Recognizing the possibility of an IEM is critical for optimal management of the child with unknown IEM. Immediate goals of treatment are to stabilize cardiopulmonary function, correct metabolic derangements, and avoid intake and/or endogenous production of potentially toxic substances. Early consultation with an IEM specialist, including prior to transport of a child being transported from an outside facility, is advised to guide treatment and collection of appropriate specimens for diagnosis.

CLINICAL PEARLS AND PITFALLS

- Recognition and treatment of a potential IEM does not require knowledge of specific IEMs but rather an understanding of the pathophysiology of categories of IEMs.
- Diseases involving the same metabolic pathways or organelle usually share similar features.
- Most IEMs with potential for acute decompensation present in neonates or infants, but may present in older children and adolescents.
- History, physical examination, and routine laboratory studies provide clues to when and which IEM should be considered. Most important in making the diagnosis of metabolic disease is a high index of suspicion.
- Any organ system can be affected depending on the IEM, manifestations are usually multiorgan. Physical examination is often normal.
- Acidosis, hypoglycemia, and/or hyperammonemia are laboratory hallmarks of IEM. Laboratory studies may be normalized by treatment, including intravenous fluids. Pretreatment samples should be sent for testing when possible.
- Prompt emergency treatment of physiologic decompensation, per PALS and APLS guidelines, metabolic derangements, as well of precipitant causes of decompensation and derangements is critical for optimizing outcome.

Current Understanding

IEMs are usually caused by single gene defects that result in abnormalities in protein, carbohydrate, fat, or complex molecule metabolism. Most are due to a defect in, or deficiency of, an enzyme, enzyme cofactor, or transport protein that results in a block in a metabolic pathway. Clinical effects are the consequence of toxic accumulations of substrates before the block or intermediates from alternative metabolic pathways and/or defects in energy production and utilization due to deficiency of products beyond the block. In the ED, evaluation and management of patients with undiagnosed suspected IEM is usually guided by the potential metabolic category of disease, and does not require a specific diagnosis. Categories of IEMs and their findings are detailed in Table 103.1. Patients with an organic acidemia, urea cycle defect, disorder of carbohydrate utilization or production, fatty acid oxidation defect, mitochondrial disorder, or peroxisomal disorder are at greatest risk of acute, life-threatening decompensation. Patients with congenital adrenal hyperplasia, detailed in Chapter 97 Endocrine Emergencies, may also present with acute critical decompensation.

TABLE 103.1

COMMON PRESENTATIONS OF INBORN ERRORS OF METABOLISM[a]

Acute neonatal catastrophe	**Gastrointestinal/hepatic dysfunction, failure**
Septic appearing	Poor feeding, food intolerances/aversion, failure to thrive
Temperature instability	Chronic intermittent vomiting, decompensation out of proportion to illness
Apnea, tachypnea, cyanosis, respiratory failure	Chronic diarrhea
Bradycardia, poor perfusion	Abdominal pain
Irritability, lethargy, coma	Pseudoobstruction
Seizures	Acute pancreatitis
Poor feeding, vomiting	Hepatomegaly
Hypertonia, hypotonia	Liver failure/hepatocellular dysfunction—jaundice (direct and/or indirect), coagulopathy, elevated liver function tests
Sudden infant death	**Myopathy**
Neurologic disturbance	Muscle weakness, pain, cramping
Developmental delay, usually progressive, with or without loss of milestones	Exercise intolerance
Autism	**Psychiatric disturbance**
Learning disabilities, behavioral and/or emotional disturbances	Anxiety
Hallucinations, delirium	Psychosis
Ataxia, dizziness, headache	Personality changes
Lethargy, coma	Behavioral disturbances
Encephalopathy	Depression
Seizures	Obsessive compulsive disorder
Movement disorder, posturing	Delirium, hallucinations, schizophrenia
Peripheral neuropathy	**Biochemical disturbance**
Stroke, stroke-like episode	Acidosis—chronic or acute recurrent
Vision, hearing, speech impairment	Hyperammonemia with or without alkalosis
Dementia	Hypoglycemia with or without ketonuria, hypoketosis
Cardiac failure/myopathy	
Failure with cardiomegaly ± skeletal muscle weakness	
Cardiac arrhythmia, syncope, sudden death	
Pericardial tamponade, effusion	

[a]Findings may be in isolation or combination and may be either intermittent or progressive over time.

Toxic accumulation of substances results from disorders of protein metabolism (i.e., aminoacidopathies, organic acidemias, urea cycle defects), carbohydrate intolerance, and lysosomal storage. Defects in energy production or utilization result from disorders of glycogenolysis and gluconeogenesis, fatty acid oxidation defects, and mitochondrial disorders. Peroxisomal disorders are a diverse group of IEMs caused by defects of single or multiple peroxisomal enzymes, or of peroxisomal biogenesis that result in toxic accumulations, energy deficiency, and/or defects in biosynthesis of complex molecules. Other categories include disorders of metal metabolism, purine, and pyrimidine biosynthesis (e.g., Lesch–Nyhan syndrome); cholesterol biosynthesis, heme, bile acid, and bilirubin metabolism, lipoprotein metabolism, and glycosylation.

Clinical Considerations

Triage

IEM should be considered in any neonate or infant who is critically ill without known etiology.

Assessment

History. Poor feeding, frequent vomiting, failure to thrive, lethargy in the morning before feeding or with delayed feeding, and onset of symptoms with change in diet and/or unusual dietary preferences, particularly protein or carbohydrate aversion, are concerning for possible IEMs. Symptoms may be episodic in an otherwise apparently normal child. Physiologic stressors such as fasting, illness, trauma, or surgery may precipitate symptoms, especially if the stressor induces a catabolic state. Intercurrent infection may result in decompensation out of proportion to the illness. A history of multiple hospitalizations for lethargy and dehydration with improvement following IV fluids and glucose is common. Psychomotor developmental delay, especially with loss of milestones, is also concerning for an IEM.

Certain findings suggest particular categories of IEMs. Vomiting occurs with many IEMs but is a prominent feature of organic acidemias and urea cycle defects. Diarrhea is also a common feature of many IEMs, particularly disorders of carbohydrate intolerance and mitochondrial disorders. Lethargy progressing to coma is common with organic acidemias, urea cycle defects, fatty acid oxidation defects, and certain disorders of carbohydrate intolerance. IEM should also be considered in any child with unexpected, unexplained sudden death, even without other history suggestive of IEM. Most IEMs are autosomal recessive in their inheritance, but they may be X-linked, mitochondrial, or uncommonly autosomal dominant. A history of suggestive findings; death due to neurologic, cardiac, and/or hepatic dysfunction; sepsis; or unexplained neonatal or sudden infant deaths in siblings or maternal male relatives are also concerning. Maternal illness during pregnancy, particularly acute fatty liver of pregnancy or HELLP (hemolysis, elevated liver enzymes, low platelets) syndrome, may be due to maternal heterozygosity for a fatty acid oxidation defect, specifically 3-hydroxyacyl-CoA dehydrogenase deficiency. A negative family history does not rule out an IEM because most carriers have no clinical manifestations of disease. A negative NBS also does not exclude the possibility of an IEM. False-negative results occur, most commonly due to screening too soon after birth (especially within the first 24 hours), prematurity, neonatal illness, medications, transfusions, inadequate samples, and inappropriate sample handling. Results are often not available in the first several days of life, and in some states, parents have the option of not having their child tested.

Neonate. Most of the IEMs that are acutely life-threatening present during the neonatal period, usually as acute encephalopathy and/or hepatic disease. Among the most common life-threatening IEMs to present in the neonate are aminoacidopathies, organic acidemias, urea cycle defects, galactosemia, and hereditary fructose intolerance. Manifestations may include poor feeding, vomiting, diarrhea, dehydration, temperature instability, tachypnea or apnea, cyanosis, respiratory failure, bradycardia, poor perfusion, hiccups, jaundice, hepatomegaly, pseudoobstruction, irritability, lethargy, coma, seizures, involuntary movements (e.g., tremors, myoclonic jerks, boxing, pedaling), posturing (e.g., opisthotonus), and abnormal tone (e.g., hypertonia or central hypotonia). These same symptoms are also manifestations of sepsis, congenital viral infections, respiratory illness, cardiac disease, gastrointestinal obstruction, hepatic dysfunction, renal disease, central nervous system (CNS) problems, and drug withdrawal. In term infants who develop symptoms of sepsis without known risk for sepsis, metabolic disease may be nearly as common as sepsis. Sepsis may be the earliest recognized clinical manifestation of an IEM. *Escherichia coli* sepsis in galactosemia is the classic example. Other IEMs with increased risk of sepsis are the organic acidemias and glycogen storage disorders.

One of the most important clues to an IEM in the neonate is a history of deterioration after an initial period of apparent good health ranging from hours to weeks. For neonates with IEMs of protein metabolism and carbohydrate intolerance disorders, onset of symptoms occurs after there has been significant accumulation of toxic metabolites following the initiation of feeding. Onset of symptoms is usually between 2 and 5 days of life. Initial symptoms often are poor feeding, vomiting, irritability, and lethargy. In the neonatal period, jaundice occurs most commonly with tyrosinemia, galactosemia, and hereditary fructose intolerance. Progression to coma, multisystem organ failure, and death is usually rapid. Neonates with tyrosinemia may present with intracranial or pulmonary hemorrhage due to coagulopathy. Patients with organic acidemias may have recurrent or chronic subdural hemorrhages, sometimes mistakenly attributed to child abuse. Fatty acid oxidation disorders, particularly very long-chain acyl-CoA dehydrogenase deficiency, may present during the neonatal period. Many of the peroxisomal disorders and some of the mitochondrial and lysosomal disorders also present in the neonatal period; these infants are less likely to have coma as an early manifestation and are more likely to have dysmorphic features, brain abnormalities, skeletal malformations, cardiopulmonary compromise, organomegaly, hepatic dysfunction, myopathy, and/or severe generalized hypotonia, usually evident at birth. Intractable seizures due to pyridoxine or folic acid responsive disorders usually begin within the first few days of life.

Infant and young child (1 month to 5 years). Infants or children with potentially acute life-threatening IEMs (most commonly partial deficiency of the urea cycle enzyme ornithine transcarbamylase, fatty acid oxidation defects, disorders of carbohydrate intolerance, and disorders of gluconeogenesis and glycogenolysis) typically present during infancy with recurrent episodes of vomiting and lethargy, ataxia, seizures, or coma. Amino and organic acidopathies also present during infancy, usually with progressive neurologic deterioration. Lysosomal storage disorders, mitochondrial disorders, and peroxisomal disorders also become apparent in infancy and early childhood, usually presenting with dysmorphism or coarse features, organomegaly, myopathy, and/or neurodegeneration. More subtle and/or progressive findings in infants and children with IEMs include failure to thrive, chronic dermatoses, dilated or hypertrophic cardiomyopathy, liver dysfunction, hepatomegaly, pancreatitis, musculoskeletal weakness, hypotonia and/or cramping, impairments of hearing and vision, and developmental delay, sometimes with loss of milestones. With routine illnesses, children with IEMs may be more symptomatic, develop symptoms more quickly, or take longer than unaffected children to recover. Children with disorders of protein metabolism may present with dietary changes. Fructose intolerance often manifests between 4 and 8 months of age when fruits are introduced. Disorders with decreased tolerance for fasting, particularly fatty acid oxidation defects and defects of gluconeogenesis and glycogenolysis, often manifest when children have poor intake due to illness or surgery and when infants begin to have longer overnight fasts, commonly between 7 and 12 months of age. The length of fasting that produces symptoms may be less than 3 hours for disorders of glyconeogenesis and glycogenolysis, and 12 to 24 hours for fatty acid oxidation defects. When patients with these disorders present with vomiting, the severity of illness, particularly lethargy, is usually out of proportion to the duration of illness and the amount of vomiting. Ketotic hypoglycemia, commonly seen in children of ages 1 to 5 years, has been shown in some cases to be caused by fatty acid oxidation defects and, less commonly, aminoacidopathies or organic acidemias. It is now recognized that Reye syndrome–like conditions are often attributable to an IEM (most often a fatty acid oxidation defect, particularly medium-chain acyl-CoA dehydrogenase deficiency, or a urea cycle defect, particularly ornithine transcarbamylase deficiency). Mortality for those with a previously undiagnosed fatty acid oxidation defect can be 40% with the first clinical decompensation. IEMs also explain sudden infant death syndrome (SIDS) in approximately 5% to 10% of cases, most commonly fatty acid oxidation defects that cause cardiac arrest due to arrhythmia and/or cardiomyopathy; the most common of these is medium-chain fatty acyl-coA dehydrogenase deficiency. Other fatty acid oxidation defects, organic acidemias, and congenital adrenal hyperplasia account for most of the remainder of SIDS cases attributable to genetic defects.

Older child, adolescent, or adult (older than 5 years). In the older child, adolescent, or even adult, undiagnosed metabolic disease should be considered in individuals with subtle neurologic or psychiatric abnormalities. Many will have had long-term manifestations believed to be due to other causes. Most typically, these individuals are diagnosed as having birth injury, behavioral problems, attention deficit hyperactivity disorder, psychiatric disorders, or atypical forms of medical diseases such as multiple sclerosis, migraines, epilepsy, or stroke. The more common findings include mild to profound developmental delay, autism, and learning disabilities. Manifestations may be intermittent, precipitated by the stress of illness or by dietary changes or fast, especially as teens take more control over their own diet, or may be progressive. Most IEMs diagnosed in this age group are not immediately life-threatening. However, even a patient with a late-onset, presumably milder, form of an IEM may die with a first metabolic crisis. An example is partial ornithine transcarbamylase deficiency, which can manifest at this time as a life-threatening encephalopathy. This is seen particularly in adolescent females with a history of protein aversion, migraine-like headaches, vomiting, abdominal pain, lethargy, and behavioral problems, particularly following protein ingestion. Fatty acid oxidation defects may also present at this time with sudden death or life-threatening cardiac arrhythmia, hypoketotic hypoglycemia, and/or rhabdomyolysis. Glycogen storage disorders that manifest as exercise intolerance, muscle weakness, cramping, and/or rhabdomyolysis often present in adolescents because of their greater participation in sports during these years. Some mitochondrial disorders present during adolescence or adulthood with loss of vision and/or hearing, cardiac dysfunction, myopathy, neurologic degeneration, and endocrine disturbances. Stroke or stroke-like episodes with or without encephalopathy may occur with aminoacidopathies, in particular homocystinuria, urea cycle defects, organic acidemias, disorders of carbohydrate metabolism, and mitochondrial disorders, most notably mitochondrial encephalomyopathy, lactic acidosis, stroke-like episodes (MELAS). Disorders in which psychiatric disturbances may be the initial presenting manifestation include homocystinuria; urea cycle defects, especially partial ornithine transcarbamylase deficiency; lysosomal storage disorders; peroxisomal disorders; and Wilson disease, a disorder of copper metabolism. Patients with phenylketonuria who are no longer on a low-protein diet may also manifest psychiatric symptoms.

Physical Examination. Clinical manifestations of IEMs vary from those of acute life-threatening decompensation to subacute progressive degenerative disease (Table 103.1). Nearly all IEMs have several variants that differ in age of clinical onset and severity. Clinical manifestations may even vary among family members. Life-threatening diseases tend to present clinically during the neonatal period or infancy, whereas those with intermittent decompensation or insidious onset and slow progression tend to become apparent later.

IEMs can affect any organ system, and often affect multiple organ systems, and therefore should be considered in patients who present with altered level of consciousness, encephalopathy, cardiac failure, hepatic failure, skeletal muscle myopathy, weakness and/or cramping, and/or neuropsychiatric disturbance. Physical examination may be normal, have subtle and/or nonspecific findings, or have findings that provide more specific diagnostic information (Table 103.2). Findings tend to be related to abnormal anatomic proportion (i.e., size and shape), rather than to major structural defects and usually become more pronounced over time. Patients tend to have characteristic facies, short stature, organomegaly, and/or musculoskeletal abnormalities. IEMs within each major category are listed in Table 103.3. Features of specific IEMs can be found in texts referenced at the end of this chapter and on various web sites, including the National Center for Biotechnology Information's "Online Mendelian Inheritance in Man" web site (http://www.ncbi.nlm.nih.gov/omim).

Laboratory Findings. In the patient with potentially life-threatening symptoms, evaluation for possible IEM should be initiated immediately.

Initial laboratory findings in the acutely ill patient that may suggest an IEM include serum electrolytes, blood gas, and lactate that detect electrolyte imbalances, an increased anion gap, and/or acid–base status abnormalities; blood urea nitrogen (BUN) and creatinine levels that reveal impaired renal function; total and direct bilirubin, aspartate transaminase (AST) and alanine transaminase (ALT) transaminases, prothrombin time (PT), partial thromboplastin time (PTT), and/or ammonia that indicate hepatic dysfunction or failure; hypoglycemia, particularly with low or absent urine ketones, that suggests inability to appropriately metabolize fatty acids or carbohydrates; or urine-reducing substances that suggest carbohydrate intolerance (Table 103.4). A complete metabolic screen may also reveal abnormalities in uric acid, calcium, phosphate, and/or magnesium. In addition to these studies, patients with history or physical examination suggestive of myopathy should have lactate dehydrogenase, aldolase, creatinine phosphokinase, and urine myoglobin measured as part of their initial screen. Although not diagnostic, IEM can lead to abnormalities of any cell line on CBC.

If a metabolic disease is suspected, consultation with an IEM specialist may be helpful in guiding further laboratory evaluation and assisting with appropriate collection and processing of specimens. Blood should be collected and, based on results of initial studies, sent for plasma amino acids and acylcarnitine profile, which reflect fatty acid oxidation and organic acid, and, indirectly, amino acid metabolisms (Table 103.5). In neonates younger than or at 14 days of age, blood on NBS filter paper can be used for tandem mass spectrometry and should be considered not only if tandem mass spectrometry was not initially performed but also if the initial screen was negative. Urine should be collected for potential analysis of organic acids, acylglycine, and/or orotic acid. Additional blood and urine for possible further testing should be obtained and stored. Cerebrospinal fluid (CSF), if obtained, should be collected at the same time as plasma and immediately frozen and stored for possible further testing for neurometabolic disorders, most commonly nonketotic hyperglycinemia, disorders of serine biosynthesis, and/or neurotransmitter disorders. Measurement of lactate and pyruvate in the acute setting may be difficult to interpret, particularly in the patient with hypoxia, poor perfusion, seizure, and/or sepsis. Plasma-free fatty acids, ketones, endocrine studies, and disease-specific tests may also be appropriate. Laboratory

TABLE 103.2

CLINICAL AND LABORATORY FINDINGS OF INBORN ERRORS OF METABOLISM

	AA	OA	UCD	FAOD	CID	CPUD	LSD	MD	PD
Clinical findings[a]									
Episodic decompensation	±	+	++	+	+	±	–	±	–
Poor feeding, vomiting, failure to thrive	±	+	++	±	+	±	+	+	+
Dysmorphic features and/or skeletal or organ abnormalities	±	±	–	±	–	±	+	+	+
Abnormal hair and/or dermatitis	–	±	±	–	–	–	±	–	±
Ophthalmologic (cataracts, corneal clouding, retinopathy, glaucoma, subluxed lens, optic atrophy, abnormal extraocular motion)	–	–	–	–	±	±	±	±	±
Cardiomegaly and/or arrhythmia, structural defect	–	±	–	±	–	±	+	±	±
Hepatomegaly and/or splenomegaly	±	+	+	+	+	+	+	±	±
Developmental delay ± neuroregression	+	+	+	±	±	±	++	+	+
Lethargy or coma	±	++	++	++	+	±	–	±	–
Seizures	±	±	+	±	±	±	+	±	+
Hypo- or hypertonia, weakness	+	+	+	+	+	±	±	±	+
Ataxia	–	±	+	±	±	±	±	±	±
Abnormal odor[b] (urine, sweat, cerumen, breath, and/or saliva)	±	±	±	–	–	–	–	–	–
Laboratory findings[a]									
Primary metabolic acidosis	±	++	–	±	+	±	–	±	–
Primary respiratory alkalosis	–	–	+	–	–	–	–	–	–
Hyperammonemia	±	+(+)	++	±	–	–	–	–	–
Hypoglycemia	±	±	–	+	+	+	–	±	–
Liver dysfunction	±	±	±	+	+	±	±	±	±
Reducing substances	±	–	–	–	+	–	–	–	–
Ketones	A/H	H	A/H	L	A/H	A/H	A	A/H	A

[a]Within disease categories, not all diseases have all findings. For disorders with episodic decompensation, clinical and laboratory findings may be present only during acute crisis. For progressive disorders, findings may not be present early in the course of disease.
[b]Urine odor best detected by drying urine on filter paper or by opening container of urine kept at room temperature for a few minutes. Urine or body odors: boiled cabbage or rancid butter—tyrosinemia; musty—phenylketonuria; sulfur—cystinuria; maple syrup—maple syrup urine disease; fruity—propionic acidemia, methylmalonic acidemia; sweaty feet—isovaleric acidemia, glutaric aciduria type II; tomcat urine—3-methylcronylCoA carboxylase deficiency, multiple carboxylase deficiency; ammonia—urea cycle defects.
AA, aminoacidopathies; OA, organic acidemias; UCD, urea cycle defects; FAOD, fatty acid oxidation defects; CID, carbohydrate intolerance disorders; CPUD, carbohydrate production/utilization disorders (glycogenolysis, gluconeogenesis); LSD, lysosomal storage disorders; MD, mitochondrial disorders; PD, peroxisomal disorders; ±, sometimes present; +, usually present; ++, always present; –, usually absent; A, appropriate; H, inappropriately high; L, inappropriately low/absent.
Adapted from Weiner DL. Inborn errors of metabolism. In: Aghababian RV, ed. *Emergency medicine: the core curriculum*. Philadelphia, PA: Lippincott-Raven, 1999:702.

abnormalities are often transient, particularly if fluids and/or glucose are administered; therefore, normal values do not rule out an IEM. It is critical to obtain pretreatment specimens, if possible. If pretreatment specimens were not obtained, as is often the case because many IEMs are first suspected based on results of routine laboratory studies, discarded pretreatment samples are likely to be more informative than those collected after therapy. Collection of samples during acute illness is usually preferred to provocative testing by metabolic challenge performed when the child is otherwise well because this method may not yield diagnostic specimens and may be dangerous.

The confirmatory specific diagnosis of most IEMs requires additional specialized tests for detection of abnormal metabolites or abnormal concentrations of metabolites in plasma, urine, and/or CSF; histochemical light and/or electron microscopic evaluation of affected tissues; and chromosome, DNA, and/or enzyme analysis in red blood cells, leukocytes, skin fibroblasts, and/or tissues from affected organs.

In the child who has died, it is still extremely important to attempt to diagnose an IEM because of the possibility that asymptomatic family members are affected or future children are at risk. Routine autopsy is usually not informative for the definitive diagnosis of IEM but may rule out other causes of death and offer clues. IEMs can be diagnosed in the child who has just died, by collecting the appropriate specimens (Table 103.6). Most IEMs can be categorized based on findings of initial laboratory evaluations. Nearly all patients with IEMs that present as acute life-threatening disease will have hypoglycemia, metabolic acidosis, and/or hyperammonemia. These initial findings will guide immediate treatment and further evaluation. Important exceptions are nonketotic hyperglycinemia (usually presents within 48 hours of birth with lethargy, coma, seizures, hypotonia, spasticity, hiccups, and

TABLE 103.3

SPECIFIC INBORN ERRORS OF METABOLISM BY CATEGORY[a]

Aminoacidopathies

Alkaptonuria
Cystinuria types I–III
Hartnup disease
Hawkinsinuria
Histidinemia
Homocystinuria types Ia, Ib, II
Nonketotic hyperglycinemia
Phenylketonuria
Tyrosinemia types I–III

Organic acidemias[b]

3-Hydroxy-3-methylglutaric aciduria
3-Methylcrotonylglycinuria
3-Methylglutaconic aciduria types I–IV
Biotinidase deficiency
Glutaric acidemia type I
Holocarboxylase synthetase deficiency
Hydroxyglutaric aciduria
Isovaleric acidemia
Maple syrup urine disease
Methylmalonic acidemia
Propionic acidemia types I, II
β-Ketothiolase deficiency

Urea cycle defects and disorders of ammonia detoxification

Urea cycle defects

Argininemia
Argininosuccinic aciduria
Carbamoyl phosphate synthetase deficiency
Citrullinemia
N-acetyl glutamate synthetase deficiency
Ornithine transcarbamylase deficiency

Hepatic amino acid transport

Homocitrullinuria, hyperornithinemia, and hyperammonemia (HHH) syndrome
Lysinuric protein intolerance

Fatty acid oxidation defects

Carnitine palmitoyltransferase deficiency types I, II
Carnitine transporter deficiency
Carnitine-acylcarnitine translocase deficiency
Hydroxymethylglutaryl-CoA (HMG-CoA) lyase deficiency, HMG-CoA synthetase deficiency
Long-chain 3-hydroxyacyl-CoA dehydrogenase (LCHAD) deficiency
Medium-chain 3-ketoacyl thiolase (MCKAT) deficiency
Medium-chain acyl-CoA dehydrogenase (MCAD) deficiency
Short-chain 3-hydroxyacyl-CoA dehydrogenase (SCHAD) deficiency
Short-chain acyl-CoA dehydrogenase (SCAD) deficiency
Very long-chain acyl-CoA dehydrogenase (VLCAD) deficiency

Disorders of carbohydrate metabolism

Carbohydrate intolerance disorders

Galactosemia
Galactokinase deficiency
Hereditary fructose intolerance
Fructosuria
Fructose-1,6-diphosphatase deficiency

Carbohydrate production/utilization disorders

Glycogen storage disorder types 0, Ia (von Gierke), Ib/c, Ic, II (Pompe), IIb, III (Cori or Forbes), IV (Anderson), V (McArdle), VI (Hers), VII (Tarui), VIII, IX, X, XI

Lysosomal storage disorders

Mucopolysaccharidosis (MPS)

MPS IH (Hurler), IH/S (Hurler–Scheie), IS (Scheie), MSII (Hunter), IIIA–D (Sanfilippo), IVA, B (Morquio), VI (Maroteaux–Lamy), VII (Sly)

Sphingolipidoses

Canavan disease
Fabry disease
Farber disease
Gaucher disease types I–III
GM1 gangliosidosis types 1–3
GM2 gangliosidosis types 1 (Tay–Sachs), 2 (Sandhoff)
GM3 gangliosidosis
Krabbe disease
Metachromatic leukodystrophy—infantile, juvenile, adult
Multiple sulfatase deficiency
Neimann–Pick disease—types IS, IC, IIA, IIS, IIC

Oligosaccharidoses (glycoproteinoses)

Aspartylglucosaminuria
Fucosidosis types I, II
Galactosialidosis
Mannosidosis α types I, II, β
Pycnodysostosis (Maroteaux–Lamy III)
Schindler disease
Sialidosis types I, II (previously mucolipidosis I)
Sialolipidosis

Mucolipidosis

Mucolipidosis types II (I-cell), III (pseudo-Hurler), IV

Mitochondrial disorders

2-Ketoglutarate dehydrogenase complex deficiency
Friedreich ataxia
Fumarase deficiency
Glutaric acidemia type II
Kearns–Sayre syndrome
Leigh disease
Mitochondrial encephalomyopathy lactic acidosis stroke-like episodes
Myoclonic epilepsy, ragged red fiber disease
Pearson syndrome
Phosphoenolpyruvate carboxylase deficiency
Pyruvate carboxylase deficiency
Pyruvate dehydrogenase complex deficiency
Succinate dehydrogenase deficiency

Peroxisomal disorders

Adrenomyeloneuropathy
Adrenoleukodystrophy in neonatal, adult
Catalase deficiency
Glutaric acidemia type III
Leber hereditary optic neuropathy
Refsum disease infantile, adult
Rhizomelic chondrodysplasia punctata
Wolfram syndrome
Zellweger syndrome

[a]Disease list is not comprehensive. Some diseases can be categorized in more than one category.
[b]Disease category and most diseases terms aciduria and acidemia are used interchangeably.

TABLE 103.4

INITIAL LABORATORY STUDIES[a]

Test	Laboratory abnormality metabolic diseases[a]	Indications, comments
Blood		
CBC (plasma)	Neutropenia (± vacuoles), anemia, and/or thrombocytopenia Organic acidemias Urea cycle defects Carbohydrate intolerance disorders Carbohydrate production/utilization disorders Lysosomal storage disorders Mitochondrial disorders	Neutropenia may be masked by infection. Patients with certain IEMs are at increased risk of infection; infection can also precipitate metabolic crisis Anemia hemolytic, megaloblastic, or normocytic, depending on specific IEM
Glucose (serum)	Hypoglycemia Aminoacidopathies Organic acidemias Fatty acid oxidation defects Carbohydrate intolerance disorders Carbohydrate production/utilization disorders Mitochondrial disorders	Hypoglycemia may be due to primary defect of gluconeogenesis or glucose consumption that exceeds production
Test of acid–base status (serum) Electrolytes Anion gap pH (arterial or venous)	Primary metabolic acidosis Aminoacidopathies Organic acidemias Fatty acid oxidation defects Carbohydrate intolerance disorders Carbohydrate production/utilization disorders Mitochondrial disorders Primary respiratory alkalosis Urea cycle defects	Na^+, K^+, Cl^- usually normal unless abnormal secondary to vomiting, which may produce hyperchloremic metabolic acidosis, or to rhabdomyolysis, which may result in hyperkalemia Normal bicarbonate does not rule out amino or organic acidemias
Ammonia (plasma)	Hyperammonemia Aminoacidopathies Organic acidemias Urea cycle defects Fatty acid oxidation defects	Obtain if altered consciousness, persistent or recurrent unexplained vomiting, recurrent dizziness or ataxia, primary metabolic acidosis with increased anion gap, primary respiratory alkalosis in the absence of toxic ingestion Must be free-flow venous (no tourniquet) or arterial. Arterial preferred because skeletal muscle releases ammonia, ice sample immediately, assay promptly Newborns 90–150 μg/dL, children 40–120 μg/dL, adults 18–54 μg/dL, (www.pediatriccareonline.org/pco/ub/view/Pediatric-drug-Lookup/153930/0/Normal-Laboratory-Values-for-Children) Normal <100 μg/dL neonate, <80 μg/dL >1 mo False positives—valproic acid
Liver function tests (serum) Bilirubin Transaminases Clotting factors	Hyperbilirubinemia Aminoacidopathies (tyrosinemia) Carbohydrate intolerance disorders Elevated transaminases Aminoacidopathies Organic acidemias Urea cycle defects Fatty acid oxidation defects Carbohydrate intolerance disorders Carbohydrate production/utilization disorders Lysosomal storage disorders Mitochondrial disorders Peroxisomal disorders	Obtain if vomiting, jaundice, and/or hepatomegaly Hyperbilirubinemia predominantly conjugated, except galactosemia first few days may be unconjugated

TABLE 103.4

INITIAL LABORATORY STUDIES[a] *(CONTINUED)*

Test	Laboratory abnormality metabolic diseases[a]	Indications, comments
Muscle function tests (serum) Lactate dehydrogenase Aldolase Creatine kinase	Abnormal muscle enzymes Carbohydrate production/utilization disorders Fatty acid oxidation defects Mitochondrial disorders	Obtain if muscle weakness, tenderness, cramping, atrophy, exercise intolerance Carnitine deficiency due to carnitine transport disorders or secondary to organic acidemias, fatty acid oxidation defects
Urine		
Reducing substances (Clinitest)	Aminoacidopathies (tyrosinemia, alkaptonuria) Carbohydrate intolerance disorders	Clinitest positive for reducing substances and dipstick negative for glucose (glucose oxidase reaction) False positives—penicillins, salicylates, ascorbic acid, drugs excreted as glucuronides Absence of reducing substances does not eliminate possibility of IEM
Ketones (Ketostix, Acetest)	Elevated ketones Aminoacidopathies Organic acidemias Carbohydrate intolerance disorders Carbohydrate production/utilization disorders Mitochondrial disorders Absent ketones, hypoketosis Fatty acid oxidation defects	Ketones detected by Ketostix, Chemstix, Acetest Inappropriate ketones Ketonuria in neonates Ketonuria, normal glucose beyond neonate Low/absent ketones, hypoglycemia beyond neonate
Myoglobin	Myoglobin present Organic acidemias Carbohydrate production/utilization disorders Mitochondrial disorders	Not always present, even with rhabdomyolysis, especially if creatinine kinase <10,000 IU

[a]Within disease categories, not all diseases have the laboratory abnormality. In disorders of protein metabolism, carbohydrate metabolism and fatty acid oxidation defects and abnormality may be present only during acute crisis.
IEM, inborn error of metabolism.
Adapted from Weiner DL. Inborn errors of metabolism. In: Aghababian RV, ed. *Emergency medicine: the core curriculum*. Philadelphia, PA: Lippincott-Raven, 1999:705.

apnea) and pyridoxine deficiency and folinic acid–responsive disorders (which present with intractable seizures with or without encephalopathy as neonate).

Hypoglycemia. Serum glucose level of less than 40 mg per dL in the neonate and less than 50 mg per dL beyond the neonatal period should be considered abnormally low. Even with poor oral intake and/or metabolic stressors, hypoglycemia less than 45 mg per dL is unusual in the normal child. Hypoglycemia may cause a decreased level of consciousness, irritability, and seizures. Newborns may also have a high-pitched cry, hypothermia, cyanosis, and poor feeding. In the older child or adult, symptoms may include headache, blurred vision, repeated yawning, diaphoresis, pallor, and nervousness. Hypoglycemia most commonly occurs with fatty acid oxidation defects, disorders of carbohydrate metabolism, and hyperinsulinemic states. Low serum glucose can also be seen with aminoacidopathies and organic acidemias due to inhibition of hepatic gluconeogenesis in these disorders. In patients with hypoglycemia, absence of ketonuria is highly suggestive of a fatty acid oxidation defect. On the other hand, neonates should never have ketonuria, and when present, it is suggestive of an IEM. Beyond the neonatal period, hypoglycemia with inappropriately low or absent ketones is also always abnormal. The presence of urinary ketones in a patient with hypoglycemia does not rule out an IEM, particularly short-chain fatty acid oxidation defects, organic acidemias, disorders of carbohydrate metabolism, or ketotic hypoglycemia of childhood. Hypoketosis, if not evident from the urine, can be determined by measuring ketones (3-hydroxybutyrate and acetoacetate) and free fatty acids in blood. In patients with hypoglycemia, the following laboratory studies should be sent: Plasma amino acids, acylcarnitine, urine organic acids and acylglycines, serum cortisol, insulin, liver function tests (LFTs), and ammonia. Growth hormone is not an informative test in the acute setting. Causes of hypoglycemia other than IEM include liver disease; hyperinsulinemia; toxic ingestions of salicylates, β-blockers, ethanol, or polyethylene glycol; maternal diabetes/gestational diabetes; prematurity or small for gestational age; asphyxia; and sepsis.

Acidosis. IEMs must be considered in patients with metabolic acidosis. Clinical manifestations of acidosis include vomiting and tachypnea. Primary metabolic acidosis is diagnosed by low pH, low P_{CO_2}, and low bicarbonate. Metabolic acidosis may also be due to dehydration, vomiting, bicarbonate loss in stool or urine, seizure, and/or hypoxia. In neonates

TABLE 103.5

SECONDARY TESTS

Test	Laboratory abnormality metabolic diseases[a]	Indications, comments
Blood		
Amino acids—quantitative (plasma or serum)	Aminoacidopathies Organic acidemias Urea cycle defects Mitochondrial disorders	Tandem mass spectrometry, requires minimum 1 mL blood, 3 mL ideal[b], heparin, or EDTA tube Obtain if metabolic catastrophe, neurologic, cardiac, GI/hepatic, musculoskeletal, psychiatric symptoms suggestive of possible IEM, metabolic acidosis, elevated anion gap, hypoglycemia, inappropriate ketonuria, hyperammonemia
Acylcarnitine profile (plasma or serum)	Organic acidemias Fatty acid oxidation defects Mitochondrial disorders Primary carnitine deficiency	Carnitine deficiency may be due to primary defect in carnitine or carnitine transporter, or secondary due to organic acidemia or fatty acid oxidation defect; can also occur in normal children during dehydration Free and total carnitine may also be helpful if carnitine deficiency is suspected
Lactate, pyruvate (deproteinized blood)	Disorders of carbohydrate utilization Mitochondrial disorders	Samples must be free flow, deproteinized at bedside—1 mL into tubes with 2 mL perchloric or trichloroacetic acid, transport on ice Evaluate lactate, pyruvate, and ratio Lactate also increased in patient with hypoxia, poor perfusion, sepsis
Urine		
Organic acids	Aminoacidopathies Organic acidemias Fatty acid oxidation defects Mitochondrial disorders Peroxisomal disorders	Urine best source for organic acids, minimum 2–5 mL, 10–20 mL ideal without preservative[c] Obtain if metabolic catastrophe, neurologic, cardiac, GI/hepatic, musculoskeletal, psychiatric, symptoms suggestive of possible IEM, metabolic acidosis, elevated anion gap, hypoglycemia, inappropriate ketonuria, hyperammonemia
Acylglycines	Organic acidemias Fatty acid oxidation defects	Should be performed only in conjunction with serum or plasma carnitines, minimum 2–5 mL without preservative[c]
Orotic acid	Urea cycle defects (ornithine transcarbamylase deficiency)	Send if hyperammonemia, minimum 1 mL without preservative
Cerebrospinal fluid		
Glucose, protein, lactate, pyruvate, glycine, serine, alanine, organic acids, neurotransmitters, folate, pterins, other disease-specific metabolites	Aminoacidopathies Organic acidemias Mitochondrial disorders Nonketotic hyperglycinemia Neurotransmitter disorders	1–4 mL, freeze −20°C or −70°C

[a]Within disease categories, not all diseases have the laboratory abnormality. In disorders of protein metabolism, carbohydrate metabolism and fatty acid oxidation defects and abnormality may be present only during acute crisis.
[b]Samples, quantities required, collection method, preparation, and storage are institution dependent. Tandem mass spectrometry measures amino acids and acylcarnitines, derived from carnitine, which combines with acyl-CoA derived from fatty acids and organic acids (which may have been derived from amino acids). Tandem mass spectrometry may be used as a screen for aminoacidopathies, organic acidemias, and fatty acid oxidation defects. Confirmation of diagnosis usually requires further testing, including plasma amino acids, urinary organic acids, histologic examination, DNA analysis, and enzyme and/or biochemical assays.
[c]Total minimum is 4 mL for organic acids and acylglycines.
EDTA, ethylenediaminetetraacetic acid; GI, gastrointestinal; IEM, inborn error of metabolism.

believed to have pyloric stenosis, the diagnosis of IEM, particularly an organic acidemia, should be considered if the patient has metabolic acidosis rather than metabolic alkalosis. An elevated anion gap acidosis (greater than 16 mmol per L) is characteristic of acute metabolic crisis with many IEMs. An elevated anion gap with a normal chloride usually reflects excess acid production, most often of lactate, ketone bodies, and/or other organic acids. Metabolic acidosis, usually severe, with marked ketonuria, with or without hyperammonemia or hypoglycemia, is a hallmark of organic acidemias. Fatty acid oxidation disorders may also present with metabolic acidosis, but usually with hypoglycemia and absent ketones or hypoketosis. The IEMs in which a primary lactic acidosis is the cause of the metabolic acidosis include disorders of gluconeogenesis and mitochondrial disorders of oxidation. Anion gap in renal tubular acidosis and acidosis from stool

TABLE 103.6

POSTMORTEM SPECIMENS COLLECTED AT AUTOPSY[a]

Postmortem specimens	Analyses	Comments on collection, storage
Blood[a]		
10-mL EDTA tube	Chromosome analysis	Obtain blood by vascular access or intracardiac puncture
4–6 filter paper spots	DNA analysis (requires PCR amplification)	For filter paper spots, apply free-flow blood to filter paper, saturate through to back, do not layer drops
5-mL heparinized tube	Tandem mass spectrometry for organic acidemias, urea cycle defects, fatty acid oxidation defects	Air-dry 3–4 hrs, do not heat. Place in envelope, refrigerate
	Acylcarnitines	Freeze plasma at −20°C or −70°C, store erythrocytes at 4°C
	Amino acids	
	Bile acids	
Urine[a]		
Urine 10 mL in 1–2-mL aliquots	Amino acids	Collect by bladder catheterization, suprapubic aspiration
	Organic acids	If unsuccessful, irrigate bladder with 20-mL normal saline and collect or perform intrabladder swabs at autopsy
	Acylcarnitines	
	Bile acids	Freeze at −20°C or −70°C
Cerebrospinal fluid (CSF)		
CSF 3–5 mL in 1-mL aliquots	Glucose	If not collected for clinical care, may be appropriate to collect postmortem
	Lactate, pyruvate	
	Glycine, serine	Freeze at −20°C or −70°C
	Neurotransmitters	
	Organic acids	
Aqueous humor		
Aqueous humor	Organic acids	May be appropriate if blood not available
		Collect by intraocular puncture at autopsy
		Freeze at −20°C or −70°C
Skin biopsy[a]		
Skin—2 samples, 3-mm diameter each	Chromosome analysis	Best collected premortem or immediately postmortem, usually viable 2–3 days, 1 wk may be helpful to discuss with specialist
	DNA analysis	
	Enzyme activity	
		Skin, punch, or incisional biopsy, sterile technique, 2 sites—flexor surface forearm, anterior thigh, transport in sterile tube completely filled with tissue culture media, viral culture media, (do not use culture media if planning for microscopic studies), normal saline without preservative, or normal saline–soaked sterile gauze in sterile tube, freeze at −70°C
		Fibroblast culture provides unlimited specimen
Organ biopsy		
Brain[b]	Histochemical light and/or electron microscopy	Biopsy potentially affected organs, collect within 1–2 hrs after death
Heart muscle[b]		
Liver[a] 1 cm^3, 10–20 mg, ≤0.5 cm thick	Enzyme activity	Needle or open incisional biopsy, sterile technique, wrap in aluminum foil, dry ice, freeze at −70°C, screw-top airtight vial
	Biochemical metabolites	
Kidney[b]	Mitochondrial studies	
Spleen[b]		Some assays may need to be performed on fresh specimens
Skeletal muscle 20–50 mg, ≤0.5 cm thick		
Bile		
Bile 2 mL	Bile acids	
	Acylcarnitines	

[a]If family declines autopsy but gives permission for specimen collection, or if unable to obtain autopsy within hours of death, collect blood, urine, and CSF; perform punch or open incisional biopsy of skin and needle biopsy of liver and skeletal muscle; take photographs of dysmorphic features; and obtain radiologic studies to evaluate for neurologic, cardiac, or skeletal abnormalities. Obtain parental permission. Tests that are not accurate using postmortem specimens are those for serum amino acids, lactate, pyruvate, and total and free carnitine assessment. Consider developing postmortem specimen collection kit for ED that contains necessary equipment, specimen containers, and institution-specific instructions.
[b]Obtain an autopsy if autopsy permission granted.
EDTA, ethylenediaminetetraacetic acid; PCR, polymerase chain reaction; ED, emergency department.

bicarbonate loss is usually normal. In patients with metabolic acidosis, concentration of serum ammonia and glucose, and presence or absence of urine ketones and reducing substances will also help direct further metabolic workup. Plasma amino acids, acylcarnitines and urine organic acids, and acylglycines should be measured. Measurement of serum lactate, pyruvate, ketones, and organic acids may also be helpful. Other causes of metabolic acidosis are hypoxia, poor perfusion, sepsis, seizures, Reye syndrome, diabetic ketoacidosis, uremia, and toxins, most notably, salicylates, ethanol, methanol, ethylene glycol, isoniazid, iron, and arsenic.

Hyperammonemia. Early manifestations of hyperammonemia are anorexia and irritability. Children and adolescents may report headache, abdominal pain, and fatigue. Progression to vomiting, lethargy, seizures, coma, and death may occur within hours. In addition to brainstem dysfunction, hyperammonemia can cause cerebral edema and intracranial hemorrhage. Some patients with chronic hyperammonemia adapt to their elevated ammonia level and may appear to have no overt symptoms despite ammonia concentrations above normal. Ammonia is an intermediary in the catabolism of nitrogen-containing compounds, particularly amino acids. Normally, ammonia is converted in the liver to either urea by the urea cycle or to glutamine by glutamine synthetase. Hyperammonemia is the hallmark of urea cycle defects. Plasma amino acids and urine orotic acid should be sent to establish the diagnosis of a urea cycle defect. Hyperammonemia also occurs with organic acidemias and fatty acid oxidation defects as a consequence of inhibition of the urea cycle. Normal ammonia levels are less than 100 μg per dL in neonates and less than 80 μg per dL beyond the neonatal period. Proper collection and handling of blood for ammonia determination is critical to prevent falsely elevated values. Abnormal levels should be confirmed immediately using proper technique for drawing and handling. Ammonia levels are typically highest in urea cycle defects and may exceed 1,000 μg per dL. Ammonia levels in organic acidemias are usually less than 500 μg per dL during decompensation but may exceed 1,000 μg per dL. Hyperammonemia in fatty acid oxidation defects, if present, is usually less than 250 μg per dL. Transient hyperammonemia of the newborn should be considered in the differential diagnosis, particularly if hyperammonemia is present on the first day of life. Hyperammonemia directly stimulates the respiratory center, resulting in tachypnea. Ammonia level higher than 250 μg per dL with respiratory alkalosis in the absence of metabolic acidosis is highly suggestive of a urea cycle defect. Patients with urea cycle defects may have compensatory metabolic acidosis. Patients with organic acidemias and fatty acid oxidation defects and hyperammonemia have primary metabolic alkalosis usually without respiratory alkalosis. Patients with hyperammonemia due to organic acidemias usually have marked ketosis and normal glucose level, whereas those with fatty acid oxidation defects usually have hypoketotic hypoglycemia. Even during minor illnesses, protein catabolism may result in hyperammonemia. In patients with hyperammonemia, liver function should be evaluated. Mild elevation of transaminases may be seen in metabolic disorders in each category. Plasma should be sent for amino acids and acylcarnitines evaluation, and urine for organic acids, acylglycines, and orotic acid evaluation. For many disorders, leukocytes, fibroblasts, or organ tissue, most often liver, is required for confirmatory enzyme or molecular assay. Liver dysfunction due to causes other than IEM, including primary liver disease, hepatic infection, toxic insult, sepsis, and asphyxia, may also cause hyperammonemia.

Imaging Studies. In the ED, imaging studies may be useful to guide management of potential acutely life-threatening organ system failure, particularly cerebral edema, hemorrhagic or thrombotic stroke, or cardiac failure. Imaging studies to aid in diagnosis and long-term management are rarely appropriate in the ED setting.

Management

Initial treatment of IEMs is aimed at correcting acute metabolic abnormalities. Even the apparently stable patient with mild symptoms may deteriorate rapidly. For patients with IEMs of amino acid or carbohydrate metabolism, treatment is aimed at elimination of toxic metabolites. For disorders of fatty acid oxidation or gluconeogenesis and glycogenolysis, therapy is aimed at correcting the energy deficiency. In patients with lysosomal, mitochondrial, and peroxisomal disorders, emergent treatment is aimed at ameliorating the effects of organ dysfunction and usually involves temporizing measures that do not have long-term impact on the inevitable progressive, degenerative course of these disorders. As always, airway, breathing, and circulation must be addressed first. Treatment for a potential IEM should be started empirically as soon as the diagnosis is considered (Table 103.7).

All oral intake should be stopped to prevent the introduction of potentially harmful protein or sugars. Fluid bolus(es), as clinically indicated, should be normal saline, 10 mL per kg for neonates or patients with concern of heart failure and 20 mL per kg for infants and children. Ringer lactate should be avoided because it can worsen acidosis.

Hypoglycemia. Hypoglycemia, if present, should be corrected by dextrose bolus instead of adding D_{10} to bolus fluid; 0.25 to 1 g per kg as 10% dextrose for neonates, and 10% or 25% dextrose for those beyond the neonatal period. Hydration after fluid/dextrose bolus should be with D_{10} to D_{15} in ½ normal saline at 1 to 1.5 times maintenance to maintain serum glucose level at 120 to 170 mg per dL, with the goal of preventing catabolism. Large, rapid fluctuations in glucose level should be avoided. Correction of hypoglycemia with glucose will improve most conditions with the exception of primary lactic acidosis due to disorders of gluconeogenesis involving pyruvate metabolism.

Acidosis. For the immediate treatment of metabolic acidosis, sodium bicarbonate may be administered but must be given cautiously. Sodium bicarbonate should not be given unless it has been determined that the patient has metabolic acidosis and is maintaining adequate ventilation. Rapid and/or overcorrection of acidosis may have adverse CNS effects. In the patient with hyperammonemia, alkalinization of the blood favors the conversion of NH_4^+ to NH_3, which crosses the blood–brain barrier more readily and may cause cerebral edema and/or hemorrhage. Furthermore, alkalinization of the urine decreases excretion of ammonia. Conservative guidelines recommend that sodium bicarbonate therapy be given for a pH of less than or equal to 7.0 at a dose of 0.25 to 0.5 mEq/kg/hr, but following these guidelines does not guarantee that complications from sodium bicarbonate therapy will be avoided. More aggressive guidelines recommend treatment of pH less than or equal to 7.2 with 1 to 2 mEq/kg/hr of

TABLE 103.7

EMERGENT TREATMENT

Access and establish airway, breathing, circulation

Fluid boluses normal saline, avoid lactated Ringer's. Avoid hypotonic fluid load due to risk of cerebral edema, particularly if hyperammonemia.

Discontinue intake of offending agents, provide adequate glucose to prevent catabolism

NPO (especially no protein, galactose, or fructose)

Glucose for hypoglycemia, 0.25–1 g/kg (i.e., D_{10} neonates; D_{10} or D_{25} infant, child).

D_{10} to D_{15} with electrolytes: 8–12 mg/kg/min IV at 1–1.5 × maintenance to maintain serum glucose level at 120–170 mg/dL.

If necessary, treat hyperglycemia with insulin to further prevent hyperglycemia.

Correct metabolic acidosis (pH <7.0–7.2) slowly, cautiously

Sodium bicarbonate and/or potassium acetate: 0.25–0.5 mEq/kg/hr (up to 1–2 mEq/kg/hr) IV; if intractable acidosis, consider hemodialysis (peritoneal dialysis, hemofiltration, exchange transfusion much less effective).

Eliminate toxic metabolites

Hyperammonemia therapy

For organic acidopathies, fatty acid oxidation defects, hyperammonemia is usually corrected by **treatment of dehydration, acidosis, and hypoglycemia. Hemodialysis** should be considered for persistent hyperammonemia for these conditions or suspected IEM.

For urea cycle defects, recommendations of the New England Consortium are to perform dialysis for ammonia >300 μg/dL if concentration is rising, prepare for possible dialysis for ammonia >200–250 μg per dL, engaging receiving dialysis unit/facility as soon as possible. If dialysis not immediately available or levels >100–125 μg/dL, use **sodium phenylacetate, sodium benzoate** as Ammonul (Ucyclyd Pharma, 1-888-829-2593). If <20 kg load 250 mg/kg (2.5 mL/kg) in 10% glucose via central line over 90–120 min, then 250 mg/kg/day (2.5 mL/kg/day) in 10% glucose via central line continuous infusion, if ≥20 kg 5.5 g/m^2 (55 mL/m^2) over 90–120 min, then 5.5 g/m^2/day (55 mL/m^2/day) via central line; **arginine HCl** 600 mg/kg (6 mL/kg) IV in 10% glucose over 90–120 min, then 600 mg/kg/day IV continuous infusion. Ammonul must be given by central line. Arginine HCl can be mixed with Ammonul. Can decrease arginine HCl doses to 200 mg/kg if carbamoyl phosphate deficiency, ornithine transcarboxylase deficiency. L-carnitine conjugates with and inactivates sodium benzoate; therefore, it must not be given with Ammonul. Has also been used for **neonatal hyperammonemic coma of unknown etiology.**

Administer cofactors if indicated

Pyridoxine (B_6) 100 mg IV for possible pyridoxine-responsive disorder (seizures unresponsive to conventional anticonvulsants)

Folic acid as leucovorin; 2.5 mg IV for possible folate-responsive disorder (seizures unresponsive to conventional anticonvulsants)

Biotin 10–40 mg NG tube for possible biotin-responsive disorder (seizures unresponsive to conventional anticonvulsants)

L-carnitine 25–50 mg/kg over 2–3 min or as an infusion added to the maintenance fluid, followed by 25–50 mg/kg over 24 hrs, max 100 mg/kg not to exceed 3 g/day for presumed carnitine deficiency if life-threatening manifestations. Use is controversial, consultation with an IEM specialist is recommended.

Adapted from Weiner DL. Inborn errors of metabolism. In: Aghababian RV, ed. *Emergency medicine: the core curriculum*. Philadelphia, PA: Lippincott-Raven, 1999:707.

bicarbonate. Continued administration of sodium bicarbonate is titrated based on acid–base status. Sodium bicarbonate may cause hypernatremia, which can in part be prevented by giving potassium as potassium acetate. When using potassium acetate, however, the infusion rate must be no more than 0.1 to 0.25 mEq/kg/hr of potassium and requires frequent analyses of serum level. Definitive treatment of acidosis requires removal of the abnormal metabolites either by restricting dietary intake, or in severe cases, by dialysis, preferably hemodialysis.

Hyperammonemia. Significant hyperammonemia is life-threatening and must be treated immediately. Treatment protocols for hyperammonemia in neonates and infants and children are detailed on the New England Consortium web site and as per their site are meant to be used in consultation with an IEM specialist: http://newenglandconsortium.org/for-professionals/acute-illness-protocols/urea-cycle-disorders/neonate-infant-child-with-hyperammonemia/. The goals of emergent treatment of hyperammonemia are to eliminate protein intake, prevent catabolism, and enhance the elimination of ammonia. Fluid containing 10% dextrose at a rate of 1 to 1.5 times maintenance to maintain serum glucose level at 120 to 170 mg per dL should be administered to prevent catabolism and enhance elimination of ammonia. Insulin can be administered to prevent hyperglycemia. Hypotonic fluid overload should be avoided, particularly in patients with hyperammonemia, because this could result in cerebral edema. Increased intracranial pressure in patients with hyperammonemia should not be treated with steroids or mannitol. Steroids increase catabolism and can therefore worsen hyperammonemia. Mannitol has not been shown to be effective.

Hemodialysis is the most rapid and effective method for removing ammonia. Extracorporeal membrane oxygenation (ECMO) is the most effective form of dialysis but has higher risks than other forms of dialysis, particularly in neonates. ECMO, which can reduce ammonia levels by more than 600 μg per dL in 1 to 2 hours, is up to 20 times more effective than hemofiltration and up to nearly 70 times more effective than peritoneal dialysis. Exchange transfusion is not effective. Consensus on ammonia concentration for which hemodialysis is indicated is lacking. Dialysis is most effective for ammonia concentrations higher than 300 μg per dL. Recommendations of the New England Consortium are to perform dialysis for ammonia >300 μg/dL if concentration is rising, prepare for possible dialysis for ammonia >200–250 μg per dL, engaging receiving dialysis unit/facility as soon as possible. If dialysis is not immediately available or levels are higher than 100 to 125 μg per dL but lower than 200 μg per dL, pharmacologic agents for ammonia removal should be administered to patients with known or suspected urea cycle defect. Sodium phenylacetate and sodium benzoate, available in combination as the preparation Ammonul, 100 mg each per mL (Ucyclyd Pharma, Inc., Scottsdale, AZ; 1-888-829-2593) eliminates nitrogen by an alternative pathway that does not rely on an intact urea cycle. Ammonul does not remove ammonia rapidly enough to serve as primary therapy in patients with severe hyperammonemia. As per the package insert (http://www.medicis.com/products/pi/pi_ammonul.pdf), Ammonul is "indicated as an adjunctive therapy for the treatment of acute hyperammonemia and associated encephalopathy in patients with deficiencies in enzymes of the urea cycle." It has also been used to treat neonatal hyperammonemic coma of unknown etiology. The dose is 2.5 mL per kg (250 mg per kg) for patients weighing less than 20 kg and 55 mL per m^2 (5.5 g per m^2) for those weighing more than 20 kg. This dose must be diluted in at least 25 mL per kg of 10% dextrose and administered as a bolus via central line over 90 to 120 minutes. The same dose in at least 25 mL per kg of 10% dextrose is then also given over a 24-hour infusion. Arginine, which enhances urea cycle activity in patients with most urea cycle defects, should be administered using arginine HCl 10% at a dose of 600 mg per kg IV over 90 to 120 minutes, followed by the same dose over 24 hours. Arginine HCl can be mixed with Ammonul. If Ammonul/arginine HCl is being administered, the hourly infusion rate of maintenance fluids should be reduced by the volume of Ammonul/arginine HCl being given. Given the high concentration of sodium in Ammonul and chloride in arginine HCl, extreme caution must be taken if administering other sodium chloride–containing fluids. Sodium phenylacetate may deplete potassium. Potassium should be replaced as potassium acetate. Ondansetron (0.15 mg per kg up to every 8 hours) should be administered for vomiting and/or prophylactically if treating with Ammonul. To assess patient response to treatment, ammonia, electrolytes, and blood gas should be monitored every 4 hours, usually, 2 to 3 days of therapy are necessary.

For seizures unresponsive to conventional anticonvulsants, empiric therapy with pyridoxine (B_6; 100 mg IV), folic acid (leucovorin; 2.5 mg IV), and/or biotin (10 to 40 mg delivered by nasogastric tube) should be considered particularly in neonates, and also in infants, to treat a possible cofactor-responsive IEM. While there are other disease-specific pharmacologic agents, their administration is rarely indicated in the ED. L-carnitine may be administered in acutely life-threatening situations for suspicion of disorders associated with carnitine deficiency, but its use is controversial and consultation with an IEM specialist is recommended. L-carnitine is given at a dose of 25 to 50 mg per kg over 2 to 3 minutes or as an infusion added to the maintenance fluid, followed by 25 to 50 mg per kg over 24 hours, maximum 3 g per day. Given that some IEMs are associated with increased risk of infection and that serious bacterial infection can precipitate metabolic crisis, antibiotics should be considered for any patient of concern for possible serious bacterial infection. Fresh frozen plasma may be indicated for patients with coagulopathy.

KNOWN IEM

Goals of Treatment

For the child with known IEM and acute decompensation, goals of treatment are to expediently and proactively evaluate for and manage cardiopulmonary decompensation and IEM-specific metabolic derangements, and restore and maintain hydration. The child with an IEM in the ED for conditions that could precipitate decompensation, such as acute infectious process, but presently without acute manifestations of their IEM should receive aggressive therapy to prevent metabolic derangements and decompensation. The family may have an emergency treatment plan with them developed by an IEM specialist, specifically for their child. Use of clinical pathways for treatment of patients with an IEM in the ED has been shown to improve timeliness and effectiveness of care. All patients with decompensation should be admitted to the hospital, and there should be a low threshold for admitting any patient at risk for acute decompensation.

Current Understanding

Manifestations of IEM are disease specific but also patient specific. Understanding of these specifics, as well as advances in treatment, will most expeditiously and effectively guide evaluation and management.

CLINICAL PEARLS AND PITFALLS

- Acute decompensations are most commonly seen with tyrosinemia, organic acidemias, urea cycle defects, fatty acid oxidation defects, and galactosemia.
- Early recognition of acute metabolic decompensation is critical for effective management of patients with known IEM.
- A history of physiologic stress, such as intercurrent illness or recent surgery, or noncompliance with diet may precipitate symptoms.

Clinical Considerations

Triage

Patients with known IEM associated with potential for acute life-threatening decompensation should be triaged expeditiously. Many families have treatment pathways in hand (or delineated in EMR) to optimize care (Table 103.8).

AMINOACIDOPATHIES

Goals of Treatment

Treatment of children with aminoacidopathy includes avoiding dietary intake of the offending amino acid(s), and correcting acute metabolic and physiologic derangements.

Current Understanding

Most aminoacidopathies do not cause acute decompensation. A notable exception is tyrosinemia type I, a disorder of phenylalanine and tyrosine metabolism that initially causes liver

TABLE 103.8

LABORATORY ABNORMALITIES, EMERGENT TREATMENT OF KNOWN IEMS

IEM category	Laboratory abnormalities	Abnormalities to treat emergently (see Table 103.7 for specifics)[a]
Aminoacidopathies	Hypoglycemia	Hypoglycemia
	Metabolic acidosis	Acidosis
	± Increased anion gap	
	± Elevated lactate	
	Elevated transaminases	
Organic acidemias	Ketonuria	
	Neutropenia, anemia thrombocytopenia	Hypoglycemia
	± Hypoglycemia	Acidosis
	Metabolic acidosis	Hyperammonemia
	Increased anion gap	
	± Elevated lactate	
	± Hyperammonemia	
	Elevated transaminases	
	Ketosis, ketonuria	
Urea cycle defects, disorders of ammonia detoxification	Myoglobinuria	
Fatty acid oxidation defects	Hyperammonemia with respiratory alkalosis	Hyperammonemia
	± Elevated transaminases	
	Hypoketotic hypoglycemia	Hypoglycemia
—	± Hyperammonemia	Acidosis
Disorders of carbohydrate intolerance	± Elevated transaminases	Hypoglycemia
	Hypoglycemia	Acidosis
	Hyperchloremic metabolic acidosis	
	Direct hyperbilirubinemia	
Disorders of carbohydrate production/ utilization	Urinary-reducing substances	Hypoglycemia
	Hypoglycemia	Acidosis
	Metabolic acidosis	
	± Increased anion gap	
	± Increased lactate, pyruvate	
	± Hyperammonemia	
	± Elevated transaminases	
	Hyperuricemia	
	Ketonuria	

[a]Treatment must also include management of airway, breathing, circulation, life-threatening organ failure, and intercurrent illness including sepsis, which is associated with galactosemia, congenital adrenal hyperplasia, and certain organic acidemias and glycogen storage disorders.
IEM, inborn error of metabolism.

failure and later hepatocellular carcinoma. It usually presents in early infancy but can present in the neonatal period.

Clinical Considerations

Assessment

Clinical features include lethargy, vomiting, diarrhea, failure to thrive, hypoglycemia, jaundice, ascites, edema, bleeding, and renal tubular acidosis. Patients, particularly neonates, may have sepsis. Infants and children, in addition to manifestations seen in the neonate, may have hepatosplenomegaly, rickets, hypotonia, and neurologic deficit. CBC, electrolytes, glucose, phosphate, calcium, albumin, PT, PTT, and blood gas should be obtained upon presentation for illness. As clinically indicated, cultures and lactate to evaluate for sepsis should be sent.

Management

To treat dehydration, normal saline bolus(es), 10 mL per kg for neonates and 20 mL per kg for infants and children should be administered. Bolus fluid should also contain 10% dextrose, unless the patient is already hypoglycemic, in which case dextrose should instead be administered separately as a bolus of 0.25 to 1 g per kg as D_{10} for neonates and D_{10} or D_{25} for infants and children. After administration of bolus fluid and correction of any hypoglycemia, D_{10} in ½ normal saline should be continued at 1 to 1.5 times maintenance to maintain serum glucose levels at 120 to 170 per mg per dL, administering insulin as needed. Stable patients without decompensation and able to feed must avoid offending amino acids. Formula brought by the family may need to be used until the appropriate formula can be obtained for the patient within the hospital.

ORGANIC ACIDEMIAS

Goals of Treatment

Goals of treatment specific to organic acidemias are to decrease organic acid production, enhance elimination of organic acids, and treat precipitating causes of decompensation, such as infection.

Current Understanding

Organic acids are intermediary products of protein, fat, and carbohydrate metabolism. Their accumulation results in metabolic acidosis, which is often very severe and usually associated with elevated anion gap. Hypoglycemia is common because metabolic stress increases metabolic demand, which induces degradation of glucose, and because toxic accumulations of organic acids inhibit gluconeogenesis. Increased metabolism of fatty acids results in ketosis in certain organic acidemias, while others are characterized by hypoketotic hyperglycemia. Hyperammonemia results from inhibition of the urea cycle by organic acids. Organic acids also cause bone marrow toxicity that inhibits leukocyte and platelet maturation, resulting in neutropenia and thrombocytopenia. Organic acidemias most likely to be associated with acute decompensation are carnitine palmitoyltransferase deficiency types I and II, and carnitine uptake deficiency, glutaric acidemia type I, holocarboxylase synthase deficiency, biotinidase deficiency, HMG-CoA lyase deficiency, maple syrup urine disease, methylmalonic acidemia, and propionic acidemia.

Clinical Considerations

Assessment

Neonatal onset forms of organic acidemias usually present within the first week with life-threatening metabolic decompensation. Clinical features include lethargy and/or encephalopathy progressing to obtundation, feeding problems, vomiting, hepatomegaly, metabolic acidosis, hyperammonemia, and neutropenia. Several of the organic acidemias result in a characteristic urine or body odor (Table 103.2). Infantile, late-onset forms tend to have a more insidious presentation with failure to thrive, seizures, spasticity, hypotonia, and developmental delay. Affected individuals may have episodic metabolic decompensation with rapid progression to coma, particularly with physiologic stressors. Many of the clinical features can be prevented by initiation of disease-specific formula free of offending metabolites, and/or disease-specific vitamin therapy for vitamin-responsive disorders, as soon as the diagnosis is made.

Evaluation of patients with organic acidemias should include assessment of vital signs, electrolytes, glucose, calcium, ammonia, AST, ALT, alkaline phosphatase, PT, PTT, plasma amino acids, serum carnitine, blood gas, lactate, CBC, differential, platelets, urine-specific gravity and ketones, urine organic acids, and as clinically indicated, tests for infection. If considering a lumbar puncture, recognize that patients may have cerebral edema due to toxic concentrations of organic acids and/or ammonia.

Management

All protein intake should be stopped for 48 to 72 hours in the acutely ill child. To treat dehydration, normal saline bolus(es), 10 mL per kg for neonates and 20 mL per kg for infants and children should be administered. Bolus fluid should contain D_{10}, unless the patient is hypoglycemic in which case dextrose should instead be administered separately as a bolus of 0.25 to 1 g per kg; D_{10} is given for neonates, and D_{10} or D_{25} for infants and children. Ringer lactate should not be used. After administration of bolus fluid, D_{10} in ½ normal saline should be continued at 1 to 1.5 times maintenance. Because of the potential for severe metabolic acidosis in these patients due to accumulation of organic acids, treatment of acidosis needs to be more aggressive than with many other types of IEMs. Sodium bicarbonate, as much as 1 to 2 mEq per kg should be administered to correct acidosis, pH less than 7.2 or bicarbonate less than 14 mmol per L, and should be titrated based on acid–base status. Patients with organic acidemias may require as much as 10 to 15 mEq/kg/day of sodium bicarbonate. Potassium given as potassium acetate may decrease the amount of sodium bicarbonate required thus decreasing the risk of hypernatremia. Treatment of acidosis and hypoglycemia usually corrects hyperammonemia. Hemodialysis is indicated to hasten clearance of metabolic toxins in the obtunded or comatose patient and to correct persistent metabolic acidosis, hyperammonemia, and/or severe electrolyte abnormalities. L-carnitine (25 to 50 mg per kg over 2 to 3 minutes or as an infusion added to the maintenance fluid, followed by 25 to 50 mg per kg over 24 hours, maximum 3 g per day) may benefit some patients with an organic acidemia but only in consultation with an IEM specialist. Glycine (150 to 300 mg/kg/day IV or PO), which enhances secretion of organic acids, should be considered for patients with isovaleric acidemia. Patients with holocarboxylase synthetase or biotinidase deficiency may improve with biotin (10 to 40 mg per day given PO or NG), those with maple syrup urine disease may benefit from hydroxocobalamin (vitamin B_{12}; 1 mg IM). It is usually not imperative that these cofactor therapies be administered in the ED. Antibiotics should be administered as clinically indicated for infection. Administration of an oral, broad-spectrum antibiotic to reduce gut flora, a significant source of organic acids, may be beneficial but usually is not initiated in the ED. Efficacy of emergent treatment is monitored by ongoing assessment of mental status, fluid and cardiovascular status, signs of bleeding, and measurement of electrolytes, glucose, ammonia, and blood gas levels every 4 to 6 hours until the patient is stabilized. Resolution of metabolic crisis usually takes days to weeks. The New England Consortium of Metabolic Programs details treatment for specific organic acidemias on their web site http://newenglandconsortium.org/for-professionals/acute-illness-protocols/organic-acid-disorders/.

UREA CYCLE DEFECTS

Goals of Treatment

For urea cycle defects the specific goals of acute treatment are to eliminate protein intake, avoid protein catabolism, and remove ammonia.

Current Understanding

Disorders of the urea cycle result in toxic accumulation of ammonia generated by the catabolism of protein. Urea cycle disorders include carbamoyl phosphate synthetase deficiency, ornithine transcarboxylase deficiency, citrullinemia, argininosuccinate lyase deficiency, and argininosuccinic aciduria. Ammonia, in excess, is a neurotoxin that results in cerebral edema as well as brainstem dysfunction.

Clinical Considerations

Assessment

Patients with severe enzyme deficiency present within the first few days of life, following consumption of protein in breast milk or formula. Those with partial deficiency usually present within the first few months of life, but may present even as adults, after intake of a quantity of protein that exceeds their metabolic capacity. Arginase deficiency typically presents later in life, ranging from infancy to adulthood, as a neurologic syndrome with developmental delay and progressive neurologic abnormalities and usually less severe hyperammonemia. Ornithine transcarboxylase deficiency, is the most common urea cycle defect, and in males (X-linked), it is the most severe. Female carriers for ornithine transcarboxylase deficiency may manifest clinical disease due to disproportionate inactivation of their normal X chromosome (lyonization), but usually present later, including during adolescence. The other urea cycle defects, of which carbamoyl phosphate synthetase deficiency is the most common, affect males and females similarly. Presentation even later in life can be acute, severe, and even life-threatening. Acute manifestations are lethargy, irritability, vomiting, hepatomegaly, ataxia, seizures, progressing to coma, and death without appropriate emergent treatment. Duration of coma is a better predictor of outcome than is serum ammonia concentration. With late-onset forms, symptoms, although similar, are usually episodic and/or less severe and may include subtle findings such as failure to thrive in infants and learning and attention deficits, personality and behavioral disturbances, and migraine-like headaches in school-age children and adolescents. Level of alertness and cardiorespiratory status must be assessed. Potential precipitating factors, such as infection, should be investigated. Hyperammonemia is a brainstem respiratory stimulant that results in tachypnea. Increased intracranial pressure due to hyperammonemia may produce bradycardia and elevated blood pressure. Electrolytes, blood gas, glucose, AST, ALT, alkaline phosphatase, bilirubin, ammonia, plasma amino acid levels, CBC, and urinalysis should be obtained. All labs except ammonia may be normal. Even patients who are not lethargic may have significant hyperammonemia, masked by acclimatization to chronic elevations of ammonia. Respiratory alkalosis is common, sometimes with secondary metabolic acidosis.

Management

Patients should be treated aggressively with fluids to correct dehydration and maintain hydration administering NS fluid bolus followed by D_{10} ½ NS, and dialysis and/or sodium benzoate, sodium phenylacetate (Ammonul), and arginine (except those with arginase deficiency) to correct hyperammonemia. Patients with urea cycle defects are usually not hypoglycemic. Although patients with urea cycle defects have low levels of carnitine and may be taking L-carnitine as a routine medication, patients should not receive L-carnitine while being treated with Ammonul because it conjugates and inactivates sodium benzoate. IV lipids can be administered to support catabolism. For treatment of seizures, valproic acid should be avoided because it decreases urea cycle activity and may therefore worsen hyperammonemia. The New England Consortium of Metabolic Programs details treatment for specific urea cycle defects on their web site http://newenglandconsortium.org/for-professionals/acute-illness-protocols/urea-cycle-disorders/.

FATTY ACID OXIDATION DEFECTS

Goals of Treatment

Goals specific for the treatment of the patient with a fatty acid oxidation defect are to correct acidosis and hypoglycemia, which should correct hyperammonemia, if present.

Clinical Understanding

Disorders include enzyme deficiencies involving metabolism of short, medium, long, and very long-chain fatty acids and carnitine transport defects. Medium-chain acyl-CoA dehydrogenase deficiency is not only the most common fatty acid oxidation defect but also one of the most common IEMs with an incidence of approximately 1 per 10,000. Patients with a fatty acid oxidation defect usually present in infancy between ages 3 months and 2 years due to longer overnight fasts as the infant begins sleeping through the night or due to increased metabolic demand caused by intercurrent illness, often gastroenteritis, recent surgery, or, particularly in children and adolescents, vigorous exercise. Hypoglycemia results in catabolism of fatty acids. Accumulation of fatty acid metabolites inhibits gluconeogenesis and has hepatotoxic effects.

Current Considerations

Assessment

Early manifestations of decompensation may include lethargy, dehydration, vomiting and/or diarrhea, hepatomegaly, and usually hypoglycemia with absent or inappropriately low ketones (except in patients with short-chain acyl-CoA deficiency who often produce ketones). Decompensation may progress within hours to encephalopathy, coma, cardiac dysfunction, liver dysfunction, hypotonia, seizures, metabolic acidosis, and hyperammonemia. Patients with very long-chain acyl-CoA dehydrogenase deficiency or long-chain L-3-hydroxyacyl-CoA dehydrogenase deficiency may have exercise-induced rhabdomyolysis. Patients may be normal between episodes of decompensation or may have chronic manifestations of disease that can include failure to thrive, developmental delay, chronic peripheral neuropathy, motor deficits (with long-chain L-3-hydroxyacyl-CoA dehydrogenase deficiency), retinitis pigmentosa (with glutaric acidemia type II), cardiac dysfunction, and dysmorphic facial features. Patients with a fatty acid oxidation defect are at risk for SIDS and cardiac arrest due to hypertrophic cardiomyopathy and/or cardiac arrhythmia. Women who are pregnant with a fetus affected with long-chain L-3-hydroxyacyl-CoA dehydrogenase deficiency are, as carriers, at risk for HELLP syndrome.

During decompensation, laboratory assessment should include electrolytes, BUN, creatinine, blood gas, glucose, AST, ALT, alkaline phosphatase, PT, PTT, bilirubin, ammonia, carnitine, and creatinine phosphokinase.

Management

After administration of bolus fluid and correction of any hypoglycemia, D_{10} in ½ normal saline should be continued at 1 to 1.5 times maintenance, along with insulin, if needed, to maintain serum glucose level at 120 to 170 mg per dL. In patients with fatty acid oxidation defects, correction of acidosis and hypoglycemia usually corrects hyperammonemia. Sodium bicarbonate should be administered for bicarbonate less than 16 mg per dL. Administration of L-carnitine is controversial because in excess, long-chain acylcarnitine may produce cardiac arrhythmias; therefore, L-carnitine should be administered only after consulting a metabolism specialist. Drugs that induce hypoglycemia and epinephrine, which stimulates lipolysis, should be avoided, and if they must be given, glucose concentration should be maintained with dextrose. Clinical and laboratory parameters should be monitored until the patient is stabilized and tolerating fluid well. Long-term, patients may be on a high-carbohydrate, low-fat diet that includes a complex carbohydrate such as cornstarch to avoid hypoglycemia. Asymptomatic siblings and parents should be tested. The New England Consortium of Metabolic Programs details treatment for specific fatty acid oxidation defects on their web site http://newenglandconsortium.org/for-professionals/acute-illness-protocols/fatty-acid-oxidation-disorders/.

CARBOHYDRATE DISORDERS

Disorders of Carbohydrate Intolerance

Galactosemia. Classic galactosemia, characterized by less than 1% galactose-1-phosphate uridyltransferase activity, results in clinical symptoms usually within the first week of life, often within the first 2 to 3 days and may be rapidly fatal.

Goals of Treatment

Treatment goals specific for galactosemia are to eliminate galactose from the diet and recognizing and treating possible sepsis.

Clinical Considerations

Assessment

Manifestations include poor feeding, vomiting, diarrhea, failure to thrive, bulging fontanelle lethargy that may progress to coma, jaundice and coagulopathy due to liver disease, and/or sepsis, classically with *E. coli,* which may be the initial manifestation. Most newborns will have cataracts although they may only be appreciated by slit lamp examination.

Urine dip will be positive for non–glucose-reducing substances, that is, positive Clinitest, and have negative or trace of glucose with glucose oxidase strip, that is, Clinistix or Glucostix. CBC will reveal hemolysis. Electrolytes may be remarkable for hyperchloremic metabolic acidosis due to renal tubular dysfunction. LFTs are expected to reveal markedly elevated bilirubin level, initially indirect and after 1 to 2 weeks direct, alkaline phosphate and mild to moderately elevated AST and ALT, and markedly elevated PT and PTT. Given that most patients present as neonates, those with known diagnosis will likely have received the diagnosis based on NBS. Definitive diagnosis requires measurement of erythrocyte enzyme activity, and particularly in patients with less severe presentation, it may reveal more benign forms.

Management

In addition to correction of dehydration, metabolic derangements, and infection, treatment requires complete lifelong exclusion of galactose from the diet. In neonates, breast milk and cow milk must be replaced with lactose-free soy formula, for example, Nutramigen, Pregestimil. Even when galactose-free diet is initiated early, those who survive the neonatal period often have developmental delay or learning disabilities.

Disorders of Carbohydrate Production or Utilization

Glycogen Storage Disorders

Goals of Treatment. Treatment goals specific for glycogen storage disorders are to correct hypoglycemia if present and provide supportive care for organ dysfunction or failure most notably for GSD II heart and liver, GSD IV liver, GSD V renal.

Current Understanding. Glycogen storage disorders are due to defects in glycogen synthesis, degradation or regulation. GSD 0, I, III, IV, VI, IX, which primarily involve liver, and GSD II, which involves skeletal and cardiac muscle, account for the vast majority of cases in the United States and Europe.

Clinical Considerations

Assessment. GSD 0 is the most likely to result in acute decompensation, usually due to hypoglycemia during intercurrent illness when patients are unable to take cornstarch, the mainstay of therapy. Presentation is similar to that for fatty acid oxidation defects. Patients with GSD I, III, VI, IX may also present with symptoms of hypoglycemia. Hepatomegaly is seen with GSD 0, I, III, IV, VI, IX. Manifestations of skeletal muscle involvement include weakness and potentially renal failure due to rhabdomyolysis. Depending on type, other findings can include cardiomyopathy, cardiac arrhythmias, hemolysis, and jaundice.

Laboratory findings, depending on the organ systems involved, may include hypoglycemia, elevated liver transaminases, ketosis, elevated CPK, myoglobinuria, elevated BUN, creatinine, anemia, neutropenia, coagulopathy, elevated LDH and bilirubin. EKG may reveal arrhythmia or findings consistent with cardiomegaly.

Management. Correction of hypoglycemia with glucose and glucose-containing fluids is the same as for fatty acid oxidation defects. Treatment for liver, skeletal muscle, cardiac, kidney, and hematologic manifestations is supportive care.

NEONATE WITH POSITIVE NEWBORN SCREEN

Goals of Treatment

Treatment goal is to confirm NBS and to prevent symptoms and metabolic derangements of IEM.

CLINICAL PEARLS AND PITFALLS

- All neonates with a positive NBS require evaluation and confirmatory testing. Those with NBS positive for a condition that may result in decompensation in the neonatal period require emergent evaluation even if they appear to be asymptomatic.
- Most neonates with a positive NBS will have a false-positive result.
- Evaluation should include history and physical examination, and IEM-specific routine laboratory tests to reveal clinical manifestation or confirm absence of findings.
- Confirmatory NBS tests should be sent even if routine laboratory tests are normal.
- Evaluation, management, and disposition should be in consultation with an IEM specialist.
- Management should include correction of any metabolic derangements, assuring adequate hydration and avoidance of potentially toxic substances even in asymptomatic patients. Neonates with even subtle clinical or metabolic abnormalities should be admitted.

Current Understanding

The American College of Medical Genetics for the Maternal and Child Health Bureau in 2005, recommends that states screen for a core panel of 29 conditions, 22 of which are IEMs, and an additional 25 conditions that are considered secondary targets on the basis of more mild symptoms and/or absence of treatment options, of which 24 are IEMs. Most, but not all states, now screen for core conditions, and at least some of the secondary targets (http://genes-r-us.uthscsa.edu/nbsdisorders.pdf).

For every true-positive NBS, there are 12 to 60 false positives. To minimize the number of false-negative NBS results, cutoff values have been deliberately set low with a national goal of an overall 0.3% false-positive rate and a 20% positive predictive value. False positives also occur because of maternal IEM, which, in some cases is undiagnosed. Even in the asymptomatic neonate, a false positive cannot be assumed. Evaluation should include history, physical examination, and routine laboratory tests to reveal clinical manifestations of disease or confirm absence of manifestations. The IEMs most likely to cause acute decompensation in neonates include certain forms of tyrosinemia, organic acidemias, urea cycle defects, galactosemia, and, less commonly, biotinidase deficiency. Manifestations and treatment of these conditions are detailed in the section of this chapter on known IEMs, and for congenital adrenal hyperplasia in Chapter 97 Endocrine Emergencies. Evaluation and management of neonates with positive NBS should be in consultation with a metabolic specialist, or endocrinologist in the case of congenital adrenal hyperplasia, and guided by American College of Medical Genetics NBS condition specific ACTion sheets and confirmatory algorithms, which provide an overview of the condition and information about potential clinical manifestations, and appropriate routine and confirmatory laboratory tests (http://www.ncbi.nlm.nih.gov/books/NBK55827/).

The New England Consortium web site includes descriptions of some of the diseases in their acute illness protocols (http://newenglandconsortium.org/for-professionals/acute-illness-protocols/). Descriptions of specific IEMs can also be found in texts referenced at the end of this chapter and on various web sites, including the National Center for Biotechnology Information's "Online Mendelian Inheritance in Man" web site (http://www.ncbi.nlm.nih.gov/omim).

Clinical Considerations

Triage

Triage should be based on symptoms. Patients with even subtle symptoms should be expedited for care.

Assessment

History should focus on details of pregnancy and delivery, including gestational age, complications, medications, exposures, route of delivery, Apgar scores, and complications; medications; family history of affected relatives, stillbirths, SIDS; and postnatal history, including fever, lethargy, feeding, vomiting, diarrhea, jaundice, abnormal movements, and abnormal odors. History may be unremarkable.

Examination should take note of level of activity, vital signs, temperature, weight, height, head circumference, dysmorphic features, skin color, fontanelle, red reflex, cataracts, heart sounds, perfusion, respiratory distress, abdominal distention, bowel sounds, hepatomegaly, splenomegaly, ambiguous genitalia, cryptorchidism, suck, grasp, Moro, deep tendon reflexes, tone, symmetry, and seizures. Physical examination may be normal.

Confirmatory testing is required for all neonates with a positive screen. Laboratory evaluation should be disease specific. Routine tests may include electrolytes, BUN, creatinine, glucose, ammonia, AST, ALT, bilirubin, PT, PTT, CBC, differential, platelets, and blood gas. Concurrent evaluation for infection should be guided by history and examination. Appropriate tests for confirmation of the NBS condition for which the patient is positive should be sent, even if all routine laboratory tests are normal. In some cases, further testing is limited, at least initially, to repeat NBS, which may include measurement of standard NBS analytes, as well as additional analytes, while in other cases, specialized tests including enzyme assays and/or molecular tests are indicated.

Management

Specifics of management depend not only on the condition for which the patient screened positive but also on the likely variant(s) of that condition, the concentration of the metabolite on NBS interpreted in the context of age at the time of screening, and other factors that could modify test results. Cardiopulmonary abnormalities and metabolic derangements must be corrected. Dietary modification, vitamin cofactors, and/or medication may be appropriate and, in many cases, can prevent clinical manifestations. Consultation with a specialist is indicated. Patients with any abnormality should, in most cases, be admitted to the hospital. For patients who are discharged, a plan for very close follow-up and genetic counseling, even though confirmatory testing may rule out true disease, should be established.

SUMMARY

Collectively IEMs are not rare, and clinical manifestations are often nonspecific. Therefore, a high index of suspicion is essential for diagnosis. A few routine tests will serve as an informative screen for most IEMs. Evaluation and treatment of patients with known IEM should be disease specific. All neonates with positive NBS, even if asymptomatic, require evaluation and confirmatory testing, and if at risk for acute decompensation emergent initiation of treatment. Rapid initiation of appropriate treatment for patients with suspected or known IEM or positive NBS may not only be lifesaving but is also critical for optimizing long-term outcome.

Suggested Readings and Key References

ACMG Newborn Screening Work Group; Metabolic Disorders. Newborn screening ACT sheets and confirmatory algorithms. http://www.acmg.net/resources/policies/ACT/condition-analyte-links.htm. Accessed January 30, 2009.[a]

Acute Illness Protocols. New England Consortium of Metabolic Programs at Children's Hospital Boston. http://www.childrenshospital.org/newenglandconsortium/NBS/Emergency_Protocols.html. Accessed January 30, 2009.[a]

Bahi-Buisson N, Dulac O. Epilepsy in inborn errors of metabolism. *Handb Clin Neurol* 2013;111:533–541.

Blau N, Duran M, Gibson KM, et al., eds. *Physicians guide to the laboratory diagnosis of metabolic diseases.* 2nd ed. Heidelberg, Germany: Springer, 2002.

Cakir B, Teksam M, Kosehan D, et al. Inborn errors of metabolism presenting in childhood. *J Neuroimaging* 2011;21(2):e117–e133. Review. Erratum in: *J Neuroimaging* 2011;21(3):306.

Calvo M, Artuch R, Macia E, et al. Diagnostic approach to inborn errors of metabolism in an emergency unit. *Pediatr Emerg Care* 2000;16(6):405–408.

Chace DH, Kalas TA, Naylor EW. Use of tandem mass spectrometry for multianalyte screening of dried blood specimens from newborns. *Clin Chem* 2003;49(11):1797–1817.

Chow SL, Gandhi V, Krywawych S, et al. The significance of a high plasma ammonia value. *Arch Dis Child* 2004;89(6):585–586.

Clarke JT. *A clinical guide to inherited metabolic diseases.* 2nd ed. Cambridge, United Kingdom: Cambridge University Press, 2002.

Enns GM, Packman S. Diagnosing inborn errors of metabolism in the newborn: clinical features. *Neoreviews* 2001;2:e183–e190.

Ezgu F. Recent advances in the molecular diagnosis of inborn errors of metabolism. *Clin Biochem* 2014;47(9):759–760.

Fernandes J, Saudubray JM, Van den Berghe G, et al. *Inborn metabolic diseases: diagnosis and treatment.* 4th ed. Heidelberg, Germany: Springer Medizin Verlag, 2006.

Ficicioglu C, An Haack K. Failure to thrive: when to suspect inborn errors of metabolism. *Pediatrics* 2009;124(3):972–979.

Garganta CL, Smith WE. Metabolic evaluation of the sick neonate. *Semin Perinatol* 2005;29(3):164–172.

Ghaziuddin M, Al-Owain M. Autism spectrum disorders and inborn errors of metabolism: an update. *Pediatr Neurol* 2013;49(4):232–236.

Hoffman GF, Nyhan WL, Zschocke J. *Inherited metabolic diseases.* Philadelphia, PA: Lippincott Williams & Wilkins, 2002.

Jalan AB. Treatment of inborn errors of metabolism. *Mol Cytogenet* 2014;7:142.

James PM, Levy HL. The clinical aspects of newborn screening: importance of newborn screening follow-up. *Ment Retard Dev Disabil Res Rev* 2006;12:246–254.

Kimonis V. Dysmorphology of inborn errors of metabolism. *Mol Cytogenet* 2014;7:139.

Krishna SH, McKinney AM, Lucato LT. Congenital genetic inborn errors of metabolism presenting as an adult or persisting into adulthood: neuroimaging in the more common or recognizable disorders. *Semin Ultrasound CT MR* 2014;35(2):160–191.

Kwon KT, Tsai VW. Metabolic emergencies. *Emerg Med Clin North Am* 2007;25(4):1041–1060, vi.

Levy PA. Inborn errors of metabolism: part 1: overview. *Pediatr Rev* 2009;30(4):131–137.

Levy PA. Inborn errors of metabolism: part 2: specific disorders. *Pediatr Rev* 2009;30(4):e22–e28.

Mak CM, Lee HC, Chan AY, et al. Inborn errors of metabolism and expanded newborn screening: review and update. *Crit Rev Clin Lab Sci* 2013;50(6):142–162.

Marsden D, Larson C, Levy HL. Newborn screening for metabolic disorders. *J Pediatr* 2006;148(5):577–584.

McKusik VA. OMIM Online Mendelian Inheritance in Man [database online]. http://www.ncbi.nlm.nih.gov/omim. Accessed January 30, 2009.[a]

National Newborn Screening and Genetics Resource Center. United States table of newborn screening tests performed by state. http://genes-r-us.uthscsa.edu/nbsdisorders.pdf. Canadian table of newborn screening tests performed by province and territory. http://genes-r-us.uthscsa.edu/nbsdisorders.pdf. Accessed January 30, 2009.[a]

Nia S. Psychiatric signs and symptoms in treatable inborn errors of metabolism. *J Neurol* 2014;261(Suppl 2):559–568.

Ozben T. Expanded newborn screening and confirmatory follow-up testing for inborn errors of metabolism detected by tandem mass spectrometry. *Clin Chem Lab Med* 2013;51(1):157–176.

Pagon RA. Gene tests. http://www.ncbi.nlm.nih.gov/sites/GeneTests/?db=GeneTests. Accessed November 10, 2009.

Parvaneh N, Quartier P, Rostami P, et al. Inborn errors of metabolism underlying primary immunodeficiencies. *J Clin Immunol* 2014;34(7):753–771.

Pasquali M, Longo N. Newborn screening and inborn errors of metabolism. *Am J Med Genet C Semin Med Genet* 2011;157C(1):1–2.

Rahman S, Footitt EJ, Varadkar S, et al. Inborn errors of metabolism causing epilepsy. *Dev Med Child Neurol* 2013;55(1):23–36.

Rinaldo P, Zafari S, Tortorelli S, et al. Making the case for objective performance metrics in newborn screening by tandem mass spectrometry. *Ment Retard Dev Disabil Res Rev* 2006;12(4):255–261.

Sahoo S, Franzson L, Jonsson JJ, et al. A compendium of inborn errors of metabolism mapped onto the human metabolic network. *Mol Biosyst* 2012;8(10):2545–2558.

Scriver CR, Sly WS, Barton C, et al., eds. *The metabolic and molecular basis of inherited disease.* 8th ed. New York, NY: McGraw-Hill, 2001.

Seashore MR, Wappner RS. *Genetics in primary care and clinical medicine.* Stamford, CT: Appleton & Lange, 1996.

Sun A, Lam C, Wong DA. Expanded newborn screening for inborn errors of metabolism: overview and outcomes. *Adv Pediatr* 2012;59(1):209–245.

The Urea Cycle Disorders Conference Group. Consensus statement from a conference for the management of patients with urea cycle disorders. *J Pediatr* 2001;138:S1–S5.

Vockley J, Chapman KA, Arnold GL. Development of clinical guidelines for inborn errors of metabolism: commentary. *Mol Genet Metab* 2013;108(4):203–205.

[a]Consider adding these URLs as bookmarks on computers where this information is needed.

Waisbren SE. Expanded newborn screening: information and resources for the family physician. *Am Fam Physician* 2008;77:987–994.

Weinstein DA, Butte AJ, Raymond K. High incidence of unrecognized metabolic and endocrinologic disorders in acutely ill children with previously unrecognized hypoglycemia. *Pediatr Res* 2001; 49:103A#578.

Wolf NI, García-Cazorla A, Hoffmann GF. Epilepsy and inborn errors of metabolism in children. *J Inherit Metab Dis* 2009;32(5):609–617.

Zand DJ, Brown KM, Lichter-Konecki U, et al. Effectiveness of a clinical pathway for the emergency treatment of patients with inborn errors of metabolism. *Pediatrics* 2008;122(6):1191–1195.

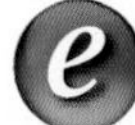

Chapter 104 appears in the eBook bundled with this text. Please see the inside front cover for eBook access instructions.

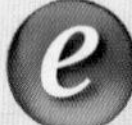

To view this chapter please access the eBook bundled with this text. Please see the inside front cover for eBook access instructions.

CHAPTER 104 ■ NEONATAL EMERGENCIES

NICKIE NIFORATOS ANDESCAVAGE, MD, DEENA BERKOWITZ, MD, MPH, AND LAMIA SOGHIER, MD, FAAP

CHAPTER 105 ■ NEUROLOGIC EMERGENCIES

MARC H. GORELICK, MD, MSCE AND MATTHEW P. GRAY, MD, MS

GOALS OF EMERGENCY CARE

Signs and symptoms of neurologic dysfunction in children are produced by either primary nervous system disorders or are secondary to systemic disease. The differential diagnosis of many such neurologic findings can be found in the second section of this book (see related chapters below). This chapter focuses on the management of conditions primarily involving the various parts of the nervous system, including the brain, spinal cord, and peripheral nerves. Most neurologic conditions present with a recognizable pattern of clinical manifestations. Goals of care in the emergency department should focus on prompt recognition of these patterns, systematic diagnostic evaluations, and appropriate subspecialist consultation.

KEY POINTS

- A detailed history and neurologic examination are imperative to identifying the etiology of most neurologic conditions.
- Anatomic localization of a neurologic injury is usually possible after evaluation of the distribution and character of the deficit.
- Neuroimaging is a useful adjunct in the diagnosis of many neurologic diseases and MRI is often the study of choice.

RELATED CHAPTERS

Signs and Symptoms
- Ataxia: Chapter 10
- Coma: Chapter 12
- Dizziness and Vertigo: Chapter 19
- Eye: Visual Disturbances: Chapter 25
- Hearing Loss: Chapter 30
- Limp: Chapter 41
- Neck Stiffness: Chapter 44
- Pain: Headache: Chapter 54
- Seizures: Chapter 67
- Vomiting: Chapter 77

Medical, Surgical, and Trauma Emergencies
- Neurotrauma: Chapter 121
- Neurosurgical Emergencies: Chapter 130

SEIZURES (SEE ALSO CHAPTER 67 SEIZURES)

Goals of Treatment

Most seizures in children are brief, lasting less than 5 minutes. *Status epilepticus* was classically defined as seizures that are continuous for 30 minutes or longer or repetitive seizures between which the patient does not regain consciousness. Many authorities now consider that seizures lasting for longer than 5 minutes or multiple seizures with no return to baseline in between constitute early status epilepticus. Initial management of the child with a seizure is directed at preventing neurologic damage through supportive care and seizure termination with timely administration of antiepileptic drugs, as well as identifying any treatable underlying cause of the seizure.

CLINICAL PEARLS AND PITFALLS

- Status epilepticus should be treated aggressively to minimize neurologic damage.
- Routine laboratory studies and acute neuroimaging are unnecessary for the majority of children with first-time seizures.

Current Evidence

Epidemiologic studies indicate that 3% to 6% of children will have at least one seizure in the first 16 years of life; most of these are simple febrile seizures, which generally occur in children 6 months to 6 years old. A *seizure* is a transient, involuntary alteration of consciousness, behavior, motor activity, sensation, and/or autonomic function caused by an excessive rate and hypersynchrony of discharges from a group of cerebral neurons. The term *convulsion* is often used to describe a seizure with prominent motor manifestations. *Epilepsy,* or seizure disorder, is a condition of susceptibility to recurrent seizures.

The basic pathophysiologic abnormality common to all seizures and convulsions is the hypersynchrony of neuronal discharges. Many precipitating factors, including metabolic, anatomic, and infectious abnormalities (see Chapter 67 Seizures), may produce seizures. Seizures that result from an identified precipitant are called *symptomatic,* or provoked, *seizures,* whereas those with no precipitating factor are called *idiopathic* or *cryptogenic.* Febrile seizures (seizures occurring in association with a febrile illness, without evidence of intracranial infection or other identified cause) are a particular type of provoked seizure seen in children between the ages of 6 months and 6 years. The exact cause of febrile seizures remains elusive. Elevated body temperature lowers the seizure threshold, and the immature brain appears to have a particular susceptibility to seizures in response to fever. Individual predisposition plays an important role.

During a seizure, cerebral blood flow, oxygen and glucose consumption, and carbon dioxide and lactic acid production increase dramatically. If the patient remains well ventilated, the increase in cerebral blood flow is sufficient to meet the increased metabolic requirements of the brain. Brief seizures rarely produce lasting deleterious effects on the brain; however, prolonged and serial seizures, especially status epilepticus, may be associated with permanent neuronal injury.

Clinical Considerations

Clinical Recognition

When the physician is examining a child with an acute paroxysmal event, the first step is to distinguish seizures from other nonepileptic phenomena. If the event is indeed a seizure, it may be classified according to type. Finally, a specific causative factor should be sought. The extent of the emergency evaluation is determined by the clinical scenario; some of the diagnostic assessment may be deferred. Of course, when a child is actively seizing, the first priority is to provide necessary resuscitation measures and control the seizures (see Chapter 67 Seizures and the following sections).

Paroxysmal events other than seizures that involve changes in consciousness or motor activity are common during childhood and may mimic epilepsy (Tables 67.1 and 105.1). Breath-holding spells occur in children 6 months to 4 years of age. Breath-holding spells take two forms: cyanotic and pallid. In the cyanotic form, the infant begins crying vigorously, often in response to an inciting event, then holds his or her breath and becomes cyanotic. After approximately 30 to 60 seconds, the child becomes rigid. As the spell ends, the child becomes limp and may have a transient loss of consciousness and twitching or jerking of the extremities, but the child quickly returns to full alertness. A pallid breath-holding spell may follow a seemingly insignificant trauma. The child may start to cry, but then turns pale and collapses. There is a brief period of apnea and limpness, followed by rapid recovery. In both types of breath-holding spells, the typical history and lack of postictal drowsiness help determine the diagnosis. Breath-holding spells may be recurrent but disappear spontaneously before school age.

Syncope is a brief, sudden loss of consciousness and muscle tone. There are numerous causes of syncope, many of which can be detected on the basis of historical information, physical examination, and simple diagnostic tests (see Chapter 71 Syncope). A syncopal episode can usually be distinguished from a seizure on the basis of the description. The child is typically upright before the event and often senses a feeling of light-headedness or nausea. The child then becomes pale and slumps to the ground. The loss of consciousness is brief, and recovery is rapid. This is in contrast to seizures, which usually have a postictal period with sleepiness. On awakening, the child is noted to have signs of increased vagal tone, such as pallor, clammy skin, dilated pupils, and relative bradycardia. Patients with narcolepsy also experience sudden alterations in alertness, with sleep occurring suddenly and uncontrollably during the daytime. In about half of the patients, narcolepsy is associated with cataplexy, an abrupt loss of muscle tone brought on by a sudden emotional outburst. Narcolepsy is far less common than syncope; both occur more often in adolescents than in younger children.

TABLE 105.1

NONEPILEPTIC EVENTS THAT MAY MIMIC SEIZURES

Breath-holding spells
Syncope
Migraine
Jitteriness
Benign myoclonus
Shuddering attacks
Tics
Acute dystonia
Gastroesophageal reflux
Night terrors
Sleep paralysis
Narcolepsy
Pseudoseizures

Single episodes of staring, involuntary movements, or eye deviation have been found to occur commonly in the first months of life, although they rarely lead to the parent seeking medical attention. In some children, however, these episodes occur frequently. Children with benign shuddering attacks have episodes of staring and rapid tremors involving primarily the arms and head, sometimes associated with tonic posturing. The episode lasts only a few seconds, and afterward, the child resumes normal activity. Acute dystonia, usually seen as a side effect of certain medications, can mimic a tonic seizure. The child having a dystonic reaction, however, does not lose consciousness and has no postictal drowsiness.

Several paroxysmal events are associated with sleep. Night terrors (see Chapter 134 Behavioral and Psychiatric Emergencies) usually begin in the preschool years. The sleeping child wakes suddenly, is confused and disoriented, and appears frightened, often screaming and showing signs of increased autonomic activity (tachycardia, tachypnea, sweating, dilated pupils). Such episodes typically last only a few minutes, and the child does not usually recall the event. Benign myoclonus is characterized by self-limited episodes of sudden jerking of the extremities, usually upon falling asleep. There is no alteration of consciousness. In sleep paralysis, there is a transient inability to move during the transition between sleeping and waking, also with no change in the level of consciousness.

Pseudoseizures are occasionally seen, often in patients with an underlying seizure disorder or in patients who have a relative

TABLE 105.2

SEIZURE TYPES

Generalized	Partial (focal)
Absence (petit mal)	Simple (no impaired consciousness)
Typical	Motor
Atypical	Sensory
Tonic–clonic (grand mal)	Autonomic
Clonic	Psychic
Tonic	Complex (impaired consciousness)
Myoclonic	Partial seizures becoming partially generalized
Akinetic/atonic (drop attacks)	

with epilepsy. Some features suggestive of pseudoseizures are suggestibility; lack of coordination of movements; moaning or talking during the seizure; lack of incontinence, autonomic changes, or postictal drowsiness; response to painful stimuli; and poor response to treatment with anticonvulsant agents.

The most important diagnostic test in distinguishing nonepileptic events from seizures is a careful history, including a detailed description of the event from the person who witnessed it. In atypical or unclear cases, referral for electroencephalogram (EEG) or video EEG monitoring may help in establishing the diagnosis.

Clinically, seizures may be divided into partial (also termed focal) and generalized seizures (Table 105.2), and partial seizures are further classified as complex or simple. Complex partial seizures imply impaired consciousness. Generalized tonic–clonic seizures (previously called *grand mal seizures*) are the type most often seen in acute pediatric care. The onset of generalized tonic–clonic seizures is usually abrupt, although 20% to 30% of children may experience a sensory or motor aura. If sitting or standing, the child falls to the ground. The face becomes pale, the pupils dilate, the eyes deviate upward or to one side, and the muscles contract. As the increased tone of the thoracic and abdominal muscles forces air through the glottis, a grunt or cry may be heard. Incontinence of urine or stool is common. After this brief tonic phase (10 to 30 seconds), clonic movements occur. The child is unresponsive during the seizure and remains so postictally for a variable period. After the seizure, there may be weakness or paralysis of one or more areas of the body (Todd paralysis). In atonic, or akinetic, seizures (drop attacks), there is abrupt loss of muscle tone and consciousness. *Myoclonic seizures* are characterized by a sudden dropping of the head and flexion of the arms (jackknifing); however, extensor posturing may also occur. The episodes occur quickly and frequently, as often as several hundred times daily.

Absence (petit mal) seizures are generalized seizures, marked by sudden and brief loss of awareness, usually lasting 5 to 30 seconds. With typical absence seizures, there is no loss of posture or tone and no postictal confusion. There may be a minor motor component such as eyelid blinking.

The child with simple partial (focal) seizures has unimpaired consciousness. Motor signs are most common in children, although sensory, autonomic, and psychic manifestations are possible. The motor activity usually involves the hands or face and spreads in a fixed pattern determined by the anatomic origin of the nerve fibers that innervate the various muscle groups. Focal seizures may become secondarily generalized, in which case there will be alteration of consciousness. Complex partial seizures, also called *psychomotor* or *temporal lobe seizures,* exhibit a diverse set of clinical features, including alterations of perception, thought, and sensation. In children, they are usually marked by repetitive and complex movements with impaired consciousness and postictal drowsiness.

An important distinction is whether the seizure is associated with fever. Simple febrile seizures are those that are single, brief (lasting less than 15 minutes), and generalized. Approximately 20% of febrile seizures are complex, meaning they are focal, prolonged (last for more than 15 minutes), or multiple episodes within 24 hours.

Triage and Initial Assessment

For an actively seizing child, initiate immediate resuscitative measures and consider administration of antiepileptic agents, as discussed below. After seizures have stopped, the first steps in the evaluation are a thorough history and a physical examination, the results of which are helpful in determining the direction of the search for a specific cause (see Table 67.1 and Fig. 67.1). Important historical items to elicit include fever, trauma, underlying illnesses, current medications, and possible toxic ingestions. A complete neurologic assessment to evaluate for signs of increased intracranial pressure (ICP), focal deficits, or signs of meningeal irritation is also essential.

Diagnostic Testing

In children older than 12 months with a typical simple febrile seizure and no signs of meningitis, generally no further evaluation of the seizure is required. However, lumbar puncture (LP) is indicated if meningitis is suspected on the basis of physical findings. An LP should be considered in children younger than 12 months, in whom signs of meningitis may be subtle, such as irritability and poor feeding; when the febrile seizure is complex; or if there has been pretreatment with antibiotics. In addition, LP should be considered for children with prolonged fever before the seizure, and for febrile children who do not return to neurologic baseline quickly. Other laboratory tests discussed in the next paragraph have been found to have little yield in the child with a typical febrile seizure and are unnecessary. Appropriate diagnostic tests to determine the source of the fever are determined by other features such as the intensity of fever, immunization status, and the child's age.

For the child who presents with a first-time, nonfebrile seizure, laboratory or radiologic evaluation to search for a specific treatable cause of the seizure may be indicated. There is little utility in extensive, routine workups; rather, ancillary test selection should be guided by the results of the history and physical examination. In young infants, children with prolonged seizures, and those with a suggestive history or physical examination, determination of serum glucose, sodium, and calcium levels are indicated. Other ancillary tests that may be indicated, depending on the clinical picture, include serum magnesium, hepatic transaminases, ammonia, serum or urine toxicology tests, electrocardiogram (ECG), and neuroimaging of the brain. LP is rarely emergently necessary in the afebrile child without meningeal signs or altered mental status, although it should be considered in neonates even without fever.

In children with a known seizure disorder, subtherapeutic anticonvulsant levels are the most common reason for breakthrough seizures. The name and dosage of anticonvulsant

TABLE 105.3

COMMONLY USED ANTICONVULSANT AGENTS

Drug	Seizure type	Daily dose (mg/kg)	Oral dosage forms	Serum half-life (hrs)	Therapeutic blood levels (μg/mL)
Carbamazepine (Tegretol)	Generalized motor, partial, complex partial	10–30	Tablets: 100, 200 mg Suspension: 100 mg/5 mL	8–24	4–12
Phenytoin (Dilantin)	Generalized motor, partial, complex partial	3–10	Capsule: 100 mg Chewable tab: 50 mg Suspension: 125 mg/5 mL	10–36	10–20
Phenobarbital	Generalized motor, partial, complex partial	3–6	Tablets: 15, 30, 60, 100 mg Elixir: 20 mg/5 mL	24–96	15–40
Valproate (Depakote)	Absence, myoclonic, partial complex, generalized motor	20–40	Tablets: 125, 250 mg Sprinkles: 125 mg Syrup: 250 mg/5 mL	6–18	50–100
Ethosuximide (Zarontin)	Absence	20–40	Capsule: 250 mg Syrup: 250 mg/5 mL	20–60	40–100
Lamotrigine (Lamictal)	Partial, atonic, myoclonic, mixed types	10–15	Tablets: 25, 100, 150 mg	24	1–5
Clonazepam (Klonopin)	Atonic, myoclonic, generalized motor	0.05–0.2	Tablets: 0.5, 1, 2 mg	18–50	0.02–0.08 (20–80 ng/mL)
Topiramate (Topamax)	Partial, Lennox–Gastaut syndrome	6–15	Tablets: 25, 100, 200 mg	19–23	2–20
Oxcarbazepine (Trileptal)	Partial	10–40	Suspension: 300 mg/5 mL Tablets: 150, 300, 600 mg	9	3–35
Tiagabine (Gabitril)	Partial	Not established for <12 yrs	Tablets: 2, 4, 12, 16 mg	2–10	2–10
Gabapentin (Neurontin)	Partial, generalized	25–35	Solution: 250 mg/5 mL Tablets: 600, 800 mg Capsules: 100, 300, 400 mg	5	Not known
Zonisamide (Zonegran)	Partial, myoclonic, Lennox–Gastaut syndrome	Not established for <12 yrs	Tablets: 25, 50, 100 mg	60	15–40
Levetiracetam (Keppra)	Partial, generalized, myoclonic	30–60	Tablets: 250, 500, 750, 1,000 mg	6–8	Not known

medications used should be elicited, as well as the time of the last dose given, any missed doses, the last change in dosage, and recent levels, if known. Intercurrent illness may also play a role because the metabolism of some medications is affected by systemic illness. Such children should have blood drawn for measurement of anticonvulsant levels. Although many drugs have a standard therapeutic range (Table 105.3), individual patients may require levels outside that range for adequate seizure control; conversely, dose-dependent toxic effects may be observed in some children even at typically therapeutic levels.

Computed tomography (CT) (or magnetic resonance imaging [MRI], if available) is indicated in the emergency evaluation of prolonged or focal seizures, when focal deficits are present, when there is a history of trauma, when the child has a ventriculoperitoneal shunt, or when there are associated signs of increased ICP. For other children with a normal neurologic examination, MRI may be useful in identifying structural anomalies and determining prognosis, but such studies may be deferred to a follow-up visit. Cranial imaging is not indicated in the evaluation of simple febrile seizures. EEG is also helpful in the evaluation of children with nonfebrile seizures. EEG is rarely beneficial in acute management, but children with nonfebrile seizures should be referred for outpatient testing.

Management

The administration of supplemental oxygen and maintenance of an adequate airway are vital parts of the initial management of the unconscious, actively convulsing child (see Chapter 67 Seizures). Trismus often occurs in generalized seizures but is transient. If the teeth are tightly clenched, even the placement of the oral airway should be deferred until it can be inserted during a phase of relaxation to avoid trauma. Seizure-associated hypoventilation and apnea are common with prolonged seizures, and may be a side effect of anticonvulsant medications; thus providers caring for such children should be prepared to offer assisted ventilation. For patients with adequate ventilatory effort but unable to fully maintain their airway, consideration should be given to airway adjuncts and airway positioning. Intravenous (IV) access should be established promptly; however, because of the potential for increased ICP, fluid therapy should be used judiciously until a more thorough evaluation is performed. The child with active convulsions should be protected from trauma.

It is unusual for the child with a brief seizure to arrive in the ED actively convulsing because, by definition, such seizures last for less than 15 minutes. Therefore, the actively convulsing child is usually already in a prolonged or serial seizure state, and pharmacologic intervention to terminate the seizure is required. Establish IV access, and draw blood for diagnostic studies. If hypoglycemia is documented by rapid glucose assay or if rapid determination is unavailable, give IV glucose in a dose of 2 to 4 mL per kg of 25% dextrose in water, or 5 to 10 mL per kg of 10% dextrose (use only the latter in infants). If hyponatremia is suspected based on a history of frequent vomiting or diarrhea or dilution of infant formula, emergent point-of-care testing for sodium should be performed. Seizures caused by hypoglycemia or hyponatremia are unlikely to be treated successfully with anticonvulsant medications without addressing the underlying cause. In neonates or in children with suspected isoniazid toxicity, IV pyridoxine 100 mg may be administered.

In most situations, benzodiazepines are the first drug of choice for acute seizures because of their rapidity of action. Overall effectiveness is approximately 70% in children. Lorazepam (Ativan) is the historically preferred agent, although recent evidence has not demonstrated superiority over Versed (midazolam) or Valium (diazepam). Given in a dose of 0.1 mg per kg IV (usual maximum 4 mg per dose), it has an onset of action of 2 to 5 minutes, and the duration of anticonvulsant effect is 12 to 24 hours. Half the dose may be repeated after 5 minutes. An alternative is diazepam (Valium), 0.2 to 0.4 mg per kg IV (usual maximum 10 mg per dose), which has a similarly rapid onset of action. If IV or intraosseous access cannot be established, diazepam may be administered rectally in a dose of 0.5 mg per kg (maximum 20 mg per dose), instilling the IV formulation with a slip-tip syringe (remove needle) or by using a specific rectal gel preparation. Intramuscular (IM) midazolam (Versed) has also been shown to be effective in a dose of 0.2 mg per kg (maximum 7 mg per dose). IV midazolam may also be given; the intranasal and buccal routes have also been described and appear to have promising initial results.

All the benzodiazepines can cause sedation and respiratory depression, which may persist for hours. Equipment for establishing an airway and supporting respiration must be available, especially if repeated doses are used. Hypotension is uncommon but may be a problem with multiple doses or when barbiturates are administered concomitantly.

If the seizures have not been controlled within 10 minutes with benzodiazepines, fosphenytoin (or phenytoin, if fosphenytoin is unavailable) should be given. Fosphenytoin is a prodrug of phenytoin, which is rapidly metabolized to the active form. It offers several advantages over phenytoin, including more rapid administration and fewer local and systemic side effects. Fosphenytoin may also be given IM, unlike phenytoin. The dose of the two drugs is identical; fosphenytoin doses are expressed as phenytoin equivalents (PE). The loading dose of fosphenytoin is 15 to 20 mg PE per kg IV, at a rate of 3 mg PE/kg/min to a maximum of 150 mg per minute. In the absence of any clinical effect, an additional 10 mg per kg IV may be administered. Cardiac monitoring is required because rapid IV infusion may lead to hypotension, QT prolongation, and cardiac dysrhythmias. (If phenytoin is used instead, the maximum rate of administration is 2 mg/kg/min in children and 50 mg per minute in an adult.) In patients known to be taking phenytoin chronically, a smaller dose of 5 to 10 mg per kg should be used initially unless the serum level is known to be very low. Each 1 mg per kg of phenytoin administered raises the serum level by approximately 1 μg per mL, although phenytoin kinetics are unpredictable. Phenytoin is highly lipid soluble and reaches therapeutic levels in the brain within 10 to 20 minutes, with duration of action of 12 to 24 hours. Unlike other anticonvulsant medications, phenytoin does not cause sedation or respiratory depression.

Phenobarbital is the next agent often added if phenytoin is not effective or contraindicated (e.g., allergy, known therapeutic level). The loading dose of phenobarbital is 20 mg per kg, sometimes given in two divided doses. The total drug dose is given over 5 to 10 minutes IV (maximum 30 mg per minute in an adult), or IM in the absence of IV access. Onset of action is usually within 15 to 20 minutes and lasts more than 24 hours. Phenobarbital, like other barbiturates, may cause significant sedation, respiratory depression, and hypotension.

IV valproate (VPA) and IV levetiracetam (Keppra) may serve as alternatives to phenobarbital or phenytoin in the treatment of SE. Valproic acid may be particularly useful for patients with a known seizure disorder, who are currently using VPA, when low serum concentrations are suspected. Effective loading dose in one study was 10 mg per kg IV when subtherapeutic levels were suspected and 25 mg per kg IV when the patient was not being treated with VPA. In this study, no adverse effects related to hypotension or heart rate were observed. The loading dose of levetiracetam is 20 to 60 mg per kg.

Patients with SE that lasts for more than 30 to 60 minutes present a special problem. Further management should be done, when possible, in conjunction with a neurologist and with EEG monitoring. Continuous infusion of benzodiazepines, barbiturate coma, or general anesthesia may be used. Previously, paraldehyde and lidocaine hydrochloride have been used to treat SE. However, these medications have not demonstrated any advantage over the conventional therapies already discussed and have more serious side effect profiles.

With prolonged seizures, the duration of postictal drowsiness and confusion may also be protracted. However, the child who fails to arouse within 15 to 30 minutes after cessation of seizures should be evaluated carefully to rule out nonconvulsive SE. Children with SE, even if successfully treated in the ED, should be admitted to the hospital for monitoring and observation. Rarely, a child may enter the ED in absence status. In this case, the child may be sitting in a confused or dreamy state. Such attacks may last for hours or even days. The drug of choice in the treatment of absence status is a benzodiazepine at the dosages outlined above.

At times, a child may present with continual focal seizure activity (with or without clouding of consciousness), a condition known as *epilepsia partialis continua.* The treatment for partial seizures is less urgent than that for generalized seizures, and such seizures are often intractable to anticonvulsant medication. In such cases, fosphenytoin in a dose of 15 to 20 mg per kg can be infused slowly. All such patients should be admitted to the hospital for further observation and evaluation. Other pharmacologic attempts to control these focal seizures should be performed in the hospital.

The decision to initiate long-term prophylactic therapy with anticonvulsant medications is based on a consideration of a number of factors, including the patient's age, type of seizure, risk of recurrence, coexisting medical conditions, and family factors. The consequences of further seizures must be balanced against the potential side effects of the anticonvulsant agents. Treatment is seldom started after a single, uncomplicated nonfebrile seizure because most such patients will not experience a seizure recurrence. It is preferable to make long-term treatment decisions in conjunction with the provider who will be responsible for ongoing follow-up of the patient, either a neurologist or the child's primary care physician. Sometimes, it may be necessary to begin prophylactic treatment in the ED, pending a more complete outpatient evaluation.

Disposition

Hospital admission is generally required for children who have had a prolonged seizure requiring acute treatment with anticonvulsant medication. With the exception of very young infants, other children, even those with a first-time seizure, can generally be followed as outpatients if they appear well after the seizure, follow-up can be ensured, and the parents are comfortable with home management. Seizure first aid should be explained to the family before discharge. Some practitioners may choose to prescribe rectal diazepam as a rescue medication until a decision is made about instituting chronic anticonvulsant therapy.

After a simple febrile seizure, hospitalization is seldom necessary, and children may be followed by their primary physician. Some useful information can be given to parents after a first febrile seizure. First, they should be informed of the benign nature of the convulsions and the lack of evidence that they cause any type of neurologic injury. Approximately one-third of children with a first febrile seizure will have another one. Of recurrences, 75% occur within 1 year, and they are uncommon beyond 2 years; fewer than 10% of children with febrile seizures have more than three. The recurrence rate is lower if the seizures begin after the first year of life, and the risk is also reduced in children with higher temperature and longer duration of fever before the initial febrile seizure. For example, the recurrence risk is about 35% when the first seizure occurs at a temperature of 38.5°C (101.3°F), compared with a risk of 13% with a temperature of 40°C (104°F). Having a complex first febrile seizure (even febrile SE) does not increase the risk of recurrence, nor does it increase the chance that a recurrent seizure, if it occurs, will be complex.

Many parents are concerned that febrile seizures will lead to future epilepsy. A child who has had a febrile seizure but no other risk factors for epilepsy may have a slightly increased risk of future nonfebrile seizures, but the magnitude of this increase is still extremely small: 1% to 2% lifetime risk versus a 0.5% to 1% lifetime risk in the general population. Several risk factors that increase the likelihood of a child experiencing future nonfebrile seizures have been identified. These risk factors include a family history of epilepsy, a complex febrile seizure, and the presence of an underlying neurologic or developmental abnormality. Importantly, even with two or more of these risk factors, the risk of epilepsy is only 10%. Thus, for most children with no risk factors, the parents may be reassured that future epilepsy, although possible, is extremely unlikely. Furthermore, there is no association between febrile seizures and any type of developmental or learning disabilities.

DISORDERS THAT PRESENT WITH HEADACHE (SEE ALSO CHAPTER 54 PAIN: HEADACHE)

Migraine

Goals of Treatment

For children with a known diagnosis of migraine, acute management is aimed at reduction of symptoms (which may include nausea and vomiting as well as pain) to a point where home management is feasible. When a diagnosis of migraine has not been established, the emergency clinician must also evaluate for other potential causes of headache.

CLINICAL PEARLS AND PITFALLS

- "Classic" findings are present in a minority of children with migraine, and clinical characteristics such as duration and laterality tend to differ from those in adult patients.
- There is limited pediatric evidence to support most commonly used acute migraine treatments. Nonsteroidal anti-inflammatory agents and prochlorperazine are the best studied.
- While commonly prescribed, opioids are not recommended as first-line treatment for migraine.

Current Evidence

Migraine—recurrent headaches separated by long, symptom-free intervals—is probably the most common specific cause of episodic headaches in afebrile children. In epidemiologic studies, prevalence estimates for migraine in children range from 3% to 10%. A number of forms of migraine are recognized. Migraine is considered *classic* when the headache is well localized and preceded by an aura and considered *common* when it is not. The common form of migraine predominates in children. Cluster headaches, which are unilateral, occur in runs and are associated with autonomic changes. They represent a rare migraine variant in childhood. Cyclic vomiting, a syndrome of recurrent, discrete attacks of abdominal pain, nausea, vomiting, and pallor, is also believed to be a migraine variant, sometimes called *abdominal migraine*.

Migraine is a result of an underlying hyperexcitable cerebral cortex. In a genetically predisposed individual, a variety of stimuli can trigger episodes of "cortical spreading depression," a slowly propagating wave of neuronal hyperpolarization followed by depolarization. This in turn triggers a neuronally mediated vascular instability that results in intracranial hypoperfusion (which may produce the migraine aura of premonitory motor, visual, or sensory symptoms), followed by vasodilation and a sterile, neurogenic inflammation, which are responsible for the headache.

Clinical Considerations

Clinical Recognition. Prolonged (up to 24 to 48 hours), moderate to severe headache is characteristic of migraine. The headaches may be pulsating and unilateral but this pattern is less common in children than in adults. Migraine is commonly associated with nausea, vomiting, abdominal pain, and photophobia or phonophobia. Auras occur in less than half of children. Occasionally, the attacks awaken the children from sleep.

A family history of migraine is helpful in diagnosis, and a disproportionate number of children who experience migraines have episodes of motion sickness, dizziness, vertigo, or frank paroxysmal events.

Initial Evaluation. The diagnosis of migraine is based almost exclusively on the history and is supported by the absence of abnormalities on examination. There are no diagnostic laboratory tests or imaging studies. The physical examination usually shows no focal neurologic deficits, although hemiplegia and ophthalmoplegia may occur in complicated migraine.

Common trigger factors for migraine in children include emotional stress, lighting changes, and minor head trauma. Particularly in adolescents, it is useful to screen for depression or other psychosocial stressors that may warrant separate treatment. Nitrates (e.g., lunch meats) and tyramine (cheeses) are less common but important food triggers.

Given an accurate history, differentiation from tension headaches, sinusitis, and headaches secondary to intracranial lesions is usually possible; studies such as EEG, CT, and MRI are rarely indicated. In children with focal neurologic deficit and no prior history of such episodes due to migraine, urgent neuroimaging should be considered.

Initial evaluation should include a determination of the level of pain using a validated scale. For patients with known migraine, establishing a target pain level for acute treatment is also helpful.

Management. A number of agents are available for the treatment of acute migraine (Table 105.4). For many children, mild oral analgesics such as acetaminophen or ibuprofen combined with bed rest may provide sufficient relief and should be considered the first-line agents of choice. Ketorolac (Toradol), a nonsteroidal anti-inflammatory agent for parenteral use, may be used when nausea or vomiting limits oral intake. A short course of a narcotic analgesic such as oxycodone may rarely be needed if nonnarcotic agents have failed, especially if the headache prevents sleep.

Dopamine receptor antagonists such as metoclopramide (Reglan), prochlorperazine (Compazine), and promethazine (Phenergan) are commonly used in the ED setting, especially in the presence of nausea and vomiting. These agents have the potential to produce dystonic reactions; it is common to prophylactically coadminister diphenhydramine. Because they have fewer side effects, ondansetron (Zofran) and granisetron (Kytril) have also become first-line agents in the treatment of nausea and vomiting associated with migraine headaches, although these medications have not been studied as primary treatment of migraine headaches.

Sumatriptan succinate (Imitrex) is a serotonergic agent available for oral, intranasal, or subcutaneous administration. Its effectiveness in relieving symptoms of acute migraine has been demonstrated in clinical trials in children and adults, but it has not been approved by the U.S. Food and Drug Administration for use in younger children. The dose for children 12 years and older is 6 mg subcutaneously or 100 mg orally. Sumatriptan is generally well tolerated; side effects include irritation at the injection site, flushing, tachycardia, disorientation, and chest tightness that last for several minutes after parenteral administration. In one trial, adverse effects were more common in younger children. A reasonable approach is to use sumatriptan after a trial of analgesics in an older child, although older children or adolescents with recurrent migraine and a history of successful treatment with sumatriptan in the past may benefit from earlier use of this agent. Other agents in this family include rizatriptan (Maxalt), almotriptan (Axert), and zolmitriptan (Zomig). Triptans should not be administered to children with complicated migraines.

Ergot preparations act primarily as cerebral vasoconstrictors and are specifically indicated for aborting acute migraine attacks. They are not typically used as a first-line treatment because of the common side effects including nausea, vomiting, cramps, and distal paresthesias, all of which may intensify the symptoms of migraine. Dihydroergotamine (DHE) is an injectable ergot derivative. It can be given to older children and adolescents in an initial dose of 0.5 mg IM or IV (no milligram per kilogram dose has been established). The initial dose of DHE may be repeated in 1 hour if necessary. Ergot preparations should not be used concomitantly with triptans. Antiemetics may be useful to control the nausea and vomiting that often occur after DHE administration. Sodium valproate, used for migraine prophylaxis, has also been reported in case series to be effective in treating migraine, but no controlled efficacy data exist.

If migraines are frequent and severe, prophylactic treatment is possible. Many drugs have been used, but because some require close, serial examination and have no effect on the acute attack, generally they should not be started in the ED. Among the medications used for chronic suppressive therapy are propranolol, tricyclic antidepressants, cyproheptadine (Periactin), valproic acid, and calcium channel blockers. More recent studies of antiepileptic medications have shown some efficacy in preventing migraine headaches in adult patients, including gabapentin, topiramate, lamotrigine, and tiagabine.

Clinical Indications for Discharge/Admission. Most patients with migraine can be successfully managed as outpatients. Admission is reserved for those in whom continued parenteral therapy is needed to control symptoms. Patients with chronic or recurrent symptoms requiring prophylactic treatment should be referred to a neurologist.

TABLE 105.4

AGENTS FOR ACUTE TREATMENT OF MIGRAINE

Drug	Usual dose
Analgesics	
Acetaminophen	10–15 mg/kg/dose PO or PR q4h
Ibuprofen	5–10 mg/kg/dose PO q6h
Ketorolac (Toradol)	30 mg initial dose, then 0.5 mg/kg (max 30 mg) IV or IM, or 10 mg/dose PO, q4–6h
Antiemetics	
Metoclopramide (Reglan)	0.5–2 mg/kg/dose PO or IV q4–6h
Prochlorperazine (Compazine)	0.1 mg/kg/dose PO, IM, or IV q6h
Promethazine (Phenergan)	0.25–1.0 mg/kg/dose PO, PR, IV, or IM q4–6h
Specific antimigraine agents	
Dihydroergotamine	0.5–1.0 mg/dose IV or IM; may repeat after 1 hr
Sumatriptan (Imitrex)	6 mg SC or 100 mg PO

PO, orally; PR, per rectum; IV, intravenously; IM, intramuscularly; SC, subcutaneously.

Idiopathic Intracranial Hypertension (Pseudotumor Cerebri)

Goals of Treatment

In addition to pain relief, initial treatment in idiopathic intracranial hypertension (IIH) is directed at preventing neurologic sequelae.

CLINICAL PEARLS AND PITFALLS

- Many children with intracranial hypertension have an identifiable cause.
- While papilledema is very commonly seen, some children may present without papilledema.

Current Evidence

IIH, also called *pseudotumor cerebri syndrome,* is a poorly understood condition of increased ICP. It may occur at any age during childhood but is more common in adolescents, especially in obese individuals. Females are more commonly affected. A number of other conditions have been reported in association with IIH; these include anatomic anomalies (cerebral venous abnormalities), infections (otitis media, mastoiditis, Lyme disease), endocrinologic conditions (hyperthyroidism, Addison disease), medications (steroid withdrawal, oral contraceptives, tetracycline, hypervitaminosis A), and mild head trauma. However, a causal relationship remains unproved, and in most cases of IIH, no cause is identified. The mechanism of increased ICP in IIH remains unknown, although several hypotheses have been postulated, including vasogenic brain edema and impaired reabsorption of cerebrospinal fluid (CSF) by the arachnoid villi.

Clinical Considerations

Clinical Recognition. Headache of variable severity and duration is the most common presenting symptom. It is typically worse in the morning. Nausea, vomiting, dizziness, and double or blurred vision also occur. If the process is long-standing, decreased visual acuity or visual field deficits can result. Infants often have nonspecific symptoms of lethargy or irritability. Papilledema is seen in virtually all cases, although a syndrome of IIH without papilledema exists. Other neurologic symptoms and signs are often absent; however, cranial nerve palsies, particularly affecting the cranial nerve VI, may be seen.

Initial Assessment. Diagnosis should be considered when a child with a prolonged history of headache is found to have evidence of papilledema without other neurologic findings. IIH is a diagnosis of exclusion, and other conditions, particularly mass lesions, must be ruled out. Because posterior fossa tumors and obstructive or nonobstructive hydrocephalus may mimic IIH early in the course of disease, neuroimaging should be obtained in all children with this constellation of findings. MRI is the study of choice, though contrast-enhanced CT may be used if MRI is unavailable or contraindicated. Magnetic resonance venography (MRV) is useful in identifying cerebral venous anomalies in atypical (i.e., younger, male, or nonobese) patients. In cases of IIH, the ventricles will appear normal or small.

If no mass lesion is present, an LP should be performed with a manometer to measure opening pressure. The patient must be in the lateral decubitus position with legs extended to ensure an accurate reading of the opening pressure. Children with idiopathic (e.g., not secondary to Lyme infection or other causes) have elevated opening pressure (greater than 250 mm H_2O) but normal CSF cell count, protein, and glucose. In children with intermittent symptoms, the opening pressure may be normal when the headache is waning, even though papilledema may persist for several weeks.

Management. For patients with visual changes or cranial nerve involvement, neurosurgical as well as ophthalmologic consultation is recommended. For the large majority of patients, removal of sufficient CSF to normalize ICP usually leads to improvement in symptoms. Treatment may then be started with acetazolamide (Diamox) to decrease CSF production (60 mg/kg/day divided four times daily). Although recommended by some, corticosteroids have not been proven to be effective in the management of this condition and should only be administered after consultation with a neurologist.

Clinical Indications for Discharge/Admission. Patients with mild symptoms and good response to LP may be discharged home with close follow-up arranged. Children with severe or persistent symptoms or those with visual changes may require hospital admission. Intracranial hypertension may be recurrent or chronic, and long-term monitoring, particularly of visual function, is important.

STROKE/CEREBROVASCULAR ACCIDENT

Goals of Treatment

The treatment of pediatric stroke remains understudied. In the absence of consensus guidelines for the primary treatment of acute stroke, the goals of treatment should focus on early recognition and prevention of secondary injury. Acute onset of a focal neurologic deficit or seizure activity in the young child should raise the clinician's level of suspicion. Early diagnosis should be made through the use of cross-sectional neuroimaging. Strategies to reduce disease progression and stroke recurrence should include maintenance of euthermia, euglycemia, and normotension, as well as the treatment of hypoxemia and seizure activity, if present.

CLINICAL PEARLS AND PITFALLS

- Presentation of stroke in children is highly variable.
- Hemorrhagic strokes are relatively more common in children than adults.
- MRI with diffusion-weighted imaging is considered the most sensitive modality for detecting early changes associated with stroke.
- Systemic thrombolysis with tPA is not routinely recommended.

Current Evidence

Stroke is defined as a syndrome of acute onset of focal neurologic deficit that persists for more than 24 hours, although some pediatric neurologists include more transient deficits. Stroke is relatively rare in healthy children but may complicate a number of other pediatric medical conditions. For example, among children with sickle cell disease, the incidence of stroke has been reported to be 6% to 9%. Others at risk are those with various forms of cardiac disease, which is one of the most common causes of stroke in children. Table 105.5 lists some of the common causes of stroke, as well as some more uncommon conditions in which stroke is a prominent clinical feature. Generally, stroke is classified as either primarily ischemic (including embolic phenomena) or hemorrhagic.

TABLE 105.5

CAUSES OF STROKE IN CHILDREN

Vascular
Arteriovenous malformation
Aneurysm
Moyamoya disease
Fibromuscular dysplasia
Cardiac
Valvular heart disease (including endocarditis)
Right-to-left shunts
Atrial tumors
Arrhythmia
Cardiomyopathy
Infectious
Meningitis (especially tuberculous)
Mycotic aneurysm
Mastoiditis, otitis media, or sinusitis leading to venous sinus thrombosis
Trauma
Intracranial hemorrhage
Cervical trauma with vertebral artery injury
Intraoral trauma with carotid injury
Brain tumor
Drugs
Cocaine
Amphetamine
Oral contraceptives
Ergot poisoning
Metabolic
Homocystinuria
Fabry disease
Mitochondrial encephalopathies (MELAS syndrome)
Organic acidemias
Hyperlipidemias
Hematologic/Autoimmune
Sickle cell disease
Coagulopathies (e.g., hemophilia)
Anticoagulant deficiency (protein C, protein S, antithrombin III)
Polycythemia
Acute myelogenous leukemia
Systemic lupus erythematosus
Neurocutaneous syndromes
Neurofibromatosis
Tuberous sclerosis
Sturge–Weber syndrome

In ischemic stroke, there is focal reduction in cerebral blood flow, with hypoxic damage to brain parenchyma, leading to neuronal injury and death. Further damage ensues from reperfusion injury of ischemic areas.

Unlike adult stroke, there is currently no consensus on primary treatment for acute stroke in childhood. This is due in large part to the lack of pediatric randomized control trials. The efficacy of systemic thrombolytic therapy is yet to be determined and safety remains a concern as a significant number of children who have undergone treatment are reported to have suffered major complications. More recently, attention has focused on secondary prevention and factors that play an important part in determining the extent of damage after acute ischemia; these include excess accumulation of excitatory amino acids and generation of free radicals. Prevention of secondary injury is essential as up to 20% of children have clinical and/or radiologic recurrence.

Clinical Considerations

Clinical Recognition

The presentation of stroke in children is highly variable, and is influenced by the portion of the cerebral vasculature affected as well as the child's age. Hemiparesis is most often observed, with facial weakness also common. In neonates and young children, however, seizure may be the only presenting symptom. Involvement of the anterior cerebral artery leads primarily to lower-extremity weakness, whereas compromise of the middle cerebral artery circulation produces hemiplegia with upper limb predominance, hemianopsia, and possibly dysphasia. Less commonly, the posterior circulation is affected, which results in vertigo, ataxia, and nystagmus, as well as hemiparesis and hemianopsia. Older children often have concomitant headache. The child with a stroke may also have a diminished level of consciousness.

Triage Considerations

Any child with an acute neurologic deficit requires prompt evaluation. Suspicion for stroke should be increased in children with predisposing medical conditions such as sickle cell disease and congenital cardiac disease.

Clinical Assessment

Because stroke can have a highly variable and at times subtle presentation, a thorough neurologic examination is necessary in any patient presenting with a neurologic deficit, seizure, or alteration of consciousness. Any new neurologic symptom or complaint in patients with underlying sickle cell disease merits close evaluation. Particular attention should be paid to identifying risk factors as the majority of children have at least one identifiable risk factor at the time of infarction. In addition, physicians need to consider other etiologies that may mimic stroke, complicated migraine, structural brain lesion, central nervous system (CNS) infection, Todd paresis, psychogenic causes, etc. (see Chapters 12 Coma and 78 Weakness).

Diagnostic Testing

Investigations in a child for whom there is a concern for stroke should be directed at confirming the diagnosis of stroke and attempting to identify an underlying cause. Cross-sectional neuroimaging is recommended for all children with suspected stroke. MRI with diffusion-weighted imaging is considered the most sensitive imaging modality and can identify ischemic changes within hours of onset. Cranial CT without contrast is the study of choice for identifying acute hemorrhage; however, CT scan may be normal in the first 12 to 24 hours after an ischemic stroke. Vascular imaging of the cervical vessels as well as proximal intracranial vessels should be included. This can be done with magnetic resonance angiography in most patients. MRV imaging should be strongly considered as a significant proportion of hemorrhages are secondary to cerebral venous sinus thrombosis.

TABLE 105.6

STUDIES TO CONSIDER IN THE EVALUATION OF THE CHILD WITH ACUTE STROKE

Brain imaging
Computed tomography (noncontrast)
Magnetic resonance imaging
Angiography (standard or magnetic resonance)
Cardiac
Electrocardiogram
Echocardiogram
Hematologic
Complete blood cell count
Prothrombin and partial thromboplastin times
Fibrinogen
Erythrocyte sedimentation rate
Hemoglobin electrophoresis
Protein C and S quantification
Antithrombin III level
Chemistry
Blood urea nitrogen
Cholesterol and triglycerides
Hepatic transaminases
Serum amino acids
Urine organic acids
Toxicology screen
Lactate
Lumbar puncture

In a child without a known predisposing condition, ancillary tests may be helpful in revealing the cause of the stroke. Studies worth considering in such patients, depending on the clinical picture, are listed in Table 105.6. In one series of 129 children with ischemic stroke, no cause was found in 35%.

Management

Initial treatment after an acute stroke should focus on stabilization and prevention of secondary neuronal injury. This includes maintenance of normotension, normothermia, euglycemia, and treatment of hypoxemia and seizures. Although evident hypotension should be treated with volume expansion, administration of free water should be restricted because of the potential for cerebral edema. Hypertension, if present, must be treated cautiously, and the blood pressure lowered gradually in order to maintain adequate cerebral perfusion. Both hypoglycemia and hyperglycemia can exacerbate ischemic stroke. Careful monitoring of serum glucose levels and judicious use of insulin are important. Fever, which can occur in children with stroke, may also contribute to ischemic damage and should be controlled with antipyretics.

Initiation of anticoagulation therapy should be strongly considered, once hemorrhagic stroke is excluded, in consultation with a pediatric hematologist. Current pediatric guidelines recommend the use of aspirin, low–molecular-weight heparin, or unfractionated heparin. The choice of acute anticoagulation treatment as well as long-term preventative therapy is influenced by stroke etiology as well as the presence of a cardioembolic cause or arterial dissection. Finally, the use of thrombolysis and mechanical thrombectomy are not routinely recommended and should only be considered with neurology consultation. If thrombolysis is considered, the timing of administration must follow adult stroke guidelines.

Further therapy is determined by the type of stroke. With hemorrhagic stroke, neurosurgical intervention may be required to evacuate a hematoma or control a bleeding arteriovenous malformation (AVM). Catheter-directed embolization may also be possible in cases of AVM. Children with sickle cell disease and stroke should have acute transfusion to decrease the level of hemoglobin S to less than 30%. Novel therapies such as calcium channel blockers and free radical scavengers have not been studied in pediatric patients and their use remains experimental.

Overall, prognosis for children with stroke is better than that in adults. However, regardless of treatment, long-term morbidity of stroke in children is high, with more than 75% of affected children experiencing sequelae such as hemiparesis, seizures, and learning difficulties.

DISORDERS THAT PRESENT WITH ENCEPHALOPATHY (SEE ALSO CHAPTER 12 COMA)

Goals of Treatment

Encephalopathy is an imprecise term that implies diffuse brain dysfunction with or without alterations in the level of consciousness. Encephalopathy may be a sign of numerous systemic disorders, or it may result from primary disorders of the CNS, the most common of which is encephalitis. The emergency physician must decide whether the child's degree of irritability, uncooperativeness, and lethargy is proportionate to the degree of systemic illness; whether it is caused by fear; or whether it represents cortical dysfunction. Encephalopathy can be associated with cardiorespiratory compromise and has a large differential, requiring prompt identification and a systematic approach to evaluation.

CLINICAL PEARLS AND PITFALLS

- A detailed clinical history is imperative to identifying a likely etiology.
- Herpes simplex virus (HSV) polymerase chain reaction testing of CSF samples is recommended for all children with suspected encephalitis.
- Empiric therapy with IV acyclovir is recommended for all patients with suspected encephalitis while confirmatory tests are pending.
- Diffusion-weighted MRI is the imaging modality of choice for the evaluation of encephalitis.

Encephalitis

Encephalitis is an inflammation of the brain parenchyma. *Meningoencephalitis* refers to additional leptomeningeal involvement, whereas *encephalomyelitis* implies involvement of the spinal cord. CNS dysfunction is caused by direct invasion of brain by a pathogen, most often a virus; is secondary to immunologic mechanisms, as in postinfectious encephalomyelitis; or is mediated by a toxic-metabolite, such as drugs and toxins.

TABLE 105.7

AGENTS OF VIRAL ENCEPHALITIS

Arboviruses
Eastern equine encephalitis
Western equine encephalitis
St. Louis encephalitis
Japanese encephalitis
California (LaCrosse) encephalitis
West Nile
Herpesviruses
Herpes simplex
Varicella-zoster
Epstein–Barr
Cytomegalovirus
Mumps
Measles
Enteroviruses
Rabies

Viral encephalitides are caused by a wide variety of viruses that lead to clinically similar illnesses (Table 105.7). Currently, an etiology is not identified in most cases, even with an extensive laboratory evaluation. Mumps was the most common cause of meningoencephalitis before the introduction of vaccination, with up to 50% of patients with mumps parotitis having CSF pleocytosis. Classically, the illness occurs several days to 2 weeks after the onset of parotitis but may precede the onset of systemic illness or occur without parotitis and tends to be mild. Measles encephalitis is less common since the advent of widespread live immunization. The onset usually occurs during the prodromal period or after the rash has appeared. Ataxia is the most common neurologic abnormality, and sequelae occur in up to 30% of cases. Varicella encephalitis occurs 2 to 9 days after the onset of the rash; severe infections are uncommon, except in the immunosuppressed host.

HSV is a relatively common cause of sporadic encephalitis. Disease in neonates is usually caused by HSV type 2, acquired from perinatal transmission. In previously healthy older children and adults, encephalitis more often results from infection with HSV type 1 and may be a complication of acute primary infection or reactivated latent infection. Recognition of herpes encephalitis is often difficult early in the course but is important because specific antiviral therapy reduces the substantial morbidity and mortality of this disease.

The arthropod-borne encephalitides—including St. Louis, Western equine, Eastern equine, and California encephalitis—occur in sporadic and epidemic forms, often in late summer or early fall, and tend to cluster in localized geographic areas. Sequelae may be severe and mortality high, especially in Eastern equine encephalitis. West Nile virus is another agent in this family that first appeared in the United States in 1999. Since then, it appears to have become endemic in large parts of North America, although clinically overt infections in children are uncommon.

Infection with rabies virus, although rare in the United States, is an important cause of encephalitis worldwide. Nonviral pathogens, including *Mycoplasma pneumoniae,* Lyme disease, and rickettsiae, may also cause encephalitis.

Viral encephalitis usually follows a viremia, although direct spread can occur less commonly via peripheral nerves or the nasal mucosa. Upon reaching the CNS, viral replication in neural cells interferes with cellular function and may lead to cell death. Cerebral edema may result from capillary leakage, with subsequent increased ICP. The degree and extent of neuronal dysfunction depends in part on the pathogen involved and also on host factors, especially immunocompetence. In general, the incidence of overt neurologic findings and sequelae is higher in children younger than 1 year.

The clinical picture of viral encephalitis ranges from a mild febrile illness associated with headache and minimal changes in mentation to a severe, fulminant presentation with coma, seizures, and death. The onset of encephalitis may be abrupt or insidious. Typical features consist of fever, headache, vomiting, and signs of meningeal irritation. Altered consciousness, ataxia, and seizures are also seen (see Chapters 10 Ataxia and 12 Coma). Focal neurologic deficits may occur in certain types of encephalitis, particularly HSV. Flaccid paralysis may be seen in cases of encephalomyelitis, and rarely, respiratory or autonomic dysfunction results from brainstem involvement. Rash or mucous membrane lesions are often seen with the exanthematous viruses such as measles and varicella; however, cutaneous findings are uncommon with HSV encephalitis.

The diagnostic evaluation of viral encephalitis should be tailored based on clinical and epidemiologic clues and requires a thorough clinical history. Determining if a patient is immunocompromised, if they have had a recent illness, as well as assessing their travel history and immunization status can help determine a likely etiology. Unless contraindicated, CSF collection for virus isolation is recommended in all patients with suspected encephalitis. Additionally, HSV PCR should be performed on all CSF samples as early identification and treatment may decrease morbidity and mortality. Viral isolation from other body sites, including the nasopharynx, skin lesions, urine, and feces, should be completed as clinically indicated. Neuroimaging is recommended in the evaluation of encephalitis in order to exclude noninfectious alternative diagnoses, and diffusion-weighted MRI is the study of choice. Additionally, certain encephalitides have characteristic patterns on MRI that may offer a diagnostic clue. Similarly, electroencephalography (EEG) is recommended as it is helpful in ruling out nonconvulsive status epilepticus and may demonstrate specific patterns of cerebral dysfunction as may be seen in HSV-associated encephalitis.

Presently, the treatment of nonherpes viral encephalitis is primarily supportive. Children with aseptic meningitis and mild manifestations may be followed at home, but those with encephalitis should be hospitalized for observation and monitoring of neurologic status, treatment of increased ICP if present, fluid restriction, and monitoring of urine output and serum sodium because of the risk for inappropriate antidiuretic hormone secretion. Recently published guidelines including those from the Infectious Disease Society of America (2008) recommend the empiric use of acyclovir for any patient with suspected encephalitis.

Herpes simplex poses a special problem because early diagnosis is important in instituting effective therapy. Polymerase chain reaction testing of CSF can yield rapid evidence of viral nucleic acid and is relatively sensitive and specific. Imaging studies, although less sensitive, may also be useful. Either CT or MRI may demonstrate focal parenchymal involvement or edema of the temporal lobes (Fig. 105.1). MRI is more sensitive than CT, although both may show normal results in the early stages of disease. Similarly, EEG may demonstrate focal slowing or epileptiform discharges localized to the temporal lobes, but absence of such findings does not rule out herpes encephalitis. Herpes simplex encephalitis causes death or neurologic sequelae

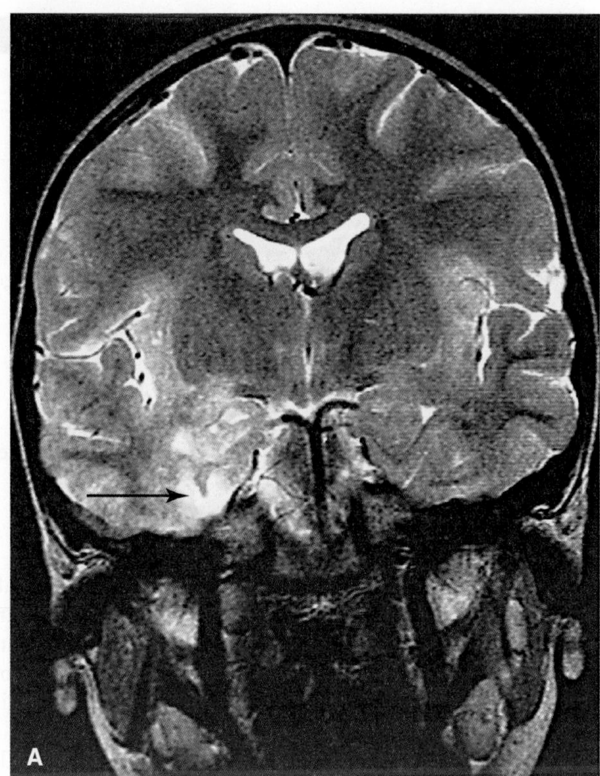

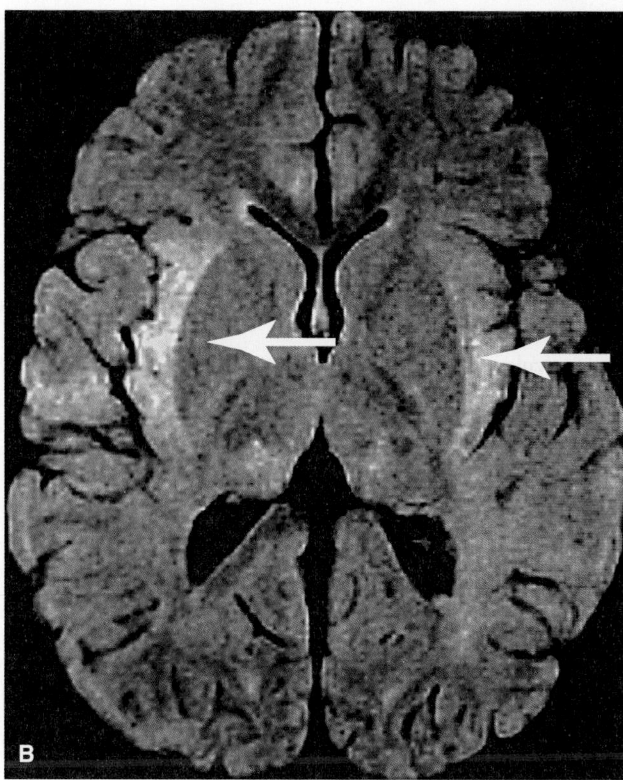

FIGURE 105.1 Coronal (**A**) and axial (**B**) T2-weighted magnetic resonance images showing multifocal areas of abnormal signal in the medial aspects of both temporal lobes (*large arrow*) and left posterior parietal lobe (*small arrows*) in a patient with herpes simplex encephalitis.

in more than 70% of patients. Treatment with acyclovir (60 mg/kg/day divided q8h daily for 14 to 21 days) has resulted in a decrease in mortality and some improvement in morbidity. Treatment should be started empirically for any patient with suspected encephalitis.

Postinfectious encephalitis may follow infection with numerous viruses, including measles, varicella, influenza, and Epstein–Barr virus. Postinfectious encephalitis is presumed to be an immune-mediated phenomenon, involving the white matter of the CNS. Demyelination, the pathologic hallmark of the disease, may be focal or widespread. The CNS involvement may be confined to a specific area, as in acute cerebellar ataxia after varicella infection, or may be widespread. The latter condition is often designated *acute disseminated encephalomyelitis (ADEM)*. A particularly virulent form with high mortality is known as *acute hemorrhagic leukoencephalitis*. A clinical syndrome of encephalopathy after immunization, particularly with whole-cell pertussis vaccine, is also described, although more recent epidemiologic evidence has called into question the association with pertussis immunization. ADEM should be suspected in the patient presenting with neurologic symptoms consistent with encephalopathy in the setting of a recent viral infection. MR imaging is the diagnostic modality of choice when postinfectious encephalitis is suspected.

Several autoimmune-mediated encephalitides have been increasingly identified in children. These include anti-N-methyl-D-aspartate receptor (anti-NMDAR) and voltage-gated potassium channel antibody-related encephalitis. Children with anti-NMDAR encephalitis often present with a constellation of symptoms consisting of psychiatric symptoms, abnormal movements, seizure, autonomic instability, and hypoventilation. If anti-NMDAR encephalitis is suspected, further evaluation is required as it can be associated with tumors, most commonly ovarian teratomas. Antibodies to voltage-gated potassium channels have been identified in children presenting with encephalopathy and status epilepticus.

DISORDERS OF MOTOR FUNCTION (SEE ALSO CHAPTER 78 WEAKNESS)

Goals of Treatment

Weakness or motor deficits are often a sign of a significant underlying illness (see Chapter 78 Weakness). The primary goals of treatment should be early recognition of life-threatening conditions such as spinal shock and ascending paralysis. Treatment should then focus on assessment of the pattern of motor deficit and anatomic localization in order to identify the underlying etiology.

Every level of the neural axis is involved in the performance of motor tasks. Paresis refers to partial or complete weakness of a part of the body. Various clinical designations are used to describe patterns of weakness: paraplegia (or paraparesis), affecting the lower half of the body; quadriplegia, affecting all limbs; and hemiplegia, referring to weakness of one side of the body. Paraplegia most often results from spinal cord involvement, whereas hemiparesis is most often a sign of cortical disease.

CLINICAL PEARLS AND PITFALLS

- Anatomic localization is usually possible after evaluation of the distribution and character of the deficit (Table 105.8).
- MRI of the spine is the imaging modality of choice to detect compressive mass lesions.

TABLE 105.8

LOCALIZING LEVEL OF NEUROMOTOR DYSFUNCTION

	Tone	Distribution	Reflexes	Babinski	Other
Upper motor neuron	Increased (may be decreased acutely)	Pattern (e.g., hemiparesis, paraparesis) Distal > proximal	Increased (may be decreased acutely)	Extensor	Cognitive dysfunction possible
Anterior horn cell	Decreased	Variable, asymmetric	Decreased to absent	Flexor	Fasciculations; no sensory involvement
Peripheral nerve	Decreased	Nerve distribution	Decreased to absent	Flexor	Sensory involvement
Neuromuscular junction	Normal	Fluctuating	Usually normal	Flexor	
Muscle	Decreased	Proximal > distal	Decreased	Flexor	Tenderness, signs of inflammation possible

Spinal Cord Dysfunction

Dysfunction of the spinal cord may result from any of a variety of disorders, either intrinsic or extrinsic to the spinal cord, with a great deal of overlap in their clinical presentation. Spinal cord dysfunction from any cause is characterized by paraplegia and hyporeflexia below the level of involvement; sensory symptoms, such as band-like pain at the level of compression; and sensory loss or paresthesias below the area of damage. If the lower spinal cord is involved (the conus), there is usually early loss of bowel and bladder control. Compression of the cauda equina usually results in asymmetric symptoms, radicular pain, and focal lower-extremity motor and sensory abnormalities.

Transverse myelitis is an intramedullary disorder, involving both halves of the cord over a variable length, with involvement of motor and sensory tracts. It occurs in children and adults, although it is rare in the first year of life. Transverse myelitis is believed to be caused by an autoimmune process, with demyelinating lesions found in the spinothalamic and pyramidal tracts as well as posterior columns of the spinal cord. During the course of the illness, the area of spinal cord inflammation may extend rostrally and caudally to involve an extensive portion of the spinal cord. Transverse myelitis may occur after a number of infections, among those commonly reported are Epstein–Barr virus, cytomegalovirus, measles, mumps, *Campylobacter jejuni,* and *M. pneumoniae.* Transverse myelitis may also result from systemic autoimmune disorders such as lupus erythematosus or scleroderma. In some older children and adolescents, transverse myelitis is a first manifestation of multiple sclerosis.

Transverse myelitis may affect any level of the spinal cord, but thoracic involvement is the most common. Initial symptoms include lower-extremity paresthesia, local back pain, unilateral or bilateral lower-extremity weakness, and urinary retention. A preceding respiratory or gastrointestinal illness is usually reported, and at the time of diagnosis, fever and meningismus are sometimes seen in children. Characteristically, the insidious onset of paresthesia or weakness of the lower extremities progresses over days or, rarely, weeks and then is replaced by the abrupt occurrence of static paraplegia or quadriplegia and, in the cooperative child, a detectable sensory level. In other children, the course of progression may be less than 12 hours. The sensory loss generally involves all modalities, although a spinothalamic deficit (pain) may occur without posterior column dysfunction (vibration). The weakness is usually symmetric but may be asymmetric. After a variable interval, initial flaccidity may be replaced by spasticity. Sphincter disturbance of the bowel and bladder occurs in most patients, bladder distention being the most common initial sign of damage.

Evaluation should consist of contrast-enhanced MRI of the entire spine. Imaging of the brain is also suggested to evaluate for lesions suggestive of multiple sclerosis. CSF evaluation should be obtained, including cell count and testing for oligoclonal bands. Serum testing for neuromyelitis optica IgG antibodies is now recommended. Presence of these antibodies can aid in determining the etiology as well as risk of recurrence.

Treatment of transverse myelitis is supportive, and some degree of recovery occurs in approximately 80% of cases. All children with this syndrome should be hospitalized. Although there are no controlled trials of their efficacy, there is a consensus supporting the use of systemic corticosteroids. Currently, there is moderate evidence to support the use of plasma exchange in patients who have failed corticosteroid therapy; however, there is insufficient evidence to support the use of IV immunoglobulin.

Acute spinal cord compression in children is usually caused by trauma, infection, or cancer. Spinal trauma may lead to contusion or concussion of the cord with hemorrhage, edema, and local mass effect, or may lead to development of a spinal epidural hematoma. Mass lesions may cause damage by direct compression of spinal cord tissues or, secondarily, by interference with the tenuous arterial (or, less commonly, venous) blood flow to the spinal cord, with resultant spinal cord infarction.

Parenchymal injury usually presents acutely, but an epidural hematoma may develop over several days after the antecedent trauma. Epidural abscess is the most common infectious cause of spinal cord compression. It is usually caused by hematogenous spread of bacteria, with *Staphylococcus aureus* being the most common pathogen. Neoplastic causes include both primary intraspinal tumors (ependymoma and astrocytoma) and extrinsic lesions such as neuroblastoma or lymphoma.

Traumatic and infectious spinal lesions are usually accompanied by relatively acute onset of local back pain, which is exacerbated by direct percussion of the area. Pain from an infectious cause occasionally may precede other symptoms for days. With tumors, however, there may be weakness in the absence of pain. Patients with epidural abscess often have systemic signs of infections such as fever, headache, vomiting, and, perhaps, neck stiffness. Bony tenderness in such a patient may indicate vertebral osteomyelitis or discitis, which can also present with weakness, although usually less severe than is seen with actual spinal cord involvement.

Diagnosis is confirmed by emergency neuroimaging, with precautions to immobilize patients with potentially unstable lesions. Plain spine films are useful initially in trauma. MRI of the spine is the procedure of choice to detect compressive mass lesions, but if not immediately available, plain or CT myelography is an alternative. LP should not be performed without first imaging the spine if a diagnosis of spinal cord compression is possible.

Treatment of children with spinal injury from trauma begins with splinting and immobilization of the spine. The role of high-dose methylprednisolone is controversial and there is a lack of controlled trials in the pediatric population. Based on a review of the literature, the American Academy of Neurological Surgeons and the Congress of Neurosurgical Surgeons no longer recommend the use of steroid therapy. Neurosurgical consultation should be obtained as soon as possible to evaluate for possible surgical decompression (see Chapter 130 Neurosurgical Emergencies).

In cases of possible epidural abscess or tumor-related masses, IV dexamethasone therapy may be beneficial, and should be considered in consultation with Neurosurgery and Oncology. IV antibiotic therapy against *S. aureus* should be started immediately. In patients with a presumed infectious cause and those with cancer of unknown origin, emergent surgical decompression is indicated to alleviate pressure and to aid in diagnosis. Further treatment depends on the specific organism or exact tumor type.

Acute Polyneuritis (Guillain–Barré Syndrome)

Acute polyneuritis, also called *Guillain–Barré syndrome,* is characterized by symmetric ascending paralysis. Pathologically, the hallmark of this disease is primary demyelination of motor and sensory nerves, believed to be caused by autoimmune mechanisms. It occurs in children in all age groups but is uncommon before 3 years of age. An antecedent respiratory or gastrointestinal infection or immunization precedes the onset of illness by 1 to 2 weeks in more than 75% of childhood cases.

Weakness, commonly with an insidious onset, is the usual presenting complaint. Paresthesias or other sensory abnormalities such as pain or numbness are prominent in up to 50% of cases, particularly in older children. The paresthesias and paralysis are usually symmetric and ascending, although variations may occur. Early in the course of illness, distal weakness is more prominent than proximal weakness. Deep tendon reflexes are depressed or absent at the time of diagnosis. Affected children often have an ataxic gait.

Cranial nerve abnormalities occur during the illness in 30% to 40% of cases and may be the predominant finding, especially in the Miller Fisher variant of this syndrome, which is characterized by oculomotor palsies, ataxia, and areflexia, without motor weakness of the extremities. The most common cranial nerve deficit is a seventh (facial) nerve palsy, followed in decreasing frequency by impairment of cranial nerves IX, X, and XI and oculomotor abnormalities. Autonomic dysfunction occurs commonly and results in blood pressure lability, postural hypotension, and cardiac abnormalities; autonomic dysfunction is a disproportionate cause of morbidity and mortality. Urinary retention, if it occurs, is usually seen late in the illness. As the paralysis ascends, muscles of breathing may become involved, leading to respiratory embarrassment.

The primary aid in diagnosis is LP, which demonstrates an elevated protein level and fewer than 10 white blood cells per cubic millimeter—the so-called albuminocytologic dissociation. CSF glucose is normal. The protein elevation occurs in almost all cases but may be delayed for weeks, usually peaking in the second or third week of illness. Emergency electromyography (EMG) and nerve conduction velocity testing are not indicated. EMG may detect the presence of nerve conduction velocity delay; however, it is usually not demonstrable until the second or third week of illness. Contrast-enhanced MRI imaging has been shown to be a sensitive and useful diagnostic adjunct, and imaging will typically demonstrate enhancement of the spinal nerve roots.

Because of the potential for progression to life-threatening respiratory compromise, the child with Guillain–Barré syndrome should be hospitalized and observed closely. Impending respiratory distress must be anticipated, and routine respiratory monitoring should be aided by specific measures of respiratory function, particularly measurement of negative inspiratory force. Because autonomic dysfunction is common, blood pressure must be monitored closely and abnormalities treated vigorously.

Acute polyneuritis is generally self-limiting, with more than 90% of children in most series having complete or near-complete recovery. In mild cases, in which children retain the ability to ambulate, only supportive care is required. However, immunomodulatory therapy may be of benefit in more severely affected children. Plasmapheresis and IV immunoglobulin both have been used. Although well-controlled, blinded studies of these treatments in children are lacking, the available data suggest that both are effective in reducing the duration and severity of illness in those most severely affected. Corticosteroids have not been shown to be beneficial in acute Guillain–Barré syndrome, and some evidence suggests they may actually delay recovery.

Myasthenia Gravis

In myasthenia gravis, antibodies directed against the acetylcholine receptor protein of the postsynaptic neuromuscular junction cause intermittent failure of neuromuscular transmission. Myasthenia manifests as fluctuating weakness of cranial and skeletal musculature, exacerbated by exertion. The onset of symptoms may be insidious or acute. Most cases affect the cranial nerves, and any cranial nerve can be involved in combination or isolation. Bilateral ptosis is the most common cranial nerve deficit, followed in incidence by oculomotor impairment. Generalized truncal and limb weakness is present at onset in up to half of cases and eventually develops in most children with myasthenia. The diagnosis should be suspected if there is a history of worsening weakness during continual activity or if fatigability of muscle strength is demonstrable.

More commonly a disease seen in adults, myasthenia gravis occurs in children in three major forms: transient neonatal, infantile (congenital), and juvenile (most common). The juvenile form of myasthenia clinically mimics the adult disease. The mean age of onset is 8 years, with a female predominance of approximately 4:1. Illnesses confused with myasthenia include the muscular dystrophies, congenital myopathies, inflammatory myopathies, acute and chronic polyneuropathies, and in the infant, botulism.

EMG can be used to provide electrophysiologic evidence for myasthenia gravis, and the Tensilon (edrophonium) test may be used, in consultation with a neurologist, to confirm the diagnosis.

Although myasthenia gravis is potentially life-threatening, specific management can usually be delayed until after diagnosis is made. Ventilatory support may be required if there is respiratory compromise. If severe weakness is present, the child should be hospitalized. Treatment is begun with the use of cholinesterase inhibitors to prolong the availability of acetylcholine at the neuromuscular junction. At present, the anticholinesterase of choice is pyridostigmine (Mestinon).

Myasthenia has a fluctuating, unpredictable course that can be exacerbated by intercurrent illness and by certain drugs, particularly the aminoglycoside antibiotics. In a known myasthenic, rapid worsening and respiratory compromise (myasthenic crises) may be difficult to differentiate from deterioration secondary to overdose of anticholinesterases (cholinergic crises) because the muscarinic side effects of the anticholinesterases, such as nausea, vomiting, cramps, and muscle fasciculations, may be absent.

Differentiation can be made by giving 1 to 2 mg of IV edrophonium after ensuring respiratory sufficiency. This should result in rapid improvement in the patient with a myasthenic crisis. This procedure may be falsely positive, however, and if the diagnosis is unclear, the patient should be withdrawn from all anticholinesterases and, if necessary, maintained on mechanical ventilation for 48 to 72 hours.

Myasthenic crises respond variably to additional anticholinesterases, and plasmapheresis or steroid therapy may be particularly useful in this situation. Cholinergic crises require the immediate withdrawal of all anticholinesterases. Both myasthenic and cholinergic crises mandate admission to the hospital.

Botulism (See Also Chapter 136 Biological and Chemical Terrorism)

Infantile botulism is a cause of acute weakness in previously well infants younger than 6 months. The illness is caused by intestinal colonization by *Clostridium botulinum,* which produces a neurotoxin that impairs acetylcholine release from the nerve terminal. Spores of *C. botulinum* are of ubiquitous origin, found in soil and agricultural products. Honey has been found to be a particularly significant reservoir. Although infant botulism occurs throughout the United States, the incidence is highest in certain areas; approximately half the cases reported have been from California, Utah, and Pennsylvania. The various host factors that predispose certain infants to intestinal colonization are poorly understood.

The initial symptom of infantile botulism is usually constipation, followed insidiously by lethargy and feeding difficulties. Physical findings at the time of presentation are hypoactive deep tendon reflexes, decreased suck and gag, poorly reactive pupils, bilateral ptosis, oculomotor palsies, and facial weakness. Differential diagnosis is broad, and infants are often misdiagnosed initially. The diagnosis is confirmed by identification of *C. botulinum* toxin (usually type A or B) in the feces or isolation of the organism in stool culture, which is less sensitive. EMG may supply more immediate information.

Affected infants require hospitalization to observe for respiratory compromise. In one large series of 57 patients, 77% required endotracheal intubation because of loss of protective airway reflexes, and 68% received mechanical ventilation for some period. Nasogastric or nasojejunal feedings are usually needed as well.

Human botulism immunoglobulin, with activity against type A and B toxins, is approved for use in infant botulism (often referred to as BabyBIG). Trials have shown a decrease in duration of illness in treated infants. Equine botulinum antitoxin has a high rate of anaphylactic reaction in infants and is not recommended. The use of cathartics or other laxatives to reduce the amount of *C. botulinum* present in the intestine has not proven beneficial. Antibiotics such as penicillin, although widely used, have not been shown to eradicate the organism from the bowel or result in clinical improvement. Aminoglycosides, which can cause neuromuscular blockade, should be avoided.

Periodic Paralysis

Familial periodic paralysis is a rare illness, inherited in an autosomal-dominant fashion, which results in episodes of severe weakness associated with an abnormality of circulating potassium during attacks. Two major forms of illness—hyperkalemic and hypokalemic—are recognized. A third type, normokalemic, has been described but most likely represents a rare variant of the hyperkalemic variety. Other disorders that can produce weakness and electrolyte abnormalities, such as use of corticosteroids or diuretics, thyrotoxicosis, hyperaldosteronism, and renal insufficiency, may mimic the periodic paralyses. The serum potassium abnormalities in familial periodic paralysis are believed to be epiphenomena of yet undelineated muscle membrane abnormalities.

Characteristically, a previously well patient develops a flaccid weakness in his or her trunk and upper thighs, and the weakness gradually involves the remainder of the skeletal muscles. Deep tendon reflexes are diminished. The attacks last from hours to days, and between the attacks, muscular strength is usually normal, although a minority of patients have residual muscular weakness. In both forms of periodic paralysis, EKG changes consistent with the serum potassium abnormality may be noted and cardiac arrhythmias may rarely arise.

Hypokalemic periodic paralysis, the most common type, occurs primarily in adolescents and young adults. Trigger factors include vigorous exercise, heavy carbohydrate meals, alcohol, and the cold. During an attack, potassium levels are usually 2 to 2.5 mEq per L. Emergency treatment of hypokalemic periodic paralysis includes oral, or rarely IV, potassium. Prophylactically, patients should avoid precipitants such as vigorous exercise or large carbohydrate loads. Recurrences may be prevented with spironolactone or acetazolamide.

The hyperkalemic form usually begins in the first decade of life, and attacks occur predominantly during the period of rest after vigorous exercise or after fasting. Attacks are typically associated with myotonia. The episodes are more common than in hypokalemic paralysis but often last less than a few hours. During the attack, plasma potassium level can be moderately elevated, although it is often in the upper normal range. Attacks of hyperkalemic periodic paralysis are often brief enough that acute treatment is unnecessary. In severe attacks, inhaled albuterol and IV calcium gluconate may be helpful. Acetazolamide, thiazide diuretics, and albuterol have been used for prevention of recurrences.

DISORDERS OF BALANCE (SEE CHAPTERS 10 ATAXIA AND 19 DIZZINESS AND VERTIGO)

Goals of Treatment

Disordered balance has a broad differential diagnosis and is often associated with symptoms such as nausea, dizziness, vertigo, and ataxia (see Chapters 10 Ataxia and 19 Dizziness and Vertigo). Ataxia is an inability to produce smooth, coordinated movements and is typically a sign of cerebellar dysfunction. Alterations of balance and ataxia can result from dysfunction of the nervous system at many levels: cerebellum, sensory pathways, posterior columns of the spinal cord. Ataxia can be a manifestation of motor weakness as seen in Guillain–Barré. Therefore, early goals of treatment should focus on identifying the level of nervous system involvement and ruling out life-threatening causes, intracranial mass lesion, stroke, CNS hemorrhage, CNS infection.

CLINICAL PEARLS AND PITFALLS

- Acute ataxia is uncommon but most cases are secondary to a benign etiology.
- Cerebellar dysfunction is the most common cause of ataxia.
- Signs of cerebellar dysfunction include the following: Gait disturbance, truncal ataxia, nystagmus, dysmetria, tremor.
- MRI is the imaging modality of choice for acute ataxia.

Acute Cerebellar Ataxia

Acute cerebellar ataxia, characterized by the acute onset of unsteadiness in a previously well child, is the most common cause of ataxia in young children. It is seen primarily between the ages of 1 and 4 years but can occur at any time during childhood. The exact cause of the illness is unclear; however, it is believed to be a parainfectious or postinfectious demyelinating phenomenon and likely represents a localized form of postinfectious encephalitis. Acute cerebellar ataxia occurs most commonly after primary varicella. Other infections implicated include infectious mononucleosis, enteroviruses, HSV, influenza, *Mycoplasma,* and Q fever. Ataxia is usually seen 5 to 10 days after the onset of illness, although symptoms may be delayed for up to 3 weeks, and there are some reports of cerebellar ataxia preceding the rash of chickenpox.

The child develops acute truncal unsteadiness with a variable degree of distal motor difficulty, such as tremor and dysmetria. Dysarthria and nystagmus are variably present. Some children have nausea and vomiting, presumably caused by vertigo. Headache is rare.

When acute ataxia follows varicella in a child with no other neurologic findings, the diagnosis may be made on clinical grounds. In atypical cases, CT or MRI may be necessary to rule out a cerebellar mass. LP is not usually necessary in typical cases; if performed, it reveals a mild CSF pleocytosis in approximately half of the cases.

Treatment is supportive. Resolution of symptoms is complete in most children within 2 weeks of onset, but mild residual neurologic deficits have been reported in 10% to 30% of cases. Varicella-associated cases appear to have the most benign prognosis.

Benign Paroxysmal Vertigo

Benign paroxysmal vertigo is an illness that affects children primarily between 1 and 4 years of age, although it can occur any time during the first decade. It manifests with acute episodes of dizziness and imbalance, lasting seconds to minutes. Between episodes, the child is asymptomatic. During the spell, the child characteristically becomes frightened and pale but does not lose consciousness. He or she may have associated nausea, vomiting, or visual disturbance. The physical examination is usually normal except for nystagmus, which may be present. Although the cause of this illness is unknown, it is believed to be a migraine variant. Many children go on to develop more typical migraine headaches later, and there is often a family history of migraine disease. As the name suggests, the course of benign paroxysmal vertigo is self-limiting and benign, and treatment is supportive.

MOVEMENT DISORDERS

Goals of Treatment

Involuntary movements are components of many CNS disorders, tend to be complex, and are diagnosed by associated neurologic findings. Classifying movements into specific subtypes, based on the character, predominant anatomic localization, rhythmicity, and frequency, can be useful in deducing the cause of the disorder. Additionally, the type of movement can suggest the location of CNS dysfunction (Table 105.9).

CLINICAL PEARLS AND PITFALLS

- Tics are the most common movement disorder in children.
- Acute dystonia in children is almost always associated with exposure to an antidopaminergic medication.
- Treatment with prednisone can decrease the duration of chorea and the time to full remission in patients with Sydenham chorea.

Acute Dystonia

Dystonia is marked by involuntary, sustained muscle contractions, typically of the neck and trunk, that cause twisting movements and abnormal postures. In generalized dystonia, the head is usually deviated to the side and there is grimacing of the face. Acute dystonia in children is nearly always the result of exposure to an antidopaminergic agent such as a neuroleptic, antiemetic, or metoclopramide. Chronic dystonias are rare but may be seen as an isolated disorder or as a manifestation of cerebral palsy. Dystonia must be differentiated from torticollis, an abnormal tilt of the head and neck usually resulting from irritation or spasm of the sternocleidomastoid muscle (see Chapter 44 Neck Stiffness). Another clinically similar condition is Sandifer syndrome, which describes intermittent arching of the back and neck in infants with gastroesophageal reflux.

Acute dystonia resulting from exposure to antidopaminergic drugs is treated with diphenhydramine (1 mg/kg/dose IV, orally [PO], or IM) or benztropine (Cogentin; 1 to 2 mg per dose IM). Because the half-life of many of the precipitating agents is fairly long, treatment should be continued for 24 to 48 hours.

TABLE 105.9

CATEGORIZATION OF MOVEMENT DISORDERS

Movement	Character	Movement location	Speed	Rhythmicity	Stereotype	Location of lesion
Chorea	Jerky	Anywhere, may be universal	Rapid	Irregular	No	Extrapyramidal
Athetosis	Writhing	Primarily distal	Slow	Irregular	At times	Extrapyramidal
Dystonia	Writhing	Primarily proximal	Slow	Irregular	At times	Extrapyramidal
Ballismus	Flailing	Proximal	Rapid	Irregular	No	Extrapyramidal
Tremor	May be resting, static, or intention	Primarily distal	Variable	Regular	Yes	Cerebellum, cerebellar outflow tract
Myoclonus	Jerky	Anywhere	Rapid	Irregular	Variable	Cerebral cortex, brainstem, spinal cord
Tic	Jerky	Anywhere (especially face, neck, hands)	Rapid	Variable	Yes	

Sydenham Chorea

Sydenham chorea, the most common form of acquired chorea seen in children, occurs primarily between the ages of 3 and 13 years. Marked by involuntary movements, coordination difficulties, and emotional lability, its onset may be abrupt or insidious. Sydenham chorea is believed to be a poststreptococcal disease and may occur months after the primary bacterial infection. It is one of the major diagnostic criteria for rheumatic fever (see Chapter 94 Cardiac Emergencies).

The involuntary movements may be subtle at first and may be exacerbated by stress. Initially, the movements classically affect the face and distal portion of the upper extremities and consist of rapid, involuntary random jerks. This results in the "milkmaid hand," in which the child's hand cannot maintain a uniform strength while grasping the examiner's hand. The involuntary movements disappear during sleep. In some cases patients have predominantly unilateral movements, hemichorea. There is usually associated muscular hypotonia and marked coordination difficulties. Speech is often jerky.

Serologic evidence for preceding streptococcal infection is absent in up to 25% of cases, and only one-third of patients have associated manifestations of rheumatic fever at the time of diagnosis. In the absence of such confirmatory evidence of a poststreptococcal cause, other disorders that may present with chorea must be considered in the differential diagnosis. These include atypical seizures, drug intoxication, choreoathetoid cerebral palsy, familial choreas, chorea gravidarum, collagen vascular disease, Wilson disease, and Lyme disease.

Evaluation should include a hematologic profile, sedimentation rate, and serologic tests performed for streptococcal infection. An ECG should also be performed to look for evidence of rheumatic carditis (e.g., prolonged P-R interval). If there is a question concerning diagnosis, further tests, such as MRI, LP, and serologic evaluation for collagen vascular disease, might be helpful, but are not usually necessary on an urgent basis. Patients should be presumptively treated with chronic prophylactic antibiotics to prevent further beta-hemolytic streptococcus infections; there is a considerable risk for reoccurrence of rheumatic fever.

Pharmacologic treatment of chorea can be difficult and unpredictable. Prednisone has been shown in both retrospective and prospective control trials to decrease overall duration of chorea and to shorten time to full remission. Haloperidol (0.5 to 1 mg PO twice daily) has been reported to result in improvement within 2 to 3 days. Multiple antiepileptic agents including valproic acid and carbamazepine have also been used. Case reports have described the use of IV immunoglobulin and plasmapheresis in refractory cases.

Tics

Tics are another form of involuntary movement that manifest as stereotyped, intermittent motor movements or vocalizations. They may be extremely difficult to distinguish from chorea and are best differentiated by their stereotypic character. In contrast to chorea, tics may persist during sleep. They probably represent the most common involuntary movement disorder but are not true neurologic emergencies. For most children, tics are transient and will not require treatment.

DISORDERS OF CRANIAL NERVE FUNCTION

Goals of Treatment

Disorders of cranial nerve function typically present with classic patterns of neurologic dysfunction. Therefore, specific attention should be paid to completing a full cranial nerve examination and obtaining a clinical history suggestive of alterations of sensation. Identifying the pattern of cranial nerve involvement will determine the necessary evaluation and the likely etiology.

CLINICAL PEARLS AND PITFALLS

- Optic neuritis is associated with both decreased visual acuity and decreased color vision.
- Facial nerve palsy with isolated upper motor neuron involvement is associated with some residual capacity to furrow the brow because of crossed innervation.
- Systemic corticosteroids have been shown to improve the likelihood of complete resolution of idiopathic facial nerve palsy.
- Lyme disease may be the most common cause of facial nerve palsy in endemic areas and testing is recommended.

Optic Neuritis

Optic neuritis is an acute inflammation or demyelination of the optic nerve, characterized by an impairment of vision, progressing over hours or days (see Chapter 25 Eye: Visual Disturbances). The disease is primarily unilateral but an increased incidence of bilateral involvement is found in children. Optic neuritis in children is thought to be an autoimmune process following a viral disease. At times, a contiguous sinusitis may cause the illness. Of patients with unilateral optic neuritis, 20% will eventually be diagnosed with multiple sclerosis.

On examination, decreased visual acuity and decreased color vision are associated with a relative afferent pupillary deficit to light and a central scotoma in the affected eye. The relative afferent pupil defect is demonstrated by the swinging flashlight maneuver. The pupil of the affected eye constricts briskly when light is shone into the contralateral eye (the consensual light reflex) and dilates when light is immediately shone into the affected eye. With bilateral disease, the change in pupillary reflexes may not be apparent. Funduscopic examination discloses a hyperemic, swollen optic disc. In rare cases of retrobulbar optic neuritis, funduscopic examination is normal.

Optic neuritis must be distinguished from papilledema, which is secondary to increased ICP. Papilledema is almost always bilateral and associated with normal vision and normal pupil reactivity until late in the disease. In cases of bilateral optic neuritis, differentiation may be impossible because funduscopic findings are identical in the two illnesses. If any doubt of increased ICP persists, the patient should undergo evaluation by CT or MRI of the brain and, if normal, CSF analysis. In optic neuritis, the opening pressure is normal, but there may be a mild lymphocytic pleocytosis or elevated CSF protein level.

The course of the illness is variable, with most patients recovering to normal or near-normal vision in 4 to 5 weeks. Treatment with high-dose systemic corticosteroids is poorly studied in the pediatric population, and has not been shown to improve the ultimate prognosis. Treatment may, however, result in a slightly faster resolution of symptoms. The efficacy of IV immunoglobulin and plasmapharesis has not been established.

Facial Nerve Palsy

Weakness in the distribution of cranial nerve VII (facial) may be produced by either central (upper motor neuron) or peripheral (lower motor neuron) dysfunction. Peripheral disease is most common in children, particularly when the facial weakness is an isolated finding. Bell palsy refers to peripheral facial nerve weakness with no identifiable underlying cause. It is believed to be caused by edema of the facial nerve as it passes through the facial canal within the temporal bone. There is often a history or preceding upper respiratory tract infection, and in at least a subset of patients, there is evidence of reactivation of infection with Epstein–Barr virus or HSV. Seventh nerve palsy may occur in association with otitis media, in which case it may indicate the presence of mastoid involvement. Facial palsy may also be a manifestation of early-disseminated Lyme disease. In general most cases of facial nerve palsy in children are of the idiopathic (or viral reactivation) type; however, in endemic areas, Lyme disease may be the most common cause.

Facial weakness may be partial or complete. On the affected side, there is flattening of the nasolabial fold at rest, and the child has difficulty closing the eye or raising the corner of the mouth to smile. With upper motor neuron involvement, there will be some residual capacity to furrow the brow because of crossed innervation, whereas the entire face is involved with peripheral disease.

The diagnosis of idiopathic facial nerve palsy is clinical and based on diffuse involvement of all distal branches of cranial nerve VII, an acute onset with progressive course, and an associated prodrome typically consisting of ear pain or dysacusis. In endemic areas, serologic testing for Lyme disease is recommended. Further evaluation with imaging and CSF is not necessary in patients with a typical presentation. Other associated neurologic abnormality, specifically involvement of other cranial nerves, or concomitant otitis media, necessitates further evaluation, including CT or MRI. Peripheral nerve palsy in association with acute otitis media may require myringotomy.

Symptomatic treatment for facial nerve palsy consists of protection of the cornea by the instillation of bland ointments (e.g., Lacri-Lube). The most recent Cochrane Review (2010) demonstrated that treatment with systemic corticosteroids significantly improves the likelihood of complete resolution for patients with idiopathic facial paralysis. A separate Cochrane Review (2009) did not demonstrate any improvement in the rate of recovery for those treated with antivirals against herpes virus alone compared to placebo or to antivirals plus corticosteroids. Patients treated with antiviral and corticosteroids did have improved rates of recovery. As such, antiretroviral therapy is not recommended without evidence of recent or active herpes infection. Regardless of treatment, complete recovery is seen in 60% to 80% of children, beginning during the second to third week of illness. Those with partial paralysis generally have a better prognosis. Patients should be referred for reexamination to ensure recovery during the expected time period.

In children with facial nerve palsy caused by Lyme disease, there may be bilateral involvement in contrast to Bell palsy, in which weakness is always unilateral. Additionally, facial nerve palsy can be the sole presenting symptom of Lyme disease. Thus, even in the absence of other findings, serologic evidence for systemic Lyme infection should be sought in all children with isolated cranial nerve VII paresis in endemic areas. The sensitivity of serologic testing increases with time after infection, so repeat titers are indicated in circumstances where suspicion is high but initial titers are negative. An LP should be performed if there is evidence of meningoencephalitis such as severe headache or nuchal rigidity; however, the need for LP in a child at risk for Lyme disease with isolated facial nerve palsy is controversial. For patients with facial nerve palsy due to Lyme disease, oral antibiotic treatment for 14 to 21 days is indicated as for other manifestations of early-disseminated Lyme disease (see Chapter 102 Infectious Disease Emergencies). Parenteral antibiotics are reserved for those with findings of meningitis. The effectiveness of steroids in such patients has not been evaluated.

Suggested Readings and Key References

Seizures

Brophy GM, Bell R, Claassen J, et al.; Neurocritical Care Society Status Epilepticus Guideline Writing Committee. Guidelines for the evaluation and management of status epilepticus. *Neurocrit Care* 2012;17:3–23.

Bye A, Kok D, Ferenschild F. Paroxysmal non-epileptic events in children: a retrospective study over a period of 10 years. *J Paediatr Child Health* 2000;36(3):244–248.

Committee on Quality Improvement, Subcommittee on Febrile Seizures. Clinical practice guideline: febrile seizures: guideline for the neurodiagnostic evaluation of the child with a simple febrile seizure. *Pediatrics* 2011;127:389–394.

Harden CL, Huff JS, Schwartz TH, et al. Reassessment: neuroimaging in the emergency patient presenting with seizure (and evidence-based review): report of the Therapeutics and Technology Assessment Subcommittee of the American Academy of Neurology. *Neurology* 2007;69:1772–1780.

Rivello JJ, Ashwal S, Hirtz D, et al. Practice parameter: diagnostic assessment of the child with status epilepticus (an evidence-based review): report of the Quality Standards Subcommittee of the American Academy of Neurology and the Practice Committee of the Child Neurology Society. *Neurology* 2006;637:1542–1550.

Migraine

Detsky ME, McDonald DR, Baerlocher MO, et al. Does this patient with headache have a migraine or need neuroimaging? *JAMA* 2005;296:1274–1283.

Gelfand A. Migraine and childhood periodic syndromes in children and adolescents. *Curr Opin Neurol* 2013;26:262–268.

Gelfand AA, Goadsby PJ. Treatment of pediatric migraine in the emergency room. *Pediatr Neurol* 2012;47:233–241.

Silver S, Gano D, Gerretsen P. Acute treatment of paediatric migraine: a meta-analysis of efficacy. *J Paediatr Child Health* 2008;44:3–9.

Idiopathic Intracranial Hypertension

Friedman DI, Liu GT, Difre KB. Revised diagnostic criteria for the pseudotumor cerebri syndrome in adults and children. *Neurology* 2013;81:1159–1165.

Rogers DL. A review of pediatric idiopathic intracranial hypertension. *Pediatr Clin North Am* 2014;61:579–590.

Stroke

Amlie-Lefond C, deVeber G, Chan AK, et al. Use of alteplase in childhood arterial ischaemic stroke: a multicentre, observational, cohort study. *Lancet Neurol* 2009;8:530–536.

Monagle P, Chan AC, Goldenberg NA, et al. Antithrombotic therapy in neonates and children. *Chest* 2012;141(2 suppl):e737S–e801S.

Roach ES, Golomb MR, Adams R, et al. Management of stroke in infants and children. *Stroke* 2008;39:2644–2691.

Royal College of Physicians, London. Paediatric Stroke Working Group. Stroke in childhood. Clinical guidelines for diagnosis, management and rehabilitation. November 2004. https://www.rcplondon.ac.uk/sites/default/files/documents/stroke-in-childhood-guideline.pdf (accessed 30 June 2015).

Shellhaas RA, Smith SE, O'Tool E, et al. Mimics of childhood stroke: characteristics of a prospective cohort. *Pediatrics* 2006;118:704–709.

Encephalitis

Campbell GL, Marfin AA, Lanciotti RS, et al. West Nile virus. *Lancet Infect Dis* 2002;2:519–529.

Dalmau J, Lancaster E, Martinez-Hernandez E, et al. Clinical experience and laboratory investigations in patients with anti-NMDAR encephalitis. *Lancet Neurol* 2011;10:63–74.

Leake JA, Albani S, Kao AS, et al. Acute disseminated encephalomyelitis in childhood: epidemiologic, clinical and laboratory features. *Pediatr Infect Dis J* 2004;23:756–764.

Thompson C, Kneen R, Riordan A, et al. Encephalitis in children. *Arch Dis Child* 2012;97:150–161.

Tunkel AR, Glaser CA, Bloch KC, et al.; Infectious Diseases Society of America. The management of encephalitis: clinical practice guidelines by the Infectious Diseases Society of America. *Clin Infect Dis* 2008;47(3):303–327.

Spinal Cord Dysfunction

Beh SC, Greenberg BM, Frohman T, et al. Transverse myelitis. *Neurol Clin* 2013;31:79–138.

Chen L, Li J, Guo Z, et al. Prognostic indicators of acute transverse myelitis in 39 children. *Pediatr Neurol* 2013;49:397–400.

Greenberg BM, Thomas KP, Krishnan C, et al. Idiopathic transverse myelitis: corticosteroids, plasma exchange, or cyclophosphamide. *Neurology* 2007;68:1614–1617.

Scott TF, Frohman EM, De Seze J, et al. Evidence-based guideline: clinical evaluation and treatment of transverse myelitis: report of the Therapeutics and Technology Assessment Subcommittee of the American Academy of Neurology. *Neurology* 2011;77: 2128–2134.

Wolf VL, Lupo PJ, Lotze TE. Pediatric acute transverse myelitis overview and differential diagnosis. *J Child Neurol* 2012;27: 1426–1436.

Acute Polyneuritis

Agrawal S, Peake D, Whitehouse WP. Management of children with Guillain-Barré syndrome. *Arch Dis Child Educ Pract Ed* 2007;92: ep161–ep168.

Hughes RA, Swan AV, van Doorn PA. Intravenous immunoglobulin for Guillain-Barré syndrome. *Cochrane Database Syst Rev* 2012;7: CD002063.

Hughes RA, van Doorn PA. Corticosteroids for Guillain-Barré syndrome. *Cochrane Database Syst Rev* 2012;8:CD001446.

Hughes RA, Wijdicks EF, Barohn R, et al. Practice parameter: immunotherapy for Guillain-Barré syndrome: report of the Quality Standards Subcommittee of the American Academy of Neurology. *Neurology* 2003;61:736–740.

Raphaël JC, Chevret S, Hughes RA, et al. Plasma exchange for Guillain-Barré syndrome. *Cochrane Database Syst Rev* 2012;7:CD001798.

Myasthenia Gravis

Andrews PI. Autoimmune myasthenia gravis in childhood. *Semin Neurol* 2004;24:101–110.

Gajdos P, Chevret S, Toyka K. Plasma exchange for myasthenia gravis. *Cochrane Database Syst Rev* 2002;(4):CD002275.

Gajdos P, Chevret S, Toyka KV. Intravenous immunoglobulin for myasthenia gravis. *Cochrane Database Syst Rev* 2012;12:CD002277.

Hetherington KA, Losek JD. Myasthenia gravis: myasthenia vs. cholinergic crisis. *Pediatr Emerg Care* 2005;21:546–548.

Patwa HS, Chaudhry V, Katzberg H, et al. Evidence-based guideline: intravenous immunoglobulin in the treatment of neuromuscular disorders: report of the Therapeutics and Technology Assessment Subcommittee of the American Academy of Neurology. *Neurology* 2012;78:1009–1015.

Botulism

Fox CK, Keet CA, Strober JB. Recent advances in infant botulism. *Pediatr Neurol* 2005;32:149–154.

Francisco AM, Arnon SS. Clinical mimics of infant botulism. *Pediatrics* 2007;119:826–828.

Long SS. Infant botulism. *Pediatr Infect Dis J* 2001;20:707–709.

Periodic Paralysis

Finsterer J. Primary periodic paralyses. *Acta Neurol Scand* 2008;117: 145–158.

Jurkat-Rott K, Lehmann-Horn F. Paroxysmal muscle weakness–the familial periodic paralyses. *J Neurol* 2006;253:1391–1398.

Venance SL, Cannon SC, Fialho D, et al. The primary periodic paralyses: diagnosis, pathogenesis and treatment. *Brain* 2006;129:8–17.

Acute Cerebellar Ataxia

Davis DP, Marino A. Acute cerebellar ataxia in a toddler: case report and literature review. *J Emerg Med* 2003;24:281–284.

Go T. Intravenous immunoglobulin therapy for acute cerebellar ataxia. *Acta Paediatr* 2003;92:504–506.

Nussinovitch M, Prais D, Volovitz B, et al. Post-infectious acute cerebellar ataxia in children. *Clin Pediatr* 2003;42:581–584.

Ryan MM, Engle EC. Acute ataxia in childhood. *J Child Neurol* 2003; 18(5):309–316.

Whelan HT, Verma S, Guo Y, et al. Evaluation of the child with acute ataxia: a systematic review. *Pediatr Neurology* 2013;49:15–24.

Benign Paroxysmal Vertigo

Tusa RJ, Saada AA, Niparko JK. Dizziness in childhood. *J Child Neurol* 1994;9:261–274.

Movement Disorder

Derinoz O, Caglar AA. Drug-induced movement disorders in children at paediatric emergency department: 'dystonia'. *Emerg Med J* 2013;30:130.

Dooley JM. Tic disorders in childhood. *Semin Pediatr Neurol* 2006;13:231–242.

Oosterveer DM, Overweg-Plandsoen WC, Roos RA. Sydenham's chorea: a practical overview of the current literature. *Pediatr Neurol* 2010;43:1.

Uddin MK, Rodnitzky RL. Tremor in children. *Semin Pediatr Neurol* 2003;10:26–34.

Wolf DS, Singer HS. Pediatric movement disorders: an update. *Curr Opin Neurol* 2008;21:491–496.

Optic Neuritis

Beck RW, Trobe JD, Moke PS, et al. High- and low-risk profiles for the development of multiple sclerosis within 10 years after optic neuritis: experience of the optic neuritis treatment trial. *Arch Ophthalmol* 2003;121:944–949.

Boomer JA, Siatkowski RM. Optic neuritis in adults and children. *Semin Ophthalmol* 2003;18:174–180.

Gal RL, Vedula SS, Beck R. Corticosteroids for treating optic neuritis. *Cochrane Database Syst Rev* 2012;4:CD001430.

Zeid NA, Bhatti MT. Acute inflammatory demyelinating optic neuritis: evidence-based visual and neurological considerations. *Neurologist* 2008;14:207–223.

Facial Nerve Palsy

Halperin JJ, Shapiro ED, Logigian E, et al. Practice parameter: treatment of nervous system Lyme disease (an evidence-based review): report of the Quality Standards Subcommittee of the American Academy of Neurology. *Neurology* 2007;69:91–102.

Kitsko DJ, Dohar JE. Inner ear and facial nerve complications of acute otitis media, including vertigo. *Curr Allergy Asthma Rep* 2007;7:444–450.

Lockhart P, Daly F, Pitkethly M, et al. Antiviral treatment for Bell's palsy (idiopathic facial paralysis). *Cochrane Database Syst Rev* 2009;4:CD001869.

Nigrovic LE, Thompson AM, Kimia A. Clinical predictors of Lyme disease among children with a peripheral facial palsy at an emergency department in a Lyme-disease endemic area. *Pediatrics* 2008;122:e1080–e1085.

Salinas RA, Alvarez G, Daly F, et al. Corticosteroids for Bell's palsy (idiopathic facial paralysis). *Cochrane Database Syst Rev* 2010;3:CD001942.

CHAPTER 106 ■ ONCOLOGIC EMERGENCIES

ALISA MCQUEEN, MD AND ANDREW E. PLACE, MD, PhD

GOALS OF EMERGENCY THERAPY

Every year in the United States, approximately 12,000 children and adolescents are diagnosed with cancer and 2,300 children die of their disease or from side effects of treatment. This chapter is organized into two major sections. The first section reviews common presenting symptoms and emergency care considerations for a child who presents to the emergency department (ED) with either a new cancer diagnosis or recurrence of disease. This section is organized by diagnosis and by location of malignancy. The second section addresses the management of complications associated with common pediatric malignancies and their treatment.

The general approach to the pediatric oncology patient in the ED is outlined in Table 106.1. When taking a history from a pediatric oncology patient, exploring the perspective of the patient and parents about the potential cause of the problem and how the patient is doing is a crucial step in the evaluative process. A detailed medication history is critical as patients are likely to be receiving multiple medications (e.g., chemotherapy, antibiotics, antiemetics) whose side effects may be contributing to their presenting symptoms. One last introductory principle is to remember the extreme psychosocial stress that a pediatric cancer diagnosis places on a family. The care of these patients requires the highest level of compassion and professionalism.

KEY POINTS

- The differential diagnosis of many common childhood complaints should include malignant processes.
- Prompt recognition of oncologic emergencies has been proven to affect outcomes.
- Early consultation with a pediatric oncologist is highly recommended.

RELATED CHAPTERS

Signs and Symptoms
- Abdominal Distension: Chapter 7
- Groin Masses: Chapter 29
- Lymphadenopathy: Chapter 42
- Neck Mass: Chapter 43
- Pain: Back: Chapter 49
- Pain: Headache: Chapter 54
- Pallor: Chapter 57

Medical, Surgical, and Trauma Emergencies
- Endocrine Emergencies: Chapter 97
- Hematologic Emergencies: Chapter 101
- Infectious Disease Emergencies: Chapter 102
- Neurologic Emergencies: Chapter 105
- Renal and Electrolyte Emergencies: Chapter 108
- Thoracic Emergencies: Chapter 132

SECTION I: INITIAL CARE OF THE CHILD WITH NEW OR RECURRENT CANCER

Childhood cancer can present with nonspecific signs and symptoms that can overlap with those of many childhood illnesses (Table 106.2). Even when the chief complaint is a localized symptom, disseminated disease may be present. Once the diagnosis of cancer is suspected, the child should be referred to a center skilled in the management of childhood cancer. However, supportive care for life-threatening complications may need to be initiated prior to referral. After stabilization, the specific workup, including obtaining tissue for diagnosis, should be carried out under the direction of a pediatric oncologist so that optimal information can be obtained. No patient should be discharged from the ED without a specific plan for definitive diagnosis and management.

The possibility of a cancer diagnosis usually causes fear and distress and requires empathic care and support from the health care team in the ED. The emergency physician should describe the findings and concern about possible cancer to the patient and family. It is appropriate to reassure them that most childhood cancer is curable. Specific details about diagnosis, treatment, and prognosis are best deferred to the pediatric oncologist once definitive information is available.

LEUKEMIA

Goals of Treatment

The primary goal of emergency management of these patients is rapid assessment and correction of hematologic, metabolic, infectious, and cardiorespiratory complications. After a patient has been stabilized, further diagnostic evaluations can be performed.

CLINICAL PEARLS AND PITFALLS

- Automated differentials may count leukemic blasts as either atypical lymphocytes or monocytes so abnormal numbers of these cell types may actually be due to leukemia.
- Avoid aggressive transfusion in severely anemic but stable patients, as this can result in rapid development of pulmonary edema and respiratory failure.

TABLE 106.1

HISTORICAL DATA NEEDED FOR EVALUATION OF PEDIATRIC ONCOLOGY PATIENTS IN THE EMERGENCY DEPARTMENT

Category	Specific history to explore
Primary diagnosis	• Tumor type • Isolated or metastatic ■ Where are sites of metastatic disease? • Date of diagnosis • Status of disease ■ In remission, on treatment ■ In remission, off treatment ■ Relapsed
Surgical history	• Date and type of surgical procedures • Surgical complications
Recent treatments	• Chemotherapy ■ Drugs and dates of most recent therapy • Radiation therapy ■ Location of radiation field(s) ■ Dates of radiation therapy • Hematopoietic stem cell transplant ■ Autologous or allogeneic ■ Use of immunosuppressants ■ History of graft-versus-host disease
Central venous access	• Type • History of infections in line
Current medications	• Chemotherapy • Prophylaxis for *Pneumocystis jirovecii* or other infections • Growth factors • Pain treatment • Antiemetics • GI acid blockade • Bowel regimen • Antihypertensives
Patient/family perspective	• How is the patient acting? • Has this problem happened before? • Are symptoms getting worse or better? • What does parent or patient believe to be the cause of the problem?

Current Evidence

Leukemia is a cancer of white blood cells (WBCs) and their precursors that proliferate in excess within the bone marrow and other hematopoietic tissues. Leukemia is the most common childhood malignancy, accounting for 29% of all cancer diagnoses in children from 0 to 14 years of age. Leukemias are classified as either acute or chronic. More than 95% of pediatric leukemias are acute, with acute lymphoblastic leukemia (ALL) accounting for the vast majority. The remaining leukemias seen in children in order of decreasing frequency include acute myeloid leukemia (AML), chronic myelogenous leukemia (CML), and juvenile myelomonocytic leukemia (JMML). Specific classification is based on morphology, immunologic surface markers, and cytogenetic abnormalities from the bone marrow aspirate. Children with trisomy 21 are at increased risk of transient myeloproliferative disorder of the newborn, AML (younger than 4 years), and ALL (older than 1 year).

Clinical Considerations

Clinical Recognition

The presentations of childhood leukemia are varied and, in some cases, the diagnosis of leukemia is not at all obvious (Table 106.2). Symptoms are usually secondary to bone marrow replacement resulting in cytopenias or from extramedullary infiltration of leukemic blast cells into tissues including the lymph nodes, testes, liver, spleen, central nervous system (CNS), and skin. Systemic symptoms such as fever and weight loss are common.

Patients with acute leukemia are at risk for serious hematologic, metabolic, infectious, and cardiopulmonary complications. The patient with suspected leukemia should be rapidly assessed for evidence of these complications.

Clinical Assessment

Table 106.3 presents assessment and management guidelines for leukemia in the ED. The evaluation should begin with a thorough history and physical examination. The history should focus on the time frame in which symptoms developed and should screen for the complications described above. Assess airway patency, which may be threatened in the setting of a mediastinal mass. Assessment of the patient's breathing should include attention to the respiratory rate and oxygenation, both of which can become compromised in the setting of anemia, leukostasis, congestive heart failure, and pulmonary infection. In assessing the patient's circulation, establish intravascular access and include an assessment for evidence of SVC syndrome. The physical examination should include an evaluation for lymphadenopathy and hepatosplenomegaly. Signs of soft tissue infiltration by leukemia cells should be explored, including skin infiltration (leukemia cutis) and testicular enlargement in male patients. A thorough neurologic examination is essential to screen for cord compression and CNS effects of the leukemia. Any abnormalities on neurologic examination warrant further imaging to determine whether a neurologic complication of the leukemia has occurred.

Laboratory evaluation should begin with a complete blood count (CBC), WBC differential, and peripheral blood smear to be reviewed by a hematologist–oncologist or pathologist. Automated differentials might count leukemic blasts as either atypical lymphocytes or monocytes so abnormal numbers of these cell types should raise concern for leukemia. Flow cytometry analysis can provide important diagnostic clues by analyzing the proteins of the blast cell surface. Specific diagnosis requires a bone marrow aspirate, which is not routinely performed in the ED and should be done in consultation with an oncologist.

In constructing a differential diagnosis, it is helpful to consider whether leukemic blasts are present in the peripheral circulation. If blasts are present in substantive quantities (greater than 20%), then leukemia is the most likely diagnosis. A smaller percentage of blasts could indicate a myelodysplastic syndrome, a myeloproliferative disorder, recovery from an aplastic process, or a leukemoid reaction. If blasts are not evident on the CBC, and the patient has pancytopenia, one must consider not only leukemia but also bone marrow failure from aplastic anemia, infection (usually viral), or marrow

TABLE 106.2

COMMON PRESENTING SYMPTOMS AND SIGNS OF PEDIATRIC CANCER

Symptoms and signs	Acute leukemia[a]	Lymphoma	Histiocytic diseases	Wilms tumor	Neuroblastoma	Hepatic tumors	Ovarian tumors	Testicular tumors	Soft tissue sarcomas	Bone tumors	Central nervous system tumors
Abdominal mass		+		+	+	+	+		+		
Anorexia	+	+	+		+	+			+		±
Back pain	+	+	+		+		±			+	+
Cord compression	±	±	±		+				±	+	+
Cranial nerve palsies	+	+	+						+		+
Diarrhea			+		+						
Diplopia											+
Epistaxis	+	±							+		
Fever	+	+	+		+	+				±	±
Failure to thrive	+	+	+		+						+
Gait abnormality	+				+					+	+
Gastrointestinal bleeding		+									
Headache	±	±									+
Head/neck mass	±	±	±		+				+		
Hepatomegaly	+	+	+		+	+					
Hypertension				+	+						+
Irritability	+		+	+	+					±	+
Limp	+		+		+					+	±
Lymphadenopathy	+	+	+		+				+		
Malaise	+	+	+		+				+		+
Nasal obstruction		+							+		
Pallor	+		+	+	+						
Petechiae	+		+		+						
Proptosis	±	±	±		+				+		+
Respiratory distress		+			+						
Testicular mass	±				±			+	+		
Seizures											+
Splenomegaly	+	+	+								
Vomiting					+	+					+
Weight loss	+	+	+		+					+	±

[a]Patients with solid tumors invading the marrow may have symptoms and signs similar to those seen in leukemia.

TABLE 106.3

EMERGENCY DEPARTMENT CARE OF PATIENT WITH SUSPECTED OR CONFIRMED ACUTE LEUKEMIA

Diagnostic evaluation

- Detailed medical history
- Complete physical examination (including testicular examination)
- CBC count with manual differential and peripheral blood smear
- Electrolytes, including potassium, calcium, phosphorus
- Uric acid
- Assessment of renal function with BUN and creatinine
- Coagulation studies, PT, PTT
- Blood group type, antibody screen
- Liver function tests
- Chest x-ray to assess for mediastinal mass
- Blood culture (if febrile or ill appearing)

Immediate supportive care

- Determine need for platelet or red blood cell transfusion
- IV fluids should run at approximately two times maintenance
- Initiation of uric acid–lowering agents (allopurinol or rasburicase)
- Consideration of broad-spectrum antibiotics in febrile or ill-appearing patients

Specific problems that require immediate intervention

Problem	Required data/findings	Therapy/management
Prevention of TLS[a]	*Frequent laboratory monitoring (q6–8h)* Uric acid Electrolytes BUN and creatinine Ca and PO_4	IV fluids run at 1.5–2 × maintenance Allopurinol Monitor urine output IV fluids as above Allopurinol or rasburicase
Hyperuricemia		Rasburicase, if renal function is impaired at presentation, if uric acid levels are rapidly rising or extremely high, or if there is a contraindication to hyperhydration
Hyperkalemia		Furosemide, insulin/glucose, kayexalate EKG
Hypokalemia		No replacement of potassium unless critical level with high risk of cardiac arrhythmia
Hyperphosphatemia		Aluminum hydroxide
Hypocalcemia		No calcium replacement unless symptomatic
Hyperleukocytosis	WBC count >100,000/mL	Ensure IV fluids are being given at maximum tolerated volume Limit transfusion of packed red blood cells, which can increase viscosity Monitor for leukostasis Prevent and monitor TLS
Leukostasis	Clinical symptoms of respiratory distress or change in neurologic status Chest x-ray findings may be present	Urgent leukopheresis Proceed with caution if PT or PTT elevated
Mediastinal mass	Chest x-ray and/or chest CT scan Echocardiogram Assessment of respiratory status while upright and supine Peak flow	Establish diagnosis as soon as possible Mass will likely shrink quickly in response to chemotherapy Support respiratory mechanics, though intubation unlikely to offer benefit No sedation/anesthesia
Fever	Blood culture (from CVL, if present) Additional culture from any site with localizing symptoms Avoid lumbar puncture	All patients should be assumed neutropenic, even if ANC >500 Empiric broad-spectrum antibiotics (see Figure 106.4) Tylenol, no NSAIDs
Anemia	Hemoglobin < 7 g/100 mL Symptoms related to low red blood cell mass	Please see Table 106.7 for special guidelines for transfusions in the oncology population If severe anemia, transfuse slowly to avoid precipitating congestive heart failure
Thrombocytopenia	Platelet count < 150,000/mL	Please see Table 106.7 for special guidelines for transfusions in the oncology population

(*continued*)

TABLE 106.3

EMERGENCY DEPARTMENT CARE OF PATIENT WITH SUSPECTED OR CONFIRMED ACUTE LEUKEMIA (*CONTINUED*)

Problem	Required data/findings	Therapy/management
Coagulopathy	PT, PTT, fibrinogen, D-dimer	Fresh frozen plasma 10 mL/kg If hypofibrinogenemia exists in isolation, treat with cryoprecipitate, 1–2 U/10 kg Platelet transfusion if count <50,000/mL Leukopheresis and lumbar puncture may be contraindicated until coagulopathy corrected
CNS symptoms	Neurologic examination WBC count to screen for hyperleukocytosis PT, PTT, fibrinogen, D-dimer to assess risk for CNS hemorrhage Serum electrolytes Head and/or spinal cord imaging with CT or MRI	Leukopheresis to decrease viscosity and leukostasis, if WBC >100,000/mL and symptomatic Correct coagulopathy (see above) Platelet transfusion if count <50,000/mL Initiation of chemotherapy is best management for CNS leukemia or chloroma Consultation with radiation oncology and neurosurgery in the setting of spinal cord compression

[a]Consider whether renal function or metabolic derangements may necessitate dialysis.
BUN, blood urea nitrogen; PT, prothrombin time; PTT, partial thromboplastin time; TLS, tumor lysis syndrome; q, every; IV, intravenous; WBC, white blood cell; CT, computed tomography; ANC, absolute neutrophil count; NSAIDs, nonsteroidal anti-inflammatory drugs; CNS, central nervous system; MRI, magnetic resonance imaging.

replacement by a solid tumor. If only one or two cell lines seem to be affected, the clinician should consider the differential diagnoses for each cytopenia individually (see Chapter 101 Hematologic Emergencies).

In addition to the laboratory investigations needed for diagnosis, screen for metabolic abnormalities due to tumor lysis by checking serum chemistries, including potassium, calcium, magnesium, phosphorus, and uric acid. Renal function should be assessed with a blood urea nitrogen (BUN) and creatinine. The results of the CBC should be reviewed to assess needs for transfusions of blood products and a prothrombin time (PT) and partial thromboplastin time (PTT) should be checked to look for coagulopathy (Table 106.3). A chest x-ray may indicate the presence of a mediastinal mass or pericardial effusion.

Management

Cytopenias. As the leukemia proliferates in the bone marrow, normal hematopoietic elements decrease, leading to anemia, thrombocytopenia, and neutropenia. This is most common in the setting of leukemia but can occur with solid tumors, such as neuroblastoma and rhabdomyosarcoma with bone marrow metastasis. Anemia can be mild or severe but is often asymptomatic because of its slow development. Anemia with associated clinical signs or symptoms should be treated with a red cell transfusion. Severely anemic but stable patients should be transfused slowly to avoid rapid development of pulmonary edema and respiratory failure. Thrombocytopenia can present with mucocutaneous bleeding such as epistaxis, gingival bleeding, petechiae, and ecchymosis. The risk of bleeding may also be compounded by coagulopathy from the leukemia itself or from disseminated intravascular coagulation (DIC) related to sepsis.

Tumor Lysis Syndrome. Tumor overproliferation or chemotherapy can lead to rapid tumor lysis, in which the release of intracellular contents increases serum levels of lactate dehydrogenase (LDH), potassium, phosphate, and uric acid with potentially severe metabolic consequences. Tumor lysis is common with acute leukemias and lymphomas but can also occur with neuroblastoma or other solid tumors with a very high tumor burden.

Calcium complexes with phosphate to form calcium phosphate crystals that can deposit in the renal tubules and other tissue sites. This can result in renal insufficiency and hypocalcemia. Urate crystals can precipitate in the acidic urine encountered in the renal tubules causing an obstructive uropathy and renal insufficiency. *Tumor lysis syndrome* (TLS) occurs when these electrolyte derangements occur with evidence of renal insufficiency or failure.

Fortunately, effective preventive strategies make clinically significant TLS a rare occurrence. Screening and preemptive therapy with hydration and allopurinol is appropriate for all patients at risk for TLS. The use of allopurinol or rasburicase (Elitek) to decrease uric acid levels is often driven by institutional protocol. A full discussion of the management of tumor lysis is found in Section II.

Hyperleukocytosis. Hyperleukocytosis is defined as WBC count above 100,000 per mm^3. When hyperleukocytosis is present, the clinical findings of leukostasis may develop from sludging of WBCs in the capillary beds. The most vulnerable beds are those in the lungs and CNS where increased viscosity can cause either thrombosis or hemorrhage. Leukostasis is much more common with myeloid leukemia than with ALL. In the setting of hyperleukocytosis, hydration should be initiated immediately to reduce viscosity. Transfusion of red blood cells and diuretics should be avoided to prevent further increases in blood viscosity, but platelet transfusion is appropriate to reduce the risk of CNS hemorrhage. Leukocytopheresis, a technique to reduce blood viscosity acutely, should be initiated immediately in the presence of respiratory or neurologic symptoms, even if mild. The use of prophylactic leukocytopheresis is controversial and should be considered only in consultation with a pediatric oncologist. Since new-onset leukemia may be associated with coagulopathy, we recommend obtaining coagulation studies to determine the risk of bleeding during leukocytopheresis.

Extramedullary Involvement. As leukemia develops, malignant cells may infiltrate nonhematopoietic tissues, producing adenopathy, hepatomegaly, and splenomegaly. Anterior mediastinal masses (AMM) occur primarily with T-lineage ALL and can lead to life-threatening airway compromise and/or superior vena cava (SVC) syndrome. The approach to the presentation and management of AMM is discussed in more detail in the section on thoracic tumors. Chloroma, a mass of leukemic blasts in the soft tissue, can occur in any body part and is much more common with AML than ALL. When this mass develops and rapidly expands near the spinal cord, compression of the cord can result (see "Tumors In and Around the Spinal Cord" section). Leukemic involvement in the spinal fluid can cause meningeal symptoms, cranial nerve palsy, headache, seizure, increased intracranial pressure (ICP), or visual disturbances (from retinal infiltrates). Boys can present with testicular enlargement. There may also be skin lesions due to leukemia cutis (more common in monocytic leukemias and infant leukemia) and gingival hypertrophy (with AML) due to leukemic infiltration.

It is not uncommon for patients with leukemia to be febrile at presentation. Although the fever may be an inflammatory reaction driven by the leukemia itself, serious infection must be explored. It is essential to determine if the febrile patient is neutropenic. If the absolute neutrophil count (ANC) is less than 500 per μL, broad-spectrum antibiotics covering gram-positive and gram-negative bacteria as well as pseudomonas should be administered in the ED. If localizing signs of a bacterial infection are evident, or if high fevers are present (>39°C), empiric therapy should be initiated even if the patient is not neutropenic. Management is summarized in Table 106.3. Patients may present with sepsis at the time of diagnosis or relapse. The increased risk of sepsis may be because of neutropenia and/or immune dysfunction caused by the underlying malignancy. Management of sepsis in the setting of leukemia is not unique and the principles are similar to those described more thoroughly in Chapters 91 Shock and 102 Infectious Disease Emergencies.

Pain. For some patients, limp or a refusal to walk or bear weight is one of the first signs of leukemia. In fact, it is not uncommon for a patient to be treated for diagnoses such as osteomyelitis or septic hip before the diagnosis of leukemia is uncovered. It is essential for the emergency physician to ensure that a refusal to walk is not because of cord compression from chloroma as discussed above. Bone pain is usually due to replacement of the bone marrow with rapidly proliferating leukemic cells causing strain on the marrow spaces. Pathologic fractures may develop as the expanding marrow compartments put strain on and weaken the bony cortex.

HISTIOCYTIC DISEASES

Goal of Treatment

Timely recognition of histiocytic diseases can be lifesaving. The most common histiocytic disease, Langerhans cell histiocytosis (LCH), rarely requires emergency care, whereas hemophagocytic lymphohistiocytosis (HLH) is a life-threatening illness that can be rapidly fatal without appropriate intervention.

CLINICAL PEARL AND PITFALLS

- Consider HLH in the acutely ill infant or young child as these patients can deteriorate quickly and require urgent oncologic consultation and ICU support.

Current Evidence

Histiocytic diseases are a complex and sometimes confusing group of disorders for two reasons. First, several different disease entities make up this group, although efforts have been made to simplify the terminology. Second, significant clinical heterogeneity exists between the major disease entities. Histiocyte is a term referring to several different cells that are thought to derive from a common CD34+ progenitor in the bone marrow. Depending on the cytokines to which the progenitors become exposed, the differentiation can yield tissue macrophages, dermal/interstitial dendritic cells, or Langerhans cells. In general, histiocytic diseases are rare; of the group, the most common is LCH, which has an incidence of three to five cases per million children.

Clinical Considerations

Clinical Recognition

LCH has clinical heterogeneity and the locations involved in the disease have implications for therapy and prognosis. Low-risk LCH may present at any age and systemic symptoms are rare. Skin, bone, lymph nodes, or a combination of these are most commonly involved. Skin involvement can present as a red papular rash, resembling a candidal diaper rash, which may appear on the groin, abdomen, back, or chest. There may also be seborrheic flaking of the scalp, often misdiagnosed as "cradle cap" in infants, draining otitis externa, or ulcerative lesions behind the ears, on the scalp, or in the genital region. Bony involvement may be asymptomatic or painful. A lytic lesion of the skull causing a tender mass is the most common but any bone may be involved. Loose teeth from involvement of the jaw may occur. Certain sites of disease have become known as "risk" organs because their involvement implies more aggressive disease. These patients are often very young with disease that involves the lung, liver, spleen, and/or bone marrow. Lung involvement is rare but worrisome and usually manifests first as hypoxia. Liver and spleen involvement is usually accompanied by enlargement of those organs, although hepatic dysfunction may also be present. Bone marrow involvement is rare, but usually presents with cytopenias, which should prompt a bone marrow aspirate and biopsy. Diabetes insipidus (DI) due to involvement of the posterior pituitary is the most frequent endocrine abnormality in LCH; some patients may present with an apparent "idiopathic" presentation of DI before other lesions are identified. A few patients may present with diarrhea or malabsorption as colitis related to LCH has been described.

HLH is a very rare but severe and life-threatening systemic disease with rapid progression from presentation to death without appropriate intervention. *Thus, consideration of this diagnosis in the ED can be critical to outcome.* For these reasons, it is essential for the emergency physician to have some familiarity with this disorder. Congenital HLH usually presents in infants and very young children. Other forms of HLH develop secondary to Epstein–Barr virus (EBV) infection, malignancy, or severe rheumatologic disorders or without a specific trigger. Regardless of etiology, HLH presents with fever, hepatosplenomegaly, adenopathy, and rash.

Clinical Assessment

All patients with suspected histiocytic disorders need a thorough history and physical examination as well as a rapid assessment of severity of illness. Patients with HLH may have significant systemic illness with organ dysfunction and even vital sign instability and will often require management in a critical care setting. At the other extreme, patients with suspected localized LCH may require little to no intervention in the ED but need only close oncologic follow-up.

Pulse oximetry should be checked to screen for hypoxia and a chest x-ray obtained if hypoxia is detected. Laboratory evaluation should include CBC, liver function testing, electrolytes to screen for DI, and inflammatory markers such as erythrocyte sedimentation rate (ESR) and C-reactive protein (CRP). If HLH is suspected, laboratory analysis may reveal a markedly high serum ferritin as well as transaminitis, hypertriglyceridemia, hypofibrinogenemia, and cytopenias. Bone marrow evaluation may show characteristic hemophagocytosis. Oncologic consultation can guide the evaluation and management of systemically ill patients, as in the case of HLH, or allow for careful follow-up of more stable patients with suspected LCH.

TUMORS OF THE CENTRAL NERVOUS SYSTEM

Goals of Treatment

CNS tumors span a wide range of clinical presentations. The most critical goal is the timely identification and management of cord compression and increased ICP. The goal of early identification of CNS tumors on initial presentation needs to be balanced against exposure to ionizing radiation from CT given that many children present with nonspecific symptoms including headache and/or vomiting. Careful recognition of atypical features and/or concerning associated signs or symptoms can assist in decision making regarding advanced imaging.

CLINICAL PEARL AND PITFALLS

- Clinical clues for increased ICP may include a bulging fontanel in infants, or headache with early morning vomiting in older children.
- Measurement of sodium levels is particularly important in patients with CNS tumors.

Current Evidence

Tumors of the CNS most commonly affect the brain and represent the most common solid tumor in the pediatric population and the second most common pediatric cancer overall. There are approximately 2,000 new malignant brain tumors diagnosed annually in children. These tumors can affect children and adolescents of any age group but the peak incidence is in school-aged children, 5 to 10 years old. Supratentorial tumors are more common in children younger than 1 year and older than 10 years. Infratentorial lesions are more common between ages 1 and 10 years. Unlike in adults, brain tumors in children are usually primary, not metastatic. Since tumor location usually drives the presenting signs and symptoms, this is the most useful categorization in the ED (Table 106.4).

Clinical Considerations

Clinical Recognition

Some of the symptoms of brain tumors in children are nonspecific, and nonlocalizing complaints occur with a variety of tumor types. Examples include headache, altered behavior, vision changes, altered growth or weight, somnolence, and altered school performance. The diagnosis of brain tumor may be delayed in such patients. Once patients develop signs and symptoms more easily referred to the CNS, their presentations tend to hinge on the tumor location (Table 106.4).

Infratentorial tumors may present with cranial nerve deficits, such as facial nerve palsies, dysphagia, or paresis of cranial nerve VI, causing diplopia or strabismus. Ependymomas of the fourth ventricle may present with hydrocephalus and increased ICP. Cerebellar lesions can elicit truncal ataxia and a reeling gait when located on the midline. When only one cerebellar hemisphere is involved, patients may display an ipsilateral hypotonia, resulting in falling to the affected side. Herniation of the cerebellar tonsil can cause head tilt toward the tumor and neck pain or stiffness.

In contrast, supratentorial masses may present with signs and symptoms derived from the involved anatomic locations. Tumors near the optic chiasm may present with vision deficits. Craniopharyngiomas, located in the pituitary gland, can cause visual disturbances, headache, and alterations in the endocrine function. Growth hormone deficiency or hypothyroidism may cause delayed growth. Pineal tumors may cause hydrocephalus by obstructing the aquaduct of Sylvius or can cause Parinaud syndrome (deficits in upward gaze, convergence nystagmus, and impaired pupillary response). Hypothalamic tumors may cause diencephalic syndrome, which includes failure to thrive, wasting, and unusual euphoria. If a tumor is located near the third ventricle, hydrocephalus and symptoms of increased ICP can result. Masses within the cerebral hemispheres themselves usually present with focal motor dysfunction or seizure.

The spinal cord may be the site of a primary tumor or, in some cases, the site of a "dropped metastasis" from a primary lesion within the brain. These can present with focal neurologic deficits attributable to areas of the spinal cord inferior to the lesion (see "Tumors In and Around the Spinal Cord" section).

Brain tumors can cause increased ICP by blocking CSF drainage. The symptoms of increased ICP vary based on patient age. Infants with an open fontanelle can sometimes present with bulging of the fontanelle as well as seizure, vomiting, irritability, or loss of acquired skills. Older children often have headache and early morning vomiting. Sixth nerve palsies are common. Sometimes increased ICP is detected only on imaging of the brain that reveals enlargement of the ventricles or effacement of the gyri.

TABLE 106.4

TUMORS AFFECTING THE CENTRAL NERVOUS SYSTEM

Location	Specific tumor types	Presenting signs and symptoms	Comments
Supratentorial hemispheric	Low-grade gliomas Pilocytic Fibrillary High-grade glioma Mixed neuronal-glial neoplasms Ganglioglioma Ependymoma Choroid plexus tumors Primitive neuroectodermal tumor (PNET)	Varies with site Hemiparesis Hemisensory deficits Seizure Hemianopsia	Outcome for these tumors usually improved by extensive resection
Supratentorial midline	Chiasmatic/hypothalamic glioma Craniopharyngioma Germinoma/malignant germ cell tumors Pineoblastoma PNET	Vision deficits Diencephalic syndrome Neuroendocrine symptoms Hydrocephalus Parinaud syndrome	Germinoma and germ cell tumors require biopsy; treatment usually chemotherapy not surgery
Infratentorial	Medulloblastoma Cerebellar astrocytoma Ependymoma Diffuse malignant brainstem glioma Benign focal brainstem glioma	Cranial nerve palsies Cerebellar signs Ataxia Dysmetria Brainstem signs Weakness Unsteady gait Increased intracranial pressure	

Seizures developing in the setting of a child with cancer, whether due to a CNS tumor or another malignancy, should be managed as described in Chapter 67 Seizures. Brain tumors should be considered in the differential diagnosis of new-onset seizures.

Patients with brain tumors are at risk for several metabolic complications. The presence of an intracranial tumor may be a cause for cerebral salt wasting or SIADH. DI can result from tumor involvement of the pituitary gland. Patients should be screened for these abnormalities with serum chemistries. However, these complications are not managed uniquely because of the brain tumors. Chapter 97 Endocrine Emergencies provides guidelines on evaluation and management.

Clinical Assessment

After ensuring the patient has a stable airway, breathing, and circulation, the evaluation in the ED should focus on a thorough history and physical examination, assessing for any neurologic symptoms and screening for complications described above. A complete physical examination should include a thorough ophthalmologic and neurologic assessment and an evaluation of the patient's external genitalia for precocious puberty or virilization, since some pediatric brain tumors may be hormone secreting. A rectal examination to evaluate the anal "wink" is also useful as a screen for spinal cord compression. If the history or physical examination raises concern for increased ICP or spinal cord compression, then therapy should be initiated as described below. A CT scan is useful to rule out hemorrhage and assess for increased ICP, and can sometimes be used to visualize a brain tumor. A CT may miss infratentorial masses so in most cases, magnetic resonance imaging (MRI) with gadolinium will ultimately be needed. Laboratory evaluation should include serum electrolytes to evaluate for SIADH, salt wasting, or DI. A CBC is also useful to ensure the patient's hematocrit and platelet count are adequate for any upcoming procedures.

Management

The emergency management of increased ICP is critical as patients often present with signs and symptoms of this condition at the time of diagnosis. If increased ICP is known or suspected, a lumbar puncture should be avoided, as this theoretically may precipitate a rapid change in ICP followed by herniation of the brain. The pressure may be relieved using steroids such as dexamethasone at a dose of 2 to 4 mg every 6 hours. Mannitol may be useful in decreasing ICP. In some situations, intubation may be needed for both airway protection and to allow for hyperventilation to lower P_{CO_2} when signs of herniation are present. Neurosurgical consultation can address the appropriateness of a ventriculostomy or debulking procedure. The decision about whether to admit a patient with a newly diagnosed brain tumor hinges primarily on the neurologic status. Patients may have altered airway, breathing, or circulation due to the tumor compressing the brainstem. Cranial nerve dysfunction may compromise a patient's ability to eat normally. The tumor may cause symptoms such as headache, nausea, or vomiting, which require inpatient management. Functional deficits may make discharge problematic. In any of these cases, patients should be admitted to the hospital with prompt consultation with pediatric oncology, pediatric neurology, and pediatric neurosurgery for definitive management.

TUMORS OF THE HEAD AND NECK

Goals of Treatment

Children with head and neck tumors should be rapidly assessed for airway impingement, breathing compromise, and cervical spinal cord compression.

CLINICAL PEARL AND PITFALLS

- Cervical lymphadenopathy is common in childhood and rarely due to cancer. Characteristics that make malignancy more likely include nontender masses, very firm/hard texture, diameter more than 3 cm, adherence to other structures, irregular margins, and absence of signs or symptoms of infection.
- Retinoblastoma often presents with leukocoria (white pupil) first noticed by parents.

Current Evidence

Head and neck tumors represent a diverse range of conditions and, with the exception of retinoblastoma and neuroblastoma, occur most commonly in older children and teenagers. Aerodigestive tract malignancies include sarcomas, lymphoid tumors, and carcinomas. While the latter are commonly seen in the adult population, carcinoma is rare in pediatrics.

Clinical Considerations

Clinical Recognition

Intraorbital tumors may involve any of the tissues contained by the orbit including bone, muscle, soft tissue, and the globe itself. Masses in these regions have a wide differential diagnosis, which includes etiologies such as infections (periorbital and orbital cellulitis), orbital myositis, benign germ cell tumors, or cystic lesions such as a dermoid cyst. Retinoblastoma is the most common intraocular malignancy in children. It occurs in 1 in 23,000 births and is usually diagnosed by age 2. Two-thirds of patients with retinoblastoma present with a white pupil (leukocoria) noted by parents. This is the tumor as seen through the vitreous. The most common malignancies affecting the *bony orbit* are LCH and neuroblastoma. Presenting symptoms usually include proptosis and strabismus. Vascular tumors including capillary hemangiomas of the orbit may present with red or purple nodular lid lesions or proptosis.

Masses in the *aerodigestive tract* may be benign, infectious, or reactive in etiology. Regardless of the tissue of origin, these masses usually present with symptoms related to their anatomic position.

Oropharyngeal tumors such as with Burkitt lymphoma can cause snoring and obstructive sleep apnea as well as chronic otitis media and unilateral tonsillar hypertrophy. Gingival hypertrophy may be a sign of a monocytic leukemia. LCH or Burkitt lymphoma of the mandible can present with loose teeth. Rhabdomyosarcoma of the salivary or parotid gland often presents with pain or a facial mass. Malignant tumors of the nose, nasopharynx, and sinuses can present with purulent or bloody rhinorrhea, epistaxis, or sinusitis. Nasopharyngeal carcinoma tends to have a long duration of symptoms before diagnosis because symptoms are rarely specific. Malignant tumors of the sinuses and base of the skull can present with cranial neuropathies such as deviation of the eyes due to compression of the cranial nerves by the tumor. Rhabdomyosarcoma of the middle ear can present with persistent otitis, pain, or cranial neuropathy. The external ear canal can be affected by LCH leading to otorrhea and otitis externa.

Neck masses due to benign congenital anomalies such as branchial cleft cysts or cystic hygromas may grow suddenly as a result of infection or bleeding. Lymphadenopathy in children is common and usually benign. It is most commonly either reactive or infectious in etiology. Bilateral nodes may be associated with viral infections such as EBV or cytomegalovirus (CMV). Unilateral lymphadenopathy, especially in infants and young children, may be associated with *Staphylococcus aureus* or group A streptococcus infections. Even lymph node enlargement with a chronic time course is still most likely infectious (e.g., mycobacteria, cat-scratch disease, toxoplasma). Lymph nodes can appear large even without infection or malignancy, as observed in Castleman's, Kikuchi's, and Rosai–Dorfman syndromes. Enlarged lymph nodes in the neck due to malignancy can be from lymphoma or leukemia or can be because of metastasis from an adjacent solid tumor such as rhabdomyosarcoma, neuroblastoma, or nasopharyngeal carcinoma. It can be difficult to distinguish the primary tumor mass from a lymph node in these circumstances.

Clinical Assessment

Children with neck tumors, regardless of etiology, must be evaluated for impact on the airway, breathing, and circulation. Clinicians should explicitly consider the following:

- Does the mass impinge upon or compress the airway?
- Does the patient experience respiratory distress or is there a compromise to breathing?
- Does the mass interfere with circulation of the head and neck leading to SVC syndrome (discussed in section on thoracic tumors)?
- Does the tumor threaten to compress the cervical spine (see "Tumors In and Around the Spinal Cord" section)?

Following this assessment, a careful history should address the duration the mass has been present and its rate of growth, any recent infectious illnesses, the patient's immunization status, cat exposure, medications, and the presence of systemic systems. Physical examination should screen for other masses or lymphadenopathy in the body. In evaluating nodes of the neck, reactive nodes are often small, mobile, and soft, or while infected nodes may be enlarged, red, and tender. Characteristics that make malignancy more likely are nontender masses, very firm/hard texture, diameter more than 3 cm, adherence to other structures, irregular margins, and absence of signs or symptoms of infection.

Management

Often radiographic imaging and laboratory evaluation is not needed. However, in the case of suspected leukemia or lymphoma, laboratory studies should be obtained to assess for hyperleukocytosis, cytopenias, and TLS (see preceding discussion on leukemia). Radiographic imaging should be pursued if more information is needed about the tumor's position in relationship to the patient's airway and other vital structures of the head and neck. A CT scan is often helpful in establishing the neck anatomy in this way. In addition, a chest x-ray should be obtained to explore whether the disease could include a mass in the anterior mediastinum. Laboratory evaluation should include a CBC with differential, ESR and LDH (which may be elevated in certain lymphomas), testing for any relevant infectious etiologies, and consideration of thyroid function testing.

Children with leukocoria should have an urgent ophthalmologic examination to help differentiate retinoblastoma from other possible etiologies such as congenital cataract, coloboma, idiopathic retinal detachment, and others. Direct extension via the optic nerve into the meninges and spinal fluid is a possible but unlikely complication of the tumor. Presentations are usually local and therefore cured by enucleation, but systemic chemotherapy, intra-arterial (ophthalmic artery) chemotherapy, cryotherapy, laser therapy, and insertion of radioactive plaques are all being explored to preserve vision. Management of retinoblastoma hinges on the probability of useful vision in the affected eye. Ophthalmology should be consulted early to determine if the patient's visual acuity has already been affected by the mass and to plan the urgency of examination under anesthesia. Management of intraorbital tumors may be possible on an outpatient basis, in conjunction with an experienced pediatric ophthalmologist, if the mass is unlikely to affect vision quickly or if vision is already profoundly impaired in the affected eye.

Management of these tumors can sometimes occur on an outpatient basis, in conjunction with a pediatric oncologist and a specialist, such as an oral surgeon or otorhinolaryngologist with expertise in the anatomic region of the tumor. However, specific symptoms such as uncontrolled pain, difficulty maintaining hydration, TLS, or any evolving threat to the airway require inpatient management.

TUMORS OF THE THORAX

Goals of Treatment

The most critical decision making and care in the ED is the differentiation of emergent from nonemergent tumors of the thorax. This difference is frequently driven by tumor location (see Figure 132.11 in Thoracic Emergencies chapter).

CLINICAL PEARL AND PITFALLS

- Children with anterior mediastinal mass must be managed with the utmost caution. Prevention of respiratory failure is critical, as these masses may be located below the carina, rendering even intubation ineffective.

Current Evidence

Thoracic tumors can be caused by a number of childhood cancers. While hematologic malignancies are common, embryonal neoplasms such as neuroblastoma, sarcomas such as primitive neuroectodermal tumor (PNET), and carcinomas can also present in the chest. In general, there are no specific predisposing conditions or factors.

The anterior mediastinum is the most common location of a thoracic tumor in children. The "4 Ts" of the anterior mediastinal tumors include "terrible lymphoma," "teratoma," "thymoma," and "thyroid carcinoma." The latter three are rare. Nonmalignant conditions with AMM include adenopathy associated with infection, sarcoid, and normal thymus. Common lymphomas (Table 106.5) in the anterior mediastinum include T-cell lymphoblastic lymphoma (or T-cell ALL with an associated AMM), Hodgkin lymphoma, and diffuse B-cell large cell lymphoma. Lymphoma can also occur in the middle mediastinum, which can also be the site of masses associated with pulmonary sequestration and other developmental anomalies. "Teratoma" of the mediastinum includes benign and malignant germ cell tumors. Posterior mediastinal masses include neuroblastoma and other neurogenic tumors such as malignant peripheral nerve sheath tumors (especially in patients with neurofibromatosis, type 1), or benign lesions such as schwannoma.

Primary lung tumors are vanishingly rare in childhood but presentation of lung metastasis at diagnosis or relapse is not uncommon. Many pediatric sarcomas, some lymphomas, germ cell tumors, Wilms tumor, and rarely neuroblastoma can present or recur with lung metastasis. These typically involve multiple small or large lung nodules in the pulmonary parenchyma or are pleural based. Askin tumor is a unique PNET chest wall tumor that occurs in children and young adults.

Clinical Considerations

Clinical Recognition

Tumors in the anterior and middle mediastinum often present with respiratory symptoms ranging from mild cough to severe respiratory distress (Fig. 106.1). These tumors can compress the great vessels and cause SVC syndrome. When asymptomatic

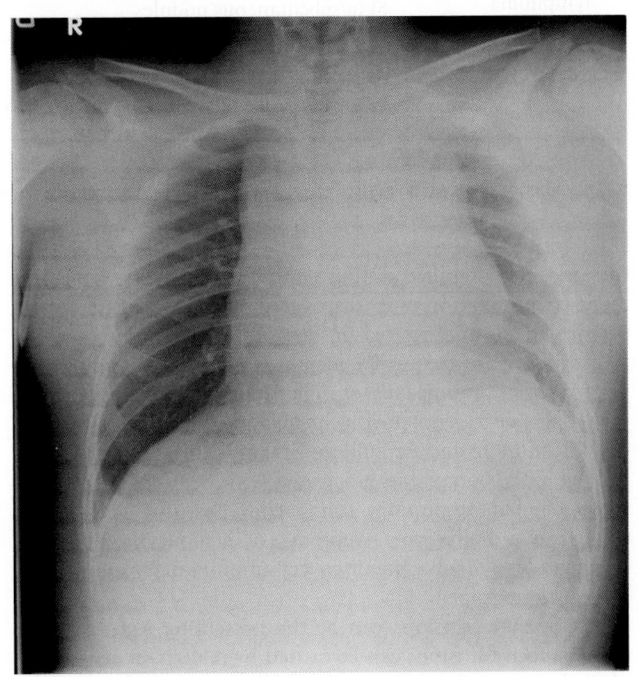

FIGURE 106.1 Chest radiograph demonstrating a large, homogenous anterior mediastinal mass. Patient presented with persistent cough and progressive orthopnea.

TABLE 106.5

LYMPHOMA PRESENTATIONS AND CONSIDERATIONS IN THE ED

Lymphoma	Typical presentation	Potential complications at diagnosis and considerations for ED management
Hodgkin disease	Painless, hard adenopathy: neck and supraclavicular common AMM common, with or without symptoms Pleural effusions uncommon May have "B" symptoms Fevers Night sweats Weight loss (at least 10% weight loss)	Superior vena cava (SVC) syndrome Tracheal obstruction
Lymphoblastic lymphoma	Painless, hard adenopathy at any site Respiratory symptoms from rapidly growing mediastinal mass, often with pleural effusions (T-lineage, advanced stage) GI tract involvement rare	Tumor lysis syndrome SVC syndrome Tracheal obstruction Pleural effusions
Burkitt lymphoma	Single site of enlarged lymphoid tissue (low stage) Incidental finding on appendectomy Asymmetric enlarged tonsil Lead point for intussusception in >3 yrs A single, painless enlarged node Painless, hard adenopathy with rapid growth (usually advanced stage) Rapidly progressing abdominal distention with diffuse involvement of the GI tract/liver with ascites and pleural effusions (advanced stage)	Rapid assessment for tumor lysis syndrome (TLS): High risk of severe tumor lysis, even prior to treatment (advanced stage) First dose rasburicase in ED if uric acid >8 and low-risk for G6PD deficiency Urgent consultation with oncology Admission to center with available pediatric dialysis
Diffuse large B-cell lymphoma	Painless, hard adenopathy at any site, neck/supraclavicular common AMM common, symptoms variable (advanced) Symptom progression can be rapid (advanced stage) Systemic symptoms of malaise, weight loss common with advanced disease GI symptoms/abdominal mass from GI tract and mesenteric nodes involvement	TLS SVC syndrome Tracheal obstruction
Anaplastic large cell lymphoma	Painless, hard adenopathy at any site Skin/subcutaneous nodules GI symptoms/abdominal mass from GI tract and mesenteric node involvement Systemic symptoms (fevers, night sweats, weight loss, malaise) common with advanced disease	TLS

AMM, anterior mediastinal mass; G6PD, glucose-6-phosphate dehydrogenase.

they may be identified during evaluation for nonspecific systemic symptoms or even discovered on a chest radiograph performed for another reason. In contrast, posterior mediastinal masses are frequently identified on a chest radiograph performed for another reason. They may, however, cause local pain from nerve root involvement and/or cord compression (see "Tumors In and Around the Spinal Cord" section).

The initial complaints associated with pulmonary metastasis may include respiratory insufficiency, postobstructive infection, foreign body–type symptoms, or hemoptysis. Presentation may also involve the discovery of pulmonary nodules on a chest radiograph.

Pulmonary effusions can be the presenting sign of childhood cancer. Effusions can be caused by malignant cells in the pleural space or from obstruction of lymphatic drainage. Effusions are common with AMM due to leukemia or lymphoma and can also occur with posterior mediastinal neuroblastoma, lung metastasis, and chest wall tumors. They may be symptomatic or asymptomatic. The effusion may obscure a mass on both chest x-ray and chest CT scan. Malignant pericardial effusions are most often associated with leukemias and lymphomas. For general diagnosis and management of pulmonary and pericardial effusions see Chapters 94 Cardiac Emergencies and 107 Pulmonary Emergencies. Askin tumor or metastatic sarcomas may present as a chest wall mass with or without pain. More commonly, it presents with respiratory symptoms from an effusion.

Clinical Assessment

There may be useful clues to the diagnosis from the history and physical examination. A recent history of new-onset asthma in an older child who responded to a course of steroids but has now returned is consistent with partial treatment of lymphoblastic leukemia or lymphoma. Many lymphomas can also present with nonspecific systemic symptoms such as weight loss, fatigue, unexplained fevers, night sweats, and malaise. Itching can be a paraneoplastic phenomenon associated with Hodgkin lymphoma. Examination should include assessment of all nodal groups (including axilla and supraclavicular) to both aid in the differential diagnosis and establish a site for possible biopsy. Of note, almost all pediatric lymphomas are high grade and have an acute to subacute course.

The initial focus should include a thorough assessment of airway, breathing, and circulation, all of which may be compromised by an AMM. When an AMM compresses the airway below the level of the carina, intubation will not be effective in managing respiratory failure. Management must focus on prevention of respiratory failure through such strategies as oxygen therapy and maximizing respiratory mechanics. Do not put the patient in a supine position if evidence of respiratory distress. Do not sedate or anesthetize the patient. Do not start empiric steroids without a discussion with an oncologist to ensure that steroids will not interfere with ability to establish the diagnosis. If there is evidence of SVC syndrome (plethora, facial edema, and jugular venous distention), ensure adequate intravascular volume to support systemic return. The patient should not receive anesthesia as it can lead to cardiovascular collapse.

Management

Diagnostic workup in the ED should always include a chest radiograph, including a lateral view, to help establish the location of the mass. Chest CT scan should only be performed in a patient who can comfortably lie supine. CT contrast should not be given without verifying adequate renal function since TLS can occur. Laboratory evaluations should include CBC to assess for evidence of marrow replacement and to identify circulating blasts. Metabolic screening for possible TLS should be performed. Patients with symptoms from an AMM must be admitted to a center with pediatric oncology expertise and may require critical care. If an effusion is drained in the ED for relief of symptoms, a fluid sample should be sent to pathology for cytology if malignancy is suspected. In general, patients who are not hemodynamically compromised by an effusion should not have fluid drained for diagnostic purposes while in the ED.

Patients who are systemically ill require admission for further evaluation and management. Those with minimal or no symptoms from the mass and no metabolic disturbances may be discharged to the care of a pediatric oncologist for further workup as an outpatient.

TUMORS OF THE HEPATOBILIARY TREE

Goals of Treatment

The most critical decision making and care in the ED is the differentiation of emergent from nonemergent. Most patients with newly diagnosed liver tumors in the ED can be managed as outpatients with close subspecialty follow-up.

CLINICAL PEARL AND PITFALLS

- Liver tumors are unusual in childhood and rarely require emergent management, except in the case of severe liver failure or tumor rupture causing hypovolemic shock.

TABLE 106.6

BENIGN AND MALIGNANT ABDOMINAL AND PELVIC MASSES IN CHILDREN

Location	Benign	Malignant
Hepatic	Adenoma Hemangioma Storage disease Hamartoma Infectious	Hepatoblastoma Hepatocellular carcinoma Sarcoma Metastatic disease Leukemia
Kidney/adrenal	Hydronephrosis Cysts Renal vein thrombosis Adrenal hemorrhage	Wilms tumor Renal cell carcinoma Rhabdoid tumor Neuroblastoma Pheochromocytoma Lymphoma
Gastrointestinal	Torsion/duplication Feces (constipation) Hernia Abscess Appendicitis	Gastrointestinal stromal tumor Lymphoma
Pancreas	Trauma Pseudocyst	Pancreatoblastoma (very rare)
Ovary	Torsion Cyst Immature teratoma	Lymphoma Germ cell tumor Sex cord/stromal tumor Carcinoma (rare)
Bladder/prostate	Duplication Cyst	Rhabdomyosarcoma

Current Evidence

Tumors of the hepatobiliary tree in children are more likely to be metastases rather than primary tumors of the liver (Table 106.6). Of the primary tumors, hepatoblastoma (HB) and hepatocellular carcinoma (HCC) are the most common (Fig. 106.2). HB usually occurs in patients younger than 6 years and is associated with risk factors such as overgrowth syndromes (e.g., Beckwith–Wiedemann), prematurity, and familial adenomatous polyposis (FAP). In contrast, HCC is more common in patients older than 6 years, particularly in children older than 10 years. Risk factors include chronic liver injury from inborn errors of metabolism such as tyrosinemia, glycogen storage disease type I, chronic hepatitis, chronic iatrogenic androgen exposure, or cirrhosis for any reason. In general, these latter risk factors rarely lead to cancer in childhood.

Clinical Considerations

Clinical Recognition

Typical presenting symptoms include abdominal mass, abdominal pain, and very rarely acute abdomen from massive hepatomegaly or tumor rupture. Other primary liver masses include embryonal sarcoma (extremely rare), nonmalignant vascular

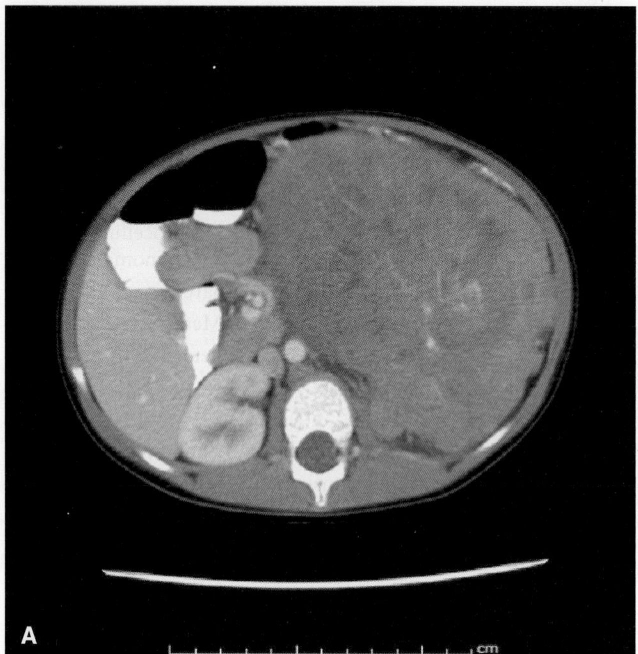

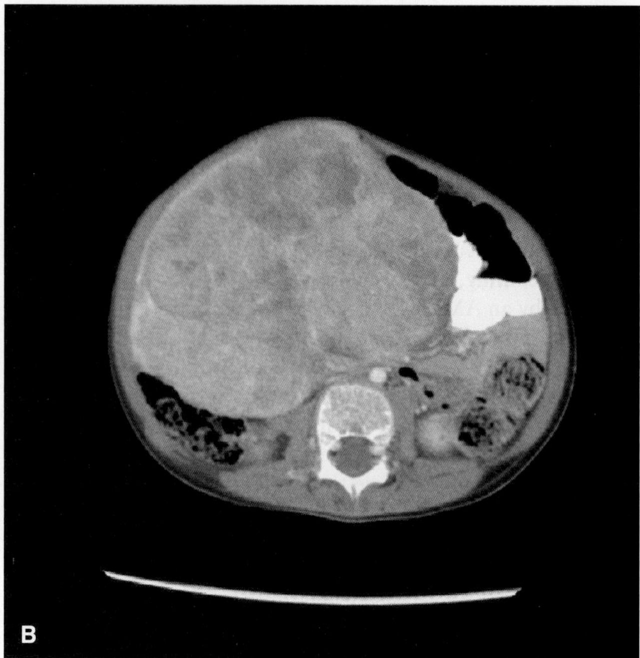

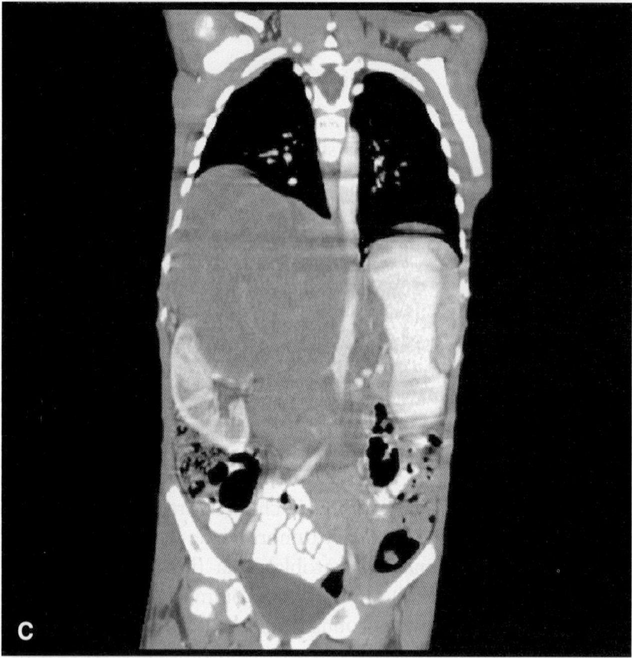

FIGURE 106.2 **A:** Wilms tumor. Computed tomography (CT) scan of the abdomen reveals a large mass entirely replacing the left kidney. **B:** Hepatoblastoma. CT scan of the abdomen reveals a large mass arising from the inferior aspect of the liver. The mass enhances heterogeneously with multiple low-density foci. **C:** Neuroblastoma. CT scan of the abdomen reveals a large mass originating from above the right kidney. The mass crosses the midline and displaces the right kidney laterally and inferiorly. The right adrenal gland is not visualized.

lesions such as infantile hemangioendothelioma, and malformations such as hamartoma. Focal nodular hyperplasia can cause a mass on liver imaging but rarely has associated symptoms or hepatic enlargement. Metastatic disease usually is characterized by diffuse nontender enlargement of the liver or multiple small nodules rather than a single dominant mass. Neuroblastoma and advanced hematologic malignancies such as ALL, AML, lymphoblastic lymphoma, and Burkitt's commonly metastasize to the liver. Although tumors may block biliary drainage, hepatic synthetic function is rarely affected by malignancy in the liver.

Clinical Assessment

Emergent management is rarely required except in the extremely rare setting of liver failure (see Chapter 99 Gastrointestinal Emergencies), tumor rupture that may require rapid repletion of intravascular volume and blood loss, or severe coagulopathy (see Chapter 101 Hematologic Emergencies). History may elicit risk factors or systemic symptoms such as malaise and anorexia that are more common with HCC than HB. Pain does not help with the differential diagnosis but does require management. Jaundice is most common with HCC but can occur with all liver tumors.

Management

Initial workup should include measurement of AST, ALT, total and direct bilirubin, CBC, PT, PTT, and fibrinogen. Alpha fetoprotein (AFP) can be elevated in both HB and HCC. It is important to note that normal AFP values are high in the first months of life, especially in premature infants. Initial diagnostic imaging should include an ultrasound, which can help identify if a palpable mass is likely to be hepatic in origin and if the liver contains one or multiple masses. If a CT scan is done in the ED, it is important to give intravenous contrast to look for intravascular extension of tumor from the hepatic veins, into the inferior vena cava, and possibly into the right atrium. Renal function should be checked before giving intravenous contrast. Since HB can metastasize to the lungs, consider performing a chest CT scan at the same time in patients younger than 10 years who have a primary liver tumor.

Children who are clinically stable and have a new liver tumor may be discharged from the ED to the care of a pediatric surgeon experienced with liver tumors or a pediatric oncologist. If the patient is unstable, they should be admitted to a center with experience in treating childhood malignancies.

TUMORS OF THE PANCREAS

Pancreatic tumors in children are very rare. They may develop in the setting of a predisposition, such as multiple endocrine neoplasias type 1 (MEN-1) syndrome, which is associated with insulinomas of the pancreas. Insulinomas will present with signs and symptoms of hypoglycemia and a history of "irrational behavior." Other tumors of the pancreas cause either an abdominal mass or vague, nonspecific abdominal symptoms. The differential diagnosis of a pancreatic mass includes nonmalignant adenoma or cystadenoma as well as malignant entities. Malignant tumors of the pancreas in children may be cystadenocarcinoma, pancreatoblastoma, an embryonal tumor, or an endocrine tumor such as insulinoma, gastrinoma, or VIPoma (Table 106.6). The pancreas may also be affected by metastatic disease from end-stage refractory cancer such as neuroblastoma or rhabdomyosarcoma.

A thorough history and physical examination should assess for endocrinologic ramifications that require medical management, such as hypoglycemia. The evaluation should include a serum AFP, which can be elevated in pancreatoblastoma. Diagnostic imaging may include a CT scan or MRI of the abdomen, but these tests are rarely needed in the ED.

The patient with a newly diagnosed pancreatic tumor may be discharged to home if the patient is otherwise well appearing and if arrangements have been made for an appropriate evaluation, including consultation with a pediatric surgeon, to continue in the outpatient setting. If the patient is ill, or if appropriate follow-up is otherwise unclear, then it is safest to admit the patient to the hospital. Surgical intervention is an important facet of the management plan for patients with pancreatic tumors, as several pancreatic tumors may be managed with just surgery alone.

TUMORS OF THE GASTROINTESTINAL TRACT

Tumors in the gastrointestinal (GI) tract in children include lymphomas, leukemias, gastrointestinal stromal tumors (GISTs), LCH, desmoplastic small round cell tumor, and colorectal carcinomas (Table 106.6). Risk factors for GI lymphomas include primary immunodeficiency. Neurofibromatosis type 1 increases the risk of GIST. FAP, Li–Fraumeni syndrome, and ulcerative colitis increase the risk of colon cancer.

Common presentations include nonspecific symptoms such as weight loss, nausea/vomiting, loss of appetite, change in bowel habits, abdominal distention, or abdominal pain. Chronic GI blood loss can cause iron deficiency anemia. Abdominal distention from masses or ascites may be present. Severe GI bleeding is a rare presentation of GI malignancy but one that requires immediate management as in Chapter 28 Gastrointestinal Bleeding. Symptoms of intermittent GI obstruction may be present. Complete obstruction is an extremely rare presentation and may require urgent surgical intervention. The lead point for intussusception in children older than 3 years may be a primary GI lymphoma. Incidental findings on appendectomies in children can include Burkitt lymphoma or carcinoid tumor.

Lymphomas involving the GI tract and/or mesenteric nodes in children include Burkitt lymphoma and large cell lymphoma (Table 106.5). Advanced Burkitt lymphoma should be suspected in patients with a rapidly evolving clinical picture of progressive abdominal distention, abdominal masses, and/or ascites. If the initial evaluation of a pediatric patient with abdominal symptoms demonstrates evidence of a very high uric acid, LDH that is many times normal, or renal insufficiency, the diagnosis of advanced Burkitt lymphoma should be suspected. Colorectal carcinoma is extremely rare in children and often presents with advanced stage disease. LCH, particularly in children younger than 1 year, can present with GI involvement manifested by formula intolerance or occult or overt lower GI blood loss. Other signs and symptoms of LCH are usually present (see section on "Histiocytic Diseases"). GISTs tend to occur in older children and adolescents and often involve the stomach and upper GI tract. This tends to be a slow-paced disease and may present with vague GI symptom and/or evidence of upper GI bleeding. Mesenteric adenopathy alone should not raise the suspicion of malignancy since a reactive process is far more likely than a malignancy in children. Mesenteric adenopathy can be associated with most of the diseases above but there is usually evidence of other abnormality on imaging. Massive adenopathy can also occur in three extremely rare nonmalignant conditions: sinus histiocytosis, Castleman disease, and Kikuchi disease.

As above, severe GI bleeding or complete GI obstruction requires rapid assessment and intervention (see Chapters 28 Gastrointestinal Bleeding and 99 Gastrointestinal Emergencies). In most patients, however, the evaluation can proceed at a more measured pace. The history and physical examination should focus on the specific findings noted above that can lead to the suspicion of a GI-based malignancy. Laboratory evaluation should include a CBC to look for evidence of blood loss, and baseline hepatic and renal function. If initial evaluation suggests advanced lymphoma, a full metabolic assessment as in the section on "Leukemia" should be completed urgently. Diagnostic imaging should be performed based on the findings and suspected diagnoses. An abdominal x-ray may reveal abnormalities of the bowel gas pattern suggestive of ascites or mass. Ultrasound can be helpful to assess the likely organ of origin of a palpable abdominal mass but rarely is sufficient to establish a diagnosis. Ultrasound findings consistent with lymphoma can include bowel wall thickening or intussusception. If a primary GI malignancy is suspected, a CT scan with both intravenous and oral contrast should be performed after establishing that renal function is adequate for intravenous contrast. In otherwise stable patients, this imaging can be performed subsequent to the ED evaluation.

Patients with evidence of high cell turnover on metabolic assessment and a suspected diagnosis of advanced Burkitt lymphoma must be admitted to a center capable of performing pediatric renal dialysis. Other patients with a suspected GI malignancy should be admitted or referred to a center with pediatric oncology expertise.

NEUROBLASTOMA

Goals of Treatment

Neuroblastoma has a wide range of clinical presentations, depending on tumor location as well as duration of symptoms. A high index of suspicion should be maintained in diagnosing these malignancies.

CLINICAL PEARL AND PITFALLS

- The periorbital ecchymoses of neuroblastoma and the subcutaneous pigmented lesions of Stage 4S neuroblastoma seen in infants can both be mistaken for child abuse.

Current Evidence

Neuroblastoma is derived from neural crest cells that exist not only within the adrenal medulla but also along the sympathetic chain. It is the most common solid tumor of childhood outside the CNS, accounting for 7% to 10% of pediatric tumors overall. With an incidence of 1 per 7,000 live births, neuroblastoma preferentially affects very young children; 50% of cases are diagnosed by age 2 and 90% by age 5. In approximately two-thirds of cases, the primary tumor is in the abdomen, specifically in the adrenal gland.

Clinical Considerations

Clinical Recognition

Neuroblastoma presentation can be clinically variable, depending on location. Bone pain may develop if the tumor involves osseous sites. Marrow replacement can cause signs or symptoms of anemia, thrombocytopenia, or neutropenia. Large masses of the chest or abdomen may impair pulmonary function and cause respiratory distress. Abdominal masses may cause GI dysmotility, such as constipation or bowel obstruction, as well as inability to tolerate oral intake and secondary cachexia.

Potentially life-threatening or organ-threatening complications of neuroblastoma include the development of SVC syndrome from a mass in the posterior mediastinum that extends anteriorly or cord compression from tumor growing through the neural foramina into the spinal canal. See sections on "Thoracic Tumors" and "Tumors In and Around the Spinal Cord" for the approach to these complications. However, at times neuroblastoma presents in a healthy, well-appearing child with an abdominal mass incidentally detected. Other unique presentations include ipsilateral Horner syndrome (ptosis, miosis, and anhydrosis) from involvement of the cervical sympathetic ganglia, "raccoon eyes" from periorbital bone and soft tissue involvement causing proptosis and ecchymosis, and opsoclonus myoclonus. This latter is a paraneoplastic syndrome characterized by "dancing eyes and dancing feet" and is associated with a favorable cancer prognosis but a poor neurocognitive outcome. Neuroblastoma can secrete catecholamines that cause hypertension and vasoactive intestinal peptide that causes secretory diarrhea. Subcutaneous nodules can occur.

Clinical Assessment

Initial assessment of a child with possible neuroblastoma should include an assessment of the patient's airway, breathing, and circulation, followed by a complete history and physical examination that focuses on the potential signs and symptoms above. Given the risk of cord compression from a retromediastinal or retroperitoneal tumor, all patients should have a thorough neurologic examination including percussing the vertebral bodies, with emergent imaging should neurologic deficits be detected. The patient's blood pressure should be measured and carefully matched against norms for age. Signs and symptoms of pain should also be explored to localize potential tumor masses and pain should be treated as needed.

Laboratory evaluation should include CBC, liver function testing, renal function testing (BUN and creatinine), and urine catecholamines. If neuroblastoma is suspected and the disease burden is high, TLS may develop (see "Leukemia" section). If the CBC shows evidence of marrow replacement, platelet and packed red blood cell transfusions may be needed (see Table 107.7). A plain film of the chest or abdomen may be useful for detecting calcifications. Abdominal ultrasound may help define the location of a mass and its relationship to other structures. CT scans should include the suspected site of the primary tumor, the surrounding lymph node groups, and the liver (a common site of metastasis).

Management

If a thorough evaluation and initial management finds no life-threatening or organ-threatening problems, no uncontrolled pain, and no evidence of severe systemic illness, discharge to the care of a pediatric oncologist may be possible. Otherwise admission is recommended.

TUMORS OF THE KIDNEY

Goals of Treatment

The most critical decision making and care in the ED is the differentiation of emergent from nonemergent. Stable patients with newly diagnosed kidney tumors can be managed as outpatients with close subspecialty follow-up.

CLINICAL PEARL AND PITFALLS

- Most patients with Wilms tumor have an asymptomatic abdominal mass, but potentially life-threatening conditions include hypertension, gross hematuria, and an acute abdomen.

Current Evidence

There are several different causes of renal tumors in children, some malignant and some benign. Wilms tumor, the most common pediatric renal tumor, arises from embryonic renal blastemal cells (see Figure 106.2). Overgrowth syndromes such as Beckwith–Wiedemann, Soto syndrome, hemihypertrophy, and Denys–Drash syndrome predispose to embryonal tumors such as Wilms'. There are 500 cases of Wilms' diagnosed annually in United States with peak incidence between the ages of 2 and 3. Eighty percent of cases are diagnosed by age 5.

The differential diagnosis of a pediatric renal mass also includes benign lesions such as hydronephrosis, multicystic or polycystic kidneys, and mesoblastic nephroma. The age of the patient can help clarify the likely etiology of a renal mass. For example, a neonatal mass is less likely to be malignant and more likely a congenital malformation of the genitourinary (GU) tract. Both neuroblastoma and Wilms tumor most commonly develop in the 1- to 5-year age range. Other less common malignant tumors include rhabdoid tumor of the kidney, clear cell sarcoma, and mesoblastic nephroma. Carcinomas, including medullary carcinoma and renal cell carcinoma, are extremely rare. Hematologic malignancies often metastasize to the kidney but rarely present with a solitary lesion.

Clinical Considerations

Clinical Recognition

Wilms tumors most commonly present with a painless mass found incidentally by either the parents or pediatrician in a child who is otherwise well appearing (see Figure 107.2). Masses are deep in the flank, smooth, and may be firm or soft. Wilms tumor may have more serious or life-threatening presentations including the following:

- Hypertension due to increased renin secretion from renal artery compression, in less than 15% of cases;
- Gross hematuria in less than 25% of cases (although microscopic hematuria is very common);
- Hematologic complications such as anemia, tumor thrombus in the renal veins with or without extension into the inferior vena cava; and
- Abdominal compartment syndrome from a massive renal tumor in a very small child.

Clinical Assessment

A thorough history and physical examination is needed, including assessment of measured blood pressure against normal values for age. Because Wilms tumor can be associated with other syndromes, such as Beckwith–Wiedemann syndrome and WAGR (Wilms tumor, aniridia, GU anomalies, mental retardation) syndrome, the physical examination should screen for physical anomalies that may signal that the renal mass is part of a larger picture. The clinician should assess and treat pain as needed. Laboratory evaluation should include a CBC to look for evidence of bleeding, a urinalysis, and liver and renal function testing (BUN and creatinine). Serum calcium may be elevated in rhabdoid tumor of the kidney or congenital mesoblastic nephroma.

Radiographic evaluation can be helpful in further defining the tumor. Ultrasound can define the anatomic position of the mass, explore whether it has cystic or solid components, and assess for any hydronephrosis or ureteral obstruction. The radiologist should assess for tumor thrombus in renal veins or inferior vena cava. Centers skilled in pediatric imaging may elect to perform a CT scan with intravenous contrast. If it is certain that the mass is renal in origin, it is appropriate to include the chest to evaluate for presence of lung metastasis.

Management

The initial management of renal masses should focus on a determination of how ill the patient is and consultation with a pediatric oncologist or pediatric surgeon. Well-appearing patients without evidence of bleeding may be discharged if appropriate follow-up with a pediatric oncologist or surgeon is arranged.

TUMORS OF THE LOWER GENITOURINARY TRACT

While tumors of the lower GU tract in adults are most commonly carcinomas, in children these tumors are more likely to be sarcomas. Their presentation is determined by their location. Vaginal tumors are most commonly rhabdomyosarcomas of the botryoid histology. These tumors classically present protruding from the vagina, accompanied by a mucous/bloody discharge. Uterine tumors more commonly present in adolescent girls and may cause a palpable mass or vaginal discharge. Tumors of the bladder may present with hematuria, urinary obstruction, or extrusion of tumor tissue from the urethra. Bladder tumors, most common in children younger than 4 years, are usually within the lumen of the bladder. Prostate tumors are usually rhabdomyosarcomas that can cause constipation, urinary obstruction, or a large pelvic mass. Paratesticular tumors present as painless unilateral scrotal enlargement or swelling (see section on "Gonadal Tumors" for details on testicular tumors).

The management of patients presenting with these tumors should begin with a thorough history and physical examination. Children are not usually acutely ill at the time of presentation. Most of the evaluation can be done on an outpatient basis, in consultation with a pediatric oncologist. The emergency physician should ensure adequate bowel, bladder, and renal function as well as appropriate analgesia. An ultrasound may be useful to determine where the tumor is located. The most common reason for admission is management of urinary obstruction.

GONADAL TUMORS

In children, most gonadal tumors are derived from malignant transformation of the primordial germ cells, although other tissues within the gonads may be the source of malignant cells. Presentation of these tumors varies based on the gender of the patient and the stage of development (i.e., the maturity) of the germ cell when the malignancy begins. During embryonic development, germ cells migrate to the gonads, but aberrant migration in the setting of malignancy can lead to extragonadal germ cell tumors. This section will focus on tumors located within the gonads themselves.

Tumors of the ovary are rare and account for only 1% of pediatric cancers overall. While they may occur at any age, the incidence begins to increase at 8 to 9 years and peaks at 19 years of age. Two-thirds of pediatric ovarian tumors are germ cell tumors. Abdominal pain is the most common presenting symptom, occurring in 80% of patients. Pain may be chronic or acute, mimicking an acute abdomen, as the tumor can cause ovarian torsion. Other presenting signs and symptoms include a palpable abdominal mass, dysfunction of the bowel or bladder, or menstrual changes. Some ovarian tumors may cause precocious puberty or virilization.

If a patient has a known or possible ovarian mass, the history and physical examination should include a thorough menstrual history as well as assessment of any virilization or precocious puberty. The differential diagnosis should include benign etiologies, such as an ovarian cyst. Laboratory evaluation should include a CBC, chemistries, quantitative beta human chorionic gonadotropin (β-HCG), AFP, LDH, and CA-125. Ultrasound can clarify whether the tumor is cystic or solid as well as location. Further imaging should generally be carried out only in conjunction with the managing oncologist or surgeon and rarely needs to be performed in the ED.

Malignant masses are most commonly germ cell derived. Of these, the more common are dysgerminoma, which may be bilateral in 20% of cases, and endodermal sinus tumor (yolk sac tumor), which presents with an elevated AFP. Malignant tumors may also be derived from nongerm cell ovarian tissue or from nonovarian tissues, as is the case for ovarian involvement in leukemia or lymphoma.

Tumors of the testicle are rare and account for only 2% of solid neoplasms in boys. While they may occur at any age, testicular tumors seen in adolescents are similar to those found in adults. Prepubertal boys have tumors with unique clinical manifestations and different prognostic implications. The major risk factor for the development of a testicular tumor is the presence of an undescended testicle, even after repair. Approximately 75% of pediatric testicular tumors are germ cell tumors (as compared with more than 90% in the adult population).

Testicular tumors commonly present as an enlarged testicle or as irregular, nontender scrotal masses that do not transilluminate. They may have minimal or no associated symptoms, which may delay the diagnosis. At the time of diagnosis, 20% of patients will also have an inguinal hernia and another 20% will have a hydrocele. About 75% of these tumors are localized at diagnosis, but sites of potential metastases include retroperitoneal lymph nodes and the chest.

The clinician in the ED should perform a thorough history and physical examination looking for evidence of virilization or precocious puberty as occurs with functional tumors. Laboratory evaluation should include a CBC, chemistries, quantitative β-HCG, and AFP. Imaging should begin with an ultrasound that can clarify the presence of a mass, and whether the tumor is cystic or solid and whether it is derived from the testicle itself or paratesticular tissues.

When evaluating scrotal enlargement, it is critical to distinguish testicular tumors from paratesticular masses, and from other etiologies such as a varicocele or scrotal edema. Almost all paratesticular tumors are rhabdomyosarcomas. Malignant tumors in the testis itself include germ cell tumors of all histologies, sex cord tumors, leukemia, lymphoma, and neuroblastoma. Teratomas, representing 10% of testicular tumors, develop mostly in children younger than 4 years. Embryonal carcinoma, the testicular tumor most commonly seen in adults, is rare in the pediatric population until late adolescence.

TUMORS IN AND AROUND THE SPINAL CORD

Tumors can come into contact with the spinal cord through various mechanisms. Those derived from tissues in close proximity can grow into and impinge upon the cord. Primary tumors from either adjacent bone (see "Tumors of Bone" section) or adjacent parameningeal soft tissues, as in neuroblastoma or soft tissue sarcomas (STSs), or from the spinal cord itself (gliomas, ependymomas) can cause cord compression. The same tumors when present at another site can also metastasize to tissue in or around the spinal cord. Tumors in the fourth ventricle can produce drop metastases that grow and compress the spinal cord. Neuroblastoma, in particular, is known for its ability to spread through spinal foramina and then expand within the spinal canal. In addition, leukemic blasts can infiltrate the paraspinal soft tissues to form a chloroma, which can enlarge to compress the spinal cord as well (see "Leukemia" section).

Evaluation of spinal cord involvement begins with a thorough history exploring whether the patient has had pain or focal neurologic symptoms including weakness or paresis which could indicate cord compression. More subtle complaints such as urinary retention, fecal incontinence, or constipation could also indicate compression of the spinal cord. A thorough neurologic examination should follow looking for loss of reflexes, focal or asymmetric weakness, sensory deficits, or an upgoing Babinski reflex. Percussion tenderness of the posterior vertebral elements should be assessed. Any abnormalities should provoke neuroimaging with a spine MRI. Management of cord compression should include analgesia, as patients are frequently in severe pain. Glucocorticoids usually improve the pain within several hours, but most patients require opiate analgesics to tolerate the physical examination and necessary diagnostic studies. Management of the compression begins with steroids, most commonly dexamethasone at a starting dose of 0.25 to 0.5 mg per kg IV (maximum dose is usually 10 mg as an initial dose followed by doses of 4 mg every 6 hours thereafter). Multispecialty consultation with neurosurgery, radiation oncology, and pediatric oncology is optimal when choosing among surgical decompression, radiation therapy, and chemotherapy. Decisions must consider both the short-term efficacy of the treatment to relieve the compression as well as the long-term consequences.

TUMORS OF BONE

Goal of Treatment

Many patients with newly diagnosed bone tumors may be able to be discharged with proper subspecialty follow-up. If discharged, consider immobilizing the affected extremity in efforts to prevent the development of a pathologic fracture.

CLINICAL PEARLS AND PITFALLS

- A history of trauma does not rule out a malignant etiology of bone pain.
- Radiographic signs of bone malignancy include periosteal elevation, ossification of soft tissue masses in a "sunburst" pattern, and lytic lesions with irregular borders.

Current Evidence

Primary bone tumors are uncommon pediatric malignancies, but bone tumors are the third most frequent malignancy of adolescent and young adults. In the United States, it is estimated that 2,400 primary bone tumors are diagnosed annually in children.

Osteosarcoma and Ewing sarcoma are the most common primary malignant bone tumors. Osteosarcoma is characterized

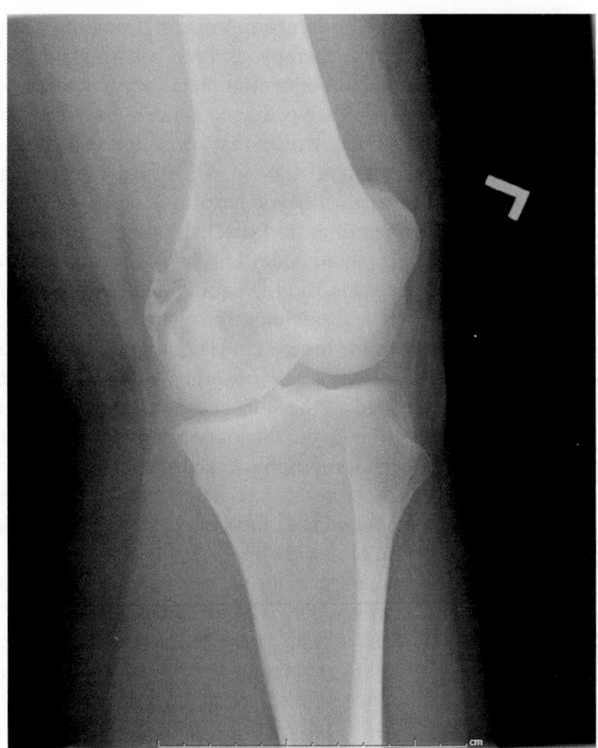
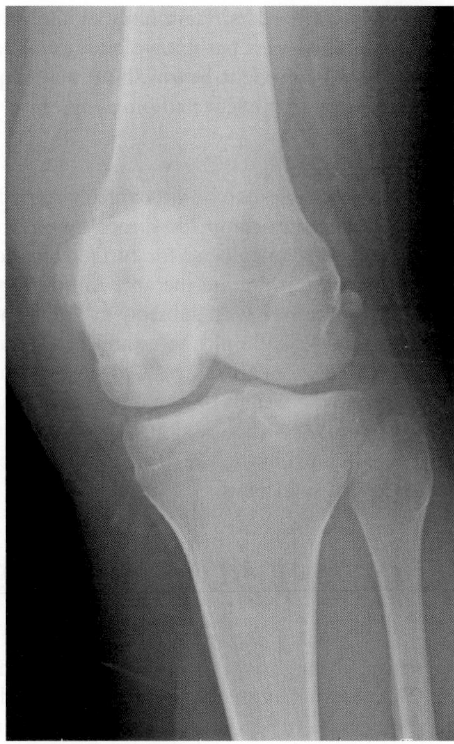

FIGURE 106.3 Two plain radiographs demonstrating osteosarcoma of the distal femur.

by its production of immature bone or osteoid. It is the most common malignant bone tumor in children and adolescents, presenting most often in the second and third decades of life. Although Ewing sarcoma is second to osteosarcoma in overall frequency, it affects children and adolescents of all ages and is more common than osteosarcoma in children younger than 10 years. Leukemia, lymphoma, LCH, and metastases from neuroblastoma, sarcomas, and other childhood tumors can all cause bone pain and abnormalities on radiograph (Fig. 106.3).

Clinical Considerations

Clinical Recognition

The differential diagnosis of a bony mass includes both benign and malignant entities. Subacute osteomyelitis can present with fever, elevated inflammatory markers, pain, and swelling over the involved bone. Benign tumors of bone account for half of the bone tumors in children and include giant cell tumor, eosinophilic granuloma, and aneurysmal bone cysts. Benign lesions usually have smooth, well-defined borders on plain radiographs and rarely have associated soft tissue masses. Presentation of malignant bone lesions commonly includes pain at the tumor site (in 80% to 90% of cases), soft tissue swelling, and/or a painful limp. The pain may wake the patient at night in some cases (less than 25%).

Clinical Assessment

Diagnostic evaluation in the ED should include a thorough history and physical examination. Though there is frequently a history of trauma in retrospect, pain may be intermittent and nondescript for weeks or months. Constitutional symptoms or signs, such as fever, fatigue, and weight loss may occur with Ewing sarcoma/PNET. If tumor is present in an extremity, a hard mass may be felt. Osteosarcoma usually involves the metaphyseal end of long bones, most commonly around the knee or proximal humerus. Ewing can occur in any bone but tends to involve the diaphysis when in a long bone. An extremity with a bony mass should be completely examined with careful attention to pulses, perfusion, range of motion, and sensation. Compartment syndrome may develop due to swelling or bleeding within the mass. Pelvic lesions often produce no specific physical findings. Lesions of the vertebral body may evoke neurologic symptoms such as neuropathic pain or cord compression. In this setting, a careful history of bowel and bladder function should be taken and a thorough neurologic examination performed. Any focal neurologic deficits should prompt immediate imaging of the spinal cord to determine if compression is present.

Laboratory evaluation should include a CBC, evaluation of renal and liver function, inflammatory markers, and serum LDH. Diagnostic imaging should begin with a plain radiograph of the affected region for characteristics concerning for tumor, as well as to assess for the presence of a pathologic fracture. Characteristic findings of primary bone tumors include a lytic lesion with cortical destruction. Early changes include loss of soft tissue fat planes and periosteal elevation (Codman triangle), which has been associated with osteosarcoma. Over time, an "onion skin" periosteal reaction develops, caused by repetitive episodes of the lesion pushing out the periosteum and followed by the periosteum responding by laying down calcium. This finding has been associated with Ewing sarcoma. Neither finding is specific. With osteosarcoma, the associated soft tissue mass is sometimes ossified in a radial or "sunburst" pattern. Benign bone tumors such as eosinophilic granuloma, aneurysmal bone cysts, and giant cell tumor of bone can present as lytic lesions that tend to have smooth, well-defined borders. Plain films should always be assessed for the presence of a pathologic fracture. A large lesion with a thin cortex in a weight-bearing bone may require immediate immobilization to prevent pathologic fracture.

Management

Often patients with bony masses can be discharged with follow-up securely arranged with an orthopedic surgeon with oncology expertise or a pediatric oncologist for further diagnostic workup and initiation of appropriate therapy. An improperly performed biopsy may interfere with subsequent limb-sparing surgery. A plan for analgesia should be established prior to discharge. Patients with tumors affecting the lower extremities should refrain from bearing weight on the affected limb so as to avoid causing a pathologic fracture. Inpatient management is appropriate for pain control or in the presence of cord compression or compartment syndrome.

TUMORS OF THE SOFT TISSUES

Tumors of the soft tissues present the clinician with a diagnostic challenge. Many of these lesions are benign. Rhabdomyosarcoma is the most common STS in children. There are many other types of STS that collectively account for less than 1% of all pediatric cancer. They can arise in any anatomic location because connective tissue is located throughout the body. Masses are frequently painless and asymptomatic. Any presenting symptoms are usually due to local nerve invasion leading to pain or weakness. Systemic symptoms are rare. The histologic variants of rhabdomyosarcoma tend to have characteristic presentations. Botryoid tumors tend to grow in potential spaces such as the bladder and vagina. Embryonal tumors often occur in the GU tract, orbit and head, neck, and parameningeal locations. Alveolar tumors often present in the extremities and have a worse prognosis. Rhabdomyosarcoma can metastasize to local lymph nodes, lungs, bone, and rarely bone marrow.

There are many benign causes of soft tissue masses in children but the emergency physician needs to consider cancer as a possible cause. Diagnostic evaluation should include a thorough history and physical examination. The history should focus on symptoms caused by the mass and other systemic or constitutional symptoms that may be present. When a reasonable suspicion for cancer exists, laboratory evaluation should include a CBC, renal and liver function tests, and serum LDH. A plain radiograph of the affected area can be useful to look for bone destruction or fracture from an underlying bone lesion. A true soft tissue mass, however, is best imaged with an MRI. Often patients can be discharged with follow-up securely arranged with a pediatric oncologist for further diagnostic workup and initiation of appropriate therapy. Inpatient management may be needed for pain control or if cord compression complicates the presentation.

CANCERS OF THE SKIN

Primary cancers of the skin, such as squamous or basal cell carcinoma or melanoma, are seen in the adult practice setting but rarely occur in children. Melanoma accounts for less than 3% of all childhood malignancies but occurs occasionally in adolescents 15 to 19 years old. There may be increased risk in the setting of immunosuppression, immunodeficiencies, history of radiation therapy or stem cell transplant, giant congenital nevi, giant congenital melanocytic nevi, or xeroderma pigmentosum. Other pediatric cancers may involve the skin, such as leukemia, which may produce leukemia cutis (particularly in infant ALL or in AML). Rash may be part of the presentation of histiocytic disorders, such as HLH or LCH. Neuroblastoma does not affect the skin but may present with subcutaneous pigmented nodules visible through the skin.

Management in the ED should begin with a thorough history and physical examination. The examination should be used to screen for other skin lesions, lymphadenopathy, hepatosplenomegaly, masses, or other signs of malignancy that might be related to the skin findings. If the history and physical examination suggest a particular diagnosis, then further laboratory or radiographic evaluation may be helpful. If not, and if the patient appears to be stable without signs or symptoms of systemic illness, then the patient can be discharged to home with follow-up secured with either oncology or dermatology. When cancer is suspected, a biopsy will aid in the diagnosis and involvement from a dermatopathologist with pediatric experience will be essential. Some melanocytic lesions in children may appear malignant to pathologists without sufficient experience with the pediatric population.

SECTION II: MANAGEMENT OF COMPLICATIONS ASSOCIATED WITH CANCER AND CANCER THERAPY

This section focuses on the complications of cancer treatment that are likely to lead to an ED visit for care. The systems-based review of management below focuses on the initial care of the patient and does not address the more detailed evaluation and management needed subsequently. Complications of specific chemotherapeutic agents are listed in Table 106.8.

HEMATOLOGIC COMPLICATIONS OF CANCER TREATMENT

Goals of Treatment

Cytopenias are common in both newly diagnosed cancer patients as well as those undergoing active therapy, and a high index of suspicion should be maintained for all of these patients.

CLINICAL PEARLS AND PITFALLS

- Patients receiving chemotherapy should be presumed to be neutropenic and isolated from the potential sources of infection that exist in the ED as soon as possible.
- Patients with thrombocytopenia requiring procedures may benefit from platelet infusion during the procedure itself.

Current Evidence

Many chemotherapeutics cause reversible myelosuppression. Neutrophils have a very short half-life and thus their numbers may drop rapidly after initiation of treatment, but also may recover quickly. Platelets have a slightly longer half-life and thus tend to drop and recover slightly more slowly. Because red blood cell half-life is over 100 days, chemotherapy effects tend to be more chronic than acute. The nadir blood counts usually occur 7 to 10 days after start of treatment and recovery usually occurs 10 to 14 days after start of treatment. The pattern of myelosuppression differs by chemotherapy regimen. For example, most solid tumor regimens allow for complete recovery within 10 to 14 days, while acute myelogenous leukemia regimens may delay recovery until 4 to 6 weeks after treatment. Even within a given regimen, there is variation both among patients and among cycles for one patient. In general, recovery is slower for patients who have already received many cycles of chemotherapy, whose course has been complicated by infection, or whose bone marrow has been extensively replaced by tumor. Radiation to the marrow cavity, especially including the spine or pelvis, can also cause myelosuppression during treatment and/or delayed recovery after treatment. In addition, cytopenias are a common finding in patients with newly diagnosed leukemia.

Significant neutropenia is usually defined as an ANC below 500 cells per μL. The ANC is calculated by multiplying the percentage of WBCs that are neutrophils or bands by the total WBC count. Patients with an ANC below 500 have an increased risk of bacterial infections due to insufficient numbers of phagocytic cells to fight bacteria. This risk increases dramatically when the ANC is below 100. Patients may develop infections with bacteria that are not pathogens in normal hosts. The risk of fungal infections increases with prolonged (more than 21 days) and severe (ANC below 500) neutropenia. The infectious risks of neutropenia are increased by a number of contributing factors. Indwelling foreign bodies such as central lines, ventriculoperitoneal shunts, and bone allografts provide a foreign surface that increases the likelihood of infection and the difficulty of treatment. The mucosal injury that typically accompanies myelosuppression increases the risk of bacteria entering the circulation through the process of translocation across disrupted mucosal surfaces. Immunosuppression decreases phagocytic function as well.

Most chemotherapy causes immunosuppression that affects WBC function, independent of WBC count. The immunosuppression persists throughout treatment and for 6 to 12 months after completion of chemotherapy, but varies by chemotherapy regimen. The impact of immunosuppression may be more profound in the patient younger than 1 year because of the immaturity of the immune system. Stem cell transplant recipients have very severe immunosuppression (see "Complications of Hematopoietic Stem Cell Transplantation" section).

Thrombocytopenia is defined as a platelet count of less than 150,000 per μL, but the risk of bleeding at a given platelet count may vary (Table 106.7). Anemia is very common in oncology patients and tends to be a chronic problem due to underproduction.

Bleeding complications are common in oncology patients. In addition to thrombocytopenia, bleeding may occur because of coagulopathy resulting from a number of different factors. Leukemia itself may cause coagulopathy. Many patients are also on anticoagulation therapy for previous clotting problems. Any bleeding risk from the anticoagulation may be exacerbated by intercurrent thrombocytopenia. Bleeding in and around solid tumors tends to be more common at diagnosis and with relapse. Bleeding can also occur after biopsy or tumor resection. Mucosal injury from treatment can contribute to bleeding throughout the GI tract.

Cancer patients have an increased risk of clotting due to a number of factors such as compression of vessels by tumor, disturbance of flow from central lines, asparaginase-induced deficiency of endogenous anticoagulants, decreased physical activity, and immobilization due to surgery. Thrombotic complications may include pulmonary emboli (PE), deep venous thromboses (DVT), or central venous sinus thrombosis, a rare complication in patients on asparaginase chemotherapy.

Clinical Considerations

Clinical Recognition

Symptoms of anemia in the cancer patient often occur at a much lower hemoglobin level compared with patients who are not receiving therapy because patients compensate for the chronic anemia. When patients become symptomatic, the signs and symptoms are typical: pallor, lethargy, headache, dizziness when rising from a supine/sitting position, and resting tachycardia. Thrombocytopenia can be accompanied by petechiae, ecchymoses, epistaxis, other mucosal bleeding and in severe cases, hemorrhage. There are no specific signs or symptoms of neutropenia and emergency physicians must assume that any patient actively receiving chemotherapy is neutropenic until proven otherwise. Bleeding can be associated with coagulopathy with or without accompanied thrombocytopenia, particularly in leukemia patients receiving asparaginase therapy. Catheter-related clots may present with line dysfunction, obvious or subtle signs of edema in the head or one upper extremity, or collateral vessels visible on the upper chest. The presentation of central venous sinus thrombosis usually consists of vague and/or nonspecific symptoms including seizure, headache, nausea, and vomiting. Physical examination may or may not have focal neurologic findings, altered mental status, or papilledema.

Clinical Assessment

A detailed history of recent chemotherapy administration can be helpful in predicting risk for cytopenias, febrile neutropenia, coagulopathies, and thrombosis. *Neutropenic patients should be isolated from the potential infectious exposures that can occur in an ED by rapid triage and placement in a private room.* In addition, routine procedures such as a rectal examination or temperature, or urinary catheterization increase the risk of bacteremia and should be avoided. Vital signs may reveal fever, hypotension, orthostasis, tachycardia, and hypoxia. Physical examination should focus on focal signs of infection, bleeding, cutaneous manifestations of thrombocytopenia and complication of thrombosis such as swelling, chest pain, headache, or altered mental status. A CBC with differential, blood cultures, PT, INR, PTT, and anticoagulant level in patients receiving therapy for thrombosis should be obtained as indicated.

Management

Management priorities are directed not toward the neutropenia itself but to the associated infectious risks (see "Infectious Complications of Cancer Treatment" section). Neutrophil and/or monocytic specific growth factors, such as filgrastim and sargramostim, can decrease the duration but not the depth of neutropenia. When neutropenia is present in the setting of sepsis, the literature does not support starting or increasing the dose of

TABLE 106.7

TRANSFUSIONS IN ONCOLOGY PATIENT IN THE EMERGENCY DEPARTMENT

Platelets	Red cells
• Platelet count <100,000/mm^3 and active bleeding or major surgery or trauma • Platelet count <50,000/mm^3 and minor surgery (e.g., lumbar puncture) or trauma or moderate mucosal bleeding (e.g., epistaxis) • Platelet count <20,000/mm^3 and mild mucosal bleeding • Platelet count <10,000/mm^3 to prevent spontaneous intracranial hemorrhage	• Hemoglobin <7 mg/dL • To support circulation in a setting of acute blood loss or sepsis • Elective transfusion of symptomatic patient to avoid admission (only if per institutional policy and feasible to transfuse in ED)

Product specifications	Platelets	Red cells	Comment
Type and cross needed	Yes[a]	Yes	
ABO matched	If product available	Yes	Slightly better response to ABO-matched platelets
Rh matched	Preferred	Yes	If Rh+ platelets to Rh donor, anti-D product within 72 hrs
Irradiated	Yes	Yes	Prevent WBCs in product from proliferating and causing graft-versus-host disease
Leukoreduced	Yes	Yes	Prevent CMV transmission in donor white cells[b]
HLA matched	Possible	No	May be useful in setting of patient refractory to platelets. Takes time to arrange; generally unable to obtain in the ED.
Single donor	Preferred[c]	No	
Premedication	Possible	Possible	Highly transfused population are at risk for reactions Acetaminophen if h/o febrile reactions Diphenhydramine if h/o allergic reaction Hydrocortisone if h/o allergic reaction despite diphenhydramine or very severe allergic reaction
Quantity	*General guidelines:* 1 unit <10 kg 3 units 10–30 kg 6 units 30–80 kg 8 units >80 kg	*pRBC elective transfusion:* 10–15 mL/kg or 2 units for >50-kg patient	Volume-reduced platelets in patients very sensitive to volume overload decrease effectiveness of transfusion Continuous infusion for platelet-refractory patient with ongoing significant bleeding

[a]Not required if type previously performed at blood bank.
[b]CMV-negative product unnecessary if product has been leukoreduced.
[c]Apheresis platelets from a single donor preferred.
ED, emergency department; ABO, blood group system; Rh, Rheus (Rh) blood group system; WBC, white blood cell; CMV, cytomegalovirus; HLA, human leukocyte antigen; h/o, history of; pRBC, packed red blood cells.

growth factor although this is the practice at some institutions. The literature is inconclusive about the use of WBC transfusions in neutropenic patients with bacteremia, if the neutrophil recovery is expected within the next 7 to 10 days.

The urgency of the need for platelet transfusion varies with the circumstance. In the ED, it may be more expedient to give platelets during a procedure rather than transfusing in advance and rechecking a platelet count prior to the procedure. Institutional guidelines should prevail regarding blood type matching, use of anti-D products in males, and prophylactic transfusion criteria. In a patient with active life-threatening bleeding, transfusion should not be delayed to await apheresis platelets. If there is severe bleeding in a patient who is refractory to platelet transfusions, the blood bank should be consulted to arrange a continuous infusion of platelets.

The need for transfusion in the ED varies with the severity of the anemia and clinical circumstances (Table 106.7). Additional information on transfusions in the actively bleeding patient and administration guidelines can be found in Chapter 101 Hematologic Emergencies. The oncology-specific history is critical to identify contributing factors. The platelet count should always be checked immediately and transfusion given as indicated (Table 106.7). Reversal of any anticoagulation should be considered in a patient with significant bleeding.

Management of thrombosis is discussed in Chapter 101 Hematologic Emergencies. If a central venous sinus thrombosis is suspected, CT scans may not be sensitive enough to secure a diagnosis, but MRI is generally reliable. Once the diagnosis is established, management consists of supportive care and initiation of anticoagulation. Of note, for patients on asparaginase receiving anticoagulation for a thrombus, the antithrombin level must be monitored regularly and should generally be replaced with antithrombin III when levels fall below 50%.

INFECTIOUS COMPLICATIONS OF CANCER TREATMENT

Goals of Treatment

Oncology patients are at high risk for life-threatening infection, and prompt initiation of volume resuscitation and antibiotic administration is critical to optimal outcome. Early administration of empiric broad-spectrum antibiotics can prevent morbidity and mortality in febrile neutropenic oncology patients.

CLINICAL PEARLS AND PITFALLS

- Administration of broad-spectrum antibiotics within 1 hour of presentation to the ED has been shown to reduce morbidity and mortality from sepsis in the setting of neutropenia.
- Digital rectal examinations and rectal temperature measurements should not be performed in neutropenic patients, as these procedures increase the risk of bacterial translocation from the intestinal tract into the bloodstream.
- Though fever should raise concern for infection, the absence of fever does not exclude the possibility of infection, particularly in patients on high-dose steroids and/or with hypothalamic dysfunction from tumor.
- Neutropenic patients may not generate erythema or purulence at the site of localized infections.

Current Evidence

Fever in a neutropenic patient is a true emergency, even in a well-appearing patient (Fig. 106.4). Identification of infection can be challenging because typical symptoms may be absent or decreased. The depth and duration of neutropenia helps to predict the risk of serious infections. All patients with an ANC below 500 or with a rapidly falling ANC that will shortly be below 500 should be considered at risk. Although fever itself can be a manifestation of some cancers, this is a diagnosis of exclusion, particularly in a patient with neutropenia. While fever should certainly raise concern for infection, the absence of fever should not overly reassure the clinician. Fever may be absent or minimized in patients on high-dose steroids and/or patients with hypothalamic dysfunction from tumor. In addition, localizing signs of infection may be blunted because the lack of neutrophils prevents many of the usual manifestations such as pus, significant local erythema, or edema.

One of the infectious risks attributable to the immunosuppression of chemotherapy is *Pneumocystis jirovecii* (formerly known as *Pneumocystis carinii*) pneumonia. Patients younger than 1 year and those receiving treatment for leukemia or high-stage lymphoma are at increased risk. Most, if not all, pediatric oncology patients are treated with prophylactic trimethoprim-sulfamethoxazole to prevent this infection. Those who do not tolerate trimethoprim-sulfamethoxazole are on second-line agents such as atovaquone, dapsone, or pentamidine.

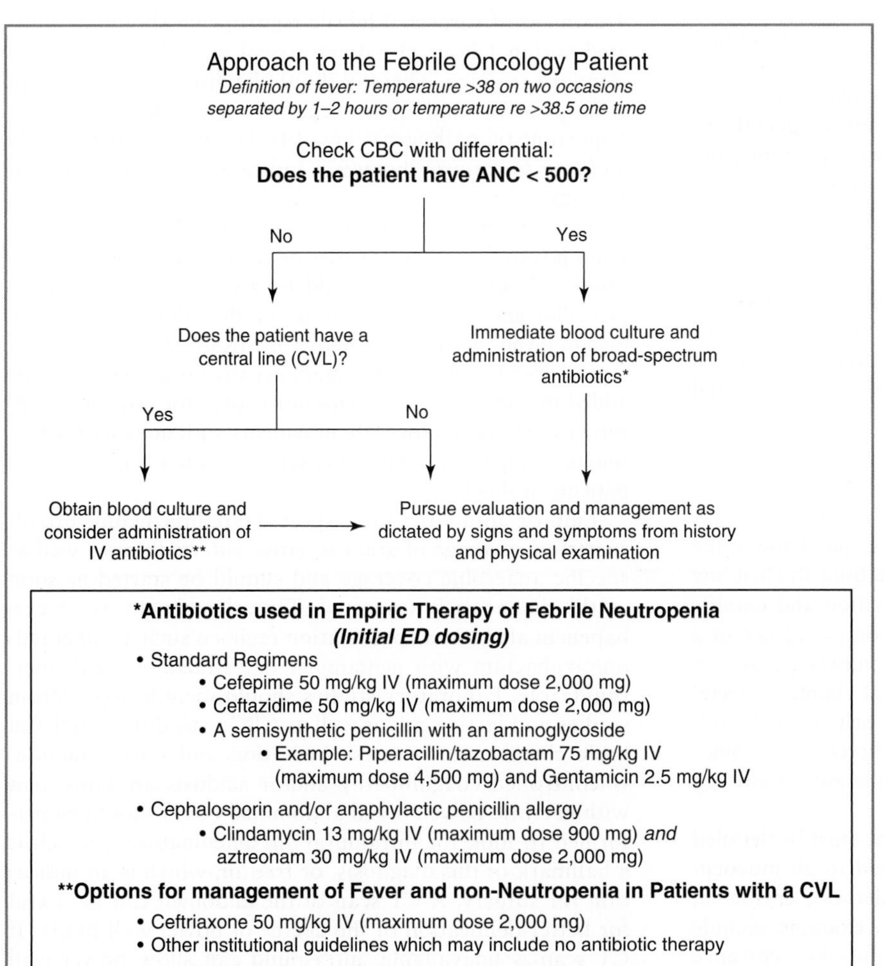
Approach to the Febrile Oncology Patient
Definition of fever: Temperature >38 on two occasions separated by 1–2 hours or temperature re >38.5 one time
Check CBC with differential:
Does the patient have ANC < 500?
No
Yes
Does the patient have a central line (CVL)?
Immediate blood culture and administration of broad-spectrum antibiotics*
Yes
No
Obtain blood culture and consider administration of IV antibiotics**
Pursue evaluation and management as dictated by signs and symptoms from history and physical examination
*Antibiotics used in Empiric Therapy of Febrile Neutropenia
(Initial ED dosing)
• Standard Regimens
• Cefepime 50 mg/kg IV (maximum dose 2,000 mg)
• Ceftazidime 50 mg/kg IV (maximum dose 2,000 mg)
• A semisynthetic penicillin with an aminoglycoside
• Example: Piperacillin/tazobactam 75 mg/kg IV (maximum dose 4,500 mg) and Gentamicin 2.5 mg/kg IV
• Cephalosporin and/or anaphylactic penicillin allergy
• Clindamycin 13 mg/kg IV (maximum dose 900 mg) and aztreonam 30 mg/kg IV (maximum dose 2,000 mg)
**Options for management of Fever and non-Neutropenia in Patients with a CVL
• Ceftriaxone 50 mg/kg IV (maximum dose 2,000 mg)
• Other institutional guidelines which may include no antibiotic therapy
See text for considerations for additional coverage

FIGURE 106.4 Management guidelines for the febrile oncology patient. Risk assessment and management hinges substantially on whether the absolute neutrophil count (ANC) is below 500, whether the patient has localizing signs or symptoms, and whether an indwelling catheter is present.

Prophylaxis for other infections varies by condition and center. Fungal prophylaxis is increasingly common with specific regimens associated with a high frequency of fungal disease. For example, many patients with acute myelogenous leukemia take prophylactic antifungals throughout their treatment. Respiratory syncytial virus (RSV) prophylaxis with RSV immunoglobulin (Palivizumab) may be used in children younger than 1 year on highly immunosuppressive regimens.

Pediatric oncology patients are also at risk for common viral infections such as RSV, CMV, EBV, influenza, and adenovirus. In general, the presentation of these infections is the same as in immunocompetent hosts. Of note, primary varicella zoster infection can rapidly progress to a life-threatening infection in an immunocompromised patient.

Typhlitis, also known as neutropenic colitis, is a potentially life-threatening infection that occurs in patients with neutropenia and GI mucosal injury. This infection occurs in the watershed regions of the cecum, appendix, and terminal ileum. It is much more common in patients with advanced hematologic malignancies but can occur in patients with solid tumors. *Clostridium difficile* colitis is relatively common in oncology patients due to treatment with broad-spectrum antibiotics that eradicates normal bowel flora.

Clinical Considerations

Clinical Recognition

In addition to sepsis, bacteremia, and soft tissue infections, the emergency physician should consider additional infectious complications not commonly encountered in noncancer patients. Initial symptoms of typhlitis can mimic appendicitis with periumbilical pain preceding right lower quadrant pain. As the infection progresses, abdominal pain can become severe and examination findings include distention and persistent right lower quadrant tenderness. *C. difficile* colitis should be considered in patients with abdominal pain and diarrhea with or without abdominal distention. Abdominal tenderness is generally minimal except in patients with very severe colitis. Perirectal pain may be the presenting symptom of perirectal abscess/cellulitis. Complaints of painful vesicular rash should raise concern for varicella infection.

Clinical Assessment

Certain elements of the history can be very helpful. Patients or family members, or referring oncologists, may know if the patient is already neutropenic. Specific questions to elicit any focal pain can direct the physical examination and empiric treatment decisions since this may be the only evidence of a localizing infection. The presence of any indwelling devices such as a central line, ventriculoperitoneal shunt, or metal hardware used for bone tumors can also help with the differential diagnosis and/or empiric antibiotic coverage. Since antibiotic allergies are common in this population, a thorough allergy history is critical.

The physical examination of the patient must be detailed and meticulous with careful attention paid to all mucocutaneous surfaces to elicit any focal tenderness, erythema, or edema, which may be slight. Sites to examine include any central venous access devices at the skin entrance site, subcutaneous reservoirs, and along the subcutaneous line tract. Nail beds on both fingers and toes should be carefully examined, and a thorough external rectal examination performed using circumferential palpation. *Do not perform an internal rectal examination* as it may increase the risk of bacteremia.

Diagnostic testing should include a CBC with differential and blood cultures from all line lumens or via venipuncture in patients without a line. Institution-specific guidelines should be followed regarding the need for peripheral blood cultures in addition to line cultures, and if additional orders or specimens are needed for anaerobic cultures. Additional diagnostic testing can be obtained as needed after empiric antibiotics are started. A chest x-ray should be obtained in patients with respiratory symptoms. A urinalysis is not valuable for screening for infection since there are too few WBCs for the leukocyte esterase to be of value. A urine culture should be obtained as long as it does not delay start of antibiotics or require catheterization, which may also increase the risk of bacteremia. If the patient has a history of urinary tract infections, the risk of urinary catheterization may be justified. Throat cultures may be of value if there are focal findings involving only the pharynx and/or tonsils but are rarely informative in a patient with diffuse mucositis. Specific imaging may be of value based on physical findings. Viral testing of vesicular lesions may identify varicella infections. Cultures of draining abscesses or wounds may help guide antibiotic choice. Diarrhea should be tested for *C. difficile* toxin.

Management

Treatment of suspected febrile neutropenia should be initiated within 1 hour of patient arrival with the institutional standard regimen. Therapy should be directed against both gram-positive and gram-negative organisms, including opportunistic pathogens (Fig. 106.4). Specific coverage, *in addition to empiric therapy,* is indicated for several clinical settings.

Third-generation cephalosporins may have inadequate gram-positive coverage for patients with soft tissue site infections and consideration should be given to a semisynthetic penicillin and an aminoglycoside or the addition of vancomycin, given the rising incidence of MRSA. With evidence of sepsis, double coverage for gram-negative organisms may be added in addition to vancomycin to cover for possible *Streptococcus viridans,* especially in patients with advanced hematologic malignancies. Fungal coverage is often considered for patients in shock.

Empiric antibiotics for suspected typhlitis include broad-spectrum coverage of gram-negative enteric flora as well as specific anaerobic coverage and should be started as soon as the diagnosis is suspected. Typical regimens are a carbapenem alone or a combination regimen such as piperacillin/tazobactam with gentamicin or ceftazidime with metronidazole. Laboratory studies should include coagulation studies and lactic acid, as well as CBC with differential and basic chemistries to assess hydration and renal function. Uncontrolled coagulopathy and/or acidosis are consistent with necrotic bowel. Serial abdominal x-rays should be performed to look for intramural air (pneumatosis), which is a hallmark of this diagnosis, or free air, which is an indication for surgery. A CT scan of the abdomen can be useful for better delineation of the degree of bowel wall injury. If CT scan is unavailable, ultrasound can show bowel wall thickening. Early surgical consultation is appropriate. Surgery itself is reserved for uncontrollable coagulopathy or acidosis as a consequence of bowel necrosis or evidence of perforation.

Treatment of confirmed or suspected *C. difficile* colitis should include empiric vancomycin (oral) or metronidazole (parenteral or oral). Imaging is rarely useful, except in the most severe cases.

As soon as characteristic vesicles on an erythematous base are seen, empiric coverage for varicella should begin with acyclovir 10 mg per kg IV every 8 hours in conjunction with appropriate hydration. The patient should be assessed for pneumonitis with a careful respiratory examination, oxygen saturation, and a chest radiograph. Liver enzymes should be measured for possible hepatic involvement.

All pediatric patients with fever and neutropenia less than 500 to 1,000 per μL should be admitted to the hospital unless there is an institutional management guideline that includes a specific follow-up plan for outpatient management of low-risk fever and neutropenia. In the case of sepsis or septic shock, acute management as described in Chapters 91 Shock and 102 Infectious Diseases Emergencies should be followed for oncology patients, with the empiric antibiotic coverage described above for neutropenia. Stress-dose steroids should be considered in patients who have received prolonged steroids recently either as part of cancer treatment or management of nausea and vomiting.

METABOLIC COMPLICATIONS OF CANCER TREATMENT

Complications affecting metabolic balance and the endocrinologic system are common in children with cancer. These may be because of the neoplastic disease itself, as has been addressed in the sections on newly diagnosed cancer, or due to complications from cancer therapy.

TLS is probably the most noteworthy example of metabolic derangement in the setting of cancer (see "Leukemia" section). TLS can be present at the time of diagnosis or develop as chemotherapy is initiated and tumor cells begin to die in response. Prevention of tumor lysis relies on protecting the function of the kidneys while preventing severe metabolic derangements (Table 106.3). Hyperhydration should be initiated to achieve brisk, dilute urine output. In addition to IV hydration, all patients should receive therapy with either allopurinol (10 mg/kg/day with maximum dose 300 mg) or rasburicase. Allopurinol is a xanthine oxidase inhibitor that impairs the production of uric acid. Rasburicase, a recombinant urate-oxidase enzyme, causes direct lysis of uric acid and leads to a rapid drop in uric acid levels. The usual starting dose is 0.2 mg per kg IV. Rasburicase is indicated in patients who are at higher risk of TLS complications such as patients with compromised renal function or an extremely elevated uric acid level; who have advanced Burkitt lymphoma; who cannot tolerate hydration (e.g., CNS hemorrhage or preexisting cardiac dysfunction); or whose uric acid is rising despite allopurinol. Rasburicase is contraindicated in glucose-6-phosphate dehydrogenase (G6PD) deficiency as it can result in oxidative stress and hemolysis. Use of alkalinized intravenous fluids is becoming less common as its efficacy is uncertain. If using rasburicase, hydration with alkalinization is unnecessary.

Of note, not all electrolyte abnormalities in the setting of TLS should be corrected (Table 106.3). Hyperphosphatemia can be treated using aluminum hydroxide as frequently as every 2 to 4 hours. Hypophosphatemia should not be corrected unless it is in a critically low range (less than 1 mEq per L). Serum potassium levels must be aggressively monitored. Hyperkalemia in the setting of TLS should be managed as it would be in other disease states (see Chapter 108 Renal and Electrolyte Emergencies) with Kayexalate, insulin and glucose, and dialysis, if needed. Hypokalemia should not be corrected unless the patient's serum potassium falls in a critically low range (less than 2 mEq per L), significant muscular weakness develops, or if hypokalemia is associated with EKG changes. Hypocalcemia should remain uncorrected as well, unless clinical signs or symptoms develop. Supplemental calcium may increase the risk of formation of calcium phosphate precipitates in the kidney.

Renal tubular dysfunction is common in oncology patients. Patients may waste electrolytes such as sodium, potassium, calcium, magnesium, and phosphorus through their kidneys as a result of specific treatment exposures or prior renal injury. Antifungal agents such as amphotericin and ambisome cause potassium wasting, which may have clinical significance. Calcineurin inhibitors, such as tacrolimus or cyclosporine, which may be used after stem cell transplantation, can cause significant magnesium wasting. Patients with hypomagnesemia are more likely to experience seizures when on calcineurin inhibitors so the magnesium should be kept more than 1.8 mEq per L in these patients. In addition, patients with tumors of the CNS may renally waste sodium so monitoring of serum sodium is crucial, especially in the postoperative period.

Patients receiving drugs that cause salt wasting are often prescribed oral electrolyte replacement. However, inability to tolerate oral medications or nonadherence may allow electrolyte abnormalities to develop. Most of these derangements are clinically asymptomatic with the notable exceptions of hypocalcemia, which can cause tetany or cardiac arrhythmias and hyponatremia resulting in refractory seizures. For the most part, management and replacement strategies for these electrolyte abnormalities do not differ from children who do not have cancer (see Chapter 108 Renal and Electrolyte Emergencies). However, when replacing calcium in pediatric oncology patients, the clinician should remember that hypomagnesemia, a common side effect of cancer therapies, could complicate efforts to address hypocalcemia.

Elevated blood sugar can be a transient side effect of corticosteroids as well as asparaginase therapy. Asparaginase affects the body's ability to make many proteins, including insulin. In ALL treatment, steroids and asparaginase may be used together and hyperglycemia may result. Treatment need not include insulin if dietary measures alone are sufficient to control the serum blood sugar. If blood glucose is greater than 250 mg per dL or is significant enough to cause glycosuria or ketonuria, treatment with small doses of insulin may be considered. However, the approach to insulin use in this setting should be conservative so as to limit the risks of hypoglycemia. Diabetic ketoacidosis is rare in this situation.

High serum calcium levels are observed commonly in the setting of adult malignancy but are rare in children with cancer. Hypercalcemia is usually related to the tumor destroying bone or to ectopic production of parathyroid hormone by the tumor itself. This complication is more common if patients are also taking calcium supplements or calcium-containing medications such as antacids. If asymptomatic, hypercalcemia does not always require intervention. When present, symptoms may include nausea/vomiting, constipation, altered mental status, and renal failure. Management in these cases is similar to strategies to address hypercalcemia outside of the oncology setting (see Chapters 97 Endocrine Emergencies and 108 Renal and Electrolyte Emergencies). However, steroids should be avoided in patients with known or suspected leukemia or lymphoma. Control of the underlying malignancy is the best way to address the hypercalcemia.

Although SIADH can develop as a result of some cancers themselves, particularly those involving the lungs or CNS, treatment with vincristine and cyclophosphamide can be associated with SIADH. Management of this complication hinges on fluid restriction and does not differ from that of SIADH developing in other settings (see Chapter 108 Renal and Electrolyte Emergencies).

PAIN

Goals of Treatment

Pain is a true emergency. The relief of pain is a critical element of caring for children with cancer, and should be addressed even in patients who present to the ED for other concerns.

CLINICAL PEARLS AND PITFALLS

- NSAIDs and aspirin are generally avoided due to their antiplatelet activity.
- Cancer patients are frequently not opioid naïve and may require higher starting doses than are standard.

Current Evidence

Unfortunately, pain is a common symptom in oncology patients with data showing that more than 30% of pediatric cancer patients have experienced pain in the previous week. When pain leads to visits to the ED, it requires careful and immediate management. Severe pain is a true emergency, in and of itself, and also may be particularly upsetting for cancer patients who may have already confronted significant pain as part of their cancer diagnosis, who may anticipate or fear future pain, and who may worry (usually needlessly) that their pain is a sign of progressive cancer.

In some cases, pain may be related to the tumor itself and therefore often will respond to chemotherapy or other cancer-directed therapies. Tumors can cause neuropathic pain when they directly invade local nerves or when they cause local edema that affects the nerves in the vicinity. Tumor infiltrating an organ may cause ill-defined pain as the organ capsule becomes stretched. Bone pain may signify a pathologic fracture from a tumor weakening the bone, as can occur with Ewing sarcoma or osteosarcoma. The bones may also hurt due to tumor invading the bone marrow space. Pain in the head and neck may result from increased ICP or tumor involvement of the meninges/cerebrospinal fluid (most common in hematologic malignancies).

On the other hand, pain may be related to cancer treatment. In these cases, the patient or family may report that this particular pain has been historically linked to a specific therapy. A particularly challenging problem is the phantom pain that can occur after limb amputation. In addition, oncology patients may experience pain of the mouth, GI tract, or even urethra as part of mucositis. Pain could also represent a focal infection, complicating the patient's compromised immune system. Bone pain may reflect recent therapy with hematopoietic growth factors to stimulate neutrophil recovery after chemotherapy. Radiation therapy can induce local tissue injury, which may be very painful.

Abdominal pain is a common complaint in cancer patients and can arise from several sources. The differential diagnosis may be very wide including pancreatitis, hepatitis, cholecystitis, constipation, mucosal injury, intra-abdominal infection, and bowel obstruction (see "Hepatic and Gastrointestinal Complications of Cancer Treatment" section).

Clinical Considerations

Clinical Assessment

An important first step in management is to explicitly address pain when taking the patient's history. Even patients who come to the ED for other reasons may have pain complicating their presentation. Upon determining that a patient is in pain, according to the patient's report as opposed to the clinician's assessment, the emergency physician must initiate immediate pain treatment. The remainder of the history and physical examination should be used to identify the cause of the pain and to explore specific treatment for that cause.

Management

Acetaminophen is a useful analgesic with minimal side effects for most patients, remembering to avoid the rectal route if the patient is neutropenic. NSAIDs and aspirin may be effective as pain relievers but are generally avoided in this patient population due to their antiplatelet effect in the setting of frequent thrombocytopenia. Opioids represent the mainstay of pain treatment for the pediatric oncology patient. General principles of dosing include the following:

- A dose that is commonly used as a standard starting dose may be insufficient to provide adequate pain relief if the patient is not opioid naïve.
- Far more important than the actual dose is the dose to *effect*. Patients may need repeated doses in order to get control of their pain and repeated doses should not be limited when analgesia has not yet been attained.
- A patient-controlled analgesia (PCA) pump is frequently needed for several types of pain, particularly mucositis where oral intake can be limited. Such pumps may be initiated in the ED using morphine, fentanyl, or hydromorphone. Small children and infants may benefit from nursing-controlled analgesia (NCA). Parents should not control analgesic pumps except in the setting of end-of-life care, per institutional policy.
- Long-acting opioids, such as MS Contin, Oxycontin, and methadone, may be appropriate in the setting of chronic pain. These medications should not be used in the setting of acute pain and are rarely initiated in the ED unless in consultation with a pain expert.

Careful consideration must be given to decisions about whether patients in pain may be discharged to home. If oral medications seem to be relieving the pain, then it is generally acceptable to discharge the patient after ensuring that he/she has an adequate supply of the analgesics for use at home. If the pain is inadequately controlled on oral medications and parenteral administration is required, then the patient will need to be admitted.

NEUROLOGIC COMPLICATIONS OF CANCER TREATMENT

Neurologic complications in children with cancer are extremely common and may relate to disease, cancer treatment, or supportive care medications. Drug-related side effects are extremely frequent. Many of the common problems are reversible but a few can lead to permanent neurologic injury. The cancer-specific history is critical to identify the likely causes of neurologic problems. The diagnosis and management of neurologic problems in children is covered in Chapter 105 Neurologic Emergencies. This section focuses on the unique considerations in the pediatric cancer patient. Both motor and sensory *peripheral neuropathies* are common in children with cancer. Vincristine and vinblastine, two chemotherapy agents used to treat many kinds of childhood cancer, cause reversible neuropathy affecting motor, sensory, and autonomic nerves. Thalidomide can also cause peripheral neuropathy, which may or may not be fully reversible.

Initial management tends to focus on establishing the diagnosis by the cancer-directed history and physical examination. Pain responds best to agents with efficacy against neuropathic pain such as gabapentin. Such drugs rarely have immediate effect and thus narcotics may be needed in the short run.

There is a wide differential to consider when evaluating a pediatric cancer patient with *new-onset cranial nerve palsy.* Symmetric involvement may reflect vincristine-induced neuropathy, particularly when it involves ptosis. Increased ICP from shunt malfunction or tumor progression should also be considered. Asymmetric involvement can occur with fatigue or vincristine-induced exacerbation of baseline weakness. Vincristine can also cause asymmetric ptosis in some patients, but this should be a diagnosis of exclusion. Increased ICP should be suspected in a child with a sixth nerve palsy. Carcinomatous meningitis should be considered in patients with a history of tumors likely to involve the cerebrospinal fluid or meninges, such as leukemia, lymphoma, parameningeal sarcomas, and meningeal seeding brain tumors, such as medulloblastoma. Patients treated with a scopolamine patch for nausea may develop pupillary asymmetry as scopolamine transferred by fingertip from the patch to the eye can elicit unilateral mydriasis.

Management in the ED requires an appropriate oncology-directed history and physical examination to establish the potential differential. Unless drug effect can be established as the most likely cause, a head CT scan to rule out increased ICP may be required. The CT scan findings may also direct the specific ED and post-ED management. Admission for observation may be required for some patients where the diagnosis or trajectory is uncertain.

The most common cause of *proximal muscle weakness* in pediatric cancer patients is prolonged steroid exposure as part of cancer treatment or management of side effects. The diagnosis can usually be established by the appropriate history and physical examination. Patients with very severe symptoms whose families cannot manage care at home may require admission for respite care or initiation of rehabilitation.

Altered mental status in pediatric cancer patients has an extremely broad differential (Table 106.9). Cerebrovascular accident (CVA) as a cause of altered mental status should be considered in patients with risk factors such as thrombocytopenia, DIC, or drug-induced coagulopathy. Somnolence can be a side effect of many supportive-care medications such as narcotics, gabapentin, antihistamines, some antiepileptics, and antidepressants. Cranial radiation causes somnolence syndrome 6 to 12 weeks after treatment that may last several weeks in duration. Typical manifestations are extreme amounts of sleep (up to 20 hours per day) with normal mental status and function when awake. Additional drug-specific CNS side effects are listed in Table 106.8.

An oncology-directed history, with particular attention to a detailed medication history, is critical to narrowing the differential diagnosis. Physical examination should look for other findings such as papilledema or focal neurologic findings that may also narrow the differential diagnosis. Laboratory evaluation should be carried out as recommended in Chapter 105 Neurologic Emergencies. If a drug-related cause is suspected, specific drug levels when available may be helpful. If a lumbar puncture is planned to look for malignant cells or an infectious etiology, the risk of herniation should be assessed. Imaging studies may be appropriate if an intracranial lesion is suspected or when the diagnosis is unclear. A CT scan without contrast can be useful to identify midline shift, increased ventricular size, or a hemorrhagic stroke. A CT scan with contrast can identify likely carcinomatous meningitis or a supratentorial mass lesion. MRI can identify mass lesions anywhere in the CNS including below the tentorium, ischemic stroke, hypertensive encephalopathy, or encephalitis.

Management of drug-related altered mental status usually involves withholding the offending agent and supporting the patient until resolution. If narcotic-related, avoid rapid reversal with standard doses of naloxone, which could cause excruciating pain that will be unresponsive to further narcotics for 2 to 3 hours. Supportive care such as stimulation should be tried prior to reversal. If reversal is required, the appropriate dose of naloxone (0.1 mg per kg) should be diluted in 10 mL of normal saline and then administered in 1-mL aliquots while titrating to effect. Alternatively, dosing can be initiated at 1 μg per kg for mild respiratory depression and 10 μg per kg for reversal of moderate to severe respiratory depression as needed. Laboratory evaluation of hepatic and renal function may identify contributing factors to increased drug effect. If ifosfamide neurotoxicity is suspected, many recommend methylene blue treatment using dosages that have been extrapolated from other settings. The usual dose for adolescents and adults is 50 mg administered orally or by slow IV push. There is no clear dosage for younger children but there are case reports using 1 to 2 mg per kg as in the treatment for methemoglobinemia. For management of hypertensive encephalopathy, see Chapter 33 Hypertension.

The presentation and management of *increased ICP* is not unique in pediatric cancer patients (see Chapter 105 Neurologic Emergencies). The differential diagnosis includes tumor (see the "Tumors of the CNS" section) or shunt malfunction more often than treatment effect. Tretinoin (all transretinoic acid), an agent uniquely used in the treatment of APML causes increased ICP. Children are particularly sensitive to this side effect. For patients with severe symptoms attributable to tretinoin, a diagnostic and therapeutic lumbar puncture may be needed. Opening pressure should be measured and cerebrospinal

TABLE 106.8

SIGNIFICANT ACUTE COMPLICATIONS OF SELECTED DRUGS

Drug	Complications
Asparaginase	• Allergy • Hemorrhage • Deep and superficial vein thrombosis (cerebral sinus venous thrombosis) • Hyperglycemia
Bleomycin	• Pulmonary fibrosis and/or pneumonitis
Anthracyclines (doxorubicin, daunorubicin)	• Cardiomyopathy
Corticosteroids	• Avascular necrosis • Hyperglycemia
Cyclophosphamide	• SIADH • Hemorrhagic cystitis
Cyclosporine	• Hypomagnesemia and seizures
Cytarabine	• Neurotoxicity (cerebellar dysfunction, onset within hours of treatment with high doses) • Eye pain, tearing, sensitivity to light and blurred vision (high doses) • Seizures (high doses) • Erythroderma, especially palmar, with resulting desquamation (high doses)
Dactinomycin	• Venoocclusive disease of the liver
Etoposide	• Hypotension (during infusion)
Ifosfamide	• Salt wasting • Neurotoxicity (confusion, inappropriate laughter, somnolence, psychosis) • Renal injury manifested as Fanconi syndrome with proximal tubular dysfunction and wasting of phosphate, glucose, potassium, and bicarbonate • Hemorrhagic cystitis
Methotrexate	• Seizures • Elevated transaminases (1–3 days after high dose administration) • Acute renal failure manifest as brisk urine output with rapidly rising creatinine • Skin rash (especially at sites of prior trauma/radiation)
Platinum-containing (carboplatin, cisplatin)	• Salt wasting • Hypomagnesemia • Chronic renal insufficiency (especially at high doses) • Delayed nausea and vomiting (2–5 days after treatment)
Tacrolimus	• Hypomagnesemia and seizures
Tretinoin	• Increased intracranial pressure
Vinca alkaloids (vincristine and vinblastine)	• SIADH • Reversible motor, sensory, and autonomic neuropathy • Cranial nerve neuropathy (ptosis, vocal cord paralysis)

TABLE 106.9

ETIOLOGY OF ACUTE ALTERATION IN MENTAL STATUS IN CHILDREN WITH CANCER

- Tumor
  - Primary CNS tumor
  - Metastatic CNS tumor
  - Leukemic or carcinomatous meningitis
  - Hyperleukocytosis
- Infection
  - Meningitis—bacterial, fungal
  - Viral encephalitis
  - Brain abscess
  - Septic shock
- Cerebrovascular accident
- Seizure/postictal state
- Increased intracranial pressure
  - Shunt malfunction
  - All transretinoic acid (Tretinoin)
- Cytotoxic chemotherapy
  - Methotrexate
  - Cytosine arabinoside
  - Ifosfamide
  - Thalidomide
- Supportive care
  - Opiates
  - Benzodiazepines
  - Gabapentin
  - Anticonvulsants
  - Tricyclic antidepressants
  - Antihistamines
  - Dronabinol
- Leukoencephalopathy
- Metabolic derangements
  - Hyponatremia/SIADH
  - Hypo/hyperglycemia
  - Hypomagnesemia
  - Uremia
- Postradiation therapy somnolence syndrome
- Hypo/hypertension
- Hypoxia
- Liver failure
- Depression

SIADH, syndrome of inappropriate antidiuretic hormone.

fluid should be withdrawn to reduce the pressure (see Chapter 105 Neurologic Emergencies).

Children with cancer are at increased risk of *seizures* from the causes summarized below and in Table 106.8. Severe metabolic disturbances can result from SIADH or from renal tubular wasting of electrolytes (see "Metabolic Complications of Cancer Treatment" section). Seizures can also be caused by primary brain tumors, particularly supratentorial, CNS metastasis of refractory solid tumors, or carcinomatous meningitis. Some chemotherapy agents can cause seizures. New-onset seizures can be a sign of a bacterial abscess (more likely with *Bacillus cereus* bacteremia), fungal abscess, or viral encephalitis such as those caused by herpes simplex virus or CMV. The approach to seizure management is not unique in patients with cancer and is addressed in Chapter 105 Neurologic Emergencies. Specific consideration should be given to assess and correct problems with metabolic abnormalities.

Children with cancer are at increased risk of *CVAs*. Specific causes in children with cancer include sagittal sinus thrombosis and intracranial bleeding with contributing factors of hypertension, coagulopathy, thrombocytopenia, intracranial tumor, prior surgery, and radiation. Spontaneous intracranial hemorrhage is extremely rare except when the platelet count is less than 5,000 per μL (see "Hematologic Complications of Cancer Treatment" section). The approach to diagnosis and management is addressed in Chapter 101 Hematologic Emergencies. Specific consideration should be given to assess and correct problems with coagulopathy and/or thrombocytopenia.

Side effects of some supportive-care medications can include extrapyramidal reactions. Symptoms of such reactions can range from oculogyric crisis with mild repetitive eye deviation and/or neck motion to severe torticollis and eye deviations. Reactions can also include tardive dyskinesia ("frozen") and akathisia (restless/agitation). The key to diagnosis involves a thorough physical examination and a thorough medication history. Dopamine-receptor antagonists used as antiemetics are the most common trigger in cancer patients. Such drugs include high-dose metoclopramide; phenothiazines such as compazine, chlorpromazine (thorazine), and thiethylperazine (Torecan); and butyrophenones such as droperidol and haldol. Since more effective antiemetics, such as serotonin-receptor antagonists, have become available, the use of these drugs has decreased along with the incidence of this side effect. If an extrapyramidal reaction is suspected, management should include diphenhydramine 1 mg per kg IV (maximum dose 50 mg). If symptoms are refractory to diphenhydramine, benztropine (Cogentin) should be given at a dosage of 0.02 mg per kg (maximum 1 mg) IV.

CARDIOVASCULAR COMPLICATIONS

Cancer treatment can affect cardiac function in patients during treatment and long after completion of therapy. Anthracycline-induced cardiomyopathy is the most common cause of cardiac damage in pediatric oncology patients although only a small percentage of them are affected. Anthracycline chemotherapy, most commonly with doxorubicin (Adriamycin) and daunorubicin (Daunomycin), is widely used in the treatment of leukemia, lymphoma, sarcoma, and embryonal tumors such as neuroblastoma and Wilms tumor. These drugs injure and potentially kill individual cardiomyocytes and can cause acute cardiomyopathy during and up to 1 year after the end of treatment. Late cardiomyopathy may develop 8 or more years after completion of therapy. Typical findings on echocardiogram include decreased shortening fraction/ejection fraction and/or increased afterload. Specific risk factors include high total dose (greater than 300 mg per m^2), high dose rate, very young age at treatment, and trisomy 21. Most regimens today are designed to minimize the risk of cardiomyopathy by limiting total dose and dose rate and/or giving dexrazoxane, a cardioprotectant.

Patients exposed to substantial doses of anthracycline are screened with echocardiograms to look for early cardiac dysfunction. Early-onset cardiomyopathy usually presents as acute cardiac failure or cardiac dysfunction out of proportion to a stressor such as sepsis. Late-onset cardiomyopathy is generally a slowly progressive process that may be detected on screening. Both forms may be associated with arrhythmias. The initial management of this problem follows the standard regimen for cardiac failure (see Chapter 94 Cardiac Emergencies).

Radiation to the heart can cause long-term injury to the endothelial surfaces leading to early onset atherosclerotic vessel and/or valve disease. The heart is exposed in mantle radiation for Hodgkin disease and total body irradiation as part of a transplant preparative regimen.

Hypertension may occur in pediatric oncology patients due to steroid exposure, salt overload, and renal injury from treatment. Most hypertension is not an emergency and is better addressed by the treating oncologist as part of long-term management. Hypertensive emergencies (see Chapter 33 Hypertension) are rare in pediatric oncology patients.

HEPATIC AND GASTROINTESTINAL COMPLICATIONS OF CANCER TREATMENT

Cancer treatment frequently affects the GI tract and liver. The majority of complications are minor and fully reversible. A few complications are potentially severe and/or have long-term consequences. Chemotherapy frequently impairs the ability of the mucosal lining of the GI tract to regenerate itself. Severity varies with different chemotherapy regimens. Time to occurrence is similar to the timing of myelosuppression with onset 7 to 10 days after treatment and recovery by 14 days. Radiation also causes temporary injury to any areas of mucosa included in the radiation field. This injury becomes evident after several weeks of treatment and will persist/worsen until treatment is complete.

Initial assessment must include a thorough oncology history to elicit chemotherapy or radiation exposures as well as localizing symptoms and a complete physical examination. *Chemotherapy-induced mucositis* can affect part of or the entire GI tract from the oropharynx to the rectum and may manifest as oral ulceration, throat pain, esophagitis, gastritis, enteritis, or rectal ulceration. Radiation-induced mucosal injury is often associated with skin manifestations in the treatment field. Oropharyngeal involvement usually includes pain and visible mucosal injury ranging from irregular mucosal surfaces to scattered ulcerations to severe diffuse ulceration with swelling of the lips and inability to open the mouth. Esophagitis may be evident only by refusal to swallow and/or retrosternal pain. Enteritis, common with radiation fields that include the intestines, may be evident with crampy watery diarrhea. Mucosal injury to the rectum leads to pain with defecation, tenesmus, or rectal pain. There may be obvious perirectal erythema or ulceration. As discussed elsewhere, avoid a digital rectal examination, which may cause an increased likelihood of bacteremia.

Management of moderate to severe mucositis usually requires pain control with parenteral narcotics. Cancer patients may require higher than standard starting doses, especially if already on narcotics at home. Patients and their families should be asked whether they have medication preferences based on prior episodes of pain. PCA with both continuous and bolus dosing should be initiated in the ED if available. Do not use NSAIDs for pain control since they usually have platelet inhibitory effects and the development of thrombocytopenia frequently coincides with mucositis. Avoid regular use of acetaminophen, which may mask fever since neutropenia also often occurs at the same time. Assess hydration and provide intravenous support as needed. Patients with adequate oral pain control and oral hydration can be discharged to home. Others will need to be admitted for pain control and/or hydration until the mucositis resolves.

Nausea and vomiting are common symptoms in oncology patients. It is critical to consider the differential diagnosis and not just attribute all such symptoms to chemotherapy-induced nausea and vomiting (CINV). CINV can be divided into three categories: acute (within 24 hours of emetogenic treatment), delayed (2 to 5 days after treatment), and anticipatory. Anticipatory symptoms are conditioned symptoms that occur without emetogenic treatment with a variety of emotional or sensory triggers. These anticipatory symptoms can become chronic in some patients. Despite appropriate prophylactic therapy, almost all cancer patients experience some nausea and vomiting. Radiation to the GI tract or the CNS is itself emetogenic. Other causes of nausea and vomiting include GI injury from a variety of causes such as gastritis from steroids, obstipation/constipation, medication side effects (e.g., narcotics), pancreatitis (from asparaginase), GI obstruction (e.g., adhesions from prior surgery), or superior mesenteric artery syndrome in patients with severe malnutrition.

Management of CINV (or radiation induced) is outlined in Table 106.10. As with pain management, all medications are less effective when treating established symptoms. Standard hydration and electrolyte management should be considered

TABLE 106.10

MANAGEMENT OF CHEMOTHERAPY-INDUCED NAUSEA AND VOMITING (CINV)

Drug class	Specific drug	Pediatric dosage and frequency (usual adult maximum)	Route	Comment
Agents with a high therapeutic index				
Serotonin-S3 receptor antagonists	Ondansetron	0.15 mg/kg (8 mg) q8h or 0.45 mg/kg (24 mg) q24h	IV/PO	Ondansetron max IV dose: 16 mg
	Granisetron	10–40 μg/kg (1 mg) q24h	IV/PO	
Steroid	Dexamethasone	10 mg/m^2 (10 mg) q12–24h	IV/PO	Should not be used in patients with steroid-sensitive malignancies without consultation with oncologist (e.g., ALL, lymphoma) Use should be avoided/minimized in patients at high risk of infection or if at increased risk of mucosal toxicity from chemotherapy (e.g., AML, advanced lymphomas, ALL during induction)
NK receptor antagonist	Aprepitant	125 mg on day 1, followed by 80 mg once daily on days 2 and 3	PO	For patients ≥20 kg May be combined with serotonin receptor antagonists
Other	Scopolamine	1.5 mg fixed-dose transdermal patch	TDP	For patients >40 kg Avoid concurrent use of anticholinergic drugs such as diphenhydramine
Agents with a low therapeutic index				
Drug class	**Specific drug**	**Pediatric dosage and frequency (usual adult maximum)**	**Route**	**Comment**
Benzodiazepine	Lorazepam	0.05 mg/kg (1 mg) q6h	IV/PO	Overdosage may be common with weight-based dosing strategies. Thus, also consider 0.25 mg for <25 kg, 0.5 mg for ≥25–50 kg, and 1 mg for ≥50 kg. More potent as an anxiolytic than as an antiemetic.
Dopamine antagonist	Metoclopramide	0.5 mg/kg q6h	IV/PO	Children are at high risk of extrapyramidal reactions. Must be given with diphenhydramine prophylaxis.
Other	Dronabinol	5 mg/m^2	PO	No data in use younger than 5 yrs
	Olanzapine	2.5–10 mg	PO	Limited data in younger patients

IV, intravenous; PO, per os; ALL, acute lymphoblastic leukemia; AML, acute myeloid leukemia; NK, neurokinin; TDP, transdermal patch.

for all patients with severe nausea/vomiting. An abdominal x-ray can be helpful if obstruction or obstipation/constipation is suspected. Amylase and lipase should be measured in patients who are being treated with asparaginase.

Constipation is very common in oncology patients. Contributing factors included decreased GI motility from vinca alkaloids, narcotics, poor oral intake, decreased activity, and/or withholding due to rectal pain from mucositis. Patients may present with complaints of nausea/vomiting, abdominal discomfort, and/or abdominal distention. The evaluation should include a detailed history to elicit any of the contributing factors as well as a specific bowel history. Physical examination should *not* include a digital rectal examination due to potential increased risk of bacteremia. Abdominal x-ray may be helpful in establishing the amount of stool. Treatment of constipation in the oncology patient should include only those agents that can be given by mouth. Rectal suppositories and enemas should be avoided except in extreme circumstances. Patients with severe symptoms may need to be admitted.

Transaminitis with elevations in AST and/or ALT is common in pediatric cancer patients. Many chemotherapy agents cause a mild reversible transaminitis. Treatment-related transaminitis is usually a laboratory-only finding without any clinical correlate. Transfusion-associated viral transaminitis can also occur in the frequently transfused oncology population, but the direct and indirect screening of donor blood has reduced the incidence of viral transmission. Immunosuppression from treatment can also increase the risk of CMV and EBV. Isolated transaminitis may be noted during an evaluation in the ED but rarely is an indication for further laboratory evaluation.

Hyperbilirubinemia is common during cancer treatment, is usually mild and reversible and rarely requires any further ED evaluation. Such elevations are likely multifactorial and may relate to chemotherapy, transfusion, or subclinical liver injury. Unexpected moderate or severe hyperbilirubinemia should be fully assessed.

Diarrhea in an oncology patient may be triggered by a variety of causes including radiation injury, chemotherapy, and *C. difficile* colitis due to prolonged hospitalizations and/or use of broad-spectrum antibiotics.

Venoocclusive disease (VOD) of the liver is a rare but important complication to recognize. Risk factors include exposure to actinomycin-D chemotherapy and liver radiation. Manifestations include hepatomegaly, transaminitis, thrombocytopenia, and ascites. The thrombocytopenia is frequently more than what would be expected from the chemotherapy alone or may occur at the wrong timing relative to chemotherapy. Once the diagnosis is suspected, a hepatic ultrasound with Doppler assessment of hepatic vein flow should be performed. Reversal of flow in the small hepatic veins establishes the diagnosis in the appropriate clinical setting. Management is supportive until the problem resolves on its own. Most patients will require admission for both observation and support.

For a discussion of typhlitis, see section on "Infectious Complications of Cancer Treatment."

RENAL COMPLICATIONS OF CANCER THERAPY

Renal injury from cancer treatment is very common and some degree of renal dysfunction is frequently present even in patients with normal creatinine for age. Other patients will have documented renal dysfunction based on elevated creatinine, decreased glomerular filtration rate (GFR), or decreased 24-hour creatinine clearance. Renal complications may also lead to metabolic disturbances (see "Metabolic Complications of Cancer Treatment" section).

Uric-acid nephropathy can occur in patients with very high cell turnover (see "Leukemia" section). *Drug-induced renal injury* is common in oncology patients (Table 106.8). *Radiation injury* to the kidney may cause renal insufficiency as well as radiation nephritis, 3 to 6 months after treatment. Typical findings include the manifestations of vasculitis with hemolytic uremic syndrome (HUS).

Oncology patients are also at risk for medical renal disease associated with poor perfusion, exposure to multiple nephrotoxic agents, and hypertension.

Since renal injury is common, it is appropriate to check BUN, creatinine, electrolytes, calcium, magnesium, and phosphate in all systemically ill oncology patients. If significant abnormalities are noted, the oncology-specific history should be reviewed to determine specific risk factors or exposures that may help explain the problem. In general, the management of significant abnormalities is not unique in patients with cancer and should follow the guidelines in Chapter 108 Renal and Electrolyte Emergencies. Consider the possibility of a decreased GFR (whether known or not) when starting antibiotics and other medications that are renally metabolized.

GENITOURINARY COMPLICATIONS OF CANCER TREATMENT

The most common form of bladder injury in cancer patients is hemorrhagic cystitis, a potential complication of exposure to cyclophosphamide or ifosfamide. Prevention of drug-induced hematuria usually includes hydration, frequent voiding, and administration of mesna (2-mercaptoethane sulfonate sodium), a drug that binds the toxic metabolite. Manifestations include dysuria, suprapubic pain, and microscopic or gross hematuria with onset within 24 hours of drug administration. Other causes of toxicity to the GU tract include infection, bladder radiation, tumor resection, or ongoing presence of tumor in the GU tract.

If a patient is complaining of bladder-related symptoms or the urinalysis shows evidence of hematuria, the oncology-specific history should be reviewed to help develop an appropriate differential diagnosis in addition to the usual causes (such as infection) that would be considered in a patient without cancer. Initial management should include initiation of one and one-half times to twice maintenance hydration and frequent voiding. Laboratory evaluation should include a urine analysis, CBC to look for anemia or thrombocytopenia, and coagulation studies. Any contribution from coagulopathy and/or thrombocytopenia should be corrected. If severe bleeding or bladder outlet obstruction from clots occurs, urology should be consulted. A bladder catheter large enough to be used for irrigation should be placed and bladder washing initiated. Packed red blood cell transfusion may be needed. In very rare cases, bleeding can be life-threatening and bladder sclerosis is indicated. Mesna has no utility once the offending drug has cleared from the system. Pain management with oxybutynin chloride and narcotics should be initiated as needed.

SKIN COMPLICATIONS OF CANCER TREATMENT

Various cancer treatments are known to have cutaneous toxicities. Radiation induces dermatitis in the treatment field that can range from mild to severe based on the total dose and any concurrent radiation sensitizers. The presentation may vary from a mild erythroderma, similar to sunburn, to severe desquamation in the treatment field. Any topical treatment must be prescribed in conjunction with the treating radiation oncologist because certain topical agents may increase the radiation dose to the skin.

Drug rashes are very common in oncology patients. Because patients tend to be on many drugs at one time, it may be difficult to identify the specific culprit. Management of a drug reaction is not unique in oncology patients. However, consultation with the oncologist may be needed to discuss if alternate treatment is needed.

Infections may be accompanied by cutaneous manifestations (see Chapter 102 Infectious Disease Emergencies). Although not unique to oncology patients, certain infections affecting the skin may be more common in this patient group. Immunosuppressed patients are at increased risk for herpes simplex and herpes zoster. Any skin lesions in a dermatomal distribution, with or without associated pain and whether or not the lesions are "classic," should be considered herpes zoster until proven otherwise. Immunocompromised patients with herpes zoster have an increased risk of disseminated disease and should be placed in respiratory isolation. Evaluation should include chest radiograph and liver function tests. If there is a vesicular lesion, it should be scraped and sent for both rapid testing and culture for herpes simplex and varicella zoster. Empiric therapy should be started with either acyclovir or one of its derivatives. Admission for intravenous therapy is indicated when there is evidence of dissemination, ophthalmologic involvement, or failure to respond to oral therapy. Oral home therapy can be considered in consultation with oncology after considering extent of involvement, degree of underlying immunosuppression, likelihood of medication compliance at home, and ability to follow-up.

COMPLICATIONS OF HEMATOPOIETIC STEM CELL TRANSPLANTATION

Bone marrow transplantation is increasingly utilized in the treatment of various hematologic, oncologic, metabolic, or immunologic diseases. In hematologic malignancies, allogeneic marrow transplantation may follow initial remission, induction, or disease relapse. The allogeneic donor may be related, usually a sibling, or unrelated to the recipient. In solid tumors and some lymphomas, patients may receive aggressive chemotherapy and radiation and then have their own stem cells infused as a "rescue" to help reconstitute their immune system following therapy (autologous transplant). Knowledge of the type of transplant a patient received (Table 106.11) can help the clinician anticipate what complications might ensue. In general, stem cell transplant recipients represent a fragile patient population at risk for many complications.

In approaching these patients, substantial immunosuppression should be presumed for at least 6 months following the transplant. For patients still receiving immunosuppressing medications, the period of immune dysfunction may be much longer. Regardless of the WBC and neutrophil counts, immune function following a stem cell transplant can be profoundly impaired.

Graft-versus-host disease (GVHD) may develop in the setting of allogeneic stem cell transplants as newly engrafted immune cells of the donor react against tissue antigens of the recipient that are perceived to be foreign (Table 106.11). Acute GVHD occurs in the first 100 days posttransplant, often when patient is still in hospital, and typically involves the skin, GI tract, or liver. Chronic GVHD presents after 100 days and is accompanied by severe immunologic dysfunction.

The evaluation of patients with known or suspected GVHD following an allogeneic stem cell transplant begins with a history to explore whether the patient could be dehydrated or anemic due to colitis or whether he/she is experiencing dyspnea due to lung involvement. Physical examination should assess the skin for rash, fibrosis, or jaundice, liver size and tenderness, and oxygen saturation, with a focus on screening for organ dysfunction serious enough to require intervention in the ED. Clinicians should have a low threshold for admitting such patients for inpatient management due to overall fragility of this patient population.

Therapy for GVHD is primarily immunosuppressive using corticosteroids, cyclosporine, and other agents directed against T cells. Specialists in hematopoietic stem cell transplant decide whether to pursue such agents and when. Often a biopsy (skin, bowel, liver, etc.) is required to diagnose GVHD on histopathology.

The management of *infectious complications* for patients following stem cell transplant is not inherently different from the oncology population overall, but the relevant organisms may vary and the clinician's level of suspicion may need to be higher (Table 106.11). Infections in these patients result from the extreme immunosuppression achieved by myeloablation, cutaneous and mucosal barrier damage intrinsic to the transplant process, and the immunologic immaturity of the transplanted marrow. Central lines exacerbate this risk.

Importantly, the types of infections patients tend to develop after hematopoietic stem cell transplant can vary based on how many days have elapsed since the transplant.

- In the first month after the transplant, as patients are hospitalized and awaiting engraftment of their bone marrow, they are vulnerable to gram-positive and gram-negative bacteria, anaerobic bacteria, respiratory viruses, reactivation of herpes simplex virus, and fungal infection with candida and aspergillus.
- After engraftment, from day 30 to 100 after the transplant, patients remain at risk for bacterial infections, particularly those related to their central lines. Aspergillus and respiratory viruses continue to be a concern. However, CMV, pneumocystis, and toxoplasma become more of a threat at this point.
- More than 100 days after the transplant, patients are at risk for encapsulated bacteria, especially if they are simultaneously affected by GVHD or ongoing immunosuppression. Aspergillus, pneumocystis, and toxoplasma continue to be a concern. Viral infections with varicella zoster virus, CMV, EBV, and respiratory viruses are also a large threat for these patients.

When patients present to the ED with fever following a hematopoietic stem cell transplant, empiric coverage with

TABLE 106.11

COMPLICATIONS OF HEMATOPOIETIC STEM CELL TRANSPLANT

Complication	Clinical findings	Management
Acute graft versus host disease (GVHD)	Skin Erythematous rash Classic involvement of palms and soles GI tract Colitis, sometimes bloody diarrhea Abdominal pain Liver Elevated bilirubin, alkaline phosphatase, transaminases Hepatomegaly Right upper quadrant tenderness	Immunosuppressive medications chosen only in consultation with experts in stem cell transplant Aggressive management of infections and fevers given immunosuppression intrinsic to GVHD Hydration as needed for dehydration from colitis Assessment of anemia secondary to bloody diarrhea Caution using drugs metabolized in the liver if hepatic GVHD present
Chronic GVHD	Pulmonary Hypoxia Shortness of breath Liver (as above) Eye dryness Mouth dryness Skin Sclerodermatous changes Contractures	
Infection	Bacterial Gram positive Gram negative Viral Endogenous Varicella zoster Herpes simplex Epstein–Barr virus Cytomegalovirus Adenovirus Exogenous Influenza Parainfluenza Respiratory syncytial virus Adenovirus Fungal Disseminated candidemia Invasive aspergillosis	Empiric broad-spectrum antibiotics for fever All patients to be considered functionally neutropenic and immunocompromised until they have been off all immunosuppressive medications for at least 6 mo Aggressive imaging to follow-up and localizing signs or symptoms elicited through history and physical examination Bacterial and fungal cultures as well as viral studies of blood, urine, sputum Spinal tap not required
Thrombotic thrombocytopenic purpura	Acute form displays classic pentad Fever Hemolytic anemia Thrombocytopenia Renal failure Neurologic symptoms Rarely can evolve into chronic hemolytic uremic syndrome–like picture	Manage as TTP would be managed outside of the stem cell transplant setting

antibiotics should be instituted at once while cultures of the blood and urine are pending. While gram-negative organisms have historically been of primary concern, gram-positive bacteria have more recently become more threatening, particularly with the emergence of MRSA in some regions. Antibiotic regimens need to broadly cover gram-positive and gram-negative bacteria (e.g., piperacillin/tazobactam and gentamicin) as well as MRSA when relevant.

Rarely seen as a complication of stem cell transplant, thrombotic thrombocytopenic purpura (TTP) can present with the classic pentad of fever, neurologic symptoms, hemolytic anemia, thrombocytopenia, and renal compromise (Table 106.11). The disorder seems to be associated with immunosuppression with cyclosporine or FK506 in the posttransplant period. In some patients, TTP may evolve into a more chronic picture with abnormal renal dysfunction and a clinical picture more consistent with HUS.

An experimental, promising new treatment for leukemia involves chimeric antigen receptor modified T-cells (CART). In this specialized therapy, a patient's T-cells are harvested and engineered to express a receptor that allows them to seek out and destroy leukemic blasts. These cells are then reinfused into the patient in an inpatient setting. Importantly for emergency physicians, steroids are contraindicated for any patients being treated with CART therapy since steroids are lymphotoxic and likely to be detrimental to this type of therapy.

CARE OF PATIENTS WITH ADVANCED CANCER

Pediatric palliative care has seen major changes in recent decades and these developments clearly impact care for children with cancer. Children with incurable cancer may still receive treatment that may be life prolonging and options for managing symptoms related to advanced disease have expanded. Also noteworthy is the increased decision-making role for the patient and family members in the setting of advanced disease. Options for patients to receive care outside of the hospital, either in hospice or at home, have greatly evolved.

Central to the mission of the emergency physician approaching a child with advanced cancer should be establishing the current goals of care. This can occur in two major ways:

- The preferences of the patient and/or family members may already be documented in the medical record. Often, these preferences have been explored during previous hospitalizations or clinic appointments with the patient's primary oncology team. In many cases, the outcome of such discussions may now be written in the form of a Do-Not-Resuscitate (DNR) order, a Seven Wish Document, or an outpatient/home form or order meant to establish limits for resuscitation. Insight into the patient's and family's goals of care may be gained by direct communication with the oncology provider who knows the patient best.
- During the visit to the ED, the clinician should ask the patient/family open-ended questions to allow for an open expression of preferences. During this conversation, if the patient has documented preferences already expressed in the medical record, the clinician should inquire whether there have been any recent changes to these preferences. Changes sometimes occur and medical staff unacquainted with the patient often feel uncomfortable embarking upon these discussions, even though patients and family members usually welcome the opportunity to communicate in this way.

Approaching patients with advanced cancer requires the clinician to acknowledge that sometimes patient/family preferences do not seem aligned with those of the healthcare team. For example, the physician may encounter a patient who is clearly within hours or days of death but who still "wants everything done," including cancer-directed therapy and aggressive management such as intubation or resuscitation. On the other hand, the clinician may instead face a patient with seemingly good functional status and quality of life who declines further disease-directed treatments. Cases may exist anywhere in between these two extremes. It is the clinician's responsibility to provide honest and complete information and elicit the patient's beliefs and wishes to facilitate decision making that most reflects the individual wishes of the patient and family. Once decisions are made, it is then the duty of the clinician to help carry out those wishes. Patients with advanced cancer may have clear preferences regarding admission to the hospital. While some patients and families may have adequate services in place to remain in their homes, some will still desire inpatient management as a form of respite.

Initiation of a management plan intended to reduce symptoms is always an appropriate step. The kind of intervention best able to reduce symptoms must be chosen based on the goals of care. Patients with advanced cancer have often received large amounts of opioids in the past and may therefore require larger doses of pain medications than routinely administered to children in the ED (see the "Pain" section). It is imperative for the clinician to increase the opioid dose until an efficacious dose is reached. Opioids may also be used to treat shortness of breath or other respiratory symptoms.

Diagnostic workup and specific management beyond symptom control should be undertaken in a manner consistent with the goals of care. If the patient's focus is only on comfort, then additional testing should be considered only if it will help identify a reasonable strategy to optimize that comfort. Consider, for example, a patient who presents for pain management but who is also cachectic and dehydrated. The clinician may wonder whether checking serum electrolytes and initiating rehydration are indicated. If the stated goals of care are comfort, then these measures should be omitted since electrolyte disturbances rarely cause pain or discomfort and hydration often will prolong the suffering associated with severe pain at the end of life. Indeed, hydration could increase edema or secretions that would actually decrease quality of life. As an additional example, consider a patient presenting with a malignant pleural effusion causing severe respiratory distress. Under other circumstances, the management of a large effusion might be immediate placement of chest tube. In this case, the clinician might instead ask, "How will a chest tube help *this* patient and does it match what he/she wants?" This change in thought process is often extremely hard for healthcare providers whose experience and training do not include care of patients with advanced disease but it is an essential element of their care.

Suggested Readings and Key References

General

Golden CB, Feusner JH. Malignant abdominal masses in children: quick guide to evaluation and diagnosis. *Pediatr Clin North Am* 2002;49:1369–1392.

Prusakowski MK, Cannone D. Pediatric oncologic emergencies. *Emerg Med Clin North Am* 2014;32:527–548.

Zojer N, Ludwig H. Hematological emergencies. *Ann Oncol* 2007;18: i45–i48.

Leukemia

Blum W, Porcu P. Therapeutic apheresis in hyperleukocytosis and hyperviscosity syndrome. *Semin Thromb Hemost* 2007;33:350–354.

Cairo MS, Coiffier B, Reiter A, et al.; TLS Expert Panel. Recommendations for the evaluation of risk and prophylaxis if tumor lysis syndrome (TLS) in adults and children with malignant diseases: an expert TLS panel consensus. *Br J Haematol* 2010;149: 1365–2141.

Cheuk DK, Chaing AK, Chan GC, et al. Urate oxidase for the prevention and treatment of tumour lysis syndrome in children with cancer. *Cochrane Database Syst Rev* 2014;8:DC006945.

Pieters R, Carroll WL. Biology and treatment of acute lymphoblastic leukemia. *Pediatr Clin North Am* 2008;55:1–20.

Pui CH, Robison LL, Look AT. Acute lymphoblastic leukemia. *Lancet* 2008;371:1030–1043.

Rubnitz JE, Gibson B, Smith FO. Acute myeloid leukemia. *Pediatr Clin North Am* 2008;55:21–51.

Histiocytic Diseases

Risma K, Jordan MB. Hemophagocytic lymphohistiocytosis: updates and evolving concepts. *Curr Opin Pediatr* 2012;24:9–15.

Weitzman S, Egeler RM. Langerhans cell histiocytosis: update for the pediatrician. *Curr Opin Pediatr* 2008;20:23–29.

Tumors of the Central Nervous System

Chintagumpala M, Gajjar A. Brain tumors. *Pediatr Clin North Am* 2015;62:167–178.

Pitfield AF, Carroll AB, Kissoon N. Emergency management of increased intracranial pressure. *Pediatr Emerg Care* 2012;28:200–204.

Ullrich NJ, Pomeroy SL. Pediatric brain tumors. *Neurol Clin* 2003;21: 897–913.

Tumors of the Head and Neck

Albright JT, Topham AK, Reilly JS. Pediatric head and neck malignancies: US incidence and trends over 2 decades. *Arch Otolaryngol Head Neck Surg* 2002;128:655–659.

Tumors of the Thorax

Allen CE, Kelly KM, Bollard CM. Pediatric lymphomas and histiocytic disorders of childhood. *Pediatr Clin North Am* 2015;62: 139–165.

Gross TG, Termuhlen AM. Pediatric non-Hodgkin's lymphoma. *Curr Oncol Rep* 2007;9:459–465.

Olson MR, Donaldson SS. Treatment of pediatric Hodgkin lymphoma. *Curr Treat Options Oncol* 2008;9:81–94.

Perger L, Lee EY, Shamberger RC. Management of children and adolescents with a critical airway due to compression by an anterior mediastinal mass. *J Pediatr Surg* 2008;43:1990–1997.

Schwartz CL. The management of Hodgkin disease in the young child. *Curr Opin Pediatr* 2003;15:10–16.

Yu JB, Wilson LD, Detterbeck FC. Superior vena cava syndrome–a proposed classification system and algorithm for management. *J Thorac Oncol* 2008;3:811–814.

Tumors of the Hepatobiliary Tree

Honeyman JN, La Quaglia MP. Malignant liver tumors. *Semin Pediatr Surg* 2012;21:245–254.

Kremer N, Walther AE, Tiao GM. Management of hepatoblastoma: an update. *Curr Opin Pediatr* 2014;26:362–369.

Neuroblastoma

De Bernardi B, Pianca C, Pistamiglio P, et al. Neuroblastoma with symptomatic spinal cord compression at diagnosis: treatment and results with 76 cases. *J Clin Oncol* 2001;19:183–190.

Kim S, Chung DH. Pediatric solid malignancies: neuroblastoma and Wilm's tumor. *Surg Clin North Am* 2006;86:469–487.

Park JR, Eggert A, Caron H. Neuroblastoma: biology, prognosis, and treatment. *Pediatr Clin North Am* 2008;55:97–120.

Tumors of the Kidney

Davenport KP, Blanco FC, Sandler AD. Pediatric malignancies: neuroblastoma, Wilm's tumor, hepatoblastoma, rhabdomyosarcoma, and sacroccygeal teratoma. *Surg Clin North Am* 2012;92: 745–767.

Kaste SC, Dome JS, Babyn PS, et al. Wilm's tumour: prognostic factors, staging, therapy, and late effects. *Pediatr Radiol* 2008;38: 2–17.

Kim S, Chung DH. Pediatric solid malignancies: neuroblastoma and Wilm's tumor. *Surg Clin North Am* 2006;86:469–487.

Malkan AD, Loh A, Bahrami A, et al. An approach to renal masses in pediatrics. *Pediatrics* 2015;135:142–158.

Gonadal Tumors

Billmire DF. Germ cell tumors. *Surg Clin North Am* 2006;86: 489–503.

Schneider DT, Calaminus G, Koch S, et al. Epidemiologic analysis of 1,442 children and adolescents registered in the German germ cell tumor protocols. *Pediatr Blood Cancer* 2004;42:169–175.

Tumors in and Around the Spinal cord

Kwok Y, DeYoung C, Garofalo M, et al. Radiation oncology emergencies. *Hematol Oncol Clin North Am* 2006;20:505–522.

Pollono D, Tomarchia S, Drut R, et al. Spinal cord compression: a review of 70 pediatric patients. *Pediatr Hematol Oncol* 2003;20: 457–466.

Tumors of Bone and Soft Tissue Tumors

Albritton KH. Sarcomas in adolescents and young adults. *Hematol Oncol Clin North Am* 2005;19:527–546.

HaDuong JH, Martin AA, Skapek SX, et al. Sarcomas. *Pediatr Clin North Am* 2015;62:179–200.

Marec-Berard P, Philip T. Ewing sarcoma: the pediatrician's point of view. *Pediatr Blood Cancer* 2004;42:477–480.

Hematologic Complications

Athale UH, Chan AK. Hemorrhagic complications in pediatric hematologic malignancies. *Semin Thromb Hemost* 2007;33: 408–415.

Wiernikowski JT, Athale UH. Thromboembolic complications in children with cancer. *Thromb Res* 2006;118:137–152.

Infectious Complications

Bremer CT, Monahan BP. Necrotizing enterocolitis in neutropenia and chemotherapy: a clinical update and old lessons relearned. *Curr Gastroenterol Rep* 2006;8:333–341.

Davila ML. Neutropenic enterocolitis. *Curr Opin Gastroenterol* 2006; 22:44–47.

Elihu A, Gollin G. Complications of implanted central venous catheters in neutropenic children. *Am Surg* 2007;73:1079–1082.

Henry M, Sung L. Supportive care in pediatric oncology: oncologic emergencies and management of fever and neutropenia. *Pediatr Clin North Am* 2015;62:27–46.

Hughes WT, Armstrong D, Bodey GP, et al. 2002 guidelines for the use of antimicrobial agents in neutropenic patients with cancer. *Clin Infect Dis* 2002;34:730–751.

McCarville MB, Adelman CS, Li C, et al. Typhlitis in childhood cancer. *Cancer* 2005;104:380–387.

Rosen GP, Nielsen K, Glenn S, et al. Invasive fungal infections in pediatric oncology patients: 11-year experience. *J Pediatr Hematol Oncol* 2005;27:135–140.

Pain

Brislin RP, Rose JB. Pediatric acute pain management. *Anesthesiol Clin North America* 2005;23:789–814.

Galloway KS, Yaster M. Pain and symptom control in terminally ill children. *Pediatr Clin North Am* 2000;47:711–746.

Levine D, Lam CG, Cunningham MJ, et al. Best practices for pediatric palliative care: a primer for clinical providers. *J Support Oncol* 2013;11:114–125.

Neurologic Complications

Sul JK, Deangelis LM. Neurologic complications of cancer chemotherapy. *Semin Oncol* 2006;33:324–332.

Cardiovascular Complications

Appel JM, Nielsen D, Zerahn B, et al. Anthracycline-induced chronic cardiotoxicity and heart failure. *Acta Oncol* 2007;46:576–580.

Hepatic and Gastrointestinal Complications

Hesketh PJ. Chemotherapy-induced nausea and vomiting. *N Engl J Med* 2008;358:2482–2494.

Complications of Stem Cell Transplantation

Barfield RC, Kasow KA, Hale GA. Advances in pediatric hematopoietic stem cell transplantation. *Cancer Biol Ther* 2008;7:1533–1539.

Munchel A, Chen A, Symons H. Emergent complications in the pediatric hematopoietic stem cell transplant patient. *Clin Pediatr Emerg Med* 2011;12:233–244.

Palliative Care

Collins JJ. Palliative care and the child with cancer. *Hematol Oncol Clin North Am* 2002;16:657–670.

Himelstein BP, Hilden JM, Boldt AM, et al. Pediatric palliative care. *N Engl J Med* 2004;350:1752–1762.

Mack JW, Wolfe J. Early integration of pediatric palliative care: for some children, palliative care starts at diagnosis. *Curr Opin Pediatr* 2006;18:10–14.

Moore D, Sheetz J. Pediatric palliative care consultation. *Pediatr Clin North Am* 2014;61:735–747.

CHAPTER 107 ■ PULMONARY EMERGENCIES

KYLE NELSON, MD, MPH, MARK I. NEUMAN, MD, MPH, AND JOSHUA NAGLER, MD, MHPEd

GOALS OF EMERGENCY THERAPY

Pulmonary emergencies are common in children, accounting for approximately 10% of pediatric emergency department (ED) visits and 20% of hospitalizations. Significant respiratory distress, particularly impending respiratory failure, must be promptly recognized and effectively managed. General approaches to improve oxygenation and ventilation are combined with therapy tailored to the underlying condition. The differential diagnosis varies by age, with many conditions unique to specific pediatric age groups. National guidelines are published for evaluation and management of asthma, bronchiolitis, and pneumonia, which have informed local clinical practice guidelines and development of measurable outcomes reflecting quality of care.

KEY POINTS

- An age-appropriate differential diagnosis must be considered when managing respiratory distress.
- Normal vital sign ranges vary according to the age of the child.
- Children with severe respiratory distress may rapidly decompensate and progress to respiratory failure.

RELATED CHAPTERS

Signs and Symptoms

- Cough: Chapter 14
- Cyanosis: Chapter 16
- Pain: Chest: Chapter 50
- Stridor: Chapter 70
- Wheezing: Chapter 80

Clinical Pathways

- Asthma: Chapter 84
- Bronchiolitis: Chapter 85
- Pneumonia, Community-Acquired: Chapter 90

Medical, Surgical, and Trauma Emergencies

- Allergic Emergencies: Chapter 93
- Thoracic Trauma: Chapter 123
- Thoracic Emergencies: Chapter 132

ACUTE RESPIRATORY FAILURE

CLINICAL PEARLS AND PITFALLS

- Impending respiratory failure must be promptly recognized and managed. Effective early intervention can limit progression, morbidity, and mortality.
- A systematic approach to prioritizing assessment and support of airway, breathing, and circulation should be employed.
- Emergency management of acute respiratory failure often involves both diagnostic testing and lifesaving therapeutic maneuvers.
- After stabilization, attention must be given to treating the underlying condition.

Current Evidence

While many cases of respiratory distress are benign and self-limited, requiring minimal or no intervention, pulmonary diseases contribute to significant morbidity and mortality in pediatrics, including 3% to 5% of deaths; some of these deaths may be preventable. Importantly, respiratory failure often precedes cardiopulmonary arrest in children; unlike adults for whom primary cardiac disease is often responsible. Therefore, careful assessment of cardiopulmonary status and anticipation of and preparation for deterioration are important aspects of care. Prompt recognition and treatment of impending respiratory failure can be lifesaving and may reduce morbidity and mortality.

By definition, there are two components to respiratory failure—inability of the respiratory system to (1) provide sufficient oxygen for metabolic needs (hypoxic respiratory failure) and (2) excrete the carbon dioxide (CO_2) produced by the body (hypercapnic or ventilatory respiratory failure). Both are often present simultaneously, but to varying degrees.

Causes of acute respiratory failure can also be categorized with consideration of location in the respiratory system (Table 107.1). In addition to primary pulmonary disease, many disorders outside the respiratory tract can lead to respiratory failure.

Primary pulmonary conditions must be considered. Parenchymal lung disease can lead to acute respiratory failure, particularly in younger children, and those with underlying cardiopulmonary disease (e.g., bronchopulmonary dysplasia [BPD] or congenital heart disease). In such cases, the additional respiratory embarrassment from acute pulmonary infection can induce respiratory failure.

Any condition that causes further narrowing or collapse of the intrinsically small pediatric airway can have a profound effect on air flow. Edema from infectious, allergic, or caustic etiologies; foreign material in the airway; or obstruction by enlarged or compressing anatomic structures can restrict airflow. These may occur in isolation or in combination.

Asthma is the most common etiology for lower airway disease, but infections such as bronchiolitis or viral pneumonia are also common. Foreign-body aspiration can present acutely with airway obstruction, or may be a delayed diagnosis

TABLE 107.1

CAUSES OF ACUTE RESPIRATORY FAILURE IN CHILDREN

Pulmonary diseases	Infectious pneumonia (bacterial, viral, fungal, and other)
	Tuberculosis
	Pertussis, parapertussis syndrome
	Cystic fibrosis
	Drug-induced pulmonary disease
	Vasculitis, collagen vascular disease
	Pulmonary dysgenesis
	Pulmonary edema
	Pneumothorax, hemothorax, chylothorax
	Drowning/near drowning
	Bronchopulmonary dysplasia
	Bronchiolitis
	Asthma
	Pulmonary hemorrhage
Airway obstruction	
Upper	Acute epiglottitis
	Laryngotracheobronchitis (croup)
	Bacterial tracheitis
	Foreign-body aspiration
	Adenotonsillar hypertrophy
	Retropharyngeal abscess
	Subglottic stenosis, web, or hemangioma
	Laryngomalacia
	Laryngeal edema
	Congenital neck anomalies (e.g., cystic hygroma, bronchial cleft abnormalities)
	Static encephalopathy
Airway obstruction	
Lower	Reactive airway disease (asthma)
	Bronchiolitis
	Foreign-body aspiration
	Cystic fibrosis
	Bronchiectasis
	Tracheobronchomalacia
	Bronchopulmonary dysplasia
	α_1-Antitrypsin deficiency
	Hydrocarbon aspiration, aspiration syndromes
	Congenital lobar emphysema
Chest wall deformity disorders	Diaphragmatic hernia
	Kyphoscoliosis (severe)
	Restrictive lung disease secondary to chest deformity
Neurologic disease	
Central nervous system	Status epilepticus
	Severe static encephalopathy
	Acute meningoencephalitis
	Brain abscess, hematoma, tumor
	Brain stem insult
	Arnold–Chiari crisis
	Drug intoxication
Spinal/anterior horn cell	Transverse myelitis
	Poliomyelitis
	Polyradiculitis (Guillain–Barré)
	Spinal muscle atrophy type 1 (Werdnig–Hoffmann syndrome)
Neuromuscular junction	Myasthenia gravis
	Botulism (e.g., infantile, food-borne, wound)
	Tetanus
	Myopathy
	Neuropathy
	Drugs (e.g., succinylcholine, curare, pancuronium, organophosphates)
Other diseases	Cardiac disease
	Anemia (severe)
	Acidemia (e.g., renal failure, diabetic ketoacidosis, hepatic disease)
	Oxygen dissociation (e.g., methemoglobinemia, carbon monoxide, or cyanide poisoning)
	Hypothermia, hyperthermia
	Sepsis
	Obstructive sleep apnea syndrome
	Acute chest syndrome in patients with sickle cell anemia

following the development of secondary postobstructive atelectasis or pneumonia.

Chest wall deformities and mechanical impairments prevent full expansion of the chest, leading to decreased vital capacity, decreased minute ventilation, and resultant hypercapnia. Inefficient respiratory efforts can cause subsequent hypoxia. Oftentimes, these patients maintain near normal respiratory function until additional physiologic compromise occurs, often from illness as minor as an upper respiratory infection.

Disruption of nonpulmonary respiratory physiology often results from either reversible or irreversible causes of central nervous system (CNS) disease. CNS disease may result in depressed respiratory drive, or inability to maintain protective airway reflexes. Alternatively, neurologic disease may directly affect the peripheral nerves or muscles, leading to either airway obstruction or inadequate excursion of the chest wall and diaphragm. The result is inadequate gas exchange and ventilation–perfusion (V/Q) mismatch.

Finally, numerous other nonpulmonary diseases may precipitate respiratory failure. Though with varied underlying pathophysiology, the diseases listed in Table 107.1 may alter the balance of O_2 consumption and CO_2 production such that gas exchange cannot be maintained by the respiratory system, leading to secondary respiratory failure.

Goals of Treatment

The goals of management of acute respiratory failure are correction of hypoxia and sufficient support of ventilation. Immediate efforts should be directed toward both lifesaving maneuvers and appropriate diagnostic testing, as establishing a diagnosis will inform disease-specific management.

Clinical Considerations

Clinical Recognition

Acute respiratory failure represents the severe end of the spectrum of respiratory disease. Though the onset can be hyperacute (e.g., complete airway obstruction from foreign-body aspiration or traumatic injury to phrenic nerve with complete loss of respiratory effort), respiratory failure more commonly results from a progression of respiratory illness and distress. The differential diagnosis is broad, though the underlying causes vary by age. While congenital anomalies are likely to present in the first several months of life, some may present in older infants and toddlers. Some progressive neurologic conditions may present in older children. It is important to appreciate that normal ranges of respiratory rate differ by age (Table 107.2). Some cases may involve patients without concerning medical history that have a severe acute condition such as upper airway obstruction from aspirated foreign body or swelling due to infection. Some cases may involve progressive deterioration of a chronic condition such as cystic fibrosis (CF). Details of management differ according to acute diagnosis and pathophysiology of underlying condition.

Patients at risk for acute respiratory failure must be quickly identified and managed to prevent deterioration. In general, patients presenting with significant respiratory distress (i.e., grunting, gasping, and severely increased work of breathing) are at risk for respiratory failure. Additionally, neonates, patients with cardiac disease, and those with worrisome trajectories and/or tiring despite therapy are considered at risk of respiratory failure. Other concerning clinical findings, blood gas abnormalities, and pulmonary function abnormalities commonly present in the setting of respiratory failure are listed in Table 107.3. Appreciation of complicating underlying conditions and the current clinical status, including response to chronic therapy and details of prior exacerbations will help to assess those at risk of deteriorating respiratory failure and inform treatment decisions.

TABLE 107.2

RESTING RESPIRATORY RATE BY AGE

Age	Breaths per minute
Neonate	30–50
2–12 mo	30–40
12 mo–2 yrs	22–30
2–12 yrs	16–24
Adolescent	12–20

TABLE 107.3

DIAGNOSIS OF ACUTE RESPIRATORY FAILURE FROM PULMONARY CAUSES IN CHILDREN

Clinical findings

Vital signs: tachycardia, tachypnea or bradypnea, hypoxemia

General appearance: cyanosis, diaphoresis, confusion, restlessness, fatigue, shortness of breath, apnea, grunting, stridor, retractions, decreased air entry, wheezing

Blood gas abnormalities

$Pa{CO_2}$ >50 mm Hg with acidosis (pH <7.25)

$Pa{CO_2}$ >40 mm Hg with severe distress

$Pa{O_2}$ <60 mm Hg (or $Sa{O_2}$ <90%) on 0.4 $F{IO_2}$

Pulmonary function abnormalities

Vital capacity (<15 mL/kg)

Inspiratory pressure (<25–30 cm H_2O)

Triage

Children with signs of impending or acute respiratory failure should be rapidly identified based on appearance or vital signs and immediately evaluated with attention to necessary lifesaving maneuvers. Supplemental oxygen and support of ventilation should be provided emergently as indicated, while additional efforts to determine underlying etiology are being addressed.

Initial Assessment/H&P

Diagnosis of acute respiratory failure is commonly made clinically, though laboratory or pulmonary function testing can be supportive. Initial assessment involves prompt appraisal of the child's appearance, level of alertness, airway patency, breathing effort, and circulation. Resuscitative efforts may be necessary to clear or support an obstructed airway, provide oxygen, and support effective ventilation. Initial history should be brief, focused, and succinct. One approach to consider is the "AMPLE" history, which involves queries into allergies, medications, pertinent medical history, last meal, and events involved in present illness including treatments already administered.

Patients with acute respiratory failure should be continually assessed using cardiopulmonary monitoring of heart rate, cardiac rhythm, respiratory rate, pulse oximetry, and blood pressure. Noninvasive monitoring of end-tidal carbon dioxide ($ETCO_2$) (i.e., capnography) is also an important adjunct, providing information about ventilatory status, including adequacy of assisted ventilation if performed.

Management

Management of acute respiratory failure is critical care in the ED. It involves performing necessary therapeutic interventions to assist oxygenation and ventilation along with close monitoring for further deterioration and consideration of appropriate diagnostic testing (Table 107.4).

Supplemental oxygen should be provided during initial assessment and any resuscitative efforts. This is most

TABLE 107.4

MANAGEMENT OF ACUTE RESPIRATORY FAILURE

Primary hypoxemia	1. High-flow supplemental oxygen (e.g., nonrebreather mask), titrate for cyanosis, or by pulse oximetry or PaO_2 2. Use PEEP through CPAP or BiPAP to further improve oxygenation 3. Consider endotracheal intubation when persistent hypoxemia on FIO_2 >0.6 or when decreased lung compliance and FIO_2 >0.4 4. Use assisted ventilation to improve gas exchange (increased inspiratory time, normal respiratory rates, tidal volume: 10–15 mL/kg; pressure cycle ventilation if wt. <10 kg, volume cycle ventilation if wt. >10 kg). If inspiratory pressure exceeds 40 cm H_2O, consider use of permissive hypercapnia to reduce barotrauma. 5. Treat underlying cause
Primary hypoventilation	1. Supplemental oxygen (as above) 2. Support ventilation a. Oral/nasal pharyngeal airway or endotracheal intubation to open the airway b. Bag-mask ventilation with high-flow oxygen c. Use assisted ventilation (normal to increased respiratory rates, increased expired time and increased flow rates with obstructive airway disease), BiPAP is favored over CPAP for noninvasive ventilation with primary hypoventilation d. Use increased tidal volume (pressure) with atelectasis e. Monitor carefully for side effects of ventilation
Adjunctive therapy	1. Intravenous fluid to achieve normal vascular volume (less fluid for child with interstitial lung disease) 2. Diuretics such as furosemide (1 mg/kg) for acute pulmonary edema or fluid overload 3. Sedatives/analgesics—morphine sulfate (0.1–0.2 mg/kg) every 1–2 hrs intravenously; midazolam (0.1–0.2 mg/kg every 2–4 hrs intravenously) 4. Muscle relaxants for intubated patients—rocuronium 1–1.2 mg/kg/dose or vecuronium bromide, starting at 0.1 mg/kg every 1–2 hrs or alternative 0.1–0.2 mg/kg/hr drip

PEEP, positive end-expiratory pressure; CPAP, constant positive airway pressure; BiPAP, bilevel positive airway pressure.

appropriately accomplished using a nonrebreather mask for spontaneously breathing patients. The goal oxygen saturation percentage may vary according to underlying and suspected acute conditions, but >90% is an appropriate initial goal for most patients. While some patients with cardiac disease may not tolerate high amounts of supplemental oxygen depending on their physiology, in general, immediate lifesaving efforts should include provision of supplemental oxygen while further details of the condition are sought and risks of overoxygenating are considered.

Clinicians should be adept at assessing airway patency and performing emergency maneuvers to optimize oxygen delivery and assisted ventilation. Use of a flow-inflating resuscitation bag (aka "anesthesia bag") can deliver 100% oxygen and continuous positive airway pressure (CPAP). Positive-pressure breaths utilizing a self-inflating or flow-inflating bag will further increase oxygen delivery. Importantly, CPAP cannot be delivered though a self-inflating (Ambu) bag. Endotracheal intubation provides the most effective means of increasing PaO_2 and is required for patients with persistent hypoxemia despite other interventions including noninvasive ventilation support such as CPAP or BiPAP.

As mentioned, support of ventilation is indicated if adequate oxygen saturation cannot be maintained in spontaneously breathing patients despite 100% oxygen delivery. Assisted ventilation may also be required to correct alveolar hypoventilation despite adequate oxygen saturation. Adequacy of ventilation should be assessed clinically by chest wall expansion with further data from either $ETCO_2$ or blood gas analysis of PCO_2. Goal tidal volumes are usually 7 to 10 mL per kg, although this will vary based on lung compliance and underlying disease.

Specific ventilation strategies will vary based on underlying disease. In children with acute respiratory failure but normal lung function (e.g., CNS depression), standard airway pressures and respiratory rates are appropriate. Positive end-expiratory pressures (PEEPs) may be useful where alveolar recruitment is important to improve gas exchange (e.g., atelectasis). This can be done manually with a bag and mask, or with CPAP or BiPAP. PEEP shifts lungs to a position on the pressure–volume curve that improves alveolar ventilation by increasing the end-expiratory lung volume or functional residual capacity. Attention must be given to minimizing the risk of barotrauma. In patients with decreased lung compliance due to either stiff lungs (e.g., fibrosis) or hyperinflation (e.g., bronchiolitis or asthma), higher pressures must be used to sufficiently ventilate the child. The inspiratory:expiratory (I:E) ratio can also be tailored to the disease process. A normal or decreased I:E ratio is used in obstructive lower airway disease to extend exhalation time to better allow elimination of CO_2. Increased I:E ratios of 1:5 to 1 should be utilized in alveolar or interstitial disorders to improve oxygenation. Permissive hypercapnia, accepting elevated PCO_2 values as long as pH is maintained, may be advantageous, as this may allow for pressure-limited ventilation, which will reduce the risk of barotrauma.

Fluid management is another important component of care for patients with respiratory failure. In general, fluids should be titrated to maintain normal intravascular volume as determined by monitoring heart rate, blood pressure, peripheral perfusion, and urine output. However, patients with significantly increased work of breathing generate high negative intrathoracic pressure which increases venous return. When these patients transition to positive-pressure ventilation, venous return rapidly decreases and may precipitate cardiovascular collapse. Therefore, unless clinical circumstances mandate more immediate action, rapid intravascular repletion before initiating positive pressure (through noninvasive ventilation or intubation) is prudent. In contrast, for patients with interstitial disease or pulmonary capillary leak, a slightly reduced intravascular volume may improve the cardiopulmonary mechanics necessary for effective ventilation. As a result, the FIO_2 requirement may be decreased and airway pressures minimized. Depending on the diagnosis, there may be other clinical indicators such as fever, vomiting, and sepsis that may affect fluid management. In severely ill or complex patients, the measurement of central venous pressure may provide a more precise guide for monitoring fluid status.

Sedation is an important adjunct to efficient assisted ventilation to reduce anxiety and increase tolerance to the presence of a tracheal tube and assisted ventilation. Morphine sulfate dosed 0.1 to 0.2 mg per kg every 1 to 2 hours or as a continuous infusion of 0.1 mg/kg/hr is often used. This is frequently combined with a benzodiazepine, such as midazolam 0.1 to 0.2 mg per kg every 1 to 2 hours or as a continuous infusion. Muscle relaxants may help optimally ventilate intubated children with severe respiratory failure, such as those with stiff lungs (e.g., severe interstitial pneumonia) or stiff chest wall (e.g., status epilepticus), by improving compliance and reducing oxygen consumption. Depolarizing agents may include repeated doses of rocuronium at 1 to 1.2 mg/kg/dose. Alternatively, vecuronium bromide can be administered starting at 0.1 mg per kg every 1 to 2 hours or as a drip at 0.1 to 0.2 mg/kg/hr.

Clinical Indications for Discharge or Admission

Patients with acute respiratory failure require hospitalization. If resuscitation efforts restore adequate oxygenation and ventilation and a stable trajectory has been established, admission to the inpatient floor for continued evaluation and management may be appropriate. However, most patients will require intensive care unit (ICU) admission, and prompt communication with the critical care team at one's institution or an appropriate transfer facility should be an early priority in management (see Chapter 6 Interfacility Transport and Stabilization).

ASTHMA

CLINICAL PEARLS AND PITFALLS

- Standard medications for acute asthma treatment include short-acting β-agonists (SABAs), anticholinergics, and systemic corticosteroids.
- Children with severe exacerbations should receive high-dose SABA mixed with ipratropium bromide in addition to prompt systemic corticosteroids. They often require continuous SABA as well, following initial treatments.
- Intravenous (IV) magnesium sulfate should be considered for patients not improving after multiple high-dose SABA or for patients with severe exacerbations.
- Emergency physicians should consider prescribing inhaled corticosteroids (ICSs) based on the degree of asthma control.

Current Evidence

Asthma is a chronic inflammatory disease of the lower airways characterized by bronchial hyperresponsiveness and reversible bronchospasm. While there is common pathophysiology for patients with asthma, the phenotype is rather heterogeneous, likely due to many interacting factors including the level of airway inflammation, degree of bronchial hyperresponsiveness, environmental exposures, and genetic differences (which may account for 60% to 80% of interindividual variance in treatment response).

The National Asthma Education and Prevention Program (NAEPP) has published guidelines outlining diagnosis and management of acute and chronic asthma. Many institutions have implemented local acute asthma clinical guidelines, which are associated with improved quality outcomes including shorter time to medication administration, shorter length of stay (LOS), and fewer medication prescription errors.

Goals of Treatment

Acute asthma management is directed at reversing bronchospasm and treating the underlying airway inflammation. Goals of treatment include prompt administration of bronchodilators and systemic corticosteroids and identification of complications.

Clinical Considerations

Clinical Recognition

Asthma is characterized clinically by a pattern of periodic episodes of cough, wheeze, respiratory distress, and reversible bronchospasm. While wheezing is the most obvious symptom, some patients may primarily have cough without significant wheeze. Asking the family about typical symptoms for the child can provide clarification.

Asthma is generally a clinical diagnosis, and some clinicians hesitate to diagnose asthma in children younger than 24 months. However, an asthma diagnosis is appropriate if the child has compatible history suggesting the characteristic features of lower airway obstruction, bronchial hyperresponsiveness, and reversible bronchospasm. Airway inflammation levels and formal pulmonary function testing are uncommonly measured in the acute setting.

The prevalence of "lifetime" asthma (ever diagnosed) is estimated at 13% of all US children, with 6.7 million having active disease, and over 3.5 million having ≥1 exacerbation per year. Children younger than 4 years old have the highest rates of ED visits, ambulatory visits, and hospitalizations. Asthma disproportionately affects minority children, those living in urban areas, and those of lower socioeconomic status.

Triage

Prompt determination of the severity of respiratory distress will help direct appropriate therapy. Level of severity can be generally categorized as mild, moderate, severe, or impending respiratory failure. There are several validated severity scoring tools, including the Pediatric Asthma Severity Score, Modified Pulmonary Index, and Pulmonary Score. Many guidelines utilize such scores and outline severity-based therapy. These scores also allow physicians and nurses to communicate about severity and response to therapy using a standard language.

Initial Assessment/H&P

In addition to determining level of severity, obtaining asthma-specific history is helpful to inform further care and disposition. Important history includes information about the current exacerbation (duration, course, home medications administered and response to treatment, and likely trigger) as well as chronic severity of asthma (number of exacerbations during prior 12 months, number of hospitalizations, number of ICU admissions, need for intubation, use of controller therapies).

Chronic asthma severity reflects asthma control, often considered to include assessment of asthma risk (prior exacerbations requiring unscheduled visits, use of systemic corticosteroids, and hospitalizations) and impairment (asthma symptom burden and rescue medication use). While such detailed assessment may not be commonly performed in a formal manner using all of the questions outlined in the NAEPP or Asthma Control Test, clinicians can query about frequency of days or nights with increased asthma symptoms and use of albuterol. Patients with 2 or more days/nights of symptoms and/or albuterol use per week likely have chronic asthma severity in the "persistent" range and prescribing or continuing inhaled steroids is recommended.

Management

Treatment involves weight-based dosing of SABA (most commonly albuterol in the United States), anticholinergics (usually ipratropium bromide), and systemic corticosteroids (prednisone, prednisolone, methylprednisolone, or dexamethasone) (see Chapter 84 Asthma).

Inhaled SABA causes bronchodilation of airway smooth muscle through activation of β2-adrenergic receptors. Albuterol is the most commonly used SABA. It is a racemic mixture of two enantiomers—R-albuterol (binds β2-receptor and causes bronchodilation and adverse effects of tachycardia and tremor) and S-albuterol (believed to have detrimental effect on airway function). Levalbuterol contains the R-enantiomer alone, and is marketed as an alternative to racemic albuterol with fewer adverse effects (e.g., tachycardia) than racemic albuterol. However, studies are inconsistent regarding clinical superiority of levalbuterol over racemic albuterol, and the increased cost of levalbuterol must be considered. The NAEPP guidelines list levalbuterol as an option for SABA treatment at half the dose of nebulized albuterol.

Albuterol can be administered using metered-dose inhalers (MDIs) with valved holding chambers (spacers) or nebulizers. Use of both requires proper technique. While there are potential differences in lung deposition between devices, studies have found equivalency or favor MDI with spacer with regard to ED LOS and tachycardia. Although nebulizers have traditionally been the preferred devices, MDI with spacer may be considered an option for children with mild and moderate exacerbations. Studies on MDI with spacer for severe asthma exacerbations are limited. Patients with severe exacerbations have significant lower airway obstruction, which limits drug deposition in the lung, and higher overall albuterol doses using nebulizer are often necessary.

For those with mild exacerbations, it is reasonable to administer one SABA treatment and reassess need for additional therapy. Patients with moderate or severe exacerbations should receive multiple doses of SABA and anticholinergics in addition to systemic steroids.

Ipratropium bromide causes bronchodilation by blocking muscarinic cholinergic receptors. Adding anticholinergics to SABA is associated with improved pulmonary function and, importantly, has been shown to reduce hospitalization rates for those with severe exacerbations, particularly using multiple-dose protocols, and many protocols recommend its use for moderate severity as well.

Corticosteroids block formation of potent inflammatory mediators and reduce airway inflammation. Systemic corticosteroids are associated with improved pulmonary function and reduced hospitalizations. The effect on reducing hospitalizations is time dependent, maximized with early administration. A common metric regarding optimal asthma care is administration of systemic corticosteroids within 60 minutes of arrival. Systemic corticosteroids are also associated with fewer ED relapse visits and hospitalization at such return visits.

Prednisone and prednisolone are the most commonly used systemic corticosteroids, and have good oral bioavailability, tolerability, and similar effectiveness compared to IV route. Methylprednisolone or dexamethasone (IV or intramuscular) are also options favored for children in severe distress in whom oral intake may not be practical, or in those who are actively vomiting or likely to do so based on prior history. Other than these exceptions, oral corticosteroids are preferred for milder exacerbations. Dexamethasone has become more popular and a recent review observed similar outcomes and less vomiting compared to prednisone or prednisolone, though there was heterogeneity among treatment regimens.

After initial therapy, it is important to reassess the need for continued and adjunctive medications. Response to therapy can be categorized as good, incomplete, and poor. Those with good response have improvement with mild features and can be observed briefly and subsequently discharged if not requiring frequent SABA or having other indications for admission. Those with incomplete response continue to have moderate or severe features. They should receive frequent and possibly continuous albuterol, and adjunctive therapies such as magnesium sulfate heliox, or parenteral bronchodilator therapy should be considered.

Many studies have evaluated use of medications considered adjunctive (e.g., continuous albuterol, magnesium sulfate, heliox) in comparison to initial standard albuterol treatment, though, in practice, most clinicians administer them after insufficient improvement with multiple albuterol treatments. Adjunctive therapies such as magnesium sulfate and heliox can be administered in conjunction with ongoing inhaled bronchodilators, and timing may vary according to severity. Frequent reassessments during initial treatment for those with severe exacerbations, and anticipating the need for adjunctive therapy are essential to avoid delays.

Continuous nebulized albuterol treatment is recommended for patients with severe exacerbations or poor response to initial inhaled bronchodilator treatment. A systematic review found that continuous albuterol was associated with greater improvement in peak expiratory flow rate (PEFR) and lower hospitalization rate, particularly among those with moderate or severe exacerbations, with no increase in adverse effects.

Magnesium sulfate causes bronchodilation by relaxing respiratory smooth muscle. It is administered as a single IV bolus with a recommended dose of 50 to 75 mg per kg (maximum 2 g). Use of this therapy has been associated with improved pulmonary function and reduced hospitalization rates.

Heliox is a mixture of helium and oxygen, thought to improve drug delivery in obstructed airways due to its lower density and airflow resistance. The commonly used mixtures (helium:oxygen) are 70:30 or 80:20, but use in patients with significant hypoxemia may be limited. Contraindication for Heliox is pneumothorax, pneumopericardium, or pneumoperitoneum, therefore a chest radiograph (CXR) should be obtained prior to initiation.

Parenteral β-agonists are also options to consider for adjunctive therapy. Epinephrine administered intramuscularly may be an option for severe exacerbations, particularly as initial treatment for patients with significant airway obstruction when delivery of inhaled medications to the lower airways may be limited. Terbutaline may be administered subcutaneously or intravenously as a bolus and continued as an IV infusion. Although commonly included in many pediatric protocols for refractory asthma, pediatric studies regarding use are limited.

Noninvasive ventilatory support (CPAP or BiPAP) may benefit patients tiring from increased work of breathing and with impending respiratory failure. Pediatric studies are limited but suggest that it is generally well tolerated. While some studies suggest that it may reduce need for ICU admission, in practice, most patients who require ventilator support are treated in an ICU setting.

Chest radiographs (CXRs) are not routinely indicated for acute asthma exacerbations in children. Wheezing is a common symptom of asthma and pneumonia in children, therefore determining which patients warrant imaging can be challenging. Data regarding children of all ages with wheezing who had CXR, suggest that approximately 5% of febrile children will have radiographic findings consistent with pneumonia. However, the potential risks of CXR include radiation exposure and false-positive results leading to unnecessary antibiotic therapy. In general, patients with a typical asthma exacerbation do not routinely warrant imaging given this low rate of abnormal findings. In a patient with mild to moderate respiratory distress, the decision to perform a CXR may be deferred until reassessment after initial treatment; focal abnormal breath sounds may have improved suggesting atelectasis as opposed to pneumonia.

Clinical Indications for Discharge or Admission

In general, children requiring frequent albuterol (generally defined as more frequent than every 2 to 4 hours) or having persistent hypoxemia require admission. Other reasons for admission include significant dehydration, infection requiring inpatient treatment or monitoring, or medical history that may impact the respiratory system (e.g., cardiac disease, neuromuscular disorder, or metabolic disorder). Most patients requiring frequent inhaled bronchodilator therapy or adjunctive therapy (e.g., parenteral bronchodilators) will require hospitalization. Protocols regarding which therapies require an ICU setting vary by institution.

Patients discharged should be encouraged to follow up with their primary care providers (PCPs) within 1 to 3 days. Discharge instructions should include information about care following the acute visit and may include formulation of an asthma action plan. This provides an opportunity to assist patients with management during future exacerbations and to encourage partnership with PCPs for ongoing discussions and modifications of asthma care.

Inhaled steroids should be continued for patients currently taking them, and clinicians should strongly consider prescribing them from the ED when indicated. Patients with 2 or more days/nights of symptoms and/or albuterol use per week likely have chronic asthma severity in the "persistent" range and inhaled steroids are recommended. Data suggest that many patients treated for acute asthma in EDs meet criteria for persistent chronic asthma severity, yet no prescription has been provided or patients are noncompliant with therapy. Therefore, the ED visit for asthma represents an opportunity to improve outcomes for these children.

ASPIRATION PNEUMONIA

CLINICAL PEARLS AND PITFALLS

- Aspiration pneumonitis refers to chemical injury and inflammation of lung tissue after inhalation of foreign material, whereas aspiration pneumonia refers to infection of lung tissue following pneumonitis.
- Patients at risk for aspiration pneumonia include those with impaired neurologic status and gastrointestinal dysmotility.
- Initial chest radiographs may be normal following aspiration episodes.
- Treatment with antibiotics is generally reserved for patients with significant respiratory impairment and signs of infection or complicating medical history.
- Treatment with corticosteroids is not routinely indicated.

Current Evidence

Aspiration of foreign material into the lung can result in inflammation and impaired lung function. *Aspiration pneumonitis* refers to chemical injury and inflammation of lung tissue from inhaled foreign material, with sterile acidic gastric contents being the most common source. *Aspiration pneumonia* refers to infection of lung tissue following inhalation of foreign material, often due to bacteria from the oropharynx.

The pathophysiology of pulmonary disease following aspiration can be classified based on the source of the foreign material. In humans, aspirate contents with a pH lower than 2.5 are considered acidic, and such material may cause a severe chemical pneumonitis with direct injury to alveolar–capillary membranes. Effects from initial injury can occur within minutes to hours, and may include reflex airway closure and destruction of surfactant resulting in atelectasis. A granulocytic, necrotizing reaction generally follows causing exudation of fluid and protein across damaged membranes creating interstitial and alveolar edema, alveolar hemorrhage, and consolidation.

Aspirates with a pH higher than 2.5 are considered nonacidic, typically arising from aspiration of contents from the oropharynx or stomach in patients taking H_2 blockers or proton-pump inhibitors. The early pathophysiologic response is similar to that seen with acidic chemical pneumonitis, with the exception of reduced alveolar neutrophilic infiltration and necrosis. The extent of lung damage from nonacid aspirates varies depending on the composition of the aspirate; clear liquid aspiration resolves quickly while sizable food particles may lead to prolonged pathologic response. Repeated aspirations occurring over an extended period may result in radiographic evidence of granuloma formation similar to that of miliary tuberculosis. Aspiration of hydrocarbons is covered separately in Chapter 110 Toxicologic Emergencies.

Goal of Treatment

Treatment of aspiration pneumonia aims at treating any underlying conditions and preventing further aspiration. Supportive measures may involve assisting ventilation and oxygenation as needed, and consideration of antibiotics.

Clinical Considerations

Clinical Recognition

Children with neurologic impairment including altered consciousness and CNS disorders that compromise normal swallowing or protective airway reflexes are at risk for aspiration. This is particularly true for chronically impaired children, although healthy children who are transiently depressed from acute neurologic deterioration, procedural sedation, or during or after seizures can also aspirate. In addition, children with decreased esophageal or intestinal motility or delayed gastric emptying are at increased risk of regurgitation of stomach contents and therefore possible aspiration. Such gastrointestinal dysmotility may be secondary to underlying disease, trauma, or medications such as opiates or those with anticholinergic properties. Similarly, anatomic narrowing or obstruction along the gastrointestinal tract can also increase the risk of aspiration.

Triage

Patients with aspiration pneumonia may present with acute severe respiratory distress, and, therefore, most will require prompt evaluation. Patients with chronic aspiration often have a more insidious course, though may have an acute event or intercurrent illness that results in more notable respiratory compromise prompting evaluation.

Initial Assessment/H&P

The reported symptoms and physical findings in patients with aspiration pneumonia are similar to patients with pulmonary infections resulting from community- or hospital-acquired bacterial or viral causes, and are further discussed in Chapter 102 Infectious Disease Emergencies.

In cases of aspiration pneumonia, a brief latent period may occur before the onset of respiratory signs and symptoms; more than 90% of patients are symptomatic within 1 hour. Fever, tachypnea, and cough are frequent findings. Hypoxia is also common, whereas apnea and shock are less likely but possible. Sputum production is usually minimal.

On examination, focal or diffuse crackles and wheezing are common. Cyanosis may appear with more severe disease. Chest radiographs (Fig. 107.1) may show either localized or diffuse infiltrates, which may be unilateral or bilateral. The chest x-ray of a patient who has aspirated may evolve from normal to complete bilateral opacification within several hours.

Management

In the acute care setting, children who aspirate require primarily supportive care. Specifically, prevention of further aspiration by gastric decompression, oropharyngeal suctioning, and proper positioning should be a goal. Supplemental oxygen should be administered as needed. Endotracheal intubation is indicated if airway reflexes are acutely compromised or for severe cases with impending respiratory failure. Children with impaired baseline pulmonary function may require significant supportive care after aspiration.

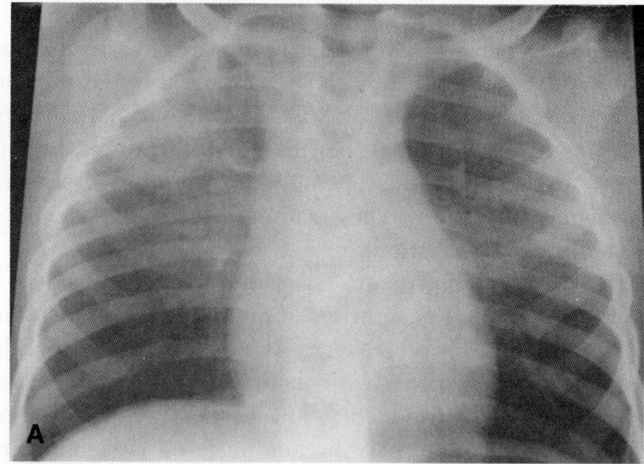

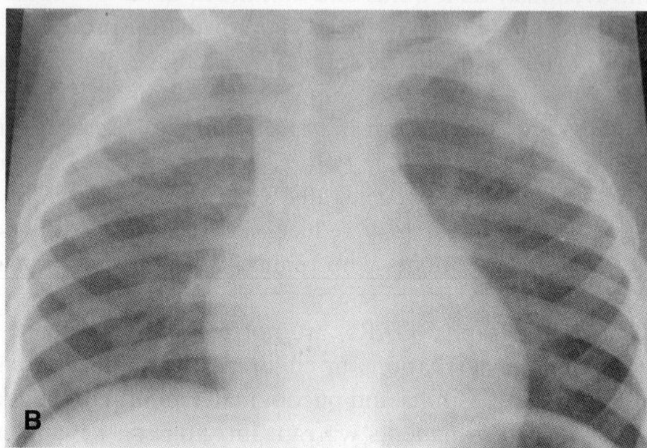

FIGURE 107.1 **A:** Blood aspiration. A 3-year-old boy with tachypnea 1 day after surgery for enlarged adenoids/tonsils. Chest film shows an infiltrate in the right upper lobe and left lower lobe. **B:** The chest film 2 days later shows clearing of the infiltrate in the right upper lobe and left lower lobe.

The suspicion of aspiration should be confirmed with a chest radiograph. Some children who aspirate may have relatively normal radiographs early in the course but significant symptomatology and findings. Conversely, radiographs may be significantly abnormal in the face of minimal clinical symptoms in patients with aspiration of hydrocarbon or other volatile agents (further discussed in Chapter 110 Toxicologic Emergencies).

The decision to initiate antibiotic therapy is challenging. Most physicians agree that infection plays little role in the initial pulmonary complications after aspiration, that is, aspiration pneumonitis. However, pathogenic bacteria from the oropharynx may accompany foreign material, resulting in direct inoculation of lung tissue. Alternatively, following acid aspiration, the injured lung is vulnerable and secondary bacterial infection may occur in up to half of these cases. There is no strong data to suggest that prophylactic antibiotic therapy will prevent subsequent infection in a patient with chemical pneumonitis. Moreover, fever, purulent sputum, leukocytosis, and pulmonary infiltrates may result from chemical inflammation alone, making the distinction between aspiration pneumonitis and aspiration pneumonia difficult. A reasonable initial approach is to defer antibiotic treatment in favor of careful observation in a well-appearing child and empirically treat only those with tenuous respiratory status or compelling clinical evidence of infection, or significant medical history that may complicate their clinical course.

For those who develop infection, two distinct patterns are possible. A localized necrotizing bacterial pneumonia, abscess, or empyema may result from a heavily infected aspirate. Although opinions vary, anaerobic organisms, either alone or as polymicrobial infection with aerobes, are likely etiologies in such cases. The second pattern of infection is that which follows large aspirates, usually of the acidic type. Aerobic rather than anaerobic organisms predominate in this case; gram-negative organisms, such as *Pseudomonas aeruginosa,* and gram-positive organisms, such as staphylococci, may be isolated.

The choice of antibiotics can be guided by the clinical setting and the results of properly obtained specimens for culture. Size and type of aspirate are considerations as are settings in which the aspiration occurs. Aspiration pneumonias developing outside the hospital generally involve aerobes and are adequately treated with ampicillin or clindamycin, whereas nosocomial infections require broader aerobic and anaerobic coverage. Clindamycin with gentamicin, or ampicillin/sulbactam, is often used. In neurologically impaired children, with either aspiration or tracheostomy-associated pneumonia, antibiotics effective against penicillin-resistant anaerobic bacteria and *P. aeruginosa* have been shown to produce superior clinical and microbiologic responses.

The use of corticosteroids in the treatment of aspiration pneumonia is controversial. Because experimental evidence indicates minimal benefit at best and because the concomitant immune suppression may contribute the development of secondary bacterial pneumonia, their administration is not usually indicated in the ED.

Clinical Indications for Discharge or Admission

Children with significant aspiration pneumonia, diagnosed either by clinical suspicion or radiograph, require admission to the hospital.

BRONCHOPULMONARY DYSPLASIA

CLINICAL PEARLS AND PITFALLS

- Diagnosis is usually established prior to presentation to the ED.
- Management involves supportive measures, including supplemental oxygen, assurance of adequate hydration, and often bronchodilators.

Current Evidence

BPD is a chronic respiratory disease, usually occurring in premature infants. BPD is a clinical diagnosis, defined as requiring supplemental oxygen at a prescribed postconceptual or chronologic age, with associated radiographic findings. The specifics of the diagnostic parameters have changed over time.

The etiology of BPD is thought to be multifactorial. While newer data suggest a genetic predisposition, previously defined risk factors include prematurity, relatively long duration of supplemental oxygen therapy after birth, requiring positive-pressure ventilation, and inadequate nutrition. The disease process is thought to begin after inflammation and injury to the lung, with resultant arrest of alveolar septation and impaired microvascular development. This occurs most commonly in infants with hyaline membrane disease or other acute perinatal lung disease. Infants with apnea, congenital heart disease, or other illnesses requiring prolonged ventilation in the first weeks of life are also at risk. Utilization of improved ventilation strategies, as well as antenatal glucocorticoids, surfactant, and improvement in nutrition, has improved outcomes in children with BPD.

In the emergency setting, patients with BPD may present with acute exacerbations of their chronic lung disease. Furthermore, BPD is a risk factor for increased severity of other respiratory illnesses.

Goals of Treatment

Treatment of BPD exacerbations involves supportive care with attention to need for supplemental oxygenation and ventilation support, as well as hydration status. Bronchodilators, ICSs, and diuretics may also be helpful.

Clinical Considerations

Clinical Recognition

BPD should be suspected among premature infants, as well as in children previously requiring either assisted ventilation and/or prolonged supplemental oxygen therapy.

Emergency physicians most often will evaluate children with BPD when their underlying disease is worsened by intercurrent acute respiratory infections. More than 50% of infants with BPD require admission for respiratory illness within a year of their diagnosis. Of particular importance is respiratory syncytial virus (RSV) infection, which typically causes bronchiolitis with fever, tachypnea, crackles, and wheezing. Patients with BPD who develop RSV bronchiolitis are prone to more severe courses, including higher rates of ICU admission, need for mechanical ventilation, and mortality.

Triage

Children with BPD exacerbations may present with significant distress and may require prompt evaluation and treatment.

Initial Assessment/H&P

Signs and symptoms of BPD exacerbations vary based on severity of the underlying disease; therefore, recognizing interim worsening of disease requires an understanding of baseline examination findings and pulmonary function.

Children with BPD are typically tachypneic at baseline, with some degree of retractions that worsen with even mild respiratory or febrile illnesses. Findings on auscultation including crackles, wheezes, or decreased breath sounds may be present at baseline and worsened with exacerbations or acute illness. Infants with BPD may have a history of failure to thrive, often resulting from concomitant nutritional issues, or from increased energy expenditure secondary to chronic increased work of breathing. Chest radiographs (Fig. 107.2) often demonstrate varying amounts of hyperinflation; several patterns occur, including cystic areas with signs of fibrosis, which are often confused with congenital lobar emphysema or severe CF. Comparison with prior CXRs is important to distinguish old changes from new infiltrates.

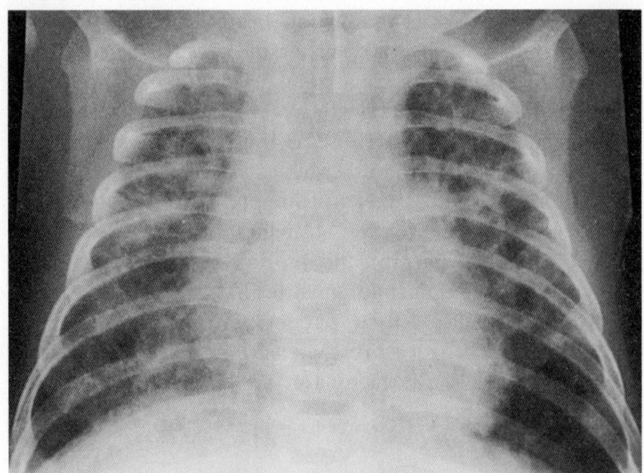

FIGURE 107.2 Bronchopulmonary dysplasia. This 2-month-old child was treated with mechanical ventilation during the first days of life for hyaline membrane disease. The chest film shows generalized overaeration and coarse nodularity with multiple cyst-like areas throughout both lung fields.

Management

Management of children with BPD and intercurrent respiratory illnesses is primarily limited to supportive care. If the exacerbation is mild, outpatient therapy may be indicated with frequent follow-up every 1 to 2 days. However, for infants with moderate to severe BPD at baseline, even mild deterioration may herald early respiratory failure. Ensuring hydration by oral or IV routes, addressing hypoxemia, and, when necessary, providing assisted ventilation for hypercarbia and respiratory acidosis are the mainstays of therapy.

Pulse oximetry is important to assess for hypoxemia. $ETCO_2$ measurement through noninvasive means or PCO_2 measurement with arterial, venous, or capillary blood gas analysis is indicated when signs and symptoms suggest hypercapnia or when cyanosis, respiratory distress, or deterioration from baseline cannot be easily reversed. A chest radiograph may provide additional information; however, given baseline abnormalities, these often need to be compared with prior films.

Bronchodilators, ICSs, and diuretics may also be helpful. Most children with BPD have had trials of β-agonist therapy. Although the use of MDIs for β-agonists is effective in older infants with asthma, the evidence for their use in young infants with BPD is less well defined. Although most acute episodes are from viral infection, antibiotic therapy should be considered when the risk of bacterial infection appears higher.

Prevention of BPD exacerbations is challenging. Although routine viral illnesses may not be avoidable, RSV and influenza are the leading preventable causes of rehospitalization in patients with BPD. Monoclonal antibody against RSV (palivizumab, Synagis) has largely replaced RSV-IVIG prophylaxis in preventing or lessening disease secondary to RSV. Such immunoprophylaxis is recommended for children less than 1 year of age who: (i) were born prior to 29 weeks gestation, (ii) were born <32 weeks with BPD (required >21% oxygen for at least 28 days after birth), (iii) have hemodynamically significant heart disease. It may also be considered in the first year of life for infants with pulmonary abnormality or neuromuscular disease that impairs the ability to clear secretions from the upper airways. Children from 1 to 2 years of age should only receive palivizumab if they required oxygen at least 28 days after birth and continue to require medical interventions for their BPD. Annual influenza vaccination should also be considered for children with BPD.

Clinical Indications for Discharge or Admission

Indications for admission generally include respiratory distress, tachypnea, increasing hypoxia or hypercarbia, poor feeding, apnea, or new radiographic infiltrates. Parental fatigue and stress are also important factors to consider in the decision to hospitalize.

CYSTIC FIBROSIS

CLINICAL PEARLS AND PITFALLS

- Patients with CF may have worsening of underlying disease due to several causes including: bacterial colonization and exacerbation, acute viral illness, acute bacterial infection, pneumothorax, hemoptysis, or allergic bronchopulmonary aspirgillosis (ABPA).
- Communication with the patient's primary CF team should occur in a timely manner.
- CXRs should be obtained in patients with increased respiratory symptoms and compared to prior studies.
- Isolation precautions should be initiated as soon as possible.

Current Evidence

CF is an autosomal recessive genetic disease, predominantly seen in Caucasians. The basic genetic defect is a mutation on the long arm of chromosome 7, resulting in an abnormal cystic fibrosis transmembrane conductance regulator (CFTR) protein with wide phenotypic variability.

These CFTR defects affect function of cells lining the respiratory tract, pancreatic exocrine system, sweat glands, and intrahepatic biliary epithelium. In the respiratory and GI tracts, this leads to dehydrated secretions that are difficult to mobilize. The manifestation in the respiratory tract is chronic inflammation and chronic infection. In the sweat glands, it produces highly concentrated sweat, which impairs electrolyte-concentrating abilities causing excessive electrolyte loss and dehydration.

While patients with CF may visit EDs for common complaints and conditions, having CF will impact even common respiratory ailments. Emergency presentations for CF patients can be grouped as pulmonary, systemic, or GI abnormalities. This section will discuss the pulmonary presentations. Some of these are single events, while others are recurrent. Knowledge of successful treatment for previous episodes will inform management.

Goals of Treatment

Treatment goals include identifying the cause of acutely worsening respiratory distress. Patients may have worsening of underlying disease due to acute viral illness, acute bacterial infection, bacterial colonization and subacute exacerbation, worsening gastroesophageal reflux disease (GERD) symptoms, pneumothorax, hemoptysis, or ABPA. Appreciation of baseline status is necessary, and communication with the patient's primary CF team should occur in a timely manner.

The possibility of renal dysfunction and impact on bowel motility must be considered when selecting medications. CF patients may not have normal renal function after years of aminoglycoside exposure and other nephrotoxic therapies. Renally excreted analgesics therefore should not be used long term without assessment of renal function. Furthermore, narcotic analgesics can cause decreased GI motility. This may, in turn, lead to constipation and bowel obstruction, which can have other implications.

Clinical Considerations

Clinical Recognition

It is rare for patients with CF to present to the ED without a known diagnosis. Newborn screening and family history often lead to early diagnosis. For those diagnosed later, nonpulmonary complaints may lead to the diagnosis. Rarely, recurrent pulmonary infections, or radiographic findings including cystic changes or bronchiectasis prompt evaluation leading to diagnosis. Most patients presenting to the ED will have established diagnoses and receive coordinated care through a CF center. The ED visit therefore most commonly focuses on identifying and treating complications from CF.

Triage

Patients with CF and worsening respiratory distress should be promptly evaluated. They also need isolation measures, often including enhanced contact and droplet precautions.

Clinical Assessment and Management

Pulmonary CF Exacerbation. Inflammation, impaired mucociliary clearance, and chronic airway infection result in pulmonary exacerbations for CF patients. These exacerbations are usually associated with declining lung function and acute worsening of respiratory symptoms. Clinical features may include increased cough, change of sputum quality or quantity, dyspnea, shortness of breath, increased work of breathing, loss of appetite, fatigue, and fever. On examination, the presence of new crackles or wheezes, increased tactile fremitus, and increased hyperinflation may be present. Pulmonary function test (PFT) changes include decrease in forced vital capacity (FVC) and/or forced expiratory volume in 1 second (FEV_1). Oxygen saturation is often decreased from baseline values. Studies including CXR, sputum culture, chemistries, and complete blood count (CBC) should be obtained. CXR should ideally be compared with prior studies to assess for new infiltrates.

For mild exacerbations, discharge with a 10- to 14-day course of oral antibiotics covering the usual organisms affecting CF patients may be appropriate. Discussion with the primary CF team is important to appreciate prior respiratory cultures and disease status. Common CF pathogens such as *Haemophilus influenzae* and *Staphylococcus aureus* (including methicillin-resistant *S. aureus*), *P. aeruginosa, Stenotrophomonas maltophilia, Achromobacter xylosoxidans,* and *Burkholderia cepacia* complex require oral and often inhaled therapy as well. Adherence to a good airway clearance regimen is necessary to optimize management.

For severe exacerbations, IV antibiotics and hospitalization are necessary. Antibiotic coverage should be based on prior respiratory culture results and should include double coverage for *Pseudomonas* to limit development of drug resistance to a single agent. Discussion with the primary CF team is important to direct coordinated care. An aggressive airway clearance regimen should be initiated. Nutritional status may have deteriorated as well and increased caloric intake may be necessary. Blood glucose levels may be more difficult to control during acute exacerbations for patients with endocrine pancreatic insufficiency and CF-related diabetes. Dehydration should be avoided, but judicious fluid use is necessary to avoid pulmonary edema, as patients with CF exacerbations may be at risk due to hyperinflation, poor oncotic pressure, and fluid administration secondary to multiple IV administrations.

Care must be given to infection control both in the ED and hospital wards. Cross infection with various organisms has been demonstrated in many studies, and policies of the Cystic Fibrosis Foundation (CFF) outline measures to decrease the chance for such transmission. Early acquisition of organisms such as *Pseudomonas* has led to more rapid decline in lung function, and thus, isolation precautions should be maintained. Gown and gloves are the minimum standard precautions for CF patient care, with mask added as required for droplet precautions with suspected viral infections.

Pneumothorax. Spontaneous pneumothorax is a complication in CF, occurring in 0.5% to 1% of patients yearly, with nearly 3.5% of all CF patients experiencing one at some point in their lives. Risk of recurrence is 20%. It is occasionally a first presentation of CF, though mean age of first pneumothorax tends to be in the late teens to early 20s.

The main risk factor for pneumothorax is CF disease severity. Mucous plugging and air trapping impose increased intrapulmonary air pressure differentials on fibroelastic lung structures weakened from chronic inflammation. Classic symptoms include sudden or subacute onset of sharp chest pain, often referred to the shoulder. Depending on the size of the pneumothorax and the patient's respiratory reserve, there can be varying degrees of dyspnea, tachypnea, hypoxemia, cyanosis, and decreased breath sounds.

Management is based on the patient's acute and chronic disease status and size of pneumothorax (see Fig. 107.3). Most patients require hospitalization and monitoring, even with small pneumothoraces. Larger and more symptomatic pneumothoraces require needle decompression acutely if signs of tension pneumothorax, are present, and chest tube insertion. Supplemental oxygen should be administered as needed to optimize oxygenation and patient comfort. Limited data exist to support faster resolution of pneumothoraces with higher FiO_2. Care must be taken to avoid excess oxygen exposure in patients with advanced disease and hypoxic ventilatory drive.

If pneumothoraces are recurrent or persistent, the patient should be evaluated for pleurodesis. While this may prevent recurrence, such intervention may have implications for lung transplant eligibility and should be discussed with physicians having experience in either CF or lung transplantation.

Daily CF therapies, such as chest percussion and postural drainage, oscillatory percussive vest therapy, other airway clearance techniques (e.g., positive expiratory pressure [PEP] mask, flutter valve), inhalation of dornase alfa (pulmozyme), and pulmonary function testing, should be suspended temporarily to avoid exacerbating the pneumothorax. Inhalational therapy with bronchodilators and/or ICSs may be continued with nebulization, but the usual inhalational maneuvers with MDIs probably should be avoided until the pneumothorax is no longer an issue. Timing for reimplementation of therapies is based on resolution of pneumothorax and discussion with the patient's CF team.

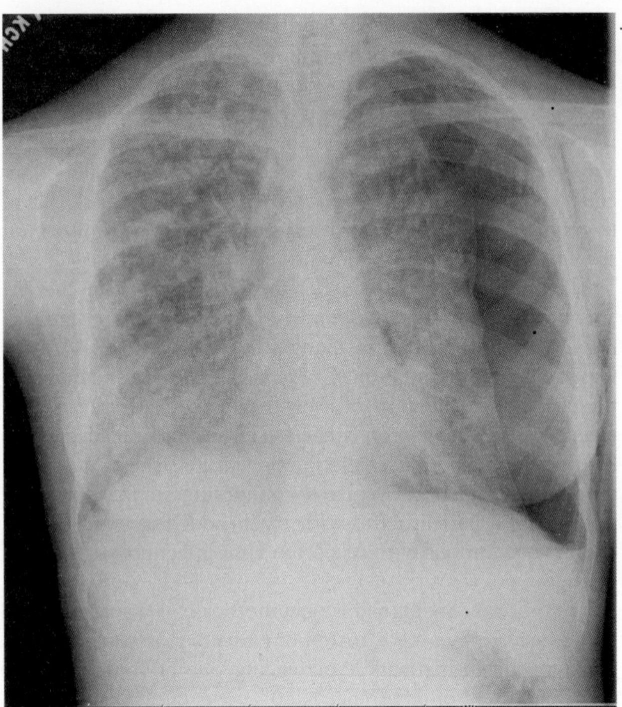

FIGURE 107.3 Chest radiograph showing pneumothorax.

Hemoptysis. Blood streaking of the sputum is common in CF patients. The CFF's Guidelines define hemoptysis as mild (less than 60 cm^3 daily), moderate (more than 60 and less than 240 cm^3 daily), and severe (more than 240 cm^3 daily or more than 100 cm^3 per day for more than 2 days). Hemoptysis should be distinguished from epistaxis or hematemesis.

Mild Hemoptysis. Mild hemoptysis requires no specific treatment other than observation. Persistent streaking may indicate a pulmonary exacerbation requiring antibiotic treatment. Other factors such as chronic use of medications with antiplatelet function activity (e.g., aspirin) or coagulopathy secondary to decreased vitamin K levels should be ruled out and treated accordingly.

Moderate/Severe Hemoptysis. Severe episodes can be life-threatening due to asphyxiation from airway obstruction, hemorrhagic shock, and/or chemical pneumonitis. Approximately 1% of CF patients experience an episode of major bleeding per year, the majority of patients being 16 years or older. The bleeding usually originates from enlarged and tortuous bronchial arteries, two-thirds of which arise from the ventral surface of the aorta. The remaining third come from the internal mammary and intercostal arteries. Onset is often abrupt.

Some patients may report localized gurgling or sensation in the specific area of lung involved. Physical examination may reveal new, localized pulmonary findings. Placing a nasogastric tube or performing endoscopy may become necessary to differentiate GI from pulmonary sources. A CXR should be obtained, though the specific area of bleeding is not often visualized.

IV access must be established and laboratory tests obtained including CBC with differential, prothrombin time, partial thromboplastin time, liver function tests, blood gas analysis, and emergency type and cross match. Sputum culture should also be obtained. Emergency bronchoscopy to localize and treat the site of bleeding should be discussed with the primary CF team. In some cases, bronchoscopy may not be helpful either because the patient has stopped bleeding or massive hemorrhage obscures visualization. Most cases of severe hemoptysis are self-limited and can be managed using vitamin K, blood products, and antibiotics in an ICU setting. Surgery or local vascular therapy with arterial embolization may be necessary for refractory bleeding. In that situation, both rigid and flexible bronchoscopy should be available during the procedure in the operating room or ICU.

Ongoing management after hemodynamic stabilization includes discontinuing medications that could interfere with coagulation (e.g., aspirin, nonsteroidal anti-inflammatory drugs [NSAIDs], inhaled drugs such as N-acetylcysteine, dornase alfa, and some aerosolized antibiotics), correcting coagulation defects with vitamin K, fresh-frozen plasma, or specific factors as indicated, and transfusions as clinically indicated, bearing in mind that patients with severe chronic disease may be awaiting lung transplantation. Whenever possible, blood products should be prepared in a manner to minimize the risk of posttransplant complications. Treatment with IV antibiotics is appropriate considering most major bleeds are associated with pulmonary exacerbations. Placing the bleeding lung in the dependent position may help to prevent aspiration into the as yet uninvolved lung. IV therapies to halt bleeding, such as pitressin or octreotide, should be discussed with the pulmonologist. Local airway treatment may be indicated in acute life-threatening situation, and include endobronchial tamponade, selective double lumen intubation, and iced saline lavage. The need for and timing of embolization and access to surgery must be determined in a timely manner. If a surgeon and interventional radiologist are not readily available, referral to another center should be considered.

Viral Respiratory Tract Infection. Simple viral respiratory infections are often inciting events for pulmonary exacerbations. CF patients will be more likely to suffer increased and/or prolonged symptoms due to impaired mucociliary clearance and decreased respiratory reserve. Whereas CXRs are routinely not indicated for most patients with what appears to be simple URIs, patients with CF with new respiratory symptoms should have CXR obtained and compared with prior studies. If there is suspicion for CF exacerbation, antibiotics should be prescribed as discussed above.

Wheezing. Patients with CF may wheeze secondary to common diagnoses such as acute viral processes, asthma, and foreign bodies. In addition, ABPA must be considered in wheezing patients with CF. ABPA occurs in 1% to 15% of patients with CF. It is an exaggerated type I hypersensitivity reaction to the ubiquitous organism *Aspergillus fumigates*. Clinically, patients present with chronic wheeze that is difficult to control, decline in pulmonary function, chronic cough, and transient infiltrates on CXR. Symptoms typically respond well to oral steroids.

Any CF patient with recurrent wheezing and cough, changes on CXR and declining lung function not responsive to antibiotic therapy and airway clearance should be evaluated for ABPA. Diagnostic criteria include elevated total serum IgE level, positive skin reactivity to *Aspergillus*, and positive specific serum antibodies to *Aspergillus*. Treatment consists of a prolonged course of oral steroids (prednisone or prednisolone), usually starting at 2 mg/kg/day, with subsequent taper and close follow-up. IgE levels should be followed at regular intervals both as indication of response to therapy and as a warning of re-exacerbation. There are no current studies to suggest a clear benefit of antifungal therapy along with steroids, although some physicians use oral itraconazole therapy as it may shorten the course of oral steroids.

Pulmonary Embolism. There is no current literature to suggest increased incidence of pulmonary embolism (PE) in children with CF. However, it should be considered in the differential diagnosis if there is acute onset of chest pain, shortness of breath, and tachypnea. Because of chronic changes seen on CXR and CT with chronic lung disease, interpretation of imaging may be challenging to unequivocally confirm or refute PE. The risks of anticoagulation or thrombolytic therapy for patients with more than mild pulmonary disease are not trivial, considering the propensity of CF patients to have hemoptysis.

Pleuritis. Pleuritic chest pain can present in CF patients during acute or subacute bacterial exacerbations or acute viral infections. The pain usually improves with oral analgesia and antibiotic treatment if bacterial exacerbation is suspected.

Gastroesophageal Reflux Disease. While many patients with CF take acid suppression medications (e.g., H_2 blocker or protein pump inhibitor [PPI]) for enhancement of exogenous pancreatic enzyme function, the incidence of GERD in children with CF is as high as 55% in some studies. Acute exacerbations of GERD can cause symptoms of gastritis and esophagitis including significant chest pain in the epigastrium and retrosternal regions. Medications, such as NSAIDs, recent dietary changes, stress, and ethanol may exacerbate GERD. An empiric trial of increased acid control may be warranted, but all patients with recurrent symptoms of GERD, including regurgitation and chest pain, should be followed closely after ED discharge. In refractory cases, referral to a gastroenterologist for a formal evaluation is appropriate to determine need for upper GI series, pH/impedance probe study, and/or endoscopy.

Other Causes of Chest Pain. Chest pain is a common complaint in patients with CF and can stem from a variety of underlying processes (Table 107.5).

Chest pain of cardiac origin is rare in the pediatric CF population. While cardiac pain is more common outside the pediatric patient age group, the rare pediatric CF patient with severe pulmonary disease, nonpulmonary pain, and borderline secondary right heart dysfunction should be evaluated with an electrocardiogram (EKG), CXR, and cardiology consultation and possible echocardiogram.

Rib fracture can occur secondary to osteopenia in patients with CF with poor nutrition, or secondary to overly aggressive chest percussion and postural drainage. Superficial ecchymoses and point tenderness along the rib margin in the setting of malnutrition and scant subcutaneous fat tissue may suggest the diagnosis of rib fracture; diagnosis can be confirmed radiologically. Treatment is complicated by the need to at least temporarily limit airway clearance, which can lead to increasing airway obstruction. History of fracture or suspicious behavior should also raise the question of child abuse in young children.

TABLE 107.5

CHEST PAIN IN CYSTIC FIBROSIS PATIENTS

Common	Uncommon	Rare
Costochondritis	Rib fracture	Cardiac disease
Pleurisy/pleuritis	Pulmonary embolism	
Pneumothorax		
Esophagitis		

Respiratory Failure. Thickened airway secretions with bacterial infection, mucous hypersecretion, bronchoconstriction, mucosal edema, inflammation, and fibrosis contribute to respiratory muscle fatigue and can lead to the development of respiratory failure in CF. The goal of treatment is to optimize gas exchange and acid–base balance, keeping in mind the patients likely have some degree of pulmonary hypertension and cor pulmonale.

Management includes maintaining adequate oxygenation and ventilation along with intensifying antibacterial treatment and airway clearance. Supplemental oxygen therapy needs to be introduced with caution in patients with chronic CO_2 retention to avoid suppressing hypoxic ventilator drive. Ventilation support may be necessary, and noninvasive means can be considered including CPAP or BiPAP. The patient should also be evaluated for comorbidities (e.g., atypical infections, ABPA, pneumothorax), which can be precipitating events for acute or subacute decompensation.

Clinical Indications for Discharge or Admission

Indications for hospitalization will vary according to the acute conditions diagnosed and underlying severity of their disease. Consultation with a pulmonologist or the patient's CF team may provide insight into the need for hospitalization.

Follow-up Care

The majority of CF patients in the United States are followed in CFF approved and supported CF centers. All centers' contact information is available at the CFF website (http://www.cff.org). Close contact between emergency physicians and the CF center team caring for this patient population facilitates continuity of care and hopefully diminishes representation to the ED for recrudescence of the presenting problem.

PULMONARY HEMORRHAGE

CLINICAL PEARLS AND PITFALLS

- Pulmonary hemorrhage may be seen in acute respiratory illnesses or after thoracic trauma, the initial presentation of a chronic vasculitic condition, or during exacerbation of a chronic condition such as CF.
- Pulmonary hemorrhage can present with significant respiratory distress and hemodynamic compromise.
- Management primarily involves assessment and support of oxygenation, ventilation, and hemodynamics, with consideration of diagnostic testing for the underlying condition.
- Bronchoscopy is generally reserved for patients with persistent bleeding or when diagnostically necessary.
- Blood products including packed red blood cells, platelets, coagulation factors, and fresh-frozen plasma should be considered if signs of significant bleeding and/or shock are present.

TABLE 107.6

CAUSES OF PULMONARY HEMORRHAGE IN CHILDREN

Primary	Associated with other organ dysfunction	Secondary	Airways	Parenchymal	Non-lung sources
Cow's milk allergy (Hiener syndrome)	Goodpasture's	Congestive heart failure	Bronchitis	Trauma (including nonaccidental)	Hematemesis/GI bleeding
Idiopathic pulmonary hemosiderosis	Wegener granulomatosis	Pulmonary hypertension	Bronchiectasis/cystic fibrosis	Infection—tuberculosis, other	Nasal or tonsillar bleeding
Acute idiopathic pulmonary hemorrhage (AIPH) among infants	Henoch–Schönlein purpura Systemic lupus erythematosus (SLE) and collagen vascular disease	Clotting disorders Malignancy Alveolar injury (e.g., drugs, radiation, smoke, acid aspiration)	Airway anomalies Vascular anomalies, (hemangioma and arteriovascular malformation [AVM]) Foreign body	Infarction Neoplasm Cavitary lesion	Factitious hemoptysis

Modified from Boat TF. Pulmonary hemorrhage and hemoptysis. In: Chernick V, Boat TF, eds. *Kendig's disorders of the respiratory tract in children*, 6th ed. Philadelphia, PA: WB Saunders, 1998:624.

Current Evidence

Pulmonary hemorrhage, or bleeding into the lung, most commonly manifests clinically with hemoptysis. Although relatively uncommon, pulmonary hemorrhage can be dramatic and life-threatening. Therefore, early evaluation and treatment is paramount.

The potential causes vary and include acute infection, exacerbation of chronic pulmonary disease, and thoracic trauma. The relative frequency of causative etiologies will vary significantly by the population being evaluated, making estimation of incidence of disease difficult. Table 107.6 provides a differential diagnosis for pulmonary hemorrhage by category.

Goals of Treatment

Management for pulmonary hemorrhage involves support of oxygenation and ventilation and attention to hemodynamics, along with appreciation of the underlying disorder for which other specific therapies may be necessary.

Clinical Considerations

Clinical Recognition

Pulmonary hemorrhage results from pathology of lung tissue which can occur in the setting of acute infection such as pneumonia, exacerbation of chronic disease such as CF, or acute localized injury after thoracic trauma. Hemoptysis is the most common symptom and finding. Patients may have significant respiratory distress and may exhibit signs of hemorrhagic shock.

Triage

Children with pulmonary hemorrhage require prompt assessment as they may present with severe respiratory distress and hemorrhagic shock.

Initial Assessment/H&P

Hemoptysis is the most common presentation of pulmonary hemorrhage. It may be necessary to distinguish this from hematemesis or blood from the nose, tonsils, pharynx, or upper airway. Findings may be mild with blood-streaked sputum, or patients may present with massive blood loss and shock. Hypoxia and shortness of breath are most likely with significant hemorrhage or as a result of exacerbation of underlying condition. Apprehension is not uncommon in these children as dyspnea is compounded by the visualization of loss of blood. Children with recurrent intrapulmonary bleeding are more likely to be anemic. As a result, they may also present with fatigue and poor weight gain as symptoms.

Examination findings are often nonspecific and include tachypnea, tachycardia, and hypoxia. Crackles may be appreciated over the affected area, although isolating the location of the bleeding by auscultation is difficult. For older patients, identifying the affected area may be best accomplished by asking the patient where they feel pain or discomfort. Other signs on examination may be helpful in elucidating an underlying diagnosis, such as abnormal cardiac sounds with heart failure, rash or joint involvement with collagen vascular disease, or external signs of thoracic injury in trauma patients. Cardiorespiratory decompensation can occur in children with severe anemia or shock from severe hemorrhage.

Radiographs will vary depending on etiology. Alveolar infiltrates may be transient localized processes, or diffuse and chronic. In idiopathic pulmonary hemosiderosis, diffuse alveolar changes are usually symmetric and spare the apices and costophrenic angles (Fig. 107.4).

Because most children swallow their sputum, a presumptive diagnosis can be made by finding hemosiderin-laden macrophages in nasogastric washings; these macrophages will stain blue with Prussian blue reaction. More definitive diagnosis, however, requires bronchoscopy and BAL. Finding similar macrophages from BAL is diagnostic, and direct visualization of the airways provides an opportunity to potentially localize the site

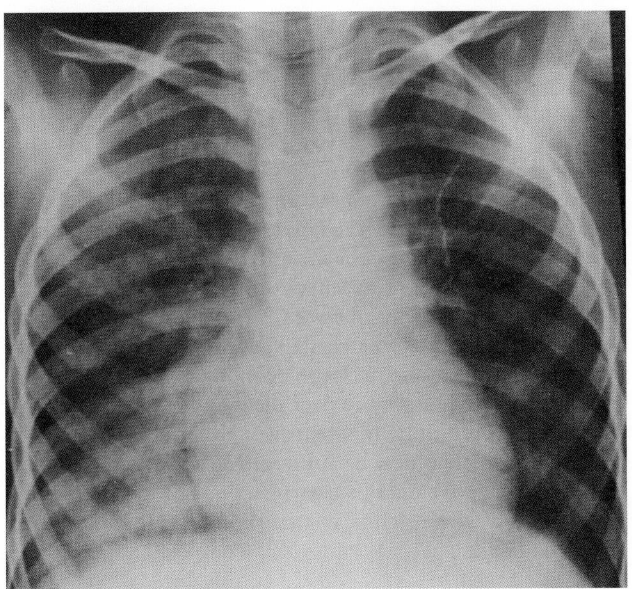

FIGURE 107.4 Idiopathic pulmonary hemosiderosis. A 5-year-old child with repeated bouts of pulmonary hemorrhage. The chest film shows diffuse radiopacities throughout both lungs (more on right side), with a well-defined alveolar opacity in the right lower lobe. Note the surgical sutures in left upper lobe.

and assess the activity of bleeding. Lung biopsy is required only for patients with recurrent bleeding in whom no diagnosis can be made on a clinical basis and alternative systemic diseases cannot be excluded.

Management

Immediate management of any patient with presumed pulmonary hemorrhage is supportive. Supplemental oxygen to correct hypoxia and intravascular volume repletion should be initiated. For those with chronic disease or large acute blood losses with resultant anemia, anticipating the need for blood transfusions is important. Occasionally, pulmonary hemorrhage is so severe that it causes respiratory insufficiency or hypotension due to hemorrhagic shock. Aggressive fluid resuscitation followed by positive-pressure ventilation with PEEP is the preferred treatment in this situation. In these severe cases, platelets and fresh-frozen plasma can also provide volume replacement and help with hemostasis.

Bronchoscopy can be diagnostically useful, usually to determine infectious causes rather than to localize a source of bleeding and control it, which can be difficult. Occasionally, for brisk bleeding in a patient with a known or likely source, such as in bronchiectasis from CF or a known vascular malformation, embolization of vessels may be employed to rapidly stop the hemorrhage.

Additional treatment is tailored to the underlying etiology of disease. In allergic, vasculitic, and idiopathic hemorrhage, the administration of methylprednisolone (2 mg/kg/day IV divided in three to four divided doses) is indicated. When hemorrhage is caused by infection, especially tuberculosis, antimicrobial therapy should be instituted and steroids avoided.

Clinical Indications for Discharge or Admission

Most patients with pulmonary hemorrhage will require hospitalization for supportive care, until the cause of the bleeding has been determined and the hemorrhage has been controlled.

PULMONARY EMBOLISM

CLINICAL PEARLS AND PITFALLS

- Most pediatric patients with PE have underlying conditions that predispose them to thrombotic events; central venous catheter (CVC) is a common predisposing factor.
- Chest computed tomography angiography (CTA) is employed more commonly than V/Q scans for diagnosis of PE in children.
- Decision to image with CTA must weigh risk of radiation exposure against pretest probability of this relatively rare condition.
- Management of PE involves supportive care and prevention of progression of thrombus.

Current Evidence

PE is the partial or complete obstruction of the pulmonary artery or its branches due to a thrombus, detached from its origination within the systemic venous system. Virchow identified stasis, venous injury, and hypercoagulabilty as the three factors contributing to thrombogenesis. A combination of environmental and genetic factors may contribute to each of these factors.

The degree of anatomic obstruction of the arterial vessel will dictate the degree of hemodynamic compromise. Increases in right-sided afterload can lead to cardiovascular pulmonary hypertension, or with concomitant reductions in left-sided preload can result in cardiovascular collapse, particularly in patients with pre-existing heart or lung disease. Beyond direct vascular obstruction, release of vasoactive and bronchoconstrictive cytokines may also lead to further V/Q mismatching and intrapulmonary shunting, which may contribute to the hypoxemia seen in greater than 80% of cases.

Although a number of diagnostic modalities exist, the most common in pediatrics is CT angiography. Validated clinical decision rules exist for use in adult populations (e.g., Wells Criteria, Geneva Score, and Pulmonary Embolism Rule-out Criteria [PERC]) though their generalizability may be limited given different risk factors. Therefore, the challenge lies in appropriately identifying those children who require further evaluation with CT, with its increased risk from ionizing radiation exposure weighted against the risk of missing this potentially serious diagnosis.

Goals of Treatment

PE is a rare, but potentially life-threatening condition in pediatrics. As an uncommon condition which often presents with nonspecific signs and symptoms, perhaps the greatest challenge is recognizing the diagnosis of PE. Once PE is diagnosed, the treatment goals are to correct hemodynamic or respiratory embarrassment when present, and prevent progression of disease and recurrence.

Clinical Considerations

Clinical Recognition

Children with PE commonly have underlying medical conditions which predispose them to thromboembolic events. CVCs have been identified as the most common, while others include malignancy, congenital heart disease, collagen vascular disease, significant trauma/surgery, and severe infection/sepsis. Available data suggests that greater than 90% of children diagnosed with PE will have at least one of these risk factors. In addition, a minority of children with PE will be diagnosed with a congenital prothrombotic condition, though the incidence is not clear. Traditional "adult" risk factors including oral contraceptives, elective abortion, prolonged immobilization, IV drug use, rheumatic heart disease, smoking, and obesity may also play a role in some older pediatric patients.

Triage

PE should be considered in the differential diagnosis for children with acute onset pleuritic chest pain, particularly those with known risk factors for thrombosis. Children presenting with significant respiratory distress require prompt evaluation. Acute circulatory collapse from massive PE is rare in children, though when present, it requires immediate resuscitative interventions.

Initial Assessment/H&P

Dyspnea, pleuritic chest pain, cough, and hemoptysis are the most common symptoms of PE in both adults and children, however children with these symptoms are more likely to have alternative diagnoses. Less frequent symptoms such as apprehension, fever, sweats, and palpitations are similarly nonspecific. Current literature in adults suggests that 25% of patients with PE will be asymptomatic which further complicates recognition. The presence of asymptomatic disease in children has not been similarly reported, however this may reflect different methodologies in available registries and studies which have not screened for subclinical disease in pediatric populations.

Abnormal physical examination findings are often absent. Tachycardia, rales, and tachypnea are the most common signs in children, though each individual finding is nondiscriminating. Significant vascular obstruction that results in pulmonary hypertension may lead to distended neck veins, a prominent S2, or a ventricular gallop. Similarly, in cases where embolism results in large pulmonary infarction, there may be decreased resonance over the lung fields and a pleural friction rub. Additionally, breath sounds may be distant or absent, and crackles may be appreciated on auscultation. The presence of hypoxemia not clearly explained by an underlying disease process or clinical state should also raise concern for possible PE.

Management

As mentioned above, the challenge is rapidly identifying the minority of patients with PE from other children who present with similar nonspecific complaints and findings, while minimizing unnecessary, higher risk, and invasive testing. To supplement initial assessment based on history, physical examination, and review of possible risk factors, some diagnostic studies may help inform the likelihood of PE. Once diagnosed, treatment involves supportive care, and prevention of thrombus progression and recurrence.

An EKG should be obtained, though, as with history and examination findings, abnormalities are rare and nonspecific when present (Table 107.7). Sinus tachycardia is the most

TABLE 107.7

CLINICAL MANIFESTATION OF PULMONARY EMBOLISM

	Nonspecific	Suggestive	Diagnostic
Symptoms	Syncope	Dyspnea out of proportion to degree of abnormal findings	
	Sweating	Hemoptysis	
	Pleuritic pain		
	Dyspnea		
	Cough		
	Apprehension		
Signs	Tachypnea	Pleural friction rub	
	Tachycardia	Unexplained cyanosis	
	Distant or absent breath sounds	Accentuated S_2	
	Crackles		
	Fever		
Laboratory/radiograph findings	Decreased PaO_2	Wedged infiltrate with ipsilateral elevated hemidiaphragm	CT angiography
		Abnormal ventilation–perfusion scan	Abnormal pulmonary angiography
EKG abnormalities	Right axis deviation	S_1-Q_3-T_3 pattern	
	ST-T wave changes		
	Right bundle branch block		

EKG, electrocardiogram.

common EKG finding, but least specific. Conversely, right axis deviation, right bundle branch block, and the classic "S1, Q3, T3" are all consistent with cor pulmonale which is seen in significantly symptomatic patients with PE, but may also be seen in nonembolic disease including pneumothorax.

Arterial blood gases will commonly reveal hypoxemia with reduced partial pressure of oxygen, which may suggest PE, but is not diagnostic. However, because 15% of patients will have a PaO_2 greater than 80 mm Hg and 5% of patients greater than 90 mm Hg, the negative predictive value of a normal partial pressure of oxygen may not justify performing this painful and occasionally difficult procedure in the diagnostic evaluation for PE in children.

The laboratory study which has traditionally played the most significant role in the evaluation of adult patients with suspected PE has been the D-dimer. Measurement of fibrin degradation products produced when plasmin splits cross-linked fibrin is a sensitive marker for intravascular clot. Such biomarkers will be positive as early as 1 hour after thrombus formation, with a circulating half-life of 4 to 6 hours. However, because of continued PE fibrinolysis, plasma D-dimer levels are commonly elevated for at least 1 week. Many different enzyme-linked immunosorbent assays (ELISA) are available to detect D-dimers in the circulation. Newer generation assays have reported sensitivities of 96% to 98% for the diagnosis of PE. Nonetheless, because of the presence of wide variability in performance of each assay, it is important for practitioners to be aware of the characteristics within their laboratory when incorporating results into their medical decision making. The applicability of D-dimer testing to evaluation and management of pediatric patients with suspected PE is discussed below in conjunction with imaging decision making.

Radiologic studies are important aspects in the evaluation of patients with possible PE. Chest radiographs are recommended because they are noninvasive, though they are rarely diagnostic. The presence of a segmental pulmonary infiltrate with an ipsilateral elevated hemidiaphragm is suggestive of a PE; however, even these radiographic findings are not pathognomonic. Occasionally, however, chest films will uncover an alternative diagnosis for a patient's symptoms, obviating the need for further evaluation of patients at low risk for PE.

For years, V/Q scans were the mainstay of imaging in patients with concern for PE. For patients without pre-existing cardiopulmonary disease, some studies can effectively rule in or out the diagnosis. A characteristic pattern of normal ventilation in a poorly perfused area of lung is considered high probability and effectively establishes the diagnosis of PE. Similarly, a normal V/Q scan essentially excludes the diagnosis. However, many patients have underlying structural lung disease or have V/Q scans reported as low or intermediate probability, making results nondiagnostic. In fact, the majority of patients ultimately diagnosed with embolic disease are classified as low or intermediate rather than high probability based on V/Q scanning alone.

In recent years, CTA has become the most common imaging modality for diagnosis of PE. Compared to V/Q scanning, it is more rapid, more readily available, and can better characterize nonvascular structures. Utilizing pulmonary angiography as the diagnostic standard, initial adult studies investigating the utility of spiral CT scanning reported sensitivities of 64% to 93% and specificity of 89% to 100%. The test performance in more recently available multidetector scanners is likely even higher. Still, CTA is likely less sensitive for emboli beyond main, lobar, or segmental pulmonary arteries. Therefore, using current technology, a negative CTA cannot definitively rule out PE, especially in any patient considered to be at high risk.

Utilizing available data from history and physical examination, as well as adjunctive testing modalities described above forms the basis for decision making regarding management of patients with suspected PE. Adults deemed to rule out for PE by PERC criteria, or have low pretest probability by Wells or Geneva scores and a negative D-dimer are felt to have a low likelihood of PE and therefore may not need further evaluation with radiologic studies. This may exempt one-third of presenting adult patients from requiring additional workup, and has been shown to have a negative predictive value of 99%. Patients with high pretest probability or an abnormal D-dimer should have additional imaging performed. Although many evaluation plans exist, the simplest has suggested that in such patients, a negative CTA was found to have an observed risk of missed diagnosis nearly identical to that identified by pulmonary arteriography.

There are a number of differences in children and adults that may make a similar approach to the evaluation for children with concern for PE less straightforward. While the Wells and Geneva scores may accurately stratify adult patients into risk categories, this may not be true for children. Risk factors in these scoring systems include age >65 years and heart rate >100 beats per minute which are less applicable in pediatrics. In addition, the majority of emboli in children originate in the upper venous system as a result of CVCs which differs dramatically from adults where over 75% of clots originate in the legs and pelvis, suggesting the need for different weighting for risk factors in children than in adults. In fact, many experts argue that all children in whom PE is being entertained as a diagnosis need to be considered high risk. Therefore, the prospect of linking pretest probability screening with D-dimer results as an initial screen may not be applicable, as a negative D-dimer in a patient who cannot be considered low risk may still not reliably exclude the possibility of PE. More data is needed before this or any other evaluative algorithm can be used safely in children. Nonetheless, the concept of utilizing available information from multiple sources to determine probability of disease in children is important. When clinical suspicion for PE is low, and all the aforementioned tests are normal and the patient's clinical condition permits, the patient may be discharged with close follow-up.

Initial therapy for patients with presumed or proven PE includes supplemental oxygen, ventilatory support as indicated, and anticoagulation. Anticoagulation with heparin is the mainstay of definitive therapy for PE because its onset of action is immediate and it is rapidly metabolized. Although unfractionated heparin has been the traditional approach, low–molecular-weight heparin (LMWH) may be advantageous. It has more predictable dosing and requires minimal monitoring which is particularly important in children in whom phlebotomy may be challenging and painful, and may have reduced risk of heparin-induced thrombocytopenia. Heparin therapy is recommended for a minimum of 5 days. Longer-term anticoagulation can be accomplished either with continuation of LMWH or oral anticoagulation with Coumadin (Table 107.8). Coumadin may be initiated either at the time of initial treatment with heparin or 1 to 2 days thereafter. The required daily dose varies, depending on concomitant

TABLE 107.8

TREATMENT FOR FIRST-TIME DVT/PE IN CHILDREN

	First line	Therapeutic goal	Duration	Notes
Immediate therapy	IV heparin	aPTT corresponding to anti-Factor Xa level 0.3–0.7 U/mL	5–10 days	Longer duration recommended for massive PE or extensive DVT
	Alternatively: LMWH	Anti-Factor Xa level 0.5–1.0 U/mL	5–10 days	
Ongoing therapy	Warfarin	INR 2.5 (2.0–3.0)	3–6 mo	Minimum 6 mo if thromboembolic event is idiopathic
	Alternatively: LMWH	Anti-Factor Xa level 0.5–1.0 U/mL	3–6 mo	For CVL-related DVT, following initial 3-mo therapy, continuation of low-dose anticoagulation (INR 1.5–1.8 or antiFactor Xa levels 0.1–0.3) until catheter is removed

IV, intravenous; aPTT, activated partial thromboplastin time; PE, pulmonary embolism; LMWH, low-molecular-weight heparin; INR, international normalized ratio; CVL, central venous line; DVT, deep vein thrombosis.
Adapted from Monagle P, Michelson AD, Bovill E, et al. Antithrombotic therapy in children. *Chest* 2001;119:344–370.

medical illness and other drug ingestion. The dose is adjusted to maintain the INR at 2.0 to 3.0. Anticoagulant therapy is usually continued for 3 to 6 months after diagnosis.

For the rare submassive or massive PE with hemodynamic compromise, fluid and inotropic support as well as immediate anticoagulation are important aspects of therapy. Thrombolytic therapy may prove helpful in cases of resultant cardiogenic shock, however the risk of intracranial or other life-threatening bleeds is not insignificant and the clinical utility in children is unknown.

Clinical Indications for Discharge or Admission

Patients who are considered clinically unlikely to have PE or in whom workup has been negative may be discharged with close outpatient follow-up. When abnormalities are uncovered, further diagnostic workup and admission to the hospital should be considered. If the clinical suspicion is high, regardless of the results, the patient should be admitted for initiation of definitive treatment. Pediatric patients who are diagnosed with PE require hospitalization for anticoagulation, and some severe cases may be candidates for thrombolytics or thrombectomy. For patients without respiratory distress or hemodynamic compromise, admission is commonly to an inpatient floor. For those with clinical or diagnostic evidence of compromise, further evaluation and management in an ICU is recommended.

PULMONARY EDEMA

CLINICAL PEARLS AND PITFALLS

- Management of pulmonary edema focuses on supplemental oxygen and providing cardiopulmonary support as needed.
- Determining the underlying cause is important to inform therapies directed at correcting abnormal plasma oncotic pressure and intrapulmonary fluid balance.

Current Evidence

Pulmonary edema is abnormal accumulation of fluid within the alveolar spaces and bronchioles. In healthy lungs, intravascular and interstitial hydrostatic and plasma oncotic pressures are relatively balanced, resulting in minimal fluid flux into the interstitium and alveoli. Pulmonary edema results from alterations in these pressures or changes in permeability of fluid-exchanging membranes in the lungs.

In adults pulmonary edema is often described as either cardiogenic pulmonary edema, due to increases in pulmonary capillary hydrostatic pressure from coronary artery disease and left-sided heart failure, or noncardiogenic edema most commonly from ARDS. In pediatrics, the etiologies are quite varied, and it is more effective to categorize according to the underlying pathophysiology.

In children, pulmonary edema can be secondary to increased hydrostatic pressure. This can be seen in cardiac conditions including congenital anomalies that are associated with left-sided heart failure, such as hypoplastic left heart syndrome, cor triatriatum, mitral stenosis, severe aortic stenosis, coarctation of the aorta, or acquired myocardial disease. Pulmonary edema from overcirculation within the pulmonary vasculature secondary to left-to-right vascular shunting can occur with patent ductus arteriosus, ventricular septal defects, and iatrogenic cardiac shunts. Beyond cardiac disease, increased hydrostatic pressures from overaggressive administration of IV fluids can also cause pulmonary edema.

Neurogenic pulmonary edema may be seen with seizure activity or increased intracranial pressure. Although the mechanism is not entirely understood, it likely results from increased capillary hydrostatic pressures after acute sympathetic discharge in these patients. The possibility of concomitant capillary leak in neurogenic pulmonary edema has also been proposed.

Decreased plasma oncotic pressure is also associated with pulmonary edema. This condition is seen with lowered levels of circulating plasma proteins, such as occurs with nephrosis, protein-losing enteropathies, massive burns, and severe malnutrition.

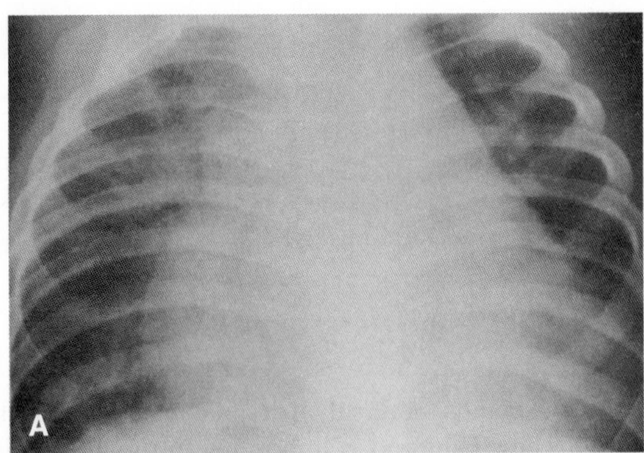

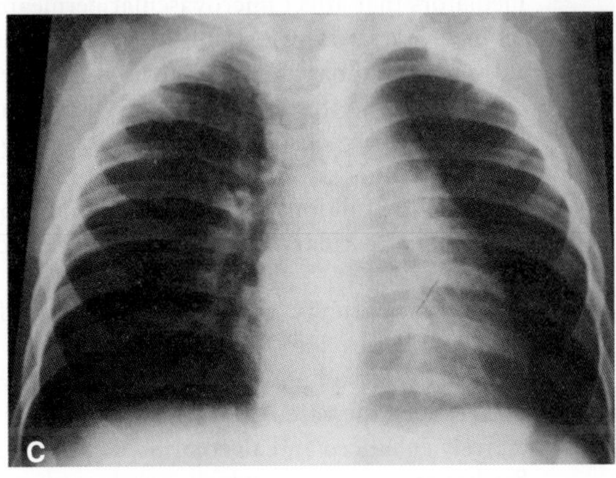

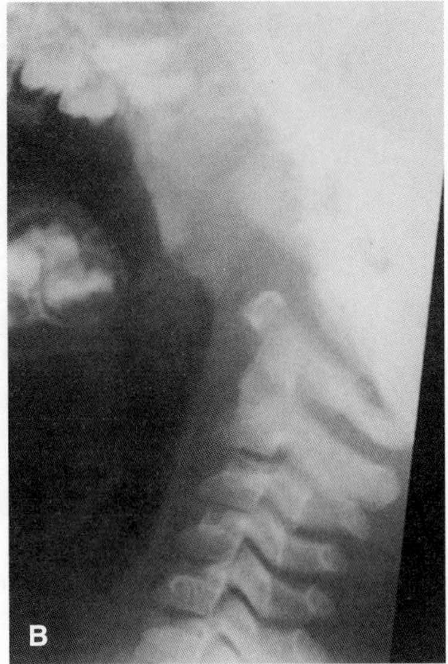

FIGURE 107.5 Cor pulmonale secondary to upper airway obstruction. **A:** This is a 2-year-old boy with tachypnea and dyspnea. The chest film shows a large heart and mild interstitial edema. **B:** The lateral view of the neck shows obstructing enlarged adenoids and tonsils. **C:** The chest film 2 days after adenoidectomy shows a decreased heart size and improvement in interstitial edema.

Any breakdown in the alveolar–capillary barrier can result in accumulation of protein-rich fluid in the interstitium. This is the initial and major manifestation of ARDS. Lung insult leads to tissue destruction and increased permeability of the alveolar–capillary membrane. In addition to ARDS, a variety of other clinical conditions can similarly lead to capillary leak syndromes. Circulating toxins, such as snake venom and endotoxins from gram-negative sepsis, are examples. In addition, altered permeability can lead to pulmonary edema from asthma, hypersensitivity pneumonitis, Goodpasture syndrome, and systemic lupus erythematosus. Inhaled environmental exposures can have a similar effect. Noxious gases from fires, hydrocarbons, oxides from sulfur and nitrogen, and inhalation of some herbicides (e.g., paraquat) can denature proteins and cause cellular damage with development of pulmonary edema.

Postobstructive pulmonary edema, also known as *negative-pressure pulmonary edema,* is associated with upper airway obstruction (Fig. 107.5A–C). It is thought to result from exaggeration of the transmural pulmonary vascular hydrostatic pressure gradient.

Pulmonary edema can also result from travel to high altitudes. This characteristically affects young people who are exposed to altitudes above 2,700 m. It generally occurs soon after arrival in high altitude locations and can occur in those who are new to such elevations or those who have returned from time spent nearer to sea level. Although the precise mechanism is unclear, cardiac catheterizations have suggested that the cause is not related to increased hydrostatic pressures.

Goals of Treatment

Management goals for patients with pulmonary edema include cardiopulmonary support which involves supplemental oxygen and may include noninvasive ventilation support and vasoactive pressor agents. Diagnosis of the underlying etiology is also an important goal, as specific targeted therapies can be utilized.

Clinical Considerations

Clinical Recognition

The onset of pulmonary edema can be variable depending on etiology but may occur rapidly (i.e., flash pulmonary edema) or more insidiously. The diagnosis of pulmonary edema involves both clinical and radiographic findings. Often children with pulmonary edema have cough, respiratory distress, hypoxia, rales on examination, and chest radiograph findings of edema. Bedside ultrasound is now also being used to identify pulmonary edema in both pediatric and adult patients. However, findings are related to the amount of edema and may not be present if edema is minimal.

Triage

Most children with pulmonary edema will have significant respiratory distress, and they should be promptly evaluated and stabilized as necessary.

Initial Assessment/H&P

Cough is the most common symptom noted in patients with pulmonary edema and may produce frothy, pink-tinged sputum. Patients may also endorse dyspnea, shortness of breath, orthopnea, and chest pain. On physical examination, the child may appear pale or cyanotic and frequently has tachycardia. Tachypnea is almost universally present. Grunting often occurs in an effort to increase airway pressure and stent open small airways and airspaces and prevent lung collapse. Auscultatory findings include decreased breath sounds and moist crackles,

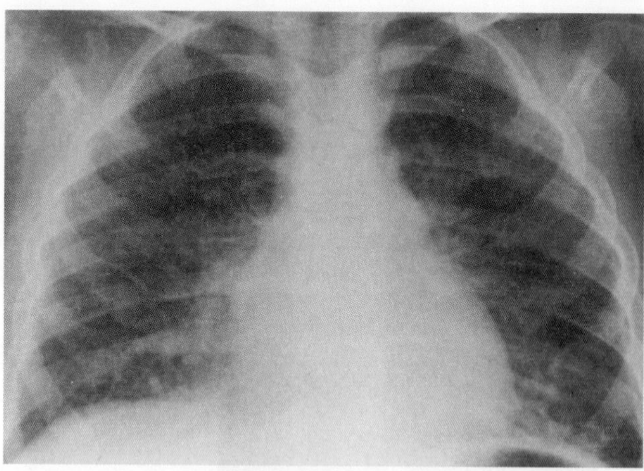

FIGURE 107.6 Interstitial fluid from volume overload. This is a 2-year-old child with paraspinal sarcoma removed 6 months earlier. Before chest radiation, he received a large fluid load. The chest film shows interstitial edema with Kerley lines.

particularly at the bases; however, these may be absent with small amounts of edema. Physical examination and radiographic findings may not manifest until the interstitial and extravascular fluid has doubled or tripled in volume.

For children with underlying conditions, it is important to understand the status of their disease and any recent changes in therapy. The possibility of acute intercurrent illness or insult should also be considered.

Chest radiographs are often diagnostic, although findings may lag behind the acute clinical process. Lymphatic and interstitial fluid accumulations may be visible as Kerley A and B lines (septal lines; Fig. 107.6), which represent interstitial edema, tangential to the radiograph beam. The B lines, which lie in the periphery, are often the first findings. Unlike blood vessels, these radiopacities will reach the lung edge. As edema progresses, Kerley A lines near the hilum may occur, and ultimately, a butterfly pattern with a central predominance of shadows can be seen. Although these findings are not specific, transient changes in an appropriate clinical context usually signify edema. Bedside ultrasound can also be very effective at identifying fluid in the lungs (see Chapter 142 Ultrasound).

The distribution, symmetry, and extent of radiographic findings may also provide helpful information regarding possible etiology and severity of edema. Patterns of radiographic findings in particular can be helpful in identifying underlying cause. Cardiac size and increased prominence of pulmonary vasculature may suggest increased hydrostatic pressure or cardiogenic edema. Conversely, presence of air bronchograms, peribronchial cuffing, and increased lung volume may suggest primary lung injury with resultant capillary leak.

If pulmonary edema is superimposed on another pulmonary process, the clinical and radiographic findings may be obscured by those of the primary illness. Similarly, once pulmonary edema is severe enough, it may be difficult to distinguish edema, atelectasis, and inflammation on the chest film.

Management

The management of patients with pulmonary edema includes supportive therapies and correction of the underlying disorder. Initial efforts (Table 107.9) should be directed toward correction of hypoxemia through the administration of supplemental oxygen. In addition to satisfying the patient's oxygen

TABLE 107.9

TREATMENT OF PULMONARY EDEMA

Oxygen	Afterload reduction
Diuresis	Morphine 0.1 mg/kg IV
Furosemide 1 mg/kg IV	

IV, intravenous.

demands, reversal of hypoxemia is often useful in relieving chest pain and is important to the metabolism of vasoactive mediators that affect microvascular permeability.

In severe cases, CPAP, BIPAP, or intubation and mechanical ventilation may be warranted. Assisted ventilation has several beneficial effects for patients with pulmonary edema. It reduces oxygen consumption by decreasing work of breathing. Oxygenation is also improved through prevention of alveolar collapse. In addition, positive intrathoracic pressures decrease pulmonary vascular volume and reduce fluid filtration in the lung.

In healthy lungs, there is a small fluid flux from pulmonary capillaries into the interstitium. This fluid is actively drained by a sodium transporter in the alveolar epithelium and reenters the vascular system as lymph. This process can be actively enhanced and alveolar fluid clearance augmented with β-adrenergic agonists, which may be utilized in some clinical circumstances.

Other therapeutic measures should be tailored to fit the patient's underlying disease process. When ventricular failure is the cause of pulmonary edema, diuretics can be used to decrease plasma volume, and inotropes can improve contractility. Morphine helps physiologically by dilating the venous system and may also relieve anxiety and dyspnea. Afterload reducers such as milrinone may also be helpful.

When decreased plasma oncotic pressure is primary, administration of colloids such as albumin is indicated. Slow infusion and concomitant diuretic use will help minimize resultant increases in pulmonary vascular pressure.

Detailed management of ARDS is beyond the scope of this chapter, though generally it is focused on addressing underlying illness and supportive ventilatory strategies. Clinical studies have shown that the use of systemic steroids does not improve outcome and may in fact increase the incidence of secondary infections and subsequent mortality.

Clinical Indications for Discharge or Admission

Most children with pulmonary edema will require hospitalization with supportive cardiopulmonary care and evaluation for underlying conditions.

PLEURITIS/PLEURAL EFFUSION

CLINICAL PEARLS AND PITFALLS

- Pleuritis without significant effusion may be associated with systemic vasculitis.
- Most pleural effusions in pediatrics are exudative.
- Management of effusions involves treating associated chest pain, and thoracentesis for diagnostic and therapeutic purposes.

Current Evidence

Pleuritis or pleurisy refers to inflammation of pleural membranes, resulting from primary pleural, adjacent pneumonic, or systemic disease. This inflammation is usually associated with an increased volume of fluid in the pleural space. Specific references to the incidence of pleural effusions in various respiratory infections are made in Chapter 102 Infectious Disease Emergencies, and the surgical approach to pleural effusions is reviewed in Chapter 132 Thoracic Emergencies.

The pleural membrane is thin and double layered, separating the lung from the chest wall, diaphragm, and mediastinum. The outer parietal pleura is adherent to the chest wall, and the inner visceral pleura completely covers the lungs except at the hila. In healthy children, the two pleural layers are opposed, separated by only a thin physiologic layer of serous fluid. This pleural fluid is constantly being turned over, entering from the parietal pleura and exiting via the lymphatics and vasculature of the visceral pleura.

Abnormal pleural fluid accumulation can result from changes in hydrostatic or oncotic pressures (such as seen with pulmonary edema) or diseases of the pleural surface that alter capillary permeability or affect lymphatic reabsorption. The underlying pathophysiology will determine if an effusion will be transudative or exudative. Transudates result from increased capillary hydrostatic pressure such as congestive heart failure or decreased oncotic pressure such as hypoproteinemic states. Exudates result from diseases of the pleural surface that produce increased capillary permeability or lymphatic obstruction, such as pleural infection or tumor.

In pediatrics, the majority of effusions are exudative. Therefore, classification focuses largely on whether pleural fluid collections are infectious or noninfectious.

Goals of Treatment

The goals of treatment for patients with pleural disease are focused on rapidly assessing and supporting respiratory function. Supporting oxygenation and ventilation may be required passively or actively. Therapeutic training of fluid may be useful for therapeutic purposes for patients with compromise respirations, and for diagnostic purposes, including identification of likely etiology, including microbiology in the case of infectious causes.

Clinical Considerations

Clinical Recognition

There exists a wide spectrum of conditions that lead to pleural inflammation (Table 107.10). Infectious etiologies are most common and may include viruses (e.g., Coxsackie virus, Epstein–Barr virus, herpes zoster), mycoplasma, bacteria (e.g., *S. aureus, Streptococcus pneumoniae, H. influenzae,* group A streptococcus, *Mycobacterium tuberculosis*), and fungi (e.g., histoplasmosis, coccidioidomycosis). Infections from pulmonary, subdiaphragmatic, or more distant sites may all eventually involve the pleura. Neoplastic involvement may also be primary or metastatic. When oncologic lesions obstruct the lymphatic drainage, accumulation of pleural fluid can occur. PE may cause pleural inflammation with or without effusion as a result of focal parenchymal necrosis. Trauma, both accidental and following diagnostic and therapeutic procedures in

TABLE 107.10

DIFFERENTIAL DIAGNOSIS OF PLEURAL EFFUSION

Transudative pleural effusions
Congestive heart failure
Cirrhosis
Nephrotic syndrome
Acute glomerulonephritis
Myxedema
Peritoneal dialysis
Hypoproteinemia
Meigs syndrome
Sarcoidosis
Vascular obstruction
Ex vacuo effusion
Exudative pleural effusions
Infectious diseases
Tuberculosis
Bacterial infections
Viral infections
Fungal infections
Parasitic infections
Neoplastic diseases
Mesotheliomas
Metastatic disease
Collagen vascular diseases
Systemic lupus erythematosus
Rheumatoid pleuritis
Pulmonary infarction/embolization
Gastrointestinal diseases
Pancreatitis
Esophageal rupture
Subphrenic abscess
Hepatic abscess
Whipple disease
Diaphragmatic hernia
Peritonitis
Trauma
Hemothorax
Chylothorax
Drug hypersensitivity
Nitrofurantoin
Methysergide
Miscellaneous diseases
Asbestos exposure
Pulmonary and lymph node myomatosis
Uremia
Postmyocardial infarction syndrome
Trapped lung
Congenital abnormalities of the lymphatics
Postradiation therapy
Drug reactions

From Light RW. Pleural effusions. *Med Clin North Am* 1977;61:1339–1352. (See text for transudate/exudate criteria.)

the chest, can irritate the pleura and lead to secondary infection. Pleuritis with or without effusion is seen in more than half of patients who have a systemic vasculitis such as systemic lupus erythematosus or sarcoidosis.

Triage

Patients with pleuritis often present with chest pain that may be severe. Depending on the amount of pleural fluid, hypoxia and significant respiratory distress may be present. Promptly addressing pain and respiratory compromise must be a priority.

Initial Assessment/H&P

The hallmarks of pleural disease are chest pain, shortness of breath, fever, and in many cases an abnormal chest radiograph. Pain with respirations, or pleuritic chest pain, is the most characteristic symptom with pleural inflammation, and may be localized. Most patients also describe some degree of dyspnea. Additional symptoms vary depending on the primary cause. In "dry" pleurisy, which is usually caused by a minor pulmonary infection, the patient is often febrile with an irritating, nonproductive cough. With oncologic etiologies, weight loss, night sweats, and fatigue may be present.

On examination, the chest wall over the involved area may be tender, and a coarse vibration may sometimes be appreciated on palpation. A pleural friction rub is most apt to be heard when pleural inflammation is associated with little or no effusion. The sound has been described as low pitched, sometimes with a grating or squeaking quality. It is usually loudest on inspiration, but often it may also be audible during expiration. Sometimes, the rub is confused with low-pitched rhonchi, produced by secretions partially blocking the airway. A vigorous cough will eliminate these secretions and sounds but will not affect the pleural friction rub. Grunting may occur, although related to pain rather than respiratory distress in most patients with dry pleurisy.

For patients with pleural effusions, characteristic physical findings include restriction of movement of the chest wall on the affected side, dullness to percussion, decreased or absent breath sounds, and diminished to absent tactile and vocal fremitus. These signs are similar to patients with large areas of atelectasis or collapse, although pleural effusions decrease the available space within the hemithorax, which may cause the trachea to deviate away from the diseased side. Conversely, atelectasis can cause the trachea to deviate toward the diseased side.

Radiographs may be used to evaluate for pleural thickening or effusion, as well as to help determine underlying etiology. Pleural inflammation alone can be difficult to appreciate on chest radiographs. Instead, effusion is the most common radiographic manifestation of pleural disease. The first radiographic sign of a pleural effusion is usually blunting of the costophrenic angles on PA or AP chest radiograph views, producing wedge-like menisci that extend upward along the lateral chest wall. Similar collections can be seen in the posterior costophrenic angles on lateral views. Larger effusions may be seen to extend up the entire lateral chest wall or retrosternally.

Pleural effusions may alternatively present with apparent prominence or thickening of the interlobar fissures or by wedge-shaped accumulations of fluid at either end of these fissures. The latter may be mistaken for focal infiltrates or segmental atelectasis on some views.

Although small effusions may be overlooked on radiograph, with proper technique, collections as small as 25 mL have been identified. In adults, pleural effusions are visible on lateral chest radiographs at a volume of approximately 50 mL. At a volume of 200 mL, the meniscus can be identified on the posteroanterior (PA) radiograph, whereas at a volume of 500 mL, the meniscus obscures the hemidiaphragm.

Management

Management of pleural disease should focus on determining the cause, treating the primary disorder, and relieving associated functional cardiopulmonary disturbances.

When no effusion is present, relief of chest pain is best accomplished with anti-inflammatory therapy and rest. Pleurisy can be significant in some children, and constant aggravation with respiration can be frustrating. Use of stronger analgesia may be required, provided comprehensive evaluation has been performed to avoid masking significant illness, and with careful attention to avoiding respiratory depression.

For patients with increased accumulation of pleural fluid, pain is usually less significant; however, respiratory compromise is more likely. Thoracentesis is indicated when fluid accumulation is extensive enough to cause dyspnea and/or for diagnostic purposes (Fig. 107.7). Ultrasound guidance for thoracentesis can be used to facilitate this procedure, particularly with small or loculated effusions. Complications of thoracentesis include pneumothorax, hemothorax, re-expansion pulmonary edema, and, rarely, air embolism. The recommended technique for thoracentesis is provided in Chapter 141 Procedures, section on Thoracentesis.

Additional means of draining pleural fluid are also available. Thoracostomy using small "pigtail" tubes placed by Seldinger technique is minimally more invasive than needle thoracentesis and allows for ongoing drainage as needed. Again, ultrasound guidance can be utilized at the bedside, or the location of maximal fluid can be marked prior to drainage. Image-guided catheter drainage is most effective in patients with short duration of symptoms, free-flowing or unilocular effusions, absence of thick pleural peel, and fluid collections that can be easily reached. Other approaches for more advanced disease include surgical tube thoracotomy; video-assisted thoracoscopic surgery (VATS), which allows directed chest tube placement and debridement; and mini thoracotomy with open pleural decortication.

Diagnostic tests of pleural fluid should include gross and microscopic examination, Gram stain, glucose, and pH determinations; cytology should be sent if malignancy is known or suspected.

For patients with exudative effusions, pleural fluid pH measurement is helpful in guiding decisions regarding drainage. In adult patients, pH values of greater than 7.2 to 7.3 are generally found in sterile pleural fluid that does not require further drainage. One exception is *Proteus mirabilis* infection, which causes an elevated pleural fluid pH. In contrast, a pH of less than 7.0 is seen only in empyema, collagen vascular disease, or esophageal rupture. With regard to management, a pleural fluid pH of less than 7.2 suggests that the effusion will likely require chest tube drainage.

A pleural fluid:serum glucose ratio less than 0.5 has a similar differential diagnosis as low pleural fluid pH. In animal studies, both leukocytes and bacteria have been shown to use glucose anaerobically, resulting in reduced glucose concentration. Diseases associated with low pleural fluid glucose (less than 60 mg per dL) include infectious causes, collagen vascular diseases, malignancies, and esophageal rupture.

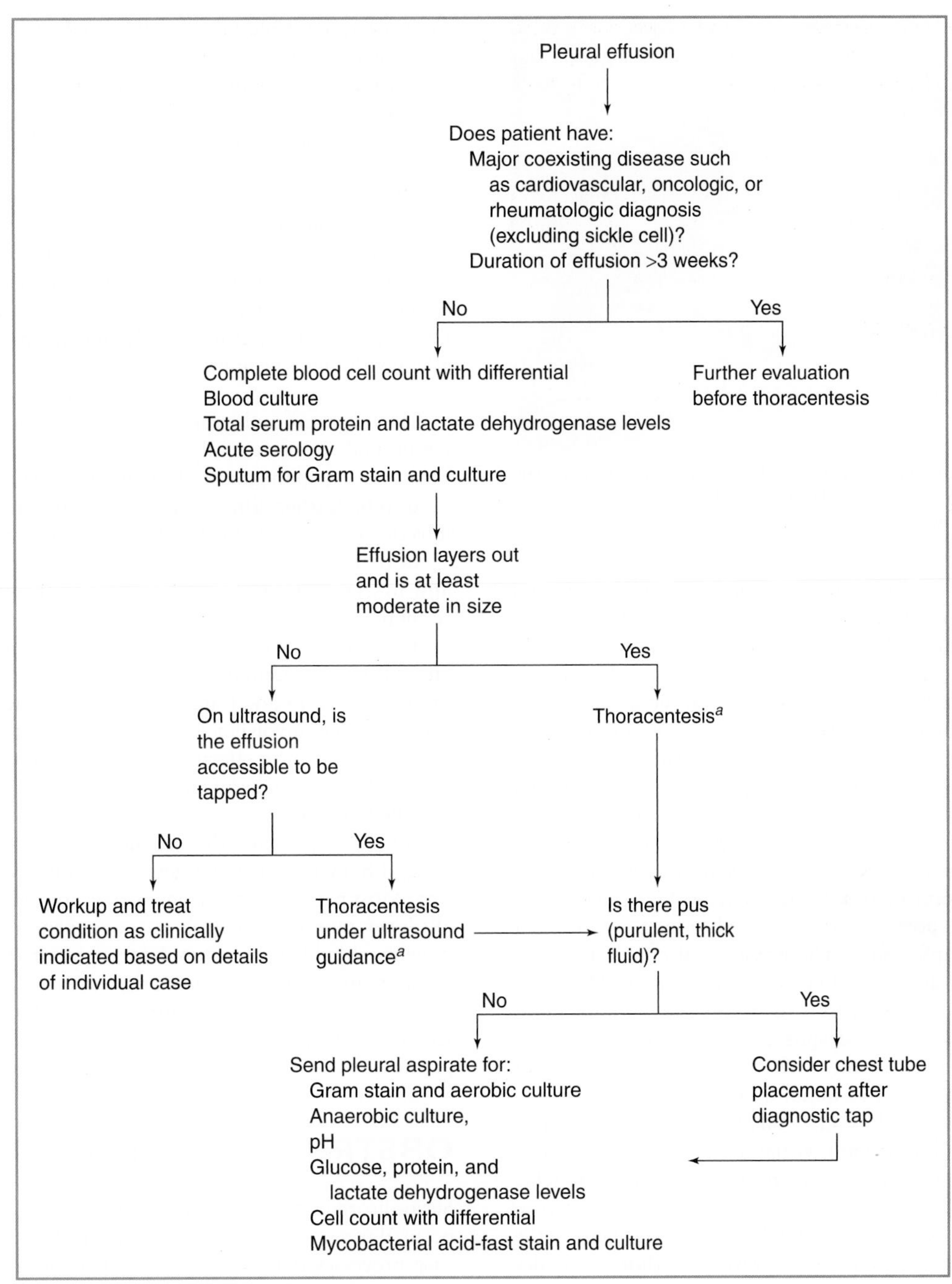

FIGURE 107.7 Approach to pleural effusion. [a]Consider simultaneous placement of small gauge (8°F to 10°F) chest tube by Seldinger technique for large, free-flowing effusions.

Clinical Indications for Discharge or Admission

Disposition for patients with pleurisy and effusion depends on the degree of pain and pulmonary compromise, as well as status of underlying condition and ability to treat as an outpatient. If imaging is negative, patients with adequate pain control and no respiratory compromise can be safely treated as outpatients. Most patients with nontrivial pleural effusions will require admission for ongoing diagnostic workup and management, and for respiratory monitoring and support. Any pediatric patient who requires fluid drainage in the ED should be admitted.

SARCOIDOSIS

Sarcoidosis is a rare, chronic, granulomatous disease of unknown cause. Lungs are the most affected organs although joints, skin, eyes, lymph nodes, liver, spleen, muscle, and brain can all be involved. Involved organs have accumulations of T lymphocytes and mononuclear phagocytes, noncaseating epithelioid granulomas, and derangements of normal tissue architecture. Although the exact cause of sarcoidosis is unknown, evidence suggests a multifactorial etiology; both environmental and genetic factors result in an exaggerated cellular immune response to an unclear antigen.

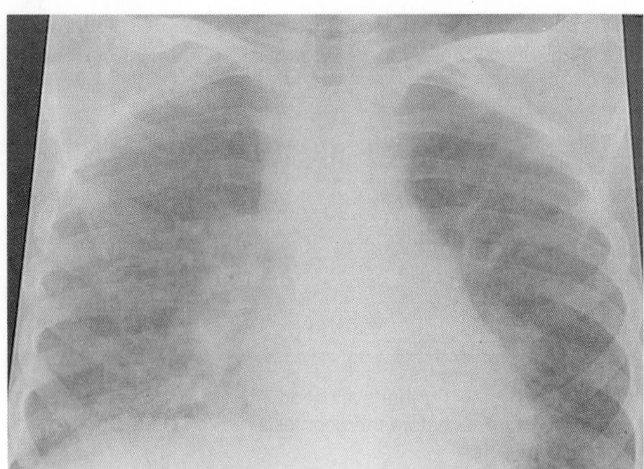

FIGURE 107.8 Sarcoid. A 9-year-old child with hepatosplenomegaly but no pulmonary complaints. The chest film shows interstitial lung disease with hilar adenopathy.

The incidence of sarcoidosis varies with age, race, and geography. The majority of those affected are adults between the ages of 20 and 40 years. Most pediatric cases present in the second decade, although cases of patients less than 1 year of age have been reported. The disease is often acute or subacute and self-limiting. However, in many, it is chronic, with waxing and waning symptoms over many years.

The most common initial symptoms in children and young adults are nonspecific and may include malaise, fatigue, fever, and weight loss. Organ-specific symptoms vary by age. Children younger than 5 years most commonly have skin, eye, and joint involvement, whereas older children are more likely to report symptoms related to lung involvement or enlarged lymph nodes. The presence of cough and dyspnea usually indicates pulmonary involvement. However, extensive pulmonary disease can be present without clinical findings. Hoarseness, dyspnea, and dysphagia can result from laryngeal involvement. Arrhythmia or congestive heart failure can also present as initial findings of cardiac disease. Other symptoms vary depending on affected systems and may include bone and joint pain, visual acuity impairment, ocular swelling or pain, parotid gland enlargement, headache, and unexplained fever.

On physical examination, lymph node enlargement is the most frequently detected abnormality. Intrathoracic nodes including hilar, paratracheal, or mediastinal chains are enlarged in 75% to 90% of patients. When present, hilar adenopathy is usually bilateral and symmetric (see Fig. 107.8).

Peripheral adenopathy is also common, particularly in cervical, axillary, and inguinal regions. Affected lymph nodes are firm, nontender, mobile, and nonulcerative. Some patients have a skin rash that is similar in appearance to erythema nodosum. Plaques, subcutaneous nodules, and maculopapular eruptions can also be seen. Uveitis is present in up to 25% of patients. Small yellow nodules are frequently found on the conjunctiva in these patients. Hepatosplenomegaly and joint effusions can also be present.

Laboratory test abnormalities in patients with sarcoidosis tend to be nonspecific. Hyperproteinemia, elevated erythrocyte sedimentation rate (ESR), hypercalciuria, eosinophilia, and rarely hypercalcemia can be seen. Although not pathognomonic, an elevated serum angiotensin-converting enzyme level in patients in whom sarcoid is suspected is strongly supportive.

On chest radiograph, between 40% and 60% of symptomatic children will have hilar adenopathy alone or in combination with parenchymal infiltrates. Pulmonary function testing usually reveals restrictive lung disease.

Diagnosis of sarcoidosis in children is challenging because it is extremely rare and oftentimes findings are subtle. For pediatric patients with multisystem complaints, however, sarcoidosis should be considered. In particular, pulmonary disease associated with rash, uveitis, or arthritis is suggestive. However, because lung disease can remain clinically silent, respiratory complaints need not be present at the time of initial presentation. Alternatively, unexplained intrathoracic adenopathy may prompt further investigation, leading to the diagnosis.

The diagnosis is ultimately made histologically. Biopsy of a lymph node or other easily accessible organ will demonstrate noncaseating epithelioid cell granulomas. These findings may need to be further differentiated from other rheumatologic or infectious diseases that can have similar histopathology.

Corticosteroid treatment is the most commonly used therapy for sarcoidosis. However, because the disease resolves spontaneously in a substantial proportion of patients, there is often debate about whether steroids are routinely indicated. Steroids may be administered to children with significant lung or eye lesions. In addition, those with cardiac, CNS, or multiorgan system involvement usually warrant therapy. Corticosteroids seem to be effective as acute therapeutic agents but have little effect on permanent organ derangements, including chronic lung disease.

For many patients, the prognosis in sarcoidosis is favorable, although clinical and genetic factors are important factors. Most patients with an acute presentation improve gradually over months and have no permanent sequelae, though patients should be monitored for signs of relapse. Younger children and those with multiorgan system involvement tend to have less favorable outcomes. Some will develop progressive cystic emphysema, bronchiectasis, or severe restrictive pulmonary disease with exercise-induced hypoxemia.

OBSTRUCTIVE SLEEP APNEA

Sleep-disordered breathing refers to respiratory disorders that occur during or are exacerbated by sleep. These include disease processes that result in central or obstructive apnea or hypoventilation. Of those with obstructive etiologies, primary habitual snoring is the most common, but also the least worrisome. On the other end of the spectrum is obstructive sleep apnea syndrome (OSAS), which can have long-term consequences, including neurocognitive deficits and cardiovascular morbidities.

The American Thoracic Society has defined OSAS in children as disordered breathing during sleep, characterized by prolonged upper airway obstruction or intermittent complete obstruction that disrupts normal ventilation during sleep and normal sleep patterns. Although the reported incidence varies depending on the data collection methodology and inclusion criteria, most studies suggest that OSAS occurs in 1% to 5% of children. It is more common in boys than girls. The peak pediatric incidence is between 2 and 8 years of age, paralleling the prominence of growth of lymphoid tissues around the airway. However, OSAS can occur in any age. Craniofacial anomalies including macroglossia and neurologic disorders affecting upper airway structure and tone predispose infants to OSAS, while obesity is often a factor in the development of the syndrome in older children.

The exact pathophysiology of OSAS is unclear. Available data suggest that upper airway resistance, from either anatomic or dynamic airway obstructions, leads to variable and abnormal breathing patterns during sleep. The limited airflow from airway obstruction prompts electrocortical arousal and autonomic activation. This response stimulates an increased respiratory effort and tachypnea in an effort to maintain normal gas exchange. Collectively, the result is disordered sleep patterns that have downstream consequences on the cardiovascular system and daytime behaviors.

In most cases, adenotonsillar hypertrophy is the major cause of airway obstruction. Obesity has become another precipitant, and a growing public health problem in this country. Of note, obese patients with OSAS tend to require less tonsillar hypertrophy to become symptomatic than do their younger, thinner counterparts.

Children with craniofacial anomalies are also at higher risk for obstruction and OSAS, oftentimes beginning shortly after birth. In children whose craniofacial anomalies reduce the size of the nasal cavity, nasopharynx, or oropharynx, the normal pharyngeal tissues or minimal hyperplasia of the lymphoid tissue of Waldeyer ring can cause varying degrees of obstruction.

Children with neuromuscular diseases are also prone to obstruction and OSAS. In these children, impaired pharyngeal tone allows posterior soft tissues to collapse into the airway during sleep. These children are likely to also have chronic pulmonary disease due to low muscle tone and impaired ability to clear pharyngeal secretions, which further complicates their evaluation and management.

Snoring and difficulty breathing are the most common complaints in children with OSAS. The snoring is described as loud, often with interspersed pauses, snorts, or gasps. Retractions during sleep are frequently noted. Episodes of obstruction may be witnessed, many of which are terminated by gasping, movement, or awakening. Children will frequently appear restless throughout the night, naturally repositioning themselves to promote airway patency. Increased autonomic tone frequently results in nighttime diaphoresis and may contribute to enuresis. Chronic nighttime cough may also be observed as a result of intermittent aspiration of small amounts of pharyngeal secretions.

Although symptoms including nasal voice and mouth breathing may be noticeable during the daytime, many children exhibit no evidence of airway compromise when awake. However, because of disrupted sleep, children with OSAS may demonstrate excessive somnolence, although this is much less common in younger children than in teens and adults. Behavioral and neurocognitive changes are relatively common, however, resembling symptoms seen in patients with attention deficit hyperactivity disorder. Other commonly associated behavioral abnormalities include fighting with peers, crying easily, withdrawal behavior, and rapid fluctuations in alertness. Older children may also experience decreased school performance, especially with regard to language acquisition. These changes may result from disrupted sleep as well as chronic, intermittent hypoxemia.

Abnormal physical findings on examination are unusual. Tonsillar enlargement may be noted; however, it is often mild to moderate rather than marked. A normal oropharyngeal examination does not exclude OSAS, given the potential for other soft tissue structures or dynamic changes to cause the airway obstruction. Other nonspecific signs might include delayed growth or impaired weight gain, from chronic increased work of breathing, intermittent hypoxia, and limited caloric intake secondary to difficulty eating and breathing comfortably at the same time. Alternatively, obesity may be noted particularly in older patients with OSAS. Abnormal facies or systemically decreased tone may be found as etiologies in young infants.

Polysomnography is gold standard for diagnosis and should be performed on children with historical and physical findings suggesting OSAS. It can distinguish primary snoring from OSAS and can determine the severity of OSAS. Although polysomnography can be performed satisfactorily in children of any age, it requires appropriate equipment and appropriately trained staff. Therefore, availability is often limited. Abbreviated or nap polysomnography in the hospital or unattended home polysomnography have been utilized in some situations.

Soft tissue radiographs of the lateral neck taken with the child lying on his/her back can be helpful but are not a definitive method of diagnosis—static images cannot replicate potential dynamic changes that may occur during sleep. Standardized recordings of breathing sounds, videotaping of a child while sleeping, or continuous overnight pulse oximetry can occur either in the hospital or in the patient's home. Evidence suggests that these screening tools can have reasonable positive predictive value; however, absence of abnormal findings cannot exclude OSAS.

Children with concern for significant apnea may warrant hospitalization until a diagnosis and severity can be determined. Historical clues will be most important in making this determination, as children with OSAS do not usually appear in extremis during wakeful periods. However, some well-appearing children may be at risk for repeated apnea and subsequent hypoxemia while sleeping.

During hospitalization, significant airway obstruction should be managed according to basic life support protocols, with airway maneuvers such as repositioning, jaw thrust, and head-tilt–chin-lift to open the upper airway as necessary. Nasal trumpets may also be helpful.

Supplemental oxygen therapy is sometimes recommended to alleviate nocturnal hypoxemia. However, it does not prevent sleep-related upper airway obstruction, sleep fragmentation, or increased work of breathing. In addition, patients with long-standing disease may chronically retain CO_2; therefore, aggressive correction of hypoxia may depress respiratory drive and potentially worsen hypoventilation. Assessing a serum HCO_3 or blood gas level may be helpful in identifying such patients.

In addition to a thorough general medical evaluation, children with OSAS will generally require otolaryngology consultation for airway evaluation and, if needed, procedures for relieving obstruction.

Numerous methods of management of OSAS have been suggested and studied. Patients with hyperplasia of the tonsils and adenoids as the primary cause for obstruction may be trialed on high-dose nasal steroids, although those who improve may not have sustained benefit. Most of these patients will have dramatic relief of symptoms following surgical resection. Postoperative polysomnography shows resolution of OSAS in 75% to 100% of patients. Patients with craniofacial anomalies and with neuromuscular disorders also usually have significant

TABLE 107.11

CAUSES OF INTERSTITIAL LUNG DISEASE

Environmental irritants	Sarcoidosis
Inorganic dusts	Inherited disorders
Organic dusts (hypersensitivity)	Neurofibromatosis
Noxious gases	Miscellaneous causes
Drugs	Celiac disease
Radiation	Whipple disease
Collagen vascular disease	Weber–Christian disease
Rheumatoid arthritis	Histiocytosis
Scleroderma	Hermansky–Pudlak syndrome
Systemic lupus erythematosus	

improvement after adenotonsillectomy or other targeted surgical procedures.

Patients with obesity hypoventilation syndrome (Pickwickian syndrome) may benefit from maintained weight reduction. Unfortunately, weight loss in these patients is often difficult to achieve or only temporarily successful. Because many obese children will be adequately treated with adenotonsillectomy, it is generally the first-line therapy for these patients.

Oral appliances have been shown to improve snoring and reduce apnea and hypopnea in adults by modifying the upper airway through changes in the posture of the mandible and tongue. Although some patients tolerate such devices well, oral discomfort probably decreases compliance rates, which may be as low as 50% in adults and would likely be even lower in children. For some OSAS patients, nasally administered CPAP or BiPAP successfully alleviates hypoventilation, although again this may be less well tolerated in pediatric population. Rarely, patients require artificial airway placement and/or supplemental ventilation.

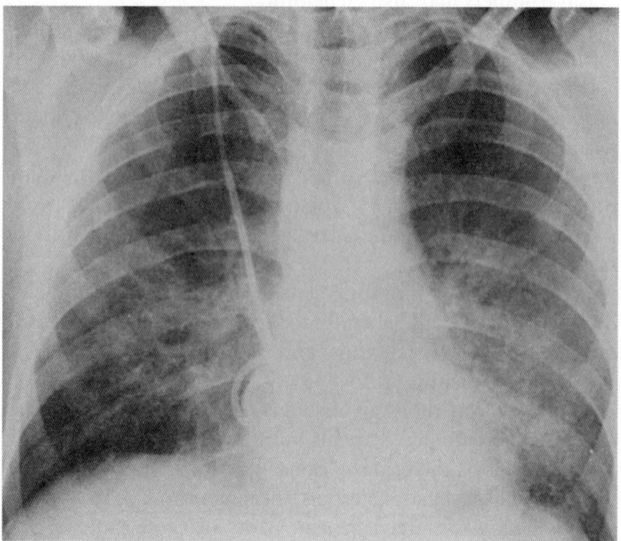

FIGURE 107.9 Idiopathic interstitial pneumonia. An 18-year-old boy with chronic granulomatous disease, after bone marrow transplant, with insidious onset of shortness of breath. The chest film shows bilateral interstitial disease in the lower lung field more on left side.

INTERSTITIAL LUNG DISEASE

Interstitial lung disease can occur from several different underlying etiologies (Table 107.11). While interstitial lung disease may present with acute respiratory distress without significant past medical history due to some inhalation injury or pneumonia (see Fig. 107.9), most patients will have underlying disorders including collagen vascular diseases and other autoimmune disorders. They may be on therapies for chronic lung disease and present with exacerbation.

Suggested Readings and References

Acute Respiratory Failure

Hansell DR. Extracorporeal membrane oxygenation for perinatal and pediatric patients. *Respir Care* 2003;48(4):352–362.

Heulitt MJ, Wolf GK, Arnold JH. Mechanical ventilation. In: Nichols DG, ed. *Textbook of Pediatric Intensive Care*, 4th ed. Baltimore, MD: Lippincott Williams & Wilkins, 2008:508–531.

Marraro GA. Innovative practices of ventilatory support with pediatric patients. *Pediatr Crit Care Med* 2003;4(1):8–20.

Asthma

Cheuk DK, Chau TC, Lee SL. A meta-analysis on intravenous magnesium sulphate for treating acute asthma. *Arch Dis Child* 2005; 90:74–77.

Gorelick M, Scribano PV, Stevens MW, et al. Predicting need for hospitalization in acute pediatric asthma. *Pediatr Emerg Care* 2008; 24:735–744.

Jia CE, Zhang HP, Lv Y, et al. The asthma control test and asthma control questionnaire for assessing asthma control: systematic review and meta-analysis. *J Allergy Clin Immunol* 2013;131:695–703.

Keeney GE, Gray MP, Morrison AK, et al. Dexamethasone for acute asthma exacerbations in children: a meta-analysis. *Pediatrics* 2014; 133(3):493–499.

Mathews B, Shah S, Cleveland RH, et al. Clinical predictors of pneumonia among children with wheezing. *Pediatrics* 2009;124(1): e29–e36.

National Asthma Education and Prevention Program. Expert panel report III: guidelines for the diagnosis and management of asthma. Bethesda, MD: National Heart, Lung, and Blood Institute, Available online at: http://www.nhlbi.nih.gov/health-pro/guidelines/current/asthma-guidelines. Accessed May 2015.

Nelson KA, Zorc JJ. Asthma update. *Pediatr Clin North Am* 2013; 60(5):1035–1048.

Ploin D, Chapuis FR, Stamm D, et al. High-dose albuterol by metered-dose inhaler plus a spacer device versus nebulization in preschool children with recurrent wheezing: a double-blind, randomized equivalence trial. *Pediatrics* 2000;106:311–317.

Qureshi F, Pestian J, Davis P, et al. Effect of nebulized ipratropium on the hospitalization rates of children with asthma. *N Engl J Med* 1998;339:1030–1035.

Qureshi F, Zaritsky A, Welch C, et al. Clinical efficacy of racemic albuterol versus levalbuterol for the treatment of acute pediatric asthma. *Ann Emerg Med* 2005;46:29–36.

Rowe BH, Spooner C, Ducharme FM, et al. Early emergency department treatment of acute asthma with systemic corticosteroids. *Cochrane Database Syst Rev* 2001;(1):CD002178.

Scarfone RJ, Fuchs SM, Nager AL, et al. Controlled trial of oral prednisone in the emergency department treatment of children with acute asthma. *Pediatrics* 1993;92:513–518.

Scarfone RJ, Zorc JJ, Angsuco CJ. Emergency physicians' prescribing of asthma controller medications. *Pediatrics* 2006;117:821–827.

Shan Z, Rong Y, Yang W, et al. Intravenous and nebulized magnesium sulfate for treating acute asthma in adults and children: a systematic review and meta-analysis. *Respir Med* 2013;107:321–330.

Zorc JJ, Pusic MV, Ogborn CJ, et al. Ipratropium bromide added to asthma treatment in the pediatric emergency department. *Pediatrics* 1999;103:748–752.

Aspiration Pneumonia

Boesch RP, Daines C, Willging JP, et al. Advances in the diagnosis and management of chronic pulmonary aspiration in children. *Eur Respir J* 2006;28:847–861.

Marik PE. Aspiration pneumonitis and aspiration pneumonia. *N Engl J Med* 2001;344:665–671.

Murray HW. Antimicrobial therapy in pneumonia aspiration. *Am J Med* 1979;66:188–190.

Platxker ACG. Gastroesophageal reflux and aspiration syndromes. In: Chernick V, Boat TF, Wilmott RW, et al., eds. *Kendig's Disorders of the Respiratory Tract in Children,* 7th ed. Philadelphia, PA: WB Saunders, 2006:592–609.

Weir K, McMahon S, Barry L, et al. Oropharyngeal aspiration and pneumonia in children. *Pediatr Pulmonol* 2007;42:1024–1031.

Bronchopulmonary Dysplasia

Abman SH, Davis JM. Bronchopulmonary dysplasia. In: Chernick V, Boat TF, Wilmott RW, et al., eds. *Kendig's Disorders of the Respiratory Tract in Children,* 7th ed. Philadelphia, PA: WB Saunders, 2006:342–358.

American Academy of Pediatrics Committee on Infectious Diseases, American Academy of Pediatrics Bronchiolitis Guidelines Committee. Updated guidance for palivizumab prophylaxis among infants and young children at increased risk of hospitalization for respiratory syncytial virus infection. *Pediatrics* 2014;134(2): 415–420.

Carpenter TC, Stenmark KR. Predisposition of infants with chronic lung disease to respiratory syncytial virus-induced respiratory failure: a vascular hypothesis. *Pediatr Infect Dis J* 2004;23:S33–S40.

Jobe AH. The new BPD. *Neoreviews* 2006;7:e531–e545.

Jobe AH, Bancalari E. Bronchopulmonary dysplasia. *Am J Respir Crit Care Med* 2001;163:1723–1729.

Walsh MC, Szefler S, Davis J, et al. Summary proceedings from the bronchopulmonary dysplasia group. *Pediatrics* 2006;117:S52–S56.

Cystic Fibrosis

Donaldson SH, Bennett WD, Zeman KL, et al. Mucus clearance and lung function in cystic fibrosis with hypertonic saline. *New Engl J Med* 2006;354(3):241–250.

Flume PA. Pulmonary complications of cystic fibrosis. *Respir Care* 2009;54(5):618–627.

Flume PA, Mogayzel PJ Jr, Robinson KA, et al. Cystic fibrosis pulmonary guidelines: treatment of pulmonary exacerbations. *Am J Respir Crit Care Med* 2009;180:802–808.

Flume PA, Strange C, Ye X, et al. Pneumothorax in cystic fibrosis. *Chest* 2005;128:720–728.

Ramsey BW, Boat TF. Outcome measures for clinical trials in cystic fibrosis: summary of a Cystic Fibrosis Foundation Consensus Conference. *J Pediatr* 1994;124:177–192.

Rommens JM, Ianuzzi MC, Bat-Sheva K, et al. Identification of the CF gene: chromosome walking and jumping. *Science* 1989;8:1059–1065.

Saiman L, Siegel J; Cystic Fibrosis Foundation. Infection control recommendations for patients with cystic fibrosis: microbiology, important pathogens, and infection control practices to prevent patient-to-patient transmission. *Infect Control Hosp Epidemiol* 2003;24:S6–S52.

Schidlow DV, Taussig LM, Knowles MR. Cystic Fibrosis Foundation Consensus Conference report on pulmonary complications of cystic fibrosis. *Pediatr Pulmonol* 1993;15:187–198.

Stevens DA, Moss RB, Kurup VP, et al. Allergic bronchopulmonary aspergillosis in cystic fibrosis—state of the art: Cystic Fibrosis Foundation Consensus Conference. *Clin Infect Dis* 2003;37(suppl 3): S225–S264.

Pulmonary Hemorrhage

Boat TF. Pulmonary hemorrhage and hemoptysis. In: Chernick V, Boat TF, Wilmott RW, et al., eds. *Kendig's Disorders of the Respiratory Tract in Children,* 7th ed. Philadelphia, PA: WB Saunders, 2006:676–685.

Brown CM, Redd SC, Damon SA. Acute idiopathic pulmonary hemorrhage among infants: recommendations from the Working Group for Investigation and Surveillance. *MMWR Recomm Rep* 2004;53:1–12.

Godfrey S. Pulmonary hemorrhage/hemoptysis in children. *Pediatr Pulmonol* 2004;37:476–484.

Susarla SC, Fan LL. Diffuse alveolar hemorrhage syndromes in children. *Curr Opin Pediatr* 2007;19:314–320.

Pulmonary Embolism

Agha BS, Sturm JJ, Simon HK, et al. Pulmonary embolism in the pediatric emergency department. *Pediatrics* 2013;132:663–667.

Chan AK, Deveber G, Monagle P, et al. Venous thrombosis in children. *J Thromb Haemost* 2003;1:1443–1455.

Johnson AS, Bolte RG. Pulmonary embolism in the pediatric patient. *Pediatr Emerg Care* 2004;20:555–560.

Monagle P, Michelson AD, Bovill E, et al. Antithrombotic therapy in children. *Chest* 2001;119:344–370.

Mullins MD, Becker DM, Hagspiel KD, et al. The role of spiral volumetric computed tomography in the diagnosis of pulmonary embolism. *Arch Intern Med* 2000;160:293–298.

Sadosty AT, Goyal DG, Boie ET, et al. Emergency department D-dimer testing. *J Emerg Med* 2001;21:423–429.

Tapson VF. Acute pulmonary embolism. *N Engl J Med* 2008;358:1037–1052.

Task Force on Pulmonary Embolism, European Society for Cardiology. Guidelines on diagnosis and management of acute pulmonary embolism. *Eur Heart J* 2000;21:1301–1336.

van Belle A, Büller HR, Huisman MV, et al. Effectiveness of managing suspected pulmonary embolism using an algorithm combining clinical probability, D-dimer testing, and computed tomography. *JAMA* 2006;295:172–179.

van Ommen CH, Heijboer H, Buller HR, et al. Venous thromboembolism in childhood: a prospective two-year registry in the Netherlands. *J Pediatr* 2001;139:676–681.

van Strijen MJ, de Monyé W, Schiereck J, et al. Single-detector helical computed tomography as the primary diagnostic test in suspected pulmonary embolism: a multicenter clinical management study of 510 patients. *Ann Intern Med* 2003;138:307–314.

Victoria T, Mong A, Altes T, et al. Evaluation of pulmonary embolism in a pediatric population with high clinical suspicion. *Pediatr Radiol* 2009;39:35–41.

Wells PS, Ginsberg JS, Anderson DR, et al. Use of a chemical model for safe management of patients with suspected pulmonary embolism. *Ann Intern Med* 1998;129:997–1005.

Pulmonary Edema

O'Brodovich H. Pulmonary edema. In: Chernick V, Boat TF, Wilmott RW, et al., eds. *Kendig's Disorders of the Respiratory Tract in Children,* 7th ed. Philadelphia, PA: WB Saunders, 2006:622–638.

Pleuritis

Bradley JS, Byington CL, Shah SS, et al.; Pediatric Infectious Diseases Society and the Infectious Diseases Society of America. The management of community-acquired pneumonia in infants and children older than 3 months of age: clinical practice guidelines by the Pediatric Infectious Diseases Society and the Infectious Diseases Society of America. *Clin Infect Dis* 2011;53:e25–e76.

Mitri RK, Brown SD, Zurakowski D, et al. Outcomes of primary image-guided drainage of parapneumonic effusions in children. *Pediatrics* 2002;110:e37–e43.

Montgomery M, Sigalet D. Air and liquid in the pleural space. In: Chernick V, Boat TF, Wilmott RW, et al., eds. *Kendig's Disorders of the Respiratory Tract in Children,* 7th ed. Philadelphia, PA: WB Saunders, 2006:368–387.

Vives M, Porcel JM, de Vera MV, et al. A study of Light's criteria and possible modifications for distinguishing exudative from transudative pleural effusions. *Chest* 1996;109:1503–1507.

Sarcoidosis

Fauroux B, Clement A. Paediatric sarcoidosis. *Paediatr Respir Rev* 2005;6:128–133.

Obstructive Sleep Apnea

Obstructive Sleep Apnea American Academy of Pediatrics, Section on Pediatric Pulmonology, Subcommittee on Obstructive Sleep Apnea Syndrome. Clinical practice guideline: diagnosis and management of childhood sleep apnea syndrome. *Pediatrics* 2002;109:704–712.

Iannuzzi MC, Rybicki BA, Teirstein AS. Sarcoidosis. *N Engl J Med* 2007;357:2153–2165.

Lumeng JC, Chervin RD. Epidemiology of pediatric obstructive sleep apnea. *Proc Am Thorac Soc* 2008;5:242–252.

Muzumdar H, Arens R. Diagnostic issues in pediatric obstructive sleep apnea. *Proc Am Thorac Soc* 2008;5:263–273.

Interstitial Lung Disease

Deutsch GH, Young LR, Deterding RR. Diffuse lung disease in young children: application of a novel classification scheme. *Am J Respir Crit Care Med* 2007;176:1120–1128.

Fan LL, Detering RR, Langston C. Pediatric interstitial lung disease revisited. *Pediatr Pulmonol* 2004;38:369–378.

Nicholson AG, Bush A. Classification of diffuse lung disease in infants: the reality of groups. *Am J Respir Crit Care Med* 2007;176: 1060–1061.

CHAPTER 108 ▪ RENAL AND ELECTROLYTE EMERGENCIES

REBEKAH A. BURNS, MD AND RON L. KAPLAN, MD

GOALS OF EMERGENCY CARE

Fluid imbalances, electrolyte abnormalities, and renal insufficiency are associated with a wide variety of conditions encountered in the pediatric ED. Severe derangements of electrolytes and renal function can lead to significant morbidity and mortality. Prompt recognition and appropriate management is necessary to ensure adequate circulating volume and prevent serious sequelae related to electrolyte and acid–base disturbances. Overly rapid correction of some electrolyte abnormalities may result in devastating consequences, so care must be taken in the management of these conditions. Patients with renal insufficiency may present with overall fluid overload but intravascular depletion, making fluid resuscitation challenging.

KEY POINTS

- Severe hypovolemia must be treated rapidly with intravenous boluses of isotonic saline.
- Once circulating volume is adequate, further treatment of hypovolemia will depend on the serum sodium.
- Overly rapid correction of hypo- or hypernatremia can lead to serious CNS complications.
- Treatment of severe hyperkalemia is aimed at stabilizing the myocardium to prevent arrhythmias and enhancing movement of potassium into the intracellular space.
- Metabolic acidosis is primarily treated by attempting to correct the underlying cause.
- Acute kidney injury may lead to severe fluid and electrolyte disturbances that require emergent intervention regardless of the underlying etiology.
- The management of many causes of acute kidney injury is supportive in nature.
- Nephrotic syndrome is often steroid responsive in children.
- Chronic kidney disease may go unrecognized prior to presentation to the emergency department.

RELATED CHAPTERS

Signs and Symptoms

- Abdominal Distension: Chapter 7
- Coma: Chapter 12
- Dehydration: Chapter 17
- Diarrhea: Chapter 18
- Edema: Chapter 20
- Hematuria: Chapter 32
- Hypertension: Chapter 33
- Pain: Abdomen: Chapter 48
- Pain: Back: Chapter 49
- Pain: Dysuria: Chapter 52
- Rash: Papulosquamous Eruptions: Chapter 65
- Respiratory Distress: Chapter 66
- Seizures: Chapter 67
- Urinary Frequency: Chapter 74
- Vomiting: Chapter 77
- Weakness: Chapter 78
- Weight Loss: Chapter 79
- Dermatologic Urgencies and Emergencies: Chapter 96

Medical, Surgical, and Trauma Emergencies

- Endocrine Emergencies: Chapter 97
- Gastrointestinal Emergencies: Chapter 99
- Hematologic Emergencies: Chapter 101
- Metabolic Emergencies: Chapter 103
- Rheumatologic Emergencies: Chapter 109
- Abdominal Trauma: Chapter 111
- Genitourinary Trauma: Chapter 116
- Genitourinary Emergencies: Chapter 127
- Transplantation Emergencies: Chapter 133

DEHYDRATION/HYPOVOLEMIA

CLINICAL PEARLS AND PITFALLS

- Oral rehydration is the treatment of choice for mild to moderate dehydration.
- In moderate to severe hypovolemia, isotonic crystalloid should be given intravenously in 20 mL per kg boluses until intravascular volume has been restored.
- Subsequent volume repletion strategies will be determined by serum sodium levels.

Current Evidence

Volume depletion occurs frequently in children and is a common finding in patients presenting to the emergency department. Hypovolemia refers to a decrease in the effective circulating volume, which can occur with salt and water loss or water loss alone. By definition, the term dehydration refers to water loss alone, but the terms hypovolemia and dehydration have been used interchangeably in the clinical literature. Children are at greater risk for hypovolemia than adults due to several factors: Gastroenteritis with significant volume loss occurs at a higher frequency in children; children have a higher surface area-to-volume ratio resulting in greater insensible losses; and children may be less able to access adequate fluids to replenish losses given their developmental limitations.

Goals of Treatment

Hypovolemia leads to a reduction in the effective circulating volume, which may compromise tissue and organ perfusion. Significant hypovolemia must be recognized and corrected rapidly in order to prevent hypoperfusion and ischemic end-organ damage and progression to hypovolemic shock, which is associated with significant morbidity and mortality. Fluid therapy is aimed at correcting existing abnormalities and maintaining normal volume and composition of body fluids. Hypovolemia may be associated with other electrolyte abnormalities or acid–base disturbances. Specific treatment will depend on associated abnormalities, particularly hyponatremia or hypernatremia.

Clinical Considerations

Clinical recognition. Concern for volume depletion should be raised in any patient presenting to the emergency department with a history of increased fluid losses or poor oral intake. Young children or children with developmental delay may also be at increased risk due to inability to communicate their needs and lack of access to fluid intake in response to thirst.

Triage considerations. Children with a history or appearance suggestive of hypovolemia should be assessed in a timely manner to evaluate their degree of hypovolemia and potential need for rapid intervention. While oral rehydration therapy may be appropriate for mild to moderate dehydration, children with severe hypovolemia require rapid resuscitation with intravenous isotonic crystalloid.

Clinical assessment. The initial assessment of a child with hypovolemia should include a medical history and thorough physical examination. A careful history should establish the cause of hypovolemia, duration of illness, approximate volume and composition of fluid taken in as well as urine output. Potential causes of increased insensible losses, such as fever and tachypnea, should be considered.

The physical assessment should include an accurate weight. A change in weight from a recent healthy baseline, if available, would provide the most accurate objective account of the degree of depletion. Assessment of intravascular volume should include the pulse quality and rate, blood pressure, hydration of mucous membranes, skin turgor and perfusion, mental status, and activity. Mild hypovolemia (3% to 5% volume loss) may be associated with minimal or absent clinical signs. Moderate hypovolemia (6% to 9% volume loss) will have clinical signs apparent, which may include tachycardia, orthostatic blood pressure changes, dry mucous membranes, and delayed capillary refill time. Several dehydration scores (Gorelick score, WHO score, and clinical dehydration score) have been proposed to aid in estimating degree of dehydration based on clinical findings, with mixed results. A systematic review of published data reported by Steiner et al. revealed that the most useful individual signs for predicting 5% hypovolemia in children were delayed capillary refill time, abnormal skin turgor, and abnormal respiratory pattern. A combination of examination signs provided the best predictive data. In the setting of severe dehydration (greater than or equal to 10% volume loss), evidence of shock may be apparent, with hypotension, poor peripheral perfusion with prolonged capillary refill time, cool or mottled extremities, lethargy, and rapid deep respirations. Severe hypovolemia requires immediate attention with aggressive isotonic fluid resuscitation (see Chapter 5 Shock).

Though laboratory assessment has been shown to be less useful than physical findings when predicting the degree of volume depletion, laboratory testing can identify associated electrolyte and acid–base abnormalities. Classification of the type of hypovolemia based upon the serum sodium may impact subsequent fluid therapy and monitoring. Solute is primarily composed of sodium salts in the extracellular fluid (ECF) and potassium salts in the intracellular fluid (ICF). The presenting serum sodium in the child with hypovolemia results from the loss of solute relative to water during the illness. Determinants of the serum sodium include the type of fluid lost, the composition of fluid provided prior to presentation, and the ability to excrete water during the illness.

Hyponatremic hypovolemia (serum sodium less than 135 mEq per L) reflects the net loss of solute in excess of water. Isonatremic hypovolemia (serum sodium 135 to 145 mEq per L) results when solute is lost in proportion to water, and hypernatremic hypovolemia (serum sodium greater than 145 mEq per L) reflects net loss of water in excess of solute.

Other biochemical abnormalities that may develop during hypovolemia include disorders of potassium homeostasis, acid–base abnormalities, and increased blood urea nitrogen and creatinine, reflecting a decline in glomerular filtration rate (GFR). Though hyperkalemia may result, hypokalemia is more commonly seen in children with gastroenteritis given the loss of potassium in diarrheal fluid and urine. Urine losses of potassium may be significant and driven by aldosterone. The effect of aldosterone is to conserve urinary sodium to maintain effective intravascular volume and promote potassium excretion.

Management. Initial management will depend on the severity of hypovolemia and presence of abnormalities of serum sodium, but the aims of treatment are to restore perfusion and maintain adequate volume in the face of ongoing losses. Oral therapy, when tolerated, is the preferred treatment of fluid and electrolyte losses in children with mild to moderate dehydration. In general, limitations to ORT include severe dehydration, altered mental status, possible surgical pathology that would mandate NPO status, abdominal ileus or disorders that limit intestinal absorption, severe and persistent vomiting, excessive stool losses, and severe electrolyte abnormalities.

Patients who have moderate or severe hypovolemia will have compromised effective circulating volume, and rapid volume resuscitation is required to restore perfusion and avoid tissue damage. Emergent intravenous fluid therapy should be provided with a rapid infusion of 20 mL per kg of isotonic crystalloid. 0.9% sodium chloride (NS) is used most frequently, but lactated Ringer (LR) solution may be appropriate as well. Patients with severe hypovolemia should receive their first bolus over 20 minutes by pressure bag or push–pull technique, and may require up to 60 mL per kg in the first hour of resuscitation (see Chapter 5 Shock). There is currently no evidence that addition of dextrose to the crystalloid provides any significant clinical benefit without evidence of hypoglycemia. The child should be reassessed during and at completion of the intravenous bolus in order to determine if additional bolus therapy is indicated. Crystalloid boluses should be repeated until adequate perfusion has been restored. Intraosseous

TABLE 108.1

WEIGHT-BASED DAILY MAINTENANCE FLUID FOR CHILDREN

Body weight (kg)	Daily fluid requirements
3.5–10 kg	100 mL/kg/day
11–20 kg	1,000 mL + 50 mL/kg (for each kg >10), maximum 1,500 mL/day
>20 kg	1,500 mL + 20 mL/kg (for each kg >20), typical maximum 2,400 mL/day

TABLE 108.2

ESTIMATED DEFICITS AND INTRAVENOUS THERAPY: 10-kg CHILD WITH 10% HYPOVOLEMIA AND SERUM SODIUM 140 mEq/L

Water and sodium (Na) deficits

Water deficit: 10 kg × 10% = 1 L

Na deficit: 1 L × 140 mEq/L = 140 mEq

Emergent fluid repletion with NS

20 mL/kg × 10 kg = 200 mL (200 mL water and ≈30 mEq sodium)

Ongoing repletion and maintenance requirements

Remaining water deficit: 1,000 mL − 200 mL = 800 mL

Daily maintenance water requirement: 100 mL/kg/day × 10 kg = 1,000 mL/day

800 mL + 1,000 mL = 1,800 mL/24 hrs = 75 mL/hr

Remaining Na deficit: 140 mEq − 30 mEq = 110 mEq

Maintenance sodium requirement: 3 mEq/100 mL water × 1,000 mL/day = 30 mEq/day

110 mEq + 30 mEq = 140 mEq/24 hrs

140 mEq/1,800 mL ≈ 0.45% sodium chloride (½ NS)

Maintenance potassium requirement: 3 mEq/100 mL water × 1,000 mL/day = 30 mEq/day

30 mEq/1,800 mL ≈ 15–20 mEq/L

Intravenous fluid based upon deficit calculations:

D5% ½ NS with 20 mEq/L KCl at 75 mL/hr

Ongoing losses

Extrarenal losses should be replaced mL-for-mL if volumes are significant.

The sodium content of the fluid lost should be estimated or measured in order to select the appropriate replacement fluid.

administration of volume replacement is an appropriate alternative if intravenous access is not available. Currently, there are inadequate data to support the use of colloid-containing solutions during resuscitation in the general population. However, if a patient with decreased oncotic pressure due to an illness such as nephrotic syndrome or cirrhosis presents with hypovolemia, he may benefit from infusion of a colloid solution such as 5% albumin when serum albumin level is less than 2.0 to 2.5 g per dL.

Once circulating volume has been adequately restored, the second phase of fluid therapy corrects persistent deficits, replaces ongoing losses, and provides maintenance fluids. The maintenance requirements for fluid in children are outlined in Table 108.1. Though common practice has been to provide relatively hypotonic maintenance fluids (D5 ¼ NS or D5 ½ NS) based upon deficit calculations and maintenance requirements, recent reports have highlighted the potential risks of acquired hyponatremia in some hospitalized patients receiving hypotonic fluids (especially in the setting on substantial ongoing losses). Some have proposed that dextrose-containing isotonic fluid be continued in the ongoing repletion and maintenance phase of therapy with periodic assessment of serum Na to determine if further adjustment in fluid composition is warranted. If isotonic fluid is used for maintenance therapy, the risks of sodium excess, inadequate free-water provision during ongoing hypotonic losses, and hypernatremia must be considered. Currently there are inadequate data to support the routine use of isotonic solutions for ongoing fluid repletion and maintenance therapy in hypovolemia. Further studies are needed to compare the efficacy and safety of differing fluid regimens.

Examples of the treatment of isonatremic, hyponatremic, and hypernatremic hypovolemia are provided in Tables 108.2 through 108.4. In all cases, the fluid of choice for the initial emergent phase of volume resuscitation is isotonic saline. In most cases, the plan for replacement usually does not need to be exact as the kidneys will correct the electrolytes once well perfused and additionally enteral feeding is often initiated.

Isonatremic hypovolemia. Table 108.2 outlines the estimated deficits and therapeutic approach to a 10-kg child with isotonic hypovolemia. In this example, the isotonic deficit is corrected by an initial bolus of isotonic saline followed by ongoing repletion. The traditional approach of deficit calculation and therapy is outlined. Replacement of ongoing extrarenal losses should be provided if the volume of losses is significant. Repeated assessment of the serum sodium may be indicated on the basis of losses and duration of intravenous therapy.

Hyponatremic hypovolemia. Children with mild to moderate hyponatremia should be provided isotonic or near-isotonic fluids to both complete the repletion phase and continue the maintenance phase of intravenous fluid therapy. Providing hypotonic fluid in the setting of persistent decreased intravascular volume and acute illness with osmotic and nonosmotic stimuli for ADH secretion may perpetuate or worsen hyponatremia. Isotonic saline will correct the volume depletion and raise the serum sodium concurrently. The therapy of asymptomatic hyponatremia requires gradual correction of the serum sodium with a target increase of less than 10 to 12 mEq/L/day.

Table 108.3 estimates the sodium and water deficits and outlines a plan for fluid management of a child with hyponatremic hypovolemia and serum sodium of 125 mEq per L. The sodium deficit is estimated by the following equation using the serum sodium concentration and estimates of total body water (TBW):

$$\text{Na deficit} = [\text{TBW(n)} \times 140\ \text{mEq/L}] - [\text{TBW(c)} \times \text{serum Na}]$$

In this calculation, TBW(n) is the estimated normal TBW, TBW(c) is the estimated current TBW, and serum sodium is the serum sodium concentration. The normal TBW in term neonates, toddlers, and older or pubertal children is approximately 75% to 80%, 65% to 70%, and 60% of body weight, respectively.

As in the previous example, circulating volume is restored with isotonic saline, and deficits are replaced over the next 24 to 48 hours. From a practical standpoint, maintenance therapy may begin with D5 NS at one-and-a-half times maintenance, and sodium concentration of subsequent fluids adjusted based on response. Care must be taken to avoid overly rapid correction

TABLE 108.3

ESTIMATED DEFICITS AND INTRAVENOUS THERAPY: 10-kg CHILD WITH 10% HYPOVOLEMIA AND SERUM SODIUM 125 mEq/L

Water and sodium deficits

Water deficit: 10 kg × 10% = 1 L

Sodium deficit: [TBW(n) × 140 mEq/L] – [TBW(c) × 125 mEq/L]

TBW(n) = 10 kg × 65% = 6.5 L

TBW(c) = TBW(n) – water deficit = 6.5 L – 1 L = 5.5 L

Sodium deficit: (6.5 L × 140 mEq/L) – (5.5 L × 125 mEq/L) ≈ 220 mEq

Emergent fluid repletion with NS

20 mL/kg × 10 kg = 200 mL (200 mL water and ≈30 mEq sodium)

Ongoing repletion and maintenance requirements

Remaining water deficit: 1,000 mL – 200 mL = 800 mL

Daily maintenance water requirement: 100 mL/kg/day × 10 kg = 1,000 mL/day

800 mL + 1,000 mL = 1,800 mL/24 hrs = 75 mL/hr

Remaining sodium deficit: 220 mEq – 30 mEq = 190 mEq

Maintenance sodium requirement: 3 mEq/100 mL water × 1,000 mL/day = 30 mEq/day

190 mEq + 30 mEq = 220 mEq

220 mEq/1,800 mL ≈ 120 mEq/L

Maintenance potassium requirement: 3 mEq/100 mL water × 1,000 mL/day = 30 mEq/day

30 mEq/1,800 mL ≈ 15–20 mEq/L KCl

Intravenous fluid based upon deficit calculations:

D5% with 120 mEq/L NaCl and 20 mEq/L KCl at 75 mL/hr

Given the availability of standard solutions in emergency departments, D5% NS *with added potassium* could be provided for the initial half of the total volume and completed with D5% ½ NS *with added potassium.*

Ongoing losses

Extrarenal losses should be replaced mL-for-mL if volumes are significant.

The sodium content of the fluid lost should be estimated or measured in order to select the appropriate replacement fluid.

TABLE 108.4

ESTIMATED DEFICITS AND INTRAVENOUS THERAPY: 10-kg CHILD WITH 10% HYPOVOLEMIA AND SERUM SODIUM 155 mEq/L

Water and sodium deficits

Total water deficit: 10 kg × 10% = 1 L

TBW(c) = TBW(n) – 1 L = (10 kg × 65%) – 1 L = 5.5 L

Free-water deficit: TBW(c)[(155/140) – 1] = 5.5[(155/140) – 1] = 0.59 L

Isotonic deficit = total water deficit – free-water deficit = 0.41 L

Sodium deficit: 0.41 L × 140 mEq/L ≈ 60 mEq

Emergent fluid repletion with NS

20 mL/kg × 10 kg = 200 mL (200 mL water and ~30 mEq sodium)

Ongoing repletion and maintenance requirements

Remaining total water deficit: 1,000 mL – 200 mL = 800 mL, plan to replace over 36–48 hrs or 400 mL/day × 2 days

Daily maintenance water requirement: 100 mL/kg/day × 10 kg = 1,000 mL/day

1,000 mL + 400 mL = 1,400/24 hrs or ≈60 mL/hr

Remaining sodium deficit: 60 mEq – 30 mEq = 30 mEq

Maintenance sodium requirement: 3 mEq/100 mL water × 1,000 mL/day = 30 mEq/day

Total sodium requirement: 30 mEq + 30 mEq = 60 mEq

60 mEq/1,400 mL or ≈0.225% sodium chloride

Maintenance potassium requirement: 3 mEq/100 mL water × 1,000 mL/day = 30 mEq/day

30 mEq/1,400 mL ≈ 20 mEq/L KCl

D5% ¼ NS with 20 mEq/L KCl at 60 mL/hr for ~36–48 hrs

Ongoing losses

Extrarenal losses should be replaced mL-for-mL if volumes are significant.

The sodium content of the fluid lost should be estimated or measured in order to select the appropriate replacement fluid.

of the serum sodium to prevent severe central nervous system (CNS) sequelae associated with osmotic demyelination. The sodium level should be rechecked 2 hours after initiation of treatment and at regular intervals thereafter to monitor the rate of correction. If the rate of rise of the serum sodium is greater than targeted (10 to 12 mEq/L/day), the concentration of sodium in the intravenous fluids should be reduced. The therapy of severe hyponatremia or symptomatic hyponatremia is discussed further in the section "Hyponatremia."

Hypernatremic hypovolemia. In children who present with hypernatremic hypovolemia, the total fluid deficit is composed of both a free-water deficit and an isotonic deficit. A pure water deficit is consistent with dehydration. Hyperosmolality initially promotes water movement out of the cells, including brain cells. Over several days, idiogenic osmoles are generated within the brain cells, prompting water movement into the intracellular space, restoring normal brain volume. Once cerebral adaptation has occurred, rapid correction of the serum sodium can result in cerebral edema and severe neurologic consequence. The goal of therapy in children with a serum sodium concentration above 150 mEq per L is to correct the hypernatremia at a rate of less than 10 to 12 mEq per L in 24 hours. The total fluid deficit can be inferred by the estimated weight loss. Calculation of the free-water deficit is based upon the serum sodium and estimated current body water:

$$\text{Free water deficit} = \text{TBW(c)} \times [(\text{serum Na}/140) - 1]$$

The difference between the total fluid deficit and the free-water deficit is the estimated isotonic deficit. Table 108.4 estimates the sodium and water deficits and outlines a plan for fluid management of a child with hypernatremic hypovolemia and serum sodium of 155 mEq per L. After the patient has received the initial isotonic fluid bolus to emergently restore intravascular volume, subsequent therapy should correct the remaining isotonic deficit, free-water deficit, ongoing losses, and maintenance requirements. Depending on the acuity and severity of the process, the free-water deficit should be replaced gradually to allow judicious correction of the serum sodium at the desired rate. In general, D5 ¼ NS at one-and-a-half times maintenance would be expected to correct deficits over 36 to 48 hours. Given the uncertainty of any correction plan and the possibility of ongoing losses, the best approach is to measure the sodium frequently as it corrects and adjust fluid content and rate as indicated.

DISORDERS OF SODIUM HOMEOSTASIS

Goals of Treatment

Hyponatremia (serum sodium less than 135 mEq per L) and hypernatremia (serum sodium greater than 150 mEq per L) are both associated with severe sequelae, and overly aggressive treatment of each can cause significant CNS complications. Treatment corrects the sodium abnormalities using estimated volume status and total body sodium content. Severe cases need to be treated at an appropriate rate in order to prevent CNS complications.

CLINICAL PEARLS AND PITFALLS

- Hyponatremia may occur secondary to increased ADH activity or in patients with hypovolemia managed with excess free water.
- Hypernatremia is usually due to excessive water loss relative to sodium and is associated with gastrointestinal illness or systemic infection.
- Hypernatremia may occur in infants due to inadequate breast-feeding or increased sodium load from improperly mixed formula.
- Clinical manifestations of hypo- or hypernatremia depend on the severity and rate of development.
- Overly rapid correction of hypo- or hypernatremia may lead to severe CNS sequelae.

Hyponatremia

When approaching a patient with hyponatremia, it is necessary to estimate the patient's total body sodium and water based on history and physical examination. There are numerous causes of hyponatremia (Table 108.5) associated with normal or increased total body sodium, including states of impaired water excretion such as renal failure and the syndrome of inappropriate antidiuretic hormone (SIADH) secretion. Release of ADH is associated with a number of clinical conditions, including hypovolemia, fever, CNS trauma, infections and tumors, pulmonary infections, hypothyroidism, and cortisol deficiency. Certain medications, including some chemotherapeutic agents and antiepileptic agents, can be associated with inappropriate ADH release. It is critical to assess for underlying causes associated with increased total body sodium and water, as in the edema-forming states. In these clinical circumstances, providing supplemental sodium would aggravate the state of volume excess.

Appropriate evaluation to determine the cause of hyponatremia begins with a thorough physical examination in order to estimate volume status. History may reveal obvious sources of sodium loss or raise the concern for water intoxication. Laboratory tests should include serum electrolytes, osmolality, and assessment of renal function. Concomitant urine studies should include osmolality, urine sodium, and urinalysis. In children with hyponatremia and concentrated urine, the urine sodium may distinguish between states of decreased effective circulating volume (urine sodium <25 mEq per L) and euvolemic hyponatremia, such as the SIADH (urine sodium >40 mEq per L).

Clinical manifestations. The symptoms of hyponatremia are primarily neurologic and due to the development of cerebral edema. The symptoms mirror the severity of cerebral edema, which in turn is related to the degree of hyponatremia and the acuity of the process. The mechanisms of cellular adaptation include movement of intracellular electrolytes to the extracellular space, which can occur within minutes. Over hours to days, organic solutes move to the extracellular space. Given the ability for cerebral adaptation, the degree of cerebral edema and neurologic symptoms are less severe in chronic hyponatremia. Early neurologic symptoms include nausea and malaise, and may be seen when the serum sodium concentration falls below 125 mEq per L. With progressive derangement of cerebral cell volume, symptoms of headache, altered mental status, lethargy, ataxia, and psychosis may ensue. Signs of severe cerebral edema include seizures, coma, and respiratory depression.

Management. For children with hyponatremia associated with hypovolemia, isotonic solutions should be provided to restore intravascular volume. Children with symptomatic hyponatremia require urgent treatment to avoid progressive neurologic complications. Symptoms are more likely to develop if hyponatremia evolves rapidly, as water will move along an osmotic gradient from the extracellular space to the

TABLE 108.5

CAUSES OF HYPONATREMIA BASED UPON TOTAL BODY SODIUM CONTENT

Low total body sodium	Normal total body sodium	High total body sodium
Diarrhea	SIADH	Congestive heart failure
Vomiting	Adrenal insufficiency	Nephrotic syndrome
Ostomy losses	Hypothyroidism	Liver failure (cirrhosis)
Bleeding	Acute renal failure	Multiorgan dysfunction
Diuretic use	Water intoxication	
Mineralocorticoid deficiency	Pseudohyponatremia	
Salt-wasting renal disease		
Cystic fibrosis		
Marathon running		

TABLE 108.6

CAUSES OF HYPERNATREMIA BASED UPON TOTAL BODY SODIUM CONTENT

Low total body sodium	Normal total body sodium	High total body sodium
Diarrhea	Increased insensible losses	Salt poisoning
Vomiting	Fever	Inappropriately mixed formula
Ostomy losses	Prematurity	Salt water drowning
Osmotic diuresis	Phototherapy	$NaHCO_3$ given with CPR
Immature renal conservation (prematurity)	Radiant warmers	
	Tachypnea	
	Nephrogenic DI	
	Central DI	

DI, diabetes insipidus; $NaHCO_3$, sodium bicarbonate; CPR, cardiopulmonary resuscitation.

intracellular space. Given the effect of cell volume regulatory mechanisms, an important goal is to control the rate of rise in serum sodium to prevent rapid fluid shifts into the extracellular space and avoid the development of osmotic demyelination. The general recommendation for a child with severe hyponatremia is to increase the serum sodium no more rapidly than 12 mEq per L in the first 24 hours or an average of 0.5 mEq/L/hr. An exception to this recommendation would be symptomatic hyponatremia and evolving cerebral edema and seizures. Symptomatic hyponatremia calls for a more aggressive initial correction of the serum sodium of approximately 2 mEq/L/hr for 2 to 3 hours, which should result in clinical improvement. This can be achieved with the administration of hypertonic 3% saline (513 mEq per L of sodium). In general, 3 mL per kg of 3% saline would be expected to raise serum sodium by approximately 3 mEq per L. A practical approach is to administer doses of 3 mL per kg (maximum dose 100 mL) until seizures stop. After the initial correction is achieved, the goal for the daily correction remains approximately 12 mEq per L in the first 24 hours (including the initial emergent correction). Frequent assessment of serum sodium is necessary to avoid rapid correction, which may lead to the osmotic demyelination syndrome.

Patients who have asymptomatic hyponatremia and euvolemia do not require urgent intervention. The care of these patients should be carefully planned and based upon the underlying diagnosis with the aim of gradual correction. If hyponatremia is associated with an edema-forming state, providing supplemental sodium will worsen the state volume excess. The goal of therapy would be to achieve negative water balance in excess of negative sodium balance. To achieve this effectively, the underlying pathophysiology must be considered, although initial water restriction is generally indicated. Sodium restriction and diuretic therapy may also be warranted. The treatment of SIADH begins with water restriction, though this may be insufficient. Some cases of SIADH require the administration of salt supplements and loop diuretics to achieve the desired negative water balance, as guided by consultation with a pediatric nephrologist.

Hypernatremia

Hypernatremia can result from an increase in the total body solutes, a decrease in body water, or a reduction of body water relatively greater than a concurrent reduction in total body solutes. Protective mechanisms to prevent the development of hypernatremia include the stimulation of thirst and the ability to excrete concentrated urine, thereby minimizing free-water loss. For these mechanisms to be effective, there must be adequate access to and the ability to retain free water. Given the potential for limited access to water, infants and children with significant developmental delay are predisposed to hypernatremic dehydration. The causes of hypernatremia based on total body sodium are outlined in Table 108.6. Hypernatremia due to isolated water deficit is termed dehydration. If both salt and water deficits are present, this condition is termed hypovolemia.

Diarrhea is a common cause of hypernatremia in the acute care setting. Although the degree of sodium deficit may vary, generally children who present for care have true hypovolemia. Breast-fed infants may be at increased risk of hypernatremia due to inadequate intake. Hypernatremia due to salt excess is rare but it can occur with the improper mixing of infant formulas or iatrogenic administration of a salt load. The latter can result after sodium bicarbonate infusion during cardiopulmonary resuscitation or during therapy of refractory metabolic acidosis. Hypernatremia secondary to nearly pure water loss may develop if replacement of insensible water loss from the skin and respiratory tract is inadequate. Central diabetes insipidus is due to insufficient release of ADH from the hypothalamus, and nephrogenic diabetes insipidus is due to a renal resistance to the effect of ADH. Most children affected with these disorders have normal thirst and free access to water and are able to maintain acceptable water balance. However, infants who do not have free access to water and children with intercurrent illness precluding adequate intake of free water are at risk for the development of hypernatremic dehydration.

The cause of hypernatremia is usually evident from the presenting history. Feeding history in breast-fed infants may reveal inadequate intake. In formula-fed infants, an accurate account of formula preparation should be pursued to evaluate for inappropriate mixing, which would result in increased renal osmotic load. Inquiries of urine volume should also be made, as the production of significant urine in a child who presents with apparent hypernatremic dehydration suggests diabetes insipidus. The physical examination should assess weight, perfusion, and mental status. During hypernatremic hypovolemia, water moves from the intracellular to the extracellular space. Given the relative preservation of the extracellular volume, the objective signs of volume depletion may develop later in the patient's course of illness. Laboratory studies should include serum electrolytes, serum osmolality, BUN, and renal serum creatinine. If the underlying diagnosis remains in question, urine studies may be informative. Urine osmolality should be compared to serum osmolality and would be elevated if renal concentrating mechanisms are intact. If the urine osmolality is inappropriately low when compared to the serum osmolality, then central or nephrogenic diabetes insipidus should be considered. The urine sodium concentration may also assist diagnosis. During hypernatremic hypovolemia, the urine sodium is generally less than 25 mEq per L due to the effect of aldosterone to maintain perfusion. If hypernatremia is due to salt excess, the appropriate renal response is to excrete sodium, and the urine sodium concentration would be elevated.

Clinical manifestations. Similar to hyponatremia, the clinical manifestations of hypernatremia are primarily neurologic. The rise in the plasma osmolality causes water movement out of the brain. The decrease in brain volume may lead to the rupture of the blood vessels contained in the membranes that tether the brain to the overlying skull and elsewhere. Early clinical manifestations can include lethargy, weakness, fever, and irritability. More severe manifestations include seizures and coma. Symptoms are more likely if the disturbance is acute and rapid. If hypernatremia evolves more slowly, there is cerebral adaptation to protect brain cell volume. Adaptive mechanisms include movement of cerebrospinal fluid into the brain, uptake of sodium and potassium into the cells, followed by intracellular accumulation of osmolytes.

Management. During sustained hypernatremia, cerebral adaptation occurs over several days to restore brain cell volume. Rapid correction of the serum sodium after cerebral adaptation occurs will result in osmotic movement of water into the brain and cerebral edema. Data suggest that the plasma sodium concentration should be lowered by less than 0.5 mEq/L/hr and no more than 12 mEq/L/day. In children with hypernatremia due to salt loading, treatment should facilitate renal excretion of sodium. This is typically achieved with salt restriction and free water and may be facilitated with diuretics. If intravenous fluids are required, the sodium plus potassium concentration of the fluid provided should be less than the sum of these electrolytes in the urine, and the fluid should be given at a rate sufficient to achieve positive water balance. Adequate intravascular volume should be assured to allow renal excretion of sodium. The therapy of children with hypernatremic hypovolemia (sodium and water deficit) was previously reviewed. In summary, children with clinical signs of decreased effective circulating volume should be provided with isotonic saline to restore perfusion. Once intravascular volume is restored, hypotonic fluids should continue to allow judicious restoration of the estimated free-water deficit, with close monitoring to avoid overly rapid correction.

DISORDERS OF POTASSIUM HOMEOSTASIS

Goals of Treatment

Potassium is the most abundant intracellular cation in the body with only approximately 2% of total body stores present in the extracellular space. Abnormalities of serum potassium are associated with abnormal neuromuscular function and risk of severe cardiac sequelae, especially with hyperkalemia. Treatment is aimed at preventing emergent cardiac complications and restoring normal serum potassium levels.

CLINICAL PEARLS AND PITFALLS

- Total body potassium depletion is present in patients with diabetic ketoacidosis (DKA) despite having normal or elevated serum potassium levels.
- Hyperkalemia should be confirmed to rule out pseudohyperkalemia due to a hemolyzed sample.
- Severe hyperkalemia may lead to cardiac arrhythmias, and initial treatment is aimed at stabilizing the myocardium with IV calcium.
- Subsequent treatment of hyperkalemia involves enhancing intracellular movement of potassium, followed by removal of excess potassium from the body.

Hypokalemia

Hypokalemia is defined as a measured serum potassium concentration below 3.5 mEq per L. Hypokalemia may result from total body deficit, transcellular shift of potassium to the intracellular space, or a combination of both processes. There are numerous causes of hypokalemia including renal loss, extrarenal loss, and increased cellular uptake, which are outlined in Table 108.7. The common causes of hypokalemia seen in pediatric emergency departments are those due to gastrointestinal loss, diuretic use, and DKA. Metabolic alkalosis will also lead to hypokalemia due to transcellular shift of potassium to the intracellular space. For every 0.1 U rise in blood pH, serum potassium would be expected to decrease by approximately 0.4 to 0.6 mEq per L.

TABLE 108.7

CAUSES OF HYPOKALEMIA

Causes
Decreased potassium intake
Increased renal excretion
Diuretics
Metabolic alkalosis (chloride deficient)
Diabetic ketoacidosis
Increased mineralocorticoid effect
Nonreabsorbable anions
Renal tubular acidosis (type 1 and type 2)
Bartter syndrome
Gitelman syndrome
Magnesium depletion
Increased gastrointestinal losses
Diarrhea
Laxatives
Ostomy losses
Increased cellular uptake (redistributive)
Acute alkalosis
Insulin therapy
Elevated β-adrenergic activity
Increase in bone marrow cell production
Hypokalemic periodic paralysis

Potassium homeostasis is complex and dynamic in the setting of DKA (see Chapter 97 Endocrine Emergencies). Urinary losses of potassium are high, so patients with DKA generally have total body potassium depletion at presentation. However, the combination of insulin deficiency, hyperosmolality, and acidosis may result in normal or elevated serum potassium at presentation. Hypokalemia in a child who presents with DKA would suggest significant potassium depletion and need for supplementation with close monitoring.

The cause of hypokalemia may be inferred after a careful history is obtained. This should include a thorough account of medications taken, such as diuretics, laxatives, and beta agonists. The laboratory assessment of hypokalemia should include serum electrolytes, magnesium, calcium, serum bicarbonate, renal function, and glucose. In addition to urinalysis and urine pH, urine electrolytes and osmolality should be submitted to assess the renal response to hypokalemia.

Clinical manifestations. The clinical manifestations of hypokalemia are generally proportionate to the severity and duration of the disorder and result from hyperpolarization of the cell membrane. Unless the serum potassium falls rapidly or is associated with digitalis use, symptoms are typically not apparent until the serum level is below 2.5 mEq per L. Symptoms may also vary dependent on the concentration of other ions, including calcium, magnesium, and hydrogen. Clinically relevant signs and symptoms of hypokalemia relate to abnormal neuromuscular function and cardiovascular effects, and monitoring of muscle strength and electrocardiogram (ECG) are indicated to assess the functional consequences of hypokalemia. Neuromuscular dysfunction typically manifests as skeletal muscle weakness in an ascending pattern with worsening hypokalemia. Lower extremity muscles are initially affected with progression to the trunk and upper extremities. Respiratory weakness may develop and lead to respiratory failure. Smooth muscle dysfunction can lead to nausea, vomiting, constipation, and voiding dysfunction with urinary retention. Significant hypokalemia produces characteristic changes on the ECG. As the serum potassium drops, T-wave amplitude declines, U waves develop, and ST segment depression may result. With more profound hypokalemia the QRS complex may widen and the PR and QT intervals may prolong. Supraventricular and ventricular dysrhythmias may develop, the likelihood being greater for patients taking digitalis and in patients with congestive heart failure and coronary ischemia. Hypokalemia may also lead to an impaired ability to concentrate urine, an acquired form of nephrogenic diabetes insipidus.

Management. The therapeutic approach to hypokalemia will depend on severity, acuity, associated clinical signs, and underlying conditions. In general, potassium replacement is indicated when there has been potassium loss. If hypokalemia is redistributive in nature but associated with either severely depressed levels or clinical signs, supplementation may be required. However, supplementation during a redistributive process should proceed with close monitoring given the risk of rebound hyperkalemia. When potassium loss is accompanied by acid–base disturbance, a redistribution effect should be factored when losses are estimated. Magnesium supplementation is indicated in hypokalemia associated with hypomagnesemia. In all cases of significant hypokalemia, monitoring for ECG changes and muscle strength is imperative, and if abnormalities are present, immediate replacement is warranted.

The choice of oral or intravenous replacement will depend on the severity of the disorder and the ability to tolerate enteral salts. If the child is clinically well, oral therapy is preferable and can be provided two to four times per day as potassium chloride. Dosing may start at 2 to 5 mEq/kg/day and be adjusted on the basis of serial laboratory assessment. If there is concurrent metabolic acidosis, potassium citrate or bicarbonate can be provided. If the child is unable to take oral medications or is symptomatic, intravenous potassium should be provided. If the child is not symptomatic, potassium can be added to the maintenance fluids. If intermittent infusion is indicated, this can begin with an intravenous dose of 0.5 to 1 mEq per kg (typical maximum 30 to 40 mEq per dose). Potassium chloride is typically used, but potassium phosphate may be used in the treatment of DKA or documented severe hypophosphatemia. Potassium acetate or its equivalent may be used if there is metabolic acidosis. The infusion rate for clinically stable patients should provide 0.25 mEq/kg/hr, though emergent conditions may warrant the maximal rate of 0.5 to 1 mEq/kg/hr (maximum 15 to 40 mEq per hour depending on local policy) with continuous ECG monitoring.

Hyperkalemia

Hyperkalemia is typically defined as serum potassium concentration exceeding 6 mEq per L in neonates or 5.5 mEq per L in children or adults. Serum potassium concentration is determined by the interplay of potassium intake, distribution between the intracellular and extracellular space, and renal excretion. Hyperkalemia can therefore result from excessive load, transcellular shift, decreased renal excretion, or a combination of these factors.

If hyperkalemia develops, both endogenous and exogenous sources of potassium should be considered. Potential sources of exogenous potassium include large volume packed red blood cell transfusion, medicines with significant potassium content, and potassium salt infusions. Given improvements in blood bank procedure, hyperkalemia is less common with transfusion of red cells. Endogenous sources of potassium may result from tissue damage, including burns, trauma, rhabdomyolysis, hemolysis, tumor lysis, and gastrointestinal bleeding with enteral reabsorption. Clinical scenarios associated with extracellular shift include metabolic acidosis, hyperosmolarity, insulin deficiency, and the use of β-adrenergic receptor antagonists. Reduced renal excretion of potassium may occur in acute or chronic renal insufficiency, hypovolemia, mineralocorticoid deficiency, inherited or acquired renal tubulopathy, and due to the use of certain medications (Table 108.8).

TABLE 108.8

MEDICATIONS ASSOCIATED WITH HYPERKALEMIA

NSAIDs
ACE inhibitors
Angiotensin II receptor blockers
Amiloride
Spironolactone
Eplerenone
Tacrolimus
Cyclosporine
Propranolol
Digitalis

Evaluation begins with a thorough history with specific inquiries regarding injuries, muscle pain, history of renal disease, and medications taken. Serum potassium should be repeated to rule out pseudohyperkalemia, which results from a hemolyzed specimen due to difficulties in obtaining the specimen. Serum sodium, chloride, calcium, phosphorus, bicarbonate levels and measures of renal function should also be obtained. Serum creatinine kinase should be submitted if there is suspicion for rhabdomyolysis. A CBC should be obtained if there is possibility of hemolysis. Urine electrolytes and osmolality should be obtained. An ECG should be obtained to monitor for cardiac effect.

Clinical manifestations. The clinical features associated with hyperkalemia are a consequence of altered cellular transmembrane potassium gradient, which reduces the resting membrane potential. Initially this increases membrane excitability, which is followed by a sustained reduction in excitability. Unless the rise is rapid, symptoms or signs generally do not become apparent until the serum potassium concentration exceeds 7 mEq per L. Clinical features predominantly involve cardiac conduction and neuromuscular disturbance. Cardiac dysrhythmias are the most serious consequence, and toxicity is exacerbated by a rapid rise in potassium concentration, acidosis, hyponatremia, and hypocalcemia. Early ECG changes include narrow, peaked T waves with shortened QT interval, which is followed by progressive lengthening of the PR interval and widening of the QRS complex. There may be loss of P-wave amplitude and eventual "sine wave" pattern when the QRS merges with the T wave. This is typically followed by ventricular fibrillation or standstill. Neuromuscular effects are rarely evident at potassium concentrations less than 8 mEq per L and include paresthesias, skeletal muscle weakness, and ascending flaccid paralysis. Respiratory muscles are typically spared.

Management. Treatment of hyperkalemia includes antagonizing the cell membrane effects of hyperkalemia, shifting potassium to the intracellular space, and removing potassium from the body (Table 108.9). The urgency of care should be based upon the degree of hyperkalemia and evidence of cardiac or neuromuscular effect. Should there be ECG changes consistent with hyperkalemia, the patient should be placed on cardiac monitor and intravenous calcium should be provided to stabilize cardiac membranes. Calcium administration is indicated only in instances of significant ECG changes, such as widening of the QRS or loss of the P wave but is not indicated in isolated peaked T waves. The effect of calcium is nearly immediate but also transient and should be coupled with other measures to shift potassium to the intracellular space and remove potassium from the body. Calcium gluconate (10% solution) 50 to 100 mg per kg IV or calcium chloride (10% solution) 20 mg per kg IV is infused over 2 to 5 minutes (never pushed rapidly) with continuous cardiac monitoring. The usual adult dose of calcium gluconate is 1,000 mg and calcium chloride is 500 to 1,000 mg. Calcium is irritating to veins and can result in tissue necrosis; therefore, central vein access is preferable for both the gluconate and chloride salts and strongly recommended if calcium chloride is infused (however, do not delay calcium administration via a peripheral vein in the setting of life-threatening hyperkalemia). In patients taking digitalis, an immediate cardiac consultation should be obtained prior to administration, if possible, as calcium therapy may precipitate other dysrhythmias.

Several therapies are aimed at shifting potassium into the intracellular space and are outlined in Table 108.6. Insulin drives movement of potassium into the cell. This can be achieved by administering a combination of 0.1 units per kg of regular insulin and 0.5 g per kg of dextrose. The time of onset is 15 to 30 minutes, peak effect at approximately 60 minutes, and duration of several hours. Providing sodium bicarbonate raises the systemic pH and promotes hydrogen movement out of the cells accompanied by potassium movement into the cells. This is most effective in patients with metabolic acidosis. In the absence of acidosis, sodium bicarbonate is not routinely recommended because it is less likely to be effective, and may lead to other complications. The onset of the effect of sodium bicarbonate is within 15 to 30 minutes and persists for several hours. β_2-Adrenergic agonists promote transcellular shift of potassium, so nebulized albuterol may provide further benefit. It is particularly useful if intravenous access is not available. Recommended doses of albuterol are 0.4 mg for neonates, 2.5 mg for infants and children under 25 kg, 5 mg for children

TABLE 108.9

THERAPIES FOR HYPERKALEMIA

Intravenous calcium to stabilize cardiac membrane
Calcium gluconate 10% solution, 50–100 mg/kg (0.5–1 mL/kg); typical adult dose 1,000 mg, max 2,000–3,000 mg
Infuse over 2–5 min, central access is preferred, may repeat in 10 min if needed
Patient must be on cardiac monitor
Effect is immediate in onset though transient (~30 min)
Measures to redistribute potassium into the intracellular space
Insulin and dextrose:
Give dextrose 0.5 g/kg and provide insulin 0.1 U/g of dextrose
Monitor blood glucose
Time to onset is ~15–30 min, duration is 2–6 hrs
β_2-agonists:
2.5–5 mg nebulized albuterol
Time to onset is 20–30 min, duration 2–4 hrs
Sodium bicarbonate:
1–2 mEq/kg IV over 5–15 min
Minimal effect if the child is not acidemic
Time to onset ~15–30 min, duration ~2 hrs
Measures to remove potassium from the body
Cation exchange resins:
Sodium polystyrene sulfonate 1 g/kg orally or per rectum, may repeat dose after 4 hrs
Do not give retention enema with sorbitol
Do not give if within 1 wk of surgery (postoperative ileus)
Time to onset is 1–2 hrs
Loop diuretics:
1–2 mg/kg furosemide IV, higher doses may be required in renal insufficiency
To avoid hypovolemia, provide appropriate non–potassium-containing fluids
Time to onset 15–60 min
Dialysis:
To be employed if conservative measures fail after discussion with nephrology consultant

25 to 50 kg, and 10 mg for patients over 50 kg. Alternatively, albuterol may be given as 4 to 8 puffs with a metered dose inhaler with a spacer.

Though slower in onset than measures applied to shift potassium into the intracellular space, efforts to remove potassium are necessary in cases of total body potassium excess. Sodium polystyrene sulfonate (Kayexalate) is a commonly used ion exchange resin. Within the intestinal lumen, the resin takes up potassium in exchange for sodium. To a lesser extent, the resin will also exchange for calcium and magnesium, and therefore, electrolytes should be monitored with frequent or prolonged dosing. In the past, the resin has been administered with sorbitol to prevent associated constipation and fecal impaction, but this combination has been associated with colonic necrosis and perforation and is no longer recommended. The pediatric oral dose is 1 g per kg provided every 4 to 6 hours as necessary, with a maximum dose of 30 g. Laxatives such as polyethylene glycol 3350 or lactulose may be given to counteract the constipating effects of the polystyrene sulfonates. Kayexalate may be given rectally at the same dose every 2 to 6 hours, though the dose must be retained for 15 to 30 minutes to be effective. Kayexalate should not be provided to patients within 1 week of bowel surgery due to risk of intestinal necrosis. In patients with normal renal function, providing isotonic saline and loop diuretics may increase potassium excretion. Isotonic expansion may be particularly effective in patients who are hypovolemic with decreased effective renal perfusion. In cases of hypovolemia, diuretics should only be provided once volume status is restored to avoid prerenal insult. Thereafter, close monitoring of volume status will allow appropriate adjustment of fluid rate and diuretic dosing. In those patients with significantly impaired renal function, dialysis may be indicated. Hemodialysis provides more rapid clearance of potassium, though peritoneal dialysis may be more practical depending on the size of the child, center preference, and comorbidities such as cardiovascular instability or congenital heart disease.

DISORDERS OF CALCIUM HOMEOSTASIS

Goals of Treatment

Calcium is the most abundant cation in the body with approximately 99% present in bone. Of the small fraction in the ECF compartment, approximately half of the calcium is free or ionized, and it is this fraction that exerts physiologic effect and is under physiologic regulation. Of note, the fraction of calcium bound to plasma proteins is affected by the extracellular pH. Acidemia causes hydrogen ions to displace calcium from proteins and increases ionized calcium levels. Alkalemia will promote the opposite effect.

Calcium homeostasis is dependent on endocrine control of three primary organ systems: intestines, kidneys, and the skeletal system. The parathyroid gland allows for the rapid regulation of ionized calcium concentration. Low concentrations of ionized calcium stimulate parathyroid hormone (PTH) secretion. PTH will increase serum calcium levels through mobilization of calcium from the bone, increased calcium reabsorption in the distal renal tubule, and stimulation of the conversion of 25-hydroxyvitamin D to 1,25-dihydroxyvitamin D, the active metabolite of vitamin D. 1,25-Dihydroxyvitamin D promotes calcium and phosphorus absorption from the gastrointestinal tract and reabsorption from the renal tubules. Calcitonin is a hormone produced by the parafollicular cells of the thyroid when calcium levels are high. Calcitonin inhibits osteoclastic activity and promotes movement of calcium from the blood into the skeletal system.

Treatment of abnormalities of serum calcium will depend on the underlying cause, with the aim of restoring normal calcium levels and preventing associated manifestations which are primarily neuromuscular and cardiac.

CLINICAL PEARLS AND PITFALLS

- Serum calcium levels are regulated by PTH; a PTH level should be considered in the evaluation of abnormal serum calcium levels.
- IV calcium is indicated for the treatment of severe hypocalcemia and in patients with ECG changes or significant neuromuscular symptoms.
- If given too rapidly, IV calcium can precipitate bradycardia or asystole.
- The presence of acidosis or abnormalities of magnesium and phosphorus have specific implications regarding treatment of hypocalcemia.
- Hypercalcemia results from increased gastrointestinal absorption, enhanced bone resorption, or impaired renal excretion of calcium.
- Treatment of hypercalcemia primarily involves volume replacement and enhancing renal excretion with loop diuretics.

Hypocalcemia

Hypocalcemia has many causes, which include PTH deficiency or resistance, vitamin D deficiency or resistance, extravascular deposition, and abnormal magnesium metabolism (Table 108.10). Abnormal serum calcium should be confirmed by repeat measurement and if confirmed, ionized serum calcium should be measured. As approximately 90% of protein-bound calcium is bound to albumin, the serum albumin concentration should also be determined. For each 1 g per dL reduction in serum albumin, the total calcium concentration will be lowered by approximately 0.8 mg per dL. Hypoalbuminemia does not affect the ionized calcium concentration, which is under hormonal regulation. If available, previous calcium levels should be reviewed to determine if the patient is experiencing an acute or chronic process. Though results will not be available during an urgent or emergent assessment period, a serum PTH level must be performed in all patients with confirmed hypocalcemia. Measurement of serum phosphate, magnesium, and creatinine should also be performed. Hyperphosphatemia increases the risk for calcium phosphate precipitation in tissues and may lead to hypocalcemia. Magnesium is required for PTH release, and hypomagnesemia results in hyporesponsiveness to the effect of PTH in target organs. Hypocalcemia is common in renal failure and is due to phosphate retention and insufficient production of 1,25-dihydroxyvitamin D. As timely serum PTH levels may not be available for review, urine calcium, phosphate, and creatinine should be submitted to assess renal tubular handling, which may suggest the PTH effect. Vitamin D metabolites should be performed in selected patients if clinically indicated.

TABLE 108.10

CAUSES OF HYPOCALCEMIA

Causes
Precipitation or altered binding
Hyperphosphatemia
Metabolic alkalosis
Citrated products
Pancreatitis
Vitamin D deficiency
Nutritional
Malabsorption
Impaired synthesis
Hepatic dysfunction
Renal dysfunction
Impaired metabolism
Vitamin D–dependent rickets
Hypoparathyroidism
Impaired synthesis
DiGeorge syndrome
Activating mutations of the calcium-sensing receptor
Pseudohypoparathyroidism
Other
Hypomagnesemia
Hungry bone syndrome
Fluoride poisoning

Clinical manifestations. The clinical manifestations of hypocalcemia are dependent on the severity of the abnormality, the rate of decline in serum calcium, and the chronicity of the underlying process. Other factors affecting the development of symptoms include acid–base balance and hypomagnesemia. Classic acute manifestations of hypocalcemia include neuromuscular instability or tetany, which affects both sensory and muscular function. Early or mild symptoms include paresthesias of the perioral region, hands and feet, and muscle cramps. More severe symptoms include seizure, laryngospasm, and bronchospasm. Classic physical findings in patients with neuromuscular instability include Trousseau sign and Chvostek sign. A positive Trousseau sign is the precipitation of carpopedal spasm by inflation of a sphygmomanometer above systolic blood pressure for 3 minutes. A positive Chvostek sign is contraction of the ipsilateral facial muscle induced by tapping of the facial nerve in front of the ear. Of note, Chvostek sign may be present in up to 10% of normal subjects. In addition to neuromuscular findings, acute hypocalcemia may result in significant cardiovascular disturbance, including hypotension, congestive heart failure, prolonged QT interval, and dysrhythmias. Papilledema may also be present and resolves with correction of hypocalcemia.

Management. Numerous forms of calcium salts are available, and therefore, attention to the salt form is critical when dosing to determine the elemental calcium dose. Calcium may be provided by either oral supplementation or intravenous solution. The appropriate choice is guided by pertinent clinical findings. In general, intravenous calcium is indicated if the patient has prolonged QT, significant symptoms (tetany, seizures, carpopedal spasm), or acute decrease in serum corrected calcium to less than or equal to 7.5 mg per dL regardless of symptoms. Oral supplementation is more appropriate when symptoms are absent or mild and corrected calcium is greater than or equal to 7.5 mg per dL. In patients with asymptomatic chronic hypocalcemia associated with CKD, oral calcium supplementation is preferred with concomitant replacement of 1,25-dihydroxyvitamin D. If hypocalcemia is associated with metabolic acidosis, correction of the acidosis will reduce the ionized calcium level. Therefore, if metabolic acidosis is not causing clinical compromise, priority should be given to increasing the serum calcium. If hypocalcemia is associated with severe hyperphosphatemia, the provision of calcium may result in the precipitation of calcium and phosphate in the tissues, a disorder known as calciphylaxis. In patients with associated hypomagnesemia, magnesium supplements should be provided, as persistent hypomagnesemia will hinder the correction of hypocalcemia.

Prompt treatment of symptomatic or severe acute hypocalcemia should be initiated intravenously with either calcium chloride or calcium gluconate. Central access is usually necessary for calcium chloride infusions, although peripheral infusions may be permissible in emergent situations. Central access is also preferred for calcium gluconate, though this salt can be infused peripherally via a large vein. The use of calcium gluconate is usually favored as it is less likely to result in tissue damage if extravasation occurs. As concentrated forms are irritating to veins, calcium salts should be diluted in dextrose and water or saline. The final concentration of calcium gluconate should be 50 mg per mL, and calcium chloride should be diluted to 20 mg per mL. Calcium should not be prepared or infused with fluids containing phosphate or bicarbonate given the risk of precipitation of insoluble salts. The dose for intravenous bolus of calcium gluconate in the setting of cardiac disturbance is 50 to 100 mg/kg/dose infused over 3 to 5 minutes and for tetany is 100 to 200 mg/kg/dose infused over 5 to 10 minutes. Intravenous calcium should not be infused more rapidly given the risk for cardiac arrhythmia, bradycardia, and arrest. Cardiac monitoring and serial monitoring of the serum calcium level should be performed. Repeat boluses should be provided until the symptoms resolve, and then a slower infusion should be continued.

For patients with either chronic hypocalcemia or milder degrees of acute hypocalcemia without severe symptoms, oral calcium is preferred. Numerous forms of oral calcium salts are available. Calcium carbonate is readily available and well tolerated. If either hypoparathyroidism or vitamin D deficiency is suspected, vitamin D replacement should be provided to optimize enteral absorption. The overall management goal of chronic hypocalcemia is to achieve acceptable serum calcium while avoiding hypercalcemia and excessive hypercalciuria.

Hypercalcemia

Hypercalcemia results when the influx of calcium into the extracellular space exceeds the rate of deposition into bone or renal capacity for excretion. This may occur due to excessive absorption from the gastrointestinal tract, accelerated bone resorption, or decreased renal excretion. Excessive exposure to vitamin D will increase intestinal calcium and phosphate absorption and would be associated with a depressed PTH level. In addition to exogenous sources of vitamin D, granulomatous disorders may be associated with increased 1,25-dihydroxyvitamin D activity and promote absorptive hypercalcemia. Accelerated bone resorption would be anticipated in primary, secondary, and tertiary hyperparathyroidism. Jansen syndrome, a genetic disorder of the PTH receptor, renders the receptor constitutively active. Children with Jansen syndrome present with hypercalcemia, undetectable levels of PTH, and skeletal changes consistent with hyperparathyroidism. Immobilization, particularly in rapidly growing adolescents, may result in significant bone resorption and hypercalcemia. Malignancy is a rare cause of hypercalcemia in children. Decreased renal excretion occurs in familial hypocalciuric hypercalcemia (FHH), an autosomal dominant disorder. FHH is characterized by mild, asymptomatic hypercalcemia, increased tubular reabsorption of calcium, and inappropriately normal PTH. Medications associated with hypercalcemia include thiazide diuretics and lithium.

The evaluation of hypercalcemia begins with a thorough assessment of symptoms, diet, medication, medical history, and family history. Laboratory evaluation should include ionized calcium, electrolytes, phosphorus, magnesium, renal function, serum albumin, and acid–base assessment. Review of previous laboratory studies, if available, should be performed. Though results will not be available to the emergency department physicians, PTH level is critical to ultimately differentiate the underlying cause. If the PTH is not elevated, vitamin D metabolites should be submitted. Assessment of urine calcium excretion via random urine calcium to creatinine ratio may also be informative. Calcium excretion is high in hyperparathyroidism but low in FHH and with thiazide therapy.

Clinical manifestations. Hypercalcemia is associated with a number of signs and symptoms depending on the acuity and severity of the disorder. Patients with mildly elevated calcium (less than 11.5 to 12 mg per dL) are often asymptomatic, especially if the elevation is chronic in onset. Patients with moderate hypercalcemia (12 to 14 mg per dL) may experience anorexia, irritability, abdominal pain, constipation, and weakness. An important renal manifestation of hypercalcemia is polyuria due to an inability to concentrate urine, an acquired form of nephrogenic diabetes insipidus. Should polyuria be associated with gastrointestinal symptoms and decreased fluid intake, dehydration will ensue and aggravate the existing hypercalcemia by reducing renal excretion of calcium. If hypercalcemia is severe, progressive weakness, confusion, seizures, and coma may develop.

Management. When hypercalcemia is mild, no specific therapy is warranted and efforts should focus on identifying the underlying condition. Chronic moderate hypercalcemia (12 to 14 mg per dL) may be well tolerated and not require immediate intervention, though thorough evaluation should be pursued. If hypercalcemia is severe (greater than 14 mg per dL) or associated with clinically significant symptoms, prompt intervention is warranted. Given the gastrointestinal and renal manifestations associated with hypercalcemia, patients may present with hypovolemia. Initial efforts should focus on restoring adequate intravascular volume with isotonic intravenous fluids, which will increase GFR and increase renal excretion of calcium. Once intravascular volume is restored, attempts to promote continued calcium excretion with intravenous saline and loop diuretics (furosemide 1 to 2 mg per kg) should be employed. Loop diuretics inhibit tubular reabsorption of calcium and enhance excretion. If the patient is in renal failure or efforts with saline diuresis are not sufficient, contacting a pediatric nephrology or endocrinology consultant is advised. Therapeutic options for cases not responsive to conventional therapies include calcitonin, bisphosphonates, and renal replacement therapy (RRT), if clinically indicated.

DISORDERS OF ACID–BASE HOMEOSTASIS

Goals of Treatment

Maintenance of normal acid–base balance involves expiration of carbon dioxide, metabolism of organic acids, and buffering and renal excretion of nonvolatile acids. Severe uncompensated acid–base disorders are associated with a variety of cardiovascular, metabolic, neurologic, and respiratory consequences. General goals include treatment of the underlying etiology and maintenance of normal pH in order to prevent potentially fatal sequelae.

CLINICAL PEARLS AND PITFALLS

- Metabolic acidosis can be categorized based on a normal or elevated anion gap (AG).
- Potentially life-threatening conditions such as septic shock and certain metabolic disorders may present with significant metabolic acidosis.
- Treatment of metabolic acidosis is primarily aimed at the underlying etiology. IV sodium bicarbonate may be indicated in the treatment of severe metabolic acidosis.
- Metabolic alkalosis in children most commonly results from diuretic therapy and H^+ loss from gastrointestinal secretions.

Metabolic Acidosis

Metabolic acidosis occurs when there is either a net gain of H^+ ions or a net loss of bicarbonate (HCO_3^-) ions. The two classes of physiologic acids are volatile acids and nonvolatile acids. The excretion of volatile acid is achieved by pulmonary ventilation, and the elimination of nonvolatile acid is achieved by renal excretion.

Clinical manifestations. The clinical manifestations of metabolic acidosis are variable and will depend on the underlying etiology and severity. Children may be asymptomatic or present with a variety of acute or chronic manifestations such as tachypnea, abdominal pain, vomiting, lethargy, neurologic abnormalities, and failure to thrive. Inquiries regarding the presence and duration of symptoms such as diarrhea, polyuria, and poor growth should be included in the historical assessment. The physical examination should include an assessment of perfusion and measurement of growth parameters to determine if growth has been impaired.

Evaluation of metabolic acidosis ideally begins with an assessment of the venous or capillary blood gas, which defines systemic pH, pulmonary compensation, and may identify the presence of complex acid–base disorders (mixed acid–base disorders). Arterial samples are discouraged in children because the information that is gained does not justify the pain of the procedure. Venous or capillary samples are sufficient in the ED setting. The serum bicarbonate is typically measured indirectly by blood gas or directly by adding a strong acid to venous blood and observing the amount of CO_2 generated. Once metabolic acidosis is diagnosed, assessment of respiratory compensation can be performed. The arterial partial pressure of

CO_2 (pCO_2) normally falls at an average of 1.2 mm Hg for every 1 mEq per L reduction in the serum HCO_3^- to a minimum pCO_2 of 10 to 15 mm Hg. The Winters' formula can also approximate the expected arterial pCO_2:

$$\text{Arterial } pCO_2 = (1.5 \times \text{measured } HCO_3^-) + 8 \pm 2$$

If the fall in pCO_2 is significantly different than the expected value, a mixed acid–base disorder is likely present.

Patients with metabolic acidosis can be classified in two groups based on the serum AG, and this determination may facilitate the diagnosis of the underlying cause. Serum electrolytes should be obtained to calculate the AG using the following formula:

$$\text{AG (mEq/L)} = Na^+ - (Cl^- + HCO_3^-)$$

The normal AG typically ranges between 7 and 13 mEq per L, and an AG greater than 14 to 16 mEq per L is elevated. In normal subjects, the AG is primarily due to negative charges from plasma proteins, particularly albumin. An elevated AG is most often due to an unmeasured anion, though can also result from a low concentration of serum cations (K^+, Ca^{2+}, Mg^{2+}). A low AG can result from an increase in serum cations or low serum albumin. For every 1 g per dL reduction in serum albumin level, the AG would be expected to be reduced by approximately 2.5 mEq per L. The causes of metabolic acidosis based on elevated or normal AG are outlined in Table 108.11. Potentially life-threatening conditions including septic shock and certain inborn errors of metabolism are important considerations in the evaluation of children with significant metabolic acidosis. Lactic acidosis has been observed in patients with severe asthma being treated with high-dose β-adrenergic agents and steroids. In addition to serum electrolytes and serum albumin, initial laboratory studies should include serum glucose, BUN, creatinine, and urinalysis with urine pH. A higher than expected urine pH in the setting of acidosis may suggest renal tubular acidosis (RTA). Further studies are based upon clinical suspicion.

TABLE 108.11

CAUSES OF METABOLIC ACIDOSIS WITH RESPECT TO THE ANION GAP

Elevated anion gap
Lactic acidosis
Hypoperfusion
Inborn errors of carbohydrate metabolism
Mitochondrial disorders
Diabetic ketoacidosis
Inborn errors of metabolism
Organic acidemias
Fatty acid oxidation defects
Ingestions
Methanol, ethanol, ethylene glycol, salicylates
Renal failure
Normal anion gap
Renal tubular acidosis
Diarrhea
Enteric fistulae
Ureterosigmoidostomy
Early renal failure

Management. The management of metabolic acidosis should focus on the identification and treatment of the underlying cause and ensuring adequate perfusion. The immediate therapy of metabolic acidosis in the emergency department generally depends on the severity of the disorder. In children with severe acidemia (serum pH less than 7.10), bicarbonate therapy is generally indicated. The basis for correcting severe acidosis is the negative impact severe acidemia has on cardiac function, including impaired cardiac contractility and increased risk for cardiac arrhythmias. Exceptions would include metabolic acidosis in patients with DKA, as lower thresholds for pH are allowed before bicarbonate is provided given the expected metabolism of ketoacid into bicarbonate with insulin and fluid repletion (see Chapter 97 Endocrine Emergencies). The role of alkali therapy remains controversial in hypoperfusion lactic acidosis and is yet to be resolved. The aim of treatment in hypoperfusion lactic acidosis is to restore intravascular volume and perfusion in a timely fashion, which will allow metabolism of lactate anions to bicarbonate. The potential complications of alkali therapy in metabolic acidosis include hypercarbia, hypernatremia, transcellular shift of potassium ion into the intracellular space resulting in hypokalemia, and alkalosis. Furthermore, alkalosis or an increase in blood pH may precipitate tetany by promoting binding of calcium to albumin, which reduces the ionized calcium concentration.

When bicarbonate therapy is to be given, estimating the necessary dose may prove to be challenging. Given the difficulty in accurately estimating the bicarbonate deficit, bicarbonate can be given at an initial dose of 0.5 to 1 mEq per kg if clinically indicated with the aim of increasing the systemic pH to more than 7.20. Further alkali therapy will depend upon the response and subsequent disease course. If the patient is asymptomatic, the underlying process can be controlled (e.g., diarrheal dehydration), and tissue perfusion can be assured, alkali therapy may not be required. In the setting of asymptomatic chronic metabolic acidosis, such as RTA and CKD, consultation with an appropriate specialist would be reasonable to guide oral therapy and avoid complications such as electrolyte derangements and volume excess.

Metabolic Alkalosis

Metabolic alkalosis is characterized by a rise in the plasma bicarbonate concentration, and causes include hydrogen loss from the gastrointestinal tract or kidneys, volume contraction around a relatively constant amount of extracellular bicarbonate (contraction alkalosis), and the administration of bicarbonate. Given the renal capacity to excrete excess bicarbonate, clinical circumstances must be present that impair bicarbonate excretion in order to develop this disorder. Therefore, when approaching the patient with metabolic alkalosis, identification of both the inciting cause and the clinical factors allowing persistence of the disorder must be pursued.

Although there are many causes (Table 108.12), metabolic alkalosis in children most commonly results from diuretic therapy and hydrogen ion loss from gastrointestinal secretions. Loop and thiazide diuretics increase distal delivery of both sodium and water and predispose to volume contraction, thereby stimulating aldosterone secretion and enhancing hydrogen ion secretion into the tubular lumen. Gastrointestinal causes of metabolic alkalosis include vomiting or nasogastric suction. Gastric secretions have high concentrations of

TABLE 108.12

CAUSES OF METABOLIC ALKALOSIS

Renal hydrogen loss
Loop or thiazide diuretics
Posthypercapnic alkalosis
Mineralocorticoid excess
Bartter and Gitelman syndromes
Gastrointestinal hydrogen loss
Vomiting
Nasogastric suction
Alkali therapy
Contraction alkalosis
Loop or thiazide diuretics
Cystic fibrosis
Congenital chloridorrhea
Intracellular movement of hydrogen
Hypokalemia

hydrogen chloride and a lesser amount of potassium chloride (5 to 10 mEq per L), and gastric losses will predispose to the development of metabolic alkalosis.

In normal subjects, the renal capacity to excrete bicarbonate prevents the development of metabolic alkalosis. The persistence of metabolic alkalosis implies a limitation of renal bicarbonate excretion, and the most common perpetuating cause is effective circulating volume depletion. In addition to volume depletion, chloride depletion will also limit renal bicarbonate excretion and is associated with gastric fluid loss and diuretic therapy. Low renal tubular concentration of chloride favors both bicarbonate reabsorption and decreases bicarbonate excretion. Hypokalemia also directly increases bicarbonate reabsorption, which is in part due to intracellular acidosis induced by the entry of hydrogen ions into the cell in exchange for potassium movement out of the cell. Intracellular acidosis induces renal acid excretion and promotes net bicarbonate reabsorption.

Clinical manifestations. Symptoms associated with metabolic alkalosis are primarily related to the underlying etiology of the alkalosis or to associated fluid and electrolyte abnormalities.

Management. The cause of metabolic alkalosis is generally evident from the history. The evaluation of metabolic alkalosis should include a thorough history to identify gastrointestinal losses and an account of medications taken, specifically diuretics and antacids. Serum studies should include assessment of renal function and electrolyte balance to evaluate for concurrent abnormalities such as hypokalemia, hypercalcemia, and abnormalities in serum magnesium, which may support a renal tubulopathy such as Gitelman syndrome. Urine electrolytes may also be informative. In patients with metabolic alkalosis and volume contraction, the urine sodium and chloride concentrations may be dissociated. If the serum bicarbonate exceeds the renal capacity to conserve, some of the excess bicarbonate will be excreted with sodium and potassium. This loss of cations will worsen the sodium deficit and may lead to potassium depletion. Despite metabolic alkalosis, the conservation of chloride is intact, and a urine chloride concentration less than 25 mEq per L would be consistent with volume depletion. A urine chloride concentration greater than 40 mEq per L in the setting of metabolic alkalosis would be consistent with disorders such as primary mineralocorticoid excess, Bartter syndrome, Gitelman syndrome, or continued diuretic therapy.

The treatment of metabolic alkalosis is supportive, and reversible underlying causes should be addressed. The focus of therapy should aim at restoring adequate circulating volume and correcting chloride and potassium deficits. Providing isotonic sodium chloride will restore intravascular volume, remove the stimulus for sodium retention, and increase distal chloride delivery. Once these results have been achieved, there will be decreased bicarbonate reabsorption, increased bicarbonate excretion, and correction of the metabolic alkalosis. Potassium chloride should be provided if depletion is suspected with close monitoring to avoid excessive replacement. Though the extracellular concentration of potassium may be low during metabolic alkalosis due to transcellular shift to the intracellular space, true potassium depletion may be present. Potassium can be lost due to impaired renal absorption from diuretic therapy, aldosterone effect associated with volume depletion, and obligatory wasting of cations (Na^+ and K^+) associated with bicarbonate excretion. In patients with metabolic alkalosis and edematous states, providing sodium chloride may be hazardous. Therapy should take into account the underlying condition and planned in concert with appropriate subspecialty care if possible.

ACUTE KIDNEY INJURY

CLINICAL PEARLS AND PITFALLS

- Children presenting with acute kidney injury (AKI) may have signs of systemic fluid overload but be intravascularly dehydrated.
- Electrolyte and acid–base abnormalities may be present upon presentation and may need to be emergently addressed.
- Patients may require RRT if intrinsic renal function is unable to maintain fluid and electrolyte balance.
- Consultation with a nephrologist will help guide evaluation and therapeutic choices.

Current Evidence

AKI, previously termed acute renal failure, is an abrupt decrease in the GFR with impairment of creatinine clearance. However, there may be a time lag between the onset of injury and clinically detectable changes in serum creatinine. Depending on the severity of the injury, there may be altered water and electrolyte excretion as well as disturbances of metabolic and acid–base regulation. In mild cases, nonoliguric AKI may be asymptomatic and only detected when serum laboratory studies are performed. When severe, oliguric AKI may result in profound derangements of electrolyte and volume balance necessitating the initiation of RRT.

The Schwartz formula allows estimation of the GFR in children based on serum creatinine, patient length, age, and gender (Table 108.13). It should be noted that this formula tends to overestimate GFR, and this overestimation increases with decreasing GFR.

TABLE 108.13

ESTIMATION OF GFR BY THE SCHWARTZ FORMULA

$$C_{cr} = k \times L/S_{cr}$$

C_{cr} = creatinine clearance in mL/min/1.73 m^2

k^a = proportionality constant

L = length (cm)

S_{cr} = serum creatinine (mg/dL)

[a]k values
Low–birth-weight infants during the first year of life = 0.33
Full-term babies during first year of life = 0.45
Children and adolescent girls = 0.55
Adolescent boys = 0.7

Adapted from Schwartz GJ, Feld LG, Langford DJ. A simple estimate of glomerular filtration rate in full-term infants during the first year of life. *J Pediatr* 1984;104:849–854; Schwartz GJ, Gauthier B. A simple estimate of glomerular filtration rate in adolescent boys. *J Pediatr* 1985;106:522–526; Schwartz GJ, Haycock GB, Edelmann CM Jr, et al. A simple estimate of glomerular filtration rate in children derived from body length and plasma creatinine. *Pediatrics* 1976;58:259–263.

AKI may be classified as prerenal, intrinsic renal, and postrenal. Prerenal AKI can result from intravascular volume depletion or reduced effective circulating volume. Volume depletion may occur in the setting of uncompensated fluid losses from a variety of sources including bleeding, cutaneous losses, urination, and gastrointestinal output. Intravascular volume depletion may also develop when fluid shifts out of the vascular space into the interstitial space such as in the setting of hypoalbuminemia or during systemic inflammatory response syndrome (SIRS). Decreased effective circulating volume may be present in heart failure or distributive shock. Intrinsic renal disease can result from insults to the renal vasculature, glomeruli, or interstitium. Causes of postrenal AKI include congenital or acquired anatomic obstructions of the urinary tract such as posterior urethral valves, stones, masses, and functional or anatomic bladder outlet obstruction.

Goals of Treatment

The goals of treatment include mitigating and/or correcting any fluid or electrolyte disturbances resulting from AKI as well as removing the underlying cause, if possible. Measures should be taken to induce nitrogenous waste elimination and achieve electrolyte homeostasis whether by the kidneys themselves or through RRT when needed.

Clinical Considerations

Clinical recognition. Children with AKI may present with a variety of complaints related either directly to kidney dysfunction or to the underlying cause itself. Patients and caregivers may notice changes in the urine output or quality. They may present with concern for changes in appearance or physical function related to volume overload. Other presenting symptoms of AKI may be nonspecific such as malaise and nausea. In other instances, the initial complaint will be related to an underlying systemic or infectious cause for the AKI.

Triage considerations. AKI includes a wide spectrum of disease and severity. Initial triage should be based on overall clinical appearance and hemodynamic stability. Patients with hypertensive crisis, respiratory distress from volume overload, or life-threatening dysrhythmias from electrolyte disturbances may warrant emergent stabilization. Children with more mild presentations may undergo further evaluation into underlying causes at the onset.

Clinical assessment. A thorough history is necessary to reveal the underlying etiology of AKI. A detailed history of fluid balance should be obtained. The quality and quantity of urine should be identified. Recent medications should be reviewed to identify potential causes of drug-induced nephrotoxicity. Important classes of medications that increase the risk for AKI include nonsteroidal anti-inflammatory drugs (NSAIDs), angiotensin-converting enzyme (ACE) inhibitors, angiotensin II receptor blockers (ARBs), and calcineurin inhibitors.

The patient should be evaluated for hypertension, and the physical examination should assess hydration status and perfusion as well as evaluate for edema and evidence of third spacing. The patient's weight should be compared to a "dry weight" or recent weight prior to the onset of illness, when possible. The examination may reveal signs of systemic vasculitis associated with nephritis, such as rashes or arthritis. The presence of a palpable bladder or mass, which may be compressing the urinary tract or stemming from the kidneys themselves, should be assessed for during the abdominal examination.

Laboratory assessment of AKI serves two purposes. First, it should determine the severity of renal dysfunction and identify associated electrolyte, metabolic or hematologic abnormalities, which may require urgent intervention. Secondly, a focused investigation should be aimed at determining the underlying cause of AKI based on the clinical presentation of the patient. Initial serum laboratory studies should include serum creatinine, electrolytes, and complete blood cell counts. Children with AKI may demonstrate hyperkalemia, hypo- or hypernatremia, AG acidosis, hypocalcemia, and/or hyperphosphatemia depending on the degree of dysfunction and the chronicity of the underlying etiology. Serial assessment of renal function and electrolytes will be required to determine the disease course and to monitor for the development of electrolyte derangements and changes in renal function. Although the results may not affect the course of management within the emergency department, laboratory studies aimed at assessing for an underlying cause may assist specialists with treatment in a more rapid fashion. In cases of suspected glomerulonephritis, serum complements, serologic testing for streptococcal infection, and autoimmune antibodies such as antinuclear antibodies, antineutrophil cytoplasmic antibodies, and antiglomerular basement (GBM) antibodies may be considered in conjunction with specialist consultation.

Initial urine studies should include urinalysis with microscopic assessment. An elevated urine specific gravity may be consistent with prerenal physiology. The presence of nitrite or leukocyte esterase suggests a urinary tract infection. Detection of large heme by dipstick is found in glomerulonephritis and myoglobinuria, and differentiation between these two disorders relies upon the presence or absence of red blood cells in the urine sediment, respectively. Heavy proteinuria by dipstick, which detects albumin excretion, would be suggestive of glomerular disease and should be followed by a quantitative urine protein to creatinine ratio (normal less than 0.2, nephrotic range greater than 2 to 3). Microscopic examination of the urine sediment may be normal or nearly normal, consistent with prerenal AKI and some cases of acute tubular necrosis (ATN). ATN may also be associated with granular, muddy brown, and/or tubuloepithelial cell casts. The finding of red blood cell casts is pathognomonic of glomerulonephritis, and concomitant white blood cells or white blood cell casts would be consistent with an exudative nephritis such as postinfectious glomerulonephritis or renal vasculitis. Urine sediment associated with acute interstitial nephritis (AIN) varies and includes microscopic hematuria, sterile pyuria, and white blood cell casts. The degree of proteinuria associated with AIN is also variable, though is typically not severe except in NSAID-induced AIN, which may be associated with nephrotic range proteinuria. If interstitial nephritis is suspected, the urine should be evaluated for the presence of eosinophils, though sensitivity and specificity of urine eosinophilia is limited.

An assessment of urine chemistries may also be useful in distinguishing prerenal AKI from ATN, and initial studies to consider include urine electrolytes and urine creatinine. The fractional excretion of sodium (FENa) is calculated as follows:

$$\text{FENa } (\%) = [(\text{urine Na} \times \text{serum creatinine})/(\text{serum Na} \times \text{urine creatinine})] \times 100$$

A value below 1% suggests prerenal disease and reflects reabsorption of almost all of the filtered sodium to maintain intravascular volume, an appropriate response to decreased renal perfusion. A value greater than 2% is consistent with ATN or other tubular disorders. Of note, the FENa may be less than 1% in normal subjects reflecting normal tubular handling of sodium in the setting of relatively low sodium intake. The fractional excretion of urea is similarly calculated as the FENa with substitution of urine urea nitrogen and blood urea nitrogen and is generally less than 35% in prerenal states. Diuretics increase urine sodium excretion but have less effect on urea excretion. Therefore, the FENa may be less reliable and the fractional excretion of urea more informative if diuretics have been provided prior to the collection of urine.

Radiographic assessment should be considered in all patients with AKI of unclear etiology. This is most certainly true in those who present with acute anuria, as urinary tract obstruction is a possible etiology and would require intervention. Given its safety and general availability, ultrasonography of the kidneys and urinary tract should be considered in all children with AKI. Ultrasound can provide assessment of renal parenchymal mass and may identify conditions of acquired or congenital obstruction of the urinary tract. Doppler investigation of the renal vessels should be performed if there is concern for vascular compromise or thrombosis, though further imaging may be necessary, given the limitations of this modality.

Management. The initial management of AKI in the emergency department is largely supportive and aimed at addressing fluid or electrolyte abnormalities while avoiding further renal insult. If prerenal physiology is suspected, appropriate volume resuscitation with isotonic fluids should be provided with frequent assessment of fluid status and urine flow. If the etiology is unclear and the patient is hemodynamically stable, gentle intravenous fluid bolus therapy starting at 10 mL per kg may be initiated with reassessment to determine if further resuscitation is indicated. Though prerenal physiology should be corrected, prevention of fluid overload should be emphasized. This balance is most challenging in those patients who present critically ill with sepsis associated with capillary leak and in those with heart failure and ineffective circulating volume. Potassium supplementation should be withheld until urine flow is established and results of serum electrolytes are available. Electrolyte and acid–base disturbances should be addressed as previously reviewed.

If AKI is associated with oligouria or anuria, the child may present in a state of volume excess. If severe, hypertension and pulmonary edema may be present and would warrant a trial of loop diuretic therapy. Intravenous furosemide given at an initial dose of 0.5 to 1 mg per kg should be provided if volume overload is causing cardiopulmonary compromise. If an adequate dose of a loop diuretic does not lead to a diuretic response, this therapy should be discontinued. Hypertension may be treated with either oral or intravenous agents. Oral calcium channel blockers and hydralazine, an arterial vasodilator, are well tolerated and do not further impair renal function like ACE inhibitors and ARB therapy. If intravenous agents are required, intermittent doses of hydralazine or labetalol are often effective. If the child remains oligouric or anuric despite diuretic challenge and has clinical evidence of volume excess, a pediatric nephrologist should be consulted given the potential need for RRT and ultrafiltration. Indications for dialysis include progressive azotemia, clinically significant volume overload, and severe electrolyte abnormalities such as hyperkalemia or acidosis that is refractory to conservative medical therapy. If medications such as antibiotics are indicated, dose adjustment based on decreased renal function must be considered. Indications for admission include hypertension and impaired renal function causing fluid or electrolyte abnormalities.

INTRINSIC CAUSES OF AKI

AKI may be caused by a wide variety of both acute and chronic processes. It may be due to a primary renal disorder or be related to a systemic disease. The differential diagnosis is broad. Table 108.14 lists some of the more common forms of glomerular disease in the pediatric population.

Hemolytic Uremic Syndrome

Goals of Treatment

The goals of treatment include supportive care and managing the consequences of microvascular endothelial cell injury in affected organs. Fluid balance, electrolyte abnormalities, and severe anemia may necessitate medical management and possible RRT. Pancreatic and hepatic injury may require close monitoring and medical support of end-organ function. Neurologic complications may be severe and require close monitoring to detect their presence.

CLINICAL PEARLS AND PITFALLS

- Hemolytic uremic syndrome (HUS) is characterized by Coombs negative hemolytic anemia, thrombocytopenia, and AKI but with normal coagulation studies, helping to differentiate it from disseminated intravascular coagulation.
- It is usually preceded by diarrhea that often becomes bloody as well as abdominal pain and emesis.
- Care is supportive and may include fluid resuscitation, blood transfusions, and RRT.
- Antibiotics are generally not indicated and may lead to recurrent HUS.

TABLE 108.14

GLOMERULAR DISEASES IN CHILDHOOD

Primary
IgA nephropathy
Focal segmental glomerulosclerosis
Membranoproliferative glomerulonephritis
Membranous glomerulonephritis
Associated with systemic disease
Henoch–Schönlein purpura
Hemolytic uremic syndrome
Goodpasture syndrome
Microscopic polyarteritis
Systemic lupus erythematosus
Wegner granulomatosis
Infectious
Poststreptococcal glomerulonephritis
Hepatitis B and C–associated nephritis
Shunt nephritis
Subacute bacterial endocarditis
Inherited
Alport syndrome
Benign familial hematuria
Thin basement membrane disease

Clinical Considerations

Clinical recognition. HUS is characterized by the clinical triad of microangiopathic hemolytic anemia, thrombocytopenia, and AKI. Its consequences are the result of microvascular endothelial cell injury. HUS can be divided into atypical cases and typical forms stemming from Shiga toxin–producing infections. Atypical HUS is a heterogenous disorder and may be precipitated by numerous triggers, including drugs, bone marrow transplantation, and nonenteric infections such as those due to *Streptococcus pneumoniae* and human immunodeficiency virus. Typical HUS accounts for approximately 90% of pediatric cases and is frequently due to infection with enterohemorrhagic *Escherichia coli* (EHEC), although other organisms such as *Shigella dysenteriae* type 1, *Salmonella,* and *Yersinia* have been implicated as well. Greater than 70% of the cases in the United States are from *E. coli* serotype O157:H7. Most cases are sporadic but outbreaks may occur and are often well publicized. HUS is most commonly seen in the summer months (see Chapter 102 Infectious Disease Emergencies).

Although children of all ages can develop typical HUS, it most commonly affects children younger than 5 years. Approximately 6% to 9% of children who develop culture confirmed *E. coli* O157:H7 gastroenteritis progress to HUS. Measures to prevent progression to postdiarrheal HUS have been unsuccessful, and the use of antibiotics and antimotility agents appear to increase the risk of subsequent HUS.

The clinical manifestations of HUS generally present 5 to 10 days after the onset of colitis. In the majority of patients, the colitis begins with watery diarrhea and evolves to hemorrhagic colitis. Vomiting and severe abdominal pain may occur. Gastrointestinal complications include bowel wall necrosis, toxic megacolon, peritonitis, intussusception, and rectal prolapse. HUS may become apparent as the diarrhea is resolving, and the evolution of the clinical signs may be rapid.

Microangiopathic injury of organs other than the kidneys and intestine may occur. Pancreatic involvement can be associated with transient or, rarely, permanent diabetes mellitus. Liver injury may manifest as hepatomegaly and elevated transaminases. Myocardial ischemia or fluid overload may lead to cardiac dysfunction. Approximately one-quarter of children demonstrate some degree of encephalopathy manifested as irritability and/or somnolence. Some may experience more severe consequences of CNS involvement including seizures, coma, stroke, hemiparesis, and cortical blindness.

Clinical assessment. The patient may present pale and lethargic. Jaundice is present in approximately one-third of patients. Given symptoms of severe diarrhea and vomiting, the child may present with evidence of hypovolemia including hypotension and signs of decreased perfusion. Alternatively, if oral intake has been maintained in the face of oliguric renal failure, signs of volume excess, including edema and hypertension, may be apparent.

A complete blood count will show microangiopathic anemia and thrombocytopenia. Assessment of the blood smear demonstrates fragmented erythrocytes, schistocytes, and helmet cells. Other studies may include increased reticulocyte count, elevated indirect bilirubin, increased lactate dehydrogenase, and decreased haptoglobin. Coagulation studies are generally normal, distinguishing HUS from sepsis and disseminated intravascular coagulation. A Coombs test will be negative. A stool culture may help identify the causative organism but will not alter medical management of AKI.

The severity of the renal involvement in typical HUS varies widely and is not related to the degree of anemia present. AKI may be mild and self-limited, associated with microscopic hematuria, mild proteinuria, and preserved renal function. When renal microangiopathy is severe, fulminant oligoanuric renal failure may ensue and necessitate RRT.

Management. Supportive care is the mainstay of therapy for typical HUS. If intravascular volume depletion is present due to gastrointestinal losses and poor intake, fluid resuscitation with isotonic saline should be provided with repeated assessment of volume status in an effort to decrease the compounding effects of prerenal AKI. Once the intravascular volume status has been restored, further fluid management should be guided by renal function and urine flow. If oliguria is present, a trial of furosemide (0.5 to 1 mg/kg/dose) may be provided to establish urine flow. If oliguria persists, fluids should be provided at a rate to ensure adequate intravascular volume but avoid volume excess. Both intravenous and oral intake should match the total of measurable output (urine and gastrointestinal losses) and insensible water losses, estimated at 300 mL/m^2/day. Frequent monitoring of fluid balance, weight, and vital signs is essential. Hypertension may be managed with calcium channel blockers.

Anemia associated with typical HUS may be severe. Packed red blood cell transfusions should be provided for symptomatic anemia or robust hemolysis with a hemoglobin <6 mg per dL or hematocrit less than 18%. Transfusions should occur slowly given the concern for fluid balance issues. If the patient is oliguric, it may need to be performed while on dialysis to avoid volume excess and hyperkalemia. Due to microangiopathy, transfused platelets will be quickly consumed and not lead to a sustained increase in the platelet count. Platelet transfusion is only indicated in patients with active bleeding or when an invasive procedure is intended.

Up to 50% of children with typical HUS will require RRT. Dialysis is also indicated to safely provide blood products and nutritional support in the setting of persistent oligoanuria. The modality of dialysis depends on the expertise of the center. However, if there are severe abdominal complications requiring surgical intervention, hemodialysis will be necessary as peritoneal dialysis will be contraindicated. Plasma exchange can be considered with expert consultation in children with severe CNS involvement such as stroke and seizures based upon reported benefits in adults with thrombotic thrombocytopenic purpura and severe neurologic dysfunction.

Postinfectious Glomerulonephritis

Goals of Treatment

The goals of treatment for postinfectious glomerulonephritis are supportive in nature. The consequences of fluid retention such as pulmonary edema and hypertension should be managed, as necessary. AKI and its complications may necessitate medical intervention such as RRT in severe cases. Children with evidence of active underlying infections should be treated appropriately.

CLINICAL PEARLS AND PITFALLS

- Clinical presentation of nephritis includes hematuria, edema, and hypertension.
- Postinfectious glomerulonephritis most often occurs after an infection with group A streptococci.
- Care is supportive, including management of fluid balance and blood pressure, and most children recover fully.

Clinical Considerations

Clinical recognition. Postinfectious glomerulonephritis is the leading cause of glomerulonephritis in children worldwide and has been associated with a multitude of bacteria, viruses, and parasites. Nephritogenic strains of group A β-hemolytic streptococci are the most frequently implicated organisms, often after a proceeding pharyngitis or cellulitis. The latent period from infection to acute poststreptococcal glomerulonephritis (APSGN) is generally 1 to 3 weeks after pharyngitis and 3 to 6 weeks with skin infections. APSGN may be sporadic or occur during an epidemic. During an epidemic of pharyngitis, the incidence of clinically detectable APSGN is 5% to 10% but can be as high as 25% with an epidemic of streptococcal skin infections. It most often affects school-age children. In recent decades, the prevalence of APSGN has declined in most industrialized nations, although it persists at high rates in some developing countries.

The clinical presentation of APSGN may vary from asymptomatic microscopic hematuria to an abrupt onset of nephritic syndrome, which can be associated with gross hematuria, proteinuria, oliguria, edema, and hypertension. Hypertension can be severe and evolve into hypertensive emergency, which typically affects the CNS in children. Symptoms include headache, seizure, and encephalopathy.

Clinical assessment. A detailed history and physical examination should be completed when there is a suspicion of APSGN. The color and quantity of urine output should be assessed by history. A history of a preceding streptococcal infection may be present, although the infection may not have been identified at the time. The physical examination should assess for the consequences of APSGN. Signs of fluid overload should be looked for. The patient should be evaluated for hypertension, and the signs and symptoms of hypertensive crisis should be addressed.

Laboratory studies during a typical episode of APSGN reflect a nephritis with activation of the alternative complement pathway. Serum studies may demonstrate reduced renal function. Associated electrolyte abnormalities include hyponatremia, reflecting an inability to excrete water, and hyperkalemia. The majority of patients have a low C3 complement, and a normal C4 complement. The C3 level normalizes in 6 to 8 weeks. If the C3 remains depressed after 3 months or the C4 is low, diagnostic considerations include chronic forms of glomerulonephritis, including membranoproliferative glomerulonephritis (MPGN) and lupus nephritis. If the complement levels are normal at presentation, APSGN is less likely, and IgA nephropathy would be a consideration.

Serologic testing to document recent streptococcal infection is helpful but does not prove causation, as a significant number of children are asymptomatic carriers. Serologic tests available include titers for antistreptolysin O (ASO), antihyaluronidase, antistreptokinase, antinicotinamide-adenine dinucleotidase, and anti-DNAse B. ASO may be negative in the setting of streptococcal cellulitis, and it is important to note that antibiotic therapy may blunt the increase in antibody titers.

The urine sediment will demonstrate glomerular erythrocytes and leukocytes, and may contain red cell casts. Proteinuria is not uncommon, though not typically in the nephrotic range.

Renal biopsy is generally not indicated for the diagnosis of APSGN. It may be considered if the clinical picture does not clearly support a diagnosis of APSGN, if renal function does not recover in an expected fashion or if C3 levels remain persistently low.

Clinical management. Therapy for APSGN is largely supportive. Given the underlying glomerular inflammation and generally intact tubular function, there is a propensity for salt and water retention leading to edema and increased blood pressure. Therefore, weight should be measured daily and blood pressure checked regularly during the early acute illness. Children with hypertension or decreased renal function should be considered for admission. If edema or hypertension is present, salt and fluid restriction should be initiated and diuretic therapy considered. Furosemide can be provided at doses of 0.5 to 1 mg per kg once to four times daily to optimize fluid balance. If the child is hypertensive, short- or long-acting calcium channel blockers can be initiated while awaiting recovery. If the blood pressure is significantly elevated, intravenous hydralazine 0.1 mg per kg can be given every 4 to 6 hours with appropriate dose adjustment until other supportive measures are effective. If a child demonstrates persistent hypertension and proteinuria and if renal function has been stable, ACE inhibitors or ARBs can be considered with close monitoring of serum creatinine and potassium.

The prognosis for complete recovery from the initial episode of APSGN is good, even for those who presented with renal insufficiency or hypertension. Generally, the clinical symptoms of APSGN begin to improve after 1 to 2 weeks. If reduced renal function and edema are evident at presentation, renal function begins to normalize and diuresis ensues within several weeks. Gross hematuria will diminish rapidly, though microscopic hematuria may persist for 6 months or longer.

Proteinuria typically improves quickly and resolves within 6 months. However, studies evaluating the long-term prognosis reveal residual signs of chronic kidney damage in some patients decades after the initial course. Late complications include proteinuria, hypertension, and decreased renal function. This underscores the importance of routine monitoring of blood pressure and urinalyses as part of health maintenance in those who have a history of APSGN.

Henoch–Schönlein Purpura

Goals of Treatment

The goals of treatment for Henoch–Schönlein purpura (HSP) are generally supportive. Analgesics and anti-inflammatory medications such as NSAIDs may help alleviate associated arthralgias and arthritis. Patients may require parenteral hydration, especially in the setting of gastrointestinal manifestations. Children with abdominal pain should be evaluated and monitored for surgical complications (see Chapter 48 Pain: Abdomen). HSP-associated nephritis rarely requires specific interventions. If there is concern for significant AKI, a nephrologist should be consulted to help determine further evaluation and management.

CLINICAL PEARLS AND PITFALLS

- Nephritis secondary to HSP may present up to 6 months after the initial presentation of rash and arthritis.
- Patients with suspected HSP should undergo urinalysis to evaluate for hematuria.
- Care is generally supportive.

Clinical Considerations

Clinical recognition. HSP is a multisystem IgA-mediated vasculitis predominantly affecting the skin, joints, gastrointestinal tract, and kidneys. The exact pathogenesis of HSP remains unclear. Though HSP can occur at any age, most cases affect children between 3 and 15 years with a peak incidence at 4 to 7 years of age. In pediatric cases, a male predominance has been noted with male-to-female ratio as high as 1.8:1. Presentation during adolescence or adulthood portends a worse prognosis. The disease is more prevalent during fall, winter, and early spring. The onset is usually sudden and frequently preceded by an acute illness, often of the upper respiratory tract.

Though the acute illness may be overshadowed by rash, joint pain, and gastrointestinal symptoms, the long-term prognosis for children with HSP depends upon the extent of the renal involvement. The exact prevalence of HSP nephritis is unknown, though rates as high as 20% to 54% have been reported. Most children who develop nephritis will have relatively mild renal involvement. Signs of mild renal involvement include asymptomatic hematuria, mild proteinuria, and preserved or mildly and transiently impaired renal function. These patients are expected to have a favorable long-term prognosis. A subset of children will develop more severe renal involvement and develop nephritic syndrome or combined nephritic–nephrotic syndrome. Severe disease can be associated with decreased renal function, hypertension, hypoalbuminemia, and edema, and severe acute involvement would increase the risk for long-term renal sequelae.

Clinical assessment. The diagnosis of HSP is clinical, and the history and physical examination should focus on evaluation for the clinical manifestations of the small-vessel vasculitis associated with HSP. The hallmark signs and symptoms include nonthrombocytopenic purpuric rash, arthralgias, nonerosive arthritis, abdominal pain, and nephritis. The rash, often the most distinctive feature of the disease, characteristically involves the buttocks and extensor surfaces of the lower extremities. Purpura and joint pain are the most common presenting symptoms, though studies have revealed that abdominal symptoms may precede the rash in as many as 15% to 35% of cases. Overall, gastrointestinal symptoms occur in approximately half of children with HSP, and the most common abdominal symptoms are periumbilical pain, vomiting, diarrhea, and hematochezia. Surgical emergencies such as intussusception and bowel perforation develop in 1% to 5% of patients.

Ninety percent of cases of nephritis will present within 6 weeks after the onset of systemic symptoms, and it is rare for nephritis to develop later than 6 months after presentation. Upon presentation to the ED, a urinalysis should be obtained to evaluate for hematuria and proteinuria. If this study is normal, no further laboratory evaluation, such as evaluation of serum electrolytes or renal function, is indicated. Patients will require regular follow-up with their primary care providers for monitoring. Generally, if the urinalyses remain normal during the initial 6-month period, there is no need to screen for renal disease thereafter. Children presenting with clinical evidence of nephritis such as hematuria, edema, and hypertension warrant laboratory evaluation including serum electrolytes, BUN, creatinine, and albumin in addition to urinalysis.

Management. Most patients with HSP and associated nephritis require only supportive care, including hydration and comfort. Hospitalization may be required for uncontrolled pain, significant gastrointestinal bleeding, surgical abdomen, or AKI. If hypertension is present, short- or long-acting calcium channel blockers can be used. Patients with HSP nephritis should undergo regular evaluation to screen for signs of progressive renal disease, such as worsening proteinuria, decreasing renal function, and hypertension.

Once HSP has developed, corticosteroids may be indicated for severe gastrointestinal symptoms. Their efficacy in preventing nephritis has not been proven, however, and should not be started for this indication.

The optimal treatment of children with extensive renal disease remains controversial. Prior to initiating therapy, a nephrologist should be consulted and a renal biopsy may need to be obtained to determine the extent of crescent formation, as this appears to be the best indicator of prognosis. Though data are limited given the rarity of severe HSP nephritis, aggressive therapy may be beneficial in patients with severe disease. These patients may benefit from treatment with steroids with or without other agents such as azathioprine, cyclophosphamide, and anticoagulants but treatment should occur under the care of a nephrologist.

In children without HSP nephritis, symptoms often resolve within 1 month. One-third of patients may have recurrent symptoms, especially within the first 4 months. The short-term outcome of childhood HSP nephritis is favorable with 94% of children demonstrating complete recovery at a mean follow-up of nearly 20 months.

Acute Interstitial Nephritis

Goals of Treatment

Patient care for AIN is primarily supportive. The symptomatic consequences such as fluid and electrolyte imbalances from

AKI and associated systemic symptoms should be mitigated. The offending agent should be identified, if possible and discontinued or treated, if not already done so. Symptomatic relief of systemic symptoms such as fever or rash may need to be provided.

Clinical Considerations

Clinical recognition. AIN is characterized by inflammatory infiltration within the interstitium of the kidney leading to AKI. It is often the result of a drug reaction but can be caused by infection or systemic processes as well. Many medications can cause AIN, and it is often difficult or impossible to identify the potential offending agent. Nonsteroidal anti-inflammatories, antibiotics (including penicillins, cephalosporins, sulfonamides, ciprofloxacin, and rifampin), proton pump inhibitors, antiretrovirals, and 5-aminosalicylates are a few of the implicated drugs. Injury is not dose dependent and may occur in the setting of previous tolerance of the medication. The onset of AIN may occur weeks to months after the first exposure to the causative agent but is usually within 3 to 5 days if it is secondary to a reexposure. Numerous infections have also been implicated including cytomegalovirus (CMV), Epstein–Barr virus (EBV), leptospira, yersinia, legionella, and mycobacterium tuberculosis. Autoimmune disorders including systemic lupus erythematosus (SLE) and Wegener granulomatosis may have AIN with or without disease-associated glomerular disease. Patients with Sjögren syndrome and sarcoidosis also have increased risk.

Presenting symptoms are often nonspecific and may indicate generalized AKI, such as nausea and malaise. Approximately 50% of patients will have oliguria. Systemic symptoms such as rash or fever may be present. A small portion of patients may complain of gross hematuria.

Clinical assessment. The clinical assessment should focus on identifying potential symptoms of kidney dysfunction and possible underlying causes for AIN. A detailed medication history including current and recently discontinued drugs should be obtained. The physical examination should look for signs of systemic infections or diseases that could act as the causative factor. Nephrotic syndrome is rare in the setting of AIN. Proteinuria and edema are unlikely to be present. Depending on the degree of underlying AKI, blood pressure may be normal.

Microscopic examination of the urine may reveal the presence of red blood cells or white blood cell casts. Eosinophiluria defined by >1% eosinophils on the urine white blood cell differential may be suggestive of AIN but is not specific. Furthermore, absence of this finding has poor negative predictive value. Eosinophilia is evident on a complete blood count in 23% of cases. Electrolytes, creatinine, and blood urea nitrogen should be obtained to evaluate for laboratory evidence of AKI.

Management. If an offending medication is identified as the likely cause, it should be discontinued immediately if not already done so. Underlying infections should be treated. Patients may require management of fluid, electrolyte, and acid–base disturbances, depending on the level of underlying renal dysfunction.

Rhabdomyolysis

Goals of Treatment

The goals of treatment for rhabdomyolysis include identifying and treating the underlying cause of the rhabdomyolysis, if possible. The prevention of AKI should be achieved via aggressive hydration and measures aimed at the mitigation of renal and electrolyte abnormalities that do occur must be taken. Pain control may be required.

CLINICAL PEARLS AND PITFALLS

- Myoglobinuria will cause a false positive for blood on urine dipstick testing, but microscopic analysis will not be consistent with hematuria.
- Hyperkalemia may result from both lysis of muscle cells as well as AKI.
- Hydration is the mainstay of management.

Clinical Considerations

Clinical recognition. Rhabdomyolysis is the necrosis of muscle cells leading to introduction of intracellular contents, including myoglobin, into the blood stream. The classic symptoms of rhabdomyolysis include myalgias, weakness, and red or brown urine, though this triad is not always present.

Rhabdomyolysis may be from traumatic or nontraumatic causes. Traumatic etiologies include crush injuries, vascular occlusions, and lower extremity compartment syndrome. Nontraumatic causes include extreme exertion, prolonged seizure, malignant hyperthermia, DKA, hypokalemia, hypophosphatemia, metabolic myopathies, neuroleptic malignant syndrome, and postarrest. It has also been associated with a variety of infections, including influenza A and B, parainfluenza, coxsackievirus, EBV, herpes simplex virus, varicella zoster, human immunodeficiency virus, pyomyositis, necrotizing fasciitis, and sepsis. Prescription medications, such as statins, antipsychotics, and colchicine, and illicit drugs such as cocaine, ecstasy, and amphetamines, may cause rhabdomyolysis as well.

AKI during rhabdomyolysis is often multifactorial, and insults include prerenal physiology, tubular cell damage, and tubular obstruction. Decreased intravascular volume and prerenal physiology develop secondary to fluid sequestration within damaged muscle and intrarenal vasoconstriction. Unlike hemoglobin, myoglobin is a monomer and is freely filtered into the urine. Rhabdomyolysis leads to AKI through formation of intratubular casts. Tubular cell injury results from tubular obstruction with heme pigment casts and lipid peroxidation from hydroxyl radicals generated by heme and free iron.

Clinical assessment. Laboratory results reflect the release of myocyte contents into the blood stream and include elevated serum creatinine kinase as well as potential electrolyte derangements such as hyperkalemia, hyperphosphatemia, and hypocalcemia which may occur independently from AKI but be further exacerbated if renal dysfunction is present. The severity of rhabdomyolysis ranges from asymptomatic elevations in serum muscle enzymes to oliguric AKI associated with life-threatening electrolyte abnormalities. AKI is generally associated with serum concentrations of creatinine kinase >5,000 units per L. Clinical factors increasing the risk for AKI at lower concentrations of serum creatinine kinase include dehydration, metabolic acidosis, and sepsis.

In the setting of myoglobinuria a urine dipstick will test positive for heme, but microscopic evaluation will be negative for red blood cells. The urine sediment may reveal pigmented granular casts and a red to brown discoloration of the urine supernatant.

Management. The mainstay of therapy for rhabdomyolysis includes early vigorous hydration to ensure adequate intravascular volume and promote urine flow. The benefit of high urine flow is the removal of obstructing pigmented casts, which initiate the cytotoxic insults. Children should be provided isotonic saline to ensure adequate renal perfusion, and intravenous fluids should continue to optimize urine flow. The intravenous fluid rate will depend on the urine flow rate and should be reevaluated regularly to avoid volume excess. A minimum urine flow rate of approximately 1 to 2 mL/kg/hr should be targeted. Should the urine flow be low despite adequate volume status, a trial of furosemide 0.5 to 1 mg per kg IV could be considered and should be continued (i.e., every 6 to 8 hours) if effective. If diuretics are used, careful attention should be given to volume balance and perfusion to avoid concomitant prerenal insult. The clinical benefits of urine alkalinization or mannitol diuresis are not proven. Should metabolic acidosis develop, this may be treated with addition of bicarbonate to intravenous fluids. The risk of providing bicarbonate is excessive alkalinization and reduction of ionized calcium in patients with evolving hypocalcemia. For those with severe AKI associated with oligoanuria and electrolyte disturbance, RRT may be required until renal recovery is achieved.

NEPHROTIC SYNDROME

CLINICAL PEARLS AND PITFALLS

- Nephrotic syndrome is characterized by edema, hypertension, proteinuria, hypoalbuminemia, and hyperlipidemia.
- The most common cause in childhood is minimal change disease (MCD).
- Patients may be intravascularly depleted despite signs of overall fluid overload.
- Children with nephrotic syndrome are at increased risk for serious bacterial infections and thrombosis.

Current Evidence

Nephrotic syndrome is the clinical expression of a variety of glomerular diseases and can be classified as primary (without evidence of systemic illness), secondary, or congenital. Primary nephrotic syndrome includes idiopathic nephrotic syndrome and nephrotic syndrome associated with primary glomerulonephritis. Secondary nephrotic syndrome is associated with systemic disorders such as HIV infection, SLE, and HSP. Intrauterine infections with syphilis, toxoplasmosis, and other organisms have been associated with congenital nephrotic syndrome. When it is diagnosed within the first 3 months, it is termed congenital nephrotic syndrome; when it is diagnosed between 3 and 12 months of life, it is called infantile nephrotic syndrome. Most of these children have a genetic basis for renal disease. Congenital nephrotic syndrome may also be due to intrauterine infection, such as congenital syphilis, toxoplasmosis, CMV, human immunodeficiency virus, and other organisms.

In children younger than 16 years, the annual incidence of nephrotic syndrome is approximately 2 per 100,000. Presentation within the first year of life is uncommon, and nephrotic syndrome within the first 3 months of life should raise the suspicion for congenital nephrotic syndrome. Idiopathic nephrotic syndrome is the most common form of childhood nephrosis with MCD causing approximately 77% of cases and focal segmental glomerulonephritis (FSGS) and MPGN the majority of the remaining occurrences. Children typically present between the ages of 2 and 6 years, and the reported ratio of boys to girls who are diagnosed at a younger age is as high has 2:1. The gender ratio is closer to 1:1 in those who present later in childhood or as adolescents.

Goals of Treatment

Many children with nephrotic syndrome present to the emergency department with signs of fluid overload. Initial management should focus on improving fluid balance while monitoring for signs of intravascular volume depletion. Children should also be assessed for underlying complications of nephrotic syndrome such as infection and thrombosis. If a diagnosis of nephrotic syndrome has not been established in the past, an initial workup for potential underlying causes may be initiated.

Clinical Considerations

Clinical recognition. Nephrotic syndrome results when there is increased permeability across the glomerular filtration barrier. It is characterized by hypoproteinemia, edema, hyperlipidemia, and massive proteinuria exceeding 50 mg/kg/day. Edema is one of the major clinical manifestations of nephrotic syndrome and represents excessive salt and water retention. Periorbital edema is often the initial finding and may be misdiagnosed as signs of allergy. The associated edema is gravity dependent and therefore will vary in location based on patient position and activity. Upon awakening, edema may be more marked in the face and then shift to the lower extremities with ambulation. It may also be notable in the scrotal or vulvar regions. Other complications of third spacing, such as ascites, pulmonary edema, and pleural effusions, may also occur.

Although children with nephrotic syndrome and edema have total body sodium and water excess, some will present with evidence of intravascular depletion. This is more likely to occur in those with severely depressed serum albumin and will be exacerbated by diuretic use, gastrointestinal losses, and restricted intake. Signs of decreased effective circulating volume include tachycardia, peripheral vasoconstriction, and oliguria.

In addition to overall volume excess with or without intravascular depletion, complications resulting from nephrotic syndrome include infection, thromboembolism, and hypovolemia. Children with nephrotic syndrome are at increased risk of developing serious bacterial infection, particularly infections with encapsulated bacteria, given urinary losses of immunoglobulins and alternative complement pathway factor B and factor D. Children who are treated with immunosuppressive agents will have additional risk. Furthermore, ascites and pleural effusions increase the risk for peritonitis, pneumonia, and empyema. Other potential complicating infections include sepsis, meningitis, cellulitis, urinary tract infection, upper respiratory tract infection, and severe acute gastroenteritis.

Thromboembolic complications are reported in 2% to 3% of children with nephrotic syndrome and may occur in either the arterial or venous circulation. The risk may be higher in children with steroid-resistant disease. Nephrotic syndrome results in a hypercoagulable state due to urinary losses of antithrombin, protein S, and plasminogen. Additional risk factors include hemoconcentration, thrombocytosis, infection, and immobility. Though many embolic events are silent, pulmonary embolism and renal vein thrombosis may result in significant morbidity. Though a much less frequent occurrence in children than in adults with nephrotic syndrome, renal vein thrombosis should be suspected in cases of sudden onset macroscopic hematuria and flank pain.

Triage considerations. Children with nephrotic syndrome may present acutely ill with signs and symptoms of fluid overload. Patients may require support of lung function due to pulmonary edema. Hypertension can be symptomatic and may require emergent management. They are at risk for serious bacterial infections as well as both venous and arterial thrombosis and may require emergent evaluation and treatment for these conditions. Other patients may present with mild symptoms related to edema and will be managed with gentle diuresis with fluid and salt restriction.

Clinical assessment. The initial assessment of a child with nephrotic syndrome should focus on the adequacy of intravascular volume and perfusion, respiratory status, and assess for evidence of infection. There should be a thorough assessment of recent fluid balance, with specific inquiries to diuretic use, urine output, and gastrointestinal losses. As some patients with nephritis will have concomitant nephrotic syndrome (secondary nephrotic syndrome), accurate measurement of blood pressure should be documented to screen for associated hypertension.

Laboratory investigation should include confirmation of nephrotic syndrome, identification of associated electrolyte abnormalities, and an evaluation for possible underlying etiologies, if clinically indicated by evidence of systemic disease. A serum albumin of less than 2.5 g per dL is suggestive of nephrotic syndrome. A freshly obtained urine sample should confirm heavy proteinuria by dipstick and be inspected for the presence of macroscopic hematuria, which may suggest glomerulonephritis. Nephrotic range proteinuria in children is defined as protein excretion greater than 50 mg/kg/day, though this would depend upon a timed 24-hour urine collection, which is prone to inaccuracies and infeasible in the emergency department. Alternatively, a urine protein to creatinine ratio can be obtained on a spot urine sample to quantify the degree of proteinuria. A normal ratio is less than 0.5 in children younger than 2 years and less than 0.2 in older children and adults. Generally, a ratio more than 2 to 3 is consistent with nephrotic range proteinuria. Idiopathic nephrotic syndrome is typically associated with bland urine sediment whereas nephrotic syndrome associated with primary glomerulonephritis, such as IgA nephropathy and MPGN, is generally associated with active urine sediment.

Serum electrolytes may reveal hyponatremia secondary to decreased intravascular volume and stimulation of ADH release. Hyponatremia in the edematous child does not reflect total body sodium depletion but water excess that is greater than sodium excess. Renal function studies may be abnormal and reflect decreased intravascular volume or the underlying renal disease. Complete blood cell counts may demonstrate elevated hemoglobin and hematocrit due to hemoconcentration. Hyperlipidemia including elevated total serum cholesterol, triglycerides, and total lipids are typical. Studies to distinguish the cause of nephrotic syndrome should be considered based on the patient's presentation. Serum complements may identify disorders associated with complement consumption such as postinfectious glomerulonephritis, MPGN, and lupus nephritis. Additional studies to be considered include serum antinuclear antibodies, especially in children 10 years or older or with symptoms of SLE, and HIV, hepatitis B and C serologies in high-risk patients.

Management. Given that there are two major processes leading to edema in nephrotic syndrome, arterial underfilling due to low oncotic pressure and primary renal sodium retention, management of fluid excess requires careful attention to the underlying causes. Diuretic therapy would be effective in reducing edema and indicated if the primary process is renal sodium retention. However, if hypoalbuminemia leads to decreased plasma volume via movement of fluid from the vascular space to the interstitium, diuretic therapy may aggravate arterial underfilling. As it may be difficult to determine intravascular volume in patients with nephrotic syndrome, clinical characteristics that may predict intravascular volume status include GFR and serum albumin level. Patients with decreased vascular volumes and severe hypoalbuminemia may require albumin infusions in conjunction with diuretics in order to maintain arterial filling pressures. Children who present with severe edema should be admitted and may be treated with furosemide and salt-poor albumin (e.g., 25% albumin) to achieve diuresis. Albumin (0.5 to 1 g per kg) infused over 4 hours with one to two doses of furosemide (0.5 to 1 mg/kg/dose) should result in fluid mobilization. Providing albumin will bolster the intravascular oncotic pressure and safeguard against volume depletion during fluid mobilization.

Once the patent is stabilized, a plan for sodium and fluid restriction should be made. Optimally, children are restricted to approximately 2 to 3 mEq/kg/day of sodium or up to a maximum of 2,000 mg per day in older children and adolescents. Water restriction should be initiated given the release and action of ADH resulting in dilutional hyponatremia. Admission for close volume management should be strongly considered if evidence of hypovolemia is apparent at presentation or uncontrolled fluid loss is anticipated (i.e., gastroenteritis) given the risk for thromboembolic complications and prerenal kidney injury.

Children who are hemodynamically stable presenting with nephrotic syndrome should be started on prednisone 2 mg per kg after consultation with a nephrologist. If they do not require hospital admission for close fluid balance monitoring, they should be followed closely as an outpatient by a specialist to monitor weight, blood pressure, and response to therapy. In children in whom infection is suspected appropriate antibiotics with coverage for *S. pneumoniae* and gram-negative bacterial infections should be provided.

Though children with nephrotic syndrome are at risk for thromboembolic complications, there is no clear evidence supporting prophylactic anticoagulation. Supportive measures to reduce the risk of thromboembolism include mobilization and avoiding intravascular volume depletion. If thrombosis does occur, anticoagulation should be initiated.

As for long-term management of nephrotic syndrome, identification of the underlying cause is necessary. Greater than 90% of patients with MCD will respond to glucocorticoid therapy. Given the high frequency of MCD as the cause of idiopathic nephrotic syndrome and the favorable response of MCD to glucocorticoid therapy, an empiric trial of glucocorticoid therapy without confirmatory pathology is often provided to prepubertal children with suggestive clinical characteristics (between 1 and 10 years of age at presentation; normal renal function, blood pressure, and complement levels; benign urine sediment). Adolescents are also considered for empiric therapy, though obtaining a renal biopsy prior to therapy or after a defined period of glucocorticoid therapy without response would be reasonable given the increased occurrence of FSGS, MPGN, and membranous nephropathy in this age group. Patients with idiopathic nephrotic syndrome are further classified on the basis of their response to glucocorticoid therapy: glucocorticoid-responsive, glucocorticoid-dependent, and glucocorticoid-resistant nephrotic syndrome. Patients with responsive disease have a favorable long-term prognosis, and those with resistant pattern have a more guarded prognosis.

CHRONIC KIDNEY DISEASE

CLINICAL PEARLS AND PITFALLS

- Children may present to the emergency department with previously undiagnosed CKD.
- Life-threatening electrolyte and acid-base disturbances may be present on presentation requiring emergent intervention.
- Management must focus on restoring homeostasis while treating any potential underlying causes.
- Patients may require emergent RRT.

Current Evidence

The definition of CKD is based upon persistent structural or functional abnormalities, which may be associated with reduced or normal GFR. It may be due to congenital or acquired pathologies. The natural history of CKD is variable and depends upon the severity of the underlying kidney damage. A significant insult or progressive loss of functioning nephron mass may lead to end-stage renal disease (ESRD). In 2002, the National Kidney Foundation Kidney Disease Outcomes Quality Initiative published diagnostic criteria and a classification scheme to define the stages of CKD in patients older than 2 years (Table 108.15).

TABLE 108.15

STAGES OF CHRONIC KIDNEY DISEASE

Stage	Description	GFR (mL/min/1.73 m^2)
1	Kidney damage with normal or increased GFR	≥90
2	Kidney damage with mildly decreased GFR	60–89
3	Moderately decreased GFR	30–59
4	Severely decreased GFR	15–29
5	Kidney failure	<15 (or dialysis)

Chronic kidney disease is defined as either kidney damage of GFR <60 mL/min/1.73 m^2 or ≥3 mo. Kidney damage is defined as pathologic abnormalities or makers of damage, including abnormalities in blood or urine tests or imaging studies.
Adapted from Hogg RJ, Furth S, LemLey KV, et al. National Kidney Foundation's Kidney Disease Outcomes Quality Initiative clinical practice guidelines for chronic kidney disease in children and adolescents: evaluation, classification, and stratification. *Pediatrics* 2003;111:1416–1421.

Goals of Treatment

Emphasis is placed on early detection and intervention, as measures to inhibit the progression of renal dysfunction include treating hypertension and reducing significant proteinuria. For children who progress to ESRD, therapies include chronic hemodialysis, peritoneal dialysis, and renal transplantation. Renal transplantation is recognized as the preferred treatment for children with ESRD, as restoration of normal renal physiologic function can greatly improve the child's quality of life.

Clinical Considerations

Clinical recognition. The clinical presentation of CKD will depend upon the severity of the renal dysfunction and the underlying cause. Children with mild CKD (stage 1 and 2) and no other comorbidities may be asymptomatic. Children with more severe CKD are at increased likelihood for associated signs and symptoms such as fatigue, anorexia, and poor growth. Furthermore, these children may present for emergent care with a variety of complaints directly related to renal dysfunction including hypertension, volume overload, anemia, and severe electrolyte or acid–base abnormalities. They may also present with illness attributable to the underlying disorder, such as urinary tract infections in those with complex urologic disease and symptoms of systemic inflammation in those with systemic vasculitis. Children with CKD have limited renal reserve and are susceptible to AKI superimposed on chronic insufficiency, which will increase the risk for metabolic derangements and volume excess.

Triage considerations. Patients with CKD may present in extremis due to fluid or electrolyte imbalances. Cardiopulmonary function may be severely compromised due to volume excess. Patients may demonstrate life-threatening dysrhythmias due to electrolyte disturbances. Altered mental status may be secondary to azotemia, electrolyte, or acid–base abnormalities. Triage will depend on the patient's clinical status at the time of presentation.

Clinical assessment. Though many children with CKD who present for emergent care have a known history of renal disease, some will present with previous unknown CKD. For those with a new diagnosis, the physician should inquire about previous episodes of urinary tract infections as well as signs of concentrating defects or urologic disease, such as polyuria, polydipsia, and enuresis. To evaluate for signs consistent with chronic glomerulonephritis, history of gross hematuria, edema, rashes, or evidence of systemic inflammation should be sought. A review of family history should include inquiries of urologic disease, vesicoureteral reflux, progressive kidney disease, cystic kidney disease, and early-onset hypertension.

The physical evaluation of a child with CKD must include accurate assessment of blood pressure, cardiopulmonary examination, volume status, and growth parameters. Initial laboratory studies should be guided by the presenting complaint and history, though assessment of blood counts, electrolytes (including calcium and phosphorus), acid–base status, and renal function should be performed. The GFR may be estimated by using the Schwartz formula (Table 108.13), which takes into account the serum creatinine and the patient's height and gender. However, it must be acknowledged that this formula overestimates GFR especially at levels of decreased function. Urinalysis should also be performed. Most patients with congenital dysplasia or reflux nephropathy will have bland urine sediments and modest amounts of proteinuria. Significant hematuria, heavy proteinuria, and active urine sediment with glomerular hematuria and cellular casts would be consistent with glomerular disease. Further laboratory studies should be guided by the presentation of illness and clinical suspicion.

For all children with newly diagnosed CKD of unknown etiology and for many children with known urologic disease, a renal ultrasound is indicated. This can provide a valuable assessment of the renal parenchyma and the urologic tract. Ultrasound can detect such disorders as renal dysplasia, renal cortical thinning consistent with reflux nephropathy, cystic kidney disease, urinary tract obstruction, and screen for renal vascular disease. Kidneys that appear relatively normal but enlarged, are more suggestive of an acute or reversible process. Small kidneys would be consistent with a chronic process and parenchymal scarring. Imaging requiring intravenous contrast including gadolinium may worsen renal injury and should be avoided when possible or used in conjunction with consultation of a pediatric nephrologist or radiologist.

Management. The treatment of children with CKD can range from routine care to intensive management. If a child with CKD presents to the emergency department with a significant illness, treatment should be coordinated with a pediatric nephrologist when possible. The initial approach should identify reversible causes of decreased renal function, such as intravascular volume depletion and use of nephrotoxic medications (i.e., NSAIDs). Children who have decreased effective circulating volume should be provided intravenous isotonic fluid if oral hydration is expected to be insufficient or not well tolerated. Bolus intravenous fluid can be provided at 10 mL per kg and should be followed by repeated assessment to determine if further intravenous fluid is warranted. Patients presenting in shock may require more aggressive fluid resuscitation. Subsequent fluid rates should be provided on the basis of ongoing losses and urine flow to ensure adequate perfusion and avoid volume excess.

With severe decline in GFR, sodium and water retention may develop and lead to clinical signs of volume overload. Diuretic therapy should be trialed for treatment of clinical volume overload, though may not be adequately effective. Furosemide at a dose of 0.5 to 2 mg per kg may be given intravenously, recognizing that higher doses may be required to achieve the desired effect for those with more severe renal dysfunction. For children with sustained hypertension, therapy will depend on the degree and the chronicity of elevation. Severe hypertension with end-organ dysfunction or concern for impending end-organ dysfunction should be treated with short-acting intravenous antihypertensive medications such as hydralazine and labetalol. The goal of therapy is to lower the blood pressure by 20% to 30% or to a range that is not acutely dangerous within the first 2 to 3 hours. Blood pressure can then be controlled gradually over the next several days or longer. ACE inhibitors and ARB therapy are generally well tolerated in early stages of CKD and may slow the progression of CKD over time, especially in those with proteinuria. However, in more severe CKD, these agents may result in dangerous elevations of serum potassium and decreased GFR. For those children with CKD on ACE inhibitor or ARB therapy chronically, these medications may need to be temporarily held during periods of acute deterioration of renal function.

Electrolyte and acid–base abnormalities are common in CKD and include hyperkalemia, hypocalcemia, hyperphosphatemia, and metabolic acidosis. The treatment of these electrolyte and acid–base disturbances was previously discussed. Of note, the metabolic disturbances associated with CKD generally develop gradually, and therefore, immediate correction may not be warranted and may, in fact, be deleterious. Given the potential for cardiac dysrhythmias, hyperkalemia should be addressed urgently. In clinically stable patients with concurrent hypocalcemia and acidosis, the potential risk for tetany with alkali therapy should be considered. If clinically reasonable, hypocalcemia should be treated initially, and this can be achieved with oral calcium if the patient is asymptomatic.

For some children with severe CKD or AKI superimposed on CKD, supportive medical management will be insufficient, and RRT will be required. Accepted indications for RRT include severe fluid overload, refractory hyperkalemia, and severe uremia. Modalities of dialysis include continuous renal replacement, intermittent hemodialysis, and peritoneal dialysis. The modality utilized will depend on the clinical circumstances, local resources, and clinician preference.

Suggested Readings and Key References

Hypovolemia and Disorders of Sodium Homeostasis

Goldman RD, Friedman JN, Parkin PC. Validation of the clinical dehydration scale for children with acute gastroenteritis. *Pediatrics* 2008;122:545–549.

Holliday MA, Friedman AL, Segar WE, et al. Acute hospital-induced hyponatremia in children: a physiologic approach. *J Pediatr* 2004; 145:584–587.

Hoorn EJ, Geary D, Robb M, et al. Acute hyponatremia related to intravenous fluid administration in hospitalized children: an observational study. *Pediatrics* 2004;113:1279–1284.

King CK, Glass R, Bresee JS, et al. Managing acute gastroenteritis among children: oral rehydration, maintenance, and nutritional therapy. *MMWR Recomm Rep* 2003;52:1–16.

Moritz ML, Ayus JC. Prevention of hospital-acquired hyponatremia: a case for using isotonic saline. *Pediatrics* 2003;111:227–230.

Moritz ML, Ayus JC. Preventing neurological complications from dysnatremias in children. *Pediatr Nephrol* 2005;20:1687–1700.

Neville KA, Verge CF, O'Meara MW, et al. High antidiuretic hormone levels and hyponatremia in children with gastroenteritis. *Pediatrics* 2005;116:1401–1407.

Neville KA, Verge CF, Rosenberg AR, et al. Isotonic is better than hypotonic saline for intravenous rehydration of children with gastroenteritis: a prospective randomised study. *Arch Dis Child* 2006; 91:226–232.

Rouhani S, Meloney L, Ahn R, et al. Alternative rehydration methods: a systematic review and lessons for resource-limited care. *Pediatrics* 2011;127:e748–e757.

Steiner MJ, DeWalt DA, Byerley JS. Is this child dehydrated? *JAMA* 2004;291:2746–2754.

Disorders of Potassium and Calcium Homeostasis

Benjamin RW, Moats-Staats BM, Calikoglu A, et al. Hypercalcemia in children. *Pediatr Endocrinol Rev* 2008;5:778–784.

Mahoney BA, Smith WA, Lo DS, et al. Emergency interventions for hyperkalemia. *Cochrane Database Syst Rev* 2005;(2):CD003235.

Masilamani K, van der Voort J. The management of acute hyperkalaemia in neonates and children. *Arch Dis Child* 2012;97:376–380.

Singh J, Moghal N, Pearce SH, et al. The investigation of hypocalcaemia and rickets. *Arch Dis Child* 2003;88:403–407.

Weisberg LS. Management of severe hyperkalemia. *Crit Care Med* 2008;36:3246–3251.

Disorders of Acid–Base Homeostasis

Aschner JL, Poland RL. Sodium bicarbonate: basically useless therapy. *Pediatrics* 2008;122:831–835.

Galla JH. Metabolic alkalosis. *J Am Soc Nephrol* 2000;11:369–375.

Kraut JA, Kurtz I. Use of base in the treatment of severe acidemic states. *Am J Kidney Dis* 2001;38:703–727.

Parker MJ, Parshuram CS. Sodium bicarbonate use in shock and cardiac arrest: attitudes of pediatric acute care physicians. *Crit Care Med* 2013;41:2188–2195.

Acute Kidney Injury

Andreoli SP. Acute kidney injury in children. *Pediatr Nephrol* 2009; 24:253–263.

Eison TM, Ault BH, Jones DP, et al. Post-streptococcal acute glomerulonephritis in children: clinical features and pathogenesis. *Pediatr Nephrol* 2011;26:165–180.

Fortenberry JD, Paden ML, Goldstein SL. Acute kidney injury in children: an update on diagnosis and treatment. *Pediatr Clin North Am* 2013;60:669–688.

Gerber A, Karch H, Allerberger F, et al. Clinical course and the role of shiga toxin-producing escherichia coli infection in the hemolytic-uremic syndrome in pediatric patients, 1997–2000, in Germany and Austria: a prospective study. *J Infect Dis* 2002;186:493–500.

Pohl M. Henoch-Schönlein purpura nephritis. *Pediatr Nephrol* 2015; 30(2):245–252.

Scharman EJ, Troutman WG. Prevention of kidney injury following rhabdomyolysis: a systematic review. *Arch Dis Child* 2010;95(11): 877–882.

Nephrotic Syndrome

Chiang CK, Inagi R. Glomerular diseases: genetic causes and future therapeutics. *Nat Rev Nephrol* 2010;6:539–554.

Eddy AA, Symons JM. Nephrotic syndrome in childhood. *Lancet* 2003;362:629–639.

Gipson DS, Massengill SF, Yao L, et al. Management of childhood onset nephrotic syndrome. *Pediatrics* 2009;124:747–757.

Hogg RJ, Portman RJ, Milliner D, et al. Evaluation and management of proteinuria and nephrotic syndrome in children: recommendations from a pediatric nephrology panel established at the National Kidney Foundation conference on proteinuria, albuminuria, risk, assessment, detection, and elimination (PARADE). *Pediatrics* 2000; 105:1242–1249.

Chronic Kidney Disease

Copelovitch L, Warady BA, Furth SL. Insights from the chronic kidney disease in children (CKiD) study. *Clin J Am Soc Nephrol* 2011;6: 2047–2053.

Hogg RJ, Furth S, LemLey KV, et al. National Kidney Foundation's Kidney Disease Outcomes Quality Initiative clinical practice guidelines for chronic kidney disease in children and adolescents: evaluation, classification, and stratification. *Pediatrics* 2003;111: 1416–1421.

Schwartz GJ, Munoz A, Schneider MF, et al. New equations to estimate GFR in children with CKD. *J Am Soc Nephrol* 2009;20:629–637.

Wong H, Mylrea K, Feber J, et al. Prevalence of complications in children with chronic kidney disease according to KDOQI. *Kidney Int* 2006;70:585–590.

Wuhl E, Schaefer F. Therapeutic strategies to slow chronic kidney disease progression. *Pediatr Nephrol* 2008;23:705–716.

CHAPTER 109 ■ RHEUMATOLOGIC EMERGENCIES

THERESA M. BECKER, DO AND MELISSA M. HAZEN, MD

GOALS OF EMERGENCY CARE

Pediatric rheumatologic conditions are rare and are typically chronic conditions with an indolent onset rather than acute conditions likely to bring a child to the emergency department (ED). Nonetheless, there are several reasons why children with rheumatologic conditions may present to the ED. First, the majority of rheumatologic conditions involve a myriad of signs and symptoms affecting many organ systems, which may bring an exasperated family to the ED searching for an elusive diagnosis. Second, arthritis, lupus, and vasculitis (especially Kawasaki disease [KD]) may have acute and life-threatening complications that require rapid initiation of appropriate therapy. Finally, the treatment of rheumatologic disorders is becoming more sophisticated and more specialized, involving combinations of anti-inflammatory, immunosuppressive, and biologic agents with a wide spectrum of undesired effects. Often a key challenge is differentiating the effects of underlying disease from the effects of therapy. Thus, the goals of emergency care are the prompt recognition of these conditions, and the expeditious use of medical therapy to treat the complications of the diseases and the side effects of drug therapy.

KEY POINTS

- Kawasaki disease requires treatment in the first 10 days of the illness in order to achieve an optimal clinical outcome.
- Many rheumatologic conditions are treated with medications that suppress the immune system.
- Stress doses of corticosteroids may be required for fever and other acute illnesses.
- Childhood vasculitis may affect any organ system and may present indolently or acutely with life-threatening end-organ involvement.
- Juvenile idiopathic arthritis subtypes are varied in their presentation and associated with different articular and extra-articular complications.
- Hemophagocytic lymphohistiocytosis (HLH) and macrophage activation syndrome (MAS) or reactive HLH should be considered in an ill child with persistent fever, organomegaly, and neurologic symptoms with systemic inflammation, cytopenias, and/or liver dysfunction.

RELATED CHAPTERS

Signs and Symptoms
- Coma: Chapter 12
- Edema: Chapter 20
- Gastrointestinal Bleeding: Chapter 28
- Hypertension: Chapter 33
- Pain: Abdomen: Chapter 48
- Seizures: Chapter 67

Medical, Surgical, and Trauma Emergencies
- Cardiac Emergencies: Chapter 94
- Gastrointestinal Emergencies: Chapter 99
- Infectious Disease Emergencies: Chapter 102
- Neurologic Emergencies: Chapter 105
- Pulmonary Emergencies: Chapter 107
- Renal and Electrolyte Emergencies: Chapter 108
- Abdominal Emergencies: Chapter 124
- Neurosurgical Emergencies: Chapter 130
- Behavioral and Psychiatric Emergencies: Chapter 134

SYSTEMIC LUPUS ERYTHEMATOSUS

CLINICAL PEARLS AND PITFALLS

- The most common initial symptoms are the gradual onset of fever, fatigue, and generalized lymphadenopathy.
- The clinical presentation is highly variable and may include diverse body systems.
- The classic malar rash is present in only one-half of pediatric patients at presentation.
- Infection is the major cause of mortality in childhood systemic lupus erythematous (SLE) because of immune dysregulation inherent in the disease and the immunosuppressant medications used to treat SLE.
- Patients taking corticosteroids may require stress doses during acute febrile illness.
- Corticosteroids may mask the symptoms of pain.

Current Evidence

SLE is a multisystem disease that is both pleomorphic in its presentation and variable in its clinical course. In many ways, it is the quintessential autoimmune disease, with antibodies to cellular constituents causing immune-mediated attack on various organs including the skin, joints, peripheral and central nervous system, kidneys, and serosal surfaces. In children, the disease is more severe, with a higher incidence of renal and neurologic involvement.

The classification system for SLE was revised in 2012, reflecting a harmonization between the newer criteria of the Systemic Lupus International Collaborating Clinics (SLICC) group and the criteria of the American College of Rheumatology (ACR), which had been the standard classification system for decades. Table 109.1 lists the ACR criteria and the updated revised SLICC criteria and definitions. This newer classification differs from the 1997 ACR criteria in two significant ways. First, the SLICC criteria were expanded to include

TABLE 109.1

CRITERIA FOR CLASSIFICATION OF SYSTEMIC LUPUS ERYTHEMATOUS

ACR criteria-1997		SLICC criteria-2012	
Criterion	**Definition**	**Criterion**	**Definition**
Malar rash	Fixed erythema, flat or raised, over the malar eminences, tending to spare the nasolabial folds	**Acute cutaneous lupus**	Lupus malar rash (do not count if malar discoid); bullous lupus; toxic epidermal necrolysis variant of SLE; maculopapular lupus rash; photosensitive lupus rash; (in the absence of dermatomyositis); *or* subacute cutaneous lupus (nonindurated psoriasiform and/or annular polycyclic lesions that resolve without scarring, although occasionally with postinflammatory dyspigmentation or telangiectasias)
Discoid rash	Erythematous raised patches with adherent keratotic scaling and follicular plugging; atrophic scaring may occur in older lesions	**Chronic cutaneous lupus**	Classic discoid rash localized (above the neck); generalized (above and below the neck); hypertrophic (verrucous) lupus; lupus panniculitis (profundus); mucosal lupus; lupus erythematosus tumidus; chilblains lupus; *or* discoid lupus/lichen planus overlap
Photosensitivity	Skin rash as a result of unusual reaction to sunlight, by patient history or physician observation		
Oral ulcers	Oral or nasopharyngeal ulceration, usually painless, observed by a physician	**Oral/nasal ulcers**	Palate, buccal, tongue, *or* nasal ulcers (in the absence of other causes, such as vasculitis, Behcet's, infection [herpes], inflammatory bowel disease, reactive arthritis, and acidic foods)
		Nonscarring alopecia	Diffuse thinning or hair fragility with visible broken hairs (in the absence of other causes such as alopecia areata, drugs, iron deficiency and androgenic alopecia)
Arthritis	Nonerosive arthritis involving two or more peripheral joints, characterized by tenderness, swelling, or effusion	**Synovitis involving two or more joints**	Characterized by swelling or effusion *or* tenderness in two or more joints and 30 minutes or more of morning stiffness
Pleuritis or pericarditis	Pleuritis—convincing history or pleuritic pain or rub heard by a physician or evidence of pleural effusion *or* Pericarditis—documented by EKG, rub, or evidence of pericardial effusion on echocardiography	**Serositis**	Typical pleurisy for more than 1 day *or* pleural effusions *or* pleural rub, *or* typical pericardial pain (pain with recumbency improved by sitting forward) for more than 1 day, *or* pericardial effusion, *or* pericardial rub or pericarditis by EKG in the absence of other causes, such as infection, uremia, and Dressler's pericarditis
Renal disorder	Persistent proteinuria >0.5 g/day or >3% if quantitation not performed *or* cellular casts—may be red cell, hemoglobin, granular, tubular, or mixed	**Renal disorder**	Urine protein-to-creatine ratio (or 24-hr urine protein) representing 500 mg protein/24 hrs *or* red blood cell casts
Neurologic disorder	Seizures *or* psychosis—in the absence of offending drugs or known metabolic derangements (uremia, ketoacidosis, or electrolyte imbalance)	**Neurologic disorder**	Seizures; psychosis; mononeuritis multiplex (in the absence of other known causes such as primary vasculitis); myelitis; peripheral or cranial neuropathy (in the absence of other causes, such as primary vasculitis, infection, and diabetes mellitus); acute confusional state (in the absence of other causes, including toxic–metabolic, uremia, drugs)
Hematologic disorder	Hemolytic anemia—with reticulocytosis *or* Leukopenia—<4,000/mm^3 total on two or more occasions *or* Lymphopenia—<1,500/mm^3 on two or more occasions *or* Thrombocytopenia—<100,000/mm^3 in the absence of offending drugs	**Hemolytic anemia**	

(continued)

TABLE 109.1

CRITERIA FOR CLASSIFICATION OF SYSTEMIC LUPUS ERYTHEMATOUS (*CONTINUED*)

ACR criteria-1997		SLICC criteria-2012	
Criterion	**Definition**	**Criterion**	**Definition**
		Leukopenia or lymphopenia	Leukopenia (<4,000/mm^3 at least once) (in the absence of other known causes, such as Felty syndrome, drugs, and portal hypertension) *or*
		Thrombocytopenia	Lymphopenia (<1,000/mm^3) at least once (in the absence of other known causes such as drugs, portal hypertension, and TTP)
		Immunologic criteria	(<100,000/mm^3) at least once (in the absence of other known causes such as drugs, portal hypertension, and TTP)
Immunologic disorders	Positive antiphospholipid antibody *or* Anti-DNA—antibody to native DNA in abnormal titer *or* Anti-Sm—presence of antibody to Sm nuclear antigen *or* False-positive serologic test for syphilis known to be positive by *Treponema pallidum* immobilization *or* fluorescent treponemal antibody absorption test	**ANA**	ANA level above laboratory reference range
Antinuclear antibody	An abnormal titer of antinuclear antibody by immunofluorescence or an equivalent assay at any point in time and in the absence of drugs known to be associated with "drug-induced lupus" syndrome	**Anti-ds DNA antibody**	Anti-ds DNA above laboratory reference range, except ELISA: Twice above laboratory reference range
		Anti-Sm	Presence of antibody to Sm nuclear antigen
		Antiphospholipid	Antiphospholipid antibody positive, by any of the following: Lupus anticoagulant; false-positive RPR; medium or high titer anticardiolipin (IgA, IgG, or IgM); or positive test result for anti–beta-2 glycoprotein I (IgA, IgG, or IgM)
		Low complement	Low C3; low C4; or low CH50
		Direct Coombs test	Direct Coombs test *in the absence of hemolytic anemia*

17 individual elements, rather than 11, thus greatly expanding the breadth of the diagnosis. Secondly, the diagnosis rests on the presence of one immunologic criterion as well as the presence of at least one clinical criterion, rather than the previous format that relied on only clinical symptoms in some cases. The SLICC criteria have improved sensitivity (97%) but decreased specificity (84%) when compared to the 1997 ACR criteria.

Although the new criteria and definitions were intended as classification symptoms to be used for research, they are often used by clinicians to establish a diagnosis. Nonetheless, patients may have SLE and not fulfill criteria, or they may meet criteria despite having another illness.

The SLICC criteria begin with four separate dermatologic manifestations and differentiates acute from chronic lesions. Acute cutaneous lupus includes the typical malar erythematous rash with butterfly distribution and sparing of the nasolabial folds, as well as photosensitivity and bullous lupus. Chronic cutaneous lupus includes classical discoid lesions both localized and generalized (Fig. 109.1). Mucosal lesions (macular and ulcerative) may involve the nose or the mouth, particularly the palate (Fig. 109.2) and are usually painless. Nonscarring alopecia in the absence of other causes such as alopecia areata, drugs, and iron deficiency is now its own separate criterion. The arthritis criteria include joint-line tenderness with 30 minutes of morning stiffness. The renal criteria now include measurement of proteinuria by the urine protein/creatinine ratio without the requirement of a time frame for collection.

In contrast to the older ACR criteria that included only seizures or psychosis as neurologic manifestations of disease, the new criteria include many other neurologic manifestations, including myelitis, peripheral or cranial neuropathy, mononeuritis multiplex, and acute confusional state. The hematologic criteria have been subdivided into three categories: hemolytic anemia, leukopenia (<4,000 per mm^3) *OR* lymphopenia (<1,000 per mm^3), and thrombocytopenia (<100,000 per mm^3). Finally, the immunologic criterion was expanded to include newly discovered antibodies present in SLE.

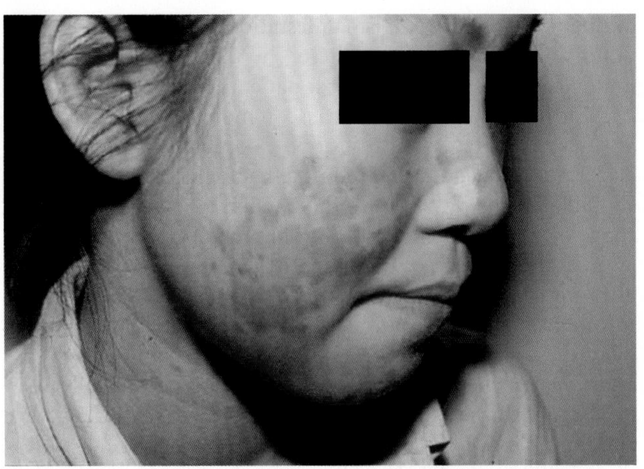

FIGURE 109.1 Adolescent girl with discoid lesions in malar distribution.

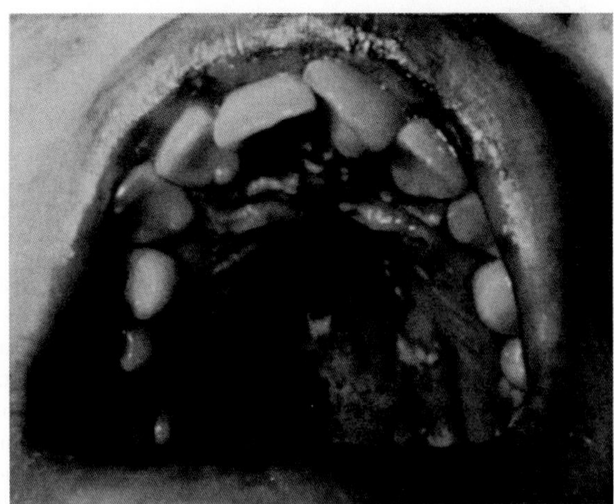

FIGURE 109.2 Mucosal lesions (macules and ulcers) of the palate in an adolescent girl with active lupus.

Goals of Treatment

SLE is often more severe in children than in adults. Although adult lupus patients are more likely to die of complications, children and adolescents with lupus are more likely to succumb earlier, during the acute stages of the disease. Common causes of death within the first 2 years of diagnosis are pancreatitis, pulmonary hemorrhage, infection, thromboembolic disease, and active neuropsychiatric disease. Delayed diagnosis and treatment are strong risk factors for morbidity and mortality in pediatric lupus. In view of the fact that cumulative disease activity over time correlates with damage from the disease, expedient diagnosis and appropriately aggressive treatment is particularly critical for children. Thus, pediatricians need to maintain a high index of suspicion for lupus, and physicians experienced in the care of children with SLE should participate in the diagnosis and management of all pediatric lupus patients.

Clinical Considerations

Clinical Recognition

Although SLE is often considered a disease of adulthood, up to 20% of lupus patients are diagnosed during the first two decades of life. Childhood SLE affects girls more often than boys but this gender difference occurs to a lesser extent than in adults. Incidence and prevalence rates vary by ethnicity and are higher in Hispanic, Asian, Native American, and African populations. The mean age of diagnosis in children is approximately 12 to 13 years. The onset of SLE may be insidious or acute. The initial presentation usually includes constitutional features, such as fever, malaise, and weight loss, in addition to manifestations of specific organ involvement such as rash, pericarditis, arthritis, or seizures. Because virtually any part of the body may be affected by SLE, patients may present with a bewildering variety of signs and symptoms. Although many of these are nonspecific, the examiner's level of suspicion for possible SLE should increase as the number of involved organ systems increases. Further, although SLE presents with a wide array of symptoms, the majority of pediatric cases present with a recognizable constellation of complaints related to musculoskeletal, cutaneous, renal, and hematologic involvement. In French and Canadian studies, the most common presenting manifestations in children are hematologic (anemia, lymphopenia, leukopenia, and/or thrombocytopenia); mucocutaneous (malar rash and/or ulcers); musculoskeletal (arthritis or arthralgia); presence of fever; and renal abnormalities (nephritis or nephritic syndrome). (Please refer to the SLICC criteria discussed above for specific details about making the diagnosis.)

Triage Considerations

Fever in a child with SLE represents a potential emergency. Children with SLE are at increased risk of infections from their disease activity and also from the immunosuppressive therapies that they receive to control their illness. Patients with fever should be evaluated rapidly and thoroughly, and often will be treated empirically with broad-spectrum antibiotics, while awaiting the results of the diagnostic evaluation. Patients taking corticosteroids may require stress doses during acute febrile illness. Children with SLE are also at increased risk for a wide variety of cardiac, pulmonary, and gastrointestinal (GI) complications, many of which are life-threatening. See Table 109.3, which describes the complications of SLE.

Clinical Assessment

Arthritis in SLE is usually symmetric, involving both large and small joints. Swollen joints may be quite painful, but they are usually not erythematous. Cutaneous lesions are present in more than 85% of patients with SLE. The typical malar rash with butterfly distribution is present at diagnosis about half the time. Features that help to distinguish it from other rashes are sparing of the nasolabial folds, extension onto the nose, and extension of the rash onto the chin. Painless oral or nasal ulcerations, alopecia, and photosensitivity are common. Discoid lesions are less frequent in children but when seen are characteristic (Fig. 109.1). Evidence of renal disease is present in approximately 50% of children with SLE at the time of presentation, with nearly 90% developing some degree of renal involvement during the course of their disease. This is significantly higher than in adult patients, in whom renal disease develops in about half. Lupus nephritis is usually asymptomatic, although close questioning often reveals nocturia due to impaired renal concentrating mechanisms. Edema or hypertension may be clues to involvement of the kidney. Despite significant improvements in treatment, the extent of renal involvement remains the single most important determinant of prognosis in SLE, and therefore will highly influence choice of immunosuppressive therapy. Thus, most children with lupus have a renal biopsy to more precisely characterize the pathology and help optimize the therapeutic regimen.

Clinical evidence of CNS involvement may occur at disease onset or later in the course. Symptoms and signs referable to the CNS include headache, seizures, polyneuropathy, hemiparesis/hemiplegia, and ophthalmoplegia. Particularly in the ED setting, the clinician should be aware of the risk of stroke (both thrombotic and hemorrhagic) and of sinus vein thrombosis in children with lupus. Chorea is the most common movement disorder and may be a presenting sign; Lyme disease (LD) and rheumatic fever must also be considered in such cases. Cranial nerve palsies most commonly involve the optic nerve, trigeminal nerve, and nerves controlling the extraocular muscles. Myasthenia gravis should be excluded if any extraocular muscles are involved. Neuropsychiatric manifestations include mood disorders, hallucinations, memory alterations, and psychosis; rarely, psychiatric symptoms may be the first clinical manifestation of childhood lupus.

Pericarditis is the most prevalent form of cardiopulmonary involvement in SLE. Myocarditis occurs less frequently. Heart murmurs caused by valvular lesions are not common, but asymptomatic vegetations on valve leaflets are seen at autopsy in most patients (Libman–Sack endocarditis), which is why patients with SLE are at increased risk for subacute bacterial endocarditis. Abnormal exercise thallium myocardial perfusion scans have been described in pediatric patients with no history of coronary symptoms, and myocardial infarctions are reported in children with lupus. Thus, the possibility of myocardial ischemia should be kept in mind if a child with lupus develops acute chest pain. Lupus patients are also at risk for early atherosclerosis, with a resultant increased risk of cardiac disease.

Pleuropulmonary involvement occurs in greater than 50% of cases of SLE. Unilateral or bilateral pleural effusions may occur, and pulmonary hemorrhage, although uncommon, also occurs in children with SLE. Pulmonary function testing (PFT) demonstrating an elevated D_{LCO} offers a readily available, noninvasive technique for identifying blood in the lungs. Pulmonary embolus, particularly in children with antiphospholipid antibodies, also must be considered in children with the acute onset of chest pain. For any SLE patient with pleuropulmonary manifestations, disease-related involvement must be distinguished from intercurrent infection, CHF, aspiration pneumonia, and renal failure.

Common GI manifestations include nausea, vomiting, and anorexia. Persistent localized abdominal pain should suggest specific organ involvement, such as pancreatitis or gastric ulcer, both of which may occur from the disease or secondary to medical therapy. Malabsorption syndrome may be a manifestation of SLE. When accompanied by melena, it suggests poorly controlled disease complicated by GI vasculitis. This is associated with a 50% mortality rate without expeditious evaluation and treatment. Of course, abdominal pain in SLE is not always related to the underlying disease but may stem from other causes, including appendicitis, ruptured ovarian cyst, or pelvic inflammatory disease. Further complicating evaluation is the fact that manifestations of any of these conditions may be masked or altered by the corticosteroids and immunosuppressive agents most patients receive.

Mild to moderate anemia is common in SLE. Hemolytic anemia associated with a positive Coombs test is most characteristic. An acute decrease in the hemoglobin or hematocrit should alert the physician to the possibility of internal hemorrhage or massive hemolysis. Autoimmune thrombocytopenia, even in the absence of offending drugs, is commonly seen in SLE; up to 20% of adults initially diagnosed with idiopathic thrombocytopenic purpura (ITP) progress to full-blown lupus over the ensuing years. Leukopenia and lymphopenia are additional hematologic abnormalities characteristically seen in SLE; apart from viral infections and drug toxicity, few other conditions cause children's lymphocyte counts to fall to less than 1,000 per mm^3. Circulating antibodies to specific clotting factors, deficiencies of one or more clotting factors, and abnormal platelet function, often lead to abnormal hemostasis in SLE. A specific circulating anticoagulant, the "lupus anticoagulant," has been described in up to 10% of patients. The antibody is so named because in vitro assays of coagulation are prolonged in its presence. In vivo, this antibody predisposes to arterial or venous thrombosis.

Proteinuria, hematuria, and cellular casts are the usual urinary abnormalities. Acute renal failure and nephrotic syndrome are possible complications of SLE (see Chapter 108 Renal and Electrolyte Emergencies).

The most important single test in children suspected of having SLE is measurement of antinuclear antibody (ANA) titers. Up to 2% of normal children have low to intermediate titers of ANA at any time; in most cases, these antibodies are transient by-products of a viral infection. In SLE, the ANA titer is typically quite high—significant levels are greater than 1:512—and often it is accompanied by antibodies to double-stranded DNA, a more specific marker for lupus. The level for the anti–double-stranded DNA (anti-ds DNA) should be above the laboratory reference range, and if tested by ELISA, should be twice that of the upper limit of the laboratory reference range. Antiphospholipid antibodies may be positive as determined by detecting any of the following: the lupus anticoagulant, false-positive RPR, medium or high titer anticardiolipin (IgA, IgG, or IgM), or presence of anti–beta-2 glycoprotein I antibodies (IgA, IgG, or IgM). Finally, low complement levels: C3, C4, or total CH50, and a direct Coombs test in the absence of hemolytic anemia, are the additional immunologic tests that may point the clinician to a diagnosis of SLE. Nonetheless, it must be remembered that SLE may only be diagnosed in the presence of evidence of multiple organ system involvement, so no laboratory study is pathognomonic.

Management

There is no specific treatment for SLE. Rather, therapy consists of immunosuppression, the type and intensity of which are dictated by the particular organ systems affected. Patients with mild disease (fever and/or arthritis) without nephritis generally receive one of the nonsteroidal anti-inflammatory drugs (NSAIDs) (e.g., naproxen sodium 15 to 20 mg/kg/day, maximum 1,000 mg). Severe systemic features, on the other hand, usually require treatment with oral or IV corticosteroids, with doses divided three or four times daily in the most florid cases. Patients with life-threatening disease,

TABLE 109.2

IMMUNOMODULATORY AGENTS FOR THE TREATMENT OF SLE IN CHILDREN

	Biologic effects	Principal toxicities	Monitor
Hydroxychloroquine	Blocks lysosome processing of autoantigens	Retinopathy, nausea, rash, agranulocytosis	Ophthalmology evaluation every 6 mo, CBC, LFTs every 3–6 mo
Azathioprine	Precursor of 6-MP; blocks purine synthesis	Bone marrow suppression, infection (especially zoster), nausea, hepatitis, rash	CBC, lymphocyte count, LFTs
Mycophenolate mofetil	Blocks purine synthesis	Bone marrow suppression, infections, nausea, diarrhea	CBC, lymphocyte count
Cyclophosphamide	Alkylates DNA leading to cytotoxicity	Bone marrow suppression, opportunistic infections, nausea, alopecia, bladder toxicity, infertility, cardiotoxicity	WBC, UA, BUN/Cr
Rituximab	Chimeric anti-CD20 monoclonal antibody that depletes B-cells	Tumor lysis syndrome, anaphylaxis, hypogammaglobulinemia, opportunistic infections	IgG level, lymphocyte count

SLE, systemic lupus erythematosus; CBC, complete blood cell count; LFT, liver function test; 6-MP, 6-mercaptopurine; DNA, deoxyribonucleic acid; WBC, white blood cells; UA, urinalysis; BUN/Cr, blood urea nitrogen/creatinine; CD20, B lymphocyte surface marker; IgG, immunoglobulin G.

particularly those with severe renal or CNS involvement, may require so-called "pulsed" doses of corticosteroids (IV methylprednisolone, 30 mg/kg/day, maximum 1.5 g), plasmapheresis, or an immunosuppressive agent (especially mycophenolate mofetil, azathioprine, rituximab, or cyclophosphamide) (Table 109.2). Symptomatic management may be necessary for the treatment of seizures, psychosis, or acute renal failure. With rare exception, patients should also receive hydroxychloroquine, which has been shown to prolong disease-free remissions once signs and symptoms of active lupus are controlled. In any event, close follow-up is mandatory to detect clinical and serologic evidence of disease flares, and to monitor drug toxicity.

Management of Complications and Emergencies

Infections in SLE. Management of emergencies in patients with SLE first and foremost involves distinguishing primary disease manifestations from secondary complications (Table 109.3). Infection is the major cause of mortality in childhood SLE. Gram-negative bacilli (especially *Salmonella*), *Listeria, Candida, Aspergillus, Cryptococcus, Toxoplasma, Pneumocystis,* and varicella-zoster virus are some of the organisms associated with severe infections in SLE. Patients with SLE who are receiving corticosteroids or cytotoxic drugs are at even higher risk for developing viral, mycotic, and other opportunistic infections. The majority of these infections are diagnosed at autopsy, so clinicians must maintain a high level of suspicion for infection in all children with SLE.

Not all patients with lupus and suspected infection require hospitalization. Patients with minor infections who are not acutely ill or neutropenic may be treated with appropriate antibiotics given orally along with close follow-up. The dose of corticosteroids should also be increased to provide stress coverage (at least three times the physiologic need) in any acutely ill child who has received more than 20 mg of prednisone daily for more than 6 weeks within the previous 12 months. Acutely ill children, those with an absolute neutrophil count of less than 1,000 per mm^3, and those with pneumonia or the possibility of meningitis, require hospitalization for IV antibiotics while awaiting culture results.

Fever. Each febrile episode in a child with SLE represents a potential emergency. It is often difficult to determine whether the fever is secondary to infection, to a flare-up of the primary disease, or to a combination of both. In addition to usual laboratory testing, urinalysis and quantitative CRP provide a rapid and general overview of the patient's well-being. CH50 (or C4), C3, ANA, and anti-ds DNA, and extractable nuclear antigen (ENA) and possibly antiphospholipid antibody titers should be obtained in order to assess the degree to which the patient's SLE is active. An elevated CRP without other evidence of active SLE is highly suggestive of bacterial infection. Blood cultures are mandatory if no source of fever is apparent after a complete physical examination, and clinicians should have a low threshold for obtaining a chest x-ray, and for culturing CSF and other fluids when indicated. In most cases, children with SLE who develop fever without a readily apparent source should be given antibiotics pending culture results; abnormal splenic function places them at increased risk of rapid development of bacteremia and overwhelming sepsis from encapsulated organisms.

Renal Complications. Renal disease is a major cause of morbidity in SLE, so it is important to establish its presence and severity at the time of diagnosis, and to regularly monitor renal function thereafter. Clinical manifestations of lupus nephritis are often minimal. Signs of nephrotic syndrome or acute renal failure require a more thorough investigation that should include estimation of the protein in a 24-hour urine collection; creatinine clearance; measurement of C3, ANA, and anti-ds DNA antibodies; and renal biopsy. In a patient with SLE and documented renal disease, hospitalization is necessary in the presence of rapidly worsening renal status, hypertensive crisis, or severe complications of therapy.

TABLE 109.3

COMPLICATIONS OF SYSTEMIC LUPUS ERYTHEMATOSUS

	Symptoms and signs	Laboratory	Treatment[a]
Fever	Malaise	CBC, urinalysis, ESR, anti-DNA antibodies CH_{50}, C3 Cultures (blood, urine, CSF, stool and appropriate secretions) Chest radiograph Gallium scan	Prednisone 1–2 mg/kg/day
Infection	Fever, headache, seizure, cough, sputum, skin lesions, arthritis, disease flare, weight loss	Same as above	Intravenous antibiotics (broad spectrum) Reevaluate prednisone dose
Renal disease	Dehydration, fever, weight gain, hypertension, decreased urine output	Urinalysis, urine culture, 24-hr urine protein Serum creatinine Creatinine clearance Anti-DNA CH_{50}, C3, C4 CBC, ESR, platelets Electrolytes, BUN	Prednisone "pulse therapy" (as needed) Cytotoxic agents (azathioprine PO or cyclophosphamide IV) Plasmapheresis
Hemolytic anemia	Fatigue, malaise, pallor, dyspnea, edema	CBC, Coombs', reticulocyte count, haptoglobin Peripheral smear Total bilirubin	Prednisone 2 mg/kg/day Transfusion, if acute emergency (may need consultation with transfusion specialist to avoid acute hemolysis of transfused blood products)
Central nervous system	Seizures, coma, cranial nerve palsies, papilledema, hypertension psychosis	EEG, MRI, CT scan CSF—opening pressure, cell count, Gram and special stains, cultures	ICU admission Prednisone 2 mg/kg/day or pulse therapy Plasmapheresis Cytotoxic agents
Pleural effusion	Fever, chest pain, dyspnea, decreased breath sounds, splinting	Chest radiograph Thoracentesis—cell count, Gram stain, protein, glucose, culture, cytology	Thoracentesis, if indicated Oxygen, prednisone, cytotoxic agents
Peritonitis	Abdominal pain, fever, vomiting, diarrhea, tenderness, rigidity, hypoactive bowel sounds, melena	Radiograph (abdominal flat plate, cross-table, upright and/or lateral decubitus) Peritoneal aspiration—cell count, special stains, cultures CBC, electrolytes, ESR, ANA Test for occult blood in gastric contents and stool, nuclear scan	Surgical consult, NPO, IV hydration, NG tube, antacids, transfusion Prednisone Interventional radiology (if available)
Pancreatitis	Same	Serum amylase/lipase	IV hydration, NPO, adjust steroid dose, hyperalimentation
Pericarditis	Fever, chest pain, distended neck veins, decreased heart sounds, hepatomegaly	Chest radiograph, EKG Echocardiogram-2d CBC, ESR, blood culture, ANA	NSAIDs Prednisone 2 mg/kg/day Pericardiocentesis as needed
Raynaud phenomenon	Triple color change of fingers and/or toes; pain, swelling in digits	CBC, ESR, ANA, cryoglobulins Doppler flow studies	Protection from cold, biofeedback, analgesia, prednisone Calcium-channel blockers Sympathetic ganglion block
Ocular	Blurring or loss of vision, headache	Funduscopic examination CT scan	Lumbar puncture (caution), prednisone
Traverse myelitis	Paraplegia, paraparesis, pain, sensory level	CT, MRI, LP (once epidural abscess excluded), antiphospholipid antibody, lupus anticoagulant	Pulse dose methylprednisolone, cytotoxic agents, anticoagulation

[a]Treatment regimens (except for infectious category) assume that an infectious etiology has been excluded.

CBC, complete blood count; ESR, erythrocyte sedimentation rate; CSF, cerebrospinal fluid; BUN, blood urea nitrogen; PO, orally; IV, intravenously; EEG, encephalogram; MRI, magnetic resonance imaging; CT, computed tomography; ICU, intensive care unit; ANA, antinuclear antibody; NPO, nothing by mouth; NG, nasogastric; EKG, electrocardiogram; NSAIDs, nonsteroidal anti-inflammatory drugs; LP, lumbar puncture.

Treatment of renal disease is aimed at preserving renal function while minimizing medication toxicity. Selection of therapeutic agents depends on biopsy results and classification of renal involvement according to the World Health Organization classification, available at http://www.wolterskluwer-india.co.in/rheumatology/Rheumatology-Issue35.html. Active disease often may be managed with pharmacologic doses of corticosteroids (prednisone 1 to 2 mg/kg/day). In the presence of progressive renal failure, the patient should be hospitalized for more aggressive therapy. This generally includes divided doses of IV corticosteroids with or without an immunosuppressive agent such as cyclophosphamide. "Pulse" therapy with methylprednisolone (30 mg per kg, 1,500 mg maximum) may be indicated in the presence of rapidly progressive renal disease. The combination of cyclophosphamide and rituximab as well as the oral agent mycophenolate mofetil have also shown promise in the treatment of lupus nephritis. Plasmapheresis has been used in the treatment of severe lupus nephritis, especially in patients who fail to respond to conventional therapy with corticosteroids and cytotoxic agents. Although this modality appears to have little effect on long-term outcome, acute disease flare-ups may be rapidly controlled by removing pathogenic autoantibodies, immune complexes, and cytokines. Such therapy may be associated with significant toxicity, so its use should be limited to centers experienced in the care of acutely ill children with SLE.

Hematologic Complications. Anemia is common in SLE and may have many causes. Most typically, patients have a nonspecific normocytic, normochromic anemia of chronic disease. Microcytic anemia, in contrast, may be a sign of GI blood loss secondary to vasculitis or gastritis, with the urgency of further investigation dependent on the severity of the bleeding and the patient's overall well-being. Hemolytic anemia in SLE may be related to the disease itself (antierythrocyte antibodies) or to medications; hemolysis may occur rapidly.

In addition to the usual laboratory tests for anemia, the antibody responsible for autoimmune hemolytic anemia is of the "warm" variety, most commonly of the IgG type; IgM-type antibody is present in only a small percentage of cases. These red cell–bound antibodies may not be demonstrated by the standard Coombs test, so more sensitive assays may be necessary.

Management of anemia will depend on the severity (see Chapter 101 Hematologic Emergencies). Corticosteroids are the most effective agents for the control of autoimmune hemolytic anemia in SLE. Prednisone at 2 mg/kg/day is the initial treatment of choice. For severe hemolytic anemia requiring transfusion, additional immune modulatory therapies may be required to ensure that red blood cells are not lysed as rapidly as they are infused. Consultation with a tertiary transfusion center as well as a hematologist and rheumatologist is recommended.

Leukopenia occurs in about 50% of patients with SLE. It may be caused by a reduction in granulocytes, lymphocytes, or both. Granulocytopenia may be caused by drugs used in the treatment of SLE or less commonly by disease-related destruction of granulocytes. As with all cases of neutropenia, febrile children with absolute granulocyte counts of less than 1,000 per mm^3 are at higher risk of severe infections and should be admitted for empiric antibiotic coverage pending results of further studies.

Thrombocytopenia occurs in approximately 25% of patients with SLE; conversely, more than 5% of children presenting with ITP eventually meet diagnostic criteria for SLE. The usual causes of thrombocytopenia are circulating antibodies to platelets or drug-induced bone marrow suppression. Infection should always be considered as a possible cause, so the presence of purpura and ecchymoses requires immediate investigation. Significant hemorrhage, a sudden drop in hemoglobin, and platelet counts of less than 20,000 per mm^3 are the usual indications for admission to the hospital. Studies should include CBC, examination of the peripheral blood smear, and appropriate cultures. At times, bone marrow examination and testing of serum for antiplatelet antibodies may be helpful in determining the cause of reduced platelet counts. Patients with SLE are at risk of bleeding from any mucosal surface because of vasculitic ulceration, impaired hemostasis, thrombocytopenia, or a combination of these factors. Patients with life-threatening *epistaxis* may require local packing and platelet replacement in addition to high-dose corticosteroids. Severe *pulmonary hemorrhage* may necessitate general supportive measures such as transfusions, ventilatory assistance, and bronchial lavage. Once infections have been excluded, treatment of the underlying condition with high-dose corticosteroids, immunosuppressive agents, and/or plasmapheresis is essential. Treatment of GI hemorrhage is described in the "Gastrointestinal Complications" section.

Although less common than in systemic juvenile idiopathic arthritis (JIA), disseminated intravascular coagulation (DIC) associated with macrophage activation syndrome (MAS) may occur in SLE, with or without an associated infection. Therefore, patients with thrombocytopenia and severe bleeding should be investigated with prothrombin time, partial thromboplastin time (PTT), fibrin split products, and examination of the peripheral smear. Lupus also appears to predispose to a particularly malignant form of thrombotic thrombocytopenic purpura. Mortality rates are high, despite general support in ICUs and aggressive treatment with pheresis and immunosuppression. Outcomes are optimal when the diagnosis is suspected early and treatment is initiated rapidly.

The presence of a circulating *lupus anticoagulant* does not lead to a bleeding diathesis unless associated with significant thrombocytopenia; on the contrary, these patients are at increased risk of deep venous or arterial thrombosis. Prolongation of PTT and chronic false-positive serologic tests for syphilis are the usual clues to the presence of these autoantibodies. Specialized studies such as mixing assays and the Russell viper venom test may confirm the diagnosis. Antiphospholipid antibodies may also be measured, and the antiphospholipid antibody syndrome is associated with significant morbidity and mortality. Significant thrombosis or pulmonary embolus in a child with SLE is an indication for immediate anticoagulation with heparin, followed by oral warfarin or subcutaneous low–molecular-weight heparin, pending assays for these circulating anticoagulants.

Neurologic Complications. *Seizures* (see Chapter 67 Seizures) and altered states of consciousness (see Chapters 12 Coma and 105 Neurologic Emergencies) are the most common manifestations of CNS involvement in SLE. Other possible causes of seizures in patients with SLE include hypertension (from the disease itself or as a complication of corticosteroid therapy), infection (meningitis, encephalitis, or abscess), and uremia. Coma is not a primary manifestation of SLE but may result from meningitis or CNS hemorrhage related to thrombocytopenia. Therefore, patients with SLE who develop seizures or altered states of consciousness require urgent imaging, specifically a Computed tomography (CT) scan, with and without contrast. Magnetic resonance imaging (MRI) may be required because the differential diagnosis includes lupus cerebritis. Patients should have repeated examinations with special attention to blood pressure and neurologic findings, as well as the following investigations: CBC with differential and platelet counts, PT/PTT, electrolytes, BUN, creatinine, and urinalysis. Once space-occupying lesions have been excluded, lumbar puncture (including measurement of opening pressure) should be performed, with CSF sent for routine studies as well as special stains to look for opportunistic organisms such as fungi and acid-fast bacilli.

No study is perfectly sensitive for detecting lupus cerebritis. An electroencephalogram (EEG), MRI study, and CT scan with contrast may facilitate elucidation of the cause of CNS signs in children with lupus. Patients with CNS lupus also demonstrate abnormal perfusion on single photon emission CT scanning.

If CNS manifestations are considered secondary to active vasculitis, IV corticosteroid therapy should be initiated. In the presence of deteriorating mental function, "pulse" methylprednisolone (30 mg per kg, 1.5 g maximum), IV cyclophosphamide, or plasmapheresis may be beneficial.

Other manifestations of CNS involvement, such as psychosis, also may need inpatient evaluation. *Listeria monocytogenes* may cause indolent meningitis that is clinically indistinguishable from organic brain syndromes. Similarly, it may be difficult to determine whether psychosis is secondary to corticosteroid therapy; steroids are most likely to induce an altered sensorium in patients with underlying psychiatric disease. Clinicians should aggressively pursue a diagnostic evaluation, including lumbar puncture and imaging procedures, so appropriate therapy may be instituted as expeditiously as possible. When psychosis due to SLE is suspected, psychotropic drugs (e.g., haloperidol 0.025 to 0.05 mg/kg/day in divided doses) may be used along with large doses of corticosteroids for 1 to 2 weeks. If there is no improvement, the steroid dose may be reduced gradually in an attempt to rule out steroid-induced psychosis.

Transverse myelitis is a rare complication of SLE believed to result from vascular compromise of the spinal cord. Patients note acute onset of pain and weakness, and they may develop incontinence. Physical examination is remarkable for weakness or flaccid paralysis below the level of the functional transection. In a high percentage of cases, the process is associated with a circulating lupus anticoagulant or antiphospholipid antibodies. Prognosis is related to the duration of symptoms prior to initiation of therapy, and favorable outcomes are only possible with urgent intervention. Thus, once infection, epidural abscess, and hematoma are excluded with appropriate imaging procedures and lumbar puncture, pulse doses of IV methylprednisolone (30 mg per kg over 1 to 2 hours), plus anticoagulation with IV heparin, are begun. Immunosuppressive agents such as cyclophosphamide, 500 to 750 mg per m^2 IV, must be added in short order.

Pulmonary Complications. *Pleural effusion* is the most common pulmonary manifestation of SLE. Pleural effusion is often bilateral and small, although occasionally it may be massive. The child is often ill with acute manifestations of systemic disease, such as fever, fatigue, and poor appetite. Symptoms may be minimal or absent; in the presence of a moderate or large effusion, the patient may have dyspnea and tachypnea.

If the child has a previous history of pleurisy and there are no concerns about infection, outpatient management may be possible for small pleural effusions. Increasing the corticosteroid dose or adding an NSAID such as indomethacin (0.5 to 2 mg/kg/day) may be adequate therapy, but arrangements must be made for close follow-up. Thoracentesis is often necessary (i) to relieve symptoms, (ii) for diagnosis, or (iii) to reveal any underlying lesions obscured by the effusion. Pleural effusions caused by SLE usually are exudative, with elevated protein levels and cell counts, primarily PMNS early and lymphocytes later, with normal glucose and the presence of ANAs.

Pulmonary hemorrhage is a potentially catastrophic complication of SLE, particularly in the pediatric age group. Early recognition and treatment are critical. A hemorrhage may be related to the disease itself (e.g., pulmonary vasculitis), to the treatment (e.g., drug-induced thrombocytopenia), or to an infection (e.g., aspergillosis). Clinical features of patients with pulmonary hemorrhage include hemoptysis, tachypnea, tachycardia, and dyspnea; respiratory function may deteriorate rapidly if the process is not controlled. Chest radiographs show fluffy infiltrates resembling pulmonary edema. CBCs often reveal a dramatic drop in hemoglobin and a low platelet count. Diagnosis of a pulmonary hemorrhage may be confirmed by PFTs, including DL_{CO}. Intra-alveolar blood increases CO absorption, making it one of the few conditions that results in an abnormally high DL_{CO}. Bronchoalveolar lavage or lung biopsy still may be needed in some patients in whom *Pneumocystis* or *Aspergillus* infection remains a concern.

Management should include ventilatory support and blood products as needed, plus high doses of IV corticosteroids. If bleeding is related to thrombocytopenia, platelet transfusion is indicated. Tracheal lavage with epinephrine may be necessary, depending on the severity and progression of the process.

Occasionally, children with lupus may develop interstitial pneumonitis. Cultures of the blood and respiratory secretions, bronchial washings, transtracheal aspirate, or lung biopsy may be necessary to exclude opportunistic infections. Supportive therapy should include increased concentrations of oxygen, adequate pulmonary toilet, and antipyretic drugs. Measures employed to control other manifestations of SLE, including corticosteroids or immunosuppressive agents, may lead to dramatic improvement once infections have been excluded.

GI Complications. Peritonitis and GI hemorrhage are emergencies associated with SLE. Drug-induced gastric ulcer and pancreatitis also occur. Often it is difficult to determine the nature of an intra-abdominal catastrophe.

Peritonitis may be a feature of the disease itself (serosal inflammation) or may be caused by secondary infection or visceral perforation. It is important to remember that clinical findings of peritoneal irritation may be masked by corticosteroid therapy. Aspiration of the peritoneal fluid under strict aseptic conditions is essential if the cause of the peritoneal effusion is in doubt. The fluid should be sent for Gram stain and culture. Cell counts higher than 300 per mm^3 should be considered indicative of infection. Peritonitis due to serositis, a feature of SLE, may be treated with one of the NSAIDs; corticosteroids may be added if there is an inadequate response to the anti-inflammatory medication or if there is additional evidence of active systemic disease. Prolonged use of both NSAIDs and corticosteroids should be avoided, however, as it increases the risk of GI irritation and/or ulceration.

An *acute abdomen* in SLE may be the result of bowel ischemia, infarction, or perforation, in addition to the occasional unrelated occurrence of intussusception or appendicitis (see Chapters 7 Abdominal Distension, 48 Pain: Abdomen, and 99 Gastrointestinal Emergencies).

Pancreatitis must be considered in children with SLE and abdominal symptoms. SLE is the most common medical cause of *pancreatitis* in children, and corticosteroids are the medication most often associated with this complication. Whether pancreatitis is truly caused by steroids or merely tends to occur in sick patients receiving steroids for the underlying disease is not entirely clear; recent evidence supports the latter. In most cases it is prudent to assume that pancreatitis is secondary to active SLE and to increase immunosuppression in order to treat it. Recovery may be protracted, during which time the patient may have to be maintained on parenteral hyperalimentation.

GI hemorrhage may be secondary to NSAIDs (stomach), vasculitis of the GI tract (small intestines), or thrombocytopenia. The patient may develop massive bleeding leading to shock. If bleeding from a gastric ulcer is suspected, endoscopy can confirm the diagnosis. Therapy for a bleeding gastric ulcer includes volume replacement, IV proton pump inhibitors, and possibly IV octeotride (1 μg per kg, maximum 100 μg, followed by an infusion of 1 to 2 μg/kg/hr [maximum 50 μg per hour]). Octeotride reduces portal venous inflow and intravariceal pressure and may reduce the risk of bleeding due to nonvariceal causes (see section on Upper GI bleeding, Chapter 28 Gastrointestinal Bleeding).

If active bleeding due to vasculitis is suspected, celiac axis angiography or endoscopy with deep intestinal biopsies is required for confirmation. GI vasculitis is rare in pediatric lupus, but when it develops, it most commonly occurs in the setting of chronically active disease. Children typically have an associated peripheral neuropathy, as well as chronic weight loss, anorexia, and inanition.

Cardiac Complications. Pericarditis and myocarditis are two of the important cardiac complications of SLE that may require emergency care (see Chapter 94 Cardiac Emergencies). Pericarditis without significant hemodynamic effects may be managed with NSAIDs or corticosteroids, whereas larger effusions may require drainage. Myocarditis is treated with corticosteroids and bed rest with monitoring.

Raynaud Phenomenon. Raynaud phenomenon (RP) is characterized by triphasic color changes of the extremities upon exposure to cold. These color changes proceed from cyanosis to blanching due to microcirculatory compromise, and resolve with erythema caused by reactive hyperemia. Severe episodes of RP may cause excruciating pain in the extremities, or even digital ulceration and autoamputation. Poor circulation impairs wound healing and clearing of infections, so patients with paronychia or digital cellulitis in the setting of acral ischemia may require admission for IV antibiotics.

Prophylactic techniques to improve digital circulation (avoidance of cold exposure, biofeedback) are the cornerstones of treatment of RP. Calcium-channel blockers (e.g., slow-release nifedipine) may decrease the frequency and severity of attacks, whereas oral (e.g., prazosin, sildenafil) and topical (e.g., nitroglycerine) vasodilators or medical or surgical sympathetic blockade may be necessary during severe episodes. Cases of impending gangrene may also be treated with prostacylin analogs such as iloprost. These medications may cause dramatic vasodilation and result in pulmonary edema or cardiac arrhythmias; therefore, they should be used only by experienced clinicians.

Hypertension. Hypertension may be a result of effects of SLE on systemic vasculature, concomitant with renal involvement, or secondary to steroid therapy.

Headaches. Up to 80% of patients with SLE develop headaches, many migrainous, and they may experience acute, incapacitating exacerbations. Meningitis (both septic and aseptic), hypertension, and pseudotumor cerebri (idiopathic intracranial hypertension) must be ruled out in children with severe headaches. They should have a complete neurologic evaluation and examination of the CSF once a space-occupying lesion has been excluded. If the headache is accompanied by blurring or loss of vision, an ophthalmologic consultation should be obtained to exclude other complications such as retinal vasculitis or retinal vascular occlusion. Gradual periodic release of CSF pressure *via* lumbar puncture is the treatment of choice for pseudotumor cerebri. High-dose corticosteroid therapy should be added if the intracranial hypertension is believed to be because of SLE, whereas it should be tapered if the pseudotumor is secondary to steroid toxicity. If other causes are excluded, a child with a severe headache may be treated for a suspected acute migraine with analgesics and antiemetics (see Chapters 54 Pain: Headache and 105 Neurologic Emergencies).

OTHER SYSTEMIC CONNECTIVE TISSUE DISEASES

Scleroderma and Mixed Connective Tissue Disease

Goals of Treatment

The goals of treatment are to control symptoms and allow the patient to maintain function while simultaneously monitoring for the development of complications.

CLINICAL PEARLS AND PITFALLS

- Complications related to systemic sclerosis (SS) should be considered if a child with localized scleroderma presents with acute clinical decompensation.
- Mixed connective tissue disease is a systemic autoimmune process similar to SLE and characterized by high titer anti-RNP antibodies and often complicated by interstitial lung disease.

Scleroderma

Scleroderma, or hardening of the skin, is most commonly a process restricted to the skin and subcutaneous tissues in children. Various conditions are included within the category of scleroderma, as listed in Table 109.4. Localized scleroderma is more common in children than in adults. The lesions may be one of the five types. Circumscribed *morphea* is a focal ivory-white patch with a violaceous or erythematous rim; it is often a single lesion on the trunk, although generalized morphea also occurs in children. Pansclerotic morphea is circumferential involvement of the limb(s) affecting the skin, subcutaneous tissue, muscle, and bone. *Linear scleroderma* causes scarring, fibrosis, and atrophy that crosses dermatomes. Involved skin develops a "hidebound" appearance due to tethering of the subcutaneous tissues to deeper structures. It may extend to involve an entire extremity (Fig. 109.3) and to affect underlying muscle and bone, leading to flexion contractures, leg-length discrepancies, and atrophy of an extremity. A variant affecting the forehead is called *scleroderma en coup de sabre;* this form may involve underlying skull and nervous tissue, as

TABLE 109.4

CLASSIFICATION OF SYSTEMIC SCLEROSIS, LOCALIZED SCLERODERMAS AND SCLERODERMA-LIKE DISORDERS

Systemic sclerosis
Cutaneous scleroderma
Diffuse
Limited
Overlap syndromes
Sclerodermatomyositis or with other connective tissue diseases
Mixed connective tissue disease (MCTD)
Localized scleroderma
Circumscribed morphea
Generalized morphea
Pansclerotic morphea
Linear (include "en coup de sabre") morphea
Mixed subtype
Graft-versus-host disease
Chemically induced scleroderma-like disease
Polyvinyl chloride
Toxic oil syndrome
Pentazocine
Bleomycin
Adjuvant disease
Pseudosclerodermas
Phenylketonuria
Syndromes of premature aging
Localized idiopathic fibroses
Scleredema
Diabetic cheiroarthropathy
Porphyria cutanea tarda

From Zulian F, Cassidy JT. The systemic sclerodermas and related disorders. In: Cassidy JT, Petty RE, Laxer RM, et al., eds. *Textbook of pediatric rheumatology*. 6th ed. Philadelphia, PA: Saunders Elsevier, 2011:414–437.

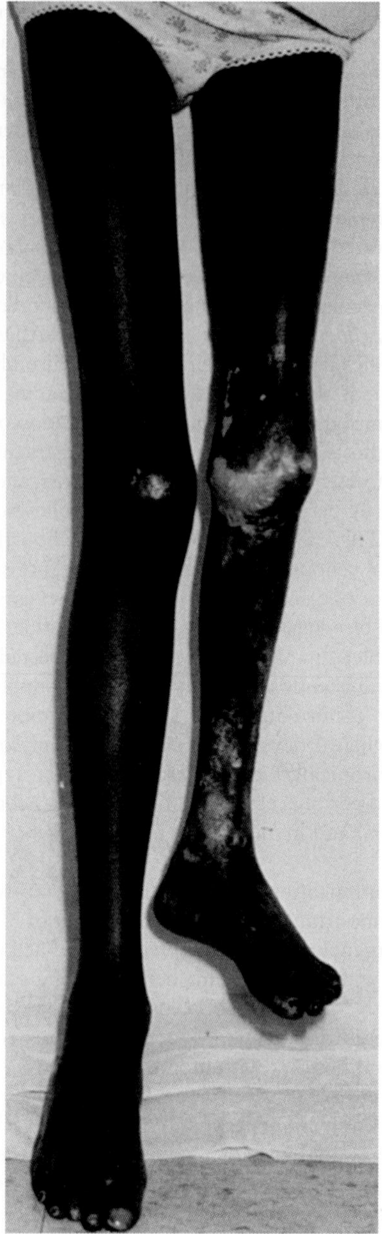

FIGURE 109.3 Linear scleroderma involving left lower extremity in a 12-year-old girl.

well as the skin. Finally, there is a mixed type which is a combination of two or more of the previous subtypes. Although localized forms of scleroderma are generally not associated with internal organ involvement, one large pediatric cohort found nearly a quarter of patients to have at least one extracutaneous manifestation. In addition, though rare, progression to SS has been reported.

The far more serious form, SS, is also rarer, occurring in fewer than 1,000 children nationwide. SS is subdivided into diffuse cutaneous SS and limited cutaneous SS, previously designated as CREST (Calcinosis cutis, Raynaud phenomenon, Esophageal dysfunction, Sclerodactyly, Telangiectasia) syndrome. SS often presents with cutaneous changes such as RP (90% of patients), edema, induration, increased pigmentation, and tightening of the skin. Some of these children may also develop arthritis resembling JIA, muscle weakness resembling juvenile dermatomyositis (JDMS), and nodules along tendon sheaths. If these features are seen, one should consider the possibility of an overlap syndrome, in which features of SLE, SS, JDMS, and JIA intermingle.

Serious illness and death can occur in SS. Severe, uncontrolled hypertension and rapidly progressive renal failure (scleroderma renal crisis) have been a major source of mortality, although the introduction of ACE inhibitors has dramatically improved short-term survival. Primary myocardial disease with conduction disturbances, pericarditis, and intractable CHF, as well as pulmonary hypertension caused by fibrosis, remains significant sources of morbidity and mortality. Additional complications of SS include (i) digital gangrene and nonhealing ulcers most frequently involving the fingers, elbows, and malleoli secondary to vascular occlusion; (ii) disordered motility of the distal esophagus with dysphagia and reflux esophagitis (60% of affected children); (iii) malabsorption syndrome; (iv) thrombocytopenia with subsequent cerebral hemorrhage; (v) interstitial lung disease; and (vi) cranial nerve involvement with trigeminal sensory neuropathy, facial weakness, and tinnitus.

TABLE 109.5

COMPLICATIONS OF SYSTEMIC SCLEROSIS

Clinical entity	Symptoms and signs	Investigations	Treatments
Myocardial fibrosis	Exertional dyspnea, orthopnea, angina pectoris Distant heart sounds, gallop rhythm, arrhythmias	Chest radiograph EKG Echocardiogram Gated nuclear-ventricular scans	Digoxin Diuretics Antiarrhythmics
Pulmonary interstitial fibrosis	Cough, dyspnea Dry crackles Cor pulmonale	Chest radiograph, EKG Pulmonary function tests, including CO diffusion High-resolution CT, bronchoalveolar lavage Lung biopsy	Corticosteroids Oxygen, bronchodilators Treatment of right-sided heart failure
Pulmonary hypertension	Acute dyspnea Increased P_2 and widely split S_2	Chest radiograph EKG Echocardiogram Right-sided heart catheterization Lung biopsy	Corticosteroids Calcium-channel blockers ACE inhibitors Direct PA installation of vasodilators
Scleroderma renal crisis	Severe headache, blurred vision, congestive heart failure, seizures Malignant hypertension, retinopathy	Electrolytes, BUN Creatinine Plasma renin activity	Captopril and other ACE inhibitors Minoxidil and other vasodilators, β-blockers Diuretics, dialysis; in refractory cases, nephrectomy
Impending gangrene	Pain, loss of sensation in distal digits Trophic changes	Cryoglobulins Doppler flow studies	Topical vasodilators Sympathetic ganglionic blockade (digital, regional), prostaglandin E_1 infusion
Esophagitis	Retrosternal pain, pyrosis, melena	CBC Barium swallow Esophageal ph probe and manometry	Antacids/cimetidine Surgical manipulation for chronic unremitting complaints

EKG, electrocardiogram; CO, carbon monoxide; CT, computed tomography; ACE, angiotensin-converting enzyme; PA, posteroanterior; BUN, blood urea nitrogen; CBC, complete blood count.

Management

Specific therapy for SS is nonexistent at present. Virtually every medication, from antihistamines to potent immunosuppressives, has been used in patients with this disease, though none shows clear benefit. During the inflammatory, prefibrotic stages of interstitial lung disease and pulmonary vascular involvement, corticosteroids (prednisone 2 mg/kg/day or the equivalent) are indicated. Cyclophosphamide appears to forestall pulmonary fibrosis if added early to the treatment regime. If the esophageal sphincter is involved, patients should be advised to sleep with the head comfortably elevated, and an antacid may be prescribed.

Minor episodes of Raynaud syndrome are managed with prophylactic measures such as the avoidance of cold exposure and the use of warm clothing, including hats and mittens. Biofeedback training and calcium-channel blockers such as nifedipine may be helpful in decreasing the frequency of attacks. Aggressive physical therapy is indicated to prevent contractures and to maintain normal function. Despite these measures, linear scleroderma with involvement of deep structures may lead to contractures of the extremities requiring surgery. Juvenile onset SS carries an approximate 5-year mortality rate of 10%.

Management of Complications and Emergencies

Cardiac Complications. Signs and symptoms of myocardial fibrosis are those of a cardiomyopathy with dyspnea, orthopnea, and fatigue (Table 109.5). Angina pectoris and myocardial infarction may occur (see also Chapters 50 Pain: Chest and 94 Cardiac Emergencies). Fibrosis of the conduction system may result in arrhythmias, presenting as palpitations, syncope, or sudden death. Pericarditis is usually silent and valvular involvement in scleroderma is rare. Even in the absence of symptoms or physical findings, cardiac involvement eventually develops in the majority of patients with SS, and sensitive imaging or functional studies reveal some cardiac involvement early in the course of disease in the majority of cases. Management of cardiac dysfunction is symptomatic, including inotropic support and afterload reduction. Extensive diuresis should be avoided because of potential adverse effects on renal perfusion. No specific drugs are available to arrest the progression of cardiac involvement.

Pulmonary Complications. Pulmonary involvement in SS may have three manifestations: pleurisy, interstitial lung disease, or pulmonary artery fibrosis. Diffuse interstitial lung disease is often asymptomatic. A dry cough may be the first symptom.

Early in the course of the disease, even before symptoms appear, pulmonary function tests show a restrictive pattern and diffusion abnormalities. Later, radiographs of the chest show increased reticulation, a so-called "honeycombed" appearance, mainly basilar and bilateral. Other diagnostic modalities, including high-resolution CT scanning, bronchoalveolar lavage, and lung biopsy, may identify earlier, prefibrotic states of disease that are more responsive to anti-inflammatory therapy. With progression of the disease, cough and dyspnea become prominent. On examination, crackles over both sides of the chest, particularly over the infrascapular area, may be the only finding. Development of right-sided heart failure is heralded by increasing dyspnea, although edema of the lower extremities may not be appreciated because of hidebound skin. Patients with right-sided heart failure generally require admission and symptomatic management.

Patients with irreversible pulmonary fibrosis and chronic respiratory failure have diminished respiratory reserve, so they must be treated promptly and aggressively when they contract intercurrent respiratory infections. Supplemental oxygen, bronchodilators, and corticosteroids may be helpful. If residual inflammation is demonstrable after further investigations such as those noted previously, these patients should receive corticosteroids (prednisone 2 mg/kg/day) for 6 to 8 weeks, although the value of this therapy is doubtful in established fibrosis. In addition, treatment of right-sided overload is indicated.

Pulmonary hypertension is the most common cause of dyspnea in patients with SS. On auscultation, there is a wide or fixed splitting of the second heart sound and the pulmonic component is accentuated. The EKG shows right ventricular hypertrophy. Echocardiography and right heart catheterization may be necessary to differentiate cardiac from pulmonary etiologies of respiratory deterioration. Corticosteroids and cyclophosphamide (50 mg per day orally or 500 to 750 mg per m^2 by monthly IV infusion) are the treatment of choice in patients without established interstitial fibrosis, in addition to supportive measures, endothelin-1 receptor antagonists such as bosentan, calcium-channel blockers, ACE inhibitors, and prostaglandin analogs (e.g., epoprostenol) may provide temporary improvement in individual cases.

Renal Complications. Sclerodermatous involvement of the vessels of the kidney is the most common cause of renal failure in adults with SS. Risk factors include proteinuria, hypertension, rapid progression of skin thickening early in the illness, anemia, pericardial effusion, and CHF. The development of a microangiopathic hemolytic anemia suggests imminent renal failure. These complications appear to be less common in children than in adults.

Renal failure may develop gradually or acutely in a patient with known renal disease, and use of corticosteroids may precipitate its appearance. Scleroderma renal crisis is characterized by a sudden rise in blood pressure to levels as high as 150 to 200 mm Hg diastolic, often with minimal or no symptoms, associated with acute renal failure. Evaluation reveals hypertensive retinopathy (flame hemorrhages, cotton wool exudates, and papilledema), elevated plasma renin activity, and rapid deterioration of renal function. Immediate investigation should include urinalysis, measurement of urine output and urinary electrolytes, serum electrolytes, BUN, creatinine, and plasma renin level.

A major advance in the pharmacologic management of scleroderma renal crisis has been the use of ACE inhibitors such as captopril. Patients who fail to respond to this drug may still respond to potent vasodilators such as minoxidil, along with β-blockers and diuretics; regimens involving multiple drugs may also be necessary (see Chapters 33 Hypertension and 108 Renal and Electrolyte Emergencies). Renal dialysis and rarely bilateral nephrectomy may be indicated in hypertension unresponsive to pharmacologic therapy. Because most patients with severe scleroderma renal disease have a component of myocarditis and ventricular stiffness, maintenance of blood volume is essential to ensure adequate preload to support the circulation.

Peripheral Vascular Complications. RP can often be incapacitating, particularly in cold weather. Symptoms include severe pain in the extremities and loss of sensation in the tips of the digits. Treatment with calcium-channel antagonists such as slow-release nifedipine may decrease the frequency or severity of attacks. In urgent cases with impending gangrene, systemic or topical vasodilators (e.g., nitroglycerine paste or intra-arterial reserpine) or sympathetic ganglion block may be tried, although these forms of therapy have not been validated in well-constructed studies. Excessive peripheral vasodilation may also precipitate cardiovascular collapse due to a "steal syndrome," so caution must be exercised to ensure cardiac filling pressures are maintained. Consequently, these procedures should be performed only with intensive monitoring. If gangrene has developed and there is no infection, spontaneous separation of the tips of the digits will occur and carries less risk and morbidity than surgical amputation.

GI Complications. Abnormal esophageal motility with reflux may result in esophagitis. The major symptom of this condition is retrosternal pain that is made worse by certain foods and recumbent positioning. The pain may be severe and incapacitating, and the risk of aspiration is increased. Although children with the complaint of retrosternal pain do not require admission to the hospital, they need an evaluation of their lower esophageal sphincter with esophageal manometry. Those with mild pain and objective manifestations of reflux (lower esophageal sphincter pressure of less than 10 mm Hg, evidence of esophagitis on endoscopy) are usually treated with simple measures, such as antacids 1 hour after meals and 1 hour before bedtime and elevation of the head during sleep. If symptoms are severe, H_2-blockers such as cimetidine (20 to 40 mg/kg/day, maximum daily dosage 1,200 mg) or proton pump inhibitors such as lansoprazole (15 to 30 mg once or twice daily) may be prescribed. Any patient with scleroderma who develops acute respiratory symptoms in association with reflux must be evaluated for possible aspiration pneumonia.

Mixed Connective Tissue Disease

Mixed connective tissue disease (MCTD) is a rare disorder among pediatric patients. The median age at onset is approximately 11 years, and like many other rheumatologic conditions occurs more frequently in girls than in boys by a ratio of 3:1. MCTD was initially described by Sharp et al. in 1972, and includes features of rheumatoid arthritis, scleroderma, SLE, and dermatomyositis (DM). RP and polyarteritis are the most common manifestations at onset. Children present with features of more than one connective tissue disease, have a speckled ANA pattern and high titers of anti-RNP.

There is no specific treatment for pediatric MCTD and treatment is typically directed at an individual's particular disease manifestations. Many patients will respond to low-dose corticosteroids, NSAIDs, hydroxychloroquine, or a combination of these medications. Patients with severe myositis, renal, or visceral disease often require high-dose corticosteroids and sometimes cytotoxic agents.

Pediatric MCTD is associated with a higher risk of nephritis than adult MCTD. Other complications include pulmonary hypertension, pulmonary fibrosis, severe thrombocytopenia, and esophageal dysfunction.

VASCULITIS

CLINICAL PEARLS AND PITFALLS

- Vasculitis may affect any body system and may lead to life-threatening complications, including stroke, myocardial infarction, hypertensive crisis, and acute renal failure.
- Systemic signs of inflammation are often present.

Current Evidence

Although the pathologic process in vasculitis is limited to the blood vessels, the presence of vasculature in every organ of the body means that virtually any symptom could be a presentation of vasculitis. Vascular inflammation and damage can lead to anything from numbness to pain, thrombosis to bleeding, aneurysm formation to vascular obstruction. Pediatric vasculitides are very rare, however, this section will be limited to a general overview of situations in which the diagnosis should be considered, followed by more detailed discussions of antinuclear cytoplasm antibody (ANCA)-associated vasculitis, polyarteritis nodosa (PAN), JDMS, and Behçet disease (BD). Along with PAN, KD is one of the most prevalent vasculitides of childhood and will be discussed separately.

Goals of Treatment

The long-term goals of treatment for the vasculitides are to minimize inflammation while monitoring for progression of disease and adverse effects of therapies. For the emergency physician, management of life-threatening emergencies will occur in the usual manner. Stress doses of corticosteroids and increases in immunosuppressant dosing may be required.

Clinical Considerations

Clinical Recognition

Early in the course of a vasculitis, findings are generally nonspecific, primarily reflecting systemic inflammation (fever, malaise, fatigue, failure to thrive, elevated acute-phase reactants). As vascular damage progresses, evidence of vascular compromise characteristic of the particular vessels involved becomes evident on physical examination. For example, hypertension may evolve as renal vascular involvement progresses. Should the diagnosis be delayed beyond this stage, irreversible tissue damage may occur; it is important that therapy be initiated while the findings remain subtle.

Despite the extreme variability of the manifestations of vasculitis, certain specific symptoms are particularly suggestive of vascular inflammation. Involvement of large- or medium-sized muscular arteries, as may be seen in Takayasu arteritis (TA) or PAN, initially causes symptoms related to the severity of the inflammatory response. As vascular compromise progresses, symptoms of arterial insufficiency begin to dominate. Involvement of large vessels to the extremities, such as the subclavian or femoral arteries, typically leads to claudication, whereas involvement of visceral vessels causes hypertension (renal arteries), abdominal pain (mesenteric and celiac axes), chest pain (aortic or coronary artery involvement), or neurologic symptoms (focal neurologic deficits or neuropathic pain).

Inflammation of smaller arteries and arterioles leads to symptoms in richly vascularized organs. Skin involvement—livedo reticularis, purpuric (generally palpable) or nonblanching lesions, and palmar or plantar rashes—is most suggestive of vascular inflammation. Pulmonary, renal, and GI arterial beds are often involved as well. Consequently, hemoptysis, hematuria, hypertension, abdominal pain, or melena may signify vascular involvement, including infarction. Capillary and venous inflammation typically involves the same organs, although the lower volume of blood flow through these vessels tends to make capillaritis and venulitis less of an acute emergency than arteritis.

Triage Considerations

Patients with a known diagnosis of a vasculitis will usually be taking immunosuppressant medications. Workup of fever should be expedited. The patient may present with life-threatening complications in any body system.

Clinical Assessment

Whenever vasculitis is considered as a diagnosis, a thorough history and careful general physical examination should be augmented by focus on clinical features of vascular disease. History should include recent illnesses, in particular infections, other exposures (including prescription and over-the-counter drugs), travel, and family history. All pulses must be palpated carefully, and bilateral Allen tests should be performed to confirm patency of the radial and ulnar arteries and volar arch. The neck, abdomen, and proximal extremities should be auscultated for bruits, and blood pressures in all four extremities should be compared for asymmetry. The skin should be examined carefully for lesions that are nodular or do not blanch, and the two other windows on small-vessel abnormalities—ocular fundi and nailbed capillaries—should be assessed as well.

Laboratory studies specific for the diagnosis of vasculitis are not yet available. When vasculitis is being considered, laboratory investigation should include a CBC and acute-phase reactants (especially erythrocyte sedimentation rate [ESR] and CRP) for evidence of systemic inflammation. Ongoing immune activation leads to hypergammaglobulinemia in many cases of systemic vasculitis. Certain small-vessel diseases (especially granulomatosis with polyangiitis [GPA, formerly Wegener granulomatosis] and eosinophilic granulomatosis with polyangiitis [EGPA, formerly Churg–Strauss syndrome]) are characterized by antinuclear cytoplasm antibodies (ANCAs). The von Willebrand factor antigen is released by damaged vascular endothelium. It is elevated in small-vessel vasculitides but also in other conditions that cause vessel damage, including stroke, trauma, and severe infections, rendering it somewhat nonspecific.

Imaging procedures should be used to confirm a clinical suspicion of vasculitis, not to hunt blindly for a diagnosis. When pulmonary involvement is suspected, pulmonary function tests and imaging of the lungs with radiographs or CT are often useful. Vascular imaging must be selected on a case-by-case basis, based on clinical and laboratory data. Doppler ultrasound studies and CT or MRI angiograms are adequate for resolving abnormalities in large- or medium-sized vessels, but conditions involving smaller vessels often can be visualized only by use of conventional angiography. Even in the hands of interventional radiologists experienced in pediatric procedures, angiography remains potentially morbid, so careful attention to history and physical examination should be relied upon to minimize the number of studies.

The reference standard for diagnosing vasculitis remains histopathologic demonstration of vascular inflammation, although tissue specimens may not be available in many cases because of the inaccessibility of lesions or patchiness of the vascular involvement. When skin lesions are present, deciding to obtain a biopsy is relatively easy; when inaccessible structures such as the brain are involved, calculating the risks and benefits of a biopsy is significantly more complicated.

Management

See sections below for PAN and KD.

POLYARTERITIS NODOSA

Current Evidence

The annual incidence of PAN in adults is approximately 0.3 per 100,000; no comparable data are available for children. Corticosteroid therapy has reduced mortality from nearly 100% to approximately 20%.

PAN is characterized by focal, pan-mural, necrotizing inflammation of small- and medium-sized muscular arteries. As the name implies, vessels affected by PAN typically develop nodules in the walls of muscular arteries. Sites of bifurcation are particularly prone to involvement, presumably because of hemodynamic turbulence at these points. Biopsies reveal a cellular infiltrate initially predominated by polymorphonuclear leukocytes and fibrinoid necrosis. As lesions mature, mononuclear cells, thrombosis, and recanalization mark the healing process.

The etiology of PAN is unknown, although it is considered to be an archetype of immune complex–mediated vascular damage. Most children with PAN have serologic evidence of an antecedent streptococcal infection; up to one-third of adults have chronic hepatitis B or C, with viral proteins demonstrable in the circulating and fixed immune complexes. The incidence of hepatitis-associated PAN in children is significantly lower, particularly in Western countries.

Clinical Considerations

Clinical Recognition

Childhood PAN occurs in both cutaneous and generalized forms, and distinguishing between them may be difficult. Both types display systemic manifestations, including fever, malaise, and myalgias. However, generalized PAN is significantly more likely to also involve the renal, GI, and central nervous systems. Common to both are rashes, although these are more likely to be nodular or lacy (so called livedo reticularis) in the cutaneous form, and urticarial, petechial, or ischemic in the systemic form. Renal involvement (including proteinuria, abnormal urinary sediment, and hypertension), abdominal pain (often a manifestation of gut vasculitis), arthritis, mononeuritis multiplex, and CNS involvement (seizures, hemiparesis) typify generalized PAN. Less commonly, children may have cardiac disease (pericarditis, cardiomegaly, EKG changes, myocardial infarction) or pulmonary involvement (diffuse infiltrates, pulmonary hemorrhage, or hemothorax). Cogan syndrome is a rare subtype of PAN characterized by interstitial keratitis and sensorineural hearing loss.

Clinical Assessment

The patient should be examined carefully for signs of end-organ involvement, including blood pressure elevation, abdominal tenderness, arthritis, CNS disease (e.g., hemiparesis), cardiac disease (e.g., pericarditis, myocardial infarction), and pulmonary involvement. Urinalysis is a useful marker for renal involvement.

Laboratory findings in polyarteritis are nonspecific. Most children have white blood cell counts higher than 15,000 per mm^3, hemoglobin less than 10 g per dL, broadly elevated acute-phase reactants, and hypergammaglobulinemia. Complement levels are usually normal or increased, and ANA and RF levels are elevated only slightly, if at all. Some children have evidence of ANCAs, although other autoantibodies are usually absent.

Diagnosis of PAN generally requires tissue confirmation. Acute necrotizing inflammation of small- and medium-sized arteries is demonstrable in renal, cutaneous, muscular, or GI tissues. At times, biopsy may not be practical, and angiographic visualization of aneurysms may provide an acceptable alternative. Other findings include visceral perfusion defects, especially in the kidneys, development of collateral arteries, and a "beaded" appearance of involved vessels as a result of alternating areas of stenosis and dilatation. Performance and interpretation of these studies requires the expertise of a radiologist experienced in pediatric angiography.

Management

The prognosis in PAN is better in patients with less disease-related organ damage, so therapy should be initiated as early as possible. The initial management of PAN includes corticosteroids (generally divided doses of prednisone, 2 mg/kg/day, to a maximum of 60 mg daily). Rash and constitutional symptoms improve first, followed by control of end-organ involvement. Pulse doses of methylprednisolone (30 mg per kg in 50 mL of 5% dextrose in water by IV infusion over 1 to 2 hours, maximum dose 1,500 mg) may offer an alternative for the treatment of acute exacerbations, provided that blood pressure and cardiac rhythm are closely monitored.

Cutaneous PAN may require lower doses of steroids to suppress disease activity, or alternative agents such as methotrexate, dapsone, or colchicine may adequately control the rash. In contrast, children with systemic PAN may not tolerate a reduction in their steroid dosage or may not respond adequately to steroids. In such cases, the addition of immunosuppressive agents (e.g., oral or IV cyclophosphamide) or biologic response modifiers (e.g., infliximab 5 to 10 mg per kg monthly) may improve the outcome or allow tapering of steroids without a disease flare. Other interventions, including NSAIDs for fever and arthritis, anticonvulsants, antihypertensives, and physical therapy, should be employed when appropriate.

Management of Complications and Emergencies

The most serious emergencies in childhood polyarteritis are (i) renal insufficiency; (ii) severe hypertension; (iii) cardiac

TABLE 109.6

COMPLICATIONS OF POLYARTERITIS NODOSA

Clinical entity	Symptoms and signs	Investigations	Treatment
Renal failure	Usually insidious; no symptoms until uremia sets in	Urinalysis (serial); BUN; creatinine; creatinine clearance; serum electrolytes	Fluid, electrolyte management Treatment of hypertension Peritoneal dialysis Hemodialysis
Renal infarction	Flank pain High blood pressure	Urinalysis; BUN; creatinine Renal arteriogram	Management of renal failure as given above, hemodialysis
Renal artery aneurysm with hemorrhage	Severe, sudden flank pain; gross hematuria; shock; palpable abdominal mass	Serial hematocrit Renal arteriogram	Management of shock Surgical consult
Hypertension	Asymptomatic or headache; retinal changes; encephalopathy	Serial measurement of BP; BUN; creatinine, creatinine clearance; IVP (or) renal arteriogram	Diuretics Antihypertensive agents
Pericarditis	Chest pain; pericardial rub; pulsus paradoxus (if tamponade)	EKG; radiograph chest; echocardiogram; removal of fluid for analysis	Rest, steroids, removal of fluid (if tamponade) *Caution:* If tamponade is sudden, it may be caused by ruptured aneurysm with blood in pericardium
Myocardial infarction	Sudden chest pain; shock; arrhythmia; dyspnea; congestive failure	EKG (continuous monitor); echocardiogram; thallium scan; coronary arteriography	Pain relief; oxygen Circulatory support Heparin, thrombolytic agents
Gastrointestinal hemorrhage	Abdominal pain; vomiting; melena, hematemesis, or hematochezia; shock; tenderness and guarding of abdomen; bowel sounds absent	Plain radiograph abdomen Peritoneal aspiration Endoscopy Celiac arteriogram	Treat shock; block bleeding vessel during angiography; surgical ligation
Gastrointestinal perforation	Sudden abdominal pain; shock; guarding, tenderness, and rigidity of abdomen; absent bowel sounds	Plain radiograph abdomen (upright)	Treat shock Surgical repair
Aneurysm with rupture (intra-abdominal)	Abdominal pain (chronic) with acute exacerbation Palpable mass Sudden onset of shock	Ultrasound Celiac arteriogram	Treat shock Surgical repair
Central nervous system lesions	Convulsions; gradual onset of loss of consciousness; hemiparesis	Exclude hypertensive encephalopathy CT scan, MRI Carotid arteriography	Supportive care Control BP Anticonvulsants High-dose corticosteroids and/ or immunosuppressives

BUN, blood urea nitrogen; BP, blood pressure; IVP, intravenous pyelogram; EKG, electrocardiogram; CT, computed tomography; MRI, magnetic resonance imaging.

complications such as CHF, myocardial infarction, and dysrhythmias; (iv) GI vasculitis resulting in bowel infarction, intestinal perforation, or cholecystitis; and (v) CNS manifestations, such as seizures and cranial nerve palsies (Table 109.6).

Renal Emergencies. Although medical management of PAN has resulted in a significantly improved prognosis, azotemia and hypertension at the time of diagnosis continue to identify children with extremely aggressive disease. Arteritis of medium-sized vessels of the kidney may lead to renal infarction and ischemia or to glomerulonephritis manifested by hematuria, hypertension, and uremia (see Chapter 108 Renal and Electrolyte Emergencies). Management of renal failure includes high doses of corticosteroids to control the underlying disease process (e.g., prednisone 2 mg/kg/day). Sudden flank pain associated with gross hematuria, falling blood pressure, and an expanding abdominal mass suggest the possibility of aneurysmal dilatation and rupture, with renal artery hemorrhage. Rupture of a renal artery aneurysm is initially managed with treatment of shock and replacement of volume, followed by surgical repair of the aneurysm once the patient is stabilized.

Hypertension. A mild to moderate elevation of blood pressure is noted in more than 90% of children with generalized PAN. Management follows the general rules for treating renovascular hypertension (see Chapter 33 Hypertension).

Cardiac Emergencies. See Chapter 94 Cardiac Emergencies. *Pericarditis* may be asymptomatic. Echocardiographic demonstration of pericardial fluid is the most sensitive means of confirming the presence of pericarditis. Patients with pericarditis with no or small effusion may be treated with bed rest, careful monitoring, and corticosteroids. Pericardiocentesis is indicated in the presence of tamponade or if infection is suspected.

Chest pain with tachycardia, arrhythmia, and dyspnea may herald the occurrence of *myocardial infarction* in a patient with PAN involving the coronary arteries. Pericardial tamponade caused by a ruptured coronary aneurysm may present similarly. Occasionally, a patient with coronary artery disease may present with CHF. Characteristic EKG changes (deep Q waves) and areas of ischemia on myocardial nuclear scanning may be seen. Echocardiography is indicated to study the function of the myocardium and the status of the valves. Coronary arteriography is essential to establish the size, location, and extent of aneurysms and occlusions.

Supportive medical management includes careful monitoring of cardiorespiratory status, judicious use of IV fluids, diuretics, and inotropes when needed. Treatment of the primary disease with steroids and immunosuppressive agents should be continued as described. If hypertension does not respond to diuretic therapy, other antihypertensive agents may be required.

GI Complications. Abdominal pain is the most common manifestation of GI involvement in PAN. It may be diffuse and nonspecific or localized and severe. Hematemesis and melena suggest ulceration and hemorrhage (see Chapter 28 Gastrointestinal Bleeding).

Visceral perforation should be suspected in cases of active systemic disease and unrelenting abdominal pain. Corticosteroid therapy may mask the usual clinical findings of peritonitis. Arteritis involving specific organs may lead to cholecystitis, pancreatitis, appendicitis, or hepatitis (see Chapters 48 Pain: Abdomen and 99 Gastrointestinal Emergencies).

Mesenteric thrombosis with infarction of the bowel may present with sudden abdominal pain, vomiting, hematemesis or hematochezia, and shock. Exquisite tenderness of the abdomen and absent bowel sounds are the major findings. Hemorrhage from a ruptured aneurysm (mesenteric, hepatic, or renal) with hemoperitoneum is heralded by sudden onset of severe pain, vomiting, tachycardia, and shock. The abdomen is tender and tense, and bowel sounds are diminished or absent.

Initial management of each of these GI catastrophes includes volume replacement, gastric decompression, and stress doses of corticosteroids. Very large volumes of IV fluids may be required. Technetium scan, angiography of the celiac axis vessels, and peritoneal aspiration may be indicated in some cases, and direct examination of the GI tract by endoscopy may yield valuable information concerning the nature, location, and extent of lesions. Surgical consultation should be obtained immediately, and in the presence of bleeding aneurysms or infarcted bowel, exploratory laparoscopy or laparotomy should be performed as soon as the patient can be stabilized.

CNS Complications. Clinical signs of CNS disease are less frequent than those of peripheral nervous system involvement. Seizures and hemiparesis are the most common manifestations of CNS involvement in PAN. CT angiogram, MRI with MRA, and/or carotid angiography may help localize the lesion.

Management of hypertensive encephalopathy and increased intracranial pressure are described elsewhere (see Chapters 105 Neurologic Emergencies and 108 Renal and Electrolyte Emergencies). Surgical correction of a ruptured aneurysm should be undertaken if the bleeding vessel can be localized and is accessible.

Miscellaneous Complications. As with all vasculitides, PAN may involve testicular vessels, leading to acute scrotal pain and purpura and accompanying dysuria. Once other causes of scrotal pain are excluded, including epididymitis and testicular torsion, treatment may proceed with steroids and immunosuppressive medications.

JUVENILE DERMATOMYOSITIS

CLINICAL PEARLS AND PITFALLS

- Patients are at risk for aspiration pneumonia and respiratory insufficiency because of muscular weakness, including weakness of the diaphragm.
- Poorly controlled disease may be associated with GI manifestations of vasculitis, including GI bleeding.
- A rare complication is the development of cardiac conduction abnormalities.

Current Evidence

JDMS is a rare rheumatic disorder characterized by inflammation of the blood vessels, skin, and striated muscle. The annual incidence rate is roughly three cases per 1 million children in the United States. Girls are more often affected than boys (~2:1), as is typical of most autoimmune conditions. The mean age of onset is estimated at 6.9 years in the United States, with almost 20% of patients diagnosed at 4 years of age or younger. Before steroid therapy was available, as many as one-third of patients died of the disease and another one-third developed permanent disabilities. More recently, the introduction of potent immunomodulators earlier in the disease course has led to improved outcomes. The mortality rate may now be as low as 1.5% in the United States, and drug- and disease-related morbidity are also improving. Despite these advances, however, JDMS remains a serious disease that requires the care of physicians experienced with its management.

Bohan and Peter's criteria for DM/polymyositis (PM) in adults are typically used for diagnosing this condition in children, and these are provided in Table 109.7. In fact, the condition

TABLE 109.7

CRITERIA FOR DIAGNOSIS OF DERMATOMYOSITIS (DM)/POLYMYOSITIS (PM)[a]

1. Symmetric weakness of the proximal limb muscles and anterior neck flexors
2. Evidence of necrosis of type I and II fibers on muscle biopsy
3. Elevation of serum levels of skeletal muscle enzymes—creatine phosphokinase and aldolase
4. Short, small, polyphasic motor unit potentials with fibrillation; insertional irritability; and high-frequency repetitive discharges on electromyography
5. Skin rash—characteristic heliotrope rash, scaly erythematous rash over extensor aspects of the joints, and periungual erythema

Definite: 4 criteria (PM)
Probable: 3 criteria (PM)
Possible: 2 criteria (PM)

[a]*N Eng J Med* 1975;292:344–347.

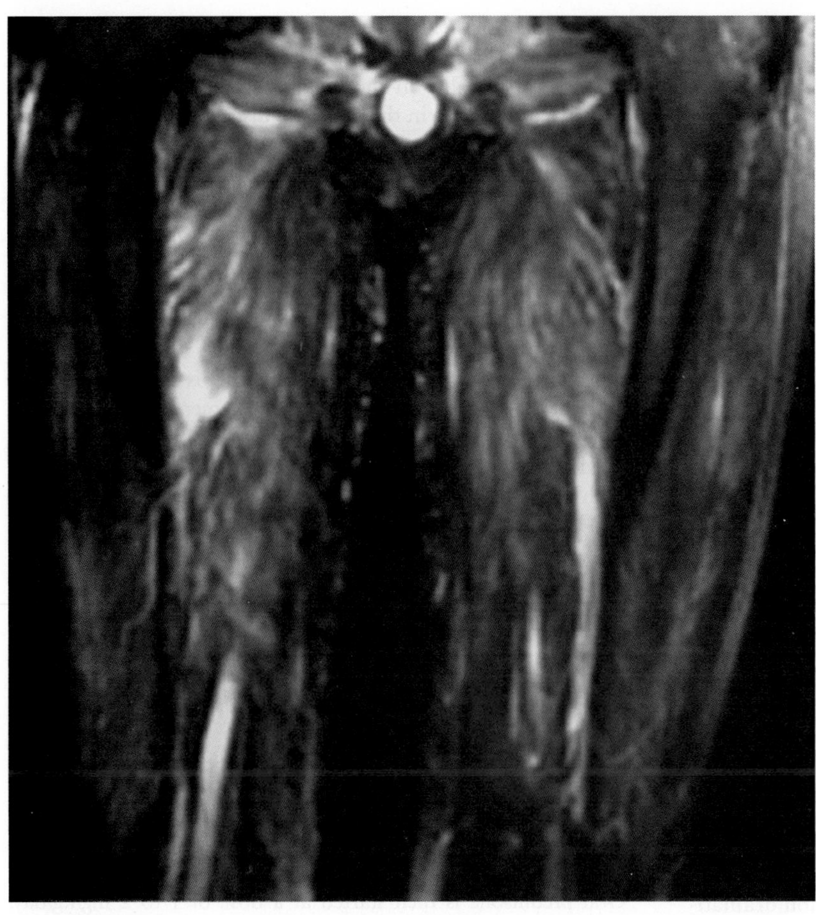

FIGURE 109.4 Coronal fast multiplanar inversion recovery image of the thighs shows areas of increased signal intensity, especially in the adductor muscle groups, in a patient with dermatomyositis.

in children differs significantly from that in adults: It includes a more prominent degree of vascular inflammation, less commonly involves detectable autoantibodies, and rarely accompanies malignancies. Further, in children, the appearance on MRI is essentially diagnostic because other causes of inflamed muscle and soft tissue are not seen in this age group (Fig. 109.4). New pediatric criteria are being developed; but until they are validated, Bohan and Peter's criteria remain the reference standard for classification of children with inflammatory myopathies.

Microscopically, the skin in JDMS shows dermal atrophy, obliteration of appendages, and lymphocytic infiltration. The muscle typically demonstrates a mixture of degenerating and regenerating muscle fibers, variations in muscle fiber size, perivascular lymphocytic infiltration, and perifascicular atrophy of muscle fibers. Small arteries, venules, and capillaries of the skin, muscle, fat, and GI tract characteristically reveal angiopathy. While the pathogenesis of JDMS has not been clearly defined, there are several models to explain its development including viral infections, particularly Coxsackie B; vasculitis caused by immune complex deposition; and cell-mediated cytotoxicity directed against muscle fibers. Certain HLA haplotypes, especially HLA-B8/DR3, may predispose to the disease. Synthesizing these findings, JDMS is thought to represent an as-yet unexplained perpetuation of muscle inflammation in susceptible hosts following what is typically a self-limited illness in most children.

Clinical Considerations

Clinical Recognition

JDMS has a wide clinical spectrum, from a mild form involving mainly the skin to a severe vasculitic type with a rapidly fulminating course. When untreated, the natural history of JDMS is to pass through four overlapping phases that typically last for 2 to 5 years but may persist indefinitely: (i) A prodromal phase of nonspecific aches and pains, (ii) a phase of progressive muscle and skin inflammation characterized by weakness and rash, (iii) a phase of persistent active disease and cumulative tissue damage, and (iv) an indolent phase with development of contractures and calcinosis but minimal ongoing inflammation. The goal of therapy is to compress this progression into a shorter time period that ends before irreversible damage occurs.

The onset of JDMS is often insidious, with aches and pains in the limbs, malaise, low-grade fever, and edema of the hands, feet, and eyelids. There may be a diffuse and nonspecific rash. This prodromal stage evolves into the acute phase, when the characteristic features of JDMS become evident. Classical skin manifestations include a violaceous heliotrope rash in the periorbital region and occasionally on the forehead; dusky red or atrophic lesions over the extensor aspects of the knees, elbows, and knuckles (Gottron papules); and periungual erythema (Fig. 109.5). Skin findings may precede or follow the onset of muscle weakness. Ulcerative skin lesions and anasarca are rare presenting manifestations of JDMS associated with a particularly severe disease course.

Muscular involvement in JDMS is characterized by pain, tenderness, and weakness of proximal muscles in a symmetric fashion. Strength of the anterior neck flexors and abdominal muscles is particularly affected, while facial muscles are spared. The disease may progress to involve the muscles of the palate and pharynx, resulting in regurgitation, nasal voice, and aspiration. Weakness of the respiratory muscles can lead

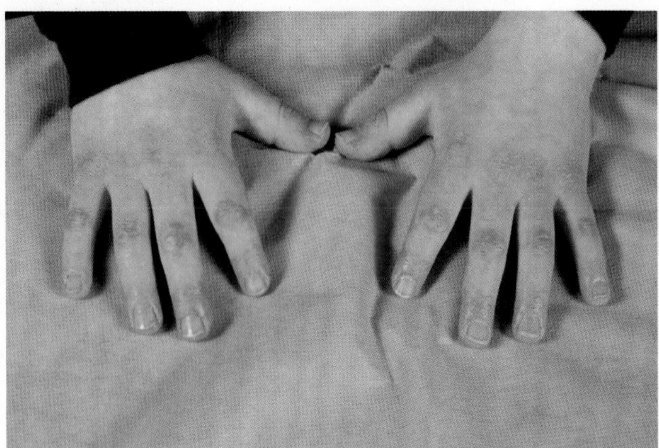

FIGURE 109.5 Gottron papules in juvenile dermatomyositis (JDMS). (Courtesy of Lisa Rider, MD.)

to a poor cough, pneumonia, and respiratory failure. Risk of GI hemorrhage and perforation are increased at this stage.

The clinical course of JDMS is variable; however, with the newer approaches to treatment, disease manifestations may be controlled within a few months in the vast majority of patients. Children with ongoing muscle inflammation for more than 6 to 12 months are at risk of developing late complications of JDMS. These include pronounced muscle wasting, contractures, lipodystrophy, and pigmentary changes of the skin. The rash over the extremities often becomes dry, scaly, and atrophic. Subcutaneous calcifications historically have occurred in up to 30% of children during this phase, although early aggressive treatment of inflammation dramatically reduces this rate. Calcifications are most typically discrete nodules around large joints, but at times they may take the form of a diffuse encasement of the soft tissues, known as calcinosis universalis. Occasionally, children pass through the early stages insidiously and come to the attention of physicians only when they develop contractures and calcinosis.

Clinical Assessment

Although skin and striated muscle are the primary targets of the inflammatory process in JDMS, typically other organ systems are also involved. Up to one-third of children develop arthritis, which may be present at diagnosis or may develop months into the disease process. The arthritis of JDMS is generally nonerosive and often improves as the primary disease is treated, although some children require specific therapy for their arthropathy. Neurologic manifestations of JDMS are extremely rare, but peripheral polyneuropathy, seizures, psychosis, and one case of suspected brainstem vasculopathy have been reported.

Weakness is a consistent manifestation of JDMS, but it is a late, variable, and subjective clinical sign. Objective evidence of muscle inflammation should also be sought by measuring serum levels of muscle enzymes that are released into the circulation when myocytes are injured. A wide variety of enzymes may be elevated in JDMS, including creatine kinase (CK), aldolase, lactate dehydrogenase (LDH), and transaminases (ALT and AST). These markers must be interpreted with caution, however, because none is specific for muscle. Elevated levels may be derived from damage to a variety of other tissues, including hepatocytes, brain cells, and the GI tract. Further, for unknown reasons many children do not reliably demonstrate elevated muscle enzymes despite significant myositis. This is particularly true during later stages of the disease, when subtle increases in LDH and aldolase may herald a disease flare-up, but CK levels often remain normal. While myositis-specific antibodies have demonstrable utility in the diagnosis of adult DM, currently they are of little use in the pediatric disease.

Because JDMS is a microangiopathic process, active disease is also characterized by elevated levels of von Willebrand factor antigen (vWFAg), which is released by damaged endothelial cells. In contrast, evidence of systemic inflammation may be absent, and acute-phase markers (including ESR and CRP) and CBCs are typically normal. MRI of the thighs may be the most sensitive method of documenting muscle inflammation (Fig. 109.4). Muscle biopsy can elucidate the diagnosis; however, given the morbidity of the procedure, the diagnosis is more often made without it. Evidence of cardiac involvement should also be sought, particularly with an EKG and an echocardiogram. Serologic markers of myocardial involvement are unreliable because both the CK-MB fraction and the troponin level are elevated in JDMS due to myoblast proliferation in skeletal muscles.

Management

General Management

The primary goal of therapy is to aggressively control muscle inflammation. The more rapidly markers of myocyte damage such as CK and aldolase can be normalized, the less the chance that acute and chronic complications will occur. Thus, virtually all children with clinical or biochemical evidence of muscle inflammation begin treatment with pulsed doses of IV methylprednisolone (30 mg per kg, maximum 1.5 g) infused over 1 to 2 hours. Oral prednisone is then started at a dose of 1 to 2 mg/kg/day. If muscle enzymes, weakness, or GI symptoms do not rapidly improve, steroid-sparing agents such as methotrexate (0.75 to 1.25 mg/kg/wk), IV immune globulin (2 g/kg/mo), or cyclosporine A (2 to 4 mg/kg/day) are introduced within 4 to 8 weeks. In more recalcitrant cases, it may be necessary to add immunosuppressive drugs such as cyclophosphamide (10 to 20 mg per m^2 every 2 to 4 weeks) or azathioprine (1 to 3 mg/kg/day). Under all circumstances, the goal is to rapidly control disease activity while minimizing toxicity from medications. Fortunately, active disease generally does not recur if a complete remission can be induced and maintained for 1 to 2 years.

During the initial evaluation of JDMS, it is essential to monitor the function of the palatopharyngeal and respiratory muscles; palatal weakness increases the risk of aspiration. Eating only in the upright position, frequent suctioning, or placement of a nasogastric tube may be necessary to avoid aspiration. Support of weak muscles, such as wearing a soft neck collar while riding in automobiles, helps minimize the risk of complications until children regain their strength.

Management of Complications and Emergencies

The most serious emergencies in JDMS relate to the respiratory and GI tracts (Table 109.8). In addition, complications may occur as a result of therapy with corticosteroids and immunosuppressive agents (e.g., infection and GI hemorrhage).

Respiratory Complications. (See also Chapters 66 Respiratory Distress and 107 Pulmonary Emergencies). Respiratory emergencies seen in childhood DM have diverse etiologies. Entities to be considered include (i) aspiration pneumonia secondary to weakness of velopalatine muscles; (ii) atelectasis and

TABLE 109.8

COMPLICATIONS OF JUVENILE DERMATOMYOSITIS

Clinical entity	Symptoms and signs	Investigations	Treatment
Respiratory failure	Air hunger, tachypnea, cyanosis, shallow respiration, alteration in mental status	Chest radiograph Arterial blood gas	Oxygen Mechanical ventilatory support Corticosteroids and immunosuppressives, plasmapheresis Antibiotics if evidence of aspiration pneumonia
Pneumothorax	Chest pain Breathlessness, tachypnea, cyanosis, diminished breath sounds, increased resonance to percussion	Chest radiograph	Chest tube
Velopalatine weakness	Pooling of secretions, drooling Nasal voice Aspiration pneumonia—recurrent	Careful barium cineradiographic study Chest radiograph	Corticosteroids Nasogastric feedings Tracheostomy
Gastrointestinal hemorrhage	Abdominal pain, nausea, vomiting Guarding, diminished bowel sounds (may be masked by corticosteroids) Hematemesis, melena, hematochezia	CBC; type and cross Abdominal radiograph: flat plate and upright Endoscopy Angiography Nuclear scan	NPO, NG tube Support of circulatory volume Antacids Corticosteroids Surgical consult Interventional radiology
Gastrointestinal perforation	May be silent (corticosteroids) or associated with abdominal pain, distention, vomiting	Abdominal radiographs: flat plate and upright	NPO, NG tube Surgical consult
Calcinosis	Swelling resembling cellulitis around large joints Fever	CBC Radiograph Aspiration	Antibiotics if superinfection suspected Pain control
Carditis	Dyspnea, tachycardia, arrhythmias	Chest radiograph EKG Echocardiogram	Digoxin, diuretics Antiarrhythmics Corticosteroids

CBC, complete blood count; NPO, nothing by mouth; NG, nasogastric; EKG, electrocardiogram.

pneumonia secondary to difficulty in clearing secretions as respiratory muscles become involved; (iii) respiratory failure secondary to profound involvement of respiratory musculature, including the diaphragm; (iv) progressive interstitial lung disease; and (v) opportunistic infection (tuberculosis, fungi, viruses, or *Pneumocystis*) in the immunosuppressed host. Because fever may also occur with active DM, it is necessary to differentiate pyrexia caused by infection from that caused by underlying disease.

In addition to usual care, preliminary investigations should include measurement of muscle enzymes (including CK, aldolase, AST, ALT, and LDH). Depending on the seriousness of the symptoms and the cooperativeness of the child, pulmonary function studies should be compared with baseline PFTs obtained previously on the same child because more than two-thirds of children with DM show restrictive disease and a diffusion abnormality.

If the etiology of the respiratory deterioration remains in doubt, more sensitive tests of disease activity, including vWFAg and MRI of the thigh muscles, may be necessary to determine whether more aggressive control of the underlying myositis is necessary. Corticosteroids are an essential component of the armamentarium for treating weakness of respiratory muscles and interstitial lung disease. If the weakness seems to be worsening, maximum efficacy may be obtained with pulsed-dose methylprednisolone. During this pulse therapy, blood pressure and cardiac rhythm should be monitored and the infusion stopped if there is sudden hyper- or hypotension or a rhythm disturbance. Plasmapheresis is reserved for children who deteriorate even after pulse steroid therapy. At best this provides temporary respite, so pheresis must be accompanied by institution of a long-term immunosuppressive regimen.

If pulmonary problems are suspected to result from infection, treatment with IV antibiotics should be initiated after appropriate cultures are obtained. In addition, sufficient corticosteroids (three times physiologic need) are given to compensate for potential iatrogenic adrenal insufficiency if the child has recently received high doses of steroids. Pneumothorax is another complication known to occur during the course of childhood DM.

GI Complications. Vasculitic changes, characterized by intimal hyperplasia and arteriolar occlusion by fibrin thrombi, are characteristic of severe or poorly controlled JDMS. Arteries and veins of the skin, muscles, and GI tract may be involved. Resultant ulcerations and perforations may occur anywhere from the esophagus to the large intestine, and they may disrupt the integrity of the integument. Symptoms and signs of these complications depend on the site of the lesion. GI hemorrhage in JDMS presents similarly to GI bleeding from other causes, and its evaluation and management are routine. The details of the management of hemorrhage from the GI tract are discussed in Chapter 28 Gastrointestinal Bleeding.

In a patient with JDMS, intestinal perforation may go unnoticed because of corticosteroid therapy and may present with pneumatosis intestinalis. This finding also may precede clinical perforation and pneumoperitoneum. Thus, any patient with JDMS and persistent abdominal pain should be examined radiographically for the presence of gas in the bowel wall.

Calcinosis. During the period of formation of subcutaneous calcification, children with JDMS may develop high fever, chills, and one or more areas of swelling under the skin. The inflammation caused by the subcutaneous calcium deposit may be indistinguishable from that of cellulitis or abscess formation, with warmth, erythema, and tenderness. Eventually, the lesion may spontaneously extrude calcium, at which time the fever often subsides. Although this is the natural history of subcutaneous calcifications, it is often hard to exclude an infectious etiology. If doubt exists, needle aspiration of the site may be performed and the fluid examined for calcium crystals and organisms. In the face of uncertainty, it is best to treat for infection with antibiotics until culture results are available. Incision and drainage or surgical debridement should be avoided, as the inflamed skin rarely heals satisfactorily. Complete control of the underlying disease offers the best hope for resolution of calcinosis, although this may be incomplete or may require many years.

Cardiac Emergencies. Although EKG abnormalities may be seen in up to 50% of children with JDMS, development of myocarditis is uncommon. Involvement of the conduction system by edema and fibrosis leads to electrical abnormalities and arrhythmias.

BEHÇET DISEASE

BD is a rare vasculitis in children, especially in nonendemic areas such as the United States. The classical description of BD is a clinical triad consisting of recurrent buccal aphthous ulcers, recurrent genital ulcers, and uveitis with hypopyon. In addition to these cardinal features of BD, there are a host of associated clinical manifestations, including arthritis, neurologic involvement, GI manifestations, vascular/thrombotic disease, and various dermatologic lesions, including erythema nodosum and necrotic folliculitis.

Clinical Considerations

Recurrent oral ulcerations are the most common presenting sign and ongoing manifestation of pediatric BD. While ulcerative mucocutaneous lesions are far from specific for BD, unlike those associated with inflammatory bowel disease, SLE, chronic oral aphthosis, and sweet syndrome, the oral lesions in BD tend to scar.

Although oral and genital ulcers can certainly be painful for the patient and problematic from a management standpoint, there are other less common but more serious complications of BD that may lead to severe morbidity and even mortality. Ocular disease can be devastating, ultimately resulting in blindness. GI disease can result in perforation. Neurologic complications are varied, including headache, meningoencephalitis, pseudotumor cerebri, and quadriparesis. Psychiatric symptoms including depression, personality changes, and memory loss are also reported. Vascular/thrombotic complications are particularly ominous development in BD patients; these can include dural sinus thrombosis and arterial lesions. In one multinational pediatric BD series, large-vessel thrombosis was the leading cause of death, carrying a 30% mortality rate.

Management

The general treatment of BD is similar to other forms of vasculitis discussed in this chapter, consisting of anti-inflammatory/immunosuppressive agents. Life-threatening cases of BD may require high-dose systemic corticosteroids and cyclophosphamide. Thrombotic disease requires anticoagulation in addition to aggressive immunosuppression.

ARTHRITIS

CLINICAL PEARLS AND PITFALLS

- Childhood arthritis lasting 6 weeks or more without alternative etiology is termed JIA.
- JIA subtypes differ in the pattern of joints involved, extra-articular manifestations, and treatment.
- MAS is a severe and potentially life-threatening complication of systemic onset JIA.
- JIA is frequently treated with disease-modifying and biologic agents that may suppress the immune system.

Arthritis is a clinical finding of persistent joint inflammation characterized by swelling or restriction of joint movement by pain. Arthritis is a common childhood finding and is caused by many factors, including infection and autoimmunity. Infectious arthritis may be caused by a multiplicity of pathogens, including bacteria, viruses, and fungi. Bacterial arthritis, also known as septic arthritis, is addressed in Chapters 41 Limp and 102 Infectious Disease Emergencies. In addition, an inappropriately self-directed immune response triggered by infection may lead to a postinfectious reactive arthritis. While this class of arthritis is typically self-limited; treatment, usually with NSAIDs, may be needed to ameliorate symptoms. On occasion postinfectious inflammatory arthritis recurs or persists, leading to a more chronic arthritis akin to more classical juvenile inflammatory arthritis. When childhood arthritis persists and no alternative etiology is discovered, it is termed JIA. In this chapter, we will focus our discussion on JIA. Lyme arthritis, a late manifestation of systemic infection with Borrelia, is discussed in Chapter 102 Infectious Disease Emergencies.

JUVENILE IDIOPATHIC ARTHRITIS

Current Evidence

JIA, formerly known as juvenile rheumatoid arthritis (JRA), is now the most common pediatric rheumatologic disease in the developed world, having replaced acute rheumatic fever. JIA occurs in all races and ethnic groups, with a reported prevalence

TABLE 109.9

CLASSIFICATION SYSTEMS FOR JUVENILE ARTHRITIS

Comparison of current classification systems for chronic arthritis in children, showing differing names for similar types of arthritis in parallel columns.

ACR	ILAR	EULAR
Juvenile rheumatoid arthritis	Juvenile idiopathic arthritis	Juvenile chronic arthritis
Systemic onset	Systemic arthritis	Systemic onset
Polyarticular onset	RF-negative polyarthritis	Polyarticular onset
	RF-positive polyarthritis	Juvenile rheumatoid arthritis
Pauciarticular onset	Oligoarthritis	Pauciarticular onset
Type 1	Persistent	
	Extended	
	Psoriatic arthritis	Juvenile psoriatic arthritis
Type 2	Enthesitis-related arthritis	Juvenile ankylosing spondylitis
	Undifferentiated arthritis	

ACR, American College of Rheumatology; ILAR, International League of Associations for Rheumatology; EULAR, European League Against Rheumatism.

that varies from 30 to 400 per 100,000 children depending upon the population studied and the diagnostic techniques used. In the United States alone, JIA affects at least 100,000 children.

A variety of different classification systems for JIA exists, but in the absence of a clear-cut understanding of the pathogenesis of arthritis, the preferred is the International League for Associations in Rheumatology (ILAR) classification system (Table 109.9). It includes the following subtypes of arthritis: polyarticular, oligoarticular (persistent and extended), and systemic onset juvenile idiopathic arthritis (soJIA) as well as psoriatic arthritis, enthesitis-related arthritis (ERA), and undifferentiated arthritis (Table 109.10). Persistent unexplained arthritis of one or more joints lasting more than 6 weeks in children younger than 16 years of age will be referred to as JIA. In all cases, because there are no laboratory abnormalities specific for JIA, the diagnosis is made clinically after exclusion of other infectious, inflammatory, and traumatic conditions.

The etiology of JIA is not known. It is useful conceptually to divide the pathogenesis of JIA into an initiating phase and a perpetuating phase. Various events, particularly viral infections, may trigger articular inflammation. For a variety of reasons related to both the host and the inciting event, a process that is self-limited in most children leads to ongoing inflammation in others. This inflammation is characterized by abnormal tissue and circulating levels of proinflammatory cytokines (including interleukin [IL]-1, IL-6, tumor necrosis factor [TNF], and interferon-γ) leading to activation of lymphocytes and infiltration of synovium. In fact, conditions labeled as JIA most likely represent a final common pathway for many different types of synovitis in view of the widely disparate characteristics of the different subtypes of JIA.

TABLE 109.10

SUBGROUPS OF JUVENILE IDIOPATHIC ARTHRITIS

Subgroup	At onset % of JIA	Gender ratio	Age at onset	Joints affected	Serologic and genetic test	Extra-articular manifestations	Prognosis
Rheumatoid-positive polyarticular	15	90% female	Late childhood	Any joints, especially hands, wrists	ANA 75% RF 100%	Low-grade fever, anemia, malaise, rheumatoid nodules	>50% Severe arthritis
Rheumatoid-negative polyarticular	20	70% female	Younger onset	Any joints	ANA 50%	Low-grade fever, mild anemia, malaise, growth retardation	20–40% Severe arthritis
Oligoarticular	50	F > M	Early childhood	Large joints	ANA often present	Uveitis	Severe arthritis uncommon
Systemic onset	15	50% female	Any age	Any joints	ANA-negative, RF-negative	High fever, rash, organomegaly, polyserositis, leukocytosis, growth retardation	30% Severe arthritis

ANA, antinuclear antibody; RF, rheumatoid factor.

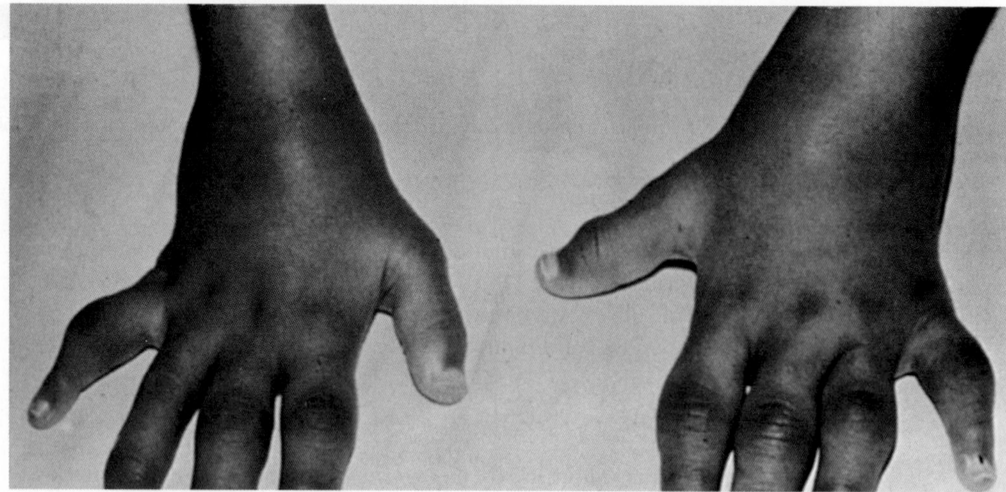

FIGURE 109.6 Symmetric involvement of large and small joints of the hands in a child with polyarticular juvenile idiopathic arthritis.

Clinical Considerations

JIA is characterized by wide demographic and clinical variety, so the condition has been divided into subtypes based on these factors and on the pattern of the disease during the first 6 months following onset (Table 109.10). These varieties, in turn, are treated in different ways, and are associated with different complications. Whereas the term JRA had previously been favored, a newer classification scheme with the umbrella term JIA has become more widely accepted in the rheumatologic literature and among rheumatologists. Until a pathophysiology-based means of classifying and distinguishing these subtypes of JIA becomes available, what is probably several discrete conditions will continue to be grouped on the basis of clinical features. The remainder of this chapter will utilize the newer JIA classification scheme.

Oligoarticular (or pauciarticular) arthritis, synovitis involving four or fewer joints, is the most common subtype of JIA and accounts for approximately half of all cases. Oligoarticular arthritis occurs more often in young girls, typically causing swelling, pain, and limitation of movement in one or more large joints. ANAs are detectable in the sera of many of these children, and their presence at any titer correlates with a higher risk for developing iridocyclitis. Polyarticular arthritis (both RF-positive and RF-negative) occurs more commonly in girls. It is characterized by the insidious onset of symmetric synovitis in both large and small joints, accompanied by low-grade fever, morning stiffness, and malaise (Fig. 109.6). The presence of RF and/or anti-CCP antibodies corresponds to an increased risk of severe, erosive arthritis. RF positivity is also associated with the development of vasculitic complications and subcutaneous nodules. Cervical spine involvement occurs in approximately 30% to 50% of patients with this variety of arthritis, resulting in neck pain, stiffness, and torticollis. Unlike oligoarticular JIA, in which ocular involvement is the cause of the most significant morbidity, polyarticular disease may result in severe musculoskeletal disability. Thus, involvement of the temporomandibular joint may result in restricted ability to open the mouth, involvement of the hips may permanently affect ambulation, and small joint arthritis of the hands may compromise manual dexterity.

The least common subtype of JIA is soJIA or Still disease. This subtype occurs most often in boys younger than 5 years of age, although it has been reported even in adults. Clinically, these children often present with a fever of unknown origin; they may have high spiking temperatures (39° to 41°C) for several weeks or months, classically in a double quotidian (twice daily) pattern. Although the child often feels stiff and does not move normally, arthritis may not be a prominent feature at the onset of the disease. Diagnosis therefore generally involves excluding infectious and malignant conditions, especially sepsis, leukemia, and neuroblastoma. A characteristic salmon-pink evanescent maculopapular rash (Fig. 109.7), diffuse lymphadenopathy, and hepatosplenomegaly (HSM) may also be present in the early stages, offering clues to the diagnosis. Arthralgias and myalgias are common, and pericarditis occurs most typically in this subtype of JIA. With time, systemic features of the disease become less prominent, and polyarticular arthritis becomes the major focus of management.

Laboratory and Radiologic Features

No laboratory test is diagnostic of JIA. Rather, it is a clinical condition diagnosed on the basis of characteristic findings on history and physical examination, although some laboratory studies may be suggestive of the diagnosis. In polyarticular JIA, one subgroup shows RF in the serum; no other pediatric rheumatologic disease typically has this marker, though the RF may be present nonspecifically in healthy children as well. Mild to moderate anemia is common in all subtypes, particularly the systemic type. The white blood count is often elevated, again most typically in the systemic type, in which leukemoid reactions may be seen. Platelet counts are often elevated indicating systemic inflammation, and urinalysis is usually normal. There is elevation of levels of acute-phase reactants in the serum, often in proportion to the number of joints involved, and most prominently in systemic onset disease. Complement levels may be normal or elevated, but immunoglobulins are typically increased, leading to a reversal of the albumin to globulin ratio.

Radiographic features of JIA include soft tissue swelling and periarticular osteopenia adjacent to affected joints (Fig. 109.8). Later, narrowing of the joint spaces, bony cysts, erosions, subluxations, and ankylosis may be seen. In children in whom physical examination is difficult or inconclusive,

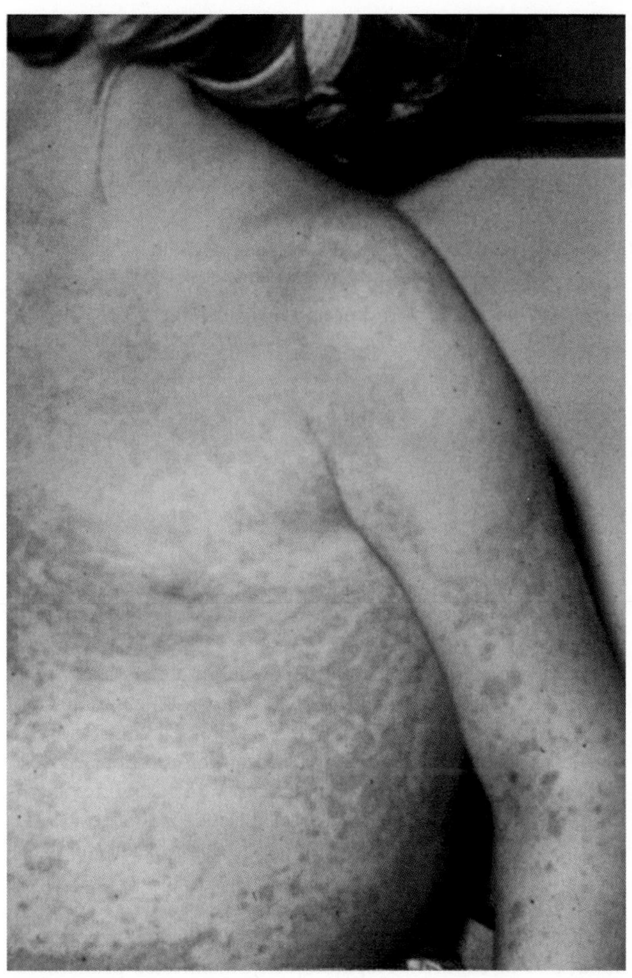

FIGURE 109.7 Macular rash in a child with systemic onset juvenile idiopathic arthritis.

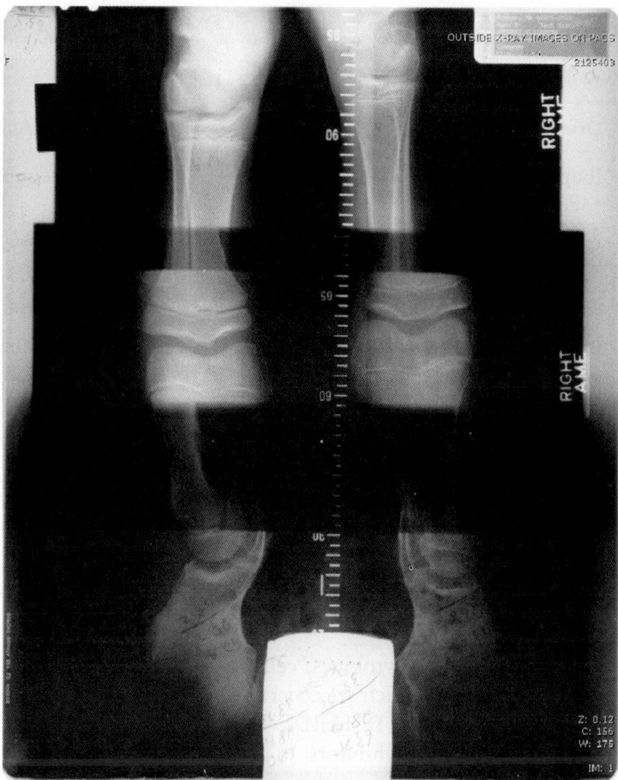

FIGURE 109.8 Radiograph showing features of juvenile idiopathic arthritis, including soft tissue swelling, bony overgrowth, and periarticular osteopenia adjacent to affected joints.

ultrasonography may confirm the presence of a joint effusion, and MRI with gadolinium enhancement may show both synovial proliferation and increased fluid in the joint space.

Management

General Management

The major goal of therapy in children with JIA is to help both the child and the family maintain as normal a life as possible. Emotional support, including the information that most children with this disease are able to lead a normal life with few long-term problems, provides reassurance. Simple measures, such as warm baths and the use of electric blankets at night, help control morning stiffness. For children with minimal joint involvement, regular daily activities, including participation in physical education classes, are to be encouraged, although direct impact on inflamed joints should be avoided. In the presence of muscle wasting, weakness, or restricted range of motion in any joint, an active physical therapy program is indicated. Splinting may be used to rest actively inflamed, painful joints and to prevent worsening of deformities, though complete disuse should be avoided in order to minimize atrophy and loss of motion.

Medications. The pharmacologic management of JIA has changed dramatically over the past two decades because of the understanding that most children continue to have active synovial inflammation for decades and do not "outgrow" their disease. Accordingly, modern therapy aims not only for relief of the symptoms of pain and stiffness, but also for joint protection through suppression of synovial inflammation. Consequently, physicians caring for these children must be familiar with the intended and unintended effects of a wide variety of anti-inflammatory and immunosuppressant medications.

NSAIDs are the initial agents used in most children with JIA. In addition to the better known NSAIDs, COX-2 inhibitors may be used to treat JIA (Table 109.11). These agents, such as celecoxib are anti-inflammatory drugs specific for the inducible isotype of the cyclooxygenase enzyme, resulting in fewer GI side effects than traditional mixed COX-1 and COX-2 inhibitors. For children who respond inadequately to NSAIDs, so-called disease-modifying antirheumatic drugs (DMARDs) must be added to control symptoms and prevent long-term complications of the arthritis. Several agents are available, including sulfasalazine, hydroxychloroquine, leflunomide, and methotrexate (Table 109.12). Practitioners choose among these agents based on a child's age, the severity of the synovitis, and the subtype of arthritis. Methotrexate is the most commonly used second-line agent and the first shown to prevent erosive changes. Even at the lower doses used for JIA, methotrexate is immunosuppressive and can be associated with bone marrow and hepatic toxicity. Sulfasalazine is most often used in children with inflammatory bowel disease and spondyloarthropathies (including ERA and psoriatic arthritis), but it also has a role in milder cases of JIA. Leflunomide inhibits *de novo* pyrimidine synthesis, especially in activated lymphocytes. The side effects of leflunomide are similar to those of methotrexate and the two agents may be used together.

The newest agents in the arthritis armamentarium are the biologic response modifiers, medications that specifically

TABLE 109.11

NSAIDs USED IN THE TREATMENT OF ARTHRITIS IN CHILDREN

Drug	Doses/day	Dose (mg/kg/day)	Side effects
Ibuprofen (Motrin, Advil, Pediaprofen)	3–4	30–40 (maximum 2,400 mg/day)	Gastric irritation, chemical hepatitis
Naproxen (Naprosyn, Aleve)	2	10–20 (maximum 1,000 mg/day)	Gastric irritation, behavioral changes, headache, photosensitivity
Meloxicam (Mobic)	1	0.25 (maximum 15 mg/day)	Gastric irritation, headache, fever
Indomethacin (Indocin)	3	1.5–3 (maximum 200 mg/day)	Gastric irritation, headache, chemical hepatitis
Celecoxib (Celebrex)	2	10–25 kg: 50 mg/dose (maximum 100 mg/day) >25 kg: 100 mg/dose (maximum 200 mg/day) >40 kg: 200 mg/dose (maximum 400 mg/day)	Gastric irritation, cough, rash (including Stevens–Johnson syndrome)

NSAIDs, nonsteroidal anti-inflammatory drugs.

target inflammatory cytokines, cellular receptors, and adhesion molecules, but which are generally more immunosuppressive than conventional DMARDs. The most widely used biologic agents are TNF inhibitors. In addition, agents that block specific proinflammatory cytokines, like anakinra (anti–IL-1 R antagonist) and tocilizumab (anti–IL-6 monoclonal antibody) may be used.

Corticosteroids must be employed judiciously in JIA due to the significant toxicity associated with their use. Systemic steroids are typically reserved for children with severe complications or time-limited flares, e.g., in the setting of systemic symptoms, pericarditis, or pleuritis, during brief flare-ups of severe arthritis, or while waiting for slower-acting agents to take effect. Intra-articular steroids may be used in patients with oligoarthritis, or in children with polyarticular disease in whom selected joints require particularly aggressive management. Topical ophthalmologic steroids are the mainstay of therapy for iridocyclitis.

Drug Toxicity. Almost all drugs used for the treatment of JIA have the potential for serious toxicity. If a child with JIA on treatment develops a new symptom, drug toxicity must always be considered as a possible cause. Tables 109.11 and 109.12 list the common adverse reactions reported with NSAIDs and DMARDs typically used in the treatment of JIA. Though new medications are more targeted in their effects on the immune system, most advanced therapies for arthritis cause at least some immunosuppression. Accordingly, physicians caring for children with JIA should be particularly vigilant for evidence of infections.

For the nonsteroidal anti-inflammatory agents, GI toxicity is the most common side effect. Nonetheless, significant NSAID gastropathy is unusual in children, and gastric or intestinal perforations, a significant problem in older adults, are rare. NSAIDs may also cause various other side effects. Reversible CNS complaints, particularly headaches, dizziness, and fatigue, occur in about 5% of children. Hepatotoxicity, manifested primarily as elevation of transaminases, and nephrotoxicity, including proteinuria and renal papillary necrosis, are rare but potentially dangerous if overlooked. Friability of the skin and a porphyria-like blistering of sun-exposed areas may be seen with these agents, especially naproxen when used in fair-skinned children.

Unlike salicylates, NSAIDs rarely cause tinnitus or hyperventilation. Reye syndrome, although far less common than with salicylates, has been reported in children receiving NSAIDs; therefore, it is prudent to consider suspension of these agents in children with influenza or varicella. Salicylates must be carefully avoided in children who are even exposed to these viruses. In any child using salicylates or other NSAIDs, development of pernicious vomiting and/or alteration in mental status warrants consideration of Reye syndrome.

TABLE 109.12

DMARDs USED IN THE TREATMENT OF JIA

Drug	Dosing schedule	Side effects
Methotrexate	Weekly	Nausea, hair loss, chemical hepatitis, hypersensitivity, pneumonitis
Leflunomide	Once a day	Nausea, diarrhea, chemical hepatitis
Sulfasalazine	Twice a day	Gastric irritation, photosensitivity, behavioral changes, hypersensitivity reaction, neutropenia
Hydroxychloroquine	Once a day	Abdominal pain, diarrhea, retinitis

DMARDs, disease-modifying antirheumatic drugs; JIA, juvenile rheumatoid arthritis.

Each of the second-line agents used in the treatment of JIA also has the potential to cause specific forms of toxicity. Despite its favorable therapeutic profile, methotrexate is an antimetabolite with the potential to cause oral ulcers, nausea, and abdominal pain. These adverse effects may be minimized by supplementation with folic acid. Children must be monitored regularly for evidence of hepatic toxicity; persistent elevation of hepatic transaminases identifies those at risk for hepatic fibrosis or cirrhosis. Methotrexate may also cause lymphopenia, especially with prolonged use, or even pancytopenia due to bone marrow suppression. Ten percent of children receiving methotrexate for arthritis may develop mild hypogammaglobulinemia, but there is no evidence that this is clinically significant. Concurrent use of other dihydrofolate reductase inhibitors, such as trimethoprim-sulfamethoxazole (Bactrim), potentiates these risks and should be avoided.

Rarely, use of methotrexate is associated with the development of pulmonary hypersensitivity. This most commonly occurs during the first 6 to 12 months of use and may be marked by dyspnea, cough, fever, and fluffy infiltrates on chest x-ray. Although such symptoms may be conclusively distinguished from viral pneumonitis only by lung biopsy, suspicion of this complication necessitates discontinuation of methotrexate and institution of treatment with systemic corticosteroids. Failure to stop the drug, or a second exposure to methotrexate, may cause fatal respiratory failure.

The biologic response modifiers are generally well tolerated, but as with all medications that target the immune response as a way of controlling inflammation, biologics are immunosuppressive. Although these effects are more limited than those of traditional cytotoxic agents, defenses against various infections are impaired. The infectious risk appears to increase significantly with use of more than one biologic agent at a time. Although most people note only an increased frequency of mild upper respiratory tract illnesses, treatment with TNF inhibitors also increases susceptibility to potentially serious mycobacterial, bacterial, fungal, and herpes viral infections.

The long-term effects of altering the immune response with anti-TNF medications are not known. In adults, new autoantibodies may develop (including ANA and anti-ds DNA), and rarely patients may develop multiple sclerosis–like CNS abnormalities. These associations should be kept in mind if a patient on anti-TNF therapy develops new neurologic or rheumatologic complaints.

Sulfasalazine is a sulfa drug, and its most severe side effects are typical of this class of medications. Headache and GI upset—especially with preparations that are not enterically coated—occur most commonly. Although rare, more concerning are bone marrow suppression, agranulocytosis, photosensitive eruptions, and hypersensitivity reactions, including Stevens–Johnson syndrome.

Antimalarial agents such as hydroxychloroquine must be administered judiciously because of their ability to cause irreversible ocular toxicity at high doses. Even at lower doses, children may develop rashes, gastric upset, or reversible visual disturbances secondary to altered accommodation. Finally, children with glucose-6-phosphate deficiency who receive hydroxychloroquine may develop hemolytic anemia, especially during intercurrent infections.

The long list of potential side effects of systemic corticosteroids is enumerated elsewhere. In the acute setting, immunosuppressive effects of systemic steroids are most salient. It is important to remember that these agents dramatically increase susceptibility to herpes viruses (especially disseminated varicella) and intracellular pathogens, such as mycobacteria and listeria. Although they have little effect on susceptibility to other bacterial pathogens, their anti-inflammatory effects tend to mask clinical signs of infection, accentuating the need for attentiveness on the part of clinicians. In addition, patients receiving chronic corticosteroid therapy are at risk for adrenal insufficiency, and treatment with stress dose steroids may be necessary in the setting of acute illness or injury.

Management of Complications and Emergencies

Patients with all subtypes of JIA may have extra-articular complications either due to their underlying disease or as a result of treatment with immunosuppressive medications. It should be noted, however, that children with soJIA are at higher risk for more severe complications of disease, including life-threatening cardiopulmonary manifestations of disease. As such, extra care to evaluate for such complications should be taken when children with soJIA present to the ED.

Fever. Marked elevation of body temperature is characteristic of soJIA, whereas a lower-grade fever often accompanies polyarticular disease. The diagnosis of soJIA is one of exclusion and fever is a common symptom, so diligent efforts should be made to rule out infectious diseases and malignancies. This may require hospitalization for a diagnostic evaluation, particularly in infants and young children. A bone marrow examination to rule out malignancy is necessary in many patients with soJIA because acute lymphoblastic leukemia may cause joint pain and swelling, fever, lymphadenopathy, and HSM that are indistinguishable from findings in JIA.

In a patient being treated for known soJIA, fever may represent recurrence of JIA, or it may be because of an intercurrent infection. Fevers in Still disease (soJIA) typically follow the classic double quotidian (twice daily) pattern, with two peaks above 39°C daily, as well as periods at or below normal without use of antipyretic medications. If there are no localizing signs of infection, if the complete blood cell count (CBC) shows the leukocytosis, thrombocytosis, and anemia typical of JIA, and if the urinalysis is normal, the child may be treated for a presumed JIA flare-up. Notably, an acute infection can cause a flare of disease and both entities may coexist. Children being treated with immunosuppressive medications may require empiric antibiotics or observation in the hospital until negative culture results allow infections to be excluded. If the patient has received more than 20 mg of prednisone daily for more than 6 weeks within the previous 12 months, appropriate coverage with stress dosages of steroids (three times the physiologic dose) is indicated while the infection is being treated.

Fever in soJIA, especially within 6 months of disease onset, occasionally may be caused by MAS, which has also been termed reactive hemophagocytic lymphohistiocytosis (HLH) as it exists on the spectrum of hemophagocytic syndromes. This spectrum of disease will be discussed in greater detail below. This life-threatening complication is characterized by systemic inflammation with disseminated intravascular coagulopathy with diffuse microthromboses, hemophagocytosis causing cytopenias, hepatic inflammation, and CNS changes progressing to seizures or coma. The cause of MAS is unknown, but it does occur more commonly during intercurrent viral illnesses, as well as in children receiving NSAIDs or DMARDs (particularly sulfasalazine) as treatment. Differentiation from sepsis or a flare of JIA may be difficult, although a sudden rise in hepatic enzymes, ferritin, and triglycerides or a sudden drop in platelets, red blood cells, or ESR (due to consumption of cellular elements and fibrinogen) are suggestive. Early diagnosis and a high level of suspicion are essential. Treatment with anakinra, pulse-dose methylprednisolone (30 mg per kg, maximum 1 g), and/or cyclosporine, as well as general support measures for DIC, often lead to full recovery. Delayed diagnosis, in contrast, is accompanied by a reported mortality rate of 20% to 50%.

Cardiac Complications. Cardiac involvement is an important feature of JIA but is uncommon in other subtypes of juvenile arthritis. Pericarditis, like other systemic manifestations of Still disease, most often occurs during the first 2 years of the illness. Fortunately, pericardial effusions in JIA rarely lead to cardiac tamponade.

Other types of cardiac involvement are unusual. Valvulitis is not typical of JIA and should suggest the possibility of acute rheumatic fever or bacterial endocarditis. Myocarditis is rare but may be seen.

Bed rest and therapy with an NSAID should be adequate for the treatment of mild to moderate pericarditis due to JIA. Corticosteroids (prednisone 1 to 2 mg/kg/day, maximum 60 to 80 mg) are indicated for the treatment of noninfectious myocarditis, for massive pericarditis causing compromise of cardiac output, or if significant symptoms persist despite therapy with NSAIDs. In the presence of tamponade or progressive deterioration, pericardiocentesis provides temporary relief, whereas anti-inflammatory medications are used to prevent reaccumulation of fluid.

Pulmonary Emergencies. Pleural effusions are a recognized manifestation of soJIA (Fig. 109.9). Occasionally, pleural fluid collections may be massive, resulting in respiratory distress. Other pleuropulmonary complications include pneumonitis, diffuse interstitial disease, lymphoid bronchiolitis, and pulmonary arteritis. In the absence of the need for thoracentesis for diagnostic or therapeutic purposes, treatment is aimed at the underlying disease process, primarily involving control of inflammation with NSAIDs, corticosteroids, or anakinra. Children with pleural effusions often require admission in order to address the overall severity of systemic features of the disease.

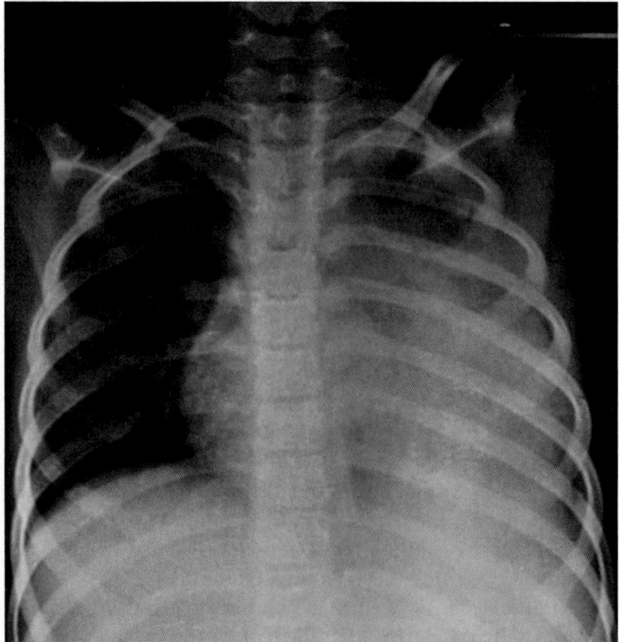

FIGURE 109.9 Pericardial and pleural effusions in a child with systemic onset juvenile idiopathic arthritis.

Iridocyclitis. Iridocyclitis (inflammation of the iris and ciliary body) occurs in approximately 10% to 20% of all children with JIA. This can be of acute or chronic onset. The chronic type of iridocyclitis occurs primarily in young children with oligoarticular JIA, especially girls with oligoarthritis and a positive ANA. In contrast, acute iridocyclitis occurs most often in older boys with oligoarticular disease.

Acute iridocyclitis is characterized by sudden onset of redness, tearing, pain, and photophobia, and urgent management may be required to preserve vision. Immediate consultation with an ophthalmologist is essential. The usual emergent treatment includes topical corticosteroids and mydriatics.

Flare of a Single Joint in a Patient with JIA. In a patient known to have JIA and receiving anti-inflammatory medication, acute swelling with pain and limitation of range of movement of a single joint raises a common management problem. Potential causes of such an acute monoarthritis include a flare of JIA versus infectious arthritis or Lyme arthritis, and careful attention to physical examination and historical features are essential to avoid misdiagnosis.

Physical findings characteristic of infection of a joint are fever, extreme pain, tenderness, erythema, and warmth over the joint. The affected joints of JIA, while often swollen, warm, and stiff, are rarely red. There is usually pronounced splinting of an infected joint due to pain; the slightest movement may cause muscle spasm. In contrast, some range of motion is usually possible even with severely inflamed joints of JIA. If the patient is taking an immunosuppressive medication, physical findings of inflammation and/or infection may be masked.

If infection cannot be excluded with confidence, joint fluid must be aspirated, and the fluid sent for cell count, Gram stain, and culture. Synovial fluid is bacteriostatic and some fastidious organisms, such as *Kingella,* may be particularly difficult to culture, so joint fluid samples should be inoculated into blood culture bottles to optimize sensitivity. If there is any doubt about the diagnosis, it is best to also obtain a blood culture (which increases diagnostic yield, as the organisms causing septic arthritis are generally spread hematogenously) and then to initiate treatment for septic arthritis.

For the acute swelling and pain in a single joint caused by a JIA flare, resting the involved extremity for 2 to 3 days may be adequate. After infection has been excluded, injection of the joint with a topical steroid preparation such as triamcinolone hexacetonide (1 mg per kg, maximum 40 to 60 mg) may provide rapid and sustained relief. If multiple joints are involved during a flare, treatment with systemic agents from NSAIDs to corticosteroids may be necessary as may escalation of the baseline anti-arthritis regimen for severe or persistently active arthritis.

Ruptured Popliteal Cyst. There are six bursae around the knee joint. Of these, the gastrocnemius semimembranosus bursa is the one that most often communicates with the synovial space. Consequently, in the presence of effusion in the knee joint, fluid may enter the bursa and produce a popliteal cyst (Baker cyst). Patients with popliteal cysts have a palpable and visible enlargement in the popliteal area, best seen while the patient is standing with knees extended.

Rupture of a popliteal cyst with drainage of fluid into the calf muscles may present as an emergency. Affected patients complain of sudden pain in the calf associated with swelling in the leg. On physical examination they have induration, erythema, warmth, and tenderness of the calf, as well as ankle edema. An effusion in the knee joint and evidence of synovial thickening are often present. Homan sign may be positive, but other signs of venous thrombosis, including palpable venous cords, dilation of collateral veins, or arterial spasm, are usually absent.

Differentiation of a ruptured popliteal cyst from thrombophlebitis may be difficult, though the latter are very rare in otherwise healthy children, and the former relatively common in children with arthritis. Elevated D-dimers and other evidence of a consumptive coagulopathy characterize venous thrombosis, while most children with soJIA do not have such abnormalities. Ultimately, ultrasonographic or MRI may be needed to establish the diagnosis. Intra-articular administration of steroids (triamcinolone hexacetonide, 1 mg per kg) is the recommended initial treatment for a ruptured Baker cyst. If there is an inadequate response or if the syndrome is chronic, surgical excision of the cyst may be necessary.

Cervical Spine Involvement. This complication usually is seen in children with established severe polyarticular JIA. Although cervical spine involvement is known to occur in 30% to 50% of patients with JIA, subluxation of the atlantoaxial (AA) joint or the lower cervical spine is less common in children than adults. Clinical evidence of pressure on the spinal cord is seen in 23% to 65% of adults with radiologic evidence of AA subluxation. Similar data are not available for children.

Neck stiffness that is worst in the morning is the most common symptom of cervical spine involvement in JIA. Occasionally, torticollis may be the presenting manifestation of cervical arthritis. Severe pain in the neck and referred pain over the occipital and retroorbital areas also may occur. The pain has a dull, aching quality and is often aggravated by neck movement. On physical examination, torticollis and/or loss of lordosis of the cervical spine, as well as limitation of range or movement of the neck, are the typical findings.

Paresthesia of the fingers is the most common symptom of spinal cord compression. Weakness of the arms and legs and inability to control the bladder or bowels are other complaints that should suggest spinal cord compression. During the initial stages, exaggerated deep tendon reflexes and an extensor plantar reflex are noted. Chronic myelopathy results in muscle atrophy and loss of deep tendon reflexes. Lateral radiographs of the neck in flexion and in extension are required for complete evaluation of the cervical spine. The patient should be asked to actively and slowly flex and extend the neck to tolerance without discomfort; care should be taken not to force these movements. On some occasions, CT or MRI may be indicated.

The distance between the anterior surface of the odontoid and the posterior surface of the anterior arch of atlas when measured in a lateral film with neck in flexion is usually 4 mm or less. In the presence of AA subluxation, this may be as wide as 10 to 12 mm (Fig. 109.10). Other radiologic abnormalities characteristic of cervical spine involvement in JIA include loss of curvature, osteoporosis, erosions and sclerosis of joints, disc-space narrowing, and altered height-to-width ratio of the vertebral bodies.

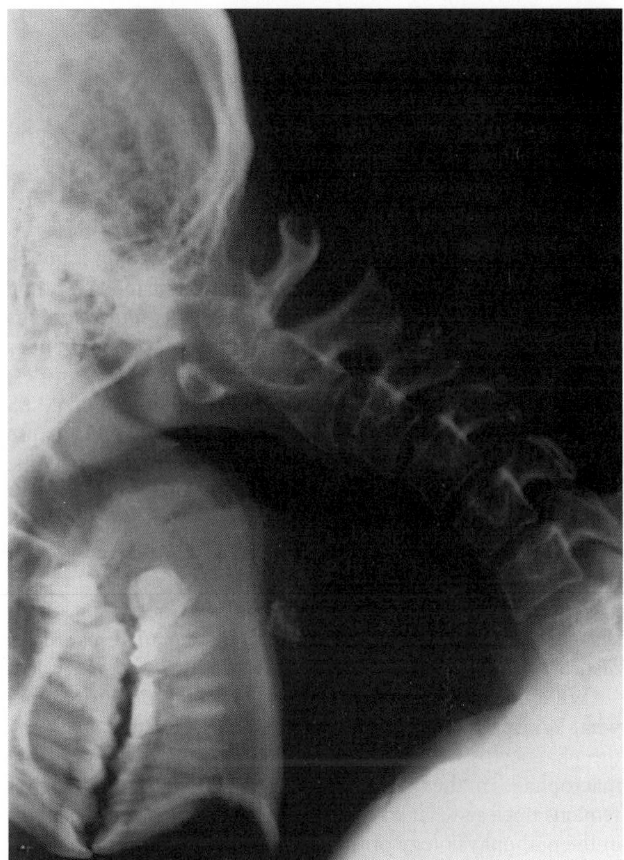

FIGURE 109.10 Atlantoaxial sublocation in a child with juvenile idiopathic arthritis. (The distance between the anterior arch of the atlas and the odontoid process in the original radiograph was 5 mm.)

Although most children with AA subluxation do not have evidence of spinal cord compression, the physician must be wary of its occurrence with excessive movement, as occurs during endotracheal intubation. Regular use of a light plastic cervical collar is often all that is required to relieve pain and prevent excessive anterior flexion, particularly during automobile rides. In the presence of spinal cord compression, surgical stabilization may be required.

Cricoarytenoid Arthritis. The cricoarytenoid joint is a diarthroidal joint with a synovial membrane. In patients with known polyarticular JIA, cricoarytenoid arthritis rarely may lead to acute airway obstruction. Clinical features of cricoarytenoid arthritis include stridor and hoarseness. The inspiratory stridor may wax and wane, and may be present only when the patient is asleep. Some of these patients also may complain of pain in the throat while swallowing, and pain in the ears. Many of these symptoms and signs are similar to those of severe acute laryngotracheobronchitis, which at times may be excluded only by direct laryngoscopy. Redness and swelling of the arytenoid eminences may be observed in cricoarytenoid arthritis, rather than the airway inflammation of croup.

Increasing airway obstruction with severe inspiratory retractions demands urgent treatment with respiratory support. Large doses of corticosteroids (methylprednisolone, 2 mg/kg/day IV) may control acute inflammation of the joints, thus avoiding emergency tracheostomy.

HEMOPHAGOCYTIC LYMPHOHISTIOCYTOSIS AND MACROPHAGE ACTIVATION SYNDROME

Current Evidence

HLH and MAS are clinically related life-threatening immune dysregulatory processes. Although rare, as our understanding of this spectrum of disease grows, more and more patients are found to suffer from these syndromes. Accordingly, it is important that the ED physician be aware of these entities, as the prompt recognition and treatment of HLH and MAS can markedly improve outcomes. Both HLH and MAS cause severe illness in children that is characterized by fever, systemic inflammation, HSM, coagulopathy, cytopenias, and neurologic complications. An ill child presenting to the ED with persistent fever and the above laboratory and physical examination findings may have hemophagocytic spectrum disease. However, because the presentation may be nonspecific, other systemic processes, including infection, malignancy, metabolic disorders, and other autoimmune disorders must be excluded.

While the clinical presentation of HLH and MAS is somewhat nonspecific, these entities are defined histologically by the phagocytosis of hematopoietic cells by normal-appearing macrophages in the bone marrow or lymphatic tissue; though it remains unclear what role, if any, this hemophagocytosis plays in the pathophysiology of these syndromes. Typically, however, this histopathologic information is not available to the ED physician at the time of acute presentation. As such, the recognition of the clinical syndrome as well as identification of at-risk children is essential to providing exceptional emergency care.

HLH may be genetic or acquired in response to infections, especially EBV. Immunocompromised children, either due to iatrogenic causes or other immune deficiency like HIV, remain at increased risk for the development of HLH.

MAS, also known as reactive HLH, can be thought of as HLH in the setting of autoimmune disease, most commonly soJIA and adult-onset Still disease. This serious complication may occur in as many as 30% to 50% of children. Children with SLE and other autoimmune disorders are also at risk for MAS, and vigilance for its evolution is advised when such children present with fever and marked laboratory and examination abnormalities. It is often challenging to differentiate a flare of underlying disease or superimposed systemic infection from MAS, and these pathologic entities may also coexist.

Clinical Considerations

The diagnosis of either HLH or MAS should be considered in an ill child with prolonged fever, HSM, elevated inflammatory markers, hematologic cytopenias, coagulopathy, neurologic symptoms, and/or evidence of liver dysfunction. A significantly elevated ferritin greater than 10,000 mg per L is a sensitive and specific marker of these processes. If HLH or MAS is suspected, additional evaluation for hypertriglyceridemia and hypofibrinogenemia should be done. Immune assays that are more specific for hemophagocytic spectrum disease, including evaluation of NK cell numbers and function, as measured in a cytotoxicity assay, can assist in identifying this disorder, though the results of these studies are often delayed.

TABLE 109.13

DIAGNOSTIC CRITERIA FOR HLH

The Diagnosis Of HLH Can Be Established If Either 1 Or 2 (Below) Is Fulfilled:

1. A molecular diagnosis consistent with HLH
2. Diagnostic criteria for HLH fulfilled (5 out of 8 criteria below)

(A) Initial diagnostic criteria

- 1. Fever
- 2. Splenomegaly
- 3. Cytopenias (affecting ≥2 of 3 lineages in the peripheral blood):
  - 1. Hemoglobin <90 g/L (in infants <4 wks: hemoglobin <100 g/L)
  - 2. Platelets <100×10^9/L
  - 3. Neutrophils <1.0×10^9/L
- 4. Hypertriglyceridemia and/or hypofibrinogenemia:
  - 1. Fasting triglycerides ≥3.0 mmol/L (i.e., ≥265 mg/dL)
  - 2. Fibrinogen ≤1.5 g/L
- 5. Hemophagocytosis in bone marrow or spleen or lymph nodes
  - 1. No evidence of malignancy

(B) New diagnostic criteria

- 6. Low or absent NK-cell activity (according to local laboratory reference)
- 7. Ferritin ≥500 mg/L
- 8. Soluble CD25 (i.e., soluble IL-2 receptor) ≥2,400 U/mL

From Henter JI, Horne A, Arico´ M, et al. HLH-2004: diagnostic and therapeutic guidelines for hemophagocytic lymphohistiocytosis. *Pediatr Blood Cancer* 2007;48:124–131.

Flow cytometric measurement of perforin, soluble CD25 (soluble IL-2 receptor alpha) and soluble CD107a expression may be helpful in making the diagnosis; though once again, these results are not usually available to the ED physician. The criteria for the diagnosis of HLH have been formalized (Table 109.13). The diagnosis of MAS can be made in the appropriate clinical setting even when HLH 2004 criteria are not met.

Management

The goal of the treatment of HLH and MAS is to suppress the hyperactive immune response. In the setting of acquired HLH or MAS, targeted treatment of the underlying triggering process is the first step. For example, if an inciting bacterial infection is suspected, then treatment with antibiotics should be initiated. When the diagnosis of HLH is made according to the HLH 2004 criteria, then treatment according to that protocol should be started, including administration of systemic corticosteroids, cyclosporine, and etoposide. In spite of these regimens, survival remains approximately 50%. In patients with familial hemophagocytic lymphohistiocytosis (FHL) and those failing the above-mentioned treatment regimen, hematopoietic stem cell transplantation (HSCT) is indicated. Because HSCT is the only chance for cure in FHL, the considerable risks of the procedure are often accepted.

As with HLH, to treat MAS one must also extinguish the rampant immune response. Systemic corticosteroids are the first line of therapy. Cyclosporine A is often used adjunctively with corticosteroids. More recently, biologic response modifiers directed against the cytokines responsible for the hyperactive response have been used successfully in the treatment of MAS. Specifically, IL1-R antagonists, like anakinra (Kineret), can lead to rapid clinical improvement in children who have not responded to the more standard therapies of corticosteroids and cyclosporine A.

HLH and MAS are severe life-threatening immune dysregulatory syndromes that may progress rapidly when untreated. As such, prompt consideration for these pathologic processes with early decision to admit to the hospital is essential to the successful care of these patients. As the process evolves, affected children may develop sepsis-like physiology with cytokine storm and ultimately cardiopulmonary collapse. Thus, they often require hemodynamic and respiratory support in addition to treatment for potential infectious complications related to both treatment with immunosuppressive medications and underlying illnesses.

KAWASAKI DISEASE

CLINICAL PEARLS AND PITFALLS

- Fever, often exceeding 40°C, is the most consistent manifestation of the disease.
- Extreme irritability is commonly observed.
- Initiation of IVIG within the first 10 days of the illness shortens disease duration and minimizes complications.
- Some children present with a clinical picture that does not fulfill the classic clinical criteria (incomplete KD).
- The majority of complications are cardiac in nature so close monitoring of the cardiac system is imperative.
- Young infants should have laboratory studies if febrile for 7 days or longer, even if there are no other clinical manifestations of KD present.

Current Evidence

KD is an acute, self-limited vasculitis that occurs in children of all ages. It is an idiopathic vasculitis of the small- and medium-sized vessels that has surpassed acute rheumatic fever to become the leading cause of acquired heart disease in children in the developed world. KD is 50% more common in boys than in girls, and it usually affects children younger than 5 years of age. The highest incidence occurs in children who live in East Asia (e.g., Japan, Korea, and Taiwan) or are of Asian ancestry living elsewhere in the world. The disease may be more difficult to diagnose in infants and adolescents, and it is more likely to cause chronic sequelae in these age groups.

Characteristically, children with KD have fever, conjunctivitis, rash, mucosal inflammation, lymphadenopathy, and extremity changes. The major morbidity of KD, however, occurs in the heart. Coronary artery aneurysms or ectasia develop in approximately 15% to 25% of untreated children and may lead to myocardial infarction, sudden death, arrhythmias, depressed myocardial contractility and heart failure, and chronic coronary artery insufficiency. IVIG decreases the incidence of coronary artery aneurysms by three- to fivefold if given within 10 days of disease onset. A recent prospective study from the Netherlands showed that male gender, delay of treatment (>10 days), and IVIG retreatment were independent risk factors for coronary artery aneurysm development. Management of children with suspected KD, therefore, requires accurate and expeditious diagnosis and close monitoring of the cardiovascular system.

In KD, as in other forms of vasculitis, blood vessel damage appears to result from an aberrant immune response leading to endothelial cell injury and vessel wall damage. A direct cell-mediated attack on endothelial cells, either because they are infected with an as-yet unidentified infectious agent, or simply as innocent bystanders, may underlie the vascular injury. The reason that KD preferentially involves coronary arteries is unknown.

The pathologic changes of the coronary arteries seen in KD have been classified by Fujiwara and Hamashima into four stages, depending on the duration of illness at the time of examination (Table 109.14). Many lines of evidence point toward a role of infections in the causation of KD. The fact that the disease often occurs in epidemics, that boys are more susceptible than girls, and that household contacts of children with KD are at increased risk for developing the disease in Japan, all point to a transmissible agent. Nonetheless, although many putative etiologies have been proposed during the past four decades, suggestions that certain viruses (EBV, human coronavirus, parvovirus, HIV-2) or bacterial toxins (streptococcal erythrogenic toxin, staphylococcal toxic shock toxin) account for the majority of cases have not been substantiated. Many researchers now believe that KD represents a final common pathway of immune-mediated vascular inflammation in genetically susceptible children triggered by any of a variety of common infections.

TABLE 109.14

PATHOLOGY OF KAWASAKI DISEASE[a]

Stage I—Disease duration <10 days
Acute perivasculitis of coronary arteries
Microvascular angiitis of coronary arteries and aorta
Pancarditis with pericardial, myocardial, endocardial inflammation
Inflammation of the atrioventricular conduction system
Stage II—Disease duration 12–28 days
Acute panvasculitis of coronary arteries
Coronary artery aneurysms present
Coronary obstruction and thrombosis
Myocardial and endocardial inflammation less intense
Stage III—Disease duration 28–45 days
Subacute inflammation in coronary arteries
Coronary artery aneurysms present
Myocardial, endocardial inflammation much decreased
Stage IV—Disease duration >50 days
Scar formation, calcification in coronary arteries
Stenosis and recanalization of coronary vessel lumen
Myocardial fibrosis without acute inflammation

[a]Duration of each stage may be decreased by prompt treatment with IVIG.
IVIG, intravenous immunoglobulin.

MEDICAL EMERGENCIES

Goals of Treatment

Early recognition of the symptoms of KD is essential to effective and timely therapy. Although no definitive test for KD exists, recognition of the constellation of signs and symptoms is instrumental in making the diagnosis. The goals of treatment are to reduce the amount of ectasia and aneurysms that occur among the coronary arteries which can be accomplished by the initiation of IVIG therapy within the first 10 days of the illness.

Clinical Considerations

Clinical Recognition

KD is a clinical syndrome diagnosed on the basis of fever and four of the five signs of mucocutaneous inflammation (Table 109.15). These diagnostic criteria should be regarded as imperfect, with less than 100% sensitivity and specificity. Children who do not meet criteria may indeed have KD, whereas some children with other conditions may nonetheless manifest all five criteria of KD. Acknowledgement of this fact was made explicit in 2004 when an expert panel published revised criteria for diagnosing and treating children with suspected KD.

Fever is probably the most consistent manifestation of KD. It reflects the elevated levels of proinflammatory cytokines (e.g., TNF-α, IL-1), which are also believed to mediate the underlying vascular inflammation. A diagnosis of KD should be considered in all children with prolonged, unexplained fever, irritability, and laboratory signs of inflammation, especially in the presence of mucocutaneous inflammation. Conversely, the diagnosis must be suspect in the absence of fever.

The remaining cardinal manifestations of KD vary considerably in frequency. Up to one-half of children with KD do not have cervical lymphadenopathy, especially children younger than 2 years of age. When present, lymphadenopathy tends to involve the anterior cervical nodes overlying the sternocleidomastoid muscle. Diffuse lymphadenopathy, as well as other signs of reticuloendothelial involvement such as splenomegaly, should prompt a search for an alternative diagnosis.

Bilateral, nonexudative conjunctivitis is present in more than 90% of patients. A predominantly bulbar injection typically begins within days of the onset of fever, and eyes eventually develop a brilliant erythema, which spares the limbus (Fig. 109.10). Children are also frequently photophobic, and five out of six patients have evidence of anterior uveitis during the first week of illness. Consequently, in ambiguous cases, slit-lamp examination may be helpful in confirming a diagnosis of KD.

Cracked, red lips and a strawberry tongue are characteristic of the mucositis typically seen during the first week of KD (Fig. 109.12). Discrete oral lesions, such as vesicles or ulcers, and tonsillar exudate, are suggestive of a viral or bacterial infection rather than KD. The cutaneous manifestations of KD are polymorphous. The rash typically begins as perineal erythema and desquamation, followed by macular, morbilliform, or targetoid lesions of the trunk and extremities. Vesicular or bullous lesions are rare. Changes in the extremities are generally the last clinical manifestation of KD to develop. Children demonstrate an indurated edema of the dorsum of their hands and feet, and a diffuse erythema of their palms and soles (Fig. 109.13). During the convalescent phase of KD,

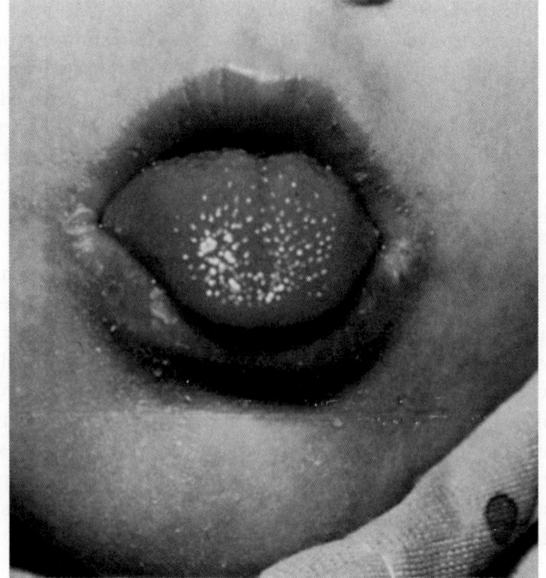

FIGURE 109.11 Cracked, erythematous lips and "strawberry" tongue in Kawasaki disease.

TABLE 109.15

DIAGNOSTIC CRITERIA FOR KAWASAKI DISEASE

Fever ≥5 days unresponsive to antibiotics
If the fever disappears because of intravenous gammaglobulin therapy before the fifth day of illness, a fever of <5 days' duration fulfills fever criterion for case definition.
At least four of the five following physical findings with no other more reasonable explanation for the observed clinical findings:
1. Bilateral conjunctival injection
2. Changes in the oropharyngeal mucous membranes (erythematous and/or fissured lips, strawberry tongue, injected pharynx)
3. Changes of peripheral extremities, including erythema and/or edema of the hands or feet (acute phase) or periungual desquamation (convalescent phase) (Fig. 109.11)
4. Polymorphous rash, primarily truncal; nonvesicular
5. Cervical lymphadenopathy ≥1.5 cm diameter

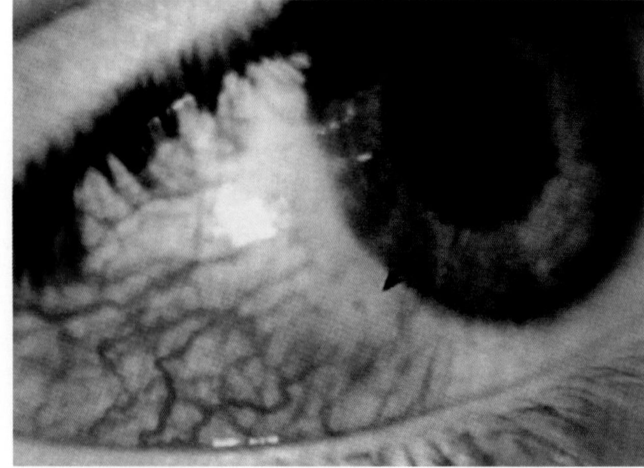

FIGURE 109.12 Bilateral, nonexudative conjunctivitis with sparing of the limbus in Kawasaki disease.

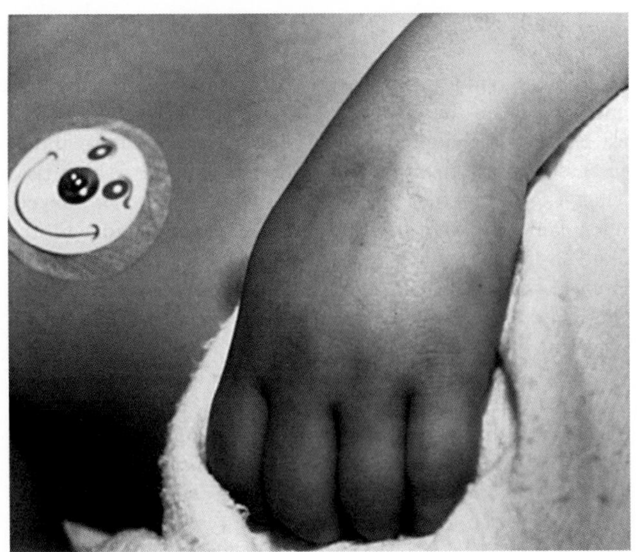

FIGURE 109.13 Brawny edema of dorsum of hand and small joint polyarthritis in Kawasaki disease.

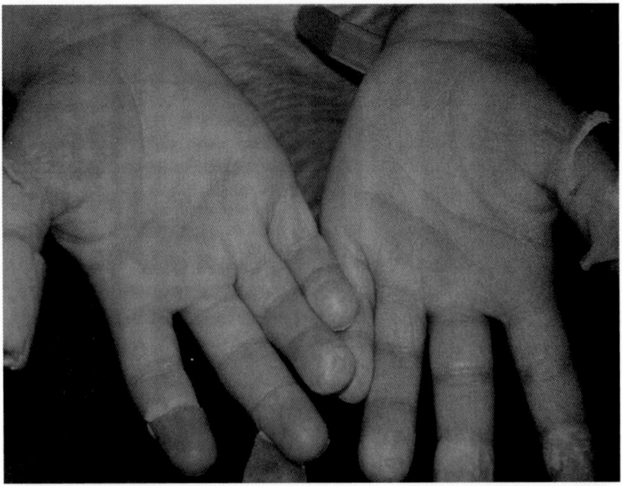

FIGURE 109.14 Periungual desquamation during the convalescent phase of Kawasaki disease.

sheet-like desquamation that begins in the periungual region of the hands and feet is characteristic (Fig. 109.14). Linear nail creases known as Beau lines are also common late manifestations of KD.

As a systemic vasculitis, KD may cause a variety of other clinical manifestations. Pulmonary involvement may lead to symptoms such as cough and infiltrates, peribronchial cuffing, and pleural effusions on chest radiographs. GI signs may range from emesis and diarrhea to findings suggestive of an acute surgical abdomen. Neurologic involvement has been reported, including aseptic meningitis, seizures, facial nerve palsies, ataxia, hemiplegia, and severe encephalopathy. In general, as with other vasculitides, manifestations of KD may be extremely variable, so clinicians should not exclude the possibility solely on the basis of atypical features.

KD is most commonly confused with exanthematous infections of childhood (Table 109.16). Measles, echovirus, and adenovirus may share many of the signs of mucocutaneous inflammation, but they typically have less evidence of systemic inflammation, and generally lack the extremity changes seen in KD. Toxin-mediated illnesses, especially β-hemolytic streptococcal infection and toxic shock syndrome, generally lack the ocular and articular involvement typical of KD. Finally, drug reactions such as Stevens–Johnson syndrome or serum sickness may mimic KD but with subtle differences in the ocular and mucosal manifestations.

TABLE 109.16

DIFFERENTIAL DIAGNOSIS OF KAWASAKI DISEASE

	Kawasaki disease	Toxic shock syndrome	Streptococcal scarlet fever	Stevens–Johnson syndrome	Systemic onset juvenile idiopathic arthritis
Age	<5 yrs	>10 yrs	2–8 yrs	All ages	2–5 yrs
Fever	≤12 days	<10 days	Variable	Prolonged	Prolonged
Eyes	Nonexudative conjunctivitis, limbal sparing, anterior uveitis	Conjunctivitis	Normal	Exudative conjunctivitis, keratitis	Normal
Oral mucosa	Erythema, "strawberry tongue"	Erythema	Pharyngitis, "strawberry tongue," circumoral pallor	Erythema, ulcerations, pseudomembrane formation	Normal
Extremities	Erythema of palms and soles, indurative edema, periungual desquamation	Peripheral edema	Fine flaking desquamation	Normal	Arthritis
Rash	Polymorphous; targetoid or purpuric in 20%	Erythroderma	Erythroderma, Pastia lines	Target lesions	Transient, salmon pink
Lymph nodes	Single anterior lymph node	Normal	Painful, diffuse cervical nodes	Normal	Diffuse
Other	Arthritis	Shock, coagulopathy, mental status changes	Positive throat culture	Arthralgia, associated herpes virus infection (30–50%)	Pericarditis

Triage Considerations

Young children with prolonged fever, especially in the setting of irritability or fussiness, in association with one or more of the following cardinal signs, conjunctivitis, rash, mucosal inflammation, cervical lymphadenopathy, or extremity changes, should lead to prompt evaluation for KD. The most serious complications of KD are cardiac and the major complication is coronary artery aneurysms. Infants younger than 1 year of age have the highest risk of developing coronary artery aneurysms. A rare but potentially life-threatening complication is KD shock syndrome. It is defined as systolic hypotension for age, a sustained decrease in systolic blood pressure from baseline of ≥20%, or clinical signs of poor perfusion.

Clinical Assessment

The conventional diagnostic criteria are particularly useful in preventing overdiagnosis, but they may result in failure to recognize incomplete forms of the illness. It should be emphasized that children who do not fulfill formal diagnostic criteria are still at risk of cardiac complications. Depending on the series, between 10% and 60% of children who develop coronary aneurysms never meet clinical criteria for KD. The guidelines of the American Heart Association Council on Cardiovascular Disease in the Young provide a useful framework for managing children with suspected KD who do not meet criteria for the diagnosis (see Fig. 109.15 and also section on Incomplete KD below).

Clinical manifestations of KD tend to be most incomplete and atypical in the youngest patients, the subgroup at highest risk for development of coronary artery abnormalities. Infants younger than 6 months are at particularly high risk. Thus, KD should be considered in any infant with prolonged, unexplained fever. In contrast, alternative explanations for the child's symptoms must be carefully excluded before treating empirically with IVIG. Consideration should be given to referring children to a regional KD center for further evaluation when the diagnosis is unclear.

At the other end of the spectrum, older children and adolescents with KD appear to be at increased risk for developing coronary aneurysms; however, older age at presentation is also associated with delayed diagnosis, which is known to incur significant risk. Unlike infants, in whom the clinical findings of KD are often incomplete, older children appear to present with fairly typical manifestations. Diagnosis may be delayed because clinicians are less likely to consider the diagnosis in older patients because most cases involve young children. Further, children older than 8 years of age frequently exhibit GI and meningeal symptoms, potentially clouding the diagnostic picture. In any event, whether KD is indeed more aggressive in older children, or simply because diagnosis is more likely to be delayed, pediatricians must consider KD as a possible cause of prolonged fever in young people of any age.

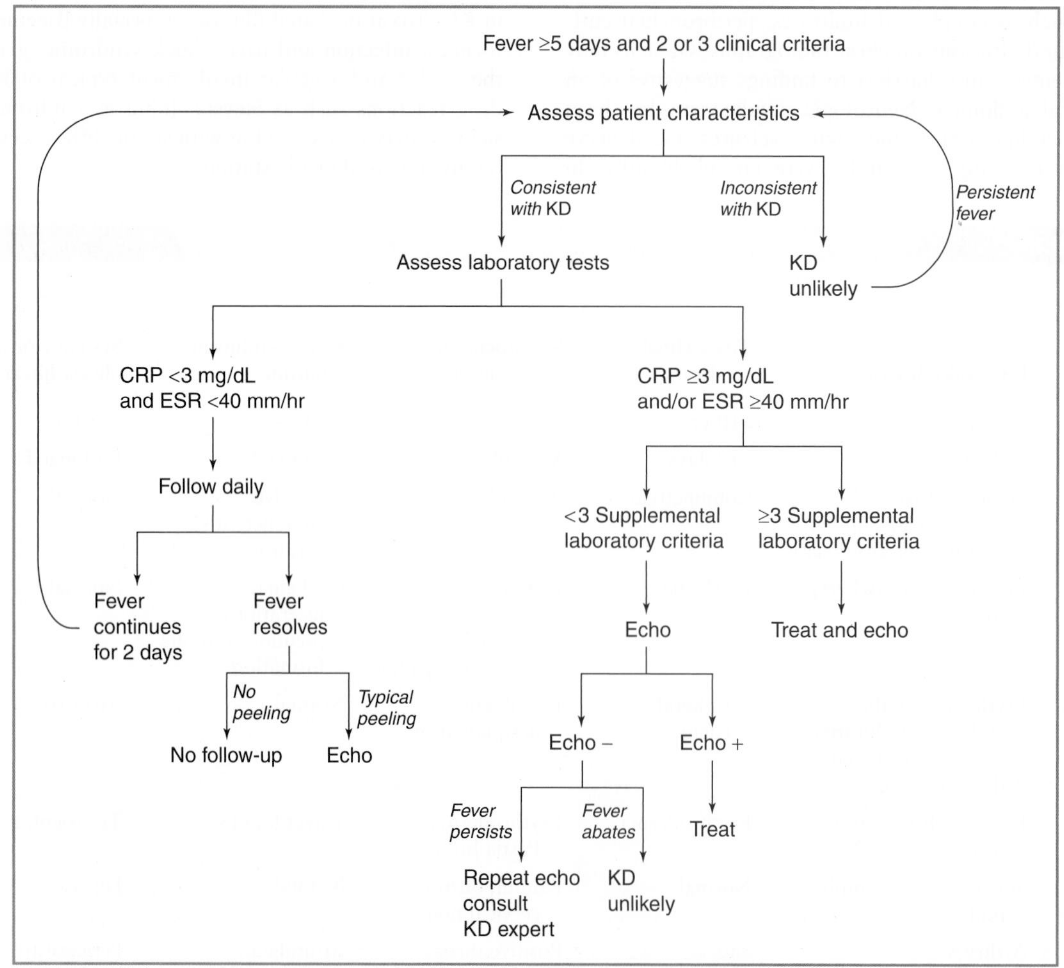

FIGURE 109.15 Evaluation of suspected incomplete Kawasaki disease (KD). (From Newburger JW, Takahashi M, Gerber M, et al. Diagnosis, treatment, and long-term management of Kawasaki disease: a statement for health professionals from the Committee on Rheumatic Fever, Endocarditis, and Kawasaki Disease, Council on Cardiovascular Disease in the Young, American Heart Association. *Pediatrics* 2004;114:1708–1733.)

No laboratory studies are included among the diagnostic criteria for KD, but certain findings may support the diagnosis. Most characteristic is systemic inflammation, with widespread elevation of acute-phase reactants (including CRP and ESR), leukocytosis, and a left shift in the white blood cell count. By the second week of illness, platelet counts also rise, reaching 1,000,000 per mm^3 in the most severe cases. Thrombocytopenia, on the other hand, is a poor prognostic factor and may indicate platelet consumption.

Children with KD often present with a normocytic, normochromic anemia; hemoglobin concentrations more than two standard deviations below the mean for age are noted in approximately one-half of patients within the first 2 weeks of illness. Urinalysis commonly reveals white blood cells on microscopic examination; the cells are mononuclear, and so are not detected by dipstick tests for leukocyte esterase. They also originate in the urethra, so they will be missed on urinalyses obtained by bladder tap or catheterization, so a clean catch is preferred. Measurement of liver enzymes often reveals elevated transaminase levels or mild hyperbilirubinemia due to intrahepatic congestion. In addition, a minority of children may develop obstructive jaundice from hydrops of the gallbladder. If sampled, other body fluids demonstrate inflammation as well: CSF typically displays a mononuclear pleocytosis (less than 100 cells per mm^3) with normal glucose and protein concentrations, whereas arthrocentesis of involved joints demonstrates 50,000 to 300,000 white blood cells per mm^3, primarily neutrophils.

Clinical Assessment of Incomplete KD

When patients do not meet the full diagnostic criteria for KD, "incomplete" KD should be considered as these patients are also at risk for coronary artery aneurysms and require prompt recognition and treatment. The term "incomplete" is preferable to "atypical." These patients lack sufficient clinical signs of the disease as opposed to demonstrating atypical features.

In 2004, the American Heart Association (AHA) put forth an algorithm suggesting an approach for evaluation of possible incomplete KD (Fig. 109.15). Unlike the classical criteria, this algorithm takes into account laboratory studies and findings on echocardiogram. A 2010 retrospective review of the 2004 criteria supports the application of the 2004 AHA recommendations, compared with the classic criteria alone.

Prolonged fever is still the cardinal manifestation of KD under the AHA algorithm. Children with 5 or more days of fever and 2 or 3 clinical criteria in which KD is being considered should be evaluated further for incomplete KD. This starts with a full assessment for possible characteristics suggesting KD, including those outlined in Table 109.17. Characteristics suggestive of an alternative diagnosis are considered as well, including exudative conjunctivitis, exudative pharyngitis, discrete intraoral lesions, bullous or vesicular rash, and generalized adenopathy. If KD appears unlikely, watchful waiting is employed, but ongoing reassessment is recommended if fevers persist. If the clinical picture is consistent with KD, laboratory tests are evaluated. If inflammatory markers are relatively unimpressive (CRP less than 3 mg per dL, ESR less than 40 mm per hour), this is less suggestive of KD, though the child should be followed daily, and formally reassessed if fever persists. Even in children with unimpressive inflammatory markers whose fever resolves, an echocardiogram should be considered if typical peeling of the skin develops.

TABLE 109.17

CLINICAL FINDINGS CONSISTENT WITH KAWASAKI DISEASE

Cardiovascular findings
Congestive heart failure, myocarditis, pericarditis, valvular regurgitation
Coronary artery abnormalities
Aneurysms of medium-size noncoronary arteries
Raynaud phenomenon
Peripheral gangrene
Musculoskeletal system
Arthritis, arthralgia
Gastrointestinal tract
Diarrhea, vomiting, abdominal pain
Hepatic dysfunction
Hydrops of gallbladder
Central nervous system
Extreme irritability
Lethargy
Aseptic meningitis
Sensorineural hearing loss
Genitourinary system
Urethritis/meatitis
Other findings
Erythema, induration at Bacille Calmette–Guerin (BCG) site
Anterior uveitis (mild)
Desquamating rash in groin

In those children with a clinical picture consistent with KD and significantly elevated inflammatory markers (CRP greater than or equal to 3 mg per dL, ESR greater than or equal to 40 mm per hour), supplemental laboratory criteria are taken into consideration. These include albumin less than or equal to 3 g per dL, anemia for age, elevated alanine aminotransferase, platelets greater than or equal to 450,000 per mm^3 after 7 days of illness, white blood cell count greater than or equal to 15,000 per mm^3, and urine greater than or equal to 10 white blood cells per high-power field. If the child has more than three supplemental laboratory criteria, treatment for KD is recommended and can be started before an echocardiogram is performed. In children with fewer than three supplemental laboratory criteria, an echocardiogram is recommended, with treatment to follow if the echocardiogram is positive (Table 109.18). Treatment is recommended even if the child is past day 10 of fever, if there are clinical and laboratory signs of continued inflammation. If the echocardiogram is negative and the fever subsides, KD is considered to have been unlikely. If the echocardiogram is negative and fever persists, a repeat echo and consultation with a KD expert are recommended.

It should be noted that special consideration is given to febrile infants less than or equal to 6 months of age. It is recommended that these young infants have laboratory studies if febrile for 7 days or longer, even if there are no other clinical manifestations of KD present. If systemic inflammation is found, it is recommended that those infants undergo echocardiogram and be treated if the echocardiogram is positive.

TABLE 109.18

ECHOCARDIOGRAPHIC CRITERIA SUGGESTIVE OF KAWASAKI DISEASE

Echocardiogram considered positive if any of the three criteria are met
I. z score of LAD or RCA of ≥2.5
II. Coronary arteries meet Japanese Ministry of Health criteria for aneurysms
III. If three or more suggestive features are present
Perivascular brightness
Lack of tapering
Decreased LV function
Mitral regurgitation
Pericardial effusion
z scores in LAD or RCA of 2–2.5

LAD, left anterior descending coronary artery; RCA, right coronary artery; LV, left ventricle.

Management

IVIG

If the clinical criteria are fulfilled, or partial clinical criteria are met with supportive supplemental laboratory criteria, then treatment should be initiated. Recommended initial therapy includes IVIG and aspirin within the first 10 days of the illness; treatment with IVIG within this time frame significantly shortens disease duration and minimizes the incidence of complications. Overall, prompt diagnosis and appropriate therapy prevent aneurysm formation in approximately 95% of children and result in rapid symptomatic improvement in about 90%. Studies in Japan were the first to suggest relative protection from coronary artery aneurysms when IVIG is administered early in the course of KD. Since then, further trials in the United States and Japan have confirmed this finding and documented the safety of high-dose infusions of immunoglobulin. At present, a single large infusion of IVIG (2 g per kg) administered over 8 to 12 hours is the standard of care for KD. This is somewhat more effective than multiple smaller infusions, and it also significantly shortens the duration of hospitalization.

Therapy with IVIG also has other benefits. Treatment results in a reduced prevalence of giant aneurysms, the most serious form of coronary abnormality caused by the disease. It also accelerates normalization of abnormalities of left ventricular systolic function and contractility. Finally, high-dose IVIG reduces fever and laboratory indices of inflammation, suggesting a rapid, generalized anti-inflammatory effect in addition to specific cardioprotective effects. Despite its advantages, IVIG is an expensive and potentially toxic intervention. The greatest long-term concern is the possible transmission of blood-borne pathogens. Elaborate sterilization procedures, including lyophilization, pasteurization, and addition of solvent detergents, are generally effective in rendering the product free of infectious agents. There have been no cases of infections transmitted by IVIG since current purification practices were initiated in 1995. Overall, significant toxicity is rare, and benefits clearly outweigh risks in children with confirmed KD.

Aspirin

Aspirin was the first medication to be used for treatment of KD, both for its anti-inflammatory and its antithrombotic effects. High-dose (greater than 80 mg/kg/day) and lower-dose regimens (30 mg/kg/day) in four divided doses are still used in conjunction with IVIG during the acute phase of the illness despite the fact that meta-analyses demonstrate no additive protection from coronary artery aneurysms from aspirin. Once fever resolves, patients are generally switched to antiplatelet doses of aspirin (3 to 5 mg/kg/day). Unless coronary artery abnormalities are detected by echocardiogram, aspirin is discontinued once laboratory studies return to normal, usually within 2 months of the onset of KD.

The risks of aspirin appear to be similar to those reported in other settings: transaminitis, chemical hepatitis, transient hearing loss, and, rarely, Reye syndrome. These risks may even be increased in KD: Aspirin-binding studies have suggested that the hypoalbuminemia of children with KD predisposes them to toxic levels of free salicylate despite measured (bound) levels within the therapeutic range. At least one case of Reye syndrome has been reported after 6 days of aspirin therapy for KD. Alternative antipyretic and anti-inflammatory agents, such as ibuprofen, may be used for treatment of arthralgias, and aspirin should be rapidly discontinued whenever intercurrent illness with varicella or influenza is possible. Influenza vaccine should be given to the patient and household contacts at the time of diagnosis according to seasonal recommendations.

Corticosteroids

Currently corticosteroids role as initial standard therapy with IVIG and aspirin remains unclear. They have largely been used as treatment for IVIG-resistant cases, but more recently have been studied for their role as possible primary adjuvant therapy in patients identified as high risk. A multicenter randomized double-blind placebo-controlled trial of pulse-dose methylprednisolone in conjunction with IVIG and ASA as initial therapy, did not find a significant difference in coronary outcome between the steroid and placebo groups. In those children who required retreatment with IVIG, however, there was improved coronary outcome in the steroid compared to the placebo group. This suggests perhaps that those children who are at risk for IVIG-resistant disease at baseline might benefit from initial use of corticosteroids. Their routine use as a primary therapy is not currently recommended. The use of corticosteroids in refractory KD is discussed below.

Tumor Necrosis Factor Inhibition

Modulation of proinflammatory cytokines, such as TNF-α, has impacted the treatment of rheumatologic conditions including vasculitis. Elevated levels of TNF-α are increased in the acute phase of KD. Currently the data do not demonstrate any benefit for the use of TNF inhibitors as adjuvant therapy for primary KD. The use of TNF inhibitors in refractory KD is discussed below.

Management of Complications and Emergencies

Cardiovascular. Cardiac abnormalities dominate the pathology of KD. Clinical examination is often remarkable for tachycardia and gallop rhythms that are more prominent than expected from the degree of fever and anemia. The EKG in acute KD may show mild abnormalities consistent with myocarditis, most commonly a prolonged PR interval and nonspecific ST- and T-wave changes. Echocardiographic evaluation of myocardial function early in the course of the disease frequently reveals reduced left ventricular function and contractility. Rarely, myocardial inflammation may progress to frank CHF. The severity of myocarditis does not correlate with the risk of coronary artery aneurysms or with other complications such as pericardial effusion, which may develop during the second week of illness. The effusion rarely progresses to tamponade and resolves spontaneously in most instances. Valvulitis presenting as either aortic or mitral regurgitation is rarely seen during the early phases of KD. Late-onset mitral regurgitation, from papillary muscle dysfunction or myocardial infarction, may also complicate the clinical course.

Most characteristic of KD is inflammation of the coronary arteries. This progresses to ectasia or aneurysm formation in 15% to 25% of untreated children. Dilatation of coronary arteries may be detected by echocardiography as early as 6 days after the onset of fever and usually peaks 3 or 4 weeks into the course of the illness. Cardiac catheterization need not be performed in patients with normal echocardiograms and EKGs throughout the disease course because the likelihood of finding unsuspected lesions is negligible.

Coronary aneurysms in early KD usually occur in the proximal segments of the major coronary vessels; abnormalities that occur distally are almost always associated with proximal coronary dilatation. Aneurysms may also occur in arteries outside the coronary system, most commonly the subclavian, brachial, axillary, iliac, or femoral vessels, and occasionally in the abdominal aorta and renal arteries. For this reason, abdominal aortography and subclavian arteriography are often performed in patients undergoing coronary angiograms for KD. For unknown reasons, visceral vessels are almost never involved.

Myocardial Disease. Myocardial infarction caused by thrombotic occlusion of an aneurysmal and/or stenotic coronary artery is the principal cause of death in KD. Rarely, dilated and weakened coronary arteries may rupture. Mortality due to KD has decreased from almost 2% to less than 0.1% as a result of improved treatment. Nonetheless, most deaths continue to occur during the first 6 months after disease onset, when myocardial and coronary artery inflammation are greatest.

In children with KD and coronary artery thrombosis, thrombolytic agents—mainly urokinase and streptokinase, either IV or intracoronary—have been used with variable success. Thrombolytic therapy for coronary artery thrombosis is most effective if begun within 3 to 4 hours of symptom onset. Immediately following clot lysis, systemic heparin is begun in combination with aspirin. Maintenance of reperfusion then requires chronic antithrombotic therapy (e.g., warfarin, low–molecular-weight heparin), although the ideal regimen has not been established.

CHF may rarely complicate the acute phase of KD. When this is because of myocarditis, routine treatment with IVIG generally results in rapid clinical improvement. Although IVIG therapy involves infusing large volumes of isotonic solution—2 g per kg of 5% IVIG delivers 40 mL per kg over 8 to 12 hours—improvements in myocardial contractility compensate for the volume load, and treatment rarely leads to circulatory deterioration. By the second week of illness, and especially in children with coronary artery dilatation, ischemia or infarction must be excluded as causes of new myocardial dysfunction.

Vascular Obstruction. Children with severe KD, especially infants or those in whom treatment is delayed, may develop other complications related to arterial occlusion. Peripheral obstruction leading to ischemia and gangrene most typically occurs in children with other manifestations of critical disease such as giant coronary artery aneurysms or aneurysms in peripheral arteries. Various therapies may restore circulation, although control of vascular inflammation with sufficient IVIG and/or other medications (e.g., corticosteroids and anti-TNF agents) is an essential prerequisite to arterial reperfusion. Thereafter, treatments may include thrombolytic therapy if arterial thrombosis is present, or vasodilators if tissue viability is primarily threatened by vasospasm. Peripheral arterial obstruction may be corrected by thrombolysis with urokinase, streptokinase, or tissue-type plasminogen activator, after which perfusion is maintained with heparin followed by a chronic oral anticoagulant regimen.

Shock Syndrome. An uncommon complication (7% in one study from a single institution), KD shock syndrome has been recognized as a complication that can occur during the acute phase of the illness, unrelated to IVIG infusion. It is defined as systolic hypotension for age, or signs of poor perfusion. It was noted that the patients who developed shock syndrome were more likely to be female, to have laboratory findings consistent with greater inflammation, and to have impaired cardiac function. All cases required fluid resuscitation and about half required inotropic support. These patients seem to have greater incidences of coronary artery abnormalities and IVIG resistance.

Other Complications. *Arthritis* occurs in approximately one-third of children with KD. Because it is rare in many of the conditions that may mimic KD, the presence of synovitis adds supportive evidence for the diagnosis in ambiguous cases. The arthritis tends to involve the small joints of the extremities during the acute phase of illness and the large joints during the second and third weeks. The arthritis of KD is always nondeforming and self-limited, generally resolving within 30 days. Anti-inflammatory medications such as ibuprofen are usually effective in relieving symptoms until spontaneous resolution occurs.

Refractory Kawasaki disease. KD may *recur* in 1% to 2% of children within 12 months of diagnosis, and an additional 5% to 10% of children treated with IVIG and aspirin may respond poorly to IVIG treatment during the initial bout of illness. In fact, patients who fail to respond completely to IVIG pose the greatest therapeutic dilemma. Prolonged fever itself correlates with increased risk of developing coronary artery abnormalities, and fever lasting for more than 14 days identifies a group of children at risk for developing giant coronary artery aneurysms (internal diameter greater than 8 mm), the group that is most susceptible to infarction and sudden death.

In cases of persistent, recurrent, or recrudescent KD, most clinicians retreat with IVIG, 2 g per kg over 8 to 12 hours. The risk of additional IVIG seems to be minimal, and several studies show a dose response to IVIG in KD. A persistent fever may be a reaction to treatment with IVIG and therefore children are not usually retreated until at least 36 hours after the initial IVIG infusion. It is, however, extremely important to confirm the diagnosis; it must be remembered that failure to respond to IVIG might indicate that the child has a different source of fever, such as a bacterial or viral infection, or a chronic inflammatory disease.

Approximately two-thirds of children with KD who fail to respond to an initial dose of IVIG improve with a second course. A small number seem to be resistant to IVIG, and they should be treated with intravenous pulsed-dose methylprednisolone (30 mg/kg/day) for 1 to 3 days. Patients who fail to respond to this regimen may be candidates for infliximab.

LYME DISEASE

Please see Chapter 102 Infectious Disease Emergencies.

Suggested Readings and Key References

Juvenile Rheumatoid Arthritis

Adams A, Lehman TJ. Update on the pathogenesis and treatment of systemic onset juvenile rheumatoid arthritis. *Curr Opin Rheumatol* 2005;17:612–616.

Bray VJ, Singleton JD. Disseminated intravascular coagulation in Still's disease. *Semin Arthritis Rheum* 1994;24:222–229.

Cassidy JT, Petty RE. Juvenile rheumatoid arthritis. In: *Textbook of pediatric rheumatology.* 3rd ed. Philadelphia, PA: WB Saunders, 1995.

Cunnane G, Doran M, Bresnihan B. Infections and biological therapy in rheumatoid arthritis. *Best Pract Res Clin Rheumatol* 2003; 17:345–363.

De Silva B, Banney L, Uttley W, et al. Psuedoporphyria and nonsteroidal antiinflammatory agents in children with juvenile idiopathic arthritis. *Pediatr Dermatol* 2000;17:480–483.

Duffy CM, Colbert RA, Laxer RM, et al. Nomenclature and classification in chronic childhood arthritis. Time for a change? *Arthritis Rheum* 2005;52:382–385.

Hashkes PJ, Laxer RM. Update on the medical treatment of juvenile idiopathic arthritis. *Curr Rheumatol Rep* 2006;8:450–458.

Ilowite NT. Current treatment of juvenile rheumatoid arthritis. *Pediatrics* 2002;109:109–115.

Ilowite NT. Update on biologics in juvenile idiopathic arthritis. *Curr Opin Rheumatol* 2008;20:613–618.

Kelly A, Ramanan AV. Recognition and management of macrophage activation syndrome in juvenile arthritis. *Curr Opin Rheumatol* 2007; 19:477–481.

Murray K, Thompson SD, Glass DN. Pathogenesis of juvenile chronic arthritis: genetic and environmental factors. *Arch Dis Child* 1997; 77:530–534.

Schneider R, Passo MH. Juvenile rheumatoid arthritis. *Rheum Dis Clin North Am* 2002;28:503–530.

Systemic Lupus Erythematosus

Aggarwal A, Srivastava P. Childhood onset systemic lupus erythematosus: how is it different from adult SLE? *Int J Rheum Dis* 2015;18(2):182–191.

Ardoin SP, Sandborg C, Schanberg LE. Management of dyslipidemia in children and adolescents with systemic lupus erythematosus. *Lupus* 2007;16:618–626.

Avcin T, Silverman ED. Antiphospholipid antibodies in pediatric systemic lupus erythematosus and the antiphospholipid syndrome. *Lupus* 2007;16:627–633.

Bader-Meunier B, Armengaud JB, Haddad E, et al. Initial presentation of childhood-onset systemic lupus erythematosus: a French multicenter study. *J Pediatr* 2005;146:648.

Benseler SM, Silverman ED. Neuropsychiatric involvement in pediatric systemic lupus erythematosus. *Lupus* 2007;16:564–571.

Brunner HI, Silverman ED, To T, et al. Risk factors for damage in childhood-onset systemic lupus erythematosus. *Arthritis Rheum* 2002;46:436–444.

Esdaile JM, Abrahamowicz M, Joseph L, et al. Laboratory tests as predictors of disease exacerbations in systemic lupus erythematosus. Why some tests fail. *Arthritis Rheum* 1996;39:370–378.

Hiraki LT, Benseler SM, Tyrrell PN, et al. Clinical and laboratory characteristics and long-term outcome of pediatric systemic lupus erythematosus: a longitudinal study. *J Pediatr* 2008;152:550–556.

Iqbal S, Sher MR, Good RA, et al. Diversity in presenting manifestations of systemic lupus erythematosus in children. *J Pediatr* 1999; 135:500–505.

Klein-Gitelman M, Reiff A, Silverman ED. Systemic lupus erythematosus in childhood. *Rheum Dis Clin North Am* 2002;28:561–577.

Lacks S, White P. Morbidity associated with childhood systemic lupus erythematosus. *J Rheumatol* 1990;17:941–945.

Lehman T. Systemic lupus erythematosus in children. In: UpToDate, Klein-Gitelman M, Tepas E, eds. UpToDate, Waltham, MA. Accessed on July 2, 2014.

MacDermott EJ, Adams A, Lehman TJ. Systemic lupus erythematosus in children: current and emerging therapies. *Lupus* 2007;16: 677–683.

Malattia C, Martini A. Paediatric-onset systemic lupus erythematosus. *Best Pract Res Clin Rheumatol* 2013;27:351–362.

Mok CC, Lau CS, Chan EY, et al. Acute transverse myelopathy in systemic lupus erythematosus: clinical presentation, treatment, and outcome. *J Rheumatol* 1998;25:467–473.

Parikh S, Swaiman KF, Kim Y. Neurologic characteristics of childhood lupus erythematosus. *Pediatr Neurol* 1995;13:198–201.

Petri M, Orbai A, Alarcon GS, et al. Derivation and validation of systemic lupus international collaborating clinics classification criteria for systemic lupus erythematosus. *Arthritis Rheum* 2012; 64(8):2677–2686.

Platt JL, Burke BA, Fish AJ, et al. Systemic lupus erythematosus in the first two decades of life. *Am J Kidney Dis* 1982;2:212–222.

Silverman E, Eddy A. Systemic lupus erythematosus. In: Cassidy JT, Petty RE, Laxer RM, et al., eds. *Textbook of pediatric rheumatology.* 6th ed. Philadelphia, PA: Saunders Elsevier, 2011:315–343.

Silverman ED, Lang B. An overview of the treatment of childhood SLE. *Scand J Rheumatol* 1997;26:241–246.

Yell JA, Mbuagbaw J, Burge SM. Cutaneous manifestations of systemic lupus erythematosus. *Br J Dermatol* 1996;135:355–362.

Dermatomyositis

Banker BQ, Victor M. Dermatomyositis (systemic angiopathy) of childhood. *Medicine (Baltimore)* 1966;45:261–289.

Bohan A, Peter JB. Polymyositis and dermatomyositis. *N Engl J Med* 1975;292:344–347, 403–407.

Pachman LM. Juvenile dermatomyositis: immunogenetics, pathophysiology, and disease expression. *Rheum Dis Clin North Am* 2002;28:579–602.

Tse S, Lubelsky S, Gordon M, et al. The arthritis of inflammatory childhood myositis syndromes. *J Rheumatol* 2001;28:192–197.

HLH/MAS

Allen CE, Yu X, Kozinetz CA, et al. Highly elevated ferritin levels and the diagnosis of hemophagocytic lymphohistiocytosis. *Pediatr Blood Cancer* 2008;50(6):1227–1235.

Behrens EM, Beukelman T, Paessler M, et al. Occult macrophage activation syndrome inpatients with systemic juvenile idiopathic arthritis. *J Rheumatol* 2007;34(5):1133–1138.

Bleesing J, Prada A, Siegel DM, et al. The diagnostic significance of soluble CD163 and soluble interleukin-2 receptor alpha-chain in macrophage activation syndrome and untreated new-onset systemic juvenile idiopathic arthritis. *Arthritis Rheum* 2007;56(3):965–971.

Cooper N, Rao K, Goulden N, et al. The use of reduced-intensity stem cell transplantation in haemophagocytic lymphohistiocytosis and Langerhans cell histiocytosis. *Bone Marrow Transplant* 2008;42(Suppl 2):S47–S50.

Henter JI, Samuelsson-Horne A, Aricò M, et al.; Histocyte Society. Treatment of hemophagocytic lymphohistiocytosis with HLH-94 immunochemotherapy and bone marrow transplantation. *Blood* 2002;100(7):2367–2373.

Janka G. Hemophagocytic lymphohistiocytosis: when the immune system runs amok. *Klin Padiatr* 2009;221(5):278–285.

Janka GE. Familial and acquired hemophagocytic lymphohistiocytosis. *Eur J Pediatr* 2007;166(2):95–109.

Loh NK, Lucas M, Fernandez S, et al. Successful treatment of macrophage activation syndrome complicating adult Still disease with anakinra. *Intern Med J* 2012;42(12):1358–1362.

Marsh RA, Vaughn G, Kim MO, et al. Reduced-intensity conditioning significantly improves survival of patients with hemophagocytic lymphohistiocytosis undergoing allogeneic hematopoietic cell transplantation. *Blood* 2010;116(26):5824–5831.

Miettunen PM, Narendran A, Jayanthan A, et al. Successful treatment of severe paediatric rheumatic disease-associated macrophage activation syndrome with interleukin-1 inhibition following conventional immunosuppressive therapy: case series with 12 patients. *Rheumatology (Oxford)* 2011;50(2):417–419.

Nagafuji K, Nonami A, Kumano T, et al. Perforin gene mutations in adult-onset hemophagocytic lymphohistiocytosis. *Haematologica* 2007;92(7):978–981.

Ravelli A, Grom AA, Behrens EM, et al. Macrophage activation syndrome as part of systemic juvenile idiopathic arthritis: diagnosis, genetics, pathophysiology and treatment. *Genes Immun* 2012;13(4): 289–298.

Risma K, Jordan MB. Hemophagocytic lymphohistiocytosis: updates and evolving concepts. *Curr Opin Pediatr* 2012;24(1):9–15.

Rohr J, Beutel K, Maul-Pavicic A, et al. Atypical familial hemophagocytic lymphohistiocytosis due to mutations in UNC13D and STXBP2 overlaps with primary immunodeficiency diseases. *Haematologica* 2010;95(12):2080–2087.

Ueda I, Kurokawa Y, Koike K, et al. Late-onset cases of familial hemophagocytic lymphohistiocytosis with missense perforin gene mutations. *Am J Hematol* 2007;82(6):427–432.

Vasculitis/Polyarteritis Nodosa

Dedeoglu F, Sundel RP. Vasculitis in children. *Pediatr Clin North Am* 2005;52:547–575.

Fink CW. Vasculitis. *Pediatr Clin North Am* 1986;33:1203–1219.

Gunal N, Kara N, Cakar N, et al. Cardiac involvement in childhood polyarteritis nodosa. *Int J Cardiol* 1997;60:257–262.

Moore PM, Cupps TR. Neurological complications of vasculitis. *Ann Neurol* 1983;14:155–167.

Sundel R, Szer I. Vasculitis in childhood. *Rheum Dis Clin North Am* 2002;28:625–654.

Ting TV, Hashkes PJ. Update on childhood vasculitides. *Curr Opin Rheumatol* 2004;16:560–565.

Kawasaki Disease

American Academy of Pediatrics. Kawasaki disease. In: Pickering LK, Baker CJ, Kimberlin DW, et al., eds. *Red Book: 2012 Report of the Committee on Infectious Diseases*. 29th ed. Elk Grove Village, IL: American Academy of Pediatrics, 2012:454–460.

Barron KS. Kawasaki disease: etiology, pathogenesis, and treatment. *Cleve Clin J Med* 2002;69:SII69–SII78.

Burns JC, Glode MP. Kawasaki syndrome. *Lancet* 2004;364:533–544.

Dimitriades VR, Brown AG, Gedalia A. Kawasaki disease: pathophysiology, clinical manifestations and management. *Curr Rheumatol Rep* 2014;16:423.

Durongpisitkul K, Gururaj VJ, Park JM, et al. The prevention of coronary artery aneurysm in Kawasaki disease: a meta-analysis on the efficacy of aspirin and immunoglobulin treatment. *Pediatrics* 1995;96:1057–1061.

Kanegaye JT, Wilder MS, Molkara D, et al. Recognition of a Kawasaki disease shock syndrome. *Pediatrics* 2009;123:e783.

Kato H, Sugimua T, Akagi T, et al. Long-term consequences of Kawasaki disease. A 10- to 21-year follow up study of 594 patients. *Circulation* 1996;94:1379–1385.

Kawasaki T, Kosaki F, Okawa S, et al. A new infantile acute febrile mucocutaneous lymph node syndrome (MLNS) prevailing in Japan. *Pediatrics* 1974;54:271–276.

Levy M, Koren G. Atypical Kawasaki disease: analysis of clinical presentation and diagnostic clues. *Pediatr Infect Dis J* 1990;9:122–126.

Newburger JW, Sleeper LA, McCrindle BW, et al. Randomized trial of pulsed corticosteroid therapy for primary treatment of Kawasaki disease. *N Engl J Med* 2007;356:663–675.

Newburger JW, Takahashi M, Gerber MA, et al. Diagnosis, treatment, and long-term management of Kawasaki disease: a statement for health professionals from the Committee on Rheumatic fever, Endocarditis, and Kawasaki disease, Council on Cardiovascular Disease in Young, American Heart Association. *Pediatrics* 2004;114:1708–1733.

Rosenfeld EA, Corydon KE, Shulman ST. Kawasaki disease in infants less than one year of age. *J Pediatr* 1995;126:524–529.

Son MF, Gauvreau K, Ma L, et al. Treatment of Kawasaki disease: analysis of 27 US pediatric hospitals from 2001 to 2006. *Pediatrics* 2009;124:1–8.

Stockheim JA, Innocentini N, Shulman ST. Kawasaki disease in older children and adolescents. *J Pediatr* 2000;137:250–252.

Sundel RP. Update on the treatment of Kawasaki disease in childhood. *Curr Rheumatol Rep* 2002;4:474–482.

Sundel RP. Kawasaki disease: Clinical features and diagnosis. In: UpToDate, Klein-Gitelman M, Kaplan SL, Tepas E, eds. UpToDate, Waltham, MA. (Accessed on July 2, 2014.)

Sundel RP, Petty RE. Kawasaki disease. In: Cassidy JT, Petty RE, Laxer RM, et al., eds. *Textbook of pediatric rheumatology.* 6th ed. Philadelphia, PA: Saunders Elsevier, 2011:505–520.

Tacke CE, Breunis WB, Pereira RR, et al. Five years of Kawasaki disease in the Netherlands: a national surveillance study. *Pediatr Infect Dis J* 2014;33(8):793–797.

Tremoulet AH, Jain S, Jaggi P, et al. Infliximab for intensification of primary therapy for Kawasaki disease: a phase 3 randomised, double-blind, placebo-controlled trial. *Lancet* 2014;383(9930): 1731–1738.

Yellen ES, Gauvreau K, Takahashi M, et al. Performance of 2004 American Heart Association Recommendations for Treatment of Kawasaki Disease. *Pediatrics* 2010;125:e234–e241.

Behçet Disease

Eldem B, Onur C, Ozen S. Clinical features of pediatric Behçet's disease. *J Pediatr Ophthalmol Strabismus* 1998;35:159–161.

Kone-Paut I, Yurdakul S, Bababri SA, et al. Clinical features of Behçet's disease in children: an international collaborative study of 86 cases. *J Pediatr* 1998;132:721–725.

Krause I, Weinberger A. Behcet's disease. *Curr Opin Rheumatol* 2008; 20:82–87.

Sakane T, Takeno M, Suzuki N, et al. Behçet's disease. *N Engl J Med* 1999;341:1284–1291.

Scleroderma

Athreya BH. Juvenile scleroderma. *Curr Opin Rheumatol* 2002;14: 553–561.

Fine LG. Systemic sclerosis: current pathogenetic concepts and future prospects for targeted therapy. *Lancet* 1996;347:1453–1458.

Foeldvari I. Update on pediatric systemic sclerosis: similarities and differences from adult disease. *Curr Opin Rheumatol* 2008;20:608–612.

Fujita Y, Yamamori H, Hiyoshi K, et al. Systemic sclerosis in children: a national retrospective survey in Japan. *Acta Paediatr Jpn* 1997;39:263–267.

Haber PL. Clinical manifestations of scleroderma. *Pediatr Rev* 1995; 16:49.

Laxer RM, Zulian F. Localized scleroderma. *Curr Opin Rheumatol* 2006;18:606–613.

Martini G, Foeldvari I, Russo R, et al. Systemic sclerosis in childhood. Clinical and immunologic features of 153 patients in an international database. *Arthritis Rheum* 2006;54:3971–3978.

Mayorquin FJ, McCurley TL, Levernier JE, et al. Progression of childhood linear scleroderma to fatal systemic sclerosis. *J Rheumatol* 1994;21:1955–1957.

Medsger TA Jr, Steen V. Systemic sclerosis and related syndromes. In: Schumacher HR, ed. *Primer on the rheumatic diseases.* 10th ed. Atlanta, GA: Arthritis Foundation, 1993.

Murray KJ, Laxer RM. Scleroderma in children and adolescents. *Rheum Dis Clin North Am* 2002;28:603–624.

Vancheeswaran R, Black CM, David J, et al. Childhood-onset scleroderma: is it different from adult-onset disease? *Arthritis Rheum* 1996;39:1041–1049.

Zulian F, Cassidy JT. The systemic sclerodermas and related disorders. In: Cassidy JT, Petty RE, Laxer RM, et al., eds. *Textbook of pediatric rheumatology.* 6th ed. Philadelphia, PA: Saunders Elsevier, 2011:414–437.

Mixed Connective Tissue Disease

Ito S, Nakamura T, Kurosawa R, et al. Glomerulonephritis in children with mixed connective tissue disease. *Clin Nephrol* 2006;66(3):160–165.

Pepmueller PH, Lindsley CB, Cassidy JT. Mixed connective tissue disease and undifferentiated connective tissue disease. In: Cassidy JT, Petty RE, Laxer RM, et al., eds. *Textbook of pediatric rheumatology.* 6th ed. Philadelphia, PA: Saunders Elsevier, 2011:448–457.

Tsai YY, Yang YH, Yu HH, et al. Fifteen-year experience of pediatric-onset mixed connective tissue disease. *Clin Rheumatol* 2010;29(1):53–58.

CHAPTER 110 ■ TOXICOLOGIC EMERGENCIES

KATHERINE A. O'DONNELL, MD, KEVIN C. OSTERHOUDT, MD, MSCE, MICHELE M. BURNS, MD, MPH, DIANE P. CALELLO, MD, AND FRED M. HENRETIG, MD

PEDIATRIC POISONINGS

Poisoning represents one of the most common medical emergencies encountered by young children and accounts for a significant fraction of emergency department (ED) visits in the adolescent population.

Estimates of poisoning episodes annually in the United States range in the millions. Poisonings may be unintentional or intentional. Unintentional or exploratory exposures to poisons make up 80% to 85% or more of all reports, whereas intentional poisonings comprise the other 10% to 15%. Persons in this latter group have much higher rates of treatment in the ED, hospitalization, and intensive care. Among children 5 years and younger, most poisoning exposures are related to exploratory behavior. Although less common, the physician must also consider the possibility of environmental exposures, therapeutic errors, suicide attempts in children, and neonates exposed to toxicants in utero. Child abuse by poisoning, while rare, should be suspected in patients outside the typical age for self-poisoning (<1 year, 5 to 11 years of age), when multiple agents or illicit drugs are involved, when siblings present with similar syndromes, and in cases of massive ingestions in a young child.

The exploratory ingestion of a drug or chemical by a toddler represents a complex interplay of host, agent, and environmental factors and may be considered a subset of the modern traumatic injury model. In this model, each factor contributes, more or less, in a given context to the probability of the injury occurring. Some children are more at risk because of peak age of 1 to 4 years, male gender, temperament that leans toward hyperactivity, and increased finger–mouth activity and/or pica. Some agents are more culpable because of ease of access, attractiveness/palatability, and toxic potential. Two classic examples are iron tablets, which may look like candy, are widely available, and are toxic in significant overdose; and mouthwash, which has a bright color, as well as a pleasant taste and smell, is often packaged in large volumes without child-safety caps, and may have surprisingly high ethanol content (15% to 25%). Typical environmental factors include an acute stressor, such as a recent move or new baby in the household, or more chronic issues, such as parental illness/disability. The young child's exploratory encounter with a poison should not be viewed as an "accident," as the combination of child, agent, and environmental factors may lead predictably to the statistical likelihood of toddler ingestion. Pediatricians have led the way in poisoning prevention strategies by modifying these risk factors with traditional anticipatory guidance and by spearheading the lobby for child-safety caps on particularly dangerous medications and household products. These efforts resulted in a dramatic decrease in childhood poisoning morbidity and mortality since the 1970s, however recent data suggests a worrisome trend. As prescribing patterns in the adult population have created an increased availability of potentially hazardous medications, there has been a clear increase in serious pharmaceutical exposures in young children. As such, pediatric poisonings continue to occur and demand the emergency physician's attention.

The scope of toxic substances involved in poisonings is broad, requiring a wide range of knowledge. Tables 110.1 and 110.2 review the categories of substances most commonly reported in human exposures in the United States for the year 2012. Table 110.3 presents the 10 most common toxic exposures involved in human deaths for the year 2012. The former listing much more closely approximates the profile of pediatric poisonings, whereas the latter is more typical of intentional adolescent and adult exposures. The most important difference between the pediatric and the adult profile by type of agent is in the higher percentage of cases in which psychopharmacologic drugs (sedatives, tranquilizers, and antidepressants) cause poisoning in adults and the much higher frequency of exposures to household and personal care products and plants in children.

There are seven basic routes of poison exposure: oral (ingestion), ocular, topical, inhalational, transplacental, parenteral, and by envenomation. Poisonings may result from acute or chronic exposures. Most poisonings treated in EDs are acute, and the patients are typified by the curious child who gains access to a medication or household cleaning product, or the adolescent who takes a massive number of pills in a fit of despair. *Chronic poisoning* refers to toxicity which develops over time as a substance accumulates in the body, and is best exemplified by environmental exposure to lead or other heavy metals. Chronic pharmaceutical toxicity also occurs. Examples of this pattern of poisoning include acetaminophen hepatotoxicity in infants and small children after repeated supratherapeutic dosing or aspirin poisoning in older adults with excessive dosing or renal impairment. Chronic toxicity can be a challenging diagnosis because the source is not always apparent, the toxicity is not always clear, and the toxic process is not often obvious until serious clinical derangements occur.

GENERAL APPROACH TO THE POISONED CHILD

Following the analogy between unintentional poisoning and traumatic injury, a similar model may be used in formulating a management approach. The poisoned patient often represents an acute-onset emergency with a broad spectrum of multiorgan system pathophysiology that shares many features with the multiple trauma patient. In essence, poisoning might be viewed as a multiple chemical trauma. The concept of a brief window of opportunity to make critical diagnostic and management decisions is likewise analogous. One may conceptualize a management approach that attempts to prioritize critical assessment and, at times, simultaneous management interventions

TABLE 110.1

SUBSTANCES MOST OFTEN REPORTED IN HUMAN EXPOSURES

Substance	Percentage of total exposures
Analgesics (including opioids)	11.6
Cosmetics/personal care products	7.8
Cleaning substances	7.2
Sedatives/hypnotics/antipsychotics	6
Foreign bodies/toys	4.1
Antidepressants	4
Cardiovascular drugs	3.9
Antihistamines	3.6
Topical preparations	3.6
Pesticides	3.3

Adapted from Mowry JB, Spyker DA, Cantilena LR Jr, et al. 2012 Annual Report of the American Association of Poison Control Centers' National Poison Data System (NPDS): 30th Annual Report. *Clin Toxicol* 2013;51:949–1229.

(Table 110.4). The initial phase (or primary survey) addresses the traditional airway, breathing, and circulation (ABCs) of airway securement and cardiorespiratory support, with a slight additional emphasis on emergent toxicologic considerations. The more specific evaluation and detoxification phase (or secondary survey) is aimed at simultaneously initiating generic treatment while assessing the actual extent of intoxication (in cases of known or presumed exposures) and/or identifying the actual toxicants involved (in unknown but highly suspected intoxications).

Initial Life Support Phase

The general approach to recognition and support of vital airway and cardiorespiratory functions (or ABCDs) is well known to most readers and is covered in detail in Chapter 1 A General Approach to Ill and Injured Children. In the context of the poisoned child, a few points deserve special emphasis. In addition to the usual signs of airway obstruction, the physician must pay special attention to evidence of disturbed airway protective reflexes, or to signs of airway injury as with a caustic ingestion. Many poisoned patients will vomit, and some may be administered charcoal, which poses an aspiration risk. Elective endotracheal intubation (Chapter 3 Airway) may thus be indicated at a slightly lower threshold in this context than in another child with comparable central nervous system (CNS) depression.

It is also particularly important to anticipate imminent respiratory failure in the deeply comatose poisoned child. Cyanosis and overt apnea are late findings with progressive drug-induced medullary depression. Thus, clinical or laboratory assessment of early ventilatory insufficiency is critical in such patients to avoid the chaos of a precipitous respiratory arrest. Likewise, it is far easier to establish intravenous (IV) access in a child with normal circulatory status than in a child in shock; early efforts to obtain a secure IV line in symptomatic overdose patients are thus well worth the time and effort.

After securing the airway, ensuring effective breathing, and supporting circulation, it is important to evaluate poisoned patients for neurologic "*d*isability," and the need for empiric "*d*rug" treatment, and emergent "*d*econtamination." Level of consciousness may be assessed rapidly with a semiquantitative scale such as the Glasgow Coma Scale or the AVPU (spontaneously *a*lert, response to *v*erbal stimulation or *p*ain, or *u*nresponsive) scale. Pupillary size and reactivity may be quickly noted. Rapid changes in mental status are common in serious intoxications and may herald precipitous cardiorespiratory failure.

Empiric drug treatment is warranted for most symptomatic poisoned children with altered mental status. All such patients may initially be given humidified *oxygen* and their blood oxyhemoglobin saturation monitored, if possible, by pulse oximetry. If available, rapid bedside blood glucose testing may be used; if low, or not readily available, a trial dosage of 0.25 to 1 g per kg glucose as 10% to 25% solution should be infused. It should be noted that drug- or toxicant-induced hypoglycemia does not present uniformly with coma or seizures. Almost any neuropsychiatric sequelae of hypoglycemia may predominate, including aphasia; slurred, dysarthric speech; and focal neurologic signs. Adrenergic signs,

TABLE 110.2

SUBSTANCES MOST OFTEN REPORTED IN PEDIATRIC EXPOSURES <5 YEARS OF AGE

Substance	Percentage of total exposures
Cosmetics/personal care products	14
Analgesics (including opioids)	10
Cleaning substances	9
Foreign bodies/toys	7
Topical preparations	6.3
Vitamins	4.3
Antihistamines	3.9
Pesticides	3.2
Plants	2.8
Antimicrobials	2.7

Adapted from Mowry JB, Spyker DA, Cantilena LR Jr, et al. 2012 Annual Report of the American Association of Poison Control Centers' National Poison Data System (NPDS): 30th Annual Report. *Clin Toxicol (Phila)* 2013;51:949–1229.

TABLE 110.3

TOXIC EXPOSURES ASSOCIATED WITH THE MOST DEATHS

Opioid analgesics	Sedative-hypnotics, antipsychotics
Antidepressants	Cardiovascular drugs
Stimulants and street drugs	Alcohols
Nonprescription analgesics	Gases and fumes (includes carbon monoxide)
Muscle relaxants	Antihistamines

Adapted from Mowry JB, Spyker DA, Cantilena LR Jr, et al. 2012 Annual Report of the American Association of Poison Control Centers' National Poison Data System (NPDS): 30th Annual Report. *Clin Toxicol (Phila)* 2013;51:949–1229.

TABLE 110.4

GENERAL APPROACH TO THE KNOWN OR SUSPECTED INTOXICATION

Initial life support phase	*Physical examination*
Airway: Maintain patency, assess protective reflexes	Vital signs
Breathing: Adequate tidal volume?	Level of consciousness, neuromuscular tone, reflexes
ABG or $ETCO_2$?	Eyes—pupil size/reactivity, extraocular movements, fundi, nystagmus
Circulation: Secure IV access, assess perfusion	Mouth—corrosive lesions, odors
Disability: Level of consciousness (AVPU or GCS)	Cardiovascular—rate, rhythm, perfusion
Pupillary size, reactivity	Respiratory—rate, chest excursion, air entry
Drugs: Dextrose (rapid bedside test)	GI—motility, corrosive effects
Oxygen	Skin—color, bullae or burns, diaphoresis, piloerection
Naloxone	Odors
(Other ALS medications)	*Laboratory* (individualize)
Decontamination: Ocular—copious saline lavage	CBC, co-oximetry
Skin—copious water, then soap and water	ABG, serum osmolarity
GI—consider options	EKG/cardiac monitor
Evaluation and detoxification phase	Chest radiograph, abdominal radiograph
History—Brief, focused	Electrolytes, BUN/creatinine, glucose, calcium, liver function panel
Known toxicant: Estimate amount	Urinalysis
Elapsed time	Urine screen for common drugs (amphetamine, benzodiazepines, barbiturates, cocaine, marijuana, opiates, phencyclidine)
Early symptoms	Quantitative toxicology tests (including acetaminophen, aspirin, ethanol)
Home treatment	*Assessment of severity/diagnosis*
Significant underlying conditions	Clinical findings
Suspected but unknown toxicant—consider poisoning if:	Laboratory abnormalities (with consideration of anion, osmolar gaps)
Patient: Acute onset of illness	Toxidromes (Table 110.6)
Pica-prone age	*Specific detoxification*
History of pica, ingestions	Reassess ABCDs
Current household "stress"	Institute appropriate GI decontamination (if not already under way)
Multiorgan system dysfunction	Urgent antidotal therapy
Significantly altered mental status	Consider excretion enhancement
Puzzling clinical picture	Continue supportive care
Family: Medications at home	
Recent illness (under treatment)	
Social: Grandparents visiting	
Holiday parties, other events, new baby	

ABG, arterial blood gas; $ETCO_2$, end-tidal carbon dioxide; AVPU, Alert, Verbal, Pain, Unresponsive; GCS, Glasgow Coma Scale; ALS, advanced life support; GI, gastrointestinal; CBC, complete blood cell count; EKG, electrocardiogram; BUN, blood urea nitrogen.

such as diaphoresis and tachycardia, are not uniformly present. Hypoglycemia is a complication seen in ingestions of ethanol, oral hypoglycemics, β-blockers (BBs), salicylates, and, of course, insulin injection. As basic as this intervention seems, in our experience, it is still one of the most often missed (or more accurately, *delayed*) critical treatments in the management of the poisoned patient. Thiamine (100 mg IV), although routinely administered to adult overdose patients who receive hypertonic glucose to obviate precipitating Wernicke encephalopathy, is not generally necessary in the pediatric population. Perhaps it should be considered in adolescent patients who may be thiamine deficient secondary to eating disorders, chronic disease (e.g., inflammatory bowel disease), or alcoholism.

Lastly, empiric naloxone therapy is just as important in potentially poisoned toddlers with altered mental status as it is in adults. As opioid prescriptions in the adult population have increased in recent years, so too has the availability of these agents to young children. Many households contain a variety of oral opioid analgesic agents, as well as cough medicines (codeine, dextromethorphan), antidiarrheal agents (paregoric, diphenoxylate), and partially naloxone-responsive antihypertensive agents such as clonidine. In addition, the possibility of exploratory ingestion of a "stash" of illicit opioids does exist. Thus, naloxone should be used as a therapeutic/diagnostic trial when there is a reasonable possibility that altered mental status is drug induced. Previous recommendations have based dosing on weight (e.g., 0.01 to 0.1 mg per kg); however, many authorities now prefer a unified pediatric dose of 0.4 to 2 mg for acute overdose patients of all ages (outside the neonatal period). Such an approach conceptualizes naloxone dosing as based on total narcotic load and number of opioid receptors that require competition for binding sites. In general, this latter approach is easier to remember and has not been associated with complication in the ED. Adolescent patients with a strong clinical picture for opioid intoxication (without habituation) may receive 2-mg bolus doses every 2 minutes, up to a total dose of 8 to 10 mg, before abandoning hope of benefit because several congeners of morphine (e.g., propoxyphene, illicit fentanyl derivatives, pentazocine, oxycodone, methadone) may require such large doses. If chronic abuse is suspected, lower initial doses (0.2 mg or less) are warranted. Administration of flumazenil to adolescents exhibiting depressed consciousness after an unknown drug overdose is not recommended as it may precipitate seizures and life-threatening benzodiazepine withdrawal (see "Central Nervous System Sedative-Hypnotics" section).

The rationale for decontamination (Decontamination) of the poisoned child is discussed in the next section. This treatment phase may begin urgently, after or in concert with attention to the ABCDs. At times, a decision to perform gastric decontamination through the preferred technique can be made almost immediately upon presentation and, if so, should be instituted as soon as possible, taking into account the patient's clinical status and the number of hands available to assist in management. For example, a toddler with coma, shock, and massive hematochezia who is rushed into the ED by the rescue squad—and for whom there is witnessed or strong circumstantial evidence of massive iron overdose—requires a concerted team effort directed toward resuscitation, stabilization, and urgent gastric decontamination. However, an asymptomatic adolescent who ingests 10 g of acetaminophen 30 minutes before arrival at the ED may be fully evaluated in a timely but orderly manner (as outlined in the next section) and considered for less emergent gastric decontamination—in this case, possibly an oral dose of activated charcoal. Significant dermal or ocular exposures require immediate copious lavage, and precautions should be taken to protect the healthcare providers tending to the patient from exposure.

At the completion of this initial life support phase, the poisoned patient should have been assessed for compromise of vital airway and cardiorespiratory function and for global neurologic status and should have had resuscitative measures instituted. Patients with significant altered mental status have been critically evaluated for respiratory status, have had IV access secured, and have had therapeutic trials of oxygen, glucose, and naloxone. Other advanced life support interventions such as anticonvulsants or antiarrhythmics have been instituted as necessary. Consideration of decontamination options has begun.

Evaluation and Detoxification Phase

History

A brief and focused *historical evaluation* should be addressed as soon as the life support phase has been completed. The primary goal is to determine the potential severity of the exposure. This assessment requires poison and patient-related data alike.

For a known or highly suspected toxic exposure, an attempt is made to estimate the total amount ingested (number of pills missing, ounces left in the bottle, dosage of pills, concentration of alcohol, and so forth). The best estimate of time elapsed since ingestion is also sought. Parents should be questioned regarding early symptoms noted at home or en route to the ED and any treatments administered before arrival. Certain underlying medical conditions may be relevant (e.g., glucose-6-phosphate dehydrogenase [G6PD] deficiency for mothball ingestions); thus, any significant medical history should be noted.

Often, children who are poisoned do not come to the ED with a clear history of exposure followed by onset of symptoms. Rather, they develop signs and symptoms that mimic other diseases and give no history of toxic exposure. Thus, the ED staff must always consider the possibility of ingestion when treating young children.

General historical features that suggest the possibility of poisoning include (i) acute onset; (ii) age range of 1 to 5 years or adolescence; (iii) history of pica or known exposure to a potential toxicant; (iv) substantial environmental stress, either acute (e.g., arrival of a new baby, serious illness in a parent) or chronic (e.g., marital conflict, parental disability); (v) multiple organ system involvement; (vi) significant alteration in level of consciousness; and (vii) a clinical picture that seems especially puzzling.

Certain family and social history variables are also important. Medications used by other household members, particularly new medications introduced into the home environment by virtue of recent illnesses or visits from grandparents and other relatives, are a common source of ingested drugs. Changes in routine and large family gatherings (e.g., holiday parties, moving to a new home) are particularly risky occasions for decreased parental supervision and new (or less carefully guarded) potentially toxic medications or household products. Although often difficult to obtain, the history of illicit drug use, manufacture, or distribution in the child's environment (the "drug-endangered child") significantly increases the risk of serious outcomes from a poison exposure as well.

Physical Examination

The focused physical examination should begin with a reassessment of vital functions and complete recording of vital signs, including core temperature. With secure airway and cardiorespiratory function confirmed, the examination should then focus on the central and autonomic nervous systems, eye findings, changes in the skin and/or oral and gastrointestinal (GI) mucous membranes, and odors (see Chapter 45 Odor: Unusual) on the breath or clothing of the patient. These features represent those areas most likely affected in toxic syndromes and, when taken together, often form a constellation of signs and symptoms referred to as toxidromes (Tables 110.5 and 110.6). Such toxidromes may be so characteristic as to provide guidance for early therapeutic management before precise historical or laboratory confirmation of a specific exposure is available.

Laboratory Evaluation

Laboratory studies may be helpful in confirming diagnostic impressions or in demonstrating toxicant-induced metabolic aberrations. However, there is no "tox panel" that is uniformly helpful or necessary. Most poisonings can be managed appropriately without extensive laboratory studies, and in particular, the reflex ordering of rapid overdose toxicology "screens" has rarely been found to be helpful in acute patient management. They have important, nonemergent roles (e.g., in resolving medicolegal issues or considering drug-induced causes of behavioral changes in a psychiatric patient). In toddlers with a known or strongly suspected specific ingestion, rapid drug screens are rarely indicated. In the adolescent intentional overdose patient who is not critically ill or who does not have a particularly puzzling clinical picture, the drug screen again is rarely helpful, although the finding of an unexpected

TABLE 110.5

CLINICAL MANIFESTATIONS OF POISONING

Vital signs

Pulse

Bradycardia

Digoxin, opioids, organophosphates, plants (lily-of-the-valley, foxglove, oleander), clonidine, β-blockers, calcium channel blockers

Tachycardia

Alcohol, amphetamines and sympathomimetics, anticholinergic agents, tricyclic antidepressants, theophylline, salicylates, phencyclidine, cocaine

Respirations

Slow, depressed

Alcohol, barbiturates (late), opioids, clonidine, sedative-hypnotics

Tachypnea

Amphetamines, barbiturates (early), methanol, ethylene glycol, salicylates, carbon monoxide

Blood pressure

Hypotension

Cellular asphyxiants (methemoglobinemia, cyanide, carbon monoxide), β-blockers, calcium channel blockers, antipsychotics, tricyclic antidepressants, barbiturates, iron, theophylline, clonidine, opioids

Hypertension

Amphetamines/sympathomimetics, phencyclidine, monoamine oxidase inhibitors (MAOIs), antihistamines, anticholinergic agents, clonidine (early)

Temperature

Hypothermia

Ethanol, barbiturates, sedative-hypnotics, opioids, phenothiazines, antidepressants, clonidine, carbamazepine

Hyperpyrexia

Sympathomimetics, anticholinergics, salicylates, neuroleptics, inhalational anesthetics, succinylcholine, serotonin reuptake inhibitors, withdrawal from sedatives/alcohol

Neuromuscular

Coma

Opioids, sedative-hypnotics, anticholinergics (antihistamines, antidepressants, phenothiazines, atropinics, OTC sleep preparations), alcohols, anticonvulsants, carbon monoxide, salicylates, organophosphate insecticides, clonidine, γ-hydroxybutyrate

Delirium/psychosis

Alcohol, phenothiazines, drugs of abuse (phencyclidine, LSD, peyote, mescaline, marijuana, cocaine, heroin, MDMA, designer drugs), sympathomimetics and anticholinergics (including prescription and OTC cold remedies), steroids, heavy metals, dextromethorphan

Convulsions

Alcohol, amphetamines, cocaine, phenothiazines, antidepressants (particularly bupropion and tricyclics), antihistamines, camphor, boric acid, lead, organophosphates, isoniazid, salicylates, plants (water hemlock), lindane, lidocaine, phencyclidine, carbamazepine, theophylline, caffeine

Ataxia

Alcohol, barbiturates, benzodiazepines, carbon monoxide, anticonvulsants, heavy metals, organic solvents, sedative-hypnotics, hydrocarbons

Paralysis

Botulism, heavy metals, plants (poison hemlock), ticks, paralytic shellfish poisoning

Eyes

Pupils

Miosis

Opioids, organophosphates, ethanol, barbiturates, phenothiazines, phencyclidine, clonidine

Mydriasis

Amphetamines, anticholinergic agents, barbiturates (if comatose), botulism, cocaine, methanol, glutethimide, LSD, marijuana, phencyclidine, antihistamines, antidepressants

Nystagmus

Phenytoin, sedative-hypnotics, carbamazepine, glutethimide, phencyclidine (both vertical and horizontal), barbiturates, ethanol, MAOIs, ketamine, dextromethorphan

Skin

Jaundice

Carbon tetrachloride, acetaminophen, naphthalene, phenothiazines, plants (hepatotoxic mushrooms, fava bean-induced hemolysis), heavy metals (iron, phosphorus, arsenic)

Cyanosis (unresponsive to oxygen, as a result of methemoglobinemia)

Aniline dyes, nitrites, benzocaine, phenacetin, nitrobenzene, phenazopyridine, dapsone

Pinkness to redness

Atropinics and antihistamines, alcohol, carbon monoxide, cyanide, boric acid

Odors

Acetone: Acetone, isopropyl alcohol, phenol, salicylates

Alcohol: Ethanol (alcoholic beverages)

Bitter almond: Cyanide

Garlic: Heavy metal (arsenic, phosphorus, thallium), selenium, organophosphates

Wintergreen: Methylsalicylates (oil of wintergreen)

Solvent: Hydrocarbons (gasoline, turpentine)

OTC, over the counter; LSD, lysergamide.
Adapted from Mofenson HC, Greensher J. The unknown poison. *Pediatrics* 1974;54:336.

toxic level of acetaminophen (which may have been omitted in the history) may impact management, and some authors recommend that quantitative acetaminophen levels (in lieu of "tox screens") be sought in all such patients.

The labor-intensive comprehensive urine drug screen may be useful for patients who are seriously ill with an occult ingestion or for the occasional intentional overdose adolescent patient whose clinical picture does not fit with the stated

TABLE 110.6

TOXIDROMES

	Sympathomimetic (amphetamines, cocaine)	Anticholinergic (antihistamines, many others)	Cholinergic (insecticides, nerve gases)	Opioids/ clonidine	Barbiturates/ sedative-hypnotics	Salicylates	Theophylline
Mental status/CNS	Agitation, delirium, psychosis, convulsions	Delirium, psychosis, coma, convulsions	Confusion, fasciculations, coma	Euphoria, somnolence, coma	Somnolence, coma	Lethargy, convulsions	Agitation, tremor, convulsions
Heart rate	Increased	Increased	Decreased (or increased)	Decreased	—	—	Increased
Blood pressure	Increased	Increased	—	Decreased	Decreased	—	Decreased
Temperature	Increased	Increased	—	Decreased	Decreased	Increased	—
Respirations	—	—	Increased	Decreased	Decreased	Increased	Increased
Pupils	Large, reactive	Large, sluggish	Small	Pinpoint	—	—	—
Bowel sounds	Present	Diminished	Hyperactive	—	—	—	—
Skin	Diaphoresis	Flushed, dry	Diaphoresis	—	—	—	—
Miscellaneous	—	—	SLUDGE[a]	—	—	Vomiting	Vomiting

[a]SLUDGE is a mnemonic representing *s*alivation, *l*acrimation, *u*rination, *d*efecation, *g*astric cramping, and *e*mesis.
CNS, central nervous system; —, minimal direct effect.

TABLE 110.7

FREQUENTLY USEFUL QUANTITATIVE TOXICOLOGY TESTS IN PEDIATRIC PATIENTS

Drug/toxin	Optimal time after ingestion (hours)
Acetaminophen	4
Carbamazepine	2–4
Carboxyhemoglobin	Immediate
Digoxin	4–6
Ethanol	½–1
Ethylene glycol	½–1
Iron	4
Lithium	2–4[a]
Methanol	½–1
Methemoglobin	Immediate
Phenobarbital	1–2
Phenytoin	1–2
Salicylate	2–4[a]
Theophylline	1–2[a]
Valproate	2–4

[a]Repeat levels over 6 to 12 hours may be necessary with sustained-release preparations.
Adapted from Weisman RS, Howland MA, Flomenbaum NE. The toxicology laboratory. In: Goldfrank LR, Flomenbaum NE, Lewin NA, et al., eds. *Toxicologic Emergencies.* Norwalk, CT: Appleton & Lange, 1990.

TABLE 110.8

IMPORTANT DRUGS AND TOXICANTS NOT DETECTED BY MOST DRUG SCREENS

Antidysrhythmics	β-Blockers[a]
Anticoagulants	Calcium channel blockers[a]
Anticonvulsants	Hypoglycemics
Antidepressants (TCAs, SSRIs)	
Antipsychotics	
Clonidine	Colchicine
Cyanide	Solvents
Designer drugs:	Toxic alcohols
MDMA, γ-hydroxybutyrate, ketamine	
Organophosphates	Synthetic opioids (i.e., methadone, buprenorphine, fentanyl, etc.)
Tetrahydrozoline (in over-the-counter eyedrops)	Plant and mushroom toxins

[a]Hypotension is often seen with bradycardia.
Adapted from Goldfrank LR, Flomenbaum NE, Lewin NA, et al., eds. *Goldfrank's toxicologic emergencies,* 9th ed. New York, NY: McGraw-Hill, 2009.

history. Often of greater help is the critical interpretation of routine measurements of serum chemistries, blood gas analysis, and osmolality in patients with altered mental status. The presence of hypoglycemia or aberrations of serum electrolytes may provide crucial information about the poisoned patient. In certain circumstances, tests of liver or renal function, urinalysis, creatine phosphokinase levels, and other select tests may be useful. Metabolic acidosis with a high anion gap is found in many clinical syndromes and toxidromes, reflected by the often-cited mnemonic *MUDPILES,* for *m*ethanol and *m*etformin; *u*remia; *d*iabetic and other ketoacidoses; *p*araldehyde; *Isoniazid* (INH), *i*ron, *i*nborn errors of metabolism and massive *i*buprofen; *l*actic acidosis (seen with hypoxia, shock, carbon monoxide, cyanide, and many drugs that cause compromised cardiorespiratory status or prolonged seizures); *e*thylene glycol; and *s*alicylates or *s*eizures. Differences between calculated and measured serum osmolarity (calculated = 2 [serum Na mEq per L] + blood urea nitrogen [BUN] mg per dL ÷ 2.8 + glucose mg per dL ÷ 18; with normal osmolarity ~290 mOsm per kg) may suggest intoxication with ethanol, isopropanol, or more rarely in pediatric patients, methanol or ethylene glycol. Blood collection tubes containing ethylenediaminetetraacetic acid (EDTA) should not be used to send samples to the laboratory because the osmolal gap will be falsely elevated.

An immediate determination of quantitative levels is helpful in making management decisions for some drugs, and these are outlined in Table 110.7. Furthermore, many important causes of coma and altered vital signs are not detected on even the most sophisticated "comprehensive" toxicology panels (which are usually biased toward psychoactive medications and illicit drugs). An overview of such agents is presented in Table 110.8. An electrocardiogram (EKG) should be performed in all seriously ill patients in whom poisoning is being considered. Detectable conduction delays (prolongation of the PR, QRS, and/or QT intervals) may provide diagnostic direction and impact management by predicting imminent life-threatening cardiac rhythm disturbances.

Assessment of Severity and Diagnosis

At this juncture, most intoxicated patients may be readily stratified by specific toxicant or category of drug(s) ingested and some judgment made as to the potential or current severity of the exposure. For some children, clinical features of a complex illness of acute onset may suggest intoxication without a specific history of such ingestion. In a few cases, some laboratory confirmation of clinical suspicion will be available on an immediate basis. Using all the clinical clues available and with some familiarity of the "toxidrome" approach to differential diagnosis as detailed previously (Tables 110.5 and 110.6) and, at times, with help from the laboratory, the emergency physician must now establish a working diagnosis and proceed with consideration of options for specific detoxification.

Specific Detoxification

Again, the proviso that the patient be continually reassessed and managed for impaired vital function is addressed. All decisions about further decontamination and/or specific antidotal therapy involve a complex interplay between the toxicant(s) ingested and the patient's condition.

GI Decontamination. The effort to "get the poison out" has long been a mainstay of the traditional discussion of toxicologic management. However, gastric emptying measures have fallen out of favor in recent years, and the routine use of activated charcoal as a poison adsorbent has been subjected to increased academic scrutiny. Unfortunately, young children have been underrepresented in clinical studies of GI decontamination. It is likely that as further research is conducted, particularly as directed toward the pediatric population, current dogma regarding optimal GI decontamination will evolve. For the sections that follow, several appropriate techniques for gastric decontamination are reviewed, all of which may be useful under certain circumstances. An approach to the overall decision process in a given patient is then offered.

Simple Dilution. Dilution may be indicated only when the toxicant produces local irritation or corrosion. Water or milk is an acceptable diluent. Dilution for caustic agents is controversial; dilution may be used in the first few minutes after an exposure but only if there is no evidence of airway compromise or significant abdominal pain/vomiting. For drug ingestion, however, dilution alone should not be used because it may increase absorption by increasing dissolution rates of the tablets or capsules or it may promote more rapid transit into the lower GI tract.

Gastric Emptying. The goal of gastric emptying is to rid the stomach of remaining poison to prevent further local effect or systemic absorption. The utility of gastric emptying diminishes with time and is most effective if done early after ingestion when unabsorbed drug is still present within the stomach (operationally, within the first 30 minutes to 1 hour). In certain circumstances, such as the delayed gastric emptying accompanying intoxication with anticholinergic drugs, benefit may be noted longer after ingestion. *Induced emesis* (with syrup of ipecac) was once a favored means of gastric emptying, but the American Academy of Pediatrics no longer recommends that syrup of ipecac be used routinely for the poisoned patient in the home or healthcare facility. This was in response to inconsistent data regarding decreased drug absorption, no evidence that it changes clinical outcomes, potential for abuse in vulnerable patients (those with eating disorders, Munchausen syndrome by proxy), and the concern that it may delay time to administration of other more effective therapies.

An alternative to ipecac-induced emesis for emptying the stomach is *gastric lavage*. This procedure has very limited indications and is usually reserved for patients who have ingested a potentially life-threatening amount of poison, in cases where the procedure can be performed safely very early after ingestion and charcoal alone is not believed to be adequate. To carry out a satisfactory lavage, the patient should be on his or her left side, head slightly lower than feet, and the largest orogastric lavage tube that can reasonably be passed should be used (e.g., 24F orogastric tube for a toddler, 36F orogastric tube for an adolescent). A smaller caliber nasogastric (NG) tube is sufficient only for some liquid toxins. Gastric contents should be aspirated initially before any lavage fluid is introduced. Normal saline aliquots of 50 to 100 mL in young children and 150 to 200 mL in adolescents can be lavaged repeatedly until the return is clear. Like induced emesis, gastric lavage's efficacy in reducing drug absorption has been reviewed critically in more recent studies. Again, the efficacy has been highly variable and lavage has not been demonstrated to improve outcome in poisoned patients. Several important risks are associated with gastric lavage, including oxygen desaturation, aspiration, and mechanical trauma to the oropharynx and esophagus. Gastric lavage is rarely recommended anymore but might be considered for patients presenting very early after very dangerous ingestions (of toxicants such as colchicine or arsenic). Contraindications to the procedure include caustic or corrosive ingestions, impending loss of airway protection, and the presence of cardiac arrhythmia.

TABLE 110.9

SUBSTANCES POORLY (OR NOT) ADSORBED BY ACTIVATED CHARCOAL

Common electrolytes
Metals—iron, lead, arsenic, lithium
Mineral acids or bases
Alcohols
Cyanide
Most solvents
Most water-insoluble compounds (e.g., hydrocarbons)

Activated Charcoal. Activated charcoal minimizes absorption of drugs by adsorbing them onto its molecular surface area. Charcoal administration has become the decontamination strategy of choice to prevent pediatric poisoning after toxicant ingestion and is most effective when used in the first hour after ingestion. Therefore, if activated charcoal is considered as a treatment option, quick triage of an exposed patient may be necessary to allow charcoal administration in a timely fashion. A number of notable compounds, such as iron and lithium, do not adsorb well to activated charcoal (Table 110.9). The usual dose of activated charcoal is 1 g per kg; adolescents and adults should receive 50 to 100 g. Most activated charcoal is now available premixed with water to make slurry that can be taken orally or administered by NG tube. Simply adding soda or another nonparticulate flavoring agent to the charcoal can improve palatability.

Activated charcoal was "rediscovered" by the toxicology community during the 1980s, with several studies finding its use to be superior to gastric emptying alone and, at least, equivalent to the combination of gastric emptying plus charcoal administration. The use of charcoal alone is less invasive and less likely to be associated with complications in the clinical setting than is gastric emptying. Aspiration of charcoal can be a serious concern among patients with poor airway protective reflexes, and vomiting remains the most common difficulty associated with its use. The use of an NG tube, which renders the esophagogastric sphincter patent, may also increase aspiration risk. Charcoal is contraindicated in patients with an unprotected airway or a disrupted GI tract (e.g., after severe caustic ingestion) or in patients in whom charcoal therapy may increase the risk and severity of aspiration (e.g., hydrocarbons). The use of multiple doses of activated charcoal to achieve enhanced drug elimination is addressed later in this chapter.

Catharsis. Little evidence exists to suggest that standard cathartics (sorbitol, magnesium citrate, magnesium sulfate) reduce drug absorption by speeding intestinal transit. It is also not established whether coadministration with activated charcoal minimizes the risk of constipation, and there does appear to be an increased risk of vomiting, cramping abdominal pain, and hypernatremic dehydration in young infants. As such, a single dose of premixed charcoal/sorbitol is safe for most pediatric ingestions, but should not be used in young infants. Oil-based cathartics (mineral oil, castor oil) are discouraged because they may be aspirated, increase absorption of some poisons, or unnecessarily extend the cathartic effect.

Whole Bowel Irrigation (WBI). An additional technique of cathartic GI decontamination is that of intestinal irrigation with large volumes and flow rates of a high–molecular-weight polyethylene glycol-balanced electrolyte solution such as GoLYTELY or Colyte. Typically, these solutions are not significantly absorbed nor do they exert an osmotic effect, so the patient's net fluid/electrolyte status is unchanged. They have a long safety track record in patient populations such as infants and in those surgical patients requiring application of preoperative bowel preparation. WBI has been found to be particularly useful in pediatric iron overdoses, in which gastric lavage may be limited by tube size, the fact that metals do not bind to charcoal, and the possibility that the ingestion is not a recent one. It has been used for other metal ingestions (e.g., lead), overdoses of sustained-release medications (e.g., lithium, theophylline, bupropion, verapamil), ingested pharmaceutical patches, and ingestions of vials or packages of illicit drugs. It might also be useful in particularly massive, dangerous, and/or late-presenting overdoses for which severe toxicity refractory to standard therapies may result and for which the efficacy of gastric emptying and/or charcoal is expected to be suboptimal. The technique may be used by mouth in cooperative patients or by NG tube; the usual recommended dosing is 500 mL per hour in toddlers and 2 L per hour in adolescents and adults.

GI Decontamination Strategies

It should be apparent that no unique approach to GI decontamination of all poisoned patients is optimal in every case. Factors to be considered include the expected degree of toxicity from the drug, the physical nature of the drug, the current location of the drug within the body, and the presence of contraindications or alternatives. A risk–benefit decision must be made before the institution of any decontamination strategy.

Due to the considerations discussed above, in the patient for whom GI decontamination is appropriate, activated charcoal and WBI are the favored procedures. Ipecac-induced emesis is no longer endorsed as appropriate home first aid for poisoning, and is not favored in the ED. Gastric lavage still has some role, albeit confined to patients with recent ingestions of extremely toxic and potentially lethal substances, especially when those substances do not bind well to charcoal. Likewise, patients with truly massive overdoses may benefit from lavage when the charcoal dose given does not achieve the ideal charcoal-to-drug ratio of 10:1. (10 g of charcoal to 1 g of drug).

The correct technique for decontamination, regardless of method, requires that careful attention be given to prevent aspiration and anatomic trauma.

Some of the patients in question would have undergone endotracheal intubation during the initial life support phase of management, as detailed previously, or they may be intubated pre-emptively because of borderline mental status and in anticipation of their ensuing critical course. Others may be awake, alert, and cooperative, with normal airway protective reflexes, and thus be given activated charcoal without prior endotracheal intubation. The combative, agitated patient poses a dilemma and must be carefully managed on an individualized basis.

An attempt to summarize these considerations is diagrammed in Figure 110.1; however, it should be reiterated that all decisions regarding gastric decontamination involve multiple patient and toxic agent-related factors and should not be made with a "cookbook" approach.

Antidotal Therapy. Beyond the setting of acetaminophen overdose, the overall number of toxic ingestions for which a specific antidote is necessary or available is small. When a specific antidote can be used, it is vital that it be administered as early as possible and in an appropriately monitored dose. Those antidotes that should be available for immediate administration include sodium bicarbonate (tricyclic antidepressants), sodium nitrite/sodium thiosulfate or hydroxocobalamin (cyanide), atropine and pralidoxime (cholinesterase inhibitors), ethanol or fomepizole (ethylene glycol and methanol), dextrose (ethanol, salicylates, oral hypoglycemics), methylene blue (methemoglobinemic agents,), oxygen (carbon monoxide), flumazenil (benzodiazepines), pyridoxine (INH and *Gyromitra* mushrooms), digoxin immune Fab (digoxin), IV lipid emulsion (local anesthetic toxicity), and naloxone (opioids). Other antidotes usually do not require such urgent administration and may be given subsequent to initiation of other management modalities. Even when available, antidotes do not diminish the need for meticulous supportive care or other therapy. Indiscriminant use of antidotes without other forms of management should be discouraged. Table 110.10 summarizes a list of commonly used antidotes, suggested doses, and their indications for use. Because of its frequent use, naloxone is discussed further here.

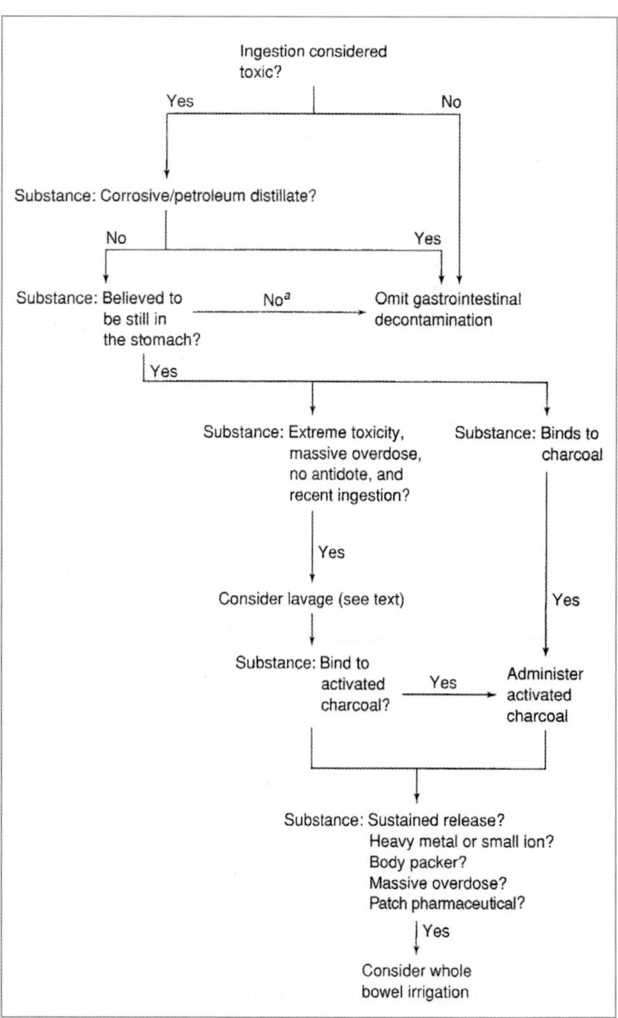

FIGURE 110.1 Approach to gastrointestinal decontamination. [a]For patients in whom the toxicant is no longer believed to be in the stomach, whole bowel irrigation might still be a valid consideration.

TABLE 110.10

SUMMARY OF ANTIDOTES

Poison	Antidote
Acetaminophen	*N*-acetylcysteine; intravenous (IV)—150 mg/kg over 1 hr, then 12.5 mg/kg/hr for 4 hrs, then 6.25 mg/kg/hr; enteral—140 mg/kg, then 70 mg/kg every 4 hrs
Anticholinergics	Physostigmine (adult, 0.5 to 2 mg; child, 0.02 mg/kg) slow IV; may repeat in 15 min until desired effect is achieved; subsequent doses every 2–3 hrs PRN (*Caution: May cause seizures, asystole, cholinergic crisis; see text*)
Anticholinesterases	Atropine, 2–5 mg (adults); 0.05–0.1 mg/kg (children) intramuscular (IM) or IV, repeated every 10–15 min until atropinization is evident
Organophosphates	Pralidoxime chloride 1–2 g (adults); 25–50 mg/kg (children) IV; repeat dose in 1 hr PRN, then every 6–8 hrs for 24–48 hrs (consider also constant infusion; see text)
Carbamates	Atropine, as above; pralidoxime for severe cases (see text)
Benzodiazepines	Flumazenil, 0.01 mg/kg IV (estimated pediatric dose; see text)
β-Adrenergic blockers	Glucagon, 0.1 mg/kg IV, followed by 0.05 mg/kg/hr
Calcium channel blockers	Calcium chloride 10%, 10 mL (adult); 0.2 mL/kg (pediatric) IV Or Calcium gluconate 10%, 30 mL (adult); 0.6 mL/kg (pediatric) IV High-dose insulin 1 unit/kg bolus followed by 0.5 units/kg/hr, with glucose infusion titrated to prevent hypoglycemia
Carbon monoxide	Oxygen 100% inhalation, consider hyperbaric for severe cases
Cyanide—nitrites/thiosulfate	*Adult:* Amyl nitrite inhalation (inhale for 15–30 s every 60 s) pending administration of 300 mg sodium nitrite (10 mL of a 3% solution) IV slowly (over 2–4 min); follow immediately with 12.5 g sodium thiosulfate (2.5–5 mL/min of 25% solution) IV over 10–30 min, or IV push in cardiac arrest *Children:* (Na nitrite should not exceed recommended dose because dangerous methemoglobinemia may result):

Hemoglobin	Initial dose 3% Na nitrite	Initial dose 25% Na thiosulfate IV (mL/kg)
8 g	0.22 mL/kg (6.6 mg/kg)	1.10
10 g	0.27 mL/kg (8.7 mg/kg)	1.35
12 g (normal)	0.33 mL/kg (10 mg/kg)	1.65
14 g	0.39 mL/kg (11.6 mg/kg)	1.95

Poison	Antidote
Cyanide—hydroxocobalamin	*Adult:* 5g IV; *Child:* 70 mg/kg IV over 30 minutes or IV push in cardiac arrest
Digitalis	Fab antibodies (Digibind): Dose based on amount ingested and/or digoxin level (see text, package insert)
Fluoride	Calcium gluconate 10%, 0.6 mL/kg IV slowly until symptoms abate, serum calcium normalizes; repeat PRN while monitoring serum calcium
Heavy metals	*BAL* (British Anti-Lewisite; dimercaprol): 300–450 mg/m^2/day (18–24 mg/kg/day) deep IM in 6 divided doses for 3–5 days[a] (*Arsenic, Mercury, Lead*) *CaNa$_2$EDTA* (ethylenediaminetetraacetic acid): 1,000–1,500 mg/m^2/day (25–75 mg/kg/day) continuous IV infusion or in 2–4 divided doses for up to 5 days; see text for further details (*Lead*) *DMSA (succimer):* 350 mg/m^2 (10 mg/kg) PO every 8 hrs for 5 days, followed by 350 mg/m^2 (10 mg/kg) PO every 12 hrs for 14 days (*Mercury, Lead*)
Iron	Deferoxamine: 5–15 mg/kg/hrs IV; use higher dosage for severe symptoms (see text) and decrease as patient recovers
Isoniazid (INH)	Pyridoxine 5–10%, 1 g per gram of INH ingested (70 mg/kg up to 5 g if dose unknown) IV slowly over 30–60 min
Local anesthetics	Intravenous lipid emulsion 20%, 1.5 mL/kg bolus followed by infusion of 0.25 mL/kg/min
Methanol/ethylene glycol	Fomepizole: Load 15 mg/kg; maintenance 10 mg/kg q12h 4 doses, then 15 mg/kg q12h (dose should be adjusted during dialysis) Ethanol loading dose: 600 mg/kg infused over 1 hr (use only if fomepizole unavailable) Ethanol maintenance: 110 mg/kg/hr infusion; adjust as needed with target level 100 mg/dL Folate 1–2 mg/kg IV every 4–6 hrs (methanol) Thiamine 0.25–0.5 mg/kg and pyridoxine 1–2 mg/kg every 6 hrs (ethylene glycol)
Methemoglobinemic agents	Methylene blue 1%, 1–2 mg/kg (0.1–0.2 mL/kg) IV slowly over 5–10 min if cyanosis is severe or methemoglobin level >40%

TABLE 110.10

SUMMARY OF ANTIDOTES (*CONTINUED*)

Poison	Antidote
Opioids	Naloxone 0.4–2 mg IV, IM, sublingual or by ETT; may repeat up to total 8–10 mg in adolescent/adult (see text)
Phenothiazines (dystonic reaction)	Diphenhydramine, 1–2 mg/kg IM or IV; or benztropine, 1–2 mg IM or IV (adolescents)
Sulfonylureas	Octreotide 1–2 μg/kg/dose subcutaneous (SC) or IV every 6–12 hrs
Tricyclic antidepressants	Sodium bicarbonate, 1–2 mEq/kg IV
Warfarin (and "superwarfarin" rat poisons)	Vitamin K_t 10 mg (adult); 1–5 mg (pediatric) IV, IM, SC, PO
Animals	Antivenin[b] For envenomation (see Chapter 91 Shock)
Snake, crotalidae (all North American rattlers and moccasins)	Crotalidae polyvalent immune Fab (BTG International)
Snake, coral	Antivenin (*Micrurus fulvius*), monovalent (Wyeth)
Spider, black widow	Antivenin *Latrodectus mactans* (Merck Sharp & Dohme)

[a]Dosing for lead poisoning/encephalopathy. Chelation regimens vary for other heavy metal poisonings.
[b]See package insert for dosage and administration.

Naloxone. Naloxone, a pure opioid receptor antagonist, is one of the broadest-acting, safest, and most effective of any true antidotes now available. It is effective against all opioids. Naloxone is a synthetic congener of oxymorphone but is devoid of morphine agonist or depressant effects. It has no significant side effects in the treatment of acute overdose except narcotic withdrawal symptoms in the addicted patient. These symptoms include GI upset, tachycardia, hyperpnea, mydriasis, piloerection, yawning, rhinorrhea, diaphoresis, sialorrhea, increased blood pressure, anxiety, restlessness, discomfort, and hyperalgesia. These symptoms are not usually life-threatening to teenagers and adults but can be potentially dangerous to an infant born to an addicted mother. Withdrawal symptoms secondary to naloxone, if observed during acute overdose treatment, would be expected to last no more than 30 minutes and should generally be treated with supportive care. The serum half-life of naloxone is 1 hour; its duration of action 1 to 4 hours. Initial reversal of narcosis may then revert to coma, requiring ongoing reassessment and readministration of naloxone. There are a few case reports of other adverse effects, including hypertension, pulmonary edema, ventricular irritability, and seizures after naloxone-induced reversal of narcosis in the perioperative setting, typically in patients with underlying cardiopulmonary disease and in the presence of additional medications or anesthetic agent use.

The mechanism of action of naloxone is by competitive displacement of narcotic analgesics at central opioid receptor sites. It can be used as a diagnostic test when faced with a questionable history. Current dosage recommendations reflect the proven safety of naloxone in large doses and the necessity of such doses to reverse effects of synthetic opioids such as propoxyphene, pentazocine, oxycodone, and methadone. If severe respiratory depression is present, the initial dose should be 2 mg IV in any patient. Repeat doses may be given every 2 minutes until 10 mg has been administered for adolescent patients with suspected opioid overdose who fail to respond to the lower dosages. Of course, concomitant airway management is vital. In patients without respiratory depression, an initial dose of 0.4 to 1 mg can be used. In adolescents suspected of chronic opiate abuse, smaller initial doses (e.g., 0.05 to 0.4 mg) are warranted. Again, if there is no response but a strong clinical suspicion, 2-mg doses can be repeated up to a total of 10 mg before concluding that further dosing will be of no benefit. Naloxone can also be given intramuscularly (IM), sublingually, intranasally, or by endotracheal tube if no IV access is available.

If a patient demonstrates a response to naloxone, naloxone will have to be repeated at the effective total dose every 20 to 60 minutes. An alternative approach is to provide a continuous IV infusion; generally about two-thirds of the total reversal dose will need to be infused per hour initially, with subsequent adjustments as necessary. This is more likely to be needed in long-acting opioid overdoses.

Nalmefene and naltrexone are longer-acting opioid antagonists that may have use in some clinical situations in which a longer duration of action (4 to 6 hours for nalmefene, 24 hours for naltrexone) is deemed beneficial, such as in reversal of procedural/postoperative opioid depression or as aids in opioid detoxification programs. However, as antidotes for acute opioid overdose in the adolescent or pediatric population, their longer duration may be problematic in assessing the actual time course for resolution of clinical toxicity and/or in precipitating prolonged withdrawal symptoms in habituated patients. Nalmefene may be a useful substitute for prolonged naloxone infusions in cases for which such opioid antagonism is necessary, but little pediatric experience and few dosing guidelines for its use are currently available.

Enhancing Excretion

The procedures available for enhancing the elimination of an absorbed poison that have the greatest value are multiple-dose activated charcoal, diuresis/urinary alkalinization, dialysis, and hemoperfusion. Because some risk is involved, these measures are indicated only in those cases in which the patient's recovery would be otherwise unlikely or in which a specific significant benefit is expected.

Diuresis/Urinary Alkalinization

Diuresis has historically been advocated in cases of poisoning with agents that are excreted primarily by the renal route. Although it is important to maintain high glomerular filtration rates in the presence of rhabdomyolysis or when chelating with agents such as EDTA, forced diuresis has limited value in the treatment of acute poisoning. Similarly, diuretic use has fallen out of favor with the possible exception of mannitol therapy for ciguatera poisoning.

Ionized diuresis takes advantage of the principle that excretion is favored when a drug is in its ionized state. Urinary alkalinization promotes excretion of salicylate (a weak acid). It may also enhance clearance of phenobarbital, chlorpropamide, and chlorophenoxy herbicides, but in these poisonings, it cannot be considered a mainstay of therapy. Urine alkalinization can be initiated with sodium bicarbonate at a dose of 1 to 2 mEq per kg per hour IV over a 1- to 2-hour period, until such time as the intoxication is resolving. Careful attention should be given to total fluid and sodium load administered, especially in patients at risk for congestive heart failure or pulmonary edema. Serum electrolytes need close monitoring; in particular, hypokalemia can interfere with the ability to achieve an alkaline urine pH and should be corrected. The rate of bicarbonate infusion can be adjusted to maintain a urinary pH of 7.5 to 8.5. Urinary acidification is never indicated because it may lead to serious side effects such as systemic acidosis and exacerbation of renal impairment in the context of myoglobinuria.

Multiple-Dose Activated Charcoal (GI Dialysis)

Several studies have shown significant increase in clearance for a number of drugs when repeated doses of 0.5 to 1 g per kg of activated charcoal are given every 4 to 6 hours. By using a nearly continuous stream of fresh charcoal that descends through the intestinal tract, a constant concentration gradient is maintained that favors the back diffusion of free drug from periluminal capillary blood into the intestinal lumen, where it may be bound immediately to the newer charcoal, so the free drug concentration in the intestinal lumen remains low. In addition, enterohepatic recirculation of some drugs may be interrupted as reabsorption from bile is prevented. To be safe and effective, this technique requires active peristalsis and an intact gag reflex or a protected airway. Common pediatric poisonings for which repetitive charcoal dosing may be considered include phenobarbital, carbamazepine, phenytoin, digoxin, salicylates, and theophylline. Cathartics, such as sorbitol, should be administered no more frequently than every third dose.

Renal Replacement Therapy

Renal replacement therapy is indicated for selected cases of severe poisoning to enhance toxin clearance and correct severe acid–base or electrolyte disturbances. High-flux hemodialysis is the modality of choice for expeditious toxin removal. Other methods such as exchange transfusion, plasmapheresis and peritoneal dialysis have little role and are much less effective in rapidly reversing the course of a given poisoning. Hemoperfusion, the process of passing blood through a dialysis circuit containing an adsorbent column, was historically used to remove higher–molecular-weight substances that could not be extracted through standard dialysis but has become obsolete since the arrival of newer "high-flux" dialysis membranes. Continuous renal replacement therapy, such as continuous venovenous hemodiafiltration (CVVHDF), also has much slower rates of toxin removal and should be reserved for the hemodynamically unstable patient who cannot tolerate conventional HD.

TABLE 110.11

A PARTIAL LISTING OF DRUGS AND THEIR PLASMA CONCENTRATIONS FOR WHICH HEMODIALYSIS SHOULD BE CONSIDERED

Lithium (acute), 4.0 mEq/L	Phenobarbital, 100 mg/L
Lithium (chronic), 2.5 mEq/L	Theophylline, 60–100 mg/L
Ethylene glycol, 50 mg/dL	Paraquat, 0.1 mg/dL
Methanol, 50 mg/dL	
Salicylates, 60 (chronic) to 80–90 (acute) mg/dL	

Adapted from Winchester JF. Active methods for detoxification. In: Hadded LM, Shannon MW, Winchester JF, eds. *Clinical management of poisoning and drug overdose,* 3rd ed. Philadelphia, PA: WB Saunders, 1998:175–187.

Acute extracorporeal removal should be considered in light of patient- and drug-related criteria. Patient-related criteria include (i) anticipated prolonged coma with the high likelihood of attendant complications, (ii) development of renal failure or impairment of normal excretory pathways, and (iii) progressive clinical deterioration despite careful medical supervision. Drug-related criteria are (i) serum concentrations in the potentially fatal range of a dialyzable substance, (ii) a correlation between serum drug concentration and toxicity, (iii) anticipated clinical benefit from faster toxin removal than what would be expected from endogenous clearance. Those xenobiotics with low volumes of distribution (less than 1 L per kg), low–molecular-weight (less than 500 Da), and low protein binding are the most amenable to enhanced clearance with dialysis. These characteristics typify the most commonly dialyzed toxicants: salicylic acid, methanol, ethylene glycol, lithium, and theophylline. Other conditions which may be amenable to extracorporeal removal or metabolic correction include poisoning by valproic acid, phenobarbital, methotrexate, and metformin-induced lactic acidosis. Table 110.11 summarizes the generally accepted common drugs and drug concentrations for which renal replacement therapy should be considered.

Risks include complications associated with central venous access, electrolyte disturbances, and hemodynamic instability. Of note, while typical dialysis patients are often hypervolemic, most poisoned dialysis patients are hypovolemic; it is incumbent upon the ED care provider to strive for euvolemia prior to hemodialysis. Very young infants in particular require extremely close attention to volume shifts. In rare neonatal cases, exchange transfusion may in fact be preferable for this reason. Nonetheless, the use of hemodialysis for other indications in pediatrics is somewhat commonplace, and in the hands of an experienced nephrologist can be safely performed. Extracorporal therapy should not be withheld even if it means transfer to another institution, as it may be essential in the critically ill poisoned child.

Supportive Care

The final step in optimizing treatment for the poisoned child is the direction of scrupulous attention to supportive care,

TABLE 110.12

PRODUCTS THAT ARE NONTOXIC WHEN INGESTED IN SMALL AMOUNTS

Abrasives	Hand lotions and creams
Adhesives	Hydrogen peroxide (medicinal 3%)
Antacids	Incense
Antibiotics	Indelible markers
Baby product cosmetics	Ink (black, blue)
Ballpoint pen inks	Laxatives
Bath oil	Lipstick
Bathtub floating toys	Lubricating oils
Bleach (household, less than 5% sodium hypochlorite)	Magic markers
Body conditioners	Matches
Bubble bath soaps	Mineral oil
Calamine lotion	Newspaper (black and white pages)
Candles (beeswax or paraffin)	Paint (indoor, latex)
Caps	Pencil (graphite)
Chalk	Perfumes
Cigarettes (less than three butts)	Petroleum jelly
Clay (modeling)	Phenolphthalein laxatives (Ex-Lax)
Colognes	Porous-tip marking pens
Contraceptive pills	Putty (less than 2 oz)
Corticosteroids	Rubber cement
Cosmetics	Shampoos (liquid)
Crayons (marked AP, CP)	Shaving creams and lotions
Dehumidifying packets (silica or charcoal)	Soap and soap products
Detergents (phosphate)	Suntan preparations
Deodorants	Sweetening agents (saccharin, cyclamates)
Deodorizers (spray and refrigerator)	Teething rings (water sterility)
Elmer Glue	Thermometers (mercury)
Etch-A-Sketch	Thyroid tablets
Eye makeup	Toothpaste
Fabric softener	Vitamins (without iron)
Fertilizer (if no insecticides or herbicides added)	Warfarin (rat poison; excludes "superwarfarins")
Glues and pastes	Watercolors
Grease	Zinc oxide (Desitin)
Hair products (dyes, sprays, tonics; excludes "relaxers")	Zirconium oxide

Adapted from Mofenson HC, Greensher J. The unknown poison. *Pediatrics* 1974;54:336.

including continued close monitoring of ABCDs, fluid and electrolyte status, urine output, and level of consciousness. The value of these efforts usually far outweighs that which may be ascribed to any specific toxicologic interventions in most cases. Severely symptomatic patients are most properly cared for in specialized facilities that have skilled pediatric critical care staff and access to toxicology consultation.

NONTOXIC INGESTION

Often, the emergency provider will be asked about a childhood ingestion of some common household products, many of which are nontoxic unless taken in huge amounts. The availability of a list of such nontoxic products often leads to immediate relief of parental anxiety and avoids the institution of unnecessary noxious interventions. Before using such a list, however, several precautions need to be kept in mind. The fact that an ingestion is nontoxic does not necessarily mean that it has no medical significance. Ingestions often occur in the context of a suboptimal environment. There may be poor supervision or unusual family stresses surrounding the incident, or the ingestion may not have been purely exploratory in nature. Several criteria have been suggested to qualify an ingestion as "nontoxic." These include the assurance that only one identifiable product is ingested in a well-approximated amount, that the product label includes no cautionary signal word, that the child is symptom free and younger than 5 years, and that an appropriate mechanism is available for telephone follow-up. When used with these criteria, Table 110.12 provides an updated list of nontoxic ingestions. In certain cases, consultation with a regional poison control center (in the United States, the phone number 1-800-222-1222 may be used nationwide) is often helpful.

PHARMACEUTICALS

Acetaminophen

Background

Acetaminophen, *N*-acetyl-*p*-aminophenol (APAP), is the most popular pediatric analgesic–antipyretic and has now become one of the most common pharmaceutical preparations ingested by young children. It is also one of the 10 most common drugs used by adolescents and adults in intentional self-poisoning. Acetaminophen also occasionally turns up as an unreported coingestant in intentional overdoses. Fortunately, exploratory ingestion in young children has been associated with low morbidity, although occasional cases of hepatotoxicity occur, particularly in the context of inadvertent repetitive overdosing.

Pathophysiology

The major toxicity of APAP is severe hepatic damage. Acetaminophen is metabolized in three ways by the liver: (i) Glucuronidation, (ii) sulfation, and (iii) metabolism through the cytochrome P-450 pathway to form a potentially toxic intermediate, which conjugates with glutathione. In a massive overdose, glutathione becomes depleted, thus allowing the undetoxified intermediate to bind to hepatocytes, leading to cellular necrosis. This damage is reflected by rising levels of liver enzymes, by hepatic dysfunction, and in severe poisonings, by hepatic failure and death. The use of *N*-acetylcysteine as an antidote relates in part to this molecule's ability to act as a glutathione precursor.

Clinical Findings

Initially, the signs and symptoms of APAP ingestion are vague and nonspecific but include nausea and vomiting, anorexia, pallor, and diaphoresis. These manifestations usually resolve within 12 to 24 hours, and the patient appears well for 1 to 4 days. During this latent period, levels of liver enzymes may rise, and jaundice with liver tenderness may ensue. Most patients have a gradual resolution of their hepatic dysfunction, although without antidotal treatment about 2% to 4% of intoxications that develop toxic plasma levels will go on to hepatic failure and death. Such patients with severe toxicity develop further clinical evidence of hepatic disease at 3 to 5 days after ingestion, and some develop renal damage. Anorexia, malaise, and abdominal pain may progress to signs of liver failure with hepatic coma.

The potential severity of an acute intoxication may be predicted by the amount ingested, if accurately known, and the plasma level of APAP. APAP in single doses of less than 200 mg per kg in young children is likely to be harmless. Severe toxicity in adolescents or adults usually occurs with overdoses of at least 7.5 to 10 g. Initial GI symptoms, although vague, are generally more pronounced when the overdose is large. However, the only reliable indication of the potential severity of the hepatic damage is the plasma APAP level, taken at least 4 hours after ingestion. After a single acute overdose at a known time of ingestion, a nomogram (Fig. 110.2) is available for using the serum APAP level in the prediction of likely toxicity. We recommend use of the lower line of the nomogram, plotted 25% below the possible toxicity line, to err on the safe side in making therapeutic decisions. Importantly, the nomogram is not validated for chronic APAP toxicity.

Management

The basic toxicologic principles of preventing absorption apply to APAP overdoses, and it is important to note that both immediate- and extended-release preparations exist. Activated charcoal therapy may be used for adsorption of gastric APAP. Many APAP-poisoned patients will benefit from the use of the oral antidote *N*-acetylcysteine (NAC), and some have speculated that activated charcoal might decrease the bioavailability of the NAC. However, studies have demonstrated clinically insignificant decreases in NAC absorption, even when using large doses of charcoal. For most cases of acetaminophen overdose per se, and particularly for those typically seen early after ingestion, charcoal alone is probably effective and should not significantly alter the ability to use NAC several hours later. In cases that present after 4 hours have elapsed, gastric decontamination is usually not warranted.

NAC, given orally or IV, is most effective at ameliorating hepatotoxicity when instituted within 8 hours of ingestion. It also lessens the severity of hepatic damage if used in the setting of clinical presentation beyond 8 hours. The major adverse reaction associated with IV NAC is the occurrence of anaphylactoid reaction, which typically occurs during the relatively higher dose loading infusion. Clinicians administering IV NAC should be skilled at recognizing and treating anaphylactoid reactions and should be particularly cautious when using this route in patients with a history of asthma. The inhalational form of NAC can be administered enterally and can be mixed with fruit juice or soda to disguise its foul smell, or it can be administered by NG tube. Only mild GI side effects result from its use, but persistent vomiting is an occasional obstacle to completing the course of therapy. This may be obviated by giving the dose slowly or by NG or duodenal tube infusion. Antiemetic therapy with metoclopramide or ondansetron may also be helpful.

The protocol for NAC therapy may be summarized as follows:

1. Consider GI decontamination options as already noted.
2. If patient presents less than 4 hours after a single acute ingestion, wait to draw 4-hour level and base therapeutic decision on nomogram (assumes rapid turnaround time so level will be available by 6 hours after ingestion); if necessary, initiate treatment as described next. For extended-release preparations, McNeil Consumer Products Co. (Fort Washington, Pennsylvania), a manufacturer of acetaminophen, suggests a second APAP level drawn 4 hours after the first; antidotal therapy is to be instituted if either level suggests possible toxicity.
3. If patient presents more than 6 to 8 hours after ingestion, initiate NAC therapy, obtain level, and base subsequent course of therapy on nomogram.
4. If level plots out above the lower line on the nomogram, admit the patient to hospital and continue NAC until APAP is not detectable in the blood and liver function is either normal or clearly recovering. Monitor complete blood cell count (CBC) and renal and liver function tests.
5. Treatment for patients who present more than 24 hours after ingestion is controversial, as is treatment for patients with subacute, repetitive overdosing over several days. We consider children who receive more than 150 mg per kg per day for 1 to 2 days to be at risk; again, a combination of a nondetectable APAP level and normal aminotransferases identifies a patient at low risk of hepatic injury from APAP.

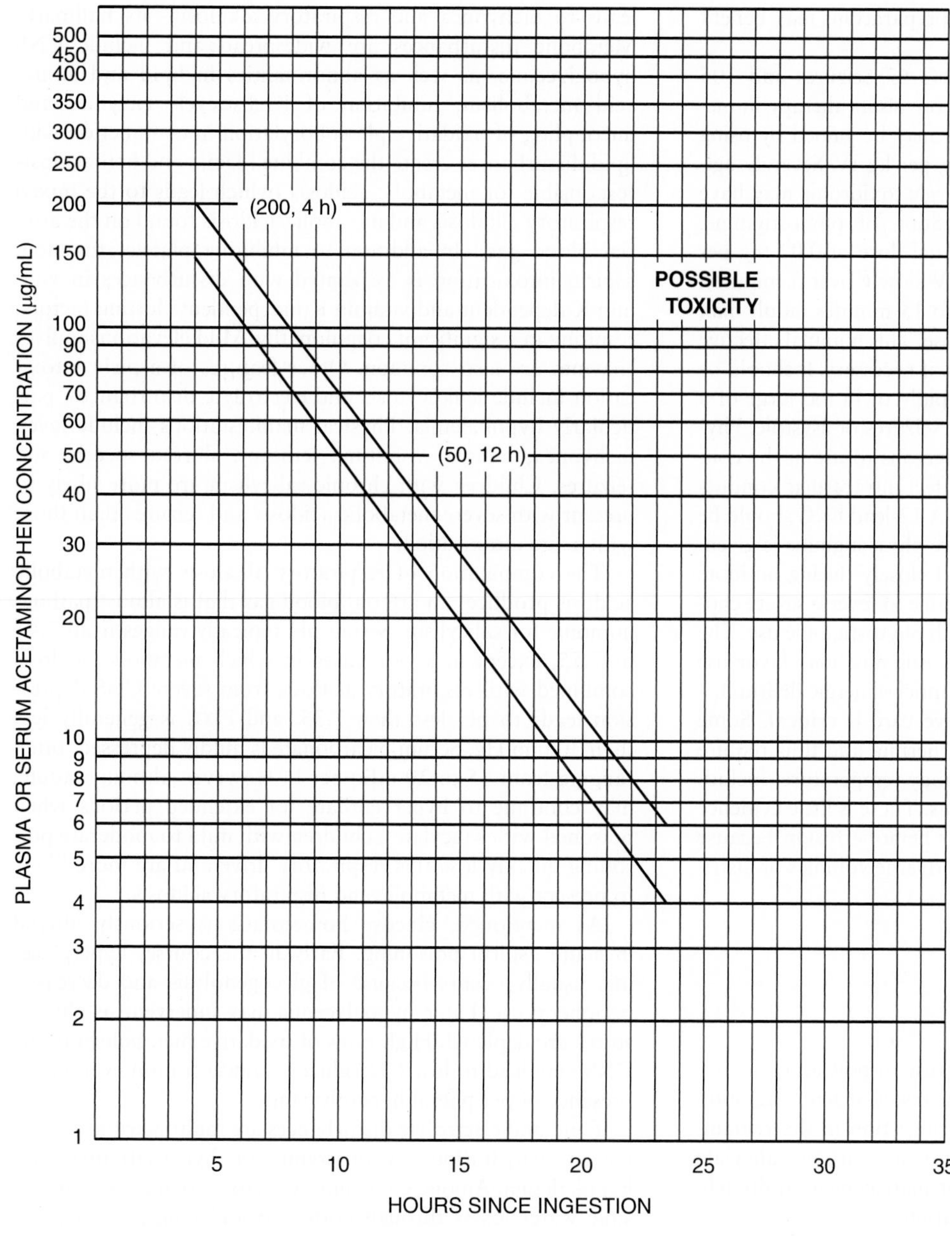

FIGURE 110.2 Nomogram for estimating severity of acute acetaminophen poisoning. (Modified from Rumack BH, Matthew H. *Pediatrics*. 1975;55:871–876. Copyright 1975, American Academy of Pediatrics. Reprinted by permission.)

Antihistamines

Antihistamines are used to treat children with allergic diseases, as sedatives and antinauseants, and to prevent motion sickness. They are present in many cough syrups, available both over the counter (OTC) and by prescription. Antihistamines may also be found in combination with analgesics, sympathomimetic amines, and caffeine for the symptomatic relief of the common cold. They are combined with analgesics, such as salicylamide, and an anticholinergic drug, such as scopolamine, for use as a nonprescription sleep medication. Finally, they are included in some liquid cough and cold preparations that may also contain ethanol as the solvent.

Antihistamines may depress or stimulate the CNS. Used therapeutically, CNS depression is most commonly seen as drowsiness or dizziness. With increasing doses, stimulation results in insomnia, nervousness, and restlessness. In antihistamine overdose, the CNS stimulatory effects of the drug predominate. In children, CNS stimulation causes excitement, tremors, hyperactivity, hallucinations, and with higher dosages, tonic–clonic convulsions. Children are also more likely to have signs and symptoms of anticholinergic poisoning: flushed skin, fever, tachycardia, and fixed dilated pupils. The nonsedating antihistamines terfenadine and astemizole (both no longer available in the United States) have caused cardiac arrhythmia after overdose and as a result of drug–drug interactions. Cetirizine, loratadine, and fexofenadine have not produced this complication. Death from antihistamine ingestion in children is usually the result of uncontrolled seizures that progress to coma and cardiorespiratory arrest.

The treatment of antihistamine poisoning requires an accurate history of the time of ingestion and the type and quantity of drug consumed. Of particular importance is the type of drug ingested because numerous sustained-release antihistamine products are available on the market. Options for GI decontamination include the use of activated charcoal, and overdoses with the sustained-release preparations may benefit from WBI.

Patients with seizures (see Chapters 67 Seizures and 105 Neurologic Emergencies) require anticonvulsant therapy immediately. Preferably, short-term control may be gained by using diazepam, in a dose of 0.1 to 0.2 mg per kg IV. Severely agitated patients with a clear anticholinergic toxidrome may have improved sensorium after administration of physostigmine. This is usually administered in an initial dose of 0.02 mg per kg (not to exceed 0.5 mg per dose) IV slowly over 3 minutes. The dose may be repeated every 10 to 15 minutes (adult max 2 mg) to establish the effective total dose. This minimal effective dose may be repeated in several hours, if necessary. It should be noted that when administered too rapidly or in too large of a dose, physostigmine might precipitate seizures or asystole. Physostigmine would be particularly dangerous to use in the context of any coingestants that might affect intracardiac conduction, such as tricyclic antidepressants. A 12-lead EKG should be examined for conduction delays before physostigmine is given. Cardiac rhythm should be monitored closely during antidote infusion, and atropine should be available to reverse severe cholinergic effects that may also occur with physostigmine use. The potential risks encountered with physostigmine may favor use of a benzodiazepine for treatment of anticholinergic delirium.

Meticulous attention to supportive care is critical. Some patients may develop extreme hyperthermia and thus require aggressive measures to reduce core body temperature, including ice water baths or misting and fans. There is little evidence for therapeutic efficacy of dialysis or hemoperfusion because of the high plasma protein binding and large volumes of distribution for most of these agents.

Aspirin

Background

Aspirin continues to be a common cause of poisoning in children and adolescents. Salicylism is the result of acute ingestion in about 60% of cases and chronic ingestion in the remaining 40%. Clinical features of acute versus chronic salicylate intoxication often require a different management approach, depending on the manner of intoxication.

Several factors work in concert to make chronic salicylate intoxication so common. The primary factor is aspirin's elimination pattern. As serum salicylate concentrations increase, the ability of the liver to metabolize the drug diminishes until predictable, first-order elimination kinetics are replaced by unpredictable, dose-dependent, zero-order elimination. Thereafter, increments in dose are associated with disproportionate increases in serum salicylate concentration. Also, much of aspirin elimination is through urinary excretion of unchanged drug. Therefore, in the face of dehydration and decreased glomerular filtration, drug clearance is impaired even more. Finally, because aspirin is often prescribed for illnesses that may be associated with hepatic dysfunction, reduced biotransformation initiates the spiraling increase in serum concentration. Unfortunately, because chronic salicylism is associated with nonspecific symptoms (e.g., fever, vomiting, tachypnea), diagnosis may be delayed until more striking signs of intoxication appear.

Pathophysiology

The direct effects of aspirin on metabolism are multiple. Aspirin stimulates the medullary respiratory center, which leads to tachypnea and respiratory alkalosis—its hallmark. Metabolic disturbances are widespread and include CNS hypoglycemia, as well as abnormalities in lipid and amino acid metabolism. Inhibition of Krebs cycle enzymes and uncoupling of oxidative phosphorylation in conjunction with lipid disturbances create the combined lactic and ketoacidosis responsible for metabolic acidosis (which leads to the mixed respiratory alkalosis and metabolic acidosis found on the arterial blood gas). In addition to inhibiting platelet function, aspirin intoxication is associated with disturbances in vitamin K-dependent and vitamin K-independent clotting factors, resulting in a significant coagulopathy. Mild elevations in liver enzymes are also common. Other features of aspirin intoxication include leukocytosis and electrolyte disturbances, particularly hypokalemia. Physical manifestations include fever, tachypnea, nausea, vomiting, lethargy, slurred speech, and seizures. Children with chronic salicylism are more likely to present with severe metabolic acidosis and seizures than those with acute intoxication.

The combination of respiratory alkalosis with metabolic acidosis produces an arterial blood gas that is almost pathognomonic for salicylism. Serum pH typically ranges from 7.41 to 7.55, except in severe cases in which metabolic acidosis combined with respiratory acidosis from severe CNS depression leads to pH less than 7.35, and P_{CO_2} is generally less than 30 mm Hg. Serum bicarbonate is mildly depressed, often ranging from 15 to 20 mEq per L. However, although adults may continue to hyperventilate for extended periods when poisoned with salicylates, children with mild to moderate poisoning quickly lose this respiratory drive and are more likely to present with metabolic and respiratory acidosis.

As mentioned, glucose homeostasis is seriously altered in acute aspirin poisoning. Early in the course, hyperglycemia usually occurs because of glycogenolysis and decreased peripheral use. Later, hypoglycemia may supervene as glucose stores are depleted. High rates of oxidative metabolism in the CNS may lead to low CNS glucose concentration even in the presence of peripheral hyperglycemia.

Fluid and electrolyte disturbances are multifactorial, resulting in dehydration, hyponatremia or hypernatremia, and hypokalemia. Among contributing factors are increased insensible water losses through both skin and lungs, emesis, and increased renal water and potassium loss. The patient with severe salicylate poisoning may lose 4 to 6 L of water per square meter.

Clinical Findings

The initial clinical signs and symptoms, the estimate of dose ingested, and the measurement of salicylate levels all serve to gauge the severity of a given acute aspirin poisoning. However, in cases of chronic therapeutic salicylism, the clinical picture is the most useful guideline. Because of the nonspecific nature of symptoms with salicylism, the initial differential diagnosis is broad and may include diabetic ketoacidosis, iron intoxication, and ethylene glycol ingestion.

Signs and symptoms of salicylism depend on the method and severity of intoxication. Acute ingestion of amounts of 150 to 300 mg per kg are associated with mild symptoms, 300 to 500 mg per kg are associated with moderate toxicity, and more than 500 mg per kg are associated with death. With mild toxicity (serum concentrations 30 to 50 mg per dL), manifestations may be confined to GI upset, tinnitus, and mild tachypnea. With moderate salicylate poisoning (serum level 50 to

100 mg per dL), more visible signs of toxicity—fever, diaphoresis, and agitation—appear. After severe salicylate poisoning (serum concentrations higher than 100 mg per dL), signs and symptoms are primarily neurologic and consist of dysarthria, coma, and seizures. Pulmonary manifestations, particularly pulmonary edema, may appear in severe cases. In patients of chronic salicylism, these same conditions appear at significantly lower serum salicylate concentrations. Death from salicylism results from severe CNS toxicity with complete loss of function in cardiorespiratory centers, leading to respiratory and/or cardiac arrest. The severity of salicylate intoxication is best assessed by physical examination, electrolytes, and blood gas level analyses rather than through use of a nomogram.

Management

Assessment of the patient of salicylate intoxication begins with an accurate history that identifies the patient as having acute or chronic poisoning. Laboratory assessment is extensive and includes serum salicylate concentration, electrolytes and arterial blood gas levels, liver function tests, CBCs, prothrombin and partial thromboplastin times, urinalysis, and an EKG. In the case of intentional ingestions by adolescents, attention to a serum acetaminophen measurement is important (because many OTC analgesics contain aspirin and acetaminophen in combination).

Supportive care includes assessment of ventilatory function, cardiac monitoring, and vascular access. Because aspirin overdose is associated with delayed gastric emptying and drug coalescence to form bezoars, GI decontamination should receive careful consideration in those patients who present within 4 to 6 hours of ingestion. In patients who present more than 6 hours after ingestion or in those with chronic salicylism, activated charcoal might still be administered because it may enhance postabsorptive elimination of salicylates (through GI dialysis).

Healthcare providers are cautioned to be wary of sedating or mechanically ventilating aspirin-poisoned patients, as depressing the spontaneous ventilation rate may worsen aspirin-induced neurotoxicity. Specific therapeutic goals in salicylate intoxication include correction of fluid and electrolyte disturbances and the enhancement of salicylate excretion.

Fluid therapy should be aimed at restoring hydration and electrolyte balance, preventing distribution of salicylate to the brain, and promoting renal salicylate excretion. Aggressive restoration of intravascular volume is advisable; however, fluids should be given prudently to prevent precipitation of pulmonary edema, particularly in patients with severe intoxication. The blood pH should be kept alkaline, pH 7.45 to 7.5. For patients with symptomatic salicylate intoxication, urine alkalinization should be combined with fluid resuscitation. The administration of sodium bicarbonate, by increasing urinary pH, ionizes filtered aspirin, increasing tubular secretion and inhibiting its tubular reabsorption (ion trapping). The initial fluid is, therefore, designed to replace both sodium and bicarbonate losses as well as promote urine alkalinization. It should contain 5% dextrose with 100 to 150 mEq per L of sodium bicarbonate. Because hypokalemia impairs the ability of the kidney to create alkaline urine and is exacerbated by administration of sodium bicarbonate, potassium must be added to IV fluids. Forced diuresis should not be used as it does not enhance salicylate excretion more than the clearance accomplished by alkalinization alone. Therefore, fluids are given as needed to restore normal hydration and to produce 1 to 2 mL per kg per hour of urine. Calcium homeostasis should also be monitored during therapy with exogenous bicarbonate. Both urine alkalinization and repetitive oral charcoal (up to every 4 hours) should be continued until salicylate concentration falls below 30 mg per dL and symptoms resolve.

Salicylate elimination can also be enhanced by hemodialysis or hemoperfusion. Although hemoperfusion results in superior clearance technique, hemodialysis is usually preferred because it permits correction of fluid and electrolyte imbalances. Hemodialysis should be reserved for seriously ill patients. Hemodialysis might be considered for patients with serum salicylate levels higher than 100 mg per dL after acute ingestion or 60 mg per dL or higher after chronic salicylism. Specific indications for hemodialysis include (i) severe acidosis or other electrolyte disturbance, (ii) renal failure, (iii) persistent neurologic dysfunction, (iv) pulmonary edema, and/or (v) progressive clinical deterioration despite standard treatment.

Cardiac Drugs

β-Adrenergic Blockers and Calcium Channel Blockers

The approaches to overdoses of these two categories of cardiovascular agents are discussed together because of similarities of clinical presentation and management approach. They both are commonly prescribed to adult patients with a variety of cardiovascular disorders, including angina and past myocardial infarction, hypertension, and arrhythmias. As such, experience with pediatric overdoses has been increasing in more recent years.

BBs vary considerably in terms of receptor specificity and pharmacokinetics, but most overdose experience is with propranolol. Similarly, the calcium channel blockers (CCBs) most commonly used in the United States (verapamil, diltiazem, nifedipine, amlodipine, etc.) are chemically dissimilar and have varied degrees of effect on vasodilation, myocardial contractility, and sinoatrial (SA)-atrioventricular (AV) node function.

Both BBs and CCBs may present with fulminant cardiovascular and neurologic findings after a large overdose. Typical presentations of both agents include marked bradycardia and hypotension; particularly with the CCBs, common additional findings are those of abnormal AV node conduction, with AV block or accelerated junctional rhythm. The CNS may also be affected, with coma and/or convulsions that occur in either category of overdoses. Metabolic disturbances include hypoglycemia with BBs and hyperglycemia and metabolic acidosis with CCBs. Bronchospasm may further complicate BB toxicity in patients with underlying reactive airway disease.

Management begins with aggressive gastric decontamination for both types of agents. Activated charcoal/cathartic should be administered to patients presenting soon after ingestion. Sustained-release preparations may cause prolonged effects, and WBI may be considered in this context. Bradycardia and hypotension may improve with standard treatment such as atropine, fluid boluses, and direct-acting vasopressors such as norepinephrine; however, many cases prove resistant to these measures.

Additional therapy includes calcium infusion for the CCBs, with the recommended adult initial dose being 10 mL of 10% calcium chloride or 30 mL of 10% calcium gluconate, which may be repeated two or three times as necessary (e.g., an initial pediatric dose of approximately 0.2 mL per kg calcium chloride or 0.6 mL per kg of calcium gluconate). Serum calcium, as well as the ionized calcium, should be monitored. Glucagon increases intracellular cyclic adenosine monophosphate (cAMP) by a mechanism independent of β receptors and has been used with success to improve heart rate and blood pressure in overdoses of BB agents. The usual adult dosing regimen is 3 to 5 mg by IV bolus, which may be repeated to a total dose of 10 mg, followed by infusion at 2 to 5 mg per hour. Such dosing translates to 50 to 150 μg per kg boluses and similar amounts per hour for pediatric patients.

For hemodynamically significant overdose of a CCB, hyperinsulinemia–euglycemia therapy is recommended; this therapy should be guided by a clinician or poison control center consultant familiar with its use. Bolus dosing of 1 unit per kg IV of regular insulin is then followed by an infusion at 0.5 units to 1 unit per kg with titration performed based on hemodynamics. Blood sugars are carefully monitored. Lipid emulsion infusion has shown promise in animal studies of verapamil toxicity as well as case reports; it is typically given if conventional therapies, including insulin are refractory or if the patient has a cardiac arrest. Severe cases may also benefit from pacemaker insertion and consideration of aortic balloon pump and/or cardiopulmonary bypass. It is unlikely that hemodialysis or hemoperfusion would benefit most of these cases.

Clonidine

Clonidine is an antihypertensive that appears to have growing popularity, part of which comes from its efficacy in illnesses other than hypertension, including opioid withdrawal and attention deficit disorder. Also, the advent of clonidine in transdermal patches has become a convenient and somewhat unique vehicle for drug administration.

Clonidine exerts its antihypertensive effect through stimulation of CNS α_2-adrenergic receptors. These receptors are located on presynaptic neurons in cardiorespiratory centers of the midbrain. Their stimulation results in decreased secretion of catecholamines into the synaptic cleft, resulting in decreased pulse and blood pressure. In addition, clonidine appears to interact with or modulate CNS opiate receptors; this interaction has been used to explain clonidine's efficacy in opiate withdrawal and the picture of coma and miosis that accompanies clonidine intoxication. An imidazoline compound, clonidine is related to other medications, including tetrahydrozoline and oxymetazoline—common vasoconstrictors found in nasal decongestants and ophthalmic agents. Brimonidine drops may be used in an ophthalmology setting and guanfacine is used also for attention deficit disorder.

Clonidine is an extremely potent drug with typical doses of 100 to 200 μg in adults. Therefore, ingestions of small amounts can potentially lead to significant toxicity in children. Initial toxic manifestations include altered mental status that may range from lethargy to coma. Patients may also develop hypothermia. In severe intoxications, coma, miosis, and respiratory depression may appear. The cardiovascular changes that accompany clonidine intoxications may range from an initial transient period of hypertension (often resolved prior to arrival in the ED) to profound hypotension and bradycardia. Clonidine-induced hypertension is believed to result from α-adrenergic effects at peripheral vascular receptors prior to the central, antihypertensive effect. The clinical picture of clonidine intoxication typically lasts 8 to 24 hours.

Management

The treatment of clonidine intoxication requires immediate assessment of the ABCs. Because patients with severe intoxication often have coma and respiratory depression, emergency endotracheal intubation may be necessary. Also, because of blood pressure instability, vascular access should be achieved immediately for better hemodynamic control. Hypotension should be treated with fluids and vasopressors as needed. Hypertension is generally uncommon, is very transient, and would rarely require specific treatment.

Activated charcoal binds clonidine. In addition to supportive care measures, other pharmacologic interventions may be effective. Naloxone has been suggested as a specific antidotal agent after clonidine intoxication, based on case reports of improved mental status and cardiorespiratory function after its administration. However, in reported case series, there have not been consistent improvements after naloxone administration.

Because naloxone is a benign agent in an opioid naïve child and may potentially improve mental status to the extent that intubation becomes unnecessary, a trial dose of 0.1 to 0.2 mg per kg should be administered. Large amounts of naloxone (up to 8 mg) must be provided before it can be concluded that the intoxication is not responsive to this therapy. If effective, repeat doses or a continuous infusion of naloxone may be useful. Other pharmacologic agents that have been used in the past include yohimbine, tolazoline, and phentolamine; but specific efficacy from these agents has not been demonstrated, and they are not considered important in the treatment of clonidine intoxication.

Digoxin

Digoxin is still widely used in young infants with congenital heart disease and elderly patients with congestive heart failure. This medication's continued popularity, its narrow therapeutic index, and the appealing color of digoxin elixir make it a source of many childhood poisoning episodes annually. Also, related agents, particularly the foxglove and oleander plants, are occasionally ingested by children, leading to a clinical picture identical to that of digoxin.

Digoxin's primary pharmacologic action is to inhibit activity of sodium–potassium adenosine triphosphatase (ATPase), which is responsible for maintaining the electrical potential of excitable tissues through transmembrane concentration of electrolytes. Therefore, the effects of digoxin are largely related to disturbances in this action.

In all patients of digoxin poisoning, two distinct pictures of toxicity exist: acute and chronic. These pictures have several differences: the patient of acute digoxin ingestion is typically a toddler who ingests a relative's medication. The toddler is generally healthy with no underlying cardiac disease. The child with chronic digoxin poisoning, however, by definition has preexisting heart disease and is likely to be taking other medications known to modulate the effects of digoxin poisoning (e.g., diuretics). Therefore, it is the latter patient who is more likely to have severe toxic manifestations after digoxin intoxication.

Digoxin pharmacokinetics are complex. After ingestion, absorption is complete within 2 to 4 hours. However, after peak serum levels are achieved, the drug is rapidly redistributed, resulting in dramatic falls in serum concentration. This principle has particular importance with the patient of acute digoxin intoxication who may have an initial serum digoxin concentration (SDC) in the highly toxic range that falls to the therapeutic range within a matter of hours. After redistribution, digoxin elimination occurs primarily through renal excretion of unchanged drug. Therefore, any condition associated with decreased renal function may be associated with the insidious development of intoxication.

The therapeutic SDC is less than 2 ng per mL. A concentration in the slightly higher range often does not correlate with clinical manifestations and may be of limited value. However, when SDC exceeds 4 ng per mL, some evidence of intoxication usually appears. This toxicity is influenced by many host factors, including patient age; underlying illness; and disturbances in serum potassium, magnesium, and calcium.

With significant intoxication, the symptoms of digoxin poisoning include nausea, vomiting, and visual disturbances. With more severe intoxication, additional symptoms, including lethargy, disorientation, electrolyte disturbances, and cardiac disturbances, appear. The hallmark of severe acute digoxin toxicity is hyperkalemia, the result of profound inhibition of sodium–potassium ATPase activity. The typical pattern of cardiac toxicity with digoxin overdose initially is prolonged AV dissociation that appears as heart block that ranges from first to third degree. These conduction disturbances can lead to the development of ventricular or supraventricular escape rhythms. In patients with chronic digoxin intoxication, these symptoms may be more striking than in those with acute, single digoxin overdoses. In fact, children with acute digoxin intoxication rarely develop life-threatening illness if their peak SDC remains below 10 ng per mL.

Management

The management of the patient with digoxin intoxication begins with evaluation of the vital signs, particularly hemodynamic status. Patients should have an EKG performed, followed by continuous cardiac monitoring. If significant cardiac arrhythmias are already present, they are treated initially according to advanced cardiac life support protocols.

GI decontamination should include administration of activated charcoal. Clinical assessment typically includes an EKG, electrolytes (including magnesium and calcium) level, urinalysis, and SDC. Electrolyte disturbances should be treated aggressively because they will aggravate any digoxin-induced arrhythmias.

Digoxin-specific antibody fragments have become specific antidotal therapy for reversing the toxic manifestations. These fragments are the result of sheep-derived immunoglobulin that is cleaved to extract only the Fab fragment. This low–molecular-weight antibody fragment is capable of avidly binding free digoxin so a gradient results that favors digoxin removal from receptor sites into interstitial water. The effect of this gradient is that sodium–potassium ATPase function is immediately restored. The digoxin–antibody complex is then rapidly excreted in the urine. Of note, after digoxin-antibody fragments are administered, SDC increases astronomically, reflecting bound, inactive digoxin that has diffused into the vascular compartment.

These antibody fragments are indicated in the following circumstances after digoxin poisoning: (i) Progressive signs and symptoms of intoxication, (ii) life-threatening cardiac arrhythmias, or (iii) severe hyperkalemia (defined as a serum potassium level of 5.5 mEq per L or higher). The dose of antibody fragments is calculated on the basis of ingested digoxin dose (in the case of acute intoxication) or on the basis of SDC (in the case of chronic intoxication). Each 40-mg vial of digoxin-Fab will bind 0.6 mg of digoxin. The total dose of Fab needed (in vials) may be estimated by dividing a known ingested dose by 0.6, or calculated for the steady-state context as body load of digoxin:

$$\text{No. of vials} = \frac{\text{SDC (ng/mL)} \times \text{wt (in kg)}}{100}$$

Complications from the administration of antibody fragments are low and consist of an allergic reaction (in approximately 0.6% of patients), precipitation of congestive heart failure (secondary to the abrupt loss of digoxin's inotropic action), and rebound hypokalemia. These complications should be anticipated and treated accordingly. Infusions should be given over 30 minutes, and some prefer to use a 0.22 μm in-line filter. If the patient is in cardiac arrest, the antibody fragments may be infused over 5 minutes.

Iron

Background

In the 1990s, iron poisoning was one of the most common, potentially fatal intoxications in children. Most serious childhood poisonings result from ingestion of prenatal vitamins or ferrous sulfate tablets (which unfortunately often look much like candy) that were intended for adults. A common scenario is that the patient is a toddler whose mother has just had a new baby; the increased demands on the mother's attention and almost universal prescription of iron to postpartum women combine to set the stage for this ingestion. In addition, numerous exposures result from ingestion of iron-fortified children's vitamins, but these tend to be far less toxic.

Sufficient data to define a safe lower limit for toxic iron ingestions are not available. As little as 20 mg per kg of elemental iron has caused GI toxicity, whereas ingestions of more than 40 mg per kg often produce moderate toxic effects with profound toxicity seen after doses of 60 mg per kg. Of course, it is often impossible to know the exact number of tablets ingested. As few as ten 300-mg $FeSO_4$ tablets have been fatal to a young child. Furthermore, the elemental iron content of whole bottles of chewable vitamins is usually about 1,200 mg. Industry standards typically lead to the use of child resistant caps for vitamin bottles that contain more than 250 mg of elemental iron. Unit dose (blister) packaging has been advised for pills with high iron content. These measures have led to a dramatic reduction in deaths due to exploratory iron poisoning.

Pathophysiology

Iron toxicity results from direct caustic effect on the GI mucosa and the presence of free iron in the circulation. Pathologic changes include hemorrhagic necrosis of stomach and intestinal mucosa and lesions in the liver that range from cloudy swelling to areas of complete necrosis. Occasionally, pulmonary congestion and hemorrhage are noted. Excess free iron is believed to act as a mitochondrial poison, particularly in the liver, with resulting changes in cellular energy metabolism and the production of metabolic acidosis.

Clinical Manifestations

The clinical effects of iron poisoning are classically divided into four phases. Phase I represents the effects of direct mucosal injury and usually lasts 6 hours. Vomiting, diarrhea, and GI blood loss are the prominent early signs; when severe, the patient may lapse into early coma and shock caused by volume loss and metabolic acidosis.

Phase II, which lasts from 6 to 24 hours after ingestion, is marked by diminution of the GI symptoms. With appropriate therapy to replace fluid and/or blood losses, the child may seem relatively well and often goes on to full recovery without any subsequent symptoms. However, this remission may be transient and may be followed by phase III, characterized by metabolic acidosis, coma, seizures, and intractable shock. This phase is believed to represent hepatocellular injury with consequent disturbed energy metabolism; elevated levels of lactic and citric acids are noted in experimental iron poisoning before cardiac or respiratory failure occurs. Jaundice and elevated transaminases are noted in this phase. A phase IV has been described in survivors of severe iron poisoning, marked by pyloric stenosis that results from scarring and consequent obstruction.

Laboratory abnormalities often associated with severe iron intoxication include metabolic acidosis, leukocytosis, hyperglycemia, hyperbilirubinemia and increased liver enzymes, and a prolonged prothrombin time. If fluid loss is significant, there will be hemoconcentration and elevated BUN. Abdominal films may show radiopaque material in the stomach, but the absence of this finding does not indicate a trivial ingestion.

Management

All children alleged to have ingested iron are potentially at significant risk for life-threatening illness. However, severe iron poisoning is uncommon compared with the number of children who develop only mild symptoms or remain entirely asymptomatic. Thus, the emergency physician needs an approach that encompasses the response to the severely poisoned child and to most who will remain well.

As noted earlier, the amount of iron ingested is often hard to quantify, and minimal "safe" amounts are not well established. Serum iron levels have been shown to correlate with the likelihood of developing symptoms (usually a reflection of the serum iron that exceeds the iron-binding capacity and results in free-circulating iron). Usually, when drawn 3 to 5 hours after ingestion, iron levels lower than 350 μg per dL predict an asymptomatic course. Patients with levels in the 350 to 500 μg per dL range often show mild phase I symptoms but rarely develop serious complications. Levels higher than 500 μg per dL suggest significant risk for phase III manifestations. However, the serum iron determination is not always available on a stat basis.

Although serum iron levels are useful, toxicity from iron overdose remains a clinical diagnosis. Ill patients require vigorous hydration and support. Children who are completely asymptomatic 6 hours after ingestion are unlikely to develop systemic illness. Among laboratory studies, the presence of metabolic acidosis or acidemia probably best correlates with toxicity. Radiopaque material on abdominal radiograph also suggests potential for significant absorption of iron (Fig. 110.3). Measurement of the total iron-binding capacity is no longer believed to be useful in acute management. With these observations in mind, it is possible to construct a protocol for the triage and initial management of the patient who has ingested a possibly toxic amount of iron (Fig. 110.4).

Categorization

Patients who arrive with severe early symptoms, including vomiting, diarrhea, GI bleeding, depressed sensorium, or circulatory compromise merit urgent, intensive treatment in the ED. The first priority is to obtain venous access.

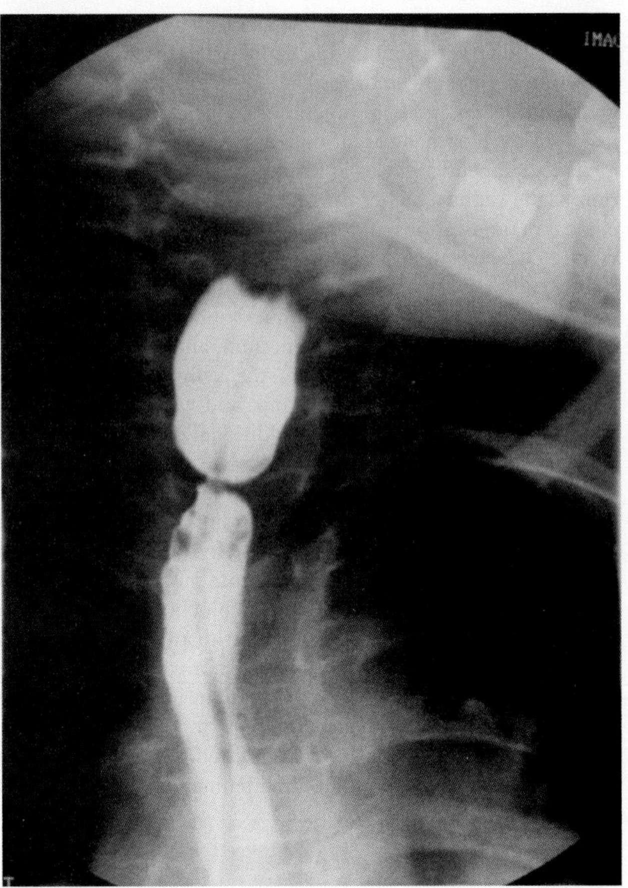

FIGURE 110.3 Intestinal iron pills evident upon abdominal radiography.

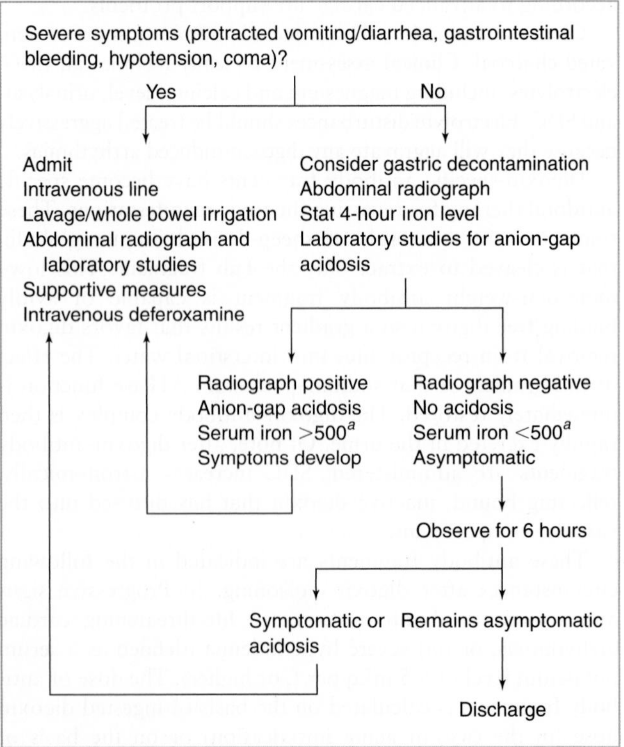

FIGURE 110.4 The initial approach to the patient ingesting a possibly toxic dose of iron. [a]Iron levels expressed in μg per dL.

Simultaneously, blood is drawn for CBC, blood glucose, electrolytes, BUN, liver function tests, serum iron, and type and cross-match analyses. GI decontamination is begun as detailed in the following section. Blood pressure should be supported with normal saline. Specific chelation therapy with IV deferoxamine is begun immediately in all severely poisoned patients. An abdominal radiograph should be obtained as soon as possible after GI decontamination to determine its efficacy and to investigate for the presence of iron pill concretions.

Patients with only mild vomiting and diarrhea in the early postingestion period still need urgent treatment but usually do well. Again, GI decontamination strategies should be promptly addressed with WBI being the preferred method. Blood studies, as previously noted, are drawn, and parenteral deferoxamine therapy is begun.

If serum iron levels are available, blood should be sent for this study, an abdominal radiograph should be obtained, and the patient should be observed for 6 hours. An iron level of less than 350 µg per dL taken 3 to 5 hours after ingestion in an asymptomatic patient with a normal radiograph suggests that the patient is at minimal risk and may be discharged. Iron levels higher than 500 µg per dL, the development of any symptoms, or a positive radiograph should lead to admission and management as previously described for the mild to moderately ill patient.

When serum iron levels are not available on an emergency basis, clinical decisions must be made based on symptoms, electrolytes, and abdominal radiography. Patients are observed for 6 hours in the ED. Those who have normal screening tests and remain asymptomatic may be discharged. Patients with abnormal screening laboratory tests should have an iron level sent for later reference. Acidotic or symptomatic patients should be admitted and treated with deferoxamine. Patients asymptomatic after 6 hours may be discharged.

Treatment

The treatment for acute iron poisoning includes efforts to decrease absorption and hasten excretion, as well as appropriate supportive care.

Most children with toxic iron exposures will exhibit spontaneous vomiting. Activated charcoal is not effective in binding iron salts. For serious poisonings, gastric lavage with normal saline can be considered in patients who present early after liquid iron ingestion, in the hope of minimizing any direct mucosal injury caused by residual particulate matter and possibly contributing to the dissolution of pill concretions.

The mainstay of GI decontamination currently for iron-poisoned patients, however, is the early and aggressive use of WBI. This approach is believed to be effective in decreasing iron absorption and in breaking up pill concretions that might be a risk for direct mucosal injury. As noted previously, an abdominal radiograph should be obtained early in the evaluation of symptomatic patients. If this study demonstrates significant radiopaque material and the patient's condition allows it, WBI should be instituted for at least 4 to 6 hours. A few hours of WBI (until rectal effluent is clear) may be indicated in symptomatic cases even without definite radiographic findings to hasten elimination of residual iron pill particles or "sludge," as long as there is no evidence of peritonitis or perforation. In patients with considerable initial radiographic findings, particularly pill concretions, a follow-up radiograph should be obtained to assess the adequacy of bowel cleansing. Further options of gastroscopy or even gastrotomy are reserved as last resorts to effect iron pill removal. Large clumps of coalesced iron tablets in the stomach or duodenum have led to severe hemorrhagic infarction of these viscera with subsequent perforation, peritonitis, and death. As previously noted, even in such patients who survive the acute phase, there is considerable risk of subsequent pyloric or bowel stenosis with obstruction, usually 4 to 6 weeks after ingestion. In this regard, we also urge early pediatric surgical consultation for patients in the first few days after ingestion who show any evidence of peritoneal irritation.

Chelation therapy with parenteral deferoxamine enhances the excretion of iron as the feroxamine complex, which turns urine an orange or *vin rose* tint. The most efficacious route is a continuous IV infusion, and the maximum recommended dose is 15 mg per kg per hour (maximum daily dose 360 mg per kg, up to 6 g total). A higher infusion rate has been associated with hypotension but may be necessary (in conjunction with blood pressure support) for severe ingestions. Chelation is continued until the serum iron level returns to normal, metabolic acidosis has resolved, the patient is clinically improved, and the urine color returns to normal. The dose of deferoxamine may be titrated down in concert with the patient's clinical response and fall in iron levels. Of note, deferoxamine is considered to be a siderophore that promotes the growth of certain bacteria such as *Yersinia enterocolitica;* therefore, monitoring for *Yersinia* sepsis is important.

Once the patient has been stabilized initially, further problems may include hypotension, profound metabolic acidosis, hypoglycemia or hyperglycemia, anemia, and colloid loss caused by GI hemorrhage (after equilibration), renal shutdown resulting from shock, and hepatic failure with an associated bleeding diathesis. The maintenance of an adequate urine output is critical to prevent renal failure and to foster excretion of the feroxamine complex. If renal failure supervenes, chelation may be continued with concurrent dialysis because the complex is dialyzable.

Isoniazid

INH is an important treatment for tuberculosis. Even when taken appropriately, INH has many actions that can lead to clinical toxicity. These include hepatic dysfunction and interactions with foods such as those containing tyramine. However, its greatest toxicity appears after acute single ingestions of more than 20 mg per kg in children or more than 1.5 g in an adult.

INH's mechanism of toxicity involves its potent effect at reversing the biologic activity of vitamin B_6 (pyridoxine). This action, as well as other effects on the synthesis of catecholamines and the neurotransmitter GABA, provides an explanation for the epileptogenic toxicity of the drug. INH also prevents hepatic conversion of lactate to pyruvate.

In overdose, the hallmark of INH poisoning is the triad of seizures, metabolic acidosis, and coma. Seizures induced by INH are typically generalized and appear to have a rhythmic recurrence. They are generally difficult to treat; patients usually remain comatose between seizures. The metabolic acidosis of INH can be severe; pH values of as low as 6.4 have been reported. As such, INH is on the list of substances associated with the development of high anion gap metabolic acidosis (see MUDPILES mnemonic). Of all these drugs, only INH possesses seizures as a prominent characteristic. Interestingly, in animal models of INH poisoning, metabolic acidosis does not occur if seizures are prevented through paralysis. Finally, the coma of INH intoxication can be severe and prolonged.

Because of the striking clinical picture of INH poisoning, diagnosis is often easily made on the basis of demographic characteristics (particularly common in patients from Southeast Asia or history of incarceration) and clinical manifestations. INH is not usually detected on routine toxicology laboratory screens, and serum concentrations are of little value in acute management. Laboratory tests that are important in initial assessment include arterial blood gas levels, electrolytes level, liver function tests, creatine kinase level, and urinalysis.

Management

Management of INH intoxication begins with advanced life support. Because of seizures and coma, airway protection and ventilation are typically necessary. Cardiac monitoring should be initiated to monitor for the development of cardiac arrhythmias (resulting from severe metabolic acidosis).

Activated charcoal may also be considered if it can be given safely. Theoretically, giving multiple doses of activated charcoal to enhance postabsorptive elimination of INH may be advantageous, but this approach must be weighed against the risk of seizure.

Pharmacologic treatment for INH intoxication includes sodium bicarbonate, anticonvulsants, and pyridoxine. Sodium bicarbonate is provided as needed to restore serum pH to normal. In treating seizures, effective anticonvulsants include the benzodiazepines or phenobarbital (both of which are GABA agonists). Either diazepam (0.1 to 0.3 mg per kg) or lorazepam (0.1 mg per kg) should be administered IV to terminate seizures.

Administration of pyridoxine has been shown to provide specific antidotal therapy for INH poisoning. After administration of vitamin B_6, seizures and metabolic acidosis promptly resolve. Pyridoxine is given as an IV dose that equals the estimated dose of INH in milligrams. In cases in which the ingested amount is unknown, a single dose of 5 g (70 mg per kg in children) of pyridoxine is administered. Rarely, repeat administration is necessary.

Although INH clearance can be enhanced by hemodialysis or hemoperfusion, these techniques are rarely necessary if pyridoxine, activated charcoal, and aggressive supportive care are provided.

Oral Hypoglycemics

Although almost all pediatric patients with diabetes mellitus require insulin therapy for control, the frequent prescription of oral hypoglycemic agents for patients with non–insulin-dependent, adult-onset diabetes has made the availability and, consequently, the ingestion of these medications commonplace among toddlers. The scenario typically involves visits to a grandparent's home (or conversely, a visit by the grandparent to the child's home). The sulfonylureas (chlorpropamide, glipizide, glyburide, glimepiride) are capable of inducing significant hypoglycemia in a toddler after the ingestion of a single tablet. In addition, the onset of hypoglycemia may be delayed up to 16 to 24 hours after ingestion. Thus, prudent management of such exposures generally implies prolonged close observation and a challenge period of fasting. Although chlorpropamide is rarely used today, it may be enhanced by urinary alkalinization. The biguanides (e.g., metformin) are unlikely to create hypoglycemia but may promote metabolic acidosis.

Maintenance of euglycemia is usually accomplished in symptomatic patients with the infusion of hypertonic glucose (e.g., 10% to 20%) solutions, supplemented as necessary by bolus doses, for acute management. Glucose cannot be used as the sole therapy, however, because the dextrose causes hyperglycemia that then leads to insulin release with resultant hypoglycemia, and a vicious cycle of unstable blood sugars ensues. Octreotide, a somatostatin analog that antagonizes insulin release, has been used effectively to stabilize any refractory hypoglycemia at a suggested dose of 1 to 2 μg per kg per dose every 6 to 12 hours via either an IV or subcutaneous route. Historically, diazoxide had been a useful adjunct in correcting refractory drug-induced hypoglycemia, but its use now has largely been replaced by octreotide.

Phenothiazines/Antipsychotics

Background and Pathophysiology

The phenothiazines are commonly prescribed major tranquilizers. Phenothiazines are also often used to treat nausea and vomiting in young children. The toxic effects of this drug class primarily involve the three components of the nervous system: central, autonomic, and extrapyramidal.

The three subgroups of phenothiazines—aliphatic, piperazine, and piperidine—vary in their effects on the different components of the CNS. In general, the aliphatic group (e.g., chlorpromazine) may cause sedation and hypotension in overdose. The piperazine group (e.g., prochlorperazine) is more likely to create extrapyramidal side effects. Several new classes of nonphenothiazine antipsychotic agents are now widely prescribed.

Clinical Findings

The manifestations of phenothiazine toxicity may be dose dependent or dose independent (idiosyncratic). These have significantly different features.

With dose-dependent effects, the manifestations of intoxication after acute ingestion vary from mild to severe. In mild intoxication, CNS signs such as sedation, ataxia, and slurred speech occur. The anticholinergic effects of these drugs may cause constipation, urinary retention, and blurred vision. Because phenothiazines have potent actions on the temperature-regulating center of the hypothalamus, temperature disturbances occur in up to 30% of patients and may consist of hypothermia or hyperthermia. Orthostatic hypotension, the probable result of peripheral vasodilation, may also be noted with mild intoxication.

In moderate intoxications, the patients may have significant depression in the level of consciousness. Extrapyramidal effects become notable at this level of intoxication with muscle stiffness or "cogwheel" rigidity seen on passive movement of the neck, biceps, or quadriceps. Anticholinergic manifestations are severe and include acute urinary retention and paralytic ileus; hypotension may be profound. Cardiac conduction disturbances may make their appearance and are often heralded by a prolonged Q-T interval.

In severe overdoses patients are unarousable. Deep tendon reflexes may be hyperactive. Dystonic reactions may occur, involving the head and neck and the cranial nerves (torticollis and opisthotonos). Arrhythmias and shock may result in death.

The dose-independent effect of the phenothiazines is the dystonic reaction. This striking clinical occurrence consists of episodic spasm of voluntary muscles, particularly those of the head and neck. Patients may develop torticollis, bruxism, tongue protrusion, or oculogyric crisis. Dystonic reactions are unrelated to the amount of ingested phenothiazine. They may or may not occur after the first dose. Their onset is 8 to 40 hours after ingestion of a single dose of phenothiazine. This marked delay between ingestion and clinical manifestations often interferes with obtaining an accurate history of ingestion. Fortunately, although painful and distressing, dystonic reactions are rarely life-threatening and usually resolve quickly after administration of anticholinergics.

The clinical chemistry of the newer antipsychotic agents is varied and complex. CNS depression, seizures, prolongation of the Q-T interval, and α-adrenergic blockade–mediated hypotension are common.

Management

Treatment of acute phenothiazine intoxication hinges on the severity of ingestion. The autonomic signs and symptoms are most often transient and require no treatment. In patients with moderate or severe overdoses, the potential for life-threatening manifestations requires prompt evaluation of vital signs, GI decontamination (if ingestion was within an hour of ED arrival), vascular access, and cardiac monitoring. Pressors such as norepinephrine (see Chapter 91 Shock) may be used to correct the hypotension. In those rare instances of hypertension, the use of nitroprusside (see Chapter 33 Hypertension) may be indicated. Severe arrhythmias should be treated aggressively, as detailed later under "Tricyclic Antidepressants". Attention should be directed to the treatment of temperature instability and other autonomic disturbances.

Dystonic reactions are effectively controlled by the IM or IV administration of diphenhydramine in a dose of 1 to 2 mg per kg (max 50 mg per dose). This dose may be repeated within 15 to 20 minutes if no effect is noted. An alternative agent is benztropine mesylate (1 to 2 mg for an older child/adolescent). This agent reportedly causes less sedation than diphenhydramine. Another potential alternative, especially in younger children, is diazepam (0.1 to 0.2 mg per kg). After resolution of the dystonic reaction, oral treatment should be continued for an additional 24 to 72 hours to prevent recurrences.

Tricyclic Antidepressants

Background

The ingestion of tricyclic antidepressant compounds is a significant problem in pediatric patients. The availability of these compounds in the household may be the result of therapy for depression for a parent or a grandparent or of treatment for enuresis in the patient, sibling, or pet.

Clinical Findings

The ingestion of 10 to 20 mg per kg of most tricyclic antidepressants represents a moderate to serious exposure, with coma and cardiovascular symptoms expected. The ingestion of 35 to 50 mg per kg may result in death. Children have been reported to be more sensitive than adults to tricyclic antidepressants and often have symptoms at lower dosages.

Cyclic antidepressants have many pharmacologic effects. Anticholinergic activity causes altered sensorium and sinus tachycardia. α-Adrenergic blockade may lead to hypotension. However, the more severe cardiovascular effects are primarily caused by the membrane-depressant or "quinidine-like" effects that depress myocardial conduction and may lead to multiple focal premature ventricular contractions and ventricular tachycardia. It has been shown that a QRS interval over 0.1 second is associated with a significant morbidity and mortality in these patients; this delay in conduction may progress to complete heart block and cardiac standstill and/or the previously mentioned ventricular arrhythmias. Another typical electrocardiographic finding suggestive of cyclic antidepressant poisoning is the finding of an R wave of greater than 3-mm amplitude in the QRS complex in lead aVR.

Neurologic findings include lethargy, disorientation, ataxia, hallucinations, and with severe overdoses, coma, and seizures. Fever is commonly present initially, but hypothermia may occur later. Additional anticholinergic symptomatology includes decreased GI motility, which delays gastric emptying time, and urinary retention. Myoclonic jerking has been observed and may be associated with increased deep tendon reflexes. Although the pupils may be dilated, they usually respond to light.

Management

Severe tricyclic antidepressant overdoses warrant gastric decontamination. Because tricyclic antidepressants decrease GI motility, unabsorbed drug may be left in the stomach for prolonged periods. Seizures should be treated aggressively with benzodiazepines and/or barbiturates, or even with neuromuscular paralysis if needed to prevent acidosis. Continuous EEG monitoring is recommended if the patient is paralyzed. Significant conduction delays or arrhythmias resulting from tricyclic antidepressants may benefit from alkalinization of the blood. A sodium bicarbonate bolus of 1 to 2 mEq per kg can be given during continuous EKG monitoring. Bicarbonate infusion can then be used to keep the serum pH at 7.45 to 7.55. These therapeutic maneuvers likely serve to decrease drug binding to the myocardium. Additional bolus doses of sodium bicarbonate may be required if the QRS interval is noted to widen. An additional benefit of the sodium cation is to overcome the sodium channel blockade that is believed to represent the biomolecular substrate of the membrane depressant effect of these agents. If arrhythmias persist, appropriate antiarrhythmic therapy should be instituted, perhaps using lidocaine (see Chapters 1 A General Approach to Ill and Injured Children and 94 Cardiac Emergencies). Quinidine or procainamide should be avoided because each may increase heart block in this situation. Physostigmine, although previously recommended for its antidotal effects on the anticholinergic aspects of these poisonings, has the potential to worsen ventricular conduction defects and to lower the seizure threshold. Its use is considered to be contraindicated in cyclic antidepressant overdoses, particularly in the setting of an abnormal EKG. In the presence of hypotension, many clinicians have advocated the use of norepinephrine infusions (0.1 to 0.3 μg per kg per minute). This approach is based on the observation that the hypotension is the result of norepinephrine depletion secondary to the block of catecholamine uptake, caused by tricyclic antidepressants. Other clinicians have reported that dopamine is as effective; however, the occurrence of ventricular arrhythmias has been reported with dopamine. Lipid emulsion therapy has shown promise in animal studies of cyclic antidepressant toxicity, as well as for calcium antagonists as noted previously. Several clinical cases of its efficacy in refractory tricyclic antidepressant cardiotoxicity and one in bupropion overdose are reported, and most experts would recommend it in cases of refractory cardiotoxicity or cardiac arrest. During the recovery period, serum electrolyte levels should also be monitored because the infusion of bicarbonate may cause hypokalemia, which may aggravate tricyclic antidepressant-induced cardiac arrhythmias. It must be remembered in the treatment of such antidepressants that these compounds have long half-lives and slow elimination rates; therefore, the therapy for these ingestions is often protracted and intensive.

Other Antidepressants

Besides the tricyclic antidepressants, numerous agents designed to elevate mood are prescribed. The chemical structure of these agents and their profile of toxicity are diverse. Major groupings of nontricyclic antidepressants include (i) the selective serotonin reuptake inhibitors (SSRIs; e.g., citalopram, fluoxetine, sertraline), (ii) the monoamine oxidase inhibitors (MAOIs; e.g., phenelzine, tranylcypromine), and (iii) other atypical antidepressants (e.g., bupropion, venlafaxine).

SSRIs most commonly produce CNS depression in overdose. Seizures may occur after large ingestions. Life-threatening events from acute overdose of these compounds rarely occur. The serotonin syndrome, manifested by the triad of autonomic instability, neuromuscular changes (myoclonus, rigidity especially in the lower extremities), and altered mental status, is potentially lethal. Citalopram and its enantiomer escitalopram cause both QTc interval prolongation as well as seizure activity that are thought to be dose related. Bupropion, prescribed for both depression and in smoking-cessation programs, prevents reuptake of biogenic amines, is highly epileptogenic, and in large overdose, may cause QRS widening and life-threatening cardiotoxicity. Bupriopion's amphetamine nucleus accounts for the positive toxicology screens seen in patients with therapeutic use as well as in overdose settings. The α-adrenergic antagonism of trazodone may lead to hypotension.

The MAOIs, although pharmacologically effective and therapeutically important, are some of the most toxic medications known. Acute single overdoses of as little as 6 mg per kg have been associated with a fatal outcome. In addition, because of their irreversible inhibition of the enzyme monoamine oxidase, which is responsible for the degradation of most biogenic amines, MAOIs possess several important interactions with foods and other medications that can lead to severe toxicity, even in the patient who takes them in appropriate doses. There are three important clinical pictures of MAOI toxicity. First, because GI tract activity of monoamine oxidase is also inhibited by these drugs, patients who take them appropriately and then ingest foods that contain biogenic amines (e.g., tyramine in wines, cheeses, or soy sauce) may develop severe hypertension with subsequent headache, seizures, or stroke. The second picture of MAOI toxicity appears when those who take the drug therapeutically are given certain sympathomimetic or serotonergic agents causing the serotonin syndrome. Important examples of such drugs include common agents in OTC cough and cold preparations such as dextromethorphan, analgesics such as meperidine, and psychotropic medications such as clomipramine and fluoxetine or other SSRIs. In these patients, this drug combination may quickly lead to hyperpyrexia, skeletal muscle rigidity, cardiac arrhythmias, and death which is one of the few fatal drug interactions known. Finally, those with acute MAOI overdoses develop a clinical syndrome that includes blood pressure instability, hyperpyrexia, skeletal muscle rigidity, opsoclonus, seizures, and death.

Because of the toxicity of these agents and the frequent delay in their onset of activity (up to 24 hours), all patients with a history of MAOI ingestion, regardless of symptoms, should be admitted to the hospital for 24 hours. Management of the patient with MAOI toxicity is largely dictated by the specific toxic manifestations. In those with hypertensive reactions, treatment consists of the immediate administration of an antihypertensive. The ideal agent may be nitroprusside because its brief duration of action permits titration of effect. In the treatment of hyperpyrexia, cooling measures are promptly instituted. Because hyperpyrexia is often accompanied by skeletal muscle rigidity and rhabdomyolysis, serum creatine kinase level should be measured and close attention should be paid to the urine for any signs of myoglobinuria. Benzodiazepines are often helpful in this situation and neuromuscular blockade may be beneficial in patients who have severe muscle rigidity with hyperthermia. In the patient with acute overdose, treatment is directed to hemodynamic stability. Because blood pressure changes occur quickly and consist of hypotension and hypertension, hypertension should be treated with short-acting agents and hypotension with fluid and vasopressor support. Intensive care unit admission is mandatory for these patients because of their clinical instability.

Drugs Dangerous in Small Doses

Toddlers often are brought to EDs for evaluation after possibly having ingested one or two doses of a medication. Most often these children will be fine with little treatment beyond reassurance. There are circumstances, however, when this situation can be life-threatening and proper intervention can be lifesaving. A large list of chemicals and poisons can be extremely toxic in small amounts; but, this is beyond the scope of this discussion. However, it is wise to be familiar with a modest list of pharmaceuticals that may cause dangerous toxicity to young children with just one or two doses (Table 110.13). Many of these agents have been discussed earlier in this chapter. The actual incidence of life-threatening toxicity of each of these drugs, when just one or two doses have been ingested, is as yet undefined.

A systematic approach to these patients includes a careful history, an examination with attention to the presence of toxidromes (Table 110.6), and a guided laboratory assessment. This approach may allow narrowing of the differential diagnosis and may allow a determination of the possible severity of the ingestion. If the differential diagnosis includes any of the drugs listed in Table 110.13, it may be prudent to consider decontamination and prolonged observation. An algorithmic approach to this situation is provided in Figure 110.5.

NONPHARMACEUTICALS

Alcohols and Glycols

The alcohols and glycols are some of the most commonly found organic compounds in the environment. Ethanol is best known as the psychoactive ingredient in beer, wine, and liquor; it is also a commonly encountered solvent and is used

TABLE 110.13

MEDICATIONS DANGEROUS TO TODDLERS IN ONE TO TWO DOSES[a]

Agent	Minimal potential fatal dose[b]	Maximal dose size	Potential fatal dose	Major toxicity
Benzocaine	<20 mg/kg	10% gel 20% spray	~2 mL Baby Orajel	Methemoglobinemia, seizures
β-Blockers (propranolol)	Unclear	160 mg	1–2 tablets	Bradycardia, hypotension, seizures, hypoglycemia
Calcium antagonists (verapamil)	<40 mg/kg	240 mg	1–2 tablets	Bradycardia, hypotension
Camphor	<100 mg/kg	1 g/5 mL	1 tsp camphorated oil 2 tsp Campho-Phenique 5 tsp Vicks Vaporub	Seizures, CNS depression
Chloroquine	<30 mg/kg	500 mg	1 tablet	Seizures, arrhythmia
Clonidine	Unclear	0.3-mg tablet 7.5-mg patch	1 tablet 1 patch	Bradycardia, CNS depression
Diphenoxylate (Lomotil)	<1.2 mg/kg	2.5 mg/tablet or tsp	2 tablets/tsp	CNS and respiratory depression
Hypoglycemics, oral (glyburide)	~1 mg/kg	5 mg	2 tablets	Hypoglycemia
Lindane	~6 mg/kg	1% lotion	2 tsp	Seizures, CNS depression
Methyl salicylate	~200 mg/kg	1.4 g/mL	½ tsp oil of wintergreen 2 tsp Icy Hot Balm	Seizures, cardiovascular collapse
Opioids	Variable by potency	Variable	1–2 tablets	CNS and respiratory depression
Phenothiazines (chlorpromazine)	~20 mg/kg	200 mg	1 tablet	Seizures, arrhythmia
Quinidine	~50 mg/kg	300 mg	2 tablets	Seizures, arrhythmia
Quinine	~80 mg/kg	650 mg	2 tablets	Seizures, arrhythmia
Theophylline	~50 mg/kg	500 mg	1 tablet	Seizures, arrhythmia
TCAs (imipramine)	~20 mg/kg	150 mg	1–2 tablets	Seizures, arrhythmia, hypotension

[a]A long list of commonly-encountered, highly toxic, *non*pharmacologic agents can be severely poisonous in 1 to 2 doses. These are not included here.
[b]For the purposes of this table, a "dose" refers to a single pill or roughly a 5-cc swallow. Calculations are based on a previously healthy toddler of 10-kg body weight.
CNS, central nervous system; TCAs, tricyclic antidepressants.

as a topical antiseptic, chemical intermediate, and in some instances, a rubbing alcohol. Methanol, or methyl alcohol, functions as an antifreeze (in windshield washers/deicers and gasoline antifreeze) and as a solvent in many industrial and home products. Isopropyl alcohol serves as a rubefacient. Ethylene glycol is used primarily as a deicer or antifreeze. A related class of compounds, the glycol ethers, is widely used in rug shampoos and brake fluids. The toxicity of these glycol ethers is complex and beyond the scope of this discussion.

Ethanol

The most commonly ingested alcohol is ethanol. After ingesting ethanol, children may develop nausea, vomiting, stupor, and ataxia. Coma and death from apnea may occur if significant quantities are consumed. In adolescents, blood concentrations of less than 50 mg per dL rarely result in overt sensory or motor impairment. Values of 80 to 150 mg per dL are consistent with intoxication and cause mild neurologic findings. Lethal blood alcohol concentrations are generally higher than 500 mg per dL. Infants and toddlers who ingest ethanol have a clinical course that is significantly different from that in adolescents and adults; a triad of coma, hypothermia, and hypoglycemia appears once ethanol levels exceed 50 to 100 mg per dL. This triad may be accompanied by metabolic acidosis. As ethanol decreases physical coordination, and increases risk taking behavior, it is important for emergency physicians to consider the possibility of head trauma in patients with coma after ethanol intoxication.

The amount of an ethanol-containing liquid that is of concern when ingested by a child depends on the alcohol concentration. However, a rough rule is that ingestion of 1 g per kg of ethanol is sufficient to raise blood alcohol to 100 mg per dL. Therefore, for a beverage such as beer (5% alcohol), approximately 10 to 15 mL per kg must be ingested before serious toxicity results. Similar estimates are 4 to 6 mL per kg for wine (14% alcohol) and 1 to 2 mL per kg for 80-proof liquor (40% alcohol).

The management of ethanol ingestion in children begins with prompt recognition and evaluation of blood glucose level. Airway or ventilatory compromise should be treated with endotracheal intubation. If seizures result from hypoglycemia, they should be promptly treated with 10% to 50% (0.25 to 1 g per kg) IV dextrose. Warming techniques should be instituted to increase core temperature. Because ethanol is rapidly absorbed from the gut and is not adsorbed by activated charcoal, there is rarely a role for GI decontamination.

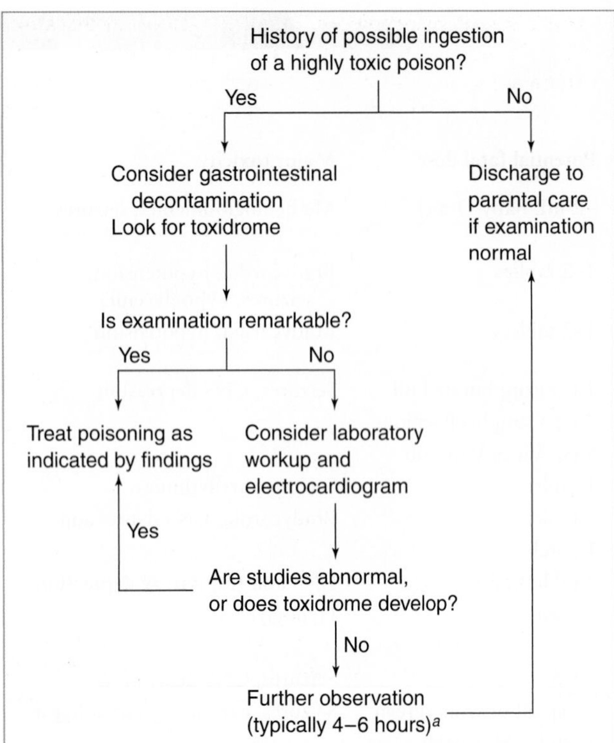
History of possible ingestion of a highly toxic poison?
Yes
No
Consider gastrointestinal decontamination
Look for toxidrome
Discharge to parental care if examination normal
Is examination remarkable?
Yes
No
Treat poisoning as indicated by findings
Consider laboratory workup and electrocardiogram
Yes
Are studies abnormal, or does toxidrome develop?
No
Further observation (typically 4–6 hours)a

FIGURE 110.5 Algorithmic approach to a toddler having ingested one to two doses (1 to 2 pills or 5- to 10-cc swallow) of a drug. [a]Medications notorious for their ability to have delayed onset in toxicity, beyond 4 to 6 hours, include oral hypoglycemic agents, sustained-release preparations, monoamine oxidase inhibitors, drugs taken concomitantly with anticholinergic agents, and acetaminophen.

Alcohol is metabolized by the hepatic enzyme alcohol dehydrogenase; its elimination rate is dose dependent. This means that the higher the blood alcohol concentrations, the longer the elimination process because the capacity of the body to produce alcohol dehydrogenase is limited. The rate of reduction in blood alcohol concentration varies from 10 to 25 mg per dL per hour. Although hemodialysis effectively enhances elimination (three- to fourfold), it is rarely necessary. The institution of hemodialysis may be useful in those patients who have impaired liver function or a blood alcohol concentration higher than 450 to 500 mg per dL.

Isopropyl Alcohol

Poisoning with isopropyl alcohol may be particularly insidious because oral ingestion is not the only route of exposure. Children may develop severe intoxication, including coma, after topical application of isopropyl alcohol for the relief of fever (although such exposure may represent inhalational exposure rather than direct, dermal absorption). Because isopropyl alcohol is usually available in a 70% concentration by volume, ingestion of 2 to 2.5 mL per kg of this solution may lead to symptoms. Ingestion of this compound causes many of the same features as ethanol ingestion, with the additional complication of severe gastritis. Unlike the other toxic alcohols, isopropyl alcohol does not lead to metabolic acidosis. This is because its metabolite, acetone, is not an acid. However, it is approximately twice as intoxicating as ethanol, leading to greater mental status impairment at comparable serum levels. The life-threatening toxicity of isopropyl alcohol is cardiac; at high serum concentrations, direct myocardial depression occurs, leading to hypotension and shock.

In any patient with coma and an unexplained osmolal gap (the difference between calculated and observed osmolarity), isopropyl alcohol should be strongly considered. The presence of ketonuria in conjunction with the absence of metabolic acidosis effectively makes the diagnosis of isopropyl intoxication.

Isopropyl alcohol is easily removed by hemodialysis. However, hemodialysis is rarely necessary because life-threatening toxicity does not occur until serum levels exceed 400 to 500 mg/dL. Therefore, the sole indication for hemodialysis is considered hemodynamic instability, regardless of serum concentration. Treatment is otherwise supportive.

Methanol

Although methanol is used primarily as a solvent for industrial purposes, it is found in other household products including fuels for stoves, paint removers, and antifreezes.

Methanol is a model for the few drugs that, rather than being detoxified, become more toxic as they are metabolized. Thus, although methanol has little or no inherent toxicity, its metabolism by alcohol and aldehyde dehydrogenase to form formaldehyde and formic acid creates highly toxic compounds. Formic acid is a potent organic acid that results in severe metabolic acidosis and ocular toxicity. Ingestions approaching 100 mg/kg should be considered dangerous.

The clinical effects of methanol ingestion usually occur after a latent period of 8 to 24 hours. This delay occurs as the result of the metabolic conversion of methanol to its toxic by-products. In large ingestions, acute methanol poisoning may cause severe CNS depression, metabolic acidosis, and a number of reversible or irreversible optic changes. In the early stages of intoxication, funduscopic examination may be remarkable for hyperemia. However, if left untreated, methanol intoxication results in blindness, with the appearance of a pale, avascular retina. In subacute ingestions, the nonspecific neurologic symptoms of methanol intoxication resemble those of ethanol with a "hangover," malaise, headache, and dizziness. During recovery from a mild ingestion, occasional paresthesias of the extremities may develop.

The most immediately significant clinical concern from methanol ingestion is severe metabolic acidosis. This acidosis is primarily the result of formic acid production. The metabolic acidosis may be intractable and results in multiorgan dysfunction, which includes cardiac arrhythmias, seizures, and pancreatitis. The ophthalmologic abnormalities that develop during methanol intoxication may be temporary or permanent. These include blurred or double vision, changes in color perception, and sharply reduced visual acuity. Permanent abnormalities may include diminished pupillary light reaction or frank blindness. The occurrence of permanent visual defects correlates directly with the degree of metabolic acidosis, the duration of the acidosis, and the quantity of methanol ingested.

Management

The treatment of methanol ingestion consists of supportive care, administration of specific therapies, and enhancement of elimination. Activated charcoal does not adsorb methanol effectively and is unnecessary.

Laboratory assessment includes serial blood gases, electrolytes, BUN, creatinine, glucose, serum osmolality, and methanol level analyses. Serum methanol concentration in milligrams per deciliter can be estimated by the formula (osmolar gap × 3).

There are three specific treatments for methanol intoxication: sodium bicarbonate, folic acid, and fomepizole (or ethanol). Sodium bicarbonate should be administered to correct metabolic acidosis: this improves physiologic functioning and may help prevent formate from reaching sensitive tissues. Folate is provided because of its role in formic acid disposition within the tetrahydrofolate cycle. Customary doses are 1 mg per kg IV every 6 hours.

Because serum methanol levels of 20 mg per dL or higher are associated with toxicity if untreated, higher levels require treatment to prevent its metabolism and/or interventions to enhance its elimination. Fomepizole, an alcohol dehydrogenase inhibitor, can prevent the metabolism of methanol to its toxic metabolites. If fomepizole is unavailable, ethanol, which has a higher affinity for alcohol dehydrogenase than methanol, may be provided to competitively "block" further production of toxic metabolites.

The loading dose of fomepizole is 15 mg per kg, which may be given IV or orally. The maintenance dose is 10 mg per kg every 12 hours for four doses, then 15 mg per kg every 12 hours thereafter. More frequent dosing is required during hemodialysis.

If fomepizole in unavailable, ethanol is administered with the goal of maintaining serum ethanol concentrations of at least 100 mg per dL. Ethanol may be given by continuous IV infusion (600 mg per kg bolus followed by 110 mg per kg per hour) or by oral administration. During dialysis, ethanol dosing may need to be doubled to maintain sufficient blood ethanol content to effectively block the metabolism of methanol. IV ethanol is preferred but has the problems of being often unavailable and hyperosmolar (precluding its administration in small veins) and of requiring large fluid volumes. When the oral route is used, it must be remembered that proof designation of a beverage is twice the alcohol concentration expressed as a percentage (e.g., 80 proof equals 40% alcohol). Children must be closely monitored for the complications of ethanol administration, including mental status depression, hypoglycemia, and hypothermia.

Hemodialysis should be strongly considered for children presenting many hours after ingestion who demonstrate significant metabolic acidosis and end-organ injury: this suggests the presence toxic metabolites which are amenable to extracorporeal removal. When alcohol dehydrogenase is blocked, methanol has a very long time to elimination, primarily via exhalation; therefore, dialysis can also be considered for high serum methanol levels (in excess of 50 mg/dL) after alcohol dehydrogenase inhibition.

Ethylene Glycol

The ingestion of ethylene glycol, although uncommon, causes significant morbidity and occasional mortality. The toxicity of ethylene glycol, like that of methanol, is the result of drug toxification; ethylene glycol has virtually no toxicity in its parent state. However, metabolism by alcohol dehydrogenase produces several toxic intermediates, including glycolaldehyde, glycolic acid, and oxalate. These metabolites result in severe metabolic acidosis and deposition of calcium oxalate crystals in all vital organs.

The clinical syndrome of ethylene glycol intoxication appears in three different stages. The first stage consists predominantly of CNS manifestations and is accompanied by a profound metabolic acidosis. In this early stage, mild hypertension, tachycardia, and leukocytosis are often present. Nausea and vomiting commonly occur, and with larger doses, coma and convulsions may appear within a few hours. Another common finding is the presence of hypocalcemia. This is believed to result from the widespread formation of calcium oxalate. Hypocalcemia may be severe enough to cause tetany and cardiac conduction disturbances. Urinalysis usually reveals a low specific gravity, proteinuria, microscopic hematuria, and crystalluria. The second distinct state is ushered in by coma and cardiopulmonary failure; it is usually the result of acidosis and hypocalcemia. The third stage usually occurs after 24 to 72 hours. Here, renal failure emerges as the dominant problem. Usually, a picture of acute tubular necrosis develops with either polyuria or anuria. Urine sediment contains blood, protein, and casts. Patients often require dialysis for extended periods and may be left with permanent renal insufficiency.

Consideration of ethylene glycol poisoning should be based either on the history or, in the absence of diabetic ketoacidosis, the presence of any of the following criteria: (i) Alcohol-like intoxication without the odor of alcohol, (ii) large anion-gap metabolic acidosis, (iii) an elevated osmolar gap in the absence of ethanol or methanol ingestion, or (iv) a urinalysis that demonstrates oxalate crystals. Another oft-mentioned diagnostic tool (with low sensitivity or specificity) is the performance of a Wood's lamp examination of urine. If the ingested substance is radiator antifreeze, the fluorescein dye that it contains will be excreted in urine and may fluoresce under Wood's lamp. Serum chemistries or blood gas levels should be obtained frequently because of the rapid evolution of metabolic acidosis. The availability of ethylene glycol levels varies by institution.

Activated charcoal negligibly adsorbs ethylene glycol and is unnecessary. As with methanol intoxication, treatment of ethylene glycol poisoning falls into three areas: supportive care, administration of pharmacologic agents, and enhancement of elimination. Supportive care includes close monitoring of vital signs and anticipation of life-threatening events, particularly cardiac arrhythmias secondary to hypocalcemia. Intravascular volume should be replenished, an EKG should be obtained, and the patient should be placed on a cardiac monitor. Intubation and mechanical ventilation should be provided as needed for airway protection and control of acid–base balance.

Correction of acidosis should begin immediately with the administration of sodium bicarbonate and appropriate ventilation. Hypocalcemia may present as skeletal muscle disturbances (tetany) or cardiac dysfunction (prolonged Q-T interval). These may be alleviated by the prompt administration of calcium (e.g., 10% calcium gluconate, 0.3 to 0.6 mL per kg). Thiamine and pyridoxine are vitamins that act as cofactors in the nontoxic metabolic pathways of ethylene glycol and, theoretically, divert its metabolism toward formation of nontoxic metabolites. Therefore, thiamine (0.25 to 0.5 mg per kg) and pyridoxine (1 to 2 mg per kg) are recommended for the first 24 hours of treatment.

Fomepizole (or ethanol) administration is an option to inhibit ethylene glycol metabolism by alcohol dehydrogenase (previously discussed under "Methanol"). Inhibition should be initiated as soon as possible to interrupt further formation of organic acids. As with methanol, alcohol dehydrogenase

TABLE 110.14

COMMON CAUSES OF DIARRHEAL FOOD POISONING IN THE UNITED STATES

Organism	Onset (hours)	Effect of heat	Typical sources
Staphylococcal	1–6	Stable	Meats, potato/egg salads, cream-filled desserts
Bacillus cereus			
Emetic type	1–6	Stable	Fried rice
Diarrheal type	12–16	Labile	Cooked meats
Clostridia	12–24	Spores, stable Toxin labile	Meats/poultry[a]
Cholera/other *Vibrio* spp.	12–24	Toxin labile	Raw shellfish

[a]In context of inadequate refrigeration.

inhibition is indicated for ethylene glycol concentrations of 20 mg per dL or higher. If a serum ethylene glycol cannot be obtained in a timely fashion, it can be estimated by the formula (osmolar gap × 6), assuming no other alcohols are contributing to the osmolar gap. Hemodialysis is indicated if there is renal failure or severe electrolyte disturbances, regardless of the serum ethylene glycol concentration. Hemodialysis may be considered for patients who are stable hemodynamically but who have very elevated blood ethylene glycol levels. The cost–benefit analysis of hemodialysis versus continued, prolonged fomepizole therapy is currently being investigated; however, recent case reports indicate that fomepizole alone can be effective for ethylene glycol ingestions when the acid–base status and renal function are normal at the time of presentation.

Foods/Fish

In addition to drugs and medications and household products and plants, toxic ingestions may occur through normal diet when the ingested product contains a toxin that is performed by microorganisms. Mycotoxins are important food contaminants worldwide. Major bacterial enterotoxins include those produced by *Shigella, Salmonella, Yersinia, Escherichia coli, Staphylococcus, Bacillus cereus, Clostridium, Vibrio,* and *Clostridium botulinum.* After this large group of toxins, the next most common cause of foodborne intoxications results from the ingestion of contaminated marine life.

When similar GI symptoms occur in a group of persons who share the same meal or the same food on separate occasions, the emergency physician may consider the possibility of foodborne disease. Detailed epidemiologic investigations are usually beyond the capacity of the ED setting, but the hospital infection control officer and/or local health department can often be helpful.

Staphylococcal food poisoning is probably the most common cause of such cases in the United States. The heat-stable toxins typically produce acute abdominal pain, nausea, vomiting, and diarrhea within 1 to 6 hours of eating the contaminated meal. The illness is usually self-limiting, although occasionally, patients develop severe symptoms and dehydration.

Other bacterial toxin-induced diarrheal food poisonings include those secondary to *B. cereus, Clostridium perfringens,* and *Vibrio* species. The onset of clinical illness and usual food sources of these and staphylococcal disease are outlined in Table 110.14. All these illnesses are generally self-limiting, and treatment is supportive, with careful attention given to fluid and electrolyte status in unusually severe cases (e.g., the rare occurrence of cholera in the United States).

Infant botulism shares many pathophysiologic and clinical features with foodborne botulism. The etiology of the foodborne disease differs, of course, in that preformed toxin is ingested at the time of consuming contaminated food, typically improperly home-canned, low-acidity vegetables (e.g., potatoes, onions, beans) or poorly refrigerated pot pies or meats. The incubation period is usually 12 to 36 hours, with initial GI symptoms soon followed by weakness, malaise, and then cranial nerve symptoms, particularly diplopia, dysphagia, and dysarthria. The neurologic examination is notable for normal mental status and symmetric ocular findings, such as ptosis, lateral rectus weakness, and pupillary abnormalities.

Diagnosis should be suspected clinically and may be buttressed with positive serum or stool analyses for botulinum toxin and suggestive electromyelograph findings. A heptavalent antitoxin for botulism is now available.

Scombroid Poisoning

Scombroid poisoning is an intoxication that occurs shortly after ingestion of spoiled fish from the Scombroidea family (e.g., tuna, bonita, skipjack), as well as ingestion of non-Scombroidea fish (e.g., bluefish, mahi mahi). The ingested toxin(s) has not been completely characterized, but large quantities of histamine-like compounds are invariably found in these fish when tissue histidine decomposes.

The clinical picture of scombroid poisoning consists of sudden-onset headache, facial flushing, a peppery taste in the mouth, dizziness, nausea, and vomiting. An urticarial eruption with pruritus may develop. In its extreme, patients may develop tachycardia, bronchospasm, respiratory distress, and hypotension.

In patients with severe symptoms, treatment is directed toward ensuring adequate ventilation and hemodynamic stability. Fluids and vasopressor support may be needed to treat hypotension. Pharmacologic treatment of scombroid poisoning includes administration of antihistamines, corticosteroids, and if necessary, adrenergic agents. Both diphenhydramine and cimetidine have been used successfully to treat the symptoms of scombroid poisoning. In the event of severe bronchospasm, other bronchodilators, including inhaled β_2 agonists may be necessary adjuncts.

Ciguatera

Ciguatera is an illness endemic to the South Pacific but is considerably less common in the continental United States, where it is largely confined to the lower Atlantic states. However, because it does occasionally appear in the United States or may occur in recent visitors from endemic areas, its clinical manifestations should be recognized.

Ciguatera results from ingestion of a toxin elaborated by the dinoflagellate, *Gambierdiscus toxicus*. This parasite is ingested by small fish, which begin to concentrate the toxin. As predators ingest those small fish, the toxin ascends the food chain until ingested by humans. The fish that most commonly harbor ciguatoxin include barracuda, grouper, red snapper, and parrot fish. The physiologic actions of ciguatoxin are primarily neurologic. The toxin decreases CNS concentrations of γ-aminobutyric acid (GABA) and dopamine. This action occurs in conjunction with sodium channels being "locked open," permitting unrestricted sodium ingress.

The clinical picture of ciguatera poisoning begins 4 to 36 hours after ingestion of contaminated fish. After a brief period of nausea and vomiting, patients develop paresthesias, particularly perioral, or weakness. A hallmark of ciguatera toxin is the reversal of hot–cold sensation. In severe cases, CNS dysfunction, including coma, may appear. Toxic manifestations may persist for days to months after significant exposure.

The diagnosis of ciguatera intoxication is clinical, based on the history of ingestion of a fish known to carry this toxin. Because symptoms appear many hours after ingestion of contaminated fish, there is no clear role for GI decontamination.

Management of ciguatera is supportive. Primary attention should be paid to CNS status and its effects on airway and ventilation. IV mannitol has shown great promise in reversing many of the neurologic manifestations, particularly coma. It is administered in a dose of 0.5 to 1 g per kg via an in-line filter.

Paralytic Shellfish Poisoning

The dinoflagellate *Gonyaulax* is responsible for elaborating the toxin (saxitoxin) that causes paralytic shellfish poisoning (PSP). The name "red tide" is based on the characteristic red pigment of the *Gonyaulax*. PSP appears in large bloom between the months of May and October and is found primarily along the eastern seaboard (although blooms have increased across the world in more recent years and may be found on either U.S. coast). The animals that ingest and concentrate this toxin are primarily bivalve shellfish, including mussels, clams, oysters, and uncommonly, scallops. The toxin, saxitoxin, is capable of reversibly binding neuronal sodium channels, resulting in depolarization disturbances. The toxin is heat stable.

After ingestion of contaminated shellfish, patients quickly develop GI distress with nausea and vomiting. This is followed by generalized paresthesias, cranial nerve disturbances, and weakness. In severe intoxications, cardiorespiratory failure may ensue.

Treatment of PSP is supportive. Patients may require ventilatory support until the intoxication resolves over hours to days.

HOUSEHOLD CLEANING PRODUCTS AND CAUSTICS

Household Cleaning Products

Background

Soaps are oil-based surface-active agents (surfactants) used to clean oil-based debri... A "detergent" is any cleansing ...n use, the word *detergent* has ...aning product that is based on ...inly for laundering and dish- ...s, "laundry pods" or "single- ...me popular commercial prod- ... include disinfectant cleaners; ...d toilet bowls; bleaches; and ... concern because their acces- ... commonly involved in human

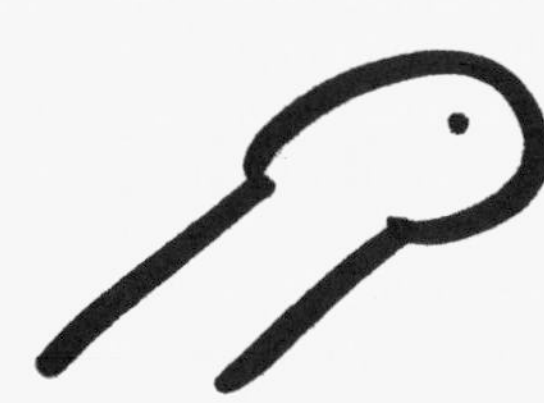

Each year, about 8% of reported pediatric exploratory ingestions involve household cleaning substances. Most of these cases involve children younger than 5 years, of whom only 1% to 2% of those ingesting noncorrosive products are hospitalized. Most such exposures occur inside the home while the product is in use. Transfer of household chemicals out of their original containers, often into empty drinking glasses or soda bottles, remains a significant risk factor for exposure.

Caustics

Background and Pathophysiology

Many agents possess corrosive potential when they are placed in direct contact with biologic tissues.

These agents, collectively referred to as *corrosives,* may be acidic, alkaline, or rarely, have neutral pH (e.g., silver nitrate, concentrated hydrogen peroxide). Essentially all corrosives found in the home are acids or alkalis. Strong alkalis and acids cause direct destruction of tissue but with differing histopathologic patterns. Acids produce coagulation necrosis that usually causes superficial damage, rather than deep, penetrating burns. Alkalis, in contrast, cause a deep and penetrating liquefaction necrosis, which often has severe consequences, such as esophageal perforation. Such deep burns are often associated with severe scarring and, ultimately, with stricture formation (Fig. 110.6). Acid corrosives include the mineral acids, such as hydrochloric, sulfuric, nitric, and hydrofluoric acids. Common household products that contain acid corrosives include toilet bowl and drain cleaners.

Alkali caustics are found in several household products. Sodium hydroxide (lye), which is available in crystalline and liquid forms, is used primarily as an oven cleaner or drain pipe cleaner. Other products may contain alkaline corrosives, including powdered laundry and dishwasher detergents.

Clinical Findings

Ingestions of acid and alkali corrosives cause immediate severe burning of exposed surfaces, usually with intense dysphagia. Associated glottic edema may cause airway obstruction

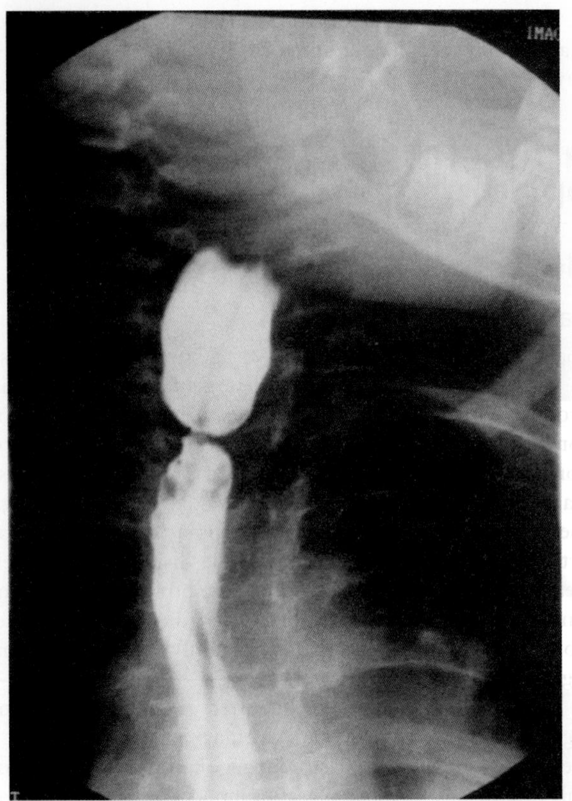

FIGURE 110.6 Barium swallow radiograph demonstrating esophageal stricture in a boy subsequent to ingestion of drain cleaner.

and asphyxia. Severe acid ingestions most often cause gastric necrosis and may be complicated by gastric perforation and peritonitis. With alkalis, severe damage is more commonly found in the esophagus; deep-tissue injury may quickly lead to esophageal perforation, mediastinitis, and death. As already noted, alkalis also produce severe esophageal strictures in survivors.

Management

The initial step in the management of a caustic ingestion is to determine whether the agent is, in fact, corrosive and, if so, whether it is an alkaline or acid corrosive. Many products that are believed to have corrosive potential (e.g., household bleach) are simple irritants and do not require intervention. Identification of ingredients and their corrosive potential can be found through consultation with a regional poison control center.

The approach to management of cleaning products and caustic ingestions, as outlined in Figures 110.7 and 110.8, begins with rapid clinical assessment of cardiorespiratory function, neurologic status, and evidence of GI hemorrhage. Life support measures may be needed emergently to secure the airway and to treat shock or metabolic acidosis. As noted previously, most patients with significant exposures develop symptoms early and may appear critically ill. However, even patients with minimal symptoms and the absence of oral lesions may have significant esophageal injury; thus, all patients with a convincing history of significant exposure to a caustic substance merit upper GI endoscopy to be evaluated

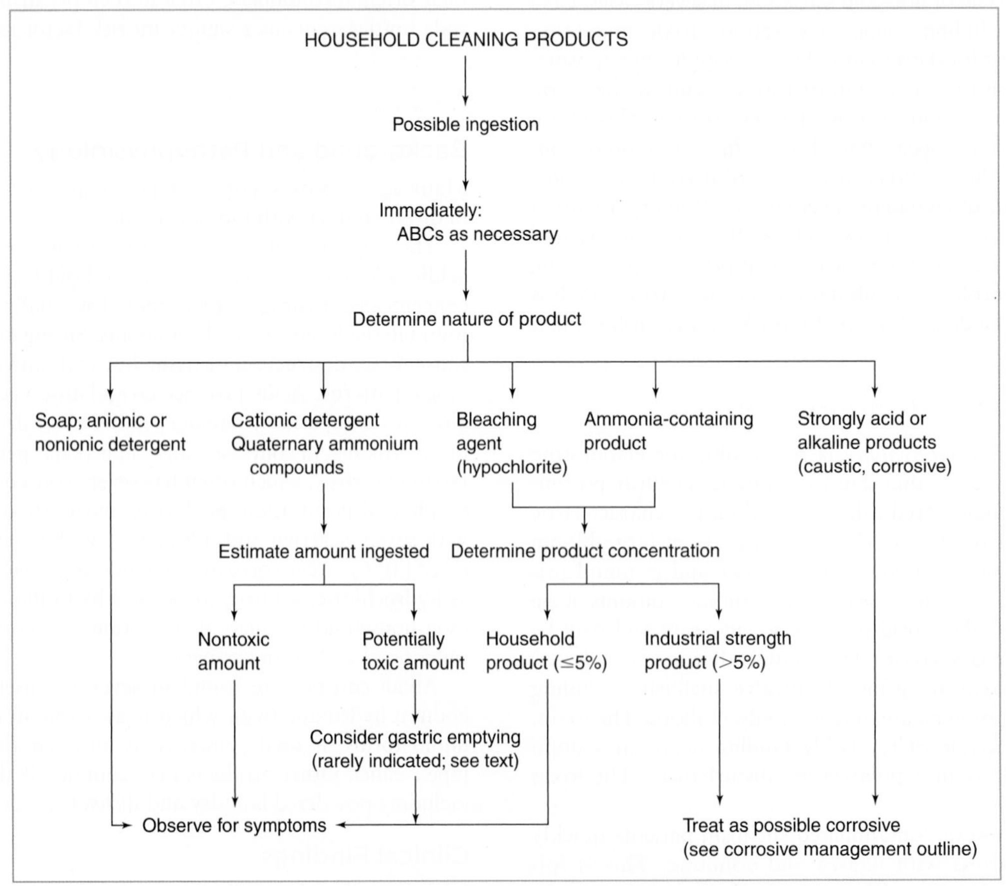

FIGURE 110.7 Algorithm for management of household cleaning product ingestion. ABC, airway, breathing, circulation. (Modified with permission from Temple AR, Lovejoy FH Jr. *Cleaning products and their accidental ingestion.* New York, NY: Soap and Detergent Association, 1980.) See text for special case of laundry "pods."

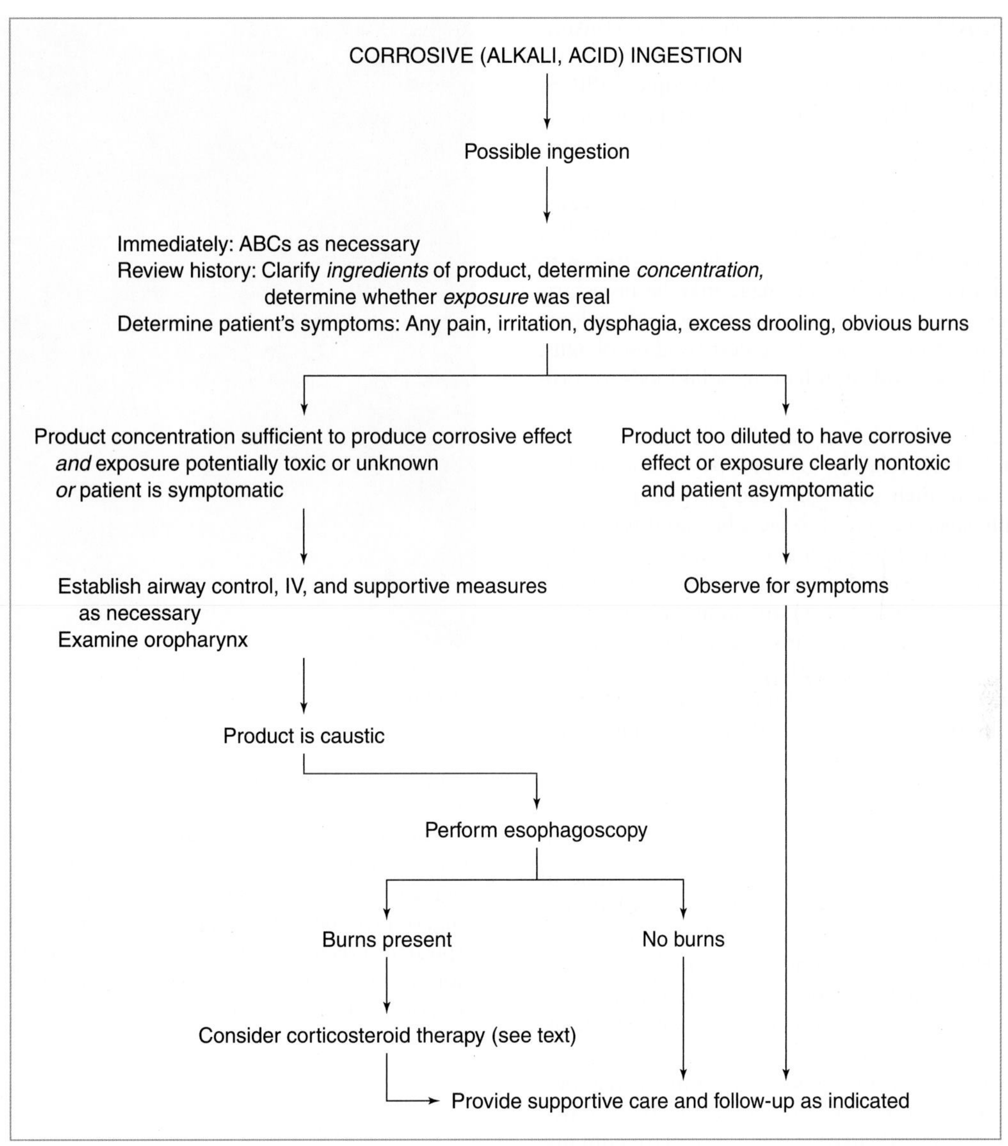
CORROSIVE (ALKALI, ACID) INGESTION
Possible ingestion
Immediately: ABCs as necessary
Review history: Clarify ingredients of product, determine concentration, determine whether exposure was real
Determine patient's symptoms: Any pain, irritation, dysphagia, excess drooling, obvious burns
Product concentration sufficient to produce corrosive effect and exposure potentially toxic or unknown or patient is symptomatic
Product too diluted to have corrosive effect or exposure clearly nontoxic and patient asymptomatic
Establish airway control, IV, and supportive measures as necessary
Examine oropharynx
Observe for symptoms
Product is caustic
Perform esophagoscopy
Burns present
No burns
Consider corticosteroid therapy (see text)
Provide supportive care and follow-up as indicated

FIGURE 110.8 Algorithm for management of corrosive ingestion. ABC, airway, breathing, circulation; IV, intravenous. (Modified with permission from Temple AR, Lovejoy FH Jr. *Cleaning products and their accidental ingestion*. New York, NY: Soap and Detergent Association, 1980.)

fully for the presence of esophageal burns. Simple dilution has been suggested as being safe and potentially diagnostic. However, there are several reasons why this should only be recommended as first aid in mildly symptomatic children. First, in the event esophageal injury or perforation has occurred, fluids may extravasate, inducing severe mediastinitis. Also, because endoscopy is the diagnostic procedure of choice in establishing the extent of injuries, an empty stomach is necessary for minimizing the risks of anesthesia. Finally, if administered fluids are alkaline or acidic, an exothermic reaction may occur that also can worsen esophageal injury. No GI decontamination is conducted after the ingestion of corrosive agents.

If the eyes are involved (something that should always be considered if a caustic has splashed on the face), copious irrigation should be provided and carried out for at least 15 minutes, with longer periods for crystalline caustics. The physician should perform pH testing of fluids in the ocular cul-de-sac after irrigation to confirm that corrosives have been neutralized; the normal pH of tears is 7. Alkali eye injuries require urgent ophthalmologic consultation. Skin contamination also deserves prolonged rinsing with water and removal of contaminated clothing. Irrigation should continue until the skin is free of alkali, as determined by disappearance of the soapy sensation.

All exposed body surfaces, especially the oropharynx, should be examined scrupulously. A CBC and chest radiograph should be obtained; the latter particularly if any respiratory signs or symptoms are noted. A lateral neck radiograph may be able to demonstrate evidence of caustic epiglottitis.

Analgesic therapy may be necessary for severe pain. An IV line should be established if not previously done for basic life support. Conflicting data regarding the role of corticosteroids in the treatment of corrosive esophageal injury exist. First-degree burns typically heal without long-term sequelae. Some evidence suggests that circumferential second-degree burns may be less likely to stricture after steroid administration but this remains controversial; thus, corticosteroids with empiric antibiotics may be considered by some providers in this scenario. Third-degree burns are likely to scar despite treatment, and administration of steroids in this situation may provide more risk than benefit. The consulting otolaryngologist or surgeon may elect to administer steroids in select patients on the basis of endoscopic findings. All patients are admitted for supportive care and monitoring for acute complications such as mediastinitis, pneumonitis, and peritonitis.

The long-term management of survivors with severe caustic esophageal burns and stricture formation is complex, involving many surgical, medical, and psychologic stresses to the patient. Years of repeated bougienage may be necessary, and some patients will require esophagectomy with colonic interposition in an effort to replace the destroyed esophagus. The patient may be incapable of tolerating solid foods for prolonged periods.

Two special household corrosive circumstances merit special discussion. Hair relaxing gels and pastes are alkaline corrosive, but due to their packaging and physical properties they are typically smeared onto the face, lips, and tongue by curious young children. These agents may cause dramatic lip swelling, but rarely cause esophageal or systemic injury. Laundry pods (single-use detergent sacs) are commonly bitten by young children due to their ubiquitous availability and colorful marketing. Asymptomatic children may be observed at home, but children with vomiting should be evaluated emergently as local corrosive injury, CNS depression, and apnea have all been described.

Hydrocarbons

Hydrocarbons are carbon compounds that become liquid at room temperature. The term *hydrocarbon* is somewhat confusing and is often used interchangeably with the term *petroleum distillates*. However, whereas all petroleum distillates are hydrocarbons, not all hydrocarbons are petroleum distillates (e.g., pine oil). Hydrocarbons can be found in solvents, fuels, household cleaners, and polishes.

Hydrocarbons are typically divided into three categories: the aliphatic hydrocarbons, the aromatics, and the "toxic" hydrocarbons. The aliphatic hydrocarbons are petroleum distillates and are found in such household products as furniture polish, lamp oils, and lighter fluids. The aromatic hydrocarbons are cyclic structures and include toluene, xylene, and benzene. These agents are found in solvents, glues, nail polish, paints, and paint removers. The "toxic" hydrocarbons consist of a broad class of substances that possesses no specific profile of toxicity. These agents include halogenated hydrocarbons and hydrocarbons that serve as vehicles for toxic substances such as pesticides.

The major toxicity of hydrocarbons varies from class to class. However, the feature that these agents have in common is a low viscosity and surface tension that permits them to spread freely over large surface areas, such as the lungs, when ingested. This property (plus their solvent actions) leads to a necrotizing, potentially fatal chemical pneumonitis (Fig. 110.9) when these compounds are aspirated. The high volatility of these substances is responsible for alterations in mental status, including narcosis, inebriation, and frank coma. In addition to these toxicities, the solvents possess additional toxicities (see "Inhalants" section), including the risk of bone marrow injury (in the case of benzene). Finally, with the toxic hydrocarbons, additional toxicities may occur as a result of actions such as cardiotoxicity or as a result of the pharmacologic properties of the other agents contained within these

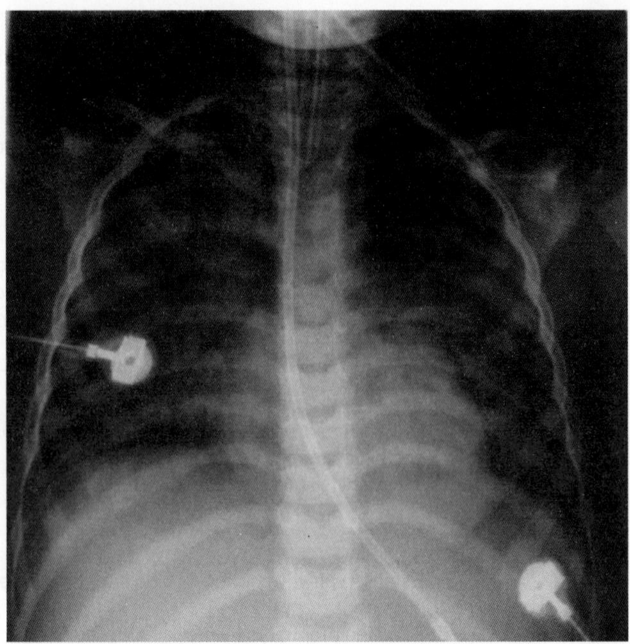

FIGURE 110.9 Chest radiographic findings in a young girl subsequent to lamp oil ingestion.

compounds. The major toxicity of hydrocarbons is classified in Table 110.15.

The amount of a hydrocarbon that has been ingested by a pediatric patient is often difficult to quantify. However, any degree of aspiration results in signs, including coughing, gagging, or tachypnea. Less than 1 mL of some compounds, when aspirated directly into the trachea, may produce severe pneumonitis and eventual death. When ingested, these compounds are poorly absorbed from the GI tract.

TABLE 110.15

CLASSIFICATION OF HYDROCARBONS

Nontoxic (unless complicated by gross aspiration)
Asphalt, tars
Mineral oil
Liquid petrolatum
Motor oil, axle grease
Baby oils, suntan oils
Systemic toxicity
Halogenated (carbon tetrachloride, trichloroethane)
Aromatic (benzene, toluene, xylene)
Additives (camphor, organophosphates, heavy metals)
Aspiration hazard **(without significant systemic toxicity unless ingested in massive quantity)**
Lamp oil/torch oil
Turpentine
Gasoline
Kerosene
Mineral seal oil (furniture polish)
Charcoal lighter fluid
Cigarette lighter fluid
Mineral spirits

The major aspiration hazard associated with hydrocarbons can be quantified by their viscosity. Products with a viscosity of 150 to 250 Saybolt seconds units (SSU), such as oils, pose a small risk of chemical pneumonitis; those with a viscosity less than 60 SSU, such as furniture oils or polishes, have a high aspiration hazard.

Clinical manifestations of hydrocarbon ingestion depend largely on the specific profile of toxicity of the ingested substances. These agents cause significant GI irritation that may be associated with nausea and bloody emesis. CNS effects may range from inebriation to coma. Hemolysis with hemoglobinuria has been reported after significant ingestions. Finally, hydrocarbon ingestion may be associated with the development of fever and leukocytosis in up to 15% of patients in the absence of clinically evident pneumonitis.

Because most hydrocarbons cause clinical toxicity only when aspirated, the mainstay of treatment is to leave ingested compounds in the gut (when possible) and to prevent emesis or reflux. Gastric emptying remains controversial for those compounds with the potential for systemic toxic effects (Table 110.15). These compounds include the halogenated hydrocarbons (e.g., trichloroethane, carbon tetrachloride) and aromatic hydrocarbons (e.g., toluene, xylene, benzene). In addition, some petroleum distillates contain dangerous additives, such as heavy metals or insecticides.

Patients who have aspirated may exhibit immediate choking, coughing, and gagging as the product is swallowed and then vomited after ingestion. Aspiration of the product may also occur at the time of the initial swallowing. ED management of these patients is outlined in Figure 110.10.. If the patient has any cough or respiratory symptoms upon arrival to the ED, a chest radiograph should be obtained immediately. Because there is a gradual evolution of abnormal radiographs, an initially negative chest radiograph should be repeated at 4 to 6 hours after ingestion. All patients with abnormal chest radiographs or persistent respiratory symptoms after 4 to 6 hours of ED observation warrant further medical observation. Patients who are asymptomatic after this period of observation may be discharged. Because pneumonitis occasionally appears 12 to 24 hours after exposure, detailed instructions should be provided for warning signs of respiratory dysfunction.

Treatment of hydrocarbon pneumonitis consists of airway control if there is mental status depression and mechanical ventilation if ventilation is impaired. Adult respiratory distress syndrome may ensue, and heroic measures such as extracorporeal membrane oxygenation have been successfully employed. Antibiotics should not be used prophylactically but should be reserved for specific infections if they develop. The use of corticosteroids in the treatment of aspiration from hydrocarbons has been associated with increased morbidity and is not recommended. In the event of hypotension or bronchospasm, epinephrine is contraindicated because hydrocarbons are known to cause ventricular irritability and predispose to fibrillation, an effect that is exacerbated by catecholamines.

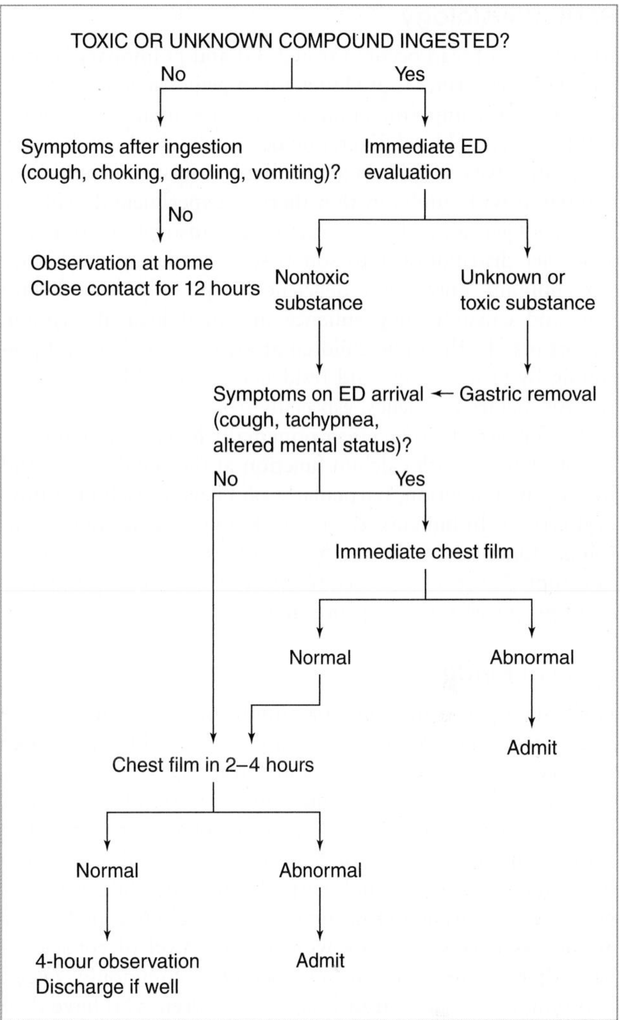

FIGURE 110.10 Management of petroleum distillate ingestion. ED, emergency department.

Lead

Background

Although lead poisoning is usually the result of chronic ingestion by pica-prone children or of occupational exposure in adults, patients with lead poisoning may come to the ED with varied complaints of recent onset that often mimic diverse acute illnesses. Fortunately, severe lead encephalopathy is now rare, attributable in large part to widespread screening programs and early recognition of asymptomatic or mildly ill children. However, the risk of lead intoxication still exists, and emergency physicians and pediatricians in every community must maintain an index of suspicion.

Sources of Lead

The major source of excess lead absorption in children is lead-based paint, widely used in home interiors through the 1950s. In addition to the ingestion of macroscopic-size chips of paint, children are often exposed to house dust with a high lead content that results from finely crumbled paint particles, which gets on their hands and toys. Repetitive mouthing can lead to increased lead exposure even in the absence of observable pica. Home renovation including anding, stripping, and burning of lead-based paint from woodwork in houses has been associated with an increased risk of lead intoxication in the occupants. Other unusual sources of lead exposure include the burning of battery casings for heat or recycling of batteries, water carried by outdated lead pipes, improperly home-glazed ceramics, lead contamination of imported spices or cosmetics, and dust or dirt contaminated by vehicles which once used leaded gasoline.

Pathophysiology

Absorption of lead occurs through GI and pulmonary routes, although the former is predominant in pediatric intoxications. Lead is then compartmentalized into three main areas: bone, soft tissues, and blood. Excretion occurs slowly through urine, feces, and sweat. Children are probably at double jeopardy as compared with adults in that there is experimental evidence that younger animals have increased absorption and also a heavier distribution into soft tissues (including the brain). Concomitant nutritional deficiency, especially low dietary iron and calcium, may enhance intestinal lead absorption. Unfortunately, the same children at greatest risk for lead poisoning by virtue of age and residence are also likely to be at risk for dietary deficiency, especially iron.

Lead exerts its toxic effect principally by two mechanisms: by interference with calcium function at the cellular level and by enzyme inhibition, particularly on enzymes rich in sulfhydryl groups. In humans, the most obvious effects are on neurologic function and on the hemesynthesis pathway, which is interrupted at several points, resulting in abnormally high levels of porphyrins and their precursors.

Clinical Findings

Early signs and symptoms of plumbism are notably vague and nonspecific. Abdominal complaints, including colicky pain, constipation, anorexia, and intermittent vomiting, are common; of course, these same symptoms are often ascribed to relatively normal 2-year-old children by their parents. The child with early plumbism may also show listlessness and irritability. When encephalopathy begins, the child develops persistent vomiting and becomes drowsy, clumsy, or frankly ataxic. As encephalopathy worsens, the level of consciousness deteriorates further, and seizures commonly occur. Pathologic examination of brains of children who have died of lead encephalopathy shows severe cerebral edema with vascular damage; intracranial pressure is often, although not invariably, increased during the encephalopathy. When spinal fluid is examined, it often reveals a picture similar to that of aseptic meningitis with a mononuclear pleocytosis and elevated protein; however, lumbar puncture should be avoided if possible because of the risk of subsequent herniation. Peripheral neuropathy often occurs in adults with lead poisoning but is rare in children, although it is seen occasionally in those with an underlying hemoglobinopathy. Other organs may be damaged by lead. The kidneys may develop disturbances that range from slight aminoaciduria to a full Fanconi syndrome with glycosuria and phosphaturia (in addition to aminoaciduria). High blood lead level (BLL) is also associated with a microcytic anemia that results from a defect in hemoglobin synthesis. However, much of the anemia seen in children with excess BLL may be caused by concurrent iron deficiency. A moderately sensitive laboratory measure of lead effect on heme synthesis is the evaluation of erythrocyte protoporphyrin (EP), a heme precursor. Moderately elevated EP levels are seen in iron deficiency, but levels above 250 to 300 μg per dL are almost always the result of chronic lead poisoning.

Management

There is no safe threshold for lead exposure and the 97.5% for BLLs among young US children is 5 μg/dL. The most important treatment for lead poisoning is to remove the lead exposure from the child's environment. The asymptomatic child discovered to have a BLL in the 5 to 44 μg per dL range, warrants environmental investigation for lead hazards and prudent follow-up by primary healthcare provider. Such children warrant thorough environmental investigation, clinical and nutritional evaluation, and case management to reduce lead exposure as expeditiously as possible. All symptomatic children and those with BLL higher than 44 μg per dL warrant urgent treatment as outlined next.

The remainder of this discussion is addressed primarily to the early recognition and treatment of plumbism, including acute lead encephalopathy. This single aspect of chronic childhood lead poisoning is focused on because it represents a true medical emergency.

Recognition

Ideally, a child's future home and school environment should be evaluated for lead hazards preconception. Children are at increased risk for asymptomatic elevation of BLLs if they spend time in a building built before 1978, have Medicaid-based health insurance, live within a community known to have a geographic epidemic of lead poisoning, have other identifiable lead exposures, or if they have immigrated to the United States from many other countries. The recognition of mildly symptomatic patients with lead poisoning (or asymptomatic children with high lead levels, who are at great risk to soon become symptomatic) requires a high index of suspicion. All children between 1 and 5 years of age are suspect if they have (i) persistent vomiting, listlessness or irritability, clumsiness, or loss of recently acquired developmental skills; (ii) afebrile convulsions; (iii) a strong tendency to pica, including a history of acute exploratory ingestions or aural or nasal foreign body; (iv) a deteriorating pre-World War II house or a parent with industrial exposures; (v) a family history of lead poisoning; (vi) iron-deficiency anemia; or (vii) evidence of child abuse or neglect.

The child between ages of 1 to 5 years who comes to the ED with an acute encephalopathy and the above-cited risk factors presents the physician with a dilemma: lead intoxication requires urgent diagnosis, but confirmation with a BLL is usually not available on an immediate basis. A constellation of historical features of lead poisoning increases the likelihood of the diagnosis. These features include (i) a prodromal illness of several days' to weeks' duration (suggestive of mild symptomatic plumbism); (ii) a history of pica; and (iii) a source of exposure to lead. Several nonspecific laboratory findings make lead poisoning likely enough to warrant presumptive chelation therapy until confirmation by lead levels is available. These findings include (i) microcytic anemia; (ii) elevated EP level, especially if higher than 250 μg per dL (conversely, a normal or minimally elevated EP level, less than 50 μg per dL, would make lead encephalopathy caused by chronic lead paint exposure unlikely); (iii) basophilic stippling of peripheral erythrocytes or, if feasible, of red blood cell precursors on bone marrow examination; (iv) glycosuria; (v) aminoaciduria; (vi) radiopaque flecks on abdominal radiographs; and (vii) dense metaphyseal bands on radiographs of knees and wrists (lead lines—Fig. 110.11).

Abnormalities on examination of cerebrospinal fluid (CSF) are also indicative of lead encephalopathy, including a lymphocytic pleocytosis, elevated protein level, and increased pressure. However, a lumbar puncture should not be performed if lead encephalopathy is strongly suspected because

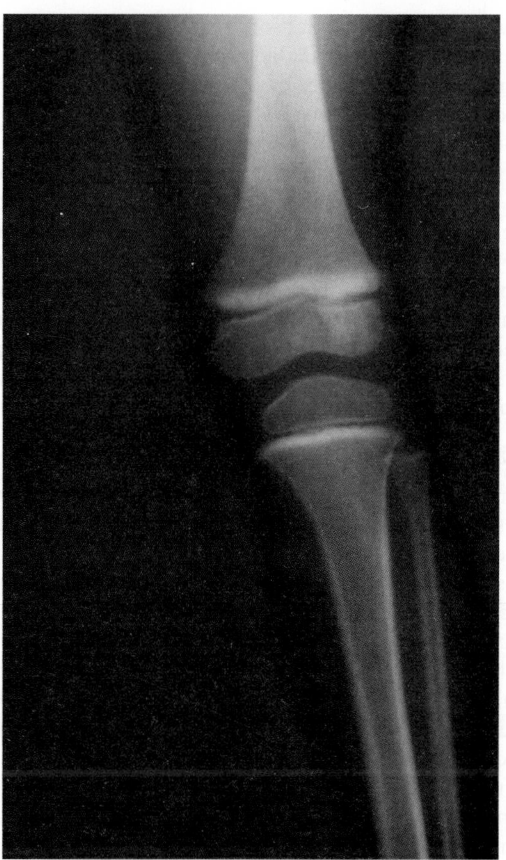

FIGURE 110.11 Knee radiograph demonstrating increased calcium deposition at metaphysis—the so-called "lead lines." (Reproduced with permission from Henretig FM. A toddler in status epilepticus. In: Osterhoudt KC, Perrone J, DeRoos F, et al., eds. *Toxicology pearls.* Philadelphia, PA: Hanley & Belfus, 2004:S2–S5.)

the risk of herniation is considerable. If CSF must be examined to rule out bacterial meningitis, the minimal amount (less than 1 mL) necessary should be obtained. Alternatively, one might institute treatment for presumed meningitis, perform a determination of BLL, and consider a delayed lumbar puncture after several days if the BLL is normal.

Treatment

The treatment of lead poisoning involves relocation of the child to a lead-free environment, consideration of chelation therapy, and appropriate supportive care. Symptomatic patients are at risk of developing encephalopathy with subsequent death or neurologic sequelae. In addition, asymptomatic patients with high BLL (especially higher than 100 μg per dL) are also at significant risk for developing CNS involvement and might require urgent treatment.

The specific chelating drugs commonly used for symptomatic lead intoxication are edetate calcium disodium (CaEDTA) and 2,4-dimercaptopropanol (British Anti-Lewisite [BAL]; Table 110.16). Side effects of CaEDTA include local reactions at injection sites, fever, hypercalcemia, and renal dysfunction manifested by rising BUN and abnormal urine sediment with proteinuria, hematuria, and/or epithelial cells. The major side effects of BAL include nausea and vomiting, so for the first day or two of BAL therapy, it is prudent to maintain the patient on IV fluids and clear liquids or nothing by mouth. BAL is formulated in peanut oil, is given only by IM injection, and also induces hemolysis in patients with G6PD deficiency. Its use is hazardous if the patient has severe hepatic dysfunction, and it forms a toxic complex if given concurrently with iron. Succimer (dimercaptosuccinic acid [DMSA]) has been approved for pediatric use in cases in which BLL exceeds 45 μg per dL (Table 110.16). This water-soluble analog of BAL may be taken orally, and several studies have found such use to be as effective as CaEDTA given parenterally. Some centers use d-penicillamine as an enteral form of chelation for elevated BLLs.

Asymptomatic children found to have BLL of 45 to 69 μg per dL should have urgent referral and treatment with oral DMSA (typically a 19-day course) or parenteral CaEDTA for 5 days (Table 110.15). If the BLL is higher than 69 μg per dL, combination therapy is initiated with both BAL and EDTA; the BAL may be discontinued in many cases after 2 to 3 days, but CaEDTA is continued for 5 days. Supportive care includes adequate hydration to promote good urine output. Symptomatic children without frank encephalopathy should receive chelation therapy with a combination of BAL for 3 to 5 days

TABLE 110.16

GUIDELINES FOR CHELATION THERAPY OF LEAD POISONING

Condition, BLL	Regimen[a]	Comment
Encephalopathy	BAL 450 mg/m^2/day +	75 mg/m^2 IM every 4 hrs for 5 days
	$CaNa_2EDTA$ 1,500 mg/m^2/day	Continuous infusion, or 2–4 divided IV doses, for 5 days (start 4 hrs after BAL)
Symptomatic, and/or BLL > 70	BAL 300–450 mg/m^2/day	50–75 mg/m^2 every 4 hrs for 3–5 days (see text)
	$CaNa_2EDTA$ 1,000–1,500 mg/m^2/day	Continuous infusion, or 2–4 divided IV doses, for 5 days (start 4 hrs after BAL)
Asymptomatic, BLL 45–69	Succimer 700–1,050 mg/m^2/day	350 mg/m^2 TID for 5 days, then BID for 14 days
	or	
	$CaNa_2EDTA$, 1,000 mg/m^2/day	Continuous infusion, or 2–4 divided IV doses, for 5 days

[a]Doses expressed in mg/kg: BAL 450 mg/m^2 (24 mg/kg), 300 mg/m^2 (18 mg/kg); $CaNa_2EDTA$ 1,000 mg/m^2 (25–50 mg/kg), 1,500 mg/m^2 (50–75 mg/kg); Succimer 350 mg/m^2 (10 mg/kg).
BLL, blood lead level (μg/dL); BAL, British Anti-Lewisite; IM, intramuscular; IV, intravenous.
Adapted from American Academy of Pediatrics, Committee on Drugs. Treatment guidelines for lead exposure in children. *Pediatrics* 1995;1996:155–160; and Henretig FM. Lead. In: Goldfrank LR, Flomenbaum NE, Lewin NA, et al., eds. *Goldfrank's toxicologic emergencies,* 9th ed. New York, NY: McGraw-Hill, 2009.

and CaEDTA for 5 days. Supportive care includes close monitoring for signs of encephalopathy and, again, maintenance of urine flow.

Patients with encephalopathy require combination chelation therapy with higher dose CaEDTA and BAL for 5 days, as well as intensive supportive care. Fluid therapy is critical and must be individualized. Adequate urine flow is needed to excrete the lead–chelate complexes; however, fluid overload must be avoided so that cerebral edema is not exacerbated. A reasonable goal is to supply basal water requirements, maintaining urine production at 0.35 to 0.5 mL per kcal per 24 hours. Basal water needs in children average 1 mL per kcal and may be calculated as 100 kcal per kg for 0 to 10 kg, plus 50 kcal per kg for 10 to 20 kg, plus 20 kcal per kg for each kilogram above 20 kg.

Seizures commonly occur in acute encephalopathy and should be controlled with anticonvulsant drugs (see Chapter 67 Seizures). Hypothetical precautions have been made about the use of phenobarbital in lead encephalopathy (i.e., synergistic disturbances in porphyrin metabolism), but its clinical use has not been associated with any noticeable deleterious effect. Recent advances have been made in the management of cerebral edema and increased intracranial pressure (see Chapter 130 Neurosurgical Emergencies), but have not been evaluated in controlled fashion in the context of lead encephalopathy.

Organophosphates

Background

Organophosphates are lipid-soluble insecticides that are commonly applied in sprayed dust or emulsion formulations. These compounds are found in agricultural and home use, and they form the basis of "nerve gases" in chemical warfare agents. Organophosphates are readily degraded in the environment and metabolized in mammals by hydraulic cleavage. Some of these chemicals are "systemic" insecticides, meaning that they are taken up by the roots of the plants and translocated into foliage, flowers, and/or fruits.

Pathophysiology

Compounds of this class can be absorbed by inhalation, ingestion, and skin penetration. They irreversibly phosphorylate the enzyme acetylcholinesterase in tissues, allowing acetylcholine accumulation at cholinergic junctions in autonomic effector sites (causing muscarinic effects), in skeletal muscle or autonomic ganglia (causing nicotinic effects), and in the CNS.

Clinical Findings

The symptoms of acute poisoning usually develop during the first 12 hours of contact. These include findings related to the CNS (dizziness, headache, ataxia, convulsions, and coma); nicotinic signs, including sweating, muscle twitching, tremors, weakness, and paralysis; and muscarinic signs characterized by the SLUDGE mnemonic (including *s*alivation, *l*acrimation, *u*rination, *d*efecation, GI cramping, and *e*mesis). In addition there may be miosis, bradycardia, bronchorrhea, and wheezing; in severe cases, pulmonary edema develops. Severe intoxications may also cause a toxic psychosis that resembles alcoholism.

A history of exposure to organophosphates and the clinical manifestations already discussed are the best clues to an organophosphate poisoning. A depression of plasma or red blood cell cholinesterase activity provides the best laboratory marker of excessive absorption of organophosphates, although it is rarely available on a stat basis. A decrease in the cholinesterase activity of the red blood cells is more specific for organophosphate inhibition than is the plasma assay. Although plasma cholinesterase is depressed by liver injury from various causes and a small percentage of the population has a genetically determined deficiency of plasma cholinesterase activity, a depression of 25% or more is a strong evidence of excessive organophosphate absorption. However, it is important that treatment not be delayed until confirmation of plasma cholinesterase is obtained. Note that children may also encounter acetylcholinesterase inhibitors if they ingest an adult's medication for Alzheimer or Parkinson disease (i.e., rivastigmine, donepezil, tacrine, and galantamine).

Management

The management of a patient who has ingested organophosphates must always include safeguards against exposure for the persons who treat the patient because the organophosphates are readily absorbed through the skin and mucous membranes. Patients who have been poisoned by the topical application of organophosphates should receive a thorough scrubbing with a soap solution on admission to prevent further absorption of organophosphates. In addition, all contaminated clothing must be removed and stored in a plastic bag to protect the institutional personnel.

After decontamination, antidotal therapy begins with the administration of atropine sulfate given in a dose of 0.05 to 0.1 mg per kg to children and 2 to 5 mg for adolescents and adults. This dose should be repeated every 10 to 30 minutes or as needed to obtain and maintain full atropinization, as indicated by an end point of clearing bronchial secretions and pulmonary rales. Therapy is continued until all absorbed organophosphate has been metabolized and may require 2 mg to more than 2,000 mg of atropine over the course of a few hours to several days. After atropinization has been instituted, severe poisonings should be treated with the addition of pralidoxime. This drug is particularly useful in poisonings characterized by profound weakness and muscle twitching. A dose of 25 to 50 mg per kg should be administered in 100 mL of saline by infusion over approximately 30 minutes; adults may receive 1 to 2 g by IV. In life-threatening situations, 50% of the initial pralidoxime dose may be infused over 2 minutes, followed by the remainder of the dose over 30 minutes. After loading, a 1% concentration may be infused continuously at the rate of 500 mg per hour in adolescents and adults, or approximately 10 mg per kg per hour in children, and can be titrated to clinical effect. Occasionally, patients may require more than 48 hours of therapy; the end point should be persistent relief of neurologic and cholinergic signs.

Organophosphates are usually dissolved in hydrocarbon bases; thus, the clinician should be prepared to treat hydrocarbon pneumonitis if it develops. Also, bronchopneumonia that complicates the pulmonary edema has been observed in acute poisonings.

Because the organophosphates cause elevated levels of acetylcholine in the plasma, compounds that affect the uptake of acetylcholine and/or its release should be avoided in the management of these patients. Specifically, aminophylline and phenothiazines are contraindicated.

Carbamate insecticides have a similar mechanism of action to organophosphate insecticides but the phosphorylation of acetylcholinesterase is reversible and temporary. Pralidoxime therapy is generally regarded as unnecessary after poisoning from carbamates.

PLANTS/MUSHROOMS

Plant Toxicity

Plants are among the more commonly reported exploratory ingestions in children. Most such ingestions involve common house and garden plants. Fortunately, of the many varieties of such plants, only a small fraction poses a serious toxic hazard (Tables 110.17 and 110.18).

When a child visits the ED after plant ingestion, a general evaluation should be performed. Activated charcoal may be useful in adsorbing plant toxins. The child who remains asymptomatic after a period of observation may then be discharged and observed at home. Children who develop symptoms or for whom there is strong suspicion or confirmation that the ingested plant poses a potentially serious intoxication should be admitted for further observation and specific or supportive treatment.

TABLE 110.17

COMMON NONTOXIC PLANTS

Abelia	Echeveria
African daisy	Eugenia
African palm	Gardenia
African violet	Grape ivy
Airplane plant	Hedge apples
Aluminum plant	Hens and chicks
Aralia	Honeysuckle
Asparagus fern (may cause dermatitis)	Hoya
Aspidistra (cast iron plant)	Impatiens
Aster	Jade plant
Baby's tears	Kalanchoe
Bachelor buttons	Lily (day, Easter, or tiger)
Begonia	Lipstick plant
Bird's nest fern	Magnolia
Blood leaf plant	Marigold
Boston ferns	Monkey plant
Bougainvillea	Mother-in-law tongue
Cactus—certain varieties	Norfolk Island pine
California holly	Peperomia
California poppy	Petunia
Camellia	Prayer plant
Christmas cactus	Purple passion
Coleus	Pyracantha
Corn plant	Rose
Crab apples	Sansevieria
Creeping Charlie	Schefflera
Creeping Jennie, moneywort, lysima	Sensitive plant
Croton (house variety)	Spider plant
Dahlia	Swedish ivy
Daisies	Umbrella
Dandelion	Violets
Dogwood	Wandering jew
Donkey tail	Weeping fig
Dracaena	Weeping willow
Easter lily	Wild onion
	Zebra plant

TABLE 110.18

COMMON PLANT TOXIDROMES

Gastrointestinal irritants
- Philodendron
- Dieffenbachia
- Pokeweed
- Wisteria
- Spurge laurel
- Buttercup
- Daffodil
- Rosary pea
- Castor bean

Digitalis effects
- Lily-of-the-valley
- Foxglove
- Oleander
- Yew

Nicotinic effects
- Wild tobacco
- Golden chain tree
- Poison hemlock

Atropinic effects
- Jimsonweed (thorn apple)
- Deadly nightshade

Epileptogenic effects
- Water hemlock

Cyanogenic effects
- Prunus species (chokecherry, wild black cherry, plum, peach, apricot, bitter almond)
- Pear (seeds)
- Apple (seeds)
- Crab apple (seeds)
- Hydrangea
- Elderberry

Specific Categories of Plant Toxidromes

Plants with GI Irritation

Plants that cause GI irritation account for most plant poisonings in the United States. The range of symptoms extends from mild oral burning to a severe gastroenteritis syndrome. Representative species include *Philodendron* and *Dieffenbachia* species (leaves), which cause minor mouth and throat burning; pokeweed (roots, stem), Wisteria (seeds), spurge laurel (berries), buttercup (leaves), and daffodil (bulbs, accidentally substituted for onions), which cause severe vomiting, colicky abdominal pain, and diarrhea; and the toxalbumin-containing plants such as rosary pea and castor bean (seeds), which can

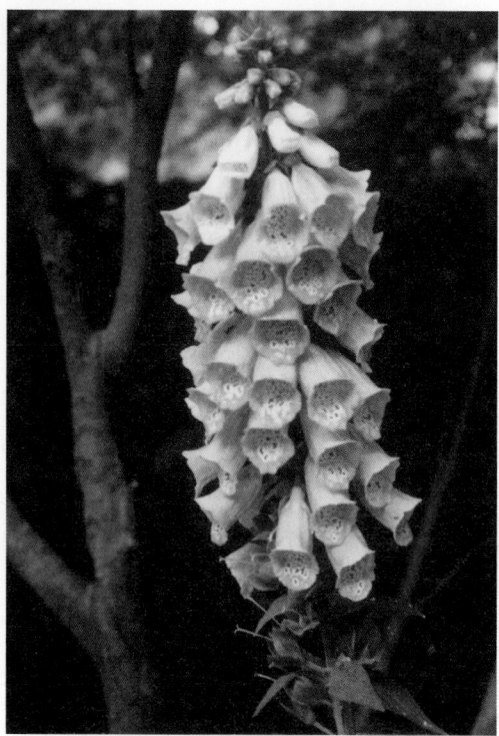
FIGURE 110.12 The foxglove plant (*Digitalis purpurea*).

cause a violent hemorrhagic gastroenteritis that leads to profound dehydration and circulatory collapse when the seeds are chewed up. The management of this group of ingestions consists essentially of fluid and electrolyte therapy.

Plants with Digitalis Effects

Several common garden or wildflowers contain digitalis, and they have been responsible for fatal ingestions. Instances of chewing on leaves or flowers or swallowing the berries of lily-of-the-valley, foxglove (Fig. 110.12), red squill, and oleander all have led to such poisonings. Intoxication has even occurred when water from a vase that contained these flowers was ingested. Early after ingestion, the child may complain of intestinal symptoms such as mouth irritation, vomiting, and diarrhea. As the digitalis is absorbed, typical digitalis effects may ensue, with conduction defects and, at times, serious arrhythmias. Treatment may include administration of digoxin-specific antibody fragments as was previously discussed.

Plants with Nicotinic Effects

Several species of plants contain nicotine or closely related alkaloids. Ingestion of wild tobacco (leaves), golden chain tree (seeds), and poison hemlock (leaves, seeds) usually leads to spontaneous vomiting within 1 hour. Salivation, headache, fever, mental confusion, and muscular weakness may follow, and the child may deteriorate to convulsions, coma, and death from respiratory failure. Inhaling vapors of concentrated nicotine liquids is rising in popularity; ingestion of these electronic cigarette nicotine liquids poses risk for exploratory or self-injurious ingestion of concentrated nicotine. Treatment consists of intensive supportive care, with anticonvulsants and ventilatory assistance.

Plants with Atropinic Effects

The most common atropine-containing plant in the United States is jimsonweed, which is widely distributed. Cases most commonly occur in rural areas but have been seen even in inner-city children who managed to find this weed growing in their neighborhoods, where flora in general is scarce.

Symptoms and signs are those of atropinization (Table 110.6) and include visual blurring, dilated pupils, dryness of the mouth, hot and dry skin, fever, delirium, and psychosis. Convulsions and coma may follow. Treatment consists of supportive care and, in severe cases, physiologic antagonism with physostigmine (Table 110.10).

Plants that Cause Convulsions

Convulsions represent the principal toxic effect of some plants. Water hemlock, with its potent cicutoxin, is the main species to cause convulsions in the United States. Within 1 hour after ingestion, nausea, vomiting, and profuse salivation occur. These initial symptoms are followed by tremors, muscle rigidity, and multiple major motor seizures. Treatment is with anticonvulsants, as for status epilepticus.

Plants that Contain Cyanogenic Glycosides

Many plants and particularly fruit seeds (pits) contain the cyanogenic glycoside amygdalin (Table 110.16). However, these glycosides are relatively protected within the seeds and would be unlikely to cause illness after an exploratory ingestion by a young child.

Symptoms and signs after ingestion are those of cyanide poisoning, with resultant cellular hypoxia. Initially, there is CNS stimulation and headache, with tachypnea, hypertension, and reflex bradycardia. Anxiety and excitation may progress to opisthotonus and seizures. Respiratory depression, with cyanosis, tachycardia, and hypotension, follows. An odor of bitter almonds may be detected. Treatment is initiated with 100% oxygen and cardiopulmonary resuscitation as necessary. Antidotal therapy for cyanide poisoning, with hydroxocobalamin, or with nitrates and sodium thiosulfate, is detailed in Table 110.10.

Mushrooms

Mushrooms cause an estimated 50% of all deaths from plant and fungi poisoning in the United States. The difficulty in accurate identification of mushrooms makes reliance on such identification for appropriate management of ingestions extremely hazardous in the ED.

Two main groups of mushrooms can be characterized on the basis of the time interval between ingestion and symptom onset: those with the immediate onset of symptoms and those with delayed onset. Regardless of the mushroom, the initial management for all suspected poisonings includes consideration of activated charcoal and other GI decontamination strategies.

Onset of symptoms within 6 hours of ingestion usually confers a benign prognosis, although careful attention to fluid and electrolyte management is critical. Most mushrooms have GI effects. There are several general classes of mushrooms in this group, each possessing a unique toxicologic feature. Some "early-onset" mushrooms cause muscarinic effects, usually within 15 minutes, such as sweating, salivation, colic, and pulmonary edema. This syndrome responds to atropine therapy. Other early-onset mushrooms cause anticholinergic effects, including drowsiness, followed by mania and hallucinations.

Another subgroup of early-onset mushrooms produces a severe gastroenteritis syndrome. Hallucinogenic mushrooms such as those containing psilocybin make up another class of mushrooms with early-onset symptoms. Finally, some mushrooms precipitate a disulfiram-like reaction if they are coingested with alcohol. Management for all these agents consists of supportive care and careful monitoring of fluid status.

The second, more important, category of mushrooms that are responsible for 90% of mushroom-related deaths are those typically associated with onset of symptoms that occur more than 6 hours after ingestion. The most important members of this group are those mushrooms that belong to the *Amanita phalloides* species. With these mushrooms, after a latent period of many hours, GI upset appears. Approximately 24 hours after ingestion, hepatic dysfunction appears, which may progress to fulminant hepatic failure. Without liver transplantation, such patients generally die.

Two compounds are known to produce the toxic effects of *A. phalloides*. Phallotoxin acts first, causing GI symptoms, including nausea, vomiting, abdominal pain, and diarrhea. Fever, tachycardia, and hyperglycemia may also occur during this stage. The other toxin, amatoxin, causes renal tubular and hepatic necrosis.

Treatment of the gastroenteric phase includes fluid and electrolyte replacement. If renal failure develops, dialysis may be necessary. Hepatic damage after *A. phalloides* ingestion may be attenuated by early use of repetitive activated charcoal, which appears to interrupt enterohepatic recirculation of amatoxin.

Additional therapies have shown mixed results in the treatment of *A. phalloides* poisoning. High-dose penicillin, cimetidine, *n*-acetylcysteine, thioctic acid, silibinin, prophylactic charcoal hemoperfusion, and other modalities await further investigation. A regional poison control center may offer guidance with experimental therapies, but multiple-dose activated charcoal and vigorous attention to supportive care remain the standard. For patients with poor prognosis, early referral for liver transplantation may be lifesaving.

SUBSTANCE ABUSE

As a special category of pediatric toxicology, exposures to psychoactive drugs are outlined in this section. In addition to the classically thought of substances of abuse, it is important to remember that misused and abused substances also include prescription medications (notably ADHD medicines and opioids), OTC medications, herbal products, supplements, and emerging synthetic agents. Three distinct age populations in the pediatric group may be placed at risk from exposures related to substance abuse and misuse: (i) The adolescent or preadolescent who abuses drugs for their mind-altering effects; (ii) the neonate who is exposed to substances of abuse during gestation and manifests signs of intoxication or abstinence after birth; and (iii) the infant or toddler who becomes exposed to drugs of abuse through either active administration by a caregiver (chemical child abuse), the ingestion of a drug left in an accessible place (e.g., the coffee table), or passive exposure created by being in an environment where drugs of abuse are used (e.g., marijuana, cocaine, phencyclidine [PCP], methamphetamine). In any of these circumstances, the exposure can be sufficient to produce severe intoxication. Thus, knowledge of the epidemiology and manifestations of substance abuse become important in the management of children of all ages.

Clinical Manifestations

The drug-abusing child or adolescent may present to the ED after an unintentional overdose, an intentional overdose, with sudden alteration of mental status or bizarre behavior, or in the setting of multiple trauma (e.g., assault, motor vehicle collision). Often, the history of drug exposure is undeclared and may not be diagnosed unless there is a high index of suspicion and appropriate diagnostic evaluation. In such cases, the patient's mental status can range from fully awake and responsive to comatose; physical examination can be without any signs of drug exposure or with overt signs of toxicity (e.g., seizures). Table 110.19 provides a summary of the common drugs of abuse, their typical routes of administration, associated symptoms, toxic levels, and duration of action.

Initial history from the patient, family, or friends must seek to clarify potentially ingested substances and estimate the quantity ingested if possible. In the absence of a history of exposure, it is important to inquire whether the patient has used any psychoactive drugs in the past. In many cases, the patient may admit to using a drug but may identify it by a street name. Although drug terminology tables are often available in pharmacology or toxicology texts or on the Internet, temporal and regional changes in street drug terminology generally make such tables of limited value. Your local poison center can be a useful source of current information and regional trends.

Management

As with any potentially poisoned patient, primary attention is initially paid toward assessment of vital signs and life support as needed to provide a patent, secure airway; to ensure adequate respiratory function; and to treat seizures, shock, or cardiorespiratory arrest. A key, but often overlooked, feature in the assessment of such patients is an accurate temperature because many drug intoxications are associated with hyperpyrexia. If there is any suspicion of hyperthermia, a rectal temperature must be obtained. In the agitated patient, physical and/or chemical restraint may be necessary to obtain vital signs. Chemical restraint should be used liberally to prevent patients from harming themselves or others. The preferred agents in such cases are diazepam (0.1 to 0.3 mg per kg IV) or midazolam (0.05 to 0.1 mg per kg IV). Haloperidol (0.05 mg per kg) given IM is also effective but reduces heat-dissipating capability and may lower the seizure threshold.

Management must also include consideration of the need for GI decontamination. With many substances of abuse, several distinct routes of exposure are possible (e.g., ingestion, inhalation, injection, and/or nasal insufflation). Therefore, GI decontamination is not always necessary or appropriate.

However, because those who abuse drugs often use more than one drug, decontamination should be considered if there is any possibility of an ingestion, utilizing the same guiding principles regarding toxin and patient characteristics detailed earlier in this chapter. In the event that decontamination seems appropriate, assessment of the patient's mental status and gag reflex must be performed. If the potential benefits of decontamination are felt to outweigh the risks in a patient with

TABLE 110.19

DRUG ABUSE: SUMMARY OF TOXICITY

Drug of abuse	Symptoms and signs of drug abuse	Diagnosis	Toxic dose	Toxic serum level	Half-life
Cannabis group (marijuana; hashish; Δ9-THC; hash oil)	Pupils unchanged; conjunctiva injected; blood pressure (BP) decreased on standing; heart rate increased; increased appetite, euphoria, anxiety; sensorium often clear; dreamy; fantasy state; time–space distortions; hallucinations rare. Significant airway obstruction with heavy smoking, decreased forced expiratory volume, and decreased vital capacity. Major psychiatric toxic effects: Panic reaction most common Psychotic reactions (especially in patients with underlying psychopathology) Toxic delirium (disorientation, confusion, memory impairment) in heavy users.	Blood, urine levels	20 mg Δ9-THC or 1 g cigarette of 2% Δ9-THC produces effects on mood, memory, motor coordination, cognitive ability sensorium, time sense		*1st phase,* minutes, distribution in lipid-rich tissues; *2nd phase,* 1½–2 days, until mobilized from lipid-rich tissue
Hallucinogens	Pupils dilated (normal or small with PCP); BP elevated, heart rate increased, hyperactive tendon reflexes, increased temperature, flushed face, euphoria, anxiety or panic, paranoid thought disorder, inappropriate affect, time and visual distortions, visual hallucinations, depersonalization.				
LSD	Psychosis with hyperalertness; changes in body image; sense of profound significance, delusions; hallucinations (also with amphetamines), visual perceptual distortions caused by peripheral effects of LSD on visual system.	Blood, urine levels	20–25 μg produce CNS effects; 0.5–2 μg/kg produce somatic symptoms; between 1 and 16 μg/kg intensity of pathophysiologic effects proportional to dose	Variable	3 h
PCP	Cyclic coma, extreme hyperactivity, violent outbursts, bizarre behavior, amnesia, analgesia, nystagmus, gait ataxia, muscle rigidity. Dystonic reactions, grand mal seizures, tardive dyskinesia, athetosis, bronchospasm, urinary retention, diaphoresis, hypoglycemia. Increased uric acid, increased creatine phosphokinase, increased creatinine, increased hepatic transaminases heralds onset of rhabdomyolysis (risk of renal failure).	Blood, gastric contents, urine (but level does not correlate with toxicity)	1 cigarette (PCP) = 1–100 mg. Psychosis may last several weeks after a dose. Fatal dose = 1 mg/kg; <5 mg = hyperactivity; 5–10 mg = stupor, coma; >10 mg = respiratory depression, convulsions	Individual variability (~0.1 μg/mL)	1–3 d
CNS stimulants					
Amphetamines	Pupils dilated and reactive. Increased BP, pulse, temperature, cardiac arrhythmias; dry mouth; sweating; tremors; sensorium hyperacute or confused; paranoid ideation; impulsivity; hyperactivity; stereotypy; convulsions; exhaustion.	Blood level, urine test	1. Variable 2. Rare under 15 mg 3. Severe reactions have occurred at 30 mg 4. 400–500 mg not uniformly fatal 5. Tolerance is striking; chronic user may take 1,700 mg/day without ill effects	Variable	3 h

Cocaine	1. Excitement, restlessness, euphoria, garrulousness. 2. Increased motor activity, physical endurance because of decreased sense of fatigue. 3. Increased tremors, convulsive movements. 4. Increased respiration, pulse, BP, temperature, chills.	Urine, serum	Fatal dose may be as low as 30 mg; ingested cocaine less toxic than by other routes		1 h (after PO or nasal route)
CNS sedatives (barbiturates, chlordiazepoxide, diazepam, flurazepam, glutethimide, meprobamate, methaqualone)	Pupils normal or small (dilated with glutethimide); BP decreased, respirations depressed; drowsy, coma, lateral nystagmus, confusion, ataxia, slurred speech, delirium; convulsions or hyperirritability with methaqualone overdosage; serious poisoning rare with benzodiazepines alone.	Serum level			
Barbiturates (Secobarbital) (Seconal)	As above.	Serum level	100 mg per dose	30 µg/mL	19–34 h
Chlordiazepoxide (Librium)	As above.	Serum level	25 mg	8 µg/mL	8–25 h
Diazepam (Valium)	As above.	Serum, urine	15 mg or greater		20–90 h
Flurazepam (Dalmane)	As above.	Serum, urine	>500 mg (acute intoxication, 3 g)	0.12 µg/mL (fatal)	47–100 h
Glutethimide (Doriden)	As above.	Serum level	>800 mg	2 mg/100 mL (but even below, full ICU support may be required)	5–22 h
Meprobamate	As above.	Serum level	200–400 mg	150 µg/mL	6–17 h
Methaqualone (Parest, Somnafae)	As above.	Serum level		10 µg/mL	20–60 h
Opioids	Pupils constricted (may be dilated with meperidine or extreme hypoxia); respiration depressed to absent with cyanosis; BP decreased, sometimes shock; temperature reduced; reflexes diminished to absent, stupor or coma; pulmonary edema; constipation; convulsions with propoxyphene or meperidine; arrhythmia with propoxyphene.	Serum, urine Serum, urine			
Heroin	As above.	Serum	—	—	1½ h[b]
Morphine	As above.	Serum	60 mg = toxic[a] 200 mg = fatal dose[a]	—	3 h[b]
Codeine	As above.	Serum	800 mg = fatal dose[a]		2 h[b]
Methadone	As above.	Serum	100 mg = fatal dose[a]	1.1 µg/mL	18–97 h[b]

(*continued*)

TABLE 110.19

DRUG ABUSE: SUMMARY OF TOXICITY (*CONTINUED*)

Drug of abuse	Symptoms and signs of drug abuse	Diagnosis	Toxic dose	Toxic serum level	Half-life
Anticholinergics (atropine, belladonna, henbane, scopolamine, trihexyphenidyl, tricyclic antidepressants, benztropine mesylate)	Pupils dilated and fixed, heart rate increased, temperature increased, BP increased; drowsy, coma, flushed, dry skin and mucous membranes, erythematous skin, amnesia, disoriented, visual hallucinations, body image alterations.	Urine test		2 µg/mL (fatal)	
Atropine	As above.		5 mg		24 h
Belladonna	As above.		5 mg		24 h
Scopolamine	As above.		5 mg		24 h
Imipramine (Tofranil)	As above.		500 mg		8–16 h
Amitriptyline (Elavil)	As above.		>500 mg	5 µg/mL	32–40 h
Desipramine	As above.		1 g	10 µg/mL	12–54 h

[a]Higher doses given for patients with addiction.
[b]Duration is for subcutaneous dose. Intravenous dose peak is more pronounced and overall effects have shorter duration.
LSD, lysergamides; ICU, intensive care unit.
Adapted from Dreisbach RH. *Handbook of poisoning*. Los Altos, CA: Lange Medical Publications, 1980.

obtundation or a diminished gag reflex, airway protection by endotracheal intubation should be accomplished before initiating decontamination measures.

Disposition

After initial assessment and medical stabilization, subsequent evaluation of any patient presenting in the setting of intentional substance use must include an estimation of the severity of the drug use problem. Although issues of patient confidentiality may require the physician to provide limited information to parents, obtaining a thorough psychosocial evaluation is necessary for complete management of the acute event. Such discussions may require or may be facilitated by an interview with a social worker or psychiatry consultant. Once the severity of the drug problem has been established, referral to a treatment program should be discussed. Primary care physicians may be comfortable managing patients without long-standing histories of drug abuse. Compulsive users or anyone who presents with a drug abstinence syndrome must be referred for intensive rehabilitation. Family therapy is often a vital component of this rehabilitation.

SPECIFIC DRUGS

The major categories of drugs of abuse that require the physician's familiarity with the whole spectrum of their physiologic effects include (i) hallucinogens (PCP, ketamine, lysergic acid diethylamide, marijuana, synthetic cannabinoids), (ii) stimulants (amphetamines, cocaine, synthetic cathinones), (iii) central anticholinergics, (iv) sedatives (benzodiazepines, barbiturates), (v) opioids (morphine, codeine, heroin, methadone, buprenorphine, oxycodone, and hydrocodone), (vi) inhalants, and (vii) alcohol.

Hallucinogens (Psychedelics)

No single characteristic distinguishes psychedelics from other classes of centrally active drugs such as anticholinergics, cocaine, and amphetamines. These drugs can produce a number of mental status changes, including illusions, hallucinations, delusions, and paranoid ideation. However, the psychedelic state is characteristically described as consisting of vivid and unusual visual experiences with diminished control over what is experienced. Images and sensations take on profound meaning, and the ability to differentiate oneself from the environment is decreased. Most drugs in this category are related to the indolealkylamines (psilocybin, dimethyltryptamine [DMT], diethyltryptamine), lysergamides (LSD), or phenylethylamines (mescaline, methylenedioxymethamphetamine [MDMA, Ecstasy, Molly], synthetic cathinones, the 2C class of drugs).

Phencyclidine, Ketamine, and Dextromethorphan

Identification

PCP was developed in the 1950s as a general anesthetic. It rapidly fell into disuse because of disturbing emergence syndromes that developed in postoperative patients. Sporadic abuse occurred in the 1960s, but its popularity peaked in the 1970s. The drug remains common in several metropolitan areas as does ketamine, a PCP analog with approximately one-tenth the potency and a shorter duration of action. Ketamine is discussed in detail in Chapter 140 Procedural Sedation. Another drug with related structure, but milder effects, is dextromethorphan, which is popular with adolescents because of its ready availability as a legal, OTC cough suppressant. PCP is easily synthesized and is often sold on the streets misrepresented as LSD, mescaline, or marijuana. It is well absorbed across all mucous membranes and is most popularly used by inhalation (often mixed into cigarettes or marijuana "joints"), but it can be ingested, injected, or insufflated.

Pharmacology

Chemically, PCP is an arylcyclohexylamine. This group of drugs has a range of CNS actions that range from hallucinations with smaller doses, to stimulation with moderate doses (occasionally associated with seizures), to profound CNS depression with respiratory arrest with large doses.

There is great variability in the metabolism of PCP. In general, 0.1 μg per mL is considered a toxic serum level. One cigarette may contain 1 to 100 mg. A dose of 5 to 10 mg may produce stupor and coma; with doses exceeding 10 mg, respiratory depression and convulsions occur. A fatal dose is in the range of 1 mg per kg. Because PCP has a long elimination half-life (18 hours), clinical symptoms may last for more than 12 hours; also, patients may have cyclic symptoms because the drug undergoes enterohepatic recirculation.

Pharmacologically, PCP acts as a dissociative anesthetic, meaning that it interferes potently with association pathways that link the cerebral cortex with deeper structures in the brain, thus diminishing the ability to integrate sensory input into meaningful behavior. Its anesthetic actions also lead to a marked diminution of pain sensation. In conjunction with bizarre behavior, this often leads patients to have feelings of invulnerability and to attempt life-threatening actions (e.g., stepping into automobile traffic).

Clinical Symptoms

Small doses of PCP produce signs and symptoms of inebriation with staggering gait, slurred speech, and nystagmus (vertical or rotatory). Users may also be diaphoretic and have catatonic muscular rigidity with a blank stare. Having sympathomimetic actions, use of PCP is often associated with hypertension and tachycardia. Dextromethorphan toxicity resembles the syndrome of low-dose PCP exposure; nystagmus and myoclonus may help distinguish this toxidrome from alcohol or sedative toxicity, and the urine drug screen may be falsely positive for PCP. Moderate doses of PCP cause other signs of intoxication, including hypersalivation, pyrexia, repetitive movements, and muscle rigidity. Larger doses can cause seizures, coma, or respiratory arrest. The typical "high" from a single dose lasts 4 to 6 hours and is followed by an extended "coming down"; PCP-induced psychotic states may be long lasting and may recur (flashbacks). Tolerance develops to the behavioral and toxic effects of the drug. Chronic users report persistent difficulties with recent memory, speech, and thinking that last from 6 months to 1 year after the last dose; they also may be left with personality changes such as withdrawal, isolation, anxiety, nervousness, and depression.

Management

PCP is easily detected through a qualitative analysis of urine. Serum levels are rarely available and do not correlate with clinical manifestations. Therefore, management must often be based solely on a history of exposure or index of suspicion. Initial treatment is directed at stabilizing vital signs and treating life-threatening events such as seizures. If exposure is the result of ingestion, GI decontamination with activated charcoal should be considered. A quiet room may be helpful, although the ability to monitor the patient cannot be compromised. Physical restraints should be avoided if possible because they may lead to significant rhabdomyolysis with resulting myoglobinuria and renal injury. For chemical restraint diazepam (0.1 to 0.3 mg per kg IV) or lorazepam (0.1 mg per kg IV) may be effective, although additional agents (e.g., haloperidol) are often necessary.

Although urine acidification (pH less than 5.0) enhances the urinary excretion of PCP, it should never be performed in these patients because it exacerbates metabolic acidosis and may promote deposition of myoglobin in renal tubules. In a review of 27 confirmed cases of PCP poisoning, three patients developed rhabdomyolysis and two progressed to acute renal failure. Both patients had received acidification measures before diagnosis. If tests for muscle enzymes and/or renal function are abnormal and the urine has a positive test for hemoglobin without red blood cells, the patient should be assumed to have rhabdomyolysis and should be treated accordingly (see Chapter 108 Renal and Electrolyte Emergencies).

LSD (Blotter, Acid)

Pharmacology. LSD and related psychedelic drugs such as psilocybin, mescaline, and DMT have actions at multiple sites in the CNS (from the cortex to the spinal cord). In addition, dozens of congeners of these agents exist in mushrooms or have been synthesized, and they also cause signs and symptoms similar to those of LSD. The pharmacologic action that these drugs seem to have in common is as agonists of presynaptic serotonin-2 receptors (which modulate serotonin release into the synaptic cleft). Most of these agents have structural similarities to serotonin (5-hydroxytryptamine).

In humans, the somatic symptoms of dizziness, weakness, drowsiness, nausea, and paresthesias may be observed after one oral dose of 0.5 to 2 μg per kg. Between the dose range of 1 to 16 μg per kg, the intensity of LSD's psychoactive effects is proportional to the dose. A typical LSD "hit" is 200 to 400 μg. A high degree of tolerance to the behavioral effects develops after three to four daily doses, with sensitivity returning after a drug-free interval. Deaths directly attributable to LSD are virtually unknown, although fatal accidents and suicides have occurred during states of intoxication.

Clinical Symptoms

In general, the somatic effects of hallucinogens are sympathomimetic and include pupillary dilation, hypertension, tachycardia, hyperreflexia, and hyperpyrexia. Doses as low as 20 to 25 μg can produce CNS effects such as euphoria, visual perceptual distortions, alteration of subjective time so time passes slowly, lability of mood, or even an acute panic episode. Hallucinations and psychosis with hyperalertness are commonly seen. The clinical duration of action of LSD is somewhat dose dependent but averages 6 to 12 hours. The psychedelic state includes a heightened awareness of sensory input, often accompanied by an enhanced sense of clarity but a diminished control over what is experienced. There is often a feeling that one part of the self is a passive observer while another part receives vivid sensory input. The ability to separate one object from another or to separate self from the environment is diminished. There is an enhanced sense of oneness with humanity.

Management

LSD intoxication is rarely associated with life-threatening events. However, vital signs should be assessed to ensure that the patient is stable in the event there has been drug coingestion. Because LSD is ingested in minuscule doses and onset of symptoms occurs hours after ingestion, GI decontamination is unnecessary, unless coingestion is suspected.

Clinical management involves placing the patient in a quiet room. Someone who knows the patient may be able to quietly "talk down" and reassure the patient. The patient's loss of boundaries and fear of fragmentation or self-disintegration create a need for a structuring or a supportive environment. Both benzodiazepines (e.g., diazepam 0.1 to 0.3 mg per kg IV or midazolam 0.05 to 0.1 mg per kg IV) and haloperidol (0.05 mg per kg IM) are effective tranquilizers in the event that anxiety or agitation persists.

Marijuana (Pot, Reefer, Smoke, Grass, Hemp)

Identification

With the exception of ethanol, marijuana remains the most popular psychoactive drug of abuse. The flowering tops of the female marijuana plant contain the highest concentration of the active constituent, tetrahydrocannabinol (THC). In the 1970s, most marijuana contained approximately 1% to 2% THC by weight. More recently, cultivated seedless varieties of marijuana (sensimilla) have become popular, and they contain 5% to 8% THC by weight. Therefore, smoking a joint is now likely to lead to a greater degree of altered mental status than previously.

Marijuana is typically sold in "nickel" bags that produce two to three joints. Marijuana is occasionally laced with other psychoactive substances, including PCP and cocaine. Marijuana may also be incorporated into various edible products, including baked goods, candies, etc. Hashish is the concentrated resin of marijuana. "Dabbing" is the process of smoking or vaporizing concentrated marijuana oil (often butane hash oil or "BHO"). With the recent decriminalization of marijuana in a number of states and the growth of the marijuana edibles industry, there has been a rise in the number of unintentional exposures in young children. The unique characteristics of synthetic cannabinoids are discussed later in this section.

Pharmacology

When smoked or vaporized, THC is absorbed via the lungs. Oral ingestion of cannabis typically results in decreased bioavailability due to hepatic first pass metabolism but more prolonged effects due to ongoing slow absorption via the GI tract. THC readily crosses the blood–brain barrier and binds to endogenous cannabinoid receptors in the CNS and periphery in order to exert its clinical effects.

It is estimated that no more than 50% of the THC inhaled in a marijuana cigarette is actually absorbed. Pharmacologic effects begin immediately. In contrast, the onset of effects after oral ingestion occurs in 30 minutes to 1 hour, and peak effects may not occur until the second and third hours after ingestion; THC is three times more potent when smoked than when taken by mouth.

Clinical Symptoms

The most prominent effects in humans are on the CNS and cardiovascular system. In doses of up to 20 mg, THC produces effects on mood, memory, motor coordination, cognitive ability, sensorium, time sense, and self-perception. There is an increased sense of well-being or euphoria accompanied by feelings of relaxation or sleepiness when subjects are alone. With greater intake of THC, short-term memory is impaired, and the capacity to carry out tasks that require multiple mental steps to reach a specific goal deteriorates. This effect on memory-dependent, goal-directed behavior has been called *temporal disintegration* and is correlated with a tendency to confuse past, present, and future. Depersonalization, a sense of strangeness and unreality about one's self, may also occur. Marijuana smokers often report a voracious appetite (the "munchies"), dry mouth and throat, more vivid visual imagery, and a keener sense of hearing. Altered time perception is a consistent effect of cannabinoids, so minutes seem like hours. Larger doses of THC can produce frank hallucinations, delusions, and paranoid feelings. Thinking becomes confused and disorganized. Anxiety that reaches panic proportions may replace euphoria, often as a feeling that the drug-induced state will never end. Because of the rapid onset of effects when marijuana is smoked, most users can regulate their intake to avoid the excessive doses that produce these unpleasant effects. Marijuana may cause an acute exacerbation of symptoms in stabilized schizophrenics. Clinical findings on exam may include tachycardia, hypertension, and marked conjunctival injection. Chronic smoking of marijuana and hashish is associated with bronchitis and asthma, even though THC is a mild bronchodilator.

Infants and toddlers passively exposed to marijuana may develop profound lethargy or coma, occasionally with tachycardia.

Management

In general, the only treatment required is discontinuation of the drug. In the adolescent patient with a psychotic reaction or acute toxic delirium, a sedative such as diazepam, 5 to 10 mg by mouth or 0.1 mg per kg IV, may be necessary. These acute symptoms should improve with drug abstinence over 4 to 6 hours.

STIMULANTS

Amphetamines (Crank, Speed, Ecstasy, Molly)

Identification

Amphetamines have been used medically to treat narcolepsy, ADHD, obesity, fatigue, and nasal congestion. Abuse and misuse of ADHD medications (dextroamphetamine, methylphenidate) is a significant problem in adolescents and young adults. Several decongestant nasal inhalers continue to add amphetamine agents that may be extracted and ingested by drug-seeking adolescents. Use of the amphetamine derivative MDMA (Ecstasy) has recently demonstrated a resurgence of use in the form of "Molly"—often sold as a white powder purported to be more "pure" and thus safer than previous iterations of the drug, however a number of deaths have been reported. Use of this form of MDMA is particularly popular at concerts, raves, and music festivals. The unique characteristics of the emerging synthetic cathinones are discussed at the end of this section.

Many drug users prefer amphetamines over cocaine because the clinical duration of action is considerably longer than that of cocaine. Also, the smokable form of methamphetamine (ice) is associated with more striking and prolonged alterations in CNS function. Children may be exposed to a myriad of dangerous chemicals when living with adults who operate clandestine methamphetamine laboratories.

Pharmacology

Amphetamines have powerful CNS stimulant actions, in addition to peripheral adrenergic actions. Unlike epinephrine, amphetamines are effective after oral administration. However, they are often taken by injection and nasal insufflation. The pharmacologic effects of amphetamines include increased blood pressure, occasionally with a reflex slowing of heart rate though more commonly with tachycardia, contraction of bladder sphincter, and dramatic CNS stimulation. Like other indirect sympathomimetics, amphetamines act by releasing endogenous biogenic amines from the presynaptic neurons. MDMA has more serotonergic activity (associated with both increased release and decreased reuptake of serotonin) which accounts for clinical effects and a toxicity profile that differ from that of traditional amphetamines.

The therapeutic dose of dextroamphetamine in adolescents is typically 5 mg three times daily. The toxic dose is variable but is rarely less than 15 mg. Severe reactions have been reported at 30 mg, yet doses up to 400 to 500 mg may cause only mild symptoms. Tolerance is striking, with chronic users taking 10 to 15 g daily without ill effects. The elimination half-life of the amphetamines is about 3 hours, with much of the drug being excreted in the urine unchanged. Timing of onset of symptoms and duration of clinical effects differs based on route of exposure and the unique characteristics of the particular formulation or amphetamine derivative utilized.

Clinical Symptoms

The psychic effect of amphetamines depends on the dose, mental state, and personality of the drug user. In general, 10 to 30 mg cause wakefulness, alertness, a decreased sense of fatigue, and an elevation of mood. Other behavioral changes may include increased initiative, self-confidence, ability to concentrate, elation, euphoria, and increased motor and speech activity. Physical performance in athletes may be improved. Prolonged use of large doses is followed by depression and fatigue. Amphetamines have an appetite-suppressant effect through an action on the lateral hypothalamic feeding center. However, tolerance to this effect also develops; thereafter, the effect is insufficient to reduce weight for a sustained period.

The acute toxic effects of amphetamine are usually extensions of its therapeutic actions. The central effects induce euphoria, restlessness, dizziness, tremor, hyperactive reflexes, talkativeness, irritability, weakness, insomnia, and fever. In addition, confusion, assaultiveness, anxiety, delirium, paranoid hallucinations, panic states, and suicidal or homicidal tendencies can occur, especially in patients who have underlying mental illnesses. However, these psychotic effects may occur in anyone who chronically abuses amphetamines. Cardiotoxic effects include palpitations, anginal pain, and rarely, hypertensive crisis or circulatory collapse. GI effects include anorexia, nausea, vomiting, diarrhea, and abdominal cramps. Severe overdoses may cause convulsions, coma, and cerebrovascular accidents. Both psychological and physical dependence occurs with chronic use. Chronic amphetamine abuse causes symptoms similar to many of those seen after acute overdose. The most common serious effect is a psychotic reaction with vivid hallucinations and paranoid delusions, often mistaken for schizophrenia. Recovery may or may not occur after withdrawal of the drug. In patients with persistent psychotic symptoms, it has been theorized that the amphetamine has hastened the onset of incipient schizophrenia. Chronic amphetamine abuse is also associated with the development of cerebral vasculitis.

In addition to the sympathomimetic features noted above, unique features of MDMA toxicity may include hyponatremia, serotonin syndrome, and hepatotoxicity.

Management

Treatment of intoxication after ingestion of these agents should include consideration of GI decontamination. For severe agitation, specific treatment consists of administration of a benzodiazepine (e.g., diazepam 0.1 to 0.2 mg per kg IV) or haloperidol (0.01 to 0.05 mg per kg IM). Severe hypertension unresponsive to benzodiazepines may be treated with such agents as phentolamine, hydralazine, or IV sodium nitroprusside. Because up to 45% of amphetamines are excreted in the urine unchanged, ample fluids are beneficial.

Cocaine

Identification

Cocaine occurs in the leaves of *Erythroxylum coca* and other species of *Erythroxylum* trees indigenous to Peru and Bolivia, where the leaves have been used for centuries by the natives to increase endurance and to promote a sense of well-being. Chemically, cocaine is benzoylmethylecgonine. Cocaine may be used by injection, inhalation (in the form of cocaine alkaloid or "crack"), nasal insufflation, and rarely, ingestion. In making crack, street cocaine (which is in the form of cocaine hydrochloride) is converted to cocaine alkaloid by removal of the salt moiety. This reaction is accomplished by mixing the cocaine with water and sodium bicarbonate. The crack is then separated from the water by filtration and drying. The paste hardens and is cut into chips that resemble soap. It is then smoked in a pipe or sprinkled onto a cigarette or joint. A small piece, called a *quarter rock,* produces a 20- to 30-minute high when smoked in a water pipe.

Although oral ingestion is uncommon, there are two circumstances under which cocaine may be ingested in toxic quantities: the "body packer" and the "body stuffer." In the body packer, large quantities of cocaine are enclosed in plastic and ingested in an attempt to smuggle the drug, usually across international boundaries. In the case of the body stuffer, the person in fear of being found with the substance suddenly ingests cocaine. Body stuffers are typically at greater risk of cocaine intoxication because they do not take sufficient care to guarantee that the cocaine does not leach from the bag.

Cocaine is reportedly used by up to 15% of women during pregnancy. Infants exposed to cocaine in utero are often preterm, small for age, irritable, and show neurodevelopmental delay. Beyond the postnatal age, passive cocaine exposure in infants and toddlers has been associated with severe intoxication, including the development of convulsions.

Pharmacology

The relief from fatigue that occurs with cocaine use results from central stimulation that masks the sensation of fatigue. Cocaine potentiates the excitatory and inhibitory responses of sympathetically innervated organs to norepinephrine and epinephrine by blocking the reuptake of catecholamines at adrenergic nerve endings. This explains why cocaine, unlike other local anesthetics, produces vasoconstriction and mydriasis. Cocaine is still occasionally used as a local anesthetic for ophthalmologic or otorhinolaryngologic procedures due to its ability to block the initiation or conduction of the nerve impulse after local application. It also can be used as a topical anesthetic for laceration repair in the form of TAC (tetracaine, adrenaline, cocaine), although this formulation has largely been replaced by the less toxic combination of lidocaine, epinephrine, and tetracaine.

Although fatalities have been associated with cocaine doses as low as 30 mg, 1 to 2 g is generally the lethal dose in adults. Ingested cocaine is less toxic than that taken by other routes because of its prolonged absorption by this route. The elimination half-life of cocaine is approximately 1 hour. Cocaine metabolism is complex and consists of nonenzymatic degradation to form benzoylecgonine and metabolism by plasma cholinesterases to form ecgonine methyl ester. A small fraction of cocaine is also metabolized through the cytochrome P-450 enzymes to form norcocaine. Individuals with congenital deficiencies in plasma cholinesterase are believed to have exaggerated responses to cocaine; cocaine abusers have been known to ingest inhibitors of cholinesterases or P-450 3A4 enzymes (e.g., organophosphate insecticides, cimetidine) to enhance the effect of the cocaine. Cocaine metabolites are readily detected in urine for approximately 3 days after exposure.

Cocaine is absorbed from all sites of application, including GI mucosa. Body packing may lead to severe toxicity (seizures and cardiorespiratory collapse) if the container ruptures. Probably because of its enhanced lipid solubility, crack crosses the blood–brain barrier rapidly, causing an intense rush of pleasure. This habit is highly addictive.

Clinical Symptoms

Cocaine's most dramatic clinical effect is CNS stimulation. In humans, this manifests in a feeling of well-being and euphoria, often accompanied by gregariousness, restlessness, excitement, and a sense of clarity. However, as the dose is increased, tremors, forced speech, agitation, and even tonic–clonic convulsions may result from excessive stimulation.

Initially, small doses (1 to 1.5 mg per kg) may slow the heart rate through central vagal stimulation. After moderate doses, pulse increases, the result of both central and peripheral adrenergic effects. Hypertension may appear abruptly and lead to cerebrovascular accidents. Fortunately, hypertension is generally short lived. Larger doses of cocaine may cause hypertension that may be followed quickly by cardiovascular collapse, often the result of myocardial ischemia and infarction. Myocardial injury that ranges from angina pectoris to massive infarction can be seen in young adults after acute cocaine exposure. With chronic cocaine use, a cardiomyopathy may develop that results in depressed cardiac function and death.

Rhythm disturbances are also characteristic of acute cocaine intoxication. These may consist of ventricular or supraventricular tachyarrhythmias and may be intractable. Arrhythmias are the most common cause of death after severe cocaine exposure.

Use of crack has been associated with a number of pulmonary disturbances, including bronchospasm, hemoptysis, pneumothorax, and pneumomediastinum. These lesions are believed to result from the barotrauma associated with inhalation of hot, particulate matter, followed by a Valsalva maneuver.

Cocaine has been associated with other syndromes of organ dysfunction, including hyperpyrexia and renal failure. *Coke fever* (or *pyrexia*) is a common occurrence after acute cocaine use. It is often associated with muscle rigidity (resembling neuroleptic malignant syndrome) or rhabdomyolysis (the result of agitation and/or physical restraint). Rhabdomyolysis may result in subsequent myoglobinuric renal failure if not promptly recognized and treated. Recent reports of cocaine adulterated with levamisole, a veterinary antihelminth that potentiates cocaine's euphoric effects, describe patients presenting with fever and reversible agranulocytosis.

Infants exposed to cocaine may also exhibit CNS excitation that includes hyperactivity, dystonic posturing, altered mental status, or frank seizures.

Management

Due to the high rate of life-threatening clinical effects, this intoxication requires rapid, thorough assessment and management. Immediate attention should be paid to the vital signs, including temperature (which should be obtained rectally). The patient who develops seizures requires immediate airway control as well as anticonvulsant therapy. Benzodiazepines (e.g., diazepam 0.1 to 0.3 mg per kg) are considered the anticonvulsants of choice because of their rapid onset of action and because animal data have associated their use with decreased mortality from cocaine intoxication. Benzodiazepines should also be administered liberally to the patient with mild to moderate toxicity (agitation, hypertension, tachycardia) because of their efficacy in reversing many of these clinical manifestations.

Because circulatory function can range from hypertensive crisis to cardiovascular collapse, early vascular access is important. Blood pressure instability should be anticipated and treated accordingly. For treatment of hypertensive crises, liberal benzodiazepine use may be combined with a short-acting antihypertensive (e.g., nitroprusside). Immediate treatment of hypertension is recommended because it may lead to cerebrovascular or myocardial injury, although the use of IV BBs alone is contraindicated. Cardiac arrhythmias are treated according to advanced cardiac life support protocols (see Chapter 4 Cardiopulmonary Resuscitation).

Hyperthermia must be recognized and treated promptly to prevent its complications. Management is discussed in Chapter 98 Environmental Emergencies, Radiological Emergencies, Bites and Stings. IV fluids should be used aggressively if urinalysis is suggestive of myoglobinuria.

Patients with CNS depression or a lateralizing neurologic examination should receive head imaging to rule out an intracranial vascular event.

Because cocaine is rarely ingested, the need for GI decontamination is confined to body packers/stuffers or when drug coingestion is suspected. With body stuffers, because bag leakage can lead to abrupt onset of severe intoxication and possibly death, activated charcoal should be administered immediately. Gastric emptying maneuvers and endoscopic removal of cocaine bags are relatively contraindicated because of the risk of bag rupture. Instead, decontamination is confined to administration of activated charcoal and WBI, though in some cases surgical removal may be indicated. Because cocaine bags and crack vials are radiopaque in up to 50% of cases, an abdominal radiograph is recommended to determine the location and extent of retained packets after decontamination has been initiated. A contrast study or computed tomography scan may be considered to improve detection.

In the event of severe intoxication or ingestion of more than 1 to 2 g of cocaine, transfer to the intensive care unit is essential for appropriate monitoring.

Central Anticholinergics

Identification

Increasingly, drugs, plants, and mushrooms with anticholinergic properties are ingested for their psychoactive effects. Because antidepressants, antihistamines, antispasmodics, and belladonna alkaloids are in widespread use, these compounds are more readily available than illicit psychoactive substances. Also, many OTC drugs possess anticholinergic activity and are ingested to get "high."

Pharmacology

These agents are competitive antagonists with acetylcholine at the neuroreceptor site (Table 110.20). The major effects of these drugs are on the myocardium, CNS, smooth muscle, and

TABLE 110.20

DRUGS AND CHEMICALS THAT MAY PRODUCE THE CENTRAL ANTICHOLINERGIC SYNDROME

- Antidepressants: Amitriptyline (Elavil), imipramine (Tofranil), doxepin (Sinequan, Adopin)
- Antihistamines: Chlorpheniramine (Ornade, Teldrin), diphenhydramine (Benadryl), orphenadrine (Norflex)
- Ophthalmologic preparations: Cyclopentolate (Cyclogyl), tropicamide (Mydriacyl)
- Antispasmodic agents: Propantheline (Probanthine), clidinium bromide (Librax)
- Antiparkinson agents: Trihexyphenidyl (Artane), benztropine (Cogentin), procyclidine (Kemadrin)
- Proprietary drugs: Sleep-Eze (scopolamine, methapyrilene), Sominex (scopolamine, methapyrilene), Asthma-Dor (belladonna alkaloids), Excedrin-PM (methapyrilene)
- Belladonna alkaloids: Atropine, homatropine, hyoscine, hyoscyamus, scopolamine
- Toxic plants: Mushroom (*Amanita muscaria*), bitter-sweet (*Solanum dulcamara*), Jimsonweed (*Datura stramonium*), potato leaves and sprouts (*Solanum tuberosum*), deadly nightshade (*Atropa belladonna*)

exocrine glands. The effects of anticholinergics vary according to the specific drug ingested, particularly because the many classes of drugs lead to secondary actions that are independent of anticholinergic actions. An important universal anticholinergic effect, however, is decreased GI motility. This is associated with delayed absorption of drug and, if GI decontamination is not performed, the appearance of severe toxicity may be delayed 12 to 24 hours after ingestion.

Clinical Symptoms

Clinical manifestations include tachycardia, mydriasis, facial flushing, hyperpyrexia, cardiac arrhythmias, urinary retention, dry mucous membranes, decreased sweating, and decreased or absent bowel sounds. CNS effects include delirium, anxiety, hyperactivity, visual hallucinations, illusions, and disorientation. These signs and symptoms lead to the common mnemonic, "Mad as a hatter, red as a beet, dry as a bone, blind as a bat, and hot as a hare." In excess, anticholinergics may lead to severe toxicity that includes cardiac arrhythmias, seizures, and death.

Management

The management of a patient with a known central anticholinergic syndrome is a challenge, particularly because one must also be prepared for the other distinct toxicities of the ingested drug or plant. Most plants and many drugs in this category are not detected on toxicology screens, so the diagnosis must rely on history and clinical suspicion. Along similar lines, serum drug levels do not predict the degree of anticholinergic symptoms.

GI decontamination may be valuable beyond an hour after anticholinergic poison ingestion because of the likelihood of drug persistence in the gut lumen for an extended time. Once again, activated charcoal remains the drug of choice.

On the basis of presenting signs and symptoms, the patient may require sedation and monitoring in an intensive care unit setting to provide ventilatory support for coma, anticonvulsants for seizures, and antiarrhythmic drugs for cardiac arrhythmias. Adequate sedation may be achieved with titrated doses of benzodiazepines. Physostigmine, a potent anticholinesterase, is a recognized antidote for anticholinergic-induced mental status alterations and can be very effective in the correct clinical setting; however, its use is controversial. Physostigmine can produce bronchospasm, bradycardia, hypotension, and seizures. It is therefore reserved for those who have normal EKGs (QRS duration less than 100 ms) and mental status dysfunction confined to hallucinations or severe agitation. The adult dose is 1 to 2 mg via slow IV infusion over 5 minutes. The trial dose can be repeated in 10 to 15 minutes up to a maximum of 4 mg. The pediatric dose is 0.5 mg IV administered slowly, with repeat every 10 minutes up to a maximum of 2 mg. The smallest effective dose may be repeated every 30 to 60 minutes if symptoms recur over 6 to 8 hours. The muscarinic toxicity of physostigmine may be treated with IV atropine at one-half the physostigmine dose given; physostigmine-related seizures may be treated with benzodiazepines.

Central Nervous System Sedative-Hypnotics

Identification

The sedative-hypnotics have tranquilizing, euphoriant effects that may be similar to morphine. With all these agents—prescribed for this tranquilizing action—it is difficult to draw the line between appropriate use, abuse, habituation, and addiction. However, for all, tolerance is common and physical dependence quickly develops. Therefore, their abuse potential is considered high. Many of these agents, including glutethimide, meprobamate, methaqualone, and barbiturates, are uncommonly available and have been replaced by the benzodiazepines. Because they have retained some popularity and still make periodic appearances on the streets, however, they should be included in discussions of such drugs.

For all sedative-hypnotics, patterns of abuse vary, ranging from infrequent sprees of intoxication to compulsive daily use. Introduction to these drugs may be through street use or drug trade (which is most common in adolescents), but, commonly, exposure is initiated through a physician's prescription to a parent for insomnia or anxiety.

Pharmacology

The sedative-hypnotics reversibly depress the activity of all excitable tissues. For most of these agents, CNS effects occur with little action on skeletal, cardiac, or smooth muscle. Uncommonly, serious depression in cardiovascular and other functions may occur. The pharmacologic characteristics of each drug are largely determined by their specific chemical nature. For example, all barbiturates are bound by plasma proteins. These characteristics have important implications in affecting their renal elimination and the effectiveness of extracorporeal drug removal techniques (hemodialysis, hemoperfusion). Because tolerance develops to most of the actions of these drugs, no signs of chronic use may be apparent.

Clinical Symptoms

After sedative-hypnotic use, the adolescent may exhibit sluggishness, difficulty in thinking, dysarthria, poor memory, faulty judgment, emotional lability, and short attention span. The classic presentation of oral sedative-hypnotic overdose is coma with relatively normal vital signs. Respiratory depression may be seen, especially with combination sedative-hypnotic ingestions (i.e., benzodiazepines and ethanol). Toddlers who unintentionally ingest benzodiazepines may present with acute-onset ataxia.

With chronic use, these drugs also lead to dependence, so a picture of abstinence may appear after their disuse, with clinical manifestations of apathy, weakness, tremulousness, agitation, or frank convulsions. In its mildest form, the abstinence syndrome may consist only of rebound increases of rapid eye movement sleep, insomnia, or anxiety.

Management

Initial attention should be directed to ensuring a patent airway and an intact gag reflex. Cardiovascular disturbances are rare after sedative use, but because of the possibility of drug coingestion, thorough hemodynamic assessment is necessary. Many sedative-hypnotics are detectable on comprehensive toxin screens, so specimens of serum and urine may be sent for analysis; however, these "send out" screens rarely come back in real time, thus minimizing their importance at the bedside. GI decontamination should be considered in select cases and can typically be confined to administration of activated charcoal. Repeated doses of charcoal have been shown to enhance clearance of certain barbiturates and benzodiazepines. Urinary alkalinization aids in the excretion of phenobarbital. In extreme cases, charcoal hemoperfusion should be considered.

Optimal treatment of significant sedative overdose often includes continuous monitoring in an intensive care unit with intubation and ventilator support as indicated. Flumazenil, a benzodiazepine antagonist, can be administered in select cases of suspected benzodiazepine ingestion. Its pediatric dose is 0.01 to 0.02 mg per kg IV (max 0.2 mg per dose) and may be repeated to a maximum of 0.05 mg per kg or 1 mg, whichever is less. Indications for flumazenil administration may be (i) to reverse a witnessed, unintentional benzodiazepine overdose in a young child or (ii) to prevent airway intubation after an iatrogenic overdose. Flumazenil must not be given empirically in unknown or intentional overdoses as it may induce potentially life-threatening seizures.

Opioids (Morphine, Codeine, Heroin, Methadone, Buprenorphine, Oxycodone, and Hydrocodone)

Identification

In the past two decades, recreational abuse of insufflated heroin and ingested prescription opioid analgesics (particularly oxycodone and hydrocodone) has risen to epidemic proportions in the United States and may be partly responsible for the first increase in overall drug-related mortality in a generation. In addition, some opioid-related deaths are likely inadvertent and represent inappropriate misuse of combinations of alcohol, sedative-hypnotic agents, and prescription analgesics.

The significant rate of opioid abuse has also given rise to the common treatment of opioid addiction by the outpatient prescription of buprenorphine (a partial opioid agonist/antagonist) which has resulted in the relatively common occurrence of an opioid syndrome in toddlers due to exploratory ingestion of this agent. Neonates may develop the neonatal abstinence syndrome due to maternal use of illicit or prescription opioids or due to treatment of maternal opioid dependence with methadone or buprenorphine during pregnancy.

Pharmacology

The opioids produce their major effects by combining with receptors in the brain and other tissues. Effects include analgesia, drowsiness, change in mood, respiratory depression, decreased GI motility, nausea, and vomiting.

Generally, the toxic opioid dose for a person who is not addicted depends on the particular drug. For example, with morphine, clinical toxicity (excessive sedation) may appear with doses that exceed 5 mg in the adolescent. Tolerance rapidly develops to many CNS effects. However, death may occur as a result of marked respiratory depression and consequent anoxia. In particular, those individuals who are ultrarapid metabolizers of codeine through CYP2D6 may have increased morbidity and mortality. Other toxicities of opiates include (neurogenic) pulmonary edema, mast cell degranulation (which leads to histamine release and an "anaphylactoid" reaction), cardiac disturbances (with propoxyphene or methadone intoxication), and neurotoxicity with seizures (with meperidine intoxication). Some opioids (i.e., methadone, buprenorphine) have particularly long half-lives.

Clinical Symptoms

Opioids invariably cause miosis, even after development of tolerance. Respiratory depression is another hallmark of opioid toxicity, due in part to decreased responsiveness of brain stem respiratory centers to increases in carbon dioxide tension. This effect is often magnified during sleep. Therapeutic doses of morphine have no effect on blood pressure or cardiac rate or rhythm. When blood pressure changes occur, they result from histamine release. Because histamine dilates capacitance blood vessels and decreases the ability of the cardiovascular system to respond to gravitational shifts, sitting or standing may produce orthostatic hypotension.

Many opioids have extensive effects on the GI tract. They decrease the secretion of hydrochloric acid, GI motility, and pancreatic secretions while increasing colonic tone to the point of spasm. In addition, the tone of the anal sphincter is augmented. Therapeutic doses of morphine and codeine can also increase biliary tract pressure, producing epigastric distress and biliary colic.

Management

The presence of coma, pinpoint pupils, and depressed respiration should suggest opioid poisoning in the absence of history. Evidence of track marks may suggest IV drug use. To confirm the diagnosis, toxicologic analysis of urine and/or serum should be considered (of note, however, several important synthetic or semisynthetic opioids such as methadone, fentanyl, and oxycodone may not be detected on routine urine drug screens).

The first management step with opioid intoxication is to ensure adequate ventilation of the patient. Endotracheal intubation may be necessary if there is severe respiratory depression or pulmonary edema. If appropriate (i.e., a large amount of oral opioids has been ingested, heroin body-packing), GI decontamination should be considered. The narcotic antagonist naloxone should be given by IV. Ideally, the dose of naloxone depends on the severity of the patient's symptoms and whether or not they chronically use opioids. Naloxone can precipitate an abstinence syndrome in those who have developed physical dependence; in such patients, smaller initial doses of 0.2 to 0.4 mg, with upward titration as needed, are preferable. A full reversal dose in a pediatric patient is 0.1 mg/kg IV. If there is no response despite the suspicion of opiate intoxication, the naloxone dose should be repeated (up to a total dose of 8 to 10 mg), depending on effect and level of suspicion.

When patients who are addicted to opiates are hospitalized, small doses of an opiate may be necessary to prevent severe withdrawal. Methadone substitution is often the preferred agent, because in small doses, it is less euphorigenic and its long elimination half-life permits once- or twice-daily dosing. Other agents, such as buprenorphine and clonidine, may also be considered.

γ-Hydroxybutyrate, γ-Hydroxybutyrolactone, and 1,4-Butanediol

Identification

The related agents, γ-hydroxybutyrate (GHB), γ-hydroxybutyrolactone (GBL), and 1,4-butanediol (1,4 BD), became popular substances of abuse among teenagers and young adults in the late 1990s and early 2000s. These agents are used for a variety of reasons, but primarily as euphoriants and aphrodisiacs at parties or all-night dance clubs (raves). GHB has gained a particular notoriety as a date-rape agent.

This class also has a reputation in the body-builder community as growth hormone stimulants and thus enhancers of muscle development and fat loss. Medically, sodium oxybate (Xyrem) is available as a schedule III substance used to treat cataplexy.

Pharmacology

GHB is an endogenous compound with neurotransmitter and/or neuromodulator function and interacts with dopamine, serotonin, GABA, and endogenous opioid-based neural systems. GBL is actually a precursor to GHB and is rapidly metabolized in vivo to GHB, thus the clinical effects of ingesting either agent are nearly indistinguishable. 1,4 BD is also metabolized to GHB via alcohol dehydrogenase.

Clinical Symptoms

GHB, GBL, and 1,4 BD are CNS depressants that cause rapid onset of deep sleep that can progress to coma and respiratory depression. Patients who have overdosed may have transient seizure activity or myoclonus and are often hypothermic and bradycardic. The coma is usually relatively short in duration, on the order of 1 to 2 hours. During emergence, transient delirium and vomiting are often observed. Depressed respiratory effort and airway-protective reflexes are common in the more severe cases, although aspiration pneumonia as a complication has been rare. Many patients are surprisingly responsive to stimulus, and attempts at laryngoscopy to effect endotracheal intubation in a seemingly deeply comatose patient may result in an angry, combative patient who sits up and swears at the endoscopist.

Management. Most patients with acute overdose can be managed with the provision of ambient oxygen, suctioning, and attention to the airway. A nasal trumpet is helpful in some cases, and endotracheal intubation may be required occasionally, although it may necessitate rapid sequence induction for the reasons previously noted. Atropine has been used for severe bradycardia with success. Blood pressure support is rarely necessary.

Inhalants

Identification

The prevalence of inhalant abuse among young children and adolescents has been related to the ready availability of these products. Patterns of abuse are also strikingly region specific, with the highest rates of abuse in the southwestern and southeastern United States. Typically, the agents are abused by "huffing" or "bagging." In huffing, the agent is placed into a rag or handkerchief, held under the nose, and then deeply inhaled. With bagging, a common method of abuse at parties, the compound is placed into a large bag (e.g., garbage bag) with the drug user placing his or her head into the bag.

Pharmacology

The psychoactive inhalants can be placed into three broad categories: (i) Hydrocarbons, (ii) nitrous oxide, and (iii) nitrites. The hydrocarbons can be subdivided further into the aliphatic hydrocarbons, the halogenated hydrocarbons, and solvents. Regardless of the class, all inhalants possess the pharmacologic property of narcosis, leading to euphoria and lightheadedness after inhalation. The halogenated hydrocarbons are particularly dangerous due to their ability to sensitize the myocardium to catecholamines, potentially leading to myocardial irritability and cardiac arrhythmias.

Clinical Symptoms

Several distinct profiles of toxicity have been described after inhalant abuse. The inebriation that these agents produce may be associated with mental status changes that include coma with respiratory arrest or aspiration. The halogenated hydrocarbons all possess potent cardiotoxicity as noted above and have been associated with many reports of spontaneous ventricular fibrillation in adolescents during a binge. A syndrome known as *sudden sniffing death* has been described in adolescents who abuse inhalants and is most commonly reported with use of halogenated hydrocarbons. Finally, the act of bagging is associated with the risk of simple asphyxia. Finally, acute exposure to those inhalants that contain nitrites may lead to methemoglobinemia, often severe.

Other toxicities are associated with chronic inhalant abuse. The solvents, particularly toluene, may lead to a syndrome that includes abdominal pain, muscle wasting, electrolyte disturbances (hypokalemia), and renal tubular acidosis. Patients of chronic solvent abuse may also develop a leukoencephalomalacia with cerebral atrophy.

Management

Because inhalant abuse may lead to the development of life-threatening symptoms, close attention should be directed to the vital signs and their stability. Patients with depressed levels of consciousness may require airway support and ventilation. Because of the risk of cardiac arrhythmias when halogenated hydrocarbons are abused, vascular access should be established early. Arrhythmias should be treated according to the standard protocol; however, the use of epinephrine is relatively contraindicated because it has been associated with worsening of rhythm disturbances. As a part of the evaluation, a complete metabolic panel that includes electrolyte levels, with calcium, phosphate, and magnesium; amylase level; liver function tests; creatine phosphokinase level; and urinalysis should be obtained. Treatment of methemoglobinemia is discussed in Chapter 101 Hematologic Emergencies.

EMERGING DRUGS OF ABUSE (SYNTHETIC CANNABINOIDS, SYNTHETIC CATHINONES)

In recent years, use of so called "designer drugs" or synthetic drugs of abuse has markedly increased, in part due to the fact that many of these substances were originally sold at head shops, convenience stores, and over the internet as "legal highs." The Synthetic Drug Abuse Prevention Act of 2012 placed many of the most commonly identified compounds into Schedule I status, though new derivatives and formulations continue to be produced and distributed. Staying up to date with these emerging substances of abuse can be challenging for providers. Your local poison control center and public health department can be helpful resources when caring for a patient with possible exposure to one of these agents. Given their particular popularity, the synthetic cannabinoids and synthetic cathinones are described in further detail below. Other important classes of these so-called designer drugs include the 2C class of drugs (phenylethylamine derivatives with sympathomimetic, hallucinogenic, and serotonergic features) and piperazines (sympathomimetic features predominate).

Synthetic Cannabinoids (Spice, K2)

Identification

In the past decade, use of synthetic cannabinoids has gained increasing popularity. Initially marketed as herbal incense or air fresheners and labeled as "not for human consumption," these compounds were sold in head shops, convenience stores, and via the internet. The term synthetic cannabinoids describes a variety of compounds (often structurally dissimilar to THC, and thus not picked up on standard urine drug screens), further subdivided into seven major structural groups, all with affinity for cannabinoid receptors and clinical effects similar to THC. Several of these compounds are now regulated as a result of the Synthetic Drug Abuse Prevention Act of 2012, but new derivatives continue to emerge onto the scene.

Pharmacology

Synthetic cannabinoids bind to cannabinoid receptors in the CNS and peripheral tissues, often with significantly higher affinity than THC. It is postulated that a combination of activity at other receptor types, active metabolites, and unique effects of various herbal compounds often mixed with synthetic cannabinoids may account for the higher reported rates of adverse effects (i.e., seizures, tachycardia, GI upset) with these compounds as compared to THC.

Users of synthetic cannabinoids typically report a faster onset of peak effects and shorter duration of effects as compared to THC. However, given the number of compounds that fall under the umbrella term of synthetic cannabinoids, there is limited published data or experience to allow us to fully characterize the pharmacodynamics of this class of compounds.

Clinical Effects

As compared to THC, use of synthetic cannabinoids is more frequently associated with tachycardia, hypertension, agitation, hallucinations, agitation, anxiety, paranoia, and vomiting. Seizures, acute kidney injury, and SVT have been reported.

Management

As with THC, treatment generally consists of discontinuation of the drug and symptom-based supportive care as needed. Benzodiazepines may be useful in managing significant paranoia, agitation, tachycardia, or seizures. Patients should be observed at least until normalization of their vital signs and improvement in their mental status.

Synthetic Cathinones ("Bath Salts")

Identification

Cathinones are naturally occurring substances found in the leaves of the khat (Catha edulis) plant. For centuries, people have chewed the leaves of this plant for the euphoric and stimulant effects. Synthetic cathinone derivatives were first synthesized in the 1920s, but use among recreational drug users noticeably escalated in 2010–11. These substances were initially sold as bath salts or plant food and labeled as "not for human consumption." Nasal insufflation and ingestion are the most common routes of administration, though inhalation, IV/IM use, and rectal administration have also been described.

Pharmacology

Cathinones are B-ketophenethylamines, structurally similar to amphetamines. The primarily pharmacologic mechanism of action is via blocking the reuptake of dopamine, norepinephrine, and serotonin. Onset of action is typically rapid, though pharmacokinetics vary depending on the particular derivative and route of administration.

Clinical Symptoms

Amphetamine-like sympathomimetic effects predominate. Desired effects include a sense of euphoria, increased energy, enhanced openness, and empathy. The most common clinical findings reported by healthcare providers include agitation, aggression, hallucinations, tachycardia, hypertension, mydriasis, and hyperthermia. Adverse effects reported by users include palpitations, chest pain, dry mouth, nausea, and vomiting. Severe sequelae of use include seizures, myocardial infarction, myocarditis, rhabdomyolysis, excited delirium syndrome, serotonin syndrome, and death. As with many ingestions, the presence of hyperthermia is typically a poor prognostic indicator.

Management

Treatment is primarily supportive, with initial attention often directed to management of agitation, aggression, tachycardia, hypertension, and hyperthermia with liberal use of IV benzodiazepines. A rectal temperature should be obtained. While benzodiazepines may effectively manage hyperthermia, consideration should be given to passive or active cooling techniques if hyperthermia persists. Further testing often includes an EKG, electrolytes, renal function, hepatic transaminases, and a CK. Standard drug screens for amphetamines are often negative in the setting of synthetic cathinone use. Appropriate IV fluids should be given, particularly in the setting of rhabdomyolysis.

Suggested Readings and Key References

Reference Toxicology Textbooks

Erickson T, Ahrens W, Aks S, et al., eds. *Pediatric toxicology: diagnosis and management of the poisoned child.* New York, NY: McGraw-Hill, 2005.

Hoffman RS, Howland MA, Lewin NA, et al., eds. *Goldfrank's toxicological emergencies,* 10th ed. New York, NY: McGraw-Hill, 2015.

Osterhoudt KC, Perrone J, DeRoos F, et al. *Toxicology pearls.* Philadelphia, PA: Hanley & Belfus, 2004.

Shannon MW, Borron SW, Burns MJ, eds. *Haddad and Winchester's clinical management of poisoning and drug overdose,* 4th ed. Philadelphia, PA: Saunders Elsevier, 2007.

General Approach and Management

Albertson TE, Dawson A, de Latorre F, et al. TOX-ACLS: toxicologic-oriented advanced cardiac life support. *Ann Emerg Med* 2001;37(4suppl):S78–S90.

American Academy of Pediatrics, Committee on Injury, Violence, and Poison Prevention. Poison treatment in the home. American Academy of Pediatrics Committee on Injury, Violence, and Poison Prevention. *Pediatrics* 2003;112:1182–1185.

Bond GR. The role of activated charcoal and gastric emptying in gastrointestinal decontamination: a state-of-the-art review. *Ann Emerg Med* 2002;39(3):273–286.

Bond GR, Woodward RW, Ho M. The growing impact of pediatric pharmaceutical poisoning. *J Pediatr* 2012;160:265–270.

Burns MM. Activated charcoal as the sole intervention for treatment after childhood poisoning. *Curr Opin Pediatr* 2000;12(2):166–171.

Calello DP, Henretig FM. Pediatric toxicology: specialized approach to the poisoned child. *Emerg Med Clin North Am* 2014;32:29–52.

Dart RC, Borron SW, Caravati EM, et al. Expert consensus guidelines for stocking of antidotes in hospitals that provide emergency care. *Ann Emerg Med* 2009;54:386–394.

Erickson TB, Thompson TM, Lu JJ. The approach to the patient with an unknown overdose. *Emerg Med Clin North Am* 2007;25:249–281.

Franklin RL, Rodgers GB. Unintentional child poisonings treated in United States hospital emergency departments: national estimates of incident cases, population-based poisoning rates, and product involvement. *Pediatrics* 2008;122:1244–1251.

Ghannoum MG, Gosselin S. Enhanced poison elimination in critical care. *Adv Chronic Kidney Dis* 2013;20:94–101.

Henretig FM, Paschall RT, Donaruma-Kwoh MM. Child abuse by poisoning. In: Reese RM, Christian CW, eds. *Child abuse: medical diagnosis and management.* Farmington Hills, MI: American Academy of Pediatrics, 2009:549–599.

Hoffman RJ, Nelson L. Rational use of toxicology testing in children. *Curr Opin Pediatr* 2001;13(2):183–188.

Litovitz TL, Manoguerra A. Comparison of pediatric poisoning hazards: an analysis of 3.8 million exposure incidents a report from the American Association of Poison Control Centers. *Pediatrics* 1992;89:999–1006.

Mowry JB, Spyker DA, Cantilena LR Jr, et al. 2012 Annual Report of the American Association of Poison Control Centers' National Poison Data System (NPDS): 30th Annual Report. *Clin Toxicol (Phila)* 2013;51:949–1229.

Osterhoudt KC, Durbin D, Alpern ER, et al. Risk factors for emesis after therapeutic use of activated charcoal in acutely poisoned children. *Pediatrics* 2004;113:806–810.

Shannon MW. Ingestion of toxic substances by children. *N Engl J Med* 2000;342(3):186–191.

Vanden Hoek TL, Morrison LJ, Schuster M, et al. Part 12: Cardiac arrest in special situations: 2010 American Heart Association guidelines for cardiopulmonary resuscitation and emergency cardiovascular care. *Circulation* 2010;122:S829–S861.

Acetaminophen

Betten DP, Cantrell FL, Thomas SC, et al. A prospective evaluation of shortened course oral N-acetylcysteine for the treatment of acute acetaminophen poisoning. *Ann Emerg Med* 2007;50:272–279.

Harrison PM, Keays R, Alexander GJ, et al. Improved outcome of paracetamol-induced fulminant hepatic failure by late administration of acetylcysteine. *Lancet* 1990;335:1572–1573.

Heard KJ. Acetylcysteine for acetaminophen poisoning. *N Engl J Med* 2008;359(3):285–292.

Henretig FM, Selbst SM, Forrest C, et al. Repeated acetaminophen overdosing causing hepatotoxicity in children. *Clin Pediatr* 1989;28:525–528.

Rumack BH, Peterson RG. Acetaminophen overdose: incidence, diagnosis and management in 416 patients. *Pediatrics* 1978;62(5 Pt 2 suppl): 898–903.

Alcohols and Glycols

Brent J. Fompizole for the treatment of pediatric ethylene and diethylene glycol, butoxyethanol, and methanol poisonings. *Clin Toxicol (phila)* 2010;48:401–406.

Ghannoum M, Hoffman RS, Mowry JB, et al. Trends in toxic alcohol exposures in the United States from 2000 to 2013: a focus on the use of antidotes and extracorporeal treatments. *Semin Dial* 2014;27(4): 395–401.

Lepik KJ, Levy AR, Sobolev BG, et al. Adverse drug events associated with the antidotes for methanol and ethylene glycol poisoning: a comparison of ethanol and fomepizole. *Ann Emerg Med* 2009;53: 439–450.

Walters D, Betensky M. An unresponsive 3-year-old girl with an unusual whine. *Pediatr Emerg Care* 2012;28:943–946.

Youssef GM, Hirsch DJ. Validation of a method to predict required dialysis time for cases of methanol and ethylene glycol poisoning. *Am J Kidney Dis* 2005;46:509–511.

Antihistamines

Baker AM, Johnson DG, Levisky JA, et al. Fatal diphenhydramine intoxication in infants. *J Forensic Sci* 2003;48(2):425–428.

Cole JB, Stellpflug SJ, Gross EA, et al. Wide complex tachycardia in a pediatric diphenhydramine overdose treated with sodium bicarbonate. *Pediatr Emerg Care* 2011;27:1175–1177.

Frascogna N. Physostigmine: is there a role for this antidote in pediatric poisonings? *Curr Opin Pediatr* 2007;19:201–205.

Nine JS, Rund CR. Fatality from diphenhydramine monointoxication: a case report and review of the infant, pediatric, and adult literature. *Am J Forensic Med Pathol* 2006;27:36–41.

Ten Eick AP, Blumer JL, Reed MD. Safety of antihistamines in children. *Drug Saf* 2001;24(2):119–147.

Aspirin Poisoning

Greenberg MI, Hendrickson RG, Hofman M. Deleterious effects of endotracheal intubation in salicylate poisoning. *Ann Emerg Med* 2003;41:583–584.

O'Malley GF. Emergency department management of the salicylate poisoned patient. *Emerg Med Clin North Am* 2007;25:333–346.

Stolbach AI, Hoffman RS, Nelson LS. Mechanical ventilation was associated with acidemia in a case series of salicylate-poisoned patients. *Acad Emerg Med* 2008;15:866–869.

β-Adrenergic Blockers

Belson MG, Sullivan K, Geller RJ. Beta-adrenergic antagonist exposures in children. *Vet Hum Toxicol* 2001;43(6):361–365.

Jovic-Stosic J, Gligic B, Putic V, et al. Severe propranolol and ethanol overdose with wide complex tachycardia treated with intravenous lipid emulsion: a case report. *Clin Toxicol* 2011;49:426–430.

Kerns W. Management of beta-adrenergic blocker and calcium channel antagonist toxicity. *Emerg Med Clin North Am* 2007;25:309–331.

Calcium Channel Blockers

Belson MG, Gorman SE, Sullivan K, et al. Calcium channel blocker ingestions in children. *Am J Emerg Med* 2000;18(5):581–586.

Durward A, Guerguerian AM, Lefebvre M, et al. Massive diltiazem overdose treated with extracorporeal membrane oxygenation. *Pediatr Crit Care Med* 2003;4(3):372–376.

Engebretsen K, Holger M. High-dose insulin therapy in beta-blocker and calcium-channel blocker poisoning. *Clin Toxicol* 2011;49:277–283.

Greene SL, Gawarammana I, Wood DM, et al. Relative safety of hyperinsulinaemia/euglycaemia therapy in the management of calcium channel blocker overdose: a prospective observational study. *Intensive Care Med* 2007;33:2019–2024.

Kerns W. Management of beta-adrenergic blocker and calcium channel antagonist toxicity. *Emerg Med Clin North Am* 2007;25:309–331.

Levine M, Boyer EW, Pozner CN, et al. Assessment of hyperglycemia after calcium channel blocker overdoses involving diltiazem or verapamil. *Crit Care Med* 2007;35:2071–2075.

Levine M, Curry SC, Padilla-Jones A, et al. Critical care management of verapamil and diltiazem overdose with a focus on vasopressors: a 25-year experience at a single center. *Ann Emerg Med* 2013;62:252–258.

Megarbane B, Karyo S, Baud FJ. Hyperinsulinaemia/euglycaemia therapy in acute calcium channel antagonist and beta-blocker poisoning. *Toxicol Rev* 2004;23:215–222.

Ranniger C, Roche C. Are one or two dangerous? Calcium channel blocker exposure in toddlers. *J Emerg Med* 2007;33:145–154.

Salhanick SD, Shannon MW. Management of calcium channel antagonist overdose. *Drug Saf* 2003;26(2):65–79.

Clonidine

Eddy O, Howell JM. Are one or two dangerous? Clonidine and topical imidazolines exposure in toddlers. *J Emerg Med* 2003;25:297–302.

Klein-Schwartz W. Trends and toxic effects from pediatric clonidine exposures. *Arch Pediatr Adolesc Med* 2002;156:392–396.

Lai Becker M, Huntington N, Woolf AD. Brimonidine tartrate poisoning in children: frequency, trends, and use of naloxone as an antidote. *Pediatrics* 2009;123:e305–e311.

Minns AB, Clark RF, Schneir A. Guanfacine overdose resulting in initial hypertension and subsequent delayed, persistent orthostatic hypotension. *Clin Toxicol* 2010;48:146–147.

Osterhoudt KC. Clonidine poisoning. In: Rose BD, ed. *UpToDate.* Waltham, MA: UpToDate.

Romano MJ, Dinh A. A 1000-fold overdose of clonidine caused by a compounding error in a 5-year-old child with attention-deficit/hyperactivity disorder. *Pediatrics* 2001;108:471–472.

Seger DL. Clonidine toxicity revisited. *J Toxicol Clin Toxicol* 2002;40(2): 145–155.

Digoxin

Thacker D, Sharma J. Digoxin toxicity. *Clin Pediatr (phila)* 2007;46:276–279.

Woolf AD, Wenger T, Smith TW, et al. The use of digoxin-specific Fab fragments for severe digitalis intoxication in children. *N Engl J Med* 1992;326:1739–1744.

Foodborne Intoxications

Donnenberg MS, Narayanan S. How to diagnose a foodborne illness. *Infect Dis Clin North Am* 2013;27:535–554.

Schmitt C, De Haro L. Clinical marine toxicology: a European perspective for clinical toxicologist and poison centers. *Toxins* 2013;5:1343–1352.

Wu F, Groopman JD, Pestka JJ. Public health impacts of foodborne mycotoxins. *Ann Rev Food Sci Technol* 2014;5:351–372.

Household Cleaning Products and Caustics

Beuhler MC, Gala P, Wolfe HA, et al. Laundry "pod" ingestions: a case series and discussion of recent literature. *Pediatr Emerg Care* 2013;29:743–747.

Salzman M, O'Malley RN. Updates on the evaluation and management of caustic exposures. *Emerg Med Clin North Am* 2007;25:459–476.

Usta M, Erkan T, Cokugras FC, et al. High doses of methylprednisolone in the management of caustic esophageal burns. *Pediatrics* 2014;133: E1518–E1524.

Hydrocarbons

Joliff HA, Fletcher E, Roberts KJ, et al. Pediatric hydrocarbon-related injuries in the United States: 2000–2009. *Pediatrics* 2013;131:1139–1147.

Mazzeo PA, Renny M, Osterhoudt KC. A toddler with curiosity and a cough. *Pediatr Emerg Care* 2010;26:232–234.

Iron

Anderson BD, Turchen SG, Manoguerra AS, et al. Retrospective analysis of ingestions of iron containing products in the United States: are there differences between chewable vitamins and adult preparations? *J Emerg Med* 2000;19(3):255–258.

Carlsson M, Cortes D, Jepsen S, et al. Severe iron intoxication treated with exchange transfusion. *Arch Dis Child* 2008;93:321–322.

Fine JS. Iron poisoning. *Curr Probl Pediatr* 2000;30(3):71–90.

Henretig FM, Drott HR, Osterhoudt KC. Acute iron poisoning. In: Shaw LM, ed. *The clinical toxicology laboratory: contemporary practice of poisoning evaluation.* Washington, DC: AACC Press, 2001:401–409.

Manoguerra AS, Erdman AR, Booze LL, et al. Iron ingestion: an evidence-based consensus guideline for out-of-hospital management. *Clin Toxicol* 2005;43:553–570.

Tenenbein M. Unit-dose packaging of iron supplements and reduction of iron poisoning in young children. *Arch Pediatr Adolesc Med* 2005;159:593–595.

Isoniazid

Geib AJ, Shannon MW. Isoniazid. In: Shannon MW, Borron SW, Burns MJ, eds. *Haddad and Winchester's Clinical management of poisoning and drug overdose.* 4th ed. Philadelphia, PA: Saunders Elsevier, 2007:919–926.

Minns AB, Ghafouri N, Clark RF. Isoniazid-induced status epilepticus in a pediatric patient after inadequate pyridoxine therapy. *Pediatr Emerg Care* 2010;26:380–381.

Morrow LE, Wear RE, Schuller D, et al. Acute isoniazid toxicity and the need for adequate pyridoxine supplies. *Pharmacotherapy* 2006;26: 1529–1532.

Orlowski FP, Paganini EP, Pippenger CE. Treatment of a potentially lethal dose isoniazid ingestion. *Ann Emerg Med* 1988;17:73–76.

Lead

CDC Advisory Committee on Childhood Lead Poisoning Prevention. Low level lead exposure harms children: a renewed call for primay prevention. *CDC Advisory Committee on Childhood Lead Poisoning Prevention. Low level lead exposure harms children: a renewed call for primay prevention.* Available at http://www.cdc.gov/nceh/lead/ACCLPP/Final_Document_030712.pdf.

Chandran L, Cataldo R. Lead poisoning: basics and new developments. *Pediatr in Rev* 2010;31:399–406.

Oral Hypoglycemics

Calello DP, Kelly A, Osterhoudt KC. Case files of the medical toxicology fellowship training program at The Children's Hospital of Philadelphia: a pediatric exploratory sulfonylurea ingestion. *J Med Toxicol* 2006;2:19–24.

Dougherty PP, Lee SC, Lung D, et al. Evaluation of the use and safety of octreotide as antidotal therapy for sulfonylurea overdose in children. *Pediatr Emerg Care* 2013;29:292–295.

Levine M, Ruha AM, Lovecchio F, et al. Hypoglycemia after accidental pediatric sulfonylurea ingestions. *Pediatr Emerg Care* 2011;27:846–849.

Lung DD, Olson KR. Hypoglycemia in pediatric sulfonylurea poisoning: an 8-year poison center retrospective study. *Pediatrics* 2011;127: e1558–e1562.

Rowden AK, Fasano CJ. Emergency management of oral hypoglycemic drug toxicity. *Emerg Med Clin North Am* 2007;25:347–356.

Phenothiazines and Other Neuroleptics

Heng Tan H, Hoppe J, Heard K. A systematic review of cardiovascular effects after atypical antipsychotic medication overdose. *Am J Emerg Med* 2009;27:607–616.

James LP, Abel K, Wilkinson J, et al. Phenothiazine, butyrophenone, and other psychotropic medication poisonings in children and adolescents. *J Toxicol Clin Toxicol* 2000;38(6):615–623.

Reilly TH, Kirk MA. Atypical antipsychotics and newer antidepressants. *Emerg Med Clin North Am* 2007;25:477–497.

Schonberger RB, Douglas L, Baum CR. Severe extrapyramidal symptoms in a 3-year-old boy after accidental ingestion of the new antipsychotic drug aripiprazole. *Pediatrics* 2004;114(6):1744–1745.

Organophosphates

Bond RG, Pieche S, Sonicki Z, et al. A clinical decision aid for triage of children younger than 5 years and with organophosphate or carbamate insecticide exposure in developing countries. *Ann Emerg Med* 2008;52:617–622.

Vates C, Osterhoudt KC. Give me three steps. *Pediatr Emerg Care* 2008; 24:389–391.

Plants/Mushrooms

Froberg B, Ibrahim D, Furbee RB. Plant poisoning. *Emerg Med Clin North Am* 2007;25:375–433.

Graeme KA. Mycetism: A review of the recent literature. *Clin Toxicol* 2014;10:173–189.

Richardson WH, Slone CM, Michels JE. Herbal drugs of abuse: an emerging problem. *Emerg Med Clin North Am* 2007;25:435–457.

Tricyclic Antidepressants/Other Antidepressants

Belson MG, Kelley TR. Bupropion exposures: clinical manifestations and medical outcome. *J Emerg Med* 2002;23(3):223–230.

Hendron D, Menagh G, Sandilands EA, et al. Tricyclic antidepressant overdose in a toddler treated with intravenous lipid emulsion. *Pediatrics* 2011;128:e1628–e1632.

Isbister GK, Bowe SJ, Dawson A, et al. Relative toxicity of selective serotonin reuptake inhibitors (SSRIs) in overdose. *J Toxicol Clin Toxicol* 2004;42:277–285.

Levine M, Brooks DE, Franken A, et al. Delayed-onset seizure and cardiac arrest after amitriptyline overdose, treated with intravenous lipid emulsion therapy. *Pediatrics* 2012;130:e432–e438.

Liebelt EL. An update on antidepressant toxicity: an evolution of unique toxicities to master. *Clin Pediatr Emerg Med* 2008;9:24–34.

Osterhoudt KC, Mistry R. A boy with tremor, diaphoresis, and altered behavior. *Pediatr Emerg Care* 2007;23:419–421.

Sirianni AJ, Osterhoudt KC, Calello DP, et al. Use of lipid emulsion in the resuscitation of a patient with prolonged cardiovascular collapse after overdose of bupropion and lamotrigine. *Ann Emerg Med* 2008;51:412–415.

Zorc JJ, Ludwig S. A 12-year-old girl with altered mental status and a seizure. *Pediatr Emerg Care* 2004;20:613–616.

Drugs Dangerous in Small Doses

Henry K, Harris CR. Deadly ingestions. *Pediatr Clin North Am* 2006; 53:293–315.

Osterhoudt KC. The toxic toddler: drugs that can kill in small doses. *Contemp Pediatr* 2000;17:73–89.

Substance Abuse

Bateman KA, Heagarty MC. Passive freebase cocaine ('crack') inhalation by infants and toddlers. *Am J Dis Child* 1989;143:25–27.

Connors NJ, Hoffman RS. Experimental treatments for cocaine toxicity: a difficult transition to the bedside. *J Pharmacol Exp Ther* 2013;347:251–257.

Dominici P, Kopec K, Manur R, et al. Phencyclidine Intoxication Case Series Study. *J Med Toxicol* 2014. [Epub ahead of print]

Gasche Y, Daali Y, Fathi M, et al. Codeine intoxication associated with ultrarapid CYP2D6 metabolism. *N Engl J Med* 2004;351:2827–2831.

Geib AJ, Babu K, Ewald MB, et al. Adverse effects in children after unintentional buprenorphine exposure. *Pediatrics* 2006;118:1746–1751.

Henretig F. Inhalant abuse in children and adolescents. *Pediatr Ann* 1996;25:47–52.

Hernandez SH, Nelson LS. Prescription drug abuse: insight into the epidemic. *Clin Pharmacol Ther* 2010;88:307–317.

Kim HK, Nelson LS. Reducing the harm of opioid overdose with the safe use of naloxone: a pharmacologic review. *Expert Opin Drug Saf* 2015;12:1–10.

Lord S, Marsch L. Emerging trends and innovations in the identification and management of drug use among adolescents and young adults. *Adolesc Med State Art Rev* 2011;22:649–669.

Meehan TJ, Bryant SM, Aks SE. Drugs of abuse: the highs and lows of altered mental states in the emergency department. *Emerg Med Clin North Am* 2010;28:663–682.

Nelson ME, Bryant SM, Aks SE. Emerging drugs of abuse. *Emerg Med Clin North Am* 2014;32:1–28.

Osterhoudt KC. A Cadillac ride to the emergency department. *Pediatr Emerg Care* 2005;21:877–879.

Osterhoudt KC, Henretig FM. Comatose teenagers at a party: what a tangled "web" we weave. *Pediatr Case Rev* 2003;3:171–173.

Ridpath A, Driver CR, Nolan ML, et al. Illnesses and deaths among persons attending an electronic dance-music festival - New York City, 2013. *MMWR Morb Mortal Wkly Rep* 2014;63:1195–1198.

Rosenbaum CD, Carreiro SP, Babu KM. Here today, gone tomorrow… and back again? A review of herbal marijuana alternatives (K2, spice), synthetic cathinones (bath salts), kratom, salvia divinorum, methoxetamine, and piperazines. *J Med Toxicol* 2012;8:15–32.

Shannon M. Methylenedioxymethamphetamine (MDMA, "Ecstasy"). *Pediatr Emerg Care* 2000;16:377–380.

Shieh-Czaja A, Calello DP, Osterhoudt KC. Sick sisters. *Pediatr Emerg Care* 2005;21:400–402.

Tancredi DN, Shannon MW. Case records of the Massachusetts General Hospital: weekly clinicopathological exercises: case 30–2003: a 21-year old man with sudden alteration of mental status. *N Engl J Med* 2003;349:1267–1275.

Traub SJ, Hoffman RS, Nelson LS. Body-packing–the internal concealment of drugs. *N Engl J Med* 2003;349:2519–2526.

Zvosec DL, Smith SW, McCutcheon R, et al. Adverse events, including death, associated with the use of 1,4-butanediol. *N Engl J Med* 2001;344:87–94.

SECTION V
Trauma

CHAPTER 111 ■ ABDOMINAL TRAUMA

RICHARD A. SALADINO, MD AND DENNIS P. LUND, MD

GOALS OF EMERGENCY CARE

Trauma is the most common cause of death in children between 1 and 18 years of age in the United States; more than 10,000 children die each year from injuries. Blunt trauma accounts for more than 90% of childhood injuries; the most common associated mechanisms are falls and motor vehicle–related trauma. Although injury to the abdomen accounts for only 10% of injuries in children with trauma, it is the most common unrecognized cause of fatal injuries. Therefore, a compulsive and systematic approach to timely identification and treatment of abdominal injuries is required.

KEY POINTS

- Children are at greater risk than adults for intra-abdominal injuries after blunt trauma because of their immature musculoskeletal system.
- The overlying muscles and associated skeleton are more pliable than in adults and, therefore, less protective; children have a higher abdominal organ-to-body mass ratio.
- A given force delivered to the abdomen is distributed over a smaller body surface area, increasing the likelihood of injury to the underlying structures.

RELATED CHAPTERS

Signs and Symptoms
- Abdominal Distension: Chapter 7
- Pain: Abdomen: Chapter 48

Medical, Surgical, and Trauma Emergencies
- Genitourinary Trauma: Chapter 116
- Musculoskeletal Trauma: Chapter 119
- Thoracic Trauma: Chapter 123

Procedures and Appendices
- Ultrasound: Chapter 142

THE APPROACH TO THE PEDIATRIC PATIENT WITH ABDOMINAL TRAUMA

CLINICAL PEARLS AND PITFALLS

- Priorities in evaluation and treatment of any child with trauma include recognition and relief of airway obstruction, appropriate protection of the cervical spine, and management of life-threatening chest injuries and shock.
- Once resuscitation and cervical spine stabilization have begun, evaluation of the abdomen is included in both the primary and secondary surveys.
- Occult abdominal trauma occurs in many settings, including children restrained only by a lap belt and in child abuse. Index of suspicion must be high in these cases.

Current Evidence

Blunt injuries account for most of the morbidity and mortality of childhood trauma, although the frequency with which penetrating injuries occur is increasing.

Goals of Treatment

The primary objective of treatment is to determine the presence or absence of intra-abdominal injury. The evaluation for intra-abdominal injuries in children starts with a determination of the mechanism of trauma, elicited from witnesses, caregivers, and emergency medical personnel. Penetrating trauma is usually evident on careful inspection of both the anterior and posterior torsi. In contrast, blunt abdominal trauma must be suspected from both historical information and careful physical examination. Children with severe multiple trauma are obviously at risk for intra-abdominal injuries, but sufficient energy to injure may also be present in apparently minor falls, direct blows to the abdomen from balls, bats, bicycle handlebars, and countless toys, and during contact sports.

Clinical Considerations

Clinical Recognition

Life-threatening abdominal injuries may be occult or manifest in several ways: abdominal ecchymoses or distention, shock, or external hemorrhage (e.g., from a penetrating injury). Historical information or physical examination findings are often subtle or lacking. Children have the capacity to maintain a normal blood pressure level in the face of significant blood loss and hence may mask major intra-abdominal bleeding. The examining physician must always keep in mind that the abdomen is a large potential reservoir for blood loss.

Triage Considerations

The American College of Surgeons suggests that triage of the trauma patient be based upon severity of the mechanism of injury and physiologic status of the patient. Clearly the patient with a mechanism associated with high velocity or with abnormal vital signs must be immediately resuscitated and evaluated for injuries. That said, even those patients with a lesser mechanism of injury and stable vital signs should be evaluated with great vigilance.

Clinical Assessment

Physical examination. A traumatized child is often difficult to examine; pain associated with extra-abdominal injuries may obscure abdominal findings. In addition, the results of physical examination may be subtle or unreliable in an unconscious, intoxicated, agitated, or fearful child. Vital signs, including blood pressure and pulse, may be normal for age, especially in children with isolated injuries of the liver and spleen. Furthermore, external signs of injury, abdominal tenderness, and absent bowel sounds seldom differentiate pediatric patients who require laparotomy from those who do not.

Careful serial examinations are critically important in maintaining the index of suspicion necessary to proceed with more sophisticated testing when appropriate. Inspection should note abrasions, lacerations, ecchymoses, penetrating wounds (including missile entry and exit sites), and telltale markings (e.g., seat belt marks, tire tracks). Attention should be paid to the anterior and posterior abdomen and to both flanks, as well as to the lower thorax, when considering abdominal injuries. Abdominal distention may be caused by hemoperitoneum or peritonitis but most often results from gastric distention from air swallowed by the crying child. Early gastric decompression may assist the abdominal examination and prevent vomiting with aspiration of gastric contents. The presence or absence of bowel sounds is generally not of much significance in the initial evaluation, but prolonged ileus may be a sign of intra-abdominal pathology. Tenderness upon palpation, percussion, or shaking may be caused by abdominal wall contusion or may indicate intra-abdominal injuries. Pelvic stability is evaluated by gently compressing and distracting the iliac wings.

Digital rectal examination should be performed; the presence of blood may indicate perforation of the bowel. A boggy or high-riding prostate, blood at the urethral meatus, or a distended bladder may be present with urethral disruption and preclude bladder catheterization until a retrograde urethrogram has been performed (see Chapter 116 Genitourinary Trauma). Diminished or absent rectal sphincter tone may indicate a spinal cord injury.

Laboratory assessment: Blood should be obtained and sent for immediate baseline hemoglobin measurement and typing and cross-matching, not only in all instances of multiple trauma but also if isolated intra-abdominal injury is suspected.

Routine multipanel laboratory testing (so-called "trauma panels") historically has been standard for patients with trauma, but more recent studies have called into question this undifferentiated approach. Nonetheless, laboratory studies that are commonly added include measurement of liver transaminases, amylase, lipase, and urinalysis.

Many recent studies indicate that, in combination with the presence of physical examination findings, abnormal laboratory findings contribute to the identification of children with intra-abdominal injuries. Elevated serum liver transaminase levels may be associated with intra-abdominal trauma, especially hepatic injuries. Screening for intra-abdominal injuries by evaluating transaminase levels is not universally accepted because sensitivity and specificity vary widely in the literature, but some data suggest that elevated transaminase levels (aspartate aminotransferase more than 200 U per L and alanine aminotransferase more than 125 U per L) correlate well with hepatic injuries. Using thresholds such as these may allow for more judicious use of computerized tomographic (CT) scan of the abdomen for children with blunt abdominal trauma.

Examination of the urine may also play a role in an increased suspicion for intra-abdominal injury after blunt force trauma to the abdomen. Grossly bloody urine indicates likely injury to the kidneys and has been shown to be associated with nonrenal intra-abdominal injuries in pediatric patients with trauma. The predictive capacity of microscopic hematuria is controversial. In one study, microscopic examination of urine that revealed more than 50 red blood cells (RBCs) per high-powered field (hpf) was 100% sensitive and 64% specific for the presence of an intra-abdominal injury (see Chapter 116 Genitourinary Trauma). A more recent study suggests consideration of CT scan of the abdomen in the context of a urinalysis demonstrating as few as five or more RBCs per hpf when the history indicates a significant force has been applied to the abdomen. In addition, clinicians must remember that major trauma may cause complete disruption of a renal pedicle without any hematuria.

Management

Basic principles of management. Airway management and cervical spine stabilization are first priorities (Fig. 111.1). Supplemental oxygen should be administered to any child with significant injuries, regardless of whether obvious signs of shock are present. Intravenous or intraosseous access should be obtained while the primary survey is completed. Immediate life-threatening injuries should be treated promptly. Hemorrhagic shock should be addressed with rapid infusion of isotonic crystalloid solution. A first intravenous administration of a bolus of 20 mL per kg may be given rapidly, followed by a second bolus of 20 mL per kg, if the pulse and blood pressure remain outside the physiologic range. If hemodynamic instability persists after 40 mL per kg of crystalloid, ongoing bleeding should be suspected and administration of blood strongly considered. The blood bank at a trauma center not only should be able to provide type-specific blood in a short time frame but must also have O-negative packed RBCs ready for resuscitation if needed. Large-bore catheters are preferable, whether in the upper or lower extremities, to allow rapid infusion of large volumes of fluid during resuscitation. Accessing the femoral

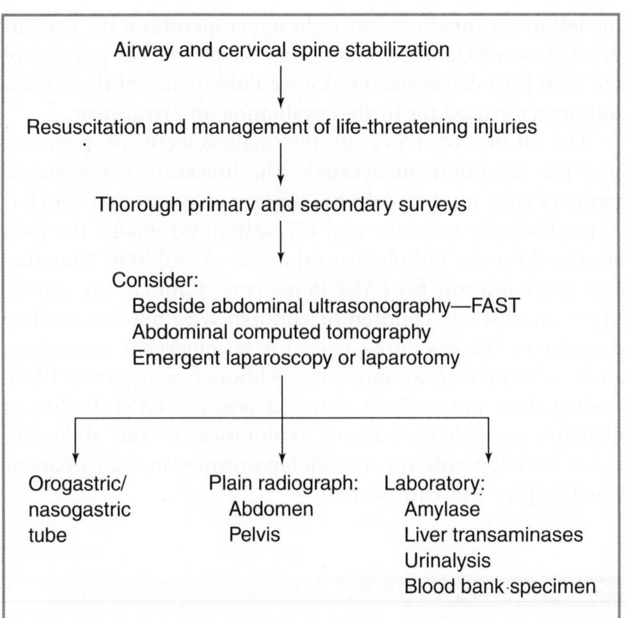

FIGURE 111.1 Initial evaluation and treatment of the child with abdominal trauma. FAST, focused abdominal sonography for trauma.

vein is acceptable and in fact is a preferred site in children when central access is needed.

The American College of Surgeons currently recommends that aggressive fluid resuscitation be pursued. Although there is some suggestion that less rigorous (hypotensive) fluid resuscitation may improve survival by limiting hemorrhage into the peritoneal space, pursuing this strategy in the management of children is still controversial and not part of the approach to the injured child with hypotension.

As the initial evaluation proceeds, the priorities of management depend on the extent of multisystem injuries and the condition of the patient (Fig. 111.2). Patients who are unstable as a result of ongoing blood loss or an expanding intracranial hemorrhage require operative intervention early in the evaluation phase.

Initial management of the unstable patient. Immediate life-threatening injuries, such as airway obstruction, tension pneumothorax, pericardial tamponade, and obvious sources of external blood loss, must be treated promptly upon detection.

If significant head trauma has occurred, a determination must be made regarding the need for immediate neurosurgical intervention. A rapidly performed CT scan of the head is usually sufficient to determine the presence of a hematoma, and the findings will dictate the next steps with regard to evaluation

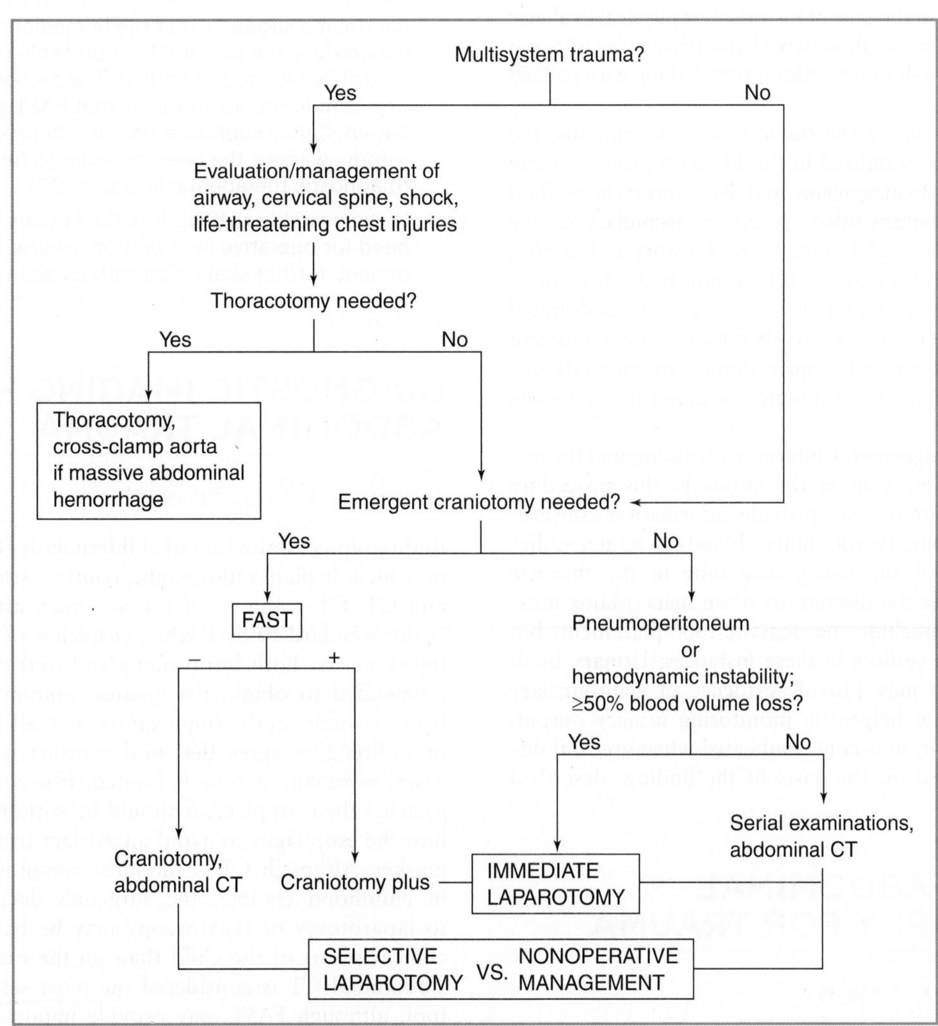

FIGURE 111.2 Management of blunt abdominal trauma. FAST, focused abdominal sonography for trauma; CT, computed tomography (Table 111.2).

TABLE 111.1

INDICATIONS FOR ABDOMINAL COMPUTED TOMOGRAPHIC SCAN IN PEDIATRIC TRAUMA PATIENTS

1. Mechanism of injury suggesting abdominal trauma
2. Slowly declining hematocrit
3. Unaccountable fluid or blood requirements
4. Neurologic injury precluding accurate abdominal examination
5. Hematuria
6. Acute "need to know" (e.g., before general anesthesia)

of the abdomen. If hemodynamic instability or the need for immediate craniotomy exists and does not allow for CT evaluation of the abdomen (Fig. 111.2), a focused abdominal sonography for trauma (FAST examination) should be performed either in the ED or in the operating suite. In the presence of a positive FAST examination, laparotomy or laparoscopy and craniotomy proceed simultaneously. Finally, if neither thoracotomy nor craniotomy is indicated, emergent laparotomy or laparoscopy is performed when pneumoperitoneum is noted on a plain radiograph or when the patient remains hemodynamically unstable in the face of historical or physical evidence of abdominal trauma. With massive hemorrhage, fresh frozen plasma and platelets should be administered along with packed RBCs.

Initial management of the stable patient. Commonly, the injured child can be stabilized in the ED with proper airway and cervical spine management, and with intravenous fluid therapy and blood transfusion. A careful secondary survey should then be performed. On the basis of history and careful, serial abdominal examinations, CT is indicated when intra-abdominal injuries are suspected (Table 111.1). An abdominal CT scan may be merited based solely on severe force inherent in a particular mechanism of injury, despite an unremarkable physical examination or the absence of abnormal screening laboratory values.

Additional management. Children with abdominal trauma often need decompression of the stomach; this procedure facilitates examination, may provide information concerning gastric or diaphragmatic injury (bloody aspirate, radiographic evidence of the nasogastric tube in the thoracic cavity), and relieves the discomfort of an ileus. Major maxillofacial trauma precludes nasogastric tube placement, but an orogastric tube suffices in these instances. Urinary bladder catheterization may provide evidence of genitourinary system injury and is helpful in monitoring urinary output. Bladder catheterization is contraindicated when urethral disruption is suspected on the basis of the findings described previously.

FOCUSED ABDOMINAL SONOGRAPHY FOR TRAUMA

Goals of Treatment

FAST is typically performed in the ED during the secondary survey. The operator looks at four windows in the abdomen: the left upper quadrant, the right upper quadrant, the pericardium via a subxiphoid window, and the pelvis. The purpose of the scan is to detect free fluid. Free fluid in any of these areas indicates the need for further evaluation and treatment.

The utility of FAST in the management of pediatric patients remains controversial. The literature for pediatric patients with intra-abdominal injuries suggests that FAST is not sufficiently sensitive and CT scanning remains the gold standard for the radiologic evaluation in children. Nonetheless, there is a role for FAST in pediatric populations, particularly in unstable children or children who need immediate transfer to the operating suite for an emergent procedure, such as cranial decompression. Although a negative FAST finding does not exclude injury, a positive FAST finding is evidence enough to warrant exploration of the abdomen, either with laparoscopy or with laparotomy, in such a patient (see Chapter 142 Ultrasound).

CLINICAL PEARLS AND PITFALLS

- While ultrasound screening (FAST) of the abdomen has been routinely utilized in adult trauma patients for many years with excellent sensitivity and specificity, the utility of FAST in children is a source of much debate.
- Review of several studies of adults with blunt abdominal trauma suggests that the immediate use of FAST may reduce the use of CT for unstable patients with a positive ultrasound finding. The preponderance of recent literature suggests that FAST (in unstable patients) may support a decision to proceed to laparotomy without the need to undergo further testing (diagnostic therapeutic lavage or CT).
- In the unstable patient, free fluid points toward the need for operative intervention, whereas in the stable patient, further evaluation with CT scan is indicated.

DIAGNOSTIC IMAGING FOR ABDOMINAL TRAUMA

Goals of Treatment

Radiographic evaluation of children with abdominal trauma may include plain radiographs, contrast studies, ultrasound, and CT. CT scanning of the abdomen after blunt trauma is the standard of care when suspicion of intra-abdominal injury exists. Both intravenous and oral contrasts are recommended to obtain the greatest amount of information from a single study. Importantly, not all trauma surgeons or radiologists agree that oral contrast is required for all cases, especially if time is limited. If a nasogastric or orogastric tube is in place, it should be withdrawn temporarily into the esophagus to avoid an artifact from its radiopaque marker. Although CT is the most common technique used in childhood trauma, the surgeon's decision to proceed to laparotomy or laparoscopy may be based more on the clinical status of the child than on the radiologic findings. Abdominal CT is considered the most sensitive diagnostic tool, although FAST may provide important data early in the course of the management of a child with suspected intra-abdominal injuries.

CLINICAL PEARLS AND PITFALLS

- Abdominal CT has low sensitivity for small gastrointestinal perforations and pancreatic injury.
- Judicious use of the combination of physical examination, laboratory screening values, and CT scanning is indicated for the stable patient. Whenever possible, protocols that use the lowest possible dose of radiation exposure for the child should be utilized.
- A FAST examination is not sufficient to exclude intra-abdominal injury.

DIAGNOSTIC PERITONEAL LAVAGE

Goals of Treatment

Diagnostic peritoneal lavage (DPL) is rarely a helpful adjunct to the management of children with abdominal trauma. The primary indication for DPL in children is an urgent "need to know" with regard to the status of the peritoneal cavity, such as in the child who is hemodynamically unstable or requires immediate craniotomy and cannot be delayed for abdominal CT. The disadvantages of DPL include the introduction of air and fluid into the abdomen (subsequent radiologic evaluations are less helpful) and peritoneal irritation caused by the procedure (subsequent physical examinations are less reliable).

If the technology is available, however, this need can be met with FAST or laparoscopy. Furthermore, laparoscopy has become readily available and most surgeons are quite facile with this technique. Laparoscopy has the advantage of direct visualization under magnification of the injury causing blood or fluid in the abdomen as well as the opportunity to look for hollow visceral injury with little to no morbidity.

CLINICAL PEARLS AND PITFALLS

- It is rarely necessary to perform laparotomy on children only for free intraperitoneal blood.
- DPL, which effectively detects small volumes of blood, is often too sensitive in children and may lead to an unnecessary operation.

EMERGENT VERSUS SELECTIVE LAPAROSCOPY OR LAPAROTOMY

Goals of Treatment

The indications for immediate laparoscopy or laparotomy are limited in blunt abdominal trauma (Table 111.2). In most cases of abdominal trauma in children (Fig. 111.2), emergency laparotomy is not necessary and further diagnostic studies direct either elective (selective) laparoscopy or observation and monitoring. In the case where there is concern for an intra-abdominal injury in a stable child, laparoscopy poses little risk and allows the trauma team to rapidly and safely "know" if there is an injury requiring surgical treatment. Further, if there is a major injury identified that cannot be treated laparoscopically, the incision can easily be converted to a laparotomy for wider exposure. The indications for emergent laparoscopy or laparotomy in children with penetrating trauma are illustrated in Figure 111.3.

TABLE 111.2

INDICATIONS FOR IMMEDIATE LAPAROSCOPY OR LAPAROTOMY FOR CHILDREN WITH ABDOMINAL TRAUMA

Multisystem injuries with indications for craniotomy in the presence of a positive diagnostic peritoneal lavage, free peritoneal fluid on ultrasonography, or strong historical, physical, or radiographic evidence of abdominal injury
Persistent and significant hemodynamic instability with evidence of abdominal injury in the absence of extra-abdominal injury
Penetrating wounds to the abdomen
Pneumoperitoneum
Significant abdominal distention associated with hypotension

CLINICAL PEARLS AND PITFALLS

- Most children with blunt abdominal trauma require only in-hospital observation and monitoring after delineation of the site and extent of their injury by abdominal CT.
- Any gunshot wound to the abdomen mandates immediate exploration.
- Other types of penetrating wounds in the presence of unexplained hemodynamic compromise, evisceration, pneumoperitoneum, or any evidence of violation of the peritoneum require prompt laparotomy.

BLUNT ABDOMINAL TRAUMA

Goals of Treatment

The goals of the evaluation and treatment of children with blunt abdominal trauma are to differentiate serious from nonthreatening injuries and determine the next steps for treatment.

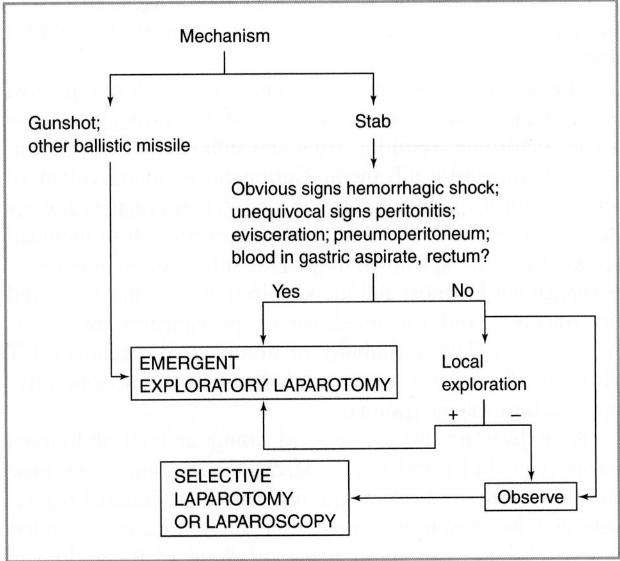

FIGURE 111.3 Management of penetrating abdominal trauma.

Suspicion for serious intra-abdominal injuries is based on the mechanism of injury and careful abdominal examination. Bilious or bloody vomiting, persistent vomiting, abdominal distention, any signs of peritoneal irritation, and rectal blood or hematuria suggest possible visceral injury, as does an elevation in amylase or liver transaminase levels in cases in which a clinical decision is made to obtain these studies. A low threshold for the use of abdominal CT should be maintained.

CLINICAL PEARLS AND PITFALLS

- Children with a troubling history or any worrisome signs should receive a diagnostic laboratory evaluation and should be observed in consultation with a surgeon.
- Children with even minor contusions of the liver, spleen, pancreas, or hollow viscera should be hospitalized.

Abdominal Wall Contusions

Many children have minor trauma to their abdomen in the course of play and as a result of minor accidental events. Balls, bats, swings, toys, and contact with other children may cause contusions of the abdominal wall. Children subjected to minor forces without signs of intra-abdominal pathology (e.g., distention, tenderness on deep palpation, peritoneal irritation) can be sent home.

Solid Organ Injuries

The spleen is the most commonly injured intra-abdominal organ, followed by the liver. Most of these injuries are the result of automobile–pedestrian trauma, although falls and bicycle accidents are also common mechanisms. The potential morbidity and mortality result from the highly vascular anatomy of this organ and hemorrhage into the large potential space of the peritoneal cavity.

Patients who have splenic injuries may present with either diffuse abdominal pain or localized tenderness. Subphrenic blood may cause referred left shoulder pain (Kehr sign). Percussion and palpation tenderness is usually of greatest magnitude in the left upper quadrant of the abdomen. Abdominal radiographs occasionally reveal a medially displaced gastric bubble. CT scan will identify the extent of injury (Figs. 111.4 and 111.5).

Management of splenic injuries has evolved during the last three decades since the recognition of the postsplenectomy sepsis syndrome, resulting from the influence of both clinical and diagnostic advances. Nonoperative management of splenic injuries with observation or interventional radiology has largely replaced the traditional treatment, which included splenectomy or splenorrhaphy. The safety of nonoperative management for most childhood spleen injuries has been well documented, and the incidence of postsplenectomy sepsis has declined. The availability of noninvasive diagnostic CT also has allowed for greater confidence in the nonoperative approach to splenic trauma.

Blunt liver trauma is the most common fatal abdominal injury (Figs. 111.6 and 111.7). Mechanisms of injury are those that are common to splenic trauma. Diffuse abdominal tenderness may be a result of hemoperitoneum, but maximal tenderness is elicited in the right upper quadrant of the abdomen. Right shoulder pain is an occasional complaint.

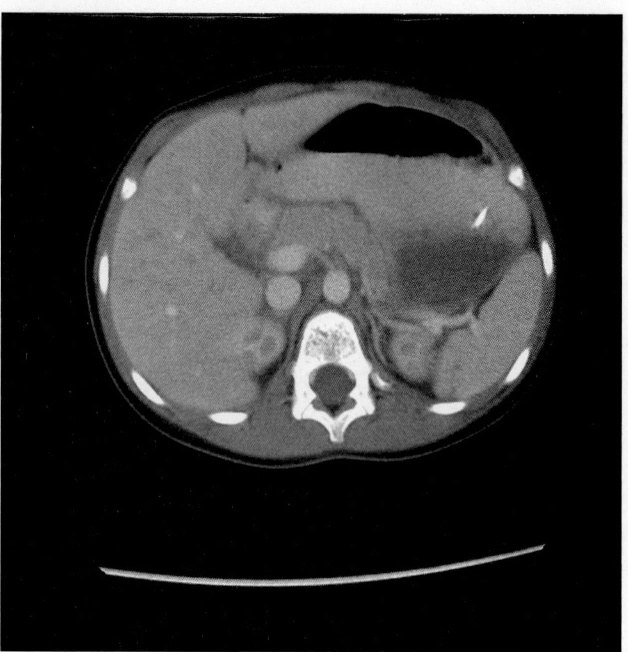

FIGURE 111.4 Abdominal computed tomography of an 8-year-old boy who was an unrestrained backseat passenger in a motor vehicle collision. The CT reveals a grade 1 splenic laceration with mild perisplenic free fluid.

As with trauma to the spleen, nonoperative management of blunt hepatic injuries has become more common and is now the rule rather than the exception. Nonoperative management of isolated spleen and liver injuries without blood transfusion is the standard of care in pediatric trauma care facilities and is successful in 95% and 90% of cases, respectively.

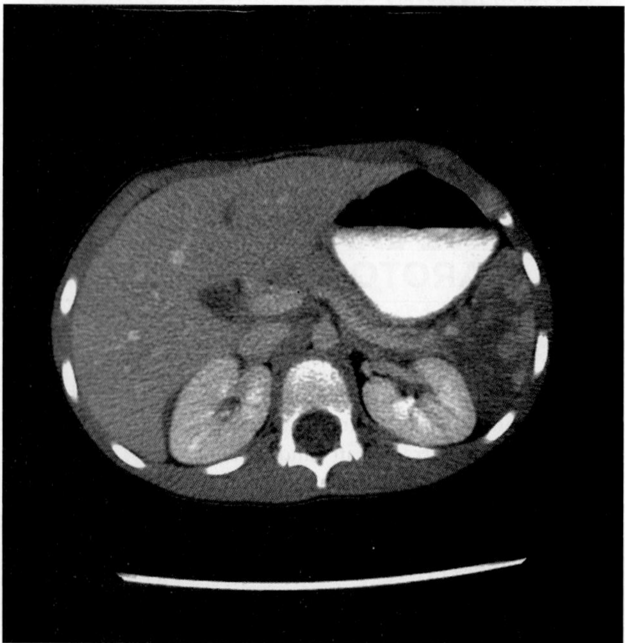

FIGURE 111.5 Abdominal computed tomography of a 5-year-old boy who jumped from a rope swing and landed on a large piece of PVC tubing, showing a grade 4 splenic laceration and hemoperitoneum.

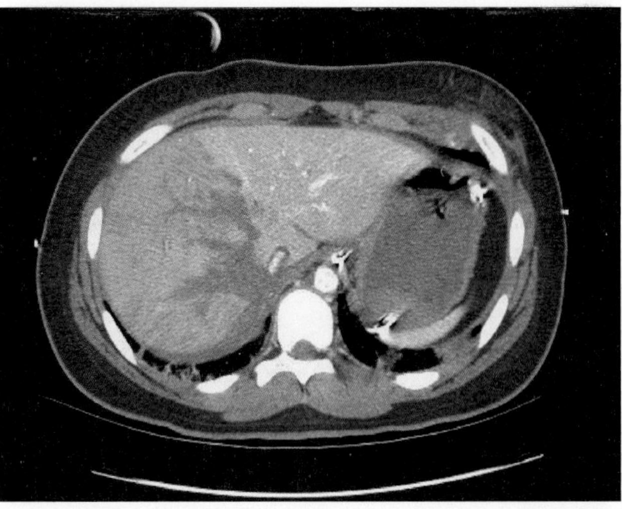

FIGURE 111.6 Abdominal computed tomography of an unrestrained 13-year-old girl in a rollover motor vehicle collision. A liver fracture is evident with differential perfusion of the lobes of the liver. Additional injuries included lung contusion.

Pancreatic Injuries

Blunt abdominal injuries, particularly from bicycle handlebars, are the most common cause of pancreatic pseudocyst formation in children, although this injury is infrequent. Diagnosis is often delayed because of the nonspecific nature of subjective complaints and physical examination findings. The classic triad of epigastric pain, a palpable abdominal mass, and hyperamylasemia are detected only rarely in children and may develop slowly. The pancreas is relatively well protected and associated trauma such as hepatic and intestinal injuries is commonly present when injury to the pancreas has occurred. Abdominal ultrasound and contrast CT (often serial examinations) are used to make the diagnosis (Fig. 111.8); however, acute pancreatic injuries may not be apparent on the initial CT scan.

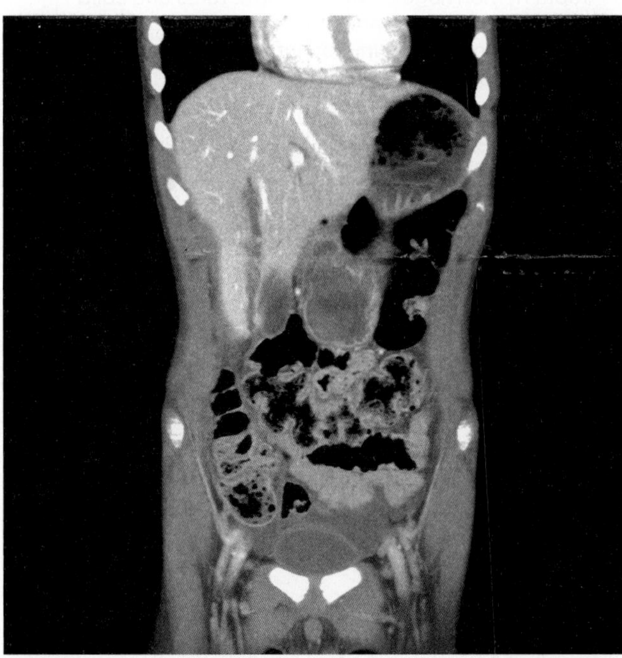

FIGURE 111.7 Abdominal computed tomography (reformat) of a 12-year-old boy who crashed his bicycle, landing on the handlebar strut, showing a grade 3 liver laceration measuring approximately 9.5 cm, and a moderate amount of free fluid indicative of hemoperitoneum.

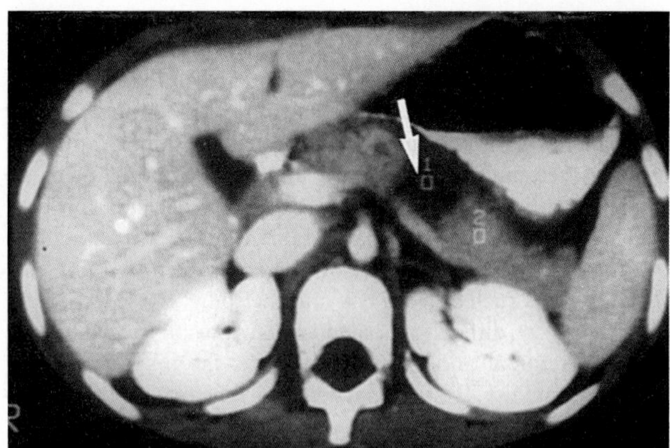

FIGURE 111.8 Abdominal computed tomography of a 6-year-old boy who fell onto the handlebar of his bicycle, showing a pancreatic hematoma and pseudocyst formation.

Severe injury of the pancreas is rare, but when it occurs, blood loss and leakage of enzyme-laden secretions may result in hypovolemia and peritonitis. Blunt abdominal trauma may also injure the ductal elements of the pancreas, and diagnosis depends on a high index of suspicion, consideration of the mechanism of injury, physical examination, serum amylase determination, and diagnostic imaging. Of note, however, is that the absence of hyperamylasemia does not preclude pancreatic trauma. Serum amylase level may be normal in 30% of patients with complete transaction, whereas elevated serum amylase level is detected in 14% to 80% of cases of blunt injury. Elevated serum amylase level should suggest the possibility of pancreatic involvement, but the absolute value does not correlate with the degree of injury.

Hyperamylasemia may be present with pancreatic injury, but its absence does not preclude injury. In one study, elevations of amylase level more than 200 U per L and lipase level more than 1,800 U per L were markers of possible major pancreatic ductal disruption. In a more recent retrospective study, elevations of amylase and lipase levels were infrequently detected in patients with blunt abdominal trauma (4% and 7%, respectively), and neither the sensitivity nor negative predictive values of elevated measurements were sufficient to be used as screening tools for pancreatic injury. Pancreatic injury is difficult to diagnose, particularly since a CT scan of the abdomen is only 60% to 70% accurate in identifying pancreatic injury.

Nasogastric decompression and bowel rest are indicated when pancreatic injury is suspected. Nonoperative therapy is normally used initially for children with isolated pancreatic pseudocyst caused by blunt trauma. Maturation of the pseudocyst may necessitate surgical drainage, although spontaneous resolution may occur in 25% of children. Experience with percutaneous drainage of pancreatic pseudocysts in children is increasing, but the traditional approach has been to use surgical internal drainage once a pseudocyst has persisted beyond 6 weeks. When severe pancreatic crush or transection is suspected, the surgeon may elect to perform immediate exploration and resection or drainage.

Hollow Abdominal Viscera Injuries

Intestinal perforation caused by blunt abdominal trauma is rare in the pediatric age group, but the most common causes of this injury are automobile–pedestrian trauma, automobile lap belt injuries, and child abuse. The mechanisms of injury usually involve rapid acceleration or deceleration of a structure near a point of anatomic fixation (e.g., ligament of Treitz), or trapping of a piece of bowel between two unyielding structures such as a lap belt and the spine. Hollow visceral injury may be difficult to diagnose because physical findings may be minimal and/or nonspecific for the first few hours, and abdominal CT is not particularly sensitive in this situation. However, bowel contents, bile, and activated pancreatic enzymes are extremely irritating to the peritoneum over time. The development of fever or worsening peritonitis on serial physical examinations should alert the examining physician to the possibility of bowel perforation.

Plain radiographs of the abdomen demonstrate free intra-abdominal air in only 30% to 50% of cases. Similarly, pneumoperitoneum or leakage of gastrointestinal contrast is only rarely seen on the CT scan. Most perforations or transections of bowel are found during laparotomy or laparoscopy which the surgeon has chosen to perform because of advancing peritonitis or unexplained persistent fever. Management depends on the site and extent of structural injury.

A significant percentage (up to 25%) of hollow visceral injuries may not be apparent on the initial CT scan of a child with blunt injury. Therefore, evaluating the mechanism of injury should lead to a high index of suspicion for this type of injury. A significant lap belt sign is a harbinger of possible bowel injury. Similarly, unexplained free fluid (e.g., not associated with a solid visceral injury) in the abdomen on CT scan should be very carefully evaluated and consideration should be given for laparoscopy or laparotomy.

Late Presentations of Intra-abdominal Trauma

Some children with abdominal trauma do not have evidence of intra-abdominal pathology on initial evaluation but may return days or weeks later with abdominal distention and/or pain, persistent emesis, or hematochezia. In particular, three injuries are characterized by late presentations: (i) Pancreatic pseudocyst (previously discussed), (ii) duodenal hematoma, and (iii) hematobilia.

Intramural duodenal hematoma is an uncommon injury that results from a direct blow to the epigastrium (blunt force delivered by a small-diameter instrument such as a broom handle or the toe of a boot) or from rapid deceleration (e.g., in the lap belt syndrome) and may cause partial or complete gastric outlet obstruction. Bleeding into the wall of the duodenum causes compression and therefore symptoms of intestinal obstruction, including pain, bilious vomiting, and gastric distention.

Diagnosis is made by ultrasonography, contrast upper gastrointestinal study, or a CT scan revealing the "coiled spring sign" or a soft tissue mass in the bowel wall. Injury of the pancreas must be suspected when duodenal hematoma is considered. Nonoperative management includes nasogastric decompression and parenteral nutrition for up to 3 weeks.

Rupture of the gallbladder is rare and is almost always associated with severe blunt trauma to the liver. It will almost always be accompanied by severe peritonitis. Likewise, hematobilia is associated with hepatic trauma and is a result of pressure necrosis from an intrahepatic hematoma or direct injury to the biliary tree. Children with hematobilia present several days to weeks after a blunt abdominal trauma with abdominal pain and upper gastrointestinal tract bleeding. Hepatic angiography confirms the diagnosis. Embolization is used to achieve hemostasis and is almost always successful, but partial hepatic resection may be necessary when this treatment fails.

PENETRATING ABDOMINAL TRAUMA

Goals of Treatment

The approach to these patients includes identification and management of all life-threatening injuries and treatment of hemorrhagic shock. The need for laparotomy must be determined quickly, and broad-spectrum antibiotics, such as cefoxitin 25 mg per kg, should be given. Intra-abdominal organs are at risk for penetrating trauma, depending on their size and location.

Hypovolemia or signs of peritonitis, or both, are the results of brisk hemorrhage and spillage of enteric contents into the peritoneal space.

CLINICAL PEARLS AND PITFALLS

- Penetrating abdominal trauma is much less common than blunt trauma in children younger than 16 years of age and accounts for less than 10% of pediatric trauma injuries.
- The high morbidity and mortality associated with penetrating trauma to the abdomen is a result of the destructive force of ballistic missiles and fragments, rapid hemorrhage of vascular structures and solid organs after missile and stab injuries, difficulty in surgical repair of grossly injured intra-abdominal organs, and postoperative complications.
- The colon and small bowel are large in volume and are the most commonly injured structures, followed by the liver, spleen, and major vessels.

Gunshot Wounds

The destructive energy of ballistic missiles and fragments is related to mass and velocity (kinetic energy = $\frac{1}{2}MV^2$, where M is the mass and V is the velocity), and more than 90% of gunshot wounds to the abdomen are associated with significant injuries. Hollow viscera and large vessels are often involved, and solid organs such as the liver and the spleen may demonstrate burst injuries. Therefore, laparotomy is mandated in virtually all gunshot wounds to the abdomen.

Stab Wounds

Stab wounds to the abdomen carry potential for devastating injury, depending on which intra-abdominal structures are involved. The extent of the injury also depends on the type, size, and length of the weapon and on the trajectory. Major vascular injuries pose the greatest threat; commonly injured vessels include the intra-abdominal aorta, the inferior vena cava, the portal vein, and the hepatic veins.

Anterior stab wounds should be explored via laparoscopy or laparotomy if hemodynamic instability or signs of peritonitis are present, if blood is noted in the gastric aspirate or on rectal examination, or if pneumoperitoneum or evisceration is noted (Fig. 111.3). Local exploration may be used to rule out penetration of the peritoneum, even in minor stab wounds, but laparoscopy is a very effective means for the evaluation of stab wounds and many minor injuries can be repaired without open surgery.

Stab wounds to the flank or back are less readily and less quickly diagnosed than anterior wounds; the retroperitoneal structures are more protected by paraspinal musculature, and bleeding is often tamponaded in this area. Dorsal stab wounds are sometimes managed nonoperatively unless hemodynamic instability or signs of peritonitis are present, although selective laparotomy is a common surgical strategy.

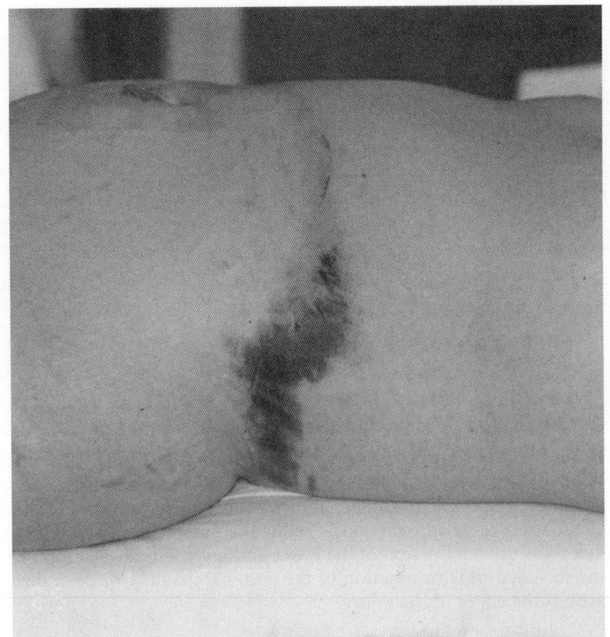

FIGURE 111.9 An 11-year-old girl with classic abdominal and flank ecchymosis in the pattern of a lap belt. Her injuries included colon perforation and a Chance fracture.

ABDOMINAL INJURIES—THE LAP BELT COMPLEX AND CHILD ABUSE

Goals of Treatment

Occult injuries in the context of motor vehicle crashes and abusive trauma are not unusual.

The goal of evaluation and treatment of such patient is detection of injuries; hence, the index of suspicion must remain high.

CLINICAL PEARLS AND PITFALLS

- Children who are too small for adult seat belts are at increased risk for injuries, including fractures of the lumbar spine in association with intra-abdominal injuries.
- Blunt abdominal trauma in children abuse is uncommon but mortality rates are as high as 50%.

LAP AND SHOULDER BELT AND AIR BAG INJURIES

Children restrained only by lap belts in motor vehicles involved in rapid deceleration crashes are at risk to sustain Chance fractures (compression or flexion–distraction fractures of the lumbar spine) in association with intra-abdominal injuries (the lap belt complex). As many as 50% of children with Chance fractures have intra-abdominal injuries, including duodenal perforation, mesenteric disruption, transection of small bowel, pancreatic injury, and bladder rupture (Fig. 111.8). Therefore, a high index of suspicion must be maintained to detect such injuries. The hallmark of the lap belt complex is abdominal or flank ecchymosis in the pattern of a strap or belt (Fig. 111.9). This is accompanied by abdominal and back pain. A normal abdominal CT scan does not rule out ruptured viscus, and laparoscopy or laparotomy should be considered for children in whom the lap belt complex is suspected strongly (Figs. 111.10 and 111.11). Carotid injuries caused by high-riding shoulder restraints in motor vehicle collisions are much less common. Consideration should be given

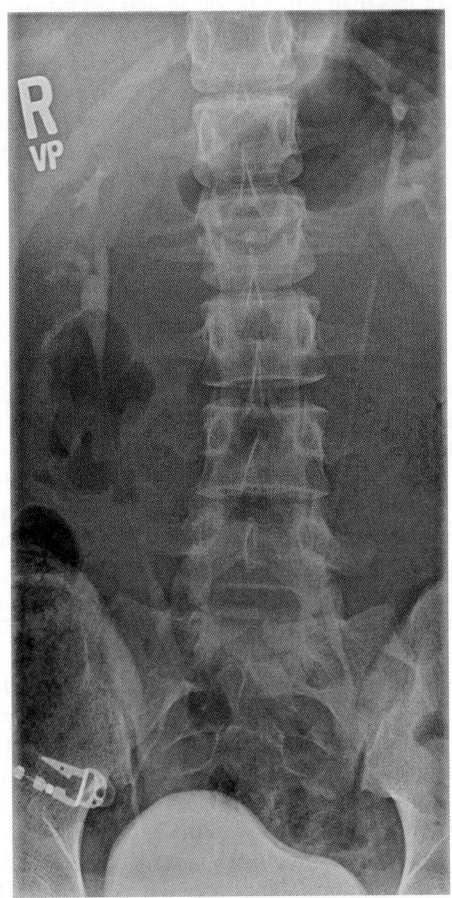

FIGURE 111.10 Plain radiograph of the lumbar spine of a 15-year-old boy lap belt only restrained passenger in a motor vehicle crash over an embankment. There is a transverse Chance fracture of the vertebral body and posterior elements of L2. The lap belt complex in this patient also included a small bowel contusion, pancreatic head contusion, a focal area of aortic disruption (dissection) just inferior to the renal arteries, and a retroperitoneal hematoma.

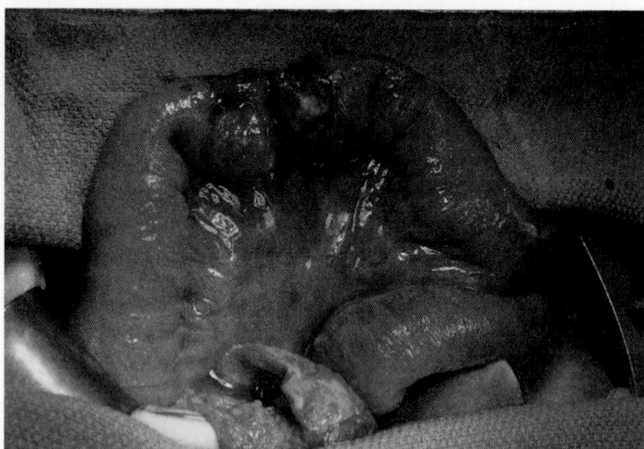

FIGURE 111.11 Intraoperative photograph of a segment of small bowel of a 15-year-old boy who was a lap and shoulder belt–restrained back seat passenger in a motor vehicle collision. Initial examination revealed ecchymosis below the umbilicus and significant tenderness upon palpation of the lower abdomen. Findings at laparotomy included near transaction of the terminal ileum with devitalized tissue at the edges of the injury.

for CT angiography of the neck vessels if there is evidence of significant neck contusion or trauma.

Although it is well publicized that children younger than 12 years or less than 5 ft in height should not ride in the front seat of a vehicle that has functioning air bag restraints, significant injuries and deaths continue to occur. Life-threatening injuries caused by air bag deployment are typically related to cervical spine injuries and closed head trauma. Less severe air bag injuries include abrasions to the face, neck, and chest; minor burns to the upper extremities; blunt ocular trauma; and chemical keratitis.

Child Abuse

The most recent report by the National Child Abuse and Neglect Data System (NCANDS) of the Children's Bureau estimated that 1,640 children died of abuse and neglect during 2012 (see Chapter 95 Child Abuse/Assault). Major blunt abdominal trauma resulting from physical abuse is uncommon but highly fatal in children; mortality rates are as high as 50%. This high fatality rate is the result of the unfortunate but typical delay with which parents or caregivers who abuse children seek treatment.

Children who are seriously injured because of physical abuse commonly have more than one site of trauma; some of the injuries can be occult, and others may have been inflicted at different times. Abdominal injuries are usually inflicted by fists, feet, or small handheld objects and are rarely penetrating. The diagnosis of blunt abdominal injury caused by battering is difficult to make unless a high index of suspicion for child abuse is maintained. An important clue is often an implausible historical account for the seriousness of the injury. As with abdominal trauma caused by other mechanisms, physical examination findings may not be obvious. Laboratory analyses and abdominal CT may be necessary to confirm the diagnosis.

Severe injuries may present with obtundation and shock, abdominal distention, and tenderness. Intra-abdominal injuries most commonly involve the liver and the spleen, as well as the pancreas–duodenum–jejunum region. In all such cases in which child battering is suspected, a child protection consultant should be involved early.

Suggested Readings and Key References

Initial Evaluation and Management of Abdominal Trauma

Holmes JF, Sokolove PE, Brant WE, et al. Identification of children with intra-abdominal injuries after blunt trauma. *Ann Emerg Med* 2002;39:500–509.

Subcommittee on Advanced Trauma Life Support of the American College of Surgeons Trauma Committee. *Advanced trauma life support for doctors*. 8th ed. Chicago, IL: American College of Surgeons, 2008.

Management of Blunt Abdominal Trauma

Cigdem MK, Onen A, Siga M, et al. Selective nonoperative management of penetrating abdominal injuries in children. *J Trauma* 2009; 67(6):1284–1286.

Gaines BA, Ford HR. Abdominal and pelvic trauma in children. *Crit Care Med* 2002;30:S416–S423.

Iqbal CQ, St. Peter SD, Tsao K, et al. Operative vs non-operative management for blunt pancreatic transection in children: multi-institutional outcomes. *J Am Coll Surg* 2014;218:157–162.

Marwan A, Harmon CM, Georgeson KE, et al. Use of laparoscopy in the management of pediatric abdominal trauma. *J Trauma* 2010;69: 761–764.

Wood JH, Partrick DA, Bruny JL, et al. Operative vs nonoperative management of blunt pancreatic trauma in children. *J Pediatr Surg* 2010;45:401–406.

Management of Penetrating Abdominal Trauma

Adesanya AA, da Rocha-Afodu JT, Ekanem EE, et al. Factors affecting mortality and morbidity in patients with abdominal gunshot wounds. *Injury* 2000;31:397–404.

Berardoni NE, Kopelman TR, O'Neill PJ, et al. Use of computed tomography in the initial evaluation of anterior abdominal stab wounds. *Am J Surg* 2011;202:690–695.

Boleken ME, Cevik M, Yagiz B, et al. The characteristics and outcomes of penetrating thoracic and abdominal trauma among children. *Pediatr Surg Int* 2013;29:795–800.

Zantut LF, Ivatury RR, Smith RS, et al. Diagnostic and therapeutic laparoscopy for penetrating abdominal trauma: a multicenter experience. *J Trauma* 1997;42:825–831.

Lap Belt Complex

Durbin DR, Arbogast KB, Moll EK. Seat belt syndrome in children: a case report and review of the literature. *Pediatr Emerg Care* 2001;17:474–477.

Le TV, Baaj AA, Deukmedjian A, et al. Chance fractures in the pediatric population. *J Neurosurg Pediatr* 2011;8:189–197.

Moremen JR, Nakayama DK, Ashley DW, et al. Traumatic disruption of the abdominal wall: lap-belt injuries in children. *J Pediatr Surg* 2013;48:e21–e24.

Newman KD, Bowman LM, Eichelberger MR, et al. The lap belt complex: intestinal and lumbar spine injury in children. *J Trauma* 1990;30:1133–1140.

Paris C, Brindamour M, Ouimet A, et al. Predictive indicators for bowel injury in pediatric patients who present with a positive seat belt sign after motor vehicle collision. *J Pediatr Surg* 2010;45: 921–924.

Child Abuse

Child maltreatment 2012. 23rd Annual Report: National Child Abuse and Neglect Data System (NCANDS) of the Children's Bureau. Available at http://www.acf.hhs.gov/programs/cb/research-data-technology/statistics-research/child-maltreatment.

Maguire SA, Upadhyaya M, Evans A, et al. A systematic review of abusive visceral injuries in childhood–their range and recognition. *Child Abuse Negl* 2013;37:430–445.

Diagnostic Laboratory in Abdominal Trauma

Capraro AJ, Mooney DP, Waltzman ML. The use of routine laboratory studies as screening tools in pediatric abdominal trauma. *Pediatr Emerg Care* 2006;22:480–484.

Karaduman D, Sarioglu-Buke A, Kilic I, et al. The role of elevated liver transaminase levels in children with blunt abdominal trauma. *Injury* 2003;34:249–252.

Lindberg DM, Shapiro RA, Blood EA, et al. Utility of hepatic transaminases in children with concern for abuse. *Pediatrics* 2013;131:268–275.

Computerized Tomography as a Diagnostic Tool for Abdominal Trauma

Chatoorgoon K, Brown RL, Garcia VF, et al. Role of computed tomography and clinical findings in pediatric blunt intestinal injury: a multicenter study. *Pediatr Emerg Care* 2012;8(12):1338–1342.

Hackam DJ, Potoka D, Meza M, et al. Utility of radiographic hepatic injury grade in predicting outcome for children after blunt abdominal trauma. *J Pediatr Surg* 2002;37:386–389.

Kerrey BT, Rogers AJ, Lee LK, et al. A multicenter study of the risk of intra-abdominal injury in children after normal abdominal computed tomography scan results in the emergency department. *Ann Emerg Med* 2013;62:319–326.

Ultrasonography as a Diagnostic Tool for Abdominal Trauma

Fox JC, Boysen M, Gharahbaghian L, et al. Test characteristics of focused assessment of sonography for trauma for clinically significant abdominal free fluid in pediatric blunt abdominal trauma. *Acad Emerg Med* 2011;18:477–482.

Richards JR, Schleper NH, Woo BD, et al. Sonographic assessment of blunt abdominal trauma: a 4-year prospective study. *J Clin Ultrasound* 2002;30:59–67.

Scaife ER, Rollins MD, Barnhart DC, et al. The role for focused abdominal sonography for trauma (FAST) in pediatric trauma evaluation. *J Ped Surg* 2013;48:1377–1383.

Sola JE, Cheung MC, Yang R, et al. Pediatric FAST and elevated liver transaminases: an effective screening tool in blunt abdominal trauma. *J Surg Res* 2009;157(1):103–107.

Williams SR, Perera P, Gharahbaghian L. The FAST and E-FAST in 2013: trauma ultrasonography: overview, practical techniques, controversies, and new frontiers. *Crit Care Clin* 2014;30(1):119–150.

CHAPTER 112 ■ BURNS

ANGELA M. ELLISON, MD, MSc AND MARGARET SAMUELS-KALOW, MD, MPhil, MSHP

GOALS OF EMERGENCY CARE

As with any emergent situation, the goals of emergency care for the burned patient include the protection of the airway, and maintenance of breathing and circulation. For the burned patient in particular, this will include attention to the potential of inhalational injury and airway edema, consideration of burn location and need for escharotomy to ensure chest wall movement, and early and careful fluid resuscitation of burn shock. Beyond immediate resuscitative interventions, rapid resuscitation and appropriate wound care can significantly improve both mortality and functional outcomes. Concomitant control of pain is also an important aspect of care for the burned patient, both to prevent unnecessary discomfort and to permit required procedures. Finally, burn management aims at decreasing the risk of infection created by disruption of the skin barrier function, and facilitating healing and optimal cosmetic outcomes.

KEY POINTS

- Burns should be described by estimated depth (superficial, partial thickness, or full thickness) and total body surface area involved (TBSA).
- Significant burns are often accompanied by other injuries (including ocular, inhalational, or traumatic) that may require emergent assessment and treatment.
- Full-thickness burns will be insensate due to destruction of the cutaneous nerves of the dermis.
- Severe burn injury requires intravenous fluid resuscitation, often calculated using the Parkland formula: IV fluid volume (mL) = (weight in kg) × (% TBSA burned) × 4. Half of this volume is given in the first 8 hours and the remaining half during the subsequent 16 hours, in addition to 24-hour maintenance fluids.

RELATED CHAPTERS

General Approach to the Ill or Injured Child
- A General Approach to Ill and Injured Children: Chapter 1
- Airway: Chapter 3
- Shock: Chapter 5

Signs and Symptoms
- Pain: Dysphagia: Chapter 51
- Respiratory Distress: Chapter 66
- Stridor: Chapter 70
- Wheezing: Chapter 80

Clinical Pathways
- Shock: Chapter 91

Medical, Surgical, and Trauma Emergencies
- Child Abuse/Assault: Chapter 95
- Toxicologic Emergencies: Chapter 110

INITIAL ASSESSMENT AND RESUSCITATION

CLINICAL PEARLS AND PITFALLS

- Consider early intubation in patients with pharyngeal or airway swelling
- Inquire about the circumstances of the burn and determine the potential for associated injuries
- Maintain cervical spine precautions when managing the airway until spinal injury has been excluded
- Remember to remove sources of continued burn

Current Evidence

Globally, burns are the 11th leading cause of death in children aged 1 to 9 and the fifth most common cause of nonlethal injury. Data from the National Burn Repository (2012) suggest that burn injuries are more prevalent in minority children than would be expected based on demographics alone. Scald and contact burns are more common in the younger ages, with fire/flame more common in adolescent and adult patients.

Recent data suggest significantly improved survival for children with careful attention to burn care. In one study, half of children with burn injuries up to 90% TBSA survived their injuries, and research is ongoing into new methods for surgical management and pharmacologic treatment of burn wounds. Burn size and inhalational injury are two key predictors of survival in children.

Major systemic physiologic effects are seen in children with burns of more than 20% of body surface area (BSA). Burn injury causes increased capillary permeability and the release of osmotically active molecules to the interstitial space resulting in extravasation of fluid. Protein is lost from the vascular space to the interstitium during the first 24 hours. In patients with large burns, vasoactive mediators are released to the circulation and result in systemic capillary leakage. Edema develops in both burned and noninjured tissues. Circulating factors that depress myocardial function decrease cardiac output. Acute hemolysis of up to 15% of red blood cells may occur both from direct heat damage and from a microangiopathic hemolytic process. The profound circulatory effects of severe burns can result in life-threatening shock early after injury.

Goals of Treatment

High quality care is key for functional outcome and survival from burn injuries. Emergency management including prehospital care, assessment, resuscitation, treatment of potential inhalational injury, wound care, infection control, and appropriate admission are the first steps in a continuum of care that extends through hospitalization, potential surgical management, and rehabilitation. The unifying goal of these treatment modalities is to compensate for the physiologic effects of the burn and promote healing.

Clinical Considerations

Clinical Recognition

During the first few seconds after arrival, the physician must determine if a patient with burn injury requires aggressive therapy for major burns. In children with severe injuries, the evaluation and initial management take place simultaneously. Smoldering clothing or other sources of continued burning must be removed. Information about the circumstances of the burn and the potential for associated injuries should be sought from prehospital care providers, police, or family members, but this should not delay the initial treatment.

It is crucial to recognize inhalational injury as a cause of impending airway obstruction or respiratory failure. Clinical signs of potential inhalational injury include smoke exposure, burns on the face, singed nasal hairs, soot in sputum or visible in the upper airway, wheezing or rales.

TABLE 112.1

BURN TRIAGE GUIDELINES

Triage level	Characteristics
Resuscitation room	Inhalational injury, altered mental status/LOC, chest pain, arrhythmias, associated major trauma
1—Critical	Facial burns with: singed nasal hairs, hoarse breath sounds, oral edema, dysphagia
	Burns >25% TBSA
	Electrical burns with hx of either altered mental status or seizure
2—Acute	Any full-thickness burn
	Partial thickness >15% TBSA
	Burns to face, genitalia
	Caustic chemicals to eyes
	Circumferential burns
	Significant burns of hands, feet
	Any burn with significant pain
	Caustic skin burns
	Electrical burns with any of:
	Loss of consciousness
	Thrown from source or frozen to source
	Entrance and exit wounds
	Concern for abuse
3—Urgent	Partial thickness >5% TBSA
	Infected burn
	Burns requiring debridement
4—Urgent	<5% partial-thickness burn
5—Nonurgent	Burn redress
	Superficial burn

Triage Considerations

All children with nontrivial burns should be rapidly transported to a hospital setting. Once in the hospital, the triage process should take into account child's age and medical history, the injury mechanism, and the surface area and depth of the burn. Children <2 years of age and those with significant comorbidities have a higher risk of burn-related complications. The physical response to burn injury and mortality prognosis appears to worsen significantly at around 30% TBSA burned, and so those children should be triaged to more rapid care.

One possible triage guideline based on a five-level emergency severity index (ESI) scale is shown in Table 112.1.

Clinical Assessment

Percentages. After the primary survey and initial stabilization, a systematic evaluation of the surface area and depth of burns follows. The rule of nines is used to estimate burn surface area in adolescents and adults. Each arm is approximately 9% TBSA, each leg is 18%, the anterior and posterior torso are each 18%, the head is 9%, and the perineum is 1%.

However, this rule cannot be applied to children because they have different body proportions. Young children have relatively larger heads and smaller extremities. Therefore, age-adjusted methods of estimating burn surface area have been developed (see Fig. 112.1). Alternatively, a child's palm including the fingers is approximately 1% of BSA and this can be used to estimate the extent of scattered, smaller burns.

Areas of partial- and full-thickness injuries should be recorded on an anatomic chart and then a percentage of TBSA computed. First-degree burns are not included. BSA calculations are inexact, and some burns may progress over time, so BSA estimates should be reassessed.

Description of Burn. The language used to describe burn severity has evolved over time, from a nomenclature of degrees to a description of the anatomic depth of the burn (see Fig. 112.2).

A superficial burn (formerly called first degree) occurs when the epidermis is injured but the dermis is intact. These burns are characterized by redness and a mild inflammatory response confined to the epidermis, without significant edema or bulla formation (see Fig. 112.3A). Superficial burns are not included in the calculation of burn surface area used for therapeutic decisions. These minor burns may be painful and usually resolve in 3 to 5 days without scarring.

In a partial-thickness burn (formerly called second degree), the dermis is partially injured and blistering is often present (see Fig. 112.3B). Increased capillary permeability, resulting from direct thermal injury and local mediator release, results in edema. These injuries are usually painful because intact sensory nerve receptors are exposed. The capillary network in the superficial dermis gives these burns a pink-red color and moist appearance. Healing occurs in about 2 weeks, and scarring is usually minimal.

Deep partial-thickness burns involve destruction of the epidermis and most of the dermis. Edema can lessen the exposure of sensory nerve receptors, making some partial-thickness burns less painful and tender, although there should

Area	Birth–1 yr	1–4 yr	5–9 yr	10–14 yr	15 yr	Adult
Head	19	17	13	11	9	7
Neck	2	2	2	2	2	2
Anterior trunk	13	13	13	13	13	13
Posterior trunk	13	13	13	13	13	13
Right buttock	2½	2½	2½	2½	2½	2½
Left buttock	2½	2½	2½	2½	2½	2½
Genitalia	1	1	1	1	1	1
Right upper arm	4	4	4	4	4	4
Left upper arm	4	4	4	4	4	4
Right lower arm	3	3	3	3	3	3
Left lower arm	3	3	3	3	3	3
Right hand	2½	2½	2½	2½	2½	2½
Left hand	2½	2½	2½	2½	2½	2½
Right thigh	5½	6½	8	8½	9	9½
Left thigh	5½	6½	8	8½	9	9½
Right leg	5	5	5½	6	6½	7
Left leg	5	5	5½	6	6½	7
Right foot	3½	3½	3½	3½	3½	3½
Left foot	3½	3½	3½	3½	3½	3½
						Total

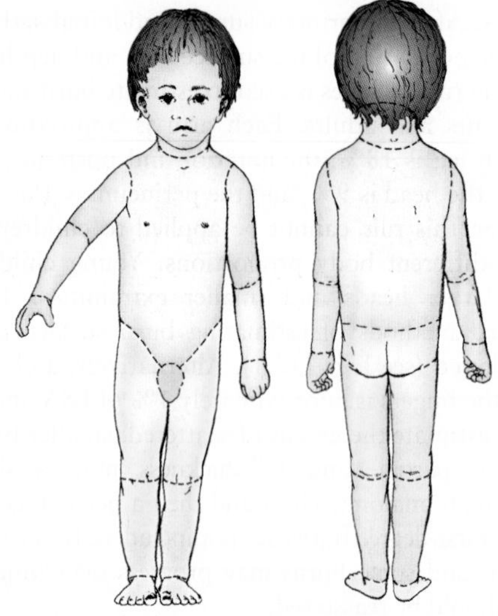

FIGURE 112.1 Estimation of surface area burned on the basis of age. This modification by O'Neill of the Brooke Army Burn Center diagram shows the change in surface of the head from 19% in an infant to 7% in an adult. Proper use of this chart provides an accurate basis for subsequent management of the child with burn injury.

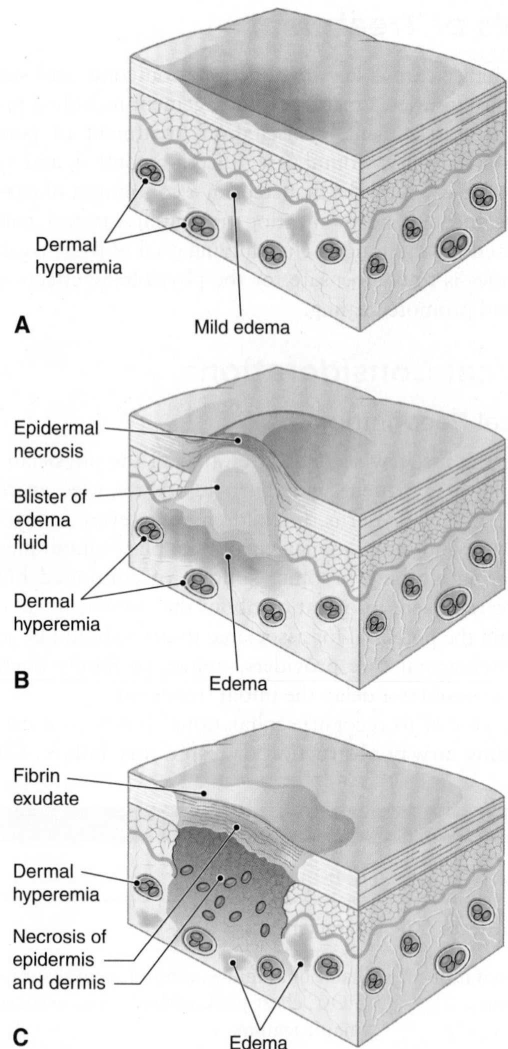

FIGURE 112.2 Skin burns are classified as superficial, partial thickness, or full thickness. **A:** Superficial burns affect only the outer layer of epidermis. **B:** Partial-thickness burns affect the lower layers of epidermis. **C:** Full-thickness burns destroy the entire layer of epidermis. (From Thomas H. McConnell. *Nature of Disease*. 2nd ed. Philadelphia, PA: Lippincott Williams & Wilkins, 2013.)

be some intact pain sensation. Deep partial-thickness burns have a paler, drier appearance than superficial injuries, at times making them difficult to distinguish from full-thickness injury (see Fig. 112.3C). Thrombosed vessels often give deep partial-thickness burns a speckled appearance. Burns evaluated immediately may appear to be partial-thickness injuries and subsequently become full-thickness injuries, especially if secondary damage from infection, trauma, or hypoperfusion ensues. Deep partial-thickness burns can take many weeks to heal completely. Significant scarring is common and skin grafting may be necessary to optimize cosmetic results.

Full-thickness burns (formerly called third degree) involve destruction of the epidermis and the entire dermis. They usually have a pale or charred color and a leathery appearance (see Fig. 112.3D). Important for recognition is the fact that destruction of the cutaneous nerves in the dermis makes them nontender, although surrounding areas of partial-thickness burns may be painful. Full-thickness burns cause a loss of skin elasticity. The burned skin cannot expand as tissue edema develops during the first 24 to 48 hours of fluid therapy. Circumferential or near-circumferential burns can therefore cause respiratory distress, abdominal compartment syndrome, and vascular insufficiency of the distal extremities. Full-thickness burns cannot reepithelialize and can heal only from the periphery. Most require skin grafting.

Management

First Aid. Early cooling is accomplished by running cold water over the injured area. If performed in the first 60 minutes after injury, it not only stops ongoing thermal damage but also prevents edema, reducing progression to full-thickness injury. Applying ice directly to the wound is painful, and the extreme cold can worsen the injury. Parents should be reminded not to put grease, butter, or any ointment on the burn because these substances do not dissipate heat well and may contaminate the area. Intact blisters should not be broken during the prehospital phase. The burn should be covered with a clean cloth or bandage.

Prehospital. Prehospital care providers should focus initially on airway, breathing, and circulation, as they would for any other patient. Rapid transport to a hospital setting is crucial. Oxygen should be administered. The trachea should be intubated if there are signs of

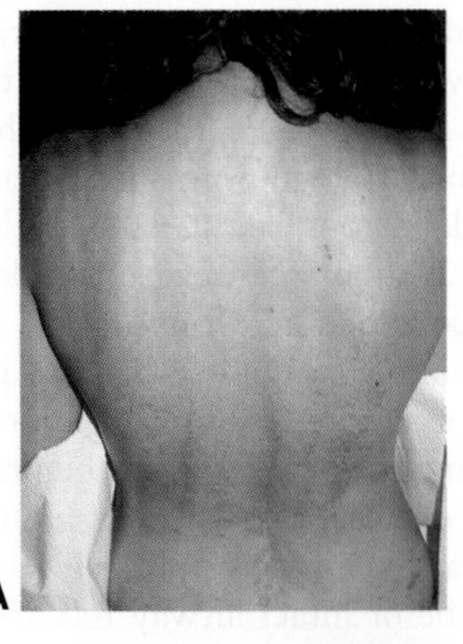

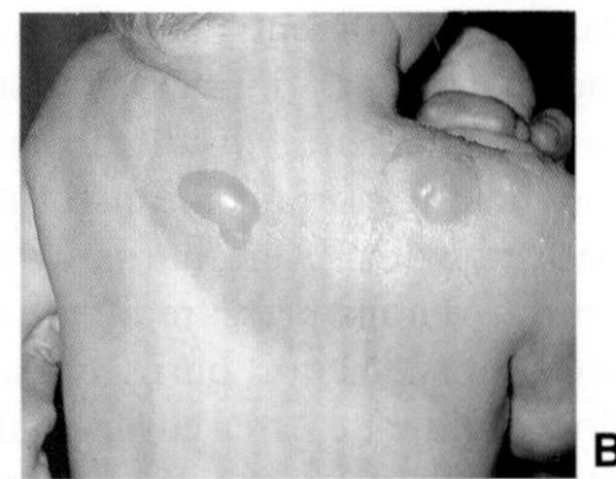

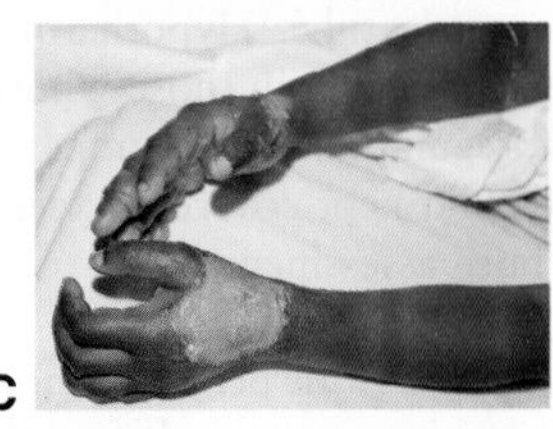

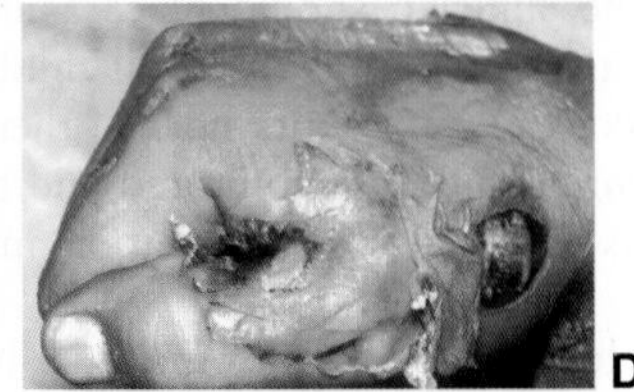

FIGURE 112.3 Examples of burns of various depths. **A:** Superficial: involves only the epidermis. **B:** Superficial partial thickness: partially injured dermis, with blistering. Note the pink-red color and moist appearance. **C:** Deep partial thickness: injury involves all of the epidermis and most of the dermis. Note the paler, drier appearance than superficial injuries. **D:** Full thickness: involves destruction of the entire epidermis and dermis. Not the area of pallor and charred color. These areas may also have a leathery appearance. (From Cohen BJ, Hull K. *Memmler's the human body in health and disease*, 13th ed. Philadelphia, PA: Wolters Kluwer, 2014.)

upper airway obstruction or impending obstruction. If transport time is likely to be prolonged, intravenous fluids should be started.

Emergency Department Management. Specific management of major and minor burns is reviewed in the sections below. The final section also addresses management of burns with specific etiologies: inflicted, chemical, and electrical burns.

Preventing Infection. Heat causes coagulation necrosis of tissue, producing a protein-rich medium that nourishes bacterial growth. Burns become colonized with potentially pathogenic organisms, primarily from the skin and intestinal flora of the patient with burn injury and not from exogenous sources. Cleansing and debridement reduce substrate for bacterial proliferation and topical antimicrobial therapy reduces the number of microorganisms, but burns are never completely sterilized so that the risk of secondary infection is always present. Burn wounds are not treated immediately with systemic antibiotics unless there is clear infection present, but must be watched closely for development of subsequent infection.

MAJOR BURNS

CLINICAL PEARLS AND PITFALLS

- The placement of a sterile sheet over burned areas can provide effective analgesia
- Consider carbon monoxide and cyanide exposure with house fires and do not delay treatment in suspected cases

Current Evidence

Risk of morbidity and mortality is associated with the size of the burn. In a large, single center, prospective study of pediatric burn patients, Kraft et al. found mortality rates ranging from 3% (30% to 39% TBSA) to 55% (90% to 100% TBSA). In this study, burn size of 62% TBSA was the marker of a significantly increased mortality risk.

Goals of Treatment

The initial management of the significantly burned patient includes protection of the airway, maintenance of breathing, and support of circulation, all with the goal of preventing mortality and disability. Initial airway assessment will need to include evaluation and management of potential direct inhalational injury and resultant airway edema, as well as inhaled toxins including carbon monoxide and cyanide. Patients should receive supplemental oxygen, as well as appropriate antidotal therapy, respiratory support as needed (potentially including escharotomy for circumferential chest burns), and appropriate intravenous fluid resuscitation to support their circulatory status. Wound care and pain management is optimized to minimize disability and improve cosmetic and functional outcomes.

Clinical Considerations

In the appropriate clinical circumstances (fire, usually in an enclosed space) it is important to consider carbon monoxide and cyanide poisoning. For carbon monoxide, one should administer 100% O_2 and send a carboxyhemoglobin level. Indications for potential hyperbaric treatment include loss of consciousness at the scene, persistent neurologic symptoms including seizure, evidence of cardiac injury, or significant elevation of carboxyhemoglobin levels (>25% to 40%). The decision to pursue hyperbaric treatment should be made in conjunction with a toxicologist, poison control center, or hyperbaric physician. Cyanide poisoning must be treated before the quantitative level is available. Indications to consider hydroxocobalamin treatment include history of CPR, abnormal vital signs, intubation, evidence of hypoxic injury, and severe metabolic acidosis.

Clinical Recognition

Recognition of the severely injured burn patient is based on a combination of the severity of burn and TBSA involved. Burn shock occurs in adults with burns over 30% of BSA but may occur in children with burns over only 20% of BSA. Circumferential burns and full-thickness burns are of the highest concern.

Triage Considerations

Please see triage guidelines in Table 112.1. Major burns should be triaged to rapid physician assessment and care.

Clinical Assessment

As part of the primary trauma survey, the clinician must be vigilant in carefully evaluating all patients for evidence of inhalational injury. Patients with a history of fire exposure in an enclosed space, soot in the nose or mouth, or facial or airway burns may require intubation for airway protection. These patients may also require treatment for carbon monoxide and cyanide exposure. In the secondary survey, it is of the greatest importance not to neglect the possibility of other injuries from the burn mechanism, or associated injuries, which may also require emergent treatment and stabilization. Finally, patients with ocular area burns will need specialized ophthalmology consultation for evaluation of corneal involvement.

Management

Airway. The inhalation of hot gases can burn the upper airway, leading to progressive edema and airway obstruction. Any child with burns of the face, singed facial hairs, or hoarseness is at high risk, but airway burns can occur in the absence of these signs. Edema of the burned airway will worsen over the first 24 to 48 hours. Knowledge of the time course of airway swelling justifies intubation of the trachea for subtle signs of airway compromise that occur shortly after the injury. Early intubation may circumvent a difficult intubation later in the course of a child with severe pharyngeal and airway edema. Endotracheal tubes of smaller diameter than expected for age should be available in anticipation of a narrowed airway. Cuffed tubes are preferred to accommodate the potential for changing airway edema over the course of the recovery.

Children who have jumped or fallen in house fires, been burned in motor vehicle accidents, or been burned by explosions are at risk for associated cervical spine and other traumatic injuries, and cervical spine precautions should be maintained during management of their airways. Furthermore, children with severe burns may have depressed levels of consciousness for many reasons and airway obstruction from the loss of pharyngeal tone is not uncommon.

Breathing. A rapid assessment of ventilation includes respiratory effort, chest expansion, breath sounds, and color. Pulse oximetry is useful, but patients with significant levels of carboxyhemoglobin will look pink and have "normal" oxygen saturation as measured by a pulse oximeter. Children with severe burn injury should receive 100% oxygen. Arterial blood gases with co-oximetry should be obtained promptly.

Inhalational injury can also cause damage to the lower airway. Chest radiographs may be normal initially, even if pulmonary injury has occurred. Mild inhalational injury can be treated with supplemental oxygen, and consideration of albuterol or racemic epinephrine nebulizer treatment. Steroids are generally not recommended for treatment of burn patients with airway injury, although a single center study showed no increased risk with a single dose. Patients should continue to be monitored closely for any deterioration in their clinical status. Significant inhalational injury will require intubation and ventilatory support.

Extensive full-thickness burns of the thorax may restrict expansion of the chest and impair ventilation. Respiratory insufficiency in this setting is an indication for escharotomy of the chest. Incision through the depth of the eschar should be performed along the anterior axillary lines to allow adequate chest expansion. If the deep burns extend to the abdomen, the escharotomies should be extended downward and connected by incision along the costal margin.

Circulation. The rapid assessment of circulation includes skin color, capillary refill time, temperature of the peripheral extremities, heart rate, and mental status. Blood pressure is often maintained until late in the course of shock, making it an unreliable early measure. Hypertension from increased systemic vascular resistance has been reported immediately after severe burns, particularly in pediatric patients, and should not be taken as an indication to discontinue proper fluid therapy.

Vascular access should be obtained soon after the arrival of the child with severe burn injury. Peripheral, large-bore intravenous catheters are favored because they have the lowest resistance. Catheters placed in the upper extremity through intact skin are preferred because they are easier to secure, but access through burned areas may be necessary. Anticipating the need for hyperalimentation, sites for central catheter placement should be saved, if possible. Attention to aseptic technique when starting intravenous catheters in the ED can prevent infectious complications during subsequent care. Circumferential taping is dangerous because the swelling that occurs during the first 24 hours can cause circulatory insufficiency distal to the constriction. Urine output is the most important means of monitoring fluid status, but in patients with severe burns with associated inhalation injury, central venous pressure monitoring may be useful in the first few hours. Major burns cause decreased splanchnic blood flow and ileus. After ensuring that the airway is protected by placement of an endotracheal tube or intact airway reflexes, the clinician should place a nasogastric tube. Hypothermia can occur rapidly in small children, especially in those whose skin injury impairs normal thermoregulation. Core temperature should be monitored and the child kept covered, except as necessary for examination and burn assessment.

Fluid Resuscitation. An initial bolus of 20 mL per kg of normal saline or Ringer's lactate solution is recommended while assessment of the extent of the burns takes place. Fluid volume from initial boluses and prehospital care should be counted when calculating fluid volumes during the first 24 hours of treatment. A urinary catheter should be placed early in the management because there are often several hours of monitoring during transport or in the ED during which urine production can provide clinicians with information about fluid status.

Rapid treatment of the hypovolemia that occurs early in children with severe thermal injuries is of prime importance. The fluid status of children with burn injury is a dynamic process that requires careful reevaluation and therapeutic adjustments. Extravasation of water, sodium, and protein through abnormally permeable capillaries continues for about 24 hours after injury. Capillary integrity then improves and intravascular volume stabilizes. Isotonic crystalloid solutions are recommended in the resuscitation phase. Potassium is released from damaged cells and may elevate measured serum levels shortly after injury; therefore, potassium replacement is not recommended during the early phase of fluid therapy.

Several formulas for the calculation of initial fluid therapy exist (see Table 112.2). The Parkland formula recommends 4 mL/kg/% of BSA of crystalloid over the first 24 hours, half during the first 8 hours from the time of injury and half during the next 16 hours. This formula underestimates the fluid needs of young children, who are also at greater risk for hypoglycemia. Maintenance requirements are added for patients with burns who are younger than 5 years using isotonic solutions with 5% dextrose. The Galveston Shriners formula uses BSA rather than weight to calculate fluid therapy. Galveston Shriners recommends 5,000 mL/m^2/% of BSA, half during the first 8 hours from the time of injury and half during the next 16 hours, plus 2,000 mL/m^2/day as maintenance.

TABLE 112.2

FLUID RESUSCITATION FORMULAS

Parkland: 4 mL/kg/% of BSA second- and third-degree burns, half in the first 8 hrs following injury, half in the next 16 hrs. Add maintenance with 5% dextrose in children <5 years old

Galveston Shriners: 5,000 mL/m^2/% of BSA second- and third-degree burns, half in the first 8 hrs, half in the next 16 hrs. Add 2,000 mL/m^2/day maintenance with 5% dextrose

Inadequate resuscitation can cause organ failure and death, while over resuscitation, or excessive fluid administration, is to be avoided because it may cause pulmonary edema and tissue edema that compromise local blood supply with resultant compartment syndrome.

A combination of endpoints is used to ensure adequate resuscitation, including urine output, mean arterial pressure, and biochemical markers such as base excess and lactate. Urine output should be measured to ensure adequate fluid resuscitation. Children should produce at least 1 mL/kg/hr of urine. Hyperglycemia may cause an osmotic diuresis and complicate care of the patient with burn injury. Before infusions are decreased in response to excessive urine output, a measurement of blood glucose should be made. Inadequate fluid resuscitation is usually manifested by oliguria. Rarely, intrinsic renal disease is responsible for oliguria, as may occur after electrical injuries because of myoglobinuria.

Trauma associated with burns may increase fluid requirements. Neurogenic shock from unrecognized cervical spine or head injury may cause hypotension, usually with a relative bradycardia. Toxins, such as cyanide, ingested before the burn or inhaled during the fire can depress myocardial function or vascular tone. Any patient with shock that appears out of proportion to the extent of the burn injury, or who is poorly responsive to fluid therapy, should have an aggressive diagnostic workup for concurrent problems.

Antibiotics. Burn sepsis continues to be the major cause of mortality after the period of resuscitation, despite improvements in topical and systemic antimicrobials. Meticulous antiseptic techniques can lessen colonization of burns with potential pathogens. Topical antibiotics further reduce bacterial number. Early streptococcal cellulitis is less common than in years before the development of topical antibiotics for burns. Most burn centers do not routinely treat patients with prophylactic systemic antibiotics given absence of data to support this practice, and the increased likelihood of inducing resistant organisms. Frequent examination of healing burns for signs of infection and cultures to monitor colonization can direct specific antibiotic therapy if documented infections were to occur.

Wound Care. Early surgical management of some partial-thickness and most full-thickness burns with excision and grafting has been an important advance in burn treatment. Initially, burns should be covered loosely with sterile sheets during the resuscitation phase in severe injuries. Once the cardiorespiratory status is stabilized, the wounds are uncovered and assessed for size and depth. The goals of burn wound care are to promote rapid healing and prevent infection. Cleansing with large volumes of lukewarm sterile saline reduces contamination. Loose tissue can often be wiped away with sterile gauze, simplifying and expediting burn debridement. Blisters should be left intact whenever possible. However, large blisters or those that obscure the assessment of the burn depth may need further debridement. Smaller blisters may be left intact to preserve the barrier to bacterial invasion. Application of temporary skin substitutes may reduce pain, expedite healing, and reduce length of hospitalization compared with topical antibiotics and conventional dressings but are often not applied in the ED. It is not necessary to apply topical antimicrobials to burns prior to transfer to a burn center or tertiary care children's hospital.

Escharotomy. First, all jewelry and watches should be removed because these may restrict distal flow of the blood. For extensive, deep upper extremity burns, the radial and ulnar pulses should be checked by Doppler ultrasound if it cannot be palpated. Posterior tibial and dorsalis pedis pulses are assessed when the lower extremity is involved. Absence of flow or progressive diminution of the pulse is an indication for escharotomy through the depth of the eschar on the medial and lateral aspects of the extremities, including the hands. Finger escharotomies are seldom necessary and should be undertaken only after consultation with a burn center surgeon. It is especially important to extend escharotomy incisions across the joints because at these locations, the skin is tightly adhered to the underlying fascia where vascular obstruction is likely to occur. The procedure does not require anesthesia because the wounds are full thickness and therefore insensate. Pulses assessed by Doppler ultrasound should immediately improve after escharotomy. If improvement is not immediate, hypovolemia should be suspected. Reperfusion of the extremities after escharotomy may abruptly reduce intravascular volume and require prompt adjustment of fluid therapy.

Tetanus. Children who have received <3 doses of tetanus toxoid or whose immunization status is unknown require tetanus toxoid-containing vaccine and tetanus immunoglobulin. Children who have had >3 doses of the vaccine require only the vaccine. Red Book Guidelines suggest giving Td to those between 7 and 10 years and Tdap to those 11 years or greater (see Chapter 118 Minor Trauma, Table 118.1 Tetanus Prophylaxis).

Pain Management. Safely reducing pain is an important consideration in the management of children with burns of all sizes. Calm, developmentally appropriate verbal reassurance, even to preverbal children, can reduce anxiety and dramatically reduce the perception of pain. The exposure of sensory nerve receptors in partial-thickness burns makes them sensitive to environmental stimuli. Movement of cool air across burned tissue increases pain significantly. The simple measure of covering burns with a sterile sheet, only exposing them when necessary for burn assessment, is an extremely effective and safe analgesia.

Many children will still have significant pain after nonpharmacologic measures are taken. Narcotic analgesics are useful when administered appropriately. Morphine may reduce the blood pressure, especially in patients who are hypovolemic. Fentanyl causes less cardiovascular effect than morphine but has a short half-life. Clinicians should be prepared to support the circulation with intravenous fluids when using opioids.

Analgesic medications administered intravenously are preferred in patients with severe burns because they are more effective and predictable. Intramuscular injections or oral doses should not be given to patients with significant burns because circulation to muscle and gut is reduced, and absorption of medication will be delayed and unpredictable. In children who do not respond well to the initial dose of pain medication, a careful assessment for other causes of pain or agitation should be sought. The possibility of compartment syndrome, hypoxemia, early shock, and occult injuries should be assessed while simultaneously preparing repeated doses of analgesics. Analgesic administration just before debridement of the burn wound is recommended.

Disposition (Transfer Criteria). Guidelines for admission must be individualized when treating children with burns.

Hospitals, physicians, and parents have varying capabilities for managing pediatric patients with burns. If a physician suspects that the burns cannot be adequately cared for in the home, admission to the hospital is warranted.

Children with burns <5% TBSA can be considered for outpatient management with close follow-up. Admission criteria include 5% to 10% TBSA burn, 2% to 5% TBSA full-thickness burn, high voltage injury, concern for inhalational injury, circumferential burn, significant associated trauma, or medical comorbidity (such as diabetes or sickle-cell disease). Burns in certain locations are at higher risk for disability or poor cosmetic outcome and should be considered for treatment in the hospital. These include more than 1% of BSA burns of the face, perineum, hands, and feet; or burns overlying joints. Children with any of the following should be considered for transfer to a burn center: >10% TBSA burn, >5% TBSA full-thickness burn, high-voltage burn, chemical burn, known inhalational injury, burn to face, hands, feet, perineum, joints, significant comorbidities that could affect treatment, intentional burns, or major associated injury.

MINOR BURNS

CLINICAL PEARLS AND PITFALLS

- Suspicious injuries should be reported to the appropriate authorities and should prompt further clinical investigation
- Assess the safety of the household and provide anticipatory guidance even in cases where there is not a suspicion of inflicted injury
- Ensure adequate wound care and follow-up

Goals of Treatment

A small minority of all burns in children requires therapy in the hospital. Once a careful assessment has led to a decision to manage a burn as an outpatient, preparations for treatment at home should begin. Parents become the physician's partner in this context and need to be instructed carefully. The goal of the treatment of minor burns is to reduce pain, decrease risk of infection, and improve functional outcome through careful home management and close outpatient follow-up.

Clinical Considerations

It is important to consider the possibility of inflicted burns and to carefully examine even minor burns for characteristic shapes and patterns. Additionally, it is crucial to perform a detailed secondary survey to ensure that no other traumatic injuries are missed.

Clinical Recognition

A child with superficial or partial-thickness burns <5% TBSA may be a suitable candidate for outpatient burn care. There should be no concern for inflicted burn, and appropriate parental and family resources need to be in place to ensure careful home care and close follow-up.

Triage Considerations

See Table 112.1 for suggested triage guidelines. Most minor burns can be triaged to the urgent or nonurgent level of care.

Clinical Assessment

Analgesia may be needed to perform a careful wound assessment. Sloughed epidermis should be removed with sterile normal saline and gauze, allowing for a detailed examination of the size and depth of the wound. A burn dressing should be placed immediately after wound assessment.

Management

Blisters. For minor burns, blisters provide a biologic dressing and intact blisters should not be ruptured, unless they are large, crossing joints or limiting activity, or those obscuring the assessment of the degree of overall injury. Once the blister has ruptured spontaneously, it will likely need debridement to improve healing and prevent infection. For these less extensive debridements, a single dose of intranasal or intramuscular opioids can be effective and avoid the need for placement of an intravenous catheter. Ruptured blisters should be unroofed using gauze and sterile saline to remove devitalized tissue, and antimicrobial ointment should be placed on the exposed wound surface.

Dressings. A superficial burn does not require dressing, and pain control with ibuprofen or acetaminophen can be given as needed. Following cleaning, a topical dressing is applied directly to the wound surface. We recommend bacitracin for the face, head, and perineum as well as the fingers and toes if there is a risk of ingestion, polysporin ophthalmic for periorbital burns, and silver sulfadiazine (silvadene) or triple antibiotic ointment for all other burns. Silvadene cannot be used in patients with a sulfa allergy. Following the topical treatment, a nonadherent dressing is placed on the burn, which can then be wrapped with gauze.

Dressings should be changed twice each day. The parent should rinse off residual antibacterial ointment with warm water and inspect the wound. Signs of infection, such as redness and tenderness around the margin of the burn, warrant immediate evaluation by a physician. A gray-greenish material formed by serous drainage from the burn mixing with the silver sulfadiazine cream is often mistaken for purulence. If the burn is healing well, the parent should reapply the antibiotic ointment and dress the wound as demonstrated by the physician or nurse in the ED. Burns should be examined by a physician every 2 or 3 days until healing is well under way. Large burns or burns of the hands, feet, perineum, or overlying joints that are managed as an outpatient should be referred for follow-up to a burn specialist and evaluated more frequently. Prophylactic antibiotics are not recommended.

Minor partial-thickness burns can be expected to have epithelial healing in 7 to 14 days.

SPECIAL CIRCUMSTANCES

Goals of Treatment

Certain types of burns require special attention. Clinicians should remain alert to historical and/or physical examination findings which suggest inflicted burn injuries, electrical injuries, and/or chemical burns. Each of these burns warrant additional work up and specific treatment.

Inflicted Burns

Child abuse must be considered in patients with specific patterns of burn injury. Between 10% and 20% of burns in children are inflicted, accounting for 10% of child abuse cases. Most inflicted burns are scalds. Forced submersion of the hands or feet often causes burns that are deep, have a clear line of immersion, and are symmetric. Scald burns of the buttocks and thighs in toddlers are frequently the result of forcible submersion in a tub of hot water as punishment for toilet-training mishaps. Inflicted contact burns also have characteristic patterns. Small, round, deep burns result from cigarettes intentionally applied to the skin. Deep injuries with distinctive patterns may be noted in children held against portable heaters or burned with irons.

In many children with inflicted burns, the pattern of injury is nonspecific and a history of abuse is not offered. A deep wound with a geometric pattern and sharply demarcated borders suggests a contact burn. Scald burns usually have scattered splash lesions. In burns from spilled hot beverages, there is often a pattern of injury spreading downward from the falling liquid. Physicians should make a judgment whether the characteristics of a burn correspond with the reported mechanism in a plausible way. Identifying suspicious injuries and consulting with child abuse specialists can prevent subsequent injuries.

Electrical Burns

Burns that result when electrical current passes through the body have unique characteristics. Each year there are more than 4,000 ED visits caused by electrical injuries, mostly in children. Electrical burns account for 3% of burn center admissions and are increasing in number. Most injuries occur in young children from contact with low-voltage (less than 120 V) alternating household current, often from mouthing plugs or extension cords. Severe high-voltage (more than 500 V) injuries are also seen, often in adolescent boys as a consequence of risk-taking behaviors.

Thermal energy is released in proportion to the amount and duration of electrical current that passes through tissue. Current flows preferentially through tissues of low electrical resistance, such as blood vessels, nerves, and muscles. Moisture on the skin decreases resistance, accounting for the greater severity of injury in the antecubital, axillary, popliteal, and inguinal areas in patients of electrical burns. Current arcing through the skin can ignite clothing and cause severe thermal burns in addition to the electrical injury. In some direct current electrical burns, a depressed entrance wound and a blown out exit wound can be identified. If the current traverses the heart, which occurs more often when the flow is arm to arm, a myocardial injury may occur. Current through the heart at certain points of the cardiac cycle can induce ventricular fibrillation or asystole. Electrical injury, especially by alternating current, can cause tetany of the musculature that may prolong the contact with the high-voltage source. Tetany of the respiratory muscles can lead to suffocation.

The initial approach to patients of electrical burns is similar to that in other children with severe burns. Electrical burns are usually more severe than they appear. Significant deep and internal injuries may occur in patients with relatively small external burns. Fluid requirements are higher than those predicted by formulas based on percentage of BSA because a larger portion of the injury is internal. Destruction of muscle often causes myoglobinuria, so serum creatine kinase and urine for myoglobin should be tested. Renal failure can usually be prevented with forced diuresis and alkalinization. Electrical injury and edema within fascial compartments can cause a compartment syndrome requiring fasciotomy. Patients with a normal electrocardiogram (rate and rhythm) in the ED do not appear to be at significant risk for later development of arrhythmias. Severe electrical injuries require extensive evaluation for internal injuries, which should be done at a children's hospital or regional burn center.

A common electrical injury occurs to the lips and mouth of toddlers who suck on plugs or extension cords. Deep burns at the corner of the mouth require specialized attention to prevent severe scarring and contracture (see Chapter 113 Dental Trauma). Bleeding from the labial artery 1 to 2 weeks after injury, when the eschar separates, can result in a significant blood loss. In previous years, children with electrical injuries were hospitalized for 2 weeks, but most burn specialists now manage these children as outpatients after giving careful instructions to children's caregivers.

Chemical Burns

More than 25,000 different caustic products are in use in the United States. Most are either acidic or alkaline. Acids cause coagulation of tissue proteins, which limit the depth of penetration. Alkali results in liquefaction and deeper injury. Some organic compounds, including petroleum products, damage tissue by dissolving the fats in cell membranes. Caustic chemicals on the skin cause a prolonged period of burning compared with most thermal burns. The patient may arrive in the ED with the chemical exposure ongoing, and so careful attention to decontamination and avoiding staff exposure is crucial.

The chemical exposure should be removed as quickly as possible, most often with irrigation. Close consultation with a toxicologist or poison control center is recommended as water irrigation can worsen some chemical burns, and a few are treated with specific antidotes (see Chapter 110 Toxicologic Emergencies for further details).

Edema of the underlying tissue can make full-thickness injuries appear deceptively superficial. A thorough examination is necessary to identify other areas of skin exposed from splashes or contact that also require irrigation. Chemical burns to the eye can threaten vision and, after starting irrigation, require prompt consultation with an ophthalmologist. Consultation with a burn specialist and admission is recommended at smaller percentages of BSA with chemical burns than with thermal injuries.

Suggested Readings and Key References

American Burn Association. 2012 National burn repository. http://www.ameriburn.org/resources_publications.php. Accessed Jul 10, 2014.

Jamshidi R, Sato TT. Initial assessment and management of thermal burn injuries in children. *Pediatr Rev* 2013;34(9):395–404.

Jeschke MG, Herndon DN. Burns in children: standard and new treatments. *Lancet* 2014;383(9923):1168–1178.

Kraft R, Herndon DN, Al-Mousawi AM, et al. Burn size and survival probability in paediatric patients in modern burn care: a prospective observational cohort study. *Lancet* 2012;379(9820):1013–1021.

Palao R, Monge I, Ruiz M, et al. Chemical burns: pathophysiology and treatment. *Burns* 2010;36(3):295–304.

Thamm OC, Perbix W, Zinser MJ, et al. Early single-shot intravenous steroids do not affect pulmonary complications and mortality in burned or scalded patients. *Burns* 2013;39(5):935–941.

Tompkins RG. Survival of children with burn injuries. *Lancet* 2012; 379(9820):983–984.

World Health Organization. Burns. http://www.who.int/mediacentre/factsheets/fs365/en. Accessed Oct 7, 2014.

CHAPTER 113 ■ DENTAL TRAUMA

ZAMEERA FIDA, DMD, LINDA P. NELSON, DMD, MScD, HOWARD L. NEEDLEMAN, DMD, AND BONNIE L. PADWA, DMD, MD

GOALS OF EMERGENCY CARE

Proper diagnosis and management of traumatic dental injuries (TDI) are essential to improve prognosis. Identifying which injuries require immediate referral to a dentist is important for emergency physicians. Since dental injuries involve the head and neck, concomitant neurologic evaluation is an important aspect of emergency care. Although the majority of injuries are the result of accidents, the patient's history must be carefully reviewed in the context of the physical findings to determine if presenting injuries could be a result of nonaccidental trauma, that is, abuse.

KEY POINTS

- TDI are common pediatric emergencies.
- Neurologic assessment is an important part of management as injury has been sustained in the head and neck region.
- Jaw fractures, avulsed and displaced teeth, and dental fractures with exposed nerves (pulp) require immediate referral to a specialist.

RELATED CHAPTERS

Resuscitation and Stabilization

- Approach to the Injured Child: Chapter 2

Medical, Surgical, and Trauma Emergencies

- Child Abuse/Assault: Chapter 95
- ENT Trauma: Chapter 114
- Facial Trauma: Chapter 115
- Minor Trauma: Chapter 118
- Dental Emergencies: Chapter 125

ASSESSMENT OF TRAUMATIC DENTAL EMERGENCIES

CLINICAL PEARLS AND PITFALLS

- In patients with TDI, carefully assess for associated injuries to the CNS, cervical spine, orbits, and jaw.
- Airway obstruction in the setting of facial trauma may be the result of an aspirated tooth or blood in the oral cavity and pharynx.
- Mucosal ecchymoses at the floor of the mouth or vestibular area are highly suggestive of mandibular fractures.
- Primary teeth in the process of exfoliation may be confused with TDI.
- Be alert to the possibility of nonaccidental trauma, that is, child abuse, if the history is not consistent with the observed injuries.

Current Evidence

The most emergent concern in a child with dental trauma is to evaluate for associated facial injuries and airway obstruction. Obstruction can result from accumulation of blood in the oral cavity and pharynx. Alternatively, the etiology may be a tooth aspirated by a child, or a fractured mandible causing the tongue to fall backward against the posterior pharynx.

Beyond airway obstruction and life-threatening injuries, trauma to the jaw, dentition, or soft tissues requires careful evaluation and treatment. Inadequate recognition and management of these injuries can lead to suboptimal cosmetic and functional outcomes.

Goals of Treatment

The care of pediatric patients with maxillofacial and dental trauma should follow the basic tenets of emergency medicine, starting with evaluation and management of airway, breathing, and circulation, as well as neurologic compromise. Once stabilized, the emergency physician should perform a thorough extraoral and intraoral examination to identify the presence of injury to the jaws, teeth, and surrounding soft tissue. Recognition of those injuries that require emergent care from a dentist is imperative.

Clinical Considerations

Clinical Assessment

Children with facial injuries are usually frightened and apprehensive. The examination should be organized to include inspection and palpation of extraoral and intraoral structures. Appropriate analgesia can facilitate the examination; procedural sedation may be required in some cases.

Extraoral examination. The extraoral examination should start with evaluating symmetry of the face in the anterior and profile views. The clinician should carefully note the location and nature of any swollen or depressed structures, the color and quality of the skin, and the presence of lacerations, hematomas, ecchymoses, foreign bodies, or ulcerations. Evaluation of the temporomandibular joints (TMJs) involves observation and gentle bilateral digital palpation while the mouth is opened and closed. There should be equal movement on both sides without major deviations. Mandibular deviation during function or limited mouth opening may signify TMJ injury. Range of motion should not be forced because it may increase the extent of injury. The infraorbital rim should be palpated to ensure it is continuous and intact all the way to the inner canthus of the eye. Examination continues across the zygoma to the nose, palpating for crepitus or mobility. The clinician should inspect for lip competency (the ability of the lips to cover the teeth) because loss of competency may indicate

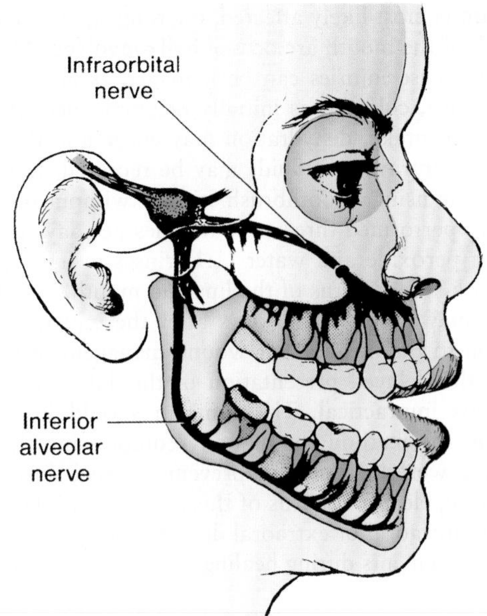

FIGURE 113.1 Infraorbital and inferior alveolar main nerve supplies the teeth.

displacement of the teeth from trauma. Attention should focus on the mandible, feeling along the posterior border of the ramus and moving anteriorly along the body to the symphysis, palpating for any discontinuity, mobility, swellings, or point tenderness. The child should be questioned and examined for any evidence of paresthesia or hypoesthesia (numbness) of the lips, nose, and cheeks, which may indicate a fracture through the bony foramen in which the nerve exits. Fig. 113.1 shows the main nerve supply to facial structures.

Intraoral examination. A good light is essential to inspect the color and quality (i.e., fluctuance or induration) of the lips, gingiva (gums), buccal mucosa, floor of the mouth, tongue, and palate. The gingiva should be pink, firm, and stippled (like a grapefruit skin). The mucosa of the cheeks and floor of the mouth should be pink, moist, and glassy in appearance. The masseter muscle should be palpated by rolling it between fingers placed intraorally and extraorally. Using a gauze pad, the clinician should hold the tongue and lift it gently to better view and examine its dorsal, ventral, and lateral surfaces. Lifting the tongue also allows for a thorough examination of the floor of mouth. Using the thumb and index finger, the clinician should palpate the alveolar ridge in all four quadrants for any swelling, discontinuity, or mobility of the soft tissues and underlying bone. The palate should be examined for any swelling or tenderness. Any soft tissue swelling, ecchymoses, and/or hematoma should be noted. Any inflamed, ulcerated, or hemorrhagic areas, as well as any foreign bodies (e.g., tooth fragments) or denuded areas of bone should be documented. Next, the oral cavity should be inspected for any missing, displaced, mobile, tender, or fractured teeth. These findings are discussed in more detail in subsequent sections.

Radiographic examination. Radiographs are a valuable supplement to the clinical examination. However, in a child with acute orofacial/dental injuries this may be difficult and reserved for a dental office. A chest radiograph may be required if an avulsed tooth is not located. Panoramic radiographs or computed tomography (CT) scans may be indicated to assess for jaw fracture.

SOFT TISSUE INJURY

CLINICAL PEARLS AND PITFALLS

- The soft tissues and bones of the lower and midface are well vascularized and bleed profusely when injured.
- Lacerated soft tissues must be evaluated for any debris, foreign body, or tooth fragment.

Current Evidence

Hemorrhage is best controlled by direct pressure and when needed, by ligating any vessels that are easily seen. However, vessels of the face often retract when severed making them difficult to visualize. If there is extensive blood loss, the patient should be assessed for signs of shock (see Chapter 5 Shock). The injured area should be thoroughly examined for a foreign body such as a tooth fragment. This may include obtaining a radiograph or bedside ultrasound before suturing when a foreign body is suspected. Infection and poor wound healing are potential sequelae of such an oversight.

Goals of Treatment

The primary goal for treatment of soft tissue injury is to achieve hemostasis. The highly vascular tissue in and around the mouth can lead to significant blood loss with seemingly mild injuries. Recognizing any embedded foreign materials (e.g., debris, or tooth fragments) is essential to allow wound healing and reduce the likelihood of complications. Injuries to the buccal mucosa and inner lip are rarely of cosmetic concern given rapid wound healing with minimal risk of scarring. Vermillion border injuries require meticulous alignment for optimal cosmetic outcome, while select intraoral lesions do not require any repair at all.

Clinical Considerations

Management of soft tissue injuries of the oral cavity follows the same emergency care principles used for extraoral soft tissue injuries. Injuries to the lip result in significant swelling after minor trauma. Lacerations of the tongue and frenum bleed profusely because of the richness of their vascularity. However, ligating specific vessels is usually unnecessary because bleeding almost always stops with direct pressure and careful suturing. Frenum lacerations often heal spontaneously without suturing. When a laceration in the oral cavity is more than 6 hours old, decisions regarding primary closure need to consider the relative risk of secondary infection.

Management

Suturing. Suturing the lip must be done carefully to achieve a precise approximation of the edges of the vermilion border to avoid a disfiguring scar. If necessary, the lip must be sparingly debrided. Wounds are generally closed with 5-0 or 6-0 sutures. Nylon sutures may be used in cooperative teenagers; however, fast-absorbing sutures are preferred in younger children given the potential challenge of subsequent suture removal. Through and through and other deep lip lacerations require closure in multiple layers, beginning with approximation of the orbicularis oris muscle using 4-0 chromic and then 5-0 or 6-0 sutures (as above) for the skin and vermilion border. Most superficial tongue lacerations heal without suturing. When necessary, tongue lacerations are usually sutured with 4-0 chromic in superficial wounds and with 3-0 chromic in deeper wounds. With tongue lacerations, it is important to consider the excessive muscular movements that pull at the sutures; therefore, tongue sutures should be made deep into the musculature (see Chapter 118 Minor Trauma).

Orthodontic trauma. Young patients are frequently undergoing orthodontic treatment, and trauma can result in loosening of wires or ligatures that are attached to orthodontic brackets or bands. Acutely, the emergency physician can bend the wire away for analgesic purposes and to avoid further soft tissue injury. Once this is temporarily addressed, arrangements for urgent dental evaluation can be pursued. Loose wires can be covered with softened wax or removed to allow the traumatized soft tissues to heal. If no discomfort is noted and no loose foreign bodies are present, definitive treatment can be delayed until the patient can be seen by an orthodontic specialist.

Postanesthesia soft tissue trauma. Young children may injure oral soft tissues (lips, intraoral mucosa, or tongue) after administration of local anesthesia for a dental procedure. The child may be numb for several hours postprocedure. This provides an opportunity for injury, which will appear as a whitish ulceration and is very painful. A common site for this is the lower lip (e-Fig. 113.1). Rarely is this type of injury associated with infection. Standard over-the-counter pain medications and keeping a bland diet are sufficient until the wound heals, typically in 1 to 2 weeks.

Electrical Burns. Electrical burns occur when children bite on electrical cords. The saliva in the mouth acts as a conductor to complete the circuit. Although the commissure of the mouth is most likely affected, the tongue, alveolar ridge, and floor of the mouth are occasionally involved. Most children with these injuries can be managed as an outpatient. A bland, soft, cold diet is initially recommended. If a child refuses oral intake, dehydration may ensue and the administration of intravenous fluids may be required. Meticulous oral hygiene using a toothbrush with or without toothpaste should be performed three to four times per day, as well as hydrogen peroxide and water (1:1) rinses in a cooperative child. With severe burns of the lips and mouth, labial artery bleeding may occur 5 to 8 days after the injury. Although admission to the hospital for wound management has been utilized, the delayed presentation of this late complication makes this impractical. The clinician should instruct the parent on the method for digitally compressing the artery if bleeding were to occur. To prevent scarring down of the commissure, electrical burns of this area require the fabrication of an intraoral or extraoral device to separate the upper and lower segments during healing (e-Fig. 113.2A,B).

TRAUMATIC DENTAL INJURIES

CLINICAL PEARLS AND PITFALLS

- Avulsed permanent teeth must be reimplanted immediately while primary teeth are generally not reimplanted.
- Displaced teeth should be repositioned as soon as possible.
- Teeth with exposed pulpal tissue require urgent dental treatment.
- Fractured posterior teeth may have an associated mandibular fracture.

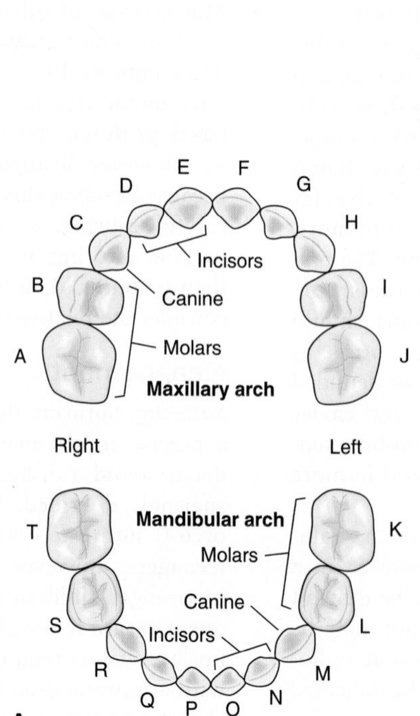

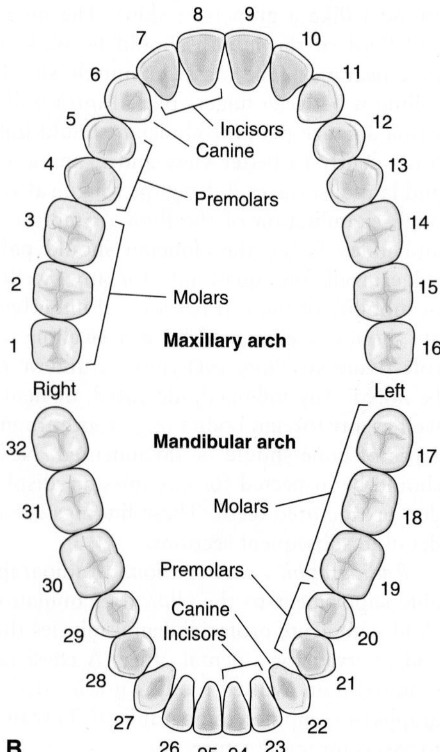

FIGURE 113.2 **A:** Primary dentition lettering system, starting with letter A in the upper right proceeding across to J in the upper left, then continuing with K in the lower left to T in the lower right. **B:** Permanent dentition number system, starting with number 1 in the upper right across to 16 in the upper left, then 17 in the lower left through 32 in the lower right. (From *Lippincott Williams & Wilkins' comprehensive dental assisting.* Philadelphia, PA: Lippincott Williams & Wilkins, 2011.)

Current Evidence

The International Association of Dental Traumatology has detailed, evidence-based guidelines for the management of dental trauma which are updated periodically and can be found online (see references). Focused recommendations within this chapter reflect current standards of care regarding management of dental injuries.

Goals of Treatment

Advocating for mouthguards, protective gear, and safe practices can help reduce the incidence of TDI. The emergency physician needs to know which injuries can be managed without dental consultation, which need follow-up care with a dentist, and which need immediate attention.

Clinical Considerations

Teeth are labeled according to their position. For older children with permanent dentition, the examiner begins on the upper right with the third molar as no. 1, proceeding across the upper arch to no. 16, and then continues on the lower left with the third molar from no. 17 across the right to no. 32. Primary dentition are labeled using letters rather than numbers, starting with letter A in the upper right proceeding across the upper arch to J then continuing on the lower left from K across to T (Fig. 113.2A,B).

Injuries to Hard Dental Tissues and Pulp

With any injury resulting in fragmentation of teeth, the emergency physician should attempt to account for all the fragments. The fragments may be embedded in a soft tissue laceration of the lip or tongue which may become infected if not debrided (see section on soft tissue injuries). Next, accessing the depth of the fracture is important. Fractures of the enamel or dentin are considered uncomplicated, while those extended into the pulp are complicated (Fig. 113.3).

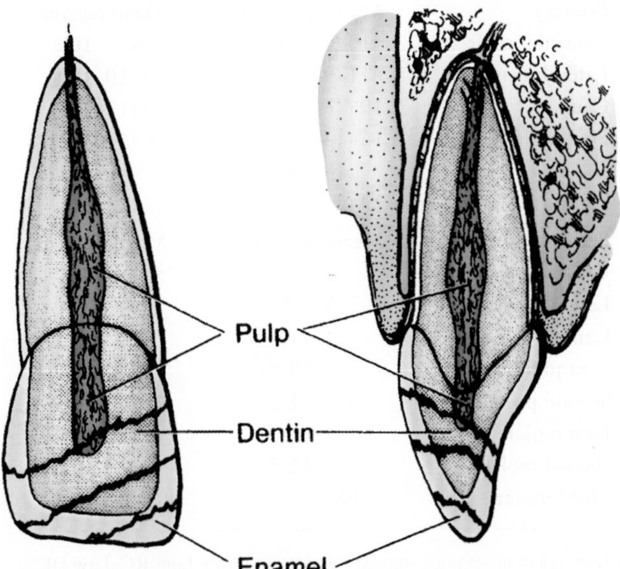

FIGURE 113.3 The anatomy of a tooth should be considered during a traumatic injury: enamel and dentin fractures are considered uncomplicated, and require dental care within 48 hours. Fractures into the pulp require emergency treatment as soon as possible.

Uncomplicated tooth fractures are confined to the enamel and the underlying dentin without pulp exposure (e-Fig. 113.3). The child may complain of sensitivity, especially to cold air and fluids. Emergency treatment is aimed at decreasing sensitivity of the involved tooth and protecting the pulp even if no frank pulp exposure is noted. The child should be seen within 48 hours by a dentist to place an insulating dressing over the exposed dentin which decreases sensitivity and minimizes the chance of pulpal necrosis. The prognosis for uncomplicated tooth fracture is good.

A complicated tooth fracture involves not only the enamel and dentin but also the pulpal tissue, which is evident by a red area within the fracture site (e-Fig. 113.4). To best preserve the viability of that tooth the exposed pulp should be treated as soon as possible. Prognosis depends on the size of the exposure, the time interval between the trauma and therapy, and the maturity of the involved tooth. Teeth with root fractures may present with mobility and/or crown displacement and can only be diagnosed with an intraoral dental radiograph. Treatment involves reduction if the tooth segments are not aligned and splinting the affected tooth to the noninjured adjacent teeth. Pulpal therapy often is necessary if physiologic healing of the fragments does not occur.

Displaced Teeth

Teeth are attached to their socket by elastic collagen fibers collectively known as the periodontal ligament (PDL). These fibers are easily injured or severed with trauma. Clinically, the emergency physician may note an increase in mobility depending on the extent of the cortical plate fracture and/or displacement of the affected teeth. TDI that involve the PDL are classified as (i) concussion, (ii) subluxation, (iii) intrusion, (iv) extrusion/lateral luxation, or (v) avulsion (Fig. 113.4).

When a traumatic blow to a tooth results in only minor damage and edema to the PDL and the tooth is sensitive to percussion, but not mobile, a concussion is diagnosed. No emergency treatment is needed although a baseline radiograph should be obtained since pulpal necrosis is possible.

Subluxation is defined as mobility of a tooth without displacement and is a result of increasing edema within the PDL. The tooth is clinically sensitive to percussion. Moderate to severely mobile teeth, especially if permanent, may require splinting for optimal dental outcome and to avoid aspiration risk. These injuries should be referred to the dental service as soon as possible. Mobile primary teeth are commonly extracted to prevent aspiration risk.

Intruded teeth are those that are displaced directly into the socket. Complete intrusion may result in the tooth not being visible, giving the false appearance of being avulsed. Thus, an intraoral dental radiograph must be obtained to make the proper diagnosis. The prognosis for maintaining pulpal vitality of an intruded tooth is poor because of the severe pulpal compression at the apex of the tooth. Intruded primary teeth can be either extracted or allowed to spontaneously reerupt, depending on the severity of the intrusion, proximity to its succedaneous tooth, and condition of the surrounding bone and soft tissues. Intrusive injuries in the permanent dentition often require repositioning and splinting; however, in some instances good outcomes are achieved if the tooth is allowed to spontaneously reerupt. Pulpal treatment (endodontics) is almost always needed because the pulp usually becomes nonvital and if left untreated the necrosis can cause root resorption and

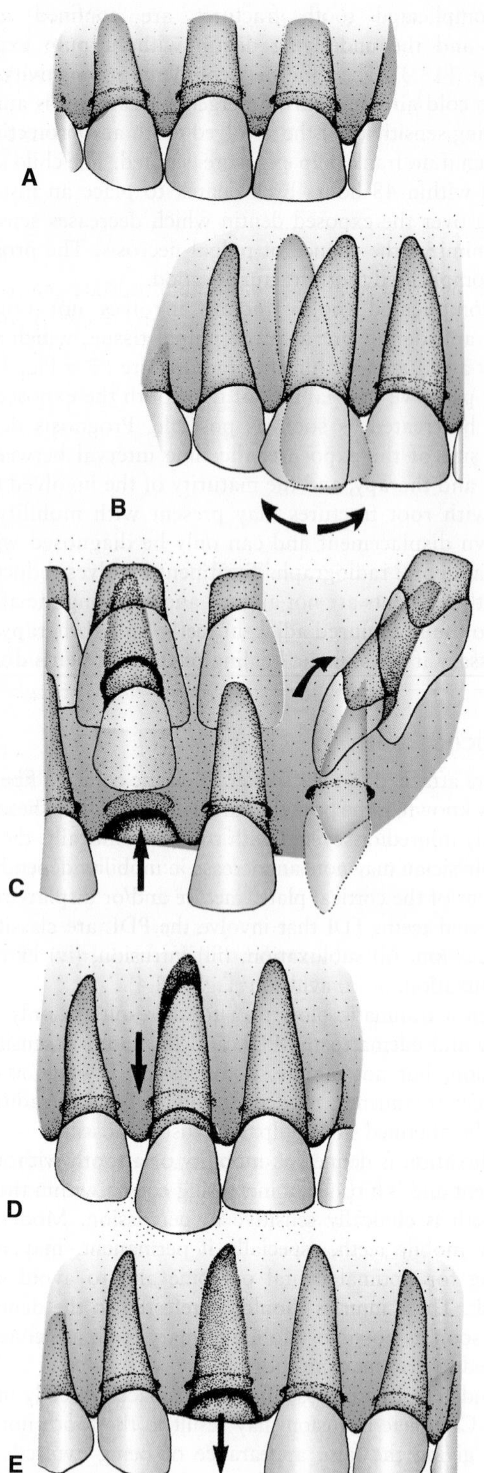

FIGURE 113.4 The various types of trauma to the periodontal structures. Concussion/subluxation (A); lateral luxation (B); intrusion (if primary tooth is intruded note location of developing permanent tooth bud) (C); extrusion (D); and avulsion (E). Refer emergencies (B) through (E) to the dental staff as soon as possible.

periapical infection. Compression fractures of the alveolar socket and anterior nasal spine may be seen radiographically and need immediate attention by a dentist.

Teeth luxated in an extrusion or lateral direction must be realigned and splinted as soon as possible. Palatally displaced teeth often prevent the child from properly occluding their upper and lower teeth. As with intrusions, endodontic treatment is usually needed since the periapical pulpal tissues that have been severed are unlikely to reanastomose in the long term. Extrusive/lateral luxations of the primary dentition usually necessitate extraction. This avoids complex treatment to a young child who will eventually lose the tooth and avoids potential injury to the succedaneous permanent tooth during realignment or as a result of eventual pulpal necrosis.

Avulsion is defined as a tooth that has been completely displaced from its alveolar socket. If the tooth was not found, radiographs are needed to confirm that the tooth was actually avulsed rather than intruded. Chest films can be obtained to assess for ingestion or aspiration of the missing tooth. The best prognosis exists when the avulsed permanent tooth is reimplanted within 15 to 30 minutes. The emergency physician or the parent needs to determine whether it is a primary or permanent tooth. If a child has missing teeth in an area of trauma, it is important to determine if any primary teeth were in the process of exfoliation. The eruption/exfoliation timetables (Tables 113.1 and 113.2) can be helpful in determining whether the loss was imminent. In addition, intraoral and/or extraoral dental radiographs such as a panoramic view can be diagnostic.

If the avulsed tooth was a permanent tooth it should be first gently rinsed under running water or saline, taking care to hold the crown of the tooth and not the root. The tooth should then be inserted into the socket in its normal position. Until splinting is achieved the tooth may extrude slightly due to pressure from the blood in the socket. Avulsed primary teeth are generally not reimplanted because of the complex treatment needed to preserve the tooth and potential damage

TABLE 113.1

CHRONOLOGY OF ERUPTION OF PRIMARY AND PERMANENT DENTITION

	Maxillary	Mandible
Primary[a]	**Mean age (mo)**	**Mean age (mo)**
Central incisor	10 (8–12)	8 (6–10)
Lateral incisor	11 (9–13)	13 (10–16)
Canine	19 (16–22)	20 (17–23)
First molar	16 (13–19 boys) (14–19 girls)	16 (14–18)
Second molar	29 (25–33)	27 (23–31)
Permanent[b]	**Mean age (yrs)**	**Mean age (yrs)**
Central incisor	7–7.5	6–6.5
Lateral incisor	8–8.5	7.2–7.7
Canine	11–11.6	9.7–10.2
First premolar	10–10.3	10–10.7
Second premolar	10.7–11.2	10.7–11.5
First molar	6–6.3	6–6.2
Second molar	12.2–12.7	11.7–12.0
Third molar	20.5	20–20.5

[a]Mean age in months ±1 standard deviation. (From Lunt RC, Law DB. A review of the chronology of eruption of deciduous teeth. *J Am Dent Assoc* 1974;89(4):872–879. Reprinted with permission.)
[b]From Baudi AR. The development and eruption of the human dentitions. In: Forrester DJ, Wagoner ML, Fleming J, eds. *Pediatric dental medicine*. Philadelphia, PA: Lea & Febiger, 1981. Reprinted with permission.

TABLE 113.2

SEQUENCE OF PRIMARY TOOTH EXFOLIATION

Rank	Mandibular arch	Maxillary arch	Mean age[a] (yrs, mo) Boys	Girls
First	Central incisors		6.0	5.7
Second		Central incisors	6.1	6.7
Third	Lateral incisors		7.2	6.1
Fourth		Lateral incisors	7.1	7.5
Fifth	Canines		10.5	9.7
Sixth	First molars		10.8	10.2
Seventh		First molars	10.1	10.6
Eighth		Canines	11.3	10.7
Ninth	Second molars	Second molars	11.9	11.5

[a]Ages are for the right side of the mouth; however, exfoliation is generally bilaterally symmetric.
From Ripa LW, Lesks GS, Sposanto AL, et al. Chronology and sequence of exfoliation of primary teeth. *J Am Dent Assoc* 1982;105:641. Reprinted with permission.

to its developing succedaneous tooth. If on-site reimplantation of an avulsed tooth is not possible, the tooth should be placed in a storage medium that preserves the vitality of the PDL of the root surface. ViaSpan or Hanks balanced salt solution is an ideal cell culture for this purpose. A commercial product such as the 3M Save-a-Tooth Emergency Tooth Preserving System (Smart Practice, Phoenix, AZ) containing Hanks solution is available to place the tooth into during transportation to the dental office. If none of these products are available, milk is an excellent alternative transport medium. Although saliva or saline are not ideal, they are alternative mediums that are preferred over water or worse allowing the root surface to air dry (Fig. 113.5). The patient should proceed directly to the dentist for radiographs, final alignment, splinting, and close follow-up.

JAW FRACTURES

CLINICAL PEARLS AND PITFALLS

- Trauma to the chin may result in a condylar fracture.
- Because the jaw is a ring structure, identification of a single fracture warrants careful examination for an accompanying injury.
- Mandibular fractures can lead to airway compromise, most commonly secondary to tongue and soft tissue falling against the posterior pharyngeal wall.

Current Evidence

Mandibular fractures are the third most common facial fractures in children (behind frontal and nasal bones). Whenever a facial fracture is present, the cervical spine, CNS, orbits, and teeth need to be carefully evaluated for associated injuries. The majority of mandibular fractures occur at the level of the condyle, which often results after trauma to the chin. Other areas of the jaw that are predisposed to fracture include the angle of the mandible where deep impacted teeth or unerupted 6-year molars make the mandible more vulnerable. Symphyseal and parasymphyseal fractures can also accompany upper mandibular fractures, as part of the closed ring of the jaw.

Goals of Treatment

History, physical examination, and appropriate radiographic evaluation should be used to establish the diagnosis of mandibular fracture. Patients should be rapidly evaluated for airway compromise and appropriate management initiated when identified. Diagnosed jaw fractures are commonly referred for outpatient treatment, although some injuries may require more urgent intervention.

Mandibular Fractures/Dislocations

Clinical recognition. The mandible can be compared with an archery bow, which is strongest at its center and weakest at its ends. Thus, most fractures occur at the neck of the condyles. Patients may present with pain or limitation when opening the mouth, or swelling at the TMJ.

Mandibular dislocation occurs when the capsule and TMJ ligaments are sufficiently stretched to allow the condyle to move to a point anterior to the articular eminence during opening. Dislocation can be unilateral or bilateral and often accompanies a history of extreme mouth opening (e.g., deep yawn) or following a prolonged dental appointment. The muscles of mastication enter a tonic contraction state, and the patient is unable to move the condyle back into the glenoid fossa and close his or her mouth.

Clinical assessment. Local bleeding, gingival/mucosal tears, or sublingual ecchymoses may be clues to underlying bony injury. Posterior tooth fractures, or evidence of malocclusion may also alert the emergency physician to the possibility of a jaw fracture. In some cases, depressed or mobile jaw fragments may be identified. A unilateral condylar fracture should be suspected if the mandible deviates toward the affected side on opening.

A panoramic radiograph or CT scan should be obtained when mandibular fractures are suspected. A panoramic radiograph may not be possible in a young or severely injured child, and may not be available in the emergency department setting.

Management. The appropriate service (dentistry, oral and maxillofacial surgery, or plastic surgery) should be consulted depending on availability. In cases where the fracture is none/minimally displaced, there is no evidence of airway obstruction, dehydration, or unremitting pain, a patient may be discharged on a soft diet with close outpatient follow-up with specialty care. For unstable or concerning fractures, specialty services are required to stabilize the fracture, using either open or closed reduction.

For a dislocation, gentle downward and backward pressure should be applied by the physician's thumb (wrapped in gauze) on the occlusal surfaces of the posterior teeth (Fig. 113.6). The downward pressure moves the dislocated condyle below the articular eminence; subsequent backward pressure on the molars shifts the condyle posteriorly into the mandibular fossa. If this approach fails, intravenous

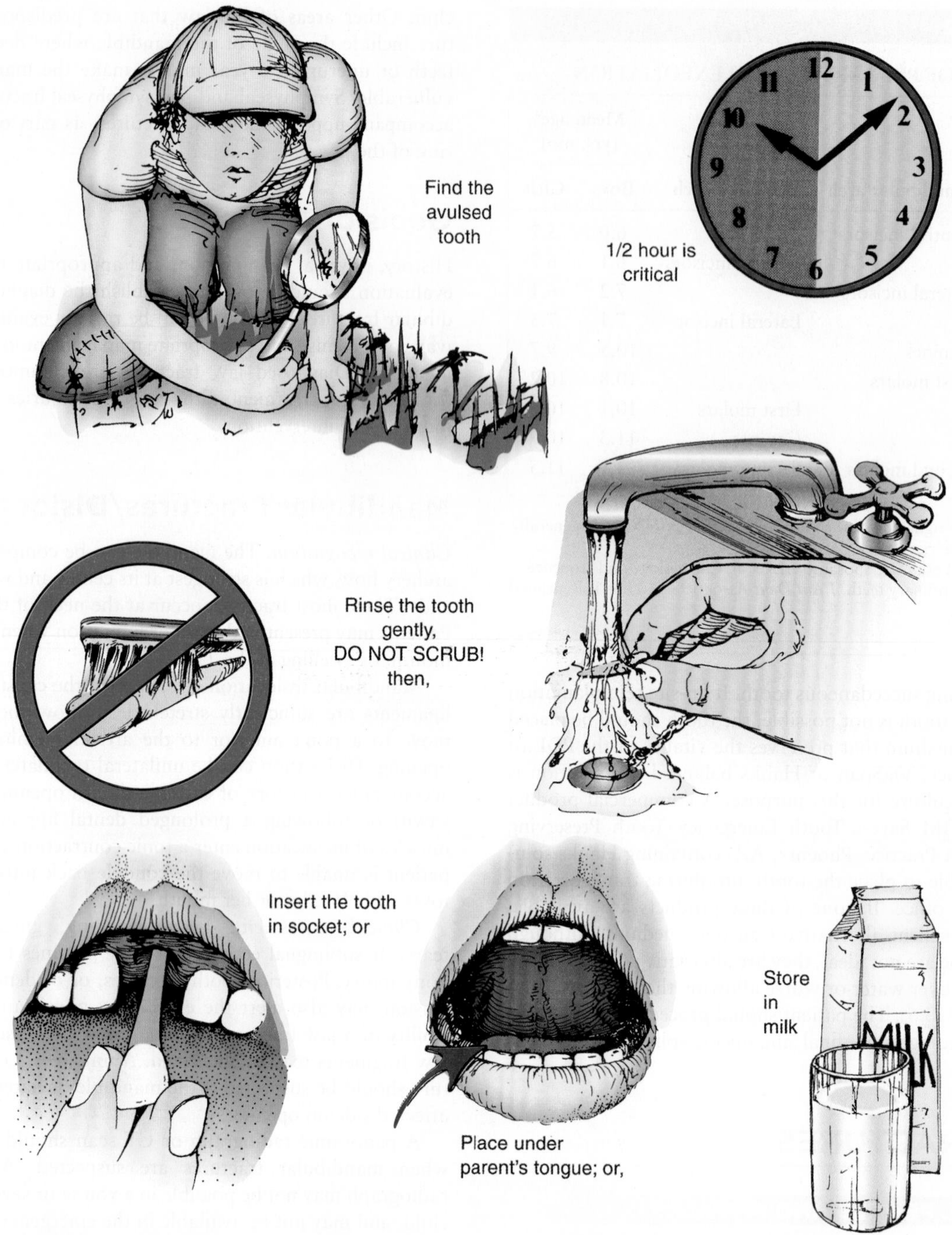
Find the
avulsed
tooth
1/2 hour is
critical
Rinse the tooth
gently,
DO NOT SCRUB!
then,
Insert the tooth
in socket; or
Place under
parent's tongue; or,
Store
in
milk
MILK

FIGURE 113.5 If a child loses or avulses a tooth, find the tooth and determine whether it is a primary or permanent tooth by checking Table 113.1. If it is a primary tooth, *do not reimplant.* Gently rinse under running water or with saline, but do not scrub the tooth. Insert the tooth back into the socket or place in milk or Hanks balanced salt solution and take immediately to the dentist. Vitality of the tooth is time dependent, with compromise starting after only 15 to 30 minutes.

diazepam (0.2 mg per kg, maximum 10 mg) can be administered as an adjunctive muscle relaxant before reattempting to relocate the condyles. Fig. 113.7 shows the anatomic landmarks and repositioning of the TMJ.

Maxillary Fractures

Premaxillary or anterior maxillary alveolar bone (commonly referred to as alveolar ridge) fractures are a common finding associated with the displacement or avulsion of maxillary anterior teeth. Acute management can be performed by the emergency physician. Gentle digital manipulation of the labial plate of bone can be guided back into position under local anesthesia. Infiltration with 2% lidocaine with 1:100,000 epinephrine is commonly used. The bone fragment can be held in place temporarily by aluminum foil (three thicknesses) molded over the teeth and alveolar ridge. This emergency splint should be held in place by having the child gently bite down. A dental consultant

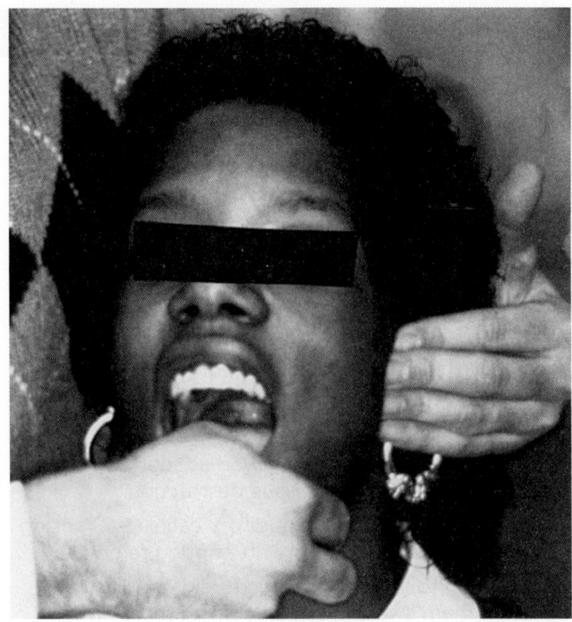

FIGURE 113.6 Position for the reduction of a dislocated mandible.

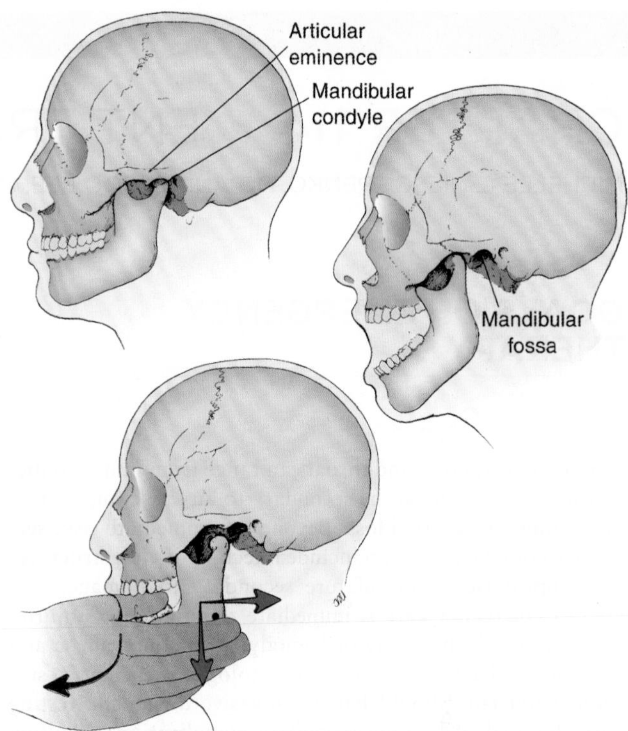

FIGURE 113.7 Dislocation of the temporomandibular joint occurs when the mandibular condyle moves to a point anterior to the articular eminence during opening. Reduction is accomplished by pushing downward and backward on the occlusal surfaces of the posterior teeth.

should be contacted as soon as possible for fabrication of a more permanent dental splint. Splinting the loose teeth and suturing the gingival tissue holds the bone fragments in place. Commonly associated mandibular and other facial fractures are covered in greater detail in Chapter 115 Facial Trauma.

Suggested Readings and Key References

Andreason JO, Andreason FM. *Textbook and color atlas of traumatic injuries to the teeth*. 4th ed. Boston, MA: Wiley-Blackwell, 2007.

Diangelis AJ, Andreasen JO, Ebeleseder KA, et al; International Association of Dental Traumatology. International Association of Dental Traumatology guidelines for the management of traumatic dental injuries: 1. Fractures and luxations of permanent teeth. *Dent Traumatol* 2012;28(1):2–12.

Fried I, Erickson P. Anterior tooth trauma in the primary dentition: incidence, classification, treatment methods, and sequelae: a review of the literature. *ASDC J Dent Child* 1995;62(4):256–261.

Kaban LB, Troulis MJ, eds. *Pediatric oral and maxillofacial surgery*. Philadelphia, PA: Saunders, 2004.

Keels MA; Section on Oral Health, American Academy of Pediatrics. Management of dental trauma in a primary care setting. *Pediatrics* 2014;133(2):e466–e476.

Layug ML, Barrett EJ, Kenny DJ. Interim storage of avulsed permanent teeth. *J Can Dent Assoc* 1998;64(5):357–363, 365–369.

Malmgren B, Andreasen JO, Flores MT, et al; International Association of Dental Traumatology. International Association of Dental Traumatology guidelines for the management of traumatic dental injuries: 3. Injuries in the primary dentition. *Dent Traumatol* 2012; 28(3):174–182.

Nelson LP, Shusterman S. Emergency management of oral trauma in children. *Curr Opin Pediatr* 1997;9(3):242–245.

Trope M. Clinical management of the avulsed tooth: present strategies and future directions. *Dent Traumatol* 2002;18(1):1–11.

Wilson S, Smith GA, Preisch J, et al. Epidemiology of dental trauma treated in an urban pediatric emergency department. *Pediatr Emerg Care* 1997;13(1):12–15.

Additional Resources

International Association of Dental Traumatology. *The dental trauma guide*. Available at: www.iadt-dentaltrauma.org/for-professionals.html.

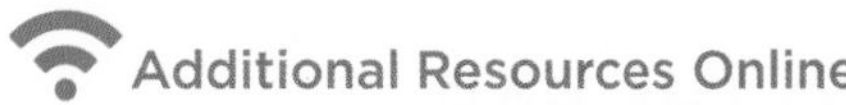

CHAPTER 114 ■ ENT TRAUMA

MICHELLE L. NIESCIERENKO, MD AND GI SOO LEE, MD, EdM

GOALS OF EMERGENCY THERAPY

General Goals

Trauma to ear, nose, and throat can range from minor to life-threatening, which can be secondary to airway compromise, or in some cases blood loss. Beyond the immediate risk, secondary complications can include infection of vital structures or compromise of vasculature secondary to damage. The goal of emergency care is immediate recognition of injuries that may result in airway or hemodynamic compromise and prompt involvement of an otolaryngologist or pediatric surgeon. Clinicians should balance invasive diagnostic testing with the goal of limiting secondary complications resulting from the injury, which include infection, hematoma, or cosmetic deformity.

RELATED CHAPTERS

Signs and Symptoms
- Dizziness and Vertigo: Chapter 19
- Epistaxis: Chapter 21
- Foreign Body: Ingestion and Aspiration: Chapter 27
- Hearing Loss: Chapter 30
- Injury: Head: Chapter 36
- Respiratory Distress: Chapter 66

Clinical Pathways
- Head Trauma: Chapter 89

Medical, Surgical, and Trauma Emergencies
- Toxicologic Emergencies: Chapter 110
- Dental Trauma: Chapter 113
- Facial Trauma: Chapter 115
- Minor Trauma: Chapter 118
- Neurotrauma: Chapter 121

TRAUMA TO THE EAR

Ear Foreign Body

Goals of Treatment

The goal of treatment is to remove the foreign body as early after it is recognized as possible. Early removal allows for the easiest possible extraction reducing risk of trauma to the external canal or tympanic membrane (TM). Removal of the foreign body prevents infection, damage to the TM and can prevent hearing compromise.

CLINICAL PEARLS AND PITFALLS

- Examine the ear with caution to avoid advancing the object further into the canal.
- Be sure to check other orifices for additional foreign bodies.
- Disk batteries should be removed as soon as they are identified to avoid rapid tissue destruction.
- Kill insects in the external auditory canal (EAC) using mineral oil or alcohol before attempting removal.
- Attempting to irrigate biologic foreign bodies can result in them swelling and becoming more firmly lodged in the auditory canal.

Current Evidence

Foreign objects in the EAC are a common occurrence in children with nearly 10,000 visits annually. Objects can cause trauma to the TM or to the sensitive canal especially the bony (medial) portion of the EAC with risk for infection or TM perforation.

Clinical Considerations

Clinical Recognition

Patients may present following a witnessed insertion of objects, the presence of ear drainage, decreased hearing, or pain. In some cases, patients are asymptomatic and the foreign body is found incidentally during physical examination. Objects can be stones, beads, foam, wax, paper, insects, beans, or other food items. Ear foreign bodies are very common in children, especially those under 5 years of age.

Triage

The majority of children are well appearing, asymptomatic, or in mild/moderate pain. Those with any bleeding from the ear or hearing loss require prompt evaluation. Live insect foreign bodies are disconcerting and mineral oil or alcohol should be immediately instilled in the canal to stop movement.

Initial Assessment

The initial assessment, history and physical examination should be focused on determining any history of object insertion, ear pain or ear drainage as well as what type of object the foreign body might be. This information is important for the removal plan.

Examination of the ear canal requires the child remain very still to avoid advancing the foreign body or local trauma to the canal. In addition to a hand held otoscope, a nasal speculum can be used to gently displace the tragus, and allow better visualization of the canal. As with the otoscope, care must be taken when inserting the tines of the nasal speculum to prevent further insertion or impaction of the foreign body or injury to the canal skin.

Management

Treatment focuses on safe removal of the foreign body (see Chapter 141 Procedures, Section on Ear Foreign Body Removal). In the emergency setting for the cooperative child, an ear curette can be used to scoop objects out, various otologic forceps (e.g., bayonette or alligator) can grasp objects. Commercially available devices (e.g., Katz extractor) are available to help remove foreign bodies from the ear or nose. These devices are designed to advance the catheter behind the object, inflate the balloon, and then pull it out of the canal. Body temperature water can be used to irrigate and remove objects against the TM, but only if the TM is intact. Avoid irrigating organic objects (e.g., food, paper) as they can swell and become further lodged in the EAC. Insects should be killed by instilling alcohol or mineral oil into the canal before attempting to remove them, provided the TM is intact. To reduce pain for these procedures a topical anesthetic can be applied in advance. If the child is uncooperative with the procedure risking further damage to the EAC or TM, procedural sedation in the emergency setting could be considered.

Following successful removal, if there is excoriation or trauma to the EAC topical otic antibiotic drops should be used to prevent otitis externa in the discharged patient. Over-the-counter pain relievers can be used for any minor discomfort. If the foreign body cannot be successfully removed, patients may be referred for removal by an otolaryngologist in a day surgery setting, provided there are no concerns for pain, bleeding, or infection.

Ear Trauma

Goals of Treatment

The primary goal of treating ear trauma is to prevent hearing loss, which is associated with lifelong disability. In addition, optimal management of ear trauma reduces local infection risk, which if left untreated could result in invasive bacterial infection, and can lead to worsened cosmetic appearance.

CLINICAL PEARLS AND PITFALLS

- Auricular hematomas should be identified and treated immediately.
- Unrecognized traumatic perforation of the TM can lead to serious complications.
- Thorough hearing assessment on children including gross hearing, whisper test, and tuning fork assessment for sensorineural hearing loss should be done for all ear injuries.

EXTERNAL EAR

Current Evidence

Injury to the external ear can include laceration to the skin, soft tissue, or cartilage, as well as hematoma with risk of cartilage necrosis. The cartilage of the ear is nourished and oxygenated by diffusion via the perichondrium. With an auricular hematoma, bleeding avulses the perichondrial layer off the cartilage as the blood collects between them. This separation of the perichondrium leads to cartilage necrosis. In addition to blunt or sharp trauma, the external ears are also susceptible to thermal injuries including both burn and frostbite.

Clinical Considerations

Clinical Recognition

Injuries to the external ear can manifest as laceration, ecchymosis, or hematoma. Thermal injury may present with bullous or peeling skin. Most commonly, there is a reported history of trauma or symptoms of pain or bleeding that prompts the emergency physician to recognize the injury. However, unwitnessed or asymptomatic injuries may also be identified during examination.

Triage

Any child with an external ear injury associated with serious trauma, active bleeding, new hearing loss, or neurologic symptoms should be evaluated emergently. Most children will present with mild to moderate discomfort without associated symptoms and can be seen urgently.

Initial Assessment

The initial assessment should focus on the mechanism and severity of the injury, where there is concern for foreign body, and the risk of other associated injuries. The ear should be inspected for any externally visible deformity/injury including lacerations, with attention to any cartilaginous laceration, ecchymosis, or hematoma. Note that isolated ecchymosis to the external ear canal without other signs of injury or with an inconsistent mechanism of injury should raise suspicion for nonaccidental trauma. Diagnostic testing is not routinely indicated for simple, isolated injuries. Imaging should be considered to evaluate for associated injuries, including closed head injury, in the setting of concerning symptoms or findings (see Chapter 89 Head Trauma).

Management

Lacerations should be repaired, with a layered repair if the ear cartilage is involved, including the ear lobe. Hematomas should be drained and a pressure dressing applied to prevent accumulation. Prompt drainage reduces the risk of permanent external ear deformity often referred to as "cauliflower ear." Ears with cold thermal injury should be rapidly rewarmed and avoid recooling. Hot thermal injuries should receive symptomatic care, avoiding excessive cooling or ice in direct contact of the ear skin. Patients with isolated minor traumatic ear injury who are discharged home should be encouraged to keep ear dressings in place to avoid infection, bleeding, or reaccumulation of hematomas. The ears should be protected from further injury and exposure until fully healed. Although data are limited, patients who have required auricular hematoma drainage may have a tenuous blood supply and therefore should receive a short course (commonly 7 to 10 days) of prophylactic antibiotics. In adolescents, a quinolone is recommended to cover for routine skin flora such as staphylococcus as well as *Pseudomonas aeruginosa*. Quinolones are also favored based on their effective penetration into cartilage. In younger children, antibiotic selection is less clear. Amoxicillin with clavulanate is commonly recommended, though others support the use of quinolones in this age group as well given the added Pseudomonas coverage. Although there are reported risks of arthropathy with quinolones, no clinical studies have demonstrated these findings in children. Even with empiric antibiotics, close monitoring for signs of chondritis including fever, erythema, or purulent drainage is important, which should prompt admission for intravenous antibiotic therapy.

MIDDLE EAR

Current Evidence

Middle ear injury is caused by barotrauma (airplane or deep water pressure including swimming pools), forced air into the ear (e.g., slap injury), or from direct contact (e.g., wave or foreign body insertion). All three mechanisms can result in TM rupture and associated injury to middle ear structures. The ossicles can be dislocated or fractured causing conductive hearing loss. Injury to the oval or round window can lead to perilymph fistula. Barotrauma is exacerbated in the child with eustachian tube dysfunction resulting in blood vessel engorgement and risk of bleeding or serous effusion into the middle ear. Because the facial nerve traverses through the middle ear, injury resulting in facial paresis is potentially associated with middle ear injuries.

Clinical Considerations

Clinical Recognition

Clinical recognition of injury occurs from identifying mechanisms consistent with middle ear injury including barotrauma, slap of air or water, or foreign object. Patients may be asymptomatic or complain of ear pain or drainage. Other symptoms may include sudden onset vertigo, nystagmus, or sensorineural hearing loss related to injury of the stapes or oval window.

Triage

At triage these patients are generally not ill appearing, although differentiation of vertigo related to middle ear injury versus posterior fossa or neurologic etiology is important.

Initial Assessment

History should focus on the mechanism of injury and any associated symptoms with detailed review of neurologic symptoms. The TM should be carefully examined for perforations. Assess the function of the facial nerve for associated injury. Hearing assessment should be done on all children with concern for a middle ear injury.

Management

Imaging is often not indicated unless the mechanism is severe enough to warrant assessment for closed head injury. Perforations with associated vertigo, nystagmus, tinnitus, or hearing loss should be immediately referred to otolaryngology. Perforations with active drainage should be treated with topical antibiotics for 5 days to help minimize infection and wash away otorrhea or bleeding. Patients with clear fluid otorrhea that may represent CSF leak, or those with vertigo or other symptoms suggestive of perilymph fistula should be evaluated by an otolaryngologist before topical antibiotics are instilled. Certain antibiotic drops will be painful due to particular ingredients or pH of the antibiotic preparation. For example, CiproHC is likely to cause burning pain, while Ciprodex is not. Cortisporin should be avoided as the neomycin may contribute to sensorineural hearing loss. Middle ear bleeding or effusions can be treated with oral antibiotics to prevent infection and generally spontaneously resolve within 3 weeks. It is critical that discharged patients with perforations follow-up for reexamination by an otolaryngologist to ensure proper healing.

INNER EAR

Current Evidence

Concussive injuries, especially with associated temporal bone fracture, can disrupt the intracochlear membrane. Children with certain bony anomalies of the inner ear, including semicircular canal dehiscence syndrome and enlarged vestibular aqueducts (EVA), collectively known as third-window lesions, are susceptible to acute sensorineural hearing loss changes with mild head trauma. Noise-induced trauma can cause also damage to the inner ear causing SNHL. Acutely, loud blasts from explosions can cause sudden loss of hearing; this is typically less common in children given their pattern of exposure.

Clinical Considerations

Clinical Recognition

Inner ear injury is recognized by sensorineural hearing loss or the onset of vertigo in the context of an appropriate history.

Triage

On presentation to triage, these children are not acutely ill appearing but have a chief complaint of hearing loss, dizziness, or tinnitus.

Initial Assessment

The history should focus on the mechanism of injury, noise exposure, and the history/progression of the hearing loss. Unless there are associated injuries there is generally nothing visible on physical examination for inner ear injuries. A thorough hearing test is a key component of the diagnostic testing. Tuning fork tests should be performed to help determine the likely etiology for any hearing loss. To evaluate for third-window lesions, a thin cut CT of the temporal bones is required. Otolaryngology should be consulted in patients with suspected inner ear injury to determine the need for further evaluation and management. Antibiotic treatment or admission is not routinely indicated. However, high dose steroids (1 mg/kg/day of prednisone or an equivalent) should be administered for new onset sudden sensorineural hearing loss.

OTHER INJURIES ASSOCIATED WITH EAR TRAUMA

Temporal Bone Fracture

Approximately 80% of temporal bone fractures are in the longitudinal orientation and 20% are transverse. This is important to predict associated ear injury. Longitudinal fractures are usually extralabyrinthine and may disrupt the bony annulus of the TM causing hemotympanum and ossicular or TM disruption. Facial nerve injury is rare with longitudinal fractures. Transverse fractures can disrupt the otic capsule, internal auditory canal, and the seventh and eighth cranial nerves. Approximately half of transverse fractures have facial nerve involvement, while sensorineural hearing loss is uncommon. Otolaryngology should be consulted for patients with traumatic facial nerve paralysis for evaluation, management, and possible exploration with nerve repair.

CSF Otorrhea

Longitudinal fractures that rupture the TM can lead to CSF otorrhea. Transverse fractures have a higher incidence of CSF leak, but are less likely to have otorrhea due to an intact TM. Clear fluid in the canal should be evaluated to determine if it is CSF. Water, tears, or home therapies can also be present. A halo of clear fluid around any red blood cells when placed on filter paper is concerning for CSF (halo test). Glucose testing can also be performed. However, beta-2-transferrin testing is considering the most specific testing for CSF otorrhea. Avoid manipulation or instrumentation when CSF otorrhea is thought to be present, to reduce risk of meningitis through the introduction of bacteria. Patients with CSF otorrhea are treated with bed rest, elevation of the head of the bed and neurosurgery consultation. Prophylactic antibiotics are controversial.

TRAUMA TO THE NOSE AND SINUSES

Nasal Foreign Body

Goals of Treatment

The goal of treatment is to identify a nasal foreign body, to allow prompt removal. Safe removal of the foreign body reduces the risk of acute aspiration, subacute local infection, sinusitis, and cartilaginous injury.

CLINICAL PEARLS AND PITFALLS

- Unilateral malodorous nasal discharge should raise suspicion for a nasal foreign body.
- Care must be taken to avoid pushing or irrigating the object during examination or removal attempts, as migration to the nasopharynx puts the child at risk for aspiration.
- Pretreatment with vasoconstrictor as well as use of a nasal speculum can improve visualization and facilitate removal.
- A known or suspected disk battery should be removed immediately to avoid caustic injury.

Current Evidence

Foreign bodies can obstruct the nares. If the object has been present for a long period of time, granulation tissue can form around the object. Either the tissue or the object itself can block the ostia and increase the risk of sinusitis.

Clinical Considerations

Clinical Recognition

Witnessed insertion or foul unilateral discharge is key to diagnosing nasal foreign body.

Triage

Children generally present to triage well appearing with a history consistent with foreign body. Rarely, associated injury may result in epistaxis that should be addressed urgently. Nasal foreign bodies can migrate posteriorly converting to aspiration symptomatology which requires emergent evaluation.

Initial Assessment

A child may be witnessed placing a foreign body in the nose. More commonly, the child will report what they have done to a parent or caregiver. Determining what type of object was placed is important to determining approaches to removal. Alternatively, when persistent nasal discharge, particularly unilaterally, is the primary complaint, gaining information about the chronicity of symptoms becomes important. On physical examination, the nare may need to be suctioned to visualize if an object is present. Sometimes, suctioning results in removal of the object. During rhinoscopy, the location of the foreign body, and any other injuries should be noted. Plain x-rays are not indicated unless there is specific concern for a radio-opaque foreign body that is not identified during direct visualization.

Management

Prior to any removal attempt, a topical nasal vasoconstricting agent such as oxymetazoline should be used to minimize bleeding, and decrease local edema which increase chances of successful removal. In the cooperative child, instruments can be used to grasp and remove the object. Alternatively, a 5 French Foley catheter or commercially available device can be inserted behind the object and the balloon inflated to pull the object out. Young or uncooperative children may require anxiolysis or procedural sedation. Otolaryngology should be consulted for longstanding foreign bodies, particularly with associated granulation tissue or obstructive sinusitis to determine acute and longer term management strategies.

After removal, antibiotic treatment is used to prevent or treat sinusitis. Children may be discharged home. Caregivers should be advised that the nose may continue to have small amounts of bleeding at home. Otolaryngology should be consulted when removal is not successful by emergency physicians. Subsequent removal may occur during the ED visit or in an outpatient setting.

Trauma to the Nose and Sinuses

Goals of Treatment

The goal of treatment for nasal trauma is to identify fractures or septal hematomas to reduce risk of cosmetic or functional deformity. Nasal septal hematomas require emergent drainage, whereas nasal fractures may require delayed repair (5 to 7 days) for improved functional or cosmetic outcomes. Detecting other injuries to the face associated with nasal injury including ocular, orbit, facial bone, or sinus injury is the secondary goal of treatment as these injuries may be life-threatening or have series sequelae if not detected.

CLINICAL PEARLS AND PITFALLS

- Septal hematomas once identified should be drained promptly to avoid necrosis of the nasal cartilage resulting in deformity.
- A thorough assessment should be done to avoid missing an associated injury resulting in CSF rhinorrhea.

Current Evidence

The nose in children is composed of prominent soft cartilage, which dissipates the force of impact across the midface. The boney components of the nose and septum can be fractured or displaced during injury. Orbital fractures, retinal detachment, or hyphema can be associated with nasal injuries. Nasal fractures that extend to the cribriform plate can result in CSF rhinorrhea. Fracture of the paranasal sinuses can occur with injury to the nose or orbit and ethmoid or anterior wall maxillary sinus fractures occur due to blunt trauma to the nose or cheek. Facial fractures/midface injuries are covered in Chapter 115 Facial Trauma.

Clinical Considerations

Nose injuries due to minor trauma or sports are commonly associated with nasal fracture and present with nosebleed, edema, ecchymosis, and occasionally clear rhinorrhea.

Triage

Children with injuries to the nose are generally in mild/moderate discomfort on presentation. For those with active nasal bleeding, direct pressure should be applied and nasal injury as part of major trauma or with neurologic changes supports urgent evaluation.

Initial Assessment

The mechanism of injury should be solicited to assess for risk of other associated conditions such as closed head injury. Physical examination should focus on a thorough assessment for nasal septal hematoma, obvious fracture/nasal deviation, and signs of associated ophthalmologic or serious head injury. CSF leak should be considered with any clear fluid drainage form the nose. Associated sinus fractures may be identified with crepitus or pain over the sinus.

Management

When the history and/or examination are concerning for a simple nasal fracture, no diagnostic imaging is indicated. If there is concern for CSF leak, fluid can be tested using the halo test (see above), or glucose concentration. Beta-2-transferrin testing is the most accurate, though results are often not available in a timeframe to be useful during acute evaluation and management. CT may be performed to assess for associated facial or orbital bone fractures (see Chapters 115 Facial Trauma and 122 Ocular Trauma) but is not indicated when concern is for isolated nasal fracture. If persistent nasal bleeding occurs in the setting of nasal trauma, apply direct pressure, topical vasoconstrictors, and ice. Once the bleeding has stopped, treatment for simple nasal fractures is supportive care with pain management and follow-up with otolaryngology or plastic surgery to assess for deformity in 4 to 7 days (see Fig. 114.1). Compound nasal fractures or those associated with sinus fracture should be treated with antibiotics for 1 week. Isolated sinus fractures

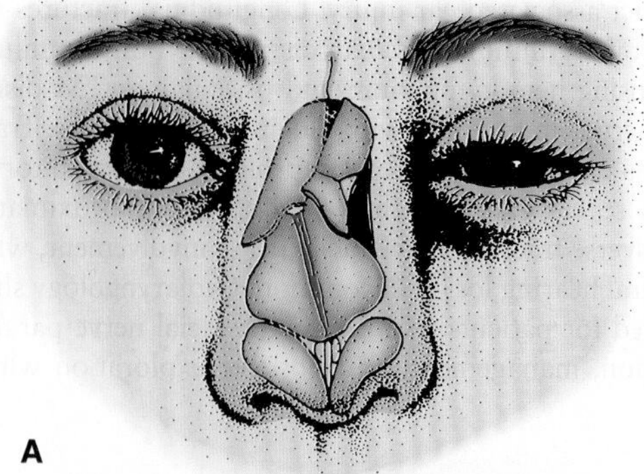

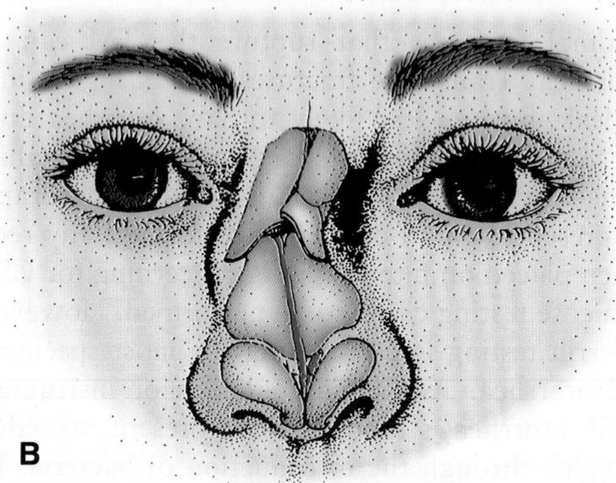

FIGURE 114.1 **A:** Postinjury edema may mask underlying nasal bone deformity. **B:** Nasal deformity manifests as edema subsides.

should be treated with antibiotics for 1 week and the patient should maintain "sinus precautions" which include avoidance of nose blowing, swimming, and use of a straw. Nasal septal hematomas should be incised and drained, and nasal packing or a pressure dressing should be left in place to avoid necrosis of the nasal septum cartilage. It is important that patients are evaluated in follow-up by an otolaryngologist or plastic surgeon within 1 week as well-healed nasal deformities are more difficult to correct, leading to more functional and cosmetic problems. Follow-up for sinus fractures should also occur at 1 week, although they rarely require subsequent intervention. Admission and elevation of head of the bed is indicated for children with suspected CSF leak.

Sinus Barotrauma

Sinus barotrauma occurs when changes in pressure are not equalized by the sinus ostia between the paranasal sinuses and maxillary sinuses. Increased pressure causes mucosal blood vessel engorgement followed by hemorrhage into the sinuses. Patients usually present with sinus pain and a history consistent with exposure to such pressure changes. The treatment for sinus barotrauma is supportive, with pain control and antimicrobials.

TRAUMA TO THE ORAL CAVITY AND PHARYNX

Goals of Treatment

The emergent goal in oral and pharyngeal injuries is to evaluate and protect the airway when at risk for compromise or obstruction. In addition, the emergency physician must identify serious injuries that may involve vascular structures or wounds that may lead to infection. Oral and pharyngeal foreign bodies should be removed promptly due to risk of aspiration. Ingestion is covered in detail in Chapters 27 Foreign Body: Ingestion and Aspiration, 99 Gastrointestinal Emergencies, and 132 Thoracic Emergencies.

CLINICAL PEARLS AND PITFALLS

- Falls with objects in the mouth may result in injuries to the vascular structures, potentially resulting in CNS complications.
- Foreign bodies may be retained in the oral cavity.

Current Evidence

A common etiology of oral cavity injury is biting of the cheek causing a laceration or hematoma. Palatal injuries are usually caused by a foreign body, often as a result of falling with something in or around the patient's mouth. Risk of associated injury can be stratified based on location of the trauma within the oral cavity. Central hard or soft palate injuries are not likely to be associated with vascular injury or associated risk of CNS complications. Lateral palate, especially soft palate or tonsillar fossa is associated with vascular injury given the close proximity of vital vessels. Posterior pharyngeal wall injuries may be associated with vascular injuries resulting in hematoma and risk of infection.

Clinical Considerations

Clinical Recognition

Oral or pharyngeal injuries in children often result from a fall, foreign body, ingestion, or blow from a projectile object such as a ball.

Triage

Children with severe intraoral injuries or punctures can present acutely ill or deteriorate quickly. Careful attention at triage should be paid and reassessment in children waiting for evaluation should occur frequently.

Initial Assessment

A history of objects in the mouth, possible foreign bodies, or bleeding from the oral cavity should raise concern for injury and a thorough oral examination for lacerations, hematomas, and foreign objects should be performed. Expanding neck hematoma, continued oral bleeding, or diminished pulses in the neck are signs of vascular injury and require immediate attention.

Management

Oral lacerations rarely require suturing unless a large flap (or defect greater than 1 to 2 cm) exists. For wounds that do not require repair, oral hygiene with warm saline rinses can keep the area clean (see Chapter 113 Dental Trauma). Antibiotics are not routinely indicated. If concern exists for a retained foreign body, imaging with CT is warranted. Any foreign bodies should be removed and frequently require OR exploration. Children with suspected vascular injury should undergo evaluation immediately either by CT or MRI with angiography.

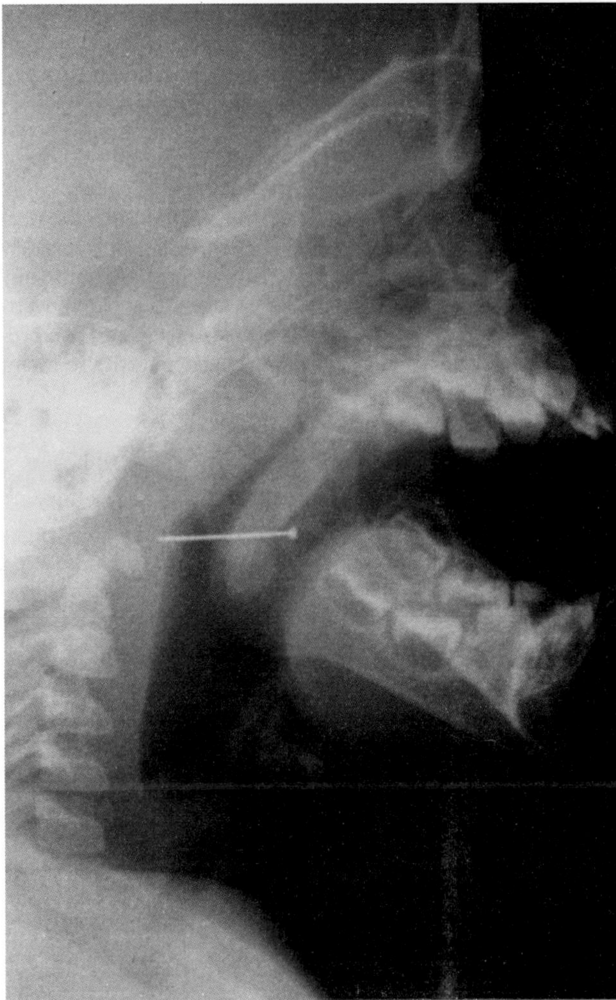

FIGURE 114.2 Lateral neck radiograph of a straight pin lodged in posterior pharyngeal wall.

Children with isolated oral injuries may be safely discharged home. Those suspected to have retained foreign body or vascular injury should be definitively imaged and admitted for further treatment if indicated (see Fig. 114.2).

Caustic Injuries

Injuries resulting from ingestion of caustic substances such as lye or acid may cause burns from the oral mucosa to the stomach. Injuries caused by basic chemicals are far more serious than those caused by acidic ones. The former creates a liquefactive necrosis that is often deeper and causes more damage than the coagulative necrosis caused by acids. Identifying the ingested agent is critical in managing the patient with caustic burns.

Skip lesions are possible, with no injuries visible on examination. Patients with definite ingestion of known caustic substances should undergo endoscopy within 12 to 24 hours to assess burns (see Chapter 110 Toxicologic Emergencies). The role of steroids has been debated, however some data suggest benefit in reducing the risk of strictures. No antidotes are available and vomiting should not be induced which may result in vomitus causing burn or aspiration. Laryngeal burns may cause edema and respiratory distress or compromise.

TRAUMA TO THE LARYNX AND TRACHEA

Foreign Body

Goals of Treatment

Laryngeal or tracheal foreign bodies can result in life-threatening partial or complete airway obstruction. The goal is to safely remove the object as soon as possible to prevent or reverse any respiratory compromise. Care must be taken to avoid converting a partial airway obstruction into complete airway compromise, and to avoid advancing the foreign material with resultant aspiration into the lung.

CLINICAL PEARLS AND PITFALLS

- Disk batteries should be removed as soon as possible to avoid caustic injury.
- Clinicians should have a high suspicion for foreign body in a child with sudden onset of stridor, persistent cough, or respiratory distress.
- Back blows and the Heimlich maneuver are not performed on the breathing child as these can cause the object to lodge further into the airway. These techniques are reserved for complete airway obstruction.

Current Evidence

Foreign bodies lodged in the laryngeal inlet or trachea cause severe distress and often present with coughing, wheezing, and inspiratory and expiratory stridor. Tracheal/bronchial foreign bodies can cause low lung volumes or hyperinflation due to check valve effect of the object.

Clinical Considerations

Clinical Recognition

Foreign bodies trapped in the laryngeal inlet will cause significant acute upper airway obstruction. The child usually presents with severe coughing, hoarseness, and significant respiratory distress. The challenge for emergency physicians is recognizing foreign body aspiration when the event was not witnessed directly and the child is not acutely compromised. Symptoms such as cough, stridor, and examination findings such as wheezing and decreased aeration are nonspecific, and seen commonly in routine pediatric illnesses such as croup, bronchiolitis, and asthma. One should be suspicious of airway foreign body in any child with sudden onset of symptoms or when there is a history consistent with ingestion or aspiration.

Triage

Children with a laryngeal or tracheal foreign body usually present in distress with hoarseness, coughing, stridor, or wheezing. If the child is able to phonate, air is moving through his or her larynx, indicating only partial obstruction. Efforts should be made to allow the child to assume a position of comfort. Invasive examination and interventions such as IV placement should be avoided when possible, as crying may result in worsening of the airway obstruction. Complete or near complete obstruction requires emergency airway management.

Initial Assessment

History may note a witnessed ingestion or sudden onset of the above symptoms with no other etiology noted. Examination findings may include stridor with upper airway foreign bodies, and wheezing, persistent cough, focal decreased aeration with lower airway foreign bodies. Asymmetric hyperinflation or areas of lung collapse are rarely detectable without radiologic evaluation.

Management

Do not perform back blows or Heimlich maneuver to treat the child who is still breathing as objects may become further lodged in the airway. Children in severe distress should be taken to the OR for emergent removal under direct laryngoscopy and bronchoscopy. For children who are not breathing, back blows or the Heimlich maneuver should be done. If unsuccessful with resultant progression to depressed mental status, laryngoscopy should be performed to assess for glottic foreign material that can be removed with forceps.

For those in mild or moderate distress, x-ray may be helpful for radiopaque objects or to show low lung volumes or hyperinflation from the check valve effect in the setting of radiolucent objects (see Fig. 114.3). A normal chest radiograph does not rule out foreign body. In stable patients, fluoroscopy or CT can add diagnostic value though this needs to be balanced against the higher doses of ionizing radiation for these studies, and the likelihood that findings will influence subsequent management. Alternatively, if there is high clinical concern for foreign body despite negative radiographs, consideration should be given to urgent bronchoscopy without further imaging. Those with low suspicion of foreign body

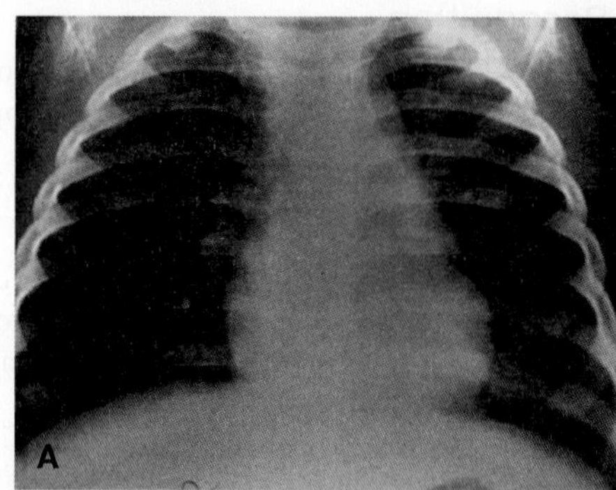

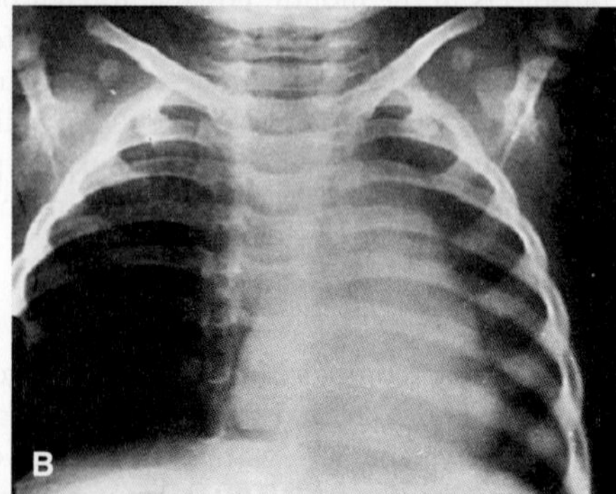

FIGURE 114.3 Chest radiograph of child with bronchial foreign body. **A:** Inspiratory film demonstrates only subtle hyperaeration of right lung. **B:** Expiratory film shows accentuated hyperaeration on the right side secondary to air trapping ("check-valve" phenomenon) by the foreign body in the right mainstem bronchus. In addition, the mediastinum is displaced to the left.

should have thorough follow-up and re-evaluation for continued possibility of foreign body.

LARYNGEAL AND TRACHEAL TRAUMA

Goals of Treatment

Blunt and penetrating laryngeal and tracheal should be promptly identified to prevent and reverse any respiratory compromise from obstruction or bleeding. The primary goal for the emergency physicians is to determine who requires urgent airway management and how to most safely accomplish this, as fiberoptic visualization or surgical intervention may be required. When acute airway management is not a concern, the aim is to identify which patient with minimal or no symptoms warrants advanced imaging and/or surgical special consultation to avoid missing injuries to these critical structures that have the potential to progress (see Chapter 120 Neck Trauma for further details).

CLINICAL PEARLS AND PITFALLS

- Patients with blunt trauma to the anterior neck should also be evaluated for cervical spine injury.
- Any patients with penetrating injuries to the central third of the neck, or zone 2 of the neck, even if stable, should be considered for surgical exploration.
- Patients with penetrating injuries to zones 1 and 3 of the neck initially should undergo MRA/MRV to assess for vascular injury.

Current Evidence

Blunt trauma can cause mucosal lacerations, laryngeal hematomas, vocal cord paralysis, or fractures of the larynx or trachea. Penetrating trauma results in additional risk to the airway and vasculature and is covered in detail in Chapter 120 Neck Trauma.

Clinical Considerations

Clinical Recognition

Blunt injuries to the neck manifest as neck pain, hoarseness, cough, hemoptysis, neck swelling, or visible injury such as ecchymosis.

Triage

Some patients will present with significant respiratory distress or with penetrating injuries to the neck and should be emergently evaluated and surgical specialty consultation should be pursued. Those with consistent history and symptoms but without acute compromise of the airway, breathing, or circulation should be seen as soon as possible and reassessed frequently as they may become unstable quickly.

Initial Assessment

History of a mechanism concerning for laryngeal trauma such as a "close line" injury or from an object across the neck should be elicited. Emergency physicians should determine if there has been any change in the quality of voice, hemoptysis, or significant neck pain. On physical examination, anterior neck tenderness, crepitus, or absence of normal thyroid cartilage contour are concerning for a larynx or trachea injury (see Fig. 114.4). Unstable patients in respiratory distress may require direct laryngoscopy, intubation, rigid bronchoscopy, or tracheotomy. An otolaryngologist should be prepared to intervene with any of these procedures. For children without distress, plain radiographs may help assess the thyroid cartilage or tracheal injury or identify subcutaneous air from these injuries. CT scans provide more details regarding the laryngeal structures in the setting of trauma. Penetrating trauma may

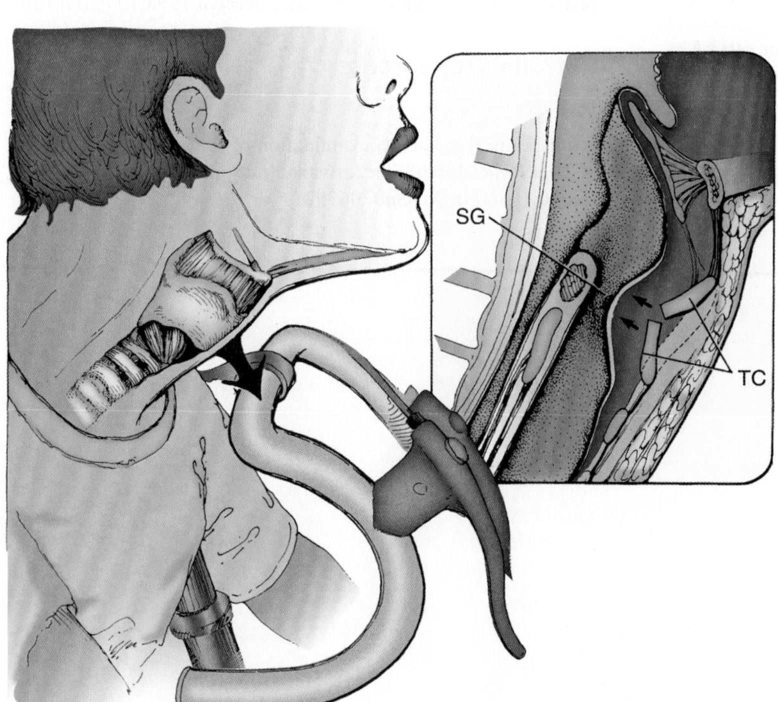

FIGURE 114.4 Loss of thyroid cartilage prominence and associated acute airway obstruction secondary to laryngeal fracture. SG, narrowed subglottic space; TC, fracture of thyroid cartilage.

require MRA/MRV to evaluate the vasculature of the neck. Surgical exploration should be considered for patients with penetrating injuries to the central third of the neck even if stable. Any patients with distress or penetrating injury should be admitted either directly to the operating room for airway management and exploration, or after complete work up in consultation with appropriate surgical specialists. Mildly symptomatic children with blunt trauma but who are otherwise stable and are determined not to have clinically significant injury by history and examination, and possibly with additional imaging and/or surgical specialty consultation, may be observed in the ED and discharged home if there is no worsening of symptoms over time.

Suggested Readings and Key References

Ear

Amadsun JE. An observational study of the management of traumatic tympanic membrane perforations. *J Laryngol Otol* 2002;116: 181–184.

Antonelli PJ, Ahmadi A, Prevatt A. Insecticidal activity of common reagents for insect foreign bodies of the ear. *Laryngoscope* 2001; 111:15–20.

Colvin IB, Beale T, Harrop-Griffiths K. Long-term follow-up of hearing loss in children and young adults with enlarged vestibular aqueducts: relationship to radiologic findings and Pendred syndrome diagnosis. *Laryngoscope* 2006;116(11):2027–2036.

Darrouzet V, Duclos JY, Liguoro D, et al. Management of facial paralysis resulting from temporal bone fractures: our experience in 115 cases. *Otolaryngol Head Neck Surg* 2001;125(1):77–84.

Greywoode JD, Pribitkin EA, Krein H. Management of auricular hematoma and the cauliflower ear. *Facial Plast Surg* 2010;26: 451–455.

Kim SH, Kazahaya K, Handler SD. Traumatic perilymphatic fistulas in children: etiology, diagnosis, and management. *Int J Ped Otorhinolaryngol* 2001;60(2):147–153.

Marin JR, Trainor JL. Foreign body removal from the external auditory canal in a pediatric emergency department. *Pediatr Emerg Care* 2006;22:630–634.

Singh GB, Sidhu TS, Sharma A, et al. Management of aural foreign body: an evaluative study in 738 consecutive cases. *Am J Otolaryngol* 2007; 28:87–90.

Svider PF, Vong A, Sheyn A, et al. What are we putting in our ears? A consumer product analysis of foreign bodies. *Laryngoscope* 2015; 125(3):709–714.

Nose and Sinuses

Fernandes SV. Nasal fractures: the taming of the shrew. *Laryngoscope* 2004;114(3):587–592.

Li S, Papsin B, Brown DH. Value of nasal radiographs in nasal trauma management. *J Otolaryngol* 1996;25:162–164.

Lin VY, Daniel SJ, Papsin BC. Button batteries in the ear, nose and upper aerodigestive tract. *Int J Pediatr Otorhinolaryngol* 2004;68: 473–479.

Sanyaolu LN, Farmer SE, Cuddihy PJ. Nasal septal haematoma. *BMJ* 2014;349:g6075.

Schlosser RJ, Bolger WE. Nasal cerebrospinal fluid leaks: critical review and surgical considerations. *Laryngoscope* 2004;114:255–265.

Svider PF, Sheyn A, Folbe E, et al. How did that get there? A population-based analysis of nasal foreign bodies. *Int Forum Allergy Rhinol* 2014;4(11):944–949.

Oral Cavity and Pharynx

Brietzke SE, Jones DT. Pediatric oropharyngeal trauma: what is the role of CT scan? *Int J Pediatr Otorhinolaryngol* 2005;69: 669–679.

Ferreira PC, Amarante JM, Silva PN, et al. Retrospective study of 1251 maxillofacial fractures in children and adolescents. *Plast Reconstr Surg* 2005;115(6):1500–1508.

Hennelly K, Kimia A, Lee L, et al. Incidence of morbidity from penetrating palate trauma. *Pediatrics* 2010;126:e1578–e1584.

Soose RJ, Simons JP, Mandell DL. Evaluation and management of pediatric oropharyngeal trauma. *Arch Otolaryngol Head Neck Surg* 2006;132:446–451.

Usta M, Erkan T, Cokugras FC, et al. High doses of methylprednisolone in the management of caustic esophageal burns. *Pediatrics* 2014; 133(6):E1518–E1524.

Larynx and Trachea

Abujamra L, Joseph MM. Penetrating neck injuries in children: a retrospective review. *Pediatr Emerg Care* 2003;19(5):308–313.

Duval EL, Geraerts SD, Brackel HJ. Management of blunt tracheal trauma in children: a case series and review of literature. *Eur J Pediatr* 2007;166:559–563.

Gold SM, Gerber ME, Shott SR, et al. Blunt Laryngotracheal Trauma in Children. *Arch Otolaryngol Head Neck Surg* 1997;123(1): 83–87.

Mace SE. Blunt laryngotracheal trauma. *Ann Emerg Med* 1986;15(7): 836–842.

Merritt RM, Bent JP, Porubsky ES. Acute laryngeal trauma in the pediatric patient. *Ann Otol Rhinol Laryngol* 1998;107:104–106.

Additional Resources

Videos

Videos in Clinical medicine: examination of the larynx and pharynx. *N Engl J Med* 2008;358:e2. Available at http://www.nejm.org/doi/full/10.1056/NEJMvcm0706392

CHAPTER 115 ■ FACIAL TRAUMA

PAUL L. ARONSON, MD AND MARK I. NEUMAN, MD, MPH

RELATED CHAPTERS

Resuscitation and Stabilization
- Airway: Chapter 3

Signs and Symptoms
- Injury: Head: Chapter 36

Trauma
- ENT Trauma: Chapter 114
- Ocular Trauma: Chapter 122

Surgical Emergencies
- Ophthalmic Emergencies: Chapter 131

Procedures and Appendices
- Procedures: Chapter 141

KEY POINTS

- Stabilization of the airway is the primary concern among children with facial trauma.
- Computerized tomography is the optimal imaging study for suspected facial fractures.
- Prompt recognition of extraocular muscle entrapment associated with orbital floor fractures is critical to prevent muscle ischemia and fibrosis.
- Displaced nasal bone fractures should be repaired within 7 days of injury.
- Fast-absorbing plain gut sutures have demonstrated similar cosmetic performance to nonabsorbable sutures for the repair of facial lacerations.

GOALS OF EMERGENCY THERAPY

Stabilization of the Airway

While injuries sustained as a result of facial trauma are rarely life-threatening, patients who have sustained enough force to cause significant facial injury may have other associated serious injuries. Stabilization of the airway is therefore the primary concern in the management of facial injuries in children. Airway obstruction may result from blood in the mouth, loose teeth, and pharyngeal edema. Thus, the airway should be cleared and examined for patency. Loss of support of subglottic musculature can result from severe mandibular fractures, and the tongue can fall posteriorly and occlude the airway in a patient with a depressed mental status. An oral or nasal airway may serve as an adjuvant to positioning in order to achieve airway patency. Tracheal intubation may be required if the airway remains unstable. Cricothyrotomy or tracheostomy may be necessary if these measures fail to secure the airway but should be attempted only as a last resort because of the technical difficulty and complications associated with such procedures, particularly in young children.

Cervical Spine Protection

Up to 10% of patients with maxillofacial trauma have an associated cervical spine injury. Patients with tenderness of the cervical spine, impaired sensorium, focal neurologic deficits, or major distracting injury should be placed in a hard cervical collar until an injury to the cervical spine can be excluded.

Identification of Specific Bony Injuries and Facial Neurologic Deficits

Following airway stabilization and cervical spine protection, examination for specific bony injuries should be performed. After careful observation for deformity and asymmetry, the clinician should palpate the facial bones in a systematic fashion (Fig. 115.1). Tenderness, crepitus, and "step off" are signs of underlying fracture. Particular attention should be paid to the malar eminences, zygomatic arches, and superior and inferior orbital rims.

Assessment for a fracture of the maxilla can be performed by grasping and attempting to move the upper central teeth. Any laxity of the maxilla or crepitus is suggestive of fracture. External and intraoral palpation of the mandibular symphysis, body, angle, and ramus can help diagnose fractures in these areas. Inspection of the mouth and oral cavity should also be performed to assess for injury to the maxilla and mandible. Occlusal disharmony is an indication of mandibular and/or maxillary displacement. Older children will be able to report if their bite "feels normal." Opposing teeth that do not come together, but that exhibit wear facets (smoothing of mammillations along the incisal surfaces of the teeth) suggest a traumatic malocclusion. An inability to hold a tongue blade between occluded teeth on each side of the mouth is suggestive of a mandibular fracture.

Examination of the eyes should include the assessment of pupillary reactivity and size, examination of extraocular movements, visual acuity, and a thorough inspection for surrounding orbital injuries. Orbital dystopia and/or enophthalmos are suggestive of a fracture of the orbit. Examination of the nose should include documentation of focal tenderness, swelling and asymmetry, bleeding, or other nasal discharge, as well as the presence or absence of a septal hematoma.

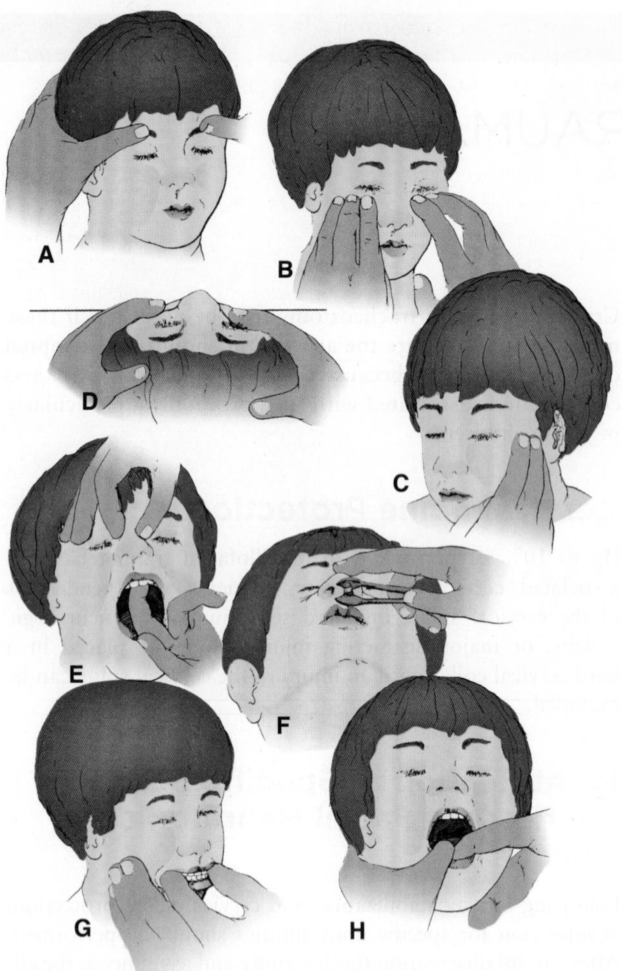

FIGURE 115.1 Sequential steps in examination for facial fractures. **A:** The supraorbital ridges are palpated while keeping the patient's head steady. **B:** The infraorbital ridges are palpated using the index, middle, and ring fingers to assess for areas of point tenderness. **C:** The zygomatic arch is palpated on each side to determine continuity and the possible presence of displaced fractures. **D:** The infraorbital rims, zygomatic bodies, and maxilla are palpated and examined from the top of the head to determine depressions and fracture displacement. **E:** The nasal bone and maxilla are examined for stability and possible fracture displacement. **F:** The nose is examined intranasally to determine the placement of the nasal septum and the possible displacement of nasal bones or disruption of nasal mucosa. **G:** The occlusion is observed to determine any disturbances of normal teeth relations. **H:** The mandible is palpated and then retracted to determine sites of discomfort and possible mandibular fractures.

Neurologic examination of the face should include evaluation of both sensory and motor functions. All three branches of the trigeminal nerve should be evaluated for sensation. Anesthesia of the cheek suggests injury to the infraorbital nerve, whereas anesthesia of the lower teeth and lower lip suggests inferior alveolar nerve involvement. The facial nerve should be evaluated by asking the patient to wrinkle the forehead, close and open the eyes fully, smile, show his or her teeth, and close the mouth tightly.

Determination of Appropriate Imaging Modality

The use of radiography in the evaluation and management of children with facial trauma should be considered if there is a concern of fracture based on history and physical examination. The complexity of bony and soft tissue facial structures can make the interpretation of plain radiographs difficult. In addition, plain radiographs are often inadequate to determine whether a patient requires operative intervention.

Computed tomography (CT) has mainly replaced plain radiographs in the definitive assessment of bony facial injuries because it has a greater ability to detect fractures and associated displacement as well as visualize soft tissue structures. Axial views demonstrate fractures of the anterior and posterior walls of the frontal sinus, medial and lateral orbital walls, posterior wall of the maxillary sinus, zygomatic arches, and mandible. Coronal views demonstrate fractures of the ethmoid, sphenoid, and paranasal sinuses; orbital floors and infraorbital rims; the nasoethmoid region; and mandibular condyles and symphyses. Coronal imaging requires hyperextension of the neck and thus requires prior exclusion of a cervical spine injury. Three-dimensional CT imaging can help guide operative repair.

Despite their limitations, there are specific plain radiograph views that may be of utility for the evaluation of facial fractures in children. The Waters view (occipitomental) is used to visualize the midface region: the orbital rims and floor of the orbit, nasal bones, zygoma, and maxilla. This view may be particularly useful in patients suspected of having a blowout fracture of the orbit, as well as for detecting fluid in the maxillary sinus. The Caldwell view supplements the Waters view for the evaluation of the upper two-thirds of the face, including visualization of the superior orbital rim, frontal sinuses, and nasoethmoid complex; however, the orbital floor is often obscured. The lateral view is useful for the detection of fractures to the anterior wall of the frontal sinus, the anterior and posterior walls of the maxillary sinus, and the nasal bones. The submentovertex view provides visualization of the zygomatic body and arch. Posterior–anterior, right and left lateral oblique, and Towne views are used to detect fractures of the mandible; however, fractures of the symphysis may be difficult to discern. Panorex views provide visualization of the entire mandible and lower teeth.

Obtain Subspecialty Consultation When Indicated

The clinician must evaluate whether subspecialist input is warranted for the management of facial trauma in children. Plastic surgeons, ophthalmologists, otorhinolaryngologists, and oral and maxillofacial surgeons have expertise in the management of patients with facial trauma. Once it is determined that subspecialist input is warranted, the decision of which subspecialist to involve will depend largely on availability and expertise of such individuals within the institution.

FACIAL FRACTURES

Mandible Fracture

Goals of Treatment

The primary goals in treatment of mandible fractures include (1) airway stabilization, (2) pain control, and (3) evaluation for the need for subspecialty consultation and possible surgical intervention.

CLINICAL PEARLS AND PITFALLS

- Clinical evaluation of any chin laceration should include palpation of the mandible, particularly the mandibular condyles, to evaluate for mandible fracture.
- The majority of mandibular fractures can be managed conservatively with closed reduction and/or maxilla-mandibular fixation.
- Preauricular swelling and inability to fully close the mouth are key features of temporomandibular joint dislocation.

Clinical Considerations

Fractures of the mandible can occur in one or more of the following regions: the symphysis, body, angle, ramus, and condyle (Fig. 115.2). The mechanism of injury often determines the site of potential fracture in patients with trauma to the mandible. Motor vehicle collisions and falls tend to cause fractures of the condyles and symphysis because the force is directed against the chin, whereas assaults tend to result in injuries to the body or angle of the mandible at the point of impact. Patients with parasymphyseal fractures resulting from falls often have an associated fracture in the contralateral subcondylar region. Pain and difficulty opening the mouth are typically present with mandibular fractures. Numbness of the lip and chin may also suggest a mandibular fracture because the inferior alveolar nerve courses through the center of the mandible, from the middle of the ramus, to its exit at the mental foramen. Mandibular fractures may result in airway obstruction due to hemorrhage either from the floor of the mouth or from a disruption in the bony support structure for the tongue.

Powerful muscles of mastication apply distracting forces to the fractured mandibular segments, often resulting in bony displacement and occlusal disharmony. The growth center for the mandible is located in the area of the condyle, and damage to this area from a fracture can cause significant growth disturbances, especially if sustained before the age of 3 years. Therefore, the clinical evaluation of any chin laceration should include palpation of the mandible, particularly the condyles. Malalignment of the lower central incisors (i.e., step off in dentition) suggests a mandibular fracture at the symphysis. Unilateral condyle fractures will most often result in the deviation of the jaw toward the side of the fracture upon mouth opening.

Temporomandibular joint dislocation may not only result from a direct blow to the chin but also may occur while yawning or opening the mouth widely. With dislocation, the condyle of the mandible is displaced anteriorly and is prevented from sliding back into place by spasm of the jaw muscles. Preauricular swelling and inability to close the mouth fully are the key features on physical examination.

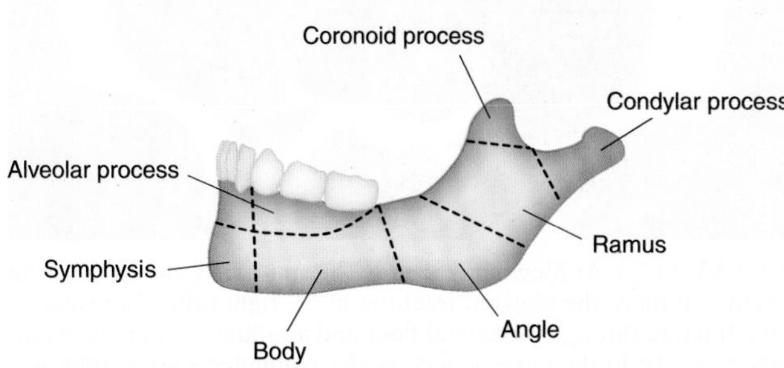

FIGURE 115.2 Anatomy of the mandible. Common sites of fracture include the condyle and subcondylar region, as well as the angle, body, and symphysis of the mandible.

Current Evidence

Mandibular fractures are treated more conservatively in children compared to adults due to the risk of injury to the permanent tooth buds and mandibular growth retardation. Most mandibular fractures can be treated with closed reduction and maxillomandibular fixation. A soft or liquid diet is recommended. Displaced fractures commonly require open reduction, internal fixation, or the use of splints. Antibiotics are generally recommended as these fractures are often in communication with the oral cavity, although there is limited data to support this recommendation.

Reduction of temporomandibular joint dislocations may be facilitated with the use of a benzodiazepine to decrease muscle spasm; procedural sedation may also be required. Downward traction is applied to the posterior aspect of the mandible. The chin is then pushed posteriorly to allow the condyle to return to its fossa.

Orbital Fracture

Goals of Treatment

The primary goals in treatment of orbital fractures are to recognize the signs of extraocular muscle entrapment, and if present, to obtain prompt ophthalmologic consultation to determine the need and timing of surgical repair to avoid muscle ischemia and fibrosis.

CLINICAL PEARLS AND PITFALLS

- In children, the floor of the orbit may fracture in a linear pattern that snaps back to create a "trapdoor" fracture. Fractures at this site can cause inferior rectus muscle entrapment, which may be identified by limitation of upward gaze.
- Decreased vision in a patient with orbital trauma may indicate a retrobulbar hemorrhage.

Clinical Considerations

Knowledge of the bony anatomy of the orbit is integral to the understanding of fractures at this site. The superior portion of the orbit is composed of the superior orbital rim and orbital roof, which is part of the thick frontal bone. The medial wall is formed by the ethmoid bone, which is adjacent to the nasal bones. The lateral wall is formed by the greater wing of the sphenoid and the zygoma, which are also quite thick. The floor and the inferior orbital rim are formed by the zygoma and the maxilla, which are relatively thin, and are further weakened by the groove for the infraorbital nerve.

Fractures of the floor of the orbit, sometimes known as "orbital blowout fractures," typically occur when a medium-sized, round, hard object, such as a baseball, strikes the eye (Fig. 115.3). The volume of the globe is fixed; thus, when an acute increase in orbital space (an opening in the floor of the orbit) occurs, the globe may be pushed posteriorly in the orbit, producing enophthalmos, a sunken appearance to the eye. A true orbital blowout fracture denotes a fracture of the floor of

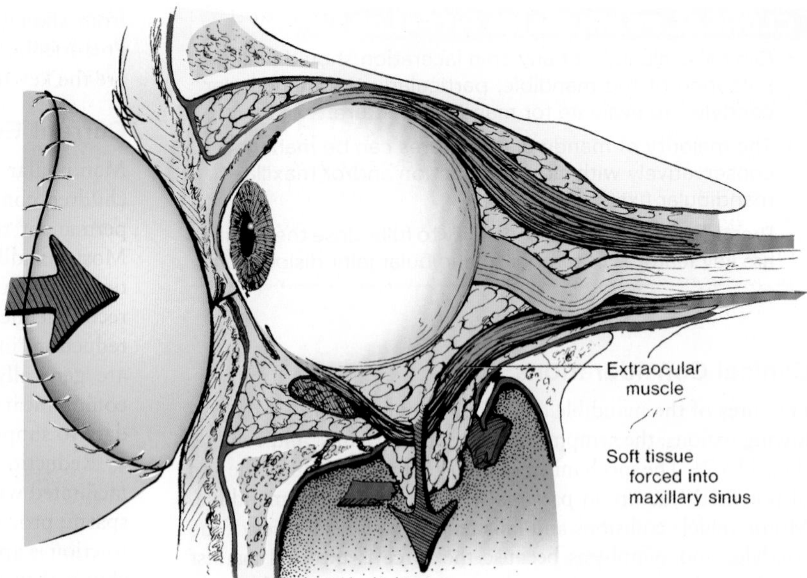

FIGURE 115.3 Mechanism of blowout fracture. In a sagittal view, a ball is shown striking the eye, deforming it, and causing increased pressure of the intraorbital contents. The periorbital fat is forced through the floor of the orbit. Retropositioning of the eye (enophthalmos), lowering of the eye, and extraocular muscle entrapment can result.

the orbit, with an intact inferior orbital rim. Although these fractures are quite rare in children, they are often due to direct trauma to the zygoma rather than a compression of the globe itself. Blood and orbital fat may sink into the maxillary sinus, clouding the sinus on radiograph (Fig. 115.4). Asymmetry in the horizontal level of the eyes (orbital dystopia) may also be present. The infraorbital nerve, the terminal branch of the maxillary division of the trigeminal nerve, exits the maxilla just below the infraorbital rim. Manifestations of injury to this nerve include decreased sensation to the cheek, upper lip, and upper gingiva on the affected side. Nausea and vomiting are often present with orbital blowout fractures and may be mistaken as symptoms of head injury.

In children, the floor of the orbit is relatively flexible. Consequently, it may fracture in a linear pattern that snaps back to create a "trapdoor" fracture. In adults, the floor of the orbit is thick and more likely to shatter when exposed to force. If the inferior rectus muscle is entrapped in the fracture gap in the floor of the orbit, voluntary upward gaze may be limited. Thin-cut coronal CT is especially valuable in detection of orbital blowout fractures and extraocular muscle entrapment. The presence of entrapment is an indication to operate on a blowout fracture on an urgent basis.

A thorough ophthalmologic examination is warranted in all patients with orbital fractures because of the high likelihood of associated eye injuries. In particular, vision should be assessed because decreased visual acuity may be an early sign of a retrobulbar hemorrhage, or injury to the optic nerve or eye itself. A retrobulbar hemorrhage can cause compression of the central retinal artery, which can threaten vision to the affected eye if not surgically decompressed. The type of eye and orbit injuries varies on the basis of the object and mechanism involved. Typically, a low-impact mechanism with a small object will result in injuries to the eye itself, such as a corneal abrasion or hyphema. Injury to the eye from a high-speed soft object such as a tennis ball will often result in a hyphema. Hard objects striking the orbit at a high speed, such as a baseball or a fist, are likely to result in an orbital blowout fracture. High-impact mechanisms, such as those encountered when the face strikes

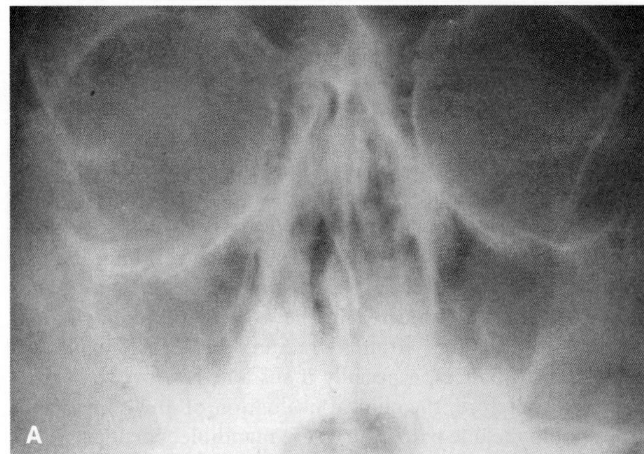

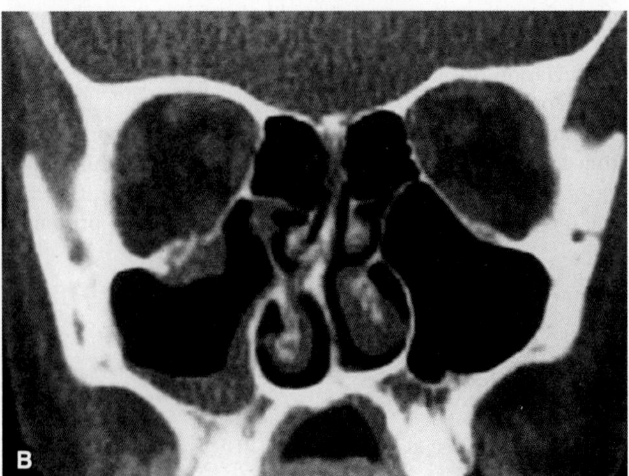

FIGURE 115.4 **A:** Blowout fracture. The sinus view shows teardrop configuration of the blowout fractures in the right orbit. Note associated fracture through the orbital floor and air–fluid level in the maxillary sinus. **B:** In the same patient as **(A)**, computed tomography section more clearly demonstrates the multiple fragment fracture through the orbital floor. Teardrop and air–fluid level are evident in the right maxillary sinus. (Courtesy of Soroosh Mahboubi, MD.)

the dashboard in a motor vehicle collision, are likely to result in complex orbital and midface fractures.

Current Evidence

Studies suggest that early repair (within 24 to 48 hours) of orbital trapdoor fracture and release of the entrapped muscles may help avoid muscle ischemia and fibrosis, and result in better functional recovery. A few studies have also demonstrated that corticosteroids may decrease swelling and hasten resolution of diplopia among patients with limitation of extraocular movement.

Nasal Fracture

Goals of Treatment

The primary goals in treatment of nasal fractures in the emergency setting are immediate recognition and drainage of septal hematoma, and in children, reduction of nasal fractures with deformity within 7 days.

CLINICAL PEARLS AND PITFALLS

- Nasal fractures may be difficult to detect clinically because of significant swelling.
- Septal hematomas require urgent incision and drainage to avoid necrosis of the avascular septal cartilage.
- Patients with nasal deformity 4 to 5 days after injury require urgent consultation with a subspecialist to restore anatomic alignment.

Clinical Considerations

The nasal bones are among the most commonly fractured bones of the facial skeleton because of their prominent location on the face. Nasal fractures may be difficult to detect because of significant swelling associated with such injuries. Plain radiographs are needed only rarely in the emergent care of children with nasal trauma because, in most cases, they do not contribute to subsequent care and management. Most nasal injuries can be managed as an outpatient, and evaluation after the swelling subsides dictates the need for further intervention.

Two particular nasal injuries that deserve specific comment are the intractable nosebleed and septal hematomas. Because of the rich vascular network in the nose, supplied by branches of both the internal (anterior ethmoidal) and external (superior labial, palatine) carotid arteries, nasal hemorrhage can be difficult to stop despite usual conservative measures (e.g., anterior compression). Treatment of persistent epistaxis may require anterior and/or posterior nasal packing with gauze or tampon, or the placement of an epistaxis balloon catheter. If a bleeding vessel can be identified, silver nitrate cauterization can be performed.

Septal hematomas arise because of hemorrhage from an artery beneath the mucoperichondrium, separating it from the septal cartilage. Because the septal cartilage is avascular and relies on the overlying mucoperichondrium for its blood supply, a hematoma may result in cartilage necrosis and eventual septal perforation. Septal hematomas require urgent incision and drainage (see Chapter 114 ENT Trauma).

Nasoorbital ethmoid fractures involve complete separation of the nasal bones and medial walls of the orbits from the stable frontal bone superiorly and infraorbital rim laterally. These injuries are usually the result of high-velocity trauma to the central midface. The bones are often fragmented and telescoped posteriorly into the ethmoid region. These patients display a characteristic flattened nose, with the loss of anterior projection on the lateral view of the face. Because the medial canthal tendons attach firmly to the medial walls of the orbits, lateral drift of the fracture segments results in traumatic telecanthus. Normal mean intercanthal distance is 16 mm at birth, which increases to 25 mm in a female and 27 mm in a male at full facial growth. A significant increase in intercanthal distance or gross asymmetry in the medial canthal to facial midline distance should raise suspicion of this fracture. Traumatic telecanthus suggests the diagnosis of a nasoorbital ethmoid fracture, which unlike a nondisplaced nasal fracture, requires urgent subspecialist input.

Current Evidence

Nasal fractures are largely a clinical diagnosis. Though rarely required for diagnosis, CT is the optimal modality for complex fractures. More recent studies suggest that high-resolution ultrasonography may be more sensitive than CT or plain radiography for the detection of simple nasal fractures.

While repair of nasal fractures can be successfully performed within a few hours after the injury, immediate repair is usually not possible because of the significant swelling that often develops rapidly with such injuries. The optimal timing after the immediate injury period is controversial. Some reports have demonstrated improved cosmetic outcome when repair is performed within 5 days of injury, while other studies have not demonstrated a difference in cosmesis with early (≤7 days) versus late (>7 days) repair. Patients suspected of having nasal fractures should be reevaluated within 4 to 5 days after the swelling subsides. Plain radiographs may be helpful at this time to determine whether malalignment exists. Patients with nasal deformity 4 to 5 days after injury require urgent consultation with a subspecialist to restore anatomic alignment.

Zygoma and Maxilla Fractures

CLINICAL PEARLS AND PITFALLS

- Particular attention to the airway is of paramount importance in children with midface fractures as significant bleeding and disruption of normal anatomic structures may compromise airway patency.

Clinical Considerations

The zygoma is composed of a body or malar eminence and the zygomatic arch. A complete fracture of the zygoma often extends through the floor of the orbit. This may result in an inferior displacement of the zygoma because of the strong inferior forces applied by the masseter muscle, which attaches to the malar eminence. Zygoma fractures often produce a flattened appearance to the cheek, with inferior displacement of the globe, and conjunctival hemorrhage. Decreased sensation along the distribution of the infraorbital nerve is also common, as zygomaticomaxillary fractures usually include the infraorbital foramen. Unilateral zygomatic arch fractures can cause a decrease in temporal width, which is best visualized when viewing the face from the front as a result of buckling of the zygomatic arch. If this buckling is severe, the mandibular

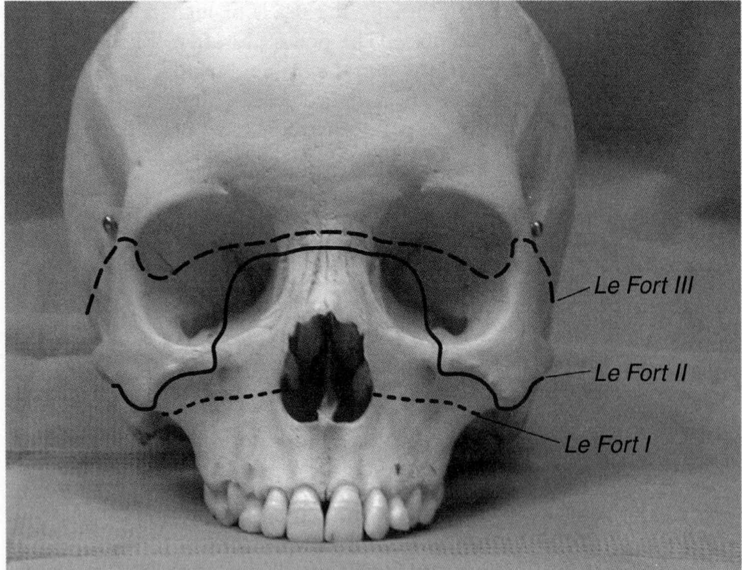

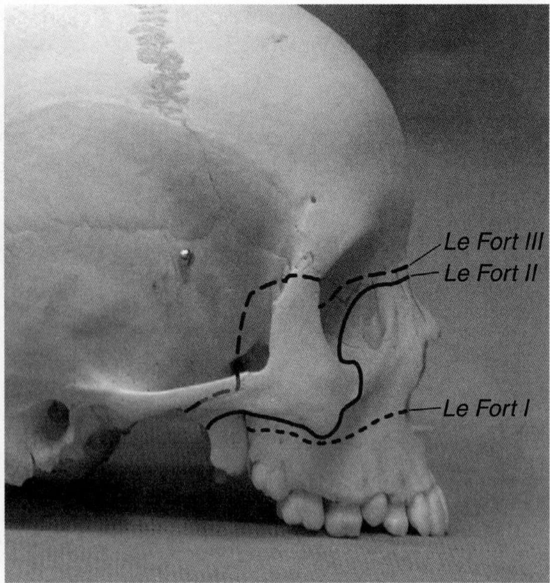

FIGURE 115.5 The Le Fort classification of fractures. With type I, the maxilla is separated from its attachments. Type II (pyramidal) produces a mobile maxilla and nose. With type III (craniofacial disjunction), all attachments of the midface to the skull have been separated. Traction on the anterior maxilla produces motion up to the inferior orbital rims and zygoma. These fractures are not mutually exclusive. For example, Le Fort II fracture may exist on the one side with type III on the other side.

condyle may be impinged, with resultant difficulty in mouth opening.

In 1901, Le Fort described three fracture patterns that occurred in patients with midface trauma (Fig. 115.5). The Le Fort I fracture pattern involves only the maxilla and extends through the zygomaticomaxillary region to the base of the pyriform aperture. It allows motion of a segment of alveolar bone and teeth when examined. The Le Fort II pattern, also called a pyramidal fracture, is similar but extends more superiorly to the infraorbital rims and across the nasofrontal sutures. The maxilla, nasal bones, and the medial orbital wall are separated from the facial skeleton. The nose and the upper jaw are movable, whereas the zygomas are stable. The Le Fort III pattern, also called craniofacial dissociation, extends across the zygomatic arch, zygomaticofrontal region, floor of the orbit, and nasofrontal sutures, effectively separating the midface from the skull base. When the nose or upper jaw is moved, the entire midface, including the zygoma, moves with it. These fractures are quite rare in children, and when they do occur, they are most often asymmetric because impact is sustained from the side rather than head on.

Patients with midface fractures typically have significant swelling over the maxilla and severe epistaxis. Particular attention to the airway is of paramount importance in these children because significant bleeding and a disruption in the normal anatomic structures may threaten the patency of the airway. Nasal manipulation should be avoided because these fractures may be associated with cribriform plate injuries and passage of a nasogastric or endotracheal tube may result in brain injury. On examination, by grasping the maxilla at the level of the central incisors, the clinician may be able to appreciate crepitus or mobility when traction is applied. Clear rhinorrhea in the setting of midface trauma may be a sign of a cerebrospinal fluid (CSF) leak and warrants neurosurgical consultation. All patients suspected of having a midface fracture require CT imaging to determine whether surgical reduction is necessary.

Frontal Bone Fractures

CLINICAL PEARLS AND PITFALLS

- Clear rhinorrhea or leakage of clear fluid from a forehead laceration should raise suspicion for fracture of the posterior wall of the frontal sinus with dural tear and CSF leak.

Clinical Considerations

Fractures of the frontal bone are rare in young children because the frontal sinuses do not develop until 8 years of age. Injury to the frontal sinus may reveal a palpable or visible depression if the anterior wall of the sinus has been compressed. Displaced fractures of the anterior wall of the frontal sinus require surgical elevation. In patients with severe frontal sinus fractures associated with forehead lacerations, a fracture of the posterior wall of the sinus and dural tear may allow CSF to leak from the wound. Leakage of clear fluid from the wound, or clear rhinorrhea, should raise suspicion for such a leak and warrant CT imaging and neurosurgical consultation.

SOFT TISSUE INJURIES

Lacerations

Goals of Treatment

The goal of laceration repair is to achieve hemostasis and provide an optimal cosmetic result.

CLINICAL PEARLS AND PITFALLS

- Deep lacerations to the cheek or lateral periorbital region should raise suspicion for facial nerve injury.
- Lacerations to the medial periorbital region near the medial canthus should be evaluated for injury to the lacrimal canaliculi.
- Fast-absorbing plain gut sutures have demonstrated equivalent cosmetic outcome compared to nonabsorbable sutures in repair of facial lacerations.

Clinical Considerations

The goal of laceration repair is to achieve hemostasis and provide an optimal cosmetic result. Knowledge of the deep structures of the face, particularly the facial nerve and the lacrimal apparatus, will aid in the evaluation and management of children with deep facial lacerations. Lateral periorbital lacerations should raise suspicion of injury to the frontal branch of the facial nerve, which travels superficially along a line from just above the tragus to a point 1.5 cm above the lateral eyebrow. Lacerations in the medial periorbital region near the medial canthus should raise suspicion for lacrimal duct injury. Because 85% of tears are drained via the lower canaliculus, failure to repair a laceration to the lacrimal duct may result in excessive tearing (epiphora). If deep lacerations are present in the cheek region, the clinician must determine whether injury to the buccal branch of the facial nerve and to the parotid duct has occurred (Fig. 115.6).

When injury to the facial nerve is suspected, function can be tested by having the patient move specific muscles of facial expression. This testing should take place before infiltration with local anesthetic. The frontal branch of the facial nerve can be tested by asking the patient to frown in order to look for symmetry of frontalis muscle action. The marginal mandibular (motor) branch may course as much as 1 to 2 cm below the border of the mandible and is responsible for the depression and eversion of the lower lip. Injury to this branch results in a characteristic inward rotation of the lower lip on the affected side as a result of unopposed orbicularis oris tone on that side. The buccal branches are in close proximity to Stensen (parotid) duct, usually close to a line between the tragus of the ear and the mid upper lip. Pure motor injuries to the facial nerve are quite amenable to microsurgical repair if detected and repaired in a timely fashion. Therefore, all suspected motor nerve injuries warrant appropriate surgical consultation to allow for the best functional recovery.

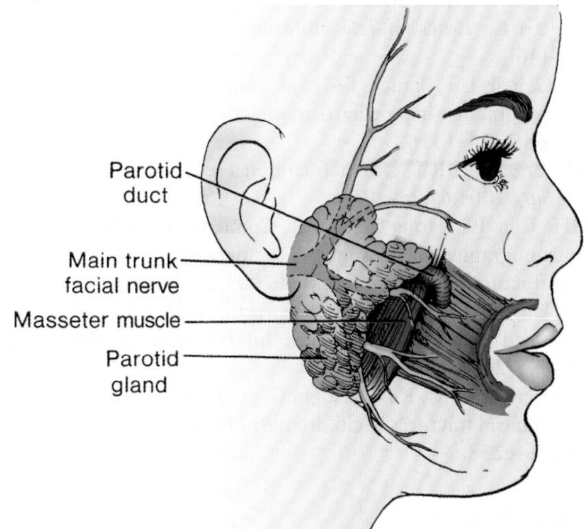

FIGURE 115.6 Deep lacerations to the cheek can injure the facial nerve, parotid gland, or parotid duct. The facial nerve becomes more superficial as it branches and proceeds distally. Distal nerve injuries can thus occur with more superficial wounds.

Examination for potential injury to Stensen duct is accomplished by grasping the commissure between the thumb and index finger and gently everting the buccal mucosa to identify Stensen duct, which lies on a vertical line along the maxillary second premolar. With the opposite hand, gentle massage of the parotid gland is accomplished by pressing in the preauricular region. The appearance of clear fluid from Stensen duct suggests an uninjured duct. The absence of fluid after several minutes of inspection, or bloody fluid, suggests injury to the gland or duct. In this case, inspection of the depth of the wound may reveal salivary fluid and severed ends of the duct may be identified. A sialogram can be a useful adjunct in the diagnosis of parotid duct injuries, as well as subspecialty consultation.

Although most lacerations should be repaired within 8 to 12 hours, clean lacerations of the face can often be reapproximated up to 24 hours after the injury was sustained. Later closure may be considered after the risks of infection in closing such a wound are weighed against the benefits of reducing the facial scarring that will result if the wound is allowed to heal secondarily. Factors such as mechanism of injury, immunocompetence, and hygiene must be considered. Anesthesia, copious irrigation, and tension-free approximation are vital to a successful closure. Subspecialty consultation may be warranted for late-presentation lacerations or heavily contaminated wounds, in which the risk of infection is high.

If possible, facial lacerations should be repaired using deep sutures to reduce tension on the wound and to help with eversion of the edges. All wounds contract as scar formation occurs and thus eversion of the skin should be achieved for facial lacerations, particularly those involving the nares, eyelids, helix of the ear, and vermillion border of the lower lip. Inadequate eversion of the wound edges at these sites may lead to a depressed scar or notching at the site of the laceration.

Repair of complex injuries to laminated structures (e.g., ear, eyelid, nose, lip) requires that each layer of the structure be reapproximated. For example, a full-thickness laceration to the nose at the nostril rim requires closure of three separate layers. The nasal lining is usually closed first with an absorbable suture material. Next, the cartilage must be repaired, also with absorbable material. Finally, the overlying skin of the nose can be reapproximated. Similarly, complex injuries of the ear, the eyelid, or the lip require layered closure to achieve the best cosmetic result. Careful attention should be paid to lip lacerations that traverse the vermillion border. Cosmetic outcome is predicated on successful alignment of tissue at this junction. Consultation with plastic surgery may be considered for lacerations involving the external ear, nasal mucosa and cartilage, as well as complex lip lacerations traversing the vermilion border.

Informed consent should be obtained from patients and families undergoing laceration repair, and this information should be documented in the medical record. The physician should provide a careful assessment and natural history of the injury if left untreated to heal on its own. The physician should also describe the recommended treatment, as well as alternative treatments, with likely outcomes and possible complications. Patients with lacerations resulting from dog bites and those who present for care after a delayed period of time should be advised of the high risk of infection. Complicated facial laceration repair and laceration repair in young children may be facilitated by the use of a short-acting benzodiazepine or procedural sedation.

Current Evidence

Randomized controlled trials that compared fast-absorbable plain catgut to nonabsorbable nylon sutures have demonstrated no significant difference in short- or long-term cosmesis or complications such as infection or wound dehiscence. Additionally, caregivers had a significantly higher future preference for the absorbable sutures. Tissue adhesives such as 2-octylcyanocrylate have similarly demonstrated similar cosmesis, less pain, and shorter procedure times when compared to sutures for simple lacerations, but may have a slightly increased risk of wound dehiscence. For deep lacerations, skin closure should be performed only after tension is relieved from wound borders, usually through the use of buried absorbable sutures. Stapling is a fast and cosmetically acceptable alternative to suturing for simple scalp lacerations.

Regional Nerve Blocks

CLINICAL PEARLS AND PITFALLS

- Important areas for regional nerve blocks on the face include the medial third of the eyebrow (supraorbital nerve), the infraorbital foramen (infraorbital nerve), and 2 to 3 cm above the inferior border of mandible (mental nerve).

Clinical Considerations

Local or regional anesthesia may be used to aid in the suturing of facial lacerations in children. Regional anesthesia has the distinct advantage of allowing the physician to perform a painless procedure, without distorting the anatomic structures under repair. In addition, regional blocks, in general, require fewer anesthetics (see Chapter 141 Procedures).

The supraorbital nerve exits the supraorbital rim in the medial third of the eyebrow approximately 2 to 3 cm from the facial midline. Local infiltration in this region can effectively provide anesthesia to the ipsilateral hemiforehead. The infraorbital nerve exits through the infraorbital foramen, approximately 5 mm inferior to the infraorbital rim. Effective block of this nerve can provide anesthesia to the ipsilateral medial cheek and upper lip. Anesthesia of the lower lip and chin may be achieved by infiltration of the ipsilateral mental (infraoral) nerve. This nerve exists approximately 2 to 3 cm superior to the inferior border of the mandible. The supraorbital and infraorbital nerves, as well as the mental nerve, exit the facial skeleton from foramen, which are inline with the first premolar tooth.

Guidelines for Subspecialty Consultation

CLINICAL PEARLS AND PITFALLS

- Lacerations that require subspecialty consultation include those with injury to deep structures such as nerves or ducts, are associated with tissue loss, or that involve the cartilage of the ear or nose.

Clinical Considerations

Most facial lacerations can be repaired by the pediatric emergency medicine physician. Injuries that require subspecialist consultation include (i) lacerations with evidence of injury to deep structures (a major motor nerve or a glandular duct), (ii) cases in which a substantial amount of devitalized tissue exists or actual tissue loss has occurred, (iii) wounds in which the amount of bleeding cannot be easily controlled, (iv) full-thickness defects of the ear and nose that involve cartilage, and (v) cases in which it is unclear exactly which tissue to approximate to restore preinjury anatomy and aesthetics (e.g., lips, eyelids, nostrils, ears).

Suggested Readings and Key References

Goals of Emergency Therapy

Druelinger L, Guenther M, Marchand EG, et al. Radiographic evaluation of the facial complex. *Emerg Med Clin North Am* 2000;18:393–410.

Eggensperger Wymann NM, Holzle A, Zachariou Z, et al. Pediatric craniofacial trauma. *J Oral Maxillofac Surg* 2008;66:58–64.

Ellis E 3rd, Scott K. Assessment of patients with facial fractures. *Emerg Med Clin North Am* 2000;18:411–448.

Holland AJ, Broome C, Steinberg A, et al. Facial fractures in children. *Pediatr Emerg Care* 2001;17:157–160.

Imahara SD, Hopper RA, Wang J, et al. Patterns and outcomes of pediatric facial fractures in the United States: a survey of the National Trauma Data Bank. *J Am Coll Surg* 2008;207: 710–716.

Ryan ML, Thorson CM, Otero CA, et al. Pediatric facial trauma: a review of guidelines for assessment, evaluation, and management in the emergency department. *J Craniofac Surg* 2011;22:1183–1189.

Shaikh ZS, Worrall SF. Epidemiology of facial trauma in a sample of patients aged 1–18 years. *Injury* 2002;33:669–671.

Vyas RM, Dickinson BP, Wasson KL, et al. Pediatric facial fractures: current national incidence, distribution, and health care resource use. *J Craniofac Surg* 2008;19:339–349.

Zimmermann CE, Troulis MJ, Kaban LB. Pediatric facial fractures: recent advances in prevention, diagnosis and management. *Int J Oral Maxillofac Surg* 2005;34:823–833.

Facial Fractures

Foulds JS, Laverick S, MacEwen CJ. "White-eyed" blowout fracture: a case series of five children. *Arch Dis Child* 2013;98: 445–446.

Gerbino G, Roccia F, Bianchi FA, et al. Surgical management of orbital trapdoor fracture in a pediatric population. *J Oral Maxillofac Surg* 2010;68:1310–1316.

Jatla KK, Enzenauer RW. Orbital fractures: a review of current literature. *Curr Surg* 2004;61:25–29.

Lee MH, Cha JG, Hong HS, et al. Comparison of high-resolution ultrasonography and computed tomography in the diagnosis of nasal fractures. *J Ultrasound Med* 2009;28:717–723.

Lee DH, Jang YJ. Pediatric nasal bone fractures: does delayed treatment really lead to adverse outcomes? *Int J Pediatr Otorhinolaryngol* 2013;77:726–731.

Yilmaz MS, Guven M, Kayabasoglu G, et al. Efficacy of closed reduction for nasal fractures in children. *Br J Oral Maxillofac Surg* 2013; 51:e256–e258.

Soft Tissue Injuries

Al-Abdullah T, Plint AC, Fergusson D. Absorbable versus nonabsorbable sutures in the management of traumatic lacerations and surgical wounds: a meta-analysis. *Pediatr Emerg Care* 2007;23: 339–344.

Farion KJ, Osmond MH, Hartling L, et al. Tissue adhesives for traumatic lacerations: a systematic review of randomized controlled trials. *Acad Emerg Med* 2003;10:110–118.

Karounis H, Gouin S, Esiman H, et al. A randomized, controlled trial comparing long-term cosmetic outcomes of traumatic pediatric lacerations repaired with absorbable plain gut versus nonabsorbable nylon sutures. *Acad Emerg Med* 2004;11:730–735.

Khan AN, Dayan PS, Miller S, et al. Cosmetic outcome of scalp wound closure with staples in the pediatric emergency department: a prospective, randomized trial. *Pediatr Emerg Care* 2002;18: 171–173.

Luck RP, Flood R, Eyal D, et al. Cosmetic outcomes of absorbable versus nonabsorbable sutures in pediatric facial lacerations. *Pediatr Emerg Care* 2008;24:137–142.

Luck R, Tredway T, Gerard J, et al. Comparison of cosmetic outcomes of absorbable versus nonabsorbable sutures in pediatric facial lacerations. *Pediatr Emerg Care* 2013;29:691–695.

CHAPTER 116 ■ GENITOURINARY TRAUMA

GREGORY E. TASIAN, MD, MSc, MSCE AND ROBERT A. BELFER, MD

Genitourinary trauma in children is common with approximately 28,000 children presenting to emergency departments in the United States annually with genitourinary injuries. Approximately 10% of patients with serious multisystem trauma have genitourinary injuries. Most injuries (90%) are the result of blunt trauma that involves crush injuries and acceleration/deceleration forces related to motor vehicle collisions, falls of high-velocity injuries such as sledding, skateboarding, or skiing.

The clinical approach to the injured child should strictly follow advanced trauma life support guidelines. Figure 116.1 provides an algorithm for diagnostic evaluation of pediatric patients with genitourinary trauma. Urologic management may be temporized to permit urinary drainage in the initial phases; the patient may subsequently require operative procedures.

KEY POINTS

- The goal of emergency therapy for genitourinary injury is to maximize organ preservation and minimize future morbidity.
- Assessment of the genitourinary system can be undertaken once life-threatening conditions have been identified and the child has been resuscitated.
- Management of hemodynamically stable children with renal injuries should proceed on the basis of radiographic staging of the traumatic injury.

RELATED CHAPTERS

Resuscitation and Stabilization
- Approach to the Injured Child: Chapter 2

Signs and Symptoms
- Groin Masses: Chapter 29
- Pain: Scrotal: Chapter 56
- Vaginal Discharge: Chapter 76
- Vaginal Bleeding: Chapter 75

Medical, Surgical and Trauma Emergencies
- Genitourinary Emergencies: Chapter 127

GOALS OF EMERGENCY THERAPY

The goal of emergency therapy for genitourinary injury is to maximize organ preservation and minimize future morbidity.

To achieve these goals, the initial management of children with genitourinary injury in the emergency department centers on prompt recognition and staging of injuries, followed by appropriate urologic consultation for management and potential surgical intervention for these injuries. The recognition and treatment of children with genitourinary injury requires an understanding of the clinical situations and signs and symptoms associated with genitourinary injury and appropriate use of diagnostic imaging. To provide a comprehensive and accessible guide for management of children with genitourinary injury, we discuss trauma of each genitourinary organ separately yet emphasize the potential for concomitant extrarenal injury and need for maintaining a high level of suspicion for these associated injuries.

KIDNEY

Goal of Treatment

The principle underlying the management of pediatric renal trauma is preservation of renal tissue and function minimizing morbidity and mortality. Patients who are hemodynamically unstable or have sustained severe intra-abdominal penetrating trauma require immediate surgical intervention. Management of hemodynamically stable children should proceed on the basis of radiographic staging of the traumatic injury.

CLINICAL PEARLS AND PITFALLS

In the adult population, radiographic evaluation is required in patients with hypotension, penetrating injuries in the vicinity of urologic organs, associated abdominal injuries, or the presence of any degree of hematuria. Criteria regarding the imaging of children with penetrating trauma are less well established.

Hypotension is not a reliable indicator of significant renal injury in children and therefore should not be used to guide management; however, most patients with multisystem trauma and hypotension undergo an abdominal computed tomographic (CT) scan screening for nonurologic injuries. Radiographic evaluation of the pediatric genitourinary tract is necessary in cases with clinical signs indicative of renal injury, gross hematuria, major associated injuries, or history of significant deceleration forces. For blunt abdominal trauma, imaging should be performed in any stable child with gross hematuria or significant microscopic hematuria (>50 red blood cells per high power field) associated with shock (systolic blood pressure <90 mm Hg). However, the late manifestations of shock in children with traumatic injuries have led some experts to recommend imaging in any stable child with microscopic hematuria >50 red blood cells with or without shock. Additionally, any child with a significant associated injury or a suspicious mechanism of injury such as a rapid deceleration, high velocity strike, fall from >15 ft, or a direct blow to the abdomen or flank should be imaged regardless of the presence of hematuria. All clinically stable children with penetrating abdominal or pelvic trauma should undergo radiographic assessment. Stable blunt trauma patients with microscopic hematuria may be observed without imaging, unless they suffered a major acceleration or deceleration injury such as a fall from a great height or high speed MVC.

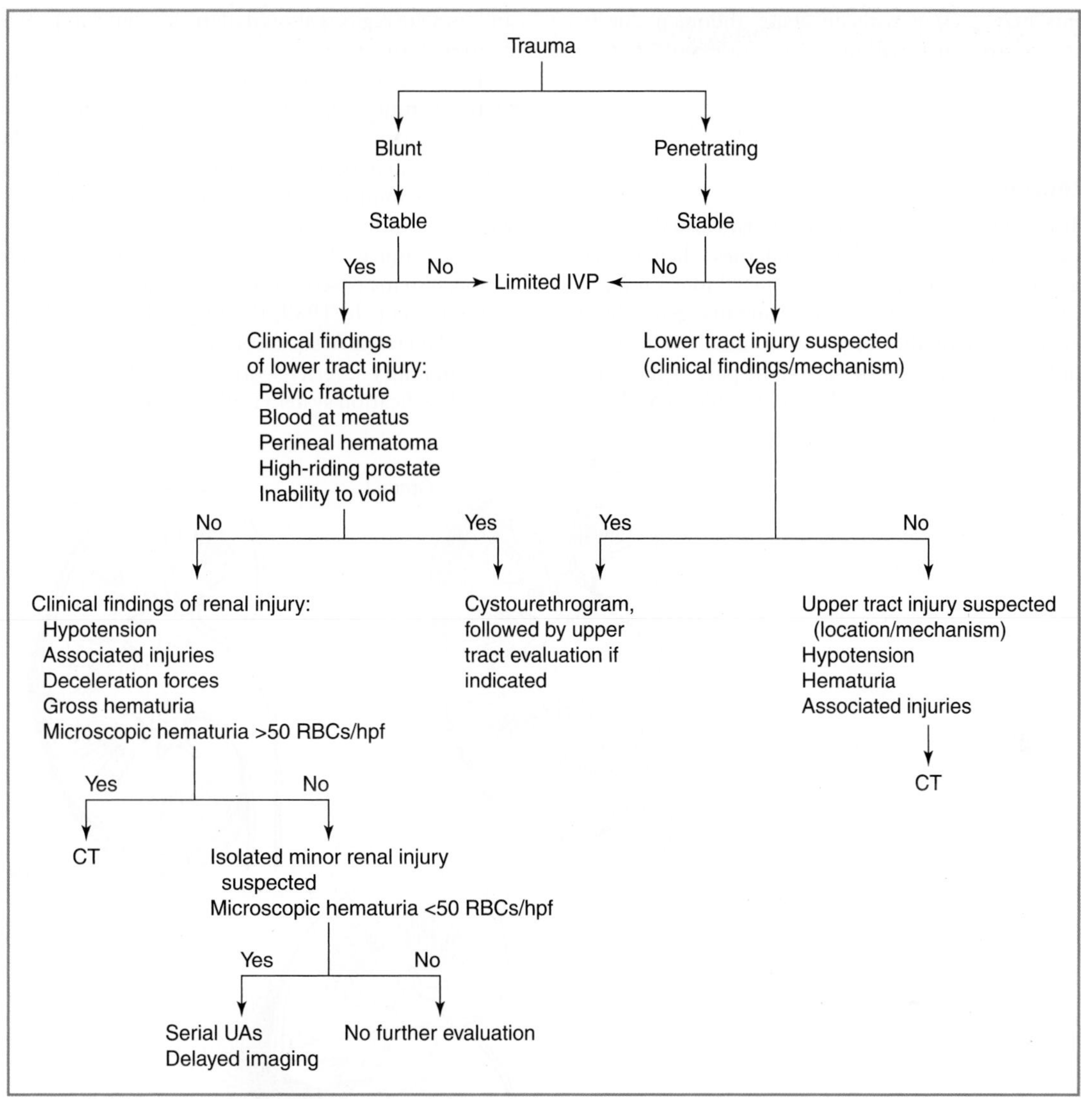

FIGURE 116.1 Algorithm for the evaluation of the pediatric patient with genitourinary trauma. IVP, intravenous pyelogram; CT, computed tomography; RBC, red blood cell; HPF, high-powered field; UAs, urinalyses.

Current Evidence

Approximately half of all genitourinary injuries involve the kidney. Children are more likely than adults to sustain renal injuries for the following reasons: The pediatric kidney is larger in proportion to the size of the abdomen than in adults; the child's kidney may retain fetal lobations which allow for easier parenchymal disruption; the pediatric kidney has inadequate protection due to weaker abdominal musculature, a less well-ossified thoracic cage, and less developed perirenal fat and fascia than in adults. Most pediatric renal trauma is minor, requiring no intervention.

Blunt trauma accounts for more than 90% of renal injuries in children. Most pediatric renal trauma is sustained in motor vehicle accidents. Falls, sports-related incidents, and direct blows are also common mechanisms of injury. In these scenarios, the kidneys are crushed against the ribs or vertebral column from their relatively fixed position within Gerota fascia. Contusions or renal lacerations can occur. In addition, the vascular pedicle can be stretched causing renal vein or artery injuries. Penetrating trauma accounts for the remaining cases. Approximately 10% of penetrating abdominal injuries involve the kidney.

Minor renal injuries account for 85% of total injuries, lacerations in 10% and severe kidney ruptures, fractures of pedicle injuries in less than 5% of cases.

Associated extrarenal injuries often occur, with head injuries being the most common. Associated intraperitoneal injuries occur in 80% of patients with penetrating renal trauma and 20% of patients with blunt renal trauma. In general, the hospital length of stay is determined by the associated injuries and not the renal injuries.

Coincidental congenital renal anomalies and intrarenal tumors have been reported in up to 20% of children with renal injuries. More accurate recent reviews show that the incidence rate is closer to 1%. Historically, pre-existing anomalies have been believed to increase the risk and severity of injury to the kidney. However, it appears that in most patients, congenital genitourinary anomalies associated with renal injury are incidental findings and do not increase morbidity. Nevertheless, a high index of suspicion should be maintained in any child who presents with gross hematuria after a relatively minor trauma.

Other patients may present with an acute abdomen due to intraperitoneal rupture of a hydronephrotic kidney.

Clinical Considerations

Clinical Recognition

Children who sustain significant renal injuries usually present with localized signs such as flank tenderness, hematoma, palpable mass, or ecchymosis. However, since kidney injuries are often associated with injuries to other organs, generalized abdominal tenderness, rigidity of the abdominal wall, paralytic ileus, and hypovolemic shock may all be part of the clinical picture. Penetrating injuries to the chest, abdomen, flank, and lumbar regions should alert the clinician to the possibility of a renal injury.

Hematuria has long been considered the cardinal marker of renal injury. However, the degree of hematuria does not correlate with the severity of the renal lesion. Additionally, hematuria may be absent in up to 50% of patients with vascular pedicle injuries and in approximately one-third of patients with penetrating injuries.

Renal injuries have been described using different classification systems based on the clinical and radiologic assessment of the patient. In 1989, the Organ Injury Scaling Committee of the American Association for the Surgery of Trauma developed an injury severity score for classification of renal trauma. This classification system is illustrated in Figure 116.2. Grade I

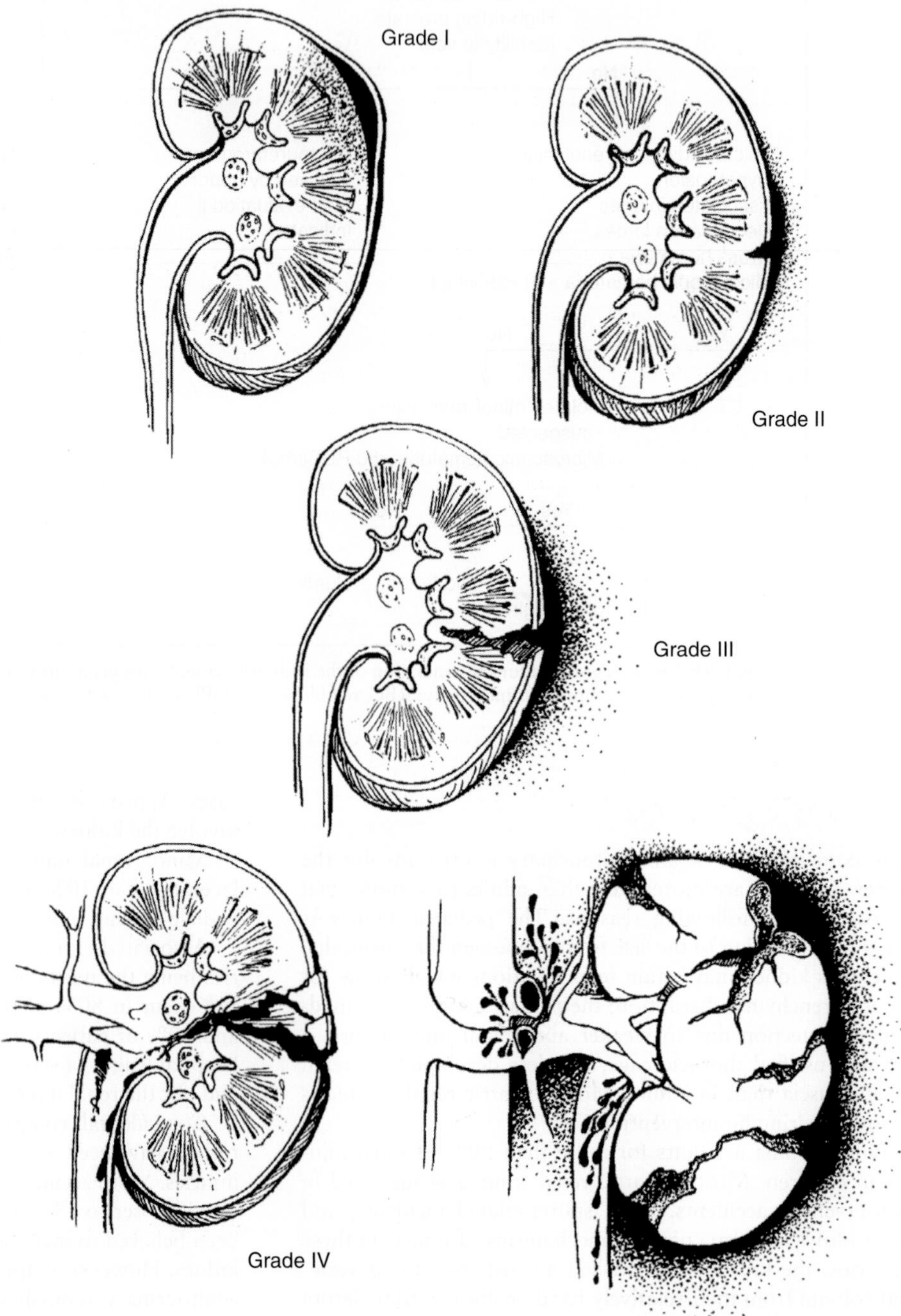

FIGURE 116.2 Classification of renal injuries as proposed by the Organ Injury Scaling Committee of the American Association for the Surgery of Trauma.

injuries include contusions or subcapsular, nonexpanding hematomas and comprise 80% of all injuries to the kidney. Grade II injuries include nonexpanding hematomas confined to the retroperitoneum or lacerations less than 1 cm in depth without urinary extravasation. Grade III injuries include lacerations extending more than 1 cm into the renal cortex without collecting system rupture or urinary extravasation. Grade IV injuries include lacerations extending into the collecting system or renal vascular injuries with contained hemorrhage. Grade V injuries include completely shattered kidneys or avulsions of renal hilum with devascularized kidneys.

Parenchymal contusions and hematomas are the most common renal injuries, accounting for 60% to 90% of all lesions from blunt trauma. Lacerations account for up to 10% of renal injuries and may involve disruption of the capsule, collecting system, or both.

Severe injuries, such as shattered kidney or pedicle avulsions, constitute approximately 3% of renal injuries. Pedicle injuries result from sheer force of the kidney with subsequent stretching of the renal vessels.

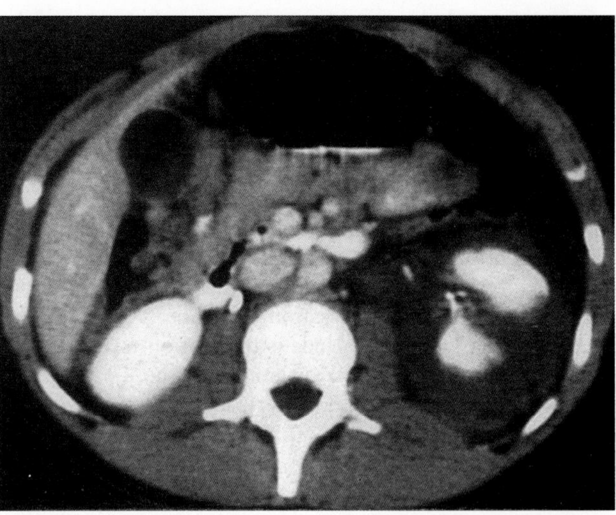

FIGURE 116.3 Renal fracture. Computed tomography section of the abdomen shows fracture of the left kidney with moderate subcapsular hematoma.

Initial Assessment

All injured children should undergo a thorough evaluation based on well-established pediatric trauma protocols. Assessment of the genitourinary system can be undertaken once life-threatening conditions have been identified and the child has been resuscitated. The flank should be inspected for ecchymosis and flank pain, and the presence of a "seat belt sign" should be noted on the abdomen, since all of these physical findings indicate significant trauma and possible renal injury. A urinalysis should be obtained in all patients with multisystem trauma or suspected isolated renal injury.

Management/Diagnostic Testing

Hemodynamically stable patients who present with suggestive clinical findings, gross hematuria, microscopic hematuria of more than 50 RBCs per hpf, major associated injuries, or a history of significant deceleration injury should undergo radiographic evaluation. These patients should have a contrast-enhanced CT scan with delayed images. Children who remain unstable despite resuscitative measures should undergo a one-shot IVP before emergency laparotomy. Children with isolated microscopic hematuria of less than 50 RBCs per hpf do not require immediate imaging. These patients may be discharged and can be evaluated on an outpatient basis with CT, IVP, or ultrasound if hematuria persists. However, in some pediatric trauma centers, management of these patients involves hospitalization for observation, followed by nonemergent radiographic evaluation.

The diagnostic performance of imaging modalities as they relate to the evaluation of renal trauma is reviewed here.

CT

Contrast-enhanced CT with additional 10-minute delayed scan is the "gold standard" imaging modality for staging a stable trauma patient. Trauma patients lacking radiographic signs of renal injury who do not have any perinephric, periureteral, or pelvic fluid collections do not require delayed imaging per expert consensus. If any of these subtle findings, especially low density fluid tracking around the kidney and down the ureter, are present on the initial contrast-enhanced CT. A UPJ or a ureteral injury can easily be missed if delayed images are not obtained.

The diagnostic accuracy of CT scan has been reported tobe as high as 98% (Fig. 116.3).

The ability of CT to quickly evaluate solid organ and vascular injuries has significantly improved the management of trauma. Important radiologic findings that should be noted when reviewing CT for renal trauma include arterial medial extravasation of contrast, denoting a severe arterial injury; medial hematoma without arterial extravasation, often secondary to a venous injury; differential contrast uptake and excretion, which is indicative of arterial injury or thrombosis; cortical rim sign, often indicative of a main renal artery injury; degree of parenchymal laceration and involvement of the collecting system; degree of devitalized tissue; and the size and location of a perinephric hematoma or fluid collection. Medial extravasation of contrast is often seen with UPJ ruptures and no contrast will be seen in the distal ureter on delayed images of complete UPJ avulsion. Historically diagnosis of UPJ injuries was delayed in 50% of cases but routine evaluation of trauma with CT, especially when delayed images are obtained, has increased the initial detection rate to almost 90%.

Ultrasound

The focused assessment by sonography for trauma (FAST) is often used to evaluate trauma patients for abdominal injuries and intra-abdominal fluid collections. Despite the availability and low risk nature of sonography, this modality has a low sensitivity (48%) for detecting renal injuries and often overlooks significant damages. The use of contrast-enhanced ultrasound has recently been reported to increase the sensitivity to 69%, which is still inferior to the >90% sensitivity of CT.

Intravenous Urography

Although almost completely replaced by CT for evaluating stable trauma patients, the intravenous urogram still maintains a role in evaluating the unstable trauma patient taken directly to the operating room by verifying the presence of a contralateral kidney (1 shot urogram with 2 mL per kg body weight bolus followed by plain film 10 minutes later). Identifying a functional contralateral kidney is important first because every possible attempt should be made to save the injured kidney if it is the only one. The injured kidney may lack contrast uptake if there is a major vascular injury or demonstrate a delayed nephrogram from significant compression from a contained hematoma. An abnormal renal outline, displacement of the bowel or ureter and loss of the psoas margin are all suggestive of renal injury and hematoma. Distinctive patterns of contrast extravasation that should raise concern of a possible UPJ injury include extravasation medial or circumferential (circumferential urinoma) to the kidney. Also, with a complete UPJ disruption, the ipsilateral ureter will lack intraluminal contrast.

Angiography

Angiography has been largely replaced by noninvasive modalities, especially in the pediatric patients in whom technical problems with vascular access result in a higher complication rate than in adults. Arteriography does not add useful information to contrast CT scanning and may increase diagnostic delay during the preoperative workup. It is useful in patients who require therapeutic embolization of an active bleeding site.

Currently, there is no role for radionuclide imaging or magnetic resonance imaging (MRI) in the acute setting for children with suspected renal trauma although there is a role in the follow-up evaluation of renal injury.

Clinical Indications for Discharge or Admission

In cases of blunt trauma, children with grade I renal injuries (contusions) can be discharged home without further imaging and followed with serial urinalyses. Patients are instructed to limit daily activity until the urinalysis is within normal limits. Outpatient radiographic evaluation is necessary if microscopic hematuria persists for more than 30 days. Grade II and III renal injuries warrant admission to the hospital for a minimum of 24 hours when the risk of bleeding is highest. Expectant treatment includes supportive care with strict bed rest, hydration, antibiotics, and serial hematocrits. Once the gross hematuria resolves, these children may be discharged home with limited activity until microscopic hematuria resolves and repeat imaging demonstrates total healing.

Management of the remaining patients (with grade IV and V injuries) evokes significant controversy. The shift from early operative intervention to a more expectant approach for most solid organ injuries has been increasingly applied to high-grade renal injuries. Advocates of early surgical exploration argue that this approach results in decreases in morbidity, hospital stay, and complications without a significant increase in the risk for nephrectomy. Opponents believe that nonoperative management of selected patients does not lead to negative consequences and may result in a higher renal salvage rate.

Nonoperative management requires admission to the hospital, serial examinations and hematocrits. Debate continues regarding the necessity of repeat CT scan 36 to 72 hours later for conservatively managed renal injuries. According to expert opinion, repeat imaging is not required for grade I and II injuries and grade III injuries without hemodynamic instability or devitalized fragments. Some authors are now beginning to advocate against routine repeat imaging for grade IV or V renal injuries when there is no clinical indication (e.g., sepsis, decrease in hematocrit, unstable blood pressure, increasing hematuria or oliguria), arguing that repeat scans rarely change the management of this population and that kidneys with stable or improved appearance on repeat CT still have a delayed complication rate of 25%.

Patients who demonstrate hemodynamic instability require surgical intervention or angiographic embolization of renal vessels. Angioembolization should be performed only in those children who have a definable segmental artery injury. Persistent urinary extravasation can be managed with percutaneous drainage or internal ureteral stenting. These procedures, as well as embolization, should be limited to institutions that can provide appropriate resources.

Operative exploration is required in 5% to 10% of cases. Absolute indications for renal exploration are life-threatening hemorrhage believed to be from renal injury, renal pedicle avulsion and expanding, pulsatile or uncontained retroperitoneal hematoma. Relative indications include incomplete radiographic staging with concurrent traumatic injuries that require repair/exploration, extensive devitalized renal parenchyma, vascular injury, and urinary extravasation. Attempts to preserve the kidney are more likely to succeed in patients with grade IV injuries. Children with grade V injuries frequently require nephrectomy. In patients with vascular injuries, chances of renal salvage are improved if renal parenchyma is minimally disrupted and revascularization is achieved within a few hours of the injury.

Penetrating renal injuries have traditionally been managed with operative intervention. Compared with blunt trauma, far less literature is available in support of nonoperative treatment after penetrating trauma. In addition, many recommendations are extrapolated from data on adult patient populations. Careful selection of hemodynamically stable patients who can tolerate CT staging may identify a cohort of children who can be safely treated conservatively. Indications for renal exploration are similar to those for injuries caused by blunt trauma. Patients with penetrating trauma have a higher need for surgical intervention.

Short-term complications of renal trauma include delayed hemorrhage, urinary extravasation, abscess formation, and ureteral obstruction secondary to clot formation. Long-term complications include compromised renal function, hypertension, and arteriovenous fistula. Chronic hypertension develops in a period ranging from 2 days to 32 years, which is why patients with a history of renal trauma should undergo long-term yearly blood pressure monitoring.

URETER

Goal of Treatment

Because ureteral injuries are uncommon in children and are often missed on initial evaluation, the goal of emergency evaluation is to recognize the clinical scenarios in which ureteral trauma is possible so as to allow prompt operative intervention. These injuries occur in less than 1% of all genitourinary traumas.

CLINICAL PEARLS AND PITFALLS

Ureteral injuries are often missed during the initial evaluation with less than 50% of patients diagnosed within 24 hours of presentation. Avulsion of the ureter should be suspected when the CT urogram demonstrates extravasation of contrast material and nonfilling of the affected ureter. CT findings suggestive of ureteral injury include medial perirenal extravasation of contrast material, a circumrenal urinoma, and the lack of opacification of the ureter distal to the injury. However, CT scan has been shown to be poorly sensitive for ureteral injury, identifying only 33% of cases in some series. In case in which suspicion for ureteral injury is high, urologic consultation is necessary as retrograde pyelogram is a more reliable examination and offers the opportunity for therapeutic intervention.

Current Evidence

Blunt trauma usually involves the ureteropelvic junction. Disruption of the ureter from the renal pelvis results from stretching of the ureter by sudden hyperextension of the trunk. Traditionally, this injury has been described more often in children. Penetrating injuries may occur at any point along the length of the ureter and are associated with injuries to other intra-abdominal organs in up to 90% of cases. Stab wounds rarely cause ureteral injuries.

Clinical Considerations

Clinical Recognition

Trauma to the ureter should be suspected in patients presenting with fracture of the transverse process of a lumbar vertebra. Pelvic fracture, hip fracture, lower rib fracture, splenic laceration, liver laceration, and diaphragmatic rupture have also been reported in association with ureteral injuries.

The physical examination may be unremarkable. However, an enlarging flank mass in the absence of signs of retroperitoneal bleeding suggests urinary extravasation. Hematuria is an unreliable sign. The urinalysis may be normal in 30% of confirmed cases. When the diagnosis has been delayed, ureteral injury may manifest with fever, chills, lethargy, leukocytosis, pyuria, bacteriuria, flank mass or pain, fistulas, and ureteral strictures.

Management/Diagnostic Testing

As mentioned above, the diagnosis of ureteral injury should be entertained when children present with penetrating abdominal injuries. A CT urogram (described in renal trauma section) can suggest the presence of ureteral injury when the ureter does not opacify with contrast on delayed images and/or there is urinary extravasation medial to the renal hilum or along the length of the ureter.

Clinical Indications for Discharge or Admission

Given the strong association of ureteral injuries with other severe abdominal injuries, most children with ureteral injury are admitted to the hospital. Urologic consultation is necessary for children with suspected ureteral injury.

BLADDER

Goal of Treatment

The goal of evaluation in the Emergency Department is recognition of bladder injuries, determining if they are extra- or intraperitoneal and obtaining prompt urologic consultation.

CLINICAL PEARLS AND PITFALLS

Bladder injuries may occur after blunt or penetrating trauma. Blunt trauma secondary to motor vehicle accidents is the leading cause of bladder injuries. More than 80% of bladder injuries are associated with pelvic fractures and penetration of the bladder by a bony fragment. However, only 10% of patients with pelvic fractures sustain lower urinary tract injury. The probability of having an associated bladder injury increases proportionally with the number of fractured pubic rami.

Current Evidence

During childhood, the bladder has a higher abdominal location, which renders the organ more susceptible to injury than in adults. The bladder can also be more easily damaged when full. The risk for this injury is especially increased in the setting of improperly fastened seat belts and lap belts. Bladder neck injuries are uncommon, but serious. Such injuries have been reported to be more common in children than in adults because of the undeveloped prostate and are often in association with a pelvic fracture. The injury may be due to longitudinal lacerations or lacerations that extend to the proximal urethra.

Bladder injuries are classified as extraperitoneal, intraperitoneal, or combined. Extraperitoneal injuries are more frequently associated with pelvic fractures of the anterior ring and may be related to either laceration or penetration from a bone spike, irrespective of bladder volume at the time of injury. In contrast, intraperitoneal injuries, which account for approximately two-thirds of major bladder injuries, are usually caused by blunt trauma, resulting in a burst mechanism to a full, distended bladder. Combined injuries are usually seen with gunshot wounds. Bladder injuries may range from contusions to rupture. Contusions are incomplete, nonperforating tears of the mucosa. Complicated injuries may involve the bladder, urethra, sacral plexus, and supporting structures of the anorectal region.

Clinical Considerations

Clinical Recognition

Hematuria and dysuria are symptoms commonly seen at presentation. Nearly 100% of patients with rupture of the bladder have gross hematuria. Microscopic hematuria is associated with less severe injuries such as contusions. Patients with intraperitoneal ruptures may develop a palpable fluid wave from extravasation of urine into the peritoneal cavity and peritoneal irritation. Elevated levels of blood urea nitrogen in the serum is out of proportion to creatinine resulting from more rapid peritoneal reabsorption of urea.

Patients with myelodysplasia who have undergone bladder augmentation may experience spontaneous bladder rupture in the presence of infection, bacteremia, or overdistension. Symptoms and signs of sepsis, as well as shoulder pain, may be encountered at presentation. Emergent exploration is indicated after a cystogram is completed.

Urethral catheterization must be avoided if physical examination reveals blood at the urethral meatus or a high-riding prostate as urethral injury is possible. Urologic consultation is required.

Initial Assessment

A large, prospective series of pelvic fractures and lower genitourinary tract injury in pediatric patients found that imaging is not required if patients are stable, have a normal genitourinary examination, do not have gross hematuria, and do not have multiple associated injuries. Diagnostic evaluation is indicated in patients who sustain pelvic or lower abdominal trauma with gross hematuria, inability to void, abnormal external genitourinary examination, or multiple associated injuries. Evaluation begins with a plain radiograph to exclude a pelvic fracture. Fracture types that have been associated with bladder injury include widening of the sacroiliac joint, symphysis pubis, and fractures of the sacrum. If a pelvic fracture is not identified, the urethra can be catheterized and a cystogram is performed.

Management/Diagnostic Testing

CT cystography should be performed for patients with suspected bladder injury after placement of a urethral catheter. Sagittal and coronal multiplanar images may be helpful in identifying most sites of bladder rupture. CT cystography does offer some advantages over plain cystography for patients undergoing CT scanning for the evaluation of other associated blunt injuries. CT scanning provides expeditious scanning of the head, chest, abdomen, and pelvis; interpretation is often less affected by overlying bone fragments from pelvic fractures and spine boards than in the plain radiographic cystogram, and the CT can detect small amounts of intra- and extraperitoneal fluid. The disadvantages of CT cystography include the much higher radiation exposure and cost than those of plain radiographs. Currently, the CT cystogram is recommended, when indicated, for patients undergoing CT scanning for other associated blunt trauma-related injuries.

With few a few exceptions, treatment of bladder rupture is determined by whether the urine extravasation is confined to the extraperitoneal space or is intraperitoneal. Extraperitoneal bladder rupture can be managed by urethral catheter or suprapubic drainage. Treatment of intraperitoneal bladder rupture involves surgical exploration and repair. Extraperitoneal injuries with a bony fragment or foreign body in the bladder also require surgical exploration.

Clinical Indications for Discharge or Admission

Children with bladder injuries should be admitted to the hospital for further operative of nonoperative care.

URETHRA

Goal of Treatment

The goals of the acute management of children with urethral injuries are recognizing children with potential urethral injury and, in consultation with urology, obtaining a retrograde urethrogram and safe drainage of the bladder.

CLINICAL PEARLS AND PITFALLS

The major sign of acute anterior injury is bleeding from the urethra. Proximal urethral injury should be suspected when there is blood at the meatus, hematuria, inability to void, displacement of the prostate on rectal examination, and/or perineal ecchymosis. Blind placement of a urethral catheter may convert a partial tear into a complete transection and therefore should be discouraged.

Current Evidence

Blunt trauma, due to motor vehicle accidents, high-velocity falls onto the perineum, and straddle injuries, accounts for most urethral injuries sustained during childhood. Injuries due to instrumentation and penetrating injuries, such as gunshot wounds, are less common. Urethral injuries occur primarily in males. In boys, the urethra is divided by the urogenital diaphragm into an anterior urethra (pendulous and bulbous) and a posterior urethra (membranous and prostatic) (Fig. 116.4). Anterior and posterior urethral injuries differ from each other by mechanism of injury, clinical presentation, and treatment.

Anterior urethral injuries result from direct trauma and are often isolated. The pendulous urethra may be damaged by blunt or penetrating forces. Bulbar injuries are commonly caused by straddle injuries, as the urethra is compressed between the symphysis pubis and a solid object. Posterior urethral injuries occur with severe trauma to the body and are usually associated with other injuries, particularly pelvic fractures. The mortality rate with fractured pelvis has been reported to be as high as 30%. Injuries to the prostatic urethra may extend to the bladder neck. Posterior urethral injuries in men almost uniformly occur distal to the prostate. In adults, the mature prostate, puboprostatic ligament, and bladder stabilize the prostatic urethra, making it less susceptible to trauma.

Female urethral injuries are commonly divided into avulsions and longitudinal tears. These injuries occur most often from blunt abdominal trauma in motor vehicle accidents and in association with pelvic fractures. Injuries may also occur after surgical procedures or instrumentation. The diagnosis is missed on initial assessment in up to 40% of patients, emphasizing the need for careful physical examination and diagnostic evaluation.

Clinical Considerations

Clinical Recognition

Blood at the meatus has been reported in up to 90% of patients sustaining anterior urethral injuries. Other findings include hematuria, inability or difficulty voiding, and periurethral or perineal edema and ecchymosis. Perineal ecchymosis in the shape of a butterfly is typical for these injuries.

Posterior urethral injury may be predicted by the location and displacement of associated pelvic fractures. There is an association between pubic arch fractures and urethral injury, with higher risk as the number of broken rami increases.

Because the female urethra is relatively mobile and short, trauma to the urethra is uncommon. It was reported in less

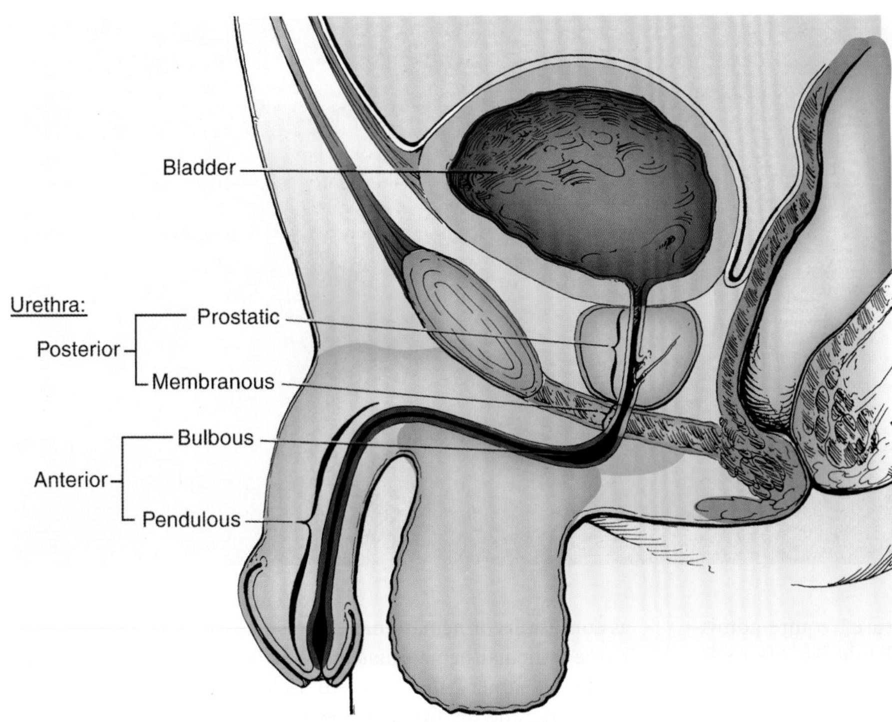

FIGURE 116.4 Sagittal section of male lower urinary tract illustrating levels of urethra.

than 6% of cases with associated pelvic fractures in one series of women and girls. When it does occur, it is found more commonly in girls than in women. In one series, every female patient with a significant urethral injury had gross hematuria or blood at the introitus and a pelvic ring fracture. Any female patient with this combination of findings should be evaluated for a urethral injury. Most serious injuries involve the vesicourethral junction and extend to the vagina.

Initial Assessment

It is recommended that, whenever possible, a full speculum examination should be performed in females with gross hematuria and pelvic ring fractures, difficulty placing a urethral catheter, and anticipated delay until the pelvic fractures is stabilized as injury often extends to the vagina.

Management/Diagnostic Testing

Urethral injuries can be diagnosed by a retrograde urethrogram. A Foley catheter appropriate for the size of the patient is inserted into the urethra to the fossa navicularis without inflating the balloon. Contrast material is injected via the catheter into the urethra and images are obtained in an oblique position. If a Foley catheter is already in place, the urethrogram can still be performed via a small feeding tube passed alongside the catheter. Retrograde urethrography should be performed under fluoroscopy with minimal pressure. Gross extravasation of the contrast agent at the site of the injury without visualization of the proximal urethra and bladder is diagnostic for complete rupture of the urethra. Partial rupture is represented by localized extravasation at the site of the injury, with some contrast passing into the proximal urethra and bladder. If no extravasation is noted, the urinary catheter can be gently advanced into the bladder. CT is not adequate for diagnosing urethral injuries and is presumptive only if extravasation is detected at the bladder neck or urethra (Fig. 116.5). MRI provides useful information in the determination of the need for surgical repair but is not helpful in the initial evaluation.

In the acute setting, anterior urethral injuries can be managed by 7 to 10 days of urethral catheterization. More severe injuries may require urinary diversion by suprapubic cystostomy. Initial management of anterior urethral injuries remains controversial. Urologic follow-up is required as the most common sequelae of anterior urethral injury, urethral stricture, may take months or longer to manifest. The acute management of posterior urethral injuries also remains controversial. The comparative effectiveness and benefits of immediate exploration and realigning the urethra over an indwelling urethral catheter versus placement of a suprapubic tube and delayed urethroplasty are debated by experts.

Penetrating wounds of the urethra demand early surgical exploration with conservative debridement and primary repair. Patients with extensive loss of urethral tissue can be managed with delayed repair and staged reconstruction.

For urethral injuries in females, most authors recommend some form of primary operative repair of the urethral rupture with closure of associated vaginal tears. Placement of a suprapubic tube and delayed repair are reserved for unstable patients, as placement has been associated with scarring, strictures, urethral obliteration, and fistulas. Long-term complications of this injury include urethrovaginal fistula, vaginal stenosis, incontinence, sexual dysfunction, and urethral stricture.

Clinical Indications for Discharge or Admission

For children with isolated straddle injuries that do not result in urethral rupture, it is necessary to ensure that the child can void and empty their bladder prior to discharge. Occasionally, a catheter may need to be placed for 5 to 7 days to allow bladder drainage while the urethral edema resolves. Follow-up with a urologist is essential. More severe urethral injuries,

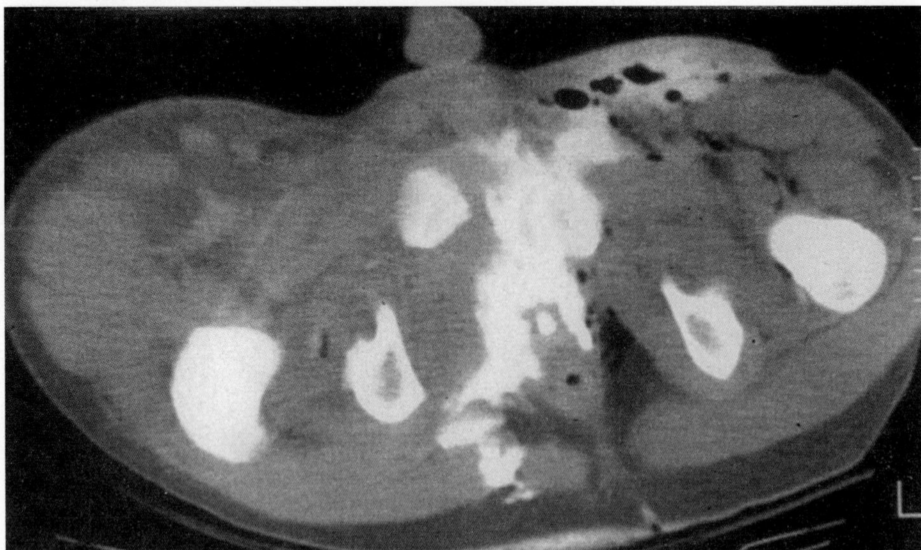

FIGURE 116.5 Posterior urethral disruption and pelvic fracture. Computed tomography of pelvis shows extravasation of contrast material from posterior urethra into the surrounding tissues.

including those that result in urethral rupture, require admission. All patients with posterior urethral injuries are to be admitted given the severity of the associated pelvic injuries.

SCROTUM

Goal of Treatment

The goals of the acute management of children with scrotal injuries are determining if there is a testicle injury and, in consultation with urology, obtaining an ultrasound to determine definitive care.

CLINICAL PEARLS AND PITFALLS

Scrotal trauma may occur as a result of straddle injuries or bicycle accidents, or during sporting events. The patient may present with scrotal tenderness, edema, and ecchymosis. Potential injuries include skin or dartos ecchymosis and lacerations, intrascrotal hematomas, testicular hematomas, testicular dislocation, and testicular rupture. In addition, a testicle may torse after trauma.

Clinical Considerations

Clinical Recognition

When inspection of the scrotum and its contents is obscured by local swelling and pain, ultrasonography is helpful to define the extent of the injury. An intratesticular hematoma may show as an echogenic or hypoechoic testicular mass. A hematocele produces a complex extratesticular fluid collection. Sonographic findings of rupture include the presence of hematocele, parenchymal heterogeneity, intraparenchymal hemorrhage, and disruption of the tunica albuginea or parenchyma. If the ultrasound examination is inconclusive, radionuclide scanning may provide additional information. Both ultrasonography and nuclear scintigraphy help in the diagnosis of testicular torsion (see Chapter 127 Genitourinary Emergencies).

Patients who sustain intrascrotal hematomas, skin ecchymosis, or skin and dartos injury without evidence of injury to the testes can be managed conservatively. Treatment consists of ice packs and scrotal support. Minor testicular injuries such as contusions or hematomas can also be treated conservatively. Large testicular hematomas may require surgical management. Delay in surgery may lead to ischemic necrosis, secondary infections, and disruption of testicular function.

Testicular dislocation may occur either as a result of an upward blow to the scrotum or, rarely, as a result of compressive displacement following severe blunt abdominal trauma. Dislocation has been described in the context of mild scrotal trauma as well.

Initial Assessment, Management and Diagnostic Testing

Diagnosis of testicular dislocation can be made by thorough physical examination, including palpation of the testes. Examination will reveal a well-developed, but empty, scrotal sac or palpation of an abnormally located testis. Severe scrotal pain, obesity, ecchymosis, swelling, or associated pelvic injuries may make examination and diagnosis difficult. In most cases, the dislocated testis lies in the inguinal canal. Associated injuries, such as pelvic fracture, are common. Operative repair is required if closed reduction fails.

Testicular rupture is a surgical emergency. It is characterized by a tear of the tunica albuginea and extravasation of testicular contents into the scrotal sac. Such injuries require early surgical exploration and repair to avoid the potential complications of atrophy and persistent pain. Ultrasonography has been demonstrated to be sensitive in the diagnosis of testicular rupture by informing the clinician of the integrity of the scrotal contents early. The high specificity of the ultrasonography may also provide information to guide the clinician on the necessity of surgical exploration. Testicular salvage is more likely when exploration is performed within 24 hours of the injury. Ultrasonography has shown poor accuracy, however, for the evaluation of isolated epididymal lesions. Other injuries requiring surgical management include tense hematoceles and torsion after trauma.

Superficial lacerations of the scrotum can be repaired using absorbable sutures. Local infiltration with lidocaine plus epinephrine provides adequate anesthesia. Urologic consultation should be obtained if the laceration extends through the dartos. Physical examination of the scrotal contents determines the need for debridement and primary closure. All penetrating testicular injuries require surgical exploration.

Degloving injuries of the scrotum can be seen after motor vehicle (particularly motorcycle), industrial, or farm machinery accidents. Scrotal injuries are associated with varying degrees of penile skin loss. The underlying penile and scrotal structures are usually spared. Management involves debridement and coverage of the defect by skin flaps or grafting.

PENIS

Clinical Recognition

The most common cause of penile trauma in infants is iatrogenic, especially at the time of circumcision. Complications include transection of the glans, urethrocutaneous fistula, deskinning of the penile shaft, and coagulation necrosis of the entire penis from electrocautery. These injuries usually require extensive surgical repair. Penile gunshot wounds are uncommon because of the position and mobility of the penis but have the potential to significantly affect quality of life. Signs that may indicate corpora cavernosa injury include uncontrolled bleeding, expanding hematoma, blood at the meatus, or a palpable corporeal defect. Urethral injury should be ruled out by retrograde urethrography if these signs are present. These injuries require urologic evaluation to determine the need and timing of surgical management.

Blunt penile trauma from toilet seats falling on the glans or distal shaft is not uncommon in toddlers. Significant injury to the corporal bodies or the urethra is rare and patients can be managed expectantly with warm soaks. Although the child does not commonly experience urinary retention, he may be more comfortable voiding in a tub of warm water.

Tourniquet injuries may result from bands, rings, or human hair. In the infant, strangulation with a fine hair may be difficult to recognize because of local edema. The initial diagnosis may be balanitis or paraphimosis. Local or general anesthesia may be required to expose and remove the hair. Complications include urethrocutaneous fistula or loss of the penis.

Fracture of the penis is produced by traumatic rupture of the corpus cavernosum. This injury usually occurs when the erect penis is forced against a hard surface. The patient may hear a cracking sound and develop pain, edema, and deformity of the penis shaft. An "eggplant deformity" of the penis is often present. The urethra may be involved. Penile fractures require surgical treatment with evacuation of the penile hematoma, repair of the torn tunica albuginea and a pressure dressing.

Superficial lacerations of the penile shaft can be repaired with absorbable sutures under local anesthesia or penile block. Lacerations extending to the corporal bodies or the urethra require urologic consultation. Diagnostic evaluation includes a retrograde urethrogram to define the extent of the injury. Injuries to the corporal bodies should be repaired primarily to prevent fibrosis and impotence. Injuries to the urethra may require urinary diversion.

Zipper entrapment of the penis or foreskin is a common complaint that can be managed in the ED. Methods of emergent release have been described in relation to the zipper parts and depending on the type of zipper. The median bar of the zipper may be cut with wire cutters and thus disassembling the zipper mechanism (Fig. 116.6). This technique may sometimes prove difficult when the metal bar is sturdy and there is edema of the entrapped penile tissue within the zipper fastener, limiting access to the metal bar. Such may be the case with heavy metal zippers such as those found on jeans and dungarees, and success may depend on the strength of the operator and the availability of bone or wire cutters. Therefore, this technique may work best with plastic or lightweight zippers. Cutting the dentition of the zipper at any position, permitting unzipping of the zipper from the rear may work best for heavy-duty metal zippers. Disengagement of the fastener by inserting a flathead screwdriver between the inner and outer faceplates and applying torque toward the median bar (Fig. 116.7) may prove helpful when it is difficult to grasp the tiny median bar with bulky cutting pliers. Elliptical incision of the entrapped foreskin or emergency circumcision can be of value when less invasive methods have failed. Regardless of technique, procedural sedation may facilitate the procedure. Edema can be treated with warm soaks.

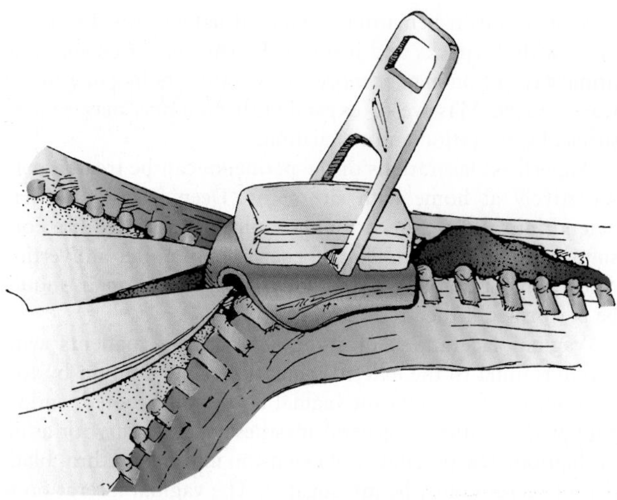

FIGURE 116.6 Penile zipper injury. A wire cutter may be used to cut the median bar of the zipper, releasing the two sides of the zipper and freeing the penis.

PERINEUM

The mechanism most commonly associated with trauma to the female perineum is a straddle-type injury. These injuries

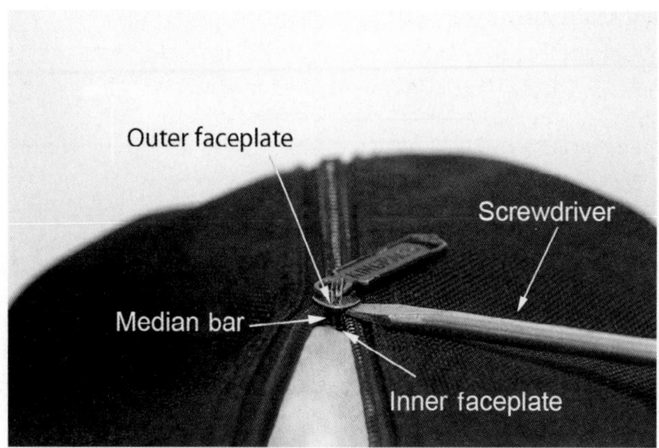

FIGURE 116.7 Screwdriver technique for the release of foreskin entrapped in the zipper. The screwdriver should be placed between the two faceplates and twisted toward the median bar.

may cause vulvar hematomas, which usually respond to treatment with ice packs and bed rest. Patients experiencing mild urinary retention may be more comfortable voiding in a tub of warm water. Massive or expanding hematomas may require surgical exploration and evacuation.

Superficial lacerations of the perineum can be treated conservatively at home with sitz baths. Deep lacerations may extend into the rectum or urethra and therefore require consultation by a surgeon. Rectal penetration requires a diverting colostomy. Suprapubic cystostomy or primary repair should be performed if the urethra is disrupted.

Vaginal lacerations must be suspected in patients with severe trauma to the external genitalia or penetration by foreign object. If a significant vaginal laceration is noted, endoscopy with sedation or general anesthesia is necessary for a full evaluation. The possibility of extension into the urethra, bladder, or rectum must be investigated. The vaginal laceration is debrided and repaired with fine absorbable sutures.

SEXUAL ABUSE

When common accidental situations fail to explain certain genitourinary injuries, the possibility of sexual abuse should be considered. Injuries resulting from sexual abuse include abrasions and hematomas in the penile shaft, vaginal lacerations, and perineal hematomas (see also Chapters 75 Vaginal Bleeding and 95 Child Abuse/Assault).

Suggested Readings and Key References

Aihara R, Blansfield J, Millham FH, et al. Fracture locations influence the likelihood of rectal and lower urinary tract injuries in patients sustaining pelvic fractures. *J Trauma* 2002;52:205–209.

Alli MO, Singh B, Moodley J, et al. Prospective evaluation of combined suprapubic and urethral catheterization to urethral drainage alone for intraperitoneal bladder injuries. *J Trauma* 2003;55:1152–1154.

Andrich D, Day AC, Mundy AR. Proposed mechanisms of lower urinary tract injury in fractures of the pelvic ring. *BJU Int* 2007; 100:567–573.

Black PC, Miller EA, Porter JR, et al. Urethral and bladder neck injury associated with pelvic fracture in 25 female patients. *J Urol* 2006;175:2140–2145.

Brandes S, Borrelli J Jr. Pelvic fracture and associated urologic injuries. *World J Surg* 2001;25:1578–1587.

Broghammer JA, Langenburg SE, Smith SJ, et al. Pediatric blunt renal trauma: its conservative management and patterns of associated injuries. *Urology* 2006;67:823–827.

Brown SL, Haas C, Dinchman KH, et al. Radiologic evaluation of pediatric blunt trauma in patients with microscopic hematuria. *World J Surg* 2001;25:1557–1560.

Buckely JC, McAninch JW. The diagnosis, management, and outcomes of pediatric renal injuries. *Urol Clin North Am* 2006;33:33–40.

Chandra RV, Dowling RJ, Ulubasoglu M, et al. Rational approach to diagnosis and management of blunt scrotal trauma. *Urology* 2007; 70:230–234.

Guichard G, El Ammari J, Del Coro C, et al. Accuracy of ultrasonography in diagnosis of testicular rupture after blunt scrotal trauma. *Urology* 2008;71:52–56.

Henderson CG, Sedberry-Ross S, Pickard R, et al. Management of high grade renal trauma: 20-year experience at a pediatric level I trauma center. *J Urol* 2006;178:246–250.

Ko SF, Ng SH, Wan YL, et al. Testicular dislocation: an uncommon and easily overlooked complication of blunt abdominal trauma. *Ann Emerg Med* 2004;43:371–375.

Nguyen MM, Das S. Pediatric renal trauma. *Urology* 2002;59:762–766.

Osman Y, El-Tabey N, Mohsen T, et al. Nonoperative treatment of isolated posttraumatic intraperitoneal bladder rupture in children—is it justified? *J Urol* 2005;173:955–957.

Parry NG, Rozycki GS, Feliciano DV, et al. Traumatic rupture of the bladder: is the suprapubic tube necessary? *J Trauma* 2003;54:431–436.

Quagliano PV, Delair SM, Malhotra AK. Diagnosis of blunt bladder injury; a prospective comparative study of computed tomography cystography and conventional retrograde cystography. *J Trauma* 2006;61:410–422.

Raveenthiran V. Releasing of zipper-entrapped skin: a novel nonsurgical technique. *Pediatr Emerg Care* 2007;23:463–464.

Rogers CG, Knight V, Macura KJ, et al. High-grade renal injuries in children—is conservative management possible? *Urology* 2004;64: 574–579.

Santucci RA, Langenburg SE, Zachareas MJ. Traumatic hematuria in children can be evaluated as in adults. *J Urol* 2004;171:822–825.

Tarman GJ, Kaplan GW, Lerman SL, et al. Lower genitourinary injury and pelvic fractures in pediatric patients. *Urology* 2002;59:123–126.

Tasian GE, Bagga HS, Fisher PB, et al. Pediatric genitourinary injuries in the United States from 2002 to 2010. *J Urol* 2013;189(1):288–293.

CHAPTER 117 ▪ HAND TRAUMA

MICHAEL WITT, MD, MPH AND JINSONG WANG, MD, PhD

GOALS OF EMERGENCY CARE

Hand trauma is extremely common in the pediatric emergency department, with a broad spectrum of clinical presentations. Injuries include fractures, sprains and soft tissue injuries, nail bed injuries, and lacerations. Understanding the anatomy, injury patterns, and necessary management and referral for ideal recovery of the hands is vital for future function. Further, the provider should recognize that injury to the hands can result from nonaccidental trauma and be vigilant for related findings and concerns.

KEY POINTS

- Lacerations and soft tissue injuries are more common in younger children and fractures are seen more frequently in older children.
- Thorough examination should include a visual examination, general alignment of the hand and digits (Fig. 117.1), focused palpation, passive and active range of motion across each joint (Fig. 117.2), and a neurovascular assessment.
- Clinical vigilance is required for possible scaphoid fractures or carpal ligamentous injuries as long-term issues can arise from inadequate care.
- Skin wounds obtained during an altercation ("fight bites") represent a risky injury with a high chance of infection due to human oral flora.
- A finger splint is not adequate immobilization for proximal phalanx fractures and a hand- or forearm-based splint is more appropriate.
- Absorbable sutures are equally effective in fingertip wounds and require less intervention on follow-up.

CARPALS

CLINICAL PEARLS AND PITFALLS

- The scaphoid is the most commonly fractured carpal bone.
- Ligamentous injuries and dislocations can be subtle but have significant morbidity.

Clinical Considerations

Clinical recognition. The incidence of carpal fractures is relatively low in children, although increasing awareness has led to improved recognition. In infancy, the carpals are completely cartilaginous and are nearly immune to injury. They progressively ossify beginning with the capitate bone. The scaphoid is by far the most common fractured carpal bone, with most fractures occurring in late childhood and adolescence. Falls are the most frequent cause.

Initial assessment. Physical examination requires attention to edema, range of motion, and point tenderness to localize carpal injuries. Snuffbox tenderness is a useful tool for detecting scaphoid fractures. Pain with axial thumb compression can also be a sign of scaphoid injury. Radiographs are obviously limited in infancy and early childhood because of the lack of ossification. As the patient ages and the carpals are progressively ossifying, comparison with the contralateral side may be of benefit. Dedicated scaphoid views or computed tomography may help to identify some fractures not seen on routine hand or wrist films. Nondisplaced scaphoid fractures may not be obvious on initial x-rays but will be visible on repeat imaging performed 2 weeks following the injury.

Management. Most suspected injuries to the carpal bones can be managed urgently with splinting and outpatient follow-up within 1 to 2 weeks. Scaphoid fractures have different patterns depending on the age of the patient. Younger patients have a significant incidence of fractures involving the distal third of the bone, although waist fractures are still the most common. Adolescents and adults tend to fracture at the waist. A unique fracture to young patients is the avulsion of the distal radial aspect of the scaphoid. This injury often is not diagnosed on first presentation and is seen on radiographs 1 to 2 weeks later. In the emergency department, scaphoid fractures should be managed with a thumb spica splint. Most scaphoid fractures are nondisplaced and managed with cast immobilization, though displaced fractures may require surgical reduction and internal fixation to prevent nonunion. In addition, those who present late with evidence of nonunion should be immobilized and referred to a hand specialist for possible surgical repair.

In addition to fractures, suspicion for ligamentous injuries should be high, particularly in late childhood and adolescence. An important radiologic concept is the distance between the scaphoid and lunate bones. In a true scapholunate dissociation, this space is widened, often called the Terry Thompson sign. This can be difficult to detect in children in whom this space is naturally widened, as the carpals are not fully ossified. It is also important to note that dynamic scapholunate instability may not be shown on routine x-ray, and may be only obvious under stressed view. Perilunate dislocation is best identified with the lateral wrist radiograph, with the bone displaced from its typical midaxial location over the radius. Concern for dissociations and dislocations requires urgent attention by a hand specialist.

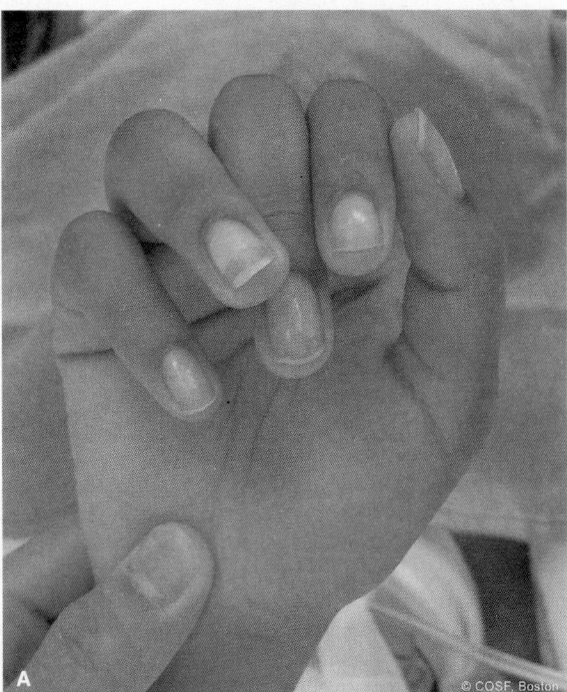

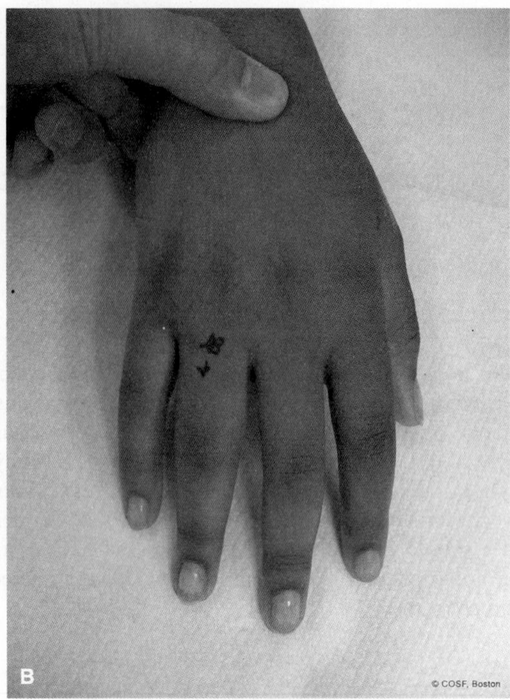

FIGURE 117.1 Abnormal tenodesis. Clinical photographs depicting abnormal rotation of the ring finger in the setting of a malrotated phalanx fracture. Note the clinical overlap of the ring finger over the long finger and increased gap between the ring finger and the small finger, with passive wrist extension (**A**) that is not clinically as apparent with the wrist in neutral position and the digits extended (**B**). (Courtesy of Children's Orthopaedic Surgery Foundation.)

METACARPALS

CLINICAL PEARLS AND PITFALLS

- Metacarpal fractures can occur at the base, shaft, or neck of the bone, with the neck of the 5th metacarpal being the most common.
- The amount of fracture angulation allowed increases across the metacarpals, from 10 to 20 degrees for the index finger up to 40 degrees for the small finger.
- MCP dislocations can be difficult to identify on radiograph and may simply appear hyperextended.

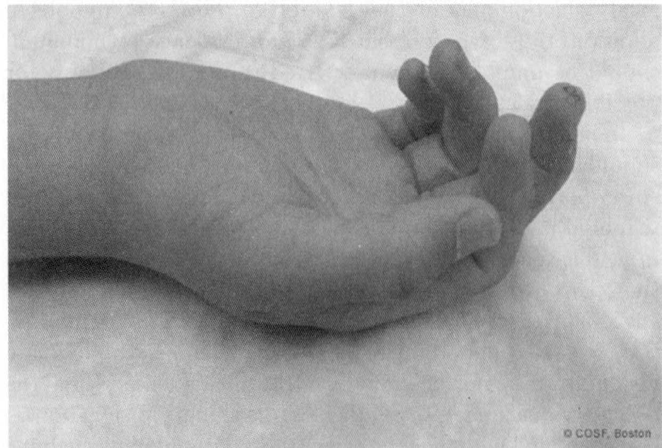

FIGURE 117.2 Clinical photograph of a patient with an isolated flexor digitorum profundus rupture of the long finger. Note the abnormal digital cascade and resting flexion posture of the long finger in relationship to the adjacent unaffected digits. (Courtesy of Children's Orthopaedic Surgery Foundation.)

Clinical Considerations

Clinical recognition. Injuries to the metacarpals include fractures and dislocations of the MCP joint. Carpometacarpal joint dislocation is rare in children, although such a dislocation may coexist with another injury. The metacarpals may be fractured at the base, shaft, or neck. These injuries often occur from crushing trauma in younger patients as well as from impact along the axis of the bones, such as in fighting, in older children and adolescents. Compartment syndrome in the hand can occur, particularly with multiple fractures and crush injury, thus careful physical examination and appropriate suspicion are required.

Initial assessment and management. Fractures of the metacarpals are least likely to occur in the base of the bone. When these occur, they usually involve the small finger. There will be significant pain and dorsal edema, which can make accurate diagnosis challenging. Minimally or nondisplaced fractures are generally managed with a splint or cast. Displaced fractures often require closed reduction, possible pinning, and subsequent casting. Carpometacarpal dislocations alone or in conjunction with a base fracture are unstable and often require operative stabilization. Bennett fractures, or intra-articular fracture of the base of the thumb metacarpal, mandate special attention, as the thumb carpometacarpal joint is critical for full use of this digit (Fig. 117.3). Similarly, Rolando fractures, comminuted fractures of the base of the thumb metacarpal, also require careful attention. These fractures can be addressed temporarily with a thumb spica splint and timely referral.

Metacarpal shaft fractures are also uncommon in the pediatric population and tend to involve the middle, ring, and small fingers. They are most often spiral in nature, indicating

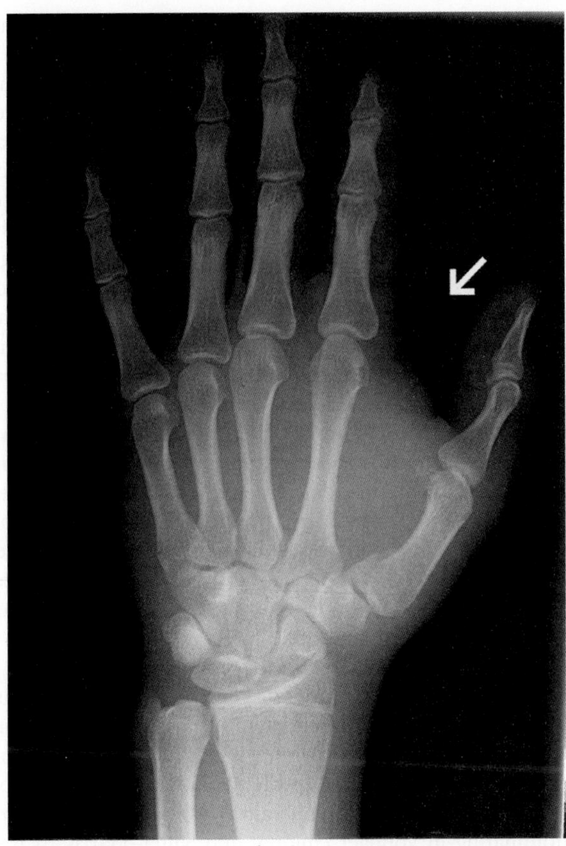

FIGURE 117.3 Anteroposterior radiograph of the hand depicting a Bennett fracture. (Courtesy of Children's Orthopaedic Surgery Foundation.)

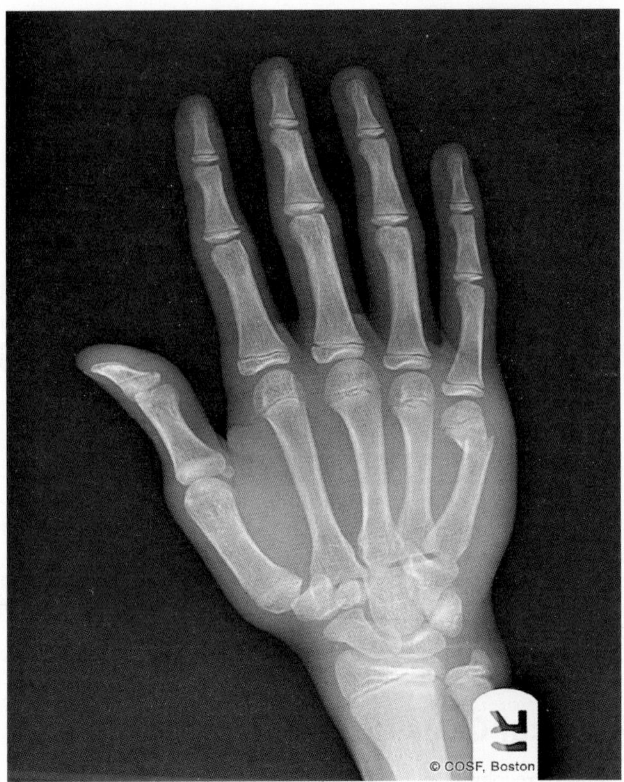

FIGURE 117.4 Anteroposterior radiograph of the hand depicting a displaced fifth metacarpal neck fracture. (Courtesy of Children's Orthopaedic Surgery Foundation.)

a rotational component to the injuring force. Careful attention to the alignment of the fingers when making a fist may demonstrate subtle rotational deformity (see Fig. 117.1 for clinical presentation of rotational deformity). These injuries also result in significant edema, but significantly angulated or displaced fractures can be suspected on examination. Most nondisplaced shaft fractures can be managed with immobilization, though fractures with significant displacement may require operative repair.

The most common metacarpal fracture occurs at the neck of the bone, with the majority involving small finger (the boxer's fracture) (Fig. 117.4). Inspection for rotational displacement of the fracture is again important, as is the evidence of skin trauma that might indicate contamination from an opponent's mouth during a fight. Any open wound with exposure to human oral secretions requires antibiotic prophylaxis, as these wounds are associated with high rates of infection. A considerable amount of angulation of the fracture can be tolerated without limiting ultimate hand function. The amount of angulation allowed increases across the metacarpals, from 10 to 20 degrees for the index finger up to 40 degrees for the small finger. Closed reduction is often all that is needed in fractures that exceed the tolerable amount of angulation, except in unstable fractures.

MCP joint dislocations are the most common dislocation among the pediatric hand injuries and most frequently involve the thumb (Fig. 117.5). These dislocations occur most often with the proximal phalanx dorsal to the metacarpal and the metacarpal head palpable in the palm. In the immature patient, these dislocations may be difficult to clarify on radiographs

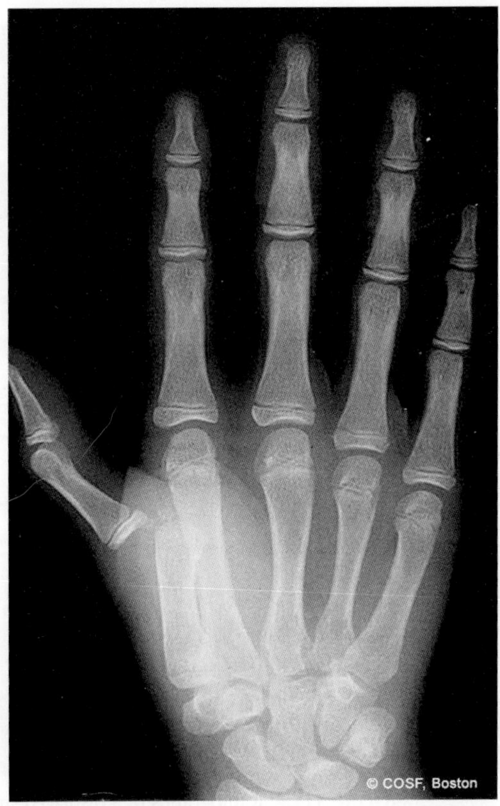

FIGURE 117.5 Anteroposterior hand radiograph depicting a dorsal complex dislocation of the thumb metacarpophalangeal joint. (Courtesy of Children's Orthopaedic Surgery Foundation.)

because of the joint consisting mainly of cartilage. Therefore, the digit may simply appear to be hyperextended. Reduction attempts should maintain or exaggerate the hyperextension while applying pressure toward the palm on the base of the phalanx. In general, straight longitudinal traction is not recommended in an effort to avoid soft tissue interposition and converting a reducible injury into an irreducible dislocation. If the joint is not easily relocated, hand specialist involvement and likely open reduction will be required because the tendons and volar plate involved may prevent reduction with inline traction.

PHALANGES

CLINICAL PEARLS AND PITFALLS

- Special attention is required for injuries to the phalanges looking for rotational deformity that can be missed with other aspects of the examination (see Fig. 117.1).
- A finger splint does not provide adequate support for a proximal phalanx fractures, therefore a wrist or forearm splint is necessary.

Clinical Considerations

Clinical recognition. Phalanx injuries are very common in children, as the fingers of a child are a first exploration into his or her world. Mechanisms of injury most frequently include: crush, hyperextension, and "jamming." Careful examination with particular attention to rotational deformity is required. Often, identifying which bone is involved in an interphalangeal joint injury can be challenging due to pain and edema.

Initial assessment and management. Proximal phalanx injuries are some of the most common pediatric hand injuries. The base of the proximal phalanx often endures a Salter–Harris II fracture (see Fig. 119.2), with the little finger being most frequent. Many are managed with splinting/casting and closed reduction if necessary. Nondisplaced shaft fractures are also generally managed with immobilization. Displaced and angulated fractures may require surgical stabilization. It is important to realize that a finger splint does not provide adequate support for a proximal phalanx fracture. A hand- or forearm-based splint is necessary. Phalangeal neck fractures can be difficult to diagnose. Oblique view radiographs may be of assistance (Fig. 117.6). These fractures require very close outpatient care, as displacement and rotation may have long-term consequences on the flexion of the adjacent interphalangeal joint. Finally, condylar fractures may involve one or both condyles and long-term management may depend on the severity of the injury (Fig. 117.7). Close follow-up is also required in these injuries, as the bone may not remodel well and may require early reduction and other intervention.

Proximal phalanx injuries to the thumb ray are unique. In adolescents and adults, a skier's or gamekeeper's thumb occurs with rupture of the ulnar collateral ligament (UCL) during stress onto the thumb away from the rest of the hand. In children, a fracture of the base of the proximal phalanx is more likely than an UCL injury, with Salter–Harris I and II fractures predominating in younger children and Salter–Harris III fractures in older children. Thumb spica splinting is appropriate for the constellation of these injuries in the emergency department.

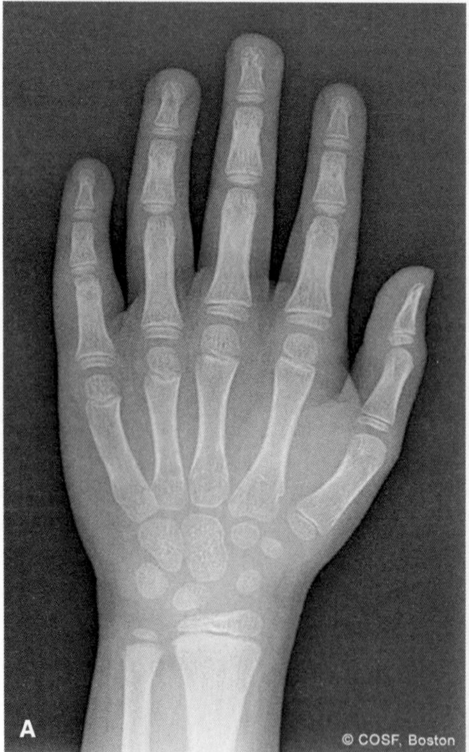

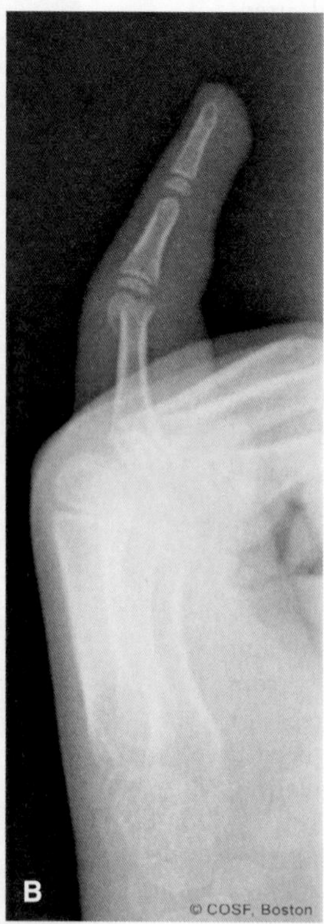

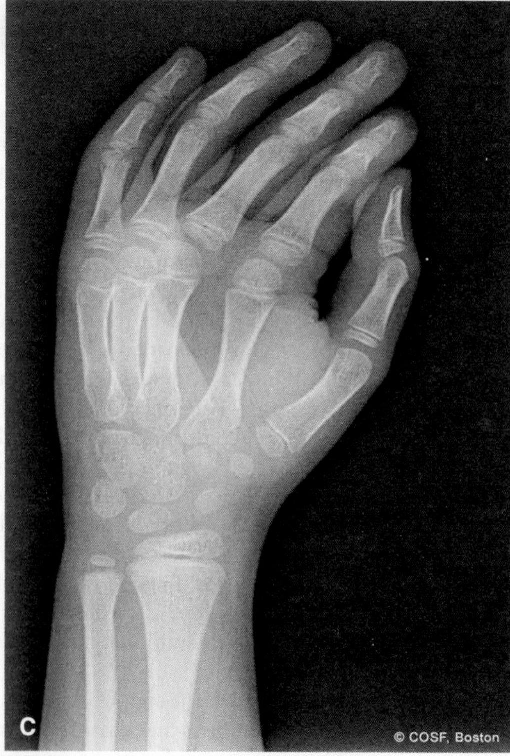

FIGURE 117.6 Radiographs of a displaced small finger proximal phalangeal neck fracture. Note the relatively subtle and benign radiographic appearance on the anteroposterior view (**A**). Fracture displacement is best seen on a dedicated lateral view (**B**) as well as on oblique projections of the small finger (**C**). (Courtesy of Children's Orthopaedic Surgery Foundation.)

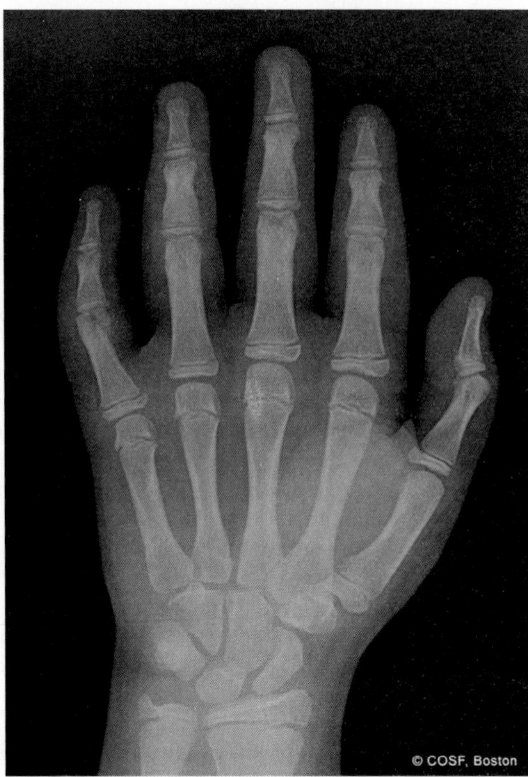

FIGURE 117.7 Anteroposterior radiograph depicting an intraarticular fracture of the head of the small finger proximal phalanx involving the radial condyle. (Courtesy of Children's Orthopaedic Surgery Foundation.)

Displaced fractures require operative management. Early hand specialist referral is appropriate.

Middle phalanx fractures are generally managed similarly to proximal phalanx injuries. Most are managed by closed management, although surgical reduction and stabilization may be required in displaced fractures. Fractures of the head of the phalanx require close management by a hand specialist because of a high rate of complications. Avulsion fractures of the middle phalanx at the insertion of the volar plate or extensor central slip are common. Avulsions on the volar side generally are from hyperextension. Often the fragment does not reattach and may result in chronic stiffness and has potential for permanent loss of range of motion. Splinting is performed initially, but early range of motion is often started a week later. Small avulsions on the extensor side are treated similarly, though larger fragments are treated with longer splinting, and displaced fractures may require open reduction.

Distal phalanx injuries are very common and often associated with nail and nail bed injuries, as discussed in the following text. When associated with nail bed injuries, after the nail is removed (if necessary), the open fracture should be copiously irrigated and the nail bed repaired, followed by splinting. These should be referred to a hand specialist for follow-up in case further intervention, such as pin fixation, is required. Seymour fractures comprise a special type of injury, with a Salter–Harris I or II fracture of the distal phalanx associated with exposure of the proximal aspect of the nail and damaged germinal matrix (Fig. 117.8). The distal interphalangeal joint is often held at some flexion. Discussion with a hand specialist is recommended, as tissue interposed into the physis may prevent the fracture from healing.

Dislocations of the MCP and interphalangeal joints are generally uncommon in younger patients, although adolescents tend to have incidence similar to adults, particularly those involved in contact sports. These dislocations most often occur with the distal bone placed dorsal to the proximal. After management of pain with either systemic analgesics or a digital block, prompt relocation is performed with inline distraction and hyperextension in the interphalangeal joints.

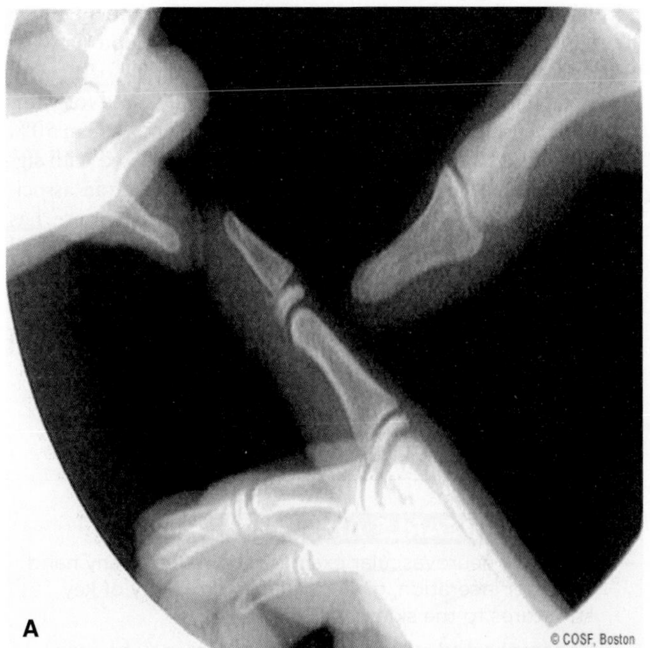

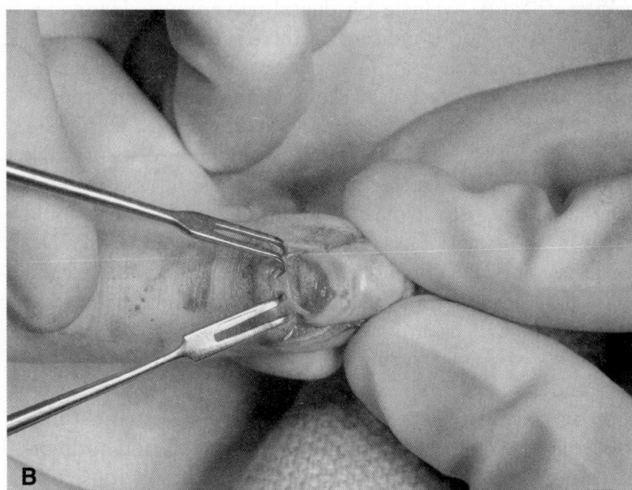

FIGURE 117.8 Seymour's fracture. **A:** Lateral radiograph depicting a displaced distal phalangeal physeal fracture in the setting of a nail bed injury. **B:** Intraoperative photograph after nail plate removal depicting the tear in the germinal matrix of the nail bed and underlying bony injury. (Courtesy of Children's Orthopaedic Surgery Foundation.)

Rapidity of relocation is particularly important when there is any concern regarding the neurovascular status. MCP dislocations are reduced by flexing the wrist to relax the tendon, hyperextending the joint, and then applying dorsal pressure both in the direction of the palm and toward the fingertip. Following relocation, these injuries should be splinted to maintain stability until reevaluation.

FINGERTIP INJURIES

CLINICAL PEARLS AND PITFALLS

- Digital block of the affected finger will likely be more successful than attempts at local anesthesia.
- Avulsed fingertips may be able to be reimplanted and should be protected in a saline-moistened gauze in a bag that is then kept cool in an ice-water mixture.
- Absorbable sutures are equally effective in fingertip wound repair and require less trauma for removal.
- Trephination for a subungual hematoma is generally indicated when it involves more than 50% of the nail bed surface.

Clinical Considerations

Clinical recognition. Fingertip injuries are very common, as the tips of the fingers are often the entry point to exploration of our surroundings. Crush injuries are the most frequent cause and can result in injuries ranging from minor lacerations and subungual hematoma to complex open fractures and tissue loss. Similarly, sharp lacerations are often simple, but particularly if the mechanism also has the force to damage the nail, complete amputations can occur. Although children often recover quite well, careful attention and care to these wounds can help reduce the risk of permanent deformity to the fingertip and nail.

Initial assessment. Although the physical examination features discussed previously hold true, fingertip injuries are often associated with significant pain and bleeding that may hamper repair efforts. Digital block of the affected digit may be required for adequate pain control. Before performing a digital block, a careful examination of fingertip sensation should be performed to evaluate for digital nerve injury. Hand specialist consultation is indicated if there is digital nerve injury. An easily removable tourniquet device is recommended if oozing from wounds precludes adequate examination and repair.

Copious irrigation is required with all wounds, with extra attention paid to open fractures. If wound debridement is felt to be required, the emergency physician should consult with a hand specialist to avoid debriding the nail bed that could result in permanent effects on subsequent nail growth. When repair is complete, a nonadherent dressing should be used and splinting considered for fracture stabilization and protection from reinjury. Petrolatum-laced mesh dressings are particularly effective at optimizing healing and minimizing discomfort and damage on removal. Prophylactic antibiotics are controversial in fingertip injuries, including open fractures. Meticulous wound care is likely most beneficial, and antibiotics should be considered in dirty wounds or those with significant devitalized tissue.

Management. Severe nail bed injuries require nail removal, if nail avulsion was not part of the initial injury. Wounds should be prepped and the often friable tissue should be repaired with 5-0 or 6-0 absorbable suture. Newer studies in adults have found equivalent outcomes using tissue adhesive. Common practice is to keep the nail fold open for the new nail to form. Several placeholders can be used. The salvaged nail can be placed, as can a sterile aluminum (from suture packaging), reinforced silicone sheeting, or a nonadhesive dressing. The nail should be tacked down with sutures proximally and distally. If nonabsorbable sutures are used, they should be removed early in the course at follow-up with a hand specialist to prevent wound tracks during nail development. Recent reports have suggested that stenting the nail fold may not be necessary, though data are limited at this time.

Fingertip lacerations are managed similarly to lacerations in other locations with a few caveats. Wound care is performed as described above. Some literature recommends nonabsorbable suture material, though we favor absorbable suture because the swelling and discomfort often preclude simple suture removal in children.

Amputations of the fingertip are not uncommon and can result in permanent deformity. The current recommendation is to transport the amputated part in saline-moistened gauze in a bag that is then kept cool in an ice–water mixture. Reimplantation has been recommended in most cases involving children provided the distal piece is available and the tissues are not damaged beyond repair. Even if the distal fragment does not remain viable, it will serve a productive function and facilitate growth of the tissue beneath it. Reimplantation may not be an option if the avulsed tip is too small, macerated, or grossly contaminated. If possible, the skin can be closed over the stump with sutures while taking care to protect the nail bed. Small avulsions are best cared for with local wound care and petroleum-based dressing until granulation and healing occur. If closure is not an option due to bone exposure or missing tissue, hand specialist consultation is indicated to determine if alternative repair techniques including rongeuring the bone or a V-Y plasty may be beneficial. Alternatively, these patients may be treated with local wound care and petroleum-based dressing until seen by a hand specialist as an outpatient.

Subungual hematomas, or the collection of blood between the nail and the nail bed, are common and generally occur with crushing injuries. Small hematomas are generally cared for without intervention, whereas hematomas involving more than 50% of the nail bed surface are more likely to be associated with significant nail bed injury, particularly in the setting of an associated distal phalanx fracture. Nevertheless, the literature has demonstrated that if the nail is intact and well adhered, then nail removal and nail bed reconstruction do not impart any improved outcome over simple trephination. Nail trephination can be performed with a heated paper clip, an electrocautery pen, or a large-bore needle drilling by rotating in a circular motion.

DEEP HAND LACERATIONS

CLINICAL PEARLS AND PITFALLS

- A careful neurovascular exam is required with any hand or finger laceration, given the close proximity of key structures to the skin in this region.
- Uncomplicated extensor tendon injuries may be managed by the emergency physician but more severe injuries or flexor tendon injuries should be managed by a hand specialist.

Deep lacerations involving the hand can be serious, related to injury to underlying structures including the neurovascular bundle, or tendons. With significant vascular injury, immediate attempts at hemostasis should be initiated with direct pressure. A careful sensory exam is required to assess for nerve involvement. A hand specialist should be involved to evaluate for potential operative repair when arterial bleeding or neurovascular compromise is identified.

Lacerations in the fingers and hands can involve underlying flexor or extensor tendons. Extensor tendon lacerations proximal to the MCP joints may be amenable to repair by the emergency physician. Extensor tendon lacerations involving the MCP joints or digits, as well as all flexor tendon lacerations, require care by a hand specialist. In consultation with the surgeon, closure of the skin and splinting may comprise appropriate care in the emergency department, with close follow-up for operative repair.

Suggested Readings and Key References

Alterfott C, Garcia FJ, Nager AL. Pediatric fingertip injuries: do prophylactic antibiotics alter infection rates? *Pediatr Emerg Care* 2008: 24(3):148–152.

Cornwall R. Finger metacarpal fractures and dislocations in children. *Hand Clin* 2006;22(1):1–10.

Gellman H. Fingertip-nail bed injuries in children: current concepts and controversies of treatment. *J Craniofac Surg* 2009:20(4):1033–1035.

Light TR. Carpal injuries in children. *Hand Clin* 2000;16(4):513–522.

Nellans KW, Chung KC. Pediatric hand fractures. *Hand Clin* 2013: 29(4):569–578.

Strauss EJ, Weil WM, Jordan C, et al. A Prospective, randomized, controlled trial of 2-octylcyanoacrylate versus suture repair for nail bed injuries. *J Hand Surg Am* 2008;33(2):250–253.

CHAPTER 118 ■ MINOR TRAUMA

MAGDY W. ATTIA, MD, FAAP, FACEP, YAMINI DURANI, MD, AND SARAH N. WEIHMILLER, MD, FAAP, FACEP

GOALS OF EMERGENCY CARE

Each year an estimated 12 million wounds are treated in emergency departments (EDs) in the United States. The first priority is stabilization of these patients who have sustained trauma who may have associated significant injuries. The care of minor injuries focuses on addressing pain, evaluating associated injuries, and wound closure. The key drivers in optimal wound repair are aimed at obtaining hemostasis, preventing infection, and achieving the best long-term cosmesis. This is performed in the context of a focus on patient and parental satisfaction, which is driven in the short term by timeliness of care and length of stay, and in the long term by avoidance of complications, including infection, hypertrophic scarring or keloid formation, and poor cosmetic results.

KEY POINTS

- Children with minor trauma should be assessed for any associated serious injuries and wound management should not preempt care of more life-threatening injuries.
- A thorough evaluation includes learning the mechanism of injury, the age of the wound, determining if there is a retained foreign body, and a careful physical examination that includes assessing for any other associated injuries.
- All wounds should be examined before and after cleansing to determine the best plan for repair.
- All wounds heal by scarring but the goal is to minimize its appearance.
- The use of absorbable sutures in pediatrics is favored in certain situations, as it avoids an additional procedure of suture removal in children.
- The use of topical anesthetics, anxiolysis, child life specialists, and distraction techniques can all be helpful and effective to facilitate wound repair.
- Patient and parent satisfaction as they apply to timeliness of care and avoidance of complications such as infection and poor cosmetic results are important factors to consider when making decisions about wound care.

RELATED CHAPTERS

Resuscitation and Stabilization
- A General Approach to Ill and Injured Children: Chapter 1
- Approach to the Injured Child: Chapter 2

Medical, Surgical, and Trauma
- Infectious Disease Emergencies: Chapter 102
- Genitourinary Trauma: Chapter 116
- Hand Trauma: Chapter 117
- Musculoskeletal Emergencies: Chapter 129

Procedures and Appendices
- Procedural Sedation: Chapter 140
- Procedures: Chapter 141

GENERAL PRINCIPLES OF MINOR WOUND REPAIR

The goals of wound repair are to obtain hemostasis, prevent infection, and achieve optimal cosmetic outcomes.

Obtaining Hemostasis

Hemostasis is important not only to prevent ongoing bleeding but also for clear wound visualization prior to any repair. Application of direct pressure with gauze is the fastest and most commonly used technique to obtain hemostasis. If there is continued bleeding, applying a blood pressure cuff or tourniquet proximal to the wound for a short period is acceptable. Injecting a local anesthetic with a vasoconstrictor such as epinephrine can help with hemostasis but should be used with caution in areas of end organ blood supply, such as digits.

Prevention of Infection

A primary goal of closure of open wounds is to prevent infection. Bacteria inhabit normal intact skin. This is the usual source of infection when skin tissue is disrupted. The amount of bacteria on the skin varies by anatomic location. High counts of bacteria are in moist areas such as the axilla and perineum, as well as in areas of exposed skin such as hand, face, and feet. Low counts of bacteria exist in dry areas such as the back, chest, and abdomen. Areas colonized with high bacterial contamination are most prone to infection. Wounds in regions of high vascularity, such as the scalp and face, more easily resist bacterial infection despite the high bacteria count. Certainly, the oral cavity is highly contaminated with bacteria, and this is an important source of infection when a child sustains a bite wound.

Wounds inflicted by shearing forces with a sharp object such as a knife cause minimal devitalization of adjacent areas and thus are less likely to lead to infection. Wounds caused by a blunt object striking the skin at an angle of less than 90 degrees result in a tension injury such as an avulsion or flap. These injuries involve a larger force applied to the skin than that of a shearing injury, and frequently there is more devitalized tissue. They are more likely to become infected than shearing injuries and are often more difficult to repair. Finally, compression injuries from blunt trauma perpendicular to the skin cause the most tissue disruption and devitalization.

These wounds are characterized by ragged edges, and lead to the highest infection rates and risk of scarring.

Cosmesis and Wound Healing

The final aim of wound repair is to optimize cosmesis. Normal skin is under constant tension due to high collagen content. Tension is also produced in part by underlying structures such as joints and muscles. The amount of tension varies by anatomic location and position of a body part. Lacerations that run parallel to joints and normal skinfolds usually heal more quickly and with better cosmetic results. Wounds under a large amount of tension, crossing joints, or perpendicular to wrinkle lines may heal with wide, more visible scars.

Lacerations regain about 5% of their previous strength 2 weeks after injury, 30% after 1 to 2 months, and full tensile strength 6 to 8 months after the original injury. Many factors, such as infection, tissue edema, and poor nutrition, may delay this progression.

All wounds deeper than the dermis have the potential for scar formation. Scar formation involves the laying down of collagen, which is a complex process essential in restoring tensile strength of the skin. Collagen synthesis begins within 48 hours of the injury and reaches a peak within the first week afterward. Anything that interferes with collagen synthesis, such as infection, may lead to wound dehiscence at this time. Tissue contraction is expected with all healing wounds through the action of fibroblasts. Therefore, eversion of suture lines is desired at the time of repair so the skin will contract to a flat surface after healing. Remodeling may occur for up to 12 months. The scar may fade and recede over the first 3 months, and the final appearance of the scar may not be apparent until 6 to 9 months after injury.

Parental Satisfaction

In general, there are many factors that influence parental and patient satisfaction with their ED experience. In the case of lacerations, as in any pain-inducing condition, parents are concerned that their child's pain, both at presentation and during any repair, is addressed properly. Additionally, parents are almost always concerned about the cosmetic outcome of the wound, particularly in the case of facial lacerations. Communicating information about the healing process, the nature of the wound, and the expected cosmetic outcome, as well as the timeline for complete healing can prevent dissatisfaction later on.

Rate of Wound Infection after Repair

The rate of wound infection is reported between 2% and 10%. Decreasing the likelihood of infection can help prevent additional morbidity, and optimize cosmesis as wounds that are infected during the healing process are more likely to scar. Efforts to reduce the risk of infection can be achieved by proper techniques discussed throughout the chapter.

Current Evidence

Lacerations account for 30% to 40% of all injuries for which care is sought in a pediatric ED. Blunt trauma with sufficient force or contact with sharp objects causes the majority of lacerations. Animal bites account for the remainder. More than 40% of the wounds involve a fall. Boys are injured twice as often as girls. The mechanism of injury varies with the patient's age. In younger children, falls and accidents are classic mechanisms; violent encounters are more likely to be the cause in older children.

Two-thirds of the injuries occur during warm weather months, although half of the injuries in an urban environment occur indoors. Deaths from minor lacerations are rare; however, complications occur in nearly 10%. Children are less likely to get wound infections compared with adults. In children, the infection rate is about 2% for all sutured wounds. The risk of infection increases if there is a delay in primary closure.

Absorbable sutures for the repair of facial lacerations in children can be used to avoid the need for suture removal. Data support that these sutures have equally acceptable cosmetic outcomes in facial lacerations.

In pediatrics, it is important to consider painless alternatives to sutures in some cases. These include tape strips and tissue adhesives (or skin glue). Tape has the advantage of not leading to marks in the skin, minimal tissue reaction, and fewer wound infections than with sutures. Multiple studies have demonstrated that the cosmetic results of skin glue are comparable to those of sutures.

The benefits of the use of routine prophylactic oral antibiotics to prevent wound infection have not been proven and their use is controversial. The risk of antibiotic use from allergic reaction to growth of resistant organisms may outweigh their benefits. Antibiotics are given for wounds with high risk of infection such as bites and heavily contaminated wounds.

The immunization and tetanus status of a patient with a wound should always be obtained and protocol followed as per administration guidelines for tetanus prophylaxis, which is discussed later in the chapter (Table 118.1).

TABLE 118.1

TETANUS PROPHYLAXIS

Prior tetanus toxoid immunization (doses)	Clean minor wound	All other wounds
Uncertain (or less than 3)	Tetanus toxoid-containing vaccine[a]	Tetanus toxoid-containing vaccine and TIG or TAT
Three or more (most recent more than 10 yrs ago)	Td	Td
Three or more (most recent between 5 and 10 yrs)	None	Td

TIG, tetanus immunoglobulin (dose: 250 to 500 units IM); TAT, tetanus antitoxin—should be used only if TIG is not available and after testing (dose: 3,000 to 5,000 units intramuscularly); Td, adult formulation of diphtheria, tetanus toxoid.

[a]If the child is <7 years give DTap. If the child is 7 to 11 years and is underimmunized give Tdap. If the child has already had a dose of Tdap between 7 and 11 years revaccination is not required at 11 years.

Clinical Considerations

Triage Considerations

Children with minor trauma should be assessed for associated significant injuries. Injuries that compromise airway, breathing or circulation (systemically or locally, such as a limb) require immediate attention.

Wound management should not preempt care of more life-threatening injuries. If there are no significant injuries, the focus should move to addressing hemostasis and pain control. Application of topical anesthetics and administration of oral analgesics can be initiated at triage. Once these measures have been initiated, the emergency physician should aim for appropriate and timely wound repair.

Clinical Assessment

History. In the evaluation of a laceration, it is important to learn the *mechanism* of the injury because this has a direct impact on management plans. For instance, if the wound was caused by an animal bite, the likelihood of infection and devitalized tissue is higher, thus wound closure may be avoided and healing by secondary intention may be preferred (Chapter 102 Infectious Disease Emergencies). Similarly, a wound caused by a blunt object may be associated with an underlying fracture or crush injury. These injuries are inherently more complicated and may require surgical consultation and hospital admission. A wound caused by a sharp or projectile object may cause deeper tissue or vascular injury. It is also important to determine the *age* of the wound, as well as the possibility of a *foreign body* in the wound, since these factors also determine the management of the wound repair.

The emergency physician should consider the *location* of the wound. If the wound is in the neck area, there may be possible extension through the platysma muscle, with potential for a serious injury to underlying structures. If the wound involves the chest, the clinician should look for crepitus in the subcutaneous tissue, suggesting injury to the underlying lung. An injury to the lower extremities is more likely to result in infection because of the relatively poor blood supply. Likewise, a wound overlying a joint space can be complicated if the joint cavity is violated. Injury to distal body parts such as the ears, nose, and fingers may threaten the viability of more distal tissues because of vascular compromise. Conversely, in areas where the vascular supply is robust, such as the face, scalp, and tongue, the infection rate is low regardless of the mechanism of injury.

Assess the *environment* in which the injury occurred. If the injury occurred on the street, it is possible that small particulate matter may be embedded in the wound. If this debris is left in place, tattooing of the skin could result, leaving an unfavorable appearance to the healed wound. Injuries that occurred in a field, farm, or a wet, swampy area may have high bacterial loads.

The patient's health status and past medical history should be addressed to determine if there are additional risk factors for poor healing. If the patient has diabetes, immunosuppression, malnutrition, or other chronic conditions, such as cyanotic heart disease, chronic respiratory problems, or renal insufficiency, higher infection rates may be anticipated. Bleeding disorders and current medications should be determined because some drugs, such as ibuprofen and corticosteroids, may also have an impact on wound healing. A history of allergies to latex, antibiotics, and local anesthetics, as well as the child's tetanus status should be determined.

Physical Examination. A careful physical examination is essential before giving local anesthesia. First, determine whether there is an associated injury distant from the obvious wound. It is important to assess the wound for *vascular damage* and to control bleeding if present. Brisk flow of blood may indicate injury to a major vessel. These vessels can usually be safely tamponaded and later ligated or sutured. The bleeding site must be identified, although it is often obscured by profuse bleeding. Pressure applied to the site or temporary use of a tourniquet or inflated blood pressure cuff (less than 2 hours) can help control hemorrhage and allow for identification of the bleeding vessel. Blind clamping of an artery should be avoided except in the scalp. Palpation of pulses and capillary refill distal to the site of injury must be checked.

Next, potential *nerve damage* must be assessed. For example, in a cooperative child, the physician should always test the median and ulnar nerve of an injured upper extremity. If a young child does not permit this, sensation may be tested with use of pinprick. Fortunately, when sensation is intact, motor function of the nerve is usually also intact.

Next, the wound must be evaluated for possible *tendon injury*. The superficial location of extensor tendons of the dorsum of the hand predisposes them to injury. Tendon injuries are sometimes visible if the wound is wide and deep. For example, a torn tendon on the flexor surface of the forearm may be seen when the patient with a laceration to the wrist is asked to flex the hand and wrist. Unless the tendon injury is obvious, wounds over joints and tendons should be put through a full range of motion. A young patient may not be cooperative enough to flex and extend the fingers on command. Therefore, it is important to inspect the resting position of the injured hand in a young child to note a flexor tendon injury to the finger. One digit may be found extended at rest, while the other uninjured digits are flexed (Fig. 118.1). Applying a noxious stimulus and noting inability to withdraw the finger that is tested may show injury to the extensor tendons.

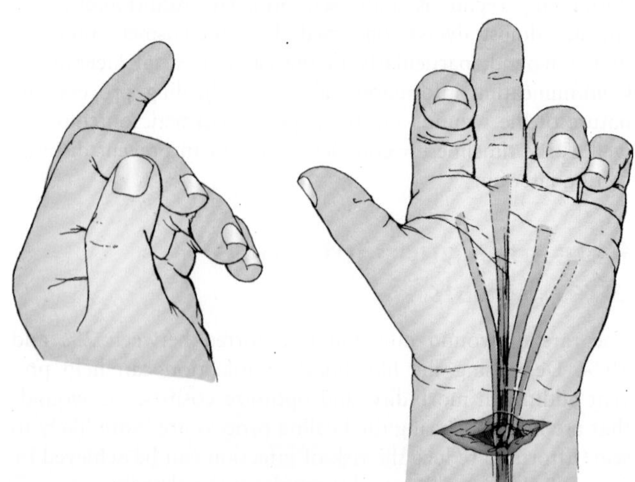

FIGURE 118.1 A seemingly superficial laceration at the wrist might be treated simply by closure of the subcutaneous tissue and skin, unless one appreciates the abnormal posture of a finger when the hand is at rest. The loss of normal flexor tone as a result of a divided superficial tendon results in the involved finger lying in a position of relative extension.

TABLE 118.2

WOUND ASSESSMENT—GENERAL PRINCIPLES

Primary survey—control bleeding	**Physical examination**
Secondary survey—other injury?	Location
	Muscle function
History	Tendon involvement
Mechanism	Vascular injury
Age of wound—time of injury	Nerve injury
	Foreign material
Possible foreign body	
Environment	
Health status—tetanus immunization	Laboratory
	Consider radiographs or ultrasound if a foreign body or fracture is suspected

Role for Imaging. If the history or physical examination raises concern for possible *foreign material* in the wound, consider obtaining a radiograph or an ultrasound of the area. This is especially important in assessing a wound caused by glass. A deeply embedded piece of glass may be missed without radiographs or ultrasound. Some recommend obtaining plain radiographs in all cases in which glass is involved, except for the most superficial wounds. Ultrasound is more sensitive in detecting and localizing foreign bodies and can identify those that are nonradiopaque, such as plastic and wood, which will not be seen on plain films. It is a good idea to further inspect for foreign material after the wound is anesthetized.

Finally, *bones* nearby the wound should be palpated for crepitus, tenderness, or deformity, which may suggest a fracture. Obtain radiographs to confirm suspicious findings. Wounds overlying a fracture may constitute an open fracture and deserve consultation with an orthopedic surgeon for possible repair in the operating room. Table 118.2 summarizes general principles of wound assessment.

Patients found to have vascular, nerve, or tendon injury or deep, extensive wounds to the face merit consideration for consultation with a surgical specialist for possible repair in the operating room.

Management

Decision to Close the Wound. Most wounds may be closed primarily, meaning the wound edges are approximated as soon as possible after the injury to speed healing and improve the cosmetic result. If primary closure is delayed, the risk of subsequent infection increases. Some authors suggest that the "golden period" for wound closure is 6 hours. However, wounds at low risk for infection (e.g., a clean kitchen knife injury) can be closed even 12 to 24 hours after the injury.

Most wounds of the face are best closed primarily, even up to 24 hours after injury to achieve an optimal cosmetic effect. If the wound is extensive or has a high potential for infection (e.g., a dog bite on the face), thorough irrigation is essential, and in some cases, the operating room may be the best site for this repair. Conversely, wounds at high risk for infection such as those in anatomic locations with poor blood supply, contaminated or crush wounds, and those involving immunocompromised hosts should be closed promptly, within 6 hours of injury. Some contaminated wounds (e.g., animal or human bites or those occurring on a farm) in an immunocompromised host should not be sutured, even if the patient presents immediately for care. Some wounds should be allowed to heal by *secondary intention* (secondary closure), although scar formation may be more unsatisfactory. Infected wounds, ulcers, and many animal bites are best left to heal by granulation and reepithelialization. Human bites over the metacarpophalangeal joints (clenched-fist bites) are especially prone to infection and risk infection with primary closure. Puncture wounds to the foot, with only a small laceration and a low concern for cosmetic results, may also be left open. A small sterile wick of iodoform gauze may be placed inside the wound to keep the edges open. This gauze can be removed after 2 to 3 days, and the subsequent granulation tissue will aid healing.

If a wound is not closed initially, *delayed primary closure* (tertiary closure) can be considered after the risk of infection decreases, about 3 to 5 days later. This is recommended for selected heavily contaminated wounds and those associated with extensive damage. These uncommon wounds in pediatrics might include: high-velocity missile injuries, crush injuries, explosion injuries of the hand, industrial wounds, those occurring on a farm and perhaps bite wounds. The wound should be cleaned and debrided and covered at the time of initial presentation, then reassessed in a few days for infection. A contaminated but healing wound may gradually gain sufficient resistance to infection to permit uncomplicated closure at a later time. This approach may reduce discomfort and lead to a better cosmetic result than no repair. Tertiary closure is used rarely in pediatrics because children have few severely contaminated wounds.

Preparing the Child and Family. It is important to reassure the child and the family that everything will be done to care for the wound appropriately and to relieve the patient's pain and anxiety. In many cases, early removal of blood and foreign material from the surface of the wound is reassuring. Also, carefully chosen words will reduce fear for the procedure. The physician must honestly warn the patient of an impending painful stimulus but may leave open the possibility that it may not hurt as much as the child thinks. Appearing unhurried and confident, giving the child some control of the situation, and explaining the upcoming procedure seems to help reduce anxiety and pain. The parent(s) and child should be informed that steps will be taken to make the procedure as quick and painless as possible, such as with the use of topical anesthetics. The clinician should provide an age-appropriate empathic explanation, to reduce anxiety. Prepare instruments that may be frightening, such as needles and scalpels, away from the child. Distraction techniques, such as allowing the child to listen to music or view age-appropriate, entertaining videos during the procedure can be quite effective (see Chapter 1 A General Approach to Ill and Injured Children). Child life specialists, if available, are also a good resource.

Inviting the parent to be in the room increases their level of confidence in the physician and can improve their overall satisfaction with the visit. Most parents want to be present during wound repair in the ED, and most can be a stabilizing force if properly oriented. The parent can reassure or distract the child with a story while maintaining physical contact under necessary drapes and restraints. It is usually best if the parent is sitting down and focusing on the child, rather than directly observing the procedure.

Appropriate use of *sedation* and *local anesthetics* is essential for successful repair of lacerations in some children. Some younger children can undergo repair after being placed in a restraining device, such as a papoose board, or wrapping the child securely but comfortably in a bedsheet for better immobilization. Restraint is needed to ensure the child's safety and allow for more rapid completion of the procedure. Because the child may get excessively warm while being restrained, it is important to ensure proper ventilation and assess the child's comfort during the restraint process. A caring, but firm nurse or assistant is often needed to further immobilize the injured body part and complete the procedure successfully. It is better to use such hospital personnel instead of parents to immobilize a child. A school-age child can usually cooperate without restraint. Some children may require procedural sedation and/or anesthesia depending on the type, extent and location of the wound, and the child's age and level of development (see Chapter 140 Procedural Sedation). Some extensive wounds may warrant more significant repair that is best accomplished with surgical consultation and possible intraoperative repair.

Minimizing Risk of Infection. Hair near the wound usually creates minimal difficulty during repair. Shaving the hair in the area of the wound may damage hair follicles and increase risk of infection. If necessary to facilitate repair, the hair should be clipped with scissors. Alternatively, petroleum jelly can be used to keep unwanted scalp hair away from the wound while suturing. Hair over the eyebrows should never be removed because this may lead to abnormal or slow regrowth.

It is essential to clean the wound periphery at the time of wound evaluation. Povidone–iodine solution (a 10% standard solution) is often used because it is a safe and effective antimicrobial with little tissue toxicity. This solution may be diluted with saline 1:10 to create a 1% solution. Use of chlorhexidine or povidone–iodine surgical scrub preparations, hydrogen peroxide, or alcohol in the wound itself is not recommended. These may be irritating to tissues and may injure white cells, increasing the risk of infection.

Wound irrigation is extremely important to reduce bacterial contamination and prevent subsequent infection. It is often necessary to anesthetize the wound before thoroughly cleansing. Using universal precautions, the wound should be irrigated with normal saline, approximately 100 mL per cm of laceration. More may be needed if the wound is unusually large or contaminated. Use a large syringe (20 to 60 mL) with a splash-guard (commonly 20-gauge bore) attached to the end to reduce splatter during the irrigation. With the splash-guard just above the skin surface, the clinician should apply firm pressure to the plunger. This technique is usually capable of generating 5 to 8 lb per square inch (PSI) which is considered ideal pressure for wound irrigation. Some institutions may have splash-guards that attach directly to the bottle of saline. Consider warming the saline before irrigation because this may be more comfortable. Tap water has been used instead of saline, and is equally effective at irrigating wounds without increasing risk for infection. Soaking the injured body part should be avoided because this may lead to maceration of the wound and edema.

Scrubbing the wound should be reserved for particularly "dirty" wounds in which contaminants are not effectively removed with irrigation alone. Use topical or infiltrative anesthetics for pain control before scrubbing. It may be necessary to extract some foreign material with fine forceps if it remains adherent after copious irrigation. This will avoid tattooing of the skin and reduce the risk of infection.

In rare cases, the wound must be extended with a scalpel to allow proper exploration and cleaning. The physician should consider trimming small amounts of tissue in irregular lacerations and excising necrotic skin but should not make dramatic changes in the wound. Devitalized tissue should be removed only if it looks ischemic or is otherwise clearly indicated. If more extensive debridement is deemed necessary, consultation with a surgical specialist is recommended. Subcutaneous fat can be safely and easily removed if it interferes with wound closure. It is wise to remove such fat carefully, in small quantities, to avoid disruption of small vessels and cutaneous nerve branches. Avoid removal of facial fat because this may leave an unsightly depression. Debridement is advantageous because it creates well-defined wound edges that can be more easily opposed. However, excessive removal of tissue can create a defect that is difficult to close or may increase tension at the wound margin such that scarring is more likely.

Examine the wound further after cleansing and debridement. After exploration, it is wise to reevaluate the decision to close the wound primarily. When proceeding further, the emergency physician should wash hands before donning sterile gloves. Although some studies report no increased risk of infection with nonsterile gloves, most still recommend using latex free, nonpowder, sterile gloves for wound repair. Sterile masks do not reduce the risk of wound infections, but a facial splash-shield is useful to protect the clinician. The area surrounding the wound should be appropriately draped before wound repair. However, if a young child is particularly upset by facial drapes, they can be omitted. Proper cleaning of the wound is more important to uncomplicated healing than meticulous attempts to avoid introduction of small numbers of bacteria by preserving a sterile field.

Type of Suture/Equipment. Suture material must have adequate strength while producing minimal inflammatory reaction. Nonabsorbable sutures such as monofilament nylon (Ethilon) or polypropylene (Prolene) retain most of their tensile strength for more than 60 days and are relatively nonreactive. Thus, they are appropriate for closing the outermost layer of a laceration. With nylon, it is important to secure the knot adequately with at least four to five throws per knot. Polypropylene is useful for lacerations in the scalp or eyebrows because it has a blue color that is more visible and thus easier to remove, although it has memory and therefore is somewhat more difficult to control while suturing. Silk is rarely used because of increased tissue reactions and infection.

Absorbable sutures are also used in some wounds. Absorbable synthetic sutures such as dexon, monocryl, or vicryl should be used in deeper, subcuticular layers. These materials may elicit an inflammatory response and may extrude from the skin before they are absorbed if they are placed too close to the skin. When subcuticular sutures are used, they should be placed on the deeper surface of the dermis, and epithelial margins may be approximated with either tape strips or cuticular sutures. Synthetic absorbable sutures are less reactive than chromic gut and retain their tensile strength for long periods, making them useful in areas with high dynamic and static tensions. Absorbable sutures are also advantageous for intraoral lacerations. Some recommend using rapidly absorbable sutures (fast-absorbing gut) for skin closure of facial wounds in children to avoid the need for subsequent suture removal. Equally acceptable cosmetic results are found with absorbable sutures compared with nonabsorbable sutures in pediatric facial laceration repair. Some hand specialists also advocate for absorbable sutures for hand lacerations in young children since removing them can be quite difficult in uncooperative young patients.

A 3-0 suture is recommended for tissues with strong tension, such as fascia, and 4-0 is recommended for deep tissues with light tension, such as subcutaneous tissue. Skin is best closed with 4-0 to 7-0 and oral mucosa with 3-0 to 4-0 sutures. The emergency physician should use the finest sutures (6-0) for wounds of the face; heavier sutures for scalp, trunk, and extremities (4-0 or 5-0); and 3-0 or 4-0 for thick skin, such as the sole of the foot, or over large joints, such as the knee.

Needles are available in various forms, including cuticular, plastics, and "reverse cutting." The reverse cutting needle is used most for laceration repair. Its outer edge is sharp to allow for atraumatic passage of the needle through the relatively tough dermis and epidermal layers; this minimizes cutting of the skin where suture tension is the greatest. A higher-grade plastic needle (designated P or PS) is often used for repairs on the face. A small needle (e.g., P3) should be used for wounds that require fine cosmesis. Needles come in various sizes such as 3/8 and 1/2 circle. Clinicians may develop a preference for a specific needle. However, in general, a 3/8 reverse cutting needle satisfies most needs.

Closure Techniques. Two of the most important goals of suturing are to match the layers of the injured tissues and to create eversion of the wound margins so they will flatten as the wound heals. Layers on one side of a wound should be sutured to the corresponding, matching layers on the other side. First, all layers of skin that have been injured should be identified. Then an attempt to oppose each layer (muscles, fascia, subcutaneous tissue, and skin) as nearly as possible back to its original location should be made. This is achieved by carefully matching the depth of the bite taken on each side of the wound when suturing.

Proper suture placement should result in slight eversion of the wound so there is not a depressed scar when remodeling takes place. Eversion may be achieved by slight thumb pressure on the wound edge as the needle is entering the opposite side. Sutures should take equal bites from both wound edges so one margin does not overlap the opposite margin when the knot is tied. Wound edge eversion is best achieved by taking proper bites while suturing, not by pulling the knot tightly (Fig. 118.2).

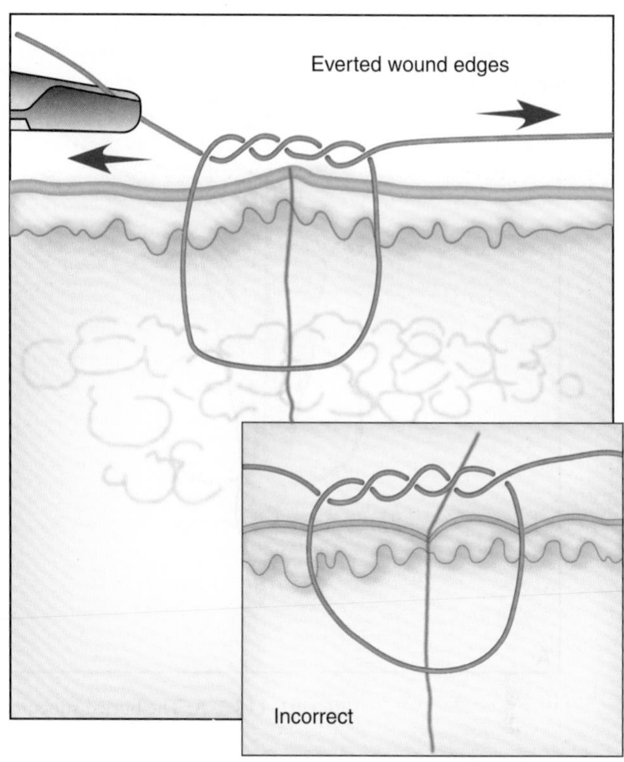

FIGURE 118.2 Suturing technique for wound edge eversion.

Suture placement may be deep or superficial. Deep sutures reapproximate the dermal layers of skin and do not penetrate the epidermis. They help relieve skin tension and improve the cosmetic appearance by reducing the width of the scar. They should be avoided in wounds prone to infection because they will further increase this risk. To place a deep suture, the needle is placed at the depth of the wound and removed at a more superficial level. The needle is then inserted superficially into the opposite side of the wound and exits deeply so the knot is buried within the wound. The needle end and free end of the suture should be on the same side of the loop before the knot is tied (Fig. 118.3). The simple interrupted technique (described next) with absorbable suture material should be used.

Superficial or percutaneous sutures are passed through the dermis and epidermis and leave the knot visible at the skin surface. Skin should be closed with a minimal amount of tension. Sutures should be pulled tightly enough to approximate the wound edges, but not so tightly that they cause tissue necrosis. Sutures that seem well placed initially may begin to cut into the tissue in the next few days because of swelling and inflammation. There is no need to tightly close the skin if other layers have been well sutured. Scalp wounds are an exception. They are under considerable tension, and the knots in this location should be pulled firmly to keep the skin together. The wound will be hidden by hair, so the skin can be pulled more tightly than elsewhere. Firm, but not strangulating, apposition of the wound will also help with hemostasis.

To ensure proper alignment, the first suture may be placed at the midpoint of the wound, with subsequent sutures then placed in a bisecting fashion lateral to the midpoint. Use of noncrushing forceps to hold tissue should be encouraged because this allows the operator to precisely pass the needle through the desired points alongside the wound edge. However, forceps use should be kept to a minimum during the repair to avoid tissue damage.

Skin wounds can generally be repaired using interrupted suturing. To place a simple interrupted suture, the needle is held pointing down toward the skin and the wrist is pronated as the needle enters the skin at a 90-degree angle. The needle tip will then move farther away from the wound margin and penetrate deeply. Thus, more tissue is at the depth of the wound, and this causes the wound to evert. Sutures should be placed about 2 mm apart and 2 mm from the wound edge on delicate areas such as the face. More sutures placed closer together decrease wound tension and leave a less noticeable scar. Larger bites should be used for body parts where cosmesis is less important.

Use an instrument tie to secure the suture (Fig. 118.4). The knots should ideally be placed on one side of the wound. Knots placed directly over the wound increase inflammation and scar

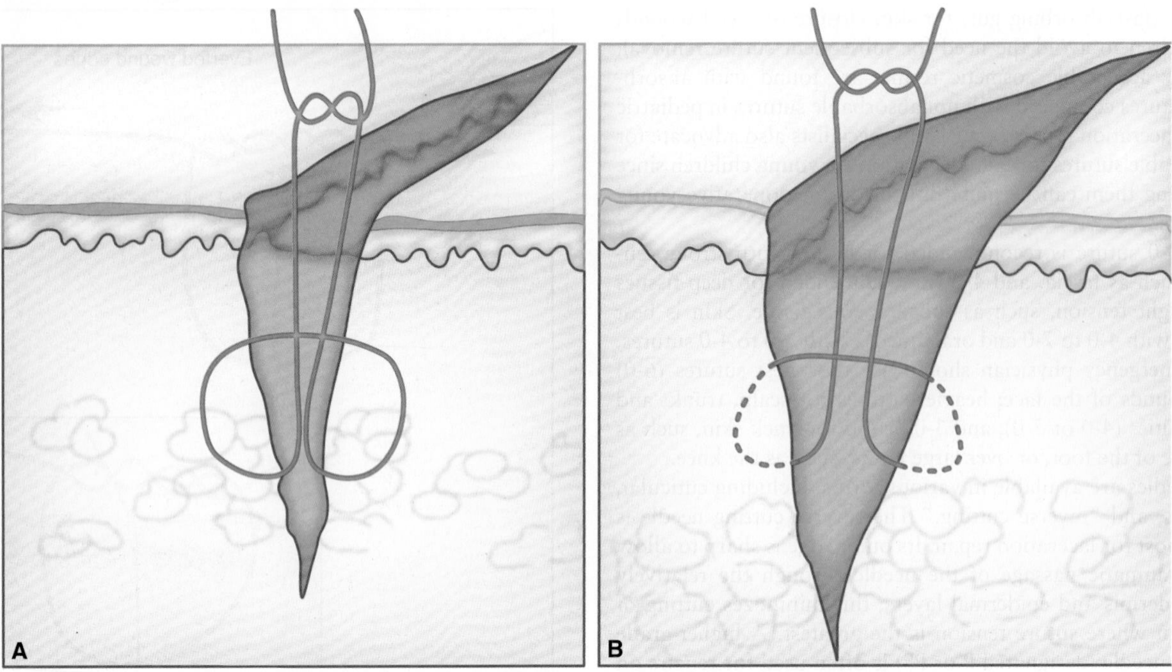

FIGURE 118.3 **A:** The buried subcutaneous suture. **B:** The horizontal dermal stitch.

formation. On the first throw, the physician should wrap the needle holder twice to create a surgeon's knot and then wrap subsequent throws a single time. The first and second throws should be snug enough to approximate the wound edges, but not so tight that tissue is strangulated. All subsequent knots are squared to maintain the closure. Four or five throws are usually required to keep the knot from unraveling. A "loop knot" is effective in apposing the wound edge with minimal tension. This involves placing a surgeon's knot, using the instrument tie, followed by a loop. The surgeon's knot will "give" slightly should edema develop subsequently. The loop knot allows easier, painless removal of sutures because it creates a free space between the suture and the skin (Fig. 118.5).

Running or continuous sutures can be applied rapidly to close large, straight wounds or multiple wounds. With this technique, the suture is not cut and tied with each stitch. The first suture is placed at one end of the wound and a knot tied, cutting only the end of thread not attached to the needle. The next loop is placed a few millimeters away and continuous loops of equal bites are made to close the wound. On the final loop, because the suture is not completely pulled through, a small loop remains on the opposite side of the wound. Now, the knot can be tied using the preceding loop of suture (Fig. 118.6). This type of stitch is more likely to leave suture marks if not removed in 5 days. Apposition of the edges and eversion is more difficult to achieve with this stitch, and the entire suture line can unravel if the suture breaks anywhere along the repair. However, the technique gives the advantage of having equal tension on the wound edges.

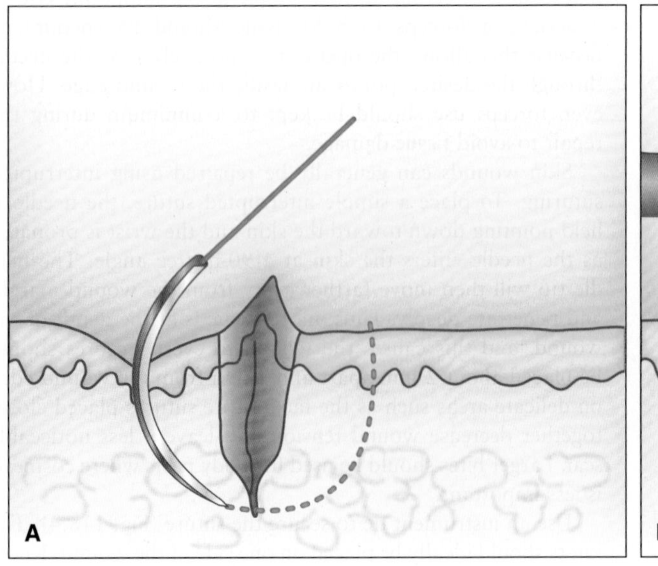

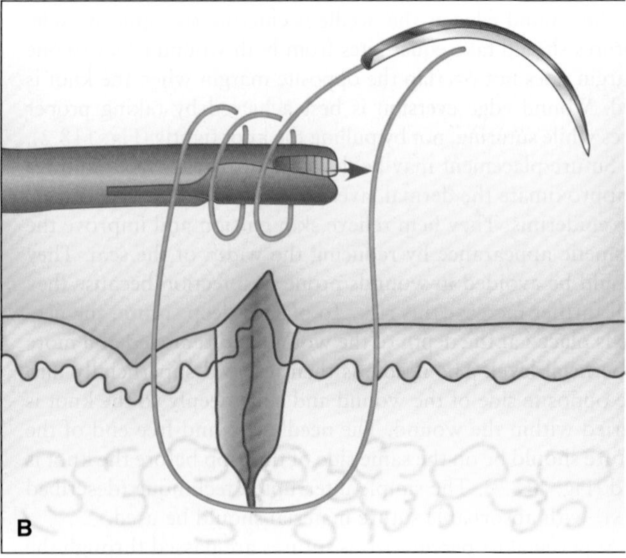

FIGURE 118.4 Simple interrupted skin suture secured with instrument tie.

TRAUMA

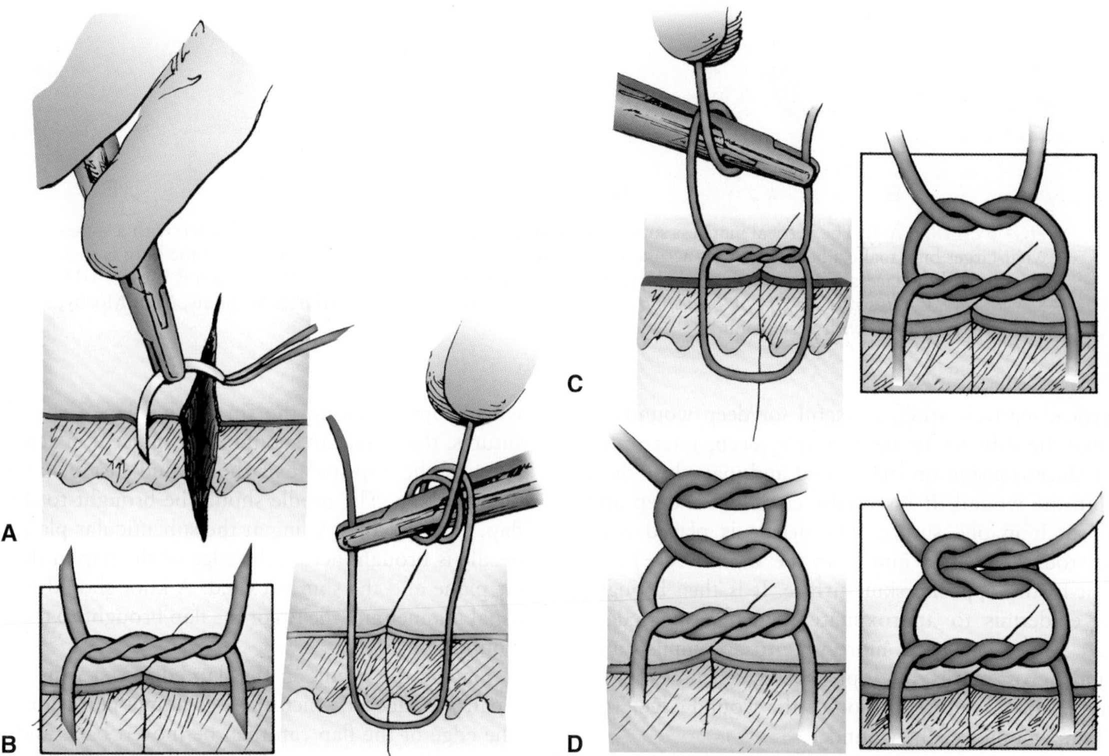

FIGURE 118.5 Placement of a "loop knot" in conjunction with simple sutures of the skin using an eversion technique. **A:** The needle enters the skin at a right angle in a way that allows somewhat less skin and more subcutaneous tissue to be caught in the passage of the needle. The needle should incorporate the same amount of skin and subcutaneous tissue on each side. The ideal suture material for placing a "loop knot" is 4-0 nylon. One can also use 5-0 nylon. **B:** The first knot should be a surgeon's knot drawn down gently to barely coapt the skin edges. **C:** The second tie should be placed to produce a square knot but should be drawn to produce an approximate 2- to 3-mm loop. **D:** The third tie should be placed to produce a square knot. This third tie can be secured tightly against the second tie, preserving the loop and allowing for some spontaneous loosening of the surgeon's knot as later edema develops.

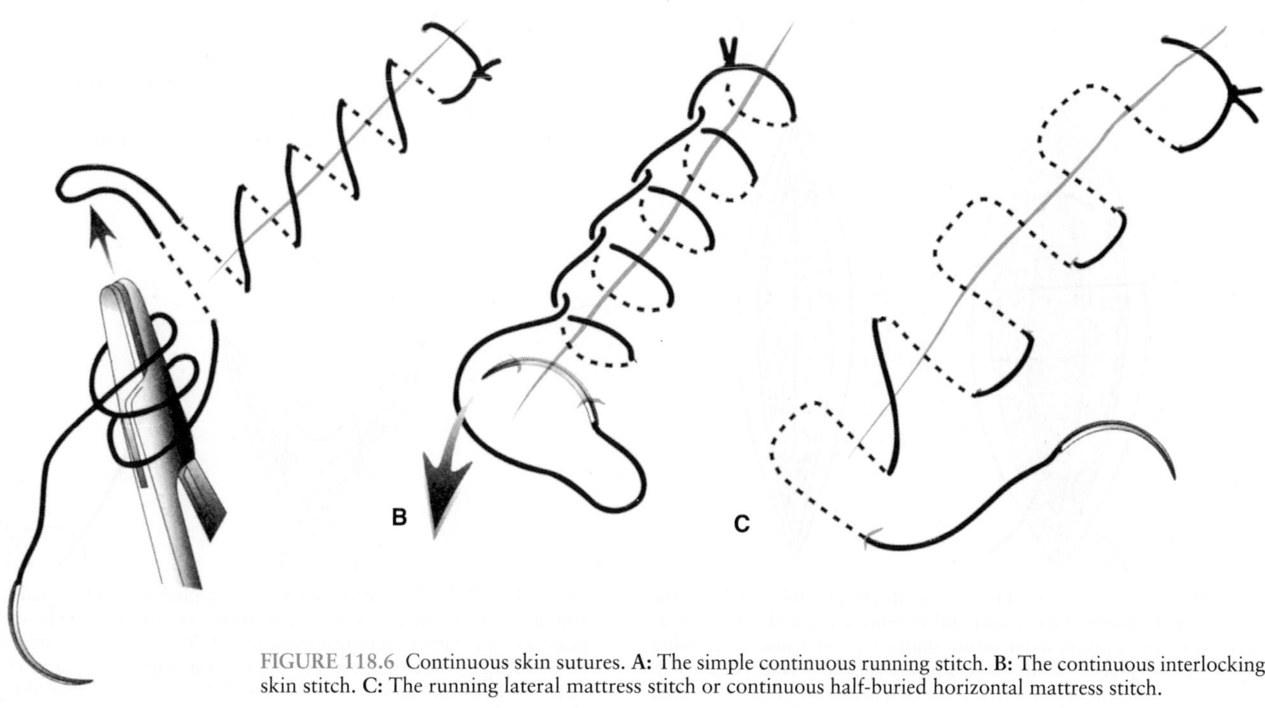

FIGURE 118.6 Continuous skin sutures. **A:** The simple continuous running stitch. **B:** The continuous interlocking skin stitch. **C:** The running lateral mattress stitch or continuous half-buried horizontal mattress stitch.

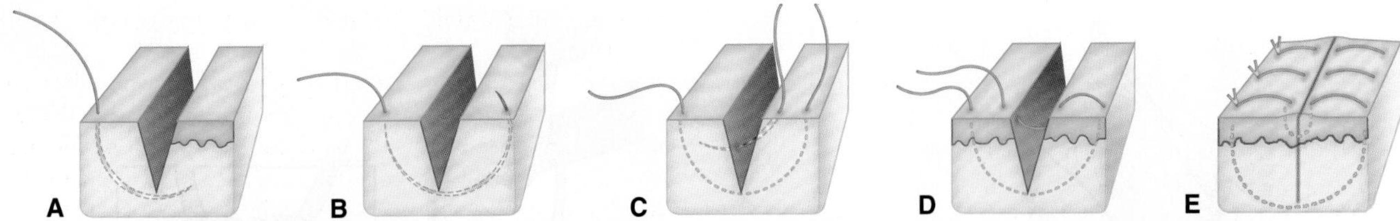

FIGURE 118.7 **A–E:** The vertical mattress suture. After initially placing a simple interrupted stitch with a somewhat larger bite, make a backhand pass across the wound, taking small, superficial bites. When the knot is tied, the edges of the laceration should evert slightly. (From Grisham J. Wound care. In: Dieckmann RA, Fiser DH, Selbst SM, eds. *Illustrated textbook of pediatric emergency & critical care procedures*. St. Louis, MO: Mosby, 1997:676, reprinted with permission.)

The vertical mattress stitch is useful for deep wounds in which it may be difficult to tie a simple, deep, interrupted suture. It reduces tension on the wound and may close dead space within the wound. It essentially combines a deep and superficial stitch in one suture. The needle is placed deep within the wound (about 3 mm from the wound edge) and brought out to the opposite skin surface. It is then brought across the epidermis to approximate the epidermal edges (Fig. 118.7). This stitch takes more time to accomplish and produces more cross marks, but it provides excellent, exaggerated wound eversion and apposition of the wound edge. Too tight of a knot can pucker the wound.

The horizontal mattress stitch reinforces the subcutaneous tissue and effectively relieves tension from the wound edges. It does not provide wound-edge approximation as well as the vertical mattress stitch. The needle is passed ½ to 1 cm away from the wound edge deeply into the wound. It is then passed through the opposite side and reenters the wound parallel to the initial suture. To avoid "buckling" and to provide some eversion of the wound edges, the skin must be entered perpendicularly, and the wound must be entered and exited at the same depth (Fig. 118.8).

The modified horizontal mattress stitch (half-buried) is often used to close a flap. It is also called the corner stitch. It relieves intrinsic tension and avoids vascular compromise when approximating the tip of the flap. Using 5-0 or 6-0 sutures, the physician should enter intact skin across from the apex of the flap and exit the wound just below the subcuticular plane. The needle should be brought to the tip of the flap, entering and exiting at the subcuticular plane. Then, the needle is brought across the edge of the flap in the subcuticular plane and the skin is exited. A knot should be tied in the usual manner and the tip of the flap brought to the apex of the wound (Fig. 118.9).

Placing the needle in the flap edge first can be utilized to repair wounds in which there is ample perfusion to the flap. The edge of the flap can then be moved back and forth until proper alignment with the opposite fixed side is obtained. After the tip of the flap is sutured, the sides of the flap are brought together. Care must be taken to ensure there is no tension on sutures at the tip of the flap. For wounds with several stellate flaps, subcuticular sutures should be used to hold the tips of the flap together. Then, a single suture at the tip will provide good apposition without further damage. Other interrupted sutures can be placed on the lateral margins of the wound to provide further support. If the wound has many narrow-based stellate flaps or necrotic flap tips, the wound may be better managed with excision and simpler repair (Fig. 118.10). Surgical specialty consultation should be considered in these complex wound repairs.

Staples can be applied more rapidly than sutures and have a lower rate of infection, with less of a foreign-body reaction. They are best for wounds of the scalp, trunk, and extremities when saving time is important and cosmesis is

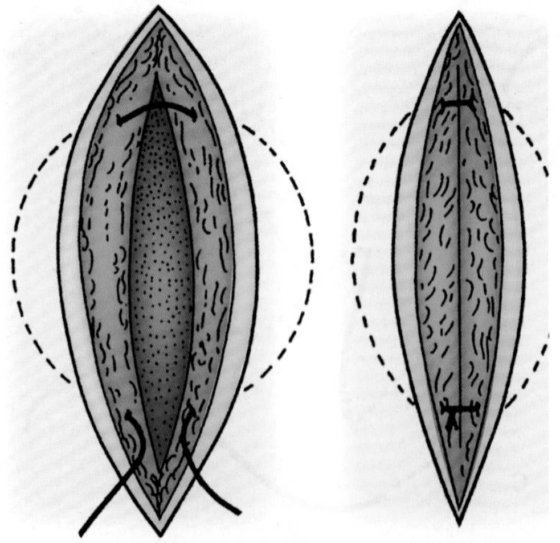

FIGURE 118.8 The horizontal mattress stitch is useful for closing the deep layer in shallow lacerations and in body areas with little subcutaneous tissue. Certain dyed suture materials may cause a tattooing of the skin if placed in such a shallow position. (From Grisham J. Wound care. In: Dieckmann RA, Fiser DH, Selbst SM, eds. *Illustrated textbook of pediatric emergency & critical care procedures*. St. Louis, MO: Mosby, 1997:678, reprinted with permission.)

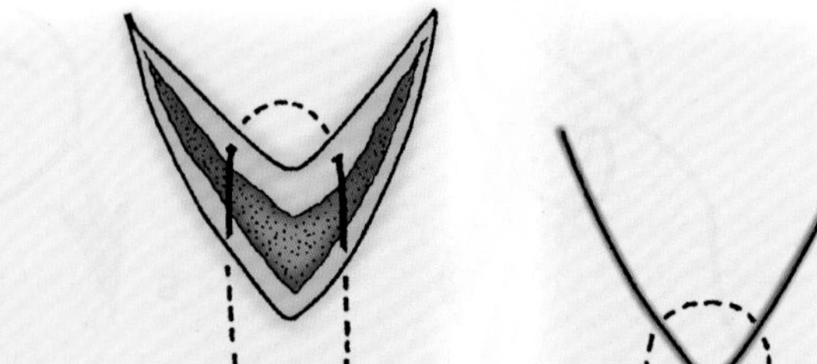

FIGURE 118.9 The corner stitch. Also called the half-buried horizontal mattress stitch, this technique allows repair of flap-type lacerations without further compromising blood flow. Place additional simple interrupted sutures along the sides of the flap if necessary. (From Grisham J. Wound care. In: Dieckmann RA, Fiser DH, Selbst SM, eds. *Illustrated textbook of pediatric emergency & critical care procedures*. St. Louis, MO: Mosby, 1997:676, reprinted with permission.)

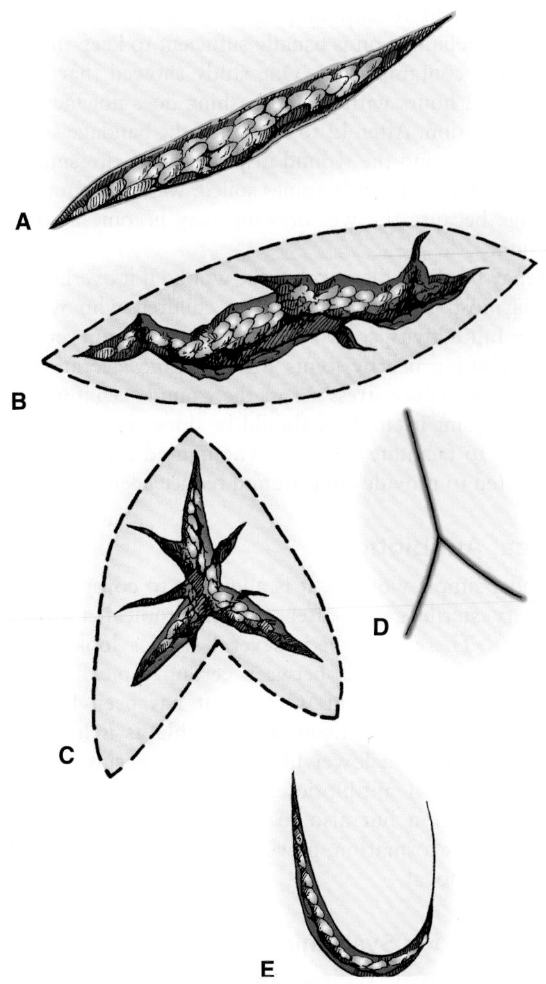

FIGURE 118.10 Variation in laceration injuries and suggestions for management: Simple laceration (**A**), elliptical excision of damaged wound margins (**B**), excision and closure of stellate laceration (**C and D**), and flap-type laceration (**E**).

less of a concern. Therefore, they are particularly helpful when treating mass casualties, or when restraining a patient with a suitable wound is challenging. Staples are left in place for the same length of time as sutures. They are somewhat more painful to remove and should be removed with a specially designed instrument to avoid tissue damage. Staples do not allow for meticulous cosmetic repair as with sutures. Thus, they should not be used for lacerations of the face, neck, hands, or feet. They should also not be used if the patient requires magnetic resonance imaging (MRI) or computed tomography (CT).

Painless Alternatives to Sutures

Skin tape causes no suture marks, minimal tissue reaction, and fewer wound infections than sutures. Tape strips, cut to size, can be used to take up tension at the wound margins and can be placed between sutures. These strips are also useful as the only means to close simple lacerations that extend just through the dermis. They may be as useful as tissue adhesives for facial lacerations in children. Multiple tangential, triangular skin flaps (e.g., those created when an unrestrained passenger hits the windshield of a car) are closed well with tape strips. Likewise, old or contaminated wounds, such as dog bites on the extremities, can be loosely approximated with skin tape.

When tape is used, the wound should be cleansed as any other wound. Care must be taken to properly realign the dermis and epithelium. If the tape is pulled too tightly, the margins of the wound may overlap, causing the wound to heal with a raised ridge-like area where the overlap occurred. The tape is applied perpendicularly across the wound with some space between to allow the wound to drain. In some cases, an adhesive such as benzoin is applied to the adjacent skin (not the wound) to keep the tape strips more securely in place. It is to be noted the benzoin can cause intense burning sensation if it comes into contact with the wound and should be applied at least 2 to 3 mm away from the wound edge but within a reaching distance of the tape. Some recommend leaving the taped wound uncovered because a bandage may increase moisture and cause the tape to fall off prematurely.

Tape strips should not be used on wounds subject to tension, such as those over flexor surfaces of joints. They should not be applied in areas of the body that are moist, such as the palms or axillae, because they will not adhere. They may be impractical for small children, who may inadvertently remove them from the face.

Tissue adhesives, or skin glues, such as octyl cyanoacrylate have become widely used for wound closure in the ED. They allow rapid and painless closure of wounds. Anesthesia is unnecessary, unless painful irrigation or exploration of the wound is anticipated. No removal is needed because the adhesives slough off after 5 to 10 days. They provide an excellent cosmetic result, comparable with sutures. One study using plastic surgeons blinded to the method of repair graded the wounds repaired with tissue adhesives to be cosmetically equal to sutured wounds at 2-month and 1-year follow-up visits.

Tissue adhesives act to decrease wound infections because they have antimicrobial effects against gram-positive organisms. Dehiscence rates (1% to 3%) are similar to that of sutured wounds. They are less expensive than sutures because little equipment is needed and personnel time is reduced. Studies have noted that some patients and families of small children prefer them to sutures. Routine follow-up is not needed for uncomplicated wounds, and no long-term complications have been reported. Newer products such as high-viscosity octyl cyanoacrylate tissue adhesives are less likely to migrate during repair, making wound repair easier to accomplish.

Before application of the tissue adhesive, the wound is cleaned and hemostasis achieved with dry gauze and pressure. The wound's edges are held together manually or with forceps while the tissue adhesive is applied along the surface of the wound. The tissue adhesive should not be applied to the inside of the wound because it will act as a foreign body and inhibit healing. The wound is then held in place for about 20 to 30 additional seconds to obtain adequate bonding. One study reported that if poor alignment of wound edges is noted, the adhesive can be removed with forceps and reapplied without further complication. The wound is then covered carefully so bandage removal will not pull off the tissue adhesive. Avoid routine application of antibiotic ointments by parents as these will dissolve the adhesive and cause dehiscence.

Tissue adhesives should be used only to close skin of superficial wounds. For many lacerations, deep absorbable sutures will also be needed because the glue has less strength than most sutures. Skin glues should not be used for wounds

TABLE 118.3

COMMON TECHNIQUES OF WOUND CLOSURE

Technique	Advantages	Disadvantages
Sutures	Greatest tensile strength	Painful
	Meticulous closure	Removal needed
	Low dehiscence rate	Slow application
		Increased tissue reaction
		Risk of needle stick (clinician)
Staples	Rapid application	Not for use on face (less meticulous closure)
	Low cost	
	Low tissue reaction	
Tissue adhesive	Rapid application	Lower tensile strength
	Painless	Not for use on joints
	No removal needed	Not for use on bite wounds
	Low cost	
	No risk of needle stick (clinician)	
Tape strips	Rapid application	High risk of dehiscence
	Painless	Not for use in moist areas, young children
	Low cost	
	Low infection risk	
	Least tissue reaction	

subject to great tension, such as on the hands or joints, or bite injuries in which occlusive closure increases the risk of infection. Table 118.3 summarizes advantages and disadvantages of several techniques available for wound closure.

Wound Care

Wound Dressing

Appropriate wound aftercare is important in preventing contamination or further injury. It is recommended that most wounds be covered with antibiotic ointment and a dressing immediately after closure. For simple lacerations, an adhesive bandage (e.g., Band-Aid) is sufficient, however larger wounds may benefit from a nonadherent sterile dressing to prevent wound edges from sticking to the dressing. This nonadherent dressing should then be covered with a layer of gauze then tape. This technique helps to protect and immobilize the wound.

For the face and trunk, a large bulky dressing is not practical. Thus, for small wounds in those areas, a clear plastic adhesive (e.g., Tegaderm) should be used to secure the bandage. Rolls of cotton or stretchable tube gauze can be used to wrap larger wounds to keep the sterile dressing in place. This keeps the young child from touching the wound. Scalp wounds are usually not dressed. Patients can generally wash their hair gently after 24 hours.

For children who are active, it may be best to keep the wound covered until sutures are removed. The original dressing should remain in place for 12 to 24 hours after which epithelialization is usually sufficient to keep the wound from gross contamination. One study showed that uncovering after 12 hours with gentle washing does not increase the risk of infection. After 12 to 24 hours, the bandage should be changed daily and the wound inspected. Any dressing should be changed sooner if it becomes soiled, wet, or saturated with drainage because the wet dressing may become a source of infection.

It may be advisable to splint the wound if it overlies a joint. This is most important for active children who will likely resume full activity soon after the injury. Some even recommend splinting nearby joints for any large laceration of an extremity to reduce stress across the wound even if it does not involve a joint itself. This should be done for no more than 72 hours to facilitate function. The injured extremity should be elevated to provide comfort and reduce edema.

Topical Antibiotics

For most simple wounds, it is adequate to cover the wound with dry sterile gauze after applying topical antibacterial ointment. There have been several studies looking at the different infection rates between certain topical antibiotics and petroleum ointment. Overall, it has been found that a triple antibiotic ointment is preferable as it has broader coverage and has a lower likelihood of causing an allergic reaction. Topical antibiotics have been noted not only to prevent infection but also to help with reepithelialization, decrease crust formation, prevent wound dehiscence, and aid in suture removal.

Guidelines for Systemic Antibiotics

Use of prophylactic systemic antibiotics for wound management is controversial. There is no data demonstrating proven benefit to the routine use of antibiotics. In addition, antibiotics may lead to allergic reactions, growth of resistant organisms, and unnecessary expense. Decontamination with proper irrigation is more efficacious than routine use of antibiotics to prevent wound infection. Antibiotic prophylaxis may be considered in certain high-risk wounds. These include heavily contaminated wound, dog and cat bites, puncture wounds of the hand, stellate lacerations, lacerations near joints, or over open fractures. Also, patients who are immunocompromised should be considered for prophylactic antibiotics. Data for the role for antibiotics in intraoral wounds is conflicting. There is less data supporting the use of antibiotics in dirty wounds, but may be considered in lacerations contaminated with soil or feces. Wounds that result in exposed cartilage of the nose or ears or extensive facial wounds that may involve contamination from adjacent nasal passages are often treated with antibiotics. It may also be reasonable to use antibiotics for wounds (other than scalp lesions) when repair takes place more than 12 hours after injury.

Usually a first-generation cephalosporin or penicillinase-resistant penicillin is used to cover staphylococci and streptococci. Amoxicillin–clavulanic acid is recommended for wounds created by mammalian bites (see Chapter 102 Infectious Disease Emergencies). Additional coverage for gram-negative organisms with an aminoglycoside is recommended for open fractures (see Chapter 119 Musculoskeletal Trauma). Methicillin-resistant *Staphylococcus aureus* (MRSA) in simple skin lacerations is less common, however if there is concern

TABLE 118.4

DISCHARGE INSTRUCTIONS FOR WOUND CARE

1. Keep the wound clean and as dry as possible for the first 24 hrs. The skin around the wound may be cleaned gently.
2. After 24 hrs the child may shower and dry the wound gently and completely.
3. Avoid any activities that will keep the wound soaked in water (e.g., swimming and a bath) until sutures are removed.
4. Consider oral pain medications.
5. Provide instructions for topical or oral antibiotics if they are recommended for the patient.
6. If a splint is applied it should be kept on, clean and dry.
7. Sunscreen may be applied after the wound heals to minimize pigment changes.
8. Watch for signs of wound infection and dehiscence.
9. Arrange follow-up for recheck as needed.

for high rates of MRSA in the community then clindamycin or trimethoprim-sulfamethoxazole should be considered.

Guidelines for Tetanus

The immunization status of all injured patients should be documented in the medical record. If the wound is clean and minor and the patient has received three previous doses of tetanus toxoid, a booster of tetanus toxoid is given only if 10 or more years have passed since the last dose. If a patient has received three or more previous tetanus immunizations but the wound is not a clean, minor laceration, tetanus toxoid is indicated if the last dose was more than 5 years prior.

In many cases, the tetanus immunization record is unknown. If tetanus status is unknown or the patient has received less than 3 doses of tetanus and the wound is not clean or minor, tetanus toxoid and tetanus immunoglobulin (TIG) are indicated. Wounds involving massive tissue destruction and contamination may also require TIG (see Table 118.1). Patients with such wounds should be admitted to the hospital.

Wound Aftercare

Careful discharge instructions, regarding wound care, covering the wound, when it is ok to get the wound wet, and how to dry it are extremely important. A summary of discharge instructions is provided in Table 118.4. The family should be informed about signs of infection. Specifically, they should be told to return for medical care if the wound develops increasing pain, redness, edema, and/or wound discharge, or if the child develops a fever. Analgesics such as ibuprofen and acetaminophen may be given for minor pain, but worsening pain should always prompt a wound check. The family should also be informed that the wound was inspected for a foreign body but that there is still a possibility of a retained foreign body or an undetected injury that may require further treatment.

Parents should be told that no matter how skillful the repair, every laceration leaves some scar. The appearance of the scar will change during the next several months, and the scar's appearance will not be complete for about 6 to 12 months.

TABLE 118.5

TIMELY SUTURE REMOVAL

Wound location	Time of removal (days)
Neck	3–4
Face	4–5
Scalp	7–10
Upper extremities, trunk	7–10
Lower extremities	8–10
Joint surface	10–14

Studies have not shown any specific ointments or creams to be helpful in scar reduction. What has been shown is that less sun exposure will help reduce scar formation and hyperpigmentation. Therefore, generous application of sunscreen is crucial for optimal results during wound healing.

Most wounds can be followed up at the time of suture removal. Those wounds requiring close follow-up (at 24 to 48 hours) include those that are contaminated, those with tenuous vascular supply, and those showing any signs of infection. Wounds closed with tape strips do not require removal of the tape because these will fall off spontaneously. Tissue adhesive also sloughs spontaneously. However, nonabsorbable sutures should be removed at the appropriate time, depending on the location of the injury. The importance of timely removal should be stressed to the patient and family. Removing sutures too early may lead to dehiscence and widening of the scar. Sutures left in too long may create an unnecessary tissue reaction and result in visible cross-hatching ("railroad ties").

Wounds on the scalp or face are nourished by a better blood supply and generally exhibit more rapid healing. Sutures in these areas are removed more quickly than other locations to avoid unsightly tracts.

When sutures are subject to considerable tension (over joints and on the hands), they should be left in place longer (Table 118.5). After removal of sutures, it may be necessary to reinforce the healing wound with tape strips to prevent dehiscence.

As discussed previously, in the first 12 to 24 hours wound dressings should be changed only if wet or soiled. After that, gentle washing can be permitted as long as the wound is then patted dry and covered again. There is no proven harm to exposing the sutures to soap and water for short periods of time.

MANAGEMENT OF SPECIFIC WOUNDS

The principles of wound care discussed earlier should be applied in repairing any of the wounds discussed in the following section. These principles include evaluation of the wound by history, physical examination, and when indicated, radiographic or ultrasound imaging. After the wound is evaluated, the feasibility of closure and the possible need for consultation with a surgical specialist should be considered. The following section discusses some of the commonly encountered wounds in children.

Facial and Oral Wounds

CLINICAL PEARLS AND PITFALLS

- Appearing unhurried and confident, giving the child, when age appropriate, some control of the situation, and explaining the upcoming procedure can help reduce anxiety.
- Use of distraction techniques and anxiolytics can avoid the need for sedation.
- Tap water can be used instead of saline, and is equally effective in reducing the risk for infection.
- Using 6-0 absorbable material is recommended for skin closure whenever possible and obviates the need for a second visit for suture removal.
- No specific ointments or creams found to be helpful in scar reduction. However, application of sunscreen may decrease hyperpigmentation of the forming scar.
- The use of epinephrine with local anesthesia during lip laceration repair could obscure the vermilion border landmark.
- Shaving the eyebrow for wound preparation may obscure landmark causing misalignment. Also, eyebrow regrowth is unpredictable.
- If the frontalis muscle is involved and is not properly approximated, its function, eyebrow elevation, could be disrupted.
- In repairing the ear lobe or auricular rim, if the skin edges are not everted at the time of closure, "notching" may occur.

Forehead Lacerations

Forehead lacerations are common in early childhood. These injuries commonly occur after falls on objects or furniture such as coffee tables. Most of these lacerations are simple and not associated with any other significant injuries. However, the head and neck requires careful evaluation for other injuries. Superficial transverse lacerations of the forehead usually have a favorable outcome. Closure with simple or continuous cuticular sutures using 6-0 absorbable material is recommended. Deeper transverse lacerations involving the deep fascia, frontalis muscle, or periosteum should be repaired in layers. Absorbable 5-0 material such as monocryl, coated vicryl, or catgut can be used. If the deeper tissue plains are not closed, the function of the frontalis muscle, eyebrow elevation, may be hampered. Other facial expressions can also be affected because the skin may tether to the scar tissue, bridging the unrepaired gaping tissues.

Vertical forehead lacerations tend to have a more visible scar because they traverse the tension lines. Complex forehead wounds, such as stellate lacerations from windshield impact and those with tissue loss, particularly secondary to animal bites, may require consultation with a plastic surgeon. Forehead lacerations are rarely associated with skull fractures, but facial or intracranial injuries should be ruled out.

Eyebrow Lacerations

Eyebrow lacerations are common. Repairing an eyebrow laceration is complicated by the presence of hair. It is advisable not to shave the eyebrow for wound preparation because it serves as a landmark during repair. Also, eyebrow regrowth is unpredictable; it may be either slow or incomplete, potentially leading to poor cosmetic outcome. Debridement, if required, should be minimal and along the same axis of the hair shafts to avoid damage to hair follicles; otherwise, alopecia of the brow will result. Closure with simple interrupted stitches using nonabsorbable material is usually sufficient. Attention must be paid to avoid inverting the hair-bearing edges into the wound. It is also important to pay attention to proper alignment of both ends of a wound along an eyebrow.

Eyelid Laceration

Most eyelid lacerations are simple transverse wounds of the upper eyelid just inferior to the eyebrow. Repairing these wounds does not require any special skills. Well-approximated lacerations in the transverse crease of the eyelid will heal well if left alone. However, recognizing complicated eyelid lacerations is crucial for proper repair and optimal outcome. Vertical lacerations involving the lid margin require precision in approximation to avoid deformity and malfunction of the eyelid. Injuries potentially involving the levator palpebrae muscle, medial canthal ligament, or lacrimal duct should be considered for ophthalmology referral. A high index of suspicion for lacrimal duct injury is particularly important when evaluating a medially positioned lower eyelid laceration. If not repaired, inferior duct injury may lead to chronic tearing as the lower lacrimal duct is the main drain of tears from the conjunctival sac. Evaluation for an associated injury of the globe is a must, particularly if periorbital fat is exposed or tarsal plate penetration is present (see Chapter 122 Ocular Trauma).

External Ear Blunt Trauma and Laceration

Although the ears are subject to trauma because of their exposed position, lacerations involving the ears are rather rare. The auricle contains a cartilaginous structure that provides the framework for the complex shape of the ear. The perichondrium covering the cartilage provides it with nutrients and oxygen. Traumatic separation of the cartilage from the perichondrium may lead to necrosis, leaving the auricle deformed. The overlying skin is thin but well vascularized. Skin flaps with small pedicles often survive and should not be hastily debrided. Simple auricular lacerations can be repaired without consultation. To avoid chondritis, approximation of the skin is important so no cartilage is exposed. It is imperative to avoid catching the auricular cartilage with the needle tip because the skin and perichondrium are in close proximity to each other. Occasionally, debridement of the cartilage is needed to obtain complete coaptation of the wound; however, cartilage debridement should be kept to a minimum and only performed by physicians comfortable with this type of repair.

Complex auricular lacerations with significant skin damage and involvement of the auricular cartilage can be difficult to repair and may require consultation with a surgical specialist. In general, when repairing auricular cartilage, 5-0 absorbable sutures should be used to approximate the edges. Landmarks of the auricle should be used for proper alignment. The perichondrium should be included in the sutures so the suture material does not tear through the friable cartilage and also to ensure restoration of nutrient and oxygen supply. For the same reason, excessive tension should be avoided. Closure of the skin should follow as described previously. If the laceration involves the anterior and posterior aspects of the ear, closure of the posterior aspect first is recommended.

To avoid a deep scar line (notching) in repairing the ear lobe or the auricular rim, the skin edges should be everted at the time of closure because fibrotic tissue will eventually pull the scar line down, leading to notching.

For partial avulsion or total amputation of the ear make every effort to reattach the amputated part because tissue survival and cosmetic outcome are often favorable. Furthermore, blunt ear trauma can lead to a simple contusion or a significant subperichondrial hematoma that can comprise the auricular cartilage. Classically, a significant perichondrial hematoma is tense and appears as smooth ecchymotic swelling that disrupts the normal contour of the auricle. This injury is particularly common among wrestlers. Auricular hematoma should be promptly drained to avoid necrosis of the cartilage and deformed auricle or cauliflower ear (see Chapter 114 ENT Trauma).

After repair of ear lacerations or evacuation of an auricular hematoma, a pressure dressing should be applied. Follow-up in 24 hours to evaluate vascular integrity to the area is recommended.

Nasal Laceration

Unlike blunt injuries, lacerations to the nose are unusual. When a laceration results from blunt trauma, careful evaluation of underlying nasal bones and examination for a nasal septal hematoma are essential. Other associated injuries, such as facial bone fractures or injuries to the orbit, should also be ruled out.

The skin overlying the nose is taut and stiff. Approximating the edges of simple, nongaping nasal wounds, mostly along the upper half of the nose, is usually straightforward. Wounds with any gaping, commonly in the lower part of the nose, can be difficult to coapt because of the nature of the skin in this location. The suture material can tear through the skin easily. Absorbable subcutaneous stitches are recommended before skin closure to relieve tension and prevent tearing through the wound edges. Skin closure should be with simple interrupted 6-0 absorbable material. Early removal of the sutures is advised for the same reason.

Full-thickness nasal lacerations involving the alae nasi or entering the vestibule require layered closure. The procedure should start with the nasal mucosa, using absorbable material and finish with the skin, preferably using continuous subcuticular suture technique.

The nasal cartilage, when involved, rarely requires sutures. When alignment is difficult, a few fine sutures (vicryl or plain catgut) will help hold it in place. When the free rim of the nares is involved, precise alignment is imperative for good cosmetic outcome. For complex nasal lacerations, lacerations associated with fractures, or when there is tissue loss, consultation with a surgical specialist is recommended.

Lip Laceration

Lip lacerations are a particular concern because of the importance of the lip as a facial landmark. The lip is a vascular structure with multiple layers. The vermilion border, the junction of the dry oral mucosa and facial skin, serves as an important landmark for proper repair when involved. The relative pallor of the vermilion border to the lip and skin easily identifies it. Therefore, the use of epinephrine with local anesthesia should be avoided so the landmark is not obscured. When parted, the vermilion border should be precisely reapposed using a 6-0 suture. The buccal mucosal surface is then closed with 5-0 absorbable material, followed by the skin, using 6-0 nonabsorbable sutures. Fast absorbing gut is also an alternative. The parents should be warned that, while the lip is still anesthetized, there is a chance that the child will bite the sutures off and that they should distract the child from doing so.

In general, lip lacerations should be closed in layers, depending on the depth of the wound. In full-thickness lip lacerations, a three-layer repair is required. The emergency physician should begin with the oral mucosa, using 5-0 absorbable material, followed by the orbicularis oris muscle layer to include the inner and outer fibrofatty layers, and finish with the skin, using 6-0 nonabsorbable or fast absorbing gut, interrupted sutures. Small wounds, less than 2 cm, on the inner aspect of the lip without communication to the skin surface need not be repaired. External lip wounds not communicating with the mucosal surface can be closed by either single- or double-layer closure, depending on the depth and degree of gaping of the wound. Absorbable sutures (5-0) for the subcutaneous layer and either absorbable or nonabsorbable (6-0) sutures for closure of the skin can be used, depending on the ease with which they can be removed.

Extensive lip injuries with tissue loss or those caused by electric burns, especially those that involve the angle of the mouth, should be referred to a plastic surgeon. Associated injuries such as dental trauma, mandibular fractures, and closed head injuries should be ruled out.

Lacerations of the Cheeks

When managing lacerations involving the cheeks, the physician must evaluate the integrity of the underlying structures. The parotid gland and duct, the facial nerve, and the labial artery are in close proximity of the surface of the skin and can be injured, often as a result of an animal bite. If parotid gland or duct injury is identified, consultation with a surgical specialist is advised. Puncture wounds resulting from animal bites should be debrided and irrigated thoroughly. Some of these puncture wounds are better off left without closure to reduce infection rate, especially if the cosmetic outcome is unlikely to be compromised. Otherwise, simple interrupted 6-0 absorbable sutures can be used to close uncomplicated lacerations of the cheeks.

Tongue Laceration

The tongue is a vascular and muscular organ. Tongue lacerations often hemorrhage excessively in the beginning, but the bleeding usually ceases quickly as the lingual muscle contracts. Controversy exists surrounding the indications for closure, which is in part related to the challenge of repair given the inaccessibility of these wounds.

Most tongue lacerations can be left alone with good results. However, large lacerations involving the free edge may heal with a notch causing dysfunction of the tongue. Generally, this type of laceration should be repaired. Large flaps and lacerations that continue to bleed or are likely to become contaminated with food should also be repaired. Assess patients with tongue lacerations requiring repair for potential airway problems, as well as the need for sedation or even general anesthesia. Often, local or regional anesthesia is sufficient. The mouth should be retained open using a padded tongue depressor placed on the side between the upper and lower teeth or by using a Denhardt–Dingman side mouth gag. The tongue can be maintained in the protruded position by a gentle pull using a towel clip or by placing a temporary suture through the tip to be used for traction. Interrupted 4-0 absorbable suture, with full-thickness bites to include the two mucosal surfaces and the lingual muscle between, will close the tongue wound and provide hemostasis. Multiple knots and inverted sutures are recommended to prevent the untying of the sutures. Some authors suggest that only deep muscle closure is required because the mucosal surface heals rapidly. As in lip lacerations, children may chew off the stitches. Parents must be warned of this possibility and should attempt to distract the child at least until the local anesthesia wears off.

Buccal Mucosa Laceration

Small, isolated lacerations of the buccal mucosa, mostly from impaction of teeth following falls, require no suturing. Lacerations 2 to 3 cm in length or with flaps are best closed with simple interrupted absorbable material. Coated vicryl (4-0) on a round needle is preferred because it is less irritating to the child and is easier to work with than chromic gut. Closure of the mucosal surface in through-and-through lip lacerations should be carried out before closure of the muscle and skin layers. After repair, a soft diet and avoidance of irritating foods should be advised, as well as vigilant mouth hygiene. Evaluation for associated injuries of the teeth or alveolar margin is imperative. Families should be alerted that buccal mucosa lacerations often develop a white ridge during the healing process which is normal and does not indicate infection.

FINGERTIP

CLINICAL PEARLS AND PITFALLS

- Fingertip injuries should be evaluated for an associated nail bed injury and for possible fractures of the phalanges.
- Under 2 years of age, conservative management of simpler injuries without repair will often yield excellent results.
- Not recognizing open fractures, injuries involving the distal interphalangeal joint space or injuries associated with tendon lacerations can lead to serious complications.
- Attempting to drain subungual hematoma after 48 hours is unlikely to be effective.

Avulsion

Fingertip injuries are rather common in children. In the young child, most of these injuries are blunt and secondary to entrapment of the finger in closing doors. Most of these injuries are contused lacerations or partial avulsions. Complete amputation of the fingertips is less common. Sharp injuries such as with knives or equipment are more common in the older child and less likely to be associated with fractures. Fingertip injuries should be evaluated clinically for an associated nail bed injury and radiographically for possible fractures of the phalanges. In general, this type of injury is managed by the emergency physician, especially in the preadolescent child, because tissue regeneration is remarkable and management is mostly conservative. Lacerations can be repaired using absorbable chromic gut.

The management of amputations of fingertips (distal to the distal interphalangeal joint) can be approached based on the absence or presence of bone exposure. If no or minimal bone is exposed, conservative management is advised. In children under 2 years of age, complete distal tip spontaneous regeneration is possible even without a surgical repair. The wound should be cleansed, dressed in nonadherent gauze, and splinted for protection. When tissue from the distal tip is available and has retained its morphology, it can be tacked on to serve as a nonsurviving biologic dressing while underlying tissue develops. Frequent dressing changes and appropriate follow-up should be planned. Antibiotic coverage is recommended. When a significant amount of bone is exposed, consultation with a hand specialist should be considered. Shortening of the distal phalanx and covering the tip with volar skin flap is usually the treatment of choice. However, some hand specialists advocate for various skin-grafting procedures to avoid permanent shortening and deformity. Consider microscopic reimplantation by a surgeon for amputations proximal to the distal interphalangeal joint (see Chapter 117 Hand Trauma).

Nail Bed

Trauma to the distal fingers is often associated with nail and nail bed (matrix) injuries. Nail avulsion can be partial or complete and may or may not be associated with nail bed laceration. An underlying fracture of the distal phalanx may also be present so an x-ray is recommended prior to any repairs. Generally, minor tuft fractures will heal with splinting and do not require an initial surgical evaluation. Injury to the fingertip is often associated with subungual hematoma. In evaluating these injuries, the emergency physician should determine the need to explore the nail bed for a laceration. Unrepaired nail bed lacerations may permanently disfigure the growth of the new nail from the cicatrix nail bed. If the nail is partially avulsed but is firmly attached to its bed, exploring the nail bed is difficult and is probably not warranted. Good outcome is expected because the nail holds the underlying lacerated nail bed tissues in place.

When the nail is completely avulsed or is attached loosely, remove the nail and assess the nail bed for laceration. If the nail bed is lacerated, repair it using 6-0 absorbable material. After cleansing and trimming its soft proximal portion, replace the nail between the nail bed and the nail fold (eponychium), and then anchor it in place with sutures. This will splint the nail fold away from the nail bed, which will prevent the obliteration of the space between the nail bed and the nail fold. If the nail itself is too damaged to replace, a nonadherent sterile gauze can be placed carefully under the nail fold. By preserving this space, the new nail is allowed to grow undisturbed. Some have used tissue adhesive (skin glue) instead of sutures to repair the nail bed and secure the nail (see Chapter 117 Hand Trauma). The preferred method of local anesthesia for nail bed repair is digital block, and the use of a finger tourniquet during the repair allows a bloodless field. The repaired fingertip can be dressed with sterile petrolatum-impregnated gauze and covered with sterile dry dressing. A finger splint after repair is recommended if there is an associated fracture or for added protection against reinjury in young children.

Consultation with a hand specialist is recommended if the fingertip injury includes a larger or complex laceration, or there is an associated tendon injury, fracture other than a minor tuft fracture, dislocation or amputation with exposure of bone or if there is any question about the optimal management. After repair of fingertip injuries, small lacerations can be followed up by the primary care provider. All other injuries should see a hand specialist to ensure appropriate healing.

Subungual Hematoma

A subungual hematoma is a collection of blood in the interface of the nail and the nail bed. It is commonly seen with blunt fingertip injuries. The usual presentation is throbbing pain and discoloration of the nail. Subungual hematomas may be associated with nail bed injury or fracture of the distal phalanx. If the injury >48 hours old the blood is typically clotted and no fluid is released with trephination. Drainage is recommended when greater than 50% of the nail bed surface area is involved, to evaluate for underlying nail bed laceration, or for symptomatic relief of pain.

Usually, drainage of the hematoma provides relief of the symptoms. Generally, no local anesthesia is required for a simple trephination by cauterization of the nail since there are no nerve endings on the nail plate. After drainage, care for simple subungual hematoma includes elevation of the hand and warm soaks for a few days. Inform the family about the possibility of nail deformity in the future. When the injury is more involved, digital block is advised. If the hematoma is large and extends to the tip of the nail, consider separating the nail from nail bed using either a sharp or blunt method to allow drainage. Outcomes with nail trephination and nail removal are similar. In the presence of a distal phalangeal fracture, the physician has to be concerned about transforming a closed fracture to an open one by communicating the subungual, and hence the fracture hematoma, to the exterior surface of the nail. If there is a possibility of an underlying fracture, consider antibiotic coverage and arrange for close follow-up.

GENITOURINARY LACERATIONS

CLINICAL PEARLS AND PITFALLS

- If needed, perform female genital examination under sedation with help from surgical specialist.
- Consider testicular ultrasound if there is suspicion of testicular injury.
- Testicular hematoma or rupture, vaginal wall lacerations, and urethral injuries may all accompany lacerations to the external genitals. Careful physical examination should be performed, and diagnostic imaging pursued as necessary.

Genitourinary lacerations can occur in children after straddle injuries. These injuries are discussed in detail in Chapter 116 Genitourinary Trauma. They typically occur in the context of falls off of climbing structures in playgrounds, sports equipment, or bicycles. When a child inadvertently straddles an object during a fall it can lead to trauma in the genitourinary area. The injuries may range from minor lacerations and hematomas to penetrating extensive lacerations. These types of injuries should also cue the emergency physician to consider sexual assault as a cause (see Chapter 95 Child Abuse/Assault).

In girls, vulvar hematomas or lacerations can occur as a result of a straddle injury. It is essential to determine the extent of the injury before determining the best repair, if any. If the injury is not fully visualized by the emergency physician, secondary to pain or blood obscuring the visualization, consultation with a surgical specialist and/or examination under anesthesia is recommended. Vulvar lacerations usually heal by secondary intention, topical antibiotics, and sitz baths help the healing process. For gaping, deeper lacerations which require primary closure, the placement of absorbable sutures under procedural sedation or general anesthesia is recommended. If a penetrating injury has led to a vaginal laceration, a surgical consultation and consideration for examination under anesthesia is recommended.

In boys, straddle injuries may lead to penile or scrotal lacerations. A thorough genitourinary examination is required to determine the extent of injury. If injury to the urethra is suspected, surgical specialty consultation is warranted and a retrograde urethrogram is required to confirm the diagnosis. Superficial lacerations to the penile shaft and scrotum can be repaired with absorbable sutures. Local anesthesia with a penile block and/or procedural sedation may be required. Urology consultation is recommended if the laceration involves the corporal body of the penile shaft or urethra. Scrotal lacerations also result from sports-related injuries. Superficial lacerations can be repaired with absorbable sutures but if the laceration extends to the dartos layer or is penetrating, there is a risk of testicular injury and this requires surgical specialty consultation in a timely manner.

VASCULAR INJURIES

CLINICAL PEARLS AND PITFALLS

- Vascular injuries may present with a large hematoma, pulsating bleeding, loss of or diminished distal pulses, and color changes.
- A thoughtful approach with adequate preparation and appropriate consultation is required before exploring a potential vascular injury.

With all lacerations, injury to the local vasculature must always be considered to prevent significant sequelae. The evaluation for vascular injury should start with a complete evaluation of pulses. Depending on the wound location, this might include the femoral, popliteal, dorsalis pedis, posterior tibial, axillary, radial, and ulnar pulses. When evaluating pulses it is important to compare the injured side and noninjured side for either absence or asymmetry of the pulse. Signs of arterial injury include, hemorrhage, hematoma, bruit over the wound, absent distal pulses, and signs of ischemia (pallor, pain, coolness).

If there is concern for vascular injury, a surgical consultation should take place. The next step in evaluation may include imaging such as an arteriography or CT angiogram, or direct exploration in the operating room.

LACERATIONS IN PROXIMITY TO JOINTS

CLINICAL PEARLS AND PITFALLS

- Keep a high index of suspicion of possible joint cavity violation when evaluating large wounds in close proximity of large joints such as the knee, elbow and ankle.
- Orthopedic consultation is required when there is concern for joint violation.
- Fluid seepage or "sucking" sound during clinical examination should raise concern immediately.
- Use 3-0 nonabsorbable sutures for noncommunicating lacerations over large joints and consider splinting the extremity to avoid wound dehiscence.

Lacerations that occur near joints need special consideration (see Chapters 37 Injury: Knee and 129 Musculoskeletal Emergencies). These most commonly include lacerations near the knee, elbow, or ankle. With even minor lacerations, if there is joint involvement, the patient may at risk for developing septic arthritis. Indications that the laceration may extend into the joint include: Fluid seepage, sucking wound sound, palpable effusion, painful range of motion, and palpable capsular defect with probing. If it is difficult to assess the penetration of the wound by clinical examination, radiographs may be helpful. Concerning signs on x-ray may include a joint effusion, foreign body near or in the joint, or air in the joint space. If there is any clinical suspicion for joint involvement, orthopedic consultation is advised and antibiotics may be indicated.

Suggested Readings and Key References

American Academy of Pediatrics Committee on Infectious Diseases. Tetanus. In: Pickering LK, ed. *Red book,* 27th ed. Elk Grove Village, IL: AAP, 2006:648–653.

Bansal BC, Wiebe RA, Perkins SD, et al. Tap water for irrigation of lacerations. *Am J Emerg Med* 2002;20:469–472.

Boutros S, Weinfeld AB, Friedman JD. Continuous versus interrupted suturing of traumatic lacerations—a time, cost, and complication rate comparison. *J Trauma* 2000;48:495–497.

Brown DJ, Jaffe JE, Henson JK. Advanced laceration management. *Emerg Med Clin N Am* 2007;25:83–99.

Callahan JM, Baker MD. General wound management. In: Henretig FM, King C, eds. *Textbook of pediatric emergency procedures,* 2nd ed. Philadelphia, PA: Wolters Kluwer Lipincott Williams & Wilkins, 2008:1005–1017.

DeBoard RH, Rondeau DF, Kang CS, et al. Principles of basic wound evaluation and management in the Emergency Department. *Emerg Med Clin North Am* 2007;25:23–29.

Dingeman RS, Mitchell EA, Meyer EC, et al. Parent presence during complex invasive procedures and cardiopulmonary resuscitation: a systematic review of the literature. *Pediatr* 2007;120:842–854.

Ernst AA, Gershoff L, Miller P, et al. Warmed versus room temperature saline for laceration irrigation—a randomized clinical trial. *South Med J* 2003;96:436–439.

Heal C, Buettner P, Raasch B, et al. Can sutures get wet? Prospective randomized control trial of wound management in general practice. *BMJ* 2006;332(7549):1053–1056.

Holger JS, Wnadersee SC, Hale DB, et al. Cosmetic outcomes of facial lacerations repaired with tissue adhesive, absorbable and non-absorbable sutures. *Am J Emerg Med* 2004;22:254–257.

Hood R, Shermock KM, Emerman C. A prospective, randomized pilot evaluation of topical triple antibiotic versus mupirocin for the prevention of uncomplicated soft tissue wound infection. *Am J Emerg Med* 2004;22(1):1–3.

Karounis H, Gouin S, Eisman H, et al. A randomized control trial comparing long-term cosmetic outcomes of traumatic pediatric lacerations repaired with absorbable plain gut versus non-absorbable nylon sutures. *Acad Emerg Med* 2004;11:730–735.

Khan AN, Dayan PS, Miller S, et al. Cosmetic outcome of scalp wound closure with staples in the pediatric emergency department: a prospective, randomized trial. *Pediatr Emerg Care* 2002;18:171–173.

Mark DG, Granquist EJ. Are prophylactic oral antibiotics indicated for the treatment of intraoral wounds? *Ann Emerg Med* 2008;52: 368–372.

Mattick A, Clegg G, Beattie T, et al. A randomized controlled trial comparing a tissue adhesive (2-octylcyanoacrylate) with adhesive strips (Steristrips) for paediatric laceration repair. *Emerg Med J* 2002;19:405–407.

McNamara R, DeAngelis M. Laceration repair with sutures, staples and wound closure tapes. In: Henretig FM, King C, eds. *Textbook of pediatric emergency procedures,* 2nd ed. Philadelphia, PA: Wolters Kluwer/Lippincott Williams & Wilkins, 2008:1018–1044.

Nakamura Y, Daya M. Use of appropriate antimicrobials in wound management. *Emerg Med Clin North Am* 2007;25(1):159–176.

Perelman VS, Francis GJ, Rutledge T, et al. Sterile versus nonsterile gloves for repair of uncomplicated laceration in the emergency department: a randomized controlled trial. *Ann Emerg Med* 2004; 43:362–370.

Singer AJ, Dagum AB. Current management of acute cutaneous wounds. *N Eng J Med* 2008;359:1037–1046.

Singer AJ, Giordano P, Fitch JL, et al. Evaluation of a new high viscosity octylcyanoacrylate tissue adhesive for laceration repair: a randomized, clinical trial. *Acad Emerg Med* 2003;10:1134–1137.

Singer AJ, Mach C, Thode HC Jr, et al. Patient priorities with traumatic lacerations. *Am J Emerg Med* 2000;18:683–686.

Singer AJ, Quinn JV, Thode HC Jr, et al. Determinants of poor outcome after laceration and surgical incision repair. *Plast Reconstr Surg* 2002;110:429–435.

Strauss EJ, Weil WM, Jordan C, et al. A prospective randomized controlled trial of 2-octylcyanoacrylate versus suture repair for nail bed injuries. *J Hand Surg AM* 2008;33:250–253.

Valente JH, Forti RJ, Freundlich LF, et al. Wound irrigation in children: saline solution or tap water? *Ann Emerg Med* 2003;41:609–616.

Weinberger LN, Chen EH, Mills AM. Is screening radiography necessary to detect retained foreign bodies in adequately explored superficial glass-caused wounds? *Ann Emerg Med* 2007;51:666–667.

Zehtabchi S. The role of antibiotic prophylaxis for prevention of infection in patients with simple hand lacerations. *Ann Emerg Med* 2007;49:682–689.

Zempsky WT, Parotti D, Grem C, et al. Randomized controlled comparison of cosmetic outcomes of simple facial lacerations closed with steri-strip skin closures or dermabond tissue adhesive. *Pediatr Emerg Care* 2004;20:519–524.

CHAPTER 119 ■ MUSCULOSKELETAL TRAUMA

RACHEL W. THOMPSON, MD, YOUNG-JO KIM, MD, PhD, AND LOIS K. LEE, MD, MPH

GENERAL PRINCIPLES OF PEDIATRIC ORTHOPEDICS

Goals of Emergency Therapy

Orthopedic trauma currently accounts for 10% to 15% of emergency department (ED) visits in urban pediatric hospitals. The number and spectrum of musculoskeletal injuries sustained by children and adolescents appear to be on the rise since the mid-1990s, in part because of the rapid growth of organized sports and other youth recreational activities. As a consequence of their skeletal immaturity and the associated anatomic and physiologic differences in bony structure, pediatric standards of care, fracture patterns, and outcomes are different than in the adult population. Thus, the emergency clinician must maintain a high level of suspicion for fracture in the child presenting with focal bony pain, even in the absence of obvious deformity. Priorities in the emergency care of these patients include the recognition and treatment of pain by both pharmacologic and other comfort measures, and the consideration of using minimal radiation when possible, given the evidence of the inverse correlation of age and risk of radiation-associated malignancy. Finally, emergency care is performed with the ultimate goal of preserving long-term function. This requires recognizing and addressing factors that may otherwise lead to complications, such as neurovascular compromise, open injuries at risk for infection, and physeal injuries that may lead to growth disturbance.

KEY POINTS

- Injury frequency increases with increasing age as children become more mobile.
- The anatomy and physiology of the immature skeleton results in unique pediatric fracture patterns including greenstick, torus (buckle), and physeal (growth plate) fractures.
- Pediatric bones have less tensile strength than the attached ligaments, resulting in higher rates of fracture from mechanisms that would produce a sprain or dislocation in skeletally mature bone.
- In addition to examination of the injured extremity with inspection, palpation, range of motion (passive and active), and neurovascular examination, there should also be a careful examination of the joints proximal and distal to the point of maximal tenderness.
- The Salter-Harris classification of physeal injuries describes five types of injuries involving the physis and provides important prognostic information.
- Weight-based dosages for pain control should be provided for all pediatric fracture patients both in the ED and once discharged home.

RELATED CHAPTERS

- Cardiopulmonary Resuscitation: Chapter 4
- Interfacility Transport and Stabilization: Chapter 6

Signs and Symptoms
- Immobile Arm: Chapter 34
- Injury: Ankle: Chapter 35
- Injury: Knee: Chapter 37
- Injury: Shoulder: Chapter 38
- Limp: Chapter 41
- Pain: Back: Chapter 49
- Pain: Joints: Chapter 55

Medical, Surgical, and Trauma Emergencies
- Child Abuse/Assault: Chapter 95
- Hand Trauma: Chapter 117
- Neck Trauma: Chapter 120
- Neurotrauma: Chapter 121
- Musculoskeletal Emergencies: Chapter 129
- Procedural Sedation: Chapter 140
- Procedures: Chapter 141

GENERAL PRINCIPLES AND PROPERTIES OF PEDIATRIC FRACTURES

Goals of Treatment

The anatomic and physiologic differences between adults and children are reflected in the different types of fractures and injuries unique to the pediatric age group, including physeal fractures, torus fractures, greenstick fractures, bowing deformities, and avulsion fractures. The emergency clinician must have an understanding of the properties of pediatric bone that result in these unique fractures. With this foundation, the provider can more accurately make the diagnosis and avoid potential complications and missed injuries.

Anatomy and Physiology of Pediatric Bone

CLINICAL PEARLS AND PITFALLS

- During periods of growth, the regions of the pediatric skeleton undergoing rapid metabolic activity are more susceptible to fracture.
- Fracture remodeling in pediatric patients is robust and allows for more angulation at the time of casting, and less frequent operative repair than adult fractures.

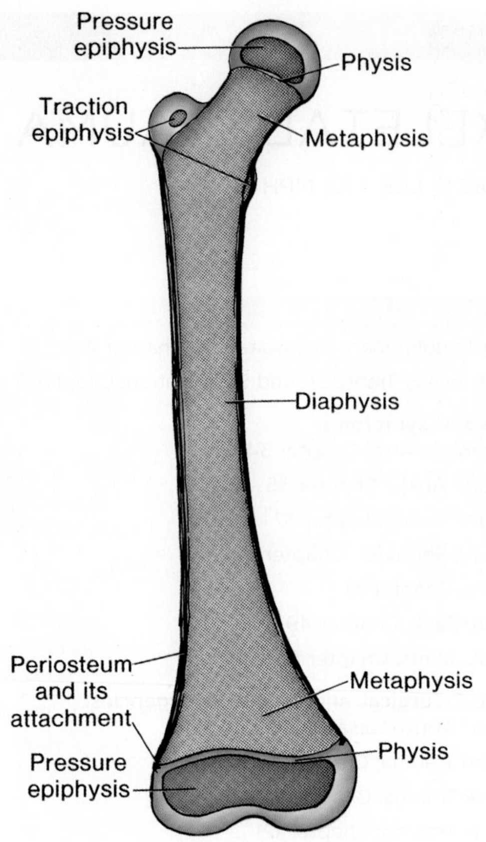

FIGURE 119.1 Diagrammatic representation of the femur in late childhood.

Current Evidence

The basic bony architecture in children includes a thick and active periosteum, a growth plate (physis), an epiphysis (secondary ossification center), and perichondrial rings (Fig. 119.1). Structurally, the bones of a child are much more porous and pliable than those of an adult. As a result, overall bony strength is less, and the incidence of fractures is greater in children than in adults. Moreover, ligaments have greater strength than the physes and perichondrial rings; thus, a child is more likely to suffer a fracture from an injury that, in a skeletally mature individual, would result in a sprain, ligamentous injury, or dislocation.

Unlike in adults, remodeling and anatomic fracture union for pediatric fractures is the expectation rather than the exception. In general, significant remodeling can be anticipated both in younger children and when the fracture occurs in the metaphysis of growing bones. The greatest degree of remodeling is anticipated with bony injuries occurring in the plane of motion of the adjacent joint. In contrast, the injuries least likely to correct without intervention include those that occur in the diaphysis of long bones in adolescents, those with bowing greater than 10 degrees, and fractures with rotational malalignment. In general, the goal is to obtain as near an anatomic reduction of the fracture fragments as possible in all age groups and not to rely on remodeling to align angulated fractures; however, relative guidelines for acceptable angulation by age are provided.

Physeal Fractures

- Salter–Harris type I injuries are frequently diagnosed clinically by point tenderness at the physis and may not be evident radiographically.
- Selective use of radiographs of the contralateral extremity may help with diagnosing physeal injury.
- An important complication of physeal fractures is growth disturbance, which may result in angular deformity, limb length discrepancy, and/or epiphyseal distortion.
- Orthopedic referral is an important component of management and follow up for these injuries.

The physis is the transition zone between the metaphysis and the epiphysis. In assessing young children with musculoskeletal trauma, the clinician must be attuned to the possibility of fractures occurring at the physis (growth plate), which may not be readily apparent on plain film. These relatively common injuries generally occur through the zone of provisional calcification, a relatively weak area of the germinal growth plate that becomes even more susceptible to injury during periods of growth in adolescence (peak incidence at 11 to 12 years of age). Most growth plate injuries occur in the upper limb, particularly in the radius and ulna.

Several classification systems have been described for physeal fractures. The most widely used is that of Salter and Harris, who described five types of growth plate fractures, each having specific prognostic and treatment implications (Fig. 119.2).

Salter–Harris type I fracture. This fracture type is a separation of the metaphysis from the epiphysis through the zone of provisional calcification resulting in a widening of the physeal space. Diagnosis may be challenging if displacement is minimal. Radiographs may only show associated soft tissue swelling. Type I fractures are generally benign, and growth disturbance is uncommon if near-anatomic reduction is achieved. Exceptions include type I injuries of the proximal and distal femur and the proximal tibia, which are subject to premature physeal closure and posttraumatic growth arrest. In general, when radiographic studies are negative, but physical examination findings are suggestive of a Salter–Harris type I injury (e.g., point tenderness over a growth plate), immobilization and a follow-up examination are essential. Imaging showing periosteal reaction along the physis 7 to 10 days after possible Salter–Harris fractures may help diagnose the occult injury.

Salter–Harris type II fracture. Type II fractures are the most common type of pediatric physeal fracture. These fractures extend through both the physis and the metaphysis. Like the type I injuries, these fractures generally carry a good prognosis and rarely cause functional deformity.

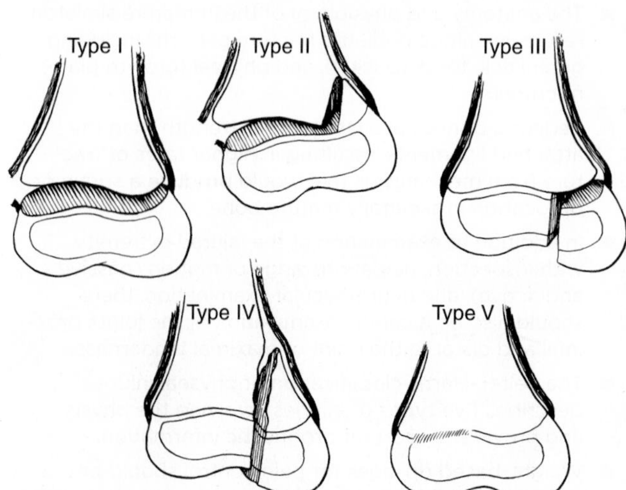

FIGURE 119.2 The Salter–Harris classification for physeal fractures. The prognosis for growth disturbance worsens from type I through type V.

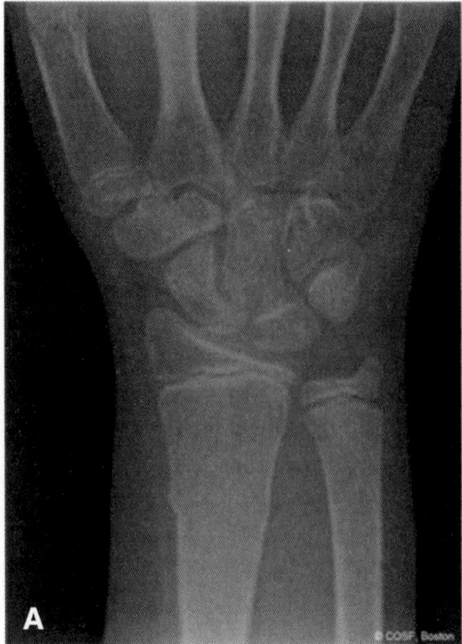

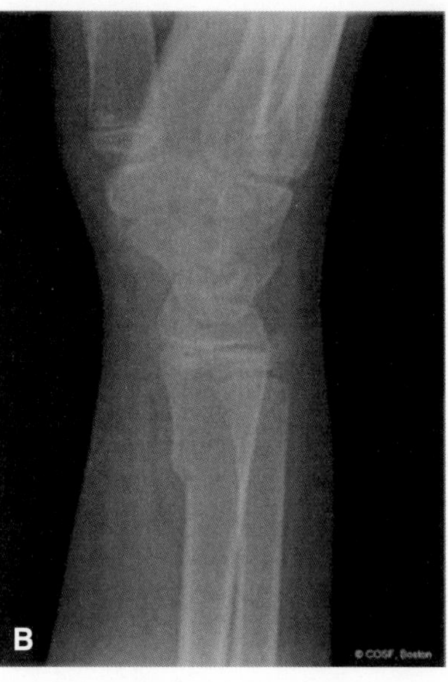

FIGURE 119.3 Anteroposterior (**A**) and lateral (**B**) radiographs of a distal radius torus fracture. (From Flynn JM, Skaggs DL, Waters PM. *Rockwood and Wilkins' fractures in children*. 8th ed. Philadelphia, PA: Wolters Kluwer, 2014.)

Salter–Harris type III and IV fractures. Type III and IV injuries are growth plate injuries that involve the intra-articular surface. In type III fractures, the fracture line typically extends from the epiphysis into the physis, resulting in a separation of the epiphysis and its associated growth plate from the rest of the epiphysis. The fracture line in type IV injuries crosses through all three regions of the bone (epiphysis, physis, and metaphysis). Anatomic position must be reestablished to restore normal joint mechanics and prevent growth disturbance. Because of these risks, which may result in functional disability, orthopedic consultation should be obtained while the patient is in the ED for all but the most minor type III and IV injuries.

Salter–Harris type V fracture. Type V fractures are the least common physeal fracture, and most commonly occur at the knee and ankle. These fractures are a crushing injury of the growth plate as a result of axial compression. It is often difficult to diagnose these injuries during the ED presentation, but a high index of suspicion should be maintained if there is a concerning mechanism or presence of a joint effusion in the absence of radiographic abnormalities of the bone. These fractures have the worst prognosis for growth disturbance as the compressive force may result in premature closure of the physis. Unfortunately, the diagnosis is often made in hindsight after a growth arrest becomes evident.

Torus Fractures

Torus (buckle) fractures are common fractures in young children. They most often occur at the junction of metaphysis and diaphysis from a compressive load. The cortex of the bone buckles in a small area, resulting in a stable fracture pattern (Fig. 119.3). As the child matures, the stiffness of the metaphyseal region increases, and the incidence of this fracture pattern decreases.

Greenstick Fractures

The composition of pediatric bones makes them less likely to propagate the force of injury into comminuted fragments. Thus, with greenstick injuries, the bone bends before it breaks, with the thick and active periosteum remaining intact on one cortex and acting like a hinge: torn on the convex side of the fracture while remaining intact on the concave side. The intact cortex thus maintains apposition at the site of fracture; however, to obtain an anatomic reduction, the fracture must often first be completed. The emergency clinician must be attuned to this injury as inadequate reduction of the deformation or bowing of the bone can result in an abnormal growth pattern and loss of function (Fig. 119.4).

Bowing Fractures

Bowing fractures occur uniquely in children. Evidence suggests that the mechanism is a longitudinal force causing "plastic" deformation (bowing), but stops short of creating a fracture (Fig. 119.4). Little remodeling can be expected from the injury, and both cosmetic and functional deficits are common. Anatomic reduction produces the most satisfactory result. All bowing deformities should be referred to an orthopedic surgeon.

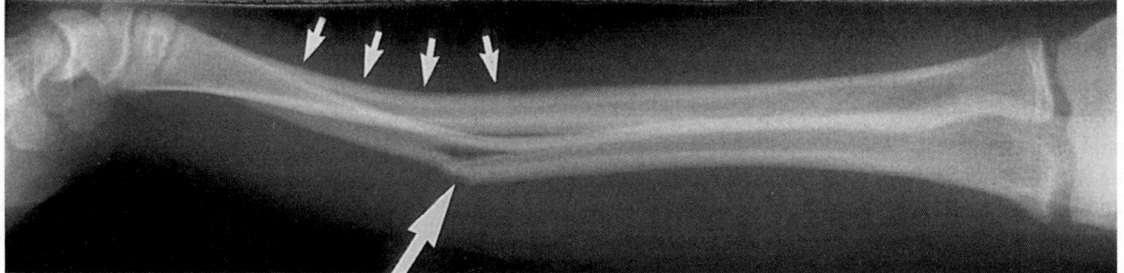

FIGURE 119.4 Greenstick fracture of the ulna (*large arrow*) and a bowing fracture (*small arrows*) of the radius. The extent of bowing can often be fully appreciated only with comparison views of the opposite extremity.

Avulsion Fractures

The frequency of avulsion fractures in pediatrics is a consequence of the strong muscular attachments to relatively weak secondary centers of ossification in the developing skeleton known as apophyses. During intense muscular contraction, fractures can occur through the apophyseal plate. Common sites include the pelvis, tibial tubercle, and the phalanges. Avulsion fractures infrequently require open or closed reduction. Conservative care is the mainstay of treatment.

GENERAL PRINCIPLES OF ACUTE ORTHOPEDIC CARE

CLINICAL PEARLS AND PITFALLS

- Any child with obvious extremity deformity should be made *nil per os* (NPO) at triage given the potential need for procedural sedation or operative management for fracture reduction and casting.
- Based on the history and mechanism of injury, the possibility of other injuries (e.g., head, chest, intra-abdominal organs) should be considered.
- Physical examination must include inspection, palpation, range of motion (passive and active), and neurovascular examination with careful examination of the joints proximal and distal to the point of maximal tenderness.
- Always carefully remove all splints, bandages, and clothing in order to perform an accurate examination with documentation of breaks in the skin, which may represent a possible open fracture.
- Splinting the injured extremity immediately after evaluation and before radiographs are taken can decrease the child's discomfort and prevent further injury.
- Neurovascular status should be assessed before and after any splinting is performed.
- If the orthopedist is not readily available, gentle longitudinal traction and gross realignment may be performed by the emergency clinician for fractures that are grossly displaced, unstable, or if there is vascular compromise.

Current Evidence

Rapid assessment and treatment of pain both in the ED and after discharge are key components of the emergency care of musculoskeletal trauma. Increasingly, triage protocols include the administration of appropriate oral analgesics prior to physician care. For significantly painful injuries, clinicians should consider intranasal fentanyl, which has the advantage of a relatively fast onset of action (<5 minutes) without requiring an IV. With this initial pain control in place, an IV can then be placed for intravenous narcotics if clinically indicated.

After discharge from the ED, children experience the most fracture pain in the first 3 days. Ibuprofen, acetaminophen, or oxycodone is recommended for pain control at home. Those requiring narcotics for pain control while in the ED and those children discharged overnight (between 10 PM and 8 AM) have an increased risk of having more pain, and these children may benefit from having a prescription for oral narcotics to be taken at home for pain. Acetaminophen with codeine is no longer recommended due to the variable metabolism of codeine in different populations, leading to either ineffective pain control or the risk of respiratory compromise.

Goals of Treatment

A systematic approach to the evaluation and management of pediatric musculoskeletal injuries is important in order to avoid overlooked injuries and prevent potential complications. The initial goals of treatment in the ED are to provide pain control, evaluate the injured extremity for any neurovascular compromise, and immobilize the injured area. Next, the specific injury must be identified with physical examination and radiologic imaging. The injured extremity should be immobilized to enhance comfort and prevent further trauma until definitive orthopedic care can be obtained. Adjunctive interventions such as elevating the injured extremity and applying a cold pack can help mitigate swelling.

Clinical Considerations

Clinical Recognition

A history of a traumatic event with physical examination findings of a painful extremity or body part with swelling, or deformity or the inability to use the extremity allows for rapid recognition of a musculoskeletal injury. Less severe injuries may be more difficult to diagnose as they may present with only mild swelling or a history of not using the extremity normally. For long bone injuries, the joints above and below the injured extremity must be examined for possible associated injuries.

Triage Considerations

Children presenting with significant pain or with a grossly deformed extremity should be evaluated immediately by the emergency clinician. A focused neurovascular assessment should be performed. Those children with a more subacute presentation (e.g., trauma occurred the day prior), and those with minimal pain may be seen less urgently.

Clinical Assessment

The injured extremity should be inspected for swelling and deformity, and the joints above and below the injury should be examined. The skin should be examined for ecchymosis, abrasions, lacerations, soft tissue defects, or exposed bone. If an open wound is present, the location, degree of contamination, and rate of active bleeding should be documented. The neurovascular status should be determined by examining the motor and sensory function distal to the fracture site. The pulses should be palpated and capillary refill assessed.

Management

Imaging. In addition to the physical examination, the history and knowledge of the most common injuries for a specific age group can guide the choice of radiographic studies. The radiographs should include the joints proximal and distal to the fracture and should include at least two views taken at 90 degrees to one another (i.e., anteroposterior and lateral views). When routine views do not identify a fracture, but clinical suspicion is high, oblique or other additional views may be useful. With the degree of normal variability, especially with the immature bone, comparison views of the contralateral extremity may be helpful to determine if a radiographic finding is a traumatic injury or normal anatomy.

In addition to plain radiography, advanced imaging may be indicated for further evaluation of the injury. For complex, intra-articular, or spine injuries, computed tomography (CT) is often used. Although not commonly used in the ED, magnetic resonance imaging (MRI) is also used for the evaluation of physeal injuries as well as the diagnosis of avulsion and stress fractures, as it can visualize cartilaginous and soft tissue structures as well as osseous ones. The use of ultrasound in the ED setting is also expanding, both for diagnosis as well as to guide closed fracture reduction.

Immobilization. Paired with pain control, immobilization is fundamental to the initial treatment of fractures. Either plaster or fiberglass may be used to immobilize the fractured bone as well as the joints above and below the fracture. Immobilization provides pain control and helps to prevent further injury. The application of several layers of padding material before the splint or cast is placed is important for comfort and to decrease neurovascular compromise from swelling of the extremity (see Chapter 141 Procedures, section on Splinting of Musculoskeletal Injuries). The decision for the emergency clinician to splint or place a circumferential cast depends on the degree of actual or anticipated swelling, the risk for compartment syndrome, and the training of the provider.

Pain Control. At triage, pain management can begin with oral analgesics (e.g., ibuprofen, acetaminophen), either given alone or in combination. For injuries with more significant pain, intranasal fentanyl or intravenous narcotics may be administered. In addition, local and regional anesthesia blocks may be used based on the injury location. When fracture reduction is performed in the ED, procedural sedation with nitrous oxide or intravenous agents should be used by appropriately trained personnel (see Chapter 140 Procedural Sedation).

Orthopedic Consultation and Referral. When consulting the orthopedic surgeon, the emergency clinician needs to present accurate and descriptive information about the injury so the orthopedist can make appropriate treatment recommendations. The initial communication should include patient's age and gender, mechanism of injury, anatomic location, neurovascular status, and extent of soft tissue injury. The radiographic description should note the anatomic location of the fracture, the type of fracture (e.g., transverse, spiral, oblique), amount of displacement, degree of angulation, shortening, or malrotation, degree of comminution, and the extent of involvement of the joint and physis (Fig. 119.5). Displacement for long bone fractures is commonly described using the approximate percentage of the shaft width displaced. Angulation is measured by drawing one line along the proximal fracture fragment as the reference and another line along the distal fracture fragment. The angle measured between the axes of those two lines describes the degree of angulation of the fracture.

Indications for orthopedic consultation will vary with the ability and experience of the emergency clinician and availability of the orthopedist. Emergent orthopedic consultation is required to evaluate open fractures, those that are significantly displaced, or if neurovascular compromise is present. Orthopedic consultation is also recommended during ED visits for pelvic fractures (other than avulsions), spinal injuries, and dislocations of major joints (other than the shoulder). Referral to see an orthopedist as an outpatient within 24 to 48 hours is recommended for any growth plate or intra-articular fractures that have more than 2 to 3 mm of displacement and for fractures of the lower extremity long bones, as long as the extremity is neurovascularly intact and pain is adequately controlled. Physeal injuries begin healing quickly; therefore, urgent orthopedic referral is important to ensure adequate reduction of any displaced fractures within a safe time period. Referral for outpatient orthopedic follow-up after initial ED management is recommended for (1) most nondisplaced Salter–Harris type I fractures, (2) nondisplaced upper extremity, foot, and phalangeal fractures, (3) incomplete, nondisplaced fractures of the lower extremity long bones, and (4) reassessment of reduced routine dislocations of the minor joints and shoulder (Table 119.1).

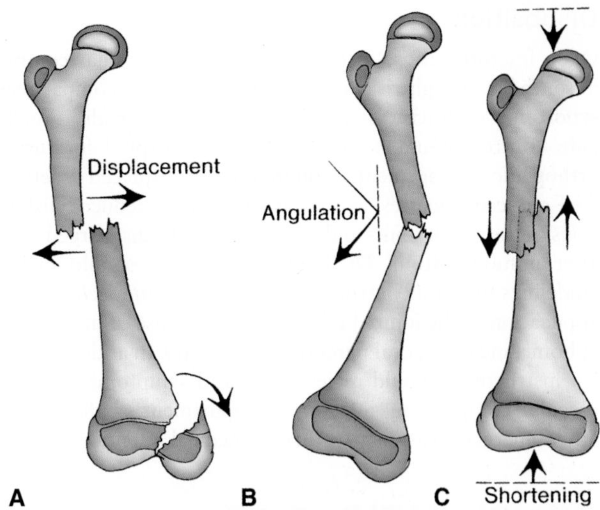

FIGURE 119.5 Diagrammatic representation of fracture deformities: displacement (**A**), angulation (**B**), and overriding with shortening (**C**).

TABLE 119.1

INDICATIONS FOR ORTHOPEDIC REFERRAL

Injuries that require immediate orthopedic referral
Open fractures
Concern for compartment syndrome
Unacceptably displaced fractures that require reduction
Significant growth plate or joint injuries
Complete or displaced fractures of the long bones of the lower extremities
Pelvic fractures (other than minor avulsions)
Spinal fractures
Dislocations of major joints other than the shoulder
Injuries that can be managed initially by the emergency clinician with outpatient orthopedic follow-up
Nondisplaced Salter–Harris type I fractures (exceptions are femur, proximal tibia)
Clavicle fractures
Nondisplaced upper extremity fractures
Routine dislocations of the shoulder and minor joints (finger) with no fracture
Nondisplaced fractures of the hand and foot
Incomplete, nondisplaced fractures of the long bones of the lower extremities

Disposition

Open fractures, those associated with neurovascular compromise, those at high risk for the development of compartment syndrome, or fractures requiring intravenous medication for pain control should be admitted to the hospital for further orthopedic management. Non/minimally displaced fractures, well-reduced fractures, as well as successfully reduced dislocations of the minor joints and shoulder, may be discharged home after immobilization. Discharge instructions should include guidelines for pain control such as elevation and ice/cold pack application to the injured extremity and the use of medications at home, including oral narcotics if necessary. In addition, written instructions should review signs and symptoms of neurovascular compromise, infection, compartment syndrome, and other emergent reasons to return to medical attention.

COMPLICATIONS OF FRACTURES: OPEN FRACTURES AND COMPARTMENT SYNDROME

Goals of Treatment

Rapid identification of a potential open fracture or compartment syndrome is important for urgent orthopedic consultation. Open fractures have an increased risk of infection; therefore, early wound management and prophylactic antibiotics in the ED are vital. Compartment syndrome, if not identified and treated, can progress to irreversible muscle and nerve damage. Early consultation with orthopedics is necessary for fasciotomy.

CLINICAL PEARLS AND PITFALLS

- The laceration associated with an open fracture should not be closed in the ED, even if the fracture is nondisplaced.
- Antibiotics should be administered as soon as possible to a patient with an open fracture to minimize risk of infection.
- Compartment syndrome associated with a fracture can occur in the forearm, hand, leg, or foot, with the leg being the most common fracture location.
- The fractures associated with compartment syndrome do not need to be severe.
- Pain out of proportion to the injury or increasing pain after analgesics, especially with passive extension, is one of the earliest signs of compartment syndrome.
- Compartment syndrome may present not only shortly after the fracture is sustained, but may also occur after reduction and casting. Therefore, neurovascular status must be checked in the injured extremity after casting.
- Fasciotomy should be considered when clinical symptoms of compartment syndrome are present and/or when compartment pressures measured in the injured extremity are within 30 mm Hg of the patient's diastolic blood pressure or the mean arterial pressure.

Current Evidence

A fracture is considered to be "open" when the injury results in disruption of the skin and underlying soft tissues overlying the fracture, thus providing a communication between the fracture and the outside environment. The organisms found to be contaminating an open fracture at the time of presentation do not represent the microbes that will eventually cause infection; therefore, wound cultures are of minimal utility. Most open fracture infections are caused by gram-negative rods and gram-positive staphylococci; however, clinicians should be mindful of a rising frequency of infections caused by methicillin-resistant *Staphylococcus aureus*. While there is consensus supporting the administration of antibiotics as soon as possible to minimize risk of infection, there are variable recommendations on the optimal regimen.

Children with compartment syndrome may present with only one associated sign or symptom, with pain being the most common presentation. In one study of compartment syndrome with tibial shaft fractures, adolescents (14 years and older) had an increased risk of compartment syndrome compared with younger children.

Clinical Considerations

Clinical Recognition

Open fractures typically occur due to a high-energy mechanism; therefore, a complete examination to identify other potentially life-threatening injuries is imperative. A fractured extremity should be carefully examined for the presence of an open wound, potentially signifying an open fracture. However, it is not always obvious if the injury is an open fracture or if it is a laceration that does not communicate with the fracture. Operative exploration by the orthopedist may be necessary to determine this.

Compartment syndrome develops when there is an accumulation of intracompartmental pressure resulting in obstruction of venous outflow and then increased pressure in the nonelastic compartment. If untreated, small arterioles and capillaries are eventually occluded, resulting in ischemia with irreversible muscle and neurovascular tissue damage. Compartment syndrome must be suspected with any fracture or blunt tissue injury when there is pain out of proportion to the injury or if the pain is increasing, despite analgesic administration. The patient may also complain of paresthesias and pain with passive extension. On physical examination the patient may have pallor and pulselessness of the injured extremity, although these may be late findings.

Triage Considerations

Children presenting with a concern for an open fracture or compartment syndrome should be evaluated immediately in the ED with urgent orthopedic consultation.

Clinical Assessment

For open fractures, the wound should be carefully examined and considered in the context of the fracture location. With compartment syndrome, the extremity may be pale and the muscular compartments may be swollen and feel hard and tense. The pulses may be diminished or absent and the limb may have paralysis or muscle weakness. Children may present with only a single sign or symptom of compartment syndrome.

Management

Open wounds should be cleaned and a sterile dressing applied. The fracture should be immobilized. Prophylactic intravenous antibiotics should be administered, and tetanus prophylaxis should be given according to the usual guidelines. Current antibiotic recommendations are for the administration of early, systemic, wide-spectrum antibiotic therapy directed at gram-positive and gram-negative organisms. A commonly recommended regimen is for a first-generation cephalosporin (e.g., cefazolin) with the addition of an aminoglycoside (e.g., gentamicin) for larger open fractures (skin laceration >1 cm with significant soft tissue damage and contamination). As an alternative to aminoglycosides, a third-generation cephalosporin or other agent with activity against gram-negative bacteria may be selected. For injuries at high risk for anaerobic infection (e.g., occurring on a farm), clinicians should add ampicillin or penicillin. Urgent orthopedic consultation is necessary for surgical debridement, irrigation, and definitive care of the wound and fracture.

If there is suspicion for compartment syndrome, compartment pressures in the injured extremity should be obtained; however, this may be difficult in an awake young child, especially if less than 5 years old. Compartment pressures >30 mm Hg have been used to diagnose compartment syndrome. Newer approaches suggest that compartment pressures should be interpreted in the context of systemic blood pressures. Compartment pressures within 30 mm Hg of either the diastolic blood pressure or the mean arterial pressure are concerning for compartment syndrome. Urgent orthopedic consultation is necessary if there is any concern for compartment syndrome, which may require treatment with fasciotomy.

Disposition

All children with open fractures or with concern for/diagnosis of compartment syndrome should be admitted to the hospital for ongoing orthopedic care given the high risks for infection and neuromuscular injury.

MULTIPLE TRAUMA

CLINICAL PEARLS AND PITFALLS

- Shock is uncommonly caused by blood loss from a fracture, except in the setting of extensive pelvic fractures or multiple long bone fractures; therefore, the presence of other injuries should be evaluated if shock is present.
- After the initial trauma evaluation and resuscitation, a thorough secondary survey is important to identify other possible orthopedic as well as nonorthopedic injuries.
- Thoracic and lumbar spine fractures are challenging to diagnose by physical examination in the setting of multisystem trauma. If the injury mechanism or examination is concerning for possible spinal injury, radiographs should be obtained and careful immobilization maintained.

In the setting of multisystem trauma, fractures may be common and sometimes are the most obvious injury, but they are rarely life-threatening. The usual trauma evaluation and resuscitation protocol should be followed for any child with concern for multisystem trauma and/or a severe mechanism of injury. After the child has been stabilized, the injured extremity should be immobilized. For unstable pelvic injuries with associated bleeding, wrapping the pelvis tightly in a sheet or the application of an external fixator device may help tamponade the bleeding.

PHYSICAL ABUSE

CLINICAL PEARLS AND PITFALLS

- Spiral fractures and metaphyseal–epiphyseal injuries in nonambulatory children are highly suspicious for nonaccidental trauma (Fig. 119.6).
- Nonaccidental trauma should be considered for children with a fracture in the absence of a history of substantial trauma, or if any of the following are present:
  - Multiple fractures, which may be in various stages of healing
  - Delayed presentation with evidence of bone healing at time of ED visit
  - Presence of rib fractures
  - Femur fracture in a nonambulatory child
  - Midshaft humeral fracture (less than 3 years old)
  - History inconsistent with the developmental stage of the child

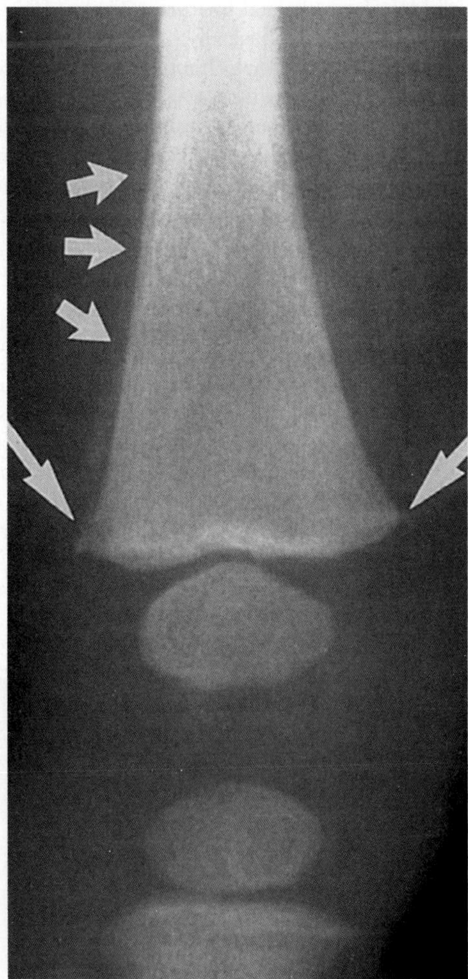

FIGURE 119.6 Radiograph of the right knee of a 3.5-month-old victim of physical abuse. The metaphyseal corner fractures (*large arrows*) are considered diagnostic of abuse. Also evident is periosteal new bone formation (*small arrows*), proof of a significant delay between injury and medical evaluation.

TABLE 119.2

FRACTURES STRONGLY SUGGESTIVE OF PHYSICAL ABUSE[a]

1. Fractures inconsistent with history
2. Fractures inconsistent with developmental stage of the child
3. Fractures with associated injuries suggestive of abuse
4. Multiple fractures, particularly in various stages of healing
5. Skull fractures (including multiple or depressed skull fractures)
6. Rib fractures
7. Fractures of the femur or tibia in a preambulatory child
8. Spiral or midshaft fractures of the humerus
9. Metaphyseal chip (corner) fractures
10. Avulsion fractures of the clavicle and acromion process

[a]Especially in children less than 18 months old.
From Kemp AM, Dunstan F, Harrison S, et al. Patterns of skeletal fractures in children abuse: systematic review. *BMJ* 2008;337:a1518.

Among all childhood fractures, nonaccidental trauma accounts for a relatively small proportion of these injuries. However, of children who have been investigated for abuse, up to a third of these children have skeletal fractures (Table 119.2). These fractures may be occult, and usually occur in infants and toddlers. The presence of multiple fractures occurs more often with nonaccidental trauma. If there is suspicion for nonaccidental trauma as the cause of the fracture, a child protection team should be consulted for further evaluation and management, including the determination of need for a skeletal survey to assess for other occult fractures (see Chapter 95 Child Abuse/Assault).

PATHOLOGIC FRACTURES

A fracture that occurs through abnormal bone is considered a pathologic fracture (Figs. 119.7 and 119.8). The predisposing condition may not become apparent until after the fracture occurs. Bony tumors, hereditary diseases, metabolic disorders, neuromuscular disease, and infections can cause focal or generalized bone weakness, making it more prone to fracture. Urgent orthopedic consultation should be obtained for all pathologic fractures with other specialists consulted based on the suspected underlying disease process (Table 119.3).

TABLE 119.3

DIFFERENTIAL DIAGNOSIS OF PATHOLOGIC FRACTURES

Tumors and cysts—benign
Aneurysmal bone cyst
Enchondroma
Eosinophilic granuloma
Fibrous dysplasia
Giant cell tumor
Nonossifying fibroma
Osteochondroma
Unicameral bone cyst

Tumors—malignant
Chondrosarcoma
Ewing sarcoma
Neuroblastoma
Osteogenic sarcoma

Hereditary diseases
Gaucher disease
Neurofibromatosis
Osteogenesis imperfecta
Osteopetrosis
Sickle cell disease

Metabolic disorders
Copper deficiency
Cushing syndrome
Hyperparathyroidism
Renal osteodystrophy
Rickets
Scurvy

Neuromuscular diseases (osteoporosis from disuse)
Cerebral palsy
Muscular dystrophy
Poliomyelitis
Severe head injury
Spina bifida with paraplegia
Traumatic paraplegia or quadriplegia

Infections
Osteomyelitis

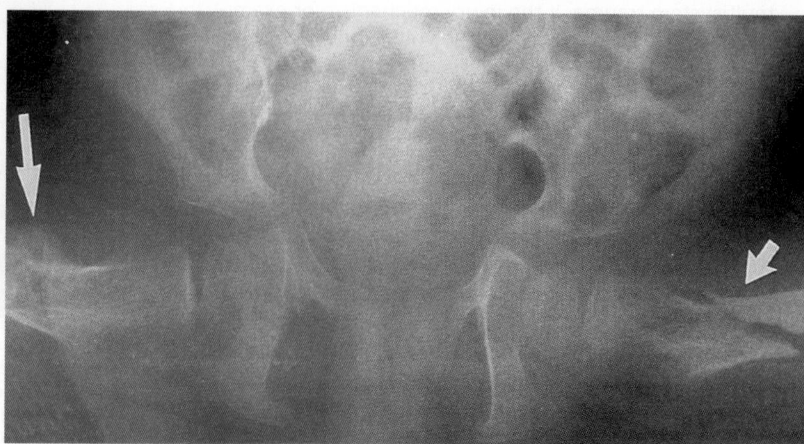

FIGURE 119.7 Radiograph of the pelvis and femur of an 18-month-old girl with osteogenesis imperfecta. There is a healing fracture of the right femur (*large arrow*), as well as an acute fracture of the left femur (*small arrow*).

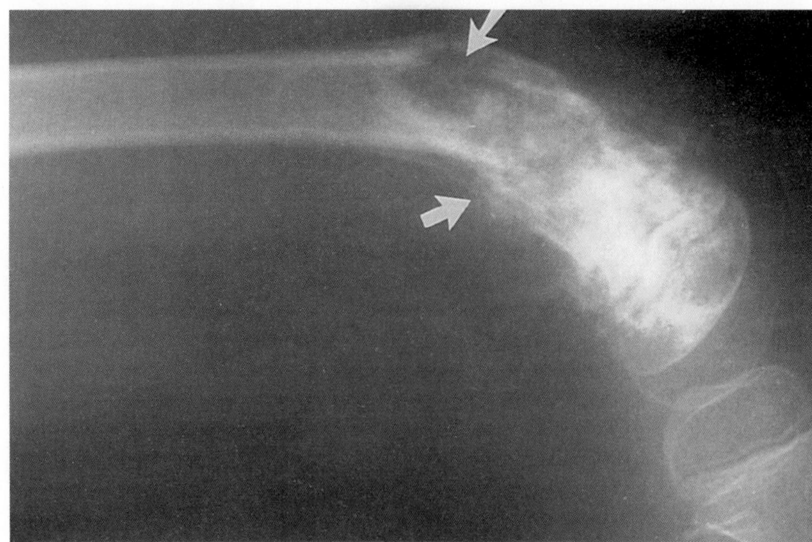

FIGURE 119.8 Radiograph of a 5-year-old girl with an osteosarcoma of the left femur showing an acute pathologic fracture (*arrows*). Amputation was ultimately necessary.

INJURIES OF THE UPPER EXTREMITIES

Injuries of the Shoulder and Humerus

Clavicle Fractures and Acromioclavicular Joint Injuries

Goals of Treatment. Fractures of the clavicle can be divided into three categories: fractures of the shaft, the medial end, and the lateral or distal portion. Injuries to the lateral aspect of the clavicle must be distinguished from acromioclavicular (AC) joint injuries. Recognition of the type of injury and location of the fracture dictates whether the fracture requires any advanced imaging, orthopedic consultation, and operative repair. The majority of fractures of the clavicle heal without complication and with full recovery of strength and range of motion. Injuries to the medial and lateral aspects of the clavicle include dislocations and physeal injuries; true medial dislocations are rare, but are important to recognize given the potential for vascular injury.

CLINICAL PEARLS AND PITFALLS

- Clavicle fractures in children less than 2 years (excluding the newborn period), particularly of the lateral end of the clavicle are uncommon, and should raise concern for possible nonaccidental trauma.
- The newborn or preverbal child who cries upon being picked up under the arms should be evaluated for possible clavicular fracture.
- Patients with sternoclavicular fractures and dislocations following blunt-force trauma to the chest, may present with referred pain to the shoulder and neck. A careful examination is critical, as posteriorly displaced sternoclavicular fractures may cause damage to the underlying neurovascular and airway structures.
- Complications in the healing of shaft fractures, such as nonunion, malunion, and refracture, can result in chronic pain, deceased range of motion, weakness, or cosmetic deformity.

Current Evidence. The clavicle is the most frequently fractured bone in children, and management considerations vary by the location of fracture (medial, shaft, or distal), age of patient, and degree of displacement. Clavicle fractures may occur in newborns as a result of birth trauma, and in ambulatory children and adolescents secondary to a fall onto the shoulder or an outstretched hand, or from a direct blow to the clavicle. Indications for operative management of clavicle fractures are evolving. While skeletally immature patients have a high rate of fracture healing and good remodeling, recent evidence in the adult literature suggests there may be superior outcomes in patients treated operatively for completely displaced midshaft fractures. Skeletally mature adolescents, with their higher activity level and functional expectations, may also potentially benefit from an interventional approach, thus challenging the traditional nonoperative approach that has been the standard in this age group.

Clinical Considerations

Clinical recognition. Children may present with shoulder pain and cradling of the injured arm, however not uncommonly, these fractures can go unnoticed until a large callus forms and then it gradually remodels over the next 6 to 12 months. The most common fracture type in younger patients is a greenstick fracture of the midshaft, attributable to the thick periosteum of this part of the bone, which is protective against significant angulation and displacement. Older children and adolescents are at higher risk for complete displacement, which is suggested on physical examination by a lowering of the affected shoulder, local swelling, and point tenderness. Medial injuries to the sternoclavicular joint, suggested by localized pain and swelling or a palpable anterior or posterior displacement, are typically physeal injuries secondary to the strong ligaments that anchor the clavicle to the sternum and the relative weakness of the physis. The lateral aspect of the clavicle is anchored by the coracoclavicular and AC ligaments, and thus, fracture through the physis is more common than dislocation (Fig. 119.9). Lateral physeal separation presents clinically as pain with all movements of the shoulder. Typically, the proximal fracture fragment is displaced superiorly, and the radiographic appearance suggests AC separation. However, the periosteum remains whole inferiorly with

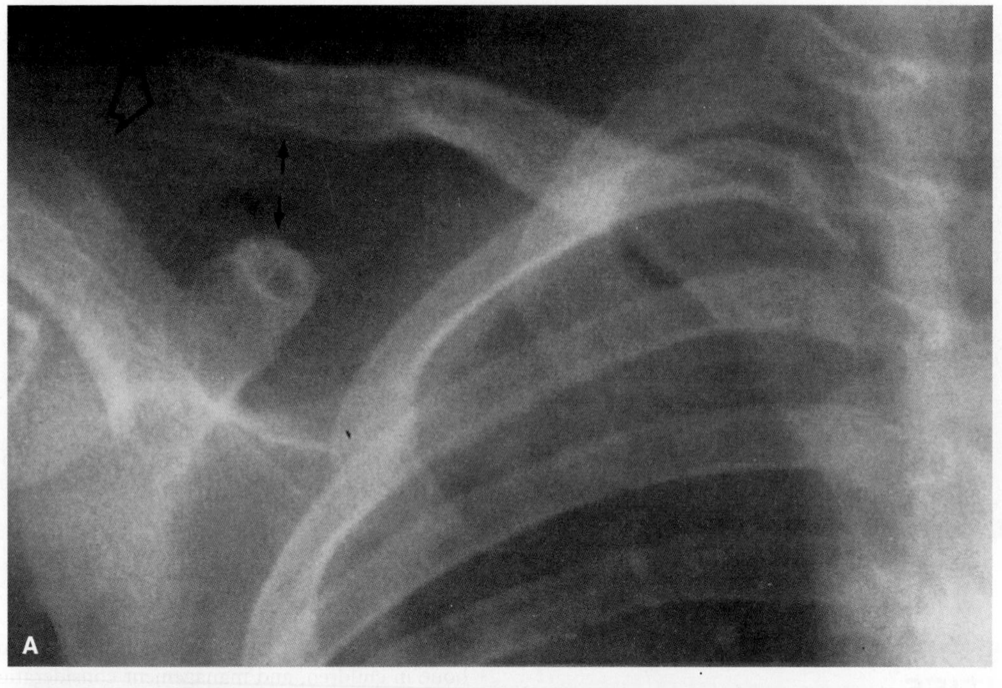

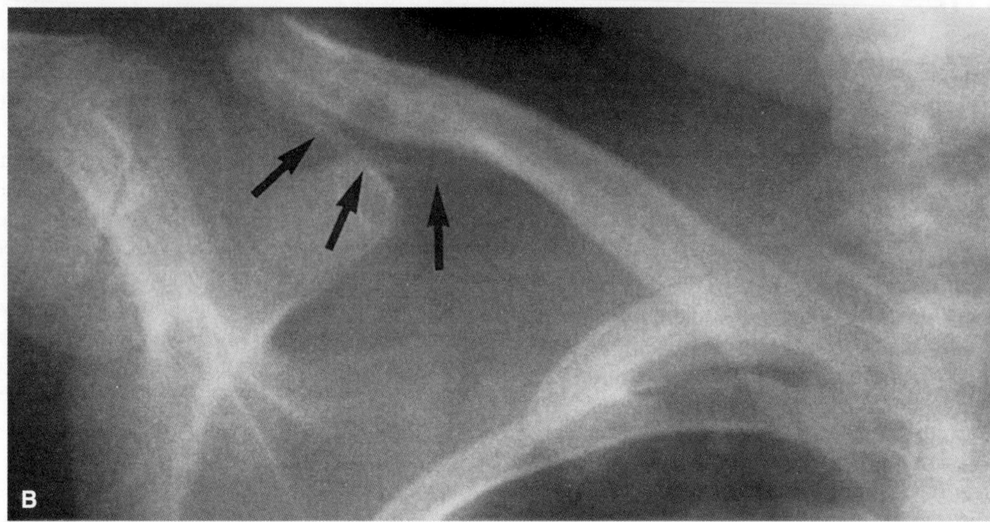

FIGURE 119.9 Radiograph of the right clavicle of a 5-year-old child. **A:** A lateral clavicular fracture (*open arrow*) and widening of the space between the clavicle and the coracoid process (*small arrows*) are evident on the initial film. **B:** The pattern of new bone formation (*arrows*) seen on the follow-up radiograph demonstrates that the periosteum and the ligaments have remained intact inferiorly.

its ligamentous connections intact. With severe displacement, the skin may be tented over the AC joint. Special note should be made of the "floating shoulder," an unstable fracture resulting from a glenoid neck fracture combined with an ipsilateral clavicle fracture, such that there is no stable bony connection between the upper extremity and the trunk.

In skeletally mature patients presenting with lateral clavicular pain, particularly young adults suffering blunt trauma such as contact sports, the emergency clinician should also consider AC joint injuries rather than physeal injuries. These injuries, classified by the Rockwood modified classification system range from low-grade (Rockwood I and II) AC joint sprains to high grade (Rockwood III, IV, V, and VI) from progressive increases in force, which result in AC ligament rupture, and then sprain and rupture of the coracoclavicular ligaments (Table 119.4).

Triage considerations. Infrequent, but serious, complications of clavicle fractures include brachial plexus injury, pneumothorax, vascular injury, and tracheal compression. Consequently, any patient with evidence of respiratory distress or neurovascular compromise requires immediate treatment and consultation. More commonly, symptom control for a suspected clavicle fracture with a sling and pain medication is the primary recommendation. With severe AC joint injuries or a forceful mechanism, examination for related cervical spine injuries or secondary neurovascular compromise should be assessed upon presentation.

Clinical assessment. In the setting of a suspected clavicle fracture, the physical examination should include both the shoulder and the arm to evaluate for possible vascular or brachial plexus injury. Visual inspection and palpation of the clavicle

TABLE 119.4

ROCKWOOD CLASSIFICATION OF ACROMIOCLAVICULAR JOINT INJURIES

Type	Description
Type I	Acromioclavicular (AC) joint sprain; ligaments intact.
Type II	AC ligament torn; coracoclavicular (CC) ligament intact. Lateral end of the clavicle may be mildly elevated.
Type III	AC and CC ligaments torn resulting in complete dislocation of the joint; >5 mm elevation of the clavicle.
Type IV	Complete dislocation of the joint with the distal clavicle displaced posteriorly into or through the trapezius muscle.
Type V	Complete dislocation with superior elevation of the clavicle one to three times above its normal position. Complete disruption of deltoid and trapezius attachments from the distal clavicle.
Type VI	Complete dislocation with the clavicle displaced inferior to the acromion and coracoid process.

for deformity or crepitus should indicate the location of the fracture. Examination for an AC injury should include visual inspection for localized bruising and swelling as well as palpation of the joint during flexion and extension of the shoulder and distraction of the arm as it is placed in adduction. If the injury is not severe and/or the diagnosis is uncertain, the Bell–van Riet test for isolated AC joint pathology is felt to be the most sensitive. For this test, the affected arm is passively raised in full adduction to 90 degrees and crossed in front of the patient toward the contralateral shoulder while maintaining full extension. The patient then attempts to elevate the arm against resistance. If this maneuver results in focal pain at the AC joint and inability to maintain the arm in the adducted and elevated position, this likely indicates an unstable AC joint.

Management. Plain radiographs with dedicated clavicle views are diagnostic in the majority of clavicular injuries (Fig. 119.9). However, radiographic visualization of medial displacement can be difficult, as this is the last physis of the body to close, and is rarely visible radiographically before age 18. Therefore, special views (e.g., the cephalic tilt view) or advanced imaging with CT may be necessary for the identification of posteriorly displaced sternoclavicular fractures (Fig. 119.10). Radiologic examination in these cases aims to identify any orthopedic injury as well as potentially lethal complications of trauma to the mediastinal structures that lie posteriorly, including the aorta and trachea. Initial imaging for suspected AC joint injury should allow for comparison of the joints either through a single anteroposterior view, which includes both AC joints, or separate radiographs of each AC joint to allow for comparison. Sensitivity for detecting injuries is increased if the x-ray is taken with the arm in internal rotation; however, stress views are no longer recommended.

Most clavicle shaft fractures in children are nondisplaced, minimally shortened or angulated, and are well treated with nonoperative management due to the ability of pediatric bones to remodel. Treatment of shaft fractures typically involves immobilization in either a sling and swathe or a simple sling for 3 weeks followed by 3 weeks of restriction from sporting activities, or until pain resolves. The figure-of-eight splint, an alternative method of immobilization, can be more uncomfortable and cumbersome than the simple sling, and without demonstrated benefit in outcomes. For newborns and toddlers, the child can be put into a long-sleeved shirt with the distal sleeve of the injured side pinned to the shoulder area of the shirt of the contralateral side.

Indications for consultation with an orthopedic surgeon for operative fixation include open fractures, impending open fractures secondary to skin tenting, and neurovascular compromise. Relative indications for operative fixation and/or orthopedic referral include fractures in multitrauma patients, floating shoulder injuries, comminuted fractures, displacement ≥2 cm in the midshaft, and shortening ≥1.5 cm. Nondisplaced fractures of the lateral end of the clavicle are generally treated with conservative measures with analgesia and sling

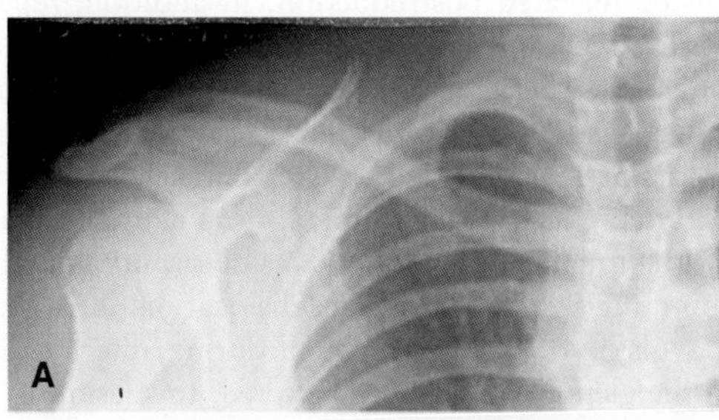

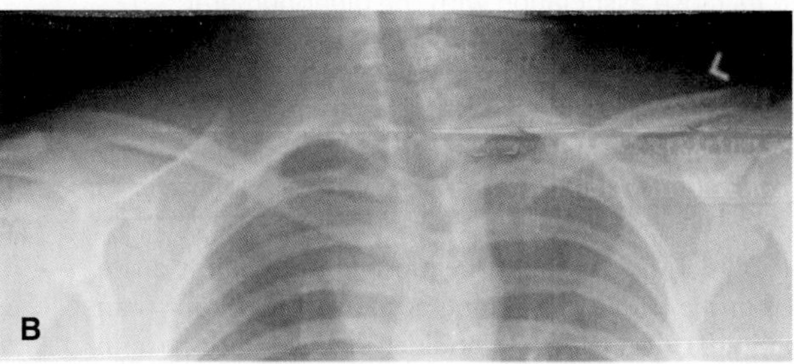

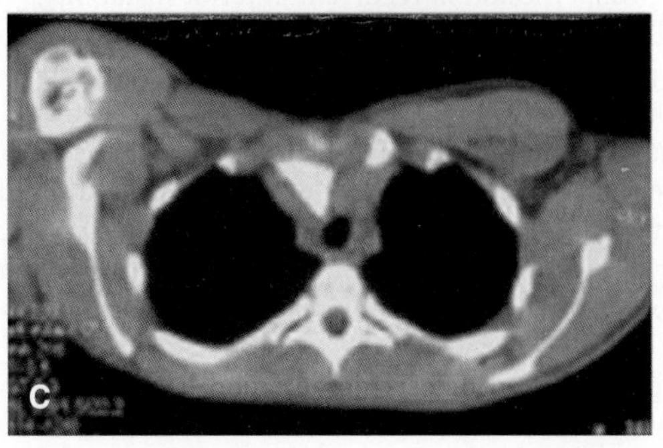

FIGURE 119.10 Three images of a patient with sternoclavicular dislocation. **A:** Apparent normal anteroposterior (AP) view of the clavicle. **B:** Serendipity view demonstrating asymmetry of the right sternoclavicular joint indicative of a posterior dislocation. **C:** CT scan showing posterior sternoclavicular dislocation on the right. (From Waters PM, Bae D, eds. *Pediatric hand and upper limb surgery: a practical guide*. Philadelphia, PA: Lippincott Williams & Wilkins, 2012, with permission.)

immobilization with good outcomes. Displaced lateral clavicle fractures are often treated operatively, due to the high rates of nonunion. Posterior sternoclavicular fracture displacement is rare in the pediatric population, representing <5% of all sternoclavicular dislocations. Surgical treatment is necessary if closed reduction fails or if there is concern for potential compromise to underlying mediastinal structures.

Management of AC joint injuries varies by severity. Typically, types I to III are nonoperative and patients are treated with rest, ice, analgesics, and support or immobilization with a sling; however operative repair of type III separations may be indicated to improve functional outcomes in children and adolescents. Types IV to VI are severe and require orthopedic evaluation and surgical treatment; emergent evaluation is required in the setting of neurovascular compromise.

Disposition. The majority of children with clavicle fractures or injuries to the AC joint can be discharged home. Fractures or injuries requiring operative intervention, including open fractures, those with substantial skin tenting, severe AC joint dislocation or any neurovascular compromise should be seen by orthopedics for possible admission.

Shoulder Dislocation

Goals of Treatment

Traumatic dislocations of the shoulder usually result from an indirect force, which overcomes the supports provided by the muscles and ligaments. This is an extremely painful injury so the initial goal of treatment is to manage the pain and expedite reduction of the shoulder dislocation after radiographs have been obtained. Postreduction radiographs should be obtained to evaluate for possible fractures after reduction.

CLINICAL PEARLS AND PITFALLS

- Complications of shoulder dislocation include fracture of the humeral head (Hill–Sachs lesion), tearing of the anteroinferior glenoid labrum with or without associated bony injury (Bankart lesion), and neurovascular injuries (Fig. 119.11).
- Due to its close association with the glenohumeral joint, the axillary nerve may be injured with shoulder dislocation, resulting in motor and sensory defects, with an estimated incidence from 19% to 55%.

Current Evidence

Anterior shoulder dislocation is the most common joint dislocation seen in the pediatric ED, and accounts for greater than 90% of shoulder dislocations. Shoulder dislocation is rare in infants, but becomes increasingly common through adolescence following physeal closure. In the skeletally immature child, fracture of the proximal humerus is more common than dislocation due to the anatomy of the physis, which largely runs external to the shoulder capsule. Shoulder dislocations are associated with a 70% to 90% recurrence rate.

Intravenous sedation and analgesia has been the mainstay of pain control for shoulder reduction; however, adult literature supports the use of intra-articular injection of lidocaine as an adjunct or possible alternative method of pain control. Although no studies in strictly pediatric populations exist, consideration of intra-articular lidocaine may be worthwhile in skeletally mature adolescents for its added benefits of shorter procedure time and potentially reduced cost.

Clinical Considerations

Clinical Recognition. The patient with a shoulder dislocation usually presents with substantial pain, holding their injured arm supported by the uninjured arm. There is often an obvious abnormality with loss of the usual rounded contour of the shoulder with the dislocation.

Triage Considerations. The patient should be given adequate pain medication, and the injured upper extremity should be placed in a sling. This injury warrants an expedited triage somore definitive management with shoulder reduction can proceed in a timely fashion.

Clinical Assessment. Findings on physical examination of an anterior dislocation include a palpable defect just inferior to the acromion, with loss of the usual rounded contour of the shoulder. On palpation, there is displacement of the humeral head most commonly anterior to the glenoid fossa, and the arm is held in abduction with external rotation. Posterior dislocations are rare, and may present with the arm held in adduction with slight internal rotation, a flattened appearance anteriorly, and prominent coracoid process. Inferior dislocations are the rarest form of shoulder dislocation, and the patient will often present with the arm maximally abducted and adjacent to the head. The complete examination should include assessment of distal neurovascular status, as injury to the axillary nerve may occur with anterior dislocations.

Management. In order to define the direction of displacement, an additional axillary (Y) view, should be obtained along with standard views (anteroposterior and axillary) of the shoulder. Treatment of anterior dislocation through closed reduction can be accomplished by numerous techniques (see Chapter 141 Procedures section on Closed Reduction of Dislocations). Pain management is fundamental for a successful reduction. A wide range of approaches have demonstrated efficacy from procedural sedation to analgesia with mild sedation to local intra-articular lidocaine injections. The neurovascular examination should be repeated postreduction. In addition, repeat radiographs are recommended after reduction to confirm anatomic placement as well as to look for any traumatic fractures such as Hill–Sachs deformities, Bankart lesions, and greater tuberosity fractures (Fig. 119.11). The Hill–Sachs deformity is a cortical depression in the humeral head caused by the glenoid rim at the time of dislocation. This deformity may destabilize the joint and result in recurrent dislocation. A Bankart lesion is an avulsion of a bony fragment during anterior dislocation when the glenoid labrum is disrupted; this lesion is felt to be the primary lesion in recurrent anterior instability.

Patients should be placed in a sling and swathe to stabilize the joint at discharge, with resumption of full activity typically within 2 to 3 weeks. Given the high rates of chronic shoulder instability and recurrent dislocation, orthopedic outpatient follow-up is recommended within 1 week after discharge. Furthermore, given the infrequency of posterior and inferior dislocations, urgent orthopedic consultation in the ED is recommended for these injuries prior to reduction.

Disposition. Once the shoulder has been reduced, the patient may be discharged provided there is no neurovascular

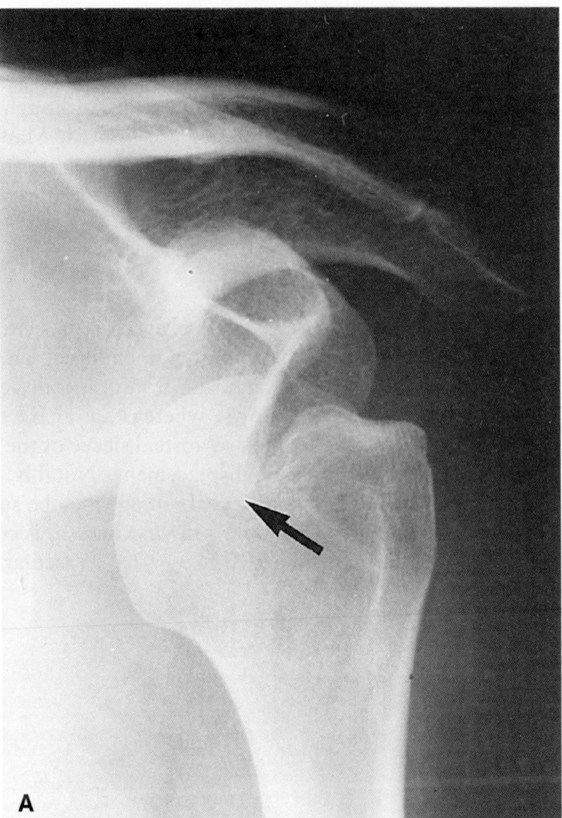

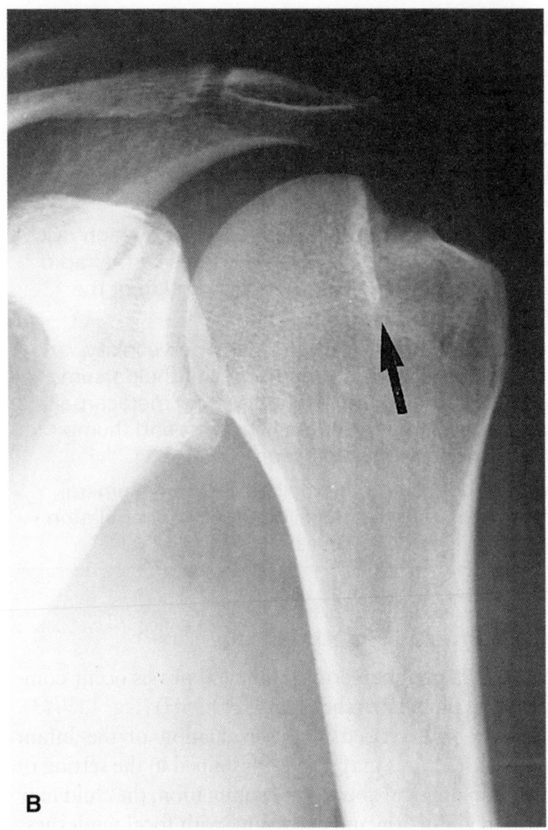

FIGURE 119.11 Hill–Sachs deformity with anterior humeral dislocation. **A:** AP shoulder demonstrating an anteroinferior dislocation of the humerus with impaction between the inferior glenoid rim and the opposing humeral head (*arrow*). The impaction produces the articular defect that has been referred to as the hatchet deformity (Hill–Sachs defect). **B:** Postreduction, AP shoulder. After repositioning the humeral head within the glenoid fossa, the residual effect of compression of the articular surface is clearly identified (*arrow*). (From Yochum TR, Rowe LJ, eds. *Yochum and Rowe's essentials of skeletal radiology*. 3rd ed. Philadelphia, PA: Liwppincott Williams & Wilkins, 2004.)

compromise. Indications for surgery include irreducible dislocations, displaced greater tuberosity fractures, and large bony glenoid lesions. Since traumatic shoulder dislocations in adolescents have a high rate of persistent instability, orthopedic follow-up is recommended for monitoring of instability and appropriate physical rehabilitation.

Injuries of the Scapula

CLINICAL PEARLS AND PITFALLS

- Scapula fractures are uncommon and generally associated with a high-energy mechanism of injury, and as such, are associated with other thoracic or potentially life-threatening injuries.

Scapula fractures are typically seen after injuries of significant force, such as a fall from a height, a motor vehicle collision or other severe direct blow (Fig. 119.12). The emergency clinician should assess for other possible associated injuries including clavicle fractures, rib fractures, pneumothorax, thoracic vertebral fractures, and fractures of the humerus. Fractures of the body and neck of the scapula are generally well visualized on plain radiographs; however, adequate definition of glenoid injuries may require a CT scan. Fracture management is often conservative, with a sling and swathe, or a shoulder immobilizer for patient comfort, graduating to gentle range-of-motion exercise after 2 weeks. Orthopedic consultation is recommended given the infrequency of this injury and its association with other injuries. Complications are not common except for possible malunion or functional impairment arising from associated thoracic injuries.

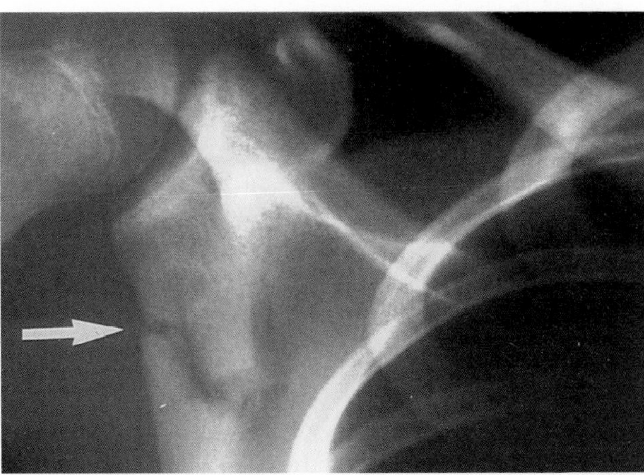

FIGURE 119.12 Radiograph of a 13-year-old boy who sustained an isolated right scapular fracture as the result of a skateboarding accident (*arrow*).

Injuries of the Humerus

CLINICAL PEARLS AND PITFALLS

- Humeral fractures are associated with high-energy direct blows; any fracture with minimal trauma should raise suspicion for pathologic fracture or abuse.
- Children in early adolescence are particularly high risk for proximal humerus physeal injuries due to the rapid growth and relative weakness of this portion of the bone.
- Humerus fractures may result in radial nerve injury, which may be identified by numbness of the dorsum of the hand between the first and second metacarpals and decreased motor strength with wrist and thumb extension and forearm supination.
- Orthopedic consultation is indicated for any humeral shaft fractures with rotational deformity or angulation greater than 15 to 20 degrees.

Proximal Humerus Fractures

Injuries to the proximal humerus or humeral physis occur commonly after a fall on outstretched hand (FOOSH) (Fig. 119.13). Caution should be exercised in the evaluation of the infant patient, as these fractures may also be sustained in the setting of birth trauma and physical abuse. On examination, the child may hold the arm in abduction and extension, with focal tenderness to palpation, localized swelling, and occasionally shortening of the affected extremity. Routine radiographs are generally sufficient for diagnosis, and comparison views may be helpful in distinguishing a fracture from the normal physeal line. The vast majority of injuries to the proximal physis are Salter–Harris types I and II. In the young infant, plain radiographs may prove inadequate to evaluate the humeral head as it is primarily cartilaginous, and therefore the distinction between a fracture and a dislocation cannot easily be determined. Ultrasonography or MRI may be necessary to make this diagnosis.

Proximal humerus fractures in skeletally immature children and adolescents are traditionally treated nonoperatively and have a tremendous capacity for remodeling. As much as 50 degrees of angulation in the proximal humerus may heal without fracture reduction in the ED. Nonunion and malunion are rare, except in adolescents with significantly displaced or angulated fractures. Adolescents with significantly displaced fractures (greater than 20 to 50 degrees) may be candidates for operative fixation, although data on whether this improves outcomes are limited. Management is typically with a sling, sling and swathe, splint, or hanging cast for several weeks. Orthopedic follow-up after discharge is recommended.

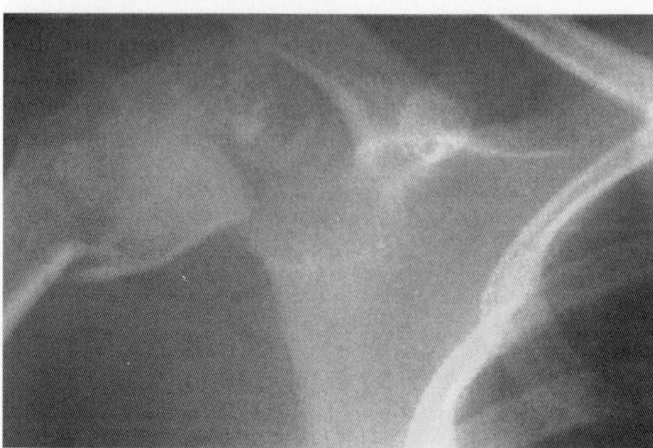

FIGURE 119.13 Impacted proximal right humeral fracture with approximately 25 degrees of angulation in a 3-year-old child. Full remodeling can be anticipated.

Humeral Shaft Fractures

Humeral shaft fractures are relatively rare, representing fewer than 10% of all humerus fractures in children. The pattern of fracture reflects the mechanism of injury; transverse fractures result from direct blows, whereas spiral fractures are caused by twisting. The thick periosteal sleeve of the humeral shaft often limits fracture displacement. Notably, a spiral fracture in a child less than 3 years of age may be suspicious for nonaccidental trauma unless the mechanism is consistent with this pattern of injury (Fig. 119.14). Vascular injuries

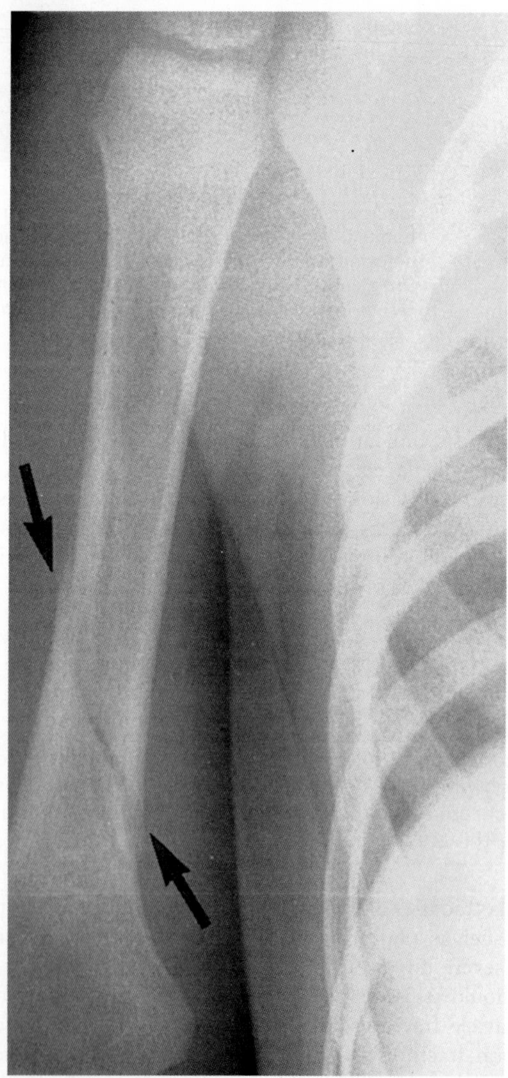

FIGURE 119.14 Spiral fracture of the right humerus in an 18-month-old girl. Although in this case the injury was accidental, spiral humeral fractures in children younger than 3 years must always evoke concerns about physical abuse.

are uncommon, but there is risk of radial nerve injury in up to 5% of fractures, particularly for fractures involving the middle and distal thirds of the humeral shaft. Fortunately, most injuries of the radial nerve represent neuropraxias, and full return of function may be expected within 3 to 4 months.

Nonoperative management is standard for uncomplicated diaphyseal fractures, using the same techniques described above for proximal humerus fractures. Alternatively, the application of a sugar tong splint to the upper arm with a sling to support the forearm is recommended for displaced fractures. Some orthopedic surgeons advise that the deformity should be reduced to less than 10 degrees before proceeding with nonoperative treatment, but this recommendation is not universal as gravity will help align the fracture over time. Indications for surgical stabilization and/or urgent orthopedic consultation for isolated humeral shaft fractures include open fractures, neurovascular compromise after reduction, completely displaced fractures, or fractures angulated more than 20 degrees in children and 10 degrees in adolescents. Children should follow-up with orthopedic surgery within 1 week of injury, and healing generally takes 4 to 6 weeks, depending upon the age of the child.

Injuries of the Elbow

Supracondylar Fractures

Goals of Treatment. Children with a mechanism and examination concerning for supracondylar fractures should have early assessment of neurovascular status to assess for neurologic or vascular compromise. Fractures associated with neurovascular compromise should have early involvement of orthopedic surgery. Management of supracondylar fractures is also aimed at preventing long-term complications including poor functional outcomes from failure to achieve anatomic alignment during reduction and immobilization.

CLINICAL PEARLS AND PITFALLS

- A radiograph with a true lateral view of the elbow is *imperative* for proper visualization of the anterior and posterior fat pads, and the anterior humeral line (Figs. 119.15 and 119.16).
- The presence of abnormalities of the fat pads or displacement of the anterior humeral line on lateral view strongly suggests presence of fracture (Fig. 119.17).
- In patients with extensive soft tissue edema, elevation of the fat pads may be obscured; therefore, relying on the clinical examination and identifying the anterior humeral line on the lateral elbow radiograph are important.
- Fractures may be complicated by vascular injury to the brachial artery, compartment syndrome or neurologic injury to the median, radial, or ulnar nerves.
- Supracondylar fractures associated with ipsilateral forearm fractures are particularly high risk for the development of ischemic injury even when pulses and capillary refill are normal on examination.

Current Evidence. Elbow fractures account for approximately 15% of all pediatric fractures but are among the most problematic pediatric fractures in terms of diagnosis, treatment, and complications. The most common mechanism of injury resulting in a supracondylar fracture is a FOOSH with the elbow in extension. The extension supracondylar fracture accounts for 95% of these injuries and is often described using the Gartland classification system (Table 119.5). The FOOSH mechanism causes the ulna and triceps muscles to exert an unopposed force on the distal humerus, causing failure of the anterior periosteum and, in more severe injuries, extending to and through the posterior cortex. This progression results in a posterior displacement of the condylar complex. Displacement of the fracture increases the risk of injury to the brachial artery and the median, radial, and ulnar nerves as the neurovascular

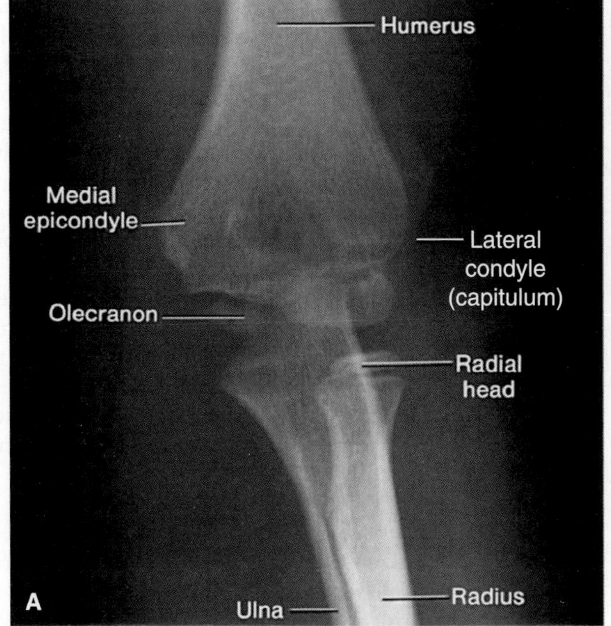

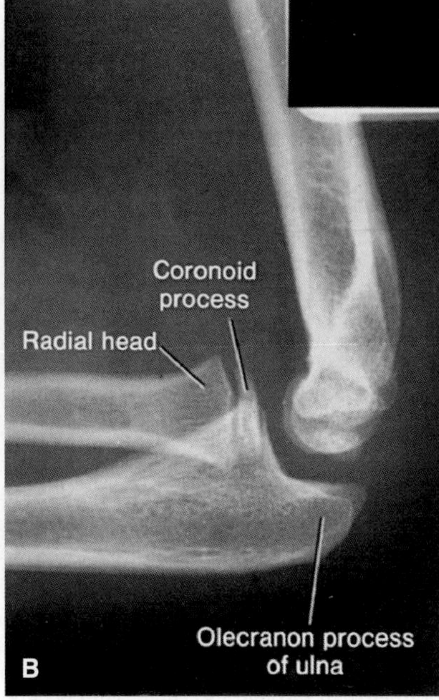

FIGURE 119.15 **A:** Anteroposterior radiograph of a normal elbow of a child. **B:** Normal lateral radiograph.

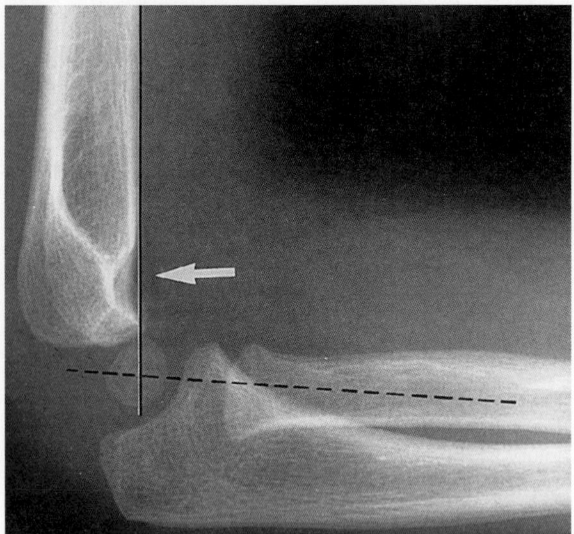

FIGURE 119.16 Normal lateral radiograph of the elbow of a 2-year-old child. The anterior fat pad is readily seen (*arrow*); the posterior fat pad is not visible. A line drawn along the anterior cortex of the humerus intersects the capitellum in its middle third (*solid line*). A line drawn along the axis of the radius also passes through the center of the capitellum (*dashed line*).

bundles are stretched and/or disrupted. Obesity in childhood and adolescence reduces bone mineral density with an increased propensity for fractures and is associated with more complex supracondylar humeral fractures, preoperative and postoperative nerve palsies, and postoperative complications.

Clinical Considerations

Clinical recognition. A child with a supracondylar fracture often presents to the ED holding the arm straight in pronation and refusing to use the arm or flex at the elbow. Supracondylar fractures occur most commonly between 3 and 10 years of age,

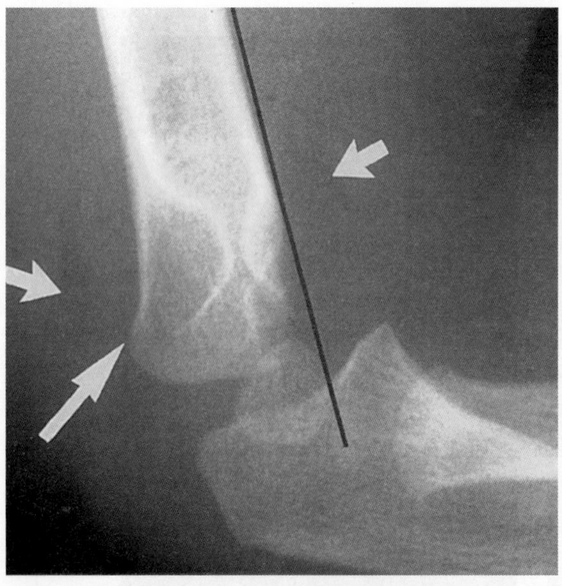

FIGURE 119.17 Lateral radiograph of the elbow of a 2-year-old girl. Both the anterior and posterior fat pads are elevated (*small arrows*). The anterior humeral line (*solid line*), passes along the anterior edge of the capitellum rather than through its center. Mild buckling of the posterior cortex of the distal humerus can be seen (*large arrow*).

TABLE 119.5

GARTLAND CLASSIFICATION FOR SUPRACONDYLAR FRACTURES

Type	Description	Radiographic findings
Type I	Nondisplaced fracture	+ posterior fat pad, "sail sign"
Type II	Displaced fracture with intact posterior cortex	Anterior humeral line is anterior to the capitellum, "hinged" or intact appearance of the posterior cortex
Type III	Completely displaced fracture with no cortical contact	Displacement of the distal fragment relative to the humeral shaft; fractures of both cortices

with a peak incidence between ages 5 and 7 due to the relative strength of the collateral ligaments and joint capsule as compared to the bone.

Clinical assessment. Typically in the setting of a supracondylar fracture, there is localized swelling and tenderness around the elbow on examination, with or without deformity of the distal humerus, depending upon the degree of displacement. The presence of extensive swelling and ecchymosis of the elbow imparts a significant risk for compartment syndrome; any progression of increasing pain, or pain with passive extension of the fingers is concerning for ischemia and requires immediate orthopedic consultation. A thorough examination of perfusion as well as motor and sensory function of the median, radial, and ulnar nerve distribution is essential (Table 119.6). The median nerve is the most commonly injured nerve—specifically the anterior interosseous branch—followed by radial and ulnar nerve injuries. Fortunately, most nerve injuries are temporary, resolving within 2 to 3 weeks after appropriate fracture reduction and immobilization.

In addition to assessing motor and sensory function, examination of skin color, temperature, capillary refill, and pulses (by palpation or Doppler) should be performed. Some children with more extensively displaced humeral fractures will not have a palpable pulse until the fracture undergoes closed reduction. If the child has a pink, warm hand with good capillary refill, a serious vascular injury is less likely; by contrast the child with a cold, pale hand with poor capillary refill is a surgical emergency. If the limb is pulseless or is cold with poor capillary refill, in the absence of the availability of emergent orthopedic consultation, immediate management includes allowing the elbow to rest in extension (avoiding hyperflexion, which may further compromise flow in the brachial artery), and applying direct anterior forward pressure on the distal fragment. If this fails to improve vascular status, immediate consultation with an orthopedic and/or vascular surgeon is indicated.

Management. Fracture diagnosis requires plain radiographs of the elbow, with both anteroposterior and lateral views. Comparison views of the elbow may be useful in diagnosis of fracture due to the complexity of the joint with its three points of articulation, numerous growth centers, and variable

TABLE 119.6

GUIDE TO THE NEUROLOGIC EXAMINATION OF THE DISTAL UPPER EXTREMITY

A. Motor function		
Nerve	**Muscles innervated**	**Motor examination**
Radial	Extensor carpi radialis longus	Wrist extension
Ulnar	Flexor carpi ulnaris	Wrist flexion and adduction
	Interosseous	Finger spread
Median	Flexor carpi radialis	Wrist flexion and abduction
	Flexor digitorum superficialis	Flexion fingers at proximal interphalangeal joint
	Opponens pollicis	Opposition thumb to base of little finger
Anterior Interosseous	Flexor digitorum profundus I and II	Flexion distal phalanx of index finger
	Flexor pollicis longus	Flexion distal phalanx of thumb (test the strength when patient is making an "ok" sign)
Nerve	**B. Sensory Innervation**	
Radial	Dorsal web space between thumb and index finger	
Ulnar	Ulnar aspect palm and dorsum of hand	
	Little finger and ulnar aspect of ring finger	
Median	Radial aspect palm of hand	
	Thumb, index, middle, radial aspect ring finger	
Anterior Interosseous	None	

timing of ossification (Table 119.7). After initial examination, patients should be splinted prior to imaging. In patients with concern for Gartland type I fractures, the lateral view should be with the elbow at 90 degrees of flexion to avoid a false-positive posterior fat pad sign, which can occur if the elbow is overly extended. In addition, radiographs of the forearm should be obtained, as there is a 10% to 15% risk of ipsilateral concurrent distal radius forearm fracture.

Interpretation of the radiographs for occult fracture requires attention to subtle changes in three regions: the anterior and posterior fat pads, the anterior humeral line, and the radiocapitellar line. In the normal lateral radiograph, the anterior fat pad is readily seen but the posterior fat pad is hidden within the olecranon fossa (Fig. 119.16). The presence of hemarthrosis and edema in the joint following trauma will elevate the anterior fat pad creating the "sail sign" and displace the posterior fat pad from the fossa creating a lucency posterior to the distal humerus on lateral view (Fig. 119.17). The presence of a posterior fat pad sign is abnormal and is 75% sensitive for the presence of an occult elbow fracture, most commonly supracondylar. The anterior humeral line is a line drawn along the anterior cortex of the humerus and should intersect the capitellum in its middle third; however, in the presence of an extension-type injury this line will pass anteriorly. Finally, a line drawn along the axis of the radius should pass through the capitellum irrespective of the degree of elbow flexion or extension on the radiograph. If this is not visualized, there may be either a lateral condyle fracture or a dislocation of the radial head (as in a Monteggia fracture) (Fig. 119.18).

The treatment of Gartland type I fractures requires splinting in a long-arm posterior splint, with the arm in pronation or neutral rotation and at 90 degrees of flexion at the elbow. Children should be referred to orthopedics for casting within 1 week, when the swelling has subsided. In some cases, casting is performed at the initial encounter in the ED. Immobilization for an additional 2 to 3 weeks is often sufficient. Displaced fractures should have urgent consultation, as they always

TABLE 119.7

GROWTH CENTERS OF ELBOW: AVERAGE AGE FOR ONSET OF OSSIFICATION

Capitellum	11 mo
Radial head	3–4 yrs
Medial epicondyle	4–6 yrs
Trochlea	6–8 yrs
Olecranon	9–10 yrs
Lateral epicondyle	10–12 yrs

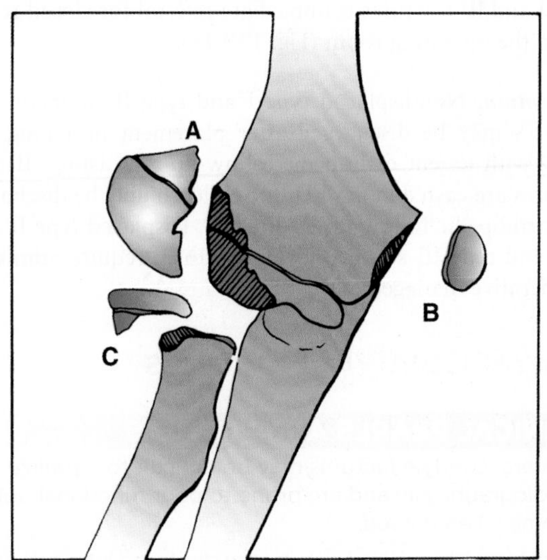

FIGURE 119.18 Common elbow fractures in children: lateral condylar fracture (A), medial epicondylar fracture (B), and radial neck fracture (C).

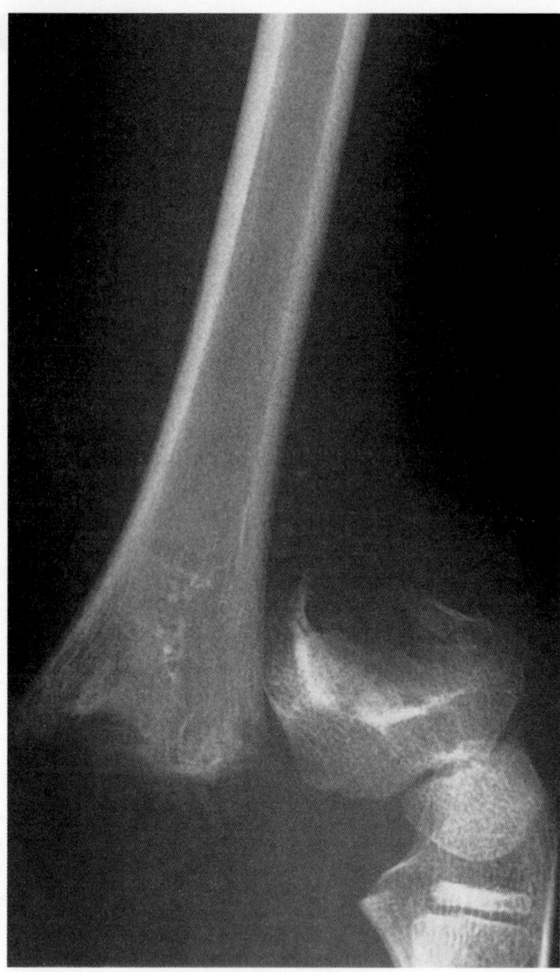

FIGURE 119.19 Displaced and rotated type III supracondylar fracture in an 8-year-old girl. The distal pulses were absent on examination, but returned with fracture reduction.

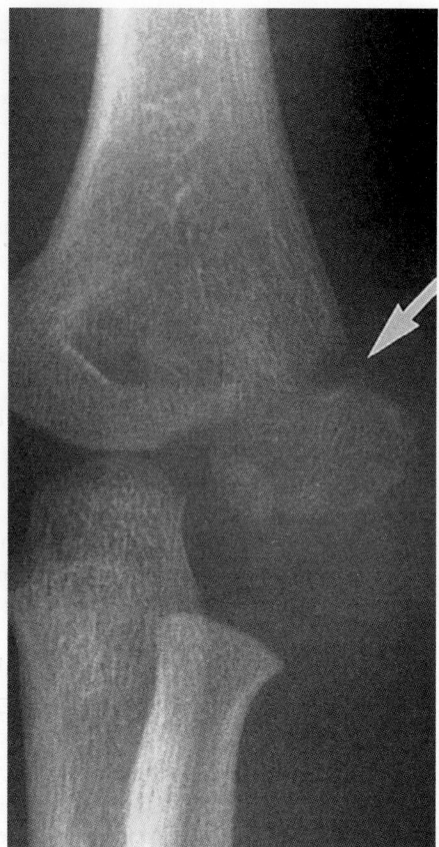

FIGURE 119.20 Lateral condylar fracture in a 2-year-old girl (*arrow*).

require a reduction to decrease the risk of cosmetic deformity or poor functional outcomes such as Volkmann contracture or cubitus varus. Unlike other injuries to the humerus, supracondylar injuries have minimal potential for remodeling. Consequently, the generally preferred treatment for all Gartland type II and III fractures is immediate referral for closed reduction in the operating room (Fig. 119.19).

Disposition. Nondisplaced type I and type II supracondylar fractures may be discharged after placement in a long arm splint, with urgent orthopedic follow-up for casting. If these fractures are casted in the ED, the children may be discharged with orthopedic follow-up as directed. Displaced type II fractures and type III supracondylar fractures require admission for operative management.

Lateral Condyle Fractures

CLINICAL PEARLS AND PITFALLS

- Lateral condyle factures may be difficult to visualize radiographically and are prone to poor functional outcome when missed.
- Most lateral condyle fractures are displaced intra-articular fractures (Salter–Harris type IV) and often require open reduction to anatomically reduce the articular surface.

Lateral condyle fractures are the second most common operative elbow fracture in children. These fractures are easily missed radiographically, and this may result in nonunion or deformity as the fracture fragment is prone to displacement. The emergency clinician should have a high level of suspicion for this diagnosis in the setting of a concerning examination. Clinically, this injury is suggested by swelling, ecchymosis, and tenderness localized over the lateral aspect of the elbow. Frequently, the lateral ligament and the common extensor tendon remain attached to the fracture fragment, which can be partially or totally avulsed from the distal humerus (Fig. 119.20). The lateral epicondyle ossifies at approximately age 13 and fuses with the capitellum around age 16. Consequently lateral condyle fractures are uncommon in the skeletally mature pediatric patient, who is more likely to sustain a T-condylar fracture of the distal humerus. Routine anteroposterior and lateral plain radiographs usually provide adequate fracture definition for severely displaced fractures; however, with less severe injuries and before the capitellum is ossified, visualization of the injury is difficult and oblique views, stress views, CT scan, or an MRI study be needed.

Given the potential complications of displacement, malunion, and nonunion, orthopedic surgery consultation is recommended for surgical management of lateral condyle injuries with displacement of 2 mm or greater. Nondisplaced or minimally displaced (<2 mm) fractures may be immobilized in the ED in a posterior splint with the elbow flexed to 90 degrees and the forearm in pronation. However, given the instability of this fracture, in addition to immobilization, orthopedic follow-up within 3 to 4 days is essential.

Medial Epicondyle Fractures

CLINICAL PEARLS AND PITFALLS

- Approximately half of all pediatric medial epicondyle fractures are associated with elbow dislocations.
- Intra-articular incarceration of the epicondylar fragment occurs in 5% to 18% of all cases of medial epicondyle fracture.
- Medial epicondyle fractures may be complicated by paresis of the ulnar nerve.
- A child presenting with acute onset of pain over the medial elbow after throwing may have an avulsion fracture of the medial epicondyle, a variant of Little League elbow.

Fractures of the medial epicondyle occur as the result of direct elbow trauma or when the elbow is subjected to a valgus stress during a fall or vigorous throwing. The medial epicondyle of the humerus is an apophysis that is the point of attachment for the forearm flexor muscles, the pronator teres, and the medial collateral ligament. As with lateral epicondyle fractures, this tends to be an avulsion injury that may be difficult to diagnose prior to ossification of the epicondyle (4 to 6 years of age), but this injury is not typically intra-articular (Fig. 119.21). Clinically, children often present with the elbow held in flexion and with swelling and tenderness localized to the medial aspect of the elbow, with valgus instability (most readily demonstrated by stress radiographs). Oblique radiograph views in addition to stress and comparison views may be needed for diagnosis. Additional imaging with MRI examination may prove useful in defining the extent of the injury. Nondisplaced fractures are managed in the emergency setting with casting or posterior splinting with the elbow in flexion and neutral position, or pronation for 3 weeks with outpatient orthopedic follow-up. Indications for surgical management include incarcerated fracture fragment within the joint, presence of neuropathy, valgus instability, and displacement of the fracture fragment. There is no consensus on what degree of displacement requires surgical intervention. Some research suggests surgery for displacement of 3 mm or more, while other studies report good long-term results, similar to those obtained with open reduction and internal fixation, with nonsurgical treatment of isolated fractures with between 5 and 15 mm of displacement.

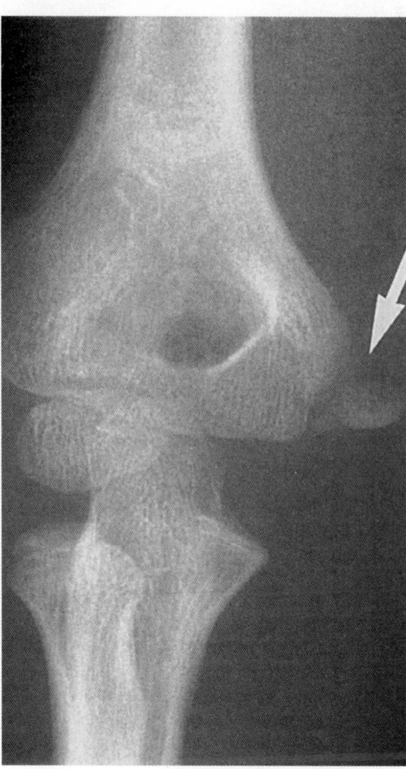

FIGURE 119.21 Displaced fracture of the medial epicondyle in an 8-year-old girl (*arrow*).

Distal Humerus Physeal Fractures

CLINICAL PEARLS AND PITFALLS

- Fractures of the distal humeral physis in children under the age of 3 years, and especially infants under the age of 1 year, should raise concern for possible abuse.
- Radiographic diagnosis of humerus physeal fractures is difficult as the distal humerus and proximal radius and ulna have not yet ossified.
- To distinguish distal humeral physeal separation from elbow dislocation, one should note that displacement of the proximal radius and ulna is usually posterior and medial in the former. With dislocation, the proximal radius and ulna are typically displaced posterolaterally, and the relationship between proximal radius and lateral condyle epiphysis is disrupted.

Separation of the distal humerus physis can be missed in the pediatric ED leading to delays in diagnosis. Most injuries involving the entire distal humeral physis occur before age 7. Recognition is both difficult and important, especially in infants, in whom this particular injury is often the result of physical abuse. The proposed mechanism in abused children is forceful twisting of the arm that shears off the distal epiphysis. Elbow swelling, pain, and disuse of the extremity, but without significant deformity, in the setting of a FOOSH are the usual history and examination; however, with significant displacement, the appearance may mimic that of an elbow dislocation. Dislocations more commonly occur in early adolescence than in children less than 7 years old. Radiographic diagnosis requires recognition of the displacement of the proximal radius and ulna, and may necessitate comparison views. Given the frequent need for reduction and pinning, all suspected epiphyseal separations of the distal humerus merit immediate orthopedic referral. MRI studies may be necessary to define the extent of damage to the cartilaginous structures. The risk of avascular necrosis increases with delay in diagnosis.

Olecranon Fractures

CLINICAL PEARLS AND PITFALLS

- Olecranon fractures typically occur in conjunction with other elbow injuries, notably a radial neck fracture or dislocation of the radial head (Monteggia variant), or lateral condyle fracture.
- Comparative views may be helpful in distinguishing the olecranon growth plate from a fracture.
- A missed fracture of the olecranon epiphysis can lead to a fixed flexion deformity resulting in significant morbidity in adulthood.
- In contrast to many elbow injuries, a nondisplaced olecranon fracture can be splinted in partial extension.

The mechanism of an isolated olecranon fracture is hypothesized to be a sudden flexion of the elbow when the triceps is strongly contracted (essentially an avulsion injury), direct trauma, or stress fracture from repeated throwing activity. Physical findings range from localized swelling to a marked hemarthrosis with weak or absent elbow extension. Nondisplaced fractures may be somewhat difficult to discern radiographically; however, the presence of an abnormal fat pad should be viewed as presumptive evidence of a bony injury (Fig. 119.22). A nondisplaced olecranon fracture can be splinted in partial extension and referred for outpatient orthopedic follow-up. Displaced fractures and stress fractures often require open reduction and internal fixation. Immediate orthopedic consultation is indicated for displaced fractures, open fractures, multiple fractures, and neurovascular injury. Isolated olecranon fractures almost invariably heal quickly and without significant complications.

Radial Head and Neck Fractures

CLINICAL PEARLS AND PITFALLS

- Radial head fractures may occur in conjunction with ulnar shaft fracture (Monteggia equivalent). Associated fractures are common, including capitellum, olecranon, and lateral humeral condyle, as well as dislocation of the distal radioulnar joint.
- When the diagnosis is uncertain, oblique, radiocapitellar, and comparison views may be useful in addition to standard AP and lateral radiographs.
- Patients with radial head and neck fractures may complain of wrist pain but have focal tenderness to palpation over the anatomic location of the injury.
- Injury may be associated with trauma to the posterior interosseous nerve.

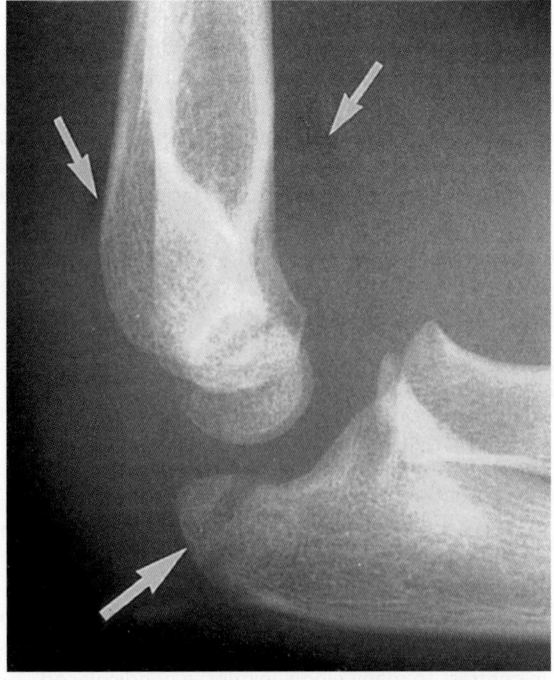

FIGURE 119.22 Nondisplaced fracture of the olecranon in an 8-year-old boy (*bottom arrow*). Note the elevated fat pads (*top arrows*).

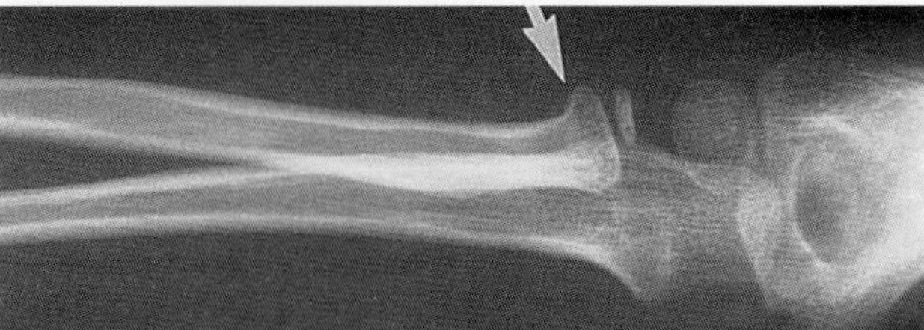

FIGURE 119.23 Buckle fracture of the radial neck in a 9-year-old girl (*arrow*). Wrist pain was the chief complaint. The treating physician failed to identify the proximal radial fracture, which was, however, noticed by the radiologist.

Radial neck fractures are far more common in children than fractures of the radial head, which tend to occur primarily in skeletally mature individuals. The cause of injury is typically a fall onto an outstretched, supinated arm. On examination, tenderness overlying the proximal radius strongly suggests the diagnosis, although it is worth noting that patients occasionally present with pain referred to the wrist (Fig. 119.23). The most common fracture pattern extends through the physis with a metaphyseal fragment (Salter–Harris II) or through the neck proper (3 to 4 mm distal to the epiphyseal plate). Imaging may also reveal a posterior fat pad on the lateral view if a hemarthrosis is present; however, when the metaphysis alone is injured, a hemarthrosis may be absent and the fat pads normal. In addition, attention should be paid on radiographs to the radiocapitellar line to pick up subtle displacement of the radius.

The majority of simple fractures of the radial head are stable, even when displaced up to 2 mm. Articular fragmentation and comminution can be seen in stable fracture patterns and are not absolute indications for operative treatment. Nonetheless, the incidence of complications, especially loss of motion and overgrowth of the radial head, is significant, making orthopedic referral advisable for all radial head and neck fractures. Injured children with minimally displaced or nondisplaced fractures should have the elbow immobilized at 90 degrees of flexion in the ED. If angulation is greater than 15 degrees in a child over the age of 10 years, immediate orthopedic consultation is indicated. In younger children, up to 30 degrees of angulation may be expected to remodel with growth, although less than 10 degrees is ideal.

Elbow Dislocations

CLINICAL PEARLS AND PITFALLS

- Fractures most commonly associated with elbow dislocation include fractures of the medial epicondyle, coronoid process, olecranon, and proximal radius.
- Posterior dislocations of the elbow must be carefully examined for neurovascular injury, with particular attention to possible median nerve entrapment, and injuries to the ulnar nerve or brachial artery. Nerve injury is more common than vascular injury.
- True arterial rupture is seen almost exclusively with open dislocations but has been described on occasion with closed injuries.

True elbow dislocation in the pediatric patient is uncommon, despite being the second most frequently dislocated joint in adolescents and adults. Dislocations of the elbow are usually accompanied by significant soft tissue and bony damage. The force and torque of the fall causing the dislocation typically results in posterior and lateral displacement of the radius and ulna, tearing of the anterior capsule, and often rupture of the medial collateral ligament as well (Fig. 119.24). In addition to obvious pain, deformity, and significant swelling, in the setting of dislocation the affected forearm may appear shortened and the humeral head can be detected as fullness in the antecubital fossa. A thorough neurovascular examination is imperative due to the risk of ulnar and median nerve injury and the potential for trauma to the brachial artery. Ulnar nerve lesions typically occur when the dislocation is complicated by intra-articular entrapment of an avulsed medial epicondyle. After initial evaluation, patients should be temporarily splinted—avoiding hyperextension—prior to imaging to ensure no further neurovascular injury occurs. The AP and lateral radiographs should be assessed for the direction of the dislocation and for the presence of associated fractures.

Although most elbow dislocations are reduced uneventfully, the risks of entrapping a fracture fragment or a nerve in the joint space during the procedure are such that immediate orthopedic consultation is recommended (see Chapter 141 Procedures, section on Closed Reduction). Open reduction may be needed in over 50% of cases. A repeat neurologic and vascular examination should be completed after ED reduction to assess for median or ulnar nerve entrapment and arterial compromise. Persistence of vascular compromise indicates the need for emergent orthopedic consultation. Postreduction radiographs are necessary to evaluate for associated fractures that may not be evident when the elbow is dislocated. The patient with a reassuring postreduction examination may be placed in a posterior splint with the elbow at 90 degrees and with the forearm in midpronation. Discharge instructions should include signs of compartment syndrome and symptoms of motor and sensory deficit that require emergent follow-up.

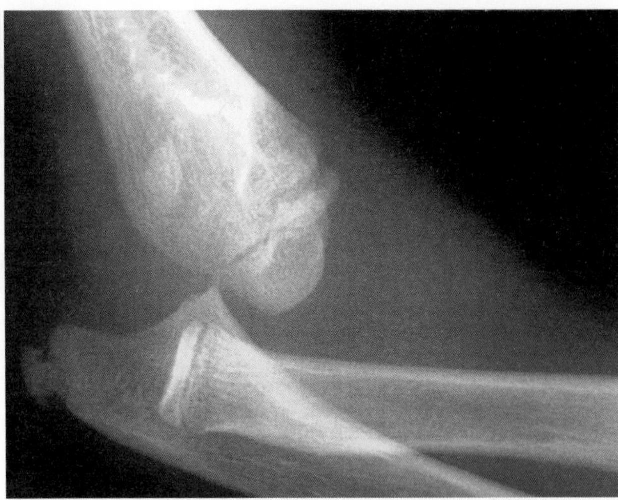

FIGURE 119.24 Elbow dislocation in an 8-year-old girl. A displaced fracture of the medial epicondyle was evident on the postreduction radiographs.

Radial Head Subluxation

CLINICAL PEARLS AND PITFALLS

- Dependent swelling of the wrist or hand may be noted in the child with a more prolonged period of subluxation.
- Recovery of function after reduction may be more prolonged in younger children and those with greater than 4 to 6 hours of subluxation.
- If reduction fails to return function, one must consider alternative diagnoses including fractures of the bones around the elbow or the clavicle, which may present similarly.

Radial head subluxation occurs when the annular ligament either tears or slips over the radial head in the setting of longitudinal traction on the arm, and then when traction is released, the ligament remains interposed between the radial head and capitellum. This injury, known more often by its moniker, the "nursemaid's elbow," is among the most common traumatic injuries to the upper extremity. It occurs most often among children from a few months to 5 years of age. After 5 years of age, the radial head becomes ossified and less spherical and the strength of the annular ligament changes, making subluxation less common.

Classically, the child will present with the injured elbow pronated, partially flexed, and held at the side with a history of refusal to use the arm after being pulled or lifted by that same arm. Frequently, however, the history is of a fall or, in infants, that the arm was trapped beneath the torso as the child is rolled over. Palpation of the elbow may elicit minimal or no pain at the radial head, but attempted supination, pronation, and elbow flexion usually elicits more discomfort. Radiographs are not routinely recommended when the history and clinical presentation are classic, as the normal and affected elbows are indistinguishable radiographically. Imaging should be obtained if the examination or history is atypical, or routine methods of reduction do not succeed.

The two most commonly used reduction techniques are supination and flexion at the elbow, or hyperpronation with an extended forearm (see Chapters 34 Immobile Arm and 141 Procedures, section on Reduction of Nursemaid's Elbow). There is some data suggesting that the pronation approach may be more effective on first attempt and less painful. When reduction succeeds, the child typically uses the arm normally within 5 to 10 minutes. There is no need for immobilization after first subluxation. With recurrent subluxations, immobilization for a few weeks in a posterior splint with the elbow at 90 degrees and with the forearm supinated may be considered. Note that even when efforts at closed reduction fail, spontaneous reduction almost invariably occurs. Once alternative diagnoses have been excluded, persistently symptomatic patients with a suspected nonreduced radial head subluxation may be discharged in a sling or posterior splint with orthopedic follow-up.

Injuries of the Forearm

Fractures of the Radial and Ulnar Shafts

Goals of Treatment. ED management should include pain control and immobilization with the arm in a position of comfort, until definitive orthopedic reduction can be achieved.

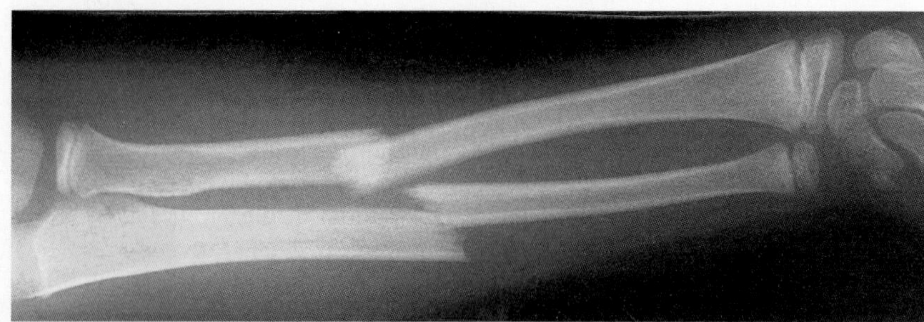

FIGURE 119.25 Complete fractures of the midshafts of the radius and ulna in a 9-year-old boy. Efforts at closed reduction failed; internal fixation was necessary.

CLINICAL PEARLS AND PITFALLS

- Plastic deformations are more common in the ulna, and are difficult to identify without comparison films of the contralateral forearm.
- Given the "ring" structure of the forearm and resulting transmission of force, the presence of an apparent single bone fracture should prompt close inspection for possible dislocation at the proximal and distal radioulnar joints.
- The potential for remodeling decreases with increasing fracture distance from the epiphysis and with the age of the child. As a result, less angulation is acceptable in midshaft fractures than in more distal injuries, and in adolescents relative to younger children.
- The incidence of neurovascular complications from forearm and wrist fractures is low.

Current Evidence. Forearm shaft fractures are the third most common fracture in children, and many require sedated reduction in the ED to obtain anatomic or near-anatomic alignment per guidelines of anticipated remodeling by age and fracture location. Unfortunately, an estimated 39% to 64% of these reduced complete shaft fractures of the ulna and radius remain unstable and will require subsequent repeat manipulation or surgical stabilization (Fig. 119.25). While closed reduction and casting remains the standard of care, recent research has questioned whether a primary surgical approach should be preferential for certain patients and fracture types. This approach is based on the potential for failed reduction and/or increased risk of permanent loss of motion secondary to waning remodeling potential of certain patients due to age or fracture location. Data suggest patients 10 years or older, those with proximal-third radius fractures, and ulna fractures with angulation greater than 15 degrees as being the highest risk for failed closed reduction. For these patients, orthopedics should be consulted as surgical management may be considered. While the standard of care has not changed, emergency clinicians should be aware of these potential complications to guide their discussions with patients.

Clinical Considerations

Clinical recognition. Radial and ulnar shaft fractures have a number of fracture patterns including greenstick, torus (buckle), plastic deformation, and complete. The management of these fractures depends on the age, type of fracture, and degree of displacement. If there is wrist or elbow pain and swelling associated with deformity suggestive of forearm fracture, the clinician must consider the possibility of Galeazzi or Monteggia fracture-dislocation pattern, respectively.

Triage considerations. These patients often present with an obvious deformity. The injured extremity should be splinted and analgesia provided while awaiting further evaluation. A focused neurovascular assessment should be performed.

Clinical assessment. In many instances, emergency clinicians can provide the satisfactory initial, if not definitive, management for many forearm injuries. However, careful history and assessment for associated fracture or dislocation is important in understanding the full complexity of the injury and determining the type of imaging and consultation necessary. The incidence of neurovascular injury is low in forearm fractures; nevertheless, the initial evaluation should include a thorough examination of circulation, sensory and motor nerve function distal to the injury.

Monteggia fractures (ulnar shaft fracture with radial head dislocation) may be diagnosed on physical examination by palpation of the dislocated radial head (Fig. 119.26). These children will frequently have considerable pain and swelling at the elbow with limited flexion and forearm supination. A palsy of the posterior interosseous nerve, a motor branch of the radial nerve, may be present with Monteggia fractures (Fig. 119.27). This may result in weakness or paralysis of the extension of the fingers or thumb (Fig. 119.28).

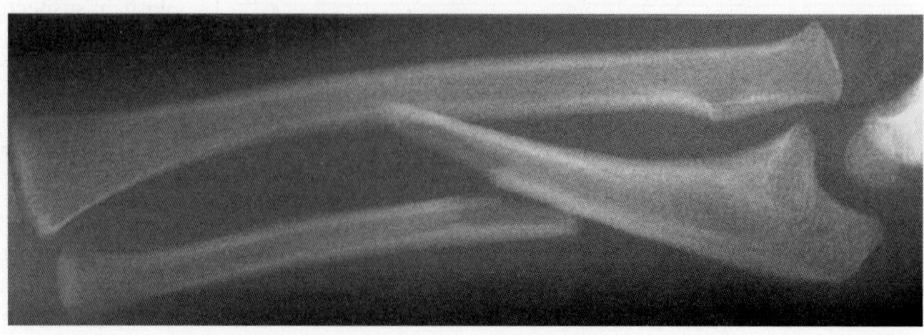

FIGURE 119.26 A Monteggia fracture in a 3-year-old boy. Note that a line drawn along the axis of the radius would fail to intersect the capitellum (compare with Fig. 119.16).

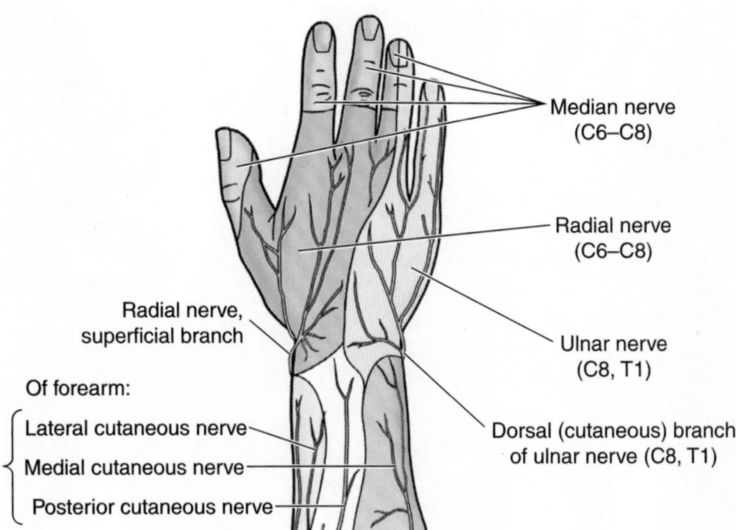

FIGURE 119.27 Sensory innervation of the wrist and hand. (From Moore KL, Dalley AF, Agur AM. *Clinically oriented anatomy*. 6th ed. Philadelphia, PA: Lippincott Williams & Wilkins, 2009.)

In the Galeazzi fracture-dislocation (fracture of the radius with dislocation of the distal radioulnar joint), the child will typically resist pronation and supination and have tenderness on examination of the wrist (Fig. 119.29). With significant dislocations, the ulnar styloid may appear prominent, but in minor dislocations the pain and examination findings can be minimal. Distal neurovascular injury is rare, but chronic pain, weakness, and limitation of supination and pronation can result from missed injuries.

Management. Standard radiographic views, including the joints above and below the fracture, are typically sufficient for diagnosis. Failure to fully evaluate the elbow and the wrist may result in missed fractures or dislocations. With suspected bowing fractures comparison views of the contralateral forearm may prove helpful. Recognition of a bowing fracture is crucial because the potential for remodeling with such injuries is minimal, and failure to correct bowing can result in permanent loss of supination and pronation (Fig. 119.4).

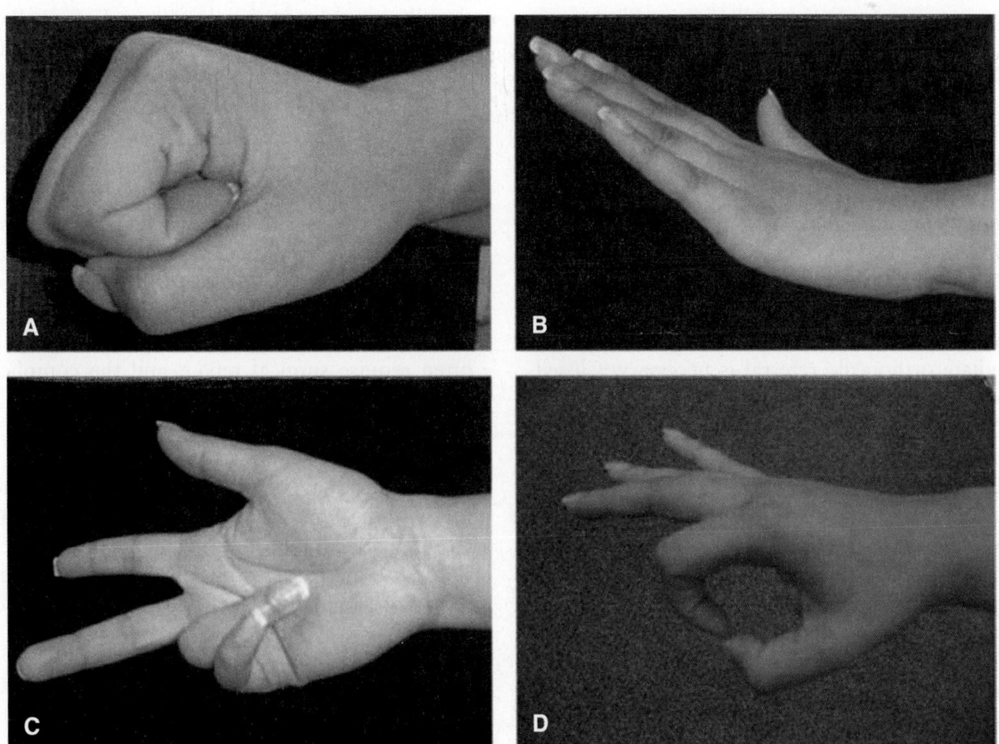

FIGURE 119.28 Upper extremity motor nerve physical examination. **A:** Rock position demonstrates median nerve motor function. **B:** Paper position demonstrates radial nerve motor function. **C:** Scissor position demonstrates ulnar nerve motor function. **D:** "OK" sign demonstrates function of the anterior interosseous nerve. (From Flynn JM, Skaggs DL, Waters PM. *Rockwood and Wilkins' fractures in children*. 8th ed. Philadelphia, PA: Wolters Kluwer, 2014.)

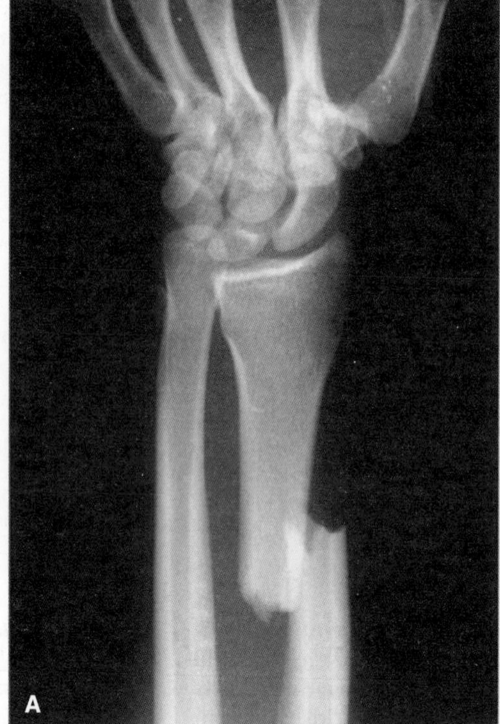

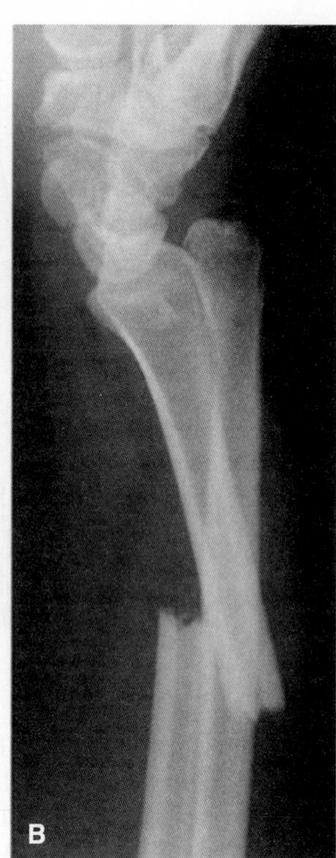

FIGURE 119.29 Galeazzi fracture-dislocation. Posteroanterior (**A**) and lateral (**B**) radiographs of the distal forearm show type I Galeazzi fracture-dislocation. Note the simple fracture of the radius affecting the distal third of the bone, with the proximal end of the distal fragment dorsally displaced and angulated. In addition, there is dislocation in the distal radioulnar joint, most clearly seen on the lateral view. (Reprinted with permission from Greenspan A. Orthopedic imaging: a practical approach. 4th ed. Philadelphia, PA: Lippincott Williams & Wilkins, 2004.)

Orthopedic consultation and closed reduction are required for a variety of forearm shaft fractures. In general, immediate orthopedic consultation is recommended for any shaft fracture angulated more than 10 to 15 degrees. It should also be noted that greenstick fractures are both unstable and have the potential for significant rotational deformity. Therefore, although the periosteum and the remaining intact cortex will limit the degree of angulation, closed reduction may be indicated irrespective of the extent of angulation. For bowing fractures, there are no strict guidelines regarding indications for closed reduction; however, any bowing fracture that presents with obvious forearm deformity or restricts pronation or supination merits immediate orthopedic referral. With complete fractures of the forearm, if the ends of the bones are well opposed and angulation and rotation are minimal, a well-applied sugar-tong splint is adequate initial treatment with outpatient orthopedic follow-up. In the setting of displaced fractures, immediate orthopedic referral is necessary. Closed reduction, although not always as simple as it may appear, is preferable. In children older than 10 to 12 years, adequate alignment is often obtained only with open reduction and internal fixation.

If only one forearm bone is fractured, radiographs of the wrist and elbow should be carefully reviewed to evaluate for a Galeazzi or Monteggia fracture-dislocation. These two injury patterns may be obvious by examination or may be subtle, and thus overshadowed by the more apparent shaft fracture of the radius or ulna. The classic Monteggia injury is a fracture of the proximal third of the ulna with an associated radial head dislocation. A Galeazzi fracture-dislocation consists most often of a radius fracture at the junction of the middle and distal third of the bone, with a dislocation at the distal radioulnar joint. These injury patterns are due to the anatomic relationship of the radius and ulna, with their points of articulation at the proximal and distal radioulnar joint and accompanying fibrous interosseous membrane. This relationship is such that when there is direct trauma to one bone, the force is transmitted to the other, typically at the points of articulation.

Monteggia and Galeazzi fractures are diagnosed by radiographs. Monteggia fractures require a true lateral view of the elbow, with attention to the radiocapitellar line. If a line drawn through the long axis of the radius fails to pass through the center of the capitellum on all projections a radial head dislocation should be considered (Fig. 119.16). It is worth noting that even bowing fractures of the ulna have been associated with radial head dislocation. Recognition of these injuries with immediate orthopedic consultation is crucial to prevent long-term disability. In pediatric patients, timely closed reduction of the fracture and dislocation followed by long arm splinting will minimize risk of permanent disability secondary to chronic irreducible radial head dislocation, limited supination and pronation, as well as nerve injury. Galeazzi fractures often require surgical repair, and the complications are few with proper management.

Disposition. Patients with adequate reduction and casting of the fracture may be discharged home with close orthopedic follow-up. Admission is necessary for any patient who will require surgical management including adolescents with fracture patterns treated primarily surgically, patients with failed reduction, and patients with Galeazzi fracture-dislocations.

Fractures of the Distal Radius and Ulna

Goals of Treatment

A key challenge facing the emergency clinicians in caring for patients with distal radius and ulna fractures is diagnosing subtle fractures and recognizing when reduction is necessary with displaced fractures. ED management should include pain control and immobilization with the arm in a position of comfort for any presumed fracture until diagnostic imaging and definitive care can be obtained.

CLINICAL PEARLS AND PITFALLS

- While the risk of growth arrest after distal radius physeal fracture is only about 4%, growth arrest of the distal ulna after physeal fracture has been reported to occur in up to 55% of cases making referral for orthopedic follow-up important.
- Fracture type varies with age and skeletal maturity: Buckle and greenstick fractures are frequent in children less than 10 years of age, growth plate fractures become increasingly common in children over 10, and complete fractures more typical in adolescents.
- Torus fractures may be subtle on radiographs; therefore, careful review in the setting of a suggestive history and physical examination is warranted.
- Ulnar styloid fractures are often accompanied by either a torus or physeal fracture of the radius.
- While there are high rates of asymptomatic nonunion in the healing of ulnar styloid fractures, fractures through the base of the styloid may interrupt the triangular fibrocartilage complex resulting in instability of the distal radial ulnar joint and requiring orthopedic follow-up.

Current Evidence

Distal forearm fractures are by far the most common of all the fractures that occur during childhood and adolescence. Fortunately, with the exception of occasional nerve entrapment at the time of reduction of a complete fracture, significant neurovascular complications are rare. The distal radial physis accounts for 60% of the growth of the radius and typically closes at 14 to 16 years of age. Consequently, the capacity for remodeling up through early adolescence for fractures of this region is significant due to proximity to the biologically active growth plates. Successful outcomes of both fracture union and full range of motion have been documented with incomplete reduction (angulation within 10 degrees of normal) of distal radial metaphyseal fractures in children under the age of 10 years—including those with translation and overriding of the fracture fragments (bayonet opposition) in the sagittal plane. The aim, however, is near-anatomic alignment whenever possible. Some cases may be managed with only gentle manipulation without sedation or through the use of local anesthetics or blocks, which eliminates the potential risks and costs associated with sedation. Distal ulnar metaphyseal fractures are typically seen in the setting of ipsilateral radial metaphyseal fractures. Complete ulnar displacement with bayonet apposition and angulation of 20 to 30 degrees are acceptable as long as radial reduction is within the accepted limits of remodeling.

Clinical Considerations

Clinical Recognition. Children with distal radius and ulna fractures will typically present with focal arm pain, swelling, or deformity. It should be noted that wrist pain may also be the chief complaint with more proximal injuries, for example, radial head fractures.

Triage Considerations. These children may present with obvious deformity and significant pain or with minimal deformity and mild pain. Patients with plastic deformities, greenstick, and buckle fractures may present several days after the injury. The injured extremity should be immobilized and pain management addressed.

Clinical Assessment. Localized swelling and tenderness commonly accompany distal radial fractures and can guide interpretation of the radiographic studies.

Management. Radiographs that include the entire forearm, including the elbow and wrist, should be obtained to identify all possible injuries to the extremity. Several common fracture patterns exist in injuries of the distal radius and ulna, and management varies by diagnosis (Fig. 119.30).

Torus fracture. In the setting of torus fractures, often the location of the soft tissue swelling on the radiographs helps highlight the position of the fracture. These fractures may be subtle, evident on only one projection and then only as a minor irregularity in the contour of the cortex. When a torus fracture is identified, a short arm volar splint or, if the swelling is minimal, a short arm cast for 3 to 4 weeks is recommended. A removable splint for 3 to 4 weeks has been shown to be as effective as casting, with the additional advantage of interfering less with physical functioning and activities. Follow-up may occur with the primary care clinician or with the orthopedic surgeon, and serial radiographs to guide management are infrequently needed.

Greenstick fractures. Greenstick fractures of the forearm, like complete fractures, have a tendency to displace if not properly immobilized. The distal fragment is angulated posteriorly in most greenstick and complete fractures of the distal forearm. Angulation of greater than 10 to 15 degrees is an indication for urgent orthopedic referral. When there is no significant angulation or displacement of greenstick and complete radial and ulnar fractures, immobilization in a neutral position with either a long arm posterior splint or a sugar-tong splint with orthopedic follow-up within 3 to 5 days is adequate emergency management.

Salter–Harris fractures. Salter–Harris types I and II injuries of the distal radial physis are common injuries among children of ages 6 to 12 years, and rarely lead to growth disturbance. The risk of growth disturbance increases with repeated and delayed manipulations. Clinicians should be prepared to make the presumptive diagnosis of a Salter–Harris type I injury when there is point tenderness on the physical examination corresponding to swelling over the distal radius on the radiograph, even when there is no obvious displacement of the epiphysis. Orthopedic consultation for closed reduction is indicated for all displaced and angulated physeal fractures, while immobilization and orthopedic referral are recommended for nondisplaced fractures of this type.

Disposition. Minimally or nondisplaced fractures may be discharged with orthopedic follow-up. Fractures that have had adequate reduction with casting may be discharged with orthopedic follow-up. Admission for surgical management may be recommended for fractures that could not be adequately reduced with procedural sedation in the ED.

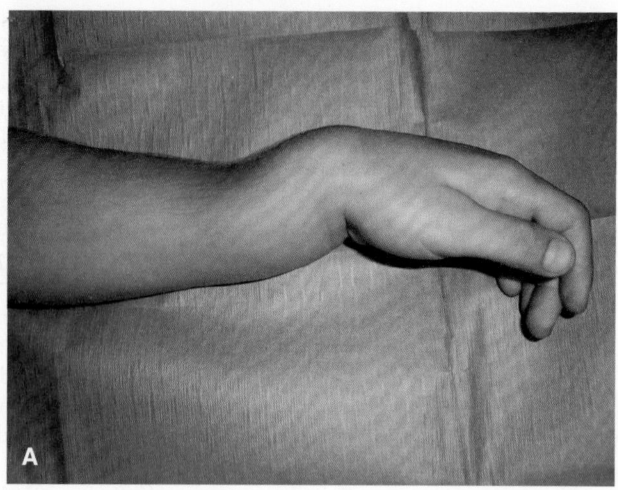

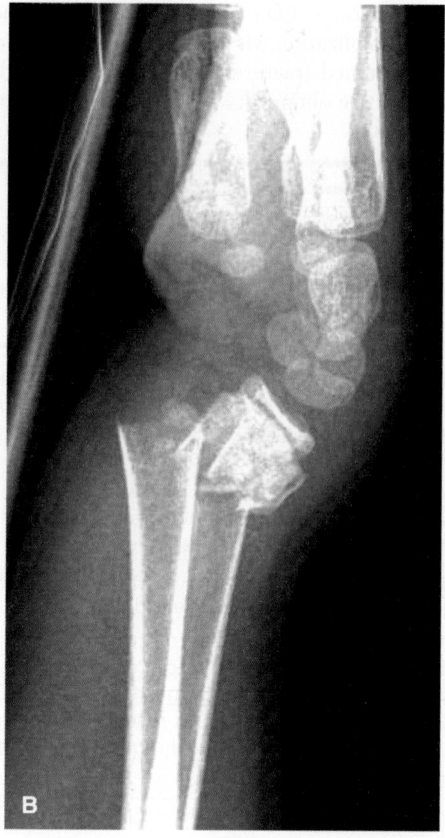

FIGURE 119.30 Colles fracture (A) shows the classic appearance on physical examination with wrist swelling and obvious deformity. B: Demonstrates the typical radiographic appearance with distal radial fracture with dorsal angulation. (Courtesy of William Phillips, MD. In: Chung EK, Atkinson-McEvoy LR, Boom JA, et al., eds. *Visual diagnosis and treatment in pediatrics*. 2nd ed. Philadelphia, PA: Lippincott Williams & Wilkins, 2010.)

INJURIES OF THE LOWER EXTREMITIES

Injuries of the Pelvis and Hip

Injuries of the Pelvis

Goals of Treatment. One of the initial goals in the treatment of pelvic fractures is the rapid identification and management of any ongoing bleeding associated with pelvic fractures or other concurrent injuries. Life-threatening hemorrhage from pelvic fractures is unusual, but if present, must be identified with timely treatment and resuscitation.

CLINICAL PEARLS AND PITFALLS

- The presence of bilateral anterior and posterior fractures is associated with the greatest risk of hemorrhage and intra-abdominal injury. Isolated pubic ramus fractures have the lowest risk for these.
- In the setting of concern for pelvic fracture, a patient with blood at the urethral meatus should be evaluated for injury to the genitourinary structures.
- In the absence of abnormalities on physical examination of the pelvis, lower extremity fracture, or other indication for abdominopelvic CT, the risk of pediatric pelvic fracture is low.

Current Evidence. Pelvic fractures are typically caused by high-energy mechanisms of injury that can be associated with multisystem trauma, including to the head, abdomen, urinary (e.g., urethra), and vascular structures. There should be a high index of suspicion for potentially life-threatening soft tissue or vascular injury. The role of routine screening pelvic x-rays in the setting of trauma has been questioned. In the conscious patient with a normal pelvis and lower extremity examination, routine x-rays of the pelvis may not be indicated, as the physical examination has a high specificity and negative predictive value for pelvic fractures, but only moderate sensitivity. Furthermore, if a patient with multisystem trauma undergoes an abdominal–pelvic CT scan for evaluation, screening radiographs are not necessary as the sensitivity of CT for detecting pelvic fractures is higher than pelvic radiographs.

Clinical Considerations

Clinical recognition. The pediatric pelvis has greater elasticity of the sacroiliac joint and the symphysis and more plasticity of the pelvic bones than the adult pelvis. As a result, a higher-energy impact is required to cause a fracture compared to the adult trauma patient. A high index of suspicion for the presence of potential pelvic fractures should be maintained for high-energy injury mechanisms, including motor vehicle collisions, pedestrians hit by a motor vehicle, and significant falls. Although the physical examination is not highly specific for pelvic fractures, those with abnormal pelvis and hip examinations with instability, pain on palpation of the pelvis, or the inability to walk due to pelvis pain should be evaluated for possible pelvic fractures.

Triage considerations. Most pelvic fractures are stable; however, those with abnormal vital signs indicating trauma-related hemorrhage require immediate resuscitative measures.

Clinical assessment. Mechanism of injury and any comorbid conditions should be emphasized in the history.

The initial assessment should include the vital signs and a thorough examination of the abdomen, pelvis, lower extremities, skin, genitourinary, and neurologic systems. Vital signs must be closely monitored and appropriate fluid resuscitation should be administered if tachycardia and/or hypotension are present. Anterior and lateral compression of the pelvis should be performed to assess pelvic stability.

Management. Pelvis and hip radiographs are the initial diagnostic test of choice. If further evaluation of the pelvis is needed, CT may be considered to further visualize the fracture(s). Immediate orthopedic consultation is required for all pelvic fractures except for minor avulsion fractures. The emergent application of an external fixator or a pneumatic antishock garment in the ED compresses the pelvis, leading to a tamponade effect to decrease the bleeding in some pelvic fractures. If commercial devices are not available, wrapping the pelvis in a sheet can provide temporary stability. Pelvic fractures can be categorized as (1) avulsion fractures, (2) pelvic ring fractures, and (3) acetabular fractures.

AVULSION FRACTURES. Sports are the most common mechanism causing avulsion fractures as they can result in strong, active contractions of the muscular attachments against resistance to the secondary centers of ossification (anterior-superior iliac spine, anterior-inferior iliac spine, and ischial tuberosity) (Fig. 119.31). The patient usually presents with localized pain and tenderness over the ossification sites (Fig. 119.32). The typical treatment is crutches with partial or no weight bearing for 4 to 6 weeks with a slow resumption of activities. The patient should be referred for outpatient orthopedic follow-up.

PELVIC RING FRACTURES. Single breaks in the pelvic ring occur with symphysis pubis diastasis, superior and inferior pubic rami fracture, and straddle fractures. These are generally considered stable fractures. One exception to this is with the open book deformity when diastasis of the pubic symphysis occurs with anterior disruption of the sacroiliac joint. With significant disruption of the symphysis pubis, closed reduction and fixation must be considered.

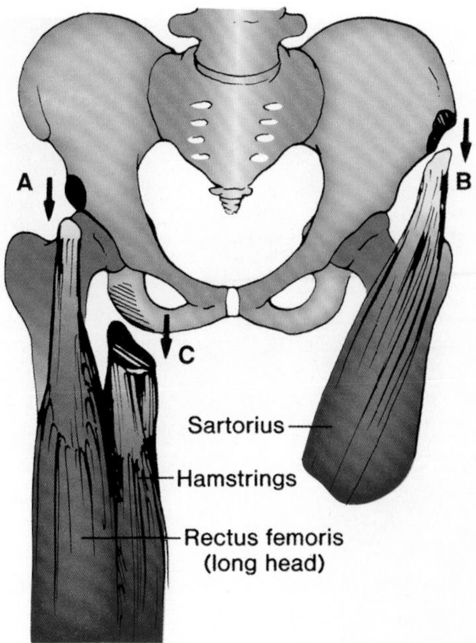

FIGURE 119.31 Common avulsion injuries of the pelvis: anterior-inferior iliac spine (**A**), anterior-superior iliac spine (**B**), and ischial tuberosity (**C**).

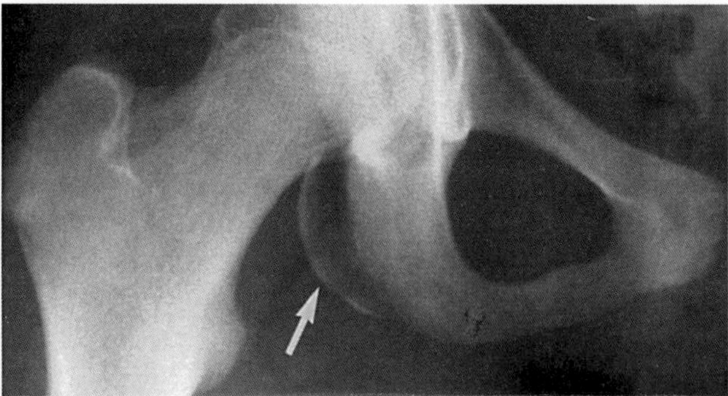

FIGURE 119.32 Avulsion fracture of the right ischial tuberosity in a 13-year-old girl (*arrow*).

Unstable fractures of the hemipelvis occur when fractures of the pubic rami or symphysis pubis are associated with a displaced sacroiliac joint dislocation or sacral fractures (Malgaigne fractures) (Fig. 119.33). These fractures are associated with a high incidence of injuries to adjacent structures, and life-threatening hemorrhage can occur from pelvic vein injury, which may require angiographic embolization for persistent bleeding. Unstable pelvic fractures are initially managed with bed rest. Urgent orthopedic consultation is recommended for pelvic ring fractures.

ACETABULAR FRACTURES. Acetabular fractures are rare in children, but may be associated with hip joint dislocation. If major pelvic disruption is present, the injury should be treated like a double break in the pelvic ring. Early orthopedic consultation should be obtained for these fractures.

Disposition. Patients with avulsion fractures may be discharged with crutches and non–weight-bearing status with orthopedic follow-up. Those with pelvic and acetabular fractures should be admitted to the hospital for further orthopedic care.

Injuries of the Hip and Proximal Femur

Goals of Treatment

Dislocations of the hip should be reduced in a timely manner, ideally within 6 hours of injury, with pre- and postreduction x-rays to identify any associated avulsion fractures. Proximal femur fractures should have urgent orthopedic consultation for reduction, as timing of surgical management (<24 hours) is associated with decreasing the risk of avascular necrosis.

CLINICAL PEARLS AND PITFALLS

- Hip dislocations should be reduced as soon as possible as the risk for avascular necrosis of the femoral head increases with each hour of delay.
- The sciatic nerve is the most common neurologic injury associated with hip dislocation.
- Complications of proximal femur fractures include nonunion, malunion, growth arrest, and avascular necrosis of the femoral head.

Current Evidence

For hip dislocations, the risk of osteonecrosis and posttraumatic arthritis is increased with delays in reduction.

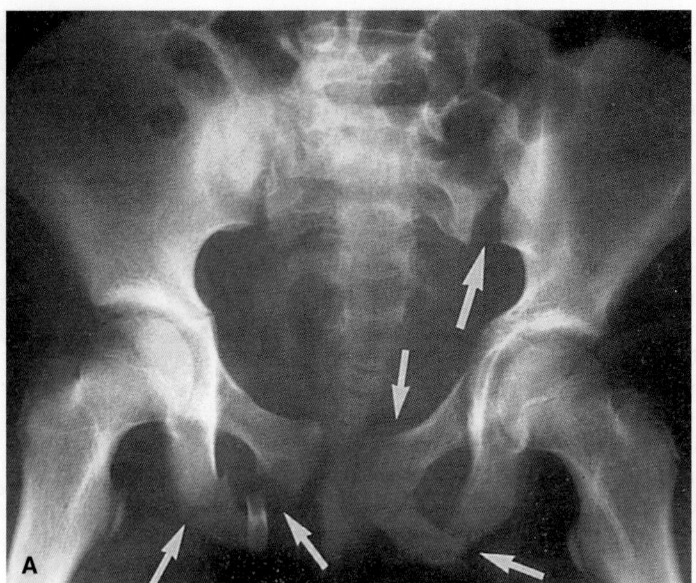

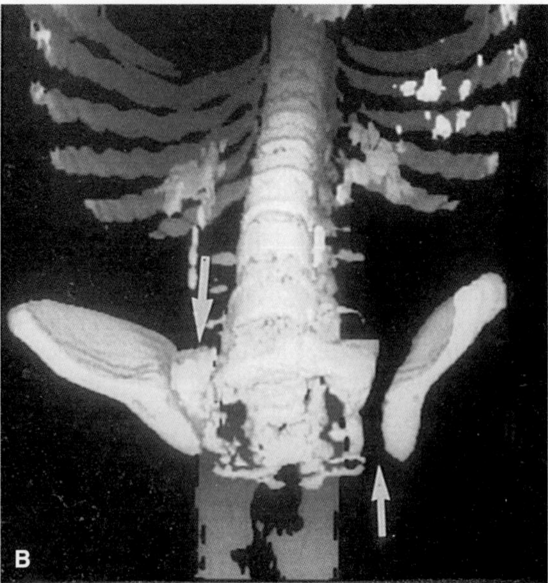

FIGURE 119.33 An unstable pelvic injury. **A:** On the plain film, multiple fractures of the pubic rami (*small arrows*) and widening of the right sacroiliac joint (*large arrow*) are apparent. **B:** On the three-dimensional reconstruction of the CT scan, the left sacroiliac fracture is even more obvious (*small arrow*), and a right-sided sacral fracture is also seen (*large arrow*).

Clinical Considerations

Clinical Recognition. Dislocations of the hip are apparent on physical examination with a painful, shortened limb. Proximal femur fractures present with hip pain, inability to bear weight, and/or limp.

Triage Considerations. Patients with injuries of the hip and proximal femur are generally hemodynamically stable, unless multisystem trauma has been sustained. As these injuries are associated with significant pain, patients should have a brief initial evaluation and then have pain medications administered.

Clinical Assessment. The initial assessment should include the vital signs and a thorough examination of the abdomen, pelvis, lower extremities, and neurologic system. A careful neurovascular examination must be performed. The presence of the dorsalis pedis and posterior tibial artery pulses should be documented, and the distal perfusion status of the limb should be examined. Sensory and motor nerve function should be evaluated as follows: The posterior tibial nerve must be assessed by evaluating sensation on the plantar aspect of the foot and by checking plantar flexion, and the peroneal nerve must be assessed by evaluating sensation over the lateral and dorsal aspects of the foot and by checking ankle eversion and dorsiflexion.

Management. X-ray is the initial imaging modality of choice for the identification of the specific fracture or dislocation (Fig. 119.34). The patient should be placed on bed rest with no weight bearing. Orthopedics should be consulted for all hip dislocations and femur fractures.

Hip dislocation. Traumatic hip dislocation in children is uncommon, though can be recognized in the child presenting with a painful, shortened, externally rotated limb. Most hip dislocations are in the posterior direction. Spontaneous reduction at the time of injury also can occur. If this is suspected, x-rays of the hips should still be obtained with attention directed to the medial clear space of the hips, which will be wider after trauma than the normal contralateral side (Fig. 119.35).

Treatment of hip dislocation is closed reduction. This will usually be done by an orthopedist under procedural sedation in the ED or in the operating room under general anesthesia. In adolescents, reduction under anesthesia is recommended as occult epiphyseal injury may be present in this age group with hip dislocation, and epiphyseal separation may occur during reduction. However, given the importance of a timely reduction, in select cases, hip reduction may be performed by

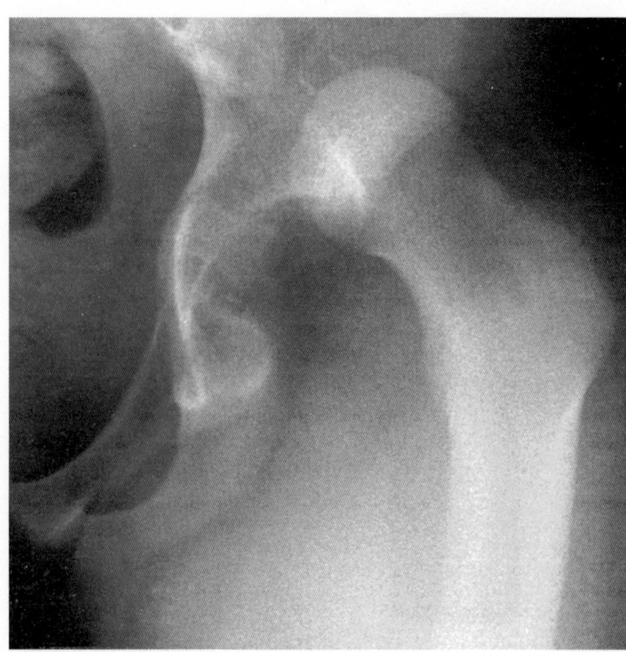

FIGURE 119.34 Dislocation of the left hip in a 9-year-old boy. If dislocation is delayed beyond 6 hours, the risk of osseous necrosis rises.

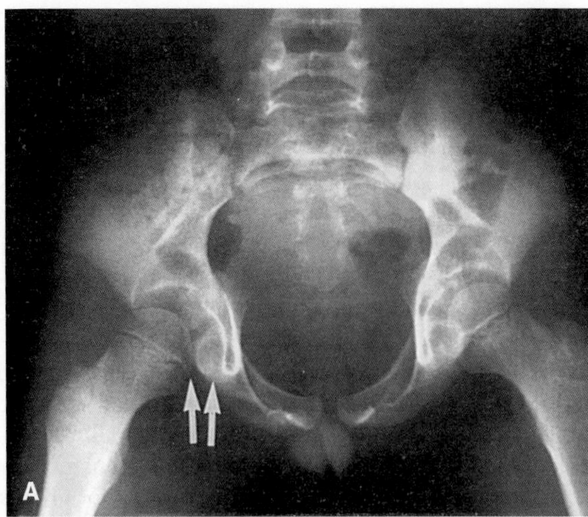

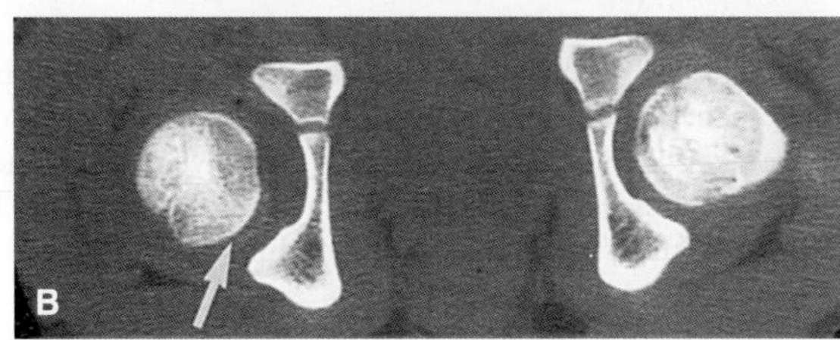

FIGURE 119.35 Radiographs taken following closed reduction of a right hip dislocation. **A:** The plain film demonstrates residual widening of the joint space (*arrows*). **B:** Widening is also apparent with magnetic resonance imaging, as is entrapment of a portion of the posterior joint capsule (*arrow*). Under general anesthesia, further efforts at closed reduction were successful.

emergency clinicians. For a posterior hip dislocation reduction, the hip and knee should be flexed to 90 degrees and with the pelvis stabilized, longitudinal traction should be applied along the axis of the femur and the femoral head gently manipulated back into the acetabulum. If closed reduction is unsuccessful, open reduction is necessary. During the dislocation, the posterior labrum and joint capsule may detach, and then become trapped in the joint space during reduction (spontaneous or closed). CT or MRI may be necessary to evaluate the adequacy of reduction if instability or joint space widening is noted, and in adolescent patients.

Proximal femoral physeal fractures. Fractures through the proximal femoral physis can have a range of displacement from minimal to complete (Fig. 119.36). Unfortunately, there is a very high risk for osteonecrosis and subsequent long-term disability for completely displaced fractures. Urgent orthopedic consultation should be obtained for surgical reduction and internal fixation. Minimally displaced fractures in children less than 2 years may be treated with closed reduction and casting.

Femoral neck fractures. Displaced femoral neck fractures are uncommon in children, but when they occur, they are considered an orthopedic emergency (Fig. 119.37). Open or closed reduction is required for treatment of these fractures. Stress fractures in the femoral neck, especially from repetitive activity sports (e.g., long distance running), can present as exercise-induced hip pain. These fractures may result in osteonecrosis if there is damage to the blood supply of the femoral head. Early recognition is important to allow activity restriction and healing, which may prevent progression to a complete fracture

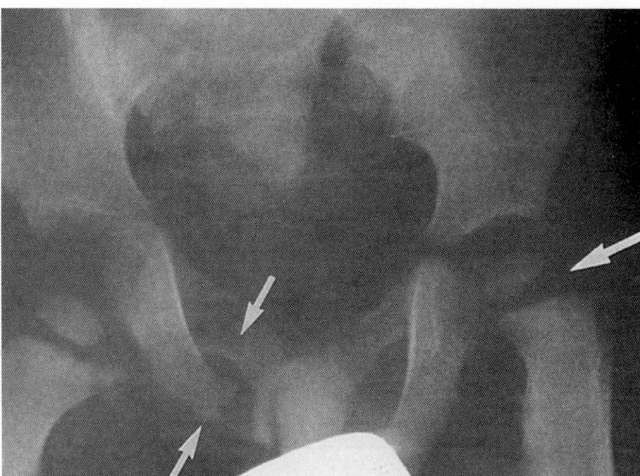

FIGURE 119.36 Displaced Salter–Harris type I fracture of the left proximal femur in a 2-year-old boy (*large arrow*). Also seen are fractures of the right pubic rami (*small arrows*). The pelvis is also disrupted posteriorly.

with displacement. Bone scan or MRI is recommended for evaluation and early diagnosis. Then open or closed reduction should be performed by the orthopedic surgeon.

Intertrochanteric fractures. These fractures are relatively uncommon in children and adolescents and have a lower risk of complications. Orthopedics should be consulted urgently. Nondisplaced or minimally displaced fractures may be treated with a spica cast for 6 to 8 weeks. With significantly displaced fractures, internal fixation may be necessary to attain appropriate alignment.

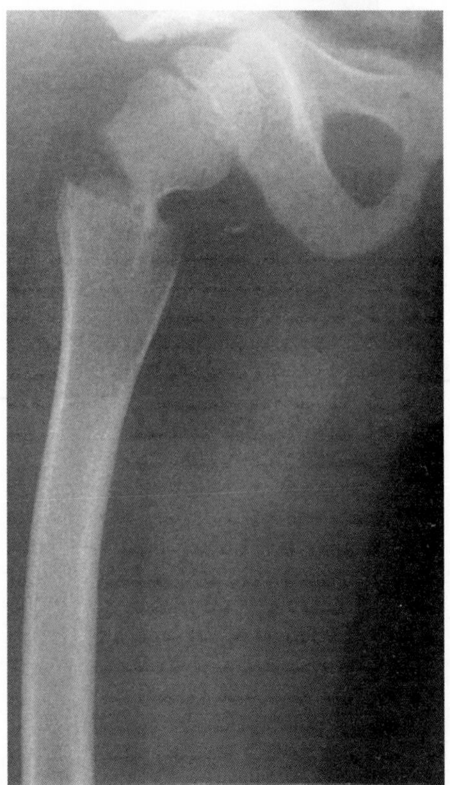

FIGURE 119.37 Fracture of the right femoral neck in a 3-year-old girl.

Disposition. Hip dislocations, proximal femur fractures, displaced femoral neck fractures, and intertrochanteric fractures should be admitted to the hospital for orthopedic management.

Injuries of the Femur and Knee

Injuries of the Shaft of the Femur

CLINICAL PEARLS AND PITFALLS

- Nonaccidental trauma should be investigated in nonambulatory children with femur fractures.
- Isolated femur fractures in children rarely result in hemodynamically significant blood loss, unlike in adults.

Femur fractures in older children and adolescents are most commonly sustained from high-energy mechanisms (e.g., motor vehicle collisions, pedestrian–motor vehicle impact) resulting in multisystem trauma involving other organ injuries. In younger children, however, less force is necessary to cause a femur fracture. A femur fracture usually presents with pain and swelling of the thigh. All patients with a femur fracture should have urgent orthopedic consultation for further management. AP and lateral radiographs of the femur, including the hip and knee, should be obtained. The extremity should be immobilized with a posterior leg splint until definitive care is obtained. Femoral shaft fractures occur in all pediatric age groups, but have different mechanisms of injury, complications, and treatments based on age.

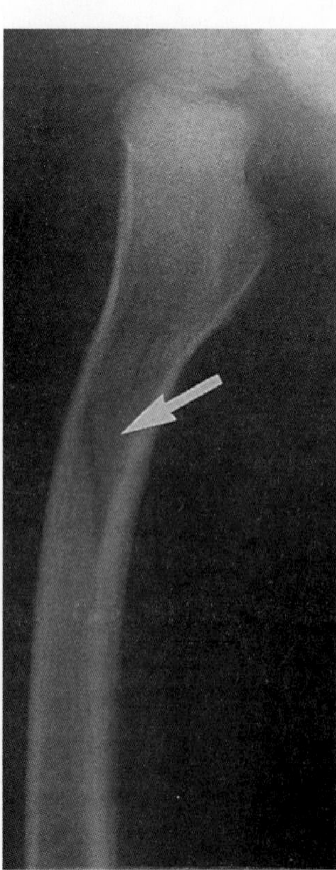

FIGURE 119.38 Spiral fracture of the right femur in a 20-month-old boy (*arrow*). In this instance, the injury occurred as the result of a motor vehicle collision. In general, spiral femur fractures in young children should prompt consideration of physical abuse.

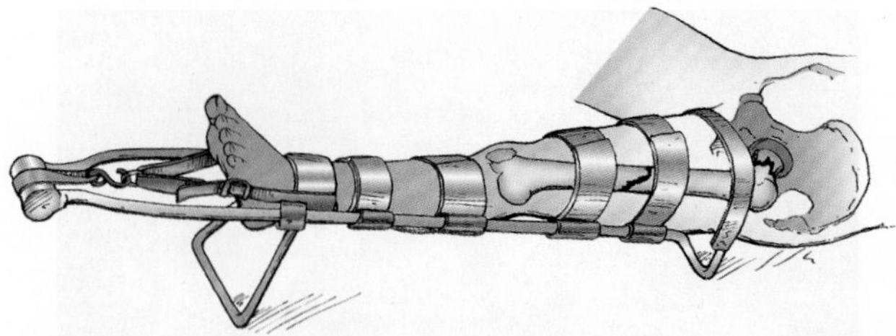

FIGURE 119.39 Use of a traction splint to stabilize femoral fractures is strongly recommended. Both adult and pediatric sizes are available.

Birth to 2 years old. Femur fractures in this young age group are typically a result of a slow twisting motion or a direct blow (Fig. 119.38). Nonaccidental trauma should always be considered in this age group, especially in the nonambulatory child. Treatment is usually with a Pavlik harness for infants or spica casting.

2 to 10 years old. Treatment is initially with traction or splinting, and then spica casting for children less than 6 years old and intramedullary nailing for those 6 to 11 years old. These fractures can result in the long-term complications of leg length discrepancy, malrotation, and malunion.

Adolescents. Femur fractures in this age group can be initially stabilized with traction splints in the field or a posterior leg splint until orthopedic consult is obtained (Fig. 119.39). Management is with surgical stabilization with internal fixation to improve alignment and promote an earlier return to activity.

Injuries of the Knee

CLINICAL PEARLS AND PITFALLS

- Skeletally immature children and adolescents are at higher risk for epiphyseal or physeal fractures around the knee; therefore, radiographs are recommended for evaluation of possible fracture after a knee injury (Fig. 119.40).
- Adolescents and teenagers more commonly sustain ligamentous injuries that may be associated with avulsion fractures.
- With distal femoral epiphyseal fractures, adequate analgesia is important to decrease muscle spasm, protecting the physis from further damage.
- Distal femoral epiphyseal fractures can be complicated by compartment syndrome or direct compression to vascular and nerve structures around the knee.
- Popliteal vessel or peroneal nerve injury can occur with distal femoral epiphyseal or proximal tibial epiphyseal fractures.

Distal Femoral Fractures

This injury is usually the result of very high shear and translational forces. These fractures are usually associated with a knee effusion, local soft tissue swelling, and physeal tenderness. On examination, tenderness and swelling may be noted proximal to the joint line, usually on bilateral sides of the distal femoral physeal site. With displaced fractures, there may be obvious deformity, and soft crepitus with motion may be felt (Fig. 119.41). If the fracture is anteriorly displaced, the

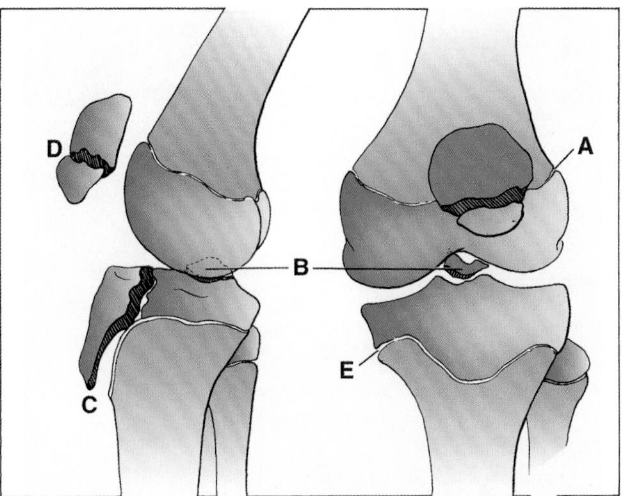

FIGURE 119.40 Common fractures of the knee in children: distal femoral physis (**A**), tibial spine (**B**), tibial tubercle (**C**), patella (**D**), and proximal tibial physis (**E**).

patella may be prominent with dimpling of the anterior skin (Fig. 119.42). If the epiphysis is posteriorly displaced, the distal metaphyseal fragment becomes prominent above the patella. These fractures can also cause damage to the popliteal vessels or peroneal nerve by direct compression. Nondisplaced fractures should be splinted in place with urgent orthopedic consultation for casting. Displaced fractures should have immediate orthopedic consultation for reduction under anesthesia. Unlike other epiphyseal fractures, even Salter type I and II injuries are associated with distal femoral growth and angular deformity.

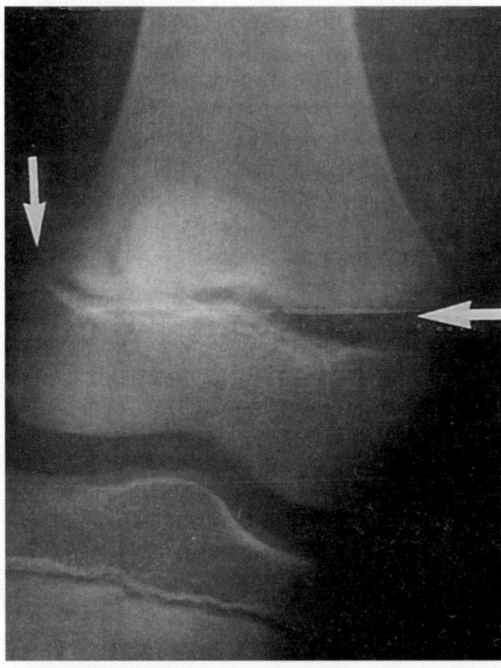

FIGURE 119.41 A Salter–Harris type II fracture of the right distal femoral physis in a 9-year-old boy. Widening of the growth plate is seen medially (*large arrow*), and a small metaphyseal fragment has been displaced laterally (*small arrow*). Closed reduction was successful. In an adult, the same mechanism of injury would have resulted in a medial collateral ligament sprain or tear.

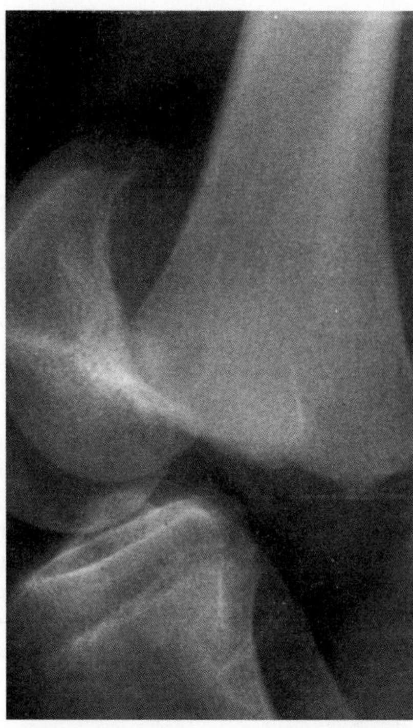

FIGURE 119.42 A Salter–Harris type I fracture of the right distal femoral physis with anterior displacement of the epiphysis in a 14-year-old boy. The injury resulted from a snowboarding accident.

Knee Dislocations

Knee dislocation, or complete dislocation of the femorotibial joint, is very uncommon in children. Hyperextension injury is more likely to result in a distal femoral epiphyseal separation. Femorotibial joint dislocation is an orthopedic emergency as there is a high risk of neurovascular compromise and/or compartment syndrome. Damage to the peroneal nerve can be assessed with having the patient dorsiflex the foot and by testing sensation to the superior and lateral aspect of the foot on the injured extremity. Reduction under procedural sedation with axial traction of the tibia and slow flexion of the knee from an extended position may be attempted in the ED.

After reduction, the ankle brachial index (ABI) should be calculated to evaluate for any vascular damage. This is the ratio of the systolic blood pressure at the ankle compared to the brachial artery in the ipsilateral arm. An ABI >0.9 has a 99% negative predictive value for ruling out a flow-limiting vascular injury requiring surgical repair; however, the patient should be observed for 24 hours with vascular checks every 2 hours. With an ABI <0.9 a CT arteriogram is recommended to assess for possible popliteal artery damage. Definitive orthopedic care includes operative repair of ligamentous injury from this dislocation.

Patellar Dislocations

The patella can be acutely dislocated when a force displaces the patella laterally while the foot is planted. It may remain dislocated or can reduce spontaneously. The child will present with an acutely swollen knee with pain to palpation especially along the medial patella retinaculum. If the patella is already reduced, displacement of the patella laterally will elicit an apprehension sign where the patient may state concern the kneecap feels like it is going to "pop out." If the patella is still dislocated, this is clinically evident with an inability to completely extend the knee and an abnormal contour of the patella. Radiograph examination can also identify patellar dislocation but is not usually required. To reduce the patella, the knee should be extended with a medial upward force on the lateral patella (see Chapter 141 Procedures, section on Closed Reduction of Dislocations). Radiographs of the knee should be obtained after reduction to evaluate for possible osteochondral fracture of the lateral femoral condyle or the medial patella facet, although these fractures are not always easily identified on x-ray. After reduction, the knee should be immobilized in an above-the-knee posterior splint or knee immobilizer for 4 weeks. Outpatient orthopedic referral is recommended for follow-up.

Patellar Fractures

Fractures of the patella are relatively uncommon in children compared to adults due to the thick cartilage covering the patella during a child's growth and development. In adolescents, fractures of the patella become more common. They may present as osteochondritis dissecans from overuse, symptomatic bipartite conditions, avulsion or "sleeve" fractures, or transverse displaced fractures. A congenital bipartite patella may be mistaken for a fracture on x-ray as an accessory ossification center is located along the superior lateral margin of the patella with smooth and rounded margins (Fig. 119.43). A sleeve fracture, which occurs when the lower half of the cartilage cap is avulsed by the patellar ligament, may also be difficult to diagnose on x-ray. It may only be apparent by a small piece of bone visualized at the superior margin of the patellar ligament as the visible bony portion of the patella is displaced superiorly by the quadriceps (Fig. 119.44). This injury presents with pain preventing active extension of the knee. A radiograph of the contralateral knee may assist in the diagnosis. Urgent orthopedic consultation should be obtained. Nondisplaced patellar fractures may be managed with a cast for 4 to 6 weeks. Displaced fractures of more than 3 to 4 mm displacement may require open reduction and internal fixation.

Ligamentous Injuries of the Knee

Ligamentous injuries to the knee are less common than fractures of the epiphyses and physes around the knee until the growth plate closes (Fig. 119.45). Most injuries occur from direct trauma to the knee or from valgus or varus stress, as experienced during athletic activities. The medial collateral and anterior cruciate ligaments (ACLs) are injured most frequently, with ACL injuries often associated with avulsion of the tibial spine. ED management often involves exclusion of a bony injury, and then outpatient referral for repeat evaluation when the swelling has improved and examination may be more reliable. Use of immobilizers is warranted for patients with significant pain with movement, but care should be taken to avoid prolonged use without repeat evaluation due to risk of quadriceps atrophy. Outpatient referral to orthopedics is recommended, and MRI may be required for further evaluation of any bony and soft tissue injuries.

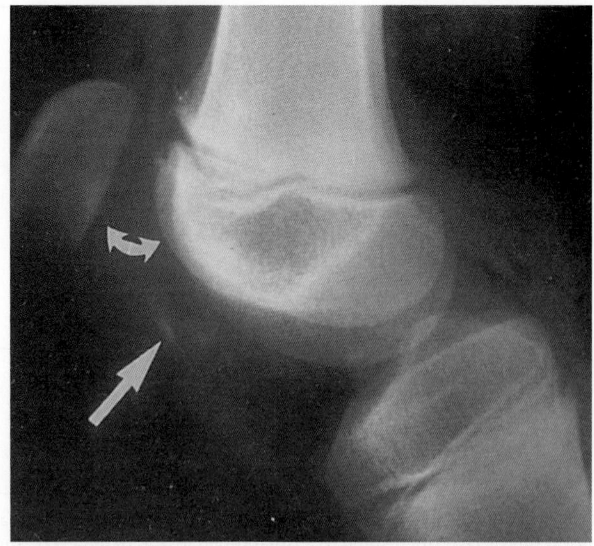

FIGURE 119.44 Radiograph demonstrating a sleeve fracture of the patella in a 10-year-old male. The inferior pole of the patella is displaced anteriorly (*curved arrow*). The bone fragment seen (*large arrow*) was avulsed by, and remains attached to, the patellar tendon.

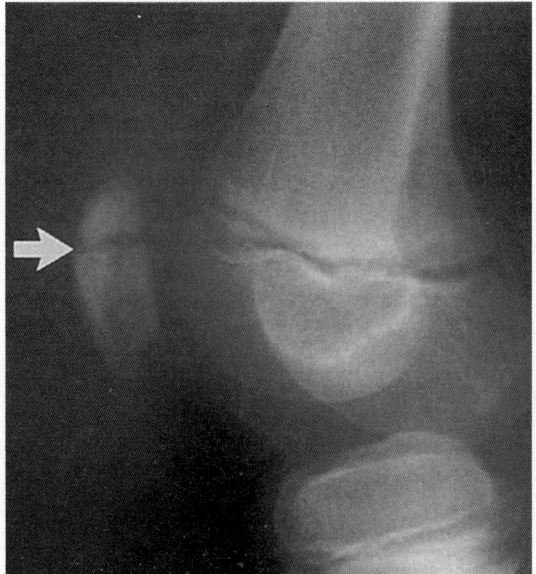

FIGURE 119.43 Transverse fracture of the patella in an 11-year-old victim of a motor vehicle collision (*arrow*).

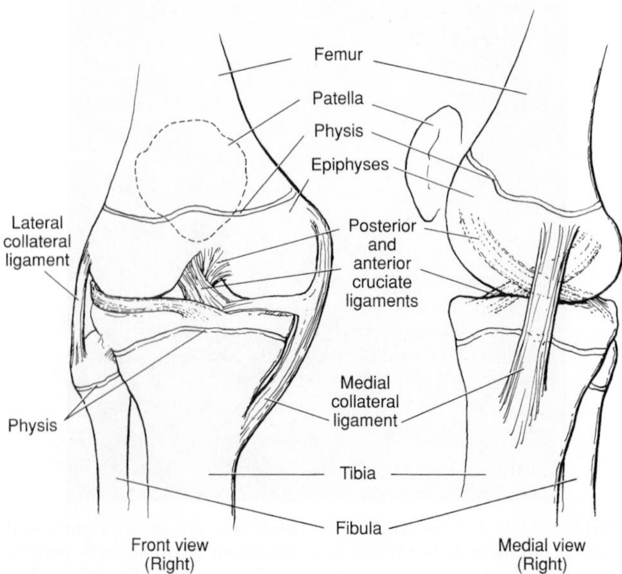

FIGURE 119.45 The ligaments of the knee. Proximally, both collateral ligaments attach to the epiphysis, whereas distally they attach to the tibia and fibula below the tibial epiphysis.

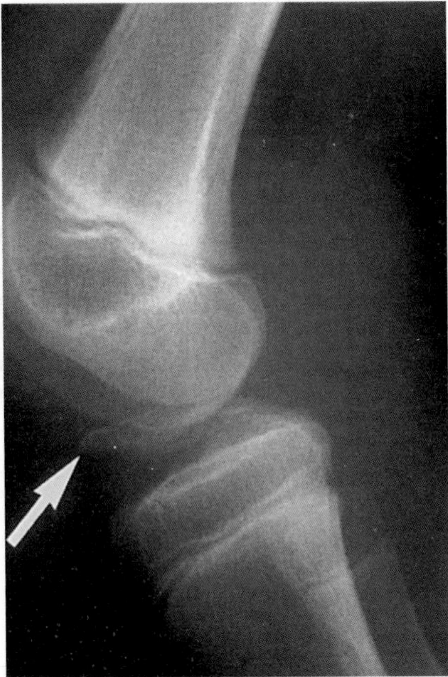

FIGURE 119.46 Avulsion fracture of the tibial spine in a 9-year-old girl (*arrow*). A significant hemarthrosis was present and was aspirated. In an adult, the same mechanism of injury would have resulted in a tear of the anterior cruciate ligament.

Tibial Tubercle and Spine Fractures

Avulsion of the tibial spine occurs with hyperflexion and presents with pain and refusal to bear weight in the presence of hemarthrosis. Radiographs should be obtained, which may reveal findings ranging from minimal elevation of the anterior portion of the tibial spine (best seen on lateral views) to complete separation (Fig. 119.46). The extremity should be splinted in extension. If the child is in significant pain, arthrocentesis of the hemarthrosis may be performed, although this must be balanced against the risk of infection from the procedure. Orthopedics should be consulted for further management. Incomplete separations may be managed with closed reduction while complete avulsion requires open repair.

Less commonly, knee injuries can also result in avulsion fractures of the tibial tuberosity. This typically occurs with jumping when the quadriceps is strongly contracted. A Salter–Harris type III fracture can result if the tibial tubercle is either partially or completely avulsed from the proximal tibial epiphysis. Orthopedics should be consulted for either closed or open reduction of the fracture, depending on its severity.

Injuries of the Proximal Tibia and Fibula and Shaft

CLINICAL PEARLS AND PITFALLS

- Proximal tibial fractures are at risk for the development of compartment syndrome and progressive posttraumatic valgus defor mity.
- A toddler (9 to 36 months old) who is nonweight bearing may not localize their tenderness; a staged approach with first imaging the tibia/fibula and progressing to imaging from foot to femur if tibia films are negative is recommended.
- Nonaccidental trauma should be investigated in nonambulatory children with spiral fractures of the tibia.

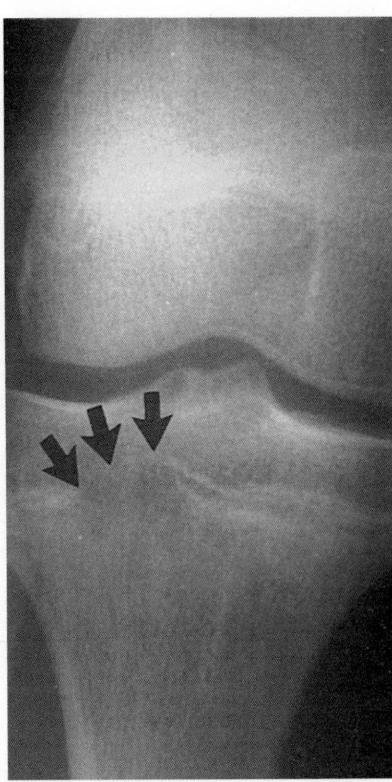

FIGURE 119.47 Although the original injury was only a Salter–Harris type I fracture of the proximal tibial physis, premature closure of the physis occurred (*arrows*). All fractures involving the proximal tibial growth plate require orthopedic referral.

Proximal Tibial Epiphyseal Fractures

Direct force to the knee is usually the mechanism of injury for this fracture, which presents with knee effusion, local soft tissue swelling, and tenderness over the proximal tibial physis (Fig. 119.47). The popliteal structures, including the popliteal artery, are tethered to the proximal tibia and are at risk for damage at the time of injury. Serial neurovascular examinations must be performed to assess for damage to these structures. Urgent orthopedic consultation should be obtained for closed reduction and internal fixation. Fractures of the proximal tibial epiphysis have a high risk for the development of recurrent deformity, growth arrest, and resultant limb length inequality.

Proximal Tibial Metaphyseal Fractures

This injury occurs when a valgus force is applied to the extended knee (Fig. 119.48). Acutely these fractures can lead to the development of compartment syndrome so orthopedic consultation and close monitoring are recommended. Closed reduction and casting is the usual management. Even with adequate reduction of the fracture, asymmetric growth of the proximal tibial physis can occur.

Tibial and Fibular Shaft Fractures

Fractures of the shaft of the tibia and fibula are the most common fractures of the lower extremity in children. In infants, the tibia is more likely to bend, buckle, or sustain a nondisplaced spiral fracture, while adolescent fractures are associated with more fracture displacement and comminution. For minimally displaced/nondisplaced fractures with no signs of compartment syndrome, the extremity may be immobilized

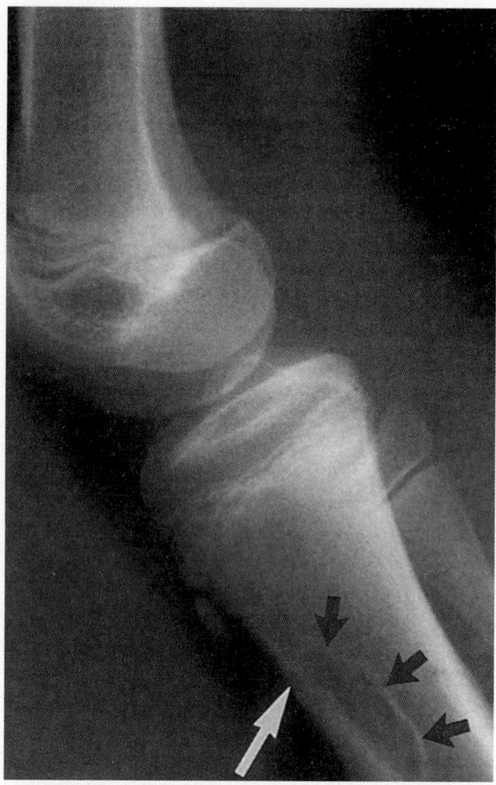

FIGURE 119.48 Nondisplaced proximal tibial metaphyseal fracture in an 11-year-old girl (*large arrow*) through a nonossifying fibroma (*small arrows*). Orthopedic consultation is mandatory both because the fracture is pathologic and because it is located in the proximal tibia.

in a posterior long leg splint with a plan for postdischarge pain control and outpatient follow-up with orthopedics. These fractures are rarely associated with delayed union or nonunion. For open fractures, ipsilateral femur fractures, or any concern for compartment syndrome, orthopedics should be consulted emergently for open treatment. Athletes older than 10 years may also sustain stress fractures of the tibia (most commonly in the proximal third) that typically present with a history of insidious leg pain that worsens with activity. Initial radiographs may be normal with radiographic changes becoming apparent about 2 weeks after symptoms. Treatment is with activity modification and a walking boot for 4 to 6 weeks. In paraplegic children, tibia and fibula fractures may present similarly to infection, with warmth and swelling over the lower leg. Fractures in these children are treated conservatively with splints or casts for 3 to 4 weeks and orthopedic follow-up.

Toddler's Fractures

Originally, a toddler's fracture referred to an oblique nondisplaced fracture of the distal tibia in children 9 to 36 months of age, but now this term is used more loosely to describe other lower extremity fractures sustained in this age group. The history typically is that of a minor fall or there may be no history of trauma at all. The physical examination may initially appear normal at rest, or there may be subtle findings of warmth or tenderness of the tibia and/or fibula. The child usually does not appear to be in pain when at rest, but may cry with manipulation of the injured extremity or when he/she tries to put weight on the lower extremity. Most often, the child refuses to bear any weight on the injured extremity and will only stand on the uninjured extremity. Radiographs may appear normal or may demonstrate a spiral or oblique fracture extending downward and medial through the distal third of the tibia (Fig. 119.49). This may be visualized on anteroposterior or lateral views, although internal oblique projections may also be useful. The extremity should be immobilized with a short leg splint or walking cast and the patient should be referred to outpatient orthopedic follow-up. If radiographs are negative, the child may be discharged home with primary care or orthopedic follow-up. X-rays after 10 days may demonstrate subperiosteal new bone formation or enough sclerosis to make the fracture visible. If no fracture is identified at this time, continued immobilization is not usually necessary.

Injuries of the Ankle and Foot

Injuries of the Ankle

Goals of Treatment. Growth plate fractures of the ankle are the third most common type of physeal fracture in children, after finger and distal radial physeal fractures. The ankle ligaments attach to the epiphysis of the tibia and fibula, and they are generally stronger than the physis. As a result, children are more likely to sustain physeal and bony injury than ligamentous injury after ankle trauma. Correctly identifying a physeal or ligamentous injury is important to ensure appropriate treatment.

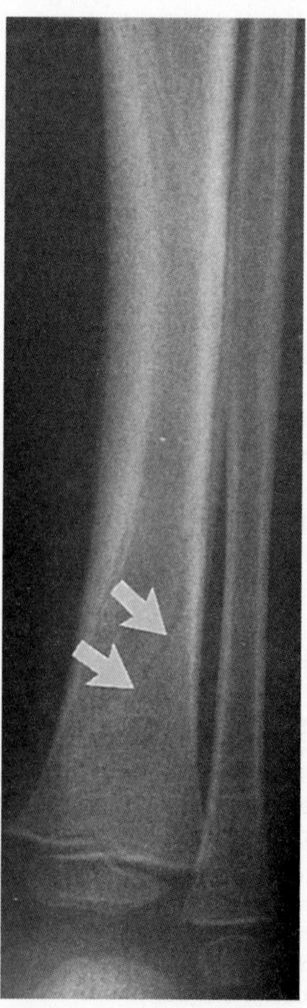

FIGURE 119.49 Toddler's fracture of the distal tibia (*arrows*). The fracture line could not be demonstrated radiographically until 2 weeks after the onset of symptoms.

CLINICAL PEARLS AND PITFALLS

- Prior to their fusion, physeal injuries are more likely than ligamentous sprains in children.
- Tenderness along the posterior aspect of the lateral malleolus can be used to distinguish a potential Salter I distal fibular fracture from an ankle sprain, which will commonly only be tender anteriorly, over the anterior talofibular ligament.
- Distal tibia/fibula and significant injuries to the foot are especially at risk for the development of compartment syndrome; therefore, the extremity should be closely monitored for increasing swelling and signs and symptoms associated with compartment syndrome.

Current Evidence. As both bony and ligamentous ankle injuries present with pain and swelling, radiographs are often used for evaluation of ankle injuries in children. The Ottawa ankle rules are a set of clinical decision rules for obtaining ankle and foot radiographs that can be useful for children over 5 years of age. They recommend that an ankle radiograph is only required if the patient has any pain in the malleolar zone, and if the patient has any of these findings: bone tenderness at the posterior edge or tip of the lateral malleolus, bone tenderness at the posterior edge or tip of the medial malleolus, or inability to bear weight both immediately and in the ED. The rules recommend a foot radiograph if there is pain in the midfoot zone and any of the following: bone tenderness at the base of the fifth metatarsal, bone tenderness over the navicular, or inability to bear weight both immediately and in the ED.

Adolescents are at risk for sustaining transitional fractures during the 18 months in which the physis begins to close (14 years in girls, 16 years in boys). While the physis is still open, the lateral aspect of the distal tibial physis is weaker and more prone to injury, leading to the specific injury patterns associated with the Tillaux fracture, involving the epiphysis only, or triplane fractures, with fracture extension into the distal tibial metaphysis. In addition, fractures of the ankle can be associated with a syndesmosis injury, seen as medial joint space widening between the distal tibia and fibula on the radiograph, which may need surgical treatment.

Clinical Considerations

Clinical recognition. After ankle trauma, the patient commonly develops pain, swelling, and ecchymosis and may be unable to bear weight. The differential diagnoses for ankle injuries include nondisplaced Salter–Harris type I fractures; ligamentous injuries; osteochondral fractures of the tibia/fibula or talus; and avulsion injuries.

Triage considerations. Pain should be addressed as appropriate and a wheelchair provided for transport if the patient is having pain with weight bearing. Significant swelling and pain associated with an ankle injury should be quickly triaged for concern of possible compartment syndrome and/or complicated ankle fracture.

Clinical assessment. Typically there is a history of a twisting mechanism to the lower leg with either eversion or inversion. The ankle and foot should be examined closely for any skin defects, deformity, degree of swelling, neurologic deficits, and vascular injury. Sensation should be evaluated on both the plantar and dorsal aspects of the foot. Toe flexion and extension can be used to evaluate motor function. The examination should include the function of the extensor hallucis longus muscle (great toe extension), ankle dorsiflexion, plantar flexion, inversion, and eversion. In addition to the capillary refill of the toes, the dorsalis pedis and posterior tibialis pulses should be assessed, and if they cannot be palpated, must be evaluated by a Doppler probe to assess for any vascular compromise. The ankle evaluation should include palpation superiorly of the tibia and fibula and inferiorly down to the proximal foot (including fifth metatarsal). Ankle sprains and fractures of the tibia may also be associated with proximal fibula fractures (Maisonneuve fracture); therefore, careful examination of the proximal fibula is important as part of the complete examination.

Management. Radiographs should be obtained if there is concern for bony injury, and the Ottawa ankle rules may be considered for use in children older than 5 years to guide the need for radiographic evaluation. Anteroposterior, mortise, and lateral x-rays should be obtained to adequately evaluate the ankle. The mortise view is especially important to evaluate fractures without obvious deformity as it may visualize a minimally displaced fracture that could be disguised by the tibiofibular overlap on the other views. Foot films are recommended to evaluate tenderness over the fifth metatarsal that may represent a Jones or pseudo-Jones fracture. Advanced imaging (CT) is recommended for the evaluation of intra-articular fractures for accurate diagnosis, preoperative planning, and assessment of reduction.

Ankle sprains. The most common mechanism for ligamentous injuries is when the foot is adducted and inverted while held in plantar flexion. Of the three lateral ankle ligaments, the anterior talofibular ligament is most commonly injured and will demonstrate tenderness with palpation just anterior to the distal fibula. Ankle sprains can be graded on three levels: (1) Grade 1 injuries have stretching of the ligaments; (2) grade 2 injuries include partial ligamentous tears without loss of stability; and (3) grade 3 injuries are complete tears of the ligamentous complex with loss of stability. Grade 1 mild sprains may be treated with an air splint or elastic wrap along with ice and elevation for 72 hours. Crutches with partial weight bearing may be used until the patient can walk without limping. Grade 2 and 3 injuries can be immobilized either in a walking cast/boot or posterior splint for up to 3 weeks with crutches for ambulation.

Distal tibial and fibular fractures. These fractures are typically classified by anatomic classification schemes, with the Salter–Harris system being used most widely. Orthopedic management depends on the child's age, fracture type, amount of displacement, and ability to restore the ankle joint. Nondisplaced fractures may be treated in the ED with a bulky posterior splint, crutches, and referral to an orthopedist as they will need cast immobilization for 3 to 6 weeks (Fig. 119.50). Open reduction and internal fixation are often needed for fractures involving both the physis and the ankle joint. The articular surface can only accept minimal displacement otherwise altered joint mechanics will develop, which can lead to complications with pain, stiffness, and arthritis. Displaced fractures should be referred urgently to the orthopedic surgeon, as they will require reduction under procedural sedation or anesthesia.

Isolated distal tibial Salter–Harris type I, type II, and type III fractures. These injuries typically occur with plantar

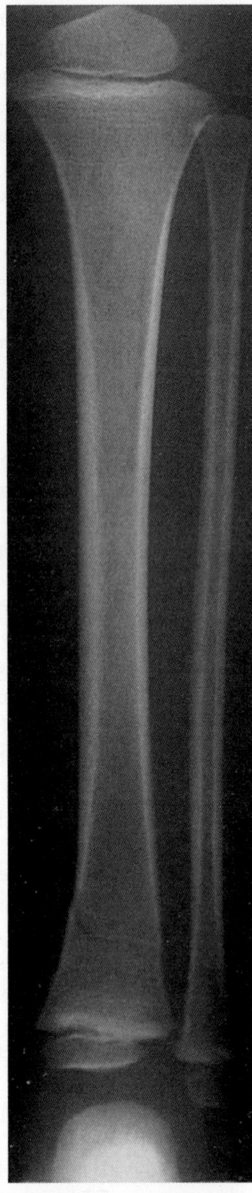

FIGURE 119.50 Nondisplaced transverse fracture of the distal tibia in a 3-year-old girl. Immobilization in a long leg posterior splint with orthopedic follow-up within 3 to 5 days would be adequate emergency treatment. The potential for growth deformity is low.

flexion with eversion. Salter I fractures may only show soft tissue swelling on the radiograph, without a clear fracture. This type of fracture should be suspected if the patient has focal tenderness only at the physis of the medial malleolus. Nondisplaced fractures may be immobilized in a short or long leg cast for 3 to 4 weeks. They should follow-up in orthopedic clinic within 1 week of injury. After casting they may be transitioned to a weight-bearing cast or walking boot for 2 to 3 weeks. Displaced fractures should have an urgent orthopedic consultation for reduction and casting under procedural sedation.

Isolated distal fibular fracture. A Salter–Harris type I or II injury occurs most commonly with isolated nondisplaced distal fibular fractures. With these types of fractures, tenderness and swelling is present over the physis of the lateral malleolus on examination, and with a type I fracture only soft tissue swelling may be apparent on radiograph (Fig. 119.51). These injuries may be treated with a short leg walking cast or boot

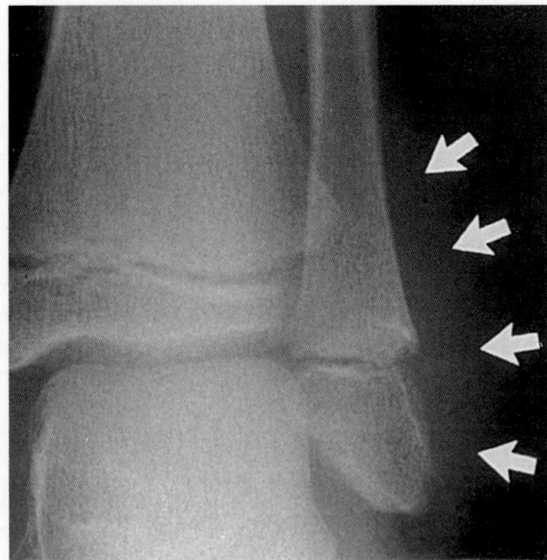

FIGURE 119.51 Radiograph of the left ankle of a 10-year-old boy notable only for soft tissue swelling localized to the distal fibula (*arrows*). The presumptive diagnosis must be a Salter–Harris type I injury of the fibula.

for 3 weeks. If the diagnosis of a Salter–Harris I injury is less certain, immobilization with a short leg cast, fiberglass/walking boot, air cast splint, or posterior splint should be applied. The patient should have a follow-up examination in 7 to 10 days. If upon repeat examination the tenderness over the physis persists, a presumptive diagnosis of a Salter–Harris I fracture should be made and immobilization should be continued for a total of 3 weeks.

Juvenile Tillaux fractures. This is a Salter–Harris type III fracture that extends through the physis and epiphysis and then exits intra-articularly. The anterior tibiofibular ligament avulses the lateral epiphysis from the medial malleolus during external rotation. This is an intra-articular fracture with the fracture line extending horizontally through the physis and vertically through the epiphysis (Fig. 119.52).

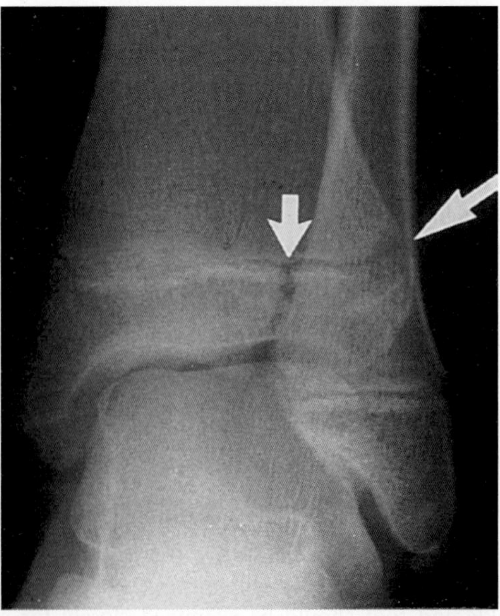

FIGURE 119.52 Classic Tillaux fracture of the distal tibia in a 14-year-old boy. The fracture line runs vertically through the epiphysis (*small arrow*) and then laterally along the physis (*large arrow*). The lateral portion of the physis is widened.

Minimally or nondisplaced fractures may be immobilized with a posterior leg splint with outpatient orthopedic referral for casting. For fractures with >2 mm displacement, CT evaluation is recommended for defining fracture displacement and for surgical planning as open reduction and internal fixation will be necessary.

TRIPLANE FRACTURES. Triplane fractures are a subgroup of Salter–Harris type IV injuries as it is a combination of a Tillaux fracture and a Salter–Harris type II fracture of the distal tibia (Fig. 119.53). These fractures result in significant growth plate damage and should have emergent orthopedic consultation. Suspected triplane fractures should be further evaluated

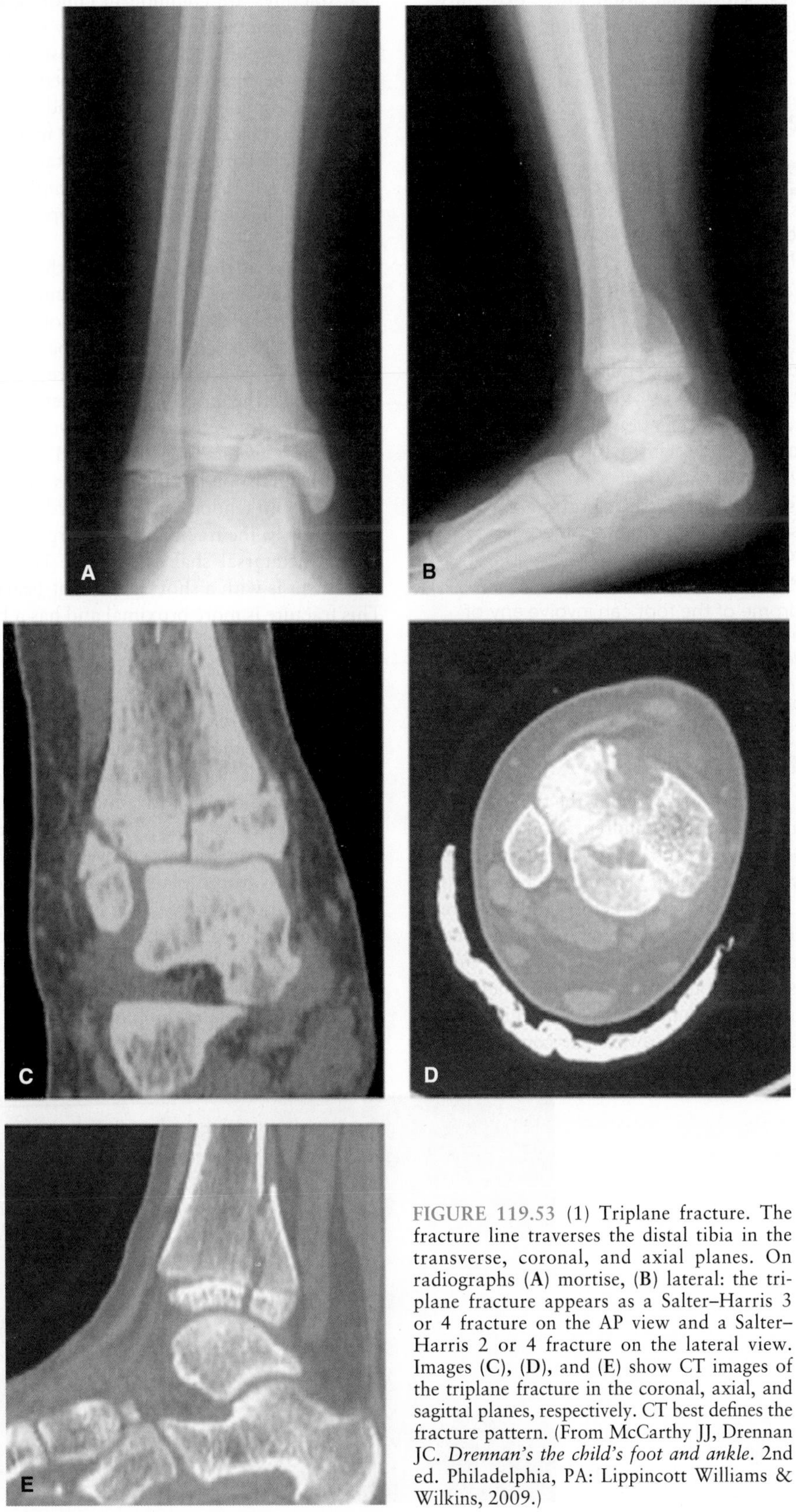

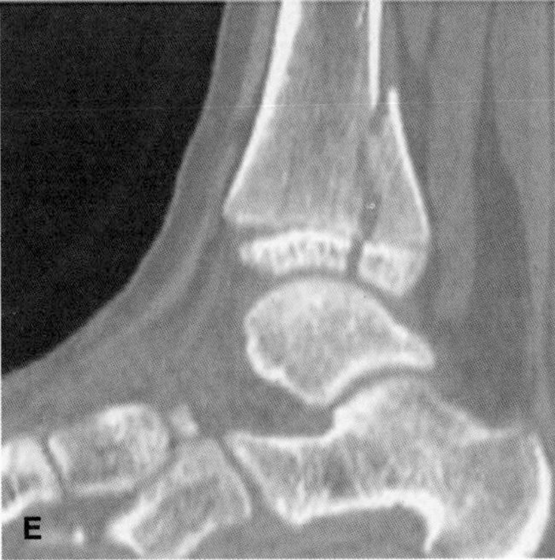

FIGURE 119.53 (1) Triplane fracture. The fracture line traverses the distal tibia in the transverse, coronal, and axial planes. On radiographs (**A**) mortise, (**B**) lateral: the triplane fracture appears as a Salter–Harris 3 or 4 fracture on the AP view and a Salter–Harris 2 or 4 fracture on the lateral view. Images (**C**), (**D**), and (**E**) show CT images of the triplane fracture in the coronal, axial, and sagittal planes, respectively. CT best defines the fracture pattern. (From McCarthy JJ, Drennan JC. *Drennan's the child's foot and ankle*. 2nd ed. Philadelphia, PA: Lippincott Williams & Wilkins, 2009.)

by CT for assessing the fracture configuration and surgical planning for fractures displaced >2 mm.

Clinical indications for discharge or admission. Children with ankle sprains may be discharged with appropriate immobilization and crutches. Those with significantly displaced physeal fractures, open fractures, substantial distal lower extremity swelling and pain should be admitted for inpatient orthopedic management.

Injuries of the Foot

CLINICAL PEARLS AND PITFALLS

- Calcaneal fractures typically occur after a fall from a height, so the spine should also be evaluated for possible compression fracture.
- Snowboarders are at risk of fractures of the lateral process of the talus.
- Avascular necrosis of the body of the talus is a serious complication that can develop depending on the location of the fracture and extent of displacement.
- CT is recommended for the evaluation of tarsometatarsal injuries and calcaneal and talar fractures, and it may also diagnose occult fractures.
- If a fracture of the second metatarsal is present, a tarsometatarsal dislocation should be considered or a Lisfranc injury should be suspected if there is also a cuboid fracture present.
- Compartment syndrome of the foot can involve any of the nine compartments and should be considered in the presence of swelling and increasing pain, especially after elevation.

Hindfoot and Midfoot Fractures

In general, fractures of the hindfoot involving the talus or calcaneus are relatively uncommon in children. Nondisplaced fractures of the hindfoot may be treated with a bulky posterior splint and crutches with no weight bearing and referral to an orthopedic surgeon. Displaced talus fractures will require reduction under anesthesia. Fractures of the midfoot involving the navicular, cuboid, and first, second, third cuneiforms and tarsometatarsal injuries are uncommon in children. They are usually caused by blunt trauma that can result in significant soft tissue damage and potential neurovascular compromise with compartment syndrome (Fig. 119.54). Nondisplaced fractures may be treated in a short leg cast. Displaced injuries of the tarsometatarsal joint will require reduction under anesthesia.

Metatarsal and Phalangeal Fractures. Metatarsal and phalangeal fractures are common in children, with fifth metatarsal fractures occurring most frequently in the foot. Radiographic evaluation should include anteroposterior, lateral, and oblique views of the foot. For nondisplaced or minimally displaced fractures, a splint can be applied and crutches given for ambulation. Phalangeal fractures can be managed with buddy taping and/or a hard sole shoe for stabilization. Intra-articular fractures of the first toe or significantly displaced fractures of the other phalanges require orthopedic referral for possible pinning.

Fractures at the base of the fifth metatarsal may be confused with accessory ossification centers that occur at this site, which are parallel to the long axis of the metatarsal shaft and are nontender to palpation. The base of the fifth metatarsal is the site of two common fractures: avulsion fractures and fractures of the proximal fifth metatarsal diaphysis, which is called the Jones fracture. The avulsion fracture of the base of the fifth metatarsal, also called a pseudo-Jones fracture, occurs from the pull of the peroneus brevis, the abductor digiti minimi quinti tendon, or lateral cord of the plantar aponeurosis. Typically, the fracture line is perpendicular to the long axis of the metatarsal shaft, and there is minimal displacement. Treatment is with a short leg weight-bearing cast for 3 weeks. This fracture is more proximal and has a better prognosis than the Jones fracture, which is associated with delayed union and nonunion. The Jones fracture occurs at the metaphyseal–diaphyseal junction at the base of the fifth metatarsal, which is a watershed area with a tenuous blood supply. Due to complications in healing, this injury should be splinted, the patient should be made nonweight bearing, and referred to the orthopedist for possible operative management.

Tarsometatarsal injuries of the foot, referred to as a Lisfranc injury, can be caused by a direct blow to the foot or when there is forced plantar flexion of the forefoot combined with a rotational force. This is more commonly seen in the skeletally mature and may be difficult to diagnose as the injuries are subtle and will present with minor pain and swelling at the base of the first and second metatarsals. Weight-bearing radiographs (AP, lateral, oblique views of the foot) are recommended to stress the joint complex. Fracture at the base of the

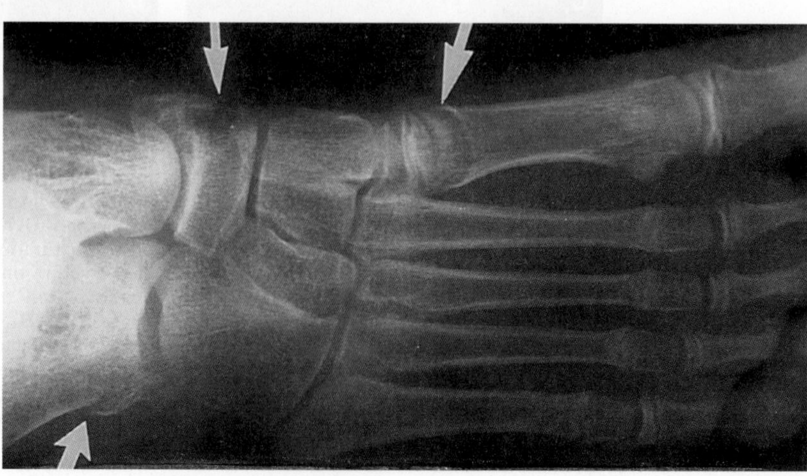

FIGURE 119.54 Radiograph of the right foot of a 13-year-old boy demonstrating fractures of the calcaneus (*small arrow*), talus (*medium arrow*), and the first metatarsal (*large arrow*).

second metatarsal should raise suspicion for a possible tarsometatarsal dislocation (Fig. 119.55). Further imaging with CT or MRI may be required to fully visualize the injury. The foot should be immobilized and the patient should follow up with outpatient orthopedics.

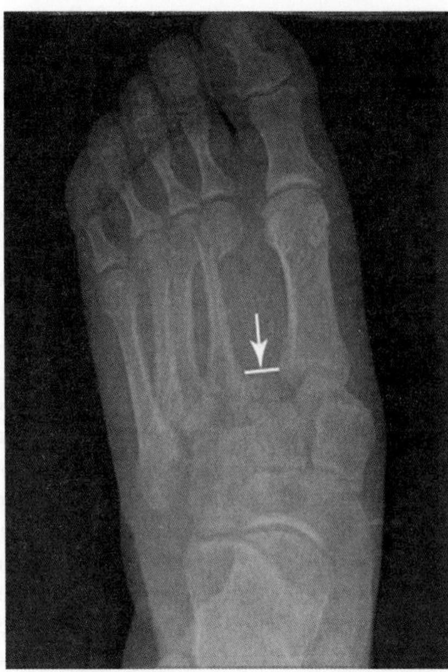

FIGURE 119.55 Lisfranc fracture, with acute fractures of the second and third metatarsals with widening of the Lisfranc interval (*arrow*). (From Bridgeforth GM. *Lippincott's primary care musculoskeletal radiology*. Philadelphia, PA: Lippincott Williams & Wilkins, 2010.)

INJURIES OF THE THORACOLUMBAR SPINE

Goals of Treatment

Injuries to the thoracolumbar spine are uncommon in children as a result of their anatomy and the biomechanics of the growing spine; however, they represent the potential for significant morbidity. An understanding of the mechanisms and energy level most likely to cause injury, as well as the key examination findings indicative of thoracolumbar injury, can prevent further incidental morbidity during evaluation in the ED. In general, any child with significant head or multisystem trauma should be assumed to have a spinal injury until proven otherwise. Diagnosis of a spinal injury in the child with a severe brain injury can be particularly problematic given that these patients are often sedated and/or paralyzed, thus limiting the examination. Therefore, initial treatment should always maintain spinal immobilization until a more detailed neurologic examination becomes possible. Injury mechanisms most commonly associated with spinal injury include motor vehicle collisions (across all age groups), falls (toddlers and school age children), sports-related trauma, and gunshot wounds (adolescents).

CLINICAL PEARLS AND PITFALLS

- Because of the overall high elasticity of the pediatric spine, significant spinal cord injury can occur in the absence of radiographic signs of bony injury.
- The risk of posttraumatic scoliosis after a complete spinal cord injury in children is high.
- Pediatric sacral injuries are rare and seldom associated with neurologic injury.
- Patients with fracture and dislocation have a higher incidence of associated neurologic injury than patients with simple fractures.
- Patients improperly restrained by a lap belt in a motor vehicle collision should be carefully evaluated for "seatbelt syndrome" with abdominal bruising ("seatbelt sign"), an associated hyperflexion-induced lumbar fracture (often a Chance fracture), and intra-abdominal injury.

Current Evidence

Structurally, the child's spine differs from the adult spine as there is increased ligamentous laxity resulting in greater mobility, more shallow angulations at the facet joints, and incomplete ossification of the vertebrae. By adolescence, the spine has mechanical qualities more like those of the adult, and the fracture patterns are similar. Injuries to the spine are rare in pediatrics; however, they contribute to a significant morbidity and mortality in children and frequently occur in association with multisystem trauma. Injuries of the lower thoracic region to upper lumbar region (T11-L1), for example, have been noted to be associated with significantly increased risk of associated gastrointestinal injury. Injuries to the lumbar and sacral regions (L2-sacral) are noted to be associated not only with abdominal injuries, but appendicular orthopedic trauma as well. Studies have indicated that high-risk mechanisms include motor vehicle crashes, falls, pedestrians or bicyclists struck by a motor vehicle, sports, recreational activities, and physical abuse.

Clinical Considerations

Clinical Recognition

Thoracolumbar spine injuries usually result from high-energy mechanisms and may have associated injuries to the torso and abdomen. Special early attention to these related injuries is paramount for the coordination of the multidisciplinary patient care.

Triage Considerations

All patients presenting with trauma after a high-energy or concerning mechanism as described above should be maintained on spine precautions until cleared by a physician. Patients presenting via EMS with spine immobilization should be removed from their backboard immediately, using standard procedure, to avoid iatrogenic injury such as pain, skin ulceration, aspiration, and respiratory compromise. Complete vital signs should be obtained to assess for spinal shock and the need for resuscitative measures.

Clinical Assessment

The initial assessment should follow trauma protocol and maintain strict spine precautions. Patients can be "logrolled" to inspect the spine as long as flexion, extension, or twisting movements do not occur. The mechanism of injury and estimated severity of the force of injury should be elicited from the family or EMS. Patient assessment should include review of vital signs and thorough examination of the back with palpation and inspection for pain, ecchymosis, abrasions, step offs, sensory changes, or other abnormalities of the neurologic examination. The most common finding on physical examination in the patients with thoracolumbar fracture is point tenderness over the fractured vertebrae. However, the sensitivity and specificity of the examination may be imperfect in pediatric patients, as the examination may be complicated by age-related reliability, referred pain, location of fracture (anterior vs. posterior), and false positives secondary to contusion. Certain physical findings can suggest the possibility of a coexisting spinal cord injury, which may or may not be associated with bony fracture. These findings include asymmetry of movement and reflexes between the arms and legs, absence of sacral reflexes, lax anal tone, priapism, spinal shock, autonomic hyperreflexia, diaphragmatic breathing, and urinary retention, as well as any evidence of a motor or sensory deficit level. There must be a careful examination for potential distracting and/or coexisting trauma to the head, chest, abdomen, pelvis, or extremities. The presence of abdominal wall ecchymosis in a patient following a motor vehicle collision has been associated with vertebral fractures, including Chance fractures, in up to 50% of patients.

Management

There is little consensus about which pediatric trauma patients warrant screening thoracolumbar radiographs in the absence of pain, tenderness, neurologic deficit, or associated cervical spine injuries. The limited data that exist suggest that selective radiographs of the thoracolumbar spine should not rely on demographic data, clinician's degree of suspicion, or injury mechanism alone. Physical examination findings have good sensitivity and fair specificity but may still miss fractures. In adults, the most common features of patients with missed injuries include high-velocity injury, decreased level of consciousness, associated head injury, and pelvis/lower extremity injury. Thus, the current adult recommendation is for thoracolumbar spine films to be obtained in all trauma patients with Glasgow Coma Scale (GCS) <15, multisystem injuries, a palpable gap or pain/tenderness in the thoracolumbar region, or a focal neurologic deficit (other than isolated head injury). Screening radiographs may also be advisable for patients with distracting injuries, those with highly suspicious mechanisms, and preverbal children, even in the absence of focal tenderness. As there is no standard for diagnostic testing, imaging that is commonly obtained includes plain radiographs with a two-view of the thoracic and lumbar vertebrae (separately) with inclusion of the thoracolumbar junction. Routine use of a spiral CT of the spine is not recommended in children. When faced with equivocal radiographs, CT scans or MRI should be considered.

After stabilization of the patient and their spinal column, those patients with documented fracture or possible spinal cord injury should have emergent orthopedic and/or neurosurgical consultation. Pediatric thoracolumbar spine trauma may result in a variety of injury patterns such as compression fractures, burst fractures, flexion-distraction injuries, fracture-dislocation injuries, apophyseal fractures/herniations, and spinous process and transverse process fractures. These fractures of the spine can be divided into the following groups based on the mechanism of injury and the radiographic appearance: (1) compression fractures, (2) flexion and distraction fractures (including Chance fractures), (3) shear fractures, and (4) neurologic injuries without fractures. The severity of the injury combined with the patient's age/skeletal maturity predicts the ability to heal and remodel. Any Chance or burst fracture associated with 15 degrees or more of kyphosis or any degree of neurologic impairment requires emergent surgical consultation, and typically is treated surgically. These injuries are associated with higher morbidity than other thoracolumbar fractures. Compression fractures and burst fractures without associated kyphosis and with normal neurologic examination typically do well without operative intervention.

Compression Fractures. Compression fractures result from hyperflexion producing an axial load and causing failure of the anterior vertebral body. The majority of spinal compression fractures occur between T11 and L2, and the presence of multiple fractures is not unusual (Fig. 119.56). On lateral plain radiographs, a typical compression fracture appears as a wedge-shaped vertebra with loss of the height of the anterior body and preservation of the height of the posterior body. The presence of posterior cortical disruption on lateral plain radiograph or interpedicular widening on the AP view should raise suspicion for burst fracture. A CT scan should be considered if there is evidence of multiple level fractures or when plain radiographs

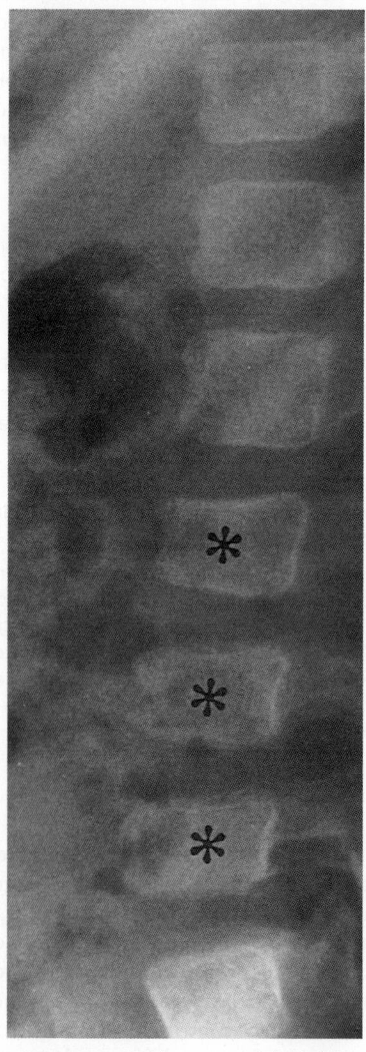

FIGURE 119.56 Compression fractures of the lumbar vertebrae in a 3-year-old boy (*asterisks*). Multiple fractures are the rule in children.

suggest the possibility of a retropulsed fragment (as in an unstable burst fracture). A compression fracture with loss of vertebral height of more than 40% may also suggest increased risk of posterior element involvement and may warrant CT imaging for evaluation. Compression fractures heal quickly in children and have little tendency to progress. Many children do not require hospitalization for compression fractures and can be treated with bed rest and symptomatic mobilization. Occasionally, a well-molded thoracolumbar sacral orthosis may be necessary for persistent pain or multiple areas of compression.

Flexion and Distraction Fractures. The most common mechanism of flexion and distraction injury is hyperflexion over a seat belt during sudden deceleration in a motor vehicle collision. The lumbar spine is most commonly injured as the result of this hyperflexion. Among the spinal injuries that can occur are distractions, subluxations, facet dislocations, and ligamentous ruptures, as well as compression fractures and Chance fractures. In simple distraction injuries, the traumatic force is typically a Salter–Harris type I fracture due to the relatively weak physeal cartilage of the maturing vertebral body. These fractures often heal well with appropriate immobilization. Chance fractures result from a combined flexion-distraction mechanism, resulting in a horizontal split through both the body and posterior elements of a vertebra, almost always a product of a seat belt injury (and, once again, often in combination with an abdominal injury) (Fig. 119.57). Chance fractures may be associated with neurologic injury, and the

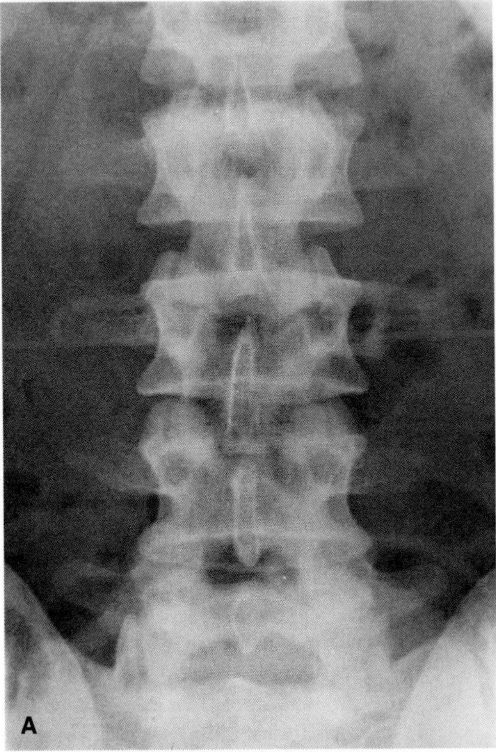

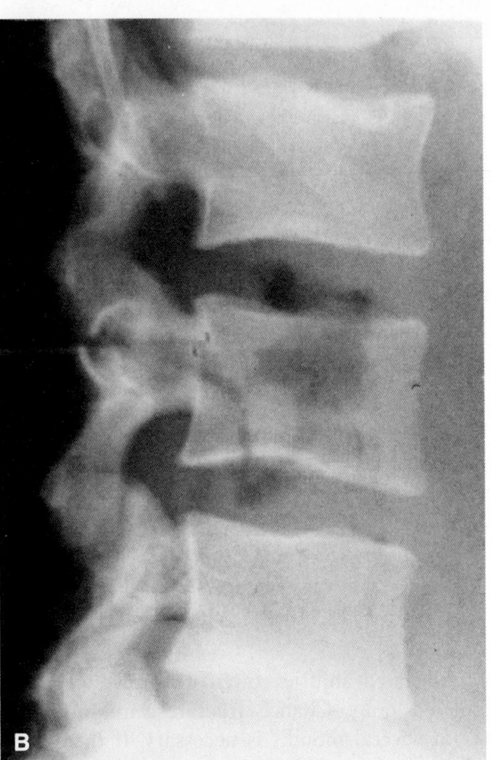

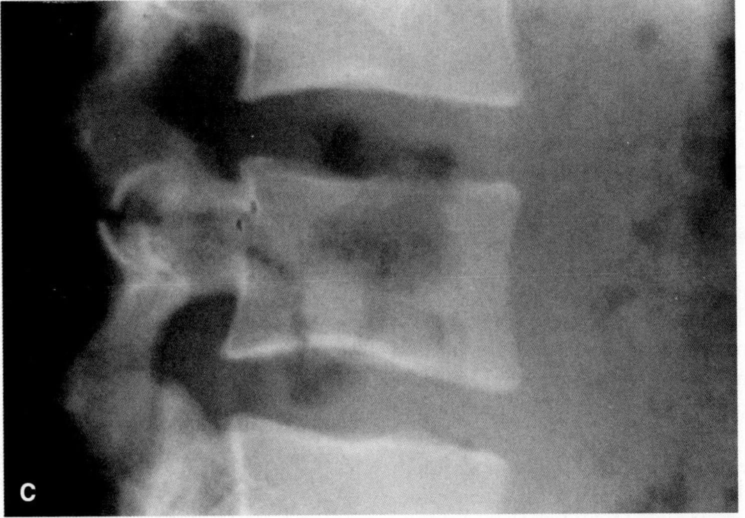

FIGURE 119.57 **A:** Anteroposterior radiograph demonstrating a Chance fracture at L3. **B:** Lateral radiograph of a Chance fracture at L3. Notice the separation at both the posterior and middle columns. There is a break in the continuity of the articular pillar and at the anterior portion of the spinal canal. **C:** Close-up of (**B**). (From Anrig CA, Plaugher G. *Pediatric chiropractic.* 2nd ed. Philadelphia, PA: Lippincott Williams & Wilkins, 2012.)

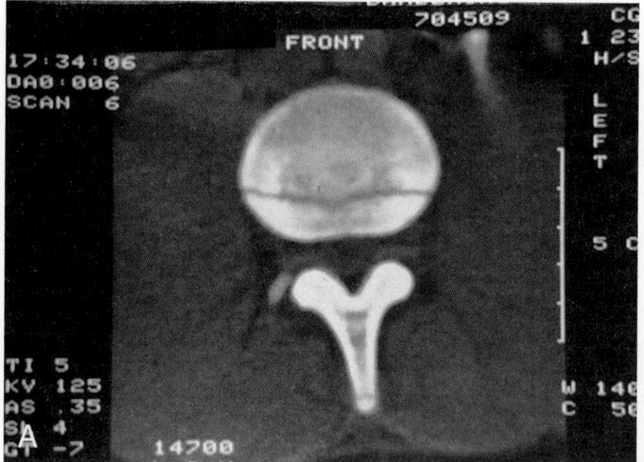

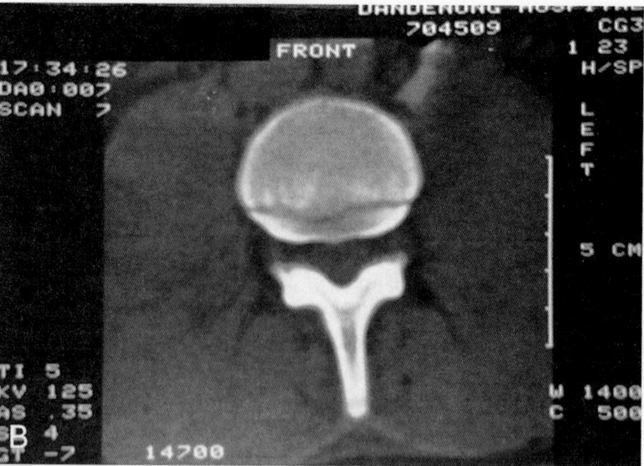

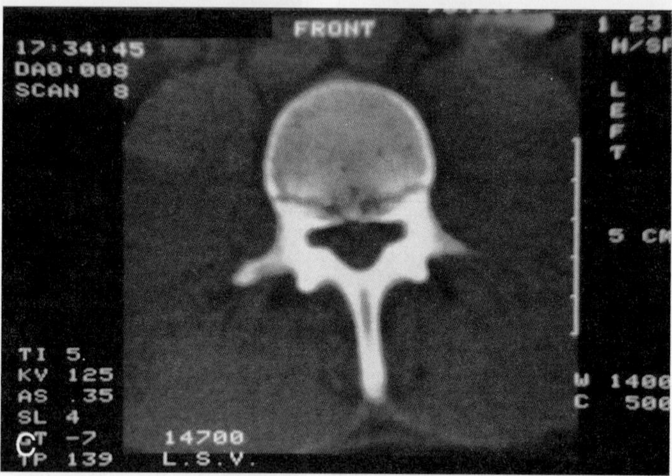

FIGURE 119.58 **A** and **B:** Fracture of the third (L3) and fourth (L4) vertebrae in a 12 year old girl, the result of a shear injury in a motor vehicle collision. **C:** Permanent paralysis of the lower extremities resulted, as suggested by the degree of spinal canal collapse seen on the computed tomography scan.

presence of associated injuries often requires hospitalization. For isolated bony Chance fractures, immobilization with a brace for several months is necessary. If there is any ligamentous involvement, definitive care requires orthopedic surgery.

Shear Fractures. Although the cervical spine is most vulnerable to shear injuries, violent trauma can also cause such injuries in the thoracic and the lumbar spine (Fig. 119.58). Unfortunately, neurologic deficits are common in this setting. All shear fractures should be considered unstable injuries that will need stabilization procedures to avoid progressive deformity and enhance any possibility of neurologic recovery.

Neurologic Injuries without Fractures. Anatomically, the immature spine is more flexible than the spinal cord. As a result, injuries causing hyperflexion or extension may induce damage to the cord and neurologic injury while leaving the bony, cartilaginous, and ligamentous structures intact. Trauma causing spinal cord injury without radiographic abnormality (SCIWORA) is much more common in children younger than 8 years, particularly affecting the cervical and thoracic spine. Both incomplete and complete neurologic deficits can occur. Any history of neurologic deficit following spinal trauma should prompt consideration of a SCIWORA and should prompt evaluation with MRI, which can best identify cord damage in the absence of a fracture.

Disposition

For any thoracolumbar spine injury with associated neurologic abnormalities, admission is recommended for serial examinations and further evaluation. Compression fractures without concern for burst injury may be discharged home with outpatient orthopedic follow-up. Arrangements for back brace fitting may be required. Referral for follow-up of thoracolumbar fractures is important because of complications that can occur related to the remaining growth potential of the spine, including deformity, instability, and neurologic injury.

Suggested Readings and Key References

General Principles of Pediatric Orthopedics

Flynn JM, Skaggs DL, Waters PM, eds. *Rockwood and Wilkins' fractures in children.* 8th ed. Philadelphia, PA: *Wolters Kluwer Health*, 2014.

Swischuk LE, Siddharth PJ. *Emergency musculoskeletal imaging in children.* New York, NY: Springer, 2014.

General Principles of Acute Orthopedic Care

Boutis K. Common pediatric fractures treated with minimal intervention. *Pediatr Emerg Care* 2010;26(2):152–157; quiz 158–162.

Kemp AM, Dunstan F, Harrison S, et al. Patterns of skeletal fractures in child abuse: systematic review. *BMJ* 2008;337:a1518.

Musgrave DS, Mendelson SA. Pediatric orthopedic trauma: principles in management. *Crit Care Med* 2002;30(11 suppl):S431–S443.

Okike K, Bhattacharyya T. Trends in the management of open fractures: a critical analysis. *J Bone Joint Surg Am* 2006;88(12):2739–2748.

Shore BJ, Glotzbecker MP, Zurakowski D, et al. Acute compartment syndrome in children and teenagers with tibial shaft fractures: incidence and multivariable risk factors. *J Orthop Trauma* 2013;27(11):616–621.

Thompson RW, Krauss B, Kim YJ, et al. Extremity fracture pain after emergency department reduction and casting: predictors of pain after discharge. *Ann Emerg Med* 2012;60(3):269–277.

Injuries of the Shoulder Region

Aronson PL, Mistry RD. Intra-articular lidocaine for reduction of shoulder dislocation. *Pediatr Emerg Care* 2014;30(5):358–362.

Carson S, Woolridge DP, Colletti J, et al. Pediatric upper extremity injuries. *Pediatr Clin North Am* 2006;53(1):41–67.

Nenopoulos SP, Gigis IP, Chytas AA, et al. Outcome of distal clavicular fracture separations and dislocations in immature skeleton. *Injury* 2011;42(4):376–380.

Pandya NK, Namdari S, Hosalkar HS. Displaced clavicle fractures in adolescents: facts, controversies, and current trends. *J Am Acad Orthop Surg* 2012;20(8):498–505.

Strauss BJ, Carey TP, Seabrook JA, et al. Pediatric clavicular fractures: assessment of fracture patterns and predictors of complicated outcome. *J Emerg Med* 2012;43(1):29–35.

Injuries of the Humerus

Gilbert SR, Conklin MJ. Presentation of distal humerus physeal separation. *Pediatr Emerg Care* 2007;23(11):816–819.

Shrader MW. Proximal humerus and humeral shaft fractures in children. *Hand Clin* 2007;23(4):431–435.

Tarallo L, Mugnai R, Fiacchi F, et al. Pediatric medial epicondyle fractures with intra-articular elbow incarceration. *J Orthop Traumatol* 2014;16(2):117–123.

Tejwani N, Phillips D, Goldstein RY. Management of lateral humeral condylar fracture in children. *J Am Acad Orthop Surg* 2011; 19(6):350–358.

Injuries of the Elbow

Aylor M, Anderson JM, Vanderford P, et al. Reduction of pulled elbow. *N Engl J Med* 2014;371:e32.

Krul M, van der Wouden JC, van Suijlekom-Smit LW, et al. Manipulative interventions for reducing pulled elbow in young children. *Cochrane Database Syst Rev* 2012;1:CD007759.

Shrader MW. Pediatric supracondylar fractures and pediatric physeal elbow fractures. *Orthop Clin North Am* 2008;39(2):163–171.

Skaggs DL, Mirzayan R. The posterior fat pad sign in association with occult fracture of the elbow in children. *J Bone Joint Surg Am* 1999; 81(10):1429–1433.

Wu J, Perron AD, Miller MD, et al. Orthopedic pitfalls in the ED: pediatric supracondylar humerus fractures. *Am J Emerg Med* 2002; 20(6):544–550.

Injuries of the Forearm

Khosla S, Melton LJ 3rd, Dekutoski MB, et al. Incidence of childhood distal forearm fractures over 30 years: a population-based study. *JAMA* 2003;290(11):1479–1485.

Pai DR, Thapa M. Musculoskeletal ultrasound of the upper extremity in children. *Pediatr Radiol* 2013;43(suppl 1):S48–S54.

Perron AD, Hersh RE, Brady WJ, et al. Orthopedic pitfalls in the ED: Galeazzi and Monteggia fracture-dislocation. *Am J Emerg Med* 2001;19(3):225–228.

Rodríguez-Merchán EC. Pediatric fractures of the forearm. *Clin Orthop Relat Res* 2005;(432):65–72.

Vopat ML, Kane PM, Christino MA, et al. Treatment of diaphyseal forearm fractures in children. *Orthop Rev (Pavia)* 2014;6(2):5325.

Injuries of the Pelvis

Kwok MY, Yen K, Atabaki S, et al. Sensitivity of plain pelvis radiography in children with blunt torso trauma. *Ann Emerg Med* 2014;65(1):63–71.e1.

Schlickewei W, Keck T. Pelvic and acetabular fractures in childhood. *Injury* 2005;36(suppl 1):A57–A63.

Wong AT, Brady KB, Caldwell AM, et al. Low-risk criteria for pelvic radiography in pediatric blunt trauma patients. *Pediatr Emerg Care* 2011;27(2):92–96.

Injuries of the Hip and Proximal Femur

Herrera-Soto JA, Price CT. Traumatic hip dislocations in children and adolescents: pitfalls and complications. *J Am Acad Orthop Surg* 2009;17(1):15–21.

Quick TJ, Eastwood DM. Pediatric fractures and dislocations of the hip and pelvis. *Clin Orthop Relat Res* 2005;(432):87–96.

Injuries of the Shaft of the Femur

Flynn JM, Schwend RM. Management of pediatric femoral shaft fractures. *J Am Acad Orthop Surg* 2004;12(5):347–359.

Rewers A, Hedegaard H, Lezotte D, et al. Childhood femur fractures, associated injuries, and sociodemographic risk factors: a population-based study. *Pediatrics* 2005;115(5):e543–e552.

Unal VS, Gulcek M, Unveren Z, et al. Blood loss evaluation in children under the age of 11 with femoral shaft fractures patients with isolated versus multiple injuries. *J Trauma* 2006;60(1):224–226; discussion 226.

Injuries of the Knee

Howells NR, Brunton LR, Robinson J, et al. Acute knee dislocation: an evidence based approach to the management of the multiligament injured knee. *Injury* 2011;42(11):1198–1204.

Zionts LE. Fractures around the knee in children. *J Am Acad Orthop Surg* 2002;10(5):345–355.

Injuries of the Proximal Tibia and Fibula and Shaft

Baron CM, Seekins J, Hernanz-Schulman M, et al. Utility of total lower extremity radiography investigation of nonweight bearing in the young child. *Pediatrics* 2008;121(4):e817–e820.

Injuries of the Ankle

Blackburn EW, Aronsson DD, Rubright JH, et al. Ankle fractures in children. *J Bone Joint Surg Am* 2012;94:1234–1244.

Dowling S, Spooner CH, Liang Y, et al. Accuracy of Ottawa Ankle Rules to exclude fractures of the ankle and midfoot in children: a meta-analysis. *Acad Emerg Med* 2009;16(4):277–287.

Wuerz TH, Gurd DP. Pediatric physeal ankle fractures. *J Am Acad Orthop Surg* 2013;13(21):234–244.

Injuries of the Foot

Ribbans WJ, Natarajan R, Alavala S. Pediatric foot fractures. *Clin Orthop Relat Res* 2005;432:107–115.

Injuries of the Thoracolumbar Spine

Achildi O, Betz RR, Grewal H. Lapbelt injuries and the seatbelt syndrome in pediatric spinal cord injury. *J Spinal Cord Med* 2007;30(suppl 1):S21–S24.

Daniels AH, Sobel AD, Eberson CP. Pediatric thoracolumbar spine trauma. *J Am Acad Orthop Surg* 2013;21(12):707–716.

Junkins EP Jr, Stotts A, Santiago R, et al. The clinical presentation of pediatric thoracolumbar fractures: a prospective study. *J Trauma* 2008;65(5):1066–1071.

CHAPTER 120 ■ NECK TRAUMA

GEORGE A. WOODWARD, MD, MBA AND LILA O'MAHONY, MD, FAAP

GOALS OF EMERGENCY CARE

Pediatric neck injuries are uncommon; but many children are routinely evaluated for injuries after trauma. Because neck injuries can be life-threatening, including those that are subtle on presentation, children with neck trauma need to be assessed in a timely and orderly manner with a high index of suspicion. The goals of emergency care are to ensure a patent airway with adequate oxygenation and ventilation, control hemorrhage, maintain spinal stability, and identify and prevent progression of all injuries. A listing of common mechanisms of neck injury is given in Table 120.1. This chapter will discuss the evaluation and management of penetrating and direct blunt injuries, as well as the evaluation of the cervical spine taking into consideration the unique features that differentiate pediatric from adult neck anatomy and physiology.

KEY POINTS

- Pediatric neck injuries are uncommon.
- Children have unique anatomical differences and mechanisms of injury that contribute to characteristic patterns of injury that vary from adults.
- Multiple structures within the neck and cervical spine are at risk for injury, knowing their anatomic relationships will help guide the emergency evaluation.
- Management priorities are first to ensure a patent airway, adequate respiration, control of hemorrhage, and spinal stabilization and second to identify and prevent progression of all injuries.

RELATED CHAPTERS

Resuscitation and Stabilization
- Approach to the Injured Child: Chapter 2
- Airway: Chapter 3

Signs and Symptoms
- Respiratory Distress: Chapter 66
- Stridor: Chapter 70

Medical, Surgical, and Trauma Emergencies
- Burns: Chapter 112
- Neurotrauma: Chapter 121

PENETRATING TRAUMA

Goals of Treatment

To anticipate, identify, manage, and prevent progression of all injuries to structures and tissues within the neck, including the airway, major blood vessels, nerves, and osseous structures.

CLINICAL PEARLS AND PITFALLS

- Penetrating trauma may be associated with extracervical injuries and involve multiple organ systems within the neck.
- Pattern of injury may not be limited to the pathway of the penetrating object.
- Injury to blood vessels can be dramatic or subtle with an initially normal examination. Vigilance and high index of suspicion is warranted.
- History of large blood loss, pulsatile lesion, rapidly expanding hematoma, hypovolemic shock, or neurologic deficits (paresis, visual loss or aphasia, altered level of consciousness) indicates possible vascular injury.
- Respiratory distress, stridor, hoarse voice, and speech difficulties may also be indicators of injury.
- Spinal cord and vertebral levels are not the same. In the cervical area, the cord level lies one segment higher than the corresponding vertebral level (C4 cord level lies opposite the C3 vertebral body). In the lower cervical area, a disparity of up to two levels may be present. This means that physical injury and objective findings may not be straightforward.
- Evaluate the chest for signs of major vessel injury, including hemothorax, widened mediastinum, and cardiac tamponade.

TABLE 120.1

COMMON MECHANISMS OF BLUNT AND PENETRATING NECK INJURIES

Penetrating trauma	Blunt trauma
High-velocity missiles	Motor vehicle accidents, including motorcycles and all-terrain vehicles; (assault) weapons with muzzle velocity >2,000 ft/s
Low-velocity missiles	Sports (hand gun) weapons with muzzle velocity <2,000 ft/s
Knives	Fights
Windshields	Falls
Sharp objects	Clothesline injuries
Explosions	Bicycle handlebars
Dog bites	Dog bites
Iatrogenic (intubation, endoscopy, gastric tubes)	Barotrauma (bottle cap under pressure or compressed air source)
	Nonaccidental (abuse)
	Exposures (fires, caustics)

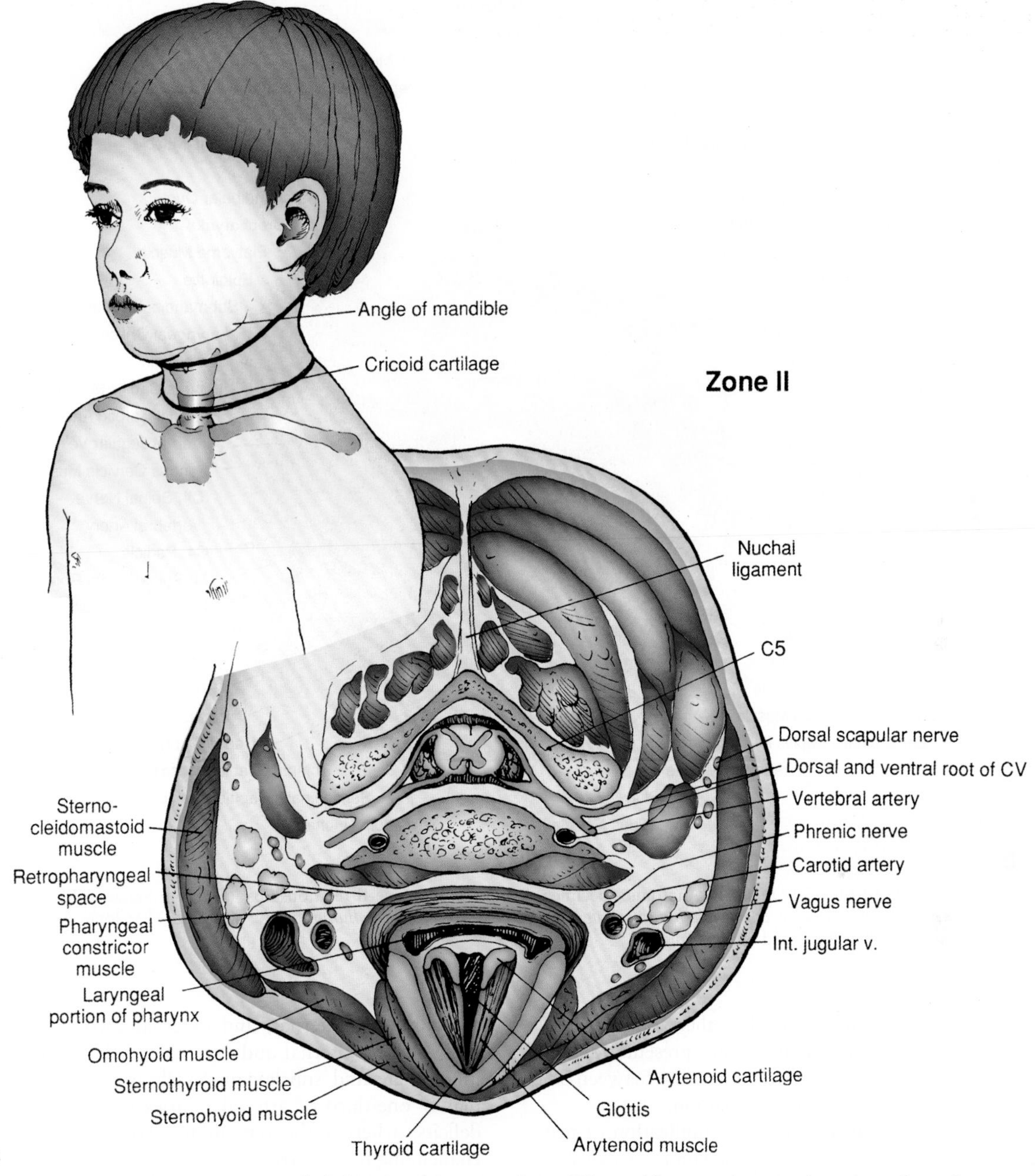

FIGURE 120.1 Anatomic neck divisions and contents of zone II located between the upper boundary of zone I and the angle of the mandible. (*continued*)

Current Evidence

Penetrating neck trauma is uncommon in children, but most often is the result of a wound from a gunshot (usually low muzzle velocity <2,000 ft per second) (Fig. 120.1), knife, broken windshield, other sharp object, or explosion (Table 120.1). The soft tissues and visceral components of the neck are protected by the spine posteriorly, the mandible anteriorly and superiorly, the shoulders and clavicles anteriorly and inferiorly, and the neck muscles. The child's relatively large head, mandible, and short neck make the anterior neck less accessible to direct trauma. However, if the neck is hyperextended, the structures of the anterior neck, including the larynx, trachea, and esophagus, are more exposed and susceptible to injury. The potential severity of direct penetrating or blunt injuries (Table 120.2) is increased because of the relatively small neck area with its large number of vital organs and structures.

Traditionally, the anterior neck has been divided into three anatomic zones (Figs. 120.2 to 120.4). Zone I encompasses the area between the thoracic inlet and the cricoid (the lower boundary of zone I is the thoracic inlet, the upper boundary is most often classified as the cricoid); zone II is the area between the cricoid and the angle of the mandible; and zone III is the area above the angle of the mandible. Knowledge of the divisions and structures they contain can be useful in the evaluation and management of neck trauma (Figs. 120.2 to 120.4). The most common site of significant penetrating injuries is

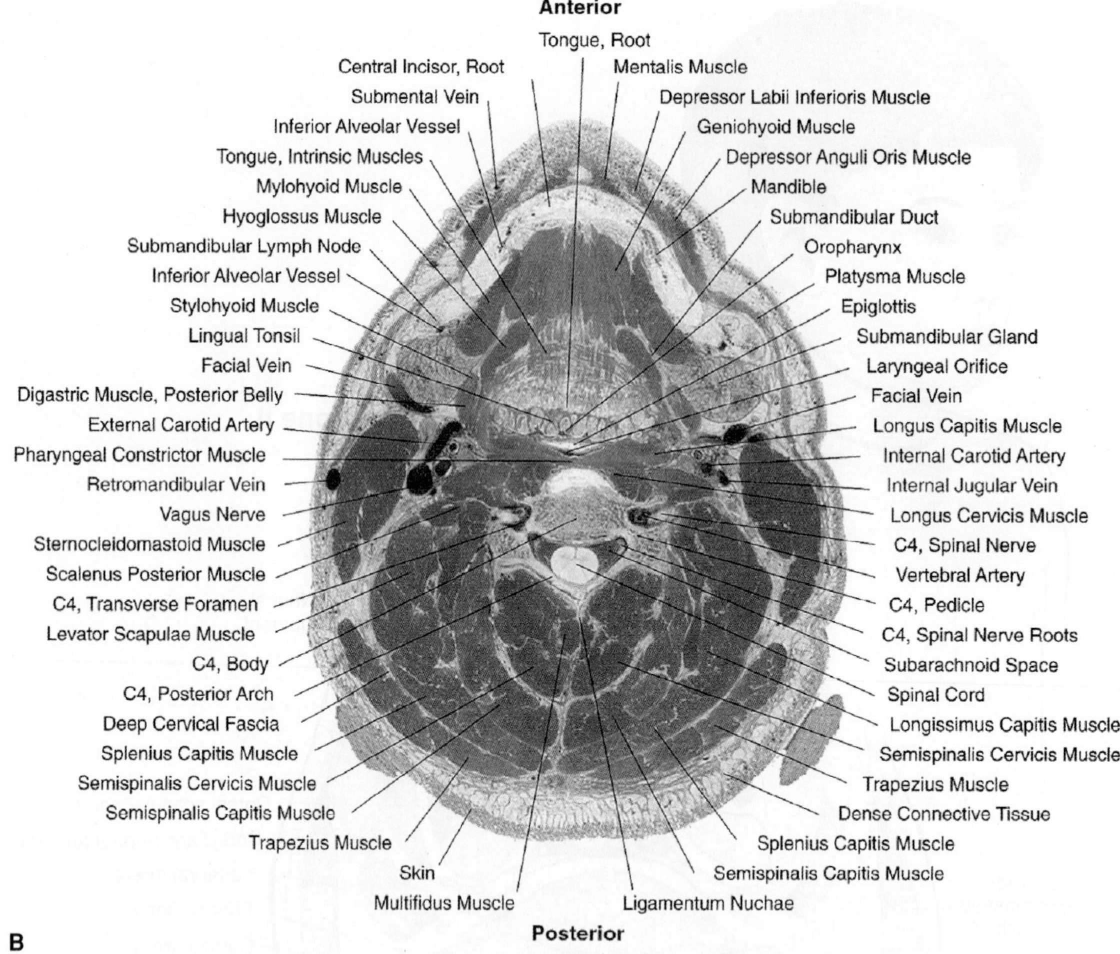

FIGURE 120.1 (*Continued*) **B:** Anatomic specimen demonstrating zone II relationships. (**B:** From Spitzer VM, Whitlock DG. *Atlas of the visible human male: reverse engineering of the human body*. Sodburg, MA: Jones & Bartlett, 1998. Reprinted with permission.)

in zone II. Compared to injuries in the other zones, zone II injuries tend to have a more straightforward presentation and surgical exploration with an associated mortality between 3% and 9%, with or without surgical intrervention.

Vascular injury is the most common complication of penetrating trauma and is the second most common cause of death. Injuries include aneurysms, dissections, occlusions, and fistulas. Major vessels that can be injured in the neck include the common, internal, and external carotid arteries; vertebral arteries; internal and external jugular veins; and nearby innominate and subclavian vessels (Table 120.2). Approximately one-third of arterial injuries present with neurologic deficits, whereas the remaining two-thirds are often more challenging to diagnose.

The subtle presentation of vascular injuries historically, led many authors to suggest mandatory exploration of all neck

TABLE 120.2

NECK CONTENTS AND CLOSELY APPROXIMATED STRUCTURES

Musculoskeletal	Vascular	Venous	Gastrointestinal	Glandular
Cervical spine	Arterial	Jugulars: internal, external	Esophagus	Thyroid
Cervical muscles	Carotids: common, internal, external	Lymphatics	**Neurologic**	Parathyroid
Ligaments		Thoracic duct	Spinal cord	Parotid
Clavicles	Vertebral	**Airway**	Cranial nerves IX–XII	Submandibular
First rib	Innominate	Larynx	Cervical nerves	
Hyoid	Subclavian	Trachea	Cervical sympathetics	
		Apices of lung	Brachial plexus	

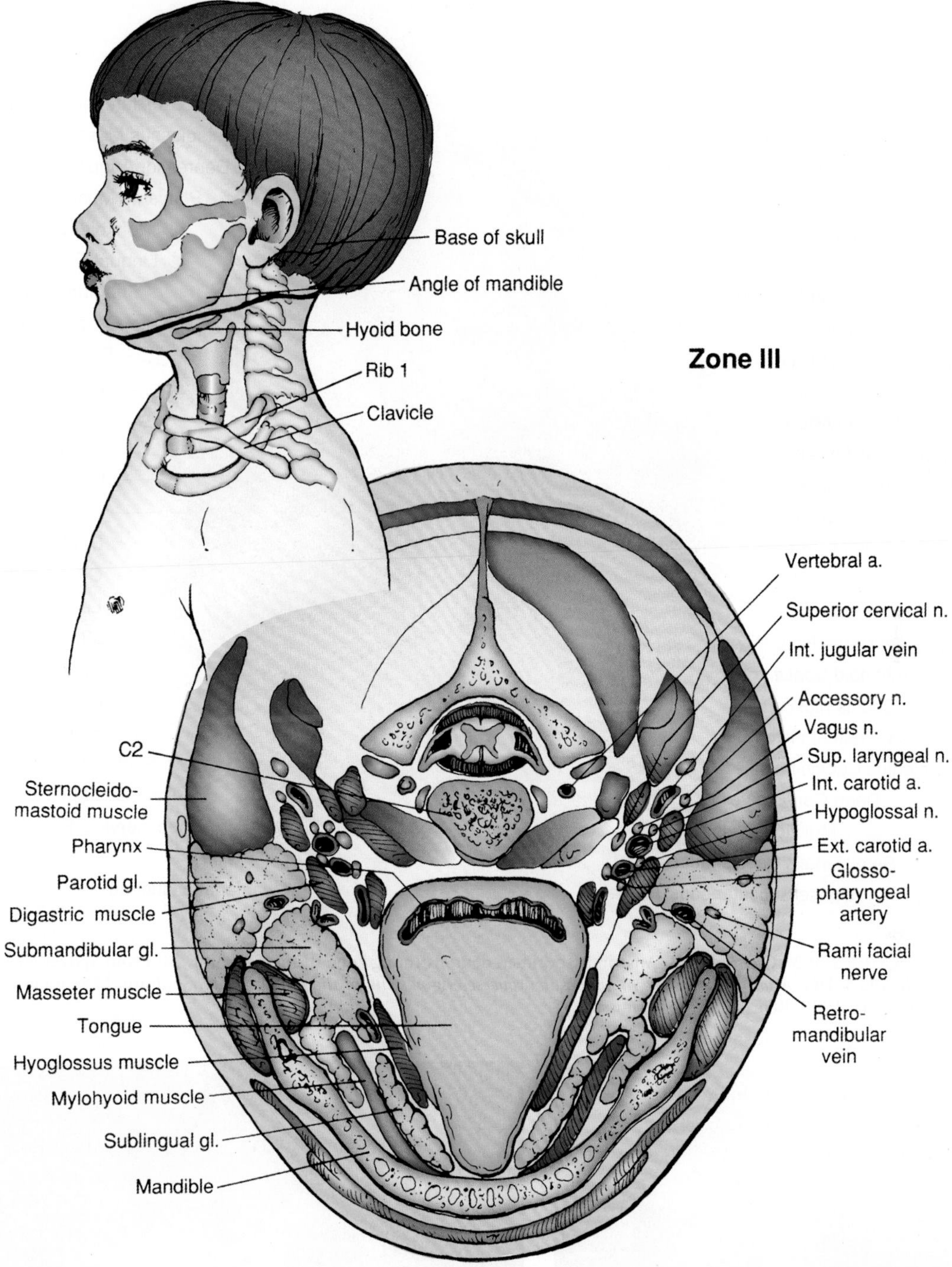

FIGURE 120.2 **A:** Anatomic neck divisions and contents of zone III. Zone III includes the area above the upper boundary of zone II. (*continued*)

injuries when the outermost muscle layer (platysma) was penetrated. More recently, the literature suggests that careful evaluation, along with ancillary studies, including arteriography, helical multislice computed tomographic (CT) scan, and color flow Doppler (CFD) coupled with the use of selective exploration, can reliably identify most significant injuries without an increase in morbidity and mortality from delays while diagnostic evaluation is being completed. The multislice helical CT scan has been noted to be a sensitive and specific diagnostic tool including the multislice helical CT angiography (CTA) in detecting vascular and aerodigestive injury with reported 100% sensitivity and 93% specificity. In some institutions, CTA has replaced conventional angiography for the vascular assessment of neck injuries, resulting in fewer neck explorations, and essentially eliminating negative exploratory surgeries. Subsequently, the use of CTA has transcribed the zone of injury into a descriptor rather than a triage tool or guide for exploratory surgery. CFD is a noninvasive, relatively sensitive screening tool with high specificity, PPV and NPV for vascular injury, but can be limited by adjacent or overlying hematomas and pneumothoraces as well as by the skill of the individual operator. The physical examination alone has been reported

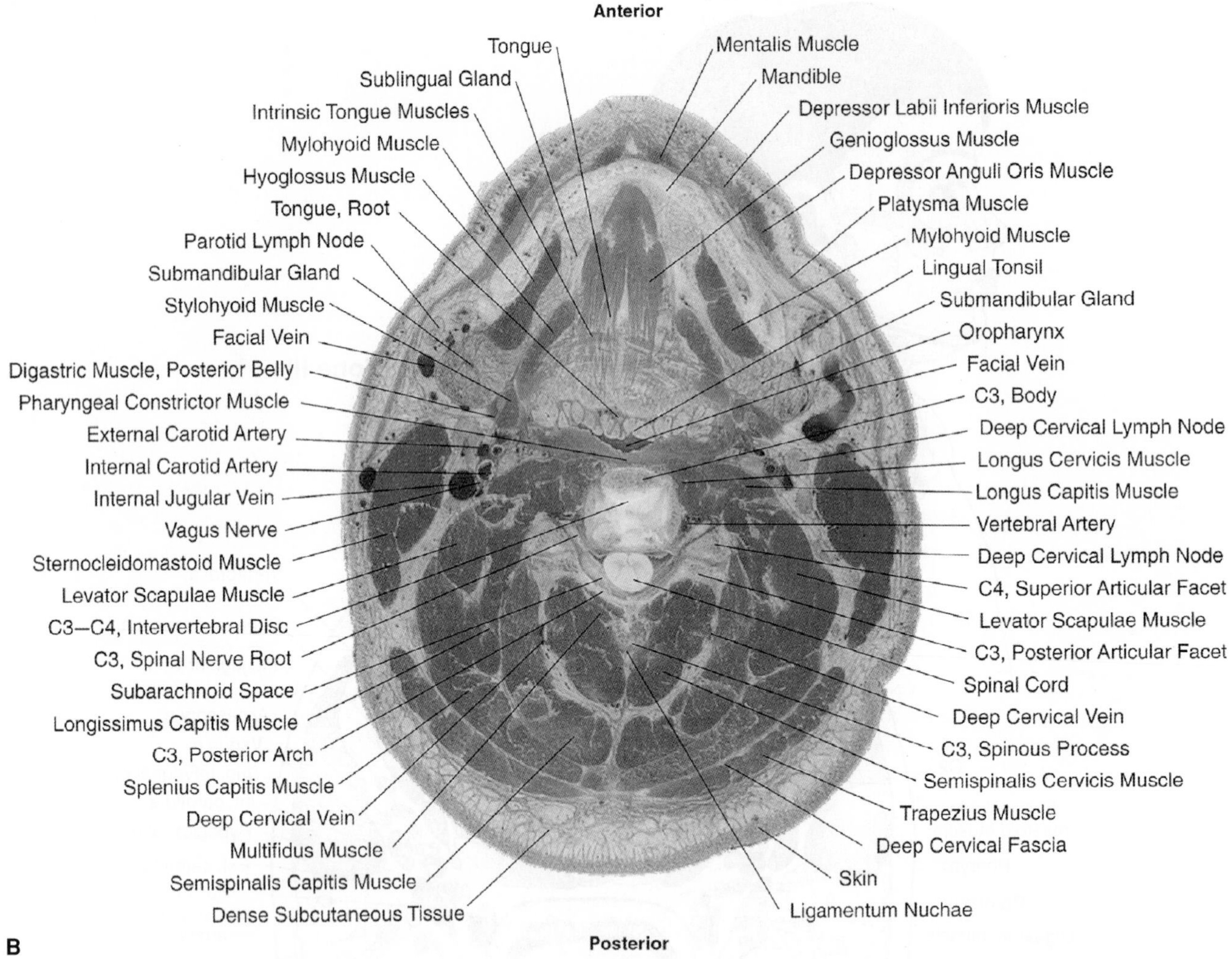

Anterior

Tongue
Sublingual Gland
Intrinsic Tongue Muscles
Mylohyoid Muscle
Hyoglossus Muscle
Tongue, Root
Parotid Lymph Node
Submandibular Gland
Stylohyoid Muscle
Facial Vein
Digastric Muscle, Posterior Belly
Pharyngeal Constrictor Muscle
External Carotid Artery
Internal Carotid Artery
Internal Jugular Vein
Vagus Nerve
Sternocleidomastoid Muscle
Levator Scapulae Muscle
C3–C4, Intervertebral Disc
C3, Spinal Nerve Root
Subarachnoid Space
Longissimus Capitis Muscle
C3, Posterior Arch
Splenius Capitis Muscle
Deep Cervical Vein
Multifidus Muscle
Semispinalis Capitis Muscle
Dense Subcutaneous Tissue

Mentalis Muscle
Mandible
Depressor Labii Inferioris Muscle
Genioglossus Muscle
Depressor Anguli Oris Muscle
Platysma Muscle
Mylohyoid Muscle
Lingual Tonsil
Submandibular Gland
Oropharynx
Facial Vein
C3, Body
Deep Cervical Lymph Node
Longus Cervicis Muscle
Longus Capitis Muscle
Vertebral Artery
Deep Cervical Lymph Node
C4, Superior Articular Facet
Levator Scapulae Muscle
C3, Posterior Articular Facet
Spinal Cord
Deep Cervical Vein
C3, Spinous Process
Semispinalis Cervicis Muscle
Trapezius Muscle
Deep Cervical Fascia
Skin
Ligamentum Nuchae

Posterior

B

FIGURE 120.2 (*Continued*) **B:** Anatomic specimen demonstrating zone III relationships. (**B:** From Spitzer VM, Whitlock DG. *Atlas of the visible human male: reverse engineering of the human body*. Sodburg, MA: Jones & Bartlett, 1998. Reprinted with permission.)

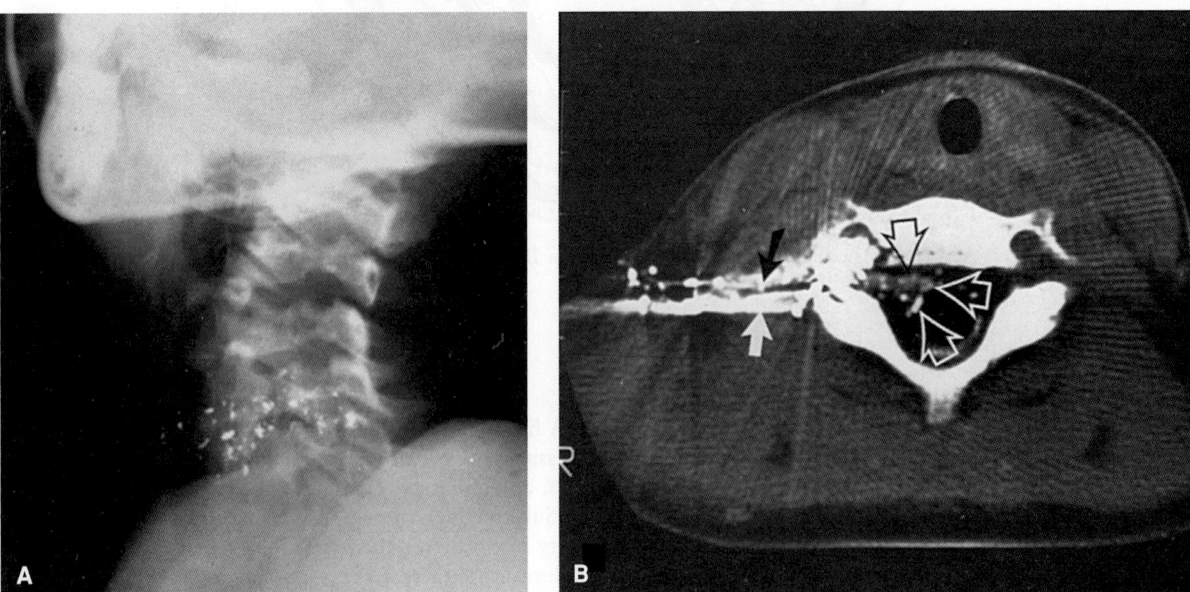

FIGURE 120.3 **A:** Gunshot wound (0.22 caliber) to the neck in a 5-year-old girl. **A:** Lateral neck radiograph showing fragmentation of bullet along path. **B:** Computed tomography (CT) scan of same patient demonstrating bullet fragments in and around the spinal canal, as well as cerebrospinal fluid and contrast leak from disruption of the dura.

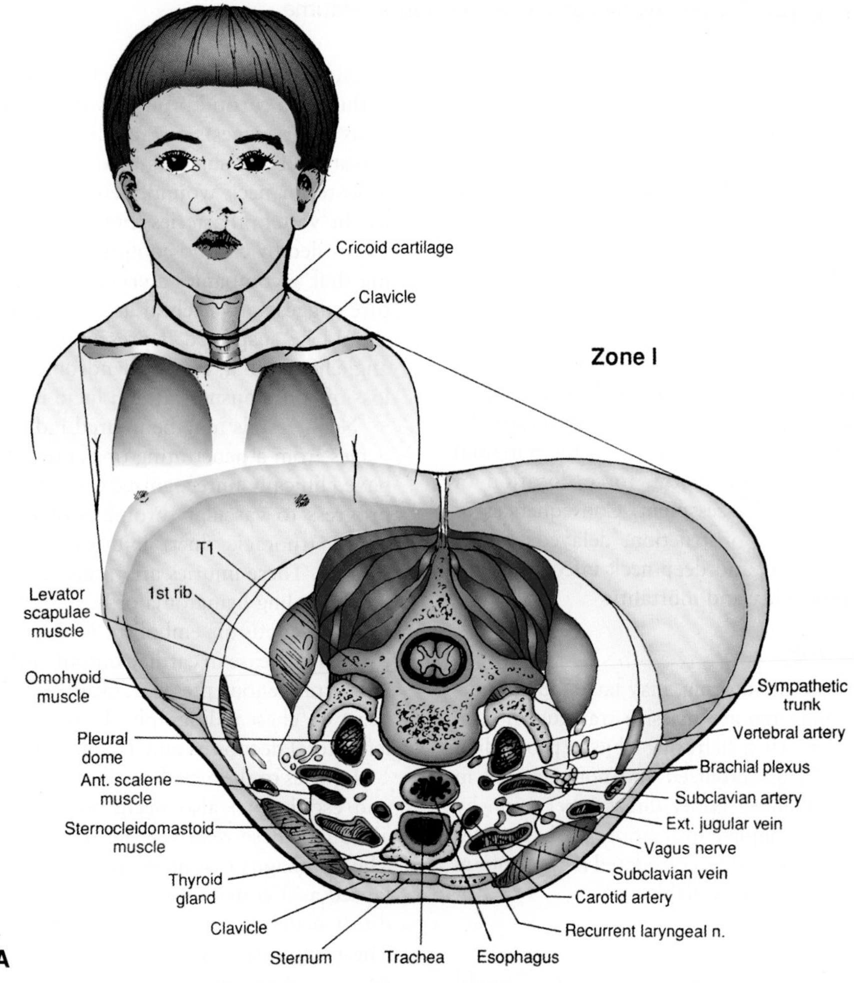

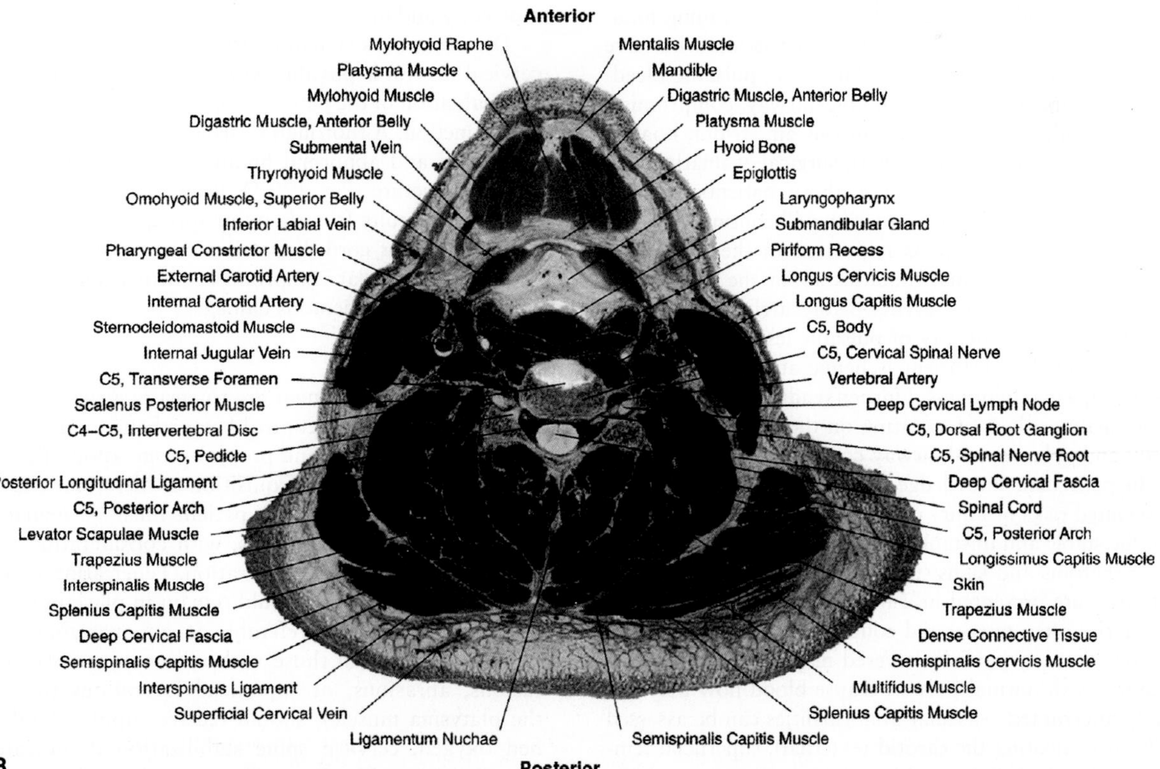

FIGURE 120.4 **A:** Anatomic neck divisions and contents of zone II located between the upper boundary of zone I and the angle of the mandible. **B:** Anatomic specimen demonstrating zone II relationships. (**B:** From Spitzer VM, Whitlock DG. Atlas of the visible human male: reverse engineering of the human body. Sodburg, MA: Jones & Bartlett, 1998. Reprinted with permission.)

to have 93% sensitivity and 87% positive predictive value in predicting vascular injuries.

Penetrating injury of the larynx and trachea occur, although blunt trauma to these areas is more common and can be associated with significant morbidity and mortality (see Chapter 126 ENT Emergencies).

Clinical Considerations

Clinical Recognition

While penetrating neck trauma is rare in children, if a child presents with a history consistent with this type of injury, the clinician should have a high index of suspicion for potential injuries based on the penetrating object, force, location of penetration, and initial clinical assessment. Consequences of missed injuries include airway obstruction, delayed hemorrhage, neurologic compromise, and deep neck infection, with potentially significant morbidity and mortality.

Triage Considerations

These patients require close monitoring, may have difficult airway management, and may require massive transfusion support for severe blood loss. All penetrating objects protruding from a child's neck should be stabilized and not removed in the emergency department unless under direct supervision by appropriate specialist after complete evaluation. Early transfer to a pediatric trauma center should be considered if appropriate surgical or critical care staff is not available.

Clinical Assessment

Rapid assessment of the patient's physiologic status should take precedence and will largely determine the ensuing management or further clinical evaluation. For patients who have "hard signs" of injury (cardiovascular shock, pulsatile bleeding or expanding hematoma, audible airway compromise, bubbling wound, extensive subcutaneous air, stridor, hoarseness, signs of intracerebral ischemia), surgical evaluation and intervention will likely ensue. For those patients without "hard signs," further clinical evaluation will continue.

The history of the event is important in the evaluation of penetrating neck trauma. Inquiries about the mechanism of injury, time of incident, events before arrival in the ED, amount of blood loss, history of pulsatile lesions, neurologic dysfunction including transient ischemic attack, limb paresthesias, hemiplegia, blindness, Horner syndrome (ptosis, miosis, enophthalmos, loss of sweating on the ipsilateral side of the face), and aphasia; and airway compromise should all be noted. In particular, knowledge of the mechanism of injury and associated risks of injury can help direct the management of both the stable and unstable patient.

The symptoms and signs suggestive of vascular and other neck injuries are presented in Table 120.3. Completely transected arteries often retract and contract with minimal bleeding. Vessels that are partially severed may continue to bleed significantly with normal pulses because blood flow may not be totally interrupted. Vascular abnormalities can be assessed partially by evaluating the carotid (external), superficial temporal, and brachial pulses, although pulses are not easily accessible to evaluate the internal carotid or vertebral arteries. Abnormal pulses suggest vascular injury, whereas normal pulses do not guarantee vascular integrity.

Auscultation of the neck is useful to identify bruits. Although a carotid bruit may be normal in children, a continuous bruit suggests a traumatic arteriovenous fistula whereas a systolic bruit suggests a partial arterial tear. Bleeding from a posterior neck wound, neurologic deficits in areas supplied by the vertebral arteries (brainstem, cerebellum), bleeding not controlled by carotid compression, a posterior bruit, or bleeding that accompanies a cervical spine transverse process fracture suggests a vertebral artery injury. Carotid artery trauma should be suspected if presentation involves an anterior triangle hematoma, Horner syndrome, transient ischemic attack, loss of consciousness after a lucid interval, or hemiplegia.

Neck vessels may be injured indirectly as a result of shock waves from a penetrating object or bullet. These patients may have clinically unrecognized vascular intimal damage that can progress to vascular thrombus or occlusion. Venous or lymphatic (thoracic duct) injuries also occur with penetrating trauma. These injuries are rarely severe and usually present as an expanding hematoma or less often with a venous air embolism. If venous air embolism is suspected because of an unexplained decrease in cardiac output and blood pressure, increase in central venous pressure, cyanosis, arrhythmias, or air in the heart on chest radiograph, the patient should be placed in the left lateral decubitus and Trendelenburg positions.

Injuries to the aerodigestive tract (pharynx, larynx, trachea, and esophagus) also occur in cases of penetrating trauma, although these relatively mobile structures are often spared. The esophagus is somewhat protected in that it is usually collapsed as it courses through the neck but it may be injured by direct penetrating objects, usually a stab or gunshot wound. These injuries can present initially in a subtle fashion, but delays in diagnosis can lead to significant increase in observed morbidity and mortality.

Direct nervous system injury (brachial plexus, spinal cord, cervical nerves) is possible with penetrating neck trauma and the evaluation of the patient should assess these structures and their function. A thorough neurologic examination should be completed and abnormal findings should correspond to the injured structure (Fig. 120.5). Primary injury to the cervical cord often results from bony or foreign-body penetration or impingement or cord distraction. Secondary cord injury can occur from vascular compromise, edema, lipid peroxidation, ischemia, and ligamentous damage.

Management

The goals of management are to ensure airway patency and adequate respiration, control hemorrhage, maintain osseous stability, and identify and prevent progression of all injuries. Methodical and timely acquisition of historical and physical findings is mandatory. The patient must be managed with strict adherence to the ABCs, with consideration of potential rapid or gradual deterioration. Penetrating objects that are lodged in the neck should remain in place until removed under surgical care, preferably in an operating room. All patients, other than those with minor injuries such as contusions, abrasions, or superficial lacerations (not through the platysma muscle), should receive supplemental humidified oxygen, cervical spine stabilization if indicated, correct airway positioning, suctioning, close observation, and monitoring. The patient should be maintained in a supine or Trendelenburg position to avoid the possibility of venous air embolism. A decision tree for the evaluation of direct blunt

TABLE 120.3

SYMPTOMS AND SIGNS OF NECK INJURIES

Laryngotracheal	Digestive	Vascular	Neurologic
Airway obstruction	Crepitus	Vigorous bleeding, internal or external	Altered consciousness
Dyspnea	Retropharyngeal air	Expansile or pulsatile hematoma	Generalized weakness
Stridor	Subcutaneous emphysema	Bruit	Hemiparesis
Retractions	Pneumomediastinum	Absent pulsations (carotid, superficial temporal, or ophthalmic artery)	Hemiplegia
Cough	Hematemesis	Unexplained hypotension	Quadriplegia
Aspiration	Chest or neck pain	Hemothorax	Seizures
Pneumomediastinum	Neck tenderness	Cardiac tamponade	Bruit
Pneumothorax	Dysphagia	Hemiplegia	Cervicosensory deficits
Crepitus	Odynophagia	Hemiparesis	Aphasia
Subcutaneous emphysema	Saliva in wound	Aphasia	Horner syndrome (ipsilateral cervical sympathetics)
Tracheal deviation	Drooling	Monocular blindness	Cranial nerve IX–XII dysfunction
Endobronchial bleeding	Fever	Loss of consciousness	Tongue deviation (hypoglossal)
Hemoptysis	Mediastinitis	Neck asymmetry, swelling, or discoloration	Drooping of corner of the mouth (mandibular branch of the facial nerve)
Epistaxis		Wide mediastinum	Hoarseness (vagus/recurrent laryngeal)
Hematemesis		Cranial nerve abnormality	Immobile vocal cords (vagus/recurrent laryngeal)
Hemothorax		Clavicle/first rib fracture	Trapezius weakness (spinal accessory)
Dysphagia			Brachial palsy (arm paresthesias)
Odynophagia			Monocular blindness (vertebral artery)
Bubbling, sucking, or hissing wound			Diaphragm paralysis (phrenic)
Neck deformity			
Asymmetry			
Loss of landmarks			
Flat thyroid prominence			
Laryngotracheal tenderness			
Dysphonia			
Aphonia			
Voice changes			
Hoarseness			
Drooling			
Neck pain, tenderness (with coughing or swallowing)			

and penetrating neck trauma is presented in Figure 120.6. Patients with "hard signs" of injury should be immediately evaluated for surgical intervention.

Airway assessment is the initial step in the evaluation of all patients with trauma. Any airway manipulation should be accomplished with consideration and prevention of possible cervical spine injury. Potential indications for an artificial airway with neck trauma include stridor, dyspnea, hypoxia, rapidly expanding hematoma, expanding crepitus, pneumothorax, hemothorax, tracheal deviation, altered mental status, quadriplegia, hemiparesis, and other signs of vascular or airway insufficiency. If the airway is unstable, intubation should be considered. Orotracheal intubation is the preferred method in children. Intubation should be attempted only after preparation for the placement of a surgical airway, if time allows. Fiber-optic intubation via the nasal route, performed by a skilled provider, may be useful. The physician must be especially careful with the use of blind nasotracheal intubation in the patient with blunt or

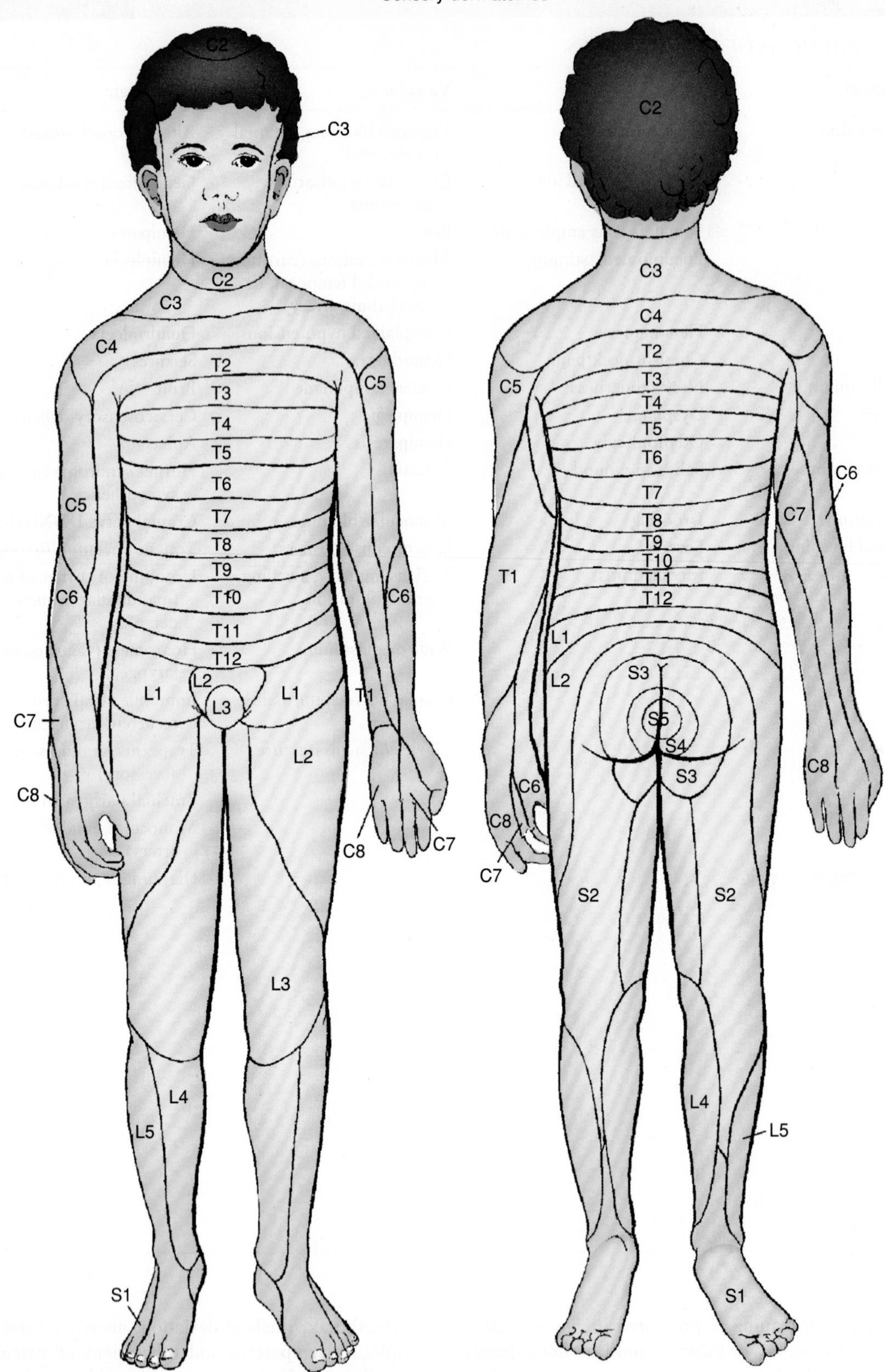

FIGURE 120.5 **A:** Sensory dermatomes.

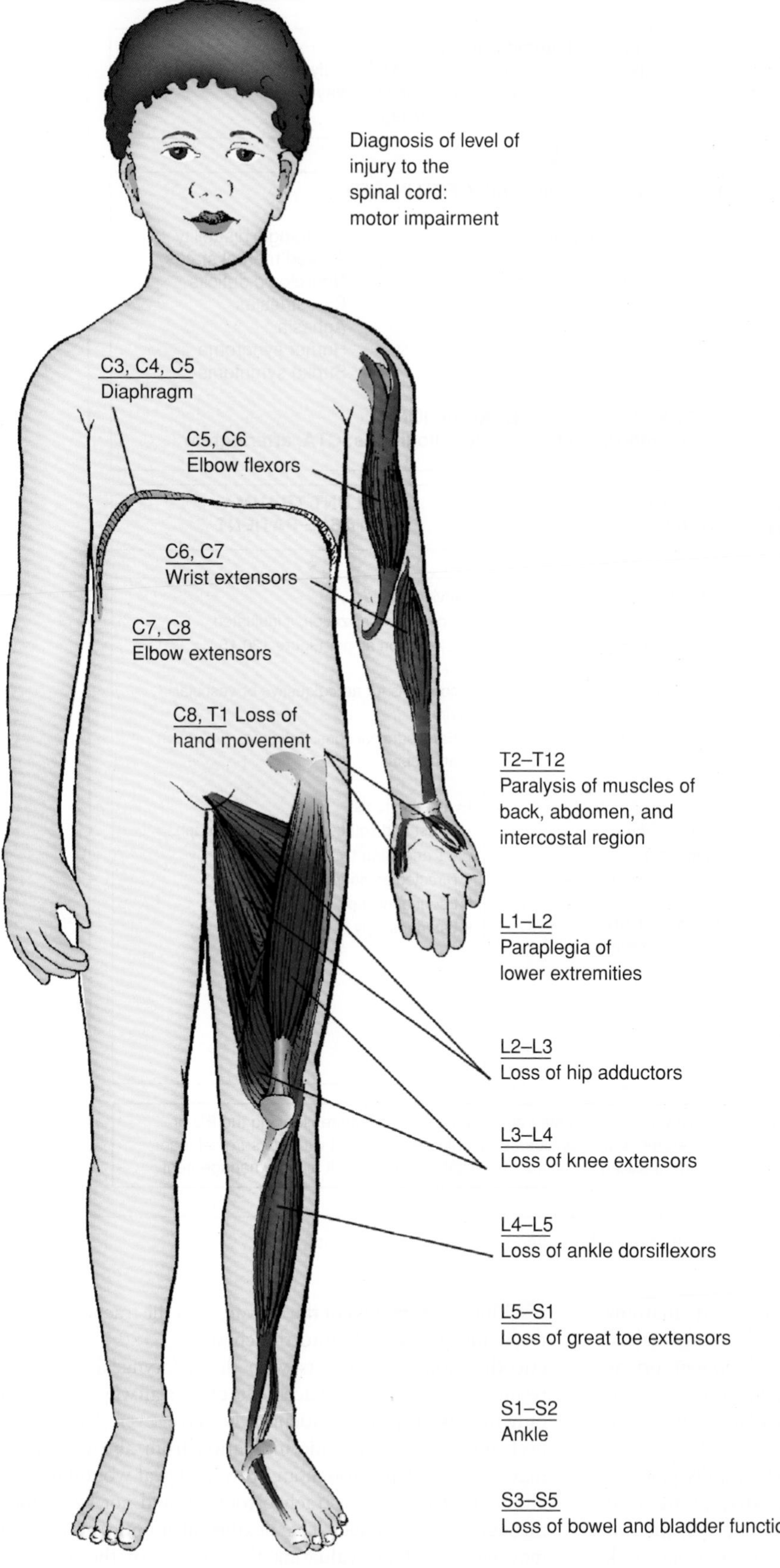

FIGURE 120.5 (*Continued*) **B:** Motor dermatomes. Knowledge of sensory and motor dermatomes can be invaluable in description of neurologic findings during initial and subsequent evaluations.

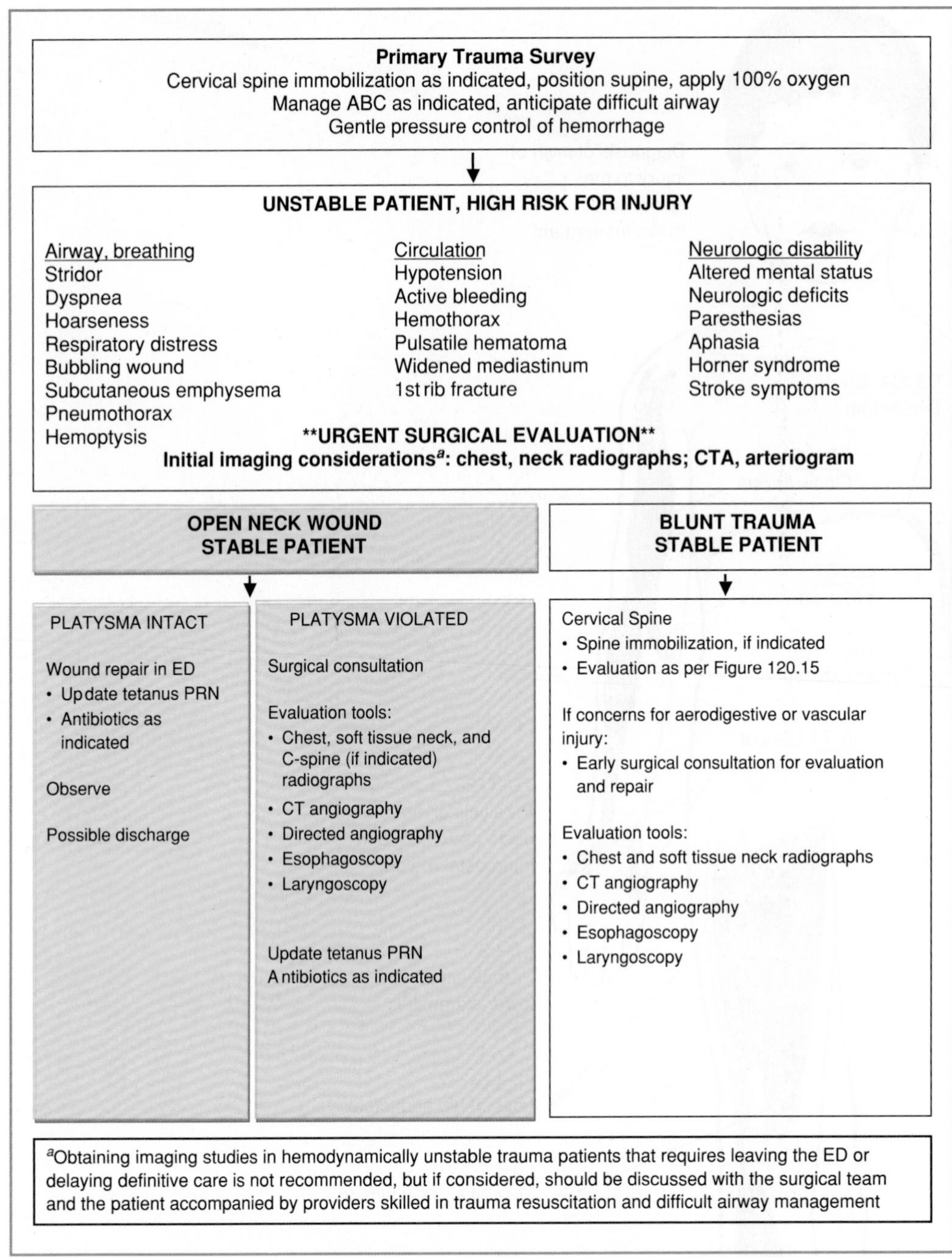

FIGURE 120.6 Evaluation of blunt and penetrating neck trauma.

penetrating neck or facial trauma because the airway anatomy may be distorted. Passage of the nasotracheal or orotracheal tube into a false or blind passage may make subsequent airway control attempts difficult, if not impossible. Therefore, considering the difficulty of emergent surgical airway placement in children, elective intubation is not recommended outside a setting where a surgical airway can be efficiently and skillfully placed.

If there is evidence of crepitus over the larynx, laryngeal or tracheal tenderness, a flattened thyroid prominence, anterior neck deformity, severe respiratory distress, an abnormal neck radiograph, or other evidence suggestive of a laryngotracheal fracture or disruption, a tracheostomy may be preferable. In this scenario, intubation should only be attempted if the airway is completely obstructed. Attempts at intubation from above may separate a tenuously attached trachea and larynx, resulting in a total loss of the airway, with the trachea commonly retracting substernally into the chest (Fig. 120.7). Attempts at cricothyrotomy in patients with direct laryngeal trauma may result in retrotracheal placement of the airway. Cricothyrotomy may be helpful in patients who have severe facial or other neck injuries that preclude intubation from above. Intubation may be attempted through an open laryngeal wound if present, although, if possible, a tracheostomy should not be performed through injured tissue. The flexible fiber-optic bronchoscope may be helpful in evaluating the patency of the airway and establishing the artificial airway. If patient condition allows, rigid bronchoscopy can also be useful in securing an airway in these patients. Care should be taken to ensure correct positioning and securing of the artificial airway, as the usual landmarks and adjacent tissues may be injured or altered.

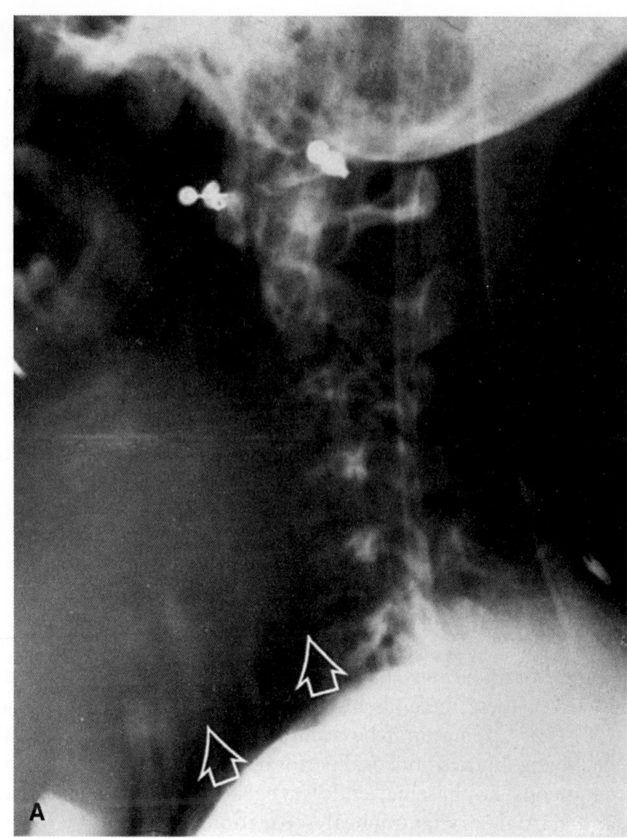

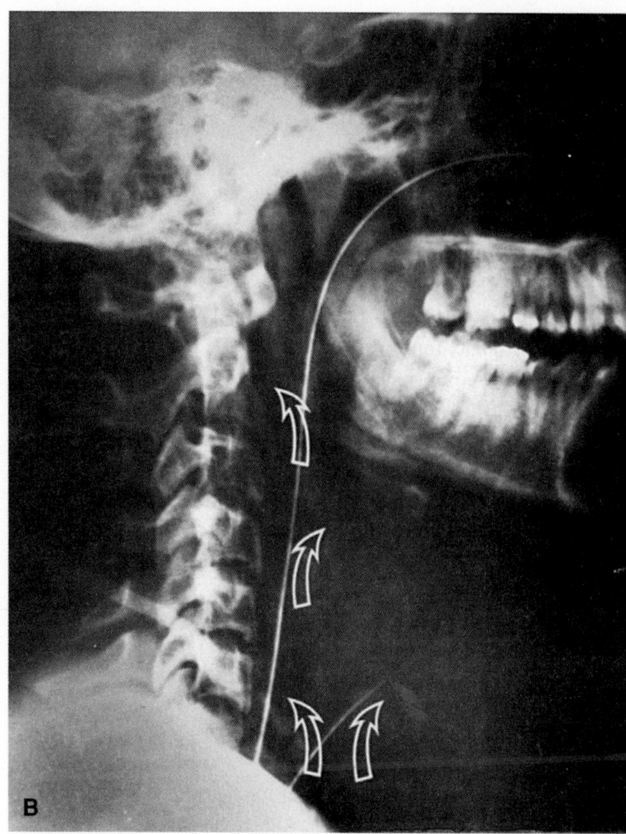

FIGURE 120.7 Tracheal injury. **A:** Initial lateral neck radiograph showing subcutaneous emphysema (*solid arrows*) in 14-year-old girl kicked in the neck by a horse. Patient's airway clinically stable at the time of this radiograph (more than 1 hour after the injury). **B:** Postcricothyrotomy radiograph in same patient demonstrating significant subcutaneous emphysema and an artificial airway in place (*open arrows*). Initial attempt at orotracheal intubation separated tenuously attached trachea, completing traumatic disruption of the trachea and requiring immediate placement of surgical airway.

Breathing abnormalities may suggest associated injuries. Missiles to the neck may also pass through or lodge in the chest. Zone I injuries of the neck can easily involve the lung apices and result in hemothorax, pneumothorax, or pneumomediastinum. Further penetration may lead to cardiac tamponade. A chest radiograph is helpful in the assessment. A normal physical examination and chest radiograph are likely sufficient to obviate the need for arteriography in this population.

In addition to the usual assessment for hypovolemia, the patient should be examined for expanding hematomas or other obvious external bleeding. External bleeding should be treated with gentle compression. Attempts to clamp bleeding vessels in the neck can injure the vessels and surrounding structures, as well as jeopardize subsequent repair attempts. Two large-bore intravenous (IV) catheters should be inserted, ideally on the side opposite to the injury if an obvious vascular abnormality is identified. If a subclavian vein injury is suspected, one of the IV catheters should be placed in the lower extremity; if there are no contraindications.

A neurologic examination for signs of cerebral injury secondary to vascular insufficiency, direct spinal cord, cranial or cervical nerve, or brachial plexus injury should be completed. An abnormal or changing neurologic examination may indicate progressive vascular insufficiency and the need for rapid surgical evaluation. Rapid assessment by CT or magnetic resonance imaging (MRI), followed by surgical intervention, will provide opportunity for optimal outcome. Direct nerve injuries may not necessitate surgical repair.

Tetanus status should be assessed in all patients with penetrating trauma. The clinician should consider a broad-spectrum antibiotic for a patient with evidence of neck trauma, especially if esophageal or pharyngeal injury seems likely. Placement of a nasogastric or an orogastric tube is controversial for the patient with cervical injury because it may worsen a pre-existing esophageal injury or dislodge clots in zone I of the neck. When placed, these tubes should be well lubricated, inserted gently and slowly, and withdrawn if difficulty in passage or evidence of obstruction occurs.

Superficial abrasions, lacerations, and puncture wounds are common in children. Wounds superficial to the platysma can be cleaned and sutured under local anesthesia in the ED. Clean wounds can be sutured as late as 12 to 18 hours after the injury because of the excellent blood flow in the neck. Closure after 72 hours is not recommended. Penetration of the platysma is an indication for surgical referral and, in some cases, surgical exploration. When neck wounds that penetrate the platysma are evaluated, exploration in the ED is discouraged because of the risk of clot dislodgement and venous air embolism. Rapid surgical exploration and repair are indicated in patients struck by a high-velocity missile, those with unstable vital signs, uncontrollable bleeding, rapidly expanding hematomas, progressive airway compromise, worsening

TABLE 120.4

INDICATIONS SUGGESTING SURGICAL EVALUATION IN PATIENTS WITH NECK TRAUMA

Unstable vital signs
Expanding or massive hematoma
Pulsatile or active bleeding
Hemorrhagic shock
Vascular deficits in the upper extremities
Abnormal distal pulses (brachial, superficial temporal, ophthalmologic, fundi)
Hematemesis, hemoptysis, epistaxis
Hemothorax
Progressive respiratory distress
Airway obstruction
Expanding subcutaneous emphysema
Bubbling or sucking wound
Pneumothorax
Progressive neurologic deficits
Hemiparesis
Horner syndrome
Cranial or cervical nerve dysfunction
Diaphragm paralysis
Decreased sensorium
Neurologic deficits in upper extremity
Increasing dysphagia
Odynophagia or dysphonia
Hoarseness
Severe neck pain or tenderness
High-velocity wounds (rifles, explosions)
Multiple low-velocity wounds
Ancillary radiographic studies not available
Experienced observation personnel not available

neurologic symptoms, increasing subcutaneous emphysema, or bubbling wounds (Table 120.4).

Surgical evaluation may give false-negative results with esophageal lacerations, small vessel lacerations, pharyngeal lacerations, or tracheal injuries. The patient who has stable vital signs, no symptoms of impaired neurologic or cardiovascular status, an intact airway, and mechanisms of injury with a low-velocity bullet or single knife wound may be managed expectantly with the use of ancillary diagnostic tests and close observation, preferably for at least 48 hours. These decisions should be made in conjunction with experienced surgical staff.

Adjuncts to the history and physical examination are given in Table 120.5. Initial evaluation should include cervical spine radiographs to detect bony or structural abnormalities, as well as a soft tissue lateral neck radiograph to assess for blood, edema, subcutaneous air, foreign bodies, and airway impingement or disruption. A chest radiograph should be evaluated for evidence of hemothorax or pneumothorax, mediastinal emphysema or widening, and heart size. If a serious injury is likely, radiographs should be obtained in the ED or the patient should be accompanied to the radiology department by someone skilled in airway management. If the patient is stable and a vascular injury is suspected, a CTA or arteriogram should be performed (Fig. 120.8). Contrast laryngography, tomography,

TABLE 120.5

ADJUNCTS TO HISTORY AND PHYSICAL EXAMINATION

Cervical spine radiographs
Soft tissue neck radiograph
Chest radiograph
Computed tomographic scan
Arteriography
Doppler
Esophagram
Contrast laryngotracheography
Indirect (mirror) laryngoscopy
Direct laryngoscopy
Flexible bronchoscopy
Direct bronchoesophagoscopy
Surgical exploration

and xeroradiography have been used for further evaluation; however, these methods have generally been replaced by the CT scan. CT may not be accurate for detection of mucosal degloving injuries, mucosal perforation in the presence of subcutaneous emphysema, endolaryngeal edema or hematoma, and partial laryngotracheal separation. Noninvasive Doppler studies and oculoplethysmography may also be useful in evaluating vascular injuries.

Contrast esophagram is helpful in evaluating the esophagus for tears or perforations, but false-negative rates of up to 50% have been reported. Evaluation can also include indirect mirror laryngoscopy to assess the larynx, vocal cord mobility, presence of mucosal edema, ecchymosis, and mucosal tears, as well as direct endoscopy to examine for tracheal, bronchial, and esophageal damage. Flexible endoscopy may be less invasive and easier to accomplish, but rigid endoscopy offers the most complete examination. Even rigid endoscopy, however, is not 100% sensitive in detecting tracheal and esophageal injuries. As mentioned, operative evaluation is mandatory for some patients and optional for others. Determinants of specific management direction include mechanism of injury, wound size and type, patient signs and symptoms, and relative stability.

Clinical Indications for Discharge or Admission

Patients can be discharged if they do not have a significant injury without platysmal penetration, are hemodynamically stable, without airway compromise, able to tolerate oral intake, and no indication or risk of abusive trauma or neglect is present. Otherwise, admission is indicated.

BLUNT TRAUMA

Goals of Treatment

To ensure airway patency, respiratory sufficiency, hemorrhage control, cervical spine stability, and identify and prevent progression of injuries to all structures and tissues within the neck, including the airway, major blood vessels, neurologic, and osseous structures.

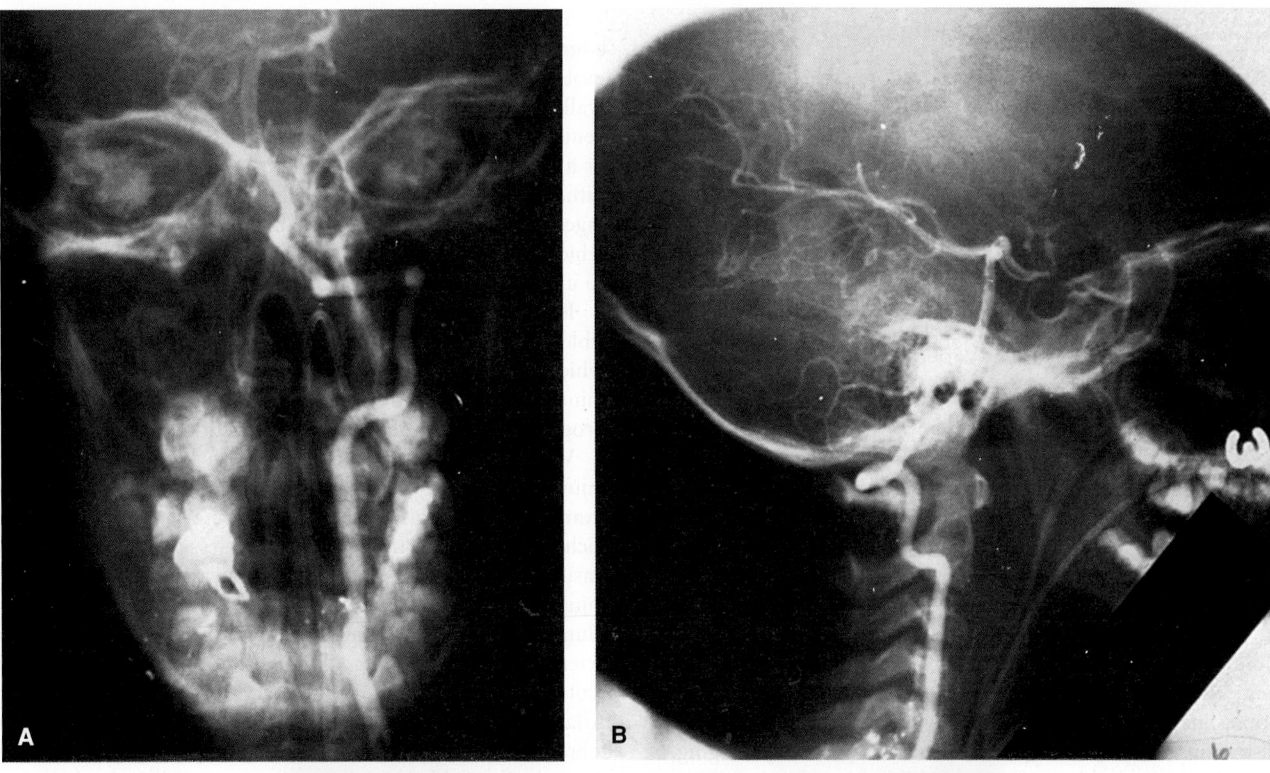

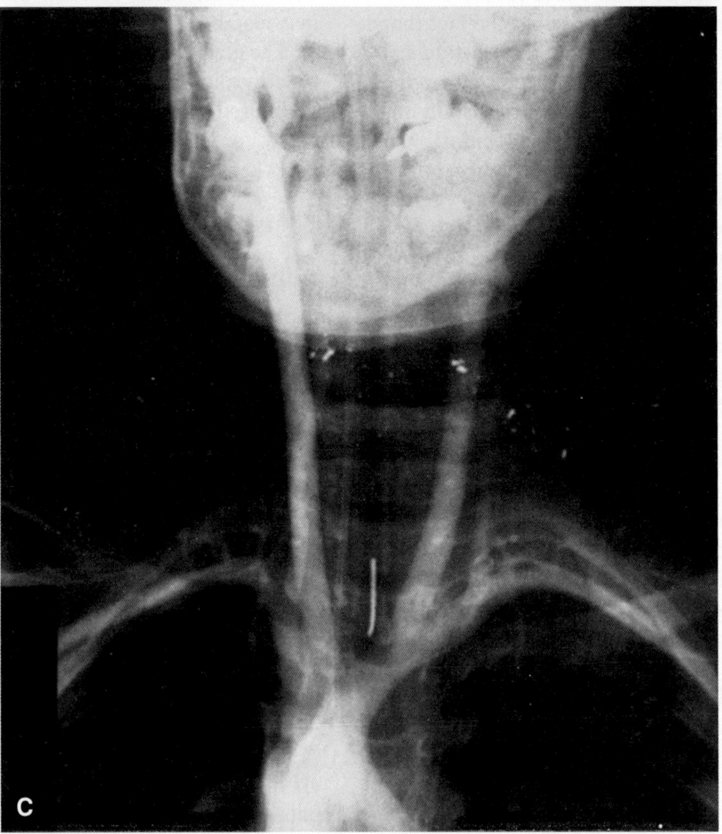

FIGURE 120.8 Angiograms in 5-year-old child shot in the neck, demonstrating normal vascular integrity. **A:** Vertebral artery angiogram (anteroposterior view). **B:** Vertebral artery angiogram (lateral view). **C:** Carotid angiogram.

CLINICAL PEARLS AND PITFALLS

- The airway may be injured with direct blunt trauma in part due to the anterior position of the larynx and trachea.
- Dyspnea, hemoptysis, and stridor suggest laryngeal airway.
- Cervical emphysema, dysphagia, and progressive airway obstruction characterize supraglottic injuries.
- Hemoptysis and persistent air leak suggest injuries inferior to the glottis.
- Early airway management should be considered for patients with facial and neck burns.
- Vascular injuries are less common compared to penetrating trauma, but are also missed on routine examination. Maintain a high index of suspicion.
- The cervical spine should be immobilized if indicated by mechanism of injury, inability to clinically clear, or in the presence of significant head/neck trauma.

Current Evidence

Blunt trauma is often the result of a motor vehicle accident, although it can also result from sports-related injuries; clothesline and handlebar injuries from bicycles, motorcycles, all-terrain vehicles, and snowmobiles; strangulation; hanging; direct blows and various forms of child abuse (Table 120.1). Pediatric-specific mechanisms of injury as well as the fact that children have a relatively short neck, mobile laryngotracheal structures, and a superior-positioned larynx protected by the mandibular arch make it less likely for children to sustain airway fractures and may impact overall severity of injury. On the other hand, the small and narrow airway increases the risk of airway-related morbidity secondary to airway edema, bleeding, swelling, and obstruction. Blunt trauma is often associated with extracervical injuries, especially maxillofacial, head, chest, and aerodigestive injuries, but is less likely than penetrating trauma to involve multiple structures within the neck or cause vascular damage.

The airway may be injured with direct blunt trauma in part as a result of the anterior and relatively fixed position of the larynx and trachea. High-impact blunt trauma to the trachea has been associated with a mortality rate of approximately 15%, although this is likely higher when one considers patients who die at the scene. The anterior neck is relatively well protected by bony structures, unless the neck is extended. With neck extension, the larynx, trachea, and esophagus are exposed to direct trauma and a blunt force may crush these structures against the posterior spinal column. A tracheal tear or rupture may occur from a sudden increase in intratracheal pressure against a closed glottis, direct blunt trauma, crush, or acceleration/deceleration injury. Shearing forces can cause edema, submucosal hematoma, laceration, perforation, vocal cord injury, and, less commonly, partial or complete airway transection. A prime target for airway fracture is the cricoid ring, which is the only complete tracheal ring.

Approximately 85% of patients with blunt tracheal injury reportedly have subcutaneous emphysema, although the onset may be delayed (Fig. 120.9). However, airway injuries may be subtle and not apparent with initial history or physical examination but progress to severe abnormalities such as airway obstruction from tracheal edema as late as 48 hours after the injury.

The esophagus is mobile and is usually collapsed as it courses through the neck but may be dilated while eating. This mobility helps protect the esophagus, but its delicate mucosal walls can be damaged easily by blunt traumatic events. Iatrogenic esophageal injuries can result from endoscopy, passage of a nasogastric or orogastric tube, vigorous suctioning, and difficult intubations. Esophageal injuries can also be seen with ingested foreign bodies and caustic chemicals. The injuries, which can be subtle, occult, and difficult to diagnose, can lead to increased morbidity and mortality if not identified.

Isolated or concurrent hyoid bone injuries are also possible, but rare. The hyoid is mobile and fairly well protected, which explains the paucity of isolated injury. As with other injuries, these symptoms and signs can be subtle initially, with progressive edema and airway obstruction.

Vascular injuries are also rare with blunt trauma. These injuries are often unsuspected and undiagnosed on routine examination. Risk factors for injury have been reported to include Glasgow Coma Scale score of less than 8; head injury; basilar skull fracture; and facial, neck, thorax, or abdominal injury. The most common vascular structure injured with blunt trauma is the common carotid artery. The vertebral arteries are rarely injured by blunt forces unless a concurrent transverse process or other cervical spine fracture occurs. Atlantooccipital dislocation can also be associated with vertebral artery injury, which if occurs frequently leads to early death in the field. Vascular contusions with intimal damage may also be seen with blunt neck trauma.

The glandular structures in the neck, including the thyroid, parathyroid, parotid, and submandibular glands, may also be injured. While these organs may be traumatized, they are rarely completely destroyed.

Clinical Considerations

Clinical Recognition

In the presence of blunt neck trauma, the triad of dyspnea, stridor, and hemoptysis suggests laryngeal injury. Injuries above the glottis often demonstrate cervical emphysema, dysphagia, hoarseness, and progressive airway obstruction, whereas those below present with hemoptysis and persistent air leak, although any or all symptoms and signs listed in Table 120.3 may be present. If a laryngeal injury is noted, the patient should be evaluated carefully for other commonly associated injuries, including in the cervical spine, chest, face, pharyngoesophageal area, and recurrent laryngeal nerve palsy.

Symptoms and signs of hyoid injury include pain in the throat that worsens with swallowing or coughing, tenderness to palpation, neck crepitus, pain on head rotation, dysphagia, dyspnea, or dysphonia.

The symptoms and signs associated with esophageal injury are listed in Table 120.3 and include neck tenderness and pain, dysphagia, odynophagia, drooling, crepitus, subcutaneous emphysema, hematemesis, fever, and mediastinitis (see Chapters 52 Pain: Dysuria, and 89 Head Trauma).

The clinician must consider subclavian or innominate vessel injuries if a fracture of the clavicle or first rib is identified.

Patients with signs or symptoms of facial or neck burns will require careful assessment, as airway edema may initially be subtle but progress rapidly. Early recognition and protection of a difficult airway is paramount.

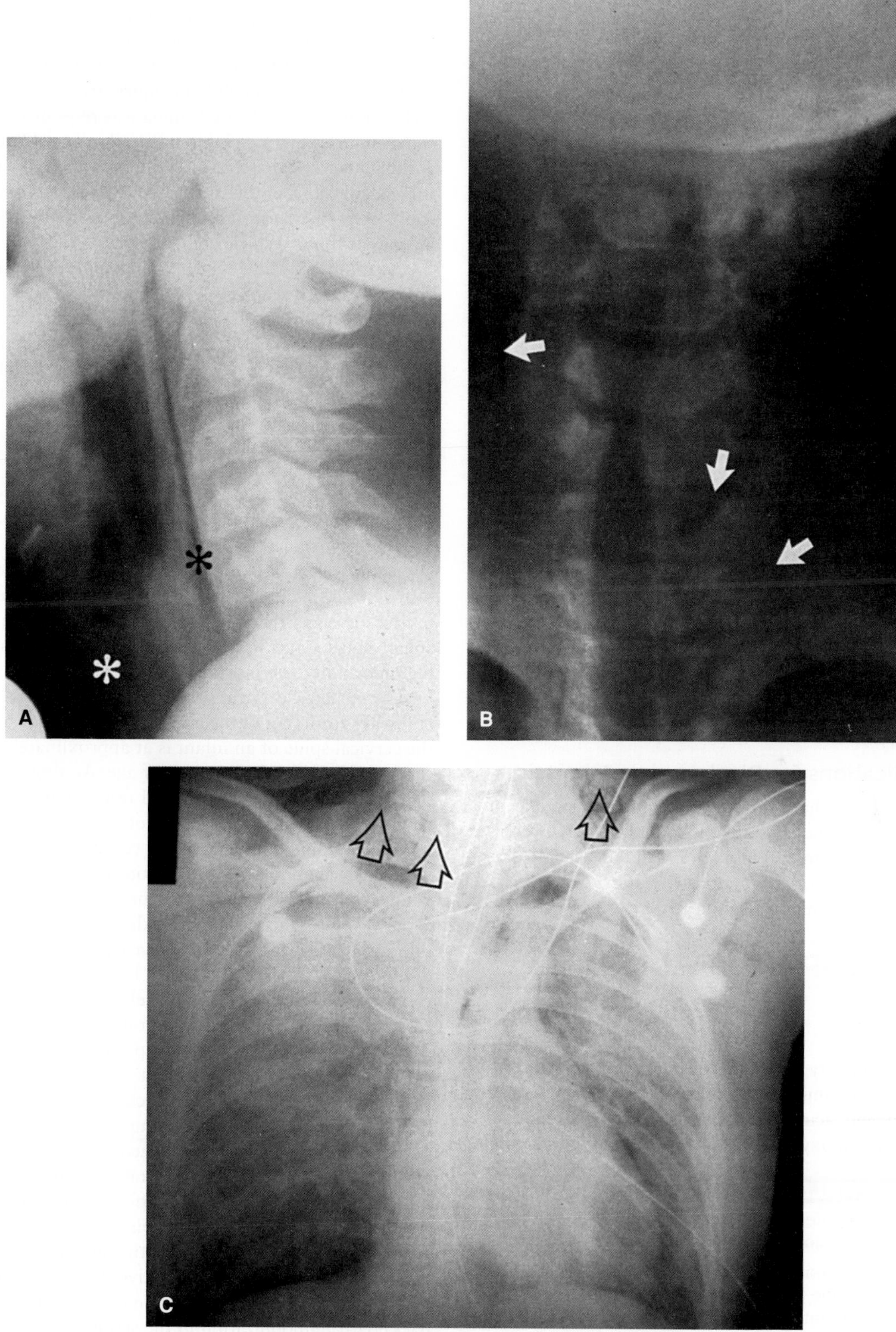

FIGURE 120.9 **A–C:** Subcutaneous emphysema (*asterisks* and *arrows*) of neck and chest in 11-year-old patient from barotrauma sustained when opening carbonated beverage container with teeth.

Triage Considerations

These patients require expedited evaluation, close monitoring and providers should anticipate difficult airway management. Early transfer to a pediatric trauma center should be considered if appropriate surgical or critical care staff is not available.

Clinical Assessment

As with all trauma patients, initial rapid assessment of their airway, breathing, and circulatory status should be completed. Given the risk of airway injury, particular attention must be paid to subtle signs and symptoms of airway injury (Table 120.3). Continued monitoring with repeat examinations is important in the recognition and identification of vascular and neurologic injuries (Table 120.3). Refer to penetrating trauma clinical assessment section for detailed recommendations.

Management

Blunt neck trauma requires similar vigilance and potentially, similar diagnostic modalities as penetrating trauma. Refer to penetrating trauma section for management recommendations. Special management considerations are included here.

Early airway management should be considered for patients with facial and neck burns, including from ingested caustic substances. For circumferential burns, an escharotomy may be indicated which involves a vertical incision from the chin to the superior aspect of the sternal notch. This should only be performed by an experienced provider familiar with pediatric neck anatomy (see Chapter 112 Burns).

In blunt trauma, progressive onset pain, irritability, and signs of cord compression may suggest a spinal (usually venous) epidural hematoma. Rapid assessment by CT or MRI, followed by surgical intervention, will help ensure optimal outcome.

Clinical Indications for Discharge or Admission

The patient can be discharged if they do not have a significant injury, are hemodynamically stable, without any airway compromise, able to tolerate oral intake to maintain their hydration, and no indication or risk of abusive trauma or neglect is present. Otherwise, admission is indicated.

CERVICAL SPINE TRAUMA

Goals of Treatment

The goals are to identify cervical spine injury and prevent progression of secondary injury by applying the principles of spine immobilization and acute trauma resuscitation to maintain adequate ventilation, oxygenation, and hemodynamic status.

CLINICAL PEARLS AND PITFALLS

- Cervical spine injuries are uncommon in children but account for the majority of vertebral injuries in children.
- Younger children tend to have higher proportion of upper cervical spine injuries (C1–C4) due to the higher fulcrum of the immature spine, dislocations instead of fractures, and spinal cord injury without radiographic abnormality (SCIWORA).
- Children with congenital spine abnormalities, osseous weakness, or ligamentous instability are at increased risk for spinal injury.
- Airway management should be accomplished with simultaneous stabilization of the cervical spine.

Current Evidence

Cervical spine injuries are uncommon in children, occurring in an estimated 1% to 2% of patients with multiple trauma. Most injuries are a result of blunt forces due to motor vehicle crashes, followed by fall, sport-related injuries, and nonaccidental trauma. Mechanism of injury also varies by age. In a 2014 study, nonaccidental trauma was responsible for 38% of spinal injuries among children 0 to 2 years of age with 73% within the cervical spine, as common a mechanism as motor vehicle collisions in this age group; where as in older children sports-related injuries accounted for as many cervical spine injuries as motor vehicle collisions.

It is estimated that 5% of all spinal injuries occur in children younger than 16 years. However, approximately 72% of spinal injuries in children younger than 8 years occur in the cervical region. Certain pre-existing conditions (Down, Maroteaux–Lamy, Morquio's, Grisel, and Klippel–Feil syndromes; achondroplasia; congenital cervical stenosis; Chiari malformation; rheumatoid disease; and acute soft tissue or bony infection or infiltration) may result in a cervical spine more predisposed to injury with minor or more significant trauma. Neurologic sequela may also occur in pediatric patients undergoing spinal manipulation for therapeutic purposes. Neonatal spinal injury may result from birth-associated trauma and is reported in approximately 1 in 60,000 births. These patients often have a history of cephalic forceps use during delivery and may have presenting signs that include weakness, flaccid quadriplegia, spinal shock, and apnea. These birth-related injuries carry high morbidity and mortality.

The pediatric cervical spine and its evaluation differ in several ways from that of the adult cervical spine. The fulcrum of the cervical spine of an infant is at approximately C2–C3 and reaches C3–C4 by 5 to 6 years of age. At about 8 to 10 years of age, the fulcrum (C5–C6) and other characteristics of the cervical spine approximate that of an adult. The higher fulcrum of a young child's spine in combination with relatively weak neck muscles and poor protective reflexes account for young children often having injuries that involve the upper cervical spine, whereas older children and adults have injuries that more often involve the lower cervical spine. Neurologic disability can occur from cervical lesions at all levels, but high cervical cord injuries are more likely to be fatal than are lower cervical cord injuries due to respiratory compromise.

Several concepts should be kept in mind concerning cervical immobilization in children. It is been estimated that 3% to 25% of spinal cord injuries occur during transit or early in the course of management, although a 2001 Cochrane report noted that there are no randomized controlled studies on the effect of immobilization on mortality, neurologic injury, spinal stability, and other adverse effects. It is also important to realize that as many as 20% of spinal injuries involve noncontiguous vertebral elements, so entire spinal column immobilization and evaluation is imperative. Currently, the Congress of Neurological Surgeons recommends a cervical collar and backboard immobilization in the setting of nonnegligible risk of injury after trauma. Soft cervical collars offer no protection to an unstable spine, and hard collars alone may allow a fair amount of flexion, extension, and lateral movement of the cervical spine. Ideal immobilization involves a hard cervical collar in conjunction with a full spine board, soft spacing devices, and securing straps (Fig. 120.10). Hard collars, including the C-Breeze and XTW (Deroyal Industries, Inc.

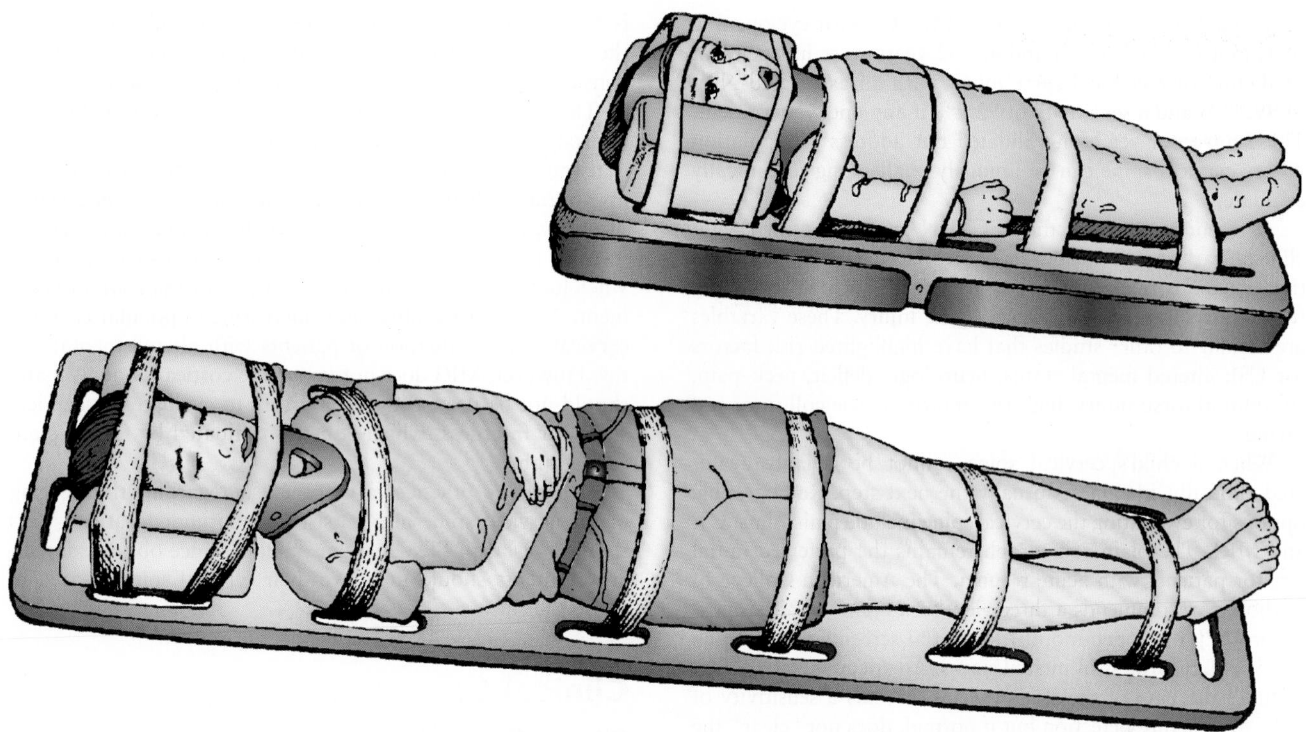

FIGURE 120.10 Cervical spine immobilization should not place the patient at an increased risk for morbidity. Securing straps should be placed around bony prominences and strap location reassessed after any movement of the patient. A neutral position of the neck should be ensured, and if necessary (younger child), a spacer can be placed underneath the child's torso and lower extremities to achieve the desired position.

Powell, TN), Miami J (Jerome Medical, Moorestown, NJ), Philadelphia (Philadelphia Collar Company, Thorofare, NJ), Stifneck (Laerdal, Stavanger, Norway), and Aspen (International Healthcare Devices, Long Beach, CA), are effective in restricting most of the range of motion in the cervical spine. Miami-J collars have been associated with lower levels of mandibular and ocular pressures, reducing the risk of occipital pressure ulcers while maintaining appropriate immobilization.

There is no standard or definitive evidence to support the practice of clinically clearing the pediatric cervical spine in the prehospital environment. Therefore, it is not recommended that prehospital providers clear a child's cervical spine if the child has experienced a potentially significant mechanism of injury. In one large study, prehospital spine immobilization for children <2 years was applied inconsistently including 25% of this age group with documented cervical spine injuries. A perceived lack of options for immobilization was cited as a reason for this practice variation. More research may help us better understand options for immobilization as well as clinical clearance guidelines for prehospital care providers. There is recent evidence to suggest better neurologic outcomes and reduced mortality among children who are transported directly to a pediatric trauma center when there is a suspected cervical spine injury.

There is also limited definitive evidence with regard to in-hospital clinical clearance and radiographic imaging of the pediatric cervical spine. Several authors have attempted to devise criteria to limit the use of cervical spine radiographs because the number of positive studies constitutes a small proportion of the total number of radiographic studies completed. The literature suggests that if the patient does not have a high-risk mechanism of injury (motor vehicle accident, fall >10 ft, dive, or sports injury), is awake and alert, can have an interactive conversation (not inebriated, no altered level of consciousness, verbal at baseline), does not complain of cervical spine pain, has no tenderness on palpation (especially in the midline), has normal neck mobility, has a completely normal neurologic examination without a history of abnormal neurologic symptoms or signs at any time after the injury, and has no other painful injuries (which may distract the patient and mask neck pain), the patient probably does not need radiographic evaluation of the cervical spine. The National Emergency X-Radiography Utilization Study (NEXUS) suggests the following criteria for the assessment of risk of spinal injury: (i) midline cervical tenderness, (ii) intoxication, (iii) alertness, (iv) focal neurologic deficit, and (v) distracting (painful) injury (i.e., long bone fracture, visceral injury, large laceration, degloving or crush injury, large burns, and injuries producing impairment in appreciation of other injuries). If these are negative, then the patient is believed to be at low risk for a spinal injury and may be able to forgo radiographic evaluation. In adults, NEXUS low-risk criteria have been reported to be 99.6% sensitive in detection of clinical important cervical spine injury and have a high negative predictive value for low-risk patients. When NEXUS criteria were applied to children <18 years, the reported sensitivity was 100% but this was in the context of a very low incidence of pediatric spinal cord injury (0.98%), an underrepresentation of children <9 years and an absence of children with injuries under 2 years of age. Therefore, caution should be had when utilizing these criteria in the evaluation of traumatized children since they may not have the same validity in young children as they do in older children and adults. A large multicenter study specifically addressed clinical clearance of the cervical spine in children

<3 years. They found that a GCS <14, a GCS for eye opening of 1, motor vehicle crash and age >2 years were independent predictors of a cervical spine injury with an associated NPV of 99.93% and a sensitivity of 92.9% if any one were present. These have not yet been validated but address a population whose cervical spine can be uniquely challenging to clinically evaluate.

A recent study from the PECARN group identified eight clinical variables for children under the age of 16 years old that when any one of them was present, had a high sensitivity for identifying potential cervical spine injury. These variables are similar to other studies that have highlighted risk factors for CSI: altered mental status, neurologic deficit, neck pain, substantial torso injury, high-risk motor vehicle collision, and diving.

When a child's cervical spine cannot be reliably evaluated clinically, imaging is usually the next step. Radiographic options for evaluating the cervical spine include plain films, CT, and MRI. The plain radiograph remains the preferred initial test for patients with acute trauma. The American College of Radiology recommends a three-view series (lateral, anteroposterior [AP], and open-mouth) for initial screening in children <14 years, regardless of mental status. An adequate lateral film includes the base of the skull and C1-T1, has a sensitivity of 79% for fracture detection but if normal, does not "clear" the cervical spine. The addition of an AP view of C3–C7 and an AP open-mouth (odontoid) view of C1–C2, increases the sensitivity of initial radiographic evaluation to more than 95%. However, the open-mouth view in young children (<8 years) has been shown to be the least useful of the three images, may not be necessary and therefore is most strongly recommended for older children or those who can readily cooperate. In one study at a combined adult and pediatric trauma center, the most common reasons for a missed injury on initial radiologic evaluation included unfamiliarity with pediatric cervical spine anatomy, failure to recognize normal developmental variants, and suboptimal conventional film techniques. Posterior elements of the cervical spine may not be well visualized with the initial radiographic series. Therefore, oblique (pillar) views are an option, but rarely add significant information to the initial radiographic assessment. Flexion and extension radiographs are accomplished in an awake patient by having the patient flex and extend the neck as far as possible without discomfort, but are not appropriate in the acute trauma evaluation and should not be obtained in a patient with pre-existing neck pain at rest. These films are best used in follow-up evaluation in children who were previously diagnosed with ligamentous injuries.

A CT scan is often used as a secondary screen, or primary in some institutions, to substantiate suspected fractures or when adequate plain radiographs cannot be obtained. A common scenario is the use of CT to supplement viewing the C1–C2 region in young children with trauma. Several studies have demonstrated the superiority of upper cervical spine CT scan versus plain radiographs in diagnosing injuries in this region. In certain circumstances, it may be indicated to obtain CT as a primary screening tool, a common approach in adult trauma patients. Benefits of primary screening with CT are most appreciable for patients with high to moderate risk of injury, where as patients with low risk of injury do not clearly benefit from this practice. In fact, obtaining unnecessary CT scans of the cervical spine introduces increased risk of malignancy due to ionizing radiation exposure, especially for the thyroid, that is 5- to 35-fold higher in children than in adults undergoing the same study. The issue of radiation exposure needs to be considered when developing institution-specific protocols.

The CT scan images soft tissue well; however, it does not approach the intrathecal, ligamentous, disc, or vascular detail that can be obtained with an MRI scan. MRI scans are more appropriate when evaluating the subacute or chronic stages of injury, ligamentous instability or disruption, or, as recommended by the American Academy of Neurological Surgeons, when looking for an acute problem with cord or root impingement. Acute MRI evaluation is increasing in popularity in the cervical spine evaluation of patients with altered mental status. However, MRI does not image the cortical bone well and should not be used as a primary tool to evaluate the cervical spine for fractures, which is better evaluated by CT or plain radiograph.

Debate and practice variation exists regarding the clearing of the cervical spine in a persistently obtunded patient. This should not be an ED debate or practice, since obtunded pediatric patients should not have their cervical spine cleared in the ED.

Clinical Considerations

Clinical Recognition

The clinician must assume that all children who sustain multiple trauma, including infants with suspected abusive head trauma, have significant head or neck injuries, possible neurologic impairment, and a cervical spine injury until proven otherwise. The devastating nature of a cervical cord injury makes it imperative not to miss a potentially unstable cervical spine injury.

Triage Considerations

Patients with potential cervical spine injury should be evaluated in an expeditious manner and placed in a hard collar to immobilize their cervical spine. Their evaluation will potentially include radiographic and laboratory studies, specialty consultation, and continued close monitoring in the ED. Removal of a hard spine board should occur as soon as possible to avoid unnecessary pain, risk of pressure sores and skin breakdown, and respiratory compromise. Early transfer to a pediatric trauma center should be considered if appropriate surgical or critical care staff is not available.

Clinical Assessment

Evaluation of a child with trauma begins with a focused history and complete physical examination. The history can be invaluable in identifying the potential for cervical spine or cord injury. The following questions should be answered: (i) What was the mechanism of injury? If a motor vehicle collision, was he or she restrained, and at what angle did the car(s) collide? (ii) Was there a sports injury? If so, did it involve a spearing motion? (iii) Did the child fall? If so, how high was the fall and how did the child land? A neurologic history should be obtained for evidence of paresthesias, paralysis, or paresis at any time after the injury. These symptoms may have been transient and may (or may not) be present at the time of the examination or volunteered by the patient, yet they are important because they may suggest cervical contusion, concussion, or SCIWORA. The answers to these and other historical questions can often be obtained from the patient,

TABLE 120.6

SYMPTOMS AND SIGNS OF CERVICAL SPINE INJURY

Abnormal motor examination (paresis, paralysis, flaccidity, ataxia, spasticity, rectal tone)
Abnormal sensory examination (pain, sensation, temperature, paresthesias, anal wink)
Altered mental status
Neck pain
Torticollis
Limitation of motion
Neck muscle spasm
Abnormal or absent reflexes
Clonus without rigidity
Diaphragmatic breathing without retractions
Spinal (neurogenic) shock (hypotension with bradycardia)
Priapism
Decreased bladder function
Fecal retention
Unexplained ileus
Autonomic hyperreflexia
Blood pressure variability with flushing and sweating
Poikilothermia
Hypothermia or hyperthermia

parents, bystanders, and EMS personnel and can help determine the potential for cervical injury. A plethora of clues can aid in the diagnosis of a cervical cord injury (Table 120.6). The symptoms and signs may be obvious or masked by other abnormalities such as altered level of consciousness, hypovolemic shock, or concurrent head injury. Head and neck injuries may present with overlapping abnormal neurologic signs, and differentiation of causation may be difficult. A thorough examination, including a complete neurologic assessment, should be completed.

Management

While attending to the basic ABCs of trauma resuscitation, the clinician should stabilize the cervical spine. An appropriately sized hard cervical collar should be chosen. The longest collar that does not hyperextend the neck is the correct choice. The choice between a one-piece collar (e.g., Stifneck) and a two-piece collar (e.g., Philadelphia) is important only in that correct fit must be ensured and the provider must understand how to apply the specific brand of collar. It is helpful to fold over the Velcro connectors on the collar before sliding it under the patient's neck to avoid Velcro attachment to the child's hair or clothing. If a patient is seated and needs to have a collar placed, this maneuver should be accomplished by positioning the collar's chin portion first, followed by the placement of the posterior portion. If the patient is wearing a helmet, it should be carefully removed. Helmet removal, if possible, should involve at least two people to avoid potential neck motion. Occasionally, mechanical bivalving of the helmet may be required for safe removal.

Caution must be exercised when applying airway maneuvers to a child with a possible cervical spine injury. Airway interventions, however, often cannot wait until the cervical spine is cleared. The clinician must prioritize and proceed with lifesaving airway maneuvers while minimizing motion of and risk to a potentially unstable cervical spine. Hyperextension of the neck to facilitate intubation should be avoided. A vigorous chin lift or jaw thrust may also inadvertently hyperextend the unstable cervical spine. Gentle cricoid pressure should not cause excessive movement to the cervical spine; however, if applied vigorously, it may cause flexion of the spine. When inline neck immobilization is used to assist with airway maneuvers, the clinician should be careful to avoid applying traction to the spine because this pressure can also stress the unstable cervical column. Tracheal intubation in a patient with a potential cervical spine injury ideally requires at least two providers to perform the procedure safely and efficiently. One provider should maintain inline immobilization of the neck while another performs the intubation. The immobilization is often best accomplished from below, allowing the intubator as much room as possible to maneuver (Fig. 120.11). The hard cervical collar should be opened anteriorly, or removed. It is difficult to intubate a child unless the reduction in mouth opening and jaw immobilization afforded by the collar is temporarily removed, as the trachea is more anterior than in an adult. Oral intubation is the preferred method because of the child's airway position and the usual experience of providers. Adjunctive airway techniques that do not require vigorous laryngoscopy, such as video fluoroscopy and optical stylets, may be useful in managing the airway of these patients. The collar should be resecured after the airway intervention is complete.

Patients often arrive in the ED with full or partial cervical spine immobilization already in place. An immediate assessment of this immobilization is imperative. Several important issues should be considered: (i) Is the patient appropriately and fully immobilized? (ii) Is the cervical collar of the correct size and type for the patient? (iii) Is the patient's neck in a neutral position? (iv) Is the patient securely strapped to a long spine board? (v) Has there been a shift in the patient or the immobilization during the prehospital or interfacility transport that might diminish effective immobilization, cause hyperflexion or hyperextension of the cervical spine, or compromise excursion of the chest with respiration? and (vi) Does the immobilization interfere with the assessment or management of the ABCs? If these or other immobilization difficulties are identified, they should be immediately addressed.

If the patient requires initiation of full spinal stabilization and use of a long spine board, he or she should be secured to the board using tape or straps that cross the forehead and chin area of the cervical collar. Appropriate straps should be used to secure the patient to the board at the bony prominences of the shoulders, pelvis, and lower extremities. Incorrect immobilization may impede respiration by obstructing chest rise or contributing to secondary spinal injury by hyperextending the neck. When a child is immobilized on a spine board, the clinician must remember that the child's head is disproportionately large compared with that of the adult. This disparate growth of the head and trunk causes the neck to be forced into relative kyphotic position when a child is placed on a hard spine board (Fig. 120.12). This is distinctly different from the adult patient whose neck is in 30 degrees of lordosis, the neutral position, when immobilized on a hard spine board. Figure 120.13 demonstrates how cervical spine alignment can be greatly affected and improved with proper positioning of the pediatric patient on the spine board. Finally, remove the spine board as soon

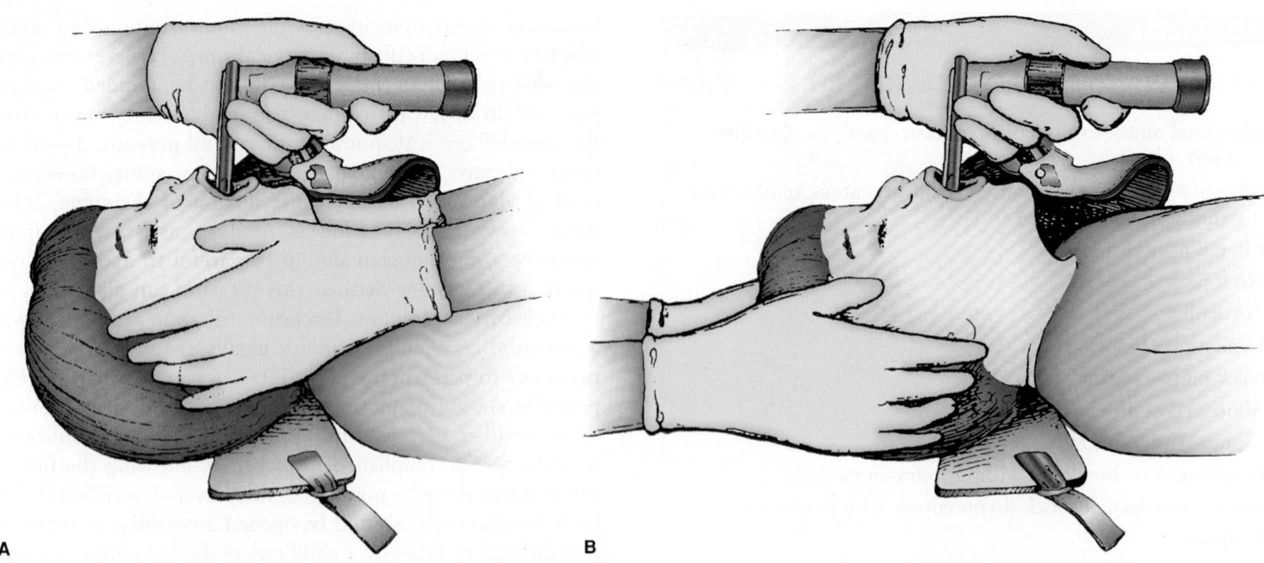

FIGURE 120.11 **A:** Manual immobilization from below. **B:** Manual immobilization from above. Adequate and expert manual cervical spine immobilization is required during airway maneuvers. The head and neck can be adequately secured from above or below. Immobilization by the second provider from below allows the airway maneuver to be accomplished without requiring a change in preferred positioning of the professional performing the maneuver.

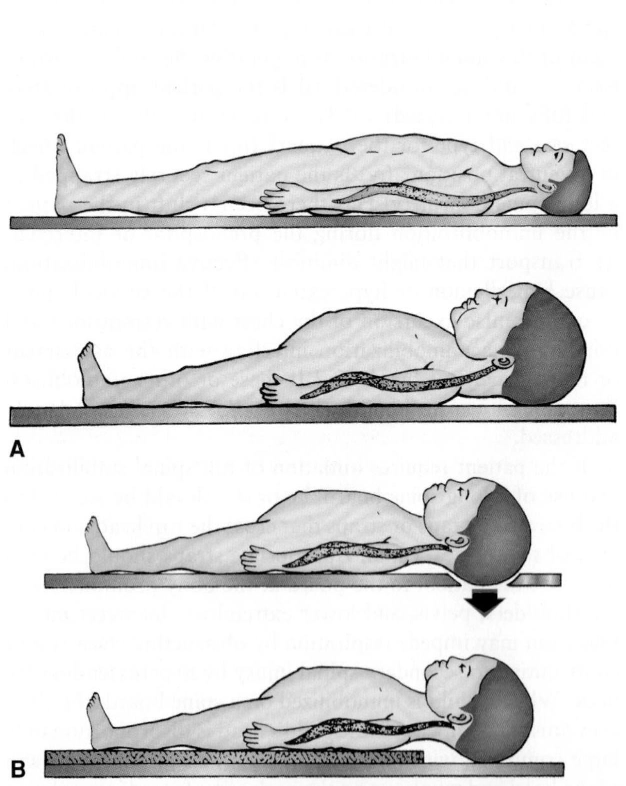

FIGURE 120.12 Effects of backboard on cervical spine position. **A:** Adult and child immobilized on standard backboard. **B:** Backboards modified with occipital recess and mattress pad to allow neutral positioning of the cervical spine in a young child. (From Herzenberg J, Hensinger R, Dedrick D, et al. Emergency transport and positioning of young children who have an injury of the cervical spine: the standard backboard may be hazardous. *J Bone Joint Surg Am* 1989;71-A:16–21. Copyright The Journal of Bone and Joint Surgery, Inc. Reprinted with permission.)

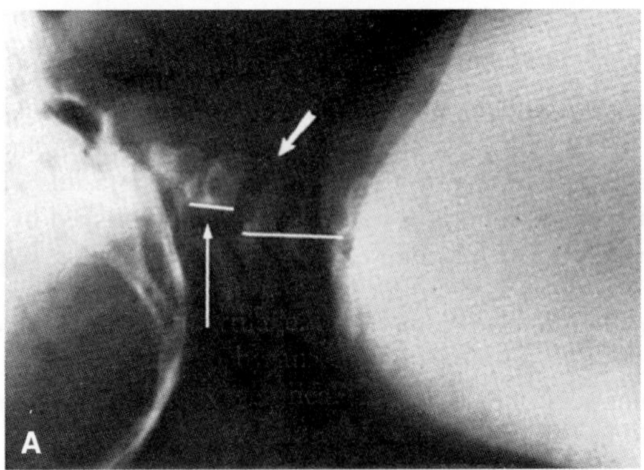

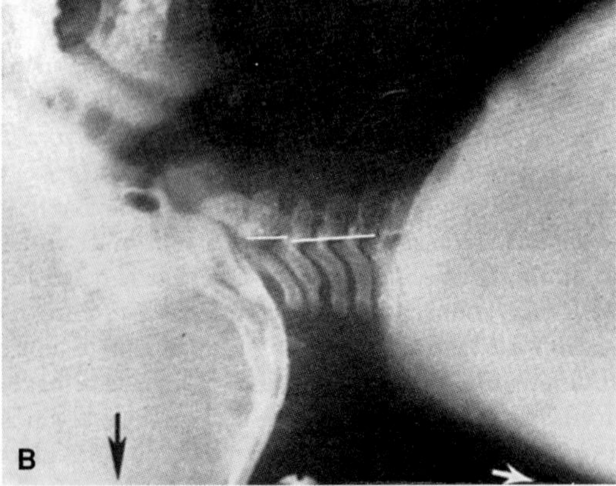

FIGURE 120.13 Effects of backboard on cervical spine position in 6-month-old child with a hangman's fracture (traumatic spondylolisthesis of posterior elements of C2) indicated by *thin arrow*. **A:** Large occiput contributes to anterior subluxation (*thick arrow*) of unstable cervical spine. **B:** Same child on backboard with occipital recess. Anterior subluxation is decreased. (From Herzenberg J, Hensiger R, Dedrick D, et al. Emergency transport and positioning of young children who have an injury of the cervical spine: the standard backboard may be hazardous. *J Bone Joint Surg Am* 1989;71-A:18. Copyright The Journal of Bone and Joint Surgery, Inc. Reprinted with permission.)

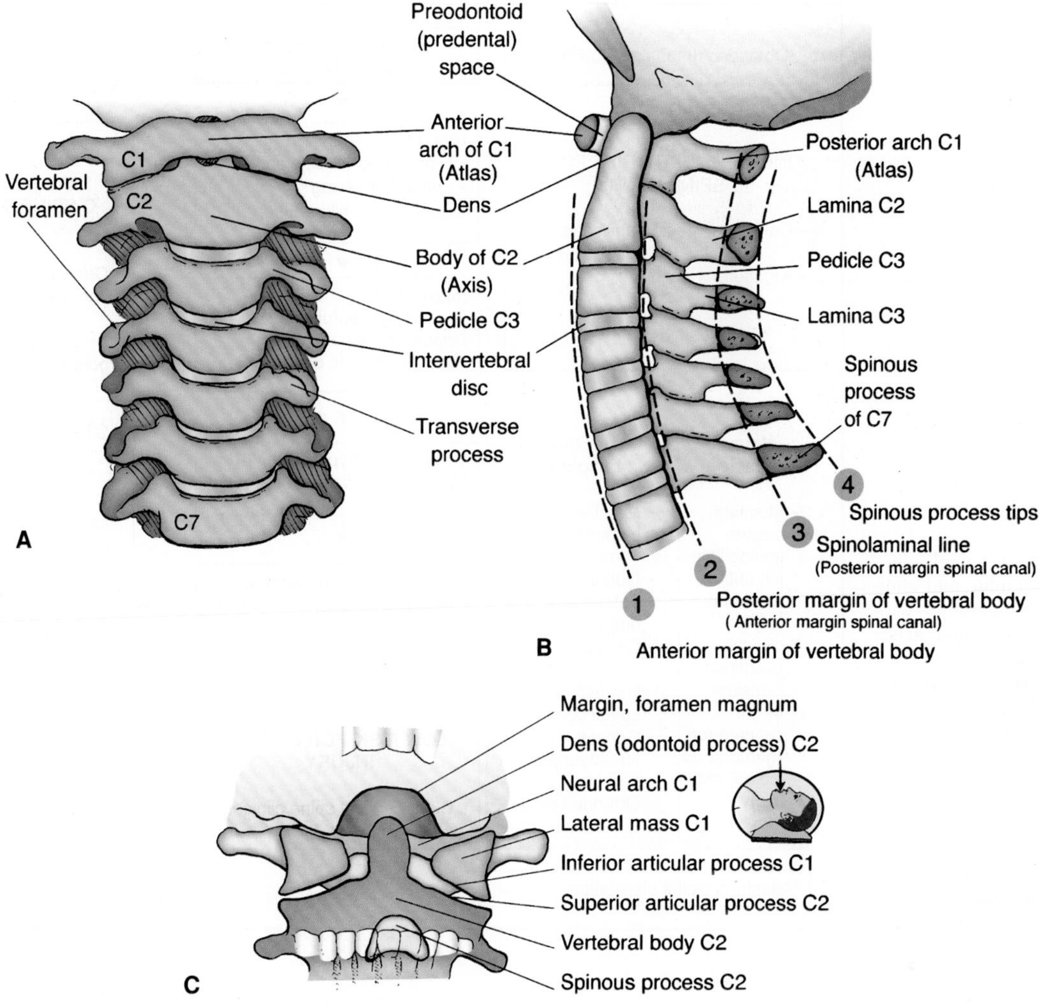

FIGURE 120.14 **A–C:** Knowledge of normal cervical spine anatomy is useful when evaluating cervical spine radiographs.

as practicable to avoid complications such as pressure sores, pain, or respiratory compromise.

Consideration of cervical spine radiographic evaluation is the next step in assessment. The cervical spine has anterior (vertebral bodies, intervertebral discs, ligaments) and posterior (lamina, pedicles, neural foramen, spinous processes, ligaments) components (Fig. 120.14) which require evaluation. The provider should be familiar with criteria to potentially clear a child's cervical spine clinically (Fig. 120.15), but recall that regardless of clearing algorithm embraced or imaging studies performed, they should never clear the cervical spine in an unconscious or obtunded patient in the ED. If one is unable to determine whether an injury (and associated pain) is indeed distracting, or if neck pain or appreciation of the pain may potentially have been diminished by medication for other injuries, cervical spine radiographic evaluation may be initiated.

When evaluating a lateral cervical spine radiograph, the clinician must ensure that C1–C7 are included as well as the C7–T1 junction. An adequate open-mouth view is often technically difficult to obtain in young children and those who are intubated. A systematic approach should be used when evaluating radiographs of the cervical spine. The ABCS method is a useful approach (Fig. 120.16). Alignment is assessed as demonstrated in Figure 120.17, keeping in mind that the spinal cord lies between the posterior spinal line and the spinolaminar line. These lordotic curves may not be present in children younger than 6 years, those on hard spine boards or in cervical collars, or those with cervical neck muscle spasm. Gross malalignment should be detectable with this assessment. Be aware of physiologic pseudosubluxation of C2 on C3 and less frequently, C3 on C4. To discern whether there is pseudosubluxation or traumatic injury, determine the distance between the posterior arch of C2 and the spinolaminar line, if it is greater than 2 mm, true injury should be considered (Fig. 120.18).

The bones should be evaluated for typical abnormalities, realizing that these may be subtle. Acute fractures are often irregular in location and appearance without sclerosis as compared with the more routine locations and appearance of cartilaginous growth areas. The clinician should be aware that structures that overlay the spine, including the skull and the teeth, might simulate fractures.

If further information about C1–C2 or any other portion of cervical spine is required, a CT scan should be considered. While it is more expensive than a plain radiograph, it is relatively

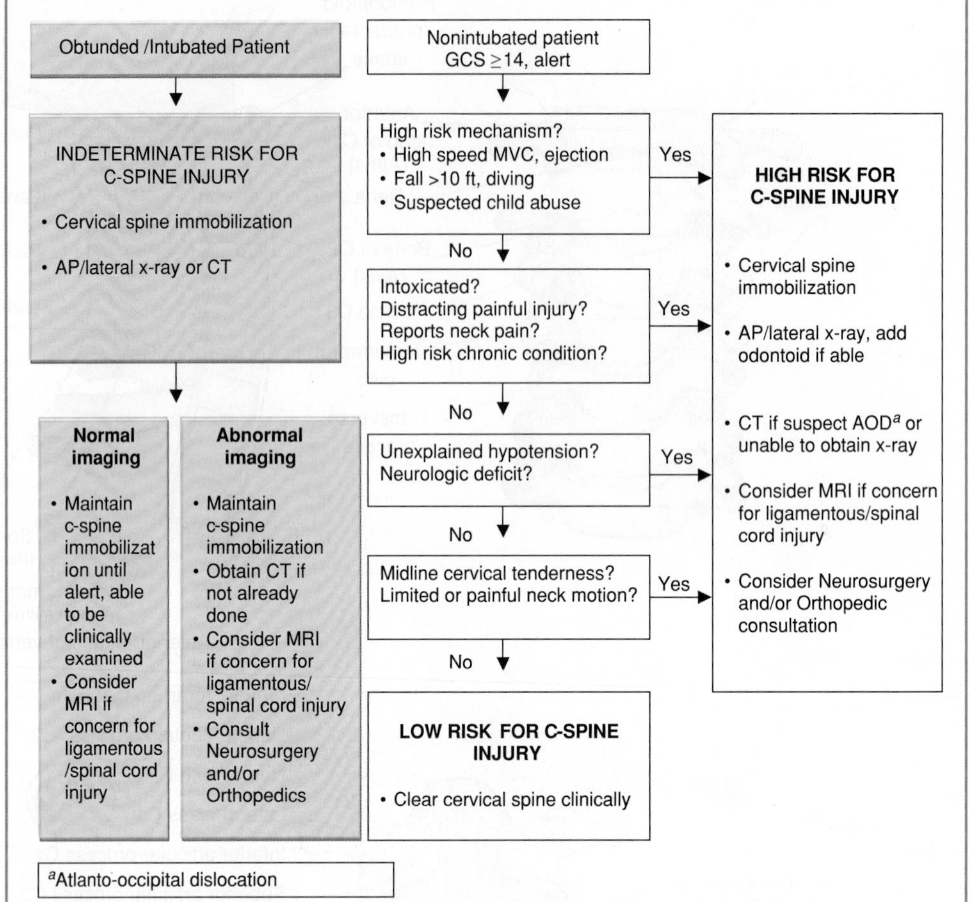

FIGURE 120.15 Clinical algorithm for radiographic and clinical evaluation of patients with possible neck injury. Emergency department evaluation if a fracture or other abnormality is identified may be limited by patient's condition, CT or MRI may be indicated when the patient is stabilized to further elucidate the identified injury. If adequate radiographs cannot be obtained, an abnormality is identified or suspected but not demonstrated or the patient is unconscious or unreliable, consider further evaluation as suggested.

easy to obtain, offers enhanced and more consistent information, and avoids the risk of missing a subtle injury. An algorithm for considering radiographic evaluation is presented in Figure 120.15. An MRI should be considered to detect ligamentous, soft tissue, and/or spinal cord injuries. Special consideration for MRI should be given to cases of nonaccidental trauma due to the increased risk of cervical spine ligamentous

A - Alignment

Lordotic curves, gross malalignment, subluxation, distraction

B - Bones

Fractures, anterior and posterior vertebral columns, ossification centers

C - Cartilage

Intervertebral disc spaces, ossification centers

S - Soft tissues

Prevertebral space, predental space

FIGURE 120.16 The ABCS of radiographic cervical spine interpretation.

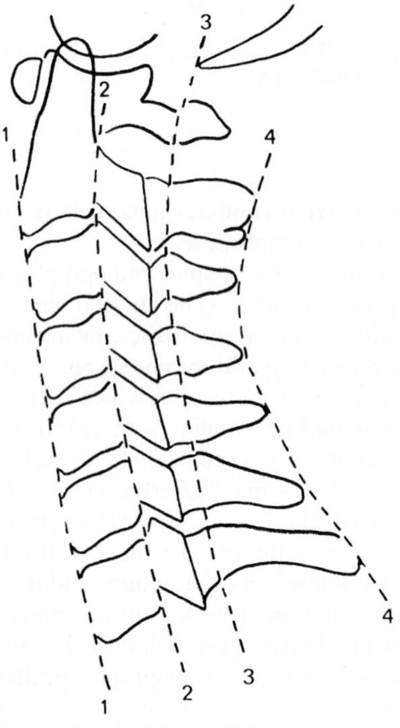

FIGURE 120.17 Four contour lines of alignment with normal cervical spine lordosis: *1*, anterior vertebral bodies; *2*, posterior vertebral bodies (anterior spinal canal); *3*, spinolaminal line (posterior spinal canal); and *4*, spinous process tips. (From Gerlock A, Kirchner S, Heller R, et al. *Advanced exercises in diagnostic radiology: the cervical spine in trauma*. Philadelphia, PA: WB Saunders, 1978:6. Reprinted with permission.)

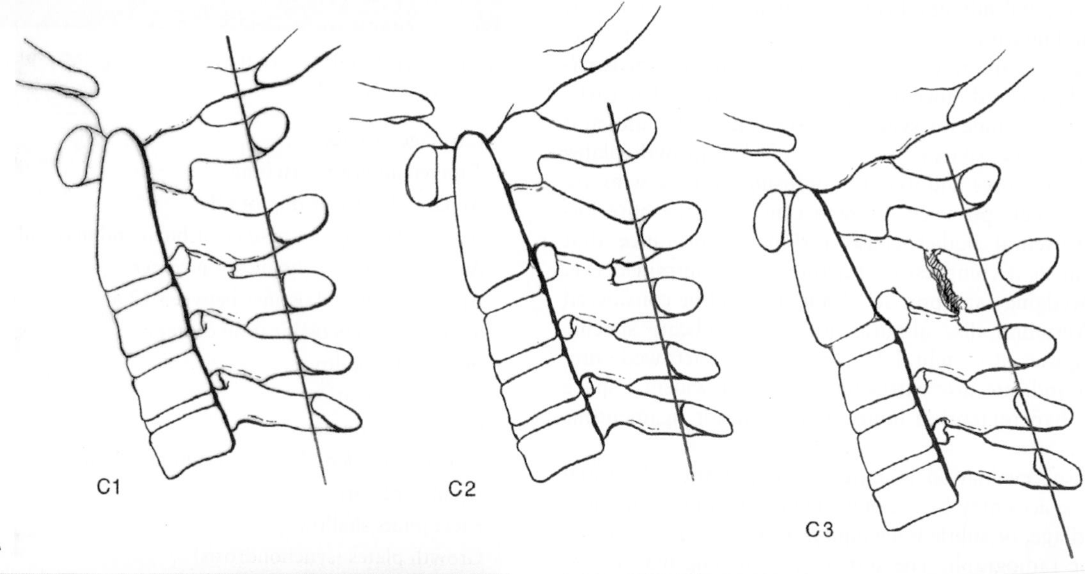

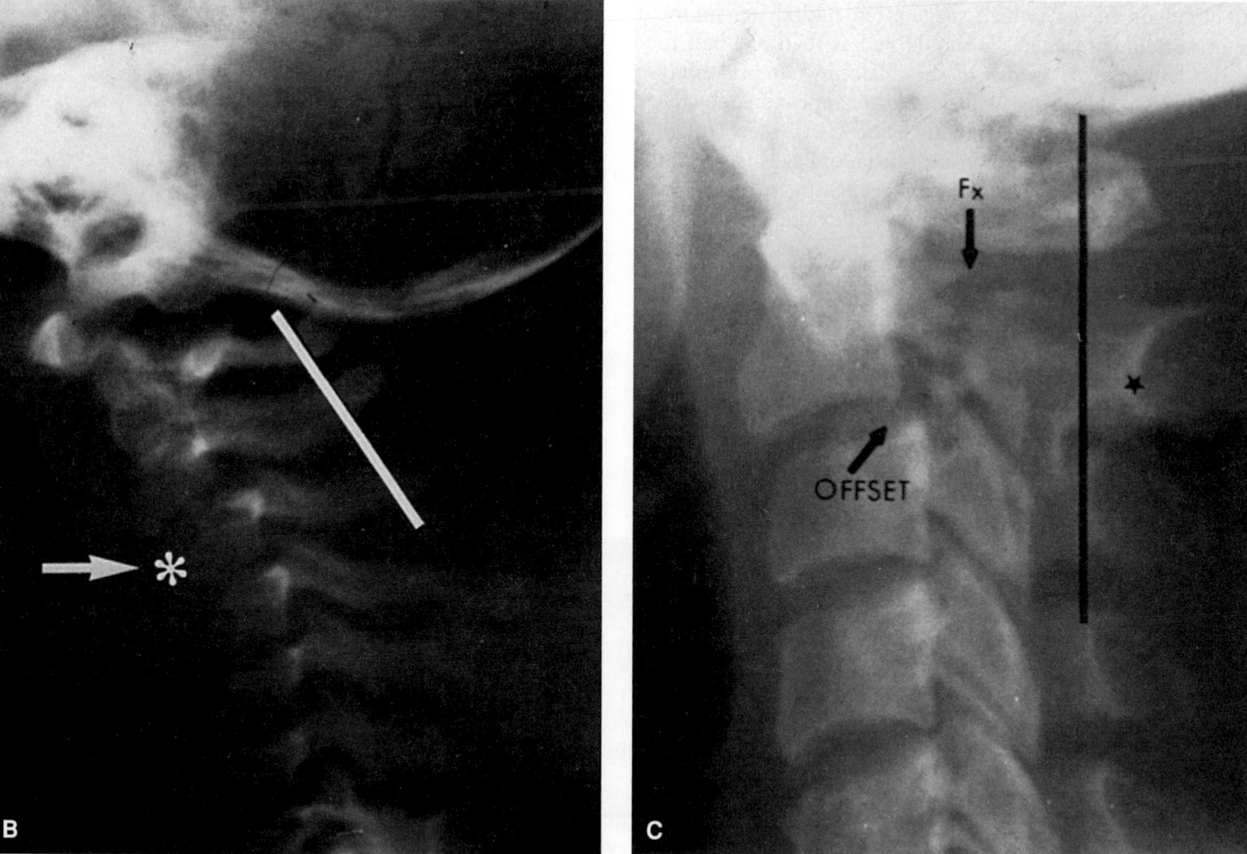

FIGURE 120.18 **A:** Posterior cervical line of Swischuk. Line is drawn from the cortex of the spinous process of C1 to the cortex of the spinous process of C3. Relationship of the line to cortex of the spinous process of C2 is noted. If the line is situated more than 2 mm anterior to the cortex of the spinous process of C2, underlying cervical pathology should be present. This line should be used only with anterior displacement of C2 on C3. **B:** Pseudosubluxation of C2 on C3 with normal posterior cervical line in a 2-year-old child. Note apparent widening of prevertebral soft tissue (*asterisk*). **C:** Abnormal posterior cervical line with an underlying hangman's fracture (star indicated anterior cortex of spinous process). Actual offset is 4 mm. (**C:** From Swischuk L. *Emergency radiology of the acutely ill or injured child*. 2nd ed. Baltimore, MD: Williams & Wilkins, 1986:562–563. Reprinted with permission.)

injuries and spinal subdural hematomas in this group compared to accidental injuries.

The next area of radiographic evaluation involves the cartilage. Cartilage is radiolucent on plain radiographs. The cartilaginous areas include the synchondroses or growth plates and intervertebral disc spaces (Table 120.7). The growth plates may mimic fractures and may be confusing to those who are unaware of their presence. Growth centers in the anterior-superior vertebral bodies cause a sloped appearance that may appear as a compression fracture to the untrained eye. Anterior wedging can approach 3 mm and still be considered normal. Vertebral disc abnormalities may indicate specific types of injuries. A vertebral disc space that is narrowed anteriorly may indicate disc extrusion, whereas a widened space suggests a hyperextension injury with posterior ligamentous disruption.

Soft tissue evaluation is extremely important. Abnormal soft tissue spaces may be the only clue to the underlying ligament, cartilage, or subtle bone injury, which may not be obvious on the radiograph. The soft tissue widening may represent blood or edema, which suggests an underlying injury. The prevertebral space at C3 should be less than one-half to two-thirds of the AP width of the adjacent vertebral body (Fig. 120.19). This space will double to approximately the width of the adjacent vertebral body below C4 (the level of the glottis) because the usually non–air-filled esophagus is present at this area. Care must be taken when evaluating the prevertebral soft tissue space because crying, neck flexion, or the expiratory phase of respiration may produce a pseudothickening in the prevertebral space (Fig. 120.20). Soft tissue abnormality should be reproducible on repeated radiographs if an actual underlying injury exists.

Many pediatric cervical spine injuries can be managed nonoperatively using immobilization techniques such as a hard

TABLE 120.7

RADIOGRAPHIC CHARACTERISTICS OF PEDIATRIC CERVICAL SPINE

Cartilage artifact
Tapered anterior vertebrae
Apparently absent ring of C1
Atlas (C1) body not ossified at birth and may fail to close
Axis (C2) has four ossification centers
Apex of odontoid ossifies between 12 and 15 yrs of age
Spinous process ossification centers
Increased mobility
Pseudosubluxation
C1 override on dens
Increased predental space (5 mm maximum)
Ligament laxity
Facet joints shallow
Growth plates (synchondrosis)
Dens ossifies between 3 and 8 yrs of age (may persist into young adults)
Posterior arch of C1 ossifies at 3 yrs of age
Anterior arch of C1 ossifies at 6–9 yrs of age
C1 reaches adult size at 3–4 yrs of age
C2 through C7 reach adult size at 5–6 yrs of age
Lack of cervical lordosis
Fulcrum varies with age
Soft tissue variability with respiration
Congenital clefts or other bony abnormalities (os odontoideum, spondylolisthesis, spina bifida, ossiculum terminale)

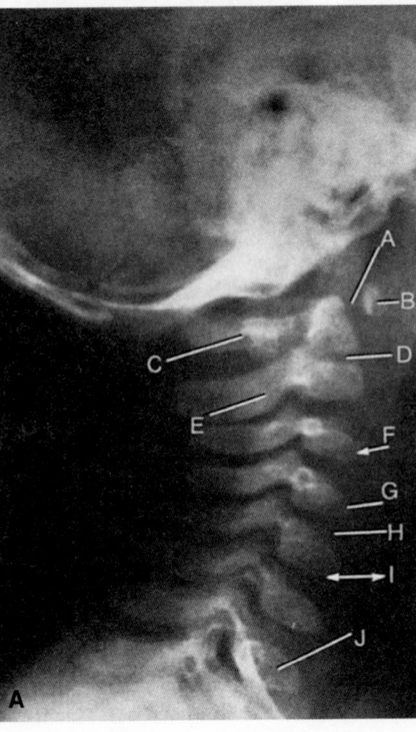

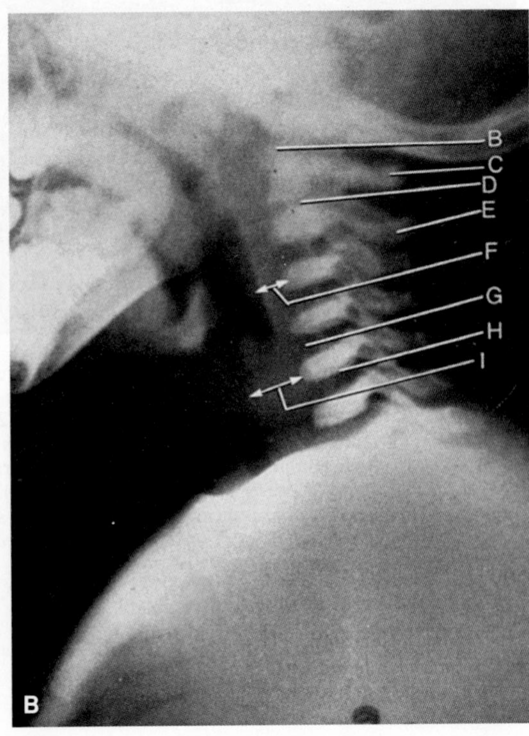

FIGURE 120.19 Normal pediatric lateral cervical spine radiographs. **A:** Three-month-old child. **B:** Twenty-month-old child. *A*, predental (predontoid) space; *B*, anterior ring of C1 (note apparent override of C1 over dens); *C*, posterior ring of C1; *D*, dens synchondrosis (growth plate); *E*, posterior elements C2; *F*, normal prevertebral space (C3 level); *G*, wedged vertebral appearance caused by cartilage artifact; *H*, intervertebral disc space; *I*, normal prevertebral space below the glottis (thickened because of radiopaque-collapsed esophagus); and *J*, vertebral body C7.

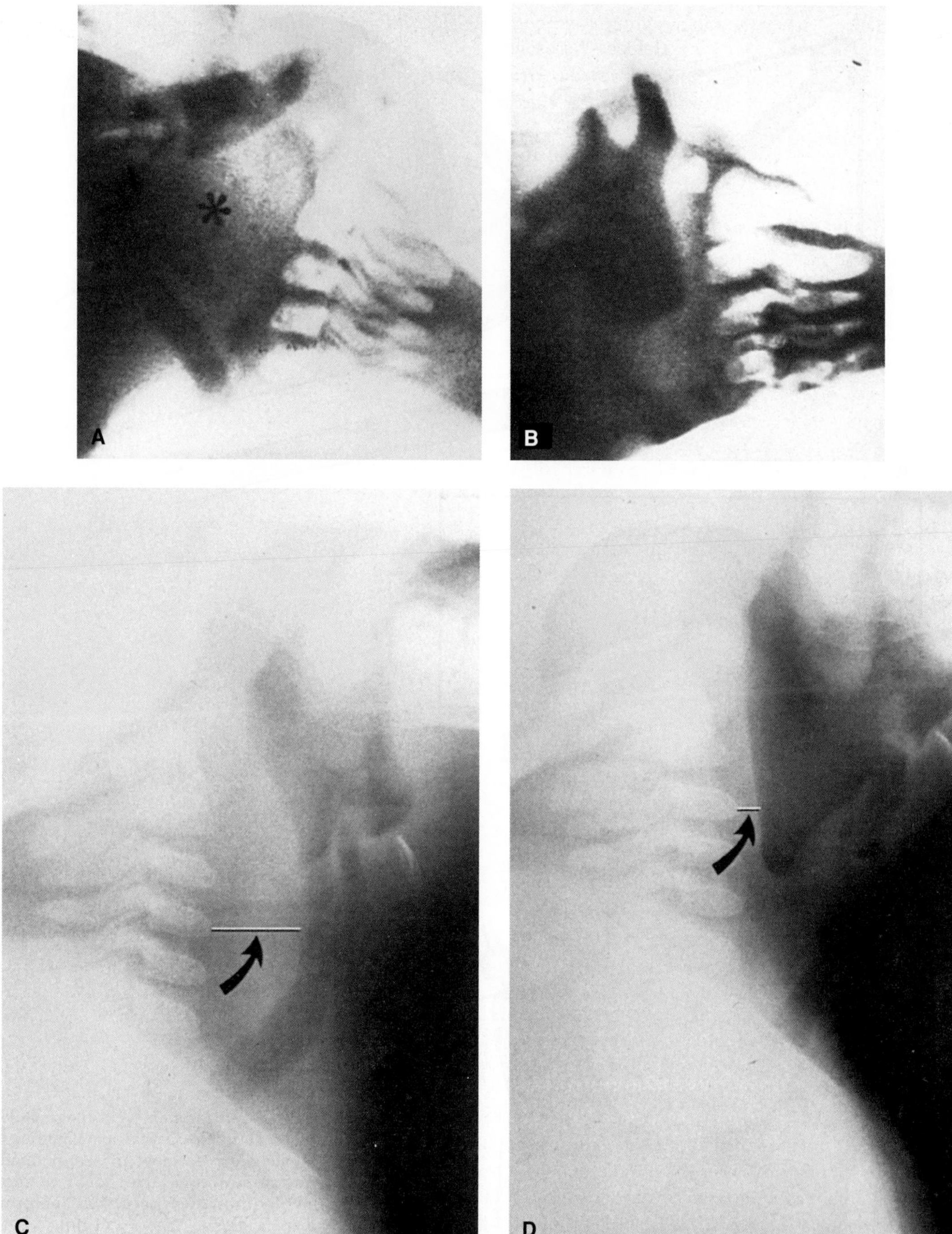

FIGURE 120.20 Effects of inspiration and positioning on prevertebral (retropharyngeal) soft tissues. **A:** Increased prevertebral space (*asterisk*) with expiration. **B:** Repeat radiograph in same patient during inspiration reveals normal prevertebral space with no suggestion of cervical spine abnormality. **C:** Increased soft tissue space (*arrow*) with expiratory phase of respiration. **D:** Normal soft tissue space (*arrow*) with inspiration in patient **C.** (**A** and **B:** From Harris J, Edeiken-Monroe B. *The radiology of acute cervical spine trauma*. 2nd ed. Baltimore, MD: Williams & Wilkins, 1987:6. Reprinted with permission.)

collar or a halo (Fig. 120.21). However, in conjunction with orthopedic and neurosurgical spine consultation, indications for operative intervention include an unstable or irreducible injury, progressive neurologic deficit(s), and progressive deformity. There are no evidence-based criteria for discharge in the presence of a cervical spine injury. Clinical judgment and specialty consultation are recommended.

SPECIFIC INJURIES

Jefferson Fracture

A Jefferson fracture is a bursting fracture of the ring of C1 as a result of an axial load. The ring of C1 is compressed between the occipital condyles of the skull and the lateral masses of C2.

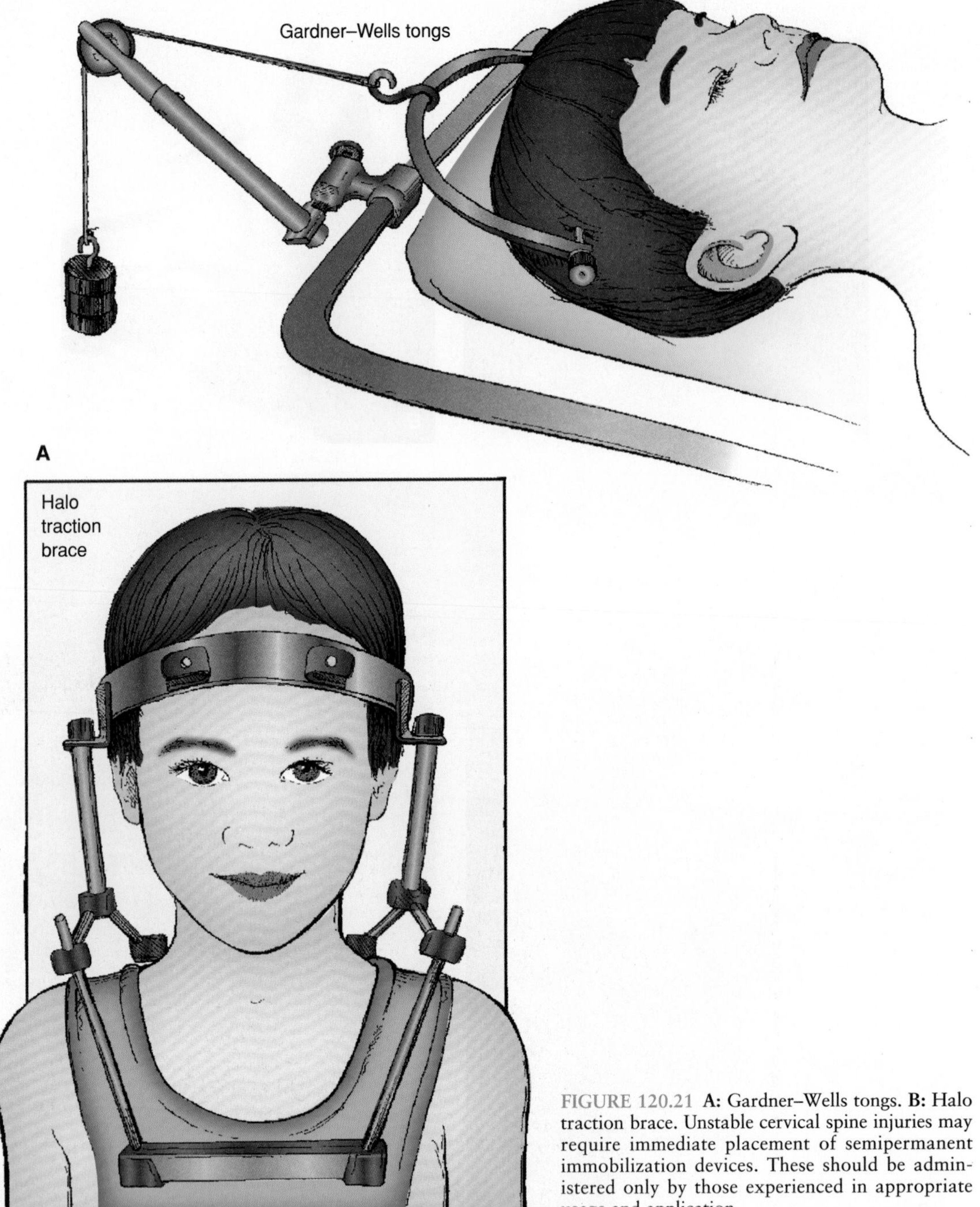

FIGURE 120.21 **A:** Gardner–Wells tongs. **B:** Halo traction brace. Unstable cervical spine injuries may require immediate placement of semipermanent immobilization devices. These should be administered only by those experienced in appropriate usage and application.

This process can cause an outward burst of C1, but it rarely causes immediate neurologic impairment because the fracture does not physically impinge on the spinal cord. The radiographic criterion for the diagnosis of a *Jefferson fracture* is lateral offset of the lateral mass of C1 of more than 1 mm from the vertebral body of C2 (Fig. 120.22). Neck rotation may give a false-positive radiographic finding. These fractures may be unstable, however, and require adequate immobilization. If the transverse ligament is intact, the fracture may be relatively stable, whereas if the transverse ligament is injured and there is an increased distance between the lateral masses and the odontoid process, it should be considered unstable. A reduced AP diameter of the cervical spinal canal is also associated with spinal cord injury. Approximately one-third of *Jefferson fractures* are associated with other cervical spine fractures, most often involving C2. The clinician must be aware of the pseudo-Jefferson fracture of childhood, which is present in 90% of children at 2 years of age and usually normalizes by 4 to 6 years of age. The pseudo-Jefferson fracture has the radiographic appearance of a *Jefferson fracture* because of increased growth of the atlas (C1) compared with the axis (C2) and radiolucent cartilage artifact. This disorder can present with unilateral or bilateral lateral mass offset. If a *Jefferson fracture* is suspected by radiographic findings and mechanism of injury in children younger than 4 years, a CT scan may be necessary to further elucidate the suspected injury (Fig. 120.23).

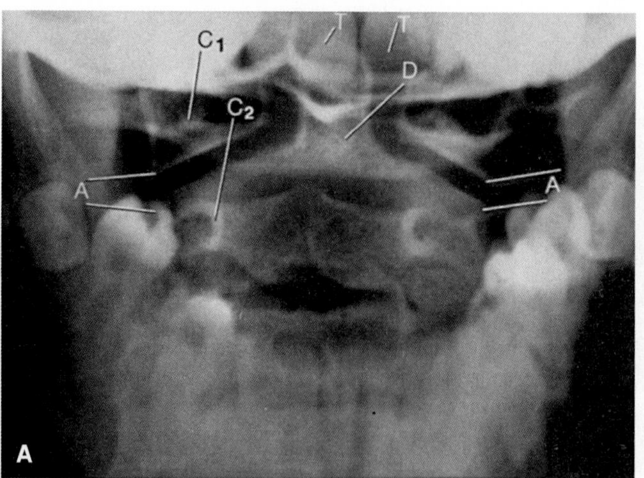

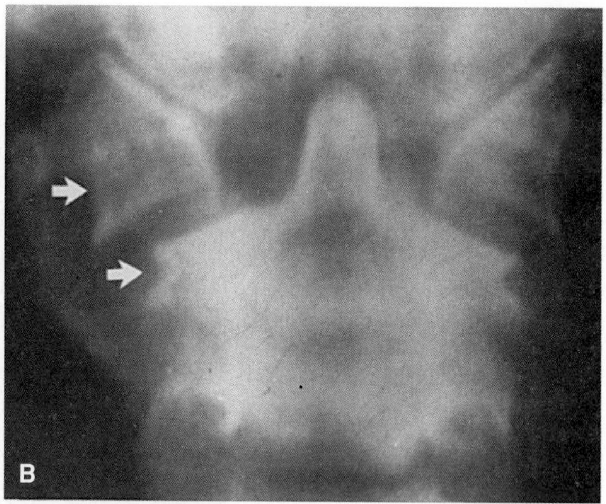

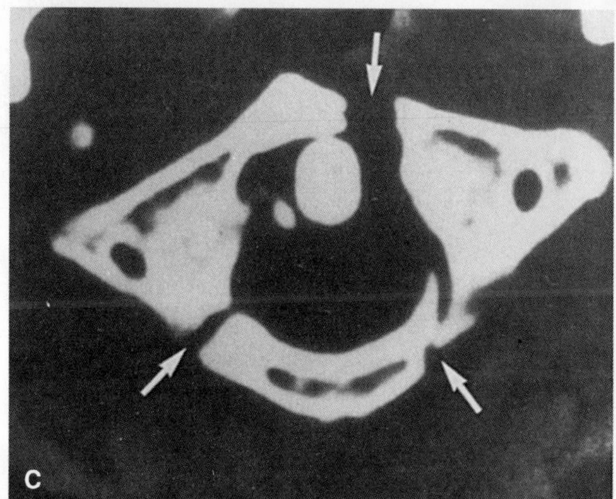

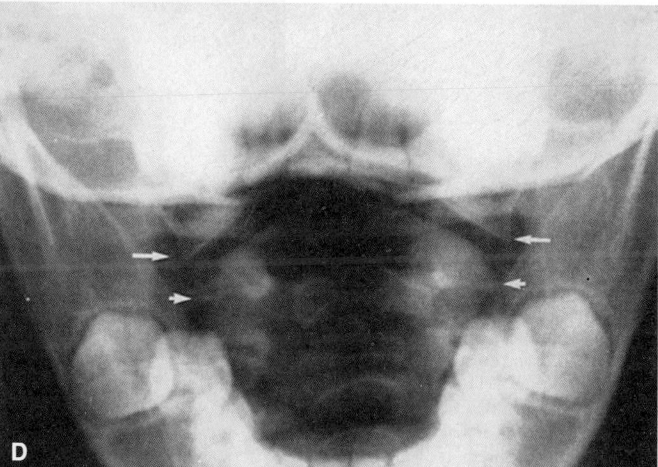

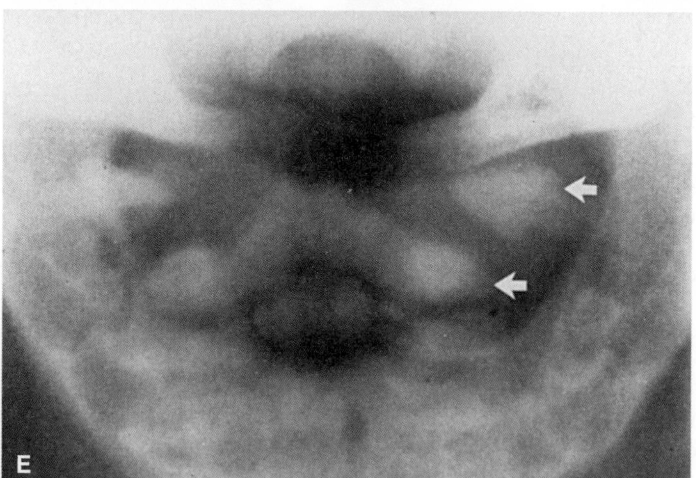

FIGURE 120.22 **A:** Normal anteroposterior (AP) (open-mouth, odontoid) view of C1 and C2. C_1, first cervical vertebra (lateral mass); C_2, second cervical vertebra; *T,* central incisors overlying dens (*D*); and *A,* normal relationship between lateral mass of C1 and vertebral body of C2. **B:** Jefferson fracture in AP view. Note lateral offset of C1 on C2 (*arrows*). **C:** Jefferson fracture. Computed tomography coronal view. Note three distinct fractures (*arrows*) and bursting nature of injury. **D:** Pseudo-Jefferson fracture of childhood in a 3-year-old child because of disparate growth of C1 and C2 and cartilage artifact (*arrows*). **E:** Pseudo-Jefferson fracture demonstrating marked offset of the lateral masses of C1 on C2 (*arrows*). (**B** and **C:** From Swischuk L. *Emergency radiology of the acutely ill or injured child.* 2nd ed. Baltimore, MD: Williams & Wilkins, 1986:591. Reprinted with permission; **D:** From Aslamy W, Danielson K, Hessel S, et al. A 3-year-old boy with neck pain after motor vehicle accident. *West Med J* 1991;155:301–302. Copyright BMJ Publishing Inc. Reprinted with permission.)

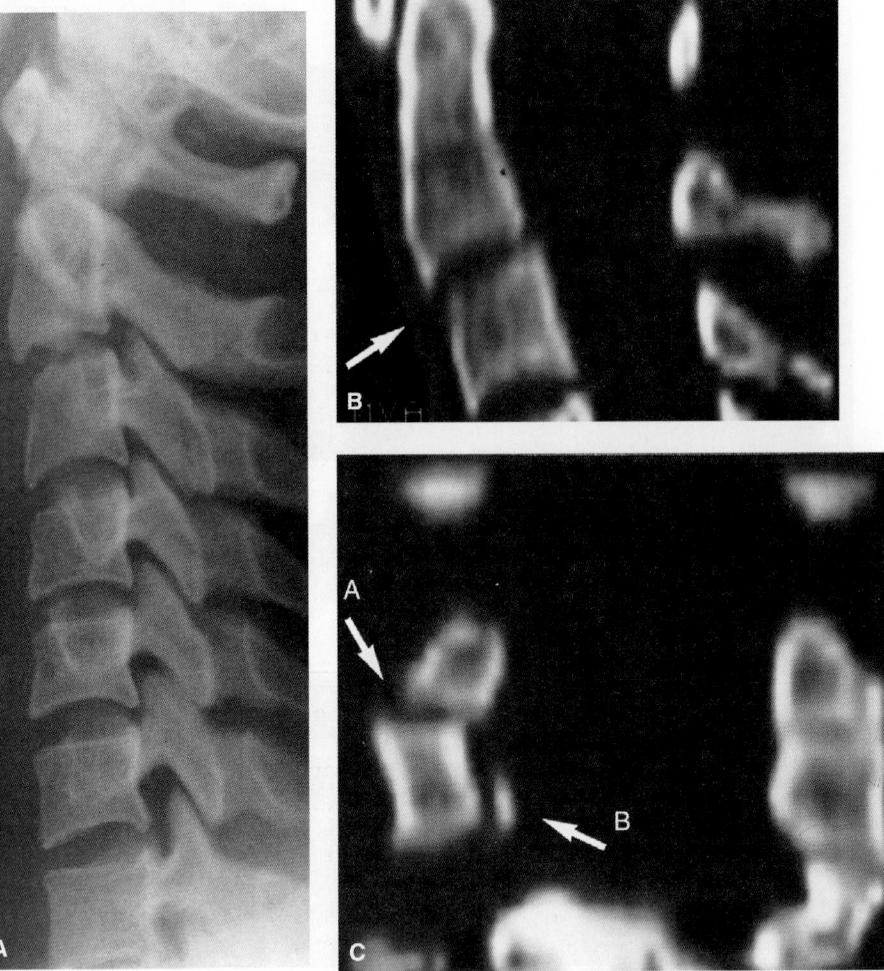

FIGURE 120.23 **A:** Apparently "normal" lateral cervical spine radiograph (16-year-old patient after motor vehicle accident). **B:** Spiral computed tomography (CT) scan demonstrating dens fracture (*arrow*). **C:** Sagittal view of spiral CT scan demonstrating dens fracture (*arrow A*) and vertebral body avulsion fracture (*arrow B*). The detail demonstrated by the spiral CT scan could help clinicians quickly identify lesions not easily visible or appreciated on conventional radiographs.

Hangman's Fracture

The hangman's fracture is a traumatic spondylolisthesis of C2. This injury occurs as a result of hyperextension, which fractures the posterior elements of C2. Hyperflexion, with resultant ligamentous damage, may follow the hyperextension or may lead to anterior subluxation of C2 on C3 and subsequent damage of the cervical cord (Fig. 120.24). The subluxation associated with a *hangman's fracture* can sometimes be mistaken for the normal or physiologic subluxation that exists in the C2–C3 or C3–C4 region in approximately 25% of children younger than 8 years and may also be seen up to 16 years of age. This radiographic pseudosubluxation is caused by ligamentous laxity, relatively horizontal facet joints, weak neck muscles, and cartilage artifact. Distinguishing between a subtle hangman's fracture and pseudosubluxation can be accomplished using Swischuk's "posterior cervical line," as described in Figure 120.18. A value of more than 1.5 to 2 mm suggests an occult *hangman's fracture* as the source of the anterior subluxation of C2 on C3. The increase in magnitude of the distance between the cortex of the spinous process of C2 and the posterior cervical line in a *hangman's fracture* is the result of anterior displacement of the skull, C1, and the anterior portion of C2 on the remainder of the lower cervical spine. Nontraumatic subluxation has also been reported at the C5/C6 and C6/C7 spinal levels, although subluxation at these

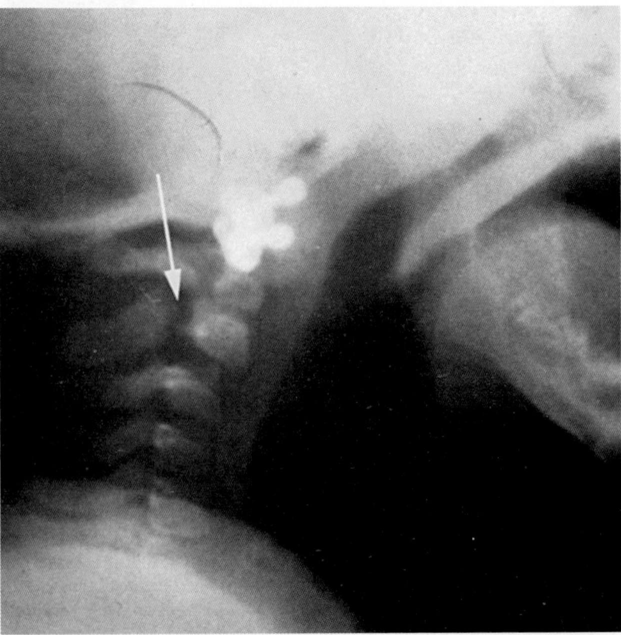

FIGURE 120.24 Hangman's fracture. A 7-week-old infant with fracture through the posterior elements of C2 as indicated by the *arrow*. (From Sumchai A, Sternback G. Hangman's fracture in a 7-week-old infant. *Ann Emerg Med* 1991;20:87. Copyright Elsevier Inc. Reprinted with permission.)

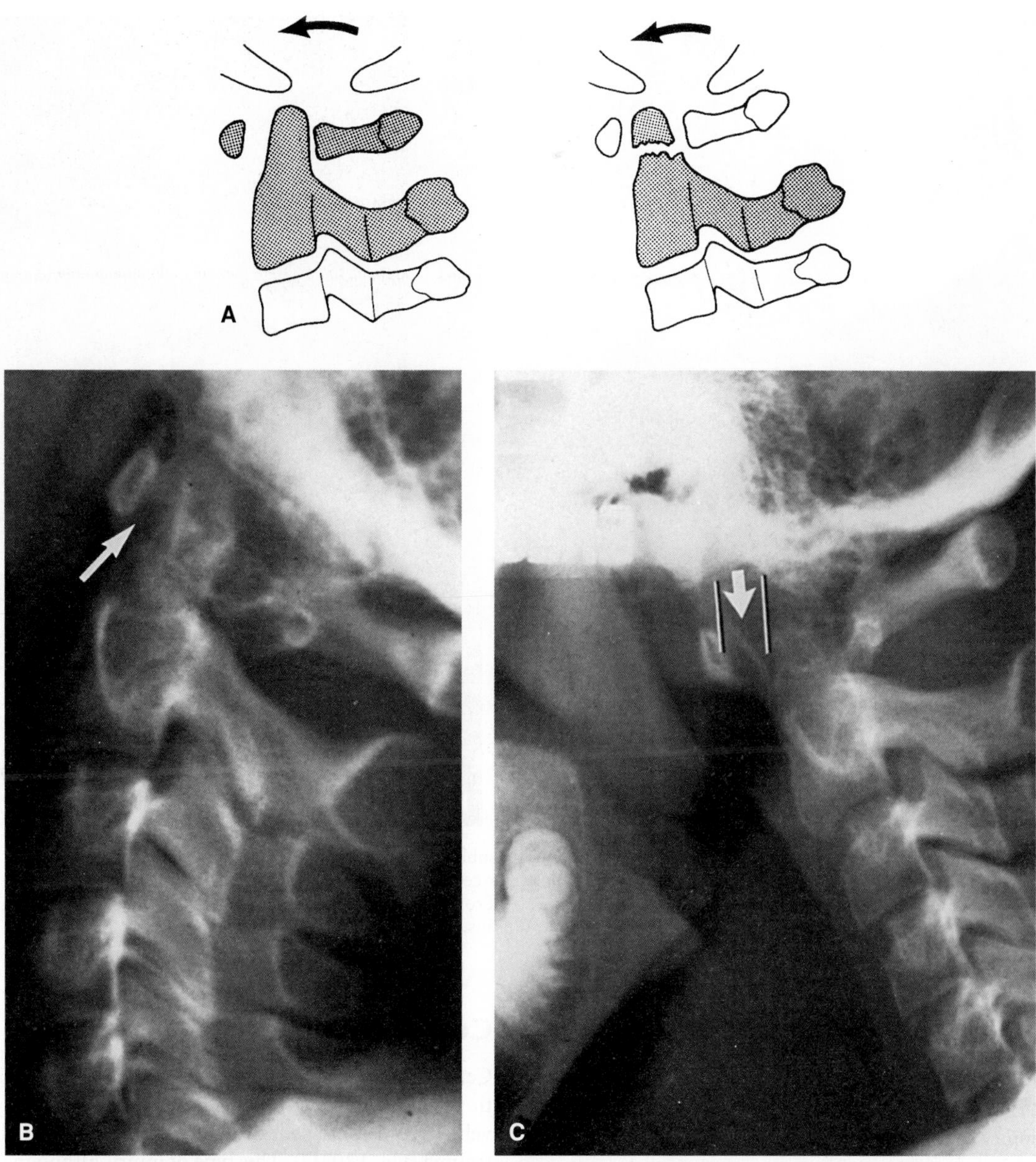

FIGURE 120.25 **A:** Diagrammatic representation of transverse ligament disruption (*left*) and dens fracture (*right*). The arrows indicate the direction of movement that resulted in the noted injury. **B:** Widened predental space on initial lateral radiograph in 15-year-old girl (actual measurement was 4 mm). **C:** Flexion radiograph in same patient demonstrating increased predental space with evidence of transverse ligament disruption. (*continued*)

lower levels should always be fully investigated for potential ligamentous injury.

Atlantoaxial Subluxation

Atlantoaxial (AA) subluxation is a result of movement between C1 and C2 secondary to transverse ligament rupture or a fractured dens (Fig. 120.25). Ligament instability may be precipitated by tonsillitis, cervical adenitis, pharyngitis, arthritis, or connective tissue disorders. Approximately 15% of patients with Down syndrome have radiographically demonstrated AA subluxation and therefore should be discouraged from contact sports. The presence or absence of AA subluxation in patients with Down syndrome, once believed to be a static phenomenon, may actually be transient and/or progressive. This ligament instability may progress to ligament rupture with minor trauma. Subluxation caused by a transverse ligament disruption is evidenced by a widened predental (periodontoid, atlantodental interval) space on a lateral radiograph (Fig. 120.25). Rotary subluxation can be classified as follows: type I (no displacement of C1), type II (3 to 5 mm C1 on C2 anterior displacement), type III (more than 5 mm C1 on C2 anterior displacement), and type IV (posterior displacement of C1 on C2). Normal predental measurement in children is less than 5 mm compared with less than 3 mm in adults. This space is wider in children than in adults for the same reasons as described for pseudosubluxation. *Steele's rule of three* states that the area within the ring of C1 consists of one-third odontoid, one-third spinal cord, and one-third connective tissue (Fig. 120.26). Therefore, limited space is available for dens movement or predental space widening without neurologic compromise. Neurologic symptoms are often not seen until the predental space exceeds 7 to 10 mm. A

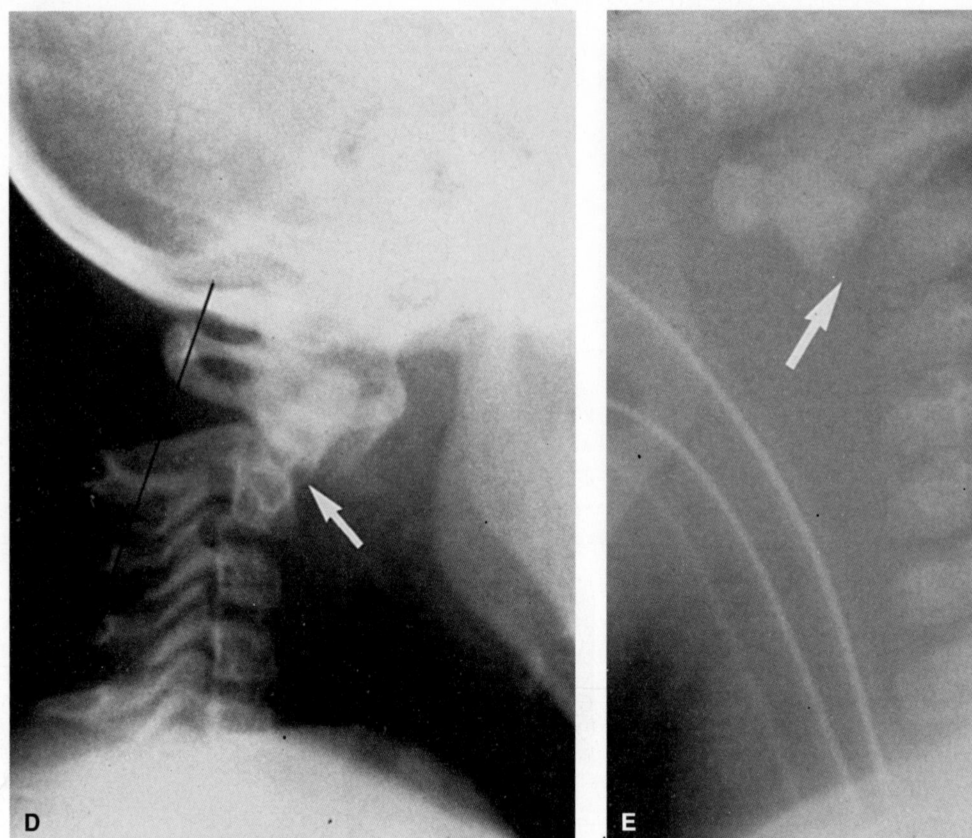

FIGURE 120.25 (*Continued*) **D:** Dens fracture with anterior subluxation of C1 and the dens on the remainder of the spinal column. *Arrow* indicates fracture. Abnormal posterior cervical *line* is also shown. **E:** Dens fracture (*arrow*) with anterior subluxation of the dens on the body of C2. (**A:** From Swischuk L. *Emergency radiology of the acutely ill or injured child*. 2nd ed. Baltimore, MD: Williams & Wilkins, 1986:572. Reprinted with permission.)

dens fracture is the cause of AA subluxation more often than ligamentous disruption in a young child because the weakest part of the musculoskeletal system in a child is the osseous component (Fig. 120.25). Neurologic damage can occur from direct spinal cord injury or secondarily from vertebral artery damage.

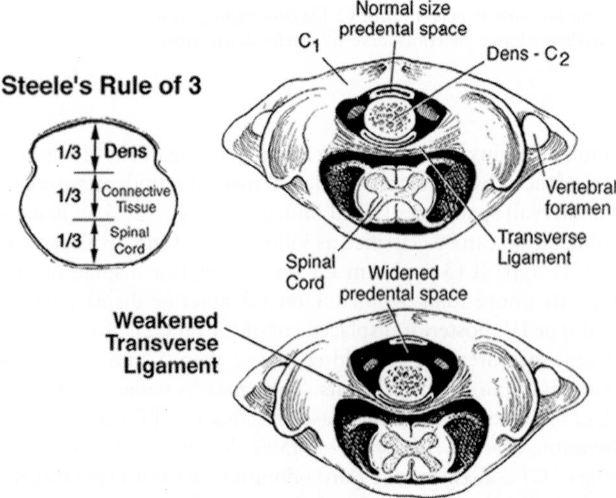

FIGURE 120.26 A cross section through the ring of C1 demonstrates Steele's rule of three. The space between the cervical cord and dens allows limited movement between C1 and C2 without immediate neurologic compromise.

Cervical Distraction Injuries

Cervical distraction injuries may result from rapid acceleration- or deceleration-type incidents, such as high-speed motor vehicle collisions, pedestrian accidents or infant abusive head trauma (Fig. 120.27). This type of injury, although uncommon, is reported to be approximately 2.5 times more common in children than in adults. Cervical distraction injuries may be obvious or subtle on the initial lateral radiograph. Measurements for potential distraction injuries include the atlantooccipital and C1–C2 interspinous distances. The atlantooccipital distance should not exceed 5 mm. The C1–C2 interspinous distance should not exceed 10 mm. Sun's ratio, C1–C2:C2–C3, >2.5 suggests potential ligamentous instability. Sun's ratio, as well as a ratio of measurements of the basion to the posterior arch of C1 (BC) and the opisthion to the anterior arch of C1 (OA), is demonstrated in Figures 120.27 and 120.28. If the BC:OA ratio is more than one, it signifies *atlantooccipital dislocation,* an often fatal injury. Neurologic deficits may develop from direct spinal damage or associated carotid or vertebral artery injury. Distraction injuries may also be seen with difficult newborn deliveries. These injuries may not be visible on a plain radiograph because the pediatric cervical spine can transiently distract 2 inches before residual radiographic evidence of spinal column separation is present. However, the spinal cord can distract only 0.25 inches before permanent neurologic damage occurs. A CT scan should be obtained in patients with potential atlantooccipital dislocation. An MRI

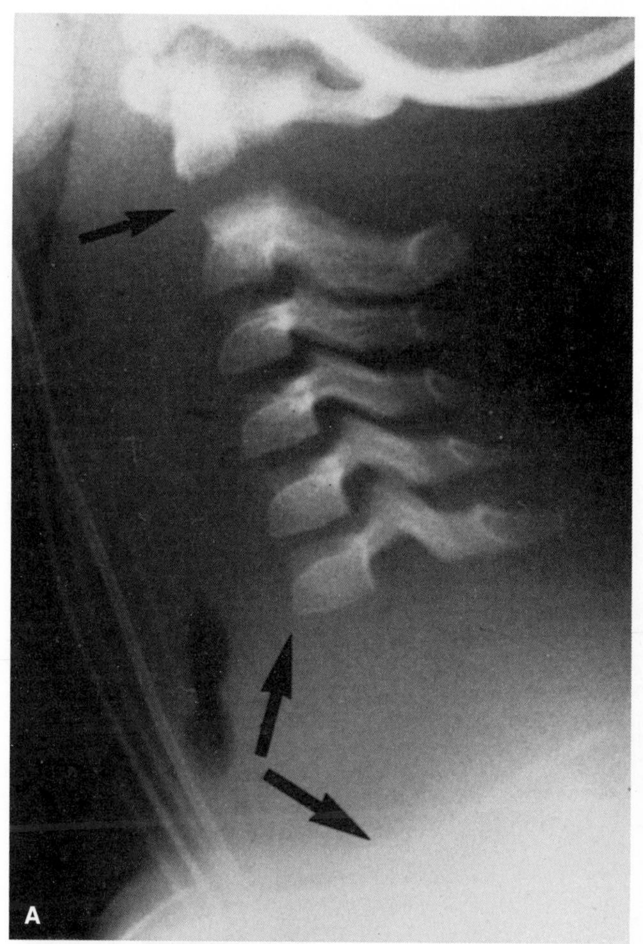

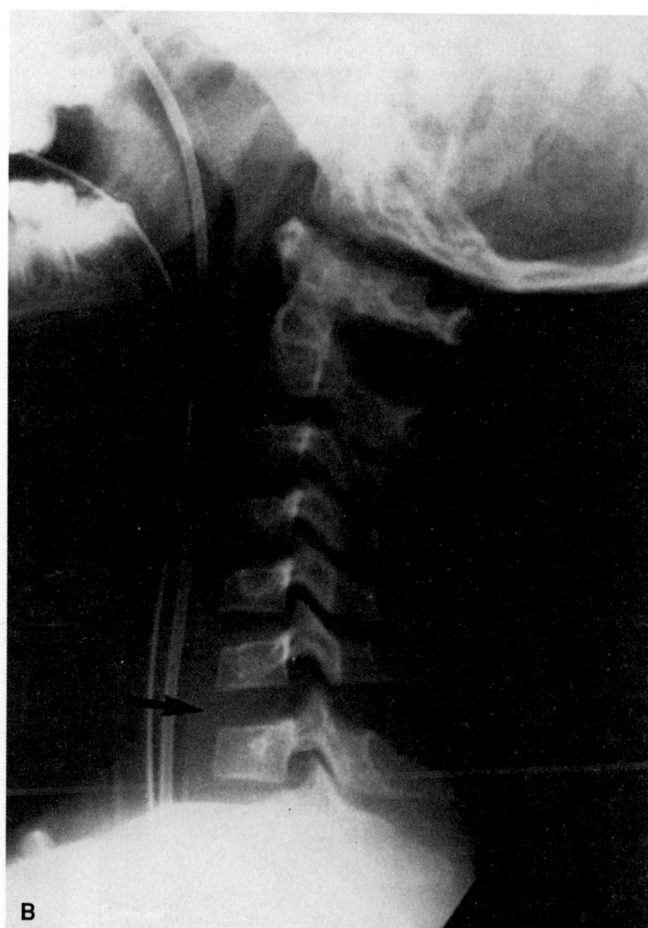

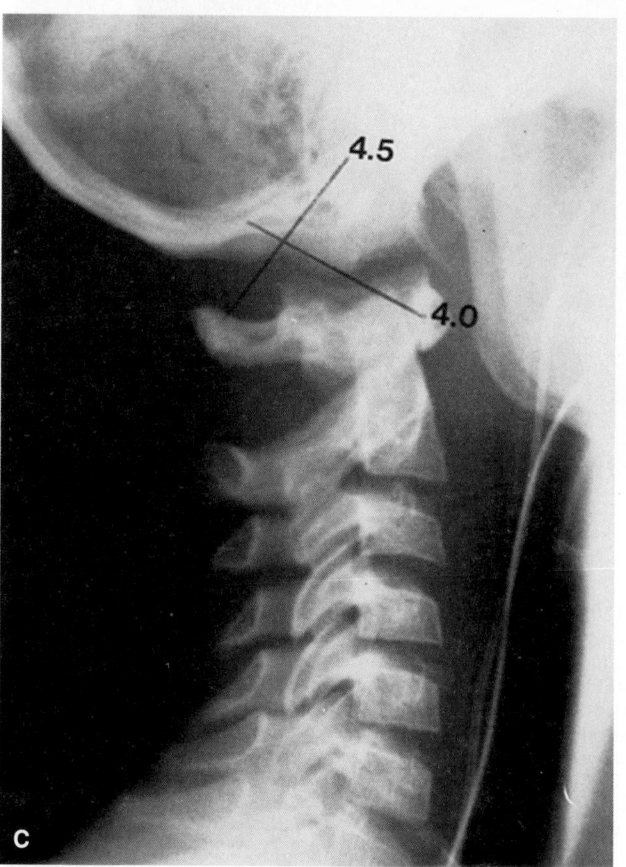

FIGURE 120.27 Distraction injuries. **A:** Dens fractures with distraction and accompanying C6–C7 distraction injury in a 3-year-old child. Injury was fatal. **B:** C6–C7 distraction injury in an 8-year-old child. **C:** BC (4.5 line): AO (4.0 line) ratio is more than 1, suggesting atlantooccipital dislocation.

FIGURE 120.28 Examples of methods to assess occipital/C1 relationships. *A*, C1 anterior arch; *B*, basion (anterior margin of foramen magnum); *C*, anterior portion of the posterior ring of C1; *O*, opisthion (posterior margin of foramen magnum); and *D*, tip of the dens (odontoid process). These landmarks may not be easily visible on all radiographs. A BC:AO ratio of more than 0.9 to 1.0 suggests anterior dislocation or subluxation of the atlantooccipital joint. A BD distance of more than 10 to 12.5 mm should be suggestive of atlantooccipital dislocation. A C1–C2:C2–C3 ratio of more than 2.5 suggests injury to the tectorial membrane and ligamentous instability.

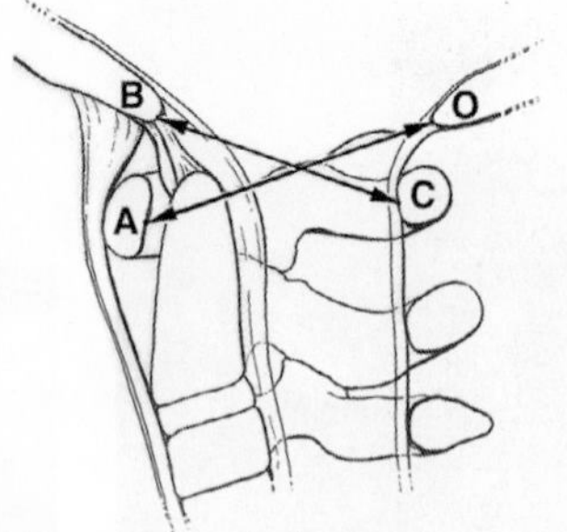

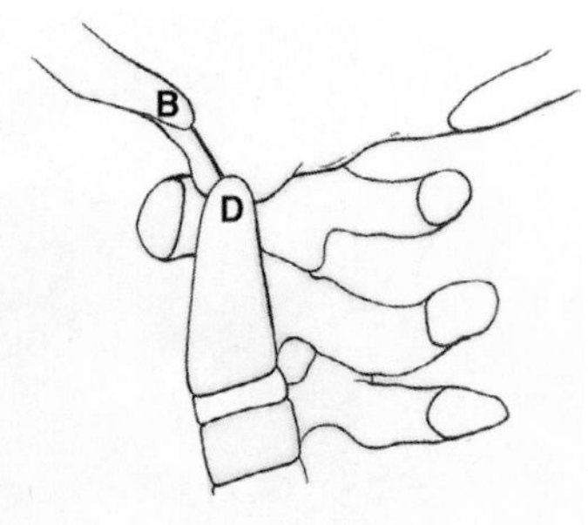

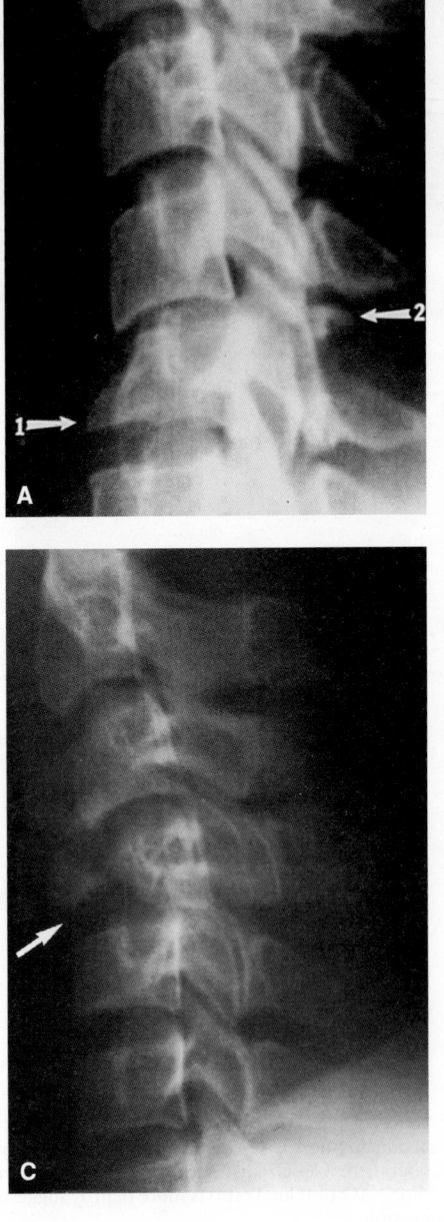

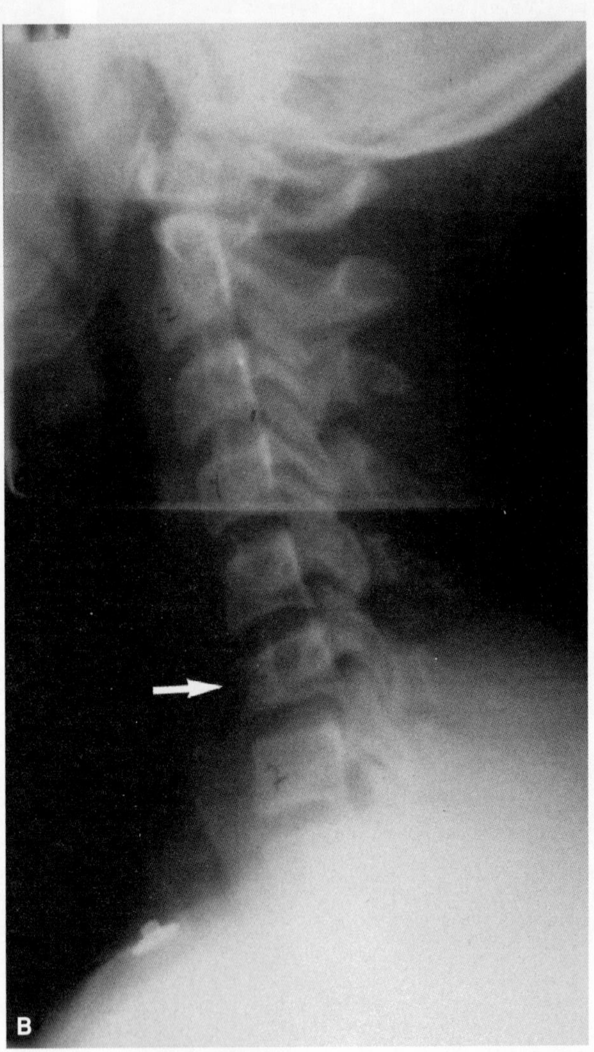

FIGURE 120.29 Examples of cervical compression injuries. **A:** Teardrop fracture. This patient sustained a whiplash injury with resultant flexion injury. A typical flexion teardrop fracture is demonstrated at (*1*). An increased interspinous distance and an associated avulsion fracture of the posterior elements of C5 are demonstrated at (*2*). **B:** Anterior C6 vertebral wedge fracture (*arrow*). **C:** Burst fracture of C4 vertebral body (*arrow*). (**A:** From Swischuk L. *Emergency radiology of the acutely ill or injured child*. 2nd ed. Baltimore, MD: Williams & Wilkins, 1986:674. Reprinted with permission.)

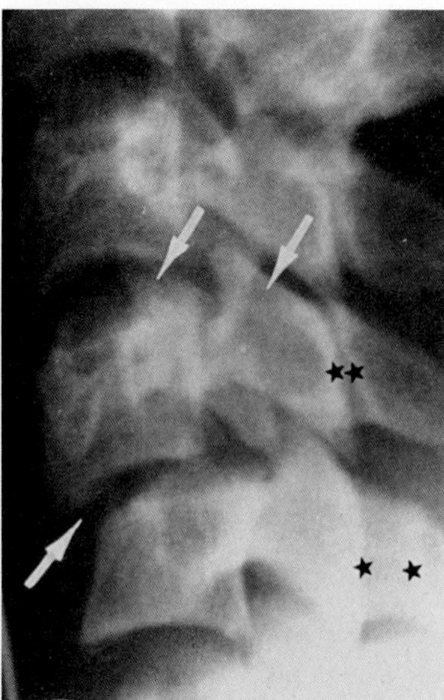

FIGURE 120.30 Unilateral facet dislocation. C4 is offset anteriorly on C5 less than 50% of the width of the vertebral body. *Arrows* denote the offset of vertebral body and apophyseal joints. The disc space between C4 and C5 is narrowed. Note that the distance between the posterior cortex of the apophyseal joint facet and the anterior cortex of the spinous process tip is wider below the level of dislocation than above the level *(stars)*. Anterior vertebral offset of more than 50% would denote a bilateral facet dislocation. (From Swischuk L. *Emergency radiology of the acutely ill or injured child*. 2nd ed. Baltimore, MD: Williams & Wilkins, 1986:697. Reprinted with permission.)

scan is useful in evaluating an infant with diminished motor activity and who is suspected of having a distraction injury.

Vertebral Compression Injuries

Vertebral compression injuries are suggested by isolated anterior wedging, teardrop fractures, or burst vertebral bodies (Fig. 120.29). The vertebral bodies should be regular, cuboid, and consistent between adjacent cervical levels (Fig. 120.29). A flexion/rotation stress can lead to anterior subluxation of one vertebral body on another with facet dislocation ("locked" or "jumped" facet) (Fig. 120.30). If the anterior displacement is less than 50% of the vertebral body width, it is consistent with a unilateral facet dislocation (Fig. 120.30). More than a 50% anterior subluxation suggests a bilateral facet dislocation (Fig. 120.30). These injuries are often accompanied by widened interspinous and interlaminar spaces, anterior soft tissue swelling, and a narrowed disc space.

Spinal Cord Injury without Radiographic Abnormality (SCIWORA)

SCIWORA was initially described as occurring in up to 67% of all children with cervical cord injuries (Fig. 120.31), and up to 25% of cervical cord injuries in children younger than 8 years. SCIWORA has been described as mainly occurring in children younger than 8 years who present with, or develop symptoms consistent with, cervical cord injuries without any radiographic or tomographic evidence of bony abnormality. Some authors have recently suggested that the diagnosis of SCIWORA be applied only to those patients who also do not have abnormal MRI findings. The original characterization of this syndrome occurred during a period when MRI was less available and

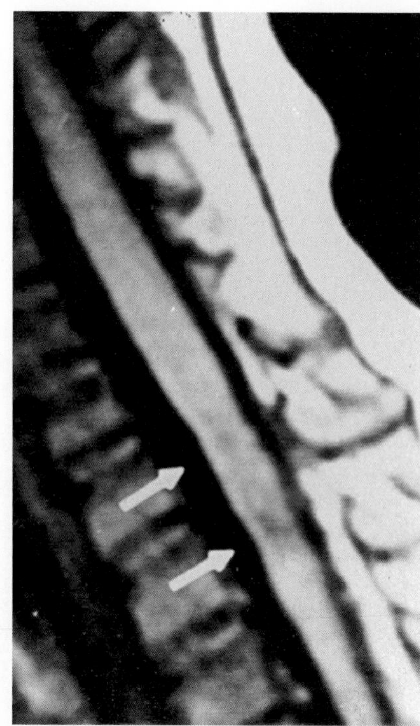

FIGURE 120.31 Magnetic resonance imaging (MRI) of SCIWORA patient. Accompanying cervical spine radiographs were normal. The MRI demonstrates an area of cord contusion in the midcervical area (*arrows*). This patient had physical evidence of a central cord syndrome. (From Swischuk L. *Emergency radiology of the acutely ill or injured child*. 2nd ed. Baltimore, MD: Williams & Wilkins, 1986:710. Reprinted with permission.)

it is important to note there are distinct differences between patients with and without MRI findings in the setting of persistent neurologic abnormalities. Regardless, this type of injury is not often seen in children older than 8 years because the forces necessary to injure the spinal cord also cause persistent spinal column abnormalities. The young child's elastic spinal column allows the spine to deform beyond physiologic extremes, injuring the cord and then reducing spontaneously without any persistent (radiographic) evidence of bone injury. The causes of the neurologic compromise can include segmental spinal instability, vascular injury (occlusion, spasm, and infarction), ligamentous injury, disc impingement, or incomplete neuronal destruction. A subset of patients has initial transient neurologic symptoms as previously described, apparently recover, and then return, on average, 1 day later with neurologic abnormalities. Therefore, hospitalization, immobilization, and further radiographic evaluation (MRI) for this group of patients may be optimal. At the least, neurosurgical consultation is recommended if the history suggests a SCIWORA-type injury in a child younger than 8 years.

Torticollis (Wry Neck)

Torticollis is a common complaint in the pediatric ED. The clinician should always inquire about traumatic events because an underlying bone injury may be present. Often, however, torticollis is caused by spasm of the sternocleidomastoid (SCM) muscle. In the patient with muscular torticollis, their chin points toward the unaffected side, while SCM spasm occurs on the affected side. This condition is different from *rotary subluxation*. *Rotary subluxation* is a cervical spine injury that is often misdiagnosed or

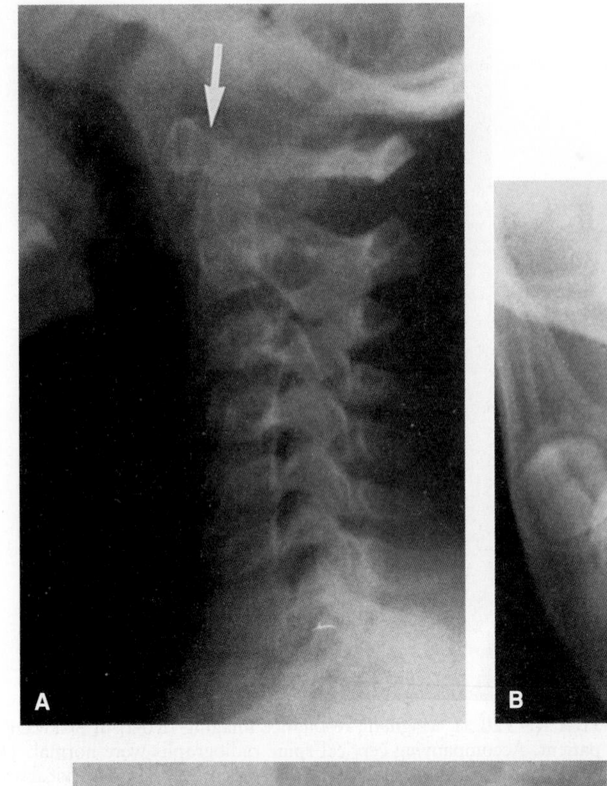

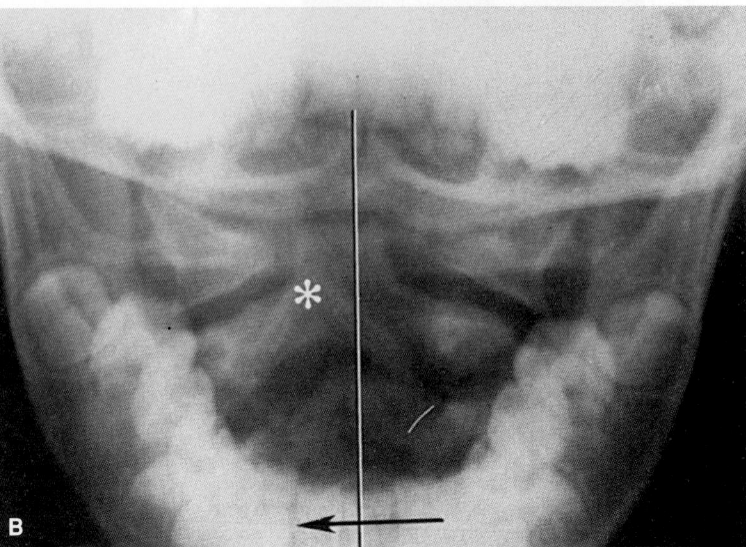

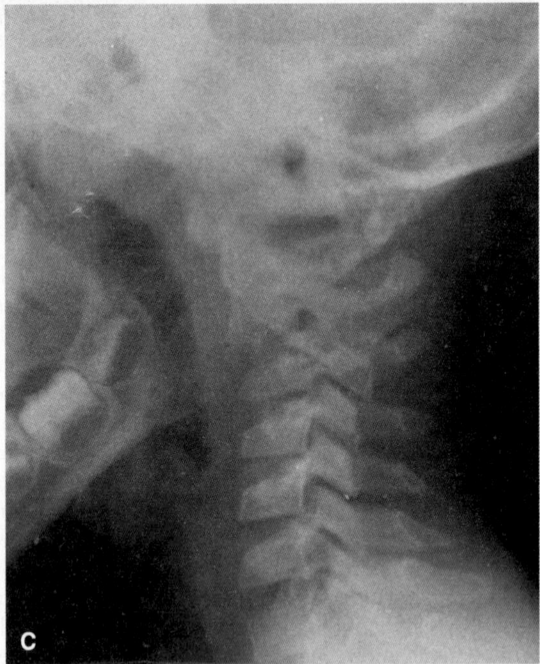

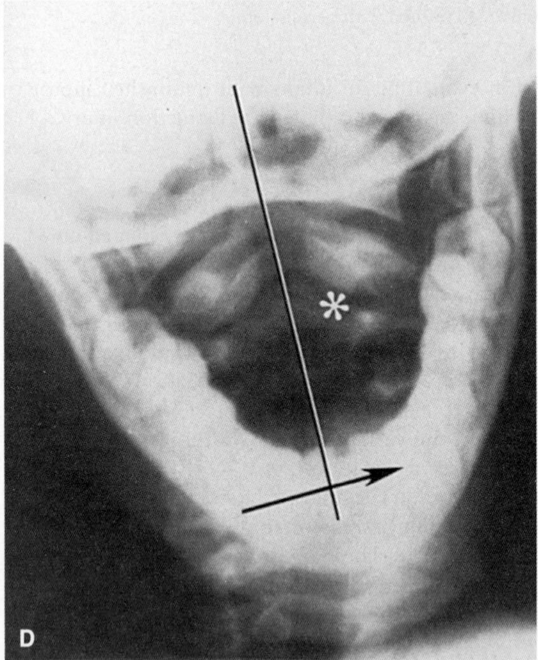

FIGURE 120.32 Torticollis (wry neck). **A:** Lateral cervical radiograph with C2 cocked forward on C3 and normal predental space (*arrow*). **B:** Anteroposterior (AP) view demonstrating spinous process of C2 (*asterisk*) on the same side of the midline as the mandible points. **C:** Difficult to interpret lateral cervical spine because of the rotation effect of torticollis. **D:** AP view demonstrating spinous process of C2 (*asterisk*) on the same side of the midline as the mandible points. (From Swischuk L. *Emergency radiology of the acutely ill or injured child.* 2nd ed. Baltimore, MD: Williams & Wilkins, 1986:588. Reprinted with permission.)

undiagnosed because of difficulty in interpreting these patient's radiographs. *Rotary subluxation* or displacement may be spontaneous or follow an upper respiratory tract infection or traumatic event with variable severity. These patients rarely present with abnormal neurologic findings. In these patients, their chin will often point to the same side as the SCM spasm giving the child the typical (cock robin) position. This presentation is logical considering that the SCM muscle is attempting to reestablish normal neck position. Radiographs may be useful to help distinguish between muscular torticollis and *rotary subluxation,* although the radiographs may be normal in both cases (Figs. 120.32 and 120.33). *Rotary subluxation* should be suspected if, on an open-mouth radiograph, one of the lateral masses of C1 appears forward and closer to the midline whereas the

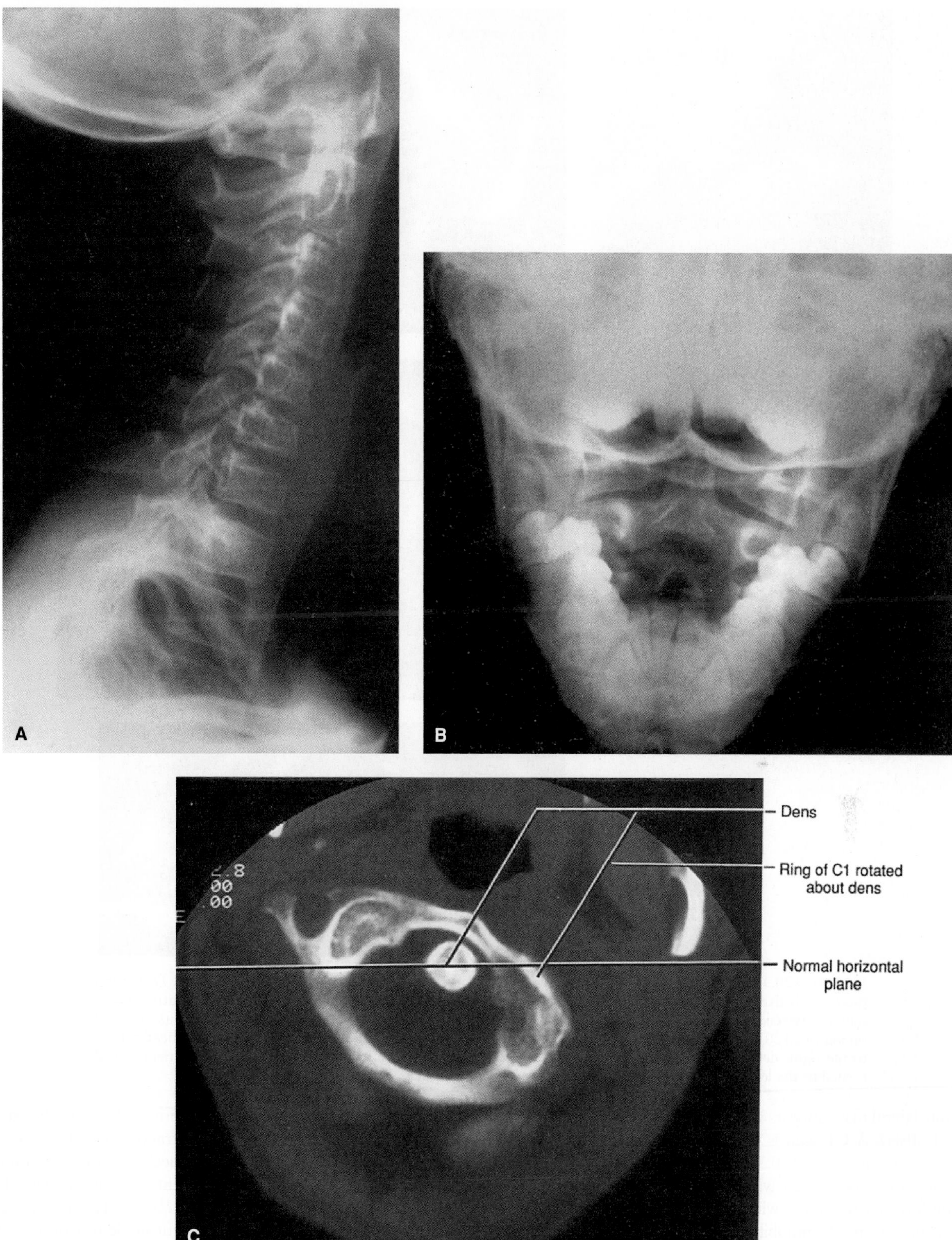

FIGURE 120.33 Rotary subluxation of C1 and C2. **A:** Grossly normal lateral neck radiograph in an 8-year-old child with rotary subluxation. **B:** Grossly normal open-mouth (odontoid) radiograph in an 8-year-old child with rotary subluxation. **C:** Computed tomographic (CT) scan demonstrating marked rotary subluxation of C1 clockwise around dens. Actual measurement was 22 degrees of rotation. (*continued*)

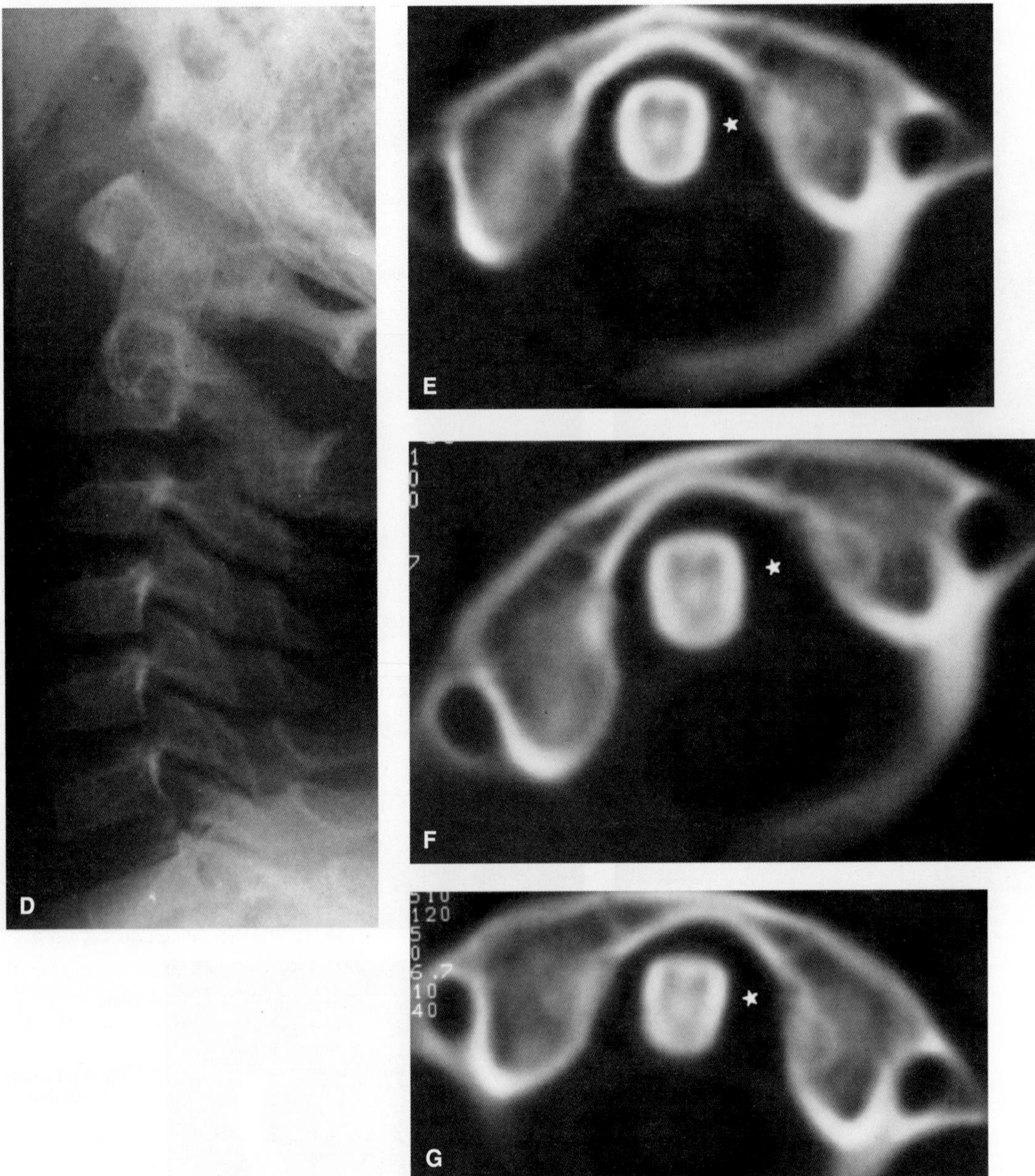

FIGURE 120.33 (*Continued*) **D–G:** CT evidence of fixed rotary subluxation in a 6-year-old child. **D:** Lateral radiograph demonstrating mild increased distance of predental space. **E:** Axial CT scan demonstrating asymmetry between right and left sides and increased distance between dens and patient's left side of C1 (star noted on Figures 120.33 D, E, F) (asymmetry between right and left sides). **F:** Axial CT scan with patient's head turned to the right, demonstrating asymmetry between the dens and ring of C1. **G:** Axial CT scan with patient's head turned to the left, demonstrating fixed asymmetry between the dens and the ring of C1.

opposite lateral mass appears narrow and away from the midline (lateral offset). A CT scan is the most useful diagnostic tool in *rotary subluxation* (Fig. 120.33). Patients with mild *rotary subluxation* should be treated with a cervical collar and analgesia for comfort, whereas those with moderate or resilient rotary displacement may need immobilization, traction or surgical intervention. If anterior displacement of C2 on C1 is present, longer immobilization may be needed to allow injured ligaments to heal.

Spinal Cord Syndromes

Several specific spinal cord syndromes may be encountered in the ED (Fig. 120.34). A spinal cord concussion (transient traumatic paresis or paralysis) involves neurologic symptoms that completely resolve over a short period. This condition can occur with or without associated fracture or dislocation. A *complete cord transection* (either mechanical or physiologic) results in immediate and permanent loss of all neurologic functions distal to that level (Fig. 120.34). The *anterior cord syndrome* results from the loss of neurologic function in those areas supplied by the anterior spinal artery (Fig. 120.34). Motor function is lost below the level of the lesion. Touch and proprioceptive functions, carried by the dorsal (posterior) columns, are preserved. The *posterior cord syndrome* is rare (Fig. 120.34). It involves the loss of proprioceptive functions, deep pressure, and pain and vibratory sense, with preservation of motor and temperature sensation. This can occur with direct posterior cord trauma or posterior spinal artery involvement. The *Brown-Séquard syndrome* (hemisection

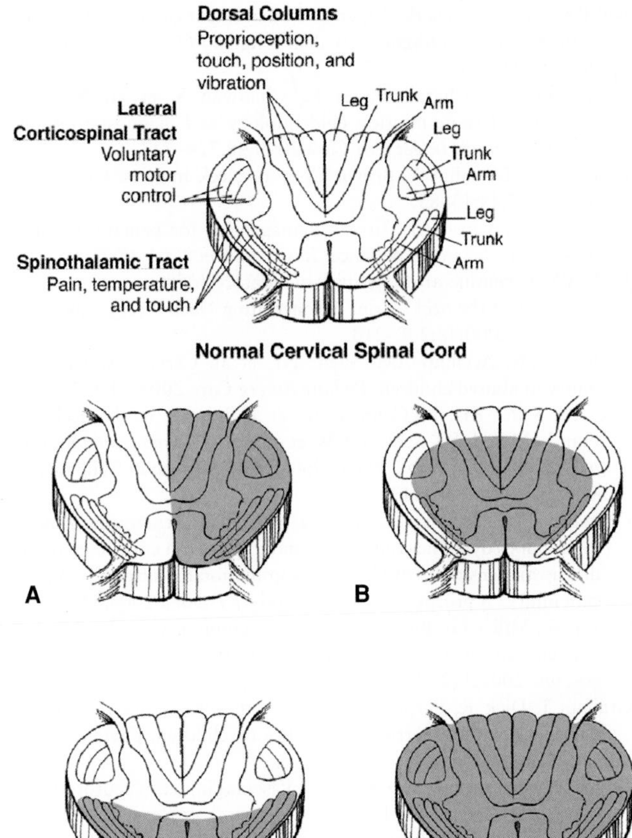

FIGURE 120.34 Graphic illustrations of a normal cervical spinal cord and specific postinjury syndromes. **A:** Brown-Séquard syndrome. **B:** Central cord syndrome. **C:** Anterior artery syndrome. **D:** Complete transection.

of the cord) involves contralateral loss of pain and temperature sensation with ipsilateral motor findings (weakness or paralysis) below the lesion (Fig. 120.34). The *central cord syndrome* signifies an injury that is most severe in the center of the cord and less so toward the periphery (Fig. 120.34). The resultant physical examination demonstrates motor strength that is more severely depressed in the arms than in the legs. These designations are useful in suggesting prognosis. Approximately two-thirds of those patients with *central cord syndrome* and one-third of those with the *Brown-Séquard syndrome* recover. *Complete transections* and *anterior cord syndrome* usually signify nonreversible lesions. Patients with *posterior cord syndrome* usually recover but may demonstrate some degree of ataxia.

The *os odontoideum* is an abnormality that may be the result of an occult flexion injury with subsequent incomplete healing and bone resorption (Fig. 120.35). It may also represent an overgrowth of the ossiculum terminale, often associated with a hypoplastic dens. This leads to a risk of increased mobility and cord injury at the C1–C2 level and may require surgical stabilization. This condition can be confused with a fracture at the base of the odontoid. The ossiculum terminale is a small ossicle at the tip of the dens (Fig. 120.36). It is seen in most children, fusing with the rest of the dens by adolescence. This ossicle can be large and associated with a hypoplastic dens, as previously described.

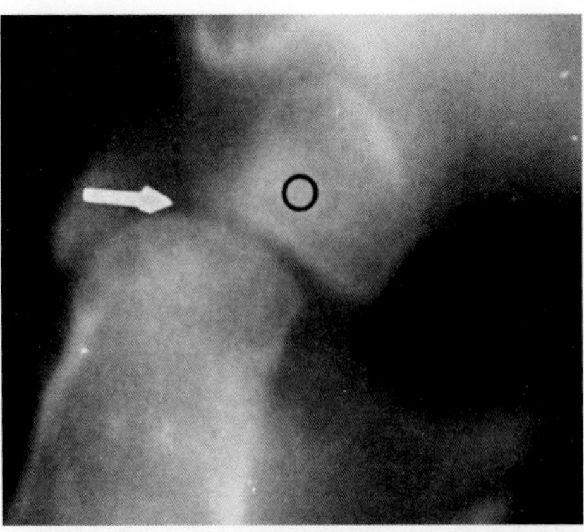

FIGURE 120.35 Example of os odontoideum. Note the hypoplastic dens and overgrown ossiculum terminale or ossiculum odontoideum (O). The *arrow* indicates posterior displacement, attesting to instability of the lesions. (From Swischuk L. *Emergency radiology of the acutely ill or injured child.* 2nd ed. Baltimore, MD: Williams & Wilkins, 1986:717. Reprinted with permission.)

Spinal epidural hematomas are also seen in the pediatric population. These hematomas are venous bleeds that compress the adjacent spinal cord and present hours or days after a sometimes minor traumatic event, with ascending neurologic symptoms as the bleed progresses. An MRI scan can be helpful in evaluating these patients (Fig. 120.37). Rapid evaluation and surgical decompression are mandatory.

Treatment of children with suspected cervical spine injuries may involve basic and advanced life-support measures, initiation and/or maintenance of immobilization, and neurosurgical or orthopedic consultation. Airway support for patients with traumatic quadriplegia should be considered because they will develop respiratory failure as they tire. Children may present in spinal shock (hypotension, bradycardia, peripheral flush) from the loss of sympathetic input to the vascular system. The physical examination may be misleading in that these patients are bradycardic (unable to mount tachycardic response to relative hypovolemia) and demonstrate warm, flushed skin in the setting of hypotension (loss of vasomotor tone). These symptoms may also be superimposed on traumatic (hypovolemic) shock. These patients need fluid resuscitation and may require inotropic (alpha agonist) support, such as norepinephrine or

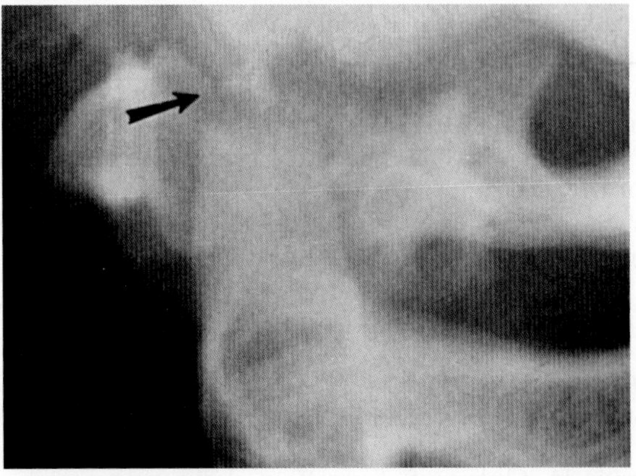

FIGURE 120.36 Normal ossiculum terminale at the tip of the dens (*arrow*). (From Swischuk L. *Emergency radiology of the acutely ill or injured child.* 2nd ed. Baltimore, MD: Williams & Wilkins, 1986:717. Reprinted with permission.)

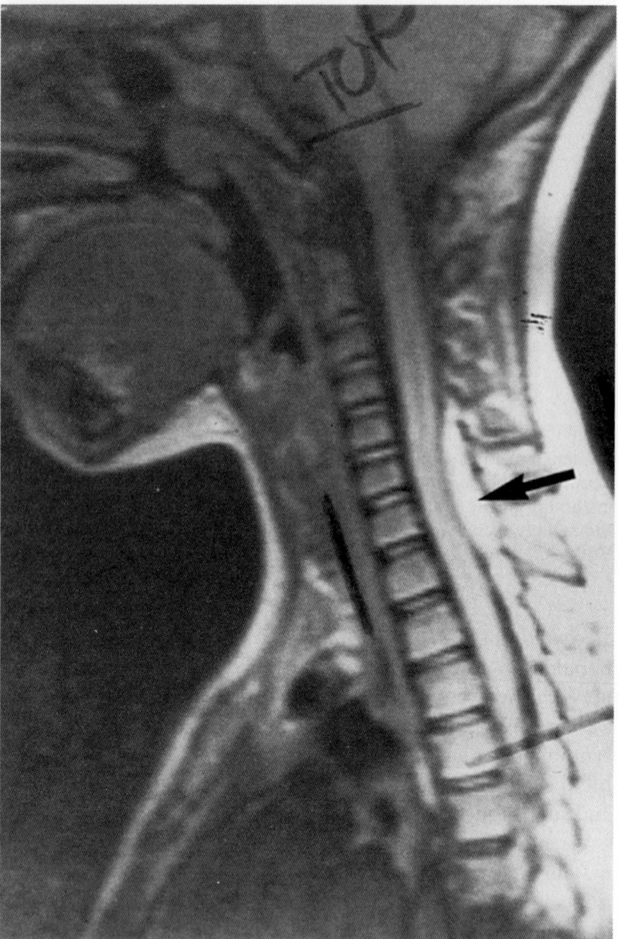

FIGURE 120.37 Magnetic resonance imaging (MRI) of cervical spine demonstrating epidural hematoma (*arrow*) from C5 to T1. Note excellent soft tissue, intervertebral disc, and fluid detail afforded by the MRI scan.

phenylephrine, to maintain adequate perfusion and avoid fluid overload. Appropriate fluid management is important in preventing hypoperfusion of the already injured spinal cord. The use of steroids for blunt cervical trauma has come under scrutiny in more recent years. Several authors suggest that steroid administration increases potential risk to the patient and does not lead to meaningful neurologic recovery and that its use as a standard of care is not justified. Steroid use for the pediatric patient with a clear or potential blunt cervical cord injury is not routinely indicated, nor well supported by available evidence and should be discussed in consultation with the treating orthopedic and neurosurgical physicians bearing in mind that it is not approved by the Federal Drug Administration for this purpose. Methylprednisolone is not recommended in conjunction with penetrating neck injuries.

Suggested Readings and Key References

Blunt and Penetrating Neck Trauma

Abujamra L, Joseph MM. Penetrating neck injuries in children: a retrospective review. *Pediatr Emerg Care* 2003;19:308–313.

Asensio JA, Chahwan S, Forno W, et al. Penetrating esophageal injuries: multicenter study of the American Association for the Surgery of Trauma. *J Trauma-Injury Infect Crit Care* 2001;50: 289–296.

Bell RB, Osborn T, Dierks EJ, et al. Management of penetrating neck injuries: a new paradigm for civilian trauma. *J Oral Maxillofac Surg* 2007;65:691–705.

Demetriades D, Charalambides K, Chahwan S, et al. Nonskeletal cervical spine injuries: epidemiology and diagnostic pitfalls. *J Trauma-Injury Infect Crit Care* 2000;48:724–727.

Demetriades D, Salim A, Brown C, et al. Neck injuries. *Curr Probl Surg* 2007;44:13–85.

Desjardins G, Varon AJ. Airway management for penetrating neck injuries: the Miami experience. *Resuscitation* 2001;48:71–75.

Eddy VA. Is routine arteriography mandatory for penetrating injury to zone 1 of the neck? Zone 1 Penetrating Neck Injury Subgroup. *J Trauma* 2000;48:208–213.

Feldman KW, Avellino AM, Sugar NF, et al. Cervical spinal cord injury in abused children. *Pediatr Emerg Care* 2008;24:222–227.

Gee AC, Salter KD, McConnell DB, et al. Injuries to the neck. In: Flint L, Meredith J, Schwab CW, et al., eds. *Trauma contemporary principles and therapy.* Philadelphia, PA: Lippincott Williams & Wilkins, 2008:335–349.

Gonzalez RP, Falimirski M, Holevar MR, et al. Penetrating zone II injury: does dynamic computed tomography scan contribute to the diagnostic sensitivity of physical examination for surgically significant injury? A prospective blinded study. *J Trauma* 2003;54:61–64.

Goudy SL, Miller FB, Bumpous JM. Neck crepitance: evaluation and management of suspected upper aerodigestive tract injury. *Laryngoscope* 2002;112:791–795.

Graham J, Dick R, Parnell D, et al. Clothesline injury mechanism associated with all-terrain vehicle use by children. *Pediatr Emerg Care* 2006;22:45–47.

Guyot LL, Kazmierczak CD, Diaz FG. Vascular injury in neurotrauma. *Neurol Res* 2001;23:291–296.

Hanson CA, Smith JA. Penetrating neck injuries in children. *J Trauma Nurs* 2007;14:12–16; quiz 17–18.

Inaba K, Munera F, McKenney M, et al. Prospective evaluation of screening multislice helical computed tomographic angiography in the initial evaluation of penetrating neck injuries. *J Trauma* 2006; 61:144–149.

Insull P, Adams D, Segar A, et al. Is exploration mandatory in penetrating zone II neck injuries? *ANZ J Surg* 2007;77:261–264.

Kim MK, Buckman R, Szeremeta W. Penetrating neck trauma in children: an urban hospital's experience. *Otolaryngol Head Neck Surg* 2000;123:439–443.

Klinkner DB, Arca MJ, Lewis BD, et al. Pediatric vascular injuries: patterns of injury, morbidity, and mortality. *J Pediatr Surg* 2007; 42:178–182; discussion 182–183.

Lee C, Woodring J, Walsh J. Carotid and vertebral artery injury in survivors of atlanto-occipital dislocation: case reports and literature review. *J Trauma* 1991;31:401–407.

Losek JD, Tecklenburg FW, White DR. Blunt laryngeal trauma in children: case report and review of initial airway management. *Pediatr Emerg Care* 2008;24:370–373.

Marathe US, Tran LP. Pediatric neck trauma causing massive subcutaneous emphysema. *J Trauma* 2006;61:440–443.

Markus-Rodden MM, Bojko T, Hauck LC. Traumatic tracheal laceration in a pediatric patient medically managed with high-frequency oscillatory ventilation. *Pediatr Emerg Care* 2008;24:236–237.

Marom T, Russo E, Ben-Yehuda Y, et al. Oropharyngeal injuries in children. *Pediatr Emerg Care* 2007;23:914–918.

Mazolewski PJ, Curry JD, Browder T, et al. Computer tomographic scan can be used for surgical decision making in zone II penetrating neck injuries. *J Trauma* 2001;51:315–319.

McKevitt EC, Kirkpatrick AW, Vertesi L, et al. Blunt vascular neck injuries: diagnosis and outcomes of extracranial vessel injury. *J Trauma* 2002;53:472–476.

Mezhir JJ, Glynn L, Liu DC, et al. Handlebar injuries in children: should we raise the bar of suspicion? *Am Surg* 2007;73:807–810.

Navsaria P, Thoma M, Nicol A. Foley catheter balloon tamponade for lifethreatening hemorrhage in penetrating neck trauma. *World J Surg* 2006;30:1265–1268.

Rathlev NK, Medzon R, Bracken ME. Evaluation and management of neck trauma. *Emerg Med Clin North Am* 2007;25:679–694, viii.

Tallon JM, Ahmed JM, Sealy B. Airway management in penetrating neck trauma at a Canadian tertiary trauma centre. *J Can Assoc Emerg Phys* 2007;9:101–104.

Verschueren DS, Bell RB, Bagheri SC, et al. Management of laryngo-tracheal injuries associated with craniomaxillofacial trauma. *J Oral Maxillofac Surg* 2006;64:203–214.

Vohra S, Johnston BC, Cramer K, et al. Adverse events associated with pediatric spinal manipulation: a systematic review. *Pediatrics* 2007;119:e275–e283. (Erratum for Vohra S, Johnston BC, Cramer K, et al. *Pediatrics* 119(1):e275–e283. Published online July 2, 2007, accessed on November 25, 2009.)

Wang BS, Smith SL, Pereira KD. Pediatric head and neck trauma from all-terrain vehicle accidents. *Otolaryngol Head Neck Surg* 2007; 137:201–205.

Williams EW, Cawich SO, James M, et al. Penetrating neck trauma and the aberrant subclavian artery. *West Indian Med J* 2007;56:288–293.

Zhang S, Michael M, Clowers K, et al. Evaluation of efficacy and 3D kinematic characteristics of cervical orthoses. *Clin Biomech (Bristol, Avon)* 2005;20(3):264–269.

Zonfrillo MR, Roy AD, Walsh SA. Management of pediatric penetrating oropharyngeal trauma. *Pediatr Emerg Care* 2008;24:172–175.

Cervical Spine

Adelgais KM, Grossman DC, Langer SG, et al. Use of helical computed tomography for imaging the pediatric cervical spine. *Acad Emerg Med* 2004;11:228–236.

Anders JF, Adelgais K, Hoyle JD, et al. Comparison of outcomes for children with cervical spine injury based on destination hospital from scene of injury. *Acad Emerg Med* 2014;21:55–64.

Anglen J, Metzler M, Bunn P, et al. Flexion and extension views are not cost-effective in a cervical spine clearance protocol for obtunded trauma patients. *J Trauma* 2002;52:54–59.

Armstrong BP, Simpson HK, Crouch R, et al. Prehospital clearance of the cervical spine: does it need to be a pain in the neck? *Emerg Med J* 2007;24:501–503.

Avellino AM, Mann FA, Grady MS, et al. The misdiagnosis of acute cervical spine injuries and fractures in infants and children: the 12-year experience of a level I pediatric and adult trauma center. *Childs Nerv Syst* 2005;21:122–127.

Barrett T, Mower W, Zucker M, et al. Injuries missed by limited computed tomographic imaging of patients with cervical spine injuries. *Ann Emerg Med* 2006;47(2):129–133.

Bell KM, Frazier EC, Shively CM, et al. Assessing range of motion to evaluate the adverse effects of ill-fitting cervical orthoses. *Spine J* 2009;9(3):225–231.

Bivins H, Ford S, Bezmalinovic Z, et al. The effects of axial traction during orotracheal intubation of the trauma victim with an unstable cervical spine. *Ann Emerg Med* 1988;17:53–57.

Bracken MB. Steroids for acute spinal cord injury. *Cochrane Database Syst Rev* 2002;(3):CD001046.

Bracken MB, Shepard MJ, Collins W, et al. A randomized, controlled trial of methylprednisolone or naloxone in the treatment of acute spinal-cord injury: results of the second national acute spinal-cord injury study. *N Engl J Med* 1990;322:1405–1411.

Bracken MB, Shepard MJ, Holford TR, et al. Administration of methylprednisolone for 24 or 48 hours or tirilazad mesylate for 48 hours in the treatment of acute spinal cord injury: results of the third national acute spinal cord injury randomized controlled trial. *JAMA* 1997;277:1597–1604.

Brenner D, Elliston C, Hall E, et al. Estimated risks of radiation-induced fatal cancer from pediatric CT. *Am J Roentgenol* 2001;176: 289–296.

Brohi K, Healy M, Fotheringham T, et al. Helical computed tomographic scanning for the evaluation of the cervical spine in the unconscious, intubated trauma patient. *J Trauma* 2005;58: 897–901.

Buhs C, Cullen M, Klein M, et al. The pediatric trauma C-spine: is the "odontoid" view necessary? *J Pediatr Surg* 2000;35:994–997.

Bulas D, Fitz C, Johnson D. Traumatic atlanto-occipital dislocation in children. *Radiology* 1993;188:155–158.

Canadian CT Head and C-Spine (CCC) Study Group. Canadian C-spine rule study for alert and stable trauma patients, part I: background and rationale. *CJEM* 2002;4:84–90.

Choudhary AK, Ishak R, Zacharia T, et al. Imaging of spinal injury in abusive head trauma: a retrospective study. *Pediatr Radiol* 2014; 44(9):1130–1140.

Cirak B, Ziegfeld S, Knight VM, et al. Spinal injuries in children. *J Pediatr Surg* 2004;39:607–612.

Citerio G, Cormio M, Sganzerla EP. Steroids in acute spinal cord injury. An unproven standard of care. *Minerva Anestesiol* 2002;68(5): 315–320.

Como J, Thompson M, Anderson J, et al. Is magnetic resonance imaging essential in cleaning the cervical spine in obtunded patients with blunt trauma? *J Trauma Injury Infect Critic Care* 2007;63(3): 544–549.

Cothren CC, Moore EE, Ray CE Jr, et al. Cervical spine fracture patterns mandating screening to rule out blunt cerebrovascular injury. *Surgery* 2007;141:76–82.

Criswell JC, Parr MJ, Nolan JP. Emergency airway management in patients with cervical spine injuries. *Anaesthesia* 1994;49(10): 900–903.

Curran C, Dietrich AM, Bowman MJ, et al. Pediatric cervical-spine immobilization: achieving neutral position? *J Trauma* 1995;39(4): 729–732.

Daffner RH, Hackney DB. ACR Appropriateness Criteria on suspected spine trauma. *J Am Coll Radiol* 2007;4:762–775.

Daffner RH, Sciulli RL, Rodriguez A, et al. Imaging for evaluation of suspected cervical spine trauma: a 2-year analysis. *Injury* 2006;37:652–658.

d'Amato C. Pediatric spinal trauma: injuries in very young children. *Clin Orthop Relat Res* 2005;(432):34–40.

Dare AO, Dias MS, Li V. Magnetic resonance imaging correlation in pediatric spinal cord injury without radiographic abnormality. *J Neurosurg* 2002;97(1 suppl):33–39.

Davis JW, Kaups KL, Cunningham MA. Routine evaluation of the cervical spine in head-injured patients with dynamic fluoroscopy: a reappraisal. *J Trauma* 2001;50:1044–1047.

Del Rossi G, Heffernan TP, Horodyski M, et al. The effectiveness of extrication collars tested during the execution of spine-board transfer techniques. *Spine J* 2004;4:619–623.

Domeier RM, Frederiksen SM, Welch K. Prospective performance assessment of an out-of-hospital protocol for selective spine immobilization using clinical spine clearance criteria. *Ann Emerg Med* 2005;46:123–131.

Dormans JP. Evaluation of children with suspected cervical spine injury. *J Bone Joint Surg Am* 2002;84-A:124–132.

Frampton A, Eynon C. High dose methylprednisolone in the immediate management of acute, blunt spinal cord injury: what is the current practice in emergency departments, spinal units, and neurosurgical units in the UK? *Emerg Med J* 2006;23:550–553.

Frank JB, Lim CK, Flynn JM, et al. The efficacy of magnetic resonance imaging in pediatric cervical spine clearance. *Spine* 2002;27(11): 1176–1179.

Fuchs S, Barthel M, Flannery A, et al. Cervical spine fractures sustained by young children in forward-facing car seats. *Pediatrics* 1989;84:348–354.

Garton HJ, Hammer MR. Detection of pediatric cervical spine injury. *Neurosurgery* 2008;62(3):700–707; comments 707–708.

Goutcher CM, Lochhead V. Reduction in mouth opening with semi-rigid cervical collars. *Br J Anaesth* 2005;95:344–348.

Griffen MM, Frykberg ER, Kerwin AJ, et al. Radiographic clearance of blunt cervical spine injury: plain radiograph or computed tomographic scan. *J Trauma* 2003;55:222–226.

Groopman J. The Reeve effect. *The New Yorker.* November 10, 2003: 83–93.

Hadley MN. Cervical spine immobilization before admission to the hospital. *Neurosurgery* 2002;50:S7–S17.

Hadley MN. Radiographic assessment of the cervical spine in asymptomatic trauma patients. *Neurosurgery* 2002;50:S30–S35.

Hadley MN. Management of pediatric cervical spine and spinal cord injuries. *Neurosurgery* 2002;50:S85–S99.

Hendey GW, Wolfson AB, Mower WR, et al. Spinal cord injury without radiographic abnormality: results of the National Emergency X-Radiography Utilization Study in blunt cervical trauma. *J Trauma* 2002;53:1–4.

Herzenberg J, Hensinger R, Dedrick D, et al. Emergency transport and positioning of young children who have an injury of the cervical spine: the standard backboard may be hazardous. *J Bone Joint Surg* 1989;71-A:15–22.

Hoffman JR, Mower WR, Wolfson AB, et al. Validity of a set of criteria to rule out injury to the cervical spine in patients with blunt trauma. National Emergency X-Radiography Study Group. *N Engl J Med* 2000;343:94–99.

Huerta C, Griffith R, Joyce S. Cervical spine stabilization in pediatric patients: evaluation of current techniques. *Ann Emerg Med* 1987; 16:55–60.

Hugenholtz H, Cass DE, Dvorak MF, et al. High-dose methylprednisolone for acute closed spinal cord injury—only a treatment option. *Can J Neurol Sci* 2002;29:227–235.

Hurlbert RJ, Hadley MN, Walters BC, et al. Pharmacological therapy for acute spinal cord injury. *Neurosurgery* 2013;72:93–105.

Insko EK, Gracias VH, Gupta R, et al. Utility of flexion and extension radiographs of the cervical spine in the acute evaluation of blunt trauma. *J Trauma* 2002;53:426–429.

Jagannathan J, Dumont AS, Prevedello DM, et al. Cervical spine injuries in pediatric athletes: mechanisms and management. *Neurosurg Focus* 2006;21:E6.

Jimenez RR, DeGuzman MA, Shiran S, et al. CT versus plain radiographs for evaluation of c-spine injury in young children: do benefits outweigh risks? *Pediatr Radiol* 2008;38:635–644.

Kaji A, Hockberger R. Imaging of spinal cord injuries. *Emerg Med Clin North Am* 2007;25:735–750, ix.

Kerr D, Bradshaw L, Kelly AM. Implementation of the Canadian C-spine rule reduces cervical spine x-ray rate for alert patients with potential neck injury. *J Emerg Med* 2005;28:127–131.

Kerwin AJ, Frykberg ER, Schinco MA, et al. The effect of early surgical treatment of traumatic spine injuries on patient mortality. *J Trauma* 2007;63:1308–1313.

Kim EG, Brown KM, Leonard JC, et al. Variability of prehospital spinal immobilization in children at risk for cervical spine injury. *Pediatr Emerg Care* 2013;29:413–418.

Knox J, Schneider J, Wimberly RL, et al. Characteristics of spinal injuries secondary to nonaccidental trauma. *J Pediatr Orthop* 2014;34: 376–381.

Kokoska ER, Keller MS, Rallo MC, et al. Characteristics of pediatric cervical spine injuries. *J Pediatr Surg* 2001;36(1):100–105.

Kriss VM, Kriss TC. Imaging of the cervical spine in infants. *Pediatr Emerg Care* 1996;13(1):44–49.

Kriss VM, Kriss TC. SCIWORA (spinal cord injury without radiographic abnormality) in infants and children. *Clin Pediatr* 1996; 35(3):119–124.

Kwan I, Bunn F, Roberts I. Spinal immobilisation for trauma patients. *Cochrane Database Syst Rev* 2001;(2):CD002803.

Lanoix R, Gupta R, Leak L, et al. C-spine injury associated with gunshot wounds to the head: retrospective study and literature review. *J Trauma* 2000;49:860–863.

Lasker M, Torres-Torres M, Green R. Neonatal diagnosis of spinal cord transection. *Clin Pediatr* 1991;30:322–324.

Leonard JR, Jaffe DM, Kupperman N, et al. Cervical spine injury patterns in children. *Pediatrics* 2014;133:e1179–e1188.

Leonard JR, Kupperman N, Olsen C, et al. Factors associated with cervical spine injury in children after blunt trauma. *Ann Emerg Med* 2011;58:145–155.

Luscombe MD, Williams JL. Comparison of a long spinal board and vacuum mattress for spinal immobilisation. *Emerg Med J* 2003; 20:476–478.

Lustrin SE, Karakas SP, Ortiz AO, et al. Pediatric cervical spine: normal anatomy, variants and trauma. *Radiographics* 2003;23: 539–560.

Mahajan P, Jaffe D, Olsen CS, et al. Spinal cord injury without radiologic abnormality in children imaged with magnetic resonance imaging. *J Trauma Acute Care Surg* 2013;75:843–847.

Manoach S, Paladino L. Manual in-line stabilization for acute airway management of suspected cervical spine injury: historical review and current questions. *Ann Emerg Med* 2007;50:236–245.

Martin B. Paediatric cervical spine injuries. *Injury* 2005;36:14–20.

Marx JA. Lateral plain films vs. helical CT for C-spine fracture: no contest. *J Watch Emerg Med* 2005;9:70–71. (Comment on: Brohi K, Healy M, Fotheringham T, et al. Helical computed tomographic scanning for the evaluation of the cervical spine in the unconscious, intubated trauma patient. *J Trauma* 2005;58:897–901.)

Menaker J, Philp A, Boswell S, et al. Computed tomography alone for cervical spine clearance in the unreliable patient—are we there yet? *J Trauma* 2008;64:898–903; discussion 903–904.

Merola A, O'Brien MF, Castro BA, et al. Histologic characterization of acute spinal cord injury treated with intravenous methylprednisolone. *J Orthopaed Trauma* 2002;16(3):155–161.

Molloy S, Middleton F, Casey AT. Failure to administer methylprednisolone for acute traumatic spinal cord injury—a prospective audit of 100 patients from a regional spinal injuries unit. *Injury* 2002;33:575–578.

Moscati RM, Lerner EB, Pugh JL. Application of clinical criteria for ordering radiographs to detect cervical spine fractures. *Am J Emerg Med* 2007;25:326–330.

Mower WR, Hoffman JR, Pollack CV, et al. Use of plain radiography to screen for cervical spine injuries. *Ann Emerg Med* 2001; 38:1–7.

Nigrovic LE, Rogers AJ, Adelgais KM, et al. Utility of plain radiographs in detecting traumatic injuries of the cervical spine in children. *Pediatr Emerg Care* 2012;28:426–432.

Panecek EA, Mower WR, Holmes JF, et al. Test performance of the individual NEXUS low-risk clinical screening criteria for cervical spine injury. *Ann Emerg Med* 2001;38:22–25.

Pang D, Nemzek WR, Zovickian J. Atlanto-occipital dislocation—part 2: the clinical use of (occipital) condyle-C1 interval, comparison with other diagnostic methods, and the manifestation, management and outcome of atlanto-occipital dislocation in children. *Neurosurgery* 2007;61(5):995–1015; discussion 1015.

Pang D, Pollack I. Spinal cord injury without radiographic abnormality in children—the SCIWORA syndrome. *J Trauma* 1989;29: 654–664.

Pang D, Wilberger J. Spinal cord injury without radiographic abnormality in children. *J Neurosurg* 1982;57:114–129.

Parent S, Mac-Thiong JM, Roy-Beaudry M, et al. Spinal cord injury in the pediatric population: a systematic review of the literature. *J Neurotrauma* 2011;28:1515–1524.

Patel JC, Tepas JJ III, Mollitt DL, et al. Pediatric cervical spine injuries: defining the disease. *J Pediatr Surg* 2001;36:373–376.

Pieretti-Vanmarcke R, Velmahos GC, Nance ML, et al. Clinical clearance of the cervical spine in blunt trauma patients younger than 3 years: a multi-center study of the American Association for the Surgery of Trauma. *J Trauma* 2009;67:543–550.

Platzer P, Jaindl M, Thalhammer G, et al. Clearing the cervical spine in critically injured patients: a comprehensive C-spine protocol to avoid unnecessary delays in diagnosis. *Eur Spine J* 2006;15: 1801–1810.

Platzer P, Jaindl M, Thalhammer G, et al. Cervical spine injuries in pediatric patients. *J Trauma* 2007;62:389–396; discussion 394–396.

Pointillart V, Petitjean ME, Wiart L, et al. Pharmacological therapy of spinal cord injury during the acute phase. *Spinal Cord* 2000;38: 71–76.

Prendergast MR, Saxe JM, Ledgerwood AM, et al. Massive steroids do not reduce the zone of injury after penetrating spinal cord injury. *J Trauma* 1994;37:576–580.

Proctor MR. Spinal cord injury. *Crit Care Med* 2002;30:S489–S499.

Qian T, Campagnolo D, Kirshblum S. High-dose methylprednisolone may do more harm for spinal cord injury. *Med Hypotheses* 2000;55(5):452–453.

Ralston ME. Physiologic anterior subluxation: case report of occurrence at C5 to C6 and C6 to C7 spinal levels. *Ann Emerg Med* 2004;44:472–475.

Richter D, Latta LL, Milne EL, et al. The stabilizing effects of different orthoses in the intact and unstable upper cervical spine: a cadaver study. *J Trauma* 2001;50:848–854.

Rozzelle CJ, Aarabi B, Dhall SS, et al. Management of pediatric cervical spine and spinal cord injuries. *Neurosurgery* 2013;72:205–226.

Schafermeyer R, Ribbeck B, Gaskins J, et al. Respiratory effects of spinal immobilization in children. *Ann Emerg Med* 1991;20:1017–1019.

Schellinger PD, Schwab S, Krieger D, et al. Masking of vertebral artery dissection by severe trauma to the cervical spine. *Spine* 2001;26:314–319.

Schenarts PJ, Diaz J, Kaiser C, et al. Prospective comparison of admission computed tomographic scan and plain films of the upper cervical spine in trauma patients with altered mental status. *J Trauma* 2001;51:663–668.

Short DJ, El Masry WS, Jones PW. High dose methylprednisolone in the management of acute spinal cord injury—a systematic review from a clinical perspective. *Spinal Cord* 2000;38(5):273–286.

Skellett S, Tibby SM, Durward A, et al. Lesson of the week: immobilisation of the cervical spine in children. *BMJ* 2002;324:591–593.

Slack SE, Clancy MJ. Clearing the cervical spine of paediatric trauma patients. *Emerg Med J* 2004;21:189–193.

Stiell IG, Wells GA, Vandemheen KL. The Canadian C-spine rule for radiography in alert and stable trauma patients. *JAMA* 2001;286: 1841–1848.

Stroh G, Braude D. Can an out-of-hospital cervical spine clearance protocol identify all patients with injuries? An argument for selective immobilization. *Ann Emerg Med* 2001;37:609–615.

Sumchai A, Sternbach G. Hangman's fracture in a 7-week-old infant. *Ann Emerg Med* 1991;20:86–89.

Sun PP, Poffenbarger GJ, Durham S, et al. Spectrum of occipitoatlantoaxial injury in young children. *J Neurosurg* 2000;93:28–39.

Swischuk L. *Emergency radiology of the acutely ill or injured child.* 3rd ed. Baltimore, MD: Williams & Wilkins, 1994:653–735.

Swischuk LE. *Imaging of the cervical spine in children.* New York, NY: Springer-Verlag, 2002.

Tescher AN, Rindflesch AB, Youdas JW, et al. Range-of-motion restriction and craniofacial tissue-interface pressure from four cervical collars. *J Trauma* 2007;63:1120–1126.

Treloar DJ, Nypaver M. Angulation of the pediatric cervical spine with and without cervical collar. *Pediatr Emerg Care* 1997;13(1):5–8.

Viccellio P, Simon H, Pressman BD, et al. A prospective multicenter study of cervical spine injury in children. *Pediatrics* 2001;108:E20, 1–6. Available at http://www.pediatrics.org/cgi/content/full/108/2/e20. Accessed November 25, 2009.

Vickery D. The use of the spinal board after the pre-hospital phase of trauma management. *Emerg Med J* 2001;18:51–54.

Vohra S, Johnston BC, Cramer K, et al. Adverse events associated with pediatric spinal manipulation: a systematic review. *Pediatrics* 2007;119:e275–e283.

Wilberger J. *Spinal cord injuries in children.* New York, NY: Futura, 1986.

Woodward GA, Kunkel CN. Cervical spine immobilization and imaging. In: King C, Henretig FM, eds. *Textbook of pediatric emergency procedures.* 2nd ed. Baltimore, MD: Wolters Kluwer Lippincott Williams & Wilkins, 2008:313–323.

Zhang S, Michael M, Clowers K, et al. Evaluation of efficacy and 3D kinematic characteristics of cervical orthoses. *Clin Biomech* 2005;20:264–269.

CHAPTER 121 ■ NEUROTRAUMA

JULIE K. MCMANEMY, MD, MPH AND ANDREW JEA, MD

GOALS OF EMERGENCY THERAPY

Head injury is a common presentation in the pediatric emergency department. The challenge is to distinguish minor head trauma from clinically important traumatic brain injury (ciTBI). Identifying which children necessitate radiographic imaging and immediate recognition of ciTBI should be the goal of the evaluation. Management of the head-injured child should focus on stabilization, recognition of clinical deterioration, and early consultation of a neurosurgeon to decrease morbidity and mortality.

KEY POINTS

- Headache is a common presenting symptom
- Most injuries are minor head trauma that do not necessitate clinical interventions
- Infants with intracranial injuries may appear to be asymptomatic due to limitations in their neurologic examination
- The most common cause of mortality from child abuse is head trauma
- Cervical spine injury in children is rare but occur with TBI 20% of the time

RELATED CHAPTERS

Resuscitation and Stabilization
- A General Approach to Ill and Injured Children: Chapter 1
- Approach to the Injured Child: Chapter 2

Signs and Symptoms
- Injury: Head: Chapter 36
- Pain: Headache: Chapter 54
- Vomiting: Chapter 77

Clinical Pathways
- Head Trauma: Chapter 89

Medical, Surgical and Trauma Emergencies
- Child Abuse/Assault: Chapter 95
- Dental Trauma: Chapter 113
- ENT Trauma: Chapter 114
- Facial Trauma: Chapter 115
- Neck Trauma: Chapter 120
  - Spinal Cord Injury covered in this chapter
- Neurosurgical Emergencies: Chapter 130

NEUROTRAUMA

Blunt Head Injury

CLINICAL PEARLS AND PITFALLS

- Infants with intracranial injuries may have limited neurologic examinations and appear asymptomatic
- Clinical assessment of infants may be challenging
- Index of suspicion for nonaccidental trauma should be low

Goal of Treatment

The primary goal in the evaluation of any patient who has sustained a blunt head injury is to determine the severity of the injury and identify ciTBI. As with all trauma evaluations, the initial goal of treatment is immediate stabilization.

Current Evidence. Neurotrauma is one of the most common reasons for emergency department evaluation with over 600,000 annual visits by children from birth to 19 years. Visits for younger children up to 4 years of age have increased significantly in the past several years, accounting for the highest rates of emergency department utilization. The age group with the highest number of fatalities continues to be adolescents ages 15 to 19. Common mechanisms of injury include falls, motor vehicle collisions either as a passenger or pedestrian struck by, bicycle accidents, sports-related, assaults and nonaccidental trauma. A detailed description of anatomy, pathophysiology, and causes of increased intracranial pressure (ICP) is included in Chapter 36 Injury: Head.

Briefly, the spectrum of traumatic brain injury (TBI) patterns ranges from minor head injury, concussion, skull fracture, pneumocephalus, intracranial hematoma, cerebral edema, diffuse axonal injury (DAI), cerebral herniation to death. Cerebral hematomas may be extra-axial, occurring in the epidural or subdural space or intra-axial, occurring within the parenchyma of the brain. Most recent studies have delineated other types of intracranial injury from ciTBI. The definition of ciTBI includes the presence of a depressed skull fracture necessitating surgical elevation, neurosurgical intervention including, but not limited to, invasive ICP monitoring, ventriculostomy, hematoma evacuation and/or decompressive craniectomy, endotracheal intubation for more than 24 hours, hospital admission for 48 hours or more, and death. Utilizing this definition, the overall incidence of ciTBI ranges from 0.02% to 4.4%.

TBI is the leading cause of acquired disability in children. Neurologic and cognitive deficits are related to patient age at time of injury, severity of injury, and degree of structural injury. Unique considerations should be given to children with shunt-dependent hydrocephalus and bleeding diatheses, platelet disorders, or coagulation disorders such as hemophilia.

Clinical Considerations (See Also Chapter 89 Head Trauma)

Clinical Recognition. The historical and physical features of TBI encompass a wide spectrum of signs and symptoms. For a detailed review of signs and symptoms, please review Chapter 36 Injury: Head. The presentation of infants may be nonspecific and include poor feeding, vomiting, irritability, a bulging anterior fontanelle, altered mental status defined as a pediatric Glasgow Coma Score of less than or equal to 14 (Table 121.1), lethargy, seizure, and presence of scalp hematoma and/or depression. Typical complaints in children include headache, progression of headache with increasing severity, vomiting, confusion, altered mental status defined as a Glasgow Coma Scale (GCS) of less than or equal to 14 (Table 121.1), seizure, lethargy, focal neurologic abnormality, obtundation, or signs of a basilar skull fracture, such as Battle sign, periorbital ecchymosis hemotympanum, and cerebral spinal fluid (CSF) otorrhea or rhinorrhea. Signs of impending cerebral herniation include altered mental status, pupillary changes, bradycardia, hypertension, and respiratory depression. Recent clinical decision rules to assist in the determination for emergent radiography have stratified ciTBI risk based on key historical and physical examination features. The clinical decision rules are applied to two separate patient populations, children less than 2 years of age and children 2 years of age and greater. Children less than 2 years of age provide a unique challenge to the clinician as they commonly present after minor trauma but may be asymptomatic or clinical assessment may be difficult. Additionally, the clinician must always have a low index of suspicion for nonaccidental trauma, as the incidence of child abuse in this age group is high. Head injury accounts for the highest mortality in nonaccidental or intentional injury. For a detailed review of inflicted injuries please refer to the Chapter 95 Child Abuse/Assault.

The features that place children less than 2 years of age at higher risk of having ciTBI include altered mental status, especially if the parent is concerned that the child is acting abnormally, parietal, temporal or occipital scalp hematoma, loss of consciousness >5 seconds, evidence of depressed or basilar skull fracture, bulging anterior fontanelle, persistent vomiting, posttraumatic seizure, focal neurologic examination findings, or suspicion of nonaccidental trauma. The features that place children 2 years of age and greater at higher risk of ciTBI include altered mental status, evidence of depressed or basilar skull fracture, posttraumatic seizure, prolonged loss of consciousness, worsening severe headache, and focal neurologic examination findings (see Table 121.2). Emergent neuroimaging should be performed for any child with one or more of these features. As certain features dictate the use of radiographic imaging, the absence of these features should compel the clinician to spare the patient unnecessary radiation exposure. Children less than the age 2 who have a normal mental status with normal behavior, lack a scalp hematoma or have a frontal scalp hematoma, without evidence of skull fracture and a normal neurologic examination should neither undergo radiographic imaging; nor should older children who have a normal mental status, no loss of consciousness, no vomiting, no severe headache, without evidence of a skull fracture and a normal neurologic examination.

The diagnostically challenging patient population is the children in the intermediate risk category. These are the children who may have isolated features indicative of ciTBI with resolution or improvement of symptoms and a normal neurologic examination. Observation for 4 to 6 hours after the injury may offer an alternative to emergent neuroimaging.

Diagnostic Imaging. Plain skull radiography has a limited role in evaluating blunt head injury as it cannot provide detail regarding intracranial injury. Because computed tomography

TABLE 121.1

GLASGOW COMA SCALE AND PEDIATRIC GLASGOW COMA SCALE

Sign	Glasgow Coma Scale [1]	Pediatric Glasgow Coma Scale [2]	Score
Eye opening	Spontaneous	Spontaneous	4
	To command	To sound	3
	To pain	To pain	2
	None	None	1
Verbal response	Oriented	Age-appropriate vocalizations, orientation to sound, follows objects, interacts, smiles	5
	Confused, disoriented	Cries, irritable	4
	Inappropriate words	Cries to pain	3
	Incomprehensible sounds	Moans to pain	2
	None	None	1
Motor response	Obeys commands	Spontaneous movements	6
	Localizes pain	Withdraws to touch (localizes pain)	5
	Withdraws	Withdraws to pain	4
	Abnormal flexion to pain	Abnormal flexion to pain (decorticate posture)	3
	Abnormal extension to pain	Abnormal extension to pain (decerebrate posture)	2
	None	None	1
Best total score			**15**

Modified with data from Teasdale G, Jennett B. Assessment of coma and impaired consciousness. A practical scale. *Lancet* 1974;2:81; Holmes JF, Palchak MJ, MacFarlane T, et al. Performance of the pediatric Glasgow coma scale in children with blunt head trauma. *Acad Emerg Med* 2005;12:814.

TABLE 121.2

CLINICAL FEATURES ASSOCIATED WITH HIGHER RISK OF CiTBI

Children <2 yrs of age	Children ≥2 yrs of age
Altered mental status or abnormal behavior per caregiver	Altered mental status
Nonfrontal location of scalp hematoma	Depressed or basilar skull fracture
Loss of consciousness >5 sec	Posttraumatic seizure
Depressed or basilar skull fracture	Loss of consciousness
Bulging anterior fontanelle	Focal neurologic findings
Persistent vomiting	Worsening severe headache
Posttraumatic seizure	
Focal neurologic findings	
Suspicion of nonaccidental trauma	

(CT) is noninvasive and widely available, it is used for screening and diagnosis of intracranial injuries. Current generation 16-detector scanners are capable of rendering very high resolution images along with high speed data acquisition. CT imaging can detect mass lesions that may be surgical, early signs of cerebral edema including compression of the ventricular system and/or perimesencephalic cisterns, midline shift, or loss of grey to white matter interface. CT is preferred for detection of fractures and subarachnoid hemorrhage.

Magnetic resonance imaging (MRI) is more sensitive than CT as it provides greater anatomical detail of the brain and ventricles, but it can be less readily available and requires longer periods of time to obtain imaging. As an alternative, "fast" MRI techniques are being used to assess TBI. This option is not the current standard protocol in many facilities. MRI utilizing T1, T2, and fluid attenuated inversion recovery (FLAIR) images is more sensitive allowing delineation of the nature and timing of hemorrhage. Additionally, diffusion-weighted imaging (DWI) outlines hypoxic-ischemic or DAI.

Management. As with any trauma evaluation, the initial assessment should focus on airway, breathing, circulation, disability and exposure per trauma guidelines. Please review the Chapters 2 Approach to the Injured Child and 89 Head Trauma for complete details as this is beyond the scope of this discussion. Management principles focus on airway management while maintaining cervical spine immobilization to provide adequate oxygenation and ventilation to prevent hypoxia and hypercarbia. Intravascular volume should be maintained to provide adequate cerebral perfusion pressure, thereby, preventing secondary brain injury. Certain adjuncts should be used in management of patients with suspected head injuries. Immobilization of the cervical spine should be maintained until it is determined that there is not a concomitant cervical spine injury (Spinal Cord Injury is covered in Chapter 120 Neck Trauma). This is accomplished with using the chin lift maneuver thus avoiding jaw thrust, application of semirigid cervical collar or inline manual stabilization. If intubation is determined to be necessary, endotracheal intubation is the preferred method. Evaluation by a neurosurgeon is preferred prior to intubation with neuromuscular blockade, but there should not be any delay in obtaining an advanced airway. Patients should be preoxygenated, and pretreatment medications that should be utilized are atropine, in all children less than 1 year of age, and lidocaine. Atropine at 0.02 mg per kg of weight with a maximum of 0.5 mg will help decrease the vagal response to intubation. Lidocaine at 1 to 2 mg per kg of weight with a maximum of 100 mg is used to prevent potential increased ICP by blunting airway reflexes. Rapid sequence intubation includes sedation and paralysis. Sedative medications should be used to decrease airway responses and keep the patient comfortable (refer to Chapter 3 Airway). Preferred medications for the child in whom a head injury is suspected include Etomidate and Midazolam. Neuromuscular blockade and paralysis may be achieved with Rocuronium or succinylcholine. There is no available outcome data regarding the use of sedatives and paralytic medications in children with ciTBI, and their use should be tailored to the individual patient.

Other noninvasive maneuvers should be a standard management to decrease ICP. The head of the bed should be elevated to 30 degrees, the head should be kept in a neutral position while maintaining cervical spine immobilization, ventilation to maintain $PaCO_2$ at 35 to 40 mm Hg, continuous sedation infusion to prevent complications after intubation and agitation. Aggressive hyperventilation should not be the standard as an initial therapy, however, it may be necessary acutely for refractory intracranial hypertension and to prevent cerebral herniation.

If the above measures are not adequate to control ICP, hyperosmolar therapy may be necessary to control cerebral perfusion pressure. Hypertonic or 3% saline may be used in the acute setting with bolus doses of 6 to 10 mL per kg of weight. Continuous infusions of hypertonic saline may be necessary to maintain ICP less than 20 mm Hg with doses starting at 0.1 mL per kg of weight per hour that may need to be increased incrementally to 1.0 mL per kg of weight per hour, titrated to keep target serum sodium levels between 145 and 155 mEq/L. Serum osmolarity should be monitored and maintained at less than 360 mOsm/L. In conjunction with hyperosmolar therapy, externalization of CSF drainage by placement of a ventricular catheter may be necessary to monitor and treat ICP. Depending on the stability of the patient, decompressive craniectomy may be necessary, especially for the evacuation of intracranial hematomas. Craniectomy is necessary for large hematomas associated with neurologic compromise or impending cerebral herniation. The timing of surgical intervention depends on the severity of the injury and stability of the patient, and should be determined in collaboration with neurosurgery.

Medications that are not routinely recommended in children with ciTBI include steroids and anticonvulsants. The use of corticosteroids has not been shown to either improve neurologic outcome or decrease ICP. When used in spinal cord injuries, there is anecdotal evidence that it may worsen outcomes for patients with ciTBI. Young children have increased risk and rate of posttraumatic seizures. The latest consensus statement advises the clinician "to consider" the use of anticonvulsants to reduce the incidence of posttraumatic seizures. Phenytoin with loading doses of 10 to 20 mg per kg of weight has been used to treat seizures acutely, and is the medication currently recommended if prophylaxis is initiated. Many centers are using other anticonvulsant medications as well, including and not limited to, phenobarbital at loading doses of 10 to 20 mg per kg of weight or Levetiracetam at loading doses of 30 mg per kg of weight.

Head trauma has been recognized as a common cause of posttraumatic hydrocephalus. As management schemes for neurotrauma have improved over recent years, more patients are surviving severe head traumas with hydrocephalus occurring as a delayed complication. About 4% of patients develop posttraumatic hydrocephalus requiring surgical CSF diversion.

Specific Brain Injury Patterns

The spectrum of brain injury patterns ranges in severity from mild and isolated to diffuse with associated hemorrhages. The continuum of injury is based upon mechanism, however, neurologic outcome is related to degree of neurologic impairment at time of presentation.

Diffuse Injury. These injury patterns include DAI, cerebral edema, hypoxic ischemia, and diffuse vascular injuries. DAI is due to shear injuries of axons and blood vessels involving the white matter of the brain. The shear occurs with acceleration and deceleration or rotational forces involving the brain matter. The degree of tissue disruption is indicative of the amount of energy dissipation. DAI may appear normal on CT scan, but as the severity of injury increases, DAI may be associated with intracerebral hemorrhages, especially multiple petechial hemorrhages in the deep white matter. MRI is more sensitive in delineating transient signal changes along white matter tracts.

Cerebral edema may be caused by a multitude of factors. Not only is edema due to direct insult to the neurons with local release of inflammatory mediators and vascular leakage, but it also may occur as a secondary injury due to hypoxemia and changes in cerebral blood flow. On CT scan, brain edema appears as an area of decreased density associated with brain shift, especially pronounced with loss of gray–white matter interface differentiation. Both DAI and cerebral edema are commonly associated with intracerebral hemorrhage and/or contusion and may lead to herniation. The component of hemorrhage or significant mass effect resulting from edema becomes a neurosurgical emergency.

Focal Injury. These injury patterns include contusions, lacerations, hemorrhage, and midline shifts. Cerebral contusions are typically due to direct impact of the brain along dural edges or intracranial bony surfaces. The presentation may be benign or symptomatic with a focal neurologic deficit or seizure. Isolated contusions with minimal localized swelling without midline shift are injuries that may be managed nonsurgically.

Subdural hemorrhage occurs when bridging vessels rupture into the potential space between the dura and arachnoid. This anatomic location allows the blood to transverse cranial sutures and accounts for the typical crescent shaped or convex appearance (Fig. 121.1). Subdural hematomas in children under the age of 2 years are more likely to be associated with child abuse than other injury patterns. Please refer to Chapter 95 Child Abuse/Assault for further discussion.

In contrast, the vascular injury causing epidural hemorrhage, typically the middle meningeal artery or dural venous sinus, allows blood to transverse the space between the dura and overlying bony surface. The accumulating epidural blood is not able to transverse the dural attachments at the sutures accounting for the lens-shaped biconvex appearance on radiographic imaging (Fig. 121.2). Venous bleeding may accumulate slowly and account for the classic presentation of patients with epidural hematomas with a period of lucidity followed by rapid clinical deterioration.

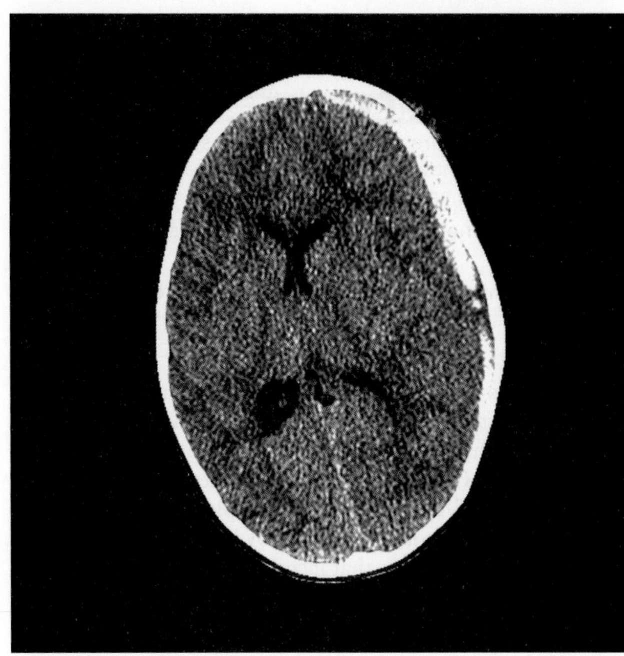

FIGURE 121.1 Traumatic subdural hemorrhage. Axial noncontrast CT shows a significant 6-mm SDH over the left hemispheric convexity with approximately 9 mm of midline shift.

Subarachnoid hemorrhage involves traumatic injury to the vessels supplying the pia mater. As the cerebral subarachnoid space extends to the spinal subarachnoid, the accumulation of blood may be extensive and layers along the bony surface.

There are no specific criteria for surgical intervention with cerebral hemorrhage. Temporizing measures described above in addition to surgical intervention, including craniotomy for hematoma evacuation or decompressive craniectomy, may be necessary to treat high ICP in a patient whose condition is deteriorating.

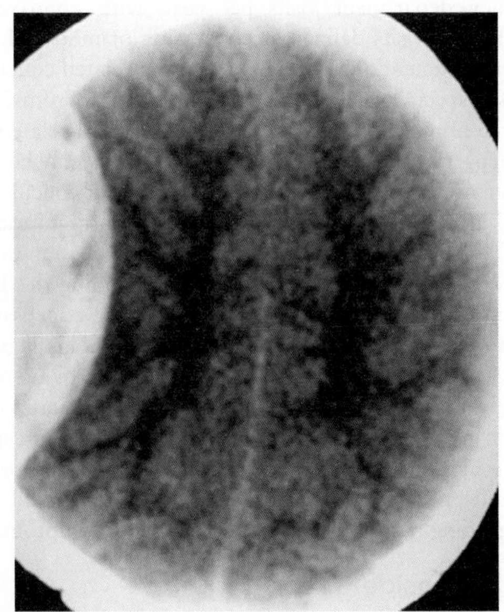

FIGURE 121.2 Epidural hematoma. A head computed tomography scan shows the classic biconvex hyperdensity of an epidural hematoma.

CONCUSSION

CLINICAL PEARLS AND PITFALLS

- Common features involve somatic symptoms, physical signs, behavioral or emotional changes, cognitive impairments, and/or sleep disturbances
- Eighty to ninety percent of symptoms resolve within 7 to 10 days
- Goal of therapy is physical and cognitive rest

Concussion is a clinical syndrome of biomechanically induced brain dysfunction without apparent radiographic injury. The panel consensus statement from the fourth International Conference on Concussion in Sport defines concussion as "a brain injury and is defined as a complex pathophysiologic process affecting the brain, induced by biomechanical forces." Several common features that incorporate clinical, pathologic, and biomechanical injury constructs that may be utilized in defining the nature of a concussive head injury include:

1. Concussion may be caused either by a direct blow to the head, face, neck, or elsewhere on the body with an "impulsive" force transmitted to the head.
2. Concussion typically results in the rapid onset of short-lived impairment of neurologic function that resolves spontaneously. However, in some cases, symptoms and signs may evolve over a number of minutes to hours.
3. Concussion may result in neuropathologic changes, but the acute clinical symptoms largely reflect a functional disturbance rather than a structural injury and, as such, no abnormality is seen on standard structural neuroimaging studies.
4. Concussion results in a graded set of clinical symptoms that may or may not involve loss of consciousness. Resolution of the clinical and cognitive symptoms typically follows a sequential course. However, it is important to note that in some cases symptoms may be prolonged.

Current Evidence. Evaluation for TBI accounts for 600,000 emergency department visits per year, with approximately 75% of those visits defined as concussion or mild TBI. There has been a tremendous emphasis on sports-related concussions and TBI, especially in children and adolescents. From 2001 to 2009, the number of sports- or recreational TBI-related emergency department visits increased by 57%. This may be due, in part, to increased identification and codifying of concussion, as well as, local and state policies regarding sports injuries. The state of Washington was the first to pass a concussion in sports law in 2009, and by 2013 all 50 states including the District of Columbia had enacted legislation regarding concussions in sports for youth and/or high school athletes. This legislation focuses on education, recommendations for removing athletes from play and permission to return to play. Many states require return to play permission be obtained by a healthcare professional, which may influence the number of TBI-related visits. Please refer to Chapter 36 Injury: Head, for a detailed discussion regarding pathophysiology and signs and symptoms.

Clinical Considerations

Clinical Recognition. The features of concussion are nonspecific and some may be indicative of ciTBI. The most common symptoms include headache, dizziness, gait abnormalities, confusion, disorientation, difficulty concentrating, nausea, vomiting, loss of consciousness, amnesia both retrograde and anterograde, light and noise sensitivity, visual changes, sleep disturbances, emotional lability, and irritability. The physical examination in patients with concussions is typically normal. The evaluation should include a comprehensive neurologic examination including mental status, gait, and cerebellar function. Any focal neurologic findings during the physical examination should alert the clinician to the potential for ciTBI and prompt the need for neuroimaging.

Multiple concussion assessment tools have been utilized in children and adolescents. The list includes, and is not limited to, the Sport Concussion Assessment Tool Version 3 (SCAT 3), Child-SCAT3, Balance Error Scoring System (BESS), Standardized Assessment of Concussion, individual sideline assessment tools, and the Centers for Disease Control and Prevention's (CDC) Acute Concussion Evaluation (ACE) tools. Many of these tools have not been validated in children which create challenges for their use in the pediatric age group. Most of these instruments are in depth, detailed, and time consuming. Their use is not conducive to the emergency department environment. While many sports personnel administer preparticipation assessments utilizing these tools, it is not standard, and those results may not be accessible to the clinician during the initial posttraumatic evaluation. A recent modification of the CDCs ACE tools for concussion diagnosis and discharge, modified for use in the ED, demonstrated improved patient follow-up and adherence to the discharge recommendations.

Diagnostic Imaging. Neuroimaging, whether CT or MRI, is not routinely performed for the child who presents with symptoms of concussion, except when the concern for ciTBI arises. As previously discussed, features that warrant emergent neuroimaging include altered mental status, evidence of depressed or basilar skull fracture, posttraumatic seizure, prolonged loss of consciousness, worsening headache, and focal neurologic examination findings. CT is widely available and quickly detects significant ciTBI. MRI may be preferred to CT to avoid radiation exposure, but is not as widely available and time may be of the essence with neurologic deterioration. MRI may be performed as an outpatient if the patient has worsening or prolonged duration of symptoms after the initial evaluation. Preliminary evidence reveals that functional MRI, as well as, proton magnetic resonance spectroscopy and diffusion tensor imaging may identify abnormalities associated with cognitive deficits. These imaging modalities are quite specific and not currently accessible at most centers.

Management. If the injury occurs during a sporting event, an on-field or sideline evaluation is done to determine disposition. If there is no licensed healthcare provider immediately available to make that determination, the patient should be removed from participation. This necessitates a complete evaluation by a physician, which may involve an emergency department visit. As with any trauma evaluation, the initial assessment should focus on airway, breathing, circulation, disability, and exposure per trauma guidelines (see Chapter 2 Approach to the Injured Child).

After excluding ciTBI or other traumatic injuries, strategic concussion management includes symptomatic relief and restriction of activity with physical and cognitive rest. Most authors recommend a graduated return to activities. Judicious use of pain medication and antiemetics should be recommended as not to mask symptoms. Their use may be necessary, but should be taken into account when recommending return to activities. An easy rule of thumb may be to restrict all physical activities until asymptomatic for 1 week. Other recommendations to improve cognitive rest should include good sleep hygiene, adequate hydration, and decreased use of electronic devices unless necessary for school performance. Then graduated return to full activity may progress slowly after patient has been asymptomatic for at least a week. This slow progression may begin with light aerobic exercise, advancing to sports-specific exercise followed by noncontact drills and full-contact practice with final advancement to full participation in all sporting activities.

SKULL FRACTURES

CLINICAL PEARLS AND PITFALLS

- Linear, parietal, nondepressed skull fractures are the most common
- Skull fractures are common in accidental and nonaccidental trauma
- Most linear, nondepressed skull fractures heal without complications

Goal of Treatment

The primary goal of treatment is to delineate simple, linear, nondepressed skull fractures from complicated skull fractures. Complicated skull fractures are more likely to be associated with intracranial injury and/or nonaccidental trauma. Early injury pattern recognition and neurosurgical consultation to determine need for surgical intervention is ideal.

Current Evidence

Unilateral, linear skull fractures account for approximately 75% of pediatric skull fractures (Fig. 121.3). This estimation applies to both accidental and nonaccidental pediatric skull fractures. The incidence of underlying intracranial injury ranges from 15% to 30%. Complicated skull fractures may include fractures that cross suture lines, complex, burst, depressed, diastatic, bilateral, multiple, or open fractures. Figure 121.4 shows a closed, depressed skull fracture. Complicated fractures have, not only an increased likelihood of underlying intracranial injury, but also an increased association with nonaccidental trauma. Of the complex fractures, ones that cross suture lines, bilateral or multiple fractures were notably more common in nonaccidental injury. The complete description and evaluation of abusive or nonaccidental head trauma is discussed separately in the Chapter 95 Child Abuse/Assault.

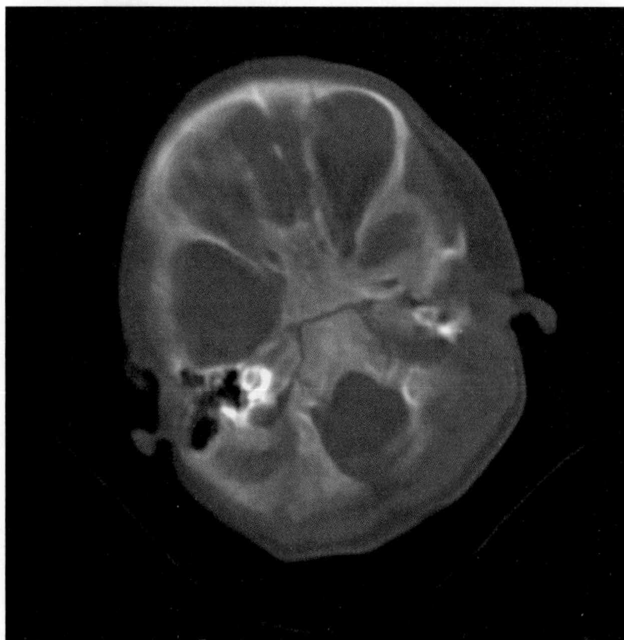

FIGURE 121.3 Linear skull fracture. An axial CT scan with bone windows demonstrates a closed linear nondisplaced skull fracture through the left orbital roof.

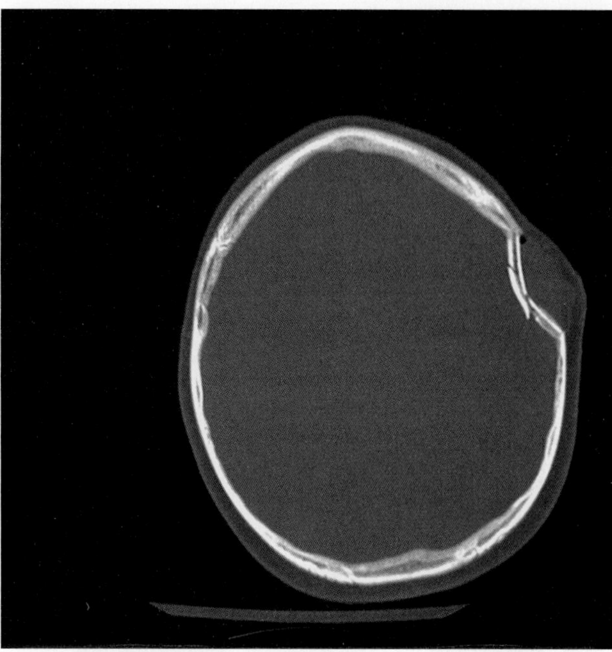

FIGURE 121.4 Depressed skull fracture. An axial CT scan with bone windows demonstrates a closed depressed skull fracture over the left parietal bone.

Clinical Considerations

Clinical Recognition

Many of the historical and physical findings suggestive of skull fracture are the same as described above for ciTBI. The history may include a witnessed fall, motor vehicle collision, or assault. However, in many instances, there is no accompanying history of a traumatic event. Many infants will present with an isolated soft tissue swelling or scalp hematoma. Other presentations may be nonspecific and include poor feeding, vomiting, irritability, a bulging anterior fontanelle, altered mental status defined as a pediatric Glasgow Coma Score of less than or equal to 14 (Table 121.1), lethargy, seizure, presence of scalp hematoma, palpable skull defect, or crepitus. Typical complaints in children include headache, localized pain or soft tissue swelling, vomiting, confusion, altered mental status defined as a GCS of less than or equal to 14 (Table 121.1), seizure, lethargy, focal neurologic abnormality, obtundation, or signs of a basilar skull fracture (Fig. 121.5).

The area of the skull most commonly involved is the parietal bone, followed by the occipital and temporal bones. The physical examination may be normal as soft-tissue swelling

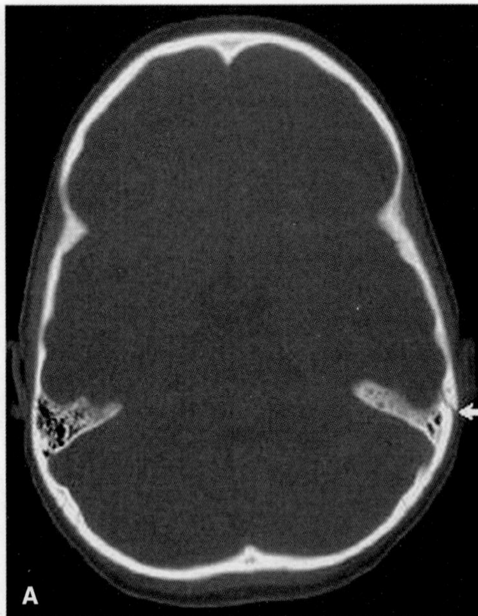

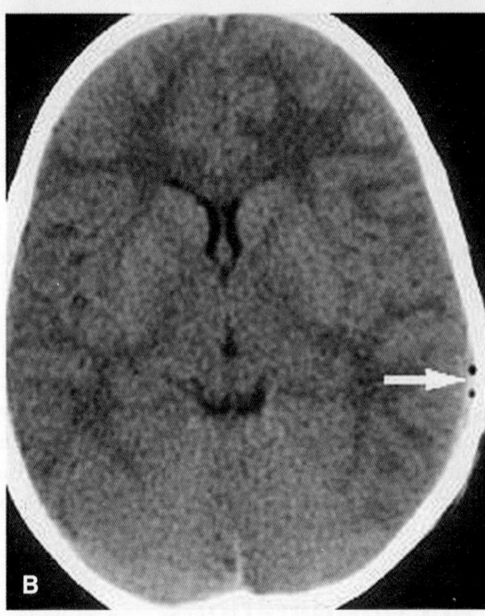

FIGURE 121.5 Basilar skull fracture. **A:** The *arrow* indicates a fracture of the left temporal bone. The adjacent mastoid air cells are somewhat opacified. **B:** A small extra-axial hematoma with associated pneumocephaly is seen (*arrow*).

may not be present at the time of evaluation, or may include a scalp hematoma or soft-tissue swelling, palpable skull defect or crepitus. Signs of a basilar skull fracture (Fig. 121.5) include Battle sign, periorbital ecchymosis, hemotympanum, and CSF otorrhea, or rhinorrhea. A full neurologic examination is mandated to isolate any focal neurologic deficits. These focal deficits are related to the underlying intracranial injury and allow for clinical detection of regional lesions. The neurologic deficits frequently identified with basilar skull fractures include anosmia, nystagmus, hearing loss (either conductive or sensorineural), abducens nerve palsy, or facial paralysis.

Diagnostic Imaging. As previously discussed, skull radiography has a limited role as it cannot provide detail regarding intracranial injury. CT is the preferred imaging modality for the initial evaluation as it allows for the detection of fractures utilizing bone windows, especially with three-dimensional reconstruction capability.

Ultrasonography has been shown to be sensitive for the detection of skull fractures. It has limited capability to detect underlying intracranial injury leading to a limited role in the initial evaluation of children with skull fractures. It may be utilized emergently if there is no availability of CT to assist in facilitating transfer to a pediatric trauma facility. Another future application may be outpatient follow-up settings monitoring skull fractures, but this is not the current standard and there is no evidence supporting this application.

Management. Unilateral, linear, nondepressed skull fractures without underlying intracranial injury typically heal spontaneously and do not necessitate immediate neurosurgical intervention. Recent evidence suggests that an increasing number of patients are managed on an outpatient basis. Less than 1% of patients who returned after initial discharge from the emergency department necessitated neurosurgical intervention. Patients with a nonfocal neurologic examination who are asymptomatic may be discharged from the emergency department if there is no concomitant intracranial injury, distracting traumatic injury, nor a concern for nonaccidental trauma.

Neurosurgical consultation is mandated in patients with complicated, basilar, and open skull fractures and when fractures are associated with underlying intracranial injury. Diastatic fractures greater than 3 mm, burst fractures and depressed skull fractures greater than 1 cm of depression are not likely to heal without surgical reconstruction due to dural injury. Elective early repair of dura and fracture fragments can prevent the late complication of a growing skull fracture. Growing skull fractures are found months to years after the initial injury and consist of craniocerebral erosion due to an enlarging leptomeningeal cyst or vascular injury which leads to an enlarging skull defect. The expanding defect may cause neurologic deterioration over time.

Early and late onset posttraumatic seizures are increased in patients with depressed skull fractures and retained bony fragments, as well as other intracranial injuries as described above. The routine use of prophylactic anticonvulsant medication is not recommended in patients with depressed skull fractures.

Basilar skull fractures should be managed in conjunction with neurosurgical consultation, but may necessitate otologic consultation as well. Despite the potential for involvement of the mastoid air cells or paranasal sinuses, the risk of meningitis in basilar skull fractures is low. There is no evidence to recommend the routine use of prophylactic antibiotics in patients with basilar skull fractures with or without CSF leakage. The risk of meningitis increased significantly in patients who had persistent CSF leakage that did not resolve within 7 days. Neurosurgical and otologic intervention may be necessary in temporal bone fractures associated with nerve palsies and persistent CSF leakage. Interventions may include external CSF drainage to decrease intrathecal pressure, operative repair of dural lacerations or fistulas.

Additional evaluation and management of children with nonaccidental head trauma are discussed separately. Please review Chapter 95 Child Abuse/Assault.

Clinical Indications for Discharge. Unilateral, linear, nondepressed skull fractures without underlying intracranial injury in patients who do not have a distracting traumatic injury with a normal neurologic examination may be discharged from the pediatric emergency department. If there is any apprehension regarding the potential for nonaccidental trauma, social work consultation, as well as neurosurgical or surgical consultation, should be obtained prior to discharge.

Suggested Readings and Key References

Anderson V, Catroppa C, Morse S, et al. Recovery of intellectual ability following traumatic brain injury in childhood: impact of injury severity and age at injury. *Pediatr Neurosurg* 2000;32(6):282–290.

Bracken MB. Steroids for acute spinal cord injury. *Cochrane Database Syst Rev* 2012;1:CD001046.

Bressan S, Romanato S, Mion T, et al. Implementation of adapted PECARN decision rule for children with minor head injury in the pediatric emergency department. *Acad Emerg Med* 2012;19(7): 801–807.

Centers for Disease Control and Prevention (CDC). *Traumatic brain injury in the United States ED visits, hospitalizations, deaths 2002–2006*. Atlanta, GA: US Department of Health and Human Services, CDC, 2010. Available at https://www.cdc.gov/traumaticbraininjury. Accessed October 15, 2014.

Centers for Disease Control and Prevention. Non-fatal traumatic brain injuries related to sports and recreational activities among persons aged ≤19 years—United States, 2001–2009. *MMWR Morb Mortal Wkly Rep* 2011;60(39):1337–1342.

Easter JS, Bakes K, Dhaliwal J, et al. Comparison of PECARN, CATCH and CHALICE rules for children with minor head injury: a prospective cohort study. *Ann Emerg Med* 2014;64(2):145–152.

Giza CC, Kutcher JS, Ashwal S, et al. Summary of evidence-based guideline update: evaluation and management of concussion in sports: Report of the Guideline Development Subcommittee of the American Academy of Neurology. *Neurology* 2013;80(24):2250–2257.

Holmes JF, Palchak MJ, MacFarlane T, et al. Performance of the pediatric Glasgow coma scale in children with blunt head trauma. *Acad Emerg Med* 2005;12(9):814–819.

Hurlbert RJ, Hamilton MG. Methylprednisolone for acute spinal cord injury: 5-year practice reversal. *Can J Neurol Sci* 2008;35(1): 41–45.

Keightley ML, Chen JK, Ptito A. Examining the neural impact of pediatric concussion: a scoping review of multimodal and integrative approaches using functional and structural MRI techniques. *Curr Opin Pediatr* 2012;24(6):709–716.

Kemp AM, Dunstan F, Harrison S, et al. Patterns of skeletal fractures in child abuse: systematic review. *BMJ* 2008;337:a1518.

Kochanek PM, Carney N, Adelson PD, et al.; American Academy of Pediatrics-Section on Neurological Surgery; American Association of Neurological Surgeons/Congress of Neurological Surgeons; Child Neurology Society, et al. Guidelines for the acute medical management of severe traumatic brain injury in infants, children, and adolescents-second edition. *Pediatr Crit Care Med* 2012;13(1): S1–S85.

Kuppermann N, Holmes JF, Dayan PS, et al.; Pediatric Emergency Care Applied Research Network (PECARN). Identification of children at very low risk of clinically important brain injuries after head trauma: a prospective cohort study. *Lancet* 2009;374(9696):1160–1170.

Mannix R, Monuteaux MC, Schutzman SA, et al. Isolated skull fractures: trends in management in US pediatric emergency departments. *Ann Emerg Med* 2013;62(4):327–331.

Mataro M, Poco MA, Sahuquillo J, et al. Neuropsychological outcome in relation to the Traumatic Coma Data Bank classification of CT imaging. *J Neurotrauma* 2001;18(9):869–879.

McCrory P, Meeuwisse WH, Aubry M, et al. Consensus statement on concussion in sport: the 4th International Conference on Concussion in Sport held in Zurich, November 2012. *Br J Sports Med* 2013; 47(5):250–258.

Missios S, Quebada PB, Forero JA, et al. Quick-brain magnetic resonance imaging for nonhydrocephalus indications. *J Neurosurg Pediatr* 2008;2(6):438–444.

National Spinal Cord Injury Statistical Center. *The 2004 annual statistical report for the model spinal cord injury care systems*. Birmingham, AL: University of Alabama, 2004.

Osmond MH, Klassen TP, Wells GA, et al. Pediatric Emergency Research Canada (PERC) Head Injury Study Group. CATCH: a clinical decision rule for the use of computed tomography in children with minor head injury. *CMAJ* 2010;182(4):341–348.

Parent S, Mac-Thiong JM, Roy-Beaudry M, et al. Spinal cord injury in the pediatric population: a systematic review of the literature. *J Neurotrauma* 2011;28(8):1515–1524.

Parri N, Crosby BJ, Glass C, et al. Ability of emergency ultrasonography to detect pediatric skull fractures: a prospective, observational study. *J Emerg Med* 2013;44(1):135–141.

Riera A, Chen L. Ultrasound evaluation of skull fractures in children: a feasibility study. *Pediatr Emerg Care* 2012;28(5):420–425.

Schutzman SA, Barnes P, Duhaime AC, et al. Evaluation and management of children younger than two years old with apparently minor head trauma: proposed guideline. *Pediatrics* 2001;107(5):983–993.

Teasdale G, Jennett B. Assessment of coma and impaired consciousness. A practical scale. *Lancet* 1974;2(7872):81–84.

Wood JN, Christian CW, Adams CM, et al. Skeletal surveys in infants with isolated skull fractures. *Pediatrics* 2009;123(2):e247–e252.

Zuckerbraun NS, Atabaki S, Collins MW, et al. Use of modified acute concussion evaluation tools in the emergency department. *Pediatrics* 2014;133(4):635–642.

CHAPTER 122 ■ OCULAR TRAUMA

CINDY G. ROSKIND, MD AND ALEX V. LEVIN, MD, MHSc, FRCSC

GOALS OF EMERGENCY CARE

The clinical evaluation of children with eye trauma should focus on the prompt recognition of the most severe eye injuries, without causing additional damage to the eye, and the initiation of timely ophthalmologic consultation. The most important goal is to quickly recognize those injuries in need of emergent consultation with ophthalmology (Table 122.1).

KEY POINTS

- Prioritize and stabilize the ABCs—the management of life-threatening injuries must be prioritized over any eye injury.
- The first step in the examination of the traumatized eye should be to assess the visual acuity of both the injured and the unaffected eye.
- Ensure the structural integrity of the eye quickly and rule out the presence of a ruptured globe.

RELATED CHAPTERS

Signs and Symptoms

- Eye: Red Eye: Chapter 22
- Eye: Strabismus: Chapter 23
- Eye: Unequal Pupils: Chapter 24
- Eye: Visual Disturbances: Chapter 25

Medical, Surgical, and Trauma Emergencies

- Child Abuse/Assault: Chapter 95
- Neurotrauma: Chapter 121
- Ophthalmic Emergencies: Chapter 131

HISTORY

When approaching a patient with eye trauma, the emergency physician should quickly assess the child's relevant past history in order to assess the expected baseline visual acuity. The mechanism of injury should also be ascertained in order to understand the risk of serious ocular pathology and predict injury patterns. Finally, the patient should be asked about current symptoms including pain, decrease in vision, foreign body sensation, photophobia, or tearing.

Assessment of Prior Eye Pathology and Relevant Medical History

It is important to quickly establish the child's prior ocular history in order to assess the anticipated baseline visual acuity. A history of prior poor vision including use of contact lenses or glasses, amblyopia, or strabismus surgery should be queried. If the child is wearing contact lenses, they should be removed. A history of systemic disorders may predispose some children to specific injuries or worse outcomes. For example, patients with collagen disorders are more prone to globe rupture, and patients with hemoglobinopathies have a higher incidence of rebleed post hyphema.

Assessment of Injury Mechanism

Clinicians should assess the exact mechanism of injury as the type of trauma and the nature of the force inflicted may predict injury patterns and prognosis. For example, significant blunt impact directly to the eyeball (e.g., baseballs), projectiles and sharp objects (e.g., sticks or pencils) have high risk of intraocular damage. Severe blunt trauma may cause orbital fractures and can also rupture the globe. Projectiles pose great risk to the globe, and globe rupture sustained following gun injury tends to lead to poor visual outcome. Hammering is a particularly high-risk behavior for intraocular foreign bodies.

PHYSICAL EXAMINATION

Every attempt should be made to examine the eye with the child in a position of comfort in order to minimize agitation, particularly if the history or gross appearance of the eye suggests the possibility of a ruptured globe. If at any point the examination is concerning for a ruptured globe, the physician should stop the examination, shield the eye, and consult with an ophthalmologist emergently.

1. Assess Visual Acuity

The first step in the examination of the eye should be an attempt to assess the visual acuity of both the injured and the unaffected eye. The presence of bilaterally poor vision in a patient with unilateral eye trauma suggests that the cause of the poor vision may be unrelated to the trauma.

Some patients may be unable to perform this task because of eye pain, noncompliance, inability to open swollen lids, or obtundation from accompanying head trauma. Even if the eyelids remain closed, the physician should test for light perception. By shining a bright light in the direction of the eyeball through the closed eyelid, the physician can ask the patient whether he or she perceives the additional light on that side. A verbal acknowledgment or a reflex contraction of the lids indicates light perception.

If the patient is able to exhibit a greater degree of compliance, the examiner may ask the patient to count fingers that are held at varying distances. The maximum distance at which these fingers can be counted should be noted on the chart (e.g., counting fingers at 4 ft). If the patient cannot stand but can identify letters or numbers, a commercially available near visual

TABLE 122.1

INDICATIONS FOR EMERGENT CONSULTATION WITH AN OPHTHALMOLOGIST

1. Ruptured globe
2. Unable to open eye and any suspicion for globe rupture
3. Visual disturbance related to ocular trauma
4. Hyphema
5. Extraocular movement disturbance
6. Foreign body not able to be removed
7. Absent red reflex
8. Papilledema
9. Retinal hemorrhages

acuity card or any other reading material can be used to assess the quality of near vision. Very few injuries cause abnormal distance vision with preservation of near vision. Therefore, normal near vision usually indicates that the patient has not sustained a significant ocular injury. If the patient is able to comply, the examiner should obtain a visual acuity using a distance chart (see Chapter 131 Ophthalmic Emergencies).

If a patient demonstrates poor vision in the traumatized eye, the clinician can readily establish whether this deficit is related to the trauma or uncorrected refractive error using the pinhole test. When a person looks through a pinhole and experiences improvement in performance on visual acuity testing, he or she must have an uncorrected refractive error as the cause of the initially tested poor vision. If the visual deficit is related to the trauma, an ophthalmologist should be consulted. The urgency of evaluation will depend on the mechanism of injury and other physical examination findings.

2. Inspect the Periorbital Tissues and Eyelids Thoroughly

The periorbital tissues and eyelids should be carefully examined for ecchymosis, laceration, deformity, swelling, tenderness, and ptosis. Palpation of the orbital bones should be performed to assess for tenderness, deformity, or step-off that may suggest orbital fracture. If crepitus is present, it may be indicative of a fracture communicating with a sinus. Laceration in the periorbital tissue should be assessed for fat prolapse, which suggests communication with the orbital compartment and need for ophthalmology consultation. Examine sensation to evaluate for infraorbital or supraorbital nerve injury secondary to laceration or blunt trauma. For eyelid lacerations, careful attention should be paid to the location of the laceration and the depth of the wound. The eyelid should be inverted to evaluate for subconjunctival involvement, indicating that the laceration may be a full-thickness, complete perforation. Further, lacerations in close proximity to the medial canthus should prompt ophthalmology consultation for evaluation of the lacrimal duct system.

3. Open the Eyelids

If the eye has been traumatized such that the patient is unable to voluntarily open the eyelids, attempts should be made to assist the patient in doing so. A warm compress may be gently

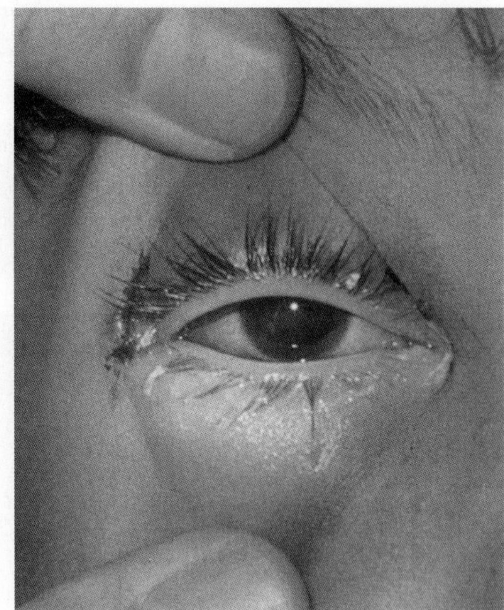

FIGURE 122.1 Opening swollen eyelids manually from the superior and inferior orbital rims.

applied to the eyelashes to loosen any crust or discharge that may be holding the eyelashes together. When opening the eyelids, avoid pressure on the eyeball, which might lead to extrusion of intraocular contents via an underlying ruptured globe. The examiner's thumbs can be placed on the supraorbital and infraorbital ridges while exerting pressure against the underlying bone, and then pulled away from each other such that the eyelids are separated (Fig. 122.1). If the eyeball cannot be readily viewed using these techniques, it is safer to refer the patient for an ophthalmology consultation. Risking the use of a speculum or retractor may upset the patient and contribute to disruption of intraocular contents if the globe is ruptured. Even the ophthalmologist may choose to avoid such attempts and proceed directly to an examination under anesthesia if the risk of ruptured globe is believed to be high.

4. Check the Red Reflex

Absence of the red reflex indicates possible corneal scar or hemorrhage within the anterior chamber or vitreous. An abnormal red reflex requires emergent ophthalmology consultation.

5. Evaluate the Pupils and the Extraocular Movements

Evaluate for pain or limitation of movement of the eye, which may suggest muscle entrapment, nerve palsy, or retrobulbar hemorrhage. Examine for symmetric shape and size of the pupil, as well as responsiveness to direct and consensual light exposure. The presence of an afferent pupillary defect suggests the possibility of serious eye injury. This can be tested with the swinging flashlight test (see Chapter 24 Eye: Unequal Pupils).

6. Evaluate the Anterior Surface of the Eye

Inspect the conjunctiva and sclera for hemorrhage, trauma, or foreign body. Examine the anterior chamber for grossly visible

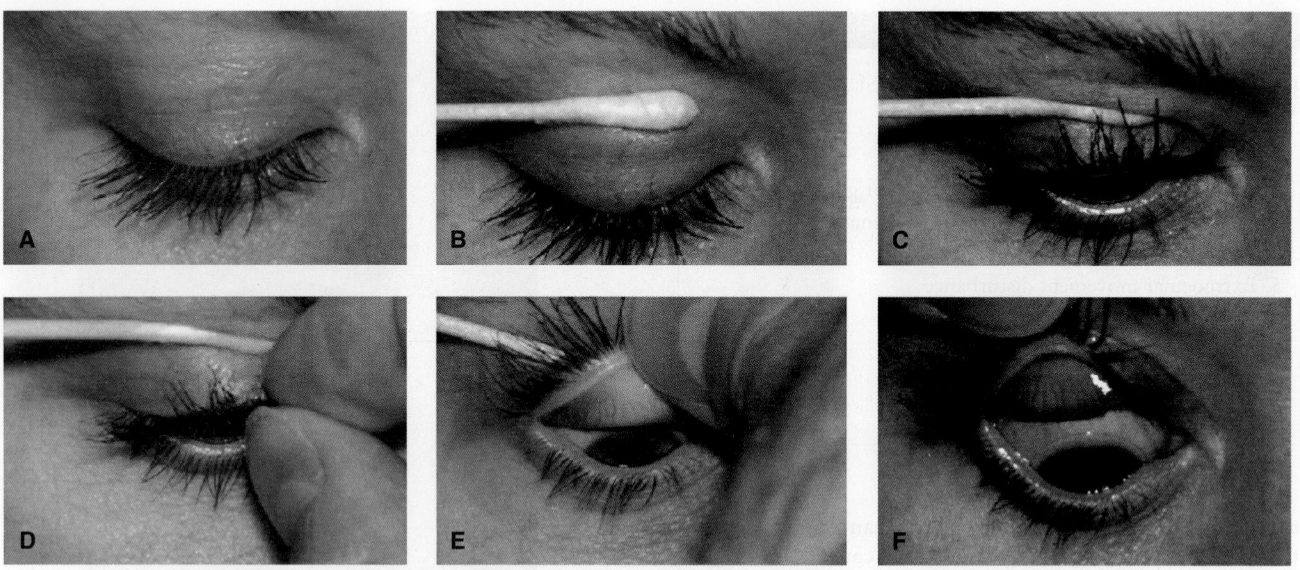

FIGURE 122.2 Upper lid eversion. Note that patient is looking down throughout procedure. In frame C, the swab is being rolled clockwise to engage skin and indirectly lift lash line. In frame E, the swab is being pushed downward as the examiner lifts the lashes upward in the opposite direction. In F, note that patient is wearing a contact lens.

layered blood. Slit lamp examination, preferably by an ophthalmologist, is required for evaluation for microhyphema.

Once a ruptured globe and a hyphema are ruled out, the administration of topical anesthetic should be considered. A drop of either proparacaine 0.5% or tetracaine 0.5% may have both diagnostic and temporary therapeutic usefulness. Any patient who is made more comfortable by the instillation of topical anesthetics must have an ocular surface problem (conjunctiva or cornea) as the cause of pain. The child who is crying and refusing to open the eyes may be compliant just a few minutes after the instillation of a topical anesthetic. Topical fluorescein is used as a diagnostic agent to stain the affected area in order to evaluate for corneal abrasions. Fluorescein is available as impregnated paper strips and as a solution combined with a topical anesthetic. When strips are used, they must be wet with either saline or topical anesthestic before instillation. Otherwise, the strip itself may cause a corneal abrasion. Fluorescein, which is orange, fluoresces yellow–green when exposed to blue light. The examiner can view through the direct ophthalmoscope, or a Wood's or Burton lamp may be used. If the staining pattern reveals one or more vertical linear abrasions, the examiner should suspect the presence of a retained foreign body under the upper lid. This foreign body may be viewed by upper lid eversion (Fig. 122.2).

7. Perform Direct Ophthalmoscopy to Evaluate for Papilledema or Retinal Hemorrhages

If either is noted, emergency consultation with ophthalmology is required. Pharmacologic dilation of the pupil may be used to assist in evaluating the posterior portion of the eye (Table 122.2).

Consider Bedside Ultrasound

Literature describing the use of emergency bedside ultrasound as an adjunct to the physical examination for the evaluation of ocular foreign body, retinal hemorrhage, papilledema, and retro bulbar hematoma is emerging.

RUPTURED GLOBE

CLINICAL PEARLS AND PITFALLS

- In order to avoid extrusion of globe contents, globe rupture requires rapid recognition and emergent evaluation by an ophthalmologist.
- Clinical findings include tear drop pupil, 360-degree subconjunctival hemorrhage, or enophthalmos (Fig. 122.3).
- If any of the above is present, immediately place an eye shield and minimize disturbing the child.

Current Evidence

Current literature related to globe rupture in children establishes that the visual prognosis is unfortunately often very poor. The following factors seem to be most predictive of poor visual outcome: blunt injury or injury resulting from a gun, young age, large wounds, wounds involving the sclera and associated injuries such as hyphema, vitreous hemorrhage, or retinal detachment. Prompt recognition and immediate referral to an ophthalmologist, ideally one with pediatric expertise, is the accepted standard of care.

TABLE 122.2

EMERGENCY DEPARTMENT OCULAR DILATING REGIMEN[a]

Phenylephrine 2.5%	For brown irides replace tropicamide with cyclopentolate 1%
Tropicamide 1%	

[a]May repeat regimen in 30 min if needed. Instilling proparacaine or tetracaine prior to these dilating drops will enhance the dilation effect.

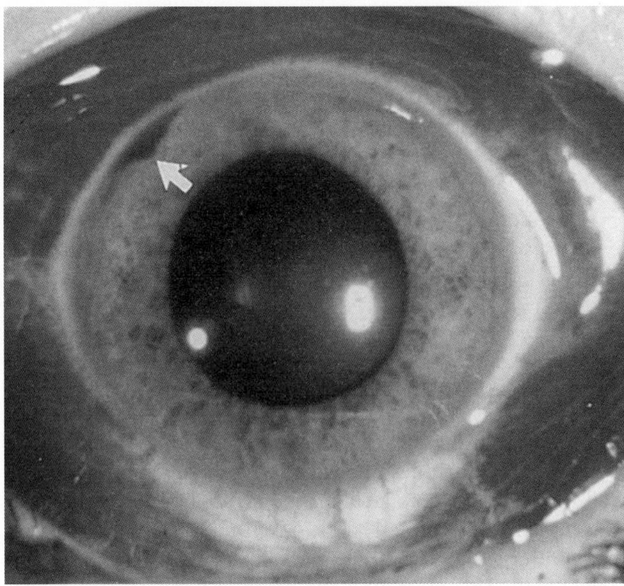

FIGURE 122.3 Subconjunctival hemorrhage extending for 360 degrees. Note the small hyphema (*arrow*).

Goals of Treatment

Globe rupture is an ominous injury that warrants emergent ophthalmology consultation. The goal of treatment in the emergency department (ED) is to avoid causing extrusion of contents from the eye, while awaiting definitive surgical repair. Further ocular examination should be stopped immediately when a globe rupture is suspected and pain control and antiemetics should be initiated.

Clinical Considerations

Clinical Recognition

A ruptured globe is defined by the presence of a corneal or scleral laceration. This condition can occur following trauma by projectile sharp implements, or blunt trauma. Sharp objects can directly penetrate the globe. In the case of blunt trauma, significant force causes compression of the globe, raising intraocular pressure and leading to rupture. Although severe intraocular disruption may occur, the eyeball has a remarkable ability to maintain its integrity. Immediately upon laceration, the iris or choroid will move forward and plug the wound at the corneoscleral junction. A blue, brown, or black material on the surface of the sclera may be visible as the iris or choroid forms a plug (Fig. 122.4). With small lacerations that are plugged by iris or choroid, the eyeball may not deflate and rather may maintain a remarkably normal external appearance. Alternatively, with the movement of the iris or choroid in more significant cases, the pupil often takes on a teardrop appearance, with the narrowest segment pointing toward the rupture (Fig. 122.5). A teardrop pupil is a worrisome indicator that a rupture may have occurred. In addition, if there is 360-degree conjunctival hemorrhage, one may be unable to see if a scleral laceration is present. Patients who present following trauma with severe 360-degree conjunctival swelling should be treated as if they have a ruptured globe and referred immediately to an ophthalmologist. Hemorrhage within the anterior chamber (hyphema) often accompanies a corneal or anterior scleral laceration (Fig. 122.4).

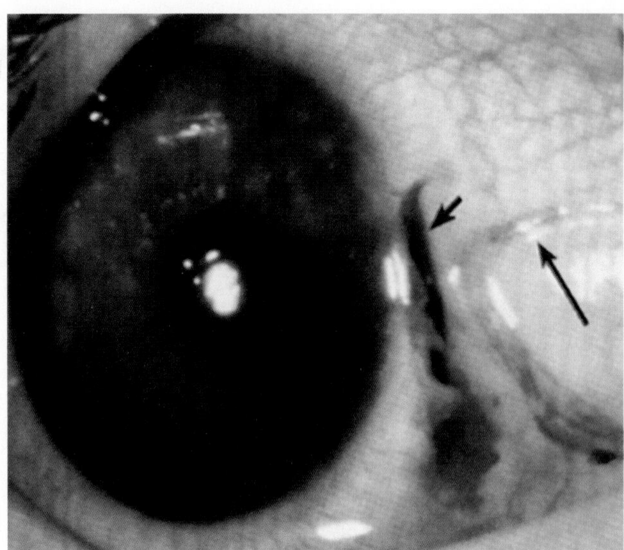

FIGURE 122.4 Ruptured globe. The scleral laceration (*short arrow*) appears as a linear brown line on the white of the eye. The pupil has a teardrop shape, the apex of which points in the direction of the rupture. The *long arrow* points to the upper border of a large conjunctival laceration. Note that the underlying sclera is intact under the conjunctival laceration. There is a diffuse hyphema in the anterior chamber, which partially obscures the pupil.

Triage Considerations

Children with eye injuries associated with severe mechanisms of injury, extreme pain, significant eyelid swelling, or visual disturbance may have globe rupture. These patients should undergo prompt evaluation in the ED with minimal interventions.

Management

If globe rupture is suspected, no eye drops should be instilled. A shield should be placed over the eye such that the edges make contact with the bony prominences above and below the eyeball (Fig. 122.6). If a commercial shield is not available, the clinician should cut off the bottom of a Styrofoam or plastic cup and use it as a shield, resting it against the bony prominences (Fig. 122.7). For multi-system trauma patients,

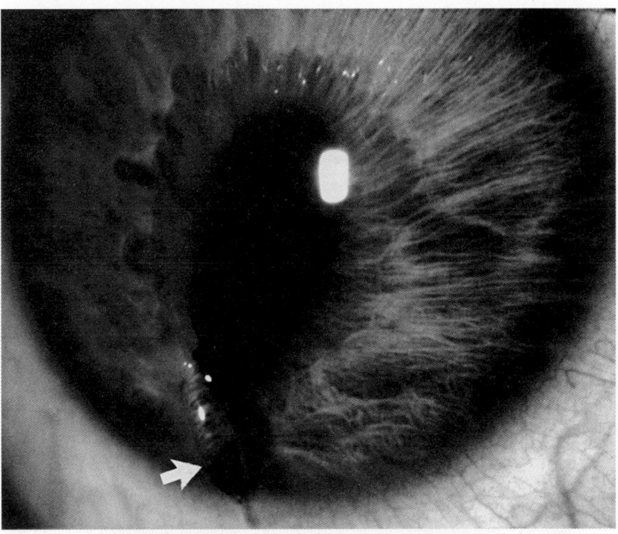

FIGURE 122.5 Corneal laceration (ruptured globe). Note iris protruding through wound (*arrow*) and teardrop-shaped pupil pointing in direction of laceration.

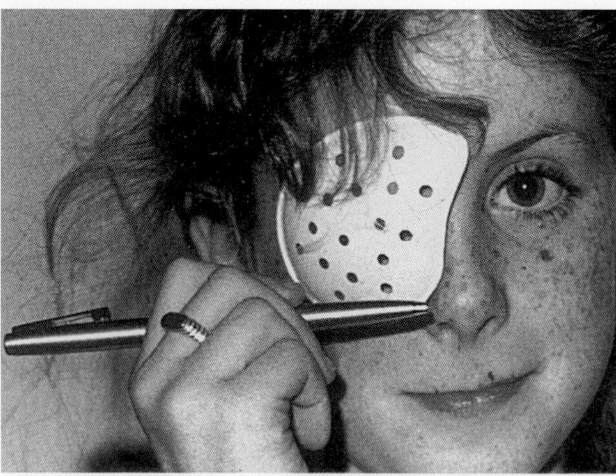

FIGURE 122.6 Patient shielded for right ruptured globe that was caused by a thrown pen.

a shield should even be placed over an obviously injured eye while other resuscitative efforts are ongoing to prevent further accidental injury or contamination by the medical staff. A patch does not provide firm protection, may place pressure on the globe, and should not be used in this circumstance.

Severe eye trauma may cause sedation or vomiting without concurrent head injury. Crying and Valsalva maneuvers such as vomiting can result in further extrusion of intraocular contents through the rupture. Every attempt should be made to keep the child calm, including analgesia and antiemetic medications. Although broad-spectrum intravenous antibiotic coverage is desirable, this treatment must be weighed against the potential aggravation of the child, which might accompany intravenous catheter placement. If an intraocular foreign body is suspected, the clinician must establish by history whether it is metallic as this may influence the choice of imaging and treatment. Even if a ruptured globe is not seen clearly on examination, any patient who has a high-risk history, severe lid swelling, and extreme resistance to examination should be given an eye shield and referred to an ophthalmologist as if a ruptured globe was confirmed.

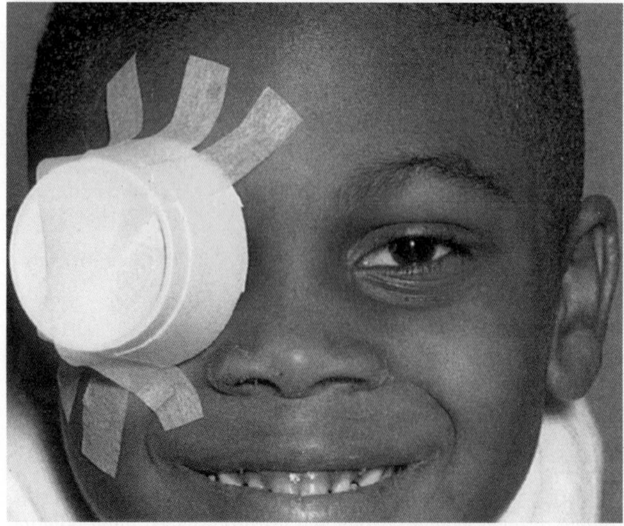

FIGURE 122.7 The bottom of a drinking cup is used as an eye shield.

BLOW-OUT FRACTURE

CLINICAL PEARLS AND PITFALLS

- Impaired extraocular movements most commonly with swelling or ecchymosis surrounding the orbit are the hallmark physical examination findings.
- Palpation of the bony rim of the orbit may not exhibit severe point tenderness even in the presence of fracture.
- Blow-out fracture requires emergent evaluation by ophthalmology.

Current Evidence

There are two proposed mechanisms for blow-out fractures. The first is that force is transmitted from the orbital rim to the medial wall or floor. The second is that force applied to the globe is transmitted to the orbital walls. Given the thicker lateral wall, the point of least resistance is the thinner bone of the floor and medial wall. This force may also result in herniation of orbital contents in the adjacent sinus cavities. Therefore, orbital fractures may occur after facial trauma with or without eyeball trauma. Computed tomography (CT) remains the imaging modality of choice, though diagnostic studies comparing ultrasound, cone beam CT, and MRI to the current gold standard are emerging.

Goals of Treatment

The primary goal of ED therapy is prompt recognition of blow-out fractures and any associated intraocular injuries, including entrapment and commonly associated globe injuries. Approximately 20% of orbital fractures are associated with eyeball injury therefore, emergent ophthalmology consultation is indicated in all cases.

Clinical Considerations

Clinical Recognition

Blow-out fracture is suggested if any of the following are present: restriction of eye movements following trauma, enophthalmos, infraorbital anesthesia, diplopia, step-off deformity, or subcutaneous emphysema. The pathophysiology and diagnosis of blow-out fractures are discussed in Chapter 23 Eye: Strabismus.

Fractures to the inferior and/or medial orbital wall are the most common. The lateral wall is the least commonly fractured. The intraocular contents often sink back into the fracture, giving an enophthalmic appearance. Conversely, proptosis can occur from orbital hemorrhage. Superior wall fracture (roof fractures) may be associated with pulsating proptosis as a result of communication between the orbit and intracranial cavity. Fractures of the inferior wall may be associated with numbness of the ipsilateral malar region caused by injury to the infraorbital nerve, which travels along the floor of the orbit. Palpation of the bony rim of the orbit is often remarkably normal, contrary to the common teaching about point tenderness and "step-off" signs.

The hallmark sign of orbital fracture is a restriction of extraocular movement. Usually, the eye is unable to look away from the fracture site because of a tethering of intraocular muscle or other orbital tissues in the fracture (see Fig. 23.6). Conversely, orbital hemorrhage at the fracture site can less commonly displace the eyeball away from the fracture and make it difficult for the eye to look in the direction of the fracture.

Axial (proptosis) or coronal displacement of the eyeball is an ominous finding because it may be a sign of orbital hemorrhage, which can cause compression of the optic nerve, requiring emergency surgical intervention. Retrobulbar hemorrhage, presenting with severe pain, vision loss, and proptosis, may also be associated with orbital fractures. Retrobulbar hemorrhage can produce central retinal artery occlusion and may require emergent canthotomy by a trained emergency physician or an ophthalmologist. Enophthalmos is also a sign that should lead to urgent radiologic evaluation and possible surgical intervention.

Triage Considerations

Children who have sustained severe blunt facial trauma and/or eye trauma should be promptly evaluated. Soft tissue swelling may increase over time, making evaluation more difficult. While the majority of orbital fractures are treated conservatively, those with associated ocular or intracranial injury require immediate intervention.

Management

Some controversy exists among ophthalmologists, otorhinolaryngologists, and craniofacial surgeons regarding the urgency for radiologic evaluation and surgical intervention in the management of orbital wall fractures. If a decision is made to proceed with radiologic imaging, CT scan of the orbit with both axial and coronal views remains the gold standard. The brain should be included, particularly when an orbital roof fracture is suspected. Plain radiographs have little role in the management of orbital wall fractures as they lack sensitivity. The necessity and timing of surgical intervention is controversial however most agree that significant extraocular restriction or persistent vomiting necessitates surgical intervention.

EYELID LACERATIONS

CLINICAL PEARLS AND PITFALLS

- The following findings require ophthalmology consultation: full-thickness laceration of the lid, ptosis, lid margin involvement, injury in close proximity to the tear duct system, tissue avulsion, and concurrent eye ball injury (Table 122.3).

Current Evidence

Simple eyelid lacerations may be managed by ED physicians with standard wound care techniques; however, it is standard of care to initiate prompt ophthalmology consultation when deeper injuries are suspected.

TABLE 122.3

EYELID LACERATIONS

Consult ophthalmology if laceration is associated with:
Full-thickness perforation of lid
Ptosis
Involvement of lid margin
Possible damage to tear drainage system
Tissue avulsion
Eyeball injury

Goals of Treatment

Similar to other lacerations, the primary goal is wound closure to achieve hemostasis, cosmesis, and prevent infection. Emergency physicians may repair simple lacerations of the eyelid and surrounding area using standard wound closure methods. However, those lacerations requiring further evaluation for possible injury to the eye itself, tear ducts, or other key structures or those requiring surgical expertise should be promptly recognized.

Clinical Considerations

Clinical Recognition

Although eyelid lacerations are usually easy to detect, the clinician must remember that the underlying eyeball might also have been lacerated or injured. Seemingly superficial lacerations of the eyelid may be associated with penetration into the orbit or intracranial cavity, particularly when a pointed implement caused the injury. Puncture wounds of the upper lid with an implement such as a stick or a pencil can result in perforation of the orbital roof and entry into the intracranial subfrontal space, with surprisingly little in the way of signs or symptoms. Oblique lacerations that extend into the medial canthal area (juncture of the upper and lower lids medially) may involve the proximal portion of the nasolacrimal system (Fig. 122.8). Sometimes, the lid margin puncta, which drains tears into the system, is displaced laterally as a result of the laceration (Fig. 122.8).

Full-thickness lid lacerations, the presence of ptosis, lid margin involvement, injury in close proximity to the tear duct system, presence of tissue avulsion, and the presence of concurrent eyeball injury should prompt ophthalmology consultation.

Triage Considerations

Children with high-risk lacerations, as detailed above, should be triaged rapidly and ophthalmology consultation initiated promptly.

Management

Lacerations of the periorbital skin and superficial eyelid may be managed by standard skin closure techniques. Tissue adhesives are widely used to close superficial, nongaping facial lacerations with good cosmetic outcomes. It is important that sutures not grasp deep tissue within the eyelid because this may result in cicatricial eversion of the eyelid margins. Table 122.3 summarizes

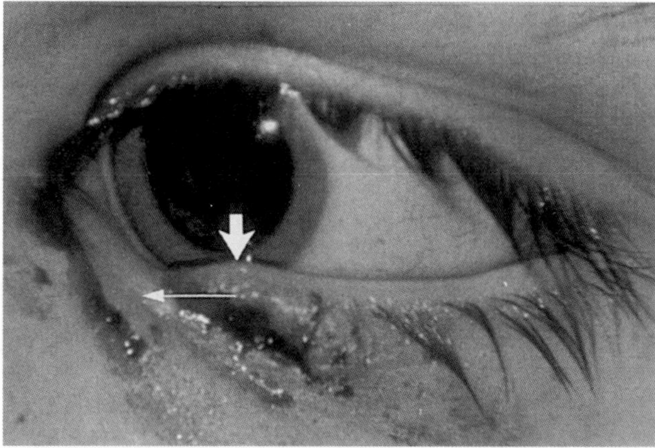

FIGURE 122.8 Lower lid laceration involving tear drainage system. *Thick arrow* indicates lower lid punctum, which has been displaced laterally. *Thin arrow* indicates normal course of canaliculus, which drains tears from the puncta to the lacrimal sac located medially.

those findings that, when associated with eyelid lacerations, should prompt ophthalmology consultation for wound closure. CT scan should be considered in all cases of full-thickness perforation of the upper lid. A perforating implement can reach the orbital apex and optic nerve, and visual field defects may be the only sign, that the nerve has been injured.

CORNEAL AND CONJUNCTIVAL INJURY

CLINICAL PEARLS AND PITFALLS

- Topical anesthetics will only improve pain if the pathology is corneal or conjunctival.
- If fluorescein staining shows one or more vertical linear abrasions, consider the presence of a foreign body.
- An ophthalmologist should see larger corneal abrasions and those involving the visual axis within 24 hours of injury.
- If a teardrop or irregular pupil is seen, the abrasion may represent penetration into the deeper corneal tissues (globe rupture) and emergent ophthalmic consultation is indicated.

Current Evidence

Recent literature has established that the use of a patch with simple corneal abrasions does not improve healing or pain control and is therefore generally not recommended. Topical antibiotic ointments are frequently prescribed although there is limited data that this practice improves outcome.

Goals of Treatment

The goals of ED treatment of corneal and conjunctival abrasions are as follows: (1) Rule out the presence of more severe ocular injury, (2) control pain, (3) facilitate corneal and conjunctival healing.

Clinical Considerations

Clinical Recognition

Corneal or conjunctival abrasions may occur even from mild surface trauma, including accidental self-inflicted injuries. Corneal abrasion can be painful and accompanied by dramatic photophobia and resistance to opening of the eyes. Patients may complain of a foreign-body sensation even though no foreign body is present. In the absence of clinical findings associated with other more severe injuries and in association with a mechanism of injury that may lead to a scratching of the cornea, abrasion should be suspected in a painful, red eye.

Triage Considerations

Patients with severe eye pain and redness should be promptly triaged and assessed. Pain control is a primary concern. Oral analgesics can be initiated if suspicion for need for sedation or systemic anesthesia is low.

Management

Literature suggests that patching corneal abrasions does not accelerate healing or decrease pain. Most physicians prefer to apply a lubricating antibiotic ointment (e.g., bacitracin, erythromycin, Polysporin) for 3 to 5 days to the ocular surface without a patch. Topical nonsteroidal anti-inflammatory agents are used for pain control in adults, though this is rarely used for children. For patients who are relatively asymptomatic with corneal or conjunctival abrasions that are small and do not involve the visual axis (i.e., not involving the central cornea over the pupil), management with antibiotic or artificial tears alone may be sufficient. The use of mydriatic drops such as cyclopentolate 1% can be instilled to relieve ciliary spasm. Ointments containing steroids or neomycin should not be used. If the patient is asymptomatic within 48 hours, no follow-up is required. Larger corneal abrasions and those involving the visual axis should be seen on the day following trauma by an ophthalmologist. For any size of corneal abrasion, if pain or foreign-body sensation continues for more than 2 to 3 days, or if there is increasing pain and redness, the patient should be instructed to seek ophthalmologic care. If a foreign body is suspected, ophthalmology should be consulted and antibiotic coverage should be tailored if contamination with *Bacillus* species from soil is suspected.

Any patient with a fluorescein-staining corneal defect who has a history of ocular herpes or who wears contact lenses should be referred urgently for ophthalmology consultation. Fluorescein should not be instilled while patients have their soft contact lens in place as this may result in permanent discoloration of the contact lens. Patients who wear contact lenses should never be patched for abrasions even if the contact lens has been removed. Patching an eye that often wears contact lenses may create a microenvironment that predisposes to bacterial ulceration of the cornea. The contact lenses should be removed immediately and not warn until the cornea is healed and topical antipseudomonal antibiotics should be prescribed.

HYPHEMA

CLINICAL PEARLS AND PITFALLS

- Patients with hyphema require emergent ophthalmology consultation.
- Patients with hyphema are at risk of increased intraocular pressure and rebleeding.
- Patients with hemoglobinopathies are at particularly high risk for rebleeding.

Current Evidence

Hyphema can result from either blunt or penetrating trauma to the globe. Traumatic forces result in tears of vessels of the iris. In most patients, bleeding stops quickly as the space is limited and clotting seals the vessel. These patients should be treated as globe rupture as described above, with shielding of the eye and emergent consultation with an ophthalmologist. Patients with clotting disorders and those who take platelet inhibiting medications may be predisposed to hyphema or subsequent spontaneous rebleeding. Patients with sickle cell disease or trait are at risk of increased intraocular pressures and rebleeding. Current evidence does not support the routine use of antifibrinolytics in the treatment of hyphema.

Goals of Treatment

The goals of treatment in the ED are as follows: (1) Prompt recognition, (2) reduce the risk of potential complications, and (3) consult ophthalmology emergently.

Clinical Considerations

Clinical Recognition

The presence of blood between the cornea and the iris is a sign of severe ocular trauma. Although the entire anterior chamber may be filled with blood (8-ball hyphema), clots may also be small, requiring careful inspection for detection (Fig. 122.3). Sometimes the blood is more diffuse throughout the anterior chamber (Fig. 122.4) or may even be microscopic, requiring slit lamp examination for detection (microhyphema). The size of the hyphema is directly proportional to the incidence of complications including increased intraocular pressure and secondary glaucoma. Visual prognosis is inversely proportional to hyphema size. Patients with hyphema are vulnerable for the first 5 days after injury when spontaneous rebleeding may occur. Patients with hemoglobinopathies are at particular risk for ocular complications of hyphema. Therefore, hemoglobin electrophoresis should be performed on all patients who are in a high-risk ethnic group at presentation.

Triage Considerations

Patients with severe eye injury and pain should be triaged and evaluated emergently.

Management

An ophthalmologist must evaluate all patients with hyphema emergently. Hospital admission is usually recommended. The eye trauma itself may result in some degree of physiologic sedation. The eye should be shielded, not patched, and the patient should be placed on bed rest with the head elevated 45 degrees. This position helps allow blood within the anterior chamber to settle inferiorly, thus allowing clearance of the visual axis, improvement of vision, and a better view for the ophthalmologist looking into the eyeball. Cycloplegic drops may have benefit in pain control and allowing improved evaluation of the posterior segment of the eye. Data supporting the use of optical steroids and/or oral antifibrinolytics is limited and should not be used without ophthalmology consultation.

TRAUMATIC IRITIS

Clinical Manifestations

Inflammation within the anterior chamber of the eye often presents 24 to 72 hours after blunt trauma. The patient may complain of eye pain, redness, photophobia, and visual loss. The pupil on the affected side may be constricted (see Chapter 24 Eye: Unequal Pupils). The ocular injection may be confined to a ring of redness surrounding the cornea (ciliary flush). Definitive recognition of traumatic iritis requires slit lamp examination. Ophthalmology consultation is recommended when the diagnosis of traumatic iritis is suspected, as it is often associated with other ocular injuries.

Management

Dilating drops and topical steroids are the mainstay of treatment for traumatic iritis. Because of the risks associated with their use, these therapies should only be prescribed in conjunction with ophthalmology consultation.

Traumatic Versus Functional Visual Loss

Occasionally, the emergency physician is faced with a child who is feigning visual loss. Functional visual loss can also be idiopathic and transient or associated with stress. In the absence of other signs of ocular or head trauma, this diagnosis should be suspected. It may become necessary to "trick" the child into demonstrating that he or she can actually see. Patients who are truly acutely blind should demonstrate some degree of anxiety and virtually complete inability to navigate in new surroundings. When asked to write their names on a piece of paper, truly blind patients can do so accurately, unlike children who are functionally blind who assume they are unable to write. Children who are feigning visual loss but not complete blindness can be more difficult to "trick." Sometimes, by placing a drop of saline or topical anesthetic in the eye while giving the child the suggestion that these "magic drops" will cause a return of vision, the child then begins to see better. The pinhole test (discussed above) can also be used in this manner. Ophthalmology consultation is sometimes critical in discovering whether a child has truly sustained visual loss.

Rarely, transient cortical visual impairment/blindness can result following direct or contrecoup blunt occipital head trauma. Despite an otherwise normal eye examination, centrally mediated vision loss may occur. Though the vision loss may be transient, ophthalmology should be consulted. Traumatic cataract, vitreous hemorrhage, commotion retinae, retinal detachment, and optic nerve injury may also cause acute traumatic vision loss. For these injuries, ophthalmology consultation is also required. The most effective screening tests for severe intraocular injury remain visual acuity testing, examination of the red reflex, and direct ophthalmoscopy.

Child Abuse

Virtually any eye injury can be the result of child abuse. Perhaps the most common ocular manifestation of child abuse is the finding of retinal hemorrhages associated with the abusive head injury (Fig. 122.9). Although these hemorrhages can be seen with the direct ophthalmoscope, ophthalmology consultation is required. Children who present to the ED before the age of 5 years with significant intracranial hemorrhage or

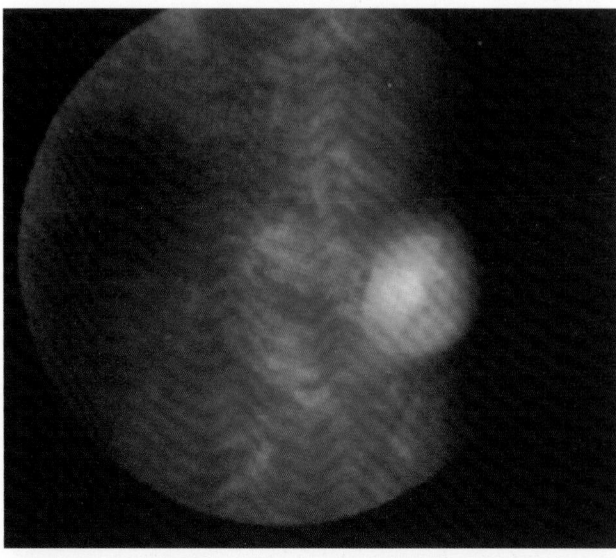

FIGURE 122.9 Retinal hemorrhages in abusive head injury.

sudden unexplained cardiorespiratory arrest should have a full dilated examination conducted by an ophthalmologist to look for retinal hemorrhages that may indicate that a non-accidental head injury has occurred.

Suggested Readings and Key References

General Approach to Ocular Trauma

Gerstenblith AT, Rabinowitz MP. *Wills Eye manual: hospital office and emergency room diagnosis and treatment of eye disease.* 6th ed. Philadelphia, PA: Lippincott Williams & Wilkins, 2012.

Levin AV. Eye emergencies: acute management in the pediatric ambulatory setting. *Pediatr Emerg Care* 1991;7:367–377.

Levin AV. General pediatric ophthalmic procedures. In: King CK, Henretig FM, eds. *Textbook of pediatric emergency procedures.* 2nd ed. Philadelphia, PA: Lippincott Williams & Wilkins, 2008: 531–544.

Levin AV. Slit lamp examination. In: King CK, Henretig FM, eds. *Textbook of pediatric emergency procedures.* 2nd ed. Philadelphia, PA: Lippincott Williams & Wilkins, 2008:545–549.

Riordan-Eva P, Whitcher JP. *Vaughan & Asbury's general ophthalmology.* 17th ed. New York, NY: McGraw-Hill, 2008.

Ultrasound

Jank S, Deibl M, Strobl H, et al. Interrater reliability in the ultrasound diagnosis of medial and lateral orbital wall fractures with a curved array transducer. *J Oral Maxillofac Surg* 2006;64(1):68–73.

Kilker BA, Holst JM, Hoffmann B. Bedside ocular ultrasound in the emergency department. *Eur J Emerg Med* 2014;21(4):246–253.

Ruptured Globe

Maw M, Pineda R, Pasquale LR, et al. Traumatic ruptured globe injuries in children. *Int Ophthalmol Clin* 2002;42(3):157–165.

Blow-out Fracture

Burnstine MA. Clinical recommendations for repair of isolated orbital floor fractures: an evidence based analysis. *Ophthalmology* 2002;109:1207–1213.

Corneal Abrasion

Calder LA, Balasubramanian S, Fergusson D. Topical nonsteroidal anti-inflammatory drugs for corneal abrasions: meta-analysis of randomized trials. *Acad Emerg Med* 2005;12(5):467–473.

Turner A, Rabiu M. Patching for corneal abrasion. *Cochrane Database Syst Rev* 2006;19(2):CD004764.

Hyphema

Gharaibeh A, Savage HI, Scherer RW, et al. Medical interventions for traumatic hyphema. *Cochrane Database Syst Rev.* 2013;12: CD005431.

Child Abuse

Levin AV, Christian CW, Committee on Child Abuse and Neglect, Section on Ophthalmology. The eye examination in the evaluation of child abuse. *Pediatrics* 2010;126:376–380.

CHAPTER 123 ■ THORACIC TRAUMA

MATTHEW EISENBERG, MD AND DAVID P. MOONEY, MD, MPH

GOALS OF EMERGENCY THERAPY

The initial goals of emergency therapy for the child with thoracic trauma, just as for all forms of major trauma, are assessment and stabilization of airway, breathing, and circulation, all of which are at increased risk due to the location of vital structures within the thorax. A thorough primary trauma survey, with immediate steps to correct any deficits in airway, breathing, and circulation before moving on to the next element of assessment, is critical. The provider should be prepared to emergently intubate the trachea, provide mechanical ventilation, administer both intravenous fluids (IVF) and red blood cells, and perform other emergency interventions such as thoracentesis, thoracostomy, and pericardiocentesis as indicated.

Respiratory compromise in children with thoracic trauma may be due to obstruction of the airway, injury to the chest wall, lung parenchyma, or central nervous system, or shock. Thoracic hemorrhage, obstruction of venous return, or direct injury to the heart may lead to circulatory compromise and shock.

The evaluation of the child with thoracic trauma is complicated by both physical and developmental differences from adults. Detailed further in the sections that follow, these include increased compliance of the thoracic cage, greater susceptibility to air and fluid in the pleural space, a shorter, more narrow trachea at greater risk of obstruction, and greater sensitivity to hypoxia. Due to fear, pain, separation from caregiver and/or young age, an injured child may not be able to articulate their complaints or comply with the examination. Therefore, attention to nonverbal cues, vital signs, and careful observation of respiratory and circulatory status are crucial. Because approximately 80% of thoracic trauma occurs as part of a multisystem injury, the physician must also consider head, neck, and intra-abdominal injuries when evaluating a child with chest trauma. An overview of the approach to the child with blunt thoracic trauma is shown in Figure 123.1.

KEY POINTS

- Significant thoracic trauma in the pediatric population is relatively uncommon, accounting for only 4% to 6% of children admitted to pediatric trauma centers.
- Despite a high rate of scene fatalities, mortality rates for children who reach the hospital with isolated thoracic trauma are low; this rate triples when thoracic trauma occurs concurrently with head or abdominal trauma.
- Blunt trauma occurs far more frequently than penetrating trauma and lung injuries outnumber those to the heart and great vessels.
- Emergency evaluation requires careful observation and examination for evidence of impaired respiration or circulation, including any abnormal vital signs.
- Be prepared to immediately secure the airway and support breathing and circulation.
- Most thoracic injuries do not require intervention and those that do most commonly require only tube thoracostomy.

RELATED CHAPTERS

Signs and Symptoms
- Cyanosis: Chapter 16
- Neck Stiffness: Chapter 44
- Pain: Chest: Chapter 50
- Pain: Dysphagia: Chapter 51
- Respiratory Distress: Chapter 66
- Stridor: Chapter 70
- Wheezing: Chapter 80

Clinical Pathways
- Shock: Chapter 91

Medical, Surgical, and Trauma Emergencies
- Approach to the Injured Child: Chapter 2
- Airway: Chapter 3
- Child Abuse/Assault: Chapter 95
- Abdominal Trauma: Chapter 111
- Musculoskeletal Trauma: Chapter 119
- Neck Trauma: Chapter 120
- Neurotrauma: Chapter 121
- Procedures: Chapter 141
- Ultrasound: Chapter 142

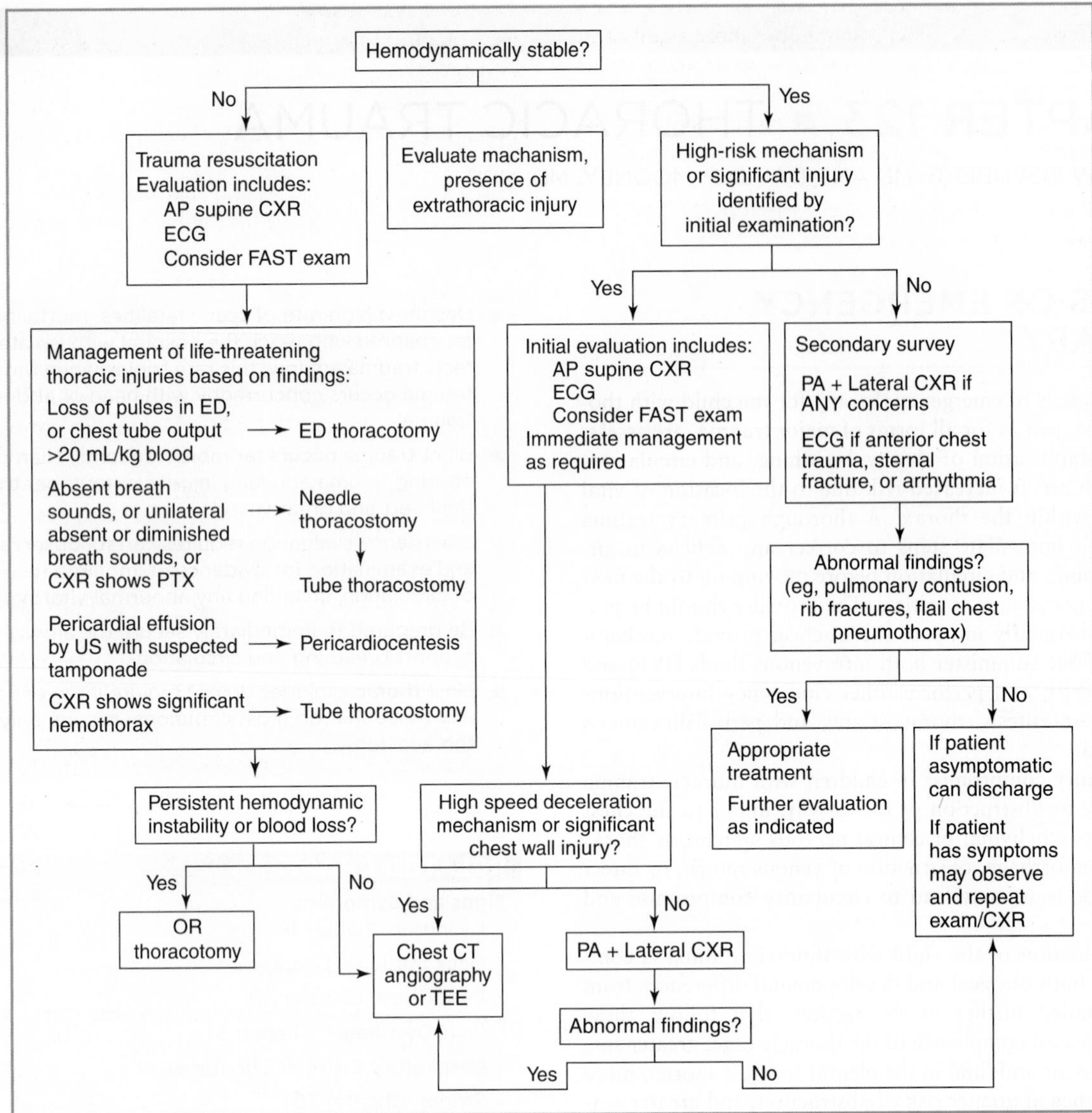

FIGURE 123.1 Algorithm showing approach to blunt thoracic trauma. Official reprint from UpToDate® "http://www.uptodate.com" © 2015 UpToDate®.

PNEUMOTHORAX AND HEMOTHORAX

CLINICAL PEARLS AND PITFALLS

- Pneumothorax is one of the most common injuries seen in thoracic trauma.
- The unstable patient with suspected tension pneumothorax requires emergent needle decompression, even before radiologic evaluation, followed by tube thoracostomy.
- The stable pediatric patient with suspected thoracic trauma may be assessed by chest radiography and bedside ultrasound (US) and without computed tomography (CT) imaging.
- Tube thoracostomy is recommended for patients with pneumothoraces that are large, associated with respiratory compromise, or when air transport is required.
- Positive pressure ventilation by itself is not an indication for tube thoracostomy in patients with a small pneumothorax detected on CT only.
- Hemothorax can lead to both respiratory and circulatory compromise, as a large volume of blood can be lost into the pleural space.
- Treatment of hemothorax includes tube thoracostomy and support of circulation with both crystalloid products and blood transfusion as needed.

Current Evidence

Pneumothorax is the second most commonly encountered injury in blunt thoracic trauma and the most common in penetrating thoracic trauma. Air within the pleural cavity can arise from penetration of the chest wall, disruption of the lung parenchyma, a tear of the tracheobronchial structures, or esophageal rupture. Hemothorax is much more common in penetrating than blunt thoracic trauma. In blunt thoracic trauma, a hemothorax can occur from rib fractures lacerating the lung, pulmonary parenchymal injuries unrelated to rib fractures, lacerations of the chest wall vessels, or disruption of the vascular structures in the mediastinum or hilum. The most common cause of a hemothorax is injury to the intercostal or internal mammary arteries, whereas injury to the lung or great vessels is less common but more significant. Intraperitoneal hemorrhage may lead to a hemothorax if associated with disruption of the diaphragm.

Air and fluid within the pleural space more easily shift the mediastinum in children, compromising venous return and cardiac output to a greater extent than in adults. Available data suggest that the mortality rate for pneumothorax (15%) is substantially lower than with hemothorax (57%). Hemothorax secondary to an injury of the great vessels usually results in death at the scene.

Goals of Treatment

Immediate recognition and stabilization of airway, breathing, and circulation is crucial to management of pneumothoraces and hemothoraces. Opening and then securing the airway with endotracheal intubation is the first step for a child with severe respiratory distress, inadequate oxygenation or ventilation, or depressed mental status after trauma. Breathing may be supported via mechanical ventilation and evacuation of intrapleural air and blood. Circulation may become impaired during tension physiology via obstruction of venous return, and evacuation of the pleura via needle or tube thoracostomy is immediately necessary. Circulation may also be affected by blood loss into the thorax necessitating volume replacement with appropriate IVF and possible blood transfusion.

For the stable patient with pneumo- or hemothorax, the focus is on careful evaluation and treatment to prevent deterioration. Chest radiograph (CXR) and US may be helpful to identify the extent of the injury and the need for intervention. Depending on the clinical progression, treatment may involve observation, tube thoracotomy, or surgical intervention.

Clinical Considerations

Clinical Recognition

Pneumothorax or hemothorax should be suspected in any child with a history of thoracic trauma who presents with chest pain, shortness of breath, respiratory distress, hypoxia, or evidence of shock. Physical examination alone may be sufficient to make the diagnosis in patients with a large hemothorax or pneumothorax or severe complications such as tension physiology, but smaller lesions may be missed by examination alone. All patients with a mechanism concerning for a thoracic injury should undergo prompt radiologic evaluation with CXR, as an initial normal physical examination may be misleading. Where available, bedside US can be used to augment the initial physical examination as it may facilitate identification of even small amounts of air or blood in the pleural space.

Triage Considerations

Children with traumatic pneumothorax or hemothorax require immediate evaluation utilizing Advanced Trauma Life Support (ATLS) protocols and activation of the appropriate local trauma response. In planning for a trauma response, preparations should be made for both needle aspiration of pleural air and placement of a chest tube, so that these procedures can be performed without delay if indicated by the patient's clinical condition or diagnostic workup.

Clinical Assessment

The child with suspected pneumothorax or hemothorax should undergo a thorough primary survey, looking for signs of compromised airway, breathing, or circulation. Careful attention to vital signs, particularly tachycardia, tachypnea, and hypoxemia, may lead to discovery of impaired physiology not otherwise detected by physical examination. It is important to recognize that due to children's excellent vascular compensation abilities, hypotension is a late finding in pediatric shock and a normal blood pressure therefore does not rule out circulatory compromise.

Some patients with a pneumothorax may be asymptomatic. Others may be tachypneic, complain of pleuritic chest pain, or be in severe respiratory distress. Physical examination may be normal or may reveal diminished or absent breath sounds, crepitus, or hyperresonance to percussion on the side of the pneumothorax. If a tension pneumothorax develops, findings may include tracheal deviation to the contralateral side and distended neck veins from impaired venous return to the heart through the deviated superior vena cava. These physical findings may be difficult to discern in a fully immobilized child in a noisy resuscitation room.

Patients with hemothorax may present in respiratory distress or profound shock secondary to obstruction of venous return or blood loss. Decreased breath sounds are noted on the affected side, and there may be tracheal or mediastinal deviation. Thirty to 40% of the patient's blood volume may be rapidly lost in the pleural cavity with major vessel lacerations. Bleeding from the intercostal or internal mammary arteries usually stops as systemic blood pressure falls and reexpansion of the lung may provide some tamponade effect.

Tension Pneumothorax

A tension pneumothorax is the most common complicated intrapleural injury. Tension pneumothorax develops in up to 20% of children after simple pneumothorax. A tension pneumothorax occurs when there is progressive accumulation of air within the pleural cavity. A laceration to the chest wall, pulmonary parenchyma, or tracheobronchial tree may function as a one-way valve, allowing air to enter but not leave the pleural space. The progressive accumulation of air within the pleural cavity not only collapses the ipsilateral lung, but it also compresses the contralateral lung (see Fig. 123.2). These patients may present in severe respiratory distress with decreased

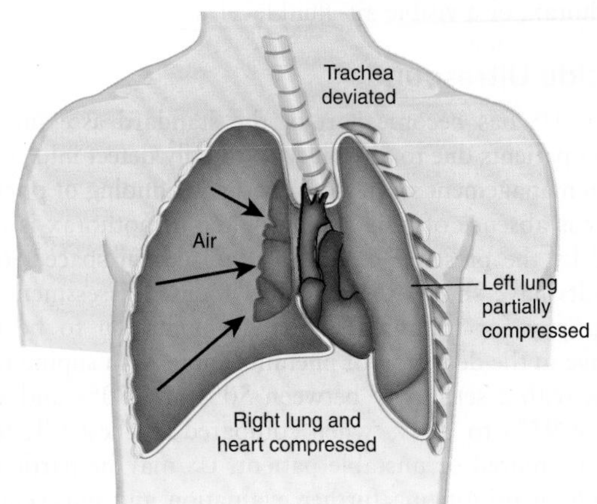

FIGURE 123.2 Tension pneumothorax with a mediastinal shift.

TRAUMA

breath sounds on the side of the pneumothorax. There is also a shift of the mediastinal structures to the contralateral side. Two-thirds of the blood supply to the body is returned to the heart via the inferior vena cava. Because the inferior vena cava is relatively fixed in place as it passes through the diaphragm and cannot shift as much as the superior vena cava, venous return to the heart is reduced.

Patients with a tension pneumothorax or hemothorax demonstrate tension physiology: tachycardia and peripheral vasoconstriction and, if left untreated, will progress to shock. Initial treatment for tension physiology consists of needle decompression. An immediate release of air should be noted and the patient's hemodynamic status should improve. The needle decompression is only a temporizing measure and must be followed by tube thoracostomy.

Open Pneumothorax

An open pneumothorax is the result of penetrating trauma. There is a direct connection between the pleural space and the atmosphere, impeding ventilation. Initial treatment includes placement of an occlusive dressing at the wound site. This is best done when the patient is in full expiration. As in a bronchial tear or lung parenchymal injury, air may enter but not leave the pleural space, creating a ball-valve effect. A chest tube should be placed immediately to prevent development of a tension pneumothorax. The chest tube should be inserted at a site different than the open wound. Larger open chest wounds may need surgical closure.

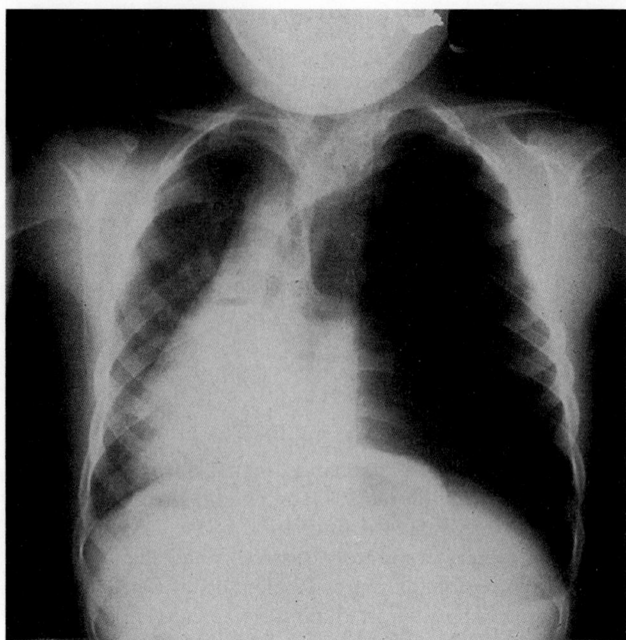

FIGURE 123.3 A 5-year-old girl fell off and was then kicked in the chest by a horse. Upon arrival of the life-flight team, the patient was found to be in both respiratory and cardiovascular distress. Chest radiograph demonstrated a left-sided tension pneumothorax. The patient was intubated, and a chest tube was placed before the patient was transported. After the intubation and chest tube insertion, both the patient's respiratory and cardiovascular status improved.

Diagnostic Testing

Chest Radiograph

A CXR remains the most widely used test for the diagnosis of hemothorax and pneumothorax. Both conditions are better visualized in the upright position than supine. Plain radiographic signs of a pneumothorax may include identification of the pleural line, a hyperlucent hemithorax, pleural air at the lung base, and/or an unusually well-defined heart and mediastinal outline due to pleural air rising anteriorly. A tension pneumothorax is indicated by the presence of midline shift to the contralateral side of the pneumothorax (see Fig. 123.3). Smaller pneumothoraces may be better visualized by positioning the patient in the lateral decubitus position with the concerning side up. Expiratory CXRs do not add significantly to the evaluation. Hemothorax on CXR may appear as blunting of the costophrenic angle, haziness or opacification of the hemithorax, or a visible air–fluid level.

Bedside Ultrasound

Bedside US has become part of the standard assessment of trauma patients due to its ability to rapidly detect injuries and inform management strategies. The major finding of pneumothorax is absence of lung sliding, while hemothorax is determined by the presence of fluid in the pleural space. Studies in adults have shown the extended focused assessment with sonography for trauma (E-FAST) examination to be more sensitive in the detection of pneumothorax than supine radiographs with a sensitivity between 50% and 80% and specificity of 95% to 100% when compared to chest CT. In the multiply injured or unstable patient, US may be particularly valuable in prioritizing further evaluation and interventions, particularly in adult patients.

Reported sensitivity of the FAST examination in children is lower than that noted in adults. In addition, children are less likely to undergo operative repair even when free fluid in the abdomen is identified, therefore the role for FAST testing is different in children than adults. Nonetheless, with thoracic trauma, identification of air or blood in the pleural space on bedside US may rapidly influence the decision for tube thoracostomy in children with respiratory or hemodynamic compromise.

Management

Needle Decompression

Initial treatment for pneumothorax may consist of observation alone, placement of a chest tube, or needle thoracentesis. Tension pneumothorax, however, should always be treated with immediate needle decompression. This is performed by insertion of a large-bore intravenous (IV) catheter in the midclavicular second intercostal space of the ipsilateral side. If there is a tension pneumothorax, an immediate release of air should be noted. Evacuation can be facilitated by attaching the catheter to a two-way stopcock and 60-cc syringe, allowing air to be continuously pulled from the pleural space although the placement of the catheter alone should temporarily resolve the tension physiology until tube thoracostomy can be performed.

Chest Tube

Tube thoracostomy is indicated in the symptomatic patient with pneumothorax or those requiring air transport. Management of asymptomatic pneumothoraces identified on CT but not visible on plain radiograph is controversial, but tube thoracostomy does not appear to be required, even in patients undergoing positive pressure ventilation.

Tube thoracostomy should be done in the midaxillary line at the level of the fifth intercostal space (nipple level). If the pneumothorax is not relieved and a significant air leak continues after chest tube placement, a tracheobronchial rupture must be considered. Evidence suggests that for a simple pneumothorax, placement of a pigtail catheter instead of a chest tube has similar efficacy while causing less pain to the patient. While data in children are lacking, pigtail catheter placement is often preferred to chest tube for management of pneumothoraces due to less need for procedural sedation and postprocedural pain medication.

Tube thoracostomy, and not pigtail catheter placement, is the treatment of choice in patients with a hemothorax in order to evacuate blood from the pleural cavity, reexpand the lung, and prevent or treat any mediastinal shift. Many hemothoraces may actually represent hemopneumothoraces. As with a pneumothorax, the chest tube is placed in the midaxillary line at the level of the fifth intercostal space (nipple level). Patients should be typed and crossed for packed red blood cells and adequately volume resuscitated, preferably with two large IV lines in place. For larger hemothoraces, donor blood should be at the patient's bedside prior to tube thoracostomy if time permits. After placement of a chest tube, blood should be slowly evacuated from the pleural space. Blood within the pleural cavity may tamponade a significant bleeding source within the chest and evacuating that blood may cause new bleeding to occur. Patients can exsanguinate rapidly, which is why IV access, adequate volume resuscitation, and blood available for transfusion should be a priority. Thoracostomy drainage needs to be closely monitored. Large ongoing blood loss from a chest tube should be collected in a system that allows autotransfusion.

Thoracotomy

Thoracotomy is indicated for bleeding that continues at a rate of greater than 1 to 2 mL/kg/hr, inability to expand the lung, or retained blood within the pleural cavity. Failure to adequately drain a hemothorax may lead to restrictive lung disease from a fibrothorax or an empyema from the clotted material becoming infected.

Disposition

All patients with a traumatic pneumothorax or hemothorax require admission to the hospital. If the pneumothorax is small and the patient is asymptomatic, hospital observation and passive administration of oxygen via a nonrebreather mask is all that is necessary. A small pneumothorax is classically described as being less than 15% of the hemithorax, although it is common to underestimate the size of a pneumothorax using plain films. An asymptomatic patient may rapidly become symptomatic if a small, simple pneumothorax progresses to a large or tension pneumothorax; therefore, even asymptomatic patients with a pneumothorax should be admitted to the hospital for observation. Patients with chest tubes should be hospitalized on a unit that is capable of monitoring and troubleshooting the tube and the collection device.

An unstable airway, respiratory distress, severe hypoxia, ongoing blood loss, and presence of other severe injuries are among the indications for admission to an intensive care unit.

PULMONARY CONTUSIONS

CLINICAL PEARLS AND PITFALLS

- Pulmonary contusion is the most common intrathoracic injury in children.
- While many contusions cause only mild symptoms such as chest pain, more severe injuries can lead to hypoxemia and respiratory failure.
- Pulmonary contusions may not show up on CXR for 4 to 6 hours after the injury, and in some cases may never be identified on plain films.
- Given the force necessary to cause a pulmonary contusion, a high index of suspicion for other associated injuries is required.

Current Evidence

Pulmonary contusion is the most common thoracic injury in children. Pulmonary contusion occurs when a blunt force is applied to the lung parenchyma, though the injury can also be seen in penetrating trauma. The pediatric thoracic cage provides less protection from blunt force impact compared to adults, secondary to greater cartilage content and the greater elasticity of the bones. Therefore, external kinetic energy applied to the thorax is transferred more readily through the chest wall to the underlying organs. Thus, a pediatric patient is more likely than an adult to have an internal injury such as a lung contusion without external evidence of trauma (rib fracture, laceration, bruising).

As in any contusion or bruise, the capillary network becomes damaged, leaking fluid into the surrounding tissues. A ventilation:perfusion mismatch will occur because of the extravasation of fluid into injured lung parenchyma, interfering with oxygenation. As the edema and swelling worsen, the patient's respiratory status will deteriorate if the contusion is large.

Clinical Considerations

Clinical Recognition

Pulmonary contusion should be suspected in any child with blunt thoracic trauma who presents with chest pain, difficulty breathing, or unexplained hypoxia. The contusion may be visualized on radiography or inferred from the absence of another explanation for these symptoms (such as pneumothorax). Due to the pliable nature of the pediatric chest wall, pulmonary contusions can often be seen in the absence of rib fracture. When present, however, rib fractures as well as chest wall ecchymosis should further raise suspicion for underlying parenchymal injury.

Triage

While a stable pulmonary contusion may not require any specific therapy, patients are at high risk of deteriorating respiratory status and therefore require an expedited evaluation. In addition, the presence of such an injury indicates that sufficient force was applied to the thorax to warrant thorough evaluation for additional injuries.

Clinical Assessment

Initial assessment should focus on assessing and stabilizing the airway, breathing, and circulation, as well as the identification

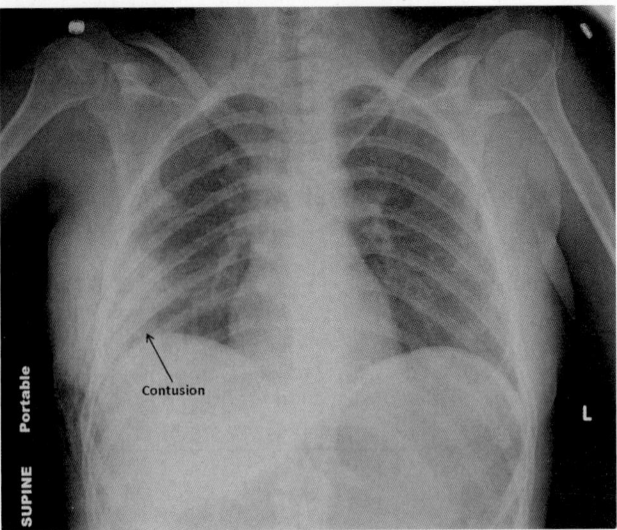

FIGURE 123.4 Right lower lobe pulmonary contusion in a patient with associated rib fractures. Subcutaneous air is also noted in the adjacent soft tissue.

of other associated injuries. Vital sign abnormalities seen with moderate-to-severe pulmonary contusions may include tachypnea and hypoxemia due to shunting within the lung. Patients may complain of chest pain or shortness of breath, and physical examination may reveal chest wall bruising and tenderness, with focally diminished breath sounds in the affected lung. These latter findings are nonspecific, however, and their absence should not be used to rule out pulmonary contusion without imaging.

Management

When pulmonary contusion is suspected, CXR is the imaging modality of choice (see Fig. 123.4). However, the contusion itself may not be visible on CXR for 4 to 6 hours after the injury, and even then false-negative rates of up to 33% have been reported.

Although more sensitive than CXR in detecting pulmonary contusion, a chest CT scan is usually unnecessary unless a significant injury to the vasculature is suspected, as management will depend on clinical condition of the patient and not the radiographic size of the contusion.

Treatment of pulmonary contusion is supportive. If required, supplemental oxygen should be administered. If the patient cannot maintain oxygenation despite passive supplemental oxygen delivery, endotracheal intubation and mechanical ventilation with positive pressure is the treatment of choice. Fluid restriction is helpful to avoid exacerbation of pulmonary edema, though must be balanced against the fluid needs arising from concurrent injuries to other organ systems and shock in the severely injured child. Patients may require high inflation pressures to maintain adequate oxygenation, which combined with injury to the lung leads to high risk of barotrauma and pneumothorax.

Disposition

Due to risk of progression of symptoms and need for increasing respiratory support, all patients with pulmonary contusion should be admitted for observation. Given the low sensitivity of CXR for pulmonary contusion, children with significant chest pain or shortness of breath or an unexplained oxygen requirement after blunt chest trauma should also be admitted even if chest imaging is normal. Admission to an intensive care unit is appropriate for patients with deteriorating vital signs, a significant oxygen requirement, worsening respiratory distress, or who otherwise appear to be at high risk of progressing to require mechanical ventilation.

BLUNT CARDIAC INJURIES

CLINICAL PEARLS AND PITFALLS

- Pericardial tamponade from blunt cardiac injury is rare but life-threatening, and requires immediate pericardiocentesis to avoid circulatory collapse.
- Any patient with suspected blunt cardiac injury who is hemodynamically unstable or has arrhythmias should undergo echocardiography and be admitted to the intensive care unit.
- All patients with suspected blunt cardiac injury need close follow-up.

Current Evidence

Cardiac injury in blunt thoracic trauma is rare. In one study of 1,288 patients with blunt thoracic trauma, only 60 (4.6%) had a blunt cardiac injury, though other smaller studies have reported higher incidence. Myocardial contusion, ventricular or atrial rupture, and valvular disruption are considered blunt cardiac injuries.

Myocardial contusion is the most common blunt cardiac injury; far outnumbering lacerations. Contusions are usually self-limited; rare complications include arrhythmia, pump failure, congestive heart failure, and shock. Also rare is commotio cordis: cardiac arrest following a single, isolated, forceful precordial blow. Prompt cardiopulmonary resuscitation/defibrillation is the only identifiable factor associated with a favorable outcome after commotio cordis.

Cardiac rupture is the most common cause of death in blunt cardiac trauma. The majority of these patients never reach a hospital because they die at the scene. The right ventricle is the chamber most commonly ruptured because of its location directly beneath the sternum. Septal rupture can also occur, with the condition of the patient correlating with the size of the rupture. Patients with cardiac rupture may present with cardiac tamponade, demonstrating one or all the components of Beck triad (jugular venous distention, low blood pressure, and muffled heart tones). Patients with valvular injury may present in congestive heart failure with a new regurgitation murmur. Coronary artery injury is rare but should be considered in patients with persistent electrocardiogram (EKG) changes consistent with ischemia following blunt thoracic trauma.

Pericardial tamponade may also occur when there is injury to the myocardium and blood accumulates in the pericardial sac. Because of the nondistensible pericardium, pressure is exerted on the heart. Cardiac output decreases secondary to a decrease in venous return and ventricular stroke volume. The body will initially compensate with an increase in the pulse rate and peripheral vascular resistance. As the pressure within the pericardial sac increases, the systolic blood pressure will decrease, causing a narrowing of the pulse pressure and subsequent hypotension and cardiogenic shock.

Clinical Considerations

Clinical Recognition

Blunt cardiac injury occurs more commonly with other associated injuries than in isolation. Unlike adults, pediatric patients with blunt cardiac injury often have few presenting signs or symptoms. In one pediatric study, less than half of the awake patients with blunt cardiac injury complained of chest pain, and external evidence of thoracic injury was present in only 60% of these patients. In the same study, cardiac examination was abnormal in less than one quarter of the patients. Additional findings that should prompt evaluation for cardiac injury include a cardiac arrhythmia, a new murmur, or evidence of congestive heart failure (an enlarged liver, a gallop heard on cardiac examination, and rales with auscultation of the lungs).

Myocardial contusion, ventricular or atrial rupture, and valvular disruption may produce cardiogenic shock. Circulatory compromise results from a decrease in cardiac output, usually from impaired myocardial contractility.

Pericardial tamponade, due to air or blood inside the pericardium, will also decrease cardiac output and cause circulatory collapse. If the patient is decompensating and a pericardial tamponade is suspected, a pericardiocentesis should be performed emergently and prior to any further diagnostic evaluation, with the exception of bedside US when available to confirm the diagnosis and facilitate the procedure (see Fig. 123.5).

Triage

Children with blunt trauma to the sternum or left hemithorax from a high-energy mechanism should be placed on a cardiac monitor and evaluated immediately. While the stable patient is unlikely to deteriorate, providers should be prepared to correct any arrhythmias by both pharmacologic and electrical means. Signs of cardiogenic shock should be addressed immediately by rapid evaluation and correction of the cause.

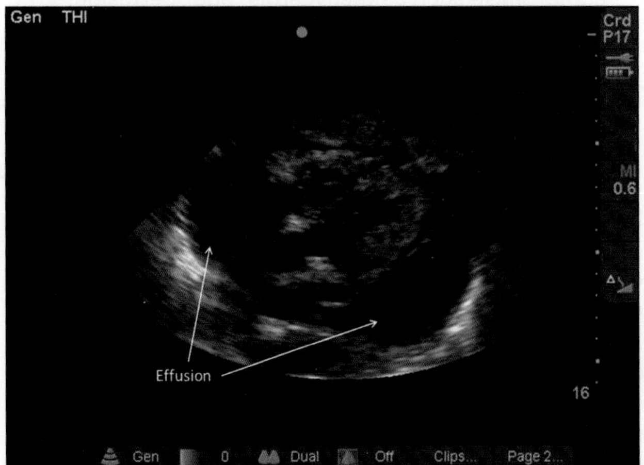

FIGURE 123.5 Bedside ultrasound showing large pericardial effusion surrounding the heart.

Initial Assessment

Patients with cardiac injuries may complain of chest or sternal pain. Physical examination may reveal tachycardia, an irregular heart rhythm, a new heart murmur, signs of congestive heart failure, or in the case of cardiac tamponade, muffled heart tones. As previously noted, however, many children with blunt cardiac injury will have neither symptoms nor abnormal physical examination findings, and therefore a high index of suspicion is required when the mechanism of injury makes cardiac injury possible.

Pericardial tamponade may initially be difficult to diagnose because of associated injuries obscuring the clinical signs and symptoms. Patients may present with distant heart sounds, low blood pressure, poor perfusion, a narrow pulse pressure, or electromechanical dissociation. Pulsus paradoxus, blood pressure falling more than 10 mm Hg during inspiration, occurs in less than one-half of patients with pericardial tamponade and should not be relied on to make the diagnosis.

Management

The evaluation for suspected blunt cardiac injury includes EKG, serum cardiac enzymes, echocardiography, and observation with continuous cardiac monitoring. A 12-lead EKG may show ST-T-wave changes or arrhythmias. The combination of a normal EKG and negative troponin is highly sensitive for ruling out myocardial contusion or other significant blunt cardiac injury. For patients with an abnormal EKG, elevated cardiac enzymes, or new findings on physical examination, echocardiography should be performed.

There is no specific therapy for myocardial contusion, other than treatment of any resultant arrhythmia and circulatory support as necessary. More significant blunt cardiac injuries, such as disruption of the atria, ventricle, or valves require emergent surgical repair.

In the unstable patient in whom pericardial tamponade is suspected, treatment includes control of the airway, intravascular volume resuscitation, and immediate pericardiocentesis (see Fig. 123.6). Bedside US may assist in both diagnosis and management and can often be performed concurrently with the physical examination. A US showing a large pericardial effusion in the clinical context of tamponade physiology should be sufficient to proceed with pericardiocentesis; additional findings, including diminished or paradoxical septal wall motion and poor cardiac output, may be evident to the more experienced sonographer.

Pericardiocentesis is performed by inserting a 20-gauge spinal needle below the xiphoid process at a 45-degree angle toward the left shoulder (see Fig. 123.7). Dynamic US guidance can help assure proper placement of the needle. Continuous EKG monitoring can be used as well, as a current should be noted on the EKG monitor if the needle touches the heart. Blood aspirated from the pericardial sac can be differentiated from intracardiac blood because pericardial blood is defibrinated and does not clot. Alternatively, pigtail catheters can be placed into the pericardial sac over a guide wire for continual drainage of blood using commercially available equipment kits designed for this purpose. Even though

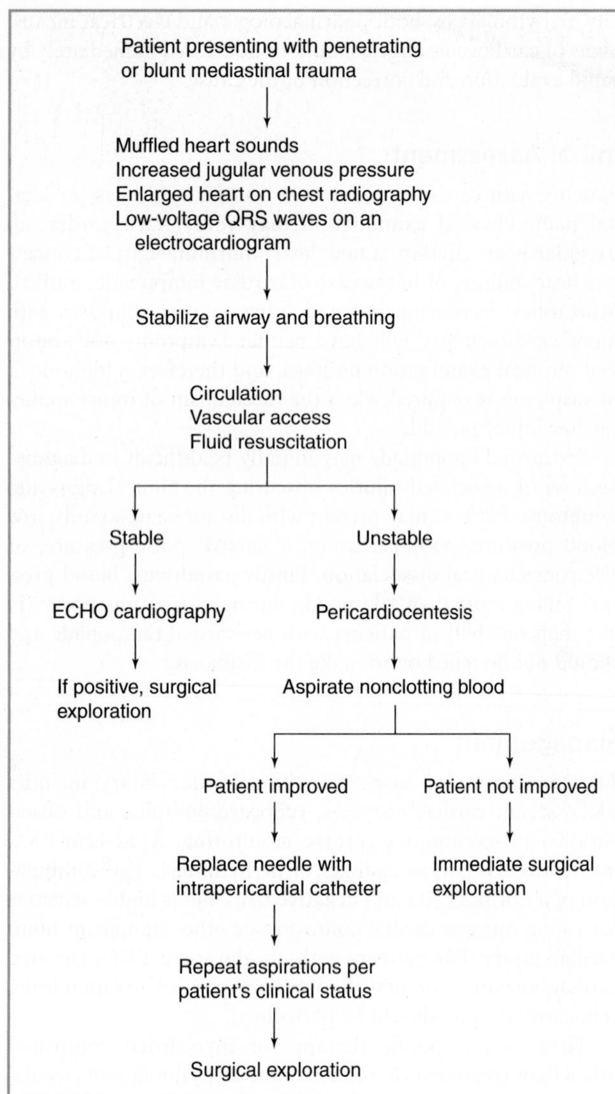

FIGURE 123.6 Algorithm for the evaluation and diagnosis of pericardial tamponade.

patients may show transient improvement after removal of blood from the pericardial sac, the patient should be taken to the operating room immediately for a pericardial window or other surgical intervention (see Chapters 141 Procedures, section on Pericardiocentesis and 142 Ultrasound).

For the stable patient with suspected pericardial tamponade, echocardiogram is the study of choice. CXR may show an enlarged heart and an EKG may show low-voltage QRS waves. While these patients will also require pericardiocentesis, consultation with an interventional cardiologist or cardiac surgeon to perform this in the operating room or cardiac catheterization laboratory is recommended provided the patient's clinical condition allows time for these resources to be mobilized.

Disposition

In one study, all children who developed heart failure or serious cardiac arrhythmias during their hospital course initially presented to the ED either in shock or with a serious arrhythmia. Based on this, patients with suspected myocardial contusion

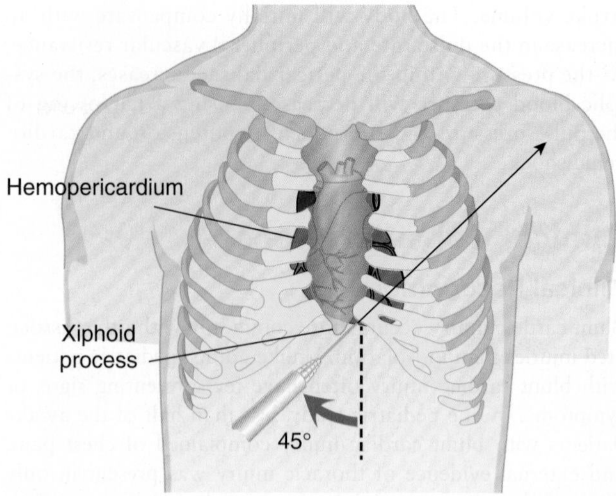

FIGURE 123.7 Pericardiocentesis is performed by inserting a 20-gauge spinal needle below the xiphoid process at a 45-degree angle toward the left shoulder.

can be monitored in the ED or hospital, and if no arrhythmias develop on EKG, can be safely sent home. Children with any arrhythmia require admission to a bed with continuous cardiac monitoring. More significant cardiac injuries necessitate admission to an intensive care unit, with interventional cardiologists or cardiac surgeons available to provide emergent interventions as needed.

INJURIES OF THE AORTA AND GREAT VESSELS

CLINICAL PEARLS AND PITFALLS

- Aortic injury should be suspected when there are severe deceleration forces; classic physical examination findings may not be present.
- Chest radiography is sensitive for the presence of aortic injury and should be followed by CT angiography when concerning.
- Aggressive resuscitation and immediate surgical intervention is necessary for patients with aortic or great vessel injuries and signs of circulatory compromise such as tachycardia, poor perfusion, or hypotension.

Current Evidence

Life-threatening injuries to the great vessels of the thorax carry a high mortality rate but are fortunately rare. The aorta is the vessel most commonly involved in both blunt and penetrating trauma. Rupture of the aorta occurs in approximately 10% to 30% of adults sustaining severe blunt trauma but is much less common in the pediatric population, affecting less than 1% of all children with blunt thoracic trauma. Early detection of such injuries is vital for survival, as overall mortality rate of aortic rupture in children is 75% to 95%, most occurring at the scene.

Clinical Considerations

Clinical Recognition

Aortic injuries are most frequently associated with high-energy deceleration forces, commonly from automobile collisions, causing a shearing stress. The descending aorta is fixed and the arch is mobile. With deceleration, shearing takes place at the level of the ligamentum arteriosum, the most superior fixation point and the most common site of aortic tears in adults and children.

When a great vessel ruptures, massive blood loss may ensue. The body's compensatory mechanisms for the blood loss include an increase in both heart rate and total peripheral vascular resistance. Relying solely on a decrease in systemic blood pressure to detect hemorrhage in children may be deceiving because children may lose up to 25% of their total blood volume before their systemic blood pressure is affected. Children with significant bleeding may have a normal systolic blood pressure but be tachycardic and poorly perfused with a prolonged capillary refill time. These findings should trigger aggressive resuscitation and urgent investigation of the source of hemorrhage, prior to the onset of hypotension.

Triage

Children with known or suspected great vessel injury should be evaluated immediately, mobilizing the highest level of trauma care available. Preparations for both radiologic evaluation and surgical intervention should begin as soon as the injury is suspected, as even the stable patient may deteriorate very rapidly.

Clinical Assessment

Children are usually symptomatic from associated injuries, and great vessel injuries can easily be missed. Clinical signs may include difference in pulse between the arms or arms and legs, thoracic ecchymosis, thoracic and back tenderness, paraplegia, and anuria. In patients with more severe injuries, hypotension or excessive bleeding from a chest tube may be seen. Patients with paraplegia and back pain may be initially diagnosed witha spinal cord injury. Unfortunately, 50% of patients with aortic injuries may have no signs pertaining directly to that injury.

Management

Early diagnosis is imperative in patients with aortic or other great vessel injuries. Morbidity and mortality increase threefold if operative intervention is delayed more than 12 hours. CXR is usually the initial study performed. Findings may include a widened mediastinum, blurred aortic knob, pleural cap, or tracheal or nasogastric tube deviation (see Fig. 123.8). While a normal CXR has been reported to have a 98% negative predictive value in excluding thoracic aortic tear, specificity of an abnormal radiograph is poor and, given sufficient clinical suspicion further imaging is required to make the diagnosis. Multidetector CT angiography has largely replaced echocardiography and aortography as the imaging modality of choice in diagnosing aortic injury, though its test characteristics in children are unknown. For the stable patient with an equivocal CT or who requires further delineation of the injury, aortography may be an appropriate follow-up study (see Fig. 123.9).

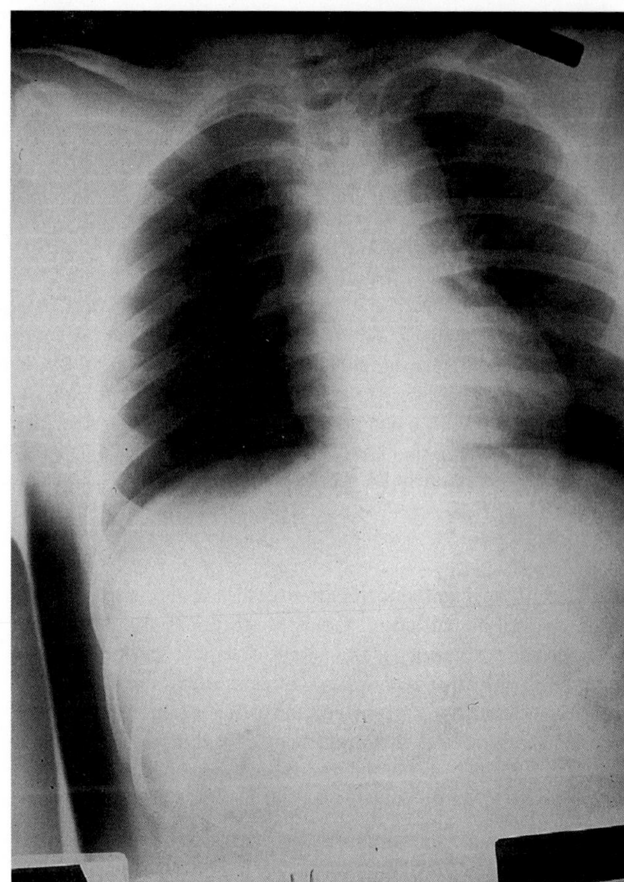

FIGURE 123.8 This 12-year-old girl was an unrestrained passenger involved in a motor vehicle accident. The patient was hypotensive at the scene and could not move her legs. In the emergency department, she had no motor or sensory function to her lower extremities and was anuric. Chest radiograph showed a widened mediastinum from traumatic rupture of the aorta.

Treatment of great vessel injuries varies based on degree and location of injury and stability of the patient. Therapeutic options include fluid resuscitation with beta blockage in hemodynamically stable patients, blood transfusion, and open or endovascular repair.

Disposition

All patients with a great vessel injury require admission to intensive care until either definitive repair of the injury or evidence that the clinical condition has stabilized and is unlikely to deteriorate.

CHEST WALL INJURIES

Goals of Treatment

The elasticity and flexibility of a child's thoracic cage make chest wall injuries less common than internal thoracic injuries such as a pulmonary contusion. When chest wall injuries do occur, the patient is at increased risk for intrathoracic injuries.

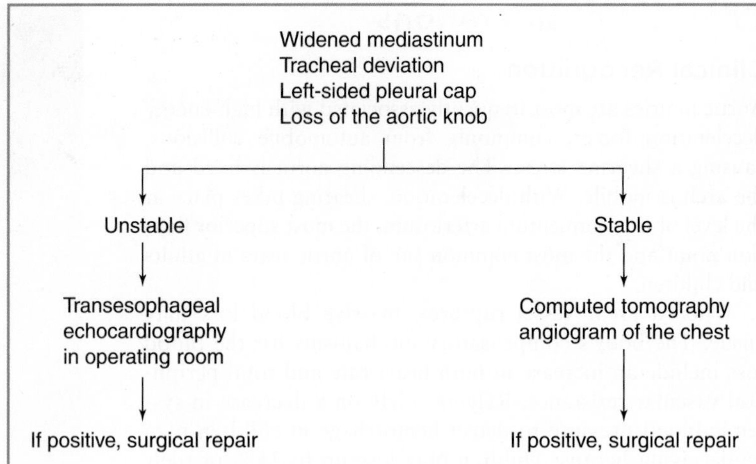

FIGURE 123.9 Algorithm for the evaluation and diagnosis of traumatic rupture of the thoracic aorta.

Included in chest wall injuries are rib, sternal, and scapular fractures, as well as flail chest. Goals of treatment should include appropriate evaluation of the extent of injury and presence of underlying intrathoracic injury. Interventions for chest wall injuries are mostly supportive, consisting of pain control to prevent splinting and encouragement of ambulation to prevent hypoventilation.

CLINICAL PEARLS/PITFALLS

- Chest wall injuries are less common in children than adults due to increased elasticity and compliance of the chest wall, and therefore their presence often indicates coincident intrathoracic injury.
- Most isolated chest wall injuries can be managed as an outpatient with adequate analgesia to prevent splinting and hypoventilation.
- Posterior rib fractures, rib fractures in infants and toddlers, fractures of different ages, and the absence of a clear mechanism of injury are all highly concerning for child abuse and should prompt further evaluation.

RIB FRACTURES

Rib fractures secondary to thoracic trauma are far less common in pediatrics than in the adult population. They may occur from either a direct blow to the rib or compression of the chest in an anterior–posterior direction. In a direct blow to the rib, the rib will fracture inward and may puncture the pleural cavity, causing a pneumothorax, or lacerate a blood vessel resulting in a hemothorax. Compression of the chest wall can cause the lateral portions of the ribs to fracture outward. Intrathoracic injury is seen less commonly with this type of fracture.

In one study, rib fractures occurred in 32% of all children admitted with thoracic trauma, with motor vehicle collisions accounting for the largest proportion of injuries. Single rib fractures did not correlate with the severity of injury, but as the number of fractures increased, so did the likelihood of multisystem and intrathoracic injuries. Although higher force mechanisms are required to injure the first rib due to its protected location, studies have shown that first rib fractures are only predictive of intrathoracic injury in the presence of other concerning symptoms. Nonetheless, a higher index of suspicion for intrathoracic injury is necessary in the presence of a first rib fracture.

The pediatric patient with a rib fracture may splint and hypoventilate secondary to pain. Physical examination may reveal point tenderness and crepitus if a pneumothorax is present. If the patient is stable, then management should focus on relief of pain, monitoring the respiratory status, and further evaluation for underlying injury. Wrapping or binding the chest wall is contraindicated because these measures may impair ventilatory function. Opiates may be required but should be used with caution because they may also cause respiratory depression. For patients requiring admission to the hospital, epidural analgesia or intercostal nerve blocks may be helpful.

Patients with multiple rib fractures should be admitted to the hospital for pain control, pulmonary physiotherapy, and observation for worsening respiratory status. Younger children may require admission to rule out child abuse. Prognosis for isolated rib fractures is excellent, with most healing within 6 weeks without any permanent disability.

RIB FRACTURES AND CHILD ABUSE

Rib fractures in young children are highly associated with child abuse. In one study, the positive predictive value of a rib fracture for nonaccidental trauma was 95% in children less than 3 years old; this number increased to 100% when there was no obvious accidental mechanism provided by the caretaker. Additionally, posterior rib fractures or fractures at multiple stages of healing in infants and toddlers are considered pathognomonic for abuse. Significant chest wall trauma in a young child should always lead the examiner to consider child abuse. If no clear mechanism of injury is presented, further diagnostic studies, such as a skeletal survey are often appropriate. Consultation with a child abuse specialist, where available, may help guide appropriate testing and management.

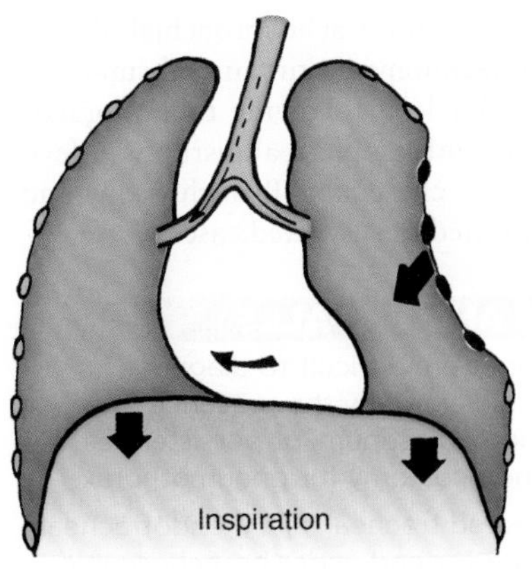

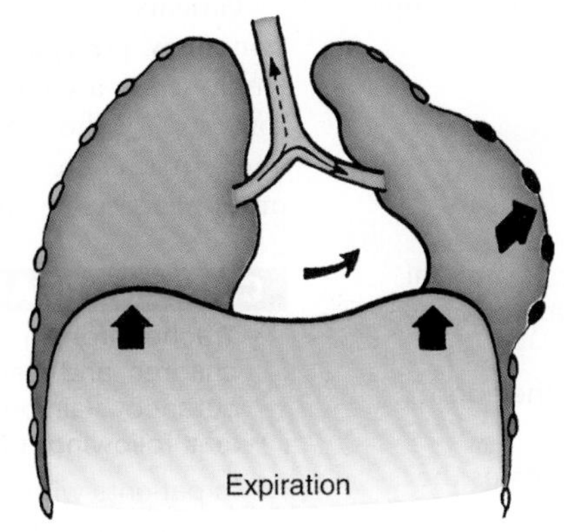

FIGURE 123.10 Pathophysiologic consequence of flail chest with paradoxical motion. (From Fleisher GR, Ludwig S, Henretig FM. *Textbook of pediatric emergency medicine*. 3rd ed. Baltimore, MD: Lippincott Williams & Wilkins, Fig. 101.4, reprinted with permission.)

FLAIL CHEST

Fracturing segments of two or more ribs on the same side may result in that particular chest wall segment losing continuity with the thoracic cage, causing a flail chest (see Fig. 123.10). Flail chest most commonly results from direct impact to the ribs, and is very uncommon in children, owing to the marked compliance of the chest wall. When a flail chest does occur, it is usually associated with an intrathoracic injury, most often pulmonary contusion, because of the force involved.

The goal of treatment should be to stabilize the involved portion of the thoracic cage. At the scene, the patient can be placed with the injured side down, thus improving tidal volume and ventilation. Any patient with respiratory distress should be intubated and managed with positive-pressure ventilation. This serves two purposes. First, the patient's airway is well protected. Second, the positive pressure provides optimal lung expansion and splinting of the injured segment. However, the high pressures necessary to inflate the underlying contused lung can cause a pneumothorax; therefore, care must be taken when delivering positive pressure to the injured child. If the patient does not require intubation, aggressive pulmonary physiotherapy, along with pain control, is the treatment of choice.

STERNAL, SCAPULAR, AND MEDIAL CLAVICLE FRACTURES

Sternal and scapular fractures are uncommon in children. When diagnosed, a thorough evaluation for other thoracic injuries is recommended because of the significant force required to fracture these bones. Fortunately, only rarely are associated vascular or brachial plexus injuries detected.

Displaced fractures of the proximal one-third of the clavicle (or sternoclavicular dislocations in older children), while uncommon, may lead to mediastinal injury from the posteriorly displaced fragment. Patients may present with neurovascular impairment of the extremity, dysphagia, hoarseness, dyspnea or even signs of circulatory compromise. Visualization of the fracture itself may be difficult on plain films of the sternum or clavicle. If a proximal clavicle fracture or dislocation is found or highly suspected on CXR, CT angiography of the chest should be performed to better characterize the injury and assess for involvement of the great vessels. Treatment will depend on the extent of the injury, but coordination between orthopedic and general or thoracic surgeons is usually necessary to ensure adequate evaluation of all possible injuries and maximize likelihood of a successful outcome (see Chapter 119 Musculoskeletal Trauma).

PENETRATING TRAUMA AND ED THORACOTOMY

Goals of Treatment

Penetrating thoracic trauma in children is less common than blunt trauma and, surprisingly, carries an overall equal risk of morbidity and mortality. Pediatric patients who die from blunt thoracic trauma are likely to perish at the scene and those who survive to ED arrival are unlikely to die from their thoracic injury, succumbing instead to associated intracranial and intra-abdominal injuries. In contrast, mortality in children with penetrating thoracic trauma who survive to ED arrival is typically related to direct injury to intrathoracic structures.

In one study, penetrating thoracic trauma occurred in 20% of pediatric patients being evaluated for thoracic injury. The most common mechanism of injury was gunshot wound, followed by stab wound. Unlike blunt thoracic trauma, where observation and supportive therapies are most common, penetrating thoracic trauma often requires invasive interventions. The most common penetrating thoracic injuries are hemothorax and pneumothorax, almost always requiring tube thoracostomy. More children with penetrating thoracic injury will require operative intervention because of the close proximity of the vital organs in the thoracic cavity in children, as compared with adults.

Evaluation and treatment includes airway stabilization, fluid resuscitation, and management of the chest wound. Radiopaque markers (such as paper clips) may be placed by the entry and exit sites to help determine the course of the missile. Penetrating injuries near the mediastinum may be critical, especially if the patient is hemodynamically unstable. Pericardial tamponade should be considered and immediately treated in the unstable patient. In the stable patient, transesophageal or transthoracic echocardiogram is helpful in evaluating the heart and determining if there is fluid within the pericardial sac. Diaphragmatic lacerations are difficult to diagnose and may require exploratory laparotomy, thoracoscopy, or laparoscopy for diagnosis and treatment.

CLINICAL PEARLS AND PITFALLS

- Penetrating trauma remains uncommon in children, but confers a high mortality risk.
- Presence of hemothorax, pneumothorax, or pericardial tamponade necessitates emergent tube thoracostomy or pericardiocentesis, respectively.
- Many patients will also have involvement of the abdomen, which requires thorough evaluation.
- Significant or fluid-resistant hypotension indicates the need for emergent thoracotomy.

Emergency Department Thoracotomy

Emergency department thoracotomy (EDT) is the most aggressive resuscitative measure for patients with thoracic trauma. With the advancement of transport systems and regionalization of trauma centers, patients who previously would have died at the scene are now surviving to arrival to trauma centers for evaluation and treatment. EDT allows the physician to evaluate and evacuate the pericardial sac, perform open cardiac massage, and temporarily control bleeding from the heart, hilum, or lung. Catheters can also be placed directly into the right atrium, helping with fluid resuscitation, and the thoracic aorta can be compressed, improving circulation to the brain and heart.

Anecdotal reports have been published suggesting EDT may be useful in the pediatric patient with penetrating trauma who has vital signs but loses them during transport or acutely deteriorates during ED resuscitation. The limited available pediatric data suggest that EDT is unlikely to be successful in blunt or penetrating trauma cases that arrive in the ED without any vital signs or EKG tracing.

Lifesaving interventions such as airway management, fluid resuscitation, and pericardiocentesis should not be delayed while waiting for EDT to be performed. The pediatric patient with vital signs, but not responding to initial treatment such as tube thoracostomy and pericardiocentesis, is a candidate for thoracotomy in the operating room, rather than the ED.

OTHER INTRATHORACIC INJURIES

Goals of Treatment

Diaphragmatic, esophageal, and tracheobronchial disruptions are rare and are often overlooked in the initial evaluation of thoracic trauma. The CXR may initially appear normal in 30% to 50% of diaphragmatic hernias. When abnormal, the CXR may show a bowel gas pattern in the lungs, a displaced nasogastric tube, or an elevated hemidiaphragm, more common on the left than the right. The patient may complain of chest pain or difficulty breathing. The examination may be normal or show decreased breath sounds, respiratory distress, or a scaphoid abdomen. Surgical exploration is indicated in all suspected cases because a diaphragmatic hernia does not improve without surgical correction.

Patients with esophageal and tracheobronchial disruptions may present with pneumomediastinum, subcutaneous emphysema, a continuous air leak following tube thoracostomy, or, for those patients with esophageal disruption, fever and gastric contents from the chest tube. Bronchoscopy and/or esophagoscopy are indicated in suspected cases.

CLINICAL PEARLS AND PITFALLS

- Tracheobronchial injuries are difficult to diagnose in children, and may be indicated by the presence of subcutaneous air, pneumomediastinum, or persistent air leak following tube thoracostomy for pneumothorax.
- In patients with suspected tracheal injury, endotracheal intubation should be performed under bronchoscopic guidance in the operating room when possible, to avoid converting a partial tracheal injury to a full tear.
- Symptoms of esophageal injury will depend on the region that perforates, and symptoms may therefore refer to the neck, chest, back, or abdomen. Delay in diagnosis has a significant impact on morbidity and mortality.
- While the finding of abdominal contents in the chest on radiograph is specific for diaphragmatic rupture, it is insensitive, and this injury must be considered any time there is significant blunt force to the abdomen or penetrating injury to the chest.
- The findings of traumatic asphyxia are dramatic, but patients who survive the initial injury are most at risk from associated intra-abdominal and intrathoracic injuries.

Tracheobronchial Injuries

Injury to the tracheobronchial tree in children occurs rarely, with an incidence of less than 1% of injured children. This injury typically results from a high-energy mechanism or a focused direct blow. Major vessels or pulmonary parenchyma are more likely to be injured in penetrating trauma than the tracheobronchial tree. Cervical tracheal rupture may be caused by a direct blow to the trachea or violent flexion and extension of the patient's head. This whiplash effect can cause a tear between two cartilaginous rings. Lower tracheobronchial injury usually occurs from a sudden increase in intrabronchial pressure. Because the child's chest wall is elastic, the trachea and main bronchi can be compressed between the chest wall and the vertebral spine. Compression of the chest against a closed glottis can cause a sudden increase in intrabronchial pressure, resulting in a tracheobronchial tear. Shear forces, traction, and crushing the airway between the chest and vertebral column may also cause a tracheobronchial injury. Approximately 80% of tracheobronchial injuries occur on the posterior wall of the airway within 2 cm of the carina.

The diagnosis of tracheobronchial injury may be difficult in the pediatric population. The mechanism of injury (fall, crush, direct blow) provides an important clue. Symptoms such as chest pain and dyspnea are common but nonspecific. Clinical signs include cyanosis, hemoptysis, tachypnea, and subcutaneous emphysema (cervical, mediastinal, or both). Pneumomediastinum and cervical subcutaneous emphysema are seen commonly in airway rupture. If a pneumothorax is present with these findings, a bronchial rupture should be suspected. A continued air leak after insertion of a thoracostomy tube should alert the physician to the possibility of a tracheobronchial disruption. Because of anatomic differences, ruptures of

TABLE 123.1

THORACIC TRAUMA INJURIES REQUIRING OPERATIVE INTERVENTION

Injury	Signs and symptoms
Tracheal/bronchial rupture	Active chest tube air leak, pneumothorax not resolved
Lung parenchyma, internal mammary artery laceration, intercostal artery laceration	Chest tube bleeding greater than 2–3 mL/kg/hr or hypotension unresponsive to transfusions
Esophageal disruption	Abnormal esophagram (uncontained leak) or esophagoscopy
	Gastric contents in the chest tube
Diaphragmatic hernia	Abnormal gas pattern in the hemithorax
	Displaced nasogastric tube in the hemithorax
Pericardial tamponade	Positive pericardiocentesis
Great vessel laceration	Widened mediastinum
	Tracheal or nasogastric tube deviation
	Blurred aortic knob
	Abnormal CT angiogram

the bronchi occur on the right side more frequently than the left. In the absence of a pneumothorax, tracheal or esophageal rupture should be suspected if a pneumomediastinum or cervical emphysema is present. However, in most patients with asymptomatic pneumomediastinum, no source is identified on evaluation.

The treatment includes initial airway stabilization and bronchoscopic evaluation of the airway. Numerous case reports describe partial tracheal tears becoming complete after endotracheal intubation. Therefore, if the airway is stable and a tear is known or strongly suspected, oral tracheal intubation should be performed in the operating room under bronchoscopic guidance. This prevents further trauma to the airway, and if a complication arises, emergency surgical access to the airway is readily available. If the airway is unstable and emergent endotracheal intubation needs to be performed, back up surgical approaches should be prepared. Emergent recruitment of a trauma or thoracic surgeon to assist if tracheal disruption worsens can be lifesaving. An advantage of early bronchoscopy is exact identification and location of the lesion. The best surgical results are achieved when operative exploration is performed early (Table 123.1). In the stable patient, CT scan of the chest can also help confirm the diagnosis and identify other injuries.

ESOPHAGEAL INJURIES

Esophageal injury is rare in children, and presents a diagnostic challenge when it does occur. Timely and accurate diagnosis of an esophageal injury is paramount. The complications of delayed diagnosis include mediastinal sepsis and death. The most common cause for esophageal perforation in the pediatric population is iatrogenic, followed by penetrating trauma (gunshot and stab wounds). Esophageal perforation can occur in blunt trauma if there is a significant amount of chest or pharyngeal compression. The cervical and thoracic regions are more commonly affected, with the thoracic region having the highest mortality rate (35%).

The patient's signs and symptoms will depend on the region injured. Patients with an esophageal rupture in the cervical region may complain of neck stiffness or neck pain. They may regurgitate bloody material and have cervical subcutaneous emphysema or odynophagia. A lateral neck radiograph may show retroesophageal emphysema. In the thoracic region, patients may present with abdominal spasms and guarding, chest pain, subcutaneous emphysema, tachycardia, or dyspnea. A CXR may show a pneumothorax, pneumomediastinum, subcutaneous emphysema in the neck, a left pleural effusion, or an air–fluid level in the mediastinum. Perforation of the intra-abdominal esophagus may cause retrosternal, epigastric, or shoulder pain.

Patients with suspected esophageal perforation should be adequately volume resuscitated and receive antibiotics covering gram-positive, gram-negative, and anaerobic organisms. The diagnosis of an esophageal perforation can be made by either an esophagram, esophagoscopy, or both. In one study, flexible esophagoscopy had a sensitivity of 100% and specificity of 96%. Depending on the expertise at each institution and the stability of the patient, these studies may be paired to lessen the chance of a misdiagnosis. Once the diagnosis is made, if the leak is large and not contained prompt surgical correction is mandatory. Smaller, contained leaks may be successfully managed nonoperatively. If the diagnosis is made within 24 hours, mortality rate is approximately 5%. Delayed diagnosis for more than 24 hours after injury is associated with a mortality rate of 70%.

DIAPHRAGMATIC INJURIES

A crushing abdominal force will produce a sudden increase in intrathoracic and intra-abdominal pressure against the fixed diaphragm. A diaphragmatic injury should also be suspected in any thoracic or upper abdominal penetrating injury. The level of the diaphragm fluctuates greatly with respirations, and injuries of the diaphragm have been reported with penetrating wounds as high as the third rib and as low as the twelfth rib. Blunt traumatic diaphragmatic rupture is more commonly left sided (80%) because the left diaphragm is relatively unprotected compared to the right, though right and bilateral diaphragmatic injuries have been reported (see Fig. 123.11). Right-sided diaphragmatic injuries are associated with increased mortality rate as these patients usually have a greater physiologic insult and associated injuries.

Motor vehicle collisions are the most common mechanism of injury. The direction of impact may play a role in the side and type of diaphragmatic rupture. A lateral torso impact has been shown to be three times more likely to result in a ruptured diaphragm than a frontal impact and the rupture tends to be on the same side as the impact. Associated injuries such as pulmonary contusions, hepatic or splenic lacerations, and fractures of the extremities are present in more than 75% of patients. Thoracic aortic injuries have been reported in up to 10% of adults with diaphragmatic injury and should be considered in children with diaphragmatic trauma.

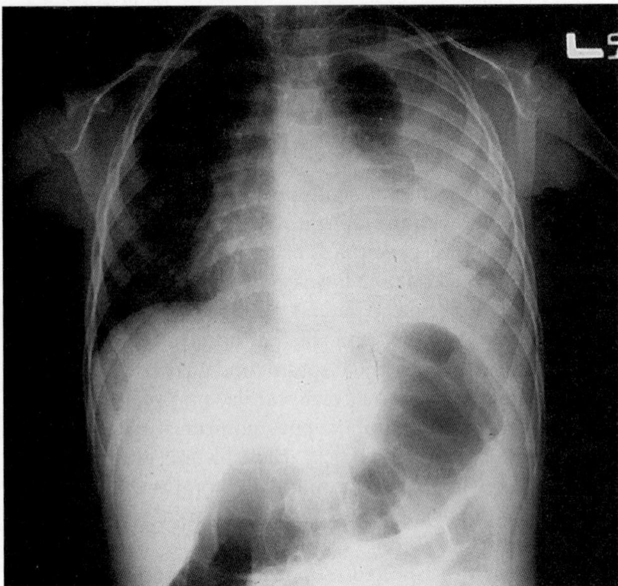

FIGURE 123.11 This 5-year-old boy was on a snowmobile when it crashed into a tree. Initially there was no respiratory distress, but upon arrival at the emergency department, the patient became tachypneic and required oxygen. Breath sounds were reportedly normal. Chest radiograph showed a left-sided diaphragmatic hernia. This injury was surgically repaired in the operating room, and the patient did well postoperatively.

Patients may present in respiratory distress and have a scaphoid abdomen, although they are more likely to be symptomatic from associated injuries than from the diaphragmatic rupture itself. The verbal child may complain of chest pain or ipsilateral shoulder pain. The presence of bowel sounds within the thoracic cavity is nonspecific because bowel sounds can be transmitted from the abdominal cavity in children. More commonly, bowel sounds are absent because of the ileus that is typically associated with the injury. A nasogastric tube may be difficult to pass in patients with a diaphragmatic injury and gastric herniation. In left-sided diaphragmatic tears, the tip of the nasogastric tube may be seen looping into the chest. Even though the diagnosis of diaphragmatic injury is usually made upon initial review of the CXR, some series reported that up to 30% to 50% of initial films were normal. Right-sided diaphragmatic injury and herniation is more difficult to diagnose because the herniated organs are more likely to be solid. The chest x-ray may just show opacification of the right lung fields. This emphasizes the importance of serial evaluations and CXRs in patients suspected of having a diaphragmatic injury. Other diagnostic studies such as chest and abdominal CT scan with contrast or upper and lower gastrointestinal tract series can help confirm the diagnosis.

Before performing a tube thoracostomy for a pneumothorax or hemothorax, diaphragmatic injury should be considered to avoid injury to herniated intra-abdominal organs. In patients who clinically appear to have a diaphragmatic injury (scaphoid abdomen, bowel sounds auscultated in the thoracic cavity), a finger should be inserted in the thoracostomy incision site and the diaphragm should be palpated before placing a chest tube.

Herniation and strangulation of bowel may result from a delayed diagnosis. Diaphragmatic defects will not spontaneously heal because of motion associated with respirations and cyclical tension. Exploratory laparotomy or laparoscopy should be performed in cases where a diaphragmatic hernia is strongly suspected.

TRAUMATIC ASPHYXIA

Traumatic asphyxia results from direct compression of the chest or abdomen. The most common mechanism is a child run over by a slowly moving motor vehicle or pinned underneath a heavy object. In anticipation of impending injury, the child may inspire, tensing the thoracoabdominal muscles and closing the glottis. Traumatic asphyxia also occurs in patients with asthma, seizures, persistent vomiting, and pertussis.

Positive pressure is transmitted to the mediastinum, and blood is forced out of the right atrium into the valveless venous and capillary systems. The clinical manifestations occur because the increase in pressure dilates the capillary and venous systems. Areas drained by the superior vena cava are particularly affected, explaining the marked difference between the patient's head and neck as opposed to the lower body. Patients with traumatic asphyxia usually present with subconjunctival and upper body petechial hemorrhages, cyanosis, periorbital edema, respiratory distress, altered mental status, and associated injuries.

The primary goal of treatment is to stabilize the patient and evaluate associated injuries. The external appearance of a child with traumatic asphyxia is quite impressive, but initial attention should be paid to the cardiopulmonary status of the child. Pulmonary contusions and hepatic injuries are commonly seen with traumatic asphyxia, and CT scan is helpful in identifying head and abdominal injuries. Because the most severe injuries cause immediate death, the prognosis is good for any patient surviving the first few hours. Cutaneous manifestations will resolve with time, and neurologic sequelae are rare.

Suggested Readings and Key References

General

Allshouse M, Eichelberger M. Patterns of thoracic injury. In: Eichelberger M, ed. *Pediatric trauma: prevention, acute care, rehabilitation*. St. Louis, MO: Mosby–Year Book, 1993:437–448.

Balci AE, Kazez A, Eren S, et al. Blunt thoracic trauma in children: review of 137 cases. *Eur J Cardiothorac Surg* 2004;26(2):387–392.

Bliss D, Silen M. Pediatric thoracic trauma. *Crit Care Med* 2002;30(11):409–415.

Cooper A. Thoracic injuries. *Semin Pediatr Surg* 1995;4(2):109–115.

Cooper A, Barlow B, DiScala C, et al. Mortality and truncal injury: the pediatric perspective. *J Pediatr Surg* 1994;29(1):33–38.

Exadaktylos AK, Sclabas G, Schmid SW, et al. Do we really need routine computed tomographic scanning in the primary evaluation of blunt chest trauma in patients with "normal" chest radiograph? *J Trauma* 2001;51(6):1173–1176.

Gittelman MA, Gonzalez-del-Rey J, Brody AS, et al. Clinical predictors for the selective use of chest radiographs in pediatric blunt trauma evaluations. *J Trauma* 2003;55(4):670–676.

Grisoni ER, Volsko TA. Thoracic injuries in children. *Respir Care Clin N Am* 2001;7(1):25–38.

Hall A, Johnson K. The imaging of paediatric thoracic trauma. *Paediatr Respir Rev* 2002;3(3):241–247.

Holmes JF, Sokolove PE, Brant WE, et al. A clinical decision rule for identifying children with thoracic injuries after blunt torso trauma. *Ann Emerg Med* 2002;39(5):492–499.

Inan M, Ayvaz S, Sut N, et al. Blunt chest trauma in childhood. *ANZ J Surg* 2007;77(8):682–685.

Peclet MH, Newman KD, Eichelberger MR, et al. Patterns of injury in children. *J Pediatr Surg* 1990;25(1):85–90.

Peclet MH, Newman KD, Eichelberger MR, et al. Thoracic trauma in children: an indicator of increased mortality. *J Pediatr Surg* 1990;25(9):961–965.

Trupka A, Waydhas C, Hallfeldt KJ. Value of thoracic computed tomography in the first assessment of severely injured patients with blunt chest trauma: results of a prospective study. *J Trauma* 1997;43(3):405–411.

Chest Wall Injury

Barsness KA, Cha ES, Bensard DD, et al. The positive predictive value of rib fractures as an indicator of nonaccidental trauma in children. *J Trauma* 2003;54(6):1107–1110.

Freedland M, Wilson RF, Bender JS, et al. The management of flail chest injury: factors affecting outcome. *J Trauma* 1990;30(12):1460–1468.

Garcia VF, Gotschall CS, Eichelberger MR, et al. Rib fractures in children: a marker of severe trauma. *J Trauma* 1990;30(6):695–700.

Harris GJ, Soper RT. Pediatric first rib fractures. *J Trauma* 1990;30(3):343–345.

Kwon A, Sorrells DL Jr, Kurkchubasche AG, et al. Isolated computed tomography diagnosis of pulmonary contusion does not correlate with increased morbidity. *J Pediatr Surg* 2006;41(1):78–82.

Landercasper J, Cogbill TH, Strutt PJ. Delayed diagnosis of flail chest. *Crit Care Med* 1990;18(6):611–613.

Sadaba JR, Oswal D, Munsch CM. Management of isolated sternal fractures: determining the risk of blunt cardiac injury. *Ann R Coll Surg Engl* 2000;82(3):162–166.

Schweich P, Fleisher G. Rib fractures in children. *Pediatr Emerg Care* 1985;1(4):187–189.

Shorr RM, Crittenden M, Indeck M, et al. Blunt thoracic trauma. Analysis of 515 patients. *Ann Surg* 1987;206(2):200–205.

Stephens NG, Morgan AS, Corvo P, et al. Significance of scapular fracture in the blunt-trauma patient. *Ann Emerg Med* 1995;26(4):439–442.

Ziegler DW, Agarwal NN. The morbidity and mortality of rib fractures. *J Trauma* 1994;37(6):975–979.

Lung Injury

Blostein PA, Hodgman CG. Computed tomography of the chest in blunt thoracic trauma: results of a prospective study. *J Trauma* 1997;43(1):13–18.

Bonadio WA, Hellmich T. Post-traumatic pulmonary contusion in children. *Ann Emerg Med* 1989;18(10):1050–1052.

Frame SB, Marshall WJ, Clifford TG. Synchronized independent lung ventilation in the management of pediatric unilateral pulmonary contusion: case report. *J Trauma* 1989;29(3):395–397.

Johnson JA, Cogbill TH, Winga ER. Determinants of outcome after pulmonary contusion. *J Trauma* 1986;26(8):695–697.

Moore MA, Wallace EC, Westra SJ. The imaging of paediatric thoracic trauma. *Pediatr Radiol* 2009;39(5):485–496.

Pneumothorax/Hemothorax

Chen SC, Markmann JF, Kauder DR, et al. Hemopneumothorax missed by auscultation in penetrating chest injury. *J Trauma* 1997;42(1):86–89.

Jalli R, Sefidbakht S, Jafari SH. Value of ultrasound in diagnosis of pneumothorax: a prospective study. *Emerg Radiol* 2013;20(2):131–134.

Kirkpatrick AW, Sirois M, Laupland KB, et al. Hand-held thoracic sonography for detecting post-traumatic pneumothoraces: the Extended Focused Assessment with Sonography for Trauma (EFAST). *J Trauma* 2004;57(2):288–295.

Kulvatunyou N, Erickson L, Vijayasekaran A, et al. Randomized clinical trial of pigtail catheter versus chest tube in injured patients with uncomplicated traumatic pneumothorax. *Br J Surg* 2014;101(2):17–22.

Kulvatunyou N, Vijayasekaran A, Hansen A, et al. Two-year experience of using pigtail catheters to treat traumatic pneumothorax: a changing trend. *J Trauma* 2011;71(5):1104–1107.

Lee LK, Rogers AJ, Ehrlich PF, et al.; Pediatric Emergency Care Applied Research Network (PECARN). Occult pneumothoraces in children with blunt torso trauma. *Acad Emerg Med* 2014;21(4):440–448.

Ma OJ, Mateer JR. Trauma ultrasound examination versus chest radiography in the detection of hemothorax. *Ann Emerg Med* 1997;29(3):312–315.

Nakayama DK, Ramenofsky ML, Rowe MI. Chest injuries in childhood. *Ann Surg* 1989;210(6):770–775.

Rowan KR, Kirkpatrick AW, Liu D, et al. Traumatic pneumothorax detection with thoracic US: correlation with chest radiography and CT—initial experience. *Radiology* 2002;225(1):210–214.

Symbas PN. Cardiothoracic trauma. *Curr Probl Surg* 1991;28(11):741–797.

Tracheal and Bronchial Injury

Baumgartner F, Sheppard B, de Virgilio C, et al. Tracheal and main bronchial disruptions after blunt chest trauma: presentation and management. *Ann Thorac Surg* 1990;50(4):569–574.

Gaebler C, Mueller M, Schramm W, et al. Tracheobronchial ruptures in children. *Am J Emerg Med* 1996;14(3):279–284.

Hancock BJ, Wiseman NE. Tracheobronchial injuries in children. *J Pediatr Surg* 1991;26(11):1316–1319.

Kadish H, Schunk J, Woodward GA. Blunt pediatric laryngotracheal trauma: case report and review of the literature. *Am J Emerg Med* 1994;12(2):207–211.

Symbas PN, Justicz AG, Ricketts RR. Rupture of the airways from blunt trauma: treatment of complex injuries. *Ann Thorac Surg* 1992;54(1):177–183.

Taskinen SO, Salo JA, Halttunnen PE. Tracheobronchial rupture due to blunt chest trauma: a follow-up study. *Ann Thorac Surg* 1989;48(6):846–849.

Esophageal Injury

Backer CL, LoCicero J, Hartz RS. Computed tomography in patients with esophageal perforation. *Chest* 1990;98(5):1078–1080.

Flowers JL, Graham SM, Ugarte MA, et al. Flexible endoscopy for the diagnosis of esophageal trauma. *J Trauma* 1996;40(2):261–265.

Jones WG, Ginsberg RJ. Esophageal perforation: a continuing challenge. *Ann Thorac Surg* 1992;53(3):534–543.

Diaphragmatic Injury

Beauchamp G, Khalfallah A, Girard R, et al. Blunt diaphragmatic rupture. *Am J Surg* 1984;148(2):292–295.

Boulanger BR, Milzman DP, Rosati C, et al. A comparison of right and left blunt traumatic diaphragmatic rupture. *J Trauma* 1993;35(2):255–260.

Brandt ML, Luks FI, Spigland NA. Diaphragmatic injury in children. *J Trauma* 1992;32(3):298–301.

Guth AA, Pachter HL, Kim U. Pitfalls in the diagnosis of blunt diaphragmatic injury. *Am J Surg* 1995;170(1):5–9.

Murray JA, Demetriades D, Cornwell EE, et al. Penetrating left thoracoabdominal trauma: the incidence and clinical presentation of diaphragm injuries. *J Trauma* 1997;43(4):624–626.

Pagliarello G, Carter J. Traumatic injury to the diaphragm: timely diagnosis and treatment. *J Trauma* 1992;33(2):194–197.

Traumatic Asphyxia

Gorenstein L, Blair GK, Shandling B. The prognosis of traumatic asphyxia in childhood. *J Pediatr Surg* 1986;21(9):753–756.

Newquist MJ, Sobel RM. Traumatic asphyxia: an indicator of significant pulmonary injury. *Am J Emerg Med* 1990;8(3):212–215.

Sklar DP, Baack B, McFeeley P, et al. Traumatic asphyxia in New Mexico: a five-year experience. *Am J Emerg Med* 1988;6(3):219–223.

Aortic and Great Vessel Injury

Dart CH Jr, Braitman HE. Traumatic rupture of the thoracic aorta. Diagnosis and management. *Arch Surg* 1976;111(6):697–702.

Eddy AC, Rusch VW, Fligner CL, et al. The epidemiology of traumatic rupture of the thoracic aorta in children: a 13-year review. *J Trauma* 1990;30(8):989–991.

Lee J, Harris JH Jr, Duke JH Jr, et al. Noncorrelation between thoracic skeletal injuries and acute traumatic aortic tear. *J Trauma* 1997; 43(4):400–404.

Saletta S, Lederman E, Fein S. Transesophageal echocardiography for the initial evaluation of the widened mediastinum in trauma patients. *J Trauma* 1995;39(1):137–141.

Smith MD, Cassidy JM, Souther S, et al. Transesophageal echocardiography in the diagnosis of traumatic rupture of the aorta. *N Engl J Med* 1995;332(6):356–362.

Blunt Cardiac Injury

Bertinchant JP, Polge A, Mohty D, et al. Evaluation of incidence, clinical significance, and prognostic value of circulating cardiac troponin I and T elevation in hemodynamically stable patients with suspected myocardial contusion after blunt chest trauma. *J Trauma* 2000;48(5):924–931.

Biffl WL, Moore FA, Moore EE, et al. Cardiac enzymes are irrelevant in the patient with suspected myocardial contusion. *Am J Surg* 1994;168(6):523–527.

Dowd MD, Krug S. Pediatric blunt cardiac injury: epidemiology, clinical features, and diagnosis. Pediatric Emergency Medicine Collaborative Research Committee: Working Group on Blunt Cardiac injury. *J Trauma* 1996;40(1):61–67.

Karalis DG, Victor MF, Davis GA, et al. The role of echocardiography in blunt chest trauma: a transthoracic and transesophageal echocardiographic study. *J Trauma* 1994;36(1):53–58.

Maron BJ, Gohman TE, Kyle SB, et al. Clinical profile and spectrum of commotio cordis. *JAMA* 2002;287(9):1142–1146.

Maron BJ, Poliac LC, Kaplan JA, et al. Blunt impact to the chest leading to sudden death from cardiac arrest during sports activities. *N Engl J Med* 1995;333(6):337–342.

Murillo CA, Owens-Stovall SK, Kim S. Delayed cardiac tamponade after blunt chest trauma in a child. *J Trauma* 2002;52(3):573–575.

Rajan GP, Zellweger R. Cardiac troponin I as a predictor of arrhythmia and ventricular dysfunction in trauma patients with myocardial contusion. *J Trauma* 2004;57(4):801–808.

Velmahos GC, Karaiskakis M, Salim A, et al. Normal electrocardiography and serum troponin I levels preclude the presence of clinically significant blunt cardiac injury. *J Trauma* 2003;54(1): 45–50.

Penetrating Thoracic Injury

Fernandez LG, Radhakrishnan J, Gordon RT, et al. Thoracic BB injuries in pediatric patients. *J Trauma* 1995;38(3):384–389.

Inci I, Ozcelik C, Nizam O. Penetrating chest injuries in children: a review of 94 cases. *J Pediatr Surg* 1996;31(5):673–676.

Nance ML, Sing RF, Reilly PM. Thoracic gunshot wounds in children under 17 years of age. *J Pediatr Surg* 1996;31(7):931–935.

Peterson RJ, Tiwary AD, Kissoon N, et al. Pediatric penetrating thoracic trauma: a five-year experience. *Pediatr Emerg Care* 1994;10(3): 129–131.

Emergency Department Thoracotomy

Beaver BL, Colombani PM, Buck JR, et al. Efficacy of emergency room thoracotomy in pediatric trauma. *J Pediatr Surg* 1987;22(1): 19–23.

Boyd M, Vanek VW, Bourguet CC. Emergency room resuscitative thoracotomy: when is it indicated? *J Trauma* 1992;33(5):714–721.

Durham LA, Richardson RJ, Wall MJ, et al. Emergency center thoracotomy: impact of prehospital resuscitation. *J Trauma* 1992;32(6): 775–779.

Esposito TJ, Jurkovich GJ, Rice CL, et al. Reappraisal of emergency room thoracotomy in a changing environment. *J Trauma* 1991; 31(7):881–885.

Langer JC, Hoffman MA, Pearl RH, et al. Survival after emergency department thoracotomy in a child with blunt multisystem trauma. *Pediatr Emerg Care* 1989;5(4):255–256.

Lorenz HP, Steinmetz B, Lieberman J. Emergency thoracotomy: survival correlates with physiologic status. *J Trauma* 1992;32(6): 780–785.

Powell RW, Gill EA, Jurkovich GJ, et al. Resuscitative thoracotomy in children and adolescents. *Am Surg* 1988;54(4):188–191.

Sheikh A, Brogan T. Outcome and cost of open- and closed-chest cardiopulmonary resuscitation in pediatric cardiac arrest. *Pediatrics* 1994;93(3):392–398.

SECTION VI
Surgical Emergencies

CHAPTER 124 ■ ABDOMINAL EMERGENCIES

RICHARD G. BACHUR, MD

GOALS OF EMERGENCY CARE

Pediatric abdominal complaints are common, and ED physicians are challenged to distinguish common, innocent gastrointestinal complaints from surgical emergencies. Logical diagnostic strategies and prompt recognition of surgical emergencies should be the goal of the evaluation. For abdominal surgical emergencies, the clinical evaluation should focus on timely recognition of a surgical condition and early involvement of a surgeon. Ideal care would limit complications such as peritonitis and ischemic bowel.

KEY POINTS

- Bilious emesis in a young infant is a surgical emergency
- Young children with appendicitis often have atypical presentations
- Intussusception can present with profound altered mental status
- Bloody stool or blood per rectum may represent ischemic bowel

RELATED CHAPTERS

Signs and Symptoms
- Abdominal Distension: Chapter 7
- Constipation: Chapter 13
- Gastrointestinal Bleeding: Chapter 28
- Pain: Abdomen: Chapter 48

Clinical Pathways
- Abdominal Pain in Postpubertal Girls: Chapter 82
- Appendicitis (Suspected): Chapter 83

Medical, Surgical, Trauma
- Gastrointestinal Emergencies: Chapter 99
- Gynecology Emergencies: Chapter 100
- Abdominal Trauma: Chapter 111

ACUTE NONPERFORATED APPENDICITIS

CLINICAL PEARLS AND PITFALLS

- Young children often have nonclassic presentations of appendicitis
- Pain and tenderness will vary based on exact location of the appendix
- Rapid improvement in pain in a child with high suspicion of appendicitis may occur at the time of perforation
- Equivocal ultrasounds for appendicitis should not lead to a CT if suspicion is relatively low

Current Evidence

Acute appendicitis is the most common, nontraumatic surgical emergency in children. Anatomic characteristics may influence the incidence and presentation of appendicitis throughout childhood. Lymphoid hyperplasia within the appendix is maximal in adolescence and might be related to the peak incidence in this age group. Generally, obstruction of the appendix (by fecal material, an appendicolith, or simply lymphoid hyperplasia) is believed to be a key step in the development of appendicitis. Once obstructed, bacterial overgrowth and invasion into the mucosal barrier leads to progressive inflammation and dilation. Localized pain and tenderness develops. Perforation rarely develops before 12 hours of pain but is common after 72 hours. Perforation can lead to generalized peritonitis or focal abscesses. Since younger children have a relatively underdeveloped omentum, they are much more likely to present with diffuse peritonitis.

Goals of Treatment

Early recognition and surgical excision prior to perforation is ideal. The clinical team should consider advanced diagnostic imaging for children without typical presentations or examination findings. Clinical outcomes for patients with suspected appendicitis include accurate identification of appendicitis over medical etiologies of focal abdominal tenderness, limiting the use of computed tomography among patients with uncomplicated acute appendicitis, minimizing the number of negative appendectomies, operative care prior to perforation,

TABLE 124.1

PROGRESSION OF SYMPTOMS AND SIGNS OF APPENDICITIS

Nonperforated appendicitis
Poorly defined midabdominal or periumbilical pain
Low-grade fever
Anorexia
Vomiting
Migration of pain to right lower quadrant
Localization depends on position of appendix
Appendix in gutter → lateral abdominal tenderness
Appendix pointing toward pelvis → tenderness near pubis may cause diarrhea or bladder irritation
Retrocecal appendix → tenderness elicited by deep palpation
Pain on coughing, hopping, or to percussion
Rectal examination: pain on palpation of right rectal wall
WBC count: 10,000–15,000/mm^3
Urinalysis: ketosis, few WBCs
Perforated appendix
Increasing signs of toxicity
Rigid abdomen with extreme tenderness
Absent bowel sounds
Dyspnea and grunting; tachycardia
Fever: 39°C–41°C (102.2°F–105.8°F)
WBC count: >15,000/mm^3 with left shift
Eventual overwhelming sepsis and shock

WBC, white blood cell.

and the consideration of serial examinations over advanced imaging for patients considered low risk for appendicitis.

Clinical Considerations

Clinical Recognition

The peak incidence of appendicitis is 9 to 12 years of age. Although neonatal cases have been reported, appendicitis rarely occurs in children younger than 2 years of age. Predictably, the diagnosis is very difficult in children younger than 5 years of age. The emergency physician must accurately evaluate the child and promptly consult a surgeon when the diagnosis is clear or when appendicitis cannot be safely ruled out. Such consultation is especially urgent in younger children, in whom perforation can occur within 8 to 24 hours of the onset of symptoms. Usually the child with appendicitis initially complains of poorly defined and poorly localized midabdominal or periumbilical pain. Unfortunately, this symptom is common to many other intra-abdominal, nonsurgical problems. In the young and, to a lesser extent, the older child, vomiting and a low-grade fever often occur. Characteristically, the pain then migrates to the right lower quadrant (Table 124.1).

Triage Considerations

Children with abdominal pain and localized right lower quadrant tenderness or guarding should be evaluated promptly for appendicitis. Associated fever, extreme pain, and ill appearance may imply perforation and demand emergent treatment and surgical consultation. Shock related to peritonitis, sepsis, or severe dehydration is rare.

Clinical Assessment

Because the position of the appendix may vary in children, the localization of the pain and the tenderness on examination may also vary. An appendix that is located in the lateral gutter may produce flank pain and lateral abdominal tenderness; an inflamed appendix pointing toward the left lower quadrant may produce hypogastric tenderness and pain with urination (from bladder contraction). An inflamed low-lying, pelvic appendix may not cause pain at McBurney's point, but instead may cause diarrhea from direct irritation of the sigmoid colon. Anorexia and nausea are common; vomiting is more common in younger children. In early stages, the patient may complain of pain with motion or walking and as peritoneal irritation worsens, the child will prefer to lay motionless in the bed.

When obtaining the history, the physician needs to consider other causes of abdominal pain, which may mimic appendicitis but, in fact, are nonsurgical (see Chapter 48 Pain: Abdomen). Concurrent GI illness in other family members or contacts suggests the possibility of an infectious gastroenteritis. Constipation, streptococcal pharyngitis, urinary tract infection, lower lobe pneumonia, mesenteric adenitis, and ovarian cyst are common conditions often masquerading as appendicitis. Although the presentation is generally more rapid and severe, torsion of the ovary and ectopic pregnancy should be considered in female patients with sudden onset of severe pain.

On examination, palpation is usually reliable in demonstrating focal tenderness at the site of the inflamed appendix. If the appendix is in the pelvis or retrocecal area, however, typical anterior peritoneal signs may be absent. When the inflamed appendix is not close to the anterior abdominal wall, as in the case of retrocecal appendix, tenderness may be more impressive on deep palpation of the abdomen or by palpating in the flank. Percussive tenderness, shake tenderness, pain with coughing or hopping suggests peritoneal irritation. Rovsing sign, pain in the right lower quadrant upon palpating the left lower quadrant, is difficult to assess in young children but when present is highly suggestive of appendicitis. A properly performed rectal examination can contribute to the clinical impression: the examining finger should be inserted as fully as possible without touching the area of presumed tenderness and then, when the child is relaxed and taking deep breaths, the examiner can indent an area high on the right rectal wall. A sudden involuntary reaction implies localized tenderness. In a child with a history of probable appendicitis for more than 2 or 3 days, a boggy, full mass may also be in this location, suggesting an abscess.

A CBC in a child with appendicitis usually shows an elevated white blood cell (WBC) count in the range of 10,000 to 15,000 per mm^3 in the first 12 to 24 hours of the illness. As the appendix becomes more gangrenous, the WBC count rises further, and the differential demonstrates more neutrophils and an increasing number of bands. The WBC or absolute neutrophil count (ANC) is elevated in 92% of cases. At a threshold value of 10,000 per mm^3 (WBC) or 6,700 per mm^3 (ANC), the sensitivity is 96% but the specificity is 51%. C-reactive protein has limited value in the evaluation of nonperforated appendicitis but when used, it has improved sensitivity after 24 hours of symptoms. Urinalysis often shows ketosis. If the inflamed appendix lies over the ureter or adjacent to the bladder, low-grade pyuria may be present. An abdominal radiograph may show an appendicolith (8% to 10%), localized

TABLE 124.2

PEDIATRIC APPENDICITIS SCORE

Clinical finding	Point
Anorexia	1
Nausea or emesis	1
Migration of pain	1
Fever >38°C	1
Pain with cough, percussion, or hopping	2
Right lower quadrant tenderness	2
White blood cell count >10,000/mm^3	1
Absolute band count >7,500/mm^3	1
Total	10

ileus with air–fluid levels, a gaseous loop in the right lower quadrant, or more commonly, a nonspecific bowel gas pattern. Subtle radiographic findings include a blurred psoas margins and thickened cecal wall. Rarely, pneumoperitoneum may be seen with perforated appendix.

Several scoring systems have been offered to help differentiate appendicitis from other causes of abdominal pain in children. Most of the scoring systems have been adapted to assign risk classifications rather than determining the need for operative care. Many departments have modified the Pediatric Appendicitis Score or Alvarado Score to guide surgical consultation and advanced imaging. The Pediatric Appendicitis Score is shown in Table 124.2. Although exact score cut-offs are not defined consistently between guidelines, children with scores less than 3 are often considered low-risk, whereas 3 to 6 and >6 are considered intermediate and high-risk respectively. See Chapter 83 Appendicitis (Suspected) for the Evaluation of Patients with Suspected Appendicitis.

Management

If the clinical and laboratory findings of acute appendicitis are convincing, no further studies are indicated and a surgeon should be consulted. Significant pain should be treated with intravenous narcotics even before surgical evaluation. Patients with equivocal findings should be monitored with serial examinations or have radiologic studies to aid diagnosis. CT and US have both been used for diagnosis. US has a reported sensitivity of 80% to 92% with a specificity of 86% to 98%. Secondary signs of appendicitis on ultrasound (focal edema of fat, free fluid, local ileus) are helpful if the appendix is not visualized. Technically, a noncompressible enlarged appendix is diagnostic of appendicitis, although the study must be considered equivocal if the appendix is not identified. Focal CT has a diagnostic sensitivity of 95% with a specificity of 96%. CT can identify an enlarged appendix, focal thickening of the cecum, periappendiceal inflammation, mesenteric nodes, and fluid collections associated with perforation. Protocols using intravenous (IV) contrast plus rectal contrast or oral contrast vary by institution. In general, US has less utility in patients with a high body mass index, and CT is most interpretable in patients with adequate periappendiceal fat. US may be preferred in adolescent females as an initial study if gynecologic conditions are suspected such as ovarian cyst, tuboovarian abscess, ovarian torsion, or ectopic pregnancy (see Chapter 82 Abdominal Pain in Postpubertal Girls for the Evaluation of Lower Abdominal Pain in Post-pubertal Girls). The management of children with nondiagnostic ultrasounds should be guided by the level of clinical suspicion; for children with lower suspicion, serial examinations and observation are indicated over CT examination. MRI has recently been introduced as another option over CT, but data are lacking on performance.

At this time, nonperforated pediatric appendicitis is primarily managed surgically although there are ongoing trials of nonoperative treatment with antibiotics for selective cases of early, uncomplicated appendicitis. The preoperative preparation of a patient with acute appendicitis should include electrolytes if the patient has been vomiting or has had poor fluid intake for more than a few hours. IV fluids should be started with the goal of rapid intravascular expansion and then correction of further fluid deficits. Protracted GI losses, as with vomiting, may lead to potassium depletion. Initial fluids should include a bolus of isotonic fluid (20 cc per kg), then changed to D5–0.5NS with 10 to 20 mEq per L of potassium. These fluids can then be altered, if necessary, once the serum chemistries are known. Antibiotics should be administered if perforation is suspected or there is any concern for peritonitis. Antibiotics are generally given perioperatively but timing should be discussed with the surgeon.

The emergency physician must keep in mind the many variations in the way appendicitis can present. Patients with equivocal findings should be admitted for monitoring and serial examinations or have imaging studies to demonstrate a normal appendix. If the imaging studies are equivocal, the surgeon will decide to operate or continue to monitor. Patients who have a typical history for appendicitis but suddenly have diminished pain may actually represent perforation of the appendix. Such patients should be observed for several hours before declaring an improved condition. Even in the presence of negative imaging studies, the emergency physician should arrange close follow-up for any patient with abdominal pain. For those patients with progressive pain, significant pain requiring narcotic medications, or persistent emesis, admission for further care and subsequent evaluation might be necessary.

PERFORATED APPENDICITIS

Goals of Treatment

When a perforated appendicitis is suspected, surgical consultation should be obtained promptly and adjusted for the stability of the patient. Early restoration of intravascular volume, correction of electrolyte derangements, pain control, and antibiotics are essential parts of early care. In collaboration with surgery colleagues, decisions about which patients need immediate operative care versus advanced imaging can be discussed. When an abscess is identified, the surgeons will determine the need for a drainage procedure in addition to antibiotic therapy prior to a delayed appendectomy. Short-term treatment outcomes include clearance of the intraperitoneal infection while limiting the duration of hospitalization and the need for repeated imaging or drainage procedures.

Clinical Considerations

Clinical Recognition

Ideally, once the diagnosis of appendicitis is considered seriously, the patient will have an accurate diagnosis and surgery before the appendix has perforated. Unfortunately, some patients, particularly younger children, may arrive for emergency care with an already perforated appendix because of a delay in seeking treatment or in making the diagnosis. Although the time to perforation is variable, the time prior to presentation is the more important determinant of perforation and not the time of evaluation in the ED. Once the appendix has perforated, there may be signs of generalized, rather than localized, peritonitis. In a young child, the omentum is thin and often incapable of walling off the inflamed appendix. As a result, perforation leads to a more disseminated infection. Although the mortality from appendicitis has decreased, the incidence of perforation in children has remained the same over the last several decades.

Clinical Assessment

Within a few hours after perforation has occurred, the child begins to develop increasing signs of peritonitis and toxicity. First, the lower abdomen and then the entire abdomen become rigid with extreme tenderness. Bowel sounds are sparse to absent. Other signs include pallor, dyspnea, grunting, significant tachycardia, and higher fever (39°C to 41°C [102.2°F to 105.8°F]). Rarely, the patient may develop septic shock from the overwhelming infection.

Initially, the findings may be confused with those of pneumonia because the extreme abdominal pain may cause rapid shallow respirations, painful respirations associated with grunting, and decreased air entry to the lower lung fields. In young children, the findings may also be confused with meningitis because of paradoxical irritability—any motion of the child, even trying to comfort the child, may cause pain and irritability.

The laboratory findings in the child with perforated appendicitis often suggest this diagnosis. The WBC count is significantly elevated, usually higher than 15,000 per mm^3, with a marked shift to left; leukopenia may be seen with perforation when associated with overwhelming sepsis.

The radiologic evaluation of suspected perforated appendicitis should include plain abdominal radiographs and either US, CT, or MRI. The plain film of the abdomen may show free air or evidence of peritonitis (Fig. 124.1). The US of the pelvis may show a complex mass with or without a calcified fecalith or free fluid within the abdominal cavity (Fig. 124.2). CT is generally performed with intravenous and enteral contrast to define the size and location of an associated abscess (Fig. 124.3). MRI is now being used by some centers although it is not well studied in pediatric appendicitis.

Management

Initially, therapy should be directed toward proper resuscitation with assessment and management of the airway, breathing, and circulation. Extremely ill children may require endotracheal intubation in cases of shock. Hypovolemia should be rapidly corrected with normal saline or Ringer lactate solution. An initial bolus of fluid starting at 20 to 60 mL per kg is given rapidly until vital signs are improved and the patient produces urine. Vasopressor therapy should be considered for patients who do not have sufficient response to 60 to 80 mL per kg of isotonic fluids. Broad-spectrum antibiotics targeting bowel flora (gram-negative enterics as well as anaerobes) should be given. Immediate surgical consultation is necessary. Placement of a bladder catheter and central venous access with measurement of central venous pressure may be necessary to monitor response to therapy. Once the patient is more stable, the surgeons generally request advanced radiologic imaging to guide next steps.

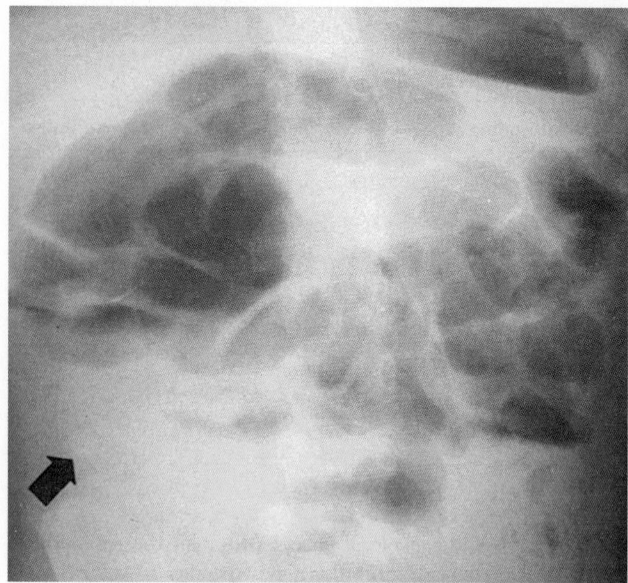

FIGURE 124.1 Perforated appendicitis with abscess and fecalith. The upright abdominal roentgenogram shows numerous dilated loops of bowel and a calcified fecalith (*arrow*). Note that the space between the individual loops indicates the presence of intraperitoneal fluid.

Once the emergency physician is certain that the airway can be controlled and the circulation is adequate, relief of pain can be accomplished by using narcotic agents (e.g., morphine 0.1 mg per kg). The patient's fever can usually be controlled by antipyretics or cooling blanket. A nasogastric tube should be placed to evacuate the contents of the stomach and to drain ongoing gastric secretions.

Children with perforated appendicitis can deteriorate quickly. Therefore, emergency resuscitation should be quickly followed by operative intervention in extremely ill patients. For patients with a perforated appendicitis with minimal systemic signs, abscesses may be treated with antibiotics and possibly drained percutaneously using radiologically guided procedures—with the expectation of a delayed appendectomy.

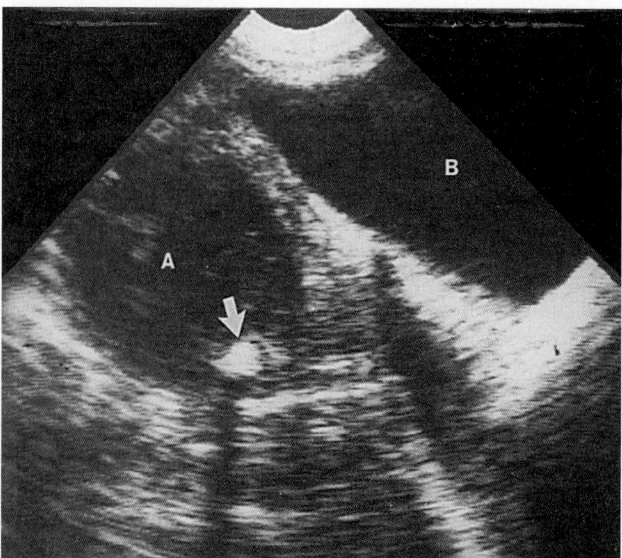

FIGURE 124.2 Perforated appendicitis with abscess and fecalith. Ultrasonography of the pelvis shows a complex mass (**A**) with a fecalith (*arrow*) producing characteristic acoustic shadowing to the right of the bladder (**B**).

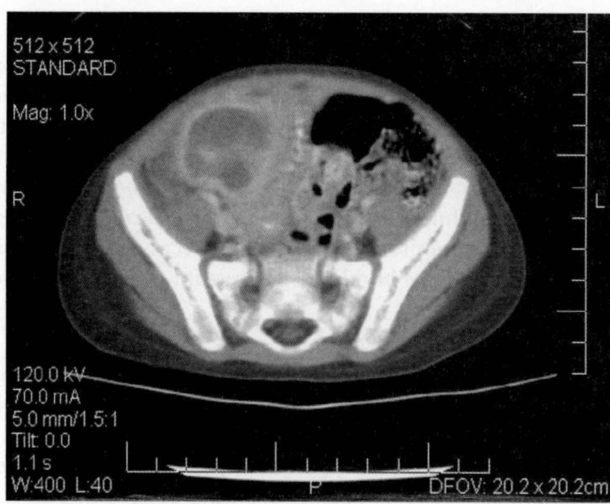

FIGURE 124.3 CT scan of perforated appendix with abscess.

ACUTE INTESTINAL OBSTRUCTION

Goals of Treatment

When intestinal obstruction is suspected, early surgical consultation should be obtained. Signs of obstruction with shock or evidence of ischemic bowel is a surgical emergency. Although diagnostic studies to identify the exact etiology of obstruction are generally valuable to direct management, a fraction of cases need exploratory surgery to rescue the bowel and prevent further deterioration of the patient.

CLINICAL PEARLS AND PITFALLS

- Bilious emesis in a neonate should be considered a surgical emergency
- Although diagnostic studies are helpful to identify the cause of obstruction, critically ill patients or those with evidence of ischemic bowel may need exploratory surgery
- Tachycardia, blood per rectum, and acidosis are potential indicators of ischemic bowel

Current Evidence

In any child with persistent emesis, especially with bilious emesis, acute intestinal obstruction must be considered. If the obstruction is high in the intestinal tract, the abdomen does not become distended; however, with lower intestinal obstruction there is generalized distension and diffuse tenderness, usually without signs of peritoneal irritation. Only if the bowel perforates or vascular insufficiency occurs will signs of peritoneal irritation be present. If complete obstruction persists, bowel habits may change, leading to complete obstipation of both flatus and stool. All patients with suspected bowel obstruction should have radiographs of the abdomen in supine and upright (or lateral decubitus) views. In patients with acute mechanical bowel obstruction, multiple dilated loops are usually seen. Fluid levels produced by the layering of air and intestinal contents are seen in the upright or lateral decubitus radiographs (Fig. 124.4).

Intussusception

CLINICAL PEARLS AND PITFALLS

- Triad of bilious emesis, abdominal mass, and blood per rectum is seen in only 20% of cases
- Intussusception should be considered in infants and toddlers with emesis and altered mental status
- Children with intussusception may arrest during a pneumatic reduction and therefore the clinical team must be prepared.
- After successful enema reduction, intussusception recurs in approximately 5% of cases in the first 48 hours.

Current Evidence

Intussusception occurs when one segment of bowel invaginates into a more distal segment. This is the leading cause of acute intestinal obstruction in infants, and it occurs most commonly between 3 and 12 months of age. The most common intussusception is ileocolic but the small bowel may intussuscept into itself. Typically, this small bowel intussusception

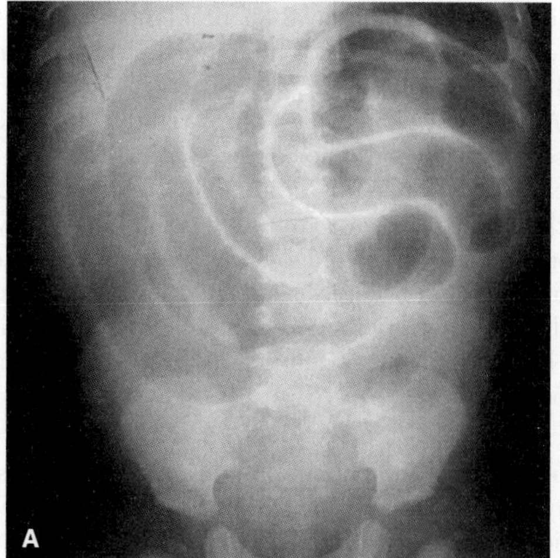

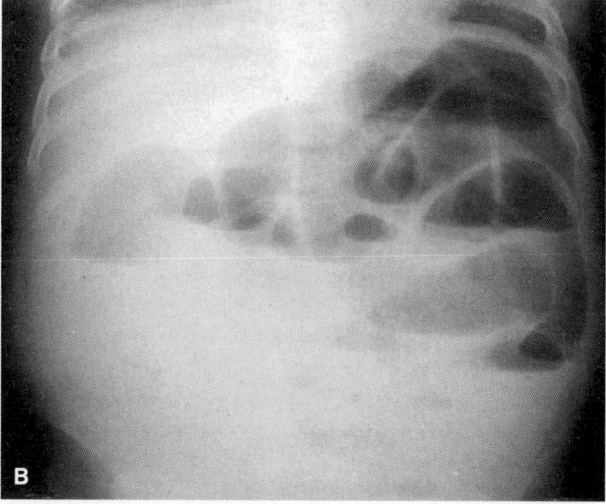

FIGURE 124.4 **A:** Small bowel obstruction. Numerous dilated small bowel loops occupy the midabdomen and have a stepladder configuration. Minimal air is seen in the rectum. **B:** Same patient as in (**A**). The upright abdominal roentgenogram shows numerous dilated loops in the small bowel with differential fluid levels in one loop indicating mechanical bowel obstruction.

SURGICAL EMERGENCIES

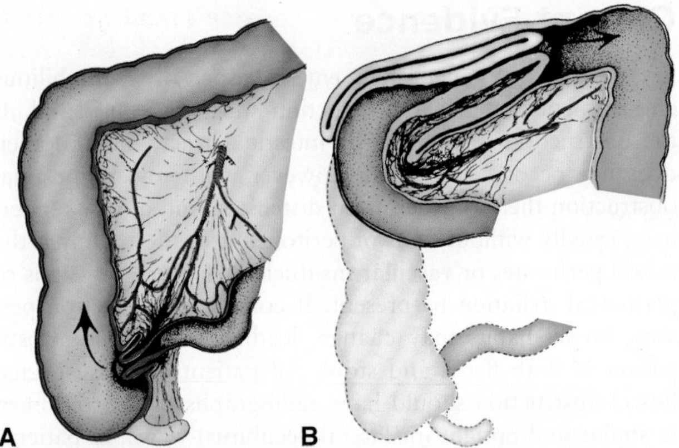

FIGURE 124.5 Ileocolic intussusception. **A:** Beginning of an intussusception in which terminal ileum prolapses through ileocecal valve. **B:** Ileocolic intussusceptum continuing through the colon. This can often be palpated as a mass in the right upper quadrant.

then prolapses through the ileocecal valve (Figs. 124.5 and 124.6). The intussusception continues through the colon a variable distance, occasionally as far as the rectum, where it can be palpated on rectal examination. Colocolic intussusceptions are rare. In infants, the lead point for the intussusception may be hypertrophied Peyer patches. In children older than 2 years of age, a specific lead point such as a polyp, a Meckel diverticulum, an intestinal duplication, or a tumor should be considered. A diarrheal illness or viral syndrome may occur several days to a week before the onset of abdominal pain and obstruction. Henoch–Schönlein purpura has been associated with intussusception (generally small bowel-small bowel).

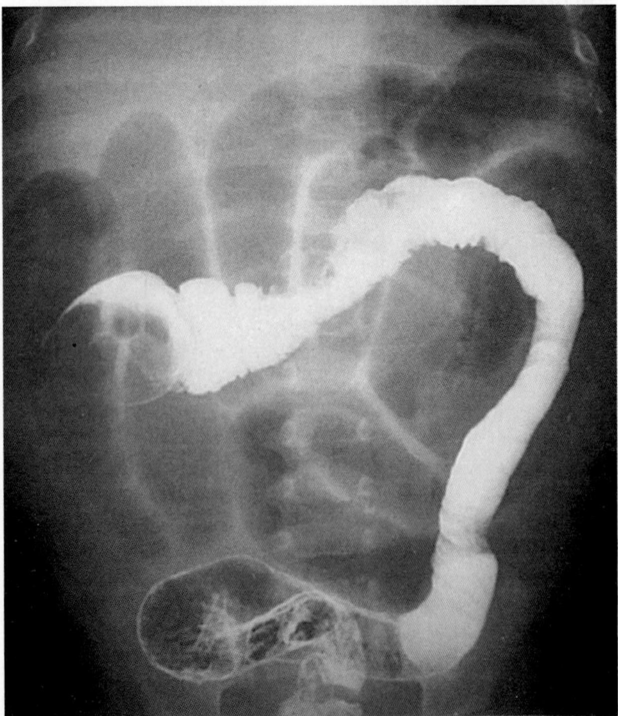

FIGURE 124.6 Ileocolic intussusception. Barium enema shows the intussusception as the filing defect within the hepatic flexure surrounded by spiral mucosal folds. Significant distended small bowel represents distal small bowel obstruction.

Clinical Considerations

Clinical Recognition. The primary manifestation of intussusception is colicky abdominal pain in an infant or toddler. Children with vomiting, especially if bilious, and intermittent abdominal pain should be evaluated for intussusception. The condition of the patient is highly variable between being happy and playful between episodes to critical ill children with evidence of peritonitis and shock. Occasionally, the primary complaint may be blood per rectum or vomiting and altered mental status.

Triage Consideration. Blood per rectum or bilious emesis in a child with possible intussusception should be triaged to an acute room with immediate assessment by the emergency department team. Children with evidence of shock or bowel obstruction may need immediate operative care.

Initial Assessment. Most children present with significant intermittent abdominal pain. This symptom may have been preceded by the symptoms and signs of a viral gastroenteritis or even an upper respiratory infection. Gradually, the child becomes more irritable and anorectic, and may vomit. The pattern of pain in a child with an intussusception is often consistent and characteristic, and the diagnosis is suggested strongly if a history of episodic pain is obtained. The child may appear to be comfortable and well between episodes. Occasionally, the infant may appear lethargic and listless. At times, patients with intussusception have been misdiagnosed as being in a postictal state or encephalopathic.

The localized portion of the intussusception leads to partial or complete obstruction and generalized abdominal distension. In some cases, the intussuscepted mass can be palpated as an ill-defined, sausage-shaped structure if the abdomen is not too distended. This mass is most often palpable in the right upper quadrant.

When children arrive in the ED early in the course of intussusception, there is often no history of having passed a currant jelly stool, although blood may be found on rectal examination (50% to 75% of cases have occult blood). However, the absence of bloody stools should not preclude making the diagnosis of a possible intussusception. Infants and young children with colicky abdominal pain and emesis should be evaluated for intussusception. Only 20% of infants with intussusception have the triad of colicky abdominal pain, abdominal mass, and bloody stools.

As the bowel becomes more tightly intussuscepted, the mesenteric veins become compressed, whereas the mesenteric arterial supply remains intact. This leads to the production of the characteristic currant jelly stool, which may be passed spontaneously or found on the rectal examination. As the intussusception becomes swollen, the pressure of entrapment occludes the arteries. At this point, the bleeding lessens, but the bowel can become gangrenous and even perforate, leading to peritonitis.

Management. The patient should receive IV fluids to correct dehydration. Surgery should be consulted immediately if the patient is critically ill or has signs of peritonitis. Nasogastric suction minimizes the risk of vomiting and aspiration if the child is critically ill. Once perfusion is improved and blood has been sent for CBC, electrolytes, and a blood bank sample, the patient should have diagnostic imaging.

Plain radiograph findings of intussusception are variable and depend primarily on the duration of the symptoms and the presence or absence of complications. In early cases, a normal gas pattern is seen. Distal colonic air cannot be interpreted as an absence of intussusception. Unless the radiograph exhibits air in the cecum, ileocolic intussusception cannot be excluded by radiograph. To improve yield, some centers utilize prone films or left lateral decubitus radiographs to enhance air movement into the cecum. In the patient with symptoms longer than 6 to 12 hours, flat and upright films often show signs of intestinal obstruction, including distended bowel with air–fluid levels (Fig. 124.4). A characteristic "target" sign may be seen or more commonly a paucity of gas in the right lower quadrant. Occasionally, the actual head of the intussusception can be seen on a plain film as a soft tissue mass.

US can be used diagnostically with reported sensitivity of 98% to 100%. Whether all patients should have plain films prior to US is debatable. If signs of intestinal obstruction or peritonitis, plain films may demonstrate pneumatosis or free air and thereby expedite operative care. Oftentimes, the radiologist may request a plain film prior to enema reduction but not necessarily before US.

Hydrostatically controlled contrast enema or air insufflation enema has been a successful therapy in up to 70% to 95% of cases with higher success rates reported with air reduction. Strict reduction guidelines must be followed to avoid perforation. The full reduction of the intussusception is confirmed only when there has been adequate reflux of barium or air into the ileum. Patients with peritonitis or free air on plain radiograph should not have an enema study or reduction attempt. In the seriously ill infant with signs of peritonitis or a frank small bowel obstruction, the diagnosis of intussusception can be made with isotonic water-soluble contrast media with no attempt at reduction. The reduction in such infants should be performed surgically. Perforation rates with enema reduction have been reported in up to 3%. Criteria that are linked to a lower reduction rate and a higher perforation rate, especially if more than one is present, are patient age younger than 3 months or older than 5 years; long duration of symptoms, especially if greater than 48 hours; hematochezia; significant dehydration; and evidence of small bowel obstruction on plain radiograph.

Many children with intussusception require emergency surgery, especially if the intussusception has been of long duration or the child shows evidence of gangrenous bowel, including high fever, leukocytosis, acidosis, significant abdominal distention, and general toxicity. If an enema reduction seems safe and appropriate, the operating room should be placed on standby and the operating team should be ready to commence immediate surgery if complications develop during the procedure or if unsuccessful. Preoperative preparation and resuscitation begins in the ED and continues during the enema. A general surgeon should be present or immediately available in case of perforation during the procedure. Air enemas can lead to massive pneumoperitoneum and cardiopulmonary arrest unless the abdomen is decompressed (by needle decompression). Sedation has been associated with decreased rates of reduction although this is not well studied. Delay in reduction can lead to gangrenous bowel.

The recurrence rate after enema reduction ranges from 3% to 5% in the first 48 hours. When there is a recurrence, a second attempt at reduction may be done by enema. This is usually successful in most cases, but with a third episode of intussusception, an exploratory laparotomy should be considered. Recurrences are more common in older children and may be caused by a lead point such as a Meckel diverticulum, an intestinal polyp, or an intraluminal tumor such as lymphoma. Therefore, it may be wise in an older child to perform a CT or operate with the first recurrence.

Incarcerated Inguinal Hernia

Goals of Treatment

The goal of treatment of an inguinal hernia is to perform a reduction before being incarcerated. Early surgical consultation is necessary in cases of incarceration with evidence of bowel obstruction or ischemia.

CLINICAL PEARLS AND PITFALLS

- Bowel obstruction or concerns for ischemic bowel should prompt emergent surgical consultation
- Procedural sedation may be necessary to facilitate reduction of a hernia
- Inguinal mass may represent a torsed ovary or testicle
- Blood per rectum with an inguinal hernia may be an indicator of gangrenous bowel

Current Evidence

Incarcerated inguinal hernia is a common cause of intestinal obstruction in the infant and young child. Approximately 60% of incarcerated hernias occur during the first year of life. Incarceration occurs more often in girls than in boys, but usually involves the ovary rather than the intestine. Often, the patient or family has no previous knowledge of the presence of a congenital hernia. Incarceration does not necessarily mean that the nonreducible portion of intestine is compromised or gangrenous. However, strangulation can occur within 24 hours of a nonreduced incarcerated hernia because of progressive edema of the bowel caused by venous and lymphatic obstruction. This obstruction then leads to occlusion of the arterial supply with resulting necrosis of the bowel and perhaps perforation.

Clinical Considerations

Triage Considerations. Children presenting with an inguinal mass should be assessed for bowel obstruction or strangulation. If the child is vomiting, has significant pain, or the hernia is discolored, the patient should be seen immediately and determine whether emergent surgical consultation is required even prior to pain control, imaging, or attempts at reduction.

Initial Assessment. The clinical presentation of a child with an incarcerated hernia is irritability due to pain, vomiting, and occasionally abdominal distension. A firm, discrete mass can be palpated at the internal ring and may or may not extend into the scrotum. Occasionally, the testicle may appear dark blue because of venous congestion, and in a prolonged incarceration, the testicle may be infarcted. Intestinal obstruction may develop quickly, and an abdominal radiograph exhibits signs of small bowel obstruction and possibly gas-filled loops of intestine in the scrotum. Lack of air in the inguinal region cannot be used to exclude a hernia because the intestine, especially when incarcerated, is often fluid filled.

It is often difficult to differentiate a tense hydrocele in the scrotum from an incarcerated hernia. If the child has had a hydrocele, a sudden increase in fluid in the tunica vaginalis may produce discomfort and concern for an incarcerated hernia. However, it is uncommon for a hernia to appear in the presence of a communicating hydrocele because of the narrowness of the patent processus vaginalis that is associated with the hydrocele. The acute hydrocele presents only in the scrotum but may extend superiorly toward the inguinal canal. With a hydrocele, however, no mass should be palpable up the inguinal canal at the level of the internal ring.

Management. Unless the child is extremely ill with signs of intestinal obstruction or toxic from gangrenous bowel, a manual reduction of the incarcerated hernia should be attempted. The child should be sedated with morphine 0.1 mg per kg intravenously with standard cardiopulmonary monitoring. The mother should then cuddle the baby until it relaxes and falls asleep. An older child may be placed in the Trendelenburg position to allow gravity to facilitate the reduction. Once the child is asleep, gentle manipulation of the incarcerated mass should be attempted. Mild pressure should be exerted at the internal ring with one hand, while the other attempts to squeeze gas or fluid out of the incarcerated bowel back into the abdominal cavity. If the reduction is unsuccessful, the child should be taken immediately to the operating room.

Disposition. After the hernia has been reduced manually, the child may be admitted for observation but not immediate repair. The hernia sac and spermatic cord are edematous after a reduction, making the repair difficult. Usually, it is done 24 hours after admission. If a child has persistent emesis after a manual reduction of a hernia, consider the possibility that the bowel was incompletely reduced. Children that develop peritoneal signs after manual reduction should be evaluated for possible perforation associated with gangrenous bowel. Rarely should a child be sent home after a manual reduction unless the parents are properly informed concerning signs of recurrence or intestinal obstruction.

Incarcerated Umbilical Hernia

Incarceration of an umbilical hernia is rare. If present, there is a persistent and tender bulge in the umbilical hernia sac. If the incarceration is of short duration, a gentle effort might be made to reduce it manually, but it is often necessary to prepare the child for urgent surgery. At the time of surgery, the loop of incarcerated bowel should be inspected, rather than letting it drop back into the abdominal cavity, to be certain there has been no vascular impairment.

Malrotation of the Bowel With Volvulus

Goals of Treatment

The goals of treatment are simple: early recognition, emergency surgical consultation, treatment of shock, and immediate operative care to preserve viability of the bowel.

CLINICAL PEARLS AND PITFALLS

- Volvulus is the most serious etiology of intestinal obstruction
- Neonates with bilious emesis should be emergently evaluated for malrotation and volvulus even if the patient appears well

Current Evidence

Malrotation of the bowel is a congenital condition associated with abnormal fixation of the mesentery of the bowel (Fig. 124.7). Therefore, the bowel has a tendency to volvulize and obstruct at points of abnormal fixation. Although malrotation with volvulus usually occurs either in utero or during early neonatal life, malrotation can be unrecognized until childhood (25% of cases present after 1 year of age). This is an extraordinarily dangerous situation because a complete volvulus of the bowel for more than an hour or two can totally obstruct blood supply to the bowel, leading to complete necrosis of the involved segment. When a volvulus involves the midgut, the entire small bowel and ascending colon may be lost. To prevent such a catastrophe, physicians should have a high index of suspicion for malrotation in any child with signs of obstruction and be prepared to get a child with a presumed volvulus to the operating room immediately.

Clinical Considerations

Initial Assessment. Any child with bile-stained vomiting and abdominal pain may have malrotation with volvulus. The pain is usually intense and constant. Blood may appear in the stool within a few hours and suggests the development of ischemia and possible necrosis of the bowel. Clinically, malrotation can present in several different ways: first, and most dangerous, is the sudden onset of abdominal pain with bilious vomiting with no prior history of GI problems; second is a similar abrupt onset of obstruction in a child who previously seemed to have "feeding problems" with transient episodes of bilious vomiting; and third is a child with failure to thrive because of alleged intolerance of feedings.

On physical examination, there may be only mild distension of the abdomen because the obstruction usually occurs high in the GI tract. On palpation, the physician may discern one or two prominently dilated loops of bowel. The abdomen may be diffusely tender and yet not have signs of peritonitis early in the course. On rectal examination, the presence of blood on the examining finger is an alarming sign of impending ischemia and gangrene of the bowel.

Management. The key to management is to be suspicious of malrotation and to obtain flat and upright radiographs of the abdomen immediately. The presence of loops of small bowel overriding the liver shadow is suggestive of an underlying malrotation. When complete volvulus has occurred, there may be only a few dilated loops of bowel with air–fluid levels. Distal to the volvulus, there may be little or no gas in the GI tract. A "double-bubble sign" is often present on an upright film because of partial obstruction of the duodenum causing distension of the stomach and first part of the duodenum (Fig. 124.8A).

When a child is being assessed for possible malrotation (with or without volvulus), an upper GI series is the study of choice. The ligament of Treitz is absent in the malrotation

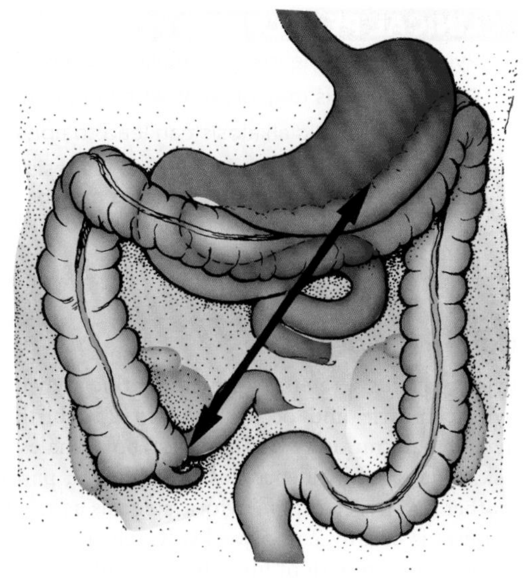

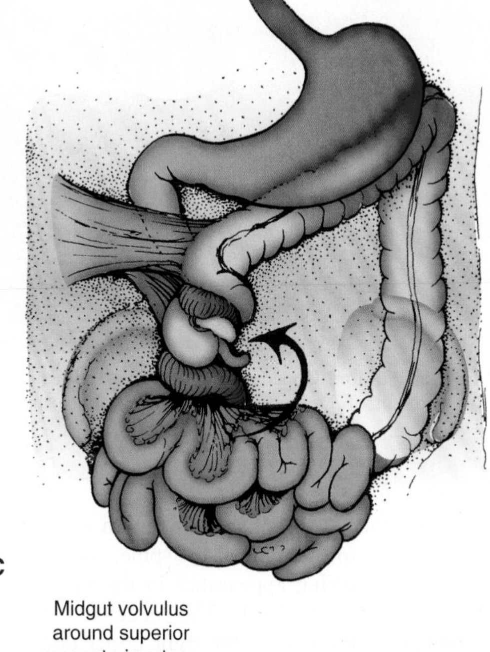

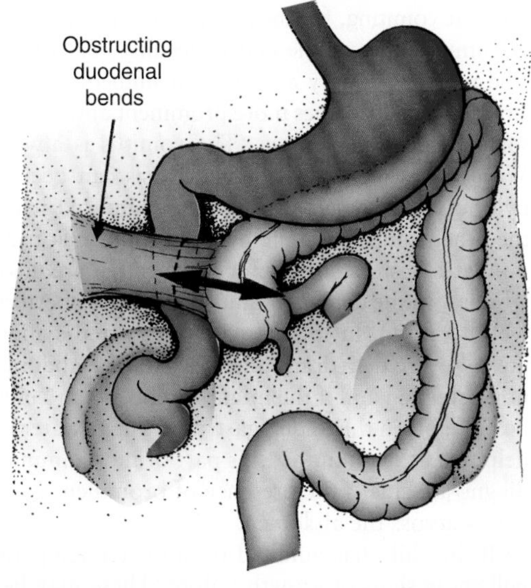

FIGURE 124.7 Malrotation with volvulus. **A:** Normal small bowel mesenteric attachment (as demonstrated by the *arrow*). This prevents twisting of small bowel because of the broad fixation of the mesentery. **B:** Malrotation of colon with obstructing duodenal bands. **C:** Midgut volvulus around the superior mesenteric artery caused by the narrow base of the mesentery.

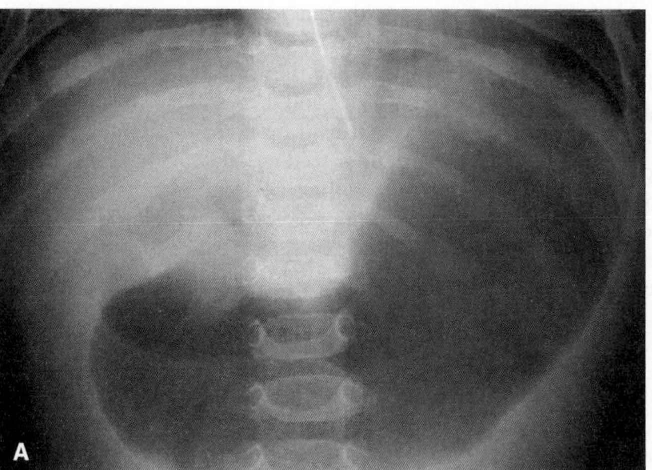

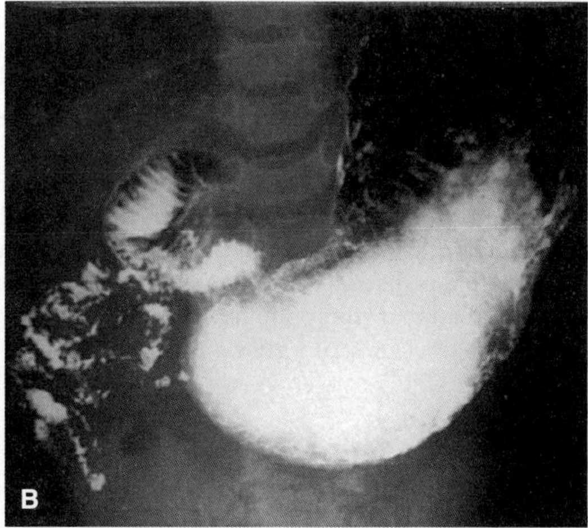

FIGURE 124.8 **A:** Malrotation of the bowel. Supine plain roentgenogram of the abdomen shows distended stomach and proximal duodenal loop. **B:** Same patient as in (**A**). Upper gastrointestinal series shows dilated proximal duodenum with abrupt transition to normal caliber of small bowel. Abnormally placed ligament of Treitz. Proximal jejunum in the right abdomen.

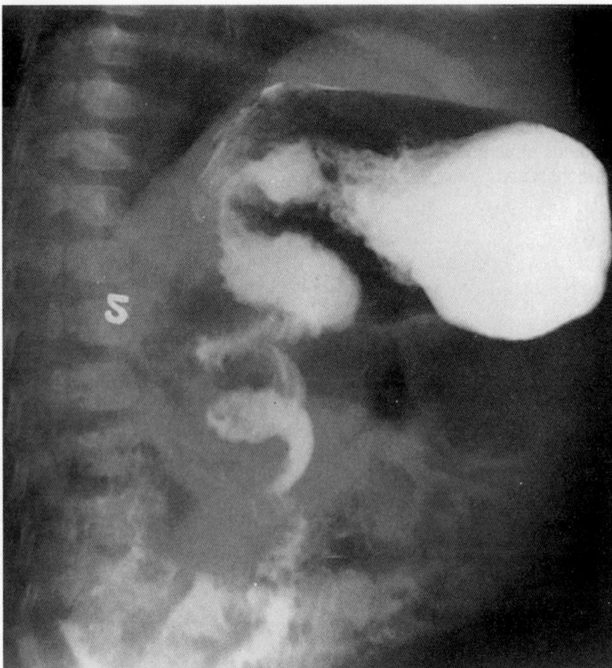

FIGURE 124.9 Malrotation. Upper gastrointestinal study showing absence of the ligament of Treitz and coiled spring appearance of jejunum.

anomaly; therefore, the C-loop of the duodenum is not present, the duodenum lies to the right of the spine, and the jejunum presents a coiled spring appearance in the right upper quadrant (Figs. 124.8B and 124.9). The cecum is not fixed and usually assumes a position in the right upper quadrant. However, because of its mobility, the cecum on barium enema may be seen in its normal position in the right lower quadrant. Therefore, a barium enema is not the most reliable study to rule out malrotation. In the neonate, the cecum sometimes takes a high position, and this could give a false impression of malrotation. If a US is obtained, as with possible pyloric stenosis or intussusception, an abnormal relationship between the superior mesenteric artery and vein should lead to an upper GI series.

As in the case of a child with an unreduced intussusception, a child with a possible volvulus should be prepared for immediate surgery. The operating room and operating team should be notified. IV fluid and electrolyte replacement should begin immediately. Laboratory studies should be obtained, but they do not add to the diagnostic evaluation. A nasogastric tube should be inserted and blood crossmatched. Because this entity can present even in adulthood, every physician should understand the pathogenesis and the need for emergency surgical treatment of vovulus. If immediate transfer to a pediatric hospital cannot be accomplished within an hour, a laparotomy should be performed without delay.

Pyloric Stenosis

Goals of Treatment

Pyloric stenosis is not a surgical emergency, but proper diagnosis and correction of electrolyte abnormalities are important for rapid recovery of the infant.

CLINICAL PEARLS AND PITFALLS

- Pyloric stenosis leads to nonbilious emesis only
- Pyloric stenosis may present with hematemesis
- Severe metabolic alkalosis can lead to apnea
- Very early in the course of pyloric stenosis, ultrasound diagnosis based on measurements may be falsely reassuring; repeat US should be performed if symptoms persist

Current Evidence

Pyloric stenosis refers to an idiopathic hypertrophy of the pyloric muscle and occurs in 1 in 250 births. There is a male:female ratio of 4:1, and first born males are at higher risk. A familial incidence has been shown, particularly if the mother had hypertrophic pyloric stenosis as an infant. The age of onset is usually 2 to 5 weeks. Rarely, the onset may be late in the second month of life. The cause of the muscle hypertrophy is unknown, but the symptoms, diagnosis, and therapy are well defined.

Clinical Considerations

Initial Assessment. Characteristically, the infant does well, without vomiting, for the first few weeks of life and then starts vomiting, either at the end of feedings or within 30 minutes. The infant is hungry and will eat immediately after vomiting. The vomiting becomes more prominent and eventually becomes forceful, projectile emesis. The vomitus is always nonbilious. With protracted emesis, hematemesis can occur. Infants with pyloric stenosis may also become jaundiced with the onset of the other symptoms. The hyperbilirubinemia usually improves or abates postoperatively for reasons that are unknown.

Early in the course, infants may appear perfectly active and well hydrated. In infants with protracted symptoms, moderate to severe dehydration may exist. The abdomen is soft and nondistended and if the infant is relaxed, an "olive" mass may be palpable in the midepigastrium. Sugar water can be used to help relax the infant for this part of the examination. Another diagnostic clue is the presence of prominent gastric peristaltic waves across the abdomen.

If the child has vomited for an extended period, he or she will show signs of growth failure. There may be loose, hanging skin and an absence of subcutaneous tissue. The infant may take on an "old man" appearance, with wrinkled skin on the face and body. Weight gain is inadequate, which may be calculated by knowing that the average child regains birth weight by 10 days of age and thereafter 15 to 30 g (0.5 to 1 oz) per day. With severe dehydration, the infant may be hypotonic and lethargic with poor feeding.

Serum electrolytes may be abnormal because of gastric losses. Accordingly, the potassium and chloride are low, and serum bicarbonate is high. This hypochloremic alkalosis may be profound with serum chlorides as low as 65 mEq per L. The patient can exhibit periods of apnea from the extreme metabolic alkalosis. When dehydration becomes severe, the patient may then develop acidosis, indicating an advanced and even more dangerous metabolic imbalance (see Chapter 108 Renal and Electrolyte Emergencies).

Management. Infants should be hospitalized and rehydrated with appropriate fluid and electrolyte replacement. Initially, IV fluids should be normal saline (lactated Ringer solution is

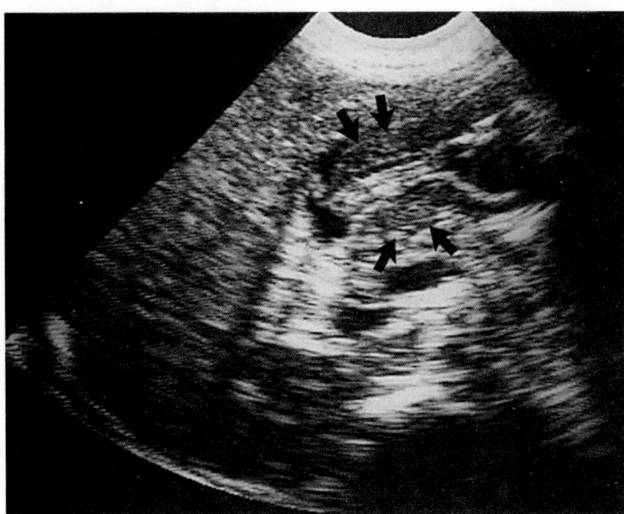

FIGURE 124.10 Hypertrophic pyloric stenosis. Ultrasonography of the abdomen shows thick pyloric muscle surrounding a centered echogenic mucosal and submucosal region (*arrows*).

contraindicated) to replenish intravascular volume and supply adequate chloride. Potassium chloride should be added once urine output has been established. If hypotonic solutions are used, there is significant risk of causing hyponatremia.

Few pediatric surgeons will operate based on a typical history without ultrasound imaging. The real-time US scanning not only increases the accuracy of the diagnosis of pyloric stenosis, but can also localize the "olive." The hypertrophic pyloric muscle is seen as a thick hypoechoic ring surrounding a central echogenic mucosal and submucosal region (Fig. 124.10). The quantitative criteria for the sonographic diagnosis of hypertrophic pyloric stenosis are 1.4 cm or longer length of the pyloric canal/channel with 0.3 cm or greater thickness of the circular muscle (institutions may vary slightly in exact measure used for diagnosis). The ability of stomach contents to pass through the pyloris can be assessed dynamically.

If the US study does not show a hypertrophic pylorus and the patient has significant forceful emesis, an upper GI series should then be done to eliminate gastroesophageal reflux, malrotation, and antral web as diagnostic possibilities. In general, pyloric stenosis can be identified by the presence of a "string sign" in the pyloric channel, seen best on oblique projections on the upper GI series (Fig. 124.11). For patients with a progressive emesis and initially normal US, repeat US should be performed even 24 to 48 hours later to remeasure the pyloris.

To lessen the risk of vomiting and aspiration, the barium should be evacuated from the stomach after the upper GI series has been completed. Surgical pyloromyotomy is standard, and such infants can usually be discharged from the hospital 2 days after surgery. Some infants will have some regurgitation postoperatively as a result of a temporary relaxation of the gastroesophageal sphincter.

Postoperative Adhesions

Prior abdominal surgery or peritonitis places a child at risk for intestinal obstruction from adhesions (Fig. 124.12). Such obstruction can occur relatively early in the postoperative course or months or even years later. The child often has the sudden onset of abdominal cramps, nausea, vomiting, and abdominal distension. Although most intestinal obstructions from adhesions do not jeopardize the perfusion of the bowel, occasionally a loop of intestine, caught under a fibrous band or herniating through the adhesion, can become gangrenous. All such patients need to be admitted to the hospital and evaluated by a surgeon who should direct the complete management.

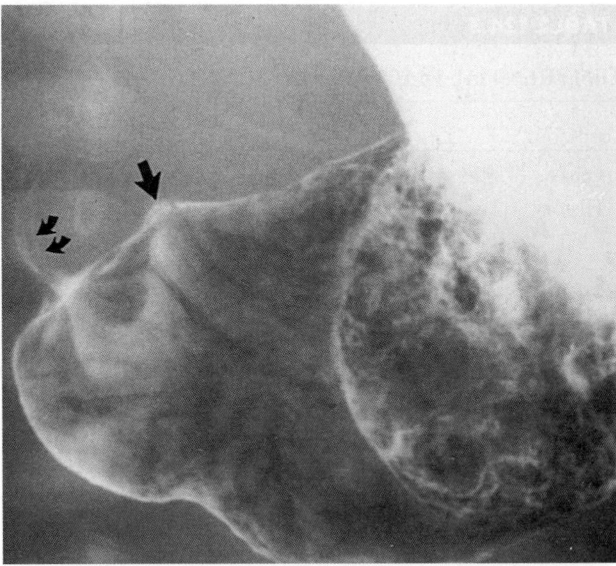

FIGURE 124.11 Pyloric stenosis. Long, narrowed, and tilting upward antropyloric canal. Parallel streaks of barium producing typical string sign with complete obstruction (*arrows*) and eccentric lesser curvature indentation pyloric tilt (*arrow*). The tilt is performed when the peristaltic wave meets the muscle mass.

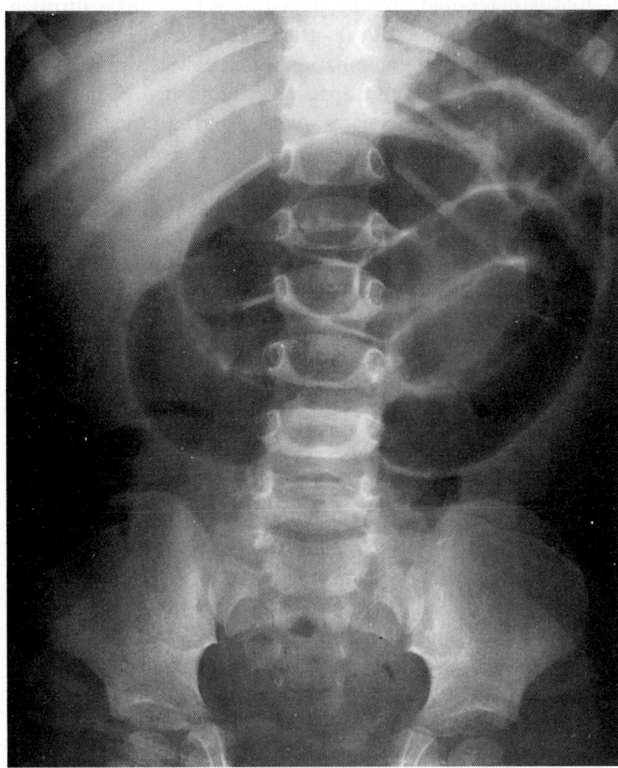

FIGURE 124.12 Dilated loops of small intestine and absence of air in lower abdomen indicating a high intestinal obstruction caused by postoperative adhesions.

TABLE 124.3

DIFFERENTIAL DIAGNOSIS OF FUNCTIONAL CONSTIPATION AND HIRSCHSPRUNG DISEASE

	Functional constipation	Hirschsprung disease
Onset	<2 yrs	Birth
History	Coercive training	Enemas necessary
	Colicky abdominal pain	No abdominal pain
	Periodic volume stools	Episodes of intestinal obstruction
Encopresis	Present	Absent
Abdominal distension	Absent or minimal	Present
Rectal examination	Feces-packed rectum	Empty rectum
Barium examination	Dilated rectum	Narrow segment
Motility	Normal	Abnormal
Biopsy	Ganglion cells	No ganglion cells

Chronic Partial Intestinal Obstruction

Any child with intermittent abdominal distension, nausea, anorexia, occasional vomiting, or chronic constipation or obstipation may have partial intestinal obstruction. A number of diagnostic considerations exist.

Chronic Constipation

Chronic constipation is probably one of the most common causes for abdominal pain, distension, and vomiting in children. The history, if available from a reliable parent, may attest to chronic constipation; however, occasionally, such a child is diagnosed only by palpating a large mass through the intact abdominal wall or a hard fecal mass blocking the anal outlet on rectal examination. Such children may have a history of encopresis and appear malnourished. Chapter 13 Constipation covers the diagnostic approach to the child with constipation.

These children should be disimpacted manually or managed with saline enemas and a rectal tube passed above the obstruction. For children unable to tolerate disimpaction, oral or nasogastric bowel evacuants such as polyethylene-glycol electrolyte solution can be used. If the process has progressed to partial bowel obstruction, either ED or inpatient management is necessary to clean out the bowel adequately.

Aganglionic Megacolon (Hirschsprung Disease)

In patients with Hirschsprung disease, the parasympathetic ganglion cells of Auerbach plexus between the circular and longitudinal muscle layers of the colon are absent. The involved segment varies in length, from less than 1 cm to involvement of the entire colon and small bowel. The effect of this absence of ganglion cells produces spasm and abnormal motility of that segment, which results in either complete intestinal obstruction or chronic constipation.

These children have a lifelong history of constipation, so it is important to obtain an accurate account of the child's stool pattern from birth. A child with Hirschsprung disease typically has never been able to stool properly without assistance (e.g., enemas, suppositories, anal stimulation). Normal stooling is not possible because of the failure of the aganglionic bowel and internal anal sphincter to relax. The child usually has no history of encopresis, as one would find in chronic functional constipation. These children have chronic abdominal distension and are often malnourished. Vomiting is uncommon, as are other symptoms. Complete intestinal obstruction in Hirschsprung disease is more likely to occur in early infancy and only rarely in the older age groups. It may present with signs and symptoms of acute bowel perforation.

Table 124.3 summarizes the pertinent diagnostic features differentiating functional constipation from Hirschsprung disease.

After flat and upright abdominal roentgenogram radiographic studies have been obtained, a properly performed barium enema with a Hirschsprung catheter is the best initial diagnostic procedure. There should be no preparation of the bowel. Ideally, the rectum should not be stimulated by enemas or digital examination for 1 to 2 days before the procedure. The key to diagnosis is seeing a "transition zone" (Fig. 124.13)

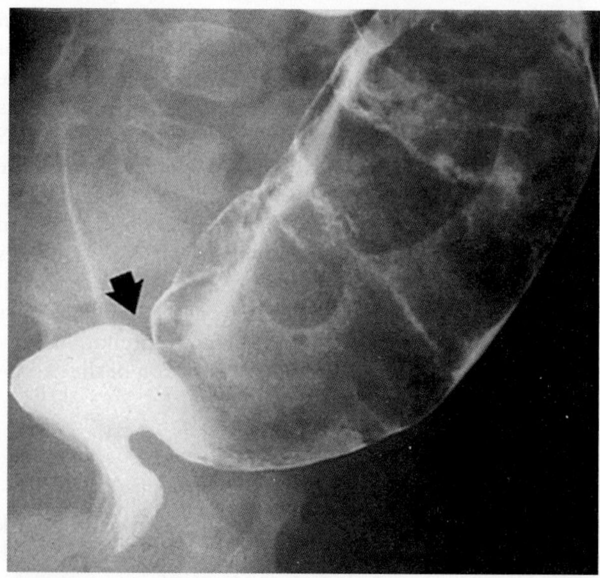

FIGURE 124.13 Hirschsprung disease. Barium enema studies in lateral view show transition zone (*arrow*) with narrow rectum but dilated sigmoid colon.

between the contracted aganglionic bowel and the proximal dilated ganglionated bowel. Stimulation of the rectum shortly before the study may result in decompression of the proximal bowel, with loss of definition of the transition zone. When a clear-cut transition zone is seen, it is not necessary to fill the colon with barium more than 12 to 18 in. above the transition point. It is important, however, not to empty the colon of barium at the end of the study. The presence of retained barium above the transition point 24 hours later strongly suggests the diagnosis of Hirschsprung disease.

Anorectal manometry to determine the presence or absence of relaxation of the internal anal sphincter is helpful in establishing the neurogenic dysfunction of the bowel. Barium enema studies and manometry are clearly complementary in the diagnosis of Hirschsprung disease. However, rectal manometric studies are more reliable than radiologic methods for short aganglionic segments that are usually not apparent on barium enema studies. Manometric studies are not dependable in infants younger than 3 weeks of age. If the barium enema and anal manometry studies indicate Hirschsprung disease, rectal biopsy is not necessary to confirm the diagnosis.

In children of all ages, an adequately performed suction mucosal biopsy of the rectum 2 cm or more above the dentate line can be reliable in diagnosing Hirschsprung disease. Because of the complicated evaluation and management of this disease, referral to a pediatric surgeon is recommended.

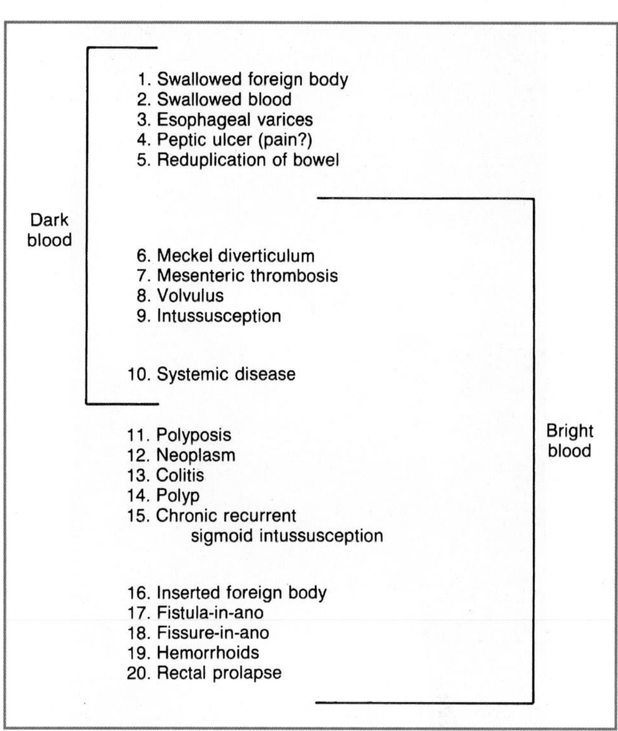

FIGURE 124.14 Causes of rectal bleeding in children.

Duplications

Duplications occur anywhere from the mouth to the anus and produce various symptoms. In the abdomen, there may be a noncommunicating cyst that gradually fills up with secretions and compresses the adjacent normal bowel, producing a palpable abdominal mass or chronic intestinal obstruction. Rarely, a marginal ulcer resulting from ectopic gastric mucosa may occur, and this produces painless bleeding. After appropriate radiographic diagnosis, surgery is indicated.

Inflammatory Bowel Disease

The older child or adolescent may develop either Crohn disease or ulcerative colitis (see Chapter 99 Gastrointestinal Emergencies), and this must be included in the differential diagnosis of chronic intestinal obstruction. Usually, the child has a history of changing bowel habits, with mucus or blood in the stools, chronic abdominal pain, and weight loss. Chapter 99 Gastrointestinal Emergencies covers inflammatory bowel disease in detail.

DISEASES THAT PRODUCE RECTAL BLEEDING

Goals of Treatment

Rectal bleeding can be a sign of a serious condition. Clinicians need to identify generally innocent etiologies from those that can be life-threatening. The primary goals should be early recognition of hemorrhagic shock and ischemic bowel. Blood on the outside of a formed stool is likely to originate from the distal large bowel, rectum, or anus. Blood mixed in the stool is generally from a higher source of bleeding. Blood associated with diarrhea is common with inflammatory bowel disease and infectious enteritis. A "tarry" stool suggests a source of bleeding in the proximal portion of the GI tract, and bright red blood suggests a more distal origin (Fig. 124.14). All patients with rectal bleeding should have a rectal examination. Those with significant hemorrhage require flexible colonoscopy. In some patients, no definite diagnosis may be reached despite extensive studies. In any patient with significant bleeding, however, surgical consultation is indicated. Chapters 28 Gastrointestinal Bleeding and 99 Gastrointestinal Emergencies further discuss the diagnosis and management of patients with GI bleeding.

CLINICAL PEARLS AND PITFALLS

- Blood per rectum can be a sign of ischemic bowel
- Meckel diverticulum can present with brisk, painless rectal bleeding
- Small amounts of blood mixed in stool of an otherwise healthy, asymptomatic infant is generally due to allergic colitis.

Fissures

An anal fissure is probably the most common cause of bleeding, especially in infants. However, fissures may occur at any age. The child usually has a history of passing a large, hard stool with anal discomfort. Often, the child has a history of chronic constipation with progressive reluctance to pass stool because of the associated discomfort. If bleeding occurs, it usually involves streaking of bright red blood on the outside of the stool or red blood on the toilet tissues. The diagnosis can easily be made by inspection or anoscopic examination and appropriate measures taken to relieve the chronic constipation (see Chapter 13 Constipation). Rarely does a child require hospitalization or surgery.

SURGICAL EMERGENCIES

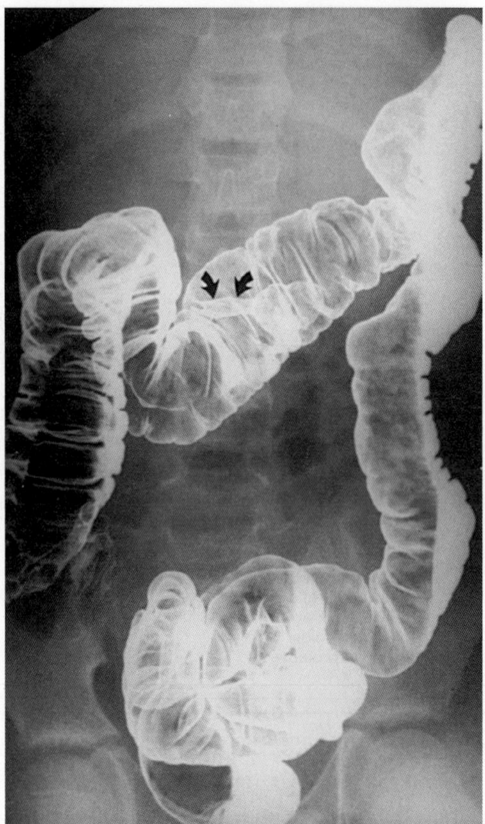

FIGURE 124.15 Juvenile polyp. Double air-contrast barium enema shows a single polyp with long stalk in transverse colon (*arrow*).

Juvenile Polyps

Older infants and children can develop either single or multiple retention polyps. Usually, the polyps occur in the lower portion of the colon and can often be palpated on rectal examination. Polyps bleed, but they rarely cause massive hemorrhage. They may intermittently prolapse at the anus or on occasion come free and be passed as a fecal mass associated with bleeding. Colonic polyps may be lead points for intussusception. Usually, however, polyps are asymptomatic except for the associated bleeding. These are not premalignant lesions, and they tend to be self-limiting (Fig. 124.15) although they can be easily removed by endoscopy.

Meckel Diverticulum

Two percent of the population is born with a Meckel diverticulum. This is the most common omphalomesenteric duct remnant. The diverticulum is usually located 50 to 75 cm proximal to the terminal ileum. Only 2% of persons with a Meckel diverticulum manifest any clinical problems. The most common complication of a Meckel diverticulum is a bleeding ulcer. Ectopic gastric mucosa in such patients is usually present in the diverticulum. The acid secretion produces ulceration at the junction of the normal ileal mucosa with the ectopic mucosa. Currant jelly stools or hemorrhage may be present. Other modes of presentation include diverticulitis, perforation with peritonitis, or intussusception as a result of the diverticulum's serving as a lead point.

Enteral contrast studies usually fail to outline a Meckel diverticulum. The imaging modality of choice for detection of ectopic gastric mucosa in a bleeding Meckel diverticulum is nuclear scintigraphy. A well-defined focal accumulation of radionuclide (99m-technetium pertechnetate) usually appears at or about the same time as activity in the stomach and gradually increases in intensity (Fig. 124.16). A duplication cyst with gastric mucosa shows the same focal accumulation of radionuclide. Preoperative differentiation between two lesions as a cause of GI bleeding is not important. The accuracy of scintigraphy in detection of ectopic gastric mucosa in Meckel diverticula is approximately 95%. False-negative results may rarely occur in patients with rapidly bleeding Meckel diverticula and with those diverticula that do not contain gastric mucosa.

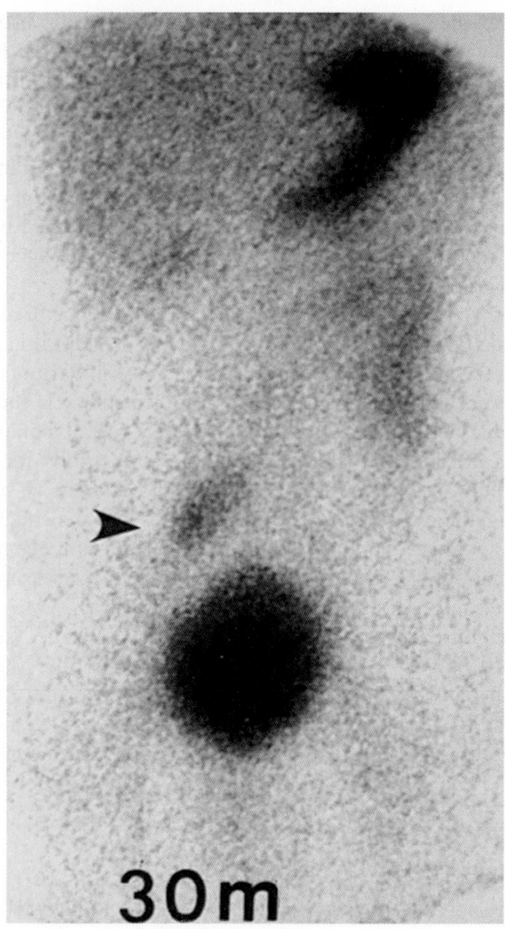

FIGURE 124.16 Meckel diverticulum. Anterior image at 30 minutes shows an oval focal accumulation of ^{99m}Tc-pertechnetate in the right lower quadrant of the abdomen (*arrowhead*).

In any child with a major rectal bleed and a negative scan, further workup, including an arteriogram if the bleeding continues to be active or colonoscopy when the bleeding is not active, is required.

INTRA-ABDOMINAL MASSES

Current Evidence

Intra-abdominal masses may be benign or malignant. Children are often asymptomatic even when the tumor is large; frequently, the mass is detected by the caregiver noticing a protuberant or lopsided abdomen.

It is difficult to feel an intra-abdominal mass, as well as outline its limits and its degree of mobility, if an infant or child

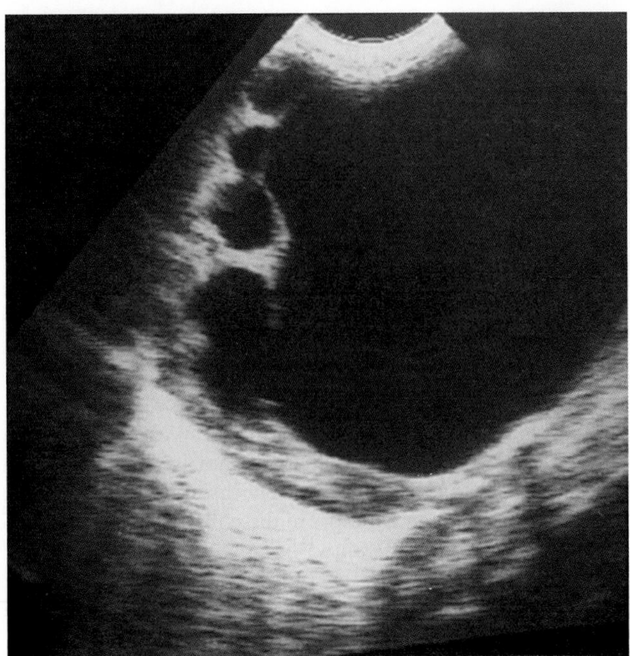

FIGURE 124.17 Ureteropelvic junction obstruction. A newborn with left flank mass. Ultrasonography of the left flank shows dilated pyelocalyceal system. The communicating dilated collecting systems are seen in the periphery of the significantly dilated renal pelvis.

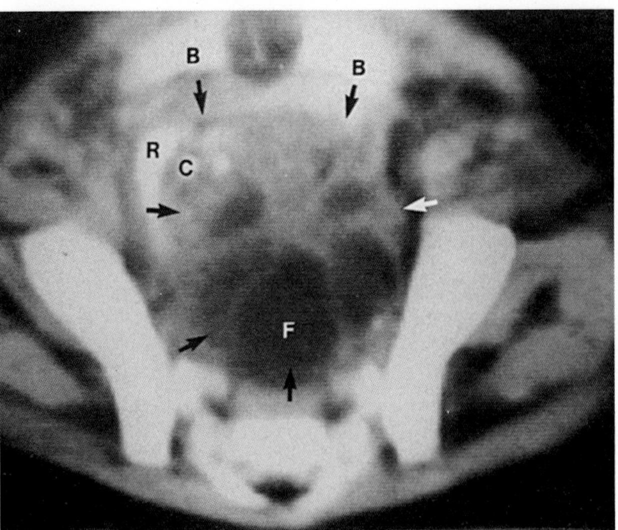

FIGURE 124.18 Presacral teratoma. Computed tomographic section of pelvis with contrast medium enhancement shows a large cystic mass (*arrows*). The mass contains both fat and calcification, and displaces the rectum anteriorly and laterally, and the bladder anteriorly. B, bladder with Foley catheter; C, calcification; F, fat; R, rectum.

is crying. The physician should then make an effort to palpate the intra-abdominal contents carefully. These masses can be fragile and prone to rupture. Therefore, palpation of the mass should be done gently and strictly limited to as few examiners as possible.

Retroperitoneal masses tend to be fixed, whereas masses attached to the mesentery or omentum are mobile and may be shifted to different locations by the examiner. Pelvic masses are commonly fixed and often can best be felt by rectal examination. A presacral mass may narrow the rectum and produce constipation. Abdominal masses present with various characteristics and may be smooth, nodular, cystic, or firm.

Initial evaluation in the ED may include plain abdominal films and an ultrasound. Ultrasonography can differentiate a cystic flank mass (Fig. 124.17) that could be a hydronephrotic kidney from a solid tumor such as an adrenal neuroblastoma, and thus, facilitate the proper referral of the child to either a urologist or a pediatric surgeon. CT and MRI are superior to other modalities for anatomic detail, and provide anatomic and physiologic information about organs and vascular structures. Renal scans are superior to excretory urography for determining renal function. Angiography is indicated for an abdominal mass only if a precise knowledge of segmental vascular anatomy is required or if interventional techniques are contemplated.

Sacrococcygeal Teratoma

The presacral sacrococcygeal teratoma is the most common tumor of the caudal region in children and is more common in females than in males (4:1). Most tumors are benign and are noted at birth. Tumors in patients beyond neonatal age have a higher incidence of malignancy. Radiography shows a soft tissue mass that arises from the ventral surface of the coccyx. Calcifications are present in 60% of presacral sacrococcygeal teratoma and are more common in benign tumors. US confirms whether presacral sacrococcygeal teratomas are cystic, solid, or mixed and can also determine impingement on the urinary tract. CT or MRI are helpful in confirming the diagnosis, particularly in older children, and demonstrates the content of a tumor, as well as its extent and bone anomalies. Tumors with more solid components are more often malignant than those with more cystic components (Fig. 124.18).

Nonmalignant Intra-Abdominal Masses

Fecaloma

A lower abdominal mass, particularly one on the left side, is most often related to retained stool and associated with chronic functional constipation than with Hirschsprung disease. If a mass is found, a careful review of bowel habits is important. If an abdominal mass is a fecaloma, a large bolus of stool can usually be felt on rectal examination just inside the anus. The evaluation of the impaction, and irrigation of the upper sigmoid colon, should cause the mass to disappear. See Chapter 13 Constipation for the causes of constipation.

Ovarian Masses

Simple ovarian cysts and solid teratomas are not uncommon and may be asymptomatic even though they have reached a large size. Occasionally, the child presents with urinary complaints from the pressure on the bladder or urethra. Granulosa cell tumors of the ovary produce precocious puberty because they are hormonally active tumors. They may be malignant. The sudden onset of severe abdominal pain may indicate torsion of an ovarian mass, with resultant ovarian infarction.

Radiographs may show calcification in about half of patients with teratomas (Fig. 124.19). Because an occasional ovarian tumor is malignant in children, children with ovarian masses should be promptly evaluated and prepared for surgery.

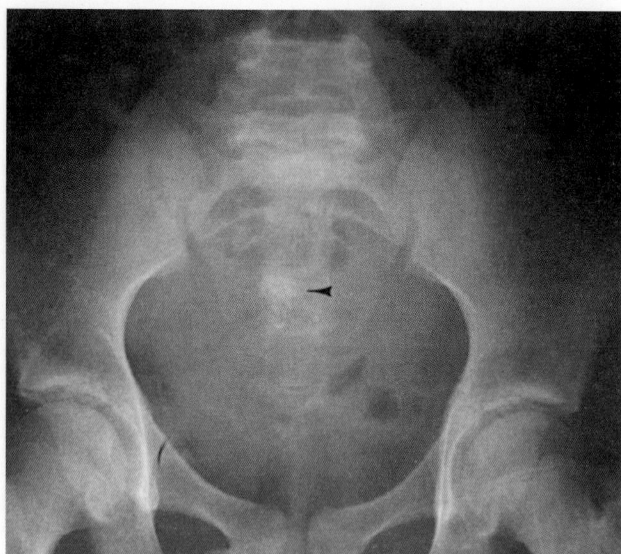

FIGURE 124.19 Ovarian dermoids. Note calcification (*arrowhead*) in superior aspect of a large pelvic mass in a 12-year-old girl.

Omental Cysts

Omental cysts are rare, are usually asymptomatic, and can fill the abdomen. It is often difficult to differentiate an omental cyst from ascites. Smaller cysts are more mobile and can be pushed freely into all quadrants of the abdomen. If a cyst volvulizes on its pedicle or has bleeding within it, it may cause abdominal pain or tenderness. Elective surgical excision is indicated.

Mesenteric Cysts

Mesenteric cysts can occur anywhere in the mesentery but are most common in the mesentery of the colon. They tend to be multilocular and are often discovered during a routine examination or after an episode of abdominal trauma with enlargement from bleeding. They are benign, but surgery is indicated, both to confirm the diagnosis and to prevent complications. They can usually be removed with sparing of the bowel, or they can be marsupialized into the general peritoneal cavity where the fluid is absorbed.

Duplications

GI duplications within the abdomen can occur anywhere along the greater curvature of the stomach, the lesser curvature of the duodenum, or the mesenteric side of either the small or large intestines. They can also be pararectal, rising up out of the pelvis. Duplications that produce abdominal masses are either noncommunicating, and hence gradually enlarge, or communicating in that their secretory lining has a distal communication with the true lumen of the bowel. Except for the rare occurrence of massive rectal bleeding in a child with a communicating duplication, most duplications do not present as emergencies. Instead, they present in children either as unexplained abdominal masses or with symptoms of intermittent colic, resulting from partial obstruction of the true lumen of the adjacent bowel. The exact diagnosis is often unclear until the time of laparotomy.

Malignant Intra-Abdominal Masses

About 50% of the solid malignant tumors seen in children occur within the abdominal cavity. Most solid masses occur in the retroperitoneum. The most common is neuroblastoma, followed by Wilms tumor and rhabdomyosarcoma. Other unusual tumors, such as embryonal cell carcinomas (yolk sac tumor) and lymphosarcoma, also occur in young children (see Chapter 106 Oncologic Emergencies). As with most malignant tumors, early diagnosis and treatment provide the best prospects for a cure.

Neuroblastoma

Neuroblastoma most often occurs as a tumor arising from the adrenal gland, but it can develop anywhere along the sympathetic chain or in the pelvis. It can grow extensively, often crossing the midline of the abdomen and enveloping key vascular and visceral structures. The best cure rates are generally in children who are younger than 1 year of age at the time of diagnosis and in whom the tumor is still localized to the point of origin. In such favorable cases, the tumor can be totally excised. When widespread dissemination occurs, complete resection is unwarranted because of the risk to other vital structures.

CT with contrast enhancement demonstrates precise anatomy, as well as renal function and organ vascularity. The CT characteristics of neuroblastoma include irregular shape, irregular margins, lack of well-defined capsules, and mixed low-density center. Neuroblastoma often displaces surrounding organs and encases vessels. Prevertebral midline extension is common. There are calcifications in at least 75% (Fig. 124.20). Ultrasonography has limitations in accurately determining tumor margins or local extension.

Wilms Tumor

Wilms tumor is the most common intrarenal tumor seen in children. The tumor can be massive before its discovery. Wilms tumor should be considered in any child who has unexplained hematuria.

A solid renal mass demonstrated by US in infants and children is usually a Wilms tumor. Because of the high frequency of tumor extension into the renal veins and inferior vena cava, these vascular structures should be examined by US. Because Wilms tumors are usually large and expansive, the inferior vena cava often is extrinsically displaced by the tumor mass. CT with bolus contrast enhancement may be required for confirmation of equivocal invasion in a patient suspected of having Wilms tumor. CT scan can define the presence of an intrarenal mass and extent of tumor, visualizes vascular structures, identifies nodal involvement, defines internal hemorrhage and necrosis, evaluates the presence or absence of liver metastases, and provides some measure of renal excretory function. Also, CT can determine whether a tumor is initially nonresectable or bilateral (Fig. 124.21). Chest CT is also performed at the initial evaluation to identify pulmonary metastases. Patients with presumed Wilms tumor require admission for coordinated approach by the surgeon and oncologists.

Rhabdomyosarcoma

Rhabdomyosarcoma can occur anywhere in the abdomen or pelvis where there is striated muscle. Tumors are particularly common in the pelvis, involving the prostate, uterus or vagina, and retroperitoneal structures, but they have also been found in the common bile duct and other unusual sites. These tumors can reach a large size before they become symptomatic, and each must be managed individually, depending on the site of origin, extent of growth, and the degree of spread.

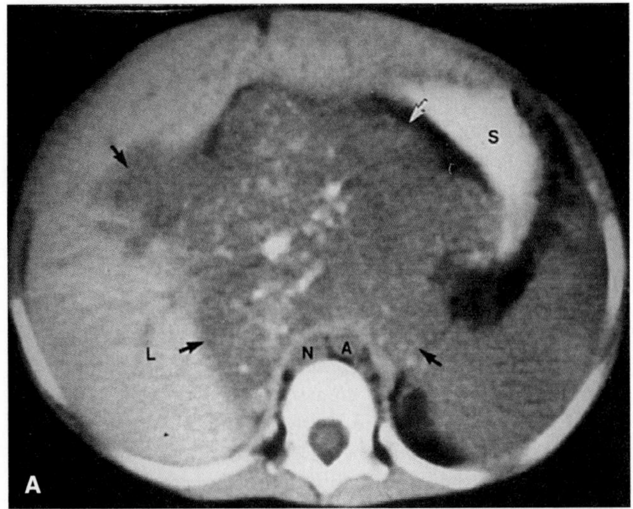

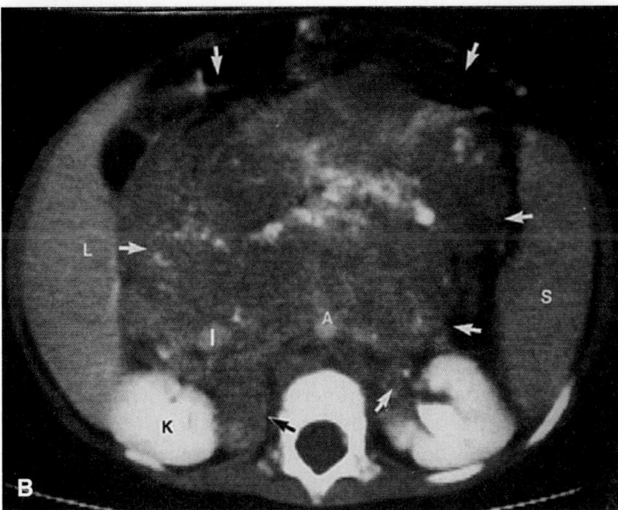

FIGURE 124.20 **A:** Celiac axis neuroblastoma. Computed tomographic (CT) section of the abdomen shows a large lobulated mass with multiple flakes of calcification displacing stomach and the liver (*white arrow*). Note presence of retrocrural node (*black arrows*). A, aorta; L, liver; N, node; S, stomach. **B:** Celiac axis neuroblastoma. Enhanced CT section of the abdomen at level of the kidney shows a large lobulated mass with irregular margins and calcification displacing the right kidney inferoposterior and laterally. Note encased inferior vena cava (IVC) and aorta. The IVC is displaced laterally and ventrally and to the right the superior mesenteric artery and celiac axis are completely surrounded by the mass. A, aorta; I, IVC; K, kidney; L, liver; S, spleen; *white arrows,* mass.

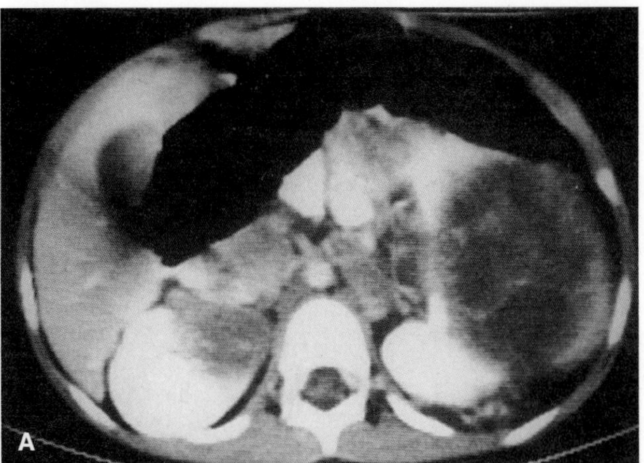

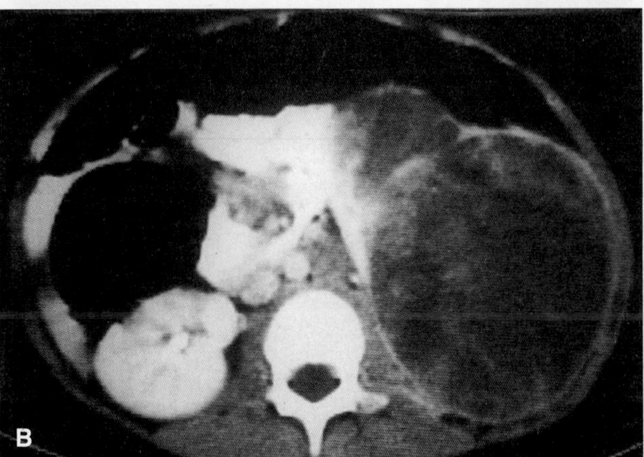

FIGURE 124.21 **A:** Bilateral Wilms tumor. A 5-year-old girl with left flank mass. Computed tomography (CT) sections of the upper abdomen with contrast medium enhancement show a necrotic mass arising from superior aspect of the left kidney. Note a small mass in the superior medial aspect of the right kidney. **B:** Bilateral Wilms tumor (same patient as in **A**). CT section of the abdomen with contrast medium enhancement shows extent of the large necrotic left Wilms tumor with periaortic adenopathy.

Hepatomas

The most common primary GI tract neoplasm is hepatic in origin. Hepatoblastoma and hepatocellular carcinoma are the two main subgroups of liver tumors; they are clinically indistinguishable at presentation. Many are asymptomatic, but symptoms such as early satiety, weight loss, and abdominal pain may be seen especially with very large tumors. More often, the tumor is discovered after caregivers notice a change in the appearance of the abdomen. They are usually seen in older infants and young children. Increased levels of alpha-fetoprotein are associated with both types. Differential diagnosis should include hemangioendothelioma, hamartoma, and renal and adrenal tumors.

Radiologic imaging is directed at diagnosis and the resectability of the tumor. CT or MRI with angiography is often required to determine surgical approach (Fig. 124.22). Long-term survival is poor unless complete resection is possible. Liver tumors commonly metastasize to the lungs, brain, and regional nodes.

ABDOMINAL WALL DEFECTS

Inguinal Hernias and Hydroceles

Indirect inguinal hernia is the most common congenital anomaly that is found in children. It is approximately 10 times more common in males than in females. There is a strong familial incidence.

Clinical Manifestations

The child with a hernia may present in different ways. The presentation is determined by the extent of obliteration of the processus vaginalis during development. A child may have a completely open hernia sac, which extends from the internal ring to the scrotum, or a segmental obliteration producing a sac that is narrow at its proximal end, creating a hydrocele of either the tunica vaginalis or the spermatic cord. The narrowing of the

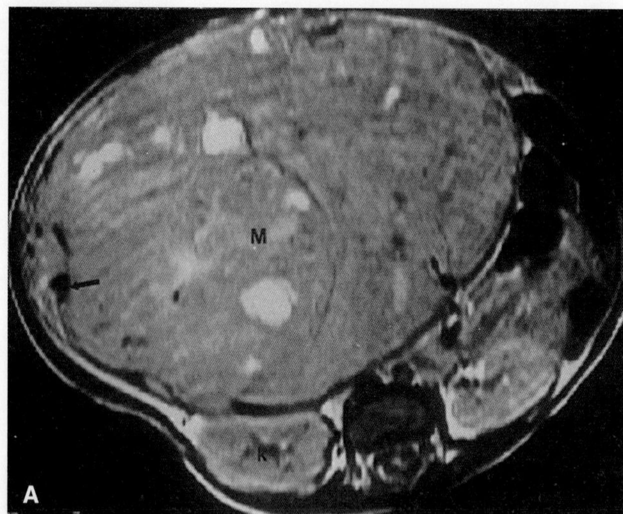

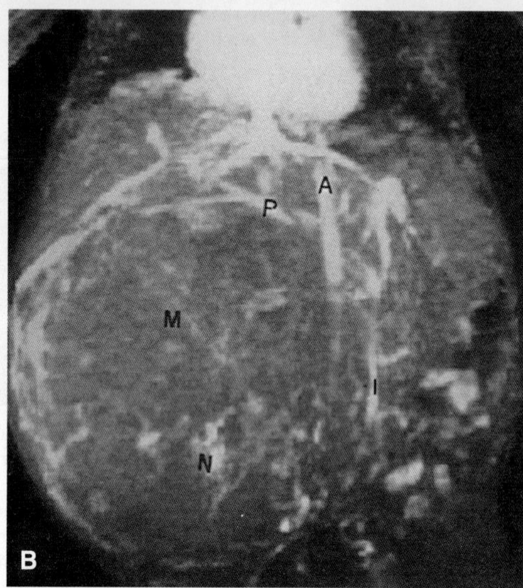

FIGURE 124.22 **A:** Hepatoblastoma in a 2-month-old boy. Axial T1 magnetic resonance imaging (MRI) shows a solid mass (M) occupying entire liver, gallbladder (*arrow*), and right kidney (K). **B:** Coronal magnetic resonance angiography shows liver mass (M), with stretching of the hepatic vessels and multiple area of neovascularity (N). Note marked stretching and displacement of the inferior vena cava (I) with patent portal vein (P). A, aorta.

processus allows the abdominal fluid to seep into the distal portion of the sac. It then becomes entrapped and produces what is clinically recognized as a hydrocele. It is often difficult for this fluid to egress through the narrow patent processus vaginalis back into the abdominal cavity.

At the time of the embryologic closure of the processus vaginalis, many fetuses will have some fluid trapped around the testicle in the tunica vaginalis. This is called a physiologic hydrocele, which is a normal newborn finding. In such cases, the fluid gradually is absorbed in the first 12 months of life. If, however, an infant or child develops a hydrocele along the cord in the tunica vaginalis sometime after birth, it must be assumed the processus vaginalis is still patent and in communication with the peritoneal cavity. This patent processus vaginalis represents a hernia sac. Surgical closure of the sac and drainage of the hydrocele are then indicated on an elective basis.

Many infants and children manifest the classical bulge in the inguinal canal that occurs during straining or crying. This is caused by a loop of intestine distending into the hernia sac (or may represent the ovary in a female). Usually, the hernia sac contents reduce into the abdominal cavity when the straining ceases. If the prolapsing loop of intestine becomes entrapped in the hernia sac, an incarceration has occurred. This is a true emergency that could eventually lead to intestinal obstruction and possibly strangulation of the bowel. For easily reduced hernias, elective herniorrhaphy should be done shortly after the hernia is diagnosed.

Hydroceles of the spermatic cord with associated communicating hernias are sometimes difficult to differentiate from an incarcerated hernia. If an empty hernia sac can be felt above the hydrocele, the physician can be assured this is an asymptomatic hernia with an associated hydrocele. However, if there is fullness above the hydrocele and the mass cannot be reduced, the child should be taken to the operating room on the assumption that it probably is an incarcerated hernia that needs to be managed surgically. If there is any uncertainty, US may be useful to define the hernia. Bowel gas in the hernia sac is not reliably present for diagnostic reasons.

Management

Fortunately, strangulation of the entrapped loop of bowel in an incarcerated hernia occurs relatively late so, contrary to adult practice, efforts to reduce the incarceration without surgery are usually warranted. When a child with an incarcerated hernia presents in the ED, the child should be given nothing to eat or drink, sedated if necessary with morphine 0.1 mg per kg, and placed in a Trendelenburg position. Often, this alone will reduce the incarceration. If it does not, bimanual reduction should be attempted. The fingers and thumb of one hand should compress the internal ring area, while an effort is made with the other hand "to milk" either gas or fluid out of the entrapped bowel back into the abdomen. This relieves the pressure and usually allows the entire loop of bowel to reduce back into the abdominal cavity. Once the incarcerated hernia is reduced, the child should be admitted or scheduled for elective surgery at the surgeon's discretion. Patients who were vomiting, had guaiac-positive stools, or had difficultly reducing hernias should be admitted for serial abdominal examinations. A day or two should be allowed to pass to lessen the edema of the area, as well as to allow an easier and safer elective herniorrhaphy.

Epiploceles (Epigastric Hernias)

If a discrete mass occurs intermittently about one-third of the distance from the umbilicus to the xiphoid, it is usually the result of a weakness of the linea alba through which properitoneal fat protrudes. This defect is called epiplocele. Such defects are fairly common in infants and usually close spontaneously. In older children, the mass may occasionally be tender. If it becomes excruciatingly tender, it is a sign that fat has become incarcerated in the hernia. Although there is no great urgency, these small midline defects should be repaired surgically when they become symptomatic.

Umbilical Hernias

Umbilical hernias are common in small infants, particularly in African-Americans. Fortunately, most of the hernias tend to close spontaneously, and only rarely does incarceration

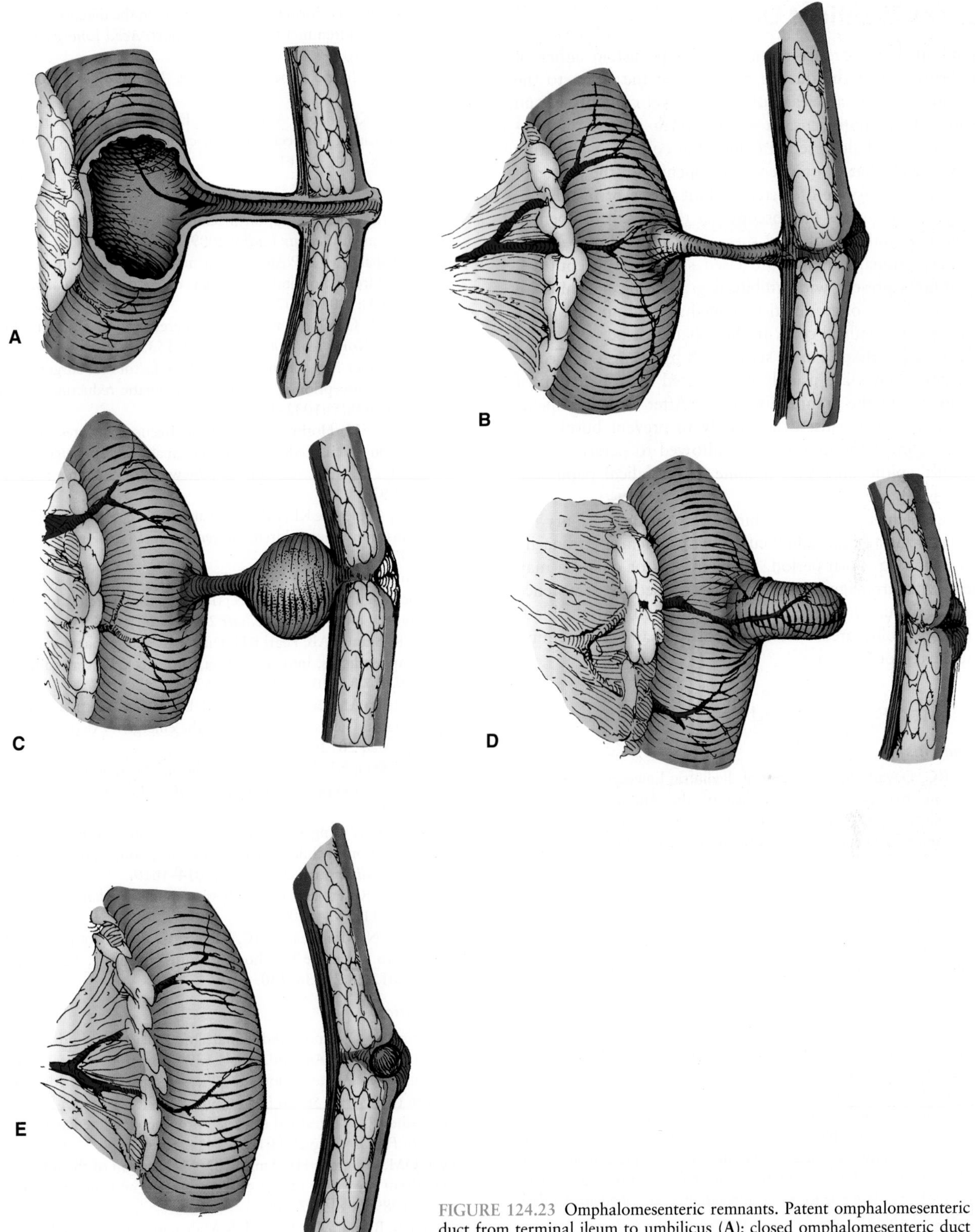

FIGURE 124.23 Omphalomesenteric remnants. Patent omphalomesenteric duct from terminal ileum to umbilicus (**A**); closed omphalomesenteric duct with mucosal patch at umbilicus (**B**); omphalomesenteric cyst below umbilicus (**C**); Meckel diverticulum (**D**); and umbilical granuloma (**E**).

occur. Umbilical hernias can be large and unsightly, and families need reassurance that watchful waiting is the best course. However, if the umbilical hernia fails to close by the age of 5 to 6 years, surgical repair is indicated. Umbilical hernias may be repaired earlier if there is a large ring that shows no signs of diminishing in size over 1 to 2 years, if there is a thinning of the umbilical skin, or if an incarceration has occurred. Hernias that have a supraumbilical component tend not to close spontaneously and may be operated on at an earlier time of life.

Other Umbilical Defects

Omphalomesenteric duct remnants may persist in either of two forms. When the duct is patent from the ileum to the umbilicus, there is a release of small bowel contents via an opening in the umbilicus. A second form involves a remnant of the omphalomesenteric duct that contains a secreting mucosal patch that is attached to an opening in the center of the umbilicus. Passage of a sterile blunt probe or instillation of contrast dye under fluoroscopy via the umbilical opening will usually confirm either of these conditions. Once identified, these remnants must be excised surgically. In contrast, some infants present with umbilical granuloma in which an excessive amount of granulation tissue has built up after separation of the umbilical cord. In these patients, no opening in the granulation tissue can be seen or felt by means of a probe. These granulomas are usually best treated by application of silver nitrate to the granulation tissue. After each treatment, the area should be rinsed thoroughly to prevent burning of adjacent skin. If the granuloma is allowed to persist, it will eventually epithelialize and become an umbilical papilloma (Fig. 124.23).

If the urachus persists after birth, it can form a urinary fistula that drains at the umbilicus. This problem is ordinarily noted in the newborn period. Older infants or children may present with drainage at the umbilicus caused by persistence of part of the urachus, even though connection with the bladder may be obliterated. These urachal remnants also require surgical excision.

Suggested Readings and Key References

Appendicitis

Bachur RG, Dayan PS, Bajaj L, et al. Pediatric Emergency Medicine Collaborative Research Committee of the American Academy of Pediatrics. The effect of abdominal pain duration on the accuracy of diagnostic imaging for pediatric appendicitis. *Ann Emerg Med* 2012;60(5):582–590.e3.

Doria AS, Moineddin R, Kellenberger CJ, et al. US or CT for diagnosis of appendicitis in children and adults? A meta-analysis. *Radiology* 2006;241(1):83–94.

Frush DP, Frush KS, Oldham KT. Imaging of acute appendicitis in children: EU versus U.S. . . . or US versus CT? A North American perspective. *Pediatric Radiol* 2009;39(5):500–505.

Hennelly KE, Bachur R. Appendicitis update. *Curr Opin Pediatr* 2011; 23(3):281–285.

Howell JM, Eddy OL, Lukens TW, et al. American College of Emergency Physicians. Clinical policy: Critical issues in the evaluation and management of emergency department patients with suspected appendicitis. *Ann Emerg Med* 2010;55(1):71–116.

Kharbanda AB, Dudley NC, Bajaj L, et al. Pediatric Emergency Medicine Collaborative Research Committee of the American Academy of Pediatrics. Validation and refinement of a prediction rule to identify children at low risk for acute appendicitis. *Arch Pediatr Adolesc Med* 2012;166(8):738–744.

Kharbanda AB, Stevenson MD, Macias CG, et al. Pediatric Emergency Medicine Collaborative Research Committee of the American Academy of Pediatrics. Interrater reliability of clinical findings in children with possible appendicitis. *Pediatrics* 2012;129(4):695–700.

Krishnamoorthi R, Ramarajan N, Wang NE, et al. Effectiveness of a Staged US and CT protocol for the diagnosis of pediatric appendicitis: reducing radiation exposure in the age of ALARA. *Radiology* 2011;259(1):231–239.

Mittal MK, Dayan PS, Macias CG, et al. Pediatric Emergency Medicine Collaborative Research Committee of the American Academy of Pediatrics. Performance of ultrasound in the diagnosis of appendicitis in children in a multicenter cohort. *Acad Emerg Med* 2013; 20(7):697–702.

Samuel M. Pediatric appendicitis score. *J Pediatr Surg* 2002;37(6): 877–881.

Schneider C, Kharbanda A, Bachur R. Evaluating appendicitis scoring systems using a prospective pediatric cohort. *Ann Emerg Med.* 2007; 49(6):778–784, 784 e1.

Intussusception

Applegate KE. Intussusception in children: evidence-based diagnosis and treatment. *Pediatr Radiol* 2009;39(2):S140–S143.

Bajaj L, Roback MG. Postreduction management of intussusception in a children's hospital emergency department. *Pediatrics* 2003; 112(6 Pt 1):1302–1307.

D'Agostino J. Common abdominal emergencies in children. *Emerg Med Clin North Am* 2002;20(1):139–153.

Fallon SC, Lopez ME, Zhang W, et al. Risk factors for surgery in pediatric intussusception in the era of pneumatic reduction. *J Pediatr Surg* 2013;48(5):1032–1036.

Gray MP, Li SH, Hoffmann RG, et al. Recurrence rates after intussusception enema reduction: a meta-analysis. *Pediatrics* 2014;134 (1):110–119. Retrieved from http://www.ncbi.nlm.nih.gov/pubmed/24935997

Kaiser AD, Applegate KE, Ladd AP. Current success in the treatment of intussusception in children. *Surgery* 2007;142(4):469–475; discussion 475–467.

Morrison J, Lucas N, Gravel J. The role of abdominal radiography in the diagnosis of intussusception when interpreted by pediatric emergency physicians. *J Pediatr* 2009;155(4):556–559.

Pepper VK, Stanfill AB, Pearl RH. Diagnosis and management of pediatric appendicitis, intussusception, and Meckel diverticulum. *Surg Clin North Am* 2012;92(3):505–526.

Riera A, Hsiao AL, Langhan ML, et al. Diagnosis of intussusception by physician novice sonographers in the emergency department. *Ann Emerg Med* 2012;60(3):264–268.

Sohoni A, Wang NE, Dannenberg B. Tension pneumoperitoneum after intussusception pneumoreduction. *Pediatr Emerg Care* 2007;23(8): 563–564.

Somme S, To T, Langer JC. Factors determining the need for operative reduction in children with intussusception: a population-based study. *J Pediatr Surg* 2006;41(5):1014–1019.

Waseem M, Rosenberg HK. Intussusception. *Pediatr Emerg Care* 2008;24(11):793–800.

Weihmiller SN, Monuteaux MC, Bachur RG. Ability of pediatric physicians to judge the likelihood of intussusception. *Pediatr Emerg Care* 2012;28(2):136–140.

Malrotation

D'Agostino J. Common abdominal emergencies in children. *Emerg Med Clin North Am* 2002;20(1):139–153.

Gauderer MW. Acute abdomen. When to operate immediately and when to observe. *Semin Pediatr Surg* 1997;6(2):74–80.

Hajivassiliou CA. Intestinal obstruction in neonatal/pediatric surgery. *Semin Pediatr Surg* 2003;12(4):241–253.

Powell OM, Othersen HB, Smith CD. Malrotation of the intestines in children: the effect of age on presentation and therapy. *J Pediatr Surg* 1989;24(8):777–780.

Spigland N, Brandt ML, Yazbeck S. Malrotation presenting beyond the neonatal period. *J Pediatr Surg* 1990;25(11):1139–1142.

Hernias

Brandt ML. Pediatric hernias. *Surg Clin North Am* 2008;88(1):27–43, vii–viii.

Chen LE, Zamakhshary M, Foglia RP, et al. Impact of wait time on outcome for inguinal hernia repair in infants. *Pediatr Surg Int* 2009;25(3):223–227.

Erez I, Rathause V, Vacian I, et al. Preoperative ultrasound and intraoperative findings of inguinal hernias in children: a prospective study of 642 children. *J Pediatr Surg* 2002;37(6):865–868.

Gill FT. Umbilical hernia, inguinal hernias, and hydroceles in children: diagnostic clues for optimal patient management. *J Pediatr Health Care* 1998;12(5):231–235.

McCollough M, Sharieff GQ. Abdominal pain in children. *Pediatr Clin North Am* 2006;53(1):107–137, vi.

Sheldon CA. The pediatric genitourinary examination. Inguinal, urethral, and genital diseases. *Pediatr Clin North Am* 2001;48(6): 1339–1380.

Miscellaneous

Dillon PW, Cilley RE. Newborn surgical emergencies. Gastrointestinal anomalies, abdominal wall defects. *Pediatr Clin North Am* 1993; 40(6):1289–1314.

Louie JP. Essential diagnosis of abdominal emergencies in the first year of life. *Emerg Med Clin North Am* 2007;25(4):1009–1040, vi.

McCollough M, Sharieff GQ. Abdominal surgical emergencies in infants and young children. *Emerg Med Clin North Am* 2003;21(4): 909–935.

Munden MM. Ultrasonography in pediatric abdominal emergencies. *Ultrasound Clin* 2013;8(3):335–353.

Van Heurn LW, Pakarinen MP, Wester T. Contemporary management of abdominal surgical emergencies in infants and children. *Br J Surg* 2014;101(1):e24–e33.

Vasavada P. Ultrasound evaluation of acute abdominal emergencies in infants and children. *Radiol Clin North Am* 2004;42(2): 445–456.

CHAPTER 125 ■ DENTAL EMERGENCIES

ZAMEERA FIDA, DMD, LINDA P. NELSON, DMD, MScD, AND STEPHEN SHUSTERMAN, DMD

GOALS OF THERAPY

Nontraumatic orofacial emergencies can appear suddenly and are frightening for children and their families. Patients may present with pain or facial swelling, complications after recent dental procedures, or with new lesions affecting the oral mucosa. Identifying the underlying etiologies, providing necessary interventions in the emergency department (ED), and recognizing indications for utilizing specialty consultation with dentistry are the aim of emergency care. Addressing symptoms and findings related to traumatic orofacial emergencies are addressed separately in Chapter 113 Dental Trauma.

KEY POINTS

- The infant or young child who may have dental pain often cannot localize the discomfort.
- An acute dental emergency may be the first opportunity for many children to receive dental care.
- The challenge with dental emergencies is recognizing which conditions can be treated primarily by emergency physicians or outpatient referral and which require urgent consultation with a dentist

RELATED CHAPTERS

Signs and Symptoms

- Oral Lesions: Chapter 47

Medical, Surgical, and Trauma Emergencies

- Infectious Disease Emergencies: Chapter 102
- Dental Trauma: Chapter 113

ODONTOGENIC OROFACIAL PAIN

CLINICAL PEARLS AND PITFALLS

- Children often cannot distinguish between tooth pain and soft-tissue pain from a lesion such as an aphthous ulcer.
- A careful intraoral examination should be performed to identify the source of the discomfort.
- In the case of significant swelling secondary to infection, consider hospitalization for parenteral antibiotics to halt the potentially dangerous spread of facial infection.
- Establishing drainage through the tooth or soft tissue is important to relieve the symptoms from abscesses, but analgesics and antibiotics are often necessary.
- Heat can be applied extraorally for symptomatic relief, without concern for resultant development of an external fistula.

Odontalgia—Simple Toothache

Toothaches are common in the pediatric population. The latest National Health and Nutrition Examination Survey (NHANES) data found that 42% of 2 to 11 year olds had caries in primary teeth and 23% have unmet dental needs. In addition, 21% of 6 to 11 year olds had caries in their permanent teeth. As low-income populations have the greatest dental needs and are also least likely to seek dental care, presentation to the emergency department with odontalgia is common.

Tooth pain may be present without associated infection. The emergency physician may note a grossly carious tooth or large restoration (i.e., filling). Swelling or inflammation in the surrounding soft tissue may be present. The tooth may be sensitive to percussion and may exhibit excessive mobility.

Oral analgesia should be provided to address pain. If symptoms can be improved and the patient is able to tolerate oral intake, a referral for outpatient dental care is appropriate. If significant swelling is noted, or pain cannot be adequately addressed with oral medications, a dental consultation is necessary.

Dentoalveolar Infection and Abscess

Odontogenic infections often results from dental caries or periodontal disease. They may also result from recurrent tooth decay, trauma, or chronic irritation from a large restoration. Dental caries develop following bacterial colonization of the tooth surface, i.e., plaque. Certain bacteria, commonly *Streptococcus mutans* and *Streptococcus sobrinus,* invade the tooth surface and can eventually infect the pulp tissue. Infected pulp causes pressure buildup in the confined space, which results in a clinical symptom of pain. Pus may egress out of the root of the infected tooth, causing local swelling. Infection can also spread and become quite extensive. Infection travels along planes of least resistance, which is predetermined by anatomic barriers, i.e., muscle, bone, and fascia. Pus perforates bone where it is thinnest and weakest: in the mandible on the lingual aspect of molars and buccal aspect of anteriors; in the maxilla on the buccal surface throughout. The infection may spread into the subperiosteal area and then to the surrounding soft tissues. If it does not drain intraorally, the infection can progress rapidly along the fascial planes of the face or neck. Resultant facial cellulitis can have severe systemic consequences, including cavernous sinus thrombosis, preseptal or orbital cellulitis, intracranial spread and meningitis, or even sepsis.

The following are clinical manifestations of a dentoalveolar abscess in a child:

- Pain: The child may present with pain or it may be elicited with percussion.
- Mobility: The tooth may have greater than normal degree of movement in the socket when palpated.
- Swelling: The soft tissues surrounding the tooth may be edematous and erythematous.
- Temperature elevation: The child may be febrile.
- Fistulous tracts: A pustule-like lesion may be noted on the gingiva (rarely on the face) when the infection has been longstanding.
- Extrusion: The tooth may become extruded because of the presence of fluid in the periradicular space.
- Lymphadenopathy: Lymph node enlargement can occur at any time during the infective process.

As with other abscesses, the treatment of choice for a localized dentoalveolar abscess is symptomatic control (oral analgesics, and moist heat) and drainage. In cases which have progressed to facial cellulitis with lymphadenopathy, antibiotics should be given. Amoxicillin or amoxicillin with clavulanate potassium are first line agents in children. Alternatively clindamycin can be used if there is a known penicillin allergy, though the palatability of the liquid preparation may make compliance challenging. Erythromycin and tetracycline are no longer recommended due to increasing resistance of some strains of bacteria.

If extensive or rapidly progressive swelling is noted, a hospital admission may be required for parenteral antibiotics. Other factors to consider in determining the need for hospital admission include the child's ability to take fluids and the likelihood of the parent's cooperation for follow-up dental care. In addition to antibiotics, warm oral saline rinses can be used (if the child is able to cooperate) or warm moist heat applied to the area of swelling. Analgesic therapy with acetaminophen or ibuprofen is usually sufficient though opiates may be required in more severe cases. Dental consultation should be obtained. As with abscesses elsewhere in the body, the basic surgical principles of treatment are to establish drainage and remove the underlying cause. For dentoalveolar abscesses specifically, definitive treatment may include venting or extraction of the offending tooth, and possibly incising any fluctuant mass when needed. Treatment of facial cellulitis is covered in Chapter 102 Infectious Disease Emergencies. In the rare case of systemic infection, blood cultures should be obtained and broad-spectrum parenteral antibiotic given.

POSTEXTRACTION COMPLICATIONS

Goals of Treatment

Children may present to the emergency department in the hours to days after dental procedures such as tooth extractions with concerns related to bleeding, swelling, pain, or fever. When these symptoms develop during hours in which their primary dentist is unavailable, the ED becomes a means of access to medical and in many cases dental providers. Emergency physicians should identify whether symptoms are related to the prior procedure and if so, treat any complications to provide relief and avoid long-term complications.

CLINICAL PEARLS AND PITFALLS

- Home remedies for postextraction bleeding including direct pressure to the site of bleeding and application of a moist tea bag. Tannic acid in tea may initiate or accelerate coagulation and assist in achieving hemostasis.
- Dry socket, or alveolar osteitis, and postextraction infections are very rare in children.

Hemorrhage

It is possible for an extraction site to ooze for 8 to 12 hours, and perhaps longer for a permanent tooth. Systemic hematologic abnormalities can often be ruled out though a thorough bleeding history (see Chapter 101 Hematologic Emergencies), though a complete blood count (CBC) and coagulation profile may be indicated in some cases. Rarely is blood loss significant enough to cause hemodynamic changes or risk of airway obstruction, however the goal of management is to achieve hemostasis as rapidly as possible. Emergency treatment to control bleeding may include the following steps:

1. Using folded gauze sponges that are placed directly over the open socket, apply biting pressure directly onto the site for 30 to 60 minutes. Avoid the temptation to remove the gauze until the bleeding has stopped, as removal of the material can disrupt any forming clot and may worsen bleeding. Most postprocedure bleeding can be successfully treated with this approach.
2. If bleeding continues despite effective direct pressure, consider the following approaches:
   A. Suture closure—The aim is to tamponade bleeding by physically closing the socket with sutures. First infiltrate local anesthesia (lidocaine with 1:100,000 epinephrine infiltration). The extraction site can then be approximated with 4-0 or 5-0 chromic gut sutures.
   B. Topical hemostatic agents or antifibrinolytic therapy can be applied to the site of bleeding. Depending on availability and practice patterns, materials such as Surgicel, Gelfoam, fibrin glue, or tranexamic acid can be used locally.

Infection

Postextraction infection is rare in children. If it occurs, it may present as localized swelling or edema surrounded by a zone of erythema, often with purulent exudate within the socket. Emergency treatment includes the application of moist heat, oral saline rinses (if the age is appropriate), and antibiotic therapy. Amoxicillin or amoxicillin with clavulanate potassium are the antibiotics of choice.

Alveolar Osteitis

Alveolar osteitis, or *dry socket*, is a painful postoperative condition produced by a disintegration of the clot in the tooth socket. This condition is usually seen in adults and only rarely in children younger than 12 years. It generally occurs approximately 72 hours after mandibular extractions. Emergency dental treatment is variable, but the immediate goal is relief of pain. Under local anesthesia, the socket may be debrided and then packed with ¼-in iodoform gauze or BIPP (bismuth, iodoform, paraffin paste). Oral analgesic and nonsteroidal anti-inflammatory (NSAID) medications should be prescribed for pain. Since it is an osteitis, antibiotics should be reserved for cases of infection rather than only inflammation.

PERIODONTAL SOFT TISSUE PATHOLOGY

Goals of Treatment

Soft tissue pathology may be painful and mistaken for odontalgia or dentoalveolar abscess. The goal is to alleviate any pain and discomfort. Referral to a dental specialist may be required. Emergency treatment for pericoronitis includes local curettage, oral rinses, heat, and scrupulous oral hygiene. Amoxicillin or amoxicillin with clavulanate may be necessary when there are systemic symptoms of infection or associated facial swelling. For patients with infection of the oral mucosa unrelated to erupting dentition, distinguishing bacterial versus viral etiology is important to direct subsequent therapies.

CLINICAL PEARLS AND PITFALLS

- The first priority is to rule out odontalgia and dentoalveolar abscess as sources of pain.
- Pericoronitis is common with the eruption of permanent molars
- Acute necrotizing ulcerative gingivitis (ANUG) is extremely rare in young children, and can be easily mistaken for primary herpetic gingivostomatitis.
- Primary herpes is usually seen in infants and toddlers, and ANUG is characteristically seen in adolescents and young adults.

Pericoronitis

Pericoronitis is a localized, acute infection surrounding an erupting tooth. It is usually associated with erupting molars in the adolescent patient, although a mild form may be associated with the eruption of the first permanent molar (Table 125.1). Symptoms usually include pain distal to the last erupted tooth in the dental arch, along with erythema and edema localized to the gingiva in the retromolar area. Localized, painful lymphadenopathy, trismus, and dysphagia may accompany these symptoms. Children may occasionally have accompanying fever. It is usual to see or palpate the cusps of the erupting tooth. The patient may complain of an inability to completely close his or her mouth because of the edematous gingiva. Exudate may be expressed from beneath the infected flap of tissue. Rarely, pain may be referred to the ear, though no pathology will be identified on otologic examination.

Acute Necrotizing Ulcerative Gingivitis, Vincent Disease, Trench Mouth

Acute necrotizing ulcerative gingivitis (ANUG), also known as Vincent disease or trench mouth, results from increases in fusiform bacillus and *Borrelia vincentii*, a spirochete, which usually coexist in a symbiotic relationship with other oral flora. Immunocompromised patients are at increased risk for this condition. Other associated risk factors include: emotional stress, malnutrition, severe dehydration, poor oral hygiene, and infectious mononucleosis.

Adolescents complain of soreness and point tenderness at the gingiva and often tell the physician that they feel as if they "cannot remove a piece of food that is painfully stuck between their teeth" (a wedging sensation). They may also complain of a metallic taste in their mouth or bleeding gums. Upon examination, the breath has an obvious fetid odor. The gingivae are hyperemic, and the usually triangular gingiva between the teeth is missing or "punched out" (Fig. 125.1). A gray, necrotic pseudomembrane may cover some areas. Intense pain is produced with probing.

The adolescent should be advised to maintain better oral hygiene, rest and reduce stress, and use oral rinses such as Peridex (0.12% chlorhexidine). Alternatively, hydrogen peroxide diluted 1:1 with warm water may be used as often as possible throughout the acute phase. Because of the rapidity of tissue destruction and the risk of secondary infection, antibiotic therapy should be initiated. Penicillin, metronidazole, tetracycline, or erythromycin should be prescribed for 7 to 10 days. When the acute phase is over, the patient should be referred to a dentist for a thorough debridement of the area.

TABLE 125.1

ERUPTION SCHEDULE FOR SPECIFIC TEETH

A. Primary teeth	Age at eruption (mo)		Age at exfoliation (yr)	
	Lower	Upper	Lower	Upper
Central incisor	6	7½	6	7½
Lateral incisor	7	9	7	8
Cuspid	16	18	9½	11½
First molar	12	14	10	10½
Second molar	20	24	11	10½
Incisors	Range ±2 mo			
Molars	Range ±4 mo		Range ±6 mo	

B. Permanent teeth[a]	Age (yr)	
	Lower	Upper
Central incisors	6–7	7–8
Lateral incisors	7–8	8–9
Cuspids	9–10	11–12
First bicuspids	10–12	10–11
Second bicuspids	11–12	10–12
First molars	6–7	6–7
Second molars	11–13	12–13
Third molars	17–21	17–21

[a]The lower teeth erupt before the corresponding upper teeth. The teeth usually erupt earlier in girls than in boys.

(Modified with permission from Massler M, Schour I. *Atlas of the mouth and adjacent parts in health and disease.* Chicago, IL: The Bureau of Public Relations Council on Dental Health, American Dental Association, 1946.)

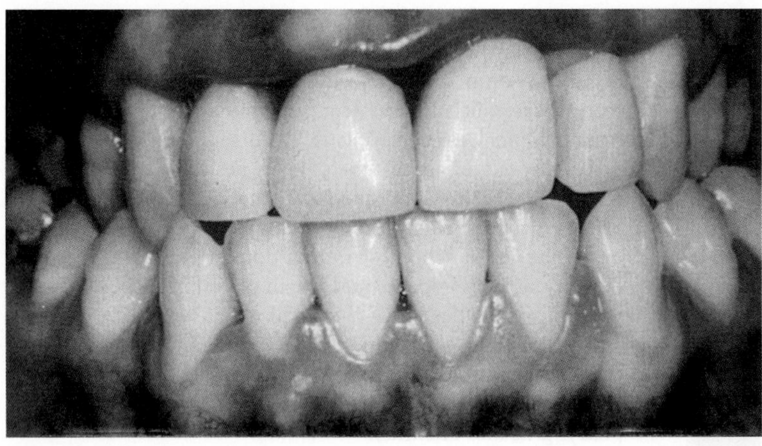

FIGURE 125.1 A child with typical "punched out" gingiva—pathognomonic for acute necrotizing ulcerative gingivitis. (Courtesy of Dr. Mark Snyder.)

Failure of response to therapy should trigger an evaluation for underlying immunosuppression.

Primary Herpetic Gingivostomatitis or Herpes Simplex Virus Type 1

Primary herpetic gingivostomatitis, or herpes simplex virus type 1, is a communicable childhood disease that is not a true dental emergency but is a common cause of ED visits. The child is usually an infant or toddler who stops eating, drinking, or talking and is often irritable. The child usually has had a fever for 3 to 5 days before any clinical oral findings. Older children may complain of headaches, malaise, nausea, regional lymphadenopathy, and/or bleeding gums. The physical examination reveals fiery red marginal gingiva with areas of spontaneous hemorrhage. Within 1 or 2 days, yellowish, fluid-filled vesicles develop on the mucosa, palate, lips, or tongue. The vesicles may coalesce or rupture spontaneously, leaving extremely painful ulcers, covered by a yellow or gray membrane and surrounded by an erythematous zone. Ulcers, especially on the lips, may become encrusted, as seen in Fig. 125.2.

If necessary, a definitive diagnosis can be made by isolation of the herpes simplex virus in tissue culture (although this is rarely indicated). Viscous lidocaine rinses or "magic mouthwash" (Maalox and Benadryl with or without lidocaine) may be helpful but may be unrealistic for children in this age range. The unpleasant taste sometimes makes administration difficult, therefore negating any benefit that the child may receive. Topical administration with a cotton swab can be accomplished in some cases. If using lidocaine, do not exceed 3 mg/kg/dose and do not give more frequently than every 3 hours.

Secondary infection, although rare, is of concern for those children who may be immunosuppressed, and in those cases, antibiotic therapy may be indicated.

Emergency treatment for primary herpetic gingivostomatitis includes support for the parent and hydration of the patient. The disease, like recurrent herpes labialis, is self-limited, with a duration of 7 to 14 days. Antiviral medication such as acyclovir have benefit if given during the prodromal phase, and may be considered for more extensive involvement, if given early in the course. Dehydration and weight loss are the major concerns; therefore, clear fluids should be encouraged. High-calorie and high-protein shakes, ice cream, and bland pureed foods may be less painful to consume and can help with satiety. The young child with extensive lesions may require hospitalization for intravenous hydration.

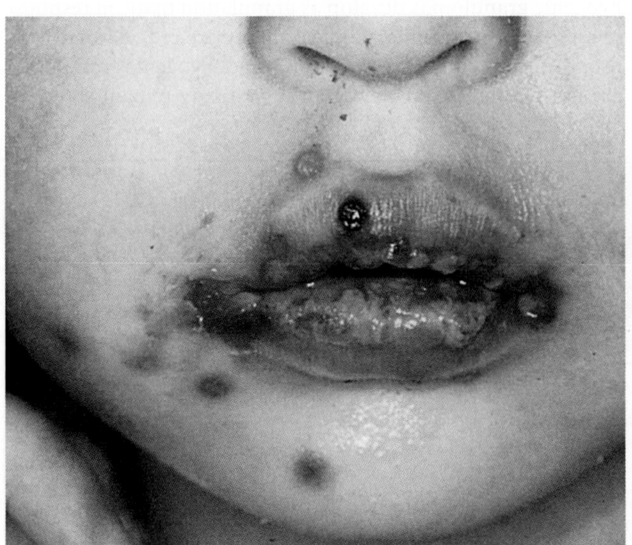

FIGURE 125.2 A child with typical crusted extraoral lesions of late primary gingivostomatitis.

ORAL MUCOSAL SOFT TISSUE PATHOLOGY

Goals of Treatment

A variety of soft tissue lesions in the mouth may prompt evaluation in the ED. The challenge for the emergency physician is to determine if the clinical picture represents a normal variant or abnormal pathology that requires further management in the ED or a referral to a dental specialist. Many of the issues described below are self-limiting and require minimal intervention.

CLINICAL PEARLS AND PITFALLS

- Eruption cysts and neonatal cysts do not require treatment.
- Treatment is palliative for HSV-1 infections, aphthous stomatitis and Riga–Fede disease.
- Mucoceles require excision when they persist or interfere with mastication.

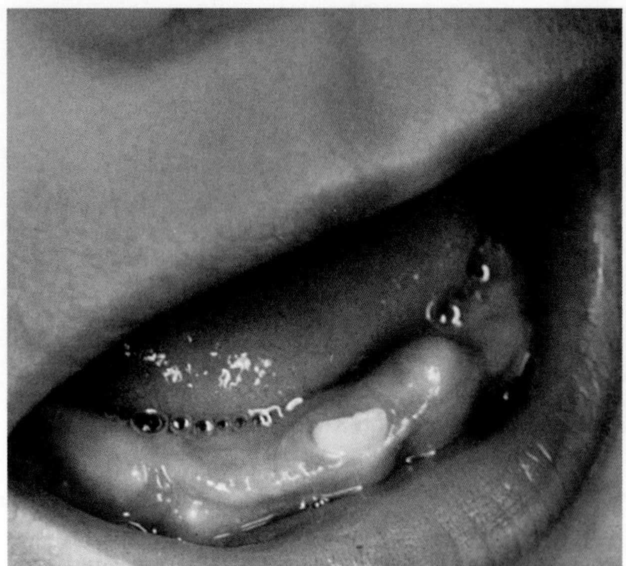

FIGURE 125.3 An eruption cyst associated with an erupting primary central incisor.

Eruption Cysts

Eruption cysts arise from the pre-eruptive dental sac and appear as a swelling of the alveolar ridge. They are associated with the eruption of primary (Fig. 125.3) and permanent teeth. Occasionally, they fill with blood and may be termed *eruption hematomas* (Fig. 125.4). Treatment is unnecessary because the erupting tooth usually emerges within several days. If treatment becomes necessary due to the size of the lesion, excision of the overlying soft tissue to expose the erupting tooth eliminates the problem.

Aphthous Stomatitis

Aphthous stomatitis is the most common disease of the oral mucosa and may affect 20% or more of the population. These painful, shallow, circular ulcerations are distinctive because of their size (2 to 4 mm), distribution, and recurrence. Clinically, the floor of the ulceration is yellowish, with a sharply defined red margin. Aphthae affect only nonkeratinized areas of the mouth, such as the tongue, cheek, or vestibule. If the hard palate or gingival margins are affected, it is unlikely to be aphthous.

Aphthous-like ulcers are often confused with HSV infection. In contrast, they are never preceded by vesicles and occur only on nonkeratinized oral mucosa. Ulcers can also be seen in systemic illnesses (e.g., inflammatory bowel disease), or in patients with neutropenia. Recurrent aphthae often start in childhood or adolescence. They peak in early adult life and then seem to spontaneously resolve. Recurrent aphthae usually occur during periods of anxiety, such as during final examinations at school or during domestic disturbances. The ulcerations may appear singly or in clusters. They are usually painful and tender, have a clinical course of 10 to 14 days, and often cause difficulties with eating. In young children, there is a syndrome of recurring aphthous ulcers and periodic fevers known as PFAPA (periodic fever, aphthous stomatitis, pharyngitis and adenitis).

Treatment of aphthous ulcers is largely empirical and also usually unsatisfactory. Drugs used in the management of aphthae have included topical local analgesics, such as lidocaine gel or benzocaine oral emollient (Orabase with benzocaine), which allow the patient enough comfort to eat. Due to the risk of methemoglobinemia secondary to benzocaine toxicity, Orabase should not be used for more than 2 days in children <2 years of age. Bland nonacidic diets to avoid further irritation may be the best recommendation.

Mucocele

The mucocele appears as a soft, raised, fluid-filled, and well-delineated nodule, most commonly on the lower lip or the mucosal lining of the lower lip (Fig. 125.5). Superficial lesions appear translucent and are bluish, whereas deep-seated lesions retain the natural color of surrounding mucosal tissue. A mucocele in the floor of the mouth is termed a *ranula* and is seen as a dome-shaped, fluid-filled lesion. Mucoceles are believed to result from severance or obstruction of a salivary gland duct, with pooling of mucin in the lamina propria. Complete excision of the mucocele or marsupialization of the ranula is indicated.

Pyogenic Granuloma

Pyogenic granulomas develop as granulation tissue in response to an irritant or trauma. Clinically, they are red, elevated, and usually ulcerated. Initial growth is rapid. Pyogenic granulomas are most common on the gingivae and may remain static for

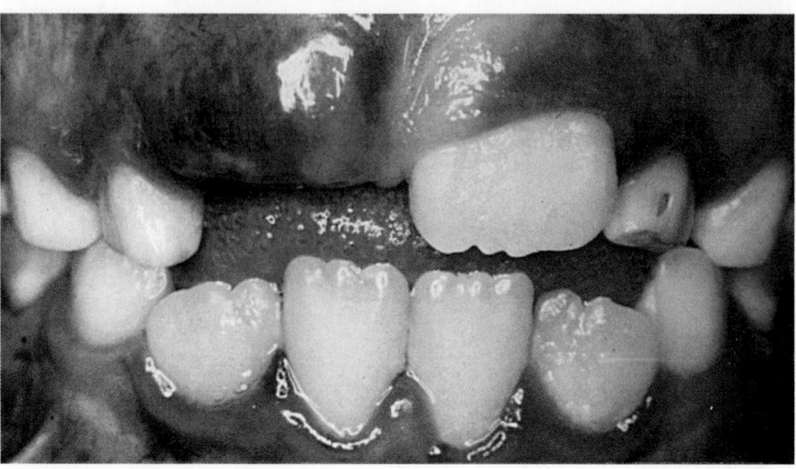

FIGURE 125.4 Erupting hematoma over erupting maxillary permanent central incisor.

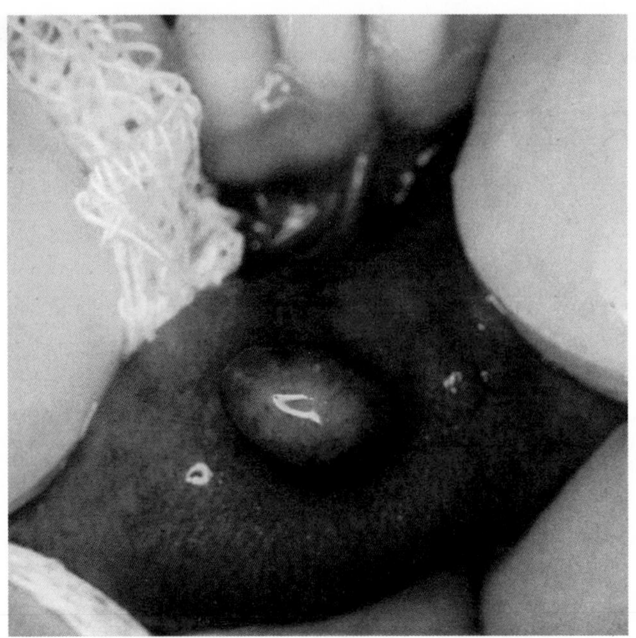

FIGURE 125.5 Mucocele associated with minor salivary gland of the lower lip.

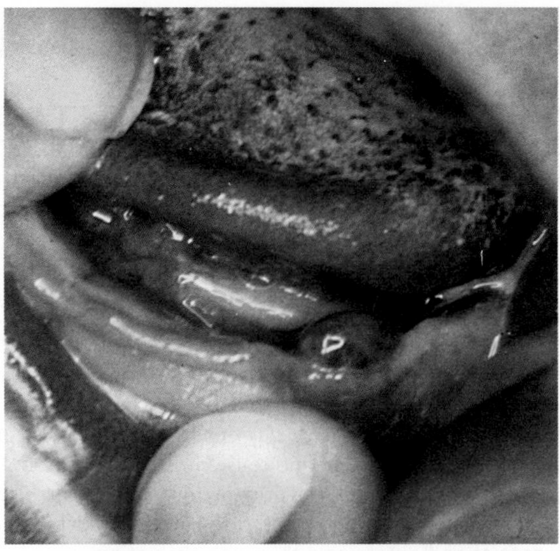

FIGURE 125.6 Dental lamina cyst in a neonate.

a time before becoming fibrotic. Treatment consists of simple excision, but recurrence is common unless the causative agent (calculus or foreign body) is removed.

Neonatal Cysts

Dental lamina cysts may be present in the newborn. Historically, they were named for the location at presentation, however terminology now groups all these lesions as dental lamina cysts. Along the midpalatine raphe, round or ovoid, white, raised nodules may be present. These are keratin-filled cystic lesions (Epstein pearls). Often, only a few can be visualized, but sometimes there are too many to count. They are believed to arise from embryologically trapped epithelium. They are present in about 80% of neonates and should be considered a normal variant. They are self-resolving and no treatment is necessary.

Remnants of the dental lamina may appear as cysts on the buccal or lingual aspect of the maxillary and mandibular dental ridges in the newborn (Bohn nodules). They may appear in the palate but are far removed from the midpalatine raphe. Although similar in shape and color, they are located differently and therefore can be easily distinguished from Epstein pearls. No treatment is necessary because they are also normal and disappear within several weeks. If present along the alveolar ridge (Fig. 125.6), they are soft and spongy, asymptomatic and tend to disappear with time of the eruption of teeth.

Riga–Fede Disease/Natal or Neonatal Teeth

Riga–Fede disease is a condition observed in infants with natal or neonatal teeth. It is characterized by ulcerations on the ventral surface of the tongue from irritation caused by the edges of lower incisors during nursing or suckling. Treatment is rarely required. The incisal edge of the erupting teeth can be smoothed off in the dental office if there is bleeding and pain associated with the lesion, and cooperation allows. In very severe cases, extraction may be necessary, but only if the natal or neonatal tooth interferes with feeding.

Suggested Readings and Key References

Cawson R, Binnie W, Barrett A, et al. *Oral disease*. 3rd ed. Edinburgh: Mosby, 2001.

Kaban L, Troulis M. *Pediatric oral and maxillofacial surgery*. Philadelphia, PA: WB Saunders, 2004.

SURGICAL EMERGENCIES

CHAPTER 126 ■ ENT EMERGENCIES

JOEL D. HUDGINS, MD AND GI SOO LEE, MD, EdM

GOALS OF EMERGENCY CARE

The ear, nose, and throat are common sites for infection and neoplasms and may be the sources of acute pain. Although the diseases prompting the emergency department (ED) visit may be distressing to the patient and cause considerable anxiety for the parents, they are rarely life-threatening. The goals of care include rapid recognition of the rare surgical and infectious emergencies and obtaining a thorough evaluation.

KEY POINTS

- New trends in treatment of otitis media center around the age of the patient and the severity of illness. Empiric treatment with antibiotics is not always warranted as this process is often self-resolving and rarely leads to complications.
- Intracranial complications of sinusitis are associated with fever, headache, vomiting, and change in mental status.
- CT scans with contrast are the diagnostic test of choice to diagnose retropharyngeal abscess.
- Life-threatening etiologies of vertigo are commonly associated with hearing loss.

RELATED CHAPTERS

Signs and Symptoms

- Dizziness and Vertigo: Chapter 19
- Epistaxis: Chapter 21
- Hearing Loss: Chapter 30
- Lymphadenopathy: Chapter 42
- Neck Mass: Chapter 43
- Oral Lesions: Chapter 47
- Pain: Earache: Chapter 53
- Sore Throat: Chapter 69

Medical, Surgical, and Trauma Emergencies

- Neurologic Emergencies: Chapter 105
- ENT Trauma: Chapter 114

ACUTE OTITIS MEDIA

Goals of Treatment

Otalgia is an exceedingly common complaint in the emergency department. Providing symptomatic relief to these patients should be a priority. Given that many cases of otitis media are viral in nature, it is important to discern which cases warrant antibiotic therapy. Judicious but appropriate antibiotic therapy may shorten duration of illness in some cases and can prevent complications such as mastoiditis, meningitis, and facial nerve paralysis.

CLINICAL PEARLS AND PITFALLS

- Children greater than 2 years of age without severe otitis media can be observed off antibiotics
- Facial nerve palsies should prompt a thorough evaluation of the middle ear
- Young children with cochlear implants are at significantly increased risk of pneumococcal meningitis secondary to acute otitis media

Current Evidence

Apart from viral infections of the upper respiratory tract, acute otitis media (AOM) is the most common head and neck infection in children and is the second most common diagnosis made in the emergency department (ED). It may occur as an isolated infection though it is commonly a complication of an upper respiratory tract infection. Children with noninfected fluid in the middle ear (also called otitis media with effusion [OME] or serous otitis media or secretory otitis media) are at increased risk for acute otitis media. Other risk factors include: day care attendance, exposure to secondhand smoke, and immunodeficiency states.

In addition to viral etiologies, the more common organisms causing acute otitis at all ages are *Streptococcus pneumoniae, Haemophilus influenzae,* and *Moraxella catarrhalis.* Group A β-hemolytic streptococci is a less common etiology. Other Gram-negative organisms may occur in hospitalized patients who are younger than 8 weeks or immunosuppressed.

Over the last decade, the American Academy of Pediatrics (AAP) and the Joint Committee of American Academy of Family Practitioners (AAFP) have developed guidelines to improve accuracy of diagnosis of AOM which were last modified in 2013. Based on the best available evidence in the literature, diagnosis of AOM can be made based on the presence of any one of the following three criteria:

1. Moderate to severe bulging of tympanic membrane
2. Acute onset otorrhea not due to otitis externa
3. Mild bulging and >48 hours of ear pain or intense erythema of tympanic membrane (TM)

Clinical Considerations

Clinical Recognition

AOM should be suspected in any child who is irritable or lethargic, has a low-grade fever, and has localized pain in the ear. Older children may have rapid onset of severe ear pain.

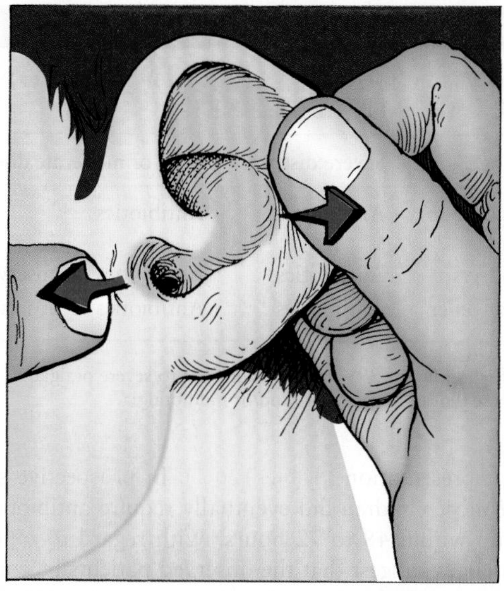

FIGURE 126.1 The external meatus is opened by pulling the auricle in the posterior-superior direction and placing traction on the skin immediately in front of the tragus.

However, younger patients may rub, tug, or hold the ear as a sign of otalgia. Spontaneous perforation of the TM with serosanguineous drainage may occur in less than 1 hour after the onset of pain. On examination, the TM is hyperemic and mobility is decreased. The strongest predictor of AOM is the presence of a bulging TM that obliterates normal landmarks, whereas isolated hyperemia is least helpful in predicting the disease. Infection with *Mycoplasma pneumoniae* and other bacteria may cause blebs on the lateral surface of the drum. The vesicles of bullous myringitis are filled with clear fluid and are painful. The appearance of the TM in AOM secondary to bacterial pathogens does not differ significantly from AOM of viral etiology.

Triage Considerations

Children with altered mental status, high fevers, extreme pain, severe headache, or neurologic abnormalities should be evaluated promptly for complications associated with otitis. Meningitis and intracranial abscesses are rare complications of otitis media.

Clinical Assessment

Acute otitis media should be suspected in any patient with low-grade fevers, ear pain, and irritability. Presentation may vary according to age, as younger patients tend to present with less-specific symptoms such as decreased oral intake and irritability, while pulling at the affected ear. Older children can typically describe otalgia.

Alternative diagnoses such as a foreign body, middle ear effusion, and otitis externa should be considered and considered during the history. A recent history of swimming or pain externally should point the clinician toward a diagnosis of otitis externa.

Examination of the ear begins by inspection of the auricle and surrounding areas. The external meatus should be visualized directly with a bright light after it is fully opened by pulling the pinna posteriorly and superiorly. The tragus may be displaced forward by traction on the skin in front of the ear with the examiner's other hand (Fig. 126.1). The ear canal can then be examined with a pneumatic otoscope, using the largest speculum that will fit in the meatus without discomfort. Wax or debris occluding the ear canal should be removed with a curette or by repeated irrigation with body-temperature water (see Chapter 141 Procedures, section on Cerumen Removal). Irrigation of the canal should not be performed if a ventilating tube is in place or if a perforation of the tympanic membrane (TM) is suspected.

The TM should be evaluated for its appearance, and part of the middle ear contents can usually be seen if the eardrum is translucent (Fig. 126.2) (see also Fig. 53.2). Mobility should

SURGICAL EMERGENCIES

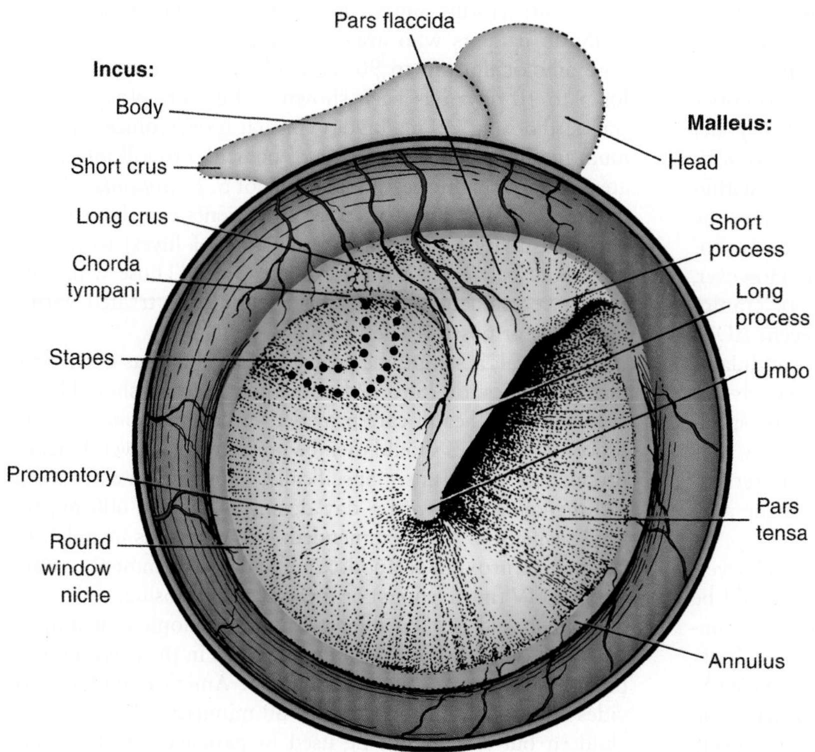

FIGURE 126.2 Right tympanic membrane.

be evaluated with the pneumatic otoscope rather than visualization alone, as this can increase the accuracy of diagnosing middle ear pathology. Pneumatic otoscopy is performed by applying positive and negative pressure to the TM, with the pneumatic otoscope fitted snugly into the ear canal. The pressure applied to the ear can be varied by squeezing a rubber bulb (see Chapter 141 Procedures, section on Pneumatic Otoscopic Examination). Middle ear effusion is more likely to be present if the TM fails to move with this technique.

The ear of a neonate requires special attention to perform an adequate otologic examination. The ear canal itself is narrow and collapsible. Often, only the otoscopic speculum can be inserted, as positive pressure from the pneumatic bulb is used to distend the canal ahead of the advancing speculum. The canal may be filled with vernix caseosa, which must be removed or irrigated out of the canal to permit visualization of the TM. The neonate's TM lies at a more oblique angle to the ear canal (compared with older children) and may make recognition of the TM and its landmarks more difficult. Amniotic fluid may be present in the middle ear cavity for days to weeks after birth and should not be confused with middle ear infection unless other symptoms such as fever and irritability are present.

A variety of scoring systems have been developed to aid in the diagnosis of AOM, though none have been formally recommended by the AAP.

Management

The clinical diagnosis of AOM is made clinically and no additional laboratory or imaging studies are necessary. Antibiotics prescribed for AOM account for 25% to 50% of all outpatient antibiotics and are partly responsible for the global finding that bacteria, especially *S. pneumoniae, H. influenzae,* and *M. catarrhalis,* are becoming increasingly resistant to these medications. As such, expert panels and various medical societies have examined the benefits and choice of antibiotics used for this disease. The AAP/AAFP guidelines stress the need to improve accuracy of diagnosis and to use antibiotics judiciously in treating AOM. Using the best available literature, including randomized clinical trials and cohort studies of patients with suspected AOM treated with antibiotics versus those treated with observation, the AAP/AAFP panel concluded that 80% of children who were not treated with antibiotics had spontaneous resolution of symptoms within a 2- to 7-day onset of symptoms. With this information, the panel suggested that a period of observation might be appropriate for otherwise healthy patients with AOM. However, very young children, those with immune, genetic, or craniofacial anomalies, known or underlying OME, or recent AOM in the previous 30 days should not be considered candidates for this option because they are more likely to suffer adverse consequences from observation alone. The panel also specified that the observation option must be used only if there is a high probability that the parent will be compliant in returning for evaluation if symptoms of AOM persist over the next 72 hours.

Specific recommendations therefore vary by age and severity of illness. Any patient younger than 6 months should be treated with antibiotics. The observation option is recommended for children 6 months to 2 years of age whose baseline health is good and who are not ill at presentation without evidence of severe disease. The option of observation is available for children older than 2 years, with nonsevere

TABLE 126.1

OPTIONS FOR THE TREATMENT OF ACUTE OTITIS MEDIA (AAP/AAFP) GUIDELINES

Child age	Severe disease[a]	Mild or moderate disease[b]
Younger than 6 mo	Antibiotics	Antibiotics
6 mo–2 yrs	Antibiotics	Antibiotics or observation
2 yrs or older	Antibiotics	Antibiotics or observation

[a]Severe disease: fever >39°C and/or moderate to severe otalgia.
[b]Non-severe illness: fever <39°C and/or mild otalgia.

illness at presentation (Table 126.1). In prospective studies, 25% of those children did eventually require antibiotic upon follow-up within 48 to 72 hours. With regard to follow-up, the guidelines suggest that the observed patients be contacted or seen within 72 hours so that they may be treated if symptoms persist. Other authors have advocated writing a "safety net prescription" to be given to parents of children who are observed at the time of the initial assessment with instructions to fill it if symptoms persist.

Guidelines for intervention for persistent or recurrent AOM vary. Patients with multiple episodes of AOM over a period of months, OME lasting more than 6 to 8 weeks, complications of middle ear disease, or associated hearing or speech concerns should be referred to an otolaryngologist for evaluation for possible surgical treatment (myringotomy and tube placement).

To effectively treat AOM, the most important pathogen to address is *S. pneumoniae* because it is less likely to resolve spontaneously without treatment compared with *H. influenzae* and *M. catarrhalis.* Although a large number of species exist that are resistant to amoxicillin and cephalosporins, evidence from the literature and guidelines suggest that no antibiotic outperforms amoxicillin as the first-line drug to treat AOM in patients who are not allergic to penicillin. Higher dose amoxicillin (80 to 90 mg/kg/day) in two divided doses for 5 to 10 days has been shown to be more effective than standard dosing (40 mg/kg/day) in that it overcomes the minimum inhibitory concentrations of penicillin to kill intermediate and some highly resistant strains of *S. pneumoniae.* Initial therapy in uncomplicated AOM in patients who have type 1 hypersensitivity (anaphylaxis or history of hives) to penicillin should be treated with a cephalosporin. Those with have similar reaction to cephalosporins should be treated with a macrolide or possibly clindamycin.

In general, if symptoms persist after a child has taken first-line antibiotics for 48 to 72 hours, then the child should be re-evaluated by a health care provider (either by phone or in the office). Antibiotics should then be prescribed to cover β-lactam producing organisms. Specifically, amoxicillin-clavulanate (90 mg/kg/day in twice a day dosing, using the 600 mg per 5 ml suspension) is recommended. Other options include oral cefdinir, cefuroxime, cefpodoxime and, less commonly, ceftriaxone in IV (intravenous) or intramuscular dosing.

Pain should be controlled with acetaminophen or ibuprofen. Oral opiates should be limited to use in those with severe pain. Topical benzocaine (Auralgan or Americaine Otic) provides additional, but brief (30 to 60 minutes), relief for some children but should not be used in patients who have TM perforations or ear tubes. Antihistamines, decongestants, and corticosteroids have shown only minimal benefit and are not recommended.

Rarely, complications of AOM may be encountered in the ED. The following changes may be noted to the TM or the middle ear:

- The purulent exudate that fills the middle ear space causes a conductive hearing loss. The congealed exudate may organize and stimulate hyalinization and calcification, leading to myringosclerosis (white patches within the TM) and sometimes tympanosclerosis (white deposits in the middle ear).
- Spontaneous perforation of the TM usually produces a small hole that heals rapidly; however, large perforations may occur that do not heal even after the infection has cleared.
- Ossicular necrosis may also occur in children who have had AOM or OME and can cause a persistent conductive hearing loss. The distal tip of the incus is most susceptible to erosion that can cause eventual disconnection of the incus from the stapes, resulting in conductive hearing loss.
- As the TM heals after a perforation, skin from the lateral surface of the TM may be trapped in the middle ear to form a cyst (cholesteatoma) that can expand and destroy the structures of the middle ear and surrounding bone.
- AOM may cause inflammation in the inner ear (serous labyrinthitis). This causes mild to moderate vertigo without a sensorineural hearing loss.

Any of these findings warrant consultation with an otolaryngologist to determine the need for acute intervention, or if the patient can be safely discharged to specialty follow-up as an outpatient.

Other complications warrant more acute intervention and urgent otolaryngology consultation:

- Facial nerve paralysis may occur suddenly during AOM. The nerve paralysis may be partial or complete when the child is first examined. The facial nerve usually recovers complete function if appropriate systemic (IV followed by oral) antibiotic therapy is administered and a wide myringotomy with or without tube placement for drainage is carried out as soon as possible.
- Bacterial invasion of the inner ear (suppurative labyrinthitis) causes severe sensorineural hearing loss and severe vertigo that is usually associated with nausea and vomiting. Early treatment with IV antibiotics and wide myringotomy with tube placement may prevent permanent inner ear damage.
- Suppurative mastoiditis (acute coalescent mastoid osteomyelitis) may develop, causing destruction of the mastoid air cell system. Temporal bone computed tomographic (CT) scans are helpful in differentiating otitis media from mastoiditis. Patients with otitis media or mastoiditis have opacified mastoid air cells when disease is present, but those with mastoiditis also have radiographic evidence of erosion of the mastoid air cells creating larger opacified spaces. As the infection spreads to the postauricular tissues, subperiosteal collection of purulent material displaces the auricle inferolaterally from its normal position. The pus may extend through air cells to the petrous portion of the temporal bone, causing a constellation of symptoms of diplopia (sixth cranial nerve palsy), severe ocular pain, and otorrhea; this trifecta is known as Gradenigo syndrome). Pus may also break through the mastoid tip, extend into the upper neck, and create a Bezold abscess.
- The most common intracranial problem associated with AOM is meningitis, which may cause severe sensorineural deafness and irreversible vestibular damage. Less commonly associated problems are cerebritis, epidural abscess, brain abscess, lateral sinus thrombosis, and otitic hydrocephalus. The child with overt or impending intracranial complications should be stabilized, be given IV antibiotics, and have a CT scan with contrast or magnetic resonance imaging (MRI) scan performed.

SINUSITIS

Goals of Treatment

The common cold and upper respiratory tract infection accounts for the majority of infections of the nose and paranasal sinuses. However, bacterial infection of the sinuses is a more serious condition that requires careful examination and prompt treatment. Differentiating bacterial from viral infections can be difficult but is an important aspect of treatment. Severe complications can also result from untreated acute bacterial rhinosinusitis (ABR), including orbital cellulitis, intracranial abscess, and meningitis. Preventing these life-threatening complications as well as prompt recognition and treatment when they do occur are important goals of treatment.

CLINICAL PEARLS AND PITFALLS

- Imaging studies are not indicated for uncomplicated acute bacterial sinusitis
- Persistence of symptoms longer than 10 days can help differentiate between bacterial sinusitis and viral upper respiratory infection
- Amoxicillin-clavulanate is an appropriate first line choice for oral antibiotic therapy in acute bacterial sinusitis

Current Evidence

Between 5% and 7% of viral upper respiratory infections are complicated by the development of secondary bacterial rhinosinusitis. Acute bacterial rhinosinusitis should be suspected when cough, halitosis, low-grade fever, and purulent rhinorrhea are present. Symptoms such as headache and facial pain may be present, but are variable, particularly in younger patients. Bacterial infection is also more likely to be present when the nasal discharge lasts more than 10 days and if the color of the discharge is thick yellow or green. Sinus imaging in uncomplicated ABR is not recommended, given the potential for false positive studies and risk of radiation exposure. Complications of ABR are estimated to occur in approximately 5% of hospitalized patients, and are a result of extension of the infection into either the orbital or intracranial space.

Clinical Considerations

Clinical Recognition

There is considerable overlap between the clinical manifestations of ABR and viral upper respiratory infections. Children will often present with cough, nasal symptoms, fever, and headache in both viral upper respiratory infections as well as ABR. The American Academy of Pediatrics (AAP) recommends a presumptive diagnosis of ABR in patients with acute upper respiratory infections with any one of the following:

- Persistent illness, such as nasal discharge or daytime cough lasting more than 10 days without improvement
- Worsening course, such as worsening or new nasal discharge, daytime cough, or fever after an initial period of improvement
- Severe onset, such as fever ≥39° Celsius and purulent nasal discharge for at least 3 consecutive days.

Triage Considerations

Children should be evaluated for complications of ABR such as orbital cellulitis or intracranial abscess. Children who present with altered mental status, vomiting associated with headache, eye swelling or pain, seizures, or focal neurologic deficits should be evaluated promptly.

Initial Assessment

Presentation of ABR may differ widely according to age. Patients that are verbal may complain of headache, facial pain/pressure and tenderness, while nonverbal patients may simply present with fussiness in addition to symptoms often found in viral upper respiratory infections. In younger verbal children, where deeper sinuses are affected, headache may be the only presenting symptom.

When obtaining the history, the provider should attempt to differentiate ABR from a viral URI, as well as screen for complications of ABR. For example, persistent headache associated with vomiting, altered mental status, or focal neurologic deficits could all be signs of intracranial extension of the infection. Periorbital swelling associated with pain with eye movement can be a sign of orbital extension.

Physical examination should focus on the head and neck, along with a detailed neurologic examination. Facial bone tenderness can be associated with sinusitis, although its absence should not dissuade one from the diagnosis. Evaluate for evidence of orbital involvement which can result from sinus infection extension into the eye or surrounding structures. A thorough neurologic examination, including detailed evaluation of the cranial nerves, is also important to evaluate for intracranial extension.

Management and Diagnostic Testing

According to recent AAP guidelines, imaging should not be routinely used to distinguish ABR from viral URIs; sinusitis is diagnosed clinically. The role for imaging remains limited to patients with features concerning for complications of sinusitis, including orbital or central nervous system involvement. The recommended imaging modality is computed tomography (CT) or magnetic resonance imaging (MRI) rather than plain radiographs. Treatment with antibiotic therapy should be initiated for patients with a diagnosis of ABR which is severe, worsening, or lasting greater than 10 days. Amoxicillin with or without clavulanate is the first line treatment for ABR, at a dose of 80 to 90 mg/kg/day, divided twice daily, with a max dose of 2 g. If there is a documented penicillin allergy, clindamycin in combination with cefixime is adequate to achieve comprehensive coverage for the suspected bacterial etiologies. IV antibiotic administration is warranted when complications of sinusitis are present. Vancomycin should be added initially when complications of sinusitis are present, given the risk of MRSA and potential increasing morbidity with inadequate coverage of these serious infections. See Table 126.2 for more details on antibiotic choices.

TABLE 126.2

ANTIBIOTIC OPTIONS FOR ACUTE BACTERIAL RHINOSINUSITIS

Age	Severity of disease	Initial antibiotic choice	Alternative antibiotic choice	Penicillin allergy	Penicillin and cephalosporin allergy
<2 yrs	Any	Amoxicillin-clavulanate (80–90 mg/kg/day divided twice daily)		Cefdinir (14 mg/kg/day div BID) or cefuroxime (15 mg/kg/dose BID)	Clindamycin (30–40 mg/kg/day div TID)
>2 yrs	Mild	Amoxicillin (80–90 mg/kg/day divided twice daily)	Amoxicillin-clavulanate (80–90 mg/kg/day divided twice daily)	Cefdinir (14 mg/kg/day div BID) or cefuroxime (15 mg/kg/dose BID)	Clindamycin (30–40 mg/kg/day div TID)
	Moderate	Amoxicillin (80–90 mg/kg/day divided twice daily)	Amoxicillin-clavulanate (80–90 mg/kg/day divided twice daily)	Cefdinir (14 mg/kg/day div BID) or cefuroxime (15 mg/kg/dose BID)	Clindamycin (30–40 mg/kg/day div TID)
	Severe[a]	Cefotaxime (100–200 mg/kg/day div q6) or ceftriaxone (100 mg/kg div BID) IV OR Ampicillin-sulbactam (200–400 mg/kg/day div q6) IV		Cefdinir (14 mg/kg/day div BID) or cefuroxime (15 mg/kg/dose BID)	Clindamycin (30–40 mg/kg/day div TID) po or IV OR Levofloxacin[b] (10–20 mg/kg/d qday or div BID)

[a]In severe disease or with complications of sinusitis, MRSA coverage should be considered in endemic areas. Treatment with vancomycin (60 mg/kg/day div q6) IV in addition to either cefotaxime or ampicillin/sulbactam is recommended.
[b]Levofloxacin should be reserved for patients with no safe or effective alternative.

For all acute sinusitis patients, 1 to 3 days of nasal vasoconstrictor sprays (e.g., oxymetazoline), and saline sprays or nasal irrigation are all part of the nasal hygiene regimen. Antihistamines are helpful if the underlying inflammatory process that resulted in sinusitis is allergic rhinitis. Decision regarding nasal steroid sprays for longer-term management can be deferred to primary care or inpatient providers, as the onset of action is 2 to 3 weeks.

Clinical Indications for Discharge or Admission

The majority of patients diagnosed with ABR can be managed as outpatients. Patients that have severe headache or clinical signs of dehydration are also potential candidates for hospital admission. Patients that fail outpatient treatment with oral antibiotics warrant admission for IV antibiotics and close observation. The indications for admission include complications such as orbital cellulitis or abscess, facial cellulitis or abscess, meningitis, or intracranial abscess. In addition to admission, these patients should have otolaryngology and potentially neurosurgery consultation as part of their evaluation, given the potential need for surgical drainage.

TONSILLITIS AND PERITONSILLAR ABSCESS/CELLULITIS

Goals of Treatment

Pharyngitis with tonsillitis is a relatively common complaint of patients presenting to the ED. Pain control is a priority for comfort as well as to facilitate oral intake. In some cases, IV hydration may be warranted. In addition, recognizing more advanced infection and differentiating between peritonsillar cellulitis and peritonsillar abscess is a key aspect of treatment. For patients diagnosed with peritonsillar abscess, the evaluation should focus on the safety of the airway and appropriate consultation, if needed, for definitive treatment with drainage.

CLINICAL PEARLS AND PITFALLS

- Peritonsillar abscess is the most common deep neck infection in adolescents
- Imaging is not necessary in most cases of peritonsillar abscess, but is occasionally warranted when the diagnosis is unclear
- Older patients that have had incision and drainage of a peritonsillar abscess can often be discharged from the ED

Current Evidence

Pharyngitis/tonsillitis (pharyngotonsillitis) may be caused by viral or bacterial organisms. Rapid strep tests have short turnaround times (5 to 10 minutes) and may be helpful in confirming a bacterial source, but may miss up to a quarter of infections. If this test result is negative and bacterial infection is still suspected, a routine throat culture is often helpful. Patients with repeated debilitating bouts of pharyngotonsillitis (five to seven in a 1-year period or several per year for several years) or complications including peritonsillar abscess should be referred to an otolaryngologist for consideration of tonsillectomy. For more information on pharyngitis, see Chapter 69 Sore Throat.

Peritonsillar abscess (PTA) or cellulitis is usually secondary to local spread from pharyngeal infections. The palatine tonsils are located between the palatoglossal arch and palatopharyngeal arches. The tonsils are surrounded by a capsule which covers part of the tonsil and is responsible for housing neurovascular structures. PTAs often develop between the tonsillar tissue and this capsule. If untreated, infection or inflammation may spread from that area to contiguous structures such as the masseter or pterygoid muscles. PTAs are more commonly seen in adolescents and young adults, though they can present in younger children as well. Infections in the peritonsillar space are usually polymicrobial, including bacteria such as group A streptococci, anaerobic bacteria, and potentially *S. aureus*.

Clinical Considerations

Clinical Recognition

Patients with tonsillitis often present with fever, sore throat, and lymphadenopathy. Patients are usually able to open their mouths fully, and have diffuse erythema and often exudate present on examination. The symptoms and examination findings are typically bilateral. When patients present with associated URI symptoms such as cough and rhinorrhea, bacterial etiologies are less common (see Chapter 69 Sore Throat).

Peritonsillar cellulitis and abscess also often present with fever and sore throat. PTA often presents with difficulty opening the mouth, or trismus, which can help the provider differentiate from simple tonsillitis or cellulitis. Additionally, the patients may have difficulty handling their secretions, and have voice changes including sounding "muffled" or speaking with a "hot-potato" voice.

Triage Considerations

Immediate assessment of the airway is paramount in patients with tonsillar infections. If patients have evidence of stridor or pooling secretions, alternative diagnoses such as epiglottitis should be considered. If the airway is in jeopardy, the patient should ideally have all airway interventions performed in the OR with an anesthesiologist and otolaryngologist present. If the patient is stable without evidence of airway compromise, triage should focus on pain control, accurate diagnosis, and appropriate consultation, if necessary.

Clinical Assessment

Peritonsillar cellulitis is characterized by erythematous, painful tonsils, with or without exudate. It may be bilateral, and is not routinely associated with uvular deviation or significant trismus. PTAs are often characterized by fever, trismus, and muffled voice. Physical examination findings consistent with a PTA include a bulging, erythematous tonsil often protruding into the uvula, causing deviation into the side of the unaffected tonsil. The tonsil may have exudate, but the symptoms are frequently unilateral (see Fig. 126.3). Bilateral PTA is rare, but may cause anterior displacement of the uvula.

Management and Disposition

Peritonsillar cellulitis should be treated with IV antibiotics, given the frequent severity of symptoms and the risk of progression to more serious illness. Common antibiotic choices include clindamycin (40 to 45 mg/kg/day div TID) or ampicillin-sulbactam (200 mg/kg/day div q6), both IV.

Peritonsillar abscess usually require surgical drainage. If the provider is experienced in performing incision and drainage

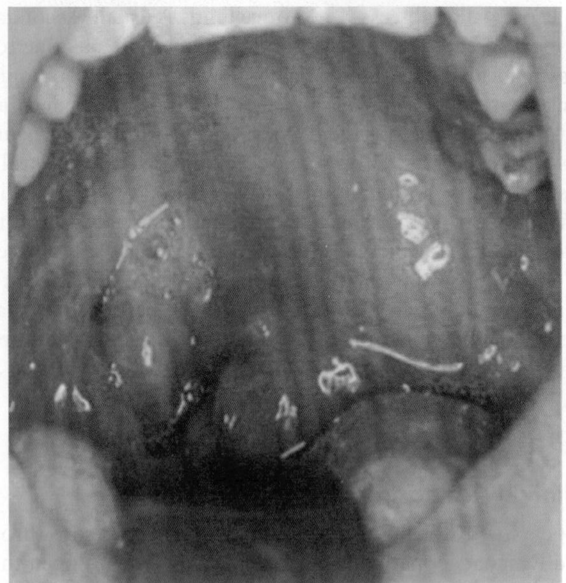

FIGURE 126.3 Peritonsillar abscess. Note the left-sided bulging, erythematous tonsil protruding into the uvula, causing deviation into the side of the unaffected tonsil. (From Jensen S. Nursing Health Assessment. 2nd ed. Philadelphia, PA: Wolters Kluwer, 2014.)

or needle aspiration, then they should perform the procedure themselves. In pediatrics, otolaryngology is frequently consulted to assist in this procedure, either in the ED or in the OR. In older, cooperative patients, the procedure can often be performed without sedation in the ED.

Following drainage or aspiration, patients should be treated with antibiotics. If patients are improved and able to tolerate oral antibiotics, discharging them on a course of amoxicillin-clavulanate (80 to 90 mg/kg/day div BID, max single dose 875 mg) or clindamycin (40 to 45 mg/kg/day div TID, max single dose 600 mg) is indicated. If they require admission, then treatment with ampicillin-sulbactam or clindamycin as with cellulitis is indicated.

RETROPHARYNGEAL AND PARAPHARYNGEAL INFECTIONS

Goals of Treatment

Deep space neck infections, such as retropharyngeal and parapharyngeal infections, can be challenging for the emergency physician as well as potentially life-threatening for the patient. Rapid and accurate identification of deep space neck infections is vital in their treatment, given the risk of upper airway obstruction or systemic illness. Providers must also provide appropriate disposition for patients with deep space neck infections, either as hospitalized inpatients or to the operating room for definitive incision and drainage.

CLINICAL PEARLS AND PITFALLS

- Patients less than one year old with deep space neck infections may present with little more than fever and fussiness
- Initial antibiotic choices for patients with deep space neck infections include ampicillin-sulbactam or clindamycin. Clindamycin has superior MRSA coverage but has a less palatable transition to oral therapy.

Current Evidence

A retropharyngeal abscess occurs in the potential space between the prevertebral fascia and the posterior pharyngeal wall. This retropharyngeal space contains two chains of lymph nodes that are prominent in younger children, but often disappear by puberty. These nodes can become enlarged and necrotic in the setting of upper respiratory tract infections, and subsequently become infected. The usual pathogens are group A streptococci, anaerobic organisms, and occasionally *S. aureus*. These infections occur most often in children younger than 4 years. A lateral pharyngeal (or parapharyngeal) abscess occurs in the deep soft-tissue space of the neck as well, but not in the midline, and is less common than a retropharyngeal infection in the younger patient population.

Clinical Considerations

Clinical Recognition

Patients with deep space neck infections often present with fever and appear quite ill. Patients presenting early in the course of illness may be diagnosed with simple pharyngitis; progression of the abscess manifests with sore throat, difficulty swallowing, stiff neck, muffled voice, and, late in the course, possibly stridor. Often, there is a history of a preceding viral upper respiratory infection.

Triage Considerations

Patients with deep space neck infections are often ill-appearing. Evidence of upper airway obstruction such as tripod positioning, difficulty with handling secretions, or stridor should be immediately evaluated by a provider. If patients are severely ill with respiratory distress, an otolaryngology evaluation should be obtained promptly.

Initial Assessment

Particular attention should be paid to signs of upper airway obstruction on physical exam. Patients may put themselves in a position of comfort. Those with more advanced disease may, show signs of severe distress such as stridor or tripod positioning. Visualization of the abscess on examination may be difficult, particularly in younger or uncooperative patients. In cooperative patients, inspection of the posterior pharyngeal wall with tongue blades and bright headlamp can reveal overt bulging or asymmetry.

Management and Diagnostic Testing

Immediate management should focus initially on maintaining a patent airway. If the diagnosis is suspected and the patient is in respiratory distress, emergent otolaryngology consultation is indicated.

Unless the airway is in immediate jeopardy, IV access should be secured to administer IV antibiotics. If the airway is a significant concern, IV access should be attempted in the operating room given the potential for destabilization and worsening of the upper airway obstruction. Laboratory evaluation will often reveal an elevated white blood cell (WBC) count. Blood cultures are frequently negative but may be useful in identifying a pathogen.

Radiographic studies are often essential in the diagnosis of deep space neck infections. In stable patients, a lateral neck radiograph is an appropriate initial choice. The radiograph

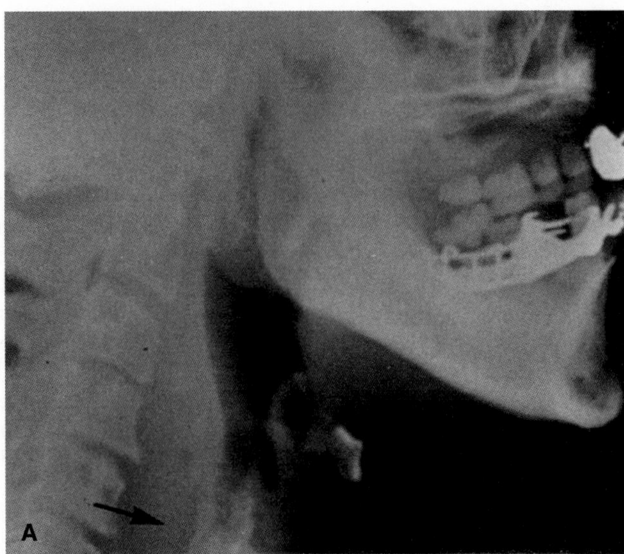

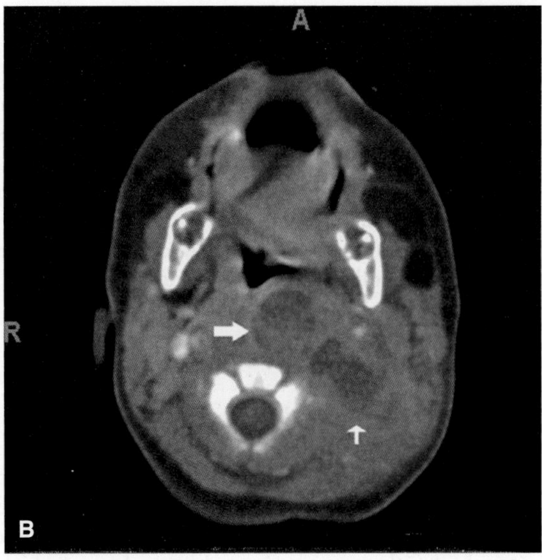

FIGURE 126.4 **A:** A lateral neck radiograph demonstrating pre-vertebral swelling (*arrow*). **B:** A computed tomographic scan of neck with contrast demonstrating a retropharyngeal abscess (*large arrow*) and smaller, contiguous parapharyngeal abscess (*small arrow*).

shows an increase in the width of the soft tissues anterior to the vertebrae and, on occasion, an air–fluid level. In the young child without retropharyngeal infection, the width of the prevertebral space is less than the width of the adjacent vertebral body at the upper cervical vertebrae (C2, C3) if the examination is performed with the neck properly extended. For children approaching school age and beyond, the width of this space is typically less than half of the adjacent vertebral body at the mid cervical spine if the neck is properly extended (Fig. 126.4A).

CT of the neck with IV contrast is the best imaging modality to identify a deep space infection. However, its use is complicated by the potential for worsening respiratory status when lying supine, coupled with the potential need for sedation to ensure an accurate study. This is particularly problematic in patients with potential airway compromise, and consideration should be given to having anesthesia or otolaryngology involved as part of the sedation process.

CT of the neck, if indicated, can often help differential cellulitis from phlegmon or abscess, as well as the extent of an abscess in the deep neck. Features that identify abscess on CT include scalloping, or irregularity of the abscess wall, as well as ring enhancement (Fig. 126.4B). It also shows the proximity of the infection to large vessels, which can be compressed by surrounding edema from an infection. This is also helpful for potential surgical planning.

Clinical Indications for Discharge or Admission

A retropharyngeal or lateral pharyngeal abscess poses a risk to the patency of the airway. All children with this infection should have careful monitoring in the ED and then be hospitalized in consultation with an otolaryngologist. Treatment should be initiated with either clindamycin (30 mg/kg/ day in four divided doses) or ampicillin/sulbactam (ampicillin 200 mg/kg/day in four divided doses). In the event of respiratory compromise, intubation or, rarely, tracheotomy becomes necessary. Patients without severe toxicity who are not imaged and those with smaller abscesses (typically less than 1 to 2 cm in greatest dimension) or phlegmon if imaged, may be treated with antibiotic therapy alone; those with larger collections or those with persistent fever despite a minimum 48 hours of IV antibiotic therapy require imaging if not done initially and may require drainage. Retropharyngeal abscesses are typically drained via a transoral approach; parapharyngeal abscesses are drained either transorally or transcervically depending on location.

CERVICAL ADENITIS AND NECK ABSCESSES

Goals of Treatment

Cervical adenitis is the most common cause of a neck mass in a child. They are commonly associated with bacterial infections of the head and neck. Differentiating from reactive lymphadenopathy and appropriately prescribing antibiotics is one goal of treatment. Additionally, treatment can prevent spread to deeper structures of the neck and development of severe illness. Surgical consultation and drainage is indicated in critically ill patients and those with a drainable collection.

CLINICAL PEARLS AND PITFALLS

- Progression to suppurative cervical adenitis is rare, but is a condition that requires hospitalization for IV antibiotics
- Cervical adenitis that does not respond to antibiotics should raise the possibility of an atypical infection such as nontuberculous mycobacterium or cat-scratch disease

Current Evidence

Cervical adenitis is the most common cause of a neck mass in a child. The lymphatic system of the neck drains the internal cavities of the head and neck (ear, nose, mouth, pharynx, sinuses, and larynx), as well as the skin and associated adnexal structures of the face and scalp. Regional cervical lymph nodes respond when there is a primary infection in any area of the head and neck. Because certain regions drain into specific groups of nodes, the location of the swollen and infected lymph node can often help the practitioner to identify the area of the primary infection. Infra-auricular nodes most often enlarge during ear infections, jugulodigastric nodes usually swell during pharyngeal infections (e.g., tonsillitis), and posterior neck nodes swell during nasopharyngeal infections (e.g., adenoiditis). Systemic illness (e.g., EBV infection) can lead to enlargement in many groups of nodes within the neck and throughout the body (see Chapter 42 Lymphadenopathy).

Clinical Considerations

Clinical Recognition

Patients with cervical adenitis often present with fever and neck swelling. Lymphadenitis is distinct from lymphadenopathy in that affected lymph nodes are inflamed and often tender to palpation, while lymphadenopathy describes painless swelling without inflammation. Acute lymphadenitis, which is commonly defined as symptoms <2 weeks, is most commonly due to bacterial or viral infections. Longer courses should raise the possibility of rarer diagnoses such as cat-scratch disease, nontuberculous mycobacterium, or neoplasm as the etiology. These conditions are almost universally painless, initially absent of overlying skin changes until far more advanced in their course (patients then present with violaceous skin discoloration), fevers, or preceding URIs.

Triage Considerations

As with other deep neck infections, care should be taken in triage to assess the patency of the airway. Patients with cervical adenitis may present with evidence of partial upper airway obstruction or respiratory distress, though that is rare. Patients that appear toxic, have high fever, malaise, or dehydration should be aggressively resuscitated. Surgical consultation, should be obtained when drainage is believed to be necessary.

Initial Assessment

The diagnosis of cervical adenitis should be suspected in any patient that presents to the emergency department with fever, neck swelling, and tenderness. A thorough evaluation of the number of nodes involved and their size is helpful. Infected nodes seen in lymphadenitis are often unilateral, warm, and tender to palpation. Erythema and warmth over the affected node should raise the possibility of an overlying cellulitis. The affected node(s) may also be fluctuant, which is common when lymphadenitis is complicated by the development of a neck abscess. The provider should also perform an oral examination, looking for dental caries or other evidence of poor dentition.

Management and Diagnostic Testing

Laboratory studies may be helpful in patients who are ill appearing or have persistent symptoms. A complete blood count (CBC), and inflammatory markers such as C-reactive protein (CRP) or erythrocyte sedimentation rate (ESR), can show evidence of acute infection. Blood culture can potentially identify a pathogen to guide therapy, though only systemically ill patients warrant evaluation for associated bacteremia. Imaging can also be helpful, particularly in identifying suppuration/abscess in the context of lymphadenitis. Ultrasound is an appropriate first choice, for its safety profile, lack of radiation, and accuracy in diagnosing abscesses. Computed tomography (CT) is also useful in diagnosis and management, particularly in patients that are anticipated to require drainage in the operating room (e-Fig. 126.1). CT may show evidence of deeper infection or loculations that could change the surgical approach.

Cervical adenitis does not usually occur following a brief, uncomplicated viral infection of the upper respiratory tract. Instead, these tender and enlarged nodes occur more often as a result of bacterial infection of the head and neck. Infections of the ear and throat are the most common source. *Streptococcus* species are the causative agents in the majority of bacterial infections of the head and neck. Infected lymph nodes usually contain the same organisms as the primary infection. Treatment with amoxicillin or penicillin usually clears the infection and causes regression of the enlarged lymph nodes. Culture of the nasopharynx, throat, or aspirate of the cervical node can assist the physician in the choice of antimicrobial agents.

Although most children respond to oral antibiotics, a small group of children develop nodes that progress to suppurative cervical adenitis that usually requires hospitalization. A recent study of children hospitalized with cervical adenitis has shown a predominance of *S. aureus* as the causative agent (63% of positive cultures were *S. aureus* and 22% were group A streptococci, respectively). Of the staphylococcal infections, 27% were MRSA and all of these were sensitive to clindamycin and trimethoprim-sulfamethoxazole, 63% were sensitive to ciprofloxacin, and 25% to erythromycin. Of the methicillin-sensitive *S. aureus* isolates, 100%, 85%, and 82% were sensitive to trimethoprim-sulfamethoxazole, clindamycin, and ciprofloxacin, respectively, though prevalence and sensitivities of MRSA will vary regionally. The high incidence of staphylococci in these hospitalized patients may occur because they have not responded to oral antimicrobials effective against the more commonly occurring *Streptococcus* species. Therefore, if cervical adenitis has not responded to the primary antimicrobial treatment, agents should be added that are effective against *S. aureus* (as well as other *Streptococcus* species).

Clinical Indications for Discharge or Admission

The majority of patients with lymphadenitis can be managed as outpatients on oral antibiotics.

A child who has demonstrated rapid enlargement of cervical nodes, poor response to oral antimicrobials, cellulitis of the overlying skin, abscess formation, or signs of toxicity (high fever, malaise, dehydration) should be admitted to the hospital for treatment with IV fluids and antimicrobials. Surgical consultation should be obtained in the management of these complicated cases in which needle aspiration, incision and drainage, or biopsy (for possible neoplasm) may be required

POSTTONSILLECTOMY HEMORRHAGE

Goals of Treatment

Hemorrhage from the oral cavity after tonsil surgery is a common and potentially life-threatening surgical complication. Expeditious triaging and accurate examination of the patient who presents with a bleed will help determine which patients are safe to be conservatively observed and which ones require urgent surgical intervention. Otolaryngology consultation is warranted for all actively bleeding patients and for those who present with fresh clots in the tonsil fossae.

CLINICAL PEARLS AND PITFALLS

- Bleeding from the inferior tonsil pole is often difficult to identify; a thorough examination of the oral cavity using tongue depressors is imperative.
- IV access and resuscitation is critical, as blood loss can be more significant than expected. This is especially important for children under age 2 years.
- If the tonsil fossae are completely void of any bleeding or clots, consider adenoid bed hemorrhage or epistaxis in the differential.

Current Evidence

Tonsil and adenoid surgery is among the most common pediatric surgeries, with over 500,000 outpatient surgeries performed annually in the US. Posttonsillectomy hemorrhage (PTH) is the most frequent serious complication and occurs in 3% to 5% of children. Bleeds are classified as either a primary or secondary PTH—a primary bleed occurs within 24 hours of the original surgery; secondary bleeds occur after 24 hours. Risk factors for hemorrhage include male gender, older age, and infectious indication for surgery.

The tonsil is a high vascular organ, with a blood supply from multiple carotid branches including the facial, lingual, ascending pharyngeal, and maxillary arteries. With the modern electrocautery device, intraoperative bleeding has been reduced to a minimum, and primary PTH rates have declined considerably compared to a cold steel technique. The rates of secondary PTH, on the other hand, have been consistent, as it is considered to be more of a function of the healing process. An eschar forms in the fossa after tonsil removal; this eschar typically sloughs off between 7 and 10 days postoperatively, and this is when most secondary PTH occurs.

Two types of tonsil surgeries are performed in the US. A total tonsillectomy involves removal of the entire tonsil with the fibromucosal capsule, leaving behind exposed muscle within the tonsil fossa. The PTH rate for a total tonsillectomy is 3% to 5%. More recently, the partial tonsillectomy, also known as *tonsillotomy* or intracapsular tonsillectomy, has been gaining popularity among surgeons, especially when operating on smaller children for obstructive sleep indications. It involves removal of most of the tonsil tissue (up to 95%), while leaving a small rind of capsule and tonsil tissue behind in the fossa. The remaining tissue behaves like a biologic dressing, and protects the underlying muscle and blood vessels. As such, the PTH rate can be as low as 1%.

Clinical Considerations

Clinical Recognition

Nearly all patients with PTH present with a history of blood-tinged sputum or discrete bleeding from the oral cavity after recent tonsil surgery, but some patients will present primarily with nausea and/or hematemesis.

Triage Considerations

Active bleeding, expulsion of fresh clots from the mouth, or any patient with hemodynamic or airway instability secondary to bleeding must be promptly evaluated and otolaryngology consultation obtained emergently. If the episode of bleeding was minor (isolated blood tinged sputum, dried blood on patient's pillow discovered in the morning, etc.), then the problem becomes less urgent, though no less important. An initial minor bleed can be an initial event (a sentinel bleed) for a more severe subsequent bleeding incident.

Initial Assessment

Obtain routine vitals and procure IV access. A careful and thorough examination of the oral cavity is performed, and both tonsil fossae must be examined. Use of a headlamp and bimanual examination of the oral cavity with tongue depressors is important when available. Alternatively, have an assistant hold an otoscope or light source, to allow freeing of both hands for positioning and using a tongue depressor. If any active bleeding or fresh clot is identified in the fossa, no further intervention is required. A clot should NOT be dislodged or irrigated, as this could cause further bleeding. If no active bleeding is identified, then other sources of bleeding must be considered, including epistaxis and adenoid bed hemorrhage.

Management/Diagnostic Testing

If active bleeding or fresh clot is identified, immediately call for otolaryngology evaluation. If profuse bleeding is encountered, obtaining a hemoglobin level or hematocrit is reasonable as is a type and cross for matching potential transfusion. Note that obtaining a blood concentration prior to adequate resuscitation will result in falsely elevated levels. Adequate pain control with judicious use of narcotic analgesics is important. Nonsteroidal analgesics (NSAIDs) should be avoided in any patient with active bleeding.

Clinical Indication for Discharge or Admission

For all PTH patients who do not require operative intervention, criteria for admission for observation will vary by institution. For nearly all patients, however, any history of bleeding from the oral cavity should be admitted for observation.

VERTIGO

Goals of Treatment

Sudden vertigo is a disturbing and often confusing symptom. Vertigo caused by middle ear pathology is often accompanied by nausea, vomiting, imbalance, and irregular gait. Correctly identifying more serious etiologies of vertigo is an important goal of treatment. Vertigo may result from dysfunction of any part of the vestibular system (from the labyrinth to the vestibular cortex), and may be associated with a number of conditions affecting the middle ear. Hearing loss is commonly associated with concerning etiologies of vertigo and should be evaluated during the visit.

CLINICAL PEARLS AND PITFALLS

- Vertigo is a symptom of underlying disease, and evaluation should always involve looking for the etiology as well as providing symptomatic treatment.
- Hearing loss often accompanies serious etiologies of vertigo.
- Vertigo in the setting of trauma should raise concern for a serious intracranial etiology and prompt additional evaluation.

Vertigo, the perception that the environment is inappropriately moving relative to the patient or that the patient is moving relative to the environment, can be immensely disturbing and frightening to patients and families. Vertigo can be rotational (sensation of spinning) or positional (sensation of horizontal or vertical displacement). Vertigo can often be confused with pseudovertigo, or symptoms that are similar to true vertigo such as light headedness or weakness. Common etiologies of vertigo are reviewed in Chapter 19 Dizziness and Vertigo, and further categorized by peripheral and central causes (see Tables 19.1 and 19.2). A thorough neurologic examination is essential to the workup of patients with vertigo, and can point to suspected vestibular or cerebellar dysfunction. Imaging needs such as MRI or CT should be guided by the history and examination. An approach to the patient with true vertigo is further delineated in Figure 19.1. Like imaging, management of patients with vertigo should be guided by the suspected underlying cause. Severe vertigo may require treatment with specific antivertiginous medications, such as dimenhydrinate (12.5 mg to 25 mg orally every 6 to 8 hours, maximum dose 75 mg per day for ages 2 to 6 years and 25 to 50 mg every 6 to 8 hours for ages 6 to 12 years, maximum dose 150 mg per day) and meclizine (12.5 mg to 25 mg orally every 12 hours in children older than 12 years of age) for symptom control.

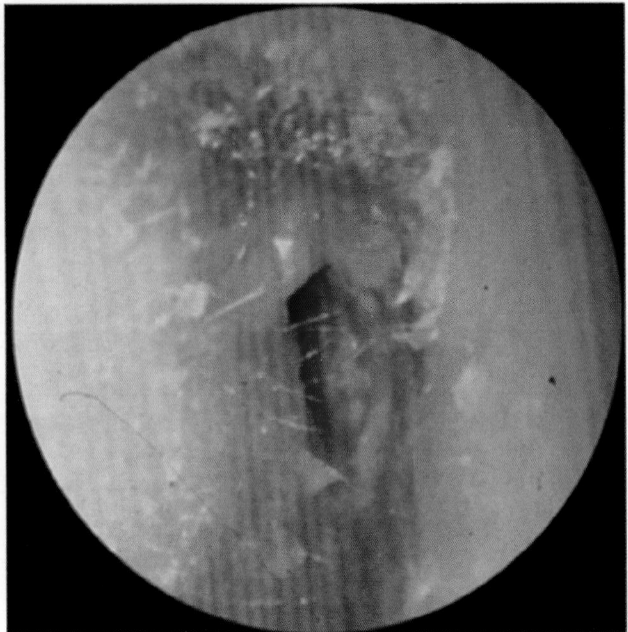

FIGURE 126.5 Otitis externa. Note the swollen, erythematous canal, filled with exudate. (From *Stedman's medical dictionary for the health professions and nursing, illustrated (standard edition)*. 6th ed. Philadelphia, PA: Lippincott Williams & Wilkins, 2007.)

OTHER CONDITIONS OF THE EXTERNAL EAR

Goals of Treatment

Chief complaints of pain or swelling of the external ear are relatively common and often benign. Recognizing conditions warranting additional therapy and evaluation should be the primary goals of treatment. Untreated infections in the external ear can progress and cause significant mortality and morbidity. Patients with immunosuppression are at particular risk for serious infections of the external ear that are rapidly progressive. Imaging should be considered for severely ill patients. Additionally, early recognition of auricular perichondritis is of particular importance, as cartilaginous infections can lead to long-term deformity if treatment is delayed.

CLINICAL PEARLS AND PITFALLS

- Otitis externa is most commonly characterized by otalgia and otorrhea
- Necrotizing otitis externa should be considered in patients that are immunocompromised with severe disease
- *Pseudomonas aeruginosa* is the most common causative agent in both otitis externa and auricular perichondritis

Otitis Externa

Otitis externa (or external otitis) is inflammation of the external auditory canal. It is particularly common in school-age children and those who participate in water sports. Most children with otitis externa present with otalgia, otorrhea, and pruritus of the external ear or canal. The diagnosis is made clinically based on symptoms, and a swollen, erythematous canal, often with exudate (Fig. 126.5). In severe or refractory cases, cultures of exudate from the canal specimens can be sent to confirm the infectious etiologic agent. Care should be taken in patients with diabetes or immunosuppression to evaluate for malignant otitis externa, which is an osteomyelitis of adjacent bony structures. Patients with malignant otitis externa are characterized by more severe pain and otorrhea, and may have cranial nerve palsies as well. Imaging is essential for diagnosis. Treatment of otitis externa involves debriding the ear canal, topical antibiotics and anti-inflammatory medications, and pain control. *P. aeruginosa* and *S. aureus* are the most common causative agents, and antibiotic therapy should be tailored to those pathogens. Topical fluoroquinolones such as ofloxacin and ciprofloxacin provide coverage against both pathogens, and are the first line therapy in most patients. If the external canal is occluded due to inflammatory swelling, an otic wick must be placed to allow medications to be drawn into the site of infection (Fig. 126.6).

Auricular Perichondritis

Auricular perichondritis is a rare but serious infection of the cartilage of the ear that can occur in the setting of trauma or surgery, or even after ear piercing. The infection is usually caused by *P. aeruginosa,* and patients present with severe swelling, erythema, and pain of the pinna (Fig. 126.7). Untreated, it can lead to permanent cartilaginous deformity. The diagnosis is made clinically, and treatment should be initiated promptly with agents that have activity against *P. aeruginosa* such as fluoroquinolones or third or fourth generation cephalosporins. Fluoroquinolones are particularly useful as they have excellent cartilage penetration. Their use in children should NOT be swayed by the minimal risk of tendon rupture complications.

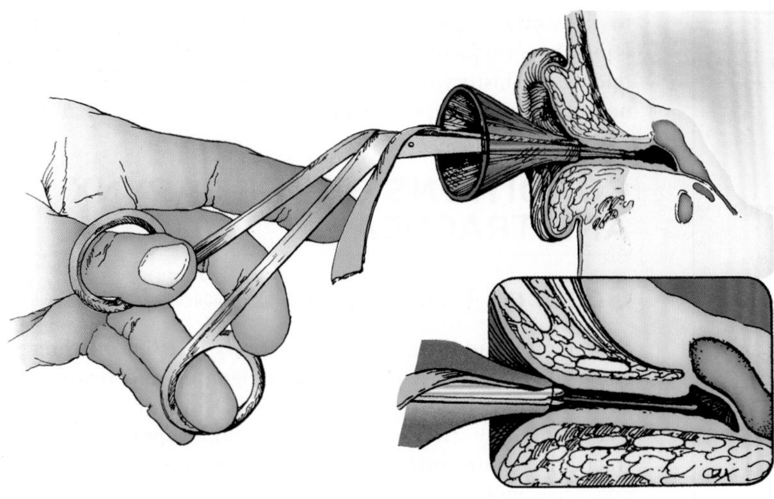

FIGURE 126.6 Gauze wick (¼ × 1½ in) being placed in ear canal to facilitate topical treatment of otitis externa.

EPISTAXIS

Goals of Treatment

Epistaxis is a common complaint of patients presenting to the emergency department. While usually self-limited, the heavily vascularized area of the anterior nose can lead to bleeding that is concerning to parents. Epistaxis is most common in school-age children, and is often the result of recurrent trauma through picking of the nose. Rarely, does epistaxis in otherwise healthy children lead to significant blood loss or airway compromise. Goals of treatment include providing appropriate reassurance to families, while also approaching the patient systematically to correctly identify those who require emergent care or consultation. Significant resuscitation with intravascular volume repletion or airway protection is extraordinarily uncommon. Avoiding costly and time consuming workups is also an important feature of optimal care in patients with epistaxis.

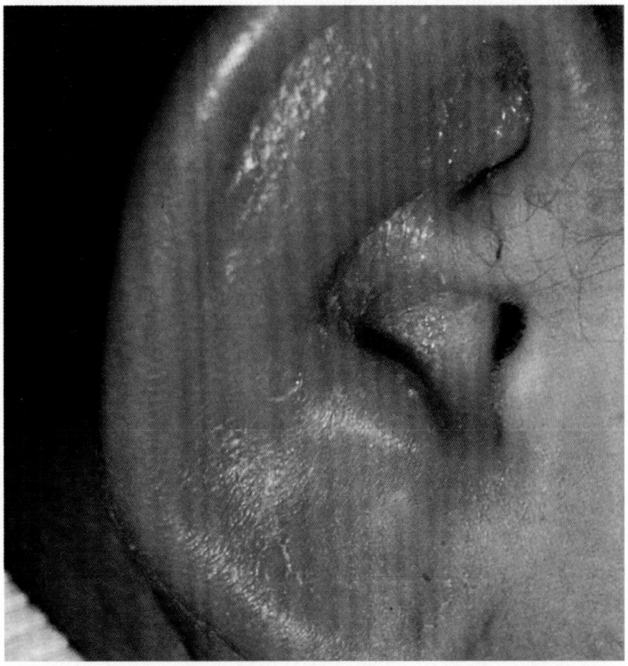

FIGURE 126.7 Perichondritis. Erythema and swelling of the pinna are consistent with perichondritis. (Used with permission from Handler SD, Myer CM. *Atlas of ear, nose and throat disorders in children*. Ontario, Canada: BC Decker, 1998:12.)

CLINICAL PEARLS AND PITFALLS

- Nosebleeds are rarely life-threatening and often need only basic measures to treat the bleeding
- Posterior nosebleeds are more difficult than anterior nosebleeds to control
- Laboratory workup is not indicated unless there is severe blood loss

Epistaxis is a relatively common presenting complaint in patients presenting to the emergency department. Most nosebleeds are a result of repetitive trauma to the anterior portion of the nose, at a vascular confluence called Kiesselbach plexus (Fig. 126.8). Additional factors such as dry ambient air, nasal congestion secondary to allergic rhinitis, nasoseptal deformities, and other infections are also related to an increased risk of nosebleeds. The physical examination is essential to identify abnormalities in general appearance, vital signs, airway,

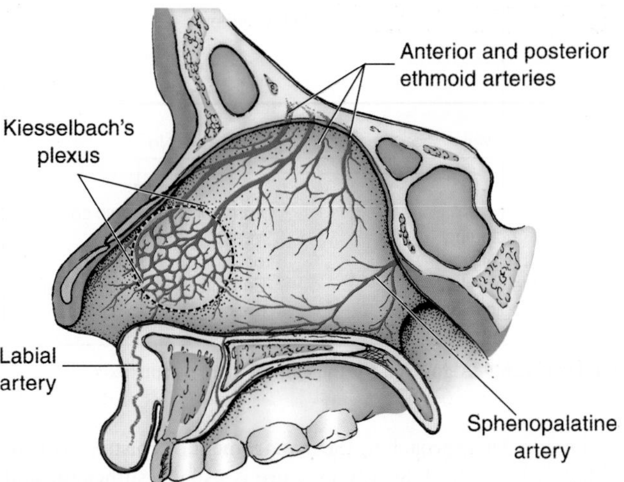

FIGURE 126.8 Vascular supply of nasal septum. Note confluence of vessels that forms Kiesselbach plexus.

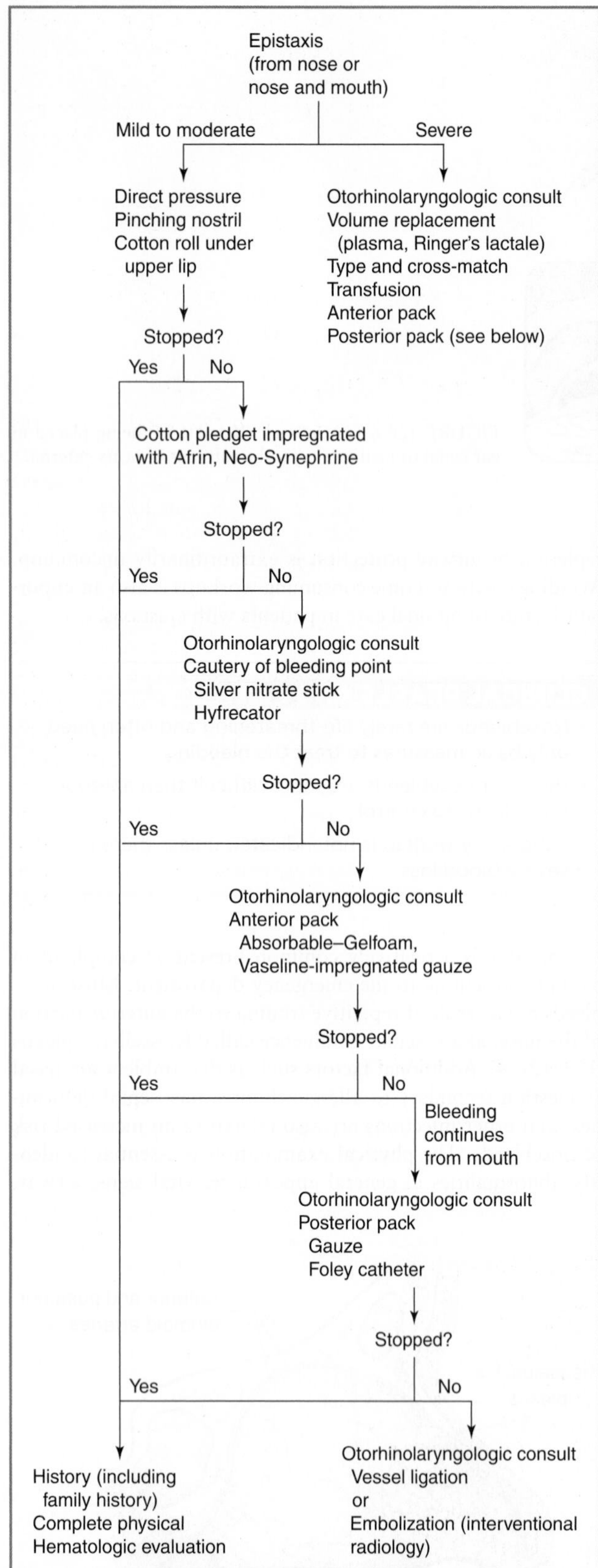

FIGURE 126.9 Algorithm for the management of epistaxis.

and color. An approach to the management of epistaxis is provided in Fig. 126.9. Steady pressure is usually sufficient, and should be applied with the patient sitting in the parent's lap, if anxious, and with the head tilted forward. Pressure is applied to the anterior portion of the nose and held continuously. Labs are infrequently indicated, unless there are concerning findings on history or examination. For more information on nosebleeds, see Chapter 21 Epistaxis.

CONDITIONS OF THE LARYNX AND TRACHEA

Goals of Treatment

Supraglottitis and tracheitis are relatively rare but life-threatening illnesses that require rapid recognition and treatment. Patients will typically present to the ED in extreme distress as evidenced by stridor and tripoding. Both supraglottitis and tracheitis require prompt consultation by otorhinolaryngology. See Chapter 102 Infectious Disease Emergencies for more details on recognition and treatment.

Suggested Readings and Key References

Center for Disease Control and Prevention (CDC). Estimated burden of acute otitis externa— United States, 2003–2007. *MMWR Morb Mortal Wkly Rep* 2011;60(19):605–609.

Centers for Disease Control and Prevention, Advisory Committee on Immunization Practices. Pneumococcal vaccination for cochlear implant candidates and recipients: updated recommendations of the Advisory Committee on Immunization Practices. *MMWR Morb Mortal Wkly Rep* 2003;52(31):739–740.

Clayman GL, Adams GL, Paugh DR, et al. Intracranial complications of paranasal sinusitis: a combined institutional review. *Laryngoscope* 1991;101(3):234–239.

Cumberworth VL, Hogarth TB. Hazards of ear-piercing procedures which traverse cartilage: a report of Pseudomonas perichondritis and review of other complications. *Br J Clin Pract* 1990;44(11):512–513.

DeSutter AI, DeMeyere MJ, Christiaens TC, et al. Does amoxicillin improve outcomes in patients with purulent rhinorrhea? A pragmatic randomized double-blind controlled trial in family practice. *J Fam Pract* 2002;51(4):317–323.

Guss J, Kazahaya K. Antibiotic-resistant Staphylococcus aureus in community-acquired pediatric neck abscesses. *Int J Pediatr Otorhinolaryngol* 2007;71(6):943–948.

Lieberthal AS, Carroll AE, Tunkel DE, et al. The diagnosis and management of acute otitis media. *Pediatrics* 2013;131(3):e964–e999.

Marchetti F, Ronfani L, Nibali SC, et al. Delayed prescription may reduce the use of antibiotics for acute otitis media. *Arch Peditr Adolesc Med* 2005;159:679–684.

McClay JE, Murray AD, Booth T. Intravenous antibiotic therapy for deep neck abscesses defined by computed tomography. *Arch Otolaryngol Head Neck Surg* 2003;129(11):1207–1212.

McEwan J, Wijayasingham G, Clarke RW, et al. Paediatric acute epiglottitis: not a disappearing entity. *Int J Pediatr Otorhinolaryngol* 2003;67:317–321.

Page NC, Bauer EM, Lieu JE. Clinical features and treatment of retropharyngeal abscess in children. *Otolaryngol Head Neck Surg* 2008;138(3):300–306.

Wald ER, Applegate KE, Bordley C, et al. American Academy of Pediatrics. Clinical practice guideline for the diagnosis and management of acute bacterial sinusitis in children aged 1 to 18 years. *Pediatrics* 2013;132(1):e262–e280.

Wald ER, Nash D, Eickhoff J, et al. Effectiveness of amoxicillin/clavulanate potassium in the treatment of acute bacterial sinusitis in children. *Pediatrics* 2009;124(1):9–15.

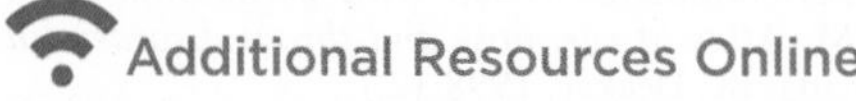

CHAPTER 127 ■ GENITOURINARY EMERGENCIES

DANA A. WEISS, MD AND CYNTHIA R. JACOBSTEIN, MD, MSCE

GOALS OF EMERGENCY CARE

Children present to the emergency department (ED) with a wide range of urologic complaints. Some are truly emergent, and some are a source of concern but can be handled with simple care and reassurance. The ability to triage and treat urologic emergencies is crucial for the ED physician. There are only a few true urologic emergencies that must be managed expeditiously: testicular torsion and a febrile obstructing kidney stone top the list. In addition, conditions such as paraphimosis and priapism warrant acute attention, while other conditions may require only assurance and close urologic follow-up.

KEY POINTS

- Identification of true urologic emergencies (testicular torsion, febrile obstructing stone).
- Judicial use of imaging in the diagnosis of urgent urologic conditions.
- The value of triage: the expedited versus routine follow-up urologic care.
- Complete genitourinary examination is crucial for all abdominal pain presentations.

RELATED CHAPTERS

Signs and Symptoms

- Constipation: Chapter 13
- Groin Masses: Chapter 29
- Hematuria: Chapter 32
- Pain: Abdomen: Chapter 48
- Pain: Back: Chapter 49
- Pain: Dysuria: Chapter 52
- Pain: Scrotal: Chapter 56
- Urinary Frequency: Chapter 74
- Vaginal Bleeding: Chapter 75
- Vaginal Discharge: Chapter 76

Clinical Pathways

- Abdominal Pain in Postpubertal Girls: Chapter 82

Medical, Surgical, and Trauma Emergencies

- Genitourinary Trauma: Chapter 116

PENILE PROBLEMS

CLINICAL PEARLS AND PITFALLS

- It is important to distinguish normal physiologic appearance from pathology.
- Paraphimosis and priapism are true emergencies.

Penile Care in the Uncircumcised Male Infant

Goals of Treatment/Clinical Assessment

With the high rate of circumcision in the United States, the recommended care of an intact foreskin is not always clear. In uncircumcised male infants, adhesions between the glans and the foreskin are normal (Fig. 127.1). The foreskin is not normally retractable in this age group. No effort should be made to strip the foreskin back in infants because this produces undue pain for the child and may result in inflammation and scarring. Between ages 2 and 4, spontaneous lysis of the adhesions occurs in 90% of boys. It is rare for the male infant to have any adverse hygienic consequence from leaving the foreskin in place until that time. The small, whitish lumps that may be seen and felt beneath the foreskin represent desquamated epithelium, smegma, and are benign. After toilet training, boys should be taught to retract the foreskin enough to expose the meatus during voids—this avoids leaving the inner foreskin wet with urine, which can lead to inflammation, mucosal abrasions, and balanoposthitis. By age 4 to 6 years, the foreskin should be drawn back as far as it can go at every bath.

Postcircumcision Concerns

Immediate Concerns

While rare, postcircumcision bleeding can be of significant concern, or it can be a minor issue. After circumcision done either with a clamp (in the newborn time period), or freehand (older boys), most postoperative bleeding will resolve with manual pressure for 5 to 10 minutes. After that, careful inspection will reveal if there is a discrete vessel bleeding, or if there is more general oozing of blood from the suture line.

Urology consultation is recommended if there is concern for injury to the glans or urethra or if bleeding does not stop with manual pressure.

Delayed Concerns

If there is concern for a skin cicatrix, a thick scar around the edge of the circumcision, encasing the urethral meatus, then the patient should be referred to the urology clinic for outpatient follow-up. This can be done as a routine visit unless there is concern for obstruction of the urinary stream, although this is very rare. If a scar is caught early it may respond to gentle release of flimsy adhesions, or, if a more robust scar, it may respond to treatment with betamethasone cream. In severe cases, a circumcision revision will have to be performed in order to release the scar around the glans.

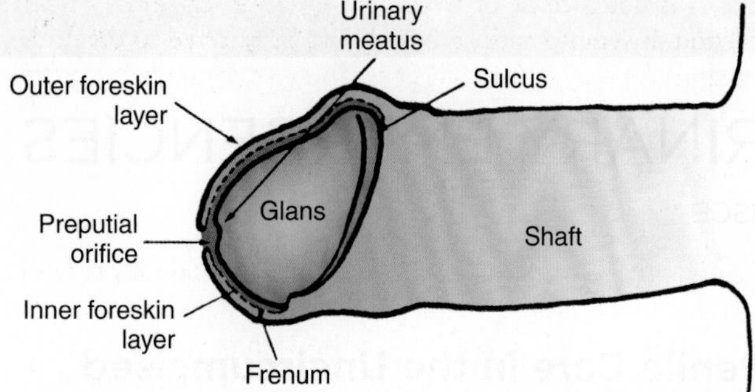

FIGURE 127.1 Anatomy of normal uncircumcised male. Adhesions between inner foreskin layer and glans are normal in newborns and prevent retraction of the foreskin. (From Wallerstein E. *Circumcision: an American health fallacy*. New York, NY: Springer, 1980:201. Reprinted with permission.)

Phimosis and Paraphimosis

Goals of Treatment

- Rule out significant skin or glans infection in cases of phimosis
- Reduce foreskin back to normal anatomic location in paraphimosis

Clinical Considerations

Phimosis exists when the distal foreskin becomes scarred so that it cannot be retracted to expose the glans. This nonretracted foreskin is a normal physiologic finding in the newborn and infant. However, this can also persist or occur later in life as a result of inflammation from chronic urine exposure, previous forceful withdrawing of the foreskin over the glans, or related to lichen sclerosus. Children may present with swelling of the foreskin, or with the complaint of seeing ballooning of the foreskin during urination.

Paraphimosis is the result of retracting foreskin behind the glans and leaving it in that position. This leads to venous congestion and edema—thus making it difficult to reduce the foreskin back to its normal position (Fig. 127.2). This often results after bathing (often by a provider not used to caring for the child), or is caused by the child himself. In iatrogenic settings, this may occur after urethral catheterization, when the foreskin is retracted for the procedure but is not returned to its normal position.

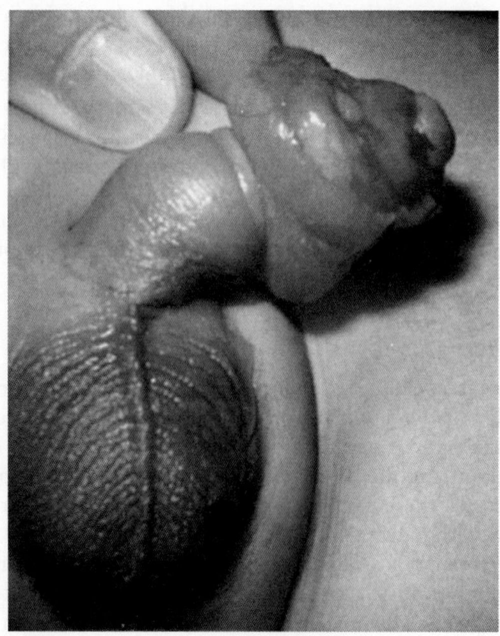

FIGURE 127.2 Paraphimosis—a foreskin that is left in a retracted position leads to venous congestion and edema of the foreskin.

Clinical Recognition. A tight phimosis can result in ballooning of the foreskin during voiding, which in turn traps urine and can lead to inflammation. In a child over 2 years old, the foreskin should be able to be retracted to the point where the urethral meatus can be visualized.

Paraphimosis is evident as a broad, edematous band of skin proximal to the glans. This skin is often erythematous and very tender to touch.

Management. Phimosis does not have to be treated emergently. Betamethasone cream, 0.05%, applied twice daily for 6 weeks, is the first-line treatment. Hydrocortisone cream is an alternative. The patient/family must be instructed to pull the foreskin back as far as it will go, then to apply a small amount directly to the tightened area.

The goal in paraphimosis is to bring the foreskin back into normal location. This requires reduction of the edema in the skin. The application of ice and steady manual compression on the inflamed ring of foreskin usually reduces the edema and permits manual reduction of the paraphimosis. Topical anesthetic cream or a dorsal penile nerve block will reduce the discomfort experienced by the child during compression of the edematous foreskin. Once a portion of the edema has been reduced, pressure on the glans (like turning a sock inside out) usually permits reduction of the foreskin back to its normal position (Fig. 127.3). If manual reduction fails, a surgical division of the foreskin to permit reduction is indicated; however it is uncommon to need to perform this (Fig. 127.4). The family should be counseled not to pull the foreskin back over the glans for at least a week. Vaseline can be applied to the raw edges of the foreskin, especially in the setting of small abrasions, to prevent infection. The family can be counseled about circumcision, although this is not required.

Meatal Stenosis

Meatal stenosis is a problem seen exclusively in circumcised males and follows an inflammatory reaction around the meatus.

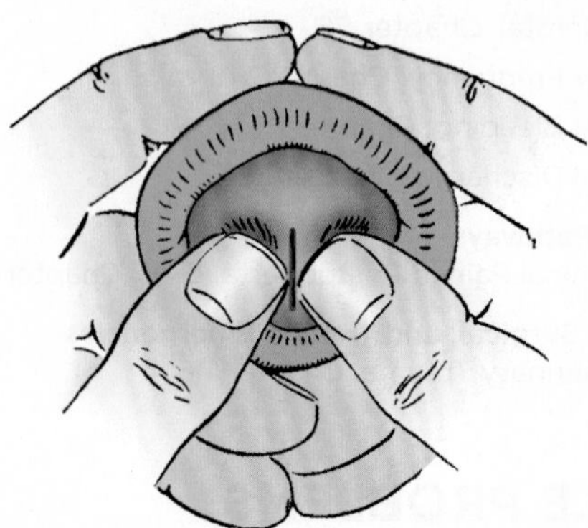

FIGURE 127.3 Manual reduction of paraphimosis. After a local anesthetic block of the dorsal nerve of the penis, the foreskin is manually compressed to reduce edema. The foreskin can be reduced by pressure on glans—like turning a sock inside out. (From Klauber GT, Sant GR. Disorders of the male external genitalia. In: Kelalis PP, King LR, Belman AB, eds. *Clinical pediatric urology*. 2nd ed. Philadelphia, PA: WB Saunders, 1985:287. Reprinted with permission.)

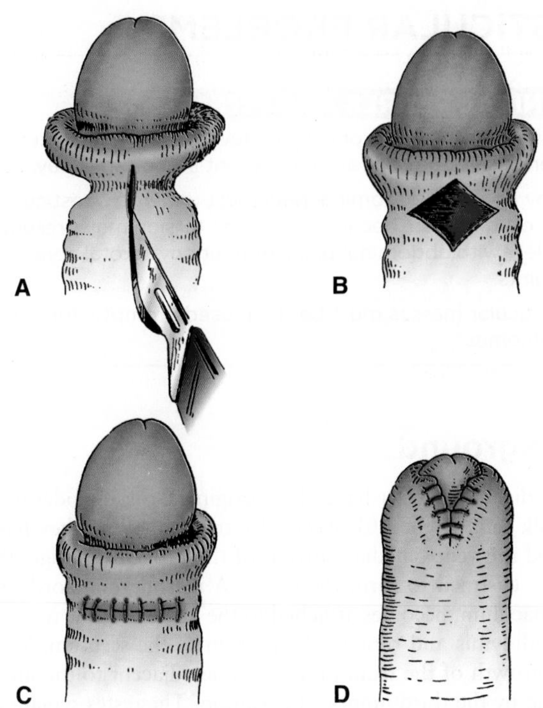

FIGURE 127.4 Surgical correction of phimosis. **A:** Constricting foreskin is incised vertically on dorsum. **B:** The incision opens laterally, relieving constriction. **C:** Incision is closed transversely with chromic catgut sutures. **D:** Foreskin can now be reduced. (From Klauber GT, Sant GR. Disorders of the male external genitalia. In: Kelalis PP, King LR, Belman AB, eds. *Clinical pediatric urology*. 2nd ed. Philadelphia, PA: WB Saunders, 1985:827. Reprinted with permission.)

This can occur from the lower edge of the meatus rubbing against a wet diaper, with inflammation of the meatus resulting from mechanical and ammoniacal chemical dermatitis. Appearances are often deceiving. The meatus may appear to be stenotic but may be functioning adequately. Significant meatal stenosis causes spraying of the urinary stream or, more commonly, dorsal deflection of the stream. Surgical treatment of the meatus is warranted only if these symptoms are present. Meatal stenosis is not a cause of frequency, enuresis, or urinary tract infection. If symptomatic, a boy should be referred to the urology clinic for evaluation and possible meatotomy in the office or a meatoplasty under anesthesia.

Balanoposthitis

Balanoposthitis is an infection of the foreskin that may extend onto the glans (Fig. 127.5). It is a form of cellulitis and has its origin from a break in the penile skin. It may be the result of local trauma or may, in the older boy, be associated with poor penile hygiene. Scarring after the inflammatory reaction may lead to true phimosis.

Goals of Treatment

- Treat active infection and establish follow-up to assess cause of infection.

Clinical Recognition

Acute swelling, blanching erythema, and pain likely indicates balanitis or balanoposthitis (infection of the foreskin and the glans). Other etiologies of penile swelling must be considered as well. Isolated penile edema that is either nontender or minimally tender can occur as a result of an insect bite, with local edema secondary to histamine release. A history of a bite or the finding of a small punctate lesion may give the clue to diagnosis. Painless penile edema may also be present with a generalized allergic reaction or as part of the manifestation of a general edematous state secondary to renal, cardiac, or hepatic problems. Here, the diagnosis is suggested by evidence of dysfunction in these organ systems on general examination.

Management

In the setting of true cellulitis, the administration of an appropriate antibiotic is warranted. The antibiotic, for example, cephalexin (clindamycin if cephalosporin allergy) should cover typical skin flora. In addition, local care may be done with warm soaks. It is unusual for a child to be unable to void as

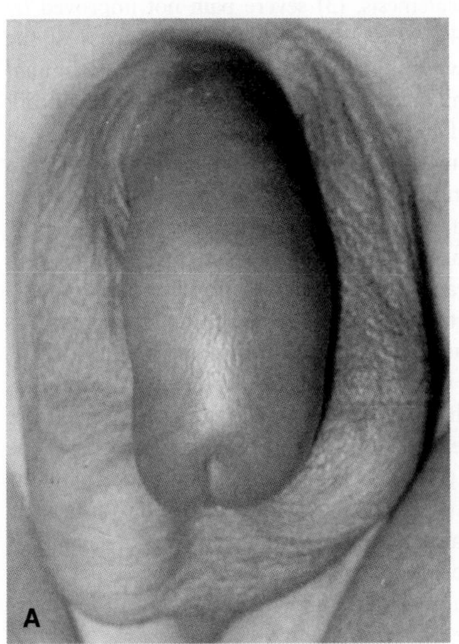

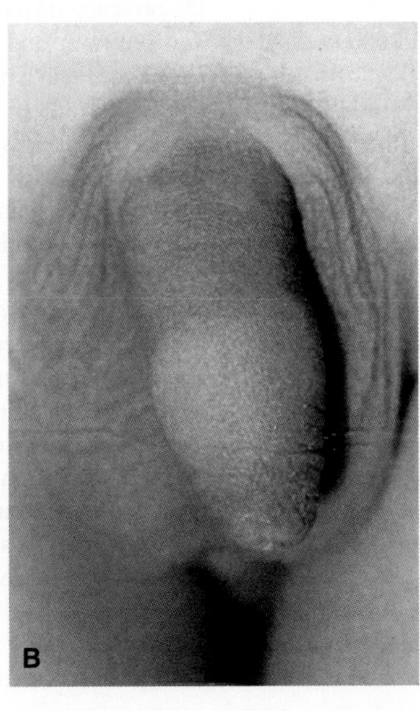

FIGURE 127.5 **A:** Balanoposthitis—cellulitis of normal foreskin with erythema, edema, and tenderness. **B:** Normal foreskin after treatment of balanoposthitis with antibiotics and warm soaks.

a result of this condition, although he may be more comfortable voiding while in a tub of warm water. After resolution of the acute infection, the boy should be reexamined for signs of phimosis. If a severe phimosis develops, or if there is a history of recurrent episodes of balanitis, then a circumcision may be recommended.

Priapism

Prolonged, painful penile erection unaccompanied by sexual stimulation is called priapism. Generally an erection lasting longer than 4 hours requires treatment. Pain that occurs prior to 4 hours is an additional indication for initiation of treatment.

Goals of Treatment

- Achieve detumescence
- Identify and/or treat underlying pathology

Clinical Recognition

In the pediatric age group, priapism may be caused by trauma or leukemic infiltration, or may be idiopathic, but it is most often seen in African-American males with sickle cell disease. Initially, priapism must be classified as ischemic (low flow) or nonischemic (high flow). A sickling crisis that involves the corporal bodies does not necessarily need to be related to symptomatic sickling elsewhere in the body. Sickling of the erythrocytes produces sludging and stasis in the erectile tissue of the corporal bodies. This stasis leads to further hypoxia, acidosis, and more sickling. The thick, dark sludge that is formed prevents detumescence of the erectile tissue, causing priapism. Pain results from ischemia. It is speculated that an inflammatory reaction to this necrotic sludge may lead to fibrosis of the erectile tissue. Impotence may result.

Triage Considerations

Treatment urgency is based on time since onset and symptoms. With ischemic priapism, delay in treatment can lead to tissue loss. Nonischemic/high-flow priapism does not require urgent treatment, but should be diagnosed.

Clinical Assessment/Management

A careful history and physical examination to determine the etiology of the priapism is the first step, and further guides evaluation and treatment. Laboratory evaluation includes urine analysis and urine culture, CBC, sickle cell screen (if not previously diagnosed), LFTs, LDH, CRP, and coagulation panel. If there is question of whether this is ischemic or nonischemic priapism, an urgent color duplex ultrasound should be obtained. If this is not conclusive, then a corporal blood gas is indicated.

The first-line treatment for priapism associated with sickle cell disease is careful hydration, oxygen, and analgesia, followed by irrigation of the corporal bodies with saline in combination with vasoactive substances (phenylephrine, 250 to 500 μg per cc). This is best performed with urologic consultation.

Untreated priapism has been documented to lead to impotence. Prompt assessment and treatment is indicated to prevent such complications.

TESTICULAR PROBLEMS

CLINICAL PEARLS AND PITFALLS

- Testicular torsion is one of the few true urologic emergencies. It does not always present in the same way.
- Any boy with abdominal pain must undergo a testicular examination, because testicular torsion may present solely with abdominal pain, without any scrotal complaints.
- Testicular masses must be diagnosed promptly for best outcomes.

Background

Primordial germ cells have their origin in the endoderm of the yolk sac. By the fifth week of intrauterine life, they have reached the ventromedial portion of the urogenital ridge, the portion destined to form the testes. A mesodermal cord, the gubernaculum, becomes attached to the bottom of the testis at the epididymis and runs to the bottom of the scrotum. With rapid growth of the trunk, the testes lie adjacent to the internal ring by the third month of gestation. The testes remain at this location until the seventh month when, preceded by a fold of peritoneum (the processus vaginalis), the testes move down the inguinal canal and reach their final scrotal position shortly before birth. This fact accounts for the higher incidence of undescended testis in premature boys.

Testicular Torsion

Goals of Treatment

Torsion of the testis is one of the few true urologic emergencies; time is of the essence. The goal in management of testicular torsion is prompt diagnosis (aided by high index of suspicion) and early consultation with a urologist for prompt surgical treatment.

Clinical Recognition

Key symptoms that should raise suspicion for testicular torsion are: (1) Acute onset, often waking a boy up from sleep, (2) presence of nausea/emesis, (3) severe pain not improved by any position, and (4) sudden enlargement and redness of the hemiscrotum in a newborn. Important signs on physical examination include (1) an enlarged, swollen hemiscrotum, (2) significant tenderness, (3) loss of cremasteric reflex, and (4) horizontal lie of the affected testis. Any boy with abdominal pain must undergo a testicular examination, because testicular torsion may present solely with abdominal pain, without any scrotal complaints.

In newborns, the testis undergoes extravaginal torsion (compared to intravaginal), and may occur prenatally or postnatally. Most often the prenatally torsed testis will present as a firm, enlarged mass in the hemiscrotum often with discoloration of the skin. On the other hand, if a normal examination is noted at birth, and a follow-up examination reveals an erythematous, tender, enlarged scrotum, the patient must be evaluated emergently and surgical intervention undertaken, as the testis may be salvaged. Many debate the need to intervene acutely in the prenatally torsed patients, however asynchronous torsion has been reported, resulting in anorchia. Thus careful balance of the risks and benefits of surgery in the newborn period must be undertaken.

Triage Considerations

Early recognition is essential. A patient presenting with scrotal pain should be evaluated immediately. Similarly, if a newborn presents with the history of a new finding of testicular swelling, he must be treated as if he had testicular torsion until proven otherwise. If symptoms are consistent with testicular torsion, urology should be consulted immediately. If there is any question, a scrotal ultrasound must be ordered on an emergent basis. Some patients will have intermittent testicular torsion—and in these cases the pain will resolve spontaneously within 30 to 45 minutes. These patients should still be evaluated with a scrotal ultrasound since a torsion may partially untwist with resolution of pain, but still have vascular compromise.

Clinical Assessment

The differential diagnosis of scrotal pain and/or swelling includes epididymitis, torsion of the testis appendix, intermittent torsion, hernia/hydrocele, trauma, cellulitis, or even vasculitis (Henoch–Schönlein purpura). Often an ultrasound is the only way to distinguish these entities. In the interest of time, some urologists will take a child to the operating room without an ultrasound; however most of the time an ultrasound is done to confirm diagnosis. Upon evaluation, the emergency physician should be able to make the diagnosis, call the consultation, and in the interim, obtain an ultrasound.

Two similar presentations that are corollaries of testicular torsion are torsion/detorsion, and intermittent torsion. If a boy presents with acute onset of pain consistent with torsion, but after 30 minutes to 1 hour (or longer), the pain abruptly resolves, and imaging shows the presence of flow to the testis, it is possible that the testis detorsed. The challenge here is that this should still be treated urgently, since (1) the testis may twist again and (2) at times there is an incomplete detorsion so that there is still a 180-degree twist, with return of some blood flow, but the testis is still compromised. Alternatively, if the patient's history is that one or two times prior to the current presentation, he has had the same type of pain, yet the pain resolved within 30 minutes each time, he may be experiencing intermittent torsion. This, too, should be treated with surgery to prevent torsion in the future, but this may be done on a semi-elective basis.

Management

The only management for testicular torsion is surgical reduction and fixation. While the testis may be able to be "detorsed" in the emergency room for temporary relief of pain, this is not adequate treatment. The patient requires exploration in the operating room. Depending on the duration of the torsion, the surgeons may find a completely nonviable testis upon evaluation, and an orchiectomy is performed. Alternatively, if there appears to be some blood flow to the testis after untwisting and allowing time for blood flow to return, then the testis will be fixed into place in the scrotum. The contralateral side will also be fixed in place to prevent torsion on the other side in the future.

Testicular Mass

Background

Pediatric (prepubertal) testicular masses account for 1% of all pediatric solid tumors, with the peak age of incidence around 2 years. Overall the most common prepubertal testicular masses are teratomas, followed by rhabdomyosarcomas, epidermoid cysts, yolk sac tumors, and germ cell tumors. Gonadoblastoma (in dysgenetic gonads), and nontesticular tumors such as lymphoma and leukemia are also possible.

Goals of Treatment

Prompt recognition, diagnosis, and referral for treatment.

Clinical Recognition

Testicular masses are often asymptomatic. These may be found as incidental findings during thorough physical examination, may present as scrotal enlargement, or may present concurrent with testicular torsion or other pathologies.

Triage Considerations

Testicular masses require early diagnosis, but treatment will not occur emergently. Once diagnosed, the urologist will typically manage the testicular mass within the next 1 to 7 days.

Clinical Assessment

If a testicular mass is palpated on examination, a scrotal ultrasound is warranted. If a mass is found incidentally on ultrasound, further workup is also warranted. All patients with a scrotal mass concerning for a tumor must undergo blood testing for AFP, bHCG, and LDH. In addition, these patients need cross-sectional imaging of the abdomen.

Management

A pediatric urologist must be consulted. Once a testicular mass is identified, it will require resection. Imaging and patient parameters will determine whether a partial orchiectomy is permissible, or a radical orchiectomy is required.

Torsion of the Appendix Testis

Clinical Recognition

A torsed appendix testis may present much like a testicular torsion by report, but the patient appears vastly different. Pain is still a presenting complaint but torsion of an appendix less often awakes a patient from sleep, and is not associated with nausea or emesis. The swelling is less pronounced, and a key finding on physical examination is focal tenderness at the superior aspect of the testis rather than the inferior testis. The "blue dot" sign, in which a bluish hue is visible through the scrotal skin at the superior aspect of the testis, is an often elusive finding.

Triage Considerations

Since the initial presentation may be similar to testicular torsion, a prompt evaluation with history and physical examination is essential to help guide evaluation and management.

Clinical Assessment

The testis may be swollen and red; thus, a scrotal ultrasound is a valid tool for diagnosis. This may identify the torsed appendage (though it does not always), but more often, and more importantly, will rule out testicular torsion.

Management

Torsion of a testicular appendage is managed with supportive care. The key component of treatment is administration of a nonsteroidal anti-inflammatory medication, such as ibuprofen, around the clock for at least 3 to 4 days, to reduce swelling and inflammation, as well as provide pain relief. This may be accompanied by ice as needed, and scrotal support, often in the form of snug underwear. If pain does not resolve in 5 to 7 days, some urologists will perform a scrotal exploration and resection of the appendage.

Epididymitis

Epididymitis can present very similarly to testicular torsion, and thus requires careful differentiation of the signs, symptoms, and examination to rule out the need for acute intervention. History often reveals a gradual increase in pain, but also may be more acute in onset. Epididymitis is usually not associated with nausea or vomiting. On examination, the scrotum will be enlarged and often erythematous. The scrotum is typically diffusely tender to palpation.

Due to the difficulty in distinguishing epididymitis from torsion in many cases, a scrotal ultrasound should be obtained if there is any question about the diagnosis. An ultrasound will show hyperemia of the epididymis.

Epididymitis in prepubertal boys is most often idiopathic, or may be due to chemical irritation. The boy should be questioned about voiding symptoms, as well as if he has to strain to urinate, because sometimes straining can cause back pressure into the ejaculatory ducts leading to irritation. Postpubertal boys with epididymitis may have a sexually transmitted infection, including *Neisseria gonorrhoeae* or *Chlamydia trachomatis*. A rare cause of epididymitis that can be mistaken for a scrotal mass is tuberculous epididymitis, so this must be on the differential for any patient who comes from areas where tuberculosis is endemic.

Treatment of chemical or reactive epididymitis includes NSAIDs, ice, and scrotal support. If a urine culture is positive, then the patient should be treated empirically with antibiotics directed at typical urinary tract pathogens. STI testing and treatment should be considered in adolescent males.

Hydrocele

Clinical Recognition

The etiologies of scrotal swelling are diverse, and some need urgent attention, while others are benign processes. Scrotal hydroceles can lead to concern as they may acutely increase in size after straining (heavy crying in an infant), and may fluctuate in size. Classically hydroceles are painless, full of fluid, and require nonurgent management.

Triage Considerations

A hydrocele presents differently than torsion of the testicle or of an appendix testis, but can strongly mimic a true hernia. It is most often a painless swelling that is noticed during a diaper change or at bath time; however, these entities may be indistinguishable until further evaluation.

Clinical Assessment

History and physical examination will quickly begin to separate a hydrocele from an emergent problem. Physical examination is often notable for a nontender scrotum, with a communicating hydrocele, in which the fluid can be compressed back into the abdomen. However, this is not always the case, and a hydrocele can have a loculated component that does not decompress. Classically, a hydrocele will transilluminate, and the testis can be seen "floating" in the middle of all the fluid.

Management

Prepubertal boys will have communicating hydroceles, whereas older boys may have loculated scrotal hydroceles. In newborns and young infants, hydroceles may resolve spontaneously. However, if they have not resolved by around 1 year of age, they are often repaired. A hydrocele and a hernia have the same pathophysiology—a persistent processus vaginalis. In a hydrocele, the opening is very small, while in a hernia it is larger. A hydrocele can turn into a hernia. Thus the family must be counseled on signs and symptoms of an incarcerated hernia, including pain, a mass that cannot be reduced, nausea, vomiting, inconsolable crying, and/or erythema. If these symptoms occur, the patient should return to the emergency room. The patient should be referred to a pediatric urologist on an outpatient basis for management of a hydrocele.

Undescended Testis

Clinical Recognition

Four percent of newborn males will have an undescended testis. The incidence decreases to 1.6% by 1 year of age, indicating that some undescended testes descend after birth. Spontaneous descent rarely occurs after 6 months of age. The child with undescended testes beyond the age of 6 months needs outpatient urologic consultation. In the physical examination of a boy, an empty scrotum on one or both sides is a common finding, but it may not always indicate a true undescended testis. Often this represents a retractile testis. In a boy with a retractile testis, the active cremaster muscle attached to the small prepubertal gonad is able to draw the testis up into a position near the pubic tubercle. There is no evidence that this causes any harm to the gonad. Imaging is not required in this setting, as scrotal ultrasounds are not indicated to locate the testis. Scrotal ultrasounds should only be obtained to evaluate for pain or mass.

Usually, an undescended testis is asymptomatic. However, in a position against the abdominal wall, it may be more subject to trauma than when freely mobile in the scrotum. The undescended testis also may undergo torsion more easily than a normally descended one. The boy who presents with an acutely tender groin mass with an ipsilateral empty scrotum may have torsion of his undescended testis. The physician must consider the differential diagnosis of an incarcerated inguinal hernia or acute hydrocele of the cord. Prompt surgical treatment may be required.

Management

Testicular malignancy and infertility are increased in the male infant with an uncorrected undescended testis. By electron microscopy, it is possible to demonstrate degenerative changes in the undescended testis by 1 year of age so referral to a urologist for orchiopexy is recommended.

If a retractile testis is identified, and the testis can definitely be brought into the scrotum without tension, then the patient can follow-up with his primary care physician for routine monitoring. If there is any question, then the patient should be referred to a pediatric urologist.

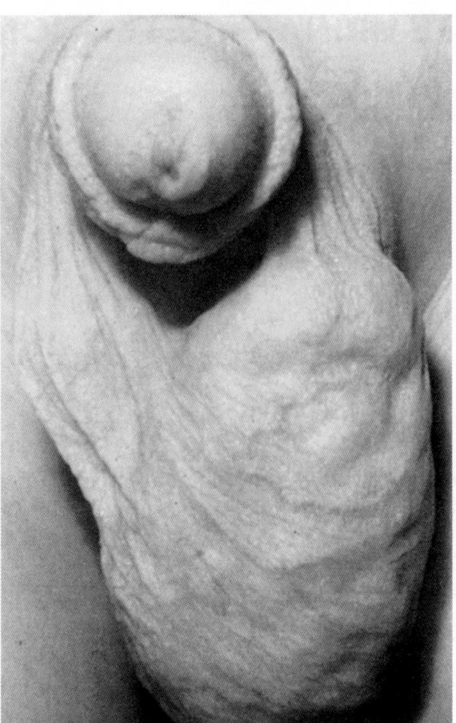

FIGURE 127.6 Varicocele—abnormal dilation of cremasteric and pampiniform venous plexuses surrounding the spermatic cord, giving the scrotum the appearance of a "bag of worms."

Varicocele

Clinical Recognition

Varicoceles are abnormal dilations of the cremasteric and pampiniform venous plexuses surrounding the spermatic cord (Fig. 127.6). They generally present as an asymptomatic scrotal swelling about the time of puberty and are rare in the prepubertal male. Almost all are of congenital origin and affect the left testis. The anatomic problem is a defect in the valves of the left spermatic vein that drains directly into the left renal vein. A higher left renal vein pressure may also play a role. Varicoceles affect about 15% of adolescent boys. If the varicocele does not disappear when the child lies down, it suggests an obstruction of the left renal vein, and a renal and bladder ultrasound is appropriate. Varicoceles are rarely symptomatic; a heavy or tugging sensation is occasionally reported. Boys may present with pain or because they notice a different feeling in the scrotum, but they do not require urgent treatment. The patient should be referred to the urology outpatient clinic for further evaluation and monitoring, although very few patients will ultimately undergo surgical treatment.

FEMALE UROLOGIC EMERGENCIES

CLINICAL PEARLS AND PITFALLS

- Most female urologic presentations are benign; however it is critical to identify the vaginal tumor on examination.
- Some vaginal cysts and masses can indicate disorders with the upper urinary tract, so a high index of suspicion is needed.

Goals of Treatment

Girls have some specific anatomic findings that may bring them in for evaluation. The key to treatment is differentiating the few true emergencies from the more benign presentations.

Clinical Recognition

The one anatomic urologic finding in a female that should cause alarm is the presence of a vaginal mass. This may represent vaginal rhabdomyosarcoma. The patient with a vaginal mass needs immediate referral to and evaluation by urology and oncology.

Some more benign vaginal "masses" may include vaginal cysts, Gartner duct cysts, Bartholin cysts, and paraurethral cysts. These cysts may represent isolated findings, or could represent an ectopic ureter draining into the introitus. Additionally, a pelvic or vaginal mass may represent hydrometrocolpos in a patient with vaginal agenesis, atresia, stenosis, or imperforate hymen.

Other female urologic issues that may present to the ER are urethral prolapse and labial adhesions.

Clinical Assessment

If there is concern for a lower abdominal or pelvic mass on history or physical examination, a renal bladder ultrasound and a pelvic ultrasound should be performed. The pelvic ultrasound will help to further define the vaginal mass, and a renal bladder ultrasound will help determine the etiology (duplicated kidney, absent kidney, hydroureteronephrosis).

Urethral prolapse typically presents in African-American girls aged ~6 to 11 years (but can occur at any time from birth to ~11 years old). This entity often presents with spotting of blood in the underwear, but is otherwise asymptomatic. On examination, a red ring of prolapsed mucosa surrounding the urethra is noticeable. The introitus must be seen to be separate and uninvolved.

Labial adhesions appear as a "median raphe" formed by the two edges of labia minora. Most commonly they begin at the posterior fourchette and extend toward the clitoris, with a pinpoint opening for urine to come out. Symptoms may include UTI symptoms, dysuria, or spraying with urination.

Management

For urethral prolapse, observation alone is often sufficient, but can be combined with estrogen cream and/or sitz baths. For recurrent cases, surgical excision of the prolapsed mucosa may prevent further episodes.

For labial adhesions, observation alone is reasonable for the asymptomatic child, as they typically resolve once the child reaches puberty and the tissues become estrogenized. If the girl is symptomatic, or the parents are concerned, the adhesions can be treated with topical estrogen cream (Premarin 0.1% twice daily for 4 to 6 weeks) followed by petroleum jelly at bedtime to keep the labia from refusing. Side effects may include hyperpigmentation and breast tenderness, which resolve after the cream is discontinued. Alternatively, after application of a topical anesthetic cream, the adhesions can be bluntly divided with a finger or a probe, and then copious petroleum jelly should be applied up to three times a day (or with every diaper change) for several months. However, adhesions can recur.

RENAL COLIC/ NEPHROLITHIASIS

CLINICAL PEARLS AND PITFALLS

- A febrile obstructing stone is a true urologic emergency, and can result in significant morbidity and even mortality, if not appropriately diagnosed in an expeditious manner.

Goals of Treatment

Determining when nephrolithiasis requires emergent treatment versus when supportive care in conjunction with medical expulsion therapy is indicated is of key importance. The primary goal in the acute setting is diagnosing obstruction, when it is present, and providing pain control, nausea control, hydration, and education.

Clinical Recognition

A kidney stone becomes a true emergency when it is associated with a fever, or if there is an obstructing stone in a solitary kidney. Aside from these two settings, management rests on symptom control and stone expulsion.

Triage Considerations

Fever in the setting of an obstructive stone is a medical and surgical emergency, and without timely treatment, a patient can progress to sepsis, with the potential for rapid decompensation. Moreover, obstruction in a solitary kidney can lead to acute renal failure. Patients with two functional kidneys who present with pain and/or nausea due to stones and without fever require only symptomatic treatment.

Management

A patient presenting with flank pain with or without the presence of hematuria should be evaluated for a kidney stone. After a history and physical examination to evaluate for a solitary kidney or chronic kidney disease and for the presence of a fever, an ultrasound is the first-line imaging that should be obtained. Initial medical management should include hydration (this should be IV until there is no chance that the child will have to undergo urgent surgical management), and pain control with narcotics and nonsteroidal anti-inflammatory medications, if there is no evidence of renal dysfunction. If a stone is suspected and the ultrasound is abnormal but does not show a stone specifically, a low-radiation noncontrast CT scan can be obtained; however this is not required. The patient can be treated with medical expulsion therapy alone, including pain medication and tamsulosin. If the patient requires surgical decompression, there are two modalities available: percutaneous nephrostomy tube placement or retrograde placement of a ureteral stent.

ACUTE URINARY RETENTION

CLINICAL PEARLS AND PITFALLS

- A seemingly benign presentation may have an underlying significant problem.
- A perforated bladder augmentation can be life-threatening, and must be diagnosed and treated on an urgent basis.
- Urinary retention in a small child may be the only presenting sign of a rhabdomyosarcoma.

Background

A patient with acute urinary retention is unable to empty the bladder even though it is full. The cause may be bladder outlet obstruction, or may be due to lack of bladder function, as a result of a neurologic problem, or may be volitional.

Goals of Treatment

Recognize the problem, and facilitate drainage of the bladder.

Clinical Recognition

Determining the underlying etiology of the urinary retention is of key importance, as is determining who is at risk for complicating factors from experiencing retention. In newborns and infants, bladder outlet obstruction due to posterior urethral valves or obstructing ureteroceles must be identified. In older children, posterior urethral valves must remain on the differential, as well as neurologic conditions such as occult tethered cord, spina bifida, or iatrogenic causes such as postoperative retention due to narcotics, fear of urination due to recent urethral manipulation, and children with severe constipation. An important uncommon etiology that cannot be missed is that of augmented bladders that cannot be catheterized, as these are at risk for perforation. Also, the practitioner should question the seemingly “simple” urinary retention with no obvious cause: rhabdomyosarcoma of the bladder or prostate may present with retention as the sole symptom.

Triage Considerations

It is essential to determine who is sick, or who can get sick very quickly. Any patient with a bladder augmentation who is in retention and unable to catheterize is at risk for bladder augment perforation—which becomes an emergent surgical matter.

Clinical Assessment

Diagnosis begins with a careful history. This will elicit not only medical history, including past surgeries, but also the history of a weak stream or difficulty initiating voiding may offer clues. Duration of retention and symptoms experienced are also important in determining the treatment plan.

Management

For the child with voluntary retention, gentle massage of the lower abdomen, combined with a soak in a warm tub, usually leads to spontaneous evacuation of the bladder. Rarely does a child's bladder become so distended, as after an outpatient surgical general anesthetic, that the child is unable to void. It should be remembered that a child is able to hold urine voluntarily for longer periods than would be suspected; up to 12 hours is not unusual.

In order to actively drain the bladder, a catheter must be placed. This can be done with a bladder catheter or small feeding tube. Once the bladder is drained, a urinalysis and urine culture should be obtained. Depending on the history, the catheter should be left indwelling, or can be removed after draining the bladder entirely. If a catheter cannot be placed (due to previous surgery, or presence of obstruction or false urethral passage), then drainage via a suprapubic approach must be undertaken. This can be performed with a needle if drainage and urine sample are needed alone, or a large tube can be placed with the assistance of interventional radiology or urology.

If a child had a history of a bladder augmentation, and they are unable to get a catheter into a catheterizable channel, a history of whether or not their urethra is open must be elicited. Urology should be consulted, and a catheter either through the channel or urethra can be attempted. If not, the bladder can be drained with a transabdominal needle. The best location for this to be placed is at the scar from a previous suprapubic catheter—this will be the safest location.

Suggested Readings and Key References

General

Lambert SM. Pediatric urological emergencies. *Pediatr Clin North Am* 2012;59:965–976.

Lao OB, Fitzgibbons RJ, Cusick RA. Pediatric inguinal hernias, hydroceles and undescended testicles. *Surg Clin North Am* 2012;92:487–504.

Leslie JA, Cain MP. Pediatric urological emergencies and urgencies. *Pediatr Clin of North Am* 2006;53:513–527.

Merriman LS, Herrel L, Kirsch AJ. Inguinal and genital anomalies. *Pediatr Clin North Am* 2012;59:769–781.

Sung EK, Setty BN, Castro-Aragon I. Sonography of the pediatric scrotum: emphasis on the Ts–torsion, trauma, and tumors. *AJR Am J Roentgenol* 2012;198:996–1003.

Penile Problems

American Academy of Pediatrics Task Force on Circumcision. Circumcision policy statement. *Pediatrics* 2012;130:585–586.

American Academy of Pediatrics Task Force on Circumcision. Male circumcision. *Pediatrics* 2012;130:e756–e785.

Brown-Trask B, Van Sell S, Carter S, et al. Circumcision care. *RN* 2009;72:22–28.

Donaldson JF, Rees RW, Steinbrecher HA. Response to commentary to priapism in children: a comprehensive review and clinical guideline. *J Pediatr Urol* 2014;10:11–25.

Rogers ZR. Priapism in sickle cell disease. *Hematol Oncol Clin North Am* 2005;19:917–928.

Testicular Problems

Barthold JS. Undescended testis: current theories of etiology. *Curr Opin Urol* 2008;18:395–400.

Da Justa DG, Granberg CF, Villanueva C, et al. Contemporary review of testicular torsion: new concepts, emerging technologies and potential therapeutics. *J Pediatr Urol* 2013;9:723–730.

Hutson JM, Clarke MC. Current management of the undescended testicle. *Semin Pediatr Surg* 2007;16:64–70.

Main KM, Skakkebaek NE, Toppari J. Cryptorchidism as part of the testicular dysgenesis syndrome: the environmental connection. *Endocr Dev* 2009;14:167–173.

Robinson SP, Hampton LJ, Koo HP. Treatment strategy for the adolescent varicocele. *Urol Clin North Am* 2010;37:269–278.

Female Emergencies

Van Eyk N, Allen L, Giesbrecht E, et al. Pediatric vulvovaginal disorders: a diagnostic approach and review of the literature. *J Obstet Gynaecol Can* 2009;31(9):850–862.

Vunda A, Vandertuin L, Gervaix A. Urethral prolapse: an overlooked diagnosis of urogenital bleeding in premenarcheal girls. *J Pediatr* 2011; 158:682–683.

Nephrolithiasis

Tasian GE, Copelovitch L. Evaluation and medical management of kidney stones in children. *J Urol* 2014;192:1329–1336.

Tasian GE, Cost NG, Granberg CF, et al. Tamsulosin and spontaneous passage of ureteral stones in children: a multi-institutional cohort study. *J Uro* 2014;192:506–511.

SURGICAL EMERGENCIES

CHAPTER 128 ■ MINOR LESIONS

SARITA CHUNG, MD

GOALS OF EMERGENCY CARE

A variety of minor lesions in children may prompt an emergency department (ED) visit. Most visits are the result of acute injury, infection, or combination of the two mechanisms (e.g., hair tourniquet, felon paronychia). Some formerly quiescent abnormalities (e.g., thyroglossal duct cyst, pyogenic granuloma) become clinically apparent after rapid enlargement secondary to infection or direct trauma. Alternatively, asymptomatic minor lesions (e.g., lipoma, pilomatrixoma) may be noted during the evaluation of an unrelated complaint. Regardless of the presentation, a systematic approach is necessary for proper diagnosis and subsequent management of these lesions. Although most "lumps and bumps" in children have a benign cause, the examiner should bear in mind the possibilities of associated systemic illness and future complications.

RELATED CHAPTERS

Signs and Symptoms

- Lymphadenopathy: Chapter 42
- Neck Mass: Chapter 43

Medical, Surgical, and Trauma Emergencies

- Dermatologic Urgencies and Emergencies: Chapter 96
- Endocrine Emergencies: Chapter 97
- Infectious Disease Emergencies: Chapter 102
- Hand Trauma: Chapter 117
- ENT Emergencies: Chapter 126
- Procedures: Chapter 141

HAND AND FOOT LESIONS

CLINICAL PEARLS AND PITFALLS

- Herpetic whitlow involving a finger is sometimes mistaken for a paronychia
- Consider hair tourniquets in the crying infant
- Ganglion cysts should not be ruptured in the ED but may require outpatient excision if painful or cosmetically concerning
- Trephination is treatment of choice for uncomplicated subungal hematomas with intact nail margins regardless of the size of the hematoma

Eponychia and Paronychia

Infections and/or minor trauma of the digits are the major etiologies of hand lesions in the emergency department (ED). The most common infections of the digits involve the eponychium (cuticle) as a result of a breakdown of the epidermal border due to trauma such as a traumatized hangnail or, particularly in children, finger sucking or nail biting. In its initial stage, the infection consists of a superficial cellulitis that remains localized to the cuticle and is termed an *eponychia*. Symptoms include erythema and localized pain at the nail margin. With progression, pus collects in a single thin-walled pocket under the cuticle, forming an acute paronychia (Fig. 128.1). Patients typically present with localized tenderness and have an area of fluctuance and purulence around the nail margin. This may progress, extending under the skin at the base of the nail, and along the nail fold. Less commonly, the pus burrows beneath the proximal nail, forming an *onychia* or subungual abscess. Causative organisms include *Staphylococcus aureus, Streptococcus pyogenes,* and anaerobic species. Chronic paronychia can be seen in patients repeatedly exposed to water or moist environments. Symptoms are present for weeks and are similar to those with acute paronychia. Eventually, the nail may become thickened and discolored. *Candida albicans* is the most frequent organism seen with chronic paronychia.

Treatment of a simple eponychia involves frequent warm soaks and attention to local hygiene. Topical antibacterial ointments may hasten resolution. Treatment of an acute paronychia is incision and drainage (Chapter 141 Procedures). If an onychia has formed, removal of the proximal portion of nail overlying the abscess is essential to ensure adequate drainage and prevent destruction of the germinal matrix. When an onychia forms under the anterolateral aspect of a nail, treatment consists of elevation and excision of the overlying portion of the nail. The role of oral antibiotics after incision and drainage has not been clearly established but does represent common practice. If the infection is due to finger biting or sucking, antibiotics providing coverage against anaerobes should be considered. Oral antimicrobial therapy is indicated for patients with associated lymphangitis. Coverage for methicillin-resistant *S. aureus* should be considered if there is clinical suspicion, high rate in the community or the infection is not improving. Treatment of chronic paronychia consists of topical steroids and/or antifungal agents.

Herpetic Whitlow

A *herpetic whitlow* involving a finger is sometimes mistaken for a paronychia and is the major differential diagnostic consideration. The majority of cases are in children younger than 2 years. Clinically, this lesion is characterized by the appearance of multiple, painful, thick-walled vesicles on erythematous bases most commonly located at the pulp space of the digits but can also occur around the nail folds and lateral aspects of the digit. During the ensuing few days, vesicles begin to coalesce and their contents become pustular (Fig. 128.2). A Gram stain of pustular fluid is negative for bacteria. If a Tzanck prep of scrapings from the base of a lesion is performed, it will reveal multinucleated giant cells. Subsequently, ulceration and crusting occur. The process initially results from inoculation of herpes simplex virus into a small break in the skin. The source may be

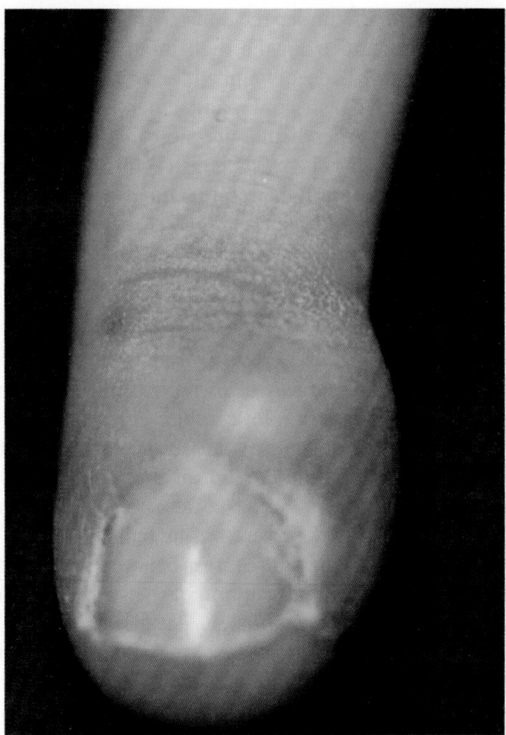

FIGURE 128.1 Paronychia of the finger. (From Salimpour RR, Salimpour P, Salimpour P. *Photographic Atlas of Pediatric Disorders and Diagnosis*, 1st ed. Philadelphia, PA: Lippincott Williams & Wilkins, 2013.)

a parent with herpes labialis, or a child with herpetic gingivostomatitis or herpes labialis may inoculate his or her own finger. With primary infection, fever and regional adenopathy are seen. With recurrences, these findings are usually absent.

The course is usually self-limited. However, oral acyclovir may be given in the first few days of the infection to shorten the course. For the immunocompromised patient, parenteral acyclovir should be considered to prevent dissemination. A complication of herpetic whitlow is bacterial superinfection.

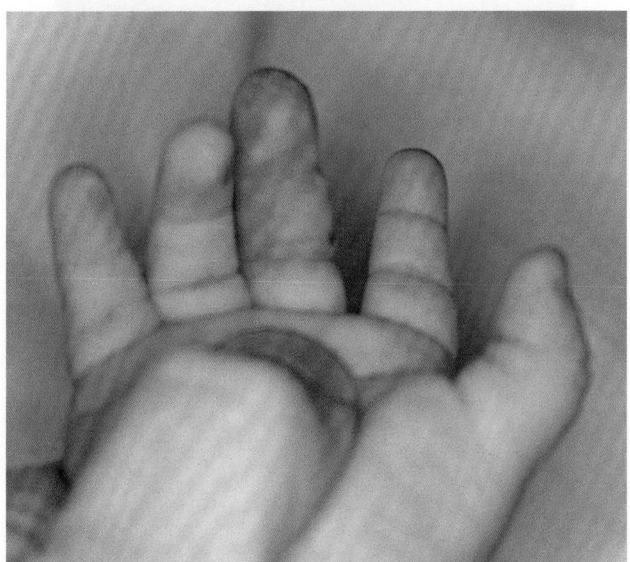

FIGURE 128.2 Herpetic whitlow. (From Fleisher GR, Ludwig W, Baskin MN. *Atlas of Pediatric Emergency Medicine*. Philadelphia, PA: Lippincott Williams & Wilkins, 2004.)

Felon

A *felon* consists of a deep infection of the distal pulp space of a fingertip. Felons are caused by introduction of bacteria into the pulp space, usually by punctures (which may be trivial) or splinters. Causative organisms are similar to those found in eponychial infections. A felon typically presents as an exquisitely tender and throbbing fingertip that is swollen, tense, warm, and erythematous. However, its evolution is usually relatively slow, beginning with mild pain and minimal swelling that progress over a few days. This process is in part caused by the anatomy of the pulp, which consists of multiple closed spaces formed by fibrous septae that connect the volar skin to the periosteum of the distal phalanx. With progression of infection, pressure buildup within these small compartments may cause local ischemia. In some cases, organisms may spread to invade the phalanx, resulting in osteomyelitis. In others, the process may point outward to the center of the touch pad, where the septae are least dense, producing an obvious area of fluctuation. Because the deep septal attachments are distal to the distal interphalangeal (DIP) joint and flexor tendon sheath, there is less risk of spread to these structures.

Treatment consists of incision, blunt dissection, and drainage. Digital blocks are favored for analgesia. A longitudinal incision over the area of maximal tension or fluctuance is the procedure of choice. If swelling is greatest laterally, an incision along the ulnar surface of the second through fourth digit or radial side of pinky or thumb may be preferred. Care should be taken to extend the incision past the DIP joint to prevent formation of a flexion contracture (see Chapter 141 Procedures). After drainage, a course of oral antibiotics is indicated. Close follow-up is essential to assess response to therapy and identify complications, such as septic arthritis and suppurative tenosynovitis. A hand specialist should be consulted for patients presenting with fever, lymphangitis, or evidence of osteomyelitis for admission, parenteral antibiotics, and definitive care.

Subungual Hematoma

A *subungual hematoma* is a collection of blood located under a nail that arises after trauma to the nail bed, typically due to a crush injury. Because this mechanism is also a common cause of phalangeal fractures, radiographs are advisable. The patient experiences throbbing pain that worsens with increasing pressure as more blood collects. If the subungual hematoma involves more than 50% of a nail surface, is associated with a distal phalanx fracture, or the nail or its margins are disrupted, the presence of a significant nail bed injury should be suspected. Nail trephination provides drainage with relief of pressure and pain. This procedure also reduces risk of secondary infection. This treatment alone suffices for uncomplicated subungual hematomas with intact nail margins, regardless of size of the hematoma. The trephined opening should be large enough (larger than 3 to 4 mm) to allow for ongoing drainage without risk of closure by a new clot. Sometimes producing two openings in the nail will promote more complete drainage (see Chapters 117 Hand Trauma and 141 Procedures). When the nail or its margins are disrupted and/or a displaced phalangeal fracture is present, the nail should be removed and the nail bed repaired. Antimicrobial prophylaxis for these injuries remains a source of controversy but is often prescribed for patients with underlying fractures and those with severe soft-tissue injuries.

Subungual Foreign Body

Foreign bodies such as a wood splinter or metallic shaving become embedded under the nail and may be the source of pain and/or infection. When the foreign body is only partially embedded, the nail can be trimmed close to the nail bed, and the object's projecting end grasped with splinter forceps and gently extracted. If a portion remains or the foreign body is deeply embedded from the outset, a digital block should be performed. Then the part of the nail overlying the object can be shaved down with a scalpel until the foreign body is exposed. Alternatively, the nail can be lifted and the object removed (see Chapter 141 Procedures). After splinter removal, the finger should be soaked in warm, soapy water, and an antibiotic ointment and protective dressing applied. Soaks should be repeated three times daily at home for the ensuing 3 to 5 days. In the unusual case of a child with multiple subungual splinters or fragments, it is best to remove the nail, clean out the foreign material, irrigate thoroughly, and then replace the nail (after trephining it to allow drainage).

Hair Tourniquet

A *hair tourniquet* injury is unique to pediatrics. It involves strangulation of a digit (or occasionally genitalia) by a hair or fine thread. It is seen most commonly in young infants and can be the cause of unexplained irritability or crying. The mechanism involves entwinement of the hair around an infant's digit. This may occur during a bath, or as a result of wiggling of the toes in a sock, bootie, or mitten that inadvertently has a hair or loose thread in it. A hair shed from a parent during diapering is the probable source of penile tourniquets. As the hair or thread becomes more tightly entwined, it produces a tourniquet effect, impairing blood flow with resultant ischemic pain and distal swelling. When noted early, the hair is often visible in a crease just proximal to the swollen area. If seen later, the hair may have cut through the skin, making it difficult to visualize (Fig. 128.3). In rare cases, frank ischemic necrosis of the distal digit may be seen on presentation. Removal requires a fine-tipped forceps and the aid of a thin loupe or probe that is inserted proximally under the constricting hair. Usually the hair can be unwound from the digit intact or cut with scissors. When the hair is deeply embedded or there is any question of a remaining constricting band, a nerve block should be performed and a perpendicular incision made over the hair. To avoid damage to neurovascular structures, such an incision should be made on the lateral or ulnar aspect of a finger or toe at 3 or 9 o'clock or at 4 or 8 o'clock along the penile shaft. When the entire hair cannot be removed with certainty, consultation with a plastic surgeon is indicated.

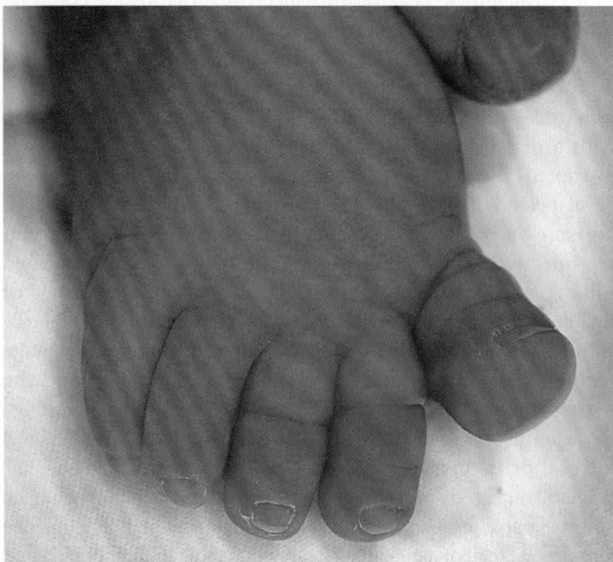

FIGURE 128.3 Hair tourniquets. (From Fleisher GR, Ludwig S, Baskin MN. *Atlas of Pediatric Emergency Medicine*. Philadelphia, PA: Lippincott Williams & Wilkins, 2004.)

Ganglion

A *ganglion* is a cystic outgrowth or protrusion of the synovial lining of a tendon sheath or joint capsule. Common locations of ganglions include the dorsal or volar surface of the wrist (usually on the radial side), the dorsum of the foot, and near the malleolus of an ankle (Fig. 128.4). Occasionally, a flexor tendon sheath ganglion may present on the palmar surface of the hand at the base of a digit. The cause is believed to involve prior trauma that causes partial disruption of the synovium and subsequent herniation of synovial tissue. The cysts are soft, slightly fluctuant, and transilluminate. Most are painless or only mildly uncomfortable. However, those on the foot or ankle may cause pain when shoes are worn. Elective surgical excision with obliteration of the base is indicated only if function is impaired or the lesion is of cosmetic significance. Even then, up to 20% recur. Striking the cyst with a heavy object, an old fashion folk remedy, should be strongly discouraged because the cystic fluid may be dispersed through the surrounding soft tissue, inciting diffuse scar formation.

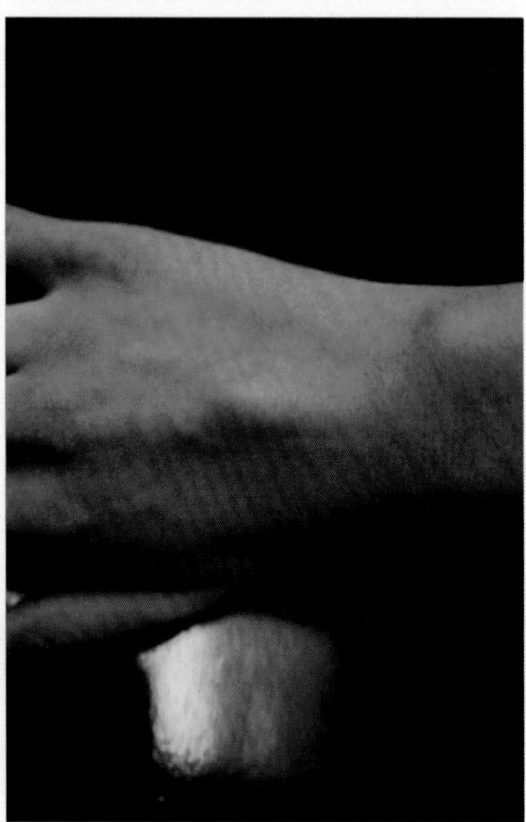

FIGURE 128.4 Ganglion cyst. (From Salimpour RR, Salimpour P, Salimpour P. *Photographic Atlas of Pediatric Disorders and Diagnosis*. 1st ed. Philadelphia, PA: Lippincott Williams & Wilkins, 2013.)

FACE AND SCALP LESIONS

CLINICAL PEARLS AND PITFALLS

- Epidermal inclusion and dermoid cyst are slow-growing nonmalignant painless lesions
- Superinfected cysts or congenital lesions may undergo incision and drainage and are treated with antibiotics before complete excision is recommended

Epidermal Inclusion Cyst

Among the most common postpubescent skin lesions is the *epidermal inclusion cyst* (EIC). These have also been termed *epithelial, sebaceous, and pilar cysts.* Most result from occlusion of pilosebaceous follicles, although some stem from inoculation of epidermal cells into the dermis via needlestick or other trauma. A few may arise from epidermal cells that become trapped along embryonic lines of closure. Lesions consist of firm, slow-growing, 1- to 3-cm, round nodules. Most are solitary lesions found about the scalp and face, although they also may be located on the trunk, neck, and scrotum. Histologically, these dermal and subcutaneous nodules consist of epidermally lined keratin-filled cysts. Presentation is that of a slow-growing painless lump that may provoke concerns of malignancy. At times, these cysts become acutely infected, and the patient complains of pain, erythema, and sudden increase in size. Infected cysts should be incised and drained, as well as treated with oral antibiotics before elective excision. Noninflamed cysts can be referred for elective excision that must include the entire sac to prevent recurrence.

When a patient presents with multiple large EICs, Gardner's syndrome should be suspected. This autosomal dominant disorder is characterized by multiple EICs, intestinal polyposis, desmoid tumors, and osseous lesions. Early diagnosis is especially important because of a 50% risk of malignant transformation of the intestinal polyps.

Dermoid Cyst

Dermoid cysts are congenital, subcutaneous nodules derived from ectoderm and mesoderm. There is a male predominance. They, too, are lined with epithelium, but unlike EICs, they may contain multiple adnexal structures such as hair, glands, teeth, bone, and neural tissue, as well as keratin. The cysts usually present as solitary, round, firm nodules with a rubbery or doughy consistency on palpation, a smooth surface, and normal overlying skin. Lesions tend to grow slowly, and malignant transformation is rare. Whereas some dermoids may be mobile, many are fixed to overlying skin or underlying periosteum. Occasionally, dermoids may have deeper attachments extending intracranially or intraspinally, along with an accompanying sinus. Because these cysts form along areas of embryonic fusion, common sites include the nasal bridge, midline neck, or scalp; the lateral brow (Fig. 128.5); anterior margin of the sternocleidomastoid; and midline scrotum or sacrum. An external ostium may or may not be visible. A small percentage of patients with dermoid cysts may have other craniofacial abnormalities. Because the sinus tract can serve as a conduit for spread of secondary infection, all midline lesions should have appropriate imaging (computed tomography [CT] and/or magnetic resonance imaging [MRI]) followed by elective excision.

Nasal Bridge Lesions

Midline nasal masses in infants and children may be acquired (e.g., EIC) or congenital, the latter stemming from improper embryologic development (e.g., dermoid cyst, encephalocele, glioma).

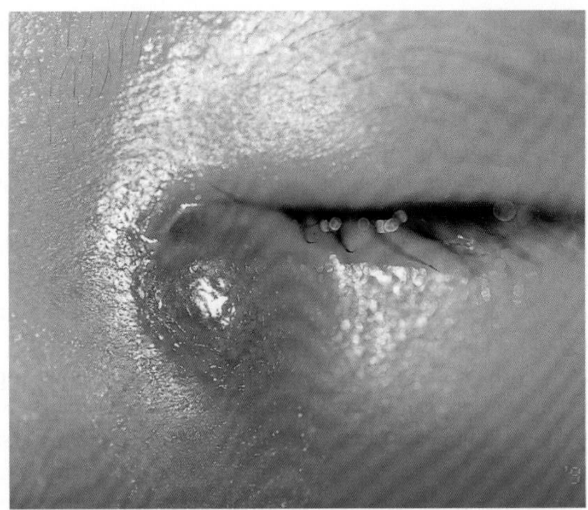

FIGURE 128.5 Dermoid cyst abscess. (From Fleisher GR, Ludwig W, Baskin MN, eds. *Atlas of pediatric emergency medicine.* Philadelphia, PA: Lippincott Williams & Wilkins, 2004. Reprinted with permission.)

Dermoids are the most common embryologically derived midline nasal lesions (see previous discussion). Clinically, a firm, round, subcutaneous mass is seen in the midline over the dorsum of the nose. Some have an overlying dimple, which may have an extruding hair (Fig. 128.6). Its attachment may extend only to the nasal septum or may go deeper through the cribriform plate into the calvarium. Because of their proximity to the nasopharynx, these dermoids are particularly prone to secondary infection and fistula formation. Hence, prompt excision is indicated after careful MRI or CT.

Gliomas are benign growths composed of ectopic neural tissue. The lesion usually consists of a firm, gray, or red–gray

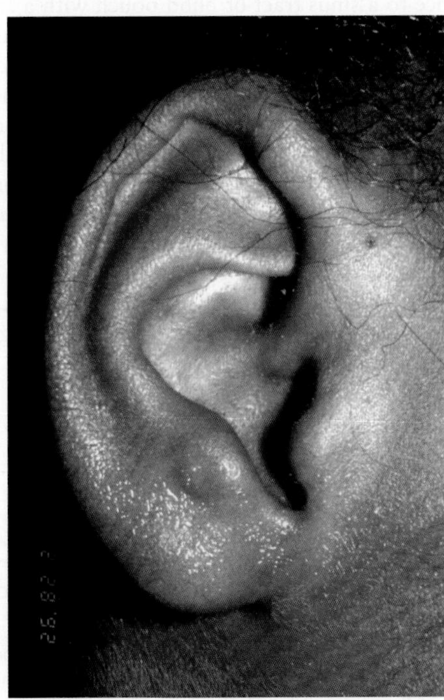

FIGURE 128.6 Preauricular surface pit. (Courtesy of David Tunkel, MD. In: Chung EK, Atkinson-McEvoy LR, Lai NL, et al., eds. *Visual Diagnosis and Treatment in Pediatrics.* 3rd ed. Philadelphia, PA: Wolters Kluwer Health, 2014.)

nodule, ranging in size from 1 to 5 cm and can be mistaken for a hemangioma. Most are extranasal (60%), occurring on the bridge of the nose. The remainders are either solely intranasal masses (30%) or have both intranasal and extranasal elements (10%). By definition, they do not have intracranial communication. They are composed of neural and fibrous tissue, covered by nasal mucosa. There is a male predominance. To prevent possible distortion of surrounding bone and cartilage, surgical excision is the treatment of choice.

Encephaloceles consist of neural tissue that has herniated through a congenital defect in the midline of the calvarium, and thus, always have an intracranial communication. Lesions appear as soft, at times pulsatile, compressible masses that enlarge with crying or straining. Compression of the jugular veins (Furstenberg test) may also cause the mass to expand in size. Some infants with nasal encephaloceles are born with overt craniofacial deformities and a rounded swelling at the base of the nose, whereas in others, the mass is confined to the nasopharynx, and external facial features are normal. The latter may present with signs of persistent nasal obstruction. In these patients, a grapelike mass is found on nasopharyngoscopy. MRI is the modality of choice for differentiating encephaloceles from other midline nasal masses and for determining their size and extent. Neurosurgical evaluation and management is indicated for all encephaloceles.

Preauricular Lesions

Preauricular lesions, located just anterior to the tragus, may be the result of imperfect fusion of the first two branchial arches (sinus tract, pit) or may consist of first arch remnants (cutaneous tag). They may be unilateral or bilateral, single or multiple. Usually, they are seen as isolated minor anomalies, but on occasion they can be found in association with other developmental anomalies involving the first branchial arch or in infants with chromosomal disorders. Most lesions are evident shortly after birth. Some individuals simply have a surface pit or dimple, whereas in others, the overlying dimple represents the entrance to a sinus tract or blind pouch with a small cyst at its base (Fig. 128.6). The latter may contain hair and other epidermal elements. Sinuses are prone to infection and abscess formation, whereupon the child presents with sudden enlargement of a painful preauricular mass and overlying erythema. When this occurs, the patient should be treated with appropriate antimicrobial therapy before elective excision of the cyst and fistula tract. Cutaneous tags, also called *accessory auricles,* are flesh-colored pedunculated lesions that may or may not have a cartilaginous component (Fig. 128.7). Some with narrow bases may simply be tied off with silk sutures. Those with wider bases and those containing cartilage can be referred for elective excision for cosmetic reasons.

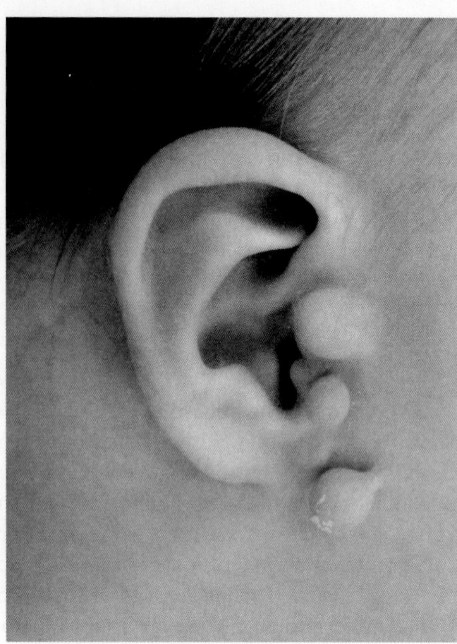

FIGURE 128.7 Multiple preauricular skin tags. (Courtesy of David Tunkel, MD.)

NECK LESIONS

CLINICAL PEARLS AND PITFALLS

- Parotitis is most commonly viral, and treatment involves supportive care including (citric or sour) food to facilitate salivary flow.
- Avoid incision and drainage of facial abscesses near the ramus of the mandible, as they may represent an infected first branchial cleft remnant.
- When torticollis is associated with a neck mass, sternocleidomastoid tumor (fibromatosis colli) should be considered in infants.
- Posterior triangle and supraclavicular masses carry a much higher risk for neoplasm than do anterior triangle masses.
- Consider treatment for methicillin resistant S. aureus in acute lymphadenitis if the infection is not improving after treatment or there is a high prevalence in the area.
- Consider an evaluation for pyriform sinus fistulas in children with acute suppurative thyroiditis.

Neck lesions in children may be of congenital origin or may be acquired as the result of an inflammatory process (Fig. 128.8). Although malignancy is a much rarer cause of neck masses in children, it must always be considered in the differential diagnosis. Neck masses or lesions are most conveniently divided into those occurring in the midline and those located in the lateral aspects of the neck (see Chapters 43 Neck Mass and 126 ENT Emergencies).

Midline Neck Lesions

Submental lymphadenitis or *lymphadenopathy* occurs in the midline just beneath the chin. Nodal enlargement stems from drainage of primary infection of the lower lip, buccal floor, or anterior tongue.

Dermoid cysts (see "Face and Scalp Lesions" section) can occur throughout the midline of the neck but are usually found above the area of the hyoid. They may also be found more laterally along the anterior border of the sternocleidomastoid.

Thyroglossal duct cysts are among the more common midline neck masses in children. Approximately 40% present before 10 years of age. They are composed of an ectodermal ductal remnant that fails to regress after fetal descent of the thyroid gland. They may occur anywhere along the path of descent of the thyroid, from the foramen cecum at the base of the tongue to the sternal notch, although most are found near the level of the hyoid bone. Presentation is usually that of a painless, smooth, mobile, cystic mass that is located in the midline or just slightly off-center (Fig. 128.9). Because of its intimate association with the hyoid, the mass moves with protrusion of the tongue or swallowing. On occasion, an

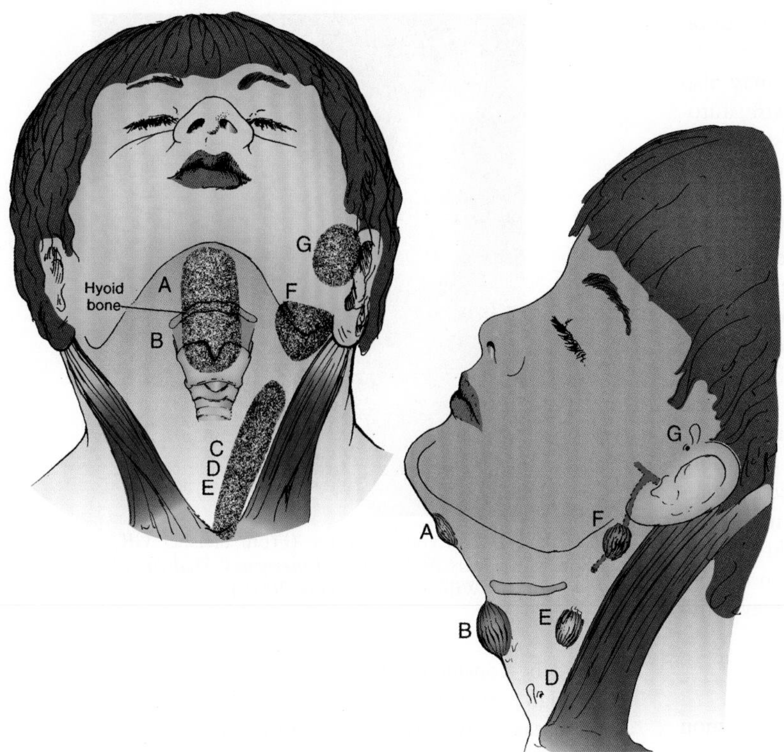

FIGURE 128.8 Head and neck congenital lesions seen in children in frontal and lateral views. The shaded areas denote the distribution in which a given lesion may be found. (**A**), dermoid cyst; (**B**), thyroglossal duct cyst; (**C**), second branchial cleft appendage; (**D**), second branchial cleft sinus; (**E**), second branchial cleft cyst; (**F**), first branchial pouch defect; (**G**), preauricular sinus or appendage.

overlying pore is present. Some cysts go unnoticed until infection occurs, causing acute swelling, pain, and erythema of the overlying skin. Patients with asymptomatic thyroglossal duct cysts should be referred for elective surgical excision. If the thyroglossal duct cyst is infected on presentation, excision is deferred until appropriate antimicrobial therapy is completed and inflammation has subsided. If incision and drainage are required during treatment, the patient should be referred to a surgeon comfortable with thyroid anatomy. Elective excision involves removal of the cyst, the entire duct to the level of the foramen cecum, and the midportion of the hyoid bone. On rare occasions, ectopic thyroid tissue in a thyroglossal duct cyst is the patient's only functioning thyroid. Therefore,

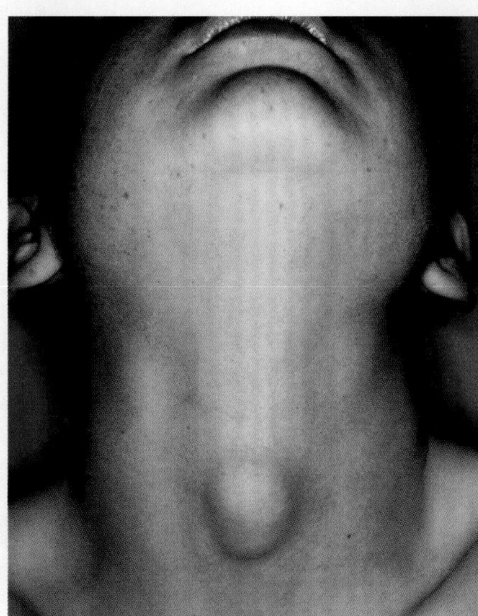

FIGURE 128.9 Thyroglossal duct cyst. (From Snell RS. *Clinical anatomy*, 7th ed. Baltimore, MD: Lippincott Williams & Wilkins; 2005:CD418. Used with permission.)

ultrasound or radioisotope scanning is recommended to confirm the presence of a normal thyroid gland before surgery.

Diffuse enlargement of the thyroid gland, or *goiter,* may be the result of infiltration, inflammation, or overstimulation of the gland. By far, the most common cause of pediatric thyroid enlargement is chronic *lymphocytic thyroiditis* (also called *Hashimoto's thyroiditis* or *autoimmune thyroiditis*). This disorder is characterized by a defect in cell-mediated immunity that results in lymphocytic infiltration of the thyroid gland. Female population is affected predominantly, and peak occurrence is during adolescence. Autoimmune thyroiditis has been associated with other autoimmune diseases such as chronic urticaria and diabetes. Usual presentation is one of a slow-growing, painless midline neck mass. Occasionally, a patient may complain of sore throat. Examination reveals a firm, nontender, diffusely enlarged gland in most affected children, but approximately one-third will have some lobular or nodular enlargement. Evaluation includes assessment of thyroid function and the detection of thyroid autoantibodies in the serum. Most patients with lymphocytic thyroiditis are euthyroid. When thyroid dysfunction is present, it usually takes the form of hypothyroidism. Any degree of nodularity of the gland warrants further investigation to rule out malignancy.

Inflammation of the thyroid gland secondary to infection, *acute suppurative thyroiditis,* is a rare cause of diffuse thyroid enlargement that can be associated with an underlying pyriform sinus fistula. Presentation usually follows an upper respiratory tract infection or otitis media and is characterized by abrupt appearance of a painful, tender, swollen mass in the region of the thyroid. Systemic illness in the form of fever and chills and severe dysphagia are often present. Flexion of the neck may alleviate pain, whereas extension worsens it. The etiologic agents include *S. aureus* and oropharyngeal flora. Appropriate broad-spectrum parenteral antimicrobial therapy is usually sufficient to eradicate the infection. Abscess formation necessitates incision and drainage by a surgeon comfortable with thyroid anatomy. Evaluation with a CT or esophagography should include identification of a pyriform sinus fistula after resolution of infection to prevent recurrences.

Acute immune stimulation of the thyroid gland may also produce diffuse thyroid enlargement. In *Graves' disease,* autoantibody attachment to the thyrotropin receptor stimulates an increase in thyroid hormone synthesis and release. Patients may initially have a history of changes of behavior, decrease in school performance, and/or increase in linear growth. On presentation, patients will have a symmetrically enlarged smooth nontender goiter and signs of thyrotoxicosis, including tachycardia, nervousness, tremor, hypertension, exophthalmos, and increased appetite. A thyroid bruit may be auscultated in 50% of patients. An elevated T_4 in the context of a low TSH level and presence of TSH receptor antibodies confirms the diagnosis. Consultation with a pediatric endocrinologist is indicated.

Solitary nodular thyroid masses deserve careful attention. Although most are secondary to chronic lymphocytic thyroiditis or consist of a benign adenoma, the incidence of malignant neoplasms is actually higher in children with thyroid nodules than in adults. Hence, every thyroid nodule found in a child merits a complete evaluation that may include a TSH level and ultrasound-guided biopsy.

Lateral Neck Lesions

Enlarged cervical lymph nodes constitute the most common lateral neck masses in children. Knowledge of the anatomy of the cervical lymphatics is of fundamental importance to understanding processes that cause enlargement of cervical lymph nodes. This section focuses mainly on local processes that cause nodal enlargement, but it is important to note that many systemic infections and inflammatory disorders can cause diffuse adenopathy that includes the cervical chain (see Chapter 42 Lymphadenopathy). Therefore, any child with a neck mass deserves a complete examination to look for the presence of generalized adenopathy and other signs of systemic disease.

Reactive cervical adenopathy refers to mild enlargement of cervical lymph nodes that accompanies a viral or bacterial upper respiratory tract infection. Involved nodes are typically located in the upper portion of the cervical chain. They are usually discrete, firm, mobile, and less than 2 cm in diameter. They may be mildly tender but have no overlying erythema, edema, or warmth. Regression within 1 to 2 weeks of resolution of the primary infection is the rule, although occasionally mild enlargement of the node may persist, if fibrosis has occurred.

Local infection of a lymph node itself is termed *acute lymphadenitis.* The involved node is solitary, typically 2 to 3 cm or larger in diameter, and extremely tender. As the infection proceeds, overlying swelling, erythema, and warmth develop and become more pronounced (Fig. 128.10). Initially the node is firm, but later it may become fluctuant if the node suppurates. Acute suppurative lymphadenitis is most often caused by streptococcal or staphylococcal organisms. Because of the high incidence of β-lactamase production by *S. aureus,* β-lactamase stable antibiotics (cephalexin or clindamycin) are the treatment of choice. Most patients respond to oral antimicrobial therapy and application of warm compresses. However, ultrasound may be indicated to establish if fluctuance has developed, and if so, if incision and drainage is warranted. Other potential causative organisms of acute, subacute, or chronic lymphadenitis include anaerobic bacteria, *Pasteurella multocida* (following animal bites), *Haemophilus influenzae, Streptococcus agalactiae, Francisella tularensis, Brucella* species, *Bartonella henselae* (cat-scratch disease), mycobacteria, and actinomycoses. Oral antimicrobial therapy for methicillin-resistant *S. aureus* (MRSA) should be considered if there is clinical suspicion, in regions with high prevalence, or if the infection is not improving. Kawasaki disease may also present with an acutely enlarged cervical node and should be considered when other clinical criteria are present (fever for more than 5 days, rash, conjunctivitis, extremity and oral changes, and hyperirritability).

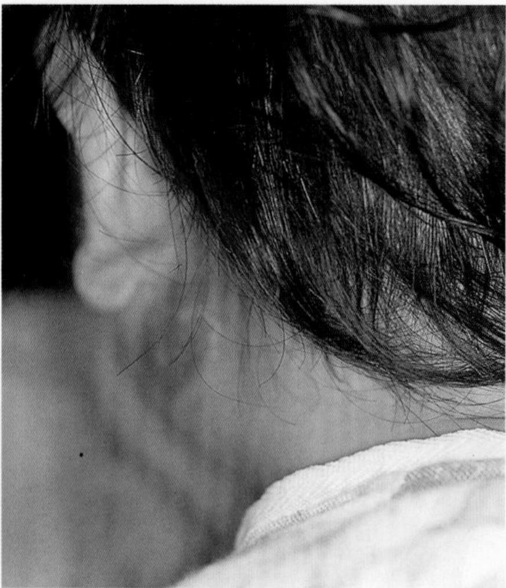

FIGURE 128.10 Lymphadenitis. (From Fleisher GR, Ludwig W, Baskin MN. *Atlas of Pediatric Emergency Medicine.* Philadelphia, PA: Lippincott Williams & Wilkins, 2004.)

Salivary gland infections, *sialadenitis,* and *parotitis,* may cause lateral neck or submental swelling. When the parotid gland is involved, firm indurated swelling is found extending in an arc from the preauricular area down under the ear and behind it. The degree of swelling is often sufficient to blunt the angle of the jaw, and the mass is usually mildly tender (Fig. 128.11). Patients complain of mild pain in the region of the pinna, which may increase with eating. Most salivary gland infections affect the parotid gland, with involvement

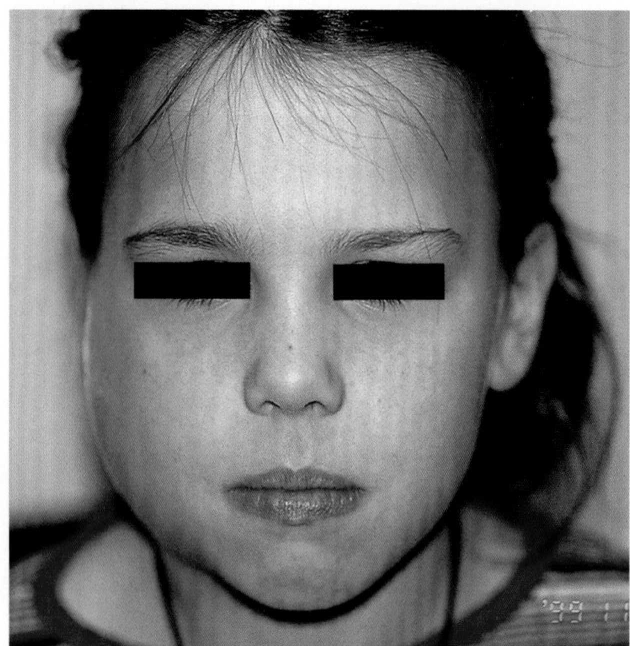

FIGURE 128.11 Parotitis. (From Fleisher GR, Ludwig W, Baskin MN. *Atlas of Pediatric Emergency Medicine.* Philadelphia, PA: Lippincott Williams & Wilkins, 2004.)

of the sublingual and submandibular glands being much less common. Viral agents (e.g., mumps virus, parainfluenza types 1 and 3, influenza A, Coxsackie virus A, and rarely, human immunodeficiency virus) cause most of these infections. Less commonly, parotitis is due to a bacterial agent such as *S. aureus*. In these cases, patients present with rapid gland enlargement and severe pain, and they often have high fever and signs of systemic toxicity. On examination, overlying erythema and exquisite tenderness are present, and purulent material can often be expressed from Stensen's duct by massaging the gland. An elevated amylase level can help confirm the diagnosis of parotitis. Symptomatic treatment of sialadenitis includes close attention to hydration and avoidance of foods that require excessive chewing. Sour foods may be used as sialogogues to hasten resolution. If bacterial sialadenitis or parotitis is suspected, β-lactamase stable parenteral antibiotics should be administered. Otolaryngologic consultation should be obtained if surgical drainage is needed because of the proximity of the facial nerve. Much less commonly, parotid gland swelling is of noninfectious origin. Causes include occlusion of Stensen's duct by a calculus and traumatic insufflation of the gland with forceful blowing (e.g., trumpet blowing) or, in rare instances, primary parotid neoplasms. Radiographs are highly sensitive for salivary stones though ultrasound can detect a range of pathologies and is radiation-sparing.

Cystic hygromas (lymphangiomas) represent malformations of the lymphatic system. They consist of dilated lymphatic channels and may be multiocular or unilocular. They occur most often in the posterior triangle of the neck (Fig. 128.12) but may be found in the axillae, groin, popliteal fossae, or on the chest or abdominal wall (Fig. 128.13). When found in the neck, extension of the mass into the anterior triangle, sublingual space, retropharyngeal space, or mediastinum is possible. Such infiltration can result in airway compromise and/or compression of vascular and neural structures. Most cystic hygromas are present at birth or become apparent shortly thereafter. Patients usually present with a slow-growing, painless neck mass that is soft and

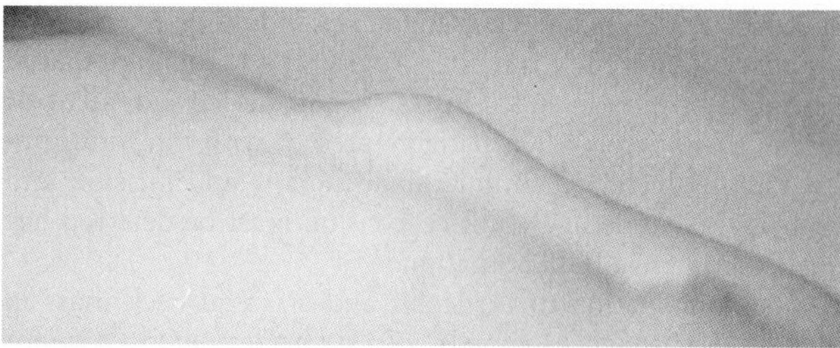

FIGURE 128.13 Lateral abdominal wall cystic hygroma (lymphangioma).

compressible, although some patients are brought for care because of sudden enlargement caused by secondary infection or hemorrhage within the lesion. Anatomic delineation of the mass is best performed with a MRI or CT. The potential risk to the airway and neurovascular structures, coupled with the possibilities of hemorrhage or lymphangitis, dictates the need for early intervention. Consultation with an otolaryngologist is indicated.

Branchial cleft anomalies consist of a group of congenital malformations, including subcutaneous cysts, sinus tracts, and cartilaginous remnants. They are caused by persistence of structures derived from the embryonic branchial arches. Of these anomalies, 90% arise from the second branchial arch and are found along the anterior border of the sternocleidomastoid muscle. Sinus tracts of second branchial arch remnants may end in an internal ostium located near the tonsillar fossa. Less commonly, first branchial arch anomalies may be noted as masses or sinus tracts near the mandibular ramus. Some first branchial arch remnants end in an internal ostium located in the external auditory canal. Branchial cleft anomalies may be noted shortly after birth either as a firm, mobile mass with or without an overlying pore, or simply as an external ostium or pore without an underlying mass (Fig. 128.14). More commonly, branchial cleft cysts are detected later in childhood when they may present as an asymptomatic mass or with acute painful enlargement as a result of secondary

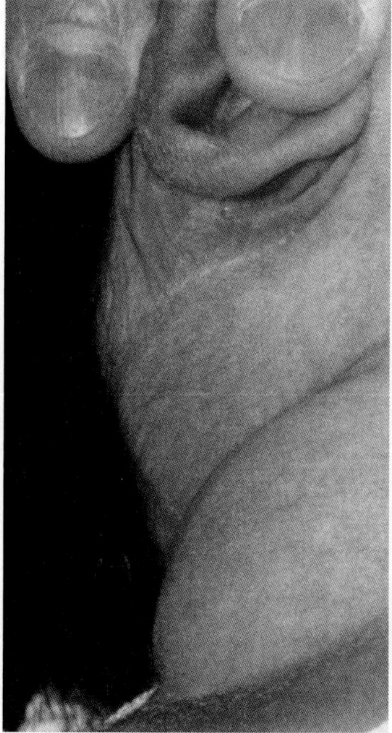

FIGURE 128.12 Lateral neck cystic hygroma (lymphangioma) in an infant.

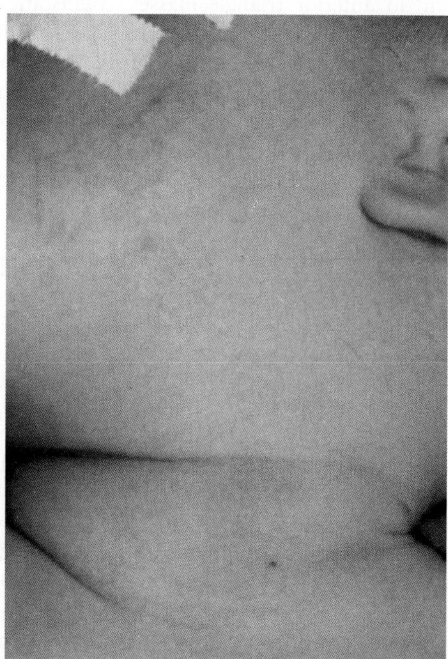

FIGURE 128.14 Second branchial cleft pit that had an underlying sinus tract.

infection. All branchial cleft anomalies should be referred for surgical excision for cosmetic purposes and to avoid potential morbidity, which includes infection and the development of carcinoma in situ. When patients present with infection, initial therapy included antimicrobial therapy and incision and drainage (if needed). Definitive excision must be deferred has quelled all signs of inflammation.

The combination of torticollis and a lateral neck mass in early infancy is highly suggestive of a *sternocleidomastoid tumor or fibromatosis colli of infancy* that can be associated with primiparous births, breech presentations, and difficult labor. Clinically, a nontender, firm, ovoid 1- to 3-cm mass is found along the middle third of the sternocleidomastoid muscle. The mass represents local muscle hemorrhage or infarction that subsequently undergoes fibrosis. It is believed to be the result of traumatic extraction of the head during delivery or secondary to fibrous dysplasia related to intrauterine positioning. Some are noted at birth, whereas others become apparent within the ensuing few weeks. The head is bent toward, and the chin away from, the affected side, and limitation of bending to the opposite side and rotation toward the involved side are noted. Initial treatment consists of passive stretching exercises and positioning of the infant so that he or she has to turn from the affected side to see others. If this fails, surgical release of the contracture is indicated to prevent secondary facial deformity with growth. Infants with this disorder should be carefully assessed for associated hip dysplasia, which coexists in up to 20% of cases.

The possibility of *malignancy* must be considered in the differential diagnosis of any child with a cervical mass. History regarding the presence of persistent fevers, malaise, night sweats, weight loss, and other constitutional symptoms should be sought, and the child assessed for presence of pallor, petechiae, generalized adenopathy, and hepatosplenomegaly. Primary lymphoid malignancies, such as leukemia and lymphoma, may present initially with a rapidly enlarging neck mass. In contrast to infectious adenopathy, involved nodes tend to be firm, matted, nontender, and poorly mobile. Posterior triangle and supraclavicular masses carry a much higher risk for neoplasm than do anterior triangle masses. Metastatic tumors, such as rhabdomyosarcoma and neuroblastoma, may also initially manifest as a neck mass. If malignancy is suspected, the ED workup should include complete blood cell count, electrolytes, uric acid, lactate dehydrogenase, liver function studies, heterophile antibody titer, and a chest radiograph. Further evaluation, including imaging and biopsy, should be performed in consultation with a pediatric oncologist.

SURFACE LESIONS

CLINICAL PEARLS AND PITFALLS

- Hemangiomas present at a young age and will initially become larger before involuting.
- While most surface lesions are not dangerous, a thorough history and physical exam should be performed to evaluate for associated systemic illnesses.
- Acute or persistent bleeding from a pyogenic granuloma often requires cauterization with silver nitrate or application of a hemostatic dressing.
- Neurofibroma can often be distinguished from other soft tissue lesion by their central invagination with digitation pressure (i.e. button holing).

Vascular Malformations

Vascular malformations result from errors in vascular morphogenesis. Unlike hemangiomas, they are present at birth, grow only in proportion to the child, and do not undergo regression. They may be of capillary, venous, or arterial origin or combinations of vessel types may exist within the same lesion. *Port-wine stains* are among the more common capillary vascular malformations. They have a characteristic deep red to purple hue (Fig. 128.15). Children with facial port-wine stains that lie in the distribution of the ophthalmic branch of the trigeminal nerve (which includes the forehead, upper eyelids, and nose) merit careful evaluation for associated anomalies. Specifically, *Sturge–Weber syndrome* is characterized by ipsilateral vascular angiomatosis of the leptomeninges and ocular vessels. Clinical manifestations may include seizures, mental retardation, hemiplegia, and glaucoma. Serial head CT scans performed on these children often demonstrate evolution of serpiginous calcifications and progressive atrophy of the cerebral cortex underlying the pial vascular malformations. Children with port-wine stains involving an extremity may develop hemihypertrophy of the affected limb because of an unusually rich underlying blood supply, known as *Klippel–Trenaunay–Weber syndrome*. All cosmetically significant port-wine lesions should be referred to a dermatologist (see Chapter 96 Dermatologic Urgencies and Emergencies).

Salmon patches, the most common form of vascular malformation seen in infancy, occur in 30% to 40% of all newborns. These flat pink lesions, which become more prominent with crying or exertion, are most commonly located on the nape of the neck (stork bites), on the glabella, or over the eyelids (angel kisses). They consist of distended dermal capillaries and almost always fade or disappear by the end of the first year of life, although nuchal salmon patches may persist into adulthood.

Hemangiomas

Hemangiomas, the most common benign neoplasm of infancy, occur in more than 10% of children younger than 1 year. Histologically, they are composed of hyperplastic vascular endothelium that develops from angioblastic tissue that has failed to connect normally with the vascular system during gestation. Although hemangiomas are rarely evident at birth (2.5%), most become apparent within the first month of life. There is an increased incidence in Caucasian, female, and premature infants.

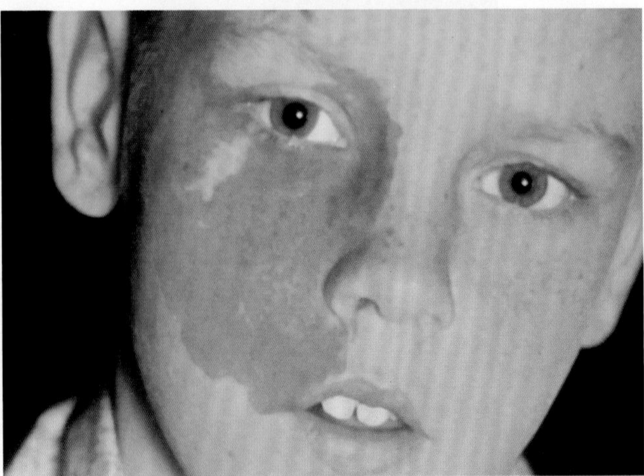

FIGURE 128.15 Facial port-wine stain. (From Weber J, Kelley J. *Health assessment in nursing*, 2nd ed. Philadelphia, PA: Lippincott Williams & Wilkins, 2003.)

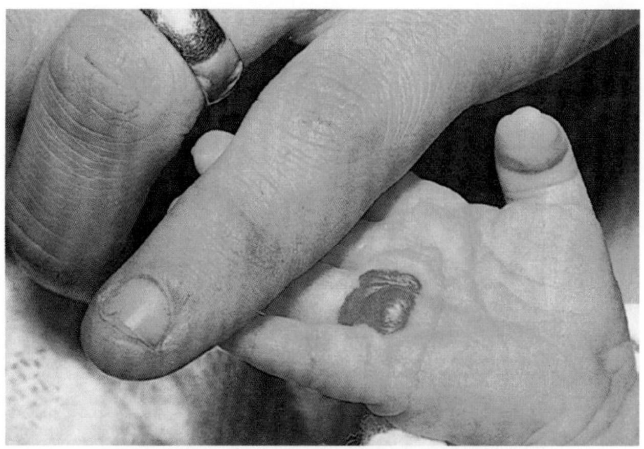

FIGURE 128.16 Superficial hemangioma of hand. (From O'Doherty N. *Atlas of the Newborn*. Philadelphia, PA: JB Lippincott, 1979.)

Sixty percent of all hemangiomas are located in the head/neck region. Lesions tend to undergo a period of rapid growth over the first 6 to 12 months, then plateau. Subsequently, a slow process of involution begins, usually by 18 months. Approximately 50% of lesions involute completely by 5 years of age, and 95% by 9 years of age. Hemangiomas can be subdivided into three types as follows:

1. *Superficial hemangiomas* are confined to the upper dermis. Formerly called *capillary* or *strawberry hemangiomas,* these lesions are red, raised, well demarcated, and compressible (Fig. 128.16).
2. *Deep hemangiomas* lie in the lower dermis or subcutaneous fat. They tend to have indistinct margins, and the overlying skin often has a bluish hue (Fig. 128.17).
3. On close inspection, many hemangiomas have a combination of both superficial and deep elements, and thus are called *mixed hemangiomas.*

Because of their natural history of ultimate regression, a combination of watchful waiting and parental reassurance remain the standard of care for most hemangiomas. However, active intervention is indicated for lesions that compromise vital structures (airway, eyes, nose); lesions that are susceptible to trauma, hemorrhage, or infection; and those that grow at an alarming rate. Infants who present with stridor at 6 to 12 weeks of age may have an undiagnosed laryngeal hemangioma. More than 50% of infants with laryngeal hemangiomas have cutaneous hemangiomas along the mandible and neck region in a "beard" distribution. Infants with large liver hemangiomas are at risk for congestive heart failure. Beta blockers may facilitate resolution, but should not be prescribed in the ED. Decisions regarding medical or interventional treatments are best made by a specialist in vascular anomalies.

Lipoma

Lipomas are benign subcutaneous tumors composed of mature adipose cells. They often present in adolescence as painless and usually solitary nodules. They may be located anywhere on the body. Clinically, lipomas are nontender and have a soft, rubbery consistency, often with lobulations. Overlying skin is normal and easily slides across the mass, which helps distinguish lipomas from other skin nodules such as pilomatricomas. *Angiolipomas* are a variant of lipoma that has a component of capillary proliferation. Unlike lipomas, they tend to be painful. Lesions that are cosmetically significant, large, or painful warrant elective surgical excision.

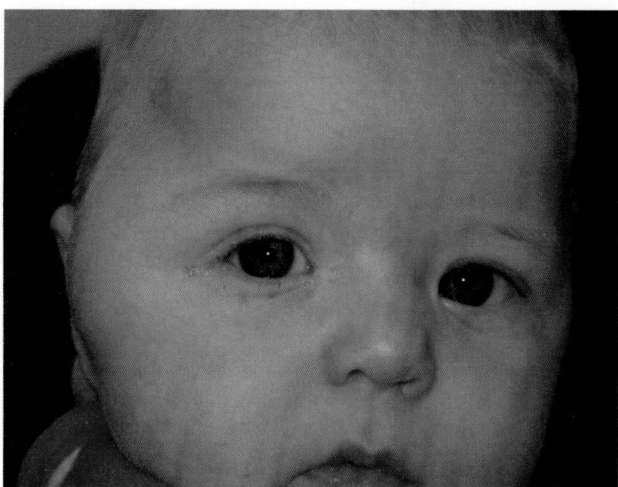

FIGURE 128.17 Deep hemangioma of face. (Courtesy of Andrea L. Zaenglein, MD. In: Chung EK, Atkinson-McEvoy LR, Lai NL, et al., eds. *Visual Diagnosis and Treatment in Pediatrics*. 3rd ed. Philadelphia, PA: Wolters Kluwer Health, 2014.)

Pilomatricoma

Pilomatricomas (calcifying epitheliomas) are relatively common lesions, accounting for 10% of superficial nodules seen in children. These benign tumors arise from cells of the hair matrix, hair cortex, or inner root sheath. Most are found on the head and neck, but some arise on the trunk and extremities. They appear as firm (resulting from calcification), solitary nodules ranging in size from 0.5 to 5 cm. An overlying bluish hue may help distinguish the lesion from other benign nodules such as epidermal or dermoid cysts. When pinched, the overlying skin "tents," providing another distinguishing feature. Multiple pilomatricomas have been associated with Gardner's syndrome, Steinert's disease, myotonic dystrophy, and sarcoidosis. Familial occurrences have been reported but are rare. If the lesion is located in a cosmetically sensitive area, elective surgical excision is the treatment of choice.

Pyogenic Granuloma

A *pyogenic granuloma* (also called *lobular capillary hemangioma*) is a benign vascular lesion most commonly found on exposed skin surfaces such as the face, hands, and forearms. Occasionally, lesions form on oral or nasal mucosal surfaces. They are composed of granulation tissue with significant vascular overgrowth and are considered the result of an exaggerated vascular growth factor response after local trauma. Lesions are usually solitary and pedunculated, measuring from 0.5 to 2 cm. At times, multiple satellite lesions are found around a central granuloma. The color and character of a pyogenic granuloma varies according to its stage of growth. Early on, the lesion appears as a glistening, red, polypoid nodule with a friable surface that bleeds easily. Later (weeks to months), the lesion becomes fibrotic and shrinks, taking on a reddish-brown hue. The most common reasons for presenting to the ED are bleeding or chronic oozing of an early lesion. Treatment in the ED consists of control of bleeding by direct pressure or silver nitrate cauterization of vessels at the base. Hemostatic dressings may also be helpful. Excision of the lesion merits referral to a dermatologist.

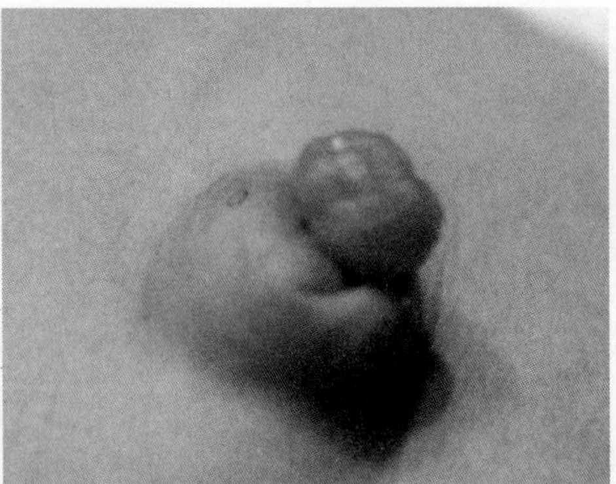

FIGURE 128.18 Large pedunculated umbilical granuloma that responded to suture ligation and repeated silver nitrate applications.

Umbilical Granuloma

An umbilical granuloma presents as a soft, friable, polypoid mass that is pink or dull red. It arises from the base of the umbilical stump and at times may be pedunculated with a short stalk (Fig. 128.18). It is the product of an exuberant granulation tissue reaction, probably secondary to excessive moisture and/or low-grade infection. Treatment of most lesions consists of cauterization with a silver nitrate stick. During this procedure, care should be taken to cover the skin of the umbilical rim with gauze to protect it from burns. Following cauterization, the lesion should be blotted dry to avoid seepage of excess silver nitrate to surrounding tissue which can lead to hyperpigmented staining. Home care consists of keeping the umbilicus clean and dry. Large granulomas may require repeated cautery at intervals of several days. Pedunculated granulomas are candidates for suture ligation (3-0 nylon). The parent is then instructed to return for follow-up for cauterization of the base (once the granuloma has necrosed and dropped off) to prevent recurrence. Umbilical granulomas must be differentiated from persistent embryonic remnants such as an *omphalomesenteric duct* or *patent urachus*. The presence of a central lumen or chronic discharge should prompt the clinician to consider these rare umbilical anomalies. The distinction is of great clinical significance because these problems may be associated with other congenital malformations, and surgical excision of the entire remnant is necessary to prevent sequelae, such as infection. Diagnosis is most commonly made by ultrasound.

Granuloma Annulare

The lesions of *granuloma annulare* are composed of infiltrates of lymphocytes and altered collagen within the dermis. They first appear as raised nodules that gradually expand centrifugally to form annular rings ranging from 1 to 5 cm in diameter. They have a firm, fibrous, sometimes-lumpy consistency on palpation. Overlying skin is usually normal or slightly hyperpigmented (Fig. 128.19). Although most are asymptomatic, a patient occasionally may report mild pruritus and present with superficial excoriation caused by scratching. The lack of an active microvesicular border, firm consistency on palpation, and the deeper dermal location of these lesions help distinguish them from *tinea corporis*. Lesions are commonly found on the extensor surfaces of the lower portions of legs and the dorsum of the hands and feet and, less often, on the trunk or abdominal wall. Although granuloma annulare may present at any age, more than 40% of cases appear before age 15. Because most lesions undergo resolution within 1 to 2 years, reassurance is usually all that is necessary. In the rare case of a patient with severe or widespread lesions, dermatologic consultation should be sought.

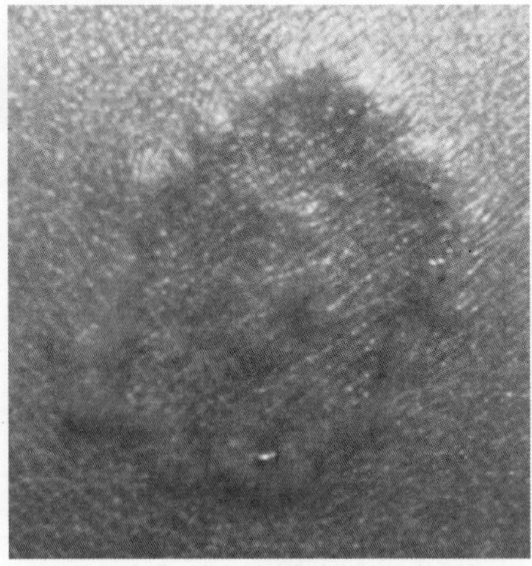

FIGURE 128.19 Granuloma annulare.

Juvenile Xanthogranuloma

Juvenile xanthogranulomas (JXG) present as nodular or plaque-like lesions with a firm or rubbery consistency. Initially reddish in color, they evolve to have a distinct yellow or orange hue (Fig. 128.20). Many are noted at birth, whereas others appear within the first several months. They range in diameter from 0.5 to 4 cm. Like hemangiomas, they tend to grow rapidly in infancy, then spontaneously regress in early childhood. Common sites include the scalp and face, proximal extremities, and occasionally, the subungual area of a digit or a mucocutaneous junction. Lesions may be solitary but are often present in groups. Histologically, xanthogranulomas are composed of lipid-laden macrophages or histiocytes within a granulomatous matrix whose inciting source is unknown. In rare cases, giant or disseminated lesions may occur. Patients who have multiple or diffuse lesions may also have ocular lesions, specifically lesions of the iris that have been associated with spontaneous anterior chamber hemorrhage and glaucoma. On occasion, ocular lesions have been misdiagnosed as

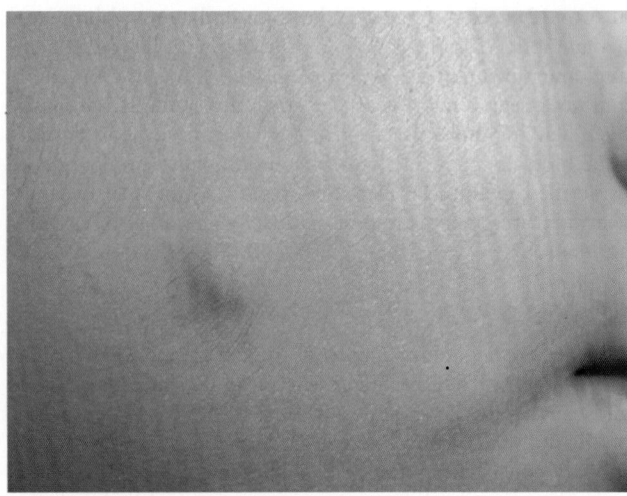

FIGURE 128.20 Yellow nodular lesion of juvenile xanthogranuloma. (From Burkhart C, Morrell D, Goldsmith LA, et al. *VisualDx: Essential Pediatric Dermatology*. Philadelphia, PA: Lippincott Williams & Wilkins, 2009.)

retinoblastoma. A systemic form of JXG exists, and affected patients may or may not have concomitant cutaneous findings. In this variant, noncutaneous lesions may involve the brain, heart, liver, spleen, and lungs. Children who have both JXG and neurofibromatosis are at a much higher risk for unusual forms of leukemia and thus should be appropriately monitored. Last, unlike children with disseminated xanthomas, there is no relationship between JXG and lipid abnormalities. All children with suspected xanthogranuloma should undergo biopsy. An ophthalmologic evaluation is necessary if JXG is confirmed, and careful observation for evidence of systemic involvement is warranted.

Neurofibroma

A neurofibroma may present as a solitary lesion in an otherwise normal patient or as a feature of neurofibromatosis type I. Cutaneous neurofibromas arise from nerve sheath cells located in the dermis. They appear as pink or flesh-colored nodules that are soft and range in size from 0.5 to 3 cm. Most do not appear until adolescence. Multiple neurofibromas should raise the suspicion for von Recklinghausen disease. Lesions may be confused with angiolipomas and hemangiomas; however, a distinguishing feature is the tendency of neurofibromas to be especially soft centrally and i[illegible] with digital pressure, described as "button-holing.[illegible] excision is indicated only if the lesion is compressin[illegible] causing nerve root pain, because excision is often fo[illegible] recurrence of an even larger lesion.

Keloid/Hypertrophic Scar

Exaggerated proliferation of fibrous connective ti[illegible] process of cutaneous wound healing results in fo[illegible] *hypertrophic scars* and *keloids*. Wounds involving areas of skin that are thick or under high tension (shoulders, back, chest, or chin) are at greatest risk. The ear lobe is another commonly affected site. Individuals with dark skin are much more susceptible to abnormal scarring, which has its highest incidence in adolescence and early adulthood. Hypertrophic scars remain confined to the area of original injury. They are rarely painful and tend to undergo slow regression over 6 to 12 months. In contrast, keloids extend beyond the original wound margins and rarely regress spontaneously. Initially, keloids may be painful and tender or pruritic. They have a rubbery consistency on palpation and a smooth pink surface (Fig. 128.21). Ear piercing, tattooing, and elective cosmetic procedures should be avoided in persons who have a tendency to form keloids. Keloids can be treated with topical or intralesional steroid injections in addition to surgical excision, though recurrence is common. Severe keloids should be referred to a dermatologist or plastic surgeon for further treatment.

Lumbosacral Lesions

Pilonidal dimples, typically located in the midline in the sacrococcygeal area, are benign lesions of no clinical significance. On close inspection, there is no evidence of a central pore or opening. In contrast, pilonidal sinuses, which are found in the same area, do have a small surface opening to a tract lined by stratified squamous epithelium that extends toward, but not into, the spinal canal. In some instances, sinuses appear to be of embryonic origin, stemming from either an abnormality of midline fusion or invagination of ectodermal elements. The base of such a lesion may consist of a small cyst containing products of skin cells and epithelial appendages, including hair. In other cases, the source may be a distorted hair follicle. Pilonidal sinuses and cysts are asymptomatic until the sinus [illegible]nd/or infected. This phenomenon is most [illegible]g adolescence or early adulthood. Male [illegible]ore commonly affected than female pop[illegible]t, hirsutism, and a sedentary lifestyle or [illegible]ires prolonged sitting also appear to be [illegible]

[illegible]ns usually gain access through the exter[illegible]e infection occurs, an abscess forms and [illegible]idly. Because the overlying skin is thick, [illegible] occur deep to the skin surface, and acquired sinus tracts may form external to the postsacral fascia. Patients typically complain of low back pain, increased on sitting, and local tenderness. On examination, a tender, indurated swelling is noted overlying the sacrococcygeal area with the original sinus at its cephalad end (Fig. 128.22). Treatment consists of incision and drainage with careful probing to break up loculations and extract any hairs present because these act

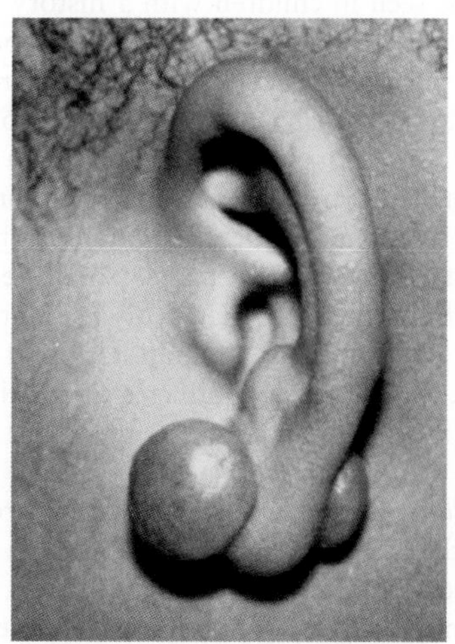

FIGURE 128.21 Large keloid that formed after ear piercing in a susceptible child.

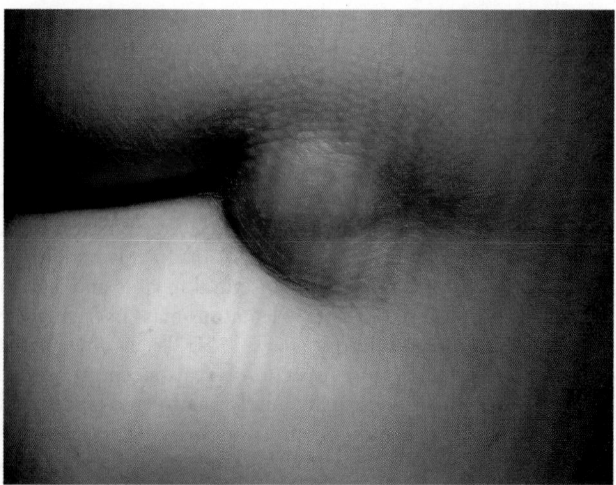

FIGURE 128.22 Infected pilonidal cyst. (Courtesy of Scott VanDuzer, MD. In: Chung EK, Boom JA, Datto GA, et al., eds. *Visual Diagnosis in Pediatrics*. Philadelphia, PA: Lippincott Williams & Wilkins, 2006.)

SURGICAL EMERGENCIES

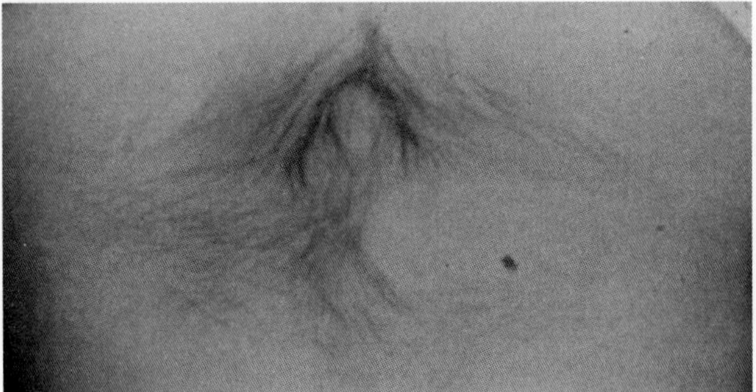

FIGURE 128.23 Lumbosacral hairy patch in a patient with diastematomyelia.

as foreign bodies. Cultures usually grow mixed organisms, including staphylococci, anaerobes, and fecal flora. Home care includes sitz baths and oral antimicrobial therapy. Elective excision of the entire cyst and all associated sinus tracts is indicated once inflammation has resolved.

Cutaneous Manifestations of Spinal Dysraphism

A number of midline cutaneous abnormalities found in the lumbosacral area are associated with underlying vertebral or spinal cord defects that are the result of defective closure of the caudal neural tube, *occult spinal dysraphism.* Skin findings include *hairy patches* (Fig. 128.23), *skin tags, port-wine stains, hemangiomas,* and *congenital dermal sinuses.* The latter tend to be more cephalad than pilonidal sinuses, and their sinus tracts often extend to the spinal column. Underlying intraspinal lesions include dermoid tumors, lipomas, and diastematomyelia. In the latter condition, the lower cord is divided sagittally by an osseous or fibrocartilaginous septum, which tethers the cord at that level, impeding its normal ascent within the spinal canal as the child grows. Patients with tethering may present with lower-extremity neurologic deficits at birth or may insidiously develop symptoms later in infancy or childhood, especially during a period of rapid growth. Complaints may include back or leg pain or stiffness, buttock pain, weakness or numbness, and bowel and bladder complaints. Physical examination may reveal decreased tone and decreased deep tendon reflexes in the lower extremities. Any child found to have one of these midline cutaneous findings should undergo radiologic imaging to detect and delineate underlying vertebrospinal defects because early neurosurgical intervention substantial reduces morbidity.

Perineal Lesions

Urethral prolapse is a phenomenon seen primarily in obese prepubescent girls (see Chapter 100 Gynecology Emergencies). Two-thirds or more are African-American. In this condition, the urethra prolapses through the urethral meatus and is seen as a red or purplish red, friable, edematous mass overlying the anterior portion of the introitus (Fig. 128.24). It often has a doughnut shape, and close inspection reveals a central orifice. The prolapsed mucosa is usually mildly painful and tender and may bleed easily. Presenting complaints may include perineal pain, dysuria, and blood spotting on underwear. Urination is not impaired. The precipitating event is often characterized by increased intraabdominal pressure, usually severe straining with constipation, a severe coughing spell, or prolonged crying. Because the red friable mass often overlies the hymenal

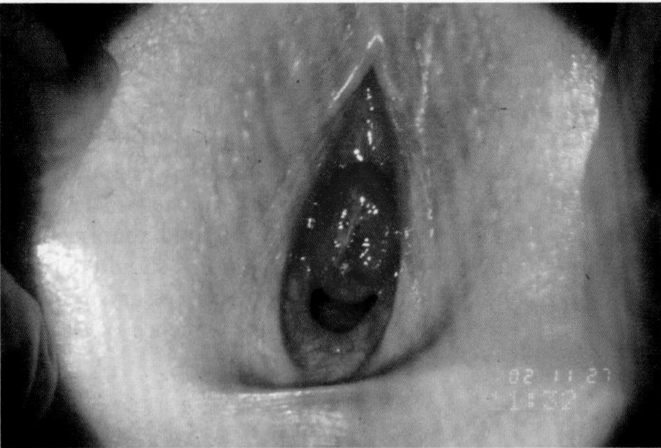

FIGURE 128.24 Urethral prolapse. (Courtesy of Tony Olsen, MD. In: Chung EK, Atkinson-McEvoy LR, Lai NL, et al., eds. *Visual Diagnosis and Treatment in Pediatrics.* 3rd ed. Philadelphia, PA: Wolters Kluwer Health, 2014.)

orifice, it can be mistaken for traumatized hymenal folds, raising suspicion of sexual abuse. Correct diagnosis often requires examination under magnification. This may require topical anesthetic to facilitate elevation of the mass to visualize the central orifice and the underlying hymen. Management consists of treating the predisposing condition, oral analgesics, and topical antibiotic creams for symptomatic relief. Twice-daily application of estrogen cream is recommended.

Hemorrhoids, internal and external, are dilated veins arising from the superior and inferior hemorrhoids veins. While very uncommon in children, incidences of hemorrhoids increase during adolescence. Development of hemorrhoids is associated with children with portal hypertension, chronic constipation, or excessive straining. Symptoms include painless bleeding (internal hemorrhoids), prolapse, pruitus, and pain secondary to vascular thrombosis. Treatment initially starts with medical management, increased fiber consumption or use of stool softeners, and topical care corticosteroids and analgesics. Refractory hemorrhoids may be managed nonoperatively with ablation or ligation. If unsuccessful, then hemorrhoidectomy should be considered. Due to the rarity of hemorrhoids in children, any presentation should prompt a careful and thorough evaluation of the underlying etiology.

Perianal skin tags are common sequelae of anal fissures and thus tend to be seen in children with a history of large, hard stools. They consist of pedunculated masses on short stalks that form during the process of healing of an anal fissure, probably in part caused by frictional forces common to this area. They are usually asymptomatic. They also can be seen in association with hypertrophic scars, another common sequela of the healing of an anal fissure. Although most patients with these lesions are otherwise normal, a small percentage have them as manifestations of perianal disease, internal fissures, and/or fistula, which may be a manifestation of inflammatory bowel disease. Management is directed at treating the predisposing or underlying condition. Bothersome pedunculated lesions can be tied off with silk suture.

Rectal prolapse, herniation of the rectum through the levator and then the anal orifice, is a phenomenon typically seen in children between 1 and 2 years of age (Fig. 128.25). The most common predisposing conditions, severe constipation and severe diarrhea, are characterized by repeated straining on defecation, which stretches pelvic suspensory structures,

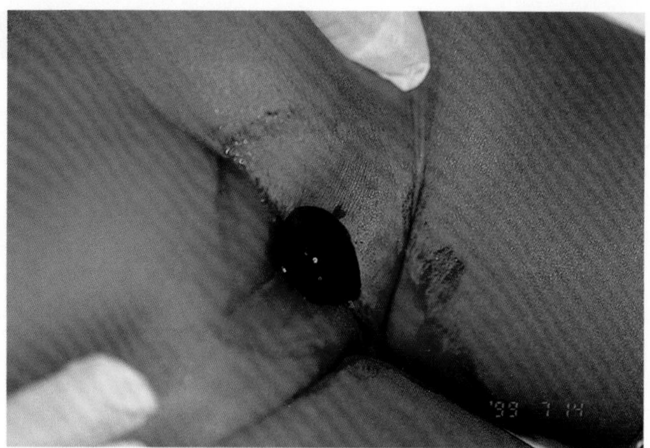

FIGURE 128.25 Rectal prolapse. (From Fleisher GR, Ludwig S, Baskin MN. *Atlas of Pediatric Emergency Medicine*. Philadelphia, PA: Lippincott Williams & Wilkins, 2004.)

facilitating herniation. Patients with spina bifida may have prolapse as a consequence of deficits in perineal innervation with attendant atrophy of the supporting perineal muscles. Rectal prolapse may be the first presenting symptom in children with cystic fibrosis. It is also associated with pinworm infection. Occasionally, an apparent rectal prolapse represents the lead end of sigmoid intussusceptions. In these cases, patients have a history of consistent with intussusception including antecedent, intermittent abdominal pain or irritability and may have vomiting, lethargy, and/or rectal bleeding. Clinically, a cylindrical mass with a central orifice and a glistening red surface is seen protruding through the anus. Acutely, the mass can be reduced with steady, gentle pressure. Applying sugar to the exposed mucosa and waiting 5 to 10 minutes can decrease edema and facilitate reduction. Attention is then directed at identifying and treating the underlying condition to prevent recurrences. The need for operative intervention for persistent recurrences is rare and is largely limited to neurodevastated patients with intractable constipation.

Suggested Readings and Key References

Ashcraft KW, Thomas MH. Acquired anorectal disorders. In: Ashcraft KW, Holcomb GW, Murphy JP, eds. *Pediatric surgery,* 6th ed. Philadelphia, PA: WB Saunders, 2014.

Barksdale Jr EM. Surgery. In: Zitelli BJ, McIntire S, Nowalk A, eds. *Atlas of pediatric physical diagnosis,* 6th ed. St. Louis, MO: Mosby, 2012:623–674.

Bellinger MF. Urologic disorders. In: Zitelli BJ, McIntire S, Nowalk A, eds. *Atlas of pediatric physical diagnosis,* 6th ed. St. Louis, MO: Mosby, 2012:535–562.

Brukner AL, Frieden IJ. Hemangiomas of infancy. *J Am Acad Dermatol* 2003;48:477–493.

Canales FL, Newmeyer WL 3rd, Kilgore ES. The treatment of felons and paronychias. *Hand Clin* 1989;5:515–523.

Chang LC, Haggstrom AN, Drolet BA, et al. Growth characteristics of infantile hemangiomas: implications for management. *Pediatrics* 2008;122:360–367.

Cohen BA, Davis HW, Gehris RP. Dermatology. In: Zitelli BJ, McIntire S, Nowalk A, eds. *Atlas of Pediatric Physical Diagnosis,* 6th ed. St. Louis, MO: Mosby, 2012:275–346.

Danielson-Cohen A, Lin SJ, Hughes CA, et al. Head and neck pilomatrixoma in children. *Arch Otolaryngol Head Neck Surg* 2001;127: 1481–1483.

Davis HW, Michaels MG. Pediatric infectious disease. In: Zitelli BJ, McIntire S, Nowalk A, eds. *Atlas of Pediatric Physical Diagnosis,* 6th ed. St. Louis, MO: Mosby, 2012:443–508.

Freyer DR, Kennedy R, Bostrom BC, et al. Juvenile xanthogranuloma: forms of systemic disease and their clinical implications. *J Pediatr* 1996;129:227–237.

Guinto-Ocampo H. Incision and drainage of a felon. In: Henretig FM, King C, eds. *Textbook of Pediatric Emergency Procedures*. Baltimore, MD: Lippincott Williams & Wilkins, 2007:1190–1194.

Henretig FM, King C, eds. *Textbook of pediatric emergency procedures,* 2nd ed. Baltimore, MD: Lipincott Williams & Wilkins, 2007.

Hermans DJ, van Beynum IM, Schultze Kool LJ, et al. Propranolol, a very promising treatment for ulceration in infantile hemangiomas: a study of 20 cases with matched historical controls. *J Am Acad Dermatol* 2011;64:833–838.

Johnson CF. Prolapse of the urethra: confusion of clinical and anatomic characteristics with sexual abuse. *Pediatrics* 1991;87(5):722–725.

Leung AK, Robson WL. Childhood cervical lymphadenopathy. *J Pediatr Health Care* 2004;18(1):3–7.

Loiselle J, Cronan KM. Hair tourniquet removal. In: Henretig FM, King C, eds. *Textbook of Pediatric Emergency Procedures*. Baltimore, MD: Lippincott Williams & Wilkins, 2007:1065–1069.

Mat Saad AZ, Purcell EM, McCann JJ. Hair-thread tourniquet syndrome in an infant with bony erosion: a case report, literature review, and meta-analysis. *Ann Plast Surg* 2006;57(4):447–452.

Mulliken JB, Fishman SJ, Burrows PE. Vascular anomalies. *Curr Probl Surg* 2000;37:517–584.

Murray PJ, Davis HW. Pediatric and adolescent gynecology. In: Zitelli BJ, McIntire S, Nowalk A eds. *Atlas of Pediatric Physical Diagnosis,* 6th ed. St. Louis, MO: Mosby, 2012:675–712.

Osterman M, Draeger R, Stern P. Acute Hand Infections. *J Hand Surg Am* 2014;39(8):1628–1635.

Paes JE, Burman KD, Cohen J, et al. Acute bacterial suppurative thyroiditis: a clinical review and expert opinion. *Thyroid* 2010;20:247–255.

Pagliai KA, Cohen BA. Pyogenic granuloma in children. *Pediatr Dermatol* 2004;21:10–13.

Paller AS, Mancini AJ, Hurwitz S, eds. *Hurwitz Clinical Pediatric Dermatology e-dition,* 3rd ed. Philadelphia, PA: WB Saunders, 2006.

Paller AS, Pensler JM, Tomita T. Nasal midline masses in infants and children. Dermoids, encephaloceles, and gliomas. *Arch Dermatol* 1991;127:362–366.

Prendville JS, Krol AL. Diseases of the dermis and subcutaneous tissues. In: Schachner LA, Hansen RC, eds. *Pediatric Dermatology,* 3rd ed. New York, NY: Churchill Livingstone, 2003.

Rahbar R, Shah P, Mulliken JB, et al. The presentation and management of nasal dermoid: a 30 year experience. *Arch Otolaryngol Head Neck Surg* 2003;129:464–471.

Raza J, Hindmarsh PC, Brook CG. Thyrotoxicosis in children: thirty years' experience. *Acta Paediatr* 1999;88:937–941.

Roberts JR, Hedges JR, eds. *Clinical Procedures in Emergency Medicine,* 5th ed. Philadelphia, PA: WB Saunders, 2009.

Roth DA, Hildesheimer M, Bardenstein S, et al. Preauricular skin tags and ear pits are associated with permanent hearing impairment in newborns. *Pediatrics* 2008;122:e884–e890.

Sampayo EM, Henretig FM. Incision and drainage of a paronychia. In: Henretig FM, King C, eds. *Textbook of Pediatric Emergency Procedures.* Baltimore, MD: Lippincott Williams & Wilkins, 2007: 1085–1089.

Stites T, Lund DP. Common anorectal problems. *Semin Pediatr Surg* 2007:16:71–78.

Varma R, Williams SD, Wessel HB. Neurology. In: Zitelli BJ, McIntire S, Nowalk A, eds. *Atlas of Pediatric Physical Diagnosis,* 6th ed. St. Louis, MO: Mosby, 2012:563–596.

Yellon RF, McBride TP, Davis HW. Otolaryngology. In: Zitelli BJ, McIntire S, Nowalk A, eds. *Atlas of Pediatric Physical Diagnosis,* 6th ed. St. Louis, MO: Mosby, 2012:889–938.

CHAPTER 129 ■ MUSCULOSKELETAL EMERGENCIES

MARK D. JOFFE, MD AND JOHN M. LOISELLE, MD

GOALS OF EMERGENCY CARE

Nonfracture related orthopedic emergencies often pose a diagnostic dilemma for even the most experienced clinician due to indolent courses and lack of distinguishing signs and symptoms. The pediatric emergency clinician is challenged to make the diagnosis and institute early therapy as outcomes often correlate with the time to institution of treatment after symptoms begin. The time to antibiotic administration and time to surgery are key goals for these disorders. A systematic approach utilizing appropriate laboratory testing, imaging, and orthopedic consultation will most often detect these conditions. Certain conditions such as septic arthritis of the hip must be diagnosed at the time of the initial visit so that surgical intervention combined with timely antibiotic therapy can minimize the likelihood of poor outcomes such as growth retardation or irreparable joint dysfunction. When unrecognized or untreated, other orthopedic conditions may lead to prolonged pain, chronic functional disorders, or a delay in the ability to return to normal activity.

KEY POINTS

- A normal plain radiograph does not rule out significant disease or pathology.
- Referred pain or the inability of the young child to localize pain can obscure the diagnosis.
- Trauma is too often assumed to be the cause of symptoms when skeletal infection is present.
- Presence of fever and significant elevations in inflammatory markers are useful when considering infectious etiologies.
- Provocative physical exam testing is helpful in distinguishing certain overuse injuries.
- Cultures should be obtained from the blood and potentially infected areas when there is concern for musculoskeletal infection.

RELATED CHAPTERS

Signs and Symptoms
- Fever: Chapter 26
- Immobile Arm: Chapter 34
- Injury: Shoulder: Chapter 38
- Limp: Chapter 41
- Pain: Back: Chapter 49
- Pain: Joints: Chapter 55

Clinical Pathways
- Fever in Children: Chapter 88

Medical, Surgical, and Trauma Emergencies
- Infectious Disease Emergencies: Chapter 102
- Musculoskeletal Trauma: Chapter 119

OSTEOMYELITIS

CLINICAL PEARLS AND PITFALLS

- Refusal to move a limb or pseudoparalysis may be a sign of osteomyelitis
- Up to 40% of children with osteomyelitis will be afebrile
- Radiographs are helpful in evaluating for alternate diagnoses but do not rule out osteomyelitis when obtained early in the course of the illness
- Osteomyelitis is frequently associated with septic arthritis in neonates
- Pathogens or etiology of musculoskeletal infection vary by age of the patient
- *Staphylococcus aureus* is the most common organism in all ages
- Magnetic resonance imaging (MRI) is the imaging study of choice
- Patients with sickle cell disease are at risk for Salmonella osteomyelitis
- Inflammatory markers are elevated in up to 90% of cases of osteomyelitis
- CRP is the most effective inflammatory marker in monitoring the response to therapy
- The lower extremity accounts for up to 70% of cases of osteomyelitis in children

Current Evidence

Osteomyelitis is an inflammation of the bone and bone marrow that is most commonly of infectious origin. Infection is confirmed by the presence of two of the following: pus on an aspirate of the bone, clinical findings consistent with the diagnosis, positive blood or bone aspirate cultures, and consistent findings on medical imaging. Osteomyelitis is more common in boys, with the highest incidence found among infants and preschool age children. Younger age and underlying disorders are associated with an increased risk for contracting osteomyelitis, as well as for the particular pathogens involved.

Bacteria gain entrance to the bone through one of three routes: hematogenous, direct spread from adjacent infection, or inoculation through a penetrating wound. Hematogenous spread is the most common route of infection in children. A transient bacteremia is believed to be the initiating event in the infection. Bacteria enter the bone at the level of the metaphysis where the predominant vascular supply is located. The sluggish blood flow within the microvasculature of the marrow predisposes to infection. Local trauma has been suggested as a possible cause of microthrombotic events further predisposing bone to infection. This is supported by an association of trauma with the occurrence of osteomyelitis and the preponderance of infections occurring within the long bones, especially those of the lower extremities. In sickle cell patients, microinfarcts within the more tenuously supplied area of the diaphysis may explain the increased occurrence in this region of the bone. As infection progresses, pressure increases and organisms penetrate up through the cortex to the subperiosteal space.

Differences in the underlying bony structure in the neonate and young infant predispose them to a higher incidence of multifocal osteomyelitis and concomitant septic arthritis. The thin cortex allows easier penetration to the subperiosteal space. The periosteum is less adherent in these ages and less effective in limiting the spread of infection. Transphyseal vessels, which are present through the first 18 months of life, allow bacteria to gain access to the adjoining epiphysis and joint space.

A less common source of osteomyelitis in children is penetration of the periosteum by adjacent infections such as a cellulitis or abscess. Inoculation of the bone from stepping on a nail, surgical instrumentation, or intraosseous line placement provides a third means for infection to gain entrance to the bone.

Goals of Treatment

Early recognition and treatment of osteomyelitis prevents the spread of infection and minimizes the risk of poor outcomes such as growth disturbance, abscess formation, sepsis, chronic osteomyelitis, or even death. The time to initiation of antibiotic administration from onset of symptoms or arrival to medical care is a key objective of care. Empiric antibiotic treatment is based on the patient's age, Gram stain of an aspirate if performed, the likely means of contracting the infection, and underlying comorbidity. The ultimate choice of antibiotic and the length of treatment are dictated by the offending organism which is identified through appropriate cultures. Although acute operative intervention is rarely necessary, timely consultation of orthopedic surgery facilitates bone aspiration when indicated and the initiation of treatment.

Clinical Considerations

Clinical Recognition

The infant or child with osteomyelitis typically presents with fever, localized musculoskeletal pain, or pain with movement. Trauma is not an obvious explanation for the symptoms. The absence of fever does not rule out the presence of osteomyelitis.

Triage Considerations

The patient with limp or localized musculoskeletal symptoms is often triaged as urgent. Those with a question of neurovascular compromise, severe pain, or who appear systemically ill should be evaluated more immediately. These patients should have their degree of pain documented and should receive analgesics on arrival.

Initial Assessment/H&P

Physical signs of osteomyelitis are age dependent and recognition requires patience and diligence on the part of the clinician. The older child is more likely to have localized infection and is more capable of expressing or identifying a site of localized pain and point tenderness. The neonate or young infant may present with a pseudoparalysis of the affected limb. Another common, although nonspecific, finding in this age group is paradoxical irritability in which the infant exhibits pain or distress upon handling and is more comfortable when left alone.

Fever and pain are highly sensitive findings but are not universally present. Fever is described in up to 90% of children with osteomyelitis upon presentation and may be quite elevated. Signs of pain may include limp, refusal to bear weight, or a decreased range of motion when a limb is involved. Erythema and swelling are less frequent but can also be observed at the site, and usually suggest more advanced periosteal involvement.

Osteomyelitis typically follows an indolent course and is less likely to present with the acute onset of symptoms that is more typical of traumatic injuries. A history of minor trauma is common and often coincidental in an active child. A history of sickle cell disease, prior surgery or skeletal manipulation places the patient at higher risk for osteomyelitis.

Management/Diagnostic Testing

In addition to clinical findings, the diagnosis of osteomyelitis depends on culture results. A blood culture and bone aspirate should be obtained in suspected cases of osteomyelitis before the initiation of antibiotics. Isolation of the causative organism is important not only for diagnosis, but also in antibiotic selection and determining the length of therapy. Reports of positive blood cultures in the setting of osteomyelitis range from 30% to 57%. An organism is recovered from a bone aspirate in 51% to 90% of cases. The combination will identify a pathogen in 75% to 80% of cases. Bone aspirates may remain positive for several days after antibiotic use, whereas blood cultures are often sterile within 24 hours of the initiation of antibiotics.

Laboratory tests vary in sensitivity. The white blood cell (WBC) count rises in only one-third of the cases of osteomyelitis, whereas both the erythrocyte sedimentation rate (ESR) and C-reactive protein (CRP) are elevated in more than 90% of the cases. The latter tests are useful in diagnosis and in monitoring the response to therapy. The CRP peaks at 2 days and gradually returns to normal over 7 to 10 days of appropriate therapy. The ESR may remain elevated for several weeks despite adequate treatment. In the setting of a low clinical suspicion for osteomyelitis, a normal CRP, ESR, and plain radiograph suggests an alternative diagnosis.

The plain radiograph is useful both in detecting early signs of osteomyelitis and excluding other diagnostic possibilities. The earliest radiographic changes suggestive of osteomyelitis include deep soft-tissue swelling with elevation of the muscle planes from the adjacent bone. These may be seen as early as 3 to 4 days after the onset of symptoms. Lytic bone changes are not detectable until 10 to 14 days. Periosteal elevation, when present, is not generally visible until 10 to 21 days after infection (Fig. 129.1). A negative radiograph in the first 10 days of illness does not rule out osteomyelitis. When suspicion remains high in the setting of a negative radiograph,

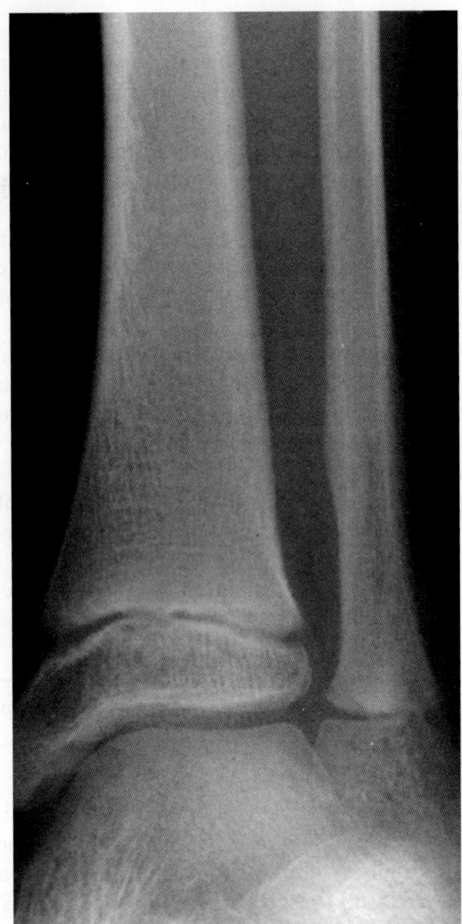

FIGURE 129.1 Periosteal activity in distal fibula in child with *Staphylococcus aureus* osteomyelitis; day 20 of illness.

further imaging studies should be obtained. The triple-phase technetium bone scan has a reported sensitivity and specificity of more than 90%, and is the test of choice when osteomyelitis is suspected but a specific site of concern cannot be identified by physical examination or when multiple foci of infection are possible. MRI is also highly sensitive in detecting osteomyelitis and does not expose the child to ionizing radiation. In addition, MRI provides a higher degree of detail than the bone scan (Fig. 129.2). This is useful in detecting suspected complications of osteomyelitis such as a subperiosteal abscess or bone sequestrum. Many orthopedic surgeons prefer this high degree of resolution to guide a bone aspirate or biopsy. Both imaging studies commonly require sedation of the young child, but the bone scan is not as affected by small movements. A bone aspirate preceding a bone scan or MRI does not alter the results and should not be delayed because of this concern.

Organisms responsible for osteomyelitis vary according to age of the patient, the route of infection, and any underlying comorbid conditions. *S. aureus* is the most common pathogen across all age groups accounting for 70% to 90% of cases. The incidence of community-acquired methicillin-resistant *S. aureus* (CA-MRSA) has increased dramatically in most areas of the United States. Some studies have found over 70% of cases due to MRSA. Osteomyelitis due to MRSA has been associated with a longer duration of fever, extended hospitalization, and increased frequency of complications. Group A β-hemolytic streptococcus and *Streptococcus pneumoniae* are the next most common organisms isolated in childhood osteomyelitis and together account for 10% of cases outside of the neonatal period. The frequency of *Kingella kingae* has been increasing and is most commonly reported in the toddler and preschool age group. It is difficult to culture and the increased incidence may be due to improved success in identification through polymerase chain reaction (PCR) and improved culture techniques. It is a gram-negative organism and therefore resistant to vancomycin and clindamycin, but sensitive to cephalosporins and β-lactam antibiotics. Bacterial isolates from neonates younger than 2 months include *S. aureus,* group B streptococcus, and *Escherichia coli* (Table 129.1).

Certain groups are at risk for particular organisms. Patients with sickle cell disease have a high incidence of osteomyelitis

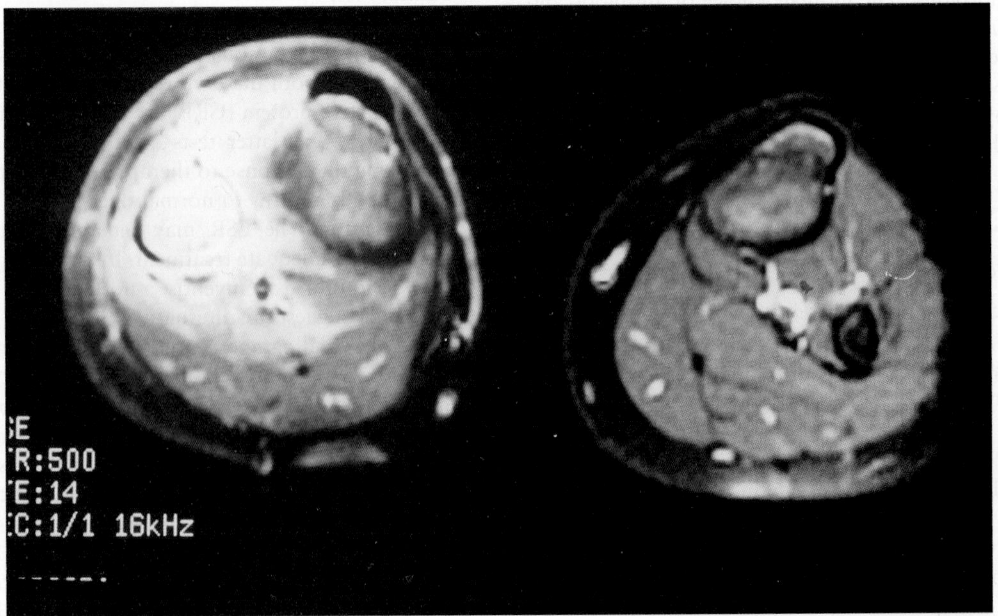

FIGURE 129.2 Magnetic resonance imaging of osteomyelitis of the proximal right fibula.

TABLE 129.1

INITIAL ANTIBIOTIC THERAPY: OSTEOMYELITIS[a]

Age	Pathogens	Antibiotics
Neonate <2 mo	*Staphylococcus aureus,* group B streptococcus, gram-negative bacilli	Vancomycin and cefotaxime
>2 mo–5 yrs	*S. aureus,* group A streptococcus, *Streptococcus pneumoniae, Kingella kingae*	Clindamycin[b,c]
>5 yrs	*S. aureus,* group A streptococcus, *S. pneumoniae*	Clindamycin[c]
Special cases		
Sickle cell disease	Salmonella, *S. aureus*	Clindamycin and ceftriaxone
Foot puncture wound	*Pseudomonas aeruginosa, S. aureus*	Cefepime or piperacillin/tazobactam

[a]Coverage modified on the basis of culture results and sensitivities.
[b]Add ceftriaxone for Gram stain negative for gram-positive cocci or culture positive for *Kingella kingae.*
[c]Vancomycin if high incidence of clindamycin resistance in community or ill appearance.

caused by salmonella. *Pseudomonas aeruginosa* is a common organism found in osteomyelitis of the foot, often resulting from a nail penetrating a sneaker.

Clinical Indications for Discharge or Admission

Initial therapy for osteomyelitis includes hospital admission with intravenous antibiotics and pain control. Empiric antibiotic therapy is based on the predominant organisms in each age group, local sensitivity patterns, the mechanism of infection, and Gram stain results. Clindamycin is the treatment of choice for osteomyelitis outside of the neonatal age range when MRSA is suspected. Vancomycin may be indicated for empiric treatment when the incidence of clindamycin resistance in the community is high or the patient is critically ill. Definitive treatment is ultimately based on the identification and sensitivity of recovered isolates. A third-generation cephalosporin or the addition of an aminoglycoside is indicated in the neonatal age group. Suggested agents are listed in Table 129.1. Early aggressive antibiotic therapy frequently prevents the need for surgical intervention. The duration of hospitalization is determined by the organism involved, the clinical response to treatment, and decreasing CRP levels.

SEPTIC ARTHRITIS

Goals of Treatment

The presence of bacterial pathogens within the articular capsule presents a true surgical emergency. Delay in the identification and treatment of an infected joint in a child can result in severe and permanent sequelae. Early initiation of treatment can preserve normal function of the joint and prevent destruction or ischemic changes due to excessive pressure buildup from the infection. Improved outcomes are associated with reduced time to initiation of antibiotic therapy and time to surgery for the septic hip. The urgency associated with this diagnosis has given rise to the maxim, "The sun should never rise or set on a septic hip." The evaluation focuses on distinguishing septic arthritis from more benign causes of joint pain that do not require invasive forms of identification and treatment.

CLINICAL PEARLS AND PITFALLS

- Resistance or pain with movement of the joint is the principal clinical finding
- A septic hip is held in abduction and external rotation
- Inflammatory markers can be helpful in distinguishing inflammatory from infectious etiologies
- Ultrasound cannot distinguish an inflammatory effusion from an infectious one, but the lack of a joint effusion can rule out septic arthritis
- Fever is more common with septic arthritis than transient synovitis
- Lyme disease most commonly manifests as monoarticular arthritis of the knee and most children are still able to ambulate
- Arthrocentesis is the definitive means of identifying septic arthritis

Current Evidence

Bacteria gain entry to the joint space through one of three means. The highly vascular synovium is most commonly infected through hematogenous seeding. The role of local injury in predisposing joints to infection by this means is unclear. Organisms from adjacent areas of infection may invade the joint, or direct inoculation can occur through penetrating injuries. Infection secondary to penetrating objects may be delayed from the actual time of injury so that external wounds may be small or healed at the time of presentation. Adjacent osteomyelitis is present in up to 10% of cases.

Eighty to 90% of septic joints occur in the lower extremities. The knee and hip are most commonly affected. The same distribution is found in the preambulatory child. Infections involve only a single joint in greater than 90% of cases. Multifocal infections are more common in neonates and infections with *Neisseria* species.

Pressure elevation within the minimally distensible joint capsule can compromise vascular flow, resulting in ischemic injury to the bone and cartilage. This is a particular concern in the hip, where avascular necrosis of the femoral head is a well-described complication of septic arthritis. Prognosis is worse in children younger than 1 year, with involvement of the hip joint, with delay to the initiation of therapy, and with infection by *S. aureus*.

Clinical Considerations

Clinical Recognition

Septic arthritis occurs in all ages. Pain is the most common presenting complaint in the child with a septic joint. Because of the predominance of septic arthritis in the lower extremities, the younger child often presents with a limp, abnormal gait, or inability to bear weight. Referred pain from the hip may manifest as groin, thigh, or knee pain. Swelling or redness of a joint is often a late finding but can be the primary reason for the patient to seek medical care. The neonate or young infant with a septic joint may display fever, asymmetric movement, or lack of movement of a limb. Recent traumatic events do not adequately explain these findings. Patients with a prior history of a rheumatologic condition or invasive procedures involving the joint are more likely to have an alternate cause for their joint pain.

Triage

Patients with complaints of joint pain and/or fever, limited range of motion of a joint, joint swelling or limp are typically categorized as urgent. The patient with severe pain, neurovascular compromise or ill appearance should be evaluated more emergently. Patients should have a temperature and pain severity documented and receive analgesics. With concern of septic arthritis, the child should be made NPO.

Initial Assessment/H&P

The history should focus on the location of joint pain, its duration, and relation to movement. Pain due to septic arthritis is typically constant or increasing over time. The clinician should inquire about local injuries that may identify a traumatic cause for the symptoms or penetrating injuries that may predispose to joint infection. A prior history of rheumatoid disorders, sickle cell disease, or joint surgery should be obtained. Sexually active teenagers are at risk for gonococcal arthritis. The presence of rash may suggest juvenile idiopathic arthritis or a viral etiology for the joint pain.

Range of motion around the affected joint is dramatically reduced. Any degree of movement causes great distress and is vigorously resisted. Many clinicians rely on this aspect of the evaluation more than any other in differentiating infection from alternative causes of joint pain.

Clinical signs are more subtle in the neonate or young infant with a septic joint. Nonspecific findings such as septic appearance, irritability, and pseudoparalysis of a limb are common presenting findings in these ages. Parents may note excessive irritability associated with diaper changes in the infant with a septic hip. The child with a septic hip will typically hold the lower extremity in abduction and external rotation in order to decrease intracapsular pressure (Fig. 129.3). Close observation, and isolated manipulation of each joint will help identify the particular area of involvement.

The skin surface should be closely evaluated for local signs of injury. Most involved joints will have obvious erythema, warmth, and swelling. The exception is the hip joint because of its deep-seated location. Swelling may be less obvious in the pudgy infant. Fever is a commonly associated sign but is absent in up to one-third of patients.

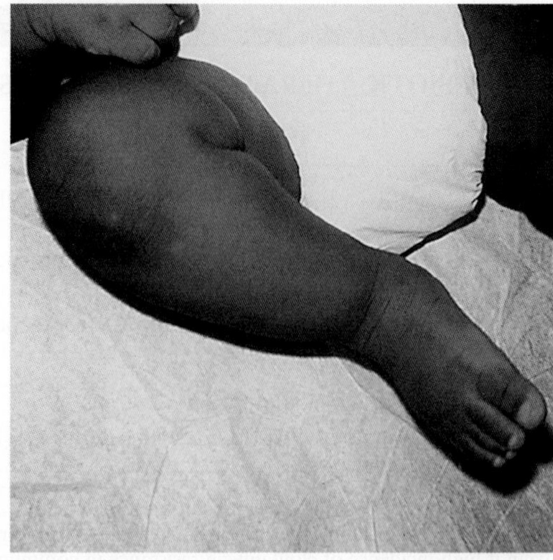

FIGURE 129.3 Five-month-old infant with septic arthritis of the right hip. Hip joint is held in flexion, abduction, and external rotation.

Management/Diagnostic Testing

The diagnosis of septic arthritis is confirmed by the identification of purulent fluid within the joint space. Arthrocentesis is a mandatory procedure in all suspected causes of septic arthritis. The decision to perform this procedure is based on the degree of clinical suspicion in combination with results of laboratory tests and imaging studies; none of these in isolation are 100% sensitive in detecting or excluding septic arthritis from other conditions. A sample of synovial fluid is often the only means of discriminating septic arthritis from less serious inflammatory processes.

The mean peripheral WBC count is generally elevated in children with septic arthritis, however, more than half of the patients will have a WBC count less than 15,000 per mm^3. The ESR and CRP are more sensitive markers and are elevated in 90% to 95% of patients. In areas endemic for Lyme disease, serum for Lyme titers (IgM and IgG; two-tiered testing) should be obtained.

Plain radiographs may demonstrate signs of an effusion ranging from subtle blurring or displacement of fascial planes to complete dislocation of the joint. The main role of the radiograph in the evaluation is to exclude fractures or other bony abnormalities that may mimic septic arthritis. Ultrasound is most useful in evaluating the hip. It is much more sensitive than the radiograph in detecting a joint effusion. Some have suggested that the absence of an effusion on an ultrasound scan effectively excludes the diagnosis of septic arthritis. The ultrasound cannot, however, distinguish between infected and sterile inflammatory effusions. Ultrasound guidance is useful in performance of a needle aspiration of the hip joint.

The isolation of a bacterial pathogen provides a definitive diagnosis and directs subsequent management. Cultures of joint fluid and blood should therefore be performed on all patients with a possible septic joint. The yield of organisms can be increased by directly inoculating joint fluid into a blood culture bottle. When indicated, cultures from additional sites should be obtained to increase the potential isolation of a pathogen. Cultures of the joint fluid demonstrate the highest yield and are positive in 50% to 80% of cases. Blood cultures identify an organism in 15% to 46% of patients with septic arthritis and are positive in many cases in which the organism is not isolated from the joint fluid. Cervical or urethral

TABLE 129.2

INITIAL ANTIBIOTIC THERAPY: SEPTIC ARTHRITIS[a]

Age	Pathogens	Antibiotics
Neonate <2 mo	*Staphylococcus aureus,* group B streptococcus, gram-negative bacilli	Vancomycin and cefotaxime
>2 mo–5 yrs	*S. aureus,* group A streptococcus, *Streptococcus pneumoniae, Kingella kingae*	Clindamycin[b,c]
>5 yrs	*S. aureus,* group A streptococcus	Clindamycin[b,c]
Adolescent	*S. aureus,* group A streptococcus, *Neisseria gonorrhoeae*	Clindamycin[c] and ceftriaxone[d]

[a]Common pathogens and empiric antibiotic coverage by age.
[b]Add ceftriaxone for Gram stain negative for gram-positive cocci or culture positive for *K. kingae,* or ill appearance.
[c]Vancomycin, if high incidence of clindamycin resistance in community or ill appearance, and consider for all hip and shoulder joints.
[d]Empiric treatment in sexually active adolescent.

cultures or urine PCR testing in sexually active adolescents with septic arthritis may identify *Neisseria gonorrhoeae* as the responsible organism. In 20% of cases, a causative organism is not recovered. Improved application of PCR techniques may increase the ability to identify pathogens in the future.

A Gram stain should be performed on joint fluid, and it occasionally provides additional assistance in identifying both the presence of an infection and the infecting organism. Although elevation of the WBC count more than 100,000 per mm^3 in the synovial fluid is considered strong evidence of infection, the actual counts are often much lower. Presence of purulent fluid, a positive Gram stain, and a highly elevated WBC count with a left shift in the synovial fluid are often used as indications for operative intervention when there is a concern of a septic hip. (See eBook link to Septic Arthritis Pathway.)

With few exceptions, bacteria found in septic arthritis are the same as those in osteomyelitis (Table 129.2). *S. aureus* is the most common reported isolate in all age groups. Prior to the introduction of the Hib vaccine, *Haemophilus influenzae type b* was the leading cause of septic arthritis in the 6-month-old to 5-year-old age group. Through immunization, this organism has now been essentially eliminated and surpassed in frequency by group A streptococcus and *S. pneumoniae. S. aureus* is also the predominant pathogen in neonatal patients. Gram-negative coliforms and Group B β-hemolytic streptococcus are also found in this age group. *N. gonorrhoeae* is found in neonates and is a frequent pathogen in sexually active teenagers. *K. kingae* is a fastidious gram-negative rod, susceptible to beta lactam antimicrobials, which has recently been isolated as a pathogen in numerous childhood bone and joint infections. It is found most commonly in children younger than 36 months. *Neisseria meningitidis* is a rare but reported cause of septic arthritis in children.

Clinical Indications for Discharge or Admission

The management of septic arthritis consists of hospitalization, parenteral administration of antibiotics (Table 129.2), and joint immobilization. Joint irrigation should be performed in selected cases. Empiric antibiotic therapy is dictated by the common organisms in the age group, local sensitivities, and by results of the synovial fluid Gram stain. Vancomycin or clindamycin is indicated depending on the incidence of clindamycin-resistant MRSA in the community; vancomycin should also be considered as part of the antimicrobial regimen for critically ill children. Gram-negative coverage should be added in neonates and adolescents. A third-generation cephalosporin should be added in patients with sickle cell disease because of susceptibility to salmonella infection.

Surgical intervention for joint irrigation is generally indicated for all cases involving the hip joint; infections in which large amounts of fibrin, debris, or loculations are found within the joint space; or when the patient fails to improve following several days of intravenous antibiotic therapy. Expeditious and aggressive management limits but does not eliminate potential sequelae of septic arthritis.

Lyme Arthritis

Lyme disease is a common cause of infectious arthritis in certain geographic locations within the United States. The infection is caused by the spirochete *Borrelia burgdorferi* which is transmitted through the bite of certain infected tick species. Arthritis is a manifestation of late disease and can occur 1 to 12 months following inoculation. Lyme arthritis is most often a monoarticular infection of the knee. If left untreated, symptoms can be episodic, lasting several days followed by several weeks to months without symptoms. Clinical and laboratory findings are similar to those for septic arthritis. Joint swelling is marked and out of proportion to the degree of pain. Fever is often absent and is generally low grade when present. Pain and limitation of movement of the affected joint is less than in septic arthritis, and patients are often able to ambulate despite the swelling. Infection can occur without a preceding known history of a tick bite or the classic skin manifestations of erythema migrans. Facial palsy or meningitis are more typical of early disseminated disease and therefore are rarely concurrent with arthritis. The ESR and CRP are elevated. When arthrocentesis is performed, the mean leukocyte count in synovial fluid is usually 10,000 to 25,000 cells per mm^3 but can exceed 50,000 cells per mm^3 with a neutrophil predominance. Routine cultures of synovial fluid are negative. In the appropriate clinical setting physical and laboratory findings may be sufficient to identify patients at low risk for septic arthritis and potentially avoid the need for arthrocentesis. Two-tiered diagnostic testing for Lyme arthritis is indicated in endemic areas. The first tier should include a serum enzyme-linked immunosorbent assay or immunofluorescence assay. Positive results should be confirmed by a Western immunoblot for IgG antibodies to *B. burgdorferi.* An IgM immunoblot assay is not necessary in late disease and may result in false-positive results. Negative serum IgG serology excludes Lyme as the cause of arthritis. Treatment for Lyme arthritis consists of a 4-week course of oral antibiotics. Doxycycline in a dose of 4 mg per kg per day divided twice daily with a maximum of 100 mg per dose is effective for children older than 8 years, whereas amoxicillin (50 mg per kg per day in three

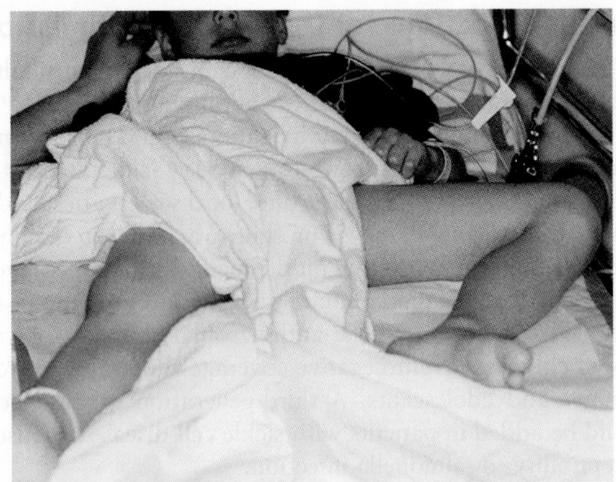

FIGURE 129.4 Seven-year-old child with transient synovitis of the left hip. Hip joint is held in same position of comfort as in septic arthritis.

divided doses with a maximum of 1.5 g per day) is sufficient in younger children. Cefuroxime (30 mg/kg/day in two divided doses with a maximum of 1,000 mg daily) is an alternative for patients with penicillin allergy. Serum antibody titers remain elevated even after adequate antibiotic treatment and should not be used as a measure of success of treatment. Persistent or recurrent joint swelling may occur 2 months beyond the initiation of treatment. Although this may represent a local autoimmune response, experts recommend retreatment with a second 4-week course of oral antibiotics or a 2- to 4-week course of parenteral ceftriaxone.

Transient Synovitis

Transient or toxic synovitis is a benign, self-limiting inflammatory condition of the hip. It afflicts males more frequently than females and is the most common cause of acute hip pain in children 3 to 10 years of age. The underlying cause is unknown, although a postinfectious inflammatory response has been suggested. Its presentation can mimic that of septic arthritis of the hip (Fig. 129.4), a distinction that is as crucial in management as it is difficult in diagnosis.

The onset of symptoms is abrupt with unilateral hip pain and limp. Fever is rare, occurring in less than 10% of cases, and when present, is usually low grade. Although patients complain of discomfort with movement of the limb, it is generally possible to gently maneuver the hip through a near full range of motion. This contrasts with the septic hip in which pain and spasm are more extreme, and patients resist a full range of motion. Additional signs of systemic illness are absent and, despite the label, the child is nontoxic appearing.

Laboratory tests are generally useful only in attempting to distinguish transient synovitis from more serious conditions. The WBC count, ESR, and CRP are generally normal or only slightly elevated. The mean WBC count, ESR, and CRP are significantly lower than in septic arthritis; however, sufficient overlap exists between values in transient synovitis and septic arthritis such that they do not reliably distinguish between the two conditions in individual patients. The Kocher criteria consist of a combination of clinical and laboratory variables which are commonly used as a clinical prediction tool to assist in distinguishing septic arthritis from transient synovitis. The four factors include a history of fever, nonweight bearing, ESR greater than 40 mm/hr, and WBC count greater than 12,000 cells/mm^3.

Radiographs may demonstrate an effusion but principally serve to exclude pathologic osseous conditions. Ultrasound is more sensitive than plain films at detecting joint effusions, although accuracy declines in patients younger than 1 year of age. Reports of an effusion of the hip by ultrasound in transient synovitis vary from 50% to 95%. The clinician must use a combination of clinical, laboratory, and radiographic findings to determine which patients require further evaluation with needle aspiration of the hip. Although patients often report relief of pain following aspiration, the procedure is unnecessary except to exclude the presence of a bacterial infection. Synovial fluid, when obtained, is sterile. The synovial fluid WBC count is typically less than 50,000 cells per mm^3.

Treatment occurs on an outpatient basis, and emphasizes rest and analgesics. Traction is of unproven benefit and is potentially harmful. Nonsteroidal anti-inflammatory medications are the first-line therapy for pain. Pain duration is typically 3 to 4 days but may last as long as 2 weeks. Exacerbations can occur if activity is resumed too early.

There is no evidence of serious sequelae resulting from transient synovitis. The relationship between transient synovitis and the subsequent development of Legg–Calvé–Perthes disease (LCPD) is unclear. Studies have been unable to demonstrate cause and effect. Some suggest that these patients are at increased risk for developing LCPD, whereas others believe only that the clinical presentations are similar. Recurrences of transient synovitis can occur up to several years later and are not associated with worse outcomes.

Penetrating Intraarticular Wounds

Penetrating intraarticular wounds are not specific to children, but they are injuries that the pediatric emergency physician must recognize and treat on an urgent basis in order to prevent serious and potentially permanent sequelae. Knees are the most commonly injured joints. Motor vehicle accidents and direct trauma from falls are the cause in the overwhelming number of cases. A penetrating joint injury commonly missed in the emergency department is the closed fist injury in which the patient strikes an opponent in the mouth. A tooth can disrupt the capsule of the metacarpophalangeal joint and introduce oral bacteria. Failure to recognize this injury can result in septic arthritis, osteomyelitis, and permanent joint damage.

An open joint may be detectable on direct visualization or by palpation through a periarticular laceration. Injuries that extend below the skin surface adjacent to a joint effusion should raise a high level of suspicion that the joint space has been violated. The presence of air in the joint on radiograph is diagnostic for joint penetration (Fig. 129.5). In less obvious cases, disruption of the joint capsule can be demonstrated by the saline load test. Arthrocentesis is performed through an uninjured site on the skin surface, and saline is injected. Extravasation of saline from the joint into the wound is diagnostic for penetrating injury. A volume of 60 mL of saline is generally adequate to evaluate knee joint integrity, 20 mL for elbow or ankle joints, and 1 to 2 mL for finger joints. The addition of a small amount (<0.1 mL) of methylene blue to the saline has historically been used to improve visualization of extravasated fluid, though it may not have clear benefit

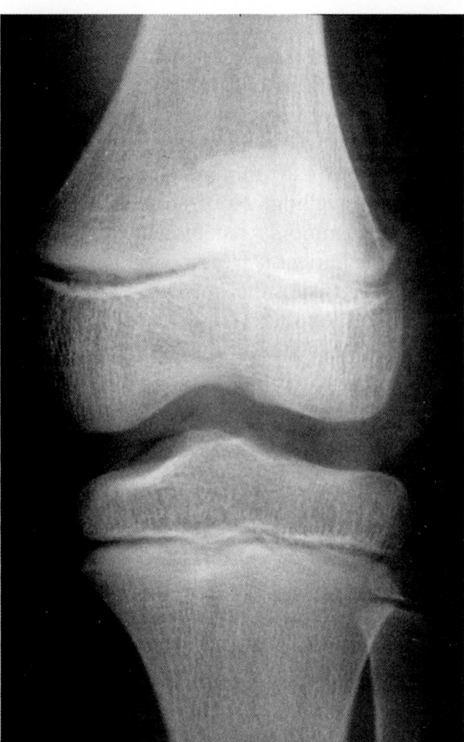

FIGURE 129.5 Intraarticular air in knee joint following penetrating injury sustained from fall on edge of stone.

over saline alone. Clinical evaluation has poor sensitivity in identifying penetrating wounds compared with saline injection. Other studies have shown that the saline load test may also miss a significant number of joint disruptions. If a question still remains regarding the integrity of the joint after such testing, then further imaging studies or surgical exploration is necessary.

Open wounds of the joint are considered contaminated and broad-spectrum antibiotics should be administered. Surgical intervention consists of vigorous irrigation and debridement, often in the operating room. Attention should be given to appropriate tetanus prophylaxis, splinting, wound dressing, and pain control while the patient remains in the emergency department.

The prognosis of penetrating intraarticular wounds is dependent on the degree of overlying soft-tissue injury and the extent of intraarticular damage. Infectious complications are the most common. Septic arthritis with a variety of both gram-positive and gram-negative organisms is an early and common outcome of inadequate early intervention. Delayed synovitis, often necessitating synovectomy, has been described after unidentified penetration of small foreign bodies.

OVERUSE SYNDROMES

Goals of Treatment

The treatment of overuse injuries strives to return the athlete rapidly and safely to full participation. Early diagnosis and initiation of appropriate therapy for overuse injuries will prevent recurrent or chronic injury as well as permanent damage to the growing musculoskeletal system.

CLINICAL PEARLS AND PITFALLS

- Initial therapy for overuse injuries includes rest, ice, and nonsteroidal anti-inflammatory medication.
- A change in biomechanics, exercise regimen, equipment, or strength and flexibility is necessary to avoid recurrence of overuse syndromes.
- Many overuse injuries have provocative clinical tests that aid in the diagnosis.
- Radiographs are indicated to rule out avulsion fractures in patients with acute or severe apophysitis.

Current Evidence

Overuse syndrome is a general term that encompasses various injuries that result from excessive and repetitive forces on susceptible structures. Children are at unique risk for such injuries, which are particularly common in adolescent athletes. There is an increased susceptibility during the growth spurt when skeletal growth exceeds the growth of the muscle–tendon unit. This results in increased stress at the apophysis, the musculotendinous origin, or insertion. In children, cartilage is interposed between the tendon and bone, and is most prone to injury from repetitive forces. Repetitive tensile forces at these sites result in chronic irritation and microfractures or avulsions of the apophysis. If allowed to progress, there is evidence that the repetitive microtrauma may weaken the bone and predispose to major avulsion fractures. Underlying anatomic variations, poor quality sporting equipment, and unforgiving playing surfaces may predispose young athletes to overuse injuries. Traction apophysitis is unique to the growing child. By adulthood, the tendon has fused to the bone and repetitive forces cause tendinitis rather than apophysitis. The late childhood and early teenage years coincide with increased participation in organized sporting activities. There is a tendency in high-intensity programs to overtrain young athletes, and at times, to encourage them to work through or ignore the early warning signs of pain.

General therapy for these injuries must emphasize several points. Rest is crucial for the specific area involved until pain has completely resolved. The athlete should be actively encouraged to use alternative activities to maintain conditioning during this time. The role of inflammation in overuse injuries is controversial, but the application of ice and use of anti-inflammatory agents is generally recommended. Directed stretching as well as strengthening exercises reduce tension on affected areas. Biomechanics should be assessed and corrected when necessary. When returning to full activity, an appropriate training regimen should emphasize a slow gradual buildup in intensity and duration and should include explicit limits. The sudden increase in intensity and duration of training that occurs with a change of sporting season is a major culprit in overuse injuries.

Numerous overuse syndromes have acquired popular eponyms. Among the most common overuse syndromes in children are Osgood–Schlatter disease, Little Leaguer elbow, and Sever disease.

Osgood–Schlatter Disease

Osgood–Schlatter disease is an apophysitis of the tibial tubercle. Repetitive stress imposed by the patellar tendon on its site

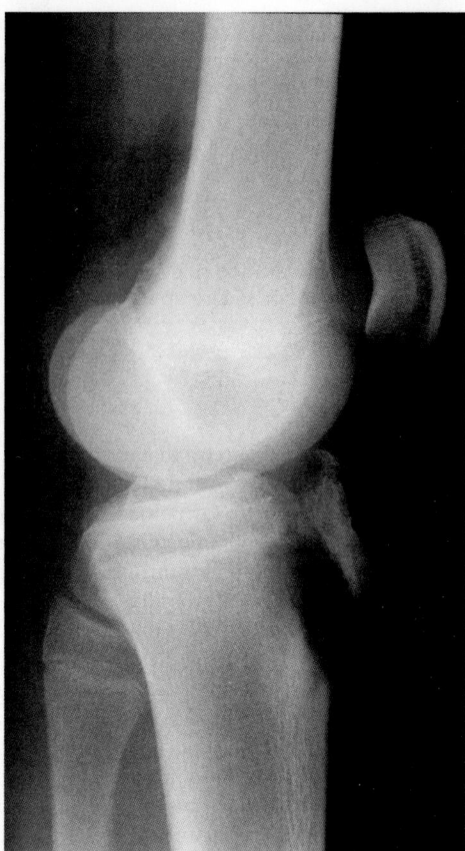

FIGURE 129.6 Acute tibial tubercle avulsion fracture in child with history of Osgood–Schlatter disease.

of insertion results in a series of microavulsions of the secondary ossification center and underlying cartilage. The condition is most common in running and jumping athletes between the ages of 11 and 15 years prior to closure of the tibial growth plate. Boys are most commonly affected, but the rising incidence among girls may be because of increased participation in previously male-dominated sports. Involvement is bilateral in a quarter of cases, although symptoms are commonly asymmetric.

The physical examination is notable for localized tenderness at the tibial tubercle. Any action that applies tension to the patellar tendon elicits pain. Placing the patient prone and flexing the knee so the heel contacts the buttocks will typically trigger pain at the tibial tubercle. Additional maneuvers likely to cause pain include forced extension of the knee, jumping, squatting, or direct pressure as when kneeling. In advanced cases, callus formation occurs, resulting in further prominence of the tubercle. Some experts have suggested a relationship between Osgood–Schlatter disease and acute avulsion fractures of the tibial tubercle (Fig. 129.6). The diagnosis is based on the clinical features. Radiographs are not necessary in typical cases. Atypical presentations including pain at night, pain unrelated to activity or sudden onset of pain should undergo imaging to rule out bony disorders that may mimic Osgood–Schlatter disease. In the early stages of the disease, radiographs are normal. Fragmentation of the tibial tubercle can be a normal finding in the adolescent and must be correlated with clinical findings. In advanced stages of the disease, avulsions from the secondary site of ossification may form ossicles that are visible on a lateral radiograph of the knee.

Management consists first and foremost of avoiding activities that place stress on the tibial tubercle. This is perhaps the most difficult instruction to enforce in young athletes. A brief period of immobilization or nonweight bearing is recommended by some as a means of ensuring compliance. Application of ice for 20 minutes at least twice daily will reduce pain and swelling. Nonsteroidal anti-inflammatory medications are commonly recommended. Activity may be resumed when the patient is free of pain. Flexibility exercises concentrate on stretching the quadriceps and hamstrings to alleviate stress on the tubercle and avoid recurrences. A neoprene sleeve on the knee or doughnut pad around the tibial tuberosity will reduce forces on the tubercle. Over 90% of cases resolve within 12 to 24 months with conservative treatment.

Sinding–Larsen–Johansson Disease

The tension in the infrapatellar tendon that causes Osgood–Schlatter disease is also transmitted proximally to the inferior pole of the patella. A traction apophysitis at this site results in pain and localized tenderness, and is known as Sinding–Larsen–Johansson disease. The predisposing factors for this injury are the same as those for Osgood–Schlatter disease, and include running and jumping activities. Sinding–Larsen–Johansson disease and Osgood–Schlatter disease can occur simultaneously. Provocative maneuvers that produce discomfort in Osgood–Schlatter disease produce pain at the distal patella. Radiographs are nonspecific but may show fragmentation or a small avulsion at the distal pole of the patella (Fig. 129.7), which must be differentiated from an acute sleeve fracture of the patella or a bipartite patella. Treatment emphasizes rest, application of ice, stretching exercises, and oral anti-inflammatory agents. Resolution occurs over a period of 12 to 18 months.

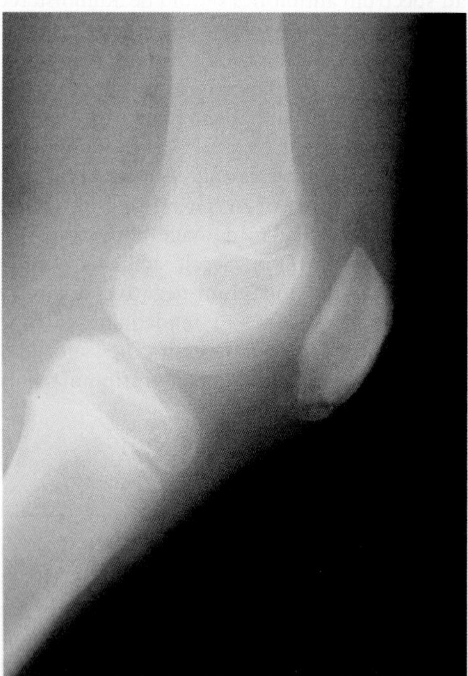

FIGURE 129.7 Avulsion of the inferior pole of the patella in a 10-year-old child with Sinding–Larsen–Johansson disease.

Little Leaguer Elbow

Little Leaguer elbow refers to a group of disorders resulting from repetitive valgus stress applied to the skeletally underdeveloped elbow. The cause of these injuries is multifactorial and includes the number of pitches thrown per outing, the number of outings, type of pitches thrown, throwing technique, and degree of skeletal maturity. Valgus force places tension on the medial collateral ligaments, which is translated to the medial epicondyle. A medial epicondylitis or apophysitis is the most commonly resulting lesion. An avulsion fracture of the medial epicondyle may result from an acute valgus force once the site has become weakened from repetitive microtrauma. Little Leaguer elbow occurs most commonly in boys aged 9 to 12 years.

Patients complain primarily of elbow pain that is exacerbated by throwing. Athletes report progressive drop off in throwing distance. Tenderness is localized over the medial elbow. Applying a valgus stress to the partially flexed elbow will reproduce the pain. Flexion of the wrist or fingers against resistance will also elicit pain. In advanced cases, extension of the elbow becomes limited.

Radiographs or MRI may reveal nonspecific changes such as an irregular or widened medial epicondylar physis, but in general an apophysitis is not visible. Any abnormalities should be correlated with clinical findings to distinguish normal musculoskeletal adaptation to stress from pathologic injury. An avulsion fracture may appear as a bony fragment separated from the medial epicondyle. Comparison views of the nonthrowing elbow may confirm asymmetric changes.

Treatment emphasizes rest for a period of at least 1 month, application of ice, and return to activity only after all pain is gone. Once activity is resumed, the athlete must concentrate on limiting the total amount of pitching, as well as minimizing stress on the medial epicondyle by employing an overhand rather than sidearm pitching motion. Routine stretching and range of motion exercises will reduce the risk of recurrence. Displacement of an avulsion fragment may require surgical repair to restore full elbow function.

Sever Disease

Sever disease is a calcaneal apophysitis occurring at the insertion of the Achilles' tendon at the posterior aspect of the calcaneus. It afflicts predominantly runners, jumpers, and soccer players. Sever disease is often bilateral, is more common in males, and has its peak incidence between 10 and 12 years of age.

Onset of pain is gradual and associated with activity. Localized tenderness occurs at the insertion of the Achilles' tendon on the calcaneus. A maneuver such as hanging the heels over the edge of a step, climbing steps, or hopping applies tension to the Achilles' tendon and exacerbates the pain. Patients are often found to have a tight gastrocnemius–soleus muscle complex and limited dorsiflexion of the foot. Radiographs of the site are usually normal and are unhelpful, except to exclude bony injuries such as stress fractures.

Management includes rest, ice, and anti-inflammatory medications. Heel padding or lifts may be helpful in relieving tension in the area. Flexibility exercises should concentrate on both the hamstrings and the calf muscles. When therapy is initiated early in the disease, most patients are able to return to normal activity by 2 months.

Bursitis

Bursa sacs are both the shock absorbers and the ball bearings of the musculoskeletal system. They disperse forces from blows on bony prominences and reduce friction where tendons or ligaments are in frequent motion.

Trauma, either in a single blow or by repetitive forces, can inflame the bursa, which responds with increased production of synovial fluid. The bursa sac subsequently swells and a cycle of swelling, irritation, and inflammation ensues. Bursitis is most commonly an overuse syndrome seen in adults and adolescents, and is less common in young children.

Injury or cellulitis of the skin overlying a bursa sac can predispose to infection. Aspiration and culture are necessary for definitive diagnosis. The organisms found in septic bursitis are the same as those in septic arthritis, with *S. aureus* accounting for more than 90% of cases. There is no consensus on the need for parenteral versus oral antibiotics. The prepatella bursa and olecranon bursa are most commonly infected.

Bursae are located throughout the body, but bursitis occurs only in a few. Prepatella bursitis, commonly called "housemaid's knee" results from frequent or prolonged kneeling. Pes anserinus bursitis occurs on the lateral aspect of the knee where the tendons of the hamstring muscles overlie the tibia. Retrocalcaneal bursitis occurs between the calcaneus and Achilles' tendon, and is often caused by direct pressure from ill-fitting footwear or high-heeled shoes. Olecranon bursitis most often results from a single direct blow to the elbow. Shoulder or subacromial bursitis is often associated with calcifications and produces severe pain with abduction. Other commonly affected bursae include the inferior calcaneal bursa and the trochanteric bursa.

An unusual form of bursitis is known as a popliteal or Baker cyst. This occurs in the bursa that cushions the tendons of the gastrocnemius and semimembranous muscles from the distal femur. The presence of this condition in adults is highly suggestive of intraarticular knee damage. In children with a Baker cyst, there is frequently a congenitally wide opening joining the bursa sac with the knee joint itself. One-way flow of synovial fluid into the bursa produces swelling just below the popliteal fossa on the medial side. Patients with chronic inflammatory conditions of the knee, such as juvenile idiopathic arthritis, are at increased risk of developing popliteal cysts. The swelling limits full flexion of the knee and produces the sensation of tension with extension. Ultrasound is suggested for confirmation, given it is noninvasive, avoids ionizing radiation, and can identify even small cysts. Plain radiographs are commonly obtained when a Baker cyst has been confirmed, to evaluate for associated bony abnormalities. MRI is more accurate than ultrasound but not as essential in children, given the lower incidence of accompanying intraarticular injury. Rarely, an arthrogram or bursagram may be used to outline the cyst, document the articular connection, and detect ruptures of the cyst.

Bursa inflammation produces swelling and localized tenderness with direct palpation. Any movement of the tendons overlying the site will reproduce the pain.

Conservative therapy consisting of restricted activity, frequent application of ice, and regular use of nonsteroidal anti-inflammatory medications is successful in most cases. Resistant cases respond well to aspiration of synovial fluid and injection of corticosteroids. Frequently recurring cases may require surgical removal of the bursa sac. A new bursa will be generated.

OSTEOCHONDRITIS DISSECANS

Current Evidence

Osteochondritis dissecans is an acquired lesion involving osteonecrosis of subchondral bone. Adults are often diagnosed with osteochondritis dissecans; however, it remains primarily a condition of the adolescent age group, with the highest incidence occurring among male athletes between 12 and 16 years of age. The term "juvenile osteochondritis dissecans" (JOCD) refers to lesions that occur prior to the closure of the growth plates, whereas "adult osteochondritis dissecans" presents after the closure of the growth plate. This distinction has important implications for prognosis and treatment because the likelihood of spontaneous healing is significantly greater in JOCD. The primary sites of osteochondritis dissecans include the medial femoral condyle in the knee, the posteromedial aspect of the talus in the ankle, and the capitellum in the elbow. It is less frequently reported in the hip, foot, and wrist. Involvement of multiple sites is rare, although some series report bilateral knee lesions in up to 30% of cases.

The underlying cause of osteochondritis dissecans remains controversial and may differ based on the anatomic location of the lesion. Trauma, vascular insult, genetic predisposition, and abnormalities of ossification have all been proposed as possible etiologies. The greatest evidence supports repetitive trauma as the sole or major contributing cause of the pathology. Overuse injury is most clearly associated with osteochondritis dissecans of the capitellum, where the majority of cases occur in Little League pitchers. Higher incidences of osteochondritis dissecans of the knee and ankle are seen in participants of activities that place increased stress on these areas, such as distance running, ballet, and basketball. Focal necrosis is suspected to follow the initial insult. Spontaneous resolution may occur at this point, or the lesion may progress with the subchondral bone undergoing various degrees of separation from the underlying epiphysis. In advanced stages, complete separation of the osteochondral fragment results in a free-floating body within the joint, which can disrupt normal mechanical function. Histologic studies have not demonstrated any evidence of inflammation.

When the disease occurs in the second decade of life, long-term outcome is generally good. Progression to osteoarthritis or other degenerative joint diseases is rare. A worse prognosis is associated with a diagnosis after skeletal maturity, a larger lesion, and complete separation of the fragment.

Clinical Considerations

Clinical Recognition

Joint pain develops gradually over several months and is worse with activity. Pain and stiffness typically improves over several hours with rest. Swelling may occasionally be present with activity.

When a free body is present, patients describe intermittent, abrupt locking of the joint. Locking in the knee or elbow prevents full extension of the extremity. This is in contradistinction to buckling, stiffness, or pain with extended range of motion.

Initial Assessment/H&P

The physical examination of the joint is frequently normal. Occasionally, a small effusion may be detectable. Lesions in the medial femoral condyle may be directly palpated and pain elicited when the knee is held in 90 degrees of flexion. The typical location of a lesion in the talus is not accessible on examination. Osteochondritis dissecans in the femoral condyle may give rise to an abnormal gait with external rotation of the affected limb.

Wilson described a clinical test for osteochondritis dissecans of the knee. Wilson sign is elicited by flexing the affected knee to 90 degrees. The tibia is held in internal rotation while the leg is slowly extended. In a positive test, pain occurs at approximately 30 degrees of flexion as the tibial spine contacts the classic location of osteochondritis dissecans in the femur. External rotation of the tibia relieves the pain. Wilson sign has demonstrated low sensitivity in validation studies but, when present, is considered specific for a medial femoral condyle lesion. Conversion from a positive sign to a negative sign over time correlates with clinical healing.

Management/Diagnostic Testing

Plain films of the joint should be obtained, and are often diagnostic when osteochondritis dissecans is suspected (Fig. 129.8). Radiographs reveal a crescentic-shaped defect within the subchondral bone. The avascular segment of subchondral bone may have increased density. A radiolucent line may demarcate the separation from the remainder of the epiphysis. A free body often includes a portion of dead subchondral bone, which appears as a radiodense object within the joint space. In addition to the standard anteroposterior (AP) and lateral views of the knee, tunnel and sunrise views are useful in detecting lesions within the femoral condyle. Lateral, AP, and mortis

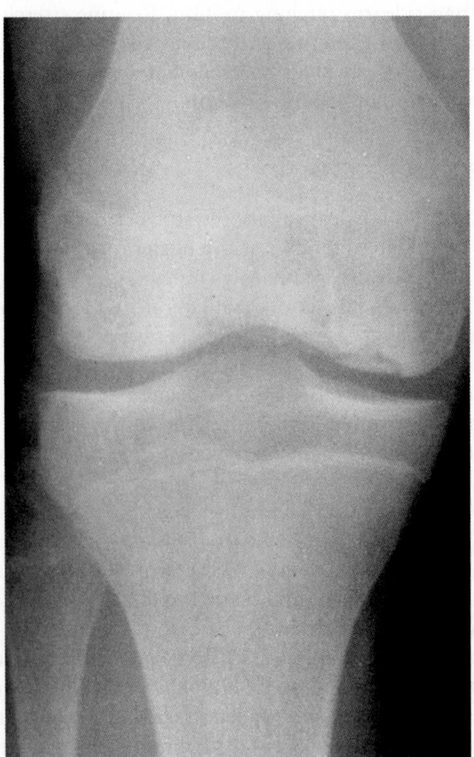

FIGURE 129.8 Osteochondritis dissecans of the medial femoral condyle. Crescentic lesion with radiolucent margin in a 14-year-old girl.

views of the ankle are adequate when a lesion of the talus is suspected, and AP and lateral views of the elbow are indicated for lesions in the capitellum.

Early lesions may not be detected on plain films, and alternate imaging modalities may improve overall sensitivity. When correlated with arthroscopic or surgical findings, MRI has been shown to have excellent ability to detect osteochondritis dissecans and accurately define the extent and stage of the lesion. Osteochondritis dissecans lesions are staged according to the degree of separation from the underlying bone. Stage three or four lesions by MRI have significant separation and are considered unstable. Most orthopedic surgeons consider MRI useful in distinguishing JOCD from other pathologic conditions, guiding therapy and monitoring healing.

The management of osteochondritis dissecans depends on the age and skeletal maturity of the patient, the location of the lesion, and the stage of the lesion. Conservative therapy consisting of restricted activity and relief of stress on the involved joint is the first line of treatment in children who have not reached skeletal maturity and for those diagnosed at an early stage of the disease. Immobilization in a cast or non-weight bearing for lower extremity lesions is often employed to enforce rest. Early return to sports may increase the risk of arthritis or further joint disease. Patients should be followed closely by an orthopedic surgeon both for resolution of clinical symptoms and evidence of healing on serial radiographs or MRIs. Most stable lesions occurring in patients prior to physeal closure go on to heal; however, a few will progress to separation. Lesions occurring in adults generally do not heal without surgery. Surgical intervention is generally recommended if lesions fail to improve clinically or radiographically after 6 months of rest. The presence of an unstable or free-floating fragment is also considered an indication for surgery. Most corrective surgical procedures can now be performed arthroscopically. Fine transarticular or retroarticular drilling through the subchondral fragment into healthy bone appears to stimulate revascularization and promote healing in stable lesions. Fragments are replaced whenever possible. Loose fragments and larger free bodies may be reduced and fixed in place with the use of screws, bioabsorbable implants, or osteochondral plugs removed from nonarticulating surfaces in the knee. When free bodies must be removed from the joint space, the resulting defects may be repaired with the use of a bone graft or through stimulation of fibrocartilage or scar tissue formation to restore congruity to the articular surface.

SLIPPED CAPITAL FEMORAL EPIPHYSIS

Goals of Treatment

Regardless of the acute or chronic nature of the presentation of a slipped capital femoral epiphysis (SCFE), the goal is to identify and stabilize the disorder early. The degree of the slip becomes progressively greater over time. The likelihood of complications and a poor outcome is directly related to the degree of displacement of the epiphysis and the time from symptom onset to intervention. Early surgical fixation of the epiphysis prevents further slippage and worse functional outcome.

CLINICAL PEARLS AND PITFALLS

- Acute (unstable) SCFE is associated with a higher rate of avascular necrosis than chronic (stable) SCFE.
- AP and frog-leg radiographs are the imaging studies of choice for SCFE.
- SCFE typically occurs during the adolescent growth spurt.
- Obesity is highly associated with SCFE.
- Presence of referred pain to the thigh or knee frequently results in delayed diagnosis.
- Flexion of the affected hip frequently results in external rotation.
- Bilateral SCFE occurs in 25% of cases and may not be detectable at the time of initial diagnosis.
- Presence of an endocrinopathy, commonly hypothyroidism, should be suspected in children with SCFE who are outside the normal age range or without the typical body habitus.

Current Evidence

SCFE is the most common hip disorder in adolescent patients and should be familiar to all who care for children in this age group. It is twice as common in males as females, and more common in African-American patients. Over 80% of patients with SCFE have body mass index above the 95th percentile, but clinicians must also consider SCFE in patients who are not obese to avoid delayed diagnosis. As expected, increasing rates of childhood obesity have been associated with an increase in the incidence of SCFE. Most children with SCFE are early adolescents in their growth spurt. Boys are most commonly affected between 13 and 15 years of age, and girls between 11 and 13 years of age because of their earlier pubertal development. SCFE onset after menarche is extremely rare.

Slippage of capital femoral epiphysis is almost always posterior and inferior relative to the proximal femoral metaphysis, however, displacement anteriorly or superiorly has been reported. The epiphysis maintains a normal relationship with the acetabulum. Although symptoms are usually unilateral, plain radiographs document bilateral slippage in about 25% of cases, computed tomographic (CT) scans and MRI in up to 50%.

The perichondrium is primarily responsible for the strength of the proximal femoral physis. SCFE differs from a displaced Salter I fracture in that the perichondrium remains intact in most cases of SCFE and is disrupted with acute Salter I fractures. Collagenous bridges that traverse the physeal cartilage and the undulating convexity of the physis toward the epiphysis contribute to the shear strength of the physis. Children with more vertically inclined physeal angles have greater shear stress across their proximal femoral physes and therefore are at greater risk for SCFE. Although it takes an enormous shearing force to produce acute slippage of an initially normal hip joint, the viscoelasticity of the physeal cartilage allows for gradual slippage. Most children with acute presentations will also have radiographic evidence of chronic slippage.

SCFE is classified by symptom duration, stability, and degree of displacement. Patients with acute SCFE have symptoms for less than 3 weeks; with chronic SCFE, symptoms are present for more than 3 weeks. Acute-on-chronic SCFE describes patients with symptoms for more than 3 weeks with a recent exacerbation. An acute slip with severe symptoms is unstable. Acute or chronic slips with mild symptoms are stable and have a more favorable prognosis.

Most patients with SCFE do not have identifiable endocrinologic problems. However, several hormonal abnormalities have been associated with increased risk. Children outside the usual age range for SCFE, and those with other signs and symptoms that suggest possible endocrine abnormalities should be referred for endocrine evaluation.

Clinical Considerations

Clinical Recognition

Pain and/or limp are the most common chief complaints in patients with SCFE. Physicians may be misled when the pain is referred to the thigh, knee, or groin. SCFE must be considered in the adolescent with these symptoms.

Triage

The presence of limp or hip pain and the potential for SCFE is rarely an emergent condition. These patients should remain nonambulatory as continued weight bearing may exacerbate the slip. The presence of fever in the setting of hip pain or limp would not be consistent with SCFE but may suggest a septic arthritis or osteomyelitis and therefore warrants a higher triage level.

Initial Assessment/H&P

The pain with SCFE is often described as dull, vague, intermittent, and oftentimes chronic in nature. The average duration of symptoms prior to diagnosis of SCFE is 2 months and slip severity is correlated with delay in diagnosis. A history of trivial injury is sometimes obtained, perhaps causing the additional slippage that precipitates a medical evaluation. Acute onset of severe symptoms suggests acute or acute-on-chronic slippage, sometimes referred to as "unstable" SCFE. These patients are often unable to bear weight and may be in significant pain.

Examination findings in patients with SCFE include a resting position with hip flexion and some external rotation. Range of motion of the hip, especially full flexion, internal rotation, and abduction, is decreased and painful. Hip flexion will often be associated with obligate external rotation. Patients with significant displacement may have evidence of limb shortening. Occasionally, there is tenderness of the hip anteriorly. Patients with more acute presentations should *not* be forced to walk as part of the evaluation. Testing for full range of motion is unnecessary once a decision to obtain radiographs has already been reached.

Diagnostic Testing

It is important for emergency physicians to have skill in interpreting plain radiographs for SCFE. Radiographs of the hip should include two views because SCFE is not apparent in one-third of cases in which a single AP view is obtained (Fig. 129.9). On the AP view, widening of the physis is usually seen, even if the displacement is absent. A line drawn along the lateral aspect of the femoral neck on the AP view (Klein line) should intersect a small portion of the femoral epiphysis in a normal hip, but will not in cases of SCFE. The epiphysis in SCFE is almost always displaced posteriorly. The externally rotated frog-leg view turns the posterior aspect medially and facilitates visualization of the offset between the epiphysis and the metaphysis in cases of SCFE. New bone formation may be visible with a chronic slip. When radiographic findings are

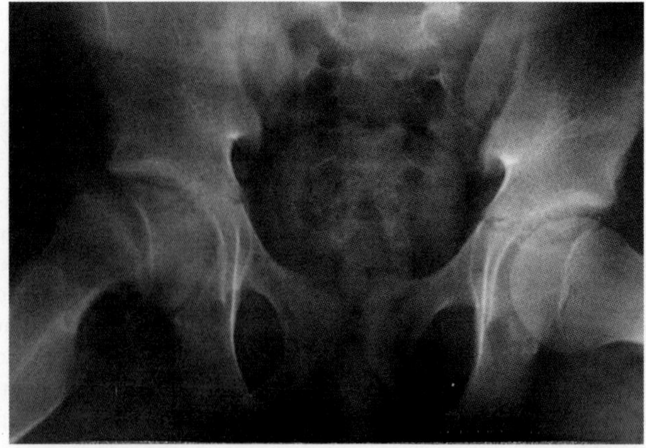

FIGURE 129.9 Slipped capital femoral epiphysis of right hip. Epiphysis is displaced medially on the frog view.

equivocal, comparison with the contralateral, asymptomatic hip should be done with caution, given the possibility of bilateral slippage with unilateral symptoms. Two radiographic views of the hip are 80% sensitive for SCFE. Those with suspicious clinical presentations but normal radiographs may have early SCFE or a "preslip" that may be detected by MRI. In experienced hands, ultrasonography may be more sensitive for SCFE than plain radiography.

The degree of slippage is expressed with a grading system: grade I or preslip with possible widening of the physis but no displacement, grade II with displacement less than one-third of the width of the metaphysis, grade III with displacement of one-third to half of the metaphyseal width, and grade IV with displacement of greater than half the metaphyseal width.

Management/Indications for Discharge or Admission

Children with SCFE who present with severe symptoms and/or acute onset should be admitted and promptly evaluated by an orthopedic surgeon. Unstable SCFE is complicated by avascular necrosis of the femoral head in up to 20% of cases. Patients with milder symptoms may be discharged on crutches, after timely orthopedic follow-up has been arranged. Treatment of SCFE is primarily surgical.

Chondrolysis, the most common complication of SCFE, occurs in about 8% of patients. Pain and persistent decreased range of motion after pinning are the usual presenting symptoms. If the pins extend into the joint space, the risk of chondrolysis is increased. Two-thirds of patients with chondrolysis have a progressive course. Ankylosis may ensue, leading to long-term disability. With a 15% risk of subsequent slippage of the contralateral hip, prophylactic pinning of the contralateral hip after unilateral SCFE is controversial. Younger chronologic age (girls younger than 10 years, boys younger than 12 years) is a very significant predictor for development of a contralateral slip.

PATELLOFEMORAL PAIN SYNDROME

Current Evidence

Patellofemoral pain syndrome describes a constellation of symptoms, principally anterior knee pain, arising from the patellofemoral joint. Chondromalacia patellae is a pathologic diagnosis referring to damage of the articular cartilage of the patella. Specific changes include softening, fissures, and erosions. Whether the two conditions are actually related is the subject of debate. They share a number of symptoms and precipitating factors. Patellofemoral pain syndrome may represent the early end of the spectrum of injury, which ultimately may or may not progress to true pathologic changes within the cartilage.

Patellofemoral pain syndrome is first seen in early adolescents. The rise in incidence tends to parallel the growth spurt. A number of underlying causes or associated factors have been identified. Malalignment of the patella and an abnormal tracking of the patella over the femoral condyles appear to be the major contributors to patellofemoral disorders. The quadriceps or Q angle is the angle between a line from the center of the tibial tubercle to the center of the patella and a second line from the center of the patella to the anterior superior iliac spine. A Q angle greater than 20 degrees has been found in a significant number of affected individuals and results in disproportionate lateral traction applied to the patella during extension. The wider pelvic bones in females result in a generally wider Q angle, which may account for the higher proportion of patellofemoral problems in females. Another contributing anatomic factor is a relative strength imbalance of the four muscles composing the quadriceps. Relative weakness of the vastus medialis is highly associated with the condition and strengthening of this muscle through rehabilitation is associated with clinical improvement. A shallow femoral intracondylar sulcus has also been associated with the disorder.

Clinical Considerations

Clinical Recognition

Patellofemoral pain syndrome is often classified as an overuse syndrome because individuals exposed to repetitive trauma are at higher risk for this disorder. Runners are particularly predisposed to develop this condition especially those running hills or stadium stairs. Poor training regimens, rapid increases in duration or intensity of training, hard or uneven running surfaces, and inadequate shoes have been blamed.

Initial Assessment/H&P

Symptoms consist mainly of anterior knee pain often described as arising from beneath or on the sides of the patella. Pain is usually of gradual onset and is exacerbated by exercise. Pain or stiffness in the knee is common after arising from prolonged sitting. Activities that involve loading of the knee when it is in flexion, such as climbing steps, are particularly painful.

The physical examination is notable for tenderness along the patellar margins or the posterior surface, which is accessible when the patella is manually displaced medially or laterally. Pain, and occasionally crepitus, are elicited with flexion and extension of the knee, or tightening the quadriceps while compressing the patella against the femoral condyles. Range of motion is not limited, and swelling is rare. The presence of an effusion is suggestive of significant cartilaginous damage. Provocative tests that reproduce the pain include climbing steps, squatting, or knee extension against resistance.

Management/Diagnostic Testing

Patellofemoral syndrome is a clinical diagnosis and imaging is not generally indicated. Radiographs may be obtained to more accurately measure the intracondylar sulcus or Q angle, or to rule out alternative diagnoses. MRI, with sensitivity greater than 80%, is considered the best noninvasive diagnostic modality for chondromalacia patellae. True confirmation of lesions requires arthroscopy but may not always be necessary.

Treatment is conservative. More than 90% of cases of patellofemoral pain syndrome resolve after instituting a program of rest, anti-inflammatory medications, and ice followed by physical therapy. Exercises that begin once the initial pain has resolved emphasize strengthening of the quadriceps muscles. Recommended exercise regimens include isometric contractions of the quadriceps with the knee in extension, straight leg raises, and knee extensions, first without and then with weights. Training routines for athletes may need modification and should emphasize soft, even running surfaces; proper biomechanics; and shoes with appropriate cushioning and support. Surgery is recommended only as a last resort in the most recalcitrant cases because results have been generally less than satisfactory. Surgery is directed at either correcting unequal tension applied to the patella or removing loose or nonviable cartilage from the posterior patellar surface.

LEGG–CALVÉ–PERTHES DISEASE

Current Evidence

LCPD is a hip disorder that affects about 1 in 1,200 children and generally has onset between the ages of 4 and 9 years. Males outnumber females by a ratio of 4:1. Most children with LCPD are short, with average or above-average weight, and often have delayed skeletal maturation.

LCPD, or osteonecrosis of the capital femoral epiphysis, is the result of ischemia. LCPD can be simulated in experimental animals by embolizing the blood supply to the femoral head. The theory that LCPD is the result of a variety of clotting abnormalities has gained support in recent years. Thrombotic venous occlusion in the proximal femur may increase intramedullary pressure and lead to ischemia.

Clinical Considerations

Clinical Recognition

Patients may remain asymptomatic despite varying degrees of necrosis and resorption of the femoral head. Some children recover completely without developing symptoms. Symptoms usually begin when routine trauma causes stress fracture of the abnormal subchondral bone. Rarefaction of the femoral head with subluxation and deformity may ensue. The process of reossification and remodeling takes 2 to 4 years.

Initial Assessment/H&P

The onset of symptoms in LCPD is usually insidious. Presentation as an acute emergency is rare. Mild hip pain and limp have usually been present for weeks to months before diagnosis. Pain is often referred in the distribution of the obturator nerve to the knee, anteromedial thigh, or groin. Physical findings include decreased hip abduction and internal rotation.

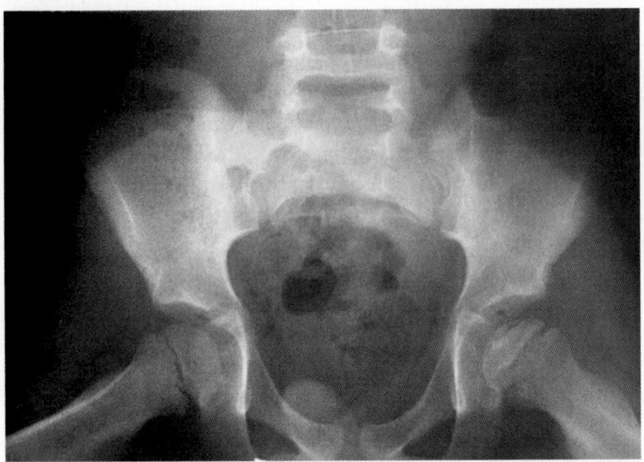

FIGURE 129.10 Legg–Calvé–Perthes disease of left hip. Epiphysis is narrowed and radiodense. A subchondral fracture is also visible.

Thigh muscle atrophy, and in advanced cases, limb shortening may also be noted.

Management/Diagnostic Testing

The sequence of radiographic changes in LCPD has been described in detail (Fig. 129.10). Gadolinium subtraction MRI may offer radiographic evidence of disease during the first 3 to 6 months of symptoms when plain radiographs are normal. At diagnosis, most patients have widening of the articular cartilage with a small, dense proximal femoral epiphysis. Subchondral fracture may be visible. Irregularity and flattening of the epiphysis develops over time. The differential diagnosis includes various bone tumors and skeletal dysplasias. As the disease progresses, anterolateral subluxation may be quantitated radiographically.

Management of LCPD requires a pediatric orthopedist who will follow and treat the child through the various stages of the disease. Prompt referral may influence long-term prognosis. Older children, obese children, girls, and those with more severe disturbance of the epiphysis on radiographs have a poorer prognosis.

ANNULAR LIGAMENT DISPLACEMENT (RADIAL HEAD SUBLUXATION)

Current Evidence

"Nursemaid's elbow" is the most common joint injury in pediatric patients, usually occurring in children between 6 months and 5 years of age. The term annular ligament displacement (ALD) is replacing radial head subluxation for this entity because it is more anatomically correct. Displacement of the annular ligament occurs as a result of traction on a pronated hand or wrist, causing the ligament to slide over the radial head and become interposed between the radius and capitellum.

Except for a very slight increase in the distance between the radial head and capitellum that can be seen on ultrasound, the relationship between radial head and capitellum remains essentially unchanged, and radiographs are normal in patients with ALD. The radial head is not abnormal and the annular ligament does not necessarily tear when this injury occurs. The left elbow is more often affected because adult caregivers tend to hold the child's left hand with their dominant right hand.

Clinical Considerations

Clinical Recognition

ALD can be strongly suspected from across the examining room. The child generally holds the arm slightly flexed, against his or her body with the forearm pronated. When left alone, the child does not appear to be in significant pain. Parents may report a problem with the wrist or shoulder because, in their attempts to assess these joints, inadvertent movement of the elbow causes pain. Physicians can be similarly fooled, especially when a classic history is not obtained.

Initial Assessment/H&P

In up to half of the cases, a history of traction on the arm is not obtained, which may suggest another mechanism for this injury or perhaps caregivers who are reluctant to volunteer self-incriminating information. Astute clinicians should suspect this injury even in the absence of the typical history.

The young child must be approached in a slow and nonthreatening manner. Examination that does not move the elbow joint at all is necessary to exclude point tenderness of the clavicle, humerus, radius, and ulna that may suggest a fracture. True tenderness and swelling at the elbow are usually absent. When disuse of the elbow is present without significant pain or bony tenderness, the clinician should perform the reduction maneuver to confirm the diagnosis of radial head subluxation.

Management/Diagnostic Testing

Radiographs of the elbow are unnecessary unless the physician suspects another injury. Swelling and localized tenderness of the distal humerus are usually apparent with supracondylar fractures, the next most common elbow injury in this age group.

Reduction of a displaced annular ligament is one of the most gratifying procedures for physicians and parents alike. Nonmedical caregivers have been instructed by telephone to reduce recurrent ALDs. Several effective reduction maneuvers have been described. In performing the traditional supination–flexion maneuver, the clinician holds the elbow with his or her thumb over the radial head (Fig. 129.11). In the majority of patients, full supination of the affected arm rotates the flared aspect of the radial head, snapping the annular ligament back to its original position with a telltale click. Flexion or extension of the elbow after supination may add to the success rate. If no click is felt, a second attempt can be made, perhaps exerting mild traction to disengage the annular ligament from between the radial head and capitellum. Forced pronation or pronation–flexion is an alternative method for reduction that appears to be more effective and less painful than the supination–flexion maneuver. Pronation–flexion sometimes succeeds after the initial attempt at reduction with supination–flexion has failed. After an attempt at reduction that does not result in a perceptible click, the child should be observed and tested for return of arm function because some successful reductions occur without a detectable click. Excessive failed attempts at reduction should be avoided. Radiographs may be useful for patients who fail reduction maneuvers.

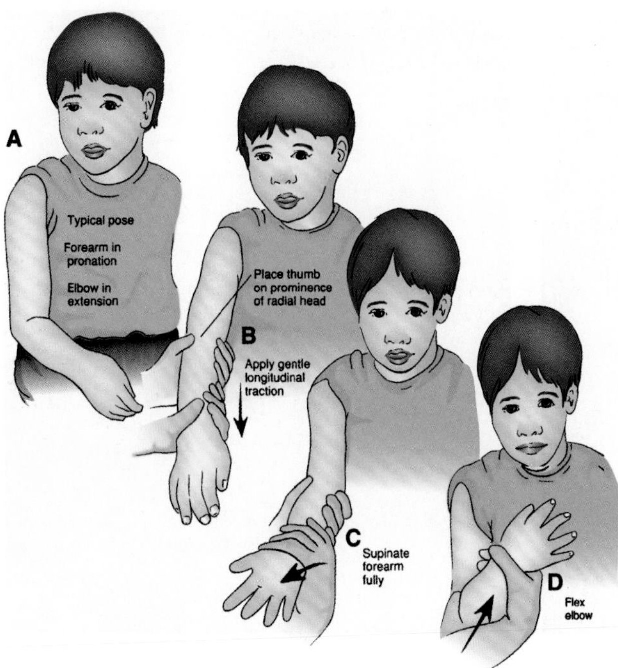

FIGURE 129.11 **A–D:** Supination–flexion maneuver for reduction of radial head subluxation (nursemaid's elbow).

Return of function after successful reduction is usually prompt, but not immediate. Toys, bottles, or interesting objects can be used to encourage the child to use the affected arm. Voluntary use of the arm will return in less than 15 minutes in almost 90% of patients. Younger children generally take longer to begin reusing the arm. Longer duration of subluxation does not appear to be associated with delayed return of function. Many clinicians relate experiences with "failed" reductions in children whose arms are better the following morning. If disuse of the arm persists and radiographs are normal, a sling should be placed and the child should be seen in follow-up by an orthopedist.

Recurrent ALDs are common, occurring in a quarter to one-third of cases. Caregivers should be counseled to lift the child from the axillae, avoiding traction on the distal extremities.

Shoulder (Glenohumeral) Subluxation/Dislocation

Shoulder dislocation is extremely uncommon in young children. Shoulder dystocia at delivery can lead to displaced Salter I fractures that look like dislocations because the unossified proximal humeral epiphysis remaining in the glenoid fossa is not visible radiographically. True dislocations become more common in adolescence, and their management is described in Chapter 141 Procedures. Intraarticular lidocaine injection is an alternative to intravenous narcotic/benzodiazepine as analgesia for reduction of shoulder dislocations that has a lower complication rate and requires less time in the emergency department.

Glenohumeral subluxation/dislocation will be recurrent in about half of all the cases, especially if the anterior glenoid rim is avulsed (Bankart lesion). Patients may report functional impairments from a shoulder that "pops out" and reduces spontaneously. Some disturbed individuals intentionally dislocate their shoulder. Arthroscopic surgery can stabilize the shoulder, reducing the likelihood of recurrent dislocation. Data are insufficient and opinion is divided on whether surgical intervention is indicated after the first shoulder dislocation or better reserved for cases that are recurrent.

DISORDERS OF THE BACK

Discitis (Diskitis)

Current Evidence

Discitis is an uncommon and poorly understood inflammatory condition involving the intervertebral disc space. Vertebral osteomyelitis with involvement of the disc space is a distinct diagnostic entity with different epidemiology and pathophysiology from discitis. The mean age of patients with discitis is less than children with vertebral osteomyelitis. No gender or racial predilection has been noted. The involved disc space is usually lumbar or lower thoracic. Most authorities believe discitis results from infection. A history of trauma is obtained in some patients with discitis, but whether the injury plays a role or is a "red herring" is unclear. The vascular anatomy of the disc space supports the notion that organisms reach the disc space via the hematogenous route. In children, the blood supply of the disc space comes from adjacent vertebral body end plates. These vascular connections are absent in older adolescents and adults, and may be the reason discitis is so rare in this age group. Discitis can also be a complication of lumbar puncture.

Bacteria are cultured from a minority of children with discitis. *S. aureus* is the predominant isolate from disc space aspirates and occasionally blood, but other organisms including *Kingella* and anaerobes have also been recovered.

Clinical Considerations

Clinical Recognition. Children with discitis are a diagnostic challenge for clinicians. The condition is uncommon and symptoms are often nonspecific and vague, especially in the younger child. They usually have been present for more than 1 week at the time of diagnosis.

Initial Assessment/H&P. Back pain is not always described. Limp, refusal to walk, leg pain, hip pain, and abdominal pain are common presenting complaints. Unlike vertebral osteomyelitis, which is usually associated with fever, only about a quarter of patients with discitis are febrile. Irritability may also be reported.

Physical findings suggesting discitis will be missed if this entity is not considered because careful examination of the spine is not performed routinely by most clinicians. Many children assume a recumbent position of comfort from which they do not want to be moved. Decreased range of motion of the spine and paravertebral muscle spasm are usually present. There is often a change in the lumbar lordosis, which may be decreased or increased. Tenderness to palpation of the disc space can usually be demonstrated. Range of motion of the hips is essentially normal, but inadvertent movement of the lumbar spine during hip examination may cause pain that is misinterpreted to suggest hip pathology. Straight leg raise may be limited by muscle spasm in the hamstrings. Neurologic assessment of the lower extremities is generally normal, but there are reports of discitis with neurologic involvement. Abnormalities in strength, sensation, and/or deep tendon

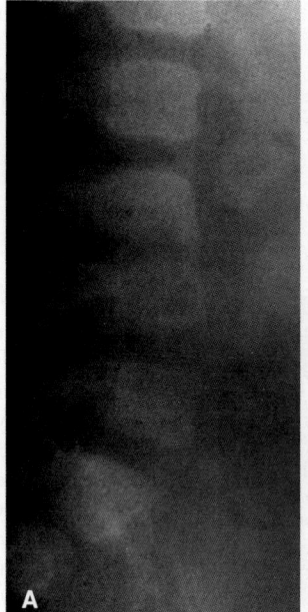

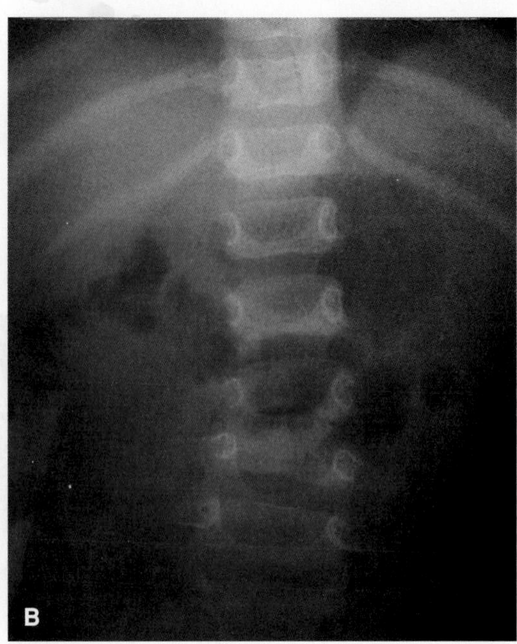

FIGURE 129.12 Discitis. L3-L4 intervertebral disc space is narrowed. Lateral (**A**) and anteroposterior (**B**) views.

reflexes suggest a spinal cord lesion, tumor, epidural abscess, or herniation of the disc (rare). Signs of discitis may vary, depending on the location of the inflamed disc. Patients with lesions of the upper spine may have meningismus.

Management/Diagnostic Testing. Imaging studies can be useful in the diagnosis of discitis. Plain radiographs may be normal initially, but intervertebral disc space narrowing develops after 2 to 3 weeks of illness (Fig. 129.12). At the time of diagnosis, 76% of children with discitis will have abnormal radiographs. Bone scan is perhaps the most sensitive imaging modality, especially early in the course of this disease. Increased uptake at the level of the involved disc can confirm the diagnosis. CT scanning can demonstrate the degree of bony erosion of the vertebral end plates and paravertebral soft-tissue involvement. MRI is 90% sensitive and can help differentiate discitis from vertebral osteomyelitis.

Laboratory testing plays a minor role. Elevation of the WBC count is sometimes noted at the time of diagnosis. ESRs of 40 to 60 mm per hour are usually noted in patients presenting with discitis and decrease with resolution of the disease. Skin testing for tuberculosis, as well as serologic testing for brucellosis and salmonellosis, are often performed but not routinely recommended. Discitis can usually be diagnosed and treated without biopsy or aspiration of the involved disc space. If the presentation is atypical, signs and symptoms severe, or response to therapy unsatisfactory, obtaining a guided needle aspiration can be helpful.

Discitis is a self-limited disease and need not be treated aggressively. Virtually all children in reported series return to normal function in a few months. Resting the spine usually results in improved symptoms in days to weeks. Immobilization with plaster has not been shown to improve outcome over bed rest alone, but therapeutic decisions should be individualized with input from an orthopedist.

Although there are no data to suggest that they speed recovery or improve outcome, antistaphylococcal antibiotics seem prudent, given the frequency of documented staphylococcal infection. When cultures demonstrate particular organisms with known antimicrobial susceptibilities, antibiotic therapy can be individualized.

Spondylolysis and Spondylolisthesis

Current Evidence

Spondylolysis, with or without spondylolisthesis, occurs in 2% to 5% of children, but the majority are asymptomatic. Most children presenting with low back pain will not receive a definitive diagnosis, but of those that do, spondylolysis is the most common condition identified. Adolescents involved in sports are at highest risk.

Spondylolysis is a defect in the pars interarticularis of the vertebral body. Spondylolisthesis is displacement of the vertebral bodies, usually involving L5 slipping anteriorly on S1. Spondylolisthesis may result from structural abnormalities of the vertebral bodies (dysplastic type) or acquired defects of the pars interarticularis (isthmic type) that allow slippage. There is a genetic predisposition to spondylolysis and spondylolisthesis. Parents of children with spondylolisthesis are found to have this condition in 28% of cases.

The cause of the defect of the pars interarticularis in spondylolysis is not fully understood. Repeated stress, such as occurs in gymnasts with frequent hyperextension of the spine, causes stress fracture. One side of the pars interarticularis fractures overtly, which adds to the stress on the contralateral side. Fracture becomes bilateral. Displacement may or may not occur. Children who play sports that stress the spine, such as gymnastics, football, rowing, diving, weight lifting, and high jumping, are at particular risk.

Clinical Considerations

Clinical Recognition. Patients who develop symptoms generally present during the adolescent growth spurt. Back pain usually has an insidious onset and worsens with activity, improves with rest. Over time, there may be pain in the buttocks and posterior thighs. Symptoms radiating down the legs suggest significant nerve root irritation. Parents may

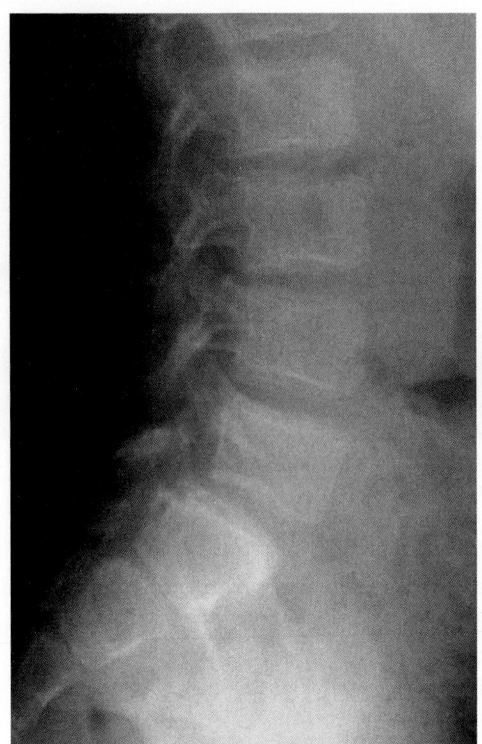

FIGURE 129.13 [illegible] iorly on S1.

describe an in [illegible] change in the child's gai[illegible]

Initial Assessn[illegible] the prone position shows [illegible] he lumbar spine and with [illegible] ually tight, with decreased [illegible] l flexion of the trunk. Children seldom have motor (10%), sensory (15%), or reflex (10%) deficits in the legs.

Management/Diagnostic Testing. Plain radiographs should include AP, lateral, and oblique views. The "scotty dog" of the oblique view will have a collar on the neck if spondylolysis is present. Spondylolisthesis can be diagnosed on the lateral view, and the degree of displacement can be quantitated relative to the width of the vertebral body (Fig. 129.13). A bone scan or MRI in children with chronic back pain and normal plain radiographs can identify spondylolysis in its early stages, when conservative therapy can result in bony union.

Treatment varies, depending on symptoms and degree of displacement, if any. Most cases of asymptomatic spondylolysis and spondylolisthesis with mild displacement will not progress. Children with displacement greater than 25% should avoid rough sports. Symptomatic children with displacement may benefit from immobilization. Decisions about treatment should be made in consultation with an orthopedic surgeon.

COMPARTMENT SYNDROME

Current Evidence

Compartment syndrome refers to vascular insufficiency caused by elevated tissue pressures that usually occurs after an injury involving hemorrhage or edema within an enclosed fascial compartment. Tight circumferential bandages or casts can also limit expansion of swollen tissues and result in elevation of tissue pressures. Fluid extravasation from intravenous or intraosseous lines, especially pressure-driven extravasation, may significantly elevate compartment pressures. Direct injury to an artery is less common as the cause of vascular insufficiency after injury but is also considered as compartment syndrome.

When compartment pressures approach the perfusion pressure of muscle, which is approximately 30 mm Hg, arterial inflow is reduced and veins and capillaries are collapsed. Ischemia of muscle leads to further swelling, and a positive feedback loop of ischemia—edema can further elevate tissue pressures and lead to complete cessation of perfusion. Muscle necrosis is irreversible after 6 to 8 hours of tissue anoxia. Fibrosis develops and ischemic contracture results in permanent disability.

Clinical Considerations

Clinical Recognition

The emergency physician must identify patients at risk for compartment syndromes, and consult with an orthopedist who can monitor tissue pressures and treat compartment syndromes before irreversible injury occurs.

Knowledge of the common pediatric injuries that are associated with compartment syndromes can raise the clinician's index of suspicion appropriately. Displaced supracondylar fractures may injure the anterior interosseous artery and the flexor compartment of the forearm causing a compartment syndrome that leads to the classic Volkmann contracture. Though controversial, some have suggested that delayed reduction is a risk factor for compartment syndrome after supracondylar fracture. Forearm fractures may also cause compartment syndromes, affecting either the flexor or extensor musculature. Fractures of the tibia and/or fibula can lead to compartment syndrome of the lower leg. Fractures that are open are at greater risk for the development of a compartment syndrome, perhaps because they result from higher-energy mechanisms. Compartment syndromes may occur from crush injuries and other soft-tissue trauma that does not necessarily involve a fracture. Poisonous snakebites, especially pit vipers, and deep tissue infections such as myositis or fasciitis may also lead to dangerous elevations of compartment pressures.

Clinical Assessment/Initial H&P

The "five Ps" of compartment syndrome is a mnemonic that can be misleading. One "P," pain, is often the only early symptom or sign of vascular insufficiency. The astute clinician would have consulted an orthopedic surgeon and suspected compartment syndrome before paresthesia, pallor, paralysis, and pulselessness are present.

Pain, the hallmark of compartment syndromes, is a symptom in almost all significant injuries. Distinguishing the pain from the injury itself from that related to the vascular insufficiency is difficult. Pain that increases over time or seems out of proportion to the injury itself suggests muscle ischemia. Full extension of the fingers or toes stretches ischemic muscles and exacerbates the pain in compartment syndromes, making this part of the examination especially important in patients at risk for compartment syndromes.

Paresthesia may be noted in the distribution of the nerves that traverse the ischemic compartment. When the flexor compartment of the forearm is involved, the median nerve is usually affected. Over time, paresthesias may progress to complete anesthesia, and pain may decrease.

Pallor from decreased perfusion may be noted distally. Sluggish circulation may cause cyanosis. Paralysis is a late finding and is probably the least sensitive marker for compartment syndrome. Pulselessness is a useful finding if present, but some physicians are falsely reassured when distal pulses are palpable. Collateral circulation can preserve pulses in larger vessels but the ischemia in compartment syndromes results from vascular occlusion of small vessels.

Management/Diagnostic Testing

Treatment of a compartment syndrome should begin from the moment it is suspected. All circumferential bandages should be removed. If symptoms persist, measurement of compartment pressures should be obtained, with by the emergency physician or in consultation with an orthopedic surgeon. Reduction of displaced fractures can improve blood flow to affected compartments. Fasciotomy in the operating room is indicated if compartment pressures remain high.

COMPLEX REGIONAL PAIN SYNDROME TYPE 1 (REFLEX SYMPATHETIC DYSTROPHY)

Current Evidence

Complex regional pain syndrome type 1 (CRPS1), formerly known as reflex sympathetic dystrophy (RSD) or reflex neurovascular dystrophy (RND), is a poorly understood disorder characterized by pain, abnormal sensation, and circulatory irregularities. Over time, atrophic changes of the extremity may develop. Initially thought to be primarily an adult disease, CRPS1 is increasingly being recognized in children. There are often delays in diagnosing children with CRPS1. Emergency physicians can play a valuable role by considering CRPS1 in children with pain and making appropriate referrals for a prompt, definitive diagnosis. In many patients symptoms of CRPS1 will eventually resolve, but early treatment may prevent prolonged disability.

Children with CRPS1 as young as 3 years have been described. The average age of children with CRPS1 is approximately 12 years, girls outnumbering boys by as much as 6:1. Most cases in children involve the lower extremity. CRPS1 usually follows minor trauma, but some cases develop without an identified precipitant.

The pathophysiology of CRPS1 is not well-understood. Early theories suggested abnormal synapses develop between sensory afferent nerves and sympathetic afferents after an injury. "Sympathetic" dystrophy is probably a misnomer, and nomenclature has changed because local epinephrine and norepinephrine levels are lower, not higher, than normal, and vasodilation, not sympathetic vasoconstriction, may predominate. Current theories include regional sensitization of the central and perhaps peripheral nervous system from an initial injury. Experimental evidence suggests involvement of glutamate and NMDA (*N*-methyl-D-aspartic acid) receptors in this process. Patients with other dysautonomic conditions, including

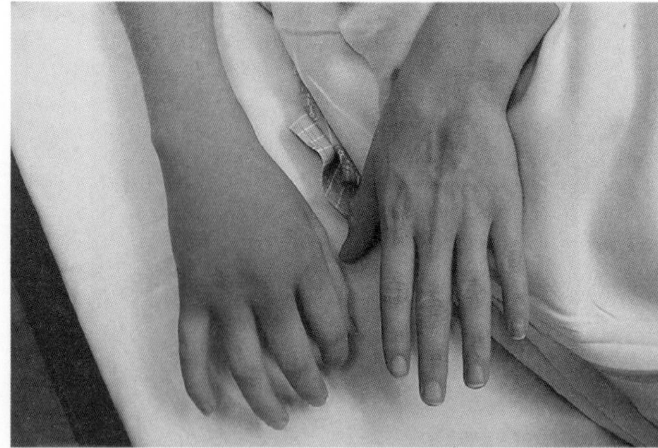

FIGURE 129.14 Reflex sympathetic dystrophy in a 10-year-old girl after a minor wrist injury.

gastrointestinal dysmotility, migraine, cyclic vomiting, and chronic fatigue, may also have CRPS1.

Clinical Considerations

Clinical Recognition

Pain is usually the presenting complaint with CRPS1. The pain is continuous, often burning in quality, with exacerbations but no complete remissions. Abnormal sensitivity is distinctive, with severe pain provoked by normally nontender touching (allodynia). The extremity is usually swollen and cool to the touch, although warmth has also been reported (Fig. 129.14). Dusky discoloration of the skin with hyperhidrosis or anhydrosis may be present. The arm or leg is not used, and atrophic muscle, skin, and bony changes develop in some patients over time. There is some evidence that demineralization of bone occurs more rapidly than would be expected from disuse alone.

Psychiatric and personality problems have been suspected in many patients with CRPS1, but controlled prospective studies are lacking. Factitious illness or conversion reactions are often considered because symptoms are out of proportion to the inciting injury.

Initial Assessment/H&P

The characteristic history and physical examination, including pain, loss of function, and evidence of autonomic dysfunction, allow for a clinical diagnosis of CRPS1 in most cases. Radiographs in children may not demonstrate the osteoporosis described in adults, especially early after the onset of symptoms. Radionuclide bone scans generally show increased blood flow and periarticular uptake in adults, but in children with CRPS1 the blood flow and osseous uptake is more often reduced. Thermography may document decreased temperature in the affected extremity.

Management

Treatment of CRPS1 focuses on early mobilization of the extremity through physical therapy to avoid atrophic changes. Physiotherapy may initially exacerbate symptoms, but experienced clinicians believe it both prevents atrophy and decreases the duration of pain. The knee-jerk response to splint for comfort may be counterproductive with CRPS1. Referral to a pediatric pain program is advisable if symptoms persist. Sympathetic block with local anesthetic is commonly performed in patients with CRPS1 but evidence of its effectiveness is lacking. There are case reports of successful treatment of CRPS1 with intravenous regional block using guanethidine, transcutaneous nerve stimulation, and sympathectomy.

Suggested Readings and Key References

Osteomyelitis

Bocchini CE, Hulten KG, Mason EO Jr, et al. Panton-Valentine leukocidin genes are associated with enhanced inflammatory response and local disease in acute hematogenous Staphylococcus aureus osteomyelitis in children. *Pediatrics* 2006;117:433–440.

Ekopimo OI, Imoisili M, Pikis A. Group A beta-hemolytic streptococcal osteomyelitis in children. *Pediatrics* 2003;112:e22–e26.

El-Shanti HI, Ferguson PJ. Chronic recurrent multifocal osteomyelitis: a concise review and genetic update. *Clin Orthop Relat Res* 2007; 462:11–19.

Gutierrez K. Bone and joint infections in children. *Pediatr Clin North Am* 2005;52:779–794.

Jacobs RF, McCarthy RE, Elser JM. Pseudomonas osteochondritis complicating puncture wounds of the foot in children: a 10-year evaluation. *J Infect Dis* 1989;160:657–661.

Martinez-Aguilar G, Avalos-Mishaan A, Hulten K, et al. Community-acquired, methicillin-resistant and methicillin-susceptible Staphylococcus aureus musculoskeletal infections in children. *Pediatr Infect Dis J* 2004;23:701–706.

Oudjhane K, Azouz ME. Imaging of osteomyelitis in children. *Radiol Clin North Am* 2001;39:251–266.

Saavedra-Lozano J, Mejias A, Ahmad N, et al. Changing trends in acute osteomyelitis in children: impact of methicillin-resistant Staphylococcus aureus infections. *J Pediatr Orthop* 2008;28:569–575.

Tuson CE, Hoffman EB, Mann MD. Isotope bone scanning for acute osteomyelitis and septic arthritis in children. *J Bone Joint Surg Br* 1994;76:306–310.

Unkila-Kallio L, Kallio MJ, Eskola J, et al. Serum C-reactive protein, erythrocyte sedimentation rate, and white blood cell count in acute hematogenous osteomyelitis of children. *Pediatrics* 1994;93:59–62.

Vazquez M. Osteomyelitis in children. *Curr Opin Pediatr* 2002;14: 112–115.

Wong M, Isaacs D, Howman-Giles R, et al. Clinical and diagnostic features of osteomyelitis occurring in the first three months of life. *Pediatr Infect Dis J* 1995;14:1047–1053.

Septic Arthritis

Arnold SR, Elias D, Buckingham SC, et al. Changing patterns of acute hematogenous osteomyelitis and septic arthritis: emergence of community-associated methicillin-resistant Staphylococcus aureus. *J Pediatr Orthop* 2006;26:703–708.

Kallio MJ, Unkila-Kallio L, Aalto K, et al. Serum C-reactive protein, erythrocyte sedimentation rate and white blood cell count in septic arthritis of children. *Pediatr Infect Dis J* 1997;16:411–413.

Kocher MS, Lee B, Dolan M, et al. Pediatric orthopedic infections: early detection and treatment. *Pediatr Ann* 2006;35:112–122.

Kocher MS, Mandiga R, Zurakowski D, et al. Validation of a clinical prediction rule for the difference between septic arthritis and transient synovitis of the hip in children. *J Bone Joint Surg Am* 2004;86: 1629–1635.

Lundy DW, Kehl DK. Increasing prevalence of Kingella kingae in osteoarticular infections in young children. *J Pediatr Orthop* 1998; 18:262–267.

Moumile K, Merckx J, Pouliquen JC, et al. Bacterial aetiology of acute osteoarticular infections in children. *Acta Pediatr* 2005;94: 419–422.

Yagupsky P, Bar-Ziv Y, Howard CB, et al. Epidemiology, etiology, and clinical features of septic arthritis in children younger than 24 months. *Arch Pediatr Adolesc Med* 1995;149:537–540.

Lyme Arthritis

Bachman DT, Srivastava G. Emergency department presentations of Lyme disease in children. *Pediatr Emerg Care* 1998;14:356–361.

Bachur RG, Adams CM, Monuteaux MC. Evaluating the child with acute hip pain ("irritable hip") in a Lyme endemic region. *J Pediatr* 2015;166(2):407–411

Deanehan JK, Nigrovic PA, Milewski MD, et al. Synovial fluid findings in children with knee monoarthritis in Lyme Disease endemic areas. *Pediatr Emerg Care* 2014;30:16–19.

Deanehan JK, Kimia AA, Tan Tanny SP, et al. Distinguishing Lyme from septic knee monoarthritis in Lyme-Disease endemic areas. *Pediatrics* 2013;131:e695–e701.

Puius YA, Kalish RA. Lyme arthritis: pathogenesis, clinical presentation, and management. *Infect Dis Clin North Am* 2008;22: 289–300.

Shapiro ED, Gerber MA. Lyme disease: fact versus fiction. *Pediatr Ann* 2002;31:170–177.

Thompson A, Mannix R, Bachur R. Acute pediatric monoarticular arthritis: distinguishing Lyme arthritis from other etiologies. *Pediatrics* 2009;123(3):959–65

Wormser GP, Dattwyler RJ, Shapiro ED, et al. The clinical assessment, treatment, and prevention of Lyme disease, human granulocytic anaplasmosis, and babesiosis: clinical practice guidelines by the Infectious Diseases Society of America. *Clin Infect Dis* 2006;43: 1089–1134.

Transient Synovitis

Caird MS, Flynn JM, Leung YL, et al. Factors distinguishing septic arthritis from transient synovitis of the hip in children. A prospective study. *J Bone Joint Surg Am* 2006;88:1251–1257.

Fink AM, Berman L, Edwards D, et al. The irritable hip: immediate ultrasound guided aspiration and prevention of hospital admission. *Arch Dis Child* 1995;72:110–114.

Kocher MS, Zurakowski D, Kasser JR. Differentiating between septic arthritis and transient synovitis of the hip in children: an evidence-based clinical prediction algorithm. *J Bone Joint Surg Am* 1999;81: 1662–1670.

Mukamel M, Litmanovitch M, Yosipovich Z, et al. Legg-Calvé-Perthes disease following transient synovitis. How often? *Clin Pediatr(Phila)* 1985;24:629–631.

Penetrating Intraarticular Injuries

Collins DN, Temple SD. Open joint injuries: classification and treatment. *Clin Orthop Relat Res* 1989;243:48–56.

Tornetta P, Boes MT, Schepsis AA, et al. How effective is a saline arthrogram for wounds around the knee? *Clin Orthop Relat Res* 2008;466:432–435.

Voit GA, Irvine G, Beals RK. Saline load test for penetration of periarticular lacerations. *J Bone Joint Surg Br* 1996;78:732–733.

Overuse Syndromes

Duri ZA, Patel DV, Aichroth PM. The immature athlete. *Clin Sports Med* 2002;21:461–482.

Dyment PG, ed. *Sports medicine: health care for young athletes.* Elk Grove Village, IL: American Academy of Pediatrics, 1991.

Gerbino PG. Elbow disorders in throwing athletes. *Orthop Clin North Am* 2003;34:417–426.

Gill TJ, Micheli LJ. The immature athlete: common injuries and overuse syndromes of the elbow and wrist. *Clin Sports Med* 1996;15: 401–423.

Gomez JE. Upper extremity injuries in youth sports. *Pediatr Clin North Am* 2002;49:593–626.

Hogan KA, Gross RH. Overuse injuries in pediatric athletes. *Orthop Clin North Am* 2003;34:405–415.

Kennedy JG, Knowles B, Dolan M, et al. Foot and ankle injuries in the adolescent runner. *Curr Opin Pediatr* 2005;17:34–42.

Purushottam AG, Scher DM, Khakharia S, et al. Osgood Schlatter syndrome. *Curr Opin Pediatr* 2007;19:44–50.

Soprano JV, Fuchs SM. Common overuse injuries in the pediatric and adolescent athlete. *Clin Pediatr Emerg Med* 2007;8:7–14.

Bursitis

Acebes JC, Sánchez-Pernaute O, Díaz-Oca A, et al. Ultrasonographic assessment of Baker's cysts after intra-articular corticosteroid injection in knee osteoarthritis. *J Clin Ultrasound* 2006;34:113.

Akagi R, Saisu T, Segawa Y, et al. Natural history of popliteal cysts in the pediatric population. *J Pediatr Orthop* 2013;33:262–268.

Harwell JI, Fisher D. Pediatric septic bursitis: case report of retrocalcaneal infection and review of the literature. *Clin Infect Dis* 2001;32: e102–e104.

Marra MD, Crema MD, Chung M, et al. MRI features of cystic lesions around the knee. *Knee* 2008;15:423–438.

Raddatz DA, Hoffman GS, Franck WA. Septic bursitis: presentation, treatment, and prognosis. *J Rheumatol* 1987;14:1160–1163.

Szer IS, Klein-Gitelman M, DeNardo BA, et al. Ultrasonography in the study of prevalence and clinical evolution of popliteal cysts in children with knee effusions. *J Rheumatol* 1992;19(3):458–462.

Osteochondritis Dissecans

Bradley J, Dandy DJ. Osteochondritis dissecans and other lesions of the femoral condyles. *J Bone Joint Surg Br* 1989;71:518–522.

Chambers HG, Shea KG, Carey JL. AAOS Clinical practice guideline: diagnosis and treatment of osteochondritis dissecans. *J Am Acad Orthop Surg* 2011;19:307–309.

Conrad JM, Stanitski CL. Osteochondritis dissecans: Wilson's sign revisited. *Am J Sports Med* 2003;31:777–778.

Letts M, Davidson D, Ahmer A. Osteochondritis dissecans of the talus in children. *J Pediatr Orthop* 2003;23:617–625.

Pill SG, Ganley TJ, Milam RA, et al. Role of magnetic resonance imaging and clinical criteria in predicting successful nonoperative treatment of osteochondritis dissecans in children. *J Pediatr Orthop* 2003;23:102–108.

Robertson W, Kelly BT, Green DW. Osteochondritis dissecans of the knee in children. *Curr Opin Pediatr* 2003;15:38–44.

Wall E, Von Stein D. Juvenile osteochondritis dissecans. *Orthop Clin North Am* 2003;34:341–353.

Slipped Capital Femoral Epiphysis

Georgiadis AG, Zaltz I. Slipped capital femoral epiphysis: how to evaluate with a review and update of treatment. *Pediatr Clin North Am* 2014;61:1119–1135.

Futami T, Suzuki S, Seto Y, et al. Sequential magnetic resonance imaging in slipped capital femoral epiphysis: assessment of preslip in contralateral hip. *J Pediatr Orthop* 2001;10:298–303.

Kocher MS, Bishop J. Delay in diagnosis of slipped capital femoral epiphysis. *Pediatrics* 2004;113:e322–e325.

Manoff EM, Banffy MB, Winell JJ. Relationship between Body Mass Index and slipped capital femoral epiphysis. *J Pediatr Orthop* 2005;25:744–746.

Mooney JF 3rd, Sanders JO, Browne RH, et al. Management of unstable/acute slipped capital femoral epiphysis: results of a survey of the POSNA membership. *J Pediatr Orthop* 2005;25:162–166.

Riad J, Bajelidze G, Gabos PG. Bilateral slipped capital femoral epiphysis: predictive factors for contralateral slip. *J Pediatr Orthop* 2007; 27:411–414.

Thawrani DP, Feldman DS, Sala DA. Current Practice in the Management of Slipped Capital Femoral Epiphysis. *J Pediatr Orthop* 2015. [Epub ahead of print]

Chondromalacia Patellae

Davidson K. Patellofemoral pain syndrome. *Am Fam Physician* 1993; 48:1254–1262.

Dyment PG, ed. *Sports medicine: health care for young athletes*. Elk Grove Village, IL: American Academy of Pediatrics, 1991.

Tria AJ Jr, Palumbo RC, Alicea JA. Conservative care for patellofemoral pain. *Orthop Clin North Am* 1992;23:545–554.

Legg–Calvé–Perthes Disease

Canavese F, Dimeglio A. Perthes' disease: prognosis in children under six years of age. *J Bone Joint Surg Br* 2008;90:940–945.

Frick SL. Evaluation of the child who has hip pain. *Orthop Clin North Am* 2006;37:133–140.

Glueck CJ, Freiberg RA, Wang P. Role of thrombosis in osteonecrosis. *Curr Hematol Rep* 2003;2:417–422.

Wall E. Legg-Calvé-Perthes disease. *Curr Opin Pediatr* 1999;11: 76–79.

Radial Head Subluxation

Green DA, Linares MY, Garcia Pena BM, et al. Randomized comparison of pain perception during radial head subluxation reduction using supination-flexion or forced pronation. *Pediatr Emerg Care* 2006;22:235–238.

Kaplan RE, Lillis KA. Recurrent nursemaid's elbow (annular ligament displacement) treatment via telephone. *Pediatrics* 2002;110:171–174.

McDonald J, Whitelaw C, Goldsmith LJ. Radial head subluxation-comparing two methods of reduction. *Acad Emerg Med* 2000;7: 207–208.

Rudloe TF, Schutzman S, Lee LK, et al. No longer a "nursemaid's" elbow: mechanisms, caregivers, and prevention. *Pediatr Emerg Care* 2012;28(8):771–774.

Schunk JE. Radial head subluxation: epidemiology and treatment of 87 episodes. *Ann Emerg Med* 1990;19:1019–1023.

Discitis

Chandrasenan J, Klezl Z, Bommireddy R, et al. Spondylodiscitis in children: a retrospective series. *J Bone Joint Surg Br* 2011;93(8): 1122–1125.

Early SD, Kay RM, Tolo VT. Childhood diskitis. *J Am Acad Orthop Surg* 2003;11:413–420.

Fernandez M, Carrol CL, Baker CJ. Discitis and vertebral osteomyelitis in children: an 18 year review. *Pediatrics* 2000;105:1299–1304.

Nussinovitch M, Sokolover N, Volovitz B, et al. Neurologic abnormalities in children presenting with diskitis. *Arch Pediatr Adolesc Med* 2002;156:1052–1054.

Spondylolysis and Spondylolisthesis

Beutler WJ, Fredrickson BE, Sweeney CA, et al. The natural history of spondylolysis and spondylolisthesis: 45-year follow-up evaluation. *Spine(Phila Pa 1976)* 2003;28:1027–1035.

Jeffries LJ, Milanese SF, Grimmer-Somers KA. Epidemiology of adolescent spinal pain: a systematic overview of the research literature. *Spine (Phila Pa 1976)* 2007;32:2630–2637.

Hirano A, Takebayashi T, Yoshimoto M, et al. Characteristics of clinical and imaging findings in adolescent lumbar spondylolysis associated with sports activities. *J Spine* 2012;1:5.

Kobayashi A, Kobayashi T, Kato K, et al. Diagnosis of radiographically occult lumbar spondylolysis in young athletes by magnetic resonance imaging. *Am J Sports Med* 2013;41:169–176.

Logroscino G, Mazza O, Aulisa G, et al. Spondylolysis and spondylolisthesis in the pediatric and adolescent population. *Childs Nerv Syst* 2001;17:644–655.

Sairyo K1, Katoh S, Takata Y, et al. MRI signal changes of the pedicle as an indicator for early diagnosis of spondylolysis in children and adolescents: a clinical and biomechanical study. *Spine(Phila Pa 1976)* 2006;31:206–211.

Sairyo K, Sakai T, Yasui N, et al. Conservative treatment for pediatric lumbar spondylolysis to achieve bone healing using a hard brace: what type and how long?: Clinical article. *J Neurosurg Spine* 2012; 16:610–614.

Compartment Syndrome

Bae DS, Kadiyala RK, Waters PM. Acute compartment syndrome in children: contemporary diagnosis, treatment and outcome. *J Pediatr Orthop* 2001;21:680–688.

Grottkau BE, Epps HR, Di Scala C. Compartment syndrome in children and adolescents. *J Pediatr Surg* 2005;40:678–682.

Ramachandran M, Skaggs DL, Crawford HA, et al. Delaying treatment of supracondylar fractures in children: has the pendulum swung too far? *J Bone Joint Surg Br* 2008;90:1228–1233.

Sharrard WJ. *Paediatric orthopaedics and fractures.* London: Blackwell Scientific, 1993.

Reflex Sympathetic Dystrophy

Cepeda MS, Carr DB, Lau J. Local anesthetic sympathetic blockade for complex regional pain syndrome. *Cochrane Database Syst Rev* 2005;19:CD004598.

Cimaz R, Matucci-Cerinia M, Zulian F, et al. Reflex sympathetic dystrophy in children. *J Child Neurol* 1999;14:363–367.

Lloyd-Thomas AR, Lauder G. Lesson of the week. Reflex sympathetic dystrophy in children. *BMJ* 1995;310:1648–1649.

Low AK, Ward K, Wines AP. Pediatric complex regional pain syndrome. *J Pediatr Orthop* 2007;27:567–572.

Schürmann M, Zaspel J, Löhr P, et al. Imaging in early posttraumatic complex regional pain syndrome: a comparison of diagnostic methods. *Clin J Pain* 2007;23:449–457.

Tan EC, Zijlstra B, Essink ML, et al. Complex regional pain syndrome type 1 in children. *Acta Paediatr* 2008;97:875–879.

Wilder RT, Berde CB, Wolohan M, et al. Reflex sympathetic dystrophy in children. Clinical characteristics and follow-up of seventy patients. *J Bone Joint Surg Am* 1992;74:910–919.

Additional Resources

Clinical Pathway

Septic Arthritis

http://www.chop.edu/clinical-pathway/suspected-septic-arthritis-clinical-pathway

CHAPTER 130 ■ NEUROSURGICAL EMERGENCIES

JULIE K. MCMANEMY, MD AND ANDREW JEA, MD

GOALS OF EMERGENCY THERAPY

A patient with a neurologic disorder is considered a neurosurgical emergency when any delay of treatment may lead to serious permanent neurologic morbidity or death. Diagnostic tests and radiographic evaluation should be tailored to early recognition of neurosurgical emergencies to assist with clinical management and appropriate neurosurgical consultation.

KEY POINTS

- Intracerebral hemorrhage may accompany cerebral vascular malformations.
- Headache is a common presenting complaint.
- Pediatric hydrocephalus often requires surgical intervention.

RELATED CHAPTERS

Signs and Symptoms

- Injury: Head: Chapter 36
- Pain: Headache: Chapter 54
- Vomiting: Chapter 77

Medical, Surgical and Trauma Emergencies

- Neurologic Emergencies: Chapter 105
- Neurotrauma: Chapter 121

SPONTANEOUS (NONTRAUMATIC) INTRACEREBRAL HEMORRHAGE

CLINICAL PEARLS AND PITFALLS

- Approximately 5% of the population have cerebrovascular malformations including arteriovenous malformations, cavernous malformations, venous angiomas, and capillary telangiectasias.
- Unruptured aneurysms and certain types of cerebral vascular malformations are asymptomatic.
- Clinical presentations in infants may be nonspecific.
- Arteriovenous malformations (AVM) typically present with spontaneous hemorrhage and/or seizure.

Clinical Considerations

The presentation of the various types of cerebral vascular malformations may be insidious. Often, these malformations are asymptomatic. The presentation of infants may be very nonspecific and include poor feeding, vomiting, irritability, bulging anterior fontanelle, and altered mental status. Typical complaints in children include headache that may be localized, early morning awakening due to headache, progression of headache with increasing severity and/or frequency, vomiting, visual changes, neck stiffness, focal neurologic findings, altered mental status, seizure, lethargy, or obtundation. Signs of impending cerebral herniation include altered mental status, pupillary changes, bradycardia, hypertension, and respiratory depression.

Aneurysm

Current Evidence. Spontaneous dissecting aneurysms comprise about 45% of all aneurysms in children <15 years of age. The most typical presentation is with ischemia; however, they may also present with subarachnoid hemorrhage (SAH) or intracerebral hematomas. Spontaneous dissection of extra- or intracranial arteries has been associated with conditions such as Marfan syndrome, fibromuscular dysplasia, artherosclerosis, and moyamoya disease. The pathophysiology of spontaneous dissecting aneurysms seems to be multifactorial, including congenital, acquired, and hemodynamic factors.

Diagnostic Imaging. Because computed tomography (CT) is noninvasive and widely available, CT angiography (CTA) has been used for the screening and diagnosis of vascular injuries (Figure 130.1). The main disadvantage of CTA is related to bony artifact limiting its ability to identify injuries in some areas such as carotid canal or transverse foramina. However, current generation 16-detector scanners are capable of rendering very high–resolution images along with high-speed data acquisition.

Magnetic resonance imaging (MRI) and angiography (MRA) offers a high-resolution noninvasive approach for diagnosis and follow-up of vascular injuries. It is helpful in visualization of the arterial wall and detection of intramural hematoma. However, the accuracy of MRA is limited in detecting small intimal injuries (<25% luminal stenosis) and early pseudoaneurysm formation. The resolution of MRA now approaches that of conventional angiography.

Cerebral angiography remains the gold standard diagnostic modality. It is currently the most accurate modality as it provides fine detail of vascular anatomy and intimal injury near bony structures such as the skull base or the transverse foramen. However, due to its invasive nature and associated risk of iatrogenic injuries, it is advisable to reserve formal angiography for confirmation of findings detected on a screening diagnostic examination.

Management. Spontaneous dissecting aneurysms presenting with bleeding are uncommon, but should be treated because of a poor natural history. Aggressive surgical management with clipping, resection, or trapping of intracranial dissecting aneurysms by surgical or endovascular methods seems the most appropriate treatment.

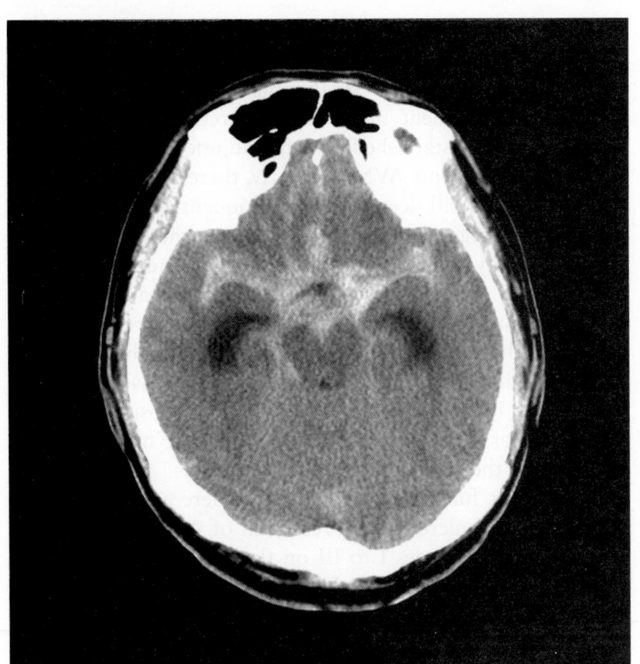

FIGURE 130.1 Axial CT of the brain shows hyperdensity consistent with aneurysm associated with acute hemorrhage in the basal cisterns.

Cavernous Malformation

Current Evidence. Cavernous malformations (CMs), also known as cavernous angiomas or cavernomas, are compact lesions comprised of sinusoidal vascular channels lined by a single layer of endothelium that lacks the full complement of mature vessel wall components. Between the vascular channels in the core of the lesion, there is loose connective tissue stroma without intervening brain parenchyma. The prevalence of CMs has been estimated to be between 0.4% and 0.9% of the population and 8% and 15% of all vascular malformations.

The majority of CMs are located supratentorially. Of the supratentorial CMs, most are located in the white matter of the cerebral hemispheres. The infratentorial CMs are located in the cerebellum, pons, midbrain, and medulla. Less frequent locations of CMs are the lateral and third ventricles, cranial nerves, and optic chiasm. Acute hemorrhage from a chiasmal CM is a rare cause of permanent visual loss. Of the extracerebral locations, the cavernous sinus, the orbits, and the spinal cord are the most common.

Diagnostic Imaging. CT is more sensitive at detecting CMs, but its specificity is low since most appear simply as high-density lesions with little or no contrast enhancement. This is in contrast to the high sensitivity and specificity of MRI for CMs. The MRI appearance of CMs has been categorized into four types: a hyperintense core on T1- and T2-weighted images representing subacute hemorrhage (Type I); a "classic" picture of mixed-signal, reticulated core surrounded by a low-signal rim (Type II); a iso- or hypointense lesion on T1 and markedly hypointense lesion with hypointense rim on T2, which corresponds to chronic hemorrhage (Type III); and punctate, poorly visualized hypointense foci, which can be visualized only on gradient echo MRI, representing tiny CM or telangiectasia (Type IV).

Management. With most asymptomatic CMs, particularly when the diagnosis is relatively clear by MRI characteristics, the right approach for the patient is conservative management with close follow-up. In contrast to a bleeding episode from an AVM, a bleeding episode from a CM is rarely life-threatening. However, there is more controversy with symptomatic cavernous malformations which hemorrhage in deep, difficult-to-access surgical locations.

AVM. Current Evidence. AVMs are vascular abnormalities leading to a fistulous connection of arteries and veins without a normal intervening capillary bed. In the cerebral hemispheres, they frequently occur as cone-shaped lesions with the apex of the cone reaching toward the ventricles. Nearly all AVMs are thought to be congenital. Supratentorial location is the most common (90%). The most common presentation of an AVM is intracerebral hemorrhage (ICH). After ICH, seizure is the second most common presentation. Other presentations of AVMs include headache and focal neurologic deficits which may be related to steal phenomena or other alterations in perfusion in the tissue adjacent to the AVM.

Size of AVM. In a series of 168 patients followed after presentation without a prior hemorrhage, the size of the AVM was not found to be predictive of future hemorrhage. However, other studies have found AVMs of small size to be at higher risk of hemorrhage.

AVMs and Aneurysms. Prevalence of the association of AVMs with aneurysms varies from 2.7% to 22.7%. This association seems to be correlated with a higher risk of hemorrhage. Brown et al. studied 91 patients with unruptured AVMs and found the risk of ICH in patients with coexisting aneurysm to be 7% at 1 year compared with 3% among those with AVM alone. At 5 years, the risk persisted at 7% per year, while it decreased to 1.7% per year in those with an AVM not associated with aneurysms.

Diagnostic Imaging. A CT scan may be used as an initial screening tool for patients presenting with neurologic sequelae related to unruptured or ruptured AVMs. This study can be used quickly to determine location of the lesion, acute hemorrhage, hydrocephalus, or areas of encephalomalacia from previous surgery or rupture. A nonenhanced CT may show irregular hyperdense areas frequently associated with calcifications in unruptured AVMs or acute hemorrhage with ruptured AVMs (Figure 130.2). A contrast enhanced CT can demonstrate the nidus, feeding vessels, or dilated draining veins.

MRI is superior to CT scan in delineating details of the macro architecture of the AVM, except in the case of acute hemorrhage. These architectural features include exact anatomic relationships of the nidus, feeding arteries, and draining veins as well as topographic relationships between AVM and adjacent brain. MRI is sensitive in revealing subacute hemorrhage. The AVM appears as a sponge-like structure with patchy signal loss, or flow voids, associated with feeding arteries or draining veins on T1-weighted sequences (Figure 130.3). MRI and angiography in combination provide complementary information that facilitates understanding the three-dimensional structure of the nidus, feeding arteries, and draining veins. MR angiography (MRA) currently cannot replace conventional cerebral angiography. In the case of acute hemorrhage, the hematoma obscures all details of the AVM making MRA virtually useless. This calls for direct use of cerebral angiography if the characteristics of the hematoma strongly suggest AVM as an etiology.

Management. The currently used treatments for AVMs include: (1) Microsurgical resection only, (2) preoperative

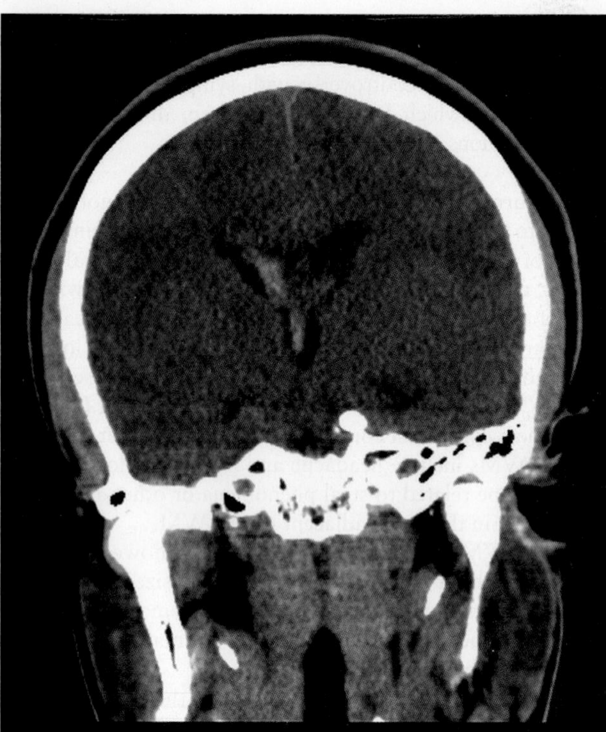

FIGURE 130.2 Coronal CT of the brain demonstrates intraventricular hemorrhage with communicating hydrocephalus with minimal interval increase in the ventricular dilatation. Diffuse cerebral edema with narrowing of the CSF space is suggestive of increased intracranial pressure.

endovascular embolization followed by microsurgical resection, (3) stereotactic radiosurgery only, (4) preprocedural endovascular embolization followed by radiosurgical treatment, (5) endovascular embolization only, and (6) observation only. The ultimate goal for all of these modalities is cure for the patient; however, the only way to achieve cure is with complete obliteration of the AVM. Microsurgery is the gold standard for resection of small superficial AVMs that other methods of treatment must be measured against. There is certainly a well-established role for adjunctive endovascular embolization of some AVM's. Clearly, there are specific situations, such as small deep AVMs in eloquent brain structures, where microsurgery should not be used as the primary treatment modality; stereotactic radiosurgery and occasionally embolization (when there is reasonable expectation of complete obliteration by embolization) are the preferred treatment options in these cases. We also make a case for observation in patients with large AVM's in or near critical areas of the brain that are not ideal for surgical resection or radiosurgery. Here, the pursuit of treatment may actually be more harmful to the patient than the natural history of the AVM.

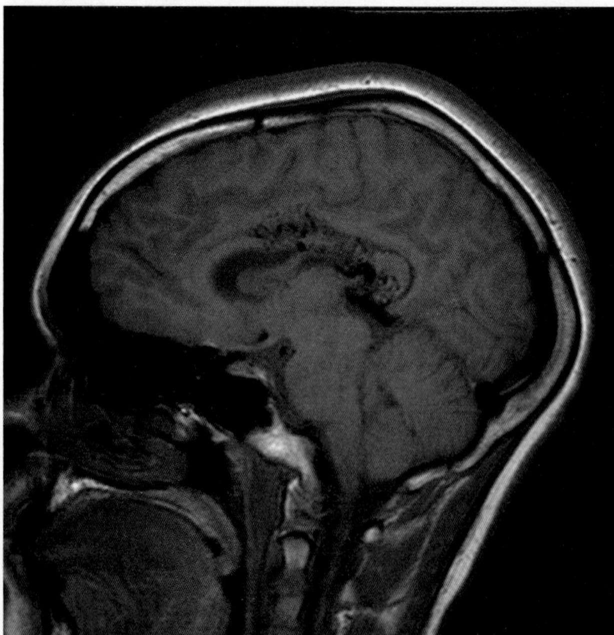

FIGURE 130.3 T1-weighted sagittal MRI demonstrates an AVM in the right corpus callosum with intraventricular hemorrhage with main feeding vessel from right pericallosal artery and draining into the right internal cerebral vein.

Indications for Surgical Resection. There are several clear indications for microsurgical resection of AVMs. AVMs with Spetzler–Martin grades I to III on the convexity should generally be resected. The Spetzler–Martin grading system takes into account three factors that greatly affect the surgical resectability of the AVM: size (<3 cm, 1 point; 3 to 6 cm, 2 points; >6 cm, 3 points), location (noneloquent cortex, 0 points; eloquent cortex, 1 point), and venous drainage (superficial only, 0 points; deep, 1 point). Patients with AVMs that present with major hemorrhage, progressive neurologic deterioration, inadequately controlled seizures, intractable headache, or venous restrictive disease should be strongly considered for surgical resection.

Cerebellar and pial brainstem AVMs should also be given strong consideration for surgical resection to prevent the higher risk of bleeding as compared to supratentorial AVMs. Some basal ganglia and thalamic AVMs should be surgically resected, as they carry a considerably higher annual bleed rate of 11.4%; in addition, morbidity and mortality with each bleed in these locations reach 7.1% and 42.9%, respectively (again, in contrast to the overall mortality rate of AVM hemorrhage of 10%).

Hence, one may justify a more aggressive approach for surgical treatment in younger patients as their cumulative risk of hemorrhage is so high. In addition, neurologic deficit caused at a young age is generally better tolerated and has a greater chance of recovery.

ACUTE HYDROCEPHALUS

CLINICAL PEARLS AND PITFALLS

- Hydrocephalus has been categorized as obstructive (noncommunicating) or nonobstructive (communicating).
- Most cases of pediatric hydrocephalus, even congenital, have a delayed diagnosis.
- Most children with hydrocephalus will need surgical treatment.

Hydrocephalus is the excess accumulation of cerebrospinal fluid (CSF), usually as the result of obstruction in CSF absorption, resulting in raised intracranial pressure (ICP). Cerebrospinal fluid is produced by the choroid plexus which is located within all four ventricles in the brain. Under normal conditions, the CSF exits the fourth ventricle to circulate in the subarachnoid space to be absorbed back into the venous system largely through arachnoid villi located at the superior sagittal sinus. Obstructive (or noncommunicating) hydrocephalus does not allow for the CSF to leave the ventricular system, and nonobstructive (or communicating) hydrocephalus occurs when the obstruction to CSF absorption lies outside the ventricular system in the subarachnoid space or at the arachnoid villi.

Common causes of obstructive hydrocephalus include stenosis of the cerebral aqueduct (from congenital causes, midbrain tumors, following hemorrhage or infection) and posterior fossa tumors. Common causes of nonobstructive hydrocephalus include scarring of the subarachnoid space and arachnoid villi following intraventricular hemorrhage (IVH) in premature infants or meningitis. In congenital conditions such myelomeningocele, the cause of hydrocephalus is likely multifactorial and may involve both obstructive and nonobstructive elements.

Current Evidence. Infections are a common cause of hydrocephalus in infants and children. An estimated 1% of pediatric patients who survive bacterial meningitis, including gram-negative organisms (particularly *Escherichia coli*) which occur most frequently in the neonatal age group, *Haemophilus influenzae, Streptococcus pneumoniae,* and group B streptococci, develop progressive hydrocephalus. Other less common infectious causes of hydrocephalus in children include tuberculosis meningitis whose worldwide prevalence is rising, toxoplasmosis (or other members of the TORCH group) usually diagnosed in the perinatal period, and viral meningitis and encephalitis. Head trauma has been recognized as a common cause of hydrocephalus. About 4% of patients develop posttraumatic hydrocephalus requiring surgical CSF diversion. True congenital hydrocephalus, meaning hydrocephalus present at birth, has an estimated incidence of 0.2 to 0.8/1,000 live births in the United States. The incidence of congenital hydrocephalus associated with conditions, such as Dandy–Walker malformation (approximately 85% to 95%), myelomeningocele (approximately 80% to 90%), and IVH of prematurity (approximately 35%), is better established.

Midline arachnoid cysts and tumors related to the ventricular system can cause hydrocephalus by obstruction of the CSF pathways. Tumors may also cause hydrocephalus by spilling blood or protein into the CSF, making the CSF more viscous, overloading the absorptive capacity of the arachnoid villi, and resulting in a communicating hydrocephalus.

Clinical Considerations

Clinical Recognition. Infants presenting symptoms include macrocephaly, bulging fontanelle, excessive irritability, lethargy, or vomiting. Sunsetting of the eyes may be present. This usually occurs later in the clinical course and consists of a spectrum of findings, including components of Parinaud syndrome (downward eye deviation, lid retraction, and convergence-retraction nystagmus). As raised ICP progresses, infants may develop bradycardia and/or apneic episodes.

In older children, the more common presenting symptoms include headache, nausea, or vomiting. These symptoms tend to be more common in the mornings, when ICP is higher after having been recumbent overnight. Other symptoms may include visual field deficits or double vision. This could be the result of severe papilledema or the because of the underlying cause of hydrocephalus, e.g., a large suprasellar tumor causing obstructive hydrocephalus and compressing the optic chiasm. Double vision might be described, usually from a unilateral or bilateral abducens nerve palsy, a classic false-localizing sign in raised ICP. Focal neurologic deficits attributable to the underlying cause of the hydrocephalus, such as ataxia from a posterior fossa tumor or bitemporal hemianopia from a suprasellar tumor, may also be present.

Clinical Pitfall. Benign macrocephaly is the most common diagnosis for an increasing head circumference. The typical infant, more commonly male, will be one whose head circumference has risen to or above the 98th percentile; but without a bulging fontanelle nor overt clinical signs of increased ICP. Brain imaging (by ultrasound, CT, or MRI) will show enlarged subarachnoid spaces over both frontal lobes. This has sometimes been termed "extraventricular obstructive hydrocephalus," although it is not truly hydrocephalus.

Diagnostic Imaging. Hydrocephalus is ultimately diagnosed with cranial imaging. A CT scan provides very good detail to make the diagnosis, is readily available, and can be done very quickly. It does, however, expose the child to radiation. Axial CT imaging will show enlarged ventricles. The pattern of enlarged ventricles, both lateral ventricles and third ventricle (or "triventricular") or all four ventricles, will vary depending on the etiology of the hydrocephalus (Figure 130.4). MRI provides greater anatomical detail of the brain and ventricles, but it can be less readily available and may require use of a general anesthetic. Depending on the results of a CT, an MRI may be necessary. Particularly if a tumor is suspected or if CT is unable to clearly elucidate the etiology. Ultrasound may be the most appropriate imaging modality for infants with suspected benign macrocephaly. This may confirm diagnosis and no further imaging may be necessary.

Management. When assessing a child with hydrocephalus, the acuity of the situation needs to be thoroughly assessed. If

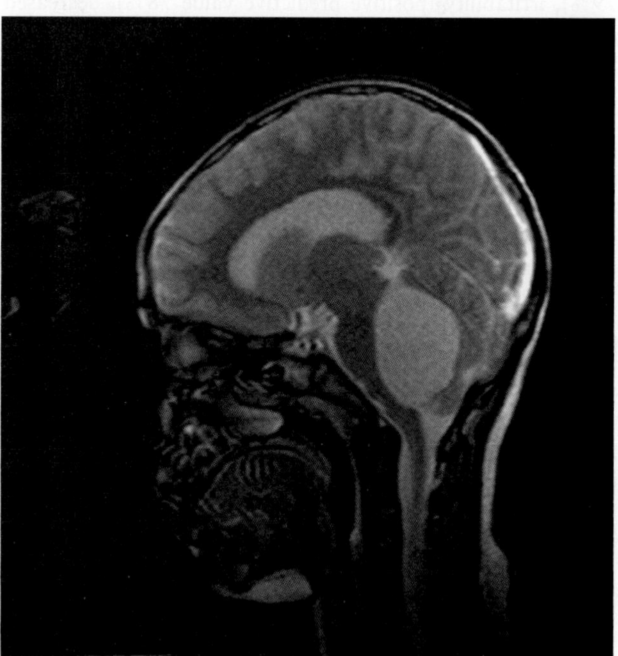

FIGURE 130.4 An approximately 4.7 × 3.3 × 3.5 cm T1 hypointense, minimally heterogeneous, circumscribed mass fills the fourth ventricle, which is effaced toward the right, and displaces the pons and medulla anteriorly. There is resultant mild-moderate dilatation of the lateral ventricles, third ventricle, and cerebral aqueduct.

SURGICAL EMERGENCIES

the child is in extremis, e.g., an obtunded child or a lethargic infant with bradycardia, the situation is emergent. After ensuring the basics of airway and cardiorespiratory maintenance, emergent cranial imaging and assessment by a neurosurgeon is essential. Definitive treatment will require some form of surgery. In some cases, there may be discreet tumor mass causing obstructive hydrocephalus and the goal of surgery will be tumor resection, which may relieve the hydrocephalus. In other situations, treatment will require diversion of the CSF itself, in the form of either a CSF shunt or an endoscopic third ventriculostomy (ETV).

SHUNT FAILURE

CLINICAL PEARLS AND PITFALLS

- Clinicians depend heavily on radiographic imaging to evaluate for shunt malfunction.
- The diagnosis may be challenging for even the most experienced clinician.

Unfortunately, shunt malfunction is one of the most common clinical problems in pediatric neurosurgery. Children with hydrocephalus, and a CSF shunt, often have significant neurologic abnormalities and developmental delays. Symptoms are nonspecific making shunt obstruction a routine consideration in this patient population. Moreover, the neurologic examination may be limited and unreliable in these patients.

Clinical Considerations

Clinical Recognition. Shunt malfunction can manifest with a multitude of acute or chronic signs and symptoms (Table 130.1). The most notable signs and symptoms of shunt failure are nausea and vomiting (positive predictive value 79%), irritability (positive predictive value 78%), decreased level of consciousness (positive predictive value 100%), and a bulging fontanel (positive predictive value 92%).

Diagnostic Imaging. CT of the brain and a shunt series x-rays are routinely used to aid in the diagnosis of shunt malfunction. More recently, brain MRI has emerged as a reasonable alternative to CT of the brain for the evaluation of ventricular morphology. The size of the ventricles may be small, normal, or enlarged in the presence of shunt malfunction. Comparing ventricular morphology on presentation to the morphology of the ventricular system at the time of the first or subsequent shunt obstructions is imperative, and may be predictive in determining the present status of the shunt system.

Management. The urgency of referral to a neurosurgeon is based on the patient's clinical presentation and radiographic signs. In general, patients should be referred for asymptomatic radiographic changes, such as mildly enlarging ventricles, in a semiurgent manner or as an outpatient. Asymptomatic patients with changes in physical examination findings, such as increasing head circumference, tense anterior fontanelle, or papilledema, require urgent neurosurgical consultation. Immediate neurosurgical consultation is mandated for symptomatic patients or the presence of radiographic changes.

TABLE 130.1

CLINICAL MANIFESTATIONS OF SHUNT MALFUNCTION

Acute	Subacute or chronic
Nausea	Change in behavior
Vomiting	Neuropsychological signs
Irritability	Change in feeding patterns
Seizures	Developmental delay
Headache	Change in school performance
Lethargy	Change in attention span
Coma	Daily headaches
Stupor	Increase in head size

SPINAL HEMORRHAGE

Spinal epidural hematoma is a rare cause of symptomatic spinal cord compression.

Spontaneous, or nontraumatic, spinal epidural hematomas are seen in association with congenital or acquired bleeding disorders, hemorrhagic tumors, spinal arteriovenous malformations, or instances of increased intrathoracic pressure. MRI of the spine is the definitive diagnostic measure for establishing the presence of spinal epidural hematoma. Decompression of the spinal cord is the key procedure for improving patient outcome. Treatment outcome was favorable for patients with incomplete preoperative sensorimotor deficit, and recovery was significantly better when decompression was performed within 36 hours in patients with complete deficits and within 48 hours in patients with incomplete deficits. There are advocates for conservative management in a very select patient population: those with no or mild deficits, those that demonstrate early, rapid, and progressive improvement in neurologic function within the first 24 hours despite an initial severe neurologic deficit, or those with small or noncompressive spinal epidural hematoma.

SPINAL INFECTION

Meningitis

Meningitis is an infection of the leptomeninges (pia, dura matter, arachnoid) and thus of the subarachnoid space. This space is continuous from the hemispheric convexities to the lumbosacral subarachnoid space (see Chapter 102 Infectious Disease Emergencies).

Current Evidence. The most common bacterial and viral pathogens are listed according to age in Table 130.2. The relative rates of meningitis, especially bacterial meningitis, remain highest in the neonatal age group.

Clinical Recognition. Most patients present with fever, evidence of meningeal irritation, and increased intracranial pressure from diffuse cerebral edema or hydrocephalus with CSF obstruction at the basilar cisterns. However, clinical manifestations may be nonspecific.

Diagnostic testing. Infection of the subarachnoid space can be diagnosed by sampling the CSF through a lumbar puncture. A CT scan or quick brain MRI should be performed prior to lumbar puncture to rule out hydrocephalus. Lumbar puncture

TABLE 130.2

PEDIATRIC MENINGITIS CAUSATIVE ORGANISMS

Age	Common pathogens
Birth to 90 days	Group B streptococcus *Escherichia coli* *Streptococcus pneumoniae* *Neisseria meningitidis* *Listeria monocytogenes* Herpes simplex virus (HSV)
≥3 months to 3 years	*Streptococcus pneumoniae* *Neisseria meningitidis* Group B streptococcus Gram-negative bacilli Herpes simplex virus
≥3 years to 10 years	*Streptococcus pneumoniae* *Neisseria meningitidis* Enterovirus
≥10 years to 18 years	*Neisseria meningitidis* Enterovirus Arboviruses

in the setting of untreated hydrocephalus may precipitate life-threatening herniation.

Management. Suspected bacterial meningitis is a medical emergency and administration of appropriate antibiotic therapy should not be deferred if lumbar puncture cannot be performed. Placement of an intracranial pressure monitor is controversial even in the presence of a poor neurologic examination or cerebral edema. Monitoring ICP has not been shown to improve outcomes in these patients. The most important prognostic factor for patients with meningitis is prompt and appropriate antimicrobial treatment.

In exceptional cases where the meningitis is complicated by hydrocephalus, an external ventricular drain may need to be placed. If the hydrocephalus is permanent from scarring of the subarachnoid spaces, a shunt for CSF diversion may need to be considered once the infection has been treated.

Discitis/Osteomyelitis

Common pathogens encountered in children include *Staphylococcus aureus,* pneumococci, and salmonella species. The prevailing hypotheses are that it is thought to arise from a prior site of infection and spread via three possible routes: hematogenously, by direct inoculation, or by direct extension. Almost 50% of children will have a prior prodromal illness related to their disc space infection. In children, blood vessels are present in the annulus fibrosus and the vessels within the vertebral body typically are anastomotic. These anatomic variations have been proposed as a reason explaining preferential localization of bacterial infections to the intervertebral disc space. Spondylodiscitis in children has a bimodal age distribution (0 to 2 years and >10 years) mostly affecting the thoracic and lumbar spine. Diagnosis can often be delayed up to 4 to 6 months secondary to the low incidence and vague presentation in children.

Clinical Recognition. Children most commonly present with back pain, but nonspecific symptoms may be the only presentation, often without fevers. Very young children with discitis often may refuse to walk, regress with ambulatory motor skills, display Gower sign, or refuse to sit. Several authors have proposed categories of symptoms for children presenting with discitis: back pain, hip and leg pain, meningeal symptoms, abdominal symptoms, or "irritable child" syndrome.

Diagnostic testing and Imaging. Laboratory values (CBC, ESR, CRP) and blood cultures should be obtained, but are often normal or only mildly elevated. Blood cultures will often be positive early in the course of the illness, but given the delay in diagnosis often only 50% are diagnostic. Very early in the course, plain radiographs may be negative as it typically takes 2 weeks to a month before disc space narrowing becomes apparent. Initial evaluation should include an MRI of the entire spine with contrast. Technetium-99, bone scans will identify the problem 7 to 12 days after onset of symptoms, but are nonspecific and require distinction between inflammatory and neoplastic etiology.

Management. Treatment is controversial as most spondylodiscitis infections have a relatively benign course. If a pathogen is not identified, a CT-guided biopsy should be considered prior to initiation of antibiotic treatment unless clinically contraindicated in the unstable or critically ill patient. More routinely however, a course of intravenous broad-spectrum antibiotics followed by oral antibiotics for 6 to 8 weeks is prescribed. Antibiotic choice should be tailored to the pathogen identified by biopsy. Surgery should be considered for refractory and progressive infections not responding to antibiotics. Epidural extension with neurologic compromise should be treated with emergent decompression and evacuation of the infection.

Clinical Pitfall. An entity known as chronic recurrent multifocal osteomyelitis (CRMO), or nonbacterial osteomyelitis (NBO), should be distinguished from spondylodiscitis or osteomyelitis. It is often associated with a syndrome of SAPHO (synovitis, acne, pustulosis, hyperostosis, and osteitis). The etiology is poorly understood. Young girls are more often affected (5:1) between the ages of 4 to 14 years. Patients are often asymptomatic between episodes, but symptoms may extend beyond 6 months. Most patients have palmoplantar pustulosis or psoriasis. Patients may have minor diagnostic criteria of normal or mildly elevated labs (CRP, ESR), hyperostosis, other autoimmune diseases, and an associated family history. Radiographic imaging can mimic osteomyelitis, but other long bones are typically involved. Bone biopsies are sterile but demonstrate evidence of inflammation and/or sclerosis or fibrosis. Standard therapy involves NSAID use, but alternate medications such as oral steroids, methotrexate, and bisphosphonates have been reported with positive early results.

Spinal Epidural Abscess

The most common anatomical site for thecal sac encroachment by epidural abscess is in the cervical spine, followed by the thoracic and lumbar spine. However, neurologic complications, paraparesis or paraplegia, as a result of thecal sac compression occurred more frequently in the thoracic and cervical regions. The most feared complication of primary or secondary spinal epidural abscess is paralysis. When paraplegia or tetraplegia is present, the prognosis is very poor.

POSTOPERATIVE COMPLICATIONS

CLINICAL PEARLS AND PITFALLS

- Common postoperative complications include mass lesions, infections, and infarctions.
- Most occur in the immediate postoperative period, however, the clinician must have a heightened clinical suspicion for weeks after surgery.

Mass Lesions

Hematoma. A postoperative hematoma may be extra-axial, occurring in the epidural or subdural space or intra-axial, occurring within the parenchyma of the brain. The clinical presentation of these lesions is not specific, and both should be included in the differential diagnosis for postoperative patients who become increasingly lethargic and exhibit focal signs such as hemiparesis, aphasia, cranial nerve palsy, or seizure. Changes in vital signs, such as Cushing triad (hypertension, bradycardia, and abnormal respiratory pattern), may reflect increasing intracranial pressure (see Chapter 54 Pain: Headache).

A CT scan should be obtained if a developing hematoma is suspected and the patient's condition is stable enough to permit a rapid work-up. Patients whose neurologic condition is deteriorating with decreasing levels of consciousness require an endotracheal tube, not only for airway protection, but to allow hyperventilation. The goal is a partial pressure of carbon dioxide (PCO_2) level between 30 and 35 torr. Hyperosmolar therapy may be necessary for the acutely decompensating patient. Evidence exists for use of hypertonic saline or mannitol to rapidly decrease ICP. Hypertonic saline may be given acutely in doses of 4 to 10 ml per kilogram of body weight. Continuous infusion of 3% saline range between 0.1 ml and 1.0 ml per kg of body weight per hour. Alternatively, Mannitol is given as an initial intravenous bolus of 1 to 1.5 g per kg body weight. Hematomas are usually treated by re-exploration and evacuation of the mass lesion.

The patient whose condition deteriorates many days or weeks after craniotomy may have a chronic subdural hematoma. Treatment is to drain by placement of burr holes with gentle aspiration, provided that the collection is not associated with enclosing membranes. A chronic subdural hematoma with membranes can be evacuated only by full craniotomy.

Brain Edema. Edema often accompanies neoplastic lesions and is more commonly associated with metastatic tumors. On CT scan, brain edema appears as an area of decreased density associated with brain shift. Brain edema is commonly associated with intracerebral hemorrhage and contusion. Edema associated with cerebral infarction generally indicates a severe stroke and may lead to herniation. The treatment of brain edema depends on the cause of the lesion. Lesions caused by neoplasia or inflammation respond to treatment with steroids. The role of steroids in treating edema caused by trauma, infarction, or anoxia is unproven. Brain edema that occurs after surgery for trauma, infarction, or hemorrhage represents increased tissue water and may require hyperosmolar therapy as described above.

Pneumocephalus. Pneumocephalus is simply the accumulation of air in the intracranial spaces. It commonly occurs after craniotomy if the air is not completely evacuated before the bone flap is replaced. It may also occur after a traumatic basilar skull fracture when air is introduced into the subarachnoid space by communication with the exterior environment, usually through the ethmoid, sphenoid, or frontal sinuses. A CT scan may show the accumulation of air beneath a bone flap or in communication with one of the sinuses. Most cases of pneumocephalus are treated with 100% oxygen by a nonrebreather mask, followed by keeping the patient in a completely prone position. Tension pneumocephalus marked by an enlarging pocket of air causing mass effect (midline shift, sulcal effacement, or both) demands more aggressive and invasive intervention. Emergency surgery is necessary to resolve the mass effect.

Pneumocephalus can be a precursor of CSF leakage. Although pneumocephalus indicates a tear in the dura, a CSF leak indicates a relatively large dural tear allowing a stream of cerebrospinal fluid to flow. CSF may drain through the ethmoid or sphenoid sinus complex, causing rhinorrhea; through the mastoid air cells, causing otorrhea; or from the scalp suture line. When rhinorrhea or otorrhea occur postoperatively, they should be treated conservatively with a lumbar drain. If a seal is not accomplished after 10 to 14 days of conservative treatment, surgical intervention is necessary. The use of antibiotics to treat either pneumocephalus or pneumocephalus with subsequent CSF leak is controversial. Treatment with antibiotics should not be initiated unless signs and symptoms of CSF infection develop.

Hydrocephalus

Types of hydrocephalus in the postoperative period include a loculated ventricle, communicating or noncommunicating. A loculated ("trapped") ventricle may cause symptoms resembling those caused by focal, expanding mass lesions. A loculated ventricle occurs when the drainage pathway from one lateral ventricle into the third ventricle is blocked. This blockage typically results from unilateral intraventricular hemorrhage or from a midline shift. Diagnosis is confirmed with CT and must be followed by permanent drainage of the loculus. The treatment of choice is emergent ventriculostomy and placement of a shunt.

The most common cause of communicating hydrocephalus is the blockage of absorption pathways by subarachnoid blood. A CT scan shows universal dilation of all ventricles. Lumbar puncture may demonstrate an elevated opening pressure. Serial lumbar punctures may be performed as a temporizing measure to diagnose and treat communicating hydrocephalus. If the patient's neurologic condition improves after lumbar puncture, definitive treatment by shunting may be required.

Any lesion that causes an obstruction at the narrow fourth ventricular inflow or outflow track can create noncommunicating or obstructive hydrocephalus. Obstructive hydrocephalus is commonly associated with lesions of the posterior fossa, and is a dreaded complication of surgical procedures to this area of the brain. Such lesions include cerebellar edema, infarct, or an intraventricular blood clot in the fourth ventricle. Patients with a noncommunicating hydrocephalus can never be safely treated with lumbar puncture, because the pressure gradient created by this procedure places the patient at risk of tonsillar herniation and sudden death. The patient may be temporarily stabilized with a ventriculostomy to provide decompression by draining CSF out of the intracranial cavity. Permanent shunt placement is the definitive treatment for obstructive or noncommunicating hydrocephalus.

Infection

Meningitis. Meningitis may occur as late as 4 weeks after surgery because of violation of mastoid air cells in the face of a

CSF leak. Unfortunately, after craniotomy the patient may normally exhibit all of the clinical signs of meningitis, including fever; therefore, the diagnosis may depend entirely upon examination of CSF and careful observation. If a shunt reservoir is present, then CSF may be obtained with a shunt tap. As mentioned in a prior section of the chapter, a CT scan or MRI of the brain should be performed prior to lumbar puncture. Lumbar puncture in the backdrop of unrecognized hydrocephalus or mass lesion may risk a potentially fatal herniation syndrome. The manifestations of postoperative meningitis are often much more subtle than those of the typical pneumococcal or meningococcal variety. If signs of meningeal irritation should occur in isolation or in association with any other changes, neurologic or metabolic, examination of the CSF is mandatory before any antibiotics are administered. Because cell count, glucose concentration, and protein concentration are abnormal after craniotomy, an absolute diagnosis must await the result of CSF culture or the demonstration of bacteria on Gram stain. Empiric treatment with broad-spectrum intravenous antibiotics should be started and directed at gram-positive cocci and gram-negative organisms, as described in the previous section. The antibiotic regimen should then be tailored once the final culture results and sensitivities have been obtained.

Ventriculitis. The clinical picture of ventriculitis differs little from that of meningitis, although the presentation is usually much more subtle. Meningeal symptoms may be minimal and fever variable, whereas alteration in mental status and neurologic function predominate. Both meningitis and ventriculitis tend to occur in the postoperative period more than 3 days after violation and contamination of the subarachnoid or ventricular space. The only diagnostic test is microscopic and bacteriologic examination of the ventricular fluid. As with meningitis, broad-spectrum antibiotics should be initiated pending gram stain and culture results.

Abscess. Brain abscess, or its immediate precursor, cerebritis, is relatively rare in the postoperative period. If an abscess does not communicate with the ventricular or subarachnoid space, meningeal signs will usually be absent. The development of meningeal signs or infected CSF in the face of focal deficits must heighten the clinician's suspicion for abscess. However, in 95% of cases of cerebral abscess, the CSF may be completely normal and the patient can be afebrile. The treatment of brain abscess is the same as that of any other abscess: incision and drainage. This procedure is diagnostic as well. Needle aspiration combined with the administration of broad-spectrum antibiotics will clear approximately 80% to 85% of abscesses. The remainder will require craniotomy for complete cure. If infection extends to the craniotomy flap; then reoperation, bone flap removal, and drainage of the abscess should be carried out for definitive therapy.

Subdural Empyema. Subdural empyema is rare after craniotomy but may follow burr hole drainage of a chronic subdural hematoma. This entity is also marked by neurologic deterioration, with the development of focal signs of hemiparesis, seizures, or both. These neurologic findings are related to mass effect from edema that unlike subdural hematomas, is out of proportion to the volume of fluid in the subdural space. Diagnosis by CT scan may be difficult, and a high index of suspicion is required. However, a parafalcine subdural collection, which can be seen on CT scan, is pathognomonic for subdural abscess. Treatment with drainage and broad-spectrum antibiotics is the gold standard. Drainage may be accomplished by reoperation or burr holes, and many surgeons recommend placing subdural catheters for irrigation of this space with antibiotic solutions such as concentrated bacitracin.

Infarctions

Arterial Infarcts. Arterial infarct is a rare complication after craniotomy but may occur if there has been substantial intraoperative manipulation of cerebral vessels. Clinically, the patient will usually exhibit focal neurologic deficits. If a large area or bilateral areas of the brain are involved, the patient may experience a global decrease in level of consciousness and more extensive neurologic deficits.

Cerebellar infarction, specifically, incurs a higher risk of obstructive hydrocephalus due to occlusion of the fourth ventricle. Symptoms and signs related to cerebellar dysfunction, such as dizziness, vertigo, nausea, vomiting, truncal ataxia, nystagmus, and dysarthria, appear first. Next, the patient may suffer from the progression of hydrocephalus with symptoms of headaches, agitation, and obtundation. The development of cranial dysfunction necessitates neurosurgical intervention for decompression of the posterior fossa with potential removal of hemorrhage.

Venous Infarcts. Venous infarcts are generally seen after craniotomy, especially if the venous sinuses are involved in the surgical field. Repair of dural sinus lacerations or prolonged compression of a sinus by an extrinsic force places the patient at risk of venous sinus thrombosis and infarction. Presenting symptoms include headache, nausea, vomiting, and seizures, often resembling those caused by pseudotumor cerebri. Cerebra venous thrombosis and/or dural sinus thrombosis can lead to venous infarction. This infarction may be hemorrhagic and often involves the subcortical white matter. CT scan reveals hemorrhage that may traverse the typical arteriovascular boundaries. The component of hemorrhage or significant mass effect resulting from cerebral edema becomes a neurosurgical emergency. Evacuation of the clot may be necessary, as may decompressive craniectomy.

Suggested Readings and References

Biffl WL, Moore EE, Offner PJ, et al. Blunt carotid and vertebral arterial injuries. *World J Surg* 2001;25(8):1036–1043.

Blumstein H, Schardt S. Utility of radiography in suspected ventricular shunt malfunction. *J Emerg Med* 2009;36(1):50–54.

Brown RD Jr, Weibers DO, Forbes GS. Unruptured intracranial aneurysms and arteriovenous malformations: frequency of intracranial hemorrhage and relationship of lesions. *J Neurosurg* 1990;73(6):859–863.

Chandrasenan J, Klezl Z, Bommireddy R, et al. Spondylodiscitis in children. *J Bone Joint Surg Br* 2011;93(8):1122–1125.

Chi JH, Fullerton HJ, Gupta N. Time trends and demographics of deaths from congenital hydrocephalus in the United States: National Center for Health Statistics data, 1979 to 1998. *J Neurosurg* 2005;103(2 Suppl):113–118.

Chun CS. Chronic recurrent multifocal osteomyelitis of the spine and mandible: case report and review of the literature. *Pediatrics* 2004;113(4):e380–e384.

Cruz J, Minoja G, Okuchi K, et al. Successful use of the new high-dose mannitol treatment in patients with Glasgow Coma Scale scores of 3 and bilateral abnormal papillary widening: a randomized trial. *J Neurosurg* 2004;100(3):376–383.

Dam-Hieu P, Mihalescu M, Tadie M. Spontaneous regression of paraplegia caused by spontaneous cervico-thoracic epidural hematoma. *Neurochirurgie* 2001;47(4):442–444.

Diringer MN, Videen TO, Yundt K, et al. Regional cerebrovascular and metabolic effects of hyperventilation after severe traumatic brain injury. *J Neurosurg* 2002;96(1):103–108.

Duffill J, Sparrow OC, Millar J, et al. Can spontaneous spinal epidural haematoma be managed safely without operation? A report of four cases. *J Neurol Neurosurg Psychiatry* 2000;69(6):816–819.

Garton HJL, Kestle JR, Drake JM. Predicting shunt failure on the basis of clinical symptoms and signs in children. *J Neurosurg* 2001; 94(2):202–210.

Gleeson H, Wiltshire E, Briody J, et al. Childhood chronic recurrent multifocal osteomyelitis: pamidronate therapy decreases pain and improves vertebral shape. *J Rheumatol* 2008;35(4):707–712.

Groen RJ, van Alphen HA. Operative treatment of spontaneous spinal epidural hematomas: a study of the factors determining postoperative outcome. *Neurosurgery* 1996;39(3):494–508.

Guyot LL, Michael DB. Post-traumatic hydrocephalus. *Neurol Res* 2000;22(1):25–28.

Hadjipavlou AG, Korovessis PG, Kakavelakis KN. Spine infection: medical versus surgical treatment options. In: Vaccaro AR, Eck JC, eds. *Controversies in spine surgery.* New York, NY: Thieme, 2010:250–260.

Haughton VM. Hydrocephalus and atrophy. In Williams AL, Haughton VM, eds. *Cranial computed tomography, a comprehensive text.* St. Louis, CV: Mosby, 1985:240–256.

Hentschel SJ, Woolfenden AR, Fairholm DJ. Resolution of spontaneous spinal epidural hematoma without surgery: report of two cases. *Spine (Phila Pa 1976)* 2001;26(22):E525–E527.

Hoh BL, Topcuoglu MA, Singhal AB, et al. Effect of clipping, craniotomy, or intravascular coiling on cerebral vasospasm and patient outcome after aneurysmal subarachnoid hemorrhage. *Neurosurgery* 2004;55(4):779–786.

Hoit DA, Schirmer CM, Weller SJ, et al. Angiographic detection of carotid and vertebral arterial injury in the high-energy blunt trauma patient. *J Spinal Disord Tech* 2008;21(4):259–266.

Holtas S, Heiling M, Lonntoft M. Spontaneous spinal epidural hematoma: findings at MR imaging and clinical correlation. *Radiology* 1996;199(2):409–413.

Hospach T, Langendoerfer M, von Kalle T, et al. Spinal involvement in chronic recurrent multifocal osteomyelitis (CRMO) in childhood and effect of pamidronate. *Eur J Pediatr* 2010;169(9):1105–1111.

Huber AM, Lam PY, Duffy CM, et al. Chronic recurrent multifocal osteomyelitis: clinical outcomes after more than five years of follow-up. *J Pediatr* 2002;141(2):198–203.

Ishikawa-Nakayama K, Sugiyama E, Sawazaki S, et al. Chronic recurrent multifocal osteomyelitis showing marked improvement with corticosteroid treatment. *J Rheumatol* 2000;27(5):1318–1319.

Iskandar BJ, McLaughlin C, Mapstone TB, et al. Pitfalls in the diagnosis of ventricular shunt dysfunction: radiology reports and ventricular size. *Pediatrics* 1998;101(6):1031–1036.

Jafar JJ, Awad IA, Huang PP. Intracranial vascular malformations: clinical decisions and multimodality management strategies. In Jafar JJ, Awad IA, Rosenwasser RH, eds. *Vascular malformations of the central nervous system.* Philadelphia, PA: Lippincott Williams and Wilkins, 1999:219–232.

Jansson A, Renner ED, Ramser J, et al. Classification of non-bacterial osteitis: retrospective study of clinical, immunological and genetic aspects in 89 patients. *Rheumatology (Oxford)* 2007;46(1):154–160.

Jung NY, Jee WH, Ha KY, et al. Discrimination of tuberculous spondylitis from pyogenic spondylitis on MRI. *AJR Am J Roentgenol* 2004;182(6):1405–1410.

Karabouta Z, Bisbinas I, Davidson A, et al. Discitis in toddlers: a case series and review. *Acta Paediatr* 2005;94(10):1516–1518.

Kayser R, Mahlfeld K, Greulich M, et al. Spondylodiscitis in childhood: results of a long-term study. *Spine (Phila Pa 1976)* 2005;30(3): 318–323.

Kim TY, Stewart G, Voth M, et al. Signs and symptoms of cerebrospinal fluid shunt malfunction in the pediatric emergency department. *Pediatr Emerg Care* 2006;22(1):28–34.

Kinouchi H, Mizoi K, Takahashi A, et al. Combined embolization and microsurgery for cerebral arteriovenous malformation. *Neurol Med Chir (Tokyo)* 2002;42(9):372–378.

Kwiatkowski S, Polak J, Uhl H, et al. Spontaneous spinal epidural hematoma. Report of two cases. *Neurol Neurochir Pol* 2001;35(4): 719–725.

Labauge P, Brunereau L, Laberge S, et al. Prospective follow-up of 33 asymptomatic patients with familial cerebral cavernous malformations. *Neurology* 2001;57(10):1825–1828.

Lasjaunias P, Wuppalapati S, Alvarez H, et al. Intracranial aneurysms in children aged under 15 years: review of 59 consecutive children with 75 aneurysms. *Childs Nerv Syst* 2005;21(6):437–450.

Lee JY, Ebel H, Ernestus RI, et al. Various surgical treatments of chronic subdural hematoma and outcome in 172 patients: is membranectomy necessary? *Surg Neurol* 2004;61(6):527–528.

Lehnert BE, Rahbar H, Relyea-Chew A, et al. Detection of ventricular shunt malfunction in the ED: relative utility of radiography, CT, and nuclear imaging. *Emerg Radiol* 2011;18(4):299–305.

Liu C, Shen C, Yang S. Diagnosis and treatment of spontaneous spinal epidural hematoma. *Zhonghua Wai Ke Za Zhi* 2001;39(8): 611–613.

Lonjon MM, Paquis P, Chanalet S, et al. Nontraumatic spinal epidural hematoma: report of four cases and review of the literature. *Neurosurgery* 1997;41(2):483–486.

Malhotra AK, Camacho M, Ivatury RR, et al. Computed tomographic angiography for the diagnosis of blunt carotid/vertebral artery injury: a note of caution. *Ann Surg* 2007;246(4):632–642; discussion 642–633.

Mater A, Shroff M, Al-Farsi S, et al. Test characterstics of neuroimaging in the emergency department evaluation of children for cerebrospinal fluid shunt malfunction. *CJEM* 2008;10(2):131–135.

Moriarity JL, Clatterbuck RE, Rigamonti D. The natural history of cavernous malformations. *Neurosurg Clin N Am* 1999;10(3):411–417.

Narayan RK, Kishore DR, Becker DP, et al. Intracranial pressure: to monitor or not to monitor? A review of our experience with severe head injury. *J Neurosurg* 1982;56:650–659.

Nigrovic LE, Kuppermann N, Malley R; Bacterial Meningitis Study Group of the Pediatric Emergency Medicine Collaborative Research Committee of the American Academy of Pediatrics. Children with bacterial meningitis presenting to the emergency department during the pneumococcal conjugate vaccine era. *Acad Emerg Med* 2008;15(6):522–528.

Oelerich M, Stogbauer F, Kurlemann G, et al. Craniocervical artery dissection: MR imaging and MR angiographic findings. *Eur Radiol* 1999;9(7):1385–1391.

Oertel M, Kelly DF, Lee JH, et al. Efficacy of hyperventilation, blood pressure elevation, and metabolic suppression therapy in controlling intracranial pressure after head injury. *J Neurosurg* 2002; 97(5):1045–1053.

Ohkuma H, Suzuki S, Shimamura N, et al. Dissecting aneurysms of the middle cerebral artery: neuroradiological and clinical features. *Neuroradiology* 2003;45(3):143–148.

Pahapill PA, Lownie SP. Conservative treatment of acute spontaneous spinal epidural hematoma. *Can J Neurol Sci* 1998;25(2): 159–163.

Peron S, Jimenez-Roldan L, Cicuendez M, et al. Ruptured dissecting cerebral aneurysms in young people: report of three cases. *Acta Neurochir (Wein)* 2010;152(9):1511–1517.

Pik JH, Morgan MK. Microsurgery for small arteriovenous malformations of the brain: results in 110 consecutive patients. *Neurosurgery* 2000;47(3):571–575.

Savitz SI. Cushing's contributions to Neuroscience, part 1: through the looking glass. *The Neuroscientist* 2000;6(5):411–414.

Savitz SI. Cushing's contributions to neuroscience, part 2: Cushing and several dwarfs. *The Neuroscientist* 2001;7(5):469–473.

Schilling F, Fedlmeier M, Eckardt A, et al. Vertebral manifestation of chronic recurrent multifocal osteomyelitis (CRMO). *Rofo* 2002; 174(10):1236–1242.

Schrot RJ, Muizelaar JP. Mannitol in acute traumatic brain injury. *Lancet* 2002;359(9318):1633–1634.

Shin M, Kawamoto S, Kurita H, et al. Retrospective analysis of a 10-year experience of stereotactic radiosurgery for arteriovenous malformation in children and adolescents. *J Neurosurg* 2002;97(4):779–784 .

Sivaganesan A, Krishnamurthy R, Sahni D, et al. Neuroimaging of ventriculoperitoneal shunt complications in children. *Pediatr Radiol* 2012;42(9):1029–1046.

Spetzler RF, Martin NA. A proposed grading system for arteriovenous malformations. *J Neurosurg* 1986;65(4):476–483.

Tew JM Jr, Lewis AI. Honored guest presentation: management strategies for the treatment of intracranial arteriovenous malformations. *Clin Neurosurg* 2000;46:267–284.

van Heesewijk JP, Casparie JW. Acute spontaneous spinal epidural haematoma in a child. *Eur Radiol* 2000;10(12):1874–1876.

Volpe JJ. Neurologic outcome in prematurity. *Arch Neurol* 1998; 55(3):297–300.

Yano M, Kobayashi S, Otsuka T. Useful ICP monitoring with subarachnoid catheter method in severe head injuries. *J Trauma* 1988; 28(4):476–480.

The Brain Trauma Foundation. The American Association of Neurological Surgeons, The joint section on neurotrauma and critical care. Recommendations for intracranial pressure monitoring technology. *J Neurotrauma* 2000;17(6-7):497–506.

The Brain Trauma Foundation. The American Association of Neurological Surgeons, The joint section on neurotrauma and critical care. Indications for intracranial pressure monitoring. *J Neurotrauma* 2000; 17:479–491.

CHAPTER 131 ■ OPHTHALMIC EMERGENCIES

DEBORAH SCHONFELD, MD, FRCPC AND ALEX V. LEVIN, MD, MHSc, FRCSC

GOALS OF EMERGENCY CARE

A wide variety of pediatric ocular complaints are first seen by the emergency room physician. A number of acute disorders such as ocular infections and exposures of a toxic nature require the immediate diagnostic workup and management that is best carried out in the emergency department (ED). While many problems can, and should be, managed by the ED physician alone, others may require immediate or expedited ophthalmologic evaluation. The ED physician must be capable of conducting an ophthalmic history and physical examination to accurately assess each ocular complaint. This chapter discusses the approach to ophthalmic emergencies commonly seen in the ED. Ocular trauma (including injuries to the globe, cornea, and eyelids) is discussed in Chapter 122 Ocular Trauma. The approach to several other common eye complaints is outlined in the related chapters mentioned below.

KEY POINTS

- The pediatric eye examination can be challenging and often requires an age-adjusted approach
- It is critical to distinguish periorbital cellulitis from the much more serious orbital cellulitis
- Patient age and associated clinical symptoms can often help the clinician differentiate between different types of conjunctivitis
- Copious ocular irrigation after caustic exposure to the eye can be vision-saving

RELATED CHAPTERS

Signs and Symptoms

- Eye: Red Eye: Chapter 22
- Eye: Strabismus: Chapter 23
- Eye: Unequal Pupils: Chapter 24
- Eye: Visual Disturbances: Chapter 25

Medical, Surgical, and Trauma Emergencies

- Ocular Trauma: Chapter 122
- Infectious Disease Emergencies: Chapter 102

EXAMINATION

Many children regard eye examinations and eye drops with the same fear that they harbor for injections. Therefore, it is important to gather as much information as possible before touching the patient or instilling eye drops.

A detailed history can be a valuable tool in focusing the examination and making a diagnosis. Questions regarding unilaterality/bilaterality, acute/chronic onset of symptoms, and prior ophthalmic care are particularly helpful. For example, a patient may be known to have an eye with poor vision, or to have had one eye patched for a visual problem suggesting amblyopia. Conversely, a child may be unaware of having poor vision in one eye because the pediatric brain is able to suppress the blurred image and focus solely on the clear image, allowing the child to proceed with normal activity unaware of the unilateral visual deficit. Importantly, an unremarkable visual screening examination at school does not necessarily imply that the vision was normal because false-negative tests are well known to occur.

It is often useful to start with assessment of the extraocular muscle movements. This procedure is discussed in Chapter 23 Eye: Strabismus. By using a toy or another interesting hand-held object, the physician can entice the child to look in the direction in which the object is placed. Both eyes should move equally in all directions. The examiner should test upward and downward gaze as well as eye movements to the left and right.

The examiner can use the direct ophthalmoscope as a tool to accomplish several tasks without touching the child. The ophthalmoscope light may be useful as a fixation target in testing eye movements, to assess whether the eyes are aligned (Hirschberg light reflex test, see Chapter 23 Eye: Strabismus), to test for a red reflex (see Chapter 122 Ocular Trauma), and as a simple hand-held magnifier. While viewing through the ophthalmoscope, the focusing wheel can be dialed in the direction of the black or green numbers to allow the eyeball to come into focus regardless of the distance between the examiner and the patient.

Visual acuity testing is usually performed at a distance of 20 ft or 10 ft. Most standard wall charts are calibrated to be read at 20 ft. If space does not permit this distance to be used, the patient can be placed 10 ft from the chart and the results interpreted with an adjustment for this distance. For example, the line marked 20/60 on the chart (a line that a person with normal sight can see at 60 ft but a person with that visual acuity would need to stand at 20 ft to see) becomes a 20/30 line when tested at a distance of 10 ft. In some centers or with some vision charts, the metric system is used with 20 ft being equivalent to 6 m. As examples, vision of 20/20 is written as 6/6, 20/30 as 6/9, and 20/200 as 6/60.

Chart selection is important when trying to obtain an accurate visual acuity. Letter charts should be used only for patients who can clearly recognize the alphabet. If there is any question by parental report, a number or picture chart (Fig. 131.1) should be used. When using picture charts that have colored figures, the examiner should avoid using those figures that are yellow because the bright illumination of the

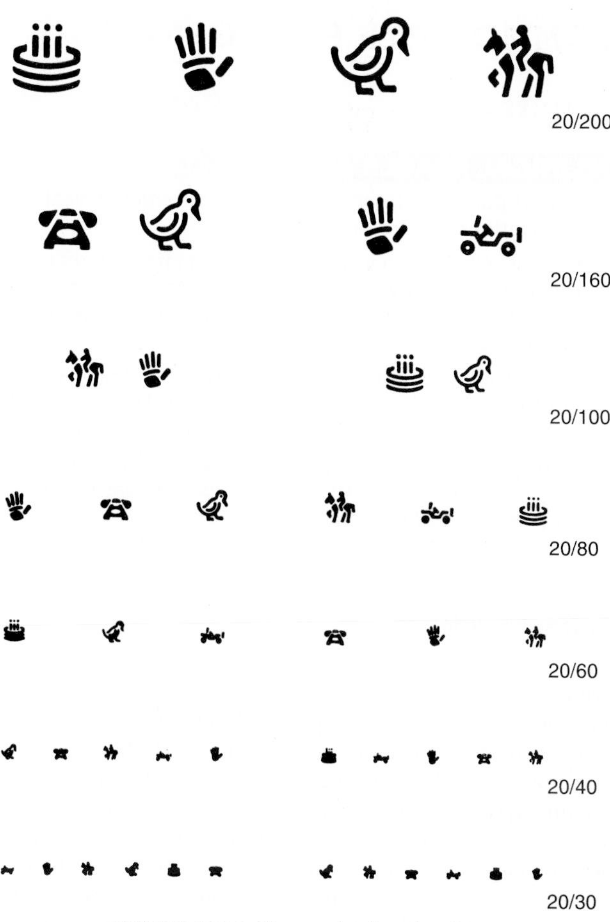

FIGURE 131.1 Picture visual acuity chart.

ED lessens the contrast between these figures and the white chart background making recognition more difficult. The "tumbling E" chart is not recommended in young children as it may be too complex for their developmental level and requires some sense of handedness, which is not developed until an age when they should easily be able to perform the other tests. This chart is more useful for older non–English-speaking children. It is sometimes referred to as the "illiterate E" test.

A useful option for children who are not "in the mood" to verbalize their responses or are very shy is the use of matching acuity chart systems. The two most common are the Sheridan Gardiner (Keeler Instruments, Inc., Broomall, PA) and HOTV (Precision Vision, La Salle, IL). In both situations, the child is holding a card that has all of the letters that are on the posted or hand-held chart 10- or 20-ft away. The child need not know letters but can identify them as shapes. For example, the H can be called a little ladder and the O a circle. Instead of verbally responding, the child points to the matching shape (letter) on the card he/she or his/her parent is holding. When using any visual acuity chart, it is not necessary to start with the largest symbol and have the patient read every symbol on every line thereafter. Doing so risks losing the child's attention. Rather, one can start with the 20/20 line and then go to larger lines if the child is having trouble. The child needs to recognize only a few letters on each line. Minor errors such as the substitution of the letter F for the letter P, or the letter C for the letter O, may be tolerated.

It is almost an instinct for young children to use their better eye and suppress the vision in their lesser eye. Therefore, children should not be allowed to cover their eye with their own hand because the small cracks between the fingers can actually allow vision out of the "covered" eye and even improve that vision by the pinhole effect (see Chapter 122 Ocular Trauma). Children may also look around commercially available occluders for the same reasons. Perhaps the best way to obstruct the vision in the eye not being tested is to use a broad piece of tape, ensuring the tape also covers the depression at the bridge of the nose (Fig. 131.2). To help ensure the patient is not "cheating," the examiner should look back directly at the child while standing by the chart indicating the letters or pictures.

Any child who can read a chart but shows reduced visual acuity should be tested using a pinhole. If vision improves with a pinhole then the patient only needs glasses and there is no organic abnormality causing the blurred vision.

After external examination and visual acuity are completed, the examiner can then proceed with other procedures as indicated, such as upper lid eversion and dilating the pupil. These techniques, along with the proper methods of examining the retina and optic nerve using the direct

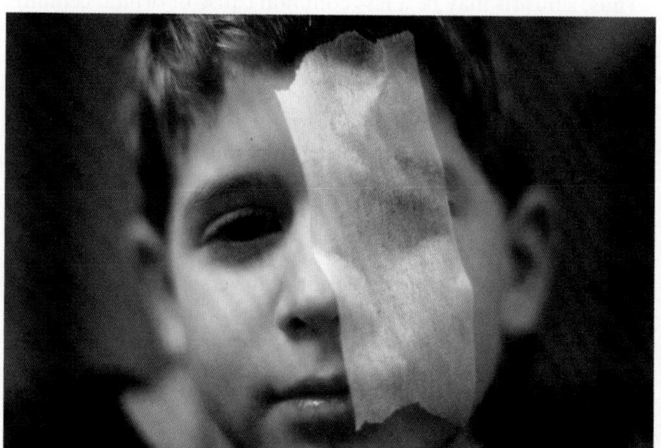

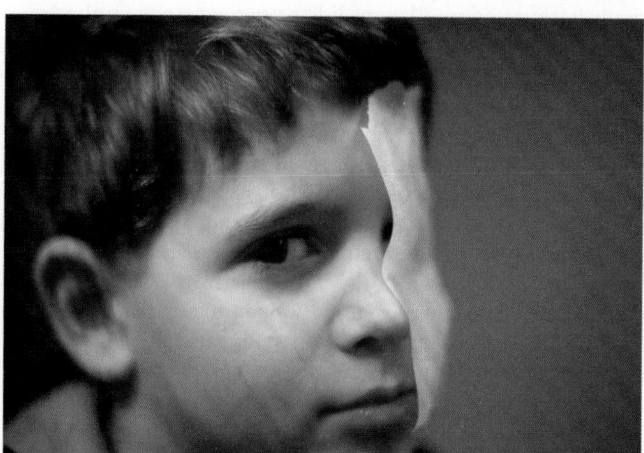

FIGURE 131.2 A broad piece of tape can be used to obstruct the vision of the eye not being tested. If the tape is not adherent to the bridge of the nose, the child can peek out by turning the face to the side (**right frame**).

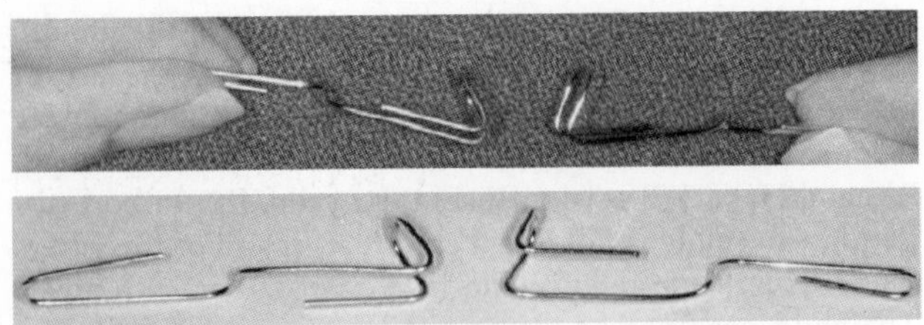

FIGURE 131.3 Paper clips can be bent into a retractor to open the eyelids.

ophthalmoscope, are discussed in Chapter 122 Ocular Trauma.

When the eyelids or periorbital tissue is edematous or the patient refuses to voluntarily open the eyelids, proper examination can be difficult. The techniques described in Chapter 122 Ocular Trauma for opening the traumatized eye may be useful. Commercially available speculums, when used in association with a topical anesthetic, are a painless and efficient way of opening the eyelids. If these are not available, a Desmarres retractor can be helpful to control the upper eyelid and can also be applied simultaneously to the lower eyelids. A similar device can be fashioned out of paper clips (Fig. 131.3). When using a paper clip, it is important to inspect it after bending. Some have a coating that may become fragmented, potentially causing particles that could be dispersed to the conjunctiva or cornea as tiny foreign bodies. In addition, the paper clip should be cleaned with an alcohol swab before starting, and should not be used on more than one patient.

In infants, the eyelids may be separated using cotton swabs. The swabs should be placed at the midbody of the upper and lower eyelids. As they are separated, pressure should be applied down against the eyelid and the swab should be rotated inward toward the eyelashes. This will keep the eyelids in place so they do not spontaneously evert and further obstruct the examiner's view. The cotton swab technique should not be used in patients being evaluated for eye trauma because pressure on the eyeball from this technique could cause further injury (see Chapter 122 Ocular Trauma).

It may be necessary to instill certain eye drops to complete the eye examination (e.g., topical anesthetics, dilating drops). Instillation of eye drops can sometimes be difficult because of swollen eyelids or patient noncompliance. Ophthalmic solutions are designed for a one-drop dose. Drops are most efficiently delivered by pulling down the lower eyelid and placing the drop in the inferior fornix. In patients who are extremely resistant, forced eyelid opening is needed to expose just a small strip of palpebral conjunctiva. The eyeball itself does not need to be visualized. An alternative technique involves placing the eye drop in the sulcus between the medial canthus and the side of the bridge of the nose while the patient is in the supine position. Every child must eventually open his or her eyes and when this happens the eye drop will naturally flow onto the conjunctiva. Topical anesthetics may be necessary to complete some parts of the examination, especially in the patient with significant pain. Topical anesthetics should never be prescribed for outpatient use. These are strictly diagnostic agents. Prolonged use of topical anesthetics may result in corneal ulceration.

COMMON EYE EMERGENCIES

Periorbital and Orbital Cellulitis

CLINICAL PEARLS AND PITFALLS

- Periorbital and orbital cellulitis have different clinical implications and treatments
- Orbital cellulitis is a vision-threatening infection that is characterized by its clinical features (pain or limitation of eye movement, optic nerve involvement, and/or proptosis)
- Since distinguishing between periorbital and orbital involvement can be difficult based on clinical observations alone, imaging may play a critical role in the diagnosis
- Many cases of orbital cellulitis can be managed medically with intravenous (IV) antibiotics, whereas other may require surgical intervention

Current Evidence

The orbital septum is an extension of periosteum from the orbital bones that inserts into the tarsal plate of the upper and lower lid to form the anterior boundary of the orbital compartment. Periorbital (or preseptal) cellulitis refers to infections limited to the soft tissues anterior to the orbital septum. Disease processes posterior to the orbital septum involve the contents of the orbit (fat, nerves, and extraocular muscles) and cause orbital (or postseptal) cellulitis. Involvement of the orbit can threaten vision and potentially result in spread to the cavernous sinus and central nervous system (CNS).

Periorbital cellulitis often has a local cause such as eyelid trauma, insect bite, or contiguous spread of an infection, such as conjunctivitis (especially neonatal gonococcal conjunctivitis) or dacryocystitis. Less commonly, it may also arise from sinusitis or an upper respiratory tract infection (URI). Orbital cellulitis most commonly results from sinusitis, which is present in up to 98% of cases. Other causes include orbital trauma and surgery, and infections of the teeth, ear, or face. It should be noted that the maxillary and ethmoid sinuses, the most likely to be involved when mucociliary clearance is impaired by a URI, are present at birth, but continue to grow and undergo pneumatization during the first few years of life. Thus, sinusitis may be a less common cause of orbital cellulitis in very young children.

The leading bacterial organisms responsible for periorbital and orbital cellulitis are *Staphylococcus aureus* and streptococcal species. Since the introduction of the *Haemophilus influenzae* type b vaccine in 1985, the incidence of this pathogen as a cause has dropped substantially.

Goals of Treatment

Accurate identification of periorbital versus orbital cellulitis is essential to proper treatment and a good clinical outcome. Timely administration of appropriate antibiotics is critical in all cases. Prompt recognition of symptoms and appropriate use of imaging allows for early diagnosis of orbital cellulitis, a potentially vision- and life-threatening condition. Ophthalmology consultation is indicated in all cases of suspected or proven orbital cellulitis. Surgical intervention may be required.

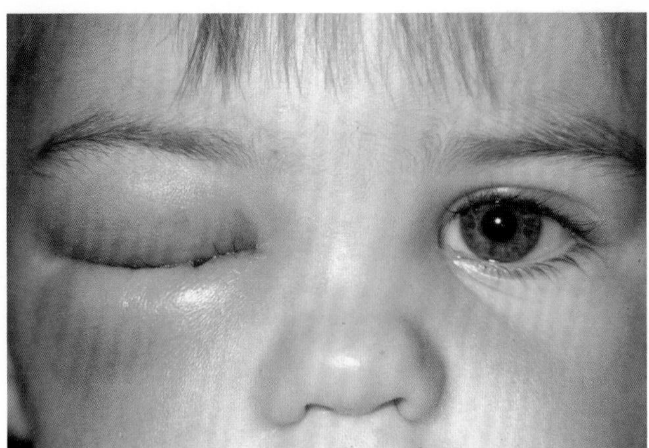

FIGURE 131.4 Periorbital cellulitis in a child with eyelid swelling, erythema, and tenderness.

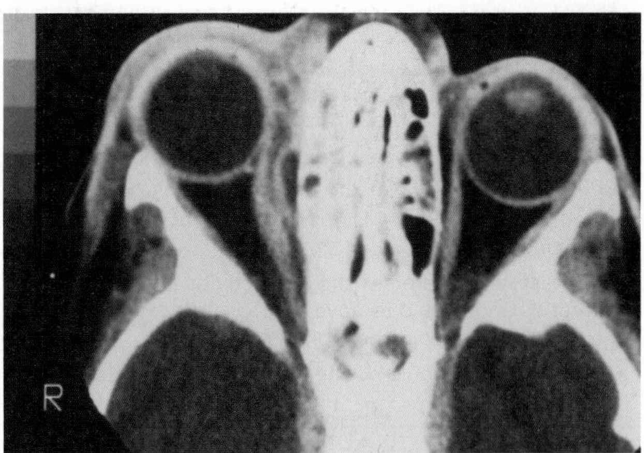

FIGURE 131.5 CT scan of a child with right-sided orbital cellulitis demonstrating retro-orbital inflammation and a subperiosteal abscess.

Clinical Considerations

Clinical Recognition. Both periorbital and orbital cellulitis are more often seen in children than adults. Both conditions commonly present with fever, and periorbital erythema and swelling (Fig. 131.4). Any pediatric patient who presents with these findings requires careful examination to rule out orbital cellulitis. The clinician should also recognize the signs of local and systemic spread of infection including visual disturbances, altered mental status, and sepsis.

Clinical Assessment. The primary concern when making the diagnosis of periorbital cellulitis is to rule out the possibility of orbital cellulitis. The cardinal signs of orbital cellulitis include decreased or painful eye movement, proptosis, decreased vision, and papilledema (or other signs of optic nerve involvement such as decreased color vision, visual field defects, or Marcus Gunn pupil). Patients with orbital cellulitis may be irritable, toxic, and have a fever, but the presence of fever and leukocytosis are not sensitive enough markers to discriminate between the two conditions.

The ED clinician should be aware that acute periorbital edema and erythema can also occur without infection. Insect bites and allergic reactions can cause dramatic acute periorbital swelling, typically with minimal induration or tenderness, but oftentimes with pruritus. These conditions are not usually associated with fever. Often, close inspection of the skin with magnification can localize a site of an insect bite. Swelling related to systemic allergic reactions is often bilateral, whereas periorbital cellulitis is rarely bilateral. Underlying sinusitis can also cause periorbital swelling without cellulitis. Conditions which may mimic some of the physical findings of orbital cellulitis include orbital tumors (rhabdomyosarcoma, neuroblastoma), orbital pseudotumor (an immune process), leukemia, and sickle cell crisis.

Diagnostic Testing. Imaging is not routinely indicated in periorbital cellulitis. Although the diagnosis of orbital cellulitis should be suspected clinically, CT or MRI scanning is used to confirm the diagnosis and detect its complications including subperiosteal abscess, orbital abscess, cavernous sinus thrombosis, and/or brain abscess. An MRI spares the patient radiation exposure and can readily identify orbital disease that can mimic orbital cellulitis such as tumor, hemorrhage, or inflammatory pseudotumor. CT imaging however is cheaper, more readily available, less likely to require sedation, and affords excellent views of the bony orbital wall (Fig. 131.5). There is some controversy over whether imaging is required in all cases of orbital cellulitis. Contrast-enhanced imaging should generally be expedited in all cases with high-risk features including limitation or pain with eye movements, vision loss, proptosis, signs of CNS involvement, inability to perform a reliable examination, and cases of presumed periorbital cellulitis which do not improve on IV antibiotics.

Management and Disposition. In otherwise well children who are beyond infancy and have mild periorbital cellulitis and no systemic signs or symptoms, oral antibiotics are appropriate. The prognosis for complete recovery without complications is excellent. The patient should be reevaluated within 24 to 48 hours to ensure improvement. If no improvement occurs, the patient should then be admitted for IV antibiotics.

All cases of orbital cellulitis should be promptly hospitalized and treated with IV antibiotics. Recent studies confirm that in the absence of acute visual compromise or other signs of disease progression, even children with small or moderate-sized abscesses deserve a trial of medical therapy before surgical intervention. Empiric broad-spectrum antibiotic treatment should be directed toward known common pathogens, including skin flora when local trauma is the likely etiology, and upper respiratory flora in cases of presumed underlying sinus disease. Blood cultures were obtained historically given the high prevalence of hematogenously spread *H. influenzae type b* as an etiology. The yield post Hib vaccine is dramatically lower, however cultures should be considered before initiating IV antibiotic therapy. Percutaneous aspiration from the area of cellulitis is not recommended. Other systemic cultures (e.g., cerebrospinal fluid, urine) may be indicated if signs of systemic toxicity or findings of CNS disease are present. The patient should be reevaluated daily looking for signs of improvement. Ophthalmic consultation and evaluation is recommended for all pediatric patients with orbital cellulitis. Otorhinolaryngology consultation should also be considered in those with extensive rhinosinusitis, and neurosurgical consultation for those with intracranial extension.

Conjunctivitis

CLINICAL PEARLS AND PITFALLS

- Not all cases of "red eye" are due to conjunctivitis
- Gonorrhea should be suspected in a neonate with purulent conjunctivitis
- Antimicrobial therapy is not indicated for cases of viral conjunctivitis
- Contact lens wearers with conjunctivitis are at risk for keratitis and should remove their contact lens and be evaluated by an ophthalmologist
- Steroid drops should not be prescribed by the ED physician

Current Evidence

The conjunctiva is the mucous membrane that lines the inner surface of the eyelids and reflects back to cover the surface of the globe up until the cornea. Conjunctivitis refers to "inflammation of the conjunctiva" and it is the most common acute eye disorder seen by pediatric ED physicians. Acute conjunctivitis is generally classified as either infectious or noninfectious. Infectious conjunctivitis may be bacterial or viral. Bacterial conjunctivitis in children is commonly caused by *Streptococcus pneumoniae, H. influenzae, S. aureus,* and *Moraxella catarrhalis.* Viral conjunctivitis is typically caused by adenovirus, although enteroviruses and herpes simplex virus are also possible pathogens. Noninfectious conjunctivitis includes both allergic conjunctivitis from airborne allergens (which may manifest as acute hypersensitivity reactions or more gradual seasonal reactions) and nonallergic conjunctivitis resulting from a mechanical or chemical insult.

Goals of Treatment

Acute conjunctivitis is typically a benign self-limited disease but can cause significant patient discomfort. Goals of treatment include symptomatic relief and shortening of the clinical course when possible. Eye lubricants (artificial tears) and/or cool compresses may provide symptomatic relief in all cases. Topical antibiotics may be used for bacterial conjunctivitis to hasten healing time and eradicate the pathogen. Cases with atypical courses and those that do not respond to treatment as expected should be referred to an ophthalmologist for further evaluation.

Clinical Considerations

Clinical Recognition. The hallmark of conjunctivitis is dilation of conjunctival blood vessels resulting in erythema and edema. Common symptoms include eye redness, irritation, tearing, discharge, and morning crusting. The patient's age is often useful in determining a specific diagnosis. Almost all newborn nurseries now use erythromycin ointment or dilute betadine solutions for prophylaxis against chlamydia and gonorrhea. However, no prophylaxis is completely effective. An infection with gonorrhea typically presents with sudden onset, severe, grossly purulent conjunctivitis, with profuse exudate and swelling of the eyelids (Fig. 131.6). Left untreated it can rapidly progress to corneal ulceration and perforation. Neonatal chlamydia trachomatis conjunctivitis, also known as inclusion conjunctivitis of the newborn (ICN), can range from mild swelling with a watery to mucopurulent discharge, to marked swelling of the eyelids with red, thickened, and friable conjunctivae. Untreated infection can cause corneal and conjunctival scarring. These two forms of conjunctivitis, as well as bacterial conjunctivitis often secondary to enteric organisms, can be difficult to distinguish clinically and may coexist.

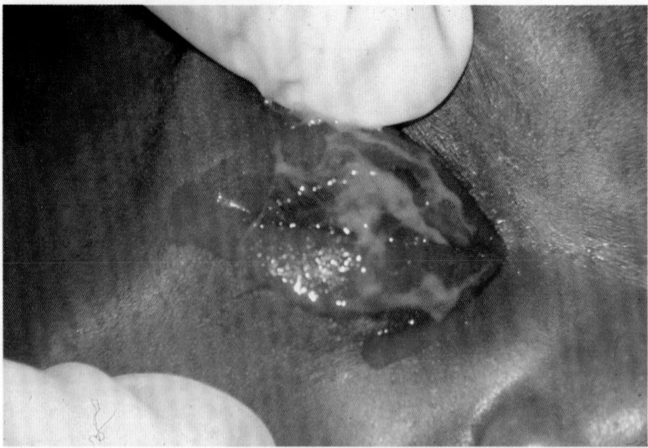

FIGURE 131.6 Neonatal gonorrheal conjunctivitis. Note the dramatic lid swelling and severe purulent discharge.

In children beyond the neonatal period, a wide range of organisms, both viral and bacterial, as well as chlamydia, can cause conjunctivitis. Clinically, these entities may be indistinguishable. Table 131.1 is designed to give some additional help in differentiating causes of conjunctivitis. In general, purulence is more characteristic of bacterial infections, whereas clear serous discharge is more characteristic of viral infection. Bacterial and viral conjunctivitis can be associated with otitis media and pharyngitis, respectively. Although both viral and bacterial conjunctivitis may be unilateral or bilateral, a history of multiple infected contacts, or consecutive involvement of one eye and then the other, argues in favor of a viral etiology. Likewise, dramatic lid swelling associated with preauricular adenopathy, mucoid or serous discharge, and perhaps an uncomfortable, sandy, foreign-body sensation is strongly suggestive of epidemic keratoconjunctivitis secondary to adenovirus. This fulminant viral infection is usually easy to recognize (Fig. 131.7). Patients with ocular HSV infection usually present with a red, painful, watery eye, often

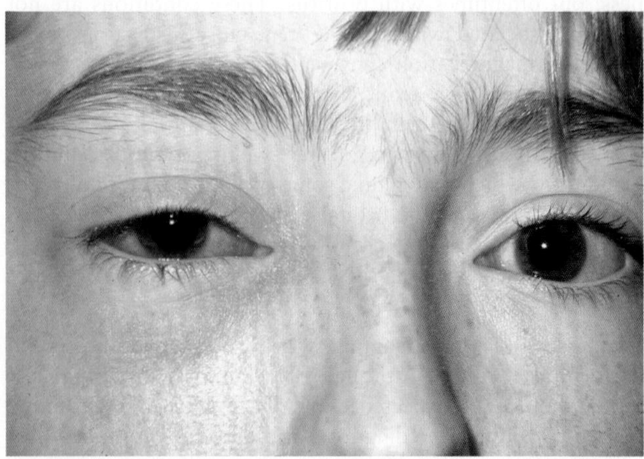

FIGURE 131.7 Patient with right epidemic keratoconjunctivitis infection. Note the lid swelling, red eye, and absence of purulent discharge. Patient also has right preauricular adenopathy (not visible). Note the early injection of left eye, representing sequential involvement.

TABLE 131.1

DIFFERENTIAL DIAGNOSIS OF CONJUNCTIVITIS

	Bacterial	Viral (Nonherpes)	Herpetic	Chlamydial	Allergic
Discharge—purulent	+++	±	—	±	—
Discharge—clear	—	+++	+++	±	+++
Swollen lids	++	+ to +++	+ to ++	+	+ to +++
Acute onset	++	++	+++	Chronic	+++ unless seasonal
Red eye	+++	+ to +++	Focally or diffuse +++	++	+
Cornea-staining with fluorescein	Nonspecific	Nonspecific	Dendrite	—	—
White cornea infiltrates	—	—	Possible	Multiple peripheral	—
Unilateral or bilateral	Uni/bi	Uni/bi	Uni	Usually bi	Usually bi
Contact history	+	+++	—	?STD	—
Preauricular node	++	+++	Usually—	±	—
Other associations	Otitis media? (*H. influenzae*)	Otitis media? Malaise, fever, pharyngitis	Prior or current skin lesions Recurrent	Genital discharge	Chemosis if acute

STD, sexually transmitted disease.
Adapted from Levin AV. Ophthalmology. In: Kropt SP, ed. The HSC handbook of pediatrics. 9th ed. Toronto: Mosby, 1997.

without concomitant vesicular lesions in the eyelid region. The conjunctival injection is usually sectoral.

Airborne or contact allergic conjunctivitis is characterized by hyperacute conjunctival injection associated with watery tearing and a blister-like swelling of the conjunctiva (chemosis) (Fig. 131.8). Itching is often a prominent symptom. The history may reveal recent exposure to an environmental allergen (cat dander). Seasonal allergic conjunctivitis, a recurrent reaction to outdoor pollens, typically has a less dramatic onset. Patients may have a history of atopy such as allergic rhinitis, asthma, or eczema.

Clinical Assessment. No child should be diagnosed or treated for conjunctivitis without a careful examination. Although conjunctivitis is characterized by ocular erythema, not all patients with a red eye have conjunctivitis. Various ophthalmic conditions, as well as many systemic processes, can be associated with a red eye. Chapter 122 Ocular Trauma outlines the evaluation and differential diagnosis of this finding. Signs and symptoms *not* typically associated with conjunctivitis that should prompt a search for a more serious condition include reduced visual acuity, significant ocular pain and/or photophobia, corneal opacities, and significant foreign-body sensations. Fluorescein instillation is recommended to fully evaluate the ocular surface in these cases. Characteristic dendritic staining patterns can be seen on the cornea or conjunctiva in herpetic infections (Fig. 131.9). Ophthalmic consultation is indicated in suspected HSV ocular disease. The clinician should also be wary of making the diagnosis of conjunctivitis in contact lens wearers. These patients are at risk for inflammation and ulceration of the cornea known as bacterial keratitis. This is a rapidly progressing sight-threatening condition characterized by pain, photophobia, and decreased vision.

Triage Considerations. Some forms of infectious conjunctivitis are highly contagious and spread by direct contact with the patient's secretions or with contaminated objects and surfaces. Potential cases of conjunctivitis should ideally

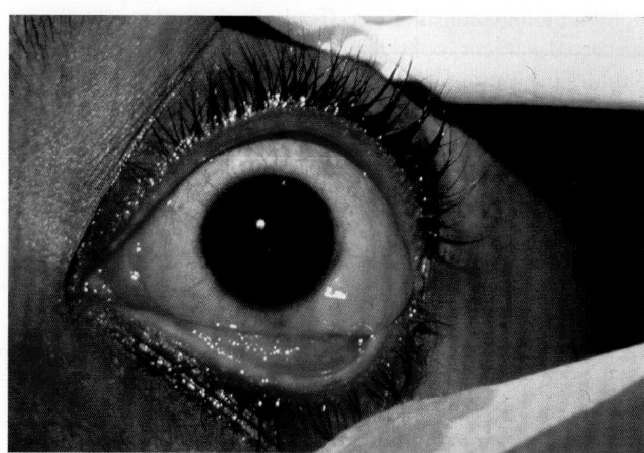

FIGURE 131.8 Nonseasonal acute allergic conjunctivitis. Acutely swollen conjunctiva (chemosis) is indicated (*arrow*).

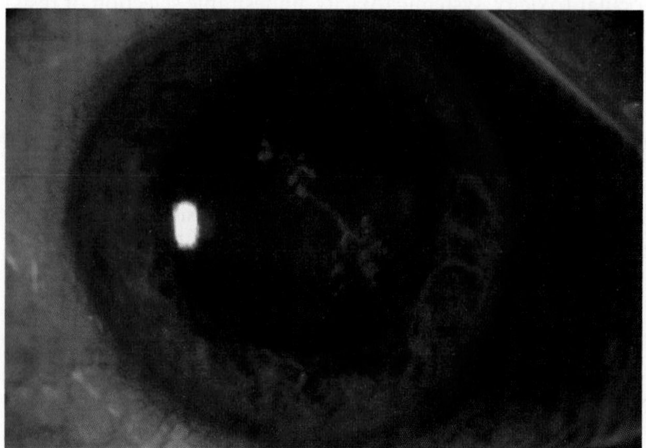

FIGURE 131.9 Fluorescein staining pattern of herpes simplex virus corneal infection. Eye is illuminated with blue light to demonstrate yellow/green branching fluorescein staining pattern of herpetic dendrite.

be identified in triage and appropriate contact precautions should be initiated. Proper hand washing is essential to prevent spread.

Diagnostic Testing. Generally, a diagnosis of conjunctivitis can be made on the clinical features alone. Urgent bacterial Gram stain and cultures should be obtained in all neonates with purulent conjunctivitis looking for gram-negative diplococci consistent with gonorrhea. Chlamydial studies may also be useful in this age group. Conjunctival specimens must contain conjunctival cells from an everted eyelid since chlamydia is an obligate intracellular organism. Although various methods of detection exist (nucleic acid amplification tests, antigen detection methods), chlamydial cultures remain the gold standard for diagnosis. Cultures should also be strongly considered in cases of conjunctivitis with severe inflammation or chronic or recurrent infections. Rapid tests for adenovirus now exist but are not universally available. Viral culturing is rarely necessary.

Management. Neonatal purulent conjunctivitis should be treated as gonorrheal conjunctivitis until proven otherwise. If a Gram stain of the purulent discharge demonstrates gram-negative diplococci, the patient should be hospitalized for parenteral ceftriaxone or cefotaxime, while awaiting results of cultures. Ophthalmology consultation is indicated. Saline ocular lavage on an hourly basis may be helpful in decreasing the amount of organisms having access to the cornea. Topical erythromycin ointment is helpful because it will also treat chlamydia, but topical treatment alone is insufficient for either organism. The neonate should be tested for chlamydial conjunctivitis as this is treated with a 14-day course of oral erythromycin, to prevent later pneumonitis, as well as topical therapy, usually with erythromycin ointment twice daily. Sexual abuse should be considered for postneonatal or prepubertal children with gonorrhea or chlamydia conjunctivitis, although there is evidence that nonsexual transmission to these sites may occur (unlike infection of the vagina, urethra, anus, or throat).

Outside the neonatal period, bacterial conjunctivitis can be treated with inexpensive nontoxic topical antimicrobials such as erythromycin or trimethoprim/polymyxin B. Table 131.2 gives ED physicians some guidelines regarding the prescription and use of ophthalmic medications. The table also includes medications that should be avoided because of problems with ocular toxicity, systemic toxicity, undesirable selection of resistant organisms, or the need for ophthalmology consultation with their use. In the first 3 months of life, topical aminoglycosides might be a reasonable choice because gram-negative and enteric organisms are more common. In older children, without strong evidence to suspect such organisms, aminoglycosides should be avoided because they may be toxic to the corneal epithelium and may select for resistant organisms. Ointment may be preferred to drops in pediatric patients in whom instillation of medication is difficult. Ophthalmic ointments are applied by placing a strip of ointment along the conjunctiva of the lower lid without touching the tip of the applicator to the eye. Antibiotic ointment doses are usually twice daily whereas drops are usually four times daily. Ultimately the choice of ointment versus drops may become a matter of patient or parental preference. Improvement should be seen within 2 days and children can return to school within 24 hours of treatment.

TABLE 131.2

PEDIATRIC EMERGENCY DEPARTMENT OPHTHALMIC DRUG GUIDELINES

Use	Avoid
Dilating drops	
Phenylephrine 2.5%	Scopolamine
Tropicamide 1%	Atropine
Cyclopentolate 1%	Homatropine
	Cyclopentolate 2%
Antibiotics	
Bacitracin ointment	Neomycin
Erythromycin ointment	Sulfacetamide
Polysporin drops or ointment	Aminoglycosides (except neonate)
Polytrim (trimethoprim/polymyxin B) drops	Quinolones
Lubricants	
Artificial tear drops or ointment	
Vasoconstrictors/antihistamines	
Naphazoline/antazoline	
Diagnostic agents	
Topical fluorescein	
Anesthetic agents	
Proparacaine, tetracaine	Cocaine
DO NOT PRESCRIBE:	
AVOID ALL ANTIVIRALS, MIOTICS, STEROIDS,[a] and ANTIGLAUCOMA AGENTS.	

[a]Including steroid-containing preparations, such as combination antibiotic-steroids.

There is no evidence to support the routine use of antimicrobials or antivirals in the majority of viral conjunctivitis cases. Contrary to popular belief, "secondary bacterial infection" is not a clinically significant problem in immunocompetent children. Rather, these patients can be treated symptomatically with cool compresses and over-the-counter lubricating agents (artificial tears) which can be used as often as hourly. Depending on the virus, symptoms may last for up to 2 to 3 weeks. Patients with symptoms that appear to be getting worse or persisting for longer than 1 week may benefit from ophthalmology consultation. If a herpetic ocular infection is suspected, urgent ophthalmologic consultation is required. Skin lesions on the lids without any conjunctival injection do not require ophthalmology consultation.

Allergic conjunctivitis is soothed by topical lubricants and cool compresses. The combination vasoconstrictor/antihistamine preparations listed in Table 131.2 may also be prescribed. Patients with recurrent allergic conjunctivitis, atopy, or asthma may benefit from long-term or seasonal topical mast cell stabilizers. A host of antiallergy eye drops are now available, the review of which is beyond the scope of this chapter. Topical glucocorticoids should not be prescribed by the ED physician without consultation with an ophthalmologist. Inappropriate use of steroids may lead to glaucoma, cataracts, and can promote herpes virus replication and corneal scarring. Finally, any patient who wears contact lenses and has conjunctivitis, should remove their contact lenses immediately and be referred for ophthalmology consultation. No topical drugs should be prescribed in these cases without the supervision and consultation of an ophthalmologist.

Ocular Chemical Injury

CLINICAL PEARLS AND PITFALLS

- Alkali ocular burns are more common and typically more severe than acid burns
- Ocular irrigation is the single most important step in the emergency treatment of all ocular chemical exposures
- Ocular irrigation should never be delayed for sedation, examination, or consultation purposes

Current Evidence

Pediatric ocular chemical exposures often occur in preschool-aged children due to accidental contact with household products such as organic solvents and other cleaning agents. Chemical burns to the eye can cause extensive damage to the ocular surface epithelium and cornea leading to blindness. The severity of damage depends on the agent involved, the duration of contact, and the depth of penetration. Acidic substances can cause significant damage on impact but ultimately produce a "coagulum" that can create a barrier to further ocular penetration. Alkaline substances tend to cause more damage as they cause saponification of fatty acids and can essentially "melt" the cornea and gain access to the internal structures of the eye.

Goals of Treatment

Chemical injury to the eyeball is a true ocular emergency requiring immediate assessment and intervention by ED personnel. Copious irrigation, even prior to ocular examination in many cases, is necessary to minimize damage to the ocular surface and is the mainstay of treatment if exposure is suspected. Emergency management may be the most important factor in determining long-term visual outcome.

Clinical Considerations

Clinical Recognition. Often, there is a clear history of a noxious substance coming in contact with the ocular surface. It may also be that the event is not witnessed and a parent may not be certain of the caustic exposure. Thus, the ED physician must maintain a high index of suspicion in children presenting with photophobia or an irritated, red or painful eye of acute onset. A prompt pH test done by touching a litmus strip to the eye can be useful in detecting acidic or alkaline conditions. It is also important to determine whether particulate matter may have been deposited on the ocular surface. Smoke can cause chemical conjunctivitis, particularly in house fires when chemicals are liberated into the air from burning plastics and other substances. Foreign bodies due to ashes and other particulate matter in the smoke are not uncommon. The examiner must also assess the degree of exposure. If a child has no symptoms (pain, photophobia) or signs (red eye, epiphora, conjunctival swelling) and a weak history of actually getting the chemical into the eye, it may be acceptable to avoid lavage.

Clinical Assessment. A thorough clinical examination of the eye is often deferred until after irrigation if there is confirmation, or strong suspicion of, chemical exposure. Immediate intervention is essential to improving the patient's prognosis.

Management. Any patient with sufficient history should be immediately placed in the supine position so ocular lavage may be started. Ocular lavage can often be frightening and anxiety provoking for a child, and some level of restraint is often needed. Sedation and topical anesthetic may be helpful, but the physician should not delay lavage while waiting for either of these adjunctive therapies. Usually, the irrigating solution itself will induce cold anesthesia. If a speculum, Desmarres retractor, or paper clip is readily available (see above), this may be used to help obtain optimal exposure of the ocular surface.

Virtually any IV fluid can be used for ocular lavage, although normal saline solution is most commonly used. The use of more pH neutral solutions (Ringer's lactate, NS with bicarbonate buffer, or a Balanced Salt Solution) may decrease ocular discomfort and irritation associated with irrigation. A standard IV bag and tubing set is used without a needle on the end. Rather, the solution is allowed to flow, with the system at its maximum flow rate, across the surface of the open eye from medial to lateral. If both eyes have been exposed, they should both be lavaged simultaneously with two separate setups. The Morgan Lens is a commercially available sterile plastic device that resembles a contact lens. It fits over the eye and can be connected to tubing that allows for continuous flow of fluid on to the ocular surface (Fig. 131.10). It is quick and easy to set up and provides a "hands-free" method of irrigating the cornea and conjunctiva. Regardless of the method used, lavage should be continued until the involved eye(s) has received either 2 L of fluid or until approximately 20 minutes have elapsed. Lid eversion should be performed (see Chapter 122 Ocular Trauma, Fig. 122.12), and lavage should be continued with the lid in this position so that the conjunctiva under the upper lid may also be cleansed. Mechanical debridement should be limited to the removal of visible particles from the ocular surface, which may contain small amounts of the offending agent or necrotic debris.

After irrigation is performed as described above, the pH should be remeasured every 15 to 30 minutes to determine whether it has normalized (pH 6.5 to 7.5) and is equal between the two eyes. The end point of equality should only be used if one eye has not been exposed to caustic chemicals. The conjunctiva under the upper lid may also be tested separately because noxious material can be harbored in the recess above the eye under the lid.

Ophthalmology consultation is usually indicated in cases of significant chemical injury. Waiting for the consultant should not delay irrigation and the ophthalmologist should be notified while lavage is ongoing. In cases of very minor exposure to substances that are clearly neither alkaline nor strongly acidic, and when the eye is not injected, an ophthalmology consultation may be deferred. The ED physicians must however be cautious about the absence of conjunctival injection because alkali burns can cause blanching of the conjunctiva, which is a poor prognostic sign.

Styes and Chalazions

A stye (external hordeolum) is a localized inflammation of the eyelid margin resulting from blocked glands in the

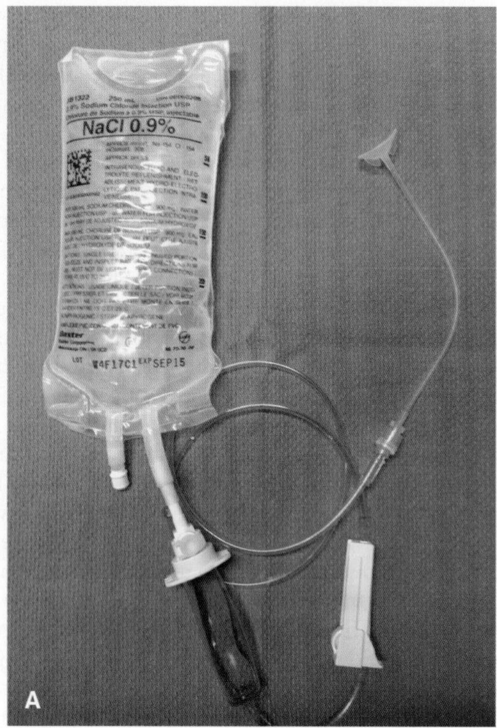

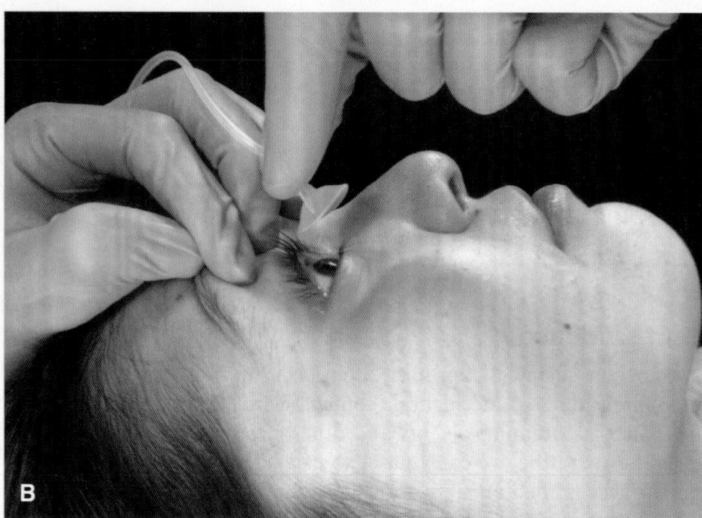

FIGURE 131.10 Irrigation set-up for ocular lavage (**A**) and the Morgan Lens (**B**).

eyelids near the lashes, while a chalazion (internal hordeolum) results from a blocked meibomian gland within the body of the eyelid. Both conditions are typically sterile but can progress to infection, most commonly with staphylococcal species.

Both conditions may present acutely with localized lid swelling, erythema, and tenderness. Styes are associated with swelling and purulent drainage at or near the lid margin (Fig. 131.11). More than one lesion may occur simultaneously, and more than one lid may be involved. An acute chalazion causes swelling and redness in the body of the eyelid and may be associated with drainage on the conjunctival surface of the eyelid with or without a red eye. It may also drain via the skin (Fig. 131.12). A chalazion may enter a chronic granulomatous phase in which there is a nontender, noninflamed, mobile pea-sized nodule within the body of the eyelid (Fig. 131.13). History can be helpful in establishing these diagnoses because patients often have had recurrent lesions in the same or other eyelid.

The treatment for both a chalazion and a stye is essentially the same. Eyelash scrubs once or twice daily are helpful in mechanically establishing drainage. Baby shampoo is applied to a washcloth and then used to gently scrub the base of the eyelashes while the eyelids are shut. Warm compresses over closed eyelids four times daily for 10 to 20 minutes may be helpful, but is rarely tolerated well by younger children. There is minimal evidence for antibiotics in the treatment of stye and chalazion in the absence of concurrent cellulitis, except in recalcitrant chronic cases. In such cases a topical antibiotic ointment with coverage for coagulase-negative staphylococcal

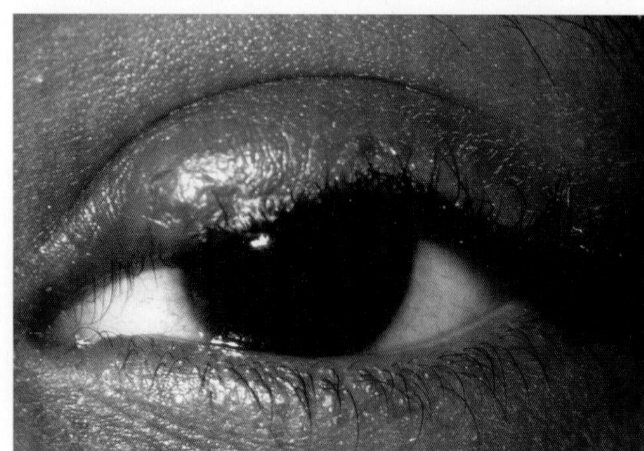

FIGURE 131.11 Acute stye (external hordeolum).

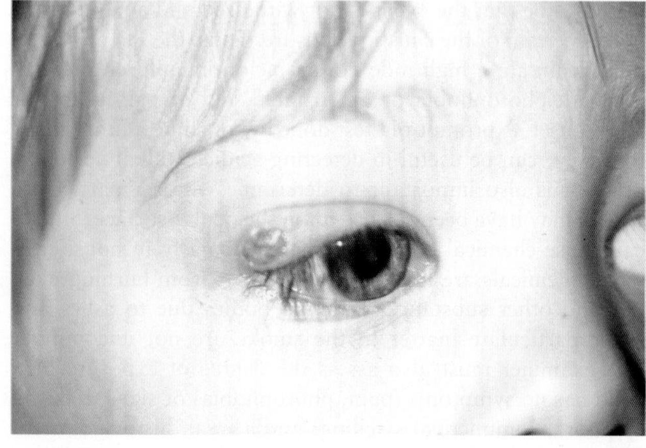

FIGURE 131.12 Chalazion draining spontaneously via skin.

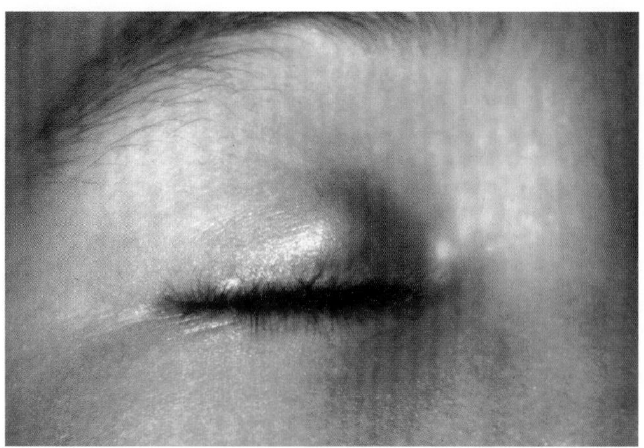

FIGURE 131.13 Chronic chalazion (*arrow*) within upper lid.

species (Table 131.2) can be applied twice daily following eyelash scrubs to help reduce staphylococcal overgrowth. If there is inadequate resolution after at least 4 to 6 weeks of medical management, incision and curettage by an ophthalmologist can be considered.

Nasolacrimal Duct Obstruction and Infection

The nasolacrimal apparatus extends from the puncta in the eyelids to the nose and is responsible for tear drainage. The most common cause of nasolacrimal duct (NLD) obstruction is incomplete canalization at the distal end of the system before it enters the nose. NLD obstruction is the most common cause of persistent tearing and ocular discharge in children, occurring in up to 20% of all normal newborns. NLD obstruction may rarely be complicated by inflammation or bacterial infection of the lacrimal sac (dacryocystitis), which is an ocular emergency.

Patients with NLD obstruction are usually younger than 1 year of age, with a history of symptoms dating back to the first weeks of life. Infants typically present with intermittent tearing and debris on the eyelashes. The discharge is mostly mucus that has precipitated out of the tear film because of stagnation of tear flow, and is usually worse on waking. In contrast to patients with conjunctivitis-associated discharge, the conjunctiva is rarely inflamed with NLD obstruction (i.e., no "red eye") (Fig. 131.14). Older children often have epiphora (excess overflow of tears) without discharge. The diagnosis can be confirmed by placing pressure on the lacrimal sac, which lies under the skin against the lacrimal bone between the medial canthus and bridge of the nose, which forces discharge out of the sac back onto the surface of the eye. Dacryocystitis is characterized by erythema, swelling, warmth and tenderness over the lacrimal sac often extending into the medial lower lid (Fig. 131.15) and may lead to periorbital or orbital cellulitis, sepsis, and meningitis. It should be noted that almost all infants with this condition have an underlying dacryocele (lacrimal duct mucocele), a cystic dilatation of the lacrimal sac which is caused by both a distal and proximal obstruction in the nasolacrimal apparatus. It often presents as a bluish mass before getting infected.

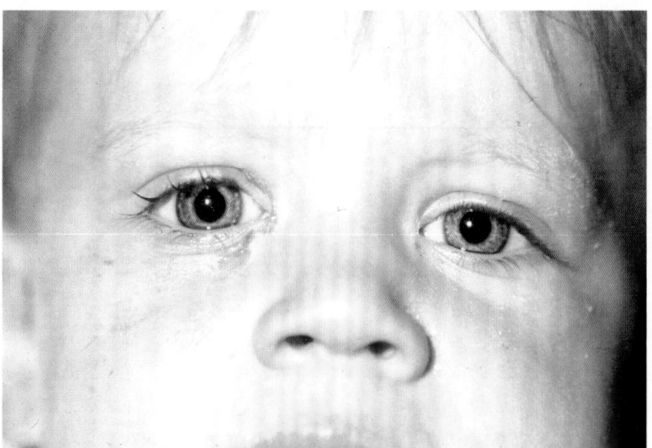

FIGURE 131.14 Left nasolacrimal duct obstruction. Note discharge on medial lower lid and wet lower lid lashes. The conjunctiva is non-inflamed (no "red eye") indicating that the child does not have conjunctivitis.

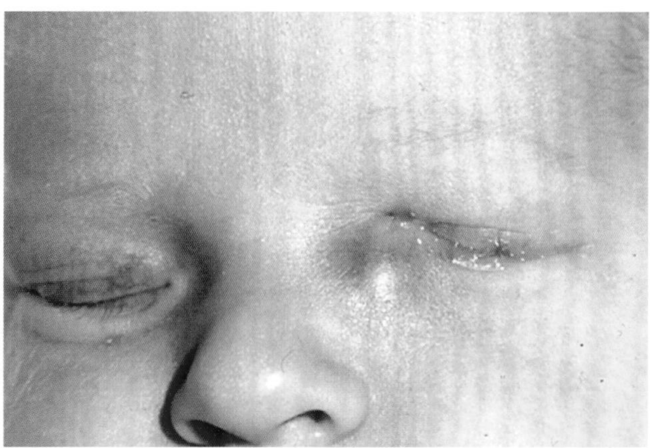

FIGURE 131.15 Dacryocystitis in an infant with a dacryocele. Erythematous, tender, swelling along the inferior medial cathal area representing inflammation of the nasolacrimal sac.

Over 90% of cases of NLD obstruction resolve spontaneously over the first year of life. Lacrimal duct massage (applying moderate pressure over the lacrimal sac) is the first line of treatment. Lacrimal duct probing or stenting may be required for select resistant cases. Acute dacryocystitis is an ocular emergency which requires immediate antibiotic treatment and ophthalmology consultation.

Suggested Readings and Key References

General

Gerstenlith AT, Rabinowitz MP, eds. *Wills Eye manual: office and emergency room diagnosis and treatment of eye disease.* 6th ed. Philadelphia, PA: Lippincott Williams & Wilkins, 2012.

Periorbital and Orbital Cellulitis

Botting AM, McIntosh D, Mahadevan M. Paediatric pre- and post-septal peri-orbital infections are different diseases. A retrospective review of 262 cases. *Int J Pediatr Otorhinolaryngol* 2008;72(3): 377–383.

Hauser A, Fogarasi S. Periorbital and orbital cellulitis. *Pediatr Rev* 2010;31(6):242–249.

SURGICAL EMERGENCIES

Rudloe TF, Harper MB, Prabhu SP, et al. Acute periorbital infections: who needs emergent imaging? *Pediatrics* 2010;125(4):e719–e726.

Vu BL, Dick PT, Levin AV, et al. Development of a clinical severity score for preseptal cellulitis in children. *Pediatr Emerg Care* 2003;19(5):302–307.

Conjunctivitis

Greenberg MF, Pollard ZF. The red eye in childhood. *Pediatr Clin North Am* 2003;50(1):105–124.

Teoh DL, Reynolds S. Diagnosis and management of pediatric conjunctivitis. *Pediatr Emerg Care* 2003;19(1):48–55.

Ocular Chemical Injury

Spector J, Fernandez WG. Chemical, thermal, and biological ocular exposures. *Emerg Med Clin North Am* 2008;26(1):125–136.

Vajpayee RB, Shekhar H, Sharma N, et al. Demographic and clinical profile of ocular chemical injuries in the pediatric age group. *Ophthalmology* 2014;121(1):377–380.

CHAPTER 132 ■ THORACIC EMERGENCIES

JOY L. COLLINS, MD, FAAP, MERCEDES M. BLACKSTONE, MD, AND MICHAEL L. NANCE, MD

INTRODUCTION

Thoracic emergencies in children often result in life-threatening alterations in cardiorespiratory physiology. A rapid, yet organized, approach to the child with a thoracic emergency is essential. The purpose of this chapter is to describe nontraumatic surgical diseases of the thorax and guide the evaluating healthcare provider in the diagnosis and treatment of these conditions. Congenital abnormalities that are usually diagnosed at birth are not included. Thoracic trauma is discussed in Chapter 123 Thoracic Trauma.

This chapter reviews the pathophysiology and clinical manifestations of thoracic emergencies, as well as the general principles of physical and laboratory assessment. Subsequent sections cover specific entities within the following categories: (i) airway obstruction, (ii) violations of the pleural space, (iii) intrinsic pulmonary lesions, (iv) mediastinal tumors, (v) diaphragmatic defects, and (vi) chest wall tumors.

GOALS OF EMERGENCY THERAPY

Children with thoracic emergencies present with a spectrum of processes and severities. Because of the potential for thoracic emergencies to be serious and even life-threatening, a rapid but organized approach to the assessment and treatment of these patients is crucial. Providers should rapidly address respiratory and hemodynamic compromise, and identify those entities that require prompt surgical consultation in the ED.

KEY POINTS

- Respiratory function requires flow of air along a pressure gradient into the tracheobronchial tree. Any compressive or obstructive force can compromise this process, resulting in a thoracic emergency.
- The emergency physician evaluating the child with a thoracic problem must attempt to determine whether the patient has evidence of airway compromise, circulatory compromise, or components of both.
- Thoracic conditions of surgical significance frequently present as a result of a mechanical or infectious complication of an *underlying anatomic abnormality.* These anatomic abnormalities may be grouped into conditions resulting in airway compromise, violations of the pleural space, intrinsic lesions of the lung, mediastinal masses, and diaphragmatic defects.
- Exceptions include pneumothorax and empyema, which can present in previously healthy children and which require prompt detection and treatment.

RELATED CHAPTERS

Resuscitation and Stabilization
- A General Approach to Ill and Injured Children: Chapter 1
- Airway: Chapter 3

Signs and Symptoms
- Foreign Body: Ingestion and Aspiration: Chapter 27
- Pain: Chest: Chapter 50
- Pain: Dysphagia: Chapter 51
- Respiratory Distress: Chapter 66
- Stridor: Chapter 70
- Wheezing: Chapter 80

Clinical Pathways
- Pneumonia, Community-Acquired: Chapter 90

Medical, Surgical, and Trauma Emergencies
- Infectious Disease Emergencies: Chapter 102
- Pulmonary Emergencies: Chapter 107
- Thoracic Trauma: Chapter 123
- Procedures: Chapter 141
- Ultrasound: Chapter 142

CLINICAL MANIFESTATIONS

Physical Examination

Evaluation of the child with a thoracic emergency requires a calm, orderly assessment of airway, breathing, and circulation (ABCs). In assessing the airway, the physician must evaluate the adequacy of air movement and gas exchange. Pulse oximetry should be performed upon the patient's arrival. Anxiety or confusion in a patient with a thoracic emergency may be evidence of hypoxemia. Increased work of breathing may indicate partial airway obstruction and can be evaluated by assessing the use of intercostal, subcostal, and supraclavicular accessory muscles. Prolonged use of these accessory muscles may result in fatigue and the most common cause of cardiac arrest in children—respiratory arrest.

Breathing is best evaluated by palpation and auscultation of the chest. The trachea should be palpated to ensure that it is midline. Any lateralization of the trachea is suggestive of either unilateral volume loss or a lateral space-occupying process, such as a pneumothorax, pleural effusion, or mass. The neck and chest should be palpated for signs of subcutaneous emphysema, suggestive of a pneumothorax or airway injury with an air leak. Finally, breath sounds should be assessed via auscultation for symmetry and adequacy of inspiratory and expiratory airflow.

Evaluation of the cardiovascular system should include an assessment of the patient's pulse for quality, rate, and regularity. The peripheral skin should be assessed for color, temperature, and capillary refill. Signs of poor perfusion often precede that of pressure instability. The neck should be assessed for signs of jugular venous distension. Finally, the heart should be examined for signs of displacement of the point of maximal impulse; shift or alteration in the heart tones; or new murmurs, gallops, or friction rubs.

Evaluation

The most important study when evaluating any patient with a thoracic emergency is a high-quality chest radiograph. The radiographs of the chest in the posteroanterior (PA) and lateral views should be performed in an upright position (unless contraindicated by the patient's condition). The width of the mediastinum and the degree of mediastinal shift are much better seen in the upright chest radiograph. Moreover, abnormalities in the lung, pleural cavity, and diaphragm are also best appreciated in this view. When a pulmonary effusion exists, lateral decubitus anteroposterior views of the chest or an ultrasound can be obtained to determine whether the effusion layers freely or is loculated.

In interpreting the chest radiograph, the physician should distinguish between a diffuse pulmonary problem and a focal lesion. Hyperaeration of one portion of the lung suggests air trapping in the involved lobe. Hyperaeration of the entire lung field on one side is usually the result of compensatory enlargement of the lung because of atelectasis and loss of lung volume on the opposite side. Depending on the condition, laboratory studies and advanced imaging modalities may be indicated.

AIRWAY COMPROMISE

Airway compromise can occur anywhere in the respiratory tract from the nose to the alveolus. Obstructive emergencies relating to the oropharynx, larynx, and proximal trachea are discussed in Chapters 114 ENT Trauma and 126 ENT Emergencies. Compromise of the more distal tracheobronchial tree may be caused by lesions in the lumen, in the wall, or extremities to the bronchus. Intrinsic bronchial obstructions may result from compression by a tumor within the bronchial lumen (e.g., carcinoid tumor), foreign body, or a mucous plug. Obstruction from lesions in the wall of the bronchus includes collapse from tracheomalacia and stenosis after tracheostomy. Extrinsic lesions (e.g., bronchogenic cyst or inflamed lymph nodes) may be symptomatic by impinging on a bronchus. Table 132.1 lists intraluminal, mural, and extrinsic conditions that produce airway obstruction.

The anatomic level of the obstruction correlates with its effects: An obstruction of the distal tracheobronchial tree may lead to segmental lung overdistension or segmental infection. An obstruction of the proximal trachea affects both lungs, with a much greater likelihood of catastrophe for the patient. Similarly, greater degrees of obstruction, as a rule, lead to greater effects on gas exchange and severity. Infection commonly follows obstruction of bronchial drainage because the clearance of bacteria or inhaled foreign materials by the mucociliary elevator is prevented.

TABLE 132.1

TRACHEOBRONCHIAL CONDITIONS ASSOCIATED WITH AIRWAY COMPROMISE

Intraluminal
Foreign bodies
Aspiration (esophageal reflux, tracheoesophageal fistula, bronchial fistula, biliary fistula, or esophageal fistula)
Mucous plugs (cystic fibrosis)
Granuloma (chronic intubation, tuberculosis)
Hemoptysis (vascular malformations, cystic fibrosis, tuberculosis, sarcoidosis, hemosiderosis, lupus)
Acute infection (tracheitis)
Mural
Tracheomalacia
Lobar emphysema
Bronchial atresia
Bronchial tumors
Extrinsic
Lymphadenopathy
Bronchogenic cyst
Cystic hygroma
Esophageal duplication
Mediastinal tumors

Tracheal Obstruction

CLINICAL PEARLS AND PITFALLS

- Although wheezing and stridor are very common presentations in children with intercurrent viral illnesses, structural problems should be considered in children with recurrent presentations or significant respiratory distress that does not respond to typical therapies.
- Radiographic studies may not reveal the cause of tracheal obstruction; since these are often dynamic processes, direct laryngoscopy or bronchoscopy may be necessary.

Current Evidence

Tracheal obstruction may be produced by stenosis or lesions within the lumen of the trachea (Fig. 132.1), in the wall of the trachea, or by extrinsic compression. One of the most common causes of intrinsic obstruction in children is an aspirated foreign body (see Chapter 27 Foreign Body: Ingestion and Aspiration for details). Other causes include congenital anomalies such as subglottic stenosis, laryngomalacia, and vocal cord paralysis; acquired subglottic stenosis after tracheostomy or prolonged intubation; viral or bacterial tracheitis or any process that causes significant mucosal edema, particularly in an infant with small baseline airway diameter; or more rarely, a space-occupying lesion such as a hemangioma. Tracheomalacia, sometimes complicating lung disease of prematurity and prolonged intubation, is characterized by a floppy trachea that collapses during expiration when the intrathoracic trachea is compressed by the positive intrathoracic pressure. Laryngomalacia, or tracheomalacia outside the thoracic inlet, may produce obstruction during inspiration

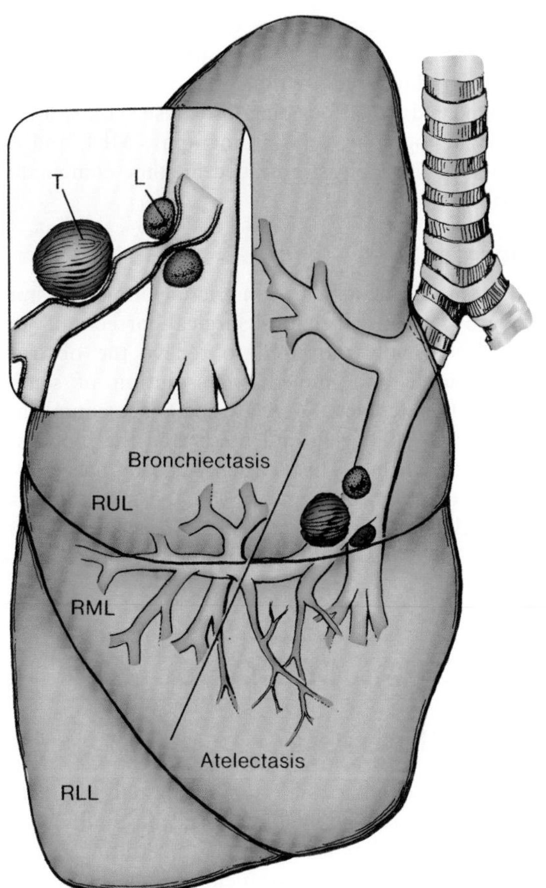

FIGURE 132.1 Acute and chronic obstruction of a bronchus owing to tumor or cyst (T) or lymph nodes (L). When the obstruction is acute, there may be bronchiectasis caused by recurrent pneumonia. The right middle lobe as shown here is particularly prone to bronchial obstruction caused by pressure from encircling lymph nodes. RUL, right upper lobe; RML, right middle lobe; RLL, right lower lobe.

when the negative intraluminal pressure transmitted from the chest causes the floppy wall to collapse. Tracheomalacia often occurs in infants born with tracheoesophageal fistula (TEF) or other intrinsic anomalies. Extrinsic compression may occur both from mass lesions (Table 132.1) and as a result of anomalous arteries.

Goals of Treatment

Tracheal obstruction can be caused by a variety of mechanical, infectious, and congenital abnormalities. Practitioners must rapidly assess the cause of obstruction while working toward stabilization of the airway. Surgical causes of obstruction require prompt consultation and coordination of care.

Clinical Considerations

Clinical Recognition. Tracheal compromise produces symptoms that vary from mild to severe, depending on the degree of obstruction present. When symptoms are mild, the underlying cause may not be evident. Occasional episodes of respiratory infection that are believed to result from croup or bronchiolitis may be the only symptom. Stridor, wheezing, or harsh barky cough occurs in patients with more significant obstruction, and a history of frequent hospitalizations for respiratory compromise may be obtained.

Severe tracheal compromise is usually manifested by a history of stridor at rest. Progressive cyanosis and apneic episodes may occur. On examination, a child with obstruction caused by extrinsic compression often has wheezing or stridor throughout the respiratory cycle. In contrast, a patient with the floppy trachea of tracheomalacia often wheezes only during expiration.

Radiographic evaluation of the stable patient should begin with PA and lateral chest radiographs, ideally obtained at full inspiration and again at full expiration. Lateral radiographs of the neck may be useful in showing an edematous epiglottis in patients with suspected epiglottitis. Mass lesions will require cross-section imaging (e.g., computed tomography [CT]) for evaluation. Bronchoscopy is often indicated to evaluate obstructive lesions, whether in the lumen, the wall, or extrinsic to the wall of the trachea.

Management. If the patient has a life-threatening airway obstruction, he or she should receive airway management as outlined in Chapters 1 A General Approach to Ill and Injured Children and 3 Airway. A coordinated effort between the emergency department (ED) physician, the surgeon, and the anesthesiologist or critical care physician may be necessary to establish an airway by endotracheal intubation, bronchoscopy, or tracheotomy. Intubation of the airway to within a short distance of the carina supports most patients with lesions extrinsic to the trachea or in the tracheal wall with a critical obstruction. Such a patient requires admission to an intensive care or other unit with ventilator capability. Lesions within the lumen will likely require endoscopic management in an operating room, and early involvement of an experienced surgeon is recommended.

Many inflammatory processes are controlled with antibiotics and respiratory care without airway manipulation or surgical intervention. Treatment in these cases includes the administration of humidified oxygen and inhaled racemic epinephrine, combined in some cases with the administration of oral, intramuscular, or intravascular dexamethasone. Although the procedure may be difficult, endotracheal intubation is well tolerated in the patient with epiglottitis, since the inflammation is supraglottic with no tracheal or lower respiratory tract involvement. Rarely is intubation necessary for more than 24 to 48 hours in these patients, after which antibiotics have begun to reduce the swelling associated with infection. In a patient with viral or bacterial tracheitis, however, intubation for more than 24 to 48 hours may produce tracheal injury and ulceration.

Tracheomalacia

Tracheomalacia, sometimes complicating lung disease of prematurity, is a relatively common cause of airway obstruction. It is characterized by a floppy trachea that collapses during expiration when the intrathoracic trachea is compressed by the positive intrathoracic pressure. It can be caused by intrinsic tracheal defects, extrinsic compression by surrounding structures, or from prolonged positive pressure ventilation. It commonly occurs in association with tracheoesophageal fistula repair (see TEF below).

Clinical Recognition

The clinical presentation of tracheomalacia depends on the severity and location of obstruction with more severe lesions presenting in infancy. Intrathoracic lesions typically cause expiratory wheeze that may be hard to distinguish from asthma. Extrathoracic lesions can progress to cause stridor at rest. Patients often have cough and evidence of respiratory distress. They may present with recurrent respiratory infections and episodes of severe obstruction and respiratory failure. Tracheomalacia is typically diagnosed using bronchoscopy during spontaneous respiration, which demonstrates the characteristic tracheal collapse with expiration. Although dynamic imaging studies may be useful, standard imaging modalities are typically not helpful in making this diagnosis.

Management

In general, children who are otherwise healthy will have resolution of symptoms by about a year of age as the cartilagenous tracheal structures mature. During episodes of acute illness, however, these children can present with severe work of breathing, cyanosis and respiratory failure. In addition to medical management, they may benefit from noninvasive or invasive ventilatory strategies. The subset of children with severe disease resulting in recurrent bouts of respiratory failure may require tracheal surgery or placement of a tracheal stent.

Vascular Rings

Vascular rings represent a rare and varied group of developmental anomalies of the aorta and great vessels. They may produce obstruction of the esophagus, trachea, or both. These rings are a result of failure of the normal involution of the appropriate segments of the six embryologic aortic arches. Vascular rings are characterized as complete when both the esophagus and trachea are fully encircled and incomplete when they are only partially encircled. Complete rings are typically caused by a double aortic arch or a right-sided aortic arch with an aberrant left subclavian artery and left ductus arteriosus or ligamentum. Incomplete rings are often caused by a pulmonary artery sling, innominate artery compression, or an aberrant right subclavian artery. The level of respiratory obstruction is usually the trachea, but compression of a bronchus by the ductus arteriosus, or by a pulmonary artery sling, may produce compression more distally.

Clinical Recognition

Vascular rings may be asymptomatic in infancy but lead to significant airway obstruction in childhood. The wide variety of anomalies produces varying degrees of symptoms with presentations ranging from incidental findings on imaging studies to neonates with critical airways. Vascular rings should be suspected in infants with stridor, dysphagia, failure to thrive associated with difficult feeding, or recurrent pneumonia. Esophageal obstruction can produce difficulty swallowing. A patient with esophageal compression may also have respiratory symptoms from compression on the trachea from a distended esophageal pouch. This may lead to reflex apnea during feeding, and eventually tracheomalacia in a more chronic setting.

Often, diagnosis is delayed by failure to consider these anatomic obstructions since their presentation can be quite varied and subtle. In a patient presenting with an acute airway obstruction or other medical problems requiring intubation and nasogastric tube placement, detection of a vascular ring can be even more difficult because of the presence of these tubes. Chest radiographs are the initial test of choice and may be supplemented by various diagnostic tests: contrast esophagography, angiography, echocardiography, MRI, and digital subtraction angiography are needed in some combination to define the anatomy.

Management

Although some patients with constricting anomalies improve as they grow, most will require surgical correction. Surgical treatment is usually indicated to relieve the obstruction, with predictable and immediate resolution of symptoms and excellent outcomes. Surgical repair is accomplished by dividing the vascular ring and preserving the blood supply to the aortic branches. This is usually accomplished by a left thoracotomy but more recently, video-assisted thoracoscopic surgical (VATS) techniques and endoscopic robotic-assisted techniques have been adopted in some centers for select patients.

BRONCHIAL LESIONS

Bronchial Atresia

Congenital bronchial atresia is a rare anomaly characterized by a bronchocele caused by a mucus-filled, blindly terminating segmental or lobar bronchus, with resulting hyperinflation of the distal obstructed segment of lung. Hyperaeration is believed to result from communication with the normally aerated lung via the pores of Kohn and the channels of Lambert.

Clinical Recognition

Neonates and infants with the lesion are usually seen for respiratory distress. In older patients, a history of episodic upper respiratory infection and wheezing may be elicited. Some older patients may complain of dyspnea on exertion or unilateral chest pain. Physical examination findings seldom suggest the diagnosis, but unilaterally decreased breath sounds may be evident.

Management

Often, the diagnosis is suggested by chest radiograph, but chest CT scan may be necessary to help more closely define the anatomy. Bronchoscopy is the most efficient way to identify the atretic opening to the involved bronchus. Bronchography has been used in the past, but high-resolution CT scan can often provide the same anatomic information noninvasively. Complete atresia of a main stem or lobar bronchus may lead to infectious complications or compression symptoms from overdistention of the affected lobe. This may require surgical management, such as lobectomy.

Right Middle Lobe Syndrome

Right middle lobe syndrome is the recurrence or persistence of atelectasis or pneumonitis of the right middle lobe, sometimes associated with bronchiectasis. It has been described in all age groups, in both the right middle and lower lobes concomitantly, and has also been observed in the lingula segment. This process can be caused by extraluminal or intraluminal obstruction, or by nonobstructive causes. The right middle lobe is anatomically predisposed to compression of its bronchus by the lymph nodes in the vicinity that encircle it, which can lead to sequestered areas of collapsed or infected lung. Since it is bordered by two fissures, it also receives less collateral ventilation than other lobes, making reinflation of collapsed lung more challenging. Because the right middle and lower lobes are favored sites for aspirated material (Fig. 132.1), recurrent inflammation caused by pneumonia can lead to chronic atelectasis and adenopathy. A similar situation can be seen with intraluminal tumors and other space-occupying lesions. In children, nonobstructive causes such as asthma, cystic fibrosis, and immobile cilia syndrome can also result in prolonged atelectasis, which promotes recurrent infection and eventual bronchiectasis.

Clinical Recognition

Right middle lobe syndrome is a radiographic diagnosis, so physical manifestations vary widely but commonly include persistent cough, intermittent wheezing, or dyspnea. Patients may have wheezing, rales, or decreased aeration on lung examination, particularly appreciated anteriorly. Chest radiographs typically reveal atelectasis of the right middle lobe, which may be recurrent or persistent. They may also show bronchiectasis or pneumonitis of the affected area. Recurrent episodes of pneumonia and associated atelectasis in the lingula or right middle (and often lower) lobes occur in these patients and are not responsive to chest percussion, postural drainage, or antibiotic treatment.

Management

Patients with right middle lobe syndrome may respond to conventional medical management along with chest physical therapy and postural drainage. When this is not the case, fiberoptic bronchoscopy and bronchoalveolar lavage may be helpful to restore patency of the bronchus, allow better postural drainage, and enhance antibiotic effectiveness. Although the need for resection is far less common than in the past, patients with systemic symptoms such as failure to thrive, obstructing lesions, bronchiectasis, bronchial stenosis, or failure to respond to medical management should be considered candidates for lobectomy.

ESOPHAGUS-RELATED CAUSES OF AIRWAY DIFFICULTIES

Goals of Treatment

Patients with congenital and acquired esophageal abnormalities may present with a variety of urgent complaints, the most concerning of which include significant dysphagia, impacted food or foreign bodies, and in some cases even respiratory symptoms or distress. In such patients, prompt evaluation and treatment is critical as with any primary airway issue. Familiarity with the common congenital esophageal anomalies acquired esophageal emergencies and urgencies are critical to arriving at a prompt diagnosis and delivering the appropriate treatment.

CLINICAL PEARLS AND PITFALLS

- Patients with a history of repaired esophageal atresia frequently have tracheomalacia. If severe, a child may present with episodes of respiratory distress or "death spells."
- Patients with an H-type esophageal fistula (patent trachea and esophagus with connection between the two structures) may present after the neonatal period with symptoms of recurrent choking and congestion with feeds, or with recurrent pneumonias.
- Patients with a history of repaired esophageal atresia may present at any age with an esophageal stricture. Typical symptoms are progressive intolerance of solid food followed later by intolerance of liquids as well. In severe cases, patients may not be able to manage oral secretions.
- Esophageal injuries in older children typically present with significant symptoms (retrosternal chest pain, dysphagia, stridor, retching). Younger children may present with more subtle or vague symptoms.

Esophageal Atresia and Tracheoesophageal Fistula

TEF is typically a congenital condition but has been rarely reported as an acquired problem after suppuration of mediastinal nodes or as a result of iatrogenic injury or a complication following foreign body ingestion. The more common congenital TEF is accompanied by atresia of the esophagus in more than 85% of patients and generally presents in the immediate perinatal period with feeding intolerance and inability to handle secretions. These patients undergo repair shortly after diagnosis, typically via a right thoracotomy or thoracoscopic approach.

Approximately 3% of all patients with TEF have an "H-type" fistula, in which both the trachea and the esophagus are intact and patent but are connected by a fistula that is frequently in the cervical region or high in the thorax (Fig. 132.2). Because there is no accompanying esophageal atresia, these patients are more likely to present later in infancy or childhood with symptoms of recurrent respiratory distress or pulmonary aspiration. The acquired form is usually in the distal trachea or proximal bronchial tree, and is extremely uncommon.

H-type fistulae are notoriously difficult to diagnose, particularly if the fistula tract is small. Children generally develop recurrent pulmonary infections with no obvious source. The characteristic history of choking or gagging with swallowing that accompanies esophageal atresia with TEF may not be present, but parents may describe excessive secretions or noisy breathing after feeds. Contrast esophagram, specifically looking for an H-type TEF is necessary. Most of these fistulae are quite small in diameter (millimeters) and short (also less than 1 cm), making radiographic identification difficult.

Following repair of esophageal atresia or fistula, patients may present at any point in life with an anastomotic stricture and/or an impacted food bolus with the site of retention typically at the site of anastomosis. Patients who present to the ED with dysphagia or intolerance of solids and/or liquids in the setting of a prior history of esophageal atresia repair should undergo contrast esophagography (e-Fig. 132.1).

SURGICAL EMERGENCIES

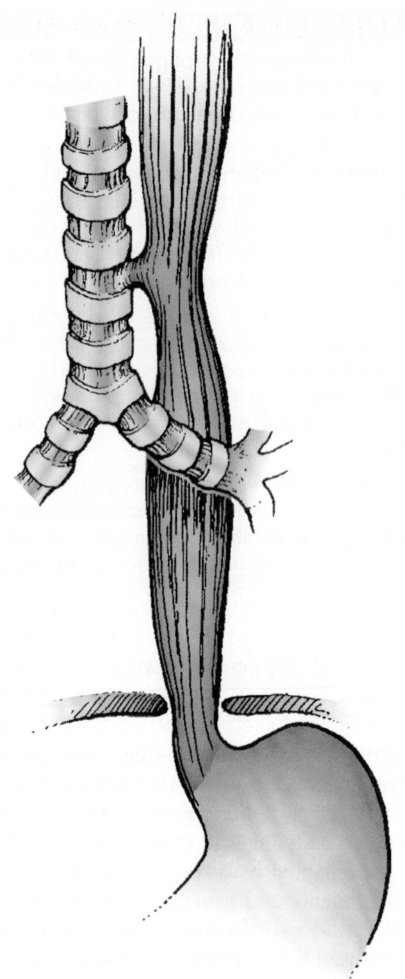

FIGURE 132.2 H-type tracheoesophageal fistula.

Patients who present with a stricture following fistula or esophageal atresia repair are typically managed with esophagoscopy under general anesthesia with removal of any impacted foreign material and bougie or balloon dilation of the stricture. Most such patients are discharged home immediately after these interventions, and some patients require multiple dilations over the course of their childhoods.

Esophageal Web

Rarely, a patient presents with symptoms caused by an esophageal web (Fig. 132.3). The membranous, congenital narrowing of unclear origin usually allows the passage of liquids, and symptoms often do not arise until the child begins to eat solid food. Patients may present with feeding intolerance or respiratory symptoms after drinking and eating. Recurrent aspiration pneumonia may also develop. Rarely, an esophageal web can present with associated anemia, in the form of Plummer–Vinson syndrome. An esophagram is usually diagnostic. Symptomatic patients who have respiratory symptoms or who are unable to achieve adequate oral intake should be admitted for observation and definitive management. Often, a thin membranous web may be split by esophageal dilators, cautery, or a hydraulic balloon placed endoscopically across the stenosis. If this approach is unsuccessful because the lumen is too small to transmit the dilator or the tissue is

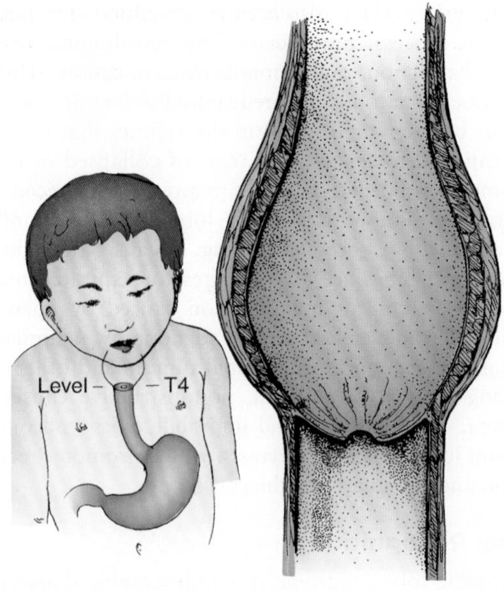

FIGURE 132.3 A child with chronic partial obstruction of the esophagus caused by a congenital web. Similar bulbous enlargement of the proximal esophagus can occur with any type of stricture and results in pressure on the trachea and recurrent regurgitation with aspiration. T4, 4th thoracic vertebrae.

unyielding, segmental esophageal resection may be necessary via thoracotomy or thoracoscopy.

Caustic Ingestion

Caustic ingestion is the leading toxic exposure in children, and can cause devastating injury to the esophagus and stomach with dire consequences. The most frequent exposures in children are to mild alkali agents such as household bleach and detergents. Button battery ingestions in children are increasingly common and can be extremely dangerous (see Chapters 99 Gastrointestinal Emergencies and 126 ENT Emergencies for a full discussion). The age distribution of pediatric ingestions is bimodal, with accidental ingestions common in children younger than 5 years and suicide attempts more common in teenagers and young adults. The extent and severity of injury depends on the type, concentration and quantity of the ingested agent, as well as the duration of exposure. Liquid agents typically cause more injury than solids, with strong alkalis being associated with very severe damage. Following the initial ingestion of an acid or alkali, a significant inflammatory response with edema, hemorrhage, and thrombosis can occur within 24 hours. Local tissue damage continues for some time after the initial exposure, causing necrosis, edema, potential perforation, and eventual fibrosis and stricture.

Clinical Recognition

Clinical findings range from a normal physical examination to respiratory distress and hemodynamic instability. Most patients will complain of oropharyngeal discomfort, odynophagia, dysphagia, and chest pain. Stridor may indicate laryngeal and epiglottic edema, and if accompanied by drooling should raise suspicion for esophageal injury. Other signs of esophageal injury include dysphagia, retrosternal pain, epigastric pain, and hematemesis. However, clinical symptoms may be poor predictors of the extent of injury. Ominous signs include hemodynamic instability, fever, tachycardia, and mental status changes; such findings raise concern for esophageal perforation and developing mediastinitis.

Management

Initial management objectives include the assessment of the severity of injury and the prevention of further injury. If possible, the type and amount of corrosive agent ingested should be identified, as this information may be useful in guiding further management. Clinicians should contact their regional Poison Control Center; this is often very helpful in determining active ingredients and the degree of concern for a given substance (see Chapter 110 Toxicologic Emergencies). The airway should be assessed and secured if necessary. Stridor should raise concern for laryngeal edema and orotracheal intubation is indicated in its presence. The airway should be visualized during this maneuver and tubes should not be passed blindly. One exception to this is in the case of ingested hydrofluoric acid, which requires immediate evacuation, best achieved by nasogastric decompression of the stomach.

Patients presenting to the ED following a caustic ingestion may become critically ill and should be closely monitored with this in mind. They should remain *nil per os* and large-bore intravenous lines should be placed for fluid administration. Measures to dilute or neutralize the ingested agent may cause further complications, and activated charcoal and emetic agents should be avoided. Two view radiographs of the chest and abdomen should be performed and reviewed carefully for evidence of pneumomediastinum, pneumoperitoneum, and pleural effusion. These findings raise concern for full-thickness esophageal or gastric injury.

Patients with suspected esophageal or gastric injury should receive prompt gastroenterology and/or surgical evaluation, as early endoscopy is the gold standard for the assessment of caustic injuries with suspected or known ingestion of caustic substances and in any symptomatic patient. This should be performed within the first 12 to 24 hours after ingestion. Patients with any concerning history or findings should be admitted to the appropriate inpatient ward for close monitoring thereafter, and patients with obvious perforation should receive broad-spectrum antibiotics and will likely require urgent operative management.

PLEURAL DISEASES

The lung is covered by the densely adherent visceral pleura, which moves smoothly over the parietal pleura of the chest wall. A thin fluid film and the friction created by apposition of the pleural layers (like two plates of glass held together by a film of water) contribute to the full expansion of the lung mechanically. When air, excess fluid, or purulent material comes between the two layers of the pleura, the lung may collapse or become significantly compressed and consideration needs to be given to drainage of the pleural space.

Pneumothorax

Goals of Treatment

Tension pneumothorax is a life-threatening emergency and needs to be evacuated immediately. Smaller pneumothoraces may be managed conservatively depending on hemodynamic and respiratory response. Once patients are stabilized, clinicians should investigate the etiology of the pneumothorax.

CLINICAL PEARLS AND PITFALLS

- Tension pneumothorax is a clinical diagnosis and does not require a radiograph for confirmation if there is hemodynamic compromise.
- Exercise caution in sedating patients with pneumothoraces or converting them to positive pressure ventilation since their hemodynamic status can be quite tenuous.
- Children with even small pneumothoraces require a period of ED observation and consideration of admission.

Current Evidence

A pneumothorax is a collection of air in the pleural space. It can occur for short- or long-term duration and can be static or accumulate progressively. Because atmospheric pressure is greater than intrapleural pressure, any mechanism that allows even momentary communication between the atmosphere outside the chest wall or within the tracheobronchial tree can result in a rapid shift of air into the pleural space. A pneumothorax may occur spontaneously, or it may be the result of trauma or a therapeutic intervention. Children with no known predisposing pulmonary conditions are diagnosed as having a primary spontaneous pneumothorax. Secondary spontaneous pneumothoraces occur in patients with underlying diseases such as asthma, cystic fibrosis, or structural abnormalities such as congenital blebs, pneumatoceles, or congenital cystic adenomatoid malformations (CCAMs).

Primary spontaneous pneumothoraces are thought to be the result of sudden increases in transpulmonary pressure resulting in alveolar rupture. Ruptured alveoli coalesce into blebs, which usually occur apically and can rupture into the pleural space. Varying amounts of entering air can lead to a small pneumothorax or complete collapse of the involved lung (Fig. 132.4). Increased intrathoracic pressure associated with the Valsalva maneuver or forceful inhalation has been associated with spontaneous pneumothorax but there may be no history of any abnormal respirations. Increasingly, genetic predisposition to spontaneous pneumothorax seems to be playing a role. Secondary spontaneous pneumothoraces often result from different pathophysiology; these may involve a defect in the visceral pleura caused by infection, inflammation, connective tissue disorders, or space-occupying lesions.

Clinical Considerations

Clinical Recognition. The peak incidence of spontaneous pneumothorax occurs in the adolescent and young adult years with a male predominance. Certain patient populations are at higher risk. Children who suffer spontaneous pneumothoraces tend to be tall and thin. Cigarette smoking is a significant risk factor in adults and illicit drugs such as marijuana and cocaine have also been associated with pneumothoraces. Patients with collagen vascular disorders such as Marfan syndrome are also at increased risk. In patients with cystic fibrosis, spontaneous pneumothorax is the second most common pulmonary complication and usually occurs in teenage or young adult patients with far advanced, diffuse disease. Another group of

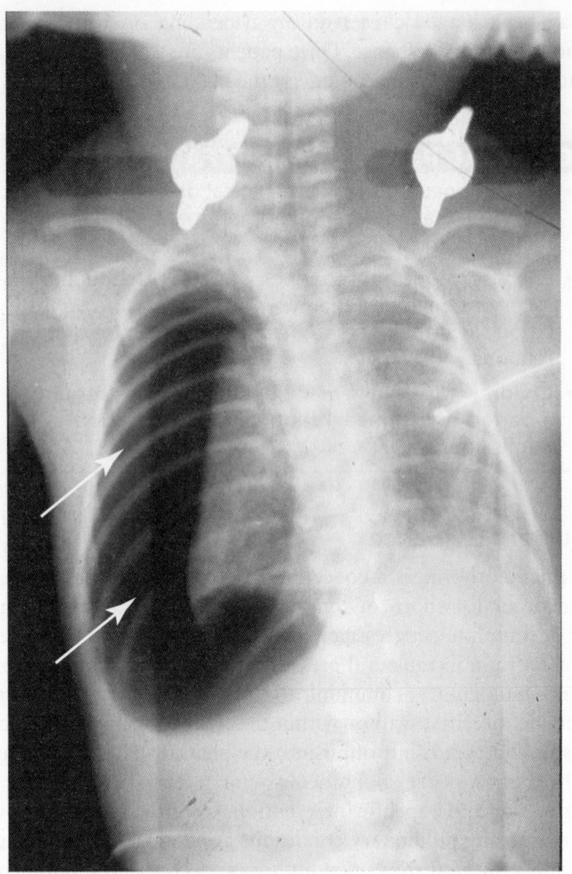

FIGURE 132.4 Large pneumothorax involving the entire thorax. Atelectatic lung border is marked by *arrows*.

children with a high incidence of spontaneous pneumothorax are those with pulmonary metastases. Children with staphylococcal pneumonia are especially prone to develop unilateral or bilateral pneumothoraces. Finally, even though only a very small proportion of asthmatics sustain pneumothoraces, given that asthma is one of the most common diagnoses encountered in the Pediatric Emergency Department, these patients represent a fair amount of cases. Iatrogenic causes of pneumothorax include thoracentesis or central venous catheter insertion, bronchoscopy, aggressive positive pressure ventilation ("barotrauma"), or cardiopulmonary resuscitation. Penetrating and blunt trauma to the chest may cause injuries to the lung, pleura, esophagus, trachea, and bronchi, all of which can result in pneumothorax. A more detailed discussion of trauma-related causes of pneumothorax can be found in Chapter 123 Thoracic Trauma.

A tension pneumothorax requires emphasis because this condition may be fatal if not recognized early and attended to rapidly. A tension pneumothorax, results not only in a complete collapse of the ipsilateral lung but also in progressive pressure across the mediastinum. This pressure impedes ventilation of the contralateral lung resulting in further compromise. Tension pneumothorax results in air accumulating in the pleural space with each inspiration. Whether the entry site of air into the pleural space is through the chest wall, a torn bronchus, or an injured lung, the physiologic result is that of a one-way valve, whereby air continues to accumulate in the pleural cavity with inspiration but cannot be expelled on expiration. This phenomenon continues until the intrathoracic pressure on the involved side is so high that no further air can enter the pleural space. This is often the point at which venous return from below the diaphragm is also impeded and circulatory failure ensues. Hemodynamic compromise may also result from rising intrathoracic pressure leading to a shift in mediastinal structures (particularly in younger children) with compression of the cardiovascular structures.

Clinical Assessment. The symptoms and signs of pneumothorax depend on the size of the pneumothorax and how rapidly it occurs. The most common presenting symptoms are unilateral chest pain and dyspnea. For example, it is common for a patient with spontaneous rupture of an emphysematous bleb to complain of sudden acute pain on the involved side of the chest followed by tachypnea, pain at the tip of the ipsilateral shoulder, and a sense of shortness of breath. Such patients usually have a small to moderate pneumothorax (less than 20% of the lung volume), often with no accompanying hypoxia. Decreased breath sounds may be heard on the ipsilateral side, and a chest radiograph will usually demonstrate the pneumothorax, particularly if taken at end expiration. Patients with a more longstanding pneumothorax may not even be in pain.

In general, a patient with a pneumothorax of 50% or more of the lung volume will exhibit signs and symptoms of ventilatory impairment: dyspnea, tachypnea, pain, splinting on the involved side, agitation, increased pulse rate, diminished breath sounds, and increased resonance to percussion on the involved side and, possibly, displacement of the trachea and heart away from the involved side. Severe dyspnea should alert the physician to the possibility of a very large or possible tension pneumothorax. A child with existing underlying lung disease may display more severe symptoms and hypoxemia with a small or moderate pneumothorax.

In addition to describing symptoms, the patient with pneumothorax should be asked about potential predisposing conditions or risk factors including asthma, foreign body aspiration, underlying infections, inhaled drug use, activities at onset of symptoms, and history of any prior pneumothoraces.

If the patient's condition is not severe, an immediate upright PA and a lateral chest radiograph should be taken. These radiographs are important to determine not only the site and extent of the pneumothorax but also any complicating features such as tumor, fluid within the pleural space, or abnormalities of the lungs, diaphragm, or mediastinum.

Management. Management depends on the extent of the pneumothorax, the severity of symptoms, ongoing expansion, presence of tension physiology, and the suspected underlying etiology or clinical condition. Small pneumothoraces that are asymptomatic can typically be managed with observation alone, either in the ED or through admission to the hospital. Supplemental oxygen may be provided to these patients to hasten the rate of pleural air absorption. Patients with larger pneumothoraces, any hypoxemia or respiratory distress, or those with evidence of ongoing leak from the lung surface usually require intervention. Options include thoracentesis, placement of a small "pigtail" catheter, or placement of a standard chest tube (see Chapter 141 Procedures). In the ED, the percutaneous, guidewire "pigtail" catheters are ideal for pneumothoraces without associated hemothorax or empyema. However, these temporary catheter devices are small gauge and thus tend to easily develop fibrin plugs. A surgical consultation is generally warranted for any patient with a pneumothorax, particularly if there is evidence of a continuing air leak or the mechanism was traumatic, or due to an underlying anatomic abnormality.

Tension pneumothoraces are a life-threatening emergency and deserve special consideration. A tension pneumothorax should be clinically obvious from absent breath sounds on the affected side, respiratory distress, hypoxia, and tracheal deviation. These patients require immediate decompression with a large-bore (14-gauge) angiocatheter into the second intercostal space anteriorly to evacuate the air and relieve the tension. Treatment should not be delayed to obtain a chest radiograph. The insertion of the needle and catheter will immediately result in release of the tension on the mediastinum and diaphragm. This maneuver should be followed by the controlled placement of an appropriate-sized chest tube. Depending on the suspected etiology, further studies such as CT may be indicated.

Definitive surgical therapy, such as VATS with pleurodesis, is typically reserved for patients who have recurrent spontaneous pneumothoraces, severe underlying lung disease, or a persistent air leak not responding to conventional chest tube drainage. Unfortunately, at least half of children who suffer from a spontaneous pneumothorax will have a recurrence.

Pneumomediastinum

Pneumomediastinum occurs when there is an abnormal collection of air in the mediastinum from either a spontaneous or traumatic mechanism. As with pneumothoraces, spontaneous pneumomediastinum tends to be found most often in tall, thin, adolescent males. Pneumomediastinum is typically caused by alveolar rupture (though air can also escape from the airways or gastrointestinal tract), resulting in free air that tracks along the bronchovascular sheath and then migrates centrally to the hilum and surrounding structures. It often dissects through soft tissues and fascial planes and can be seen in the neck and chest. Most of the time, due to this dissection into the soft tissues, there is no significant buildup of pressure in the mediastinum. In extreme cases, however, the tension produced in the mediastinum can be great enough to impair both circulation and ventilation. Although rare, this phenomenon is most likely to occur in a patient who is receiving positive-pressure ventilation, which enhances escape of air from the bronchial tree into the mediastinum (e-Fig. 132.2A).

Clinical Recognition

Pneumomediastinum is most commonly associated with asthma exacerbations, but can also be identified in cases of Valsalva maneuver, severe cough, barotrauma, forceful emesis, foreign body aspiration, and inhalational drugs. The predominant symptom is pleuritic chest pain, which may radiate and be accompanied by dyspnea and/or dysphagia. Crepitus over the neck or upper thorax may be appreciated on physical examination. Auscultation over the heart may reveal Hamman sign, which is a crunching sound that may obscure the heart sounds. In the rare cases of tension pneumomediastinum, patients may be in severe distress with distended neck veins, tachypnea, and cyanosis.

Management

Pneumomediastinum is diagnosed on chest radiography, which demonstrates air tracking around and outlining mediastinal structures on both frontal and lateral views. Subcutaneous emphysema is often appreciated as well. These findings may be quite subtle (e-Fig. 132.2B). Management of pneumomediastinum depends largely on the suspected etiology. In the vast majority of cases of spontaneous pneumomediastinum, conservative treatment with rest, observation, and analgesia is appropriate since most of these self-resolve over several days. If esophageal perforation is suspected due to an esophageal foreign body or a significant history of forceful emesis, an esophogram using water-soluble contrast may be helpful. In the extremely rare case of a tension pneumomediastinum, surgical drainage of the accumulated air in the mediastinum is necessary.

Pleural Effusion

Pleural fluid in excess amount is not a disease per se, but it indicates the presence of pulmonary or systemic illness. The classification of the fluid into transudate, which accumulates when the normal pressure relationships between the capillary pressure in the lung, the pleural pressure, and the lymphatic drainage pressure are disturbed, or exudate, an inflammatory collection, has less utility today than in previous years because of other diagnostic tools presently available. Nevertheless, an awareness that an increased pulmonary capillary pressure (as in congestive heart failure), a decreased colloid osmotic pressure (as in renal disease), increased intrapleural negative pressure (as in atelectasis), or impaired lymphatic drainage of the pleural space (e.g., from surgical trauma to the thoracic duct) may result in transudative effusion is important. In children, the inflammatory cause of effusion is most commonly a result of pneumonia, with accumulation of infected fluid in the pleural space, or empyema (see below). Malignant effusions from associated oncologic diagnoses are much less common than in adults, but also occur in children. The accumulation of blood in the pleural space because of trauma is discussed in Chapter 123 Thoracic Trauma. Hemothorax may also result from nontraumatic conditions. Necrotizing pulmonary infections, tuberculosis, pulmonary arteriovenous (AV) malformation, torn pleural adhesions, hemophilia, thrombocytopenia, systemic anticoagulation, and pleural tumors have all been reported to cause hemothorax. Chylothorax, or the accumulation of lymphatic fluid in the pleural space, has increased in frequency as thoracic, especially complex cardiac, surgical operations have become more common in children.

Clinical Recognition

Small, sterile collections, as well as large, chronic collections, may be asymptomatic. Acute collections produce symptoms by compressive effects on the lung, with resultant atelectasis, and right-to-left shunting, with resultant hypoxia and hypercapnia. Respiratory distress may follow, marked by dyspnea, tachypnea, increased use of accessory muscles of respiration, and even cyanosis. Small to moderate effusions may not be evident on physical examination, with most effusions detected by chest radiograph. Larger effusions will cause dullness to percussion and decreased breath sounds.

Small effusions can be quite subtle and may manifest as slight blunting of the costophrenic angle on chest x-ray. Larger effusions may cause significant opacification of a hemithorax and may layer out on an upright view of the chest, creating the so-called "meniscus sign." Chest radiographs may also demonstrate the likely etiology of the effusion since cardiomegaly, mediastinal masses, hilar lymphadenopathy may all be appreciated. Moderate to large effusions on chest x-ray merit further evaluation by ultrasound to further characterize the effusion and determine whether it is comprised of free fluid or a loculated collection. In skilled hands, ultrasound provides more information than either decubitus radiographs or CT and has the obvious advantages of not requiring sedation or exposing the child to radiation.

Management

Children with pleural effusions should have peripheral blood counts and blood cultures obtained since parapneumonic collections are the most likely culprit. Drainage of pleural fluid, or thoracentesis (see Chapter 141 Procedures), should be performed if it is therapeutically necessary due to the degree of respiratory distress or if there is concern for a noninfectious cause of the collection. Gram stain and culture should always be sent when pleural fluid is available. Nucleic acid amplification testing through polymerase chain reaction (PCR) or specific antigen testing of pleural fluid may increase the likelihood of pathogen detection, particularly in patients who have been partially treated with antibiotics. Fluid should be sent for a cell count with differential since this can help distinguish between various infectious pathogens and malignancy. Cytology should be sent as well when malignancy is suspected. Analysis of other pleural fluid parameters that have historically been assessed such as pH, LDH, glucose, and protein have been used to predict the need for further interventions, but may not be routinely required.

Many pleural effusions do not require drainage. Small effusions often resolve with treatment of the underlying disease. Moderate to large effusions significant enough to cause respiratory distress, and purulent effusions typically require drainage. Thin free-flowing fluid may sometimes be managed by intermittent thoracentesis or the effusion may resolve as the underlying condition is treated. If not, a small-diameter tube, such as an 8F pigtail percutaneous tube, can be placed in the anterior or midaxillary line. Thick fluid, such as blood, pus, and sometimes chyle, requires the placement of a larger diameter tube. Either tube must be attached to a pleural drainage system. When the drainage decreases significantly, to approximately 1 mL per pound of body weight per day, the drain may be removed. The drain should not be removed in the presence of an accompanying "air leak" caused by a bronchopleural connection. See section below on empyema for discussion of further drainage modalities.

Disposition

Pleural effusions that require drainage or further diagnostic evaluation clearly warrant inpatient admission. There is a role for outpatient antibiotic therapy in the setting of very small effusion in the well-appearing child who has close follow-up. Please refer to pneumonia clinical pathway (Chapter 90 Pneumonia, Community-Acquired) for suggested empiric antibiotic therapy. This should be tailored, however, to local sensitivities for common pathogens.

Empyema

Goals of Treatment

The goals of treatment for empyema include the provision of adequate antibiotic treatment for the underlying infection and evacuation of significant pleural collections to allow for lung re-expansion. Patients who develop small parapneumonic effusions will frequently improve clinically with appropriate antibiotic therapy, and small- to moderate-sized simple effusions may resorb as the underlying intraparenchymal infection resolves. Large effusions that compress the lung or complex, loculated effusions are best treated with drainage. Simple layering effusions may be effectively evacuated with tube thoracostomy alone, while large or complex, loculated effusions and simple effusions not effectively managed with tube thoracostomy may require chemical fibrinolysis or surgical drainage and debridement. Surgical drainage and debridement, which can typically be done via a minimally invasive thoracoscopic approach, serves to relieve acute lung compression and to prevent a complex parapneumonic effusion from organizing and establishing a thick pleural peel, which could entrap the lung and result in chronic restriction on the affected side.

CLINICAL PEARLS AND PITFALLS

- Utilize ultrasound for moderate to large pleural effusions to better characterize the fluid collection and identify loculations
- Involve surgical consultants early on since patients with empyema may need surgical intervention

Current Evidence

An empyema is the presence of infected fluid within the pleural cavity and is typically a sequela of an underlying pneumonia. Unfortunately, despite a decrease in invasive pneumococcal disease with widespread vaccination, there has been an increase in the incidence of children hospitalized with empyemas over the past decades. Emyemas seem to have seasonal variation, being more common in the winter and spring months. While chronic medical problems do predispose children to having more complicated pneumonias and empyemas, they also affect previously healthy children. The predominant organisms implicated in empyemas have varied over time with vaccination and resistance patterns but they generally include *Streptococcus pneumoniae, Staphylococcus aureus,* group A streptococci, and *Haemophilus influenza* among others. When empyema follows accidental trauma or surgery, other bacterial organisms may be involved. Viruses and mycoplasma pneumonia infections can also cause parapneumonic effusions but these rarely require intervention and patients are generally less severely ill than with traditional bacterial collections.

Clinical Considerations

Clinical Recognition. Empyema is most common in children 2 to 9 years of age, though children under 2 years tend to have the highest mortality. Presentation with a pneumonia that fails to improve after about 48 hours of appropriate antibiotic treatment should lead to the consideration of a complication like empyema. High fever is common, as are the symptoms of pneumonia: cough, pleuritic chest pain, malaise, and shortness of breath. Children are typically ill appearing and may demonstrate tachypnea, respiratory distress, and hypoxia. Examination findings may include decreased breath sounds on the affected side and dullness to percussion.

Please refer to Chapter 90 Pneumonia, Community-Acquired for the pneumonia clinical pathway. Plain radiographs of the chest should be obtained. Lateral decubitus films (or ultrasound) can be used to delineate if the fluid in the pleural space layers. Children with a moderate (opacification of more than ¼ of the thorax) to large (opacification of more than ½ of the thorax) effusion should undergo ultrasound to better characterize the fluid. Ultrasound has several advantages over CT in terms of lack of radiation and need for sedation as well as earlier detection of septae and loculations, as well as superior ability to describe the nature of the fluid collection. Furthermore it can be used therapeutically to help with chest tube placement when necessary.

Management

Children with empyemas are more likely to be bacteremic and they should all have a blood culture drawn in order to help direct antimicrobial therapy. Empyema in healthy children may respond to prolonged IV antibiotic therapy and chest tube drainage, if the fluid is thin and not loculated. Initial antibiotics should be broad spectrum and based on local resistance patterns and can be narrowed later if a pathogen is identified. If a patient fails to respond to this management, loculation of thick purulent material should be suspected. In such cases, both thoracostomy drainage with the addition of fibrinolytic agents and VATS have been shown to be effective in hastening recovery and reducing morbidity. Choice of therapy is often dictated by regional expertise. Regardless of treatment modality, early surgical consultation is warranted for significant empyemas.

VATS allows for thoracoscopic debridement of the infected fibrinous peel that encases the lung and prevents its full expansion. A chest tube is then placed to drain the pleural cavity and left in place for a period of days. Studies suggest that early surgical intervention likely decreases duration of IV antibiotics, days with a chest tube, and hospitalization. In centers where a chest tube and fibrinolytic therapy is the initial treatment of choice, patients who fail to improve clinically after a few days should progress to VATS. Seldom is open thoracotomy now necessary to resolve empyema. It should be remembered that VATS will aid in the resolution of the pleural space disease but not necessarily the parenchymal disease which will need ongoing therapy.

Solid Lung and Pleural Lesions

A number of solitary lesions are benign, with the most common being inflammatory pseudotumor and hamartoma, both of which may become quite large and cause symptoms of respiratory distress, cough, airway obstruction, or mediastinal compression. Solid lesions in the pleural space occur uncommonly in children. A localized, pleural-based mass should suggest neoplasm, which may be primary or metastatic. The most common primary lung tumors are bronchial adenomas, and the most common metastatic lesions are Wilms tumor and osteogenic sarcoma. They may encase the lung and produce restrictive lung disease.

It is impossible to generalize the mode of presentation of such rare processes. Focal lesions may be expected to be found in the investigation of symptoms caused by local compression or erosion; because of the large functional pulmonary reserve of children, restrictive lung disease caused by a diffuse process is distinctly uncommon; or by serendipity. A full radiographic evaluation, including a CT scan, should be obtained, admission to the hospital strongly considered, and appropriate consultation sought. Focal lesions should be considered malignant until proven otherwise; thus, operation for biopsy or excision will likely be required.

LUNG LESIONS

Goals of Treatment

Since patients with lung lesions typically present with respiratory symptoms and even distress, prompt evaluation and treatment is critical. Familiarity with normal variations and potential pathologic abnormalities is necessary to arriving at a prompt diagnosis and delivering the appropriate treatment, as patients with space-occupying lung lesions may require quite different management than patients with more common respiratory illnesses.

CLINICAL PEARLS AND PITFALLS

- Airway and lung lesions are uncommon in children, but can present with common respiratory symptoms and signs.
- Chest radiographs are the initial diagnostic modality of choice, and should be obtained promptly in patients with respiratory distress when such lesions are suspected.
- Patients with large cystic lesions or hyperinflation may develop air trapping and worsened respiratory compromise if positive-pressure ventilation is applied.
- Prompt surgical consultation may be needed in cases of respiratory distress caused by a lung lesion.

Current Evidence

Most lung lesions in children are congenital, with the majority comprised of CCAMs (also known as congenital pulmonary adenomatoid malformations or CPAMs), bronchogenic cysts, bronchopulmonary sequestrations (BPSs), and congenital lobar emphysema (CLE). Many lesions are discovered prenatally and are asymptomatic after birth, while some cause clear early signs of respiratory distress or circulatory impairment. Complications associated with the above-mentioned lesions include compression of critical structures, infection, pneumothorax, or rarely, malignant degeneration; therefore, surgical intervention is frequently warranted in the care of children with lung lesions.

Cystic Lung Disorders—CCAM and BPS

Cystic lesions of the lung are congenital processes that can present with pulmonary infection, a mass or tension effect causing respiratory distress, or an abnormal chest radiograph in an otherwise asymptomatic patient. CCAM lesions are the result of an overgrowth of bronchioles (e-Fig. 132.3) and an increase in terminal respiratory structures and mucous cells lining the cyst walls. These lesions are generally supplied solely by the pulmonary arterial system, and are present in more than one lobe of the lung in up to 3% of cases. If a

CCAM lesion also receives systemic blood supply, which is a characteristic of BPS, it is termed a *hybrid lesion*. The tissue within a CCAM does not function in normal gas exchange but is connected with the tracheobronchial tree; therefore, these lesions can lead to air trapping and recalcitrant pulmonary infections. Rarely, patients may develop malignant degeneration within the lesion (pleuropulmonary blastoma, rhabdomyosarcoma).

BPSs arise from an accessory bronchopulmonary bud of the foregut. Histologically, they consist of pulmonary tissue; however, they are not connected with the normal bronchial tree or pulmonary vessels (and hence, the pulmonary tissue is "sequestered"). Occasionally, sequestrations have a connection with the esophagus or stomach, because of their foregut derivation. They have a systemic rather than pulmonary blood supply. A sequestration is described as *intralobar* if it is contained within the normal pleura, or *extralobar* if it has its own pleural investment and is separated from the normal lung parenchyma. Sequelae of BPS can be respiratory, with symptoms of respiratory distress or feeding intolerance, or circulatory, in which substantial arteriovenous shunting can occur within the sequestered lobe, leading to high-output cardiac failure. Case reports of associations between BPS and diaphragmatic abnormalities have been described.

Clinical Recognition

Recurrent respiratory infections often lead to a chest radiograph, which demonstrates an abnormal lesion. These lesions can appear as hyper-aerated segments of lung, lung containing air–fluid levels in the instance of CCAM (e-Fig. 132.4), or as solid masses in BPS. As mentioned, clinical findings may be identical to those of a lobar pneumonia. Occasionally, a lesion is discovered in older patients in the setting of recurrent lobar pneumonia or after an empyema fails to recover with appropriate management.

Management

Chest radiographs in the PA, lateral, and decubitus positions should be obtained to evaluate any areas with air–fluid levels. Patients with significant respiratory symptoms, fever, or significant abnormality on chest film should be admitted for further evaluation and treatment. When a CCAM or BPS is suspected, a CT scan with IV contrast should be obtained to better delineate the lesion and to identify any possible systemic blood supply. Because the blood supply may arise from below the diaphragm in up to 20% of cases of BPS, the scan should include both the chest and the upper abdomen. Arteriography is seldom necessary with currently available imaging techniques. The CT scan will likely exclude other conditions that may present similarly, such as a diaphragmatic hernia, postpneumonic pneumatoceles, or esophageal duplication. In the setting of infection, any pathogens identified in the sputum should be treated with appropriate antibiotics. After control of superimposed infection, the lesion should be resected to prevent recurrent infection. Attempted aspiration of the cystic lesions or placement of a chest tube is to be avoided because it may lead to spread of infection into the pleural space.

Surgical resection is indicated for all CCAM and BPS lesions. For young, asymptomatic patients resection can occur electively. For patients who present with infection, resection is typically deferred until 6 to 8 weeks after the resolution of the infection. Resection can be accomplished with low morbidity and mortality; thoracoscopic resection is feasible for some lesions, with the remainder approached via traditional thoracotomy.

Bronchogenic Cyst

Bronchogenic cysts are believed to result from aberrant budding from the primitive foregut or tracheobronchial tree. They arise from the trachea or a bronchus and may be found anywhere along the tracheobronchial tree, in the lung substance, adjacent to the esophagus or in other ectopic locations.

Clinical Recognition

Centrally located cysts may present with symptoms caused by compression of an airway or the esophagus. Wheezing, persistent cough, fever, recurrent pneumonia, and dysphagia may result in such children. In infants and smaller children, large airway compression can lead to significant and life-threatening air trapping and CLE. In contrast, patients with peripherally located cysts are more likely to be asymptomatic or present with milder, nonspecific symptoms, such as cough, dyspnea, tachypnea, or wheezing. Physical examination is often unrevealing, but in patients with large, centrally located lesions, tracheal deviation may be present.

Management

Initial detection of bronchogenic cysts almost always occurs by radiograph. Chest radiograph may demonstrate findings of a smooth paratracheal or hilar mass, airway displacement and/or air trapping, or a structure containing an air–fluid level if there is communication with the airway or gastrointestinal tract (e-Fig. 132.4). CT scan and magnetic resonance imaging (MRI) are helpful in identifying and delineating the anatomic relations of these lesions to surrounding structures. Cysts with turbid, mucoid fluid may appear solid on CT scan.

The standard treatment of bronchogenic cysts is surgical resection, even if asymptomatic. Active infection, if present, should be brought under control before resection. Typically, this is done in the inpatient setting with intravenous antibiotics and close observation. Asymptomatic cysts should be removed to establish the diagnosis and to prevent the complications of secondary bronchial communication, bleeding, or perforation into the pleural cavity. Carcinomas and fibrosarcomas have been reported to arise in benign-appearing bronchogenic cysts.

Congenital Lobar Emphysema

Congenital lobar emphysema (CLE), also known as congenital lobar hyperinflation (CLH), is caused by overexpansion of the air spaces of a segment or lobe of histologically normal lung (Fig. 132.5). Operative findings can reveal large blebs protruding from the lung parenchyma (e-Fig. 132.5), but often the lobe is anatomically normal in appearance, with the exception of massive overdistention. Compression of adjacent normal lung and mediastinal structures frequently occurs, and may result in potentially life-threatening respiratory and hemodynamic compromise. This process is caused by air trapping from either a developmental deficiency of supporting cartilage in the bronchus of a particular lobe or

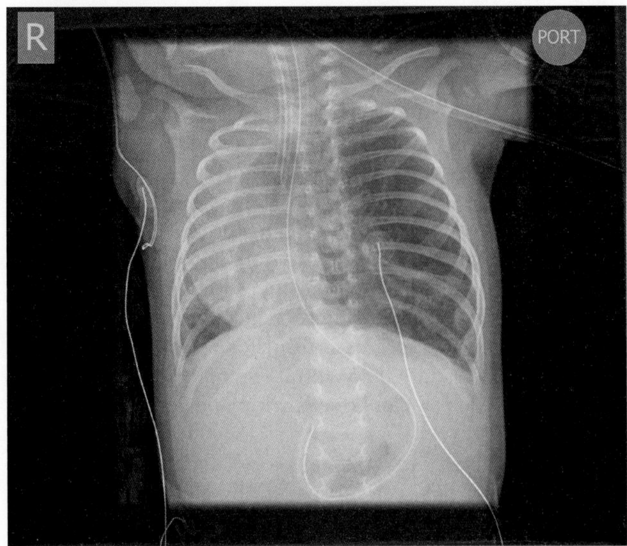

FIGURE 132.5 Congenital lobar emphysema of the left upper lobe in a 3-month-old girl who presented with decreased breath sounds and rales in this area. Note the left-sided secondary compression atelectasis of the lower lobe.

a partially obstructing bronchial lesion, either endobronchial or from external compression (as with a bronchogenic cyst).

Clinical Recognition

Infants with CLE are often normal in appearance at birth, but develop tachypnea, cough, wheezing, dyspnea, and/or cyanosis within a few days. The onset of symptoms may be more gradual; nevertheless, 80% of patients are symptomatic by 6 months of age. The upper lobes are involved in about two-thirds of patients; less commonly, the lower lobes are involved. Chest radiographs show striking radiolucency in the involved lobe with mediastinal shift to the opposite side. The diaphragm is usually flattened on the affected side. It can be difficult to tell whether pulmonary markings are present in the involved lobe, and pneumothorax may be suspected. The compressed normal lung may be erroneously believed to be atelectatic with the emphysematous lobe compensatory.

Management

Initially, the clinical presentation and physiologic derangements may be similar to that of tension pneumothorax, and the two entities should be distinguished. Physical examination may reveal an asymmetric thorax, unilateral hyperresonance and decreased breath sounds on the affected side, and evidence of mediastinal shift. Typical findings on chest radiograph include lobar overinflation, contralateral shift of the mediastinum, and collapse of lung tissue on the contralateral side, with flattening of the ipsilateral hemidiaphragm (Fig. 132.5). In a stable patient, CT or ventilation/perfusion scanning can be helpful in establishing the diagnosis.

If a patient is asymptomatic or minimally symptomatic, bronchoscopy may be helpful in identifying and relieving a reversible cause of bronchial obstruction, such as a mucous plug or granulation tissue. However, pulmonary lobectomy is most commonly required and may be needed acutely if symptoms are progressive. The diseased lobe is evident at thoracotomy because of its overdistended state, often billowing out of the chest. Lobectomy is curative if the cause of the obstruction is also relieved.

Congenital Pulmonary Arteriovenous Fistula

Congenital pulmonary AV fistula is a congenitally occurring communication between a major pulmonary artery and a vein within the lung, usually with an aneurysmal sac. Fistulae vary in size from a few millimeters to several centimeters and can be multiple. At times, a systemic artery may also be involved. Direct right-to-left shunting leads to hypoxemia, and the size of the fistula correlates with the degree of desaturation.

Clinical Recognition

As the initial presentation of this disorder is frequently that of wheezing and desaturation, the child may be initially diagnosed with asthma. Clubbing and cyanosis may demonstrate the hypoxemia. Examination of the chest may reveal a palpable thrill or murmur. If there are symptoms of hemoptysis and epistaxis, one may find telangiectasias or hemangiomas of the skin and mucous membranes. Evaluation of the family may also reveal the presence of hereditary hemorrhagic telangiectasia (Rendu–Osler–Weber disease), which is present in more than half the patients with congenital pulmonary AV fistula.

Management

Children who are symptomatic from this condition are best evaluated by CT scan, contrast echocardiography, perfusion scintigraphy, and arteriogram of the pulmonary artery and aorta. Chest radiographs may demonstrate the aneurysmal areas as rounded or lobulated discrete lesions in the parenchyma. Often, tortuous vessels trace from these rounded areas to the hilum. Symptomatic patients should be admitted to the hospital while a definitive management course is decided. Resection of the fistula, often involving lobectomy, is indicated if the lesion is localized, and may be curative. Multiple small lesions may be amenable to embolization. Unfortunately, some patients have such diffuse disease that such intervention is impossible.

Rare Lesions

Unusual lung lesions encountered in the pediatric population include certain rare tumors and uncommon infections. Rare solid tumors, often identified incidentally on radiographs, include primary sarcoma, pulmonary blastoma, hamartomas, and teratomas. Fungal infections, including actinomycosis, histoplasmosis, mucormycosis, and coccidioidomycosis, may look like tumors on chest radiograph. Atresia of the bronchus or pulmonary artery is rare and will produce differences in the density of the two lungs. The reader is referred to texts of pulmonary medicine or thoracic surgery for further discussion.

MEDIASTINAL TUMORS

See Chapter 106 Oncologic Emergencies.

Goals of Treatment

Since mediastinal lesions frequently cause compression in the limited and confined space of the mediastinum, respiratory and circulatory compromise may occur and may be the presenting symptoms. Prompt identification of a space-occupying mediastinal mass and an awareness of the relevant anatomy are critical. These patients require careful attention and early consultation with appropriate specialists for complete workup and expeditious treatment.

CLINICAL PEARLS AND PITFALLS

- Symptoms of mediastinal lesions are frequently respiratory in nature.
- Orthopnea is a worrisome sign, particularly with anterior mediastinal masses. Such patients may experience respiratory or circulatory collapse with sedation or anesthesia.
- Chest x-ray is the initial diagnostic study of choice and will demonstrate most significant mediastinal masses.
- Anterior mediastinal tumors are frequently neoplastic and middle mediastinal tumors are often cystic.
- Prompt surgical consultation may be needed in cases of respiratory distress or circulatory compromise.

Current Evidence

At least one-third of all mediastinal lesions occur in children younger than 15 years of age and are of varied pathology. Half of these masses are symptomatic, and half of the symptomatic masses are malignant tumors, with the likelihood of malignancy increasing with the age of the patient. More than 90% of asymptomatic masses are benign.

The mediastinum is commonly divided into anterior, superior, middle, and posterior compartments (Fig. 132.6), and the location of a lesion can help to limit its differential diagnosis. The superior mediastinal compartment contains germ cell tumors of the thymus, thymomas, and lymphangiomas. The anterior compartment contains thymic tumors and lymphangiomas as well as lymphomas and teratomas. Bronchogenic cysts in the area of the hilum are located in the middle mediastinum, and frequently have a cystic appearance on cross-sectional imaging. Esophageal cysts and most neurogenic tumors, such as neuroblastomas and ganglioneuromas, are found in the posterior compartment. Neurogenic tumors are the most common cause of mediastinal masses, with lymphomas and germ cell tumors being second and third in frequency. Infection is an uncommon cause of mediastinal node enlargement, but when present, is largely caused by histoplasmosis. Thymic enlargement may mimic an anterior mediastinal mass.

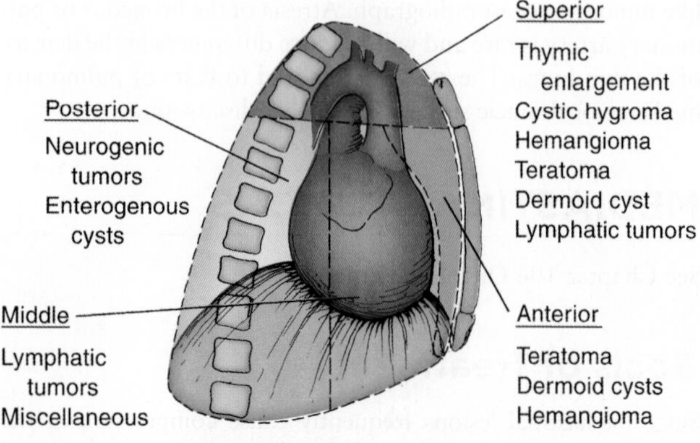

FIGURE 132.6 Mediastinal tumors in children. Differential diagnosis is based on anatomic location within the mediastinum.

Clinical Considerations

Clinical Recognition

Mediastinal masses frequently present with chest pain or respiratory symptoms as a result of airway compression. Patients may present with cough, wheezing, recurrent respiratory infections, bronchitis, atelectasis, and hemoptysis. Dysphagia and hematemesis may occur with compression of the esophagus. Superior vena cava syndrome is a rare complication, usually in association with a rapidly growing tumor, but orthopnea may occur with vascular compression. If the recurrent laryngeal nerve is compressed as a result of the mass, hoarseness and inspiratory stridor may result. Spinal cord compression and vertebral erosion can be seen with a posterior mediastinal tumor.

A careful history may reveal more subtle symptoms, and families should be queried specifically about fever, chills, weight loss, and night sweats. Physical examination should be thorough. It is important to focus on a careful respiratory and cardiac examination, evaluation of the head and neck for palpable masses or venous distention, palpation of the abdomen for organomegaly or masses, and examination of the various nodal basins for adenopathy.

Solid Mediastinal Masses

Children with tumors of the anterior or superior mediastinum should be admitted to an inpatient ward for urgent evaluation because these tumors may pose an immediate threat to life. CT scan or MRI of the chest is generally needed to supplement plain radiographs, in order to further define the location and extent of the mass, and to potentially provide details that may help establish the diagnosis. Much of the management depends upon whether the lesion is cystic or solid. Solid masses raise concern for oncologic pathology, particularly if located in the anterior mediastinum. In the appropriate clinical setting, tumor markers should be obtained, including serum alpha fetoprotein (AFP) and beta-human chorionic gonadotropin (bHCG) levels, and urine catecholamine and metanephrine levels. Lymphomas and teratomas are the most common solid mediastinal tumors in children, with other solid masses occurring more rarely. Thymomas comprise less than 1% of mediastinal tumors in children, with multimodal therapy the mainstay. Benign thymic hyperplasia typically does not cause respiratory compromise, but rapid enlargement often warrants intervention, such as steroid therapy or resection.

When biopsy of a large mediastinal mass is necessary, the logistics of the procedure require careful, thoughtful evaluation, ideally involving the pediatrician or emergency physician, surgeon, oncologist, and anesthesiologist. Airway and cardiac compression by large mediastinal masses can be significant. Large mediastinal masses should be evaluated by CT scan of the chest to assess the presence and extent of tracheal compression. MRI may be a better diagnostic modality for posterior mediastinal masses because many of them are neurogenic in origin and may have extension into the spinal canal. An echocardiogram should also be obtained prior to surgery, to assess the extent of mediastinal shift and the degree of atrial or ventricular compression by the mass. Endotracheal intubation and delivery of general anesthesia may decrease negative intrathoracic pressure leading to occlusion of the thoracic trachea by the tumor. This situation can be challenging to manage; passage of a rigid bronchoscope may be necessary to stent the trachea open to allow gas exchange. If significant tracheal compression is present, consideration should be given to the feasibility of biopsy under local anesthesia. The anesthesiologist should be apprised of the nature of the tumor, and a bronchoscope should be at hand if a general anesthetic is needed. Tissue may be obtained in numerous ways, with the location of the tumor dictating the approach.

Cystic Mediastinal Lesions

The differential diagnosis of cystic mediastinal lesions is large, with the various subtypes arising in predictable anatomic locations of the mediastinum. The most common of these lesions will be discussed in this section.

Thymic cysts are seen in the anterior mediastinum and neck and can cause symptoms if they become infected or hemorrhagic. These cysts are lined with ciliated respiratory epithelium, and contain thymic tissue and lymphocytes. When enlarged and symptomatic, resection is curative.

Pericardial cysts arise in the middle mediastinum. These are benign, thin-walled cysts lined with mesothelium. These lesions are typically asymptomatic and are seen on routine chest films. CT scan can confirm the diagnosis, and unless these lesions are symptomatic or large, no intervention is warranted.

Foregut duplications are cystic or tubular structures found in the posterior mediastinum, and are believed to arise from the original primitive foregut. They can frequently be categorized as *enteric duplications and cysts* lined by intestinal epithelium, *bronchogenic cysts* lined by respiratory epithelium, or *neurenteric cysts* with associated vertebral anomalies or having a connection with the nervous system. Enteric duplications can be located throughout the neck and mediastinum, though the majority (60%) are intrathoracic. Duplication cysts may communicate with the lumen of the airway or esophagus, though most commonly they exist completely separately from the structure of origin. Most are asymptomatic at presentation and are discovered incidentally on chest films obtained for an unrelated reason. Occasionally, these lesions can enlarge and cause compression of the airways and esophagus, leading to dyspnea, cough, wheezing and in some cases, respiratory distress. Rarely, mucosal bleeding in a foregut duplication will create enlargement of the lesion and compression of surrounding structures or hemoptysis/hematemesis if there is connection with a patent lumen. Chest x-ray and CT are the main initial diagnostic modalities, with foregut duplications appearing as well-defined, tissue-density structures with smooth borders. Contrast studies, abdominal ultrasound, and MRI may also be useful adjuncts in the diagnosis of these lesions. Definitive treatment consists of complete surgical excision, which can frequently be accomplished without injury to the bronchial or esophageal walls. In cases of long tubular foregut duplications that share a wall with the aerodigestive tract, the mucosal lining may be stripped, leaving the common muscular wall intact and preserving the integrity of nearby critical structures.

If an asymptomatic cystic mediastinal mass is discovered incidentally in the ED, the child may be discharged home for further outpatient evaluation after surgical consultation. If any symptoms are present or if there is concern for compression of critical structures, however, the patient should be admitted to the hospital for further workup and management by the surgical team.

DIAPHRAGMATIC PROBLEMS

Goals of Treatment

Diaphragmatic hernia and dysfunction are concerning because of potential associated abnormalities of the lung and respiratory dynamics, causing symptoms that range from feeding difficulty and persistent or recurrent respiratory infections to overt respiratory distress. The primary goals of the clinician are recognition of the diaphragmatic abnormality (which can be difficult to distinguish acutely from a primary lung lesion), administration of respiratory support if needed, and consultation of appropriate subspecialty services for long-term management.

CLINICAL PEARLS AND PITFALLS

- Congenital diaphragmatic hernia (CDH) occurs most commonly on the left side.
- Infants with congenital diaphragmatic abnormalities have a 10% to 50% risk of associated anomalies.
- Diaphragmatic hernia may have a similar radiographic appearance to a primary lung lesion such as a CCAM or sequestration.
- Diaphragmatic eventration can be either congenital or acquired, and can present later in infancy or childhood.

Current Evidence

The development of the diaphragm remains incompletely understood and is the result of complex tissue interactions during embryogenesis. The diaphragm is composed of four distinct components, the precursors of which begin to form during the fourth week of gestation and fuse centrally during week 6. These four components merge to close the pleuroperitoneal canal during week 8 of gestation, with the right side closing before the left. Delay or failure of muscular fusion in certain areas of the diaphragm predisposes to weakness or diaphragmatic defects.

Congenital Diaphragmatic Hernia

Congenital diaphragmatic hernia (CDH) is a defect in the diaphragm with resultant protrusion of abdominal viscera into the chest. CDH is estimated to occur in 1:2,000 to 1:5,000 live births, with approximately 80% to 90% of defects on the left side through the area known as the foramen of Bochdalek. Herniation may also occur through the foramen of Morgagni, which lies just posterior to the sternum, comprising 2% or 3% of all diaphragmatic hernias. CDH may be associated with a variety of genetic conditions, including trisomy 21, 18, 13, and Cornelia de Lange, Fryns, and Beckwith–Wiedemann syndromes. Diaphragmatic hernias may be acquired through traumatic rupture of any portion of the diaphragm and may present in a delayed fashion. Information in this chapter will focus largely on diaphragmatic hernias diagnosed in stable older babies and children, who are more likely to present to the ED than those in whom the diagnosis is made in the perinatal period.

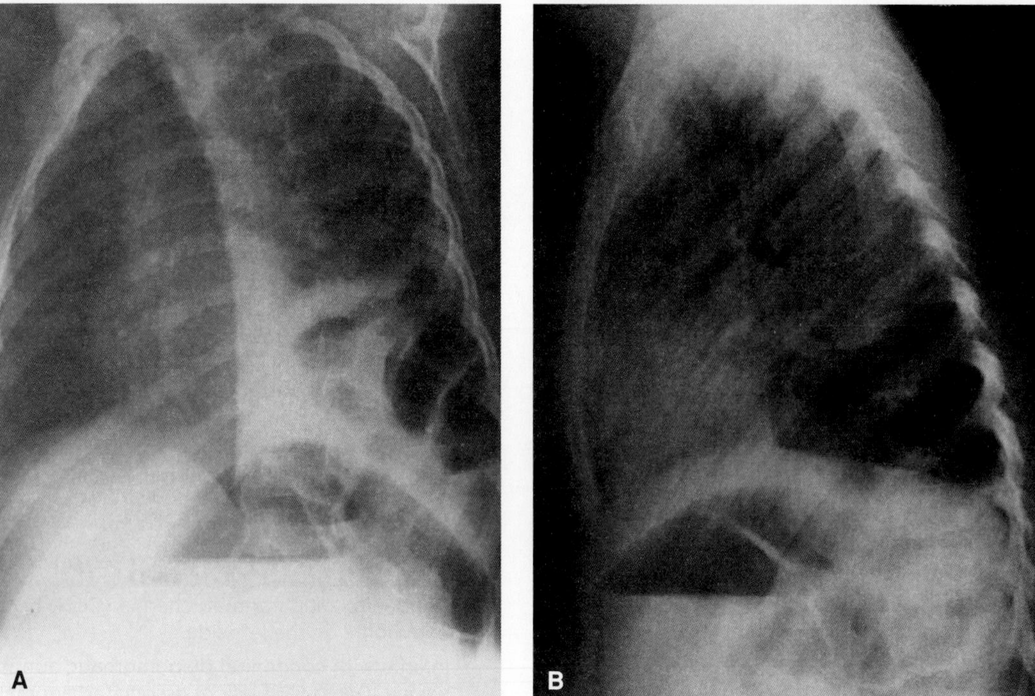

FIGURE 132.7 A 4-year-old boy admitted with 1-day history of recurrent severe upper abdominal colicky pain with dyspnea and decreased breath sounds in the left base. Posteroanterior (**A**) and lateral (**B**) chest films demonstrate multiple bowel loops in the lower, posterior, left side of chest, indicative of a foramen of Bochdalek hernia that was subsequently repaired without difficulty.

Most children with CDH become symptomatic as newborns, when profound respiratory compromise leads to diagnosis. Until recent years, it was believed that the respiratory difficulties of babies with CDH were caused by mechanical compression of the lung by the intestinal viscera herniated through the diaphragmatic opening into the chest. It has become clear in recent years, however, that the situation is more complex. Lung development in infants with CDH is quite abnormal, with associated pulmonary hypoplasia and abnormal vasculature leading to pulmonary hypertension of varying severity. The physiologic consequence of these changes can lead to a life-threatening vicious cycle of hypoxia, acidosis, and intrapulmonary shunting in newborns with this diagnosis. More rarely, CDH may also be identified after the neonatal period. Older infants and children are less likely to present with this form of respiratory distress but may present with features of bowel obstruction, visceral ischemia, or pleural inflammation arising from sudden shift of abdominal viscera into the chest.

Clinical Recognition

When found in older babies and children, identification is usually by a chest radiograph obtained for nonspecific symptoms such as fever, cough, chest or abdominal pain, or vomiting. The presence of loops above the diaphragm may be seen on chest radiograph, and passage of a nasogastric tube may demonstrate an intra-thoracic stomach. Loops of intrathoracic intestine on the chest radiograph may be mistaken for pneumonia with pneumatocele formation (Fig. 132.7). A gastrointestinal contrast study or preferably a chest and abdominal CT scan may provide clarity if the diagnosis is uncertain. Potential intestinal or visceral ischemia caused by obstruction and strangulation is one of the reasons operative repair is undertaken emergently.

Management

In the stable but symptomatic patient, surgical repair should be undertaken soon after the diagnosis is made, but may be elective in the asymptomatic patient. Because the diagnosis may be made incidentally during evaluation for a condition such as pneumonia, which would increase risk of elective operation, the timing of surgery must be tailored to the individual situation. Certainly the pediatric surgeon should be consulted as soon as the diagnosis is suspected, and symptomatic patients are admitted to the surgical ward. If a patient is symptomatic from acute ischemia of the herniated viscera, an urgent operation may be required. Usually, a transverse or subcostal abdominal incision is used but in selected patients, thoracoscopic repair has been performed safely and effectively.

Foramen of Morgagni Hernias

Frequently asymptomatic or presenting with vague symptoms of abdominal discomfort, a Morgagni diaphragmatic hernia results from a defect in the anterior diaphragm just behind the sternum. Substernal or epigastric pain and bowel obstruction resulting from a narrow defect may occur spontaneously or be precipitated by any condition that increases intra-abdominal pressure (Fig. 132.8). A lateral chest radiograph should clarify the abnormality as anterior and demonstrate that the herniation is not through the esophageal hiatus. In stable patients, a contrast enema to evaluate for transverse colon involvement or a CT scan should be considered if doubt remains. Surgical repair, indicated to prevent incarceration of bowel even in

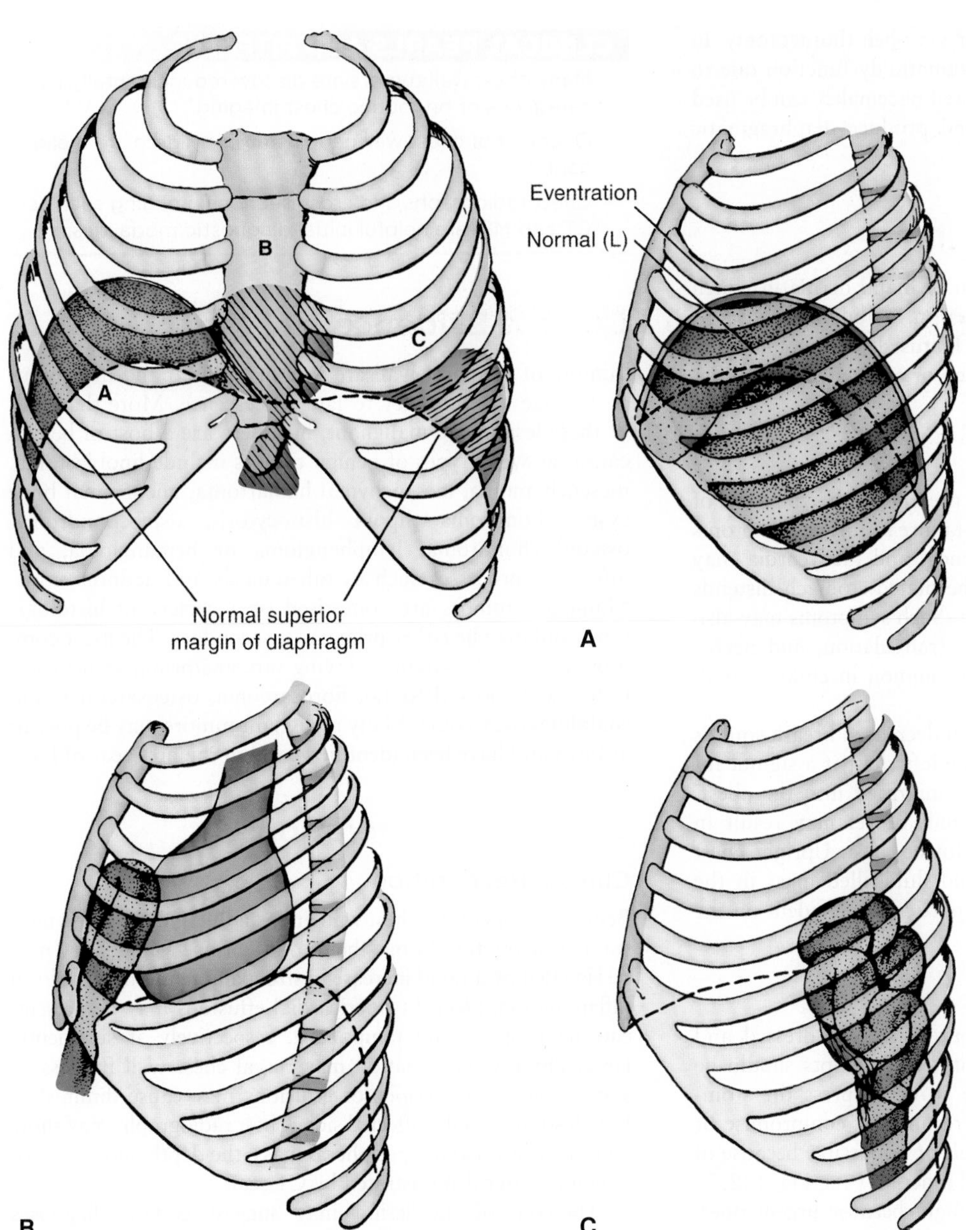

FIGURE 132.8 Diaphragmatic defects in infants and children. The nature of these defects is often better appreciated on a lateral view of the chest. Eventration of the diaphragm (**A**); foramen of Morgagni hernia (**B**); and left foramen of Bochdalek hernia (**C**).

asymptomatic patients, may be performed laparoscopically or through an upper abdominal incision.

Diaphragmatic Eventration

Eventration is an abnormal elevation of one or both hemidiaphragms, and may present to the emergency physician as an unexpected finding on a chest radiograph obtained for another reason. Eventration may be congenital or acquired. Acquired diaphragmatic eventration is commonly the result of a phrenic nerve paralysis, which may be caused by birth, operative, or other trauma. Neoplastic or inflammatory processes in close proximity to the phrenic nerve can also lead to eventration.

Diaphragmatic eventration occurs most commonly on the left side, but may be bilateral. The affected hemidiaphragm moves paradoxically during inspiration and expiration, with compromise of pulmonary mechanics and function. A large enough congenital eventration may affect prenatal and postnatal lung development, potentially resulting in pulmonary hypoplasia.

Clinical Recognition

Patients with eventration may be asymptomatic, but potentially will exhibit respiratory distress as a result of alveolar hypoventilation and paradoxical diaphragmatic movement. This frequently manifests as tachypnea, pallor, and feeding difficulties. Physical examination findings of nonaerated lung, including absent breath sounds and dullness to percussion, should be investigated by chest radiograph. Chest radiographs usually confirm the presence of an elevated hemidiaphragm (e-Fig. 132.6). This finding may be confirmed by fluoroscopy or ultrasound, which will demonstrate paradoxical motion of the hemidiaphragm and mediastinal shift with inspiration and expiration.

Management

Minor, asymptomatic eventrations may be observed. The need for repair is based on the severity of the eventration and the degree of pulmonary dysfunction. Treatment consists of plication of the attenuated portion of diaphragm, and can be performed thoracoscopically or via open thoracotomy. In selected cases of acquired diaphragmatic dysfunction due to phrenic nerve paralysis, an implanted pacemaker can be used to stimulate the phrenic nerve and produce diaphragmatic motion.

Paraesophageal Hernia

A paraesophageal hernia is a form of hiatal hernia in which the stomach and potentially other intra-abdominal organs protrude through the esophageal hiatus. It is uncommon in children, and may be congenital and/or associated with other anomalies.

Clinical Recognition

A paraesophageal hernia typically presents with symptoms of respiratory distress, vomiting, and failure to thrive. Symptoms of upper abdominal pain, tachypnea, and tachycardia may accompany the condition as the herniated stomach distends with swallowed air inside the chest. Such symptoms may also be indicative of gastric volvulus, strangulation, and necrosis, although these findings are uncommon in children with paraesophageal hernia.

Physical examination may reveal decreased breath sounds and dullness to percussion over the left chest if a significant amount of abdominal viscera has migrated into the chest. Rarely, herniation of colon or small bowel may result in bowel sounds heard over the left lower chest. Upright chest radiographs may show an air- and fluid-filled mass in the left lower chest, which should be particularly evident on the lateral view.

Management

Respiratory distress should be appropriately addressed and the patient should be fluid resuscitated. Attempts should be made to place a nasogastric tube to decompress the stomach in the patient with associated respiratory compromise or abdominal pain, but may be difficult or impossible because of angulation of the gastroesophageal junction (e-Fig. 132.7). Surgical consultation should be sought because urgent operative intervention may be necessary if the patient has signs of obstruction or strangulation. If symptoms are significant or if concern for strangulated viscera exists, patients should be admitted to the inpatient ward for observation and acute management. Symptomatic paraesophageal hernias warrant surgical repair, which can be done via laparoscopic or open abdominal approach.

CHEST WALL TUMORS

Goals of Treatment

Although tumors of the chest wall rarely present with symptoms requiring truly emergent intervention, large masses or those with associated effusion may cause respiratory symptoms or significant pain. Timely diagnosis of a chest wall mass is of great value as a significant percentage of these tumors are malignant. Patients in whom such a lesion is discovered in the ED will benefit from prompt characterization of the mass and involvement of appropriate subspecialty services, such as the oncology and pediatric surgery teams.

CLINICAL PEARLS AND PITFALLS

- Many chest wall tumors are discovered incidentally by caregivers or on routine chest imaging.
- Over half of chest wall neoplasms in children are malignant.
- Chest radiographs and cross-sectional imaging such as CT and MRI are helpful initial diagnostic modalities.

Current Evidence

Tumors of the chest wall are rare in children and may occur at any age from infancy to late adolescence. More than half of these lesions are malignant, but there are a host of benign causes as well. Types of benign tumors include lipoblastoma, mesenchymoma, mesenchymal hamartoma, aneurysmal bone cysts, chondroma, lipoid histiocytosis, osteochondroma, osteoid chondroma, lymphangioma or hemangioma, and infectious processes such as tuberculosis and actinomycosis. Malignant tumors are comprised of a variety of histologic types and may be either primary or secondary. The most common are chondrosarcoma, Ewing sarcoma/primitive neuroectodermal tumors (PNETs), fibrosarcoma, osteosarcoma, and rhabdomyoscarcoma. Many malignant tumors may be present at birth and have been identified early in the first year of life.

Clinical Considerations

Clinical Recognition

Benign tumors of the chest wall are usually asymptomatic until trauma or fracture brings them to attention. Malignancy may be signaled by a rapid increase in size, pain, tenderness, or local inflammation. Pleural or pericardial effusions may be present, causing dyspnea and tamponade, respectively, if sufficiently large. Physical examination may reveal chest wall fullness or a mass, and large lesions or effusions may cause diminished breath sounds on the affected side. Chest radiographs may show pleural effusion and a peripheral mass, the depth and extent of which is better demonstrated by CT scan.

The site of the lesion may suggest certain diagnoses (Fig. 132.9). Ewing tumor typically involves the lateral aspects of the ribs. Chondrosarcoma typically involves the costal cartilages between the sternum and the distal rib end. The sternum

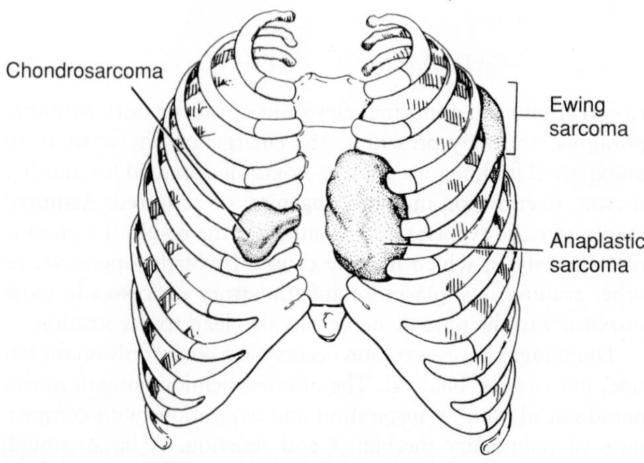

FIGURE 132.9 Malignant chest wall tumors in children. Most common lesions and their usual sites of origin are shown.

is a favored site for anaplastic sarcomas. These last two tumors may extend into the thoracic cavity, as well as outside the bony thorax.

Management

If the clinical and radiologic picture clearly indicates a benign, self-limited process, observation may be appropriate. However, if there is concern that the lesion is not benign, even a small chest mass in a child should be considered malignant and biopsy is appropriate.

Initial management of patients presenting with respiratory distress includes supplemental oxygen administration, evaluation for pleural and pericardial effusions with aspiration or tube thoracostomy drainage if present, and pain management if clinically indicated. Radiographic evaluation should include a CT scan of the pertinent area and a metastatic bone survey. If a malignant process is suspected, oncology and surgical consultations are warranted.

Multimodal, coordinated treatment is frequently required involving surgery, chemotherapy, and radiotherapy. Initial biopsy should be done using a core needle technique or a limited open approach, with care to place and orient the incision so as not to compromise the subsequent resection and chest wall reconstruction. Preoperative chemotherapy and radiotherapy may be useful to shrink selected lesions. Resection of the tumor and subsequent recurrences have resulted in disease-free survivals of 15 years or more. Extensive chest wall resections may result in thoracic instability and paradoxical chest wall motion. Technical advances have included the use of rigid materials such as mesh and methylmethacrylate, and together with improvements in surgical technique and postoperative care, significant resections including sternectomy or vertebrectomy can be done safely with excellent preservation of chest contour and respiratory function.

Suggested Readings and Key References

General

Holcomb GW III, Murphy JP, Ostlie DJ, eds, St. Peter SD, assoc ed. *Ashcraft's Pediatric surgery.* 6th ed. London: Elsevier Saunders, 2014.

Sellke FW, del Nido PJ, Swanson SJ. *Sabiston & Spencer Surgery of the chest.* 8th ed, 2 vols. Philadelphia, PA: Elsevier Saunders, 2010.

Townsend CM, Beauchamp RD, Evers BM, et al. *Sabiston textbook of surgery.* 19th ed. Philadelphia, PA: Elsevier Saunders, 2012.

Wilmott RW, Boat TF, Bush A, et al., *Kendig and Chernick's disorders of the respiratory tract in children.* 8th ed. Philadelphia, PA: Elsevier Saunders, 2012.

Tracheal Obstruction

Bove T, Demanet H, Casimir G, et al. Tracheobronchial compression of vascular origin. Review of experience in infants and children. *J Cardiovasc Surg (Torino)* 2001;42(5):663–666.

Holcomb GW III, Murphy JP, Ostlie DJ, eds, St. Peter SD, assoc ed. *Ashcraft's pediatric surgery,* 6th ed. London: Elsevier Saunders, 2014.

Stroud RH, Friedman NR. An update on the inflammatory disorders of the pediatric airway: epiglottitis, croup, and tracheitis. *Am J Otolaryngol* 2001;22:268–275.

Wenig BL, Abramson AL. Tracheal bronchogenic cyst: a new clinical entity? *Ann Otol Rhinol Laryngol* 1987;96:58–60.

Bronchial Obstruction

Ahrens B, Wit J, Schmitt M, et al. Symptomatic bronchogenic cyst in a six-month-old infant: case report and review of the literature. *J Thorac Cardiovasc Surg* 2001;122(5):1021–1023.

Augustin N, Hofmann V Kap-herr S, Wurnig P. Endotracheal and endobronchial tumors in childhood. *Prog Pediatr Surg* 1987;21: 136–144.

Ayed AK. Resection of the right middle lobe and lingula in children for right middle lobe/lingula syndrome. *Chest* 2004;125:38–42.

Bailey PV, Tracy T Jr, Connors RH, et al. Congenital bronchopulmonary malformations. Diagnostic and therapeutic considerations. *J Thorac Cardiovasc Surg* 1990;99:597–603.

Bonnard A, Auber F, Fourcade L, et al. Vascular ring abnormalities: a retrospective study of 62 cases. *J Pediatr Surg* 2003;38(4):539–543.

Chouabe S, Becquart LA, Lepoulain M, et al. [Bronchial atresia. A case report]. *Rev Pneumol Clin* 2002;58(1):27–30.

Horak E, Bodner J, Gassner I, et al. Congenital cystic lung disease: diagnostic and therapeutic considerations. *Clin Pediatr (Phila)* 2003; 42(3):251–261.

Livingston GL, Holinger LD, Luck SR. Right middle lobe syndrome in children. *Int J Pediatr Otorhinolaryngol* 1987;13:11–23.

Priftis KN, Mermiri D, Papadopoulou A, et al. The role of timely intervention in right middle lobe syndrome in children. *Chest* 2005;128(4):2504–2510.

Ramenofski ML, Leape LL, McCauley RG, et al. Bronchogenic cyst. *J Pediatr Surg* 1979;14:219–224.

Schwartz DS, Reyes-Mugica M, Keller MS. Imaging of surgical disease of the newborn chest. Intrapleural mass lesions. *Radiol Clin North Am* 1999;37(6):1067–1078, v.

Wesley JR, Heidelberger KP, DiPietro MA, et al. Diagnosis and management of congenital cystic disease of the lung in children. *J Pediatr Surg* 1986;21:202–207.

Esophagus-related Causes of Airway Difficulties

Brookes JT, Smith MC, Smith RJ, et al. H-type congenital tracheoesophageal fistula: University Of Iowa experience 1985 to 2005. *Ann Otol Rhinol Laryngol* 2007;116(5):363–368.

Chao HC, Chen SY, Kong MS. Successful treatment of congenital esophageal web by endoscopic electrocauterization and balloon dilatation. *J Pediatr Surg* 2008;43(1):e13–e15.

Fiorino KN, Mamula P. Esophageal injuries. In: Mattei P, ed. *Fundamentals of pediatric surgery.* Springer, 2011.

Ioannides AS, Copp AJ. Embryology of oesophageal atresia. *Semin Pediatr Surg* 2009;18(1):2–11.

Konkin DE, O'Hali WA, Webber EM, et al. Outcomes in esophageal atresia and tracheoesophageal fistula. *J Pediatr Surg* 2003;38(12): 1726–1729.

Laberge J-M. Esophageal atresia and trachea-esophageal fistula. In: Mattei P, ed. *Fundamentals of pediatric surgery.* Springer 2011.

Lugo B, Malhotra A, Guner Y, et al. Thoracoscopic versus open repair of tracheoesophageal fistula and esophageal atresia. *J Laparoendosc Adv Surg Tech A* 2008;18(5):753–756.

Ng J, Antao B, Bartram J, et al. Diagnostic difficulties in the management of H-type tracheoesophageal fistula. *Acta Radiol* 2006;47(8): 801–805.

Pleural Disease

Avansino JR, Goldman B, Sawin RS, et al. Primary operative versus nonoperative therapy for pediatric empyema: a meta-analysis. *Pediatrics* 2005;115:1652–1659.

Bradley JS, Byington CL, Shah SS, et al. The management of community-acquired pneumonia in infants and children older than 3 months of age: clinical practice guidelines by the Pediatric Infectious Diseases Society and the Infectious Diseases Society of America. *Clin Infect Dis* 2011;53:e25–e76.

Cohen G, Hjortdal V, Ricci M, et al. Primary thoracoscopic treatment of empyema in children. *J Thorac Cardiovasc Surg* 2003;125(1): 79–83.

Islam S, Calkins CM, Goldin AB, et al. The diagnosis and management of empyema in children: a comprehensive review from the APSA Outcomes and Clinical Trials Committee. *J Pediatr Surg* 2012;47:2101–2110.

Kurt BA, Winterhalter KM, Connors RH, et al. Therapy of parapneumonic effusions in children: video-assisted thoracoscopic surgery versus conventional thoracostomy drainage. *Pediatrics* 2006; 118(3):e547–e553.

Li ST, Tancredi DJ. Empyema hospitalizations increased in US children despite pneumococcal conjugate vaccine. *Pediatrics* 2010;125(1): 26–33.

McLaughlin FJ, Goldmann DA, Rosenbaum DM, et al. Empyema in children: clinical source and long-term follow-up. *Pediatrics* 1984;73:587–593.

Pugligandla PS, Laberge JM. Respiratory infections: pneumonia, lung abscess, and empyema. *Semin Pediatr Surg* 2008;17(1):42–52.

Pugligandla PS, Laberge JM. Infections and Diseases of the Lungs, Pleura, and Mediastinum. In: Coran AG, Adzick NS, Krummel TM, et al., eds. *Pediatric surgery.* 7th ed. Philadelphia, PA: Elsevier Saunders, 2012.

Ramnath RR, Heller RM, Ben-Ami T, et al. Implications of early sonographic evaluation of parapneumonic effusions in children with pneumonia. *Pediatrics* 1998;101:68–71.

Shaw KS, Prasil P, Nguyen LT, et al. Pediatric spontaneous pneumothorax. *Semin Pediatr Surg* 2003;12(1):55–61.

Stiles QR, Lindesmith GG, Tucker BL, et al. Pleural empyema in children. *Ann Thorac Surg* 1970;10:37–44.

Yang PC, Luh KT, Chang DB, et al. Value of sonography in determining the nature of pleural effusion: analysis of 320 cases. *Am J Roentgenol*1992;159(1):29–33.

Lung Lesions

Adzick NS, Flake AW, Crombleholme TM. Management of congenital lung lesions. *Semin Pediatr Surg* 2003;12:10–16.

Chiu B, Flake AW. Congenital lung lesions. In: Mattei P, ed. *Fundamentals of pediatric surgery.* Springer, 2011.

Fraga JC, Favero E, Contelli F, et al. Surgical treatment of congenital pulmonary arteriovenous fistula in children. *J Pediatr Surg* 2008;43(7):1365–1367.

Hendren WH, McKee DM. Lobar emphysema of infancy. *J Pediatr Surg* 1966;1:24–39.

Liechty KW, Flake AW. Pulmonary vascular malformations. *Semin Pediatr Surg* 2008;17(1):9–16.

Shanti CM, Klein MD. Cystic lung disease. *Semin Pediatr Surg* 2008; 17(1):2–8.

Tsai AY, Liechty KW, Hedrick HL, et al. Outcomes after postnatal resection of prenatally diagnosed asymptomatic cystic lung lesions. *J Pediatr Surg* 2008;43:513–517.

Weldon CB, Shamberger RC. Pediatric pulmonary tumors: primary and metastatic. *Semin Pediatr Surg* 2008;17(1):17–29.

Mediastinal Tumors

Azizkhan RG, Dudgeon B. Life threatening airway obstruction and a complication to the management of mediastinal masses in children. *J Pediatr Surg* 1985;20:816–822.

Azzie G, Beasley S. Diagnosis and treatment of foregut duplications. *Semin Pediatr Surg* 2003;12(1):46–54.

Grosfeld JL, Weinberger M, Kilman JW, et al. Primary mediastinal neoplasms in infants and children. *Ann Thorac Surg* 1971;12:179–190.

Mehta RP, Faquin WC, Cunningham, MJ. Cervical bronchogenic cysts: a consideration in the differential diagnosis of pediatric cervical cystic masses. *Int J Pediatr Otorhinolaryngol* 2004;68(5):563–568.

Takeda S, Miyoshi S, Minami M, et al. Clinical spectrum of mediastinal cysts. *Chest* 2003;124(1):125–132.

Enterogenous Cysts

Azzie G, Beasley S. Diagnosis and treatment of foregut duplications. *Semin Pediatr Surg* 2003;12(1):46–54.

Berrocal T, Madrid C, Novo S, et al. Congenital anomalies of the tracheobronchial tree, lung, and mediastinum: embryology, radiology, and pathology. *Radiographics* 2004;24(1):e17.

Ildstad ST, Tollerud DJ, Weiss RG, et al. Duplications of the alimentary tract. Clinical characteristics, preferred treatment, and associated malformations. *Ann Surg* 1988;208:184–189.

Mehta RP, Faquin WC, Cunningham MJ. Cervical bronchogenic cysts: a consideration in the differential diagnosis of pediatric cervical cystic masses. *Int J Pediatr Otorhinolaryngol* 2004;68(5): 563–568.

Perger L, Azzie G, Watch L, et al. Two cases of thoracoscopic resection of esophageal duplication in children. *J Laparoendosc Adv Surg Tech A* 2006;16(4):418–421.

Tessier N, Elmaley-Berges M, Ferkdadji L, et al. Cervical bronchogenic cysts: usual and unusual clinical presentations. *Arch Otolaryngol Head Neck Surg* 2008;134(11):1165–1169.

Diaphragmatic Defects

Al-Salem AH. Congenital hernia of Morgagni in infants and children. *J Pediatr Surg* 2007;42(9):1539–1543.

Harting MT, Lally KP. Surgical management of neonates with congenital diaphragmatic hernia. *Semin Pediatr Surg* 2007;16(1): 109–114.

Hedrick HL. Evaluation and management of congenital diaphragmatic hernia. *Pediatr Case Rev* 2001;1:25–36.

Scott DA. Genetics of congenital diaphragmatic hernia. *Semin Pediatr Surg* 2007;16(2):88–93.

Yazici M, Karaca I, Arikan A, et al. Congenital eventration of the diaphragm in children: 25 years experience in three pediatric surgery centers. *Eur J Pediatr Surg* 2003;13(5):298–301.

Chest Wall Tumors

Hines MH. Video-assisted diaphragm plication in children. *Ann Thorac Surg* 2003;76(1):234–236.

Hwang Z, Shin JS, Cho YH, et al. A simple technique for the thoracoscopic plication of the diaphragm. *Chest* 2003;124(1): 376–378.

LaQuaglia MP. Chest wall tumors in childhood and adolescence. *Semin Pedatr Surg* 2008;17(3):173–180.

Saenz NC, Hass DJ, Meyers P, et al. Pediatric chest wall Ewing's sarcoma. *J Pediatr Surg* 2000;35(4):550–555.

Soyer T, Karnak I, Ciftci AO, et al. The results of surgical treatment of chest wall tumors in childhood. *Pediatr Surg Int* 2006;22(2):135–139.

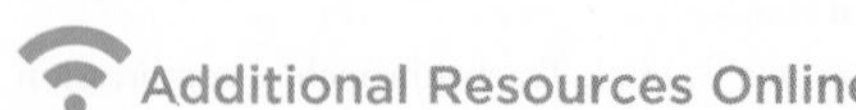

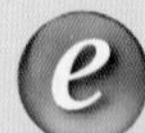

To view this chapter please access the eBook bundled with this text. Please see the inside front cover for eBook access instructions.

CHAPTER 133 ■ TRANSPLANTATION EMERGENCIES

HEIDI C. WERNER, MD, MSHPEd, KARAN McBRIDE EMERICK, MD, MSCI, HENRY C. LIN, MD, AND MARYANNE R.K. CHRISANT, MD

SECTION VII
Behavioral Health Emergencies

CHAPTER 134 ▪ BEHAVIORAL AND PSYCHIATRIC EMERGENCIES

EMILY R. KATZ, MD, LAURA L. CHAPMAN, MD, ERON Y. FRIEDLAENDER, MD, MPH, JOEL A. FEIN, MD, MPH, AND THOMAS H. CHUN, MD, MPH

The emergency department (ED) is frequently the setting for the initial evaluation of emotional and psychiatric difficulties of children and their families. As such, ED physicians must be proficient in psychiatric evaluation, crisis intervention, and disposition planning, regardless of whether a mental health professional is consulted. Even when a consultant is involved, the ED physician still shares responsibility for the patient's care and disposition. As in any other situation involving a consultant, it is critical that the ED physician and the consultant agree on a treatment plan, both from a patient care perspective and from a medicolegal standpoint.

GOALS OF EMERGENCY MENTAL HEALTH ASSESSMENT AND CRISIS INTERVENTION

First and foremost, the assessment and management of psychiatric emergencies requires that the ED establish and maintain a safe environment for the patient, family members, and staff. Systems/protocols must be in place to enable early identification of patients at high risk of violence toward self and/or others, to provide adequate observation, to immediately intervene for unsafe behaviors, and to prevent further harm. ED physicians must be facile in evaluating for underlying causes of emotional/behavioral disturbances, including potential medical etiologies for the patient's symptoms, assessing the risk for further decompensation and future harm, and developing adequate disposition and aftercare plans. Additional goals include providing support and stabilization for the patient's family and offering adequate guidance around prevention/management of any future unsafe behaviors, means restriction, and indications for return to care.

KEY POINTS

- ED physicians must be competent at assessing and managing psychiatric emergencies and have systems in place to safely manage acutely suicidal or aggressive patients.
- All patients with mental health complaints should receive a medical evaluation to identify significant underlying or comorbid illnesses.
- Verbal de-escalation and trauma-informed care are key components to managing agitation. Specific techniques are available to help limit the distress of children with autism and other developmental disabilities.
- All suicidal comments and acts should be taken seriously. Means restriction is an essential component of disposition planning.
- ED physicians are typically best served using their usual "pretest probability threshold" for ordering testing/interventions on children with suspected somatization/conversion disorder.

REQUIREMENTS OF THE EMERGENCY DEPARTMENT

The ability to respond effectively to psychiatric emergencies of children and families requires special capacities of the ED and its staff. Ensuring safety includes not only the physical characteristics of the patient room but also the access to medical and hospital security personnel, as well as appropriate safety procedures and policies.

It is vitally important to ensure patients do not bring weapons or other dangerous objects into the ED. Procedures to achieve this end may include use of metal detectors or a physical search of the patient and their belongings. Some EDs use a protocol whereby all patients must wear a hospital gown and slippers while in the ED. This separates the patient from their belongings and can facilitate a search for harmful objects. Such a policy may also theoretically reduce the risk of patient elopement.

A safe and adequate physical space is an absolute requirement of the ED. Patients with high risk of harm to self/others need to be under constant supervision by either ED medical or security staff via direct visualization of the patient or by continuous video monitoring. At a minimum, the patient room should be free of objects that could cause harm including objects used for strangulation (e.g., medical tubing, electrical or equipment cords). Such objects should be either inaccessible to the patient (e.g., in locked cabinets) or physically removed from the room.

The optimal setting for a psychiatric evaluation is a quiet and low-stimulus environment in which interruptions are infrequent, and privacy and confidentiality are assured; ideally this environment would be a separate, distinct area from the main ED with direct access to medical and security staff and capacity for using restraints.

Clinicians in the ED should have a pre-existing relationship with a mental health team that is committed to providing child psychiatric consultation at all times. The ED should also have relationships with (a) psychiatric inpatient unit(s), for efficient transfers and hospitalizations when needed. The staff should be thoroughly familiar with the procedures for psychiatric hospitalization, including the specific legal requirements for involuntary commitment. The hospital should have specific guidelines or protocols for the management of psychiatric patients requiring admission for treatment of medical conditions.

Finally, the ED should have relationships with other social agencies and an awareness of relevant laws. The police should be aware of which children to bring to the ED for psychiatric assessment and should be prepared to remain in the ED until adequate security has been arranged. Relationships should be developed with community mental health resources, temporary shelters, and other crisis intervention centers, ensuring effective referrals when necessary. Staff should be aware of child protection laws and the procedures for emergency intervention in situations of abuse and neglect.

EVALUATION

The evaluation of the psychiatric patient should include a medical history, physical examination including a detailed neurologic examination, mental status examination, and an interview of family members.

Medical History and Physical Examination

"Medical clearance" of psychiatric patients is one of the prime reasons children with psychiatric emergencies are referred to EDs. As with all ED patients, unstable medical conditions or acute injuries are identified and treated first. Most psychiatric facilities do not have the capacity to care for acute medical problems; thus they must be stabilized prior to transfer to the psychiatric facility. The second aim is to consider possible medical causes for psychiatric symptoms. Many medical conditions, as well as acute intoxications, can mimic psychiatric disorders (Table 134.1).

TABLE 134.1

MEDICAL CONDITIONS THAT MAY MANIFEST WITH NEUROPSYCHIATRIC SYMPTOMS

Neurologic	**Toxic**
Cerebrovascular disorder (hemorrhage, infarction)	Intoxication or withdrawal associated with drug or alcohol abuse
Head trauma (concussion, posttraumatic hematoma)	Adverse effects of prescribed and over-the-counter medications
Epilepsy (especially complex partial seizures)	Environmental toxins (volatile hydrocarbons, heavy metals, carbon monoxide, organophosphates)
Narcolepsy	**Nutritional**
Brain neoplasms (primary or metastatic)	Vitamin B_{12} deficiency (pernicious anemia)
Normal-pressure hydrocephalus	Nicotinic acid deficiency (pellagra)
Multiple sclerosis	Folate deficiency (megaloblastic anemia)
Metachromatic leukodystrophy	Thiamine deficiency (Wernicke–Korsakoff syndrome)
Migraine	Trace metal deficiency (zinc, magnesium)
Endocrine	Nonspecific malnutrition and dehydration
Hypothyroidism	Celiac disease
Hyperthyroidism	**Infectious**
Hypoadrenalism	AIDS
Hyperadrenalism	Viral meningitides and encephalitides (e.g., herpes simplex)
Hypoparathyroidism	Brain abscess
Hyperparathyroidism	Viral hepatitis
Hypoglycemia	Infectious mononucleosis
Hyperglycemia	Tuberculosis
Diabetes mellitus	Systemic bacterial infections (especially pneumonia) and viremia
Panhypopituitarism	Streptococcal infections
Pheochromocytoma	Pediatric infection-triggered, autoimmune neuropsychiatric disorders
Gonadotropic hormonal disturbances	**Autoimmune**
Pregnancy	Systemic lupus erythematosus
Metabolic and systemic	**Neoplastic**
Fluid and electrolyte disturbances (e.g., syndrome of inappropriate antidiuretic hormone secretion)	Central nervous system primary and metastatic tumors
Hepatic encephalopathy	Endocrine tumors
Uremia	Pancreatic carcinoma
Porphyria	Paraneoplastic syndromes
Hepatolenticular degeneration (Wilson disease)	
Hypoxemia (chronic pulmonary disease)	
Hypotension	
Hypertensive encephalopathy	

Adapted from Sadock BJ, Sadock VA, eds. *Kaplan & Sadock's synopsis of psychiatry*. 9th ed. Philadelphia, PA: Lippincott Williams & Wilkins, 2003:2.

TABLE 134.2

SCREENING TESTS FOR MEDICAL ILLNESS

1. Complete blood cell count with differential
2. Complete blood chemistries (including measurements of electrolytes, glucose, calcium, and magnesium levels and tests of hepatic and renal function)
3. Thyroid function tests
4. Pregnancy test
5. Urinalysis
6. Urine and serum toxicology screen
7. EKG
8. Plasma levels of any drugs being taken, if appropriate
9. Head CT (if clinically indicated)
10. Lumbar puncture (if clinically indicated)

EKG, electrocardiogram; CT, computed tomography.
Adapted from Sadock BJ, Sadock VA, eds. *Kaplan & Sadock's synopsis of psychiatry*. 9th ed. Philadelphia, PA: Lippincott Williams & Wilkins, 2003:24.

Failing to diagnose an underlying medical condition may result in significant morbidity to the patient. It is important to note that psychiatrically ill children may also have concomitant medical problems and, in fact, are at greater risk for presenting with emergent medical conditions such as injuries and ingestions than are nonpsychiatrically ill children.

A thorough medical history, including current medication and possible ingestions, followed by a complete physical examination, including a complete neurologic examination is all that is required on the majority of patients. There is no "standard" set of laboratory evaluations that must be obtained to "clear" a psychiatric patient. Patients with new onset of or acute change in psychiatric symptoms, especially psychosis or alterations in mental status, must be carefully evaluated for possible underlying medical conditions. These patients may require additional laboratory evaluation or subspecialist consultation. In addition, some psychiatric facilities may request or require baseline laboratory data before accepting a transfer.

Toxicologic screens and pregnancy tests in postpubertal teens are the most frequently obtained laboratory tests. Table 134.2 lists laboratory evaluations that may be considered for psychiatric patients.

Mental Status of the Child

Evaluation of the child's mental status takes place throughout the entire ED visit. The mental status examination provides a psychological profile of the child and contributes to the assessment of psychiatric diagnoses. Frequently much of the relevant data often emerges during the history, physical examination, and interactions with the child and family members. The emergency physician should have a systematic and thorough understanding of the mental status examination and should follow up any areas of concern with more specific questions. Table 134.3 lists the major categories of the mental status examination, with a focus on the aspects most relevant to emergency psychiatric assessment.

Family Evaluation

The mental status of the family can be assessed while observing the presentation of the history and the interactions of caregivers with the patient during the emergency department visit. The presentation of caregivers should be coherent and logical and should follow a temporal sequence. Family members under the influence of drugs or alcohol may not be fully alert and oriented. Depressed parents may appear withdrawn and downcast and may be so preoccupied with their depression that they do not focus effectively on the child's problem or may blame the child for their own problems. Families that do not present with organized mental and social functioning may have serious difficulties resolving crises (Table 134.4).

The goal of a family evaluation for childhood psychiatric emergencies is to determine the methods they use to help the child when distressed, how well these work, and gauge the willingness to try new strategies to help with the current crisis. When the physician approaches parents as partners, the likelihood of an effective collaboration between parents and medical staff is maximized.

TABLE 134.3

CHILDHOOD/ADOLESCENT PSYCHIATRIC EMERGENCIES: CHILD MENTAL STATUS EXAMINATION

- Orientation
- Appearance
- Memory
- Cognition
- Behavior
- Speech
- Mood and affect
- Thought process
- Thought content (including suicidal ideation, homicidal ideation, obsessions, delusions, hallucinations)
- Insight and judgment

Using Social Support

Some families come to the ED feeling isolated, overwhelmed, and exhausted. Often, such families have not used all the family

TABLE 134.4

CHILDHOOD/ADOLESCENT PSYCHIATRIC EMERGENCIES: FAMILY ASSESSMENT

Signs of competence and strength
- Level of concern
- Verbal communication
- Problem-solving ability

Relationships
- Parents and child
- Parents or caregivers
- Parents and physician

Danger signs with parents/caregivers
- Psychosis
- Intoxication/drug abuse
- Depression
- Violence
- History of abuse (physical, emotional, sexual) and/or neglect

and community resources available to them. Effective crisis intervention for psychiatric emergencies involves not only emergency treatment but also effective disposition planning for the family. The ED staff should determine what other family members and community resources are available to the family.

GOALS OF TREATMENT FOR AGITATED OR VIOLENT BEHAVIOR

The goals of treatment for a patient presenting with agitated or violent behavior includes de-escalation of active unsafe behavior, avoiding unnecessary physical or chemical restraints, assuring a secure setting, a process for observation of signs of increasing agitation, and establishing a safe, appropriate disposition plan that includes guidance on means restriction.

CLINICAL PEARLS AND PITFALLS

Pediatric emergency providers are called upon to assess potentially violent individuals. EDs may also find themselves on the front lines of violence or possibly active shooter scenarios, and thus need adequate screening and response policies in place to manage acute safety.

Remember that agitated or violent behavior may be situation dependent; once removed from the situation, the patient's behavior may significantly improve. In fact, the behavior may appear to be normal by the time they arrive at the ED. It is potentially a mistake to equate the lack of significant symptoms in the ED with the absence of a significant problem. The problematic behavior may easily reoccur if the patient is returned to the same situation without any appropriate intervention(s). In assessing the potentially violent patient obtain thorough collateral information, as patients themselves may not be fully forthcoming about their thought content or plans.

There are important medicolegal considerations in caring for these patients. The ED physician may have Tarasoff obligations to warn and protect identified targets of violence and must also consider their obligations to protect society at large. Every state has laws regarding involuntary admission of patients at imminent risk for harm to self and/or others. It is incumbent upon ED physicians to familiarize themselves with their state's laws and regulations.

A significant percentage of patients with psychiatric complaints have experienced trauma in the past. Treatment in the ED can be retraumatizing in numerous ways, including having their clothing and belongings removed, having a security guard present, being confined to a single room, and receiving chemical and/or physical restraints. For some patients, these factors may be the underlying or contributing cause for their agitated or aggressive behavior. Chronically traumatized children often have an elevated stress response and live in a state of constant alarm; the ED experience may be difficult for them to handle. "Trauma-informed care" assumes that all patients have trauma in their past, the clinician's approach should allow patients to feel some control over their current situation. Creating a space where the child feels safe, giving them choices when possible, and actively listening may improve care. It helps providers maintain compassion when dealing with children that, on the surface, seem challenging or antagonistic. Implementing such care usually requires careful negotiations with patient, as well as planning and flexibility by ED clinicians.

Clinical Considerations

Clinical Recognition

Agitation may manifest in a wide variety of behaviors, depending on the patient's age and developmental and physical state. Signs and symptoms may include restlessness, hyperactive motor activity, confusion or disorientation, uncontrollable crying, verbal threats, and overt physical violence toward oneself, others, or physical property.

Triage

A patient who is mildly agitated or who presents for evaluation of threats of harm may be able to wait safely in an ED waiting room and may benefit from de-escalating strategies. However, care should be taken to monitor these patients for signs of escalation and to prevent elopement. A thorough search of persons and belongings should be performed.

Actively/potentially violent or highly agitated patients require immediate transition to a secure area of the ED that is under the constant observation of hospital personnel. Security officers should be used whenever patients have the potential for significant violence or aggression.

Initial Assessment

Agitation or violence is a symptom of various psychological, medical, and toxicologic disturbances. The ED physician's assessment should focus on differentiating among the many possible causes.

Assessment and frequent reassessment signs and symptoms for violence and danger to others are important (Tables 134.5 and 134.6). Patients should be asked if they currently have any violent or homicidal thoughts, if they have specific plans or thoughts, if they have access to firearms or other weapons. Unfortunately, no single sign, symptom, or set of criteria successfully identifies all patients with significant risks for violence.

Management

Verbal De-escalation. Studies have shown that when hospital staff are trained in verbal restraint techniques, there is significant decrease in the use of chemical and physical restraint in the care of psychiatric patients. Ideally, all ED staff participating in the care of psychiatric patients should have training in verbal de-escalation techniques (Table 134.7).

All verbal de-escalation techniques share common features. Strategies include approaching the patient with a calm, nonjudgmental manner, and being empathetic. The simple act of listening can have a powerful effect. The patient should be reassured that the ED staff is there to help and work with them. Frequent updates about the care plan can help the patient stay calm.

Patients should be given as much autonomy as possible; try to present a few reasonable treatment options and allow them to choose. Patients often feel empowered and are better able to control themselves. It is equally important to set clear limits with the patient to maintain safety. Limit setting, done in a nonpunitive manner, may include discussing acceptable and unacceptable behaviors as well as consequences for these behaviors. With few exceptions, one should avoid "bargaining" with patients as this may encourage limit testing. Feeling threatened or punished may exacerbate a patient's agitation and/or behavior.

TABLE 134.5

ASSESSING AND PREDICTING VIOLENT BEHAVIOR

Signs of impending violence
Recent acts of violence, including property violence
Verbal or physical threats
Carrying weapons or other objects that may be used as weapons (e.g., forks, ashtrays)
Progressive psychomotor agitation
Alcohol or other substance intoxication
Paranoid features in a psychotic patient
Command violent auditory hallucinations—some but not all patients are at high risk
Brain diseases, global or with frontal lobe findings; less commonly with temporal lobe findings (controversial)
Catatonic excitement
Certain manic episodes
Certain agitated depressive episodes
Personality disorders (rage, violence, or impulsivity)
Assess the risk for violence
Consider violent ideation, wish, intention, plan, availability of means, implementation of plan, wish for help
Consider demographics—gender (male), age (15–24), socioeconomic status (low), social supports (few)
Consider the patient's history—violence, nonviolent antisocial acts, impulsivity (e.g., gambling, substance abuse, suicide or self-injury, psychosis)
Consider overt stressors (e.g., parental/peer conflict, real or symbolic loss)

From Sadock BJ, Sadock VA, eds. *Kaplan & Sadock's synopsis of psychiatry*. 9th ed. Philadelphia, PA: Lippincott Williams & Wilkins, 2003.

TABLE 134.6

PREDICTORS OF DANGEROUSNESS TO OTHERS

High degree of intent to harm
Presence of a victim
Frequent and open threats
Concrete plan
Access to instruments of violence
History of loss of control
Chronic anger, hostility, or resentment
Enjoyment in watching or inflicting harm
Lack of compassion
Self-view as victim
Resentful of authority
Childhood brutality or deprivation
Decreased warmth and affection in home
Early loss of parent
Fire setting, bed-wetting, and cruelty to animals
Prior violent acts
Reckless driving

From Sadock BJ, Sadock VA, eds. *Kaplan & Sadock's synopsis of psychiatry*. 9th ed. Philadelphia, PA: Lippincott Williams & Wilkins, 2003.

TABLE 134.7

VERBAL DE-ESCALATION/CALMING TECHNIQUES

Clearly introduce yourself
Use simplified language, a soft voice, and slow movements
Explain what will happen in the ED
Reduce environmental stimulation, if possible (less noise or light, fewer people)
Remove access to breakable objects/equipment
Allow room for pacing, if possible
Offer food or drink, which is inherently calming
Reassure child that you are there to keep him or her safe, that this is your job
Listen and empathize (a treatment cornerstone)
Tell child how you plan to honor his or her reasonable requests
Clarify the child's goal and then try to link his or her cooperation to that goal
Find things for the child to control, like choice of drinks
Engage available consultants: security, social work, psychiatry
Offer distracting toys/sensory modalities
Remain engaged; perceived ignoring may encourage escalations
Remember not to take their anger personally

ED, emergency department.
From Hilt RJ, Woodward TA. Agitation treatment for pediatric emergency patients. *J Am Acad Child Adolesc Psychiatry* 2008;47(2): 132–138.

Restraints. Physical and chemical restraint may be necessary to contain the patient's violent behavior. However, controversy exists regarding in what situations and when restraint is indicated. While the use of restraints can prevent significant and potentially life-threatening violent outbursts and can help an out-of-control patient calm down, restraints can also be physically harmful and traumatizing to the patient, the family, and the staff.

Restraint has the potential to harm patients. Adverse reactions to chemical restraint, physical harm and death due to physical restraint, as well as psychological harm (e.g., feelings of shame and/or of being personally violated, frank symptoms of posttraumatic stress disorder [PTSD]) have all been reported. Both the Centers for Medicare and Medicaid Services (CMS) and the Joint Commission mandate that healthcare institutions monitor their use of restraints, and develop and maintain protocols in which patients are treated in the least restrictive manner possible. ED physicians and staff thus need to be familiar with their institution's restraint policies, practices, and guidelines.

Medications for Agitation. Medications can be a useful tool in helping to manage unsafe behaviors in the pediatric emergency setting and can be used to treat agitation related to the patient's underlying condition. This is distinct from the concept of chemical restraint, which CMS defines as "a medication used to control behavior or to restrict a patient's freedom of movement and not standard treatment for the patient's medical or psychiatric condition." Although medications are extensively used to treat agitation and there are numerous published studies of their use in the adult ED and psychiatric settings, there is scant literature on their use in pediatric populations. In addition, as is the case with many medications

TABLE 134.8

CHEMICAL RESTRAINT MEDICATIONS

Medication	Initial dose[a]	Onset of action (min)	Half-life, $t_{1/2}$ (h)	Comments/adverse effect
Diphenhydramine	1.25 mg/kg[b]	5–15 (IM/IV)	2–8	Paradoxical reaction[a]
	Teen: 50 mg	20–30 (PO)	2–8	
Hydroxyzine	1.25 mg/kg[b]	5–15 (IM/IV)	7–10	Paradoxical reaction[a]
	Teen: 50 mg	20–30 (PO)	7–10	Paradoxical reaction[a]
Lorazepam	0.05–0.1 mg/kg[b]	5–15 (IM/IV)	12	Paradoxical reaction[a]; respiratory depression
	Teen: 2–4 mg	20–30 (PO)	12	
Midazolam	0.05–0.15 mg/kg[b]	5–15 (IM/IV)	3–4	Paradoxical reaction[a]; respiratory depression
	0.2–0.4 mg/kg[c]	5–10 (intranasal)[c]	0.5	
	Teen: 2–4 mg	20–30 (PO)	3–6	
Haloperidol[d]	0.1 mg/kg[b]	15–30 (IM)	21	EPS/NMS
	Teen: 2–5 mg	30–60 (PO)	21	Transient hypotension, may prolong QTc[e]
Chlorpromazine	0.5 mg/kg	15–30 (IM)	30	Transient hypotension
		30–60 (PO)	30	
Clonidine	0.05–0.1 mg	120 (PO)	12	Hypotension
Risperidone[f,g]	<12 yrs: 0.5 mg	45–60 (PO)	20	EPS/NMS may prolong QTc[e]
	Teen: 1 mg	45–60 (PO)	20	
Olanzapine[f]	<12 yrs: 2.5 mg	30–60 (IM)	30	EPS/NMS may prolong QTc[e]
	Teen: 5–10 mg	45–60 (PO)	30	
Quetiapine	25 mg	45–60 (PO)	6	EPS/NMS may prolong QTc[e]
Ziprasidone	<12 yrs: 5 mg	30–60 (IM)	2–5	EPS/NMS may prolong QTc[e]
	Teen: 10–20 mg	60 (PO)	7	

IM, intramuscular; IV, intravenous; PO, oral; EPS, extrapyramidal symptoms; NMS, neuroleptic malignant syndrome.
[a]A paradoxical reaction, such as behavioral disinhibition, agitation, hyperexcitability, and insomnia may occur.
[b]Round dose to nearest milligram or half milligram.
[c]Intranasal route: maximum dose: 10 mg; use IV formulation via an atomizer.
[d]Although not U.S. Food and Drug Administration approved, haloperidol lactate has been used IV (with dosage usually approximated at PO dose × 0.625).
[e]Relative risk for QTc prolongation: ziprasidone > quetiapine > risperidone, olanzapine, haloperidol.
[f]Rapidly disintegrating oral tablet available.
[g]Liquid formulation available.

and pediatric populations, few of the medications have FDA approved indications for treating agitation associated with pediatric mental health conditions, and none are approved for the purpose of chemical restraint in children and adolescents. Any medication used for chemical restraint is thus an "off-label" use of the medication. Although there are multiple published studies using the oral forms of the newer, atypical antipsychotics in children and adolescents, there is scant published evidence regarding the parenteral forms of these medications. These limitations aside, it is widely held by experienced psychiatric and pediatric emergency physicians that these medications are both safe and efficacious. Adverse reactions to these medications in the acute setting are rare and usually easily managed when they arise.

Medications that are commonly used for agitation and the appropriate initial dose of these medications are listed in Table 134.8. It is acceptable to round the dose to the nearest half or whole milligram or the nearest whole pill dose. Alternatively, for patients already on psychiatric medications, their current dose or an increased dose of one of their medications may be appropriate.

The choice of medication(s) should be based on the level of the patient's agitation or dangerousness. For mild agitation, antihistamines, alpha-adrenergic agents such as clonidine, or benzodiazepines are the first line of treatment. For moderate to severe agitation, possible medications include benzodiazepines, alpha-adrenergic agents, typical antipsychotics, and atypical antipsychotics. The ED physician should choose between these different agents on the basis of the degree of agitation, the patient's willingness to take oral medications, and the medication side effect profile. The newer, atypical antipsychotics may have fewer adverse effects than traditional antipsychotics (e.g., extrapyramidal symptoms [EPS], dystonic reactions, neuroleptic malignant syndrome [NMS]). However, their use in the ED may be limited in that ziprasidone, aripiprazole, and olanzapine are the only atypical antipsychotics that have an immediate release parenteral form, and there is limited experience using these medications in pediatric populations. The rapidly dissolving oral forms of olanzapine, aripiprazole, and risperidone may be an acceptable alternative to physicians and patients.

For patients with severe agitation, *rapid tranquilization* is the strategy favored by many experts. In this approach, a dose of a benzodiazepine and an antipsychotic are given simultaneously. These medications can be given orally but often will need to be given parenterally. If needed, subsequent doses can be given 60 and 120 minutes after the initial dose. This approach may be more effective than a single agent alone and may result in the use of less total medication. A variation of this approach is to alternate medications, that is, give a dose of one medication and reassess the patient 30 minutes later. If the patient's agitation has not sufficiently resolved, a dose of the other medication is given. The patient is reassessed every 30 minutes and redosed with the appropriate medication as needed.

Both haloperidol and the atypical antipsychotics, ziprasidone to the largest degree, may cause QTc prolongation. As such, patients receiving these medications should be closely monitored. There is no consensus regarding the prophylactic use of benztropine (1 mg oral (PO)/intramuscular [IM]) or other anticholinergic agents in patients receiving antipsychotics. Some experts favor giving such medications to all patients receiving antipsychotics, for the prevention of EPS. Others prefer to use these medications only if and when EPS develop.

NMS is a rare complication of antipsychotic use. It is more commonly seen in young, muscular males, although it may occur in patients of any age, gender, and body habitus. Preexisting dehydration and chronic antipsychotic use are other risk factors for developing NMS. Because there is no test that absolutely confirms it, NMS can be vexing to diagnose. In addition, the clinical picture of fever, altered mental status, and autonomic hyperactivity may be difficult to differentiate from meningoencephalitis, intracranial injury, various toxins, serotonin syndrome, or an underlying psychiatric condition. It should be strongly considered in any agitated patient whose condition worsens or does not resolve when given antipsychotic medication.

Of note, two antipsychotics, thioridazine and droperidol, currently carry FDA "black box" warnings as they may cause fatal arrhythmias.

Physical restraint. Any device that restricts a patient's mobility is a physical restraint. Theoretically, a bed rail is a form of restraint. In the treatment of agitated patients, however, physical restraints specifically refer to devices used with the express purpose of restraining a patient's limbs. Only such approved devices should be used for physical restraint.

The Joint Commission analyzed cases of physical restraint and identified several risk factors associated with patient deaths. Asphyxiation was associated with excess weight being placed on the back of prone patients, a towel or sheet being placed over the patient's head to protect against spitting or biting, and airway obstruction due to placing the patient's arm across the neck area.

A minimum of five trained staff are needed to restrain a patient, one to control each limb and one for the patient's head. For extremely violent or agitated patients, the prone position, although more restrictive, is safer for both the patient and the care provider. Physically restrained patients need constant observation by medically trained. The Joint Commission mandates documentation of patient's vital signs, assessment of behavioral status, and offering of food, water, and access to bathroom facilities at regular intervals. These standards also mandate a face-to-face evaluation of the patient by the ordering physician within 1 hour of the patient being placed in restraints. Orders for restraint can be renewed, but each order cannot exceed 1 hour for children younger than 9 years, 2 hours for children and adolescents between 9 and 17 years, or 4 hours for adults.

Restraints should be removed as soon as possible in an organized manner, taking into account the severity of the patient's agitation. The same number of personnel needed to place the restraints should be present when the restraints are removed, in case the restraints need to be reapplied. There is no consensus as to the optimal method; some remove all restraints once the patient is judged to be safe. Others prefer a stepwise approach, releasing an arm first, then the opposite leg, and finally the remaining limbs. Between each step, the patient is informed that if they remain under control, the removal process will continue. Patients should not be left with only one limb restrained. They have too much mobility and could injure themselves or others if they become combative.

Disposition

Patients who are at imminent risk of serious harm to others and who cannot be safely maintained in lower levels of care require admission to an inpatient psychiatric facility. Alternatives to inpatient admission include partial-hospitalization programs, acute residential treatment, in-home services, routine outpatient care, and, in rare circumstances, placement in the juvenile justice system. Outpatient and in-home services may be of particular use when family issues are playing a significant role in the unsafe behaviors. Brief placements in respite care or alternative placements for those in foster care may also be considered as a diversion from inpatient hospitalization. Special efforts should be made to avoid inpatient hospitalization in very young children, children with reactive-attachment disorders, or those with personality disorders; for these populations in particular, admission may be countertherapeutic.

Caregivers of those being discharged home should be counseled regarding means restriction of potential weapons, provided with de-escalation strategies, and instructed on indications for return. ED physicians may also use this opportunity to help parents establish, present, and/or reinforce any pertinent behavioral rules, rewards, consequences, etc. for the child.

In the event that an ED physician is evaluating and managing a truly homicidal patient, the ED physician has a duty to both warn the potential victim (typically via contacting local police) and to take actions to protect the potential victim from harm (e.g., by psychiatrically hospitalizing the patient). This duty was established in the landmark case of *Tarasoff* versus *the University of California* and has withstood numerous court challenges. This duty to warn and protect the potential victim supersedes the physician's duty to maintain patient confidentiality.

SUICIDE ATTEMPTS

Goals of Emergency Evaluation and Treatment

The goal of emergency evaluation and treatment of patients presenting in the wake of a suicide attempt are to identify and treat any potential medical sequelae of the attempt, to maintain the patient's safety in the ED, and to establish an adequate disposition plan.

CLINICAL PEARLS AND PITFALLS

Suicide is the final common pathway for various situations in which the child experiences a pervasive sense of helplessness, with a perceived absence of alternative solutions. To the distressed child, suicide appears to be the only solution to his or her problems and the family's problems. Most suicide attempts occur in depressed children; others occur with children experiencing major losses, such as serious illness or death in the family or in children with depression with associated impulsivity. A small but significant percentage of suicide attempts occur in psychotic children and adolescents (Table 134.9).

Children have differing conceptions of death at various ages. Up to age 5, death is seen as a reversible process in which the activities of life still occur. From 5 to 9 years, the irreversibility of death is beginning to be understood, but death is personified rather than seen as an independent event. It is not until about age 9 that death is seen as irreversible in the adult sense of being both final and inevitable. Even then, however, the child may imagine his or her own death as being reversible. Under such circumstances, a suicide attempt may have a different meaning than for an adult, where suicide corresponds to a definite end of one's life.

While it is common for psychiatric symptoms to be present for weeks to months before an attempt and the vast majority of patients who suicide meet criteria for a psychiatric or substance abuse diagnosis at the time of their death, the time between a patient deciding to kill themselves and carrying out the act is often quite short and often occurs in the midst of an acute crisis. Studies of survivors of potentially lethal attempts suggest that close to 25% act on their decision within 5 minutes, another nearly 25% act between 5 and 19 minutes, while another nearly 25% act between 20 minutes and 1 hour. This means that effective prevention efforts include the strategies of identifying and treating psychiatric disorders prior to the development of suicidal ideation as well as efforts to restrict access to the most lethal and common means of suicide attempts.

Emergency physicians must provide clear guidance around means restriction including firearms and potentially dangerous medications. Over 80% of pediatric patients who suicided by firearm use a family member's firearm. Of those, over two-thirds used guns that were unlocked and the remainder either knew how to open the gun safe or were able to break in. In one study, nearly a quarter of children whose parents believed they had never handled their firearms were mistaken. Removal of firearms (and potentially dangerous medications) from the home—at least temporarily—is ideal; safe storage is a minimum.

The dichotomy sometimes drawn between suicide "attempts" and suicide "gestures" is ill conceived, and the lethality of attempt does not always correlate with lethality of intent. As a corollary, minimizing a suicidal act as "just cry for help" by not responding adequately only invites a potentially far-more-lethal "scream for help."

Suicidal ideation is common enough that EDs could consider screening all teens for suicidal ideations or attempts, especially ones engaging in any high-risk behaviors or with other identifiable risk factors. Several screening tools, such as the Risk of Suicide Questionnaire (RSQ) and briefer 2- and 4-question screening tools are effective and accurate in screening for suicidality in patients presenting with nonpsychiatric complaints.

TABLE 134.9

POTENTIAL SOURCES OF ADOLESCENT SUICIDE ATTEMPTS

Developmental stress—identity crisis
Dependence/independence
Accepting disappointments/limitations
Planning for future
Body changes and self-image
Physical growth
Onset of puberty
Awareness of sexuality/need to look attractive
Peer pressures
Friendships and competition with peers of same gender
Dating, romantic involvements, dealing with sexuality
Rejection by special person or peer group
School pressures
Academic competition
Personal need to succeed
Meeting parental expectations
Family pressures
Parent–child expectations/problems
Parental impairment (medical, psychiatric, drug or alcohol)
Parental conflict or divorce
Financial/job-related crises
Societal influences
Mobility and social isolation
Romanticizing of violence and suicide
Lack of confidence in secure future
Adolescent depression
Physiologic vulnerability
Situational stresses
Sexual orientation and/or gender identity

Clinical Considerations

Suicidal behavior involves thoughts or actions that may lead to self-inflicted death or serious injury. A distinction is made between suicidal ideation and suicidal attempts in which deliberate attempts to take one's life occurred. The increasing trend toward suicidal behavior by children and adolescents is alarming (Table 134.10).

Clinical Recognition

Table 134.11 indicates the high-risk situations for suicidal behavior in which direct questioning about suicide should occur. The first two situations immediately alert the physician to the danger of suicidal behavior. The other situations involve a different chief complaint, masking possible suicidal ideation or behavior. All ingestions that are not clearly accidental, intoxicated drivers, drivers involved in single vehicle crashes, and patients who present with trauma from engaging in high-risk behaviors should be screened for suicidal behavior. Overtly depressed children, depressed children who present with somatic complaints, and children who have acted violently are also at risk. Psychotic children present a special

TABLE 134.10

CHILDHOOD AND ADOLESCENT SUICIDE: NATURE OF THE PROBLEM

Adolescent suicide
44% rise in suicide rate, adolescents ages 15–19 yrs, since 1970
4,000 completed adolescent and young adult suicides, 2000
Estimated 400,000 adolescent attempts, 2000 (1:50–1:100 attempts succeed)
Suicide is the third leading cause of death, ages 15–24 yrs (after accidents, homicides)
Childhood suicide
Serious problem
Younger children attempt suicide as a result of depression and/or poor judgment
Increase in attempted and completed suicides, children ages 6 yrs and older
Suicide attempts via ingestions (children ages 5–14 yrs) five times more common than all forms of meningitis
Additional data
Girls *attempt* at least three times more often than boys
Boys *succeed* at least two times more often than girls
80% of attempts are pill ingestions
More lethal means—gun, knife, jumping, running into car—more common with boys
Many car "accidents" are not accidents

problem and may present with inadvertent suicide attempts as the result of impaired judgment, hallucinations, and delusions of persecution. The isolated, withdrawn child may harbor suicidal thoughts that are uncovered only by direct questioning.

In school-aged children, certain risk factors have been identified that distinguish children with suicidal behavior from other children with emotional problems (Table 134.12). Suicidal children are likely to be depressed and hopeless. Self-esteem is low, and they see themselves as worthless. The want to die is present, as are preoccupations with death. The family history may include past episodes of parental depression and suicidal behavior. Suicidal children tend to view death as temporary and pleasant rather than irreversible.

TABLE 134.11

CHILDHOOD AND ADOLESCENT SUICIDE: HIGH-RISK SITUATIONS FOR SUICIDE ATTEMPTS

Suicide attempt just made
Suicidal threat made
"Accidental" ingestion
Child complains of depression
Psychotic child
Significant withdrawal by child
History of aggressive or violent behavior
History of substance abuse
History of previous suicide attempt(s)
Medical concerns, but child appears depressed
Highly lethal method of suicide attempt
Availability of or access to firearms

TABLE 134.12

CHARACTERISTICS ASSOCIATED WITH CHILDHOOD AND ADOLESCENT SUICIDE ATTEMPTS

Positive family history
Hopelessness
Low self-esteem
Active desire to die
Depression
Anger/desire for revenge

Assessment

All patients require a thorough medical assessment in order to identify and treat any potential physical sequelae. Consider obtaining urine toxicology for drugs of abuse and serum screens for acetaminophen and salicylates on all suicidal teenage patients, as a concealed ingestion may be present or the patient may be self-medicating with drugs of abuse.

The psychiatric evaluation should include an assessment of the actual and believed medical lethality of the act, the suicidal intent, the impulsivity of the act, and the strengths and supports within the family (Table 134.13). The lethality of a suicide attempt by itself may be misleading because suicidal children may over- or underestimate the harm intended. In general, more violent methods of attempted suicide (e.g., hanging, shooting, jumping) often reflect greater suicidal intent (Table 134.14). However, the physician cannot conclude that attempts with low lethality are not serious attempts until they have specifically asked about and assessed the child's suicidal intent, that is, determined how seriously the child wanted to end their life (Table 134.15). These questions should be asked of the child without the parents in the room.

The physician should gather as much information as possible about the attempt itself to help infer the degree of suicidal intent on the part of the child. (What did the child think or hope would happen? Did the child take all the pills that were available? Did he or she expect to wake up? Did he or she tell anyone after taking the pills? Did he or she leave a suicide note? Now that he or she is awake, is the child pleased or displeased to be alive? Does he or she intend to try again?)

Children who threaten suicide without making an actual attempt should also be questioned carefully about suicidal intent. (How long has the child considered suicide? What methods? When will this take place? Previous attempts? How about other family members?) Psychotic and depressed children, especially when the parents appear unable to supervise the child, should elicit particular concern.

Assessment of the child's level of impulsivity is also important (Table 134.16). Does the attempt appear to have been

TABLE 134.13

ASSESSING CHILDHOOD/ADOLESCENT SUICIDE ATTEMPTS: FOUR MAJOR DIMENSIONS

Medical lethality
Suicidal intent
Impulsivity
Strengths/supports

TABLE 134.14

CHILD AND ADOLESCENT SUICIDE: ASSESSING MEDICAL LETHALITY

Vital signs
Level of consciousness
Evidence of drug/alcohol intoxication (e.g., pupils, smell on breath)
Need for emesis, lavage, or catharsis
Acute medical complications (cardiac, respiratory, renal, neurologic)
Indications for medical hospitalization, including intensive care
Residual abnormalities

TABLE 134.15

CHILDHOOD AND ADOLESCENT SUICIDE: ASSESSING SUICIDE INTENT

Circumstances of suicide attempt
Nature of suicide attempt (e.g., ingestion vs. violent means)
Use of multiple methods
Method used to extreme (all vs. some pills ingested)
Suicide note written
Secrecy of attempt (attempt concealed vs. revealed)
Premeditation (long planned vs. impulsive attempt)
History of prior attempts
Child self-report
Premeditation of attempt
Anticipation of death
Desire for death
Attempt to conceal attempt
Nature of precipitating stresses
Child's mental status
Orientation/cognitive intactness
Presence/absence of psychosis
Manner of relating to physician
Current suicidality
Response to being saved/being unsuccessful in attempt
Active plan for another attempt
Readiness to discuss stresses
Readiness to accept external and family support
Nature of orientation toward future

TABLE 134.16

CHILDHOOD AND ADOLESCENT SUICIDE: ASSESSING IMPULSIVITY

Evidence of impulsive suicide attempt
History of prior impulsive behaviors
Evidence of impulsivity during interview

TABLE 134.17

CHILDHOOD AND ADOLESCENT SUICIDE: ASSESSING STRENGTHS AND SUPPORTS

Strengths and assets of child
Ability to relate to physician
Ability to rely on parents in crisis
Ability to acknowledge problem
Positive orientation toward future
Strengths and assets of family
Commitment to child
Ability to unite during crisis
Problem-solving abilities
Capacity to supervise child (support *and* limits)
Ability to use external supports
Nature of external supports
Outpatient psychiatrist/family physician
Extended family
Neighbors/other significant adults
Religious community
Self-help groups

impulsive rather than planned? Is there a history of prior impulsive behaviors? Is there evidence of impulsivity during the ED interview?

The physician should ask the child and family about possible precipitating events to determine what changes in the environment may be needed. The strengths of the family should be assessed to determine whether sufficient social support exists to allow for outpatient management (Table 134.17).

Management

Evaluation for Hospitalization. No universally agreed-on criteria have been established for when to hospitalize a child with suicidal behavior and when they can be safely managed on an outpatient basis. Garfinkel and Golombek identified seven areas to assess to determine whether hospitalization is indicated (Table 134.18).

The degree to which the family can commit to support the child's safety and well-being and other resources (extended family, neighbors, peers, and teachers) must be assessed. The decision to hospitalize the child is made when the child's safety is still in doubt after these questions have been answered.

TABLE 134.18

AREAS TO ASSESS FOLLOWING A SUICIDE ATTEMPT

Social set
Intent
Method
History
Stress
Mental status
Support

TABLE 134.19

INDICATIONS FOR PSYCHIATRIC HOSPITALIZATION FOLLOWING CHILDHOOD/ADOLESCENT SUICIDE ATTEMPT

1. Failure of rapport among physician, child, and family
2. Serious suicide attempt (lethality and intent)
3. Continuing active suicidality
4. Inability to engage in safety planning
5. Psychosis of child
6. Divisive/disturbed family, incapable of support and supervision
7. Denial of significance of suicide attempt

Any suicide attempt deserves a thorough assessment by the emergency physician and a complete psychiatric consultation. Hospitalization should be used in the circumstances listed in Table 134.19.

Initiating Treatment. If inpatient treatment is required, the child and family should be informed about the goals of hospitalization and the active role of the family in the treatment emphasized. In instances in which the child or parents do not agree to hospitalization, involuntary commitment may be needed as a last resort.

Outpatient management of suicidal behavior becomes feasible when (i) the child and family are cooperative and engageable; (ii) the attempt is determined not to have been too serious in terms of intent/medical lethality; (iii) the child is not actively suicidal or psychotic; (iv) the child can earnestly engage in safety planning; (v) the family can take responsibility for safely managing the child until formal psychiatric treatment is begun; and (vi) adequate means restriction can be carried out. Before sending a family home, the family should formulate an acceptable, concrete plan for how it will manage the child.

Parents should be given guidelines for the prevention of suicide (Table 134.20) and instruction in the early warning signs (Table 134.21).

TABLE 134.20

PREVENTION OF CHILDHOOD AND ADOLESCENT SUICIDE: GUIDELINES FOR PARENTS

- Understand nature of parent—child dilemma during adolescence
- Maintain physical contact—be around, combat tendency toward isolation
- Maintain emotional contact—stay involved, show positive regard
- Listen to child before responding—promote safety in talking
- Respond to child once child has finished—take child seriously, do not dismiss or attack
- Encourage choices by adolescent
- Acknowledge child and provide respect
- Restrict means to suicide (such as firearms, knives, drugs/alcohol, motor vehicles, toxins) as indicated

TABLE 134.21

PREVENTION OF CHILDHOOD AND ADOLESCENT SUICIDE: WARNING SIGNS FOR PARENTS

- Withdrawal (peers, parents, siblings)
- Somatic complaints
- Irritability
- Crying
- Diminished school performance
- Sad or anxious appearance
- Significant loss (rejection by peer group, breakup of romance, poor grades, failure to achieve important goal)
- Major event or change within family
- Casual mention of suicide or being "better off dead"
- Explicit suicide threat
- Giving away of possessions
- Abrupt improvement in mood (which may represent relief upon deciding to carry out suicidal act)
- Minor, seemingly unimportant suicide "gestures"
- Apparent "accidents"
- Other unusual behavior pattern—housebound behavior, breaking curfew, running away, drug or alcohol abuse, bizarre or antisocial actions

DEPRESSION

Goals of Treatment

The goals of emergency treatment of the depressed pediatric patient are to establish a safe and appropriate disposition plan and to provide brief psychoeducational and therapeutic interventions to the patient and their family.

CLINICAL PEARLS AND PITFALLS

Depression in pediatric patients may present with either sad or irritable mood as its predominant symptom. Unlike depressed adults, who tend to be consistently down or sad, depressed pediatric patients will often have moments in which they seem happy—often when they are engaged in a preferred activity. Clinicians should not rule out depression based on these moments of what is referred to as mood reactivity.

Clinical Considerations

Depression involves a pervasive inflexibility of sad or irritable mood, accompanied frequently by self-deprecation and suicidal ideation. Depression also implies a change in functioning from an earlier state of relatively good adjustment. The depressed child typically experiences a profound sense of helplessness, feeling unable to improve an unsatisfactory situation.

Estimates of the incidence of depression in children and adolescents vary between 20% and 33%. It is higher in children with school problems, including learning disabilities and attention-deficit hyperactivity disorder (ADHD), and in children with significant medical problems. Most children with depression come to the ED with other chief complaints (somatic symptoms, school or behavior problems); this ED clinicians must consider the possibility of depression in all children seen with recurrent or vague somatic complaints. A large body of evidence suggests that a genetic predisposition exists for depression, particularly severe depression. Depressive episodes may be triggered by environmental events of significance to the child.

Depression manifests differently, depending on the stage of development. In infancy, depression is usually the result of loss of important attachments and/or nurturance and is seen as a global interference of normal growth and physiologic functioning, including apathy, listlessness, staring, hypoactivity, poor feeding and weight loss, and increased susceptibility to infection.

In school-aged children key features include dysphoric mood, irritability, and self-deprecatory ideation. Dysphoric mood is manifested by looking or feeling sad and forlorn, being moody and irritable, and crying easily. Self-deprecatory thoughts are reflected by low self-esteem, feelings of worthlessness, and suicidal ideation. Depression in this age can also appear as other common symptoms, including multiple somatic complaints, school avoidance, or underachievement, including learning disabilities or ADHD, angry outbursts, runaway behavior, phobias, and fire setting.

Symptoms of depression during adolescence are more similar to those seen in adult-onset depression. The major symptom is a sad, unhappy or irritable mood, and/or a pervasive loss of interest and pleasure. Other symptoms may include a change in appetite, change in a sleep behavior, and psychomotor retardation or agitation. Also present in many depressed teenagers are loss of energy, feelings of worthlessness or excessive guilt, decreased ability to concentrate, indecisiveness, and recurrent thoughts of death or suicide. Depressed teenagers can also present with somatic complaints, academic problems, promiscuity, drug or alcohol use, aggressive behavior, and stealing. Many teenagers with behaviors such as these are unaware of their depression, others simply deny it. In talking with these patients about their lives at home, at school, and with peers, the underlying depression usually becomes apparent.

A medical evaluation is needed to rule out potential medical causes, concurrent medical illness, and to assess for self-injurious/suicidal behaviors and side effects of prescribed medications. See Table 134.2.

Management

The three major goals in the management of depression involve (i) determining suicidal potential, (ii) uncovering acute precipitants, and (iii) making an appropriate disposition.

The emergency treatment of depression includes prevention of suicide attempts. ED physicians screen for suicide attempts or whether suicidal ideation is present. Direct questions about suicidal thoughts represent a positive confrontation of the problem of depression, are unlikely to catalyze suicide attempts, and may actually provide a sense of relief for the depressed child.

The physician should attempt to determine possible acute precipitants to guide subsequent recommendations. The duration of the depression should be determined, as well as the family response. Assessing overall adjustment at home, in school, and with peers is important, as well as looking for the strengths of child and family for use in the treatment plan.

Outpatient management may be considered when adequate social support is present. Parental acknowledgment of the severity of and risk associated with their child's symptoms as well as a strong commitment to participating in the child's care are important first steps. Cognitive behavioral therapy is a well-studied therapeutic intervention for pediatric depression. In moderate to severe depression, therapy is most effective when combined with antidepressant medications. Psychotropic medications should be prescribed in the outpatient setting.

The emergency physician should be familiar with commonly used antidepressants. Over the past several decades, the selective serotonin reuptake inhibitors (SSRIs) have displaced TCAs as first-line medications. Advantages of SSRIs over TCAs include a decreased likelihood of cardiotoxicity, the absence of anticholinergic side effects, and the relative safety of these medications when taken in overdose. Another commonly prescribed antidepressant is bupropion, which is chemically distinct from other agents and primarily acts on the dopaminergic system. Seizure is a potential side effect. Newer mixed mechanism agents such as duloxetine, venlafaxine, and mirtazapine are also being used in children and adolescents. Paroxetine, an SSRI, is generally avoided in pediatric patients due to its short half-life and heightened concern for inducing suicidal ideation.

In December 2004, the FDA mandated a "Black Box" warning label on all antidepressants. The labels warn about possible increased risk of suicidality with these drugs and about the need to monitor patients for the worsening of depression and the emergence of suicidal ideation. The agency advises that children and adolescents on antidepressants should be closely monitored, particularly after starting or increasing the dose of medication. Subsequent research have supported the conclusion that, when prescribed appropriately and with appropriate monitoring, SSRIs such as fluoxetine can be safe and effective treatments for adolescent depression and their use correlates with decreased suicide rates in the pediatric population.

MANIA/BIPOLAR DISORDER

Goals of Emergency Treatment

The goals of emergency treatment of mania include identifying and treating any medical etiologies, providing acute pharmacologic interventions, and a safe and appropriate disposition plan.

CLINICAL PEARLS AND PITFALLS

Unlike adults, mania in childhood may not always include euphoric mood; irritable mood is much more common. Emotional lability is common and can be disorienting to parents, who cannot understand why the child changes so much and so dramatically. Unlike the older adolescent, the child often does not have a clear recovery from identified episodes but rather may exhibit continued irritability. Explosive, disorganized behavior may also be seen. True psychotic features are rare and the course of childhood bipolar disorder tends to be chronic and continuous, rather than episodic.

Symptoms of bipolar disorder in adolescents are more similar to the adult form. Psychotic symptoms, suicide attempts, inappropriate sexual behavior, and a "stormy" first year of illness may be typical of adolescent mania. However, when compared with adults, adolescents may have a more prolonged early course and be less responsive to treatment.

The adolescent with mania has a distinct period of predominantly elevated, expansive, and/or irritable mood (Table 134.22). The patient has a significant decrease in

TABLE 134.22

ACUTE MANIA IN ADOLESCENCE: MOST COMMON FEATURES

Pressured speech
Grandiosity
Apparent "high" (euphoria)
Rapid shifts of emotion
Euphoria
Anxiety/irritability
Combativeness/panic
Hypersexuality

need for sleep, high distractibility, hyperactivity, pressured speech, and emotional lability. Patients may also exhibit *flight of ideas.* The manic patient may have inflated self-esteem, self-confidence, and grandiosity which may also include delusional ideas. The person may be aggressive and combative, go on buying sprees, pursue other reckless behaviors, or be hypersexual. Manic patients usually have a history of previous depressive episodes, but may present with an acute manic episode. A family history of psychiatric disturbance usually exists in patients with manic–depressive disorder. Typically, manic patients report feeling extremely well, and they are often brought to the ED against their will.

Sometimes, patients present with *mixed episodes* and have symptoms of both mania and depression. Irritability is usually the prominent manic symptom. Mixed episodes are particularly dangerous with a significantly increased risk for suicidal behaviors.

Initial Assessment

Children presenting with symptoms suggestive of mania need a thorough medical evaluation to rule out any potential medical causes of their symptoms including possible toxin exposure (Table 134.1). Assess for potential medical sequelae of impaired judgment, such as sexually transmitted infections, need for emergency contraception, or occult head trauma. Laboratory and imaging workup should be based on history and clinical findings.

Management

Psychiatric consultation is indicated if a new diagnosis of bipolar disorder is suspected, a manic/mixed episode is present, or if the patient is engaging in any unsafe behaviors. In younger children, outpatient management—with the combination of mood-stabilizing medications and intensive behavioral treatment—may be sufficient. Inpatient hospitalization is often required to maintain the patient's safety while effective treatments are being initiated. Patients who are manic can have severely impaired insight and judgment. This can lead to dangerous behaviors that can have lifelong consequences including unprotected sex, unsafe driving, engaging in felony-level criminal offenses, or even death. Involuntary commitment may be necessary.

Initial emergency treatment of the agitated manic patient may require the use of restraints and the administration of medications for acute agitation (Table 134.8). Of note, benzodiazepines can have antimania effects and atypical antipsychotics are often used as first-line mood-stabilizing agents in bipolar patients.

PSYCHOSIS

Goals of Emergency Treatment

The goals of emergency treatment of psychosis include identifying and treating any medical etiologies of the psychosis, providing acute pharmacologic and de-escalation interventions when indicated, maintaining the safety of the patient and others, and identifying a safe and appropriate disposition plan.

CLINICAL PEARLS AND PITFALLS

It is more common for pediatric patients presenting with psychotic features to have underlying mood, anxiety, or trauma disorders, rather than schizophrenia or a brief psychotic episodes. True psychotic symptoms in children must be distinguished from developmentally appropriate experiences such as imaginary friends and culturally normative experiences.

Clinical Considerations

Psychosis is a severe disturbance in a patient's mental functioning; manifested by aberrations in cognition, perception, mood, impulses, and reality testing. Behavior may range from agitated to excessively withdrawn to the extent that the patient does not attend to physical needs. The subjective experience of psychotic patients is often one of helplessness and extreme anxiety.

Psychosis in children and adolescents is caused by medical or psychiatric etiologies. Psychiatrically based psychosis has several major causes: (i) Primary psychotic disorders such as schizophreniform disorder and schizophrenia; (ii) brief psychotic episode; and (iii) mood, anxiety, or trauma disorders. Developmental and cultural factors contribute to the difficulty in accurately diagnosing psychosis. Hallucinations can be seen in various normal developmental conditions and cultural and religious beliefs, taken out of context may be misconstrued as psychotic symptoms. Patients with new onset or sudden change in psychotic symptoms need careful evaluation for underlying medical conditions in addition to psychiatry consultation.

Clinical Recognition: Psychosis due to a Medical Condition

Psychosis caused by medical conditions indicates that the underlying etiology is known, and resolution depends on improvement in the underlying medical problem. Psychiatrically based psychoses, in contrast, are those in which specific medical causes have not yet been determined. Differentiating between medical and psychiatric psychoses can be difficult. Certain features of the history and physical and mental status examinations are often helpful (Table 134.23). Psychosis caused by medical conditions include acute or chronic illnesses, trauma, or intoxications with an exogenous substance (Tables 134.24 to 134.26).

TABLE 134.23

MEDICALLY VERSUS PSYCHIATRICALLY BASED PSYCHOSIS: MAJOR DIFFERENTIATING FEATURES

Assessment feature	Medically based psychosis	Psychiatrically based psychosis
History		
Nature of onset	Acute	Insidious
Preillness history	Prior illness/drug use	Prior psychiatric history (self or family)
Medical evaluation		
Vital signs	May be impaired	Usually normal
Level of consciousness	May be impaired	Normal
Pathologic autonomic signs	May be present	Normal
Laboratory studies	May be abnormal	Normal
Mental status evaluation		
Orientation	May be impaired	Intact
Recent memory	May be impaired	Intact
Cognitive/intellectual functioning	May be impaired	Intact
Nature of hallucinations	Usually not auditory (e.g., visual, tactile)	Auditory
Response to support and medication	Often dramatic	Often limited

Patients with psychosis due to a medical condition often present in an agitated, confused state. The patient's orientation to time and place is often disturbed; they may be highly distractible, with significant disturbance of recent memory. Evidence of bizarre and distorted thoughts is apparent, and disconnected ideas may be juxtaposed. The child may have significant difficulty controlling behavior and has little regard for personal safety. Intellectual functioning may also be impaired. Visual and/or tactile hallucinations may be present. Auditory hallucinations are less common in medically based psychoses. As a result of impaired reality testing, these patients are often extremely difficult to control and may strike out at family or staff when attempts are made to control their behavior.

TABLE 134.24

CAUSES OF MEDICALLY BASED PSYCHOSIS

- Medical conditions (acute and chronic)
- Trauma (acute and chronic)
- Prescribed medications (toxicity/side effects/withdrawal)
- Drug intoxications
  - Accidental including misuse of proprietary medication
  - Drug abuse/experimentation
  - Alcohol abuse (alone or with drugs)
  - Deliberate suicide attempt

TABLE 134.25

MEDICAL CONDITIONS THAT MAY LEAD TO PSYCHOSIS

Central nervous system lesions
- Tumors
- Brain abscess
- Cerebral hemorrhage
- Meningitis or encephalitis (including autoimmune encephalitis)
- Temporal lobe epilepsy

Cerebral hypoxia
- Pulmonary insufficiency
- Severe anemia
- Cardiac failure
- Carbon monoxide poisoning

Metabolic and endocrine disorders
- Celiac disease
- Electrolyte imbalance
- Hypoglycemia
- Hypocalcemia
- Thyroid disease (hyper and hypo)
- Adrenal disease (hyper and hypo)
- Uremia
- Hepatic failure
- Diabetes mellitus
- Porphyria

Rheumatic diseases
- Systemic lupus erythematosus
- Polyarteritis nodosa

Infections
- Malaria
- Typhoid fever
- Subacute bacterial endocarditis
- Subacute sclerosing panencephalitis

Miscellaneous conditions
- Wilson disease
- Reye syndrome

A thorough history and physical examination is essential looking for underlying disease. A complete medical history helps determine whether the psychosis is a concomitant feature of an already existing chronic illness (e.g., lupus cerebritis), a result of medication or toxin exposure, elevated intracranial pressure, seizure, trauma, or infections. No specific features of the mental status examination differentiate the various causes of psychosis.

Patients with psychosis due to a medical condition require hospitalization for further evaluation and subspecialty consultation.

Clinical Recognition: Psychosis Due to Psychiatric Causes

Brief Psychotic Episode. *Brief psychotic episode* is a time-limited loss of reality, caused by the accumulated effects of externally imposed traumatic events. The acuteness of the

TABLE 134.26

EXOGENOUS SUBSTANCES THAT CAUSE PSYCHOSIS FOLLOWING INGESTION OF SIGNIFICANT QUANTITY

Alcohol
Barbiturates
Antipsychotics (e.g., phenothiazines)
Amphetamines
Hallucinogens—lysergic acid diethylamide (LSD) peyote, mescaline
Marijuana
Phencyclidine (PCP)
Quaalude
Anticholinergic compounds
Heavy metals
Cocaine and crack
Corticosteroids
Reserpine
Opiates (e.g., heroin, methadone)

clinical presentation and its precipitating events differentiates brief psychotic episode from PTSD. Different traumatic experiences, including physical or sexual abuse, rape, homelessness, and running away, may elicit a reactive psychosis. Diagnosis is made after complete medical evaluation and psychiatry consultation.

Schizophrenia. Schizophrenia may present in adolescence occurring in 0.5% of the population. It is equally common in male and female patients, although males present at an earlier age; and is more prevalent among patients who have family members with the disease. Schizophreniform disorder denotes similar symptomatology that is present for less than 6 months. Symptoms of schizophrenia involve impairment of basic psychological processes, including perception, thinking, affect, capacity to relate, and behavior (Table 134.27). Impaired thought content includes delusions, illogical thinking, and loose associations. Auditory hallucinations are common and may include direct commands for suicide or violence to others. Typically, but not always, the voices talk to the patient in the third person, with a highly critical and demeaning message. Affect may be blunted and flat or inappropriate and bizarre. Sudden and unpredictable changes in mood may occur. These teenagers may appear extremely agitated or may be withdrawn, speaking only in monosyllables and describing only concrete objects. Schizophrenic patients typically have significant distortions of their identity and their abilities and demonstrate behavior that is not goal directed.

TABLE 134.27

ACUTE SCHIZOPHRENIA IN ADOLESCENCE: MOST COMMON FEATURES

Flat affect
(Patient uninvolved and without emotion)
Auditory hallucinations
(Physician: "Have you been hearing voices even when no one is there?")
Thoughts spoken aloud
(Physician: "Can other people read your mind? Can you read their minds?")
Delusions of external control
(Physician: "Is anyone trying to kill you?. .. trying to control your mind or your body?")

The history often reveals a prodromal phase that includes social withdrawal, peculiar behavior, failure to look after one's appearance, and significant reduction in performance in school or work. An acute phase follows in which the previously described symptoms develop, sometimes as a result of an acutely stressful event. The overall course of schizophrenia is often chronic and associated with remissions and exacerbations. Exacerbations often occur when treatment, including medication, is suspended. However, other individuals experience a schizophrenic-like acute psychosis and recover completely with appropriate treatment, experiencing no further deterioration.

Other Psychiatric Causes. Schizophrenia and brief psychotic episodes are relatively rare in pediatric patients; underlying mood, anxiety, or trauma disorders are the most common causes of psychosis in children. Patients with depression or mania with psychotic features typically have severe mood symptoms and impairment of functioning. When present, psychotic symptoms tend to occur when mood symptoms are at their most severe and are "mood congruent." Patients suffering from anxiety disorders typically have delusions or hallucinations related to their specific fears. Patients with PTSD may also report hallucinatory experiences such as seeing scary people in the corner of the room or hearing their abuser call out to them. Typically, these cases can be distinguished from primary psychotic disorders as the symptoms are placed within the greater clinical context of the patient's presentation.

Management

Psychosis Due to a Medical Condition. Any child with psychosis in which an underlying medical condition is suspected requires medical admission for diagnostic evaluation and treatment. Other important management involves controlling the child's behavior, preventing injury to self/others, and alleviating the child's fear and anxiety. This should be attempted first with supportive statements acknowledging the child's condition and distress, and using distractions that allow the child to have some control, such as offering choices of food or drink or safe toys. As the child is distractible and anxious, instructions may need to be repeated frequently.

Brief Psychotic Episode. When a brief psychotic episode is suspected, the emergency physician should appreciate that these children may not have a permanent psychiatric disorder. The emergency management is similar to that of other psychotic states, including psychiatric consultation. Efforts to avoid antipsychotic medication should be made in the beginning, but, when necessary, low-dose antipsychotic medication can be used.

After emergency treatment, the prognosis of the child depends in large measure on the restoration or creation of a safe and dependable family support system. Referral for outpatient family therapy should be made unless the child requires psychiatric hospitalization for further evaluation or treatment. In the absence of adequate family support, some of these children may eventually require foster placement, residential treatment, or other placements.

Schizophrenia. The management of an acute schizophrenic episode requires psychiatric consultation. Patients with suicidal or homicidal ideation require psychiatric hospitalization. Psychotic patients from disorganized home environments should also be hospitalized for initial treatment. In general, the approach to the psychotic patient in the ED depends on the condition of the patient and the anticipated site of the ongoing treatment. For agitation and dangerous thoughts or behaviors, approaches include reassurance and a quiet setting, psychotropic medication, and/or physical restraint. The patient's vital signs, general condition, and possible side effects should be monitored frequently. If the patient does not respond to medication, inpatient psychiatric hospitalization is necessary. If significant improvement occurs, suicidality and homicidality are absent, and side effects do not occur, the patient can be considered for discharge to outpatient psychiatric treatment with careful follow-up, as long as the parents or caregivers are well organized, appreciate the child's condition, and feel capable of managing the child at home.

Long-standing antipsychotic medications, referred to as *typical antipsychotics,* exert their influence primarily on dopaminergic neurons. The newer class of antipsychotic medications referred to as *atypical antipsychotics,* is now the mainstay of treatment. These medications affect multiple neurotransmitter systems, most frequently dopamine and serotonin. In this class are risperidone (Risperdal), clozapine (Clozaril), olanzapine (Zyprexa), aripiprazole (Abilify), quetiapine (Seroquel), ziprasidone (Geodon). Recently additions that are not yet commonly used in pediatric patients include Iloperidone (Fanapt), lurasidone (Latuda), asenapine (Saphris), and paliperidone (Invega). Clinical advantages offered by this new class of medications include clinical effects on the "positive symptoms" of schizophrenia (e.g., an improvement in the ability of the individual to relate to the environment and to others, not just a positive effect on hallucinations and delusions) and a decreased likelihood of EPS and long-term tardive dyskinesia.

The major side effects of typical antipsychotic medications are EPS, including acute dystonic reactions (abnormal muscle tone or posturing), akathisia (motor restlessness), and parkinsonian effects (rigidity, tremor, slowed movement, and loss of balance). Acute dystonic reactions are best treated by PO, intravenous, or IM administration of diphenhydramine (25 to 50 mg) or PO or IM administration of benztropine (1 to 2 mg per day).

CONVERSION AND OTHER SOMATIC DISORDERS

Goals of Treatment

The goals of emergency treatment of conversion disorder and other psychosomatic symptoms are to assess for underlying emergent/common medical etiologies, limit unnecessary medical workup and treatment as much as possible, identify possible contributing stressors, provide the family and patient with empathic, supportive, and therapeutic information about the psychological contributors to the patient's symptoms, and to provide appropriate referrals and guidance about how families can best support the patient's return to function.

CLINICAL PEARLS AND PITFALLS

Children with psychiatric illnesses can be medically ill. Assuming a patient's symptoms are psychosomatic without first performing an appropriate medical assessment is ill-advised. Conversely, it is relatively rare for a pediatric patient who is given the diagnosis of conversion disorder to be subsequently diagnosed with an underlying medical condition.

ED physicians are typically best served by maintaining their usual "pretest probability threshold" for ordering tests, consultations, and medical interventions based on the clinical presentation at hand. Expanding the scope of evaluation and/or treatment to reassure parents or to accede to their demands is often both ineffective at calming parents and countertherapeutic for the patient.

Conversion disorder and other psychosomatic symptoms are not consciously produced. Patients are truly experiencing the symptoms and functional impairment that they are reporting. ED clinicians should be clear that they believe that the patient is truly suffering from the symptoms/impairment that they are reporting, that they are not "making it up," and that it is not "all in their head." Patients cannot get well if they still need to convince people that they are sick.

Patients with conversion disorder and other psychosomatic symptoms are typically in significant distress; they are often trapped in seemingly unsolvable dilemmas, and are very much in need of appropriate and supportive care.

Placebo trials without the family's consent should typically be avoided. Even when "successful," they tend to make families feel betrayed.

How physicians discuss psychosomatic symptoms with patients and families can have a major impact on the clinical outcome.

Family beliefs about psychological versus medical illness typically play a significant role in the development and perpetuation of psychosomatic symptoms and must be addressed as part of effective treatments.

ED physicians should frame the negative findings and lack of need for further medical intervention as "good news." For example, the fact that a patient's MRI shows that they do not have a brain tumor is good news, even if the patient and family seem disappointed or frustrated by the negative result. Being able to stop or avoid initiation of medications that have real and potentially significant side effects is also "good news."

A patient's presentation is very rarely ever 100% due to medical factors or 100% due to psychological factors. Psychological factors commonly impact the onset, severity, perpetuation, and/or recovery from medical illness and psychological stressors often have physiologic consequences. ED physicians may want to take as much of an "agnostic" view of the cause of the symptoms as possible (and acknowledging that a nonemergent medical illness may have helped triggered the patient's course) and focus instead on the ways to promote recovery and return to functioning. The framing of treatment interventions using the model of physical rehabilitation can be particularly effective.

Clinical Considerations

Conversion disorder is defined by one or more symptoms of altered voluntary motor or sensory function that are incompatible with recognized neurologic or medical conditions and that cause significant distress and/or impairment in functioning. The term "psychosomatic" symptoms or "functional" medical disorders can be used to refer to symptoms in other systems that meet similar criteria. Psychological factors can also frequently contribute to the development, perpetuation, or exacerbation of the suffering from underlying medical illnesses. In fact, it should be considered the exception, rather than the rule, when there are NO psychological factors impacting a patient's illness.

Initial Assessment

There is no single finding or test result that can definitively rule in or out conversion disorder or other psychosomatic symptoms. Clinical recognition must be based on a thorough review of the history including prior testing results, close observation and examination of the patient, and any further testing as indicated. Conversion disorder and other psychosomatic symptoms should also not be considered a diagnosis of exclusion. ED physicians should look for risk factors, signs, and symptoms that positively support the diagnosis.

Patients and their families may not often acknowledge significant stressors. In some cases, the patient might not be fully aware of the presence or impact of a potential stressor. That being said, a thorough history including a detailed psychosocial assessment can often help the ED physician identify likely contributing factors. Patients and their families should be interviewed individually and together. Information gathered from the interview that would support a diagnosis of conversion disorder are listed in Table 134.29.

Management

As noted above, ED physicians should adhere to their normal clinical decision-making processes when working up a patient's symptoms. Symptoms that could legitimately have an emergent underlying medical etiology should be assessed accordingly. Conversely, ED physicians should avoid performing unnecessary tests, especially for nonemergent diagnoses. Unnecessary testing rarely reassures families; it overmedicalizes patients, strengthens the reinforcement of the symptoms/impairment, places patients at risk for the sequelae of false-positive or incidental findings, confers iatrogenic risk and discomfort without clear benefit, and distracts attention away from interventions that are more likely to be successful. The same concept holds true for prescribing medications or other treatment interventions.

Efforts should focus on relaying the "good news" of the negative findings and the lack of need for further intervention at this time. Education about the nature of psychosomatic symptoms should be given in a supportive and nonjudgmental way. Treatment recommendations should focus on referrals for psychological support, providing anticipatory guidance and advice to parents around supporting return to function (including the use of physical therapy when indicated).

In some circumstances, inpatient medical admission may be necessary, including in cases where video EEG monitoring is indicated or patients are unable to orally hydrate themselves or ambulate. It can be helpful at these times for the ED physician to try to "set up" the admission as one that may very well not lead to the identification of an underlying medical illness or alleviate all of the symptoms but rather to facilitate further workup, specialists consultation to put an appropriate aftercare plan into place. Psychiatric etiologies should be listed in a nonjudgmental fashion as part of the differential and involvement of the mental health team for diagnostic purposes and support of recovery should be presented, whenever possible, from the start.

TABLE 134.28

GUIDELINES FOR MANAGEMENT OF ACUTE ADOLESCENT PSYCHOSIS

Diagnose underlying cause.
Request immediate psychiatric consultation.
Use medical hospitalization, if clinically indicated, with medically based psychosis.
Request psychiatric consultation with psychotic drug intoxications, either immediately or when mental status stabilizes.
Use quiet room, family and friends, and constant medical supervision.
Use restraints, if necessary.
Recognize clinical variations of extrapyramidal reactions to antipsychotic medications.

TABLE 134.29

HISTORICAL FEATURES OF A PSYCHOSOMATIC DIAGNOSIS

Temporal relationship between onset of symptoms and psychosocial stressor
Families who accept physical illness but not psychological symptoms as a cause for disability, have a strong belief that there is a single undiagnosed explanation for the symptoms, and/or lack faith in the medical system
Reinforcement of the medical symptoms and functional impairment via increased sympathy and attention from family/ friends, increased attention from medical providers, and/or avoidance of stressful situations such as school attendance
Traumatic life events or significant family or psychosocial stressors
Physical illness/disability in the family (which can provide an "illness model" to the patient)
Personality/coping styles that include a difficulty or avoidance of verbalizing feelings; introspectiveness; poor self-concept; pessimism; "Good kids" who are people pleasers and reluctant to burden others with their stress
Comorbid psychiatric illnesses such as depression and anxiety
History of prior unexplained or functional medical symptoms

POSTTRAUMATIC STRESS DISORDERS

PTSD can occur in childhood and adolescence, and is usually due to severe trauma during earlier years. Children may be more sensitive to the effects of trauma than are adults and thus may have higher rates of PTSD. Either the reemergence of the old trauma, the emergence of a new similar one, or the recollection of the original trauma can activate a PTSD.

Traumatic events involve situations where there was threatened or actual death, serious injury, or disease to someone. Highly stressful experiences leading to PTSD in children may include but are not limited to any of the following: physical violence, verbal threats, sexual abuse, long-standing hunger and poverty, as well as medical interventions such as bone marrow transplant, and injury such as burns and motor vehicle accidents. Children may respond to traumatic events with intense fear, helplessness or horror, or even disorganized or agitated behavior. In addition, the traumatic event is persistently reexperienced in one or more ways, for example, persistent avoidance of stimuli associated with the trauma, numbing of general responsiveness, and persistent hyperarousal.

With children, PTSD probably emerges through a combination of traumatic events, along with a silent or nonaccepting environment that fails to provide the child with adequate protection and support. A child's PTSD symptoms may be observed through repetitive play by which themes or aspects of the trauma are expressed. Recurrent and distressing dreams of the event may also occur. Hallucinations and flashbacks may follow the child's sudden reliving of the experience. In addition, events that symbolize or resemble some aspect of the traumatic event may produce intense anxiety and distress; the connection between precipitating event and distress is not always evident to parents or child.

Other PTSD symptoms experienced by children include generalized numbing of responsiveness to events and people. Stimuli associated with the trauma may be consistently avoided. The emergency physician should also be alert for signs of increased arousal—anxiety and agitation, difficulty falling asleep, irritability or anger, suspiciousness, difficulty concentrating—and various physiologic complaints in response to events that resemble or symbolize the traumatic event. The key task for the emergency physician is to recognize PTSD in the differential diagnosis of an agitated, confused, or even psychotic child or adolescent. A careful history usually provides clues to this diagnosis. Supportive management in the ED, including using family and friends, is often sufficient. Low-dose antipsychotic medication may be recommended after psychiatry consultation for those who are frankly psychotic and who do not respond to reality-based support. Often, an antihistamine or anxiolytic medication may suffice.

The ED physician may also have an important role in the prevention of PTSD. When patients are being treated for an acute traumatic episode, refer a patient for mental health counseling.

When parents dismiss or doubt the child's symptoms or worries, the emergency physician can encourage the parents to respond supportively to their child. When the physician suspects parental abuse, this concern must be addressed directly with the family. Many children with PTSD benefit significantly from individual and family therapy. If child and family are not already in treatment, a referral is appropriate.

PANIC ATTACKS

Children experiencing panic attacks commonly present to the ED. After ruling out any medical cause for the child's symptoms, the ED physician should educate the patient and their family about the nature of panic attacks and discuss use of relaxation techniques. Benzodiazepines should be avoided when possible, so as to help the patient and their family recognize that the symptoms of a panic attack are time limited and self-resolving. If the panic attacks are frequent, cause significant distress, or are leading the patient/family to repeatedly seek medical care, referral to an outpatient mental health provider is indicated. If left untreated, panic attacks can blossom into lifelong and severely impairing anxiety disorders. However, with appropriate and early treatment, future panic attacks and their sequelae can be prevented.

CARING FOR CHILDREN WITH AUTISM SPECTRUM DISORDERS IN THE EMERGENCY DEPARTMENT

Autism spectrum disorder (ASD) is a neurodevelopmental disorder defined by difficulties in social communication and restricted or repetitive behaviors and interests. Individuals with ASD demonstrate challenges engaging in social reciprocity, appreciating nonverbal social behaviors, and establishing social relationships. Characteristically, this population exhibits highly fixed interests and adherence to strict routines. Revealing clinical signs typically manifest by 3 years of age, although core deficits in communication, social responsiveness, and play present as early as 6 to 12 months of age.

Significant heterogeneity exists in clinical phenotype, severity, type, and frequency of symptoms. Children with ASD may lack attention, avoid eye contact, struggle to talk about feelings, prefer not to be touched, repeat or echo words said to them, engage repetitive actions, have trouble expressing needs in typical words or behaviors, display anxiety with changes in routine, and demonstrate exaggerated distress to modest sensory experiences. Many relate degree of disability to the level of support needed in school and with daily functioning.

The biology of ASD is incompletely understood as a disorder of neuronal-cortical organization reflecting both genetics and environmental influences. ASD affects all racial, ethnic, and sociodemographic populations, with disproportionately higher rates among boys. A 2014 prevalence study by the Centers for Disease Control reports overall 1 in 68 children (1 in 42 boys) carries a diagnosis of ASD. Thirty percent to 40% have associated intellectual disability.

Clinical Considerations

Predictable patterns of comorbid medical conditions have been described in those with ASD. Investigators identify significantly higher rates of healthcare utilization among children with ASD for psychiatric, gastrointestinal, neurologic, and allergic complaints. Eighty percent of children with ASD report at least one psychiatric diagnosis, including inattention and hyperactivity, anxiety, depression, or movement disorders. Thirteen percent of emergency care among this population relates to psychiatric-related concerns as compared to 2% in children without ASD. Among those with ASD, families seek care most often for management of externalizing behaviors, such as physical aggression and disruptive conduct.

Similarly, many children with ASD require care for gastrointestinal and neurologic complaints. Although 9% to 70% of individuals with ASD report concerning abdominal pain, constipation, chronic diarrhea, and symptoms of gastroesophageal reflux disease; there is no evidence for pathogenic mechanisms specific to ASD. Importantly, children with ASD and common gastrointestinal disorders may present atypically with behavior changes, irritability, disordered sleep, or new noncompliance with previously mastered demands. Many individuals with ASD have restricted or selective diets and may be at risk for nutritional deficiencies causing illness or sequelae. Children with ASD frequently seek neurologic intervention for impaired motor development and seizure management. Notably, epilepsy occurs in 25% to 46% of individuals with ASD.

Children with ASD in general have significantly higher rates of poisonings, self-injury, traumatic brain injuries, injuries to the face and neck, contusions, fractures, open wounds, and burns with lower rates of sprains and strains than peers without ASD.

Self-injury is most common in patients with associated intellectual disability or limited functional communication abilities. Such behavior may be a means of seeking attention, avoiding nonpreferred activities, mediating pain, expressing frustration, or displaying anxiety. Addressing what motivates these behaviors allows for appropriate targeted interventions. As with any other vulnerable population, give thought to signs suggestive of abuse and consider that challenging behaviors during examination may be defensive responses.

Management

There are no effective medical treatments for the core deficits of ASD, however medications are used to help ameliorate some of the symptoms of comorbid conditions and complement standard behavioral and educational interventions. Pharmacotherapy most successfully temporizes concerns related to inattention, hyperactivity, aggression, repetitive activity, anxiety, depression, disordered sleep, and seizures. The most widely studied medications with greatest effect are methylphenidate for inattention and hyperactivity and risperidone and aripiprazole for aggression and challenging behaviors.

Challenges in Healthcare Environment

People with ASD have unusual ways of learning, paying attention, or reacting to different sensations. These vulnerabilities may interfere with the ability of an individual with ASD to understand what is happening during a hospital visit and to communicate with medical staff, while a disrupted routine and noxious sensory experiences may stress any ability to self-regulate and cooperate with physical examinations and procedures. Many patients with ASD require no additional supports or adaptations during medical encounters other than provider awareness of how and why they interact and communicate differently. A small population of individuals with ASD benefit from simple environmental adaptations and communication tools that support compliance. A minority of children with ASD demonstrate escalating behaviors that prohibit successful interactions with medical staff and require reactive measures to ensure patient safety and promote delivery of optimal care.

Engaging caregivers is the most successful way to facilitate care with individuals with ASD. Quickly appreciating how best to communicate, how hard it might be for a particular child to maintain composure in a medical setting, and particularly what reduces anxiety and what provokes escalating behaviors allows for simple accommodations and flexibility among medical providers to enable successful interactions. In general, communicate directly with the child using simple, concrete language. Give brief instructions, warn about transitions, offer positive reinforcement, allow for frequent breaks, recognize when tasks are overwhelming, and attempt to limit unstructured time.

For children with limited verbal abilities and those with significant anxiety and escalating behaviors, consider using visual supports to help communicate expectations and structure the encounter. Some children use specific picture systems at home. Others are familiar with tools used in many other treatment and educational settings which are easily adapted to hospital-based care. Among these are if/then cards, visual schedules, and social stories. These can be quickly sketched at the bedside or printed from on-line templates. If/then cards display two images revealing an action and then a reward if the action is completed. Visual schedules organize a series or words or pictures representing the steps of an event. Social stories explain the sequence of an action or activity in simple illustrations with or without accompanying text.

Just as a highly structured encounter offers significant support to individuals with ASD, flexibility and at times, simple accommodations to the care environment, often reduce anxiety enough to gain compliance and safe interactions. For example, the core deficits of ASD significantly interfere with this population's ability to effectively utilize traditional pain assessment tools. Encouraging children to describe their pain and looking to caregivers to help interpret behaviors as a means to communicate best enable an understanding of pain among this population. In addition, some children with ASD seek out certain sensations that are comforting and others avoid specific exposures. Respecting and working around triggers for agitation often facilitates a safe and cooperative experience. Importantly, recognize many behaviors are a reflection of significant anxiety and consider anxiolysis with diphenhydramine or a benzodiazepine to minimize distress.

SCREENING FOR MENTAL HEALTH PROBLEMS IN THE EMERGENCY DEPARTMENT

Many children with psychiatric illness do not present to the ED with overt psychiatric symptoms. It is also clear that many patients with psychiatric disorders exhibit somatic symptoms, such as headache and abdominal pain; some chronic medical illnesses, such as asthma and diabetes, can also be exacerbated by stress and anxiety. Because the ED may be the only point of contact for children with undiagnosed psychiatric illness, the American Academy of Pediatrics (AAP) has acknowledged the role of the ED as a safety net for children and adolescents with unmet mental health needs.

Several challenges are important to consider when screening for behavioral disorders or psychiatric illness in acute care settings. Lack of an ongoing therapeutic relationship and fear of stigma may prevent an adolescent from reporting depression, substance use, or suicidal thoughts and behaviors. The high stimulus setting of the ED may also discourage the disclosure of sensitive mental health matters. Screening instruments need to be valid when administered by clinicians who do not have specific training in psychology or psychiatry. Oftentimes the behavioral health system, particularly for low-income patients, leaves physicians with limited referral options. Ethical and legal concerns are also of consideration, including the need for standardized, confidential documentation for positive screens, misperceptions about mandated reporting requirements, and legal limitations of communication options with parents and other family members. It is very helpful if ED and hospital leadership understand the legislative and local policies around these issues and make their faculty and staff aware of the standard of care in this regard.

While there are culturally sensitive and developmentally appropriate screening tools that promote the accurate detection of suicide, depression, and other psychiatric illnesses as well as substance use, the need for efficiency in the acute care setting creates an extra challenge. In the current medical and economic climate, busy clinicians prefer clinical innovations to be "pushbutton" in nature, creating added value while minimizing time and effort. Computer technology offers some solutions to these barriers, and also offers the potential for skip-logic and "computerized adaptive testing" that can maximize accuracy by adding follow-up questions only when initial, more sensitive questions are answered positively.

Of all screening domains, suicidality is a paramount concern for ED clinicians. The key question is often distinguishing between self-harm and intent to die. It should be noted, however, that previous acts of self-harm that may not have required medical attention might also be a potent indicator of suicide risk. An adolescent who divulges that he/she had specific plans for suicide or a suicide attempt and a desire to kill him/herself within the past week should be deemed imminent risk and will likely require psychiatric hospitalization or rapid, intense outpatient therapy. In addition, although simply stating a belief that "life is not worth living" without having a suicide plan rarely leads to psychiatric hospitalization, these adolescents may still benefit from outpatient mental health services to prevent escalation of symptoms and subsequent suicide attempts. Recent innovations have produced efficient screening instruments and processes that can be used in the acute care setting. The RSQ is a brief screening tool for screening for suicidal ideation in the ED that assesses major facets for suicide risk, present and past suicidal ideation, previous self-destructive behavior, and current stressors. The Behavioral Health Screen is a computerized version of the questions: "In the past week including today, have you felt like life is not worth living?" and "In the past week including today, have you wanted to kill yourself?" Positive endorsement of the second question leads to these follow-up questions: "Have you ever tried to kill yourself?" and "In the past week including today, have you made plans to kill yourself?" Any one positive answer to these questions should prompt consultation by social worker or psychiatrist, or referral to a crisis intervention team.

Similar developments have occurred in the real-time assessment of other mental health domains such as traumatic stress in pediatric ED patients. Brief screening tools for acutely injured children and their families can assess previous adverse experiences as well as immediate response to an acute illness and the ED visit itself. There are also resources that provide education on what to expect, how to parent a traumatized child, how to know when additional help is needed, and where to find it. Information such as this can be found at sites for the National Traumatic Stress Network (http://www.nctsnet.org) and The Center for Pediatric Traumatic Stress at The Children's Hospital of Philadelphia (http://www.healthcaretoolbox.org).

Ultimately, the ED physician bears the burden of responsibility to consult with necessary mental health and crisis professionals and make the appropriate discharge decisions. Notably, the family's experience in the ED may impact the outpatient referral process. The establishment of realistic expectations about treatment follow-up and a commitment from the adolescent and his/her family to return for treatment may enhance initial compliance with treatment recommendations.

Suggested Readings and Key References

General

American Psychiatric Association. *Diagnostic and statistical manual of mental disorders*. 5th ed., text rev. (DSM-V). Washington, DC: American Psychiatric Association Press, 2013.

Bath H. The three pillars of trauma-informed care. *Reclaiming Children and Youth* 2008;17(3):17–21.

Green WH. *Child and adolescent clinical psychopharmacology*. 3rd ed. Philadelphia, PA: Lippincott Williams & Wilkins, 2001.

McClellan JM, Werry JS. Evidence-based treatments in child and adolescent psychiatry: an inventory. *J Am Acad Child Adolesc Psychiatry* 2003;42:1388–1400.

Riddle MA, Kastelic EA, Frosch E. Pediatric psychopharmacology. *J Child Psychol Psychiatry* 2001;42:73–90.

Agitated or Violent Behavior and the Use of Restraint

Hilt RJ, Woodward TA. Agitation treatment for pediatric emergency patients. *J Am Acad Child Adolesc Psychiatry* 2008;47(2):132–138.

Masters KJ, Bellonci C, Bernet W, et al.; American Academy of Child and Adolescent Psychiatry. Practice parameter for the prevention and management of aggressive behavior in child and adolescent psychiatric institutions, with special reference to seclusion and restraint. *J Am Acad Child Adolesc Psychiatry* 2002;41(2 suppl):4S–25S.

Sorrentino A. Chemical restraints for the agitated, violent, or psychotic pediatric patient in the emergency department: controversies and recommendations. *Curr Opin Pediatr* 2004;16:201–205.

Suicide

Achilles J, Gray D, Moskos M. Adolescent suicide myths in the United States. *Crisis* 2004;25(4):176–182.

Baxley F, Miller M. Parental misperceptions about children and firearms. *Arch Pediatr Adolesc Med* 2006;160(5):542–547.

Gould M, Greenberg T, Velting D, et al. Youth suicide risk and preventive interventions: a review of the past 10 years. *J Am Acad Child Adolesc Psychiatry* 2003;42(4):386–405.

Grossman DC, Mueller BA, Riedy C, et al. Gun storage practices and risk of youth suicide and unintentional firearm injuries. *JAMA* 2005;293(6):707–714.

Horowitz LM, Wang PS, Koocher GP, et al. Detecting suicide risk in a pediatric emergency department: development of a brief screening tool. *Pediatrics* 2001;107(5):1133–1137.

Rutman MS, Shenassa E , Becker BM. Brief screening for adolescent depressive symptoms in the emergency department. *Acad Emerg Med* 2008;15(1):17–22.

Depression and Bipolar Disorder

Bridge JA, Iyengar S, Salary CB, et al. Clinical response and risk for reported suicidal ideation and suicide attempts in pediatric antidepressant treatment: a meta-analysis of randomized controlled trials. *JAMA* 2007;297:1683–1696.

Gibbons RD, Hur K, Bhaumik DK, et al. The relationships between antidepressant prescription rates and rate of early adolescent suicide. *Am J Psychiatry* 2006;163(11):1898–1904.

Birmaher B, Brent D and the AACAP Work Group of Quality Issues. Practice parameters for the assessment and treatment of children and adolescents with depressive disorders: AACAP. *J Am Acad Child Adolesc Psychiatry* 2007;46(11):1503–1526.

Pavuluri M, Birmaher B, Naylor M. Pediatric bipolar disorder: a review of the past 10 years. *J Am Acad Child Adolesc Psychiatry* 2005;44(9):846–871.

Psychosis

Edelson GA. Hallucinations in children and adolescents: considerations in the emergency setting. *Am J Psychiatry* 2006;163:781–785.

Hollis C, Rapoport J. Child and adolescent schizophrenia. In: Weinberger DR, Harrison PJ, eds. *Schizoprenia.* 3rd ed. Oxford, UK: Blackwell Publishing, 2011:24–46.

Pao M, Lohman C, Gracey D, et al. Visual, tactile, and phobic hallucinations: recognition and management in the emergency department. *Pediatr Emerg Care* 2004;20:30–34.

Posttraumatic Stress Disorder

Gerson R, Rappaport N. Traumatic stress and posttraumatic stress disorder in youth: recent research findings on clinical impact, assessment, and treatment. *J Adolesc Health* 2013;52(2):137–143.

Ursano RJ. Post-traumatic stress disorder. *N Engl J Med* 2002;346: 130–132.

Conversion Disorder and Other Psychosomatic Symptoms

Ghaffar O, Staines R, Feinstein A. Functional MRI changes in patients with sensory conversion disorder. *Neurology* 2006;67:2036–2038.

Harwick PJ. Engaging families who hold strong medical beliefs in a psychosomatic approach. *Clin Child Psychol Psychiatry* 2005;10(4): 601–616.

Shaw RJ, Spratt EJ, Bernard RS, et al. Somatoform disorders. In: Shaw RJ, DeMaso DR, eds. *Textbook of pediatric psychosomatic medicine.* Washington, DC: American Psychiatric Press, 2010:121–139.

Autism Spectrum Disorders

Anagostou E, Hansen R. Medical treatment overview: traditional and novel psycho-pharmacological and complementary medications. *Curr Opin Pediatr* 2011;23:621–627.

Chun TH, Katz ER, Duffy SJ. Pediatric mental health emergencies and special health care needs. *Pediatr Clin N Am* 2013;60:1185–1201.

Kalb LG, Stuart EA, Freedman B, et al. Psychiatric-related emergency department visits among children with an autism spectrum disorder. *Pediatr Emerg Care* 2012;28:1269–1276.

Levy SE, Mandell DS, Schultz RT. Autism. *Lancet* 2009;374:1627–1638.

McDermott S, Zhou L, Mann J. Injury treatment among children with autism or pervasive developmental disorder. *J Autism Dev Disord* 2008;38:626–633.

Nazeer A, Ghaziuddin M. Autism spectrum disorders: clinical features and diagnosis. *Pediatr Clin N Am* 2012;59:19–25.

Scarpinato N, Bradley J, Kurbjun K, et al. Caring for the child with an autism spectrum disorder in the acute care setting. *J Spec Pediatr Nurs* 2010;15:244–254.

Wong C, Odom SL, Hume K, et al. *Evidence-based practice for children, youth, and young adults with autism spectrum disorder.* Autism Evidence-Based Practice Review Group. Frank Porter Graham Child Development Institute, University of Chapel Hill. 2014. Available at http://autismpdc.fpg.unc.edu/sites/autismpdc.fpg.unc.edu/files/2014-EBIP-Report.pdf. Accessed on August 10, 2015.

Screening for Mental Health Problems in the Emergency Department

Fein JA, Pailler M, Diamond G, et al. Feasibility and effects of a Web-based adolescent psychiatric assessment administered by clinical staff in the pediatric emergency department. *Arch Pediatr Adolesc Med* 2010;164(12):1112–1117.

Horowitz LM, Bridge JA, Teach SJ, et al. Ask Suicide-Screening Questions (ASQ): a brief instrument for the pediatric emergency department. *Arch Pediatr Adolesc Med* 2012;12:1170–1176.

Pena JB, Caine ED. Screening as an approach for adolescent suicide prevention. *Suicide Life Threat Behavior* 2006;36:614–637.

Wintersteen MB, Diamond GS, Fein JA. Screening for suicide risk in the pediatric emergency and acute care setting. *Curr Opin Pediatr* 2006;19:398–404.

CHAPTER 135 ■ SEXUAL ASSAULT: CHILD AND ADOLESCENT

MONIKA K. GOYAL, MD, MSCE, PHILIP SCRIBANO, DO, MSCE, JENNIFER MOLNAR, MSN, RN, PNP-BC, CPNP-AC, SANE-P, AND CYNTHIA J. MOLLEN, MD, MSCE

GOALS OF EMERGENCY CARE

- Treat life-threatening or limb-threatening injuries first, although the vast majority of sexually assaulted patients will not require such immediate intervention.
- Determine best location and care team for the patient. All patients presenting to the ED must have a medical screening examination to determine whether an emergency medical condition exists that requires further treatment. If there is no urgency for evaluation of possible injury, forensic evidence collection, or acute or prophylaxis treatment, a complete and thorough examination can be scheduled for a later date with a child abuse expert.
- An emergency examination is indicated if the alleged assault occurred within the preceding 72 hours, if the patient has genital complaints or other symptoms requiring medical attention, or if the safety of the child is in question.
- A coordinated, multidisciplinary team approach to the evaluation provides victims with access to comprehensive care, minimizes any potential trauma, encourages the use of community resources, and may help facilitate legal investigations.
- Comprehensive care includes history and physical examination documentation, photo documentation of injury, forensic evidence collection, STI screening and prophylaxis (including HIV), pregnancy prophylaxis, crisis management, reporting to CPS and law enforcement, and assuring medical and psychosocial follow-up care.
- A successful sexual assault response team (SART) Program requires ongoing team education, case review for quality management, and significant institutional resources.

OVERVIEW OF APPROACH

Team Composition

A sexual assault response team (SART) is a multidisciplinary team of specially trained professionals devoted to the care of the pediatric victim of sexual assault. Team composition includes, but is not limited to, members of the emergency department, general pediatrics, child abuse, HIV, and trauma surgery specialists, social work, and child life specialists. Collaboration between all team members is best accomplished by designating a team coordinator and a lead support person from each clinical area. The multidisciplinary nature of the team allows for sharing of best practice, provides a common mental model for patient care, organizes communication, supports important processes such as in-house 24/7 coverage for victims of sexual assault, and provides a forum for continued quality improvement. In settings where a dedicated SART is not available, a multidisciplinary, team approach, based on available resources, is ideal.

Training

Recruitment, initial and ongoing training of all team members (MD, CRNP, RN) are critical steps in building an effective SART. Identifying nursing professionals who have a passion for serving the special needs of this unique patient population adds to the success of the program. Specialized training prepares practitioners to respond to the acute sexual assault pediatric victim and includes an initial minimum of 40 educational hours spent in didactics and mentored clinical experience, as recommended by national standards. In settings without a SART, attention to specific training, with ongoing review of cases and review of skills, remains essential.

Assessing and Maintaining Competency

Yearly updates, refresher workshops with simulation, and real-time feedback are critical to continued SART training. Throughout the year, real-time chart reviews including photo documentation of each case allow for timely feedback and targeted education. Monthly team meetings, quarterly skill-building sessions with simulations, literature review, and case review are essential to advancing clinical care for the pediatric sexual assault victim. Strong partnerships with local law enforcement, child advocacy, and child protective services (CPS) include key stakeholders as part of the SART team ongoing education.

Professional development is strongly encouraged. Certification by the International Association of Forensic Nurses (IAFN) is recognized as the highest validation of competency for sexual assault nurse examiners (SANE) with the designation SANE-A for adult/adolescent specialization or SANE-P for pediatric/adolescent specialization. Membership to a local chapter of IAFN is also encouraged.

Assessing and Maintaining Quality

Technologic advances in photo documentation and telemedicine change rapidly; SART members must stay abreast of trends and new developments in the specialty. Maintaining a database of all patients' cases, performing group literature reviews, and meeting with key players within the local community allow the SART mission to be enhanced through collaboration and advocacy across the community and its services. Significant institutional support and strong leadership are required to put these processes into place.

KEY POINTS

- Timely care for the victim of sexual assault is crucial.
- A multidisciplinary team approach is best, with ongoing case review and targeted education provides opportunity for continued quality improvement.
- Partnership with CPS, law enforcement, Forensic Crime Laboratory and community services including child advocacy, WOAR (women organized against rape), and Behavioral Health Agencies is important.

CLINICAL PEARLS AND PITFALLS

- First and foremost, assure that the child is provided optimal comfort during what can be an anxiety provoking clinical encounter. Efforts to gauge the child's level of anxiety prior to conducting the examination will guide approach to the examination. If a nonoffending caregiver is available, and is able to provide comfort and reassurance to the child, maintaining contact with that adult during the assessment can be very beneficial.
- Second, prepare all necessary equipment, supplies and specimen and testing swabs and collection kits prior to positioning the child for the examination. If a colposcope or some other related equipment for visualization and photo documentation is used for these examinations, allow the child to become acclimated with the equipment to alleviate anxiety.
- Third, utilize child life specialists or other personnel to provide distraction techniques and additional comfort and support to the child. While the optimal examination position is a supine frog-leg position using stirrups on an examination table, for the younger child, positioning the child on the lap of a trusted caregiver facilitates cooperation with the examination.
- A head-to-toe examination is conducted to looking for signs of physical abuse or neglect. Given the importance of the child's cooperation to adequately visualize all of the genital structures, avoidance of any potentially noxious examination experiences should be a priority. When obtaining specimens for testing and/or evidence collection, avoidance of any direct contact of the hymenal tissue reduces discomfort.

CURRENT EVIDENCE

The majority of children will have a normal anogenital examination. In studies evaluating acute injuries of child sexual assault, as many as 75% to 80% of examinations can be normal. This rate approaches 96% in children which the examination was conducted well beyond the 72-hour timeframe after which evidence collection is not indicated. It is important to reassure the child and caregiver that the examination is normal, and to emphasize that the lack of injury does not mean that the assault did not occur. It is equally important to recognize that there are anogenital conditions that can be misinterpreted as trauma. A list of common mimickers of sexual abuse trauma are listed in Table 135.1.

CLINICAL CONSIDERATIONS

Given the acute nature of sexual assault, emergency medicine (EM) providers are often the first clinicians to care for a victim. EM providers should be familiar with institutional and local protocols for the evaluation of acute sexual assault victim including jurisdictional policies regarding forensic evidence submission, law enforcement and CPS reporting requirements, and available community advocacy and mental health services.

Emergency departments should have guidelines detailing the care of these patients; ideally, trained sexual assault forensic examiners conduct the forensic medical examination. Many studies have documented improved quality of care when evaluations are conducted by specially trained personnel. As this is not always possible, it is important for pediatric emergency providers to be knowledgeable about genital examination and forensic evidence collection. A comprehensive medical evaluation conducted by a skilled provider can have important implications for the patient's medical and psychological care, legal proceedings, and provide important reassurance to the child and family.

The child/adolescent present to the ED in the following ways: (1) a disclosure of abuse is made or abuse has been witnessed; (2) CPS and/or law enforcement referral for medical evaluation, evidence collection, and crisis management; (3) caregiver or other individual who suspects abuse because of behavioral or physical symptoms brings the child; or (4) child has an unrelated complaint and during the course of the

TABLE 135.1

CONDITIONS MISTAKEN FOR SEXUAL ABUSE TRAUMA

Variants of normal anatomy	Vestibular bands (periurethral, hymenal); hymenal skin tags, septa, clefts; median raphe; linea vestibularis (hymen, posterior fourchette); perianal erythema; anal dilation; failure of midline fusion
Nonabusive trauma	Straddle injuries; impalement to anogenital structures; zipper injuries; suction drain injury; toilet seat injury
Dermatologic	Lichen sclerosus; seborrheic, atopic, or contact dermatitis; psoriasis; hemangioma
Infectious	*Staphylococcus aureus* (impetigo); Group A streptococcus (balanitis, vaginitis, anal); shigella; human papilloma virus (perinatal and horizontal transmission); molluscum contagiosum; autoinoculation of oral HSV infection or herpetic whitlow; scabies; diaper candidiasis; parasitic (pinworms)
Inflammatory/allergic	Crohn disease; Kawasaki disease; Behçet syndrome; erythema multiforme; Stevens–Johnson syndrome
Miscellaneous	Idiopathic thrombocytopenic purpura; prolapse (urethral, rectal); labial fusion; hair tourniquet; retained foreign body

examination behavioral and/or physical signs of abuse are observed.

Clinical Recognition

While many patients will present to the ED with a chief complaint of assault or abuse, the ED clinician should consider the potential for sexual assault in patients with injuries that do not match the provided history.

Triage

Patients are triaged based on injury/symptom severity and the potential need for ED resources. Patients presenting after sexual assault with any of the following should be triaged as ESI level 2: acute assault within 72 hours; evidence/concern for trauma; and complaint of abdominal pain or genital symptoms. Patients should be instructed to remain clothed, refrain from eating or drinking, and avoid urination if possible until decision is made regarding forensic evidence collection.

Initial Assessment

A team approach limits the number of times a history is given and the number of times a patient is examined. Unstable patients or patients with significant injuries should be treated as any other trauma patient, with an attempt to preserve clothing and other potential evidence if possible. For stable patients, the evaluation begins with history taking, ideally with all relevant team members (physician, nurse, sexual assault examiner, social worker) present.

A minimal fact interview assessing the types of sexual contact guides forensic evaluation decisions and assists with interpretation of physical examination findings and treatment. Victims will likely be interviewed in detail by law enforcement, forensic interviewers, and CPS personnel, and so it is unnecessary to obtain great detail about the event in the ED setting. Avoiding repetitive, detailed interviews minimizes the potential for inconsistent or confusing stories. In younger patients, much or all of the history of the assault can be obtained from family members, police, and CPS workers. Adolescent patients can provide the relevant details themselves, and should be interviewed alone, unless the patient objects to the parent leaving the room. In fact, it is ideal to interview children of all ages alone when possible, in order to minimize the influence of parental presence. Important tips for interviewing include the use of open-ended questions, developmentally appropriate language; and use of the child's own words for their body parts. The history should focus on identifying the location of the assault, the alleged perpetrator, the details of the type of sexual contact, and the time elapsed since the event. However, when making a determination about forensic evidence collection, remember that the details of the event can become more specific over time. The provider should document the history source, a description of the event, and use quotations when documenting the exact words from patient's disclosure when possible. Witnesses to the interview should be documented in the medical record.

A full physical examination is documented including injuries sustained during the assault. The examinations should be performed with a chaperone, regardless of the gender of the patient or provider. This chaperone should be a trained member of the medical staff who can assist in examination procedures and serves as an unbiased witness. A parent or another familiar adult can remain with the child to provide support and comfort. Pain control, anxiolysis, or sedation may be required in some situations. The genital examination follows and includes careful inspection of the penis and scrotum in males, the labia, vaginal opening, and hymen in females, and the anus in all patients. A speculum or bimanual examination is rarely required in adolescent patients, it is indicated if there is significant vaginal bleeding, or concern for a retained vaginal foreign body. It should be avoided in prepubertal patients. Photo documentation of all injuries is recommended. It may be useful to photo document a normal genital examination as well. A colposcope provides magnification for optimal visualization and high-quality photo documentation. Documentation should also include detailed written examination descriptions and diagrams in the medical record.

Of note, urgent physical examination is not required if the assault occurred >72 hours prior to presentation, unless the child has ongoing symptoms such as genital pain, bleeding, or discharge. If that is not the case, it may be preferable to refer the child for an outpatient examination with a specialist in child sexual assault.

As stated previously, the vast majority of children have normal genital examinations, in part due to the rapid healing of the mucosa as well as the nonviolent nature of child sexual abuse. A normal physical examination does not rule out sexual assault. Many studies have documented the examination findings that are indicative of sexual abuse, including lacerations of posterior aspect of the hymen and posterior fourchette, ecchymosis of the hymen, or perianal lacerations. Other acute genital injuries are concerning, though not diagnostic of sexual abuse, and include bruising or lacerations of the vulva, penis, scrotum, or perineum. These injuries can be caused by accidental mechanisms, but the history provides the context for interpretation.

Management/Diagnostic Testing

Acute Medical Management

Medical or surgical treatment of associated injuries should follow standard procedure with immediate consultation by specialty services as indicated to manage significant trauma. During initial medical evaluation and stabilization, all reasonable attempts should be made to preserve potential evidence, if possible. Avoiding cutting through holes found in clothing, collect all clothing and place in paper bags and leaving it with the patient until chain of custody can be confirmed. Avoid washing away potential DNA evidence. The management of serious coexisting injuries or other acute medical conditions takes precedence over preservation of forensic evidence. If needed, a forensic examination can be completed in the operating room while other serious injuries are being managed.

Forensic Evidence Collection

Studies in prepubertal children have shown that the yield of forensic evidence collection diminishes rapidly with time, and is low for children presenting more than 24 hours after assault. However, a few recent studies have documented few findings of DNA evidence outside of the 24-hour window in prepubertal victims and these authors postulate that as the field of DNA technology continues to advance, consideration

TABLE 135.2

FORENSIC EVIDENCE COLLECTION KIT

Use a standardized forensic evidence kit that meets the requirements of the police authority in your location. The exact content of the kit may vary based on the jurisdiction but in general most kits will include the following items: • Container in which most of the evidence will be placed • Form for obtaining authorization to collect and release evidence and information to law enforcement • Checklists to guide history taking, physical examination, and specimen collection • Evidence seals • Form for documenting chain of custody • Labels for identifying information and evidence • Paper bags to hold clothing and other bulky items that do not fit in container[a] • Envelopes or other containers for collection of debris, nail scrapings, hair, etc. • Several cotton swabs for collection of specimens plus or minus glass slides[b] • Tubes or containers for collection of secretions • Buccal swabs and/or blood sample tubes for blood typing and DNA analysis • Combs for scalp and/or pubic hair combings • Instrument for obtaining nail scrapings and/or cuttings • Gauze or swabs for saliva sample Other items that may be needed but that are not necessarily in the kit include: • Camera or colposcope for photographic documentation • Alternate light source • Forensic swab dryer and rack

[a]Plastic bags should not be used for evidence collection because they retain moisture which can lead to degradation of evidence.
[b]Slides may be included if the forensic laboratory prefers that the swabs be made into slides at the hospital. Other forensic laboratories may prefer that the swabs be placed in envelopes or containers without slides being made.

of collection outside of the current time recommendations should be considered in some cases. For adolescent patients presenting within 72 hours of assault, the collection of forensic evidence has significantly high yield. Upon ED entry, victims should be advised not to undress, eat or drink, and avoid urination if possible. The patient's clothes should be stored in a paper bag. A significant amount of forensic evidence has been retrieved from linens and clothing. Tables 135.2 and 135.3 provide details about forensic evidence collection.

Drug-Facilitated Sexual Assault

Alcohol or other drugs play an important role in many sexual assaults, whether voluntarily ingested by the victim, surreptitiously given by the assailant, or ingested under force or coercion. Adolescents often report using alcohol and/or drugs immediately before a sexual assault. Increasing rates of drug-facilitated rape have been associated with the availability of alcohol and benzodiazepines. While "date-rape" drugs (e.g., flunitrazepam [Rohypnol], Y-hydroxybutyrate [GHB], ketamine) have received much recent attention, these are rarely identified as the offending agent. Drug testing should be performed if a patient appears intoxicated, reports drug-facilitated assault, or cannot recall details of the assault. In addition, patients should be reminded that even if drug use was voluntary, it is important to provide history of intoxication preceding assault. Protocols with the toxicology laboratory at each institution are necessary as date-rape drugs and many other drugs of abuse are not included in standard drug-screening panels.

Pregnancy Testing

Pregnancy testing should be performed in all pubertal females.

STI Testing

With rare exception, the identification of sexually transmitted infections (STIs) in children beyond the neonatal period suggests sexual abuse. Postnatally acquired gonorrhea (GC), chlamydia (CT), syphilis, and nontransfusion-acquired HIV are usually diagnostic of sexual abuse. Sexual abuse should also be suspected when genital herpes is diagnosed. Although genital warts are found in sexually abused children, they can also be present in children in whom there is no suspicion of abuse due to the high prevalence of human papillomavirus in the population. The possibility of sexual abuse must be investigated thoroughly if no conclusive explanation for nonsexual transmission of an STI can be identified. The recommended action by the American Academy of Pediatrics (AAP) regarding the reporting of suspected child sexual abuse varies by the specific organism and is outlined in Table 135.4.

The decision to evaluate STIs is made on an individual basis. Most experts recommend that pubertal victims of sexual assault undergo STI testing as the prevalence of preexisting asymptomatic infection in this group is high. Therefore, although the identification of an STI may represent an infection acquired prior to the assault, laws in all 50 states strictly limit the evidentiary use of a survivor's previous sexual history, including evidence of previously acquired STIs, as part of an effort to undermine the credibility of the survivor's testimony. In addition, STI tests have been found to be positive as a result of an assault even when obtained within 72 hours of the assault. Alternatively, because the prevalence of STIs in prepubertal patients is quite low, occurring in less than 10% of prepubertal victims, the AAP and Centers for Disease Control and Prevention (CDC) recommend targeted

TABLE 135.3

GUIDELINES FOR FORENSIC EVIDENCE COLLECTION

General

1. Obtain consent to collect forensic evidence in adolescent sexual assault cases. In cases of child sexual abuse, consent is not needed.
2. Instruct patient not to wash, change clothes, urinate, defecate, smoke, drink, or eat until evaluated by examiners, unless medically necessary.
3. Wash your hands and wear gloves.
4. Use photographs to document physical findings
   a. The first photograph should be that of the child's ID label with full name, date of birth, and medical record number.
   b. Take as many photographs as needed to document injuries.
   c. Document each injury separately with ruler/color guide in photographs.
5. Use anatomical diagrams to document findings including location, size, and appearance.

Initial debris and clothing collection

1. Debris collection: Carefully inspect patient's head, hands, and other exposed skin surfaces, as well as outer surface of clothing, for any loose debris including hairs, grass, leaves, fibers, threads, etc. Using one piece of clean white copy paper carefully remove the loose material and place it inside the unfolded paper. Refold paper to retain material; indicate location on patient's body or clothing from which material was collected. Repeat as necessary. Place folded paper into envelope marked "Miscellaneous," seal, and label envelope as indicated.
2. Clothing collection: Spread clean sheet on floor, place large paper sheet from "Foreign Material" envelope in the middle of the cloth sheet. Have patient stand in the middle of the sheet and remove clothing one piece at a time, careful not to shake the clothing. If parents or the nurse is helping patient, advise them not to stand on the sheet with the patient. Ask the patient to remove one article of clothing at a time. If the article of clothing has wet stains of potential biologic material (blood, saliva, semen, etc.), lay flat to dry. Place each article of clothing in a separate paper bag, labeled with patient identification sticker, date, time, and forensic examiner's initials.
   a. Underpants and/or diapers should be collected even if they are not the pair worn during or immediately after the incident. Vaginal secretions may accumulate, even if the patient has bathed or showered.
   b. Collect all clothing if worn during assault or immediately after assault. If patient is not wearing the same underwear from the assault, the examiner should inquire about the location of the garment and instruct patient or family to save the garment for police/SVU (ideally unlaundered in a paper bag).

Physical examination evidence collection

1. Skin surface assessment: Carefully perform a visual inspection of the patient's external skin surfaces. Locate, describe, and photograph any evidence of trauma or adherent foreign matter.
   a. If areas of dried secretions are noted on external skin surfaces, document findings on anatomical diagrams.
2. Secretions collection: Prior to any swabs or evidence collection, an alternative light source should be utilized in a dark room over the patient's entire body. If there is a positive (fluorescent specimen), a sterile swab moistened with sterile water should be used to swab area. Allow to air dry. Place in "Debris or Miscellaneous" envelope—noting where specimens were collected.
   a. Use extra swabs to collect specimens if needed. Be sure to label the "Debris or Miscellaneous" envelopes carefully to what evidence is inside and where it was obtained.
3. Bite mark evidence: Document location of bite mark(s) on anatomical diagram form and, where possible, photograph the bite mark with and without scale. With 2 premoistened swabs, simultaneously rub swabs over area of potential/actual bite mark in order to collect any dried saliva left by the offender.
4. Examination of hands: Carefully inspect dorsal and palmar surface of hands for any signs of trauma. Document all findings on anatomical diagram. Swab only fingernails if there are dried secretions, if so, follow directions for dried secretions.
5. Oral swabs: Open the swab packet from the envelope marked "Oral Swabs," grasp both swabs together by the shaft, and swab the area between the patient's cheek and gum, and behind the back molars on both the upper and lower jaws.
   a. Mucosal membranes swabs do not need to be moistened.
6. Genital inspection: Carefully inspect entire external genital area for signs of trauma. Use colposcope or other light source to examine for injuries. Document findings, including size, shape, color and location, on anatomical diagrams of genitalia.
7. Pubic hair combings: Remove paper fold from envelope marked "Pubic Hair Combings." Ask patient to sit on unfolded paper so that the paper protrudes between the thighs; comb downward on pubic hair to dislodge any debris or loose hairs onto the paper. Place comb on paper and fold paper to retain debris; place paper in the envelope marked "Pubic Hair Combings," seal, and label as indicated.
8. Perianal swabs: Carefully evaluate the anus and buttocks for signs of injury. Document positive findings on gender-appropriate anatomical diagrams. Using two moistened swabs simultaneously, gently rub swabs on anal folds and anal opening. Dry completely and place in the envelope marked "Perianal Swabs."
9. Rectal swabs: After external anal swabs have been collected, the anal area should be cleansed by wiping carefully with a moistened gauze pad. Simultaneously insert two sterile cotton swabs approximately 2 cm into the rectum and swab rectal walls. Remove swabs, avoiding contact with the external anal tissue. Dry completely and place in the envelope marked "Rectal Swabs."

TABLE 135.3

GUIDELINES FOR FORENSIC EVIDENCE COLLECTION (*CONTINUED*)

10. External genital swabs: Use swabs in external genital envelope. For male patients, wipe the surface of the glans and shaft; for female patients, wipe the inner surfaces of the labia minora with a downward motion. After drying, place in a marked envelope.
11. Vaginal swabs: Using two swabs simultaneously, collect secretions from the vagina near the vaginal fornix (area below the cervix). (This step may be performed with a speculum in place in postpubertal children, or by blind sweep without the use of a speculum.)
12. Cervix swabs: Using two swabs simultaneously, collect secretions from cervical os. This step should be performed only with the use of a speculum to ensure visualization of the cervix and thus should not be performed in prepubertal children unless under anesthesia. Dry completely and place in envelope marked "Cervix Swabs."
    a. If using a speculum for cervical examination, after evidence is collected, use the aptima cervical swab to obtain specimen for STIs.
13. All tampons, pads, pantyliners should be collected and dried. Once dry, place in the "Miscellaneous" envelope.
14. All evidence should be dry before packaging. To dry swabs, place swabs in swab drying machine, with cotton tip pointing upward to promote drying.
15. Do not allow cotton tip of swabs to contact other objects or surfaces during drying process. (Use the test tube rack not allowing it to touch any other swabs.)
16. After drying, swabs should be placed in swab boxes and then into the envelopes provided for each specimen. (If additional specimens were collected and no swab box or evidence envelope is available for packaging, dried swabs may be placed in a plain envelope.)
17. All envelopes and boxes should be labeled with patient's name, case number, date, and name of the examiner.
18. Seal enveloped: Do not lick envelopes to seal them. Use a clean gauze or cotton and wet with sterile water to moisten adhesive on collection envelopes.
19. All envelopes containing evidence specimens should be placed inside the evidence kit box. The sealed bag containing underpants may be placed inside evidence kit box if space permits; all other clothing bags should remain outside of evidence box. Each item collected must be noted on the evidence receipt form.

Adapted from *Forensic Exam Checklist*, Children's Hospital of Philadelphia, Philadelphia, PA.

screening in this age group. It is recommended that prepubertal victims be screened for STIs if signs or symptoms of an STI are present; there is history and/or evidence of ejaculation or oral/genital penetration; the suspected assailant is known to have an STI; if there is a high community prevalence of STIs; or if the patient or parent requests STI testing. Signs or symptoms of an STI include vaginal discharge or pain, genital itching or odor, urinary symptoms, and genital ulcers or other lesions.

If STI testing is obtained, testing should occur prior to the initiation of any treatment. Furthermore, if a patient is thought to have an STI, tests should be sent for all common STIs. Because of the legal and psychosocial consequences of a false-positive diagnosis, only tests with high specificities should be used (see discussion below).

For all patients, determination of which sites to sample is based on areas of possible contact with assailant's bodily fluids and includes vaginal, urethral, anorectal, oropharyngeal,

TABLE 135.4

IMPLICATIONS OF COMMONLY ENCOUNTERED SEXUALLY TRANSMITTED (ST) OR SEXUALLY ASSOCIATED (SA) INFECTIONS FOR DIAGNOSIS AND REPORTING OF SEXUAL ABUSE AMONG INFANTS AND PREPUBERTAL CHILDREN[a]

ST/SA confirmed	Evidence for sexual abuse	Suggested action
Gonorrhea[a]	Diagnostic	Report[b]
Syphilis[a]	Diagnostic	Report[b]
Human immunodeficiency virus[c]	Diagnostic	Report[b]
Chlamydia trachomatis[a]	Diagnostic	Report[b]
Trichomonas vaginalis	Highly suspicious	Report[b]
Condylomata acuminata[a] (anogenital warts)	Suspicious	Consider report[b]
Genital herpes[a]	Suspicious	Consider report[b,d]
Bacterial vaginosis	Inconclusive	Medical follow-up

[a]If not likely to be perinatally acquired and rare nonsexual, vertical transmission is excluded.
[b]Reports should be made to the agency in the community mandated to receive reports of suspected child abuse or neglect.
[c]If not likely to be acquired perinatally or through transfusion.
[d]Unless there is a clear history of autoinoculation.
Adapted from Kellogg N; American Academy of Pediatrics Committee on Child Abuse and Neglect. The evaluation of sexual abuse in children. *Pediatrics* 2005;116(2):506–512.

TABLE 135.5

SEXUAL ASSAULT PROPHYLAXIS BY WEIGHT GROUP[a]

For prevention of		Weight <45 kg	Weight ≥45 kg
Gonorrhea and chlamydia	Ceftriaxone	25–50 mg/kg IV or IM in a single dose (not to exceed 125 mg)	250 mg IM or IV in a single dose
	AND		
	Azithromycin	Azithromycin 20 mg/kg orally in a single dose (maximum 1 g)	1 g orally in a single dose
	Or		
	Doxycycline	n/a	100 mg orally twice per day for 7 days (if age ≥8 yrs)
Trichomoniasis	Metronidazole	15 mg/kg/day orally divided three times a day for 7 days	2 g orally in a single dose
Hepatitis B virus (if not fully immunized)	Hepatitis B vaccine		

[a]Adapted from Centers for Disease Control and Prevention. Sexually transmitted diseases treatment guidelines, 2015.

and/or blood. As the history of the assault provided or recalled may change with time, the clinician should consider testing for STIs from multiple sources. Nucleic acid amplification tests (NAATs) on urine specimens for GC and CT have essentially replaced vaginal/cervical/urethral culture in both prepubertal and pubertal female and male patients. In addition, while NAATs are not FDA approved for extragenital sites, the extensive use and reliability of this technology has resulted in its use testing on pharyngeal and rectal specimens. Culture may be used; however, compared to NAATs, it is an inferior testing method for chlamydia detection. If NAAT testing is performed, all positive tests should be confirmed by a second NAAT that targets a different genomic sequence to increase specificity of the test; most commercial test kits include a second DNA probe for this purpose. Cervical specimens are not recommended for prepubertal girls. All vesicular or ulcerative genital or perianal lesions should be sent for viral culture to test for genital herpes. The preferred testing method for Trichomonas vaginalis is rapid antigen testing or NAAT; given the poor sensitivity and specificity of wet mount. The wet mount can also be used to evaluate for BV and candidiasis, if vaginal discharge, malodor, or itching is evident. Syphilis testing should be performed using rapid plasma reagin (RPR) test and Hepatitis B testing is indicated if the patient has not been fully immunized against this infection. HIV serum testing should be performed using a fourth-generation p-24antigen/HIV-1 and HIV-2 antibody combination (preferred) or a third-generation HIV-1/2 antibody immunoassay. HIV testing should be performed after appropriate counseling emphasizing that the test result will only provide evidence of infection acquired prior to 6 months, although the new fourth-generation HIV immunoassays can detect more acute HIV-1 infection.

Post-Exposure Prophylaxis

The risk of a child acquiring an STI as a result of sexual assault/abuse has not been well studied. In prepubertal patients, prophylaxis is not recommended because the incidence of infection is low after assault/abuse as is the risk for ascending infection, and regular follow-up of children can usually be ensured. All pubertal patients should be offered STI prophylaxis due to poor follow-up rates among this patient population. Empiric antibiotics for GC, CT, and TV are given. See Table 135.5 for recommended treatments and doses; please refer to the CDC STD treatment guidelines for those requiring alternative regimens. Patients who have not been previously vaccinated against Hepatitis B should receive the Hepatitis B vaccination, without Hepatitis B immunoglobulin (HBIG). Finally, consider Hepatitis C testing based on risk assessment of assault.

HIV Prophylaxis

HIV prophylaxis is not universally recommended because although HIV seroconversion has occurred in people whose only risk factor was sexual assault, the frequency of this occurrence is extremely low. Several factors impact the medical recommendation for HIV post-exposure prophylaxis (PEP). These include the likelihood of the assailant having HIV; any exposure characteristics that might increase the risk for HIV transmission based on type of sexual contact (e.g., single episode vs. multiple/chronic); the time elapsed after the event; and the potential benefits and risks associated with the PEP. Often, an assailant's HIV status at the time of the assault examination is unknown. It is therefore important to consider any known HIV-risk behaviors of the perpetrator, local epidemiology of HIV/AIDS, and exposure characteristics of the assault. Higher-risk exposures include vaginal or anal penetration, ejaculation on any mucous membrane, history of multiple assailants, and whether mucosal lesions are present in the assailant or patient.

The rationale for HIV PEP assumes a window of time in which the viral load can be controlled by the immune system. The addition of antiretroviral medications during this window may then stop replication. Although a definitive statement of benefit cannot be made regarding PEP after sexual assault, the possibility of HIV exposure should be assessed at the time of the postassault examination. If PEP is offered to a patient, it is important to discuss the relative risks and benefits of antiretroviral medications, the importance of close follow-up, and strict adherence to the recommended dosing so an informed decision about prophylaxis can be made by the patient and caregiver. PEP should be given within 72 hours of the assault, and is more effective as soon as possible following the exposure. Providers should emphasize that PEP is usually well tolerated and serious adverse effects are rare. If initiating PEP, specialist consultation is recommended regarding treatment if a local protocol is

TABLE 135.6

GUIDELINES FOR MAKING THE DECISION TO REPORT SEXUAL ABUSE OF CHILDREN

Data available				Response	
History	**Behavioral symptoms**	**Physical examination**	**Diagnostic tests**	**Level of concern about sexual abuse**	**Report decision**
Clear statement	Present or absent	Normal or abnormal	Positive or negative	High	Report
None or vague	Present or absent	Normal or nonspecific	Positive for *Chlamydia trachomatis*, gonorrhea, *Trichomonas vaginalis*, syphilis, or herpes[a]	High	Report
None or vague	Present or absent	Concerning or diagnostic findings	Negative or positive	High[b]	Report
Vague or history by parent only	Present or absent	Normal or nonspecific	Negative	Indeterminate	Refer when possible
None	Present	Normal or nonspecific	Negative	Indeterminate	Possible report,[c] refer, or follow

[a]If nonsexual transmission is unlikely or excluded.
[b]Confirmed with various examination techniques and/or peer review with expert consultant.
[c]If behaviors are rare/unusual in normal children.
Reproduced with permission from Kellogg N; American Academy of Pediatrics Committee on Child Abuse and Neglect. The evaluation of sexual abuse in children. *Pediatrics* 2005;116(2):506–512, Copyright 2005 by the AAP.

not established. No large studies examining different treatment regimens have been performed with sexual assault victims, but on the basis of current occupational-exposure guidelines, two nucleoside reverse-transcriptase inhibitors and one of either a nonnucleoside reverse-transcriptase inhibitor or protease inhibitor for 4 weeks are typically recommended. Since these medications may not be readily available at some pharmacies, patients in whom PEP is initiated should be given a minimum of a 3- to 5-day supply of PEP at discharge. A follow-up visit or some method of care coordination should be scheduled for several days after the initial visit to allow for additional counseling, to assure that the patient has filled the prescription and to assess tolerance of medications. In addition, if PEP is started, a complete blood cell count and serum chemistry should be performed for baseline levels (including liver transaminases) as well as an HIV antibody test.

Pregnancy Prophylaxis

Emergency contraception should be offered to every pubertal female; consent includes risks of prophylaxis, failure and options for pregnancy management. A pregnancy test must be performed and negative prior to administration. It is offered within 120 hours of assault where vaginal penetration or genital contact with ejaculation occurred. Progestin-only emergency contraceptive pills are most favorable in terms of safety, adverse effects, and efficacy. A total of 1.5 mg of levonorgestrel can be taken once, with or without ondansetron to mitigate nausea and/or vomiting. Emergency contraception is up to 90% effective in pregnancy prevention. No studies to date show untoward effects on the fetus should pregnancy occur; it does not disrupt an already implanted pregnancy. Pregnancy testing should be repeated at 2 weeks.

Reporting

Physicians and other healthcare professionals are mandated reporters under United States law, and therefore, are required to report suspected as well as known cases of child abuse (Table 135.6). In many states, the suspicion of child sexual abuse as a possible diagnosis requires a report to both the appropriate law enforcement and CPS agencies. For many children who present with complaints of sexual assault, CPS and the police have already been involved; however, some children present prior to contact with these agencies. Medical providers need to be aware of their mandated reporter status and the associated obligation to report any suspicions of child abuse. The threshold for reporting is low; if there is a reasonable suspicion of sexual abuse a report is indicated. The CPS agency then has the responsibility to conduct a thorough investigation to determine whether the abuse has occurred. Mandated reporters are protected against criminal or civil repercussions for any report made in good faith, no matter the eventual outcome of that investigation.

The majority of adolescent sexual assaults are perpetrated by an acquaintance or relative of the adolescent. Depending on the patient's age, the identity of the alleged perpetrator, and state law, the assault may have to be reported. Statutory rape, defined as consensual sexual intercourse between an older person and a person younger than the state-mandated age of consent, continues to be a controversial issue. In these cases, the assault may have to be reported, even if the adolescent does not want it to be reported. Furthermore, sexual assault patients may also be victims of intimate partner violence and healthcare providers must be sensitive to this association and screen patients for associated physical and psychological abuse and address their safety.

Clinical Indications for Discharge or Admission

Disposition

In most cases, the sexual assault victim may be discharged from the ED in the care of relatives. On occasion, hospitalization

TABLE 135.7

APPROACH TO INTERPRETING PHYSICAL AND LABORATORY FINDINGS IN SUSPECTED CHILD SEXUAL ABUSE

Findings documented in newborns or commonly seen in nonabused children (the presence of these findings generally neither confirms nor discounts a child's clear disclosure of sexual abuse)	
Normal variants	**Findings commonly caused by other medical conditions**
1. Periurethral or vestibular bands 2. Intravaginal ridges or columns 3. Hymenal bumps or mounds 4. Hymenal tags or septal remnants 5. Linea vestibularis (midline avascular area) 6. Hymenal notch/cleft in the anterior (superior) half of the hymenal rim (prepubertal girls), on or above the 3–9 o'clock line, patient supine 7. Shallow/superficial notch or cleft in inferior rim of hymen (below 3–9 o'clock line) 8. External hymenal ridge 9. Congenital variants in appearance of hymen, including: Crescentic, annular, redundant, septate, cribriform, microperforate, imperforate 10. Diastasis ani (smooth area) 11. Perianal skin tag 12. Hyperpigmentation of the skin of labia minora or perianal tissues in children of color, such as Mexican-American and African-American children 13. Dilation of the urethral opening with application of labial traction 14. "Thickened hymen" (may be due to estrogen effect, folded edge of hymen, swelling from infection, or swelling from trauma. The latter is difficult to assess unless follow-up examination is done)	15. Erythema (redness) of the vestibule, penis, scrotum, or perianal tissues. (May be due to irritants, infection, or trauma.[a]) 16. Increased vascularity ("dilatation of existing blood vessels") of vestibule and hymen. (May be due to local irritants, or normal pattern in nonestrogenized state.) 17. Labial adhesions. (May be due to irritation or rubbing.) 18. Vaginal discharge. (Many infectious and noninfectious causes, cultures must be taken to confirm if it is caused by sexually transmitted organisms or other infections.) 19. Friability of the posterior fourchette or commissure. (May be due to irritation, infection, or may be caused by examiner's traction on the labia majora.) 20. Excoriations/bleeding/vascular lesions. (These findings can be due to conditions such as lichen sclerosus, eczema or seborrhea, vaginal/perianal Group A streptococcus, urethral prolapse, hemangiomas.) 21. Perineal groove (failure of midline fusion), partial or complete 22. Anal fissures (Usually due to constipation, perianal irritation.) 23. Venous congestion or venous pooling in the perianal area. (Usually due to positioning of child, also seen with constipation.) 24. Flattened anal folds. (May be due to relaxation of the external sphincter or swelling of the perianal tissues due to infection or trauma.[a]) 25. Partial or complete anal dilatation to less than 2 cm (anterior–posterior dimension), with or without stool visible. (May be a normal reflex, or have other causes, such as severe constipation or encopresis, sedation, anesthesia, neuromuscular conditions.)
Indeterminate findings: Insufficient or conflicting data from research studies. (May require additional studies/evaluation to determine significance. These physical/laboratory findings may support a child's clear disclosure of sexual abuse, if one is given, but should be interpreted with caution if the child gives no disclosure. In some cases, a report to Child Protective Services may be indicated to further evaluate possible sexual abuse.)	
Physical examination findings	**Lesions with etiology confirmed: Indeterminate specificity for sexual transmission (report to protective services recommended by AAP Guidelines unless perinatal or horizontal transmission is considered likely)**
26. Deep notches or clefts in the posterior/inferior rim of hymen in prepubertal girls, located between 4 and 8 o'clock, in contrast to transections (see 41) 27. Deep notches or complete clefts in the hymen at 3 or 9 o'clock in adolescent girls 28. Smooth, noninterrupted rim of hymen between 4 and 8 o'clock, which appears to be less than 1 mm wide, when examined in the prone knee–chest position, or using water to "float" the edge of the hymen when the child is in the supine position. 29. Wart-like lesions in the genital or anal area. (Biopsy and viral typing may be indicated in some cases if appearance is not typical of *Condyloma acuminata*.) 30. Vesicular lesions or ulcers in the genital or anal area (viral and/or bacterial cultures, or nucleic acid amplification tests may be needed for diagnosis). 31. Marked, immediate anal dilation to an AP diameter of 2 cm or more, in the absence of other predisposing factors.	32. Genital or anal *Condyloma acuminata* in a child, in the absence of other indicators of abuse 33. Herpes Type 1 or 2 in the genital or anal area in a child with no other indicators of sexual abuse.

TABLE 135.7

APPROACH TO INTERPRETING PHYSICAL AND LABORATORY FINDINGS IN SUSPECTED CHILD SEXUAL ABUSE (*CONTINUED*)

Findings Diagnostic of trauma and/or sexual contact (The following findings support a disclosure of sexual abuse, if one is given, and are highly suggestive of abuse even in the absence of a disclosure, unless the child and/or caretaker provides a clear, timely, plausible description of accidental injury. It is recommended that diagnostic quality photo documentation of the examination findings be obtained and reviewed by an experienced medical provider, before concluding that they represent acute or healed trauma. Follow-up examinations are also recommended.)	
Acute trauma to external genital/anal tissues	**Residual (healing) injuries. (These findings are difficult to assess unless an acute injury was previously documented at the same location.)**
34. Acute lacerations or extensive bruising of labia, penis, scrotum, perianal tissues, or perineum. (May be from unwitnessed accidental trauma, or from physical or sexual abuse.) 35. Fresh laceration of the posterior fourchette, not involving the hymen. (Must be differentiated from dehisced labial adhesion or failure of midline fusion. May also be caused by accidental injury or consensual sexual intercourse in adolescents.)	36. Perianal scar (rare, may be due to other medical conditions such as Crohn disease, accidental injuries, or previous medical procedures) 37. Scar of posterior fourchette or fossa. (Pale areas in the midline may also be due to linea vestibularis or labial adhesions.)
Injuries indicative of blunt force penetrating trauma (or from abdominal/pelvic compression injury if such history is given)	**Presence of infection confirms mucosal contact with infected and infective bodily secretions, contact most likely to have been sexual in nature**
38. Laceration (tear, partial, or complete) of the hymen, acute. 39. Ecchymosis (bruising) on the hymen (in the absence of a known infectious process or coagulopathy). 40. Perianal lacerations extending deep to the external anal sphincter (not to be confused with partial failure of midline fusion). 41. Hymenal transection (healed). An area between 4 and 8 o'clock on the rim of the hymen where it appears to have been torn through, to or nearly to the base, so there appears to be virtually no hymenal tissue remaining at that location. This must be confirmed using additional examination techniques such as a swab, prone knee–chest position or Foley catheter balloon (in adolescents), or prone knee–chest position or water to float the edge of the hymen (in prepubertal girls). This finding has also been referred to as a "complete cleft" in sexually active adolescents and young adult women. 42. Missing segment of hymenal tissue. Area in the posterior (inferior) half of the hymen, wider than a transection, with an absence of hymenal tissue extending to the base of the hymen, which is confirmed using additional positions/methods as described above.	43. Positive confirmed culture for gonorrhea, from genital area, anus, and throat, in a child outside the neonatal period. 44. Confirmed diagnosis of syphilis, if perinatal transmission is ruled out. 45. Trichomonas vaginalis infection in a child older than 1 year of age, with organisms identified by culture or in vaginal secretions by wet-mount examination by an experienced technician or clinician. 46. Positive culture from genital or anal tissues for Chlamydia, if child is older than 3 years at time of diagnosis, and specimen was tested using cell culture or comparable method approved by the Centers for Disease Control. 47. Positive serology for HIV, if perinatal transmission, transmission from blood products, and needle contamination has been ruled out. **Diagnostic of sexual contact** 48. Pregnancy 49. Sperm identified in specimens taken directly from a child's body.

[a]Follow-up examination is necessary before attributing these findings to trauma.
Reprinted with minor adaptations from Adams JA, Kaplan RA, Starling SP, et al. Guidelines for medical care of children who may have been sexually abused. *J Pediatr Adolesc Gynecol* 2007;20:163–172, with permission from Elsevier.

is necessary for treatment or observation of injuries, exacerbation of pre-existing or new medical conditions; or suicidal, homicidal, or psychotic reactions. If the patient is deemed medically stable for discharge and has a safe place to go once leaving the ED, follow-up care should be arranged before final discharge with appropriate referrals provided in written form.

Follow-up

Victims of sexual assault must be discharged with a specific plan of care that includes adequate follow-up with their primary care provider or child abuse specialist, child advocacy center, and psychological/mental health services. Patients should be counseled to follow-up with their primary care provider or child abuse specialist within 1 week to assess healing and sooner, if symptoms occur. Victims of sexual abuse are at risk for short- and long-term psychological disturbances, such as posttraumatic stress disorder, depression, and suicidality. Law enforcement contact information should also be provided so that the patient can determine the status of their report.

Because infectious agents acquired through assault may not produce sufficient concentrations of organisms to be detected during initial testing, evaluation for STIs can be repeated within 1 to 2 weeks of the assault if treatment was not initially provided, and/or there is the onset of STI symptoms. Serologic tests for syphilis are repeated 6 weeks, 3 months, and 6 months after the assault if initial test results were negative and infection in the assailant cannot be ruled out. Completion of the Hepatitis B vaccine series is also considered at 1 to 2 and 4 to 6 months after the first dose, if the patient was not previously vaccinated and had received the first dose during the initial evaluation. If initial HIV testing was negative and a third-generation test (as described above) was performed, repeat testing should occur at 6 weeks, 3 months, and 6 months; if a fourth-generation test was performed, repeat testing should occur at 4 and 12 weeks. Finally, if HIV PEP was initiated, follow-up to monitor side effects and adherence to regimen is recommended.

NONACUTE SEXUAL ABUSE

Children presenting >72 hours after alleged sexual abuse may be referred to child sexual abuse clinic or child advocacy center for medical evaluations. A screening evaluation to satisfy EMTALA requirements is indicated. Assessment of the child's safety including the need for reporting to the CPS agency and/or law enforcement agency (based upon specific jurisdiction laws of your state) is required as part of this abbreviated emergency department visit.

If there are medical concerns which warrant an immediate medical examination in the ED (i.e., pain, dysuria, bleeding), a complete medical evaluation is warranted, with follow-up care at the child sexual abuse clinic or child advocacy center medical clinic. The interpretation of nonacute sexual abuse examination findings requires significant knowledge of normal anatomy, including normal variants, and examination findings which could be considered supportive of healed penetrating trauma (Table 135.7). Over- and underinterpretation of nonacute findings may cause undue harm to child and family and forensic interpretations should be referred to those clinicians with appropriate expertise.

Follow-up should include assessment of mental health needs and victim support services to assist navigating the challenges ahead during the investigation and legal actions.

Suggested Readings and Key References

Adams JA, Kaplan RA, Starling SP, et al. Guidelines for medical care of children who may have been sexually abused. *J Pediatr Adolesc Gynecol* 2007;20(3):163–172.

American College of Obstetricians and Gynecologists. ACOG practice bulletin. Emergency oral contraception. Number 25, March 2001. (Replace practice pattern number 3, December 1996). American College of Obstetricians and Gynecologists. *Int J Gynaecol Obstet* 2002;78(2):191–198.

Bechtel K. Sexual abuse and sexually transmitted infections in children and adolescents. *Curr Opin Pediatr* 2010;22(1):94–99.

Bechtel K, Ryan E, Gallagher D. Impact of sexual assault nurse examiners on the evaluation of sexual assault in a pediatric emergency department. *Pediatr Emerg Care* 2008;24(7):442–447.

Black CM, Driebe EM, Howard LA, et al. Multicenter study of nucleic acid amplification tests for detection of Chlamydia trachomatis and Neisseria gonorrhoeae in children being evaluated for sexual abuse. *Pediatr Infect Dis J* 2009;28(7):608–613.

Christian CW, Lavelle JM, De Jong AR, et al. Forensic evidence findings in pre-pubertal victims of sexual assault. *Pediatrics* 2000;106(1 Pt 1): 100–104.

DeVore HK, Sachs CJ. Sexual assault. *Emerg Med Clin North Am* 2011; 29(3):605–620.

Girardet RG, Lahoti S, Howard LA, et al. Epidemiology of sexually transmitted infections in suspected child victims of sexual assault. *Pediatrics* 2009;124(1):79–86.

Hornor G, Thackeray J, Scribano P, et al. Pediatric sexual assault nurse examiner care: trace forensic evidence, ano-genital injury, and judicial outcomes. *J Forensic Nurs* 2012;8(3):105–111.

Jenny C, Crawford-Jakubiak JE. The evaluation of children in the primary care setting when sexual abuse is suspected. *Pediatrics* 2013;132(2):e558–e567.

Kaufman M. Care of the adolescent sexual assault victim. *Pediatrics* 2008;122(2):462–470.

Mollen CJ, Goyal MK, Frioux SM. Acute sexual assault: a review. *Pediatr Emerg Care* 2012;28(6):584–590; quiz 591–593.

Palusci VJ, Cox EO, Shatz EM, et al. Urgent medical assessment after child sexual abuse. *Child Abuse Negl* 2006;30(4):367–380.

Thackeray JD, Hornor G, Benzinger EA, et al. Forensic evidence collection and DNA identification in acute child sexual assault. *Pediatrics* 2011;128(2):227–232.

Workowski KA, Bolan GA, Centers for Disease Control and Prevention. Sexually transmitted diseases treatment guidelines, 2015. *MMWR Recomm Rep* 2015;64(3):1–138.

Young KL, Jones JG, Worthington T, et al. Forensic laboratory evidence in sexually abused children and adolescents. *Arch Pediatr Adolesc Med* 2006;160(6):585–588.

Chapters 136–143 appear in the eBook bundled with this text. Please see the inside front cover for eBook access instructions.

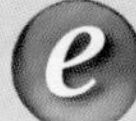

To view these chapters please access the eBook bundled with this text. Please see the inside front cover for eBook access instructions.

SECTION VIII
Procedures and Appendices

CHAPTER 136 ■ BIOLOGICAL AND CHEMICAL TERRORISM

RICHARD J. SCARFONE, MD, JAMES M. MADSEN, MD, MPH, FCAP, FACOEM COL, MC-FS, THEODORE J. CIESLAK, MD, FRED M. HENRETIG, MD, AND EDWARD M. EITZEN JR., MD, MPH

CHAPTER 137 ■ EQUIPMENT

RICHARD G. BACHUR, MD

CHAPTER 138 ■ INSTRUCTIONS FOR PARENTS

HILARY A. HEWES, MD AND NANETTE C. DUDLEY, MD

CHAPTER 139 ■ PREHOSPITAL CARE

TONI K. GROSS, MD, MPH AND GEORGE A. WOODWARD, MD, MBA

CHAPTER 140 ■ PROCEDURAL SEDATION

JEANNINE DEL PIZZO, MD, JOEL A. FEIN, MD, MPH, AND STEVEN M. SELBST, MD

CHAPTER 141 ■ PROCEDURES

MATTHEW R. MITTIGA, MD AND RICHARD M. RUDDY, MD

CHAPTER 142 ■ ULTRASOUND

JASON LEVY, MD, RDMS, JOANNA S. COHEN, MD, ALYSSA M. ABO, MD, RACHEL REMPELL, MD, RDMS, AND J. KATE DEANEHAN, MD, RDMS

CHAPTER 143 ■ TECHNOLOGY ASSISTED CHILDREN

JOEL A. FEIN, MD, MPH, KATHLEEN M. CRONAN, MD, AND JILL C. POSNER, MD, MSCE, MSEd

INDEX

Note: Pages followed by f indicate figures; pages followed by t indicate tables. Those followed by e indicate for web chapters.

C

D

G

H

J

M

N

P

U

V